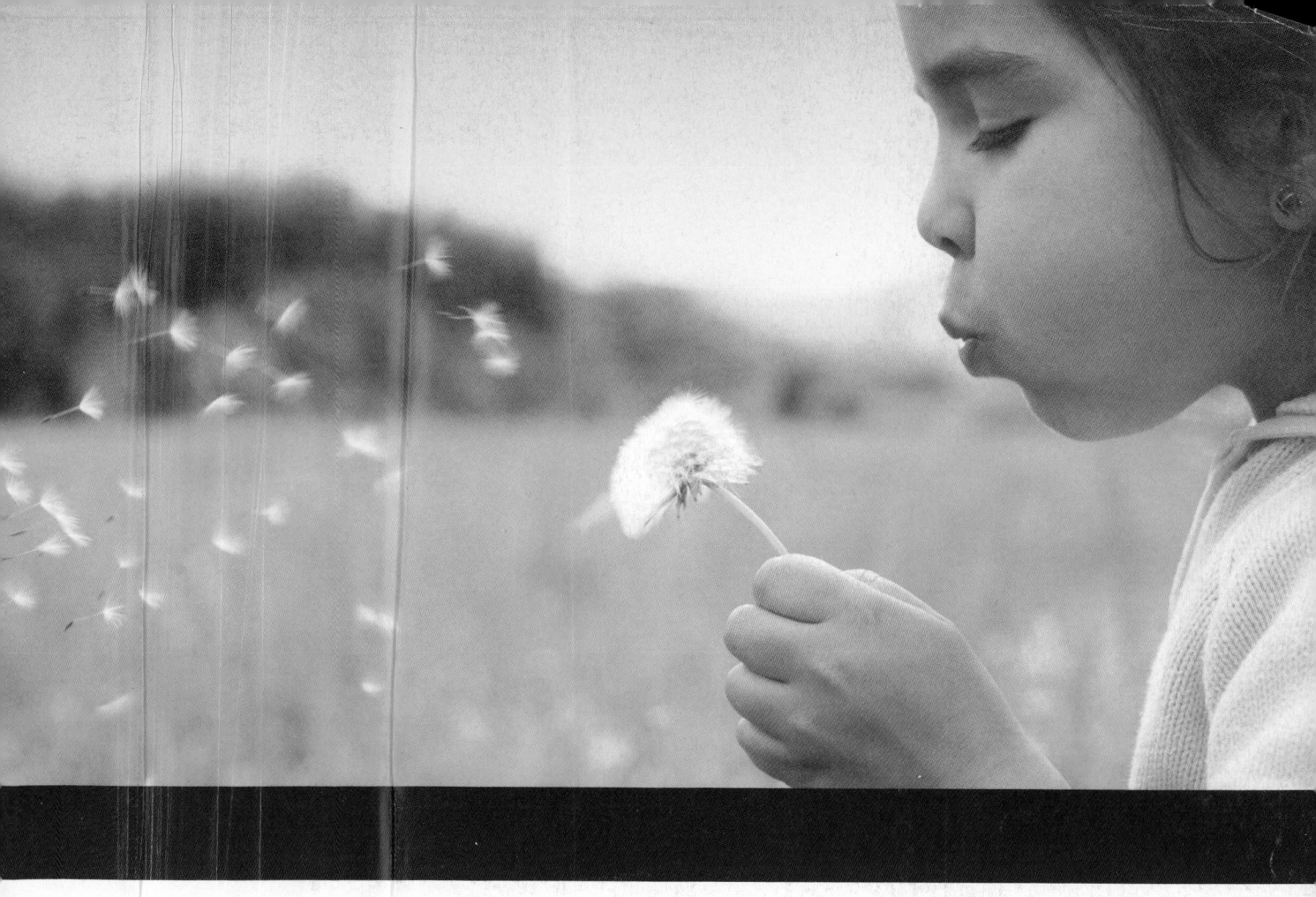

MATERNITY AND
PEDIATRIC NURSING

MATERNITY AND PEDIATRIC NURSING

Susan Scott Ricci, ARNP, MSN, MEd
Nursing Faculty
University of Central Florida
Orlando, Florida
Former Nursing Program Director and Faculty
Lake Sumter Community College
Leesburg, Florida

Terri Kyle, MSN, CPNP
Nursing Faculty
Herzing College
Orlando, Florida

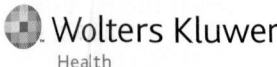
Wolters Kluwer | Lippincott Williams & Wilkins
Health

Philadelphia • Baltimore • New York • London
Buenos Aires • Hong Kong • Sydney • Tokyo

Acquisitions Editor: Jean Rodenberger
Development Editor: Danielle DiPalma
Editorial Assistant: Erin Sweeney
Senior Production Editor: Tom Gibbons
Director of Nursing Production: Helen Ewan
Senior Managing Editor/Production: Erika Kors
Art Director, Design: Joan Wendt
Art Director, Illustration: Brett MacNaughton
Manufacturing Coordinator: Karin Duffield
Indexer: Katherine Pitcoff
Compositor: Circle Graphics

9 8 7 6 5 4 3 2 1

Printed in China

Library of Congress Cataloging-in-Publication Data

Ricci, Susan Scott.
    Maternity and pediatric nursing / Susan Scott Ricci, Terri Kyle.
        p. ; cm.
    Includes bibliographical references and index.
    ISBN 978-0-7817-8055-1 (cloth : alk. paper) 1. Maternity nursing—Textbooks. 2. Pediatric nursing—Textbooks. I. Kyle, Terri. II. Title.
    [DNLM: 1. Maternal-Child Nursing. 2. Pediatric Nursing. 3. Women's Health. WY 157.3 R4912e 2009]
    RG951.R538 2009
    618.92'00231—dc22

                                                                2008025030

ISBN-13: 978-0-7817-8055-1

LWW.com

This book is dedicated to my loving husband Glenn, who has shown me the joy of learning,—and living—who continues to support me in all of my professional pursuits and whose patience and understanding have meant the world to me. And also to my children, Brian and Jennifer, who have always inspired me throughout their lives.

Susan Scott Ricci

This text is dedicated to my awesome family. My husband John has consistently encouraged and persuaded me to continue moving forward. My wonderful children, Christian and Caitlin, constantly delight and surprise me. I thank them for their support and faith in me.

Terri Kyle

ACKNOWLEDGMENTS

We would like to thank so many people who have helped bring the exciting prospect of this textbook into being. Our appreciation goes to Jean Rodenberger for her ongoing leadership and Elizabeth Nieginski for approaching us with this project and believing that we could assist in achieving her vision. We would also like to especially thank Danielle DiPalma for her editorial expertise and for her steadfastness to this project. She has been ever patient through chapter drafts and revisions. In addition, we would like to thank Maryann Foley for her professional collaboration and attention to detail within the chapters. Her nursing background has been invaluable from the start. Special thanks also to Sarah Kyle for her continued dedication to the vision and format of this textbook, as well as for her expert editing, and to Erin Sweeney for gently prodding us to complete revisions.

We would like to thank Tom Gibbons for his skillful production of the text. We would also like to thank Brett MacNaughton for his role in the beautiful illustrations and photographs, as well as photographer Gus Freedman and photo producer Amy Geller for their dedicated work on the photo shoot. We would like to thank the following institutions for their help in obtaining the photos for this book:

Boston Shriners Hospital
UMass Memorial Health Care
The Birthplace at Wellesley
Brigham and Women's Hospital
Newton-Wellesley Hospital

Also thanks to the many nurses, midwives, doctors, and families for their participation in this book, especially Debbie Turner, Paula McGarr, Susan Martinson, Grace Jackson, and Marianne Cummings. As always, special thanks to Terri's close friend and colleague Susan Carman for all of the physical work she performed on this text and, even more importantly, the emotional and moral support she so unfailingly provides.

S.S.R., T. K.

ABOUT THE AUTHORS

Susan Scott Ricci has a diploma from Washington Hospital Center School of Nursing, with a BSN, MSN, from Catholic University of America in Washington, D.C., and an M.Ed. in Counseling from the University of Southern Mississippi. She has worked in numerous women's health care settings, including labor and delivery, postpartum, prenatal, and family planning ambulatory care clinics. Susan is a women's health care nurse practitioner who has spent 30+ years in nursing education teaching in LPN, ADN, and BSN programs. She is involved in several professional nursing organizations and holds memberships in Sigma Theta Tau International Honor Society of Nursing, National Association of Ob/Gyn Nurses, Who's Who in Professional Nursing, American Nurses Association, and the Florida Council of Maternal-Child Nurses.

With Susan Scott Ricci's wealth of practical and educational experience, the time has come for her to concentrate on the "essential facts" of nursing instruction and reduce the amount of "nice to know" information that is presented to students. As an educator, she recognized the tendency for nursing educators to want to "cover the world" when teaching rather than focusing on the facts that students need to know to practice nursing. With this thought, Susan has directed her energy to the *birth* of this essentials textbook.

She recognizes that instructional time is shrinking as the world of health care is expanding exponentially. Therefore, with the valuable instructional time allotted, she has recognized the urgent need to present pertinent facts as concisely as possible to promote application of knowledge within nursing practice.

Terri Kyle earned a Bachelor of Science in Nursing from the University of North Carolina at Chapel Hill and a Master of Science in Nursing from Emory University in Atlanta, Georgia. She is a certified pediatric nurse practitioner and is currently enrolled in the Doctor of Nursing Practice program at the University of Florida. Practicing pediatric nursing for over 20 years, Terri has had the opportunity to serve children and their families in a variety of diverse settings.

She has experience in inpatient pediatrics in pediatric and neonatal intensive care units, newborn nursery, specialized pediatric units, and community hospitals. She has worked as a pediatric nurse practitioner in pediatric specialty clinics and primary care. She has been involved in teaching nursing for over 15 years with experience in both graduate and undergraduate education. Terri is a fellow in the National Association of Pediatric Nurse Practitioners and a member of the Sigma Theta Tau International Honor Society of Nursing, the National League for Nursing, the Society of Pediatric Nurses, and the Association of Camp Nurses.

With the limited time allotted in schools to the topic of maternity and pediatric nursing, Terri recognized the need for a textbook that "got to the point." She strongly believes in a concepts-based approach for learning nursing—that is, to teach the basics to students in a broad, contextual format so that they can apply that knowledge in a variety of situations. The concepts-based approach to nursing education is time efficient for nursing educators and fosters the development of critical thinking skills in student nurses.

Contributing Editor and Reviewers

CONTRIBUTING EDITOR

Susan Carman, BSN, MSN, MBA
Hubertus, Wisconsin

REVIEWERS

Virgie Barnes
Somerset Community College
Somerset, Kentucky

Kathleen Barta
University of Arkansas, Fayetteville
Fayetteville, Arkansas

Peggy Bozarth
Hopkinsville Community College
Hopkinsville, Kentucky

Marie Bright-Cobb
University of Akron
Akron, Ohio

Michele Brimeyer
University of Florida
Gainesville, Florida

Darlene Cantu
San Antonio College
San Antonio, Texas

Angelina Chambers
University of Texas Health Sciences, Houston
Houston, Texas

Patricia Coyne
Cochran School of Nursing
Yonkers, New York

Karen Davis
University of Arkansas Medical Sciences
Little Rock, Arkansas

Karen DeBoer
Macomb City CC Center
Clinton Township, Michigan

Carol Deresz
University of Texas Health Sciences, San Antonio
San Antonio, Texas

Patricia DuClos-Miller
Capital Community College
Hartford, Connecticut

Linda Dunn
University of Alabama, Tuscaloosa
Tuscaloosa, Alabama

Bernadette Emerick
Indian River Community College
Fort Pierce, Florida

Mary-Margaret Finney
North Georgia College
Dahlongea, Georgia

Jamie Flower
University of Arkansas, Fort Smith
Fort Smith, Arkansas

Rosa Garces
University of Puerto Rico Medical Sciences
Mercedita, Puerto Rico

Susan Gauthier
University of Alberta
Edmonton, Alberta

Julie Greenwalt
Indiana University of Pennsylvania
Indiana, Pennsylvania

Teresa James
University of Texas Health Science Center
San Antonio, Texas

Gloria Johns
Georgia Perimeter College
Clarkston, Georgia

Kathy Johnson
University of South Dakota
Sioux Falls, South Dakota

Linda Kapinos
Capital Community College
Hartford, Connecticut

Sandy Kluka
University of Manitoba
Winnipeg, Manitoba

Karen Knowles
Crouse Hospital School of Nursing
Syracuse, New York

Sue Koos
Heartland Community College, Normal
Normal, Illinois

Rochelle Kuhn
Frankford Hospital School of Nursing
Philadelphia, Pennsylvania

Robyn Leo
Worcester State College
Worcester, Massachusetts

Diwana Lowe
Georgia Perimeter College
Lawrenceville, Georgia

Deborah Lyons
Henry Ford Community College
Dearborn, Michigan

Maria Marconi
University of Rochester
Rochester, New York

Cindy Morgan
University of Tennessee, Chattanooga
Chattanooga, Tennessee

Sandra Nadelson
University of Nevada, Las Vegas
Las Vegas, Nevada

Valerie O'Dell
Youngstown State University
Youngstown, Ohio

Michelle Offutt
St. Petersburg College
Pinellas Park, Florida

Cynthia Payne
Georgia Perimeter College
Clarkston, Georgia

Gena Porter-Lankist
Chipola Junior College
Marianna, Florida

Sherri St. Pierre
Boston College
Chestnut Hill, Massachusetts

Ann Schide
Chattanooga State Tech CC
Chattanooga, Tennessee

Joy Shewchuk
Humber College
Toronto, Ontario

Cordia Starling
Dalton State College
Dalton, Georgia

Lois Tate
Union University
Germantown, Tennessee

Rosalie Tierney-Gumaer
University of Texas, San Antonio
San Antonio, Texas

Mareen Tippen
University of Michigan, Flint
Flint, Michigan

Alison Trider
St. Joseph College, West Hartford
West Hartford, Connecticut

Jennifer Visbisky
Jamestown Community College
Jamestown, New York

Bobbie Walker
Montgomery College, Takoma Park
Silver Spring, Maryland

Robin Wilson
Lincoln Memorial University
Harrogate, Tennessee

Barbara Wilson
Arizona State University
Mesa, Arizona

PREFACE

Many nursing curricula combine and teach maternity and pediatrics in tandem. This can be viewed as a *natural fit* of two content areas that belong together. Nursing education in general is founded upon the principle of mastering simpler concepts first and incorporating those concepts into the student's knowledge base. The student is then able to progress to problem solving in more complex situations. In today's education climate with reduced class time devoted to specialty courses, it is particularly important for nursing educators to focus on key concepts, rather than attempting to cover everything within a specific topic.

The intent of *Maternity and Pediatric Nursing* is to provide the nurse the basis needed for sound nursing care of women and children. The content in the book will enable the reader to guide women and children toward higher levels of wellness throughout the life cycle. In addition, the focus of the textbook will allow the reader to anticipate, identify, and address common problems and provide timely, evidence-based interventions to reduce long-term sequelae.

This textbook is designed as a practical approach to understanding the health of women and children. The main objective is to help the student build a strong knowledge base and assist with the development of critical thinking skills. Women in our society are becoming empowered to make informed and responsible choices regarding their health and that of their children, but to do so they need the encouragement and support of nurses who care for them. This textbook focuses on women and children throughout their lifespan, covering a broad scope of topics with emphasis placed upon common issues. Maternity nursing content coverage is comprehensive, yet presented in a concise and straightforward manner. The pediatric nursing content presents the important differences when caring for children compared with caring for adults. A nursing process approach provides relevant information in a concise and non-redundant manner. The content covered in the text arms the student or practicing nurse with essential information to care for women and their families, to assist them to make the right choices safely, intelligently, and with confidence.

Organization

Each chapter of *Maternity and Pediatric Nursing* focuses on a different aspect of maternity and/or pediatric nursing care. The book is divided into eleven units, beginning with general concepts related to maternity and pediatric nursing care, progressing from women's health, pregnancy and birth, through child health promotion and nursing management of alterations in children's health.

Unit 1: Introduction to Maternity and Pediatric Nursing

Unit 1 helps build a foundation for the student beginning the study of the care of women, infants, and children. This unit explores contemporary issues and trends in maternity and pediatric nursing. Perspectives on women's health and pediatric nursing, use of the nursing process, family-centered and atraumatic care, communication, and community-based nursing are addressed.

Unit 2: Women's Health Throughout the Lifespan

Unit 2 introduces the student to selected women's health topics, including structure and function of the reproductive system, common reproductive concerns, sexually transmitted infections, problems of the breast, and benign disorders and cancers of the female reproductive tract. This unit encourages the student to assist women in maintaining their quality of life, reducing their risk of disease, and becoming active partners with their health care professional.

Unit 3: Pregnancy

Unit 3 addresses topics related to normal pregnancy, including fetal development, genetics, and maternal adaptation to pregnancy. Nursing management during normal pregnancy is addressed, encouraging application of basic knowledge to nursing practice. Nursing management includes maternal and fetal assessment throughout pregnancy, interventions to promote self-care and minimize common discomforts, and patient education.

Unit 4: Labor and Birth

Unit 4 begins with an explanation of the normal labor and birth process, including maternal and fetal adaptations. This is followed by content focusing on the nurse's role during normal labor and birth, which includes maternal and fetal assessment, pharmacologic and non-pharmacologic comfort measures and pain management, and specific nursing interventions during each stage of labor and birth.

Unit 5: Postpartum Period

Unit 5 focuses on maternal adaptation during the normal postpartum period. Both physiologic and psychological aspects are explored. Paternal adaptation is also considered. This unit also presents related nursing management, including assessment of physical and emotional status, promoting comfort, assisting with elimination, counseling about sexuality and contraception, promoting nutrition, promoting family adaptation, and preparing for discharge.

Unit 6: The Newborn

Unit 6 covers physiologic and behavioral adaptations of the normal newborn. It also delves into nursing management of the normal newborn, including immediate assessment and specific interventions as well as ongoing assessment, physical examination, and specific interventions during the early newborn period.

Unit 7: Childbearing at Risk

Unit 7 shifts the focus to at-risk pregnancy, childbirth, and postpartum care. Pre-existing conditions of the woman, pregnancy-related complications, at-risk labor, emergencies associated with labor and birth, and medical conditions and complications affecting the postpartum woman are all covered. Treatment and nursing management are presented for each medical condition. This organization allows the student to build on a solid foundation of normal material when studying the at-risk content.

Unit 8: The Newborn at Risk

Unit 8 continues to center on at-risk content. Issues of the newborn with birth-weight variations, gestational age variations, congenital conditions, and acquired disorders are explored. Treatment and nursing management are presented for each medical condition. This organization helps cement the student's understanding of the material.

Unit 9: Health Promotion for the Growing Child and Family

Unit 9 provides information related to growth and development expectations of the well child from newborn through adolescence. Although not exhaustive in nature, this unit provides a broad knowledge base related to normal growth and development that the nurse can draw on in any situation. Common concerns related to growth and development and client/family education are included in each age-specific chapter.

Unit 10: Foundations of Pediatric Nursing

Unit 10 covers broad concepts that provide the foundation for providing nursing care for children. Rather than reiterating all aspects of nursing care, the unit focuses on specific details needed to provide nursing care for children in general. The content remains focused upon differences in caring for children compared with adults. Topics covered in this unit include anticipatory guidance and routine well child care (including immunization and safety), health assessment, nursing care of the child in the hospital, concerns common to special needs children, pediatric variations in medication and intravenous fluid delivery and nutritional support, and pain management in children.

Unit 11: Nursing Care of the Child With a Health Disorder

Unit 11 focuses on children's responses to health disorders. This unit provides comprehensive coverage of illnesses affecting children and is presented according to broad topics of disorders organized with a body systems approach. It also includes infectious, genetic, and mental health disorders as well as pediatric emergencies. Each chapter follows a similar format in order to facilitate presentation of the information as well as reduce repetition. The chapters begin with a nursing process overview for the particular broad topic, presenting differences in children and how the nursing process applies. The approach provides a general framework for addressing disorders within the chapter. Individual disorders are then addressed with attention to specifics related to pathophysiology, nursing assessment, nursing management, and special considerations. Common pediatric disorders are covered in greater depth than less common disorders. The format of the chapters allows for the building of a strong knowledge base and encourages critical thinking. Additionally, the format is nursing process driven and consistent from chapter to chapter, providing a practical and sensible presentation of the information.

Recurring Features

In order to provide the instructor and student with an exciting and user-friendly text, a number of recurring features have been developed.

Key Terms

A list of terms that are considered essential to the chapter's understanding is presented at the beginning of each chapter. Each key term appears in boldface, with the definition included in the text. Key terms may also be accessed on thePoint.

Learning Objectives

Learning Objectives included at the beginning of each chapter guide the student in understanding what is important and why, leading the student to prioritize information for learning. These valuable learning tools also provide opportunities for self-testing or instructor evaluation of student knowledge and ability.

WOW

Each chapter opens with inspiring Words of Wisdom, which offer helpful, timely, or interesting thoughts. These WOW statements set the stage for each chapter and give the student valuable insight into nursing care of women, children, and their families.

Case Studies

Real-life scenarios present relevant woman, child, and family information that is intended to perfect the student's caregiving skills. Questions about the scenario provide an opportunity for the student to critically evaluate the appropriate course of action.

Watch and Learn Icon

A special icon **WATCH&LEARN** throughout the book directs the student to free video clips that highlight maternity nursing care, childhood growth and development, communication with children, and provision of nursing care to children in the hospital. These clips can be viewed on thePoint website and also on the Student Resource CD.

Evidence-Based Practice

The consistent promotion of evidence-based practice is a key feature of the text. Throughout the chapters, pivotal questions addressed by current research have been incorporated into Evidence-Based Practice displays, which cite studies relevant to chapter content.

Healthy People 2010

Throughout the textbook, relevant *Healthy People 2010* objectives are outlined in box format. The nursing implications or guidance provided in the box serve as a roadmap for improving the health of women, mothers, and children.

Teaching Guidelines

An important tool for achieving health promotion and disease prevention is health education. Throughout the textbook, Teaching Guidelines raise awareness, provide timely and accurate information, and are designed to ensure the student's preparation for educating women, children, and their families about various issues.

Drug Guides

Drug guide tables summarize information about commonly used medications. The actions, indications, and significant nursing implications presented assist the student in providing optimum care to women, children, and their families.

Common Laboratory and Diagnostic Tests

The Common Laboratory and Diagnostic Tests tables in many of the chapters provide the student with a general understanding of how a broad range of disorders is diagnosed. Rather than reading the information repeatedly throughout the narrative, the student is then able to refer to the table as needed.

Common Medical Treatments

The Common Medical Treatments tables in many of the nursing management chapters provide the student with a broad awareness of how a common group of disorders is treated either medically or surgically. The tables serve as a reference point for common medical treatments.

Nursing Care Plans

Nursing Care Plans provide concrete examples of each step of the nursing process and are included in numerous chapters. The Nursing Care Plans summarize issue- or system-related content, thereby minimizing repetition.

Comparison Charts

These charts compare two or more disorders or other easily confused concepts. They serve to provide an explanation that clarifies the concepts for the student.

Nursing Procedures

Step-by-step Nursing Procedures are presented in a clear, concise format to facilitate competent performance of relevant procedures as well as to clarify pediatric variations when appropriate.

Consider This!

In every chapter the student is asked to *Consider This!* These first-person narratives engage the student in real-life scenarios experienced by their patients. The personal accounts evoke empathy and help the student to perfect caregiving skills. Each box ends with an opportunity for further contemplation, encouraging the student to think critically about the scenario.

Take Note!

The *Take Note!* feature draws the student's attention to points of critical emphasis throughout the chapter. This feature is often used to stress life-threatening or otherwise vitally important information.

Tables, Boxes, Illustrations, and Photographs

Abundant tables and boxes summarize key content throughout the book. Additionally, beautiful illustrations and photographs help the student to visualize the content. These features allow the student to quickly and easily access information.

Key Concepts

At the end of each chapter, Key Concepts provide a quick review of essential chapter elements. These bulleted lists help the student focus on the important aspects of the chapter.

References and Websites

References and websites that were used in the development of the text are provided at the end of each chapter. These listings enable the student to further explore topics of interest. Many online resources are provided as a means for the student to electronically explore relevant content material. These resources can be shared with women, children, and their families to enhance patient education and support.

Chapter Worksheets

Chapter worksheets at the end of each chapter assist the student in reviewing essential concepts. Chapter worksheets include:

• **Multiple Choice Questions**—These review questions are written to test the student's ability to apply chapter material. Questions cover maternal-newborn and women's health content that the student might encounter on the national licensing exam (NCLEX).

- **Critical Thinking Exercises**—These exercises challenge the student to incorporate new knowledge with previously learned concepts and reach a satisfactory conclusion. They encourage the student to think critically, problem solve, and consider his or her own perspective on given topics.
- **Study Activities**—These interactive activities promote student participation in the learning process. This section encourages increased interaction/learning via clinical, on-line, and community activities.

Teaching-Learning Package

Instructor's Resource DVD

This valuable resource for instructors includes all the materials instructors need to teach the maternity-pediatric course, including:

- PowerPoint presentations that correspond to each chapter and serve as a supplement to the instructor's course development
  - A Test Generator that features hundreds of questions within a powerful tool to help the instructor create quizzes and tests
- An Image Bank that provides access to photographs and illustrations from the text in a convenient, searchable format
- Lecture Outlines for organizing classroom instruction
- Sample syllabi for setting up the maternity-pediatric nursing course
- Assignments and reading comprehension quizzes, designed to test the student's understanding

Student Resource CD-ROM

The student resource CD-ROM, which is included for free in the front of the book, features video clips highlighting the developmental stages of pregnancy, vaginal labor and birth, scheduled cesarean section, breastfeeding assistance, developmental considerations, and nursing care of the child in the hospital. The CD-ROM also includes a Spanish-English audio glossary and an NCLEX alternate-item format tutorial.

ThePoint Solution

ThePoint Solution, http://thepoint.lww.com, a trademark of Wolters Kluwer Health, is a web-based course and content management system providing every resource that the instructor and student need in one easy-to-use site. Advanced technology and superior content combine at ThePoint to allow instructors to design and deliver online and offline courses, maintain grades and class rosters, and communicate with students. Students can visit ThePoint to access supplemental multimedia resources, such as Answers to Worksheets, a Glossary, and NCLEX-style student review questions to enhance their learning experience. ThePoint Solution package also includes an EBook, so students can search their text electronically, and journal articles to help students understand evidence-based practice. Students can also check the course syllabus, download content, upload assignments, and join an online study group. For instructors, a wealth of information can be found at ThePoint, all designed to make teaching easier, for example:

- Pre-lecture quizzes, made of five true/false and five fill-in-the-blank questions, are meant to be given at the beginning of class and help evaluate whether students are keeping up with the reading and the material it covers.
- Assignments, broken into four types—written, group, clinical, and Web—and organized by learning objective, provide opportunities for in- or after-class activities.
- Discussion topics, also organized by learning objective, allow students to critically

think through scenarios and discuss their ideas with other students. Case studies help bring the discussion topics and critical thinking exercises to life by presenting realistic and challenging situations in which to apply new skills.

• Guided lecture notes organize the chapter objective by objective and provide references to appropriate PowerPoint slides and figures from the text.

• Sample syllabi assist instructors with setting their courses and are provided for four different course lengths: 6, 8, 10, and 15 weeks.

ThePoint . . . where teaching, learning and technology click!

Susan Scott Ricci and Terri Kyle

CONTENTS

CHAPTER *9*

Violence and Abuse 242

U N I T   T H R E E
PREGNANCY 263

CHAPTER *10*

Fetal Development and Genetics 265

CHAPTER *11*

Maternal Adaptation During Pregnancy 288

CHAPTER *12*

Nursing Management During Pregnancy 313

UNIT FOUR
LABOR AND BIRTH 357

CHAPTER 13
Labor and Birth Process 359

CHAPTER 14
Nursing Management During Labor and Birth 385

UNIT FIVE
POSTPARTUM PERIOD 427

CHAPTER 15
Postpartum Adaptations 429

CHAPTER *16*

Nursing Management During the Postpartum Period 443

UNIT SIX
THE NEWBORN 477

CHAPTER *17*

Newborn Adaptation 479

CHAPTER *18*

Nursing Management of the Newborn 497

UNIT SEVEN
CHILDBEARING AT RISK 547

CHAPTER *19*

Nursing Management of Pregnancy at Risk: Pregnancy-Related Complications 549

CHAPTER *20*

Nursing Management of the Pregnancy at Risk: Selected Health Conditions and Vulnerable Populations 588

CHAPTER *21*

Nursing Management of Labor and Birth at Risk 634

CHAPTER *22*

Nursing Management of the Postpartum Woman at Risk 671

Wound Infections 680
Urinary Tract Infections 680
Mastitis 680
Therapeutic Management 681
Nursing Assessment 681
Nursing Management 682

Postpartum Affective Disorders 683
Postpartum or Baby Blues 685
Postpartum Depression 685
Postpartum Psychosis 686
Nursing Assessment 687
Nursing Management 688

UNIT EIGHT
THE NEWBORN AT RISK 693

CHAPTER 23
Nursing Care of the Newborn
With Special Needs 695

Birthweight Variations 696
Small-for-Gestational-Age Newborns 697
Large-for-Gestational-Age Newborns 698
Nursing Assessment 702
Nursing Management 702

Gestational Age Variations 703
Postterm Newborn 703
Preterm Newborn 704
Late Preterm Newborn 720

CHAPTER 24
Nursing Management of the Newborn
at Risk: Acquired and Congenital
Newborn Conditions 724

Acquired Disorders 726
Neonatal Asphyxia 726
Transient Tachypnea of the Newborn 727
Respiratory Distress Syndrome 728
Meconium Aspiration Syndrome 731
Persistent Pulmonary Hypertension of the
Newborn 732
Periventricular–Intraventricular Hemorrhage 733
Necrotizing Enterocolitis 734
Infants of Diabetic Mothers 735
Birth Trauma 740
Newborns of Substance-Abusing Mothers 743
Hyperbilirubinemia 750
Newborn Infections 755

Congenital Conditions 758
Esophageal Atresia and Tracheoesophageal Fistula 759

Omphalocele and Gastroschisis 760
Imperforate Anus 762
Bladder Exstrophy 762

UNIT NINE
HEALTH PROMOTION FOR THE GROWING CHILD
AND FAMILY 767

CHAPTER 25
Growth and Development of the
Newborn and Infant 769

Growth and Development Overview 770
Physical Growth 770
Weight 770
Height 770
Head and Chest Circumference 770
Organ System Maturation 771
Neurologic System 771
Respiratory System 771
Cardiovascular System 775
Gastrointestinal System 775
Genitourinary System 776
Integumentary System 776
Hematopoietic System 776
Immunologic System 777
Psychosocial Development 777
Cognitive Development 777
Motor Skill Development 777
Gross Motor Skills 777
Fine Motor Skills 779
Sensory Development 779
Sight 779
Hearing 780
Smell and Taste 780
Touch 780
Communication and Language Development 780
Social and Emotional Development 782
Stranger Anxiety 783
Separation Anxiety 783
Temperament 783
Cultural Influences on Growth and Development 783

The Nurse's Role in Newborn and Infant Growth
and Development 784
Nursing Process Overview 784
Promoting Healthy Growth and Development 784
Promoting Growth and Development Through Play 784
Promoting Early Learning 787
Promoting Safety 787
Promoting Nutrition 789
Promoting Healthy Sleep and Rest 793
Promoting Healthy Teeth and Gums 793

UNIT TEN
FOUNDATIONS OF PEDIATRIC NURSING 903

CHAPTER *30*
Health Supervision 905

CHAPTER *31*
Health Assessment of Children 938

UNIT ELEVEN
NURSING CARE OF THE CHILD WITH A HEALTH DISORDER 1097

CHAPTER *36*
Nursing Care of the Child With an Infectious or Communicable Disorder 1099

CHAPTER *37*
Nursing Care of the Child With a Neurologic Disorder 1138

CHAPTER *38*

Nursing Care of the Child With a Disorder
of the Eyes or Ears 1187

CHAPTER *39*

Nursing Care of the Child With a Respiratory Disorder 1219

CHAPTER *40*

Nursing Care of the Child With a Cardiovascular Disorder 1280

CHAPTER *41*

Nursing Care of the Child With a Gastrointestinal Disorder 1327

CHAPTER *51*

Nursing Care of the Child With a Cognitive or Mental Health Disorder 1694

CHAPTER *52*

Nursing Care During a Pediatric Emergency 1718

UNIT ONE

INTRODUCTION TO MATERNITY AND PEDIATRIC NURSING

PERSPECTIVES ON MATERNAL AND CHILD HEALTH CARE

KEY TERMS

atraumatic care
case management
certified nurse
   midwife (CNM)
childhood mortality rate
cultural competence
culture
discipline
doula

emancipated minor
ethnicity
ethnocentrism
evidence-based nursing
   practice
family
family-centered care
family structure
fetal mortality rate

foster care
infant mortality rate
maternal mortality rate
morbidity
mortality
neonatal mortality rate
religion
social capital
spirituality

LEARNING OBJECTIVES

Upon completion of the chapter, the learner will be able to:

1. Identify the key milestones in the evolution of maternal and child health nursing.
2. Describe the major components, concepts, and influences associated with the nursing management of women, children, and families.
3. Compare the past definitions of health and illness to the current definitions, as well as the measurements used to assess health and illness in children.
4. Identify the factors that affect maternal and child health.
5. Delineate the structures, roles, and functions of the family and how they affect the health of women and children.
6. Evaluate how society and culture can influence the health of women, children, and families.
7. Appraise the health care barriers affecting women, children, and families.
8. Discuss the ethical and legal issues that may arise when caring for women, children, and families.

*S*ophia Greenly, a 38-year-old woman pregnant with her third child, comes to the prenatal clinic for a routine follow-up visit. Her mother, Betty, accompanies her because Sophia's husband is out of town. Sophia lives with her husband and two children, ages 4 and 9. She works part-time as a lunch aide in the local elementary school. What factors may play a role in influencing the health of Sophia and her family?

Wow

Being pregnant and giving birth is like crossing a narrow bridge: people can accompany you to the bridge, and they can greet you on the other side, but you walk that bridge alone. And the journey doesn't end there: children are the future of a society and special gifts to the world. Changes in our society and world require us to be attentive to and value them and their health.

A person's ability to lead a fulfilling life and to participate fully in society depends largely on his or her health status. Although the overall health of children has improved and the rates of death and illness in some areas have decreased, the need to focus on the health of women and children remains. Habits and practices established during pregnancy and early during childhood can have profound effects on a person's health and illness throughout life. As a society, creating a population that cares about women, children, and families and promotes solid health care and lifestyle choices is crucial.

Maternal and newborn nursing encompasses a wide scope of practice typically associated with childbearing. It includes care of the woman before pregnancy, care of the woman and her fetus during pregnancy, care of the woman after pregnancy, and care of the newborn, usually during the first 6 weeks after birth. The overall goal of maternal and newborn nursing is to promote and maintain optimal health of the woman and her family. Child health nursing, commonly referred to as pediatric nursing, involves the care of the child from infancy through adolescence. In the United States, the number of children under age 18 years is approximately 73.5 million, accounting for 25% of the population (Child Trends, 2006a, 2006b). The overall goal of pediatric nursing practice is to promote and assist the child in maintaining optimal levels of health, while recognizing the influence of the family on the child's well-being. This goal involves health promotion and disease and injury prevention as well as assisting with care during illness. The common thread in both of these is the care of the family.

Now more than ever, nurses contribute to nearly every health care experience. Events from birth to death, and every health care emergency in between, will likely involve the presence of a nurse. Involvement of a knowledgeable, supportive, comforting nurse often leads to a positive health care experience. Skilled nursing practice depends on a solid base of knowledge and clinical expertise delivered in a caring, holistic manner. Nurses, using their knowledge and passion, help meet the health care needs of their clients throughout the life span, whether the client is a pregnant woman, a fetus, a partner, a child, or the parents or family members of a child. Nurses fill a variety of roles in helping clients to live healthier lives by providing direct care, emotional support, comfort, information, advice, advocacy, support, and counseling. Nurses are often "in the trenches" advocating for issues, drawing attention to the importance of health care for the client, and dealing with the lack of resources, the lack of access to health care, and the focus on acute care rather than education and prevention.

This chapter presents a general overview of the health care of women, children, and families and describes the major factors affecting maternal and child health. Nurses need to be knowledgeable about these concepts and factors to ensure that they provide professional care.

Historical Development

The health care of children has changed over the years due in part to devastating epidemics, social trends in our country, changes in the health care system, and federal and state regulations. By reviewing historical events, nurses can gain a better understanding of the current and future status of maternal and child health nursing.

Evolution of Maternal and Newborn Nursing

Childbirth in colonial America was a difficult and dangerous experience. During the 17th and 18th centuries, women giving birth often died as a result of exhaustion, dehydration, infection, hemorrhage, or seizures (Cassidy, 2006). Approximately 50% of all children died before age 5 (Brodsky, 2006; Jolivet, 2006), compared with the 0.06% infant mortality rate of today (World Factbook, 2006).

Centuries ago, "granny midwives" handled the normal birthing process for most women. They learned their skills through an apprenticeship with a more experienced midwife. Physicians usually were called only in extremely difficult cases, and all births took place at home.

During the early 1900s, physicians attended about half the births in the United States. Midwives often cared for women who could not afford a doctor. Many women were attracted to hospitals because this showed affluence and they provided pain management, which was not available in home births. In the 1950s, "natural childbirth" practices advocating birth without medication and focusing on relaxation techniques were introduced. These techniques opened the door to childbirth education classes and helped bring the father back into the picture. Both partners could participate by taking an active role in pregnancy, childbirth, and parenting (Fig. 1.1).

Box 1.1 shows a timeline of childbirth in America. In many ways, childbirth practices in the United States have come full circle, as we see the return of nurse midwives and doulas. The concept of women helping other women during childbirth is not new: women who labored and gave birth at home were traditionally attended to by relatives and midwives (see Evidence-Based Practice box). A **certified nurse midwife** (**CNM**) has postgraduate training in the care of normal pregnancy and delivery and is certified by the American College of Nurse Midwives (ACNM). A **doula** is a birth assistant who provides emotional, physical, and educational support to the woman and family during childbirth and the postpartum period. Many nurses working in labor and birth areas today are credentialed in their specialty so that they can provide optimal care to the woman and her newborn. Childbirth

FIGURE 1.1 Today fathers and partners are welcome to take an active role in the pregnancy and childbirth experience. (**A**) A couple can participate together in childbirth education classes. (Photo by Gus Freedman.) (**B**) Fathers and partners can assist the woman throughout her labor and delivery. (Photo by Joe Mitchell.)

choices are often based on what works best for the mother, child, and family.

Evolution of Child Health Nursing

In the 17th and 18th centuries in the United States, the overall health of the country was poorer than it is today, as demonstrated by the high mortality rates and shorter life spans. Beginning in the early 19th century, a flood of immigrants left the eastern American cities, which had high rates of infectious diseases as a result of the crowded living conditions, inadequate and unsanitary food such as contaminated milk, and harsh working conditions, including child labor. The devastating epidemics of small-pox, diphtheria, scarlet fever, and measles hit the young the hardest. During this period, society viewed children as a commodity to increase the population and share in the work to be done.

Over time, changes have focused attention on the health of children. During the 19th century, public schools were developed in this country and the court system began viewing children as minors. In 1870, the first pediatric pro-fessorship for a physician was awarded in the United States to Abraham Jacobi, who is known as the father of pedi-atrics. This event was a major change in the United States because it underlined the importance of providing special-ized training and education about children to health care providers. In 1889 Jacobi started milk distribution centers, which provided mothers with uncontaminated milk for their sick infants as well as information about the impor-tance of pasteurization. This one intervention decreased the number of infant deaths.

In the early 1900s, Lillian Wald established the Henry Street Settlement House in New York City; this is consid-ered the start of public health nursing. This facility pro-vided medical and other services to the poor families. Services included home nurse visits to mothers to provide instruction and nursing care. As hospitals developed dur-ing this time, health care personnel were trained to take care of children in this setting. Parents of hospitalized chil-dren were actually discouraged from visiting their children to prevent the spread of infection or transmission of dis-ease. Health care personnel also thought that restricted parental involvement would minimize emotional stress.

Nursing in public schools began in 1902 with the ap-pointment of Lina Rogers as a full-time public school nurse in New York. A professional course in pediatric nursing started in the early 1900s at Teachers' College of Columbia University.

The turn of the 20th century brought new knowledge about nutrition, sanitation, bacteriology, pharmacology, medication, and psychology. Penicillin, corticosteroids, and vaccines, which were developed during this time, as-sisted with the fight against communicable diseases. By the end of the 20th century, technological advances signifi-cantly affected all aspects of health care. These trends have led to increased survival rates in children; however, many of these survivors have chronic disabilities. For example, mechanical ventilation and medications to foster lung de-velopment in premature infants have increased their sur-vival rate, but the survivors are often faced with a myriad of chronic illnesses such as bronchopulmonary dysplasia, retinopathy of prematurity, cerebral palsy, or developmen-tal delay.

In the 1960s, changes in the health care delivery sys-tem and shifts in the population's health status led to the development of the nurse practitioner role. The 1970s saw the introduction of cost-control systems from the federal government because of rapid escalation of health care ex-penditures. The significant changes in the U.S. health care system in the 1980s have affected pediatric nursing and child health care, as outcomes and cost containment were emphasized. Some of these changes brought more ad-vanced practice nurses into the field of pediatrics. Mod-ern maternal–child advanced practice nursing includes nurse practitioners, nurse midwives, clinical nurse spe-cialists, and case managers. In the 1980s, the Division of

---

BOX 1.1   Childbirth in America: A Time Line

1700s   Men did not attend births because it was considered indecent.

Women faced birth not with joy and ecstasy but with fear of death.

Female midwives attended the majority of all births at home.

1800s   There is a shift from using midwives to doctors among middle-class women.

The word *obstetrician* was formed from the Latin, meaning "to stand before."

Puerperal (childbed) fever was occurring in epidemic proportions.

Louis Pasteur demonstrated that streptococci were the major cause of puerperal fever that was killing mothers after delivery.

The first cesarean section was performed in Boston in 1894.

The x-ray was developed in 1895 and was used to assess pelvic size for birthing purposes (Feldhusen, 2003).

1900s   Twilight sleep (a heavy dose of narcotics and amnesiacs) was used on women during childbirth in the United States.

The United States was 17th out of 20 nations in infant mortality rates.

Fifty percent to 75% of all women gave birth in hospitals by 1940.

Nurseries were started because mothers could not care for their baby for several days after receiving chloroform gas.

Dr. Grantley Dick–Reed (1933) wrote *Childbirth Without Fear*, which reduced the "fear–tension–pain" cycle women experienced during labor and birth.

Dr. Fernand Lamaze (1984) wrote *Painless Childbirth: The Lamaze Method*, which advocated distraction and relaxation techniques to minimize the perception of pain.

Amniocentesis was first performed to assess fetal growth in 1966.

In the 1970s the cesarean section rate was about 5%. By 1990 it rose to 24%, where it stands currently (Martin, 2002).

The 1970s and 1980s see a growing trend to return birthing back to the basics—nonmedicated, nonintervening childbirth.

In the late 1900s, freestanding birthing centers—LDRPs—were designed, and the number of home births began to increase.

2000s   One in four women undergo a surgical birth (cesarean).

CNMs once again assist couples at home, in hospitals, or in freestanding facilities with natural childbirths. Research shows that midwives are the safest birth attendants for most women, with lower infant mortality and maternal rates, and fewer invasive interventions such as episiotomies and cesareans (Keefe, 2003).

Childbirth classes of every flavor abound in most communities.

According to the latest available data, the United States ranks 21st in the world in maternal deaths. The maternal mortality rate is approximately 7 in 1,000 live births.

According to the latest available data, the United States ranks 27th in the world in infant mortality rates. The infant mortality rate is approximately 7 in 1,000 live births (United Nations, 2003).

Maternal–Child Health Nursing Practice of the American Nurses Association developed maternal–child health standards to provide important guidelines for delivering nursing care.

Core Concepts of Maternal and Child Health Nursing

Maternal and child health nursing focuses on providing evidence-based care to the client within the context of the family. This care involves the implementation of an interdisciplinary plan in a collaborative manner to ensure continuity of care that is cost-effective, quality-oriented, and outcome-focused. Maternal and child health nursing involves family-centered, evidence-based, case-managed care. Children should receive atraumatic care to minimize the stress associated with health care procedures or situations.

Family–Centered Care

Family-centered care is the delivery of safe, satisfying, high-quality health care that focuses on and adapts to the physical and psychosocial needs of the family. It is a cooperative effort of families and other caregivers that recognizes the strength and integrity of the family. The basic principles of family-centered care are:

- Childbirth is considered a normal, healthy event in the life of a family.
- Childbirth affects the entire family, and relationships will change.
- Families are capable of making decisions about their own care if given adequate information and professional support (Roudebush et al., 2006).

The philosophy of family-centered care recognizes the family as the constant. The health and functioning of the family affect the health of the client and other mem-

EVIDENCE-BASED PRACTICE 1.1
How Do Women in Childbirth Respond to Continuous Labor Support?

● Study

Throughout history, women have been helping other women in labor by providing emotional support, comfort measures, information, and advocacy. However, in recent years this practice has waned, and facilities frequently adhere to strict specific routines that may leave women feeling "dehumanized." A study was done to assess the effects on mothers and their newborns of continuous, one-to-one intrapartum care in comparison to usual care. The study also evaluated routine practices and policies in the birth environment that might affect a woman's autonomy, freedom of movement, and ability to cope with labor; who the caregiver was, whether or not a staff member of the facility; and when the support began, early or late in labor.

All published and unpublished randomized clinical trials comparing continuous support during labor with usual care were examined. One author and one research assistant used standard methods for data collection and analysis and extracted the data independently. Clinical trial authors provided additional information. The researchers used relative risk for categorical data and weighted mean difference for continuous data. Sixteen trials from 11 countries involving 13,391 women were examined to provide the data.

▲ Findings

Women receiving continuous intrapartum support had a greater chance of a spontaneous vaginal delivery (includ-

ing without forceps or vacuum extraction). They also had a slight decrease in the length of labor and required less analgesia during this time. These women also reported increased satisfaction with their labor and childbirth experience. Overall, the support, when provided by someone other than a facility staff member and initiated early in labor, proved to be more effective.

■ Nursing Implications

Based on this research, it is clear that women in labor benefit from one-to-one support during labor. Nurses can use the information gained from this study to educate women about the importance of support persons during labor and delivery. Nurses can also act as client advocates in facilities where they work to foster an environment that encourages the use of support persons during the intrapartum period. The focus of nursing needs to be individualized, supportive, and collaborative with the family during their childbearing experience. In short, nurses should place the needs of the mother and her family first in providing a continuum of care.

Although the study found that support is more effective when provided by someone other than a staff member, support from an individual is key. Assigning the same nurse to provide care to the couple throughout the birthing experience also fosters a one-to-one relationship that helps meet the couple's needs and promotes feelings of security. By meeting the couple's needs, the nurse is enhancing their birthing experience.

Source: Hodnett, E. D., Gates, S. Hofmeyr, G. J., & Sakata, C. Continuous support for women during childbirth. *Cochrane Database of Systematic Reviews* 2007. Issue 3. Art No.: CD003766.DOI:10.1002/14651858.CD003766.pub2.

bers of the family. Family members support one another well beyond the health care provider's brief time with them, such as during the childbearing process or during a child's illness. Birth is viewed as a normal life event rather than a medical procedure.

With family-centered care, support and respect for the uniqueness and diversity of families are essential, along with encouragement and enhancement of the family's strengths and competencies. It is important to create opportunities for families to demonstrate their abilities and skills. Families also can acquire new abilities and skills to maintain a sense of control and empowerment in meeting the needs of the client. Family-centered care promotes greater family self-determination, decision-making abilities, control, and self-efficacy, thereby enhancing the client's and family's sense of empowerment. When implementing family-centered care, nurses seek caregiver input; these suggestions and advice are incorporated into the client's plan of care as the nurse counsels and teaches the family appropriate health care interven-

tions. Today, as nurses partner with various experts to provide high-quality and cost-effective care, one expert partnership that nurses can make is with the client's family.

The impact of family-centered care can be seen in the models of care delivery for women. From the 1980s to the present, there have been increased access to care for all women (regardless of their ability to pay) and hospital redesigns (labor, delivery, and recovery [LDR] rooms; labor, delivery, recovery, and postpartum [LDRP] spaces) aimed at keeping families together during the childbirth experience. This impact also can be seen in the care of children: rooming-in and liberal visiting policies allow parents and other family members to participate in the child's care (Fig. 1.2).

Evidence-Based, Case-Managed Care

Evidence-based nursing practice involves the use of research or evidence in establishing a plan of care and

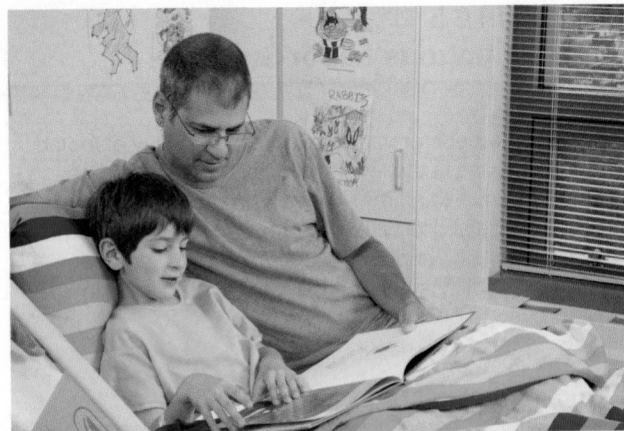

FIGURE 1.2 Providing an opportunity for the parent to interact with the child is an important component of family-centered nursing care.

implementing that care. Evidence-based practice is a problem-solving approach to making nursing clinical decisions (Newhouse, 2006). This model of nursing practice includes the use of the best current evidence in making decisions about care. Widespread use of evidence-based practice may lead to a decrease in variation of care while at the same time increasing quality.

Modern health care focuses on an interdisciplinary plan of care designed to meet a client's physical, developmental, educational, spiritual, and psychosocial needs. This interdisciplinary collaborative type of care is termed **case management**, a collaborative process involving assessment, planning, implementation, coordination, monitoring, and evaluation. It involves the following components:

• Advocacy, communication, and resource management
• Client-focused comprehensive care across a continuum
• Coordinated care with an interdisciplinary approach (Commission for Case Management Certification, n.d.)

When the nurse effectively functions in the role as a case manager, client and family satisfaction is increased, fragmentation of care is decreased, and outcome measurement for a homogenous group of clients is possible.

Atraumatic Pediatric Care

Children undergo a wide range of interventions, many of which can be traumatic, stressful, and painful. The various settings where the child receives care can be scary and overwhelming to the child and family. The child and family interact with various health care personnel, which leads to an increased potential for anxiety. A major component of the child health nursing philosophy is the importance of providing **atraumatic care**. This involves the use of interventions that minimize physical and psychological distress for children and families. Nurses must be ever-vigilant for any situation that has the potential for causing

distress and should be able to identify potential stressors. Pediatric nurses should minimize separation of the child from the family, should decrease the child's exposure to stressful situations, and should strive to prevent or minimize pain and injury. The importance of providing atraumatic care to children is integrated throughout this text.

Think back to Sophia and her mother, Betty, who were described at the beginning of the chapter. Sophia and her husband are planning to use natural childbirth and to have their children present for the birth. While Sophia is waiting to be called for her appointment, Betty says, "Things have changed so much since I was pregnant. It's amazing what happens nowadays." Explain how things have changed in maternal and child health care, focusing on the concept of family-centered care.

Health Status

At one time, health was defined simply as the absence of disease; health was measured by monitoring the mortality and morbidity of a group. Over the past century, however, the focus on health has shifted to disease prevention, health promotion, and wellness. The World Health Organization defines health as "a state of complete physical, mental, and social well-being, and not merely the absence of disease or infirmity" (WHO, 2008). The definition of health is complex; it is not merely the absence of disease or an analysis of mortality and morbidity statistics.

In 1979, the Surgeon General's Report, *Healthy People*, presented a prevention agenda for the nation that identified the most significant preventable threats to the health of the United States. Through a series of reports (the current report is *Healthy People 2010: National Health Promotion and Disease Prevention Objectives*), the country now has a comprehensive, nationwide health promotion and disease prevention agenda that includes emphasis on children's health (U.S. Department of Health & Human Services [DHHS], 2000). Ten specific health indicators serve as a way to evaluate progress made in the public health arena and to coordinate the national health improvement efforts. The *Healthy People 2010* Box 1.1 highlights the major health indicators of the 21st century that need to be addressed.

HEALTHY PEOPLE *2010*

Major Health Concerns of the 21st Century

• Physical activity	• Mental health
• Overweight and obesity	• Injury and violence
• Tobacco use	• Environmental quality
• Substance abuse	• Immunizations
• Responsible sexual behavior	• Access to health care

Healthy People 2010 also outlines major goals intended to increase the quality and years of healthy life and to eliminate health disparities between ethnic groups by targeting the lifestyle choices and environmental conditions that cause 70% of premature deaths in the United States. The *Healthy People 2010* Box 1.2 identifies specific national health goals related to maternal, infant, and child health.

Measuring health status is not a simple or convenient process. For example, some individuals with chronic illnesses do not see themselves as ill if they can control their condition through self-management. A traditional method used in this country to measure health is to examine mortality and morbidity data. Information is collected and analyzed to provide an objective description of the nation's health.

Mortality

Mortality is the incidence or number of individuals who have died over a specific period. This statistic is presented as rates per 100,000 and is calculated from a sample of death certificates. The National Center for Health Statistics, under the DHHS, collects, analyzes, and disseminates the data on America's mortality rates.

HEALTHY PEOPLE 2010

National Health Goals—Maternal, Infant, and Child Health

- Reduce fetal and infant deaths.
- Reduce maternal deaths.
- Reduce maternal illness and complications resulting from pregnancy.
- Increase the proportion of pregnant women who receive early and adequate prenatal care.
- Increase the proportion of pregnant women who attend a series of prepared childbirth classes.
- Increase the proportion of very low-birth weight (VLBW) infants born at level III hospitals or subspecialty perinatal centers.
- Reduce cesarean births among low-risk (full-term, singleton, vertex presentation) women.
- Reduce low birth weight (LBW) and VLBW.
- Reduce preterm births.
- Increase the proportion of mothers who achieve a recommended weight gain during their pregnancies.
- Increase the percentage of healthy, full-term infants who are laid down to sleep on their backs.
- Reduce the occurrence of developmental disabilities.
- Reduce the occurrence of spina bifida and other neural tube defects (NTDs).
- Increase the proportion of pregnancies begun with an optimum folic acid level.
- Increase abstinence from alcohol, cigarettes, and illicit drugs among pregnant women.
- Reduce the occurrence of fetal alcohol syndrome (FAS).
- Increase the proportion of mothers who breast-feed their babies.
- Ensure appropriate newborn bloodspot screening, follow-up testing, and referral to services.

Maternal Mortality

The **maternal mortality rate** is the number of deaths from any cause during the pregnancy cycle per 100,000 live births. In the United States, the maternal mortality rate is 7.5 (McClure, Goldenberg & Bann, 2007). The federal government has pledged to improve maternal–child care outcomes and thus reduce mortality rates for women and children.

During the past several decades, mortality and morbidity have dramatically decreased as a result of an increased emphasis on hygiene, good nutrition, exercise, and prenatal care for all women. However, women are still experiencing complications at significant rates. The United States is one of the most medically and technologically advanced nations and has the highest per capita spending on health care in the world, but our current mortality rates indicate the need for improvement. For example:

- Two to three women die in the United States every day from pregnancy complications, and more than 30% of pregnant women (1.8 million women annually) experience some type of illness or injury during childbirth (Centers for Disease Control and Prevention [CDC], 2006b, 2006e, 2006f).
- The United States ranks 21st (in other words, below 20 other countries) in rates of maternal deaths (deaths per 100,000 live births).
- Most pregnancy-related complications are preventable. The most common are ectopic pregnancy, preterm labor, hemorrhage, emboli, hypertension, infection, stroke, diabetes, and heart disease. The leading causes of pregnancy-related mortality for the year 2003 (the last year for which data are available) are embolism (20%), hemorrhage (17%), pregnancy-related hypertension (16%), and infection (13%; CDC, 2006b, 2006e, 2006f).

The maternal mortality and morbidity rates for African-American women have been three to four times higher than for whites (Matthews & MacDorman, 2006). Researchers do not entirely understand what accounts for this disparity, but some suspected causes of the higher maternal mortality rates for minority women include low socioeconomic status, limited or no insurance coverage, bias among health care providers (which may foster distrust), and quality of care available in the community. Language and legal barriers may also explain why some immigrant women do not receive good prenatal care.

Lack of care during pregnancy is a major factor contributing to a poor outcome. Prenatal care is well known to prevent complications of pregnancy and to support the birth of healthy infants, and not all women receive the same quality and quantity of health care during a pregnancy. More than 40% of African-American, Native American, and Latino women do not obtain prenatal care during their first trimester of pregnancy (Hollander, 2006).

The CDC has noted that the disparity in maternal mortality rates between women of color and white women represent one of the largest racial disparities among public health indicators. Eliminating racial and ethnic disparities in maternal–child health care requires enhanced efforts at preventing disease, promoting health, and delivering appropriate and timely care (CDC, 2006b, 2006e, 2006f). The CDC has called for more research and monitoring to understand and address racial disparities, along with increased funding for prenatal and postpartum care. Research is needed to identify causes and to design initiatives to reduce these disparities, and the CDC is calling on Congress to expand programs to provide preconception and prenatal care to underserved women.

The Health Resources and Services Administration (HRSA)'s Maternal and Child Health Bureau (MCHB) has primary federal responsibility for improving the health of mothers and children in the United States. More than 28 million infants, children, and pregnant women are served by an MCHB program annually (CDC, 2006e).

Fetal Mortality

The **fetal mortality rate** or fetal death rate refers to the intrauterine death of a fetus who is 20 weeks of gestation or more per 1,000 live births. Fetal mortality may be attributable to maternal factors (e.g., malnutrition, disease, or preterm cervical dilation) or fetal factors (e.g., chromosomal abnormalities or poor placental attachment). Fetal mortality provides an overall picture of the quality of maternal health and prenatal care.

Neonatal and Infant Mortality

The **neonatal mortality rate** is the number of infant deaths occurring in the first 28 days of life per 1,000 live births. The **infant mortality rate** is the number of deaths occurring in the first 12 months of life. It also is documented as the number of deaths of infants younger than 1 year of age per 1,000 live births. The infant mortality rate is used as an index of the general health of a country. Generally, this statistic is one of the most significant measures of children's health. In the United States, the infant mortality rate is 6.0 (CDC, 2006e; National Center for Health Statistics [NCHS], 2006) (Fig. 1.3).

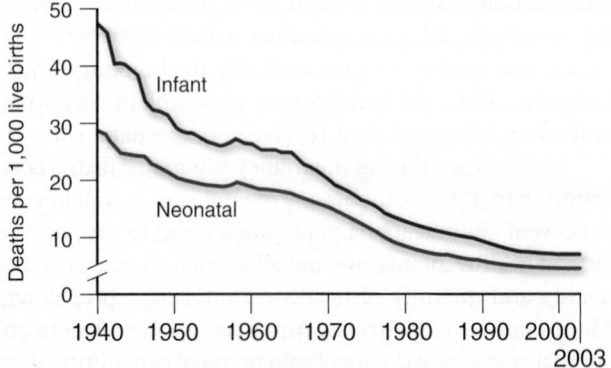

FIGURE 1.3 Infant and neonatal mortality, 1940–2003.

The infant mortality rate varies greatly from state to state as well as between ethnic groups. The United States has one of the highest gross national products in the world and is known for its technological capabilities, but in 2000 it ranked 27th in infant mortality rates among industrialized nations (U.S. Department of Health and Human Services, 2006). The main causes of early infant death in this country include problems occurring at birth or shortly thereafter. These include prematurity, low birthweight, congenital anomalies, sudden infant death syndrome, and respiratory distress syndrome.

> ▶ **Take** NOTE!
>
> *African-American and American Indian/ Alaska Native infants have consistently had higher infant mortality rates than other ethnic groups (Federal Interagency Forum on Child and Family Statistics, 2006).*

Congenital anomalies remain the leading cause of infant mortality in the United States. Low birthweight and prematurity are major indicators of infant health and significant predictors of infant mortality (Hoyert et al., 2006). The lower the birthweight, the higher the risk of infant mortality; thus, the high incidence of low birthweight (<2,500 g) in the United States is a significant reason why its infant mortality rate is higher than that of other countries (Ogbolu, 2007).

After birth, other health promotion strategies can significantly improve an infant's health and chances of survival. Breastfeeding has been shown to reduce rates of infection in infants and to improve their long-term health. Emphasizing the importance of placing an infant on his or her back to sleep will reduce the incidence of sudden infant death syndrome (SIDS). Encouraging mothers to join support groups to prevent postpartum depression and learn sound child-rearing practices will improve the health of both mothers and their infants.

Childhood Mortality

The **childhood mortality rate** is the number of deaths per 100,000 population in children 1 to 14 years of age. The childhood mortality rate in the United States has decreased by about 50% since 1980: in 2003, the mortality rate for children ages 1 to 4 years was 31 per 100,000, and the rate for children ages 5 to 14 years was 17 per 100,000 (Child Trends, 2006b). The leading cause of death in children is motor vehicle accidents. Many of these deaths could be prevented by educating parents about the value of car seats and seat belt use, the dangers of driving under the influence of alcohol and other substances, and the importance of pedestrian safety. Other causes of childhood mortality are suicide, homicide, and AIDS.

Morbidity

Morbidity is the measure of the prevalence of a specific illness in a population at a particular time. It is presented in rates per 1,000 population. Morbidity is often difficult to define and record because the types of measurement used vary widely—for example, visits to the physician or diagnosis for hospital admission. Information may be difficult to obtain, such as that gathered by household interviews from research studies. Morbidity statistics are revised less frequently because of this difficulty in defining or obtaining the information.

Women's Health Indicators

Women today face not only diseases of genetic origin but also diseases that arise from poor personal habits. Even though women represent 51% of the population, only recently have researchers and the medical community focused on their special health needs. A recent significant study identified an urgent need to improve women's access to health insurance and health care services, place a stronger emphasis on prevention, and invest in more research on women's health (National Women's Law Center [NWLC] et al., 2007). It identified indicators of women's access to health care services, measuring the degree to which women receive preventive health care and engage in health-promoting activities (Box 1.2). The report card gave the nation an overall grade of "unsatisfactory," and not a single state received a grade of "satisfactory." Other substandard findings included the following:

- No state has focused enough attention on preventive measures, such as smoking cessation, exercise, nutrition, and screening for diseases.

BOX 1.2 **The National Indicators of Women's Health**

- Lung cancer death rate
- Diabetes
- Heart disease death rate
- Binge drinking
- High school completion
- Poverty
- Wage gap
- Rate of AIDS
- Maternal mortality rate
- Rate of *Chlamydia* infection
- Breast cancer death rate
- Heart disease death rate

- Smoking
- Being overweight
- No physical activity during leisure time
- Eating five fruits and vegetables daily
- Colorectal screening
- Mammograms
- Pap smears
- First-trimester prenatal care
- Access to health insurance

Adapted from National Women's Law Center, FOCUS/University of Pennsylvania, the Lewin Group. (2007). *Making the grade on women's health: a national state-by-state report card.* Washington, DC: National Women's Law Center.

- Too many women lack health insurance coverage: nationally, nearly one in seven women (14%) has no health insurance.
- No state has adequately addressed women's health needs in the areas of reproductive health, mental health, and violence against women.
- Limited research has been done on health conditions that primarily affect women and that affect women differently than men (NWLC et al., 2007).

Poor health habits can have a negative impact on all women. Smoking, drug abuse, high cholesterol levels, and obesity lead to high mortality and morbidity rates in our nation. Cardiovascular disease (CVD) is the number-one cause of death of women, regardless of racial or ethnic group. More than 500,000 women die annually in the United States of CVD—about one death per minute (Alexander et al., 2007) Women who have a heart attack are more likely than men to die. Heart attacks in women are often more difficult to diagnose than in men because of their vague and varied symptoms. Heart disease is still thought of as a "man's disease" and thus a heart attack may not be considered in the differential diagnosis when a woman presents to the emergency room. Nurses need to look beyond the obvious "crushing chest pain" textbook symptom that heralds a heart attack in men. Manifestations of heart disease are different between men and women in several other ways—for example, menopause (associated with a significant rise in coronary events); diabetes, high cholesterol levels, and left ventricular hypertrophy; and repeated episodes of weight loss and gain (increased coronary morbidity and mortality) (Framingham Heart Study [FHS], 2007).

Cancer is the second leading cause of death among women (American Cancer Society [ACS], 2007a, 2007b; Wong, Chung, Boscardin, et al., 2006). Women have a one-in-three lifetime risk of developing cancer, and one out of every four deaths is from cancer (Alexander et al., 2007). Although much attention is focused on cancer of the reproductive system, lung cancer is the number-one killer of women. This is largely the result of smoking and second-hand smoke. Lung cancer has no early symptoms, making early detection almost impossible. Thus, lung cancer has the lowest survival rate of any cancer: more than 90% of people who get lung cancer die of it (ACS, 2007).

Breast cancer occurs in one in every seven women in a lifetime, with more than 213,000 women diagnosed annually in the United States. It is the most common malignancy in women and second only to lung cancer as a cause of cancer mortality in women (ACS, 2007). Although a positive family history of breast cancer, aging, and irregularities in the menstrual cycle at an early age are major risk factors, others risk factors include excess weight, not having children, oral contraceptive use, excessive alcohol consumption, a high-fat diet, and long-term use of hormone replacement therapy (ACS, 2007). Breast cancer rates have dropped recently, possibly due to the decreased use of long-term hormone replacement therapy that occurred after the Women's Health Initiative (WHI) report was released in 2002 (Pace, 2006). However, early detection and treatment continue to offer the best chance for a cure, and reducing the risk of cancer by decreasing avoidable risks continues to be the best preventive plan.

Women's health is a complex issue, and no single policy is going to change the overall dismal state ratings. Although progress in science and technology has helped reduce the incidence of and improve the survival rates for several diseases, women's health issues continue to have an impact on our society. By eliminating or decreasing some of the risk factors and causes for prevalent diseases and illnesses, society and science could minimize certain chronic health problems. Focusing on the causes and effects of particular illnesses could help resolve many women's health issues of today.

Childhood Morbidity

According to a 2002 summary of children's health statistics, 56% of children had excellent health and 28% had very good health (Dey, Schiller & Tai, 2004). Factors that may increase morbidity include homelessness, poverty, low birthweight, chronic health disorders, foreign-born adoption, attending a daycare center, and barriers to health care. For example, 16% of children live in poverty. These children have a higher incidence of disease, limited coordination of health services, and limited access to health care except for visits to the emergency department (Federal Interagency Forum on Child and Family Statistics, 2006). Although the poverty rate has declined from 22% in 1993 to 18% in 2005, 35% of African-American children live in poverty; these children are at an increased risk for illness and disease (Federal Interagency Forum on Child and Family Statistics, 2007).

The most important aspect of morbidity is the degree of disability it produces, which is measured in children as the number of days missed from school or confined to bed. In 2005, only 25% of children did not miss any school due to illness or injury; however, 5% missed more than 11 days of school because of injury or illness (Bloom et al., 2006). In the United States during 2003, there were 3.7 million hospitalizations in children 1 to 21 years of age (U.S. Department of Health and Human Services, Health Resources and Services Administration, Maternal and Child Health Bureau, 2005). Figure 1.4 shows the major causes of hospitalization by age in the United States during this period.

Common health problems in children include respiratory disorders, such as asthma and allergies; gastrointestinal disturbances, which lead to malnutrition and dehydration; and injuries. In the United States, 12.7% of children have asthma and 11.7% of children have respiratory allergies. Diseases of the respiratory system were the major cause of hospitalization for children 1 to 9 years of age (Bloom et al., 2006). As more immunizations become available, common childhood communicable diseases affect fewer children. Tracking the leading indicators from *Healthy People 2010* provides information about how children's health is improving.

One trend in the United States is an increase in the number of children with mental health disorders and other emotional, social, or behavioral problems. According to the Methodology for Epidemiology of Mental Disorders in Children and Adolescents (MECA) Study, as many as 20% of children have mental health problems (InCrisis, 2007). These problems may reduce the child's educational success and may also increase his or her risk for significant mental health problems later in life and the chance of firearms use, reckless driving, promiscuous sexual activity,

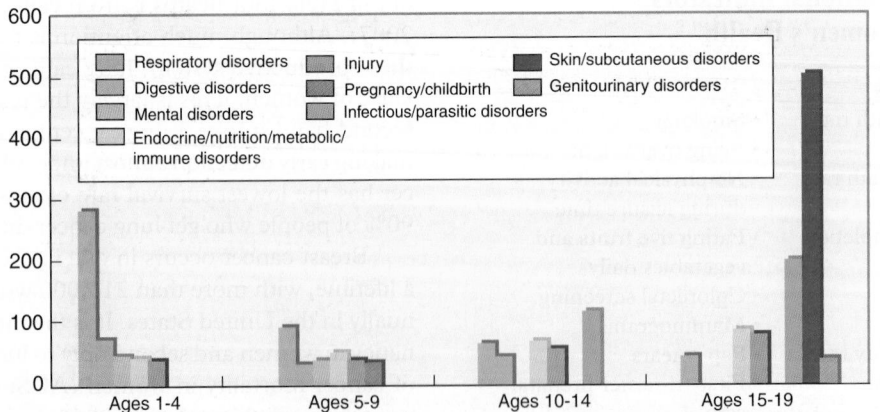

FIGURE 1.4 Major causes of hospitalization (number of hospital discharges, in thousands), by age, for the year 2002. (Adapted from U.S. Department of Health and Human Services, Health Resources and Services Administration, Maternal and Child Health Bureau. *Child health USA 2004.* Rockville, MD: U.S. Department of Health and Human Services, 2004.)

and substance abuse during adolescence. Overall, these behavioral, social, and educational problems can interfere with children's social and academic development.

The incidence of mental health disorders and other emotional, social, or behavioral problems can range from 5% to 30%, depending on how the problems are defined. In addition to HIV/AIDS, experts now identify the "new morbidity" in children as including academic difficulties, mental health disorders, harm to self and others, firearms use, school hostility, substance abuse, and adverse media influence (Reasor & Farrell, 2004). Often insurance does not pay for treatment of these problems, so they may go untreated.

> ▶ *Take* NOTE!
>
> *Environmental and psychosocial factors are now an identified area of concern in the morbidity of children. The "new morbidity" in children includes academic difficulties, complex psychiatric disorders, increased incidence of self-harm and harm to others, use of firearms, hostility at school, substance abuse, HIV/AIDS, and adverse media influences.*

Factors Affecting Maternal and Child Health

From conception, children are shaped by a myriad of factors such as genetics and the environment. As members of a family, they are also members of a specific population, community, culture, and society. As they learn and grow, they are affected by multiple, complex, and ever-changing influences around them. For example, dramatic demographic changes in the United States have led to shifts in majority and minority population groups. Globalization has led to an international focus on health. Access to and the types of health care available have changed due to modifications in health care delivery and financing. In addition, the United States is still grappling with issues such as immigration, poverty, homelessness, and violence.

These factors may affect the person positively, promoting healthy growth and development, or negatively, increasing the person's health risks. Nurses, especially those working with women and children, need to understand how these influences affect the quality of nursing care and health outcomes. They must examine the impact of these variables to gain the knowledge and skills needed to plan effective care, thereby achieving the best possible outcomes for women, children, and families.

Family

The **family** is considered the basic social unit. The way that families are defined has changed. The U.S. Census Bureau (2007) defines family as a group of two or more persons related by birth, marriage, or adoption and living together. Earlier definitions of family emphasized the legal ties or genetic relationships of people living in the same household with specific roles. The American Academy of Family Physicians recognizes that family may be considered as "a group of intimates with a history and a future" and that it may be seen as more or less inclusive (Ventres & Gobbo, 2005). Today's multiple types of families do not fall under a single definition, and the definition of family is changing to reflect today's structural and functional changes.

The family greatly influences the development and health of its members. For example, children learn health care activities, health beliefs, and health values from their family. The family's structure, the roles assumed by family members, and social changes that affect the family's life can influence the child and his or her health status. Families are unique: each one has different views and requires distinct methods for support.

Various theories and models have been generated to explain the concept of family. They have influenced the definition of family, the understanding of the structure and function of the family, and the way family coping and adaptation are assessed. Table 1.1 summarizes some of the major theories related to family.

> ▶ *Take* NOTE!
>
> *The lifestyle of the parents basically is the lifestyle of the children. For instance, parents who are inactive and eat poorly will have children who do the same, and the problems associated with these unhealthy habits, such as diabetes, obesity, and early heart disease, are showing up earlier in children and adolescents. It is important for parents to serve as role models for proper nutrition and physical activity (through sports, hobbies, or other activities).*

Family Structure

Family structure is the composition of individuals who interact with one another on a regular, recurring basis in socially sanctioned ways. It involves how the family unit is organized, which often influences the relationship of the members of the family. Family members are gained or lost through events such as divorce, marriage, birth, death, abandonment, and incarceration. All of these events can

TABLE 1.1 SUMMARY OF MAJOR THEORIES RELATED TO FAMILY

Theory	Description	Key Components
Friedman's (2002) structural functional theory	Emphasizes the social system of family such as the organization or structure of the family and how the structure relates to the function	Identified five functions of families: • Affective function: meeting the love and belonging needs of each member • Socialization and social placement function: teaching children how to function and assume the adult roles in society • Reproductive role: continuing the family and society in general • Economic function: ensuring the family has necessary resources with appropriate allocation • Health care function: involving the provision of physical needs to keep the family healthy
Duvall's (1977) developmental theory	Emphasizes the developmental stages that all families evolve through beginning with marriage; the longitudinal career of the family, also known as the family life cycle	Described eight chronological stages with specific predictable tasks that each family completes: • Marriage: beginning of family • Childbearing stage • Family with preschool children • Family with school-aged children • Family with adolescents • Family with young adults • Middle-aged parents • Family in later years
Von Bertalanffy's (1968) general systems theory applied to families	Emphasizes the family as a system with interdependent, interacting parts that endure over time to ensure the survival, continuity, and growth of its components; the family is not the total sum of its parts but is characterized by wholeness and unity	Used to define how families interact with and are influenced by the members of their family and society and how to analyze the interrelationships of the members and the impact that change affecting one member will have on the other members
Family stress theory (Boss, 2002)	Addresses the way families respond to stress and how the family copes with the stress as a group and as individuals	Described elements of stress as occurring within the family (such as values, beliefs, structure), which the family can control or change, or from outside the family (such as the culture of the surrounding community, genetics, the family's current time or place), over which the family has no control. Mobilization of family resources results in either a positive response of constructive coping or a negative response of a crisis. Identified the main determinant of adequate coping based on the meaning of the stressful event to the family and its members
Resiliency model of family stress, adjustment, and adaptation	Addresses the way families adapt to stress and can rebound from adversity	Identified the elements of risks and protective factors that aid a family in achieving positive outcomes

alter the family structure, leading to roles being redefined or redistributed. Table 1.2 provides examples of the types of family structures found in today's society.

The traditional nuclear family is no longer considered the dominant family structure (Fig. 1.5). From 1970 to 1996, the percentage of children under age 18 who were living with two married parents decreased steadily from 85% to 68%; in 2005, this percentage was 67% (Child Trends, 2005). By understanding clients' family structure and any changes that may occur, nurses can provide them with support to alleviate or prevent dysfunctional alterations in family coping and adaptation.

TABLE 1.2   EXAMPLES OF FAMILY STRUCTURES IN TODAY'S SOCIETY

Theory	Description	Key Components
Nuclear family	Husband, wife, and children living in same household	May include natural or adopted children Once considered the traditional family structure; now less common due to increased divorce rates and child-rearing by unmarried persons
Binuclear family	Child who is a member of two families due to joint custody; parenting is considered a "joint venture"	Always works better when the interests of the child are put first and above the parents' needs and desires
Single-parent family	One parent is responsible for care of children	May result from death, divorce, desertion, birth outside marriage, or adoption These families are likely to face challenges because of economic, social, and personal restraints; one person serves as homemaker, caregiver, and financial provider.
Commuter family	Adults in the family live and work apart for professional or financial reasons, often leaving the daily care of children to one parent.	Similar to single-parent family
Step- or blended family	Adults with children from previous marriages or from the new marriage	May lead to family conflict due to different expectations on the part of the child and adults; they may have different views and practices related to childcare and health
Extended family	Nuclear family and grandparents, cousins, aunts, and uncles	Need to identify decision-maker and primary caretaker of the children Popular in some cultures, such as Hispanic and Asian cultures
Same-sex family (also called homosexual or gay/lesbian family)	Adults of the same sex living together with or without children	May face negative attitudes about their "different" lifestyle
Communal family	Group of people living together to raise children and manage household; unrelated by blood or marriage	May face negative attitudes about their "different" lifestyle Need to determine the decision-maker and caretaker of the children
Foster family	A temporary family for children who are placed away from their parents to ensure their emotional and physical well-being	May include the foster family's children and other foster children in the home Foster children are more likely to have unmet health needs and chronic health problems because they may have been in a variety of health systems (AAP, 2000).
Grandparents-as-parent families	Grandparents raising their grandchildren due to the inability or absence of the parents	May increase the risk for physical, financial, and emotional stress on older adults May lead to confusion and emotional stress for child if biological parents are in and out of child's life
Adolescent families	Young parents who are still mastering the developmental tasks of their childhood	Are at greater risk for health problems in pregnancy and delivery; more likely to have premature infants, which then leads to risk of subsequent health and developmental problems Probably still need support from their family related to financial, emotional, and school issues

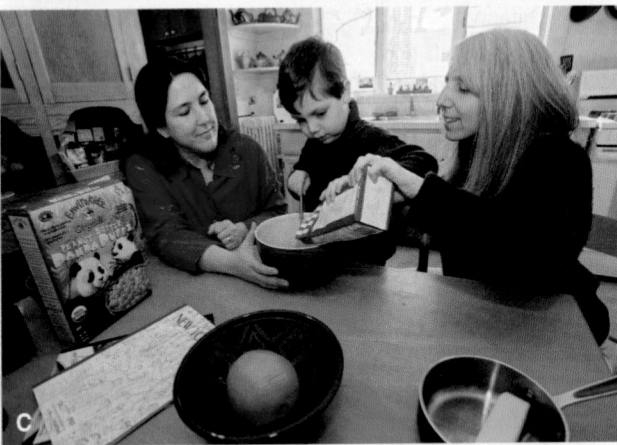

FIGURE 1.5 Nurses must take into account family dynamics when providing health care. There are many different family structures, and they influence the client's needs. (**A**) The traditional nuclear family is composed of two parents and their biological or adopted children. (**B**) The extended family includes the nuclear family plus other family members, such as grandparents, aunts, uncles, and cousins. (**C**) Gay and lesbian families comprise two people of the same sex sharing a committed relationship with or without children.

Family Roles and Functions

Within a family, each member has a specific position or status and role when interacting with other members of the family. Typical family roles and their functions include:

- Nurturer: the primary caregiver
- Provider: the person who is primarily responsible for generating the family's income
- Decision maker: the person who is responsible for making choices, especially related to lifestyle and leisure time
- Financial manager: the person who works with the money, such as paying bills and saving
- Problem solver: the person to whom other members go for help in solving problems
- Health manager: the person responsible for maintaining the family members' health, such as scheduling visits and ensuring that immunizations or screenings are up to date
- Gatekeeper: the person who manages information inflow and outflow (Pillitteri, 2007)

Roles and functions are further defined by each family using its own traditions and values and the set of standards for interacting within and outside the family. For example, birth order may affect roles and relationships. First-born children are typically different from those born later. The older child may feel that he or she is in a position of greater power and may attempt to control younger siblings. The youngest child, in response, may learn how to bargain and interact effectively to deal with the situation.

Parental Roles

The parents or caregivers are of utmost importance for the survival and healthy development of a young child (WHO, 2004). The parents or caregivers provide the physical and emotional care of the child and also impart the rules and expected behaviors of a society. These expected behaviors depend on the culture of the family, the child's developmental stage and physical and cognitive abilities, and the values and beliefs of the family. The parents should nurture their children and provide them with the environmental influences to become competent, productive, self-directed members of society. Young children are particularly dependent on the care they receive; their growth, health, and personhood depend on the capacity of the adults in their life to understand, perceive, and respond to their bids for assistance and support (WHO, 2004).

Parenting Styles

The three major parenting styles are authoritarian, authoritative, and permissive. These three styles differ in the amount of control exerted over the child during parenting. Whatever the style, however, sensitive and responsive care is needed for appropriate physical, neurophysiologic, and psychological development (WHO, 2004).

Authoritarian parents expect unquestioning obedience from the child. The parents' rules and standards are strictly enforced and firm. Parents also expect the children to accept the family's beliefs and values and demand respect for these beliefs. The parents are the ultimate authority on matters and behaviors and allow little if any participation by the child in making decisions. Behavior that does not adhere to the family rules and standards is forcibly punished.

Authoritative or democratic parents show some respect for the opinions of children. Although parents have the ultimate authority and expect adherence to rules, authoritative parents allow children to be different and believe that each child is an individual. They employ consistent, firm enforcement of the family rules and standards but without the emphasis on punishment of the child.

Permissive or laissez-faire parents exert little control over the behavior of their children. Rules or standards may be inconsistent, unclear, or nonexistent. Permissive parents allow their children to set their own standards and rules for behavior. Discipline can be lax, inconsistent, or absent.

Discipline

Much of parenting involves increasing desirable behaviors and decreasing or eliminating undesirable behaviors, a process known as **discipline**. People in our society have various beliefs about the best or most effective method of discipline. Discipline should be based on expectations that are appropriate for the child's age and should be used to set reasonable, consistent limits while permitting choices among acceptable alternatives (Banks, 2002). Discipline is an ongoing learning process, and if it is to be effective, the child needs to feel secure and loved.

The American Academy of Pediatrics (1998) suggests three strategies for effective discipline:

• Maintaining a positive, supportive, nurturing caregiver–child relationship
• Using positive reinforcement techniques to increase the desirable behaviors
• Removing positive reinforcements or using punishment to reduce or eliminate undesirable behaviors (Fig. 1.6)

Teaching Guidelines 1.1 gives advice about appropriate discipline.

Changes in Parental Roles Over Time

Parental roles have evolved over time due to social and economic changes as well as family changes. Traditionally, the role of provider was assigned to the father. However, with increased numbers of women in the workplace and more households with two parents working, today both parents are often the providers as well as the nurturers for the children. Technological expansion has provided parents with opportunities to work at home, allowing some parents to maintain the provider role while simultaneously

FIGURE 1.6 Although he might not like it, quiet solitude helps the child develop inner control.

fulfilling the nurturer and health manager roles. Fathers also are taking on greater responsibilities related to household management and child care. Additionally, the number of single-father parent families and grandparent families are increasing.

Recall Sophia, the pregnant woman described at the beginning of the chapter. Identify the parental roles assumed by Sophia. How might these roles be different from those of her mother when she was Sophia's age?

Changes in Family Structure and Roles

Families today face complex challenges as they try to nurture, develop, and socialize their members. Family structure changes such as divorce, blending families, adoption, or foster care can have wide-ranging and lifelong effects.

Divorce

As many as 50% of marriages end in divorce (Hetherington, 2005). Conflict between the parents and family dysfunction may exert a significant stress on children. Parents need to understand the impact that divorce can have on their children, placing the children's interest first. Parents can use the rules given in Teaching Guidelines 1.2 to help reduce the tension and conflict associated with divorce.

Single Parenting

Single-parent families may result from divorce or separation, death of a spouse, childbearing by an unmarried woman, or adoption by an unmarried man or woman. For

TEACHING GUIDELINES 1.1

Promoting Effective Discipline

- Set clear, consistent, and developmentally appropriate expected behaviors; offer choices whenever possible.
- Maintain consistency in responding to behaviors; provide encouragement and affection.
- Role-model appropriate behaviors.
- Provide an age-appropriate explanation of the consequence if the child demonstrates unacceptable behavior.
- Always administer the consequence soon after the unacceptable behavior.
- Keep the consequence appropriate to the age of the child and the situation.
- Stay calm but firm without showing anger when administering the consequence.
- Always praise the child for displaying appropriate behavior (positive reinforcement).
- Set the environment to assist the child in accomplishing the appropriate behavior; remove temptations that may lead to inappropriate behavior.
- Reinforce that the child's behavior was "bad" but the child was not "bad."
- Use extinction to reduce or eliminate reinforcement for an inappropriate behavior (for example, ignore a temper tantrum).
- When using time-out, use 1 minute per year of the child's age (a 3-year-old would have time-out for 3 minutes). Do not exceed 5 minutes.

TEACHING GUIDELINES 1.2

Guidelines for Divorcing Parents

- Tell your children about the divorce and the reasons for the divorce in terms that they can understand. Be sure that you and your spouse are present together when telling the children; tell all the children at the same time.
- Reassure your children that the divorce is not their fault. Repeat this as often as possible and as necessary.
- Inform the children well in advance before anyone moves out of the house (except when abuse is present or there are concerns for immediate safety).
- Clearly inform the children about the family structure after the divorce, such as who will live with whom and where; also discuss visitation clearly and honestly.
- Do not make your children be or act like adults.
- Do not discuss money or finances with your children.
- Maintain rules and be consistent in this area.
- Never force or allow your children to take sides.
- Avoid belittling your spouse with earshot of the children. However, do not lie to cover up for irresponsible behavior by the other parent.
- Never put your children in the middle between you and your spouse.

Adapted from Bryner, C. L. (2001). Children of divorce. *Journal of the American Board of Family Practice, 14*(3), 176–183.
Accessed 9/21/06 Available at: http://www.medscape.com/viewarticle/405852

several reasons, this family structure can affect the health of family members. Life in a single-parent household can be stressful for the adult and children. The single parent may feel overwhelmed by the responsibility of juggling child care, maintaining a job, and keeping up with the bills and household chores (American Psychological Association, 2008). These issues may be compounded by other pressures, such as custody problems, decreased time available to spend with children, continuing conflicts between separated or divorced parents, or changes in relationships with extended family members. Communication and support are essential to the optimal functioning of the single-parent family. The parent and children need to be able to discuss their feelings and work through the problems together.

Blending Families

The creation of a blended family can be a stressful time for the parents and children involved. Although it creates a structure and stability and reduces some of the financial stresses of single parenthood, making the transition

to a blended family takes time. Children may feel jealous of the stepparent or feel disloyal to the biological parent. There may be competition or rivalry among the stepchildren. The child may fear that the stepparent is interfering with the child's relationship with the parent or taking away his or her source of love, affection, and attention. Mutual respect is necessary to ease the transition to a blended family, as is open, honest communication among all individuals involved—and this includes the biological parent when possible.

Adoption

Adopted families are created in a number of different ways. The parents may contact an agency or intermediary such as an attorney in their own area or country to seek a child. Families may adopt a child from another country (intercountry or international adoption). The child may be of a different culture, race, or ethnicity (Fig. 1.7). Some children may have complex medical, developmental, behavioral, educational, and psychological issues. Children may be adopted after spending time in foster care. An increas-

FIGURE 1.7 An adoptive family in which the child is from a different culture.

ing number of single-parent families, blended families, families with gay or lesbian partners, and families with older parents are providing homes to children through adoption (American Psychological Association, 2005).

The amount of contact between the adoptive parents and the birth mother can vary greatly. There may be no contact at all (closed adoption) or there may be as much direct contact as desired (open adoptions). Regardless of the method used to adopt a child, adoptive families may be faced with unique issues that can affect the health of the family members, such as:

• The adopted child may have been exposed to risk factors (e.g., poverty; neglect; infectious diseases; lack of adequate food, clothing, shelter, and consistent caregivers), increasing the child's risk for problems.
• Information about the adopted child's family medical history may be lacking.
• Parents may not know when to tell a child that he or she was adopted.
• The adopted child may be troubled about his or her loss of a "birth family" or the reason for the birth mother's decision for an adoption plan. He or she may have feelings of abandonment, emotional uncertainty, and identity conflict.
• The child and family may face racism or bigotry if the child is from a different culture or race.

Foster Care

Foster care refers to the care given to a child who is placed in an alternative living situation apart from his or her parents of origin or legal guardians. The child typically is placed in this living situation due to some difficulty in the family situation such as abuse, neglect, abandonment, or the parent's inability to meet the child's needs such as from illness, substance abuse, or death. The living situation may be with relatives (termed kinship care) or foster parents, who are strangers providing protection and shelter in a state-approved foster home.

Many children who are placed in foster care have been the victims of abuse or neglect. In addition, 30% of children in foster care have severe emotional, behavioral, or developmental problems (AACAP, 2008). Children who are placed in foster care may have a wide range of problems, including:

• Physical health problems
• Self-blame and feelings of guilt
• Feelings of being unwanted
• Feelings of helplessness
• Insecurity and uncertainty about the future
• Ambivalent feelings related to foster parents; feelings of being disloyal to birth parents (AACAP, 2008)

Genetics

Genetics (the study of heredity and its variations) has implications for all stages of life and all types of diseases. The child's biological traits, including gender, race, some behavioral traits, and the presence of certain diseases or illnesses, are directly linked to genetic inheritance. New technologies in molecular biology and biochemistry have led to a better understanding of the mechanisms involved in hereditary transmission, including those associated with genetic disorders. These advances are leading to better diagnostic tests and better management options.

Gender

Gender is established when the sex chromosomes join. A person's gender can influence many aspects, such as physical characteristics and personal attributes, attitudes, and behaviors (Fig. 1.8). Some diseases or illnesses are more common in one sex; for example, scoliosis is more common in females and color blindness in males.

Race

Race refers to the physical features that distinguish members of a particular group, such as skin color, bone structure, or blood type. Some physical features that are normal in a particular race may be considered a sign of a disorder in other races. For example, epicanthal folds (the vertical folds of skin that partially or completely cover the inner canthi of the eye) are normal in Asian children but may occur with Down syndrome or renal agenesis in other races. In addition, certain malformations and diseases are found more commonly in specific races. For example, sickle cell anemia occurs more often in African and Mediterranean population groups, and cystic fibrosis is

FIGURE 1.8 Interactions with family members and peers as well as activities and societal values affect how children perceive themselves as a certain gender.

seen more often in individuals from the Northwestern European population group.

Society

Society has a major impact on the health of women, children, and families. Major influences include social roles, socioeconomic status, the media, and the expanding global nature of society. Each of these may influence a person's self-concept, where he or she lives, the lifestyle he or she leads—and thus his or her health.

Social Roles

Society often prescribes specific patterns of behaviors: certain behaviors are permitted and others are prohibited. These social roles are often an important factor in the development of self-concept. Social roles influence a person's ideas about himself or herself. Social roles are generally carried out in groups with which the individual has intimate daily contact, such as the family, school, workplace, or peer groups.

Socioeconomic Status

Another dominant influence is a person's socioeconomic status, his or her relative position in society. This includes the family's economic, occupational, and educational levels. Children are raised differently by parents of different educational levels, occupations, and incomes. Low socioeconomic status typically has an adverse influence on an individual's health. Health care costs are continuing to rise, as are health insurance premiums. The family may not be able to afford food, health care, and housing; meals may be unbalanced, erratic, or insufficient. Housing may be overcrowded or have poor sanitation. These families may not understand the importance of preventive care or may simply not be able to afford it. As a result, they may be exposed to health risks such as lead poisoning or may not be immunized against communicable diseases.

Poverty

Poverty is a measurement based on the specific monetary income of a family. The poverty threshold is the dollar amount that the U.S. Census Bureau uses to determine whether a family is living in poverty. If the individual's or family's income is below the threshold, then that person or family is said to be living in poverty. According to the Census Bureau, about 18.5% of children under age 18 years live in poverty. Although the rates have stabilized somewhat after several years of consecutive increases, more children live in poverty than all other Americans, and these rates are highest among minority groups.

Despite the many global economic gains that have been made during the past century, poverty continues to grow and the gap between rich and poor is widening. Major gaps continue between the economic opportunities and status afforded to women and those offered to men. A disproportionate share of the burden of poverty rests on women's shoulders, and this undermines their health. However, poverty, particularly for women, is more than monetary deficiency. Women continue to lag behind men in control of cash, credit, and collateral. Other forms of impoverishment may include deficiencies in literacy, education, skills, employment opportunities, mobility, and political representation, as well as pressures on time and energy linked to their responsibilities. These poverty factors may affect a woman's health (WHO, 2007a, 2007b, 2007c).

The effects of poverty on children's health can be wide-ranging. The child may live in substandard housing or housing that poses a threat to the child (e.g., unsanitary conditions, exposure to toxins, or exposure to violence). Poverty may lead to homelessness for the family. Children living in poverty are more likely than other children to be poorly nourished, to have inadequate health care, to become teen parents, and to have insufficient education. Children living in poverty are also at increased risk for experiencing abuse and violence (Children's Defense Fund, 2005).

Homelessness

Families with children are the fastest-growing segment of the homeless population. Homeless families commonly are victims of violence and may have mental health challenges. According to the National Coalition for the Homeless, approximately 1.35 million children are homeless on any given night (National Center on Family Homelessness, 2008). Children make up 39% of the homeless population; 42% of these children are under age 5 years (National Coalition for the Homeless, 2006). Homelessness occurs in large urban areas and midsize cities as well as suburban and rural areas.

Homelessness can have a negative impact on health and well-being in numerous ways, including:

- Increased mental health issues such as anxiety, depression, or aggressive behavior

- Higher incidence of chronic health problems and trauma-related injuries
- Problems related to nutritional deficiencies, affecting fetal or child growth and development
- Participation in behaviors such as illegal substance use or unprotected sex with multiple partners
- Limited access to health care services such as preventive care, prenatal care, or dental care

Media

Today's children are inundated with various forms of media, such as television, the Internet, videos, movies, magazines, books, and newspapers (Fig. 1.9). Some of these present images and information that may not be in the child's best interest. Children may identify with and mimic characters who engage in risky behaviors or lifestyles. They may believe that those lifestyles or behaviors are the norm and acceptable. Research has demonstrated that exposure to media violence is linked to increased aggression in children (Bushman & Huesmann, 2006) and that television viewing places young adolescents at risk for sexual initiation (Ashby et al., 2006).

The images that children view every day will affect their behaviors and may influence their health. For instance, magazines, movies, and television shows portray thinness as a body type to be emulated, and boys and girls may take up unhealthy dieting or other behaviors to develop that body type. Those whose body type does not fit the ideal may develop depression or self-esteem issues.

The media's influence relates not only to its content but also to the total viewing time. For example, excessive television viewing has been linked to lack of exercise, weight gain, and obesity (Lumeng et al., 2006).

However, the media may also exert positive influences. Public service messages about the negative effects of substance abuse, smoking, or gang involvement or about teenage pregnancy and birth control are two examples of the media's positive influence. In addition, positive television programs can serve as valuable educational resources.

The Internet has fostered closer connections between distant areas of the world. Individuals are no longer limited to their immediate surroundings. The Internet can be a valuable resource for people to access information, learn new things, and communicate, but it also brings threats to health and safety (American Academy of Pediatrics, 2006). Online exposure to sexual predators, illicit sex, pornography, violence, and racism are a few of the potential threats. Parents need to be alert to these hazards and safeguard their children (Teaching Guidelines 1.3).

Violence

Violence can occur in any setting and can involve any individual. Violence against women is a major health

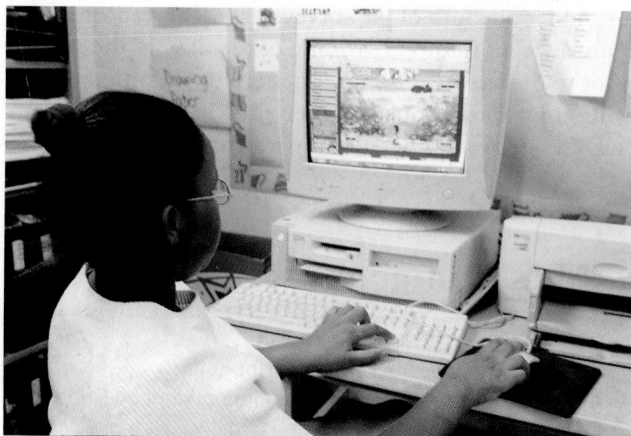

FIGURE 1.9 Computer games can be fun and educational, but the child should be monitored while using the computer and other forms of media to minimize negative effects.

TEACHING GUIDELINES 1.3

Promoting Safe Internet Use

- Determine a specific time limit that your child can spend online each day or week. Be consistent in enforcing this time limit.
- Ensure that Internet use does not replace or interfere with homework, friends, or household or school activities.
- Tell your child NEVER to share personal information with anyone online unless you are sure of the person and the child has your permission to do so.
- Tell your child NEVER to share his or her password with anyone, even friends.
- Review Internet sites with your child, and explain what information and websites are appropriate. Use safety and parental controls offered by your Internet service provider.
- Avoid placing the computer in the child's room. Instead, place the computer in a public area of your home, such as the den or kitchen, so that you can monitor your child's use.
- Discuss with your child the need for maintaining safety while using the Internet. Explain potential hazards in terms the child can understand.
- Advise your child to immediately close any sites or stop any communication that makes him or her confused or uncomfortable. Tell your child NEVER to arrange any face-to-face meeting with persons he or she meets online. Urge your child to seek you out if he or she encounters such a situation.
- Teach the child NEVER to open e-mail from any unknown senders.
- Be aware of computer use policies in your child's school.

concern—it affects thousands of lives and costs the health care system millions of dollars. Violence affects families, women, and children of all ages, ethnic backgrounds, races, educational levels, and socioeconomic levels. Pregnancy is often a time when physical abuse starts or escalates, resulting in poorer outcomes for the mother and the baby. The nurse is responsible for assessing for and following up on any abuse.

Domestic Violence

Violence in the home environment, known as domestic violence, affects many lives in the United States. The U.S. Bureau of Justice estimates that 1 million violent crimes are committed by former spouses, boyfriends, or girlfriends each year; about 85% of the victims are women (Rennison & Welchans, 2000). This violence is known as intimate partner abuse, family violence, wife beating, battering, marital abuse, or partner abuse, but regardless of the term used, its effects are widespread.

Children often witness domestic violence, and they may be physically, sexually, or emotionally abused themselves (Abell & Ey, 2008). The federal Child Abuse Prevention and Treatment Act (CAPTA) defines child abuse and neglect as any recent act or failure to act on the part of a parent or caretaker that results in death, serious physical or emotional harm, sexual abuse or exploitation, or an act or failure to act that presents an imminent risk of serious harm to a child (Child Welfare Information Gateway, 2007). Of the children identified as being maltreated, 61% were victims of neglect, 19% were victims of physical abuse, 10% were victims of sexual abuse, and 5% were victims of emotional or psychological abuse (CDC, 2006a, 2006c, 2006d, 2006g). According to Prevent Child Abuse America (2008), four children die in America every day as a result of child abuse or neglect. About 78% of these deaths occur in infants and children younger than 3 years of age.

Domestic violence is often accompanied by other major risk factors for children, such as poverty, female-headed households, and low education level of the primary caregiver. Children may feel the need to call for help or to blame themselves for the dispute that led to the abuse (Hornor, 2005). Children who experience domestic violence or child abuse are at risk for problems such as sleep disturbances, headaches, stomach aches, depression, enuresis, aggressive behaviors, decreased social competencies, withdrawal, developmental regression, fears, anxiety, and learning problems (Children's Defense Fund; 2005, CDC, 2006a, 2006c, 2006d, 2006g). Additional risks include poor academic outcomes, teenage prostitution, substance abuse, and conducting abuse or sexual assault as an adult (National Coalition Against Domestic Violence, 2005).

Nurses serve their clients best not by trying to rescue them, but by helping them build on their strengths and providing support, thereby empowering them to help themselves. All nurses need to include "RADAR" in every client visit (Box 1.3).

Youth Violence

Although the new century has shown an overall decline in violence by and against children, youth violence is still an important public health problem. Violent crimes include those such as murder, rape, robbery, and aggravated assault. CDC (2006d) statistics revealed that for young people between 10 and 24 years of age:

- Approximately 5,570 individuals were murdered; of those murders, firearms accounted for 82% of the deaths in 2003.
- More than 750,000 individuals were treated in emergency departments for injuries due to violence in 2004.
- Homicide was the leading cause of death for African Americans, the second leading cause of death for Hispanics, and the third leading cause of death for American Indians, Alaska Natives, and Asian/Pacific Islanders.

Youth violence affects not only the child and family in terms of injury and death, but also the entire community. Studies have shown that youth violence is associated with a disruption in social services, an increase in health care costs, and a decline in property values.

In recent years, school violence has received much attention, resulting in an increased concern for student safety, which in turn has led to a decline in school violence (Children's Defense Fund, 2005). Students are more likely to be victims of violent crimes away from school, but physical fights, thefts, weapon carrying, teacher victimization, and fear of school environments have increased (National Youth Violence Prevention Resource Center, 2005). For example, in a nationwide CDC survey of high school students about risk behavior, approximately 36% of the students reported that they had been involved in a physical altercation at least once in the previous year, and just under one fifth of the surveyed students reported carrying a weapon for at least one of the days in the month prior to the survey. Of the students who admitted to carrying a weapon, approximately 5% had carried a gun (CDC, 2006g). The continued coordination among

---

BOX 1.3 **RADAR**

R–Routinely screen every patient for abuse.
A–Ask direct, supportive, and nonjudgmental questions.
D–Document all findings.
A–Assess your client's safety.
R–Review options and provide referrals.

schools, law enforcement, social services, and mental health systems and the development of effective programs will help to reduce these risk behaviors.

Due to the potential impact of violence on children and families, it is essential to identify any violent situation via a thorough assessment. Providing referrals to shelters and child advocacy centers and intervening to assist children in dealing with this issue are key.

> ▶ *Take* NOTE!
>
> *Not all children exposed to violence suffer negative consequences. Children have resiliency, and preliminary studies indicate that protective factors, such as involvement in social activities, a strong commitment to school and academic performance, and ability to discuss problems with a supportive adult, can buffer children from the effects of violence, thereby helping to reduce the risk of developing violent behaviors.*

Community

Community encompasses a broad range of concepts, from the nation where a person lives down to a particular neighborhood or group. The surrounding community affects many aspects of a person's health and general welfare. The quality of life within the community has a great influence on an individual's ability to develop and become a functional member of society. Community influences include the school, which is a community in itself, and peer groups. The support and assistance offered to women, children, and families from other areas of the community, such as school programs and community centers, can improve the individual's overall health and well-being.

Schools

Over the past century, major societal changes have led to children starting school earlier, spending more time in child care settings, and being involved in various community centers and activities. By age 4, many children spend several hours a day in a preschool setting; some children spend more time in school and child care settings than they do at home. As many as 63% of children under age 5 years attend child care regularly (Child Trends, 2005). As a result, schools serve as major influences on children.

Although the primary role of schools has always been academic education, today they are performing more health-related functions. School also serves as a means of socialization. School rules about attendance and authority relationships and the system of sanctions and rewards based on achievement transmit to children behavioral expectations that will help them succeed in employment and relationships in the adult world. Schools can also

play a major role in improving health and encouraging healthy behaviors. Academic success is linked to healthy behaviors, good mental health, and avoidance of pregnancy and juvenile justice problems, as well as health, jobs, and self-sufficiency in adult life.

Because of social changes in America, more children are in child care and after-school programs than ever before. Thus, the socialization process begins earlier and involves a larger percentage of the child's waking hours (Fig. 1.10). Community centers and after-school programs can provide support, empowerment, boundaries and expectations, and constructive use of time (Search Institute, 2007).

Peer Groups

Peer groups can have a great impact on children. Relationships with peers often begin early, and they continue to be a large part of the child's world, particularly in school-age children and adolescents. This influence starts in the play groups in early preschool or elementary school. The child comes into contact with a variety of values and belief systems from interactions with peer groups. When these values and beliefs differ from those of the child's family, conflicts can occur, possibly separating children from parents and strengthening the bond with the peer group. When the peer group is involved with school activities, athletics, or other healthy behaviors, the influence is very positive, but the opposite is also true: peer groups can exert negative influences on the child. Thus, it is vital to identify the important peer groups in a child's life and the positive or negative behaviors associated with these groups.

Community and Neighborhood Connectedness

Social capital refers to the bonds between individuals that assist social networks in communities to achieve a variety of goals. Basically, it is a mechanism by which resources in a community can be mobilized by and from the

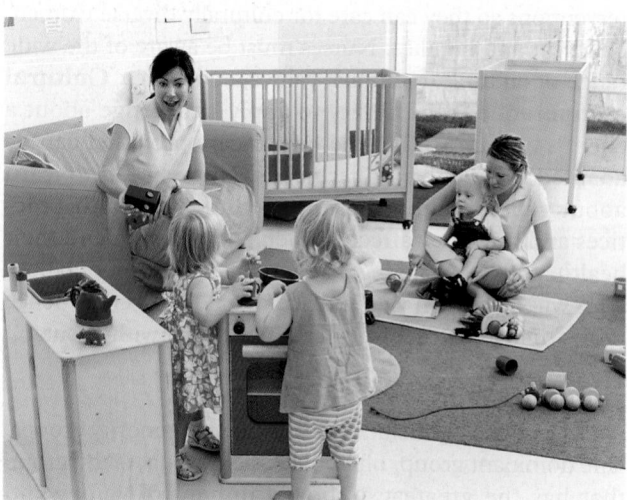

FIGURE 1.10 Daycare centers provide socialization and support for young children.

people, not for them (Looman & Lindeke, 2005). Such connectedness, relationships, and common interests propel neighborhoods and communities toward engagement. Connected communities support an environment that makes it easy for people to engage in health-promoting behaviors. Looman and Lindeke (2005) believe that asking a simple question such as, "How is your relationship with your neighbors?" can help give an understanding of a client's social milieu. They suggest three areas to include in nursing interventions and strategies:

• Bringing families together in communities to set the stage for networking
• Disseminating knowledge about what helps create healthy, supported communities
• Thinking of relationships as investments, with social interactions as the processes by which resources for health are exchanged (Looman & Lindeke, 2005)

Culture

Culture is a view of the world and a set of traditions that are used by a specific social group and are transmitted to the next generation. It plays a critical role with women, children, and families. A person's culture influences not only socialization but also his or her experiences related to health and specific health practices (Pillitteri, 2007). Culture is a complex phenomenon involving many components, such as beliefs, values, language, time, personal space, and view of the world, all of which shape a person's actions and behavior. Individuals learn these patterns of cultural behaviors from their family and community through a process called enculturation, which involves acquiring knowledge and internalizing values. Culture influences every aspect of development and is reflected in child-bearing and child-rearing beliefs and practices designed to promote healthy adaptation.

With today's changing demographic patterns, nurses must be able to assimilate cultural knowledge into their interventions so they can care for culturally diverse women, children, and families. Nurses must be aware of the wide range of cultural traditions, values, and ethics. **Cultural competence** is the ability to apply knowledge about a client's culture so that the health care provided can be adapted to meet his or her needs. Nurses need to learn about general cultural groups, ethnicity, health practices and how they affect women and children and their health, and the changing demographics of the population. This will help them view culture as a point of congruence rather than as a potential source of conflict with clients.

Cultural Groups

A society typically includes dominant and minority groups. The dominant group, often the largest group, is the group that has the greatest authority to control values and sanctions of the society (Taylor et al., 2005). As a result, the dominant or majority culture may have the largest impact on health. The minority cultural groups may remain in their own communities and maintain some of their traditions and values while mainstreaming into American society. A culture may contain many subcultures, and geographic differences also can occur: for example, Latin Americans living in New York may be quite different from Latin Americans living in Florida. Being aware of these differences is essential in providing culturally competent care.

Ethnicity is sometimes used synonymously with culture; the definition basically involves group membership by virtue of common ancestry. The basic groups or divisions are differentiated by customs, characteristics, language, or similar distinguishing factors. Ethnic groups can be identified by their specific family structures, languages, food preferences, moral codes, and health care practices. Children learn the group's mode of behavior by observing and imitating those around them. Many Americans in the dominant culture do not view themselves as belonging to any specific ethnic group, though some persons may closely identify with their ethnicity. The influences of culture and ethnicity on women and children and families are highly variable, and traditional behaviors can change based on new circumstances and a dynamic environment.

Ethnocentrism is a belief that one's own ethnic group is superior to other groups, and thus one's one way of living, ideas, and practices are the best. This attitude can lead to a slanted view of the world and may hinder a nurse's ability to give culturally competent care.

Nurses need to be aware of the health care values and practices that are passed along from one generation to the next. For example, the belief in folk healers relates to how the culture interprets illness and health. Some of these parts of the culture may have major influences on an individual's health. Table 1.3 highlights some major cultural groups and their common health beliefs and practices.

> ► **Take** NOTE!
>
> *Nurses can have a lifelong influence on an individual's perceptions of health and use of health services. By understanding how the child's and family's culture influences their health practices, nurses can enhance the family's traditional practices, and different cultural practices can become sources of strength rather than areas of conflict.*

Spirituality and Religion

Spirituality is a basic human quality involving the belief in something greater than oneself and a faith that affirms life. It is a major influence for many people, providing a meaning or purpose to life and a foundation for and source of love, relationships, and service. Spirituality is considered a universal human phenomenon. During life-changing events and crises, such as a serious illness or the birth of a

TABLE 1.3 BELIEFS AND PRACTICES OF SELECTED CULTURAL GROUPS

Cultural Group	Beliefs and Practices Affecting Maternal and Children's Health
African Americans	Strong extended family relationships; mother as head of household; older family members valued and respected Food as a symbol of health and wealth View of health as harmony with nature; illness as disruption in harmony Use of folk healing and home remedies common View of pregnancy as a state of wellness Emotional support during labor commonly from other women, primarily the woman's own mother Liberal use of oil on newborn's and infant's scalp and skin Belief in illnesses as natural (due to natural forces person hasn't protected self against) and unnatural (due to person or spirit) Illness commonly associated with pain Pain and suffering inevitable; relief achieved through prayers and laying on of hands Individuals vulnerable to external forces
Asian Americans	Strong loyalty to the family Family as the center, with members expected to care for one another Use of complementary modalities with Western health care practices View of life as a cycle with everything connected to health Pain described by diverse body symptoms Health viewed as a balance between the forces of yang and yin Respect for authority emphasized View of pregnancy as a natural process and happy time for woman Little involvement of the father during labor; quiet, stoic appearance of woman during labor Protection of woman from cold forces for 30 days after birth of newborn
Arab Americans	Women subordinate to men; young individuals subordinate to older persons Family loyalty is primary Good health associated with eating properly, consuming nutritious foods, and fasting to cure disease Illness is due to inadequate diet, shifts in hot and cold, exposure of stomach while sleeping, emotional or spiritual distress, and 'evil eye' Little emphasis on preventive care View of pain as unpleasant, requiring immediate control or relief Birthmarks on newborn due to unsatisfied maternal cravings Pain of labor demonstrated via facial expressions, verbalizations, and body movements; reluctant to use breathing and relaxation techniques during labor Wrapping of newborn's stomach at birth to prevent cold or wind from entering baby's body Breastfeeding often delayed for 2 to 3 days after birth Cleanliness important for prayer
Native Americans	High value on family and tribe; respect for elders Family as an extended network providing care for newborns and children Women as the verbal decision-makers View of pregnancy as normal and natural process; entire family may be present at birth Newborn not given colostrum Celebrations to mark the stages of growth and development Use of food to celebrate life events and in healing and religious ceremonies Health as harmony with nature; illness due to disharmony, evil spirits Restoration of physical, mental, and spiritual balance through healing ceremonies View of pain as something to be tolerated
Hispanic	Family important; father as the source of strength, wisdom, and self-confidence Mother as the caretaker and decision-maker for health View of children as persons to continue the family and culture Birthmark on baby due to unsatisfied food cravings during pregnancy Mother's legs brought together after birth of newborn to prevent air from entering uterus Possibly boisterous and loud during labor Bedrest for first 3 days postpartum; no bathing for 14 days Newborn protection from the evil eye Use of food for celebrations and socialization Health as God's will, maintainable with a balance of hot and cold food intake Freedom from pain indicative of good health; pain tolerated stoically due to belief that it is God's will Folk medicine practices and prayers, herbal teas and poultices for illness treatment

child with a congenital defect, families often turn to spirituality for hope, comfort, and relief.

Though the word "religion" is often used interchangeably with spirituality in our society, they are distinctly different. Spirituality is considered private and individual. **Religion,** in contrast, is an organized way of sharing beliefs and practicing worship. Over 95% of parents in America believe in God. Their spiritual or religious beliefs and views can provide strength and support during times of stress and illness. In some religions, illness is seen as a punishment for sin or wrongdoing. Others religions view illness as a test of strength that allows them to strive for faithfulness.

Identifying a client's religious beliefs and customs is important. Families appreciate recognition of and respect for their beliefs. Dietary restrictions, rituals such as baptism or communion, use of amulets or icons, or practices related to birth or newborn care can be incorporated into the plan of care.

▶ *Take* NOTE!

Never make assumptions about a family's religious or spiritual affiliation. Although they may belong to a particular religion, they may not adhere to all of its beliefs or participate in all aspects of the religion. Be alert for clues that would provide insight into their specific beliefs.

Diversity of Client Populations

The United States is no longer a melting pot of various cultures and ethnicities but a society with each individual bringing a diversity and richness that enriches the country as a whole. According to the U.S. Census Bureau reports, the Hispanic population is now the fastest-growing population group, increasing by 3.3% from July 1, 2004, to July 1, 2005, and accounting for almost half of the total population growth during that time frame. At the same time, non-Hispanic whites accounted for less than one fifth of the total population growth (U.S. Census Bureau, 2006). In addition, the increasing number of intermarriages between individuals from different ethnic origins is producing an increasing number of children who have a heritage that represents more than one cultural group.

The United States is also viewed as a place of employment and economic opportunities, expanded human rights, educational opportunities, and other types of freedoms and opportunities, thus inspiring many individuals to move to the United States from other countries. Immigration significantly affects the health, educational, and social services offered in this country. It also presents issues related to access to care and the types of care that need to be offered. The United States is currently evaluating, enforcing, and changing many of its immigration laws.

Immigration imposes unique stresses on women, children and families, including:

• Depression, grief, or anxiety associated with migration and acculturation
• Separation from support systems
• Inadequate language skills in a society that is not tolerant of linguistic differences
• Disparities in social, professional, and economic status between the country of origin and the United States
• Traumatic events such as war or persecution that may have occurred in their native country (American Academy of Pediatrics Committee on Community Health Services, 2005)

Immigrant families may face financial, language, cultural, and other type of barriers that reduce their ability to receive preventive care, and care for minor conditions may be delayed until they become more serious. Stresses experienced by immigrant children and their families, such as those associated with relocation, separation, and traumatic events, also can affect their psychological health.

Health Status and Lifestyle

An individual's chronic health conditions and his or her lifestyle can increase or decrease the risk of health problems. Chronic health conditions can begin soon after birth. For example, the incidence of multiple births has been increasing in this country due to the increased use of in vitro fertilization and other assisted technologies (Reynolds et al., 2003). The complications associated with multiple births include intrauterine growth retardation and prematurity (Reynolds et al., 2003). These complications may lead to chronic health problems that can hinder the child's growth and development. Children with chronic health conditions may experience developmental delays, especially in acquiring skills related to cognition, communication, adaptation, social functioning, and motor functioning. Thus, the beginning health status of a child may affect his or her long-term health and development.

Developmental Level and Disease Distribution

Developmental level has a major impact on an individual's health status. In general, the distribution of diseases or illnesses varies with age. For example, adolescents who become pregnant are at a higher risk for certain complications, such as anemia, hypertension, preterm labor, cephalopelvic disproportion, and postpartum hemorrhage. Pregnant adolescents also experience higher rates of intimate partner violence and substance abuse. Moreover, substance abuse can contribute to low birthweight, intrauterine growth restriction, preterm births, newborn addiction, and sepsis (Mittendorfer-Rutz & Wasserman, 2008). Women who become pregnant after age 35 are at risk for hypertension, dystocia, and postpartum hemorrhage. Older pregnant women are also more likely to have a pre-existing condition that could complicate the pregnancy. Moreover, fetuses of older pregnant women are at risk for chromosomal abnormalities.

Certain communicable diseases are more commonly associated with certain age groups. Before the use of routine immunizations, conditions such as measles and mumps were more commonly seen in younger school-age children. The physiologic immaturity of an infant's body systems increases the risk for infection. Ingestion of toxic substances and poisoning are major health concerns for toddlers as they become more mobile and inquisitive. Adolescents are establishing their identity, which may lead them to distance themselves from their family values and traditions for a period of time and conform more with their peers. This journey may lead to risky behaviors, resulting in injuries or other health problems.

Nutrition

Nutrition provides the body with the calories and nutrients to sustain life and promote growth, as well as the essentials required to maintain health and prevent illness. Nutritional deficiencies or excesses are common problems in the United States, as evidenced by the persistent problem of iron-deficiency anemia and the increasing incidence of childhood obesity. Inadequate food intake, social and cultural food practices or habits that may be nutritionally unsound, the availability of processed and nutritionally inadequate foods, lack of nutrition education in homes and schools, and the presence of illness that interferes with the ingestion, digestion, and absorption of food are factors that can affect an individual's nutrition.

During pregnancy, a woman needs additional calories to support fetal growth and development as well as to support her own needs, and an adequate intake of folic acid is important to prevent neural tube defects (Fig. 1.11). For the child, inadequate nutrition is associated with lowered cognitive ability, poor or altered emotional and mental health, increased susceptibility to childhood illnesses, and stunted physical growth. The "fast food" or "junk food" that is prevalent in today's society is a key factor in the epidemic of childhood obesity and increases in the prevalence of childhood type 2 diabetes. Nutrition and its effects on health status are integrated throughout this text.

Lifestyle Choices

Lifestyle choices that affect an individual's health include patterns of eating, exercise, use of tobacco, drugs, or alcohol, and methods of coping with stress. Most health problems that arise today are due to an individual's lifestyle. For children, the lifestyle of the parents basically is the lifestyle of the child, so parents need to set a good example in terms of nutrition and physical activity.

Environmental Exposure

Some environmental exposures can jeopardize health. In utero, the child can be affected by lack of maternal nutri-

FIGURE 1.11 (**A**) The dietary habits established early in life can have a long-lasting impact on the child's health and quality of life. (**B**) This pregnant client is eating a healthy meal to ensure adequate nutrition.

tion, maternal infections, or maternal use of alcohol, tobacco, and drugs. Nurses caring for pregnant women should be aware of the risks to the fetus posed by certain drugs, chemicals, and dietary agents, as well as maternal illnesses. These agents, known as teratogens, may be linked to birth defects in children. Not all drugs or agents have fetal effects, however, and research is necessary to identify the correlations between teratogens and other variables.

The environment continues to affect a child's health after birth. Exposure to lead, air pollution, tobacco, and water or food contaminants can impair a child's health. Exposure to safety hazards in the home or community can lead to falls, burns, drowning, or other accidents. Statistically, more drownings occur in children in warmer states because more homes have pools. Exposure to secondhand smoke, radiation, or chemicals is another health hazard for children. Because children are smaller and still developing, environmental exposures can cause more health problems, both in the short and long term, for them than for adults.

Stress and Coping

Disasters such as the terrorist attacks of Sept. 11, 2001, the killings at Columbine High School, or Hurricane Katrina can have a significant impact on the well-being of women, children, and families. Stressors such as war, terrorism, school violence, and natural disasters may decrease a person's coping ability (Ryan-Wenger, Sharrer, & Campbell, 2005) and lead to alterations in growth and development (Crane & Clements, 2005). Exposure to traumatic events and violence may have long-term effects on an individual's psychosocial development and status. Children who have experienced these events are at risk for the development of post-traumatic stress disorder, behavioral issues, and depression (Wexler, Branski, & Kerem, 2006).

Exposure to stress is not limited to disasters or traumatic events, however. Stress can also include areas such as inadequate finances, family crises, inadequate support systems, or domestic violence. Like disasters and traumatic events, the effects of these stressors can dramatically affect the health status of a woman, child, or family.

Recall Sophia, the 38-year-old pregnant woman who has come to the prenatal clinic for a visit. While talking with the nurse, Sophia mentions that her children are very involved in activities. She says, "My husband is busy at work, so I do most of the running around. Sometimes I feel like the people at the drive-through know me by name! My husband helps out on the weekends, but during the week, it's all me." What factors may be influencing Sophia's health? How might these factors be influencing the health of the children and the family?

Health Care Cost Containment

The health care system functions within a market setting, offering goods and services that carry a cost to health care consumers and clients. The advent of managed care has led to a trend of attempting to reduce health care costs. These efforts have led to shorter hospital stays and increased awareness on the part of nurses of the costs of supplies and services. The overall challenge is to maintain the quality of care while reducing its cost. For example, if a pregnant diabetic woman needs to go to an endocrinologist, she has very little choice except to purchase the services needed or go without care. In today's managed care environment, the woman will need to go through her "primary health care professional" or "gatekeeper" to receive a referral to a specialist. Often she must trust her primary provider to make that choice for her instead of making that decision on her own.

Although cost containment is important to restrain health care spending, such efforts should not reduce the quality or safety of care delivered. Preventive care (remember the old saying "an ounce of prevention is worth a pound of cure") has been shown to lower costs significantly. Mammograms, cervical cancer screenings, prenatal care, smoking cessation programs, and immunizations are a few examples of preventive care that yield positive outcomes and reduce overall health care costs. Using technological advances to diagnose and treat diseases early saves lives as well as money.

Nurses can be leaders in providing quality care within a limited-resource environment by emphasizing to their clients the importance of making healthy lifestyle and food choices, seeking early interventions for minor problems before they become major ones, and learning about health-related issues that affect them so they can select the best option for themselves and their families. Prevention services and health education are the cornerstones of delivering quality maternal and child health care.

Access to Health Care

The health care system continues to change. In the United States, changes in the health care system result from pressures coming from many directions. These changes reflect shifts in social and economic realities and the results of the biomedical and technological progress that has been made over the past several decades. The effects are felt by every individual who seeks health care in any form. The system of providing medical care in a hi-tech environment has changed to providing health care in an environment with limited resources and access to services. Ways to allocate our limited health care resources continue to be the focus.

A major factor involved access to care is health insurance. People without health insurance typically cannot afford to seek health care for maintenance and prevention interventions, and 11.7% of children lack health insurance; many of them are minority children, children in immigrant families, and adolescents (Future of Children, 2004). The "working poor" may not earn enough money to afford health insurance or medical care, and part-time workers do not always receive benefits such as health insurance.

Preventive Care Focus

The emphasis on cost reduction also led to an emphasis on preventive care and services. Anticipatory guidance is vital during each health contact with women, children, and families. Education of the family includes everything from keeping the home safe to ways to prevent illness.

The Continuum of Care Emphasis

A "continuum of care" strategy is cost-effective and provides more efficient and effective services. This continuum extends from acute care settings such as hospitals to outpatient settings such as ambulatory care clinics, primary care offices, rehabilitative units, community care settings, long-term facilities, homes, and even schools. For example, the hospital stay is now integrated into a continuum that allows the client to complete therapy at home, school, or other community settings, while re-entering the hospital for short periods for specific treatments or illnesses.

Improvements in Diagnosis and Treatments

Because of the tremendous improvements that have been made in technology and biomedicine, disorders and diseases are being diagnosed and treated earlier. The 1990s witnessed a remarkable and productive connection between genetics and various pathophysiologic processes. For example, female fetuses with congenital adrenal hyperplasia, a genetic disorder resulting in a steroid enzyme deficiency that can lead to disfiguring anatomic abnormalities, are beginning to receive treatment before birth. In addition, many genetic defects are being identified so counseling and treatment may occur early. With these improved diagnoses and treatments, nurses may now be caring for individuals who have survived situations that once would have been fatal, who are living well beyond their life expectancy for a specific illness, or who are functioning with chronic disabilities. For example, at one time women with congenital heart disease did not live long enough to become pregnant. However, with new surgical techniques to correct the defects, many of these women survive and become pregnant, progressing through their pregnancy without significant problems.

While positive and exciting, these advances and trends also pose new challenges for the health care community. For example, as health care for premature newborns improves and survival rates increase, the incidence of long-term chronic conditions such as respiratory airway dysfunction or developmental delays has also increased. As a result, nurses are faced with caring for clients at all stages along the health–illness continuum, such as well children, those who are occasionally ill, and women, children, and families with chronic and sometimes disabling conditions.

Empowerment of Health Care Consumers

Due to the influence of managed care, the focus on prevention, a more educated population, and technological advances, individuals and families have taken an increased responsibility for their own health. Health consumers are now better informed, and they want to play a greater role in managing health and illness. Families want information about illnesses and they want to participate in making decisions about treatment options. As client advocates valuing family-centered care, nurses are instrumental in promoting this empowerment. To do this, the nurse should respect the family's views and concerns, address all issues and concerns, consider the family members as important participants, and always include the woman, child, and family in the decision-making process.

Barriers to Health Care

Women are major consumers of health care services, in many cases arranging not only their own care but also that of family members. Compared with men, women have more health problems, longer life spans, and more significant reproductive health needs. Access to care can be jeopardized by lower incomes and greater responsibilities (juggling work and family). Lack of finances or transportation, language or cultural barriers, inconvenient clinic hours, and poor attitudes by health care workers often discourage clients from seeking health care.

Finances

Financial barriers are one of the most important factors that limit care. Many women have limited or no health insurance and cannot afford to pay for care. Although Medicaid covers prenatal care in most states, the paperwork and enrollment process can be so overwhelming that many women do not register.

Although the poverty rate is declining in this country, 36% of America's households with children had inadequate or crowded housing, or the housing cost more than 30% of the household income in 2001 (Federal Interagency Forum on Child and Family Statistics, 2006). The percentage of children covered by health insurance was 88% (leaving 12% of children without insurance). The majority of coverage since 1999 has not been from private health insurance but from government-supported plans (Federal Interagency Forum on Child and Family Statistics, 2006). Many children and families do not have health insurance, do not have enough insurance to cover services obtained, or cannot pay for services.

Transportation

Getting to and from appointments can be challenging for clients who do not drive or own a car or cannot use public transportation (if there is public transportation in the area). It can be difficult for these clients to attend all recommended prenatal health care visits or well-child visits, especially if the woman has other small children who must be taken along on the visit. These challenges can reduce the adherence to scheduled appointments and follow-up.

Language and Culture

Language is how people communicate with each other to increase their understanding or knowledge. If a health care worker cannot speak the same language as the client or does not have a trained interpreter available, a barrier is created. The client's complaints can be misinterpreted or ignored or their significance can be misconstrued. The language barrier might prevent the client from accessing the necessary care, such as prenatal care or preventative care.

Sociocultural and ethnic factors also pose barriers to health care. These factors may involve the lack of transportation, financial situations that require both parents to work, or genetic factors. Knowledge barriers (e.g., lack of understanding or awareness of the importance of prenatal care or child health promotion) and spiritual barriers (e.g., some forms of treatment are proscribed by religions) also cross all ethnic groups.

Health Care Delivery System

The health care delivery system itself can create barriers. Eighty-five percent of employed families with insurance are covered by some type of managed health care plan or health maintenance organization (HMO). This prospective payment system based on diagnosis-related groups (DRGs) limits the amounts of health care the family may receive. This also includes Medicaid reimbursement. Due to cost-containment efforts, the trend is to discharge clients as soon as possible from the hospital and to deliver care in the home or through community-based services. Although overall insurance plans may improve access to preventive services, they may limit access to specialty care—which greatly impacts clients with chronic or long-term illnesses.

Clinic hours must meet the needs of the clients, not the health care providers who work there. Evening or weekend hours might be needed to meet the schedules of working clients. Clinic personnel should evaluate the availability and accessibility of the services they offer.

Unfortunately, some health care workers exhibit negative attitudes toward poor or culturally diverse families, and this could deter these clients from seeking health care. Long delays, hurried examinations, and rude comments by staff discourage clients from returning.

▶ **Consider** THIS!

I was a 17-year-old pregnant migrant worker needing prenatal care. Although my English wasn't good, I was able to show the receptionist my "big belly" and ask for services. All the receptionist seemed interested in was a social security number and health insurance—neither of which I had. She proceeded to ask me personal ques-

(continued)

▶ **Consider** THIS! (continued)

tions concerning who the father was and commented on how young I looked. The receptionist then "ordered" me in a loud voice to sit down and wait for an answer by someone in the back, but never contacted anyone that I could see. It seemed to me like all eyes were on me while I found an empty seat in the waiting room. After sitting there quietly for over an hour without any attention or answer, I left.

Thoughts: Why did she leave before receiving any health care service? What must she have been feeling during her wait? Would you come back to this clinic again? Why or why not?

Legal and Ethical Issues in Maternal and Child Health Care

Law and ethics are interrelated and affect all of nursing. Professional nurses must understand their scope of practice, standards of care, institutional or agency policies, and state laws. Every nurse is responsible for knowing current information regarding ethics and laws related to their practice.

Numerous federal programs have had a major impact on women's and children's health (Table 1.4).

Several areas are of particular importance to the health care of women and children. These include abortion, substance abuse, fetal therapy, informed consent, client rights, and confidentiality.

Abortion

Abortion was a volatile legal, social, and political issue even before *Roe v. Wade*, the 1973 Supreme Court decision that legalized abortion. Forty-nine percent of pregnancies in American women are unintended, and 40% of them are terminated by abortion (Alan Guttmacher Institute, 2007).

Abortion is one of the most common procedures performed in the United States. It has become a hotly debated political issue that separates people into two camps: pro-choice and pro-life. The pro-choice group supports the right of any woman to make decisions about her reproductive functions based on her own moral and ethical beliefs. The pro-life group feels strongly that abortion is murder and deprives the fetus of the basic right to life. Both sides will continue to debate this very emotional issue for years to come.

Medical and surgical modalities are available to terminate a pregnancy, depending on how far the pregnancy has developed. A surgical intervention can be performed up to 14 weeks' gestation; a medical intervention can be performed up to 9 weeks' gestation (Gan et al., 2008). All women undergoing abortion need emotional support,

TABLE 1.4 MILESTONES IN FEDERAL PROGRAMS IN SUPPORT OF THE HEALTH OF WOMEN AND CHILDREN

Date	Action	Impact
1909	First White House Conference on Care of Dependent Children (convened by President Theodore Roosevelt)	Addressed the poor working and living conditions of many children in the United States
1912	U.S. Children's Bureau	First governmental agency to oversee children's health and environmental conditions
1921	Maternity & Infancy (Sheppard-Towner) Act	Provided grants to states to establish maternal and child health divisions in state health departments
1930	White House Conference on Child Welfare Standards and American Academy of Pediatrics	Produced the Children's Charter, documenting the child's need for health, education, welfare, and protection
1935	Title V of the Social Security Act	Established federal–state partnership and provided Aid to Families with Dependent Children (AFDC), maternal–child health services, and child welfare services
1959	14th General Assembly of United Nations	Approved the Declaration of the Rights of the Child
1965	Medicaid Program under Title XIX of Social Security Act; special programs such as Child Health Assessment Program	Provided state block grants to reduce financial barriers to health care for the poor and special services to pregnant women and young children
1966/1974	Women, Infants, Children (WIC) Program	Provided nutritional supplements and education to low-income families, pregnant, postpartum, and lactating women, and infants and children up to age 5
1969	U.S. Children's Bureau moved to Office of Health, Education, & Welfare (HEW)	Established greater presence for the programs
1975	Education for All Handicapped Children Act (Public Law 94-142) Title XX Social Services	Established federally mandated special education in public schools; provided block grants to day care, emergency shelters, counseling, family planning, and other services for children
1981	Alcohol, Drug Abuse & Mental Health block grants	Began funding services for children and adolescents with mental health issues
1986	Education of Handicapped Act Amendments (Public Law 99-457)	Established federal funding for states to create statewide, comprehensive, coordinated, and multidisciplinary early intervention services for handicapped infants and toddlers
1990	Omnibus Budget Reconciliation Act	Extended Medicaid coverage to all children (6–18 years) with family income below 133% of poverty level
1993	Family & Medical Leave Act (FMLA)	Allowed eligible employees to take up to 12 weeks of unpaid leave from their jobs every year to care for newborns or newly adopted children or children, parents, or spouses with serious health condition; employee can return to previous job or an comparable job with the same conditions

a stable environment in which to recover, and nonjudgmental care throughout.

Abortion is a complex issue, and the controversy is not only in the public arena: many nurses struggle with the conflict between their personal convictions and their professional duty. Nurses are taught to be supportive client advocates and to interact with a nonjudgmental attitude under all circumstances. However, nurses have their own personal and political views, which may be very different from those of their clients. Nurses need to clarify their personal values and beliefs on this issue and must be able to provide nonbiased care before assuming responsibility for clients who might be in a position to consider abortion. Their decision to care for or refuse to care for such clients affects staff unity, influences staffing decisions, and challenges the ethical concept of duty (Trybulski, 2006).

The ANA's Code of Ethics for Nurses upholds the nurse's right to refuse to care for a client undergoing an abortion if the nurse ethically opposes the procedure (ANA, 2001). Nurses need to make their values and beliefs known to their managers before the situation occurs so that alternative staffing arrangements can be made. Open communication and acceptance of the personal beliefs of others can promote a comfortable working environment.

Substance Abuse

Substance abuse for any person is a problem, but when it involves a pregnant woman, substance abuse can cause fetal injury and thus has legal and ethical implications. In some instances, courts have issued jail sentences to pregnant women who caused harm to their fetuses. Many state laws require reporting evidence of prenatal drug exposure, which may lead to charges of negligence and child endangerment against the pregnant woman. This punitive approach to fetal injury raises ethical and legal questions about the degree of governmental control that is appropriate in the interests of child safety.

Fetal Therapy

Intrauterine fetal surgery is a procedure that involves opening the uterus during pregnancy, performing a surgery, and replacing the fetus in the uterus. Although the risks to the fetus and the mother are both great, fetal therapy may be used to correct anatomic lesions (Noble & Rodeck, 2008). Some argue that medical technology should not interfere with nature, and thus this intervention should not take place. Others would argue that the surgical intervention improves the child's quality of life. For many people, these are the subjects of debates and intellectual discussions, but for nurses, these procedures may be part of their daily routine.

Nurses play an important supportive role in caring and advocating for clients and their families. As the use of technology grows, situations will surface more frequently that test a nurse's belief system. Encouraging open discussions to address emotional issues and differences of opinion among staff members is healthy and increases tolerance for differing points of view.

Informed Consent

Informed consent has four key components: disclosure, comprehension, competency, and voluntariness (Taylor et al., 2005). It occurs prior to initiation of the procedure or specific care and addresses the legal and ethical requirement of informing the client about the procedure. The physician or advanced practice nurse is responsible for informing the client about the procedure and obtaining consent by providing a detailed description of the procedure or treatment, its potential risks and benefits,

and alternative methods available. If the client is a child, typically this information is provided to the parents or legal guardian. The nurse's responsibility related to informed consent includes:

- Ensuring that the consent form is completed with signatures from the client (or parents or legal guardians if the client is a child)
- Serving as a witness to the signature process
- Determining whether the client or parents or legal guardians understand what they are signing by asking them pertinent questions

Although laws vary from state to state, certain key elements are associated with informed consent (Box 1.4). Nurses need to be familiar with their specific state laws as well as the policies and procedures of the health care agency. Treating clients without obtaining proper consent may result in charges of assault, and the health care provider and/or facility may be held liable for any damages.

Generally, only people over the age of majority (18 years of age) can legally provide consent for health care. Since children are minors, when care is rendered to them, the process involves obtaining written permission from a parent or legal guardian. In cases requiring a signature for consent, usually the parent provides consent for care for children less than 18 years of age, except in certain situations (see further discussion below).

▶ **Take** NOTE!

Allow older children and adolescents to be involved in the decision-making process to the extent possible. However, keep in mind that the parent is still ultimately responsible for giving consent to treatment.

BOX 1.4 **Key Elements of Informed Consent**

- The decision-maker must be of legal age in that state, with full civil rights, and must be competent (have the ability to make the decision).
- Information is presented in a manner that is simple, concise, and appropriate to the level of education and language of the individual responsible for making the decision.
- The decision must be voluntary, without coercion or force or under duress.
- There must be a witness to the process of informed consent.
- The witness must sign the consent form.

Most care rendered in a health care setting is covered by the initial consent for treatment signed when the individual becomes a client at that office or clinic or by the consent to treatment signed upon admission to the hospital or other inpatient facility. Certain procedures, however, require a specific process of informed consent: major and minor surgery; invasive procedures such as amniocentesis, internal fetal monitoring, lumbar puncture (LP), or bone marrow aspiration; treatments placing the client at higher risk, such as chemotherapy or radiation therapy; procedures or treatments involving research; and photography involving the client. Applying restraints to children now requires consent.

If the client cannot provide consent or, in the case of a child, the parent is not available, then the person closest to the client or in charge of the child (relative, babysitter, or teacher) may give consent for emergency treatment if he or she has a signed form from the parent or legal guardian allowing him or her to do so. During an emergency situation, a verbal consent, via the telephone, may be obtained. Two witnesses must also be listening simultaneously and must sign the consent form, indicating that consent was received via telephone. Health care providers can provide emergency treatment to a child without consent if they have made reasonable attempts to contact the child's parent or legal guardian (AAP, 2005). Table 1.5 provides additional information about the informed consent process with children.

▶ *Take* NOTE!

Never assume that the adult accompanying the child is the parent or legal guardian. Always clarify the relationship of the accompanying adult.

Refusal of Medical Treatment

All clients have the right to refuse medical treatment, based on the American Hospital Association's Bill of Rights. In the case of a child, parental autonomy (the right to decide for or against medical treatment) is a constitutionally protected right (Linnard-Palmer & Kools, 2004). Ideally, medical care without informed consent should be used only when the life of a client is in danger. Refusal of treatment may occur when the treatment conflicts with religious or cultural beliefs. In these cases, it is important to educate the client and family about the importance of the recommended treatment without coercing or forcing the client to agree. Sometimes common ground may be reached between the family's religious or cultural beliefs and the health care team's recommendations. Communication and education are the keys in this situation.

If providing medical treatment may save a child's life, health care providers and the judicial system strive to advocate for the child. The state has an overriding interest

TABLE 1.5 SPECIAL CONSIDERATIONS RELATED TO INFORMED CONSENT WITH CHILDREN

Issue	Definition	Nursing Considerations
Child not living with biological or adoptive parents	Child is living: • In foster care • With potential adoptive parent • With a relative	– Legally appointed guardian is responsible for providing consent – Verification of authority of legally appointed guardian – Documentation of the legal guardian in the child's medical record (AAP, 2003)
Parental consent after divorce	Ability to give consent for health care rests with parent who has legal custody by divorce degree	– Determination of joint custody or sole custody by one parent – Parent with only physical custody may give consent for emergency care. Court involvement may be needed if there is joint legal custody but parents disagree on care.
Consent for organ donation	For a minor to donate, the parents must be aware of the risks and benefits and must provide emotional support to child; there should be a close relationship between the donor and recipient.	– Referral of potential donors to local organ procurement organization – Family education about policies related to organ donation – Legal guardian or parental consent to organ donation (AAP, 2002)
Consent for medical experimentation	Requirements include consent of parents, assent of child, and a perceived benefit to the child	Need to comply with all federal regulations if federal funds received (see discussion of assent in text)

in the health and welfare of the child and can order that medical treatment proceed without a signed informed consent. This is referred to as *parens patriae* (the state has a right and a duty to protect children).

Parents may refuse treatment if they perceive that their child's quality of life will be significantly impaired by the medical care that is offered. If the parents refuse treatment but the health care team feels the treatment is reasonable and warranted, the case should be referred to the institution's ethics committee. If the issue remains unresolved, then the judicial system becomes involved (Kon, 2006a, 2006b).

Exceptions to Required Parental Consent for Children

The **emancipated minor** is considered to have the legal capacity of an adult and may make health care decisions (AAP, 2003). State laws vary in relation to the definition of an emancipated minor and the types of treatment that may be obtained as an emancipated minor (without parental consent). Emancipation may be considered in any of the following situations, depending upon the state's laws:

• Membership in a branch of the armed services
• Marriage
• Court-determined emancipation
• Financial independence and separate living arrangement from parents
• College attendance
• Pregnancy
• Mother less than 18 years of age
• Runaway

Nurses must be familiar with laws of the state where they work so they can be in compliance when rendering health care and treatment.

In some states, a minor may give consent to certain medical treatments. A mature minor is usually an adolescent over 14 years of age and is considered sufficiently mature and intelligent to make the decision for treatment. The provider considers the complexity of the treatment and the risks and benefits, as well as whether the treatment is necessary or elective, prior to obtaining consent from a mature minor (AAP, 2003).

In addition, many states do not require consent or notification of parents or legal guardians when providing specific types of care to minors. According to the state law, health care may be provided to minors for certain conditions, in a confidential manner, without notifying the parents. These types of care may include pregnancy counseling, prenatal care, contraception, testing and treatment for sexually transmitted infections and communicable diseases (including HIV), substance abuse and mental illness counseling and treatment, or health care required as a result of a crime-related injury (AAP, 2003). These exceptions provide a confidential environment for children who would avoid care if they were required to inform their parents or legal guardian. Again, the laws vary

by state, so nurses must be knowledgeable about the laws in the state where they practice.

Assent

Assent may be defined as agreeing to something. In the care of children, the term refers to the child's participation in the decision-making process about his or her health care (McCullough & Stein, 2007). The age of assent depends on the child's developmental level and maturity. The American Academy of Pediatrics recommends the age of 7 years (Bray, 2007; Broome & Richards, 2003). Certainly, the older the child is, the stronger the ethical obligation is to include the child in the decision-making process (Olechnowicz et al., 2002). The Society of Pediatric Nurses (2006) makes the following recommendations related to assent:

• Child 4 to 6 years of age: Use developmentally appropriate materials to inform the child about the participation in research or treatment.
• Child 7 to 12 years of age: Obtain assent for non-therapeutic research.
• Adolescent 13 to 17 years of age: Obtain assent for therapeutic and non-therapeutic research.

The AAP recommends that if a health care provider solicits the child's opinion about the direction of treatment or participation in research, then the child's views and desires should be seriously considered.

The converse of assent is dissent (disagreeing with the treatment plan), and dissent by an adolescent 13 to 17 years of age is considered binding in some states. The Society of Pediatric Nurses (2006) believes that dissent in the 7- to 12-year-old should also be considered binding. If the decision is made to move forward with treatment despite the child's dissent, this decision must be explained to the child in developmentally appropriate terms. In the case of research studies, the study itself must specifically ascertain if child assent is necessary, and at what age (Kimberly et al., 2006). Prior to recruitment for a research study, the researchers must also decide if the child's objection to participation will be honored (Kon, 2006a).

Clients' Rights

The American Hospital Association first established a Patient's Bill of Rights in 1972 as a way to promote the value and dignity of the client. This information is updated periodically. Most health care agencies and professional organizations have developed some type of document that addresses clients' rights.

Ensuring that clients' rights are upheld is a key aspect in the care of any client. For the pregnant woman, two clients must be considered—the pregnant woman and her fetus. The American Foundation for Maternal and Child Health developed the Pregnant Patient's Bill of Rights to address specific concerns and situations involving the health and well-being of the mother and her fetus. A child, due to his or her age and developmental level, may lack mature decision-making abilities. Many pediatric institutions have adopted a bill of rights for children's health care specific to that institution (Box 1.5).

The U.S. Department of Health and Human Services has issued laws related to protecting the welfare of newborns ("Baby Doe" law). Parents ultimately are the decision-makers for their children. In ethical dilemmas such as babies born with brain damage or extremely preterm birth, parents must be accurately informed about the risks and benefits of treatment before giving consent to treatment or deciding to withdraw or forego treatment (Hurst, 2006). Some professionals are advocating for prenatal advance directives that would guide care from the time of birth of an extremely premature or otherwise impaired term infant (Catlin, 2005).

A number of national and international organizations have been formed in recent years to protect the rights of women and children in the United States and worldwide. These organizations focus on issues such as violence and abuse, child labor and soldiering, juvenile justice, child immigrants and orphans, abandoned children, and homeless women, children, and families. All of these issues can have negative impacts on the health of women, children, and families. As client advocates, nurses need to support policies that protect their clients' rights and improve health care.

Confidentiality

With the establishment of the Health Insurance Portability and Accountability Act (HIPAA) of 1996, the confidentiality of health care information is now mandated by law. The primary intent of the law is to protect health insurance coverage for workers and their families when they change or lose jobs. Another aspect of the law requires the

Department of Health and Human Services to establish national standards for electronic transmission of health information. The plan also addresses the security and privacy of health information. For example, no information that clearly identifies a client can be in public display, including information on a client's chart. In maternal and child health care, information is shared only with the client, legal partner, parents, legal guardians, or individuals as established in writing by the client or the child's parents. This law promotes the security and privacy of health care and health information for all clients. Client information should always be kept confidential in the context of the state law, as well as the institution's policies.

Exceptions to confidentiality exist. For example, suspicion of physical or sexual abuse and injuries caused by a weapon or criminal act must be reported to the proper authorities. Abuse cases are reported to the appropriate welfare authorities, whereas criminal acts are reported to the police. The health care provider must also follow public health laws related to reporting certain infectious diseases to the local health department (e.g., tuberculosis, hepatitis, HIV, and other sexually transmitted diseases). Finally, there is a duty to warn third parties when there is a specific threat to an identifiable person. There must be a balance between confidentiality and required disclosure. If health care information must be disclosed by law, the client must be informed that this will occur (Feldman-Winter & McAbee, 2002).

Implications for Nurses

The health care system is intricately woven into the political and social structure of our society, and nurses should understand social, legal, and ethical health care issues so that they can play an active role in meeting the health care needs of women, children, and families. Nurses need to take a proactive role in advocating for and empowering their clients. For example, nurses can help women to increase control over the factors that affect health, thereby improving their health status. A woman may become empowered by developing skills not only to cope with her environment, but also to change it. Nurses also can assume this mentoring role with children and families, thus helping them to improve their overall health status and health outcomes.

Nurses must have a solid knowledge base about the factors affecting maternal and child health and barriers to health care. They can use this information to provide anticipatory guidance, health counseling, and teaching for women, children, and families. It also is useful in identifying high-risk groups so that interventions can be initiated early on, before problems occur.

When caring for women, children, and families, the nurse operates within the framework of the nursing process, which is applicable to all health care settings. Maternal and child health nursing is ever-changing as globalization and the exchange of information expands. Nurses must remain up to date about new technologies and treatments

---

BOX 1.5 A Child's Bill of Rights

- To be called by name
- To receive compassionate health care in a careful, prompt, and courteous manner
- To know the names of all providers caring for the child
- To have basic needs met and usual schedules or routines honored
- To be kept without food or drink when necessary for the shortest time possible
- To be unrestrained if able
- To have parents or other important persons with the child
- To have an interpreter for the child and family when needed
- To object noisily if desired
- To be educated honestly about the child's health care
- To be respected as a person—not having people talk about the child within earshot unless the child knows what is happening
- For all health care providers to respect the child's confidentiality about his/her illness at all times

Adapted from UCI University Children's Hospital, 2006.

and integrate high-quality, evidence-based interventions into the care they provide.

■■■ Key Concepts

■ Maternal and child health nurses provide care using a philosophy that focuses on the family as the emphasis of care, providing atraumatic care and using evidence-based practice in a case management environment to provide quality, cost-effective care.

■ Healthy People 2010 presents a national set of health goals and objectives for adults and children that focuses on health promotion and disease prevention.

■ One method to establish the aggregate health status of women, infants, and children is with statistical data, such as mortality and morbidity rates.

■ The infant mortality rate is the lowest in the history of the United States, but it is still higher when compared with other industrialized countries. This high rate may be the result of the increase in low-birth-weight infants born in this country.

■ The family is considered the basic social unit. The family greatly influences the development and health of its members. Members learn health care activities, health beliefs, and health values from their family.

■ Social roles are often an important factor in the development of one's self-concept, which can have a very positive influence on health or present various limitations and problems, possibly resulting in a negative influence on health.

■ Culture influences every aspect of development and is reflected in childbearing and childrearing beliefs and practices designed to promote healthy adaptation.

■ Spirituality, a major influence for many individuals, provides a meaning and purpose to life and is a foundation for and a source of love, relationships, and service. Spiritual and religious beliefs and views can provide strength and support to women, children, and their families during times of stress and illness.

■ Other factors impacting the health of women and children include health status and lifestyles, health care cost containment, improved diagnosis and treatment, and health care consumer empowerment. Finances, transportation, language, culture, and the health care delivery system can provide barriers to health care.

■ Advances in science and technology have led to increased ethical dilemmas in health care.

■ All clients have the right to refuse medical treatment based on the American Hospital Association's Bill of Rights. For a child, the parents have the legal right to decide for or against medical treatment. Minor children (under the age of 18 years) must have their parents or legal guardians provide consent for health care in most cases.

■ In certain states, mature minors and emancipated minors may consent to their own health care and certain health care may be provided to adolescents without parental notification, including contraception, preg-

nancy counseling, prenatal care, testing and treatment of sexually transmitted infections and communicable diseases (including HIV), substance abuse and mental illness counseling and treatment, and health care required as a result of a crime-related injury.

■ The nurse must be knowledgeable about the laws related to health care of women and children in the specific state of nursing practice as well as the specific policies of the health care institution.

REFERENCES

Abell, S., & Ey, J. L. (2008). Domestic violence: Its impact on children. *Clinical Pediatrics, 47*(4), 413–415.

Alexander, L. L., LaRosa, J. H., Bader, H., & Garfield, S. (2007). *New dimensions in women's health* (3rd ed.). Sudbury, MA: Jones & Bartlett Publishers.

Alan Guttmacher Institute. (2007) *Facts in brief: Induced abortion.* Available at: www.agi-usa.org/pubs/fb_induced_abortion.html

American Academy of Child & Adolescent Psychiatry (AACAP). (2008). *Foster care* [Online]. Available at: http://www.aacap.org/cs/root/facts_for_families/foster_care.

American Academy of Pediatrics, Committee on Bioethics. (1995). Informed consent, parental permission, and assent in pediatric practice. *Pediatrics, 95*, 314–317.

American Academy of Pediatrics Committee on Community Health Services. (2005). Providing care for immigrant, homeless, and migrant children. *Pediatrics, 115*(4), 1095–1100.

American Academy of Pediatrics Committee on Psychosocial Aspects of Child and Family Health. (1998). Guidance for effective discipline. *Pediatrics, 101*(4), 723–728; reaffirmed 2004.

American Academy of Pediatrics. (2006). *Setting rules for Internet use.* Accessed 9/26/06. Available at: www.aap.org/pubed/ZZZQJ9C0B7C.htm?&sub_cat=17

American Academy of Pediatrics. (2003). Consent by proxy for nonurgent pediatric care. *Pediatrics, 112*, 1186–1195.

American Cancer Society. (2007a). *Breast cancer facts and figures.* Available at www.cancer.org/docroot/STT/stt_0.asp.

American Cancer Society. (2007b). *What are the risk factors for breast cancer? Cancer Reference Information.* Available at: www.cancer.org/docroot/CRI/content/CRI_2_4_2X_What_are_the_risk_factors_for_breast_cancer_5.asp?sitearea=.

American Nurses Association. (2001). *Code of ethics for nurses with interpretive statements.* Washington, D.C.: American Nurses Publishing.

American Nurses Association (ANA). (2002). *Code of ethcis for nurses* [Online]. Available at: http://www.linfield.edu/portland/documents/manuals/PDXStudent/StudentHandbook/CodeofEthicsforNurses.pdf.

American Pediatric Association (APA). (2005). Joint position statement on emergency care of children. *Ambulatory Pediatrics, 3*(6), 283.

American Psychological Association. (2005). *Lesbian and gay parenting.* Washington, DC: American Psychological Association.

American Psychological Association. (2004). *Single parenting and today's family.* Retrieved June 3, 2008 from http://apahelpcenter.org/articles/article.php?id=16.

American Psychological Association (APA). (2008). *Doing it alone* [Online]. Available at: http://www.americanpregnancy.org/unplannedpregnancy/doingitalone.html.

Ashby, S. L., Arcari, C. M., & Edmonson, B. (2006). Television viewing and risk of sexual initiation by young adolescents. *Archives of Pediatric and Adolescent Medicine, 160*, 375–380.

Banks, J. B. (2002). Childhood discipline: Challenges for clinicians and parents. *American Family Physician, 66*(8), 1447–1452.

Behrman, R., et al. (2004). *Nelson textbook of pediatrics* (17th ed.). Philadelphia: W. B. Saunders.

Bloom, B., Dey, A. N., & Freeman, G. (2006). Summary health statistics for U.S. children: National Health Interview survey, 2005. *Vital Health Statistics, 10*(231), 1–93.

Boss, P. (2001). *Family stress management* (2nd ed.). Thousand Oaks, CA: Sage.

Bray, L. (2007). Developing an activity to aid informed assent when interviewing children and young people. *Journal of Nursing Research, 12*(5), 447–457.

Brodsky, P. L. (2006). Childbirth. A journey through time. *International Journal of Childbirth Education, 21*(3), 10–15.

Broome, M. E., & Richards, D. J. (2003). The influence of relationships on children's and adolescents' participation in research. *Nursing Research, 52*(3), 191–197.

Bryner, C. L. (2001). Children of divorce. *Journal of the American Board of Family Practice, 14*(3), 176–183. Accessed 9/21/06. Available at: http://www.medscape.com/viewarticle/405852

Bushman, B. J., & Huesmann, R. (2006). Short-term and long-term effects of violent media on aggression in children and adults. *Archives of Pediatric and Adolescent Medicine, 160,* 348–352.

Cassidy, T. (2006). *Birth: The surprising history of how we are born.* Berkeley, CA: Grove/Atlantic, Inc.

Catlin, A. J. (2005). Thinking outside the box: Prenatal care—the call for a prenatal advance directive. *Journal of Perinatal & Neonatal Nursing, 19*(2), 169–176.

Centers for Disease Control and Prevention, National Center for Health Statistics, National Vital Statistics System. *National Vital Statistics Reports, 54*(16), 1–29.

Centers for Disease Control and Prevention. (2006a). *Adverse Childhood Experiences Study* (2006). Major findings. Accessed 10/5/06. Available at: http://www.cdc.gov/NCCDPHP/ACE/findings.htm

Centers for Disease Control and Prevention. (2006b). *Fact sheet: Pregnancy-related mortality surveillance—United States, 1991–1993.* Available at www.cdc.gov/od/oc/media/pressrel/fs030220.htm. Accessed January 2007.

Centers for Disease Control and Prevention. (2006c). *National Center for Injury Prevention and Control Child Maltreatment: Fact sheet.* Accessed 10/5/06. Available at: http://www.cdc.gove/ncipc/factsheets.cmfacts.htm

Centers for Disease Control and Prevention. (2006d). *National Center for Injury Prevention and Control Youth Violence: Fact sheet.* Accessed 10/5/06. Available at: http://www.cdc.gov/ncipc/factsheets/yvfacts.htm

Centers for Disease Control and Prevention. (2006e). *Safe motherhood: Promoting health for women before, during and after pregnancy.* Atlanta: CDC, Division of Reproductive Health.

Centers for Disease Control and Prevention. (2006f). State-specific maternal mortality among black and white women—United States, 1987–1996. *MMWR, 48,* 492–496. Also available at www.cdc.gov/epo/mmwr/preview/mmwrhtm/mm4823a3.htm.

Centers for Disease Control and Prevention. (2006g). Youth risk behavior surveillance—United States, 2005. *MMWR, 55*(SS-5), 1–112. Accessed 10/5/06. Available at: www.dcde/gov/mmwr/PDF/SS/SS5505.pdf

Children's Defense Fund. (2005). *The state of American's children 2005.* Washington, DC: Author.

Child Trends. (2005). Child Trends calculations of U.S. Census Bureau, Current Population Survey, 2005 Annual Social and Economic supplement. "America's Families and Living Arrangements: 2005." Accessed 9/18/06. Available at: http://www.census.gov/population/www/socdemo/hh-fam/cps2005.html

Child Trends. (2006a). *Child trends data bank.* Accessed 8/30/06. Available at http://www.childtrendsdatabank.org/indicators/53NumberofChildren.cfm.

Child Trends. (2006b). *Infant, child and youth death rates.* Accessed 8/23/06. Available at http://www.childtrendsdatabank.org/indicators/63ChildMortality.cfm.

Child Welfare Information Gateway. (2007). *Definitions in federal law.* Retrieved June 3, 2008 from http://www.childwelfare.gov/can/defining/federal.cfm.

Commission for Case Management Certification. (n.d.). *Case management practice.* Retrieved June 3, 2008 from http://www.ccmcertification.org/pages/13frame_set.html.

Crane, P. A., & Clements, P. T. (2005). Psychological response to disasters: Focus on adolescents. *Journal of Psychosocial Nursing & Mental Health Services, 43*(8), 31–38.

Dey, A. N., Schiller, J. S., & Tai, D. A. (2004). Summary health statistics for U.S. children: National Health Interview Survey, 2002. *Vital and Health Statistics, 10*(221), 1–78.

DiLauro, M. D. (2004). Psychosocial factors associated with types of child maltreatment. *Child welfare, 83*(1), 69–99.

Duvall, E. (1997). *Marriage and family development* (5th ed.). Philadelphia: J. B. Lippincott.

Federal Interagency Forum on Child and Family Statistics. (2006). America's children: Key national indicators of well-being, 2007. Retrieved June 3, 2008 from http://www.childstats.gov/americaschildren/index.asp

Feldman-Winter, L., & McAbee, G. N. (2002). Legal issues in caring for adolescent patients: Physicians can optimize healthcare delivery to teens. *Postgraduate Medicine, 111*(5), 15. Retrieved from Proquest database June 1, 2006, at http://proquest.umi.com/pqdweb?did=121957428&sid=2&Fmt=3&clientld=2157&RQT=309&VName=PQD.

Framingham Heart Study (FHS). (2007). *Through the looking glass: Women and heart disease.* Available at: http://www.framingham.com/heart/4stor_04.htm

Friedman, M. M. (2002). *Family nursing: Theory and practice* (5th ed.). Norwalk, CT: Appleton & Lange.

Friedman, M., Bowden, V., & Jones, E. (2003). *Family nursing: Research, theory, and practice* (5th ed.). Upper Saddle River, NJ: Prentice Hall.

Future of Children. (2004). *Children of immigrant families.* Washington, DC: The David and Lucile Packard Foundation.

Gan, C., Zou, Y., Wu, S., Li, Y. & Liu, Q. (2008). The influence of medical abortion compared with surgical abortion on subsequent pregnancy outcome. *International Journal of Gynecology and Obstetrics, 101*(3), 231–238.

Guardianship of Children Resource Center. (2008). *Guardianship of children* [Online]. Available at http://www.nolo.com/resource.cfm/catID/5F2ECF95-E8DD-4A04-A0A6FEB1213633FE/118/122/186/.

Hetherington, E. M. (2005). Divorce and the adjustment of children. *Pediatrics in Review, 26,* 13–169.

Hodnett, E. D., Gates, S., Hofmeyr, G. J., & Sakata C. (2007). Continuous support for women during childbirth. *Cochrane Database of Systematic Reviews* 2007. Issue 3. Art. No.: CD003766.DOI: 10.1002/14651858.CD003766.pub2.

Hollander, D. (2006). Early prenatal care does not close racial gaps in perinatal mortality. *Perspectives on Sexual & Reproductive Health, 38*(3), 174–177.

Hornor, G. (2005). Domestic violence and children. *Journal of Pediatric Health Care, 19*(4), 206–212.

Howard, E. D. (2006). Family-centered care in the context of fetal abnormality. *Journal of Perinatal & Neonatal Nursing, 20*(3), 237–242.

Hoyert, D. L., Matthews, T. J., Menacker, F., Strobino, D. M., & Guyer, B. (2006). Annual summary of vital statistics: 2004. *Pediatrics, 117*(1), 168–183.

Hurst, I. (2006). The legal landscape at the threshold of viability for extremely premature infants: A nursing perspective, part I. *JONA's Healthcare Law, Ethics, and Regulation, 8*(1), 20–28.

InCrisis. (2007). *The prevalence of mental health and addictive disorders.* Retrieved March 22, 2007, from www.incrisis.org/Articles/Prevalence MHProblems.htm.

Jolivet, R. (2006). Nurse-midwives committed to women throughout the lifespan. *The Nurse Practitioner, 9,* 10–13.

Kimberly, M. B., Hoehn, S., Feudtner, C., Nelson, R. M., & Schreiner, M. (2006). Variations in standards of research compensation and child assent practices: A comparison of 69 institutional review board-approved informed permission and assent forms for 3 multicenter pediatric clinical trials. *Pediatrics, 117*(5), 1706–1711.

King, D., & White, M. (2005). Infant and neonatal mortality rates in the United States. *International Journal of Childbirth Education, 20*(4), 26–27.

Kon, A. A. (2006a). Assent in pediatric research. *Pediatrics, 117*(5), 1806–1810.

Kon, A. A. (2006b). When parents refuse treatment for their child. *JONA's Healthcare Law, Ethics, and Regulation, 8*(1), 5–9.

Linnard-Palmer, L., & Kools, S. (2004). Parents' refusal of medical treatments based on religious and/or cultural beliefs: The law, ethical principles, and clinical implications. *Journal of Pediatric Nursing, 19*(5), 351–356.

London, M. L., Ladewig, P. A., Ball, J. W., & Bindler, R. M. (2007). *Maternal and child nursing care* (2nd ed.). Upper Saddle River, NJ: Pearson Education.

Looman, W. S., & Lindeke, L. L. (2005). Health and social context: Social capital's utility as a construct for nursing and health promotion. *Pediatric Health Care, 19*(2), 90–94.

Lumeng, J. C., Rahnama, S., Appugliese, D., Kaciroti, N., & Bradley, R. H. (2006). Television exposure and overweight risk in preschoolers. *Archives of Pediatric and Adolescent Medicine, 160,* 417–422.

Matthews, T. J., & MacDorman, M. F. (2006) Infant mortality statistics from the 2003 period linked birth/infant death data set. *National Vital Statistics Reports, 54*(16), 1–30.

McClure, E. M., Goldenberg, R. L., & Bann, C. M. (2007). Maternal mortality, stillbirth and measures of obstetric care in developing and developed countries. *International Journal of Gynecology & Obstetrics, 96*(2), 139–146.

McCullough, L. B., & Stein, F. (2007). *Pediatric assent and confidentiality in clinical practice.* Retrieved June 3, 2008, from http://www.baylorcme.org/assent/.

Mittendorfer-Rutz, E., & Wasserman, D. (2008). Pregnancies in high psychosocial risk groups: Research findings and implications for early intervention. *Psychiatric Clinics of North America, 31*(2), 205–212.

National Center for Health Statistics. (2006). More babies born at very low birthweight: linked to rise in infant mortality in 2004. In NCHS news release fact sheets. Available at: www.cdc.gov/nchs/pressroom/05news/lowbirthwt.htm.

Montgomery, K. S. (2003). Nursing care for pregnant adolescents. *JOGNN, 32*(2), 249–257.

National Center on Family Homelessness. (2008). *Homeless children: America's new outcasts.* Retrieved June 3, 2008 from http://www.familyhomelessness.org/pdf/fact_outcasts.pdf.

National Center on Family Homelessness. (2008). *The characteristics and needs of the families experiencing homelessness* [Online]. Available at: http://www.familyhomelessness.org/pdf/Characteristics_Needs_Homeless_Families.pdf.

National Clearinghouse of Child Abuse and Neglect (NCCAN). (2008). *Child abuse and neglect* [Online]. Available at: http://www.happinessonline.org/LoveAndHelpChildren/p7.htm.

National Coalition Against Domestic Violence. (2005). *Children and domestic violence facts.* Retrieved March 27, 2007, from http://www.ncadv.org/files/Children_.pdf

National Coalition for the Homeless. (2006). Who is homeless? NCH Fact Sheet #3. Accessed 10/9/06. Available at: http://www.nationalhomeless.org/publications/facts/Whois.pdf

National Women's Law Center, FOCUS/University of Pennsylvania, and the Lewin Group. (2007). *Making the grade on women's health: A national state-by-state report card.* Washington, DC: National Women's Law Center.

National Youth Violence Prevention Resource Center. (2005). *School violence.* Retrieved March 27, 2007, from http://www.safeyouth.org/scripts/teens/school.asp.

Newhouse, R. P. (2006). Examining the support for evidence-based nursing practice. *Journal of Nursing Administration, 36*(7/8), 337–340.

Noble, R. & Rodeck, C. H. (2008). Ethical considerations of fetal therapy. *Bailliere's Best Practice & Research in Clinical Obstetrics & Gynecology, 22*(1), 219–231.

Ogbolu, Y. (2007). Neonatal mortality: A critical global issue. *Neonatal Network, 26*(6), 357–360.

Olechnowicz, J. Q., Eder, M., Simon, C., Zyzanski, S., & Kodish, E. (2002). Assent observed: Children's involvement in leukemia treatment and research discussions. *Pediatrics, 109*(5), 806–814.

Pace, D. T. (2006). Menopause: Studying the research. *Nurse Practitioner, 31*(8), 16–23.

Pillitteri, A. (2007). *Maternal and child health nursing* (5th ed.). Philadelphia: Lippincott Williams & Wilkins.

Prevent Child Abuse America (PCAA). (2007). *Promoting healthy families in your communities* [Online]. Available at http://www.preventchildabuse.org/publications/cap/index.shtml.

Prevent Child Abuse America. (2008). *2006 child maltreatment statistics.* Retrieved June 3, 2008 from http://member.preventchildabuse.org/site/DocServer/Child_Maltreatment_Fact_Sheet_2005.pdf?docID=221.

Reasor, J. E., & Farrell, S. P. (2004). Early childhood mental health: Services that can save a life. *Journal of Pediatric Nursing, 19*(2), 140–144.

Rennison, C. M., & Welchans, S. (2000). *Intimate partner violence: Bureau of Justice Statistics special report.* Washington, DC: U.S. Department of Justice.

Reynolds, M. A., et al. (2003). Trends in multiple births conceived using assisted reproductive technology, US, 1997–2000. *Pediatrics, 111*, 1159.

Roudebush, J. R., Kaufman, J., Johnson, B. H., Abraham, M. R., & Clayton, S. R. (2006). Patient- and family-centered perinatal care. *Journal of Perinatal & Neonatal Nursing, 20*(3), 201–209.

Ryan-Wenger, N. A., Sharrer, V. W., & Campbell, K. K. (2005). Changes in children's stressors over the past 30 years. *Pediatric Nursing, 31*(4), 282–291.

Search Institute. (2007). *Developmental assets: An overview, 2007.* Available at www.search-institute.org/assets

Society of Pediatric Nurses. (2006). *The role of the staff nurse in protecting children and families involved in research.* Retrieved July 1, 2006, from www.pedsnurses.org/pdfs

Taylor, C., Lillis, C., & LeMone, P. (2005). *Fundamentals of nursing: The art and science of nursing care* (5th ed.). Philadelphia: Lippincott Williams & Wilkins.

Trupin, S. R. (2006). *Common pregnancy complaints and questions.* Retrieved June 3, 2008 from http://www.emedicine.com/med/topic3238.htm.

Trybulski, J. (2006) Women and abortion: The past reaches into the present. *Journal of Advanced Nursing, 54*(6), 683–690.

U.S. Census Bureau. (2006). Nation's population one third minority. Press release, May 10, 2006. Accessed 10/2/06. Available at: http://www.census.gov/Press-Release/www/releases/archieves/population/006808.html

U.S. Census Bureau. (2007). *American fact finder.* Retrieved March 22, 2007, from http://factfinder.census.gov/home/en/epss/glossary_f.html

U.S. Department of Health & Human Services. (2000). *Healthy people 2010.* Retrieved August 23, 2006, from http://www.healthypeople.gov/Publications/

U.S. Department of Health & Human Services. (2006). *Preventing infant mortality.* Retrieved August 23, 2006, from http://www.hhs.gov/news/factsheet/infant.html

U.S. Department of Health and Human Services, Health Resources and Services Administration. (2006). *Women's Health USA 2006.* Rockville, MD: U.S. Department of Health and Human Services.

U.S. Department of Health and Human Services, Health Resources and Services Administration, Maternal and Child Health Bureau. (2005). *Child health USA 2005.* Rockville, MD: U.S. Department of Health and Human Services.

U.S. Department of Health & Human Services, Public Health Service. (1979). *Healthy people: The Surgeon General's report on health promotion and disease prevention* (DHEW publication No. PHS 79-5507). Washington, DC: U.S. Government Printing Office.

Ventres, W., & Gobbo, R. (2005). The A to Z of cross-cultural medicine. *Family Practice Management, 12*(7), 57–58.

Von Bertalanffy, L. (1968). *General systems theory.* London: Penguin Press.

Von Hertzen, H., & Baird, D. (2006). Frequently asked questions about medical abortion. *Contraception, 74*(1), 3–10.

Wexler, I. D., Branski, D., & Kerem, E. (2006). War and children. *JAMA, 296*(5), 579–581.

Wong, M. D., Chung, A. K., Boscardin, W., et al. (2006). The contribution of specific causes of death to sex differences in mortality. *Public Health Reports, 121*(6), 746–754.

World Factbook. (2006). *Infant mortality rate.* Washington, DC: Central Intelligence Agency.

World Health Organization. (2004). *Child health in the community.* Geneva, Switzerland: Department of Child and Adolescent Health and Development.

World Health Organization. (2007a). *Statistical information system.* Available at: http://www.who.int/whosis/indicatordefinitions/en/print.html

World Health Organization. (2007b). *Integrating poverty and gender into health programs: A sourcebook for health professionals.* Available at: http://www.wpro.who.int/publications/pub_9290612126.htm

World Health Organization. (2007c). *Gender, health and poverty fact sheet.* Available at: www.who.int/inf-fs/en/fact251.html

World Health Organization. (2008). *Frequently asked questions.* Retrieved June 3, 2008 from http://www.who.int/suggestions/faq/en/.

WEBSITES

American Academy of Pediatrics: http://www.aap.org
Centers for Disease Control National Center for Injury Prevention and Control: http://www.cdc.gov/ncipc
Children's Defense Fund: www.childrensdefense.org
Family Violence Prevention Fund: http://www.endabuse.org
Global Health Council: www.globalhealth.org
National Coalition Against Domestic Violence: http://www.ncadv.org
National Coalition for the Homeless: http://www.nationalhomeless.org
National Institute of Mental Health: http://www.nimh.nih.gov
National Safety Council: www.nsc.org
Office of Juvenile Justice and Delinquency Prevention: www.usdoj.gov
Raising Resilient Children Foundation: www.raisingresilientkids.com
Save the Children: www.savethechildren.org/publications
UNICEF: www.unicef.org
United Nations Development Program: www.undo.org
World Health Organization (WHO): www.who.int

CHAPTER WORKSHEET

MULTIPLE CHOICE QUESTIONS

1. When preparing a presentation for a local woman's group on women's health problems, what would the nurse include as the number-one cause of mortality for women in the United States?

   a. Breast cancer

   b. Childbirth complications

   c. Injury resulting from violence

   d. Heart disease

2. Which factor would most likely be responsible for a pregnant women's failure to receive adequate prenatal care in the United States?

   a. Belief that it is not necessary in a normal pregnancy

   b. Use of denial to cope with pregnancy

   c. Lack of health insurance to cover expenses

   d. Inability to trust traditional medical practices

3. When caring for children, how should the nurse best incorporate the concept of family-centered care?

   a. Encouraging the family to allow the physician to make health care decisions for the child

   b. Using the concepts of respect, family strengths, diversity, and collaboration with family

   c. Advising the family to choose a pediatric provider who is on the covered child's health care plan

   d. Recognizing that families undergoing stress related to the child's illness cannot make good decisions

4. When caring for an adolescent, in which instance must the nurse share information with the parents, no matter which state care is provided in?

   a. Pregnancy counseling

   b. Depression

   c. Contraception

   d. Tuberculosis

5. The following events were milestones in the support of women's and children's health. Place the events in the correct sequence, from oldest to most recent.

   ____a. Declaration of the Rights of the Child approved

   ____b. WIC program established

   ____c. U.S. Children's Bureau established

   ____d. Sheppard-Towner Act passed

   ____e. Family and Medical Leave Act passed

   ____f. Education for all Handicapped Children Act passed

6. The nurse is preparing a class for a group of students about homelessness. Which factors contribute to homelessness? Select all that apply.

   ____a. Decrease in the number of people living in poverty

   ____b. Rises in unemployment

   ____c. Exposure to abuse or neglect

   ____d. Cutbacks in public welfare programs

   ____e. Development of community crisis centers

CRITICAL THINKING EXERCISES

1. As a nurse working in a federally funded low-income clinic offering women's health services, you are becoming increasingly frustrated with the number of "no-shows" or appointments missed in your maternity clinic. Some clients come for their initial prenatal intake appointment and never come back. You realize that some just forget their appointments, but most don't even call to notify you. Many of the clients are high risk and thus are jeopardizing their health and the health of their future child.

   a. What changes might be helpful to address this situation?

   b. Outline what you might say at your next staff meeting to address the issue of clients making one clinic visit and then never returning.

   c. What strategies might you use to improve attendance and notification?

   d. Describe what cultural and customer service techniques might be needed.

2. A couple has adopted an 11-month-old infant girl from China and have brought her to the health care facility for a checkup. The couple had no contact with the infant's birth parents. The infant spent 7 months in an orphanage before being adopted. Describe the family structure and the issues that may affect this family.

3. You have been asked by the local school district to speak to a group of middle-school children and their parents about Internet safety. Describe the topics that you should address.

4. A 12-year-old is to undergo research treatment for a serious illness. Explain the concept of assent as it relates to this situation.

STUDY ACTIVITIES

1. Research a current policy, bill, or issue being debated on the community, state, or national level that pertains to the health and welfare of women or children. Summarize the major facts and supporting and opposing arguments and prepare an oral report on your findings.

2. Interview a child life specialist about the effects of using the atraumatic approach or the traditional approach for restraining children during procedures. Compare and contrast the effects on children at various developmental stages.

3. Within your clinical group, debate the following statement: Should access to health care be a right or a privilege?

4. Visit a local community health center that offers services to women and children from various cultures. Interview the staff about any barriers to health care that they have identified. Investigate what the staff has done to minimize these barriers.

FAMILY-CENTERED COMMUNITY-BASED CARE

KEY TERMS

community
cultural competence
epidemiology

Individualized Health Plan
(IHP)
health literacy

medically fragile children
respite care

LEARNING OBJECTIVES

Upon completion of the chapter, the learner will be able to:

1. Examine the major components and key elements of family-centered home health care.
2. Explain the reasons for the increased emphasis on community-based care.
3. Differentiate community-based nursing from nursing in acute care settings.
4. Explain the different levels of prevention in community-based nursing, providing examples of each.
5. Give examples of cultural issues that may be faced when providing community-based nursing.
6. Provide culturally competent care to women, children, and families.
7. Identify the variety of settings where community-based care can be provided to women, children, and families.
8. Outline the various roles and functions assumed by the community health nurse.
9. Demonstrate the ability to use excellent therapeutic communication skills when interacting with women, children, and families.
10. Explain the process of health teaching as it relates to women, children, and families.
11. Examine the importance of discharge planning and case management in providing community-based care.

M aria was home a few days after giving birth to her first child. She had just changed her newborn son and placed him on his stomach for a nap when the community health nurse arrived for a postpartum visit. Because the nurse didn't speak Spanish and Maria didn't speak English, a great deal of gesturing followed. After examining Maria, the nurse then picked up her son and placed him on his back in the crib. How might the nurse have prepared for this home visit? What message did the nurse convey in changing the newborn's position?

Wow

To recognize diversity in others and respect it, we must first have some awareness of who we are.

Women, children, and families receive most of their health care, both well and ill care, in the community setting. During the past several years, the health care delivery system has changed dramatically. With a focus on cost containment, people are spending less time in the hospital. Clients are being discharged "sicker and quicker" from their hospital beds. The health care system has moved from reactive treatment strategies in hospitals to a proactive approach in the community. This has resulted in an increasing emphasis on health promotion and illness prevention within the community.

Nurses play an important role in the health and wellness of a community. They not only meet the health care needs of the individual but also go beyond that to implement interventions that affect the community as a whole. Nurses practice in a variety of settings within a community, such as clinics and physician offices, schools, shelters, churches, health departments, community health centers, and homes. They promote the health of individuals, families, groups, communities, and populations and promote an environment that supports health.

This chapter describes the concepts of community and community-based nursing, addressing the varied settings where such care is provided to women, children, and families. The chapter also highlights the major roles and functions of community-based nurses, emphasizing their role as educators in health promotion and maintenance.

Family-Centered Care

Family-centered cares refers to the collaborative partnership among the individual, family, and caregivers to determine goals, share information, offer support, and formulate plans for health care (Chia-Chen & Thompson, 2007). Key elements in the provision of family-centered care include demonstrating interpersonal sensitivity, providing general health information and being a valuable resource, communicating specific health information, and treating people respectfully (Grindel, 2006). The philosophy of family-centered care recognizes the family as the constant: the health of all the family members and their functional abilities influence the health of the client and other members of the family. Family-centered care works well in all arenas of health care, from preventive care to long-term care. Family-centered care enhances the confidence of all those involved about their skills and helps to prepare children and young adults for assuming responsibility for their own health care needs. It is vital for the nurse to assess how much knowledge the family has about the client's health or illness.

Using a family-centered approach is associated with positive outcomes such as decreased anxiety, improved pain management, shortened recovery times, and enhanced confidence and problem-solving skills. Communication between the health care team and the family is also improved, leading to greater satisfaction for both health care providers and health care consumers (families). Practicing true family-centered care may empower the family, strengthen family resources, and help the woman or child feel more secure throughout the process.

Community-Based Care

Community may be defined as a "specific group of people, often living in a defined geographical area, who share a common culture, values, and norms and who are arranged in a social structure according to relationships the community has developed over a period of time" (Canadian Community Health Nursing Standards of Practice, 2003, p. 18). The common features of a community may be common rights and privileges as members of a certain city or common ties of identity, values, norms, culture, language, or social support. Women are caregivers to children, parents, spouses, and neighbors and provide important social support in these roles. The child's community consists of the family, school, neighborhood, youth organizations, and other peer groups.

A person can be a part of many communities during the course of daily life. Examples might include area of residence (home, apartment, shelter), gender, place of employment (organization or home), language spoken (Spanish, Chinese, English), educational background or student status, culture (Italian, African-American, Indian), career (nurse, businesswoman, housewife), place of worship (church or synagogue), and community memberships (garden club, YMCA, support group, school PTA, youth organizations, athletic teams).

In community-based care, the community is the unit of service. The providers of care are concerned not only with the clients who present for service but also with the larger population of potential or at-risk clients.

Community Health Nursing

Community health nursing focuses on preventing illness and improving the health of populations and communities. Population is defined as "a collection of individuals who have one or more personal or environmental characteristics in common" (Canadian Community Health Nursing Standards of Practice, 2003, p. 20). Community health nurses work in geographically and culturally diverse settings. They address current and potential health needs of the population or community. They promote and preserve the health of a population and are not limited to particular age groups or diagnoses. Public health nursing is a specialized area of community health nursing.

Epidemiology (the study of the causes, distribution, and control of disease in populations) can help determine the health and health needs of a population and assist in planning health services. Community health nurses perform epidemiologic investigations to help analyze and develop health policy and community health initiatives. Community health initiatives can be focused on the community as a whole or a specific target population with specific needs. *Healthy People 2010* (HP 2010) is an example of national health initiatives developed using the epidemiological process. HP 2010 ensures that health care professionals evaluate the individual as well as the community. It emphasizes the ever-present link between the individual's health and the health of the community (Clark, 2007; Zahner & Block, 2006). HP 2010 identifies two major goals: to increase the quality of life and the life expectancy of individuals of all ages and to decrease health disparities among different populations. The focus of health care initiatives today is on people and their needs, strengthening their abilities to shape their own lives. The emphasis has shifted away from dependence on health professionals toward personal involvement and personal responsibility, and this gives nurses the opportunity to interact with individuals in a variety of self-help roles. Nurses in the community can be the primary force in identifying the challenges and implementing changes in women's and children's health for the future. (Relevant HP 2010 objectives are highlighted throughout this text, and HP 2010 is available online at www.healthypeople.gov.)

Community-Based Nursing

In the past, the only community-based roles for nurses were community health nurses or public health nurses. This is now a subset of what is considered community-based nursing. The health needs of the society and consumer demand brought about community-based and community-focused services. The movement from an illness-oriented "cure" perspective in hospitals to a focus on health promotion and primary health care in community-based settings has dramatically changed employment opportunities for today's nurses. This shift in emphasis to primary care and outpatient treatment and management will likely continue. As a result, employment growth in a variety of community-based settings can be expected for properly educated nurses.

The 2004 National Sample Survey of Registered Nurses (U.S. Department of Health and Human Services [USDHHS], Bureau of Health Professions, 2004) found the following trends in registered nurse (RN) employment settings:

- 44% of RNs work outside the hospital setting.
- The number of RNs employed in community-based settings showed a 35% increase between 2000 and 2004; this was largely the result of an increase in nurses working in home health care and managed care organizations.

Community-based nursing settings include ambulatory care, home health care, occupational health, school

health, and hospice settings (Table 2.1). Clinical practice within the community may also include case management, research, quality improvement, and discharge planning. Nurses with advanced practice and experience may be employed in areas of staff development, program development, and community education.

Community-Based Nursing Interventions

Nursing interventions involve any treatment that the nurse performs to enhance the client's outcome. Nursing practice in the community uses the nursing process and is similar to that in the acute care setting, because assessing, performing procedures, administering medications, coordinating services and equipment, counseling clients and their families, and teaching about care are all part of the care administered by nurses in the community. Box 2.1 highlights the most common nursing interventions used in community-based nursing practice.

Community-Based Nursing Challenges

Despite the benefits achieved by caring for families in their own homes and communities, challenges also exist. Clients are being discharged from acute care facilities very early in their recovery course and present with more

TABLE 2.1 COMMUNITY-BASED PRACTICE SETTINGS

Setting	Description
Ambulatory care settings	Doctor's offices Health maintenance organizations (HMOs) Day surgery centers Freestanding urgent care centers Family planning clinics Mobile mammography centers
Home health care services	High-risk pregnancy/neonate care Maternal/child newborn care Skilled nursing care Hospice care
Health Department services	Maternal/child health clinics Family planning clinics Sexually transmitted infection programs Immunization clinics Substance abuse programs Jails and prisons
Long-term care	Skilled nursing facilities Nursing homes Hospices Assisted living
Other community-based settings	Parish nursing programs Summer camps Childbirth education programs School health programs Occupational health programs

BOX 2.1 Community-Based Nursing Interventions

- Health screening—detecting unrecognized or preclinical illness among individuals so they can be referred for definitive diagnosis and treatment (e.g., mammogram or Pap smear, well-child vision and hearing checks)
- Health education programs—assisting clients in making health-related decisions about self-care, use of health resources, and social health issues such as smoking bans and motorcycle helmet laws (e.g., childbirth education or breast self-examination, child safety programs, poisoning prevention, youth drug awareness programs)
- Medication administration—preparing, giving, and evaluating the effectiveness of prescription and over-the-counter drugs (e.g., hormone replacement therapy in menopausal women, childhood immunizations)
- Telephone consultation—identifying the problem to be addressed; listening and providing support, information, or instruction; documenting advice/instructions given to concerns raised by caller (e.g., consultation for a mother with a newborn with colic, interaction with a parent whose child has a fever or is vomiting)
- Health system referral—passing along information about the location, services offered, and ways to contact agencies (e.g., referring a woman for a breast prosthesis after a mastectomy, arranging for home tutoring for a child with a long-term illness)
- Instructional—teaching an individual or a group about a medication, disease process, lifestyle changes, community resources, or research findings concerning their environment (e.g., childbirth education class, basic life support classes for parents, child safety education classes)
- Nutritional counseling—demonstrating the direct relationship between nutrition and illness while focusing on the need for diet modification to promote wellness (e.g., Women, Infants, and Children [WIC] program; counselor interviewing a pregnant woman or a child and parents who have anemia; eating disorders program)
- Risk identification—recognizing personal or group characteristics that predispose people to develop a specific health problem, and modifying or eliminating them (e.g., genetic counseling of an older pregnant woman at risk for a Down syndrome infant; genetic screening of family members for cystic fibrosis or Huntington's disease.

Source: Dochterman, J. M., & Bulechek, G. M. (2004). *Nursing interventions classification* (NIC) (4th ed.). St. Louis: Mosby.

health care needs than in the past. As a result, nursing care and procedures in the home and community are becoming more complex and time-consuming. Consider the example of a woman who developed a systemic infection, a pelvic abscess, and deep vein thrombosis in her leg after a cesarean birth who is being discharged from the hospital. The nurse's primary focus of care in this situation would be to administer heparin and antibiotics intravenously rather than educating her about childcare and follow-up appointments. In the past, this woman would have remained hospitalized for treatment, but home infusion therapy is now less costly and allows the client to be discharged sooner.

This demand on the nurse's time may limit the amount of time spent on prevention measures, education, and the family's psychosocial issues. More time may be needed to help families deal with these issues and concerns. With large client caseloads, nurses may find it difficult to spend the time needed while meeting the time restrictions dictated by their health care agencies.

Nurses working in the community have fewer resources available to them compared with the acute care setting. Decisions often have to be made in isolation. The nurse must possess excellent assessment skills and the ability to communicate effectively with the family to be successful in carrying out the appropriate plan of care.

Nurses interested in working in community-based settings must be able to apply the nursing process in an environment that is less structured or controlled than that associated with acute care facilities. Nurses must be able to assimilate information well beyond the immediate physical and psychosocial needs of the client in a controlled acute care setting and deal with environmental threats, lifestyle choices, family issues, different cultural patterns, financial burdens, transportation problems, employment hazards, communication barriers, limited resources, and client acceptance and compliance.

Although opportunities for employment in community-based settings are plentiful, many positions require a baccalaureate degree. Previous medical-surgical experience in an acute care setting is typically required by home health agencies because these nurses must function fairly independently within the home environment.

The nurse must also be familiar with and respectful of many different cultures and socioeconomic levels, remaining objective in dealing with such diversity and demonstrating an understanding of and appreciation for cultural differences. Interventions must be individualized to address the cultural, social, and economic diversity among clients in their own environment (Papadopoulos, 2006).

Shift in Responsibilities from Hospital-Based to Community-Based Nursing

Community care, especially home care, is a rapidly growing service in the United States. Community-based care has been shown to be a cost-effective method for providing care. An increase in disposable income and the increased longevity of children with chronic and debilitating health conditions have also contributed to the continued shift of health care to the community and home setting. Technology has advanced, allowing for improved monitoring of clients in community settings and at home as well as allowing complicated procedures to be done at home, such as intravenous administration of antibiotics. A major cause for the increase in community care, especially home care in the pediatric population, is the understanding that an acute care setting is not an appropriate environment for children to grow (Hewitt-Taylor, 2005). Caring for children at home not only improves their physical health but also allows for adequate growth and development within their family. They are in a familiar environment with the comfort and support of family, which leads to improved care and quality of life.

Levels of Prevention in Community-Based Nursing

The concept of prevention is a key part of community-based nursing practice. The emphasis on health care delivery in community-based settings has moved beyond primary preventive health care (e.g., well-child checkups, routine physical examinations, prenatal care, and treat-

ment of common acute illnesses) and now encompasses secondary and tertiary care.

Primary Prevention

The concept of primary prevention involves preventing the disease or condition before it occurs through health promotion activities, environmental protection, and specific protection against disease or injury. It encompasses a vast array of areas, including nutrition, good hygiene, sanitation, immunization, adequate shelter, smoking cessation, family planning, and the use of seat belts (Fig. 2.1; Stanhope & Lancaster, 2008).

Prevention of neural tube defects (NTDs), such as anencephaly and spina bifida, in children is an example of primary prevention. The use of folic acid supplementation daily for 3 months before and 3 months after conception reduces the risk of first occurrence of NTD (American College of Obstetricians and Gynecologists [ACOG], 2007). All women of childbearing age should take 0.4 mg folic acid daily as soon as they plan to become pregnant and should

FIGURE 2.1 Levels of prevention in community-based nursing. (A) At the primary prevention level, the nurse provides anticipatory guidance and family teaching. (B) At the secondary level of prevention, a woman undergoes a mammography screening for early detection of breast problems. (C) At the tertiary level of prevention, a child with a developmental disability participates in a rehabilitation program.

continue taking it throughout the pregnancy to prevent this devastating condition. Giving anticipatory guidance to parents about poison prevention and safety during play is another example of primary prevention.

Secondary Prevention

Secondary prevention is the early detection and treatment of adverse health conditions. Health screenings are the mainstay of secondary prevention. Pregnancy testing, blood pressure evaluations, cholesterol monitoring, fecal occult blood testing, breast examinations, mammography screening, hearing and vision examinations, and Papanicolaou (Pap) smears are examples of this level of prevention. Such interventions do not prevent the health problem but are intended for early detection and prompt treatment to prevent complications (Anderson & McFarlane, 2007).

Tertiary Prevention

Tertiary prevention is designed to reduce or limit the progression of a disease or disability. The purpose of tertiary prevention is to restore individuals to their maximum potential (Anderson & McFarlane, 2007). Tertiary prevention measures are supportive and restorative. For example, tertiary prevention efforts would focus on minimizing and managing the effects of a chronic illness, such as a spinal cord injury or cerebral palsy, or the chronic effects of sexually transmitted infections such as herpes, human immunodeficiency virus (HIV), and untreated syphilis. Another example would involve working with women who have suffered long-term consequences of violence. The focus of the nurse would be to maximize the woman's strengths, to help them recover from the trauma and loss, and to build support systems.

The Nurse's Role in Community-Based Preventive Care

All health professionals have a special role in health promotion, health protection, and disease prevention. Much of community nursing involves prevention, early identification, and prompt treatment of health problems and monitoring for emerging threats that might lead to health problems. Community-based nurses provide health care for women and children at all three levels of prevention. This care often involves advocacy for services to meet their needs.

Cultural Issues in Community-Based Nursing

The United States contains an ever-changing mix of cultural groups. The Yearbook of Immigration Statistics (United States Department of Homeland Security [USDHS], 2006) reports that the U.S. immigrant population has reached 38 million, with people arriving from every corner of the world. One million immigrants come to the United States each year, and more than half are of child-bearing age. Latin America accounts for more than 50% of immigrants to the United States. By the year 2050, people of African, Asian, and Latino backgrounds will make up one half of our population (U.S. Census Bureau, 2007).

This growing diversity has strong implications for the health care system. For years nurses have struggled with the issues of providing optimal health care that meets the needs of women, children, and families from varied cultures and ethnic groups. In addition to displaying competence in technical skills, nurses must also become competent in caring for clients from varied ethnic and racial backgrounds. Adapting to different cultural beliefs and practices requires flexibility and acceptance of others' viewpoints. Nurses must listen to clients and learn about their beliefs about health and wellness. To provide culturally appropriate care to diverse populations, nurses need to know, understand, and respect culturally influenced health behaviors. Chapter 1 provides a more detailed discussion of culture and its impact on the health of women, children, and families.

Nurses must research and understand the cultural characteristics, values, and beliefs of the various people to whom they deliver care so that false assumptions and stereotyping do not lead to insensitive care. Time orientation, personal space, family orientation (patriarchal, matriarchal, or egalitarian), and language are important cultural concepts.

Culturally Competent Nursing Care

Cultural competence is defined as the knowledge, willingness, and ability to adapt health care to enhance its acceptability to and effectiveness with clients from diverse cultures (Clark, 2007). Cultural competence is a dynamic process during which nurses obtain and then apply cultural information. Nurses must look at clients through their own eyes and the eyes of clients and family members. Nurses must develop nonjudgmental acceptance of cultural differences in clients, using diversity as a strength that empowers them to achieve mutually acceptable health care goals (Kersey–Matusiak, 2006). This cultural awareness allows nurses to see the entire picture and improves the quality of care and health outcomes.

Cultural competence does not appear suddenly; it must be developed through a series of steps (Box 2.2).

Barriers to Cultural Competence

Barriers to cultural competence can be grouped into two categories: those related to providers and those related to systems (Godfrey, 2006). When a health care provider lacks knowledge of a client's cultural practices and beliefs or when the provider's beliefs differ from those of the client, the provider may be unprepared to respond when the client makes unexpected health care decisions. System-related barriers can occur if agencies that have not been designed for cultural diversity want all clients to conform to the established rules and regulations and attempt to fit everyone into the same mold.

BOX 2.2 Steps to Developing Cultural Competence

1. Cultural Self-Awareness
   - Become aware of, appreciate, and become sensitive to the values, beliefs, customs, and behaviors that have shaped one's own culture.
   - Engage in self-exploration beyond one's own culture and "see" clients from different cultures.
   - Examine personal biases and prejudices toward other cultures.
   - Become aware of differences in personal and clients' backgrounds.
2. Cultural Knowledge
   - Obtain knowledge about various worldviews of different cultures, such as through reading about different cultures, attending continuing education courses on different cultures, accessing websites, and attending cultural diversity conferences.
   - Become familiar with culturally/ethnically diverse groups, worldviews, beliefs, practices, lifestyles, and problem-solving strategies.
3. Cultural Skills
   - Learn how to perform a competent cultural assessment.
   - Assess each client's unique cultural values, beliefs, and practices without depending solely on written facts about specific cultural groups.
4. Cultural Encounter
   - Engage in cross-cultural interactions with people from culturally diverse backgrounds, such as attending religious services or ceremonies and participating in important family events.
   - Participate in as many cultural encounters as possible to avoid cultural stereotyping.

Cultural competence does not mean replacing one's own cultural identity with another, ignoring the variability within cultural groups, or even appreciating the cultures being served. Instead, nurses skilled at cultural competence show a respect for difference, an eagerness to learn, and a willingness to accept multiple views of the world (Godfrey, 2006; Laveist, 2005).

Community-Based Nursing Care Settings for Women and Children

Community-based nursing takes place in a variety of settings, including physician's offices, clinics, health departments, urgent care centers, hospital outpatient centers, schools, camps, churches, shelters, and clients' homes. Nurses provide well care, episodic ill care, and chronic care. They work to promote, preserve, and improve the health of the women, children, and families in these settings.

Due to technological advances, cost containment, and shortened hospital stays, the home is a common care setting for women, children, and families today. Home care is geared toward the needs of the client and family. Private-duty nursing care is used when more extensive care is needed; it may be delivered hourly (several hours per day) or on a full-time, live-in basis. Periodic nursing visits may be used for intermittent interventions, such as IV antibiotic administration, follow-up with client teaching, and monitoring. The goals of nursing care in the home setting include promoting, restoring, and maintaining the health of the client.

Home care focuses on minimizing the effects of the illness or disability along with providing the client with the means to care for the illness or disability at home. Nurses in the home care setting are direct care providers, educators, advocates, and case managers.

Prenatal Care

Early, adequate prenatal care has long been associated with improved pregnancy outcomes (March of Dimes, 2007). Adequate prenatal care is a comprehensive process in which any problems associated with pregnancy are identified and treated. Basic components of prenatal care are early and continuing risk assessment, health promotion, medical and psychosocial interventions, and follow-up. Within the community setting, several services are available to provide health care for pregnant women (Box 2.3).

Not all women are aware of the community resources available to them. Most public health services are available for consultation, local hospitals have "hotlines" for questions, and public libraries have pregnancy-related resources as well as Internet access. Nurses can be a very helpful link to resources for all women regardless of their economic status.

Technologically advanced care has been shown to improve maternal and child outcomes. Regionalized high-risk care, recommended by the American Academy of Pediatrics in the late 1970s, aimed to promote uniformity nationwide, covering the prenatal care of high-risk pregnancies and high-risk newborns. The advanced technology found in level III perinatal regional centers and community-based prenatal surveillance programs have resulted in better risk-adjusted mortality rates (Britt, Edean & Evans, 2006; Martin & Foley, 2006). For example, fetal monitoring and ultrasound technology have traditionally been used in acute care settings to monitor the progress of many high-risk pregnancies. However, with the increased cost of hospital stays, many services were moved to outpatient facilities and into the home. The intent was to reduce health care costs and to monitor women with complications of pregnancy in the home rather than in the hospital. Examples of services offered in the home setting might include:

- Infusion therapy to treat infections or combat dehydration
- Hypertension monitoring for women with gestational hypertension

---

BOX 2.3   Maternal/Child Community Health Care Services

- State public health prenatal clinics provide access to care based on a sliding scale payment schedule or have services paid for by Medicaid.
- Federally funded community clinics typically offer a variety of services, which may include prenatal, pediatric, adult health, and dental services. A sliding scale payment schedule or Medicaid may cover costs.
- Hospital outpatient health care services offer maternal–child health services. Frequently they are associated with a teaching hospital in which medical school students, interns, and OB/GYN residents rotate through the clinic services to care for patients during their education process.
- Private OB/GYN offices are available for women with health insurance seeking care during their pregnancies. Some physicians in private practice will accept Medicaid patients as well as private patients.
- Community free clinics offer maternal–child services in some communities for women with limited economic resources (homeless, unemployed).
- Freestanding birth centers offer prenatal care for low-risk mothers as well as childbirth classes to educate couples regarding the birthing process. Most centers accept private insurance and Medicaid for reimbursement services.

- Midwifery services are available in many communities where midwives provide women's health services. They usually accept a multitude of payment plans from private pay to health insurance to Medicaid for reimbursement purposes.
- WIC provides food, nutrition counseling, and access to health services for low-income women, infants, and children. WIC is a federally funded program and is administered by each state. All persons receiving Aid to Families with Dependent Children (AFDC), food stamps, or Medicaid are automatically eligible for WIC. An estimated 45% of the infants born in the United States are served by WIC (USDA Food and Nutrition Service, 2004; Fig. 2-1).
- Childbirth classes offer pregnant women and their partners a series of educational classes on childbirth preparation. Women attend them during their last trimester of pregnancy. Some classes are free and some have a fee.
- Local La Leche League groups provide mother-to-mother support for breast-feeding, nutrition, and infant care problem-solving strategies. All women who have an interest in breast-feeding are welcome to participate in the meetings, which are typically held in the home of a La Leche member.

- Uterine monitoring for mothers who are at high risk for preterm labor
- Fetal monitoring to evaluate fetal well-being
- Portable ultrasound to perform a biophysical profile to assess fetal well-being

As a result, home care has the potential to produce cost savings compared to inpatient care.

Labor and Birth Care

Pregnancy involves numerous choices: cloth or disposable diapers, breastfeeding or bottle feeding, doctor or midwife, and where to give birth—at a birthing center, at home, or at a hospital. Deciding where to give birth depends on the woman's pregnancy risk status. For the pregnant woman who is at high risk as a result of medical or social factors, the hospital is considered the safest place for birth. Potential complications can be addressed because medical technology, skilled professionals, and neonatal services are available. For low-risk women, a freestanding birthing center or a home birth is an option.

The choice between a birthing center, home birth, or hospital depends on the woman's preferences, her risk status, and her distance from a hospital. Some women choose an all-natural birth with no medications and no medical intervention, whereas others would feel more comfortable in a setting in which medications and trained staff are avail-

able if needed. Presenting the facts to women and allowing them to choose in collaboration with their health care provider is the nurse's role. Safety is paramount, but at the same time nurses must protect the woman's right to select birth options and should promote family-centered care in all maternity settings (see Evidence-Based Practice box).

Birthing Center

A birthing center is a cross between a home birth and a hospital. Birthing centers offer a homelike setting but with close proximity to a hospital in case of complications. Midwives often are the sole care providers in freestanding birthing centers, with obstetricians as backups in case of emergencies. Birthing centers usually have fewer restrictions and guidelines for families to follow and allow for more freedom in making decisions about labor. The rates of cesarean birth and the costs are much lower than those of a hospital (Steppe, 2006). The normal discharge time after birth is usually measured in hours (4 to 24 hours), not days.

Birthing centers aim to provide a relaxing home environment and promote a culture of normalcy. Birth is considered a normal physiologic process, and most centers use a non-interventional view of labor and birth. The range of services for the expectant family often includes prenatal care, childbirth education, intrapartum care, and postpartum care, including home follow-up and family plan-

EVIDENCE-BASED PRACTICE 2.1
Is a Home-Like Institutional Birth Setting Better for Women Than a Conventional Institutional Birth Setting?

● Study

Women have been giving birth to newborns in the home setting since the beginning of time. Births occurring in a facility or institution became the norm during the early 20th century. These institutions continue to be the primary setting for birth. However, with the growing emphasis of the client as a consumer of health care and the desire for family-centered care, greater numbers of facilities and institutions are attempting to incorporate some of the home birth components into their delivery of care. A study was done to compare the effect of care in a home-like institutional birth setting and a conventional institutional birth setting.

Two researchers using standard methods for data collection and analysis compiled information from all randomized and quasi-randomized controlled trials involving a comparison of home-like institutional and conventional institutional birth settings. In addition, the researchers evaluated eight journals and two published conference proceedings. Six trials that involved 8,677 women were included. The researchers were unable to include information related to freestanding birthing centers because they found no trials on this topic. The researchers reported the results using relative risk and 95% confidence intervals.

▲ Findings

The results showed that women giving birth in home-like institutional birth settings were less likely to receive or require intrapartum analgesia or anesthesia, less likely to have an episiotomy, and more likely to experience a spontaneous vaginal birth. Other benefits identified included a greater chance for choosing the same setting for future births, greater satisfaction with intrapartum care, and a greater likelihood for initiating breastfeeding with continuation for the next 6 to 8 weeks. Unfortunately, women giving birth in a home-like institutional birth setting had an increased risk for vaginal or perineal tears. Additionally, the risks for perinatal mortality were increased.

▪ Nursing Implications

The study did identify several important benefits that nurses can integrate into their practice when counseling and teaching pregnant women about available birthing options. However, nurses need to underscore the increased risk for perinatal mortality when providing this education so that women can make informed decisions about their choice of birth setting.

Nurses also can provide input about incorporating a more "home-like" atmosphere when their facilities are constructing and designing birthing areas. In addition, nurses can advocate for the pregnant woman in labor to ensure that she has freedom to move about the birthing area, allowing her to feel more "at home."

Source: Hodnett, D. D., Downe, S., Edwards, N., & Walsh, D. Home-like versus conventional institutional settings for birth. *Cochrane Database of Systematic Reviews* 2005. Issue 1. Art. No.: CD000012. DOI:10.1002/14651858.CD000012.pub2.

ning (Fig. 2.2). One of the hallmarks of the freestanding birthing center is that it can provide truly family-centered care by approaching pregnancy and birth as a normal family event and encouraging all family members to participate. Education is often provided by such centers, encouraging families to become informed and self-reliant in the care of themselves and their families (Bainbridge, 2006).

Birthing centers provide an alternative for women who are uncomfortable with a home birth but who do not want to give birth in a hospital. Advantages of birthing centers include a non-interventional approach to obstetric care, freedom to eat and move around during labor, ability to give birth in any position, and the right to have any number of family and friends attend the birth. Disadvantages are that some centers have rigid screening criteria, which may eliminate healthy mothers from using birth centers; many have rigid rules concerning transporting the mother to the hospital (e.g., prolonged labor, ruptured membranes); and many have no pediatrician on staff if the new-born has special needs after birth (Clarke, Bowcock & Gales, 2007; Downe, 2006).

Home Birth

For centuries women have been giving birth to babies in their home. Many feel more comfortable and relaxed when giving birth in their own environment. Women who want no medical interventions and a very family-centered birth often choose to have a home birth. Home births are recommended for pregnant women who are considered to be at low risk for complications during labor and birth. Home birth is advantageous because it:

• Is the least expensive
• Allows the woman to experience labor and birth in the privacy, comfort, and familiarity of home while surrounded by loved ones
• Permits the woman to maintain control over every aspect affecting her labor (e.g., positions, attire, support people)

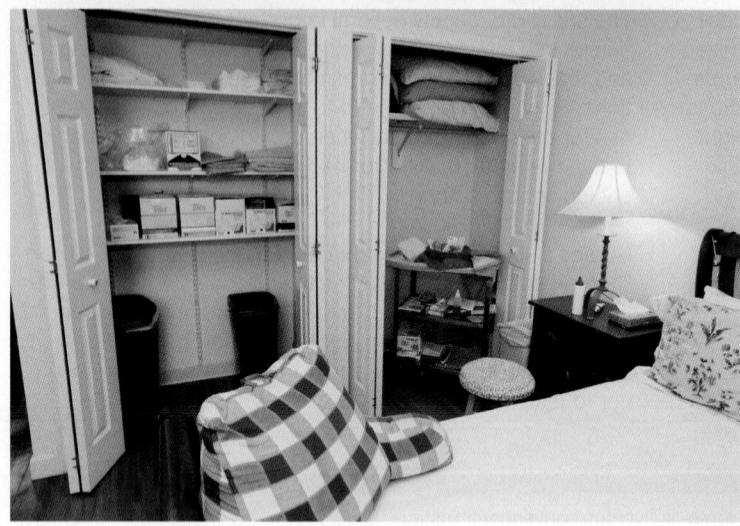

FIGURE 2.2 Birthing centers aim to provide a relaxing home environment and promote a culture of normality while offering a full range of health care services to the expectant family. (Photos by Gus Freedman.)

• Minimizes interference and unnecessary interventions, allowing labor to progress normally
• Provides continuous one-on-one care by the midwife throughout the childbirth process
• Promotes the development of a trusting relationship with the nurse midwife (American Pregnancy Association [APA], 2007)

A home birth does have some disadvantages, including the limited availability of pain medication and danger to the mother and baby if an emergency arises (e.g., placenta abruptio, uterine rupture, cord prolapse, or a distressed fetus). Delay in getting to the hospital could jeopardize the life of the child or the mother. A backup plan for a health care provider and nearby hospital on standby must be established should an emergency occur (Ramsey, 2007).

Postpartum and Newborn Care

Recent reforms in health care financing have reduced hospital stays significantly for women after giving birth. As a result, community-based nurses play a major role in extending care beyond the hospital setting. When new mothers are discharged from the hospital, most are still experiencing perineal discomfort and uterine cramping. They may still have pain from an episiotomy. They are fatigued and may be constipated. They may feel uncertain about feeding and caring for their newborn. These new mothers need to be made aware of community resources such as telephone consultation by nurses, outpatient clinics, and home visits.

Telephone Consultation

Many hospitals offer telephone consultation services by their maternity nurses. The discharged mother is given the phone number of the nursing unit on the day of discharge and is instructed to call if she has any questions or concerns. Because the nurses on the unit are familiar with her birth history and the newborn, they are in a good position to assist her in adjusting to her new role. Although this service is usually free, not all families recognize a problem early or use this valuable informational resource.

Outpatient Clinics

Outpatient clinics offer another community-based site where the childbearing family can obtain services. Usually the mother has received prenatal care before giving birth and thus has established some rapport with the nursing staff there. The clinic staff is usually willing to answer any questions she may have about her health or that of her newborn. Appointments usually include an examination of the mother and newborn and instructions about umbilical cord care, postpartum and infant care, and nutrition for both mother and infant.

Postpartum Home Visits

Home visits offer services similar to those offered at a scheduled clinic visit, but they also give the nurse an opportunity to assess the family's adaptation and dynamics and the home environment. During the past decade, hospital stays have averaged 24 to 48 hours or less for vaginal births and 72 to 96 hours for cesarean births (Centers for Disease Control [CDC], 2007a). Federal legislation went into effect in 1998 that prohibited insurers from restricting hospital stays for mothers and newborns to less than 2 days for vaginal births or 4 days for cesarean births (CDC, 2007a). These shortened stays have reduced the time available for educating mothers about caring for themselves and their newborns.

Postpartum care in the home environment usually includes:

- Monitoring the physical and emotional well-being of the family members (Fig. 2.3)
- Identifying potential or developing complications for the mother and newborn
- Bridging the gap between discharge and ambulatory follow-up for mothers and their newborns (Rice, 2005)

High-Risk Newborn Home Care

With the reduced lengths of stay, high-risk newborns are also being cared for in community settings. Hi-tech care

FIGURE 2.3 The nurse makes a postpartum home visit to assess the woman and her newborn. During the visit, the nurse assists the mother with breastfeeding.

once was provided only in the hospital. Now, however, the increasing cost of complex care and the influences of managed care have led to the provision of hi-tech care at home. Families have become "health care systems" by providing physical, emotional, social, and developmental home care for their technology-dependent infants. Suitable candidates for home care may include preterm infants who continue to need oxygen, low-birthweight infants needing nutritional or hypercaloric formulas or adjunct feeding methods (e.g., tube feedings), or infants with hydrocephalus or cerebral palsy. A wide range of equipment may be used, including mechanical ventilation, electronic apnea monitors, home oxygen equipment, intravenous infusions, respiratory nebulizers, phototherapy, and suction equipment.

All family members must work together to provide 24-hour care. The parents must negotiate with insurers for reimbursement for durable medical equipment, must be able to troubleshoot equipment problems, and must be able to manage inventories of supplies and equipment. In addition, they must be able to assess the infant for problems, determine the problem, decide when to call the nurse, pharmacist, or physical therapist, and interpret and implement prescriptions. Technology in the home requires nurses to focus on the family "home care system" to provide total care to the infant.

Nurses can play a key role in assisting families by preparing them for and increasing their confidence in caring for their infants at home. This adaptation begins before discharge from the hospital. Family members are active participants in the transition-to-home plan. Recognition of parental needs and addressing each area in the discharge plan will ease the transition home.

Assessment of the family's preparedness is essential. The following questions can provide valuable information about this area:

- How well prepared are you to take care of your infant's physical, emotional, and equipment needs?
- How well prepared are you to obtain the home services you need for your infant?
- How well prepared are you to manage the stress of home care?

These simple questions convey the nurse's concern for the infant and family while obtaining a thorough assessment of the family's learning needs.

Once preparedness has been assessed, the nurse can intervene as necessary. For example, if the caretakers do not think they are prepared to maintain machinery, technology, medication, or developmental therapy, then the nurse can demonstrate the care to the family. The nurse provides instructions and hands-on experience within a supportive environment until the family's confidence increases. The nurse can also assist the family to anticipate the common problems that might occur (e.g., advising them to avoid running out of supplies, to have enough medication or special formula mixture to last throughout the weekend, and to keep backup batteries for powering machines or portable oxygen). The outcome of the preparedness assessment and intervention is that the safety of the infant is established and maintained.

Nursing for families who are using complex home care equipment requires caring for the infant and family members' physical and emotional well-being as well as providing effective solutions to problems they may encounter. Home health nurses need to identify, mobilize, and adapt a myriad of community resources to support the family in giving the best possible care in the home setting. Preparing families for hi-tech care before hospital discharge, with home health nurses continuing and reinforcing that focus, will help ease the burden of managing hi-tech equipment in the home.

Women's Health Care

A woman's reproductive years span half her lifetime, on average. This is not a static period, but rather one that encompasses several significant stages. As her reproductive goals change, so do a woman's health care needs. Because of these changing needs, comprehensive community-centered care is critical.

Community-based women's health services have received increased emphasis during the past few decades simply because of economics. Women use more health care services than men, they make as many as 90% of health care decisions, and they represent the majority of the population (CDC, 2007b). Women spend 66 cents of every health care dollar, and 7 of the 10 most frequently performed surgeries in the United States are specific to women (Alexander et al., 2007). Examples of community-based women's health care services that can be freestanding or hospital-based include:

- Screening centers that offer mammograms, Pap smears, bone density assessments, genetic counseling, ultrasound, breast examinations, complete health risk appraisals, laboratory studies (complete blood count, cholesterol testing, thyroid testing, glucose testing for diabetes, follicle-stimulating hormone [FSH] levels), and electrocardiograms
- Educational centers that provide women's health lectures, instruction on breast self-examinations and Pap smears, and computers for research
- Counseling centers that offer various support groups: genetics, psychotherapy, substance abuse, sexual assault, and domestic violence
- Wellness centers that offer stress reduction techniques, massage therapy, guided imagery, hypnosis, smoking cessation, weight reduction, tai chi, yoga, and women's fitness/exercise classes
- Alternative/wholeness healing centers that provide acupuncture, aromatherapy, biofeedback, therapeutic touch, facials, reflexology, and herbal remedies
- Retail centers that offer specialty equipment for rental and purchase, such as breast prostheses

Women have multiple choices regarding services, settings, and health care providers. In the past most women received health care services from physicians such as obstetricians, gynecologists, and family physicians, but today nurse midwives and nurse practitioners are becoming more prevalent in providing well-women care.

Nurses who work in community-based settings need to be familiar with the many health issues commonly encountered by women within their communities. All nurses who work with women of any age in community-based settings, including the workplace, schools, practitioner offices, and clinics, should possess a thorough understanding of the scope of women's health care and should be prepared to intervene appropriately to prevent problems and to promote health.

Child Health Care

The majority of care for a child occurs in the community setting. The numerous settings may be broad or highly specialized. For example, one setting may provide well-child care as well as illness-related care. Another setting may be limited to providing well-child care; a third setting may be limited to diagnostic evaluation, emergency care, or surgical intervention. Other settings may focus on caring for children with specific conditions or diagnosis, such as diabetes or cancer.

Outpatient and Ambulatory Care

Outpatient and ambulatory care is health care provided to individuals who do not require care in an acute setting. Due to advances in medical technology, more medical procedures, such as diagnostic tests and treatments and surgeries, can be performed on an outpatient basis, thereby minimizing the need for the child to be hospitalized. Outpatient and ambulatory care offers convenient and cost-effective access to health care for children and their families, many times right within their own community. These settings allow for increased independence and permit children to return to their normal routine as quickly as possible. More and more outpatient and ambulatory care centers are developing; they are associated with health maintenance organizations (HMOs), physician offices, community agencies and public health departments, and hospitals (Hunt, 2005).

Physician Offices, Clinics, and Urgent Care Centers

Physician offices, clinics, and urgent care centers are used by children and their families for well care, episodic ill care, acute care, and care of chronic conditions. For well care and illness or injury, children are often seen by their primary care physician. They may use a physician office or clinic. In more acute situations or for after-hours issues that cannot wait until clinic operating hours, a child may be seen in an urgent care center or may be referred to the emergency department. The American Academy of Pediatrics does not encourage the use of urgent care centers or the emergency department for routine care since it is difficult to provide coordinated, comprehensive family-centered care consistent with a "medical home" concept (refer to Chapter 30 for more information on medical homes)(Krug et al., 2005).

The nurse's role in these settings includes preparing clients, collecting pertinent health information, performing assessments, assisting the physician with diagnostic testing and procedures, administering injections and medications, changing dressings, assisting with minor surgery, helping to maintain records, and educating the child and family about follow-up care, including when to call the physician or return to be seen.

Outpatient Units

Outpatient units are used to keep hospital stays short and decrease the cost of hospitalization. Outpatient units may be a part of the hospital or a freestanding facility. The child and family arrive in the morning; the child has the procedure, test, or surgery and then goes home later in the day. Examples of surgeries and procedures performed in outpatient units include tympanostomy tube placement, hernia repair, tonsillectomy, cystoscopy, bronchoscopy, blood transfusions, dialysis, and chemotherapy. This setting is advantageous because there is minimal separation of the child from the family, minimal disruption of the family pattern, a decreased risk of infection, and decreased cost. However, the unit does not have the equipment for overnight stays. Thus, if the child develops a complication, he or she will need to be transported to the acute care facility.

Many centers offer presurgery health assessment and teaching sessions, which allows the parent and child opportunities to voice questions and concerns so that they can be resolved before the procedure or surgery. On the day of the procedure or surgery, parents usually are allowed to remain with their child until the procedure or surgery begins. Parents should also be allowed to be with their child in the post-anesthesia care unit (PACU) as soon as possible. Minimizing separation between the parents and the child provides reassurance, promotes comfort, and meets the physical and emotional needs of the child and family.

Nurses working in the outpatient unit setting are involved with admission and assessment, preoperative teaching and preparation, client assessment and support, postoperative monitoring, case management, discharge planning, and teaching. Before the procedure or surgery, the nurse commonly reviews the routine to be followed and any special instructions such as nothing by mouth (NPO) orders and familiarizes the child and family with the setting.

> ▶ **Take** NOTE!
>
> *Encourage the parent to bring a favorite toy, blanket, or game to make the child feel more comfortable.*

The nurse performs any surgical preparation and discusses intraoperative procedures as necessary. The nurse also provides provide postprocedural or postoperative care and assessment of the child. Once the child is stable and meets the discharge criteria of the facility, the nurse reviews instructions, including pain management, care of the incision if appropriate, diet, and activity, including the time frame for returning to school, necessary follow-up, and when to call the physician.

Medically Fragile Day Care Centers

The number of **medically fragile children**, children who have complex medical needs that require skilled nursing interventions, is growing. Reasons include the increased sophistication of medical technology, the increase in preterm births, and the increase in childhood trauma (Mentro, 2003). It is estimated that 1 million children in the United States have complex, disabling, and costly health conditions (Anonymous, 2000). For many years these children lived in hospital settings their entire lives. Due to concerns about the high cost of long-term hospitalization and the quality of life for these children, alternative care settings in the community, such as medically fragile day care centers, are being developed.

Medically fragile day care centers are designed to meet the needs of these children. Most centers accept children who have complicated medical needs or are technology-dependent. Examples include children with multiple congenital anomalies, children who are ventilator-dependent, children with respiratory conditions, children with cardiac conditions, and children with cancer. Some centers will accept children with less complicated needs, such as cardiorespiratory monitoring or asthma. Some centers include children without health care needs to promote peer relationships and acceptance.

Medically fragile day care centers are similar to typical day care centers. Parents or caregivers can drop off the child in the morning and pick up the child in the afternoon. Some centers offer after-school, weekend, or respite services. The centers usually have indoor and outdoor play areas, educational activities, arts and crafts, and needed therapies.

Health care professionals are present to provide for the child's medical, emotional, and developmental needs. Nurses trained in pediatric and neonatal care, physical therapists, occupational therapists, speech therapists, child life specialists, and social workers staff the centers; some centers also have respiratory therapists on site. Children can receive all of their prescribed therapies while at the center.

Nurse provide direct care such as medication administration and dressing changes, assess and evaluate the child's overall condition, identify potential medical emergencies, determine the need for changes in care or treatment and monitoring, and provide the necessary treatments or interventions to maintain life and health. Most centers are located in the community to help ease transportation issues. Some centers will provide transportation to and from home or school. Centers are licensed by the state day care licensing authorities or, in some states, Physician Prescribed Extended Care (PPEC) agencies. Families may be eligible for financial assistance from their private insurance or Medicaid. The cost of this type of community-based service, on average, is one third that of inpatient hospitalization (Anonymous, 2000). Additionally, there appear to be decreases in the number of rehospitalizations and in family stress (Anonymous, 2000).

Telephone Triage

Telephone triage constitutes a large percentage (more than 25%) of child health treatment (Simonsen-Anderson, 2002). Up to 380 calls per week are received in the average pediatric office (Corjulo, 2005). When parents feel comfortable with the providers in their child's medical home office, they often call for advice to treat their child at home. This practice saves health care dollars by keeping stable or less ill children at home rather than seeking care in an emergency department or urgent care center. If the call is received during office hours and the child's condition warrants evaluation, then the child can be seen in the pediatric primary care office. Telephone triage also is used extensively by pediatric specialty practices.

While telephone triage can be a money-saving and even life-saving intervention, it cannot be used without caution. Triage nurses must be able to determine from the call whether the child needs to be evaluated and if that evaluation should be made emergently. The nurse must carefully question the parent or caregiver about the specifics of the child's condition to determine whether it fits into a low or high risk category. When counseling a parent over the phone, obtain the following information:

- Signs and symptoms; their onset and progression; and characteristics such as location, severity, and aggravating or relieving factors
- History of the child's present illness, including onset and duration, progression of symptoms, any care given at home, and whether this condition is related to a recent diagnostic procedure, surgery, or hospitalization
- The child's health history, including chronic illnesses and routine medications or alternative treatments
- The child's current status in relation to eating, drinking, elimination, and energy and activity level
- Degree and effectiveness of coping by the child and family to this health alteration (adapted from Simonsen-Anderson, 2002)

After obtaining this thorough assessment, the nurse must use critical thinking skills, experience, and established telephone triage protocols to determine the severity and risk of the child's situation. Pediatric telephone protocols are available for purchase through the American Academy of Pediatrics (http://www.aap.org). If the child's situation is determined to be low risk, then home care instruction and advice is appropriate. Children with moderate risk should be seen in the office that day or within 24 hours; advise the family on appropriate care while awaiting the office visit. High-risk children should be evaluated immediately, either in the office or emergency department. Certain high-risk situations warrant activation of the emergency medical system and immediate paramedic evaluation.

> ▶ *Take* NOTE!
>
> *Parents or caregivers often can pick up on subtle problems or cues. Although they may not be able to describe the signs and symptoms accurately, they do know that their child is not acting right. Nurses must listen carefully and act on the parents' or caregivers' concerns.*

Schools

School nursing is a specialized practice of professional nursing and focuses on improving student health to enhance the achievement and success of students. School nurses work to remove or minimize health barriers to learning, thereby providing students with the best opportunity at academic success. The National Association of School Nurses defines school nursing as "a specialized practice of professional nursing that advances the well-being, academic success, and life-long achievement of students. To that end, school nurses facilitate positive student responses to normal development; promote health and safety; intervene with actual and potential health problems; provide case management services; and actively collaborate with others to build student and family capacity for adaptation, self management, self-advocacy, and learning" (*Pediatrics*, 2008). A goal of HP 2010 speaks directly to students and school nurses (Healthy People 2010 2.1).

At the heart of school nursing is the belief that all children have the ability to learn and a right to an education, and that society is best served if children are educated (*Pediatrics*, 2008). School nurses coordinate school health programs and link health service programs within the school and community. School nurses carry out a variety of roles in providing healthcare to children (Fig. 2.4). Box 2.4 provides examples of activities performed by the school nurse.

HEALTHY PEOPLE *2010*

Objective	Significance
Increase the proportion of middle, junior high, and senior high schools that provide school health education to prevent health problems in the following areas: unintentional injury; violence; suicide; tobacco use and addiction; alcohol and other drug use; unintended pregnancy, HIV/AIDS, and STD infection; unhealthy dietary patterns; inadequate physical activity; and environmental health.	• Provide education and training to school staff in health problem areas. • Work with schools to develop appropriate health education with focus on health problem areas.

FIGURE 2.4 The school nurse provides nursing assessment as well as health education to students in the school setting.

BOX 2.4 Examples of Activities of the School Nurse

• Conducting health screenings (e.g., vision, hearing, and scoliosis)
• Assessing growth and development
• Providing emergency first aid
• Training and educating staff on CPR and first aid and health issues
• Assessing, monitoring, and referring students with communicable diseases
• Educating on health promotion and disease prevention (e.g., immunizations, bike and car safety, and decreasing high-risk behaviors, such as smoking, drinking, drug use, and sexual activity)
• Acting as a resource for health issues and education
• Acting as a liaison between home, school, and community and between health care provider and school
• Reinforcing client and family health education (e.g., discharge instructions, self-care measures such as catheterization)
• Monitoring long-term illness in students
• Networking with community agencies and making necessary referrals

The population of students has changed over the years. Access to public schools for children with disabilities is mandated. Because of advances in technology, children with chronic conditions or special needs live longer and enter school. Schools are seeing an increased number of children with psychiatric conditions such as depression, attention-deficit/hyperactivity disorder, and bipolar disorder. All of these factors have contributed to an increase of children with diverse and sometimes complex health needs in the school system.

Although the essential role of the school nurse has not changed, the responsibilities and expectations have. School nurses are challenged to meet the growing needs of this changing school population.

Just as nurses in the acute care setting develop nursing care plans, nurses in the school setting develop **Individualized Health Plans (IHPs)**. An individual health plan formalizes the plan of support for a student with complex health care needs. It is a written agreement developed by an interdisciplinary collaboration of school staff along with the student, the student's family, and the student's health care provider. The plan will describe the student's needs and how the school plans to meet them. The nurse plays a critical role in developing these plans, using the nursing process to develop goals and interventions based on the nursing assessment and diagnosis to ensure that the needs of the child are being met. Examples of students who may need an IHP include students with asthma, serious allergies, chronic conditions such as type I diabetes, physical disabilities, attention-deficit/hyperactivity disorder, and medication needs. Figure 2.5 gives an example of an IHP for a child with asthma.

> ▶ **Take** NOTE!
>
> *The IHP needs to include directions for care while the child is at school and also must take into account variations in school routine, absence of staff, field trips and extracurricular activities, and emergency plans.*

Childcare Centers, Camps, Health Department Clinics, and Shelters

Other settings in the community, such as childcare centers, camps, health department clinics, and shelters, also focus on promoting health, preventing disease and injury, and ensuring a safe environment. Nurses play important roles in these settings. In childcare centers nurses address infection control issues and assess for a safe environment. They provide education and training to staff members. Camp nurses ensure a safe environment for all campers and provide first aid and acute illness care as needed. Camps for children with special health care needs employ specially trained nurses (Fig. 2.6). These camps cater to children with complex health care needs, such as diabetes, head injuries, and physical disabilities, and allow the children the opportunity to experience camp while providing a safe environment and necessary medical care while there. Nurses working in health department clinics and shelters focus on health supervision services and connecting clients to needed community resources.

> ▶ **Take** NOTE!
>
> *Nurses have a unique opportunity to give back to their community by volunteering their services in various settings, such as shelters and clinics in medically underserved areas.*

Pediatric Home Care

Pediatric home care provides short- or long-term services for children and their families in their home. It also is used for medically needy and technology-dependent children, such as children requiring mechanical ventilation. Children with acute illnesses, such as a child with osteomyelitis requiring intravenous antibiotics, or chronic health care issues, such as a child with bronchopulmonary dysplasia, that traditionally would have required inpatient care can often benefit from home care.

Pediatric home care can be advantageous for the child and family, minimizing the separation of the child from the family and allowing the child to remain in an environment that is familiar and comfortable. However, pediatric home health care does have some disadvantages. The presence of health care professionals in the home can be an intrusion on family privacy. Also, caring for children with complex medical needs can be overwhelming for some families. Financial issues can become a burden, as families may have higher out-of-pocket costs due to lack of reimbursement from a third party for home care. Having one parent or caregiver at home full time and not earning an income can contribute to increased financial strain, not to mention the social isolation of that person. All of these situations can lead to increased stress on family members. Nurses need to be aware of these potential disadvantages, work in partnership with the family, and provide support and resources as necessary.

Responsibilities of the Pediatric Home Care Nurse

As the provider of care, the home health care nurse uses the nursing process. Assessment in the home is similar to that in the acute care setting, but it will involve obtaining first-hand data about the family and family functioning. The nurse needs to assess growth and development and thoroughly assess the home environment (refer to Chapter 33 for additional information). The nurse should ensure that the home provides a safe and nurturing environment for the child by assessing the following:

- Availability of resources, such as necessary equipment (e.g., hospital bed, oxygen)
- Suitable physical and emotional surroundings (can the family members deal with the stress of the situation?)
- Ability to contact emergency services
- Power backup if needed
- Ease of evacuation of the child in case of a fire

The nurse also needs to ensure that adequate electricity, sanitary conditions, heat, possibly air conditioning, and telephone access exist in the home. If there is no phone in the home, the family needs to have plans for how to access a phone in case of emergency. This may include use of a neighbor's phone or relying on a pay phone near the home. The nurse should identify areas of priority and provide appropriate referrals to resources.

During the assessment phase, the nurse identifies the primary caregiver, who must be included in the plan of care. This person may be the mother, father, grandparent, or older sibling. The primary caregiver should be considered the expert about the child and family, providing valuable insights into direct care and the strategies that will be most effective with this child. The primary caregiver can also give key information about the physical layout of the home, the financial ability of the family, and the family's functioning.

The environment differs greatly between the acute setting and the home setting. In the acute setting the nurse

Example Individualized Healthcare Plan

Name:

Address:
Home Phone:
Parent/Guardian:
Day/Work Phone:
Healthcare Provider:
Provider's Phone:
IHP Written by:

Birthdate:

School:
Teacher/Counselor:
Grade:
IHP Date:
IEP Date:
Review Dates:
ICD-9 Codes:

Assessment Data	Nursing Diagnosis	Student Goals	Interventions	Outcomes
	Risk for Ineffective Breathing (NANDA 1.5.1.3)		**Airway Management (NIC 2K-3140)** **Activities:**	Symptom Control Behavior (NOC 4Q-1608) Indicators:
12-year-old diagnosed asthma at age 9	Characterized by shortness of breath, coughing, and/or wheezing related to asthma	Student will demonstrate appropriate use of inhaler at the beginning of school year.	Review use of inhaler with student at the beginning of the school year (Nurse).	Recognizes symptom onset Never 1 Rarely 2 Sometimes 3 Often 4 Consistently 5
Carries Proventil inhaler at all times		Student will initiate treatment when symptoms appear throughout the school year.	At the beginning of the school year, review with teacher, and other appropriate staff, the signs and symptoms of asthma exacerbation and when student should use inhaler (Nurse).	Uses preventative measures Never 1 Rarely 2 Sometimes 3 Often 4 Consistently 5
Independent in identifying symptoms and need for treatment		Student will keep record of peak flow meter readings if required throughout the school year.	Every two months obtain student's record of inhaler use for documentation in health file. Report increased use of inhaler to parents/physician (Nurse).	Uses relief measures Never 1 Rarely 2 Sometimes 3 Often 4 Consistently 5
M.D. order normal P.E. program		Student will keep record of use of inhaler for health office throughout the school year. Student will avoid having an emergency asthma attack during this school year.	**Emergency plan:** See STUDENT ASTHMA ACTION CARD located in the classroom, locker room, and health office.	Reports controlling symptoms Never 1 Rarely 2 Sometimes 3 Often 4 Consistently 5

I have read and approve of the above plan for school healthcare:

Parent signature

Nurse signature

Date reviewed by the educational team

Physician signature (optional)

FIGURE 2.5 Example of an IHP.

FIGURE 2.6 The camp nurse may care for typical healthy children or may work at a camp for children with special needs or chronic illness.

is in control of the environment, while in the home setting the nurse is a guest in the home. It is important for the nurse to establish a trusting relationship with both the child and family (Fig. 2.7), because a trusting therapeutic relationship will enhance all aspects of care.

The pediatric home care nurse assesses the family's teaching and learning needs. In many situations, care such as frequent dressing changes must be learned immediately so that the child can be cared for at home. This teaching should begin prior to hospital discharge. However, teaching is ongoing, with teaching and learning needs shifting as the child grows and his or her condition changes. The nurse empowers the child and family through education.

After the assessment is complete, the nurse develops and implements a plan of care. This will include the frequency and duration of the home visits. The nurse adheres to agency policies, certification standards, and private insurance and/or Medicaid regulations to assist in the development of the plan (Thompson, 2000). The nurse may provide direct care to the child or may plan and supervise the care given by others, such as unlicensed personnel and family caregivers.

Nursing care in the home requires excellent assessment and critical thinking skills. The nurse has a great deal of independence since there are no other nurses, supervisors, or physicians on site. Also, due to the potential complexity of care being provided, the nurse needs to adjust procedures to fit the setting. For example, feeding schedules may be adjusted to fit a child's school schedule, or equipment may be adjusted to allow a child to receive feedings continuously while at school (Fig. 2.8).

Home Care of the Technology-Dependent Child

Due to advances in medicine and technology, a new population of children with chronic disease and disability has emerged. Some of these children are considered technology-dependent, meaning they need medical or technical assistance to remain alive or avoid further disability. To improve the quality of life for these children and to reduce health care costs, more and more families are providing care for these children at home.

Meeting the needs of these children usually requires an interdisciplinary team approach. The team may consist of a specialty physician, occupational therapist, speech therapist, physical therapist, nutritionist, special educators, psychologist, social worker, and nurse. Studies have shown that families of technology-dependent children experience increased emotional, physical, psychological, and financial stress (Fleming, 2004). Nurses need to assess the family for these stressors and assist them in finding appropriate resources for assistance.

Due to the intensive, around-the-clock care that many of these children require, physical and emotional exhaustion can occur. Therefore, **respite care**, the provision of

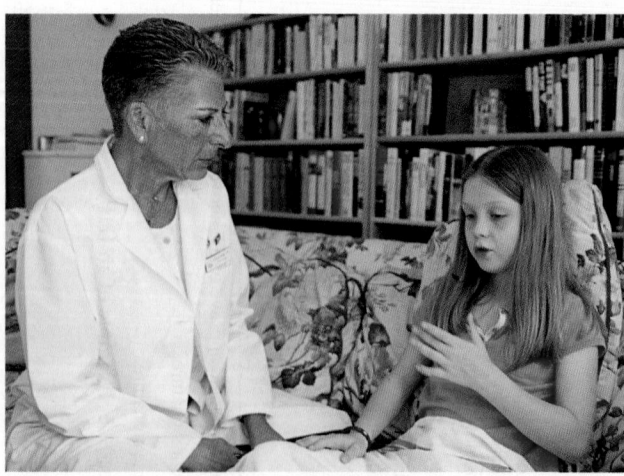

FIGURE 2.7 Listening to the child helps to develop a trusting relationship between the home care nurse and the child and her family.

FIGURE 2.8 The home care nurse may have to adjust procedures and equipment to fit the home setting. Placing a feeding pump in a backpack allows this child to receive feedings continuously while at school.

support services to temporarily relieve the caregiver from responsibility of providing care, is crucial. Nurses must assess the need for respite care and assist families in finding appropriate resources. (Refer to Chapter 33 for additional information about respite care.)

Roles and Functions of the Community-Based Nurse

Many nurses find the shift from acute care to community settings a challenge. With the shift in responsibilities from hospital care to community care, changes in nursing care have resulted. Nurses working in community-based settings share many of the same roles and responsibilities as their colleagues in acute care settings, but there are some differences. For example, in the community or home care setting the nurse will provide direct client care but will spend more time in the role of educator, communicator, and manager than the nurse in the acute care setting. In home care the nurse will spend a significant amount of time in the supervision or management role.

Communicator

Effective therapeutic communication with women, children, and families is critical to the provision of quality nursing care. Client- and family-centered communication increases satisfaction with nursing care and aids in improving knowledge and health care skills (Sobo, 2004).

Communicating with children can be more difficult than communicating with adults. However, children are able to inform nurses of their experiences reliably and accurately, and nurses need to be able to discern this information from communication with the child. Children may be more apt to communicate if they are engaged in another activity, may use fewer words than adults, and tend to rely more upon nonverbal communication and silence (Curtin, 2001). Parents and adults more often require neutral communication—that is, verbal communication that is related to assessing and solving problems. On the other hand, children usually desire affective communication (establishment of rapport and trust, giving comfort). Therefore, nurses need to find a balance between neutral and affective communication, communicating on multiple levels with children of different ages and on a supportive level with adolescents and adults (Shin & White-Traut, 2005).

Verbal and Nonverbal Communication

Nurses use verbal communication continuously throughout the day when interacting with their clients. Good verbal communication skills are necessary for excellent nursing assessment and teaching. Nonverbal communication, also referred to as body language, includes attending to others and active listening. When clients and families feel they are being heard, trust and rapport are established.

Recall Maria, who recently was discharged from the hospital with her newborn son. How did the nurse communicate with Maria? Did the nurse's actions during the visit promote the development of trust between Maria and the nurse? What might have been done differently to foster trust?

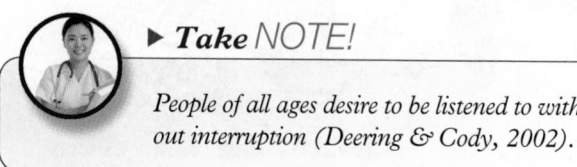

▶ ***Take*** NOTE!

People of all ages desire to be listened to without interruption (Deering & Cody, 2002).

Active listening is critical to the communication process. Listening may uncover fears or concerns that the nurse may not have discovered through questioning. By not listening, critical information may be missed. The client or family may sense that the nurse is not listening and thus may be reluctant to share further information. During the interaction, determine whether the client's verbal communication is congruent with his or her nonverbal communication.

Communication With Children

To communicate effectively with children, it is necessary to use a variety of age-appropriate methods. Encourage children to actively participate to promote feelings of control over the interaction (Shin & White-Traut, 2005). Talk to the parents first if the child is shy to allow the child time to become comfortable. Spending time with younger children (even just a few moments) may help them adapt and feel more at ease with the nurse (Donate-Bartfield & Passman, 2000). Use specific and clear phrases in an unhurried, quiet yet confident manner. Communicate at the child's eye level. Instead of direct questioning, use dolls, puppets, or stuffed animals to question younger children (Fig. 2.9). Using metaphors (such as referring to white blood cells as "bad guy fighters") helps to illustrate concepts to young and school-age children (Fleitas, 2003).

Older children need privacy. Provide the child or adolescent with honest answers at a developmentally appropriate level. Allow children to express their thoughts and feelings. Offer the child choices only when they truly exist (Mandleco, 2005). Box 2.5 highlights some guidelines for effective communication with children.

Children will be empowered when they are communicated with directly. Children may also desire advice about their health care and reassurance about their health status. To be effective when communicating with children of different developmental stages, the nurse must become familiar with how children of different ages communicate and then use age-appropriate techniques for effective communication. Table 2.2 provides some

FIGURE 2.9 Sitting at the child's level and allowing the child time for self-expression provide for improved therapeutic communication.

suggestions for developmentally appropriate communication techniques.

Communication With Families

When communicating with families, always be honest. Families desire to be valued and should be equal partners

---

BOX 2.5 Guidelines for Effective Communication with Children

- Introduce yourself and explain your role.
- Position yourself at the child's level.
- Allow the child to remain near the parent if needed, so the child can remain comfortable and relaxed.
- Smile and make eye contact with the child if culturally appropriate.
- Direct your questions and explanations to the child.
- Listen attentively and pause to allow time for the child to formulate his or her thoughts.
- Use the child's or family's terms for body parts and medical care when possible.
- Speak in a calm, quiet, confident, and unhurried voice.
- Use positive rather than negative statements and directions.
- Encourage the child to express his or her feelings and ask questions.
- Observe for nonverbal cues.
- Ask for permission if you need to approach the child to avoid appearing threatening.

TABLE 2.2 DEVELOPMENTALLY APPROPRIATE COMMUNICATION TECHNIQUES FOR CHILDREN

Age	Techniques
Infants	• Respond to crying in a timely fashion. • Allow the infant time to warm up to you. • Use play and playful persuasion. • Use a soothing and calming tone when speaking to the infant. • Talk to the baby directly.
Toddlers	• Approach toddlers carefully, as they often are fearful and quite resistant. • Use the toddler's particular words for objects or actions so that he or she is better able to understand. • Use storytelling, dolls, and books. • Prepare toddlers for procedures just before they are about to occur.
Preschoolers	• Use play, puppetry, or storytelling for a "third-party" approach. • Speak honestly. • Use simple, concrete terms. • Allow the child to have choices as appropriate. • Prepare preschoolers about 1 hour prior to a procedure.
School-age children	• Use diagrams, illustrations, books, and videos. • Allow the child to express feelings honestly. • Use third-party stories to elicit desired information. • Allow the child to ask questions related to care and treatment, and allow adequate time for all of the questions to be answered. • Prepare the child a few days in advance for a procedure.
Adolescents	• Always respect the teenager's need for privacy. • Ensure confidentiality. • Use appropriate medical terminology, defining words as necessary. • Use creativity. • Prepare the teen up to 1 week before a procedure.

in the health care team. Allow family members to verbalize concerns and questions. Explain the use of equipment and the correct sequence of procedures thoroughly. Help the members understand the long-term as well as short-term effects of the health treatment. Teach them what the client will feel like and how he or she will look during a procedure or treatment. When interacting with families, remember to ask the members how they are doing and to provide positive reinforcement as well as reassurance (Mandleco, 2005).

When the client is a child, encourage parents to perform as much of the child's care as is reasonable, teaching them how to perform treatments as permitted. Inquire about the parents' perception of the child's progress. Allowing the parents to be involved in the care of their child gives them a sense of control and lets them know that they are valued by the health care team.

Working With an Interpreter

Attempting to communicate with a family who does not speak English can be a highly frustrating situation for health care providers. Interpreters are an invaluable aid and an essential component of client and family education. Working with an interpreter, whether in person or over the phone, requires coordination of efforts so that both the family and the interpreter understand the information to be communicated. Working as a team, the nurse questions or informs and the interpreter conveys the information completely and accurately. Box 2.6 presents tips for working with an interpreter to maximize teaching efforts.

Healthy People 2010 also addresses the topic of language differences (Healthy People 2010 2.2). In addition, many health care facilities subscribe to Language Line (http://www.languageline.com/), which offers telephone access to interpretation of 150 languages. Numerous other interpreters, translators, and language resources are available online.

*R*ecall Maria, the woman with the newborn who is receiving home care. One the second visit to Maria's home, the nurse brought a Spanish-speaking interpreter who explained the reason for the "back to sleep" position and demonstrated to Maria several other useful positions for feeding and holding. Maria was smiling when the nurse left and asking when she would be back. What made the difference in their relationship the second visit? What interventions demonstrate culturally competent care?

Communicating With Deaf or Hearing-Impaired Clients and Families

For the hearing-impaired, determine the method of communication used: lip reading, American Sign Language (ASL), another method, or some combination. If the nurse is not proficient in ASL and the client or family uses it, then an ASL interpreter must be available if another adult

---

BOX 2.6 Tips for Working With Interpreters

- **Help the interpreter prepare and understand what needs to be done ahead of time.** A few minutes of preparation may save a lot of time and help communication flow more smoothly in the long run.
- **Remember, the interpreter is the "communication bridge" and not the "content expert."** The nurse's presence at teaching sessions is vital.
- **Be patient. The interpreter's timing may not match that of others involved.** It often takes longer to say in some languages what has already been said in English; therefore, plan for more time than you normally would.
- **Speak slowly and clearly.** Avoid jargon. Use short sentences and be concise. Avoid interrupting the interpreter.
- **Pause every few sentences so the interpreter can translate your information.** After 30 seconds of speaking, stop and let the interpreter express the information. Talk directly to the family, not the interpreter.
- **Give the family and the interpreter a break.** Sessions that last longer than 20 or 30 minutes are too much for anyone's attention span and concentration.
- **Express the information in two or three different ways if needed.** There may be cultural barriers as well as language and dialect differences that interfere with understanding. Interpreters may often know the correct communication protocols for the family.
- **Use an interpreter to help ensure the family can read and understand translated written materials.** The interpreter can also help answer questions and evaluate learning.
- **Avoid side conversations during sessions.** These can be uncomfortable for the family and jeopardize client–provider relationships and trust.
- **Remember, just because someone speaks another language doesn't mean that he or she will make a good interpreter.** An interpreter who has no medical background may not understand or interpret correctly, no matter how good his or her language skills are.
- **Do not use children as interpreters.** Doing so can affect family relationships, proper understanding, and compliance with health care issues.

Adapted from Weech, W. A. (1999). *Tips for using interpreters.* Foreign Service Institute of the U.S. Department of State.

---

family member is not present for translation. According to federal law, deaf clients and deaf family members must be given the ability to communicate effectively with healthcare providers (Sheehan, 2000).

Maintenance of Confidentiality and Privacy

Electronic medical records (EMR) improve efficiency and accuracy in a variety of clinical settings and may also improve the quality of client care by simplifying the function

Objective	Significance
Increase the proportion of local health departments that have established culturally appropriate and linguistically competent community health promotion and disease prevention programs.	• Work with professionals and individuals from various cultures to develop materials and programs for health promotion that are culturally competent. • Ensure teaching materials are provided in the appropriate language.

of recording complete data (Roukema et al., 2006). The EMR also simplifies sharing of client information across health care disciplines (Adams, Mann & Bauchner, 2003). Client confidentiality and privacy must be maintained in the EMR in a similar fashion as is required with paper documentation. At each point of electronic transmission, client data must remain secure and Health Insurance Portability and Accountability Act (HIPAA) guidelines must be followed (Flores & Dodier, 2005). When using computerized documentation and an EMR, continuously ensure that the client's and family's privacy and confidentiality are maintained.

Direct Care Provider

The community-based nurse typically performs less direct physical care than the nurse in the acute care setting. Many times the nurse may observe the client or caregiver performing physical care tasks. Excellent assessment skills are especially important in the community care setting. The nurse often is functioning in a more autonomous role, and after data collection, the community-based nurse will often decide whether to initiate, continue, alter, or end physical nursing care. Assessment extends beyond physical assessment of the client to include the environment and the community.

Management of the Perinatal Client

The nurse provides direct care to the perinatal client, beginning with the woman's first visit to the health care provider and extending through the pregnancy and birth. In addition, the nurse provides direct care involving the following areas:

- Contraception
- Abortion
- Infertility
- Screening for sexually transmitted infections
- Preconceptual risk assessment and care

Provision of Atraumatic Care for Children

To minimize the stress experienced by children and their families in relation to health care, nurses, child life specialists, and other health care professionals advocate for the provision of atraumatic care. Atraumatic care refers to the delivery of health care in a manner that eliminates or minimizes psychological and physical distress to children and families (Wong, 2002). The key principles of atraumatic care include:

- Preventing or minimizing physical stressors
- Preventing or minimizing separation of the child from the family
- Promoting a sense of control

Table 2.3 provides suggestions for incorporating the principles of atraumatic care into nursing care for the child and family.

Educator

Due to shortened hospital stays and decreased admissions, providing client and family education is a key role for nurses in the community. Many times teaching begins in the community setting, especially the home. In the community-based setting, client teaching is often focused on assisting the client and family to achieve independence.

Regardless of the type of setting, nurses are in a unique position to help clients and families manage their own health care needs. Clients and families need to be knowledgeable about areas such as their condition, the health care management plan, and when and how to contact health care providers. With the limited time available in all health care arenas, nurses must focus on teaching goals and begin teaching at the earliest opportunity (London, 2004).

▶ **Take** NOTE!

There is no prescription more valuable than knowledge. (C. Everett Koop, MD, Former Surgeon General of the United States)

Client education occurs when nurses share information, knowledge, and skills with clients and families, thus empowering them to take responsibility for their health care. Through client education, clients and families can overcome feelings of powerlessness and helplessness and gain the confidence and capability to be active members in their plan of care. According to the Joint Commission on the Accreditation of Healthcare Organizations (JCAHO) standards, the goals of client and family education are to:

- Promote interactive communication with providers
- Improve understanding of health status and health care options
- Encourage decision making about care
- Improve compliance with the plan of care
- Reduce anxiety

TABLE 2.3   SUGGESTIONS FOR PROVIDING ATRAUMATIC CARE

Principle	Suggestions for Nursing Care
Preventing or minimizing physical stressors	• For painful injections, use numbing techniques. • During painful or invasive procedures, avoid traditional restraint or "holding down" of the child. Use alternative positioning such as "therapeutic hugging." • If these positions are not an option, have the parent stand near the child's head to provide comfort. • Insert a saline lock if the child will require multiple doses of parenteral medications. • Advocate for minimal laboratory blood specimen collections. • Avoid use of or minimize intramuscular or subcutaneous injections. • Provide appropriate pain management.
Preventing or minimizing child and family separation	• Promote family-centered care. • Allow the family the choice about whether to stay for invasive procedures, and support them in their decision.
Promoting a sense of control	• Maintain the child's home routine related to ADLs. • Encourage the child to have a security item with him or her if desired. • Involve the child and family in planning of care from the first moment of the first encounter. • Empower the family and child by providing knowledge. • Allow the child and family choices when they are available. • Make the environment more inviting, less intimidating.

• Return a sense of autonomy and control
• Promote healthy lifestyles (JCAHO, 2004)

Overall, client and family education allows clients and families to make informed decisions, ensures the presence of basic health care skills, promotes recognition of problem situations, promotes appropriate responses to problems, and allows for questions to be answered (London, 2004). Client and family education is a priority and is addressed in Healthy People 2010 2.3.

▶ **Take** NOTE!

To cope effectively with illness, understand and participate in decisions about treatment plans, and maintain and improve health after treatment, clients and their families must have access to the specific knowledge and skills relevant to their conditions (JCAHO, 2004).

HEALTHY PEOPLE 2010

Objective	Significance
Increase the proportion of persons appropriately counseled about health behaviors. (Developmental) Increase the proportion of health care organizations that provide client and family education; increase the proportion of clients who report that they are satisfied with the client education they receive from their health care organization.	• Assess health learning needs of women, children, and their families. • Plan health care education in collaboration with clients and their families. • Provide health education at each client encounter.

Steps of Client and Family Education

The steps of client and family education are similar to the steps of the nursing process. The nurse must assess, plan, implement, evaluate, and finally document education. Once a level of comfort and experience are obtained with each of these steps, they all blend together into one harmonious whole that becomes an everyday part of nursing practice. Client education begins with the first client encounter and proceeds through discharge and beyond. Reassessment after each step or change in the process is critical to ensuring success.

Assessing Teaching and Learning Needs

Client education begins with a learning needs assessment that includes the client's and family's learning needs, learning styles, and potential barriers to learning. A learning needs assessment also is a good time to establish rapport with the family to demonstrate interest in them and confidence in their ability to learn.

Based on the results of the assessment, an individualized plan can be developed to reduce the time and effort required for nurses to teach while maximizing learning for the client and family. When caring for children, the educational process is targeted at both the child, when developmentally appropriate, and the adult members of the family. Therefore, it is advisable to conduct a learning needs assessment on both the adult caregivers and the child when appropriate.

The assessment, when completed, should be shared with all members of the interdisciplinary team so that the entire team can facilitate the learning. Although assessment generally takes place during the first or second meeting with the client and family, it should also occur with each encounter to check for any changes to ensure the success of the education across the continuum of care.

Cultural Impact on Assessment of Learning Needs

Culture can have a significant impact on learning. During the learning needs assessment, determine the language spoken in the home and the use of eye and physical contact. Also investigate the following:

- Person responsible for caring for the client and person considered the authority figure in the family
- The social support structure
- Special dietary needs and concerns during illness
- Traditional health practices, such as the use of healers, shamans, talismans, folk remedies, and herbs
- Special clothes or other items that help to maintain health
- Religious beliefs, ceremonies, and spiritual practices

Culture also influences the interpretation and meaning of illness to a client and family. Question them about their thoughts or ideas, such as the cause, effects, severity, and hopes for treatment. Then an individualized teaching plan can be negotiated with the client and family.

> ► **Consider** THIS!
>
> Our medical mission took a team of nurse practitioners into the rural mountains of Guatemala to offer medical services to people who had never had any. One day, a distraught mother brought her 10-year-old daughter to the mission clinic, asking me if there was anything I could do about her daughter's right wrist. She had sustained a fracture a year ago and it had not healed properly. As I looked at the girl's malformed wrist, I asked if it had been splinted to help with alignment, knowing what the answer was going to be. The
>
> *(continued)*

> ► **Consider** THIS! *(continued)*
>
> interpreter enlightened me by saying that this young girl would never marry and have children because of this injury. I appeared puzzled at the interpreter's prediction of this girl's future. It was later explained to me that if the girl couldn't make tortes from corn meal for her husband because of her wrist disability, she would not be worthy of becoming someone's wife and thus would probably live with her parents the rest of her life.
>
> I reminded myself during the week of the medical mission not to impose my cultural values on the women for whom I was caring and to accept their cultural mores without judgment. These silent self-reminders served me well throughout the week, for I was open to learning about their lifestyles and customs.
>
> Thoughts: What must the young girl be feeling at the age of 10, being rejected for a disability that wasn't her fault? What might have happened if I had imposed my value system on this patient? How effective would I have been in helping her if she didn't feel accepted? This incident ripped my heart out, for this young girl will be deprived of a fulfilling family life based on a wrist disability. This is just another example of female suppression that happens all over the world—such a tragedy—and yet a part of their culture, on which nurses should not pass judgment.

Nurses involved in teaching immigrant or refugee families may encounter specific issues, such as:

- Use of the English versus the metric system for measurement
- Use of measurements such as a "a handful" or "a pinch" rather than specific measurements such as a measuring device
- Lack of access to refrigeration for liquid medications
- Breastfeeding practices

Literacy Issues

Health literacy is the ability to read, understand, and use health care information. The inability to read and comprehend health care information or materials is an enormous problem in America today. Low health literacy affects people of all ages, races, and educational and income levels. Even persons with adequate literacy skills may have difficulty reading and understanding health care information.

Adequate literacy skills are essential for client and family education, yet many people in America today have marginal reading abilities. The average adult in America reads at an eighth-grade level, and approximately 20% read and understand only information written below a fifth-grade level. For the English-speaking Medicaid population, the average reading level is fifth grade; for native Spanish-speaking persons, the average reading level is third grade (Schillinger, 2002). Studies have reported that literacy skills are a stronger predictor of health status than age, income, employment, education, or racial or ethnic group (Weiss, 2003).

When new and unfamiliar information is disseminated or when emotional distress is present, reading ability and understanding are further reduced. In addition, the last grade completed in school does not equate with reading ability: poor readers often read three to five grade levels below their grade completion. Most health care materials are written at a tenth-grade level. Moreover, medical information is becoming increasingly complex, while the amount of time clients have to spend with nurses and other health care providers is decreasing. As a result, many studies have shown that persons with limited literacy skills cannot understand basic medical words and health concepts, whether verbal or written.

Unfortunately, recognizing poor health literacy skills is difficult: appearance, verbal ability, employment status, and educational level cannot be used to identify persons who do not read well. People who do not read well often go to great lengths to hide their disability: 68% of persons with limited literacy skills have never told their spouse and 75% have never told their health care provider (Weiss, 2003).

▶ *Take* NOTE!

Watch for these red flags that may indicate poor literacy skills:
- *Difficulty filling out registration forms, questionnaires, and consents*
- *Frequently missed appointments*
- *Noncompliance and lack of follow-up with treatment regimens*
- *Responses such as, "I forgot my glasses" or "I'll read this when I get home"*
- *Inability to answer common questions about their treatment or medicines*
- *Avoidance of asking questions for fear of looking "stupid"*

Planning Education

Once the assessment is completed, plan mutually agreed-upon achievable learning goals and objectives. It is important that achievement of goals is possible from both the caregiver's and the learner's perspective. Finding common ground and building a bridge between the client's and family's concerns and what the health care team believes they need to know is a critical part of an education plan. This also is an excellent time to consider client education materials and resources that can be used to maximize learning and retention.

Planning client education should involve input from the entire interdisciplinary team when appropriate. Through good communication and collaboration, team members can work together to empower the client and family to become knowledgeable and skilled. Overriding the traditional path of teacher-centered education by providing family-centered education requires thought and skill.

To achieve maximum success with education, it is beneficial to know how people learn. Edgar Dale (1969) suggested that people learn best when actively involved in the learning process. Figure 2.10 provides a summary of his principles, known as the "cone of learning." The implications for client education are clear: the more senses employed and the more actively involved the learner is, the better he or she will remember what was taught.

Intervening to Enhance Learning

Nurses are in an excellent position to foster an environment that is conducive to learning. For example, it is entirely appropriate to say to the client, "Many people have a problem reading and remembering the information on this paper (booklet, manual). Is this ever a problem for you?" Once a problem is acknowledged, the nurse is free to adjust verbal communication techniques and written materials to assist with learning and to communicate this need to the entire interdisciplinary healthcare team.

Nurses implement individualized teaching techniques based on the assessment information and identified goals. In general, the following techniques can facilitate learning:

- Slow down and repeat information often.
- Speak in conversational style using plain, nonmedical language.
- "Chunk" information and teach it in small bites using logical steps.
- Prioritize information and teach "survival skills" first.
- Use visuals, such as pictures, videos, and models.
- Teach using an interactive, "hands-on" approach.

If the client or family has poor health literacy skills, learning can be fostered by the use of pictures or illustrations, videos or audio tapes, or color coding (such as medication bottles or steps of a procedure). In addition, teaching can include a "back-up" family member.

Children and adolescents have a great need for information about their illness as they attempt to master feelings of anxiety and restore feelings of competency, self-confidence, and hope for the future. As with adults, they learn best when their input is valued and they are actively included and involved in the learning process. The age and developmental level of the child will determine the amount, format, and timing of the information given. Table 2.4 provides some guidelines to keep in mind when teaching children. Before beginning to teach a child, it is important to establish rapport and lay the foundation for good communication.

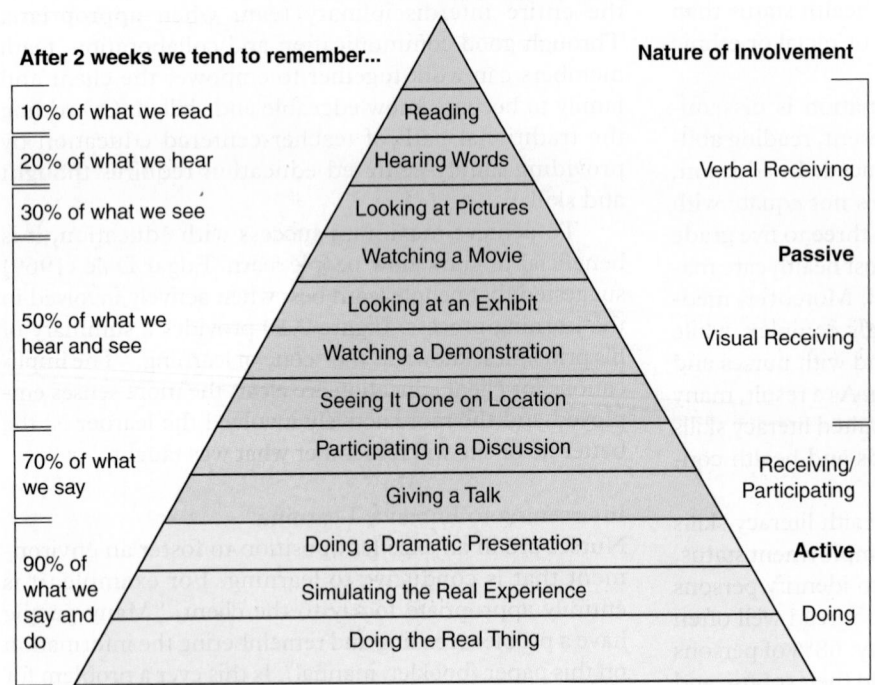

FIGURE 2.10 Cone of Learning (adapted from Dale).

When teaching preschoolers, the nurse or family assumes part or all of the responsibility for what is learned, how it is learned, and when it is learned. Employing their vivid imaginations, young children often attempt to invent pieces of information, or pick up bits and pieces of misinformation that can lead to false assumptions. Skillfully delivered and timed information as well as proper preparation can help encourage trust, calm, and control for an otherwise apprehensive and uncooperative preschooler.

Unless they are quite ill, school-age children need to cooperate and achieve and usually want to participate in their care. When teaching, speak directly to them and include them in the education plan. Parents can often learn by listening to and observing the care being given to their child (Fig. 2.11).

Adolescents are particularly sensitive about maintaining body image and feelings of control and autonomy. This is especially important with health care processes and decisions that affect them. Education is an essential aspect of care for the adolescent who is pregnant.

Evaluating Learning

Teaching, even when done well, does not necessarily mean that learning has occurred. Evaluation of learning is critical to ensure that the client and family have actually learned what the nurse tried to teach. Evaluation should occur with each educational encounter and goals and interventions should be adjusted accordingly. The nurse, along with the rest of the interdisciplinary team, is responsible for client and family learning. If they have not learned, the health care team must adjust teaching strategies so that the client and family do learn.

▶ **Take** NOTE!

The ultimate goal of education is a change in behavior on the part of the client and family; this change can occur in their level of knowledge, skills, or both.

Evaluation of learning can occur in several different ways, depending on the topic and the method of teaching. The client or family may:

• Demonstrate a skill. Learning can quickly and easily be identified using this method.
• Repeat back or teach back information using their own words.
• Answer open-ended questions. Open-ended questions provide an opportunity to assess for missing or incorrect information. Open-ended questions are those that cannot be answered with a simple "yes" or "no."

Another option to evaluate learning is to provide a "pretend" scenario for the client or family, having them verbalize all the steps related to care from the routine measures to those for handling an emergency situation. Information must be conveyed accurately as the client or family walks through the necessary steps.

Documenting Teaching and Learning

Documenting client care and education is part of every nurse's professional practice and serves four main purposes. First and foremost, the client's medical record serves

TABLE 2.4 GUIDELINES FOR TEACHING CHILDREN

Teaching Tips	Practical Applications
Preschoolers	
Offer simple, concise, concrete explanations based on the assessed needs, questions, and developmental level of the child.	Use a child's senses and relate what a procedure will look, sound, smell, taste, or feel like ("The MRI machine will sound very loud, like a big train").
Be honest, even when the information you need to convey is not positive. This helps the child to form a bond of trust and confidence with caregivers.	Use the family's words that the child understands; use "soft words" ("This will feel warm" instead of "This will burn").
Time explanations to decrease anxiety and excess worry before the event. Avoid telling unpleasant news close to bedtime.	As a general rule, give toddlers information about procedures, medicines, and other interventions immediately beforehand; give 4- to 7-year-olds information 1 or 2 days in advance.
Enlist the aid of the parents because they know their child best. Eliciting information from them about their child's past behaviors and coping skills can often mean the difference between a positive and negative experience for their child.	Teach parents how to coach their child with pain management, visualization, or other methods of distraction when appropriate ("Remember when we went to the beach. . . .").
Provide an active role for the child. This helps to foster a child's sense of self-confidence and control over the situation.	Allow the child to help with simple self-care activities such as holding a dressing or piece of tape. Provide props and dolls to touch and feel as much as possible ("Your job is to keep your hands still").
Respect the child's wishes when he or she verbalizes or demonstrates that he or she does not want more information.	Keep explanations short and simple; know when to stop teaching.
Praise children and let them know how much you appreciate their help and cooperation.	Use "please" and "thank you" often ("Thank you. I like the way you held still for me.").
School-age children	
Allow the child some control and involvement in the decision-making process.	Offer choices whenever possible (taking the medicine with juice or milk), but don't offer choices when there are no alternatives (taking the medicine vs. not taking the medicine).
Know that children can relate current happenings to past experiences.	Use examples and past experiences that are familiar to the child ("Remember when you were learning to swim?").
Allow children to be actively involved when possible; achievement and accomplishment are very important to children at this age, so anything they can be actively involved in will help them adjust and learn.	Provide an active role and allow the child to do as much care as possible. Use props, dolls, games, and computers to enhance learning.
Remember that at this age, most children are able to sequence, understand cause-and-effect, and make sense of time.	Teach children the steps involved and how long they will take ("Today I'm going to teach you how to change your dressing. This will help keep your cut clean. First, wash your hands. . . .").
Enhance self-confidence by allowing the child to gain control over the situation and prepare for it mentally.	Provide information 3 to 7 days in advance, depending on the child's age and developmental level.
Praise children and let them know how much you appreciate their help and cooperation.	Use "please" and "thank you" often ("Thanks! You did a great job using your inhaler").
Adolescents	
Allow teens to be in control and involved in the decision-making process.	Speak directly to teens; consider their input in all decisions about their care and education.

(continued)

TABLE 2.4 GUIDELINES FOR TEACHING CHILDREN (continued)

Teaching Tips	Practical Applications
Keep in mind that adolescents can process abstract information and understand how their actions affect long-term outcomes.	Provide reasons why something is important and discuss how their lives will be affected by their decision to take care of their health needs ("If you eat a nutritious diet, you'll help your baby grow").
Remember that adolescents are very concerned about how they look and how they fit in with their peers.	Collaborate with the teen to develop acceptable solutions and strategies for dealing with health issues that affect personal appearance and peer acceptance (wig vs. head scarves for hair loss from chemotherapy).
Know that adolescents strive for independence and have personal values and ideologies that may conflict with those of their parents and the medical community.	Expect some noncompliance with care, despite your best educational efforts. Work together to achieve win–win outcomes of educational goals.

as a communication tool that the entire interdisciplinary team can use to keep track of what the client and family has learned already and what learning still needs to occur. Next, it serves to testify to the education the family has received if and when legal matters arise. Thirdly, it verifies standards set by the JCAHO, Centers for Medicare and Medicaid Services (CMS), and other accrediting bodies that hold health care providers accountable for client education activities. And lastly, it informs third-party payers of goods and services provided for reimbursement purposes.

Documentation of client and family education is imperative. It is the only means available to ensure that the family's educational plan and objectives have been completed.

Discharge Planner and Case Manager

Due to the short length of stays in acute settings and the shift to community settings for clients with complex health needs, discharge planning and case management have become an important nursing role in the community. Discharge planning involves the development and implementation of a comprehensive plan for the safe discharge of a client from a health care facility and for continuing safe and effective care in the community and at home. Case management focuses on coordinating health care services while balancing quality and cost outcomes. Often clients requiring community-based care, especially home care, have complex medical needs that require an interdisciplinary team to meet their physical, psychosocial, medical, nursing, developmental, and education needs. The nurse plays an important role in initiating and maintaining the link between team members and the client to ensure that the client and family are receiving comprehensive, coordinated care.

Advocate and Resource Manager

Client advocate is another important role of the community-based nurse to ensure that the client's and family's needs are being met. Advocacy also helps ensure that the client and family have available resources and appropriate health care services. For example, the pregnant woman on bed rest at home may need help in caring for her other children, maintaining the household, or getting to her appointments. Children with complex medical needs may require financial assistance through Medicaid or Medicaid waivers (state-run programs that use federal and state money to pay for the health care of individuals with certain medical conditions). They may also need assistance in obtaining needed equipment, additional services, and transportation. Community-based nurses need a basic understanding of community, state, and federal resources to ensure that clients and their families have access to those necessary for them.

FIGURE 2.11 Nurses need to adapt teaching to the child's developmental level. For the school-age child, teaching the child and parents together fosters the child's need for achievement.

■■■ Key Concepts

■ Family-centered care recognizes the concept of the family as the constant. The health and functioning ability of the family influences and impacts the health of the patient and other members of the family. Family-centered care recognizes and respects family strengths and individuality, encourages referrals for family support, and facilitates collaboration. It ensures flexible, accessible, and responsive health care delivery while incorporating developmental needs and implementing policies to provide emotional and financial support to women, children, and their families.

- Health care delivery has moved from acute care settings out into the community, with an emphasis on health promotion and illness prevention. Community health nursing focuses on prevention and improvement of the health of populations and communities, addressing current and potential health needs of the population or community, promoting and preserving the health of a population regardless of a particular age group or diagnosis. Community health nurses perform epidemiologic investigations to help analyze and develop health policy and community health initiatives.

- Community-based nurses focus on providing personal care to individuals and families in the community. They center on promoting and preserving health as well as preventing disease or injury. They help women, children, and their families cope with illness and disease. Community-based nurses are direct care providers as well as advocators and educators. They focus on minimizing and removing barriers to allow the patient to develop to his or her full potential.

- Community-based nursing uses the nursing process in caring for patients within community settings and applies primary, secondary, and tertiary prevention levels. Nursing interventions in community-based settings include health screening, education, medication administration, telephone consultation, health system referral, instruction, nutritional counseling, and risk identification.

- Nurses working in the community need to develop cultural competence. Steps to gaining cultural competence include cultural self-awareness, cultural knowledge, cultural skills, and cultural encounters.

- Settings for community-based nursing including physicians' offices, clinics, health departments, urgent care centers, clients' homes, schools, camps, churches, and shelters such as abuse, homeless, and disaster shelters. Nurses provide both well, episodic ill care, and chronic care to women, children, and their families.

- There has been a rise in home health care due to shorter hospital stays and cost containment along with an increase in income and longevity of children with chronic and debilitating health conditions. Technology also has improved, which allows for better monitoring of patients at home and for performing complicated procedures at home.

- Roles and functions of the community-based nurse include communicator, direct care provider, educator, discharge planner and case manager, and advocate and resource manager.

- Open, honest lines of communication are essential for community-based nurses. The use of an interpreter may be necessary to ensure effective communication with women, children, and their families in the community setting. Maintaining confidentiality and privacy are key.

- A family's knowledge related to the patient's health or illness is vitally important. Nurses working in the community play a major role in educating women, children, and their families. For children, teaching is provided based on the child's developmental level.

- Discharge planning provides a comprehensive plan for the safe discharge of a client from a health care facility and for continuing safe and effective care in the community. Case management focuses on coordinating health care services while balancing quality and cost outcomes. Both contribute to improved transition from the hospital to the community for women, children, their families, and the health care team.

- Community-based nurses act as advocates and resource managers to help ensure that the patient and family have the necessary resources and appropriate health care services available to them.

REFERENCES

Adams, W. G., Mann, A. M., & Bauchner, H. (2003). Use of an electronic medical record improves the quality of urban pediatric primary care. *Pediatrics, 111*(3), 626–632.

Alexander, L. L., LaRosa, J. H., Bader, H., & Garfield, S. (2007). *New dimensions in women's health* (4th ed.). Sudbury, MA: Jones and Bartlett Publishers.

American College of Obstetricians and Gynecologists (ACOG). (2007). National Folic Acid Awareness Week. Available at: www.acog.org

American Pregnancy Association (APA). (2007). Birthing choices: Care providers and labor locations. Available at: http://www.americanpregnancy.org/labornbirth/birthingchoices.html

Anderson, E. T., & McFarlane, J. (2007). *Community as partner: Theory and practice in nursing* (5th ed.). Philadelphia: Lippincott Williams & Wilkins.

Anonymous. (2000). Exceptional Professionals techno-daycare [Electronic Version]. *The Exceptional Parent, 30*(2), 28–31.

Bainbridge, J. (2006). Birth centers: What price maternal choice and professional autonomy. *British Journal of Midwifery, 14*(1), 40–41.

Britt, D. W., Edean, R. D., & Evans, M. I. (2006) Matching risk and resources in high-risk pregnancies. *Journal of Maternal-Fetal Medicine, 19*(10), 645–650.

Canadian Community Health Nursing Standards of Practice. (2003). Community Health Nursing Association of Canada [Electronic Version].

Centers for Disease Control & Prevention (CDC). (2007a). *Longer hospital stays for childbirth*. National Center for Health Statistics. Available at www.cdc.gov/nchs/products/pubs/pubd/hestats/hospbirth.htm

CDC. (2007b). *New study profiles women's use of health care*. Available at: www.cdc.gov/od/oc/media/pressrel/r010725.htm

Chia-Chen, A., & Thompson, E. A. (2007). Family-centered care. *Journal for Specialists in Pediatric Nursing, 12*(2), 119–122.

Clark, M. J. (2007). *Community health nursing: Advocating for healthy populations* (5th ed.). Upper Saddle River, NJ: Prentice Hall.

Clarke, P., Bowcock, M., & Gales, P. (2007). Development of an integrated care pathway for natural birth. *British Journal of Midwifery, 15*(1), 12–15.

Corjulo, M. T. (2005). Telephone triage for asthma medication refills. *Pediatric Nursing, 31*(2), 116–120, 124.

Curtin, C. (2001). Eliciting children's voices in qualitative research. *American Journal of Occupational Therapy, 55*, 295–302.

Dale, E. (1969). *Audio-visual methods in teaching* (3rd ed.). Austin, TX: Holt, Rinehart, and Winston.

Deering, C. G., & Cody, D. J. (2002). Communicating with children and adolescents. *American Journal of Nursing, 102*(3), 34–41.

Dochterman, J. M., & Bulechek, G. M. (2004). *Nursing interventions classification* (NIC) (4th ed.). St. Louis: Mosby.

Donate-Bartfield, E., & Passman, R. H. (2000). Establishing rapport with preschool-age children: implications for practitioners. *Children's Health Care, 29*(3), 179–188.

Downe, S. (2006) Normal birth focus: Engaging with the concept of unique normality in childbirth. *British Journal of Midwifery, 14*(6), 352–354.

Fleitas, J. (2003). The power of words: Examining the linguistic landscape of pediatric nursing. *MCN, 28*(6), 384–390.

Fleming, J. (2004). *Home health care for children who are technology dependent*. New York: Springer.

Flores, J., & Dodier, A. (2005). HIPAA: Past, present and future implications for nurses. *Online Journal of Issues in Nursing, 10*(2), 1–12. Available at: www.nursingworld.org/ojin/topic27/tpc27_4.htm

Godfrey, J. R. (2006). Toward optimal health: The need for cultural competence in the healthcare of women. *Journal of Women's Health, 15*(5), 480–484.

Grindel, C. (2006) Fostering a nurse, client, and family partnership in care. *MedSurg Nursing, 15*(2), 58–59.

Hewitt-Taylor, J. (2005). Caring for children with complex and continuing health needs. *Nursing Standard, 19*(42), 41–47.

Hewitt-Taylor, J. (2005). Children with complex needs: Training for care staff. *Journal of Community Nursing, 19*(8), 8–12.

Hodnett, D. D., Downe, S., Edwards, N., & Walsh, D. (2005). Home-like versus conventional institutional settings for birth. *Cochrane Database of Systematic Reviews.* Issue 1.Art.No.: CD000012. DOI:10.1002/14651858.CD000012.pub2.

Hunt, R. (2005). *Introduction to community-based nursing* (3rd ed.). Philadelphia: Lippincott Williams & Wilkins.

Joint Commission on Accreditation of Healthcare Organizations. (1998–2004). *Comprehensive accreditation manual for hospitals.* Oakbrook Terrace, IL: JCAHO.

Kersey–Matusiak, G. (2006). An action plan for cultural competence. *Nursing Spectrum.* Available at http://nsweb.nursingspectrum.com/ce/ce255.htm

Krug, S. E., Bojko, T., Dolan, M. A., Frush, K. S., et al. (2005). Pediatric care recommendations for freestanding urgent care facilities [Electronic Version]. *Pediatrics, 116*(1), 258–260.

Laveist, T. (2005) *Minority populations and health: An introduction to health disparities in the U.S.* Indianapolis: Wiley & Sons.

London, F. (2004). How to prepare families for discharge in the limited time available. *Pediatric Nursing, 30*(3), 212–214, 227.

Mandleco, B. (2005). *Pediatric nursing skills and procedures.* Clifton Park, NY: Thomson Delmar.

March of Dimes. (2007). *Why prenatal care? March of Dimes Birth Defect Prevention Foundation.* Available at www.modimes.org

Martin, S. R., & Foley, M. R. (2006), Intensive care in obstetrics: An evidence-based review. *American Journal of Obstetrics & Gynecology, 195*(3), 673–689.

Mentro, A. (2003). Health care policy for medically fragile children. *Journal of Pediatric Nursing, 18*(4), 225–232.

Papadopoulos, I. (2006) *Transcultural health and social care: Development of culturally competent practitioners.* St. Louis, MO: Elsevier Health Sciences

Ramsey, L. (2007). Birthing options: Birthing center, home, and hospitals. *PageWise.* Available at http://ncnc.essortment.com/birthingoptions_rikm.html

Rice, R. (2005). *Home care nursing practice: Concepts and applications* (4th ed.). St. Louis: Elsevier Health Sciences.

Roukema, J., Los, R. K., Bleeker, S. E., van Ginneken, A. M., van der Lei, J., & Moll, H. A. (2006). Paper versus computer: Feasibility of an electronic medical record in general pediatrics. *Pediatrics, 117*(1), 15–21.

Schillinger, D. (2002). Association of health literacy with diabetes outcomes. *Journal of the American Medical Association, 288*(4), 475–482.

Sheehan, J. P. (2000). Caring for the deaf: Do you do enough? *RN, 63*(3), 69–70, 72.

Shin, H., & White-Traut, R. (2005). Nurse–child interaction on an inpatient paediatric unit. *Journal of Advanced Nursing, 52*(1), 56–62.

Simonsen-Anderson, S. (2002). Safe and sound: Telephone triage and home recommendations save lives and money. *Nursing Management, 33*(6), 41–43.

Sobo, E. J. (2004). Pediatric nurses may misjudge parent communication preferences. *Journal of Nursing Care Quality, 19*(3), 253–262.

Staff. (2008). Role of the school nurse in providing school health services. *Pediatrics, 121*(5), 1052–1056.

Stanhope, M., & Lancaster, J. (2006). *Foundations of community health nursing: Community-oriented practice* (2nd ed.). St. Louis: Mosby.

Stanhope, M., & Lancaster, J. (2008). *Public health nursing: Population-centered health care in the community* (7th ed.). St. Louis: Mosby Elsevier.

Steppe, B. (2006). Experience the experience. *International Journal of Childbirth Education, 21*(3), 33.

Thompson, J. M. (2000). Pediatric assessment in the home [Electronic Version]. *Home Healthcare Nurse, 18*(10), 639–646.

U.S. Census Bureau. (2007). *The 2007 statistical abstract: the national data book.* Available at: http://www.census.gov/compendia/statab/brief.html

U.S. Department of Health and Human Services. (2000). *Healthy People 2010.* Available at www.healthypeople.gov

U.S. Department of Health and Human Services, Health Resources and Services Administration, Bureau of Health Professions. (2004). *National sample survey of RNs, final report.* Available at: ftp://ftp.hrsa.gov/bhpr/rnsurvey2000/rnsurvey00-1.pdf

U.S. Department of Homeland Security. (USDHS). (2006) *Yearbook of immigration statistics: 2005.* Washington, DC: U.S. Department of Homeland Security, Office of Immigration Statistics.

Weech, W. A. (1999). *Tips for using interpreters.* Foreign Service Institute of the U.S. Department of State.

Weiss, B. D. (2003). *Health literacy: A manual for clinicians.* Chicago: American Medical Association Foundation.

Wolfe, L. C., & Selekman, J. (2002). School nurses: What it was and what it is. *Pediatric Nursing, 28*(4), 403–407.

Wong, D. L. (2002). *Beyond first do no harm: Principles of atraumatic care.* Retrieved June 25, 2006 from http://www3.us.elsevierhealth.com/WOW/op022a.html

Zahner, S. J., & Block, D. E. (2006). The road to population health: Using Healthy People 2010 in nursing education. *Journal of Nursing Education, 45*(3), 105–108.

WEBSITES

American Academy of Pediatrics: www.aap.org
American Translators Association (ATA): www.atanet.org
Association of Camp Nurses: www.campnurse.org
Association for Women's Health, Obstetrics, and Neonatal Nursing: www.awhonn.org
Center for Applied Linguistics: www.cal.org
Centers for Disease Control and Prevention: www.cdc.gov
Child Health Information Center: www.childhealthinfo.com/
Children's Healthcare is a Legal Duty (CHILD, Inc.): www.childrens healthcare.org/
Guide to Children's Health and Safety: www.keepkidshealthy.com
Institute for Family-Centered Care: www.familycenteredcare.org/
Language Line: www.languageline.com/
National Association of School Nurses: www.nasn.org/Default.aspx
Northwest Translators and Interpreters Society: www.notis.net
Office of Minority Health, U.S. Department of Health and Human Services: www.omhrc.gov
Transcultural Nursing Society: www.tcns.org

CHAPTER WORKSHEET

MULTIPLE CHOICE QUESTIONS

1. A community-based nurse is involved in secondary prevention activities. Which activities might be included? Select all that apply.

    a. Fecal occult blood testing

    b. Hearing screening

    c. Smoking cessation program

    d. Cholesterol testing

    e. Hygiene program

    f. Pregnancy testing

2. A woman is to undergo a colonoscopy at a freestanding outpatient surgery center. Which would the nurse identify as a major disadvantage associated with this community-based setting?

    a. Increased risk for infection

    b. Increased health care costs

    c. Need to be transferred if overnight stay is required

    d. Increased disruption of family functioning

3. A 2-year-old boy is scheduled to undergo an endoscopic procedure. His parents are asking when they should tell him about it. Based on the nurse's understanding of the child's developmental stage, when would be the most appropriate time to prepare the child for the procedure?

    a. About 1 week before the scheduled date

    b. A few days in advance of the scheduled date

    c. About an hour before the procedure is to occur

    d. Just before the procedure is to be performed

4. When developing a teaching plan for a child and his parents, which action would the nurse do first?

    a. Decide which procedures and medications the child will be discharged on.

    b. Determine the child's and family's learning needs and styles.

    c. Ask the family if they have ever performed this type of procedure.

    d. Tell the child and family what the goals of the teaching session are.

CRITICAL THINKING EXERCISES

1. A 3-year-old girl from Saudi Arabia has become seriously ill while on a visit to the United States. It is projected that she will require a lengthy hospitalization. Describe the steps the nurse should take to communicate with and provide extensive health care teaching to this child's family.

2. A pregnant woman is discharged home from the hospital after admission due to preterm labor. The woman is to be on complete bed rest and will receive home health care through a local agency to assist her and her family and to monitor her health status. As the home health nurse assigned to this woman, what should your nursing assessment include?

STUDY ACTIVITIES

1. Describe health education topics that would be appropriate in a school setting for elementary students.

2. Shadow a nurse working in a community setting, such as a women's health clinic, birthing center, camp, home care, or health department. Identify the role the nurse plays in the health of women, children, and families in the setting and the community.

3. Arrange for a visit to a community health center that offers services to various cultural groups. Interview the staff about the strategies used to overcome communication barriers and different health care practices for the women and children in these groups.

4. Select one of the websites listed on page 70 and explore the information provided. How could a community-based nurse use this information?

UNIT TWO

WOMEN'S HEALTH THROUGHOUT THE LIFESPAN

ANATOMY AND PHYSIOLOGY OF THE REPRODUCTIVE SYSTEM

KEY TERMS

breasts
cervix
endometrium
estrogen
fallopian tubes
follicle-stimulating
   hormone (FSH)

luteinizing hormone (LH)
menarche
menstruation
ovaries
ovulation
penis
progesterone

testes
uterus
vagina
vulva

LEARNING OBJECTIVES

Upon completion of the chapter, the learner will be able to:

1. Define the key terms used in this chapter.
2. Explain the structure and function of the major external and internal female genital organs.
3. Outline the phases of the menstrual cycle, the dominant hormones involved, and the changes taking place in each phase.
4. Classify external and internal male reproductive structures and the function of each in hormonal regulation.

Linda, 49, started menstruating when she was 12 years old. Her menstrual periods have always been regular, but now she is experiencing irregular, heavier, and longer ones. She wonders if there is something wrong, or if this is normal.

Wow

All nurses should take care of and respect the human body, for it is a wondrous, precision machine.

The reproductive system consists of organs that function in the production of offspring. The female reproductive system produces the female reproductive cells (the eggs, or ova) and contains an organ (uterus) in which development of the fetus takes place; the male reproductive system produces the male reproductive cells (the sperm) and contains an organ (penis) that deposits the sperm within the female. Nurses need to have a thorough understanding of the anatomy and physiology of the male and female reproductive systems to be able to assess the health of these systems, to promote reproductive system health, to care for conditions that might affect the reproductive organs, and to provide client teaching concerning the reproductive system. This chapter will review the female and male reproductive systems and the menstrual cycle as it relates to reproduction.

Female Reproductive Anatomy and Physiology

The female reproductive system is composed of both external and internal reproductive organs.

External Female Reproductive Organs

The external female reproductive organs collectively are called the **vulva** (which means "covering" in Latin). The vulva serves to protect the urethral and vaginal openings and is highly sensitive to touch to increase the female's pleasure during sexual arousal (Coad & Dunstall, 2005). The structures that make up the vulva include the mons pubis, the labia majora and minora, the clitoris, the structures within the vestibule, and the perineum (Fig. 3.1).

Mons Pubis

The mons pubis is the elevated, rounded fleshy prominence over the symphysis pubis. This fatty tissue and skin

is covered with pubic hair after puberty. It protects the symphysis pubis during sexual intercourse.

Labia

The labia majora (large lips), which are relatively large and fleshy, are comparable to the scrotum in males. The labia majora contain sweat and sebaceous (oil-secreting) glands; after puberty, they are covered with hair. Their function is to protect the vaginal opening. The labia minora (small lips) are the delicate hairless inner folds of skin; they can be very small or up to 2 inches wide. They lie just inside the labia majora and surround the openings to the vagina and urethra. The labia minora grow down from the anterior inner part of the labia majora on each side. They are highly vascular and abundant in nerve supply. They lubricate the vulva, swell in response to stimulation, and are highly sensitive.

Clitoris and Prepuce

The clitoris is a small, cylindrical mass of erectile tissue and nerves. It is located at the anterior junction of the labia minora. There are folds above and below the clitoris. The joining of the folds above the clitoris forms the prepuce, a hood-like covering over the clitoris; the junction below the clitoris forms the frenulum.

> ▶ **Take** NOTE!
>
> *The hood-like covering over the clitoris is the site for female circumcision, which is still practiced in some countries by some cultures.*

A rich supply of blood vessels gives the clitoris a pink color. Like the penis, the clitoris is very sensitive to touch, stimulation, and temperature and can become erect. For its small size, it has a generous blood and nerve supply.

FIGURE 3.1 (**A**) The external female reproductive organs. (**B**) Normal appearance of external structures. (Photo by B. Proud.)

There are more free nerve endings of sensory reception located on the clitoris than on any other part of the body, and it is, unsurprisingly, the most erotically sensitive part of the genitalia for most females. Its function is sexual stimulation (Katz, 2007).

▶ *Take* NOTE!

The word "clitoris" is from the Greek word for key; in ancient times the clitoris was thought to be the key to a woman's sexuality.

Vestibule

The vestibule is an oval area enclosed by the labia minora laterally. It is inside the labia minora and outside of the hymen and is perforated by six openings. Opening into the vestibule are the urethra from the urinary bladder, the vagina, and two sets of glands. The opening to the vagina is called the introitus, and the half-moon–shaped area behind the opening is called the fourchette. Through tiny ducts beside the introitus, Bartholin's glands, when stimulated, secrete mucus that supplies lubrication for intercourse. Skene's glands are located on either side of the opening to the urethra. They secrete a small amount of mucus to keep the opening moist and lubricated for the passage of urine (Schuiling & Likis, 2006).

The vaginal opening is surrounded by the hymen (maidenhead). The hymen is a tough, elastic, perforated, mucosa-covered tissue across the vaginal introitus. In a virgin, the hymen may completely cover the opening, but it usually encircles the opening like a tight ring. Because the degree of tightness varies among women, the hymen may tear at the first attempt at intercourse, or it may be so soft and pliable that no tearing occurs. In a woman who is not a virgin, the hymen usually appears as small tags of tissue surrounding the vaginal opening, but the presence or absence of the hymen can neither confirm nor rule out sexual experience (Mattson & Smith, 2004).

▶ *Take* NOTE!

Heavy physical exertion, use of tampons, or injury to the area can alter the appearance of the hymen in girls and women who have not been sexually active.

Perineum

The perineum is the most posterior part of the external female reproductive organs. This external region is located between the vulva and the anus. It is made up of skin, muscle, and fascia. The perineum can become lacerated or incised during childbirth and may need to be repaired with sutures. Incising the perineum area to provide more space for the presenting part is called an episiotomy. Although still a common obstetric procedure, the use of episiotomy has decreased over the past 25 years. The procedure should be applied selectively rather than routinely. An episiotomy can add to postpartum discomfort and perineal trauma and can lead to fecal incontinence (Cunningham et al., 2005).

Internal Female Reproductive Organs

The internal female reproductive organs consist of the vagina, uterus, fallopian tubes, and ovaries. These structures develop and function according to the specific hormone influences that affect fertility and childbearing (Fig. 3.2).

Vagina

The **vagina** is a highly distensible musculomembranous canal situated in front of the rectum and behind the bladder. It is a tubular, fibromuscular organ lined with mucous membrane that lies in a series of transverse folds called rugae. The rugae allow for extreme dilatation of the canal during labor and birth. The vagina is a canal that connects the external genitals to the uterus. It receives the penis and the sperm ejaculated during sexual intercourse, and it serves as an exit passageway for menstrual blood and for the fetus during childbirth. The front and back walls normally touch each other so that there is no space in the vagina except when it is opened (e.g., during a pelvic examination or intercourse). In the adult, the vaginal cavity is 3 to 4 inches long. Muscles that control its diameter surround the lower third of the vagina. The upper two thirds of the vagina lies above these muscles and can be stretched easily. During a woman's reproductive years, the mucosal lining of the vagina has a corrugated appearance and is resistant to bacterial colonization. Before puberty and after menopause (if the woman is not taking estrogen), the mucosa is smooth due to lower levels of estrogen (Dorland, 2007).

The vagina has an acidic environment, which protects it against ascending infections. Antibiotic therapy, douching, perineal hygiene sprays, and deodorants upset the acid balance within the vaginal environment and can predispose women to infections.

Uterus

The **uterus** is a pear-shaped muscular organ at the top of the vagina. It lies behind the bladder and in front of the rectum and is anchored in position by eight ligaments, although it is not firmly attached or adherent to any part of the skeleton. A full bladder tilts the uterus backward; a distended rectum tilts it forward. The uterus alters its position by gravity or with change of posture, and is the size and shape of an inverted pear. It is the site of menstruation, implantation of a fertilized ovum, development of the fetus during pregnancy, and labor. Before the first pregnancy, it measures approximately 3 inches long, 2 inches wide, and 1 inch thick. After a pregnancy, the uterus remains larger than before the pregnancy. After menopause, it becomes smaller and atrophies.

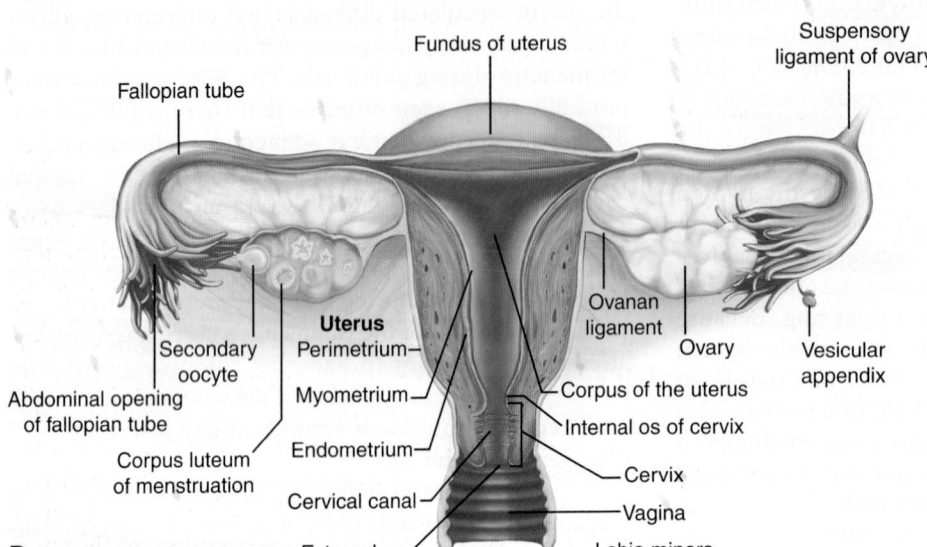

FIGURE 3.2 The internal female reproductive organs. (**A**) Lateral view. (**B**) Anterior view. (Source: Anatomical Chart Company [2001]. *Atlas of human anatomy.* Springhouse, PA: Springhouse.)

The uterine wall is relatively thick and composed of three layers: the endometrium (innermost layer), the myometrium (muscular middle layer), and the perimetrium (outer serosal layer that covers the body of the uterus). The **endometrium** is the mucosal layer that lines the uterine cavity in nonpregnant women. It varies in thickness from 0.5 mm to 5 mm and has an abundant supply of glands and blood vessels (Cunningham et al., 2005). The myometrium makes up the major portion of the uterus and is composed of smooth muscle linked by connective tissue with numerous elastic fibers. During pregnancy, the upper myometrium undergoes marked hypertrophy, but there is limited change in the cervical muscle content.

Anatomic subdivisions of the uterus include the convex portion above the uterine tubes (the fundus); the central portion (the corpus or body) between the fundus and the cervix; and the cervix, or neck, which opens into the vagina.

Cervix

The **cervix**, the lower part of the uterus, opens into the vagina and has a channel that allows sperm to enter the uterus and menstrual discharge to exit. It is composed of fibrous connective tissue. During a pelvic examination, the part of the cervix that protrudes into the upper end of the vagina can be visualized. Like the vagina, this part of the cervix is covered by mucosa, which is smooth, firm, and doughnut-shaped, with a visible central opening called the external os (Fig. 3.3). Before childbirth, the external cervical os is a small, regular, oval opening.

FIGURE 3.3 Appearance of normal cervix. Note: This is the cervix of a multipara female. (Photo by B. Proud.)

FIGURE 3.4 (**A**) Nulliparous cervical os. (**B**) Parous cervical os.

After childbirth, the opening is converted into a transverse slit that resembles lips (Fig. 3.4). Except during menstruation or ovulation, the cervix is usually a good barrier against bacteria. The cervix has an alkaline environment, which protects the sperm from the acidic environment in the vagina.

The canal or channel of the cervix is lined with mucus-secreting glands. This mucus is thick and impenetrable to sperm until just before the ovaries release an egg (**ovulation**). At ovulation, the consistency of the mucus changes so that sperm can swim through it, allowing fertilization. At the same time, the mucus-secreting glands of the cervix actually become able to store live sperm for 2 or 3 days. These sperm can later move up through the corpus and into the fallopian tubes to fertilize the egg; thus, intercourse 1 or 2 days before ovulation can lead to pregnancy. Because some women do not ovulate consistently, pregnancy can occur at varying times after the last menstrual period. The channel in the cervix is too narrow for the fetus to pass through during pregnancy, but during labor it stretches to let the newborn through.

Corpus

The corpus, or the main body of the uterus, is a highly muscular organ that enlarges to hold the fetus during pregnancy. The inner lining of the corpus (endometrium) undergoes cyclic changes as a result of the changing levels of hormones secreted by the ovaries: it is thickest during the part of the menstrual cycle in which a fertilized egg would be expected to enter the uterus and is thinnest just after menstruation. If fertilization does not take place

during this cycle, most of the endometrium is shed and bleeding occurs, resulting in the monthly period. If fertilization does take place, the embryo attaches to the wall of the uterus, where it becomes embedded in the endometrium (about 1 week after fertilization); this process is called implantation (Heffner & Schust, 2006). Menstruation then ceases during the 40 weeks (280 days) of pregnancy. During labor, the muscular walls of the corpus contract to push the baby through the cervix and into the vagina.

Fallopian Tubes

The **fallopian tubes** are hollow, cylindrical structures that extend 2 to 3 inches from the upper edges of the uterus toward the ovaries. Each tube is about 7 to 10 cm long (4 inches) and approximately 0.7 cm in diameter. The end of each tube flares into a funnel shape, providing a large opening for the egg to fall into when it is released from the ovary. Cilia (beating, hair-like extensions on cells) line the fallopian tube and the muscles in the tube's wall. The fallopian tubes convey the ovum from the ovary to the uterus and sperm from the uterus toward the ovary. This movement is accomplished via ciliary action and peristalsis. If sperm is present in the fallopian tube as a result of sexual intercourse or artificial insemination, fertilization of the ovum can occur in the distal portion of the tube. If the egg is fertilized, it will divide over a period of 4 days while it moves slowly down the fallopian tube and into the uterus.

Ovaries

The **ovaries** are a set of paired glands resembling unshelled almonds set in the pelvic cavity below and to either side of the umbilicus. They are usually pearl-colored and oblong. They are homologous to the testes. Each ovary weighs from 2 to 5 grams and is about 4 cm long, 2 cm wide, and 1 cm thick (Speroff & Fritz, 2005). The ovaries are not attached to the fallopian tubes but are suspended nearby from several ligaments, which help hold them in position. The development and the release of the ovum and the secretion of the hormones estrogen and progesterone are the two primary functions of the ovary. The ovaries link the reproductive system to the body's system of endocrine glands, as they produce the ova (eggs) and secrete, in cyclic fashion, the female sex hormones estrogen and progesterone. After an ovum matures, it passes into the fallopian tubes.

Breasts

The two mammary glands, or **breasts**, are accessory organs of the female reproductive system that are specialized to secrete milk following pregnancy. They overlie the pectoralis major muscles and extend from the second to the sixth ribs and from the sternum to the axilla. Each breast has a nipple located near the tip, which is surrounded by a circular area of pigmented skin called the areola. Each breast is composed of approximately 9 lobes (the number can range between 4 and 18), which contain glands (alveolar) and a duct (lactiferous) that leads to the nipple and opens to the outside (Fig. 3.5). The lobes are separated by dense connective and adipose tissues, which also help support the weight of the breasts (Ramsay, Kent, Hartmann & Hartmann, 2005).

During pregnancy, placental estrogen and progesterone stimulate the development of the mammary glands. Because of this hormonal activity, the breasts may double in size during pregnancy. At the same time, glandular tissue replaces the adipose tissue of the breasts.

Following childbirth and the expulsion of the placenta, levels of placental hormones (progesterone and lactogen) fall rapidly, and the action of prolactin (milk-producing hormone) is no longer inhibited. Prolactin stimulates the production of milk within a few days after childbirth, but in the interim, a dark yellow fluid called colostrum is secreted. Colostrum contains more minerals and protein, but less sugar and fat, than mature breast milk. Colostrum secretion may continue for approximately a week after childbirth, with gradual conversion to mature milk. Colostrum is rich in maternal antibodies, especially immunoglobulin A (IgA), which offers protection for the newborn against enteric pathogens.

Female Sexual Response

With sexual stimulation, tissues in the clitoris and breasts and around the vaginal orifice fill with blood and the erectile tissues swell. At the same time, the vagina begins to expand and elongate to accommodate the penis. As part of the whole vasocongestive reaction, the labia majora and minor swell and darken. As sexual stimulation intensifies, the vestibular glands secrete mucus to moisten and lubricate the tissues to facilitate insertion of the penis.

Hormones play an integral role in the female sexual response as well. Adequate estrogen and testosterone must be available for the brain to sense incoming arousal stimuli. Research indicates that estrogen preserves the vascular function of female sex organs and affects genital sensation. It also is believed to promote blood flow to these areas during stimulation. Testosterone is thought to be the hormone of sexual desire in women (McKinney, 2007).

The zenith of intense stimulation is orgasm, the spasmodic and involuntary contractions of the muscles in the region of the vulva, the uterus, and the vagina that produce a pleasurable sensation to the woman. Typically the woman feels warm and relaxed after an orgasm. Within a short time after orgasm, the two physiologic mechanisms that created the sexual response, vasocongestion and muscle contraction, rapidly dissipate.

The Female Reproductive Cycle

The female reproductive cycle is a complex process that encompasses an intricate series of chemical secretions and reactions to produce the ultimate potential for fertility and birth. The female reproductive cycle is a general term encompassing the ovarian cycle, the endometrial cycle, the hormonal changes that regulate them, and the cyclical changes in the breasts. The endometrium, ovaries, pituitary gland, and hypothalamus are all involved in the cyclic changes that help to prepare the body for fertilization. Absence of fertilization results in menstruation, the monthly shedding of the uterine lining. Menstruation

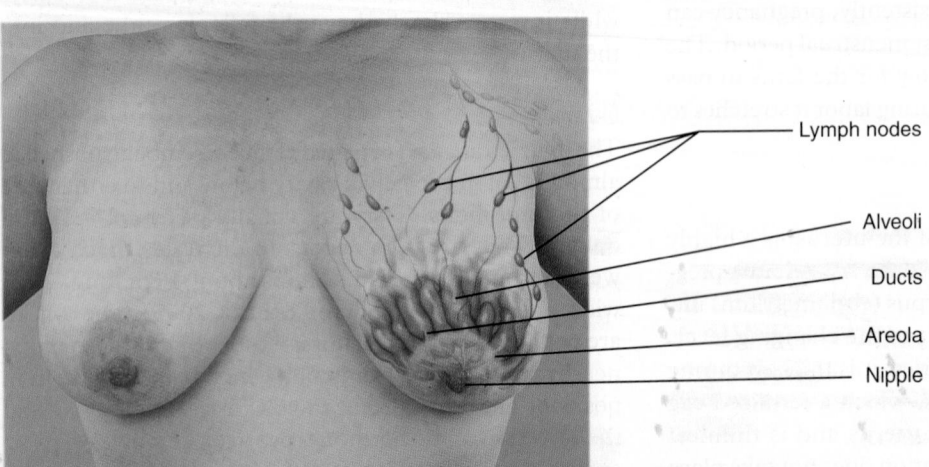

Lymph nodes

Alveoli

Ducts

Areola

Nipple

FIGURE 3.5 Anatomy of the breasts. (Photo by B. Proud.)

marks the beginning and end of each menstrual cycle. Menopause is the naturally occurring cessation of regular menstrual cycles.

Menstruation

Menstruation is the normal, predictable physiologic process whereby the inner lining of the uterus (endometrium) is expelled by the body. Typically, this occurs monthly. Menstruation has many effects on girls and women, including emotional and self-image issues. In the United States, the average age at **menarche** (the start of menstruation in females) is 12.8 years, with a range between 8 and 18. Genetics is the most important factor in determining the age at which menarche starts, but geographic location, nutrition, weight, general health, nutrition, and psychological factors are also important (Shelby & Ruocco, 2007). Pubertal events preceding the first menses have an orderly progression: thelarche, the development of breast buds; adrenarche, the appearance of pubic and then axillary hair, followed by a growth spurt; and menarche (occurring about 2 years after the start of breast development). In healthy pubertal girls, the menstrual period varies in flow heaviness and may remain irregular in occurrence for up to 2 years following menarche. After that time, the regular menstrual cycle should be established. Most women will experience 300 to 400 menstrual cycles within their lifetime (Diaz, Laufer & Breech, 2006). Normal, regular menstrual cycles vary in frequency from 21 to 36 days (with the average cycle lasting 28 days), bleeding lasts 3 to 7 days, and blood loss averages 20 to 80 mL (Schuiling & Likis, 2006). Irregular menses can be associated with irregular ovulation, stress, disease, and hormonal imbalances (Cunningham et al., 2005).

*T*hink back to Linda, who was introduced at the beginning of the chapter. What questions might need to be asked to assess her condition? What laboratory work might be anticipated to validate her heavier flow?

Although menstruation is a normal process, various world cultures have taken a wide variety of attitudes toward it, seeing it as everything from a sacred time to an unclean time. In a society where menstruation is viewed negatively, nurses can help women develop a more positive image of this natural physiologic process.

▶ *Take* NOTE!

Knowledge about menstruation has increased significantly and attitudes have changed since early times, when many cultures saw it as "unclean." What was once discussed only behind closed doors is discussed openly today.

Reproductive Cycle

The reproductive cycle, also referred to as the menstrual cycle, results from a functional hypothalamic–pituitary–ovarian axis and a precise sequencing of hormones that lead to ovulation. If conception doesn't occur, menses ensues. The ranges of normal menstrual cycles are as follows:

- Cycle length: 21 to 36 days
- Duration of flow: 3 to 7 days
- Amount of flow: 20 to 80 mL

The female reproductive cycle involves two cycles that occur simultaneously: the ovarian cycle, during which ovulation occurs, and the endometrial cycle, during which menstruation occurs. Ovulation divides these two cycles at midcycle. Ovulation occurs when the ovum is released from its follicle; after leaving the ovary, the ovum enters the fallopian tube and journeys toward the uterus. If sperm fertilizes the ovum during its journey, pregnancy occurs. Figure 3.6 summarizes the menstrual cycle.

Ovarian Cycle

The ovarian cycle is the series of events associated with a developing oocyte (ovum or egg) within the ovaries. While men manufacture sperm daily, often into advanced age, women are born with a single lifetime supply of ova that are released from the ovaries gradually throughout the childbearing years. In the female ovary, 2 million oocytes are present at birth, and about 400,000 follicles are still present at puberty. The excess follicles are depleted during the childbearing years, with only 400 follicles ovulated during the reproductive period (Speroff & Fritz, 2005). The ovarian cycle begins when the follicular cells (ovum and surrounding cells) swell and the maturation process starts. The maturing follicle at this stage is called a graafian follicle. The ovary raises many follicles monthly, but usually only one follicle matures to reach ovulation. The ovarian cycle consists of three phases: the follicular phase, ovulation, and the luteal phase.

Follicular Phase

This phase is so named because it is when the follicles in the ovary grow and form a mature egg. This phase starts on day 1 of the menstrual cycle and continues until ovulation, approximately 10 to 14 days later. The follicular phase is not consistent in duration because of the time variations in follicular development. These variations account for the differences in menstrual cycle lengths (Hackley, Kriebs & Rousseau, 2007). The hypothalamus is the initiator of this phase. Increasing levels of estrogen secreted from the maturing follicular cells and the continued growth of the dominant follicle cell induce proliferation of the endometrium and myometrium. This thickening of the uterine lining supports an implanted ovum if pregnancy occurs.

Prompted by the hypothalamus, the pituitary gland releases follicle-stimulating hormone (FSH), which stimulates the ovary to produce 5 to 20 immature follicles. Each follicle houses an immature oocyte or egg. The follicle that

FIGURE 3.6 Menstrual cycle summary based on a 28-day (average) menstrual cycle.

is targeted to mature fully will soon rupture and expel a mature oocyte in the process of ovulation. A surge in luteinizing hormone (LH) from the anterior pituitary gland is actually responsible for affecting the final development and subsequent rupture of the mature follicle.

Ovulation

At ovulation, a mature follicle ruptures in response to a surge of LH, releasing a mature oocyte (ovum). This usually occurs on day 14 in a 28-day cycle. When ovulation occurs, there is a drop in estrogen. Typically ovulation takes place approximately 10 to 12 hours after the LH peak and 24 to 36 hours after estrogen levels peak (Speroff & Fritz, 2005). The distal ends of the fallopian tubes become active near the time of ovulation and create currents that help carry the ovum into the uterus. The lifespan of the ovum is only about 24 hours; unless it meets a sperm on its journey within that time, it will die.

During ovulation, the cervix produces thin, clear, stretchy, slippery mucus that is designed to help the sperm travel up through the cervix to meet the ovum for fertil-

ization. The one constant, whether a women's cycle is 28 days or 120 days, is that ovulation takes place 14 days before menstruation (Shelby & Ruocco, 2007).

▶ *Take* NOTE!

Some women can feel a pain on one side of the abdomen around the time the egg is released. This midcycle pain is called mittelschmerz.

Luteal Phase

The luteal phase begins at ovulation and lasts until the menstrual phase of the next cycle. It typically occurs day 15 through day 28 of a 28-day cycle. After the follicle ruptures as it releases the egg, it closes and forms a corpus luteum. The corpus luteum secretes increasing amounts of the hormone progesterone, which interacts with the endometrium to prepare it for implantation. At the beginning of the luteal phase, progesterone induces the endometrial glands to secrete glycogen, mucus, and other substances. These glands become tortuous and have large lumens due to increased secretory activity. The progesterone secreted by the corpus luteum causes the temperature of the body to rise slightly until the start of the next period. A significant increase in temperature, usually 0.5 to 1 degrees Fahrenheit, is generally seen within a day or two after ovulation has occurred; the temperature remains elevated for 12 to 16 days, until menstruation begins (Chandran, 2007). This rise in temperature can be plotted on a graph and gives an indication of when ovulation has occurred. In the absence of fertilization, the corpus luteum begins to degenerate and consequently ovarian hormone levels decrease. As estrogen and progesterone levels decrease, the endometrium undergoes involution. In a 28-day cycle, menstruation then begins approximately 14 days after ovulation in the absence of pregnancy. FSH and LH are generally at their lowest levels during the luteal phase and highest during the follicular phase.

▶ *Consider* THIS!

We had been married 2 years when my husband and I decided to start a family. I began thinking back to my high-school biology class and tried to remember about ovulation and what to look for. I also used the Internet to find the answers I was seeking. As I was reading, it all started to come into place. During ovulation, a woman's cervical mucus increases and she experiences a wet sensation for several days midcycle. The mucus also becomes stretchable during this time. In addition, body temperature rises slightly and then falls if no conception takes place. Armed with this knowledge, I began to check my temperature daily before arising and began to monitor the consistency of my cervical mucus. I figured that monitoring these two signs of ovulation could help me discover the best time to conceive. After 6 months of trying without results, I wondered what I was doing wrong. Did I really understand my body's reproductive activity?

What additional suggestions might the nurse offer this woman in her journey to conception? What community resources might be available to assist this couple? How does knowledge of the reproductive system help nurses take care of couples who are trying to become pregnant?

Endometrial Cycle

The endometrial cycle occurs in response to cyclic hormonal changes. The four phases of the endometrial cycle are the proliferative phase, secretory phase, ischemic phase, and menstrual phase.

Proliferative Phase

The proliferative phase starts with enlargement of the endometrial glands in response to increasing amounts of estrogen. The blood vessels become dilated and the endometrium increases in thickness dramatically from 0.5 to 5 mm in height and increases eight-fold in thickness in preparation for implantation of the fertilized ovum (Heffner & Schust, 2006). Cervical mucus becomes thin, clear, stretchy, and more alkaline, making it more favorable to sperm to enhance the opportunity for fertilization. The proliferative phase starts on about day 5 of the menstrual cycle and lasts to the time of ovulation. This phase depends on estrogen stimulation resulting from ovarian follicles, and this phase coincides with the follicular phase of the ovarian cycle.

Secretory Phase

The secretory phase begins at ovulation to about 3 days before the next menstrual period. Under the influence of progesterone released by the corpus luteum after ovulation, the endometrium becomes thickened and more vascular (growth of the spiral arteries) and glandular (secreting more glycogen and lipids). These dramatic changes are all in preparation for implantation, if it were to occur. This phase typically lasts from day 15 (after ovulation) to day 28 and coincides with the luteal phase of the ovarian cycle. The secretory phase doesn't take place if ovulation has not occurred.

Ischemic Phase

If fertilization does not occur, the ischemic phase begins. Estrogen and progesterone levels drop sharply during this phase as the corpus luteum starts to degenerate. Changes in the endometrium occur with spasm of the arterioles, resulting in ischemia of the basal layer. The ischemia leads to shedding of the endometrium down to the basal layer, and menstrual flow begins.

Menstrual Phase

The menstrual phase begins as the spiral arteries rupture secondary to ischemia, releasing blood into the uterus, and the sloughing of the endometrial lining begins. If fertilization does not take place, the corpus luteum degenerates. As a result, both estrogen and progesterone levels fall and the thickened endometrial lining sloughs away from the uterine wall and passes out via the vagina. The beginning of the menstrual flow marks the end of one menstrual cycle and the start of a new one. Most women report bleeding for an average of 3 to 7 days. The amount of menstrual flow varies, but approximately 6 to 8 ounces in volume per cycle is average (Alexander et al., 2007).

Menstrual Cycle Hormones

The menstrual cycle involves a complex interaction of hormones. The predominant hormones include gonadotropin-releasing hormone, FSH, LH, estrogen, progesterone, and prostaglandins. Box 3.1 summarizes menstrual cycle hormones.

- Luteinizing hormone (LH) rises and stimulates the follicle to produce estrogen.
- As estrogen is produced by the follicle, estrogen levels rise, inhibiting the output of LH.
- Ovulation occurs after an LH surge damages the estrogen-producing cells, resulting in a decline in estrogen.
- The LH surge results in establishment of the corpus luteum, which produces estrogen and progesterone.
- Estrogen and progesterone levels rise, suppressing LH output.
- Lack of LH promotes degeneration of the corpus luteum.
- Cessation of the corpus luteum means a decline in estrogen and progesterone output.
- The decline of the ovarian hormones ends their negative effect on the secretion of LH.
- LH is secreted, and the menstrual cycle begins again.

Gonadotropin-Releasing Hormone

Gonadotropin-releasing hormone (GnRH) is secreted from the hypothalamus in a pulsatile manner throughout the reproductive cycle. It pulsates slowly during the follicular phase and increases during the luteal phase. GnRH induces the release of FSH and LH to assist with ovulation.

Follicle-Stimulating Hormone

Follicle-stimulating hormone (FSH) is secreted by the anterior pituitary gland and is primarily responsible for the maturation of the ovarian follicle. FSH secretion is highest and most important during the first week of the follicular phase of the reproductive cycle.

Luteinizing Hormone

Luteinizing hormone (LH) is secreted by the anterior pituitary gland and is required for both the final maturation of preovulatory follicles and luteinization of the ruptured follicle. As a result, estrogen production declines and progesterone secretion continues. Thus, estrogen levels fall a day before ovulation, and progesterone levels begin to rise.

Estrogen

Estrogen is secreted by the ovaries and is crucial for the development and maturation of the follicle. Estrogen is predominant at the end of the proliferative phase, directly preceding ovulation. After ovulation, estrogen levels drop sharply as progesterone dominates. In the endometrial cycle, estrogen induces proliferation of the endometrial glands. Estrogen also causes the uterus to increase in size and weight because of increased glycogen, amino acids, electrolytes, and water. Blood supply is expanded as well.

Progesterone

Progesterone is secreted by the corpus luteum. Progesterone levels increase just before ovulation and peak 5 to 7 days after ovulation. During the luteal phase, progesterone induces swelling and increased secretion of the endometrium. This hormone is often called the hormone of pregnancy because of its calming effect (reduces uterine contractions) on the uterus, allowing pregnancy to be maintained.

Prostaglandins

Prostaglandins are a closely related group of oxygenated fatty acids that are produced by the endometrium, with a variety of effects throughout the body. Although they have regulatory effects and are sometimes called hormones, prostaglandins are not technically hormones because they are produced by all tissues rather than by special glands (Speroff & Fritz, 2005). Prostaglandins increase during follicular maturation and play a key role in ovulation by freeing the ovum inside the graafian follicle. Large amounts of prostaglandins are found in menstrual blood. Research is ongoing as to the various roles prostaglandins have on the menstrual cycle (Cunningham et al., 2005).

Menopause

Perimenopause and menopause are biologic markers of the transition from young adulthood to middle age. Neither of these is a symptom or disease, but rather a natural maturing of the reproductive system.

During the perimenopausal years (2 to 8 years prior to menopause) women may experience physical changes associated with decreasing estrogen levels, which may include vasomotor symptoms of hot flashes, irregular menstrual cycles, sleep disruptions, forgetfulness, irritability, mood disturbances, decreased vaginal lubrication, fatigue, vaginal atrophy, and depression (Shifren & Schiff, 2007).

Menopause refers to the cessation of regular menstrual cycles. This naturally occurring phase of every woman's life marks the end of menstruation and childbearing capacity. The average age of natural menopause—defined as 1 year without a menstrual period—is 51 (Alexander et al., 2007). As the average life expectancy for women increases, the number of women reaching and living in menopause has escalated. Most women can expect to spend more than one third of their lives beyond menopause. It is usually marked by atrophy of the breasts, uterus, fallopian tubes, and ovaries (Curran & Bachmann, 2006).

Many women pass through menopause without untoward symptoms. These women remain active and in good health with little interruption of their daily routines. Other women experience vasomotor symptoms, which give rise to sensations of heat, cold, sweating, headache, insomnia, and irritability (Kessenich, 2007). Until recently, hormone therapy was the mainstay of menopause pharmacotherapy, but with the recent results of the Women's Health Initiative trial, the use of hormone therapy has become controversial. Many women have turned to nontraditional remedies to manage their menopausal symptoms. Common herbal remedies used include Dong Quai, black cohosh, melatonin, ginseng, and St. John's wort. Research to validate their efficacy, safety, and potential harmful effects is lacking at this time, and much of the efficacy is largely anecdotal (Kessenich, 2007). Nurses can play a major role in assisting menopausal women by educating and counseling them about the multitude of options available for disease prevention, treatment for menopausal symptoms, and health promotion during this time of change in their lives. Menopause should be an opportunity for women to strive for a healthy, long life, and nurses can help to make this opportunity a reality. (See Chapter 4 for more information about menopause.)

Recall Linda, who was experiencing changes in her menstrual patterns. Which hormones might be changing, and which systems might they affect? What approach should the nurse take to enlighten Linda about what is happening to her?

Male Reproductive Anatomy and Physiology

The male reproductive system, like that of the female, consists of those organs that facilitate reproduction. The male organs are specialized to produce and maintain the male sex cells, or sperm; to transport them, along with supporting fluids, to the female reproductive system; and to secrete the male hormone testosterone. The organs of the male reproductive system include the two testes (where sperm cells and testosterone are made), the penis, the scrotum, and the accessory organs (epididymis, vas deferens, seminal vesicles, ejaculatory duct, urethra, bulbourethral glands, and prostate gland).

External Male Reproductive Organs

The penis and the scrotum form the external genitalia in the male (Fig. 3.7).

Penis

The **penis** is the organ for copulation and serves as the outlet for both sperm and urine. The skin of the penis is thin, with no hairs. The prepuce (foreskin) is a circular fold of skin that extends over the glans unless it is removed by circumcision shortly after birth. The urinary meatus, located at the tip of the penis, serves as the external opening to the urethra (Fig. 3.8). The penis is composed mostly of erectile tissue. Most of the body of the penis consists of three cylindrical spaces (sinuses) of erectile tissue. The two larger

FIGURE 3.7 The external male reproductive organs. (Photo by B. Proud.)

ones, the corpora cavernosa, are side by side. The third sinus, the corpus spongiosum, surrounds the urethra. Erection results when nerve impulses from the autonomic nervous system dilate the arteries of the penis, allowing arterial blood to flow into the erectile tissues of the organ.

Scrotum

The scrotum is the thin-skinned sac that surrounds and protects the testes. The scrotum also acts as a climate-control system for the testes, because they need to be slightly cooler than body temperature to allow normal sperm development. The cremaster muscles in the scrotal wall relax or contract to allow the testes to hang farther from the body to cool or to be pulled closer to the body for warmth or protection (Ceo, 2006). A medial septum divides the scrotum into two chambers, each of which encloses a testis.

Internal Male Reproductive Organs

The internal structures include the testes, the ductal system, and accessory glands (Fig. 3.9).

FIGURE 3.8 The urinary meatus. (Photo by B. Proud.)

FIGURE 3.9 Lateral view of the internal male reproductive organs. (Source: Anatomical Chart Company. [2001]. *Atlas of human anatomy.* Springhouse, PA: Springhouse.)

Testes

The **testes** are oval bodies the size of large olives that lie in the scrotum; usually the left testis hangs a little lower than the right one. The testes have two functions: producing sperm and synthesizing testosterone (the primary male sex hormone). Sperm is produced in the seminiferous tubules of the testes. Similar to the female reproductive system, the anterior pituitary releases the gonadotropins, FSH and LH. These hormones stimulate the testes to produce testosterone, which assists in maintaining spermatogenesis, increases sperm production by the seminiferous tubules, and stimulates production of seminal fluid (London, Ladewig, Ball & Bindler 2007). The epididymis, which lies against the testes, is a coiled tube almost 20 feet long. It collects sperm from the testes and provides the space and environment for sperm to mature (Fig. 3.10).

The Ductal System

The vas deferens is a cordlike duct that transports sperm from the epididymis. One such duct travels from each testis up to the back of the prostate and enters the urethra to form the ejaculatory ducts. Other structures, such as blood vessels and nerves, also travel along with each vas deferens and together form the spermatic cord. The urethra is the terminal duct of the reproductive and urinary systems, serving as a passageway for semen (fluid containing sperm) and urine. It passes through the prostate gland and the penis and opens to the outside.

Accessory Glands

The seminal vesicles, which produce nutrient seminal fluid, and the prostate gland, which produces alkaline prostatic fluid, are both connected to the ejaculatory duct leading into the urethra. The paired seminal vesicles are

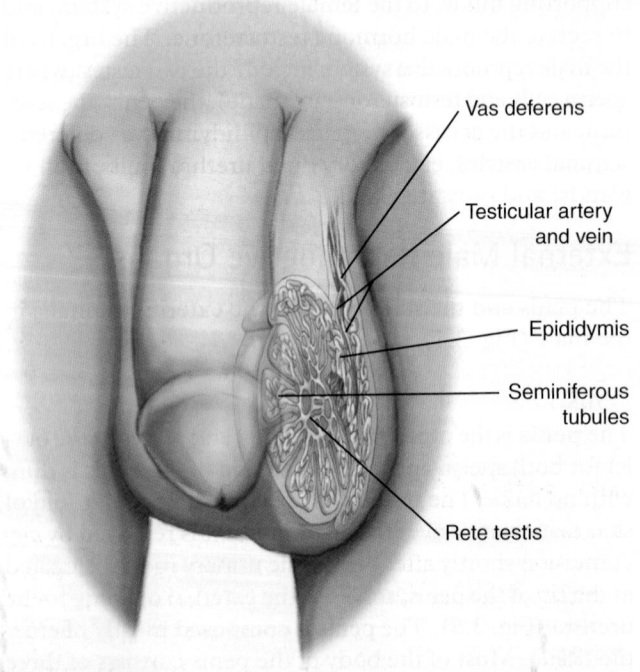

FIGURE 3.10 Internal structures of a testis.

convoluted pouch-like structures lying posterior to, and at the base of, the urinary bladder in front of the rectum. They secrete an alkaline fluid that contains fructose and prostaglandins. The fructose supplies energy to the sperm on its journey to meet the ovum, and the prostaglandins assist in sperm mobility.

The prostate gland lies just under the bladder in the pelvis and surrounds the middle portion of the urethra. Usually the size of a walnut, this gland enlarges with age. The prostate and the seminal vesicles above it produce fluid that nourishes the sperm. This fluid provides most of the volume of semen, the secretion in which the sperm is expelled during ejaculation. Other fluid that makes up the semen comes from the vas deferens and from mucous glands in the head of the penis.

The bulbourethral glands (Cowper's glands) are two small structures about the size of peas, located inferior to the prostate gland. They are composed of several tubes whose epithelial linings secrete a mucus-like fluid. It is released in response to sexual stimulation and lubricates the head of the penis in preparation for sexual intercourse. Their existence is said to be constant, but they gradually diminish in size with advancing age.

Male Sexual Response

With sexual stimulation, the arteries leading to the penis dilate and increase blood flow into erectile tissues. At the same time, the erectile tissue compresses the veins of the penis, reducing blood flow away from the penis. Blood accumulates, causing the penis to swell and elongate and producing an erection. As in women, the culmination of sexual stimulation is an orgasm, a pleasurable feeling of physiologic and psychological release.

Orgasm is accompanied by emission (movement of sperm from the testes and fluids from the accessory glands) into the urethra, where it is mixed to form semen. As the urethra fills with semen, the base of the erect penis contracts, which increases pressure and forces the semen through the urethra to the outside (ejaculation). During ejaculation, the ducts of the testes, epididymis, and vas deferens contract, causing expulsion of sperm into the urethra, where the sperm mixes with the seminal and prostatic fluids. These substances, together with mucus secreted by accessory glands, form the semen, which is discharged from the urethra.

■■■ Key Concepts

■ The female reproductive system produces the female reproductive cells (the eggs, or ova) and contains an organ (uterus) where the fetus develops. The male reproductive system produces the male reproductive cells (the sperm) and contains an organ (penis) that deposits the sperm within the female.

■ The internal female reproductive organs consist of the vagina, the uterus, the fallopian tubes, and the ovaries. The external female reproductive organs make up the vulva. These include the mons pubis, the labia majora and minora, the clitoris, structures within the vestibule, and the perineum.

■ The breasts are accessory organs of the female reproductive system that are specialized to secrete milk following pregnancy.

■ The main function of the reproductive cycle is to stimulate growth of a follicle to release an egg and prepare a site for implantation if fertilization occurs.

■ Menstruation, the monthly shedding of the uterine lining, marks the beginning and end of the cycle if fertilization does not occur.

■ The ovarian cycle is the series of events associated with a developing oocyte (ovum or egg) within the ovaries.

■ At ovulation, a mature follicle ruptures in response to a surge of LH, releasing a mature oocyte (ovum).

■ The endometrial cycle is divided into four phases: the follicular or proliferative phase, the luteal or secretory phase, the ischemic phase, and the menstrual phase.

■ The menstrual cycle involves a complex interaction of hormones. The predominant hormones are gonadotropin-releasing hormone (GnRH), follicle-stimulating hormone (FSH), luteinizing hormone (LH), estrogen, progesterone, and prostaglandins.

■ The organs of the male reproductive system include the two testes (where sperm cells and testosterone are made), penis, scrotum, and accessory organs (epididymis, vas deferens, seminal vesicles, ejaculatory ducts, urethra, bulbourethral glands, and prostate gland).

REFERENCES

Alexander, L. L., LaRosa, J. H., Bader, H., & Garfield, S. (2007). *New dimensions in women's health* (4th ed.). Boston: Jones and Bartlett.

Ceo, P. D. (2006) Assessment of the male reproductive system. *Urologic Nursing, 26*(4), 290–296.

Chandran, L. (2007) Menstruation disorders. *eMedicine.* Available at: http://www.emedicine.com/ped/topic2781.htm

Coad, J., & Dunstall, M. (2005). *Anatomy and physiology for midwives* (2nd ed.). St. Louis, MO: Elsevier Health Sciences.

Cunningham, F. G., Leveno, K. J., Bloom, S. L., et al. (2005). *Williams obstetrics* (22nd ed.). New York: McGraw-Hill.

Curran, D., & Bachmann, G. (2006). Menopause. *eMedicine.* Available at: http://www.emedicine.com/med/topic3289.htm

Diaz, A., Laufer, M. R., & Breech, L. L. (2006). Menstruation in girls and adolescents: Using the menstrual cycle as a vital sign. *Pediatrics, 118*(5), 2245–2250.

Dorland, D. (2007) *Dorland's illustrated medical dictionary* (31st ed.). St. Louis, MO: Elsevier Saunders.

Hackley, B., Kriebs, J. M., & Rousseau, M. E. (2007). *Primary care of women: A guide for midwives and women's health providers.* Sudbury, MA: Jones and Bartlett Publishers.

Heffner, L. J., & Schust, D. J. (2006). *Reproductive system at a glance* (2nd ed.). Ames, IA: Blackwell Publishing Professional.

Katz, A. (2007) Sexuality and women. *Nursing for Women's Health, 11*(1), 37–43.

Kessenich, C. R. (2007). Inevitable menopause. *Nursing Spectrum*. Available at: http://nsweb.nursingspectrum.com/ce/ce232c.htm

London, M. L., Ladewig, P. W., Ball, J. W., & Bindler, R. C. (2007). *Maternal and child nursing care* (2nd ed.). Upper Saddle River, NJ: Pearson Prentice Hall.

Mattson, S., & Smith, J. E. (2004). *Core curriculum for maternal-newborn nursing* (3rd ed.). St Louis: Elsevier Saunders.

McKinney, L. N. (2007). Low libido in postmenopausal women. *Advance for Nurse Practitioners, 15*(1), 28–35.

Ramsay, D. T., Kent, J. C., Hartmann, R. A., & Hartmann, P. E. (2005). Anatomy of the lactating human breast redefined with ultrasound imaging. *Journal of Anatomy, 206*(6), 525–534.

Schuiling, K. D., & Likis, F. E. (2006). *Women's gynecologic health*. Sudbury, MA: Jones and Bartlett Publishers.

Shelby, K., & Ruocco, E. (2007). Women's hormones across the life span. *Nursing Spectrum*. Available at: http://www.nurse.com/ce/course.html?CCID=2199

Shifren, J. L., & Schiff, I. (2007). Menopause. In R. E. Rakel & E. T. Bope, eds., *Conn's current therapy 2007* (Chapter 16, pp. 1243–1244). Philadelphia: Saunders Elsevier.

Speroff, L., & Fritz, M. A. (2005). *Clinical gynecologic endocrinology and infertility* (7th ed.). Philadelphia: Lippincott Williams & Wilkins.

WEBSITES

Alan Guttmacher Institute: www.agi-usa.org
American Society for Reproductive Medicine: www.asrm.com
Kinsey Institution: www.indiana.edu/~kinsey/index.html
National Women's Health Information Center: www.4woman.gov
National Women's Health Resource Center: www.healthywomen.org
Sexuality Information of the United States: www.siecus.org
Society for Women's Health Research: www.womens-health.org

CHAPTER WORKSHEET

MULTIPLE CHOICE QUESTIONS

1. The predominant anterior pituitary hormones that orchestrate the menstrual cycle include:

   a. Thyroid-stimulating hormone (TSH)

   b. Follicle-stimulating hormone (FSH)

   c. Corticotropin-releasing hormone (CRH)

   d. Gonadotropin-releasing hormone (GnRH)

2. Which glands are located on either side of the female urethra and secrete mucus to keep the opening moist and lubricated for urination?

   a. Cowper's

   b. Bartholin's

   c. Skene's

   d. Seminal

3. What event occurs during the proliferative phase of the menstrual cycle?

   a. Menstrual flow starts

   b. Growth hormone is secreted

   c. Ovulation occurs

   d. Progesterone secretion peaks

4. Which hormone is produced in high levels to prepare the endometrium for implantation just after ovulation by the corpus luteum?

   a. Estrogen

   b. Prostaglandins

   c. Prolactin

   d. Progesterone

5. Sperm maturation and storage in the male reproductive system occurs in the:

   a. Testes

   b. Vas deferens

   c. Epididymis

   d. Seminal vesicles

CRITICAL THINKING EXERCISE

1. The school nurse was asked to speak to a 10th-grade biology class about menstruation. The teacher felt that the students don't understand this monthly event and wanted to dispel some myths about it. After the nurse explains the factors influencing the menses, one girl asks, "Could someone get pregnant if she had sex during her period?"

   a. How should the nurse respond to this question?

   b. What factor regarding the menstrual cycle was not clarified?

   c. What additional topics might this question lead to that might be discussed?

STUDY ACTIVITIES

1. Select a website from the list above and visit it to find information concerning a topic of interest regarding women's health. Be prepared to discuss it in class.

2. List the predominant hormones and their function in the menstrual cycle.

3. The ovarian cycle describes the series of events associated with the development of the _____ within the ovaries.

4. Sperm cells and the male hormone testosterone are made in which of the following structures? Select all that apply.

   a. Vas deferens

   b. Penis

   c. Scrotum

   d. Ejaculatory ducts

   e. Prostate gland

   f. Testes

   g. Seminiferous tubules

   h. Bulbourethral glands

COMMON REPRODUCTIVE ISSUES

KEY TERMS

abortion
abstinence
amenorrhea
basal body temperature (BBT)
cervical cap
cervical mucus ovulation method
coitus interruptus
condoms
contraception
contraceptive sponge
Depo-Provera

diaphragm
dysfunctional uterine bleeding (DUB)
dysmenorrhea
emergency contraception (EC)
endometriosis
fertility awareness
implant
infertility
lactational amenorrhea method (LAM)
Lunelle injection

menopause
oral contraceptives
premenstrual syndrome (PMS)
Standard Days Method (SDM)
sterilization
symptothermal method
transdermal patch
tubal ligation
vaginal ring
vasectomy

LEARNING OBJECTIVES

Upon completion of the chapter, the learner will be able to:

1. Define the key terms used in this chapter.
2. Examine common reproductive concerns in terms of symptoms, diagnostic tests, and appropriate interventions.
3. Identify risk factors and outline appropriate client education needed in common reproductive disorders.
4. Compare and contrast the various contraceptive methods available and their overall effectiveness.
5. Explain the physiologic and psychological aspects of menopause.
6. Delineate the nursing management needed for women experiencing common reproductive disorders.

Izzy, a 27-year-old, presents to her health care provider complaining of progressive severe pelvic pain associated with her monthly periods. She has to take off work and "dope up" with pills to endure the pain. In addition, she has been trying to conceive for over a year without any luck.

Wow

When women bare their souls to us, we must respond without judgment.

ood health throughout the life cycle begins with the individual. Women today can expect to live well into their 80s and need to be proactive in maintaining their own quality of life. Women need to take steps to reduce their risk of disease and need to become active partners with their health care professional to identify problems early, when treatment may be most successful (Teaching Guidelines 4.1). Nurses can assist women in maintaining their quality of life by helping them to become more attuned to their body and its clues and can use the assessment period as an opportunity for teaching and counseling.

Common reproductive issues addressed in this chapter that nurses might encounter in caring for women include menstrual disorders, infertility, contraception, abortion, and menopause.

Menstrual Disorders

Many women sail through their monthly menstrual cycles with little or no concern. With few symptoms to worry about, their menses are like clockwork, starting and stopping at nearly the same time every month. For others, the menstrual cycle causes physical and emotional symptoms that initiate visits to their health care provider for consultation. The following menstruation-related conditions will be discussed in this chapter: amenorrhea, dysmenorrhea, dysfunctional uterine bleeding (DUB), premenstrual syndrome (PMS), premenstrual dysphoric disorder (PMDD), and endometriosis. To gain an understanding of menstrual disorders, it is important to know the terms used in describing them (Box 4.1).

TEACHING GUIDELINES 4.1

Tips for Being an Active Partner in Managing Your Health

- Become an informed consumer. Read, ask, and search.
- Know your family history and know factors that put you at high risk.
- Maintain a healthy lifestyle and let moderation be your guide.
- Schedule regular medical checkups and screenings for early detection.
- Ask your health care professional for a full explanation of any treatment.
- Seek a second medical opinion if you feel you need more information.
- Know when to seek medical care by being aware of disease symptoms.

BOX 4.1 **Menstrual Disorder Vocabulary**

- Meno = menstrual-related
- Metro = time
- Oligo = few
- A = without, none or lack of
- Rhagia = excess or abnormal
- Dys = not or pain
- Rhea = flow

▶ AMENORRHEA

Amenorrhea is the absence of menses during the reproductive years. Amenorrhea is normal in prepubertal, pregnant, and postmenopausal females. The two categories of amenorrhea are primary and secondary amenorrhea. Primary amenorrhea is defined as either:

1. Absence of menses by age 14, with absence of growth and development of secondary sexual characteristics, or
2. Absence of menses by age 16, with normal development of secondary sexual characteristics (Bielak & Harris, 2006)

Ninety-eight percent of American girls menstruate by age 16 (Krantz, 2007a, 2007b). Secondary amenorrhea is the absence of menses for three cycles or 6 months in women who have previously menstruated regularly.

Etiology

There are multiple causes of primary amenorrhea:

- Extreme weight gain or loss
- Congenital abnormalities of the reproductive system
- Stress from a major life event
- Excessive exercise
- Eating disorders (anorexia nervosa or bulimia)
- Cushing's disease
- Polycystic ovary syndrome
- Hypothyroidism
- Turner syndrome
- Imperforate hymen
- Chronic illness
- Pregnancy
- Cystic fibrosis
- Congenital heart disease (cyanotic)
- Ovarian or adrenal tumors (Master-Hunter & Heiman, 2006)

Causes of secondary amenorrhea might include:

- Pregnancy
- Breastfeeding

- Emotional stress
- Pituitary, ovarian, or adrenal tumors
- Depression
- Hyperthyroid or hypothyroid conditions
- Malnutrition
- Hyperprolactinemia
- Rapid weight gain or loss
- Chemotherapy or radiation therapy to the pelvic area
- Vigorous exercise, such as long-distance running
- Kidney failure
- Colitis
- Use of tranquilizers or antidepressants
- Postpartum pituitary necrosis (Sheehan syndrome)
- Early menopause (Bielak & Harris, 2006)

Therapeutic Management

Therapeutic intervention depends on the cause of the amenorrhea. The treatment of primary amenorrhea involves the correction of any underlying disorders and estrogen replacement therapy to stimulate the development of secondary sexual characteristics. If a pituitary tumor is the cause, it might be treated with drug therapy, surgical resection, or radiation therapy. Surgery might be needed to correct any structural abnormalities of the genital tract. Therapeutic interventions for secondary amenorrhea may include:

- Cyclic progesterone, when the cause is anovulation, or oral contraceptives
- Bromocriptine to treat hyperprolactinemia
- Nutritional counseling to address anorexia, bulimia, or obesity
- Gonadotropin-releasing hormone (GnRH), when the cause is hypothalamic failure
- Thyroid hormone replacement, when the cause is hypothyroidism (Schuiling & Likis, 2006)

Nursing Assessment

Nursing assessment for the young girl or woman experiencing amenorrhea includes a thorough health history and physical examination and several laboratory and diagnostic tests.

Health History and Physical Examination

A thorough history and physical examination is needed to determine the etiology. The history should include questions about the women's menstrual history; past illnesses; hospitalizations and surgeries; obstetric history; use of prescription and over-the-counter drugs; recent or past lifestyle changes; and history of present illness, with an assessment of any bodily changes.

The physical examination should begin with an overall assessment of the woman's nutritional status and general health. A sensitive and gentle approach to the pelvic examination is critical in young women. Height and weight should be taken, along with vital signs. Hypothermia,

bradycardia, hypotension, and reduced subcutaneous fat may be observed in women with anorexia nervosa. Facial hair and acne might be evidence of androgen excess secondary to a tumor. The presence or absence of axillary and pubic hair may indicate adrenal and ovarian hyposecretion or delayed puberty. A general physical examination may uncover unexpected findings that are indirectly related to amenorrhea. For example, hepatosplenomegaly, which may suggest a chronic systemic disease or an enlarged thyroid gland, might point to a thyroid disorder as well as a reason for amenorrhea (Nelson & Bakalov, 2006).

Laboratory and Diagnostic Tests

Common laboratory tests that might be ordered to determine the cause of amenorrhea include:

- Karyotype (might be positive for Turner syndrome)
- Ultrasound to detect ovarian cysts
- Pregnancy test to rule out pregnancy
- Thyroid function studies to determine thyroid disorder
- Prolactin level (an elevated level might indicate a pituitary tumor)
- Follicle-stimulating hormone (FSH) level (an elevated level might indicate ovarian failure)
- Luteinizing hormone (LH) level (an elevated level might indicate gonadal dysfunction)
- 17-ketosteroids (an elevated level might indicate an adrenal tumor)
- Laparoscopy to detect polycystic ovary syndrome
- CT scan of head if a pituitary tumor is suspected (Pagana & Pagana, 2007)

Nursing Management

Counseling and education are primary interventions and appropriate nursing roles. Address the diverse causes of amenorrhea, the relationship to sexual identity, possible infertility, and the possibility of a tumor or a life-threatening disease. In addition, inform the woman about the purpose of each diagnostic test, how it is performed, and when the results will be available to discuss with her. Sensitive listening, interviewing, and presenting treatment options are paramount to gain the woman's cooperation and understanding.

Nutritional counseling is also vital in managing this disorder, especially if the woman has findings suggestive of an eating disorder. Although not all causes can be addressed by making lifestyle changes, emphasize maintaining a healthy lifestyle (Teaching Guidelines 4.2).

▶ DYSMENORRHEA

Dysmenorrhea refers to painful menstruation. This condition has also been termed cyclic perimenstrual pain (CPPD) (Taylor, 2005). The term **dysmenorrhea** is derived from

TEACHING GUIDELINES 4.2

Tips for Maintaining a Healthy Lifestyle

- Balance energy expenditure with energy intake.
- Modify your diet to maintain ideal weight.
- Avoid excessive use of alcohol and mood-altering or sedative drugs.
- Avoid cigarette smoking.
- Identify areas of emotional stress and seek assistance to resolve them.
- Balance work, recreation, and rest.
- Maintain a positive outlook regarding the diagnosis and prognosis.
- Participate in ongoing care to monitor any medical conditions.
- Maintain bone density through:
  - Calcium intake (1,200 to 1,500 mg daily)
  - Weight-bearing exercise (30 minutes or more daily)
  - Hormone therapy

Source: Nelson & Bakalov, 2006.

the Greek words "dys," meaning difficult, painful, or abnormal, and "rrhea," meaning flow. It may affect more than half of menstruating women (Smith, 2006). Uterine contractions occur during all periods, but in some women these cramps can be frequent and very intense. Dysmenorrhea is categorized as primary or secondary.

Etiology

Primary dysmenorrhea is caused by increased prostaglandin production by the endometrium in an ovulatory cycle. This hormone causes contraction of the uterus, and levels tend to be higher in women with severe menstrual pain than women who experience mild or no menstrual pain. These levels are highest during the first 2 days of menses, when symptoms peak (Doty & Attaran, 2006). This results in increased rhythmic uterine contractions from vasoconstriction of the small vessels of the uterine wall. This condition usually begins within a few years of the onset of ovulatory cycles at menarche.

Secondary dysmenorrhea is painful menstruation due to pelvic or uterine pathology. It may be caused by endometriosis, adenomyosis, fibroids, pelvic infection, an intrauterine device, cervical stenosis, or congenital uterine or vaginal abnormalities. Adenomyosis involves the ingrowth of the endometrium into the uterine musculature. Endometriosis involves ectopic implantation of endometrial tissue in other parts of the pelvis. It occurs most commonly in the third or fourth decades of life and affects 10% of women of reproductive age (Hompes &

Mijatovic, 2007). Endometriosis is the most common cause of secondary dysmenorrhea and is associated with pain beyond menstruation, dyspareunia, and infertility (Speroff & Fritz, 2005). Treatment is directed toward removing the underlying pathology.

Think back to Izzy from the chapter opener. Is her pelvic pain complaint a common one with women?

Therapeutic Management

Therapeutic intervention is directed toward pain relief and building coping strategies that will promote a productive lifestyle. Treatment measures usually include treating infections if present; suppressing the endometrium if endometriosis is suspected by administering low-dose oral contraceptives; administering prostaglandin inhibitors to reduce the pain; administering Depo-Provera; and initiating lifestyle changes. Table 4.1 lists selected treatment options for dysmenorrhea.

Nursing Assessment

As with any gynecologic complaint, a thorough focused history and physical examination is needed to make the diagnosis of primary or secondary dysmenorrhea. In primary dysmenorrhea, the history usually reveals the typical cramping pain with menstruation, and the physical examination is completely normal. In secondary dysmenorrhea, the history discloses cramping pain starting after 25 years old with a pelvic abnormality, a history of infertility, heavy menstrual flow, irregular cycles, and little response to nonsteroidal anti-inflammatory drugs (NSAIDs), oral contraceptives, or both (Harel, 2006).

Health History and Clinical Manifestations

Note past medical history, including any chronic illnesses and family history of gynecologic concerns. Determine medication and substance use, such as prescription medications, contraceptives, anabolic steroids, tobacco, and marijuana, cocaine, or other illegal drugs. A detailed sexual history is essential to assess for inflammation and scarring (adhesions) secondary to pelvic inflammatory disease (PID). Women with a previous history of PID, sexually transmitted infections (STIs), multiple sexual partners, or unprotected sex are at increased risk.

During the initial interview, the nurse might ask some of the following questions to assess the woman's history of dysmenorrhea:

- "At what age did you start your menstrual cycles?"
- "Have your cycles always been painful, or did the pain start recently?"
- "When in your cycle do you experience the pain?"
- "How would you describe the pain you feel?"

TABLE 4.1 TREATMENT OPTIONS FOR DYSMENORRHEA

Therapy Options	Dosage	Comments
Nonsteroidal anti-inflammatory agents (NSAIDs)		
Ibuprofen (Ibuprin, Advil, Motrin)	400–800 mg TID	Take with meals. Don't take with aspirin. Avoid alcohol. Watch for signs of GI bleeding.
Naproxen (Anaprox, Naprelan, Naprosyn, Aleve)	250–500 mg TID	Same as above
Hormonal contraceptives		
Low-dose oral contraceptives	Taken daily (42/7 days; 63/7 or 84/7)	Take active pills for an extended time to reduce number of monthly cycles (Archer, 2006).
Depo-medroxyproges-terone (DMPA), Depo-Provera	150 mg IM every 12 wks	Within 9–12 months of DMPA therapy, 75% of women will be amenorrheic (Schuiling & Likis, 2006).
Lifestyle changes Daily exercise Limit salty foods Weight loss Smoking cessation Relaxation techniques		Gives sense of control over life

- "Are you sexually active?"
- "What impact does your cycle have on your physical and social activity?"
- "When was the first day of your last menstrual cycle?"
- "Was the flow of your last menstrual cycle a normal amount for you?"
- "Do your cycles tend to be heavy or last longer than 5 days?"
- "Are your cycles generally regular and predictable?"
- "What have you done to relieve your discomfort? Is it effective?"
- "Has there been a progression of symptom severity?"
- "Do you have any other symptoms?"

Assess for clinical manifestations of dysmenorrhea. Affected women experience sharp, intermittent spasms of pain, usually in the suprapubic area. Pain may radiate to the back of the legs or the lower back. Pain usually develops within hours of the start of menstruation and peaks as the flow becomes heaviest during the first day or two of the cycle (Edmundson & Erogul, 2006). Systemic symptoms of nausea, vomiting, diarrhea, fatigue, fever, headache, or dizziness are fairly common. Explore the history for physi-cal symptoms of bloating, water retention, weight gain, headache, muscle aches, abdominal pain, food cravings, or breast tenderness.

Physical Examination

The physical examination performed by the health care provider centers on the bimanual pelvic examination. This examination is done during the nonmenstrual phase of the cycle. Explain to the woman how it is to be performed, especially if is her first pelvic examination. Prepare the woman in the examining room by offering her a cover gown to put on and covering her lap with a privacy sheet on the examination table. Remain in the examining room throughout the examination to assist the health care provider with any procedures or specimens and to offer the woman reassurance.

Laboratory and Diagnostic Tests

Common laboratory tests that may be ordered to determine the cause of dysmenorrhea might include:

- Complete blood count to rule out anemia
- Urinalysis to rule out a bladder infection

- Pregnancy test (human chorionic gonadotropin level) to rule out pregnancy
- Cervical culture to exclude STI
- Erythrocyte sedimentation rate to detect an inflammatory process
- Stool guaiac to exclude gastrointestinal bleeding or disorders
- Pelvic and/or vaginal ultrasound to detect pelvic masses or cysts
- Diagnostic laparoscopy and/or laparotomy to visualize pathology that may account for the symptoms

What diagnostic tests might be ordered to diagnose Izzy's pelvic pain?

Nursing Management

Educating the client about the normal events of the menstrual cycle and the etiology of her pain is paramount in achieving a successful outcome. Explaining the normal menstrual cycle will teach the woman the correct terms so she can communicate her symptoms more accurately and will help dispel myths. Provide the woman with monthly graphs or charts to record menses, the onset of pain, the timing of medication, relief afforded, and coping strategies used. This involves the woman in her care and provides objective information so that therapy can be modified if necessary.

The nurse should explain in detail the dosing regimen and the side effects of the medication therapy selected. Commonly prescribed drugs include NSAIDs such as ibuprofen (Motrin), naproxen (Naprosyn), and Advil. They alleviate dysmenorrhea symptoms by decreasing intrauterine pressure and inhibiting prostaglandin synthesis, thus reducing pain (Skidmore-Roth, 2007). If pain relief is not achieved in two to four cycles, a low-dose combination oral contraceptive may be initiated. Client teaching and counseling should include information about how to take pills, side effects, and danger signs to watch for.

Encourage the woman to apply a heating pad or warm compress to alleviate menstrual cramps. Additional lifestyle changes that the woman can make to restore some sense of control and active participation in her care are listed in Teaching Guidelines 4.3.

◆ DYSFUNCTIONAL UTERINE BLEEDING

Dysfunctional uterine bleeding (DUB) is a disorder that occurs most frequently in women at the beginning and end of their reproductive years. Defined as irregular, abnormal bleeding that occurs with no identifiable anatomic

TEACHING GUIDELINES 4.3

Tips to Manage Dysmenorrhea

- Exercise to increase endorphins and suppress prostaglandin release.
- Limit salty foods to prevent fluid retention.
- Increase water consumption to serve as a natural diuretic.
- Increase fiber intake with fruits and vegetables to prevent constipation.
- Use heating pads or warm baths to increase comfort.
- Take warm showers to promote relaxation.
- Sip on warm beverages, such as decaffeinated green tea.
- Keep legs elevated while lying down or lie on side with knees bent.
- Use stress management techniques to reduce emotional stress.
- Practice relaxation techniques to enhance ability to cope with pain.
- Stop smoking and decrease alcohol use.

Source: Nasir, 2007.

pathology, it affects 33% to 50% of women (Rackow & Arici, 2007). It is frequently associated with anovulatory cycles, which are common for the first year after menarche and later in life as women approach menopause.

The pathophysiology of DUB is related to a hormone disturbance. With anovulation, estrogen levels rise as usual in the early phase of the menstrual cycle. In the absence of ovulation, a corpus luteum never forms and progesterone is not produced. The endometrium moves into a hyperproliferative state, ultimately outgrowing its estrogen supply. This leads to irregular sloughing of the endometrium and excessive bleeding (Aeby & Frattarelli, 2006). If the bleeding is heavy enough and frequent enough, anemia can result.

DUB is similar to several other types of uterine bleeding disorders and sometimes overlaps these conditions. They include:

- Menorrhagia (abnormally long, heavy periods)
- Oligomenorrhea (bleeding occurs at intervals of more than 35 days)
- Metrorrhagia (bleeding between periods)
- Menometrorrhagia (bleeding occurs at irregular intervals with heavy flow lasting more than 7 days)
- Polymenorrhea (too frequent periods)

Etiology

The possible causes of DUB may include:

- Adenomyosis
- Pregnancy

- Hormonal imbalance
- Fibroid tumors (see Chapter 7)
- Endometrial polyps or cancer
- Endometriosis
- Intrauterine device (IUD)
- Polycystic ovary syndrome
- Morbid obesity
- Steroid therapy
- Hypothyroidism
- Blood dyscrasias/clotting disorder

Therapeutic Management

Treatment of DUB depends on the cause of the bleeding and the age of the client. When known, the underlying cause of the disorder is treated. Otherwise, the goal of treatment is to relieve the symptoms so that uterine bleeding does not interfere with a woman's normal activities or cause anemia (Dodds & Sinert, 2006).

Management of DUB might include medical care with pharmacotherapy or insertion of an IUD. Oral contraceptives are used for cycle regulation as well as contraception. They help prevent the risks associated with prolonged unopposed estrogen stimulation of the endometrium. NSAIDs and the levonorgestrel-releasing IUD (Mirena) decrease menstrual blood loss significantly (Lethaby, Cooke & Rees, 2006). The drug categories used in the treatment of DUB are:

- Estrogens: cause vasospasm of the uterine arteries to decrease bleeding
- Progestins: used to stabilize an estrogen-primed endometrium
- Oral contraceptives: regulate the cycle and suppress the endometrium
- NSAIDs: inhibit prostaglandins
- Levonorgestrel-20 Intrauterine System: suppresses endometrial growth
- Iron salts: replenish iron stores lost during heavy bleeding

If the client does not respond to medical therapy, surgical intervention might include dilation and curettage (D&C), endometrial ablation, or hysterectomy. Endometrial ablation is an alternative to hysterectomy. A thermal balloon or a laser is used to ablate the tissue, producing improvement in 90% of women (Speroff & Fritz, 2005).

Nursing Assessment

A thorough history should be taken to differentiate between DUB and other conditions that might cause vaginal bleeding, such as pregnancy and pregnancy-related conditions (abruptio placentae, ectopic pregnancy, abortion, or placenta previa); systemic conditions such as Cushing disease, blood dyscrasias, liver disease, renal disease, or thyroid disease; and genital tract pathology such as infections, tumors, or trauma (Hackley, Kriebs & Rousseau, 2007).

Assess for clinical manifestations of DUB, which commonly include vaginal bleeding between periods, irregular menstrual cycles (usually less than 28 days between cycles), infertility, mood swings, hot flashes, vaginal tenderness, variable menstrual flow ranging from scanty to profuse, obesity, acne, and diabetes. Signs of polycystic ovary syndrome might be present, since it is associated with unopposed estrogen stimulation, elevated androgen levels, and insulin resistance and is a common cause of anovulation (Torpy, 2007).

Measure orthostatic blood pressure and orthostatic pulse; a drop in pressure or pulse rate may occur with anemia. The health care provider, with the nurse assisting, performs a pelvic examination to identify any structural abnormalities.

Common laboratory tests that may be ordered to determine the cause of DUB include:

- Complete blood count to detect anemia
- Prothrombin time (PT) to detect blood dyscrasias
- Pregnancy test to rule out a spontaneous abortion or ectopic pregnancy
- Thyroid-stimulating hormone (TSH) level to screen for hypothyroidism
- Transvaginal ultrasound to measure endometrium
- Pelvic ultrasound to view any structural abnormalities
- Endometrial biopsy to check for intrauterine pathology
- D&C for diagnostic evaluation

Nursing Management

Educate the client about normal menstrual cycles and the possible reasons for her abnormal pattern. Inform the woman about treatment options. Do not simply encourage the woman to "live with it": complications such as infertility can result from lack of ovulation; severe anemia can occur secondary to prolonged or heavy menses; and endometrial cancer can occur associated with prolonged buildup of the endometrial lining without menstrual bleeding (Rackow & Arici, 2007). Instruct her about any prescribed medications and potential side effects. For example, if high-dose estrogens are prescribed, the woman may experience nausea. Teach her to take antiemetics as prescribed and encourage her to eat small, frequent meals to alleviate nausea. Adequate follow-up and evaluation for women who do not respond to medical management is essential. See Nursing Care Plan 4.1: Overview of a Woman With Dysfunctional Uterine Bleeding (DUB).

▶ PREMENSTRUAL SYNDROME

Premenstrual syndrome (PMS) describes a wide range of recurrent symptoms that occur during the luteal phase or last half of the menstrual cycle and resolve with the onset of menstruation (Braverman & Neinstein,

Nursing Care Plan 4.1

OVERVIEW OF A WOMAN WITH DYSFUNCTIONAL UTERINE BLEEDING (DUB)

Stacy, a 52-year-old obese woman, comes to her gynecologist with the complaint of heavy erratic bleeding. Her periods were fairly regular until about 4 months ago, and since that time they have been unpredictable, excessive, and prolonged. Stacy reports she is tired all the time, can't sleep, and feels "out of sorts" and anxious. She is fearful she has cancer.

NURSING DIAGNOSIS: Fear related to current signs and symptoms possibly indicating a life-threatening condition

Outcome Identification and Evaluation
The client will acknowledge her fears as evidenced by statements made that fear and anxiety have been lessened after explanation of diagnosis.

Interventions: Reducing Fear and Anxiety
- Distinguish between anxiety and fear to determine appropriate interventions.
- Check complete blood count and assess for possible anemia secondary to excessive bleeding to determine if fatigue is contributing to anxiety and fear. Fatigue occurs because the oxygen-carrying capacity of the blood is reduced.
- Reassure client that symptoms can be managed to help address her current concerns.
- Provide client with factual information and explain what to expect to assist client with identifying fears and help in her coping with her condition.
- Provide symptom management to reduce concerns associated with the cause of bleeding.
- Teach client about early manifestations of fear and anxiety to aid in prompt recognition and to minimize escalation of anxiety.
- Assess client's use of coping strategies in the past and reinforce use of effective ones to help control anxiety and fear.
- Instruct client in relaxation methods, such as deep breathing exercises and imagery, to provide her with additional methods for controlling anxiety and fear.

NURSING DIAGNOSIS: Deficient knowledge related to perimenopause and its management

Outcome Identification and Evaluation
The client will demonstrate understanding of her symptoms as evidenced by making health-promoting lifestyle choices, verbalizing appropriate health care practices, and adhering to measures to comply with therapy.

Interventions: Providing Patient Education
- Assess client's understanding of perimenopause and its treatment to provide a baseline for teaching and developing a plan of care.
- Review instructions about prescribed procedures and recommendations for self-care, frequently obtaining feedback from the client to validate adequate understanding of information.
- Outline link between anovulatory cycles and excessive buildup of uterine lining in perimenopausal women to assist client in understanding the etiology of her bleeding.
- Provide written material with pictures to promote learning and help client visualize what is occurring to her body during perimenopause.
- Inform client about the availability of community resources and make appropriate referrals as needed to provide additional education and support.
- Document details of teaching and learning to allow for continuity of care and further education, if needed.

2007). The American College of Obstetricians and Gynecologists (ACOG) defines premenstrual syndrome as "the cyclic occurrence of symptoms that are sufficiently severe to interfere with some aspects of life, and that appear with consistent and predictable relationship to menses" (ACOG, 2000). A woman experiencing PMS may have a wide variety of seemingly unrelated symptoms; for that reason, it is difficult to define and more challenging to diagnose. PMS affects millions of women during their reproductive years: up to 85% of menstruating women report having one or more premenstrual symptoms, and up to 10% report disabling, incapacitating symptoms

(Campagne & Campagne, 2007). The exact cause of PMS is not known. It is thought to be related to the interaction between hormonal events and neurotransmitter function, specifically serotonin. Not all women respond to serotonin reuptake inhibitors (SSRIs), however, which implies that other mechanisms may be involved (Braverman & Neinstein, 2007).

As defined by the American Psychological Association, premenstrual dysphoric disorder (PMDD) is a more severe variant of PMS. Experts compare the difference between PMS and PMDD to the difference between a mild tension headache and a migraine (Giulio & Reissing, 2006). PMDD markedly interferes with work and school, or with social activities and relationships with others.

Therapeutic Management

Treatment of PMS is often frustrating for both patients and health care providers. Clinical outcomes can be expected to improve as a result of recent consensus on the diagnostic criteria for PMS and PMDD, data from clinical trials, and the availability of evidence-based clinical guidelines.

The management of PMS or PMDD requires a multidimensional approach because these conditions are not likely to have a single cause, and they appear to affect multiple systems within a woman's body; therefore, they are not likely to be amenable to treatment with a single therapy. To reduce the negative impact of premenstrual disorders on a woman's life, education, along with reassurance and anticipatory guidance, are needed for women to feel they have some control over their condition.

> ▶ **Take** NOTE!
>
> *Because there are no diagnostic tests that can reliably determine the existence of PMS or PMDD, it is the woman herself who must decide that she needs help during this time of the month. The woman must embrace multiple therapies and become an active participant in her treatment plan to find the best level of symptom relief.*

Therapeutic interventions for PMS and PMDD address the symptoms because the exact cause of this condition is still unknown. Treatments may include vitamin supplements, diet changes, exercise, lifestyle changes, and medications (Box 4.2). Medications used in treating PMDD may include antidepressant and antianxiety drugs, diuretics, anti-inflammatory medications, analgesics, synthetic androgen agents, oral contraceptives, or GNrH agonists to regulate menses (Pavlovich-Danis, 2007).

BOX 4.2 **Treatment Options for PMS and PMDD**

- Lifestyle changes:
  Reduce stress.
  Exercise three to five times each week.
  Eat a balanced diet and increase water intake.
  Decrease caffeine intake.
  Stop smoking.
  Limit intake of alcohol.
  Attend a PMS/women's support group.
- Vitamin and mineral supplements
  Multivitamin daily
  Vitamin E, 400 units daily
  Calcium, 1,200 mg daily
  Magnesium, 200 to 400 mg daily
- Medications
  NSAIDs taken a week prior to menses
  Oral contraceptives (low dose)
  Antidepressants (SSRIs)
  Anxiolytics (taken during luteal phase)
  Diuretics to remove excess fluid
  Progestins
  Gonadotropin-releasing hormone (GnRH agonists)
  Danazol (androgen hormone inhibits estrogen production)

Many women use dietary supplements and herbal remedies for their menstrual health and treating their bleeding disorders, although there has been little research to demonstrate their efficacy. Some alternative therapies used might include calcium, magnesium, vitamin B6, evening primrose oil, vitex agnus castus, ginkgo biloba, viburnum, dandelion, stinging nettle, burdock, raspberry leaf, skullcap, and St. John's wort (Canning, Waterman & Dye, 2006). Although research hasn't validated alternative therapy's efficacy, it is important for the nurse to be aware of the alternative products that many women choose to use.

Nursing Assessment

Although little consensus exists in the medical literature and among researchers about what constitutes PMS and PMDD, the physical and psychological symptoms are very real. The extent to which the symptoms debilitate or incapacitate a woman is highly variable.

There are more than 200 symptoms assigned to PMS, but irritability, tension, and dysphoria are the most prominent and consistently described (Moreno & Giesel, 2006). To establish the diagnosis of PMS, elicit a description of cyclic symptoms occurring before the woman's menstrual period. The woman should chart her symptoms daily for two cycles. These data will help demonstrate symptoms clustering around the luteal phase of ovulation, with resolution after bleeding starts. Ask the woman to bring her list of symptoms to the next appointment. Symptoms can be categorized using the following:

- A: anxiety: difficulty sleeping, tenseness, mood swings, clumsiness
- C: craving: headache, cravings for sweets, salty foods, chocolate
- D: depression: feelings of low self-esteem, anger, easily upset
- H: hydration: weight gain, abdominal bloating, breast tenderness
- O: other: hot flashes or cold sweats, nausea, change in bowel habits, aches or pains, dysmenorrhea, acne breakout (Pavlovich-Danis, 2007)

The ACOG diagnostic criteria for PMS consist of having at least one of the following affective and somatic symptoms during the 5 days before menses in each of the three previous cycles:

- Affective symptoms: depression, angry outbursts, irritability, anxiety
- Somatic symptoms: breast tenderness, abdominal bloating, edema, headache
- Symptoms relieved from days 4 to 13 of the menstrual cycle (ACOG, 2000)

In PMDD, the main symptoms are mood disorders such as depression, anxiety, tension, and persistent anger or irritability. Physical symptoms such as headache, joint and muscle pain, lack of energy, bloating, and breast tenderness are also present (Hsiao & Liu, 2007). It is estimated that 20% to 40% of reproductive-age women experience premenstrual symptoms that meet the ACOG criteria for PMS and up to 10% meet the diagnostic criteria for PMDD (Futterman & Rapkin, 2006).

According to the American Psychiatric Association, a woman must have at least five of the typical symptoms to be diagnosed with PMDD (Andoisek & Rapkin, 2007). These must occur during the week before and a few days after the onset of menstruation and must include one or more of the first four symptoms:

1. Affective lability: sadness, tearfulness, irritability
2. Anxiety and tension
3. Persistent or marked anger or irritability
4. Depressed mood, feelings of hopelessness
5. Difficulty concentrating
6. Sleep difficulties
7. Increased or decreased appetite
8. Increased or decreased sexual desire
9. Chronic fatigue
10. Headache
11. Constipation or diarrhea
12. Breast swelling and tenderness (Htay & Aung, 2006)

Nursing Management

Educate the client about the management of PMS or PMDD. Advise her that lifestyle changes often result in significant symptom improvement without pharmacotherapy. Encourage women to eat a balanced diet that includes nutrient-rich foods to avoid hypoglycemia and associated mood swings. Encourage adolescent girls to participate in aerobic exercise three times a week to promote a sense of well-being, decrease fatigue, and reduce stress. Administer calcium (1,200 to 1,600 mg/day), magnesium (400 to 800 mg/day), and vitamin B6 (50 to 100 mg/day) as prescribed. In some studies, these nutrients have been shown to decrease the intensity of PMS symptoms. NSAIDs may be useful for painful physical symptoms and spironolactone (Aldactone) may help with bloating and water retention. Herbs such as Vitex (chaste tree berry), evening primrose, and SAM-e may be recommended; although not harmful, not all herbs have enough clinical or research evidence to document their safety or efficacy (Schuiling & Likis, 2006).

A recent research study proposes calcium (1,600 mg/day) and vitamin D (400 IU/day) supplementation in adolescents and women in an effort to prevent PMS (Clayton, 2008).

Explain the relationship between cyclic estrogen fluctuation and changes in serotonin levels and how the different management strategies help maintain serotonin levels, thus improving symptoms. It is important to rule out other conditions that might cause erratic or dysphoric behavior. If the initial treatment regimen does not work, explain to the woman that she should return for further testing. Behavioral counseling and stress management might help women regain control during these stressful periods. Reassuring the woman that support and help are available through many community resources/support groups can be instrumental in her acceptance of this monthly disorder. Nurses can be a very calming force for many women experiencing PMS or PMDD.

▶ *Take* NOTE!

Adolescents and women who experience more extensive emotional symptoms with PMS should be evaluated for PMDD, as they may require antidepressant therapy.

▶ ENDOMETRIOSIS

Endometriosis is one of the most common gynecologic diseases, affecting more than 5.5 million women in the United States. In this condition, bits of functioning endometrial tissue are located outside of their normal site, the uterine cavity. This endometrial tissue is commonly found attached to the ovaries, fallopian tubes, the outer surface of the uterus, the bowels, the area between the vagina and the rectum (rectovaginal septum), and the pelvic side wall (Fig. 4.1). The places where the tissue attaches are called implants, or lesions. Endometrial tissue found outside the uterus responds to hormones released during the menstrual cycle in the same way as endometrial lining within the uterus.

At the beginning of the menstrual cycle, when the lining of the uterus is shed and menstrual bleeding begins, these abnormally located implants swell and bleed also. In short, the woman with endometriosis experiences several "mini-periods" throughout her abdomen, wherever this endometrial tissue exists.

Think back to Izzy, with her progressive pelvic pain and infertility concerns. After a pelvic examination, her health care provider suspects she has endometriosis.

Etiology and Risk Factors

It is not currently known why endometrial tissue becomes transplanted and grows in other parts of the body. Several theories exist, but to date none has been scientifically proven. However, several factors that increase a woman's risk of developing endometriosis have been identified:

- Increasing age
- Family history of endometriosis in a first-degree relative
- Short menstrual cycle (less than 28 days)
- Long menstrual flow (more than 1 week)
- Young age of menarche (younger than 12)
- Few (one or two) or no pregnancies (Speroff & Fritz, 2005)

Therapeutic Management

Therapeutic management of the client with endometriosis needs to take into consideration the following factors: severity of symptoms, desire for fertility, degree of disease, and the client's therapy goals. The aim of therapy is to suppress levels of estrogen and progesterone, which cause the endometrium to grow. Treatment can include surgery or medication (Table 4.2).

Nursing Assessment

Nurses encounter women with endometriosis in a variety of settings: community health settings, schools, clinics, day surgical centers, and hospitals. Health care professionals must not trivialize or dismiss the concerns of these women, because early recognition is essential to preserve fertility.

Health History
Obtain a health history and elicit a description of signs and symptoms to determine risk factors. Endometriosis is often asymptomatic, but it can be a severe and debilitating condition. It typically is chronic and progressive. Assess the client for clinical manifestations, which include:

- Infertility
- Pain before and during menstrual periods
- Pain during or after sexual intercourse
- Painful urination
- Depression
- Fatigue
- Painful bowel movements
- Chronic pelvic pain
- Hypermenorrhea (heavy menses)
- Pelvic adhesions

FIGURE 4.1 Common sites of endometriosis formation.

TABLE 4.2   TREATMENT OPTIONS FOR ENDOMETRIOSIS

Therapy Options	Comment
Surgical intervention	
Conservative surgery	Removal of implants/lesions using laser, cautery, or small surgical instruments. This intervention will reduce pain and allows pregnancy to occur in the future.
Definitive surgery	Abdominal hysterectomy, with or without bilateral salpingo-oophorectomy. Will eliminate pain but will leave a woman unable to become pregnant in the future.
Medication therapy	
NSAIDs	First-line treatment to reduce pain; taken early when premenstrual symptoms are first felt
Oral contraceptives	Suppresses cyclic hormonal response of the endometrial tissue
Progestogens	Used to cast off the endometrial cells and thus destroy them
Antiestrogens	Suppresses a woman's production of estrogen, thus stopping the menstrual cycle and preventing further growth of endometrium
Gonadotropin-releasing hormone analogues (GnRH-a)	Suppresses endometriosis by creating a temporary pseudomenopause
Danazol (Danacrine)	A synthetic androgen (male sex hormone) used typically as a second-line treatment of endometriosis. Disrupts the action of the pituitary gland by suppressing the output of some hormones, thus reducing estrogen, halting menstruation, and resulting in the growth of facial hair and acne.

• Irregular and more frequent menses
• Premenstrual vaginal spotting (Schuiling & Likis, 2006)

The two most common symptoms are infertility and pain. Endometriosis occurs in 38% of infertile women and in 71% to 87% of women with chronic pelvic pain (Aeby & Hraoka, 2006). About 30% to 40% of women with this condition are infertile, making it one of the top three causes of female infertility (NICHD, 2006).

What are the two most common symptoms experienced by women with endometriosis? Is Izzy's profile typical? As a nurse, what would be your role in Izzy's continued workup?

Physical Examination and Laboratory and Diagnostic Tests

The pelvic examination typically correlates with the extent of the endometriosis. The usual finding is nonspecific pelvic tenderness. The hallmark finding is the presence of tender nodular masses on the uterosacral ligaments,

the posterior uterus, or the posterior cul-de-sac (Saul & Dave, 2006).

After a thorough history and a pelvic examination, the health care practitioner may suspect endometriosis, but the only certain method of diagnosing it is by seeing it. Pelvic or transvaginal ultrasound is used to assess pelvic organ structures. However, a laparoscopy is needed to diagnose endometriosis. Laparoscopy is the direct visualization of the internal organs with a lighted instrument inserted through an abdominal incision. A tissue biopsy of the suspected implant taken at the same time and examined microscopically confirms the diagnosis.

Nurses can play a role by offering a thorough explanation of the condition and explaining why tests are needed to diagnose endometriosis. The nurse can set up appointments for imaging studies and laparoscopy.

Nursing Management

In addition to the interventions outlined above, the nurse should encourage the client to adopt healthy lifestyle habits with respect to diet, exercise, sleep, and stress management. Referrals to support groups and Internet resources can help the woman to understand this condition and to cope with chronic pain. A number of organizations provide information about the diagnosis and treatment of endometriosis and offer support to women and their families (Box 4.3). See Evidence-Based Practice 4.1.

fter completing several diagnostic tests, Izzy is diagnosed with endometriosis. She asks you about her chances of becoming pregnant and becoming pain-free. What treatment options would you explain to Izzy? What information can you give about her future childbearing ability?

Infertility

Infertility is defined as the inability to conceive a child after 1 year of regular sexual intercourse unprotected by contraception, or the inability to carry a pregnancy to term (Covington & Burns, 2006). Secondary infertility is the inability to conceive after a previous pregnancy. Many people take the ability to conceive and produce a

---

| BOX 4.3 | **Organizations and Web Resources to Assist the Client With Endometriosis** |

- American College of Obstetricians and Gynecologists (ACOG): www.acog.org or e-mail at resources@acog.org
- American Society of Reproductive Medicine: www.asrm.org or e-mail at asrm@asrm.org
- Center for Endometriosis Care: http://www.centerforendo.com/
- Endometriosis Association: www.endometriosisassn.org or www.KillerCramps.org
- Endometriosis Association support groups: e-mail at support@endometriosisassn.org
- NICHD Information Resource Center: www.nichd.nih.gov or e-mail at NICHDClearinghouse@mail.nih.gov
- National Women's Health Information Center (Dept. of Health and Human Services): http://www.4women.gov

---

EVIDENCE-BASED PRACTICE 4.1
The Effectiveness of Danazol Compared to Placebo or No Treatment in the Treatment of the Symptoms and Signs (Other than Infertility) of Endometriosis in Women of Reproductive Age

● Study
Endometriosis is defined as the presence of endometrial tissue (stromal and glandular) outside the normal uterine cavity. Conventional medical and surgical treatments for endometriosis aim to remove or decrease deposits of ectopic endometrium. The observation that hyperandrogenic states (an excess of male hormone) induce atrophy of the endometrium has led to the use of androgens in the treatment of endometriosis. Danazol is one of these treatments. The efficacy of danazol is based on its ability to produce a high-androgen/low-estrogen environment (a pseudomenopause), which results in the atrophy of endometriotic implants and thus an improvement in painful symptoms.

Only four trials met the inclusion criteria, and two authors independently extracted data from these trials. All four trials compared danazol to placebo. Two trials used danazol as sole therapy and two trials used danazol as an adjunct to surgery. Although the main outcome was pain improvement, other data relating to laparoscopic scores and hormonal parameters were also collected.

▲ Findings
Treatment with danazol was effective in relieving painful symptoms related to endometriosis when compared to placebo. Laparoscopic scores were improved with danazol treatment when compared with either placebo or no treatment. Side effects were more commonly reported in the patients receiving danazol than those receiving placebo. Thus, danazol is effective in treating the symptoms and signs of endometriosis. However, its use is limited by the occurrence of androgenic side effects.

■ Nursing Implications
According to the results of the study, danazol is an effective treatment for relieving painful symptoms of endometriosis, but it has side effects. As a nurse, it is important to educate the patient about these; they may include clitoral enlargement and masculinization. In addition, the response to the drug may take several weeks or months. Women should be cautioned to report yellowing of the skin (jaundice), fluid retention, shortness of breath, and changes in vaginal bleeding. It is important to stress that there are several effective therapies to treat endometriosis if the side effects are problematic with danazol.

Source: Selak, V., Farquhar, C., Prentice, A., & Singla, A. (2006). Danazol for pelvic pain associated with endometriosis. *Cochrane Library,* Retrieved Feb. 14, 2007, from the CINAHL Plus with Full Text database.

child for granted, but infertility affects over 6 million Americans, or 15% of the reproductive-age population, according to the American Society for Reproductive Medicine (ASRM, 2007). Infertility is a widespread problem that has an emotional, social, and economic impact on couples. Nurses must recognize infertility and understand its causes and treatment options so that they can help couples understand the possibilities as well as the limitations of current therapies. Recent studies found that women wished to be treated with respect and dignity and given appropriate information and support. They wanted their distress recognized and they wanted to feel cared for and to have confidence in health care professionals in situations where outcomes were uncertain. The caring aspect of professional nursing is an essential component of meeting the special needs of these couples (Redshaw, Hockley & Davidson, 2007). Prevention of infertility through education should also be incorporated into any client–nurse interaction.

Cultural Considerations

Cross-culturally, the expectation for couples to reproduce is an accepted norm and the inability to conceive may be considered a violation of this cultural norm. In this context, infertility represents a crisis for the couple. The manner in which different cultures, ethnic groups, and religious groups perceive and manage infertility may be very different. For example, many African-Americans believe that assisted reproductive techniques are unnatural and that they remove the spiritual or divine nature of creation from conception. For this reason, they may seek spiritual rather than medical assistance when trying to conceive. The Hispanic culture believes that children validate the marriage, so families are typically large. Like the African-American culture, Hispanics are very spiritual and may consider infertility a test of faith and seek spiritual counseling.

Religion often influences cultural factors and for this reason may also be considered when pursuing treatment for infertility. In the Jewish religion procreation is felt to be an obligation and a responsibility. Roman Catholics have a very restrictive view on the use of assisted reproductive technologies since in their view procreation cannot be separated from the relationship between parents. Thus, children must be created by the physical union between husband and wife and conceived through sexual intercourse (Schenker, 2005). Nurses must be cognizant of the client's cultural and religious background and how it may dictate which, if any, reproductive treatment options are chosen. Nurses need to include this awareness in their counseling of infertile couples.

Etiology and Risk Factors

Multiple known and unknown factors affect fertility. Female-factor infertility is detected in about 40% of cases, male-factor infertility in about 40% of cases. The remaining 20% fall into a category of combined (both male and female factors) or unexplained infertility. In women, ovarian dysfunction (40%) and tubal/pelvic pathology (40%) are the primary contributing factors to infertility (ASRM, 2007).

Risk factors for infertility include:

- For women:
  - Overweight or underweight (can disrupt hormone function)
  - Hormonal imbalances leading to irregular ovulation
  - Fibroids
  - Tubal blockages
  - Reduced oocyte quality
  - Chromosomal abnormalities
  - Congenital anomalies of the cervix and uterus
  - Immune system disorders
  - Chronic illnesses such as diabetes, thyroid disease, asthma
  - STIs
  - Age older than 27
  - Endometriosis
  - History of PID
  - Smoking and alcohol consumption
  - Multiple miscarriages
  - Psychological stress (Kelly-Weeder & O'Conner, 2006)
- For men:
  - Exposure to toxic substances (lead, mercury, x-rays)
  - Cigarette or marijuana smoke
  - Heavy alcohol consumption
  - Use of prescription drugs for ulcers or psoriasis
  - Exposure of the genitals to high temperatures (hot tubs or saunas)
  - Hernia repair
  - Frequent long-distance cycling
  - STI
  - Undescended testicles (cryptorchidism)
  - Mumps after puberty (Ficorelli & Weeks, 2007)

Therapeutic Management

The test results are presented to the couple and different treatment options are suggested. The majority of infertility cases are treated with drugs or surgery. Various ovulation-enhancement drugs and timed intercourse might be used for the woman with ovulation problems. The woman should understand the drug's benefits and side effects before consenting to take them. Depending on the type of drug used and the dosage, some women may experience multiple births. If the woman's reproductive organs are damaged, surgery can be done to repair them. Still other couples might opt for the hi-tech approaches of artificial insemination (Fig. 4.2), in vitro fertilization (IVF; Fig. 4.3), and egg donation or contract for a gestational

A **B**

FIGURE 4.2 Artificial insemination. Sperm are deposited next to the cervix (**A**) or injected directly into the uterine cavity (**B**).

carrier or surrogate (Grainger, Frazier & Rowland, 2006). Table 4.3 lists selected infertility options.

Nursing Assessment

Infertile couples are under tremendous pressure and often keep the problem a secret, considering it to be very personal. The couple is often beset by feelings of inadequacy and guilt, and many are subject to pressures from both family and friends. As their problem becomes more chronic, they may begin to blame one another, with consequent marital discord. Seeking help is often a very difficult step for them, and it may take a lot of courage to discuss something about which they feel deeply embarrassed or upset. The nurse working in this specialty setting must be aware of the conflict and problems couples present with and must be very sensitive to their needs.

A full medical history should be taken from both partners, along with a physical examination. The data needed for the infertility evaluation are very sensitive and of a personal nature, so the nurse must use very professional interviewing skills.

There are numerous causes of and contributing factors to infertility, so it is important to use the process of elimination, determining what problems don't exist to better comprehend the problems that do exist. At the first visit, a plan of investigation is outlined and a complete health history is taken. This first visit forces many couples to confront the reality that their desired pregnancy may not occur naturally. Alleviate some of the anxiety associated with diagnostic testing by explaining the timing and reasons for each test.

Assessing Male Factors

The initial screening evaluation for the male partner should include a reproductive history and a semen analysis. From the male perspective, three things must happen for conception to take place: there must be an adequate number of sperm; those sperm must be healthy and mature; and the sperm must be able to penetrate and fertilize the egg. Normal males need to have more than 20 million sperm per milliliter with greater than 50% motility (WHO, 2007). Semen analysis is the most important indicator of male fertility. The man should abstain from

A **B** **C** **D**

FIGURE 4.3 Steps involved in in vitro fertilization. (**A**) Ovulation. (**B**) Capture of the ova (done here intra-abdominally). (**C**) Fertilization of ova and growth in culture medium. (**D**) Insertion of fertilized ova into uterus.

TABLE 4.3   SELECTED TREATMENT OPTIONS FOR INFERTILITY

Procedure	Comments	Nursing Considerations
Fertility drugs		
Clomiphene citrate (Clomid)	A nonsteroidal synthetic antiestrogen used to induce ovulation	Nurse can advise the couple to have intercourse every other day for 1 week starting after day 5 of medication.
Human menopausal gonadotropin (HMG); Pergonal	Induces ovulation by direct stimulation of ovarian follicle	Same as above
Artificial insemination	The insertion of a prepared semen sample into the cervical os or intrauterine cavity Enables sperm to be deposited closer to improve chances of conception Husband or donor sperm can be used	Nurse needs to advise couple that the procedure might need to be repeated if not successful the first time.
Assisted reproductive technologies*		
In vitro fertilization (IVF)	Oocytes are fertilized in the lab and transferred to the uterus. Usually indicated for tubal obstruction, endometriosis, pelvic adhesions, and low sperm counts	Nurse advises woman to take medication to stimulate ovulation so the mature ovum can be retrieved by needle aspiration.
Gamete intrafallopian transfer (GIFT)	Oocytes and sperm are combined and immediately placed in the fallopian tube so fertilization can occur naturally. Requires laparoscopy and general anesthesia, which increases risk	Nurse needs to inform couple of risks and have consent signed.
Intracytoplasmic sperm injection (ICSI)	One sperm is injected into the cytoplasm of the oocyte to fertilize it. Indicated for male factor infertility.	Nurse needs to inform the male that sperm will be aspirated by a needle through the skin into the epididymis.
Donor oocytes or sperm	Eggs or sperm are retrieved from a donor and the eggs are inseminated; resulting embryos are transferred via IVF. Recommended for women older than 40 and those with poor-quality eggs.	Nurse needs to support couple in their ethical/religious discussions prior to deciding.
Gestational carrier (surrogacy)	Laboratory fertilization takes place and embryos are transferred to the uterus of another woman, who will carry the pregnancy. Medical-legal issues have resulted over the "true ownership" of the resulting infant.	Nurse should encourage an open discussion regarding implications of this method with the couple.

*When other options have been exhausted, these are considered.

sexual activity for 24 to 48 hours before giving the sample. For a semen examination, the man is asked to produce a specimen by ejaculating into a specimen container and delivering it to the laboratory for analysis within 1 to 2 hours. When the specimen is brought to the laboratory, it is analyzed for volume, viscosity, number of sperm, sperm viability, motility, and sperm shape. If semen parameters are normal, no further male evaluation is necessary (Quallich, 2006).

The physical examination routinely includes:

• Assessment for appropriate male sexual characteristics, such as body hair distribution, development of the Adam's apple, and muscle development

- Examination of the penis, scrotum, testicles, epididymis, and vas deferens for abnormalities (e.g., nodules, irregularities, varicocele)
- Assessment for normal development of external genitalia (small testicles)
- Performance of a digital internal examination of the prostate to check for tenderness or swelling (DeMasters, 2004)

Assessing Female Factors

The initial assessment of the woman should include a thorough history of factors associated with ovulation and the pelvic organs. Diagnostic tests to determine female infertility may include:

- Assessment of ovarian function
  - Menstrual history: regularity of cycles
  - Ovulation predictor kits used midcycle
  - Urinary LH level
  - Clomiphene citrate challenge test
  - Endometrial biopsy to document luteal phase
- Assessment of pelvic organs
  - Papanicolaou (Pap) smear to rule out cervical cancer or inflammation
  - Cervical culture to rule out Chlamydia infection
  - Postcoital testing to evaluate sperm–cervical mucus interaction
  - Ultrasound to assess pelvic structures
  - Hysterosalpingography to visualize structural defects
  - Laparoscopy to visualize pelvic structures and diagnose endometriosis

Laboratory and Diagnostic Testing

The diagnostic procedures that should be done during an infertility workup should be guided by the couple's history. They generally proceed from less to more invasive tests.

Home Ovulation Predictor Kits

Home ovulation predictor kits contain monoclonal antibodies specific for LH and use the ELISA test to determine the amount of LH present in the urine. A significant color change from baseline indicates the LH surge and presumably the most fertile day of the month for the woman.

Clomiphene Citrate Challenge Test

The clomiphene citrate challenge test is used to assess a woman's ovarian reserve (ability of her eggs to become fertilized). FSH levels are drawn on cycle day 3 and on cycle day 10 after the woman has taken 100 mg clomiphene citrate on cycle days 5 through 9. If the FSH level is greater than 15, the result is considered abnormal and the likelihood of conception with her own eggs is very low (Schuiling & Likis, 2006).

Endometrial Biopsy

Another assessment of ovulation that indicates whether the secretion of progesterone is adequate is an endometrial biopsy. A strip of endometrial tissue is removed just before menstruation. Histologic documentation of secretory endometrial development implies that ovulation has taken place. An endometrium that does not conform to the normal histologic pattern indicates a defect in the luteal phase.

Postcoital Testing

Postcoital testing is done to assess the receptivity of the cervical mucus to sperm. Cervical mucus from the woman is examined 2 to 8 hours after intercourse during the expected time of ovulation, and the number of live, motile sperm present is assessed. Cervical mucus is also evaluated for stretchability (spinnbarkeit) and consistency (Alexander et al., 2007). The results are described in Comparison Chart 4.1.

Hysterosalpingogram

In a hysterosalpingogram, 3 to 10 mL of an opaque contrast medium is slowly injected through a catheter into the endocervical canal so that the uterus and tubes can be visualized during fluoroscopy and radiography. If the fallopian tubes are patent, the dye will ascend upward to distend the uterus and the tubes and will spill out into the peritoneal cavity (Fig. 4.4).

Laparoscopy

A laparoscopy is usually performed early in the menstrual cycle. During the procedure, an endoscope is inserted through a small incision in the anterior abdominal wall. Visualization of the peritoneal cavity in an infertile woman may reveal endometriosis, pelvic adhesions, tubal occlusion, fibroids, or polycystic ovaries (DeSutter, 2006).

Nursing Management

Nurses play an important role in the care of infertile couples. They are pivotal educators about preventive health care. There are a number of potentially modifiable risk

COMPARISON CHART 4.1 NORMAL VERSUS ABNORMAL POSTCOITAL TEST RESULTS

Normal	Abnormal
Normal amounts of sperm are seen in the sample.	No sperm or a large percentage of dead sperm are seen in the sample.
Sperm are moving forward through the cervical mucus.	Sperm are clumped.
The mucus stretches at least 2 in (5 cm).	Mucus cannot stretch 2 in (5 cm).
The mucus dries in a fernlike pattern.	Mucus does not dry in a fernlike pattern.

Source: DeSutter, 2006.

FIGURE 4.4 Insertion of a dye for a hystero-salpingogram. The contrast dye outlines the uterus and fallopian tubes on an x-ray to demonstrate patency.

factors associated with the development of impaired fertility in women, and women need to be aware of these risks to institute change. The nurse is most effective when he or she offers care and treatment in a professional manner and regards the couple as valued and respected individuals. The nurse's focus must encompass the whole person, not just the results of the various infertility studies. Throughout the entire process, the nurse's role is to provide information, anticipatory guidance, stress management, and counseling. The couple's emotional distress is usually very high, and the nurse must be able to recognize that anxiety and provide emotional support. The nurse may need to refer couples to a reproductive endocrinologist or surgeon, depending on the problem identified.

There is no absolute way to prevent infertility per se because so many factors are involved in conception. Nurses can be instrumental in educating men and women about the factors that contribute to infertility. The nurse can also outline the risks and benefits of treatments so that the couple can make an informed decision.

With advances in genetics and reproductive medicine also come a myriad of ethical, social, and cultural issues that will affect the couple's decisions. With this in mind, provide an opportunity for the couple to make informed decisions in a nondirective, nonjudgmental environment. It is important to encourage couples to remain optimistic throughout investigation and treatment. Through the use of advocacy and anticipatory guidance, assist and support couples through the diagnosis and treatment of infertility (Jenkins & Jenkins, 2006).

Finances and insurance coverage often dictate the choice of treatment. Help couples decipher their insurance coverage and help them weigh the costs of various procedures by explaining what each will provide in terms of information about their infertility problems. Assisting them to make a priority list of diagnostic tests and potential treatment options will help the couple plan their financial strategy.

Many infertile couples are not prepared for the emotional roller coaster of grief and loss during infertility treatments. Financial concerns and coping as a couple are

---

two major areas of stress when treatment is undertaken. During the course of what may be months or even years of infertility care, it is essential to develop a holistic approach to nursing care. Stress management and anxiety reduction need to be addressed, and referral to a peer support group such as Resolve might be in order (Box 4.4).

▶ *Consider* THIS!

We had been married for 3 years and wanted to start a family, but much to our dismay nothing happened after a year of trying. I had some irregular periods and was finally diagnosed with endometriosis and put on Clomid. After 3 years of taking Clomid on and off, I went to a fertility expert. The doctor lasered the endometriosis tissue, sent air through my tubes to make sure they were patent, and put me back on Clomid, but still with no luck. Finally, 2 years later, we were put on an IVF waiting list and prayed we would have the money for the procedure when we were chosen. By then I felt a failure as a woman. We then decided that it was more important for us to be parents than it was for me to be pregnant, so we considered adoption. We tried for another year without any results.

We went to the adoption agency to fill out the paperwork for the process to begin. Our blood was

(continued)

▶ *Consider THIS!* *(continued)*

taken and we waited for an hour, wondering the whole time why it was taking so long for the results. The nurse finally appeared and handed a piece of paper to me with the word "positive" written on it. I started to cry tears of joy, for a pregnancy had started and our long journey of infertility was finally ending.
Thoughts: For many women the dream of having a child is not easily realized. Infertility can affect self-esteem, disrupt relationships, and result in depression. This couple experienced many years of frustration in trying to have a family. What help can be offered to couples during this time? What can be said to comfort the woman who feels she is a failure?

Contraception

In the United States, there are approximately 62 million women in their childbearing years, ages 15 to 44. Overall, 64% of those 60 million women use contraception, but still more than 3 million unintended pregnancies occur every year (CDC, 2006). Although numerous fertility control methods are available, the United States continues to have a higher unintended pregnancy rate than other Western countries. Every minute of every day, 10 people become infected with HIV, most through heterosexual contact; 190 women conceive an unwanted pregnancy; 1 woman dies from a pregnancy-related cause; and 40 women undergo unsafe abortions, as outlined in the UNFPA State of the World Population 2006 Report. Much of this suffering could be prevented by access to safe, efficient, appropriate, modern contraception for everyone who wants it (UNFPA, 2007).

Contraception is any method that prevents conception or childbirth. A woman's reproductive life spans almost 40 years, and throughout those years, a variety of contraceptive methods may be used. Oral contraceptives, sterilization of the female, and the male condom are the most popular methods in the United States (Alan Guttmacher Institute, 2007).

Couples must decide which method is appropriate for them to meet their changing contraceptive needs throughout their life cycles. Nurses can educate and assist couples during this selection process. This part of the chapter will outline the most common birth control methods available.

In an era when many women wish to delay pregnancy and avoid STIs, choices are difficult. There are numerous methods available today, and many more will be offered in the near future. The ideal contraceptive method for many women would have to have the following characteristics: ease of use, safety, effectiveness, minimal side effects, "naturalness," nonhormonal method, and immediate reversibility (Samra & Wood, 2006). Currently, no one contraceptive method offers everything. Box 4.5 out-

---

> ### BOX 4.5 Outline of Contraceptive Methods
>
> **Reversible Methods**
> Behavioral
> • Abstinence
> • Fertility awareness
> • Withdrawal (coitus interruptus)
> • Lactational amenorrhea method (LAM)
>
> Barrier
> • Condom (male and female)
> • Diaphragm
> • Cervical cap
> • Sponge
>
> Hormonal
> • Oral contraceptives
> • Injectable contraceptive
> • Transdermal patches
> • Vaginal ring
> • Implantable contraceptives
> • Intrauterine systems
> • Emergency contraceptives
>
> **Permanent Methods**
> • Tubal ligation for women
> • Vasectomy for men

---

lines the contraceptive methods available today. Table 4.4 provides a detailed summary of each type, including information on failure rates, advantages, disadvantages, STI protection, and danger signs.

Types of Contraceptive Methods

Contraceptives methods can be divided into three types: behavioral methods, barrier methods, and hormonal methods.

Behavioral Methods

Behavioral methods refer to any natural contraceptive method that does not require hormones, pharmaceutical compounds, physical barriers, or surgery to prevent pregnancy. These methods require couples to take an active role in preventing pregnancy through their sexual behaviors.

Abstinence

Abstinence (not having vaginal or anal intercourse) is one of the least expensive forms of contraception and has been used for thousands of years. Basically, pregnancy cannot occur if sperm is kept out of the vagina. It also reduces the risk of contracting HIV/AIDS and other STIs, unless body fluids are exchanged through oral sex; however, some infections, like herpes and HPV, can be passed by skin-to-skin contact. There are many pleasurable

(text continues on page 114)

TABLE 4.4 SUMMARY OF CONTRACEPTIVE METHODS

Type	Description	Failure Rate	Pros	Cons	STI Protection	Danger Signs	Comments
Abstinence	Refrain from sexual activity	None	Costs nothing	Difficult to maintain	100%	None	Must be joint couple decision
Fertility awareness	Refrain from sex during fertile period	25%	No side effects; acceptable to most religious groups	High failure rate with incorrect use	None	None	Requires high level of couple commitment
Withdrawal (coitus interruptus)	Man withdraws before ejaculation	27%	Involves no devices and is always available	Requires considerable self-control by the man	None	None	Places woman in trusting and dependent role
Lactational amenorrhea method (LAM)	Uses lactational infertility for protection from pregnancy	1–2% chance of pregnancy in first 6 months	No cost; not coitus-linked	Temporary method; effective for only 6 months after giving birth	None	None	Mother must breastfeed infant on demand without supplementation for 6 months
Male condom	Thin sheath placed over an erect penis, blocking sperm	15%	Widely available; low cost; physiologically safe	Decreased sensation for man; interferes with sexual spontaneity; breakage risk	Provides protection against STIs	Latex allergy	Couple must be instructed on proper use of condom
Female condom	Polyurethane sheath inserted vaginally to block sperm	21%	Use controlled by woman; eliminates postcoital drainage of semen	Expensive for frequent use; cumbersome; noisy during sex act; for single use only	Provides protection against STIs	Allergy to polyurethane	Couple must be instructed on proper use of condom
Diaphragm with spermicide	Shallow latex cup with spring mechanism in its rim to hold it in place in the vagina	16%	Does not use hormone; considered medically safe; provides some protection against cervical cancer	Requires accurate fitting by health care professional; increase in UTIs	None	Allergy to latex, rubber, polyurethane, or spermicide. Report symptoms of toxic shock syndrome. Change size if excessive weight gain or loss.	Woman must be taught to insert and remove diaphragm correctly

(continued)

TABLE 4.4 SUMMARY OF CONTRACEPTIVE METHODS (continued)

Type	Description	Failure Rate	Pros	Cons	STI Protection	Danger Signs	Comments
Cervical cap with spermicide	Soft cup-shaped latex device that fits over base of cervix	24%	No use of hormones; provides continuous protection while in place	Requires accurate fitting by health care professional; odor may occur if left in too long	None	Irritation, allergic reaction; abnormal Pap test; risk of toxic shock syndrome	Instructions on insertion and removal must be understood by client
Sponge with spermicide	Disk-shaped polyurethane device containing a spermicide that is activated by wetting it with water	25%	Offers immediate and continuous protection for 24 hours; OTC	Can fall out of vagina with voiding; is not form-fitting in the vagina	None	Irritation, allergic reactions; toxic shock syndrome can occur if sponge left in too long	Caution woman not to leave sponge in beyond 24 hours
Oral contraceptives (combination)	A pill that suppresses ovulation by combined action of estrogen and progestin	8%	Easy to use; high rate of effectiveness; protection against ovarian and endometrial cancer	User must remember to take pill daily; possible undesirable side effects; high cost for some women; prescription needed	None	Dizziness, nausea, mood changes, high blood pressure, blood clots, heart attacks, strokes	Each woman must be assessed thoroughly to make sure she is not a smoker and does not have a history of thromboembolic disease
Oral contraceptives (progestin-only minipills)	A pill containing only progestin that thickens cervical mucus to prevent sperm from penetrating	8%	No estrogen-related side effects; may be used by lactating women; may be used by women with history of thrombophlebitis	Must be taken with meticulous accuracy; may cause irregular bleeding; less effective than combination pills	None	Irregular bleeding, weight gain, increased incidence of ectopic pregnancy	Women should be screened for history of functional ovarian cysts, previous ectopic pregnancy, hyperlipidemia prior to giving prescription

Method	Description	Failure rate	Advantages	Disadvantages		Special considerations	Teaching
Lunelle injectable	An injectable form of progestin and estrogen given monthly	3%	Woman will regain fertility 2–3 months after last injection; no need for daily pill taking	Must make arrangements for monthly injection; possible weight gain	None	Irregular spotting; similar to oral combination pills	Screen woman's ability to schedule monthly appointment for injection
Patch (Ortho Evra)	Transdermal patch that releases estrogen and progestin into circulation	8%	Easy system to remember; very effective	May cause skin irritation where it is placed; may fall off and not be noticed and thus provide no protection	None	Less effective in women weighing more than 200 pounds	Instruct woman to apply patch every week for 3 weeks and then not to wear one during week 4
Ring (NuvaRing)	Vaginal contraceptive ring about 2 inches in diameter that is inserted into the vagina; releases estrogen and progestin	8%	Easy system to remember; very effective	May cause a vaginal discharge; can be expelled without noticing and not offer protection	None	Similar to oral contraceptives	Instruct woman to use a backup method if ring is expelled and remains out for more than 3 hours
Depo-Provera injection	An injectable progestin that inhibits ovulation	3%	Long duration of action (3 months); highly effective; estrogen-free; may be used by smokers; can be used by lactating women	Menstrual irregularities; return visit needed every 12 weeks; weight gain, headaches, depression; return to fertility delayed up to 12 months	None	If depression is a problem, this method may increase the depression.	Inform woman that fertility is delayed after stopping the injections

(continued)

TABLE 4.4   SUMMARY OF CONTRACEPTIVE METHODS (continued)

Type	Description	Failure Rate	Pros	Cons	STI Protection	Danger Signs	Comments
Implant (Implanon)	A time-release implant (one rod) of levo-norgestrel for 3 years	0.05%	Long duration of action; low dose of hormones; reversible; estrogen-free	Irregular bleeding; weight gain; breast tenderness; headaches; difficulty in removal	None	If bleeding is heavy, anemia may occur.	Before insertion, assess woman to make sure she is aware that this method will produce about 3–5 years of infertility
Intrauterine systems (IUSs)	A T-shaped device inserted into the uterus that releases copper or progesterone or levo-norgestrel	1%	It is immediately and highly effective; allows for sexual spontaneity; can be used during lactation; return to fertility not impaired; requires no motivation by the user after insertion	Insertion requires a skilled professional; menstrual irregularities; prolonged amenorrhea; can be unknowingly expelled; may increase the risk of pelvic infection; user must regularly check string for placement; no protection against STIs; delay of fertility after discontinuing for possibly 6 to 12 months	None	Cramps, bleeding, pelvic inflammatory disease; infertility; perforation of the uterus	Instruct woman how to locate string to check monthly for placement

Postcoital emergency contraceptives (ECs)	Combination of progestin-only pills taken within 72 hours after unprotected intercourse	80%	Provides a last chance to prevent a pregnancy	Risk of ectopic pregnancy if EC fails	None	Nausea, vomiting, abdominal pain, fatigue, headache	Inform woman that ECs do not interrupt an established pregnancy, and the sooner they are taken the more effective they are
Permanent sterilization			One-time decision provides permanent sterility; short recovery time; low long-term risks	Procedures are difficult to reverse; initial cost may be high; chance of regret; some pain/discomfort after procedures	None for both	Postoperative complications: pain, bleeding, infection	Counsel both as to permanence of procedure and urge them to think it through prior to signing consent
Male	Sealing, tying, or cutting the vas deferens	<1%					
Female	Fallopian tubes are blocked to prevent conception	<1%					

Sources: Samra, 2006; FDA, 2006; Youngkin & Davis, 2004; Hatcher, 2004.

options for sex play without intercourse ("outercourse"), such as kissing, masturbation, erotic massage, sexual fantasy, sex toys such as vibrators, and oral sex.

Many people have strong feelings about abstinence based on religious and moral beliefs. There are many good and personal reasons to choose abstinence. For some it is a way of life, while for others it is a temporary choice. Some people choose abstinence because they want to:

• Wait until they are older
• Wait for a long-term relationship
• Avoid pregnancy or STIs
• Follow religious or cultural expectations

Fertility Awareness

Fertility awareness is a natural method of contraception in which no contraceptive devices are used; instead, certain observations, techniques, and calculations are used to determine the "fertile" and the "safe" periods in a monthly menstrual cycle. There are normal physiologic changes caused by hormonal fluctuations during the menstrual cycle that can be observed and charted. This information can be used to avoid or promote pregnancy. Fertility awareness methods rely upon the following assumptions:

• A single ovum is released from the ovary 14 days before the next menstrual period. It lives approximately 24 hours.
• Sperm can live up to 5 days after intercourse. The "unsafe period" during the menstrual cycle is thus approximately 6 days: 3 days before and 3 days after ovulation. Since bodily changes start to occur before ovulation, the woman can become aware of them and not have intercourse on these days or use another method to prevent pregnancy.
• The exact time of ovulation cannot be determined, so 2 to 3 days are added to the beginning and end to avoid pregnancy.

Techniques used to determine fertility include the cervical mucus ovulation method, the basal body temperature (BBT) method, and the symptothermal method (Hatcher et al., 2004). Fertility awareness methods are moderately effective but are very unforgiving if not carried out as prescribed: not following the guidelines might cause a 27% failure or pregnancy rate per cycle (Murphy, Morgan & Likis, 2006). Fertility awareness can be used in combination with coital abstinence or barrier methods during fertile days if pregnancy is not desired.

Cervical Mucus Ovulation Method

The **cervical mucus ovulation method** is used to assess the character of the cervical mucus. Cervical mucus changes in consistency during the menstrual cycle and plays a vital role in fertilization of the egg. In the days preceding ovulation, fertile cervical mucus helps draw sperm up and into the fallopian tubes, where fertilization usually takes place. It also helps maintain the survival of sperm.

As ovulation approaches, the mucus becomes more abundant, clear, slippery, and smooth; it can be stretched between two fingers without breaking. Under the influence of estrogen, this mucus looks like egg whites. It is called spinnbarkeit mucus (Fig. 4.5). After ovulation, the cervical mucus becomes thick and dry under the influence of progesterone.

The cervical position can also be assessed to confirm changes in the cervical mucus at ovulation. Near ovulation, the cervix feels soft and is high/deep in the vagina, the os is slightly open, and the cervical mucus is copious and slippery (Hatcher et al., 2004).

This method works because the woman becomes aware of her body changes that accompany ovulation. When she notices them, she abstains from sexual intercourse or uses another method to prevent pregnancy. Each woman is an individual, so each woman's unsafe time of the month is unique and thus must be individually assessed and determined.

Basal Body Temperature

The **basal body temperature** (BBT) refers to the lowest temperature reached upon wakening. The woman takes her temperature orally before rising and records it on a chart. Preovulation temperatures are suppressed by estrogen, whereas postovulation temperatures are increased under the influence of heat-inducing progesterone. Temperatures typically rise within a day or two after ovulation and remain elevated for approximately 2 weeks (at which point bleeding usually begins). If using this method by itself, the woman should avoid unprotected intercourse until the BBT has been elevated for 3 days. Other fertility awareness methods should be used along with BBT for better results (Fig. 4.6).

FIGURE 4.5 Spinnbarkeit is the ability of cervical mucus to stretch a distance before breaking.

Basal body temperature

A

B

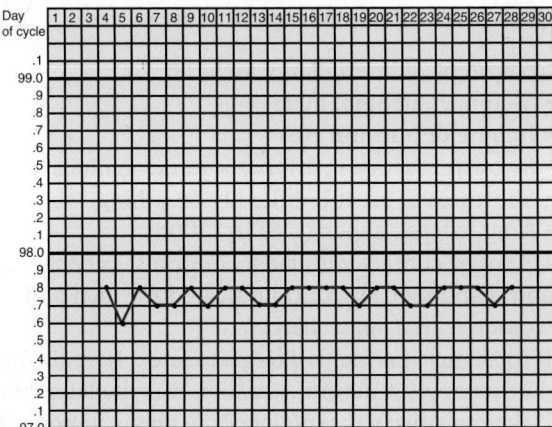

C

FIGURE 4.6 Basal body temperature graph. (**A**) The woman's temperature dips slightly at midpoint in the menstrual cycle, then rises sharply, an indication of ovulation. Toward the end of the cycle (the 24th day), her temperature begins to decline, indicating that progesterone levels are falling and that she did not conceive. (**B**) The woman's temperature rises at the midpoint in the cycle and remains at that elevated level past the time of her normal menstrual flow, suggesting that pregnancy has occurred. (**C**) There is no preovulatory dip and no rise of temperature anywhere during the cycle. This is the typical pattern of a woman who does not ovulate.

Symptothermal Method

The **symptothermal method** relies on a combination of techniques to recognize ovulation, including BBT, cervical mucus changes, alterations in the position and firmness of the cervix, and other symptoms of ovulation, such as increased libido, mittelschmerz, pelvic fullness or tenderness, and breast tenderness (Dirubbo, 2006). Combining all these predictors increases awareness of when ovulation occurs and increases the effectiveness of this method. A home predictor test for ovulation is also available in most pharmacies. It measures LH levels to pinpoint the day before or the day of ovulation. These tests are widely used for fertility and infertility regimens.

The Standard Days Method and the Two-Day Method

The **Standard Days Method (SDM)** and the Two-Day Method are both natural methods of contraception developed by Georgetown University Medical Center's Institute for Reproductive Health. Both methods provide women with simple, clear instructions for identifying fertile days. Women with menstrual cycles between 26 and 32 days long can use the SDM to prevent pregnancy by avoiding unprotected intercourse on days 8 through 19 of their cycles. An international clinical trial of the SDM showed that the method is more than 95% effective when used correctly (Sinai, Arevalo & Jennings, 2006). SDM identifies the 12-day "fertile window" of a woman's menstrual cycle. These 12 days takes into account the lifespan of the women's egg (about 24 hours) and the viability of the sperm (about 5 days) as well as the variation in the actual timing of ovulation from one cycle to another. For the Two-Day Method, women observe the presence or absence of cervical secretions by examining toilet paper or underwear or by monitoring their physical sensations. Every day, the woman asks two simple questions "Did I note any secretions yesterday?" and "Did I note any secretions today?" If the answer to either question is yes, she considers herself fertile and avoids unprotected intercourse. If the answers are no, she is unlikely to become pregnant from unprotected intercourse on that day (Sinai, Arevalo & Jennings, 2006).

To help women keep track of the days on which they should avoid unprotected intercourse, a string of 32 color-coded beads (CycleBeads) is used, with each bead representing a day of the menstrual cycle. Starting with the red bead, which represents the first day of her menstrual period, the woman moves a small rubber ring one bead each day. The brown beads are the days when pregnancy is unlikely, and the white beads represent her fertile days (Arevalo, 2007). This method has been used in underdeveloped countries for women with limited educational resources (Fig. 4.7).

Withdrawal (Coitus Interruptus)

In **coitus interruptus**, also known as withdrawal, a man controls his ejaculation during sexual intercourse and ejaculates outside the vagina. It is better known colloquially as

If your period does not start by the day after you move the ring to the last BROWN bead, your cycle is longer than 32 days.

The RED bead marks the first day of your menstrual period. On the day your period starts, move the ring to the red bead. Continue to move the ring one bead each day.

The DARK BROWN bead helps you know if your cycle is less than 26 days long. If your period starts before you move the ring to the dark brown bead, your cycle is shorter than 26 days.

All BROWN beads mark the days when you are not likely to get pregnant if you have unprotected sex.

All WHITE beads mark the days when you are likely to get pregnant. Do not have unprotected sex on the white bead days if you do not want to get pregnant.

FIGURE 4.7 CycleBeads help women use the Standard Days Method.

"pulling out in time" or "being careful." It is one of the oldest and most widely used means of preventing pregnancy in the world (Murphy, Morgan & Likis, 2006). The problem with this method is that the first few drops of the true ejaculate contain the greatest concentration of sperm, and if some pre-ejaculatory fluid escapes from the urethra before orgasm, conception may result. This method requires that the woman rely solely on the cooperation and judgment of the man.

Lactational Amenorrhea Method

The **lactational amenorrhea method (LAM)** is an effective temporary method of contraception used by breastfeeding mothers. Continuous breastfeeding can postpone ovulation and thus prevent pregnancy. Breastfeeding stimulates the hormone prolactin, which is necessary for milk production, and also inhibits the release of another hormone, gonadotropin, which is necessary for ovulation.

Breastfeeding as a contraceptive method can be effective for 6 months after delivery only if a woman:

- Has not had a period since she gave birth
- Breastfeeds her baby at least six times daily on both breasts
- Breastfeeds her baby "on demand" at least every 4 hours
- Does not substitute other foods for a breast-milk meal
- Provides nighttime feedings at least every 6 hours
- Does not rely on this method after 6 months (Planned Parenthood, 2007)

Barrier Methods

Barrier contraceptives are forms of birth control that prevent pregnancy by preventing the sperm from reaching the ovum. Mechanical barriers include condoms, diaphragms, cervical caps, and sponges. These devices are placed over the penis or cervix to physically obstruct the passage of sperm through the cervix. Chemical barriers called spermicides may be used along with mechanical barrier devices. They come in creams, jellies, foam, suppositories, and vaginal films. They chemically destroy the sperm in the vagina. These contraceptives are called barrier methods because they not only provide a physical barrier for sperm, but also protect against STIs. Since the HIV/AIDS epidemic started in the early 1980s, these methods have become extremely popular.

Many of these barrier methods contain latex. Allergy to latex was first recognized in the late 1970s, and since then it has become a major health concern, with increasing numbers of people affected. According to the American Academy of Allergy, Asthma and Immunology (2007), 6% of the general population, 10% of health care workers, and 50% of spina bifida patients are sensitive to natural rubber latex. Since the late 1980s, with the establishment of policies dictating barrier requirements resulting from the HIV/AIDS epidemic, there has been an exponential increase in the use of latex gloves and condoms (Lenehan, 2004). Teaching Guidelines 4.4 provides tips for individuals with latex allergy.

TEACHING GUIDELINES 4.4

Tips for Individuals Allergic to Latex

- Symptoms of latex allergy include:
  - Skin rash, itching, hives
  - Itching or burning eyes
  - Swollen mucous membranes in the genitals
  - Shortness of breath, difficulty breathing, wheezing
  - Anaphylactic shock (OSHA, 2006)
- Use of or contact with latex condoms, cervical caps, and diaphragms is contraindicated for men and women with a latex allergy.
- If the female partner is allergic to latex, have the male partner apply a natural condom over the latex one.
- If the male partner experiences penile irritation after condom use, try different brands or place the latex condom over a natural condom.
- Use polyurethane condoms rather than latex ones.
- Use female condoms; they are made of polyurethane.
- Switch to another birth control method that isn't made with latex, such as oral contraceptives, intrauterine systems, Depo-Provera, fertility awareness, and other non-barrier methods.
  However, these methods do not protect against sexually transmitted infections.

Condoms

Condoms are barrier methods of contraceptives made for both males and females. The male condom is made from latex or polyurethane or natural membrane and may be coated with spermicide. Male condoms are available in many colors, textures, sizes, shapes, and thicknesses. When used correctly, the male condom is put on over an erect penis before it enters the vagina and is worn throughout sexual intercourse (Fig. 4.8). It serves as a barrier to pregnancy by trapping seminal fluid and sperm and offers protection against STIs. Condoms are not perfect barriers, though, because breakage and slippage can occur. In addition, the non-latex condoms have a higher risk of pregnancy and STIs than latex condoms (Gallo, Grimes, Lopez & Schultz, 2006).

The female condom is a polyurethane pouch inserted into the vagina. It consists of an outer and inner ring that is inserted vaginally and held in place by the pubic bone. Some women complain that the female condom is cumbersome to use and makes noise during intercourse. Female condoms are readily available, are inexpensive, and can be carried inconspicuously by the woman. The female condom was the first woman-controlled method that offered protection against pregnancy and some STIs.

Diaphragm

The **diaphragm** is a soft latex dome surrounded by a metal spring. Used in conjunction with a spermicidal jelly or cream, it is inserted into the vagina to cover the cervix (Fig. 4.9). The diaphragm may be inserted up to 4 hours before intercourse but must be left in place for at least 6 hours afterwards. Diaphragms are available in a range of sizes and styles. The diaphragm is available only by prescription and must be professionally fitted by

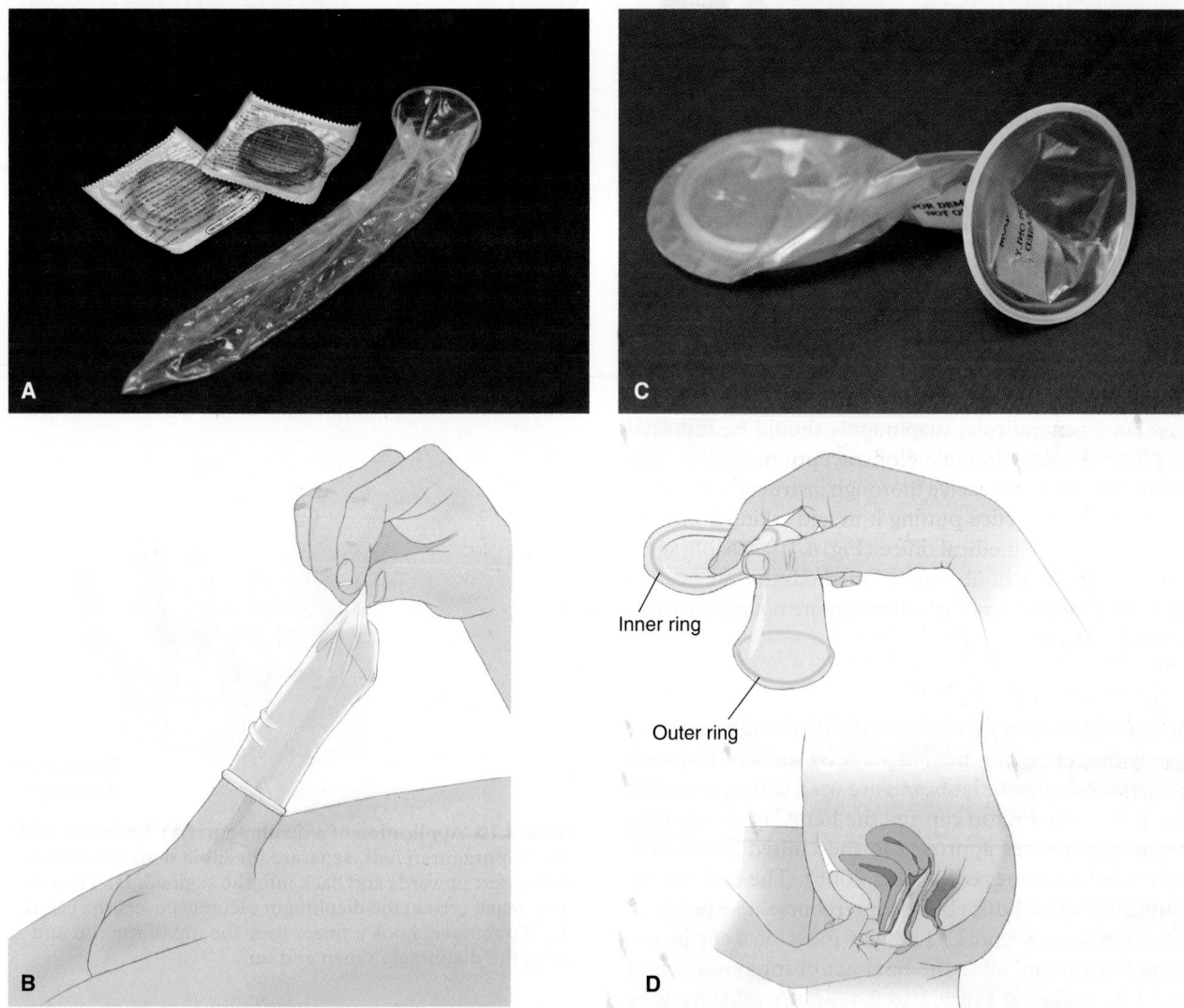

FIGURE 4.8 (**A**) Male condom. (**B**) Applying a male condom. Leaving space at the tip helps to ensure the condom will not break with ejaculation. (**C**) The female condom. (**D**) Insertion technique.

FIGURE 4.9 Sample diaphragm used for measuring.

a health care professional. Women may need to be refitted with a different-sized diaphragm after pregnancy, abdominal or pelvic surgery, or weight loss or gain of 10 pounds or more. As a general rule, diaphragms should be replaced every 1 to 2 years (Female Contraception, 2006). The woman also needs to receive thorough instruction about its use and should practice putting it in and taking it out before she leaves the medical office (Fig. 4.10). Diaphragms are user-controlled, nonhormonal methods that are needed only at the time of intercourse, but they are not effective unless used correctly.

Cervical Cap

The **cervical cap** is smaller than the diaphragm and covers only the cervix; it is held in place by suction. Caps are made from silicone or latex and are used with spermicide (Fig. 4.11). The Prentif cap and the FemCap are the only cervical cap devices approved in the United States currently (Gallo, Grimes & Schultz, 2006). The cap may be inserted up to 12 hours before intercourse and provides protection for 48 hours. The cap must be kept in the vagina for 8 hours after the final act of intercourse and should be replaced every 1 to 2 years. A refitting may also be necessary when a women experiences pregnancy, abortion, or weight changes. The dome of the cap is filled about one-third full with spermicide. Spermicide should

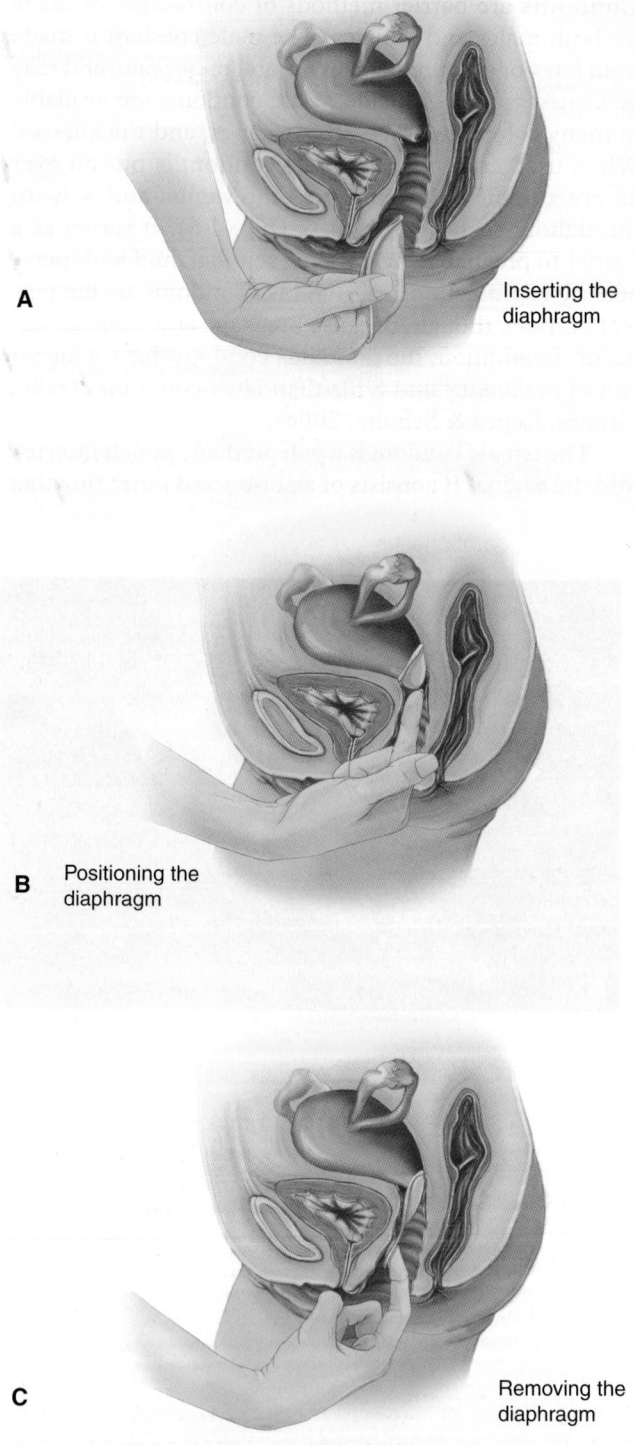

A Inserting the diaphragm

B Positioning the diaphragm

C Removing the diaphragm

FIGURE 4.10 Application of a diaphragm. (**A**) To insert, fold the diaphragm in half, separate the labia with one hand, then insert upwards and back into the vagina. (**B**) To position, make certain the diaphragm securely covers the cervix. (**C**) To remove, hook a finger over the top of the rim and bring the diaphragm down and out.

FIGURE 4.11 A cervical cap is placed over the cervix and used with a spermicidal jelly, the same as a diaphragm.

not be applied to the rim because it might interfere with the seal that must form around the cervix. The cap is available only by prescription and must be fitted by a health care professional.

Contraceptive Sponge

The **contraceptive sponge** is a nonhormonal, non-prescription device that includes both a barrier and a spermicide. When it was removed from the market in 1995, it was the most popular over-the-counter female contraceptive in America (Brucker, 2006). The manufacturer, Wyeth, stopped making the sponge rather than upgrade its manufacturing plant after the FDA found deficiencies, but the device's effectiveness and safety were never questioned. After receiving re-approval from the FDA in 2005, the contraceptive sponge is once again being marketed to women.

The contraceptive sponge is a soft polyurethane concave device that prevents pregnancy by covering the cervix and releasing spermicide. While it was less effective than several other methods and does not offer protection against STIs, the sponge achieved a wide following among women who appreciated the spontaneity with which it could be used and its easy availability. To use the sponge, the woman first wets it with water, then inserts it into the vagina with a finger, using a cord loop attachment. It can be inserted up to 24 hours before intercourse and should be left in place for at least 6 hours following intercourse. The sponge provides protection for up to 12 hours, but should not be left in for more than 30 hours after insertion to avoid the risk of toxic shock syndrome (Brucker, 2006). The sponge is a contraceptive method but does not protect against STIs.

Hormonal Methods

Several options are available to women who want long-term but not permanent protection against pregnancy. These methods of contraception work by altering the hormones within a woman's body. They rely on estrogen and progestin or progestin alone to prevent ovulation. When used consistently, these methods are a most reliable way to prevent pregnancy. Hormonal methods include oral contraceptives, injectables, implants, vaginal rings, and transdermal patches.

Oral Contraceptives

As early as 1937, scientists recognized that the injection of progesterone inhibited ovulation in rabbits and provided contraception. Breakthrough bleeding was reported in early clinical trials in women, and the role of estrogen in cycle control was launched. This established the rationale for modern combination **oral contraceptives (OCs)** that contain both estrogen and progesterone (Roederer, Blackwell & Blenning, 2006). In 1960 the FDA approved the first combination OC, Enovid-10 (150 mcg estrogen and 9 mg progesterone), for use in the United States. Today, nearly 50 combination OCs are available in the United States. The most notable change in over 40 years of OC improvement has been the lowering of the estrogen dose to as low as 20 mcg and the introduction of new progestins.

Oral contraceptives are the most popular method of nonsurgical contraception, used by approximately 18 million women in the United States (Dirubbo, 2006) (Fig. 4.12). Unlike the original OCs that women took decades ago, the new low-dose forms carry fewer health risks.

OCs, while most commonly prescribed for contraception, have long been used in the management of a wide range of conditions and have many health benefits, such as:

- Reduced incidence of ovarian and endometrial cancer
- Prevention and treatment of endometriosis
- Decreased incidence of acne and hirsutism

FIGURE 4.12 Oral contraceptive.

- Decreased incidence of ectopic pregnancy
- Decreased incidence of acute PID
- Reduced incidence of fibrocystic breast disease
- Decreased perimenopausal symptoms
- Increased menstrual cycle regularity
- Lower incidence of colorectal cancer
- Reduced iron-deficiency anemia by treating menorrhagia
- Reduced incidence of dysmenorrhea (Roederer, Blackwell & Blenning, 2006)

OCs work primarily by suppressing ovulation by adding estrogen and progesterone to a woman's body, thus mimicking pregnancy. This hormonal level stifles gonadotropin-releasing hormone (GnRH), which in turn suppresses FSH and LH and thus inhibits ovulation. Cervical mucus also thickens, which hinders sperm transport into the uterus. Implantation is inhibited by suppression of the maturation of the endometrium and alterations of uterine secretions (Trussell, 2004).

The combination pills are prescribed as monophasic pills, which deliver fixed dosages of estrogen and progestin, or as multiphasic ones. Multiphasic pills (e.g., biphasic and triphasic OCs) alter the amount of progestin and estrogen within each cycle. To maintain adequate hormonal levels for contraception and enhance compliance, OCs should be taken at the same time daily.

OCs that contain progestin only are called minipills. They are prescribed for women who cannot take estrogen. They work primarily by thickening the cervical mucus to prevent penetration of the sperm and make the endometrium unfavorable for implantation. Progestin-only pills must be taken at a certain time every 24 hours. Breakthrough bleeding and a higher risk of pregnancy have made these OCs less popular than combination OCs (Mishell et al., 2007).

Extended OC regimens have been used for the management of menstrual disorders and endometriosis for years but now are attracting wider attention. Surveys asking women about their willingness to reduce their menstrual cycles from 12 to 4 annually were returned with a resounding "yes!" (Archer, 2006). Recent studies confirm that the extended use of active OC pills carries the same safety profile as the conventional 28-day regimens (Anderson et al., 2006; Edelman et al., 2006; Grimes, 2006). The extended regimen consists of 84 consecutive days of active combination pills, followed by 7 days of placebo. The woman has four withdrawal-bleeding episodes a year. Seasonale, a combination OC, is on the market for women who choose to reduce the number of periods that they have. There is no physiologic requirement for cyclic hormonal withdrawal bleeds while taking OCs (Wysocki, 2007).

The balance between the benefits and the risks of OCs must be determined for each woman when she is being assessed for this type of contraceptive. It is a highly effective contraceptive when taken properly but can ag-

gravate many medical conditions, especially in women who smoke. Comparison Chart 4.2 lists advantages and disadvantages of OCs. A thorough history and pelvic examination, including a Pap smear, must be completed before the medication is prescribed and yearly thereafter. Women should also be counseled that the effectiveness of OCs is decreased when the woman is taking antibiotics; thus, the woman will need to use an alternative or secondary method during this period to prevent pregnancy.

Nurses need to provide OC users with a great deal of education before they leave the health care facility. They need to be able to identify early signs and symptoms that might indicate a problem.

▶ **Take** NOTE!

The mnemonic "ACHES" can help women remember the early warning signs that necessitate a return to the health care provider (Box 4.6).

Injectable Contraceptives

The **Lunelle injection** is a long-term reversible contraceptive for women. It contains the same hormones as the

COMPARISON CHART 4.2 **ADVANTAGES AND DISADVANTAGES OF ORAL CONTRACEPTIVES**

Advantages	Disadvantages
Regulate and shorten menstrual cycle	Offer no protection against STIs
Decrease severe cramping and bleeding	Pose slightly increased risk of breast cancer
Reduce anemia	Modest risk for vein thrombosis and pulmonary emboli
Reduce ovarian and colorectal cancer risk	
Decrease benign breast disease	Increased risk for migraine headaches
Reduce risk of endometrial cancer	Increased risk for myocardial infarction, stroke, and hypertension for women who smoke
Improve acne	
Minimize perimenopausal symptoms	
Decrease incidence of rheumatoid arthritis	May increase risk of depression
Improve PMS symptoms	User must remember to take pill daily
Protect against loss of bone density	High cost for some women

Source: Dirubbo, 2006

combination OCs. It is administered once every 28 to 33 days by intramuscular injection. It provides immediate, very effective contraception if given within 5 days after the last normal menses. Its mechanism of action, contraindications, and side effects are similar to those of OCs (Murphy, Morgan & Likis, 2006).

Depo-Provera is the trade name for an injectable form of a progesterone-only contraceptive given every 12 weeks. Depo-Provera works by suppressing ovulation and the production of FSH and LH by the pituitary gland, by increasing the viscosity of cervical mucus and causing endometrial atrophy. A single injection of 150 mg into the buttocks acts like other progestin-only products to prevent pregnancy for 3 months at a time (Fig. 4.13). The primary side effect of Depo Provera is menstrual cycle disturbance.

Recent clinical studies have raised concerns about whether Depo-Provera reduces bone mineral density. This evidence has prompted the manufacturer and the FDA to issue a warning about the long-term use of Depo-Provera and bone loss (Robinson, 2005). It is not entirely clear if this loss in bone mineral density is reversible because there haven't been any long-term prospective studies in current and past users.

Transdermal Patches

A **transdermal patch**, Ortho Evra, is also available. It is a matchbox-sized patch containing hormones that are absorbed through the skin when placed on the lower abdomen, upper outer arm, buttocks, or upper torso (avoiding the breasts). The patch is applied weekly for 3 weeks, followed by a patch-free week during which withdrawal bleeding occurs. The patch delivers continuous levels of progesterone and estrogen. Transdermal absorption allows the drug to enter the bloodstream directly, avoiding rapid inactivation in the liver known as first-pass metabolism. Since estrogen and progesterone are metabolized by liver enzymes, avoiding first-pass metabolism was thought to reduce adverse effects. However, recent evidence suggests that the risk of venous thrombosis and embolism is increased with the patch (Courtney, 2006). Additional studies are underway to understand the clinical significance of these latest findings, but in the interim nurses need to focus on ongoing risk assessment and should be prepared to discuss current research findings with clients.

Compliance with combination contraceptive patch use has been shown to be significantly greater than compliance with OCs (Graziottin, 2006). The patch provides combination hormone therapy with a side effect profile similar to that of OCs. The manufacturer is currently evaluating extended regimens for the patch (Stewart et al., 2006) (Fig. 4.14).

Vaginal Rings

The contraceptive **vaginal ring**, NuvaRing, is a flexible, soft, transparent ring that is inserted by the user for a 3-week period of continuous use followed by a ring-free week to allow withdrawal bleeding (Fig. 4.15). The ring can be inserted by the woman and does not have to be

FIGURE 4.13 Injectable contraceptive.

FIGURE 4.14 Transdermal patch.

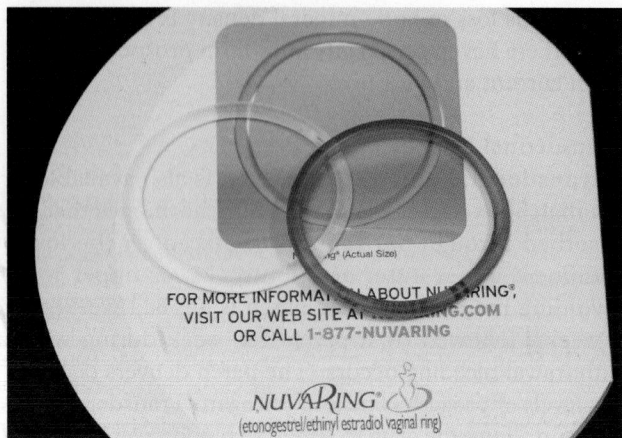

FIGURE 4.15 Vaginal ring.

fitted. The woman compresses the ring and inserts it into the vagina, behind the pubic bone, as far back as possible, but precise placement is not critical. The hormones are absorbed through the vaginal mucosa. It is left in place for 3 weeks and then removed and discarded. Effectiveness and adverse events are similar to those seen with combination OCs. Clients need to be counseled regarding timely insertion of the ring and what to do in case of accidental expulsion. This device is also being tested for extended regimens to reduce menstrual bleeding.

Implantable Contraceptives

The **implant** is a subdermal time-release method that delivers synthetic progestin. Once in place, it delivers several years of continuous, highly effective contraception. Like progestin-only pills, implants act by inhibiting ovulation and thickening cervical mucus so sperm cannot penetrate. A single-rod progestin implant (Implanon) received FDA approval in 2006 (Tolaymat & Kaunitz, 2007). The side effects are also similar to progestin-only pills: irregular bleeding, headaches, weight gain, breast tenderness, and depression. Fertility is restored quickly after it is removed. Implants require a minor surgical procedure for both insertion and removal. The implants don't offer any protection against STIs.

Intrauterine Systems

Intrauterine systems are small plastic T-shaped objects that are placed inside the uterus to provide contraception (Fig. 4.16). They prevent pregnancy by making the endometrium of the uterus hostile to implantation of a fertilized ovum by causing a nonspecific inflammatory reaction (Hearton, 2006). Monthly periods become lighter, shorter, and less painful, making this a useful method for women with heavy, painful periods. Some implants may contain copper or progesterone to enhance their effectiveness. One or two attached strings protrude into the vagina so that the user can check for placement.

Currently there are three intrauterine systems available in the United States: the copper ParaGard-T-380A; Progestasert, a progesterone device; and the levonorgestrel intrauterine system (LNG-IUS) Mirena, a levonorgestrel-releasing device. The ParaGard-T-380A is approved for 10 years of use. The Progestasert may stay in place 1 year, then must be removed and replaced. Mirena provides intrauterine conception for up to 5 years. An advantage of these hormonally impregnated intrauterine systems is that they are relatively maintenance-free: users must consciously discontinue using them to become pregnant rather than making a daily decision to avoid conception (French et al., 2006). Box 4.7 highlights warning signs of complications.

Emergency Contraception

Unplanned pregnancy is a major health, economic, and social issue for women. Approximately half of all unplanned pregnancies end in abortion (CDC, 2006). **Emergency contraception (EC)** reduces the risk of pregnancy after unprotected intercourse or contraceptive failure such as condom breakage (Lever, 2005). It is used within 72 hours of unprotected intercourse to prevent pregnancy. The sooner ECs are taken, the more effective

Drug reservoir (progesterone)

Rate controlling membrane

Monofilament thread (string)

FIGURE 4.16 (**A**) Intrauterine system. (**B**) An IUS in place in the uterus.

BOX 4.7 Warnings for Intrauterine System Users of Potential Complications

P: Period late, pregnancy, abnormal spotting or bleeding
A: Abdominal pain, pain with intercourse
I: Infection exposure, abnormal vaginal discharge
N: Not feeling well, fever, chills
S: String length shorter or longer or missing

Source: Hatcher et al., 2004.

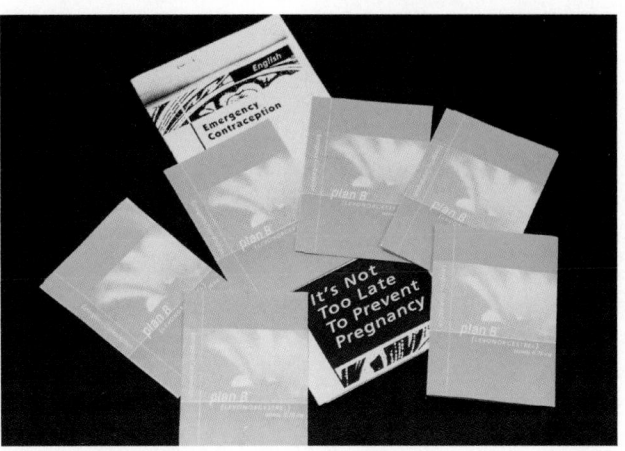

FIGURE 4.17 Emergency contraceptive kit.

they are. They reduce the risk of pregnancy for a single act of unprotected sex by almost 80% (Cheng et al., 2006). The methods available in the United States are progestin-only OCs, combination OCs, EC kit (Plan B) (Fig. 4.17), or insertion of a copper-releasing intrauterine system up to 7 days after unprotected intercourse (Lever, 2005). The FDA recently approved Plan B (levonorgestrel) to be sold over the counter to women aged 18 and older; it is still available by prescription to women younger than 18 years (U.S. Food & Drug Administration, 2006). Table 4.5 lists recommended oral medication and intrauterine regimens.

Prime points to stress concerning ECs are:

• ECs do not offer any protection against STIs or future pregnancies.
• ECs should not be used in place of regular birth control, as they are less effective.
• ECs are regular birth control pills given at higher doses and more frequently.
• ECs are contraindicated during pregnancy because they are considered to be teratogenic (Ravin, 2006).

Contrary to popular belief, ECs do not induce abortion and are not related to mifepristone or RU-486, the so-called abortion pill approved by the FDA in 2000. Mifepristone chemically induces abortion by blocking the body's progesterone receptors, which are necessary for pregnancy maintenance. ECs simply prevent embryo creation and uterine implantation from occurring in the first place. There is no evidence that ECs have any effect on an already-implanted ovum. The side effects are nausea and vomiting.

Sterilization

Sterilization is an attractive method of contraception for those who are certain they do not want any, or any more, children. **Sterilization** refers to surgical procedures intended to render the person infertile. It is one of the most popular methods of contraception in the United States and worldwide (Swica & Westhoff, 2006). More women than men undergo surgical sterilization. According to the

TABLE 4.5 EMERGENCY CONTRACEPTION (EC) OPTIONS

Product	First Dose (Within 72 Hours)	Second Dose (Taken 12 Hours Later)
Combined OCs		
Preven	2 tablets	2 tablets
Ovral		
Lo/Ovral, Nordette Levlen, TriLevlen	4 tablets	4 tablets
Triphasil		
Progestin-Only OCs		
Ovrette	20 tablets	20 tablets
Plan B	1 tablet	1 tablet
Intrauterine Devices		
Copper-containing IUD such as Paragard-T-380A	Inserted within 7 days after unprotected sexual episode	Can be left in for long-term contraception

FIGURE 4.18 Laparoscopy for tubal sterilization.

CDC, approximately 18% of women undergo female sterilization in comparison to 7% of men in the United States (CDC, 2006). Sterilization should be considered a permanent end to fertility because reversal surgery is difficult, expensive, and not highly successful.

Tubal Ligation

Tubal ligation, the sterilization procedure for women, can be performed postpartum, after an abortion, or as an interval procedure unrelated to pregnancy. A laparoscope is inserted through a small subumbilical incision to provide a view of the fallopian tubes. They are grasped and sealed with a cauterizing instrument or with rings, bands, or clips or cut and tied (Fig. 4.18).

A new approach used to visualize the fallopian tubes is through the cervix instead of the abdominal incision. This procedure, called transcervical sterilization, offers several advantages over conventional tubal ligation: general anesthesia and incisions are not needed, thereby increasing safety, lowering costs, and improving access to sterilization. A tiny coil (Essure) is introduced and released into the fallopian tubes through the cervix. The coil promotes tissue growth in the fallopian tubes, and over a period of 3 months, this growth blocks the tubes (Valle, 2006). This less-invasive technique has become increasingly popular.

Vasectomy

Male sterilization is accomplished with a surgical procedure known as a **vasectomy**. It is usually performed under local anesthesia in an urologist's office, and most men can return to work and normal activities in a day or two. The procedure involves making a small incision into the scrotum and cutting the vas deferens, which carries sperm from the testes to the penis (Fig. 4.19). After vasectomy, semen no longer contains sperm. This is not immediate, though, and the man must submit semen specimens for analysis until two specimens show that no sperm is present. When the specimen shows azoospermia, the man's sterility is then confirmed (Dassow & Bennett, 2006).

Nursing Management of the Woman Choosing a Contraceptive Method

The choice of a contraceptive method is a very personal one involving many factors. What makes a woman choose one contraceptive method over another? In making contraceptive choices, couples must balance their sexual

FIGURE 4.19 Vasectomy. (**A**) Site of vasectomy incisions. (**B**) The vas deferens is cut with surgical scissors. (**C**) Cut ends of the vas deferens are cauterized to ensure blockage of the passage of sperm. (**D**) Final skin suture.

lives, their reproductive goals, and each partner's health and safety. The search for a choice that satisfies all three objectives is challenging. A method that works for a sexually active teenage girl may not meet her needs later in life. Several considerations influence a person's choice of contraceptives:

- Motivation
- Cost
- Cultural and religious beliefs (Box 4.8)
- Convenience
- Effectiveness
- Side effects
- Desire for children in the future
- Safety of the method
- Comfort level with sexuality
- Protection from STIs
- Interference with spontaneity

If a contraceptive is to be effective, the woman must understand how it works, must be able to use it correctly and consistently, and must be comfortable and confident with it. If a patient cannot comply with taking a pill daily, consider a method used once a week (transdermal patches), once every 3 weeks (transvaginal ring), or once every 3 months (Depo-Provera injection). Another option may be a progesterone intrauterine device that lasts 3 to 5 years and reduces menstrual flow significantly.

Regardless of which method is chosen, the client's needs should be paramount in the discussion. The nurse can educate clients about which methods are available and their advantages and disadvantages, efficacy, cost, and safety. Counseling can help the woman choose a contraceptive method that is efficacious and fits her preferences and lifestyle.

Nursing Assessment

When assessing which contraceptive method might meet the client's needs, the nurse might ask:

- Do your religious beliefs interfere with any methods?
- Will this method interfere with your sexual pleasure?
- Are you aware of the various methods currently available?
- Is cost a major consideration, or does your insurance cover it?
- Does your partner influence which method you choose?
- Have you heard anything troubling about any of the methods?
- How comfortable are you touching your own body?
- What are your future plans for having children?

Although deciding on a contraceptive is a very personal decision between a woman and her partner, nurses can assist in this process by performing a complete health history and physical examination, and by educating the woman and her partner about necessary laboratory and diagnostic testing. Areas of focus during the nursing assessment are as follows:

- Medical history: smoking status, cancer of reproductive tract, diabetes mellitus, migraines, hypertension, thromboembolic disorder, allergies, risk factors for cardiovascular disease
- Family history: cancer, cardiovascular disease, hypertension, stroke, diabetes
- OB/GYN history: menstrual disorders, current contraceptive, previous STIs, PID, vaginitis, sexual activity
- Personal history: use of tampons and female hygiene products, plans for childbearing, comfort with touching herself, number of sexual partners and their involvement in the decision
- Physical examination: height, weight, blood pressure, breast examination, thyroid palpation, pelvic examination
- Diagnostic testing: urinalysis, complete blood count, Pap smear, wet mount to check for STIs, HIV/AIDS tests, lipid profile, glucose level

Figure 4.20 shows an example of a family planning flow record that can be used during the assessment. After collecting the assessment data above, consider the medical factors to help decide if she is a candidate for all methods or whether some should be eliminated. For example, if she reports she has multiple sex partners and has a lengthy history of various pelvic infections, she would not be a good candidate for an intrauterine system, based on her infection history. Barrier methods (male or female

---

BOX 4.8 Selected Religious Choices for Family Planning and Abortion

- Roman Catholic—Abstinence and natural family planning; no abortion
- Judaism—Family planning and abortion accepted in first trimester
- Islam—Family planning accepted; abortion only for serious reasons
- Protestant Christianity—Firmly in favor of family planning; mixed on abortion
- Buddhism—Long experience with family planning and abortion
- Hinduism—Accept both family planning and abortion
- Native American religions—Accept both family planning and abortion
- Chinese religions—Taoism and Confucianism accept both

Source: Maguire, 2004.

FAMILY PLANNING FLOW (VISIT) RECORD

Name: _____
ID #: _____
Date of Birth: _____

	Date:			Date:	
Current Method					
Reason for Visit					
LMP					
SUBJECTIVE DATA	**Pt.**	**Comments**		**Pt.**	**Comments**
Severe headaches					
Depression					
Visual abnormalities					
Dyspnea/chest pain					
Breast changes					
SBE					
Abdominal pain					
Nausea and vomiting					
Dysuria/frequency					
Menstrual irregularities					
Vaginal discharge/infections					
Leg pain					
Surgery, injury, infections, or serious illness since last visit					
Allergic reaction					
Pregnancy plans					
Other					
OBJECTIVE DATA	**Weight**	**B.P.**		**Weight**	**B.P.**
Other					
Lab					
ASSESSMENT					
Check here if assessment continues on progress notes	O			O	
PLAN					
Type of contraceptive given					
COUNSELING/EDUCATION					
Next appointment					
SIGNATURE/TITLE					
SIGNATURE/TITLE					

O = normal   ✓ = abnormal

FIGURE 4.20 Family planning flow (visit) record.

condoms) of contraception might be recommended to this client to offer protection against STIs.

Nursing Diagnoses

A few nursing diagnoses that might be appropriate based on the nurse's assessment during the decision-making process include:

- Deficient knowledge related to:
  - Methods available
  - Side effects/safety
  - Correct use of method chosen
  - Previous myths believed
- Risk for infection related to:
  - Unprotected sexual intercourse
  - Past history of STIs
  - Methods offering protection

Nursing diagnoses applicable to the contraceptive would be:

- Health-seeking behaviors related to:
  - Perceived need for limiting number of children
  - Overall health relative to contraceptives
- Risk for ineffective health maintenance related to:
  - Not being familiar with the various contraceptive methods
  - Being unaware of high-risk sexual behavior leading to STIs
- Fear related to:
  - Not understanding the correct procedure to use
  - Unintended pregnancy occurring if not used correctly
  - General health concerning the long-term side effects

Nursing Interventions

Contraception is an important issue for all couples, and the method used should be decided by the woman and her partner jointly. Facilitate this process by establishing a trusting relationship with the client and by providing unbiased, accurate information about all methods available. As a nurse, reflect honestly on your feelings towards contraceptives while allowing the client's feelings to be central. Be aware of the practical issues involved in contraceptive use, and avoid making assumptions, making decisions on the woman's behalf, and making judgments about her and her situation. To do so, it is important to keep up to date on the latest methods available and convey this information to clients. Encourage female clients to take control of their lives by sharing information that allows them to plan their futures.

The following guidelines are helpful in counseling and educating the client or couple about contraceptives:

- Encourage the client/couple to participate in choosing a method.
- Provide client education. The client/couple must be informed users before the method is agreed upon. Education should be targeted to the client's level so it

is understood. Provide step-by-step teaching and an opportunity for practice for certain methods (cervical caps, diaphragms, vaginal rings, and condoms). See Teaching Guidelines 4.5 and Figure 4.21.
- Obtain written informed consents, which are needed for intrauterine systems, implants, abortion, or sterilization. Informed consent implies that the client is making a knowledgeable, voluntary choice; has received complete information about the method, including the risks; and is free to change her mind before using the method or having the procedure (Youngkin & Davis, 2004).
- Discuss contraindications for all selected contraceptives.
- Consider the client's cultural and religious beliefs when providing care.
- Address myths and misperceptions about the methods under consideration in your initial discussion of contraceptives.

It is also important to clear up common misconceptions about contraception and pregnancy. Clearing up misconceptions will permit new learning to take hold and a better client response to whichever methods are explored and ultimately selected. Some common misconceptions include:

- Breastfeeding protects against pregnancy.
- Pregnancy can be avoided if the male partner "pulls out" before he ejaculates.
- Pregnancy can't occur during menses.
- Douching after sex will prevent pregnancy.
- Pregnancy won't happen during the first sexual experience.
- Taking birth control pills protects against STIs.
- The woman is too old to get pregnant.
- Irregular menstruation prevents pregnancy.

When discussing in detail each method of birth control, focus on specific information for each method outlined. Include information such as how this particular method works to prevent pregnancy under normal circumstances of use; the noncontraceptive benefits to overall health; advantages and disadvantages of all methods; the cost involved for each particular method; danger signs that need to be reported to the health care provider; and the required frequency of office visits needed for the particular method.

In addition, outline factors that place the client at risk for method failure. There are several reasons why there are contraceptive failures. Use Table 4.6 to provide patient education concerning a few of the reasons for contraceptive failure. Help clients who have chosen abstinence or fertility awareness methods to define the sexual activities in which they want and don't want to participate. This helps them set sexual limits or boundaries. Help them to develop communication and negotiation skills that will allow them to be successful. Supporting, encouraging, and respecting a couple's choice of abstinence is vital for nurses.

TEACHING GUIDELINES 4.5

Tips for Cervical Caps, Diaphragms, Vaginal Rings, and Condoms

Cervical Cap Insertion/Removal Technique

- It is important to be involved in the fitting process.
- To insert the cap, pinch the sides together, compress the cap dome, insert into the vagina, and place over the cervix.
- Use one finger to feel around the entire circumference to make sure there are no gaps between the cap rim and the cervix.
- After a minute or two, pinch the dome and tug gently to check for evidence of suction. The cap should resist the tug and not slide off easily.
- To remove the cap, press the index finger against the rim and tip the cap slightly to break the suction, and gently pull out the cap.
- The woman should practice inserting and removing the cervical cap three times to validate her proficiency with this device.

Client teaching and counseling regarding the cervical cap

- Fill the dome of the cap up about one-third full with spermicide cream or jelly. Do not apply spermicide to the rim, since it may interfere with the seal.
- Wait approximately 30 minutes after insertion before engaging in sexual intercourse to be sure that a seal has formed between the rim and the cervix.
- Leave the cervical cap in place for a minimum of 6 hours after sexual intercourse. It can be left in place for up to 48 hours without additional spermicide being added.
- Do not use during menses due to the potential for toxic shock syndrome. Use an alternative method such as condoms during this time.
- Inspect the cervical cap prior to insertion for cracks, holes, or tears.
- After using the cervical cap, wash it with soap and water, dry thoroughly, and store in its container.

Diaphragm Insertion/Removal Technique

- Always empty the bladder prior to inserting the diaphragm.
- Inspect diaphragm for holes or tears by holding it up to a light source, or fill it with water and check for a leak.
- Place approximately a tablespoon of spermicidal jelly or cream in the dome and around the rim of the diaphragm.
- The diaphragm can be inserted up to 6 hours prior to intercourse.

- Select the position that is most comfortable for insertion:
  - Squatting
  - Leg up, raising the nondominant leg up on a low stool
  - Reclining position, lying on her back in bed
  - Sitting forward on the edge of a chair
- Hold the diaphragm between the thumb and fingers and compress it to form a "figure-eight" shape.
- Insert the diaphragm into the vagina, directing it downward as far as it will go.
- Tuck the front rim of the diaphragm behind the pubic bone so that the rubber hugs the front wall of the vagina.
- Feel for the cervix through the diaphragm to make sure it is properly placed.
- To remove the diaphragm, insert the finger up and over the top side and move slightly to the side, breaking the suction.
- Pull the diaphragm down and out of the vagina.

Client Teaching and Counseling Regarding the Diaphragm

- Avoid the use of oil-based products such as baby oil, since this may weaken the rubber.
- Wash the diaphragm with soap and water after use and dry thoroughly.
- Place the diaphragm back into the storage case.
- The diaphragm may need to be refitted after weight loss or gain or childbirth.
- Diaphragms should not be used by women with latex allergies.

Vaginal Ring Insertion/Removal Technique and Counseling

- Each ring is used for one menstrual cycle, which consists of 3 weeks of continuous use followed by a ring-free week to allow for menses.
- No fitting is necessary—one size fits all.
- The ring is compressed and inserted into the vagina, behind the pubic bone, as far back as possible.
- Precision placement is not essential.
- Backup contraception is needed for 7 days if the ring is expelled for more than 3 hours during the 3-week period of continuous use.
- The vaginal ring is left in place for 3 weeks, then removed and discarded.
- The vaginal ring is not recommended for women with uterine prolapse or lack of vaginal muscle tone (Youngkin & Davis, 2004).

(continued)

TEACHING GUIDELINES 4.5

Tips for Cervical Caps, Diaphragms, Vaginal Rings, and Condoms (continued)

Male Condom Insertion/Removal Technique and Counseling

- Always keep the condom in its original package until ready to use.
- Store in a cool, dry place.
- Spermicidal condoms should be used if available.
- Check expiration date before using.
- Use a new condom for each sexual act.
- Condom is placed over the erect penis prior to insertion.
- Place condom on the head of the penis and unroll it down the shaft.
- Leave a half-inch of empty space at the end to collect ejaculate.
- Avoid use of oil-based products, because they may cause breakage.
- After intercourse, remove the condom while the penis is still erect.
- Discard condom after use.

Female Condom Insertion/Removal Technique and Counseling

- Practice wearing and inserting prior to first use with sexual intercourse.
- Condom can be inserted up to 8 hours before intercourse.
- Condom is intended for one-time use.
- It can be purchased over the counter—one size fits all.
- Avoid wearing rings to prevent tears; long fingernails can also cause tears.
- Spermicidal lubricant can be used if desired.
- Insert the inner ring high in the vagina, against the cervix.
- Place the outer ring on the outside of the vagina.
- Make sure the erect penis is placed inside the female condom.
- Remove the condom after intercourse. Avoid spilling the ejaculate.

After clients have chosen a method of contraception, it is important to address the following:

- Emphasize that a second method to use as a backup is always needed.
- Provide both oral and written instructions on the method chosen.
- Discuss the need for STI protection if not using a barrier method.
- Inform the client about the availability of ECs.

FIGURE 4.21 The nurse demonstrates insertion of a vaginal ring during client teaching.

Abortion

Abortion is defined as the expulsion of an embryo or fetus before it is viable (Alexander et al., 2007). Abortion can be a medical or surgical procedure. The purpose of abortion is to terminate a pregnancy. Surgical abortion is the most common procedure performed in the United States (approximately 1.6 million annually) and might be the most common surgical procedure in the world (Speroff & Fritz, 2005). Both medical and surgical abortions are safe and legal in the United States; an abortion is considered a woman's constitutional right based on the fundamental right to privacy (Curlin et al., 2007).

Since the landmark U.S. Supreme Court decision *Roe v. Wade* legalized abortion in 1973, debate has continued over how and when abortions are provided. Every state has laws regulating some aspects of the provision of abortion, and many have passed restrictions such as parental consent or notification requirements, mandated counseling and waiting periods, and limits on funding for abortion. Each state addresses these matters independently, and the laws that are passed or enforced are a legislative decision and a function of the political system. Although opponents of abortion continue to be very much a part of the current debates, recently they have refocused their attention on "regulation legislation" to reduce the number of abortions not medically necessary.

TABLE 4.6　CONTRACEPTIVE PROBLEMS AND EDUCATIONAL NEEDS

Contraceptive Failure Problem	Client Education Needed
Not following instructions for use of contraceptive correctly	Take pill the same time every day. Use condoms properly and check condition before using. Make sure diaphragm or cervical cap covers cervix completely. Check IUD for placement monthly.
Inconsistent use of contraceptive	Contraceptives must be used regularly to achieve maximum effectiveness. All it takes is one unprotected act of sexual intercourse to become pregnant. 2% to 5% of condoms will break or tear during use.
Condom broke during sex	Check expiration date. Store condoms properly. Use only a water-based lubricant. Watch for tears caused by long fingernails. Use spermicides to decrease possibility of pregnancy if failure occurs.
Use of antibiotics or other herbs taken with OCs	Use alternative methods during the antibiotic therapy, plus 7 additional days. Implement on day 1 of taking antibiotics.
Belief that you can't get pregnant during menses or that it is safe "just this one time"	It may be possible to become pregnant on almost any day of the menstrual cycle.

Surgical Abortion

Surgical abortion is usually carried out by vacuum aspiration or suction curettage. It is an ambulatory procedure done under local anesthesia. The cervix is dilated prior to surgery and then the products of conception are removed by suction evacuation. The uterus may gently be scraped by curettage to make sure that it is empty. The entire procedure lasts about 10 minutes.

HEALTHY PEOPLE 2010

Objective	Significance
Reduce pregnancies among adolescent females. Increase the proportion of sexually active, unmarried adolescents age 15–17 years who use contraception that both effectively prevents pregnancy and provides barrier protection against disease.	Would reduce number of unplanned pregnancies and girls not finishing their education. This would in turn reduce the number of single parents on state financial assistance.
Increase the proportion of young adults who have received formal instruction before turning age 18 years on reproductive health issues, including all of the following topics: birth control methods, safer sex to prevent HIB, prevention of sexually transmitted disease, and abstinence.	Awareness of contraceptive methods brings about better compliance and prevention of unintended pregnancies in this age group.
Reduce AIDS and the number of HIV infections among adolescents and adults.	Reduce the number of HIV/AIDS victims by using barrier methods to prevent the transmission of this fatal STI.
Reduce the proportion of adolescents and young adults with *Chlamydia trachomatis* infections.	Reduce the number of women with infertility issues secondary to *Chlamydia* infections.

Medical Abortion

In a medical abortion, the woman takes certain medications to induce a miscarriage to remove the products of conception. There are two methods currently used to terminate a pregnancy during the first trimester. The first method uses methotrexate (an antineoplastic agent) followed by misoprostol (a prostaglandin agent) given as a vaginal suppository or in oral form 3 to 7 days later. Methotrexate induces abortion because of its toxicity to trophoblastic tissue, the growing embryo. Misoprostol works by causing uterine contractions, which helps to expel the products of conception. This method is 90% to 98% successful in completing an abortion (Hatcher et al., 2004).

The second method used to induce first-trimester abortions involves using mifepristone (a progesterone antagonist) followed 48 hours later by misoprostol (a prostaglandin agent), which causes contractions of the uterus and expulsion of the uterine contents. Mifepristone, the generic name for RU-486, is sold under the brand names Mifeprex and Early Option. Mifepristone is a potent oral anti-progestogen; it blocks the action of progesterone that prepares the endometrium for implantation and then maintains the pregnancy. This method is 95% effective when used within 49 days after the last menstrual cycle (Hatcher et al., 2004).

Abortion is a very emotional, deeply personal issue. Give support and accurate information. If for personal, religious, or ethical reasons you feel unable to actively participate in the care of a woman undergoing an abortion, you still have the professional responsibility to ensure that the woman receives the nursing care and help she requires. This may necessitate a transfer to another area or a staffing reassignment.

Menopause

The change of life. The end of fertility. The beginning of freedom. Whatever people call it, menopause is a unique and personal experience for every woman. **Menopause** refers to the cessation of regular menstrual cycles. It is the end of menstruation and childbearing capacity. The average age of natural menopause—defined as 1 year without a menstrual period—is 51 years old (Alexander et al., 2007). With current female life expectancy at 80, this event comes in the middle of a woman's adult life.

▶ *Take* NOTE!

Humans are virtually the only species to outlive their reproductive capacities.

Menopause signals the end of an era for many women. It concludes their ability to reproduce, and some women find advancing age, altered roles, and these physiologic changes to be overwhelming events that may precipitate depression and anxiety (Kessenich, 2007). Menopause does not happen in isolation. Midlife is often experienced as a time of change and reflection. Change happens in many arenas: children are leaving or returning home, employment pressures intensify as career moves or decisions are required, elderly parents require more care or the death of a parent may have a major impact, and partners are retrenching or undergoing their own midlife crises. Women must negotiate all these changes in addition to menopause. Managing these stressful changes can be very challenging for many women as they make the transition into midlife.

A woman is born with approximately 500,000 ova, but only 300 to 400 ever mature fully to be released during the menstrual cycle. The absolute number of ova in the ovary is a major determinant of fertility. Over the course of her premenopausal life there is a steady decline in the number of immature ova. No one understands this depletion, but it does not occur in isolation. Maturing ova are surrounded by follicles that produce two major hormones: estrogen, in the form of estradiol, and progesterone. The cyclic maturation of the ovum is directed by the hypothalamus. The hypothalamus triggers a cascade of neurohormones, which act through the pituitary and the ovaries as a pulse generator for reproduction.

This hypothalamic-pituitary-ovarian axis begins to break down long before there is any sign that menopause is imminent. Some scientists believe that the pulse generator in the hypothalamus simply degenerates; others speculate that the ovary becomes more resistant to the pituitary hormone FSH and simply shuts down (Krantz, 2007b). The final act in this well-orchestrated process is amenorrhea.

As menopause approaches, more and more of the menstrual cycles become anovulatory. This period of time, usually 2 to 8 years before cessation of menstruation, is termed perimenopause (Manson, 2006). In perimenopause, the ovary begins to sputter, producing irregular and missed periods and an occasional hot flash. When menopause finally appears, viable ova are gone. Estrogen levels plummet by 90%, and estrone, produced in fat cells, replaces estradiol as the body's main form of estrogen. The major hormone produced by the ovaries during the reproductive years is estradiol; the estrogen found in postmenopausal women is estrone. Estradiol is much more biologically active than estrone (Krantz, 2007). In addition, testosterone levels decrease with menopause.

Menopause, with its dramatic decline in estrogen, affects not only the reproductive organs, but also other body systems:

- Brain: hot flashes, disturbed sleep, mood and memory problems
- Cardiovascular: lower levels of high-density lipoprotein (HDL) and increased risk of cardiovascular disease
- Skeletal: rapid loss of bone density increases the risk of osteoporosis
- Breasts: duct and glandular tissues are replaced by fat
- Genitourinary: vaginal dryness, stress incontinence, cystitis
- Gastrointestinal: less calcium is absorbed from food, increasing the risk for fractures
- Integumentary: skin becomes dry and thin, and collagen levels decrease
- Body shape: more abdominal fat; waist size swells relative to hips

Therapeutic Management

Menopause should be managed individually. In the past, despite the wide diversity of symptoms and risks, the traditional reaction was to reach for the one-size-fits-all therapy: hormone therapy. Today the medical community is changing its thinking in light of the Women's Health Initiative (WHI) study and the Heart and Estrogen/Progestin Replacement Study Follow-Up (HERS II), which reported that long-term hormone therapy (HT) increased the risks of heart attacks, strokes, and breast cancer; in short, the overall health risks of HT exceeded the benefits (Writing Group, 2002, p. 321). In addition, HT didn't protect against the development of coronary artery disease, nor did it prevent the progression of coronary artery disease, as it was previously touted to do (Shelby & O'Hair, 2007). As expected, the fallout from this study and others forced practitioners to re-evaluate their usual therapies and tailor treatment to each client's history, needs, and risk factors.

There is a universe of treatment options out there, but factors in the client's history should be the driving force when determining therapy. Women need to educate themselves about the latest research findings and collaborate with their health care provider on the right menopause therapy. The following factors should be considered in management:

- HT is not indicated to treat or prevent cardiovascular disease, according to WHI. Instead, consider lipid-lowering agents and lifestyle changes if risk or disease is present.
- HT should not be taken for more than 5 years for vasomotor symptoms. Use the lowest dose possible for any hormone therapy.
- HT is acceptable as long as there is a clear indication for use, the woman is under medical supervision, and she is aware of the risks and benefits (North American Menopause Society, 2004).
- Consider nonhormonal therapies such as bisphosphonates and selective estrogen receptor modulators (SERMs).
- Consider weight-bearing exercises, calcium, vitamin D, smoking cessation, and avoidance of alcohol to treat or prevent osteoporosis.
- Annual breast examinations and mammograms are essential.
- Local estrogen creams can be used for vaginal atrophy.
- Consider herbal therapies for symptoms (Krantz, 2007).

Although numerous symptoms have been attributed to menopause (Box 4.9), some of them are more closely related to the aging process than to estrogen deficiency. A few of the more common menopausal conditions and their management will be discussed.

Managing Hot Flashes and Night Sweats

Hot flashes and night sweats are classic signs of estrogen deficiency and the predominant complaint of perimenopausal women. A hot flash is a transient and sudden sensation of warmth that spreads over the body, particularly the neck, face, and chest. Hot flashes are caused by vasomotor instability. Nearly 85% of menopausal women experience them (Alexander et al., 2007). Hot flashes are an early and acute sign of estrogen deficiency. These flashes

---

BOX 4.9 **Common Symptoms of Menopause**

- Hot flashes or flushes of the head and neck
- Dryness in the eyes and vagina
- Personality changes
- Anxiety and/or depression
- Loss of libido
- Weight gain and water retention
- Night sweats
- Fatigue
- Irritability
- Insomnia
- Stress incontinence
- Heart palpitations

Source: Chedraui et al., 2007.

---

can be mild or extreme and can last from 2 to 30 minutes (Grady, 2006).

There are many options for treating hot flashes. Treatment must be based on symptom severity, the client's medical history, and the client's values and concerns. Although the gold standard in the treatment of hot flashes is estrogen, this is not recommended for all women. The following are suggestions for the management of hot flashes:

- Pharmacologic options
  - HT unless contraindicated
  - Androgen therapy (potentiates estrogen)
  - Estrogen and androgen combinations
  - Progestin therapy (Depo-Provera injection every 3 months)
  - Clonidine (central alpha-adrenergic agonist) weekly patch
  - Neurontin (anti-seizure) decreased hot flashes
  - Acupuncture reduced frequency of hot flashes
  - Propranolol (beta-adrenergic blocker)
  - Gabapentin (Neurontin): antiseizure drug
  - SSRIs: venlafaxine (Effexor) and sertraline (Zoloft) have shown promise
  - Vitamin E: 100 mg daily (Rubin, 2007)
- Lifestyle changes
  - Lower room temperature; use fans.
  - Wear clothing in layers for easy removal.
  - Limit caffeine and alcohol intake.
  - Drink 8 to 10 glasses of water daily.
  - Stop smoking or cut back.
  - Avoid hot drinks and spicy food.
  - Take calcium (1,200 to 1,500 mg) and vitamin D (400 to 600 IU).
  - Try relaxation techniques, deep breathing, and meditation.
  - Exercise daily, but not just before bedtime.

- Maintain a healthy weight.
- Identify stressors and learn to manage them.
- Keep a diary to identify triggers of hot flashes.
- Alternative therapies
  - Phytoestrogens: isoflavones, ligands, coumenstrols
  - Black cohosh
  - Chamomile: mild sedative to alleviate insomnia
    - Unopposed transdermal progesterone
    - Compounded bioidentical hormones
      - Estrogen
      - Progesterone
      - Testosterone
      - Dehydroepiandrosterone (DHEA)
      - Pregnenolone (Campbell, 2006)
  - Chasteberry (vitex): balances progesterone and estrogen
  - Dong quai: acts as a form of phytoestrogen
  - Ginseng: purported to improve memory
  - St. John's wort: reduces depression and fatigue
  - Valerian root: induces sleep and relaxation (AAFP, 2006)

Many women are choosing alternative treatments for managing menopausal symptoms. Because of their natural origin, women perceive that alternative treatments are safer. The interest in phytoestrogens came about because of the low prevalence of hot flashes in Asian women, which was attributed to their diet being rich in phytoestrogens (Manson, 2006). Recent studies have found that black cohosh, multibotanical herbs, and increased soy intake do not reduce the frequency or severity of menopausal hot flashes or night sweats (ACOG, 2005; Huntzinger, 2006; Newton et al., 2006; Seppa, 2007). Other remedies for easing menopausal symptoms might include red clover, motherwort, ginseng, sarsaparilla root, valerian root, L-tryptophan, calcium-magnesium, and kelp tablets (Haas, 2007). Again, research thus far has been skeptical about their efficacy, but many women report they ease their symptoms and their use has skyrocketed. While there might be some benefits to their use, evidence of the efficacy of alternative products in menopause is largely anecdotal. Small, preliminary clinical trials might demonstrate the safety of some of the nonpharmacologic products. Nurses should be aware of the purported action of these agents as well as any adverse effects or drug interactions.

Managing Urogenital Changes

Menopause can be a physically and emotionally challenging time for women. In addition to the psychological burden of leaving behind the reproductive phase of life and the stigma of an "aging" body, sexual difficulties due to urogenital changes plague most women but are frequently not addressed.

Vaginal atrophy occurs during menopause because of declining estrogen levels. These changes include thinning of the vaginal walls, an increase in pH, irritation, increased susceptibility to infection, dyspareunia, loss of lubrication with intercourse, vaginal dryness, and a decrease in sexual desire related to these changes. Decreased estrogen levels can also influence a woman's sexual function as well. Delayed clitoral reaction, decreased vaginal lubrication, diminished circulatory response during sexual stimulation, and reduced contractions during orgasm have all been linked to low estrogen levels (McKinney, 2007).

Management of these changes might include the use of estrogen vaginal tablets (Vagifem) or Premarin cream; Estring, an estrogen-releasing vaginal ring that lasts for 3 months; testosterone patches; and over-the-counter moisturizers and lubricants (Astroglide). A positive outlook on sexuality and a supportive partner are also needed to make the sexual experience enjoyable and fulfilling.

> ▶ **Take** NOTE!
>
> *Sexual health is an important aspect of the human experience. By keeping an open mind, listening to women, and providing evidence-based treatment options, the nurse can help improve quality of life for menopausal women.*

Preventing and Managing Osteoporosis

Women are greatly affected by osteoporosis after menopause. Osteoporosis is a condition in which bone mass declines to such an extent that fractures occur with minimal trauma. Bone loss begins in the third or fourth decade of a woman's life and accelerates rapidly after menopause. It affects 8 million women, with millions more at high risk for developing it. This translates to 1 in 2 women over the age of 50 having an osteoporosis-related fracture in their lifetime (Alexander et al., 2007). This condition puts many women into long-term care, with a resulting loss of independence. Figure 4.22 shows the skeletal changes associated with osteoporosis.

Most women with osteoporosis don't know they have the disease until they sustain a fracture, usually of the wrist or hip. Risk factors include:

- Increasing age
- Postmenopausal status without hormone replacement
- Small frame, thin-boned
- Caucasian or Asian
- Impaired eyesight
- Rheumatoid arthritis
- Family history of osteoporosis
- Sedentary lifestyle
- History of treatment with:
  - Antacids with aluminum
  - Heparin
  - Steroids
  - Thyroid replacement drugs

FIGURE 4.22 Skeletal changes associated with osteoporosis. (John Radcliffe Hospital/ Photo Researcher Inc.)

- Smoking and consuming alcohol
- Low calcium and vitamin D intake
- Excessive amounts of caffeine
- Anorexia nervosa or bulimia (Hansberger, 2007)

Screening tests to measure bone density are not good predictors for young women who might be at risk for developing this condition. Dual-energy x-ray absorptiometry (DXA or DEXA) is a screening test that calculates the mineral content of the bone at the spine and hip. It is highly accurate, fast, and relatively inexpensive (McNally, Kenny & Smith, 2007).

The best management for this painful, crippling, and potentially fatal disease is prevention. Women can modify many risk factors by doing the following:

- Engage in daily weight-bearing exercise, such as walking.
- Increasing calcium and vitamin D intake.
- Avoid smoking and excessive alcohol.
- Discuss your bone health with your health care provider.
- When appropriate, have a bone density test and take medication if needed (National Osteoporosis Foundation, 2007).

Medications that can help in preventing and managing osteoporosis include:

- HT (Premarin)
- SERMs (Evista)
- Calcium and vitamin D supplements (Tums)
- Bisphosphonates (Actonel or Fosamax)
- Calcitonin (Miacalcin) (Hansberger, 2007)

Preventing and Managing Cardiovascular Disease

Although cardiovascular disease is still thought of as a "man's disease," it is the major killer of postmenopausal women 50 to 75 years of age (Rosano et al., 2007). Half a million women die annually in the United States of cardiovascular disease, with strokes accounting for about 20% of the deaths (Alexander et al., 2007). This translates into approximately one death every minute. Coronary heart disease accounts for the majority of cardiovascular deaths in women, with nearly two thirds of these women dying suddenly without any previously recognized symptoms (Hackley, Kriebs & Rousseau, 2007).

For the first half of a woman's life, estrogen seems to be a protective substance for the cardiovascular system by smoothing, relaxing, and dilating blood vessels. It even helps boost HDL and lower LDL levels, helping to keep the arteries clean from plaque accumulation. But when estrogen levels plummet as women age and experience menopause, the incidence of cardiovascular disease increases dramatically.

Menopause is not the only factor that increases a woman's risk for cardiovascular disease. Lifestyle and medical history factors such as the following play a major role:

- Smoking
- Obesity
- High-fat diet
- Sedentary lifestyle
- High cholesterol levels
- Family history of cardiovascular disease
- Hypertension
- Apple-shaped body
- Diabetes

Two of the major risk factors for coronary heart disease are hypertension and dyslipidemia. Both are modifiable and can be prevented by lifestyle changes and, if needed, controlled by medication. This is why prevention is essential. In addition, women who experience early menopause lose the protection afforded by endogenous estrogen to the cardiac system and are at greater risk for more extensive atherosclerosis. Major preventive strategies include a healthy diet, increased activity, exercise, smoking cessation, decreased alcohol intake, and weight reduction.

Raising awareness of heart disease in women is an essential role for nurses. Lifestyle interventions are effective in preventing cardiovascular disease in all individuals regardless of their underlying risk (Hackley, Kriebs & Rousseau, 2007). Stressing the importance of lifestyle modifications must begin early in life and should be reinforced from the beginning of a young woman's reproductive years through menopause. Nurses are in an ideal position to teach the importance of good nutrition, healthy weight, and daily exercise before cardiovascular disease becomes clinically evident.

Nursing Assessment

Menopause is a universal and irreversible part of the overall aging process involving a woman's reproductive system. While not a disease state, menopause does place women at greater risk for the development of many conditions of aging. Nurses can help the woman become aware of her risk for postmenopausal diseases, as well as strategies to prevent them. The nurse can be instrumental in assessing risk factors and planning interventions in collaboration with the client. These might include:

• Screening for osteoporosis, cardiovascular disease, and cancer risk
  • Assessment of blood pressure to identify hypertension
  • Blood cholesterol to identify hyperlipidemia risk
  • Mammogram to find a cancerous lesion
  • Pap smear to identify cervical cancer
  • Pelvic examination to identify endometrial cancer or masses
  • Digital rectal examination to assess for colon cancer
  • Bone density testing as a baseline at menopause to identify osteopenia (low bone mass), which might lead to osteoporosis
• Assessing lifestyle to plan strategies to prevent chronic conditions:
  • Dietary intake of fat, cholesterol, and sodium
  • Weight management
  • Calcium intake
  • Use of tobacco, alcohol, and caffeine
  • Performance of breast self-examinations

Nursing Management

There is no "magic bullet" in managing menopause. Nurses can counsel women about their risks and help them to prevent disease and debilitating conditions with specific health-maintenance education. Women should make their own decisions, but the nurse should make sure they are armed with the facts to do so intelligently. Nurses can offer a thorough explanation of the menopausal process, including the latest research findings, to help women understand and make decisions about this inevitable event.

If the woman decides to use HT to control her menopausal symptoms, after being thoroughly educated, she will need frequent reassessment. There are no hard-and-fast rules that apply to meeting a woman's individual needs. The nurse can provide realistic expectations of the therapy to reduce the woman's anxiety and concern.

It is also useful to emphasize the value of friends to gain support and share information and resources. Often just talking about emotional difficulties like a death of a parent or problematic relationships helps solve problems. It also shows the woman that her emotional responses are valid.

Healthy lifestyles and stress management techniques are vital to health and longevity, and it is important to keep these on the client's agenda when discussing menopause (Staff of Boston Women's Health Book Collective, 2007).

Evidence-based interventions include lifestyle modifications, risk management therapies, and preventive drug interventions, such as the following:

• Participate actively in maintaining health.
• Exercise regularly.
• Take supplemental calcium and eat appropriately to prevent osteoporosis.
• Stop smoking to prevent lung and heart disease.
• Reduce caffeine and alcohol intake to prevent osteoporosis.
• Monitor blood pressure, lipids, and diabetes (drug therapy management).
• Use low-dose aspirin.
• Reduce dietary intake of fat, cholesterol, and sodium to prevent cardiovascular disease.
• Maintain a healthy weight for body frame.
• Perform breast self-examinations to detect breast lesions.
• Control stress (Dormire & Becker, 2007).

These life approaches may seem low-tech, but they can stave off menopause-related complications such as cardiovascular disease, osteoporosis, and depression. These tips for healthy living work well, but the client needs to be motivated to stick with them.

■■■ Key Concepts

■ Establishing good health habits and avoiding risky behaviors early in life will prevent chronic conditions later on.
■ There are more than 200 symptoms of PMS, and at least two different syndromes have been recognized: PMS and premenstrual dysphoric disorder (PMDD).
■ Endometriosis is a condition in which bits of functioning endometrial tissue are located outside their normal site, the uterine cavity.
■ Infertility is a widespread problem that has an emotional, social, and economic impact on couples.
■ More than half (53%) of all unintended pregnancies occur in women who report using some method of birth control during the month of conception.
■ Hormonal methods include oral contraceptives, injectables, implants, vaginal rings, and transdermal patches.
■ Recent studies have shown that the extension of active oral contraceptive pills carries the same safety profile as the conventional 28-day regimens.
■ Currently there are three IUSs available in the United States: the copper ParaGard-T-380A; Progestasert, a progesterone device; and the levonorgestrel intrauterine system (LNG-IUS) Mirena, a levonorgestrel-releasing device.
■ Sterilization is the most popular method of contraception in the United States and worldwide.
■ Menopause, with a dramatic decline in estrogen levels, affects not only the reproductive organs but also other bodily systems.

- Most women with osteoporosis do not know they have the disease until they sustain a fracture, usually of the wrist or hip.
- Half a million women die annually in the United States of cardiovascular diseases, with strokes accounting for about 20% of the deaths.
- Nurses should aim to have a holistic approach to the sexual health of women from menarche through menopause.

REFERENCES

AAFP (2006). Evidence-based complementary and alternative medicine (CAM): What should physicians know? *Medscape.* Available at: http://www.medscape.com/viewarticle/549067

ACOG Practice Bulletin (2000). Clinical management guidelines for obstetricians-gynecologists, number 15: Premenstrual syndrome. *Obstetrics & Gynecology, 95,* 1–9.

ACOG (2005). ACOG's Hormone Therapy report. *Obstetrics & Gynecology,* ACOG Task Force, (Supplement to October issue), 1–131.

Aeby, T. C., & Frattarelli, L. C. (2006). Dysfunctional uterine bleeding. *eMedicine Journal.* Available at: http://www.emedicine.com/ped/topic628.htm

Aeby, T. C., & Hraoka, M. R. (2006). Endometriosis. *Emedicine.* Available at: http://www.emedicine.com/ped/topic677.htm

Alan Guttmacher Institute (2007). Get "in the know": 20 questions about pregnancy, contraception and abortion. Available at: http://www.guttmacher.org/in-the-know/index.html

Alexander, L. L., LaRosa, J. H., Bader, H., & Garfield, S. (2007). *New dimensions in women's health* (4th ed.). Boston: Jones and Bartlett.

American Academy of Allergy, Asthma, and Immunology (AAAAI) (2007). Tips to remember: Latex allergy. Available at: http://www.aaaai.org/patients/publicedmat/tips/latexallergy.stm

American Society for Reproductive Medicine (ASRM) (2007). Frequently asked questions about infertility. Available at: http://www.asrm.org/Patients/faqs.html

Anderson, F. D., Gibbons, W., & Portman, D. (2006). Long-term study of an extended-cycle oral contraceptive (Seasonale): A 2-year multicenter open-label extension trial. *American Journal of Obstetrics & Gynecology, 195*(1), 92–96.

Andoisek, K. M., & Rapkin, A. J. (2007). Contraceptive use in women with premenstrual disorders. *USC Dialogues in Contraception, 10*(4), 4–7.

Archer, D. F. (2006). Menstrual-cycle-related symptoms: A review of the rationale for continuous use of oral contraceptives. *Contraception, 74*(5), 359–366.

Arevalo, M. (2007). CycleBeads: Easy, effective natural family planning. Available at: http://www.cyclebeads.com

Bielak, K. M., & Harris, G. S. (2006). Amenorrhea. *eMedicine.* Available at: http://www.emedicine.com/ped/topic2779.htm

Braverman, P. K., & Neinstein, L. S. (2007). Dysmenorrhea and premenstrual syndrome. In L. S. Neinstein (Ed.), *Adolescent health care, a practical guide* (5th ed., pp. 952–965). Philadelphia: Lippincott Williams & Wilkins.

Brucker, M. C. (2006). Return of the sponge: Will consumers return to a worthy old favorite? *AWHONN Lifelines, 10*(1), 74–76.

Campagne, D. M., & Campagne, G. (2007). The premenstrual syndrome revisited. *European Journal of Obstetrics & Reproductive Biology, 130*(1), 4–17.

Campbell, S. (2006) Bioidentical hormones: Achieving the perfect fit. *Advance for Nurse Practitioners, 14*(2), 25–30.

Canning, S., Waterman, M., & Dye, L. (2006). Dietary supplements and herbal remedies for premenstrual syndrome (PMS): A systematic review of the evidence for their efficacy. *Journal of Reproductive & Infant Psychology, 24*(4), 363–378.

Centers for Disease Control and Prevention (CDC) (2006). Contraceptive use. National Center for Health Statistics. Available at: http://www.cdc.gov/women/natstat/reprhlth.htm#contraception

Chedraul, P., Hidalgo, L., Chavez, D., Morocho, N., Alvarado, M., & Huc, A. (2007). Menopausal symptoms and associated risk factors among postmenopausal women screened for the metabolic syndrome. *Archives of Gynecology & Obstetrics, 275*(3), 161–168.

Cheng, L., Gulmezogulu, A. M., Van Oel, C. J., Piaggio, G., Ezcurra, E., & Van Look, P. F. A. (2006). Interventions for emergency contraception. *Cochrane Library:* CD001324, 2009357452.

Clayton, A. H. (2008). Symptoms related to the menstrual cycle: Diagnosis, prevalence, and treatment. *Journal of Psychiatric Practice, 14*(1), 13–21.

Courtney, K. (2006). The contraceptive patch: Latest developments. *AWHONN Lifelines, 10*(3), 250–253.

Covington, S., & Burns, L. H. (2006). *Infertility counseling: A comprehensive handbook for clinicians* (2nd ed.). Cambridge, UK: Cambridge University Press.

Curlin, F. A., Lawrence, R. E., Chin, M. H., & Lantos, J. D. (2007). Religion, conscience, and controversial clinical practice. *New England Journal of Medicine, 356*(6), 593–600.

Dassow, P., & Bennett, J. M. (2006). Vasectomy: An update. *American Family Physician, 74*(12), 2069–2074.

DeMasters, J. (2004). Male infertility. *Advance for Nurses, 6*(1), 19–25.

DeSutter, P. (2006). Rational diagnosis and treatment in infertility. *Best Practice & Research: Clinical Obstetrics & Gynecology, 20*(5), 647–664.

Dirubbo, N. E. (2006). Counsel your patients about contraceptive options. *Nurse Practitioner, 31*(4), 40–44.

Dodds, N., & Sinert, R. (2006). Dysfunctional uterine bleeding. *eMedicine.* Available at: http://www.emedicine.com/emerg/topic155.htm

Dormire, S., & Becker, H. (2007). Menopause health decision support for women with physical disabilities. *JOGNN, 36*(1), 97–104.

Doty, E., & Attaran, M. (2006). Managing primary dysmenorrhea. *Journal of Pediatric & Adolescent Gynecology, 19*(5), 341–344.

Edelman, A. B., Gallo, M. F., Jensen, J. T., Nichols, M. D., Schulz, K. F., & Grimes, D. A. (2006). Continuous or extended cycle versus cyclic use of combined oral contraceptives. *Cochrane Library:* CD004695

Edmundson, L. D., & Erogul, M. (2006) Dysmenorrhea. *eMedicine.* Available at: http://www.emedicine.com/emerg/topic156.htm

Female Contraception (2006). *Contraception: Female, annual report.* ADAM. Available at: http://search.ebscohost.com/login.aspx?direct=true&db=aph&AN=20517070&site=ehost-live

Ficorelli, C. T., & Weeks, B. (2007). Untangling the complexities of male infertility. *Nursing2007, 37*(1), 24–26.

French, R., Vliet, H., Cowan, F., Mansour, D., Morris, S., Hughes, D., Robinson, A., Proctor, T., Summerbell, C., Logan, S., Helmerhorst, F., & Guillebaud, J. (2006). Hormonally impregnated intrauterine systems (IUSs) versus other forms. *Cochrane Library.* CD001776: 2009357603.

Futterman, L. A., & Rapkin, A. J. (2006). Diagnosis of premenstrual disorders. *Journal of Reproductive Medicine, 51*(4), 349–358.

Gallo, M. F., Grimes, D. A., Lopez, L. M., & Schultz, K. F. (2006). Nonlatex versus latex condoms for contraception. *Cochrane Library.* Available at: www.cinahl.com/cgi-bin/refsvc?jid=3053&accno=2009358379

Gallo, M., Grimes, D., & Schultz, K. (2006). Cervical cap versus diaphragm for contraception. *Cochrane Library.* Available at: http://search.ebscohost.com/login.aspx?direct=true&db=rzh&AN=2009358282&site=ehost-live

Giulio, G. D., & Reissing, E. D. (2006). Premenstrual dysphoric disorder: Prevalence, diagnostic considerations, and controversies. *Journal of Psychosomatic Obstetrics & Gynecology, 27*(4), 201–210.

Grady, D. (2006). Management of menopausal symptoms. *New England Journal of Medicine, 355*(22), 2338–2347.

Grainger, D. A., Frazier, L. M., & Rowland, C. A. (2006) Preconception care and treatment with assisted reproductive technologies. *Maternal & Child Health,* (Supplement 10), 161–164.

Graziottin, A. (2006). A review of transdermal hormone contraception: Focus on the ethinyl estradiol/norelgestromin contraceptive patch. *Treatments in Endocrinology, 5*(6), 359–365.

Haas, E. (2007). Easing menopause symptoms naturally. *Share Guide, 89,* 29–78.

Hackley, B., Kriebs, J. M., & Rousseau, M. E. (2007). *Primary care of women: A guide for midwives and women's health providers.* Sudbury, MA: Jones and Bartlett Publishers.

Hansberger, J. (2007). Osteoporosis: Review of disease, diagnosis, and treatments for the advanced practice nurse. *Journal of Advanced Nursing Practice, 8*(1), 5–6.

Harel, Z. (2006). Dysmenorrhea in adolescents and young adults. *Journal of Pediatric & Adolescent Gynecology, 19*(6), 363–371.

Hatcher, R. A., et al. (2004). *Contraceptive technology* (18th ed.). New York: Ardent Media, Inc.

Hearton, L. (2006). Long-acting methods of reversible contraception. *Primary Health Care, 16*(4), 21–22.

Hompes, P. G., & Mijatovic, V. (2007). Endometriosis: The way forward. *Gynecological Endocrinology, 23*(1), 5–12.

Hsiao, M., & Liu, C. (2007). Unusual manifestations of premenstrual syndrome. *Psychiatry & Clinical Neurosciences, 61*(1), 120–123.

Htay, T. T., & Aung, K. (2006). Premenstrual dysphoric disorder. *Emedicine.* Available at: http://www.emedicine.com/med/topic3357.htm

Huntzinger, A. (2006). ACOG reports on compounded bioidentical hormones. *American Family Physician, 73*(12), 2242–2245.

Jenkins, G., & Jenkins, J. (2006). Issues relating to infertility. *Practice Nurse, 32*(4), 14–22.

Kelly-Weeder, S., & O'Conner, A. (2006). Modifiable risk factors for impaired fertility in women: What nurse practitioners need to know. *Journal of the American Academy of Nurse Practitioners, 18*(6), 268–276.

Kessenich, C. R. (2007). Inevitable menopause. *Nursing Spectrum.* Available at: http://www.nurse.com/ce/course.html?CCID=3183ce232.htm

Krantz, C. (2007a). Amenorrhea. In R. E. Rakel (Ed.), *Conn's current therapy 2007.* Philadelphia: Elsevier W. B. Saunders.

Krantz, C. (2007b). Menstrual cycle. In R. E. Rakel (Ed.), *Conn's current therapy 2007.* Philadelphia: Elsevier W. B. Saunders.

Lenehan, G. P. (2004). Latex allergy: Separating fact from fiction. *Travel Nursing,* pp. 12–17.

Lethaby, A., Cooke, I., & Rees, M. (2006). Progesterone/progestogen releasing intrauterine systems versus either placebo or any other medication for heavy menstrual bleeding. *Cochrane Database Systematic Review* (4), CD002126.

Lever, K. A. (2005) Emergency contraception. *AWHONN Lifelines, 9*(3), 218–225.

Manson, J. E. (2006) Perimenopause, hormones, and midlife health. *Harvard Women's Health Watch, 14*(3), 1–3.

Master-Hunter, T., & Heiman, D. L. (2006). Amenorrhea: Evaluation and treatment. *American Family Physician, 73*(8), 1374–1382.

McKinney, L. N. (2007). Low libido in postmenopausal women. *Advance for Nurse Practitioners, 15*(1), 28–36.

McNally, D. N., Kenny, A. M., & Smith, J. A. (2007), Adherence of academic geriatric practitioners to osteoporosis screening guidelines. *Osteoporosis International, 18*(2), 177–183.

Mishell, D. R., Guillebaud, J., Westoff, C., Nelson, A. L., Kaunitz, A. M., Trussell, J., & Davis, A. J. (2007). Combined hormonal contraceptive traits: Variable data collection and bleeding assessment methodologies influence study outcomes and physician perception. *Contraception, 75*(1), 4–10.

Moreno, M. A., & Giesel, A. E. (2006). Premenstrual syndrome. *Emedicine.* Available at: http://www.emedicine.com/ped/topic1890.htm

Murphy, P. A., Morgan, K., & Likis, F. E. (2006). Contraception. In K. D. Schuiling & F. E. Likis (Eds.), *Women's gynecologic health* (pp. 169–228). Sudbury, MA: Jones and Bartlett Publishers.

Nasir, L. S. (2007). Dysmenorrhea. In R. E. Rakel & E. T. Bope (Eds.), *Conn's current therapy 2007* (pp. 1238–1240). Philadelphia: Saunders.

National Institute of Child Health and Human Development (NICHD) (2006). Endometriosis. NICHD Information Resource Center, NIH Pub. No. 02-2413. Available at: http://www.nichd.nih.gov/health/topics/Endometriosis.cfm

National Osteoporosis Foundation (NOF) (2007). Steps to prevent osteoporosis. Available at: http://www.nof.org/prevention/index.htm

Nelson, L. M., & Bakalov, V. (2006). Amenorrhea. *eMedicine.* Available at: http://www.emedicine.com/med/topic117.htm

Newton, K. M., Reed, S. D., LaCroix, A. Z., Grothaus, L. C., Ehrlich, K., & Guiltinan, J. (2006). Treatment of vasomotor symptoms of menopause with black cohosh, multibotanicals, soy, hormone therapy, or placebo. A randomized trial. *Annals of Internal Medicine, 145,* 869–879.

North American Menopause Society (NAMS) (2004). Recommendations for estrogen and progesterone use in peri-menopausal and post-menopausal women. *Menopause, 11*(6), 589–600.

OSHA (2006). Latex allergy. U.S. Department of Labor, Occupational Safety & Health Administration. Available at: http://www.osha.gov/SLTC/latexallergy

Pagana, K. D., & Pagana, T. J. (2007). *Mosby's diagnostic and laboratory test reference* (8th ed.). Philadelphia: Elsevier Mosby.

Pavlovich-Danis, S. J. (2007). Cyclic upheaval: Premenstrual syndrome and premenstrual dysphoric disorder. *Nursing Spectrum.* Available at: http://www.nurse.com/ce/course.html?CCID=3297

Planned Parenthood (2007). Facts about birth control. Available at: http://www.plannedparenthood.org/bc/bcfacts4.html

Quallich, S. (2006). Examining male infertility. *Urologic Nursing, 26*(4), 277–288.

Rackow, B. W., & Arici, A. (2007). Dysfunctional uterine bleeding. In R. E. Rakel & E. T. Bope (Eds.), *Conn's current therapy 2007* (pp. 1230–1232). Philadelphia: Saunders.

Ravin, C. R. (2006). Considering contraception: What practitioners are saying. *AWHONN Lifelines, 10*(2), 122–128.

Redshaw, M., Hockley, C., & Davidson, L. L. (2007). A qualitative study of the experience of treatment for infertility among women who successfully become pregnant. *Human Reproduction, 22*(1), 295–304.

Robinson, K. (2005). Depo-Provera: New concerns—same issues? *AWHONN Lifelines, 9*(3), 214–217.

Roederer, M. W., Blackwell, J., & Blenning, C. (2006). Risks and benefits of combination contraceptives. *American Family Physician, 74*(11), 1915–1916.

Rosano, G. M., Vitale, C., Marazzi, G., Voltazzi, G., & Volterrani, M. (2007). Menopause and cardiovascular disease: The evidence. *Climacteric* (Supplement 1, 10), 19–24.

Rubin, R. (2007). A herbal menopause therapy: Get a closer look. *USA Today,* Jan. 11, 2007, p. 7.

Samra, O. M., & Wood, E. (2006). Contraception. *Emedicine.* Available at: http://www.emedicine.com/med/topic3211.htm

Saul, T., & Dave, A. K. (2006) Endometriosis. *Emedicine.* Available at: http://www.emedicine.com/EMERG/topic165.htm

Schenker, J. G. (2005). Assisted reproductive practice: Religious perspectives. *Reproductive BioMedicine, 10*(3), 310–319.

Schuiling, K. D., & Likis, F. E. (2006). *Women's gynecologic health.* Sudbury, MA: Jones and Bartlett Publishers.

Seppa, N. (2007). Putting the kibosh on black cohosh. *Science News, 171*(2), 29–30.

Shelby, K., & O'Hair, K. (2007). Hormone replacement therapy: What we know now. *Nursing Spectrum.* Available at: http://www.nurse.com/ce/course.html?CCID=2325&PageNum=3&Begin=11545

Sinai, I., Arevalo, M., & Jennings, V. (2006). Fertility awareness-based methods of family planning: Predictors of correct use. *International Family Planning Perspectives, 32*(2), 94–100.

Skidmore-Roth, L. (2007). *Mosby's drug guide for nurses* (7th ed.). St. Louis, MO: Elsevier Mosby.

Smith, R. P. (2006) Finding the best approach to dysmenorrhea. *Contemporary OB/GYN, 51*(11), 54–62.

Speroff, L., & Fritz, M. A. (2005). *Clinical gynecologic endocrinology and fertility* (7th ed.). Philadelphia: Lippincott Williams & Wilkins.

Staff of the Boston Women's Health Book Collective (2007). *Our bodies, ourselves: Menopause.* New York: Simon & Schuster Trade.

Stewart, F. H., Kaunitz, A. M., LaGuardia, K. D., Karvois, D. L., Fisher, A. C., & Friedman, A. J. (2006). Extended use of transdermal norelgestromin/ethinyl estradiol: A randomized trial. *Obstetrics & Gynecology, 105*(6), 1389–1396.

Swica, Y., & Westhoff, C. (2006). Update on new contraceptive choices. *Journal of Clinical Outcomes Management, 13*(8), 447–455.

Taylor, D. (2005). Perimenstrual symptoms and syndromes: Guidelines for symptom management and self-care. *Advanced Studies in Medicine, 5*(5), 228–241.

Tolaymat, L. L., & Kaunitz, A. M. (2007). Contraceptive methods. In R. E. Rakel & E. T. Bope (Eds.), *Conn's current therapy 2007* (pp. 882–885). Philadelphia: Saunders.

Torpy, J. M. (2007). Polycystic ovary syndrome. *JAMA, 297*(5), 554–557.

Trussell, J. (2004). Contraceptive efficacy. In R. Hatcher, et al. (Eds.), *Contraceptive technology* (18th rev. ed.). New York: Ardent Media, Inc.

UNFPA (2007). *The state of the world population 2006 report.* Available at: http://www.unfpa.org/swp/swpmain.htm

U.S. Bureau of the Census (2006). *National population estimates-characteristics.* Available at: http://eire.census.gov/popest/data/national/tables/asro/NA-EST2002-ASRO-01.php

U.S. Food & Drug Administration (FDA) (2006). FDA approves over-the-counter access for Plan B for women 18 and older; prescription remains required for those 17 and younger. *FDA News* (August 24, 2006). Available at: www.fda.gov/bbs/topics/NEWS/2006/New01436.html

Valle, R. F. (2006). Combination of tubal sterilization and endometrial ablation is safe and effective. *Fertility and Sterility, 86*(1), 152–158.

World Health Organization (WHO) (2007). Infertility in developing countries. *Reproductive Health.* Available at: http://www.who.int/reproductive-health/infertility/index.htm

Writing Group for the Women's Health Initiative Investigators (2002). Risks and benefits of estrogen plus progestin in healthy post-menopausal women: Principal results from the Women's Health Initiative randomized controlled trial. *JAMA, 288*(3), 321–333.

Wysocki, S. (2007). Clinical rationale for continuous oral contraception. *American Journal for Nurse Practitioners, 11*(3), 57–67.

Youngkin, E. Q., & Davis, M. S. (2004). *Women's health: A primary care clinical guide* (3rd ed.). New Jersey: Prentice Hall.

WEBSITES

American College of Obstetricians and Gynecologists (ACOG): (202) 863-2518, http://www.acog.org

American Psychiatric Association: (202) 682-6000, http://psych.org

American Society for Reproductive Medicine: (205) 978-5000, http://www.asrm.org

Centers for Disease Control and Prevention: (202) 329-1819, http://www.cdc.gov

Consortium for Emergency Contraceptive: http://www.cecinfo.org

Center for Reproductive Rights: http://www.crlp.org

Emergency Contraception Hotline: (888) 668-2528, http://www.not-2-late.com

Endometriosis Association: (414) 355-2200, http://www.ovf.com/endohtml.html

FDA's Office of Women's Health: http://www.fda.gov/womens

Hormone Foundation: (800) 467-6663, http://hormone.org

International Counsel on Infertility Information Dissemination: (703) 379-9178, http://www.inciid.org

National Institute of Mental Health: (301) 443-4513, http://www.nimh.nih.gov

National Women's Health Resource Center: (877) 986-9472, http://www.healthywomen.org

National Women's Information Center (NWHIC): (800) 994-9662, http://www.4women.gov

North American Menopause Society: http://www.menopause.org

Planned Parenthood Federation of America, Inc.: (800) 669-0156, http://www.plannedparenthood.org

Premenstrual Institute: (248) 624-3366, http://www.pmsinst.com

Resolve, The National Infertility Association: (617) 623-0744, http://www.resolve.org

CHAPTER WORKSHEET

MULTIPLE CHOICE QUESTIONS

1. A couple is considered infertile after how many months of trying to conceive?

   a. 6 months

   b. 12 months

   c. 18 months

   d. 24 months

2. A couple reports that their condom broke while they were having sexual intercourse last night. What would you advise to prevent pregnancy?

   a. Inject a spermicidal agent into her vagina immediately.

   b. Obtain emergency contraceptives and take them immediately.

   c. Douche with a solution of vinegar and hot water tonight.

   d. Take a strong laxative now and again at bedtime.

3. Which of the following combination contraceptives has been approved for extended continuous use?

   a. Seasonale

   b. NuvaRing

   c. Ortho Evra

   d. Mirena

4. Which of the following measures helps prevent osteoporosis?

   a. Iron supplementation

   b. Sleeping 8 hours nightly

   c. Eating lean meats only

   d. Walking 3 miles daily

5. Which of the following activities will increase a woman's risk of cardiovascular disease if she is taking oral contraceptives?

   a. Eating a high-fiber diet

   b. Smoking cigarettes

   c. Taking daily multivitamins

   d. Drinking alcohol

6. Hormone therapy taken by menopausal women reduces:

   a. Weight gain

   b. Bone density

   c. Hot flashes

   d. Heart disease

7. Throughout life, a woman's most proactive activity to promote her health would be to engage in:

   a. Consistent exercise

   b. Socialization with friends

   c. Quality quiet time with herself

   d. Consuming water

8. What comment by a woman would indicate that a diaphragm is not the best contraceptive device for her?

   a. "My husband says it is my job to keep from getting pregnant."

   b. "I have a hard time remembering to take my vitamins daily."

   c. "Hormones cause cancer and I don't want to take them."

   d. "I am not comfortable touching myself down there."

CRITICAL THINKING EXERCISE

1. Ms. London, 25, comes to your family planning clinic requesting to have an intrauterine system (IUS) inserted because "birth control pills give you cancer." In reviewing her history, you note she has been into the STI clinic three times in the past year with vaginal infections and was hospitalized for pelvic inflammatory disease (PID) last month. When you question her about her sexual history, she reports having sex with multiple partners and not always using protection.

   a. Is an IUS the most appropriate method for her? Why or why not?

   b. What myths/misperceptions will you address in your counseling session?

   c. Outline the safer sex discussion you plan to have with her.

STUDY ACTIVITIES

1. Develop a teaching plan for an adolescent with premenstrual syndrome and dysmenorrhea.

2. Arrange to shadow a nurse working in family planning for the morning. What questions does the nurse ask to ascertain the kind of family planning method that is right for each woman? What teaching goes along with each method? What follow-up care is needed? Share your findings with your classmates during a clinical conference.

3. Surf the Internet and locate three resources for infertile couples to consult that provide support and resources.

4. Sterilization is the most prevalent method of contraception used by married couples in the United States. Contact a local urologist and gynecologist to learn about the procedure involved and the cost of a male

and female sterilization. Which procedure poses less risk to the person and costs less?

5. Take a field trip to a local drugstore to check out the variety and costs of male and female condoms. How many different brands did you find? What was the range of costs?

6. Noncontraceptive benefits of combined oral contraceptives include which of the following? Select all that apply.

   a. Protection against ovarian cancer

   b. Protection against endometrial cancer

   c. Protection against breast cancer

   d. Reduction in incidence of ectopic pregnancy

   e. Prevention of functional ovarian cysts

   f. Reduction in deep venous thrombosis

   g. Reduction in the risk of colorectal cancer

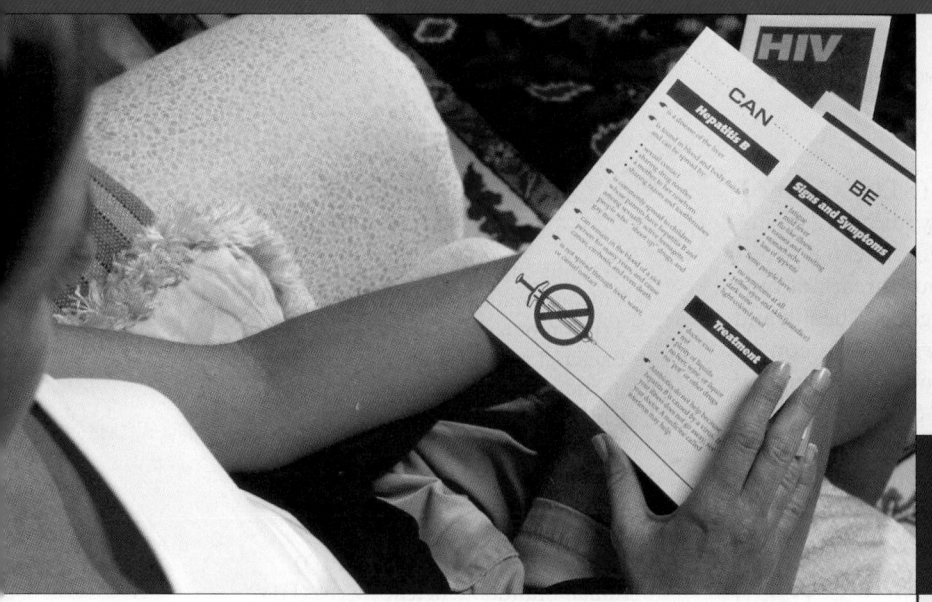

CHAPTER 5

SEXUALLY TRANSMITTED INFECTIONS

KEY TERMS

bacterial vaginosis
gonorrhea
pelvic inflammatory
  disease (PID)

sexually transmitted
  infection (STI)
syphilis

trichomoniasis
vulvovaginal candidiasis

LEARNING OBJECTIVES

Upon completion of the chapter, the learner will be able to:

1. Define the key terms used in this chapter.
2. Discuss the spread and control of sexually transmitted infections.
3. Identify risk factors and outline appropriate client education needed in common sexually transmitted infections.
4. Discuss how contraceptives can play a role in the prevention of sexually transmitted infections.
5. Analyze the physiologic and psychological aspects of sexually transmitted infections.
6. Delineate the nursing management needed for women with sexually transmitted infections.

Sandy, a 19-year-old, couldn't imagine what these "things" were that appeared "down there" in her genital area last week. She was too embarrassed to tell anyone, so she stopped by the college health service today to find out what they were.

WOW

Unconditional self-acceptance in clients is the core to reducing risky behavior and fostering peace of mind.

141

Sexually transmitted infections (STIs) are infections of the reproductive tract caused by microorganisms transmitted through vaginal, anal, or oral sexual intercourse (CDC, 2006). STIs pose a serious threat not only to women's sexual health but also to the general health and well-being of millions of people worldwide. STIs constitute an epidemic of tremendous magnitude. An estimated 65 million people live with an incurable STI, and another 15 million are infected each year (CDC, 2006). The incidence of STIs continues to rise in the United States.

STIs are biologically sexist, presenting greater risk and causing more complications among women than among men. Women are diagnosed with two thirds of the estimated 15 million new cases of STIs annually in the United States. After only a single exposure, women are twice as likely as men to acquire infections from pathogens causing gonorrhea, chlamydia infection, hepatitis B, and syphilis (Johnson-Mallard et al., 2007). STIs may contribute to cervical cancer, infertility, ectopic pregnancy, chronic pelvic pain, and death. Certain infections can be transmitted in utero to the fetus or during childbirth to the newborn (Table 5.1). STIs know no class, racial, ethnic, or social barriers—all individuals are vulnerable if exposed to the infectious organism. The problem of STIs has still not been tackled adequately on a global scale, and until this is done, numbers worldwide will continue to increase.

A special section on STIs and adolescents is presented below. This is followed by discussion of specific STIs categorized according to the CDC framework, which groups STIs according to the major symptom manifested (Box 5.1). A section on preventing STIs is included at the end of the chapter.

BOX 5.1 CDC Classification of STIs

- Infections characterized by vaginal discharge
  - Vulvovaginal candidiasis
  - Trichomoniasis
  - Bacterial vaginosis
- Infections characterized by cervicitis
  - Chlamydia
  - Gonorrhea
- Infections characterized by genital ulcers
  - Genital herpes simplex
  - Syphilis
- Pelvic inflammatory disease (PID)
- Human immunodeficiency virus (HIV)
- Human papillomavirus infection (HPV)
- Vaccine-preventable STIs
  - Hepatitis A
  - Hepatitis B
- Ectoparasitic infections
  - Pediculosis pubis
  - Scabies

Sexually Transmitted Infections and Adolescents

An estimated two thirds of all STIs occur among persons under the age of 25 (Waugh, 2007). Each year there are 4 million cases of STIs among teenagers. In the United States, teens who are sexually active experience high rates of STIs, and some groups are at higher risk, including African-American youths, abused youths, homeless youths,

---

TABLE 5.1 **STIs AND EFFECTS ON THE FETUS OR NEWBORN**

STI	Effects on Fetus or Newborn
Chlamydia	Can be infected during delivery Eye infections (neonatal conjunctivitis), pneumonia, low birthweight, preterm birth, stillbirth
Gonorrhea	Can be infected during delivery Rhinitis, vaginitis, urethritis, inflammation of sites of fetal monitoring Ophthalmia neonatorum can lead to blindness and sepsis (including arthritis and meningitis).
Herpes type II (genital herpes)	Contamination can occur during birth. Mental retardation, premature birth, low birthweight, death
Syphilis	Can be passed in utero Can result in fetal or infant death Congenital syphilis symptoms include skin ulcers, rashes, fever, weakened or hoarse cry, swollen liver and spleen, jaundice and anemia, various deformations.
Trichomoniasis	Fever, irritability, preterm birth, low birthweight
Venereal warts	May develop warts in throat (laryngeal papillomatosis); uncommon but life-threatening

young men having sex with men, and gay, lesbian, bisexual, and transgendered youths.

> ▶ *Take* NOTE!
>
> *It is estimated that before graduating from high school, 25% of adolescents will contract an STI (Pickering, 2006).*

Biological and behavioral factors place teenagers at high risk. Female adolescents are more susceptible to STIs due to their anatomy. During adolescence and young adulthood, women's columnar epithelial cells are especially sensitive to invasion by sexually transmitted organisms, such as chlamydia and gonococci, because they extend out over the vaginal surface of the cervix, where they are unprotected by cervical mucus; these cells recede to a more protected location as women age. Behaviorally, adolescent and young adults tend to think they are invincible and deny the risks of their behavior. This risky behavior exposes them to STIs and HIV/AIDS. Adolescents frequently have unprotected intercourse, they engage in partnerships of limited duration, and they face many obstacles that prevent them from using the health care system.

Nursing Assessment

Many health care providers fail to assess adolescent sexual behavior and STI risks, to screen for asymptomatic infection during clinic visits, or to counsel adolescents on STI risk reduction. Nurses need to remember that they play a key role in the detection, prevention, and treatment of STIs in adolescents. All states allow adolescents to give consent to confidential STI testing and treatment. Table 5.2 discusses clinical manifestations of common STIs in adolescents.

Nursing Management

Encourage the client to complete the antibiotic prescription (specific management for each type of STI is discussed below).

Prevention of STIs among adolescents is critical. Health care providers have a unique opportunity to provide counseling and education to their clients. Adapt the style, content, and message to the client's developmental level. Identify risk factors and risk behaviors and guide the client to develop specific individualized actions of prevention. Your interaction with the client needs to be direct and nonjudgmental.

Encourage adolescents to postpone initiation of sexual intercourse for as long as possible, but if they choose to have sexual intercourse, explain the necessity of using barrier methods, such as male and female condoms (Teaching

Guidelines 5.1). For teens who have already had sexual intercourse, the clinician can encourage abstinence at this point. If adolescents are sexually active, they should be directed to teen clinics and contraceptive options should be explained. In areas where specialized teen clinics are not available, nurses should feel comfortable discussing sexuality, safety, and contraception with teens. Encourage adolescents to minimize their lifetime number of sexual partners, to use barrier methods consistently and correctly, and to be aware of the connection between drug and alcohol use and the incorrect use of barrier methods. Table 5.3 discusses barriers to condom use and means to overcome them.

*T*hink back to Sandy, who was introduced at the beginning of the chapter. How should the nurse handle Sandy's anxious state? What specific questions should the nurse ask Sandy to determine the source of the possible infection in her genital area?

Infections Characterized by Vaginal Discharge

Vaginitis is a generic term that means inflammation and infection of the vagina. There can be hundreds of causes for vaginitis, but more often than not the cause is infection by one of three organisms:

- Candida, a fungus
- Trichomonas, a protozoan
- Gardnerella, a bacterium

The complex balance of microbiological organisms in the vagina is a key element in the maintenance of health. Subtle shifts in the vaginal environment may allow organisms with pathologic potential to proliferate, causing infectious symptoms.

The nurse's role in managing vaginitis is one of primary prevention and education to limit recurrences of these infections. Primary prevention begins with changing the sexual behaviors that place women at risk for infection. In addition to assessing women for the common signs and symptoms and risk factors, the nurse can help women to avoid vaginitis or to prevent a recurrence by teaching them to take the precautions highlighted in Teaching Guidelines 5.2.

▶ VULVOVAGINAL CANDIDIASIS

Vulvovaginal candidiasis is one of the most common causes of vaginal discharge. It is also referred to as yeast, monilia, and a fungal infection. It is not considered an

(text continues on page 148)

TABLE 5.2 STIs COMMON IN ADOLESCENTS

Disease	Causative Organism	Transmission Mode	Diagnostic Testing	Female Symptoms	Male Symptoms	Treatment
Chlamydia Curable STI Seen frequently among sexually active adolescents and young adults Sexually active adolescents should be screened at least annually.	Chlamydia trachomatis (bacteria)	Vaginal, anal, oral sex, and by childbirth	Culture fluid from urethral swabs in males or endocervical swabs for females and conjunctival secretions in neonates	May be asymptomatic Dysuria Vaginal discharge (mucus or pus) Endocervicitis May lead to pelvic inflammatory disease, ectopic pregnancy, and infertility Can cause inflammation of the rectum and lining of the eye (conjunctivitis) Can infect the throat from oral sexual contact with an infected partner	May be asymptomatic Dysuria Penile discharge (mucus or pus) Urethral tingling May lead to epididymitis (inflammation of the epididymis, the tubular structure that connects the testicle with the vas deferens) and sterility Can cause inflammation of the rectum and lining of the eye (conjunctivitis) Can infect the throat from oral sexual contact with an infected partner	Azithromycin (Zithromax) Doxycycline (Vibramycin) Erythromycin (EES) Ofloxacin (Floxin) Sexual partners need evaluation, testing, and treatment also.
Gonorrhea Curable STI Client is often co-infected with Chlamydia trachomatis	Neisseria gonorrhoeae (bacteria)	Vaginal, anal, oral sex, and by childbirth	Staining samples directly for the bacterium, detection of bacterial genes or DNA in urine, and growing the bacteria in laboratory cultures More than one test may be used.	May be asymptomatic or no recognizable symptoms until serious complications such as pelvic inflammatory disease Dysuria Urinary frequency Vaginal discharge (yellow, foul) Dyspareunia Endocervicitis Arthritis May lead to pelvic inflammatory disease, ectopic pregnancy, and infertility Symptoms of rectal infection include discharge, anal itching, and occasional painful	Most produce symptoms but can be asymptomatic Dysuria Penile discharge (pus) Arthritis May lead to epididymitis and sterility Symptoms of rectal infection include discharge, anal itching, and occasional painful bowel movements with fresh blood.	Usually a single dose of one of the following: Cefiximine (Suprax) Ciprofloxacin (Cipro) Ceftriaxone (Rocephin) Ofloxacin (Floxin) Levofloxin (Levaquin) **No Floxin or Cipro if <18 years or pregnant!** Azithromycin (Zithromax) Doxycycline (Vibramycin) Usually will be treated for co-infection with chlamydia, so a combination is given (e.g., ceftriaxone and doxycycline). Sexual partners need evaluation, testing, and treatment also.

Herpes Type II (Genital Herpes)	Herpes simplex virus II (HSV II)	Having sexual contact (vaginal, oral, or anal) with someone who is shedding the herpes virus either during an outbreak or during a period with no symptoms. Can be transmitted through close skin-to-skin contact	Visual inspection and symptoms or culture. Virologic and type-specific serologic tests can tell if herpes simplex virus II is present but does not confirm genital herpes, though most providers will assume a positive HSV II means genital herpes.	bowel movements with fresh blood. Blister-like genital lesions. Dysuria. Fever, headache, muscle aches	Blister-like genital lesions. Dysuria. Fever, headache, muscle aches	Acyclovir (Zovirax). Other antivirals. DOES NOT CURE, just controls symptoms. Sexual partners benefit from evaluation and counseling. If symptomatic, they need treatment. If asymptomatic, offer testing and education.
Herpes Type II (Genital Herpes) Lifelong recurrent viral disease. Most people have not been diagnosed. There is no cure.						
Syphilis	*Treponema pallidum* (spirochete bacteria)	Sexual contact with an infected person	Blood tests. Venereal Disease Research Laboratory (VDRL), Rapid Plasma Reagin (RPR), and treponemal tests (e.g., fluorescent treponemal antibody absorbed [FTA-ABS]) can lead to a presumptive diagnosis. Darkfield examination and direct fluorescent antibody tests	Disease is divided into four stages. *Primary infection* • Chancre on place of entrance of bacteria (usually vulva or vagina but can develop in other parts of the body) *Secondary infection* • Maculopapular rash (hands & feet) • Sore throat • Lymphadenopathy • Flu-like symptoms *Latent infection* • No symptoms • No longer contagious • Many people if not treated will suffer no further signs and symptoms.	Disease is divided into four stages. *Primary infection* • Chancre on place of entrance of bacteria (usually on penis but can develop in other parts of the body) *Secondary, latent, and tertiary infections* All similar to female symptoms	Penicillin G inj. (if penicillin allergy, doxycycline or erythromycin). Sexual partners need evaluation and testing.

(continued)

TABLE 5.2 STIs Common in Adolescents (continued)

Disease	Causative Organism	Transmission Mode	Diagnostic Testing	Female Symptoms	Male Symptoms	Treatment
			of lesion exudate or tissue provide definitive diagnosis of early syphilis.	Some people will go on to develop tertiary or late syphilis. *Tertiary infections* • Tumors of skin, bones & liver • CNS symptoms • CV symptoms • Usually not reversible at this stage		
Trichomoniasis	*Trichomonas vaginalis* (protozoan)	Vaginal intercourse with an infected partner May be picked up from direct genital contact with damp or moist objects, such as towels, wet clothing, or a toilet seat	Microscopic evaluation of vaginal secretions or culture	Many women have symptoms but some may be asymptomatic. Dysuria Urinary frequency Vaginal discharge (yellow, green, or gray & foul odor) Dyspareunia Irritation or itching of genital area	Most infected men are asymptomatic. Dysuria Penile discharge (watery, white)	Metronidazole (Flagyl) Sexual partners need evaluation, testing, and treatment also.

Venereal Warts	Cause	Transmission	Diagnosis	Signs and Symptoms	Treatment
Venereal Warts (condylomata acuminata) One of the most common STIs in the United States Could lead to cancers of the cervix, vulva, vagina, anus, or penis No cure; warts can be removed but virus remains	Human papillomavirus	Vaginal, anal, or oral sex with an infected partner	Visual inspection Abnormal Pap smear may indicate cervical infection of HPV.	Wart-like lesions that are soft, moist, or flesh-colored and appear on the vulva and cervix and inside and surrounding the vagina and anus Sometimes appear in clusters that resemble cauliflower-like bumps, and are either raised or flat, small or large	May disappear without treatment Treatment is aimed at removing the lesions rather than HPV itself No optimal treatment has been identified, but there are several ways to treat them depending on size and location. Most methods rely on chemical or physical destruction of the lesion: Imiquimod cream 20% Podophyllin anti-mitotic solution 0.5% Podofilox solution 5% 5-fluorouracil cream Trichloroacetic acid (TCA) Small warts can be removed by: • Freezing (cryosurgery) • Burning (electro-cautery) • Laser treatment Large warts that have not responded to treatment may be removed surgically.
				Wart-like lesions that are soft, moist, or flesh-colored and appear on the scrotum or penis Sometimes appear in clusters that resemble cauliflower-like bumps, and are either raised or flat, small or large	

TEACHING GUIDELINES 5.1

Proper Condom Use

- Use latex condoms.
- Use a new condom with each act of sexual intercourse. Never reuse a condom.
- Handle condoms with care to prevent damage from sharp objects such as fingernails and teeth.
- Ensure condom has been stored in a cool, dry place away from direct sunlight. Do not store condoms in wallet or automobile or anywhere they would be exposed to extreme temperatures.
- Do not use a condom if it appears brittle, sticky, or discolored. These are signs of aging.
- Put condom on before any genital contact.
- Put condom on when penis is erect. Ensure it is placed so it will readily unroll.
- Hold the tip of the condom while unrolling. Ensure there is a space at the tip for semen to collect, but make sure no air is trapped in the tip.
- Ensure adequate lubrication during intercourse. If external lubricants are used, use only water-based lubricants such as KY jelly with latex condoms. Oil-based or petroleum-based lubricants, such as body lotion, massage oil, or cooking oil, can weaken latex condoms.
- Withdraw while penis is still erect, and hold condom firmly against base of penis.

Adapted from Pickering, L. K. (Ed.) (2006). *Red book: 2006 report of the committee on infectious diseases* (27th ed.). Elk Grove Village, IL: American Academy of Pediatrics; and Public Health Agency of Canada (2006). *Canadian guidelines on sexually transmitted infections.* Ottawa, ON: Author.

STI because Candida is a normal constituent in the vagina and becomes pathologic only when the vaginal environment becomes altered. An estimated 75% of women will have at least one episode of vulvovaginal candidiasis, and 40% to 50% will have two or more episodes in their lifetime (CDC, 2006).

Therapeutic Management

Treatment of candidiasis includes one of the following medications:

- Miconazole (Monistat) cream or suppository
- Clotrimazole (Mycelex) tablet or cream
- Terconazole (Terazol) cream or intravaginal suppository
- Fluconazole (Diflucan) oral tablet (CDC, 2006, p. 55)

Most of the above medications are used intravaginally in the form of a cream, tablet, or suppository used for 3 to 7 days. If fluconazole (Diflucan) is prescribed, a 150-mg oral tablet is taken as a single dose.

Topical azole preparations are effective in the treatment of vulvovaginal candidiasis, relieving symptoms and producing negative cultures in 80% to 90% of women who complete therapy (CDC, 2006). If vulvovaginal candidiasis is not treated effectively during pregnancy, the newborn can develop an oral infection known as thrush during the birth process; that infection must be treated with a local azole preparation after birth.

Nursing Assessment

Assess the patient's health history for predisposing factors for vulvovaginal candidiasis, which include:

- Pregnancy
- Use of oral contraceptives with a high estrogen content
- Use of broad-spectrum antibiotics
- Diabetes mellitus
- Obesity
- Use of steroid and immunosuppressive drugs
- HIV infection
- Wearing tight, restrictive clothes and nylon underpants
- Trauma to vaginal mucosa from chemical irritants or douching

Assess the patient for clinical manifestations of vulvovaginal candidiasis. Typical symptoms, which can worsen just before menses, include:

- Pruritus
- Vaginal discharge (thick, white, curd-like)
- Vaginal soreness
- Vulvar burning
- Erythema in the vulvovaginal area
- Dyspareunia
- External dysuria

Figure 5.1 shows the typical appearance of vulvovaginal candidiasis.

Speculum examination will reveal white plaques on the vaginal walls. The vaginal pH remains within normal range. Definitive diagnosis is made by a wet smear, which reveals the filamentous hyphae and spores characteristic of a fungus when viewed under a microscope.

Nursing Management

Teach preventive measures to women with frequent vulvovaginal candidiasis infections, including:

- Reduce dietary intake of simple sugars and soda.
- Wear white, 100% cotton underpants.
- Avoid wearing tight pants or exercise clothes with spandex.
- Shower rather than taking tub baths.
- Wash with a mild, unscented soap and dry the genitals gently.
- Avoid the use of bubble baths or scented bath products.
- Wash underwear in unscented laundry detergent and hot water.

TABLE 5.3 BARRIERS TO CONDOM USE AND MEANS TO OVERCOME THEM

Perceived Barrier	Intervention Strategy
Decreases sexual pleasure (sensation) Note: Often perceived by those who have never used a condom.	• Encourage patient to try. • Put a drop of water-based lubricant or saliva inside the tip of the condom or on the glans of the penis before putting on the condom. • Try a thinner latex condom or a different brand or more lubrication.
Decreases spontaneity of sexual activity	• Incorporate condom use into foreplay. • Remind patient that peace of mind may enhance pleasure for self and partner.
Embarrassing, juvenile, "unmanly"	• Remind patient that it is "manly" to protect himself and others.
Poor fit (too small or too big, slips off, uncomfortable)	• Smaller and larger condoms are available.
Requires prompt withdrawal after ejaculation	• Reinforce the protective nature of prompt withdrawal and suggest substituting other postcoital sexual activities.
Fear of breakage may lead to less vigorous sexual activity.	• With prolonged intercourse, lubricant wears off and the condom begins to rub. Have a water-soluble lubricant available to reapply.
Non-penetrative sexual activity	• Condoms have been advocated for use during fellatio; unlubricated condoms may prove best for this purpose due to the taste of the lubricant. • Other barriers, such as dental dams or an unlubricated condom, can be cut down the middle to form a barrier; these have been advocated for use during certain forms of non-penetrative sexual activity (e.g., cunnilingus and anolingual sex).
Allergy to latex	• Polyurethane male and female condoms are available. • A natural skin condom can be used together with a latex condom to protect the man or woman from contact with latex.

From Public Health Agency of Canada. (2006). *Canadian guidelines on sexually transmitted infections.*

• Dry underwear in a hot dryer to kill the yeast that clings to the fabric.
• Remove wet bathing suits promptly.
• Practice good body hygiene.
• Avoid vaginal sprays/deodorants.
• Avoid wearing pantyhose (or cut out the crotch to allow air circulation).
• Use white, unscented toilet paper and wipe from front to back.
• Avoid douching (which washes away protective vaginal mucus).
• Avoid the use of super-absorbent tampons (use pads instead).

▶ TRICHOMONIASIS

Trichomoniasis is another common vaginal infection that causes a discharge. The woman may be markedly symptomatic or asymptomatic. Men are asymptomatic carriers. Although this infection is localized, there is increasing evidence of preterm birth and postpartum endometritis in women with this vaginitis (CDC, 2006). *Trichomonas vaginalis* is an ovoid, single-cell protozoan parasite that can be observed under the microscope making a jerky swaying motion.

Therapeutic Management

A single 2-gram dose of oral metronidazole (Flagyl) or tinidazole (Tindamax) for both partners is a common treatment for this infection. Sex partners of women with trichomoniasis should be treated to avoid recurrence of infection.

Nursing Assessment

Assess the patient for clinical manifestations of trichomoniasis, which include:

• A heavy yellow/green or gray frothy or bubbly discharge
• Vaginal pruritus and vulvar soreness
• Dyspareunia
• Cervix may bleed on contact
• Dysuria
• Colpitis macularis ("strawberry" look on cervix)

Figure 5.2 shows the typical appearance of trichomoniasis.

The diagnosis is confirmed when a motile flagellated trichomonad is visualized under the microscope. In addition, a vaginal pH of greater than 4.5 is a typical finding.

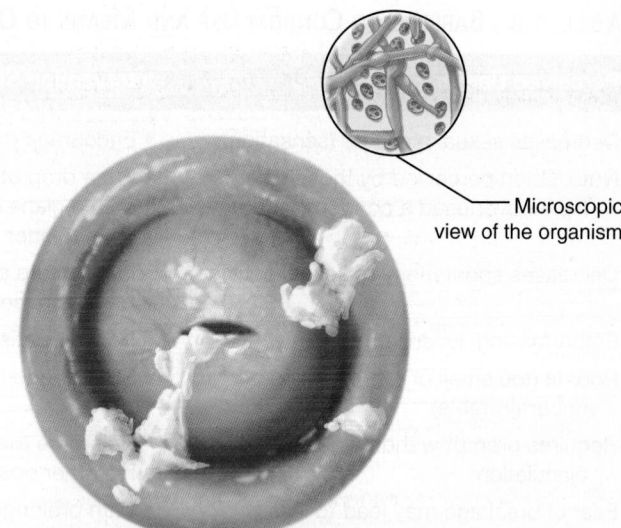

Healthy People 2010 Objectives 25–1, 2, 3, 5, 11, & 19	Significance
Reduce the proportion of adolescents and young adults with *Chlamydia trachomatis* infections. Reduce gonorrhea. Eliminate sustained domestic transmission of primary and secondary syphilis. (Developmental) Reduce the proportion of persons with human papillomavirus (HPV) infection. Increase the proportion of adolescents who abstain from sexual intercourse or use condoms if currently sexually active. (Developmental) Increase the proportion of all sexually transmitted disease clinic patients who are being treated for bacterial STDs (chlamydia, gonorrhea, and syphilis) and who are offered provider referral services for their sex partners.	Provide confidential care to all adolescents. Assess for sexual behaviors and STI risks during clinic visits; take every opportunity to educate on risks of STIs and risk reduction. Be direct and nonjudgmental and tailor your approach to the client. Encourage adolescents to postpone initiation of sexual intercourse for as long as possible. For teens who have already had sexual intercourse, encourage abstinence at this point. Encourage adolescents to minimize their lifetime number of sexual partners. Educate about the importance of correct and consistent condom use.

— Microscopic view of the organism

FIGURE 5.1 Vulvovaginal candidiasis. (Source: The Anatomical Chart Company. [2002]. *Atlas of pathophysiology.* Springhouse, PA: Springhouse.)

Nursing Management

Instruct clients to avoid sex until they and their sex partners are cured (i.e., when therapy has been completed and both partners are symptom-free) and also to avoid consuming alcohol during treatment because mixing the medications and alcohol causes severe nausea and vomiting (CDC, 2006).

▶ BACTERIAL VAGINOSIS

A third common infection of the vagina is **bacterial vaginosis,** caused by the gram-negative bacillus *Gardnerella vaginalis.* It is the most prevalent cause of vaginal discharge or malodor, but up to 50% of women are asymptomatic. Bacterial vaginosis is a sexually associated infection characterized by alterations in vaginal flora in which lactobacilli

TEACHING GUIDELINES 5.2

Preventing Vaginitis

- Avoid douching to prevent altering the vaginal environment.
- Use condoms to avoid spreading the organism.
- Avoid tights, nylon underpants, and tight clothes.
- Wipe from front to back after using the toilet.
- Avoid powders, bubble baths, and perfumed vaginal sprays.
- Wear clean cotton underpants.
- Change out of wet bathing suits as soon as possible.
- Become familiar with the signs and symptoms of vaginitis.
- Choose to lead a healthy lifestyle.

— Microscopic view of the organism

— Greenish-grey cervical discharge

FIGURE 5.2 Trichomoniasis. (Source: The Anatomical Chart Company. [2002]. *Atlas of pathophysiology.* Springhouse, PA: Springhouse.)

EVIDENCE-BASED PRACTICE 5.1
Interventions for Trichomoniasis in Pregnancy

● **Study**

Trichomoniasis is a very common sexually transmitted infection. Symptoms include vaginal itching and discharge. It is not clear whether pregnant women with trichomoniasis are more likely to give birth preterm or to have other pregnancy complications. The review of trials found that the drug metronidazole is effective against trichomoniasis when taken by women and their partners during pregnancy, but it may harm the baby. Of the two clinical trials reviewed, one was stopped early because women taking metronidazole were more likely to give birth preterm and have low-birthweight babies. Further research into trichomoniasis treatments for pregnant women is needed.

▲ **Findings**

Metronidazole is effective against a trichomoniasis infection during pregnancy but may increase the risk of preterm and low-birthweight babies.

■ **Nursing Implications**

The nurse's role concerning this study's results is to counsel women diagnosed with trichomoniasis during pregnancy about the potential risks of treatment. The woman should be cautioned about taking this medication if she has a previous history of preterm births, is carrying twins, or is experiencing preterm contractions. In addition, an ultrasound should validate the fetal weight linked to the gestational age to make sure it is within normal range before this medication is prescribed.

Source: Gülmezoglu A. M. (2007). Interventions for trichomoniasis in pregnancy. *Cochrane Database of Systematic Reviews* 2006, Issue 3. Art. No.: CD000220. DOI: 10.1002/14651858.CD000220.

---

in the vagina are replaced with high concentrations of anaerobic bacteria. The cause of the microbial alteration is not fully understood but is associated with having multiple sex partners, douching, and lack of vaginal lactobacilli (CDC, 2006). Research suggests that bacterial vaginosis is associated with preterm labor, premature rupture of membranes, chorioamnionitis, postpartum endometritis, and pelvic inflammatory disease (CDC, 2006).

Therapeutic Management

Treatment for bacterial vaginosis includes oral metronidazole (Flagyl) or clindamycin (Cleocin) cream. Treatment of the male partner has not been beneficial in preventing recurrence because sexual transmission of bacterial vaginosis has not been proven (CDC, 2006).

Nursing Assessment

Assess the patient for clinical manifestations of bacterial vaginosis. Primary symptoms are a thin, white homogeneous vaginal discharge and a characteristic "stale fish" odor. Figure 5.3 shows the typical appearance of bacterial vaginosis.

To diagnose bacterial vaginosis, three of the four criteria must be met:

• Thin, white homogeneous vaginal discharge
• Vaginal pH > 4.5
• Positive "whiff test" (secretion is mixed with a drop of 10% potassium hydroxide on a slide, producing a characteristic stale fishy odor)

• The presence of clue cells on wet-mount examination (CDC, 2006)

Nursing Management

The nurse's role is one of primary prevention and education to limit recurrences of these infections. Primary prevention begins with changing the sexual behaviors that place women at risk for infection. In addition to assessing women for common signs, symptoms, and risk factors,

Clue cell seen in bacterial vaginosis caused by *Gardnerella vaginalis*

Discharge with fishy odor

FIGURE 5.3 Bacterial vaginosis. (Source: The Anatomical Chart Company. [2002]. *Atlas of pathophysiology.* Springhouse, PA: Springhouse.)

the nurse can help women to avoid vaginitis or to prevent a recurrence by teaching them to take the precautions highlighted in Teaching Guidelines 5.2.

Infections Characterized by Cervicitis

Cervicitis is a catchall term that implies the presence of inflammation or infection of the cervix. It is used to describe everything from symptomless erosions to an inflamed cervix that bleeds on contact and produces quantities of purulent discharge containing organisms not ordinarily found in the vagina. Cervicitis is usually caused by gonorrhea or chlamydia, as well as almost any pathogenic bacterial agent and a number of viruses. The treatment of cervicitis involves the appropriate therapy for the specific organism that has caused it.

▶ CHLAMYDIA

Chlamydia is the most common bacterial STI in the United States. The CDC estimates that there are 4 million new cases each year; the highest predictor for the infection is age. The highest rates of infection are among those ages 15 to 19, mainly because their sexual relations are often unplanned and are sometimes the result of pressure or force, and typically happen before they have the experience and skills to protect themselves. The rates are highest among this group regardless of demographics or location (CDC, 2006). The young have the most to lose from acquiring STIs, since they will suffer the consequences the longest and might not reach their full reproductive potential.

Asymptomatic infection is common among both men and women. Men primarily develop urethritis. In women, chlamydia is linked with cervicitis, acute urethral syndrome, salpingitis, ectopic pregnancy, pelvic inflammatory disease (PID), and infertility (Marrazzo & Martin, 2007). Chlamydia causes half of the 1 million recognized cases of PID in the United States each year, and treatment costs run over $1 billion yearly.

Chlamydia trachomatis is the bacterium that causes chlamydia. It is an intracellular parasite that cannot produce its own energy and depends on the host for survival. It is often difficult to detect, and this can pose problems for women due to the long-term consequences of untreated infection. Moreover, lack of treatment provides more opportunity for the infection to be transmitted to sexual partners. Newborns delivered to infected mothers may develop conjunctivitis or pneumonitis and have a 50% to 70% risk of acquiring the infection (Glasier et al., 2006).

Therapeutic Management

Antibiotics are usually used in treating this STI. The CDC treatment options for chlamydia include doxycy-

cline (Vibromycin) 100 mg orally twice a day for 7 days or azithromycin (Zithromax) 1 gram orally in a single dose. Because of the common co-infection of chlamydia and gonorrhea, a combination regimen of ceftriaxone (Rocephin) with doxycycline or azithromycin is prescribed frequently (CDC, 2006). Additional CDC guidelines for patient management include annual screening of all sexually active women aged 20 to 25 years old; screening of all high-risk people; and treatment with antibiotics effective against both gonorrhea and chlamydia for anyone diagnosed with a gonococcal infection (CDC, 2006).

Nursing Assessment

Assess the health history for significant risk factors for chlamydia, which may include:

• Being an adolescent
• Having multiple sex partners
• Having a new sex partner
• Engaging in sex without using a barrier contraceptive (condom)
• Using oral contraceptives
• Being pregnant
• Having a history of another STI (Geisler, 2007)

Assess the client for clinical manifestations of chlamydia. The majority of women (70% to 80%) are asymptomatic (CDC, 2006). If the client is symptomatic, clinical manifestations include:

• Mucopurulent vaginal discharge → *mucus w/ pus*
• Urethritis
• Bartholinitis
• Endometritis
• Salpingitis
• Dysfunctional uterine bleeding

The diagnosis can be made by urine testing or swab specimens collected from the endocervix or vagina. Culture, direct immunofluorescence, EIA, or nucleic acid amplification methods by polymerase chain reaction or ligase chain reaction (DNA probe, such as GenProbe or Pace2) are highly sensitive and specific when used on urethral and cervicovaginal swabs. They can also be used with good sensitivity and specificity on first-void urine specimens (Mehta, 2007). The chain reaction tests are the most sensitive and cost-effective. The CDC strongly recommends screening of asymptomatic women at high risk in whom infection would otherwise go undetected (CDC, 2006).

▶ GONORRHEA

Gonorrhea is a serious and potentially very severe bacterial infection. It is the second most commonly reported infection in the United States. Gonorrhea is highly contagious and is a reportable infection to the health department authorities. Gonorrhea increases the risk for PID, infertility, ectopic pregnancy, and HIV acquisition and transmission (CDC, 2007a, 2007b, 2007d). It is rapidly becoming more and more resistant to cure. In the United States, an estimated 600,000 new gonorrhea infections occur annually (CDC, 2006). In common with all other STIs, it is an equal-opportunity infection—no one is immune to it, regardless of race, creed, gender, age, or sexual preference.

The cause of gonorrhea is an aerobic gram-negative intracellular diplococcus, *Neisseria gonorrhoeae*. The site of infection is the columnar epithelium of the endocervix. Gonorrhea is almost exclusively transmitted by sexual activity. In pregnant women, gonorrhea is associated with chorioamnionitis, premature labor, premature rupture of membranes, and postpartum endometritis (Peterson et al., 2007). It can also be transmitted to the newborn in the form of ophthalmia neonatorum during birth by direct contact with gonococcal organisms in the cervix. Ophthalmia neonatorum is highly contagious and if untreated leads to blindness in the newborn.

Therapeutic Management

The treatment of choice for uncomplicated gonococcal infections is cefixime (Suprex) 400 mg orally in a single dose or ceftriaxone (Rocephine) 125 mg intramuscularly in a single dose. Azithromycin (Zithromax) orally or doxycycline (Vibromycin) should accompany all gonococcal treatment regimens if chlamydial infection is not ruled out (CDC, 2006). Pregnant women should not be treated with quinolones or tetracyclines. Cephalosporins or a single 2-gram intramuscular dose of spectinomycin should be used during pregnancy (CDC, 2006). To prevent gonococcal ophthalmia neonatorum, a prophylactic agent should be instilled into the eyes of all newborns; this procedure is required by law in most states. Erythromycin or tetracycline ophthalmic ointment in a single application is recommended (CDC, 2006).

Nursing Assessment

Assess the client's health history for risk factors, which may include low socioeconomic status, living in an urban area, single status, inconsistent use of barrier contraceptives, age under 20 years old, and multiple sex partners. Assess the client for clinical manifestations of gonorrhea, keeping in mind that between 50% and 90% of women infected with gonorrhea are totally symptom-free (Glasier et al., 2006). Because women are so frequently asymptomatic, they are regarded as a major factor in the spread of gonorrhea. If symptoms are present, they might include:

• Abnormal vaginal discharge
• Dysuria
• Cervicitis
• Abnormal vaginal bleeding

• Bartholin's abscess
• PID
• Neonatal conjunctivitis in newborns
• Mild sore throat (for pharyngeal gonorrhea)
• Rectal infection (asymptomatic)
• Perihepatitis (Bennett & Domachowske, 2007)

Sometimes a local gonorrhea infection is self-limiting (there is no further spread), but usually the organism ascends upward through the endocervical canal to the endometrium of the uterus, further on to the fallopian tubes, and out into the peritoneal cavity. When the peritoneum and the ovaries become involved, the condition is known as PID. The scarring to the fallopian tubes is permanent. This damage is a major cause of infertility and is a possible contributing factor in ectopic pregnancy (Mehta, 2007).

If gonorrhea remains untreated, it can enter the bloodstream and produce a disseminated gonococcal infection. This severe form of infection can invade the joints (arthritis), the heart (endocarditis), the brain (meningitis), and the liver (toxic hepatitis). Figure 5.4 shows the typical appearance of gonorrhea.

The CDC recommends screening for all women at risk for gonorrhea. Pregnant women should be screened at the first prenatal visit and again at 36 weeks of gestation. Nucleic acid hybridization tests (GenProbe) are used for diagnosis. Any woman suspected of having gonorrhea should be tested for chlamydia also because co-infection (45%) is extremely common (CDC, 2006).

Nursing Management of Chlamydia and Gonorrhea

The prevalence of chlamydia and gonorrhea is increasing dramatically, and these infections can have long-term effects on people's lives. Sexual health is an important part of a person's physical and mental health, and nurses have a professional obligation to address it. Be particularly sensitive when addressing STIs because women are often embarrassed or feel guilty. There is still a social stigma attached to STIs, so women need to be reassured about confidentiality.

FIGURE 5.4 Gonorrhea.

The nurse's knowledge about chlamydia and gonorrhea should include treatment strategies, referral sources, and preventive measures. It is important to be skilled at patient education and counseling and to be comfortable talking with, and advising, women diagnosed with these infections.

Provide education about risk factors for these infections. High-risk groups include single women, women younger than 25 years, African-American women, women with a history of STIs, those with new or multiple sex partners, those with inconsistent use of barrier contraception, and women living in communities with high infection rates (Bennett & Domachowske, 2007). Assessment involves taking a health history that includes a comprehensive sexual history. Ask about the number of sex partners and the use of safer sex techniques. Review previous and current symptoms. Emphasize the importance of seeking treatment and informing sex partners. The four-level P-LI-SS-IT model (Box 5.2) can be used to determine interventions for various women because it can be adapted to the nurse's level of knowledge, skill, and experience. Of utmost importance is the willingness to listen and show interest and respect in a nonjudgmental manner.

In addition to meeting the health needs of women with chlamydia and gonorrhea, the nurse is responsible for educating the public about the increasing incidence of these infections. This information should include high-risk behaviors associated with these infections, signs and symptoms, and the treatment modalities available. Stress that both of these STIs can lead to infertility and long-term sequelae. Teach safer sex practices to people in nonmonogamous relationships. Know the physical and psychosocial responses to these STIs to prevent transmission and the disabling consequences.

▶ **Take** NOTE!

If the epidemic of chlamydia and gonorrhea is to be halted, nurses must take a major front-line role now.

Infections Characterized by Genital Ulcers

In the United States, the majority of young, sexually active patients who have genital ulcers have genital herpes, syphilis, or chancroid. The frequency of each condition differs by geographic area and patient population; however, genital herpes is the most prevalent of these diseases. More than one of these diseases can be present in a patient who has genital ulcers. All three of these diseases have been associated with an increased risk for HIV infection. Not all genital ulcers are caused by STIs.

▶ GENITAL HERPES SIMPLEX

Genital herpes is a recurrent, lifelong viral infection. The CDC estimates that 50 million Americans have genital herpes simplex (HSV) infection, with a half million new cases annually (CDC, 2006). Two serotypes of HSV have been identified: HSV-1 (not sexually transmitted) and HSV-2 (sexually transmitted). Today, approximately 10% of genital herpes infections are thought to be caused by HSV-1 and 90% by HSV-2 (Paz-Baily et al., 2007). HSV-1 causes the familiar fever blisters or cold sores on the lips, eyes, and face. HSV-2 invades the mucous membranes of the genital tract and is known as herpes genitalis. Most persons infected with HSV-2 have not been diagnosed.

The herpes simplex virus is transmitted by contact of mucous membranes or breaks in the skin with visible or nonvisible lesions. Most genital herpes infections are transmitted by individuals unaware that they have an infection. Many have mild or unrecognized infections but still shed the herpes virus intermittently. HSV is transmitted primarily by direct contact with an infected individual who is shedding the virus. Kissing, sexual contact, and vaginal delivery are means of transmission.

Having sex with an infected partner places the individual at risk for contracting HSV. After the primary outbreak, the virus remains dormant in the nerve cells for life, resulting in periodic recurrent outbreaks. Recurrent genital herpes outbreaks are triggered by precipitating factors such as emotional stress, menses, and sexual intercourse, but more than half of recurrences occur without a precipitating cause. Immunocompromised women have more

---

BOX 5.2 **The P-LI-SS-IT Model**

P   Permission—gives the woman permission to talk about her experience

LI Limited Information—information given to the woman about STIs

• Factual information to dispel myths about STIs
• Specific measures to prevent transmission
• Ways to reveal information to her partners
• Physical consequences if the infections are untreated

SS Specific Suggestions—an attempt to help women change their behavior to prevent recurrence and prevent further transmission of the STI

IT Intensive Therapy—involves referring the woman or couple for appropriate treatment elsewhere based on their life circumstances frequent and more severe recurrent outbreaks than normal hosts (Paz-Bailey et al., 2007).

Living with genital herpes can be difficult due to the erratic, recurrent nature of the infection, the location of the lesions, the unknown causes of the recurrences, and the lack of a cure. Further, the stigma associated with this infection may affect the individual's feelings about herself and her interaction with partners. Potential psychosocial consequences may include emotional distress, isolation, fear of rejection by a partner, fear of transmission of the disease, loss of confidence, and altered interpersonal relationships (Alexander et al., 2007).

Along with the increase in the incidence of genital herpes has been an increase in neonatal herpes simplex viral infections, which are associated with a high incidence of mortality and morbidity. The risk of neonatal infection with a primary maternal outbreak is between 30% and 50%; it is less than 1% with a recurrent maternal infection (CDC, 2006).

Therapeutic Management

No cure exists, but antiviral drug therapy helps to reduce or suppress symptoms, shedding, and recurrent episodes. Advances in treatment with acyclovir (Zovirax) 400 mg orally three times daily for 7 to 10 days, famciclovir (Famvir) 250 mg orally three times daily for 7 to 10 days, and valacyclovir (Valtrex) 1 gram orally twice daily for 7 to 10 days have resulted in an improved quality of life for those infected with HSV. However, these drugs neither eradicate latent virus nor affect the risk, frequency, or severity of recurrences after the drug is discontinued (CDC, 2006). Suppressive therapy is recommended for individuals with six or more recurrences per year. The natural course of the disease is for recurrences to be less frequent over time.

The management of genital herpes includes antiviral therapy. The safety of antiviral therapy has not been established during pregnancy. Therapeutic management also includes counseling regarding the natural history of the disease, the risk of sexual and perinatal transmission, and the use of methods to prevent further spread.

Nursing Assessment

Assess the client for clinical manifestations of HSV. Clinical manifestations can be divided into the primary episode and recurrent infections. The first or primary episode is usually the most severe, with a prolonged period of viral shedding. Primary HSV is a systemic disease characterized by multiple painful vesicular lesions, mucopurulent discharge, superinfection with candida, fever, chills, malaise, dysuria, headache, genital irritation, inguinal tenderness, and lymphadenopathy. The lesions in the primary herpes episode are frequently located on the vulva, vagina, and perineal areas. The vesicles will open and weep and finally crust over, dry, and disappear without scar formation

FIGURE 5.5 Genital herpes simplex.

(Fig. 5.5). This viral shedding process usually takes up to 2 weeks to complete.

Recurrent infection episodes are usually much milder and shorter in duration than the primary one. Tingling, itching, pain, unilateral genital lesions, and a more rapid resolution of lesions are characteristics of recurrent infections. Recurrent herpes is a localized disease characterized by typical HSV lesions at the site of initial viral entry. Recurrent herpes lesions are fewer in number and less painful and resolve more rapidly (Sharma & Brilliant, 2007).

Diagnosis of HSV is often based on clinical signs and symptoms and is confirmed by viral culture of fluid from the vesicle. Papanicolaou (Pap) smears are an insensitive and nonspecific diagnostic test for HSV and should not be relied on for diagnosis.

▶ SYPHILIS

Syphilis is a complex, curable bacterial infection caused by the spirochete *Treponema pallidum*. It is a serious systemic disease that can lead to disability and death if untreated. Rates of syphilis in the United States were declining, but they remain high among young adults and African-Americans in urban areas and in the south (CDC, 2006). It continues to be one of the most important STIs both because of its biological effect on HIV acquisition and transmission and because of its impact on infant health (Stoner, 2007).

The spirochete rapidly penetrates intact mucous membranes or microscopic lesions in the skin and within hours enters the lymphatic system and bloodstream to produce a systemic infection long before the appearance of a primary lesion. The site of entry may be vaginal, rectal, or oral (Ferguson & Varnado, 2006). The syphilis spirochete can cross the placenta at any time during pregnancy. One out of every 10,000 infants born in the United States has congenital syphilis (CDC, 2006). Maternal infection consequences include spontaneous abortion, prematurity, stillbirth, and multisystem failure of the heart, lungs, spleen, liver, and pancreas, as well as structural bone damage and nervous system involvement and mental retardation (Gilbert, 2007).

Therapeutic Management

Fortunately, there is effective treatment for syphilis. Penicillin G, administered by either the intramuscular or intravenous route, is the preferred drug for all stages of syphilis. For pregnant or nonpregnant women with syphilis of less than 1 year's duration, the CDC recommends 2.4 million units of benzathine penicillin G intramuscularly in a single dose. If the syphilis is of longer duration (more than 1 year) or of unknown duration, 2.4 million units of benzathine penicillin G is given intramuscularly once a week for 3 weeks. The preparations used, the dosage, and the length of treatment depend on the stage and clinical manifestations of disease (CDC, 2006). Other medications, such as doxycycline, are available if the client is allergic to penicillin.

Women should be re-evaluated at 6 and 12 months after treatment for primary or secondary syphilis with additional serologic testing. Women with latent syphilis should be followed clinically and serologically at 6, 12, and 24 months (McGregor & Richard, 2007).

Nursing Assessment

Assess the client for clinical manifestations of syphilis. Syphilis is divided into four stages: primary, secondary, latency, and tertiary. Primary syphilis is characterized by a chancre (painless ulcer) at the site of bacterial entry that will disappear within 1 to 6 weeks without intervention (Fig. 5.6). Motile spirochetes are present on darkfield examination of ulcer exudate. In addition, painless bilateral adenopathy is present during this highly infectious period. If left untreated, the infection progresses to the secondary stage. Secondary syphilis appears 2 to 6 months after the initial exposure and is manifested by flu-like symptoms and

FIGURE 5.6 Chancre of primary syphilis.

a maculopapular rash of the trunk, palms, and soles. Alopecia and adenopathy are both common during this stage. In addition to rashes, secondary syphilis may present with symptoms of fever, pharyngitis, weight loss, and fatigue (Waugh, 2007). The secondary stage of syphilis lasts about 2 years. Once the secondary stage subsides, the latency period begins. This stage is characterized by the absence of any clinical manifestations of disease, although the serology is positive. This stage can last as long as 20 years. If not treated, tertiary or late syphilis occurs, with life-threatening heart disease and neurologic disease that slowly destroys the heart, eyes, brain, central nervous system, and skin.

Clients with a diagnosis of HIV or another STI should be screened for syphilis, and all pregnant women should be screened at their first prenatal visit. Darkfield microscopic examinations and direct fluorescent antibody tests of lesion exudate or tissue are the definitive methods for diagnosing early syphilis. A presumptive diagnosis can be made by using two serologic tests:

- Nontreponemal tests (Venereal Disease Research Laboratory [VDRL] and rapid plasma reagin [RPR])
- Treponemal tests (fluorescent treponemal antibody absorbed [FTA-ABS] and *T. pallidum* particle agglutination [TP-PA]) (CDC, 2006)

Nursing Management of Herpes and Syphilis

Genital ulcers from either herpes or syphilis can be devastating to women, and the nurse can be instrumental in helping her through this difficult time. Referral to a support group may be helpful. Address the psychosocial aspects of these STIs with women by discussing appropriate coping skills, acceptance of the lifelong nature of the condition (herpes), and options for treatment and rehabilitation. Teaching Guidelines 5.3 highlights appropriate teaching points for the patient with genital ulcers.

Pelvic Inflammatory Disease

Pelvic inflammatory disease refers to an inflammatory state of the upper female genital tract and nearby structures. The fallopian tubes, ovaries, or peritoneum may be involved and endometriosis may also be present. PID results from an ascending polymicrobial infection of the upper female reproductive tract, frequently caused by untreated chlamydia or gonorrhea (Fig. 5.7). An estimated 1.5 million cases are diagnosed annually, resulting in over 250,000 hospitalizations (CDC, 2006). It is a serious health problem in the United States, costing an estimated $10 billion annually in terms of hospitalizations and surgical procedures (Crossman, 2006). Complications include ectopic pregnancy, pelvic abscess, infertility, recurrent or chronic episodes of the disease, chronic abdominal pain, pelvic adhesions, and depression (Glasier et al., 2006).

TEACHING GUIDELINES 5.3

Caring for Genital Ulcers

• Abstain from intercourse during the prodromal period and when lesions are present.
• Wash hands with soap and water after touching lesions to avoid autoinoculation.
• Use comfort measures such as wearing nonconstricting clothes, wearing cotton underwear, urinating in water if urination is painful, taking lukewarm sitz baths, and air-drying lesions with a hair dryer on low heat.
• Avoid extremes of temperature such as ice packs or hot pads to the genital area as well as application of steroid creams, sprays, or gels.
• Use condoms with all new or noninfected partners.
• Inform health care professionals of your condition.

Because of the seriousness of the complications of PID, an accurate diagnosis is critical.

Therapeutic Management

Treatment of PID must include empiric, broad-spectrum antibiotic coverage of likely pathogens. The client is treated on an ambulatory basis with oral antibiotics or is hospitalized and given antibiotics intravenously. The decision to hospitalize a woman is based on clinical judgment and the severity of her symptoms (e.g., severely ill with high fever or with protracted vomiting). Frequently, oral antibiotics are initiated, and if no improvement is seen within 72 hours, the woman is admitted to the hospital. Treatment then includes intravenous antibiotics, increased oral

Spread of gonorrhea or chlamydia

FIGURE 5.7 Pelvic inflammatory disease. Chlamydia or gonorrhea spreads up the vagina into the uterus and then to the fallopian tubes and ovaries.

fluids to improve hydration, bed rest, and pain management. Follow-up is needed to validate that the infectious process is gone to prevent the development of chronic pelvic pain.

Nursing Assessment

Nursing assessment of the woman with PID involves a complete health history and assessment of clinical manifestations, physical examination, and laboratory and diagnostic testing.

Health History and Clinical Manifestations

Explore the client's current and past medical health history for risk factors for PID, which may include:

• Adolescence or young adulthood
• Nonwhite female
• Having multiple sex partners
• Early onset of sexual activity
• History of PID or STI
• Sexual intercourse at an early age
• Alcohol or drug use
• Having intercourse with a partner who has untreated urethritis
• Recent insertion of an intrauterine device (IUD)
• Nulliparity
• Cigarette smoking
• Engaging in sex during menses (Reyes & Abbuhl, 2007)
• Lack of consistent condom use
• Lack of contraceptive use
• Douching
• Prostitution

Assess the client for clinical manifestations of PID, keeping in mind that, because of the wide variety of clinical manifestations of PID, clinical diagnosis can be challenging. To reduce the risk of missed diagnosis, the CDC has established criteria to establish the diagnosis of PID. Minimal criteria (all must be present) are lower abdominal tenderness, adnexal tenderness, and cervical motion tenderness. Additional supportive criteria that support a diagnosis of PID are:

• Abnormal cervical or vaginal mucopurulent discharge
• Oral temperature above 101°F
• Elevated erythrocyte sedimentation rate (inflammatory process)
• Elevated C-reactive protein level (inflammatory process)
• *N. gonorrhoeae* or *C. trachomatis* infection documented (causative bacterial organism)
• White blood cells on saline vaginal smear (CDC, 2006)
• Prolonged or increased menstrual bleeding
• Dysmenorrhea
• Dysuria
• Painful sexual intercourse
• Nausea
• Vomiting

Physical Examination and Laboratory and Diagnostic Tests

Inspect the client for presence of fever (usually over 101°F) or vaginal discharge. Palpate the abdomen, noting tenderness over the uterus or ovaries. However, the only way to diagnose PID definitively is through an endometrial biopsy, transvaginal ultrasound, or laparoscopic examination.

Nursing Management

If the woman with PID is hospitalized, maintain hydration via intravenous fluids if necessary and administer analgesics as needed for pain. Semi-Fowler's positioning facilitates pelvic drainage. A key element to treatment of PID is education to prevent recurrence. Depending on the clinical setting (hospital or community clinic) where the nurse encounters the woman diagnosed with PID, a risk assessment should be done to ascertain what interventions are appropriate to prevent a recurrence. To gain the woman's cooperation, explain the various diagnostic tests needed. Discuss the implications of PID and the risk factors for the infection; her sexual partner should be included if possible. Sexual counseling should include practicing safer sex, limiting the number of sexual partners, using barrier contraceptives consistently, avoiding vaginal douching, considering another contraceptive method if she has an IUD and has multiple sexual partners, and completing the course of antibiotics prescribed (Reyes & Abbuhl, 2007). Review the serious sequelae that may occur if the condition is not treated or if the woman does not comply with the treatment plan. Ask the woman to have her partner go for evaluation and treatment to prevent a repeat infection. Provide nonjudgmental support while stressing the importance of barrier contraceptive methods and follow-up care. Teaching Guidelines 5.4 gives further information related to PID prevention.

Human Papillomavirus

Human papillomavirus (HPV) is the most common viral infection in the United States (CDC, 2007c). Genital warts

---

TEACHING GUIDELINES 5.4

Preventing Pelvic Inflammatory Disease

- Advise sexually active girls and women to insist their partners use condoms.
- Discourage routine vaginal douching, as this may lead to bacterial overgrowth.
- Encourage regular sexually transmitted infection screening.
- Emphasize the importance of having each sexual partner receive antibiotic treatment.

HEALTHY PEOPLE 2010

Healthy People 2010 Objectives 25-6,7	Significance
Reduce the proportion of females who have ever required treatment for pelvic inflammatory disease (PID). Reduce the proportion of childless females with fertility problems who have had a sexually transmitted disease or who have ever required treatment for pelvic inflammatory disease (PID).	Educate women that abstinence is the only way to completely avoid contracting sexually transmitted infections. Encourage women always to use condoms if participating in any sexual act. Provide an open and confidential environment so women will report symptoms and seek treatment earlier.

---

or condylomata (Greek for warts) are caused by HPV. Conservative estimates suggest that in the United States, approximately 20 million people have productive HPV infection, and 5.5 million Americans acquire it annually (CDC, 2007c). Clinical studies have confirmed that HPV is the cause of essentially all cases of cervical cancer, which is the fourth most common cancer in women in the United States, following lung, breast, and colorectal cancer (ACS, 2007). HPV-mediated oncogenesis is responsible for up to 95% of cervical squamous cell carcinomas and nearly all preinvasive cervical neoplasms (Gearhart & Randall, 2007). More than 30 types of HPV can infect the genital tract. HPV is most prevalent in young women between the ages of 20 and 24 years old, followed closely by the 15-to-19-year-old age group (Hackley et al., 2007).

▶ *Take* NOTE!

The lifetime risk of HPV infection is estimated to be as high as 80% in sexually active individuals.

Nursing Assessment

Nursing assessment of the woman with HPV involves a complete health history and assessment of clinical manifestations, physical examination, and laboratory and diagnostic testing.

Health History and Clinical Manifestations

Assess the client's health history for risk factors for HPV, which include having multiple sex partners, age (15 to 25), sex with a male who has had multiple sexual partners, and first intercourse at 16 or younger (Moore & Seybold, 2007). Risk factors contributing to the development of cervical cancer include smoking, few or no screenings for cervical cancer, multiple sex partners, immunosuppressed state, long-term contraceptive use (more than 2 years), co-infection with another STI, pregnancy, nutritional deficiencies, and early onset of sexual activity (Dunne et al., 2007).

Assess the client for clinical manifestations of HPV. Most HPV infections are asymptomatic, unrecognized, or subclinical. Visible genital warts usually are caused by HPV types 6 or 11. In addition to the external genitalia, genital warts can occur on the cervix and in the vagina, urethra, anus, and mouth. Depending on the size and location, genital warts can be painful, friable, and pruritic, although most are typically asymptomatic (Fig. 5.8). The strains of HPV associated with genital warts are considered low risk for development of cervical cancer, but other HPV types (16, 18, 31, 33, and 35) have been strongly associated with cervical cancer (CDC, 2006).

Physical Examination and Laboratory and Diagnostic Tests

Clinically, visible warts are diagnosed by inspection. The warts are fleshy papules with a warty, granular surface. Lesions can grow very large during pregnancy, affecting urination, defecation, mobility, and descent of the fetus (CDC, 2006). Large lesions, which may resemble cauliflowers, exist in coalesced clusters and bleed easily.

Serial Pap smears are performed for low-risk women. These regular Pap smears will detect the cellular changes associated with HPV. The FDA has recently approved an HPV test as a follow-up for women who have an ambiguous Pap test. In addition, this HPV test may be a helpful addition to the Pap test for general screening of women age 30 and over. The HPV test is a diagnostic test that can determine the specific HPV strain, which is useful in discriminating between low-risk and high-risk HPV types. A specimen for testing can be obtained with a fluid-phase collection system such as Thin Prep. The HPV test can identify 13 of the high-risk types of HPV associated with the development of cervical cancer and can detect high-risk types of HPV even before there are any conclusive visible changes to the cervical cells. If the test is positive for the high-risk types of HPV, the woman should be referred for colposcopy.

U *pon physical examination, it is determined that Sandy has genital warts. The nurse finds out that Sandy engaged in high-risk behavior with a stranger she "hooked up" with recently at college. She couldn't imagine that he would give her a STI because "he looked so clean-cut." She wonders how she could possibly have genital warts. What information should be given to Sandy about STIs in general? What specific information about HPV should be stressed?*

Therapeutic Management

There is currently no medical treatment or cure for HPV. Instead, therapeutic management focuses heavily on prevention through the use of the HPV vaccine and education and on the treatment of lesions and warts caused by HPV. In summer 2006, the FDA approved the HPV vaccine (Gardasil) to prevent cervical cancer. The CDC's Advisory Committee on Immunization Practices (ACIP) has recommended the vaccine for routine administration to 11- and 12-year-old girls. The ACIP also endorsed the use of Gardasil for girls as young as 9 and recommended that women between the ages of 13 and 26 receive the vaccination series, which consists of three injections over 6 months. The vaccine has been found 100% effective in preventing precancerous lesions of the cervix and genital warts (Wald, 2007). The duration of protection afforded by this vaccine, as well as its impact on long-term outcomes, is not yet known (Kennedy, 2007).

The vaccine is administered intramuscularly in three separate 0.5-mL doses. The first dose may be given to any individual 9 to 26 years old prior to infection with HPV. The second dose is administered 2 months after the first, and the third dose is given 6 months after the initial dose. The deltoid region of the upper arm or anterolateral area of the thigh may be used (Leggatt & Frazer, 2007).

If the woman doesn't receive primary prevention with the vaccine, then secondary prevention would focus on education about the importance of receiving regular Pap smears and, for women over 30, including an HPV test to determine whether the woman has a latent high-risk virus that could lead to precancerous cervical changes. Finally, treatment options for precancerous cervical lesions or genital warts caused by HPV are numerous and may include:

- Topical trichloroacetic acid (TCA) 80% to 90%
- Liquid nitrogen cryotherapy
- Topical imiquimod 5% cream (Aldara)
- Topical podophyllin 10% to 25%
- Laser carbon dioxide vaporization
- Client-applied Podofilox 0.5% solution or gel
- Simple surgical excision
- Loop electrosurgical excisional procedure (LEEP)

FIGURE 5.8 Genital warts.

• Intralesional interferon therapy (National Institute of Allergy and Infectious Diseases, 2007b)

The goal of treating genital warts is to remove the warts and induce wart-free periods for the client. Treatment of genital warts should be guided by the preference of the client and available resources. No single treatment has been found to be ideal for all clients, and most treatment modalities appear to have comparable efficacy. Because genital warts can proliferate and become friable during pregnancy, they should be removed using a local agent. A cesarean birth is not indicated solely to prevent transmission of HPV infection to the newborn, unless the pelvic outlet is obstructed by warts (Gearhart & Randall, 2007).

Nursing Management

An HPV infection has many implications for the woman's health, but most women are unaware of HPV and its role in cervical cancer. The average age of sexual debut is in early adolescence; therefore, it is important to target this population for use of the HPV/cervical cancer vaccine.

Key nursing roles are teaching about prevention of HPV infection and patient education and promotion of vaccines and screening tests in order to reduce the morbidity and mortality associated with cervical cancer caused by HPV infection. Teach all women that the only way to prevent HPV is to refrain from any genital contact with another individual. Although the effect of condoms in preventing HPV infection is unknown, latex condom use has been associated with a lower rate of cervical cancer. Teach women about the link between HPV and cervical cancer. Explain that, in most cases, there are no signs or symptoms of infection with HPV. Strongly encourage all young women between 9 and 26 to consider getting Gardasil, the vaccine against HPV. For all women, promote the importance of obtaining regular Pap smears and, for women over 30, suggest an HPV test to rule out the presence of a latent high-risk strain of HPV.

Education and counseling are important aspects of managing women with genital warts. Teach the woman that:

• Even after genital warts are removed, HPV still remains and viral shedding will continue.
• The likelihood of transmission to future partners and the duration of infectivity after treatment for genital warts are unknown.
• The recurrence of genital warts within the first few months after treatment is common and usually indicates recurrence rather than reinfection (CDC, 2006).

Sandy is being treated for HPV and is anxious for her "things" to disappear and never return. What education is needed to prevent further transmission from Sandy to any future sexual partners?

Vaccine–Preventable STIs: Hepatitis A and B

Hepatitis is an acute, systemic, viral infection that can be transmitted sexually. The viruses associated with hepatitis or inflammation of the liver are hepatitis A, B, C, D, E, and G. Hepatitis A (HAV) is spread via the gastrointestinal tract. It can be acquired by drinking polluted water, by eating uncooked shellfish from sewage-contaminated waters or food handled by a hepatitis carrier with poor hygiene, and from oral/anal sexual contact. Approximately 33% of the U.S. population has serologic evidence of prior hepatitis A infection; the rate increases directly with age (Wasley et al., 2007). A person with hepatitis A can easily pass the disease to others within the same household.

Hepatitis B (HBV) is transmitted through saliva, blood serum, semen, menstrual blood, and vaginal secretions (Assan & Kraszewski, 2006). In the early 2000s, transmission among heterosexual partners accounted for 40% of infections, and transmission among men who have sex with men accounted for 20% of infections. The World Health Organization (WHO) estimates the prevalence of hepatitis B worldwide is 350 million chronically infected people. Worldwide, hepatitis B has the highest death rate of any STI except HIV (WHO, 2007a). Risk factors for infection include having multiple sex partners, engaging in unprotected receptive anal intercourse, and having a history of other STIs (CDC, 2006). The most effective means to prevent the transmission of hepatitis A or B is pre-exposure immunization. Vaccines are available for the prevention of HAV and HBV, both of which can be transmitted sexually. Every person seeking treatment for an STI should be considered a candidate for hepatitis B vaccination, and some individuals (e.g., men who have sex with men, and injection-drug users) should be considered for hepatitis A vaccination (CDC, 2006).

Therapeutic Management

Unlike other STIs, HBV and HAV are preventable through immunization. HAV is usually self-limiting and does not result in chronic infection. HBV can result in serious, permanent liver damage. Treatment is generally supportive. No specific treatment for acute HBV infection exists.

Nursing Assessment

Assess the client for clinical manifestations of hepatitis A and B. Hepatitis A produces flu-like symptoms with malaise, fatigue, anorexia, nausea, pruritus, fever, and upper right quadrant pain. Symptoms of hepatitis B are similar to those of hepatitis A, but with less fever and skin involvement. The diagnosis of hepatitis A cannot be made based on clinical manifestations alone and requires serologic testing. The presence of IgM antibody to HAV is diagnostic of acute HAV infection. Hepatitis B is detected by a blood test that looks for antibodies and proteins produced by the virus and is positively diagnosed by the presence of hepatitis B surface antibody (HBsAg) (Pyrsopoulos & Reddy, 2007).

Nursing Management

Nurses should encourage all women to be screened for hepatitis when they have their annual Pap smear, or sooner if high-risk behavior is identified. Nurses should also encourage women to undergo HBV screening at their first prenatal visit and repeat screening in the last trimester for women with high-risk behaviors (Assan & Kraszewski, 2006). Nurses can also explain that hepatitis B vaccine is given to all infants after birth in most hospitals. The vaccination consists of a series of three injections given within 6 months. The vaccine has been shown to be safe and well tolerated by most recipients (CDC, 2006). Hepatitis A vaccine is strongly encouraged for children between 12 and 23 months; persons 1 year of age and older traveling to countries with a high prevalence of hepatitis A, such as Central or South America, Mexico, Asia, Africa, and eastern Europe; men who have sex with men; persons who use street drugs; and persons with chronic liver disease (CDC, 2007c). For others, hepatitis A vaccine series (two doses 6 months apart) may be started whenever a person is at risk of infection.

Ectoparasitic Infections

Ectoparasites are a common cause of skin rash and pruritus throughout the world, affecting persons of all ages, races, and socioeconomic groups. Overcrowding, delayed diagnosis and treatment, and poor public education contribute to the prevalence of ectoparasites in both industrial and nonindustrial nations. Approximately 300 million cases of ectoparasitic cases are reported worldwide each year (CDC, 2006). These infections include infestations of scabies and pubic lice. Since these parasites are easily passed from one person to another during sexual intimacy, clients should be assessed for them when receiving care for other STIs. Scabies is an intensely pruritic dermatitis caused by a mite. The female mite burrows under the skin and deposits eggs, which hatch. The lesions start as a small papule that reddens, erodes, and sometimes crusts. Diagnosis is based on history and appearance of burrows in the webs of the fingers and the genitalia (Cordoro & Wilson, 2007). Aggressive infestation can occur in immunodeficient, debilitated, or malnourished people, but healthy people do not usually suffer sequelae.

Clients with pediculosis pubis (pubic lice) usually seek treatment because of the pruritus, because of a rash brought on by skin irritation from scratching, or because they notice lice or nits in their pubic hair, axillary hair, abdominal and thigh hair, and sometimes in the eyebrows,

FIGURE 5.9 Pubic lice. A small brown living crab louse is seen at the base of hairs (*arrow*). (Source: Goodheart, H. [2003]. *Goodheart's photoguide of common skin disorders.* Philadelphia: Lippincott Williams & Wilkins.)

eyelashes, and beards. Infestation is usually asymptomatic until after a week or so, when bites cause pruritus and secondary infections from scratching (Fig. 5.9). Diagnosis is based on history and the presence of nits (small, shiny, yellow, oval, dewdrop-like eggs) affixed to hair shafts or lice (a yellowish, oval, wingless insect) (Wolfram, 2007).

Treatment is directed at the infested area, using permethrin cream or lindane shampoo (CDC, 2006). Bedding and clothing should be washed in hot water to decontaminate it. Sexual partners should be treated also, as well as family members who live in close contact with the infected person.

Nursing care of a woman infested with lice or scabies involves a three-tiered approach: eradicating the infestation with medication, removing nits, and preventing spread or recurrence by managing the environment. Over-the-counter products containing pyrethrins (RID, Triple X, Pronto, and Kwell) are safe for use and kill the active lice or mites. Nurses should provide education about these products (Teaching Guidelines 5.5). The nurse can follow these same guidelines to prevent the health care facility from becoming infested.

TEACHING GUIDELINES 5.5

Treating and Minimizing the Spread of Scabies and Pubic Lice

• Use the medication according to the manufacturer's instructions.
• Remove nits with a fine-toothed nit comb.
• Do not share any personal items with others or accept items from others.
• Treat objects, clothing, and bedding and wash them in hot water.
• Meticulously vacuum carpets to prevent a recurrence of infestation.

Human Immunodeficiency Virus (HIV)

An estimated 1 million people currently live with HIV and an estimated 50,000 new HIV infections have occurred annually in the United States (CDC, 2007b). In terms of epidemiology, fatality rate, and its social, legal, ethical, and political aspects, HIV/AIDS has become a public health crisis and has generated more concern than any other infectious disease in modern medical history (Mullan, 2007). To date, there is no cure for this fatal viral infection.

The HIV virus is transmitted by intimate sexual contact, by sharing needles for intravenous drug use, from mother to fetus during pregnancy, or by transfusion of blood or blood products. Men who have sex with men represent the largest proportion of new infections, followed by men and women infected through heterosexual sex (CDC, 2007b).

The number of women with HIV infection and AIDS has been increasing steadily worldwide. WHO estimates that over 25 million women are living with HIV/AIDS worldwide, accounting for approximately 50% of the 40 million adults living with HIV/AIDS (National Institute of Allergy and Infectious Diseases, 2007a). HIV disproportionately affects African-American and Hispanic women: together they represent less than 25% of all U.S. women, yet they account for more than 82% of AIDS cases in women (CDC, 2007b). Worldwide, more than 90% of all HIV infections have resulted from heterosexual intercourse. Women are particularly vulnerable to heterosexual transmission of HIV due to substantial mucosal exposure to seminal fluids. This biological fact amplifies the risk of HIV transmission when coupled with the high prevalence of nonconsensual sex, sex without condoms, and the unknown and/or high-risk behaviors of their partners (National Institute of Allergy and Infectious Diseases, 2007a). Therefore, the face of HIV/AIDS is becoming the face of young women. That shift will ultimately exacerbate the incidence of HIV because women spread it not only through sex, but also through nursing and childbirth.

AIDS is a breakdown in the immune function caused by HIV, a retrovirus. The infected person develops opportunistic infections or malignancies that become fatal. Progression from HIV infection to AIDS occurs a median of 11 years after infection (Mullan, 2007).

Twenty years have passed since HIV/AIDS began to affect our society. Since then, 50 million people have been infected by the virus, with AIDS being the fourth leading cause of death globally (CDC, 2007b). The morbidity and mortality of HIV continue to hold the attention of the medical community. While there has been a dramatic improvement in both morbidity and mortality with the use of highly active antiretroviral therapy (HAART), the incidence of HIV infection continues to rise.

> ▶ *Take* NOTE!
>
> *More than 90% of individuals infected with HIV worldwide do not know they are infected (Dubin, 2007).*

The fetal and neonatal effects of acquiring HIV through perinatal transmission are devastating and eventually fatal. An infected mother can transmit HIV infection to her newborn before or during birth and through breastfeeding. Most cases of mother-to-child HIV transmission, the cause of more than 90% of pediatric-acquired infections worldwide, occur late in pregnancy or during delivery. Transmission rates vary from 25% in untreated non-breastfeeding populations in industrialized countries to about 40% among untreated breastfeeding populations in developing countries (National Institute of Allergy and Infectious Diseases, 2007a). Despite the dramatic reduction in perinatal transmission, hundreds of infants will be born infected with HIV.

HIV and Adolescents

The effects of HIV and AIDS on adolescents and young adults is of increasing concern, but it is difficult to get accurate data due to varying ways this population seeks health care services. Some adolescents continue to receive care through pediatricians and adult services, but many do not have access to health care. HIV infections are increasing in adolescents and young adults (13 to 24 years). Also, the proportion of adolescents diagnosed with AIDS has increased from 4% in 1999 to 6% in 2006 (NIH, 2008). At least one adolescent in the United States is infected with HIV each hour. Since it takes an average of 10 years for AIDS symptoms to appear when HIV is left untreated, it is obvious that many adults with AIDS were infected as adolescents.

Most HIV-infected adolescents are exposed to the virus though sexual intercourse. Recent data suggest that the majority of HIV-infected adolescent males are infected through sex with men. A small number of adolescent males appear to be exposed through injection of drugs or heterosexual contact. Adolescent females are mostly exposed through heterosexual contact, with a small percentage becoming infected through injected drug use (www.niaid.hih.gov/factsheets/hivadolescent.htm). African-American and Hispanic adolescents between the ages of 13 and 19 account for 66% and 21%, respectively, of reported AIDS cases in 2003. Because adolescents think they are invincible, they may delay testing, and if they test positive, they may delay treatment or refuse treatment. The inability to trace this population for medical care can lead to increased transmission of HIV.

► *Consider* THIS!

I was thinking of my carefree college days, when the most important thing was having an active sorority life and meeting guys. I had been raised by very strict parents and was never allowed to date under their watch. Since I attended an out-of-state college, I figured that my parents' outdated advice and rules no longer applied. Abruptly, my thoughts of the past were interrupted by the HIV counselor asking about my feelings concerning my positive diagnosis. What was there to say at this point? I had a lot of fun but never dreamed it would haunt me for the rest of my life, which was going to be shortened considerably now. I only wish I could turn back the hands of time and listen to my parents' advice, which somehow doesn't seem so outdated now.

Thoughts: All of us have thought back on our lives to better times and wondered how our lives would have changed if we had made better choices or gone down another path. It is a pity that we have only one chance to make good, sound decisions at times. What would you have changed in your life if given a second chance? Can you still make a change for the better now?

Clinical Manifestations

When a person is initially infected with HIV, he or she goes through an acute primary infection period for about 3 weeks. The HIV viral load drops rapidly because the host's immune system works well to fight this initial infection. The onset of the acute primary infection occurs 2 to 6 weeks after exposure. Symptoms include fever, pharyngitis, rash, and myalgia. Most people do not associate this flu-like condition with HIV infection. After initial exposure, there is a period of 3 to 12 months before seroconversion. The person is considered infectious during this time.

After the acute phase, the infected person becomes asymptomatic, but the HIV virus begins to replicate. Even though there are no symptoms, the immune system runs down. A normal person has a CD4 T-cell count of 450 to 1,200 cells per microliter. When the CD4 T-cell count reaches 200 or less, the person has reached the stage of AIDS. The immune system begins a constant battle to fight this viral invasion, but over time it falls behind. A viral reservoir occurs in T cells that can store various stages of the virus. The onset and severity of the disease correlate directly with the viral load: the more HIV virus that is present, the worse the person will feel.

As profound immunosuppression begins to occur, an opportunistic infection will occur, qualifying the person for the diagnosis of AIDS. The diagnosis is finally confirmed when the CD4 count is below 200. As of now, AIDS will eventually develop in everyone who is HIV-positive.

Because HIV over time depletes the CD4 cell population, infected people become more susceptible to opportunistic infections. Currently, the AIDS virus and response to treatment are tracked based on CD4 count rather than viral load. Untreated HIV will progress to AIDS in about 11 years, but this progression can be delayed by antiretroviral therapy (Dubin, 2007).

Diagnosis

Newly approved quick tests for HIV produce results in 20 minutes and also lower the health care worker's risk of occupational exposure by eliminating the need to draw blood. The CDC's Advancing HIV Prevention initiative, launched in 2003, has made increased testing a national priority. The initiative calls for testing to be incorporated into routine medical care and to be delivered in more nontraditional settings.

Fewer than half of adults between the ages of 18 and 64 have ever had an HIV test, according to the CDC. The agency estimates that one fourth of the million HIV-infected people in the United States do not know they are infected. This means they are not receiving treatment that can prolong their lives, and they may be unknowingly infecting others. In addition, even when people do get tested, one in three failed to return to the testing site to learn their results when there was a 2-week wait. The CDC hopes that the new "one-stop" approach to HIV testing changes that pattern. About 50,000 new HIV cases are reported each year in the United States, and that number has held steady for the past few years despite massive efforts in prevention education (CDC, 2007b).

The OraQuick Rapid HIV-1 Antibody Test detects the HIV antibody in a blood sample taken with a fingerstick or from an oral fluid sample. Both can produce results in as little as 20 minutes with more than 99% accuracy (Aaron et al., 2006). The FDA has approved two other rapid blood tests: the Reveal Rapid HIV-1 Antibody Test and the Uni-Gold Recombigen HIV Test.

Testing for HIV should be offered to anyone seeking evaluation and treatment for STIs. Counseling before and after testing is an integral part of the testing procedure. Informed consent must be obtained before an HIV test is performed. HIV infection is diagnosed by tests for antibodies against HIV-1 and HIV-2 (HIV-1/2). Antibody testing begins with a sensitive screening test (e.g., the enzyme immunoassay [ELISA]). This is a specific test for antibodies to HIV that is used to determine whether the person has been exposed to the HIV retrovirus. Reactive screening tests must be confirmed by a more specific test (e.g., the Western blot [WB]) or an immunofluorescence assay (IFA). This is a highly specific test that is used to validate a positive ELISA test finding. If the supplemental test (WB or IFA) is positive, it confirms that the person is infected with HIV and is capable of transmitting the virus to others. HIV antibody is detectable in at least 95% of people within 3 months after infection (CDC, 2006).

Therapeutic Management

The goals of HIV drug therapy are to:

• Decrease the HIV viral load below the level of detection
• Restore the body's ability to fight off pathogens
• Improve the client's quality of life
• Reduce HIV morbidity and mortality (Cressey & Lallemant, 2007)

Highly active antiretroviral therapy (HAART), which combines at least three antiretroviral drugs, has dramatically improved the prognosis of HIV/AIDS. Often treatment begins with combination HAART therapy at the time of the first infection, when the person's immune system is still intact. The current HAART therapy standard is a triple combination therapy, but some clients may be given a fourth or fifth agent.

There are obvious challenges involved in meeting these goals. The viral load can be reduced much more quickly than the T-cell count can be increased, and this disparity leaves the woman vulnerable to opportunistic infections.

Current therapy to prevent the transmission of HIV to the newborn includes a three-part regimen of having the mother take an oral antiretroviral agent at 14 to 34 weeks of gestation; it is continued throughout pregnancy. During labor, an antiretroviral agent is administered intravenously until delivery. An antiretroviral syrup is administered to the infant within 12 hours after birth.

Dramatic new treatment advances with antiretroviral medications have turned a disease that used to be a death sentence into a chronic, manageable one for individuals who live in countries where antiretroviral therapy is available. Despite these advances in treatment, however, only a minority of HIV-positive Americans who take antiretroviral medications are receiving the full benefits because they are not adhering to the prescribed regimen. Successful antiretroviral therapy requires nearly perfect adherence to a complex medication regimen; less-than-perfect adherence leads to drug resistance (Battaglioli-Denero, 2007).

Adherence is difficult because of the complexity of the regimen and the lifelong duration of treatment. A typical antiretroviral regimen may consist of three or more medications taken twice daily. Adherence is made even more difficult because of the unpleasant side effects, such as nausea and diarrhea. Women in early pregnancy already experience these, and the antiretroviral medication only exacerbates them.

Nursing Management

Nurses can play a major role in caring for the HIV-positive woman by helping her accept the possibility of a shortened life span, cope with others' reactions to a stigmatizing illness, and develop strategies to maintain her physical and emotional health. Educate the woman about changes she can make in her behavior to prevent spreading HIV to others, and refer her to appropriate community resources such as HIV medical care services, substance abuse, mental health services, and social services. See Nursing Care Plan 5.1: Overview for the Woman With HIV.

Providing Education About Drug Therapy

The goal of antiretroviral therapy is to suppress viral replication so that the viral load becomes undetectable (below 400). This is done to preserve immune function and delay disease progression but is a challenge because of the side effects of nausea and vomiting, diarrhea, altered taste, anorexia, flatulence, constipation, headaches, anemia, and fatigue. Although not everyone experiences all of the side effects, the majority do have some of them. Current research hasn't documented the long-term safety of exposure of the fetus to antiretroviral agents during pregnancy, but collection of data is ongoing.

Help to reduce the development of drug resistance and thus treatment failure by identifying the barriers to adherence; identifying these barriers can help the woman to overcome them. Some of the common barriers exist because the woman:

• Does not understand the link between drug resistance and nonadherence
• Fears revealing her HIV status by being seen taking medication
• Hasn't adjusted emotionally to the HIV diagnosis
• Doesn't understand the dosing regimen or schedule
• Experiences unpleasant side effects frequently
• Feels anxious or depressed (Dubin, 2007)

Depending on which barriers are causing nonadherence, work with the woman by educating her about the dosing regimen, helping her find ways to integrate the prescribed regimen into her lifestyle, and making referrals to social service agencies as appropriate. By addressing barriers on an individual level, the nurse can help the woman to overcome them.

Educate the woman about the prescribed drug therapy and stress that it is very important to take the regimen as prescribed. Offer suggestions about how to cope with anorexia, nausea, and vomiting by:

• Separating the intake of food and fluids
• Eating dry crackers upon arising
• Eating six small meals daily
• Using high-protein supplements (Boost, Ensure) to provide quick and easy protein and calories
• Eating "comfort foods," which may appeal when other foods don't

Promoting Compliance

Remaining compliant with drug therapy is a huge challenge for many HIV-infected people. Compliance becomes diffi-

Nursing Care Plan 5.1

OVERVIEW OF THE WOMAN WHO IS HIV-POSITIVE

Annie, a 28-year-old African-American woman, is HIV-positive. She acquired HIV through unprotected sexual contact. She has been inconsistent in taking her antiretroviral medications and presents today stating she is tired and doesn't feel well.

NURSING DIAGNOSIS: Risk for infection related to positive HIV status and inconsistent compliance with antiretroviral therapy

Outcome Identification and Evaluation

Client will remain free of opportunistic infections as evidenced by temperature within acceptable parameters and absence of signs and symptoms of opportunistic infections.

Interventions: Minimizing the Risk of Opportunistic Infections

- Assess CD4 count and viral loads *to determine disease progression* (CD4 counts <500/L and viral loads >10,000 copies/L = increased risk for opportunistic infections).
- Assess complete blood count *to identify presence of infection* (>10,000 cells/mm³ may indicate infection).
- Assess oral cavity and mucous membranes for painful white patches in mouth *to evaluate for possible fungal infection.*
- Teach client to monitor for general signs and symptoms of infections, such as fever, weakness, and fatigue, *to ensure early identification.*
- Provide information explaining the importance of avoiding people with infections when possible *to minimize risk of exposure to infections.*
- Teach importance of keeping appointments so her CD4 count and viral load can be monitored *to alert the health care provider about her immune system status.*
- Instruct her to reduce her exposure to infections via:
  - Meticulous handwashing
  - Thorough cooking of meats, eggs, and vegetables
  - Wearing shoes at all times, especially when outdoors
- Encourage a balance of rest with activity throughout the day *to prevent overexertion.*
- Stress importance of maintaining prescribed antiretroviral drug therapies *to prevent disease progression and resistance.*
- If necessary, refer Annie to a nutritionist to help her understand what constitutes a well-balanced diet with supplements *to promote health and ward off infection.*

NURSING DIAGNOSIS: Knowledge deficit related to HIV infection and possible complications

Outcome Identification and Evaluation

Client will demonstrate increased understanding of HIV infection as evidenced by verbalizing appropriate health care practices and adhering to measures to comply with therapy and reduce her risk of further exposure and reduce risk of disease progression.

Interventions: Providing Patient Education

- Assess her understanding of HIV and its treatment *to provide a baseline for teaching.*
- Establish trust and be honest with Annie; encourage her to talk about her fears and the impact of the disease *to provide an outlet for her concerns.* Encourage her to discuss reasons for her noncompliance.
- Provide a nonjudgmental, accessible, confidential, and culturally sensitive approach *to promote Annie's self-esteem and allow her to feel that she is a priority.*
- Explain measures, including safer sex practices and birth control options, to prevent disease transmission; determine her willingness to practice safer sex to protect others *to determine further teaching needs.*
- Discuss the signs and symptoms of disease progression and potential opportunistic infections *to promote early detection for prompt intervention.*
- Outline with the client the availability of community resources and make appropriate referrals as needed *to provide additional education and support.*
- Encourage Annie to keep scheduled appointments *to ensure follow-up and allow early detection of potential problems.*

cult when the same pills that are supposed to thwart the disease are making the person sick. Nausea and diarrhea are just two of the possible side effects. It is often difficult to increase the client's quality of life when so much oral medication is required. The combination medication therapy is challenging for many people, and staying compliant over a period of years is extremely difficult. Stress the importance of taking the prescribed antiretroviral drug therapies by explaining that they help prevent replication of the retroviruses and subsequent progression of the disease, as well as decreasing the risk of perinatal transmission of HIV. In addition, provide written materials describing diet, exercise, medications, and signs and symptoms of complications and opportunistic infections. Reinforce this information at each visit.

Preventing HIV Infection

The lack of information about HIV infection and AIDS causes great anxiety and fear of the unknown. It is vital to take a leadership role in educating the public about risky behaviors in the fight to control this disease. The core of HIV prevention is to abstain from sex until marriage, to be faithful, and to use condoms. This is all good advice for many women, but some simply do not have the economic and social power or choices or control over their lives to put that advice into practice. Recognize that fact, and address the factors that will give women more control over their lives by providing anticipatory guidance, giving ample opportunities to practice negotiation techniques and refusal skills in a safe environment, and encouraging the use of female condoms to protect against this deadly virus. Prevention is the key to reversing the current infection trends.

Providing Care During Pregnancy and Childbirth

Voluntary counseling and HIV testing should be offered to all pregnant women as early in the pregnancy as possible to identify HIV-infected women so that treatment can be initiated early. Once a pregnant woman is identified as being HIV-positive, she should be informed about the risk for perinatal infection. Current evidence indicates that in the absence of antiretroviral medications, 25% of infants born to HIV-infected mothers will become infected with HIV (CDC, 2007b). If women do receive a combination of antiretroviral therapies during pregnancy, however, the risk of HIV transmission to the newborn drops below 2% (National Institute of Allergy and Infectious Disease, 2007a). In addition, HIV can be spread to the infant through breastfeeding, and thus all HIV-infected pregnant women should be counseled to avoid breastfeeding and use formula instead. A recent maternal infection with HIV may raise the risk of transmission through breastfeeding to twice that of a woman with earlier established infection, owing probably to the high viral load associated with recent infection (WHO, 2007b).

In addition, the woman needs instructions on ways to enhance her immune system by following these guidelines during pregnancy:

- Getting adequate sleep each night (7 to 9 hours)
- Avoiding infections (e.g., staying out of crowds, handwashing)
- Decreasing stress in her life
- Consuming adequate protein and vitamins
- Increasing her fluid intake to 2 liters daily to stay hydrated
- Planning rest periods throughout the day to prevent fatigue

Despite the dramatic reduction in perinatal transmission, hundreds of infants will be born infected with HIV. The birth of each infected infant is a missed prevention opportunity. To minimize perinatal HIV transmission, identify HIV infection in women, preferably before pregnancy; provide information about disease prevention; and encourage HIV-infected women to follow the prescribed drug therapy.

Providing Appropriate Referrals

The HIV-infected woman may have difficulty coping with the normal activities of daily living because she has less energy and decreased physical endurance. She may be overwhelmed by the financial burdens of medical and drug therapies and the emotional responses to a life-threatening condition, as well as concern about her infant's future, if she is pregnant. A case management approach is needed to deal with the complexity of her needs during this time. Be an empathetic listener and make appropriate referrals for nutritional services, counseling, homemaker services, spiritual care, and local support groups. Many community-based organizations have developed programs to address the numerous issues regarding HIV/AIDS. The national AIDS hotline (1-800-342-AIDS) is a good resource.

Preventing Sexually Transmitted Infections

Education about safer sex practices—and the resulting increase in the use of condoms—can play a vital role in reducing STI rates all over the world. Clearly, knowledge and prevention are the best defenses against STIs. The prevention and control of STIs is based on the following concepts (CDC, 2006):

1. Education and counseling of persons at risk about safer sexual behavior
2. Identification of asymptomatic infected individuals and of symptomatic individuals unlikely to seek diagnosis and treatment
3. Effective diagnosis and treatment of infected individuals

4. Evaluation, treatment, and counseling of sex partners of people who are infected with an STI
5. Pre-exposure vaccination of people at risk for vaccine-preventable STIs

Nurses play an integral role in identifying and preventing STIs. They have a unique opportunity to educate the public about this serious public health issue by communicating the methods of transmission and symptoms associated with each condition, tracking the updated CDC treatment guidelines, and offering clients strategic preventive measures to reduce the spread of STIs.

It is not easy to discuss STI prevention when globally we are failing at it. Knowledge exists on how to prevent every single route of transmission, but the incidence continues to climb. Challenges to prevention of STIs include lack of resources and difficulty in changing the behaviors that contribute to their spread. Regardless of the challenging factors involved, nurses must continue to educate and to meet the needs of all women to promote their sexual health. Successful treatment and prevention of STIs is impossible without education. Successful teaching approaches include giving clear, accurate messages that are age-appropriate and culturally sensitive.

Primary prevention strategies include education of all women, especially adolescents, regarding the risk of early sexual activity, the number of sexual partners, and STIs. Sexual abstinence is ideal but often not practiced; therefore, the use of barrier contraception (condoms) should be encouraged (see Teaching Guidelines 5.1).

Secondary prevention involves the need for annual pelvic examinations with Pap smears for all sexually active women, regardless of age. Many women with STIs are asymptomatic, so regular screening examinations are paramount for early detection. Understanding the relationship between poor socioeconomic conditions and poor patterns of sexual and reproductive self-care is significant in disease-prevention and health-promotion strategies.

Every successful form of prevention requires a change in behavior. The nursing role in teaching and rendering quality health care is invaluable evidence that the key to reducing the spread of STIs is through behavioral change. Nurses working in these specialty areas have a responsibility to educate themselves, their clients, their families, and the community about STIs and to provide compassionate and supportive care to clients. Some strategies nurses can use to prevent the spread of STIs are detailed in Box 5.3.

Behavior Modification

Research validates that changing behaviors does result in a decrease in new STI infections, but it must encompass all levels—governments, community organizations, schools, churches, parents, and individuals (Peterson et al., 2007). Education must address ways to prevent becoming infected, ways to prevent transmitting infection, symptoms

---

BOX 5.3 **Selected Nursing Strategies to Prevent the Spread of STIs**

- Provide basic information about STI transmission.
- Outline safer sexual behaviors for people at risk for STIs.
- Refer clients to appropriate community resources to reduce risk.
- Screen asymptomatic persons with STIs.
- Identify barriers to STI testing and remove them.
- Offer pre-exposure immunizations for vaccine-preventable STIs.
- Respond honestly about testing results and options available.
- Counsel and treat sexual partners of persons with STIs.
- Educate school administrators, parents, and teens about STIs.
- Support youth development activities to reduce sexual risk-taking.
- Promote the use of barrier methods (condoms, diaphragms) to prevent the spread of STIs.
- Assist clients to gain skills in negotiating safer sex.
- Discuss reducing the number of sexual partners to reduce risk

---

of STIs, and treatment. At this point in the STI epidemic, nurses do not have time to debate the relative merits of prevention versus treatment: both are underused and underfunded, and one leads to the other. But being serious about prevention and focusing on the strategies outlined above will bring about a positive change on everyone's part.

Contraception

The spread of STIs could be prevented by access to safe, efficient, appropriate, modern contraception for everyone who wants it. Nurses can play an important role in helping women to identify their risk of STIs and to adopt preventive measures through the dual protection that contraceptives offer. Traditionally, family planning and STI services have been separate entities. Family planning services have addressed a woman's need for contraception without considering her or her partner's risk of STI; meanwhile, STI services have been heavily slanted toward men, ignoring the contraceptive needs of men and their partners.

Many women are at significant risk for unintended pregnancy and STIs, yet with this separation of services, there is limited evaluation of whether they need dual protection—that is, concurrent protection from STIs and unintended pregnancy. This lack of integration of services represents a missed opportunity to identify many at-risk women and to offer them counseling on dual protection (Hogben, 2007).

Nurses can expand their scopes in either setting by discussing dual protection by use of a male or female condom alone or by use of a condom along with a nonbarrier contraceptive. Because barrier methods are not the most effective means of fertility control, they have not been typically recommended as a method alone for dual protection. Unfortunately, the most effective pregnancy prevention methods—sterilization, hormonal methods, and intrauterine devices—do not protect against STIs. Dual-method use protects against STIs and pregnancy.

■■■ Key Concepts

■ Avoiding risky sexual behaviors may preserve fertility and prevent chronic conditions later in life.

■ An estimated 65 million people live with an incurable STI, and another 15 million are infected each year.

■ The most reliable way to avoid transmission of STIs is to abstain from sexual intercourse (i.e., oral, vaginal, or anal sex) or to be in a long-term, mutually monogamous relationship with an uninfected partner.

■ Barrier methods of contraception are recommended because they increase protection from contact with urethral discharge, mucosal secretions, and lesions of the cervix or penis.

■ The high rate of asymptomatic transmission of STIs calls for teaching high-risk women the nature of transmission and how to recognize infections.

■ The CDC and ACOG recommend that all women be offered group B streptococcal screening by rectovaginal culture at 35 to 37 weeks of gestation, and that colonized women be treated with intravenous antibiotics at the time of labor or ruptured membranes.

■ Nurses should practice good handwashing techniques and follow standard precautions to protect themselves and their patients from STIs.

■ Nurses are in an important position to promote the sexual health of all women. Nurses should make their clients and the community aware of the perinatal implications and life-long sequelae of STIs.

REFERENCES

Aaron, E., Levine, A. B., Monahan, K., & Biondo, C. P. (2006). A rapid HIV testing program for labor and delivery in an inner city teaching hospital. *AIDS Reader, 16*(1), 22–37.

Alexander, L. L., LaRosa, J. H., Bader, H., & Garfield, S. (2007). *New dimensions in women's health* (4th ed.). Sudbury, MA: Jones and Bartlett Publishers.

American Cancer Society (ACS). (2007). American Cancer Society Guideline for HPV vaccine use to prevent cervical cancer and its precursors. *CA: A Cancer Journal for Clinicians, 57*(1), 7–28.

Assan, S., & Kraszewski, S. (2006). Sexually transmitted infections: Hepatitis B. *Practice Nurse, 32*(7), 58–62.

Battaglioli-Denero, A. M. (2007). Strategies for improving adherence to therapy and long-term patient outcomes. *Journal of the Association of Nurses in AIDS Care, 18*(1), S17–22.

Bennett, N. J., & Domachowske, J. (2007). Gonorrhea. *eMedicine.* Available at: http://www.emedicine.com/PED/topic886.htm

Centers for Disease Control and Prevention (CDC). (2006). Sexually transmitted diseases treatment guidelines 2006. *MMWR, 55*(RR-11), 1–89.

Centers for Disease Control and Prevention (CDC). (2007a). Increases in gonorrhea 2000–2006. *MMWR, 56*(10), 222–225.

Centers for Disease Control and Prevention (CDC). (2007b). A glance at the HIV/AIDS epidemic. Available at: http://www.cdc.gov/hiv/resources/factsheets/print/At-A-Glance.htm

Centers for Disease Control and Prevention (CDC). (2007c). Genital HPV infection—CDC fact sheet. Available at: http://www.cdc.gov/std/HPV/STDFact-HPV.htm

Centers for Disease Control and Prevention (CDC). (2007d). Pelvic inflammatory disease—CDC fact sheet. Available at: http://www.cdc.gov/std/PID/STDFact-PID.htm

Cordoro, K. M., & Wilson, B. B. (2007). Scabies. *eMedicine.* Available at: http://www.emedicine.com/DERM/topic382.htm

Cressey, T. R., & Lallemant, M. (2007). Pharmacogenetics of antiretroviral drugs for the treatment of HIV-infected patients: An update. *Infection, Genetics & Evolution, 7*(2), 333–342.

Crossman, S. H. (2006). The challenge of pelvic inflammatory disease. *American Family Physician, 73*(5), 859–864.

Dubin, J. (2007). HIV infection and AIDS. *eMedicine.* Available at: http://www.emedicine.com/EMERG/topic253.htm

Dunne, E. F., Unger, E. R., Sternberg, M., McQuillan, G., Swan, D. C., Patel, S. S., & Markowitz, L. E. (2007). Prevalence of HPV infection among females in the United States. *JAMA, 297*(8), 813–819.

Ferguson, L. A., & Varnado, J. W. (2006) Syphilis: An old enemy still lurks. *Journal of the American Academy of Nurse Practitioners, 18,* 49–55.

Gearhart, P. A., & Randall, T. C. (2007). Human papillomavirus. *eMedicine.* Available at: http://www.emedicine.com/med/topic1037.htm

Geisler, W. M. (2007). Management of uncomplicated *Chlamydia trachomatis* infections in adolescents and adults. *Clinical Infectious Diseases, 44*(3), S77–83.

Gilbert, E. S. (2007). *Manual of high-risk pregnancy and delivery* (4th ed.). St. Louis, MO: Mosby Elsevier

Glasier, A., Gulmezoglu, A. M., Schmid, G. P., Moreno, C. G., & Van Look, P. F. A. (2006). Sexual reproductive health: A matter of life and death. *Lancet, 368*(9547), 1595–1607.

Hackley, B., Kriebs, J. M., & Rousseau, M. E. (2007). *Primary care of women: A guide for midwives and women's health providers.* Sudbury, MA: Jones and Bartlett Publishers.

Hogben, M. (2007). Partner notification for sexually transmitted disease. *Clinical Infectious Disease, 44*(3), S160–174.

Johnson-Mallard, V., Lengacher, C. A., Kromroy, J. D., Campbell, D. W., Jevitt, C. M., Daley, E., & Schmitt, K. (2007). Increasing knowledge of sexually transmitted infection risk. *Nurse Practitioner, 32*(2), 26–33.

Kennedy, M. S. (2007). In the clinical arena. *AJN, 107*(1), 22.

Leggatt, G. R., & Frazer, I. H. (2007). HPV vaccines: The beginning of the end for cervical cancer. *Current Opinion in Immunology, 19*(2), 232–238.

Marrazzo, J. M., & Martin, D. H. (2007). Management of women with cervicitis. *Clinical Infectious Diseases, 44*(3), S102–110.

McGregor, T. A., & Richard, A. J. (2007). Syphilis. *eMedicine.* Available at: http://www.emedicine.com/EMERG/topic563.htm

Mehta, S. D. (2007). Gonorrhea and chlamydia in emergency departments: Screening, diagnosis and treatment. *Current Infectious Diseases, 9*(2), 134–142.

Moore, S. L., & Seybold, V. K. (2007). HPV vaccine. *Clinical Reviews, 17*(1), 36–42.

Mullan, F. (2007). Responding to the global HIV/AIDS crisis. *Journal of the American Medical Association, 297*(7), 744–746.

National Institute of Allergy and Infectious Disease. (2006a). Chlamydia. Retrieved Sept. 15, 2007, from http://www.niaid.nih.gov/factsheets/stdclam.htm

National Institute of Allergy and Infectious Disease. (2006b). Gonorrhea. Retrieved Sept. 15, 2007, from http://www.niaid.nih.gov/factsheets/stdgon.htm

National Institute of Allergy and Infectious Diseases. (2007a). HIV infection in women. National Institutes of Health. Available at: http://www.niaid.nih.gov/factsheets/womenhiv.htm

National Institute of Allergy and Infectious Diseases. (2007b). Human papillomavirus and genital warts. National Institutes of Health. Available at: http://www.niaid.nih.gov/factsheets/stdhpv.htm

National Institute of Allergy and Infectious Disease. (2007c). Syphilis. Retrieved Sept. 15, 2007, from http://www3.niaid.nih.gov/health science/healthtopics/syphilis/default.htm.

National Institutes of Health (NIH). (2008). *HIV/AIDS among youth* [Online]. Available at http://www.cdc.gov/hiv/resources/factsheets/youth.htm

Paz-Bailey, G., Ramaswamy, M., Hawkes, S., & Geretti, A. (2007). Herpes simplex virus type 2: Epidemiology and management options in developing countries. *Sexually Transmitted Infections, 83*(1), 16–22.

Peterson, R., Albright, J., Garrett, J., & Curtis, K. (2007). Pregnancy and STD prevention counseling using an adaptation of motivational interviewing: A randomized controlled study. *Perspectives on Sexual & Reproductive Health, 39*(1), 21–28.

Pickering, L. K. (Ed.) (2006). *Red book: 2006 report of the committee on infectious diseases* (27th ed.). Elk Grove Village, IL: American Academy of Pediatrics.

Public Health Agency of Canada. (2006). *Canadian guidelines on sexually transmitted infections.* Ottawa, ON: Author.

Pyrsopoulos, N. T., & Reddy, K. R. (2007). Hepatitis B. *eMedicine.* Available at: http://www.emedicine.com/MED/topic992.htm

Reyes, I., & Abbuhl, S. (2007). Pelvic inflammatory disease. *eMedicine.* Available at: http://emedicine.com/emerg/topic410.htm

Sharma, R., & Brilliant, L. C. (2007). Herpes simplex. *eMedicine.* Available at: http://www.emedicine.com/EMERG/topic246.htm

Stoner, B. P. (2007). Current controversies in the management of adult syphilis. *Clinical Infectious Diseases, 44*(3), S130–146.

Wald, A. (2007). The CDC releases its HPV vaccine recommendations. *Journal Watch Women's Health.* Available at: http://womens-health.jwatch.org/cgi/content/full/2007/824/1

Wasley, A., Miller, J. T., & Finelli, L. (2007). Surveillance for active viral hepatitis—United States, 2005. *MMWR, 56*(3), 1–24.

Waugh, M. (2007). Sexual health medicine 2007. *Skinmed, 6*(2), 88–90.

Wolfram, W. (2007). Pediculosis (lice). *eMedicine.* Available at: http://www.emedicine.com/ped/topic1304.htm

World Health Organization (WHO). (2007a). Hepatitis B fact sheet. Available at: http://www.who.int/mediacentre/factsheets/fs204/en/

World Health Organization (WHO). (2007b). HIV transmission through breastfeeding. Available at: http://www.who.int/reproductive-health/docs/hiv_infantfeeding/breastfeeding.html

Workowski, K. A., & Berman, S. M. (2006). Sexually transmitted diseases treatment guidelines, 2006. *MMWR Recommendations Report, 55*(RR11), 1–94.

WEBSITES

American College of Obstetricians and Gynecologists (ACOG): (202) 863-2518, http://www.acog.org

American Psychiatric Association: (202) 682-6000, http://psych.org

American Society for Reproductive Medicine: (205) 978-5000, http://www.asrm.org

Centers for Disease Control and Prevention: (202) 329-1819, http://www.cdc.gov

CDC National AIDS hotline: 1-800-342-2437

Herpes Resource Center: www.ashastd.org/herpes/hrc

National Institute of Allergy and Infectious Disease: Human papillomavirus and genital warts, http://www.niaid.hih.gov/factsheets/stdhpv.htm

National Institute of Allergy and Infectious Disease: Chlamydia, http://www.niaid.nih.gov/factsheets/stdclam.htm

National Institute of Allergy and Infectious Disease: Gonorrhea, http://www.niaid.nih.gov/factsheets/stdgon.htm.

National Institute of Allergy and Infectious Disease: Syphilis, http://www.niaid.nih.gov/factsheets/stdsyph.htm.

National Institute of Mental Health: (301) 443-4513, http://www.nimh.nih.gov

National Women's Health Resource Center: http://www.healthy-women.org

National Women's Information Center (NWHIC): 1-800-994-9662, http://www.4women.gov

Resolve, Inc. (impaired fertility): (617) 623-0744, http://www.resolve.org

Teen Source (STI information for teens): www.teensource.org

CHAPTER WORKSHEET

MULTIPLE CHOICE QUESTIONS

1. Which of the following contraceptive methods offers protection against sexually transmitted infections (STIs)?

   a. Oral contraceptives

   b. Withdrawal

   c. Latex condom

   d. Intrauterine device

2. In teaching about HIV transmission, the nurse explains that the virus cannot be transmitted by:

   a. Shaking hands

   b. Sharing drug needles

   c. Sexual intercourse

   d. Breastfeeding

3. A woman with HPV is likely to present with which nursing assessment finding?

   a. Profuse, pus-filled vaginal discharge

   b. Clusters of genital warts

   c. Single painless ulcer

   d. Multiple vesicles on genitalia

4. The nurse's discharge teaching plan for the woman with PID should reinforce which of the following potentially life-threatening complications?

   a. Involuntary infertility

   b. Chronic pelvic pain

   c. Depression

   d. Ectopic pregnancy

5. To confirm a finding of primary syphilis, the nurse would observe which of the following on the external genitalia?

   a. A highly variable skin rash

   b. A yellow-green vaginal discharge

   c. A nontender, indurated ulcer

   d. A localized gumma formation

CRITICAL THINKING EXERCISE

1. Sally, age 17, comes to the teen clinic saying that she is in pain and has some "crud" between her legs. The nurse takes her into the examining room and questions her about her symptoms. Sally states she had numerous genital bumps that had been filled with fluid, then ruptured and turned into ulcers with crusts. In addition, she has pain on urination and overall body pain. Sally says she had unprotected sex with several men when she was drunk at a party a few weeks back, but she thought they were "clean."

   a. What STI would the nurse suspect?

   b. The nurse should give immediate consideration to which of Sally's complaints?

   c. What should be the goal of the nurse in teaching Sally about STIs?

STUDY ACTIVITIES

1. Select a website at the end of the chapter to explore. Educate yourself about one specific STI thoroughly and share your expertise with your clinical group.

2. Contact your local health department and request current statistics regarding three STIs. Ask them to compare the current number of cases reported to last year's. Are they less or more? What may be some of the reasons for the change in the number of cases reported?

3. Request permission to attend a local STI clinic to shadow a nurse for a few hours. Describe the nurse's counseling role with patients and what specific information is emphasized to patients.

4. Two common STIs that appear together and commonly are treated together regardless of identification of the secondary one are _____ and _____.

5. Genital warts can be treated with which of the following? Select all that apply.

   a. Penicillin

   b. Podophyllin

   c. Imiquimod

   d. Cryotherapy

   e. Antiretroviral therapy

   f. Acyclovir

CHAPTER 6

DISORDERS OF THE BREASTS

KEY TERMS

benign breast disorder
breast cancer
breast-conserving surgery
breast self-examination
carcinoma
chemotherapy

duct ectasia
endocrine therapy
fibroadenomas
fibrocystic breast changes
intraductal papilloma
mammography

mastitis
modified radical
  mastectomy
simple mastectomy

LEARNING OBJECTIVES

Upon completion of the chapter, the learner will be able to:

1. Define the key terms used in this chapter.
2. Identify the incidence, risk factors, screening methods, and treatment modalities for benign breast conditions.
3. Outline preventive strategies for breast cancer through lifestyle changes and health screening.
4. Explain the incidence, risk factors, treatment modalities, and nursing considerations related to breast cancer.
5. Develop an educational plan to teach breast self-examination to a group of young women.

Nancy hasn't been able to sleep well since she felt the lump in her left breast over a month ago, just after her 60th birthday. She knows she is at high risk because her mother died of breast cancer, but she can't bring herself to have it checked out.

Wow

Focus on reducing fear, anxiety, pain, and aloneness in all women diagnosed with a breast disorder.

The female breast is closely linked to womanhood in American culture. Women's breasts act as physical markers for transitions from one stage of life to another, and although the primary function of the breasts is lactation, they are perceived as a symbol of beauty and sexuality.

This chapter will discuss assessments, screening procedures, and management of specific benign and malignant breast disorders. Nurses play a key role in helping women maintain breast health by education and screening. A good working knowledge of early detection techniques, diagnosis, and treatment options is essential.

Benign Breast Disorders

A **benign breast disorder** is any noncancerous breast abnormality. Though not life-threatening, benign disorders can cause pain and discomfort, and they account for a large number of visits to primary care providers.

Depending on the type of benign breast disorder, treatment might or might not be necessary. Although these disorders are benign, the emotional trauma women experience is phenomenal. Fear, anxiety, disbelief, helplessness, and depression are just a few of the reactions that a woman may have when she discovers a lump in her breast. Many women believe that all lumps are cancerous, but actually more than 90% of the lumps discovered are benign and need no treatment (Alexander et al., 2007). Patience, support, and education are essential components of nursing care.

▶ *Consider* THIS!

It was pouring down rain and I was driving alone along dark wet streets to my 8 a.m. appointment for a breast ultrasound. I recently had my annual mammogram and the radiologist thought he saw something suspicious on my right breast. I was on my way to confirm or refute his suspicions, and I couldn't keep focused on the road ahead. For the past few days I had been a basket case, fearing the worst. I was playing in my mind, what I would do if . . . ? What changes would I make in my life and how would I react when told? I have been through such personal turmoil since that doctor announced he wanted "more tests."

Thoughts: This woman is worrying and is emotionally devastated before she even has a conclusive diagnosis. Is this a typical reaction to a breast disorder? Why do women fear the worst? Many women use denial to mask their feelings and hope against hope the doctor made a mistake or misread their mammogram. How would you react if you or your sister, girlfriend, or mother were confronted with a breast disorder?

The most commonly encountered benign breast disorders in women include fibrocystic breasts, fibroadenomas, intraductal papilloma, mammary duct ectasia, and mastitis. Although these breast disorders are considered benign, fibrocystic breasts and intraductal papillomas carry a cancer risk, with prolific masses and hyperplastic changes within the breasts. Generally speaking, fibroadenomas, mastitis, and mammary duct ectasia carry little cancer risk (Sukumvanich & Borgen, 2007). Table 6-1 summarizes benign breast conditions.

▶ FIBROCYSTIC BREAST CHANGES

Fibrocystic breast changes do not refer to a disease; rather, they represent a variety of changes in the glandular and structural tissues of the breast. Because this condition affects many women at some point, it is more accurately defined as a "change" rather than a "disease." The cause of fibrocystic changes is related to the way breast tissue responds to monthly levels of estrogen and progesterone. During the menstrual cycle, hormonal stimulation of the breast tissue causes the glands and ducts to enlarge and swell. One or both breasts can be involved, and any part of the breast can become tender (Hackley, Kriebs, & Rousseau, 2007). Fibrocystic changes do not increase the risk of breast cancer for most women except when the breast biopsy shows "atypia" or abnormal breast cells. The cause for concern for many women with fibrocystic changes is that breast examinations and mammography become more difficult to interpret with multiple cysts present, and early cancerous lesions that occur may occasionally be overlooked (American Cancer Society [ACS], 2007a).

Fibrocystic breast changes are most common in women between the ages of 30 and 50. The condition is rare in postmenopausal women not taking hormone replacement therapy. According to the ACS, fibrocystic breast changes affect at least half of all women at some point in their lives and are the most common breast disorder today (ACS, 2007a).

Therapeutic Management

Management of the symptoms of fibrocystic breast changes begins with self-care. In severe cases drugs, including bromocriptine, tamoxifen, or danazol, can be used to reduce the influence of estrogen on breast tissue. However, several undesirable side effects, including masculinization, have been documented. Aspiration or surgical removal of breast lumps will reduce pain and swelling by removing the space-occupying mass.

Nursing Assessment

Nursing assessment consists of a health history, physical examination, and laboratory and diagnostic tests.

TABLE 6.1 SUMMARY OF BENIGN BREAST DISORDERS

Breast Condition	Nipple Discharge	Site	Characteristics/ Age of Client	Tenderness	Diagnosis & Treatment
Fibrocystic breast changes	+ or −	Bilateral; upper outer quadrant	Round, smooth Several lesions Cyclic, palpable 30 to 50 years old	+	Aspiration and biopsy Limit caffeine; ibuprofen; supportive bra
Fibroadenomas	−	Unilateral; nipple area or upper outer quadrant	Round, firm, movable Palpable, rubbery Well delineated Single lesion 15 to 30 years old	−	Mammogram "Watchful waiting" Aspiration and biopsy Surgical excision
Intraductal papilloma	+	Unilateral; near nipple	Small, wart-like Poorly delineated Nonpalpable Can become large 40 to 60 years old	+	Culture discharge Mammogram Ultrasound Surgical excision
Duct ectasia	+	Unilateral; behind nipple	Inflammation Pasty, greenish discharge Nonmobile Burning, itching Perimenopausal women	+	Mammogram Ultrasound Culture Antibiotics Surgical excision
Mastitis	−	Unilateral; outer quadrant	Wedge-shaped Warmth, redness Swelling Nipple cracked Breast engorged	+	Antibiotics Warm shower Supportive bra Breastfeeding Increase fluids

Sources: ACS, 2007a; Alexander et al., 2007; Blackburn, 2007; Sukumvanich & Borgen, 2007

Health History

Ask the woman about common clinical manifestations, which include lumpy, tender breasts, particularly during the week before menses. Changes in breast tissue produce pain by nerve irritation from edema in connective tissue and by fibrosis from nerve pinching. The pain is cyclic and frequently dissipates after the onset of menses. The pain is described as a dull, aching feeling of fullness. Masses or nodularities usually appear in both breasts and are often found in the upper outer quadrants. Some women also experience spontaneous clear to yellow nipple discharge when the breast is squeezed or manipulated.

Physical Examination

It is best to examine a woman's breast a week after menses, when swelling has subsided. Observe the breasts for fibrosis, or thickening of the normal breast tissues, which occurs in the early stages. Cysts form in the later stages and feel like multiple, smooth, well-delineated tiny pebbles or bumpy oatmeal under the skin (Fig. 6.1). On physical examination of the breasts, a few characteristics might be helpful in differentiating a cyst from a cancerous lesion. Cancerous lesions typically are fixed and painless and may cause skin retraction (pulling). Cysts tend to be mobile and tender and do not cause skin retraction in the surrounding tissue.

Laboratory and Diagnostic Tests

Mammography can be helpful in distinguishing fibrocystic changes from breast cancer. Ultrasound is a useful adjunct to mammography for breast evaluation because it helps to differentiate a cystic mass from a solid one (Aliotta & Schaeffer, 2006). Ultrasound produces images of the breasts by sending sound waves through a gel applied to the breasts. Fine-needle aspiration biopsy can also be done to differentiate a solid tumor, cyst, or malignancy. A fine-needle aspiration biopsy uses a thin needle guided by ultrasound to the mass. In a method called stereotactic needle biopsy, a computer maps the exact location of the mass using mammograms taken from two angles, and the map is used to guide the needle.

A

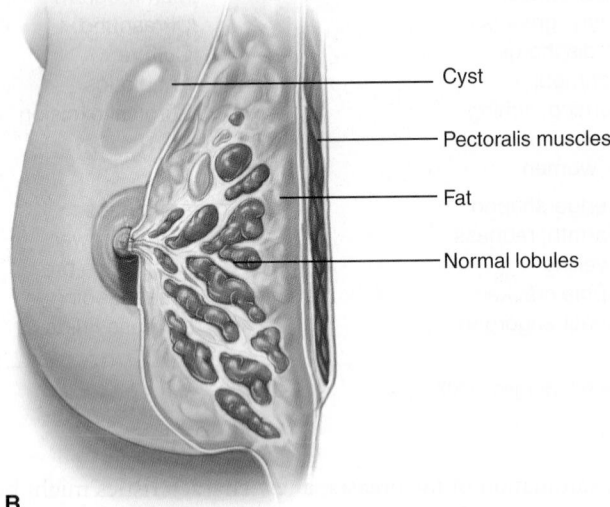

B

FIGURE 6.1 (**A**) Fibrocystic breast changes. (**B**) Cysts. (Source: The Anatomical Chart Company. [2002]. *Atlas of pathophysiology.* Springhouse, PA: Springhouse Corporation.)

Nursing Management

A nurse caring for a woman with fibrocystic breast changes can teach her about the condition, provide tips for self-care (Teaching Guidelines 6.1), suggest lifestyle changes, and demonstrate how to perform monthly breast self-examination after her menses to monitor the changes. Nursing Care Plan 6.1 presents a plan of care for a woman with fibrocystic breast changes.

▶ FIBROADENOMAS

Fibroadenomas are common benign solid breast tumors that occur in about 10% of all women and account for up

Relieving Symptoms of Fibrocystic Breast Changes

- Wear an extra-supportive bra to prevent undue strain on the ligaments of the breasts to reduce discomfort.
- Avoid caffeine, which is a stimulant. This reduces discomfort for some women.
- Take oral contraceptives, as recommended by a health care practitioner, to stabilize the monthly hormonal levels.
- Eat a low-fat diet rich in fruits, vegetables, and grains to maintain a healthy nutritional lifestyle and ideal weight.
- Apply heat to the breasts to help reduce pain via vasodilation of vessels.
- Take diuretics, as recommended by a health care practitioner, to counteract fluid retention and swelling of the breasts.
- Reduce salt intake to reduce fluid retention and swelling in the breasts.
- Take OTC medications, such as aspirin or ibuprofen (Motrin, Advil, Nuprin), to reduce inflammation and discomfort.
- Use thiamine and vitamin E therapy. This has been found helpful for some women, but research has failed to demonstrate a direct benefit from either therapy.
- Take medications as prescribed (e.g., bromocriptine, tamoxifen, or danazol).
- Discuss the possibility of aspiration or surgical removal of breast lumps with a health care practitioner.

to half of all breast biopsies. They are the most common mass in women (Harris, 2007). They are considered hyperplastic lesions associated with an aberration of normal development and involution rather than a neoplasm. Fibroadenomas can be stimulated by external estrogen, progesterone, lactation, and pregnancy (Sukumvanich & Borgen, 2007). They are composed of both fibrous and glandular tissue and usually occur in women between 20 and 40 years of age (Alexander et al., 2007). Giant fibroadenomas account for approximately 10% of cases. These masses are frequently larger than 5 cm and occur most often in pregnant or lactating women. These large lesions may regress in size once hormonal stimulation subsides (Hackley, Kriebs, & Rousseau, 2007). Fibroadenomas are rarely associated with cancer.

Therapeutic Management

Treatment may include a period of "watchful waiting" because many fibroadenomas stop growing or shrink on their own without any treatment. Other growths may need to be

Nursing Care Plan 6.1

OVERVIEW OF THE WOMAN WITH FIBROCYSTIC BREAST CHANGES

Sheree Rollins is a 37-year-old woman who comes to the clinic for her routine check-up. During the examination, she says, "Sometimes my breasts feel so heavy and they ache a lot. I noticed a couple of lumpy areas in my breast last week just before I got my period. Is this normal? Now they feel like they're almost gone. Should I be worried?" Clinical breast examination reveals two small (pea-sized), mobile, slightly tender nodules in each breast bilaterally. No skin retraction noted. Previous mammogram revealed fibrocystic breast changes.

NURSING DIAGNOSIS: Pain related to changes in breast tissue

Outcome Identification and Evaluation
Client will demonstrate a decrease in breast pain as evidenced by a pain rating of 1 or 2 on a pain rating scale of 0 to 10 and statements that pain is lessened.

Interventions: Relieving Pain
* Ask client to rate her pain using a numeric pain rating scale *to establish a baseline.*
* Discuss with client any measures used to relieve pain *to determine effectiveness of the measures.*
* Encourage use of a supportive bra *to aid in reducing discomfort.*
* Instruct client in use of over-the-counter analgesics *to promote pain relief.*
* Advise the client to apply warm compresses or allow warm water from the shower to flow over her breasts *to promote vasodilation and subsequent pain relief.*
* Tell client to reduce her intake of salt to reduce risk of fluid retention and swelling leading *to increased pain.*

NURSING DIAGNOSIS: Deficient knowledge related to fibrocystic breast changes and appropriate care measures

Outcome Identification and Evaluation
Client will verbalize understanding of condition as evidenced by statements about the cause of breast changes and appropriate choices for lifestyle changes, and demonstration of self-care measures.

Interventions: Providing Patient Education
* Assess client's knowledge of fibrocystic breast changes *to establish a baseline for teaching.*
* Explain the role of monthly hormonal level changes and describe the signs and symptoms *to promote understanding of this condition.*
* Teach the client how to perform breast self-examination after her menstrual period *to monitor for changes.*
* Encourage client to report any changes promptly *to ensure early detection of problems.*
* Suggest client speak with her primary care provider about the use of oral contraceptives *to help stabilize monthly hormonal levels.*
* Review lifestyle choices, such as avoiding caffeine, eating a low-fat diet rich in fruits, vegetables, and grains, and adhering to screening recommendations *to promote health.*
* Discuss measures for pain relief *to minimize discomfort associated with breast changes.*

---

surgically removed if they do not regress or if they remain unchanged. Cryoablation, an alternative to surgery, can also be used to remove a tumor. In this procedure, extremely cold gas is piped into the tumor using ultrasound guidance. The tumor freezes and dies. The current trend is toward a more conservative approach to treatment after careful evaluation and continued monitoring.

Nursing Assessment

Ask the woman about clinical manifestations of fibroadenomas. These lumps are felt as firm, rubbery, well-circumscribed, freely mobile nodules that might or might not be tender when palpated.

Breast fibroadenomas are usually detected incidentally during clinical or self-examinations and are usually located in the upper outer quadrant of the breast; more than one may be present (Fig. 6.2). Several other breast lesions have similar characteristics, so every woman with a breast mass should be evaluated to exclude cancer. A clinical breast examination by a health care professional is critical. In addition, diagnostic studies include imaging studies (mammography, ultrasound, or both) and some form of biopsy, most often a fine-needle aspiration, core needle biopsy, or stereotactic needle biopsy. The core needle biopsy removes a small cylinder of tissue from the breast mass, more than the fine-needle aspiration biopsy.

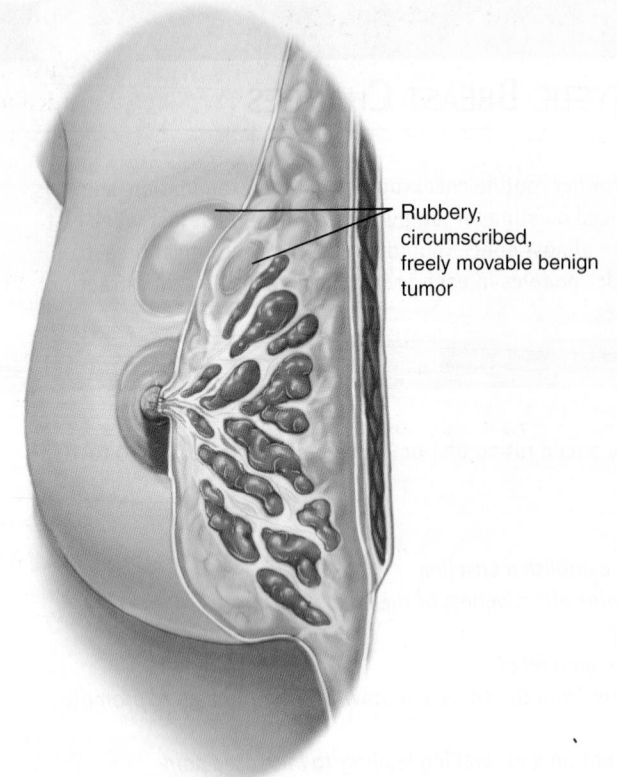

Rubbery,
circumscribed,
freely movable benign
tumor

FIGURE 6.2 Fibroadenoma. (Source: The Anatomical Chart Company. [2002]. *Atlas of pathophysiology*. Springhouse, PA: Springhouse Corporation.)

If additional tissue needs to be evaluated, the advanced breast biopsy instrument (ABBI) is used. This instrument removes a larger cylinder of tissue for examination by using a rotating circular knife. The ABBI procedure removes more tissue than any of the other methods except a surgical biopsy (ACS, 2007b).

Nursing Management

The nurse should urge the client to return for re-evaluation in 6 months, perform monthly breast self-examinations, and return annually for a clinical breast examination.

▶ INTRADUCTAL PAPILLOMA

An **intraductal papilloma** is a benign, wart-like growth found in the mammary ducts, usually near the nipple. This benign growth is thought to be caused by a proliferation and overgrowth of ductal epithelial tissue. An intraductal papilloma is generally less than 1 cm in diameter and might not be palpable. It produces a spontaneous serous, serosanguineous, or watery nipple discharge (Graham, 2006). It mostly affects women between the ages of 40

and 60. A single duct or several ducts may be involved. Women with solitary papilloma without atypia carry a minimal increase of developing breast cancer over the general population. These women are not classified as high risk. However, the risk of subsequent breast cancer is increased by four- to fivefold in the presence of atypia (Sukumvanich & Borgen, 2007).

Therapeutic Management

Treatment consists of surgical removal of the papilloma and a part of the duct it is found in, usually through an incision at the edge of the areola. The excised papilloma and duct are sent to the pathology laboratory to rule out cancer (ACS, 2007a).

Nursing Assessment

The woman might report a feeling of fullness in the breast and may state that she can manually express a serous, serosanguineous, or watery discharge from the nipple. If the papilloma is large enough, it can be palpated in the nipple area as a soft, nontender, mobile, poorly delineated mass.

Laboratory and diagnostic testing is important to rule out cancer. The nipple discharge is evaluated for the presence of occult blood using a Hemoccult card; a blue coloration on the card indicates the presence of blood. In addition, a sample of the discharge may be sent for cytologic evaluation to screen for cancer cells. Mammography, ultrasound, or ductography (radiographic dye is instilled into a duct; it outlines the breast ductal system on radiographs) is used to diagnose or differentiate this lesion from a cancerous one. An intraductal papilloma appears as a smooth, lobulated filling defect or a solitary obstructed duct on ductography (Aliotta & Schaeffer, 2006).

Nursing Management

The nurse should advise the woman to continue monthly breast self-examinations and yearly clinical breast examinations.

▶ DUCT ECTASIA

Duct ectasia is a dilation and inflammation of the ducts behind the nipple. It is most common in perimenopausal women. This benign condition frequently occurs in women who have breastfed their children. The cause is unclear; however, chronic periductal inflammation, fibrosis, and ductal dilatation are associated factors. This condition results in noncyclic breast pain, nipple retraction, and discharge (Hackley, Kriebs, & Rousseau, 2007).

Therapeutic Management

This condition frequently improves without any specific treatment, or with warm compresses and antibiotics. If symptoms persist, the abnormal duct is removed through a local incision at the border of the areola. The tissue is sent to the pathology laboratory for evaluation.

Nursing Assessment

Assess the patient for clinical manifestations of duct ectasia. If the ducts have been chronically infected, an erythematous lesion will be present at the edge of the nipple area (ACS, 2007a). The woman may complain of nipple discharge, which can be green, brown, straw-colored, reddish, gray, or cream-colored, with the consistency of toothpaste. In addition, the woman may report a dull nipple pain, subareolar swelling, or a burning sensation accompanied by pruritus around the nipple (Richards et al., 2007).

Physical examination of the breasts might reveal subareolar redness and swelling, with mild to moderate tenderness on palpation. In addition, palpation will reveal the presence of tortuous tubular swellings beneath the areola, along with nipple retraction and dimpling in some postmenopausal women (Graham, 2006). Diagnostic and laboratory testing includes mammography, ultrasound, and cytology and testing for occult blood on a nipple discharge sample, and ductography may be used to assist in the diagnosis of this lesion.

Nursing Management

The nurse should reassure the woman that this condition is benign and should reinforce the importance of monthly self-examinations as well as annual clinical breast examinations by the woman's health care provider. This benign breast condition is typically self-limiting; the only intervention needed is reassurance.

▶ MASTITIS

Mastitis is an infection of the connective tissue in the breast that occurs primarily in lactating or engorged women. Mastitis is divided into lactational or nonlactational. The usual causative organisms for lactational mastitis are *Staphylococcus aureus, Haemophilus influenzae,* and *Haemophilus* and *Streptococcus* species, the source of which is the baby's flora. One or more of the ducts drain poorly or become blocked, resulting in bacterial growth in the retained milk (Sukumvanich & Borgen, 2007).

Nonlactational mastitis can be caused by duct ectasia, which occurs when the milk ducts become congested with secretions and debris, resulting in periductal inflammation. These women present with greenish nipple discharge, nipple retraction, and noncyclical pain.

Therapeutic Management

Management of both types of mastitis involves the use of oral antibiotics (usually a penicillinase-resistant penicillin or cephalosporin) and acetaminophen (Tylenol) for pain and fever.

Nursing Assessment

Assess the patient's health history for risk factors for mastitis, which include poor handwashing, ductal abnormalities, nipple cracks and fissures, lowered maternal defenses due to fatigue, tight clothing, poor support of pendulous breasts, failure to empty the breasts properly while breastfeeding, or missing breastfeedings.

Assess the patient for clinical manifestations of mastitis, which include flu-like symptoms of malaise, leukocytosis, fever, and chills. Physical examination of the breasts reveals increased warmth, redness, tenderness, and swelling. The nipple is usually cracked or abraded and the breast is distended with milk (Fig. 6.3). The diagnosis is made based on history and examination.

Nursing Management

Teach the woman about the etiology of mastitis and encourage her to continue to breastfeed, emphasizing that the prescribed medication is safe to take during lactation. Continued emptying of the breast or pumping improves the outcome, decreases the duration of symptoms, and decreases the incidence of breast abscess. Thus, continued breastfeeding is recommended in the presence of mastitis (Reddy et al., 2007). Instructions for the woman with mastitis are detailed in Teaching Guidelines 6.2.

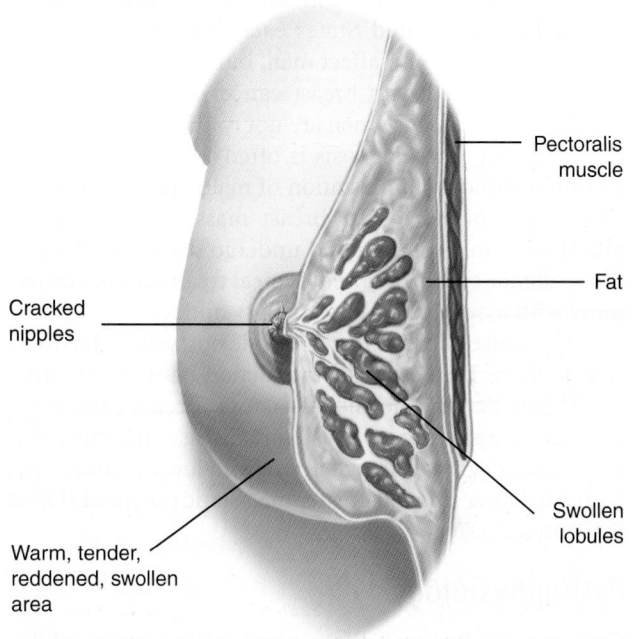

FIGURE 6.3 Mastitis.

Pectoralis muscle

Fat

Cracked nipples

Swollen lobules

Warm, tender, reddened, swollen area

TEACHING GUIDELINES 6.2

Caring for Mastitis

- Take medications as prescribed.
- Continue breastfeeding, as tolerated.
- Wear a supportive bra 24 hours a day to support the breasts.
- Increase fluid intake.
- Make sure infant is positioned correctly on the nipple.
- Practice good handwashing techniques.
- Apply warm compresses to the affected breast or take a warm shower before breastfeeding.
- Frequently change positions while nursing.
- Get adequate rest and nutrition to support or improve the immune system.

Sources: ACS, 2007a; Blackburn, 2007; Eglash, Plane, & Mundt, 2006.

Malignant Breast Disorders

Breast cancer is a neoplastic disease in which normal body cells are transformed into malignant ones (Opatt & Chung, 2007). It is the most common cancer in women and the second leading cause of cancer deaths (lung cancer is first) among American women. Breast cancer accounts for one of every three cancers diagnosed in the United States (ACS, 2007c). A new case is discovered every 2 minutes. It is estimated that one out of every seven women will develop the disease at some time during her life, and the mortality rate of those with breast cancer is 1 in 30 (National Cancer Institute [NCI], 2007b).

Over 200,000 cases of invasive breast cancer are diagnosed in the United States each year (ACS, 2007c). Breast cancer can also affect men, but only 1% of all individuals diagnosed with breast cancer annually are men (ACS, 2007). Because men are not routinely screened for breast cancer, the diagnosis is often delayed. The most common clinical manifestation of male breast cancer is a painless, firm, subareolar breast mass. Any suspicious breast mass in a male should undergo diagnostic biopsy. If a malignancy is diagnosed, typical treatment is mastectomy with assessment of the axillary nodes.

The cause of breast cancer, while not well understood, is thought to be a complex interaction between environment, genetic, and hormonal factors. Breast cancer is a progressive rather than a systemic disease, meaning that most cancers grow from small size with low metastatic potential to larger size and greater metastatic potential (Opatt & Chung, 2007).

Pathophysiology

Cancer is not just one disease, but rather a group of diseases that result from unregulated cell growth. Without regulation, cells divide and grow uncontrollably until they eventually form a tumor. Extensive research has determined that all cancer is the result of changes in DNA or chromosome structure that cause the mutation of specific genes. Most genetic mutations that cause cancer are acquired sporadically, which means they occur by chance and are not necessarily due to inherited mutations (Law & Alcamo, 2007). Cancer development is thought to be clonal in nature, which means that each cell is derived from another cell. If one cell develops a mutation, any daughter cell derived from that cell will have that same mutation, and this process continues until a malignant tumor forms.

Breast cancer starts in the epithelial cells that line the mammary ducts within the breast. The growth rate depends on hormonal influences, mainly estrogen and progesterone. The two major categories of breast cancer are noninvasive and invasive. Noninvasive, or in situ, breast cancers are those that have not extended beyond their duct, lobule, or point of origin into the surrounding breast tissue. Conversely, invasive, or infiltrating, breast cancers have extended into the surrounding breast tissue, with the potential to metastasize. Many researchers believe that most invasive cancers probably originate as noninvasive cancers (Underwood, 2006).

By far the most common breast cancer is invasive ductal carcinoma, which represents 85% of all cases (ACS, 2007f). **Carcinoma** is a malignant tumor that occurs in epithelial tissue; it tends to infiltrate and give rise to metastases. The incidence of this cancer peaks in the sixth decade of life (>60 years old). It spreads rapidly to axillary and other lymph nodes, even while small. Infiltrating ductal carcinoma may take various histologic forms—well differentiated and slow-growing, poorly differentiated and infiltrating, or highly malignant and undifferentiated with numerous metastases. This common type of breast cancer starts in the ducts, breaks through the duct wall, and invades the fatty breast tissue (Aliotta & Schaeffer, 2006).

Invasive lobular carcinomas, which originate in the terminal lobular units of breast ducts, account for 10% to 15% of all cases of breast cancer. The tumor is frequently located in the upper outer quadrant of the breast, and by the time it is discovered the prognosis is usually poor (Underwood, 2006). Other invasive types of cancer include tubular carcinoma (29%), which is fairly uncommon and typically occurs in women aged 55 and older. Colloid carcinoma (2% to 4%) occurs in women 60 to 70 years of age and is characterized by the presence of large pools of mucus interspersed with small islands of tumor cells. Medullary carcinoma accounts for 5% to 7% of malignant breast tumors; it occurs frequently in younger women (<50 years of age) and grows into large tumor masses. Inflammatory breast cancer (<4%) often presents with skin edema, redness, and warmth and is associated with a poor prognosis. Paget's disease (2% to 4%) originates in the nipple and typically occurs with invasive ductal carcinoma (Sukumvanich & Borgen, 2007).

Breast cancer is considered to be a highly variable disease. While the process of metastasis is a complex and poorly understood phenomenon, there is evidence to suggest that new vascularization of the tumor plays an important role in the biological aggressiveness of breast cancer (Hackley, Kriebs, & Rousseau 2007). Breast cancer metastasizes widely and to almost all organs of the body, but primarily to the bone, lungs, lymph nodes, liver, and brain. The first sites of metastases are usually local or regional, involving the chest wall or axillary supraclavicular lymph nodes or bone (ACS, 2007f).

Breast cancers are classified into three stages based on:

1. Tumor size
2. Extent of lymph node involvement
3. Evidence of metastasis

The purposes of tumor staging are to determine the probability the tumor has metastasized, to decide on an appropriate course of therapy, and to assess the client's prognosis. Table 6.2 gives details and characteristics of each stage. The overall 10-year survival rate for a woman with stage I breast cancer is 80% to 90%; for a woman with stage II, it is about 50%. The outlook is not as good for women with stage III or IV disease (Alexander et al., 2007).

There is no completely accurate way to know whether the cancer has micrometastasized to distant organs, but certain tests can help determine if the cancer has spread. A bone scan can be performed to assess the bones. Magnetic resonance imaging (MRI) can be used to detect metastases to the liver, abdominal cavity, lungs, or brain.

Risk Factors

An estimated 80% of women in whom breast cancer develops have no documented risk factors (Sukumvanich & Borgen, 2007). Breast cancer is thought to develop in response to a number of related factors: aging, delayed childbearing or never bearing children, high breast density, family history of cancer, late menopause, and hormonal factors (ACS, 2007e). Other factors might contribute to breast cancer but have not been scientifically proven.

In 1970, the lifetime risk for developing breast cancer was one in ten; since then, the risk has gradually risen (NCI, 2007b). This slight increase in incidence might be explained in a variety of ways—better detection and screening tools are available, which have identified more cases; women are living to an older age, when their risk increases; and lifestyle changes in American women (having their first pregnancy at an older age, having fewer children, and using hormonal therapy to treat the symptoms of menopause) might have produced the higher numbers. Age is a significant risk factor. Because rates of breast cancer increase with age, estimates of risk at specific ages are more meaningful than estimates of lifetime risk. The estimated chances of a woman being diagnosed with breast cancer between the ages of 30 and 70 are detailed in Table 6.3.

Risk factors for breast cancer can be divided into those that cannot be changed (nonmodifiable risk factors) and those that can be changed (modifiable risk factors). Nonmodifiable risk factors (ACS, 2007e) are:

- Gender (female)
- Aging (>50 years old)
- Genetic mutations (BRCA-1 and BRCA-2 genes)
- Personal history of ovarian or colon cancer
- Increased breast density
- Family history of breast cancer (mother, sister, daughter, grandmother, or aunt)
- Personal history of breast cancer (three- to fourfold increase in risk for recurrence)
- Race (higher in Caucasian women, but African-American women are more likely to die of it)
- Previous abnormal breast biopsy (atypical hyperplasia)
- Exposure to chest radiation (radiation damages DNA)
- Previous breast radiation (12 times normal risk)
- Early menarche (<12 years old) or late onset of menopause (>55 years old), which represents increased estrogen exposure over the lifetime

Modifiable risk factors related to lifestyle choices (ACS, 2007e) include:

- Not having children at all or not having children until after age 30—this increases the risk of breast cancer by not reducing the number of menstrual cycles
- Postmenopausal use of estrogens and progestins—the Women's Health Initiative study (2002) reported increased risks with long-term (>5 years) use of hormone replacement therapy

TABLE 6.2 STAGING OF BREAST CANCER

Stage	Characteristics
0	In situ, early type of breast cancer
I	Localized tumor <1 inch in diameter
II	Tumor 1–2 inches in diameter; spread to axillary lymph nodes
III	Tumor 2 inches or larger; spread to other lymph nodes and tissues
IV	Cancer has metastasized to other body organs

Source: ACS, 2007c.

TABLE 6.3 ESTIMATED RISK OF BREAST CANCER AT SPECIFIC AGES

Age 30 to 40	1 out of 262
Age 40 to 50	1 out of 68
Age 50 to 60	1 out of 35
Age 60 to 70	1 out of 27

Modified from National Cancer Institute (NCI). (2007). Probability of breast cancer in American women. Available at: http://cis.nci.nih.gov/fact/5_6.htm

• Failing to breastfeed for up to a year after pregnancy—increases the risk of breast cancer because it does not reduce the total number of lifetime menstrual cycles
• Alcohol consumption—boosts the level of estrogen in the bloodstream
• Smoking—exposure to carcinogenic agents found in cigarettes
• Obesity and consumption of high-fat diet—fat cells produce and store estrogen, so more fat cells create higher estrogen levels
• Sedentary lifestyle and lack of physical exercise—increases body fat, which houses estrogen

The presence of risk factors, especially several of them, calls for careful ongoing monitoring and evaluation to promote early detection. Even though risk factors are important considerations, many women with newly diagnosed breast cancer have no known risk factors. While routine mammography and self-examination are prudent for everyone, these precautions may become lifesavers for at-risk individuals.

Diagnosis

There are many studies performed to make an accurate diagnosis of a malignant breast lump. Diagnostic tests may include:

• Diagnostic mammography
• Magnetic resonance mammography (MRM)
• Fine-needle aspiration
• Stereotactic needle-guided biopsy
• Sentinel lymph node biopsy
• Hormone receptor status
• DNA ploidy status
• Cell proliferative indices
• HER-2/neu genetic marker (Opatt & Chung, 2007)

Mammography

Mammography involves taking x-ray pictures of the bare breasts while they are compressed between two plastic plates. This procedure is performed to identify and characterize a breast mass and to detect an early malignancy.

EVIDENCE-BASED PRACTICE 6.1
Can a Low-Fat Diet Reduce Breast Cancer Risk in Postmenopausal Women?

The hypothesis that a low-fat diet can reduce breast cancer risk has existed for decades but has never been tested in a controlled intervention trial.

● Study
To assess the effects of a low-fat diet on breast cancer incidence, a randomized, controlled, primary prevention trial was conducted at 40 U.S. clinical centers from 1993 to 2005. A total of 48,835 postmenopausal women, aged 50 to 79 years, without prior breast cancer, including 18.6% of minority race/ethnicity, were enrolled. Women were randomly assigned to the dietary modification intervention group (40% [n = 19,541]) or the comparison group (60% [n = 29,294]). The intervention was designed to promote dietary change with the goals of reducing intake of total fat to 20% of energy and increasing consumption of vegetables and fruit to at least five servings daily and grains to at least six servings daily. Comparison group participants were not asked to make dietary changes.

Dietary fat intake was significantly lower in the dietary modification intervention group compared with the comparison group. Vegetable and fruit consumption was higher in the intervention group by at least one serving per day and a smaller, more transient difference was found for grain consumption.

▲ Findings
The number of women who developed invasive breast cancer (annualized incidence rate) over the 8-year average follow-up period was 655 (0.42%) in the intervention group and 1,072 (0.45%) in the comparison group (hazard ratio, 0.91; 95% confidence interval, 0.83–1.01 for the comparison between the two groups). Secondary analyses suggested a lower hazard ratio among adherent women, provided greater evidence of risk reduction among women who ate a high-fat diet at baseline, and suggested a dietary effect that varies by hormone receptor characteristics of the tumor. Among postmenopausal women, a low-fat diet did not result in a statistically significant reduction in invasive breast cancer risk over an 8-year average follow-up period.

■ Nursing Implications
Although the results didn't confirm that eating a low-fat diet reduces the risk of breast cancer, nurses need to counsel their patients about the other benefits derived from a low-fat diet: weight loss, lower cholesterol levels, and decreased risk for cardiovascular disease. These additional benefits should be emphasized as part of an overall healthy lifestyle.

Source: Prentice RL, Caan B, Chlebowski RT, et al. (2006). Low-fat dietary pattern and risk of invasive breast cancer: The Women's Health Initiative Randomized Controlled Dietary Modification Trial. *JAMA, 295*(6), 629–642.

A screening mammogram typically consists of four views, two per breast (Fig. 6.4). It can detect lesions as small as 0.5 cm (the average size of a tumor detected by a woman practicing occasional breast self-examination is approximately 2.5 cm) (Kubota et al., 2007). A diagnostic mammogram is performed when the woman has suspicious clinical findings on a breast examination or an abnormality has been found on a screening mammogram. A diagnostic mammogram uses additional views of the affected breast as well as magnification views. Diagnostic mammography provides the radiologist with additional detail to render a more specific diagnosis. A digital mammography, which records images in computer code instead of on x-ray film, can also be used so that images can be transmitted and easily stored.

Most women find the 10-minute mammography procedure uncomfortable but not painful. Teaching Guidelines 6.3 offers tips for a patient to follow before she undergoes this procedure.

Magnetic Resonance Mammography

MRM is a relatively new procedure that might allow for earlier detection because it can detect smaller lesions and provide finer detail. MRM is a highly accurate (>90%

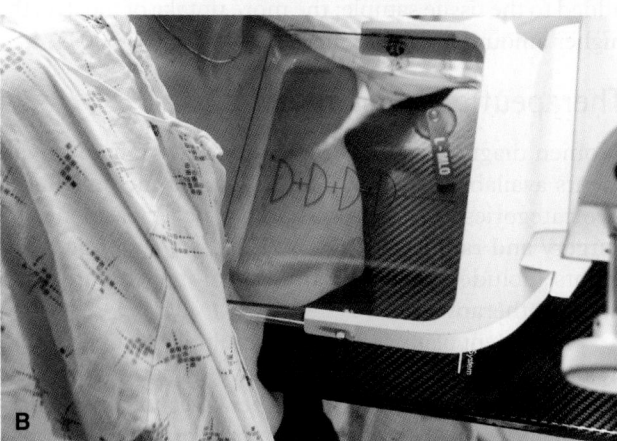

FIGURE 6.4 Mammography. (**A**) A top-to-bottom view of the breast. (**B**) A side view of the breast.

TEACHING GUIDELINES 6.3

Preparing for a Screening Mammogram

- Schedule the procedure just after menses, when breasts are less tender.
- Don't use deodorant or powder the day of the procedure, because they can appear on the x-ray film as calcium spots.
- Acetaminophen (Tylenol) or aspirin can relieve any discomfort after the procedure.
- Remove all jewelry from around your neck, because the metal can cause distortions on the film image.
- Select a facility that is accredited by the American College of Radiology (ACR) to ensure appropriate credentialed staff.

sensitivity for invasive carcinoma) but costly tool. Contrast infusion is used to evaluate the rate at which the dye initially enters the breast tissue. The basis of the high sensitivity of MRM is the tumor angiogenesis (vessel growth) that accompanies a majority of breast cancers, even early ones. Malignant lesions tend to exhibit increased enhancement within the first 2 minutes (Preda et al., 2006). Currently MRM is used only as a complement to mammography and clinical breast examination because it is expensive, but it may move into the diagnostic arena in the near future (Smith, 2007).

Fine-Needle Aspiration

Fine-needle aspiration (FNA) is done to identify a solid tumor, cyst, or malignancy. It is a simple office procedure that can be performed with or without anesthesia. A small (20- to 22-gauge) needle connected to a 10-cc or larger syringe is inserted into the breast mass and suction is applied to withdraw the contents. The aspirate is then sent to the cytology laboratory to be evaluated for abnormal cells.

Stereotactic Needle-Guided Biopsy

This diagnostic tool is used to target and identify mammographically detected nonpalpable lesions in the breast. This procedure is less expensive than an excisional biopsy. The procedure takes place in a specially equipped room and generally takes about an hour. When proper placement of the breast mass is confirmed by digital mammograms, the breast is locally anesthetized and a spring-loaded biopsy gun is used to obtain two or three core biopsy tissue samples. After the procedure is finished, the biopsy area is cleaned and a sterile dressing is applied.

Sentinel Lymph Node Biopsy

The status of the axillary lymph nodes is an important prognostic indicator in early-stage breast cancer. The presence or absence of malignant cells in lymph nodes is highly significant: the more lymph nodes involved and the more aggressive the cancer, the more powerful chemotherapy will have to be, both in terms of the toxicity of drugs and the duration of treatment (Teal, Tabbara, & Kelly, 2007). With a sentinel lymph node biopsy, the clinician can determine whether breast cancer has spread to the axillary lymph nodes without having to do a traditional axillary lymph node dissection. Experience has shown that the lymph ducts of the breast typically drain to one lymph node first before draining through the rest of the lymph nodes under the arm. The first lymph node is called the sentinel lymph node.

This procedure can be performed under local anesthesia. A radioactive blue dye is injected 2 hours before the biopsy to identify the afferent sentinel lymph node. The surgeon usually removes one to three nodes and sends them to the pathologist to determine whether cancer cells are present. The sentinel lymph node biopsy is usually performed before a lumpectomy to make sure the cancer has not spread. Removing only the sentinel lymph node can allow women with breast cancer to avoid many of the side effects (lymphedema) associated with a traditional axillary lymph node dissection (Underwood, 2006).

Hormone Receptor Status

Normal breast epithelium has hormone receptors and responds specifically to the stimulatory effects of estrogen and progesterone. Most breast cancers retain estrogen receptors, and for those tumors estrogen will retain proliferative control over the malignant cells. It is therefore useful to know the hormone receptor status of the cancer to predict which women will respond to hormone manipulation. Hormone receptor status reveals whether the tumor is stimulated to grow by estrogen and progesterone. Tumors that have estrogen receptors are said to be "ER positive" (ER+) and tumors that do not have estrogen receptors are "ER negative" (ER–). The same terminology applies to progesterone (PR+ or PR–). ER+ and PR+ tumors have a better than 75% response to endocrine therapy in comparison to tumors that are ER+ and PR–, whose response rate is under 35%. Postmenopausal women tend to be ER+; premenopausal women tend to be ER– (Opatt & Chung, 2007). To determine hormone receptor status, a sample of breast cancer tissue obtained during a biopsy or a tumor removed surgically during a lumpectomy or mastectomy is examined by a cytologist.

DNA Ploidy Status

DNA ploidy status, which correlates with tumor aggressiveness, indicates the amount of DNA in cancer cells. Cancer cells that have the correct amount of DNA (diploid) in contrast with too much or too little DNA (aneuploid) tend not to spread. An aneuploid DNA pattern denotes a greater tendency to metastasize than a diploid one (Sukumvanich & Borgen, 2007). A sample of breast cancer tissue obtained during a biopsy or a tumor removed surgically during a lumpectomy or mastectomy is examined for abnormal amounts of DNA. Using flow cytometry (process of counting and measuring cells), it is possible to measure the DNA content and proliferative activity of a tumor. The number of chromosome sets in the nucleus indicates the speed of cell replication and tumor growth; a high number predicts a poor outcome.

Cell Proliferative Indices

Research indicates that cell proliferation potential may have prognostic significance. Cell proliferative indices indirectly measure the rate of cell division, which is an indication of how fast the cancer is growing. Flow and image cytometry techniques are used to measure the tumor's cell cycle rate. The percentage of tumor cells in S phase (synthesis stage of cell division) of the cell cycle is assessed. S-phase percentages below 10% are considered low, and the tumor has less of a chance of spreading than one with a higher percentage. A tumor with high proliferative activity has a more aggressive metastatic potential (ACS, 2007f).

HER-2/neu Genetic Marker

Molecular and biologic factors are increasingly being used as indicators for prognosis and treatment. HER-2 is a human epidermal growth factor receptor whose biological function is associated with cell growth, resulting in loss of cell regulation and uncontrolled cell proliferation.

HER-2/neu oncoprotein is a protein that is significant, especially in large tumors. Overexpression of this protein results from an acquired genetic mutation and occurs in approximately 30% of women with metastatic breast cancer. Women whose tumors have high levels of HER-2/neu oncoprotein have a poor prognosis: they have rapid tumor progression, an increased rate of recurrence, a poor response to standard therapies, and a lower survival rate (Chernecky & Berger, 2007). The presence or absence of this oncoprotein helps determine which chemotherapy treatment will be most effective. A breast tissue sample is obtained by a fine-needle or open biopsy and treated with a material that binds to HER-2/neu oncoprotein. A dye is added to the tissue sample: the more uptake of the dye, the higher amount present (Chernecky & Berger, 2007).

Therapeutic Management

Women diagnosed with breast cancer have many treatments available to them. Generally, treatments fall into two categories: local and systemic. Local treatments are surgery and radiation therapy. Effective systemic treatments include chemotherapy, hormonal therapy, and immunotherapy.

Treatment plans are based on multiple factors, primarily on whether the cancer is invasive or noninvasive, the tumor's size and grade, the number of cancerous axillary lymph nodes, the hormone receptor status, and the ability to obtain clear surgical margins (ACS, 2007f). A combination of surgical options and adjunctive therapy is often recommended.

Another consideration in making decisions about a treatment plan is genetic testing for BRCA-1 and BRCA-2. This genetic testing became available in 1995 and can pinpoint women who have a significantly increased risk for breast and ovarian cancer: individuals with BRCA-1 and BRCA-2 mutations have a 75% lifetime risk of breast cancer and a 30% lifetime risk of ovarian cancer. Most cases of breast and ovarian cancer are sporadic in nature, but approximately 7% of breast cancers and 10% of ovarian cancers are thought to result from genetic inheritance (Kell & Burke, 2007).

Testing positive for a BRCA-1 or BRCA-2 mutation can significantly alter health care decisions. In some cases, before genetic testing was available, lumpectomy with radiation or mastectomy was the treatment most often recommended. However, if the woman is found to have a BRCA-1 mutation, she is most likely to be offered the option of contralateral prophylactic mastectomy and possible bilateral oophorectomy (Kell & Burke, 2007).

Severe psychological distress can occur as a result of genetic testing. Also, many women perceive their breasts as intrinsic to their femininity, self-esteem, and sexuality, and the risk of losing a breast can provoke extreme anxiety (Alexander et al., 2007). Nurses need to address the physical, emotional, and spiritual needs of the women they care for, as well as their families, since this mutation is inherited in an autosomal dominant fashion. Based on Mendelian genetics, first-degree relatives of affected women have a 50% risk of having inherited the mutation (Kell & Burke, 2007).

Surgical Options

Generally, the first treatment option for the woman diagnosed with breast cancer is surgery. A few women with tumors larger than 5 cm or inflammatory breast cancer may undergo neoadjuvant chemotherapy or radiotherapy to shrink the tumor before surgical removal is attempted (Opatt & Chung, 2007). The surgical options depend on the type and extent of cancer. The choices are typically either breast-conserving surgery (lumpectomy with radiation) or mastectomy with or without reconstruction. The overall survival rate with lumpectomy and radiation is about the same as that with modified radical mastectomy (ACS, 2007f). Research has shown that the survival rates in women who have had mastectomies versus those who have undergone breast-conserving surgery followed by radiation are the same. However, lumpectomy may not be an option for some women, including those:

- Who have two or more cancer sites that cannot be removed through one incision
- Whose surgery will not result in a clean margin of tissue
- Who have active connective tissue conditions (lupus or scleroderma) that make body tissues especially sensitive to the side effects of radiation
- Who have had previous radiation to the affected breast
- Whose tumors are larger than 5 cm (2 inches)
(National Comprehensive Cancer Network, 2007)

These decisions are made jointly between the woman and her surgeon. If mastectomy is chosen, either by tumor characteristics or patient preference, then discussion needs to include breast reconstruction and regional lymph node biopsy versus sentinel lymph node biopsy. The mastectomy techniques are a simple mastectomy with sentinel node biopsy or a radical mastectomy with regional node biopsy. Removal of numerous lymph nodes places the patient at high risk for lymphedema.

Breast-Conserving Surgery

Breast-conserving surgery, the least invasive procedure, is the wide local excision (or lumpectomy) of the tumor along with a 1-cm margin of normal tissue. A lumpectomy is often used for early-stage localized tumors. The goal of breast-conserving surgery is to remove the suspicious mass along with tissue free of malignant cells to prevent recurrence. The results are less drastic and emotionally less scarring to the woman. Women undergoing breast-conserving therapy receive radiation after lumpectomy with the goal of eradicating residual microscopic cancer cells to limit locoregional recurrence. In women who do not require adjuvant chemotherapy, radiation therapy typically begins 2 to 4 weeks after surgery to allow healing of the lumpectomy incision site. Radiation is administered to the entire breast at daily doses over a period of several weeks (Rao et al., 2007).

A sentinel lymph node biopsy may also be performed since the lymph nodes draining the breast are located primarily in the axilla. Theoretically, if breast cancer is to metastasize to other parts of the body, it will probably do so via the lymphatic system. If malignant cells are found in the nodes, more aggressive systemic treatment may be needed.

Mastectomy

A **simple mastectomy** is the removal of all breast tissue, the nipple, and the areola. The axillary nodes and pectoral muscles are spared. This procedure would be used for a large tumor or multiple tumors that have not metastasized to adjacent structures or the lymph system.

A **modified radical mastectomy** is another surgical option; survival rates are comparable to those of radical mastectomy, but it is more conducive to breast reconstruction and results in greater mobility and less lymphedema (Alexander et al., 2007). This procedure involves removal of breast tissue, the axillary nodes, and some chest muscles, but not the pectoralis major, thus avoiding a concave anterior chest (DiSaia & Creasman, 2007).

In conjunction with the mastectomy, lymph node surgery (removal of underarm nodes) may need to be done to reduce the risk of distant metastasis and improve a woman's chance of long-term survival. For women with a positive sentinel node biopsy, 10 to 20 underarm lymph nodes may need to be removed. Complications associated with axillary lymph node surgery include nerve damage during surgery, causing temporary numbness down the upper aspect of the arm; seroma formation followed by wound infection; restrictions in arm mobility (some women need physiotherapy); and lymphedema. In many women lymphedema can be avoided by:

• Avoiding using the affected arm for drawing blood, inserting intravenous lines, or measuring blood pressure (can cause trauma and possible infection)
• Seeking medical care immediately if the affected arm swells
• Wearing gloves when engaging in activities such as gardening that might cause injury
• Wearing a well-fitted compression sleeve to promote drainage return

Women having mastectomies must decide whether to have further surgery to reconstruct the breast. If the woman decides to have reconstructive surgery, it ideally is performed immediately after the mastectomy. The woman must also determine whether she wants the surgeon to use saline implants or natural tissue from her abdomen (TRAM flap method) or back (LAT flap method).

In the transverse rectus abdominis myocutaneous (TRAM) flap method, the rectus abdominis muscle is transferred from the abdomen via a tunnel under the skin and brought out through a new excision in the breast area. The blood supply is maintained. This tissue is used to reconstruct the breast that has been removed. In the latissimus dorsi (LAT) flap method, tissue from the latissimus dorsi muscle in the upper back is tunneled subcutaneously up to the chest area.

If reconstructive surgery is desired, the ultimate decision regarding the method will be determined by the woman's anatomy (e.g., is there sufficient fat and muscle to permit natural reconstruction) and her overall health status. Both procedures require a prolonged recovery period.

Some women opt for no reconstruction, and many of them choose to wear breast prostheses. Some prostheses are worn in the bra cup and others fit against the skin or into special pockets made into clothing.

Whether to have reconstructive surgery is an individual and very complex decision. Each woman must be presented with all of the options and then allowed to decide. The nurse can play an important role here by presenting the facts to the woman so that she can make an intelligent decision to meet her unique situation.

Adjunctive Therapy

Adjunctive therapy is supportive or additional therapy that is recommended after surgery. Adjunctive therapies include local therapy such as radiation therapy and systemic therapies using chemotherapy, hormonal therapy, and immunotherapy.

Radiation Therapy

Radiation therapy uses high-energy rays to destroy cancer cells that might have been left behind in the breast, chest wall, or underarm area after the tumor has been removed surgically. Usually serial radiation doses are given 5 days a week to the tumor site for 6 to 8 weeks postoperatively. Each treatment takes only a few minutes, but the dose is cumulative. Women undergoing breast-conserving therapy receive radiation to the entire breast after lumpectomy with the goal of eradicating residual microscopic cancer cells to reduce the chance of recurrence (Holcomb, 2006).

Side effects of traditional radiation therapy include inflammation, local edema, anorexia, swelling, and heaviness in the breast; sunburn-like skin changes in the treated area; and fatigue. Changes to the breast tissue and skin usually resolve in about a year (Willett, Czito, & Tyler, 2007). This type of therapy can be given several ways: external beam radiation, which delivers a carefully focused dose of radiation from a machine outside the body, or internal radiation, in which tiny pellets that contain radioactive material are placed into the tumor.

Several advances have taken place in the field of radiation oncology for the treatment of women with early-stage breast cancer that assist in reducing the side effects. The treatment position for external radiation has changed from supine to prone, with the arm on the affected side raised above the head, so that the treated breast hangs dependently through the opening of the treatment board. Treatment in the prone position improves dose distribution within the breast and allows for a decrease in the dose delivered to the heart, lung, chest wall, and other breast (National Comprehensive Cancer Network, 2007).

High-dose brachytherapy is another advance that is an alternative to traditional radiation treatment. A balloon catheter is used to insert radioactive seeds into the breast after the tumor is removed surgically. The seeds deliver a concentrated dose directly to the operative site; this is important because most cancer recurrences in the breast (67% to 100%) occur at or near the lumpectomy site. This allows a high dose of radiation to be delivered to a small target volume with a minimal dose to the surrounding normal tissue. This procedure takes 4 to 5 days as opposed to the 4 to 6 weeks that traditional radiation therapy takes; it also eliminates the need to delay radiation therapy to allow for wound healing. Brachytherapy is now used as a primary radiation treatment after breast-conserving surgery in selected women as an alternative to whole breast irradiation (Sanders et al., 2007). Side effects of brachytherapy include redness or discharge around catheters, fever, and infection. Daily cleansing of the catheter insertion site with a mild soap and application of an antibiotic ointment will minimize the risk of infection.

Intensity-modulated radiation therapy (IMRT) offers still another new approach to the delivery of treatment to reduce the dose within the target area while sparing surrounding normal structures. A computed tomography scan is used to create a three-dimensional model of the breast. Based on this model, a series of intensity-modulated beams are produced to the desired dose distribution to reduce radiation exposure to underlying structures. Acute toxicity is thus minimized (Willett, Czito, & Tyler, 2007). Research is ongoing to evaluate the impact of all of these advances in radiation therapy.

Chemotherapy

Chemotherapy refers to the use of drugs that are toxic to all cells and interfere with a cell's ability to reproduce. They are particularly effective against malignant cells but affect all rapidly dividing cells, especially those of the skin, the hair follicles, the mouth, the gastrointestinal tract, and the bone marrow. Breast cancer is a systemic disease in which micrometastases are already present in other organs by the time the breast cancer is diagnosed. Chemotherapeutic agents perform a systemic "sweep" of the body to reduce the chances that distant tumors will start growing.

Chemotherapy may be indicated for women with tumors larger than 1 cm, positive lymph nodes, or cancer of an aggressive type. Chemotherapy is prescribed in cycles, with each period of treatment followed by a rest period. Treatment typically lasts 3 to 6 months, depending on the dose used and the woman's health status.

Different classes of drugs affect different aspects of cell division and are used in combinations or "cocktails." The most active and commonly used chemotherapeutic agents for breast cancer include alkylating agents, anthracyclines, antimetabolites, and vinca alkaloids. Fifty or more chemotherapeutic agents can be used to treat breast cancer; however, a combination drug approach versus a single drug treatment appears to be more effective (ACS, 2007f).

Side effects of chemotherapy depend on the agents used, the intensity of dosage, the dosage schedule, the type and extent of cancer, and the client's physical and emotional status (Boehmke & Dickerson, 2006). However, typical side effects include nausea and vomiting, diarrhea or constipation, hair loss, weight loss, stomatitis, fatigue, and immunosuppression. The most serious is bone marrow suppression (myelosuppression). This causes an increased risk of infection, bleeding, and a reduced red-cell count, which can lead to anemia. Treatment of the side effects can generally be addressed through appropriate support medications such as antinausea drugs like granisetron hydrochloride (Kytril) or ondansetron (Zofran). In addition, growth-stimulating factors, such as epoetin alfa (Procrit) and filgrastim (Neupogen), help keep blood counts from dropping too low. Counts that are too low would stop or delay the use of chemotherapy.

An aggressive systemic option, when other treatments have failed or when there is a strong possibility of relapse or metastatic disease, is high-dose chemotherapy with bone marrow and/or stem cell transplant. This therapy involves the withdrawal of bone marrow before the administration of toxic levels of chemotherapeutic agents. The marrow is frozen and then returned to the client after the high-dose chemotherapy is finished. Clinical trials are still researching this experimental therapy (Guarneri et al., 2007).

Endocrine Therapy

One of estrogen's normal functions is to stimulate the growth and division of healthy cells in the breasts. However, in some women with breast cancer, this normal function contributes to the growth and division of cancer cells.

The objective of **endocrine therapy** is to block or counter the effect of estrogen. Estrogen plays a central role in the pathogenesis of cancer, and treatment with estrogen deprivation has proven to be effective (Bush, 2007). Several different drug classes are used to interfere or block estrogen receptors. They include selective estrogen receptor modulators (SERMs), estrogen receptor down-regulators, aromatase inhibitors, luteinizing hormone-releasing hormone, progestin, and biologic response modifiers (Underwood, 2006). Current recommendations for most women with ER+ breast cancer are to take a hormone-like medication—known as a SERM anti-estrogenic agent—daily for up to 5 years after initial treatment. Certain areas in the female body (breasts, uterus, ovaries, skin, vagina, and brain) contain specialized cells called hormone receptors that allow estrogen to enter the cell and stimulate it to divide. SERMs enter these same receptors and act like keys, turning off the signal for growth inside the cell (Bush, 2007). The best-known SERM is tamoxifen (Nolvadex, 20 mg daily for 5 years). Although it works well in preventing further spread of cancer, it is also associated with an increased incidence of endometrial cancer, pulmonary embolus, deep vein thrombosis, hot flashes, vaginal discharge and bleeding, stroke, and cataract formation (Bush, 2007).

A relatively new SERM is the anti-osteoporosis drug raloxifene (Evista), which has shown promising results. It has anti-estrogen effects on the breast and uterus. In a recent study involving more than 20,000 postmenopausal women at high risk for breast cancer, raloxifene worked as well as tamoxifen in preventing breast cancer, but with fewer serious adverse effects. Both drugs cut the cancer risk in half (Medical Letter, 2006). It was originally marketed solely for the prevention and treatment of osteoporosis but is now used as adjunctive breast cancer therapy.

Another class of endocrine agents, aromatase inhibitors, work by inhibiting the conversion of androgens to estrogens. Aromatase inhibitors include letozole (Femara, 2.5 mg daily), exemestane (Aromasin, 25 mg daily), and anastrozole (Arimidex, 1 mg daily for 5 years), all of which are taken orally. These are usually given to women with advanced breast cancer or cancer that recurs despite the use of tamoxifen (Holcomb, 2006).

The side effects associated with these endocrine therapies include hot flashes, bone pain, fatigue, nausea, cough, dyspnea, and headache (Hackley, Kriebs, & Rousseau, 2007). Women with hormone-sensitive cancers can live for long periods without any intervention other than hormonal manipulation, but quality-of-life issues need to be addressed in the balance between treatment and side effects.

Immunotherapy

Immunotherapy, used as an adjunct to surgery, represents an attempt to stimulate the body's natural defenses to recognize and attack cancer cells. Trastuzumab (Herceptin, 2- to 4-mg/kg intravenous infusion) is the first monoclonal antibody approved for breast cancer (National Comprehensive Cancer Network, 2007). Some tumors produce excessive amounts of HER-2/neu protein, which regulates cancer cell growth. Breast cancers that overexpress the protein HER-2/neu are associated with a more aggressive form of disease and a poorer prognosis. Trastuzumab blocks the effect of this protein to inhibit the growth of cancer cells. It can be used alone or in combination with other chemotherapy to treat clients with metastatic breast disease (Opatt & Chung, 2007). Adverse effects of trastuzumab include cardiac toxicity, vascular thrombosis, hepatic failure, fever, chills, nausea, vomiting, and pain with first infusion (Skidmore-Roth, 2007).

NURSING PROCESS FOR THE PATIENT WITH BREAST CANCER

When a woman is diagnosed with breast cancer, she faces treatment that may alter her body shape, may make her feel unwell, and may not carry a certainty of cure. Nurses can support women from the time of diagnosis, through the treatments, and through follow-up after the surgical and adjunctive treatments have been completed. Allowing patients time to ask questions and to discuss any necessary preparations for treatment is critical. As our understanding of breast disorders keeps improving, treatments continue to change. Although the goal of treatment remains improved survival, increasing emphasis is focused on prevention (Stephenson, 2007). Nurses can have an impact on early detection of breast disorders, treatment, and symptom management (Underwood, 2006). A nurse who is involved in the woman's treatment plan from the beginning can effectively offer support throughout the whole experience.

Teamwork is important in breast screening and caring for women with breast disorders. Treatment is often fragmented between the hospital and community treatment centers, which can be emotionally traumatic for the woman and her family. The advances being made in the diagnosis and treatment of breast disorders mean that guidelines are constantly changing, requiring all health care professionals to keep up to date. Informed nurses can provide support and information and, most importantly, continuity of care for the woman undergoing treatment for a breast problem.

The nurse plays a particularly important role in providing psychological support and self-care teaching to patients with breast cancer. Nurses can influence both physical and emotional recovery, which are both important aspects of care that help in improving the woman's quality of life and the ability to survive. The nurse's role should extend beyond helping clients; spreading the word in the community about screening and prevention is a big part in the ongoing fight against cancer. The community should see nurses as both educators and valued sources of credible information. This role will help improve clinical outcomes while achieving high levels of client satisfaction.

Remember Nancy from the chapter opener? Is her response typical of many women upon discovering a lump in their breast? Nancy confides her discovery of the lump and her worries to you. What advice would you give her?

Assessment

Early breast cancer has no symptoms. The earliest sign of breast cancer is often an abnormality seen on a screening mammogram before the woman or the health care professional feels it. In the woman presenting with a breast disorder, take a thorough history of the problem and explore the woman's risk factors for breast cancer. Assess the woman for clinical manifestations of breast cancer, such as changes in breast appearance and contour, which become apparent with advancing breast cancer (ACS, 2007d). These changes include:

- Continued and persistent changes in the breast
- A lump or thickening in one breast
- Persistent nipple irritation
- Unusual breast swelling or asymmetry
- A lump or swelling in the axilla
- Changes in skin color or texture
- Nipple retraction, tenderness, or discharge (Fig. 6.5)

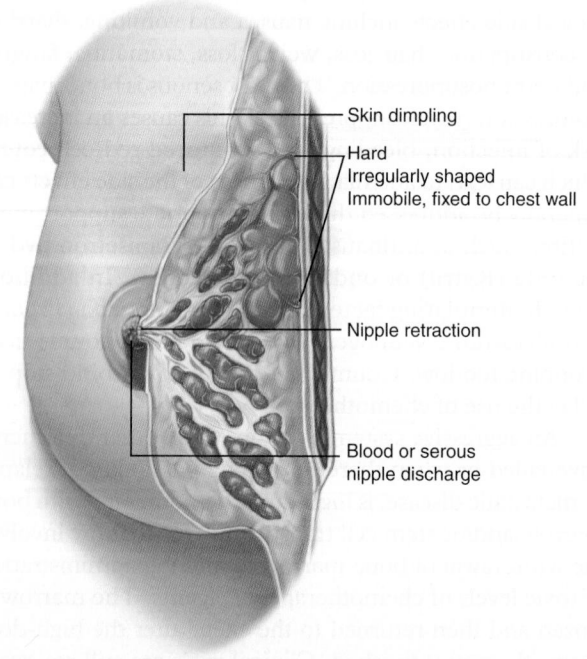

FIGURE 6.5 Malignant breast tumor.

Complete a breast examination to validate the clinical manifestations and findings of the health history and risk factor assessment. The clinical breast examination involves both inspection and palpation (Nursing Procedure 6.1). Helpful characteristics in evaluating palpable breast masses are described in Box 6.1. If a lump can be palpated, the cancer has been there for quite some time.

Be cognizant of the impact that breast cancer has on a woman's emotional state, coping ability, and quality of life. Women may experience sadness, anger, fear, and guilt as a result of breast cancer. However, despite potential negative outcomes, many women have a positive outlook for their futures and adapt to treatment modalities with a good quality of life (Holcomb, 2006). Closely monitor clients for their psychosocial adjustment to diagnosis and treatment and be able to identify those who need further psychological intervention. By giving practical advice, the nurse can help the woman adjust to her altered body image and to accept the changes to her life.

Because family members play a significant role in supporting women through breast cancer diagnosis and treatment, assess the emotional distress of both partners during the course of treatment and, if needed, make a referral for psychological counseling. By identifying interpersonal strains, negative psychosocial side effects of cancer treatment can be minimized.

Nursing Diagnosis

Appropriate nursing diagnoses for a woman with a diagnosis of breast cancer might include:

- Disturbed body image related to:
  - Loss of body part (breast)
  - Loss of femininity
  - Loss of hair due to chemotherapy
- Fear related to:
  - Diagnosis of cancer
  - Prognosis of disease
- Educational deficit related to:
  - Cancer treatment options
  - Reconstructive surgery decisions
  - Breast self-examination

Nursing Interventions

Offer information, support, and perioperative care to women diagnosed with breast cancer who are undergoing treatment. Implement health-promotion and disease-prevention strategies to minimize the risk for developing breast cancer and to promote optimal outcomes.

Remember Nancy, who discovered a breast lump? You offer to go with her to the doctor. After a full examination and several diagnostic tests, the results come back positive for breast cancer. What treatment options does Nancy have, and what factors need to be considered in selecting those options?

Providing Patient Education

Help the woman and her partner to prioritize the voluminous amount of information given to them so that they can make informed decisions. Explain all treatment options in detail so the patient and her family understand them. By preparing an individualized packet of information and reviewing it with the woman and her partner, the nurse can help them understand her specific type of cancer, the diagnostic studies and treatment options she may choose, and the goals of treatment. For example, nurses play an important role in educating women about the use of endocrine therapies, observing women's experiences with treatment, and communicating those observations to their primary care professionals to make dosage adjustments, in addition to contributing to the knowledge base of endocrine therapy in the treatment of breast cancer.

Providing information is a central role of the nurse in caring for the woman with a diagnosis of breast cancer. This information can be given via telephone counseling, one-to-one contact, and pamphlets. Telephone counseling with women and their partners may be an effective method to improve symptom management and quality of life (Knobf, 2007).

Providing Emotional Support

The diagnosis of cancer affects all aspects of life for a woman and her family. The threatening nature of the disease and feelings of uncertainty about the future can lead to anxiety and stress. Address the woman's needs for:

- Information about diagnosis and treatment
- Physical care while undergoing treatments
- Contact with supportive people
- Education about disease, options, and prevention measures
- Discussion and support by a caring, competent nurse

Reassure the client and her family that the diagnosis of breast cancer does not necessarily mean imminent death, a decrease in attractiveness, or diminished sexuality. Encourage the woman to express her fears and worries. Be available to listen and address the woman's concerns in an open manner to help her toward recovery. All aspects of care must include sensitivity to the patient's personal efforts to cope and heal. Some women will become involved in organizations or charities that support cancer research; they may participate in breast cancer walks to raise awareness or become a Reach for Recovery volunteer to help others. Each woman copes in her own personal manner, and all of these efforts can be positive motivators for her own healing.

To help women cope with the diagnosis of breast cancer, the American Cancer Society launched Reach to Recovery more than 30 years ago. Specially trained breast cancer survivors give women and their families opportunities to express their feelings, verbalize their fears, and get answers. Most importantly, Reach to Recovery vol-

(text continues on page 190)

Nursing Procedure 6.1

CLINICAL BREAST EXAMINATION

Purpose: To Assess Breasts for Abnormal Findings

1. Inspect the breast for size, symmetry, and skin texture and color. Inspect the nipples and areola. Ask the client to sit at the edge of the examination table, with her arms resting at her sides.

2. Inspect the breast for masses, retraction, dimpling, or ecchymosis.
   - The client places her hands on her hips.

   - She then raises her arms over her head so the axillae can also be inspected.

   - The client then stands, places her hands on her hips, and leans forward.

3. Palpate the breasts. Assist the client into a supine position with her arms above her head. Place a pillow or towel under the client's head to help spread the breasts. Three patterns might be used to palpate the breasts:

   - Spiral

Nursing Procedure 6.1 (continued)

- Pie-shaped wedges

- Vertical strip

4. Compress the nipple gently between the thumb and index finger to evaluate for masses and squeeze to check for any discharge.

5. Palpate the axillary area for any tenderness or lymph node enlargement. Have the client sit up and move to the edge of the examination table. While supporting the client's arm, palpate downward from the armpit, palpating toward the ribs just below the breast.

Adapted from Rhoads, J. (2006). *Advanced health assessment and diagnostic reasoning.* Philadelphia: Lippincott Williams & Wilkins.

BOX 6.1 **Characteristics of Benign vs. Malignant Breast Masses**

- **Benign breast masses are described as:**
  - Frequently painful
  - Firm, rubbery mass
  - Bilateral masses
  - Induced nipple discharge
  - Regular margins (clearly delineated)
  - No skin dimpling
  - No nipple retraction
  - Mobile, not affixed to the chest wall
  - No bloody discharge

- **Malignant breast masses are described as:**
  - Hard to palpation
  - Painless
  - Irregularly shaped (poorly delineated)
  - Immobile, fixed to the chest wall
  - Skin dimpling
  - Nipple retraction
  - Unilateral mass
  - Bloody, serosanguineous, or serous nipple discharge
  - Spontaneous nipple discharge

unteers offer understanding, support, and hope through face-to-face visits or by telephone; they are proof that people can survive breast cancer and live productive lives. National contact information is 1-800-ACS-2345.

Providing Postoperative Care

For the woman who has had surgery to remove a malignant breast lump or an entire breast, excellent postoperative nursing care is crucial. Tell the woman what to expect in terms of symptoms and when they usually occur during treatment and after surgery. This allows women to anticipate these symptoms and proactively employ management strategies to improve their cancer experience. Postoperative care includes immediate postoperative care, pain management, care of the affected arm, wound care, mobility care, respiratory care, emotional care, educational needs, and referrals.

Immediate Postoperative Care

Assess the client's respiratory status by auscultating the lungs and observing the breathing pattern. Assess circulation; note vital signs, skin color, and skin temperature. Observe the client's neurologic status by evaluating the level of alertness and orientation. Monitor the wound for amount and color of drainage. Monitor the intravenous lines for patency, correct fluid, and rate. Assess the drainage tube for amount, color, and consistency of drainage.

Pain Management

Provide analgesics as needed. Reassure the woman that her pain will be controlled. Teach the woman how to communicate her pain intensity on a scale of 0 to 10, with 10 being the worst pain imaginable. Assess the client's pain level frequently and anticipate pain before assisting the woman to ambulate.

Affected Arm Care

Elevate the affected arm on a pillow to promote lymph drainage. Make sure that no treatments are performed on the affected arm, including laboratory draws, intravenous lines, blood pressures, and so on. Place a sign above the bed to warn others not to touch the affected arm.

Wound Care

Observe the wound often and empty drainage reservoirs as needed. Tell the client to report any evidence of infection early, such as fever, chills, or any area of redness or inflammation along the incision line. Also tell the client to report any increase in drainage, foul odor, or separation at the incision site.

Mobility Care

Perform active range-of-motion and arm exercises as ordered. Encourage self-care activities for successful rehabilitation. Perform dressing and drainage care; explain the care during the procedure.

Respiratory Care

Assist with turning, coughing, and deep breathing every 2 hours. Explain that this helps to expand collapsed alveoli in the lungs, promotes faster clearance of inhalation agents from the body, and prevents postoperative pneumonia and atelectasis.

Emotional Care and Referrals

Encourage the client to participate in her care. Assess her coping strategies preoperatively. Explain possible body image concerns after discharge. Promote the ACS websites, which provide the latest cancer therapy news. Encourage the client to attend local support groups for breast cancer survivors, such as Reach to Recovery, an ACS program in which trained volunteers provide support and up-to-date information for spouses, children, friends, and other loved ones. Reach to Recovery volunteers can also, when appropriate, provide a temporary breast form and give information on types of permanent prostheses, as well as lists of where those items are available in the community.

Educational Needs

Provide follow-up information about adjunctive therapy. Explain that radiation therapy may start within weeks postoperatively. Discuss chemotherapy, its side effects and cycles, home care during treatment, and future monitoring strategies. Explain hormonal therapy, including antiestrogens or aromatase inhibitors. Teach progressive arm exercises to minimize lymphedema. Explain that ongoing surveillance is needed to detect recurrence of cancer or a new primary site and that the patient will typically see the health care provider every 6 months.

Nancy underwent a mastectomy with radiation and chemotherapy. What follow-up care is needed? How can the nurse assist Nancy to cope with her uncertain future? What community resources might help her?

Implementing Health-Promotion and Disease-Prevention Strategies

In the past, most women assumed that there was little they could do to reduce their risk of developing breast cancer. However, research has found that the daily choices women make concerning breast cancer screening, diet, exercise, and other health practices have a profound impact on cancer risk. In the fight against cancer, nurses often assume a variety of roles, such as educator, counselor, advocate, and role model. Nurses can offer education about the following:

- Prevention
- Early detection
- Screening
- Dispelling myths and fears

• Self-examination techniques
• Individual risk status and strategies for risk reduction

It is important to be knowledgeable about the most current evidence-based practices and cognizant of how the media presents this information. Offer prevention strategies within the context of a woman's life. Factors such as lifestyle choices, economic status, and multiple roles need to be taken into consideration when counseling women. Advocate for healthy lifestyles and making sound choices to prevent cancer. Nurses, like all health care professionals, should offer guidance from a comprehensive perspective that acknowledges the unique needs of each individual (Banning, 2007).

Breast cancer is a frightening experience for women. Like a black cloud hanging over their heads, with little regard for any victim, breast cancer stalks women everywhere they go. Many have a close friend or relative who is battling the disease; many have watched their mothers and sisters die of this dreaded disease. Those with risk factors live with even greater anxiety and fear. No woman wants to hear those chilling words: "The biopsy is positive. You have breast cancer." Provide women with information about detection and risk factors, inform them about the new ACS screening guidelines, instruct them on breast self-examination, and outline dietary changes that might reduce their risk of breast cancer.

Awareness is the first step toward a change in habits. Raising the level of awareness about breast cancer is of paramount importance, and nurses can play an important role in health promotion, disease prevention, and education.

Breast Cancer Screening

The three components of early detection are breast self-examination, clinical breast examination, and mammography.

The ACS (2007b) has issued breast cancer screening guidelines that, for the first time, offer specific guidance for the women and greater clarification of the role of breast examinations (Table 6.4). ACS screening guidelines are revised about every 5 years to include new scientific findings and developments.

Women are exposed to multiple sources of cancer prevention information, and much of it may not be sound. Discuss the benefits, risks, and potential limitations of breast self-examination, clinical breast examination, and mammography with each woman and tailor the information to her specific risk factors (ACS, 2007b). Based on the new guidelines, make clinical judgments as to the appropriateness of recommending breast self-examination, and re-evaluate the need to teach the procedure to all women; the focus might instead be on encouraging regular mammograms (depending, of course, on the woman's individual risk factors).

TABLE 6.4 AMERICAN CANCER SOCIETY BREAST CANCER SCREENING GUIDELINES

Woman's Age	Screening Activity
20–39	Breast self-examination (BSE) is optional Clinical breast examination every 3 years
40+	BSE every month is optional Clinical breast examination every year Mammogram every year, continuing for as long as the woman is in good health

Women at increased risk (e.g., family history, genetic tendency, past history of cancer) should discuss with their health care professionals the pros and cons of starting mammography screening earlier, undergoing additional diagnostic tests (e.g., ultrasound or MRI), or increasing the frequency of examinations.

Source: ACS, 2007c.

Breast self-examination is a technique that enables a woman to detect any changes in her breasts; this could result in early cancer detection. The emphasis is now on awareness of breast changes, not just discovery of cancer. Research has shown that breast self-examination plays a small role in detecting breast cancer compared with self-awareness. However, doing breast self-examination is one way for a woman to know how her breasts normally feel so that she can notice any changes that do occur (ACS, 2007g).

There are two steps to conducting breast self-examination: visual inspection and tactile palpation. The visual part should be done in three separate positions: with the arms up behind the head, with the arms down at the sides, and bending forward. Instruct the woman to look for:

• Changes in shape, size, contour, or symmetry
• Skin discoloration or dimpling, bumps/lumps
• Sores or scaly skin
• Discharge or puckering of the nipple

In the second part, the tactile examination, the woman feels her breasts in one of three specific patterns: spiral, pie-shaped wedges, or up and down. When using any of the three patterns, the woman should use a circular rubbing motion (in dime-sized circles) without lifting the fingers. She checks not only the breasts but also between the breast and the axilla, the axilla itself, and the area above the breast up to the clavicle and across the shoulder. The pads of the three middle fingers on the right hand are used to assess the left breast; the pads of the three middle fingers on the left hand are used to assess the right breast. Instruct the woman to use three different degrees of pressure:

• Light (move the skin without moving the tissue underneath)
• Medium (midway into the tissue)
• Hard (down to the ribs)

Once the tactile examination has been completed while standing in front of a mirror, it should be repeated while lying down. Teaching Guidelines 6.4 details breast self-examination.

Nutrition

Nutrition plays a critical role in health promotion and disease prevention (Escott-Stump, 2007). Being overweight or obese is a risk factor for breast cancer in postmenopausal women (Wright, 2007). *Healthy People 2010* identified being overweight or obese as one of the 10 leading health indicators and a major health concern (USDHHS, 2000). Almost 62% of women over the age of 20 years are overweight; of these, 33.4% are obese (Smith-Warner & Stampfer, 2007). A diet high in fruits, vegetables, and high-fiber carbohydrates and low in animal fats seems to offer protection against breast cancer as well as weight control. Women who followed these dietary guidelines decreased their risk of breast cancer (Escott-Stump, 2007).

The Women's Health Initiative Dietary Modification Trial (Prentice et al., 2006) was designed to study a low-fat diet, a nutritional approach to prevention of chronic diseases. It found a marginally statistically significant reduction in breast cancer incidence among women in the low-fat dietary pattern group.

The American Institute for Cancer Research (AICR), which conducts extensive research, made the following

---

TEACHING GUIDELINES 6.4

How to Perform Breast Self-Examination

Step 1

• Stand before a mirror.
• Check both breasts for anything unusual.
• Look for discharge from the nipple and puckering, dimpling, or scaling of the skin.

The next two steps check for any changes in the contour of your breasts. As you do them, you should be able to feel your muscles tighten.

Step 2

• Watch closely in the mirror as you clasp your hands behind your head and press your hands forward.
• Note any change in the contour of your breasts.

TEACHING GUIDELINES 6.4 (continued)

How to Perform Breast Self-Examination

Step 3

- Next, press your hands firmly on your hips and bow slightly toward the mirror as you pull your shoulders and elbows forward.
- Note any change in the contour of your breasts.

Some women perform the next part of the examination in the shower. Your fingers will glide easily over soapy skin, so you can concentrate on feeling for changes inside the breast.

Step 4

- Raise your left arm.
- Use 3 or 4 fingers of your right hand to feel your left breast firmly, carefully, and thoroughly.
- Beginning at the outer edge, press the flat part of your fingers in small circles, moving the circles slowly around the breast.
- Gradually work toward the nipple.
- Be sure to cover the whole breast.

- Pay special attention to the area between the breast and the underarm, including the underarm itself.
- Feel for any unusual lumps or masses under the skin.
- If you have any spontaneous discharge during the month—whether or not it is during your BSE—see your doctor.
- Repeat the examination on your right breast.

Step 5

- Lie flat on your back with your left arm over your head and a pillow or folded towel under your left shoulder. (This position flattens your breast and makes it easier to check.)
- Repeat the actions of Step 4 in this position for each breast.

Source: American Cancer Society. (2007). *How to perform a breast self exam.* Available online at http://www.cancer.org/docroot/cri/content/cri_2_6x_how_to_perform_a_breast_self_exam_5.asp

recommendations to reduce a woman's risk for developing breast cancer:

- Engaging in daily moderate exercise and weekly vigorous physical activity
- Consuming at least five servings of fruits and vegetables daily
- Not smoking or using any tobacco products
- Keeping a maximum body mass index (BMI) of 25 and limiting weight gain to no more than 11 pounds since age 18
- Consuming seven or more daily portions of complex carbohydrates, such as whole grains and cereals

- Limiting intake of processed foods and refined sugar
- Restricting red meat intake to approximately 3 ounces daily
- Limiting intake of fatty foods, particularly those of animal origin
- Restricting intake of salted foods and use of salt in cooking (Wright, 2007)

The medical community is also starting to study the role of phytochemicals in health. The unique geographic variability of breast cancer around the world and the low rate of breast cancer in Asian compared to Western countries prompted this interest. This area of research appears hopeful for women seeking to prevent breast cancer as well as those recovering from it. Although the mechanism isn't clear, certain foods demonstrate anticancer properties and boost the immune system. Phytochemical-rich foods include:

- Green tea and herbal teas
- Garlic
- Whole grains and legumes
- Onions and leeks
- Soybeans and soy products
- Fruits (citrus, apricots, pumpkin, berries)
- Green leafy vegetables (spinach, collards, romaine)
- Colorful vegetables (carrots, squash, tomatoes)
- Cruciferous vegetables (broccoli, cabbage, cauliflower)
- Flax seeds (Escott-Stump, 2007)

Adopt a holistic approach when addressing the nutritional needs of women with breast cancer. Incorporate nutritional assessment into the general overall assessment of all women. Culturally sensitive nutritional assessment tools need to be developed and used to enhance this process. Providing examples of appropriate foods associated with the woman's current dietary habits, relating current health status to nutritional intake, and placing proposed modifications within a realistic personal framework may increase a woman's willingness to incorporate needed changes in her nutritional behavior. Be able to interpret research results and stay up to date on nutritional influences so that you can transmit this key information to the public.

■■■ Key Concepts

- Many women believe that all lumps are cancerous, but actually more than 90% of the lumps discovered are benign and need no treatment.
- The most commonly encountered benign breast disorders in women include fibrocystic breasts, fibroadenomas, intraductal papilloma, mammary duct ectasia, and mastitis.
- Current research suggests that women with fibrocystic breast disease or other benign breast conditions are more likely to develop breast cancer later only if a breast biopsy shows "atypia" or abnormal breast cells.
- Fibroadenomas are common benign solid breast tumors that can be stimulated by external estrogen, progesterone, lactation, and pregnancy.
- An intraductal papilloma is generally less than 1 cm in diameter, not palpable, and produces a spontaneous serous, serosanguineous, or watery nipple discharge.
- Duct ectasia is a dilation and inflammation of the ducts behind the nipple that results in noncyclic breast pain, nipple retraction, and discharge.
- Mastitis is an infection of the connective tissue in the breast that occurs primarily in lactating or engorged women; it is divided into lactational or nonlactational types.

- Management of both types of mastitis involves the use of oral antibiotics (usually a penicillinase-resistant penicillin or cephalosporin) and acetaminophen (Tylenol) for pain and fever.
- Breast cancer is the most common cancer in women and the second leading cause of cancer deaths (lung cancer is first) among American women.
- Breast cancer metastasizes widely and to almost all organs of the body, but primarily to the bone, lungs, lymph nodes, liver, and brain.
- The etiology of breast cancer is unknown, but the disease is thought to develop in response to a number of related factors: aging, delayed childbearing or never bearing children, high breast density, family history of cancer, late menopause, and hormonal factors.
- Breast cancer treatments fall into two categories: local and systemic. Local treatments are surgery and radiation therapy. Effective systemic treatments include chemotherapy, hormonal therapy, and immunotherapy.
- Women perceive their breasts as intrinsic to their femininity, self-esteem, and sexuality, and the risk of losing a breast can provoke extreme anxiety.
- Nurses can influence both physical and emotional recovery, which are both important aspects of care that help in improving the woman's quality of life and the ability to survive.
- Providing up-to-date information and emotional support are central roles of the nurse in caring for the woman with a diagnosis of breast cancer.

REFERENCES

Alexander, L. L., LaRosa, J. H., Bader, H., & Garfield, S. (2007). *New dimensions in women's health* (4th ed.). Boston: Jones and Bartlett Publishers.
Aliotta, H. M., & Schaeffer, N. J. (2006). Breast conditions. In K. D. Schuiling & F. E. Likis (Eds.), *Women's gynecologic health* (pp. 321–342). Sudbury, MA: Jones and Bartlett Publishers.
American Cancer Society. (2007a). Benign breast conditions. Available at: http://www.cancer.org/docroot/CRI/content/CRI_2_6X_Benign_Breast_Conditions_59.a.
American Cancer Society. (2007b). Updated breast cancer screening guidelines released. Available at: http://www.cancer.org/docroot/MED/content/MED_2_1x_American_Cancer_Society_Is.
American Cancer Society. (2007c). *Cancer facts and figures 2006.* Atlanta, GA: Author.
American Cancer Society (2007d). Screening guidelines for the early detection of cancer in asymptomatic people. *Cancer prevention and early detection facts & figures 2006* (p. 31). Atlanta, GA: Author.
American Cancer Society. (2007e). What are the risk factors for breast cancer? Cancer Reference Information. Available at: http://www.cancer.org/docroot/CRI_2_4_2X_What_are_the_risk_factors_fo.
American Cancer Society. (2007f). *Breast cancer clear and simple.* Atlanta, GA: Author.
American Cancer Society (2007g). How to perform a breast self-exam. Available at: http://www.cancer.org/docroot/cri/content/cri_2_6x_how_to_perform_a_breast_self_exam_5.asp
Banning, M. (2007). Advanced breast cancer: Etiology, treatment and psychosocial features. *British Journal of Nursing, 16*(2), 86–90.
Boehmke, M. M., & Dickerson, S. S. (2006). The diagnosis of breast cancer: Transition from health to illness. *Oncology Nursing Forum, 33*(6), 1121–1127.
Bush, N. J. (2007). Advances in hormonal therapy for breast cancer. *Seminars in Oncology Nursing, 23*(1), 46–54.

Chernecky, C. C., & Berger, B. J. (2007). *Laboratory tests and diagnostic procedures* (5th ed.). Philadelphia: Elsevier Health Sciences.

DiSaia, P. J., & Creasman, W. T. (2007). *Clinical gynecologic oncology* (7th ed.). St. Louis, MO: Elsevier Health Sciences.

Eglash, A., Plane, M. B., & Mundt, M. (2006). History, physical and laboratory findings, and clinical outcomes of lactating women treated with antibiotics for chronic breast and/or nipple pain. *Journal of Human Lactation, 22*(4), 429–438.

Escott-Stump, S. (2007). *Nutrition and diagnosis-related care* (6th ed.). Philadelphia: Lippincott Williams & Wilkins.

Graham, H. (2006). Understanding benign breast conditions. *Practice Nurse, 32*(2), 29–32.

Guarneri, V., Frassoldati, A., Giovannelli, S., Borghi, F., & Conte, P. (2007). Primary systemic therapy for operable breast cancer: A review of clinical trials and perspectives. *Cancer Letters, 248*(2), 175–185.

Hackley, B., Kriebs, J. M., & Rousseau, M. E. (2007). *Primary care of women: A guide for midwives and women's health providers.* Sudbury, MA: Jones and Bartlett Publishers.

Harris, J. (2007). How to help women understand benign breast conditions. *Nursing in Practice: The Journal for Today's Primary Care Nurse,* Mar (33), 78–81.

Holcomb, S. S. (2006). Breast cancer therapy and treatment guidelines. *Nurse Practitioner, 31*(10), 59–63.

Kell, M. R., & Burke, J, P. (2007), Management of breast cancer in women with BRCA gene mutation. *British Medical Journal, 334*(7591), 437–438.

Knobf, M. T. (2007). Psychosocial responses in breast cancer survivors. *Seminars in Oncology Nursing, 23*(1), 71–83.

Kubota, K., Ogawa, Y., Nishioka, A., et al. (2007). Diagnostic accuracy of mammography, ultrasonography and magnetic resonance imaging in the detection of intraductal spread of breast cancer following neoadjuvant chemotherapy. *Oncology Reports, 17*(4), 915–918.

Law, M. P., & Alcamo, I. E. (2007). *Breast cancer.* New York: Chelsea House Publishers.

Mattson, S., & Smith, J. E. (2004). *Core curriculum for maternal-newborn nursing* (3rd ed.). St. Louis, MO: Elsevier Saunders.

Medical Letter. (2006). Raloxifene (Evista) for breast cancer prevention in postmenopausal women. *Obstetrics & Gynecology, 108*(4), 1023–1024.

National Cancer Institute. (NCI) (2007a). Breast cancer: treatment. Available at: http://cancer.gov/cancertopics/pdq/treatment/breast/healthprofessional

National Cancer Institute. (NCI) (2007b). Probability of breast cancer in American women. Available at: http://cis.nci.nih.gov/fact/5_6.htm

National Comprehensive Cancer Network (NCCN). (2007). Breast cancer treatment guidelines. NCCN patient guidelines. Available at: http://www.nccn.org/patients/patient_gls/_english/_breast/5_treatment.asp

Opatt, D. M., & Chung, C. (2007). Breast cancer. *eMedicine.* Available at: http://www.emedicine.com/plastic/topic521.htm

Ottoboni, A., & Ottoboni, F. (2007). Low-fat diet and chronic disease prevention: The Women's Health Initiative and its reception. *Journal of American Physicians & Surgeons, 12*(1), 10–13.

Preda, L., Villa, G., Rizzo, S., Bazzi, L., Origgi, D., Cassano, E., & Bellomi, M. (2006). Magnetic resonance mammography in the evaluation of recurrence at the prior lumpectomy site after conservative surgery and radiotherapy. *Breast Cancer Research, 8*(5), R53–55.

Prentice, R. L., Caan, B., Chlebowski, R. T., et al. (2006). Low-fat dietary pattern and risk of invasive breast cancer: The Women's Health Initiative Randomized Controlled Dietary Modification Trial. *JAMA, 295*(6), 629–642.

Rao, V. S., Garimella, V., Hwang, M., & Drew, P. (2007). Management of early breast cancer in the elderly. *International Journal of Cancer, 120*(6), 1155–1160.

Reddy, P., Chao, Q., Zembower, T., Noskin, G., & Bolon, M. (2007). Postpartum mastitis and community-acquired methicillin-resistant *Staphylococcus aureus. Emerging Infectious Diseases, 13*(2), 298–301.

Richards, T., Hunt, A., Courtney, S., & Umeh, H. (2007). Nipple discharge: A sign of breast cancer? *Annals of the Royal College of Surgeons of England, 89*(2), 124–126.

Sanders, M. E., Scroggins, T., Ampil, F. L., & Li, B. D. (2007). Accelerated partial breast irradiation in early-stage breast cancer. *Journal of Clinical Oncology, 25*(8), 996–1002.

Skidmore-Roth, L. (2007). *Mosby's drug guide for nurses with 2008 update* (7th ed.). St. Louis, MO: Elsevier Health Sciences

Smith, R. A. (2007). The evolving role of MRI in the detection and evaluation of breast cancer. *New England Journal of Medicine, 356,* 1362–1364.

Smith-Warner, S. A., & Stampfer, M. J. (2007). Fat intake and breast cancer. *Journal of the National Cancer Institute, 99*(6), 418–419.

Stephenson, J. (2007). Reducing breast cancer risk. *JAMA, 297*(11), 1182–1184.

Sukumvanich, P., & Borgen, P. (2007). Diseases of the breast. In R. E. Rakel & E. T. Bope (Eds.), *Conn's current therapy 2007* (pp. 1214–1225). Philadelphia: Saunders Elsevier.

Teal, C. B., Tabbara, S., & Kelly, T. A. (2007). Evaluation of intraoperative scrape cytology for sentinel lymph node biopsy in patients with breast cancer. *Breast Journal, 13*(2), 155–157.

Underwood, S. M. (2006). Breast cancer in African American women: Nursing essentials. *ABNF Journal,* Jan/Feb (1), 3–13.

U.S. Department of Health and Human Services (USDHHS). (2000). *Healthy people 2010.* Rockville, MD: Author.

Willett, C. G., Czito, B. G., & Tyler, D. S. (2007). Intraoperative radiation therapy. *Journal of Clinical Oncology, 25*(8), 971–977.

Wright, H. (2007). Getting physically active may increase your chances of surviving cancer. *Environmental Nutrition, 30*(3), 1–4.

Writing Group for Women's Health Initiative Investigators (WHI). (2002). Risks and benefits of estrogen plus progestin in healthy menopausal women: Principal results for the Women's Health Initiative randomized controlled trial. *JAMA, 288*(3), 321–333.

WEBSITES

American Cancer Society (ACS): 1-800-ACS-2345: http://www.cancer.org

Facing Our Risk of Cancer Empowered: www.facingourrisk.org

International Society of Nurses in Genetics: http://nursing.creighton.edu/isong

Living Beyond Breast Cancer, 1-888-753-5222: http://www.lbbc.org

National Alliance of Breast Cancer Organizations, 1-888-80-NABCO: http://www.nabco.org

National Cancer Institute (NCI), 1-800-422-6327: http://www.nci.nih.gov

Oncology Nursing Society (ONS), 1-866-257-4ONS: http://www.ons.org

Susan G. Komen Breast Cancer Foundation, 1-800-462-9273: http://www.komen.org

Y-me National Breast Cancer Organization, 1-800-221-2141: http://www.Y-me.org

CHAPTER WORKSHEET

MULTIPLE CHOICE QUESTIONS

1. Breast self-examinations involve both touching of breast tissue and:

   a. Palpation of cervical lymph nodes

   b. Firm squeezing of both breast nipples

   c. Visualizing both breasts for any change

   d. A mammogram to evaluate breast tissue

2. Which of the following is the strongest risk factor for breast cancer?

   a. Advancing age and being female

   b. High number of children

   c. Genetic mutations in BRCA-1 and BRCA-2

   d. Family history of colon cancer

3. A biopsy procedure that traces radioisotopes and blue dye from the tumor site through the lymphatic system into the axillary nodes is:

   a. Stereotactic biopsy

   b. Sentinel node biopsy

   c. Axillary dissection biopsy

   d. Advanced breast biopsy

4. The most serious potential adverse reaction from chemotherapy is:

   a. Thrombocytopenia

   b. Deep vein thrombosis

   c. Alopecia

   d. Myelosuppression

5. What suggestion would be helpful for the client experiencing painful fibrocystic breast changes?

   a. Increase her caffeine intake.

   b. Take a mild analgesic when needed.

   c. Reduce her intake of leafy vegetables.

   d. Wear a bra bigger than she needs.

6. A postoperative mastectomy client should be referred to which of the following organizations for assistance?

   a. National Organization for Women (NOW)

   b. Food and Drug Administration (FDA)

   c. March of Dimes Foundation (MDF)

   d. Reach to Recovery volunteers

CRITICAL THINKING EXERCISES

1. Mrs. Gordon, 48, presents to the women's community clinic where you work as a nurse. She is very upset and crying. She tells you that she found lumps in her breast: "I know that it's cancer and I will die." When you ask her about her problem, she says she does not check her breasts monthly and hasn't had a mammogram for years because "they're too expensive." She also describes the intermittent pain she experiences.

   a. What specific questions would you ask this client to get a clearer picture?

   b. What education is needed for this client regarding breast health?

   c. What community referrals are needed to meet this client's future needs?

2. Ruth Davis, 51, stops in at the urgent care facility with an anxious look on her face. She tells the nurse practitioner that she has green discharge coming from her right breast and discomfort intermittently. She can't understand how this would happen since she hasn't previously had any nipple discharge or pain.

   a. What benign breast condition might the nurse practitioner suspect based on her description?

   b. What specific information should the nurse practitioner give Mrs. Davis about duct ectasia?

   c. The typical treatment of this benign breast condition would include what?

STUDY ACTIVITIES

1. Discuss with a group of women what their breasts symbolize to them and to society. Do they symbolize something different to each one?

2. When a woman experiences a breast disorder, what feelings might she be experiencing and how can a nurse help her sort them out?

3. Interview a woman who has fibrocystic breast changes and find out how she manages this condition.

4. An infection of the breast connective tissue that frequently occurs in the lactating woman is _____.

BENIGN DISORDERS OF THE FEMALE REPRODUCTIVE TRACT

KEY TERMS

cystocele

enterocele

Kegel exercises

ovarian cyst

pelvic organ prolapse

pessary

polyps

polycystic ovary syndrome

rectocele

urinary incontinence

uterine fibroids

uterine prolapse

LEARNING OBJECTIVES

Upon completion of the chapter, the learner will be able to:

1. Define the key terms.
2. Identify the major pelvic relaxation disorders in terms of etiology, management, and nursing interventions.
3. Outline the nursing management needed for the most common benign reproductive disorders in women.
4. Discuss urinary incontinence in terms of pathology, clinical manifestations, treatment options, and effect on quality of life.
5. Compare the various benign growths in terms of their symptoms and management.
6. Discuss the emotional impact of polycystic ovarian syndrome and the nurse's role as a counselor, educator, and advocate.

Liz, a 26-year-old, overweight woman, presented to the clinic with hirsutism and facial acne and told the nurse she was concerned about her irregular menstrual periods. She also said her hair seemed to be falling out on top of her head recently. What diagnostic tests might the nurse anticipate with this patient? How can the nurse prepare Liz for them?

Wow

Women can influence their aging process by making wise lifestyle choices early on.

The incidence of several benign pelvic disorders increases as women age. For instance, women may experience pelvic support disorders related to pelvic relaxation or urinary incontinence. These disorders generally develop after years of wear and tear on the muscles and tissues that support the pelvic floor—such as that which occurs with childbearing, chronic coughing, straining, surgery, or simply aging. In addition to pelvic support disorders, woman may also experience various benign neoplasms of the reproductive tract, such as cervical polyps, uterine leiomyomas (fibroids), ovarian cysts, genital fistulas, and Bartholin's cysts. This chapter provides an overview of various pelvic support disorders and benign neoplasms, discussing the assessment, treatment, and prevention strategies for each.

Pelvic Support Disorders

Pelvic support disorders such as pelvic organ prolapse (POP) and urinary and fecal incontinence are common in aging women. The majority of the more than 13 million people in the United States who experience urinary incontinence are women with POP (Smith, 2007). Pelvic support disorders cause significant physical and psychological morbidity and can diminish women's social interactions, emotional well-being, and overall quality of life. Because pelvic support disorders increase with age, the problem will grow worse as our population ages. These disorders occur as a result of weakness of the connective tissue and muscular support of pelvic organs due to a number of factors: vaginal childbirth, obesity, lifting, chronic cough, straining at defecation secondary to constipation, and estrogen deficiency (ACOG, 2007). The bony pelvis has an exaggerated lumbar spine curve and downward tilt to it. The bladder rests on the symphysis and the posterior organs rest on the sacrum and coccyx. The pelvis holds the organs, but a woman's erect posture causes a funneling effect and constant downward pressure.

▶ PELVIC ORGAN PROLAPSE

Pelvic organ prolapse (from the Latin *prolapsus,* a slipping forth) refers to the abnormal descent or herniation of the pelvic organs from their original attachment sites or their normal position in the pelvis. POP occurs when structures of the pelvis shift and protrude into or outside of the vaginal canal. The Egyptians were the first to describe prolapse of the genital organs. Hippocrates made reference to placing a pomegranate half into the vagina to treat organ prolapse. A disorder exclusive to women, POP rarely results in severe morbidity or mortality but can affect a woman's daily activities and quality of life.

It is difficult to determine the incidence of POP, as the disorder is often asymptomatic and many women do not seek treatment. It has been estimated, however, that up to 75% of all women who have given birth experience POP (ACOG, 2007). With the aging of the population, POP and its associated symptoms are becoming increasingly common (Bartoletti, 2007).

The treatment and diagnosis of POP is challenging and problematic.

Types of Pelvic Organ Prolapse

The four most common types of genital prolapse are cystocele, rectocele, enterocele, and uterine prolapse (Fig. 7.1):

- **Cystocele** occurs when the posterior bladder wall protrudes downward through the anterior vaginal wall.
- **Rectocele** occurs when the rectum sags and pushes against or into the posterior vaginal wall.
- **Enterocele** occurs when the small intestine bulges through the posterior vaginal wall (especially common when straining).
- **Uterine prolapse** occurs when the uterus descends through the pelvic floor and into the vaginal canal. Multiparous women are at particular risk for uterine prolapse.

The extent of uterine prolapse is described in terms of degree:

- First degree: prolapse of the organ into the vaginal canal
- Second degree: cervix descends to the vaginal introitus
- Third degree: cervix is below the vaginal introitus (Berzuk, 2007)

Etiology

Anatomic support of the pelvic organs is mainly provided by the levator ani muscle complex and the connective tissue attachments of the pelvic organ fascia. Dysfunction of one or both of these components can lead to loss of support and eventually POP. Weakened pelvic floor muscles also prevent complete closure of the urethra, resulting in urine leakage during physical stress. This problem is not limited to older women: urinary incontinence has been documented in women of varying ages, including very young women (Smith, 2007).

Many risk factors for POP have been suggested, but the true cause is likely to be multifactorial. Causes might include:

- Constant downward gravity because of erect human posture
- Atrophy of supporting tissues with aging and decline of estrogen levels
- Weakening of pelvic support related to childbirth trauma
- Reproductive surgery
- Family history of POP
- Young age at first birth

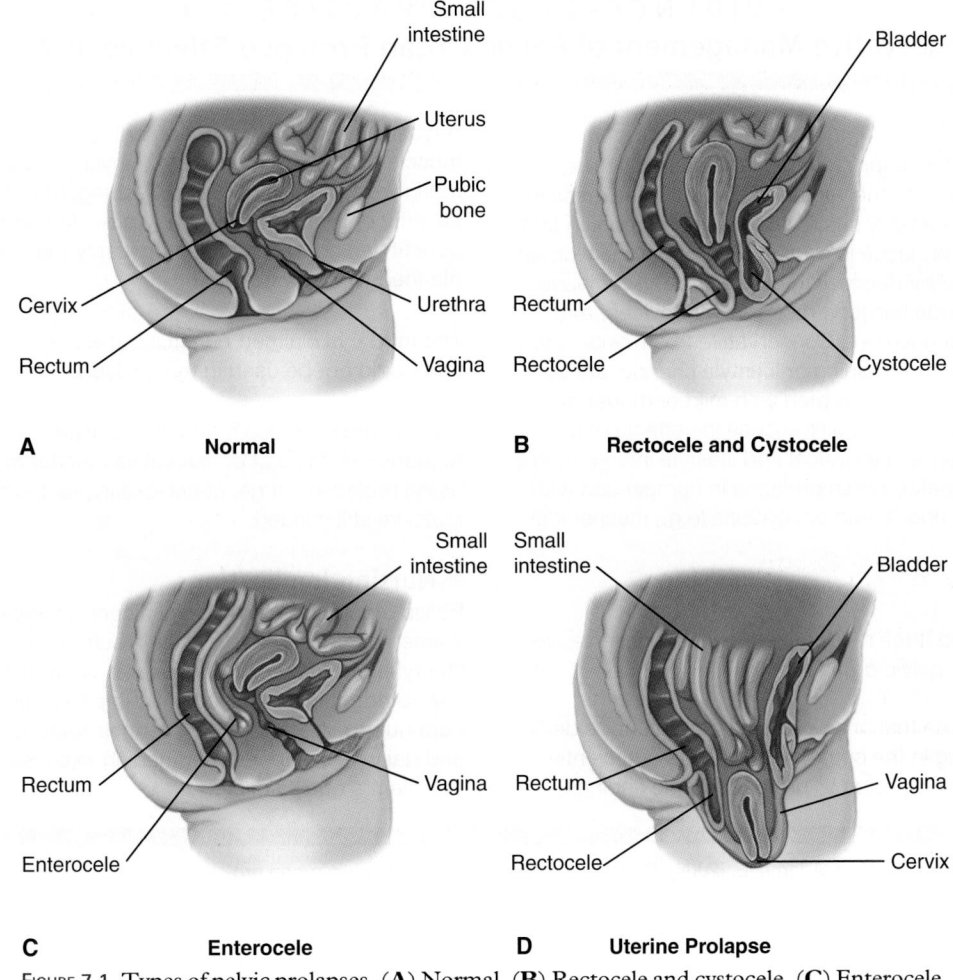

FIGURE 7.1 Types of pelvic prolapses. (**A**) Normal. (**B**) Rectocele and cystocele. (**C**) Enterocele. (**D**) Uterine prolapse.

- Connective tissue disorders
- Infant birthweight of more than 4,500 g
- Pelvic radiation
- Increased abdominal pressure secondary to:
  - Lifting of children or heavy objects
  - Straining due to chronic constipation
  - Respiratory problems or chronic coughing
  - Obesity (Jelovsek, Maher, & Barber, 2007)

Therapeutic Management

Treatment options for POP depend on the symptoms and their effect on the woman's quality of life. Important considerations when deciding on nonsurgical or surgical options include the severity of symptoms, the woman's preferences, the woman's health status, age, and suitability for surgery, and the presence of other pelvic conditions (urinary or fecal incontinence). When surgery is being considered, the nature of the procedure and the likely outcome must be fully explained and discussed with the woman and her partner. Treatment options

for POP include Kegel exercises, estrogen replacement therapy, dietary and lifestyle modifications, use of pessaries or the Colpexin Sphere, and surgery (see Evidence-Based Practice 7.1).

Kegel Exercises

Kegel exercises strengthen the pelvic floor muscles to support the inner organs and prevent further prolapse. The purpose of pelvic floor exercises is to increase the muscle volume, which will result in a stronger muscular contraction. Kegel exercises might limit the progression of mild prolapse and alleviate mild prolapse symptoms, including low back pain and pelvic pressure. They will not, however, help severe uterine prolapse.

Hormone Replacement Therapy

Hormone replacement therapy (orally, transdermally, or vaginally) may improve the tone and vascularity of the supporting tissue in perimenopausal and menopausal women by increasing blood perfusion and the elasticity of the vaginal wall.

EVIDENCE-BASED PRACTICE 7.1
Is Conservative Management of Pelvic Organ Prolapse Effective in Women?

● Study

Pelvic organ prolapse (protrusion of the uterus, cervix, bladder, or bowel into the vagina because of weakness in the tissues that normally support them) is common; in fact, some degree of prolapse is seen in 50% of parous women. The symptoms vary depending on the type of prolapse. Treatments include surgery, mechanical devices, and conservative management. Conservative treatments, such as pelvic floor muscle training or lifestyle change, are commonly recommended for women with mild or moderate prolapse. A study was done to assess the effects of conservative management (physical and lifestyle interventions) for women with pelvic organ prolapse in comparison with no treatment or other treatment options (e.g., mechanical devices or surgery).

▲ Findings

This review found three randomized trials of conservative management for pelvic organ prolapse.

One relatively large trial of an exercise program for elderly Thai women living in the community was not sufficiently well conducted or reported to provide reliable findings.

A feasibility study (n = 47 women) found that pelvic floor muscle training, delivered by a physiotherapist to symptomatic women in an outpatient setting, may reduce the severity of prolapse. The study provided some evidence of benefit, which was sufficient to justify the large trial that is planned to follow it.

The third trial claimed benefits but was reported in a way that could not be used in the analysis.

Overall, the evidence found in this review was not sufficient to judge the value of conservative management of pelvic organ prolapse. Large, better-quality, randomized controlled trials are still needed.

■ Nursing Implications

Pelvic organ prolapse is a significant clinical issue among women of all ages, and it often results in discomfort, altered lifestyle, and urinary incontinence. Although this review did not identify a clear-cut first-line treatment, nurses can continue to stress lifestyle changes such as weight loss and daily pelvic floor strengthening exercises to improve the client's quality of life.

Hagen, S., Stark, D., Maher. C., & Adams, E. (2006). Conservative management of pelvic organ prolapse in women. *Cochrane Database of Systematic Reviews* 2006, Issue 4. Art. No.: CD003882. DOI: 10.1002/14651858.CD003882.pub3.

▶ *Take* NOTE!

Before hormone therapy is considered, a thorough medical history must be taken to assess her risk for complications (e.g., endometrial cancer, myocardial infarction, stroke, breast cancer, pulmonary emboli, and deep vein thrombosis). Because of these risks, estrogens, with or without progestins, should be given at the lowest effective dose and for the shortest duration consistent with the treatment goals and risks for the individual woman (ACOG, 2007).

Dietary and Lifestyle Modifications

Dietary and lifestyle modifications may help prevent pelvic relaxation and chronic problems later in life. Dietary habits can exacerbate the prolapse by causing constipation and consequently chronic straining. The stools of a constipated woman are hard and dry, and typically she must strain while bearing down to defecate. This straining to pass a hard stool increases intra-abdominal pressure, which over time causes the pelvic organs to prolapse. Dietary mod-

ifications can help to establish regular bowel movements without discomfort and eliminate flatus and bloating.

Pessaries

A **pessary** is a silicone or plastic device that is placed into the vagina to support the uterus, bladder, and rectum as a space-filling device, replacing normal pressure on the vaginal walls when levator ani support is unreliable (Fig. 7.2). Although there are many types and shapes, the most commonly used pessary is a firm ring that presses against the wall of the vagina and urethra to help decrease leakage and support a prolapsed vagina or uterus. Pessaries are of two main types:

- Support pessaries, which rest under the symphysis and sacrum and elevate the vagina (e.g., Ring, Gehrung, and Hodge pessaries)
- Space-occupying pessaries, which are designed to manage severe prolapse by supporting the uterus even with a lack of vaginal tone (e.g., cube, doughnut, and inflatable Gellhorn pessaries)

Indications for pessary use include uterine prolapse or cystocele, especially among elderly clients for whom surgery is contraindicated; younger women with prolapse

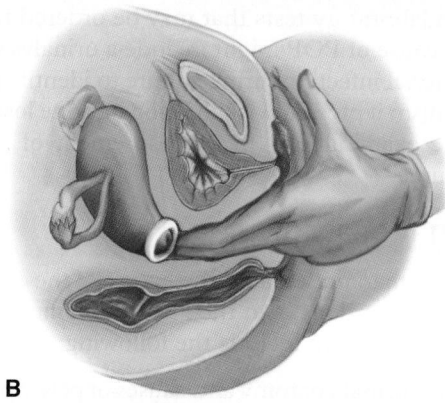

FIGURE 7.2 Examples of pessaries. (**A**) Various shapes and sizes of pessaries available. (**B**) Insertion of one type of pessary.

who plan to have additional children; and women with marked prolapse who prefer to use a pessary rather than undergo surgery (Newman, 2007). Many women use pessaries for only a short period of time and become free of symptoms. Long-term use can lead to pressure necrosis in some women; in this situation other methods of support should be explored.

Pessaries are fitted by trial and error; the woman often needs to try several sizes or styles. The largest pessary that the woman can wear comfortably is generally the most effective. The woman should be instructed to report any discomfort or difficulty with urination or defecation while wearing the pessary.

Colpexin Sphere

A new intravaginal device, the Colpexin Sphere, which became available in 2006, supports the pelvic floor muscle and facilitates rehabilitation of the pelvic floor muscles. Although pessaries may support a prolapsed pelvic organ,

they do not allow for concomitant strengthening of pelvic floor musculature and they do not reduce urine leakage (Smith, 2007). The Colpexin Sphere is a polycarbonate sphere with a locator string that is fitted above the hymenal ring to support the pelvic floor muscle. The sphere is used in conjunction with pelvic floor muscle exercises, which should be performed daily.

Surgical Interventions

Surgical interventions for genital organ prolapse are designed to correct specific defects, with the goals being to restore normal anatomy and to preserve function (ACOG, 2007). Surgery is not an option for all women. Women who are at high risk of suffering recurrent prolapse after a surgical repair or who have morbid obesity, chronic obstructive pulmonary disease, or medical conditions in which general anesthesia would be risky are not good candidates for surgical repair (Bartoletti, 2007), and noninvasive treatment strategies should be discussed with them.

Surgical interventions might include anterior or posterior colporrhaphy (to repair a cystocele or rectocele) and vaginal hysterectomy (for uterine prolapse).

An anterior and posterior colporrhaphy may be effective for a first-degree prolapse. This surgical procedure tightens the anterior and posterior vaginal wall, thus repairing a cystocele or rectocele. The pubocervical fascia (supportive tissue between the vagina and bladder) is folded and sutured to bring the bladder and urethra in proper position (Lazarou & Scotti, 2007).

A vaginal hysterectomy is the treatment of choice for uterine prolapse because it removes the prolapsed organ that is bringing down the bladder and rectum with it. It can be combined with an anterior and posterior repair if a cystocele or rectocele is present.

Nursing Assessment

Nursing assessment for women with POP includes a thorough health history and physical examination and several laboratory and diagnostic tests.

Health History and Clinical Manifestations

The cause of prolapse is multifactorial, with vaginal childbirth, advancing age, and increasing body mass index as the most consistent risk factors (Jelovsek, Maher, & Barber, 2007). Assessment of risk factors (chronic straining, hysterectomy, normal aging, and abnormalities of connective tissue) in the woman's history will assist the health care provider in the diagnosis and treatment of POP. The history should include questions about:

• The woman's obstetrical history (number of pregnancies, weight of newborns, pregnancy spacing)
• Chronic respiratory condition (chronic coughing)
• Menopausal status
• Weight history (loss or gain)

- Constipation (frequency and chronicity)
- Age
- Family history (family member with POP)
- Urinary incontinence
- Previous pelvic surgeries

Assess for clinical manifestations of POP. POP is often asymptomatic, but when symptoms do occur, they are often related to the site and type of prolapse. Symptoms common to all types of prolapses are a feeling of dragging, a lump in the vagina, or something "coming down." Women with POP can present either with one symptom, such as vaginal bulging or pelvic pressure, or with several complaints, including many bladder, bowel, and pelvic symptoms. Symptoms associated with POP are summarized in Box 7.1.

Women present with varying degrees of descent. Uterine prolapse is the most troubling type of pelvic relaxation because it is often associated with concomitant defects of the vagina in the anterior, posterior, and lateral compartments (Lazarou & Scotti, 2007).

BOX 7.1 **Symptoms Associated With Pelvic Organ Prolapse**

- Urinary symptoms
  - Stress incontinence
  - Frequency (diurnal and nocturnal)
  - Urgency and urge incontinence
  - Hesitancy
  - Poor or prolonged stream
  - Feeling of incomplete emptying
- Bowel symptoms
  - Difficulty in defecation
  - Incontinence of flatus or liquid or solid stool
  - Urgency of defecation
  - Feeling of incomplete evacuation
  - Rectal protrusion or prolapse after defecation
- Sexual symptoms
  - Inability to have frequent intercourse
  - Dyspareunia
  - Lack of satisfaction or orgasm
  - Incontinence during sexual activity
- Other local symptoms
  - Pressure or heaviness in the vagina
  - Pain in the vagina or perineum
  - Low back pain after long periods of standing
  - Palpable bulge in the vaginal vault
  - Difficulty walking due to a protrusion from the vagina
  - Difficulty inserting or keeping a tampon in place
  - Vaginal-cervical mucosa hypertrophy, excoriation, ulceration, and bleeding
  - Abdominal pressure or pain (Jelovsek, Maher, & Barber, 2007; Smith, 2007)

Physical Examination

The pelvic examination performed by the health care provider includes an external genital inspection to visualize any obvious protrusion of the uterus, bladder, urethra, or vaginal wall occurring at the vaginal opening. Usually the woman is asked to perform the Valsalva maneuver (bearing down) while the examiner notes which organ prolapses first and the degree to which it occurs. Any urine leakage during the examination is important to note. The woman is asked to contract the pubococcygeal muscles (Kegel exercise); the health care provider inserts two fingers into the vagina to assess the strength and symmetry of the contraction. Since genital organ prolapse can cause urinary symptoms such as incontinence, bladder function should be assessed by determining postvoid residual with a catheter. If the woman has more than 100 mL of retained urine, she should be referred for further urodynamic evaluation and testing.

Laboratory and Diagnostic Tests

Common laboratory tests that may be ordered to determine the cause of POP might include a urinalysis to rule out a bacterial infection, urine culture to identify the specific organism if present, visualization of urine loss during the pelvic examination, and measurement of postvoid urine volume.

Nursing Management

Help the woman understand the nature of the condition, the treatment options, and the likely outcomes. Nursing considerations might include the following:

- Describe normal anatomy and causes of pelvic prolapse.
- Assess how this condition has affected the woman's life.
- Outline the options, with the advantages and disadvantages of each.
- Allow the client to make the decision that is right for her.
- Provide education.
- Schedule preoperative activities needed for surgery.
- Reassure the client that there is a solution for her symptoms.
- Provide community education about genital prolapse.

Nursing Care Plan 7.1 provides an overview of care for a woman with POP.

Encourage Pelvic Floor Muscle Training

Encourage the woman to perform Kegel exercises daily (Teaching Guidelines 7.1). Discuss current research findings and educate the woman about hormone therapy, allowing the woman to make her own decision on whether to use hormones. Controversy still exists regarding the benefits versus the risks of taking hormones, so the woman must weigh this option carefully (Luft, 2006).

Encourage Dietary and Lifestyle Modifications

Instruct clients to increase dietary fiber and fluids to prevent constipation. A high-fiber diet with an increase in

Nursing Care Plan 7.1

OVERVIEW OF A WOMAN WITH PELVIC ORGAN PROLAPSE (POP)

Katherine, a 62-year-old multiparous woman, came to her gynecologist with complaints of a chronic dragging or heavy painful feeling in her pelvis, lower backache, constipation, and urine leakage. Her symptoms increase when she stands for long periods. She hasn't had menstrual cycles for at least a decade. She tells you, "I'm not taking any of those menopausal hormones."

NURSING DIAGNOSIS: Pain related to relaxation of pelvic support and elimination difficulties

Outcome Identification and Evaluation
Client will report an acceptable level of discomfort within 1 to 2 hours of intervention as evidenced by a rating of less than 4 on a 0-to-10 pain scale.

Interventions: Providing Pain Management
- Obtain a thorough pain history, including ongoing pain experiences, methods of pain control used, what worked, what didn't, any allergies to pain medications, and the effect of pain on her activities of daily living *to provide a baseline and enable a systematic approach to pain management.*
- Assess the location, frequency, severity, duration, precipitating factors, and aggravating/alleviating factors *to identify characteristics of the client's pain to plan appropriate interventions.*
- Educate client about any medications prescribed (correct dosage, route, side effects, and precautions) *to increase the client's understanding of the therapy and promote compliance.*
- Assess problematic elimination patterns *to identify underlying factors from which to plan appropriate prevention strategies.*
- Encourage client to increase fluids and fiber in diet and increase physical activity daily *to promote peristalsis.*
- Assist client with establishing regular toileting patterns by setting aside time daily for bowel elimination *to promote regular bowel function and evacuation.*
- Urge client to avoid the routine use of laxatives *to reduce risk of compounding constipation.*

NURSING DIAGNOSIS: Knowledge deficit related to causes of structural disorders and treatment options

Outcome Identification and Evaluation
Client will demonstrate understanding of current condition and treatments as evidenced by identifying treatment options, making health-promoting lifestyle choices, verbalizing appropriate health care practices, and adhering to treatment plan.

Interventions: Provide Client Education
- Assess client's understanding of pelvic organ prolapse and its treatment options *to provide a baseline for teaching.*
- Review information provided about surgical procedures and recommendations for healthy lifestyle, obtaining feedback frequently, *to validate client's understanding of instructions.*
- Discuss association between uterine, bladder, and rectal prolapse and symptoms *to help client understand the etiology of her symptoms and pain.*
- Have client verbalize and discuss information related to diagnosis, surgical procedure, preoperative routine, and post-operative regimen *to ensure adequate understanding and provide time for correcting or clarifying any misinformation or misconceptions.*
- Provide written material with pictures *to promote learning and help client visualize what has occurred to her body secondary to aging, weight gain, childbirth, and gravity.*
- Discuss pros and cons of hormone replacement therapy, osteoporosis prevention, and cardiovascular events common in postmenopausal women *to promote informed decision making by the client about available menopausal therapies.*
- Inform client about the availability of community resources and make appropriate referrals as needed *to provide additional education and support.*
- Document details of teaching and learning *to allow for continuity of care and further education, if needed.*

TEACHING GUIDELINES 7.1

Performing Kegel Exercises

- Squeeze the muscles in your rectum as if you are trying to prevent passing flatus.
- Stop and start urinary flow to help identify the pubococcygeus muscle.
- Tighten the pubococcygeus muscle for a count of three, and then relax it.
- Contract and relax the pubococcygeus muscle rapidly 10 times.
- Try to bring up the entire pelvic floor and bear down 10 times.
- Repeat Kegel exercises at least five times daily.

fluid intake alleviates constipation by increasing stool bulk and stimulating peristalsis. It is accomplished by replacing refined, low-fiber foods with high-fiber foods. The recommended daily intake of fiber for women is 25 g (Dudek, 2006). In addition to increasing the amount of fiber in her diet, also encourage the woman to drink eight 8-oz glasses of fluid daily and to engage in regular aerobic exercise, which promotes muscle tone and stimulates peristalsis.

Educate the client about other lifestyle changes that will assist with prolapse, such as:

- Achieve ideal weight to reduce intra-abdominal pressure and strain on pelvic organs, including pressure on the bladder.
- Wear a girdle or abdominal support to support the muscles surrounding the pelvic organs.
- Avoid lifting heavy objects to reduce the risk of increasing intra-abdominal pressure, which can push the pelvic organs downward.
- Avoid high-impact aerobics, jogging, or jumping repeatedly to minimize the risk of increasing intra-abdominal pressure, which places downward pressure on the organs.
- Give up smoking to minimize the risk for a chronic "smoker's cough," which increases intra-abdominal pressure and forces the pelvic organs downward.

Provide Teaching for Pessary Use

Educate the woman about pessary use. Discuss complications as part of the instruction. Although the pessary is a safe device, it is still a foreign body in the vagina. Because of this, the most common side effects of the pessary are increased vaginal discharge, urinary tract infections, vaginitis, and odor. This can be reduced by douching with dilute vinegar or hydrogen peroxide. Postmenopausal women with thin vaginal mucosa are susceptible to vaginal ulceration with the use of a pessary. Advise the woman to use

estrogen cream to make the vaginal mucosa more resistant to erosion and to strengthen the vaginal walls.

The woman must be capable of managing use of the pessary, either alone or with the help of a caretaker. The most common recommendations for pessary care include removing the pessary twice weekly and cleaning it with soap and water; using a lubricant for insertion; and having regular follow-up examinations every 6 to 12 months after an initial period of adjustment. Educate the woman in the care of her pessary so she feels comfortable with all aspects of care before leaving the health care facility.

Provide Perioperative Care

Prepare the woman for surgery by reinforcing the risks and benefits of surgery and describing the postoperative course. Explain that a Foley catheter will be in place for up to 1 week, and that she might not be able to urinate due to the swelling after the catheter has been removed. Provide home care instructions for the Foley catheter. She should cleanse the perineal area daily with mild soap and water, especially around where the catheter enters the urinary meatus. If the woman is provided with a leg bag to be worn during waking hours, instruct her to empty it frequently and keep it below the level of the bladder to prevent backflow. The same principles are applied to the primary Foley bag when emptying.

During the recovery period, instruct the client to avoid for several weeks activities that cause an increase in abdominal pressure, such as straining, sneezing, and coughing. In addition, advise her to avoid lifting anything heavy or straining to push anything. Explain to the woman that stool softeners and gentle laxatives might be prescribed to prevent constipation and straining with bowel movements. Pelvic rest will be prescribed until the operative area is healed in 6 weeks.

Promote Prevention Strategies

Limited data are available on ways to prevent POP. Approaches include lifestyle changes that reduce modifiable risk factors, such as losing weight, avoiding heavy lifting, and relieving constipation. Explore with the woman what factors in her lifestyle might be modified to reduce her risk of developing POP (primary prevention), or improve her quality of life after receiving treatment (secondary prevention).

► URINARY INCONTINENCE

Urinary incontinence is the involuntary loss of urine sufficient enough to be a social or hygiene problem (Reena, Kekre, & Kekre, 2007). This disorder affects approximately 25 million people in the United States, about 12 million of them women (Berzuk, 2007). It has been estimated that one in four women experience urinary incontinence at some time in their life, varying in severity from mild to severe (Selby, 2006). It is more common than diabetes and Alzheimer's disease, both of which receive a great deal of press attention. About half the women with incontinence have never discussed the problem with their health care provider because they feel ashamed, embarrassed, guilty, or lacking control (Wallace, 2007).

> ▶ *Take* NOTE!
>
> *Incontinence is preventable, treatable, and often curable. However, many women believe that loss of bladder function is a normal and expected part of aging.*

Incontinence can have far-reaching effects. Some women experience anxiety, depression, social isolation, and disruptions in their self-esteem and dignity. It can cause the woman to stop working, traveling, socializing, and enjoying sexual relationships. In addition, incontinence can create a tremendous burden for caretakers and is a common reason for admission to a long-term care facility (Lemack, 2007).

The three most common types of incontinence are urge incontinence (overactive bladder caused by detrusor muscle contractions), stress incontinence (inadequate urinary sphincter function), and mixed incontinence (involves both stress and urge incontinence) (Ogundele & Silverberg, 2007). Comparison Chart 7.1 details these types.

Pathophysiology and Etiology

Urinary continence requires several factors, including effective functioning of the bladder, adequate pelvic floor muscles, neural control from the brain, and integrity of the neural connections that facilitate voluntary control.

The bladder neck and proximal urethra function as a sphincter. During urination the sphincter relaxes and the bladder empties. The ability to control urination requires the integrated function of numerous components of the lower urinary tract, which must be structurally sound and function normally. Incontinence can develop if the bladder muscles become overactive due to weakened sphincter muscles, if the bladder muscles become too weak to contract properly, or if signals from the nervous system to the urinary structures are interrupted. A major factor in women that contributes to urinary continence is the estrogen level, because this hormone helps maintain bladder sphincter tone. In perimenopausal or menopausal women, incontinence can be a problem as estrogen levels begin to decline and genitourinary changes occur. In simple terms, the bladder is the reservoir, the urethra is the seal, and the levator ani muscle is the gate that holds pressure against the outflow of urine by supporting the urethra and bladder from below. When there is a dysfunction of any of the three structures, incontinence occurs.

Contributing factors in urinary incontinence include:

- Fluid intake, especially alcohol, carbonated drinks, and caffeinated beverages
- Constipation: alters the position of the pelvic organs and puts pressure on the bladder
- Habitual "preventive" emptying: may result in training the bladder to hold only small amounts of urine
- Advancing age: age-related anatomic changes provide less pelvic support
- Pregnancy and childbirth: damage to pelvic structures during childbirth
- Obesity: increases abdominal pressure (Hines & Miller, 2006)

Therapeutic Management

Treatment options depend on the type of urinary incontinence. In general, the least invasive procedure with the

COMPARISON CHART 7.1 **Urge Incontinence vs. Stress Incontinence**

	Urge Incontinence	Stress Incontinence
Description	Precipitous loss of urine, preceded by a strong urge to void, with increased bladder pressure and detrusor contraction	Accidental leakage of urine that occurs with increased pressure on the bladder from coughing, sneezing, laughing, or physical exertion
Etiology	Causes might be neurologic, idiopathic, or infectious	Develops commonly in women in their 40s and 50s, usually as the result of weakened muscles and ligaments in the pelvis following childbirth
Signs and Symptoms	Urgency, frequency, nocturia, and a large amount of urine loss	Involuntary loss of a small amount of urine in response to physical activity that raises intra-abdominal pressure

fewest risks is the first choice for treatment. Surgery is used only if other methods have failed. There is a widespread belief that urinary incontinence is an inevitable problem of getting older and that little or nothing can be done to relieve symptoms or reverse it. Nothing is further from the truth, and attitudes must change so that women feel comfortable seeking help for this embarrassing condition.

For many women with urge incontinence, simple reassurance and lifestyle interventions might help. However, if more than simple lifestyle measures are needed, effective treatments might include:

- Bladder training to establish normal voiding intervals (every 3 to 5 hours)
- Kegel exercises to strengthen the pelvic floor musculature
- Pessary ring to support pelvic structures that have weakened
- Pharmacotherapy to reduce the urge to void. Anticholinergic agents such as oxybutynin (Ditropan) or tolterodine (Detrol) might be prescribed. The most common side effects of anticholinergic agents are dry mouth, blurred vision, constipation, nausea, dizziness, and headaches (Lemack, 2007).

For women with stress incontinence, treatment is not always a cure, but it can minimize the impact of this condition on the woman's quality of life. Some treatment options for stress incontinence might include:

- Weight loss if needed
- Avoidance of constipation
- Smoking cessation
- Kegel exercises to strengthen the pelvic floor
- Pessaries
- Weighted vaginal cones to improve the tone of pelvic floor muscles
- Periurethral injection (injecting a bulking agent [collagen] to form a bulge that brings the urethral walls closer together to achieve a better closure)
- Medications such as duloxetine (Cymbalta, Yentreve) to increase urethral sphincter contractions during the storage phase of the urination cycle
- Estrogen replacement therapy to improve bladder sphincter tone
- Surgery to correct genital prolapse and improve urethral and bladder tone

Nursing Assessment

The assessment of the incontinent woman includes a history, physical examination, laboratory tests, and possibly urodynamic testing. The onset, frequency, severity, and pattern of incontinence should be determined, as well as any associated symptoms such as frequency, dysuria, urgency, and nocturia. Incontinence may be quantified by asking the woman if she wears a pad and how often the pad is changed. A review of the woman's current medica-

tions, including over-the-counter medications, should be included in the history.

A complete physical examination should be carried out by the health care provider; it should include a neurologic assessment and pelvic and rectal examinations. The presence of associated POP should be noted because it can contribute to the woman's voiding problems and may have an impact on diagnosis and treatment. A rectal examination is done to evaluate sphincter tone and perineal sensation.

A urinalysis is performed to look for hematuria, pyuria, glucosuria, or proteinuria. A urine culture is done if there is pyuria or bacteriuria. Postvoid residual should be measured either with pelvic ultrasound or directly with a catheter. If the residual exceeds the limit set, urodynamic testing is then used to diagnose the incontinence.

Nursing Management

Incontinence can be devastating and can cause psychosocial concerns and isolation. Nurses can encourage women with troublesome symptoms to seek help. Discuss the treatment options with the client, including benefits and potential outcomes, and encourage her to select the continence treatment best for her lifestyle. Provide education about good bladder habits and strategies to reduce the incidence or severity of incontinence (Teaching Guidelines 7.2). Provide support and encouragement to ensure compliance. Remember that aging can increase the risk of incontinence,

TEACHING GUIDELINES 7.2

Managing Urinary Incontinence

- Avoid drinking too much fluid (i.e., 1.5 L total daily limit), but do not decrease your intake of fluids.
- Reduce intake of fluids and foods that are bladder irritants and precipitate urgency, such as chocolate, caffeine, sodas, alcohol, artificial sweetener, hot spicy foods, orange juice, tomatoes, and watermelon (Lemack, 2007).
- Increase fiber and fluids in your diet to reduce constipation.
- Control blood glucose levels to prevent polyuria.
- Treat chronic cough.
- Remove any barriers that delay you from reaching the toilet.
- Practice good perineal hygiene by using mild soap and water. Wipe from front to back to prevent urinary tract infections.
- Become aware of adverse drug effects.
- Take your medications as prescribed.
- Continue to do pelvic floor (Kegel) exercises.

but incontinence is not an inevitable part of aging. Review the anatomy and physiology of the urinary system and offer simple explanations to help the woman cope with urinary alterations. Therapeutic listening is important. Be aware of the courage it takes for a woman to disclose an embarrassing condition.

▶ *Consider* THIS!

Life can be complicated and embarrassing at times when we least expect it. I met a man in church who seemed interested in me, and he asked me out for coffee after Sunday services. I have been alone for 10 years and this prospect seemed exciting to me. We talked for hours over coffee and seemed to have a great deal in common, especially since both of us had lost our spouses to cancer. He asked me to go square dancing with him, since that was an activity we both had enjoyed in the past with our spouses. I hadn't been out or physically active for ages and didn't realize how my body had changed with age.

It was during the first dance that I noticed a wet sensation between my legs, which I was unable to control. I managed to continue on and pretend that all was fine, but then realized what many of my friends were talking about—stress incontinence. Not being able to control one's urine is very embarrassing and it complicates your life, but I made up my mind that it wasn't going to control me!

Thoughts: Gravity and childbirth take a toll on women's reproductive organs by bringing them downward. This woman is not going to let stress incontinence curtail her outside activity, which demonstrates a good attitude. What can be done about her embarrassing accidents? Were there any preventive strategies she could have used at an earlier age?

▶ *Take* NOTE!

Simple diet and lifestyle alterations, combined with a proper pelvic floor muscle strengthening program, can often produce significant improvements for women of all ages.

Benign Growths

The most common benign growths of the reproductive tract include cervical, endocervical, and endometrial polyps; uterine fibroids (leiomyomas); ovarian cysts; genital fistulas; and Bartholin's cysts.

▶ POLYPS

Polyps are small benign growths. The cause of polyp growth is not well understood, but they are frequently the result of infection. Polyps might be associated with chronic inflammation, an abnormal local response to increased levels of estrogen, or local congestion of the cervical vasculature (Kaminski & Hoffman, 2007). Single or multiple polyps might occur. They are most common in multiparous women. Polyps can appear anywhere but are most common on the cervix and in the uterus (Fig. 7.3).

Cervical polyps often appear after menarche. They occur in 2% to 5% of women, and approximately 2% of these polyps have cancerous changes (Verga, 2006). Endocervical polyps are commonly found in multiparous women age 40 to 60. Endocervical polyps are more common than cervical polyps, with a stalk of varied width and length. Endometrial polyps are benign tumors or localized overgrowths of the endometrium. Most endometrial polyps are solitary, and they rarely occur in women younger than 20 years of age. The incidence of these polyps rises steadily with increasing age, peaks in the fifth decade of life, and gradually declines after menopause. They are present in up to 25% of women being seen for abnormal bleeding (Verga, 2006).

Therapeutic Management

Treatment of polyps usually consists of simple removal with small forceps done on an outpatient basis, removal during hysteroscopy, or dilatation and curettage (D&C). The polyp base can be removed by laser vaporization. Because many polyps are infected, an antibiotic may be

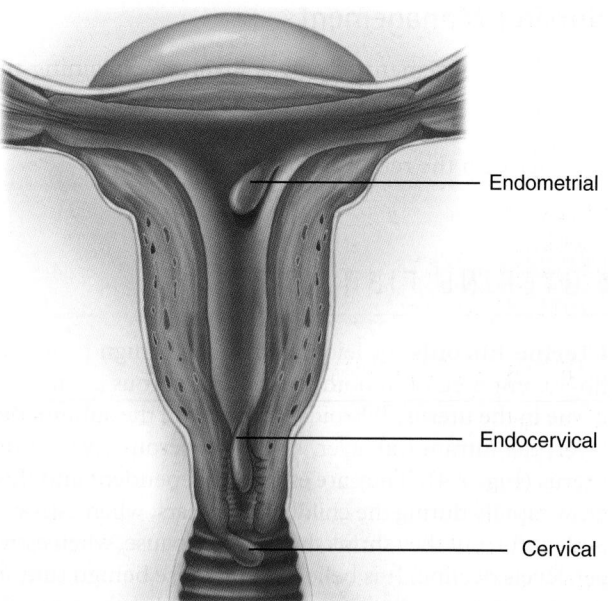

FIGURE 7.3 Cervical, endocervical, and endometrial polyps.

ordered after removal as a preventive measure or to treat early signs of infection.

Although polyps are rarely cancerous, a specimen should be sent after surgery to a pathology laboratory to exclude malignancy. A cervical biopsy typically reveals mildly atypical cells and signs of infection. Polyps rarely return after they are removed. Regularly scheduled Pap smears are suggested for women with cervical polyps to detect any future abnormal growths that may be malignant.

Nursing Assessment

Nursing assessment for a woman with polyps includes assisting with the physical examination and preparing the collected specimen to be sent to the cytologist.

Clinical Manifestations

Assess for clinical manifestations of polyps. Most endocervical polyps are cherry red, while most cervical polyps are grayish-white (Verga, 2006). Cervical and endocervical polyps are often asymptomatic, but they can produce mild symptoms such as abnormal vaginal bleeding (after intercourse or douching, between menses) or discharge. The most common clinical manifestation of endometrial polyps is metrorrhagia (irregular, acyclic uterine bleeding).

Physical Examination and Laboratory and Diagnostic Studies

Typically, cervical polyps are diagnosed when the cervix is visualized through a speculum during the woman's annual gynecologic examination (Kaminski & Hoffman, 2007). Endometrial polyps are not detected on physical examination, but rather with ultrasound or hysteroscopy (introduction of a small camera through the cervix to visualize the uterine cavity).

Nursing Management

Nursing management of polyps involves explaining the condition and the rationale for removal and giving follow-up care instructions. The nurse also assists the health care provider with the removal procedure.

▶ UTERINE FIBROIDS

Uterine fibroids, or leiomyomas, are benign proliferations composed of smooth muscle and fibrous connective tissue in the uterus. Fibroids can occur in the submucous layer, the intramural layer, or the subserous layer of the uterus (Fig. 7.4). They are estrogen-dependent and thus grow rapidly during the childbearing years, when estrogen is plentiful, but they shrink during menopause, when estrogen levels decline. It is believed that these benign tumors develop in up to 50% of all women older than age 30 (Thomason, 2007). Fibroids are the most common indi-

FIGURE 7.4 Submucosal, intramural, and subserosal fibroids.

cation for hysterectomy in the United States. The peak incidence occurs around the age of 45, and they are two to three times more prevalent in African-American women (Verga, 2006).

Etiology

Although the cause of fibroids is unknown, several predisposing factors have been identified, including:

• Age (late reproductive years)
• Genetic predisposition
• African-American ethnicity
• Nulliparity
• Obesity (Alexander et al., 2007)

Therapeutic Management

Treatment depends on the size of the fibroids and the woman's symptoms. There are several options, from watchful waiting to surgery.

Medical Management

The goals of medical therapy are to reduce symptoms and to reduce the tumor size. This can be accomplished with gonadotropin-releasing hormone (GnRH) agonists such as Lupron (leuprolide), Synarel (nafarelin), or Zoladex (goserelin), which induce reversible menopause, or low-dose mifepristone, a progestin antagonist. Both have produced regression and reduced the size of the tumors without surgery, but long-term therapy is expensive and not tolerated by most women. The side effects of GnRH medications include hot flashes, headaches, mood changes, vaginal dryness, musculoskeletal malaise, bone loss, and depression (Thomason, 2007). Long-term mifepristone therapy can result in endometrial hyperplasia, which increases the risk of endometrial malignancy. Once either therapy is stopped, the fibroids typically recur.

Uterine artery embolization (UAE) is an option in which polyvinyl alcohol pellets are injected into selected blood vessels via a catheter to block circulation to the fibroid, causing it to shrink and producing symptom resolution. After treatment, most fibroids are reduced by 50% within 3 months, but they might recur (Edwards et al., 2007). The failure rate is approximately 10% to 15%, and this therapy should not be performed on women desiring to retain their fertility.

Surgical Management

For women with large fibroids or severe menorrhagia, surgery is preferred over medical treatment. Surgical management might involve myomectomy, laser surgery, or hysterectomy.

Myomectomy involves removing the fibroid alone. A myomectomy is performed via laparoscopy, through an abdominal incision, or through a vaginal approach. The advantage is that only the fibroid is removed; fertility is not jeopardized because this procedure leaves the uterine muscle walls intact. Myomectomy relieves symptoms but does not affect the underlying process; thus, fibroids grow back and further treatment will be needed in the future.

Laser surgery (or electrocauterization) involves destroying small fibroids with lasers. Laser therapy can be done using a vaginal approach or laparoscopically. The laser treatment preserves the uterus, but the process may cause scarring and adhesions, thus impairing fertility (Verga, 2006). Fibroids can return after this procedure. Controversy remains as to whether laser treatment weakens the uterine wall and thus may contribute to uterine rupture in the future.

A hysterectomy is the surgical removal of the uterus. After cesarean section, it is the second most frequently performed surgical procedure for women in the United States. Approximately 600,000 hysterectomies are performed annually in the United States (CDC, 2007). The top three conditions associated with hysterectomies are fibroids, endometriosis, and uterine prolapse (CDC, 2007). A hysterectomy to remove fibroids eliminates both the symptoms and the risk of recurrence, but it also terminates the woman's ability to bear children. Three types of hysterectomy surgeries are available: vaginal hysterectomy, laparoscopically assisted vaginal hysterectomy, and abdominal hysterectomy.

In a vaginal hysterectomy, the uterus is removed through an incision in the posterior vagina. Advantages include a shorter hospital stay and recovery time and no abdominal scars. Disadvantages include a limited operating space and poor visualization of other pelvic organs.

In a laparoscopically assisted vaginal hysterectomy, the uterus is removed through a laparoscope, through which structures within the abdomen and pelvis are visualized. Small incisions are made in the abdominal wall to permit the laparoscope to enter the surgical site. Advantages include a better surgical field, less pain, lower cost, and a shorter recovery time. Disadvantages include potential injury to the bladder and the inability to remove enlarged uteruses and scar tissue.

In abdominal hysterectomy, the uterus and other pelvic organs are removed through an incision in the abdomen. This procedure allows the surgeon to visualize all pelvic organs and is typically used when a malignancy is suspected or a very large uterus is present. Disadvantages include the need for general anesthesia, a longer hospital stay and recovery period, more pain, higher cost, and a visible scar on the abdomen.

Nursing Assessment

Nursing assessment for the woman with uterine fibroids includes a thorough health history and physical examination.

Health History and Clinical Manifestations

The history should include questions about the woman's menstrual cycle, including alterations in the menstrual pattern (e.g., pain or pressure, aggravating and alleviating factors), history of infertility, and any history of spontaneous abortion, which might indicate a space-occupying uterine lesion. Ask if any female relatives have had fibroids, as there is a familial predisposition. Assess for clinical manifestations of uterine fibroids. Symptoms of fibroids depend on their size and location and may include:

• Chronic pelvic pain
• Low back pain
• Iron deficiency anemia secondary to bleeding
• Bloating
• Infertility (with large tumors)
• Dysmenorrhea
• Dyspareunia
• Urinary frequency, urgency, incontinence
• Irregular vaginal bleeding (menorrhagia)
• Feeling of heaviness in the pelvic region

Physical Examination and Laboratory and Diagnostic Studies

The bimanual examination performed by the health care provider typically shows an enlarged, irregular uterus. The uterus may be palpable abdominally if the fibroid is very large. Ultrasound may be used to confirm the diagnosis.

Nursing Management

Provide information about surgery so the woman can make an informed decision. Offer a thorough explanation of the

---

BOX 7.2 **Nursing Interventions for a Woman Undergoing a Hysterectomy**

Preoperative Care
- Instruct the patient and her family about the procedure and aftercare.
- Provide interventions to reduce anxiety (due to perceived threats to the woman's self-concept and role functioning) and fear of alteration in body image, complications, and pain. Prepare the woman so she knows what to expect throughout her perioperative experience. Explain postoperative pain management procedures that will be used. Identify the high-risk woman early to reduce her stress.
- Teach turning, deep breathing, and coughing before surgery to prevent postoperative atelectasis and respiratory complications such as pneumonia.
- Encourage the woman to discuss her feelings. Some women equate their femaleness with their reproductive capability, and loss of the uterus could evoke grieving.
- Complete all preoperative orders in a timely manner to allow for rest.

Postoperative Care
- Provide comfort measures.
- Administer analgesics promptly or use a PCA pump.
- Administer antiemetics to control nausea and vomiting per order.
- Change the client's linens and gown frequently to promote hygiene.
- Change the client's position frequently and use pillows for support to promote comfort and pain management.
- Assess the incision, the dressing, and vaginal bleeding and report if bleeding is excessive (soaking perineal pad within an hour).

- Monitor elimination and provide increased fluids and fiber to prevent constipation and straining.
- Encourage ambulation and active range-of-motion exercises when in bed to prevent thrombophlebitis and venous stasis.
- Monitor vital signs to detect early complications.
- Be comfortable discussing sexual concerns with the client.

Discharge Planning
- Advise the client to reduce her activity level to avoid fatigue, which might inhibit healing.
- Advise the client to rest when she is tired and to increase her activity level slowly.
- Educate the client on the need for pelvic rest (nothing in the vagina) for 6 weeks.
- Instruct the client to avoid heavy lifting or straining for about 6 weeks to prevent an increase in intra-abdominal pressure, which could weaken her sutures.
- Teach the client the signs and symptoms of infection.
- Advise the woman to take showers instead of tub baths to reduce the risk for infection.
- Encourage the client to eat a healthy diet with increased intake of fluids to prevent dehydration and fluid and electrolyte imbalance.
- Instruct the client to change her perineal pad frequently to prevent infection.
- Explain and schedule follow-up care appointments as needed.
- Provide information about community resources for support/help.

---

procedure and aftercare (Box 7.2). A woman undergoing a hysterectomy for the treatment of fibroids often needs special care.

▶ GENITAL FISTULAS

Genital fistulas are abnormal openings between a genital tract organ and another organ, such as the urinary tract or the gastrointestinal tract. A fistula can result from a congenital anomaly, surgical complications, Bartholin's gland abscesses, radiation, or malignancy, but the majority of fistulas that occur worldwide are related to obstetric trauma (Husain et al., 2007). During normal labor, the bladder is displaced upward into the abdomen and the anterior vaginal wall, the base of the bladder, and the urethra are compressed between the fetal head and the posterior pubis. When labor is obstructed or prolonged, this unrelieved compression causes ischemia, which causes pressure necrosis and subsequent fistula formation.

Common types of fistulas include:

- Vesicovaginal: communication between the bladder and genital tract
- Urethrovaginal: communication between the urethra and the vagina
- Rectovaginal: communication between the rectum or sigmoid colon and the vagina

The direct consequences of this damage include urinary incontinence and fecal incontinence if the rectum is involved. This tragic condition has plagued women since the beginning of history (Hamilton, Spencer, & Evans, 2007).

Therapeutic Management

Many small fistulas will heal without treatment, but large fistulas often require surgical repair; surgery may be postponed until the edema or inflammation in the surrounding tissues has dissipated. Surgical repair of fistulas is associated with a high success rate if it is done in a timely manner, but larger fistulas and those of long duration have a poorer prognosis (Kriplani et al., 2007).

Nursing Assessment

The history should include questions about any changes in the woman's urinary and bowel patterns. Assess for common signs and symptoms of fistulas, which are related to the type of fistula. If the opening involves the rectum, feces and flatus will leak through the vagina. If it involves the bladder, urine will leak from the vagina. Depending on the location and size of the fistula, the woman may or may not experience discomfort. The health care provider can detect these abnormal openings through inspection and palpation during the pelvic examination. Diagnostic or laboratory tests are generally not ordered once this condition is found.

Nursing Management

Provide guidance and support. Offer information to help the woman learn about her condition and, with appropriate intervention, to improve her quality of life. Begin by making sure the woman understands her anatomy and why she is having such symptoms. Provide a thorough explanation of the treatment options so that she can make an informed decision. Be sensitive to the woman's feeling of shame and fear about her incontinence; these feelings may be why she delayed seeking treatment. Address all of the woman's needs, both physical and emotional.

▶ BARTHOLIN'S CYSTS

A Bartholin's cyst is a swollen, fluid-filled, sac-like structure that results when one of the ducts of the Bartholin's gland becomes blocked. The cyst may become infected and an abscess may develop in the gland. The Bartholin's glands are two mucus-secreting glandular structures with duct openings bilaterally at the base of the labia minora near the opening of the vagina that provide lubrication during sexual arousal. Bartholin's cysts are the most common cystic growths in the vulva, affecting approximately 2% of women at some time in their life (Patil, Sultan, & Thakar, 2007).

Therapeutic Management

Treatment can be conservative or surgical depending on the symptoms, the size of the cyst, and whether it is infected or not. Small asymptomatic cysts do not require treatment. Sitz baths along with analgesics are used to reduce discomfort. Antibiotics are prescribed if the gland is infected. The aim of treatment for a cyst or abscess is to create a fistulous tract from the dilated duct to the outside vulva by incision and drainage (I&D). However, cysts or abscesses tend to return if this option is used.

Other treatment options beyond I&D include placement of a Word catheter to prevent closure and to allow drainage and use of a carbon dioxide laser to remove the cyst. After the Word catheter is inserted, the balloon tip is inflated and it is left in place for 4 to 6 weeks. This procedure is a safe and effective alternative to surgery (Haider et al., 2007). Treatment for a pregnant woman with a Bartholin's cyst depends on the severity of the symptoms and whether an infection is present. Surgery may be delayed until after the woman gives birth if there are no symptoms.

Nursing Assessment

Nursing assessment for the woman with a Bartholin's cyst includes a thorough health history and physical examination and laboratory and diagnostic tests.

Health History

The history should include questions about the woman's sexual practices and protective measures used. Assess for common signs and symptoms of Bartholin's cysts. The woman may be asymptomatic if the cyst is small (less than 5 cm) and not infected. If infection is present, symptoms include varying degrees of pain, especially when walking or sitting; unilateral edema; redness around the gland; and dyspareunia. Extensive inflammation may cause systemic symptoms. Abscess formation occurs when the cystic fluid becomes infected. An abscess usually develops rapidly over a 2- to 3-day period and may spontaneously rupture. A history of sudden relief of pain following profuse discharge is highly suggestive of spontaneous rupture (Schuiling & Likis, 2006).

Physical Examination and Laboratory and Diagnostic Studies

The diagnosis of Bartholin's cysts or abscesses is primarily made during a physical examination when a protruding tender labial mass is located. In women over the age of 40, there is an increased risk of malignancy, accounting for 2% to 7% of all invasive vulvar malignancies (Patil, Sultan, & Thakar, 2007). Cultures of the purulent abscess fluid and of the cervix should be obtained for *Neisseria gonorrhea* and *Chlamydia trachomatis* to rule out a sexually transmitted infection.

Nursing Management

Nurses must be aware of and knowledgeable about vulvar cysts and treatment options. The woman may be aware of a vulvar cyst secondary to the pain or may be unaware of it if it is asymptomatic. A Bartholin's cyst may be an incidental finding during a routine pelvic examination. Explain the cause of the cyst and assist with cultures if needed. Provide reassurance and support.

▶ OVARIAN CYSTS

An **ovarian cyst** is a fluid-filled sac that forms on the ovary (Fig. 7.5). These very common growths are benign 90% of the time and are asymptomatic in many women (Hackley, Kriebs, & Rousseau, 2007). Ovarian cysts occur in 30% of women with regular menses, 50% of women with irregular menses, and 6% of postmenopausal women (Verga, 2006). When the cysts grow large and exert pressure on surrounding structures, women often seek medical help.

Types of Ovarian Cysts

The most common benign ovarian cysts are follicular cysts, corpus luteum (lutein) cysts, theca-lutein cysts, and polycystic ovarian syndrome (PCOS).

Follicular Cysts
Follicular cysts are caused by the failure of the ovarian follicle to rupture at the time of ovulation. Follicular cysts seldom grow larger than 5 cm in diameter; most regress and require no treatment. They can occur at any age but are more common in reproductive-aged women and are rare after menopause. They are detected by vaginal ultrasound.

Corpus Luteum (Lutein) Cysts
A corpus luteum cyst forms when the corpus luteum becomes cystic or hemorrhagic and fails to degenerate after 14 days. These cysts might cause pain and delay the next menstrual period. A pelvic ultrasound helps to make this diagnosis. Typically these cysts appear after ovulation and resolve without intervention.

Theca-Lutein Cysts
Prolonged abnormally high levels of human chorionic gonadotropin (hCG) stimulate the development of theca-lutein cysts. Although rare, these cysts are associated with hydatidiform mole, choriocarcinoma, PCOS, and Clomid therapy.

FIGURE 7.5 Ovarian cyst.

Polycystic Ovarian Syndrome
Polycystic ovary syndrome (PCOS) involves the presence of multiple inactive follicle cysts within the ovary that interfere with ovarian function. It is associated with obesity, hyperinsulinemia, elevated luteinizing hormone levels (linked to ovulation), elevated androgen levels (virilization), hirsutism (male-pattern hair growth), follicular atresia (ovarian growth failure), ovarian growth and cyst formation, anovulation (failure to ovulate), and amenorrhea (absence of menstruation or irregular periods). Recent studies also indicate that PCOS is associated with an increase in the risk of uterine fibroids (Wise et al., 2007). It is the most common endocrine disorder in reproductive-age women, affecting 1 in 15 women in the United States (Panidis & Farmakiotis, 2007).

▶ **Take** NOTE!

Careful attention should be given to this condition because affected women are at increased risk for long-term health problems such as cardiovascular disease, hypertension, dyslipidemia, type 2 diabetes (half of all women), and cancer (endometrial, breast, and ovarian) (Lorenz & Wild, 2007).

Initially PCOS was called Stein-Leventhal syndrome after its researchers, but it is now recognized to be an anabolic syndrome (Vignesh & Mohan, 2007). Its etiology is not clearly understood, but studies suggest a genetic (autosomal-dominant) component (Speroff & Mishell, 2007).

Therapeutic Management

Treatment of ovarian cysts focuses on differentiating a benign cyst from a solid ovarian malignancy. Transvaginal ultrasound is useful in distinguishing fluid-filled cysts from solid masses. Laparoscopy may be needed to remove the cyst, if it is large and pressing on surrounding structures. For smaller cysts, monitoring with repeat ultrasounds every 3 to 6 months might be in order (Helm, 2007). Oral contraceptives are often prescribed to suppress gonadotropin levels, which may help resolve the cysts. Pain medication is also prescribed if needed.

Management of PCOS includes both drug and nondrug therapy, along with lifestyle modifications. Goals of therapy focus on reducing the production and circulating levels of androgens, protecting the endometrium against the effects of unopposed estrogens, supporting lifestyle changes to achieve ideal body weight, lowering the risk of cardiovascular disease, avoiding the effects of hyperinsulinemia on the risk of cardiovascular disease and diabetes, and inducing ovulation to achieve pregnancy if desired (see Evidence-Based Practice 7.2). Treatment modalities for PCOS are highlighted in Box 7.3.

EVIDENCE-BASED PRACTICE 7.2
Are Insulin-Sensitizing Drugs More Effective Than the Combined Oral Contraceptive Pill in Minimizing Hirsutism, Acne, Risk of Diabetes, Cardiovascular Disease, and Endometrial Cancer in PCOS?

● Study

Women with polycystic ovary syndrome (PCOS) have excessive hairiness (hirsutism), irregular periods, and acne. They are also at greater risk of developing diabetes, cardiovascular disease, and endometrial cancer. Insulin-sensitizing drugs (ISDs) have recently been advocated as a safer and more effective long-term treatment than the oral contraceptive pill (OCP) in women with PCOS. A study was conducted to assess the effectiveness and safety of ISDs versus the OCP (alone or in combination) in improving clinical, hormonal, and metabolic features of PCOS.

▲ Findings

In women with PCOS, the OCP is more effective than ISDs in improving menstrual pattern and reducing serum androgen (male hormone) levels, whereas the ISD metformin is more effective than the OCP in reducing fasting insulin levels and not increasing triglyceride levels. There is insufficient

evidence in favor of either metformin or the OCP in treating hirsutism or acne, or in preventing diabetes, heart disease, or endometrial cancer. The limited data available do not support the preferential use of either ISDs or the OCP (alone or in combination) for the long-term medical management of PCOS.

■ Nursing Implications

Oral contraceptives have been the mainstay of long-term management of PCOS by decreasing LH and FSH secretion and ovarian production of androgens to reduce symptoms. This study compared the ISD metformin to the traditional therapy without conclusive results. PCOS is associated with increased insulin resistance and increased unbound androgen levels. Since this study was inconclusive, nurses can continue to counsel women to improve their lifestyle (e.g., diet, exercise, weight management) to avoid health problems later in life related to diabetes and heart disease.

Costello, M., Shrestha, B., Eden, J., Sjoblom, P., & Johnson, N. (2007). Insulin-sensitizing drugs versus the combined oral contraceptive pill for hirsutism, acne and risk of diabetes, cardiovascular disease, and endometrial cancer in polycystic ovary syndrome. *Cochrane Database of Systematic Reviews* 2007, Issue 1. Art. No.: CD005552. DOI: 10.1002/14651858.CD005552.pub2.

Nursing Assessment

Nursing assessment for the woman with PCOS includes a thorough health history and physical examination and laboratory and diagnostic tests.

Health History

The history should include questions about the woman's symptoms, including onset, location, frequency, quality,

---

BOX 7.3 Treatment Modalities for PCOS

- Oral contraceptives to treat menstrual irregularities and acne
- Mechanical hair removal (shaving, waxing, plucking, or electrolysis) to treat hirsutism
- Glucophage (metformin), which improves insulin uptake by fat and muscle cells, to treat hyperinsulinemia; thiazolinediones (Actos, Avandia) to decrease insulin resistance
- Ovulation induction agents (Clomid) to treat infertility
- Lifestyle changes (e.g., weight loss; exercise; balanced, low-fat diet)
- Referral to support groups to help improve emotional state and build self-esteem

Sources: ACOG, 2006; Dronavalli & Ehrmann, 2007; Barron & Falsetti, 2008.

---

intensity, and aggravating and alleviating factors of her discomfort. Note the last menstrual period and whether or not her cycles are regular. Ask about her overall general health and any changes recently noticed, such as a change in abdominal girth without a concomitant weight gain.

Assess for common signs and symptoms of ovarian cysts. Findings might include:

- Hirsutism (face and chin, upper lip, areola, lower abdomen and perineum)
- Alopecia (frontal region and crown of head)
- Virilization (clitoral hypertrophy, deepening of voice, increased muscle mass, breast atrophy, male-pattern baldness)
- Menstrual irregularity and infertility (menorrhagia, anovulation)
- Polycystic ovaries (12 or more follicles on ovaries)
- Obesity (occurs in more than 50% of women with PCOS; occurs in abdominal region, with an increase in the waist–hip ratio)
- Insulin resistance (chronic hyperinsulinemia leads to type 2 diabetes)
- Metabolic syndrome (elevated cholesterol, triglycerides, low-density lipoprotein; risk of cardiovascular disease)
- Increased risk for endometrial cancer, ovarian cancer, breast cancer
- Psychological impact (depression, frustration, anxiety, eating disorders)
- Acne (face and shoulders) (Krantz, 2007)

Physical Examination and Laboratory and Diagnostic Studies

The physical examination includes inspection, auscultation, and palpation of the abdomen because large ovarian masses may cause visible changes in the abdomen. A complete pelvic examination is performed to assess the location, size, shape, texture, mobility, and tenderness of any palpable mass.

Diagnostic tests include a pregnancy test to rule out ectopic pregnancy. Gonorrhea and chlamydia testing is warranted if an ovarian abscess is suspected. An ultrasound may be ordered to differentiate between functional or simple ovarian cysts and a solid tumor. Additional tests may be performed depending on the findings.

Remember Liz, the client with irregular menses, facial hair, and acne? Her glucose level is elevated, multiple cysts were felt on her ovaries during the pelvic examination, and laboratory tests found elevated lipid and lipoprotein levels. What education should the nurse provide Liz regarding her PCOS diagnosis? What medications might be prescribed to address her abnormal laboratory values?

Nursing Management

Nursing care should include education about the condition, treatment options, diagnostic test arrangements, and referral for surgery if needed. Provide support and reassurance during the diagnostic period to allay anxiety in the client and her family. Reassure the woman that the majority of ovarian cysts are benign, but regardless stress the importance of follow-up care. Listen to the woman's concerns about her appearance, infertility, and facial hair growth. Offer suggestions to help the woman feel better about herself and her health.

Nurses can have a positive impact on women with PCOS through counseling and education. Provide support for women dealing with negative self-image secondary to the physical manifestations of PCOS. Through education, help the woman understand the syndrome and its associated risk factors to prevent long-term health problems. Encourage the woman to make positive lifestyle changes. Make community referrals to local support groups to help the woman build her coping skills.

Liz returns to the clinic a month later for re-evaluation of her PCOS. She has been taking metformin to reduce her insulin resistance and has followed her exercise regimen and reduced her caloric intake to lose weight, but she still complains about her facial hair and acne. What interventions might be helpful to address this problem? What medication might also be prescribed to regularize her menses and relieve the hirsutism?

■■■ Key Concepts

- Pelvic support disorders such as pelvic organ prolapse and urinary and fecal incontinence are prevalent conditions in aging women. They cause significant physical and psychological morbidity, with obvious detriment to women's social interactions, emotional well-being, and overall quality of life.
- The four most common types of genital prolapse are cystocele, rectocele, enterocele, and uterine prolapse.
- The purpose of pelvic-floor exercises is to increase the muscle volume, which will result in a stronger muscular contraction. Kegel exercises might limit the progression of mild prolapse and alleviate mild prolapse symptoms, including low back pain and pelvic pressure.
- Urinary incontinence is the involuntary loss of urine sufficient enough to be a social or hygiene problem. It affects approximately 18 million people in the United States, about 11 million of them women.
- The three most common types of incontinence are urge incontinence (overactive bladder caused by detrusor muscle contractions), stress incontinence (inadequate urinary sphincter function), and mixed incontinence (involves both stress and urge incontinence).
- The most common benign growths of the reproductive tract include cervical, endocervical, and endometrial polyps; uterine fibroids (leiomyomas); and ovarian cysts.
- PCOS involves the presence of multiple inactive follicle cysts within the ovary that interfere with ovarian function. Hyperandrogenism, insulin resistance, and chronic anovulation characterize PCOS. Careful attention should be given to this condition because women with it are at increased risk for long-term health problems such as cardiovascular disease, hypertension, dyslipidemia, type 2 diabetes, and cancer (endometrial, breast, and ovarian).

REFERENCES

Alexander, L. L., LaRosa, J. H., Bader, H., & Garfield, S. (2007). *New dimensions in women's health* (4th ed.). Sudbury, MA: Jones and Bartlett Publishers.

American College of Obstetrics and Gynecology (ACOG). (2006). ACOG Committee opinion number 351. The overweight adolescent: Prevention, treatment, and obstetric-gynecologic implications. *Obstetrics & Gynecology, 108*(5), 1337–1348.

American College of Obstetrics and Gynecology (ACOG). (2007). Pelvic organ prolapse. *Obstetrics & Gynecology, 109*(2), 461–473.

Barron, A. M., & Falsetti, D. (2008). Polycystic ovary syndrome in adolescents. *Advance for Nurse Practitioners, 16*(3), 49–54.

Bartoletti, R. (2007) Pelvic organ prolapse: A challenge for the urologist. *European Urology, 51*(4), 884–886.

Berzuk, K. (2007). A strong pelvic floor: How nurses can spread the word. *Nursing for Women's Health, 11*(1), 54–61.

Centers for Disease Control and Prevention (CDC). (2007). *Women's reproductive health: Hysterectomy.* CDC Reproductive Health. [Online] Available at: http://www.cdc.gov/reproductivehealth/WomensRH/Hysterectomy.htm.

Dronavalli, S., & Ehrmann, D. A. (2007). Pharmacologic therapy of polycystic ovary syndrome. *Clinical Obstetrics & Gynecology, 50*(1), 244–254.

Dudek, S. G. (2006). *Nutrition essentials for nursing practice* (5th ed.). Philadelphia: Lippincott Williams & Wilkins.

Edwards, R. D., Moss, J. G., Lumsden, M. A., Wu, O., & Murray, L. S. (2007). Uterine-artery embolization versus surgery for symptomatic uterine fibroids. *New England Journal of Medicine, 356*(4), 360–370.

Hackley, B., Kriebs, J. M., & Rousseau, M. E. (2007). *Primary care of women: A guide for midwives and women's health providers.* Sudbury, MA: Jones and Bartlett Publishers.

Haider, Z., Condous, G., Kirk, E., Mukri, F., & Bourne, T. (2007). The simple outpatient management of Bartholin's abscess using the Word catheter: A preliminary study. *Australian & New Zealand Journal of Obstetrics & Gynecology, 47*(2), 137–140.

Hamilton, S., Spencer, C., & Evans, A. (2007). Vagino-rectal fistula caused by Bartholin's abscess. *Journal of Obstetrics & Gynecology, 27*(3), 325–326.

Helm, C. W. (2007). Ovarian cysts. *eMedicine.* Available at: http://emedicine.com/med/topic1699.htm.

Hines, S. H., & Miller, J. M. (2006). Urinary incontinence. In K. D. Schuiling & F. E. Likis (Eds.), *Women's gynecologic health* (Chapter 24; pp. 635–658). Sudbury, MA: Jones and Bartlett Publishers.

Husain, A., Johnson, K., Glowacki, C. A., Osias, J., Wheeless, C. R., Asrat, K., Ghebrekidan, A., & Polam, M. L. (2007). Surgical management of complex obstetric fistulas in Eritrea. *Journal of Women's Health, 14*(9), 839–844.

Jelovsek, J. E., Maher, C., & Barber, M. D. (2007). Pelvic organ prolapse. *Lancet, 369*(9566), 1027–1038.

Kaminski, P., & Hoffman, M. (2007). Benign cervical lesions. *eMedicine.* Available at: http://www.emedicine.com/med/topic3297.htm.

Krantz, C. A. (2007). Amenorrhea. In R. E. Rakel & E. T. Bope (Eds.), *Conn's current therapy 2007* (Section 16, pp. 1235–1238). Philadelphia: Saunders Elsevier.

Kriplani, A., Agarwai, N., Gupta, A., & Bhatla, N. (2007). Observations on etiology and management of genital fistulas. *Archives of Gynecology & Obstetrics, 271*(1), 14–18.

Lazarou, G., & Scotti, R. J. (2007). Uterine prolapse. *eMedicine.* Available at: http://emedicine.com/med/topic3291.htm.

Lemack, G. E. (2007). Incontinence: Helping women stay in control. *Cortlandt Forum, 20*(1), 53–54.

Lorenz, L. B., & Wild, R. A. (2007). Polycystic ovarian syndrome: An evidence-based approach to evaluation and management of diabetes and cardiovascular risks for today's clinician. *Clinical Obstetrics & Gynecology, 50*(1), 226–243.

Luft, J. (2006). Pelvic organ prolapse: Current state of knowledge about this common condition. *Journal for Nurse Practitioners, 2*(3), 170–177.

Newman, D. (2007). Nonsurgical solutions for pelvic organ prolapse. *Nursing Spectrum, 16*(1), 12–13.

Ogundele, O., & Silverberg, M. A. (2007). Urinary incontinence. *eMedicine.* Available at: http://www.emedicine.com/emerg/topic791.htm.

Panidis, D., & Farmakiotis, D. (2007). Treatment of infertility in the polycystic ovary syndrome. *New England of Medicine, 356*(19), 1999–2001.

Patil, S., Sultan, A. H., & Thakar, R. (2007). Bartholin's cysts and abscesses. *Journal of Obstetrics & Gynecology, 27*(3), 241–245.

Reena, C., Kekre, A. N., & Kekre, N. (2007). Occult stress incontinence in women with pelvic organ prolapse. *International Journal of Gynecology & Obstetrics, 97*(1), 31–34.

Schuiling, K. D., & Likis, F. E. (2006). *Women's gynecologic health.* Sudbury, MA: Jones and Bartlett Publishers.

Selby, M. (2006). Dealing with incontinence. *Practice Nurse, 32*(8), 33–38.

Smith, D. A. (2007). Pelvic organ prolapse. *Advance for Nurse Practitioners, 15*(8), 39–42.

Speroff, L., & Fritz, M. A. (2005). *Clinical gynecologic endocrinology and infertility* (7th ed.). Philadelphia: Lippincott Williams & Wilkins.

Speroff, L., & Mishell, D. R. (2007). Polycystic ovary syndrome: Management and contraception. *Dialogues in Contraception, 11*(1), 5–10.

Thomason, P. (2007). Leiomyoma, uterus (fibroid). *eMedicine.* Available at: http://www.emedicine.com/radio/topic777.htm.

Verga, C. A. (2006). Benign gynecologic conditions. In K. D. Schuiling & F. E. Likis (Eds.), *Women's gynecologic health* (Chapter 22, pp. 561–594). Sudbury, MA: Jones and Bartlett Publishers.

Vignesh, J. P., & Mohan, V. (2007). Polycystic ovary syndrome: A component of metabolic syndrome? *Journal of Postgraduate Medicine, 53*(2), 128–134.

Wallace, J. D. (2007). Woman with incontinence and a history of childhood sexual abuse. *Urologic Nursing, 27*(1), 38–39.

Wise, L. A., Palmer, J. R., Stewart, E. A., & Rosenberg, L. (2007). Polycystic ovary syndrome and the risk of uterine leiomyomata. *Fertility and Sterility, 87*(5), 1108–1115.

WEBSITES

American Cancer Society: (800)-ACS-2345, www.cancer.org

American College of Obstetricians and Gynecologists: (202) 863-2518, www.acog.org

American Urological Association: (410) 727-1100, www.auanet.org

Fibroid Treatment Collective: (310) 794-6645, www.fibroid.org

Hysterectomy Educational Resource and Services (HERS): (215) 667-7757, www.ccon.com/hers

National Association for Continence: (800) 252-3337, www.nafc.org

National Women's Health Information Center: (800) 994-9662, www.4women.gov

Polycystic Ovarian Syndrome Association: www.pcossupport.org

Sexuality Information and Education Council of the United States: (212) 819-9770, www.siecus.org

CHAPTER WORKSHEET

MULTIPLE CHOICE QUESTIONS

1. When you are interviewing a patient with uterine fibroids, what subjective data would you expect to find in her history?

   a. Cyclic migraine headaches

   b. Urinary urgency

   c. Chronic pelvic pain

   d. Chronic constipation

2. Treatment options available for women with pelvic organ prolapse are:

   a. Pessaries and Kegel exercises

   b. External pelvic fixation devices

   c. Weight gain and yoga

   d. Firm panty-and-girdle garments

3. Which of the following dietary and lifestyle modifications might the nurse recommend to help prevent pelvic relaxation as women age?

   a. Eat a high-fiber diet to avoid constipation and straining.

   b. Avoid sitting for long periods; get up and walk around frequently.

   c. Limit the amount of exercise to prevent over-developing muscles.

   d. Space children a year apart to reduce wear and tear on the uterus.

4. Women with polycystic ovarian syndrome (PCOS) are at increased risk for developing which of the following long-term health problems?

   a. Osteoporosis

   b. Lupus

   c. Type 2 diabetes

   d. Migraine headaches

5. Side effects experienced by women taking gonadotropin-releasing hormone (GnRH) agonists for the treatment of fibroids closely resemble those of:

   a. Osteoporosis

   b. Osteoarthritis

   c. Depression

   d. Menopause

CRITICAL THINKING EXERCISE

1. Faith, a 42-year-old multiparous woman, presents to the women's health clinic complaining of pelvic pain, menorrhagia, and vaginal discharge. She says she has been having these problems for several months. On examination, her uterus is enlarged and irregular in shape. Her blood studies reveal anemia.

   a. What condition might Faith have, based on her symptoms?

   b. What treatment options are available to address this condition?

   c. What educational interventions should the nurse discuss with Faith?

STUDY ACTIVITIES

1. Prepare an educational session to teach women how to do Kegel exercises to prevent stress incontinence and pelvic floor relaxation.

2. In a small group, discuss the personal, social, and sexual issues that might affect a woman with pelvic organ prolapse. How might these issues affect her socialization? How might a support group help?

3. List the symptoms that a woman with uterine fibroids might have. Discuss how these symptoms might mimic a more frightening condition and why the woman might delay seeking treatment.

4. A bladder that herniates into the vagina is a
   _____.

5. A rectum that herniates into the vagina is a
   _____.

CANCERS OF THE FEMALE REPRODUCTIVE TRACT

KEY TERMS

cervical cancer
cervical dysplasia
colposcopy
cone biopsy

cryotherapy
endometrial cancer
human papillomavirus
ovarian cancer

Papanicolaou (Pap) test
vaginal cancer
vulvar cancer

LEARNING OBJECTIVES

Upon completion of the chapter, the learner will be able to:

1. Define the key terms in the chapter.
2. Identify the major modifiable risk factors for reproductive tract cancers.
3. Discuss the risk factors, screening methods, and treatment modalities for cancers of the female reproductive tract.
4. Outline the nursing management needed for the most common malignant reproductive tract cancers in women.
5. Discuss lifestyle changes and health screenings that can reduce the risk of or prevent reproductive tract cancers.
6. List the community resources available for a woman undergoing surgery for cancer of the reproductive tract.
7. Explain the psychological distress felt by women diagnosed with cancer, and outline information that can help them to cope.

Carmella is an obese, 55-year-old woman who presents to her woman's health care provider with vaginal bleeding. She has been through menopause and wonders why she is having a period again. Her history includes infertility and hypertension. Three years ago she had a mastectomy for breast cancer, and she has been taking tamoxifen (Nolvadex) to prevent recurrent breast cancer since her surgery. What risk factors in Carmella's history might predispose her to a reproductive tract cancer? What additional information is needed to make a diagnosis?

The word "cancer" can strike fear into anyone who hears it. But when it involves a reproductive organ, this fear is often magnified.

Cancer is the second leading cause of death for women in the United States, surpassed only by cardiovascular disease (Centers for Disease Control and Prevention [CDC], 2007b). Cardiovascular disease is and should continue to be a major focus of efforts in women's health. However, this should not overshadow the fact that many women between the ages of 35 and 74 are developing and dying of cancer (National Cancer Institute [NCI], 2007a). Women have a one-in-three lifetime risk of developing cancer, and one out of every four deaths is from cancer (Alexander et al., 2007). African-American women have the highest death rates from both heart disease and cancer (CDC, 2007b). According to the American Cancer Society (2008), it is estimated that over 39,000 new cases of uterine cancer (6% of all cancers) and over 22, 000 cases of ovarian cancer (3% of all cancers) will be diagnosed in 2007, with the number of estimated deaths to be over 7,000 and 15,000 respectively.

It has been estimated that in the United States half of all premature deaths, one third of acute disabilities, and one half of chronic disabilities are preventable (NCI, 2007a). Nurses need to focus their energies on screening, education, and early detection to reduce these numbers. Because cancer risk is strongly associated with lifestyle and behavior, screening programs are of particular importance for early detection. There is evidence that prevention and early detection have reduced cancer mortality rates and prevented reproductive cancers (CDC, 2007b).

This chapter begins with a nursing process overview of the care of women with reproductive cancer. It then describes selected cancers of the reproductive system—ovarian, endometrial, cervical, vaginal, and vulvar cancer. The chapter discusses the nurse's role through diagnosis, intervention, and follow-up care. Cancer management requires a multidisciplinary approach, including specialists in surgical, medical, and radiation oncology. The nurse can provide guidance and support to the client as she finds her way through the health care maze.

NURSING PROCESS OVERVIEW FOR THE WOMAN WITH CANCER OF THE REPRODUCTIVE TRACT

The word "cancer" is laden with fear and dread. These feelings may be worsened when the cancer involves a woman's reproductive tract. The diagnosis of a reproductive tract cancer can have a profound impact on a woman's sexuality because it affects the very core of her identity as a female. The loss of the reproductive body part as well as the possible loss of childbearing ability can have a significant effect on women and their partners. Nurses need to remember this impact when counseling women and their partners about cancer treatment and side effects and changes in gender roles and sexuality.

When a woman is first diagnosed with a reproductive tract cancer, two primary needs arise: information and emotional support. When the diagnosis is made, the woman typically has many questions, such as, "What is going to happen to me?", "How will this change my life?," and "Will I survive?" Nurses can play a major role in helping women find the answers to their questions and directing them to the resources they need. Two reliable sources of general cancer information are the National Cancer Institute (NCI) and the American Cancer Society (ACS). They can be reached via the Internet or by phone.

The nurse also plays a key role in offering emotional support, determining appropriate sources of support, and helping the woman use effective coping strategies. Many research studies have found that social support from the woman's family, friends, and coworkers is one of the strongest predictors of how well she will cope (Fieler & Henry, 2007). Women without a social support network may need a social work referral or may need to be guided toward support groups to receive the emotional support they need.

In addition, cancer clients have a strong need for hope. Strategies for inspiring hope may include active listening, touch, presence, and helping clients overcome communication barriers. Often it is not what nurses say or do but just their presence that counts.

Assessment

Assessment of a woman with cancer of the reproductive tract involves a thorough history and physical examination. In addition, various laboratory and diagnostic tests may be done to evaluate for a malignancy.

Health History and Physical Examination

Interview the woman carefully to determine any current or past factors that might increase her risk of cancer, such as early menarche, late menopause, sexually transmitted infections, use of hormonal agents, or infertility. Find out if the woman has a family history of cancer. Be thorough in obtaining the woman's past medical history, especially her reproductive, obstetric, and gynecologic history. Ask about her lifestyle and behaviors, including risky behaviors such as engaging in unprotected sexual intercourse or sexual intercourse with multiple partners. Find out if she has had routine or recommended screening procedures.

Ask if the woman has had any symptoms, such as abnormal vaginal bleeding or discharge or vaginal discomfort. Often the symptoms of cancer are vague and nonspecific and the woman may attribute them to another problem, such as aging, stress, or improper diet.

Perform a complete physical examination, including a review of body systems and a pelvic examination. Observe for lesions or masses in the perineal area. Note any masses when palpating the abdomen or when performing the pelvic examination.

Laboratory and Diagnostic Testing

Some of the laboratory and diagnostic tests used to help diagnose cancer of the reproductive tract are discussed in Common Laboratory and Diagnostic Tests 8.1.

Nursing Diagnoses and Related Interventions

Upon completion of a thorough assessment, the nurse might identify several nursing diagnoses, including:

- Deficient knowledge
- Disturbed body image
- Anxiety
- Fear
- Pain

Nursing goals, interventions, and evaluation for the woman with a reproductive cancer are based on the nursing diagnoses. Nursing Care Plan 8.1 may be used as a guide in planning nursing care for the woman with a reproductive cancer. It should be individualized based on the woman's symptoms and needs.

Nurses have traditionally served as advocates in the health care arena and should continue to be on the forefront of health education and diagnosis, acting as leaders in the fight against cancer. Over a half-million women in the United States will be diagnosed with cancer this year alone, and more than half will die of it. The public needs to know that not only are these deaths preventable, but many of the cancers themselves are preventable. Nurses need to work to improve the availability and quality of cancer-screening services, making them accessible to underserved and socioeconomically disadvantaged clients. Through a unified effort by health care professionals, health policy experts, government agencies, health insurance companies, the

COMMON LABORATORY TESTS 8.1

Test	Explanation	Indications	Nursing Implications
Clinical breast examination	Assessment of the breast for abnormal findings; patient may discover lump herself; high-risk history for breast cancer	Identifies palpable mass, skin change, inverted nipple, or unresolved rash	• Educate client to perform breast self-examination and report any abnormalities. • Reinforce need for frequent clinical breast examinations if risk factors are present.
Mammography	Screening modality for breast cancer or any distortion in breast tissue architecture	Detects calcifications, densities, and nonpalpable cancer lesions	Stress importance of annual mammograms for all women after the age of 40 or 50, depending on their risk history.
Pap smear	Cervical cytology screening to diagnose cervical cancers	Aids in detecting abnormal cells of the cervix (from squamocolumnar junction of the cervix; most cervical cancers arise here)	Encourage all sexually active women to receive an annual pelvic examination, including a Pap smear, to promote early detection of cervical cancer.
Transvaginal ultrasound	Screening for pelvic pathology to assist in diagnosing endometrial cancers	Allows measurement of endometrial thickness to determine if endometrial biopsy is needed for postmenopausal bleeding	• Review the risk factors for the development of endometrial cancer and reason for this screening test. • Assist in preparing the patient for this examination.
CA-125	Nonspecific blood test used as a tumor marker	Elevation of marker suggests malignancy but is not specific to ovarian cancer.	• Review risk factors for ovarian cancer and explain that a series of diagnostic tests may be performed (transvaginal ultrasound, CT scan, CA-125) to assist in the diagnosis and treatment plan. • Elevated marker levels are not specific to ovarian cancer; they can be elevated in other types of cancer.

Nursing Care Plan 8.1

OVERVIEW OF A WOMAN WITH A REPRODUCTIVE TRACT CANCER

Molly, a thin 28-year-old woman, comes to the free health clinic complaining of a thin, watery vaginal discharge and spotting after sex. She says she is homeless and has lived "on the streets" for years. Molly says she has had multiple sex partners to pay for her food and cigarettes. She had an abnormal Pap smear "a while back" but didn't return to the clinic for follow-up. She hopes nothing "bad" is wrong with her because she just found a job that will allow her to get off the streets. "I'm worried that I won't be the same if there is something wrong. I don't know what I'd do if there is a problem," she tells you. Cervical cancer is suspected.

NURSING DIAGNOSIS: Anxiety related to uncertainty of diagnosis, possible diagnosis of cancer, and eventual outcome as evidenced by client's report of signs and symptoms, statements of being worried and not knowing what she would do

Outcome Identification and Evaluation
Client will demonstrate measures to cope with anxiety *as evidenced by statements acknowledging anxiety, use of positive coping strategies, and verbalization that anxiety has decreased.*

Interventions: Reducing Anxiety
- Encourage client to express her feelings and concerns *to reduce her anxiety and to determine appropriate interventions.*
- Assess the meaning of the diagnosis to the client, clarify misconceptions, and provide reliable, realistic information *to enhance her understanding of her condition, subsequently reducing her anxiety.*
- Assess client's psychological status *to determine degree of emotional distress related to diagnosis and treatment options.*
- Identify and address verbalized concerns, providing information about what to expect *to decrease uncertainty about the unknown.*
- Assess the client's use of coping mechanisms in the past and their effectiveness *to foster use of positive strategies.*
- Teach client about early signs of anxiety and help her recognize them (e.g., fast heartbeat, sweating, or feeling flushed) *to minimize escalation of anxiety.*
- Provide positive reinforcement that the client's condition can be managed *to relieve her anxiety.*

NURSING DIAGNOSIS: Deficient knowledge related to diagnosis, prevention strategies, disease course, and treatment as evidenced by client's statements about hoping nothing bad is wrong, lack of follow-up for previous abnormal Pap test, and high-risk behaviors

Outcome Identification and Evaluation
Client will demonstrate understanding of diagnosis, *as evidenced by making health-promoting lifestyle choices, verbalizing appropriate health care practices, describing condition once diagnosed, and adhering to measures to comply with therapy.*

Interventions: Providing Client Teaching
- Assess client's current knowledge about her diagnosis and proposed therapeutic regimen *to establish a baseline from which to develop a teaching plan.*
- Review contributing factors associated with development of reproductive tract cancer, including lifestyle behaviors, *to foster an understanding of the etiology of cervical cancer.*
- Review information about treatments and procedures and recommendations for healthy lifestyle, obtaining feedback frequently *to validate adequate understanding of instructions.*
- Discuss strategies, including using condoms and limiting the number of sexual partners, *to reduce the risk of transmission of STIs,* including human papillomavirus (HPV), which is associated with cervical cancer.
- Encourage client to obtain prompt treatment of any vaginal or cervical infections *to minimize the risk for cervical cancer.*
- Urge the client to have an annual Pap smear *to allow screening and early detection.*
- Describe the treatment measures used *to provide client with knowledge of what may be necessary.*
- Provide written material with pictures *to allow for client review and help her visualize what is occurring in her body.*
- Inform client about available community resources and make appropriate referrals as needed *to provide additional education and support.*
- Document details of teaching and learning *to allow for continuity of care and further education, if needed.*

Nursing Care Plan 8.1 (continued)

NURSING DIAGNOSIS: Disturbed body image related to suspected reproductive tract cancer and impact on client's sexuality and sense of self as evidenced by statement of being worried about not being the same

Outcome Identification and Evaluation
Client will verbalize or demonstrate a positive self-esteem in relation to body image as evidenced by positive statements about self, sexuality, and participation in activities with others.

Interventions: Promoting Healthy Body Image
* Assess client's use of self-criticism *to determine client's current state of coping and adjustment.*
* Determine if the client's change in body image has contributed to social isolation *to provide a direction for care.*
* Provide opportunities for client to explore her feelings related to issues of sexuality, including past behaviors that may have placed her at risk, *to minimize feelings of guilt about her condition.*
* Acknowledge the client's feelings about possible changes in her body and sexuality and her illness *to foster trust and allow client to ventilate feelings and concerns.*
* Facilitate contact with other clients with the same type of cancer *to promote sharing of feelings and decrease feelings of isolation.*
* Initiate referrals for counseling and community support groups as necessary *to assist client in gaining a positive image of herself.*

media, educational institutions, and women themselves, along with consistency and continuity, nurses can offer quality care to all women with cancer.

Educating to Prevent Cancer
Nurses need to provide clients with information to help prevent disease and enhance quality of life. Educate women about the importance of consistent and timely screenings to identify cancer early. Emphasize the importance of having an annual pelvic examination. Also stress the need for follow-up screenings as recommended. Provide clients with information if further diagnostic testing is required.

Nurses also play a key role in promoting cancer awareness, prevention, and control. Advocate to improve the availability of cancer-screening services and work to provide public education about risk factors for cancer.

Nurses can be instrumental in helping women to identify and change behaviors that put them at risk for various reproductive tract cancers (Teaching Guidelines 8.1). Do not limit your interventions to providing preventive education only: inform women about the consequences of doing nothing about their conditions and what the long-range outcomes might be without treatment. For example, stress the importance of visiting a health care professional if certain signs and symptoms appear:

* Blood in a bowel movement
* Unusual vaginal discharge or chronic vulvar itching
* Persistent abdominal bloating or constipation
* Irregular vaginal bleeding
* Persistent low backache not related to standing
* Elevated or discolored vulvar lesions
* Bleeding after menopause
* Pain or bleeding after sexual intercourse

Teaching the Client About Her Diagnosis
Provide information about tests that may be required to confirm or rule out the diagnosis. Review with the woman what she has been told about her diagnosis and her understanding of her condition. It is not unusual for the woman to hear the diagnosis and then become overwhelmed by the thought of cancer, blocking out whatever is said after

---

TEACHING GUIDELINES 8.1

Reducing Your Risk for Cancer

* Don't smoke.
* Drink alcohol only in moderation (no more than one drink daily).
* Be physically active daily.
* Eat a healthy diet.
* Stay current with immunizations.
* Reach and maintain a healthy weight.
* Take preventive medicines if needed.
* Get recommended screening tests:
  * Body mass index (BMI) to identify obesity
  * Mammogram every 1 to 2 years starting at age 40
  * Pap smear every 1 to 3 years if sexually active, between the ages of 21 and 65
  * Cholesterol checked annually starting at age 45
  * Blood pressure checked at least every 2 years
  * Diabetes test if hypertensive or hypercholesterolemic
  * Check for sexually transmitted infections (STIs) if sexually active

Sources: AHRQ, 2007; Mayo Clinic, 2008; WHO, 2008.

that. Answer any questions she may have. Go slowly and repeat the information as necessary. Use written materials to explain and reinforce the teaching. Provide information about her condition and recommended therapies. For example, if a client is undergoing surgery, discuss postoperative issues such as incision care, pain, and activity level. Instruct the client on health maintenance activities after treatment, and inform her and her family about available support resources.

Providing Emotional Support

Once the diagnosis is made, provide the woman and her family with emotional support. Validate the client's feelings and provide realistic hope, using a nonjudgmental approach and therapeutic communication skills during all interactions. Individualize the care based on the client's cultural traditions and beliefs.

Ensuring Culturally Competent Cancer Care

Cultural diversity in America is increasing, and as diverse cultures interact, conflicts inevitably ensue. These conflicts can affect health care outcomes. Providing culturally competent cancer care can improve outcomes and decrease disparities in care. Work to develop cultural competence by learning about and showing respect for all cultures. Be aware of the client's cultural background, religion, migration history, degree of acculturation, living conditions, educational level, and legal status, because each of these factors can affect the client's understanding of her diagnosis and the eventual outcome (Jenko & Moffitt, 2006).

In some cultures, sharing news of a serious illness like cancer is considered disrespectful and impolite. For example, some Europeans view such sharing as inhumane; the Asian culture views a cancer diagnosis as unnecessarily cruel. The Chinese, out of respect for aging family members, withhold discussions of serious illness to avoid causing unnecessary anxieties (Surbone, 2006). Integrate this knowledge in your care to ensure a culturally competent approach.

▶ **Take** NOTE!

When a diagnosis of cancer is made, assessing an individual's strengths and weaknesses from a cultural perspective will help the nurse to provide culturally competent care.

As life becomes increasingly multilingual, multicultural, and multi-faith, learning about clients' values and cultural beliefs becomes challenging. Be willing to learn about client preferences; doing so promotes caring and nurturing.

Supporting the Pregnant Woman With Cancer

Theoretically, changes in the mother's immune system during pregnancy can increase the risk of malignancy because cell-mediated immunity, which is suppressed in pregnant women, normally protects against cancerous tumors (Blackburn, 2007). Some research has hinted at an increased rate of progression and decreased survival times in women who develop breast and cervical cancer and then become pregnant, but this generally has not been validated by research studies.

Ovarian cancer during pregnancy is rare because the disease typically occurs in older women. Because most pregnant women receive frequent medical care, including pelvic examinations, most ovarian cancers in pregnant women are found at early stages; this carries a good prognosis for both the mother and the newborn (Machado et al., 2007). Since routine screening for endometrial cancer is currently not recommended in the general population, few cases would be detected in the relatively young pregnant population (Sonoda & Barakat, 2006). Cervical cancer is more common in the pregnant population than other reproductive malignancies, and it can affect the woman's health status and the pregnancy.

Women diagnosed with any malignancy during pregnancy must confront the reality of the disease and its impact on their future fertility and live with the risk of recurrence (Roberts, Rezai, & Edmondson, 2007). The wishes of the pregnant woman and her family are of paramount importance when making decisions about continuing the pregnancy and undergoing cancer treatment. Some women will decide to terminate the pregnancy for the sake of their own health; others will undergo treatment during the pregnancy to preserve the life of the unborn child. Regardless of the woman's decision, provide support and education during treatment, birth, and beyond.

Ovarian Cancer

Ovarian cancer is malignant neoplastic growth of the ovary (Fig. 8.1). It is the eighth most common cancer among women and the fifth most common cause of cancer deaths for women in the United States. It accounts for more deaths than any other cancer of the reproductive system (ACS, 2007c). The ACS estimates that about 23,000 new cases of ovarian cancer will be diagnosed in the United States during 2007 and 15,000 deaths will occur. A woman's risk of getting ovarian cancer during her lifetime is 1.5%, or about 1 in 67. About 76% of women with ovarian cancer survive 1 year after diagnosis; only 45% survive longer than 5 years (ACS, 2007c). Older women are at highest risk. Ovarian cancer occurs most frequently in women between 55 and 75 years of age, and approximately 25% of ovarian cancer deaths occur in women between 35 and 54 years old (ACS, 2007c).

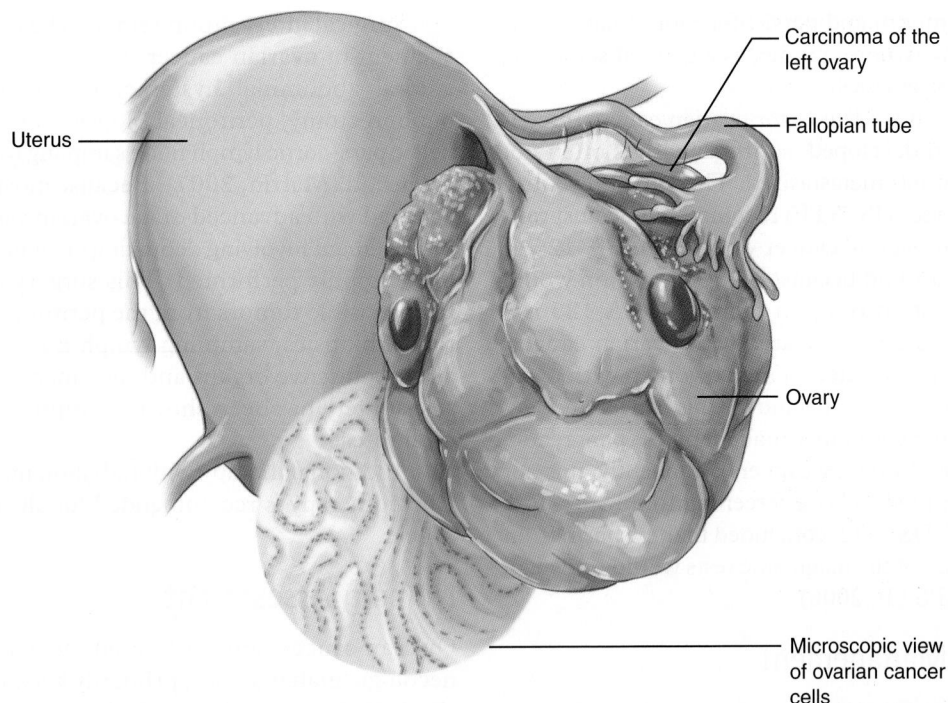

FIGURE 8.1 Ovarian cancer. (The Anatomical Chart Company. [2005]. *Atlas of pathophysiology* [2nd ed.]. Philadelphia: Lippincott Williams & Wilkins.)

The most important variable influencing the prognosis is the extent of the disease. Survival depends on the stage of the tumor, grade of differentiation, gross findings at surgery, amount of residual tumor after surgery, and effectiveness of any adjunct treatment postoperatively. Many women with ovarian cancer will experience recurrence despite the best efforts of eradicating the cancer through surgery, radiation, or chemotherapy to eliminate residual tumor cells. The likelihood of long-term survival in the event of recurrence is dismal (Eaton, 2007). The 5-year survival rates (the percentage of women who live at least 5 years after their diagnosis) are shown in Table 8.1 according to stage.

TABLE 8.1 FIVE-YEAR SURVIVAL RATES FOR OVARIAN CANCER

Stage	Five-Year Relative Survival Rates
I	80% to 90%
II	65% to 70%
III	30% to 60%
IV	20%

American Cancer Society (ACS). (2007c). *What are the key statistics about ovarian cancer?* American Cancer Society, Inc. [Online] Available at: http://www.cancer.org/docroot/CRI/content/CRI_2_4_1X_What_are_the_key_statistics_for_ovarian_cancer_33.asp?sitearea=&level=.

Pathophysiology

Ovarian cancer, the cause of which is unknown, can originate from different cell types. Most ovarian cancers originate in the ovarian epithelium. They usually present as solid masses that have spread beyond the ovary and seeded into the peritoneum prior to diagnosis. An inherited genetic mutation is the causative factor in 5% to 10% of cases of epithelial ovarian cancer.

Screening and Diagnosis

Seventy-five percent of ovarian cancers are not diagnosed until the cancer has advanced to stage III or IV, primarily because there is still no adequate screening test. Two genes, BRCA-1 and BRCA-2, are linked with hereditary breast and ovarian cancers. Blood tests can be performed to assess DNA in white blood cells to detect mutations in the BRCA genes. These genetic markers do not predict whether the person will develop cancer; rather, they provide information regarding the risk of developing cancer: a woman who is BRCA positive may have up to an 80% chance of developing breast cancer and a 40% chance of developing ovarian cancer (Eaton, 2007).

To assist in screening, researchers have been developing an ovarian cancer symptom index that includes pelvic and abdominal pain, urinary frequency and urgency, increased abdominal size (bloating), and difficulty eating (feeling full) (Goff et al., 2007). The symptom index is considered positive if any of these symptoms occur more than 12 times a month and persist for more than 1 year. The utility of this symptom index as a general screening tool remains to be assessed.

Specific clinical guidelines for ovarian cancer screening have not been developed, so the disease is often not diagnosed until it has metastasized. The U.S. Preventive Services Task Force (USPSTF) recommends against routine screening for ovarian cancer with serum CA-125 or transvaginal ultrasound because earlier detection would have a small effect, at best, on mortality. CA-125 is a biologic tumor marker associated with ovarian cancer. Although levels are elevated in many women with ovarian cancer, CA-125 is not specific for this cancer and levels may be elevated with other malignancies (pancreatic, liver, colon, breast, and lung cancers). Currently, it is not sensitive enough to serve as a screening tool (Speroff & Fritz, 2005). The USPSTF concluded that the harm from the invasive nature of the diagnostic tests would outweigh the benefits (USPSTF, 2006).

Therapeutic Management

Treatment options for ovarian cancer vary depending on the stage and severity of the disease. Usually a laparoscopy (abdominal exploration with an endoscope) is performed for diagnosis and staging, as well as evaluation for therapy. In stage I the cancer is limited to the ovaries. In stage II the growth involves one or both ovaries, with pelvic extension. Stage III cancer has spread to the lymph nodes and other organs or structures inside the abdominal cavity. In stage IV, the cancer has metastasized to distant sites (Alexander et al., 2007). Figure 8.2 shows the likely metastatic sites for ovarian cancer.

Surgical intervention remains the mainstay of management of ovarian cancer. Surgery generally includes a total abdominal hysterectomy, bilateral salpingo-oophorectomy, peritoneal biopsies, omentectomy, and pelvic para-aortic lymph node sampling to evaluate cancer extension (Martin, 2007). Because most women are diagnosed with advanced-stage ovarian cancer, aggressive management involving debulking or cytoreductive surgery is commonly performed. This surgery involves resecting all visible tumors from the peritoneum, taking peritoneal biopsies, sampling lymph nodes, and removing all reproductive organs and the omentum. This aggressive surgery has been shown to improve long-term survival rates.

Additional therapy with radiation may be warranted. Chemotherapy is recommended for all stages of ovarian cancer.

Nursing Assessment

Ovarian cancers are considered the worst of all the gynecologic malignancies, primarily because they develop slowly and remain silent and without symptoms until the cancer is far advanced. It has been described as "the overlooked disease" or "the silent killer" because women and health care practitioners often ignore or rationalize early symptoms. For example, women may attribute gastrointestinal problems to stress and midlife changes. However, these vague complaints may precede more obvious symptoms by months. The most common early symptoms include abdominal bloating, early satiety, fatigue, vague abdominal pain, urinary frequency, diarrhea or constipation, and unexplained weight loss or gain. The later symptoms include anorexia, dyspepsia, ascites, a palpable abdominal mass, pelvic pain, and back pain (Wallace & Sanford, 2006).

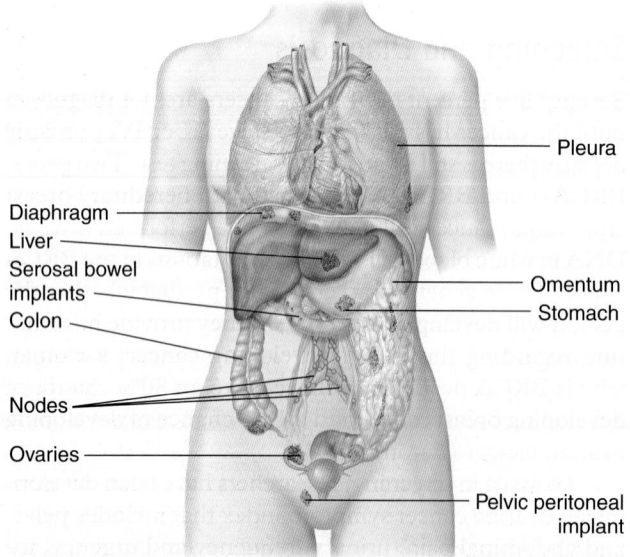

FIGURE 8.2 Common metastatic sites for ovarian cancer. (The Anatomical Chart Company. [2005]. *Atlas of pathophysiology* [2nd ed.]. Philadelphia: Lippincott Williams & Wilkins)

▶ *Consider THIS!*

I felt I was a lucky woman because I had been in remission from breast cancer for 12 years, and I had been given the gift of life to share with my beloved family. Recently I became ill with stomach problems: pain, indigestion, bloating, and nausea. My doctor treated me for GERD (acid reflux disease), but the symptoms persisted. I then was referred to a gastroenterologist, an urologist, and then a gynecologist, who did an ultrasound, which was negative. I received reassurance from all three that there was nothing wrong with me. As time went by, I experienced more pain, more symptoms, and increased frustration. Six months after seeing all three specialists, a repeat ultrasound revealed I had ovarian cancer, and I needed surgery as soon as possible. I underwent a complete hysterectomy

(continued)

► *Consider* THIS! *(continued)*

and my surgeon found I was in stage 3. Since then, I have undergone chemotherapy and participated in a clinical cancer study that wasn't successful for me, and now I am facing the fact that I am going to die soon.

Thoughts: This woman has tried everything to save her life, but, alas, time has run out for her with advanced ovarian cancer. Women diagnosed with breast cancer are at a significant risk for developing ovarian cancer later in life. Of the string of doctors she saw, one has to ponder why none ordered a CA-125 blood test with her history of breast cancer. We are haunted with the question: If they had and it was elevated, would she be in stage 3 now? I guess we will never know.

Obtain a thorough history of the woman's symptoms, including their onset, duration, and frequency. Review the woman's history for risk factors such as:

• Nulliparity
• Early menarche (before 12 years old)
• Late menopause (after 55 years old)
• Increasing age (over 50 years of age)
• High-fat diet
• Obesity
• Persistent ovulation over time
• First-degree relative with ovarian cancer
• Use of perineal talcum powder or hygiene sprays
• Older than 30 years at first pregnancy
• Positive BRCA-1 and BRCA-2 mutations
• Personal history of breast, bladder, or colon cancer
• Hormone replacement therapy for more than 10 years
• Infertility (CDC, 2007c)

Perform a complete physical examination. Inspect the abdomen, noting any distention or bloating. Palpate the abdomen. Be alert for a mass or pain on palpation. Anticipate further testing to confirm the diagnosis.

Nursing Management

The complexities of ovarian cancer make a multidisciplinary approach necessary for optimal management. With the subtle nature and high risk of recurrence and mortality of this condition, most women find it an emotionally exhausting and devastating experience. Nursing management focuses on measures to promote early detection, educate the woman about the disease and its treatments, and provide emotional support. Nurses should show a positive attitude that communicates understanding and reassurance.

Promoting Early Detection

Nurses need to ensure that women are aware of the risk factors for ovarian cancer. Urge women not to dismiss

seemingly innocuous symptoms as "just a part of aging." Encourage women to describe such nonspecific complaints at health visits.

Assess the woman's family and personal history for risk factors and encourage genetic testing for women with affected family members. Outline screening guidelines for women with hereditary cancer syndrome and inform women at high risk about the appropriate screening strategies.

Urge women to have yearly bimanual pelvic examinations and a transvaginal ultrasound to allow identification of ovarian masses in their early stages. After menopause, a mass on an ovary is not a cyst: physiologic cysts can arise only from a follicle that has not ruptured or from the cystic degeneration of the corpus luteum.

► *Take* NOTE!

A small ovarian "cyst" found on ultrasound in an asymptomatic postmenopausal woman should arouse suspicion. Any mass or ovary palpated in a postmenopausal woman should be considered cancerous until proven otherwise (Cherry, DeGaetano, & Martin, 2007).

Educating the Client

Education is a major focus of nursing care. This teaching involves risk reduction and health promotion. Teach the woman about risk-reduction strategies; for instance, pregnancy, use of oral contraceptives, and breastfeeding reduce the risk of ovarian cancer. Instruct women to avoid using talc and hygiene sprays on their genitals. Review the lifetime risks related to BRCA-1 and BRCA-2 genes and options available should the woman test positive for these genes. Help to promote community awareness of ovarian cancer by educating the public about risk-reducing behaviors.

Instruct the woman about the importance of healthy lifestyles. Stress the importance of maintaining a healthy weight to reduce risk. Encourage women to eat a low-fat diet.

For the woman who is diagnosed with ovarian cancer, describe in simple terms the tests, treatment modalities, and follow-up needed. For example, if the woman will be having surgery, provide thorough teaching about what to expect before, during, and after surgery. Outline treatment options and the implications of choices. Assist the woman and her family to decipher the myriad of information related to staging, tests, and treatments. Teach the woman about additional treatment measures, such as radiation therapy or chemotherapy, including how to handle the common adverse effects of treatment.

Supporting the Client and Family

The diagnosis of ovarian cancer, like any cancer, can be overwhelming. In addition, the treatments and their effects can be highly stressful, both physically and emotionally. Provide one-to-one support for women facing treatment for ovarian cancer. Ovarian cancer involves the reproductive system, which has a direct impact on the woman's view of herself. Encourage open discussion of sexuality and the impact of cancer. Listen and support the woman and her family as they try to cope with this disease. Encourage the use of appropriate coping strategies to allow for the best quality of life. Try to restore hope to women with ovarian cancer, and stress treatment compliance. If appropriate, encourage participation in clinical trials to offer hope for all women. Continue to offer support to the woman and her family members as they experience sadness and grief.

Endometrial Cancer

Endometrial cancer (also known as uterine cancer) is malignant neoplastic growth of the uterine lining. It is the most common gynecologic malignancy and accounts for 6% of all cancers in women in the United States. The NCI estimates that there will be over 40,000 new cases in 2007; approximately 8,000 of these women will die (NCI, 2007b). It is uncommon before the age of 40, but as women age, their risk of endometrial cancer increases. Approximately 95% of these malignancies are carcinomas of the endometrium. Because endometrial cancer is usually diagnosed in the early stages, it has a better prognosis than cervical or ovarian cancer (ACS, 2007f).

Pathophysiology

Two mechanisms are believed to be involved in the development of endometrial cancer. A history of exposure to unopposed estrogen is the cause in 75% of women. Those that are spontaneous and are unrelated to estrogen or endometrial hyperplasia represent the other 25% of endometrial cancers.

Endometrial cancer may originate in a polyp or in a diffuse multifocal pattern. The pattern of spread partially depends on the degree of cellular differentiation. Well-differentiated tumors tend to limit their spread to the surface of the endometrium. Metastatic spread occurs in a characteristic pattern and most commonly involves the lungs, inguinal and supraclavicular nodes, liver, bones, brain, and vagina (NCI, 2007b). Early tumor growth is characterized by friable and spontaneous bleeding. Later tumor growth is characterized by myometrial invasion and growth toward the cervix (Fig. 8.3).

Adenocarcinoma of the endometrium is typically preceded by hyperplasia. Carcinoma in situ is found only on the endometrial surface. In stage I, it has spread to the muscle wall of the uterus. In stage II, it has spread to the cervix. In stage III, it has spread to the bowel or vagina, with metastases to pelvic lymph nodes. In stage IV, it has invaded the bladder mucosa, with distant metastases to the lungs, liver, and bone (Burke & Gallup, 2007).

Type I carcinomas, the most common, begin as endometrial hyperplasia and progress to carcinomas. Giving estrogen preparations without progestin for hormone replacement therapy leads to an increased risk for endometrial cancer. Type I is generally found at an earlier stage and treatment results are more favorable.

Unlike type I endometrial carcinoma, type II carcinomas appear spontaneously, are associated with a poorly differentiated cell type, and have a poor prognosis (Burke & Gallup, 2007). They account for less than 10% of all endometrial cancers but contribute to the majority of all endometrial deaths.

Screening and Diagnosis

Remember Carmella, the woman with postmenopausal bleeding? In postmenopausal women, any bleeding is abnormal and warrants further assessment. What testing would the nurse anticipate as being ordered to confirm the diagnosis? What would be the nurse's role during this testing?

Screening for endometrial cancer is not routinely done because it is not practical or cost-effective. The ACS recommends that women should be informed about the risks and symptoms of endometrial cancer at the onset of menopause and strongly encouraged to report any unexpected bleeding or spotting to their health care provider (ACS, 2007f). A pelvic examination is frequently normal in the early stages of the disease. Changes in the size, shape, or consistency of the uterus or its surrounding support structures may exist when the disease is more advanced.

An endometrial biopsy is the diagnostic procedure of choice. It can be done in the health care provider's office without anesthesia. A slender suction catheter is used to obtain a small sample of tissue for pathology. This test can detect up to 90% of cases of endometrial cancer in women with postmenopausal bleeding, depending on the technique and experience of the health care provider (Wallace & Sanford, 2006). The woman may experience mild cramping and bleeding after the procedure for about 24 hours, but typically mild pain medication will reduce this discomfort.

Transvaginal ultrasound can be used to evaluate the endometrial cavity and measure the thickness of the endometrial lining. It can be used to detect endometrial hyperplasia. If the endometrium measures less than 4 mm, then the client is at low risk for malignancy (Sonoda & Barakat, 2006).

Therapeutic Management

Typically, the stage of the disease directs treatment. It usually involves surgery with adjunct therapy based on pathologic findings. Surgery most often involves removal

FIGURE **8.3** Progression of endometrial cancer. (The Anatomical Chart Company. [2005]. *Atlas of pathophysiology* [2nd ed.]. Philadelphia: Lippincott Williams & Wilkins)

of the uterus (hysterectomy) and the fallopian tubes and ovaries (salpingo-oophorectomy). Removal of the tubes and ovaries is recommended because tumor cells spread early to the ovaries, and any dormant cancer cells could be stimulated to grow by ovarian estrogen. In more ad- vanced cancers, radiation and chemotherapy are used as adjuncts to surgery. Routine surveillance intervals for follow-up care are typically every 3 to 4 months for the first 2 years, since 85% of recurrences occur in the first 3 years after diagnosis (Burke & Gallup, 2007).

Nursing Assessment

Obtain a thorough history from the woman, ascertaining her primary complaint. Most commonly, the major initial symptom of endometrial cancer is abnormal and painless vaginal bleeding.

▶ *Take* NOTE!

Any episode of bright-red bleeding that occurs after menopause should be investigated. Abnormal uterine bleeding is rarely the result of uterine malignancy in a young woman, but in the postmenopausal woman it should be regarded with suspicion.

Also review the woman's history for any risk factors, including:

- Nulliparity
- Obesity (more than 50 pounds overweight)
- Liver disease
- Infertility
- Diabetes mellitus
- Hypertension
- History of pelvic radiation
- Polycystic ovary syndrome
- Infertility
- Early menarche (before 12 years old)
- High-fat diet
- Use of prolonged exogenous unopposed estrogen with an intact uterus
- Endometrial hyperplasia
- Family history of endometrial cancer
- Personal history of hereditary nonpolyposis colon cancer
- Personal history of breast or ovarian cancer
- Late onset of menopause (after age 52 years)
- Tamoxifen use
- Chronic anovulation (Tiffen & Mahon, 2006)

Assess the woman for additional manifestations, such as dyspareunia, low back pain, purulent genital discharge, dysuria, pelvic pain, weight loss, and a change in bladder and bowel habits. These may suggest advanced disease.

Perform a physical examination and assist with or perform, as appropriate, a pelvic examination. Observe for vaginal discharge. Note any changes in the size, shape, or consistency of the uterus or surrounding structures or client reports of pain during examination. Anticipate the need for transvaginal ultrasound to identify endometrial hyperplasia (usually greater than 4 mm) and endometrial biopsy to identify malignant cells.

Nursing Management

Ensure that the woman understands all the treatment options. Address any concerns the woman expresses, including those of a sexual nature. Ensure that follow-up appointments are scheduled appropriately. Refer the client to a support group. Offer the woman and family explanations and emotional support throughout.

Educate the client about preventive measures or follow-up care if she has been treated for cancer. Education may be the most important tool currently available for the early detection of endometrial cancer. Many risk factors for endometrial cancer are modifiable, including obesity, hypertension, and diabetes. Educating women about risk factors and ways to decrease the risks is essential so that women can learn about their own risk and can become partners in the fight against the number-one gynecologic cancer (Teaching Guidelines 8.2).

TEACHING GUIDELINES 8.2

Preventive and Follow-Up Measures for Endometrial Cancer

- Schedule regular pelvic examinations after the age of 21.
- Visit health care practitioner for early evaluation of any abnormal bleeding after menopause.
- Maintain a low-fat diet throughout life.
- Exercise daily.
- Manage weight to discourage hyperestrogenic states, which predispose to endometrial hyperplasia.
- Pregnancy serves as a protective factor by reducing estrogen.
- Ask your doctor about the use of combination estrogen and progestin pills.
- When combination oral contraceptives are taken to facilitate the regular shedding of the uterine lining, take risk-reduction measures.
- Be aware of risk factors for endometrial cancer and make modifications as needed.
- Report any of the following symptoms immediately:
  - Bleeding or spotting after sexual intercourse
  - Bleeding that lasts longer than a week
  - Reappearance of bleeding after 6 months or more of no menses
- After cancer therapy, schedule follow-up appointments for the next few years.
- After cancer therapy, frequently communicate with your health care provider concerning your status.
- After surgery, maintain a healthy weight.

*C*armella's endometrial biopsy indicates endometrial adenocarcinoma. Her health care provider recommends surgery and adjuvant radiation therapy. How long will Carmella need to follow up after surgery? What lifestyle changes will the nurse need to stress with Carmella?

Cervical Cancer

Cervical cancer is cancer of the uterine cervix. The ACS estimates that over 12,000 cases of invasive cervical cancer will be diagnosed in the United States in 2007; approximately 3,000 of these women will die. Some researchers estimate that noninvasive cervical cancer (carcinoma in situ) is about four times more common than invasive cervical cancer. The 5-year survival rate for all stages of cervical cancer is 72% (ACS, 2007a). It is five to eight times more common in women affected with HIV or AIDS than those who do not have this virus. The probability of a woman in the United States developing cervical cancer is approximately 1 in 120, but this statistic is age-dependent; the highest incidence is in women 40 to 49 years of age (Hopkins & Sawa, 2007).

The incidence and mortality rates of cervical cancer have decreased noticeably in the past several decades, with most of the reduction attributed to the **Papanicolaou (Pap) test**, which detects cervical cancer and precancerous lesions. Cervical cancer is one of the most treatable cancers when detected at an early stage (ACS, 2007a). *Healthy People 2010* identifies two goals that address cervical cancer (Healthy People 2010 8.1; USDHHS, 2000).

HEALTHY PEOPLE 2010

Objective	Significance
Reduce the death rate from cancer of the uterine cervix from 3 per 100,000 females (1998) to 2 per 100,000 females in 2010. Increase the proportion of women who received a Pap smear within the preceding 3 years from 79% to 90% by 2010.	• Will help improve mortality rates and quality of life for women, and reduce health care costs related to treatment of malignancies. • Will help to promote screening and early detection. The National Institutes of Health (NIH) reported that half of women diagnosed with invasive cervical cancer have never had a Pap smear and 10% have not had Pap smears during the past 5 years (NIH, 2007).

Pathophysiology

Cervical cancer starts with abnormal changes in the cellular lining or surface of the cervix. Typically these changes occur in the squamous–columnar junction of the cervix. Here, cylindrical secretory epithelial cells (columnar) meet the protective flat epithelial cells (squamous) from the outer cervix and vagina in what is termed the transformation zone. The continuous replacement of columnar epithelial cells by squamous epithelial cells in this area makes these cells vulnerable to take up foreign or abnormal genetic material (ACS, 2007a). Figure 8.4 shows the pathophysiology of cervical cancer.

FIGURE 8.4 Cervical cancer. (The Anatomical Chart Company. [2005]. *Atlas of pathophysiology* [2nd ed.]. Philadelphia: Lippincott Williams & Wilkins)

The development of cervical cancer has been linked to the **human papillomavirus (HPV)**, which is acquired through sexual activity (Torpy, 2007). More than 90% of squamous cervical cancers contain HPV DNA, and the virus is now accepted as a major causative factor in the development of cervical cancer and its precursor, **cervical dysplasia** (disordered growth of abnormal cells).

Screening and Diagnosis

Screening for cervical cancer is very effective because the presence of a precursor lesion, cervical intraepithelial neoplasia (CIN), helps determine whether further tests are needed. Lesions start as dysplasia and progress in a predictable fashion over a long period, allowing ample opportunity for intervention at a precancerous stage. Progression from low-grade to high-grade dysplasia takes an average of 9 years, and progression from high-grade dysplasia to invasive cancer takes up to 2 years (Hopkins & Sawa, 2007).

Widespread use of the Pap test (also known as a Pap smear), a procedure used to obtain cells from the cervix for cytology screening, is credited with saving tens of thousands of women's lives and decreasing deaths from cervical cancer by more than 70% (ACS, 2007a). Despite its outstanding record of success as a screening tool for cervical cancer (it detects approximately 90% of early cancer changes), the conventional Pap smear has a 20% false-negative rate. High-grade abnormalities missed by human screening are frequently detected by computerized instruments (NCI, 2007a). Thus, many technologies have been developed to improve the sensitivity and specificity of Pap testing, including:

- Thin-Prep: In this liquid-based technique, the cervical specimen is placed into a vial of preservative solution rather than on a glass slide.
- Computer-assisted automated Pap test rescreening (Autopap): An algorithm-based decision-making technology identifies slides that should be rescreened by cytopathologists by selecting samples that exceed a certain threshold for the likelihood of abnormal cells.
- HPV-DNA typing (Hybrid Capture): This system uses the association between certain types of HPV (16, 18, 31, 33, 35, 45, 51, 52, and 56) and the development of cervical cancer. This system can identify high-risk HPV types and improves detection and management.
- Computer-assisted technology (Cytyc CDS-1000, AutoCyte, AcCell): These computerized instruments can detect abnormal cells that are sometimes missed by technologists (Wallace & Sanford, 2006).

The high rate of false-negative results may also be due to other factors, including errors in sampling the cervix, in preparing the slide, and in client preparation.

Although professional medical organizations disagree as to the recommended frequency of screening for cervi-

cal cancer, the ACS 2007 guidelines suggest that women should begin annual screening for cervical cancer via a Pap test after they initiate sexual activity or at 21 years of age, whichever comes first. If three consecutive Pap smears are negative, a trained health care provider may suggest that screening can be performed less frequently. Women ages 65 to 70 with no abnormal tests in the previous 10 years may choose to stop screenings (ACS, 2007a). High-risk women should continue to have annual Pap smears throughout their life (Table 8.2).

Pap smear results are classified using the Bethesda System (Box 8.1), which provides a uniform diagnostic terminology that allows clear communication between the laboratory and the health care provider. The information provided by the laboratory is divided into three categories: specimen adequacy, general categorization of cytologic findings, and interpretation/result (ACS, 2007b).

Therapeutic Management

Treatment for abnormal Pap smears depends on the severity of the results and the health history of the woman. Therapeutic choices all involve destroying as many affected cells as possible. Box 8.2 describes treatment options.

Using the Bethesda system, the following management guidelines for abnormal Pap results were developed by the NCI to provide direction to health care providers and clients:

- ASC-US: Repeat the Pap smear in 4 to 6 months or refer for colposcopy.
- ASC-H: Refer for colposcopy without HPV testing.
- Atypical glandular cells (AGC) and adenocarcinoma in situ (AIS): Immediate colposcopy; follow-up is based on the findings.

Colposcopy is a microscopic examination of the lower genital tract using a magnifying instrument called a colposcope. Specific patterns of cells that correlate well with certain histologic findings can be visualized.

TABLE 8.2 **PAP SMEAR GUIDELINES**

First Pap	Age 21 or within 3 years of first sexual intercourse
Until age 30	Yearly—using glass slide method Every 2 years—using liquid-based method
Age 30–70	Every 2–3 years if last 3 Paps were normal
After age 70	May discontinue if: - Past 3 Paps were normal and - No Paps in the past 10 years were abnormal

American Cancer Society (ACS). (2007b). *How Pap test results are reported.* American Cancer Society, Inc. [Online] Available at: http://www.cancer.org/docroot/PED/content/PED_2_3X_Pap_Test.asp.

BOX 8.1 The 2001 Bethesda System for Classifying Pap Smears

Specimen Type: Conventional Pap smear vs. liquid-based

Specimen Adequacy: Satisfactory or unsatisfactory for evaluation

General Categorization: (optional)
• Negative for intraepithelial lesion or malignancy
• Epithelial cell abnormality. See interpretation/result

Automated Review: If case was examined by automated device or not

Ancillary Testing: Provides a brief description of the test methods and report results so health care provider understands

Interpretation/Result:
• Negative for intraepithelial lesion or malignancy
• Organisms: *Trichomonas vaginalis;* fungus; bacterial vaginosis; herpes simplex
• Other non-neoplastic findings: Reactive cellular changes associated with inflammation, radiation, IUDs, atrophy
• Other: Endometrial cells in a woman >40 years of age
• Epithelial cell abnormalities:
• *Squamous cell*
  - Atypical squamous cells
    - Of undetermined significance (ASC-US)
    - Cannot exclude HSIL (ASC-H)
  - Low-grade squamous intraepithelial lesion (LSIL)
    - Encompassing HPV/mild dysplasia/CIN-1
  - High-grade squamous intraepithelial lesion (HSIL)
    - Encompassing moderate and severe dysplasia CIS/CIN-2 and CIN-3
    - With features suspicious for invasion
  - Squamous cell carcinoma
• *Glandular Cell:* Atypical
  - Endocervical, endometrial, or glandular cells
    - Endocervical cells—favor neoplastic
    - Glandular cells—favor neoplastic
    - Endocervical adenocarcinoma in situ
  - Adenocarcinoma
    - Endocervical, endometrial, extrauterine
• Other malignant neoplasms (specify)

Educational Notes and Suggestions: (optional)

Sources: NIH, 2007; ACS, 2007b; Schuiling & Likis, 2006; Sherman et al., 2007.

Nursing Assessment

Obtain a thorough history and physical examination of the woman. Investigate her history for risk factors such as:

• Early age at first intercourse (within 1 year of menarche)
• Lower socioeconomic status
• Promiscuous male partners
• Unprotected sexual intercourse

BOX 8.2 Treatment Options for Cervical Cancer

• *Cryotherapy*—destroys abnormal cervical tissue by freezing with liquid nitrogen, Freon, or nitrous oxide. Studies show a 90% cure rate (Persinger & Beal, 2007). Healing takes up to 6 weeks, and the client may experience a profuse, watery vaginal discharge for 3 to 4 weeks.

• *Cone Biopsy* or *conization*—removes a cone-shaped section of cervical tissue. The base of the cone is formed by the ectocervix (outer part of the cervix) and the point or apex of the cone is from the endocervical canal. The transformation zone is contained within the cone sample. The cone biopsy is also a treatment and can be used to completely remove any precancers and very early cancers. There are two methods commonly used for cone biopsies:
  • LEEP (loop electrosurgical excision procedure) or LLETZ (large loop excision of the transformation zone)—the abnormal cervical tissue is removed with a wire that is heated by an electrical current. For this procedure, a local anesthetic is used. It is performed in the health care provider's office in approximately 10 minutes. Mild cramping and bleeding may persist for several weeks after the procedure.
  • Cold knife cone biopsy—a surgical scalpel or a laser is used instead of a heated wire to remove tissue. This procedure requires general anesthesia and is done in a hospital setting. After the procedure, cramping and bleeding may persist for a few weeks.

• *Laser therapy*—destroys diseased cervical tissue by using a focused beam of high-energy light to vaporize it (burn it off). After the procedure, the woman may experience a watery brown discharge for a few weeks. Very effective in destroying precancers and preventing them from developing into cancers.

• *Hysterectomy*—removes the uterus and cervix surgically

• *Radiation therapy*—delivered by internal radium applications to the cervix or external radiation therapy that includes lymphatics of the pelvis

• *Chemoradiation*—weekly cisplatin therapy concurrent with radiation. Investigation of this therapy is on-going (ACS, 2007).

• Family history of cervical cancer (mother or sisters)
• Sexual intercourse with uncircumcised men
• Female offspring of mothers who took diethyl-stilbestrol (DES)
• Infections with genital herpes or chronic chlamydia
• Multiple sex partners
• Cigarette smoking
• Immunocompromised state
• HIV infection
• Oral contraceptive use

• Moderate dysplasia on Pap smear within past 5 years
• HPV infection (CDC, 2007b)

Question the woman about any signs and symptoms. Clinically, the first sign is abnormal vaginal bleeding, usually after sexual intercourse. Also be alert for reports of vaginal discomfort, malodorous discharge, and dysuria.

In some cases the woman is asymptomatic, with detection occurring at an annual gynecologic examination and Pap test.

Perform a physical examination. Inspect the perineal area for vaginal discharge or genital warts. Perform or assist with a pelvic examination, including the collection of a Pap smear as indicated (Nursing Procedure 8.1).

Nursing Procedure 8.1

ASSISTING WITH COLLECTION OF A PAP SMEAR

Purpose: To Obtain Cells From the Cervix for Cervical Cytology Screening

1. Explain procedure to the client (Fig. A).
2. Instruct client to empty her bladder.
3. Wash hands thoroughly.
4. Assemble equipment, maintaining sterility of equipment (Fig. B).
5. Position client on stirrups or foot pedals so that her knees fall outward.
6. Drape client with a sheet for privacy, covering the abdomen but leaving the perineal area exposed.
7. Open packages as needed.
8. Encourage client to relax.
9. Provide support to client as the practitioner obtains a sample by spreading the labia; inserting the speculum;

inserting the cytobrush and swabbing the endocervix; and inserting the plastic spatula and swabbing the cervix (Fig. C–H).
10. Transfer specimen to container (Fig. I) or slide. If a slide is used, spray the fixative on the slide.
11. Place sterile lubricant on the practitioner's fingertip when indicated for the bimanual examination.
12. Wash hands thoroughly.
13. Label specimen according to facility policy.
14. Rinse reusable instruments and dispose of waste appropriately (Fig. J).
15. Wash hands thoroughly.

A

B

C

D

Nursing Procedure 8.1 (continued)

Used with permission from Klossner, N. J. (2006). *Introductory maternity nursing.* Philadelphia: Lippincott Williams & Wilkins.

> ▶ **Take** NOTE!
>
> *Suspect advanced cervical cancer in women with pelvic, back, or leg pain, weight loss, anorexia, weakness and fatigue, and fractures.*

Prepare the woman for further diagnostic testing if indicated, such as a colposcopy. In a colposcopy, the woman is placed in the lithotomy position and her cervix is cleansed with acetic acid solution. Acetic acid makes abnormal cells appear white, which is referred to as acetowhite. These white areas are then biopsied and sent to the pathologist for assessment. Although this test is not painful, has no side effects, and can be performed safely in the clinic or office setting, women may be apprehensive or anxious about it because it is done to identify and confirm potential abnormal cell growth. Provide appropriate physical and emotional preparation for this test (Evidence-Based Practice 8.1).

Nursing Management

The nurse's role involves primary prevention by educating women about risk factors and ways to prevent cervical

EVIDENCE-BASED PRACTICE 8.1
Anxiety Reduction for Women Undergoing a Colposcopy

● Study

Getting abnormal Pap smear results can be upsetting for a woman. A colposcopy is a follow-up examination that is commonly used to identify these suspicious cells and obtain a specimen for biopsy. A woman's anxiety about this examination is increased by the possibility of a cancer diagnosis. Studies have shown that anxiety can heighten discomfort, so researchers sought to discover which method of preparation for colposcopy best reduces a woman's anxiety. They conducted a detailed search of databases, clinical trial registers, and protocols to evaluate all randomized and quasi-randomized controlled trials involving interventions to reduce anxiety during colposcopy. Eleven trials involving 1,441 women were identified. The trials compared the anxiety levels of the intervention group with those of a control group. The methods used to reduce anxiety were informational leaflets, counseling, informational videos, video during colposcopy, music, and verbal information.

▲ Findings

Three methods were found to significantly reduce anxiety during colposcopy: listening to music, watching informational videos, and viewing the video during the procedure. Other methods, such as informational leaflets, counseling, and verbal information, were not found to reduce anxiety vs. control groups.

■ Nursing Implications

Nurses can use the information from this study to design appropriate strategies for client teaching and can encourage women to use these measures to reduce anxiety. For example, the nurse can suggest that the client listen to her favorite music during the procedure to help her relax. Nurses can urge women to seek agencies or settings that include these measures as part of their procedure, and nurses can work with their facilities to ensure that music, informational videos, and videotape equipment are available for use during this procedure.

Galaal, K. A., Deane, K., Sangal, S., & Lopes, A. D. (2007). Interventions for reducing anxiety in women undergoing colposcopy. *Cochrane Database of Systematic Reviews 2007,* Issue 3, Art.No.: CD006013.DOI:10.1002/14651858.CD006013.pub2.

dysplasia. Cervical cancer rates have decreased in the United States because of the widespread use of Pap testing, which can detect precancerous lesions of the cervix before they develop into cancer. Nevertheless, during 2007, an estimated 12,000 new cases will be diagnosed and approximately 3,800 women will die from cervical cancer (CDC, 2007a, 2007b; Advisory Committee on Immunization Practices [ACIP], 2007).

Gardasil, the first vaccine developed to protect girls and women from HPV, is now available. The vaccine prevents infection from four HPV types: HPV 6, 11, 16, and 18. Theses types are responsible for 70% of cervical cancers and 90% of genital warts (Snow, 2007). Clinical trials indicate that the vaccine has high efficacy in preventing persistent HPV infection, cervical cancer precursor lesions, vaginal and vulvar cancer precursor lesions, and genital warts (Bryan, 2007). The vaccine is administered by intramuscular injection, and the recommended schedule is a three-dose series with the second and third doses administered 2 and 6 months after the first dose. The recommended age for vaccination of females is 11 to 12 years old, but the vaccine can be administered to girls as young as 9 years old (Pichichero, 2007). The long-term efficacy of HPV vaccines remains to be determined. Sustained efficacy up to 4.5 years has been documented, but it could be that boosters will be needed (CDC, 2007a). However, the vaccine is not a substitute for routine cervical cancer screening, and vaccinated women should have Pap smears as recommended.

Focus primary prevention education on the following:

- Identify high-risk behaviors in clients and teach them how to reduce them:
  - Take steps to prevent STIs.
  - Avoid early sexual activity.
  - Faithfully use barrier methods of contraception.
  - Avoid smoking and drinking.
  - Receive the HPV vaccine.
- Instruct women on the importance of screening for cervical cancer by annual Pap smears. Outline the proper preparation before having a Pap smear (Teaching Guidelines 8.3). Reinforce specific guidelines for screening.

Nurses also can advocate for clients by making sure that the Pap smear is sent to an accredited laboratory for interpretation. Doing so reduces the risk of false-negative results.

Secondary prevention focuses on reducing or limiting the area of cervical dysplasia. Tertiary prevention focuses on minimizing disability or spread of cervical cancer. Explain in detail all procedures that might be needed. Encourage the client who has undergone any cervical treatment to allow the pelvic area to rest for approximately 1 month. Discuss this rest period with the client and her partner to gain his cooperation. Outline alternatives to vaginal intercourse, such as cuddling, holding hands, and kissing. Remind the woman about any follow-up procedures that are needed and assist her with scheduling if necessary.

Throughout the process, provide emotional support to the woman and her family. During the decision-making process, the woman may be overwhelmed by the diagnosis and all the information being presented. Refer the woman and her family to appropriate community resources and support groups as indicated.

Vaginal Cancer

Vaginal cancer is malignant tissue growth arising in the vagina. It is rare, representing less than 3% of all genital cancers. The ACS estimates that in 2007, over 2,000 new cases of vaginal cancer will be diagnosed in the United States, and approximately 800 will die of this cancer (ACS, 2007d). The peak incidence of vaginal cancer occurs at 60 to 65 years of age. The prognosis of vaginal cancer depends largely on the stage of disease and the type of tumor. The overall 5-year survival rate for squamous cell carcinoma is about 42%; that for adenocarcinoma is about 78% (NCI, 2007c). Vaginal cancer can be effectively treated, and when found early it is often curable.

Pathophysiology

The etiology of vaginal cancer has not been identified. Malignant diseases of the vagina are either primary vagi-

nal cancers or metastatic forms from adjacent or distant organs. About 80% of vaginal cancers are metastatic, primarily from the cervix and endometrium. These cancers invade the vagina directly. Cancers from distant sites that metastasize to the vagina through the blood or lymphatic system are typically from the colon, kidneys, skin (melanoma), or breast. Tumors in the vagina commonly occur on the posterior wall and spread to the cervix or vulva (NCI, 2007c).

Squamous cell carcinomas that begin in the epithelial lining of the vagina account for about 85% of vaginal cancers. This type of cancer usually occurs in women over age 50. They develop slowly over a period of years, commonly in the upper third of the vagina. They tend to spread early by directly invading the bladder and rectal walls. They also metastasize through blood and lymphatics. The remaining 15% are adenocarcinomas, which differ from squamous cell carcinoma by an increase in pulmonary metastases and supraclavicular and pelvic node involvement (ACS, 2007d).

Therapeutic Management

Treatment of vaginal cancer depends on the type of cells involved and the stage of the disease. If the cancer is localized, radiation, laser surgery, or both may be used. If the cancer has spread, radical surgery might be needed, such as a hysterectomy, or removal of the upper vagina with dissection of the pelvic nodes in addition to radiation therapy.

Nursing Assessment

Begin the history and physical examination by reviewing for risk factors. Although direct risk factors for the initial development of vaginal cancer have not been identified, associated risk factors include advancing age (over 60 years old), previous pelvic radiation, exposure to diethylstilbestrol (DES) in utero, vaginal trauma, history of genital warts (HPV infection), HIV infection, cervical cancer, chronic vaginal discharge, smoking, and low socioeconomic level (ACS, 2007d).

Question the woman about any complaints. Most women with vaginal cancer are asymptomatic. Those with symptoms have painless vaginal bleeding (often after sexual intercourse), abnormal vaginal discharge, dyspareunia, dysuria, constipation, and pelvic pain (NCI, 2007c). During the physical examination, observe for any obvious vaginal discharge or genital warts, or changes in the appearance of the vaginal mucosa. Anticipate colposcopy with biopsy of suspicious lesions to confirm the diagnosis.

Nursing Management

Nursing management for this cancer is similar to that for other reproductive cancers, with emphasis on sexuality counseling and referral to local support groups. Women undergoing radical surgery need intensive counseling about the nature of the surgery, risks, potential complications, changes in physical appearance and physiologic function, and sexuality alterations.

Vulvar Cancer

Vulvar cancer is an abnormal neoplastic growth on the external female genitalia (Fig. 8.5). It is responsible for 0.6% of all malignancies in women and 4% of all female genital cancers. It is the fourth most common gynecologic cancer, after endometrial, ovarian, and cervical cancers (Naumann & Higgins, 2007). The ACS estimates that in 2007, about 4,000 cancers of the vulva will be diagnosed in the United States and over 900 women will die of this cancer (ACS, 2007e). When detected early, it is highly curable.

Vulvar cancer is found most commonly in older women in their mid-60s to 70s, but the incidence in women younger than 35 years old has increased over the past few decades. The overall 5-year survival rate when lymph nodes are not involved is 90%, but it drops to 50% to 70% when the lymph nodes have been invaded (ACS, 2007e).

Pathophysiology

Approximately 90% of vulvar tumors are squamous cell carcinomas. This type of cancer forms slowly over several years and is usually preceded by precancerous changes. These precancerous changes are termed vulvar intraepithelial neoplasia (VIN). The two major types of VIN are classic (undifferentiated) and simplex (differentiated). Classic VIN, the more common one, is associated with HPV infection (genital warts due to types 16, 18, 31, 33, 35, and 51) and smoking (Wallace & Sanford, 2006). It typically occurs in women between 30 and 40 years old. In contrast to classic VIN, simplex VIN usually occurs in

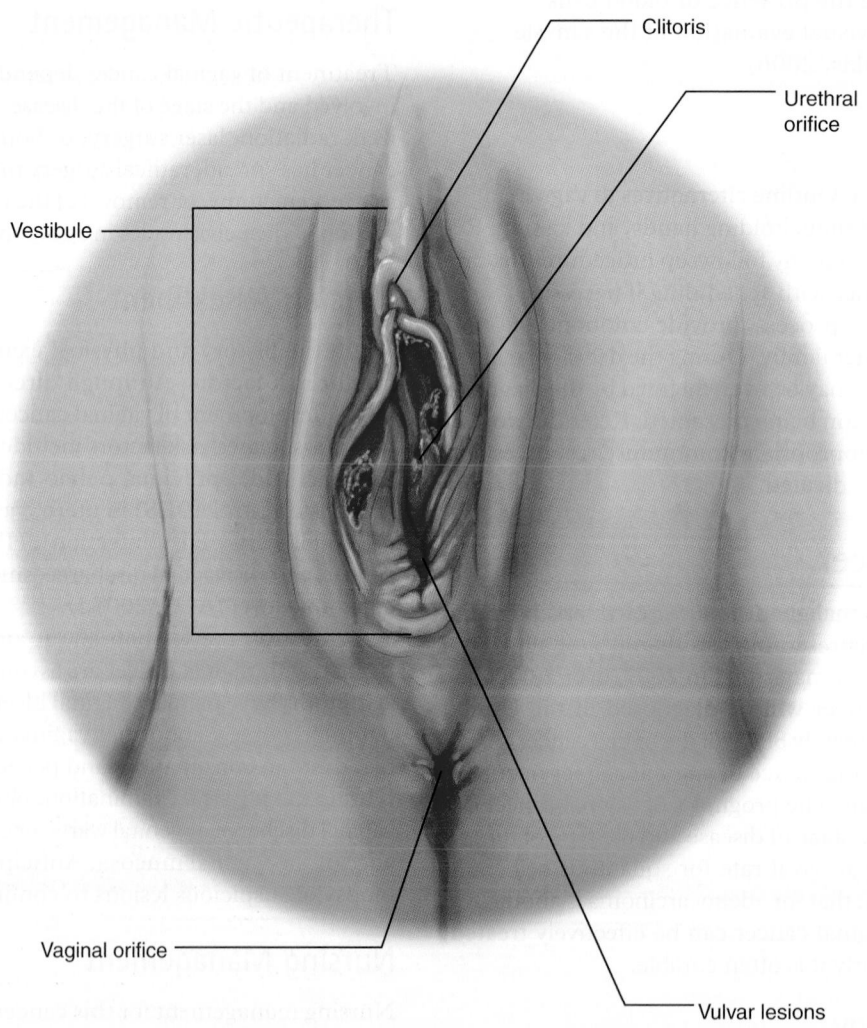

FIGURE 8.5 Vulvar cancer. (The Anatomical Chart Company. [2005]. *Atlas of pathophysiology* [2nd ed.]. Philadelphia: Lippincott Williams & Wilkins)

postmenopausal women and is not associated with HPV (Davidson, 2007).

Screening and Diagnosis

Annual vulvar examination is the most effective way to prevent vulvar cancer. Careful inspection of the vulva during routine annual gynecologic examinations remains the most productive diagnostic technique. Liberal use of biopsies of any suspicious vulvar lesion is usually necessary to make the diagnosis and to guide treatment. However, many women do not seek health care evaluation for months or years after noticing an abnormal lump or lesion.

The diagnosis of vulvar cancer is made by a biopsy of the suspicious lesion, which is usually found on the labia majora.

> ▶ *Take* NOTE!
>
> *Vulvar pruritus or a lump is present in the majority of women with vulvar cancer. Lumps should be biopsied even if the woman is asymptomatic.*

Therapeutic Management

Treatment varies depending on the extent of the disease. Laser surgery, cryosurgery, or electrosurgical incision may be used. Larger lesions may need more extensive surgery and skin grafting. The traditional treatment for vulvar cancer has been radical vulvectomy, but more conservative techniques are being used to improve psychosexual outcomes.

Nursing Assessment

Typically, no single specific clinical symptom heralds this disease, so diagnosis is often delayed significantly. Therefore, it is important to review the woman's history for risk factors such as:

• Exposure to HPV type 16
• Age over 50
• HIV infection
• VIN
• Lichen sclerosus
• Melanoma or atypical moles
• Exposure to HSV II
• Multiple sex partners
• Smoking
• History of breast cancer
• Immune suppression
• Hypertension
• Diabetes mellitus
• Obesity (ACS, 2007e)

In most cases, the woman reports persistent vulvar itching that does not improve with the use of creams or ointments. During the physical examination, observe for any masses or thickening of the vulvar area. A vulvar lump or mass most often is noted. The vulvar lesion is usually raised and may be fleshy, ulcerated, leukoplakic, or warty (Naumann & Higgins, 2007). Less commonly, the woman may present with vulvar bleeding, discharge, dysuria, and pain.

Nursing Management

Women with vulvar cancer must clearly understand their disease, treatment options, and prognosis. To accomplish this, provide information and establish effective communication with the client and her family. Act as an educator and advocate.

Teach the woman about healthy lifestyle behaviors, such as smoking cessation and measures to reduce risk factors. For example, instruct the woman how to examine her genital area, urging her to do so monthly between menstrual periods. Tell her to look for any changes in appearance (e.g., whitened or reddened patches of skin); changes in feel (e.g., areas of the vulva becoming itchy or painful); or the development of lumps, moles (e.g., changes in size, shape, or color), freckles, cuts, or sores on the vulva. Urge the woman to report these changes to the health care provider (ACS, 2007e).

Teach the woman about preventive measures such as not wearing tight undergarments and not using perfumes and dyes in the vulvar region. Also educate her about the use of barrier methods of birth control (e.g., condoms) to reduce the risk of contracting HIV, HSV, and HPV.

For the woman diagnosed with vulvar cancer, provide information and support. Discuss potential changes in sexuality if radical surgery is performed. Encourage her to communicate openly with her partner. Refer her to appropriate community resources and support groups.

■■■ Key Concepts

■ Women have a one-in-three lifetime risk of developing cancer, and one out of every four deaths is from cancer; thus, nurses must focus on screening and educating all women regardless of risk factors.

■ The nurse plays a key role in offering emotional support, determining appropriate sources of support, and helping the woman use effective coping strategies when facing a diagnosis of cancer of the reproductive tract. Although reproductive tract cancer is rare during pregnancy, the woman's vigilance and routine screenings should continue throughout.

■ A woman's sexuality and culture are inextricably interwoven, and it is essential that nurses working with women of various cultures recognize this and remain sensitive to the vast changes that will take place when the diagnosis of cancer is made.

■ Ovarian cancer is the eighth most common cancer among women and the fourth most common cause of cancer deaths for women in the United States, accounting for more deaths than any other cancer of the reproductive system.

■ Ovarian cancer has been described as "the overlooked disease" or "silent killer," because women and/or health care practitioners often ignore or rationalize early symptoms. It is typically diagnosed in advanced stages.

■ Unopposed endogenous and exogenous estrogens, obesity, nulliparity, menopause after the age of 52 years, and diabetes are the major etiologic risk factors associated with the development of endometrial cancer.

■ The American Cancer Society (ACS) recommends that women should be informed about risks and symptoms of endometrial cancer at the onset of menopause and strongly encouraged to report any unexpected bleeding or spotting to their health care providers.

■ Malignant diseases of the vagina are either primary vaginal cancers or metastatic forms from adjacent or distant organs. Vaginal cancer tumors can be effectively treated and, when found early, are often curable.

■ Cervical cancer incidence and mortality rates have decreased noticeably in the past several decades, with most of the reduction attributed to the Pap test, which detects cervical cancer and precancerous lesions.

■ The nurse's role involves primary prevention of cervical cancer through education of women regarding risk factors and preventive techniques to avoid cervical dysplasia.

■ Diagnosis of vulvar cancer is often delayed significantly because there is no single specific clinical symptom that heralds it. The most common presentation is persistent vulvar itching that does not improve with the application of creams or ointments.

REFERENCES

Advisory Committee on Immunization Practices (ACIP). (2007). Quadrivalent human papillomavirus vaccine. *MMWR, 56*(RR-2), 1–24.

Agency for Healthcare Research and Quality (AHRQ). (2007). *Women: Stay healthy at any age—Your checklist for health.* AHRQ Publications No. 07-IP005-A. Available at: http://www.ahrq.gov/ppip/healthywom.htm.

Alexander, L. L., LaRosa, J. H., Bader, H., & Garfield, S. (2007). *New dimensions in women's health* (4th ed.). Sudbury, MA: Jones and Bartlett Publishers.

American Cancer Society (ACS). (2007a). *What are the key statistics about cervical cancer?* Available at: http://www.cancer.org/docroot/CRI/content/CRI_2_4_1X_What_are_the_key_statistics_for_cervical_cancer_8.asp?sitearea=.

American Cancer Society (ACS). (2007b). *How Pap test results are reported.* Available at: http://www.cancer.org/docroot/PED/content/PED_2_3X_Pap_Test.asp.

American Cancer Society (ACS). (2007c). *What are the key statistics about ovarian cancer?* Available at: http://www.cancer.org/docroot/CRI/content/CRI_2_4_1X_What_are_the_key_statistics_for_ovarian_cancer_33.asp?sitearea=&level=.

American Cancer Society (ACS). (2007d). *What are the key statistics about vaginal cancer?* Available at: http://www.cancer.org/docroot/CRI/content/CRI_2_4_1X_What_are_the_key_statistics_for_vaginal_cancer_55.asp?sitearea=.

American Cancer Society (ACS). (2007e). *What are the key statistics about vulvar cancer?* Available at: http://www.cancer.org/docroot/cri/content/cri_2_4_1x_what_are_the_key_statistics_for_vulvar_cancer_45.asp?sitearea=&level=.

American Cancer Society (ACS). (2007f). *Endometrial cancer.* Available at: http://www.cancer.org/docroot/CRI/CRI_2_1x.asp?rnav=criov&dt=11.

American Cancer Society (ACS). (2007g). *Cancer prevention and early detection: Cancer facts and figures 2007.* Atlanta: ACS.

American Cancer Society. (2008). *Cancer facts and figures 2007.* Atlanta: ACS.

Blackburn, S. T. (2007). *Maternal, fetal and neonatal physiology: A clinical perspective* (3rd ed.). St. Louis, MO: Saunders Elsevier.

Bryan, J. T. (2007). Developing an HPV vaccine to prevent cervical cancer and genital warts. *Vaccine, 25*(16), 3001–3006.

Burke, J. J., & Gallup, D. G. (2007). Endometrial cancer. In R. E. Rakel & E. T. Bope (Eds.), *Conn's current therapy 2007* (Section 16, pp. 1261–1264). Philadelphia: Saunders Elsevier.

Centers for Disease Control and Prevention (CDC). (2007a). Quadrivalent human papillomavirus vaccine: Recommendations of the Advisory Committee on Immunization Practices (ACIP). *MMWR, 56*(RR-2), 1–24.

Centers for Disease Control and Prevention (CDC). (2007b). *Cancer A-Z.* Available at: http://www.cdc.gov/cancer/healthdisparities/statistics/ethnic.htm.

Centers for Disease Control and Prevention (CDC). (2007c). *Ovarian cancer.* Available at: http://www.cdc.gov/cancer/ovarian/basic_info/.

Cherry, C., DeGaetano, C., & Martin, V. (2007). Ovarian cancer: Awareness is key. *Nursing Spectrum.* Available at: http://www.nurse.com/ce/print.html?CCID=3193.

Davidson, S. A. (2007). Neoplasms of the vulva. In R. E. Rakel & E. T. Bope (Eds.), *Conn's current therapy 2007* (Section 16; pp. 1268–1271). Philadelphia: Saunders Elsevier.

Eaton, L. A. (2007). Ovarian cancer. In R. E. Rakel & E. T. Bope (Eds.), *Conn's current therapy 2007* (Section 16, pp. 1259–1261). Philadelphia: Saunders Elsevier.

Fieler, V., & Henry, B. (2007). How to give psychological support to clients with cancer. *Nursing Spectrum.* Available at: http://www.nurse.com/ce/print.html?CCID=3309.

Galaal, K. A., Deane, K., Sangal, S., & Lopes, A.D. (2007). Interventions for reducing anxiety in women undergoing colposcopy. *Cochrane Database of Systematic Reviews 2007,* Issue 3, Art. No.: CD006013.DOI:10.1002/14651858.CD006013.pub2.

Goff, B. A., Mandel, L. S., Drescher, C. W., Urban, N., Gough, S., Schurman, K. M., Patras, J., Mahony, B. S., & Andersen, M. R. (2007). Development of an ovarian cancer symptom index: Possibilities for earlier detection. *Cancer, 109*(2), 221–227.

Hopkins, M. P., & Sawa, W. (2007). Cancer of the uterine cervix. In R. E. Rakel & E. T. Bope (Eds.), *Conn's current therapy 2007* (Section 16, pp. 1264–1267). Philadelphia: Saunders Elsevier.

Jenko, M., & Moffitt, S. R. (2006). Transcultural nursing principles. *Journal of Hospice and Palliative Nursing, 8*(3), 172–181.

Machado, F., Vegas, C., Leon, J., Perez, A., Sanchez, R., Parrilla, J., & Abad, L. (2007). Ovarian cancer during pregnancy: Analysis of 15 cases. *Gynecologic Oncology, 105*(2), 446–450.

Martin, V. R. (2007). Ovarian cancer: An overview of treatment options. *Clinical Journal of Oncology Nursing, 11*(2), 201–207.

Mayo Clinic. (2008). *Cancer prevention: 7 steps to reduce your risk* [Online]. Available at: http://www.mayoclinic.com/health/cancer-prevention/CA00024.

National Cancer Institute (NCI). (2007a). *Annual report on the status of cancer.* U.S. National Institutes of Health. Available at: http://www.nci.nih.gov/newscenter/pressreleases/ReportNation2007Release.

National Cancer Institute (NCI). (2007b). *Endometrial cancer: treatment.* U.S. National Institutes of Health. Available at: http://www.nci.hih.gov/cancertopics/pdq/treatment/endometrial/HealthProfessional/page1/.

National Cancer Institute (NCI). (2007c). *Vaginal cancer.* Available at: http://www.cancer.gov/cancertopics/types/vaginal/.

National Institutes of Health (NIH). (2007). *Cervical cancer: Prevention.* National Cancer Institute. Available at: http://www.nci.nih.gov/cancertopics/pdq/prevention/cervical/HealthProfessional/page2.

Naumann, R. W., & Higgins, R. V. (2007). Surgical treatment of vulvar cancer. *eMedicine.* Available at: http://www.emedicine.com/med/topic3328.htm.

Persinger, M. F., & Beal, M. W. (2007). Cervical and ovarian cancer screening. In B. Hackley, J. M. Kriebs, & M. E. Rousseau (Eds.), *Primary care of women: A guide for midwives and women's health providers.* Sudbury, MA: Jones and Bartlett Publishers.

Pichichero, M. E. (2007). Who should get the HPV vaccine? *Journal of Family Practice, 56*(3), 197–202.

Roberts, K., Rezai, N., & Edmondson, R. J. (2007). Cervical cancer in pregnancy: An assault on family and fertility. *British Journal of Midwifery, 15*(3), 1320–1326.

Schuiling, K. D., & Likis, F. E. (2006). *Women's gynecologic health.* Sudbury, MA: Jones and Bartlett Publishers.

Sherman, M. E., Dasgupta, A., Schiffman, M., Nayar, R., & Solomon, D. (2007). The Bethesda Interobserver Reproducibility Study (BIRST): A Web-based assessment of the Bethesda 2001 system for classifying cervical cytology. *Cancer, 111*(1), 15–25.

Snow, M. (2007). HPV vaccine: New treatment for an old disease. *Nursing2007, 37*(3), 67–68.

Sonoda, Y., & Barakat, R. R. (2006). Screening and the prevention of gynecologic cancer: Endometrial cancer. *Bailliere's Best Practice & Research in Clinical Obstetrics & Gynecology, 20*(2), 363–377.

Speroff, L., & Fritz, M. A. (2005). *Clinical gynecologic endocrinology and infertility* (7th ed.). Philadelphia: Lippincott Williams & Wilkins.

Surbone, A. (2006). Cultural aspects of communication in cancer care. *Recent Results in Cancer Research, 168*(1), 91–104.

Tiffen, J. M., & Mahon, S. M. (2006). Educating women regarding the early detection of endometrial cancer—What is the evidence? *Clinical Journal of Oncology Nursing, 10*(1), 102–105.

Torpy, J. M. (2007). Human papillomavirus infection. *Journal of the American Medical Association, 297*(8), 912–913.

U.S. Department of Health and Human Services (USDHHS), Public Health Service. (2000). *Healthy people 2010* (conference edition, in two volumes). Washington, DC: U.S. Government Printing Office.

U.S. Preventive Services Task Force (USPSTF). (2006). *Screening for ovarian cancer. U.S. Preventive Services Task Force Summary of Recommendations.* Available at: http://www.ahrq.gov/clinic/uspstf/uspsovar.htm.

Wallace, M., & Sanford, A. (2006). Gynecologic cancers. In K. D. Schuiling & F. E. Likis (Eds.), *Women's gynecologic health* (Chapter 23, pp. 595–633). Sudbury, MA: Jones and Bartlett Publishers.

World Health Organization (WHO). (2008). *Cancer prevention* [Online]. Available at: http://www.who.int/cancer/prevention/en/.

WEBSITES

American Cancer Society: 1-800-ACS-2345, www.cancer.org
American Urological Association: (410) 727-1100, www.auanet.org
Cancer Care, Inc.: (212) 712-8080, www.cancercare.org
Gilda Radner Familial Ovarian Cancer Registry: (800) OVARIAN, www.ovariancancer.com
Gynecologic Cancer Foundation: (800) 444-4441, www.wcn.org
Hysterectomy Educational Resource and Services (HERS): (215) 667-7757, www.ccon.com/hers
National Ovarian Cancer Coalition: (888) 682-7426. www.ovarian.org
National Women's Health Information Center: (800) 994-9662, www.4women.gov
Oncology Nursing Society (ONS): (866) 257-4ONS, www.ons.org
Ovarian Cancer Research Fund, Inc.: (800) 873-9569, www.ocrf.org
Sexuality Information and Education Counsel of the United States: (212) 819-9770, www.siecus.org
SHARE: Self-Help for Women with Breast or Ovarian Cancer: (866) 891-3431, www.sharecancersupport.org
Vulvar Health: www.vulvarhealth.org
Women's Cancer Network: (312) 644-6610, www.wcn.org

CHAPTER WORKSHEET

MULTIPLE CHOICE QUESTIONS

1. When describing ovarian cancer to a local women's group, the nurse states that ovarian cancer often is not diagnosed early because:

   a. The disease progresses very slowly.

   b. The early stages produce very vague symptoms.

   c. The disease usually is diagnosed only at autopsy.

   d. Clients don't follow up on acute pelvic pain.

2. A postmenopausal woman reports that she has started spotting again. Which of the following would the nurse do?

   a. Instruct the client to keep a menstrual diary for the next few months.

   b. Tell her not to worry, since this a common but not serious event.

   c. Have her start warm-water douches to promote healing.

   d. Anticipate that the doctor will do an endometrial biopsy.

3. Which of the following would the nurse identify as the priority psychosocial need for a women diagnosed with reproductive cancer?

   a. Clear information

   b. Hand-holding

   c. Cheerfulness

   d. Offering of hope

4. When teaching a group of women about screening and early detection of cervical cancer, the nurse would include which of the following as most effective?

   a. Fecal occult blood test

   b. CA-125 blood test

   c. Pap smear

   d. Sigmoidoscopy

5. After teaching a group of students about reproductive tract cancers, the nursing instructor determines that the teaching was successful when the students identify which of the following as the deadliest type of female reproductive cancer?

   a. Vulvar

   b. Ovarian

   c. Endometrial

   d. Cervical

CRITICAL THINKING EXERCISES

1. Tammy Scott, a 27-year-old sexually active Caucasian woman, visits the Health Department family planning clinic and requests information about the various methods available. In taking her history, the nurse learns that she started having sex at age 15 and has had multiple sex partners since then. She smokes two packs of cigarettes daily. Because she has been unemployed for a few months, her health insurance policy has lapsed. She has never previously obtained any gynecologic care.

   a. Based on her history, which risk factors for cervical cancer are present?

   b. What recommendations would you make for her, and why?

   c. What are this client's educational needs concerning health maintenance?

2. Jennifer Nappo, a 60-year-old nulliparous woman, presents to the gynecologic oncology clinic after her health care provider palpated an adnexal mass on her right ovary. In taking her history, the nurse learns that she has experienced mild abdominal bloating and weight loss for the past several months but felt fine otherwise. She was diagnosed with breast cancer 15 years ago and was treated with a lumpectomy and radiation. She has occasionally used talcum powder in her perineal area over the past 20 years.

   A transvaginal ultrasound reveals a complex mass in the right adnexa. She undergoes a total abdominal hysterectomy and bilateral salpingo-oophorectomy and lymph node biopsy. Pathology confirms a diagnosis of stage III ovarian cancer with abdominal metastasis and positive lymph nodes.

   a. Is this client's profile typical for a woman with this diagnosis?

   b. What in her history might increase her risk for ovarian cancer?

   c. What can the nurse do to increase awareness of this cancer for all women?

STUDY ACTIVITIES

1. During your surgical clinical rotation, interview a female client undergoing surgery for cancer of her reproductive organs. Ask her to recall the symptoms that brought her to the health care provider. Ask her what thoughts, feelings, and emotions went through her mind before and after her diagnosis. Finally, ask her how this experience will change her life in the future.

2. Visit an oncology and radiology treatment center to find out about the various treatment modalities available for reproductive cancers. Contrast the various treatment methods and report your findings to your class.

3. Visit one of the websites listed at the end of the chapter to explore a topic of interest concerning reproductive cancers. How correct and current is the content? What is its level? Share your assessment with your classmates.

4. Taking oral contraceptives provides protection against _____ cancer.

5. Two genes, BRCA-1 and BRCA-2, are linked with hereditary _____ and _____ cancers.

CHAPTER 9

VIOLENCE AND ABUSE

KEY TERMS

acquaintance rape
battered women
    syndrome
cycle of violence
date rape

female genital mutilation
human trafficking
incest
intimate partner
    violence

post-traumatic stress
    disorder
rape
sexual abuse
statutory rape

LEARNING OBJECTIVES

After completion of the chapter, the student should be able to:

1. Define the key terms.
2. Discuss the incidence of violence in women.
3. Outline the cycle of violence and appropriate interventions.
4. Discuss the myths and facts about violence.
5. Analyze the dynamics of rape and sexual abuse.
6. Describe the resources available to women experiencing abuse.
7. Discuss the role of the nurse who cares for abused women.

Dorothy came to the prenatal clinic with a complaint of recurring headaches. She had been in twice this week already, but insisted she be seen today and started to cry. When the nurse called her into the examination room, Dorothy's cell phone rang. She hurried to answer it and told the person on the other end that she was at the store. When the nurse asked if she was afraid at home, Dorothy answered "at times." What cues did the nurse pick up on to ask that question? How frequent is this problem in women?

WOW After being traumatized, women can decide to stay in the shallow end of the pool or they can find support and swim in the ocean.

Violence against women is a significant health and social problem affecting virtually all societies, but often it goes unrecognized and unreported. For all the strides American women have made in the past 100 years, obliterating violence against themselves isn't one of them. Violence against women is a growing problem. In many countries it is still accepted as part of normal behavior. According to the Federal Bureau of Investigation, one third to one half of all women in the United States will experience some form of physical violence during their lifetime (FBI, 2007). Forty percent to 60 percent of murders of women in North America are committed by intimate partners (FBI, 2007). Federal funding for the problem is trickling down to local programs, but it isn't reaching victims fast enough. In the United States, there are three times more shelters for animals than for battered women (Dutton, 2007). In many cases, a victim escapes her abuser only to be turned away from a local shelter because it is full. The number of abused women is staggering: one woman is being battered every 12 seconds in the United States (CDC, 2007a).

Nurses play a major role in assessing women who have suffered some type of violence. Often, after a woman is victimized, she will complain about physical ailments that will give her the opportunity to visit a health care setting. A visit to a health care agency is an ideal time for women to be assessed for violence. Because nurses are viewed as trustworthy and sensitive about very personal subjects, women often feel comfortable in confiding or discussing these issues with them.

> ▶ *Take* NOTE!
>
> *Nurses will come in contact with violence and sexual abuse no matter what health care setting they work in. Nurses must be ready to ask the right questions and to act on the answers, because such action could be life-saving.*

This chapter will address two types of violence against women: intimate partner violence and sexual abuse. Both types of violence against women have devastating and costly consequences for all of society.

Intimate Partner Violence

Intimate partner violence is actual or threatened physical or sexual violence or psychological/emotional abuse. It includes threats of physical or sexual violence when the threat is used to control a person's actions (CDC, 2007a). Intimate partners include individuals who are currently in dating, cohabitating, or marital relationships, or those who have been in such relationships in the past. Some of the common terms used to describe intimate partner violence are domestic abuse, spouse abuse, domestic violence, battering, and rape. Intimate partner violence affects a distressingly high percentage of the population and has physical, psychological, social, and economic consequences (Fig. 9.1).

A nurse may be the first health care professional to assess and identify the signs of intimate partner violence and can have a profound impact on a woman's decision to seek help. Thus, it is important for nurses to be able to identify abuse and aid the victim. Intimate partner violence can leave significant psychological scars, and a well-trained nurse can have a positive impact on the victim's mental and emotional health.

Incidence

Although estimates vary, as many as 6 million women are abused annually (CDC, 2007a). Even more shocking, 75% of the abused women initially identified in a medical setting go on to suffer repeated abuse, including homicide (CDC, 2007a). This may include physical violence, emotional abuse, sexual assault, rape, incest, or elder abuse. Each year, intimate partner violence results in an estimated 1,200 deaths and 2 million injuries among women (CDC, 2008).

Women are at risk for violence at nearly every stage of their lives. Old, young, beautiful, unattractive, married, single—no woman is completely safe from the risk of intimate partner violence. Current or former husbands or lovers kill over half of the murdered women in the United States. Intimate partner violence against women causes more serious injuries and deaths than automobile accidents, rapes, and muggings combined. The medical cost of intimate partner violence approaches $6 billion each year to pay for medical and surgical care, counseling, child care, incarceration, attorney fees, and loss of work productivity (Kelly, 2007).

Abuse occurs in both heterosexual and homosexual relationships. Violence within gay and lesbian relationships may go unreported for fear of harassment or ridicule. In addition, since gay and lesbian partnerships are not seen

FIGURE 9.1 Intimate partner violence has significant physical, psychological, social, and economic consequences. An important role of the health care provider is to identify abusive or potentially abusive situations as soon as possible and provide support for the victim.

as legal in many states, there are few statistics gathered on incident rates.

Background

Until the mid-1970s, our society tended to legitimize a man's power and control over a woman. The U.S. legal and judicial systems considered intervention into family disputes wrong and a violation of the family's right to privacy. Intimate partner violence was often tolerated and even socially acceptable. Fortunately, attitudes and laws have changed to protect women and punish abusers. In *Healthy People 2010*, two key objectives address violence against women.

Characteristics of Intimate Partner Violence

Although more research is needed in this area, studies have found certain risk factors for intimate partner violence:

• Use and abuse of substances such as alcohol (this increases the risk of perpetration and victimization for both men and women)
• Negative affect (e.g., hostility and depression)
• History of childhood abuse
• History of antisocial behavior
• Current unemployment
• Neighborhood norms that accept violence and drug use
• Traditional gender role expectations (Herrenkohl et al., 2007)

Generation-to-Generation Continuum of Violence

Violence is a learned behavior that, without intervention, is self-perpetuating. It is a cyclical health problem. The long-term effects of violence on victims and children can be profound. Children who witness one parent abuse another are more likely to become delinquents or batterers themselves because they see abuse as an integral part of a close relationship. Thus, an abusive rela-

---

HEALTHY PEOPLE 2010

Objective	Significance
1. Reduce the rate of physical assault by current or former intimate partners. 2. Reduce the annual rate of rape or attempted rape.	• Will increase women's quality and years of healthy life • Eliminate health disparities for survivors of violence • Goal is to have 90% compliance in screening for intimate partner violence by health professionals. • Meeting these objectives will reflect the importance of early detection, intervention, and evaluation.

Available at www.healthypeople.gov/

---

tionship between father and mother can perpetuate future abusive relationships. Research has found that children who witness intimate partner violence are at risk for developing psychiatric disorders, developmental problems, school failure, violence against others, and low self-esteem (Paluzzi, 2007).

Childhood maltreatment is a major health problem that is associated with a wide range of physical conditions and leads to high rates of psychiatric morbidity and social problems in adulthood. Women who were physically or sexually abused as children have an increased risk of victimization and experience adverse mental health conditions such as depression, anxiety, and low self-esteem as adults (Ferris, 2007).

In 50% to 75% of the cases when a parent is abused, the children are abused as well (Paluzzi, 2007). Exposure to violence has a negative impact on children's physical, emotional, and cognitive well-being. The cycle continues into another generation through learned responses and violent acting out. While there are always exceptions, most children deprived of their basic physical, psychological, and spiritual needs do not develop healthy personalities. They grow up with feelings of fear, inadequacy, anxiety, anger, hostility, guilt, and rage. They often lack coping skills, blame others, demonstrate poor impulse control, and generally struggle with authority. Unless this cycle is broken, more than half become abusers themselves (CDC, 2007a).

The Cycle of Violence

In an abusive relationship, the **cycle of violence** comprises three distinct phases: the tension-building phase, the acute battering phase, and the honeymoon phase (Dutton, 2007). The cyclical behavior begins with a time of tension-building arguments, progresses to violence, and settles into a making-up or calm period. This cycle of violence increases in frequency and severity as it is repeated over and over again. The cycle can cover a long or short period of time. The honeymoon phase gradually shortens and eventually disappears altogether. Abuse in relationships typically becomes accelerated and thus more dangerous over time. The abuser no longer feels the need to apologize and indulge in a honeymoon phase as the woman becomes increasingly disempowered in the relationship.

Phase 1: Tension-Building

During the first—and usually the longest—phase of the cycle, tension escalates between the couple. Excessive drinking, jealousy, or other factors might lead to name-calling, hostility, and friction. The woman might sense that her partner is reacting to her more negatively, that he is on edge and reacts heatedly to any trivial frustration. A woman often will accept her partner's building anger as legitimately directed toward her. She internalizes what she perceives as her responsibility to keep the situation from exploding. In her mind, if she does her job well, he remains calm. But if she fails, the resulting violence is her fault.

Phase 2: Acute Battering

The second phase of the cycle is the explosion of violence. The batterer loses control both physically and emotionally. This is when the victim may be assaulted or murdered. After a battering episode, most victims consider themselves lucky that the abuse was not worse, no matter how severe their injuries. They often deny the seriousness of their injuries and refuse to seek medical treatment.

Phase 3: Honeymoon

The third phase of the cycle is a period of calm, loving, contrite behavior on the part of the batterer. He may be genuinely sorry for the pain he caused his partner. He attempts to make up for his brutal behavior and believes he can control himself and never hurt the woman he loves. The victim wants to believe that her partner really can change. She feels responsible, at least in part, for causing the incident, and she feels responsible for her partner's well-being (Box 9.1).

Types of Abuse

Abusers may use whatever it takes to control a situation—from emotional abuse and humiliation to physical assault. Victims often tolerate emotional, physical, financial, and sexual abuse. Many remain in abusive relationships because they believe they deserve the abuse.

Emotional Abuse

Emotional abuse includes:

- Promising, swearing, or threatening to hit the victim
- Forcing the victim to perform degrading or humiliating acts
- Threatening to harm children, pets, or close friends
- Humiliating the woman by name-calling and insults
- Threatening to leave her and the children
- Destroying valued possessions
- Controlling the victim's every move

BOX 9.1 **Cycle of Violence**

- Phase 1: Tension-building: Verbal or minor battery occurs. Almost any subject, such as housekeeping or money, may trigger the buildup of tension. The victim attempts to calm the abuser.
- Phase 2: Acute battering: Characterized by uncontrollable discharge of tension. Violence is rarely triggered by the victim's behavior: she is battered no matter what her response.
- Phase 3: Reconciliation (honeymoon)/calm phase: The batterer becomes loving, kind, and apologetic and expresses guilt. Then the abuser works on making the victim feel responsible.

Sources: AWHONN, 2007; Aggeles, 2007; Burgess, 2007.

Physical Abuse

Physical abuse includes:

- Hitting or grabbing the victim so hard that it leaves marks
- Throwing things at the victim
- Slapping, spitting at, biting, burning, pushing, choking, or shoving the victim
- Kicking or punching the victim, or slamming her against things
- Attacking the victim with a knife, gun, rope, or electrical cord
- Controlling access to health care for injury

Financial Abuse

Financial abuse includes:

- Preventing the woman from getting a job
- Sabotaging a current job
- Controlling how all money is spent
- Failing to contribute financially

Sexual Abuse

Sexual abuse includes:

- Forcing the woman to have vaginal, oral, or anal intercourse against her will
- Biting the victim's breasts or genitals
- Shoving objects into the victim's vagina
- Forcing the victim to perform sexual acts on other people or animals

Myths and Facts About Intimate Partner Violence

There are many myths about intimate partner violence (Table 9.1). Health care providers should take steps to dispel these myths.

Abuse Profiles

Victims

Ironically, victims rarely describe themselves as abused. In **battered woman syndrome**, the woman has experienced deliberate and repeated physical or sexual assault by an intimate partner. She is terrified and feels trapped, helpless, and alone. She reacts to any expression of anger or threat by avoidance and withdrawal behavior.

Some women believe that the abuse is caused by a personality flaw or inadequacy in themselves (e.g., inability to keep the man happy). These feelings of failure are reinforced and exploited by their partners. After being told repeatedly that they are "bad," some women begin to believe it. Many victims were abused as children and may have poor self-esteem, depression, insomnia, or a history of suicide attempts, injury, or drug and alcohol abuse (Aggeles, 2007).

Abusers

Abusers come from all walks of life and often feel insecure, powerless, and helpless, feelings that are not in line with the macho image they would like to project. The abuser

TABLE 9.1 COMMON MYTHS AND FACTS ABOUT VIOLENCE

Myths	Facts
Battering of women occurs only in lower socioeconomic classes.	Violence occurs in all socioeconomic classes.
Substance abuse causes the violence.	Violence is a learned behavior and can be changed.
Violence occurs to only a small percentage of women.	The presence of drugs and alcohol can make a bad problem worse.
Women can easily choose to leave the abusive relationship.	One in four women will be victims of violence.
Only men with mental health problems commit violence against women.	Women stay in the abusive relationship because they feel they have no options.
Pregnant women are protected from abuse by their partners.	Abusers often seem normal and don't appear to suffer from personality disorders or other forms of mental illness.
Women provoke their partners to abuse them.	One in five women is physically abused during pregnancy.
Violent tendencies have gone on for generations and are accepted.	The effects of violence on infant outcomes can include preterm delivery, fetal distress, low birthweight, and child abuse.
	Women may be willing to blame themselves for someone else's bad behavior, but nobody deserves to be beaten.
	The police, justice system, and society are beginning to make domestic violence socially unacceptable.

Sources: Aggeles, 2007; AWHONN, 2007; Giardino, 2007; Kelly, 2007.

expresses his feelings of inadequacy through violence or aggression toward others (Du Plat-Jones, 2006).

Violence typically occurs at home and is usually directed toward the man's intimate partner or the children who live there. Abusers refuse to share power and choose violence to control their victims. They often exhibit child-like aggression or antisocial behaviors. They may fail to accept responsibility or blame others for their own problems. They might also have a history of substance abuse problems, mental illness, arrests, troubled relationships, obsessive jealousy, controlling behaviors, erratic employment history, and financial problems.

Violence Against Pregnant Women

Many think of pregnancy as a time of celebration and planning for the unborn child's future, but in a troubled relationship it can be a time of escalating violence. The strongest predictor of abuse during pregnancy is prior abuse (Giardino, 2007). For women who have been abused before, beatings and violence during pregnancy are "business as usual" for them.

Women are at a higher risk for violence during pregnancy. Pregnant women are vulnerable during this time, and abusers can take advantage of it. An estimated 325,000 pregnant women are abused by their partners each year (CDC, 2007a). Abuse during pregnancy poses special risks and dynamics.

Various factors may lead to battering during pregnancy, including:

- Inability of the couple to cope with the stressors of pregnancy
- Resentment toward the interference of the growing fetus and change in the woman's shape

- Doubts about paternity or the expectant mother's fidelity during pregnancy
- Perception that the baby will be a competitor
- Outside attention the pregnancy brings to the woman
- Unwanted pregnancy
- The woman's new interest in herself and her unborn baby
- Insecurity and jealousy about the pregnancy and the responsibilities it brings
- Financial burden related to expense of pregnancy and loss of income
- Stress of role transition from adult man to becoming the father of a child
- Physical and emotional changes of pregnancy that make the woman vulnerable
- Previous isolation from family and friends that limit the couple's support system

Abuse during pregnancy threatens the well-being of the mother and fetus. Physical violence may involve injuries to the head, face, neck, thorax, breasts, and abdomen (Casanueva & Martin, 2007). The mental health consequences are also significant. Several studies have confirmed the relationship between abuse and poor mental health, especially depression (Giardino, 2007). For the pregnant woman, this most often manifests itself as postpartum depression.

 ▶ *Take* NOTE!

Frequently the fear of harm to her unborn child will motivate a woman to escape an abusive relationship.

Women assaulted during pregnancy are at risk for:

- Injuries to themselves and the fetus
- Depression
- Chronic anxiety
- Miscarriage
- Stillbirth
- Poor nutrition
- Insomnia
- Placental abruption
- Uterine rupture
- Excessive weight gain or loss
- Smoking and substance abuse
- Delayed or no prenatal care
- Preterm labor
- Chorioamnionitis
- Vaginitis
- Sexually transmitted infections
- Urinary tract infections
- Premature and low-birthweight infants (Sharps, Laughon, & Giangrande, 2007)

Signs of abuse can emerge during pregnancy and may include poor attendance at prenatal visits, unrealistic fears, weight fluctuations, difficulty with pelvic examinations, and noncompliance with treatment.

Uncovering abuse in pregnant women requires a consistent and direct approach to every client by the nurse. Multiple assessments may enhance reporting by enabling the nurse to establish trust and rapport with the woman and identify changes in her behavior. Once abuse is discovered in a pregnant woman, interventions should include safety assessment, emotional support, counseling, referral to community services, and ongoing prenatal care (Burgess, 2007).

Violence Against Older Women

Intimate partner violence affects women of all ages, but often the literature focuses on women in the childbearing years, ignoring the problems of aging women experiencing abuse. There are laws in all 50 states requiring health care professionals to report elder or vulnerable person abuse. Estimates suggest that 500,000 to 1.5 million cases of elder abuse and neglect occur annually in the United States (Bonomi et al., 2007).

Although an injury may bring the older woman into the health care system, the physical and emotional sequelae of intimate partner violence may be more subtle: they may include depression, insomnia, chronic pain, atypical chest pain, or other kinds of somatic symptoms (Thackeray et al., 2007). Accurate detection and assess-

---

EVIDENCE-BASED PRACTICE 9.1
Nurse Case Management for Pregnant Women Experiencing or at Risk for Abuse

The goal of this randomized controlled trial was to determine whether individualized nursing case management can decrease stress among pregnant women at risk for abuse or in abusive relationships.

● Study
The study was conducted at two prenatal clinics in the Pacific Northwest and rural Midwest. Participants were 1,000 women who spoke English and were 13 to 23 weeks pregnant at time of recruitment. All intervention group women (n = 499) were offered an abuse video and had access to a nurse case manager 24/7. Participants at risk for abuse or in abusive relationships also received individualized nursing care management throughout the pregnancy.

▲ Findings
The most common nursing activities were providing support (38%) and assessing needs (32%). The nursing care management group received an average of 22 contacts,

most (80%) by telephone, and had a significant reduction in stress scores as measured by the Prenatal Psychosocial Profile. Compared to the control group, the differences were in the predicted direction but were not statistically different. A major finding was the choice by abused women to focus on basic needs and their pregnancies rather than the abuse, although all received safety planning.

■ Nursing Implications
Pregnant women at risk for abuse or in abusive relationships experience very stressful and complex lives. Nurses need to focus on the needs they identify, which may not be the abusive relationship.

Curry, M. A., Durham, L., Bullock, L., Bloom, T., & Davis, J. (2006). Nurse case management for pregnant women experiencing or at risk for abuse. *Journal of Obstetric, Gynecologic, and Neonatal Nursing, 35*(2), 181–192.

ment of abuse in elderly women are essential duties of all nurses.

Nursing Management

Nurses encounter thousands of abuse victims each year in their practice settings, but many victims slip through the cracks. There are many things that nurses can do to help victims. Early recognition and intervention can significantly reduce the morbidity and mortality associated with intimate partner violence. To stop the cycle of violence, nurses need to know how to assess for and identify violence and implement appropriate actions. The key is astute assessment and identification.

Assessment

Routine screening for intimate partner violence is the first way to detect abuse. The nurse should build rapport by showing an interest in the concerns of the woman, listening, and creating an atmosphere of openness. Communicating support through a nonjudgmental attitude, or telling her that no one deserves to be abused, is the first step toward establishing trust and rapport. Rather than overlooking abused women as "chronic complainers," astute nurses need to be vigilant for subtle clues of abuse.

Learning how to assess for abuse is critical. Some basic assessment guidelines follow.

Screen for Abuse During Every Health Care Visit

Screening for violence takes only a few minutes and can have an enormously positive effect on the outcome for the abused woman. Any woman could be a victim; no single sign marks a woman as an abuse victim, but the following clues may be helpful:

- Injuries: bruises, scars from blunt trauma, or weapon wounds on the face, head, and neck
- Injury sequelae: headaches, hearing loss, joint pain, sinus infections, teeth marks, clumps of hair missing, dental trauma, pelvic pain, breast or genital injuries
- Reported history of injury that is not consistent with the actual presenting problem
- Mental health problems: depression, anxiety, substance abuse, eating disorders, suicidal ideation or suicide attempts
- Frequent health care visits for chronic, stress-related disorders such as chest pain, headaches, back or pelvic pain, insomnia, and gastrointestinal disturbances
- Partner's behavior at the health care visit: appears overly solicitous or overprotective, is unwilling to leave her alone with the health care provider, answers questions for her, and attempts to control the situation (Aggeles, 2007)

Look for the following indicators of abuse:

- Previous history of assault
- Previous injuries inflicted by weapons

- Multiple medical visits for injuries or anxiety symptoms
- History of depression, substance use, or suicide attempts
- Tranquilizer or sedative use
- Sexually transmitted infections or pelvic inflammatory disease
- Bruises to the upper arm, neck and face, abdomen, or breasts
- Comments about emotional or physical abuse of "a friend"
- Hovering behavior of male partner during visit (Aggeles, 2007; Giardino, 2007)

*D*orothy, who you met at the beginning of the chapter, has been frequenting the clinic with vague somatic complaints in recent weeks and admits she is sometimes afraid at home. She tells the nurse her partner doesn't want her to work, even though he was only sporadically employed at low-paying jobs. What cues in her assessment might indicate abuse? What physical signs might the nurse observe?

Isolate Patient Immediately From Family

If abuse is detected, immediately isolate the woman to provide privacy and to prevent potential retaliation from the abuser. Asking about abuse in front of the perpetrator may trigger an abusive episode during the interview or at home. Ways to ensure the woman's safety would be to take the victim to an area away from the abuser to ask questions. The assessment can take place anywhere— x-ray area, ultrasound room, elevator, ladies' room, laboratory—that is private and away from the abuser.

If abuse is detected, the nurse can do the following to enhance the nurse–client relationship:

- Educate the woman about the connection between the violence and her symptoms.
- Help the woman acknowledge what has happened to her and begin to deal with the situation.
- Offer her referrals so she can get the help that will allow her to begin to heal.

*D*orothy returns to the prenatal clinic a month later with anemia, inadequate weight gain, bruises on her face and neck, and second-trimester bleeding. This time she is accompanied by her partner, who stays close to Dorothy. What questions should the nurse ask to assess the situation? Where is the appropriate location to ask these questions? What legal responsibilities does the nurse have concerning her observations?

Ask Direct or Indirect Questions About Abuse

Questions to screen for abuse should be routine and handled just like any other question. Many nurses feel uncomfortable asking questions of this nature, but broaching the subject is important even if the answer comes later. Just knowing that someone else knows about the abuse offers a victim some relief.

Ask difficult questions in an empathetic and nonthreatening manner and remain nonjudgmental in all responses and interactions. Choose the type of question that makes you most comfortable. Direct and indirect questions produce the same results. "Does your partner hit you?" or "Have you ever been or are you now in an abusive relationship?" are direct questions. If that approach feels uncomfortable, try indirect questions: "We see many women with injuries or complaints like yours and often they are being abused. Is that what is happening to you?" or "Many women in our community experience abuse from their partners. Is anything like that happening in your life?" With either approach, nurses need to maintain a nonjudgmental acceptance of whatever answer the woman offers.

The SAVE Model is a screening protocol that nurses can use when assessing women for violence (Box 9.2).

BOX 9.2 SAVE Model

SCREEN all of your patients for violence by asking:
- Do you feel safe in your home?
- Do you feel you are in control of your life?
- Have you ever been sexually or physically abused?
- Can you talk about your abuse with me now?

ASK direct questions in a nonjudgmental way:
- Begin by normalizing the topic to the woman.
- Make continuous eye contact with the woman.
- Stay calm; avoid emotional reactions to what she tells you.
- Never blame the woman, even if she blames herself.
- Don't dismiss or minimize what she tells you, even if she does.
- Wait for each answer patiently. Don't rush to the next question.
- Do not use formal, technical, or medical language.
- Use a nonthreatening, accepting approach.

VALIDATE the patient by telling her:
- You believe her story.
- You do not blame her for what happened.
- It is brave of her to tell you this.
- Help is available for her.
- Talking with you is a hopeful sign and a first big step.

EVALUATE, educate, and refer this patient by asking her:
- What type of violence was it?
- Is she now in any danger?
- How is she feeling now?
- Does she know that there are consequences to violence?
- Is she aware of community resources available to help her?

Sources: Dutton, 2007; Du Plat-Jones, 2006; Thackeray et al., 2007.

Assess Immediate Safety

The Danger Assessment Tool helps women and health care providers assess the potential for homicidal behavior in an ongoing abusive relationship. It is based on research that showed several risk factors for abuse-related murders:

- Increased frequency or severity of abuse
- Presence of firearms
- Sexual abuse
- Substance abuse
- Generally violent behavior outside of the home
- Control issues (e.g., daily chores, friends, job, money)
- Physical abuse during pregnancy
- Suicide threats or attempts (victim or abuser)
- Child abuse (Kelly, 2007)

Document and Report Your Findings

If the interview reveals a history of abuse, accurate documentation is critical because this evidence may support the woman's case in court. Documentation must include details about the frequency and severity of abuse; the location, extent, and outcome of injuries; and any treatments or interventions. When documenting, use direct quotes and be very specific: "He choked me." Describe any visible injuries, and use a body map (outline of a woman's body) to show where the injuries are. Obtain photos (with informed consent) or document her refusal if the woman declines photos. Pictures or diagrams can be worth a thousand words. Figure 9.2 shows a sample documentation form for intimate partner violence.

Laws in many states require health care providers to alert the police to any injuries that involve knives, firearms, or other deadly weapons or that present life-threatening emergencies. If assessment reveals suspicion or actual indication of abuse, you can explain to the woman that you are required by law to report it.

Nursing Diagnosis

When violence is suspected or validated, the nurse needs to formulate nursing diagnoses based on the completed assessment. Possible nursing diagnoses related to violence against women might include the following:

- Deficient knowledge related to understanding the cycle of violence and availability of resources
- Fear related to possibility of severe injury to self or children during cycle of violence
- Low self-esteem related to feelings of worthlessness
- Hopelessness related to prolonged exposure to violence
- Compromised individual and family coping related to persistence of victim–abuser relationship

Interventions

If abuse is identified, nurses can undertake interventions that can increase the woman's safety and improve her health. The goal of intervention is to enable the victim to gain control of her life. Provide sensitive, predictable care

INTIMATE PARTNER VIOLENCE DOCUMENTATION FORM

Explain to Client: The majority of what you tell me is confidential and cannot be shared with anyone without your written permission. However, I am required by law to report information pertaining to child or adult abuse and gunshot wounds or life-threatening injuries.

STEP 1–Establish total privacy to ask screening questions. Safety is the first priority. Client must be alone, or if the client has a child with her, the child must not be of verbal age. ONLY complete this form if YOU CAN assure the client's safety, privacy, and confidentiality.

STEP 2–Ask the client screening questions.

"Because abuse is so common, we are now asking all of our female clients:

Are you in a relationship in which you are being hurt or threatened, emotionally or physically?
___Yes ___ No

Do you feel unsafe at home?"
___Yes ___ No

If both screening questions are NO in STEP 2, and you are not concerned that the client may be a victim, sign and date the form in the signature block directly below. Provide information and resources as appropriate.

Signature _____ **Title** _____ **Date** _____

If both screening answers are NO and you are concerned that the client may be a victim, go to STEP 5. If the client answers YES to either question, proceed to STEP 3 below. Sign and date the signature block on the back of the form after completing STEP 6.

STEP 3–Assess the abuse and safety of the client and any children.

Say to client: "From the answers you have just given me, I am worried for you."

    "Has the relationship gotten worse, or is it getting scarier?"   ___Yes ___ No

    "Does your partner ever watch you closely, follow you, or stalk you?"   ___Yes ___ No

Ask the following question in clinic settings only. Do not ask in home settings:

"If your partner is here with you today, are you afraid to leave with him/her?"   ___Yes ___ No

"Is there anything else you want to tell me?" _____
_____
_____
_____

Name: _____

ID No: _____

Date of Birth: _____

DH 3202, 2/03
Stock Number: 5744-000-3202-2

FIGURE **9.2** Intimate partner violence documentation form. (Florida Department of Health) *(continued)*

"Are there children in the home?" ___Yes ___ No

If the answer to the question above is "yes," say to client: "I'm concerned for your safety and the safety of your children. You and your children deserve to be at home without feeling afraid."

"Have there been threats of abuse or direct abuse of the children?" ___Yes ___ No

STEP 4–Assess client's physical injuries and health conditions, past and present.

Observations/Comments/Interventions:

STEP 5–If both screening answers are NO, and you ARE CONCERNED that the client may be a victim:

a. Say to the client: "All of us know of someone at some time in our lives who is abused. So, I am providing you with information in the event you or a friend may need it in the future."

b. Document under comments in Step 6.

STEP 6–Information, referrals or reports made

Yes   No

___   ___   1. Client given domestic violence information including safety planning
___   ___   2. Reviewed domestic violence information including safety planning
___   ___   3. State Abuse Hotline (1-800-96-ABUSE) and State Domestic Violence
            Hotline number (1-800-500-1119) given to the client
___   ___   4. Client called hotline during visit
___   ___   5. Client seen by advocate during visit
___   ___   6. Report made. If yes, to whom: _____

Comments

Signature _____ Title _____ Date _____

FIGURE 9.2 (continued) Intimate partner violence documentation form. (Florida Department of Health) in an accepting setting. Offer step-by-step explanations of procedures. Provide educational materials about violence. Allow the victim to actively participate in her care and have control over all health care decisions. Pace your nursing interventions and allow the woman to take the lead. Communicate support through a nonjudgmental attitude. Carefully document assessment findings and nursing interventions.

Depending on when in the cycle of violence the nurse encounters the abused woman, goals may fall into three groups:

- Primary prevention: aimed at breaking the abuse cycle through community educational initiatives by nurses, physicians, law enforcement, teachers, and clergy
- Secondary prevention: focuses on dealing with victims and abusers in early stages, with the goal of preventing progression of abuse
- Tertiary prevention: activities are geared toward helping severely abused women and children recover and become productive members of society and rehabilitating abusers to stop the cycle of violence. These activities are typically long term and expensive.

A tool developed by Holtz and Furniss (1993)—the ABCDES—provides a framework for providing sensitive nursing interventions to abused women (Box 9.3).

Specific nursing interventions for the abused woman include educating her about community services, providing emotional support, and offering a safety plan.

BOX 9.3 The ABCDES of Caring for Abused Women

- **A** is reassuring the woman that she is not alone. The isolation by her abuser keeps her from knowing that others are in the same situation and that health care providers can help her.
- **B** is expressing the belief that violence against women is not acceptable in any situation and that it is not her fault.
- **C** is confidentiality, since the woman might believe that if the abuse is reported, the abuser will retaliate.
- **D** is documentation, which includes the following:
  1. A clear quoted statement about the abuse
  2. Accurate descriptions of injuries and the history of them
  3. Photos of the injuries (with the woman's consent)
- **E** is education about the cycle of violence and that it will escalate.
- **S** is safety, the most important aspect of the intervention, to ensure that the woman has resources and a plan of action to carry out when she decides to leave.

Educate the Woman About Community Services

A wide range of support services are available to meet the needs of victims of violence. Nurses should be prepared to help the woman take advantage of these opportunities. Services will vary by community but might include psychological counseling, legal advice, social services, crisis services, support groups, hotlines, housing, vocational training, and other community-based referrals.

Give the woman information about shelters or services even if she initially rejects it. Give the woman the National Domestic Violence hotline number: (800) 799-7233. Since 1992, guidelines from the Joint Commission on Accreditation of Healthcare Organizations (JCAHO) have required emergency departments to maintain lists of community referral agencies that deal with the victims of intimate partner violence (JCAHO, 2007).

Provide Emotional Support

Providing reassurance and support to a victim of abuse is key if the violence is to end. Nurses in all clinical settings can help victims to feel a sense of personal power and provide them with a safe and supportive environment. Appropriate action can help victims to express their thoughts and feelings in constructive ways, manage stress, and move on with their lives. Appropriate interventions are:

- Strengthen the woman's sense of control over her life by:
  - Teaching coping strategies to manage her stress
  - Assisting with activities of daily living to improve her lifestyle
  - Allowing her to make as many decisions as she can
  - Educating her about the symptoms of post-traumatic stress disorder and their basis
- Encourage the woman to establish realistic goals for herself by:
  - Teaching problem-solving skills
  - Encouraging social activities to connect with other people
- Provide support and allow the woman to grieve for her losses by:
  - Listening to and clarifying her reactions to the traumatic event
  - Discussing shock, disbelief, anger, depression, and acceptance
- Explain to the woman that:
  - Abuse is never OK. She didn't ask for it and she doesn't deserve it.
  - She is not alone and help is available.
  - Abuse is a crime and she is a victim.
  - Alcohol, drugs, money problems, depression, or jealousy does not cause violence, but these things can give the abuser an excuse for losing control and abusing her.
  - The actions of the abuser are not her fault.
  - Her history of abuse is believed.
  - Making a decision to leave an abusive relationship can be very hard and takes time.

Offer a Safety Plan

The choice to leave must rest with the victim. Nurses cannot choose a life for the victim; they can only offer choices. Leaving is a process, not an event. Victims may try to leave their abusers as many as seven or eight times before succeeding. Frequently, the final attempt to leave may result in the death of the victim. Women planning to leave an abusive relationship should have a safety plan, if possible (Teaching Guidelines 9.1).

Sexual Violence

Sexual violence is both a public health problem and a human rights violation. More than once every 3 minutes, 78 times an hour, 1,871 times a day, girls and women in America are raped (Medicine Net, 2007). Rape has been reported against females from age 6 months to 93 years, but it still remains one of the most underreported violent crimes in the United States. Estimates suggest that, somewhere in the United States, a woman is sexually assaulted every 2.5 minutes (RAINN, 2007). The National Center for Prevention and Control of Sexual Assault estimates that one out of three women will be sexually assaulted sometime in her life, and two thirds of these assaults will not be reported (CDC, 2007b). Over the course of their lives, women may experience more than one type of violence.

Sexual violence can have a variety of devastating short- and long-term effects. Women can experience psychological, physical, and cognitive symptoms that affect them daily. They can include chronic pelvic pain, headaches, backache, sexually transmitted infections, pregnancy, anxiety, denial, fear, withdrawal, sleep disturbances, guilt, nervousness, phobias, substance abuse, depression, sexual dysfunction, and post-traumatic stress disorder (CDC, 2007b). A traumatic experience not only damages a woman's sense of safety in the world, but it can also reduce her self-esteem and her ability to continue her education, to earn money and be productive, to have children and, if she has children, to nurture and protect them (Macy et al., 2007).

> ▶ **Take** NOTE!
>
> *Sexual violence has been called a "tragedy of youth." More than half of all rapes (54%) of women occur before age 18 (Medicine Net, 2007).*

Assailants, like their victims, come from all walks of life and all ethnic backgrounds; there is no typical profile. More than half are under 25, and the majority are married and leading "normal" sex lives. Why do men rape? No theory provides a satisfactory explanation. So few assailants are caught and convicted that a clear profile remains elusive. What is known is that many assailants have trouble dealing with the stresses of daily life. Such men become angry and experience feelings of powerlessness. They commit a sexual assault as an expression of power and control (Macy et al., 2007).

Sexual violence is a broad term that can be used to describe sexual abuse, incest, rape, female genital mutilation, and human trafficking.

Sexual Abuse

Sexual abuse occurs when a woman is forced to have sexual contact of any kind (vaginal, oral, or anal) without her consent. Marriage does not constitute a tacit agreement for a spouse to inflict one's demands on the other without permission. Childhood sexual abuse is any type of sexual exploitation that involves a child younger than 18 years old; it might include disrobing, nudity, masturbation, fondling, digital penetration, and intercourse (Alekseeva, 2007).

Childhood sexual abuse has a lifelong impact on its survivors. Women who were sexually abused during childhood are at a heightened risk for repeat abuse. This is because the early abuse lowers their self-esteem and their ability to protect themselves and set firm boundaries. Childhood sexual abuse is a trauma that influences the way victims form relationships, deal with adversity, cope with daily problems, relate to their children and peers, protect their health, and live. Studies have shown that the more victimization a woman experiences, the more likely it is she will be re-victimized (Kristensen & Lau, 2007).

TEACHING GUIDELINES 9.1

Safety Plan for Leaving an Abusive Relationship

- When leaving an abusive relationship, take the following items:
  - Driver's license or photo ID
  - Social security number or green card/work permit
  - Birth certificates for you and your children
  - Phone numbers for social services or women's shelter
  - The deed or lease to your home or apartment
  - Any court papers or orders
  - A change of clothing for you and your children
  - Pay stubs, checkbook, credit cards, and cash
  - Insurance cards (Du Plat-Jones, 2006; Dutton, 2007)
  - If you need to leave a domestic violence situation immediately, turn to authorities for assistance in gathering this material.
- Develop a "game plan" for leaving and rehearse it.
- Don't use phone cards—they leave a trail to follow.

EVIDENCE–BASED PRACTICE 9.2
Cognitive-Behavioral Interventions for Children Who Have Been Sexually Abused

Despite different perceptions as to what constitutes child sexual abuse, there is a consensus among clinicians and researchers that this is a substantial social problem that affects large numbers of children and young people worldwide. The effects of sexual abuse manifest themselves in a wide range of symptoms, including fear, anxiety, post-traumatic stress disorder and behavior problems such as externalizing or internalizing, or inappropriate sexual behaviors. Child sexual abuse is associated with an increased risk of psychological problems in adulthood. Knowing what is most likely to benefit children already traumatized by these events is important.

● Study
The aim of this review was to assess the efficacy of cognitive-behavioral therapy (CBT) in addressing the immediate and longer-term sequelae of sexual abuse in children. Ten studies comprising 847 children were identified that met the inclusion criteria.

▲ Findings
The evidence suggests that CBT may have a positive impact on the sequelae of child sexual abuse, but most results were statistically nonsignificant.

● Nursing Implications
The review confirms CBT's potential for addressing the adverse consequences of child sexual abuse but highlights the tenuousness of the evidence base and the need for more carefully conducted and better reported trials.

Macdonald, G. M., Higgins, J. P. T., & Ramchandani, P. (2006). Cognitive-behavioral interventions for children who have been sexually abused. *Cochrane Database of Systematic Reviews* 2006, Issue 4. Art. No.: CD001930. DOI: 10.1002/14651858.CD001930.pub2.

Incest

Childhood sexual abuse involves any kind of sexual experience between a child and another person that violates the social taboos of family roles; children cannot yet understand these activities and cannot give informed consent (Alekseeva, 2007). **Incest** is any type of sexual exploitation between blood relatives or surrogate relatives before the victim reaches 18 years of age. Such sexual abuse is not only a crime but also a symptom of acute and irreversible family dysfunction. Survivors of incest are often tricked, coerced, or manipulated. All adults appear to be powerful to children. Perpetrators might threaten victims so that they are afraid to disclose the abuse or might tell them the abuse is their fault. Often these threats serve to silence victims.

Incestual relationships in the home endanger not only the child's intellectual and moral development, but also the health of the child. Many children don't ask for help because they don't want to expose their "secret." For this reason, just the tip of the iceberg is statistically visible—serious injuries, internal damage, sexually transmitted infections, or pregnancy. Incest can have serious long-term effects on its victims, which may include eating disorders, sexual problems in their adult life, post-traumatic stress disorder, intense guilt and shame, low self-esteem, depression, and self-destructive behavior (NCVC, 2007).

Whether an incest victim endured an isolated incident of abuse or ongoing assaults over an extended period, recovery can be painful and difficult. The recovery process begins with admission of abuse and the recognition that help and services are needed. Resources for incest victims include books, self-help groups, workshops, therapy programs, and possibly legal remedies. In addition to listening to and believing incest victims, nurses need to search for ways to prevent future generations from enduring such abuse and from continuing the cycle of abuse in their own family and relationships.

▶ *Consider* THIS!

At 53 years old, I stood and looked at myself in the mirror. The image staring back at me was one of a frightened, middle-aged, cowardly woman hiding her past. I had been sexually abused by my father for many years as a child and never told anyone. My mother knew of the abuse but felt helpless to make it stop. I married right out of high school to escape and felt I lived a "happy normal life" with my husband and three children. My children have left home and live away, and my husband recently died of a sudden heart attack. I am now experiencing dreams and thoughts about my past abuse and feeling afraid again.

Thoughts: This woman suppressed her abusive past for most of her life and now her painful experience has surfaced. What can be done to reach out to her at this point? Did her health care providers miss the "red flags" that are common to women with a history of childhood sexual abuse all those years?

▶ *Take* NOTE!

Childhood sexual abuse is a trauma that can affect every aspect of the victim's life.

Rape

Rape is an expression of violence, not a sexual act. It is not an act of lust or an overzealous release of passion: it is a violent, aggressive assault on the victim's body and integrity. Rape is a legal rather than a medical term. It denotes penile penetration of the vagina, mouth, or rectum of the female or male without consent. It may or may not include the use of a weapon. **Statutory rape** is sexual activity between an adult and a person under the age of 18 and is considered to have occurred even if the underage person was willing (Kandakai & Smith, 2007). Nine out of every 10 rape victims are female (Alexander et al., 2007). Enforcement of laws, education, and community empowerment are all needed to prevent rape.

Many people believe that rape usually occurs on a dark night when a stranger assaults a provocatively dressed, promiscuous woman. They believe that rapists are sex-starved people seeking sexual gratification. Such myths and the facts are presented in Table 9.2.

Acquaintance Rape

In **acquaintance rape**, someone is forced to have sex by a person he or she knows. Rape by a coworker, a teacher, a husband's friend, or a boss is considered acquaintance rape. **Date rape**, an assault that occurs within a dating relationship or marriage without consent of one of the par-

ticipants, is a form of acquaintance rape. Acquaintance and date rapes commonly occur on college campuses. One in four college women has been raped—that is, has been forced, physically or verbally, actively or implicitly, to engage in sexual activity (Elliott, 2008).

These forms of rape are physically and emotionally devastating for the victims. Research has indicated that the survivors of acquaintance rape report similar levels of depression, anxiety, complications in subsequent relationships, and difficulty attaining pre-rape levels of sexual satisfaction to what survivors of stranger rape report. Acquaintance rape remains a controversial topic because there is lack of agreement on the definition of consent (Sampson, 2007).

Although acquaintance rape and date rape do not always involve drugs, a rapist might use alcohol or other drugs to sedate his victim. In 1996 the federal government passed a law making it a felony to give an unsuspecting person a "date rape drug" with the intent of raping him or her. Even with penalties of large fines and up to 20 years in prison, the use of date rape drugs is growing (U.S. DHHS, 2007).

Date rape drugs are also known as "club drugs" because they are often used at dance clubs, fraternity parties, and all-night raves. The most common is Rohypnol (also known as roofies, forget pills, and the drop drug). It comes in the form of a liquid or pill that quickly dissolves in liquid with no odor, taste, or color. This drug is 10 times as strong as diazepam (Valium) and produces memory loss for up to 8 hours. Gamma hydroxybutyrate (GHB; called liquid ecstasy or easy lay) produces euphoria, an out-of-body high, sleepiness, increased sex drive, and memory loss. It comes in a white powder or liquid and may cause unconsciousness, depression, and coma.

TABLE 9.2 **COMMON MYTHS AND FACTS ABOUT RAPE**

Myths	Facts
Women who are raped get over it quickly.	It can take several years to recover emotionally and physically from rape.
Most rape victims tell someone about it.	The majority of women never tell anyone about it. In fact, almost two thirds of victims never report it to the police.
Once the rape is over, a survivor can again feel safe in her life.	The victim feels vulnerable, betrayed, and insecure afterwards.
If a woman does not want to be raped, it cannot happen.	A woman can be forced and overpowered by most men.
Women who feel guilty after having sex then say they were raped.	Few women falsely cry "rape." It is very traumatizing to be a victim.
Victims should report the violence to the police and judicial system.	Only 1% of rapists are arrested and convicted.
Women blame themselves for the rape, believing they did something to provoke the rape.	Women should never blame themselves for being the victim of someone else's violence.
Women who wear tight, short clothes are "asking for it."	No victim invites sexual assault, and what she wears is irrelevant.
Women have rape fantasies and want to be raped.	Reality and fantasy are different. Dreams have nothing to do with the brutal violation of rape.
Medication can help women forget about the rape.	Initially medication can help, but counseling is needed.

Sources: CDC, 2007b; Dutton, 2007; Medicine Net, 2007.

TEACHING GUIDELINES 9.2

Protecting Yourself Against Date Rape Drugs

• Avoid parties where alcohol is being served.
• Never leave a drink of any kind unattended.
• Don't accept a drink from someone else. Accept drinks from a bartender or in a closed container only.
• Don't drink from a punch bowl or a keg.
• If you think someone drugged you, call 911.

The third date rape drug, ketamine (known as Special K, vitamin K, or super acid), acts on the central nervous system to separate perception and sensation. Combining ketamine with other drugs can be fatal.

Date rape drugs can be very dangerous, and there are a variety of ways that women can protect themselves (Teaching Guidelines 9.2).

Rape Recovery

Rape survivors take a long time to heal from their traumatic experience. Some women never heal and never get professional counseling, but most can cope. Rape is viewed as a situational crisis that the survivor is unprepared to handle because it is an unforeseen event. Survivors typically go through four phases of recovery following rape (Table 9.3).

A significant proportion of women who are raped also experience symptoms of **post-traumatic stress disorder** (PTSD). PTSD develops when an event outside the range of normal human experience occurs that produces marked distress in the person. Symptoms of PTSD are divided into three groups:

• Intrusion (re-experiencing the trauma, including nightmares, flashbacks, recurrent thoughts)
• Avoidance (avoiding trauma-related stimuli, social withdrawal, emotional numbing)
• Hyperarousal (increased emotional arousal, exaggerated startle response, irritability)

Nursing Management

Research has found that rape survivors undergo a profound and complex trauma. The survivor should be provided with a safe and comfortable environment for a forensic examination. Nursing care of the rape survivor should focus on providing supporting care, collecting and documenting evidence, assessing for sexually transmitted infections, preventing pregnancy, and assessing for PTSD. Once initial treatment and evidence collection are completed, follow-up care should include counseling, medical treatment, and crisis intervention. There is mounting evidence that early intervention and immediate counseling speed a rape survivor's recovery. Nursing Care Plan 9.1 highlights a sample plan of care for a victim of rape.

> ▶ *Take NOTE!*
>
> *Many rape survivors seek treatment in the hospital emergency room if there are no rape crisis centers available. Unfortunately, many emergency room doctors and nurses have little training in how to treat rape survivors or in collecting evidence. To make matters worse, if they have to wait for hours in public waiting rooms, survivors may leave the hospital, never to receive treatment or supply the evidence needed to arrest and convict their assailants.*

Providing Supporting Care

Establishing a therapeutic and trusting relationship will help the survivor describe her experience. Take the woman to a secure, isolated area away from family, friends, and other patients and staff so she can be open and honest when asked about the assault. Provide a change of clothes, access to a shower and toiletries, and a private waiting area for family and friends.

Collecting and Documenting Evidence

The victim should be instructed to bring all clothing, especially undergarments, worn at the time of the assault to the medical facility. The victim should not shower or bathe before presenting for care. Typically a specially trained nurse will collect the evidence from the victim.

TABLE 9.3 FOUR PHASES OF RAPE RECOVERY

Phase	Survivor's Response
Acute phase (disorganization)	Shock, fear, disbelief, anger, shame, guilt, feelings of uncleanliness; insomnia, nightmares, and sobbing
Outward adjustment phase (denial)	Appears outwardly composed and returns to work or school; refuses to discuss the assault and denies need for counseling
Reorganization	Denial and suppression don't work, and the survivor attempts to make life adjustments by moving or changing jobs and uses emotional distancing to cope.
Integration and recovery	Survivor begins to feel safe and starts to trust others. She may become an advocate for other rape victims.

Nursing Care Plan 9.1

OVERVIEW OF THE WOMAN WHO IS A VICTIM OF RAPE

Lucia, a 20-year-old college junior, was admitted to the emergency room after police found her when a passerby called 911 to report an assault. She stated, "I think I was raped a few hours ago while I was walking home through the park." Assessment reveals the following: numerous cuts and bruises of varying sizes on her face, arms, and legs; lip swollen and cut; right eye swollen and bruised; jacket and shirt ripped and bloodied; hair matted with grass and debris; vital signs within acceptable parameters; client tearful, clutching her clothing, and trembling; perineal bruising and tearing.

NURSING DIAGNOSIS: Rape-trauma syndrome related to report of recent sexual assault

Outcome Identification and Evaluation

Client will demonstrate adequate coping skills related to effects of rape as evidenced by her ability to discuss the event, verbalize her feelings and fears, and exhibit appropriate actions to return to her pre-crisis level of functioning.

Interventions: Promoting Adequate Coping Skills

- Stay with the client *to promote feelings of safety.*
- Explain the procedures to be completed based on facility's policy *to help alleviate client's fear of the unknown.*
- Assist with physical examination for specimen collection *to obtain evidence for legal proceedings.*
- Administer prophylactic medication as ordered *to prevent pregnancy and sexually transmitted infections.*
- Provide care to wounds as ordered *to prevent infection.*
- Assist client with hygiene measures as necessary *to promote self-esteem.*
- Allow client to describe the events as much as possible *to encourage ventilation of feelings about the incident;* engage in active listening and offer nonjudgmental support *to facilitate coping and demonstrate understanding of the client's situation and feelings.*
- Help the client identify positive coping skills and personal strengths used in the past *to aid in effective decision making.*
- Assist client in developing additional coping strategies and teach client relaxation techniques *to help deal with the current crisis and anxiety.*
- Contact the rape counselor in the facility *to help the client deal with the crisis.*
- Arrange for follow-up visit with rape counselor *to provide continued care and to promote continuity of care.*
- Encourage the client to contact a close friend, partner, or family member to accompany her home *to provide support.*
- Provide the client with the telephone number of a counseling service or community support groups *to help her cope and obtain ongoing support.*
- Provide written instructions related to follow-up appointments, care, and testing *to ensure adequate understanding.*

Assessing for Sexually Transmitted Infections

As part of the assessment, a pelvic examination will be done to collect vaginal secretions to rule out any sexually transmitted infections. This examination is very emotionally stressful for most women and should be carried out very gently and sensitively.

Preventing Pregnancy

An essential element in the care of rape survivors involves offering them pregnancy prevention. After unprotected intercourse, including rape, pregnancy can be prevented by using emergency contraceptive pills, sometimes called postcoital contraception. Emergency contraceptive pills involve high doses of the same oral contraceptives that millions of women take every day. The emergency regimen consists of two doses: the first dose is taken within 72 hours of the unprotected intercourse and the second dose is taken 12 hours after the first dose or sooner. Emergency contraception works by preventing ovulation, fertilization, or implantation. It does not disrupt an established pregnancy and should not be confused with mifepristone (RU-486), a drug approved by the Food and Drug Administration for abortion in the first 49 days of gestation. Emergency contraception is most effective if the first dose is taken within 12 hours of the rape; it becomes less effective with every 12 hours of delay thereafter.

Assessing for PTSD

Nurses can begin to assess the extent to which a survivor is suffering from PTSD by asking the following questions:

- To assess the presence of intrusive thoughts:
  - Do upsetting thoughts and nightmares of the trauma bother you?

- Do you feel as though you are actually reliving the trauma?
- Does it upset you to be exposed to anything that reminds you of that event?
- To assess the presence of avoidance reactions:
  - Do you find yourself trying to avoid thinking about the trauma?
  - Do you stay away from situations that remind you of the event?
  - Do you have trouble recalling exactly what happened?
  - Do you feel numb emotionally?
- To assess the presence of physical symptoms:
  - Are you having trouble sleeping?
  - Have you felt irritable or experienced outbursts of anger?
  - Do you have heart palpitations and sweating?
  - Do you have muscle aches and pains all over? (Kiump, 2006)

Female Genital Mutilation

Female genital mutilation, also known as female circumcision, is a cultural practice carried out predominantly in countries of southern Africa and in some areas of the Middle East and Asia. The World Health Organization (WHO) defines female genital mutilation as all procedures involving the partial or total removal or other injury to the female genital organs, whether for cultural or other nontherapeutic purposes (WHO, 2007). More than 140 million girls are estimated to have undergone female genital mutilation and another 2 million are at risk annually, approximately 6,000 daily (WHO, 2007).

This issue has drawn increasing global attention over the past several years. Nongovernmental organizations such as Amnesty International are conducting research and campaign work on the practice. The U.S. government has taken steps to criminalize the practice in America and now considers asylum applications in light of mutilation practices in the country of origin (WHO, 2007). WHO is fighting tirelessly to eradicate this practice through advocacy, policy development, research, and training for health care providers (Zaidi et al., 2007). In fact, WHO, the United Nations Population Fund, and the United Nations Children's Fund have issued a joint plea for the eradication of the practice, saying it would be a major step forward in the promotion of human rights worldwide (WHO, 2007).

> ▶ *Take NOTE!*
>
> *From a Western perspective, female genital mutilation is hard to comprehend. Because it is not talked about openly in communities that practice it, women who have undergone it accept it without question and assume it is done to all girls (Wakabi 2007).*

Background

Reasons for performing the ritual reflect the ideology and cultural values of each community that practices it. Some consider it a rite of passage into womanhood; others use it as a means of preserving virginity until marriage. In cultures where it is practiced, it is an important part of culturally defined gender identity. In any case, all the reasons are cultural and traditional and are not rooted in any religious texts (RAINBO, 2007). Female genital mutilation causes injury to women and does not benefit them.

Female genital mutilation is usually performed when the girl is between 4 and 10 years old, an age when she cannot give informed consent for a procedure with lifetime health consequences (WHO, 2007). In its mildest form, the clitoris is partially or totally removed. In the most extreme form, called infibulation, the clitoris, labia minora, labia majora, and the urethral and vaginal openings are cut away. The vagina is then stitched or held together, leaving a small opening for menstruation and urination. Cutting and restitching may be necessary to permit the woman to have sexual intercourse and bear children. Box 9.4 lists types of female genital mutilation procedures.

Untrained village practitioners, using no form of anesthesia, generally perform the operation. Cutting instruments may include broken glass, knives, tin lids, scissors, unspecialized razors, or other crude instruments. In addition to causing intense pain, the procedure carries with it a number of health risks, including:

- Pelvic infections
- Hemorrhage
- HIV infection
- Damage to the urethra, vagina, and anus
- Recurrent vaginitis
- Urinary tract infections
- Incontinence
- Post-traumatic stress disorder
- Panic attacks

(BOX 9.4) **Four Major Types of Female Genital Mutilation Procedures**

Type I: Excision of the prepuce with or without excision of part or all of the clitoris

Type II: Excision of the clitoris and part or all of the labia minora

Type III (Infibulation): Excision of all or part of the external genitalia and stitching/narrowing of the vaginal opening

Type IV: Pricking, piercing, or incision of the clitoris or labia

    Stretching of the clitoris and/or labia

    Cauterizing by burning the clitoris and surrounding tissues

    Scraping or cutting the vaginal orifice

    Introduction of a corrosive substance into the vagina

    Placing herbs into the vagina to narrow it

Sources: WHO, 2007; Keleher & Franklin, 2008.

- Keloid formation
- Dermoid cysts
- Vulvar abscesses
- Dysmenorrhea
- Dyspareunia
- Psychosomatic illnesses
- Depression
- Feelings of betrayal
- Bitterness and anger towards family members who allowed it
- Increased morbidity and mortality during childbirth (WHO, 2007)

Nursing Management

Because of increasing migration, nurses throughout the world are increasingly exposed to women who have suffered these procedures and thus need to know about its impact on women's reproductive health. Helping women who have had one of these procedures requires good communication skills and often an interpreter, since many may not speak English. Nurses have the opportunity to educate patients by providing accurate information and positive health care experiences. Make sure that you are comfortable with your own feelings about this practice before dealing with patients. Some guidelines are as follows:

- Let the client know you are concerned and interested and want to help.
- Speak clearly and slowly, using simple, accurate terms.
- Use the term or name for this practice the recipient uses, not "female genital mutilation."
- Use pictures and diagrams to help the woman understand what you are saying.
- Be patient in allowing the client to answer questions.
- Repeat back your understanding of the client's statements.
- Always look and talk directly to the client, not the interpreter.
- Place no judgment on the cultural practice.
- Encourage the client to express herself freely.
- Maintain strict confidentiality.
- Provide culturally competent care to all women.

Human Trafficking

A girl who was just 14 years old was held captive in a tiny trailer room, where she was forced to have sex with as many as 30 men a day. On her night stand was a teddy bear that reminded her of her childhood in Mexico.

This scenario describes **human trafficking**, the enslavement of immigrants for profit in America. Human trafficking is both a global problem and a domestic problem. The United States is a major receiver of trafficked persons. Human trafficking is a modern form of slavery that affects nearly 1 million people worldwide and approximately 20,000 persons in the United States annually

(U.S. Department of State, 2007). Women and children are the primary victims of human trafficking, many in the sex trade as described above and others through forced-labor domestic servitude.

Trafficking persons is hugely profitable: one estimate places global profits at approximately $32 billion annually. Among illegal enterprises, trafficking is second only to drug dealing and is tied with the illegal arms industry in its ability to generate dollars (Jones et al., 2007).

The United States is a profitable destination country for traffickers, and these profits contribute to the development of organized criminal enterprises worldwide. According to findings of the Victims of Trafficking and Violence Protection Act of 2000:

- Victims are primarily women and children who lack education, employment, and economic opportunities in their own countries.
- Traffickers promise victims employment as nannies, maids, dancers, factory workers, sales clerks, or models in the United States.
- Traffickers transport the victims from their counties to unfamiliar destinations away from their support systems.
- Once they are here, traffickers coerce them, using rape, torture, starvation, imprisonment, threats, or physical force, into prostitution, pornography, sex trade, forced labor, or involuntary servitude.

These victims are exposed to serious and numerous health risks, such as rape, torture, HIV/AIDS, sexually transmitted infections, cervical cancer, violence, hazardous work environments, poor nutrition, and drug and alcohol addiction (Hodge & Lietz, 2007). Health care is one of the most pressing needs of these victims, and there isn't any comprehensive care available for undocumented immigrants. As a nurse it is important to be alert for trafficking victims in any setting and to recognize cues (Box 9.5).

Human trafficking is a violation of human rights. If you suspect a trafficking situation, notify local law enforcement and a regional social service organization that has experience in dealing with trafficking victims. It is imperative to reach out to these victims and stop the cycle of abuse by following through on your suspicions.

Summary

The causes of violence against women are complex. Many women will experience some type of violence in their lives, and it can have a debilitating affect on their health and future relationships. Violence frequently leaves a "legacy of pain" to future generations. Nurses can empower women and encourage them to move forward and take control of their lives. When women live in peace and security and free from violence, they have an enormous potential to contribute to their own communities and to the

BOX 9.5 **Identifying Victims of Human Trafficking**

Cues

Look beneath the surface and ask yourself: Is this person. . . .

- A female or a child in poor health?
- Foreign-born and doesn't speak English?
- Lacking immigration documents?
- Giving an inconsistent explanation of injury?
- Reluctant to give any information about self, injury, home, or work?
- Fearful of authority figure or "sponsor" if present? ("Sponsor" might not leave victim alone with health care provider.)
- Living with the employer?

Sample questions to ask the potential victim of human trafficking:

- Can you leave your job or situation if you wish?
- Can you come and go as you please?
- Have you been threatened if you try to leave?
- Has anyone threatened your family with harm if you leave?
- What are your working and living conditions?
- Do you have to ask permission to go to the bathroom, eat, or sleep?
- Is there a lock on your door so you cannot get out?
- What brought you to the United States? Are your plans the same now?
- Are you free to leave your current work or home situation?
- Who has your immigration papers? Why don't you have them?
- Are you paid for the work you do?
- Are there times you feel afraid?
- How can your situation be changed?

Sources: http://www.rainn.org/statistics.html; Jones et al., 2007.

national and global society. Violence against women is not normal, legal, or acceptable and it should never be tolerated or justified. It can and must be stopped by the entire world community.

■■■ Key Concepts

- Violence against women is a major public health and social problem because it violates a woman's very being and causes numerous mental and physical health sequelae.
- Every woman has the potential to become a victim of violence.
- Several *Healthy People 2010* objectives focus on reducing the rate of physical assaults and the number of rapes and attempted rapes.

- Abuse may be mental, physical, or sexual in nature or a combination.
- The cycle of violence includes three phases: tension-building, acute battering, and honeymoon.
- Many women experience post-traumatic stress disorder (PTSD) after being sexually assaulted. PTSD can inhibit a survivor from adapting or coping in a healthy manner.
- Pregnancy can precipitate violence toward the woman to start or escalate.
- The nurse's role in dealing with survivors of violence is to establish rapport; open up lines of communication; apply the nursing process to assess and screen all patients in all settings; and implement and intervene as appropriate.

REFERENCES

Aggeles, T. B. (2007). *Domestic violence advocacy, Florida, update.* Available at: http://nsweb.NursingSpectrum.com/ce/ce60133.html

Alekseeva, L. S. (2007). Problems of child abuse in the home. *Russian Education and Society, 49*(5), 6–18.

Alexander, L. L., LaRosa, J. H., Bader, H., & Garfield, S. (2007). *New dimensions in women's health* (4th ed.). Sudbury, MA: Jones and Bartlett Publishers.

Association of Women's Health, Obstetric and Neonatal Nurses (AWHONN). (2007). *Violence against women: Identification, screening and management of intimate partner violence.* Available at: http://www.awhonn.org.

Bonomi, A. E., Anderson, M. L., Reid, R. J., Carrell, D., Fishman, P. A., Rivara, F. P., & Thompson, R. S. (2007). Intimate partner violence in older women. *Gerontologist, 47*(1), 34–41.

Burgess, A. W. (2007) How many red flags does it take? *American Journal of Nursing, 107*(1), 28–31.

Casanueva, C. E., & Martin, S. L. (2007). Intimate partner violence during pregnancy and mother's child abuse potential. *Journal of Interpersonal Violence, 22*(5), 603–622.

Centers for Disease Control and Prevention (CDC). (2007a). *Intimate partner violence: Fact sheet.* National Center for Injury Prevention and Control. Available at: http://www.cdc.gov/ncipc/factsheets/ipvfacts.htm.

Centers for Disease Control and Prevention (CDC). (2007b). *Sexual violence: Fact sheet.* National Center for Injury Prevention and Control. Available at: http://www.cdc.gov/ncipc/factsheets/svfacts.htm.

CDC/National Center for Injury Prevention and Control. (2007). *Tips for handling domestic violence.* Available at: http://www.cdc.gov/communication/tips/domviol.htm.

Centers for Disease Control and Prevention (CDC). (2008). Adverse health conditions and health risk behaviors associated with intimate partner violence—United States. *MMWR, 57*(5), 113–117.

Du Plat-Jones, J. (2006). Domestic violence: The role of health professionals. *Nursing Standard, 21*(14), 44–48.

Dutton, D. G. (2007). *Rethinking domestic violence.* Vancouver, British Columbia, Canada: University of British Columbia Press.

Elliott, S. M. (2008). Drug-facilitated sexual assault: Educating women about the risks. *Nursing for Women's Health, 12*(1), 30–37.

Federal Bureau of Investigation (FBI). (2007). *Intimate partner violence.* Available at: http://www.ojp.usdoj.gov/bjs/pub/ascii/ipv.txt.

Ferris, L. E. (2007). Intimate partner violence. *British Medical Journal, 334*(7596), 706–707.

Giardino, E. R. (2007). Uncovering abuse in the pregnant woman. *Nursing Spectrum.* Available at: http://www.nurse.com/ce/print.html?CCID=3141.

Healthy People 2010 (2000). Available at: http://www.healthypeople.gov/document/HTML/Volume2/15Injury.htm#_Toc490549392.

Herrenkohl, T. I., Kosterman, R., Mason, W. A., & Hawkins, J. D. (2007). Youth violence trajectories and proximal characteristics of intimate partner violence. *Violence and Victims, 22*(3), 259–274.

Hodge, D. R., & Lietz, C. A. (2007). The international sexual trafficking of women and children: A review of the literature. *Journal of Women & Social Work, 22*(2), 163–174.

Holtz, H., & Furniss, K. K. (1993). The health care provider's role in domestic violence. *Trends in Health Care Law and Ethics, 15*, 519–522.

Joint Commission on Accreditation of Healthcare Organizations. (2007). *The Joint Commission accreditation manual for hospitals.* Chicago: JCAHO.

Jones, L., Engstrom, D. W., Hilliard, T., & Diaz, M. (2007). Globalization and human trafficking. *Journal of Sociology & Social Welfare, 24*(2), 107–122.

Kandakai, T. L., & Smith, L. C. (2007). Denormalizing a historical problem: Teen pregnancy, policy, and public health action. *American Journal of Health Behavior, 31*(2), 170–180.

Keleher, H., & Franklin, L. (2008). Changing gendered norms about women and girls at the level of household and community: A review of the evidence. *Global Public Health, Suppl. 1*(3), 42–57.

Kelly, P. J. (2007). Integrating intimate partner violence prevention into daily practice. *Journal of Psychosocial Nursing, 45*(4), 8–10.

Kiump, M. C. (2006). Posttraumatic stress disorder and sexual assault in women. *Journal of College Student Psychotherapy, 21*(2), 67–83.

Kristensen, E., & Lau, M. (2007). Women with a history of childhood sexual abuse. Long-term social and psychiatric aspects. *Nordic Journal of Psychiatry, 61*(2), 115–120.

Macy, R. J., Nurius, P. S., & Norris, J. (2007). Latent profiles among sexual assault survivors. *Journal of Interpersonal Violence, 22*(5), 543–565.

Medicine Net. (2007). *Sexual assault.* Available at: http://www.medicinenet.com/script/main/art.asp?articlekey=46498&pf=3.

National Center for Victims of Crime (NCVC). (2007). *Incest.* Available at: http://www.ncvc.org/ncvc/main.aspx?dbName=DocumentViewer&DocumentID=32360.

Paluzzi, P. A. (2007). Violence against women and children. In B. Hackley, J. M. Kriebs, & M. E. Rousseau (Eds.), *Primary care of women: A guide for midwives and women's health providers* (Chapter 7, pp. 193–212). Sudbury, MA: Jones and Bartlett Publishers.

Research Action and Information Network for the Bodily Integrity of Women (RAINBO). (2007). *Caring for women with circumcision: Fact sheet for physicians.* Available at: http://www.rainbo.org/factsheet.html.

Rape, Abuse, and Incest National Network (RAINN). (2007). *RAINN statistics.* Available at: http://www.rainn.org/statistics.html.

Sampson, R. (2007). *Acquaintance rape of college students.* U.S. Department of Justice COPS. Available at: http://www.cops.usdoj.gov.

Sharps, P. W., Laughon, K., & Giandrande, S. K. (2007). Intimate partner violence and the childbearing year. *Trauma, Violence & Abuse, 8*(2), 105–116.

Thackeray, J., Stelzner, S., Downs, S. M., & Miller, C. (2007). Screening for intimate partner violence. *Journal of Interpersonal Violence, 22*(6), 659–670.

U.S. Department of Health and Human Services (U.S. DHHS). (2007). *Frequently asked questions about date rape drugs.* The National Women's Health Information Center. Available at: http://www.4woman.gov/faq/rohypnol.pdf.

U.S. Department of State. (2007). *Trafficking in persons report.* U.S. Department of State Publication No. 11057, p. 7. Washington, DC: Author.

Victims of Trafficking and Violence Protection Act of 2000, Pub. Law No. 106-386 [H.R. 3244] (2000). Available at: http://ojp.gov/vawo/laws/vawo2000/stitle_a.htm.

Wakabi, W. (2007). Africa battles to make female genital mutilation history. *Lancet, 369*(9567), 1069–1070.

World Health Organization (WHO). (2007). *Female genital mutilation.* Available at: http://www.who.int/mediacentre/factsheets/fs241/en/print.html.

Zaidi, N., Khalil, A., Roberts, C., & Browne, M. (2007). Knowledge of female genital mutilation among healthcare professionals. *Journal of Obstetrics & Gynecology, 27*(2), 161–164.

WEBSITES

Boat People S.O.S., Inc.: www.bpsos.org

Center for the Prevention of Sexual and Domestic Violence: (206) 634-1903, www.cpsdv.org

Centers for Disease Control and Prevention: Intimate Partner Violence: www.cdc.gov/ncipc/factsheets/ipvfacts.htm

Coalition to Abolish Slavery and Trafficking: www.trafficked-women.org

Domestic Violence Handbook: www.domesticviolence.org

Immigrant & Refugee Community Organization: www.irco.org/irco

National Coalition Against Sexual Assault (NCADV): (303) 839-1852, www.ncadv.org

National Domestic Violence Hotline: (800) 799-SAFE (7233), www.ndvh.org

Nursing Network on Violence Against Women, International: Resources for Health Care Professionals: http://www.nnvawi.org/links.htm#professional

Protection Project: www.protectionproject.org

Rape, Abuse, and Incest National Network (RAINN): (800) 656-HOPE, www.rainn.org

SAGE Project: www.sageinc.org

Trafficking Information and Referral Hotline: (888) 373-7888, www.acf.hhs.gov/trafficking

U.S. Department of Health Human Services: aaqui@acf.hhs.gov

U.S. Department of Labor, Women's Bureau: www.dol.gov.dol/wb

Violence Against Women Office, U.S. Department of Justice: (202) 616-8894, www.raw.umn.edu

CHAPTER WORKSHEET

MULTIPLE CHOICE QUESTIONS

1. The primary goal of intervention in working with abused women is to:

   a. Set up an appointment with a mental health counselor for the victim

   b. Convince them to set up a safety plan to use when they leave

   c. Help them to develop courage and financial support to leave the abuser

   d. Empower them and improve their self-esteem to regain control of their lives

2. The first phase of the abuse cycle is characterized by:

   a. The woman provokes the abuser to bring about battering

   b. Tension-building and verbal or minor battery

   c. A honeymoon period that lulls the victim into forgetting

   d. An acute episode of physical battering

3. Women recovering from abusive relationships need to learn ways to improve their:

   a. Cooking skills and provide more nutritious meals for their children

   b. Creativity so as to improve their decorating skills within the home

   c. Communication and negotiation skills to increase their assertiveness

   d. Personal appearance by losing weight and exercising more

4. Which of the following statements might empower abuse victims to take action?

   a. "You deserve better than this."

   b. "Your children deserve to grow up in a two-parent family."

   c. "Try to figure out what you do to trigger his abuse and stop it."

   d. "Give your partner more time to come to his senses about this."

CRITICAL THINKING EXERCISE

1. Mrs. Boggs has three children under the age of 5 and is 6 months pregnant with her fourth child. She has made repeated unscheduled visits to your clinic with vague somatic complaints regarding the children as well as herself, but has missed several scheduled prenatal appointments. On occasion she has worn sunglasses to cover bruises around her eyes. As a nurse you sense there is something else bothering her, but she doesn't seem to want to discuss it with you. She appears sad and the children cling to her.

   a. Outline your conversation when you broach the subject of abuse with Mrs. Boggs.

   b. What is your role as a nurse in caring for a family in which you suspect abuse?

   c. What ethical/legal considerations are important in planning care for this family?

STUDY ACTIVITIES

1. Visit the BellaOnline website for victims of violence (www.bellaonline.com). Discuss what you discovered on this site and your reactions to it.

2. Research the statistics about violence against women in your state. Are law enforcement and community interventions reducing the incidence of sexual assault and intimate partner violence?

3. Attend a dorm orientation at a local college to hear about measures in place to protect women's safety on campus. Find out the number of sexual assaults reported and what strategies the college uses to reduce this number.

4. Volunteer to spend a weekend evening at the local sheriff's department 911 hotline desk to observe the number and nature of calls received reporting domestic violence. Interview the dispatch operator about the frequency and trends of these calls.

5. Identify three community resources that could be useful to a victim of violence. Identify their sources of funding and the services they provide.

UNIT THREE

PREGNANCY

FETAL DEVELOPMENT AND GENETICS

CHAPTER 10

KEY TERMS

allele
blastocyst
embryonic stage
fertilization
fetal stage
genes
genetic counseling
genetics
genome

genotype
heterozygous
homozygous
karyotype
mosaicism
monosomies
morula
mutation
phenotype

placenta
polyploidy
preembryonic stage
trisomies
trophoblast
umbilical cord
zona pellucida
zygote

LEARNING OBJECTIVES

Upon completion of the chapter, the learner will be able to:

1. Describe the process of fertilization, implantation, and cell differentiation.
2. Explain the functions of the placenta, umbilical cord, and amniotic fluid.
3. Outline normal fetal development from conception through birth.
4. Compare the various inheritance patterns, including nontraditional patterns of inheritance.
5. Give examples of ethical and legal issues surrounding genetic testing.
6. Explain the role of the nurse in genetic counseling and genetic-related activities.

Robert and Kate Shafer have just received the good news that Kate's pregnancy test was positive. It had been a long and anxious 3 years of trying to start a family. Although both were elated about the prospect of becoming parents, they were concerned about the possibility of a genetic problem because Kate was 38 years old. What might be their first step in looking into their genetic concern? As a nurse, what might raise concerns for you?

Wow

Being a nurse without awe is like food without spice. Nurses only have to witness the miracle of life to find their lost awe.

265

Human reproduction is one of the most intimate spheres of an individual's life. For conception to occur, a healthy ovum from the woman is released from the ovary, passes into an open fallopian tube, and starts its journey downward. Sperm from the male is deposited into the vagina and swims approximately 7 inches to meet the ovum at the outermost portion of the fallopian tube, the area where fertilization takes place (Gilbert, 2007). When one spermatozoon penetrates the ovum's thick outer membrane, pregnancy begins. All this activity takes place within a 5-hour time span.

Nurses caring for the childbearing family need to have a basic understanding of conception and prenatal development so they can identify problems or variations and can initiate appropriate interventions should any problems occur. This chapter presents an overview of fetal development, beginning with conception. It also discusses hereditary influences on fetal development and the nurse's role in genetic counseling.

Fetal Development

Fetal development during pregnancy is measured in number of weeks after fertilization. The duration of pregnancy is about 40 weeks from the time of fertilization. This equates to 9 calendar months or approximately 266 to 280 calendar days. The three stages of fetal development during pregnancy are:

1. **Preembryonic stage**: fertilization through the second week
2. **Embryonic stage**: end of the second week through the eighth week
3. **Fetal stage**: end of the eighth week until birth

Fetal circulation is a significant aspect of fetal development that spans all three stages.

Preembryonic Stage

The preembryonic stage begins with **fertilization**, also called *conception*. Fertilization is the union of ovum and sperm, which is the starting point of pregnancy. Fertilization typically occurs around 2 weeks after the last normal menstrual period in a 28-day cycle (Dillon, 2007). Fertilization requires a timely interaction between the release of the mature ovum at ovulation and the ejaculation of enough healthy, mobile sperm to survive the hostile vaginal environment through which they must travel to meet the ovum. All things considered, the act of conception is difficult at best. To say merely that it occurs when the sperm unites with the ovum is overly simple because this union requires an intricate interplay of hormonal preparation and overcoming an overwhelming number of natural barriers. A human being is truly an amazing outcome of this elaborate process.

Prior to fertilization, the ovum and the spermatozoon undergo the process of meiosis. The primary oocyte completes its first meiotic division before ovulation. The secondary oocyte begins its second meiotic division just before ovulation. Primary and secondary spermatocytes undergo meiotic division while still in the testes (Fig. 10.1).

Although more than 200 million sperm/mL are contained in the ejaculated semen, only one is able to enter the ovum to fertilize it. All others are blocked by the clear protein layer called the **zona pellucida**. The zona pellucida disappears in about 5 days. Once the sperm reaches the plasma membrane, the ovum resumes meiosis and forms a nucleus with half the number of chromosomes (23). When the nucleus from the ovum and the nucleus of the sperm make contact, they lose their respective nuclear membranes and combine their maternal and paternal chromosomes. Because each nucleus contains a haploid number of chromosomes (23), this union restores the diploid number (46). The resulting **zygote** begins the process of a new life. The genetic information from both ovum and sperm establishes the unique physical characteristics of the individual. Sex determination is also determined at fertilization and depends on whether the ovum is fertilized by a Y-bearing sperm or an X-bearing sperm. An XX zygote will become a female and an XY zygote will become a male (Fig. 10.2).

Fertilization takes place in the outer third of the ampulla of the fallopian tube. When the ovum is fertilized by the sperm (now called a zygote), a great deal of activity immediately takes place. Mitosis, or *cleavage,* occurs as the zygote is slowly transported into the uterine cavity by tubal muscular movements (Fig. 10.3). After a series of four cleavages, the 16 cells appear as a solid ball of cells or **morula**, meaning "little mulberry." The morula reaches the uterine cavity about 72 hours after fertilization (Johnson, 2007).

With additional cell division, the morula divides into specialized cells that will later form fetal structures. Within the morula, an off-center, fluid-filled space appears, transforming it into a hollow ball of cells called a **blastocyst** (Fig. 10.4). The inner surface of the blastocyst will form the embryo and amnion. The outer layer of cells surrounding the blastocyst cavity is called a **trophoblast**. Eventually, the trophoblast develops into one of the embryonic membranes, the chorion, and helps to form the placenta.

At this time, the developing blastocyst needs more food and oxygen to keep growing. The trophoblast attaches itself to the surface of the endometrium for further nourishment. Normally, implantation occurs in the upper uterus (fundus), where a rich blood supply is available. This area also contains strong muscular fibers, which clamp down on blood vessels after the placenta separates from the inner wall of the uterus. Additionally, the lining is thickest here so the placenta cannot attach so strongly that it remains attached after birth (Alvero & Schlaff, 2006). Figure 10.5 shows the process of fertilization and implantation.

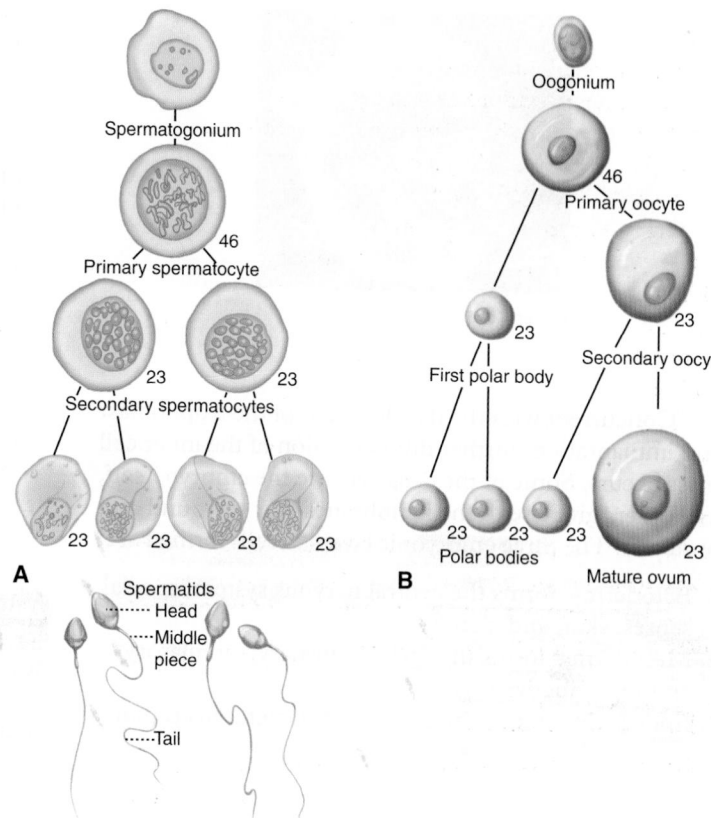

A

B

FIGURE 10.1 The formation of gametes by the process of meiosis is known as gametogenesis. (**A**) Spermatogenesis. One spermatogonium gives rise to four spermatozoa. (**B**) Oogenesis. From each oogonium, one mature ovum and three abortive cells are produced. The chromosomes are reduced to one-half the number characteristic for the general body cells of the species. In humans, the number in the body cells is 46, and that in the mature spermatozoon and secondary oocyte is 23.

FIGURE 10.2 Inheritance of gender. Each ovum contains 22 autosomes and an X chromosome. Each spermatozoon (sperm) contains 22 autosomes and either an X chromosome or a Y chromosome. The gender of the zygote is determined at the time of fertilization by the combination of the sex chromosomes of the sperm (either X or Y) and the ovum (X).

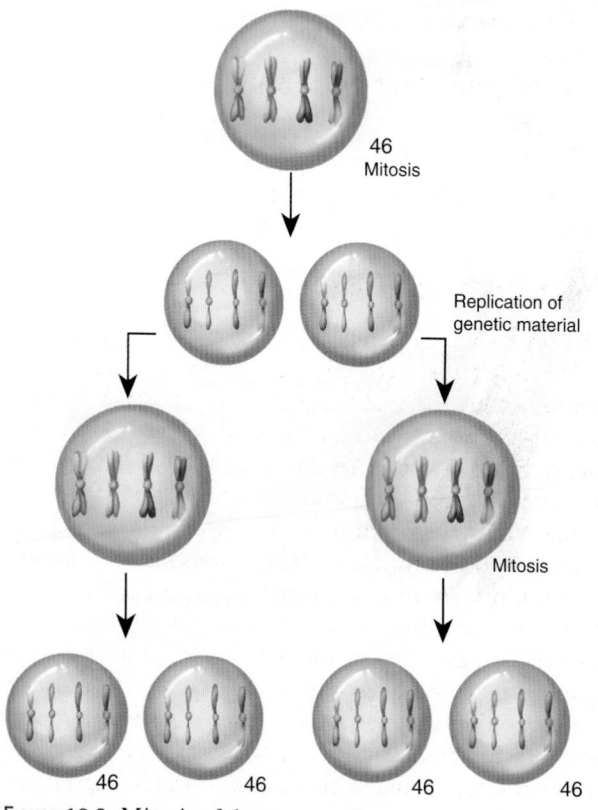

FIGURE 10.3 Mitosis of the stoma cells.

FIGURE 10.4 Blastocyst.

Concurrent with the development of the trophoblast and implantation, further differentiation of the inner cell mass occurs. Some of the cells become the embryo itself, and others give rise to the membranes that surround and protect it. The three embryonic layers of cells formed are:

1. Ectoderm—forms the central nervous system, special senses, skin, and glands
2. Mesoderm—forms the skeletal, urinary, circulatory, and reproductive organs
3. Endoderm—forms the respiratory system, liver, pancreas, and digestive system

These three layers are formed at the same time as the embryonic membranes, and all tissues, organs, and organ

---

BOX 10.1 **Summary of Preembryonic Development**

- Fertilization takes place in ampulla of the fallopian tube.
- Union of sperm and ovum forms a *zygote* (46 chromosomes).
- Cleavage cell division continues to form a *morula* (mass of 16 cells).
- The inner cell mass is called *blastocyst,* which forms the embryo and amnion.
- The outer cell mass is called *trophoblast,* which forms the placenta and chorion.
- Implantation occurs 7 to 10 days after conception in the endometrium.

---

systems develop from these three primary germ cell layers (Dillon, 2007). Box 10.1 summarizes preembryonic development.

Despite the intense and dramatic activities going on internally to create a human life, many women are unaware that pregnancy has begun. Several weeks will pass before even one of the presumptive signs of pregnancy—missing the first menstrual period—will take place.

FIGURE 10.5 Fertilization and tubal transport of the zygote. From fertilization to implantation, the zygote travels through the fallopian tube, experiencing rapid mitotic division (cleavage). During the journey toward the uterus the zygote evolves through several stages, including morula and blastocyst.

Embryonic Stage

The embryonic stage of development begins at day 15 after conception and continues through week 8. Basic structures of all major body organs and the main external features are completed during this time period. Table 10.1 and Figure 10.6 summarize embryonic development.

The embryonic membranes (Fig. 10.7) begin to form around the time of implantation. The chorion consists of trophoblast cells and a mesodermal lining. It has finger-like projections called *chorionic villi* on its surface. The amnion originates from the ectoderm germ layer during the early stages of embryonic development. It is a thin protective membrane that contains amniotic fluid. As the embryo grows, the amnion expands until it touches the chorion. These two fetal membranes form the fluid-filled amniotic sac, or bag of waters, that protects the floating embryo (Creatsas, Chrousos, & Mastorakos, 2007).

Amniotic fluid surrounds the embryo and increases in volume as the pregnancy progresses, reaching approximately a liter at term. Amniotic fluid is derived from two sources: fluid transported from the maternal blood across the amnion and fetal urine. Its volume changes constantly as the fetus swallows and voids. Sufficient amounts of amniotic fluid help maintain a constant body temperature for the fetus, permit symmetric growth and development, cushion the fetus from trauma, allow the **umbilical cord** to be relatively free from compression, and promote fetal movement to enhance musculoskeletal development. Amniotic fluid is composed of 98% water and 2% organic matter. It is slightly alkaline and contains albumin, urea, uric acid, creatinine, bilirubin, lecithin,

TABLE 10.1 EMBRYONIC AND FETAL DEVELOPMENT

Week 3
Beginning development of brain, spinal cord, and heart
Beginning development of the gastrointestinal tract
Neural tube forms, which later becomes the spinal cord
Leg and arm buds appear and grow out from body

Week 4
Brain differentiates
Limb buds grow and develop more

4 weeks

Week 5
Heart now beats at a regular rhythm
Beginning structures of eyes and ears
Some cranial nerves are visible
Muscles innervated

Week 6
Beginning formation of lungs
Fetal circulation established
Liver produces RBCs
Further development of the brain
Primitive skeleton forms
Central nervous system forms
Brain waves detectable

Week 7
Straightening of trunk
Nipples and hair follicles form
Elbows and toes visible
Arms and legs move
Diaphragm formed
Mouth with lips and early tooth buds

Week 8
Rotation of intestines
Facial features continue to develop
Heart development complete
Resembles a human being
  (Ratner, 2002)

8 weeks

Weeks 9–12
Sexual differentiation continues
Buds for all 20 temporary teeth laid down
Digestive system shows activity
Head comprises nearly half the fetus size
Face and neck are well formed
Urogenital tract completes development
Red blood cells are produced in the liver
Urine begins to be produced and excreted
Fetal gender can be determined by week 12
Limbs are long and thin; digits are well formed

12 weeks

(continued)

T A B L E 10.1 EMBRYONIC AND FETAL DEVELOPMENT (continued)

Weeks 13–16
A fine hair develops on the head called lanugo
Fetal skin is almost transparent
Bones become harder
Fetus makes active movement
Sucking motions are made with the mouth
Amniotic fluid is swallowed
Fingernails and toenails present
Weight quadruples
Fetal movement (also know as quickening) detected
  by mother

16 weeks

Weeks 17–20
Rapid brain growth occurs
Fetal heart tones can be heard with stethoscope
Kidneys continue to secret urine into amniotic fluid
Vernix caseosa, a white greasy film, covers the fetus
Eyebrows and head hair appear
Brown fat deposited to help maintain temperature
Nails are present on both fingers and toes
Muscles are well developed

20 weeks

Weeks 21–24
Eyebrows and eyelashes are well formed
Fetus has a hand grasp and startle reflex
Alveoli forming in lungs
Skin is translucent and red
Lungs begin to produce surfactant

25 weeks

Weeks 25–28
Fetus reaches a length of 15 inches
Rapid brain development
Eyelids open and close
Nervous system controls some functions
Fingerprints are set
Blood formation shifts from spleen to bone marrow
Fetus usually assumes head-down position

28 weeks

Weeks 29–32
Rapid increase in the amount of body fat
Increased central nervous system control over body
  functions
Rhythmic breathing movements occur
Lungs are not fully mature
Fetus stores iron, calcium, and phosphorus

32 weeks

Weeks 33–38
Testes are in scrotum of male fetus
Lanugo begins to disappear
Increase in body fat
Fingernails reach the end of fingertips
Small breast buds are present on both sexes
Mother supplies fetus with antibodies against disease
Fetus is considered full term at 38 weeks
Fetus fills uterus (Bailey, 2003)

37 weeks

FIGURE 10.6 Embryonic development. (**A**) 4-week embryo. (**B**) 5-week embryo. (**C**) 6-week embryo.

sphingomyelin, epithelial cells, vernix, and fine hair called lanugo (Johnson, 2007).

The volume of amniotic fluid is important in determining fetal well-being. It gradually fluctuates throughout the pregnancy. Alterations in amniotic fluid volume can be associated with problems in the fetus. Too little amniotic fluid (<500 mL at term), termed *oligohydramnios*, is associated with uteroplacental insufficiency and fetal renal abnormalities. Too much amniotic fluid (>2,000 mL at term), termed *hydramnios*, is associated with maternal diabetes, neural tube defects, chromosomal deviations, and

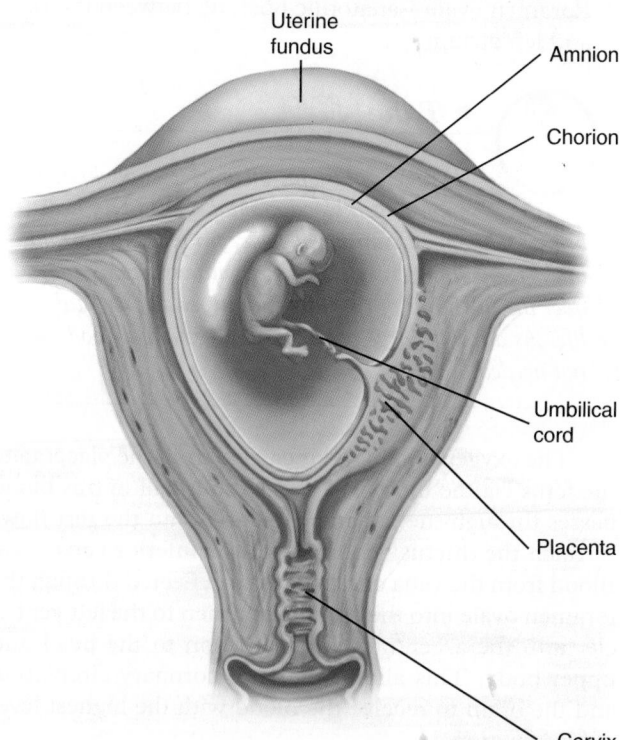

FIGURE 10.7 The embryo is floating in amniotic fluid, surrounded by the protective fetal membranes (amnion and chorion).

malformations of the central nervous system and/or gastrointestinal tract that prevent normal swallowing of amniotic fluid by the fetus (Gilbert, 2007).

While the placenta is developing (end of the second week), the umbilical cord is also formed from the amnion. It is the lifeline from the mother to the growing embryo. It contains one large vein and two small arteries. Wharton's jelly (a specialized connective tissue) surrounds these three blood vessels in the umbilical cord to prevent compression, which would cut off fetal blood and nutrient supply. At term, the average umbilical cord is 22 inches long and about an inch wide (Johnson, 2007).

The precursor cells of the placenta—the trophoblasts—first appear 4 days after fertilization as the outer layer of cells of the blastocyst. These early blastocyst trophoblasts differentiate into all the cells that form the **placenta**. When fully developed, the placenta serves as the interface between the mother and the developing fetus. As early as 3 days after conception, the trophoblasts make human chorionic gonadotropin (hCG), a hormone that ensures that the endometrium will be receptive to the implanting embryo. During the next few weeks the placenta begins to make hormones that control the basic physiology of the mother in such a way that the fetus is supplied with the nutrients and oxygen needed for growth. The placenta also protects the fetus from immune attack by the mother, removes waste products from the fetus, induces the mother to bring more food to the placenta, and, near the time of delivery, produces hormones that ready fetal organs for life outside the uterus (Johnson, 2007).

At no time during pregnancy does the mother's blood mix with fetal blood because there is no direct contact between their bloods; layers of fetal tissue always separate the maternal blood and the fetal blood. These fetal tissues are called the *placental barrier*. Materials can be interchanged only through diffusion. The maternal uterine arteries deliver the nutrients to the placenta, which in turn provides nutrients to the developing fetus; the mother's uterine veins carry fetal waste products away. The structure of the placenta is usually completed by week 12.

The placenta is not only a transfer organ but a factory as well. It produces several hormones necessary for normal pregnancy:

- hCG—preserves the corpus luteum and its progesterone production so that the endometrial lining of the uterus is maintained; this is the basis for pregnancy tests
- Human placental lactogen (hPL)—modulates fetal and maternal metabolism, participates in the development of maternal breasts for lactation, and decreases maternal insulin sensitivity to increase its availability for fetal nutrition
- Estrogen (estriol)—causes enlargement of a woman's breasts, uterus, and external genitalia; stimulates myometrial contractility
- Progesterone (progestin)—maintains the endometrium, decreases the contractility of the uterus, stimulates maternal metabolism and breast development, provides nourishment for the early conceptus
- Relaxin—acts synergistically with progesterone to maintain pregnancy, causes relaxation of the pelvic ligaments, softens the cervix in preparation for birth (Alvero & Schlaff, 2006)

The placenta acts as a pass-through between the mother and fetus, not a barrier. Almost everything the mother ingests (food, alcohol, drugs) passes through to the developing conceptus. This is why it is so important to advise pregnant women not to use drugs, alcohol, and tobacco, because they can be harmful to the conceptus.

During the embryonic stage, the conceptus grows rapidly as all organs and structures are forming. During this critical period of differentiation the growing embryo is most susceptible to damage from external sources, including teratogens (substances that cause birth defects, such as alcohol and drugs), infections (such as rubella or cytomegalovirus), radiation, and nutritional deficiencies.

Fetal Stage

The average pregnancy lasts 280 days from the first day of the last menstrual period. The fetal stage is the time from the end of the eighth week until birth. It is the longest period of prenatal development. During this stage, the conceptus is mature enough to be called a fetus. Although all major systems are present in their basic form, dramatic growth and refinement of all organ systems take place during the fetal period (see Table 10.1). Figure 10.8 depicts a 12- to 15-week-old fetus.

Fetal Circulation

The circulation through the fetus during uterine life differs from that of a child or an adult. Fetal circulation involves the circulation of blood from the placenta to and through the fetus, and back to the placenta. A properly functioning fetal circulation system is essential to sustain the fetus. Before it develops, nutrients and oxygen diffuse through the

FIGURE 10.8 Fetal development: 12- to 15-week fetus.

extraembryonic coelom and the yolk sac from the placenta. As the embryo grows, its nutrient needs increase and the amount of tissue easily reached by diffusion increases. Thus, the circulation must develop quickly and accurately (Blackburn, 2007).

The circulatory system of the fetus functions much differently from that of a newborn. The most significant difference is that oxygen is received from the placenta during fetal life and via the lungs after birth. In addition, the fetal liver does not perform the metabolic functions that it will after birth because the mother's body performs these functions. Three shunts also are present during fetal life:

1. Ductus venosus—connects the umbilical vein to the inferior vena cava
2. Ductus arteriosus—connects the main pulmonary artery to the aorta
3. Foramen ovale—anatomic opening between the right and left atrium

▶ *Take* NOTE!

Fetal circulation functions to carry highly oxygenated blood to vital areas (e.g., heart, brain) while first shunting it away from less important ones (e.g., lungs, liver). The placenta essentially takes over the functions of the lungs and liver during fetal life. As a result, large volumes of oxygenated blood are not needed.

The oxygenated blood is carried from the placenta to the fetus via the umbilical vein. About half of this blood passes through the hepatic capillaries and the rest flows through the ductus venosus into the inferior vena cava. Blood from the vena cava is mostly deflected through the foramen ovale into the left atrium, then to the left ventricle, into the ascending aorta, and on to the head and upper body. This allows the fetal coronary circulation and the brain to receive the blood with the highest level of oxygenation.

Deoxygenated blood from the superior vena cava flows into the right atrium, the right ventricle, and then the pulmonary artery. Because of high pulmonary vascular resistance, only a small percentage (5% to 10%) of the blood in the pulmonary artery flows to the lungs; the majority is shunted through the patent ductus arteriosus and then to the descending aorta (Blackburn, 2007). The fetal lungs are essentially nonfunctional because they are filled with fluid, making them resistant to incoming blood flow. They receive only enough blood for proper nourishment. Finally, two umbilical arteries carry the unoxygenated blood from the descending aorta back to the placenta.

At birth, a dramatic change in the fetal circulatory pattern occurs. The foramen ovale, ductus arteriosus, ductus venosus, and umbilical vessels are no longer needed. With the newborn's first breath, the lungs inflate, which leads to an increase in blood flow to the lungs from the right ventricle. This increase raises the pressure in the left atrium, causing a one-way flap on the left side of the foramen ovale, called the septum primum, to press against the opening, creating a functional separation between the two atria. Blood flow to the lungs increases because blood entering the right atrium can no longer bypass the right ventricle. As a result, the right ventricle pumps blood into the pulmonary artery and on to the lungs. The ductus venosus closes with the clamping of the umbilical cord and inhibition of blood flow through the umbilical vein. The ductus arteriosus constricts partly in response to the higher arterial oxygen levels that occur after the first few breaths. This closure prevents blood from the aorta from entering the pulmonary artery (Blackburn, 2007). All of these changes leave the newborn with the typical adult pattern of circulation. Figure 10.9 shows fetal circulation.

Genetics

Genetics is the study of heredity and its variation (Slee, Slee, & Schmidt, 2008). According to the Centers for Disease Control and Prevention (CDC), birth defects and genetic disorders occur in about 3% of all infants born in the United States (CDC, 2007). Traditionally, genetics has been associated with making decisions about childbearing and caring for children with genetic disorders. Recently, genetic and technologic advances are expanding our understanding of how genetic changes affect human diseases such as diabetes, cancer, Alzheimer's disease, and other multifactorial diseases that are prevalent in adults (Dolan, Biermann, & Damus, 2007). Our ability to diagnose genetic conditions is more advanced than our ability to cure or treat the disorders. However, accurate diagnosis has led to improved treatment and outcomes for those affected with these disorders.

▶ *Take* NOTE!

Genetic science has the potential to revolutionize health care with regard to national screening programs, predisposition testing, detection of genetic disorders, and pharmacogenetics.

Today, nurses are required to have basic skills and knowledge in genetics, genetic testing, and genetic counseling so they can assume new roles and provide information and support to women, children, and families.

Advances in Genetics

Recent advances in genetic knowledge and technology have affected all areas of health. These advances have increased the number of health interventions that can be undertaken with regard to genetic disorders. For example, genetic diagnosis is now possible before conception and very early in pregnancy (see Evidence-Based Practice). Genetic testing can now identify presymptomatic conditions in children and adults. Gene therapy can be used to replace or repair defective or missing genes with normal ones. Gene therapy has been used for a variety of disorders, including cystic fibrosis, melanoma, diabetes, HIV, and hepatitis (Newman & Bettinger, 2007). The potential exists for creation of increased intelligence and size through genetic intervention. Genetic agents may replace drugs, general surgery may be replaced by gene surgery, and genetic intervention may replace radiation (Erlen, 2006). It may also be used to treat many chronic illnesses. See Evidence-Based Practice.

The Human Genome Project (HGP) was an international 13-year effort to produce a comprehensive sequence of the human genome. It was started in 1990 by the Department of Energy and the National Institutes of Health and was completed in May 2003. It has brought advances to the field of genetics and genetic testing (Jenkins & Calzone, 2007). An individual's **genome** represents his or her genetic blueprint, which determines **genotype** (the gene pairs inherited from parents; the specific genetic makeup) and **phenotype** (observed outward characteristics of an individual) (Edgar, 2004).

A primary goal of the HGP was to translate the findings into new strategies for the prevention, diagnosis, and treatment of genetic diseases and disorders. Two key findings from the project were that all human beings are 99.9% identical at the DNA level, and approximately 30,000 genes make up the human genome (International Human Genome Sequencing Consortium, 2004). More information about the HGP may be accessed at: http://www.ornl.gov/sci/techresources/Human_Genomehome.shtml#index.

Current and potential applications for the HGP to health care include rapid and more specific diagnosis of disease, with hundreds of genetic tests available in research or clinical practice; earlier detection of genetic predisposition to disease; less emphasis on treating the symptoms of a disease and more emphasis on looking at the fundamental causes of the disease; new classes of drugs; avoidance of environmental conditions that may trigger disease; and possible augmentation or replacement of defective genes through gene therapy. This new genetic knowledge and technology, along with the commercialization of this

To head

To arm

Superior vena cava

Right lung

Right atrium

Foramen ovale

Inferior vena cava

Portal vein

Umbilicus

Umbilical vein

From placenta

To placenta

Aorta

Ductus arteriosus

Left lung

Left atrium

Aorta

Liver

Ductus venosus

To leg

Umbilical arteries

FIGURE 10.9 Fetal circulation. Arrows indicate the path of blood. The umbilical vein carries oxygen-rich blood from the placenta to the liver and through the ductus venosus. From there it is carried to the inferior vena cava to the right atrium of the heart. Some of the blood is shunted through the foramen ovale to the left side of the heart, where it is routed to the brain and upper extremities. The rest of the blood travels down to the right ventricle and through the pulmonary artery. A small portion of the blood travels to the nonfunctioning lungs, while the remaining blood is shunted through the ductus arteriosus into the aorta to supply the rest of the body.

knowledge, will change both professional and parental understanding of genetic disorders.

The potential benefits of these discoveries are vast, but so is the potential for misuse. These advances challenge all health care professionals to consider the many ethical, legal, and social ramifications of genetics in human lives. In the near future, individual risk profiling based on an in-

dividual's unique genetic makeup will be used to tailor prevention, treatment, and ongoing management of health conditions. This profiling will raise issues associated with patient privacy and confidentiality related to workplace discrimination and access to health insurance. Issues of autonomy are equally problematic as society considers how to address the injustices that will inevitably surface when

EVIDENCE-BASED PRACTICE 10.1
Preimplantation Genetic Screening and Promoting Pregnancy With Assisted Reproductive Technologies

● Study

Assisted reproductive technologies such as in vitro fertilization (IVF) and intracytoplasmic sperm injection (ICSI) involve the transfer of an embryo to the mother to achieve pregnancy. The physician selects the embryos for transfer based on specific criteria related to their structure and form. These "good-quality" embryos are then implanted in the mother in the hopes of achieving a pregnancy. Unfortunately, many women do not experience a pregnancy. The reasons for these failures are not known. One belief is that the embryos being transferred, although they meet the criteria for structure and form, may have an abnormal number of chromosomes, which affects implantation and the development of a pregnancy. Preimplantation genetic screening (PGS) is a tool being used to identify embryos of good quality with the normal number of chromosomes. Based on the screening, only these embryos are implanted; in theory, this would increase the rate of pregnancy. However, there are questions as to how effective PGS is in improving the rates of pregnancy and live birth.

Two independent authors used predetermined quality criteria to collect and analyze data from numerous databases, registers, and reference lists of articles. The researchers also gathered additional data from other authors as necessary. The researchers selected all relevant randomized controlled trials dealing with IVF or ICSI with and without PGS. The researchers measured the outcome based primarily on the live birth rate.

The researchers reviewed two randomized controlled trials. Both trials involved IVF or ICSI with and without the use of PGS. The group without PGS was considered the control group. The trials also involved women of advanced maternal age (over age 35).

▲ Findings

Compared with the control group, the PGS group did not show significant differences in the live birth rate. There were also no significant differences in the rates for ongoing pregnancy. The researchers noted that these findings are limited by the small number of trials (two trials), the advanced maternal age, and the sample size of the one trial (39 women). Based on this study, the researchers could not find evidence to support routine use of PGS to facilitate pregnancy. They recommended more in-depth randomized trials to evaluate this technology.

■ Nursing Implications

Although the study failed to support the effectiveness of PGS, nurses need to be aware of the emerging technology and techniques associated with genetics so that they can provide women and their families with the most appropriate information about available options and therapies. Nurses can incorporate information from this study in their teaching, anticipatory guidance, and counseling activities related to options so that couple can make the best-informed decision possible.

Twisk, M., Mastenbroek, S., van Wely, M., Heineman, M. J., Van der Veen, F., & Repping, S. (2006). Preimplantation genetic screening for abnormal number of chromosomes (aneuploidies) in in vitro fertilization or intracytoplasmic sperm injection. *Cochrane Database of Systematic Reviews,* Issue 1. Art. No.: CD005291.DOI:10.1002/14651858.CD005291.pub2.

disease risk can be determined years in advance of its occurrence. Nurses will play an important role in developing policies and providing direction and support in this arena, and to do so they will need a basic understanding of genetics, including inheritance and inheritance patterns. (For more information on the ethical, social, and legal issues surrounding human genetic research and advances, go to: http://www.ornl.gov/sci/techresources/Human_Genome/research/elsi.shtml.)

Inheritance

The nucleus within the cell is the controlling factor in all cellular activities because it contains chromosomes, long continuous strands of deoxyribonucleic acid (DNA) that carry genetic information. Each chromosome is made up of **genes**. Genes are individual units of heredity of all traits and are organized into long segments of DNA that occupy

a specific location on a chromosome and determine a particular characteristic in an organism.

DNA stores genetic information and encodes the instructions for synthesizing specific proteins needed to maintain life. DNA is double-stranded and takes the form of a double helix. The side pieces of the double helix are made up of a sugar, deoxyribose, and a phosphate, occurring in alternating groups. The cross-connections or rungs of the ladder are attached to the sides and are made up of four nitrogenous bases: adenine, cytosine, thymine, and guanine. The sequence of the base pairs as they form each rung of the ladder is referred to as the genetic code (Fig. 10.10; Wright & Hastie, 2007).

Each gene has a segment of DNA with a specific set of instructions for making proteins needed by body cells for proper functioning. Genes control the types of proteins made and the rate at which they are produced (Dolan, Biermann, & Damus, 2007). Any change in gene structure

Cell

Nucleus

Chromosomes

DNA molecule

Gene

Chemical bases

FIGURE 10.10 DNA is made up of four chemical bases. Tightly coiled strands of DNA are packaged in units called chromosomes, housed in the cell's nucleus. Working subunits of DNA are known as genes. (From the National Institute of Health and National Cancer Institute [1995]. *Understanding gene testing* [NIH Pub. No. 96-3905]. Washington, DC: U.S. Department of Human Services.)

or location leads to a **mutation**, which may alter the type and amount of protein produced (Fig. 10.11). Genes never act in isolation; they always interact with other genes and the environment. They are arranged in a specific linear formation along a chromosome.

The genotype, the specific genetic makeup of an individual, usually in the form of DNA, is the internally coded inheritable information. It refers to the particular **allele**, which is one of two or more alternative versions of gene at a given position or locus on a chromosome that imparts the same characteristic of that gene. For instance, each human has a gene that controls height, but there are variations of these genes, which are alleles, in accordance with the specific height for which the gene codes. A gene that controls eye color may have an allele that can produce blue eyes or an allele that produces brown eyes. The genotype, together with environmental variation that influences the individual, determines the phenotype, or the observed, outward characteristics of an individual. A human inherits two genes, one from each parent. Therefore, one allele comes from the mother and one from the father. These alleles may be the same for the characteristic (**homozygous**) or different (**heterozygous**). For example, WW stands for homozygous dominant; ww stands for homozygous recessive. Heterozygous would be indicated as Ww. If the two alleles differ, such as Ww, the dominant one will usually be expressed in the phenotype of the individual.

Human beings typically have 46 chromosomes. This includes 22 pairs of non-sex chromosomes or autosomes and 1 pair of sex chromosomes (two X chromosomes in females, and an X chromosome and a Y chromosome in males). Offspring receive one chromosome of each of the 23 pairs from each parent.

Regulation and expression of the thousands of human genes is very complex and is the result of many intricate interactions within each cell. Alterations in gene structure,

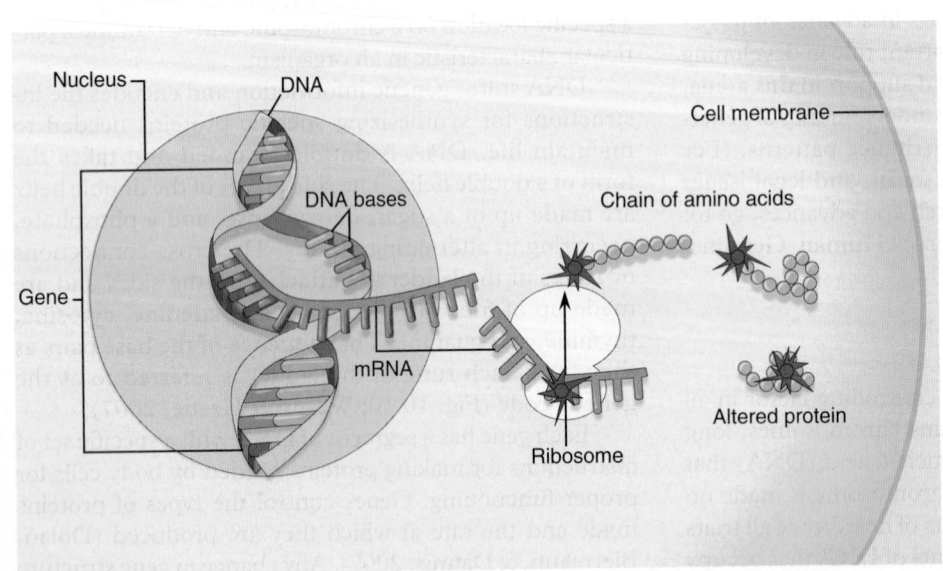

Nucleus

DNA

Cell membrane

DNA bases

Chain of amino acids

Gene

mRNA

Ribosome

Altered protein

FIGURE 10.11 When a gene contains a mutation, the protein encoded by that gene will be abnormal. Some protein changes are insignificant, while others are disabling. (From the National Institutes of Health and National Cancer Institute. [1995]. *Understanding gene testing* [NIH Pub. No. 96-3905]. Washington, DC: U.S. Department of Human Services.)

function, transcription, translation, and protein synthesis can influence an individual's health (Wright & Hastie, 2007). Gene mutations are a permanent change in the sequence of DNA. Some mutations have no significant effect, whereas others can have a tremendous impact on the health of the individual. Several genetic disorders can result from these mutations, such as cystic fibrosis, sickle-cell disease, phenylketonuria, or hemophilia.

The pictorial analysis of the number, form, and size of an individual's chromosomes is termed the **karyotype**. This analysis commonly uses white blood cells and fetal cells in amniotic fluid. The chromosomes are numbered from the largest to the smallest, 1 to 22, and the sex chromosomes are designated by the letter X or Y. A female karyotype is designated as 46,XX and a male karyotype is designated as 46,XY. Figure 10.12 illustrates an example of a karyotyping pattern.

Patterns of Inheritance

A genetic disorder is a disease caused by an abnormality in an individual's genetic material or genome. Diagnosis of a genetic disorder is usually based on clinical signs and symptoms or on laboratory confirmation of an altered gene associated with the disorder. Accurate diagnosis can be aided by the recognition of the pattern of inheritance within a family. The pattern of inheritance is also vital to understand when teaching and counseling families about the risks in future pregnancies. Some genetic disorders occur in multiple family members, while others may occur in only a single family member. A genetic disorder is caused by completely or partially altered genetic material, while a familial disorder is more common in relatives of the affected individual but may be caused by environmental influences and not genetic alterations. For a more detailed discussion of specific types of genetic disorders, see Chapter 50.

Monogenic Disorders

Patterns of inheritance demonstrate how a genetic disorder can be passed on to offspring. Principles of genetic disease inheritance of single gene disorders are the same principles that govern the inheritance of other traits, such as eye and hair color. These are known as Mendel's laws of inheritance, named for the genetic work of Gregor Mendel, an Austrian naturalist. These patterns occur due to a single gene being defective and are referred to as monogenic or sometimes Mendelian disorders. If the defect occurs on the autosome, the genetic disorder is termed autosomal; if the defect is on the X chromosome, the genetic disorder is termed X-linked. The defect also can be classified as dominant or recessive. Monogenic disorders include autosomal dominant, autosomal recessive, X-linked dominant, and X-linked recessive patterns.

FIGURE 10.12 Karyotype pattern. (**A**) Normal female karyotype. (**B**) Normal male karyotype.

Autosomal Dominant Inheritance Disorders

Autosomal dominant inherited disorders occur when a single gene in the heterozygous state is capable of producing the phenotype. In other words, the abnormal or mutant gene overshadows the normal gene and the individual will demonstrate signs and symptoms of the disorder. The affected person generally has an affected parent, and an affected person has a 50% chance of passing the abnormal gene to each of his or her children (Fig. 10.13). Affected individuals are present in every generation. Males and family members who are phenotypically normal (do not show signs or symptoms of the disorder) do not transmit the condition to their offspring. Females and males are equally affected and a male can pass the disorder on to his son. This male-to-male transmission is important in distinguishing autosomal dominant inheritance from X-linked inheritance. There are varying degrees of presentation among individuals in a family. Therefore, a parent with a mild form could have a child with a more severe form. Common types of genetic disorders that follow the autosomal dominant pattern of inheritance include neurofibromatosis, Huntington's disease, achondroplasia, and polycystic kidney disease.

Autosomal Recessive Inheritance Disorders

Autosomal recessive inherited disorders occur when two copies of the mutant or abnormal gene in the homozygous state are necessary to produce the phenotype. In other words, two abnormal genes are needed for the individual to demonstrate signs and symptoms of the disorder. These disorders are generally less common than autosomal dominant disorders (Behrman et al., 2007). Both parents of the affected person must be heterozygous carriers of the gene (clinically normal but carry the gene), and their offspring have a 25% chance of being homozygous (a 50% chance of getting the mutant gene from each parent and therefore a 25% chance of inheriting two mutant genes). If the child is clinically normal, there is a 50% chance the child is a carrier (Fig. 10.14). Affected individuals are usually present in only one generation of the family. Females and males are equally affected and a male can pass the disorder on to his son. The chance that any two parents will both be carriers of the mutant gene is increased if the couple is consanguineous (having a common ancestor). Common types of genetic disorders that follow the autosomal recessive inheritance pattern include cystic fibrosis, phenylketonuria, Tay-Sachs disease, and sickle-cell disease.

X-linked Inheritance Disorders

X-linked inherited disorders are those associated with altered genes present on the X chromosome. They differ in characteristic from autosomal disorders. If a male inherits an X-linked altered gene, he will express the condition. Since a male has only one X chromosome, all the genes on his X chromosome will be expressed (the Y chromosome carries no normal allele to compensate for the altered gene). Because females inherit two X chromosomes, they can be either heterozygous or homozygous for any allele. Therefore, X-linked disorders in females are expressed similarly to autosomal disorders.

Most X-linked disorders demonstrate a recessive pattern of inheritance. Males are more affected than females. A male has only one X chromosome and all the genes on his X chromosome will be expressed, whereas a female will

FIGURE 10.13 Autosomal dominant inheritance.

FIGURE 10.14 Autosomal recessive inheritance.

usually need both X chromosomes to carry the disease. There is no male-to-male transmission (since no X chromosome from the male is transmitted to male offspring), but any man who is affected will have carrier daughters. If a woman is a carrier, there is a 50% chance that her sons will be affected and a 50% chance that her daughters will be carriers (Fig. 10.15). Common types of genetic disorders that follow X-linked recessive inheritance patterns include hemophilia, color blindness, and Duchenne muscular dystrophy.

X-linked dominant inheritance is present if heterozygous female carriers demonstrate signs and symptoms of the disorder. All of the daughters and none of the sons of an affected male have the condition, while both male and female offspring of an affected woman have a 50% chance of inheriting and presenting with the condition (Fig. 10.16). X-linked dominant disorders are rare. The most common is hypophosphatemic (vitamin D–resistant) rickets.

Multifactorial Inheritance Disorders

Multifactorial inherited disorders are those disorders thought to be caused by multiple gene (polygenic) and environmental factors. Many of the common congenital malformations, such as cleft lip, cleft palate, spina bifida, pyloric stenosis, clubfoot, congenital hip dysplasia, and cardiac defects, are attributed to multifactorial inheritance. A combination of genes from both parents, along with unknown environmental factors, produces the trait or condition. An individual may inherit a predisposition to a particular anomaly or disease. The anomalies or diseases

FIGURE 10.16 X-linked dominant inheritance.

vary in severity, and often a sex bias is present. For example, pyloric stenosis is seen more often in males, while congenital hip dysplasia is much more likely to occur in females. Multifactorial conditions tend to run in families, but the pattern of inheritance is not as predictable as with single-gene disorders. The chance of recurrence is also less than in single-gene disorders, but the degree of risk is related to the number of genes in common with the affected individual. The closer the degree of relationship, the more genes an individual has in common with the affected family member, resulting in a higher chance the individual's offspring will have a similar defect. In multifactorial inheritance the likelihood that both identical twins will be affected is not 100%, indicating that there are non-genetic factors involved.

Nontraditional Inheritance Patterns

Molecular studies have revealed that some genetic disorders are inherited in ways that do not follow the typical patterns of dominant, recessive, X-linked, or multifactorial inheritance. Examples of nontraditional inheritance patterns include mitochondrial inheritance and genomic imprinting (Box 10.2). As the science of molecular genetics advances and more is learned about inheritance patterns, other nontraditional patterns of inheritance may be discovered or found to be relatively common.

Chromosomal Abnormalities

In some cases of genetic disorders, the abnormality occurs due to problems with the chromosomes. Chromosomal abnormalities do not follow straightforward patterns of

FIGURE 10.15 X-linked recessive inheritance.

BOX 10.2   Nontraditional Inheritance Patterns

Mitochondrial Inheritance

Certain diseases result from mutations in the mitochondrial DNA. Mitochondria, which are the part of the cell responsible for energy production, are inherited almost exclusively from the mother. Therefore, mitochondrial inheritance is usually passed from the mother to the offspring, regardless of the offspring's sex (differentiating mitochondrial inheritance from X-linked recessive inheritance). These mutations are often deletions and abnormalities of these disorders and are often seen in one or more specific organs, such as the brain, eye, and skeletal muscle. They are often associated with energy deficits in cells with high energy requirements, such as nerve and muscle cells. These disorders tend to be progressive, and the age of onset can vary from infancy to adulthood. There is an extreme amount of variability in symptoms within a family. Examples of disorders that follow mitochondrial inheritance include Kearns-Sayre syndrome, which is a neuromuscular disorder, and Leber's hereditary optic neuropathy, which causes progressive visual impairment.

Genomic Imprinting

Another nontraditional inheritance pattern results from a process called genomic imprinting. Genomic imprinting plays a critical role in fetal growth and development and placental functioning. In genomic imprinting, the expression of a gene is determined by its parental origin. In genomic imprinting both the maternal and paternal alleles are present, but only one is expressed; the other is inactive. Genomic imprinting does not alter the genetic sequence itself but affects the phenotype observed. In these cases the altered genes in a certain region of the genome have very different expressions depending on whether they were inherited from the mother or the father. Several human syndromes are known to be associated with defects in gene imprinting. Disorders that result from a disruption of imprinting usually involve a growth phenotype and include varying degrees of developmental problems. Common examples include Prader-Willi syndrome (a condition resulting in severe hypotonia and hyperphagia leading to obesity and mental retardation), Angelman syndrome (a neurodevelopmental disorder associated with mental retardation, jerky movements, and seizures), and Beckwith-Wiedemann syndrome (characterized by somatic overgrowth, congenital malformations, and a predisposition to embryonic neoplasia).

---

inheritance. Sperm and egg cells each have 23 unpaired chromosomes. When they unite during pregnancy they form a fertilized egg with 46 chromosomes. Sometimes before pregnancy begins, an error has occurred during the process of cell division, leaving an egg or sperm with too many or too few chromosomes. If this egg or sperm cell joins with a normal egg or sperm cell, the resulting embryo has a chromosomal abnormality. Chromosomal abnormalities can also occur due to an error in the structure of the chromosome. Small pieces of the chromosome may be deleted, duplicated, inverted, misplaced, or exchanged with part of another chromosome. Most chromosomal abnormalities occur due to an error in the egg or sperm. Therefore, the abnormality is present in every cell of the body. However, some abnormalities can happen after fertilization during mitotic cell division and result in **mosaicism**. Mosaicism or mosaic form refers to when the chromosomal abnormalities do not show up in every cell and only some cells or tissues carry the abnormality. In mosaic forms of the disorder, the symptoms are usually less severe than if all the cells were abnormal.

About 1 in 150 live-born infants is born with a chromosomal abnormality (March of Dimes, 2007a). These often cause major defects because they involve added or missing genes. Congenital anomalies and mental retardation are often associated with chromosomal abnormalities. These abnormalities occur on autosomal as well as sex chromosomes and can result from changes in the number of chromosomes or changes in the structure of the chromosomes.

Numerical Abnormalities

Chromosomal abnormalities of number often result due to nondisjunction, or failure of the chromosome pair to separate during cell division, meiosis, or mitosis. Few chromosomal numerical abnormalities are compatible with full-term development and most result in spontaneous abortion. There are some numerical abnormalities that do support development to term because the chromosome on which the abnormality is present carries relatively few genes (such as chromosome 13, 18, 21, or X). Two common abnormalities of chromosome number are monosomies or trisomies. In **monosomies** there is only one copy of a particular chromosome instead of the usual pair (an entire single chromosome is missing). In these cases, all fetuses spontaneously abort in early pregnancy. Survival is seen only in mosaic forms of these disorders. In **trisomies**, there are three of a particular chromosome instead of the usual two (an entire single chromosome is added). The most common trisomies include trisomy 21 (Down syndrome), trisomy 18, and trisomy 13. Figure 10.17 shows the karyotype of a child with Down syndrome. (See Chapter 50 for a detailed discussion of these disorders.) Trisomies may be present in every cell or may present in the mosaic form.

Another type of abnormal chromosome number is **polyploidy**. Polyploidy causes an increase in the number of haploid sets (23) of chromosomes in a cell. Triploidy refers to three whole sets of chromosomes in a single cell (in humans, a total of 69 chromosomes per cell); tetraploidy refers to four whole sets of chromosomes in a

FIGURE 10.17 Karyotype of a child with Down syndrome.

single cell (in humans, a total of 92 chromosomes per cell). Polyploidy usually results in an early spontaneous abortion and is incompatible with life.

Structural Abnormalities

Chromosome abnormalities of structure usually occur when there is a breakage and loss of a portion of one or more chromosomes and during the repair process the broken ends are rejoined incorrectly. Structural abnormalities usually lead to having too much or too little genetic material. Altered chromosome structure can take on several forms. Deletions occur when a portion of the chromosome is missing or deleted, resulting in a loss of that portion of the chromosome. Duplications are seen when a portion of the chromosome is duplicated and an extra chromosomal segment is present. Clinical findings vary depending on how much chromosomal material is involved. Inversions occur when a portion of the chromosome breaks off at two points and is turned upside down and reattached; therefore, the genetic material is inverted. With inversion, there is no loss or gain of chromosomal material and carriers are phenotypically normal, but they do have an increased risk for miscarriage and chromosomally abnormal offspring. Ring chromosomes are seen when a portion of a chromosome has broken off in two places and formed a circle or ring.

The most clinically significant structural abnormality is a translocation. This occurs when a potion of one chromosome is transferred to another chromosome and an abnormal rearrangement is present.

Structural abnormalities can be balanced or unbalanced. Balanced abnormalities involve the rearrangement of genetic material with neither an overall gain nor loss. Individuals who inherit a balanced structural abnormality are usually phenotypically normal but are at a higher risk for miscarriages and having chromosomally abnormal offspring. Examples of structural rearrangements that can be balanced include inversions, translocation, and ring chromosomes. Unbalanced structural abnormalities are similar to numerical abnormalities because genetic material is either gained or lost. Unbalanced structural abnormalities

can encompass several genes and result in severe clinical consequences.

Sex Chromosome Abnormalities

Chromosomal abnormalities can also involve sex chromosomes. These cases are usually less severe in their clinical effects than autosomal chromosomal abnormalities. Sex chromosome abnormalities are gender-specific and involve a missing or extra sex chromosome. They affect sexual development and may cause infertility, growth abnormalities, and possibly behavioral and learning problems. Many affected individuals lead essentially normal lives. Examples are Turner syndrome (in females) and Klinefelter's syndrome (in males; see Chapter 50 for a more detailed discussion of these disorders).

Genetic Evaluation and Counseling

Genetic counseling has been defined as "an educational process that seeks to assist affected and/or at risk individuals to understand the nature of a genetic disorder, its transmission, and the options available to them in management and family planning" (Behrman et al., 2004, p. 395). There are a variety of reasons an individual should be referred for genetic counseling. Box 10.3 lists those who may benefit from genetic counseling. In many cases, geneticists and genetic counselors provide information to families regarding genetic diseases. However, an experienced family physician, pediatrician, or nurse who has received special training in genetics may also provide the information.

BOX 10.3 **Those Who May Benefit From Genetic Counseling**

- Maternal age 35 years or older when the baby is born
- Paternal age 50 years or older
- Previous child, parents, or close relatives with an inherited disease, congenital anomalies, metabolic disorders, developmental disorders, or chromosomal abnormalities
- Consanguinity or incest
- Pregnancy screening abnormality, including alpha-fetoprotein, triple screen, amniocentesis, or ultrasound
- Stillborn with congenital anomalies
- Two or more pregnancy losses
- Teratogen exposure or risk
- Concerns about genetic defects that occur frequently in their ethnic or racial group (for instance, those of African descent are most at risk for having a child with sickle-cell anemia)
- Abnormal newborn screening
- Child born with one or more major malformations in a major organ system
- Child with abnormalities of growth
- Child with developmental delay, mental retardation, blindness, or deafness

A genetic consultation involves evaluation of an individual or a family. Its purposes are to confirm, diagnose, or rule out genetic conditions; to identify medical management issues; to calculate and communicate genetic risks to a family; to discuss ethical and legal issues; and to provide and arrange psychosocial support. Genetic counselors serve as educators and resource persons for other health care providers and the general public.

The ideal time for genetic counseling is before conception. Preconception counseling gives couples the chance to identify and reduce potential pregnancy risks, plan for known risks, and establish early prenatal care. Unfortunately, many woman delay seeking prenatal care until their second or third trimester, after the crucial time of organogenesis. Therefore, it is important that preconception counseling is offered to all women as they seek health care throughout their childbearing years, especially if they are contemplating pregnancy. This requires health care providers to take an active role.

Preconception screening and counseling can raise serious ethical and moral issues for a couple. The results of prenatal genetic testing can lead to the decision to terminate a pregnancy, even if the results are not conclusive but indicate a strong possibility that the child will have an abnormality. The severity of the abnormality may not be known, and some may find the decision to terminate unethical. Another difficult situation that provides an example of the ethical and moral issues surrounding genetic screening and counseling involves disorders that affect only one gender of offspring. A mother may find she is a carrier of a gene for a disorder for which there is no prenatal screening test available. In these cases the couple may decide to terminate any pregnancy where the fetus is the affected sex, even though there is a 50% chance that the child will not inherit the disorder. In these situations, the choice is the couple's and information and support must be provided in a nondirective manner.

Genetic counseling is particularly important if a congenital anomaly or genetic disease has been diagnosed prenatally or if a child is born with a life-threatening congenital anomaly or genetic disease. In these cases families need information urgently so they can make immediate decisions. If a diagnosis with genetic implications is made later in life, if a couple with a family history of a genetic disorder or a previous child with a genetic disorder is planning a family, or if there is suspected teratogen exposure, urgency of information is not such an issue. In these situations, the family needs time to ponder all their options. This may involve several meetings over a longer period of time.

Genetic counseling involves gathering information regarding birth history, past medical history, and current health status as well as a family history of congenital anomalies, mental retardation, genetic diseases, reproductive history, general health, and causes of death. A detailed family history is imperative and in most cases will include the development of a pedigree, which is like a family tree (Fig. 10.18). Information is ideally gathered on three gen-

FIGURE 10.18 A pedigree is a diagram made using symbols that demonstrates the links between family members and focuses on medical and health information for each relative.

erations, but if the family history is complicated, information from more distant relatives may be needed. Families receiving genetic counseling may benefit from being told in advance that this information will be necessary; they may need to discuss these sensitive, private issues with family members to obtain the needed facts. When necessary, medical records may be requested for family members, especially those who have a genetic disorder, to help ensure accuracy of the information. Sometimes a pedigree may reveal confidential information not known by all family members, such as an adoption, a child conceived through in vitro fertilization, or a husband not being the father of a baby. Therefore, maintaining confidentiality is extremely important. After careful analysis of the data obtained, referral to a genetic counselor when indicated is appropriate.

Medical genetic knowledge has increased dramatically over the past few decades. Not only is it possible to detect specific diseases with genetic mutations, but it is also possible to test for a genetic predisposition to various diseases or conditions and certain physical characteristics. This leads to complex ethical, moral, and social issues. Maintaining client privacy and confidentiality and administering care in a nondiscriminatory manner are essential while maintaining sensitivity to cultural differences. It is essential to respect client autonomy and present information in a nondirective manner.

Nursing Roles and Responsibilities

The nurse is likely to interact with the client in a variety of ways related to genetics—taking a family history, scheduling genetic testing, explaining the purposes of all screening and diagnostic tests, answering questions, and addressing concerns raised by family members. Nurses are often the first health care providers to encounter women with preconception and prenatal issues. Nurses play an important role in beginning the preconception counseling process and referring women and their partners for further genetic testing when indicated.

An accurate and thorough family history is an essential part of preconception counseling. Nurses in any practice setting can obtain a patient's history during the initial encounter. The purpose is to gather patient and family information that may provide clues as to whether the patient has a genetic trait, inherited condition, or inherited predisposition (Erlen, 2006). At a basic level, all nurses should be able to take a family medical history to help identify those at risk for genetic conditions, and then initiate a referral when appropriate. Box 10.4 presents examples of focused assessment questions that can be used. Based on the information gathered during the history, the nurse must decide whether a referral is necessary to a genetic specialist or whether further evaluation is needed. Prenatal testing to assess for genetic risks and defects might be used to identify genetic disorders. These tests are described in Common Laboratory and Diagnostic Tests 10.1.

*R*emember Robert and Kate Shafer? Based on the information gathered from their genetic history, they were referred to a genetic specialist. What prenatal tests might be ordered to assess their risk for genetic disorders? What would be the nurse's role related to genetic counseling?

BOX 10.4   **Focused Health Assessment: Genetic History**

What was the cause and age of death for deceased family members?

Does any consanguinity exist between relatives?

Do any serious illnesses or chronic conditions exist? If so, what was the age of onset?

Do any female family members have a history of miscarriages, stillbirths, or diabetes?

Do any female members have a history of alcohol or drug use during pregnancy?

What were the ages of female members during childbearing, especially if older than 35?

Do any family members have mental retardation or developmental delays?

Do any family members have a known or suspected metabolic disorder such as PKU?

Do any family members have an affective disorder such as bipolar disorder?

Have any close relatives been diagnosed with any type of cancer?

What is your ethnic background (explore as related to certain disorders)?

Do any family members have a known or suspected chromosomal disorder?

Do any family members have a progressive neurologic disorder?

Source: Kumar & Burton, 2007.

Nurses working with families involved with genetic counseling typically have certain responsibilities. These include:

- Using interviewing and active listening skills to identify genetic concerns
- Knowing basic genetic terminology and inheritance patterns
- Explaining basic concepts of probability and disorder susceptibility
- Safeguarding the privacy and confidentiality of patients' genetic information
- Providing complete informed consent to facilitate decisions about genetic testing
- Discussing costs of genetic services and the benefits and risks of using health insurance to pay for genetic services, including potential risks of discrimination
- Recognizing and defining ethical, legal, and social issues
- Providing accurate information about the risks and benefits of genetic testing
- Providing culturally appropriate methods to convey genetic information
- Monitoring patients' emotional reactions after receiving genetic analysis
- Providing information on appropriate local support groups
- Knowing their own limitations and making appropriate referrals (Jenkins & Calzone, 2007)

Talking with families who have recently been diagnosed with a genetic disorder or who have had a child born with congenital anomalies is very difficult. Many times the nurse may be the one who has first contact with these parents and will be the one to provide follow-up care.

Genetic disorders are significant, life-changing, and possibly life-threatening situations. The information is highly technical and the field is undergoing significant technologic advances. Nurses need an understanding of who will benefit from genetic counseling and must be able to discuss the role of the genetic counselor with families. The nurse wants to ensure that families at risk are aware that genetic counseling is available before they attempt to have another baby.

*B*ased on the results of their genetic tests, Robert and Kate are placed at moderate risk for having an infant with an autosomal recessive genetic disorder. The couple asks the nurse what all of this means. What information should the nurse provide about concepts of probability and disorder susceptibility for this couple? How can the nurse help this couple to make knowledgeable decisions concerning their reproductive future?

Nurses play an essential role in providing emotional support to the family through this challenging time. This

COMMON LABORATORY AND DIAGNOSTIC TESTS 10.1
PRENATAL TESTS TO ASSESS RISK FOR GENETIC DISORDERS

Test	Description	Indication	Timing
Alpha-fetoprotein	A sample of the woman's blood is drawn to evaluate plasma protein that is produced by the fetal liver, yolk sac, and GI tract, and crosses from the amniotic fluid into the maternal blood.	Increased levels might indicate a neural tube defect, Turner syndrome, tetralogy of Fallot, multiple gestation, omphalocele gastroschisis, or hydrocephaly. Decreased levels might indicate Down syndrome or trisomy 18.	Typically performed between 15 and 18 weeks' gestation
Amniocentesis	Amniotic fluid aspirated from the amniotic sac; safety concerns include infection, pregnancy loss, and fetal needle injuries	To perform chromosome analysis, alpha-fetoprotein, DNA markers, viral studies, karyotyping; and identify inborn errors of metabolism	Usually performed between 15 and 20 weeks' gestation to allow for adequate amniotic fluid volume to accumulate; results take 2 to 4 weeks
Chorionic villus sampling	Removal of small tissue specimen from the fetal portion of the placenta, which reflects the fetal genetic makeup; main complications include severe transverse limb defects and spontaneous pregnancy loss	To detect fetal karyotype, sickle-cell anemia, phenylketonuria, Down syndrome, Duchenne muscular dystrophy, and numerous other genetic disorders	Typically performed between 10 and 12 weeks' gestation, with results available in less than a week
Percutaneous umbilical blood sampling	Insertion of a needle directly into a fetal umbilical vessel under ultrasound guidance; two potential complications: fetal hemorrhage and risk of infection	Used for prenatal diagnosis of inherited blood disorders such as hemophilia A, karyotyping, detection of fetal infection, determination of acid–base status, and assessment and treatment of isoimmunization	Generally performed after 16 weeks' gestation
Fetal nuchal translucency (FNT)	An intravaginal ultrasound that measures fluid collection in the subcutaneous space between the skin and the cervical spine of the fetus	To identify fetal anomalies; abnormal fluid collection can be associated with genetic disorders (trisomies 13, 18, and 21), Turner syndrome, cardiac deformities, and/or physical anomalies. When the FNT is greater than 2.5 mm, the measurement is considered abnormal.	Performed between 10 and 14 weeks' gestation
Level II ultrasound/ fetal scan	Use of high-frequency sound waves to visualize the fetus	Enables evaluation of structural changes to be identified early	Typically performed after 18 weeks' gestation
Triple marker test	Serum screening test using the levels of three maternal serum markers—MSAFP, unconjugated estriol, and hCG—in combination with maternal age to calculate risk	To identify risk for Down syndrome, neural tube defects, and other chromosomal disorders. Elevated hCG combined with lower than normal estriol and MSAFP levels indicate increased risk for Down syndrome or other trisomy condition.	Performed between 16 and 18 weeks' gestation

Sources: Kumar & Burton, 2007; Wynbrandt, 2008; Leveno, Cunningham, Alexander, et al., 2007; Gilbert, 2007.

is especially important with follow-up counseling after the couple or family has been to the genetic specialist.

▶ **Take** NOTE!

Nurses need to be actively engaged with patients and their families and help them consider the facts, values, and context in which they are making decisions. Nurses need to be open and honest with families as they discuss these sensitive and emotionally laden choices.

The nurse is in an ideal position to help families review what has been discussed during the genetic counseling sessions and to answer any additional questions they might have. Referral to appropriate agencies, support groups, and resources, such as a social worker, a chaplain, or an ethicist, is another key role when caring for families with suspected or diagnosed genetic disorders.

▶ **Consider** THIS!

As I waited for the genetic counselor to come into the room, my mind was filled with numerous fears and questions. What does an inconclusive amniocentesis really mean? What if this pregnancy produced an abnormal baby? How would I cope with a special child in my life? If only I had gone to the midwife sooner when I thought I was pregnant, but still in denial. Why did I wait so long to admit this pregnancy and get prenatal care? If only I had started to take my folic acid pills when prescribed. Why didn't I research my family's history to know of any hidden genetic conditions? What about my sister with a Down syndrome child? What must I have been thinking? I guess I could play the "what-if" game forever and never come up with answers. It was too late to do anything about this pregnancy because I was in my last trimester. I started to pray silently when the counselor opened the door. . . .

Thoughts: This woman is reviewing the last several months, looking for answers to her greatest fears. Inconclusive screenings can introduce emotional torment for many women as they wait for validating results. Are these common thoughts and fears for many women facing potential genetic disorders? What supportive interventions might the nurse offer?

■■■ Key Concepts

- Fertilization, which takes place in the outer third of the ampulla of the fallopian tube, leads to the formation of a zygote. The zygote undergoes cleavage, eventually implanting in the endometrium about 7 to 10 days after conception.

- Three embryonic layers of cells are formed and include the ectoderm, which forms the central nervous system, special senses, skin, and glands; the mesoderm, which forms the skeletal, urinary, circulatory, and reproductive systems; and the endoderm, which forms the respiratory system, liver, pancreas, and digestive system.

- Amniotic fluid surrounds the embryo and increases in volume as the pregnancy progresses, reaching approximately a liter in volume by term.

- At no time during pregnancy is there any direct connection between the blood of the fetus and the blood of the mother, so there is no mixing of blood.

- A specialized connective tissue known as Wharton's jelly surrounds the three blood vessels in the umbilical cord to prevent compression, which would choke off the supply of blood and nutrients to the growing life inside.

- The placenta protects the fetus from immune attack by the mother, removes waste products from the fetus, induces the mother to bring more food to the placenta, and, near the time of delivery, produces hormones that mature fetal organs in preparation for life outside the uterus.

- The purpose of fetal circulation is to carry highly oxygenated blood to vital areas (heart and brain) while first shunting it away from less vital ones (lungs and liver).

- Humans have 46 paired chromosomes that are found in all cells of the body, except the ovum and sperm cells, which have just 23 chromosomes. Each person has a unique genetic constitution, or genotype.

- Research from the Human Genome Project has provided a better understanding of the genetic contribution to disease.

- Genetic disorders can result from abnormalities in patterns of inheritance or chromosomal abnormalities involving chromosomal number or structure.

- Autosomal dominant inheritance occurs when a single gene in the heterozygous state is capable of producing the phenotype. Autosomal recessive inheritance occurs when two copies of the mutant or abnormal gene in the homozygous state are necessary to produce the phenotype. X-linked inheritance disorders are those associated with altered genes present on the X chromosome. They can be dominant or recessive. Multifactorial inheritance is thought to be caused by multiple genetic and environmental factors.

- In some cases of genetic disorders, a chromosomal abnormality occurs. Chromosomal abnormalities do not follow straightforward patterns of inheritance. These abnormalities occur on autosomal as well as sex chromosomes and can result from changes in the number or structure of the chromosomes.

- Genetic counseling involves evaluation of an individual or a family. Its purpose is to confirm, diagnose, or rule out genetic conditions; identify medical management issues; calculate and communicate genetic risks to a family; discuss ethical and legal issues; and assist in providing and arranging psychosocial support.

■ Legal, ethical, and social issues can arise related to genetic testing and may include the privacy and confidentiality of genetic information, who should have access to personal genetic information, psychological impact and stigmatization due to individual genetic differences, use of genetic information in reproductive decision making and reproductive rights, and whether testing should be performed if no cure is available.

■ Preconception screening and counseling can raise serious ethical and moral issues for a couple. Prenatal genetic testing can lead to the decision to terminate a pregnancy based on the results.

■ Nurses play an important role in beginning the preconception counseling process and referring women and their partners for further genetic information when indicated. Many times the nurse is the one who has first contact with these women and will be the one to provide follow-up care.

■ Nurses need to have a solid understanding of who will benefit from genetic counseling and be able to discuss the role of the genetic counselor with families, ensuring that families at risk are aware that genetic counseling is available before they attempt to have another baby.

■ Nurses play an essential role in providing emotional support and referrals to appropriate agencies, support groups, and resources when caring for families with suspected or diagnosed genetic disorders. Nurses can assist patients with their decision making by referring them to a social worker, a chaplain, or an ethicist.

REFERENCES

Alvero, R., & Schlaff, W. D. (2006). *Reproductive endocrinology and infertility: The requisites in obstetrics and gynecology.* St. Louis: Mosby, Inc.

Behrman, R. E., Kliegman, R. M., & Jenson, H. B. (2007). *Nelson's textbook of pediatrics* (18th ed.). Philadelphia: Elsevier Health Sciences.

Blackburn, S. T. (2007). *Maternal, fetal and neonatal physiology* (3rd ed.). Philadelphia: Saunders.

Centers for Disease Control and Prevention (CDC) (2007). *Frequently asked questions about birth defects.* Available at: http://www.cdc.gov/ncbddd/bd/faq1.htm#Whatisabirthdefect

Creatsas, G., Chrousos, G. P., & Mastorakos, G. (2007). *Women's health and disease: Gynecologic and reproductive issues.* Malden, MA: Blackwell Publishers.

Dillon, P. M. (2007). *Nursing health assessment: A critical thinking, case studies approach* (2nd ed.). Philadelphia: F. A. Davis.

Dolan, S., Biermann, J., & Damus, K. (2007). Genomics for health in preconception and prenatal periods. *Journal of Nursing Scholarship, 39*(1), 4–9.

Edgar, D. A. (2004). Advances in genetics: Implications for children, families and nurses. *Paediatric Nursing, 16,* 26–29.

Erlen, J. A. (2006). Genetic testing and counseling: Selected ethical issues. *Orthopedic Nursing, 25*(6), 423–427.

Gilbert, E. S. (2007). *Manual of high-risk pregnancy and delivery* (4th ed.). St. Louis: Mosby Inc.

Human Genome Management Information System. (2006). *Human Genome Project information.* Available at http://www.ornl.gov/sci/techresources/Human_Genome/home.shtml#index.

International Human Genome Sequencing Consortium. (2004). Finishing the euchromatic sequence of the human genome. *Nature, 431,* 931–945.

Jenkins, J., & Calzone, K. A. (2007). Establishing the essential nursing competencies for genetics and genomics. *Journal of Nursing Scholarship, 39*(1), 10–16.

Johnson, M. H. (2007). *Essential reproduction* (6th ed.). Malden, MA: Blackwell Publishers.

Leveno, K. J., Cunningham, F. G., Alexander, J. M., et al. (2007). *Williams manual of obstetrics: Pregnancy and complications* (22nd ed.). New York: McGraw-Hill.

March of Dimes. (2007a). *Quick reference and fact sheet: Chromosomal abnormalities.* Retrieved April 7, 2007, from http://www.marchofdimes.com/professionals/681_1209.asp.

March of Dimes. (2007b). *Recommended newborn screening tests: 29 disorders.* Retrieved April 23, 2007, from http://www.marchofdimes.com/professionals/14332_15455.asp

Newman, C. M., & Bettinger, T. (2007). Gene therapy progress and prospects. *Gene Therapy, 14*(6), 465–475.

Twisk, M., Mastenbroek, S., van Wely, M., Heineman, M. J., Van der Veen, F., & Repping, S. (2006). Preimplantation genetic screening for abnormal number of chromosomes (aneuploidies) in in vitro fertilization or intracytoplasmic sperm injection. *Cochrane Database of Systematic Reviews,* Issue 1. Art. No.: CD005291. DOI:10.1002/14651858.CD005291.pub2.

Venes, D. (2005). *Taber's cyclopedic medical dictionary* (20th ed.). Philadelphia: F. A. Davis.

Wright, A., & Hastie, N. (2007). *Genes and common diseases.* New York: Cambridge University Press.

Wynbrandt, J. (2008). *Genetic disorders and birth defects.* New York: Facts on File, Incorporated.

WEBSITES

American Society of Human Genetics: www.faseb.org/genetics/ashg/ashgmenu.htm

CDC, Office of Genetics: www.cdc.gov/genetics/activities/ogdp.htm

Gene Clinics: www.geneclinics.org

Gene Tests: www.genetests.org

Genetic Alliance: www.geneticalliance.org

Human Genome Project of the U.S. Department of Energy: www.ornl.gov/hgmis

International Society of Nurses in Genetics: www.nursing.creighton.edu/isong

March of Dimes: www.marchofdimes.com

National Coalition for Health Professional Education in Genetics: www.nchpeg.org

National Human Genome Research Institute: www.nhgri.gov

Virtual Library on Genetics: www.ornl.gov/TechResources/Human_Genome/genetics.html

Visible Embryo: www.visembryo.ucsf.edu

CHAPTER WORKSHEET

MULTIPLE CHOICE QUESTIONS

1. After teaching a group of students about fertilization, the instructor determines that the teaching was successful when the group identifies which as the usual site of fertilization?

   a. Fundus of the uterus

   b. Endometrium of the uterus

   c. Upper portion of fallopian tube

   d. Follicular tissue of the ovary

2. A client comes to the clinic for pregnancy testing. The nurse explains that the test detects the presence of which hormone?

   a. hPL

   b. hCG

   c. FSH

   d. TSH

3. The nurse is counseling a couple, one of whom is affected by an autosomal dominant disorder. They express concerns about the risk of transmitting the disorder. What is the best response by the nurse regarding the risk that their baby may have for the disease?

   a. "You have a one in four (25%) chance."

   b. "The risk is 12.5%, or a one in eight chance."

   c. "The chance is 100%."

   d. "Your risk is 50%, or a one in two chance."

4. What is the first step in determining a couple's risk for a genetic disorder?

   a. Observing the patient and family over time

   b. Conducting extensive psychological testing

   c. Obtaining a thorough family health history

   d. Completing an extensive exclusionary list

5. A nurse is working in a women's health clinic. Genetic counseling would be most appropriate for the woman who:

   a. Just had her first miscarriage at 10 weeks

   b. Is 30 years old and planning to conceive

   c. Has a history that reveals a close relative with Down syndrome

   d. Is 18 weeks pregnant with a normal triple screen result

CRITICAL THINKING EXERCISE

1. Mr. and Mrs. Martin wish to start a family, but they can't agree on something important. Mr. Martin wants his wife to be tested for cystic fibrosis (CF) to see if she is a carrier. Mr. Martin had a brother with CF and watched his parents struggle with the hardship and the expense of caring for him for years, and he doesn't want to experience it in his own life. Mr. Martin has found out he is a CF carrier. Mrs. Martin doesn't want to have the test because she figures that once a baby is in their arms, they will be glad, no matter what.

   a. What information/education should this couple consider before deciding whether to have the test?

   b. How can you assist this couple in their decision-making process?

   c. What is your role in this situation if you don't agree with their decision?

STUDY ACTIVITIES

1. Obtain the video "Miracle of Life," which shows conception and fetal development. What are your impressions? Is the title of this video realistic?

2. Select one of the websites listed above to explore the topic of genetics. Critique the information presented. Was it understandable to a layperson? What specifically did you learn? Share your findings with your classmates during a discussion group.

3. Draw your own family pedigree, identifying inheritance patterns. Share it with your family to validate its accuracy. What did you discover about your family's past health?

4. Select one of the various prenatal screening tests (alpha-fetoprotein, amniocentesis, chorionic villus sampling, or fetal nuchal translucency) and research it in depth. Role-play with another nursing student how you would explain its purpose, the procedure, and potential findings to an expectant couple at risk for a fetal abnormality.

MATERNAL ADAPTATION DURING PREGNANCY

KEY TERMS

ballottement
Braxton Hicks contractions
Chadwick's sign
dietary reference intakes (DRIs)

Goodell's sign
Hegar's sign
linea nigra
physiologic anemia of pregnancy

pica
quickening
trimester

LEARNING OBJECTIVES

Upon completion of the chapter, the learner will be able to:

1. Define the key terms used in this chapter.
2. Differentiate between subjective (presumptive), objective (probable), and diagnostic (positive) signs of pregnancy.
3. Explain maternal physiologic changes that occur during pregnancy.
4. Summarize the nutritional needs of the pregnant woman and her fetus.
5. Identify the emotional and psychological changes that occur during pregnancy.

*M*arva, age 17, appeared at the health department clinic complaining that she had a stomach virus and needed to be seen today. When the nurse asked her additional questions about her illness, Marva reported that she had been sick to her stomach and "beat tired" for days. She had stopped eating to avoid any more nausea and vomiting.

Wow

When a woman discovers that she is pregnant, she must remember to protect and nourish the fetus by making wise choices.

Pregnancy is a normal life event that involves considerable physical and psychological adjustments for the mother. A pregnancy is divided into three **trimesters** of 13 weeks each (Arenson & Drake, 2007). Within each trimester, numerous adaptations take place that facilitate the growth of the fetus. The most obvious are physical changes to accommodate the growing fetus. However, pregnant women also undergo psychological changes as they prepare for parenthood.

Signs and Symptoms of Pregnancy

Traditionally, signs and symptoms of pregnancy have been grouped into the following categories: presumptive, probable, and positive (Box 11.1). The only signs that can determine a pregnancy with 100% accuracy are positive signs.

What additional information is necessary to complete the assessment of Marva, the 17-year-old with nausea and vomiting? What diagnostic tests might be done to confirm the nurse's suspicion that she is pregnant?

Subjective (Presumptive) Signs

Presumptive signs are those signs experienced by the woman herself. The most obvious presumptive sign of pregnancy is the absence of menstruation. Skipping a period is not a reliable sign of pregnancy by itself, but if it is accompanied by consistent nausea, fatigue, breast tenderness, and urinary frequency, pregnancy would seem very likely.

Presumptive changes are the least reliable indicators of pregnancy because any one of them can be caused by conditions other than pregnancy (Walsh, 2007). For example, amenorrhea can be caused by early menopause,

endocrine dysfunction, malnutrition, anemia, diabetes mellitus, long-distance running, cancer, or stress. Nausea and vomiting can be caused by gastrointestinal disorders, food poisoning, acute infections, or eating disorders. Fatigue could be caused by anemia, stress, or viral infections. Breast tenderness may result from chronic cystic mastitis, premenstrual changes, or the use of oral contraceptives. Urinary frequency could have a variety of causes other than pregnancy, such as infection, cystocele, structural disorders, pelvic tumors, or emotional tension (Frieden & Chan, 2007).

▶ *Consider THIS!*

Jim and I decided to start our family, so I stopped taking the Pill 3 months ago. One morning when I got out of bed to take the dog out, I felt queasy and lightheaded. I sure hoped I wasn't coming down with the flu. By the end of the week, I was feeling really tired and started taking naps in the afternoon. In addition, I seemed to be going to the bathroom frequently, despite not drinking much fluid. When my breasts started to tingle and ache, I decided to make an appointment with my doctor to see what "illness" I had contracted.

After listening to my list of physical complaints, the office nurse asked me if I might be pregnant. My eyes opened wide: I had somehow missed the link between my symptoms and pregnancy. I started to think about when my last period was, and it had been 2 months ago. The office ran a pregnancy test and much to my surprise it was positive!

Thoughts: Many women stop contraceptives in an attempt to achieve pregnancy but miss the early signs

(continued)

BOX 11.1 Signs and Symptoms of Pregnancy

Presumptive (Time of Occurrence)	Probable (Time of Occurrence)	Positive (Time of Occurrence)
Fatigue (12 wk)	Braxton Hicks contractions (16–28 wk)	Ultrasound verification of embryo or fetus (4–6 wk)
Breast tenderness (3–4 wk)	Positive pregnancy test (4–12 wk)	Fetal movement felt by experienced clinician (20 wk)
Nausea and vomiting (4–14 wk)	Abdominal enlargement (14 wk)	Auscultation of fetal heart tones via Doppler (10–12 wk)
Amenorrhea (4 wk)	Ballottement (16–28 wk)	
Urinary frequency (6–12 wk)	Goodell's sign (5 wk)	
Hyperpigmentation of the skin (16 wk)	Chadwick's sign (6–8 wk)	
Fetal movements (quickening; 16–20 wk)	Hegar's sign (6–12 wk)	
Uterine enlargement (7–12 wk)		
Breast enlargement (6 wk)		

Sources: Blackburn, 2007; Frieden and Chan, 2007; Torgersen and Curran 2006.

▶ *Consider THIS!* (continued)

of pregnancy. This woman was experiencing several signs of early pregnancy—urinary frequency, fatigue, morning nausea, and breast tenderness. What advice can the nurse give this woman to ease these symptoms? What additional education related to her pregnancy would be appropriate at this time?

imately 60 to 70 days after fertilization; they then decrease to a plateau at 100 to 130 days of pregnancy (Likes & Rittenhouse, 2007).

▶ *Take* NOTE!

This elevation of hCG corresponds to the morning sickness period of approximately 6 to 12 weeks during early pregnancy.

Objective (Probable) Signs

Probable signs of pregnancy are those that are apparent on physical examination by a health care professional. Common probable signs of pregnancy include softening of the lower uterine segment or isthmus (Hegar's sign), softening of the cervix (Goodell's sign), and a bluish-purple coloration of the vaginal mucosa and cervix (Chadwick's sign). Other probable signs include changes in the shape and size of the uterus, abdominal enlargement, Braxton Hicks contractions, and **ballottement** (the examiner pushes against the woman's cervix during a pelvic examination and feels a rebound from the floating fetus).

Along with these physical signs, pregnancy tests are also considered a probable sign of pregnancy. Several pregnancy tests are available (Table 11.1). The tests vary in sensitivity, specificity, and accuracy and are influenced by the length of gestation, specimen concentration, presence of blood, and the presence of some drugs (Likes & Rittenhouse, 2007).

Human chorionic gonadotropin (hCG) is the earliest biochemical marker for pregnancy, and many pregnancy tests are based on the recognition of hCG or a beta subunit of hCG. hCG levels in normal pregnancy usually double every 48 to 72 hours until they peak approx-

Home pregnancy tests are available over the counter and have become quite popular since their introduction in 1975. These tests are very sensitive, cost-effective, and faster than traditional laboratory pregnancy tests. Enzyme-linked immunosorbent assay (ELISA) technology is the basis for most home pregnancy tests.

Although probable signs suggest pregnancy and are more reliable than presumptive signs, they still are not 100% reliable in confirming a pregnancy. For example, uterine tumors, polyps, infection, and pelvic congestion can cause changes to uterine shape, size, and consistency. And although pregnancy tests are used to establish the diagnosis of pregnancy when the physical signs are still inconclusive, they are not completely reliable, because conditions other than pregnancy (e.g., ovarian cancer, choriocarcinoma, hydatidiform mole) can also elevate hCG levels.

Positive Signs

Usually within 2 weeks after a missed period, enough subjective symptoms are present so that a woman can be reasonably sure she is pregnant. However, an experienced health care professional can confirm her suspicions by

TABLE 11.1 SELECTED PREGNANCY TESTS

Type	Specimen	Example	Remarks
Agglutination inhibition tests	Urine	Pregnosticon, Gravindex	If hCG is present in urine, agglutination does not occur, which is positive for pregnancy; reliable 14–21 days after conception; 95% accurate in diagnosing pregnancy
Immunoradiometric assay	Blood serum	Neocept, Pregnosis	Measures ability of blood sample to inhibit the binding of radiolabeled hCG to receptors; reliable 6–8 days after conception; 99% accurate in diagnosing pregnancy
Enzyme-linked immunosorbent assay (ELISA)	Blood serum or urine	Over-the-counter home/office pregnancy tests; precise	Uses an enzyme to bond with hCG in the urine if present; reliable 4 days after implantation; 99% accurate if hCG specific

Sources: Hackley, Kriebs, & Rousseau, 2007; Likes & Rittenhouse, 2007.

identifying positive signs of pregnancy. The positive signs of pregnancy confirm that a fetus is growing in the uterus. Visualizing the fetus by ultrasound, palpating for fetal movements, and hearing a fetal heartbeat are all signs that make the pregnancy a certainty.

Once pregnancy is confirmed, the health care professional will set up a schedule of prenatal visits to assess the woman and her fetus throughout the entire pregnancy. Assessment and education begins at the first visits and continues throughout the pregnancy (see Chapter 12).

Remember Marva, who thought she had a stomach virus? Her pregnancy test was positive. On questioning by the nurse, she acknowledged missing two menstrual periods and being sexually active with her boyfriend without using protection. What is the nurse's role at this point with Marva? What instructions might be given to her while she waits for her first prenatal visit?

Physiologic Adaptations During Pregnancy

Every system of a woman's body changes during pregnancy to accommodate the needs of the growing fetus, and with startling rapidity. The physical changes of pregnancy can be uncomfortable, although every woman reacts uniquely.

Reproductive System Adaptations

Significant changes occur throughout the woman's body during pregnancy to accommodate the growing human being within her. Many have a protective role for maternal homeostasis and are essential to meet the demands of both the mother and the fetus. Many adaptations are reversible after the woman gives birth, but some persist for life.

Uterus

During the first few months of pregnancy, estrogen stimulates uterine growth, and the uterus undergoing a tremendous increase in size, weight, length, width, depth, volume, and overall capacity throughout pregnancy. The weight of the uterus increases from 70 g to about 1100 g at term; its capacity increases from 10 mL to 5000 mL or more at term (Levano, Cunningham, Alexander, et al., 2007). The uterine walls thin to 1.5 cm or less; from a solid globe, the uterus becomes a hollow vessel.

Uterine growth occurs as a result of both hyperplasia and hypertrophy of the myometrial cells, which do not increase much in number but do increase in size. Blood vessels elongate, enlarge, dilate, and sprout new branches to support and nourish the growing muscle tissue, and the increase in uterine weight is accompanied by a large increase in uterine blood flow necessary to perfuse the uterine muscle and accommodate the growing fetus (Frieden & Chan, 2007).

Uterine contractility is enhanced as well. Spontaneous, irregular, and painless contractions, called **Braxton Hicks contractions**, begin during the first trimester. These contractions continue throughout pregnancy, becoming especially noticeable during the last month, when they function to thin out or efface the cervix before birth (see Chapter 12 for more information).

Changes in the uterus occurring during the first 6 to 8 weeks of gestation produce some of the typical findings, including a positive **Hegar's sign**. This softening and compressibility of the lower uterine segment results in exaggerated uterine anteflexion during the early months of pregnancy, which adds to urinary frequency (Arenson & Drake, 2007).

The uterus remains in the pelvic cavity for the first 3 months of pregnancy, after which it progressively ascends into the abdomen (Fig. 11.1). As the uterus grows, it presses on the urinary bladder and causes the increased frequency of urination experienced during early pregnancy. In addition, the heavy gravid uterus in the last trimester can fall back against the inferior vena cava in the supine position, resulting in vena cava compression, which reduces venous return and decreases cardiac output and blood pressure, with increasing orthostatic stress. This occurs when the woman changes her position from recumbent to sitting to standing. This acute hemodynamic change, termed supine hypotensive syndrome, causes the woman

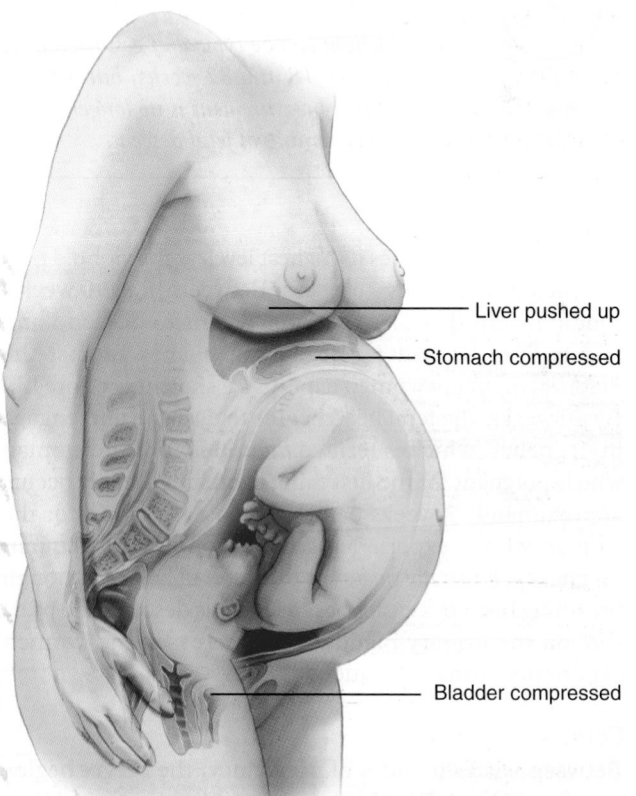

Liver pushed up
Stomach compressed
Bladder compressed

FIGURE 11.1 The growing uterus in the abdomen.

Supine position   Side-lying position

FIGURE 11.2 Supine hypotensive syndrome.

to experience symptoms of weakness, lightheadedness, nausea, dizziness, or syncope (Fig. 11.2). These changes are reversed when the woman is in the left lateral position, which displaces the uterus to the left and off the vena cava.

The uterus, which starts as a pear-shaped organ, becomes ovoid as length increases over width. By 20 weeks' gestation, the fundus, or top of the uterus, is at the level of the umbilicus and measures 20 cm. A monthly measurement of the height of the top of the uterus in centimeters, which corresponds to the number of gestational weeks, is commonly used to date the pregnancy.

▶ *Take* NOTE!

Fundal height can be typical of gestational weeks between 18 and 32 weeks, but after 36 weeks' gestation, this measurement is no longer reliable because of the beginning of fetal descent.

The fundus reaches its highest level, at the xiphoid process, at approximately 36 weeks. Between 38 to 40 weeks, fundal height drops as the fetus begins to descend and engage into the pelvis. Because it pushes against the diaphragm, many women experience shortness of breath. By 40 weeks, the fetal head begins to descend and engage in the pelvis, which is termed *lightening*. For the woman who is pregnant for the first time, lightening usually occurs approximately 2 weeks before the onset of labor; for the woman who is experiencing her second or subsequent pregnancy, it usually occurs at the onset of labor. Although breathing becomes easier because of this descent, the pressure on the urinary bladder now increases and women experience urinary frequency again.

Cervix

Between weeks 6 and 8 of pregnancy, the cervix begins to soften (**Goodell's sign**) due to vasocongestion. Along with the softening, the endocervical glands increase in size and number and produce more cervical mucus. Under the influence of progesterone, a thick mucus plug is formed that blocks the cervical os and protects the opening from bacterial invasion. At about the same time, increased vascularization of the cervix causes **Chadwick's sign**. Cervical ripening (softening, effacement, and increased distensibility) begins about 4 weeks before birth. Ripening is an inflammatory process and is not dependent on uterine contractions (Blackburn, 2007).

Vagina

During pregnancy, there is increased vascularity because of the influences of estrogen, resulting in pelvic congestion and hypertrophy of the vagina in preparation for the distention needed for birth. The vaginal mucosa thickens, the connective tissue begins to loosen, the smooth muscle begins to hypertrophy, and the vaginal vault begins to lengthen (Frieden & Chan, 2007).

Vaginal secretions become more acidic, white, and thick. Most women experience an increase in a whitish vaginal discharge, called leukorrhea, during pregnancy. This is normal except when it is accompanied by itching and irritation, possibly suggesting *Candida albicans*, a monilial vaginitis, which is a very common occurrence in this glycogen-rich environment (Mashburn, 2006). Monilial vaginitis is a benign fungal condition that is uncomfortable for the woman, but it can be transmitted from an infected mother to her newborn at birth. Neonates develop an oral infection known as thrush, which presents as white patches on the mucous membranes of their mouths. It is self-limiting and is treated with local antifungal agents.

Ovaries

The increased blood supply to the ovaries causes them to enlarge until approximately the 12th to 14th week of gestation. The ovaries are not palpable after that time because the uterus fills the pelvic cavity. Ovulation ceases during pregnancy because of the elevated levels of estrogen and progesterone, which block secretion of follicle-stimulating hormone (FSH) and luteinizing hormone (LH) from the anterior pituitary. The ovaries are very active in hormone production to support the pregnancy until about weeks 6 to 7, when the corpus luteum regresses and the placenta takes over the major production of progesterone.

Breasts

The breasts increase in fullness, become tender, and grow larger throughout pregnancy under the influence of estrogen and progesterone. The breasts become highly vascular, and veins become visible under the skin. The nipples become larger and more erect. Both the nipples and the areola become deeply pigmented, and tubercles of Montgomery (sebaceous glands) become prominent. These sebaceous glands keep the nipples lubricated for breastfeeding.

Changes that occur in the connective tissue of the breasts, along with the tremendous growth, lead to striae (stretch marks) in approximately half of all pregnant women (Graham, 2007). Initially they appear as pink to purple lines on the skin, but they eventually fade to a silver color. Although they become less conspicuous in time, they never completely disappear.

Creamy, yellowish breast fluid called colostrum can be expressed by the third trimester. This fluid provides nourishment for the breastfeeding newborn during the first few days of life (see Chapters 15 and 16 for more information).

Table 11.2 summarizes reproductive system adaptations.

General Body System Adaptations

In addition to changes in the reproductive system, the pregnant woman also experiences changes in virtually every other body system in response to the growing fetus.

Gastrointestinal System

The gastrointestinal (GI) system begins in the oral cavity and ends at the rectum. During pregnancy, the gums become hyperemic, swollen, and friable and tend to bleed easily. This change is influenced by estrogen and increased proliferation of blood vessels and circulation to the mouth. In addition, the saliva produced in the mouth becomes more acidic. Some women complain about excessive salivation, termed ptyalism, which may be caused by the decrease in unconscious swallowing by the woman when nauseated (Cunningham et al., 2005). Dental plaque,

calculus, and debris deposits increase during pregnancy and are all associated with gingivitis. Recent studies have linked periodontal disease with preterm birth and low-birthweight risk (Pretorius, Jagatt, & Lamont, 2007).

Smooth muscle relaxation and decreased peristalsis occur related to the influence of progesterone. Elevated progesterone levels cause smooth muscle relaxation, which results in delayed gastric emptying and decreased peristalsis. Transition time of food throughout the GI tract may be so much slower that more water than normal is reabsorbed, leading to bloating and constipation. Constipation can also result from low-fiber food choices, reduced fluid intake, use of iron supplements, decreased activity level, and intestinal displacement secondary to a growing uterus. Constipation, increased venous pressure, and the pressure of the gravid uterus contribute to the formation of hemorrhoids.

The slowed gastric emptying combined with relaxation of the cardiac sphincter allows reflux, which causes heartburn. Acid indigestion or heartburn (pyrosis) seems to be a universal problem for pregnant women. It is caused by regurgitation of the stomach contents into the upper esophagus and may be associated with the generalized relaxation of the entire digestive system. Over-the-counter antacids will usually relieve the symptoms, but they should be taken with the health care provider's knowledge and only as directed.

The emptying time of the gallbladder is prolonged secondary to the smooth muscle relaxation from progesterone. Hypercholesterolemia can follow, increasing the risk of gallstone formation. Other risk factors for

TABLE 11.2 SUMMARY OF REPRODUCTIVE SYSTEM ADAPTATIONS

Reproductive Organ	Adaptations
Uterus	Size increases 20 times that of nonpregnant size. Capacity increases by 2,000 times to accommodate the developing fetus. Weight increases from 2 oz to approximately 2 lb at term. Uterine growth occurs as a result of both hyperplasia and hypertrophy of the myometrial cells. Increased strength and elasticity allow uterus to contract and expel fetus during birth.
Cervix	Increases in mass, water content, and vascularization Changes from a relatively rigid to a soft, distensible structure that allows the fetus to be expelled Under the influence of progesterone, a thick mucus plug is formed, which blocks the cervical os and protects the developing fetus from bacterial invasion.
Vagina	Increased vascularity because of estrogen influences, resulting in pelvic congestion and hypertrophy Increased thickness of mucosa, along with an increase in vaginal secretions to prevent bacterial infections
Ovaries	Increased blood supply to the ovaries causes them to enlarge until approximately the 12th to 14th week of gestation, when the placenta takes over their function. Ovulation ceases during pregnancy because of the elevated levels of estrogen and progesterone.
Breasts	Breast changes begin soon after conception; they increase in size and areolar pigmentation. The tubercles of Montgomery enlarge and become more prominent, and the nipples more erect. The blood vessels become more prominent, and blood flow to the breast doubles.

gallbladder disease include obesity, Hispanic ethnicity, and increasing maternal age (Ko, 2006).

Nausea and vomiting, better known as morning sickness, plagues about 50% to 80% of pregnant women (Lane, 2007). Although it occurs most often in the morning, the nauseated feeling can last all day in some women. The highest incidence of morning sickness is between 6 and 12 weeks. The physiologic basis for morning sickness is still debatable. It has been linked to the high levels of hCG, high levels of circulating estrogens, reduced stomach acidity, and the lowered tone and motility of the digestive tract (Lane, 2007).

Cardiovascular System

Cardiovascular changes occur early during pregnancy to meet the demands of the enlarging uterus and the placenta for more blood and more oxygen. Perhaps the most striking cardiac alteration occurring during pregnancy is the increase in blood volume.

Blood Volume

Blood volume increases by approximately 1,500 mL, or 50% above nonpregnant levels (Cunningham et al., 2005). The increase is made up of 1,000 mL plasma plus 450 mL red blood cells (RBCs). It begins at weeks 10 to 12, peaks at weeks 32 to 34, and decreases slightly at week 40.

▶ *Take* NOTE!

The rise in blood volume correlates directly with fetal weight.

This increase in blood volume is needed to provide adequate hydration of fetal and maternal tissues, to supply blood flow to perfuse the enlarging uterus, and to provide a reserve to compensate for blood loss at birth and during postpartum (Martin & Foley, 2006). This increase is also necessary to meet the increased metabolic needs of the mother and to meet the need for increased perfusion of other organs, especially the woman's kidneys, because she is excreting waste products for herself and the fetus.

Cardiac Output and Heart Rate

Cardiac output is the product of stroke volume and heart rate. It increases from 30% to 50% over the nonpregnant rate by the 32nd week of pregnancy and declines to about a 20% increase at 40 weeks' gestation. The increase in cardiac output is associated with an increase in venous return and greater right ventricular output, especially in the left lateral position (Blackburn, 2007). Heart rate increases by 10 to 15 bpm between 14 and 20 weeks of gestation, and this persists to term. There is slight hypertrophy or enlargement of the heart during pregnancy. This is probably to accommodate the increase in blood volume

and cardiac output. The heart works harder and pumps more blood to supply the oxygen needs of the fetus as well as those of the mother. Both heart rate and venous return are increased in pregnancy, contributing to the increase in cardiac output seen throughout gestation. A woman with preexisting heart disease may become symptomatic and begin to decompensate during the time the blood volume peaks. Close monitoring is warranted during 28 to 35 weeks' gestation.

Blood Pressure

Blood pressure, especially the diastolic pressure, declines slightly during pregnancy as a result of peripheral vasodilation caused by progesterone. It reaches a low point at midpregnancy and thereafter increases to prepregnant levels until term (Blackburn, 2007). During the first trimester, blood pressure typically remains at the prepregnancy level. During the second trimester, the blood pressure decreases 5 to 10 mmHg and thereafter returns to first-trimester levels (Blackburn, 2007). Any significant rise in blood pressure during pregnancy should be investigated to rule out gestational hypertension.

Blood Components

The number of RBCs also increases throughout pregnancy to a level 25% to 33% higher than nonpregnant values, depending on the amount of iron available. This increase is necessary to transport the additional oxygen required during pregnancy. Although there is an increase in RBCs, there is a greater increase in the plasma volume as a result of hormonal factors and sodium and water retention. Because the plasma increase exceeds the increase of RBC production, normal hemoglobin and hematocrit values decrease. This state of hemodilution is referred to as **physiologic anemia of pregnancy**. Changes in RBC volume are due to increased circulating erythropoietin and accelerated RBC production. The rise in erythropoietin in the last two trimesters is stimulated by progesterone, prolactin, and human placental lactogen (Blackburn, 2007).

Iron requirements during pregnancy increase because of the demands of the growing fetus and the increase in maternal blood volume. The fetal tissues take predominance over the mother's tissues with respect to use of iron stores. With the accelerated production of RBCs, iron is necessary for hemoglobin formation, the oxygen-carrying component of RBCs.

▶ *Take* NOTE!

Many women enter pregnancy with insufficient iron stores and thus need supplementation to meet the extra demands of pregnancy.

Both fibrin and plasma fibrinogen levels increase, along with various blood-clotting factors. These factors make pregnancy a hypercoagulable state. These changes, coupled with venous stasis secondary to venous pooling, which occurs during late pregnancy after long periods of standing in the upright position with the pressure exerted by the uterus on the large pelvic veins, contribute to slowed venous return, pooling, and dependent edema. These factors also increase the woman's risk for venous thrombosis (Martin & Foley, 2006).

Respiratory System

The growing uterus and the increased production of the hormone progesterone cause the lungs to function differently during pregnancy. During the pregnancy, the amount of space available to house the lungs decreases as the uterus puts pressure on the diaphragm and causes it to shift upward by 4 cm above its usual position. The growing uterus does change the size and shape of the thoracic cavity, but diaphragmatic excursion increases, chest circumference increases by 2 to 3 in, and the transverse diameter increases by an inch, allowing a larger tidal volume, as evidenced by deeper breathing (Blackburn, 2007). Tidal volume or the volume of air inhaled increases gradually by 30 to 40% (from 500 to 700 mL) as the pregnancy progresses. As a result of these changes, the women's breathing becomes more diaphragmatic than abdominal (Torgersen & Curran, 2006).

A pregnant woman breathes faster and more deeply because she and the fetus need more oxygen. Oxygen consumption increases during pregnancy as airway resistance and lung compliance remain unchanged. Changes in the structures of the respiratory system take place to prepare the body for the enlarging uterus and increased lung volume (Alexander et al., 2007). As muscles and cartilage in the thoracic region relax, the chest broadens, with a conversion from abdominal breathing to thoracic breathing. This leads to a 50% increase in air volume per minute. All these structural alterations are temporary and revert back to their prepregnant state at the end of the pregnancy.

Increased vascularity of the respiratory tract is influenced by increased estrogen levels, leading to congestion. This congestion gives rise to nasal and sinus stuffiness, epistaxis (nosebleed), and changes in the tone and quality of the woman's voice (Martin & Foley, 2006).

Renal/Urinary System

The renal system must handle the effects of increased maternal intravascular and extracellular volume and metabolic waste products as well as excretion of fetal wastes. The predominant structural change in the renal system during pregnancy is dilation of the renal pelvis and uterus. Changes in renal structure occur from hormonal influences of estrogen and progesterone, pressure from an enlarging uterus, and an increase in maternal blood volume.

Like the heart, the kidneys work harder throughout the pregnancy. Changes in kidney function occur to accommodate a heavier workload while maintaining a stable electrolyte balance and blood pressure. As more blood flows to the kidneys, the glomerular filtration rate (GFR) increases, leading to an increase in urine flow and volume, substances delivered to the kidneys, and filtration and excretion of water and solutes (Jeyabalan & Lain, 2007).

Anatomically, the kidneys enlarge during pregnancy. Each kidney increases in length and weight as a result of hormonal effects that cause increased tone and decreased motility of the smooth muscle. The renal pelvis becomes dilated. The ureters (especially the right ureter) elongate, widen, and become more curved above the pelvic rim as early as the 10th gestational week (Jeyabalan & Lain, 2007). Progesterone is thought to cause both these changes because of its relaxing influence on smooth muscle.

Blood flow to the kidneys increases by 50% to 80% as a result of the increase in cardiac output. This in turn leads to an increase in the GFR by as much as 40% to 60% starting during the second trimester. This elevation continues until birth (Blackburn, 2007).

The activity of the kidneys normally increases when a person lies down and decreases on standing. This difference is amplified during pregnancy, which is one reason a pregnant woman feels the need to urinate frequently while trying to sleep. Late in the pregnancy, the increase in kidney activity is even greater when the woman lies on her side rather than her back. Lying on the side relieves the pressure that the enlarged uterus puts on the vena cava carrying blood from the legs. Subsequently, venous return to the heart increases, leading to increased cardiac output. Increased cardiac output results in increased renal perfusion and glomerular filtration (Fitzgerald & Graziano, 2007).

Musculoskeletal System

Changes in the musculoskeletal system are progressive, resulting from the influence of hormones, fetal growth, and maternal weight gain. Pregnancy is characterized by changes in posture and gait. By the 10th to 12th week of pregnancy, the ligaments that hold the sacroiliac joints and the pubis symphysis in place begin to soften and stretch, and the articulations between the joints widen and become more movable (Frieden & Chan, 2007). The relaxation of the joints peaks by the beginning of the third trimester. The purpose of these changes is to increase the size of the pelvic cavity and to make delivery easier.

The postural changes of pregnancy—an increased swayback and an upper spine extension to compensate for the enlarging abdomen—coupled with the loosening of the sacroiliac joints may result in lower back pain. The woman's center of gravity shifts forward, requiring a realignment of the spinal curvatures. An increase in the normal lumbosacral curve (lordosis) occurs and a compensatory curvature in the cervicodorsal area develops

A. Early pregnancy

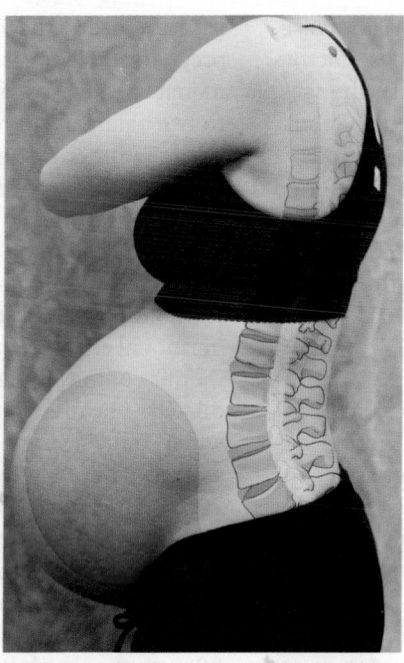

B. Late pregnancy

FIGURE 11.3 Postural changes during (**A**) the first trimester and (**B**) the third trimester.

to assist her in maintaining her balance (Fig. 11.3). In addition, relaxation and increased mobility of joints occur because of the hormones progesterone and relaxin, which lead to the characteristic "waddle gait" that pregnant women demonstrate toward term. Increased weight gain can add to this discomfort by accentuating the lumbar and dorsal curves (Torgersen & Curran, 2006).

Integumentary System

The skin of pregnant women undergoes hyperpigmentation primarily as a result of estrogen, progesterone, and melanocyte-stimulating hormone levels. These changes are mainly seen on the nipples, areola, umbilicus, perineum, and axilla. Although many integumentary changes disappear after giving birth, some only fade. Many pregnant women express concern about stretch marks, skin color changes, and hair loss. Unfortunately, little is known about how to avoid these changes.

Complexion changes are not unusual. The increased pigmentation that occurs on the breasts and genitalia also develops on the face to form the "mask of pregnancy," or facial melasma. It occurs in up to 70% of pregnant women. There is a genetic predisposition toward melasma, which is exacerbated by the sun; it tends to recur in subsequent pregnancies. This blotchy, brownish pigment covers the forehead and cheeks in dark-haired women. Most fade as the hormones subside at the end of the pregnancy, but some may linger. The skin in the middle of the abdomen may develop a pigmented line called **linea nigra**, which extends from the umbilicus to the pubic area (Fig. 11.4).

Striae gravidarum, or stretch marks, are irregular reddish streaks that appear on the abdomen, breasts, and buttocks in about half of pregnant women. Striae are

most prominent by 6 to 7 months. They result from reduced connective tissue strength resulting from the elevated adrenal steroid levels and stretching of the structures secondary to growth (Tunzi & Gray, 2007). They are more common in younger women, women with larger infants, and women with higher body mass indices. Nonwhites and women with a history of breast or thigh striae or a family history of striae gravidarum also are at higher risk (Osman et al., 2007).

FIGURE 11.4 Linea nigra.

Vascular changes during pregnancy manifested in the integumentary system include varicosities of the legs, vulva, and perineum. Varicose veins commonly are the result of distention, instability, and poor circulation secondary to prolonged standing or sitting and the heavy gravid uterus placing pressure on the pelvic veins, preventing complete venous return. Interventions to reduce the risk of developing varicosities include:

- Elevating both legs when sitting or lying down
- Avoiding prolonged standing or sitting; changing position frequently
- Resting in the left lateral position
- Walking daily for exercise
- Avoiding tight clothing or knee-high hosiery
- Wearing support hose if varicosities are a preexisting condition to pregnancy

Another skin manifestation, believed to be secondary to vascular changes and high estrogen levels, is the appearance of small blood vessels called vascular spiders. They may appear on the neck, thorax, face, and arms. They are especially obvious in white women and typically disappear after childbirth (Tunzi & Gray, 2007). Palmar erythema is a well-delineated pinkish area on the palmar surface of the hands. This integumentary change is also related to elevated estrogen levels (Tunzi & Gray, 2007).

Some women also notice a decline in hair growth during pregnancy. The hair follicles normally undergo a growing and resting phase. The resting phase is followed by a loss of hair; the hairs are then replaced by new ones. During pregnancy, fewer hair follicles go into the resting phase. After delivery, the body catches up with subsequent hair loss for several months. Nails typically grow faster during pregnancy. Pregnant women may experience increased brittleness and transverse grooves on the nails, but most of these conditions resolve in the postpartum period (Tunzi & Gray, 2007).

Endocrine System

The endocrine system undergoes many changes during pregnancy because hormonal changes are essential in meeting the needs of the growing fetus. Hormonal changes play a major role in controlling the supplies of maternal glucose, amino acids, and lipids to the fetus. Although estrogen and progesterone are the main hormones involved in pregnancy changes, other endocrine glands and hormones also change during pregnancy.

Thyroid Gland

The thyroid gland enlarges slightly and becomes more active during pregnancy as a result of increased vascularity and hyperplasia. Increased gland activity results in an increase in thyroid hormone secretion starting during the first trimester; levels taper off within a few weeks after birth and return to normal limits (Poppe, Velkeniers, & Glinoer, 2007). With an increase in the secretion of thyroid hormones, the basal metabolic rate (BMR; the amount of oxygen consumed by the body over a unit of time in milliliters per minute) progressively increases by 25%, along with heart rate and cardiac output (Blackburn, 2007).

Pituitary Gland

The pituitary gland, also known as the hypophysis, is a small, oval gland about the size of a pea that is connected to the hypothalamus by a stalk called the infundibulum. During pregnancy, the pituitary gland enlarges; it returns to normal size after birth.

The anterior lobe of the pituitary is glandular tissue and produces multiple hormones. The release of these hormones is regulated by releasing and inhibiting hormones produced by the hypothalamus. Some of these anterior pituitary hormones induce other glands to secrete their hormones. The increase in blood levels of the hormones produced by the final target glands (e.g., the ovary or thyroid) inhibits the release of anterior pituitary hormones. Changes in levels of pituitary hormones are discussed in the following paragraphs.

FSH and LH secretion are inhibited during pregnancy, probably as a result of hCG produced by the placenta and corpus luteum, and the increased secretion of prolactin by the anterior pituitary gland. Levels remain decreased until after delivery.

Thyroid-stimulating hormone (TSH) is reduced during the first trimester but usually returns to normal for the remainder of the pregnancy. Decreased TSH is thought to be one of the factors, along with elevated hCG levels, associated with morning sickness, nausea, and vomiting during the first trimester.

Growth hormone (GH) is an anabolic hormone that promotes protein synthesis. It stimulates most body cells to grow in size and divide, facilitating the use of fats for fuel and conserving glucose. During pregnancy, there is a decrease in the number of GH-producing cells and a corresponding decrease in GH blood levels. The action of human placental lactogen (hPL) is thought to decrease the need for and use of GH.

During pregnancy, prolactin is secreted in pulses and increases ten-fold to promote breast development and the lactation process. High levels of progesterone secreted by the placenta inhibit the direct influence of prolactin on the breast during pregnancy, thus suppressing lactation. At birth, as soon as the placenta is expelled and there is a drop in progesterone, lactogenesis can begin (Cunningham et al., 2005).

Melanocyte-stimulating hormone (MSH), another anterior pituitary hormone, increases during pregnancy. For many years, its increase was thought to be responsible for many of the skin changes of pregnancy, particularly changes in skin pigmentation (e.g., darkening of the areola, melasma, and linea nigra). However, currently it is thought that the skin changes are due to estrogen (and possibly progesterone) as well as the increase in MSH.

The two hormones oxytocin and antidiuretic hormone (ADH) released by the posterior pituitary are actually synthesized in the hypothalamus. They migrate along nerve fibers to the posterior pituitary and are stored until stimulated to be released into the general circulation.

Oxytocin is released by the posterior pituitary gland, and its production gradually increases as the fetus matures (Ochedalski et al., 2007). Oxytocin is responsible for uterine contractions, both before and after delivery. The muscle layers of the uterus (myometrium) become more sensitive to oxytocin near term. Toward the end of a term pregnancy, levels of progesterone decline and contractions that were previously suppressed by progesterone begin to occur more frequently and with stronger intensity. This change in the hormonal levels is believed to be one of the initiators of labor.

Oxytocin is responsible for stimulating the uterine contractions that bring about delivery. Contractions lead to cervical thinning and dilation. They also exert pressure, helping the fetus to descend in the pelvis for eventual delivery. After delivery, oxytocin secretion continues, causing the myometrium to contract and helping to constrict the uterine blood vessels, decreasing the amount of vaginal bleeding after delivery.

Oxytocin is also responsible for milk ejection during breastfeeding. Stimulation of the breasts through sucking or touching stimulates the secretion of oxytocin from the posterior pituitary gland. Oxytocin causes contraction of the myoepithelial cells in the lactating mammary gland. With breastfeeding, "after pains" often occur, which signals that oxytocin is being released.

Vasopressin (ADH) functions to inhibit or prevent the formation of urine via vasoconstriction, which results in increased blood pressure. Vasopressin also exhibits an antidiuretic effect and plays an important role in the regulation of water balance (Fitzgerald & Graziano, 2007).

Pancreas

The pancreas is an exocrine organ, supplying digestive enzymes and buffers, and an endocrine organ. The endocrine pancreas consists of the islets of Langerhans, which are groups of cells scattered throughout, each containing four cell types. One of the cell types is the beta cell, which produces insulin. Insulin lowers blood glucose by increasing the rate of glucose uptake and utilization by most body cells. The growing fetus needs significant amounts of glucose, amino acids, and lipids. Even during early pregnancy the fetus makes demands on the maternal glucose stores. Ideally, hormonal changes of pregnancy help meet fetal needs without putting the mother's metabolism out of balance.

A woman's insulin secretion works on a "supply-versus-demand" mode. As the demand to meet the needs of pregnancy increases, more insulin is secreted. Maternal insulin does not cross the placenta, so the fetus must produce his or her own supply to maintain glucose con-

---

BOX 11.2 Pregnancy, Insulin, and Glucose

- During early pregnancy, there is a decrease in maternal glucose levels because of the heavy fetal demand for glucose. The fetus is also drawing amino acids and lipids from the mother, decreasing the mother's ability to synthesize glucose. Maternal glucose is diverted across the placenta to assist the growing embryo/fetus during early pregnancy, and thus levels decline in the mother. As a result, maternal glucose concentrations decline to a level that would be considered "hypoglycemic" in a nonpregnant woman. During early pregnancy there is also a decrease in maternal insulin production and insulin levels.
- The pancreas is responsible for the production of insulin, which facilitates entry of glucose into cells. Although glucose and other nutrients easily cross the placenta to the fetus, insulin does not. Therefore, the fetus must produce its own insulin to facilitate the entry of glucose into its own cells.
- After the first trimester, hPL from the placenta and steroids (cortisol) from the adrenal cortex act against insulin. hPL acts as an antagonist against maternal insulin, and thus more insulin must be secreted to counteract the increasing levels of hPL and cortisol during the last half of pregnancy.
- Prolactin, estrogen, and progesterone are also thought to oppose insulin. As a result, glucose is less likely to enter the mother's cells and is more likely to cross over the placenta to the fetus (Cunningham et al., 2005).

---

trol (Box 11.2 gives information about pregnancy, glucose, and insulin).

During the first half of pregnancy, much of the maternal glucose is diverted to the growing fetus, and thus the mother's glucose levels are low. hPL and other hormonal antagonists increase during the second half of pregnancy. Therefore, the mother must produce more insulin to overcome the resistance by these hormones.

If the mother has normal beta cells of the islets of Langerhans, there is usually no problem meeting the demands for extra insulin. However, if the woman has inadequate numbers of beta cells, she may be unable to produce enough insulin and will develop glucose intolerance during pregnancy. If the woman has glucose intolerance, she is not able to meet the increasing demands and her blood glucose level increases.

Adrenal Glands

Pregnancy does not cause much change in the size of the adrenal glands themselves, but there are changes in some secretions and activity. One of the key changes is the marked increase in cortisol secretion, which regulates carbohydrate and protein metabolism and is helpful in times of stress. Although pregnancy is considered a normal condition, it is a time of stress for a woman's body. Cortisol increases in response to increased estrogen levels throughout pregnancy and returns to normal levels within 6 weeks postpartum (Blackburn, 2007).

During the stress of pregnancy, cortisol:

• Helps keep up the level of glucose in the plasma by breaking down noncarbohydrate sources, such as amino and fatty acids, to make glycogen. Glycogen, stored in the liver, is easily broken down to glucose when needed so that glucose is available in times of stress.
• Breaks down proteins to repair tissues and manufacture enzymes
• Has anti-insulin, anti-inflammatory, and antiallergic actions
• Is needed to make the precursors of adrenaline, which the adrenal medulla produces and secretes (Cunningham et al., 2005)

Aldosterone, also secreted by the adrenal glands, is increased during pregnancy. It normally regulates absorption of sodium from the distal tubules of the kidney. During pregnancy, progesterone allows salt to be "wasted" (or lost) in the urine. Aldosterone is produced in increased amounts by the adrenal glands as early as 15 weeks of pregnancy (Jeyabalan & Lain, 2007).

Prostaglandin Secretion During Pregnancy

Prostaglandins are not protein or steroid hormones; they are chemical mediators, or "local" hormones. Although hormones circulate in the blood to influence distant tissues, prostaglandins act locally on adjacent cells. The fetal membranes of the amniotic sac—the amnion and chorion—are both believed to be involved in the production of prostaglandins. Various maternal and fetal tissues, as well as the amniotic fluid itself, are considered to be sources of prostaglandins, but details about their composition and sources are limited. It is widely believed that prostaglandins play a part in softening the cervix and initiating and/or maintaining labor, but the exact mechanism is unclear.

Placental Secretion

The placenta has a feature possessed by no other endocrine organ—the ability to form protein and steroid hormones. Very early during pregnancy, the placenta begins to produce the following hormones:

• hCG
• hPL
• Relaxin
• Progesterone
• Estrogen

Table 11.3 summarizes the role of these hormones.

Immune System

The immune system is made up of organs and specialized cells whose primary purpose is to defend the body from foreign substances (antigens) that may cause tissue injury or disease. The mechanisms of innate and adaptive immunity work cooperatively to prevent, control, and eradicate foreign antigens in the body.

A general enhancement of innate immunity (inflammatory response and phagocytosis) and suppression of adaptive immunity (protective response to a specific foreign antigen) takes place during pregnancy. These immunologic alterations help prevent the mother's immune system from rejecting the fetus (foreign body), increase her risk of developing certain infections such as urinary tract infections, and influence the course of chronic disorders such as autoimmune diseases. Some chronic conditions worsen (diabetes) while others seem to stabilize (asthma) during pregnancy, but this is individualized and not predictable. In general, immune function in pregnant women is similar to immune function in nonpregnant women.

Marva returns for her first prenatal appointment and tells the nurse that her whole body is "out of sorts." She is overwhelmed and feels poorly. Outline the bodily changes Marva can expect each trimester to help her understand the adaptations taking place. What guidance can the nurse give Marva to help her understand the changes of pregnancy?

Table 11.4 summarizes the general body systems adaptations to pregnancy.

Changing Nutritional Needs of Pregnancy

Healthy eating during pregnancy enables optimal gestational weight gain and reduces complications, both of which are associated with positive birth outcomes. During pregnancy, maternal nutritional needs change to meet the demands of the pregnancy. Healthy eating can help ensure that adequate nutrients are available for both mother and fetus.

Nutritional intake during pregnancy has a direct effect on fetal well-being and birth outcome. Inadequate nutritional intake, for example, is associated with preterm birth, low birthweight, and congenital anomalies. Excessive nutritional intake is connected with fetal macrosomia (>4,000 g), leading to a difficult birth, neonatal hypoglycemia, and continued obesity in the mother (Blackburn, 2007).

Since the requirements for so many nutrients increase during pregnancy, pregnant women should take a vitamin and mineral supplement daily. Prenatal vitamins are prescribed routinely as a safeguard against a less-than-optimal diet. In particular, iron and folic acid need to be supplemented because their increased requirements during pregnancy are usually too great to be met through diet alone

TABLE 11.3 PLACENTAL HORMONES

Hormone	Description
hCG	• Responsible for maintaining the maternal corpus luteum, which secretes progesterone and estrogens, with synthesis occurring before implantation • Production by fetal trophoblast cells until the placenta is developed sufficiently to take over that function • Basis for early pregnancy tests because it appears in the maternal bloodstream soon after implantation • Production peaks at 8 weeks and then gradually declines.
hPL (also known as human chorionic somatomammotropin [hCS])	• Preparation of mammary glands for lactation and involved in the process of making glucose available for fetal growth by altering maternal carbohydrate, fat, and protein metabolism • Antagonist of insulin because it decreases tissue sensitivity or alters the ability to use insulin • Increase in the amount of circulating free fatty acids for maternal metabolic needs and decrease in maternal metabolism of glucose to facilitate fetal growth
Relaxin	• Secretion by the placenta as well as the corpus luteum during pregnancy • Thought to act synergistically with progesterone to maintain pregnancy • Increase in flexibility of the pubic symphysis, permitting the pelvis to expand during delivery • Dilation of the cervix, making it easier for the fetus to enter the vaginal canal; thought to suppress the release of oxytocin by the hypothalamus, thus delaying the onset of labor contractions (Blackburn, 2007)
Progesterone	• Often called the "hormone of pregnancy" because of the critical role it plays in supporting the endometrium of the uterus • Supports the endometrium to provide an environment conducive to fetal survival • Produced by the corpus luteum during the first few weeks of pregnancy and then by the placenta until term • Initially, causes thickening of the uterine lining in anticipation of implantation of the fertilized ovum. From then on, it maintains the endometrium, inhibits uterine contractility, and assists in the development of the breasts for lactation (Graham, 2007).
Estrogen	• Promotes enlargement of the genitals, uterus, and breasts, and increases vascularity, causing vasodilatation. • Relaxation of pelvic ligaments and joints (Blackburn, 2007) • Associated with hyperpigmentation, vascular changes in the skin, increased activity of the salivary glands, and hyperemia of the gums and nasal mucous membranes (Tunzi & Gray, 2007) • Aids in developing the ductal system of the breasts in preparation for lactation (Graham, 2007)

(Blackburn, 2007). Iron and folic acid are needed to form new blood cells for the expanded maternal blood volume and to prevent anemia. Folic acid is essential before pregnancy and in the early weeks of pregnancy to prevent neural tube defects in the fetus. For most pregnant women, supplements of 30 mg of ferrous iron and 600 mcg of folic acid per day are recommended by the **dietary reference intakes (DRIs)** (Institute of Medicine [IOM], 2006a, 2006b, 2006c, 2006d, 2006e, 2006f). Women with a previous history of a fetus with a neural tube defect are often prescribed a higher dose.

There is an abundance of conflicting advice about nutrition during pregnancy and what is good or bad to eat. Overall, the following guidelines are helpful:

• Increase your consumption of fruits and vegetables.
• Replace saturated fats with unsaturated ones.
• Avoid hydrogenated or partially hydrogenated fats.

• Use reduced-fat spreads and dairy products instead of full-fat ones.
• Eat at least two servings of fish weekly, with one of them being an oily fish.
• Consume at least 2 quarts of water daily (Arenson & Drake, 2007).

In the months before conception, food choices are key. The foods and vitamins consumed can ensure that the woman and her fetus will have the nutrients that are essential for the very start of pregnancy.

While most women recognize the importance of healthy eating during pregnancy, some find it challenging to achieve. Many women say they have little time and energy to devote to meal planning and preparation. Another barrier to healthy eating is conflicting messages from various sources, resulting in a lack of clear, reliable, and relevant information. Moreover, many women

TABLE 11.4 SUMMARY OF GENERAL BODY SYSTEM ADAPTATIONS

System	Adaptation
Gastrointestinal system	*Mouth and pharynx:* Gums become hyperemic, swollen, and friable and tend to bleed easily. Saliva production increases. *Esophagus:* Decreased lower esophageal sphincter pressure and tone, which increases the risk of developing heartburn *Stomach:* Decreased tone and mobility with delayed gastric emptying time, which increases the risk of gastroesophageal reflux and vomiting. Decreased gastric acidity and histamine output, which improves symptoms of peptic ulcer disease. *Intestines:* Decreased intestinal tone motility with increased transit time, which increases risk of constipation and flatulence *Gallbladder:* Decreased tone and motility, which may increase risk of gallstone formation
Cardiovascular system	*Blood volume:* Marked increase in plasma (50%) and RBCs (25% to 33%) compared to nonpregnant values. Causes hemodilution, which is reflected in a lower hematocrit and hemoglobin. *Cardiac output and heart rate:* CO increases from 30% to 50% over the nonpregnant rate by the 32nd week of pregnancy. The increase in CO is associated with an increase in venous return and greater right ventricular output, especially in the left lateral position. Heart rate increases by 10 to 15 bpm between 14 and 20 weeks of gestation, and this increase persists to term. *Blood pressure:* Diastolic pressure decreases typically 10 to 15 mmHg to reach its lowest point by mid-pregnancy; it then gradually returns to nonpregnant baseline values by term. *Blood components:* The number of RBCs increases throughout pregnancy to a level 25% to 33% higher than nonpregnant values. Both fibrin and plasma fibrinogen levels increase, along with various blood-clotting factors. These factors make pregnancy a hypercoagulable state.
Respiratory system	Enlargement of the uterus shifts the diaphragm up to 4 cm above its usual position. As muscles and cartilage in the thoracic region relax, the chest broadens, with conversion from abdominal breathing to thoracic breathing. This leads to a 50% increase in air volume per minute. Tidal volume, or the volume of air inhaled, increases gradually by 30% to 40% (from 500 to 700 mL) as the pregnancy progresses.
Renal/Urinary system	The renal pelvis becomes dilated. The ureters (especially the right ureter) elongate, widen, and become more curved above the pelvic rim. Bladder tone decreases and bladder capacity doubles by term. GFR increases 40% to 60% during pregnancy. Blood flow to the kidneys increases by 50% to 80% as a result of the increase in cardiac output.
Musculoskeletal system	Distention of the abdomen with growth of the fetus tilts the pelvis forward, shifting the center of gravity. The woman compensates by developing an increased curvature (lordosis) of the spine. Relaxation and increased mobility of joints occur because of the hormones progesterone and relaxin, which lead to the characteristic "waddle gait" that pregnant women demonstrate toward term.
Integumentary system	Hyperpigmentation of the skin is the most common alteration during pregnancy. The most common areas include the areola, genital skin, axilla, inner aspects of the thighs, and linea nigra. Striae gravidarum, or stretch marks, are irregular reddish streaks that may appear on the abdomen, breasts, and buttocks in about half of pregnant women. The skin in the middle of the abdomen may develop a pigmented line called linea nigra, which extends from the umbilicus to the pubic area. Melasma ("mask of pregnancy") occurs in 45% to 70% of pregnant women. It is characterized by irregular, blotchy areas of pigmentation on the face, most commonly on the cheeks, chin, and nose.
Endocrine system	Controls the integrity and duration of gestation by maintaining the corpus luteum via hCG secretion; production of estrogen, progesterone, hPL, and other hormones and growth factors via the placenta; release of oxytocin (by the posterior pituitary gland), prolactin (by the anterior pituitary), and relaxin (by the ovary, uterus, and placenta).
Immune system	A general enhancement of innate immunity (inflammatory response and phagocytosis) and suppression of adaptive immunity (protective response to a specific foreign antigen) takes place during pregnancy. These immunologic alterations help prevent the mother's immune system from rejecting the fetus (foreign body), increase her risk of developing certain infections, and influence the course of chronic disorders such as autoimmune diseases.

are eating less in an effort to control their weight, putting them at greater risk of inadequate nutrient intake.

Nutritional Requirements During Pregnancy

Pregnancy is one of the most nutritionally demanding periods of a woman's life. Gestation involves rapid cell division and organ development, and an adequate supply of nutrients is essential to support this tremendous fetal growth.

Most women are usually motivated to eat properly during pregnancy for the sake of the fetus. The Food and Nutrition Board of the National Research Council has made recommendations for nutrient intakes for people living in the United States. The DRIs are more comprehensive than previous nutrient guidelines issued by the board. They have replaced previous recommendations because they are not limited to preventing deficiency diseases; rather, the DRIs incorporate current concepts about the role of nutrients and food components in reducing the risk of chronic disease, developmental disorders, and other related problems. The DRIs can be used to plan and assess diets for healthy people (Dudek, 2006).

These dietary recommendations also include information for women who are pregnant or lactating, because growing fetal and maternal tissues require increased quan-

tities of essential dietary components. For example, the current DRIs suggest an increase in the pregnant woman's intake of protein from 60 to 80 g per day, iron from 18 to 27 g per day, and folate from 400 to 600 mcg per day, along with an increase of 300 calories per day over the recommended intake of 1,800 to 2,200 calories for nonpregnant women (IOM, 2006a, 2006b, 2006c, 2006d, 2006e, 2006f) (Table 11.5).

For a pregnant woman to meet recommended DRIs, it is important for her to eat according to the USDA's Food Guide Pyramid (Fig. 11.5). The 2005 Dietary Guidelines for Americans are the basis for federal nutrition policy. The Food Guide Pyramid provides guidance to help implement these guidelines. A summary of the new guidelines is as follows:

- Eat a variety of food from all food groups using portion control.
- Increase intake of vitamins, minerals, and dietary fiber.
- Lower intake of saturated fats, trans fats, and cholesterol.
- Consume adequate synthetic folic acid from supplements or from fortified foods.
- Increase intake of fruits, vegetables, and whole grains.
- Balance calorie intake with exercise to maintain ideal healthy weight (USDA, 2005).

An eating plan that follows the pyramid should provide sufficient nutrients for a healthy pregnancy. Except

TABLE 11.5 DIETARY RECOMMENDATIONS FOR THE PREGNANT AND LACTATING WOMAN

Nutrient	Nonpregnant Women	Pregnant Woman	Lactating Woman
Calories	2,200	2,500	2,700
Protein	60 g	80 g	80 g
Water/fluids	6–8 glasses daily	8 glasses daily	8 glasses daily
Vitamin A	700 mcg	770 mcg	1,300 mcg
Vitamin C	75 mg	85 mg	120 mg
Vitamin D	5 mcg	5 mcg	5 mcg
Vitamin E	15 mcg	15 mcg	19 mcg
B1 (thiamine)	1.1 mg	1.5 mg	1.5 mg
B2 (riboflavin)	1.1 mg	1.4 mg	1.6 mg
B3 (niacin)	14 mg	18 mg	17 mg
B6 (pyridoxine)	1.3 mg	1.9 mg	2 mg
B12 (cobalamin)	2.4 mcg	2.6 mcg	2.8 mcg
Folate	400 mcg	600 mcg	500 mcg
Calcium	1,000 mg	1,000 mg	1,000 mg
Phosphorus	700 mg	700 mg	700 mg
Iodine	150 mcg	220 mcg	290 mcg
Iron	18 mg	27 mg	9 mg
Magnesium	310 mg	350 mg	310 mg
Zinc	8 mg	11 mg	12 mg

Sources: Institute of Medicine, 2006a, 2006b, 2006c, 2006d, 2006e, 2006f.

MyPyramid Plan for Moms

Food Group	1st Trimester	2nd and 3rd Trimesters	What counts as 1 cup or 1 ounce?	Remember to...
	Eat this amount from each group daily.*			
Fruits	2 cups	2 cups	1 cup fruit or juice, ½ cup dried fruit	*Focus on fruits—* Eat a variety of fruit.
Vegetables	2½ cups	3 cups	1 cup raw or cooked vegetables or juice, 2 cups raw leafy vegetables	*Vary your veggies—* Eat more dark green and orange vegetables and cooked dry beans.
Grains	6 ounces	8 ounces	1 slice bread; ½ cup cooked pasta, rice, cereal; 1 ounce ready-to-eat cereal	*Make half your grains whole—* Choose whole instead of refined grains.
Meat and Beans	5½ ounces	6½ ounces	1 ounce lean meat, poultry, fish; 1 egg; ¼ cup cooked dry beans; ½ ounce nuts; 1 tablespoon peanut butter	*Go lean with protein—*Choose low-fat or lean meats and poultry.
Milk	3 cups	3 cups	1 cup milk, 8 ounces yogurt, 1½ ounces cheese, 2 ounces processed cheese	*Get your calcium-rich foods—*Go low-fat or fat-free when you choose milk, yogurt, and cheese.

*These amounts are for an average pregnant woman. You may need more or less than the average. Check with your doctor to make sure you are gaining weight as you should.

FIGURE 11.5 Food Guide Pyramid for pregnancy.

for iron, folic acid, and calcium, most of the nutrients a woman needs during pregnancy can be obtained by making healthy food choices. However, a vitamin and mineral supplement is generally prescribed.

> ▶ *Take* NOTE!
>
> *Good food sources of folic acid include dark green vegetables, such as broccoli, romaine lettuce, and spinach; baked beans; black-eyed peas; citrus fruits; peanuts; and liver.*

Fish and shellfish are an important part of a healthy diet because they contain high-quality protein, are low in saturated fat, and contain omega-3 fatty acids. However, nearly all fish and shellfish contain traces of mercury and some contain higher levels of mercury that may harm a developing fetus if ingested by pregnant women in large amounts. With this in mind, the FDA and the Environmental Protection Agency (EPA) are advising women who may become pregnant, pregnant women, and nursing mothers to do the following:

- Avoid eating shark, swordfish, king mackerel, and tilefish.
- Eat up to 12 ounces (two average meals) weekly of these fish:
  - Shrimp, canned light tuna, salmon
  - Pollock and catfish
- Check local advisories about the safety of fish caught by family and friends in local lakes, rivers, and coastal areas (Hibbeln et al., 2007)

EVIDENCE-BASED PRACTICE 11.1
Effects of Zinc Supplementation in Pregnancy on Maternal, Fetal, Neonatal, and Infant Outcomes

● **Study**

It has been suggested that low serum zinc levels may be associated with suboptimal outcomes of pregnancy such as prolonged labor, atonic postpartum hemorrhage, pregnancy-induced hypertension, preterm labor, and post-term pregnancies, although many of these associations have not yet been established.

Many women of childbearing age may have mild to moderate zinc deficiency. Low zinc levels may cause preterm birth or may prolong labor. It is also possible that zinc deficiency may affect infant growth.

A review of 17 trials, involving over 9,000 women and their babies, found that although zinc supplementation has a small effect on reducing preterm births, it does not help to prevent low-birthweight babies. Finding ways to improve women's overall nutritional status, particularly in low-income areas, will do more to improve the health of mothers and babies than giving pregnant women zinc supplements.

▲ **Findings**

The 14% relative reduction in preterm birth for zinc compared with placebo was primarily in the group of studies involving women of low income, and this has some relevance in areas of high perinatal mortality. There was no convincing evidence that zinc supplementation during pregnancy results in other important benefits. Since the preterm association could well reflect poor nutrition, studies to address ways of improving the overall nutritional status of populations in impoverished areas, rather than focusing on micronutrient and/or zinc supplementation in isolation, should be a priority.

■ **Nursing Implications**

Nurses can dispel any myths associated with the use of zinc as a preventive measure for preterm births, since research doesn't seem to validate this. Encouraging better nutrition, increasing water consumption, and taking rest periods throughout the day are all associated with longevity of pregnancy. At this point, the exact triggering mechanism for preterm labor is not known.

Mahomed, K., Bhutta, Z., & Middleton, P. (2007). Zinc supplementation for improving pregnancy and infant outcome. *Cochrane Database of Systematic Reviews,* Issue 2. Art. No.: CD000230. DOI: 10.1002/14651858.CD000230.pub3.

Maternal Weight Gain

The amount of weight that a woman gains during pregnancy is not as important as what she eats. A woman can lose extra weight after a pregnancy, but she can never make up for a poor nutritional status during the pregnancy. Currently, the American College of Obstetricians & Gynecologists (2005) recommends a 25- to 35-pound weight gain during pregnancy. Table 11.6 summarizes the distribution of weight gain during pregnancy.

The best way to assess whether a pregnant woman is consuming enough calories is to follow her pattern of weight gain. If she is gaining in a steady, gradual manner, then she is taking in enough calories. However, consuming an adequate amount of calories doesn't guarantee that her nutrients are sufficient. It is critical to evaluate both the quantity and the quality of the foods eaten.

The IOM has issued recommendations for weight gain during pregnancy based on prepregnancy body mass index (BMI; Box 11.3). A woman who is underweight before pregnancy or who has a low maternal weight gain pattern should be monitored carefully because she is at risk of giving birth to a low-birthweight infant (<2,500 g or 5.5 pounds). Frequently these women simply need advice on what to eat to add weight. Encourage the woman to eat snacks that are high in calories such as nuts, peanut butter, milkshakes, cheese, fruit, yogurt, and ice cream. Any woman who has a prepregnancy BMI of less than 19.8 is considered to be high risk and should be referred to a nutritionist. These women are encouraged to gain 28 to 40 pounds during the pregnancy (IOM, 2006a).

Conversely, women who start a pregnancy while overweight (BMI >25 to 29) run the risk of having a high-

TABLE 11.6 **NORMAL DISTRIBUTION OF WEIGHT GAIN DURING PREGNANCY**

Component	Weight
Fetus	7.5–8.5 pounds
Blood	4 pounds
Uterus	2 pounds
Breasts	1 pound
Placenta and umbilical cord	1.5 pounds
Fat and protein stores	7.5 pounds
Tissue fluids	2.7 pounds
Amniotic fluid	1.8 pounds
Approximate total weight gain	29 pounds

Sources: ACOG, 2005; Blackburn, 2007; Dudek, 2006.

Body Mass Index

Body Mass Index (BMI) provides an accurate estimate of total body fat and is considered a good method to assess overweight and obesity in people. BMI is a weight-to-height ratio calculation that can be determined by dividing a woman's weight in kilograms by her height in meters squared. BMI can also be calculated by weight in pounds divided by the height in inches squared, multiplied by 704.5.

The Centers for Disease Control and Prevention (CDC) categorizes BMI as follows:
- Underweight: less than 18.5
- Healthy weight: 18.5 to 24.9
- Overweight: 25 to 29.9
- Obese: 30 or higher (CDC, 2007)

Use this example to calculate BMI:

Mary is 5-foot-5 tall and weighs 150 pounds.
1. Convert weight into kilograms 150 divided by 2.2 lb/kg = 68.18 kg.
2. Convert height into meters:
   a. 5-foot-5 = 65 inches times 2.54 cm/in = 165.1 cm
   b. 165.1 cm/100 cm = 1.65 m
3. Then square the height in meters: 1.65 times 1.65 = 2.72
4. Calculate BMI 68.18 divided by 2.72 = 25

---

birthweight infant, with resulting cephalopelvic disproportion and, potentially, a surgical birth. Dieting during pregnancy is never recommended, even for women who are obese. Severe restriction of caloric intake is associated with a decrease in birthweight. Because of the expansion of maternal blood volume and the development of fetal and placental tissues, some weight gain is essential for a healthy pregnancy. Women who gain more than the recommended weight during pregnancy and who fail to lose this weight 6 months after giving birth are at much higher risk of being obese nearly a decade later (ACOG, 2005). Women who are overweight when beginning a pregnancy should gain no more than 15 to 25 pounds during the pregnancy, depending on their nutritional status and degree of obesity (ACOG, 2005).

All pregnant women should aim for a steady rate of weight gain throughout pregnancy. During the first trimester, for women whose prepregnant weight is within the normal weight range, weight gain should be about 3.5 to 5 pounds. For underweight women, weight gain should be at least 5 pounds. For overweight women, weight gain should be about 2 pounds. Much of the weight gained during the first trimester is caused by growth of the uterus and expansion of the blood volume.

During the second and third trimesters, the following pattern is recommended. For women whose prepregnant weight is within the normal weight range, weight gain should be about 1 pound per week. For underweight women, weight gain should be slightly more than 1 pound per week. For overweight women, weight gain should be about two thirds of a pound per week (Blackburn, 2007).

Nutrition Promotion

Through education, nurses can play an important role in ensuring adequate nutrition for pregnant women. During the initial prenatal visit, health care providers conduct a thorough assessment of a woman's typical dietary practices and address any conditions that may cause inadequate nutrition, such as nausea and vomiting or lack of access to adequate food. Assess and reinforce dietary information at every prenatal visit to promote good nutrition. A normal pregnancy and a well-balanced diet generally provide most of the recommended nutrients except iron and folate, both of which must be supplemented in the form of prenatal vitamins.

The Food Guide Pyramid, developed in 1992 and revised in 2005 by the U.S. Department of Agriculture, is the typical tool used for nutritional education and is recognized by the general population as the gold standard for healthy eating patterns (Dudek, 2006). Use this well-known tool as a basis for dietary instruction and tailor it to meet each woman's individual needs (Teaching Guidelines 11.1).

Special Nutritional Considerations

Many factors play an important role in shaping a person's food habits, and these factors must be taken into account

TEACHING GUIDELINES 11.1

Teaching to Promote Optimal Nutrition During Pregnancy

- Follow the Food Guide Pyramid and select a variety of foods from each group.
- Gain weight in a gradual and steady manner as follows:
  a. Normal-weight woman—25 to 35 pounds
  b. Underweight woman—28 to 40 pounds
  c. Overweight woman—15 to 25 pounds
  d. Obese woman—15 pounds
- Take your prenatal vitamin/mineral supplementation daily.
- Avoid weight-reduction diets during pregnancy.
- Do not skip meals; eat three meals with one or two snacks daily.
- Limit the intake of sodas and caffeine-rich drinks.
- Avoid the use of diuretics during pregnancy.
- Do not restrict the use of salt unless instructed to do so by your health care provider.
- Engage in reasonable physical activity daily.

if nutritional counseling is to be realistic and appropriate. Nurses need to be aware of these factors to ensure individualized teaching and care.

Cultural Variations and Restrictions

Food is important to every cultural group. It is often part of celebrations and rituals. When working with women from various cultures, the nurse needs to adapt American nutritional guidelines to meet their nutritional needs within their cultural framework. Food choices and variations for different cultures might include the following:

- Bread, cereal, rice and pasta group:
  - Bolello
  - Couscous
  - Hau juan
  - Flaxseed
- Vegetable group:
  - Agave
  - Bok choy
  - Jicama
  - Okra
  - Water chestnuts
- Protein group:
  - Bean paste
  - Blood sausage
  - Legumes
  - Shellfish
- Fruit group:
  - Catabopy
  - Kumquats
  - Plantain
  - Yucca fruit
  - Zapate
- Milk and dairy:
  - Buttermilk
  - Buffalo milk
  - Soybean milk

Lactose Intolerance

The best source of calcium is milk and dairy products, but for women with lactose intolerance, adaptations are necessary. Women with lactose intolerance lack an enzyme (lactase) needed for the breakdown of lactose into its component simple sugars, glucose, and galactose. Without adequate lactase, lactose passes through the small intestine undigested and causes abdominal discomfort, gas, and diarrhea. Lactose intolerance is especially common among women of African, Asian, and Middle Eastern descent (Dudek, 2006).

Additional or substitute sources of calcium may be necessary. These may include peanuts, almonds, sunflower seeds, broccoli, salmon, kale, and molasses (Escott-Stump, 2007). In addition, encourage the woman to drink lactose-free dairy products or calcium-enriched orange juice or soy milk.

Vegetarians

Vegetarian diets are becoming increasing prevalent in the United States. People choose a vegetarian diet for various reasons, including environmental, animal rights, philosophical, religious, and health beliefs (Hughes & Brown, 2006). Vegetarians choose not to eat meat, chicken, and fish. Their diets consist mostly of plant-based foods, such as legumes, vegetables, whole grains, nuts, and seeds. Vegetarians fall into groups defined by the types of foods they eat. Lacto-ovo-vegetarians omit red meat, fish, and poultry but eat eggs, milk, and dairy products, in addition to plant-based foods. Lacto-vegetarians consume milk and dairy products along with plant-based foods; they omit eggs, meat, fish, and poultry. Vegans eliminate all foods from animals, including milk, eggs, and cheese, and eat only plant-based foods (Dudek, 2006).

The concern with any form of vegetarianism, especially during pregnancy, is that the diet may be inadequate in nutrients. Other risks of vegetarian eating patterns during pregnancy may include low gestational weight gain, iron-deficiency anemia, compromised protein utilization, and decreased mineral absorption (Dudek, 2006). A diet can become so restrictive that a woman is not gaining weight or is consistently not eating enough from one or more of the food groups. Generally, the more restrictive the diet, the greater the chance of nutrient deficiencies.

Well-balanced vegetarian diets that include dairy products provide adequate caloric and nutrient intake and do not require special supplementation; however, vegan diets do not include any meat, eggs, or dairy products. Pregnant vegetarians must pay special attention to their intake of protein, iron, calcium, and vitamin B12. Suggestions include:

- For protein: substitute soy foods, beans, lentils, nuts, grains, and seeds.
- For iron: eat a variety of meat alternatives, along with vitamin C-rich foods.
- For calcium: substitute soy, calcium-fortified orange juice, and tofu.
- For vitamin B12: eat fortified soy foods and a B12 supplement.

The woman may also take a multivitamin prenatal supplement (Hughes & Brown, 2006).

Pica

Many women experience unusual food cravings during their pregnancy. Having cravings during pregnancy is perfectly normal. Sometimes, however, women crave substances that have no nutritional value and can even be dangerous to themselves and their fetus. **Pica** is the compulsive ingestion of nonfood substances. Pica is derived from the Latin term for magpie, a bird that is known to consume a variety of nonfood substances. Unlike the bird, however, pregnant women who develop a pica habit typically have one or two specific cravings.

The exact cause of pica is not known. Many theories have been advanced to explain it, but none has been proven scientifically. The incidence of pica is difficult to determine, since it is underreported. It is more common in the United States among African-American women compared to other ethnicities, but the practice of pica is not limited to any one geographic area, race, creed, or culture. In the United States, pica is also common in women from rural areas and women with a family history of it (Mikkelsen, Andersen, & Olsen, 2007)

The three main substances consumed by women with pica are soil or clay (geophagia), ice (pagophagia), and laundry starch (amylophagia). Nutritional implications include:

- Soil: replaces nutritive sources and causes iron-deficiency anemia
- Clay: produces constipation; can contain toxic substances and cause parasitic infection
- Ice: can cause iron-deficiency anemia, tooth fractures, freezer burn injuries
- Laundry starch: replaces iron-rich foods, leads to iron deficiencies, and replaces protein metabolism, thus depriving the fetus of amino acids needed for proper development (Blackburn, 2007)

Clinical manifestations of anemia often precede the identification of pica because it is rarely addressed by the health care provider and the woman does not usually volunteer such information (Cunningham et al., 2005). Secrecy surrounding this habit makes research and diagnosis difficult because some women fail to view their behavior as anything unusual, harmful, or worth reporting. Because of the clinical implications, pica should be discussed with all pregnant women as a preventive measure. The topic can be part of a general discussion of cravings, and the nurse should stress the harmful effects outlined above.

Suspect pica when the woman exhibits anemia although her dietary intake is appropriate. Ask about her usual dietary intake, and include questions about the ingestion of nonfood substances. Consider the potential negative outcomes for the pregnant woman and her fetus, and take appropriate action.

Psychosocial Adaptations During Pregnancy

WATCH & LEARN

Pregnancy is a unique time in a woman's life. It is a time of dramatic alterations in her body and her appearance, as well as a time of change in her social status. All these changes occur simultaneously. Concurrent with the physiologic changes within her body systems are psychosocial changes within the mother and family members as they face significant role and lifestyle changes.

Maternal Emotional Responses

Motherhood, perhaps more than any role in society, has acquired a special significance for women. Women are taught they should find fulfillment and satisfaction in the role of the "ever-bountiful, ever-giving, self-sacrificing mother" (Thies & Travers, 2006). With such high expectations, many pregnant women experience various emotions throughout their pregnancy. The woman's approach to these emotions is influenced by her emotional makeup, her sociologic and cultural background, her acceptance or rejection of the pregnancy, whether the pregnancy was planned, if the father is known, and her support network (Alexander et al., 2007).

Despite the wide-ranging emotions associated with the pregnancy, many women experience similar responses. These responses commonly include ambivalence, introversion, acceptance, mood swings, and changes in body image.

Ambivalence

The realization of a pregnancy can lead to fluctuating responses, possibly at the opposite ends of the spectrum. For example, regardless of whether the pregnancy was planned, the woman may feel proud and excited at her achievement while at the same time fearful and anxious of the implications. The reactions are influenced by several factors, including the way the woman was raised, her current family situation, the quality of the relationship with the expectant father, and her hopes for the future. Some women express concern over the timing of the pregnancy, wishing that goals and life objectives had been met before becoming pregnant. Other women may question how a newborn or infant will affect their career or their relationships with friends and family. These feelings can cause conflict and confusion about the pregnancy.

Ambivalence, or having conflicting feelings at the same time, is a universal feeling and is considered normal when preparing for a lifestyle change and new role. Pregnant women commonly experience ambivalence during the first trimester. Usually ambivalence evolves into acceptance by the second trimester, when fetal movement is felt. The woman's personality, her ability to adapt to changing circumstances, and the reactions of her partner will affect her adjustment to being pregnant and her acceptance of impending motherhood.

Introversion

Introversion, or focusing on oneself, is common during the early part of pregnancy. The woman may withdraw and become increasingly preoccupied with herself and her fetus. As a result, her participation with the outside world may be less, and she will appear passive to her family and friends.

This introspective behavior is a normal psychological adaptation to motherhood for most women. Introversion seems to heighten during the first and third trimesters, when the woman's focus is on behaviors that will ensure a safe and health pregnancy outcome. Couples need to be aware of this behavior and should be informed about measures to maintain and support the focus on the family.

Acceptance

During the second trimester, the physical changes of the growing fetus with an enlarging abdomen and fetal movement bring reality and validity to the pregnancy. There are many tangible signs that someone separate from herself is present. The pregnant woman feels fetal movement and may hear the heartbeat. She may see the fetal image on an ultrasound screen and feel distinct parts, recognizing independent sleep and wake patterns. She becomes able to identify the fetus as a separate individual and accepts this.

Many women will verbalize positive feelings about the pregnancy and will conceptualize the fetus. The woman may accept her new body image and talk about the new life within. Generating a discussion about the woman's feelings and offering support and validation at prenatal visits are important.

Mood Swings

Emotional lability is characteristic throughout most pregnancies. One moment a woman can feel great joy, and within a short time she can feel shock and disbelief. Frequently, pregnant women will start to cry without any apparent cause. Some women feel as though they are riding an "emotional roller-coaster." These extremes in emotion can make it difficult for partners and family members to communicate with the pregnant woman without placing blame on themselves for their mood changes. Clear explanations about how common mood swings are during pregnancy are essential.

Change in Body Image

The way in which pregnancy affects a woman's body image varies greatly from person to person. Some women feel as if they have never been more beautiful, whereas others spend their pregnancy feeling overweight and uncomfortable. For some women pregnancy is a relief from worrying about weight, whereas for others it only exacerbates their fears of weight gain. Changes in body image are normal but can be very stressful for the pregnant woman. Offering a thorough explanation and initiating discussion of the expected bodily changes may help the family to cope with them.

Maternal Role Tasks

Reva Rubin (1984) identified maternal tasks that a woman must accomplish to incorporate the maternal role into her personality. Accomplishing these tasks helps the expectant mother to develop her self-concept as a mother and

---

BOX 11.4 **Maternal Role Tasks**

- **Ensuring safe passage throughout pregnancy and birth**
  - Primary focus of the woman's attention
  - First trimester: woman focuses on herself, not on the fetus
  - Second trimester: woman develops attachment of great value to her fetus
  - Third trimester: woman has concern for herself and her fetus as a unit
  - Participation in positive self-care activities related to diet, exercise, and overall well-being
- **Seeking acceptance of infant by others**
  - First trimester: acceptance of pregnancy by herself and others
  - Second trimester: family needs to relate to the fetus as member
  - Third trimester: unconditional acceptance without rejection
- **Seeking acceptance of self in maternal role to infant ("binding in")**
  - First trimester: mother accepts idea of pregnancy, but not of infant
  - Second trimester: with sensation of fetal movement (quickening), mother acknowledges fetus as a separate entity within her
  - Third trimester: mother longs to hold infant and becomes tired of being pregnant
- **Learning to give of oneself**
  - First trimester: identifies what must be given up to assume new role
  - Second trimester: identifies with infant, learns how to delay own desires
  - Third trimester: questions her ability to become a good mother to infant (Rubin, 1984)

---

to form a mutually gratifying relationship with her infant. These tasks are listed in Box 11.4.

Pregnancy and Sexuality

The way a pregnant woman feels and experiences her body during pregnancy can affect her sexuality. The woman's changing shape, emotional status, fetal activity, changes in breast size, pressure on the bladder, and other discomforts of pregnancy result in increased physical and emotional demands. These can produce stress on the sexual relationship between the pregnant woman and her partner. As the changes of pregnancy ensue, many partners become confused, anxious, and fearful of how the relationship may be affected.

Sexual desire of pregnant women may change throughout the pregnancy. During the first trimester, the woman may be less interested in sex because of fatigue, nausea, and fear of disturbing the early embryonic development. During the second trimester, her interest may increase because of the stability of the pregnancy. During the third trimester, her enlarging size may produce discomfort during sexual activity (Frieden & Chan, 2007).

A woman's sexual health is intimately linked to her own self-image. Sexual positions to increase comfort as the pregnancy progresses as well as alternative noncoital modes of sexual expression, such as cuddling, caressing, and holding, should be discussed. Giving permission to talk about and then normalizing sexuality can help enhance the sexual experience during pregnancy and, ultimately, the couple's relationship. If avenues of communication are open regarding sexuality during pregnancy, any fears and myths the couple may have can be dispelled.

Pregnancy and the Partner

Nursing care related to childbirth has expanded from a narrow emphasis on the physical health needs of the mother and infant to a broader focus on family-related, social and emotional needs. One prominent feature of this family-centered approach is the recent movement toward promoting the mother–infant bond. To achieve a truly family-centered practice, nursing must make a comparable commitment to understanding and meeting the needs of the partner in the emerging family. Recent studies suggest that the partner's potential contribution to the infant's overall development has been misperceived or devalued and that the partner's ability and willingness to assume a more active role in the infant's care may have been underestimated.

Reactions to pregnancy and to the psychological and physical changes by the woman's partner vary greatly. Some enjoy the role of being the nurturer, whereas others experience alienation and may seek comfort or companionship elsewhere. Some expectant fathers may view pregnancy as proof of their masculinity and assume the dominant role, whereas others see their role as minimal, leaving the pregnancy up to the woman entirely. Each expectant partner reacts uniquely.

Emotionally and psychologically, expectant partners may undergo less visible changes than women, but most of these changes remain unexpressed and unappreciated (Thies & Travers, 2006). Expectant partners also experience a multitude of adjustments and concerns. Physically, they may gain weight around the middle and experience nausea and other GI disturbances—what is termed couvade syndrome, a sympathetic response to their partner's pregnancy. They also experience ambivalence during early pregnancy, with extremes of emotions (e.g., pride and joy versus an overwhelming sense of impending responsibility).

During the second trimester of pregnancy, partners go through acceptance of their role of breadwinner, caretaker, and support person. They come to accept the reality of the fetus when movement is felt, and they experience confusion when dealing with the woman's mood swings and introspection. During the third trimester, the expectant partner prepares for the reality of this new role and negotiates what the role will be during the labor and birthing process. Many express concern about being the primary support person during labor and birth and worry how they will react when faced with their loved one in pain. Expectant partners share many of the same anxieties as their pregnant partners. However, it is uncommon for them to reveal these anxieties to the pregnant partner or health care professionals. Often, how the expectant partner responds during the third trimester depends on the state of the marriage or partnership. When the marriage or partnership is struggling, the impending increase in responsibility toward the end of pregnancy acts to drive the expectant partner further away. Often it manifests as working late, staying out late with friends, or beginning new or superficial relationships. In the stable marriage or partnership, the expectant partner who may have been struggling to find his or her place in the pregnancy now finds concrete tasks to do—for example, painting the nursery, assembling the car seat, attending Lamaze classes, and so on.

Pregnancy and Siblings

A sibling's reaction to pregnancy is age-dependent. Some children might express excitement and anticipation, whereas others might have negative reactions. A young toddler might regress in toilet training or ask to drink from a bottle again. An older school-aged child may ignore the new addition to the family and engage in outside activities to avoid the new member. The introduction of an infant into the family is often the beginning of sibling rivalry, which results from the child's fear of change in the security of the relationship with his or her parents (Thies & Travers, 2006). Preparation of the siblings for the anticipated birth is imperative and must be designed according to the age and life experiences of the sibling at home. Constant reinforcement of love and caring will help to reduce the older child's fear of change and worry about being replaced by the new family member.

If possible, parents should include siblings in preparation for the birth of the new baby to help them feel as if they have an important role to play (Fig. 11.6). Parents must also continue to focus on the older sibling after the birth to reduce regressive or aggressive behavior toward the newborn.

■■■ Key Concepts

- Pregnancy is a normal life event that involves considerable physical, psychosocial, emotional, and relationship adjustments.
- The signs and symptoms of pregnancy have been grouped into those that are subjective (presumptive)

FIGURE 11.6 Parents preparing sibling for the birth of a new baby.

and experienced by the woman herself, those that are objective (probable) and observed by the health care professional, and those that are the positive, beyond-the-shadow-of-a-doubt signs.

- Physiologically, almost every system of a woman's body changes during pregnancy with startling rapidity to accommodate the needs of the growing fetus. A majority of the changes are influenced by hormonal changes.

- The placenta is a unique kind of endocrine gland; it has a feature possessed by no other endocrine organ—the ability to form protein and steroid hormones.

- Occurring in conjunction with the physiologic changes in the woman's body systems are psychosocial changes occurring within the mother and family members as they face significant role and lifestyle changes.

- Commonly experienced emotional responses to pregnancy in the woman include ambivalence, introversion, acceptance, mood swings, and changes in body image.

- Reactions of expectant partners to pregnancy and to the physical and psychological changes in the woman vary greatly.

- A sibling's reaction to pregnancy is age dependent. The introduction of a new infant to the family is often the beginning of sibling rivalry, which results from the established child's fear of change in security of their relationships with their parents. Therefore, preparation of the siblings for the anticipated birth is imperative.

REFERENCES

Alexander, L. L., et al. (2007). *New dimensions in women's health* (4th ed.). Sudbury, MA: Jones and Bartlett Publishers.

American College of Obstetricians and Gynecologists (ACOG). (2005). Body mass index. Provider advice, and target gestational weight gain. *Obstetrics & Gynecology, 105*(3), 633–638.

Arenson, J., & Drake, P. (2007). *Maternal and newborn health.* Sudbury, MA: Jones and Bartlett Publishers.

Blackburn, S. T. (2007). *Maternal, fetal, and neonatal physiology: A clinical perspective* (3rd ed.). St. Louis, MO: Saunders Elsevier.

Centers for Disease Control and Prevention (CDC). (2007). BMI for adults: Body mass index calculator. Available at: http://www.cdc.gov/nccdphp/dnpa/bmi/calc-bmi.htm

Cunningham, F., et al. (2005). *William's obstetrics* (22nd ed.). New York: McGraw-Hill.

Dudek, S. G. (2006). *Nutrition essentials for nursing practice* (5th ed.). Philadelphia: Lippincott Williams & Wilkins.

Escott-Stump, S. (2007). *Nutrition and diagnosis-related care* (6th ed.). Philadelphia: Lippincott Williams & Wilkins.

Fitzgerald, M. P., & Graziano, S. (2007). Anatomic and functional changes in the lower urinary tract during pregnancy. *Urologic Clinics of North America, 34*(1), 7–12.

Frieden, F. J., & Chan, Y. (2007). Antepartum care. In R. E. Rakel & E. T. Bope (Eds.), *Conn's current therapy* (Section 16; pp. 1169–1175). Philadelphia: Saunders Elsevier.

Graham, H. (2007). Breast health and pregnancy. *British Journal of Midwifery, 15*(3), 137–140.

Hackley, B., Kriebs, J. M., & Rousseau, M. E. (2007). *Primary care of women: A guide for midwives and women's health providers.* Sudbury, MA: Jones and Bartlett Publishers.

Hibbeln, J. R., Davis, J. M., Steer, C., Emmett, P., Rogers, I., Williams, C., & Golding, J. (2007). Benefits may outweigh risks of maternal seafood consumption in pregnancy. *Lancet, 369*(9561), 578–585.

Hughes, J. V., & Brown, J. (2006). A meat-free pregnancy. *Vegetarian Times,* April (340), 23–25.

Institute of Medicine (IOM). (2006a). *Nutrition during pregnancy. Part I: Weight gain. Part II: Nutrient supplements.* National Academy of Sciences. Washington, DC: National Academy Press.

Institute of Medicine (IOM). (2006b). *Dietary reference intakes for calcium, phosphorus, magnesium, vitamin D and fluoride.* Washington, DC: National Academy Press.

Institute of Medicine (IOM). (2006c). *Dietary reference intakes for thiamine, riboflavin, niacin, vitamin B6, vitamin B 12, pantothenic acid, biotin, and choline.* Washington, DC: National Academy Press.

Institute of Medicine (IOM). (2006d). *Dietary reference intakes for vitamin C, vitamin E, selenium, and carotenoids.* Washington, DC: National Academy Press.

Institute of Medicine (IOM). (2006e). *Dietary reference intakes for vitamin A, vitamin K, arsenic, boron, chromium, copper, iodine, manganese, molybdenum, nickel, silicon, vanadium, and zinc.* Washington, DC: National Academy Press.

Institute of Medicine (IOM). (2006f). *Dietary reference intakes for energy, carbohydrates, fiber, protein and amino acids.* Washington, DC: National Academy Press.

Jeyabalan, A., & Lain, K. Y. (2007). Anatomic and functional changes in the upper urinary tract during pregnancy. *Urologic Clinics of North America, 34*(1), 1–6.

Ko, C. W. (2006). Risk factors for gallstone-related hospitalization during pregnancy and the postpartum. *American Journal of Gastroenterology, 101*(10), 2263–2268.

Lane, C. A. (2007). Nausea and vomiting in pregnancy: A tailored approach to treatment. *Clinical Obstetrics & Gynecology, 50*(1), 100–111.

Levano, K. J., Cunningham, F. G., Alexander, J. M., et al. (2007). *Williams' manual of obstetrics: Pregnancy complications* (22nd ed.). New York: McGraw-Hill.

Likes, R. L., & Rittenhouse, E. (2007). Pregnancy diagnosis. *eMedicine.* Available at: http://www.emedicine.com/med/topic3277.htm

Martin, S. R., & Foley, M. R. (2006). Intensive care in obstetrics: An evidence-based review. *American Journal of Obstetrics & Gynecology, 195*(3), 673–689.

Mashburn, J. (2006). Etiology, diagnosis, and management of vaginitis. *Journal of Midwifery & Women's Health, 51*(6), 423–430.

National Academy of Sciences. (2007). *Dietary reference intakes for energy, carbohydrates, fiber, fat, protein and amino acids (macronutrients).* Washington, DC: National Academies Press, pp. 5–64.

Ochedalski, T., Subburaju, S., Wynn, P. C., & Aguilera, G. (2007). Interaction between estrogen and oxytocin on hypothalamic-pituitary-adrenal axis activity. *Journal of Neuroendocrinology, 19*(3), 189–197.

Osman, H., Rubeiz, N., Tamim, H., & Nassar, A. H. (2007). Risk factors for the development of striae gravidarum. *American Journal of Obstetrics & Gynecology, 196*(1), 62–65.

Poppe, K., Velkeniers, B., & Glinoer, D. (2007). Thyroid disease and female reproduction. *Clinical Endocrinology, 66*(3), 309–321.

Pretorius, C., Jagatt, A., & Lamont, R. F. (2007). The relationship between periodontal disease, bacterial vaginosis, and preterm birth. *Journal of Perinatal Medicine, 35*(2), 93–99.

Rubin, R. (1984). *Maternal identity and the maternal experience.* New York: Springer.

Thies, K. M., & Travers, J. F. (2006). *Handbook of human development for health care professionals.* Sudbury, MA: Jones and Bartlett Publishers.

Torgersen, K. L., & Curran, C. A. (2006). A systematic approach to the physiologic adaptations of pregnancy. *Critical Care Nursing Quarterly, 29*(1), 2–19.

Tunzi, M., & Gray, G. R. (2007). Common skin conditions during pregnancy. *American Family Physician, 75*(2), 211–218.

United States Department of Agriculture (USDA). (2005). *Dietary guidelines for Americans 2005.* Center for Nutrition Policy and Promotion. Available: http://www.mypyramid.gov/

Walsh, D. (2007). *Evidence-based care for normal labor and birth: A guide for midwives.* London: Taylor & Francis, Inc.

WEBSITES

American College of Nurse Midwives: 202-347-5445, www.acnm.org

American College of Obstetricians and Gynecologists: www.acog.com

Association of Women's Health: Obstetrics & Neonatal Nurses: www.awhonn.org

Dietary Guidelines for Americans: http://www.nal.usda.gov/fnic/dga

International Childbirth Education Association: www.icea.org

March of Dimes: www.modimes.org

Mayo Clinic Pregnancy Center: www.mayoclinic.org

National Center for Education in Maternal and Child Health: www.ncemch.org

Nutrition during pregnancy and breastfeeding: www.nal.usda.gov/fnic/pubs/topics/pregnancy/precom.html

Vegan diet during pregnancy: www.vrg.org/nutrition/veganpregnancy.htm

Weight gain during pregnancy: www.marchofdimes.com/pnhec/159_153.asp

CHAPTER WORKSHEET

MULTIPLE CHOICE QUESTIONS

1. What factors would change during a pregnancy if the hormone progesterone were reduced or withdrawn?

   a. The woman's gums would become red and swollen and would bleed easily.

   b. The uterus would contract more and peristalsis would increase.

   c. Morning sickness would increase and would be prolonged.

   d. It would inhibit the secretion of prolactin by the pituitary gland.

2. Which of the following is a presumptive sign or symptom of pregnancy?

   a. Restlessness

   b. Elevated mood

   c. Urinary frequency

   d. Low backache

3. When obtaining a blood test for pregnancy, which hormone would the nurse expect the test to measure?

   a. hCG

   b. hPL

   c. FSH

   d. LH

4. During pregnancy, which of the following should the expectant mother reduce or avoid?

   a. Raw meat or uncooked shellfish

   b. Fresh, washed fruits and vegetables

   c. Whole grains

   d. Protein and iron from meat sources

5. A feeling expressed by most women upon learning they are pregnant is:

   a. Acceptance

   b. Depression

   c. Jealousy

   d. Ambivalence

6. Reva Rubin identified four major tasks that the pregnant woman undertakes to form a mutually gratifying relationship with her infant. What is "binding in"?

   a. Ensuring safe passage through pregnancy, labor, and birth

   b. Seeking acceptance of this infant by others

   c. Seeking acceptance of self as mother to the infant

   d. Learning to give of oneself on behalf of the infant

CRITICAL THINKING EXERCISES

1. When interviewing a woman at her first prenatal visit, the nurse asks about her feelings. The woman replies, "I'm frightened and confused. I don't know whether I want to be pregnant or not. Being pregnant means changing our whole life, and now having somebody to care for all the time. I'm not sure I would be a good mother. Plus I'm a bit afraid of all the changes that would happen to my body. Is this normal? Am I okay?"

   a. How should the nurse answer this question?

   b. What specific information is needed to support the client during this pregnancy?

2. Sally, age 23, is 9 weeks pregnant. At her clinic visit she says, "I'm so tired I can barely make it home from work. Then once I'm home, I don't have the energy to make dinner." She says she is so sick in the morning that she is frequently late to work and spends much of the day in the bathroom. Sally's current lab work is within normal limits.

   a. What explanation can the nurse offer Sally about her discomforts?

   b. What interventions can the nurse offer to Sally?

3. Bringing a new infant into the family affects the siblings. What strategies can a nurse discuss when a mother asks how to deal with this?

STUDY ACTIVITIES

1. Go to your local health department's maternity clinic and interview several women regarding their feelings and the bodily changes that have taken place since they became pregnant. Based on your findings, place them into appropriate trimesters of their pregnancy.

2. Search the Internet for information about the psychological changes that occur during pregnancy. Share your websites with your clinical group.

3. During pregnancy, the plasma volume increases by 50% but the RBC volume increases by only 25% to 33%. This disproportion is manifested as

   _____.

4. When a pregnant woman in her third trimester lies on her back and experiences dizziness and lightheadedness, the underlying cause of this is

   _____.

CHAPTER 12

NURSING MANAGEMENT DURING PREGNANCY

KEY TERMS

alpha–fetoprotein
amniocentesis
biophysical profile
chorionic villus
   sampling (CVS)

gravida
high–risk pregnancy
linea nigra
natural childbirth

para
perinatal education
preconception care

LEARNING OBJECTIVES

Upon completion of the chapter, the learner will be able to:

1. Define the key terms used in this chapter.
2. Identify the information typically collected at the initial prenatal visit.
3. Explain the assessments completed at follow-up prenatal visits.
4. Describe the tests used to assess maternal and fetal well-being, including nursing management for each.
5. Outline appropriate nursing management to promote maternal self-care and to minimize the common discomforts of pregnancy.
6. List the key components of perinatal education.

Linda and her husband, Rob, are eager to start a family within the next year. They are stable in their careers and financially secure. They decide to check out a new nurse-midwife practice associated with the local hospital, and they go for a preconception appointment. They leave their appointment overwhelmed with all the information they were given about having a healthy pregnancy.

Wow

The secret of human touch is simple: showing a sincere liking and interest in people. Nurses need to use touch often.

Pregnancy is a time of many physiologic and psychological changes that can positively or negatively affect the woman, her fetus, and her family. Misconceptions, inadequate information, and unanswered questions about pregnancy, birth, and parenthood are common. The ultimate goal of any pregnancy is the birth of a healthy newborn, and nurses play a major role in helping the pregnant woman and her partner achieve this goal. Ongoing assessment and education are essential.

This chapter describes the nursing management required during pregnancy. It begins with a brief discussion of preconception care and then describes the assessment of the woman at the first prenatal visit and on follow-up visits. The chapter discusses tests commonly used to assess maternal and fetal well-being, including specific nursing management related to each test. The chapter also identifies important strategies to minimize the common discomforts of pregnancy and promote self-care. Lastly, the chapter discusses perinatal education, including childbirth education, birthing options, care provider options, preparation for breastfeeding or bottle feeding, and final preparation for labor and birth.

Preconception Care

Ideally, couples thinking about having a child should schedule a visit with their health care provider for preconception counseling to ensure that they are in the best possible state of health before pregnancy. **Preconception care** is the promotion of the health and well-being of a woman and her partner before pregnancy. The goal of preconception care is to identify any areas such as health problems, lifestyle habits, or social concerns that might unfavorably affect pregnancy (Dunlop, Jack, & Frey, 2007).

Risk Factors for Adverse Pregnancy Outcomes

Preconception care is just as important as prenatal care to reduce adverse pregnancy outcomes such as maternal and infant mortality, preterm births, and low-birthweight infants. Adverse pregnancy outcomes constitute a major public health challenge: 12% of infants are born premature; 8% are born with low birthweight; 3% have major birth defects; and 32% of women suffer pregnancy complications (Centers for Disease Control & Prevention [CDC], 2007b).

Risk factors for these adverse pregnancy outcomes are prevalent among women of reproductive age, as demonstrated by the following statistics:

- 12% of women smoke during pregnancy, contributing to fetal addiction to nicotine.
- 13% consume alcohol during pregnancy, leading to fetal alcohol spectrum disorder.

- 70% of women do not take folic acid supplements, increasing the risk of neural tube defects in the newborn. Taking folic acid reduces the incidence of neural tube defects by two thirds.
- 32% of women starting a pregnancy are obese, which may increase their risk of developing hypertension, diabetes, and thromboembolic disease and may increase the need for cesarean birth.
- 3% take prescription or over-the-counter drugs that are known teratogens (substances harmful to the developing fetus).
- 5% of women have preexisting medical conditions that can negatively affect pregnancy if unmanaged (CDC, 2007b).

All of the factors above pose risks to pregnancy and could be addressed with early interventions if the woman sought preconception health care. Specific recognized risk factors for adverse pregnancy outcomes that fall into one or more of the above categories are listed in Box 12.1.

The period of greatest environmental sensitivity and consequent risk for the developing embryo is between days 17 and 56 after conception. The first prenatal visit, which is usually a month or later after a missed menstrual period, may occur too late to affect reproductive outcomes associated with abnormal organogenesis secondary to poor lifestyle choices. In some cases, such as with unplanned pregnancies, women may delay seeking health care, denying that they are pregnant. Thus, commonly used prevention practices may begin too late to avert the morbidity and mortality associated with congenital anomalies and low birthweight (Atrash et al., 2006). Therefore, it is best that the woman and her partner seek preconception care.

What is the purpose of couples like Linda and Rob going for preconception counseling? What are the goals of preconception care for this couple?

BOX 12.1 **Risk Factors for Adverse Pregnancy Outcomes**

- Taking retinoic acid (Accutane) to clear cystic acne
- Alcohol use
- Anti-epileptic drugs
- Autoimmune disorders
- Diabetes (preconception)
- Folic acid deficiency
- HIV/AIDS
- Maternal phenylketonuria (PKU)
- Rubella seronegativity
- Obesity
- STI
- Smoking (CDC, 2006)
- Underweight

Sources: CDC (2008); NIH (2008); March of Dimes (2008).

Nursing Management

Preconception care involves obtaining a complete health history and physical examination of the woman and her partner. Key areas include:

- Immunization status of the woman
- Underlying medical conditions, such as cardiovascular and respiratory problems or genetic disorders
- Reproductive health data, such as pelvic examinations, use of contraceptives, and sexually transmitted infections (STIs)
- Sexuality and sexual practices, such as safer-sex practices and body image issues
- Nutrition history and present status
- Lifestyle practices, including occupation and recreational activities
- Psychosocial issues such as levels of stress, exposure to abuse and violence
- Medication and drug use, including use of tobacco, alcohol, over-the-counter and prescription medications, and illicit drugs
- Support system, including family, friends, and community (Fig. 12.1 gives a sample preconception screening tool)

This information provides a foundation for planning health-promotion activities and education. For example, to have a positive impact on the pregnancy:

- Ensure that the woman's immunizations are up to date.
- Take a thorough history of both partners to identify any medical or genetic conditions that need treatment or a referral to specialists.
- Identify history of STIs and high-risk sexual practices so they can be modified.
- Complete a dietary history combined with nutritional counseling.
- Gather information regarding exercise and lifestyle practices to encourage daily exercise for well-being and weight maintenance.
- Stress the importance of taking folic acid to prevent neural tube defects.
- Urge the woman to achieve optimal weight before a pregnancy.
- Identify work environment and any needed changes to promote health.
- Address substance use issues, including smoking and drugs.
- Identify victims of violence and assist them to get help.
- Manage chronic conditions such as diabetes and asthma.
- Educate the couple about environmental hazards, including metals and herbs.
- Offer genetic counseling to identify carriers.
- Suggest the availability of support systems, if needed (Graham, 2006).

Nurses can act as advocates and educators, creating healthy, supportive communities for women and their partners in the childbearing phases of their lives. It is important to enter into a collaborative partnership with the woman and her partner, enabling them to examine their own health and its influence on the health of their future baby. Provide information to allow the woman and her partner to make an informed decision about having a baby, but keep in mind that this decision rests solely with the couple.

> ▶ *Take* NOTE!
>
> *"Preconception care should be integrated into the women's health care continuum to achieve high levels of lifetime wellness for all women"* (Dunlop, Jack, & Frey, 2007).

*L*inda and Rob decide to change several aspects of their lifestyle and nutritional habits before conceiving a baby, based on advice from the nurse-midwife. They both want to lose weight, stop smoking, and increase their intake of fruits and vegetables. How will these lifestyle and dietary changes benefit Linda's future pregnancy? What other areas might need to be brought up to date to prepare for a future pregnancy?

The First Prenatal Visit

Once a pregnancy is suspected and, in some cases, tentatively confirmed by a home pregnancy test, the woman should seek prenatal care to promote a healthy outcome. Although the most opportune window (preconception) for improving pregnancy outcomes may be missed, appropriate nursing management starting at conception and continuing throughout the pregnancy can have a positive impact on the health of pregnant women and their unborn children.

The assessment process begins at this initial prenatal visit and continues throughout the pregnancy. The initial visit is an ideal time to screen for factors that might place the woman and her fetus at risk for problems such as preterm delivery. The initial visit also is an optimal time to begin educating the client about changes that will affect her life.

Counseling and education of the pregnant woman and her partner are critical to ensure healthy outcomes for mother and her infant. Pregnant women and their partners frequently have questions, misinformation, or misconceptions about what to eat, weight gain, physical discomforts, drug and alcohol use, sexuality, and the birthing process. The nurse needs to allow time to answer questions and provide anticipatory guidance during the pregnancy and to make appropriate community referrals to meet the needs of these clients. To address these issues and foster the

PRECONCEPTION SCREENING AND COUNSELING CHECKLIST

NAME	BIRTHPLACE	AGE

DATE: / /   ARE YOU PLANNING TO GET PREGNANT IN THE NEXT SIX MONTHS? ___Y ___N

IF YOUR ANSWER TO A QUESTION IS YES, PUT A CHECK MARK ON THE LINE IN FRONT OF THE QUESTION. FILL IN OTHER INFORMATION THAT APPLIES TO YOU.

DIET AND EXERCISE

What do you consider a healthy weight for you?_____
___Do you eat three meals a day?
___Do you follow a special diet (vegetarian, diabetic, other)?
___Which do you drink (__ coffee __ tea __ cola __ milk __ water __ soda/pop
other_____)?
___Do you eat raw or undercooked food (meat, other)?
___Do you take folic acid?
___Do you take other vitamins daily (__ multivitamin __ vitamin A __ other)?
___Do you take dietary supplements (__ black cohosh __ pennyroyal __ other)?
___Do you have current/past problems withh eating disorders?
___Do you exercise? Type/frequency:_____

Notes:

LIFESTYLE

___Do you smoke cigarettes or use other tobacco products?
How many cigarettes/packs a day?_____
___Are you exposed to second-hand smoke?
___Do you drink alcohol?
What kind?_____How often?_____How much?_____
___Do you use recreational drugs (cocaine, heroin, ecstasy, meth/ice, other?
List:_____
___Do you see a dentist regularly?
What kind of work do you do?_____
___Do you work or live near possible hazards (chemicals, x-ray or other radiation,
lead)? List:_____
___Do you use saunas or hot tubs?

Notes:

MEDICATION /DRUGS

___Are you taking prescribed drugs (Accutane, valproic acid, blood thinners)? List
them_____
___Are you taking non-prescribed drugs?
List them:_____
___Are you using birth control pills?
___Do you get injectable contraceptives or shots for birth control?
___Do you use any herbal remedies or alternative medicine?
List:_____

NOTES:

MEDICAL/FAMILY HISTORY

Do you have or have you ever had:
___Epilepsy?
___Diabetes?
___Asthma?
___High blood pressure?
___Heart disease?
___Anemia?
___Kidney or bladder disorders?
___Thyroid disease?
___Chickenpox?
___Hepatitis C?
___Digestive problems?
___Depression or other mental health problem?
___Surgeries?
___Lupus?
___Scleroderma?
___Other conditions?
Have you ever been vaccinated for:
___Measles, mumps, rubella?
___Hepatitis B?
___Chickenpox?

NOTES:

WOMEN'S HEALTH

___Do you have any problems with your menstrual cycle?
___How many times have you been pregnant?
What was/ were the outcomes(s)?_____
___Did you have difficulty getting pregnant last time?
___Have you been treated for infertility?
Have you had surgery on your uterus, cervix, ovaries, or tubes?
___Did you mother take the hormone DES during pregnancy?
Have you ever had HP V, genital warts or chlamydia?
___Have you ever been treated for a sexually transmitted infection (genital herpes,
gonorrhea, syphilis, HIV/AIDS, other)? List:_____

NOTES:

GENETICS

Does your family have a history of   Or   Your partner's family
___Hemophilia?   ___
___Other bleeding disorders?   ___
___Tay-Sachs disease?   ___
___Blood diseases (sickle cell, thalassemia, other)?   ___
___Muscular dystrophy?   ___
___Down syndrome/mental retardation?   ___
___Cystic fibrosis?   ___
___Birth defects (spine/heart/kidney)?   ___
Your ethnic background is:_____
Your partner's ethnic background is: _____

NOTES:

HOME ENVIRONMENT

___Do you feel emotionally supported at home?
___Do you have help from relatives or friends if needed?
___Do you feel you have serious money/financial worries?
___Are you in a stable relationship?
___Do you feel safe at home?
___Does anyone threaten or physically hurt you?
___Do you have pets (cats, rodents, exotic animals)? List:_____
___Do have any contact with soil, cat litter, or sandboxes?

Baby preparation (if planning pregnancy):
___Do you have a place for a baby to sleep?
___Do you need any baby items?

NOTES:

OTHER

IS THERE ANYTHING ELSE YOU'D LIKE ME TO KNOW?

ARE THERE ANY QUESTIONS YOU'D LIKE TO ASK ME?

FIGURE 12.1 Sample preconception screening tool. (Used with permission. Copyright March of Dimes.)

overall well-being of pregnant women and their fetuses, specific National Health Goals have been established (see the Healthy People 2010 box).

Comprehensive Health History

During the initial visit, a comprehensive health history is obtained, including age, menstrual history, prior obstetric history, past medical and surgical history, family history, genetic screening, medication or drug use, and history of exposure to infections (STIs) (Frieden & Chan, 2007). Often, using a prenatal history form (Fig. 12.2) is the best way to document the data collected.

The initial health history typically includes questions about three major areas: the reason for seeking care; the client's past medical, surgical, and personal history, including that of the family and her partner; and the client's reproductive history. During the history-taking process, the nurse and client establish the foundation of a trusting relationship and jointly develop a plan of care for the pregnancy. Tailor this plan to the client's lifestyle as much as possible and focus primarily on education for overall wellness during the pregnancy. The ultimate goal is early detection and prevention of any problems that occur during the pregnancy (Frieden & Chan, 2007).

HEALTHY PEOPLE 2010

Objective	Nursing Implications
Increase the proportion of pregnant women who receive early and adequate prenatal care: • Increase the number of women receiving maternal prenatal care beginning in the first trimester of pregnancy from a baseline of 83% to 90% of live births. • Increase the number of women receiving early and adequate prenatal care from a baseline of 74% to 90% of live births.	Will contribute to reduced rates of perinatal illness, disability, and death by helping to identify possible risk factors and implementing measures to lessen these factors that contribute to poor outcomes
Increase the proportion of pregnant women who attend a series of prepared childbirth classes.	Will contribute to a more pleasant birthing experience because women will be prepared for what they will face; also help in reducing pain and anxiety
Increase abstinence from alcohol, cigarettes, and illicit drugs among pregnant women.	Will help to reduce the wide-ranging effects, such as spontaneous abortion, low birthweight, and preterm birth, associated with prenatal substance use

Source: U.S. Department of Health & Human Services, 2000.

Reason for Seeking Care

The woman commonly comes for prenatal care based on the suspicion that she is pregnant. She may report that she has missed her menstrual period or has had a positive result on a home pregnancy test. Ask the woman for the date of her last menstrual period (LMP). Also ask about any presumptive or probable signs of pregnancy that she might be experiencing. Typically a urine or blood test to check for evidence of human chorionic gonadotropin (hCG) is done to confirm the pregnancy.

Past History

Ask about the woman's past medical and surgical history. This information is important because conditions that the woman experienced in the past (e.g., urinary tract infections) may recur or be exacerbated during pregnancy. Also, chronic illnesses, such as diabetes or heart disease, can increase the risk for complications during pregnancy for the woman and her fetus. Ask about any history of allergies to medications, foods, or environmental substances. Ask about any mental health problems, such as depression or anxiety. Gather similar information about the woman's family and her partner.

The woman's personal history also is important. Ask about her occupation, possible exposure to teratogens, exercise and activity level, recreational patterns (including the use of substances such as alcohol, tobacco, and drugs), use of alternative and complementary therapies, sleep patterns, nutritional habits, and general lifestyle. Each of these may have an impact on the outcome of the pregnancy. For example, if the woman smokes during pregnancy, nicotine in the cigarettes causes vasoconstriction in the mother, leading to reduced placental perfusion. As a result, the newborn may be small for gestational age. The newborn will also go through nicotine withdrawal soon after birth. In addition, no safe level of alcohol ingestion in pregnancy has been determined. Many fetuses exposed to heavy alcohol levels during pregnancy develop fetal alcohol syndrome, a collection of deformities and disabilities.

Reproductive History

The woman's reproductive history includes a menstrual, obstetric, and gynecologic history. Typically, this history begins with a description of the woman's menstrual cycle, including her age at menarche, number of days in her cycle, typical flow characteristics, and any discomfort experienced. The use of contraception also is important, including when the woman last used any contraception.

Ask the woman the date of her LMP to determine the estimated or expected date of birth (EDB) or delivery (EDD). Several methods may be used to estimate the date of birth. Nagele's rule can be used to establish the EDD or EDB. Using this rule, subtract 3 months and then add 7 days to the first day of the LMP. Then correct the year by adding 1 to it. This date has a margin of error of plus or minus 2 weeks. For instance, if a woman reports that her LMP was Oct. 14, 2007, you would subtract 3 months

(text continues on page 320)

Health History Summary
Maternal/Newborn Record System

Page 1 of 2

Patient's name _____

ID. No. _____

_____

_____

Demographic data

Date of birth _____ Age ____ Language ☐ _____ English ☐   Interpreter ☐ _____ None ☐
☐ N/A

Religion ☐ _____   Race/ethnicity _____

Marital status S M SEP D W   Name of baby's father _____

Education	Occupation	Full	Part	Self	Unemp	Work Tel No	Home Tel No
Patient		☐	☐	☐	☐		
Father of baby		☐	☐	☐	☐		

Allergy/sensitivity
☐ None ☐ Latex

☐ Other _____

Primary/referring physician

Menstrual history

	Menarche yrs	Interval days	Length days	Abnormalities ☐ None		

Certain ☐ Yes ☐ No   Positive pregnancy test ___/___/___
LMP ___/___/___   Normal ☐ Yes ☐ No

☐ Blood
☐ Urine

EDD
By dates ___/___/___
By ultrasound ___/___/___
Date of ultrasound ___/___/___

Pregnancy history	Gravida	Full term	Premature	Spontaneous Ab	Induced Ab	Ectopic	Multiple births	Live

No	Month/year	Infant sex	Weight at birth	Wks gest	Hours in labor	Type of delivery	Anesthesia	Comments/complications
1								
2								
3								
4								
5								
6								
7								

Medical history
Obstetric   Patient

Check and detail positive findings below. Use reference numbers.

1. Anemia _____ ☐
2. Fetal/neonatal death or anomaly _____ ☐
3. Gestational diabetes _____ ☐
4. Hemorrhage _____ ☐
5. Hyperemesis _____ ☐
6. Incompetent cervix _____ ☐
7. Intrauterine growth retardation _____ ☐
8. Isoimmunization _____ ☐
9. Polyhydramnios _____ ☐
10. Postpartum depression _____ ☐
11. Pregnancy-induced hypertension _____ ☐
12. Preterm labor or birth _____ ☐
13. PROM-chorioamnionitis _____ ☐
14. Rhogam given _____ ☐
15. RH neg _____ ☐

Gynecologic
16. Contraceptive use _____ ☐
17. Abnormal PAP _____ ☐
18. Fibroids _____ ☐
19. Gyn· surgery _____ ☐

Gynecologic (cont'd.)   Patient
20. Infertility _____ ☐
21. In utero exposure to DES _____ ☐
22. Uterine/cervical anomaly _____ ☐

Sexually transmitted diseases
23. Chlamydia _____ ☐
24. Gonorrhea _____ ☐
25. Herpes (HSV) _____ ☐
26. Syphilis _____ ☐

Vaginal/genital infections
27. Trichomonas _____ ☐
28. Condylomata _____ ☐
29. Candidiasis _____ ☐

Other infections
30. Toxoplasmosis _____ ☐
31. Group B streptococcus _____ ☐
32. Rubella or immunization _____ ☐
33. Varicella or immunization _____ ☐
34. Cytomegalovirus (CMV) _____ ☐
35. AIDS (HIV) _____ ☐
36. Hepatitis (type ____) _____ ☐
   or immunization (type ____)

FIGURE 12.2 Sample prenatal history form. (Used with permission. Copyright Briggs Corporation, 2001.)

Health History Summary
Maternal/newborn record system

Page 2 of 2

Patient's name _____

ID. No. _____

_____

_____

Check and detail positive findings below. Use reference numbers.

Cardiovascular

	Patient	Family
37. Myocardial infarction	☐	☐
38. Heart disease	☐	☐
39. Rheumatic fever	☐	
40. Valve disease	☐	
41. Chronic hypertension	☐	☐
42. Disease of the aorta	☐	☐
43. Varicosities Thrombophlebitis	☐	☐
44. Previous pulmonary embolism	☐	
45. Blood disorders	☐	☐
46. Anemia/ hemoglobinopathy	☐	☐
47. Blood transfusions	☐	
48. Other	☐	

Pulmonary

	Patient	Family
49. Asthma	☐	
50. Tuberculosis	☐	☐
51. Chronic obstructive pulmonary disease	☐	☐

Endocrine

	Patient	Family
52. Diabetes	☐	☐
53. Thyroid dysfunction	☐	☐
54. Maternal PKU	☐	
55. Endocrinopathy	☐	☐
56. Gastrointestinal	☐	
57. Liver disease	☐	

Renal disease

	Patient	Family
58. Cystitis	☐	
59. Pyelonephritis	☐	
60. Asymptomatic bacteriuria	☐	
61. Chronic renal disease	☐	☐
62. Autoimmune disease	☐	☐
63. Cancer	☐	☐

Neurologic disease

	Patient	Family
64. Cerebrovascular accident	☐	☐
65. Seizure disorder	☐	☐
66. Migraine headaches	☐	☐
67. Degenerative disease	☐	☐
68. Other	☐	

Psychological/surgical

	Patient	Family
69. Psychiatric disease Mental illness	☐	☐
70. Physical abuse or neglect	☐	☐
71. Emotional abuse or neglect	☐	☐
72. Addiction (drug, alcohol, nicotine)	☐	☐
73. Major accidents	☐	
74. Surgery	☐	
75. Anesthetic complications	☐	
76. Non-surgical hospitalization	☐	
77. Other	☐	
78. **No known disease/problems**	☐	

Genetic history

	Patient	Father of baby	Family
79. Age 35 or older (female) 50 or older (male)	☐	☐	☐
80. Cerebral palsy	☐	☐	☐
81. Cleft lip/palate	☐	☐	☐
82. Congenital anomalies	☐	☐	☐
83. Congenital heart disease	☐	☐	☐
84. Consanguinity	☐	☐	☐
85. Cystic fibrosis	☐	☐	☐
86. Down's syndrome	☐	☐	☐
87. Hemophilia	☐	☐	☐
88. Huntington's chorea	☐	☐	☐

	Patient	Father of baby	Family
89. Mental retardation	☐	☐	☐
90. Muscular dystrophy	☐	☐	☐
91. Neural tube defect	☐	☐	☐
92. Sickle cell disease or trait	☐	☐	☐
93. Tay-sachs disease	☐	☐	☐
94. Test for fragile X	☐	☐	☐
95. Thalassemia A or B	☐	☐	☐
96. Other	☐	☐	☐
97. Other	☐	☐	☐
98. Other	☐	☐	☐

Historical risk status   ☐ No risk factors noted
☐ At risk (identify)

Signature

FIGURE 12.2 (continued)

(July) and add 7 days (21), then add 1 year (2008). The woman's EDD or EDB is July 21, 2008.

Because of the normal variations in women's menstrual cycles, differences in the normal length of gestation between ethnic groups, and errors in dating methods, there is no such thing as an exact due date. In general, a birth 2 weeks before or 2 weeks after the EDD or EDB is considered normal. Nagele's rule is less accurate if the woman's menstrual cycles are irregular, if the woman conceives while breastfeeding or before her regular menstrual cycle is established, if she is ovulating although she is amenorrheic, or after she discontinues oral contraceptives (Hackley, Kriebs, & Rousseau, 2007).

A gestational or birth calculator or wheel can also be used to calculate the due date (Fig. 12.3). Some practitioners use ultrasound to more accurately determine the gestational age and date the pregnancy.

Typically, an obstetric history provides information about the woman's past pregnancies, including any problems encountered during the pregnancy, labor, delivery, and afterward. Such information can provide clues to problems that might develop in the current pregnancy. Some common terms used to describe and document an obstetric history include:

- Gravid: the state of being pregnant
- **Gravida**: a pregnant woman; gravida I (primigravida) during the first pregnancy, gravida II (secundigravida) during the second pregnancy, and so on

- **Para**: The number of pregnancies that a woman has, regardless of whether the newborn is born alive or dead. Thus, a primipara is a woman who has given birth once after a pregnancy of at least 20 weeks, commonly referred to as a "primip" in clinical practice. A multipara is a woman who has had two or more pregnancies resulting in viable offspring, commonly referred to as a "multip." Nullipara (para 0) is a woman who has not produced a viable offspring.

Other systems may be used to document a woman's obstetric history. These systems often break down the category of para more specifically (Box 12.2).

Information about the woman's gynecologic history is important. Ask about any reproductive tract surgeries the woman has undergone. For example, surgery on the uterus may affect its ability to contract effectively during labor. A history of tubal pregnancy increases the woman's risk for another tubal pregnancy. Also ask about safe-sex practices and any history of STIs.

Physical Examination

The next step in the assessment process is the physical examination, which detects any physical problems that may affect the pregnancy outcome. The initial physical examination provides the baseline for evaluating changes during future visits.

FIGURE 12.3 EDB using a birth wheel. The first day of the woman's last normal menstrual period was October 1. Using the birth wheel, her EDB would be approximately July 8 of the following year. (Used with permission. Copyright March of Dimes, 2007.)

BOX 12.2   Obstetric History Terms

GTPAL or TPAL

G = gravida, T = term births, P = preterm births,
  A = abortions, L = living children
  G—the current pregnancy
  T—the number of pregnancies ending >37 weeks'
    gestation, at term
  P—the number of preterm pregnancies ending
    >20 weeks or viability but before completion of
    37 weeks
  A—the number of pregnancies ending before
    20 weeks or viability
  L—the number of children currently living

Consider this example:

Mary Johnson is pregnant for the fourth time. She
  had one abortion at 8 weeks' gestation. She has a
  daughter who was born at 40 weeks' gestation and a
  son born at 34 weeks. Mary's obstetric history would
  be documented as follows:

Using the gravida/para method: gravida 4, para 2
Using the TPAL method: 1112 (T = 1 [daughter born
  at 40 weeks]; P = 1 [son born at 34 weeks], A = 1
  [abortion at 8 weeks]; L = 2 [two living children])

Preparation

Instruct the client to undress and put on a gown. Also ask her to empty her bladder and, in doing so, to collect a urine specimen. Typically this specimen is a clean-catch urine specimen that is sent to the laboratory for a urinalysis to detect a possible urinary tract infection.

Begin the physical examination by obtaining vital signs, including blood pressure, respiratory rate, temperature, and pulse. Also measure the client's height and weight. Abnormalities such as an elevated blood pressure may suggest pregestational hypertension, requiring further evaluation. Abnormalities in pulse rate and respiration require further investigation for possible cardiac or respiratory disease. If the woman weighs less than 100 pounds or more than 200 pounds or there has been a sudden weight gain, report these findings to the primary care provider; medical treatment or nutritional counseling may be necessary.

Head-to-Toe Assessment

A complete head-to-toe assessment is usually performed by the health care professional. Every body system is assessed. Some of the major areas are discussed here. Throughout the assessment, be sure to drape the client appropriately to ensure privacy and prevent chilling.

Head and Neck

Assess the head and neck area for any previous injuries and sequelae. Evaluate for any limitations in range of motion. Palpate for any enlarged lymph nodes or swelling. Note any edema of the nasal mucosa or hypertrophy of gin-

gival tissue in the mouth; these are typical responses to increased estrogen levels in pregnancy. Palpate the thyroid gland for enlargement. Slight enlargement is normal, but marked enlargement may indicate hyperthyroidism, requiring further investigation.

Chest

Auscultate heart sounds, noting any abnormalities. A soft systolic murmur caused by the increase in blood volume may be noted. Anticipate an increase in heart rate by 10 to 15 beats per minute (starting between 14 and 20 weeks of pregnancy) secondary to increases in cardiac output and blood volume. The body adapts to the increase in blood volume with peripheral dilatation to maintain blood pressure. Progesterone causes peripheral dilatation.

Auscultate the chest for breath sounds, which should be clear. Also note symmetry of chest movement and thoracic breathing patterns. Estrogen promotes relaxation of the ligaments and joints of the ribs, with a resulting increase in the anteroposterior chest diameter. Expect a slight increase in respiratory rate to accommodate the increase in tidal volume and oxygen consumption.

Inspect and palpate the breasts. Increases in estrogen and progesterone and blood supply make the breasts feel full and more nodular, with increased sensitivity to touch. Blood vessels become more visible and there is an increase in breast size. Striae gravidarum (stretch marks) may be visible in women with large breasts. Darker pigmentation of the nipple and areola is present, along with enlargement of Montgomery's glands.

▶ *Take* NOTE!

Use this opportunity to reinforce and teach breast self-examination.

Abdomen

The appearance of the abdomen depends on the number of weeks of gestation. The abdomen enlarges progressively as the fetus grows. Palpate the abdomen, which should be rounded and nontender. A decrease in muscle tone may be noted due to the influence of progesterone. Inspection also may reveal striae gravidarum (stretch marks) and linea nigra, depending on the duration of the pregnancy.

Typically, the height of the fundus is measured when the uterus arises out of the pelvis to evaluate fetal growth. At 12 weeks' gestation the fundus can be palpated at the symphysis pubis. At 16 weeks' gestation the fundus is midway between the symphysis and the umbilicus. At 20 weeks the fundus can be palpated at the umbilicus and measures approximately 20 cm from the symphysis pubis. By 36 weeks the fundus is just below the ensiform cartilage and measures approximately 36 cm. The uterus maintains a globular/ovoid shape throughout pregnancy (Frieden & Chan, 2007).

Extremities

Inspect and palpate both legs for dependent edema, pulses, and varicose veins. If edema is present in early pregnancy, further evaluation may be needed to rule out gestational hypertension. Ask the woman if she has any pain in her calf that increases when she ambulates. This might indicate a deep vein thrombosis (DVT). High levels of estrogen during pregnancy place women at higher risk for DVT.

Pelvic Examination

The pelvic examination provides information about the internal and external reproductive organs. In addition, it aids in assessing some of the presumptive and probable signs of pregnancy and allows for determination of pelvic adequacy. During the pelvic examination, remain in the examining room to assist the health care provider with any specimen collection, fixation, and labeling. Also provide comfort and emotional support for the woman, who might be anxious. Throughout the examination, explain what is happening and why, and answer any questions as necessary.

External Genitalia

After the client is placed in the lithotomy position and draped appropriately, the external genitalia are inspected visually. They should be free from lesions, discharge, hematomas, varicosities, and inflammation upon inspection. A culture for STIs may be collected at this time.

Internal Genitalia

Next, the internal genitalia are examined via a speculum. The cervix should be smooth, long, thick, and closed. Because of increased pelvic congestion, the cervix will be softened (Goodell's sign), the uterine isthmus will be softened (Hegar's sign), and there will be a bluish coloration of the cervix and vaginal mucosa (Chadwick's sign).

The uterus typically is pear-shaped and mobile, with a smooth surface. It will undergo cell hypertrophy and hyper-plasia so that it enlarges throughout the pregnancy to accommodate the growing fetus.

During the pelvic examination, a Papanicolaou (Pap) smear may be obtained. Additional cultures, such as for gonorrhea and chlamydia screening and group B streptococcus screening, also may be obtained. Ensure that all specimens obtained are labeled correctly and sent to the laboratory for evaluation. A rectal examination is done last to assess for lesions, masses, prolapse, or hemorrhoids.

Once the examination of the internal genitalia is completed and the speculum is removed, a bimanual examination is performed to estimate the size of the uterus to confirm dates and to palpate the ovaries. The ovaries should be small and nontender, without masses. At the conclusion of the bimanual examination, the health care professional reinserts the index finger into the vagina and the middle finger into the rectum to assess the strength and regularity of the posterior vaginal wall.

Pelvic Size, Shape, and Measurements

The size and shape of the women's pelvis can affect her ability to deliver vaginally. Pelvic shape is typically classified as one of four types: gynecoid, android, anthropoid, and platypelloid. Refer to Chapter 13 for an in-depth discussion of pelvic size and shape.

Taking internal pelvic measurements determines the actual diameters of the inlet and outlet through which the fetus will pass. This is extremely important if the woman has never given birth vaginally. Taking pelvic measurements is unnecessary for the woman who has given birth vaginally before (unless she has experienced some type of trauma to the area) because vaginal delivery demonstrates that the pelvis is adequate for the passage of the fetus.

Three measurements are assessed: diagonal conjugate, true conjugate, and ischial tuberosity (Fig. 12.4). The diagonal conjugate is the distance between the anterior surface of the sacral prominence and the anterior surface

A   **B**

FIGURE 12.4 Pelvic measurements. (**A**) Diagonal conjugate (solid line) and true conjugate (dotted line). (**B**) Ischial tuberosity diameter.

of the inferior margin of the symphysis pubis (Frieden & Chan, 2007). This measurement, usually 12.5 cm or greater, represents the anteroposterior diameter of the pelvic inlet. The diagonal conjugate is the most useful measurement for estimating pelvic size because a misfit with the fetal head occurs if it is too small.

The true conjugate, also called the obstetric conjugate, is the measurement from the anterior surface of the sacral prominence to the posterior surface of the inferior margin of the symphysis pubis. This diameter cannot be measured directly; rather, it is estimated by subtracting 1 to 2 cm from the diagonal conjugate measurement. The average true conjugate diameter is at least 11.5 cm (Cunningham et al., 2005). This measurement is important because it is the smallest front-to-back diameter through which the fetal head must pass when moving through the pelvic inlet.

The ischial tuberosity diameter is the transverse diameter of the pelvic outlet. This measurement is made outside the pelvis at the lowest aspect of the ischial tuberosities. A diameter of 10.5 cm or more is considered adequate for passage of the fetal head (Blackburn, 2007).

Laboratory Tests

A series of tests are generally ordered during the initial visit so that baseline data can be obtained, allowing for early detection and prompt intervention if any problems occur. Tests that are generally conducted for all pregnant women include urinalysis and blood studies. The urine is analyzed for albumin, glucose, ketones, and bacteria casts. Blood studies usually include a complete blood count (hemoglobin, hematocrit, red and white blood cell counts, and platelets), blood typing and Rh factor, a rubella titer, hepatitis B surface antibody antigen, HIV, VDRL, and RPR tests, and cervical smears to detect STIs (Common Laboratory and Diagnostic Tests 12.1). In addition, most offices and clinics have ultrasound equipment available to validate an intrauterine pregnancy and assess early fetal growth.

The need for additional laboratory studies is determined by a woman's history, physical examination findings, current health status, and risk factors identified in the initial interview. Additional tests can be offered, but ultimately the woman and her partner make the decision about undergoing them. Educate the client and her partner about the tests, including the rationale. In addition, support the client and her partner in their decision-making process, regardless of whether you agree with the couple's decision. The couple's decisions about their health care are based on the ethical principle of autonomy, which allows an individual the right to make decisions about his or her own body.

COMMON LABORATORY AND DIAGNOSTIC TESTS 12.1

Test	Explanation
Complete blood cell count (CBC)	Evaluates hemoglobin (12–14 g) and hematocrit (42% +/– 5) levels and red blood cell count (4.2–5.4 million/mm³) to detect presence of anemia; identifies WBC (5,000–10,000/mm³), which if elevated may indicate an infection; determines platelet count (150,000–450,000 cubic mL) to assess clotting ability
Blood typing	Determines woman's blood type and Rh status to rule out any blood incompatibility issues early; Rh-negative mother would likely receive RhoGAM (at 28 weeks) if she is Rh sensitive via indirect Coombs test
Rubella titer	Detects antibodies for the virus that causes German measles; if titer is 1:8 or less, the woman is not immune, requires immunization after birth, and is advised to avoid people with undiagnosed rashes
Hepatitis B	Determines if mother has hepatitis B by detecting presence of hepatitis antibody surface antigen (HbsAg) in her blood
HIV testing	Detects HIV antibodies and if positive requires more specific testing, counseling, and treatment during pregnancy with antiretroviral medications to prevent transmission to fetus
STI screening: Venereal Disease Research Laboratory (VDRL) or rapid plasma reagin (RPR) serologic tests	Detects STIs (such as syphilis, herpes, HPV, gonorrhea) so that treatment can be initiated early to prevent transmission to fetus
Cervical smears	Detects abnormalities such as cervical cancer (Pap test) or infections such as gonorrhea, chlamydia, or group B streptococcus so that treatment can be initiated if positive

Sources: Skidmore-Roth 2004; Spratto and Woods, 2004

Remember Linda and Rob, the couple who want to start a family? Ten months after the preconception appointment, Linda calls to make a first prenatal appointment. What key areas will be addressed at this first prenatal visit? What interventions might be suggested for Linda to implement in order to ensure a healthy newborn?

Follow-Up Visits

Continuous prenatal care is important for a successful pregnancy outcome. The recommended follow-up visit schedule for a healthy pregnant woman is as follows:

- Every 4 weeks up to 28 weeks (7 months)
- Every 2 weeks from 29 to 36 weeks
- Every week from 37 weeks to birth

At each subsequent prenatal visit the following assessments are completed:

- Weight and blood pressure, which are compared to baseline values
- Urine testing for protein, glucose, ketones, and nitrites
- Fundal height measurement to assess fetal growth
- Assessment for quickening/fetal movement to determine fetal well-being
- Assessment of fetal heart rate (should be 110 to 160 bpm)

At each follow-up visit, answer questions, provide anticipatory guidance and education, review nutritional guidelines, and evaluate the client for compliance with prenatal vitamin therapy. Throughout the pregnancy, encourage the woman's partner to participate if possible.

Fundal Height Measurement

Fundal height is the distance (in cm) measured with a tape measure from the top of the pubic bone to the top of the uterus (fundus) with the client lying on her back with her knees slightly flexed (Fig. 12.5). Measurement in this

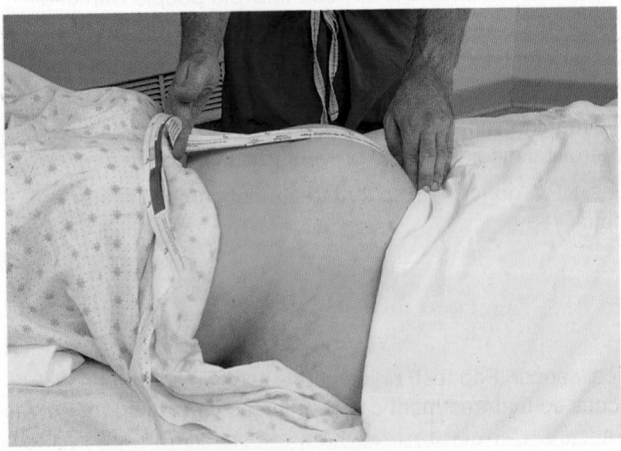

FIGURE **12.5** Fundal height measurement.

way is termed the McDonald's method. Fundal height typically increases as the pregnancy progresses; it reflects fetal growth and provides a gross estimate of the duration of the pregnancy.

Between 12 and 14 weeks' gestation, the fundus can be palpated above the symphysis pubis. The fundus reaches the level of the umbilicus at approximately 20 weeks and measures 20 cm. Fundal measurement should approximately equal the number of weeks of gestation until week 36. For example, a fundal height of 24 cm suggests a fetus at 24 weeks' gestation. After 36 weeks, the fundal height then drops due to lightening and may no longer correspond with the week of gestation.

It is expected that the fundal height will increase progressively throughout the pregnancy, reflecting fetal growth. However, if the growth curve flattens or stays stable, it may indicate the presence of intrauterine growth restriction (IUGR). If the fundal height measurement is greater than 4 cm from the estimated gestational age, further evaluation is warranted if a multifetal gestation has not been diagnosed or hydramnios has not been ruled out (Dillon, 2007).

Fetal Movement Determination

Fetal movement is usually perceived by the client between 16 and 20 weeks' gestation. Perceived fetal movement is most often related to trunk and limb motion and rollovers, or flips (Arenson & Drake, 2007). Fetal movement is a gross indicator of fetal well-being. Decreased fetal movement may indicate asphyxia and IUGR. If compromised, the fetus decreases its oxygen requirements by decreasing activity (Mangesi & Hofmeyr, 2007). A decrease in fetal movement may be related to other factors as well, such as maternal use of central nervous system depressants, fetal sleep cycles, hydrocephalus, bilateral renal agenesis, and bilateral hip dislocation (Arenson & Drake, 2007).

Two suggested techniques for determining fetal movement, also called fetal movement counts, are the Cardiff technique and the Sadovsky technique (Box 12.3). Fetal movement is a noninvasive method of screening and can be easily taught to all pregnant women. Both techniques require client participation.

Instruct the client about how to count fetal movements, the reasons for doing so, and the significance of decreased fetal movements. Urge the client to perform the counts in a relaxed environment and a comfortable position, such as semi-Fowler's or side-lying. Provide the client with detailed information concerning fetal movement counts and stress the need for consistency in monitoring (at approximately the same time each day) and the importance of informing the health care provider promptly of any reduced movements. Providing clients with "fetal kick count" charts to record movement helps promote compliance. There is no established number of fetal movements that indicates fetal well-being, but instruct the

BOX 12.3 Techniques for Fetal Movement Counts

Maternal perception of fetal movements or counting fetal movements is an inexpensive, noninvasive method of assessing fetal well-being. Several different techniques, two of which are described below, can be used. Scientific evidence has not shown that one technique is better than another. However, the amount of time required for the client to complete the count varies. Additionally, because counts are highly subjective on the mother's part, consistency is essential when performing fetal movement counts. Fetal movement counts should be done at approximately the same time each day, and further testing should be initiated within 12 hours of a client's perception of decreased activity (Mangesti & Hofmeyr, 2007).

Cardiff Technique
The woman lies or sits and concentrates on fetal movements until she records 10 movements. She must record the length of time during which the 10 movements occurred. She is instructed to notify her health care provider if she doesn't feel at least 10 movements within 1 hour. Further follow-up testing is indicated.

Sadovsky Technique
The woman lies down on her left side for 1 hour after meals and concentrates on fetal movement. Four movements should be felt within 1 hour. If four movements have not been felt within 1 hour, then the woman should monitor movement for a second hour. If after 2 hours four movements haven't been felt, the client should contact her health care provider.

Nursing Procedure 12.1

MEASURING FETAL HEART RATE

Purpose: To assess fetal well-being
1. Assist the woman onto the examining table and have her lie down.
2. Cover her with a sheet to ensure privacy, and then expose her abdomen.
3. Palpate the abdomen to determine the fetal lie, position, and presentation.
4. Locate the back of the fetus (the ideal position to hear the heart rate).
5. Apply lubricant gel to abdomen in the area where the back has been located.
6. Turn on the handheld Doppler device and place it on the spot over the fetal back.
7. Listen for the sound of the amplified heart rate, moving the device slightly from side to side as necessary to obtain the loudest sound. Assess the woman's pulse rate and compare it to the amplified sound. If the rates appear the same, reposition the Doppler device.
8. Once the fetal heart rate has been identified, count the number of beats in 1 minute and record the results.
9. Remove the Doppler device and wipe off any remaining gel from the woman's abdomen and the device.
10. Record the heart rate on the woman's medical record.
11. Provide information to the woman regarding fetal well-being based on findings.

woman to report a count of less than three fetal movements within an hour. Further investigation with a nonstress test or biophysical profile is usually warranted (Mangesi & Hofmeyr, 2007).

Fetal Heart Rate Measurement

Fetal heart rate measurement is integral to fetal surveillance throughout the pregnancy. Auscultating the fetal heart rate with a handheld Doppler at each prenatal visit helps confirm that the intrauterine environment is still supportive to the growing fetus. The purpose of assessing fetal heart rate is to determine rate and rhythm. Nursing Procedure 12.1 lists the steps in measuring fetal heart rate.

Follow-Up Visit Intervals and Assessments

Up to 28 weeks' gestation, follow-up visits involve assessment of the client's blood pressure and weight. The urine is tested for protein and glucose. Fundal height and fetal heart rate are assessed at every office visit. Between weeks 24 and 28, a blood glucose level is obtained using a 50-g glucose load followed by a 1-hour plasma glucose determination. If the result is more than 140 mg/dL, further testing, such as a 3-hour 100-g glucose tolerance test, is warranted to determine whether gestational diabetes is present.

During this time, review the common discomforts of pregnancy, evaluate any client complaints, and answer questions. Reinforce the importance of good nutrition and use of prenatal vitamins, along with daily exercise.

Between 29 and 36 weeks' gestation, all the assessments of previous visits are completed, along with assessment for edema. Special attention is focused on the presence and location of edema during the last trimester. Pregnant women commonly experience dependent edema of the lower extremities from constriction of blood vessels secondary to the heavy gravid uterus. Periorbital edema around the eyes, edema of the hands, and pretibial edema are abnormal and could be signs of gestational hypertension. Inspecting and palpating both extremities, listening for complaints of tight rings on fingers, and observing for swelling around the eyes are important assessments. Abnormal findings in any of these areas need to be reported.

If the mother is Rh negative, her antibody titer is re-evaluated. RhoGAM is given if indicated. The client also is evaluated for risk of preterm labor. At each visit, ask if she is experiencing any common signs or symptoms of preterm labor (e.g., uterine contractions, dull backache, feeling of pressure in the pelvic area or thighs, increased vaginal discharge, menstrual-like cramps, vaginal bleeding). A pelvic examination is performed to assess the cervix for position, consistency, length, and dilation. If the woman has had a previous preterm birth, she is at risk for another and close monitoring is warranted.

Counsel the woman about choosing a health care provider for the newborn, if she has not selected one yet. Along with completion of a breast assessment, discuss the choice of breastfeeding versus bottle-feeding. Reinforce the importance of daily fetal movement monitoring as an indicator of fetal well-being. Re-evaluate hemoglobin and hematocrit levels to assess for anemia.

Between 37 and 40 weeks' gestation, the same assessments are done as for the previous weeks. In addition, screening for group B streptococcus, gonorrhea, and chlamydia is done. Fetal presentation and position (via Leopold's maneuvers) are assessed. Review the signs and symptoms of labor and forward a copy of the prenatal record to the hospital labor department for future reference. Review the client's desire for family planning after birth as well as her decision to breastfeed or bottle-feed. Remind the client that an infant car seat is required by law and must be used to drive the newborn home from the hospital or birthing center.

Teaching About the Danger Signs of Pregnancy

It is important to educate the client about danger signs during pregnancy that require further evaluation. Explain that she should contact her health care provider immediately if she experiences any of the following:

- During the first trimester: spotting or bleeding (miscarriage), painful urination (infection), severe persistent vomiting (hyperemesis gravidarum), fever higher than 100°F (infection), and lower abdominal pain with dizziness and accompanied by shoulder pain (ruptured ectopic pregnancy)
- During the second trimester: regular uterine contractions (preterm labor); pain in calf, often increased with foot flexion (blood clot in deep vein); sudden gush or leakage of fluid from vagina (premature rupture of

membranes); and absence of fetal movement for more than 24 hours (possible fetal distress or demise)
- During the third trimester: sudden weight gain; periorbital or facial edema, severe upper abdominal pain, or headache with visual changes (pregnancy-induced hypertension); and a decrease in fetal daily movement for more than 24 hours (possible demise). Any of the previous warning signs and symptoms can also be present in this last trimester (March of Dimes, 2008c).

One of the warning signs that should be emphasized is early contractions, which can lead to preterm birth. All pregnant women need to be able to recognize early signs of contractions to prevent preterm labor, which is a major public health problem in the United States. Approximately 12% of all live births—or one out of eight babies—is born too soon (March of Dimes, 2008c). These preterm infants (born at less than 37 weeks' gestation) can suffer lifelong health consequences such as mental retardation, chronic lung disease, cerebral palsy, seizure disorders, and blindness, among other problems (March of Dimes, 2008c). Preterm labor can happen to any pregnant women at any time. In many cases it can be stopped with medications if it is recognized early, before significant cervical dilation has taken place. If the woman experiences menstrual-like cramps occurring every 10 minutes accompanied by a low, dull backache, she should stop what she is doing and lie down on her left side for 1 hour and drink two or three glasses of water. If the symptoms worsen or don't subside after 1 hour, she should contact her health care provider.

Assessment of Fetal Well-Being

During the antepartum period, several tests are performed routinely to monitor fetal well-being and to detect possible problems. When a high-risk pregnancy is identified, additional antepartum testing can be initiated to promote positive maternal, fetal, and neonatal outcomes. **High-risk pregnancies** include those that are complicated by maternal or fetal conditions (coincidental with or unique to pregnancy) that jeopardize the health status of the mother and put the fetus at risk for uteroplacental insufficiency, hypoxia, and death (Gilbert, 2007). However, additional antepartum fetal testing should take place only when the results obtained will guide future care, whether it is reassurance, more frequent testing, admission to the hospital, or the need for immediate delivery (Gilbert, 2007).

Ultrasonography

Since its introduction in the late 1950s, ultrasonography has become a very useful diagnostic tool in obstetrics. Real-time scanners can produce a continuous picture of the fetus on a monitor screen. A transducer that emits high-frequency sound waves is placed on the mother's abdomen and moved to visualize the fetus (Fig. 12.6). The fetal

FIGURE 12.6 Ultrasound. (**A**) Ultrasound device being applied to client's abdomen. (**B**) View of monitor.

heartbeat and any malformations in the fetus can be assessed and measurements can be made accurately from the picture on the monitor screen.

Ultrasound, which is noninvasive, is considered a safe, accurate, and cost-effective tool. It provides important information about fetal activity, growth, and gestational age, assesses fetal well-being, and determines the need for invasive intrauterine tests (Valley & Fly, 2006).

There are no hard-and-fast rules as to the number of ultrasounds a woman should have during her pregnancy. An ultrasound usually is performed in the first trimester to confirm pregnancy, exclude ectopic or molar pregnancies, and confirm cardiac pulsation. A second scan may be performed at about 18 to 20 weeks to look for congenital malformations, exclude multifetal pregnancies, and verify dates and growth. A third scan may be done at around 34 weeks to evaluate fetal size, assess fetal growth, and verify placental position (Valley & Fly, 2006). An ultrasound is used to confirm placental location during amniocentesis and to provide visualization during chorionic villus sampling. An ultrasound is also ordered whenever an abnormality is suspected based on clinical grounds.

Nursing management during the ultrasound focuses on educating the woman about the ultrasound test and reassuring her that she will not experience any sensation from the sound waves during the test. No special client preparation is needed before performing the ultrasound, although in early pregnancy the woman may need to have a full bladder. Inform her that she may experience some discomfort from the pressure on the full bladder during the scan, but it will last only a short time. Tell the client that the conducting gel used on the abdomen during the scan may feel cold initially.

Doppler Flow Studies

Doppler flow studies can be used to measure the velocity of blood flow via ultrasound. Doppler flow studies can detect fetal compromise in high-risk pregnancies. The test is noninvasive and has no contraindications. The color images produced help to identify abnormalities in diastolic flow within the umbilical vessels. The velocity of the fetal red blood cells can be determined by measuring the change in the frequency of the sound wave reflected off the cells. Thus, Doppler flow studies can detect the movement of red blood cells in vessels (Gilbert, 2007). In pregnancies complicated by hypertension or IUGR, diastolic blood flow may be absent or even reversed (Gilbert, 2007). Doppler flow studies also can be used to evaluate the blood flow through other fetal blood vessels, such as the aorta and those in the brain. Research continues to determine the indications for Doppler flow studies to improve pregnancy outcomes. Nursing management of the woman undergoing Doppler flow studies is similar to that described for an ultrasound.

Alpha–Fetoprotein Analysis

Alpha-fetoprotein (AFP) is a substance produced by the fetal liver between weeks 13 and 20 of gestation. About 30 years ago, elevated levels of maternal serum AFP or amniotic fluid AFP were first linked to the occurrence of fetal neural tube defects. This biomarker screening test is now recommended for all pregnant women (Alexander et al., 2007; ACOG, 2007a).

AFP is present in amniotic fluid in low concentrations between 10 and 14 weeks of gestation and can be detected in maternal serum beginning approximately at 12 to 14 weeks of gestation (Gilbert, 2007). If there is a developmental defect, such as failure of the neural tube to close, more AFP escapes into amniotic fluid from the fetus. AFP then enters the maternal circulation by crossing the placenta, and the level in maternal serum can be measured. The optimal time for AFP screening is 16 to 18 weeks of gestation (ACOG, 2007a). Correct information about gestational dating, maternal weight, race, number of fetuses, and insulin dependency is necessary to ensure the accuracy of this screening test. If incorrect maternal information is submitted or the blood specimen is not drawn during the appropriate time frame, false-positive results may occur, increasing the woman's anxiety. Subsequently, further testing might be ordered based on an inaccurate interpretation, resulting in additional financial and emotional costs to the woman.

A variety of situations can lead to elevation of maternal serum AFP, including open neural tube defect, underestimation of gestational age, the presence of multiple fetuses, gastrointestinal defects, low birthweight, oligohydramnios, and decreased maternal weight (Frieden & Chan, 2007). Lower-than-expected maternal serum AFP levels are seen when fetal gestational age is overestimated or in cases of fetal death, hydatidiform mole, increased maternal weight, maternal type I diabetes, and fetal trisomy 21 (Down syndrome) or trisomy 18 (Edward's syndrome) (Gilbert, 2007).

Measurement of maternal serum AFP is minimally invasive, requiring only a venipuncture for a blood sample. It detects approximately 80% of all open neural tube defects and open abdominal wall defects in early pregnancy (Dashe et al., 2006). AFP has now been combined with other biomarker screening tests to determine the risk of neural tube defects and Down syndrome.

Nursing management for AFP testing consists of preparing the woman for this screening test by gathering accurate information about the date of her LMP, weight, race, and gestational dating. Accurately determining the window of 16 to 18 weeks' gestation will help to ensure that the test results are correct. Also explain that the test involves obtaining a blood specimen.

Marker Screening Tests

Two additional blood screening tests may be used to determine the risk of open neural tube defects and Down syndrome: the triple-marker screen and the addition of a fourth marker, inhibin A, which is used to enhance the accuracy of screening for Down syndrome in women younger than 35 years of age. Low inhibin A levels indicate the possibility of Down syndrome (Frieden & Chan, 2007). These tests combine three or four procedures to enhance the ability to make a diagnosis. These biomarkers are merely screening tests and identify women who need further definitive procedures (i.e., amniocentesis and genetic counseling) to make a diagnosis of neural tube defects (anencephaly, spina bifida, and encephalocele) or Down syndrome in the fetus. Most screening tests are performed between 15 to 22 weeks of gestation (16 to 18 weeks is ideal) (Blackburn, 2007).

The triple-marker screening or triple screening test is performed at 16 to 18 weeks of gestation. It uses the levels of three maternal serum markers (AFP, unconjugated estriol, and hCG), in combination with maternal age, to calculate risk (Frieden & Chan, 2007). With this screening, low maternal serum AFP and unconjugated estriol levels and a high hCG level suggests the possibility of

Down syndrome. Elevated levels of maternal serum AFP are associated with open neural tube defects, ventral wall defects, some renal abnormalities, multiple gestation, certain skin disorders, fetal demise, and placental abnormality. The addition of the other two markers enhances the detection rate, from 25% using AFP alone to approximately 69% using all three (Frieden & Chan, 2007).

The screening test using four maternal markers (i.e., quadruple-marker screening) is also used to screen for Down syndrome. It uses maternal age at term and the concentration of four biomarkers in maternal serum: AFP, unconjugated estriol, hCG, and inhibin A. This test is done at 14 to 22 weeks of pregnancy and is reported to detect 85% of trisomy 21 cases; the triple screen was reported to detect only 69% (Hackley, Kriebs, & Rousseau, 2007). AFP and inhibin A levels are decreased in infants with trisomy 21 (Down syndrome).

Nursing management related to marker screening tests consists primarily of providing education about the tests. Prenatal screening has become standard in prenatal care. However, for many couples it remains confusing, emotionally charged, and filled with uncertain risks. Offer a thorough explanation of the test, reinforcing the information given by the health care professional. Provide couples with a description of the risks and benefits of performing these screens, emphasizing that these tests are for screening purposes only. Remind the couple that a definitive diagnosis is not made without further tests such as an amniocentesis. Answer any questions about these prenatal screening tests and respect the couple's decision if they choose not to have them done. Many couples may choose not to know because they would not consider having an abortion regardless of the test results.

Nuchal Translucency Screening

Nuchal translucency screening (ultrasound) is also done in the first trimester between 11 and 14 weeks. This allows for earlier detection and diagnosis of some fetal chromosomal and structural abnormalities. Ultrasound is used to identify an increase in nuchal translucency, which is due to the subcutaneous accumulation of fluid behind the fetal neck. Increased nuchal translucency is associated with chromosomal abnormalities such as trisomy 21, 18, and 13. Infants with trisomies tend to have more collagen and elastic connective tissue, allowing for accumulation (Caughey et al., 2007).

Amniocentesis

Amniocentesis involves a transabdominal puncture of the amniotic sac to obtain a sample of amniotic fluid for analysis. The fluid contains fetal cells that are examined to detect chromosomal abnormalities and several hereditary metabolic defects in the fetus before birth. In addition, amniocentesis is used to confirm a fetal abnormality when other screening tests detect a possible problem.

Amniocentesis is performed in the second trimester, usually between weeks 16 and 18. It can be done as early as week 14 or as late as week 20 (Singh & Singh, 2007). Over 40 different chromosomal abnormalities, inborn errors of metabolism, and neural tube defects can be diagnosed with amniocentesis. It can replace a genetic probability with a diagnostic certainty, allowing the woman and her partner to make an informed decision about the option of therapeutic abortion.

Amniocentesis can be performed in any of the three trimesters of pregnancy. An early amniocentesis (performed between weeks 11 and 14) is done to detect genetic anomalies. However, early amniocentesis has been associated with a high risk of spontaneous miscarriage and postprocedural amniotic fluid leakage compared with transabdominal chorionic villus screening (Singh & Singh, 2007). ACOG (2004) has issued a position statement on first-trimester screening methods, recommending chorionic villus sampling and nuchal translucency to detect Down syndrome rather than amniocentesis because of the increased risks associated with the early procedure. However, early screening and diagnosis can provide the couple with time to make decisions about the pregnancy outcome.

In the second trimester the procedure is performed between 15 and 20 weeks to detect chromosomal abnormalities, evaluate the fetal condition when the woman is sensitized to the Rh-positive blood, diagnose intrauterine infections, and investigate amniotic fluid AFP when the maternal serum AFP level is elevated (Gilbert, 2007).

In the third trimester amniocentesis is most commonly indicated to determine fetal lung maturity after the 35th week of gestation via analysis of lecithin-to-sphingomyelin ratios (L/S ratio) and to evaluate the fetal condition with Rh isoimmunization. Table 12.1 lists amniotic fluid analysis findings and their implications.

The second trimester is the most common time to have an amniocentesis for any prenatal diagnosis since it carries such high risk if done earlier. By week 14 to 16 of gestation, there is sufficient amniotic fluid for sampling yet enough time for a safe abortion, if desired. Amniocentesis is offered to women who are 35 years of age or older, women who have a child with a neural tube defect, and women with elevated maternal serum AFP levels. It also

TABLE 12.1 AMNIOTIC FLUID ANALYSIS AND IMPLICATIONS

Test Component	Normal Findings	Fetal Implications of Abnormal Findings
Color	Clear with white flecks of vernix caseosa in a mature fetus	Blood of maternal origin is usually harmless. "Port wine" fluid may indicate abruptio placentae. Fetal blood may indicate damage to the fetal, placental, or umbilical cord vessels.
Bilirubin	Absent at term	High levels indicate hemolytic disease of the neonate in isoimmunized pregnancy.
Meconium	Absent (except in breech presentation)	Presence indicates fetal hypotension or distress.
Creatinine	More than 2 mg/dL in a mature fetus	Decrease may indicate immature fetus (less than 37 weeks).
Lecithin–sphingomyelin ratio (L/S ratio)	More than 2 generally indicates fetal pulmonary maturity.	A ratio of less than 2 indicates pulmonary immaturity and subsequent respiratory distress syndrome.
Phosphatidylglycerol	Present	Absence indicates pulmonary immaturity.
Glucose	Less than 45 mg/dL	Excessive increases at term or near term indicate hypertrophied fetal pancreas and subsequent neonatal hypoglycemia.
Alpha-fetoprotein	Variable, depending on gestation age and laboratory technique; highest concentration (about 18.5 µg/mL) occurs at 13 to 14 weeks	Inappropriate increases indicate neural tube defects such as spina bifida or anencephaly, impending fetal death, congenital nephrosis, or contamination of fetal blood.
Bacteria	Absent	Presence indicates chorioamnionitis.
Chromosomes	Normal karyotype	Abnormal karyotype may indicate fetal sex and chromosome disorders.
Acetylcholinesterase	Absent	Presence may indicate neural tube defects, exomphalos, or other serious malformations.

Sources: Blackburn, 2007; Dillon, 2007; Frieden & Chang, 2007.

may be used to detect chromosomal aberrations when a parent has a chromosomal abnormality or is a carrier for a metabolic disease (Cunningham et al., 2005).

Procedure

Amniocentesis is performed after an ultrasound examination identifies an adequate pocket of amniotic fluid free of fetal parts, the umbilical cord, or the placenta (Fig. 12.7). The health care provider inserts a long pudendal or spinal needle, a 22-gauge, 5-inch needle, into the amniotic cavity and aspirates amniotic fluid, which is placed in an amber or foil-covered test tube to protect it from light. When the desired amount of fluid has been withdrawn, the needle is removed and slight pressure is applied to the site. If there is no evidence of bleeding, a sterile bandage is applied to the needle site. The specimens are then sent to the laboratory immediately for the cytologist to evaluate.

Examining a sample of fetal cells directly produces a definitive diagnosis rather than a "best guess" diagnosis based on indirect screening tests. It is an invaluable diagnostic tool, but the risks include spontaneous abortion (1 in 200), maternal or fetal infection, fetal-maternal hemorrhage, leakage of amniotic fluid, and maternal discomfort after the procedure. The test results may take up to 3 weeks.

Nursing Management

When preparing the woman for an amniocentesis, explain the procedure and encourage her to empty her bladder just before the procedure to avoid the risk of bladder puncture.

FIGURE 12.7 Technique for amniocentesis: Inserting needle.

Inform her that a 20-minute electronic fetal monitoring strip usually is obtained to evaluate fetal well-being and obtain a baseline to compare after the procedure is completed. Obtain and record maternal vital signs.

After the procedure, assist the woman to a position of comfort and administer RhoGAM intramuscularly if the woman is Rh negative to prevent potential sensitization to fetal blood. Assess maternal vital signs and fetal heart rate every 15 minutes for an hour after the procedure. Observe the puncture site for bleeding or drainage. Instruct the client to rest after returning home and remind her to report fever, leaking amniotic fluid, vaginal bleeding, or uterine contractions or any changes in fetal activity (increased or decreased) to the health care provider.

When the test results come back, be available to offer support, especially if a fetal abnormality is found. Also prepare the woman and her partner for the need for genetic counseling. Trained genetic counselors can provide accurate medical information and help couples to interpret the results of the amniocentesis so they can make the decisions that are right for them as a family.

Chorionic Villus Sampling

Chorionic villus sampling (CVS) is a procedure for obtaining a sample of the chorionic villi for prenatal evaluation of chromosomal disorders, enzyme deficiencies, and fetal gender determination and to identify sex-linked disorders such as hemophilia, sickle cell anemia, and Tay-Sachs disease (Blackburn, 2007). Chorionic villi are finger-like projections that cover the embryo and anchor it to the uterine lining before the placenta is developed. Because they are of embryonic origin, sampling provides information about the developing fetus. CVS can be used to detect numerous genetic disorders, with the exception of neural tube defects (Jenkins et al., 2007).

There has been an impetus to develop earlier prenatal diagnostic procedures so that couples can make an early decision to terminate the pregnancy if an anomaly is confirmed. Early prenatal diagnosis by CVS was proposed as an alternative to routine amniocentesis, which carries fewer risks if done later in the pregnancy. In addition, results of CVS testing are available sooner than those of amniocentesis, usually within 48 hours.

Procedure

CVS is generally performed 10 to 13 weeks after the LMP. Earlier, chorionic villi may not be sufficiently developed for adequate tissue sampling and the risk of limb defects is increased (Kenner & Lott, 2007). First, an ultrasound is done to confirm gestational age and viability. Then, under continuous ultrasound guidance, CVS is performed using either a transcervical or transabdominal approach. With the transcervical approach, the woman is placed in the lithotomy position and a sterile catheter is introduced through the cervix and inserted in the placenta, where a sample of chorionic villi is aspirated. This approach requires the client to have a full bladder to push the uterus and placenta into a position that is more accessible to the catheter. A full bladder also helps in better visualization of the structures. With the transabdominal approach, an 18-gauge spinal needle is inserted through the abdominal wall into the placental tissue and a sample of chorionic villi is aspirated. Regardless of the approach used, the sample is sent to the cytogenetics laboratory for analysis.

Potential complications of CVS include mild vaginal bleeding and cramping, spontaneous abortion, limb abnormalities, rupture of membranes, infection, chorioamnionitis, and fetal-maternal hemorrhage (Blackburn, 2007). The pregnancy loss rate is approximately 1.3%, which is somewhat higher than with traditional amniocentesis (Walling, 2007). In addition, women who are Rh negative should receive immune globulin (RhoGAM) to avoid isoimmunization (Gilbert, 2007).

Nursing Management

Explain to the woman that the procedure will last about 15 minutes. An ultrasound will be done first to locate the embryo, and a baseline set of vital signs will be taken before starting. Make sure she is informed of the risks related to the procedure, including their incidence.

If a transabdominal CVS procedure is planned, advise her to fill her bladder by drinking increased amounts of water. Inform her that a needle will be inserted through her abdominal wall and samples will be collected. Once the samples are collected, the needle will be withdrawn and the samples will be sent to the genetics laboratory for evaluation.

For transcervical CVS, inform the women that a speculum will be placed into the vagina under ultrasound guidance. Then the vagina is cleaned and a small catheter is inserted through the cervix. The samples obtained through the catheter are then sent to the laboratory.

After either procedure, assist the woman to a position of comfort and clean any excess lubricant or secretions from the area. Instruct her about signs to watch for and report, such as fever, cramping, and vaginal bleeding. Urge her not to engage in any strenuous activity for the next 48 hours. Assess the fetal heart rate for changes and administer RhoGAM to an unsensitized Rh-negative woman after the procedure.

Percutaneous Umbilical Blood Sampling

Percutaneous umbilical blood sampling (PUBS) permits the collection of a blood specimen directly from the fetal circulation (Fig. 12.8). This test allows for rapid chromosomal analysis to achieve a timely diagnosis. It is done

FIGURE 12.8 Collecting blood sample for PUBS.

specifically for women at risk for genetic anomalies and those with potential blood disorders, such as blood incompatibility or hemoglobinopathies.

Procedure

Under continuous ultrasound guidance, a fine needle is inserted through the mother's abdomen and uterine wall into an umbilical cord vessel. Specimens can be evaluated for coagulation studies, blood group typing, complete blood count, karyotyping, and blood gas analysis (Singh & Singh, 2008). Fetal infection, Rh incompatibility, and fetal acid–base status can be determined. The blood sample is usually drawn late in the second trimester to assist in medical management, but PUBS can be done anytime after 16 weeks of gestation.

Although the information gained from this procedure is valuable and can be life-saving for many fetuses, PUBS is not without risks. Potential complications include leakage of blood from the puncture site, cord laceration, cord hematomas, transient fetal bradycardia, infection, thromboembolism in the umbilical cord, preterm labor, infection, and premature rupture of membranes (Blackburn, 2007).

Nursing Management

Explain the procedure thoroughly to the woman. Position her properly on the examination table and help clean the area for needle insertion. Monitor vital signs and fetal heart rate throughout the procedure. At the conclusion of the procedure, closely monitor the mother and fetus for changes. Assess fetal heart rate continuously and perform external fetal monitoring for up to 2 hours before the woman is discharged from the outpatient area. A repeat ultrasound is usually done within an hour after the procedure to rule out bleeding or hematoma formation.

Prior to discharge, instruct the woman to report signs of infection, an increase in contractions, or a change in fetal activity level from normal. Reinforce the need to count fetal movements, and review the technique so she can assess them when she is discharged home.

Nonstress Test

The nonstress test (NST) is an indirect measurement of uteroplacental function. Unlike the fetal movement counting done by the mother alone, this procedure requires specialized equipment and trained personnel. The basis for the nonstress test is that the normal fetus produces characteristic fetal heart rate patterns in response to fetal movements. In the healthy fetus there is an acceleration of the fetal heart rate with fetal movement. Currently, an NST is recommended twice weekly (after 28 weeks of gestation) for clients with diabetes and other high-risk conditions, such as IUGR, preeclampsia, postterm pregnancy, renal disease, and multifetal pregnancies (Cunningham et al., 2005).

NST is a noninvasive test that requires no initiation of contractions. It is quick to perform and there are no known side effects. However, it is not as sensitive to fetal oxygen reserves as the contraction stress test, and there is a high false-positive rate (Gilbert, 2007).

Procedure

Before the procedure the client eats a meal to stimulate fetal activity. Then she is placed in the left lateral recumbent position to avoid supine hypotension syndrome. An external electronic fetal monitoring device is applied to her abdomen. The device consists of two belts, each with a sensor. One of the sensors records uterine activity; the second sensor records fetal heart rate. The client is handed an "event marker" with a button that she pushes every time she perceives fetal movement. When the button is pushed, the fetal monitor strip is marked to identify that fetal movement has occurred. The procedure usually lasts 20 to 30 minutes.

Nursing Management

Prior to the NST, explain the testing procedure and have the woman empty her bladder. Position her in a semi-Fowler's position and apply the two external monitor belts. Document the date and time the test is started, patient information, the reason for the test, and the maternal vital signs. Obtain a baseline fetal monitor strip over 15 to 30 minutes.

During the test, observe for signs of fetal activity with a concurrent acceleration of the fetal heart rate. Interpret the NST as reactive or nonreactive. A "reactive" NST includes at least two fetal heart rate accelerations from the baseline of at least 15 bpm for at least 15 seconds within the 20-minute recording period. If the test does not meet these criteria after 40 minutes, it is considered nonreactive. A "nonreactive" NST is characterized by the absence of two fetal heart rate accelerations using the 15-by-15 cri-

terion in a 20-minute time frame. A nonreactive test has been correlated with a higher incidence of fetal distress during labor, fetal mortality, and IUGR. Additional testing, such as a contraction stress test or biophysical profile, should be considered (Frieden & Chan, 2007).

After the NST procedure, assist the woman off the table, provide her with fluids, and allow her to use the restroom. Typically the results are discussed with the woman at this time by the health care provider. Provide teaching about signs and symptoms to report. If serial NSTs are being done, schedule the next testing session.

Contraction Stress Test

Because blood flow to the uterus and placenta is slowed during uterine contractions, the contraction stress test (CST), formerly called the oxytocin-challenge test, is a diagnostic procedure performed to determine the fetal heart rate response under stress, such as during contractions. The goal of the test is to achieve three uterine contractions in a 10-minute period. This can occur spontaneously with the aid of nipple stimulation, which causes the release of endogenous oxytocin, or through the use of an oxytocin infusion. Its use has been indicated in pregnancies in which placental insufficiency is suspected—preeclampsia, IUGR, diabetes mellitus, postterm pregnancy, a previous stillbirth—or when an irregularity of the fetal heart rate has been observed. However, the CST has given way to the biophysical profile and has limited use today (Blackburn, 2007).

Biophysical Profile

A **biophysical profile** uses a real-time ultrasound to allow assessment of various parameters of fetal well-being: fetal tone, breathing, motion, and amniotic fluid volume. These four parameters, together with the NST, constitute the biophysical profile. Each parameter is controlled by a different structure in the fetal brain: fetal tone by the cortex; fetal movements by the cortex and motor nuclei; fetal breathing movements by the centers close to the fourth ventricle; and the NST by the posterior hypothalamus and medulla. The amniotic fluid is the result of fetal urine volume. Not all facilities perform an NST unless other parameters of the profile are abnormal (Gilbert, 2007). The biophysical profile is based on the concept that a fetus that experiences hypoxia loses certain behavioral parameters in the reverse order in which they were acquired during fetal development (normal order of development: tone at 8 weeks; movement at 9 weeks; breathing at 20 weeks; and fetal heart rate reactivity at 24 weeks).

Scoring and Interpretation

The biophysical profile is a scored test with five components, each worth 2 points if present. A total score of 10 is possible if the NST is used. Thirty minutes are allotted for testing, although fewer than 10 minutes are usually needed. The following criteria must be met to obtain a score of 2; anything less is scored as 0 (Gilbert, 2007):

- Body movements: three or more discrete limb or trunk movements
- Fetal tone: one or more instances of full extension and flexion of a limb or trunk
- Fetal breathing: one or more fetal breathing movements of more than 30 seconds
- Amniotic fluid volume: one or more pockets of fluid measuring 2 cm
- NST: normal NST = 2 points; abnormal NST = 0 points

Interpretation of the biophysical profile score can be complicated, depending on several fetal and maternal variables. Because it is indicated as a result of a non-reassuring finding from previous fetal surveillance tests, this test can be used to quantify the interpretation, and intervention can be initiated if appropriate. One of the important factors is the amniotic fluid volume, taken in conjunction with the results of the NST. Amniotic fluid is largely composed of fetal urine. As placental function decreases, perfusion of fetal organs, such as kidneys, decreases, and this can lead to a reduction of amniotic fluid. If oligohydramnios or decreased amniotic fluid is present, the potential exists for antepartum or intrapartum fetal compromise (Gearhart & Sehdev, 2007).

Overall, a score of 8 to 10 is considered normal if the amniotic fluid volume is adequate. A score of 6 or below is suspicious, possibly indicating a compromised fetus; further investigation of fetal well-being is needed.

Because the biophysical profile is an ultrasonographic assessment of fetal behavior, it requires more extensive equipment and more highly trained personnel than other testing modalities. The cost is much greater than with less sophisticated tests. It permits conservative therapy and prevents premature or unnecessary intervention. There are fewer false-positive results than with the NST alone or CST (Gearhart & Sehdev, 2007).

Nursing Management

Nursing management focuses primarily on offering the client support and answering her questions. Expect to complete the NST before scheduling the biophysical profile, and explain why further testing might be needed. Tell the woman that the ultrasound will be done in the diagnostic imaging department.

Nursing Management for the Common Discomforts of Pregnancy

Most women experience common discomforts during pregnancy and ask a nurse's advice about ways to minimize them. However, other women will not bring up their concerns unless asked. Therefore, the nurse needs to address the common discomforts that occur in each trimester at each prenatal visit and provide realistic measures to help the client deal with them (Teaching Guidelines 12.1). Nursing Care Plan 12.1 applies the nursing process to the care of a woman experiencing some discomforts of pregnancy.

First-Trimester Discomforts

During the first 3 months of pregnancy, the woman's body is undergoing numerous changes. Some women experience many discomforts, but others have few. These discomforts are caused by the changes taking place within the body and pass as the pregnancy progresses.

Urinary Frequency or Incontinence

Urinary frequency or incontinence is common in the first trimester because the growing uterus compresses the bladder. This also is a common complaint during the third trimester, especially when the fetal head settles into the pelvis. However, the discomfort tends to improve in the second trimester, when the uterus becomes an abdominal organ and moves away from the bladder region.

After infection and gestational diabetes have been ruled out as causative factors of increased urinary frequency, suggest that the woman decrease her fluid intake 2 to 3 hours before bedtime and limit her intake of caffeinated beverages. Increased voiding is normal, but encourage the client to report any pain or burning during urination. Also explain that increased urinary frequency may subside as she enters her second trimester, only to recur in the third trimester. Teach the client to perform Kegel exercises throughout the day to help strengthen perineal muscle tone, thereby enhancing urinary control and decreasing the possibility of incontinence.

Fatigue

Fatigue plagues all pregnant women, primarily in the first and third trimesters (the highest energy levels typically occur during the second trimester), even if they get their normal amount of sleep at night. First-trimester fatigue most often is related to the many physical changes (e.g., increased oxygen consumption, increased levels of progesterone and relaxin, increased metabolic demands) and psychosocial changes (e.g., mood swings, multiple role demands) of pregnancy. Third-trimester fatigue can be caused by sleep disturbances from increased weight (many women cannot find a comfortable sleeping position due to the enlarging abdomen), physical discomforts such as heartburn, and insomnia due to mood swings, multiple role anxiety, and a decrease in exercise (Trupin, 2006).

Once anemia, infection, and blood dyscrasias have been ruled out as contributing to the client's fatigue, advise

TEACHING GUIDELINES 12.1

Teaching to Manage the Discomforts of Pregnancy

Urinary Frequency or Incontinence

- Try Kegel exercises to increase control over leakage.
- Empty your bladder when you first feel a full sensation.
- Avoid caffeinated drinks, which stimulate voiding.
- Reduce your fluid intake after dinner to reduce nighttime urination.

Fatigue

- Attempt to get a full night's sleep, without interruptions.
- Eat a healthy balanced diet.
- Schedule a nap in the early afternoon daily.
- When you are feeling tired, rest.

Nausea and Vomiting

- Avoid an empty stomach at all times.
- Munch on dry crackers/toast in bed before arising.
- Eat several small meals throughout the day.
- Drink fluids between meals rather than with meals.
- Avoid greasy, fried foods or ones with a strong odor, such as cabbage or Brussels sprouts.

Backache

- Avoid standing or sitting in one position for long periods.
- Apply heating pad (low setting) to the small of your back.
- Support your lower back with pillows when sitting.
- Stand with your shoulders back to maintain correct posture.

Leg Cramps

- Elevate legs above heart level frequently throughout the day.
- If you get a cramp, straighten both legs and flex your feet toward your body.
- Ask your health care provider about taking additional calcium supplements, which may reduce leg spasms.

Varicosities

- Walk daily to improve circulation to extremities.
- Elevate both legs above heart level while resting.
- Avoid standing in one position for long periods of time.
- Don't wear constrictive stockings and socks.
- Don't cross the legs when sitting for long periods.
- Wear support stockings to promote better circulation.

Hemorrhoids

- Establish a regular time for daily bowel elimination.
- Prevent straining by drinking plenty of fluids and eating fiber-rich foods and exercising daily.
- Use warm sitz baths and cool witch hazel compresses for comfort.

Constipation

- Increase your intake of foods high in fiber and drink at least eight 8-ounce glasses of fluid daily.
- Exercise each day (brisk walking) to promote movement through the intestine.
- Reduce the amount of cheese consumed.

Heartburn/Indigestion

- Avoid spicy or greasy foods and eat small frequent meals.
- Sleep on several pillows so that your head is elevated.
- Stop smoking and avoid caffeinated drinks to reduce stimulation.
- Avoid lying down for at least 2 hours after meals.
- Try drinking sips of water to reduce burning sensation.
- Take antacids sparingly if burning sensation is severe.

Braxton Hicks Contractions

- Keep in mind that these contractions are a normal sensation.
- Try changing your position or engaging in mild exercise to help reduce the sensation.
- Drink more fluids if possible.

her to arrange work, childcare, and other demands in her life to permit additional rest periods. Work with the client to devise a realistic schedule for rest. Using pillows for support in the side-lying position relieves pressure on major blood vessels that supply oxygen and nutrients to the fetus when resting (Fig. 12.9). Also recommend the use of relaxation techniques, providing instructions as necessary, and suggest she increase her daily exercise level.

Nausea and Vomiting

Nausea and vomiting are common discomforts during the first trimester: at least 50% of women experience nausea during pregnancy (Hackley, Kriebs, & Rousseau, 2007). The physiologic changes that cause nausea and vomiting are unknown, but research suggests that unusually high levels of estrogen, progesterone, and hCG and a vitamin B6 deficiency may be contributing factors. Symp-

Nursing Care Plan 12.1

OVERVIEW OF THE WOMAN EXPERIENCING COMMON DISCOMFORTS OF PREGNANCY

Alicia, a 32-year-old, G1 P0, at 10 weeks' gestation, comes to the clinic for a visit. During the interview she tells you, "I'm running to the bathroom to urinate it seems like all the time, and I'm so nauseous that I'm having trouble eating." She denies any burning or pain on urination. Vital signs are within acceptable limits.

NURSING DIAGNOSIS: Impaired urinary elimination related to frequency secondary to physiologic changes of pregnancy

Outcome Identification and Evaluation

Client will report a decrease in urinary complaints, as evidenced by a decrease in the number of times she uses the bathroom to void, reports that she feels her bladder is empty after voiding, and use of Kegel exercises.

Interventions: Promoting Normal Urinary Elimination Patterns

- Assess client's usual bladder elimination patterns to establish a baseline for comparison.
- Obtain a urine specimen for analysis to rule out infection or glucosuria.
- Review with client the physiologic basis for the increased frequency during pregnancy; inform client that frequency should abate during the second trimester and that it most likely will return during her third trimester. This will promote understanding of the problem.
- Encourage the client to empty her bladder when first feeling a sensation of fullness to minimize risk of urinary retention.
- Suggest client avoid caffeinated drinks, which can stimulate the need to void.
- Encourage client to drink adequate amounts of fluid throughout the day; however, have client reduce her fluid intake before bedtime to reduce nighttime urination.
- Urge client to keep perineal area clean and dry to prevent irritation and excoriation from any leakage.
- Instruct client in Kegel exercises to increase perineal muscle tone and control over leakage.
- Teach client about the signs and symptoms of urinary tract infection and urge her to report them should they occur to ensure early detection and prompt intervention.

NURSING DIAGNOSIS: Imbalanced nutrition, less than body requirements, related to nausea and vomiting

Outcome Identification and Evaluation

Client will ingest adequate amounts of nutrients for maternal and fetal well-being as evidenced by acceptable weight gain pattern and statements indicating an increase in food intake with a decrease in the number of episodes of nausea and vomiting.

Interventions: Promoting Adequate Nutrition

- Obtain weight and compare to baseline to determine effects of nausea and vomiting on nutritional intake.
- Review client's typical dietary intake over 24 hours to determine nutritional intake and patterns so that suggestions can be individualized.
- Encourage client to eat five or six small frequent meals throughout the day to prevent her stomach from becoming empty.
- Suggest that she munch on dry crackers, toast, cereal, or cheese or drink a small amount of lemonade before arising to minimize nausea.
- Encourage client to arise slowly from bed in the morning and avoid sudden movements to reduce stimulation of the vomiting center.
- Advise client to drink fluids between meals rather than with meals to avoid overdistention of the abdomen and subsequent increase in abdominal pressure.
- Encourage her to increase her intake of foods high in vitamin B6 such as meat, poultry, bananas, fish, green leafy vegetables, peanuts, raisins, walnuts, and whole grains, as tolerated, to ensure adequate nutrient intake.
- Advise the client to avoid greasy, fried, or highly spiced foods and to avoid strong odors, including foods such as cabbage, to minimize gastrointestinal upset.
- Encourage the client to avoid wearing tight or restricting clothes to minimize pressure on the expanding abdomen.
- Arrange for consultation with nutritionist as necessary to assist with diet planning.

FIGURE 12.9 Using pillows for support in the side-lying position.

toms generally last until the second trimester and are generally associated with a positive pregnancy outcome (Cunningham et al., 2005).

To help alleviate nausea and vomiting, advise the woman to eat small, frequent meals (five or six a day) to prevent her stomach from becoming completely empty. Other helpful suggestions include eating dry crackers, Cheerios, lemonade, or cheese before getting out of bed in the morning and increasing her intake of foods high in vitamin B6, such as meat, poultry, bananas, fish, green leafy vegetables, peanuts, raisins, walnuts, and whole grains, or making sure she is receiving enough vitamin B6 by taking her prescribed prenatal vitamins. Other helpful tips to deal with nausea and vomiting include:

• Get out of bed in the morning very slowly.
• Avoid sudden movements.
• Open a window to remove odors of food being cooked.
• Limit intake of fluids or soups during meals (drink them between meals).
• Avoid fried foods and foods cooked with grease, oils, or fatty meats, for they tend to upset the stomach.
• Avoid highly seasoned foods such as those cooked with garlic, onions, peppers, and chili.
• Drink a small amount of caffeine-free carbonated beverage (ginger ale) if nauseated.
• Avoid strong smells.
• Avoid wearing tight or restricting clothes, which might place increased pressure on the expanding abdomen.
• Avoid stress (Lane, 2007).

Breast Tenderness

Due to increased estrogen and progesterone levels, which cause the fat layer of breasts to thicken and the number of milk ducts and glands to increase during the first trimester, many women experience breast tenderness. Offering a thorough explanation to the woman about the reasons for the breast discomfort is important. Wearing a larger bra with good support can help alleviate this discomfort.

Advise her to wear a supportive bra, even while sleeping. As her breasts increase in size, advise her to change her bra size to ensure adequate support.

Constipation

Increasing levels of progesterone during pregnancy lead to decreased contractility of the gastrointestinal tract, slowed movement of substances through the colon, and a resulting increase in water absorption. All of these factors lead to constipation. Lack of exercise or too little fiber or fluids in the diet can also promote constipation. In addition, the large bowel is mechanically compressed by the enlarging uterus, adding to this discomfort. The iron and calcium in prenatal vitamins can also contribute to constipation during the first and third trimesters.

Explain how pregnancy exacerbates the symptoms of constipation and offer the following suggestions:

• Eat fresh or dried fruit daily.
• Eat more raw fruits and vegetables, including their skins.
• Eat whole-grain cereals and breads such as raisin bran or bran flakes.
• Participate in physical activity every day.
• Eat meals at regular intervals.
• Establish a time of day to defecate, and elevate your feet on a stool to avoid straining.
• Drink six to eight glasses of water daily.
• Decrease your intake of refined carbohydrates.
• Drink warm fluids on arising to stimulate bowel motility.
• Decrease your consumption of sugary sodas.
• Avoid eating large amounts of cheese.

If the suggestions above are ineffective, suggest that the woman use a bulk-forming laxative such as Metamucil.

Nasal Stuffiness, Bleeding Gums, Epistaxis

Increased levels of estrogen cause edema of the mucous membranes of the nasal and oral cavities. Advise the woman to drink extra water for hydration of the mucous membranes or to use a cool mist humidifier in her bedroom at night. If she needs to blow her nose to relieve nasal stuffiness, advise her to blow gently, one nostril at a time. Advise her to avoid the use of nasal decongestants and sprays.

If a nosebleed occurs, advise the woman to loosen the clothing around her neck, sit with her head tilted forward, pinch her nostrils with her thumb and forefinger for 10 to 15 minutes, and apply an ice pack to the bridge of her nose.

If the woman has bleeding gums, encourage her to practice good oral hygiene by using a soft toothbrush and flossing daily. Warm saline mouthwashes can relieve discomfort. If the gum problem persists, instruct her to see her dentist.

Cravings

Desires for certain foods and beverages are likely to begin during the first trimester but do not appear to reflect any physiologic need. Foods with a high sodium or sugar content often are the ones craved. At times, some women crave non-food substances such as clay, cornstarch, laundry detergent, baking soda, soap, paint chips, dirt, ice, or wax. This craving for non-food substances, termed pica, may indicate a severe dietary deficiency of minerals or vitamins, or it may have cultural roots (Lynch, 2007). Pica is discussed in Chapter 11.

Leukorrhea

Increased vaginal discharge begins during the first trimester and continues throughout pregnancy. The physiologic changes behind leukorrhea arise from the high levels of estrogen, which cause increased vascularity and hypertrophy of cervical glands as well as vaginal cells (Cunningham et al., 2005). The result is progressive vaginal secretions throughout pregnancy.

Advise the woman to keep the perineal area clean and dry, washing the area with mild soap and water during her daily shower. Also recommend that she avoid wearing pantyhose and other tight-fitting nylon clothes that prevent air from circulating to the genital area. Encourage the use of cotton underwear and suggest wearing a nightgown rather than pajamas to allow for increased airflow. Also instruct the woman to avoid douching and tampon use.

Second-Trimester Discomforts

A sense of well-being typically characterizes the second trimester for most women. By this time, the fatigue, nausea, and vomiting have subsided and the uncomfortable changes of the third trimester are a few months away. Not every woman experiences the same discomforts during this time, so nursing assessments and interventions must be individualized.

Backache

Backache, experienced by many women during the second trimester, is due to a shift in the center of gravity caused by the enlarging uterus. Muscle strain results. In addition, a high level of circulating progesterone softens cartilage and loosens joints, thus increasing discomfort. Upper back pain also can be caused by increased breast size (ACOG, 2007b).

After exploring other reasons that might cause backache, such as uterine contractions, urinary tract infection, ulcers, or musculoskeletal back disorders, the following instructions may be helpful:

- Maintain correct posture, with head up and shoulders back.
- Wear low-heeled shoes with good arch support.
- When standing for long periods, place one foot on a stool or box.
- Use good body mechanics when lifting objects.
- When sitting, use foot supports and pillows behind the back.

- Try pelvic tilt or rocking exercises to strengthen the back (ACOG, 2007b).

The pelvic tilt or pelvic rock is used to alleviate pressure on the lower back during pregnancy by stretching the lower back muscles. It can be done sitting, standing, or on all fours. To do it on all fours, the hands are positioned directly under the shoulders and the knees under the hips. The back should be in a neutral position with the head and neck aligned with the straight back. The woman then presses up with the lower back and holds this position for a few seconds, then relaxes to a neutral position. This action of pressing upward is repeated frequently throughout the day to prevent a sore back (ACOG, 2007b). See Evidence-Based Practice 12.1.

Leg Cramps

Leg cramps occur primarily in the second and third trimesters and could be related to the pressure of the gravid uterus on pelvic nerves and blood vessels (Arenson & Drake, 2007). Diet can also be a contributing factor if the woman is not consuming enough of certain minerals, such as calcium and magnesium. The sudden stretching of leg muscles may also play a role in causing leg cramps (Trupin, 2006).

Encourage the woman to gently stretch the muscle by dorsiflexing the foot up toward the body. Wrapping a warm, moist towel around the leg muscle can also help the muscle to relax. Advise the client to avoid stretching her legs, pointing her toes, and walking excessively. Stress the importance of wearing low-heeled shoes and support hose and arising slowly from a sitting position. If the leg cramps are due to deficiencies in minerals, the condition can be remedied by eating more foods rich in these nutrients. Also instruct the woman on calf-stretching exercises: have her stand 3 feet from the wall and lean toward it, resting her lower arms against it, while keeping her heels on the floor. This may help reduce cramping if it is done before going to bed.

Elevating the legs throughout the day will help relieve pressure and minimize strain. Wearing support hose and avoiding curling the toes may help to relieve leg discomfort. Also instruct the client to avoid standing in one spot for a prolonged period or crossing her legs. If she must stand for prolonged periods, suggest that she change her position at least every 2 hours by walking or sitting to reduce the risk of leg cramps. Encourage her to drink eight 8-ounce glasses of fluid throughout the day to ensure adequate hydration.

Varicosities of the Vulva and Legs

Varicosities of the vulva and legs are associated with the increased venous stasis caused by the pressure of the gravid uterus on pelvic vessels and the vasodilation resulting from increased progesterone levels. Progesterone relaxes the vein walls, making it difficult for blood to return to the heart from the extremities; pooling can result. Genetic predispo-

EVIDENCE-BASED PRACTICE 12.1
Interventions for Preventing and Treating Pelvic and Back Pain in Pregnancy

● Study

More than two thirds of pregnant women experience back pain and almost one fifth experience pelvic pain. The pain increases with advancing pregnancy and interferes with work, daily activities, and sleep. Many women experience back or pelvic pain during pregnancy. This pain generally increases as pregnancy advances and it interferes with daily activities (like carrying, cleaning, sitting, and walking), can prevent women from going to work, and sometimes disturbs sleep. Suggestions to help manage the pain are varied and include special pregnancy exercises, frequent rest, hot and cold compresses, a supportive belt, massage, acupuncture, chiropractic, aromatherapy, relaxation, herbs, yoga, and Reiki. Sometimes drugs like acetaminophen have also been suggested. No studies were found dealing with the prevention of back and pelvic pain.

For treatment, the review of trials found eight studies, involving 1,305 participants, that examined the effects of various pregnancy-specific exercises, physiotherapy programs, acupuncture, and using special pillows added to usual prenatal care. They were compared to usual pregnancy care or other treatments. The quality of the studies was not the best, and so the findings should be treated with caution.

▲ Findings

The review found that specifically tailored strengthening exercises, sitting pelvic tilt exercise programs, and water gymnastics all reported beneficial effects. In addition, acupuncture seemed more effective than physiotherapy. Adverse effects, when reported, appeared minor and transient. More research is needed on this widespread problem of pregnancy.

■ Nursing Implications

Nurses can apply these findings to help pregnant women cope with and actively participate in their therapy to relieve their pelvic and back discomfort. The nurse should offer a thorough explanation of the reasons for the discomfort and then proceed to outline the effective therapies. In addition, the nurse can provide instruction and demonstrate how to go through each exercise.

Source: Pennick, V. E., & Young, G. (2007). Interventions for preventing and treating pelvic and back pain in pregnancy. *Cochrane Database of Systematic Reviews* 2007, Issue 2. Art. No.: CD001139. DOI: 10.1002/14651858.CD001139.pub2.

sition, inactivity, obesity, and poor muscle tone are contributing factors.

Encourage the client to wear support hose and teach her how to apply them properly. Advise her to elevate her legs above her heart while lying on her back for 10 minutes before she gets out of bed in the morning, thus promoting venous return before she applies the hose. Instruct the client to avoid crossing her legs and avoid wearing knee-high stockings. They cause constriction of leg vessels and muscles and contribute to venous stasis. Also encourage the client to elevate both legs above the level of the heart for 5 to 10 minutes at least twice a day (Fig. 12.10); to wear low-heeled shoes; and to avoid long periods of standing or sitting, frequently changing her position. If the client has vulvar varicosities, suggest she apply ice packs to the area when she is lying down. See Evidence-Based Practice 12.2.

Hemorrhoids

Hemorrhoids are varicosities of the rectum and may be external (outside the anal sphincter) or internal (above the sphincter) (ACOG, 2007d). They occur as a result of progesterone-induced vasodilation and from pressure of the enlarged uterus on the lower intestine and rectum.

Hemorrhoids are more common in women with constipation, poor fluid intake or poor dietary habits, smokers, or those with a previous history of hemorrhoids (Arenson & Drake, 2007).

Instruct the client in measures to prevent constipation, including increasing fiber intake and drinking at least 2 liters of fluid per day. Recommend the use of topical anesthetics (e.g., Preparation H, Anusol, witch hazel compresses) to reduce pain, itching, and swelling, if permitted by the health care provider. Teach the client about local comfort measures such as warm sitz baths, witch hazel compresses, or cold compresses. To minimize her risk of straining while defecating, suggest that she elevate her feet on a stool. Also encourage her to avoid prolonged sitting or standing (ACOG, 2007d).

Flatulence With Bloating

The physiologic changes that result in constipation (reduced gastrointestinal motility and dilation secondary to progesterone's influence) may also result in increased flatulence. As the enlarging uterus compresses the bowel, it delays the passage of food through the intestines, thus allowing more time for gas to be formed by bacteria in

FIGURE 12.10 Woman elevating her legs while working.

the colon. The woman usually reports increased passage of rectal gas, abdominal bloating, or belching. Instruct the woman to avoid gas-forming foods, such as beans, cabbage, and onions, as well as foods that have a high content of white sugar. Adding more fiber to the diet, increasing fluid intake, and increasing physical exercise are also helpful in reducing flatus. In addition, reducing the swallowing of air when chewing gum or smoking will reduce gas build-up. Reducing the intake of carbonated beverages and cheese and eating mints can also help reduce flatulence during pregnancy (Trupin, 2006).

Third-Trimester Discomforts

As women enter their third trimester, many experience a return of the first-trimester discomforts of fatigue, urinary frequency, leukorrhea, and constipation. These discomforts are secondary to the ever-enlarging uterus compressing adjacent structures, increasing hormone

---

EVIDENCE-BASED PRACTICE 12.2
Interventions for Varicose Veins and Leg Edema in Pregnancy

● **Study**

Pregnancy is presumed to be a major contributory factor in the increased incidence of varicose veins in women, which can in turn lead to venous insufficiency and leg edema. The most common symptom of varicose veins and edema is substantial pain, as well as night cramps, numbness, and tingling; also, the legs may feel heavy and achy and the veins may be unsightly.

Varicose veins, sometimes called varicosity, occur when a valve in the blood vessel walls weakens and the blood stagnates. This leads to problems with the circulation in the veins and to edema or swelling. The vein then becomes distended and its walls stretch and sag, allowing the vein to swell into a tiny balloon near the surface of the skin. The veins in the legs are most commonly affected as they are working against gravity, but the vulva (vaginal opening) or rectum, resulting in hemorrhoids (piles), can be affected too.

Treatment of varicose veins is usually divided into three main groups: surgery, pharmacological, and non-pharmacological treatments. Treatment for leg edema mostly involves symptom reduction rather than cure and uses pharmacological and non-pharmacological approaches.

The review identified three trials involving 159 women. Although the drug rutoside seemed to be effective in

reducing symptoms, the study was too small to be able to say this with real confidence. Similarly, with compression stockings and reflexology, there were insufficient data to be able to assess benefits and harms, but they looked promising. More research is needed.

▲ **Findings**

Rutoside appears to relieve the symptoms of varicose veins in late pregnancy. However, this finding is based on one small study (69 women), and there are not enough data presented in the study to assess its safety in pregnancy. It therefore cannot be routinely recommended. Reflexology appears to improve symptoms for women with leg edema, but again this is based on one small study (43 women). External compression stockings do not appear to have any advantages in reducing edema.

■ **Nursing Implications**

Nurses can use this evidence to instruct women about varicose veins and outline the various therapies available to treat them. It is not clear that any of the therapies are totally successful in relieving the discomfort associated with varicose veins, based on this analysis, but comfort therapies can be covered to help with the discomfort. Maintaining an ideal weight gain throughout the pregnancy will also help reduce the risk of varicose vein formation.

Source: Bamigboye, A. A., & Smyth, R. (2007). Interventions for varicose veins and leg edema in pregnancy. *Cochrane Database of Systematic Reviews* 2007, Issue 1. Art. No.: CD001066. DOI: 10.1002/14651858.CD001066.pub2.

levels, and the metabolic demands of the fetus. In addition to these discomforts, many women experience shortness of breath, heartburn and indigestion, swelling, and Braxton Hicks contractions.

Shortness of Breath and Dyspnea

The increasing growth of the uterus prevents complete lung expansion late in pregnancy. As the uterus enlarges upward, the expansion of the diaphragm is limited. Dyspnea can occur when the woman lies on her back and the pressure of the gravid uterus against the vena cava reduces venous return to the heart (Arenson & Drake, 2007).

Explain to the woman that dyspnea is normal and will improve when the fetus drops into the pelvis (lightening). Instruct her to adjust her body position to allow for maximum expansion of the chest and to avoid large meals, which increase abdominal pressure. Raising the head of the bed on blocks or placing pillows behind her back is helpful too. In addition, stress that lying on her side will displace the uterus off the vena cava and improve her breathing. Advise the woman to avoid exercise that precipitates dyspnea, to rest after exercise, and to avoid overheating in warm climates. If she still smokes, encourage her to stop.

Heartburn and Indigestion

Heartburn and indigestion result when high progesterone levels cause relaxation of the cardiac sphincter, allowing food and digestive juices to flow backward from the stomach into the esophagus. Irritation of the esophageal lining occurs, causing the burning sensation known as heartburn. It occurs in up to 70% of women at some point during pregnancy, with an increased frequency seen in the third trimester (Blackburn, 2007). The pain may radiate to the neck and throat. It worsens when the woman lies down, bends over after eating, or wears tight clothes. Indigestion (vague abdominal discomfort after meals) results from eating too much or too fast; from eating when tense, tired, or emotionally upset; from eating food that is too fatty or spicy; and from eating heavy food or food that has been badly cooked or processed (Trupin, 2006). In addition, the stomach is displaced upward and compressed by the large uterus in the third trimester, thus limiting the stomach's capacity to empty quickly. Food sits, causing heartburn and indigestion.

Review the client's usual dietary intake and suggest that she limit or avoid gas-producing or fatty foods and large meals. Encourage the client to maintain proper posture and remain in the sitting position for 1 to 3 hours after eating to prevent reflux of gastric acids into the esophagus by gravity. Urge the client to eat slowly, chewing her food thoroughly to prevent excessive swallowing of air, which can lead to increased gastric pressure. Instruct the client to avoid highly spiced foods, chocolate, coffee, alcohol, sodas, and spearmint or peppermint. These items stimulate the release of gastric digestive acids, which may cause reflux into the esophagus. Avoid late-night or large meals and gum chewing.

Dependent Edema

Swelling is the result of increased capillary permeability caused by elevated hormone levels and increased blood volume. Sodium and water are retained and thirst increases. Edema occurs most often in dependent areas such as the legs and feet throughout the day due to gravity; it improves after a night's sleep. Warm weather or prolonged standing or sitting may increase edema. Generalized edema, appearing in the face, hands, and feet, can signal preeclampsia if accompanied by dizziness, blurred vision, headaches, upper quadrant pain, or nausea (Trupin, 2006). This edema should be reported to the health care provider.

Appropriate suggestions to minimize dependent edema include:

- Elevate your feet and legs above the level of the heart.
- Wear support hose when standing or sitting for long periods.
- Change position frequently throughout the day.
- Walk at a sensible pace to help contract leg muscles to promote venous return.
- When taking a long car ride, stop to walk around every 2 hours.
- When standing, rock from the ball of the foot to the toes to stimulate circulation.
- Lie on your left side to keep the gravid uterus off the vena cava to return blood to the heart.
- Avoid foods high in sodium, such as lunch meats, potato chips, and bacon.
- Avoid wearing knee-high stockings.
- Drink six to eight glasses of water daily to replace fluids lost through perspiration.
- Avoid high intake of sugar and fats, because they cause water retention.

Braxton Hicks Contractions

Braxton Hicks contractions are irregular, painless contractions that occur without cervical dilation. Typically they intensify in the third trimester in preparation for labor. In reality, they have been present since early in the pregnancy but may have gone unnoticed. They are thought to increase the tone of uterine muscles for labor purposes (ACOG, 2007e).

Reassure the client that these contractions are normal. Instruct the client in how to differentiate between Braxton Hicks and labor contractions. Explain that true labor contractions usually grow longer, stronger, and closer together and occur at regular intervals. Walking usually strengthens true labor contractions, whereas Braxton Hicks contractions tend to decrease in intensity and taper off. Advise the client to keep herself well hydrated and to rest in a side-lying position to help relieve the discomfort. Suggest that she use breathing techniques such as Lamaze techniques to ease the discomfort.

▶ *Consider* THIS!

One has to wonder sometimes why women go through what they do. During my first pregnancy I was sick for the first 2 months. I would experience waves of nausea from the moment I got out of bed until midmorning. Needless to say, I wasn't the happiest camper around. After the third month, my life seemed to settle down and I was beginning to think that being pregnant wasn't too bad after all. For the moment, I was fooled. Then, during my last 2 months, another wave of discomfort struck—heartburn and constipation—a double whammy! I now feared eating anything that might trigger acid indigestion and also might remain in my body too long. I literally had to become the "fiber queen" to combat these two challenges. Needless to say, my "suffering" was well worth our bright-eyed baby girl in the end.

Thoughts: Despite the various discomforts associated with pregnancy, most women wouldn't change their end result. Do most women experience these discomforts? What suggestions could be made to reduce them?

Nursing Management to Promote Self-Care

Pregnancy is considered a time of health, not illness. Health promotion and maintenance activities are key to promoting an optimal outcome for the woman and her fetus.

Pregnant women commonly have many questions about the changes occurring during pregnancy, how these changes affect their usual routine, such as working, traveling, exercising, or engaging in sexual activity, how the changes influence their typical self-care activities, such as bathing, perineal care, or dental care, and whether these changes are signs of a problem.

▶ *Take* NOTE!

Women may have heard stories about or been told by others what to do and what not to do during pregnancy, leading to many misconceptions and much misinformation.

Nurses can play a major role in providing anticipatory guidance and teaching to foster the woman's responsibility for self-care, helping to clarify misconceptions and correct any misinformation. Educating the client to identify threats to safety posed by her lifestyle or environment

and proposing ways to modify them to avoid a negative outcome are important. Counseling should also include healthy ways to prepare food, advice to avoid medications unless they are prescribed for her, and advice on identifying teratogens within her environment or at work and how to reduce her risk from exposure. The pregnant client can better care for herself and the fetus if her concerns are anticipated and identified by the nurse and are incorporated into teaching sessions at each prenatal visit.

Personal Hygiene

Hygiene is a necessity for the maintenance of good health. Cleansing the skin removes dirt, bacteria, sweat, dead skin cells, and body secretions. Counsel women to wash their hands frequently throughout the day to lower the bacterial count on their hands and under their fingernails. During pregnancy a woman's sebaceous (sweat) glands become more active under the influence of hormones, and sweating is more profuse. This increase may make it necessary to use a stronger deodorant and shower more frequently. The cervical and vaginal glands also produce more secretions during pregnancy. Frequent showering helps to keep the area dry and promotes better hygiene. Encourage the use of cotton underwear to allow greater air circulation. Taking a tub bath in early pregnancy is permitted, but closer to term, when the woman's center of gravity shifts, it is safer to shower to prevent the risk of slipping.

Hot Tubs and Saunas

Caution pregnant women to avoid using hot tubs, saunas, whirlpools, and tanning beds during pregnancy. The heat may cause fetal tachycardia as well as raise the maternal temperature. Exposure to bacteria in hot tubs that have not been cleaned sufficiently is another reason to avoid them during pregnancy.

Perineal Care

The glands in the cervical and vaginal areas become more active during pregnancy secondary to hormonal influences. This increase in activity will produce more vaginal secretions, especially in the last trimester. Advise pregnant women to shower frequently and wear all-cotton underwear to minimize the effects of these secretions. Caution pregnant women not to douche, because douching can increase the risk of infection, and not to wear panty liners, which block air circulation and promote moisture. Explain that they should also avoid perfumed soaps, lotions, perineal sprays, and harsh laundry detergents to help prevent irritation and potential infection.

Dental Care

Research has established that the elevated levels of estrogen and progesterone during pregnancy cause women to be more sensitive to the effects of bacterial dental plaque, which can cause gingivitis, an oral infection characterized by swollen and bleeding gums (Hackley, Kriebs, & Rousseau, 2007). Brushing and flossing teeth twice daily will help reduce bacteria in the mouth. Advise the woman to visit her dentist early in the pregnancy to address any dental caries and have a thorough cleaning to prevent possible infection later in the pregnancy. Advise her to avoid exposure to x-rays by informing the hygienist of the pregnancy. If x-rays are necessary, the abdomen should be shielded with a lead apron.

Researchers are exploring a link between prematurity and periodontitis, an oral infection that spreads beyond the gum tissues to invade the supporting structures of the teeth. Periodontitis is characterized by bleeding gums, loss of tooth attachment, loss of supporting bone, and bad breath due to pus formation. Unfortunately, because this infection is chronic and often painless, women frequently don't realize they have it. Additional guidelines that the nurse should stress regarding maintaining dental health include:

- Seek professional dental care during the first trimester for assessment and care.
- Obtain treatment for dental pain and infection promptly during pregnancy.
- Brush twice daily for 2 minutes, especially before bed, with fluoridated toothpaste and rinse well. Use a soft-bristled toothbrush and be sure to brush at the gum line to remove food debris and plaque to keep gums healthy.
- Eat healthy foods, especially those high in vitamins A, C, and D and calcium.
- Avoid sugary snacks.
- Chew sugar-free gum for 10 minutes after a meal if brushing isn't possible.
- After vomiting, rinse your mouth immediately with baking soda ($\frac{1}{4}$ teaspoon) and warm water (1 cup) to neutralize the acid (Hackley, Kriebs, & Rousseau, 2007).

Breast Care

Since the breasts enlarge significantly and become heavier throughout pregnancy, stress the need to wear a firm, supportive bra with wide straps to balance the weight of the breasts. Instruct the woman to anticipate buying a larger-sized bra about halfway through her pregnancy because of the increasing size of the breasts. Advise her to avoid using soap on the nipple area because it can be very drying. Encourage her to rinse the nipple area with plain water while bathing to keep it clean. The Montgomery glands secrete a lubricating substance that keeps the nipples moist and discourages growth of bacteria, so there is no need to use alcohol or other antiseptics on the nipples.

If the mother has chosen to breastfeed, nipple preparation is unnecessary unless her nipples are inverted and do not become erect when stimulated. Breast shells can be worn during the last 2 months to address this issue (Alexander et al., 2007).

Around week 16 of pregnancy, colostrum secretion begins, which the woman may notice as moisture in her bra. Advise the woman to place breast pads or a cotton cloth in her bra and change them frequently to prevent build-up, which may lead to excoriation.

Clothing

Many contemporary clothes are loose-fitting and layered, so the woman may not need to buy an entirely new wardrobe to accommodate her pregnancy. Some pregnant women may continue to wear tight clothes. Point out that loose clothing will be more comfortable for the client and her expanding waistline.

Advise pregnant women to avoid wearing constricting clothes and girdles that compress the growing abdomen. Urge the woman to avoid knee-high hose, which might impede lower-extremity circulation and increase the risk of developing deep vein thrombosis. Low-heeled shoes will minimize pelvic tilt and possible backache. Wearing layered clothing may be more comfortable, especially toward term, when the woman may feel overheated.

Exercise

Exercise is well tolerated by a healthy woman during pregnancy. It promotes a feeling of well-being, improves circulation, helps reduce constipation, bloating, and swelling, increases energy level, improves posture, helps sleep, promotes relaxation and rest, and relieves the lower back discomfort that often arises as the pregnancy progresses (ACOG, 2007h). However, the duration and difficulty of exercise should be modified throughout pregnancy because of a decrease in performance efficiency with gestational age. Some women continue to push themselves to maintain their prior level of exercise, but most find that as their shape changes and their abdominal area enlarges, they must modify their exercise routines. Modification also helps to reduce the risk of injury caused by laxity of the joints and connective tissue due to the hormonal effects (ACOG, 2007h).

Exercise during pregnancy is contraindicated in women with preterm labor, poor weight gain, anemia, facial and hand edema, pain, hypertension, threatened abortion, dizziness, shortness of breath, incompetent cervix, multiple gestation, decreased fetal activity, cardiac disease, and palpitations (Trupin, 2006).

ACOG has stated that healthy pregnant women can perform the same activity recommended for the general population: 30 minutes or more of moderate exercise every day (ACOG, 2007h; Fig. 12.11). It is believed that pregnancy is a unique time for behavior modification and that healthy behaviors maintained or adopted during

FIGURE 12.11 Exercising during pregnancy.

pregnancy may improve the woman's health for the rest of her life. The excess weight gained in pregnancy, which some women never lose, is a major public health problem (Trupin, 2006). Exercise helps the woman avoid gaining excess weight during pregnancy.

Exercise during pregnancy helps return a woman's body to good health after the baby is born. The long-term benefits of exercise that begin in early pregnancy include improved posture, weight control, and improved muscle tone; exercise also aids in the prevention of osteoporosis after menopause and assists in keeping the birthweight of the fetus within the normal range (Perkins et al., 2007). Teaching Guidelines 12.2 highlights recommendations for exercise during pregnancy.

Sleep and Rest

Getting enough sleep helps a person feel better and promotes optimal performance levels during the day. The body releases its greatest concentration of growth hormone during sleep, helping the body to repair damaged tissue and grow. Also, with the increased metabolic demands during pregnancy, fatigue is a constant challenge to many pregnant women, especially during the first and third trimesters.

The following tips can help promote adequate sleep:

• Stay on a regular schedule by going to bed and waking up at the same times.
• Eat regular meals at regular times to keep external body cues consistent.
• Take time to unwind and relax before bedtime.
• Establish a bedtime routine or pattern and follow it.
• Create a proper sleep environment by reducing the light and lowering the room temperature.

TEACHING GUIDELINES 12.2

Teaching to Promote Exercise During Pregnancy

• Consume liquids before, during, and after exercising.
• Exercise three or four times each week, not sporadically.
• Engage in brisk walking, swimming, biking, or low-impact aerobics; these are considered ideal activities.
• Avoid getting overheated during exercise.
• Reduce the intensity of workouts in late pregnancy.
• Avoid jerky, bouncy, or high-impact movements.
• Avoid lying flat (supine) after the fourth month because of hypotensive effect.
• Use pelvic tilt and pelvic rocking to relieve backache.
• Start with 5 to 10 minutes of stretching exercises.
• Rise slowly following an exercise session to avoid dizziness.
• Avoid activities such as skiing, surfing, scuba diving, and ice hockey.
• Never exercise to the point of exhaustion.

Sources: ACOG (2007b); AAFP (2008); APA (2008).

• Go to bed when you feel tired; if sleep doesn't occur, read a book until you are sleepy.
• Reduce caffeine intake later in the day.
• Limit fluid intake after dinner to minimize trips to the bathroom.
• Exercise daily to improve circulation and well-being.
• Use a modified Sims position to improve circulation in the lower extremities.
• Avoid lying on your back after the fourth month, which may compromise circulation to the uterus.
• Avoid sharply bending your knees, which promotes venous stasis below the knees.
• Keep anxieties and worries out of the bedroom. Set aside a specific area in the home or time of day for them.

Sexual Activity and Sexuality

Pregnancy is characterized by intense biological, psychological, and social changes. These changes have direct and indirect, conscious and unconscious effects on a woman's sexuality. The woman experiences dramatic alterations in her physiology, her appearance, and her body, as well as her relationships. A woman's sexual responses during pregnancy vary widely. Common symptoms such as fatigue, nausea, vomiting, breast soreness, and urinary frequency may reduce her desire for sexual intimacy. However, many women report enhanced sexual desire due to increasing levels of estrogen.

> ▶ **Take** NOTE!
>
> *Fluctuations in sexual desire are normal and a highly individualized response throughout pregnancy.*

The physical and emotional adjustments of pregnancy can cause changes in body image, fatigue, mood swings, and sexual activity. The woman's changing shape, emotional status, fetal activity, changes in breast size, pressure on the bladder, and other common discomforts of pregnancy result in increased physical and emotional demands. These can produce stress on the sexual relationship of the pregnant woman and her partner. However, most women adjust well to the alterations and experience a satisfying sexual relationship (ACOG, 2007c).

Often pregnant women ask whether sexual intercourse is allowed during pregnancy or whether there are specific times when they should refrain from having sex. This is a good opportunity to educate clients about sexual behavior during pregnancy and also to ask about their expectations and individual experience related to sexuality and possible changes. It is also a good time for nurses to address the impact of the changes associated with preg-

nancy on sexual desire and behavior. For example, some women experience increased sexual desire while others experience less. Couples may enjoy sexual activity more because there is no fear of pregnancy and no need to disrupt spontaneity by using birth control. An increase in pelvic congestion and lubrication secondary to estrogen influence may heighten orgasm for many women. Some women have a decrease in desire because of a negative body image, fear of harming the fetus by engaging in intercourse, and fatigue, nausea, and vomiting (Trupin, 2006). A couple may need assistance to adjust to the various changes brought about by pregnancy.

Reassure the women and her partner that sexual activity is permissible during pregnancy unless there is a history of any of the following:

• Vaginal bleeding
• Placenta previa
• Risk of preterm labor
• Multiple gestation
• Incompetent cervix
• Premature rupture of membranes
• Presence of infection (Trupin, 2006)

Inform the couple that the fetus will not be injured by intercourse. Suggest that alternative positions may be more comfortable (e.g., woman on top, side-lying), especially during the later stages of pregnancy.

Many women feel a particular need for closeness during pregnancy, and the woman should communicate this need to her partner (Thies & Travers, 2006). Emphasize to the couple that closeness and cuddling need not culminate in intercourse, and that other forms of sexual expression, such as mutual masturbation, foot massage, holding hands, kissing, and hugging can be very satisfying (Thies & Travers, 2006).

Women will experience a myriad of symptoms, feelings, and physical sensations during their pregnancy. Having a satisfying sexual relationship during pregnancy is certainly possible, but it requires honest communication between partners to determine what works best for them, and a good relationship with their health care provider to ensure safety (March of Dimes, 2007a).

Employment

For the most part, women can continue working until delivery if they have no complications during their pregnancy and the workplace does not present any special hazards (ACOG, 2007a). Hazardous occupations include health care workers, daycare providers, laboratory technicians, chemists, painters, hairstylists, veterinary workers, and carpenters (ACOG, 2007a). Jobs requiring strenuous work such as heavy lifting, climbing, carrying heavy objects, and standing for prolonged periods place a pregnant woman at risk if modifications are not instituted.

Assess for environmental and occupational factors that place a pregnant women and her fetus at risk for injury. Interview the woman about her employment environment. Ask about possible exposure to teratogens (substances with the potential to alter the fetus permanently in form or function) and the physical demands of employment: Is she exposed to temperature extremes? Does she need to stand for prolonged periods in a fixed position? A description of the work environment is important in providing anticipatory guidance to the woman. Stress the importance of taking rest periods throughout the day, because constant physically intensive workloads increase the likelihood of low birthweight and preterm labor and birth (Cunningham et al., 2005).

Due to the numerous physiologic and psychosocial changes that women experience during their pregnancies, the employer may need to make special accommodations to reduce the pregnant woman's risk of hazardous exposures and heavy workloads. The employer may need to provide adequate coverage so that the woman can take rest breaks; remove the woman from any areas where she might be exposed to toxic substances; and avoid work assignments that require heavy lifting, hard physical labor, continuous standing, or constant moving. Some recommendations for working while pregnant are given in Teaching Guidelines 12.3.

Travel

Pregnancy does not curtail a woman's ability to travel in a car or in a plane. However, women should follow a few safety guidelines to minimize risk to themselves and their fetuses. According to ACOG, pregnant women can travel safely throughout their pregnancy, although the second trimester is perhaps the best time to travel because there is the least chance of complications (ACOG, 2007f). Pregnant women considering international travel should evaluate the problems that could occur during the journey as well as the quality of medical care available at the destination.

▶ *Take* NOTE!

In general, pregnant women with serious underlying illnesses should not travel to developing countries (CDC, 2007c).

Advise pregnant women to be aware of the potential for injuries and trauma related to traveling, and teach women ways to prevent these from occurring. Teaching Guidelines 12.4 offers tips for safe travel on planes and to foreign areas.

When traveling by car, the major risk is a car accident. The impact and momentum can lead to traumatic separation of the placenta from the wall of the uterus. Shock and massive hemorrhage might result (Trupin, 2006). Tips that nurses can offer to promote safety during ground travel include:

- Always wear a three-point seat belt, no matter how short the trip, to prevent ejection or serious injury from collision.
- Apply a nonpadded shoulder strap properly; it should cross between the breasts and over the upper abdomen, above the uterus (Fig. 12.12).
- If no seat belts are available (buses or vans), ride in the back seat of the vehicle.
- Use a lap belt that crosses over the pelvis below the uterus.
- Deactivate the airbag if possible. If you can't, move the seat as far back from the dashboard as possible to minimize impact on the abdomen.
- Avoid using a cellular phone while driving to prevent distraction.
- Avoid driving when very fatigued in the first and third trimesters.
- Avoid late-night driving, when visibility might be compromised.
- Direct a tilting steering wheel away from the abdomen (Hackley, Kriebs, & Rousseau, 2007).

Immunizations and Medications

Ideally, clients should receive all childhood immunizations before conception to protect the fetus from any risk of congenital anomalies. If the client comes for a preconception visit, discuss immunizations such as measles, mumps, and rubella (MMR), hepatitis B, and diphtheria/tetanus (every 10 years); administer them at this time if needed.

TEACHING GUIDELINES 12.3

Teaching for the Pregnant Working Woman

- Plan to take two 10- to 15-minute breaks within an 8-hour workday.
- Be sure there is a place available for you to rest, preferably in the side-lying position, with a restroom readily available.
- Avoid jobs that require strenuous workloads; if this is not possible, then request a modification of work duties (lighter tasks) to reduce your workload.
- Change your position from standing to sitting or vice versa at least every 2 hours.
- Ensure that you are allowed time off without penalty, if necessary, to ensure a healthy outcome for you and your fetus.
- Make sure the work environment is free of toxic substances.
- Ensure the work environment is smoke-free so passive smoking isn't a concern.
- Minimize heavy lifting if associated with bending.

TEACHING GUIDELINES 12.4

Teaching to Promote Safe Travel on Planes and in Foreign Countries

• Bring along a copy of the prenatal record if your travel will be prolonged in case there is a medical emergency away from home.
• When traveling abroad, carry a foreign dictionary that includes words or phrases for the most common pregnancy emergencies.
• Travel with at least one companion at all times for personal safety.
• Check with your health care provider before receiving any immunizations necessary for foreign travel; some may be harmful to the fetus.
• When in a foreign country, avoid fresh fruit, vegetables, and local water.
• Avoid any milk that is not pasteurized.
• Eat only meat that is well cooked to avoid exposure to toxoplasmosis.
• Request an aisle seat and walk about the airplane every 2 hours.
• While sitting on long flights, practice calf-tensing exercises to improve circulation to the lower extremities.
• Be aware of typical problems encountered by pregnant travelers, such as fatigue, heartburn, indigestion, constipation, vaginal discharge, leg cramps, urinary frequency, and hemorrhoids.
• Always wear support hose while flying to prevent the development of blood clots.
• Drink plenty of water to keep well hydrated throughout the flight.

Sources: ACOG (2007f); APA (2008).

The risk to a developing fetus from vaccination of the mother during pregnancy is primarily theoretical. Routine immunizations are not usually indicated during pregnancy. However, no evidence exists of risk from vaccinating pregnant women with inactivated virus or bacterial vaccines or toxoids. A number of other vaccines have not been adequately studied, and thus theoretical risks of vaccination must be weighed against the risks of the disease to mother and fetus (Hackley, Kriebs, & Rousseau, 2007).

▶ **Take** NOTE!

Advise pregnant women to avoid live virus vaccines (MMR and varicella) and to avoid becoming pregnant within 1 month of having received one of these vaccines because of the theoretical risk of transmission to the fetus (CDC, 2007a).

FIGURE 12.12 Proper application of a seat belt during pregnancy.

CDC guidelines for vaccine administration are highlighted in Box 12.4.

It is best for pregnant women not to take any medications. At the very least, encourage them to discuss with the health care provider their current medications and any herbal remedies they take so that they can learn about any potential risks should they continue to take them during pregnancy. Generally, if the woman is taking medicine for seizures, high blood pressure, asthma, or depression,

---

BOX 12.4 **CDC Guidelines for Vaccine Administration During Pregnancy**

Vaccines That Should be Considered If Otherwise Indicated
• Hepatitis B
• Influenza (inactivated)
• Tetanus/diphtheria
• Meningococcal
• Rabies

Vaccines Contraindicated During Pregnancy
• Influenza (live, attenuated vaccine)
• Measles
• Mumps
• Rubella
• Varicella

Sources: CDC (2007a); March of Dimes (2008); Future Medicine (2007).

the benefits of continuing the medicine during pregnancy outweigh the risks to the fetus. The safety profile of some medications may change according to the gestational age of the fetus (Trupin, 2006).

The Food and Drug Administration has developed a system of ranking drugs that appears on the labels and in the package inserts. These risk categories are summarized in Box 12.5. Always advise women to check with the health care provider for guidance.

A common concern of many pregnant women involves the use of over-the-counter medications and herbal agents. Many women consider these products benign simply because they are available without a prescription (Cragan et al., 2006). While herbal medications are commonly thought of as "natural" alternatives to other medicines, they can be just as potent as some prescription medications. A major concern about herbal medicine is the lack of consistent potency in the active ingredients in any given batch of product, making it difficult to know the exact strength by reading the label. Also, many herbs contain chemicals that cross the placenta and may cause harm to the fetus.

> **BOX 12.5 FDA Pregnancy Risk Classification of Drugs**
>
> - Category A: These drugs have been tested and found safe during pregnancy. Examples: folic acid, vitamin B6, and thyroid medicine.
> - Category B: These drugs have been used frequently during pregnancy and do not appear to cause major birth defects or other fetal problems. Examples: antibiotics, acetaminophen (Tylenol), aspartame (artificial sweetener), famotidine (Pepcid), prednisone (cortisone), insulin, and ibuprofen.
> - Category C: These drugs are more likely to cause problems and safety studies have not been completed. Examples: prochlorperazine (Compazine), fluconazole (Diflucan), ciprofloxacin (Cipro), and some antidepressants.
> - Category D: These drugs have clear health risks for the fetus. Examples: alcohol, lithium (treats bipolar disorders), phenytoin (Dilantin); all chemotherapeutic agents used to treat cancer.
> - Category X: These drugs have been shown to cause birth defects and should never be taken during pregnancy. Examples: Accutane (treats cystic acne), androgens (treat endometriosis), Coumadin (prevents blood clots), antithyroid medications for overactive thyroid; radiation therapy (cancer treatment), Tegison or Soriatane (treats psoriasis), streptomycin (treats tuberculosis); thalidomide (treats insomnia), diethylstilbestrol (DES) (treats menstrual disorders), and organic mercury from contaminated food.

Sources: Trupin (2006); USDHHS (2007).

Nurses are often asked about the safety of over-the-counter medicines and herbal agents. Unfortunately, many drugs have not been evaluated in controlled studies, and it is difficult to make general recommendations for these products. Therefore, encourage pregnant women to check with their health care provider before taking anything. Questions about the use of over-the-counter and herbal products are part of the initial prenatal interview.

Nursing Management to Prepare the Woman and Her Partner for Labor, Birth, and Parenthood

Childbirth today is a very different experience from childbirth in previous generations. In the past, women were literally "put to sleep" with anesthetics, and they woke up with a baby. Most women never remembered the details and had a passive role in childbirth as the physician delivered the newborn. In the 1950s, consumers began to insist on taking a more active role in their health care, and couples desired to be together during the extraordinary event of childbirth. Beginning in the 1970s, the father or significant other support person remained with the mother throughout labor and birth (Lleras, 2007).

Childbirth education began because women demanded to become more involved in their birthing experience rather than simply turning control over to a health care provider. Nurses played a pivotal role in bringing about this change by providing information and supporting clients and their families, fostering a more active role in preparing for the upcoming birth.

Traditional childbirth education classes focused on developing and practicing techniques for use in managing pain and facilitating the progress of labor. Recently, the focus of this education has broadened: it now encompasses not only preparation for childbirth, but also preparation for breastfeeding, infant care, transition to new parenting roles, relationship skills, family health promotion, and sexuality (Risica & Phipps, 2007). The term used to describe this broad range of topics is **perinatal education**. Subjects commonly addressed in perinatal education include:

- Anatomy and physiology of reproduction
- Fetal growth and development
- Prenatal maternal exercise
- Physiologic and emotional changes during pregnancy
- Sex during pregnancy
- Infant growth and development
- Nutrition and healthy eating habits during pregnancy
- Teratogens and their impact on the fetus
- Signs and symptoms of labor
- Preparation for labor and birth (for parents, siblings, and other family members)
- Options for birth
- Infant nutrition, including preparation for breastfeeding
- Infant care, including safety, CPR, and first aid
- Family planning (March of Dimes, 2007b)

Childbirth Education Classes

Childbirth education classes teach pregnant women and their support person about pregnancy, birth, and parenting. The classes are offered in local communities or online and are usually taught by certified childbirth educators.

Most childbirth classes support the concept of **natural childbirth** (a birth without pain-relieving medications) so that the woman can be in control throughout the experience as much as possible. The classes differ in their approach to specific comfort techniques and breathing patterns. The three most common childbirth methods are the Lamaze (psychoprophylactic) method, the Bradley (partner-coached childbirth) method, and the Dick-Read (natural childbirth) method.

Lamaze Method

Lamaze is a psychoprophylactic ("mind prevention") method of preparing for labor and birth that promotes the use of specific breathing and relaxation techniques. Dr. Fernand Lamaze, a French obstetrician, popularized this method of childbirth preparation in the 1960s. Lamaze believed that conquering fear through knowledge and support was important. He also believed women needed to alter the perception of suffering during childbirth. This perception change would come about by learning conditioned reflexes that, instead of signaling pain, would signal the work of producing a child, and thus would carry the woman through labor awake, aware, and in control of her own body (Leonard, 2007). Lamaze felt strongly that all women have the right to deliver their babies with minimal or no medication while maintaining their dignity, minimizing their pain, maximizing their self-esteem, and enjoying the miracle of birth.

Lamaze classes include information on toning exercises, relaxation exercises and techniques, and breathing methods for labor. The breathing techniques are used in labor to enhance relaxation and to reduce the woman's perception of pain. The goal is for women to become aware of their own comfortable rate of breathing in order to maintain relaxation and adequate oxygenation of the fetus. Breathing techniques are an effective attention-focusing strategy to reduce pain.

Paced breathing involves breathing techniques used to decrease stress responses and therefore decrease pain. This type of breathing implies self-regulation by the woman. The woman starts off by taking a cleansing breath at the onset and end of each contraction. This cleansing breath symbolizes freeing her mind from worries and concerns. This breath enhances oxygenation and puts the woman in a relaxed state.

Slow-paced breathing is associated with relaxation and should be half the normal breathing rate (six to nine breaths per minute). This type of breathing is the most relaxed pattern and is recommended throughout labor.

Abdominal or chest breathing may be used. It is generally best to breathe in through the nose and breathe out either through the nose or mouth, whichever is more comfortable for the woman.

Modified-paced breathing can be used for increased work or stress during labor to increase alertness or focus attention or when slow-paced breathing is no longer effective in keeping the woman relaxed. The woman's respiratory rate increases, but it does not exceed twice her normal rate. Modified-paced breathing is a quiet upper chest breath that is increased or decreased according to the intensity of the contraction. The inhalation and the exhalation are equal. This breathing technique should be practiced during pregnancy for optimal use during labor.

Patterned-paced breathing is similar to modified-paced breathing but with a rhythmic pattern. It uses a variety of patterns, with an emphasis on the exhalation breath at regular intervals. Different patterns can be used, such as 4/1, 6/1, 4/1. A 4/1 rhythm is four upper chest breaths followed by an exhalation (a sighing out of air, like blowing out a candle). Random patterns can be chosen for use as long as the basic principles of rate and relaxation are met.

Couples practice these breathing patterns typically during the last few months of the pregnancy until they feel comfortable using them. Focal points (visual fixation on a designated object), effleurage (light abdominal massage), massage, and imagery (journey of the mind to a relaxing place) are also added to aid in relaxation. From the nurse's perspective, encourage the woman to breathe at a level of comfort that allows her to cope. Always remain quiet during the woman's periods of imagery and focal point visualization to avoid breaking her concentration.

Bradley Method (Partner-Coached)

The Bradley method uses various exercises and slow, controlled abdominal breathing to accomplish relaxation. Dr. Robert Bradley, a Denver-based obstetrician, advocated a completely unmedicated labor and birth experience. The Bradley method emphasizes the pleasurable sensations of childbirth, teaching women to concentrate on these sensations while "turning on" to their own bodies (Leonard, 2007). In 1965, he wrote *Husband-Coached Childbirth*, which advocated the active participation of the husband as labor coach.

A woman is conditioned to work in harmony with her body using breath control and deep abdominopelvic breathing to promote general body relaxation during labor. This method stresses that childbirth is a joyful, natural process and emphasizes the partner's involvement during pregnancy, labor, birth, and the early newborn period. Thus, the training techniques are directed toward the coach, not the mother. The coach is educated in massage/comfort techniques to use on the mother throughout the labor and birth process.

Dick-Read Method

In 1944 Grantly Dick-Read, a British obstetrician, wrote *Childbirth Without Fear.* He believed that the attitude of a woman toward her birthing process had a considerable influence on the ease of her labor, and he believed that fear is the primary pain-producing agent in an otherwise normal labor. He felt that fear builds a state of tension, creating an antagonistic effect on the laboring muscles of the uterus, which results in pain. Pain causes more fear, which further increases the tension, and the vicious cycle of "fear–tension–pain" is established (Leonard, 2007). Dick-Read sought to interrupt the circular pattern of fear, tension, and pain during the labor and birthing process. He promoted the belief that the degree of fear could be diminished with increased understanding of the normal physiologic response to labor (Alexander et al., 2007).

Dick-Read believed that prenatal instruction was essential for pain relief and that emotional factors during labor interfered with the normal labor progression. The woman achieves relaxation and reduces pain by arming herself with the knowledge of normal childbirth and using abdominal breathing during contractions.

Nursing Management and Childbirth Education

Childbirth education is less about methods than about mastery. The overall aim of any of the methods is to promote an internal locus of control that will enable each woman to yield her body to the process of birth. As the woman gains success and tangible benefits from the exercises she is taught, she begins to reframe her beliefs and gains practical knowledge, and the impetus will be there for her to engage in the conscious use of the techniques (Fig. 12.13). Nurses play a key role in supporting and encouraging each couple's use of the techniques taught in childbirth education classes.

Every woman's labor is unique, and it is important for nurses not to generalize or stereotype women. The most effective support a nurse can offer couples using prepared childbirth methods is encouragement and presence. These nursing measures must be adapted to each individual throughout the labor process. Offering encouraging phrases such as "great job" or "you can do it" helps to reinforce their efforts and at the same time empowers them to continue. Using eye-to-eye contact to engage the woman's total attention is important if she appears overwhelmed or appears to lose control during the transition phase of labor.

Nurses play a significant role in enhancing the couple's relationship by respecting the involvement of the partner and demonstrating concern for his needs throughout labor. Offering to stay with the woman to give him a break periodically allows him to meet his needs while at the same time still actively participating. Offer anticipatory guidance to the couple and assist during critical times in labor. Demonstrate many of the coping techniques to the partner and praise their successful use, which increases self-esteem. Focus on their strengths and the positive elements of the labor experience. Congratulating the couple for a job well done is paramount.

Throughout the labor experience, demonstrate personal warmth and project a friendly attitude. Frequently, a nurse's touch may help to prevent a crisis by reassuring the mother that she is doing fine.

Options for Birth Settings and Care Providers

From the moment a woman discovers she is pregnant, numerous decisions await her—where the infant will be born, what birth setting is best, and who will assist with the birth. The great majority of women are well and healthy and can consider the full range of birth settings—hospital, birth center, or home setting—and care providers. They should be given information about each to ensure the most informed decision.

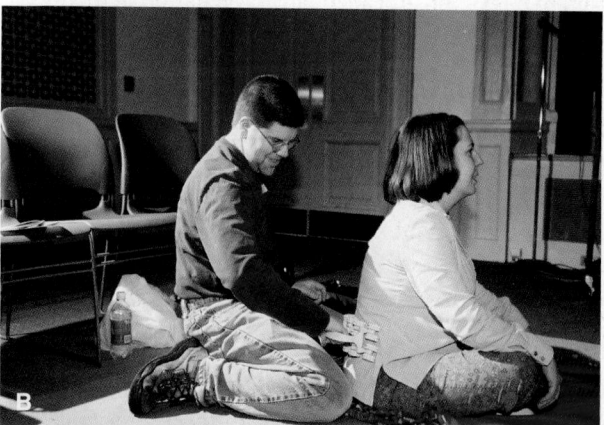

FIGURE **12.13** A couple practicing the techniques taught in a childbirth education class.

Birth Settings

Hospitals are the most common site for birth in the United States. If the woman has a serious medical condition or is at high risk for developing one, she will probably need to plan to give birth in a hospital setting under the care of an obstetrician. Giving birth in a hospital is advantageous for several reasons. Hospitals are best equipped to diagnose and treat women and newborns with complications; trained personnel are available if necessary; and no transportation is needed if a complication should arise during labor or birth. Disadvantages include the high-tech atmosphere; strict policies and restrictions that might limit who can be with the woman; and the medical model of care.

Within the hospital setting, however, choices do exist regarding birth environments. The conventional delivery room resembles an operating room, where the health care professional delivers the newborn from the woman, who is positioned in stirrups. The woman is then transferred to the recovery area on a stretcher and then again to the postpartum unit. The birthing suite is the other option within the hospital setting. In the birthing suite, the woman and her partner remain in one place for labor, birth, and recovery. The birthing suite is a private room decorated to look as homelike as possible. For example, the bed converts to allow for various birthing positions, and there may be a rocking chair or an easy chair for the woman's partner. Despite the homey atmosphere, the room is still equipped with emergency resuscitative obstetric equipment and electronic fetal monitors in case they are needed quickly (Fig. 12.14A). Such settings provide a more personal childbirth experience in a less formal and intimidating atmosphere compared to the traditional delivery room.

A freestanding birth center (Fig. 12.14B) can be a good choice for a woman who wants more personalized care than in a hospital but does not feel comfortable with a home birth. In contrast to the institutional environment in hospitals, most freestanding birth centers have a homelike atmosphere, and many are, in fact, located in converted homes. Some are located on hospital property and are affiliated with them. Birth centers are designed to provide maternity care to women judged to be at low risk for obstetric complications. Women are allowed and encouraged to give birth in the position most comfortable for them. Care in birth centers is often provided by midwives and is more relaxed, with no routine intravenous lines, fetal monitoring, and restrictive protocols. A disadvantage of the birth center is the need to transport the woman to a hospital quickly if an emergency arises, because emergency equipment is not readily available. In a research study comparing homelike to conventional institutional settings, the author concluded that there appeared to be some benefits from homelike settings for childbirth, although increased support from caregivers may be more important (Walsh, 2007).

Most women who choose a home birth believe that birth is a natural process that requires little medical intervention (Mayor, 2007). Home births can be safe if there are qualified, experienced attendants and an emergency transfer system in place in case of serious complications. Many women choose the home setting out of a strong desire to control their child's birth and to give birth surrounded by family members. Most home birth caregivers are midwives who have provided continuous care to the woman throughout the pregnancy. Disadvantages include the need to transport the woman to the hospital during or after labor if a problem arises, and the limited pain management available in the home setting.

Care Providers

While most women in the United States still receive pregnancy care from an obstetrician, an increasing number are choosing a midwife for their care. The difference is a matter of degrees. Obstetricians must finish a 4-year residency in obstetrics and gynecology in addition to medical school. Certified nurse-midwives complete 1 to 2 years of graduate work in midwifery following nursing school. Obstetricians can handle high-risk pregnancies and delivery emergencies; can administer or order pain-relief

FIGURE 12.14 (**A**) Birthing suite. (**B**) Birthing center.

drugs; and are assisted by a support staff in the hospital setting. Midwives work in hospitals, birthing centers, and home settings to deliver care. They believe in the normalcy of birth and tolerate wide variations of what is considered normal during labor, which leads to fewer interventions applied during the childbirth process (Knowlton, 2007). They are not able to handle high-risk births and some birth emergencies.

In addition to the woman's primary health care professional, some women hire a doula to be with them during the childbearing process. Doula is a Greek word that means "woman's servant." A doula is a laywoman trained to provide women and their families with encouragement, emotional and physical support, and information through late pregnancy, labor, birth, and postpartum. Doulas provide the woman with continuous support throughout labor but do not perform any clinical procedures.

Preparation for Breastfeeding or Bottle-Feeding

Pregnant women are faced with a decision about which method of feeding to choose. Educate the pregnant client about the advantages and disadvantages of each method, allowing the woman and her partner to make an informed decision about the best method for their situation. Providing the client and her partner with this information will increase the likelihood of a successful experience regardless of the method of feeding chosen.

Breastfeeding
Substantial scientific evidence exists documenting the health benefits of breastfeeding for newborns. Human milk provides an ideal balance of nutrients for newborns (ACOG, 2006). Breastfeeding is advantageous for the following reasons:

- Human milk is digestible and economical and requires no preparation.
- Bonding between mother and child is promoted.
- Cost is less than purchasing formula.
- Ovulation is suppressed (however, this is not a reliable birth control method).
- The risk of ovarian cancer and the incidence of premenopausal breast cancer are reduced for the woman.
- Extra calories are used, which promotes weight loss gradually without dieting.
- Oxytocin is released to promote more rapid uterine involution with less bleeding.
- Sucking helps to develop the muscles in the infant's jaw.
- Absorption of lactose and minerals in the newborn is improved.
- The immunologic properties of breast milk help prevent infections in the baby.
- The composition of breast milk adapts to meet the infant's changing needs.

- Constipation in the baby is not a problem with adequate intake.
- Food allergies are less likely to develop in the breast-fed baby.
- The incidence of otitis media and upper respiratory infections in the infant is reduced.
- Breastfed babies are less likely to be overfed, thus reducing the risk of adult obesity.
- Breastfed newborns are less prone to vomiting (ACOG, 2006).

One could say that lactation and breastfeeding are so natural that they should just happen on their own accord, but this is not the case. Learning to breastfeed takes practice, requires support from the partner, and requires dedication and patience on the part of the mother; it may be necessary to work closely with a lactation consultant to be successful and comfortable in doing it.

Breastfeeding also has disadvantages. These include breast discomfort, sore nipples, mastitis, engorgement, milk stasis, vaginal dryness, and decreased libido (Blackburn, 2007). Some mothers feel it is inconvenient or embarrassing, limits other activities, limits partner involvement, increases their dependency by being tied to the infant all the time, and restricts their use of alcohol or drugs. Nurses can help mothers to cope with their fear of dependency and feelings of obligation by emphasizing the positive aspects of breastfeeding and encouraging bonding experiences.

Nipple preparation is not necessary during the prenatal period unless the nipples are inverted and do not become erect when stimulated. Assess for this by placing the forefinger and thumb above and below the areola and compressing behind the nipple. If it flattens or inverts, advise the client to wear breast shields during the last 2 months of pregnancy. Breast shields exert a continuous pressure around the areola, pushing the nipple through a central opening in the inner shield (ACOG, 2006). The shields are worn inside the bra. Initially the shields are worn for 1 hour, and then the woman progressively increases the wearing time up to 8 hours daily. The client maintains this schedule until after delivery, and then she wears the shield 24 hours a day until the infant latches on easily (ACOG, 2006). In addition, suggest that the woman wear a supportive nursing bra 24 hours a day.

Encourage the woman to attend a breastfeeding support group (e.g., La Leche League), provide her with sources of information about infant feeding, and suggest that she read a good reference book about lactation. All of these activities will help in her decision-making process and will be invaluable to her should she choose to breastfeed her newborn.

Bottle Feeding
Bottle-feeding an infant isn't just a matter of "open, pour, and feed." Parents need information on types of

formulas, preparation and storage of formula, equipment, and feeding positions. It is recommended that normal full-term infants receive conventional cow's milk-based formula; the physician should direct this choice. If the infant has a reaction (diarrhea, vomiting, abdominal pain, excessive gas) to the first formula, another formula should be tried. Sometimes a soy-based formula is substituted. In terms of preparation of formula and its use, the following guidelines should be stressed:

• Obtain adequate equipment (six 4-ounce bottles, eight 8-ounce bottles, and nipples).
• Consistency is important. Stay with a nipple that is comfortable to the infant.
• Frequently assess nipples for any loose pieces of rubber at the opening.
• Correct formula preparation is critical to the health and development of the infant. Formula is available in three forms: ready-to-feed, concentrate, and powder.
• Read the formula label thoroughly before mixing.
• Correct formula dilution is important to avoid fluid imbalances. For ready-to-use, use as is without dilution. For concentrated formulas, dilute with equal parts of water. For powdered formulas, mix one scoop of powder with 2 ounces of water.
• If the water supply is safe, sterilization is not necessary.
• Bottles and nipples should be washed in hot, sudsy water using a bottle brush.
• Formula should be served at room temperature.
• If the water supply is questionable, water should be boiled for 5 minutes before use.
• Formula should not be heated in a microwave oven, because it is heated unevenly.
• Formula can be prepared 24 hours ahead of time and stored in the refrigerator.

Teach the woman and other caretakers to feed the infant in a semi-upright position using the cradle hold in the arms. This position allows for face-to-face contact between the infant and caretaker. Advise the caretaker to hold the bottle so that the nipple is kept full of formula to prevent excessive air swallowing. Instruct the caretaker to feed the infant every 3 to 4 hours and adapt the feeding times to the infant's needs. Frequent burping of the infant (every ounce) helps prevent gas from building up in the stomach. Caution the caretaker not to prop the bottle; propping the bottle can cause choking (Lawson, 2007).

Bottle-feeding should mirror breastfeeding as closely as possible. While nutrition is important, so are the emotional and interactive components of feeding. Encourage the caretaker to cuddle the infant closely and position the infant so that his or her head is in a comfortable position. Also encourage communication with the infant during feedings.

▶ **Take** NOTE!

Warn the caretaker about the danger of putting the infant to bed with a bottle; this can lead to "baby bottle tooth decay" because sugars in the formula stay in contact with the infant's developing teeth for prolonged periods.

Final Preparation for Labor and Birth

The nurse has played a supportive/education role for the couple throughout the pregnancy and now needs to assist in preparing them for their "big event" by making sure they have made informed decisions and completed the following checklist:

• Attended childbirth preparation classes and practiced breathing techniques
• Selected a birth setting and made arrangements there
• Know what to expect during labor and birth
• Toured the birthing facility
• Packed a suitcase to take to the birthing facility when labor starts
• Made arrangements to have siblings and/or pets taken care of during labor
• Have been instructed on signs and symptoms of labor and what to do
• Know what to do if membranes rupture prior to going into labor
• Know how to reach their health care professional when labor starts
• Communicated their needs and desires concerning pain management
• Discussed the possibility of a cesarean birth if complications occur
• Discussed possible names for the newborn
• Selected a feeding method (bottle or breast) with which they feel comfortable
• Made a decision regarding circumcision if they have a boy
• Purchased an infant safety seat in which to bring their newborn home
• Decided on a pediatrician
• Have items needed to prepare for the newborn's homecoming:
  • Infant clothes in several sizes
  • Nursing bras
  • Infant crib with spaces between the slats that are 2⅜ inches or less apart
  • Diapers (cloth or disposable)
  • Feeding supplies (bottles and nipples if bottle-feeding)
  • Infant thermometer
• Selected a family planning method to use after the birth

At each prenatal visit the nurse has had the opportunity to discuss and reinforce the importance of being prepared for the birth of the child with the parents. It is now up to the parents to use the nurse's guidance and put it into action to be ready for their upcoming "big event."

▰▰▰ Key Concepts

▰ Preconception care is the promotion of the health and well-being of a woman and her partner before pregnancy. The goal of preconception care is to identify any areas such as health problems, lifestyle habits, or social concerns that might unfavorably affect pregnancy.

▰ A thorough history and physical examination is performed on the initial prenatal visit.

▰ A primary aspect of nursing management during the antepartum period is counseling and educating the pregnant women and her partner to promote healthy outcomes for all involved.

▰ Nagele's rule can be used to establish the estimated date of birth. Using this rule, subtract 3 months, add 7 days to the first day of the last normal menstrual period, then correct the year by adding 1 to it. This date is within plus or minus 2 weeks (margin of error).

▰ Pelvic shape is typically classified as one of four types: gynecoid, android, anthropoid, and platypelloid. The gynecoid type is the typical female pelvis and offers the best shape for a vaginal delivery.

▰ Continuous prenatal care is important for a successful outcome. The recommended schedule is every 4 weeks up to 28 weeks (7 months); every 2 weeks from 29 to 36 weeks; and every week from 37 weeks to birth.

▰ The height of the fundus is measured when the uterus arises out of the pelvis to evaluate fetal growth.

▰ The fundus reaches the level of the umbilicus at approximately 20 weeks and measures 20 cm. Fundal measurement should approximately equal the number of weeks of gestation until week 36.

▰ At each visit the woman is asked whether she is having any common signs or symptoms of preterm labor, which might include uterine contractions, dull backache, pressure in the pelvic area or thighs, increased vaginal discharge, menstrual-like cramps, and vaginal bleeding.

▰ Prenatal screening has become standard in prenatal care to detect neural tube defects and genetic abnormalities.

▰ The nurse should address common discomforts that occur in each trimester matter-of-factly at all prenatal visits and should provide realistic measures to help the client deal with them effectively.

▰ The pregnant client can better care for herself and the fetus if her concerns are anticipated by the nurse and incorporated into guidance sessions at each prenatal visit.

▰ Iron and folic acid need to be supplemented because their increased requirements during pregnancy are usually too great to be met through diet alone.

▰ The American College of Obstetricians and Gynecologists recommends a 25- to 35-pound weight gain during pregnancy.

▰ For a pregnant woman to meet recommended dietary reference intakes (DRIs), it is important for her to eat according to the USDA's Food Guide Pyramid.

▰ Throughout pregnancy, a well-balanced diet is critical for a healthy baby.

▰ Perinatal education has broadened its focus to include preparation for pregnancy and family adaptation to the new parenting roles. Childbirth education began because of increasing pressure from consumers who wanted to become more involved in their birthing experience.

▰ Three common childbirth education methods are Lamaze (psychoprophylactic), Bradley (partner-coached childbirth), and Dick-Read (natural childbirth).

▰ The great majority of women in the United States are well and healthy and can consider the full range of birth settings: hospital, birth center, or home setting.

▰ All pregnant women need to be able to recognize early signs of contractions to prevent preterm labor.

REFERENCES

Alexander, L. L., LaRosa, J. H., Bader, H., & Garfield, S. (2007). *New dimensions in women's health* (4th ed.). Sudbury, MA: Jones and Bartlett Publishers.

American Academy of Family Physicians (AAFP). (2008). Pregnancy and exercise: What you can do for a healthy pregnancy. Available at: http://familydoctor.org/online/famdocen/home/women/pregnancy/basics/305.html

American College of Obstetricians and Gynecologists (ACOG). (2004). *ACOG issues position on first-trimester screening methods.* ACOG News Release. Available at: http://acog.org/from_home/publications/press_releases/nr06-30-04.cfm

American College of Obstetricians and Gynecologists (ACOG). (2006). *Breastfeeding your baby.* Available at: http://www.acog.org/publications/patient_education/bp029.cfm

American College of Obstetricians and Gynecologists (ACOG). (2007a). *Planning for your pregnancy and birth* (4th ed.). Washington, DC: Author.

American College of Obstetricians and Gynecologists (ACOG). (2007b). *Easing back pain during pregnancy.* Available at: http://www.acog.org/publications/patient_education/bp115.cfm

American College of Obstetricians and Gynecologists (ACOG). (2007c). *Sexuality and sexual problems.* Available at: http://www.acog.org/publications/patient_education/bp072.cfm

American College of Obstetricians and Gynecologists (ACOG). (2007d). *Problems of the digestive system.* Available at: http://www.acog.org/publications/patient_education/bp120.cfm

American College of Obstetricians and Gynecologists (ACOG). (2007e). *How to tell when labor begins.* Available at: http://www.acog.org/publications/patient_education/bp004.cfm

American College of Obstetricians and Gynecologists (ACOG). (2007f). *Air travel during pregnancy* (ACOG Committee Opinion No. 264). Washington, DC: Author.

American College of Obstetricians and Gynecologists (ACOG). (2007g). *Neural tube defects* (ACOG Practice Bulletin No. 44). Available at http://www.guideline.gov/summary/summary.aspx?ss=15&doc_id=3994&nbr=3131

American College of Obstetricians and Gynecologists (ACOG). (2007h). *Exercise during pregnancy.* Available at: http://www.acog.org/publications/patient_education/bp119.cfm

American Pregnancy Association (APA). (2008). Effect of exercise on pregnancy. Available at: http://www.americanpregnancy.org/pregnancy/health/effectsofexerciseonpreg.html

American Pregnancy Association (APA). (2008). Pregnancy and travel. Available at: http://www.americanpregnancy.org/pregnancyhealth/travel.html

Arenson, J., & Drake, P. (2007). *Maternal and newborn nursing.* Sudbury, MA: Jones and Bartlett Publishers.

Atrash, H. K., Johnson, K., Adams, M., Cordero, J. F., & Howse, J. (2006). Preconception care for improved perinatal outcomes: The time to act. *Maternal & Child Health, 10*(5), Supplement: S3–11.

Blackburn, S. T. (2007). *Maternal, fetal, and neonatal physiology: A clinical perspective* (3rd ed.). St. Louis, MO: Saunders Elsevier.

Caughey, A. B., Musci, T. J., Belluomini, J., Main, D., Otto, C., & Goldberg, J. (2007). Nuchal translucency screening: How do women actually utilize the results? *Prenatal Diagnosis, 27*(2), 119–123.

Centers for Disease Control and Prevention (CDC). (2006). *Recommendations to improve preconception health and health care—United States.* Atlanta, GA: CDC.

Centers for Disease Control and Prevention (CDC). (2007a). *Guidelines for vaccinating pregnant women.* Recommendations of the Advisory Committee on Immunization Practices (ACIP). Atlanta, GA: CDC.

Centers for Disease Control and Prevention (CDC). (2007b). *Preconception health and care.* Available at: http://www.cdc.gov/ncbddd/preconception/default.htm

Centers for Disease Control and Prevention (CDC). (2007c). *Pregnancy, breast-feeding and travel: Factors affecting the decision to travel.* Traveler's Health. Available at: http://www.cdc.gov/travel/pregnant.htm

Centers for Disease Control and Prevention (CDC). (2008). Having a healthy pregnancy. Available at: http://www.cdc.gov/ncbdd/bd.abc.htm

Cragan, J. D., Friedman, J. M., Holmes, L. B., Uhl, K., Green, N. S., & Riley, L. (2006). Ensuring the safe and effective use of medications during pregnancy: Planning and prevention through preconception care. *Maternal & Child Health Journal,* Supplement, Vol. 10, 129–135.

Cunningham, F., et al. (2005). *William's obstetrics* (22nd ed.). New York: McGraw-Hill.

Dashe, J. S., Twickler, D. M., Santos-Ramos, R. McIntire, D. D., & Ramus, R. M. (2006). Alpha-fetoprotein detection of neural tube defects and the impact of standard of ultrasound. *American Journal of Obstetrics & Gynecology, 195*(6), 1623–1628.

Dillon, P. M. (2007). *Nursing health assessment: A critical thinking, case studies approach.* Philadelphia: F. A. Davis Company.

Dunlop, A. L., Jack, B., & Frey, K. (2007). National recommendations for preconception care: The essential role of the family physician. *Journal of the American Board of Family Medicine, 20*(1), 81–84.

Frieden, F. J., & Chan, Y. (2007). Antepartum care. In R. E. Rakel & E. T. Bope (Eds.), *Conn's current therapy 2007* (Section 16; pp. 1169–1174), Philadelphia: Saunders Elsevier.

Future Medicine. (2007). Vaccination during pregnancy. Available at: http://futuremedicine.com/doi/abs/10.2217/17455057.3.2.227

Gearhart, P. A., & Sehdev, H. M. (2007). Biophysical profile. *eMedicine.* Available at: http://emedicine.com/radio/topic758.htm

Gilbert, E. S. (2007). *Manual of high-risk pregnancy and delivery* (4th ed.). St. Louis, MO: Mosby.

Graham, L. (2006). CDC releases guidelines on improving preconception health care. *American Family Physician, 74*(11), 1967–1970.

Hackley, B., Kriebs, J. M., & Rousseau, M. E. (2007). *Primary care of women: A guide for midwives and women's health practitioners.* Sudbury, MA: Jones and Bartlett Publishers.

Jenkins, T. M., Caughey, A. B., Hopkins, L. M., & Norton, M. E. (2007). Chorionic villus sampling compared with amniocentesis and the difference in the rate of pregnancy loss. *Obstetrics & Gynecology, 109*(1), 204–206.

Kenner, C., & Lott, J. W. (2007). *Comprehensive neonatal care: An interdisciplinary approach* (4th ed.). St. Louis, MO: Saunders Elsevier.

Knowlton, L. (2007). Labor of love: Nurse midwife Ruth Watson Lubic. *American Journal of Nursing, 107*(4), 86–87.

Lane, C. A. (2007). Nausea and vomiting in pregnancy: A tailored approach treatment. *Clinical Obstetrics & Gynecology, 50*(1), 100–111.

Lawson, M. (2007). Contemporary aspects of infant feeding. *Pediatric Nursing, 19*(2), 39–44.

Leonard, P. (2007). Childbirth education: A handbook for nurses. *Nursing Spectrum.* Available at: http://nsweb.nursingspectrum.com/ce/m350a.htm

Lleras, D. (2007). The childbirth experience: An obstetrical nurse's experience. *International Journal of Childbirth Education, 22*(1), 19–21.

Lynch, S. W. (2007). Greater expectations. *Alternative Medicine Magazine,* March (95), 64–71.

Mangesi, L., & Hofmeyr, G. (2007). Fetal movement counting for assessment of fetal well-being. *Cochrane Database of Systematic Reviews.* (Cochrane Database Syst Rev) 2007(1). Cochrane AN: CD004909.

March of Dimes. (2007a). The joy of sex during pregnancy. Available at: http://www.marchofdimes.com/printableArticles/159_516.asp?printable=true

March of Dimes. (2007b). Childbirth educational classes. Available at: http://www.marchofdimes.com/pnhec/159_12929.asp

March of Dimes. (2007c). Prematurity: The answers can't come soon enough. Available at: http://www.marchofdimes.com/prematurity

March of Dimes. (2008). Before pregnancy: Preconception. Available at: http://www.marchofdimes/com/pnhec/173.asp

March of Dimes. (2008). Vaccination during pregnancy. Available at: http://www.marchofdimes.com/pnhec/159_16189.asp

Mayor, S. (2007). NICE recommends women should choose where to give birth after discussing the risks. *British Medical Journal, 334*(7295), 654–660.

Mikkelsen, T. B., Andersen, A. N., & Olsen, S. F. (2007). Pica in pregnancy in a privileged population: Myth or reality? *Obstetrical & Gynecological Survey, 62*(2), 94–95.

National Institutes of Health (NIH). (2008). High-risk pregnancy. Available at: http://www.nichd.nih.gov/healthtopics/high_risk_pregnancy.cfm

Perkins, C., Pivarnik, J. M., Paneth, N., & Stein, A. D. (2007). Physical activity and fetal growth during pregnancy. *Obstetrics & Gynecology, 109*(1), 81–87.

Risica, P. M., & Phipps, M. G. (2007). Educational preferences in a prenatal clinic population. *International Journal of Childbirth Education, 21*(4), 4–7.

Singh, D., & Singh, J. R. (2008). Prenatal diagnosis for congenital malformations and genetic disorders. *eMedicine.* Available at: http://www.emedicine.com/oph/topic485.htm

Thies, K. M., & Travers, J. F. (2006). *Handbook of human development for health care professionals.* Sudbury, MA: Jones and Bartlett Publishers.

Trupin, S. R. (2006). Common pregnancy complaints and questions. *eMedicine.* Available at: http://emedicine.com/med/topic3238.htm

U.S. Department of Health and Human Services. (2000). *Healthy People 2010.* Washington, DC: US Department of Health and Human Services.

U.S. Department of Health and Human Services (USDHHS). (2007). Pregnancy and medicines. Available at: http://www.4women.gov/faq/pregmed.htm

Valley, V. T., & Fly, C. A. (2006). Pelvic ultrasonography. *eMedicine.* Available at: http://www.emedicine.com/emerg/topic622.htm

Walling, A. D. (2007). Pregnancy loss after amniocentesis and CVS. *American Family Physician, 75*(2), 258–259.

Walsh, D. J. (2007). A birth center's encounters with discourses of childbirth: how resistance led to innovation. *Sociology of Health & Illness, 29*(2), 216–232.

WEBSITES

American Academy of Husband-Coached Childbirth: www.bradleybirth.com

American College of Nurse Midwives: (202) 347-5445, www.acnm.org

American College of Obstetricians and Gynecologists (ACOG): www.acog.org

Association of Women's Health, Obstetrics & Neonatal Nurses: www.awhonn.org

Doulas of North America (DONA): (206) 324-5440, www.dona.com

International Childbirth Education Association: www.icea.org

International Lactation Consultation Association (ILCA): www.ilca.org

La Leche League International: (800) 525-3243, www.lalacheleague.org

Lamaze International: (800) 368-4404, www.lamaze-childbirth.com

March of Dimes: www.modimes.org

Mayo Clinic Pregnancy Center: www.mayoclinic.org

National Center for Education in Maternal and Child Health: www.ncemch.org

Prepared Childbirth Education: www.childbirtheducation.org

Special Supplemental Nutrition Program for Women, Infants, and Children (WIC): www.usda.gov/fns/wic.html

CHAPTER WORKSHEET

MULTIPLE CHOICE QUESTIONS

1. Which of the following biophysical profile findings indicate poor oxygenation to the fetus?

   a. Two pockets of amniotic fluid

   b. Well-flexed arms and legs

   c. Nonreactive fetal heart rate

   d. Fetal breathing movements noted

2. The nurse teaches the pregnant client how to perform Kegel exercises as a way to accomplish which of the following?

   a. Prevent perineal lacerations

   b. Stimulate postdates labor

   c. Increase pelvic muscle tone

   d. Lose pregnancy weight quickly

3. During a clinic visit, a pregnant client at 30 weeks' gestation tells the nurse, "I've had some mild cramps that are pretty irregular. What does this mean?" The cramps are probably:

   a. the beginning of labor in the very early stages

   b. an ominous finding indicating that the client is about to have a miscarriage

   c. related to overhydration in the client

   d. Braxton Hicks contractions, which occur throughout pregnancy

4. The nurse teaches a pregnant woman about exercise and activity, including activities not recommended during pregnancy. The nurse determines that the teaching was effective when the pregnant woman states that which of the following activities is not recommended during pregnancy?

   a. Swimming

   b. Walking

   c. Scuba diving

   d. Bike riding

5. A pregnant client's last normal menstrual period was on August 10. Using Nagele's rule, the nurse calculates that her estimated date of birth (EDB) will be which of the following?

   a. June 23

   b. July 10

   c. July 30

   d. May 17

CRITICAL THINKING EXERCISES

1. Mary Jones comes to the Women's Health Center, where you work as a nurse. She is in her first trimester of pregnancy and tells you her main complaints are nausea and fatigue, to the point that she wants to sleep most of the time and eats one meal daily. She appears pale and tired. Her mucous membranes are pale. She reports that she gets 8 to 9 hours of sleep each night but still can't seem to stay awake and alert at work. She tells you she knows that she is not eating as she should, but she isn't hungry. Her hemoglobin and hematocrit are low.

   a. What subjective and objective data do you have to make your assessment?

   b. What is your impression of this woman?

   c. What nursing interventions would be appropriate for this client?

   d. How will you evaluate the effectiveness of your interventions?

2. Monica, a 16-year-old African-American high school student, is here for her first prenatal visit. Her last normal menstrual period was 2 months ago, and she states she has been "sick ever since." She is 5 feet, 6 inches tall and weighs 110 pounds. In completing her dietary assessment, the nurse asks about her intake of milk and dairy products. Monica reports that she doesn't like "that stuff" and doesn't want to put on too much weight because it "might ruin my figure."

   a. In addition to the routine obstetric assessments, which additional ones might be warranted for this teenager?

   b. What dietary instruction should be provided to this teenager based on her history?

   c. What follow-up monitoring should be included in subsequent prenatal visits?

3. Maria, a 27-year-old Hispanic woman in her last trimester of pregnancy (34 weeks), complains to the clinic nurse that she is constipated and feels miserable most of the time. She reports that she has started taking laxatives, but mostly they don't help her. When questioned about her dietary habits, she replies that she eats beans and rice and drinks tea with most meals. She says she has tried to limit her fluid intake so she doesn't have to go to the bathroom so much because she doesn't

want to miss any of her daytime soap operas on television.

a. What additional information would the nurse need to assess her complaint?

b. What interventions would be appropriate for Maria?

c. What adaptations will Maria need to make to alleviate her constipation?

STUDY ACTIVITIES

1. Visit a freestanding birth center and compare it to a traditional hospital setting in terms of restrictions, type of pain management available, and costs.

2. Arrange to shadow a nurse-midwife for a day to see her role in working with the childbearing family.

3. Select two of the websites supplied at the end of this chapter and note their target audience, the validity of information offered, and their appeal to expectant couples. Present your findings.

4. Request permission to attend a childbirth education class in your local area and help a woman without a partner practice the paced breathing exercises. Present the information you learned and think about how you can apply it while taking care of a woman during labor.

5. A laywoman with a specialized education and experience in assisting women during labor is a _____.

UNIT FOUR

LABOR AND BIRTH

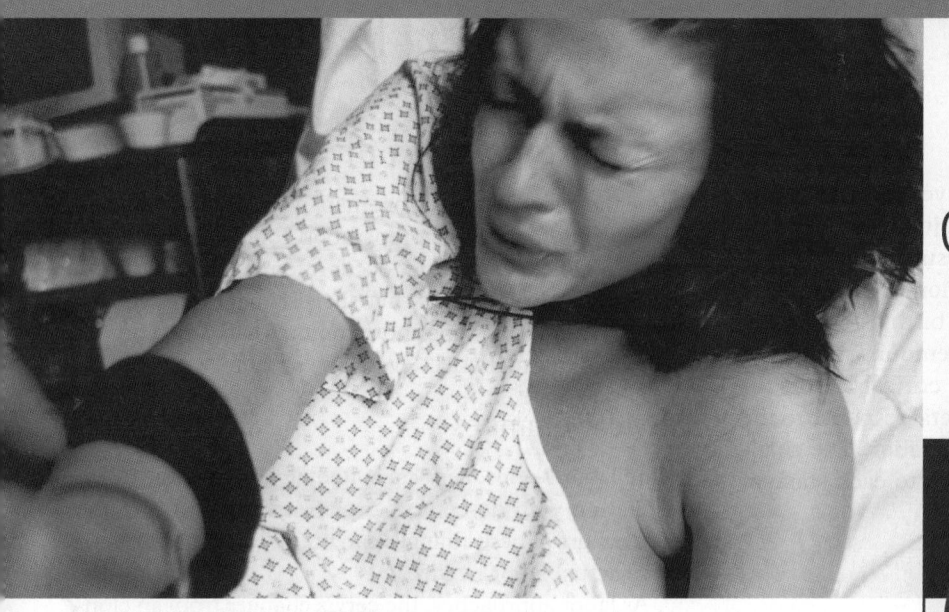

LABOR AND BIRTH PROCESS

KEY TERMS

attitude	engagement	molding
dilation	frequency	position
doula	intensity	presentation
duration	lie	station
effacement	lightening	

LEARNING OBJECTIVES

Upon completion of the chapter, the learner will be able to:

1. Outline premonitory signs of labor.
2. Compare and contrast true versus false labor.
3. Categorize the critical factors affecting labor and birth.
4. Analyze the cardinal movements of labor.
5. Identify the maternal and fetal responses to labor and birth.
6. Classify the stages of labor and the critical events in each stage.
7. Explain the normal physiologic/psychological changes occurring during all four stages of labor.
8. Formulate the concept of pain as it relates to the woman in labor.

*K*athy and Chuck have been eagerly awaiting the birth of their first child for what seems to them an eternity. When Kathy finally feels contractions in her abdomen, she and Chuck rush to the birthing center. After the OB nurse completes a complete history and physical assessment, she informs Kathy and her husband that she must have experienced "false labor" and that they should return home until she starts true labor.

Wow
Intense physical and emotional support promotes a positive and memorable birthing experience.

The process of labor and birth involves more than the birth of a newborn. Numerous physiologic and psychological events occur that ultimately result in the birth of a newborn and the creation or expansion of the family.

This chapter describes labor and birth as a process. It addresses initiation of labor, the premonitory signs of labor, including true and false labor, critical factors affecting labor and birth, maternal and fetal response to the laboring process, and the four stages of labor. The chapter also identifies critical factors related to each stage of labor: the "10 P's" of labor.

Initiation of Labor

Labor is a complex, multifaceted interaction between the mother and fetus. It is a series of processes by which the fetus is expelled from the uterus. It is difficult to determine exactly why labor begins and what initiates it. Although several theories have been proposed to explain the onset and maintenance of labor, none of these has been proved scientifically. It is widely believed that labor is influenced by a combination of factors, including uterine stretch, progesterone withdrawal, increased oxytocin sensitivity, and increased release of prostaglandins.

One theory suggests that labor is initiated by a change in the estrogen-to-progesterone ratio. During the last trimester of pregnancy, estrogen levels increase and progesterone levels decrease. This change leads to an increase in the number of myometrium gap junctions. Gap junctions are proteins that connect cell membranes and facilitate coordination of uterine contractions and myometrial stretching (Gilbert, 2007).

Although physiologic evidence for the role of oxytocin in the initiation of labor is inconclusive, the number of oxytocin receptors in the uterus increases at the end of pregnancy. This creates an increased sensitivity to oxytocin. Estrogen, the levels of which are also rising, increases myometrial sensitivity to oxytocin. With the increasing levels of oxytocin in the maternal blood in conjunction with fetal production, initiation of uterine contractions can occur. Oxytocin also aids in stimulating prostaglandin synthesis through receptors in the decidua. Prostaglandins lead to additional contractions, cervical softening, gap junction induction, and myometrial sensitization, thereby leading to a progressive cervical **dilation** (the opening or enlargement of the external cervical os) (Blackburn, 2007).

Prostaglandins are produced in the decidua and fetal membranes and have a central role in the initiation of labor. Prostaglandin levels increase late during pregnancy secondary to elevated estrogen levels. Prostaglandins stimulate smooth muscle contraction of the uterus. An increase in prostaglandins leads to myometrial contractions and a reduction in cervical resistance. Subsequently, the cervix softens, thins out, and dilates during labor.

Premonitory Signs of Labor

Before the onset of labor, a pregnant woman's body undergoes several changes in preparation for the birth of the newborn. The changes that occur often lead to characteristic signs and symptoms that suggest that labor is near. These premonitory signs and symptoms can vary, and not every woman experiences every one of them.

Cervical Changes

Before labor begins, cervical softening and possible cervical dilation with descent of the presenting part into the pelvis occurs. These changes can occur 1 month to 1 hour before actual labor begins.

As labor approaches, the cervix changes from an elongated structure to a shortened, thinned segment. Cervical collagen fibers undergo enzymatic rearrangement into smaller, more flexible fibers that facilitate water absorption, leading to a softer, more stretchable cervix. These changes occur secondary to the effects of prostaglandins and pressure from Braxton Hicks contractions (Blackburn, 2007).

Lightening

Lightening occurs when the fetal presenting part begins to descend into the maternal pelvis. The uterus lowers and moves into a more anterior position. The shape of the abdomen changes as a result of the change in the uterus. With this descent, the woman usually notes that her breathing is much easier. However, she may complain of increased pelvic pressure, cramping, and low back pain. She may notice an increase in vaginal discharge and more frequent urination. Also, edema of the lower extremities may occur as a result of the increased stasis of pooling blood. In primiparas, lightening can occur 2 weeks or more before labor begins; among multiparas it may not occur until labor (Walsh, 2007).

Increased Energy Level

Some women report a sudden increase in energy before labor. This is sometimes referred to as nesting, because many women will focus this energy toward childbirth preparation by cleaning, cooking, preparing the nursery, and spending extra time with other children in the household. The increased energy level usually occurs 24 to 48 hours before the onset of labor. It is thought to be the result of an increase in epinephrine release caused by a decrease in progesterone (Cheng & Caughey, 2007).

Bloody Show

At the onset of labor, the mucous plug that fills the cervical canal during pregnancy is expelled as a result of cervical softening and increased pressure of the presenting part. These ruptured cervical capillaries release a small amount of blood that mixes with mucus, resulting in the pink-tinged secretions known as bloody show.

Braxton Hicks Contractions

Braxton Hicks contractions, which the woman may have been experiencing throughout the pregnancy, may become stronger and more frequent. Braxton Hicks contractions are typically felt as a tightening or pulling sensation of the top of the uterus. They occur primarily in the abdomen and groin and gradually spread downward before relaxing. In contrast, true labor contractions are more commonly felt in the lower back. These contractions aid in moving the cervix from a posterior position to an anterior position. They also help in ripening and softening the cervix. However, the contractions are irregular and can be decreased by walking, voiding, eating, increasing fluid intake, or changing position.

Braxton Hicks contractions usually last about 30 seconds but can persist for as long as 2 minutes. As birth draws near and the uterus becomes more sensitive to oxytocin, the frequency and intensity of these contractions increase. However, if the contractions last longer than 30 seconds and occur more often than four to six times an hour, advise the woman to contact her health care provider so that she can be evaluated for possible preterm labor, especially if she is less than 38 weeks pregnant.

▶ *Take* NOTE!

An infant born between 34 and 36 completed weeks of gestation is identified as "late preterm" and experiences many of the same health issues as other preterm birth infants (AWHONN, 2007).

Spontaneous Rupture of Membranes

One in four women will experience spontaneous rupture of the membranes before the onset of labor (Institute of Medicine, 2007). The rupture of membranes can result in either a sudden gush or a steady leakage of amniotic fluid. Although much of the amniotic fluid is lost when the rupture occurs, a continuous supply is produced to ensure protection of the fetus until birth.

After the amniotic sac has ruptured, the barrier to infection is gone and an ascending infection is possible. In addition, there is a danger of cord prolapse if engagement has not occurred with the sudden release of fluid and pressure with rupture. Due to the possibility of these complications, advise women to notify their health care provider and go in for an evaluation.

▶ *Consider* THIS!

I always pictured myself a dignified woman and behaved in ways to demonstrate that, for that was the way I was raised. My mother and grandmother always stressed that you should look good, dress well, and do nothing to embarrass yourself in public. I did a fairly good job of living up to their expectations until I become pregnant. I recall I was overdue according to my dates and was miserable in the summer heat. I decided to go to the store for some ice cream. As I waddled down the grocery aisles, all of a sudden my water broke and came pouring down my legs all over the floor. Not wanting to make a spectacle of myself and remembering what my mother always said about being dignified at all times in public, I quickly reached up onto the grocery shelf and "accidentally" knocked off a large jar of pickles right where my puddle was. As I walked hurriedly away from that mess without my ice cream, I heard on the store loudspeaker, "Clean-up on aisle 13!"

Thoughts: We tend to live by what we are taught, and in this case, this woman needed to save face from her ruptured membranes. Many women experience ruptured membranes before the onset of labor, so it is not out of the ordinary for this to happen in public. What risks can occur when membranes do rupture? What action should this woman take now to minimize these risks? How will the nurse validate this woman's ruptured membranes?

True Versus False Labor

False labor is a condition occurring during the latter weeks of some pregnancies in which irregular uterine contractions are felt, but the cervix is not affected. In contrast, true labor is characterized by contractions occurring at regular intervals that increase in frequency, duration, and intensity. True labor contractions bring about progressive cervical dilation and effacement. Table 13.1 summarizes the differences between true and false labor. False labor, prodromal labor, and Braxton Hicks contractions are all names for contractions that do not contribute in a measurable way toward the goal of birth.

Many women fear being sent home from the hospital with "false labor." All women feel anxious when they feel contractions, but they should be informed that labor could be a long process, especially if it is their first pregnancy. Encourage the woman to think of false labor or "pre-labor signs" as positive, as they are part of the entire labor continuum. With first pregnancies, the cervix can take up to 20 hours to dilate completely (Cunningham et al., 2005).

TABLE 13.1 DIFFERENCES BETWEEN TRUE AND FALSE LABOR

Parameters	True Labor	False Labor
Contraction timing	Regular, becoming closer together, usually 4–6 minutes apart, lasting 30–60 seconds	Irregular, not occurring close together
Contraction strength	Become stronger with time, vaginal pressure is usually felt	Frequently weak, not getting stronger with time or alternating (a strong one followed by weaker ones)
Contraction discomfort	Starts in the back and radiates around toward the front of the abdomen	Usually felt in the front of the abdomen
Any change in activity	Contractions continue no matter what positional change is made	Contractions may stop or slow down with walking or making a position change
Stay or go?	Stay home until contractions are 5 minutes apart, last 45–60 seconds, and are strong enough so that a conversation during one is not possible—then go to the hospital or birthing center.	Drink fluids and walk around to see if there is any change in the intensity of the contractions; if the contractions diminish in intensity after either or both—stay home.

Sources: Arenson & Drake, 2007; Blackburn, 2007; Cunningham et al., 2005.

Remember Kathy and Chuck, the anxious couple who came to the hospital too early? Kathy felt sure she was in labor and is now confused. What explanations and anticipatory guidance should be offered to this couple? What term would describe her earlier contractions?

Factors Affecting the Labor Process

In many references, the critical factors that affect the process of labor and birth are outlined as the "five P's":

1. Passageway (birth canal)
2. Passenger (fetus and placenta)
3. Powers (contractions)
4. Position (maternal)
5. Psychological response

These critical factors are commonly accepted and discussed by health care professionals. However, five additional "P's" can also affect the labor process:

1. Philosophy (low-tech, high-touch)
2. Partners (support caregivers)
3. Patience (natural timing)
4. Patient preparation (childbirth knowledge base)
5. Pain control (comfort measures)

These five additional "P's" are helpful in planning care for the laboring family. These patient-focused factors are an attempt to foster labor that can be managed through the use of high touch, patience, support, knowledge, and pain management.

Passageway

The birth passageway is the route through which the fetus must travel to be born vaginally. The passageway consists of the maternal pelvis and soft tissues. Of the two, however, the maternal bony pelvis is more important because it is relatively unyielding (except for the coccyx). Typically the pelvis is assessed and measured during the first trimester, often at the first visit to the health care provider, to identify any abnormalities that might hinder a successful vaginal birth. As the pregnancy progresses, the hormones relaxin and estrogen cause the connective tissues to become more relaxed and elastic and cause the joints to become more flexible to prepare the mother's pelvis for birth. Additionally, the soft tissues usually yield to the forces of labor.

Bony Pelvis

The maternal bony pelvis can be divided into the true and false portions. The false (or greater) pelvis is composed of the upper flared parts of the two iliac bones with their concavities and the wings of the base of the sacrum. The false pelvis is divided from the true pelvis by an imaginary line drawn from the sacral prominence at the back to the superior aspect of the symphysis pubis at the front of the pelvis. This imaginary line is called the linea terminalis. The false pelvis lies above this imaginary line; the true pelvis lies below it (Fig. 13.1). The true pelvis is the bony passageway through which the fetus must travel. It is made up of three planes: the inlet, the mid-pelvis (cavity), and the outlet.

Pelvic Inlet

The pelvic inlet allows entrance to the true pelvis. It is bounded by the sacral prominence in the back, the ilium on the sides, and the superior aspect of the symphysis pubis in

False pelvis

Pelvic outlet

True pelvis   Linea terminalis   Pelvic inlet

Anterior view   Superior view   Inferior view

FIGURE 13.1 The bony pelvis.

the front (Edmonds, 2007). The pelvic inlet is wider in the transverse aspect (sideways) than it is from front to back.

Mid-Pelvis

The mid-pelvis (cavity) occupies the space between the inlet and outlet. It is through this snug, curved space that the fetus must travel to reach the outside. As the fetus passes through this small area, its chest is compressed, causing lung fluid and mucus to be expelled. This expulsion removes the space-occupying fluid so that air can enter the lungs with the newborn's first breath.

Pelvic Outlet

The pelvic outlet is bound by the ischial tuberosities, the lower rim of the symphysis pubis, and the tip of the coccyx. In comparison with the pelvic inlet, the outlet is wider from front to back. For the fetus to pass through the pelvis, the outlet must be large enough.

To ensure the adequacy of the pelvic outlet for vaginal birth, the following pelvic measurements are assessed:

• Diagonal conjugate of the inlet (distance between the anterior surface of the sacral prominence and the anterior surface of the inferior margin of the symphysis pubis)
• Transverse or ischial tuberosity diameter of the outlet (distance at the medial and lowest aspect of the ischial tuberosities, at the level of the anus; a known hand span or clenched-fist measurement is generally used to obtain this measurement)
• True or obstetric conjugate (distance estimated from the measurement of the diagonal conjugate; 1.5 cm is subtracted from the diagonal conjugate measurement)

For more information about pelvic measurements, see Chapter 12.

If the diagonal conjugate measures at least 11.5 cm and the true or obstetric conjugate measures 10 cm or more (1.5 cm less than the diagonal conjugate, or about 10 cm), then the pelvis is large enough for a vaginal birth of what would be considered a normal-size newborn.

Pelvic Shape

In addition to size, the shape of a woman's pelvis is a determining factor for a vaginal birth. The pelvis is divided into four main shapes: gynecoid, anthropoid, android, and platypelloid (Fig. 13.2).

The gynecoid pelvis is considered the true female pelvis, occurring in about 50% of all women; it is less common in men (Leonard, 2007). Vaginal birth is most favorable with this type of pelvis because the inlet is round and the outlet is roomy. This shape offers the optimal diameters in all three planes of the pelvis. This type of pelvis allows early and complete fetal internal rotation during labor.

The anthropoid pelvis is common in men and occurs in 20% to 30% of women (Billington & Stevenson, 2007). The pelvic inlet is oval and the sacrum is long, producing a deep pelvis (wider front to back [anterior to posterior] than side to side [transverse]). Vaginal birth is more favorable with this pelvic shape compared to the android or platypelloid shape (Frieden & Chan, 2007).

The android pelvis is considered the male-shaped pelvis and is characterized by a funnel shape. It occurs in approximately 20% of women (Cunningham et al., 2005). The pelvic inlet is heart-shaped and the posterior segments are reduced in all pelvic planes. Descent of the fetal head into the pelvis is slow, and failure of the fetus to rotate is common. The prognosis for labor is poor, subsequently leading to cesarean birth.

The platypelloid or flat pelvis is the least common type of pelvic structure among men and women, with an approximate incidence of 5% (Billington & Stevenson, 2007). The pelvic cavity is shallow but widens at the pelvic outlet, making it difficult for the fetus to descend through

FIGURE 13.2 Pelvic shapes. (**A**) Gynecoid. (**B**) Android. (**C**) Anthropoid. (**D**) Platypelloid.

the mid-pelvis. It is not favorable for a vaginal birth unless the fetal head can pass through the inlet. Women with this type of pelvis usually require cesarean birth.

An important principle is that most pelves are not purely defined but occur in nature as mixed types. Many women have a combination of these four basic pelvis types, with no two pelves being exactly the same. Regardless of the shape, the newborn will be born if size and positioning remain compatible. The narrowest part of the fetus attempts to align itself with the narrowest pelvic dimension (e.g., biparietal to interspinous diameters, which means the fetus generally tends to rotate to the most ample portion of the pelvis).

Soft Tissues

The soft tissues of the passageway consist of the cervix, the pelvic floor muscles, and the vagina. Through **efface-ment,** the cervix effaces (thins) and dilates (opens) to allow the presenting fetal part to descend into the vagina.

▶ *Take* NOTE!

Cervical effacement and dilation is similar to pulling a turtleneck sweater over your head.

The pelvic floor muscles help the fetus to rotate anteriorly as it passes through the birth canal. The soft tissues of the vagina expand to accommodate the fetus during birth.

Passenger

The fetus (with placenta) is the passenger. The fetal head (size and presence of molding), fetal attitude (degree of body flexion), fetal lie (relationship of body parts), fetal presentation (first body part), fetal position (relationship to maternal pelvis), fetal station, and fetal engagement are all important factors that have an impact on the ultimate outcome in the birthing process.

Fetal Head

The fetal head is the largest and least compressible fetal structure, making it an important factor in relation to labor and birth. Considerable variation in the size and diameter of the fetal skull is often seen.

Compared with an adult, the fetal head is large in proportion to the rest of the body, usually about one quarter of the body surface area (Kenner & Lott, 2007). The bones that make up the face and cranial base are fused and essentially fixed. However, the bones that make up the rest of the cranium (two frontal bones, two parietal bones, and the occipital bone) are not fused; rather, they are soft and pliable, with gaps between the plates of bone. These gaps, which are membranous spaces between the cranial bones, are called sutures, and the intersections of these sutures are called fontanelles. Sutures are important because they allow the cranial bones to overlap in order for the head to adjust in shape (elongate) when pressure is exerted on it by uterine contractions or the maternal bony pelvis. Some diameters shorten whereas others lengthen as the head is molded during the labor and birthing process. This malleability of the fetal skull may decrease fetal skull dimensions by 0.5 to 1 cm (Blackburn, 2007). After birth, the sutures close as the bones grow and the brain reaches its full growth.

The changed (elongated) shape of the fetal skull at birth as a result of overlapping of the cranial bones is known as **molding**. Along with molding, fluid can also collect in the scalp (caput succedaneum) or blood can collect beneath the scalp (cephalohematoma), further distorting the shape and appearance of the fetal head. Caput succedaneum can be described as edema of the scalp at the presenting part. This swelling crosses suture lines and disappears within 3 to 4 days. Cephalhematoma is a collection of blood between the periosteum and the bone. It does not cross suture lines and is generally reabsorbed over the next 4 to 6 weeks (Arenson & Drake, 2007).

> ▶ *Take* NOTE!
>
> *Parents may become concerned about the distortion of their newborn's head. However, reassurance that the oblong shape is only temporary is usually all that is needed to reduce their anxiety.*

Sutures also play a role in helping to identify the position of the fetal head during a vaginal examination. Figure 13.3 shows a fetal skull. The coronal sutures are located between the frontal and parietal bones and extend transversely on both sides of the anterior fontanelles. The frontal suture is located between the two frontal bones. The lambdoidal sutures are located between the occipital bone and the two parietals, extending transversely on either side of the posterior fontanelles. The sagittal suture is located between the parietal bones and divides the skull into the right and left halves. During a pelvic examination, palpation of these sutures by the examiner reveals the position of the fetal head and the degree of rotation that has occurred.

The anterior and posterior fontanelles are also useful in helping to identify the position of the fetal head, and they allow for molding. In addition, the fontanelles are important when evaluating the newborn. The anterior

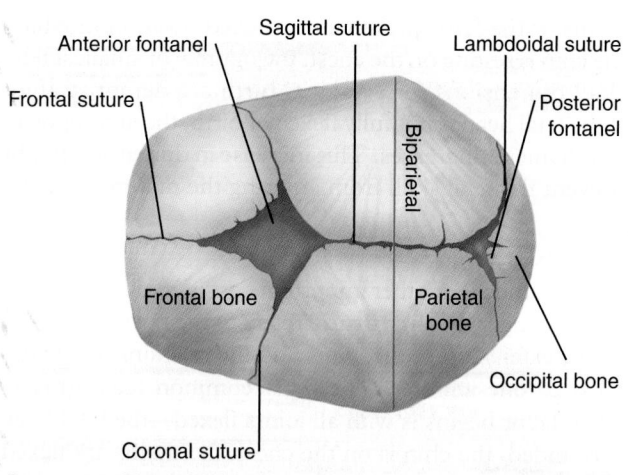

FIGURE 13.3 Fetal skull.

fontanelle is the famous "soft spot" of the newborn's head. It is diamond-shaped and measures about 2 to 3 cm. It remains open for 12 to 18 months after birth to allow for growth of the brain (Edmonds, 2007). The posterior fontanelle corresponds to the anterior one but is located at the back of the fetal head; it is triangular. This one closes within 8 to 12 weeks after birth and measures, on average, 0.5 to 1 cm at its widest diameter (Kenner & Lott, 2007).

The diameter of the fetal skull is an important consideration during the labor and birth process. Fetal skull diameters are measured between the various landmarks of the skull. Diameters include occipitofrontal, occipitomental, suboccipitobregmatic, and biparietal (Fig. 13.4). The two most important diameters that can affect the birth process are the suboccipitobregmatic (approximately 9.5 cm at term) and the biparietal (approximately 9.25 cm at term) diameters. The suboccipitobregmatic diameter, measured from the base of the occiput to the center of the anterior fontanelle, identifies the smallest anteroposterior diameter of the fetal skull. The biparietal diameter measures the largest transverse diameter of the fetal skull: the distance between the two parietal bones. In a cephalic (headfirst) presentation, which occurs in 95% of all term

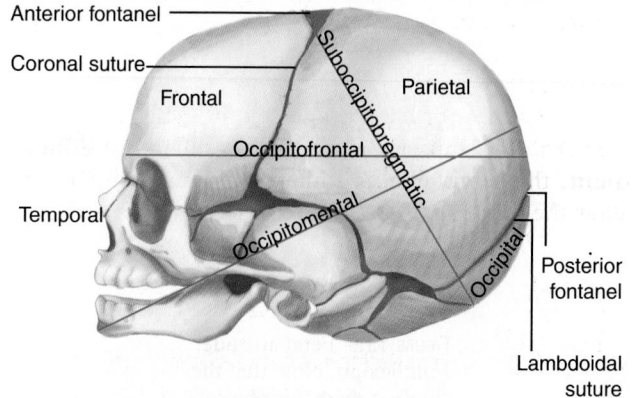

FIGURE 13.4 Fetal skull diameters.

births, if the fetus presents in a flexed position in which the chin is resting on the chest, the optimal or smallest fetal skull dimensions for a vaginal birth are demonstrated. If the fetal head is not fully flexed at birth, the anteroposterior diameter increases. This increase in dimension might prevent the fetal skull from entering the maternal pelvis.

Fetal Attitude

Fetal attitude is another important consideration related to the passenger. Fetal **attitude** refers to the posturing (flexion or extension) of the joints and the relationship of fetal parts to one another. The most common fetal attitude when labor begins is with all joints flexed—the fetal back is rounded, the chin is on the chest, the thighs are flexed on the abdomen, and the legs are flexed at the knees (Fig. 13.5). This normal fetal position is most favorable for vaginal birth, presenting the smallest fetal skull diameters to the pelvis.

When the fetus presents to the pelvis with abnormal attitudes (no flexion or extension), the diameter can increase the diameter of the presenting part as it passes through the pelvis, increasing the difficulty of birth. An attitude of extension tends to present larger fetal skull diameters, which may make birth difficult.

Fetal Lie

Fetal **lie** refers to the relationship of the long axis (spine) of the fetus to the long axis (spine) of the mother. There are two primary lies: longitudinal (which is the most common) and transverse (Fig. 13.6).

A longitudinal lie occurs when the long axis of the fetus is parallel to that of the mother (fetal spine to maternal spine side-by-side). A transverse lie occurs when the long axis of the fetus is perpendicular to the long axis of the mother (fetus spine lies across the maternal abdomen and crosses her spine). A fetus in a transverse lie position cannot be delivered vaginally (Billington & Stevenson, 2007).

FIGURE 13.5 Fetal attitude: Full flexion. Note that the smallest diameter presents to the pelvis.

A. Longitudinal lie

B. Transverse lie
FIGURE 13.6 Fetal lie.

Fetal Presentation

Fetal **presentation** refers to the body part of the fetus that enters the pelvic inlet first (the "presenting part"). This is the fetal part that lies over the inlet of the pelvis or the cervical os. Knowing which fetal part is coming first at birth is critical for planning and initiating appropriate interventions.

The three main fetal presentations are cephalic (head first), breech (pelvis first), and shoulder (scapula first). The majority of term newborns (95%) enter this world in a cephalic presentation; breech presentation accounts for 3% of term births, shoulder presentations for approximately 2% (Edmonds, 2007).

In a cephalic presentation, the presenting part is usually the occiput portion of the fetal head (Fig. 13.7). This presentation is also referred to as a vertex presentation. Variations in a vertex presentation include the military, brow, and face presentations.

Breech presentation occurs when the fetal buttocks or feet enter the maternal pelvis first and the fetal skull enters last. This abnormal presentation poses several challenges at birth. Primarily, the largest part of the fetus (skull) is born last and may become "hung up" or stuck in the pelvis. In addition, the umbilical cord can become compressed between the fetal skull and the maternal pelvis after the fetal chest is born because the head is the last to exit. Moreover, unlike the hard fetal skull, the buttocks are soft and are not as effective as a cervical dilator during labor compared with a cephalic presentation. Finally, there is the possibility of trauma to the head as a result of the lack of opportunity for molding.

FIGURE 13.7 Fetal presentation: cephalic presentations. (**A**) Vertex. (**B**) Military. (**C**) Brow. (**D**) Face.

The types of breech presentations are determined by the positioning of the fetal legs (Fig. 13.8). In a frank breech (50% to 70%), the buttocks present first with both legs extended up toward the face. In a full or complete breech (5% to 10%), the fetus sits crossed-legged above the cervix. In a footling or incomplete breech (10% to 30%), one or both legs are presenting. Breech presentations are associated with prematurity, placenta previa, multiparity, uterine abnormalities (fibroids), and some congenital anomalies such as hydrocephaly (Fischer, 2007). A frank breech can result in a vaginal birth, but complete, footling, and incomplete breech presentations generally necessitate a cesarean birth.

A shoulder presentation occurs when the fetal shoulders present first, with the head tucked inside. Odds of a shoulder presentation are one in 1,000 (Cunningham et al., 2005). The fetus is in a transverse lie with the shoulder as the presenting part. Conditions associated with shoulder presentation include placenta previa, multiple gestation, or fetal anomalies. A cesarean birth is typically necessary (Edmonds, 2007).

Fetal Position

Fetal **position** describes the relationship of a given point on the presenting part of the fetus to a designated point of the maternal pelvis (Walsh, 2007). The landmark fetal presenting parts include the occipital bone (O), which designates a vertex presentation; the chin (mentum [M]), which designates a face presentation; the buttocks (sacrum [S]), which designate a breech presentation; and the scapula (acromion process [A]), which designates a shoulder presentation.

In addition, the maternal pelvis is divided into four quadrants: right anterior, left anterior, right posterior, and left posterior. These quadrants designate whether the presenting part is directed toward the front, back, left, or right side of the pelvis. Fetal position is determined first by identifying the presenting part and then the maternal quadrant the presenting part is facing (Fig. 13.9). Position is indicated by a three-letter abbreviation as follows:

• The first letter defines whether the presenting part is tilted toward the left (L) or the right (R) side of the maternal pelvis.

FIGURE 13.8 Breech presentations. (**A**) Frank breech. (**B**) Complete breech. (**C**) Single footling breech. (**D**) Double footling breech.

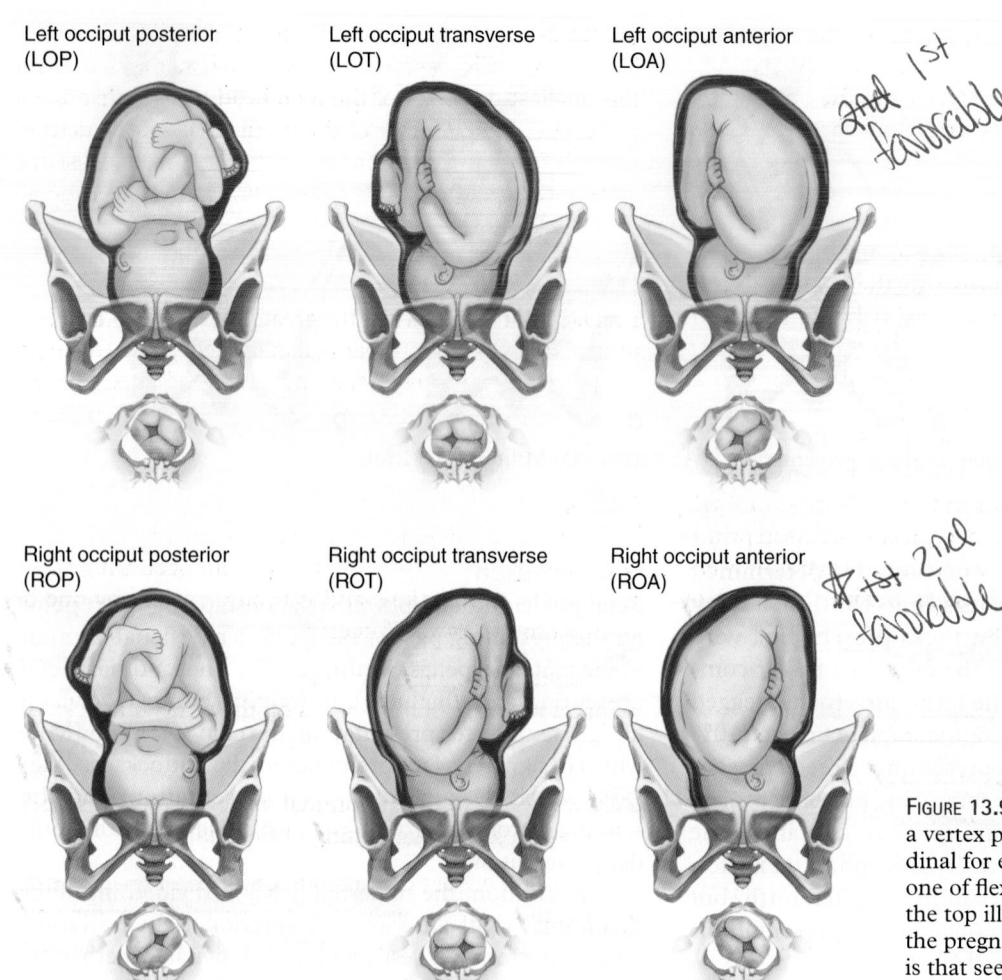

Left occiput posterior (LOP)

Left occiput transverse (LOT)

Left occiput anterior (LOA)

Right occiput posterior (ROP)

Right occiput transverse (ROT)

Right occiput anterior (ROA)

FIGURE 13.9 Examples of fetal positions in a vertex presentation. The lie is longitudinal for each illustration. The attitude is one of flexion. Notice that the view of the top illustration is seen when facing the pregnant woman. The bottom view is that seen with the woman in a dorsal recumbent position.

- The second letter represents the particular presenting part of the fetus: O for occiput, S for sacrum (buttocks), M for mentum (chin), A for acromion process, and D for dorsal (refers to the fetal back) when denoting the fetal position in shoulder presentations (Cheng & Caughey, 2007).
- The third letter defines the location of the presenting part in relation to the anterior (A) portion of the maternal pelvis or the posterior (P) portion of the maternal pelvis. If the presenting part is directed to the side of the maternal pelvis, the fetal presentation is designated as transverse (T).

For example, if the occiput is facing the left anterior quadrant of the pelvis, then the position is termed left occipitoanterior and is recorded as LOA. LOA is the most common (and most favorable) fetal position for birthing today, followed by right occipitoanterior (ROA).

The positioning of the fetus allows the fetal head to contour to the diameters of the maternal pelvis. LOA and ROA are optimal positions for vaginal birth. An occiput posterior position may lead to a long and difficult birth, and other positions may or may not be compatible with vaginal birth.

Fetal Station

Station refers to the relationship of the presenting part to the level of the maternal pelvic ischial spines. Fetal station is measured in centimeters and is referred to as a minus or plus, depending on its location above or below the ischial spines. Typically, the ischial spines are the narrowest part of the pelvis and are the natural measuring point for the birth progress.

Zero (0) station is designated when the presenting part is at the level of the maternal ischial spines. When the presenting part is above the ischial spines, the distance is recorded as minus stations. When the presenting part is below the ischial spines, the distance is recorded as plus stations. For instance, if the presenting part is above the ischial spines by 1 cm, it is documented as being a −1 station; if the presenting part is below the ischial spines by 1 cm, it is documented as being a +1 station. An easy way to understand this concept is to think in terms of meeting the goal, which is the birth. If the fetus is descending downward (past the ischial spines) and moving toward meeting the goal of birth, then the station is positive and the centimeter numbers grow bigger from +1 to +4. If the fetus is not descending past the ischial spines, then the station is negative and the centimeter numbers grow bigger from −1 to −4. The farther away the presenting part from the outside, the larger the negative number (-4 cm). The closer the presenting part of the fetus is to the outside, the larger the positive number (+4 cm). Figure 13.10 shows stations of presenting part.

Fetal Engagement

Engagement signifies the entrance of the largest diameter of the fetal presenting part (usually the fetal head) into the smallest diameter of the maternal pelvis (Blackburn, 2007). The fetus is said to be "engaged" in the pelvis when the presenting part reaches 0 station. Engagement is determined by pelvic examination.

The largest diameter of the fetal head is the biparietal diameter. It extends from one parietal prominence to the other. It is an important factor in the navigation through the maternal pelvis. Engagement typically occurs in primigravidas 2 weeks before term, whereas multiparas may experience engagement several weeks before the onset of labor or not until labor begins.

> ▶ **Take** NOTE!
>
> *The term* floating *is used when engagement has not occurred, because the presenting part is freely movable above the pelvic inlet.*

Cardinal Movements of Labor

The fetus goes through many positional changes as it travels through the passageway. These positional changes are known as the cardinal movements of labor. They are deliberate, specific, and very precise movements that allow the smallest diameter of the fetal head to pass through a corresponding diameter of the mother's pelvic structure. Although cardinal movements are conceptualized as separate and sequential, the movements are typically concurrent (Fig. 13.11).

Engagement

Engagement occurs when the greatest transverse diameter of the head in vertex (biparietal diameter) passes through the pelvic inlet (usually 0 station). The head usually enters the pelvis with the sagittal suture aligned in the transverse diameter.

Descent

Descent is the downward movement of the fetal head until it is within the pelvic inlet. Descent occurs intermittently with contractions and is brought about by one or more of the following forces:

• Pressure of the amniotic fluid
• Direct pressure of the fundus on the fetus' buttocks or head (depending on which part is located in the top of the uterus)
• Contractions of the abdominal muscles (second stage)
• Extension and straightening of the fetal body

Descent occurs throughout labor, ending with birth. During this time, the mother experiences discomfort, but she is unable to isolate this particular fetal movement from her overall discomfort.

Flexion

Flexion occurs as the vertex meets resistance from the cervix, the walls of the pelvis, or the pelvic floor. As a result, the chin is brought into contact with the fetal thorax and the presenting diameter is changed from occipitofrontal to suboccipitobregmatic (9.5 cm), which achieves the smallest fetal skull diameter presenting to the maternal pelvic dimensions.

Internal Rotation

After engagement, as the head descends, the lower portion of the head (usually the occiput) meets resistance from one side of the pelvic floor. As a result, the head rotates about 45 degrees anteriorly to the midline under the symphysis. This movement is known as internal rotation. Internal rotation brings the anteroposterior diameter of the head in line with the anteroposterior diameter of the pelvic outlet. It aligns the long axis of the fetal head with the long axis of the maternal pelvis. The widest portion of the maternal pelvis is the anteroposterior diameter, and thus the fetus must rotate to accommodate the pelvis.

Extension

With further descent and full flexion of the head, the nucha (the base of the occiput) becomes impinged under

FIGURE 13.10 Fetal stations.

-4
-3
-2
-1
0
+1
+2
+3
+4

Engagement, Descent,
Flexion

Internal Rotation

Extension Beginning
(rotation complete)

Extension Complete

External Rotation
restitution)

External Rotation
(shoulder rotation)

Expulsion

FIGURE 13.11 Cardinal movements
of labor.

the symphysis. Resistance from the pelvic floor causes the fetal head to extend so that it can pass under the pubic arch. Extension occurs after internal rotation is complete. The head emerges through extension under the symphysis pubis along with the shoulders. The anterior fontanel, brow, nose, mouth, and chin are born successively.

External Rotation (Restitution)
After the head is born and is free of resistance, it untwists, causing the occiput to move about 45 degrees back to its original left or right position (restitution). The sagittal suture has now resumed its normal right-angle relationship to the transverse (bisacromial) diameter of the shoulders (i.e., the head realigns with the position of the back in the birth canal). External rotation of the fetal head allows the shoulders to rotate internally to fit the maternal pelvis.

Expulsion
Expulsion of the rest of the body occurs more smoothly after the birth of the head and the anterior and posterior shoulders (Cheng & Caughey, 2007).

Powers

The primary stimulus powering labor is uterine contractions. Contractions cause complete dilation and effacement of the cervix during the first stage of labor. The secondary powers in labor involve the use of intra-abdominal pressure (voluntary muscle contractions) exerted by the woman as she pushes and bears down during the second stage of labor.

Uterine Contractions

Uterine contractions are involuntary and therefore cannot be controlled by the woman experiencing them, regardless of whether they are spontaneous or induced. Uterine contractions are rhythmic and intermittent, with a period of relaxation between contractions. This pause allows the woman and the uterine muscles to rest. In addition, this pause restores blood flow to the uterus and placenta, which is temporarily reduced during each uterine contraction.

Uterine contractions are responsible for thinning and dilating the cervix, and they thrust the presenting part toward the lower uterine segment. With each uterine contraction, the upper segment of the uterus becomes shorter and thicker, whereas the lower passive segment and the cervix become longer, thinner, and more distended. The division between the contractile upper portion (fundus) of the uterus and the lower portion is described as the physiologic retraction ring. Longitudinal traction on the cervix by the fundus as it contracts and retracts leads to cervical effacement and dilation. Uterine contractions cause the upper uterine segment to shorten, making the cervix paper-thin when it becomes fully effaced.

The cervical canal reduces in length from 2 cm to a paper-thin entity and is described in terms of percentages from 0 to 100%. In primigravidas, effacement typically starts before the onset of labor and usually begins before dilation; in multiparas, however, neither effacement nor dilation may start until labor ensues. On clinical examination the following may be assessed:

• Cervical canal 2 cm in length would be described as 0% effaced.
• Cervical canal 1 cm in length would be described as 50% effaced.

• Cervical canal 0 cm in length would be described as 100% effaced.

Dilation is dependent on the pressure of the presenting part and the contraction and retraction of the uterus. The diameter of the cervical os increases from less than 1 cm to approximately 10 cm to allow for birth. When the cervix is fully dilated, it is no longer palpable on vaginal examination. Descriptions may include the following:

• External cervical os closed: 0 cm dilated
• External cervical os half open: 5 cm dilated
• External cervical os fully open: 10 cm dilated

During early labor, uterine contractions are described as mild, they last about 30 seconds, and they occur about every 5 to 7 minutes. As labor progresses, contractions last longer (60 seconds), occur more frequently (2 to 3 minutes apart), and are described as being moderate to high in intensity.

Each contraction has three phases: increment (buildup of the contraction), acme (peak or highest intensity), and decrement (descent or relaxation of the uterine muscle fibers; Fig. 13.12).

Uterine contractions are monitored and assessed according to three parameters: frequency, duration, and intensity.

1. **Frequency** refers to how often the contractions occur and is measured from the increment of one contraction to the increment of the next contraction.
2. **Duration** refers to how long a contraction lasts and is measured from the beginning of the increment to the end of the decrement for the same contraction.
3. **Intensity** refers to the strength of the contraction determined by manual palpation or measured by an internal intrauterine catheter (IUPC). The catheter is positioned in the uterine cavity through the cervix after the membranes have ruptured. It reports intensity by measuring the pressure of the amniotic fluid inside the uterus in millimeters of mercury (Edmonds, 2007).

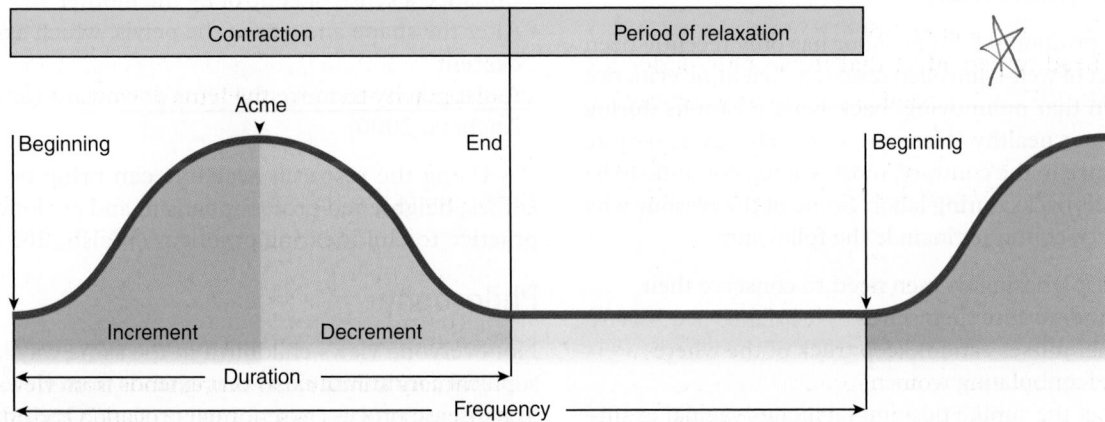

FIGURE 13.12 The three phases of a uterine contraction.

Intra-Abdominal Pressure

Increased intra-abdominal pressure (voluntary muscle contractions) compresses the uterus and adds to the power of
the expulsion forces of the uterine contractions (Blackburn,
2007). Coordination of these forces in unison promotes
birth of the fetus and expulsion of the fetal membranes and
placenta from the uterus. Interference with these forces
(such as when a woman is highly sedated or extremely anxious) can compromise the effectiveness of these powers.

Psychological Response

Childbearing can be one of the most life-altering experiences for a woman. The experience of childbirth goes
beyond the physiologic aspects: it influences her self-
confidence, self-esteem, and view of life, relationships,
and children. Her state of mind (psyche) throughout the
entire process is critical to bring about a positive outcome for her and her family. Factors promoting a positive birth experience include:

• Clear information about procedures
• Support; not being alone
• Sense of mastery, self-confidence
• Trust in staff caring for her
• Positive reaction to the pregnancy
• Personal control over breathing
• Preparation for the childbirth experience

Having a strong sense of self and meaningful support
from others can often help women manage labor well.
Feeling safe and secure typically promotes a sense of control and ability to withstand the challenges of the childbearing experience. Anxiety and fear, however, decrease
a woman's ability to cope with the discomfort of labor.
Maternal catecholamines secreted in response to anxiety
and fear can inhibit uterine blood flow and placental perfusion. In contrast, relaxation can augment the natural
process of labor (Leonard, 2007). Preparing mentally for
childbirth is important so that the woman can work with,
rather than against, the natural forces of labor.

Position (Maternal)

Maternal positioning during labor has only recently been
the subject of well-controlled research. Scientific evidence
has shown that nonmoving, back-lying positions during
labor are not healthy (Hanson 2006). However, despite
this evidence to the contrary, most women continue to lie
flat on their backs during labor. Some of the reasons why
this practice continues include the following:

• Belief that laboring women need to conserve their
  energy and not tire themselves
• Belief that nurses cannot keep track of the where-
  abouts of ambulating women
• Belief that the supine position facilitates vaginal examinations and external belt adjustment

• Belief that a bed is "where one is supposed to be" in a
  hospital setting
• Belief that the position is more convenient for the
  delivering health professional
• Belief that laboring women are "connected to things"
  that impede movement (Hanson, 2006)

Although many labor and birthing facilities claim
that all women are allowed to adopt any position of comfort during their laboring experience, the great majority
of women spend their time on their backs during labor
and birth.

> ▶ **Take** NOTE!
>
> *If the only furniture provided is a bed, this
> is what the woman will use. Furnishing
> rooms with comfortable chairs, beanbags, and other
> birth props allows a woman to choose from a variety of
> positions and to be free to move during labor.*

Changing positions and moving around during labor
and birth offer several benefits. Maternal position can influence pelvic size and contours. Changing position and
walking affect the pelvis joints, which may facilitate fetal
descent and rotation. Squatting enlarges the pelvic outlet
by approximately 25%, whereas a kneeling position removes pressure on the maternal vena cava and helps to rotate the fetus in the posterior position (Terry et al., 2006).
The use of any upright or lateral position, compared with
supine or lithotomy positions, may:

• Reduce the length of the first stage of labor
• Reduce the duration of the second stage of labor
• Reduce the number of assisted deliveries (vacuum and
  forceps)
• Reduce episiotomies and perineal tears
• Contribute to fewer abnormal fetal heart rate patterns
• Increase comfort/reduce requests for pain medication
• Enhance a sense of control by the mother
• Alter the shape and size of the pelvis, which assists in
  descent
• Assist gravity to move the fetus downward (Simkin &
  Ancheta, 2006)

Using the research available can bring better outcomes, heightened professionalism, and evidence-based
practice to childbearing practices (Walsh, 2007).

Philosophy

Not everyone views childbirth in the same way. A philosophical continuum exists that extends from viewing labor
as a disease process to a normal process. One philosophy
assumes that women cannot manage the birth experience

EVIDENCE-BASED PRACTICE 13.1
Continuous Support for Women During Childbirth

● Study

Historically, women have been attended and supported by other women during labor. However, in recent decades in hospitals worldwide, continuous support during labor has become the exception rather than the rule. Concerns about the consequent dehumanization of the birth experiences have led to calls for a return to continuous support by women for women during labor.

This review of studies included 16 trials, from 11 countries, involving over 13,000 women in a wide range of settings and circumstances. The primary outcome was to assess the effects, on mothers and their babies, of continuous, one-to-one intrapartum support compared with usual care. The secondary outcome was to determine whether the effects of continuous support are influenced by (1) routine practices and policies in the birth environment that may affect a woman's autonomy, freedom of movement, and ability to cope with labor; (2) whether the caregiver is a member of the staff of the institution; and (3) whether the continuous support begins early or later in labor.

▲ Findings

Women who received continuous labor support were more likely to give birth "spontaneously" (vaginally, without vacuum or forceps). They were less likely to use pain medications, were more likely to be satisfied with their experience, and had slightly shorter labors. In general, labor support appeared to be more effective when it was provided by women who were not part of the hospital staff. It also appeared to be more effective when it started early in labor. No adverse effects were identified.

■ Nursing Implications

Knowing the results of this evidence-based study, all nurses should strive to be a real "presence" for all of their laboring couples. Based on the findings, continuous nursing support promotes positive birthing outcomes and fewer technical/surgical interventions. Both maternal and fetal well-being is preserved when nurses are present and involved during the childbirth experience.

Hodnett, E. D., Gates, S., Hofmeyr, G. J., & Sakala, C. (2007). Continuous support for women during childbirth. *Cochrane Database of Systematic Reviews* 2007, 3. Art. No.: CD003766. DOI: 10.1002/14651858.CD003766.pub2.

adequately and therefore need constant expert monitoring and management. The other philosophy assumes that women are capable, reasoning individuals who can actively participate in their birth experience.

The health care system in the United States today appears to be leaning toward the former philosophy, applying technological interventions to most mothers who enter the hospital system. Giving birth in a hospital in the 21st century for many women has become "intervention intensive"—designed to start, continue, and end labor through medical management rather than allowing the normal process of birth to unfold. Advances in medical care have improved the safety for women with high-risk pregnancies. However, the routine use of intravenous therapy, electronic fetal monitoring, augmentation, and epidural anesthesia has not necessarily improved birth outcomes for all women (Leonard, 2007). Perhaps a middle-of-the-road philosophy for intervening when circumstances dictate, along with weighing the risks and benefits before doing so, may be appropriate.

During the 1970s, family-centered maternity care was developed in response to the consumer reaction to the depersonalization of birth. The hope was to shift the philosophy from "technologization" to personalization to humanize childbirth. The term "family-centered birthing" is more appropriate today to denote the low-tech, high-touch approach requested by many childbearing women, who view childbirth as a normal process.

Certified nurse midwives (CNMs) are champions of family-centered birthing, and their participation in the childbirth process is associated with fewer unnecessary interventions when compared to obstetricians. CNMs subscribe to a normal birth process where the woman uses her own instincts and bodily signs during labor. In short, midwives empower women within the birthing environment (Russell, 2007; Steppe, 2007).

No matter what philosophy is held, it is ideal if everyone involved in the particular birth process—from the health care provider to the mother—shares the same philosophy toward the birth process.

Partners

Women desire support and attentive care during labor and birth. Caregivers can convey emotional support by offering their continued presence and words of encouragement. Throughout the world, few women are left to labor totally alone: emotional, physical, or spiritual support during labor is the norm for most cultures (Ballen & Fulcher, 2006). A caring partner can use massage, light touch, acupressure, hand-holding, stroking, and relaxation, can help the woman communicate her wishes to the staff, and can provide a continuous, reassuring presence, all of which bring some degree of comfort to the laboring woman (Ballen & Fulcher, 2006). Although the presence of the baby's father at the birth provides special emotional support, a partner can be anyone who is present to support the woman throughout the experience.

Worldwide, women usually support other women in childbirth. Hodnett et al. (2003) reported that the continuous presence of a trained female support person (**doula**) reduced the need for medication for pain relief, the use of vacuum or forceps delivery, and the need for cesarean births. Continuous support was also associated with a slight reduction in the length of labor. The doula, who is an experienced labor companion, provides the woman and her partner with emotional and physical support and information throughout the entire labor and birth experience.

A similar study in the United States found that nursing care decreases the likelihood of negative evaluations of the childbirth experience, feelings of tenseness during labor, and finding labor worse than expected. Also reported were less perineal trauma, reduced difficulty in mothering, and reduced likelihood of early cessation of breastfeeding (Ballen & Fulcher, 2006).

Given the many benefits of intrapartum support, laboring women should always have the option to receive partner support, whether from nurses, doulas, significant others, or family. Whoever the support partner is, he or she should provide the mother with continuous presence and hands-on comfort and encouragement.

Patience

The birth process takes time. If more time were allowed for women to labor naturally without intervention, the cesarean birth rate would most likely be reduced (Simkin & Ancheta, 2006). The literature suggests that delaying interventions can give a woman enough time to progress in labor and reduce the need for surgical intervention (American College of Obstetricians and Gynecologists [ACOG], 2007). *Healthy People 2010* has two goals related to cesarean births in the United States:

1. Reduce the rate of cesarean births among low-risk (full-term, singleton, vertex presentation) women having their first child to 15% of live births, from a baseline of 18%.
2. Reduce the rate of cesarean births among women who have had a prior cesarean birth to 63% of live births, from a baseline of 72% (USDHHS, 2000).

We are a long way from achieving these goals, since the current cesarean birth rate in the United States—30%—is the highest since these data first became available from birth certificates in 1989. Cesarean birth is associated with increased morbidity and mortality for both mother and infant, as well as increased inpatient length of stay and health care costs (CDC, 2007).

It is difficult to predict how a labor will progress and therefore equally difficult to determine how long a woman's labor will last. There is no way to estimate the likely strength and frequency of uterine contractions, the extent to which the cervix will soften and dilate, and how much the fetal head will mold to fit the birth canal. We cannot know beforehand whether the complex fetal rotations needed for an efficient labor will take place properly. All of these factors are unknowns when a woman starts labor.

There is a trend in health care, however, to attempt to manipulate the process of labor through medical means such as artificial rupture of membranes and augmentation of labor with oxytocin (Walsh, 2007). The labor induction rate has increased dramatically in the United States since the 1980s (Gulmezoglu, Crowther, & Middleton, 2007).

Approximately one in five women are induced or have labor augmented with uterine-stimulating drugs or artificial rupture of membranes to accelerate their progress (Bricker & Luckas, 2007). An amniotomy (artificial rupture of the fetal membranes) may be performed to augment or induce labor when the membranes have not ruptured spontaneously. Doing so allows the fetal head to have more direct contact with the cervix to dilate it. This procedure is performed with the fetal head at −2 station or lower, with the cervix dilated to at least 3 cm. Synthetic oxytocin (Pitocin) is also used to induce or augment labor by stimulating uterine contractions. It is administered piggybacked into the primary intravenous line with an infusion pump titrated to uterine activity.

There is compelling evidence that elective induction of labor significantly increases the risk of cesarean birth, especially for nulliparous women (Simkin & Ancheta, 2006). The belief is that many cesarean births could be avoided if women were allowed to labor longer and if the natural labor process were allowed to complete the job. The longer wait (using the intervention of patience) usually results in less intervention.

The ACOG attributes the dramatic increase in inductions in part to pressure from women, convenience for physicians, and liability concerns. They recommend a "cautious approach" regarding elective induction until clinical trials can validate a more liberal use of labor inductions (ACOG, 2002). There are medical indications for inducing labor, such as spontaneous rupture of membranes and when labor does not start; a pregnancy more than 42 weeks' gestation; maternal hypertension, diabetes, or lung disease; and a uterine infection (ACOG, 2006).

When the laboring woman feels the urge to bear down, pushing begins. Most women respond extremely well to messages from their body without being directed by the nurse. A more natural, undirected approach allows the woman to wait and bear down when she feels the urge to push. Having patience and letting nature take its course will reduce the incidence of physiologic stress in the mother, resulting in less trauma to her perineal tissue.

Patient Preparation

Basic prenatal education can help women manage their labor process and feel in control of their birthing experience. The literature indicates that if a woman is prepared before the labor and birth experience, the labor is more likely to remain normal or natural (without the need for medical intervention) (Gagnon, 2006). An increasing body of evidence also indicates that the well-prepared woman, with good labor support, is less likely to need analgesia or anesthesia and is unlikely to require cesarean birth (Risica & Phipps, 2006).

Prenatal education teaches the woman about the childbirth experience and increases her sense of control. She is then able to work as an active participant during the labor and birth experience (Brodsky, 2006). The research also suggests that prenatal preparation may affect intrapartum and postpartum psychosocial outcomes. For example, prenatal education covering parenting communication classes had a significant effect on postpartum anxiety and postpartum adjustment. Prenatal education should be viewed as an opportunity to strengthen families by providing anticipatory guidance and improve family members' life skills. In short, prenatal education helps to promote healthy families during the transition to parenthood and beyond (Polomeno, 2006).

> ▶ *Take* NOTE!
>
> *Learning about labor and birth allows women and couples to express their needs and preferences, enhances their confidence, and improves communication between themselves and the staff.*

Pain Management

Labor and birth, although a normal physiologic process, can produce significant pain. Pain during labor is a nearly universal experience. Controlling the pain without harm to the fetus or labor process is the major focus of pain management during childbirth.

Pain is a subjective experience involving a complex interaction of physiologic, spiritual, psychosocial, cultural, and environmental influences (Smith et al., 2006). Cultural values and learned behaviors influence perception and response to pain, as do anxiety and fear, both of which tend to heighten the sense of pain (Walsh, 2007). The challenge for care providers is to find the right combination of pain management methods to keep the pain manageable while minimizing the negative effect on the fetus, the normal physiology of labor, maternal–infant bonding, breastfeeding, and a woman's perception of the labor itself (Wood, 2007). Chapter 14 presents a full discussion of pain management during labor and birth.

Physiologic Responses to Labor

Labor is the physiologic process by which the uterus expels the fetus and placenta from the body. During pregnancy, progesterone secreted from the placenta suppresses the spontaneous contractions of a typical uterus, keeping the fetus within the uterus. In addition, the cervix remains firm and noncompliant. At term, however, changes occur in the cervix that make it softer. In addition, uterine contractions become more frequent and regular, signaling the onset of labor.

The labor process involves a series of rhythmic, involuntary, usually quite uncomfortable uterine muscle contractions. They bring about a shortening that causes effacement and dilation of the cervix and a bursting of the fetal membranes. Then, accompanied by both reflex and voluntary contractions of the abdominal muscles (pushing), the uterine contractions result in the birth of the baby (Blackburn, 2007). During labor, the mother and fetus make several physiologic adaptations.

Maternal Responses

As the woman progresses through childbirth, numerous physiologic responses occur that assist her to adapt to the laboring process. The labor process stresses several of the woman's body systems, which react through numerous compensatory mechanisms. Maternal physiologic responses include:

- Heart rate increases by 10 to 20 bpm.
- Cardiac output increases by 10% to 15% during the first stage of labor and by 30% to 50% during the second stage of labor.
- Blood pressure increases by 10 to 30 mm Hg during uterine contractions in all labor stages.
- The white blood cell count increases to 25,000 to 30,000 cells/mm^3, perhaps as a result of tissue trauma.
- Respiratory rate increases and more oxygen is consumed related to the increase in metabolism.
- Gastric motility and food absorption decrease, which may increase the risk of nausea and vomiting during the transition stage of labor.
- Gastric emptying and gastric pH decrease, increasing the risk of vomiting with aspiration.
- Temperature rises slightly, possibly due to an increase in muscle activity.
- Muscular aches/cramps occur as a result of the stressed musculoskeletal system.
- Basal metabolic rate increases and blood glucose levels decrease because of the stress of labor (Blackburn, 2007; Cheng & Caughey, 2007).

A woman's ability to adapt to the stress of labor is influenced by her psychological and physical state. Among the many factors that affect her coping ability are:

• Previous birth experiences and their outcomes
• Current pregnancy experience (planned versus unplanned, discomforts experienced, age, risk status of pregnancy, chronic illness, weight gain)
• Cultural considerations (values and beliefs about health status)
• Support system (presence and support of a valued partner during labor)
• Childbirth preparation (attended childbirth classes and has practiced paced breathing techniques)
• Exercise during pregnancy
• Expectations of the birthing experience
• Anxiety level
• Fear of labor and loss of control
• Fatigue and weariness (Edmonds, 2007)

Fetal Responses

Although the focus during labor may be on assessing the mother's adaptations, several physiologic adaptations occur in the fetus as well. The fetus is experiencing labor along with the mother. If the fetus is healthy, the stress of labor usually has no adverse effects. The nurse needs to be alert to any abnormalities in the fetus' adaptation to labor. Fetal responses to labor include:

• Periodic fetal heart rate accelerations and slight decelerations related to fetal movement, fundal pressure, and uterine contractions
• Decrease in circulation and perfusion to the fetus secondary to uterine contractions (a healthy fetus is able to compensate for this drop)
• Increase in arterial carbon dioxide pressure (PCO_2)
• Decrease in fetal breathing movements throughout labor
• Decrease in fetal oxygen pressure with a decrease in the partial pressure of oxygen (PO_2) (Kenner & Lott, 2007)

► **Take** NOTE!

Respiratory changes during labor help to prepare the fetus for extrauterine respiration immediately after birth.

Stages of Labor

Labor is typically divided into four stages: dilation, expulsive, placental, and restorative. Table 13.2 summarizes the major events of each stage.

The first stage is the longest: it begins with the first true contraction and ends with full dilation (opening) of the cervix. Because this stage lasts so long, it is divided into three phases, each corresponding to the progressive dilation of the cervix.

Stage two of labor, or the expulsive stage, begins when the cervix is completely dilated and ends with the birth of the newborn. The expulsive stage can last from minutes to hours.

The third stage, or the placental stage, starts after the newborn is born and ends with the separation and birth of the placenta. Continued uterine contractions typically cause the placenta to be expelled within 5 to 30 minutes.

The fourth stage, or the restorative stage, lasts from 1 to 4 hours after birth. This period is when the mother's body begins to stabilize after the hard work of labor and the loss of the products of conception. The fourth stage is often not recognized as a true stage of labor, but it is a critical period for maternal physiologic transition as well as new family attachment (Arenson & Drake, 2007).

First Stage

During the first stage of labor, the fundamental change underlying the process is progressive dilation of the cervix. Cervical dilation is gauged subjectively by vaginal examination and is expressed in centimeters. The first stage ends when the cervix is dilated to 10 cm in diameter and is large enough to permit the passage of a fetal head of average size. The fetal membranes, or bag of waters, usually rupture during the first stage, but they may have burst earlier or may even remain intact until birth. For the primigravida, the first stage of labor lasts about 12 hours. However, this time can vary widely: for the multiparous woman, it is usually only half that.

During the first stage of labor, women usually perceive the visceral pain of diffuse abdominal cramping and uterine contractions. Pain during the first stage of labor is primarily a result of the dilation of the cervix and lower uterine segment, and the distention (stretching) of these structures during contractions. The first stage is divided into three phases: latent or early phase, active phase, and transition phase.

Latent or Early Phase

The latent or early phase gives rise to the familiar signs and symptoms of labor. This phase begins with the start of regular contractions and ends when rapid cervical dilation begins. Cervical effacement occurs during this phase, and the cervix dilates from 0 to 3 cm.

Contractions usually occur every 5 to 10 minutes, last 30 to 45 seconds, and are described as mild by palpation. Effacement of the cervix is from 0% to 40%. Most women are very talkative during this period, perceiving their contractions to be similar to menstrual cramps. Women may remain at home during this phase, contacting their health care professional about the onset of labor.

For the nulliparous woman, the latent phase typically lasts about 9 hours; in the multiparous woman, it lasts about 6 hours (Cheng & Caughey, 2007). During this phase, women are apprehensive but excited about the start of their labor after their long gestational period.

TABLE 13.2 STAGES AND PHASES OF LABOR

	First Stage	Second Stage	Third Stage	Fourth Stage
Description	From 0–10 cm dilation; consists of three phases	From complete dilation (10 cm) to birth of the newborn; lasts up to 1 hour	Separation and delivery of the placenta	1–4 hours after the birth of the newborn; time of maternal physiologic adjustment
Phases	**Latent phase** (0–3 cm dilation) – Cervical dilation from 0 to 3 cm – Cervical effacement from 0% to 40% – Nullipara, lasts up to 9 hours; multipara, lasts up to 5–6 hours – Contraction frequency every 5–10 minutes – Contraction duration 30–45 seconds – Contraction intensity mild to palpation **Active phase** (4–7 cm dilation) – Cervical dilation from 4 to 7 cm – Cervical effacement from 40% to 80% – Nullipara, lasts up to 6 hours; multipara, lasts up to 4 hours – Contraction frequency every 2–5 minutes – Contraction duration 45–60 seconds – Contraction intensity moderate to palpation **Transition phase** (8–10 cm dilation) – Cervical dilation from 8 to 10 cm – Cervical effacement from 80% to 100% – Nullipara lasts up to 1 hour; multipara, lasts up to 30 minutes – Contraction frequency every 1–2 minutes – Contraction duration 60–90 seconds – Contraction intensity strong by palpation	**Pelvic phase** (period of fetal descent) **Perineal phase** (period of active pushing) – Nullipara, lasts up to 1 hour; multipara, lasts up to 30 minutes – Contraction frequency every 2–3 minutes or less – Contraction duration 60–90 seconds – Contraction intensity strong by palpation – Strong urge to push during the later perineal phase	**Placental separation:** detaching from uterine wall **Placental expulsion:** coming outside the vaginal opening	

Think back to the couple who were sent home from the hospital birthing center. Three days later Kathy awoke with a wet sensation and intense discomfort in her back, spreading around to her abdomen. She decided to go for a walk, but her contractions didn't diminish; instead, they continued to occur every few minutes and grew stronger in intensity. She and Chuck decided to go back to the hospital birthing center. Was there a difference in the location of Kathy's discomfort this time? What changes will the admission nurse find in Kathy if this is true labor?

Active Phase

Cervical dilation begins to occur more rapidly during the active phase. The cervix usually dilates from 4 to 7 cm, with 40% to 80% effacement taking place. This phase can last up to 6 hours for the nulliparous woman and 4.5 hours for the multiparous woman (Simkin & Ancheta, 2006). The fetus descends farther in the pelvis. Contractions become more frequent (every 2 to 5 minutes) and increase in duration (45 to 60 seconds). The woman's discomfort intensifies (moderate to strong by palpation). She becomes more intense and inwardly focused, absorbed in the serious work of her labor. She limits interactions with those in the room. If she and her partner have attended childbirth education classes, she will begin to use the relaxation and paced breathing techniques that they learned to cope with the contractions. The typical dilation rate for the nulliparous woman is 1.2 cm/hour; for the multiparous woman, it is 1.5 cm/hour (Cunningham et al., 2005).

Transition Phase

The transition phase is the last phase of the first stage of labor. During this phase, dilation slows, progressing from 8 to 10 cm, with effacement from 80% to 100%. The transition phase is the most difficult and, fortunately, the shortest phase for the woman, lasting approximately 1 hour in the first birth and perhaps 15 to 30 minutes in successive births (Walsh, 2007). During transition, the contractions are stronger (hard by palpation), more painful, and more frequent (every 1 to 2 minutes), and they last longer (60 to 90 seconds). The average rate of fetal descent is 1 cm/hour in nulliparous women and 2 cm/hour in multiparous women. Pressure on the rectum is great, and there is a strong desire to contract the abdominal muscles and push.

Other maternal features during the transitional phase include nausea and vomiting, trembling extremities, backache, increased apprehension and irritability, restless movement, increased bloody show from the vagina, inability to relax, diaphoresis, feelings of loss of control, and being overwhelmed (the woman may say, "I can't take it any more"). This phase should not last longer than 3 hours for nulliparas and 1 hour for multiparas (Cunningham et al., 2005).

In assessing Kathy, the nurse finds she is 4 cm dilated and 50% effaced with ruptured membranes. In what stage and phase of labor would this assessment finding place Kathy?

Second Stage

The second stage of labor begins with complete cervical dilation (10 cm) and effacement and ends with the birth of the newborn. Although the previous stage of labor primarily involved the thinning and opening of the cervix, this stage involves moving the fetus through the birth canal and out of the body. The cardinal movements of labor occur during the early phase of passive descent in the second stage of labor.

Contractions occur every 2 to 3 minutes, last 60 to 90 seconds, and are described as strong by palpation. The average length of the second stage of labor in a nullipara is approximately 1 hour and less than half that time for the multipara. During this expulsive stage, the mother usually feels more in control and less irritable and agitated. She is focused on the work of pushing. Traditionally, women have been taught to hold their breath to the count of 10, inhale again, push again, and repeat the process several times during a contraction. This sustained, strenuous style of pushing has been shown to lead to hemodynamic changes in the mother and interfere with oxygen exchange between the mother and the fetus. In addition, it is associated with pelvic floor damage: the longer the push, the more damage to the pelvic floor (Hanson, 2006). The newest protocol from the Association of Women's Health and Newborn Nursing (AWHONN) recommends an open-glottis method in which air is released during pushing to prevent the buildup of intrathoracic pressure. Doing so also supports mother's involuntary bearing-down efforts (Roberts, Gonzalez, & Sampselle, 2007).

During the second stage of labor, pushing can either follow the mother's spontaneous urge or be directed by the caregiver. Much debate still exists between spontaneous and directed pushing during the second stage of labor. Although directed pushing is common practice in hospitals, there is evidence to suggest that directed pushing should be avoided. Research seems to support spontaneous pushing—when the woman is allowed to follow her own instincts (Hanson, 2006). Evidence is mounting that the management of the second stage, particularly pushing, is a modifiable risk factor in long-term perinatal outcomes. Valsalva (holding breath) bearing down and supine maternal positions are linked to negative maternal–fetal hemodynamics and outcomes. The adoption of a physiologic, woman-directed approach to bearing down is advocated (Roberts, Gonzalez, & Sampselle, 2007).

Evidence-based practice focuses on a physiologic approach to the second stage of labor. Behaviors demonstrated by laboring women during this time include pushing at the onset of the urge to bear down; using their own pattern and technique of bearing down in response to sensations they experience; using open-glottis bearing down with contractions; pushing with variations in strength and duration; pushing down with progressive intensity; and using multiple positions to increase progress and comfort. This approach is in stark contrast to management by arbitrary time limits and the directed bearing-down efforts seen in practice today (Hanson, 2006).

Laboring down (promotion of passive descent) is an alternative strategy for second-stage management in women with epidurals. Using this approach, the fetus descends and is born without coached maternal pushing.

The second stage of labor has two phases (pelvic and perineal) related to the existence and quality of the maternal urge to push and to obstetric conditions related to fetal descent. The early phase of the second stage is called the pelvic phase, because it is during this phase that the fetal head is negotiating the pelvis, rotating, and advancing in descent. The later phase is called the perineal phase, because at this point the fetal head is lower in the pelvis and is distending the perineum. The occurrence of a strong urge to push characterizes the later phase of the second stage and has also been called the phase of active pushing (Roberts, Gonzalez, & Sampselle, 2007).

The later perineal phase occurs when the mother feels a tremendous urge to push as the fetal head is lowered and is distending the perineum. The perineum bulges and there is an increase in bloody show. The fetal head becomes apparent at the vaginal opening but disappears between contractions. When the top of the head no longer regresses between contractions, it is said to have crowned. The fetus rotates as it maneuvers out. The second stage commonly lasts up to 3 hours in a first labor and up to an hour in subsequent ones (Fig. 13.13).

Third Stage

The third stage of labor begins with the birth of the newborn and ends with the separation and birth of the placenta. It consists of two phases: placental separation and placental expulsion.

Placental Separation

After the infant is born, the uterus continues to contract strongly and can now retract, decreasing markedly in size. These contractions cause the placenta to pull away from the uterine wall. The following signs of separation indicate that the placenta is ready to deliver:

• The uterus rises upward.
• The umbilical cord lengthens.
• A sudden trickle of blood is released from the vaginal opening.
• The uterus changes its shape to globular.

Spontaneous birth of the placenta occurs in one of two ways: the fetal side (shiny gray side) presenting first (called Schultz's mechanism or more commonly called "shiny Schultz's") or the maternal side (red raw side) presenting first (termed Duncan's mechanism or "dirty Duncan").

Placental Expulsion

After separation of the placenta from the uterine wall, continued uterine contractions cause the placenta to be expelled within 2 to 30 minutes unless there is gentle external traction to assist. After the placenta is expelled, the uterus is massaged briefly by the attending physician or midwife until it is firm so that uterine blood vessels constrict, minimizing the possibility of hemorrhage. Normal blood loss is approximately 500 mL for a vaginal birth and 1,000 mL for a cesarean birth (Arenson & Drake, 2007).

If the placenta does not spontaneously deliver, the health care professional assists with its removal by manual extraction. On expulsion, the placenta is inspected for its intactness by the health care professional and the nurse to make sure all sections are present. If any piece is still attached to the uterine wall, it places the woman at risk for postpartum hemorrhage because it becomes a space-occupying object that interferes with the ability of the uterus to contract fully and effectively.

Fourth Stage

The fourth stage begins with completion of the expulsion of the placenta and membranes and ends with the initial physiologic adjustment and stabilization of the mother (1 to 4 hours after birth). This stage initiates the postpartum period. The mother usually feels a sense of peace and excitement, is wide awake, and is very talkative initially. The attachment process begins with her inspecting her newborn and desiring to cuddle and breastfeed him or her. The mother's fundus should be firm and well contracted. Typically it is located at the midline between the umbilicus and the symphysis, but it then slowly rises to the level of the umbilicus during the first hour after birth (Walsh, 2007). If the uterus becomes boggy, it is massaged to keep it firm. The lochia (vaginal discharge) is red, mixed with small clots, and of moderate flow. If the woman has had an episiotomy during the second stage of labor, it should be intact, with the edges approximated and clean and no redness or edema present.

The focus during this stage is to monitor the mother closely to prevent hemorrhage, bladder distention, and venous thrombosis. Usually the mother is thirsty and hungry during this time and may request food and drink. Her bladder is hypotonic and thus she has limited sensation to acknowledge a full bladder or to void. Vital signs, the amount and consistency of the vaginal discharge (lochia), and the uterine fundus are usually monitored every 15 minutes for at least 1 hour. The woman will be

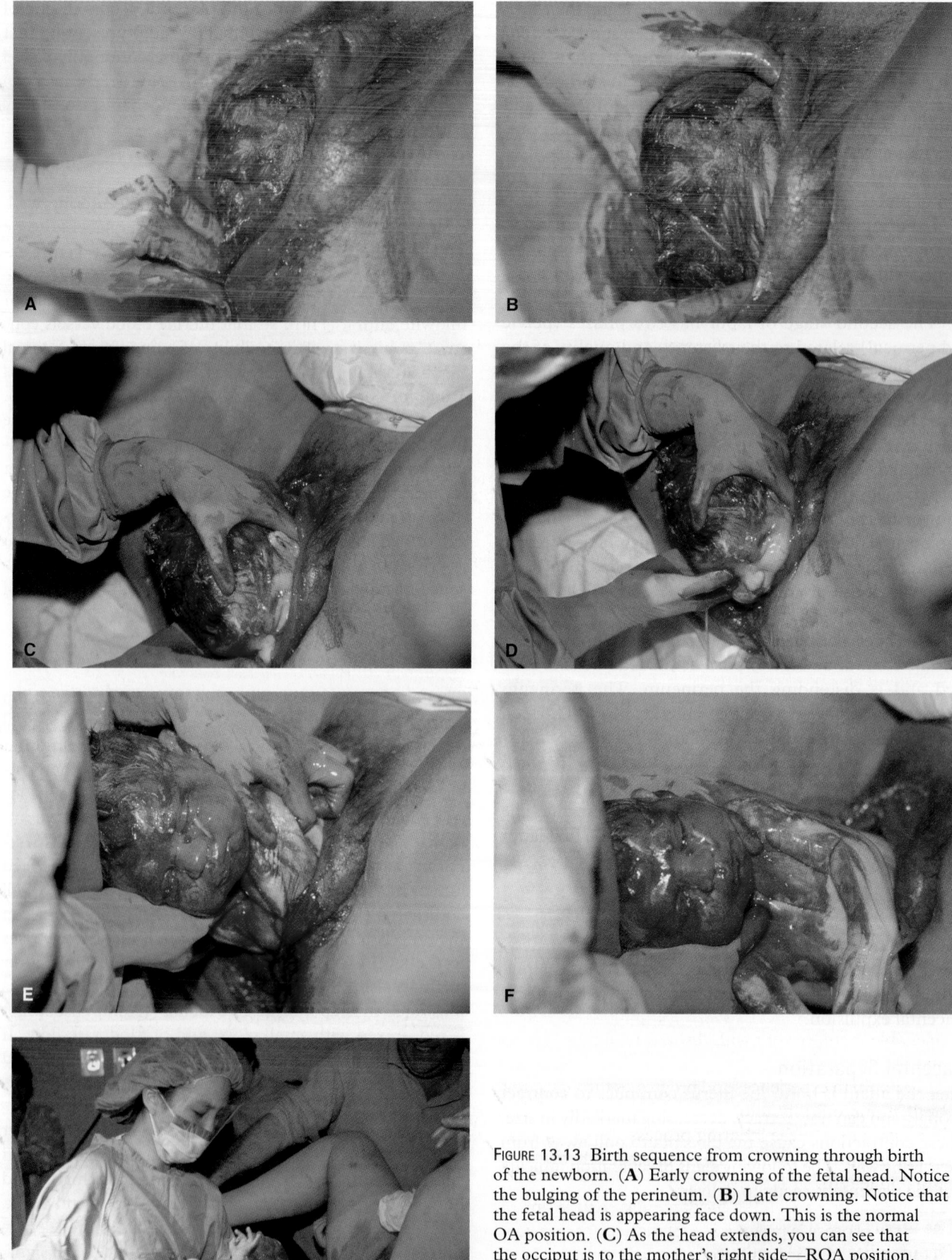

FIGURE 13.13 Birth sequence from crowning through birth
of the newborn. (**A**) Early crowning of the fetal head. Notice
the bulging of the perineum. (**B**) Late crowning. Notice that
the fetal head is appearing face down. This is the normal
OA position. (**C**) As the head extends, you can see that
the occiput is to the mother's right side—ROA position.
(**D**) The cardinal movement of extension. (**E**) The shoulders
are born. Notice how the head has turned to line up with the
shoulders—the cardinal movement of external rotation.
(**F**) The body easily follows the shoulders. (**G**) The newborn
is held for the first time! (© B. Proud.)

feeling cramp-like discomfort during this time due to the contracting uterus.

■■■ Key Concepts

- Labor is a complex, multifaceted interaction between the mother and fetus. Thus, it is difficult to determine exactly why labor begins and what initiates it.
- Before the onset of labor, a pregnant woman's body undergoes several changes in preparation for the birth of the newborn, often leading to characteristic signs and symptoms that suggest that labor is near. These changes include cervical changes, lightening, increased energy level, bloody show, Braxton Hicks contractions, and spontaneous rupture of membranes.
- False labor is a condition seen during the latter weeks of some pregnancies in which irregular uterine contractions are felt, but the cervix is not affected.
- The critical factors in labor and birth are designated as the 10 P's: passageway (birth canal), passenger (fetus and placenta), powers (contractions), psychological response, maternal position, philosophy (low tech, high touch), partners (support caregivers), patience (natural timing), patient preparation (childbirth knowledge base), and pain control (comfort measures).
- The size and shape of a woman's pelvis are determining factors for a vaginal birth. The female pelvis is classified according to four main groups: anthropoid, android, gynecoid, and platypelloid.
- The labor process is comprised of a series of rhythmic, involuntary, usually quite uncomfortable uterine muscle contractions that bring about a shortening (effacement) and opening (dilation) of the cervix, and a bursting of the fetal membranes. Important parameters of uterine contractions are frequency, duration, and intensity.
- The diameters of the fetal skull vary considerably, with some diameters shortening and others lengthening as the head is molded during the labor and birth process.
- Pain during labor is a nearly universal experience for childbearing women. Having a strong sense of self and meaningful support from others can often help women manage labor well and reduce their sensation of pain.
- Preparing mentally for childbirth is important for women to enable them to work with the natural forces of labor and not against them.
- As the woman experiences and progresses through childbirth, numerous physiologic responses occur that assist her adaptation to the laboring process.
- Labor is typically divided into four stages that are unequal in length.
- During the first stage, the fundamental change underlying the process is progressive dilation of the cervix. It is further divided into three phases: latent phase, active phase, and transition.
- The second stage of labor is from complete cervical dilation (10 cm) and effacement through the birth of the infant.
- The third stage is that of separation and birth of the placenta. It consists of two phases: placental separation and placental expulsion.
- The fourth stage begins after the birth of the placenta and membranes and ends with the initial physiologic adjustment and stabilization of the mother (1–4 hours).

References

American College of Obstetricians and Gynecologists (ACOG). (2002). *ACOG news release commentary—Nonmedical indications help fuel rise in induction rate.* [Released June 30, 2002.] Washington, DC: ACOG.

American College of Obstetricians and Gynecologists (ACOG). (2006). *Planning your pregnancy and birth.* Washington, DC: ACOG.

American College of Obstetricians and Gynecologists (ACOG). (2007). *Evaluation of cesarean birth.* Washington, DC: ACOG.

Arenson, J., & Drake, P. (2007) *Maternal and newborn health.* Sudbury, MA: Jones and Bartlett Publishers.

Association of Women's Health, Obstetric and Neonatal Nurses (AWHONN). (2007). The late preterm infant assessment guide. *AWHONN News,* Spring 2007, p. 11.

Ballen, L. E., & Fulcher, A. J. (2006). Nurses and doulas: Complementary roles to provide optimal maternity care. *Journal of Obstetrics, Gynecologic & Neonatal Nursing,* 35(2), 304–311.

Billington, M., & Stevenson, M. (2007). *Critical care in childbirth for midwives.* Malden, MA: Blackwell Publishers.

Blackburn, S. T. (2007). *Maternal, fetal and neonatal physiology: A clinical perspective* (3rd ed.). St. Louis, MO: Saunders Elsevier.

Bricker, L., & Luckas, M. (2007). Amniotomy alone for induction of labor updated. *Cochrane Database of Systematic Reviews,* 2. Art No.: CD002862. DOI: 1002/14651858.CD002862.

Brodsky, P. L. (2006). Childbirth: A journey through time. *International Journal of Childbirth Education,* 21(3), 10–15.

Centers for Disease Control and Prevention (CDC). (2007). Quick-Stats: Percentage of all live births by cesarean delivery—National Vital Statistics, United States. *MMWR,* 56(15), 373.

Cheng, Y. W., & Caughey, A. B. (2007). Normal labor and delivery. *eMedicine.* Available at: http://www.emedicine.com/MED/topic3239.htm

Cunningham, G., Gant, N. F., Leveno, K. J., Gilstrap, L. C., Hauth, J. C., & Wenstrom, K. D. (2005). *Williams' obstetrics* (22nd ed.). New York: McGraw-Hill.

Edmonds, K. (2007). *Dewhurst's textbook of obstetrics and gynecology* (7th ed.). Oxford, UK: Blackwell Publishers Limited.

Fischer, R. (2007). Breech presentation. *eMedicine.* Available at www.emedicine.com/med/topic3272.htm

Gagnon, A. J. (2006). Individual or group antenatal education for childbirth/parenthood. *Cochrane Library* 2006(4), CD002869.

Gulmezoglu, A. M., Crowther, C. A., & Middleton, P. (2007). Induction of labor for improving birth outcomes for women at or beyond term. *Cochrane Database of Systematic Reviews 2007,* 4. Art. No. CD004945. DIO: 10.1002/14651858.CD004945.pub2.

Gilbert, E. S. (2007). *Manual of high-risk pregnancy and birth.* St. Louis: Mosby.

Hanson, L. (2006). Pushing for change. *Journal of Perinatal & Neonatal Nursing,* 20(4), 282–284.

Hodnett, E. D., Gates, S., Hofmeyr, G. J., & Sakala, C. (2003). Continuous support for women during childbirth. *Cochrane Database of Systematic Reviews,* 3. Art. No. CD003766 DOI: 10.1002/14651858.CD003766.

Institute of Medicine (IOM). (2007). *Preterm birth: Causes, consequences, and prevention.* Washington, DC: National Academies Press.

Kenner, C., & Lott, J. W. (2007). *Comprehensive neonatal care: An interdisciplinary approach* (4th ed.). St. Louis: Saunders Elsevier.

Leonard, P. (2007). Childbirth education: A handbook for nurses. *Nursing Spectrum.* Available at: http://nsweb.nursingspectrum.com/ce/m350b.htm.

Polomeno, V. (2006). Relationship or content? Which is more important in perinatal education? *International Journal of Childbirth Education,* 22(1), 4–16.

Risica, P. M., & Phipps, M. G. (2006). Educational preferences in a prenatal clinic. *International Journal of Childbirth Education, 21*(4), 4–7.

Roberts, J. M., Gonzalez, C. B., & Sampselle, C. (2007). Why do supportive birth attendants become directive of maternal bearing-down efforts in second-stage labor? *Journal of Midwifery & Women's Health, 52*(2), 134–141.

Russell, K. E. (2007). Mad, bad or different? Midwives and normal birth in obstetric-led units. *British Journal of Midwifery, 15*(3), 128–131.

Simkin, P., & Ancheta, R. S. (2006). *The labor progress handbook* (2nd ed.). Malden, MA: Blackwell Publishers.

Smith, C. A., Collins, C. T., Cyna, A. M., & Crowther, C. A. (2006). Complementary and alternative therapies for pain management in labor. *Cochrane Library, 2006*(4), CD003521: 2009358378.

Steppe, B. (2007). In honor of the midwife. *International Journal of Childbirth Education, 22*(1), 39–40.

Terry, R. R., Westcott, J., O'Shea, L., & Kelly, F. (2006). Postpartum outcomes in supine delivery by physicians vs. nonsupine delivery by midwives. *Journal of the American Osteopathic Association, 106*(4), 199–205.

U.S. Department of Health and Human Services (USDHHS). (2000). *Healthy people 2010.* Washington, DC: Author.

Walsh, D. (2007). *Evidence-based care for normal labor and birth.* Andover, UK: Taylor & Francis, Inc.

Wood, S. (2007). Coping with labor pain. *March of Dimes.* Available at: http://www.marchofdimes.com/printableArticles/240_12936.asp

WEBSITES

Academy for Guided Imagery, Inc.: www.interactiveimagery.com/
American College of Obstetricians and Gynecologists: www.acog.org
American College of Nurse Midwives: www.midwife.org
American Public Health Association: www.apha.org
Association of Labor Assistants and Childbirth Educators: www.alace.org
Association of Women's Health, Obstetric and Neonatal Nurses (AWHONN): www.awhonn.org
Birthworks: www.birthworks.org
Childbirth Organization: www.childbirth.org
Diversity Rx: www.diversityrx.org
Doulas of North America: www.dona.org
Evidence-Based Nursing: www.evidencebasednursing.com
HypnoBirthing Institute: www.hypnobirthing.com
International Childbirth Education Association: www.icea.org
Lamaze International: www.lamaze-childbirth.com
National Association of Childbearing Centers: www.birthcenters.org

CHAPTER WORKSHEET

MULTIPLE CHOICE QUESTIONS

1. When determining the frequency of contractions, the nurse would measure which of the following?

   a. Start of one contraction to the start of the next contraction

   b. Beginning of one contraction to the end of the same contraction

   c. Peak of one contraction to the peak of the next contraction

   d. End of one contraction to the beginning of the next contraction

2. Which fetal lie is most conducive to a spontaneous vaginal birth?

   a. Transverse

   b. Longitudinal

   c. Perpendicular

   d. Oblique

3. Which of the following observations would suggest that placental separation is occurring?

   a. Uterus stops contracting altogether.

   b. Umbilical cord pulsations stop.

   c. Uterine shape changes to globular.

   d. Maternal blood pressure drops.

4. As the nurse is explaining the difference between true versus false labor to her childbirth class, she states that the major difference between them is:

   a. Discomfort level is greater with false labor.

   b. Progressive cervical changes occur in true labor.

   c. There is a feeling of nausea with false labor.

   d. There is more fetal movement with true labor.

5. The shortest but most intense phase of labor is the:

   a. Latent phase

   b. Active phase

   c. Transition phase

   d. Placental expulsion phase

6. A laboring woman is admitted to the labor and birth suite at 6 cm dilation. She would be in which phase of the first stage of labor?

   a. Latent

   b. Active

   c. Transition

   d. Early

7. Which assessment would indicate that a women is in true labor?

   a. Membranes are ruptured and fluid is clear

   b. Presenting part is engaged and not floating

   c. Cervix is 4 cm dilated, 90% effaced

   d. Contractions last 30 seconds, every 5 to 10 minutes

CRITICAL THINKING EXERCISES

1. Cindy, a 20-year-old primipara, calls the birthing center where you work as a nurse and reports she thinks she is in labor because she feels labor pains. Her due date is this week. The midwives have been giving her prenatal care throughout this pregnancy.

   a. What additional information do you need to respond appropriately?

   b. What suggestions/recommendations would you make to her?

   c. What instructions need to be given to guide her decision making?

   d. What other premonitory signs of labor might the nurse ask about?

   e. What manifestations would be found if Cindy is experiencing true labor?

2. You are assigned to lead a community education class for women in their third trimester of pregnancy to prepare them for their upcoming birth. Prepare an outline of topics that should be addressed.

STUDY ACTIVITIES

1. During clinical post-conference, share with the other nursing students how the critical forces of labor influenced the length of labor and the birthing process for a laboring woman assigned to you.

2. The cardinal movements of labor include which of the following? Select all that apply.

   a. Extension and rotation

   b. Descent and engagement

   c. Presentation and position

   d. Attitude and lie

   e. Flexion and expulsion

3. Interview a woman on the mother–baby unit who has given birth within the past few hours. Ask her to describe her experience and examine psychological factors that may have influenced her laboring process.

4. On the following illustration, identify the parameters of uterine contractions by marking an "X" where the nurse would measure the duration of the contraction.

NURSING MANAGEMENT DURING LABOR AND BIRTH

KEY TERMS

accelerations
artifact
baseline fetal heart rate
baseline variability
crowning

deceleration
electronic fetal
    monitoring
episiotomy
Leopold's maneuvers

neuraxial analgesia/
    anesthesia
periodic baseline changes

LEARNING OBJECTIVES

Upon completion of the chapter, the learner will be able to:

1. Define the key terms related to the labor and birth process.
2. Discuss the measures used to evaluate maternal status during labor and birth.
3. Explain the advantages and disadvantages of external and internal fetal monitoring, including the appropriate use for each.
4. Choose appropriate nursing interventions to address nonreassuring fetal heart rate patterns.
5. Outline the nurse's role in fetal assessment.
6. Explain the various comfort-promotion and pain-relief strategies used during labor and birth.
7. Summarize the assessment data collected on admission to the perinatal unit.
8. Discuss the ongoing assessments involved in each stage of labor and birth.
9. Explain the nurse's role throughout the labor and birth process.

Sheila is admitted in active labor (5 cm dilated) to the labor and birth suite at term. This is her second pregnancy and she is prepared to avoid pain medications this time so she can be more involved with the birthing process. She has been using modified-paced breathing with success thus far.

Wow

Wise nurses are not always silent, but they know when to be during the miracle of birth.

The laboring and birthing process is a life-changing event for many women. Nurses need to be respectful, available, encouraging, supportive, and professional in dealing with all women. Nursing management for labor and birth involves assessment, comfort measures, emotional support, information and instruction, advocacy, and support for the partner (Sauls, 2007).

The health of mothers and their infants is of critical importance, both as a reflection of the current health status of a large segment of our population and as a predictor of the health of the next generation. *Healthy People 2010* (USDHHS, 2000) addresses maternal health in two objectives: reducing maternal deaths and reducing maternal illness and complications due to pregnancy. In addition, another objective addresses increasing the proportion of pregnant women who attend prepared childbirth classes. (See Chapters 12 and 22 for more information on these objectives.)

This chapter provides information about nursing management during labor and birth. First, the essentials for in-depth assessment of maternal and fetal status during labor and birth are discussed. This is followed by a thorough description of the major methods of promoting comfort and providing pain management. The chapter concludes by putting all the information together with a discussion of the nursing care specific to each stage of labor, including the necessary data to be obtained with the admission assessment, methods to evaluate labor progress during the first stage of labor, and key nursing measures that focus on maternal and fetal assessments and pain relief for all stages of labor.

Maternal Assessment During Labor and Birth

During labor and birth, various techniques are used to assess maternal status. These techniques provide an ongoing source of data to determine the woman's response and her progress in labor. Assess maternal vital signs, including temperature, blood pressure, pulse, respiration, and pain, which are primary components of the physical examination and ongoing assessment. Also review the prenatal record to identify risk factors that may contribute to a decrease in uteroplacental circulation during labor. If there is no vaginal bleeding on admission, a vaginal examination is performed to assess cervical dilation, after which it is monitored periodically as necessary to identify progress. Evaluate maternal pain and the effectiveness of pain-management strategies at regular intervals during labor and birth.

Vaginal Examination

Although not all nurses perform vaginal examinations on laboring women in all practice settings, most nurses working in community hospitals do so because physicians are not routinely present in labor and birth suites. Since most newborns in the United States are born in community hospitals, nurses are performing vaginal examinations (American Hospital Association, 2007). Vaginal examinations are also performed by midwives and physicians.

▶ **Take** NOTE!

A vaginal examination is an assessment skill that takes time and experience to develop; only by doing it frequently in clinical practice can the practitioner's skill level improve.

The purpose of performing a vaginal examination is to assess the amount of cervical dilation, the percentage of cervical effacement, and the fetal membrane status and to gather information on presentation, position, station, degree of fetal head flexion, and presence of fetal skull swelling or molding (Fig. 14.1). Prepare the woman by informing her about the procedure, what information will be obtained from it, how she can assist with the procedure, how it will be performed, and who will be performing it.

The woman is typically on her back during the vaginal examination. The vaginal examination is performed gently, with concern for the woman's comfort. If it is the initial vaginal examination to check for membrane status, water is used as a lubricant. If the membranes have already ruptured, an antiseptic solution is used to prevent an ascending infection. After donning sterile gloves, the examiner inserts his or her index and middle fingers into the vaginal introitus. Next, the cervix is palpated to assess dilation, effacement, and position (e.g., posterior or an-

FIGURE 14.1 Vaginal examination to determine cervical dilation and effacement.

terior). If the cervix is open to any degree, the presenting fetal part, fetal position, station, and presence of molding can be assessed. In addition, the membranes can be evaluated and described as intact, bulging, or ruptured.

At the conclusion of the vaginal examination, the findings are discussed with the woman and her partner to bring them up to date about labor progress. In addition, the findings are documented either electronically or in writing and reported to the primary health care professional in charge of the case.

Cervical Dilation and Effacement

The amount of cervical dilation and the degree of cervical effacement are key areas assessed during the vaginal examination as the cervix is palpated with the gloved index finger. Although this finding is somewhat subjective, experienced examiners typically come up with similar findings. The width of the cervical opening determines dilation, and the length of the cervix assesses effacement. The information yielded by this examination serves as a basis for determining which stage of labor the woman is in and what her ongoing care should be.

Fetal Descent and Presenting Part

In addition to cervical dilation and effacement findings, the vaginal examination can also determine fetal descent (station) and presenting part. During the vaginal examination, the gloved index finger is used to palpate the fetal skull (if vertex presentation) through the opened cervix or the buttocks in the case of a breech presentation. Station is assessed in relation to the maternal ischial spines and the presenting fetal part. These spines are not sharp protrusions but rather blunted prominences at the midpelvis. The ischial spines serve as landmarks and have been designated as zero station. If the presenting part is palpated higher than the maternal ischial spines, a negative number is assigned; if the presenting fetal part is felt below the maternal ischial spines, a plus number is assigned, denoting how many centimeters below zero station.

Progressive fetal descent (−5 to +4) is the expected norm during labor—moving downward from the negative stations to zero station to the positive stations in a timely manner. If progressive fetal descent does not occur, a disproportion between the maternal pelvis and the fetus might exist and needs to be investigated.

Rupture of Membranes

The integrity of the membranes can be determined during the vaginal examination. Typically, if intact, the membranes will be felt as a soft bulge that is more prominent during a contraction. If the membranes have ruptured, the woman may have reported a sudden gush of fluid. Membrane rupture also may occur as a slow trickle of fluid. When membranes rupture, the priority focus should be on assessing fetal heart rate (FHR) first to identify a deceleration, which might indicate cord compression secondary to cord prolapse. If the membranes are ruptured

when the woman comes to the hospital, it is important to ascertain when it occurred. Prolonged ruptured membranes increase the risk of infection as a result of ascending vaginal organisms for both mother and fetus. Signs of intrauterine infection to be alert for include maternal fever, fetal and maternal tachycardia, foul odor of vaginal discharge, and an increase in white blood cell count.

To confirm that membranes have ruptured, a sample of fluid is taken from the vagina and tested with Nitrazine paper to determine the fluid's pH. Vaginal fluid is acidic, whereas amniotic fluid is alkaline and turns Nitrazine paper blue. Sometimes, however, false-positive results may occur, especially in women experiencing a large amount of bloody show, because blood is alkaline. The membranes are most likely intact if the Nitrazine test tape remains yellow to olive green, with pH between 5 and 6. The membranes are probably ruptured if the Nitrazine test tape turns a blue-green to deep blue, with pH ranging from 6.5 to 7.5 (Frieden & Chan, 2007).

If the Nitrazine test is inconclusive, an additional test, called the fern test, can be used to confirm rupture of membranes. With this test, a sample of fluid is obtained, applied to a microscope slide, and allowed to dry. Using a microscope, the slide is examined for a characteristic fern pattern that indicates the presence of amniotic fluid.

Assessing Uterine Contractions

The primary power of labor is uterine contractions, which are involuntary. Uterine contractions increase intrauterine pressure, causing tension on the cervix. This tension leads to cervical dilation and thinning, which in turn eventually forces the fetus through the birth canal. Normal uterine contractions have a contraction (systole) and a relaxation (diastole) phase. The contraction resembles a wave, moving downward to the cervix and upward to the fundus of the uterus. Each contraction starts with a building up (increment), gradually reaching an acme (peak intensity), and then a letting down (decrement). Each contraction is followed by an interval of rest, which ends when the next contraction begins. At the acme (peak) of the contraction, the entire uterus is contracting, with the greatest intensity in the fundal area. The relaxation phase follows and occurs simultaneously throughout the uterus.

Uterine contractions during labor are monitored by palpation and by electronic monitoring. Assessment of the contractions includes frequency, duration, intensity, and uterine resting tone (see Chapter 13 for a more detailed discussion).

Uterine contractions with an intensity of 30 mm Hg or greater initiate cervical dilation. During active labor, the intensity usually reaches 50 to 80 mm Hg. Resting tone is normally between 5 and 10 mm Hg in early labor and between 12 and 18 mm Hg in active labor (Gilbert, 2007).

To palpate the fundus for contraction intensity, place the pads of your fingers on the fundus and describe how

FIGURE 14.2 Nurse palpating the woman's fundus during a contraction.

it feels: like the tip of the nose (mild), like the chin (moderate), or like the forehead (strong). Palpation of intensity is a subjective judgment of the indentability of the uterine wall; a descriptive term is assigned (mild, moderate, or strong) (Fig. 14.2).

▶ *Take NOTE!*

Frequent clinical experience is needed to gain accuracy in assessing the intensity of uterine contractions.

The second method used to assess the intensity of uterine contractions is electronic monitoring, either external or internal. Both methods provide an accurate measurement of the actual intensity of uterine contractions. Although the external fetal monitor is sometimes used to estimate the intensity of uterine contractions, it is not as accurate an assessment tool.

For woman at risk for preterm birth, home uterine activity monitoring can be used to screen for prelabor uterine contractility so that escalating contractility can be identified, allowing earlier intervention to prevent preterm birth. The home uterine activity monitor consists of a pressure sensor attached to a belt that is held against the abdomen and a recording/storage device that is carried on a belt or hung from the shoulder. Uterine activity is typically recorded by the woman for one hour twice daily, while she is performing routine activities. The stored data are transmitted via telephone to a perinatal nurse, and a receiving device prints out the data. The woman is contacted if there are any problems.

Although in theory identifying early contractions to initiate interventions to arrest the labor sounds reasonable, research shows that uterine activity monitoring in asymptomatic high-risk women is inadequate for predicting preterm birth (Herbst & Nilsson, 2006). This practice continues even though numerous randomized trials have found no relationship between monitoring and actual reduction of preterm labor. In more recent research findings, cervical length is predictive of preterm birth in all populations studied. A cervical length less than 25 mm warrants intervention to improve the health outcomes of pregnant women and their infants (Grimes-Dennis & Berghella, 2007).

Performing Leopold's Maneuvers

Leopold's maneuvers are a method for determining the presentation, position, and lie of the fetus through the use of four specific steps. This method involves inspection and palpation of the maternal abdomen as a screening assessment for malpresentation. A longitudinal lie is expected, and the presentation can be cephalic, breech, or shoulder. Each maneuver answers a question:

• What fetal part (head or buttocks) is located in the fundus (top of the uterus)?
• On which maternal side is the fetal back located? (Fetal heart tones are best auscultated through the back of the fetus.)
• What is the presenting part?
• Is the fetal head flexed and engaged in the pelvis?

Leopold's maneuvers are described in Nursing Procedure 14.1.

Fetal Assessment During Labor and Birth

A fetal assessment identifies well-being or signs that indicate compromise. The character of the amniotic fluid is assessed, but the fetal assessment focuses primarily on determining the FHR pattern. Fetal scalp sampling, fetal pulse oximetry, and fetal stimulation are additional assessments performed as necessary in the case of questionable FHR patterns.

Analysis of Amniotic Fluid

Amniotic fluid should be clear when the membranes rupture, either spontaneously or artificially through an amniotomy (a disposable plastic hook [Amnihook] is used to perforate the amniotic sac). Cloudy or foul-smelling amniotic fluid indicates infection. Green fluid may indicate that the fetus has passed meconium secondary to transient hypoxia; however, it is considered a normal occurrence if the fetus is in a breech presentation. If it is determined that meconium-stained amniotic fluid is due to fetal hypoxia, the maternity and pediatric teams work together to prevent meconium aspiration syndrome. This would necessitate suctioning after the head is born before the infant takes a breath and perhaps direct tracheal suctioning

Nursing Procedure 14.1

PERFORMING LEOPOLD'S MANEUVERS

Purpose: To Determine Fetal Presentation, Position, and Lie

1. Place the woman in the supine position and stand beside her.
2. Perform the first maneuver to determine presentation.
   a. Facing the woman's head, place both hands on the abdomen to determine fetal position in the uterine fundus.
   b. Feel for the buttocks, which will feel soft and irregular (indicates vertex presentation); feel for the head, which will feel hard, smooth, and round (indicates a breech presentation).

3. Complete the second maneuver to determine position.
   a. While still facing the woman, move hands down the lateral sides of the abdomen to palpate on which side the back is located (feels hard and smooth).
   b. Continue to palpate to determine on which side the limbs are located (irregular nodules with kicking and movement).

4. Perform the third maneuver to confirm presentation.
   a. Move hands down the sides of the abdomen to grasp the lower uterine segment and palpate the area just above the symphysis pubis.
   b. Place thumb and fingers of one hand apart and grasp the presenting part by bringing fingers together.
   c. Feel for the presenting part. If the presenting part is the head, it will be round, firm, and ballottable; if it is the buttocks, it will feel soft and irregular.

(continued)

Nursing Procedure 14.1 (continued)

5. Perform the fourth maneuver to determine attitude.
   a. Turn to face the client's feet and use the tips of the first three fingers of each hand to palpate the abdomen.
   b. Move fingers toward each other while applying downward pressure in the direction of the symphysis pubis. If you palpate a hard area on the side opposite the fetal back, the fetus is in flexion, because you have palpated the chin. If the hard area is on the same side as the back, the fetus is in extension, because the area palpated is the occiput.

Also, note how your hands move. If the hands move to-gether easily, the fetal head is not descended into the woman's pelvic inlet. If the hands do not move together and stop because of resistance, the fetal head is engaged into the woman's pelvic inlet (Dillon, 2007).

---

after birth if the Apgar score is low. In some cases an am-nioinfusion (introduction of warmed, sterile normal saline or Ringer's lactate solution into the uterus) is used to di-lute moderate to heavy meconium released in utero to as-sist in preventing meconium aspiration syndrome.

Analysis of the FHR

Analysis of the FHR is one of the primary evaluation tools used to determine fetal oxygen status indirectly. FHR assessment can be done intermittently using a fetoscope (a modified stethoscope attached to a headpiece) or a Doppler (ultrasound) device, or continuously with an electronic fetal monitor applied externally or internally.

Intermittent FHR Monitoring

Intermittent FHR monitoring involves auscultation via a fetoscope or a hand-held Doppler device that uses ultrasound waves that bounce off the fetal heart, produc-ing echoes or clicks that reflect the rate of the fetal heart (Fig. 14.3). Traditionally, a fetoscope was used to assess fetal heart rate, but the Doppler device has been found to have a greater sensitivity than the fetoscope (Edmonds, 2007); thus, at present it is more commonly used.

> ▶ *Take* NOTE!
>
> *Doppler devices are relatively low in cost and are not used only in hospitals. They are used in home births and birthing centers, and pregnant women can also purchase them to help reduce anxiety between clinical examinations if they had a previous problem during pregnancy (Walsh, 2007).*

Intermittent FHR monitoring allows the woman to be mobile in the first stage of labor. She is free to move around and change position at will since she is not attached to a stationary electronic fetal monitor. How-ever, intermittent monitoring does not provide a con-tinuous FHR recording and does not document how the fetus responds to the stress of labor (unless listening is done during the contraction). The best way to assess fetal well-being would be to start listening to the FHR at the end of the contraction (not after one) so that late decelerations could be detected. However, the pressure of the device during a contraction is uncomfortable and can distract the woman from using her paced-breathing patterns.

Intermittent FHR auscultation can be used to detect FHR baseline and rhythm and changes from baseline. However, it cannot detect variability and types of deceler-ations, as electronic fetal monitoring can (Murray, 2007).

FIGURE 14.3 Auscultating fetal heart rate.

During intermittent auscultation to establish a baseline, the FHR is assessed for a full minute after a contraction. From then on, unless there is a problem, listening for 30 seconds and multiplying the value by two is sufficient. If the woman experiences a change in condition during labor, auscultation assessments should be more frequent. Changes in condition include ruptured membranes or the onset of bleeding. In addition, more frequent assessments occur after periods of ambulation, a vaginal examination, admin-

istration of pain medications, or other clinically important events (Hale, 2007).

The FHR is heard most clearly at the fetal back. In a cephalic presentation, the FHR is best heard in the lower quadrant of the maternal abdomen. In a breech presentation, it is heard at or above the level of the maternal umbilicus (Fig. 14.4). As labor progresses, the FHR location will change accordingly as the fetus descends into the maternal pelvis for the birthing process. To ensure that

A   B   C

D   E

FIGURE 14.4 Locations for auscultating fetal heart rate based on fetal position. (**A**) Left occiput anterior (LOA). (**B**) Right occiput anterior (ROA). (**C**) Left occiput posterior (LOP). (**D**) Right occiput posterior (ROP). (**E**) Left sacral anterior (LSA).

the maternal heart rate is not confused with the FHR, palpate the client's radial pulse simultaneously while the FHR is being auscultated through the abdomen.

The procedure for using a fetoscope or Doppler device to assess FHR is similar (see Nursing Procedure 12.1 in Chapter 12). The main difference is that a small amount of water-soluble gel is applied to the woman's abdomen or ultrasound device before auscultation with the Doppler device to promote sound wave transmission. This gel is not needed when a fetoscope is used. Usually the FHR is best heard in the woman's lower abdominal quadrants; if it is not found quickly, it may help to locate the fetal back by performing Leopold's maneuvers.

Although the intermittent method of FHR assessment allows the client to move about during labor, the information obtained fails to provide a complete picture of the well-being of the fetus moment to moment. This leads to the question of what the fetal status is during the times that are not assessed. For women who are considered at low risk for complications, this period of non-assessment is not a problem. However, for the undiagnosed high-risk woman, it might prove ominous.

National professional organizations have provided general guidelines for the frequency of assessments based on existing evidence. The American College of Obstetricians and Gynecologists (ACOG), the Institute for Clinical Systems Improvement (ICSI), and the Association of Women's Health, Obstetric, and Neonatal Nurses (AWHONN) have published guidelines designed to assist clinicians in caring for laboring clients. Their recommendations are supported by large controlled studies. They recommend the following guidelines for assessing FHR:

- Initial 10- to 20-minute continuous FHR assessment on entry into labor/birth area
- Completion of a prenatal and labor risk assessment on all clients
- Intermittent auscultation every 30 minutes during active labor for a low-risk woman and every 15 minutes for a high-risk woman
- During the second stage of labor, every 15 minutes for the low-risk woman and every 5 minutes for the high-risk woman and during the pushing stage (ACOG, 2005; AWHONN, 2006; ICSI, 2007).

In several randomized controlled studies comparing intermittent auscultation with electronic monitoring in both low- and high-risk clients, no difference in intrapartum fetal death was found. However, in each study a nurse–client ratio of 1:1 was consistently maintained during labor (ICSI, 2007). This suggests that adequate staffing is essential with intermittent FHR monitoring to ensure optimal outcomes for the mother and fetus. There is insufficient evidence to indicate specific situations where continuous electronic fetal monitoring might result in better outcomes when compared to intermittent assess-

ment. However, in pregnancies involving an increased risk of perinatal death, cerebral palsy, or neonatal encephalopathy and when oxytocin is used for induction or augmentation, it is recommended that continuous electronic fetal monitoring be used rather than intermittent fetal auscultation (Society of Obstetricians and Gynecologists of Canada, 2006).

Continuous Electronic Fetal Monitoring

Electronic fetal monitoring uses a machine to produce a continuous tracing of the FHR. When the monitoring device is in place, a sound is produced with each heartbeat. In addition, a graphic record of the FHR pattern is produced.

Current methods of continuous electronic fetal monitoring were introduced in the United States during the 1960s, specifically for use in clients considered to be at high risk. However, the use of these methods gradually increased and they eventually came to be used for women other than just those at high risk. This increased use has become controversial because it is suspected of being associated with the steadily increasing rates of cesarean births. Many studies suggest that when compared with standardized intermittent auscultation, the use of intrapartum electronic fetal monitoring seems to increase the number of preterm and surgical births but has no significant effect on reducing the incidence of intrapartum death or long-term neurologic injury (Lockwood, 2007).

With electronic fetal monitoring, there is a continuous record of the FHR: no gaps exist, as they do with intermittent auscultation. The concept of hearing and evaluating every beat of the fetus's heart to allow for early intervention seems logical. On the downside, however, using continuous monitoring can limit maternal movement and encourages the woman to lie in the supine position, which reduces placental perfusion. Despite the criticisms, electronic fetal monitoring remains an accurate method for determining fetal health status by providing a moment-to-moment printout of FHR status.

Various groups within the medical community have criticized the use of continuous fetal monitoring for all pregnant clients, whether high risk or low risk. Concerns about the efficiency and safety of routine electronic fetal monitoring in labor have led expert panels in the United States to recommend that such monitoring be limited to high-risk pregnancies. However, its use in low-risk pregnancies continues globally (Gagnon, Meier, & Waghorn, 2007). This remains an important research issue.

Continuous electronic fetal monitoring can be performed externally (indirectly), with the equipment attached to the maternal abdominal wall, or internally (directly), with the equipment attached to the fetus. Both methods provide a continuous printout of the FHR, but they differ in their specificity. The efficacy of electronic fetal monitoring depends on the accurate interpretation of the tracings, not necessarily which method (external vs. internal) is used.

Continuous External Monitoring

In external or indirect monitoring, two ultrasound transducers, each of which is attached to a belt, are applied around the woman's abdomen. They are similar to the hand-held Doppler device. One transducer, called a toco-transducer, detects changes in uterine pressure and converts the pressure registered into an electronic signal that is recorded on graph paper (Murray, 2007). The toco-transducer is placed over the uterine fundus in the area of greatest contractility to monitor uterine contractions. The other ultrasound transducer records the baseline FHR, long-term variability, accelerations, and decelerations. It is positioned on the maternal abdomen in the midline between the umbilicus and the symphysis pubis. The diaphragm of the ultrasound transducer is moved to either side of the abdomen to obtain a stronger sound and is then attached to the second elastic belt. This transducer converts the fetal heart movements into beeping sounds and records them on graph paper (Fig. 14.5).

Good continuous data are provided on the FHR. External monitoring can be used while the membranes are still intact and the cervix is not yet dilated. It is non-invasive and can detect relative changes in abdominal pressure between uterine resting tone and contractions. External monitoring also measures the approximate duration and frequency of contractions, providing a permanent record of FHR (Murray, 2007).

However, external monitoring can restrict the mother's movements. It also cannot detect short-term variability. Signal disruptions can occur due to maternal obesity, fetal malpresentation, and fetal movement, as well as by artifact. **Artifact** describes irregular variations or absence of FHR on the fetal monitor record that result from mechanical limitations of the monitor or electrical interference. For instance, the monitor may pick up transmissions from CB radios used by truck drivers on nearby roads and translate them into a signal. Additionally, gaps in the monitor strip can occur periodically without explanation.

Continuous Internal Monitoring

Continuous internal monitoring is usually indicated for women or fetuses considered to be at high risk. Possible conditions might include multiple gestation, decreased fetal movement, abnormal FHR on auscultation, intrauterine growth restriction (IUGR), maternal fever, pre-eclampsia, dysfunctional labor, preterm birth, or medical conditions such as diabetes or hypertension. It involves the placement of a spiral electrode into the fetal presenting part, usually the head, to assess FHR and a pressure transducer placed internally within the uterus to record uterine contractions (Fig. 14.6). The fetal spiral electrode is considered the most accurate method of detecting fetal heart characteristics and patterns because it involves receiving a signal directly from the fetus (Murray, 2007). Trained labor and birth nurses can place the spiral electrode on the fetal head when the membranes rupture in some health care facilities, but they do not place the intrauterine pressure catheter in the uterus. Internal monitoring does not have to include both an intrauterine pressure catheter and a scalp electrode. A fetal scalp electrode can be used to monitor the fetal heartbeat without monitoring the maternal intrauterine pressure.

Both the FHR and the duration and interval of uterine contractions are recorded on the graph paper. This method permits evaluation of baseline heart rate and changes in rate and pattern.

Four specific criteria must be met for this type of monitoring to be used:

• Ruptured membranes
• Cervical dilation of at least 2 cm

FIGURE 14.5 Continuous external electronic fetal monitoring device applied to the woman in labor.

Intrauterine pressure catheter

Internal fetal monitor
Electrode
Scalp

FIGURE 14.6 Continuous internal electronic fetal monitoring.

• Presenting fetal part low enough to allow placement of the scalp electrode
• Skilled practitioner available to insert spiral electrode (ICSI, 2007)

Compared to external monitoring, continuous internal monitoring can accurately detect both short-term (moment-to-moment) changes and long-term variability (fluctuations within the baseline) and FHR dysrhythmias. In addition, maternal position changes and movement do not interfere with the quality of the tracing.

Determining FHR Patterns

Assessment parameters of the FHR are classified as baseline rate, baseline variability (long-term and short-term), and periodic changes in the rate (accelerations and decelerations). The nurse must be able to interpret the various FHR parameters to determine if the pattern is reassuring (indicating fetal well-being) or nonreassuring (indicating fetal problems) to care for the woman effectively during labor and birth. Table 14.1 summarizes these patterns.

Baseline FHR

Baseline fetal heart rate refers to the average FHR that occurs during a 10-minute segment that excludes periodic or episodic rate changes, such as tachycardia or bradycardia. It is assessed when the woman has no contractions and the fetus is not experiencing episodic FHR changes. The normal baseline FHR ranges between 110 and 160 beats per minute (bpm) (National Institute of Child Health and Human Development [NICHD], 2006). The normal baseline FHR can be obtained by auscultation, ultrasound, or Doppler, or by a continuous internal direct fetal electrode.

Fetal bradycardia occurs when the FHR is below 110 bpm and lasts 10 minutes or longer (NICHD, 2006).

It can be the initial response of a healthy fetus to asphyxia. Causes of fetal bradycardia might include fetal hypoxia, prolonged maternal hypoglycemia, fetal acidosis, administration of drugs to the mother, hypothermia, maternal hypotension, prolonged umbilical cord compression, and fetal congenital heart block (Arenson & Drake, 2007). Bradycardia may be benign if it is an isolated event, but it is considered an ominous sign when accompanied by a decrease in long-term variability and late decelerations.

Fetal tachycardia is a baseline FHR greater than 160 bpm that lasts for 10 minutes or longer (NICHD, 2006). It can represent an early compensatory response to asphyxia. Other causes of fetal tachycardia include fetal hypoxia, maternal fever, maternal dehydration, amnionitis, drugs (e.g., cocaine, amphetamines, nicotine), maternal hyperthyroidism, maternal anxiety, fetal anemia, prematurity, fetal heart failure, and fetal arrhythmias. Fetal tachycardia is considered an ominous sign if it is accompanied by a decrease in variability and late decelerations (Hale, 2007).

Baseline Variability

Baseline variability is defined as normal physiologic variations in the time intervals that elapse between each fetal heartbeat observed along the baseline in the absence of contractions, decelerations, and accelerations (Menihan & Kopel, 2008). It represents the interplay between the parasympathetic and sympathetic nervous systems. The constant interplay (push-and-pull effect) on the FHR from the parasympathetic and sympathetic systems produces a moment-to-moment change in the FHR. Because variability is in essence the combined result of autonomic nervous system branch function, its presence implies that the both branches are working and receiving adequate oxygen (Hale, 2007). Thus, variability is one of the most important characteristics of the FHR.

Variability is described in three ways: minimal or absent, moderate, and marked. Minimal or absent variability typically is caused by uteroplacental insufficiency, cord compression, maternal hypotension, uterine hyperstimulation, abruptio placentae, or a fetal dysrhythmia. Interventions to improve uteroplacental blood flow and perfusion through the umbilical cord include lateral positioning of the mother, increasing the IV fluid rate to improve maternal circulation, administering oxygen at 8 to 10 L/min by mask, considering internal fetal monitoring, documenting findings and reporting to the health care provider. Preparation for a surgical birth may be necessary if no changes occur after attempting the interventions.

Moderate viability indicates that the autonomic and central nervous systems of the fetus are well developed and well oxygenated. It is considered a good sign of fetal well-being and correlates with the absence of significant metabolic acidosis (Fig. 14.7).

Marked variability occurs when there are more than 25 beats of fluctuation in the FHR baseline. Causes of this include cord prolapse or compression, maternal hypotension, uterine hyperstimulation, and

TABLE 14.1   INTERPRETING FHR PATTERNS

Reassuring FHR signs	• Normal baseline (110–160 bpm) • Moderate bradycardia (100–110 bpm); good variability • Good beat-to-beat variability and fetal accelerations
Nonreassuring signs	• Fetal tachycardia (>160 bpm) • Moderate bradycardia (100–110 bpm); lost variability • Absent beat-to-beat variability • Marked bradycardia (90–100 bpm) • Moderate variable decelerations
Ominous signs	• Fetal tachycardia with loss of variability • Prolonged marked bradycardia (<90 bpm) • Severe variable decelerations (<70 bpm) • Persistent late decelerations

Sources: Hale, 2007; Lockwood, 2007; Murray, 2007, NICHD, 2006.

FIGURE 14.7 Long-term variability (average or moderate).

abruptio placentae. Interventions include determining the cause if possible, lateral positioning, increasing IV fluid rate, administering oxygen at 8 to 10 L/min by mask, discontinuing oxytocin infusion, observing for changes in tracing, considering internal fetal monitoring, communicating an abnormal pattern to the health care provider, and preparing for a surgical birth if no change in pattern is noted (Menihan & Kopel, 2008).

FHR variability is an important clinical indicator that is predictive of fetal acid–base balance and cerebral tissue perfusion (Bakker et al., 2007). As the central nervous system is desensitized by hypoxia and acidosis, FHR decreases until a smooth baseline pattern appears. Loss of variability may be associated with a poor outcome. Some causes of decreased variability include fetal hypoxia/acidosis, drugs that depress the central nervous system, congenital abnormalities, fetal sleep, prematurity, and fetal tachycardia (Walsh, 2007).

> ▶ *Take* NOTE!
>
> *External electronic fetal monitoring cannot assess short-term variability. Therefore, if external monitoring shows a baseline that is smoothing out, use of an internal spiral electrode should be considered to gain a more accurate picture of the fetal health status.*

Periodic Baseline Changes

Periodic baseline changes are temporary, recurrent changes made in response to a stimulus such as a contraction. The FHR can demonstrate patterns of acceleration or deceleration in response to most stimuli. Fetal **accelerations** are transitory increases in the FHR above the baseline associated with sympathetic nervous stimulation. They are visually apparent, with elevations of FHR of more than 15 bpm above the baseline, and their duration is less than 2 minutes (NICHD, 2006). They are generally considered reassuring and require no interventions. Accelerations denote fetal movement and fetal well-being and are the basis for nonstress testing.

A **deceleration** is a transient fall in FHR caused by stimulation of the parasympathetic nervous system. Decelerations are described by their shape and association to a uterine contraction. They are classified as early, late, variable, and prolonged (Fig. 14.8).

Early decelerations are characterized by a gradual decrease in the FHR in which the nadir (lowest point) occurs at the peak of the contraction. They rarely decrease more than 30 to 40 bpm below the baseline. Typically, the onset, nadir, and recovery of the deceleration occur at the same time as the onset, peak and recovery of the contraction. They are most often seen during the active stage of any normal labor, during pushing, crowning, or vacuum extraction. They are thought to be a result of fetal head compression that results in a reflex vagal response with a resultant slowing of the FHR during uterine contractions. Early decelerations are not indicative of fetal distress and do not require intervention.

Late decelerations are transitory decreases in FHR that occur after a contraction begins. The FHR does not return to baseline levels until well after the contraction has ended. Delayed timing of the deceleration occurs, with the nadir of the uterine contraction. Late decelerations are associated with uteroplacental insufficiency, which occurs when blood flow within the intervillous space is decreased to the extent that fetal hypoxia exists (Bakker et al., 2007). Conditions that may decrease uteroplacental perfusion with resultant decelerations include maternal hypotension, gestational hypertension, placental aging secondary to diabetes and postmaturity, hyperstimulation via oxytocin infusion, maternal smoking, anemia, and cardiac disease. They imply some degree of fetal hypoxia. Repetitive late decelerations and late decelerations with decreasing baseline variability are nonreassuring signs. Box 14.1 highlights interventions for decelerations.

Variable decelerations present as visually apparent abrupt decreases in FHR below baseline and have an unpredictable shape on the FHR baseline, possibly demonstrating no consistent relationship to uterine contractions. The shape of variable decelerations may be U, V, or W, or they may not resemble other patterns (Hale, 2007). Variable decelerations usually occur abruptly with quick deceleration. They are the most common deceleration pattern

FIGURE 14.8 Decelerations. (**A**) Early. (**B**) Variable. (**C**) Late.

found in the laboring woman and are usually transient and correctable (Murray, 2007). Variable decelerations are associated with cord compression. However, they become a nonreassuring sign when the FHR decreases to less than 60 bpm, persists at that level for at least 60 seconds, and is repetitive (ICSI, 2007). The pattern of variable deceleration consistently related to the contractions with a slow return to FHR baseline is also nonreassuring.

Prolonged decelerations are abrupt FHR declines of at least 15 bpm that last longer than 2 minutes but less than 10 minutes (NICHD, 2006). The rate usually drops to less than 90 bpm. Many factors are associated with this pattern, including prolonged cord compression, abruptio placentae, cord prolapse, supine maternal position, vaginal examination, fetal blood sampling, maternal seizures, regional anesthesia, or uterine rupture (Murray, 2007). Prolonged decelerations can be remedied by identifying the underlying cause and correcting it.

Combinations of FHR patterns obtained by electronic fetal monitoring during labor are not infrequent. Nonreassuring patterns are more significant if they are mixed and persist for long periods. Other nonreassuring patterns include prolonged late decelerations, absent or minimal variability, bradycardia or tachycardia, and prolonged variable decelerations lower than 60 bpm. The likelihood of fetal compromise is increased if various nonreassuring patterns coexist, particularly those associated with decreased baseline variability or abnormal contraction patterns (ICSI, 2007).

Other Fetal Assessment Methods

In situations suggesting the possibility of fetal compromise, such as inconclusive or nonreassuring FHR patterns, further ancillary testing such as fetal scalp sampling, fetal pulse oximetry, and fetal stimulation may be used to validate the FHR findings and assist in planning interventions.

Fetal Scalp Sampling

Fetal scalp sampling was developed as a means of measuring fetal distress in conjunction with electronic fetal monitoring to make critical decisions about the management of labor and to prevent unnecessary operative interventions resulting from the use of electronic fetal monitoring alone. Nonreassuring FHR patterns may not necessarily indicate fetal hypoxia or acidosis. Therefore, assessing fetal acid–base status through fetal scalp sampling may help to prevent unnecessary surgical intervention.

A sample of fetal scalp blood is obtained to measure the pH. Sampling requires that the woman have ruptured membranes, cervical dilation of at least 3 to 5 cm, and a vertex presentation at −1 station (Moses, 2007). Normal fetal blood pH is 7.25 to 7.35. When the fetal scalp pH is below 7.15, this is a nonreassuring finding indicating acidosis (Moses, 2007).

> **BOX 14.1 Interventions for Nonreassuring Decelerations**
>
> If a patient develops a nonreassuring deceleration pattern such as late or variable decelerations:
> • Notify the health care provider about the pattern and obtain further orders, making sure to document all interventions and their effects on the FHR pattern.
> • Reduce or discontinue oxytocin as dictated by the facility's protocol, if it is being administered.
> • Provide reassurance that interventions are being done to effect a pattern change.
> Additional interventions specific for a late deceleration FHR pattern would include:
> • Turning the client on her left side to increase placental perfusion
> • Administering oxygen by mask to increase fetal oxygenation
> • Increasing the IV fluid rate to improve intravascular volume
> • Assessing client for any underlying contributing causes
> • Providing reassurance that interventions are to effect pattern change
> Specific interventions for a variable deceleration FHR pattern would include:
> • Changing the client's position to relieve compression on the cord
> • Providing reassurance that interventions are to effect pattern change
> • Giving oxygen and IV fluids as ordered

▶ **Take** NOTE!

During the past decade, the use of fetal scalp sampling has decreased, being replaced by less invasive techniques that yield similar information.

Fetal Oxygen Saturation Monitoring (Fetal Pulse Oximetry)

Fetal pulse oximetry measures fetal oxygen saturation directly and in real time. It is used with electronic fetal monitoring as an adjunct method of assessment when the FHR pattern is nonreassuring or inconclusive. Normal oxygen saturation of a healthy fetus is 30% to 70% (Miller, 2007). If the fetal oxygen saturation is reassuring (a trend of more than 30% between contractions), unnecessary cesarean births, invasive procedures such as fetal blood sampling, and operative vaginal births can be minimized (Peek, Condous, & Nanan, 2007). Any reduction in un-

necessary interventions during labor and birth has the potential to improve maternal and fetal outcomes and reduce costs.

Adequate maintenance of fetal oxygenation is necessary for fetal well-being. Fetal oxygen saturation monitoring is used for a singleton term fetus in a vertex presentation, at a −2 station or below, and with a nonreassuring FHR pattern. In addition, the fetal membranes must be ruptured and the cervix dilated at least 2 cm (Gilbert, 2007). A soft sensor is introduced through the dilated cervix and placed on the cheek, forehead, or temple of the fetus. It is held in place by the uterine wall. The sensor then is attached to a special adaptor on the fetal monitor that provides a real-time recording that is displayed on the uterine activity panel of the tracing. It is a noninvasive, safe, and accurate method for assessing fetal oxygenation.

The fetal pulse oximetry traces along the contraction portion of the monitoring strip, so it is easy to see how the saturation changes with the contraction. This adjunct test can help support decisions to allow labor to continue or to intervene surgically. Observing the trend of oxygen saturation on the tracing and documenting the values on the labor flow sheet or other medical record forms is crucial. The physician or midwife must be notified if the fetal oxygen saturation becomes nonreassuring (less than 30% between contractions) in conjunction with a nonreassuring FHR pattern. Ongoing communication is needed between the nurse and the primary care provider to enhance the maternal–fetus status.

Fetal Stimulation

An indirect method used to evaluate fetal oxygenation and acid–base balance to identify fetal hypoxia is fetal scalp stimulation and vibroacoustic stimulation. If the fetus does not have adequate oxygen reserves, carbon dioxide builds up, leading to acidemia and hypoxemia. These metabolic states are reflected in nonreassuring FHR patterns as well as fetal inactivity. Fetal stimulation is performed to promote fetal movement with the hope that FHR accelerations will accompany the movement.

Fetal movement can be stimulated with a vibroacoustic stimulator (artificial larynx) applied to the woman's lower abdomen and turned on for a few seconds to produce sound and vibration or by tactile stimulation via pelvic examination and stimulation of the fetal scalp with the gloved fingers. A well-oxygenated fetus will respond when stimulated (tactile or by noise) by moving in conjunction with an acceleration of 15 bpm above the baseline heart rate that lasts at least 15 seconds. This FHR acceleration reflects a pH of more than 7 and a fetus with an intact central nervous system. Fetal scalp stimulation is not done if the fetus is preterm, or if the woman has an intrauterine infection, a diagnosis of placenta previa (which could lead to hemorrhage), or a fever (which increases the risk of an ascending infection) (Gilbert, 2007).

Promoting Comfort and Providing Pain Management During Labor

Pain during labor is a universal experience, although the intensity of the pain may vary. Although labor and childbirth are viewed as natural processes, both can produce significant pain and discomfort. The physical causes of pain during labor include cervical stretching, hypoxia of the uterine muscle due to a decrease in perfusion during contractions, pressure on the urethra, bladder, and rectum, and distention of the muscles of the pelvic floor (Leonard, 2007). A woman's pain perception can be influenced by her previous experiences with pain, fatigue, pain anticipation, positive or negative support system, labor and birth environment, cultural expectations, and level of emotional stress and anxiety (Albers, 2007).

The techniques used to manage the pain of labor vary according to geography and culture. For example, some Appalachian women believe that placing a hatchet or knife under the bed of a laboring woman may help "cut the pain of childbirth," and a woman from this background may wish to do so in the hospital setting (Bowers, 2007). Asian, Latino, and Orthodox Jewish women may request that their own mothers, not their husbands, attend their births; husbands do not actively participate in the birthing process. Cherokee, Hmong, and Japanese women will often remain quiet during labor and birth and not complain of pain because outwardly expressing pain is not appropriate in their cultures. Never interpret their quietness as freedom from pain (Bowers, 2007).

Culturally diverse childbearing families present to the labor and birth suites with the same needs and desires of all families. Give them the same respect and sense of welcome shown to all families. Make sure they have a high-quality birth experience: uphold their religious, ethnic, and cultural values and integrate them into care.

Today, women have many safe nonpharmacologic and pharmacologic choices for the management of pain during labor and birth, which may be used separately or in combination with one another.

Nurses are in an ideal position to provide childbearing women with balanced, clear, concise information about effective nonpharmacologic and pharmacologic measures to relieve pain. Pain management standards issued by JCAHO mandate that pain be assessed in all clients admitted to a health care facility. Thus, it is important for nurses to be knowledgeable about the most recent scientific research on labor pain-relief modalities, to make sure that accurate and unbiased information about effective pain-relief measures is available to laboring women, to be sure that the woman determines what is an acceptable labor pain level for her, and to allow the woman the choice of pain-relief method.

Nonpharmacologic Measures

Nonpharmacologic measures may include continuous labor support, hydrotherapy, ambulation and position changes, acupuncture and acupressure, attention focusing and imagery, therapeutic touch and massage, breathing techniques, and effleurage. Most of these methods are based on the "gate control" theory of pain, which proposes that local physical stimulation can interfere with pain stimuli by closing a hypothetical gate in the spinal cord, thus blocking pain signals from reaching the brain (Arenson & Drake, 2007). It has long been a standard of care for labor nurses to first provide or encourage a variety of nonpharmacologic measures before moving to the pharmacologic interventions.

Nonpharmacologic measures are usually simple, safe, and inexpensive to use. Many of these measures are taught in childbirth classes, and women should be encouraged to try a variety of methods prior to the real labor. Many of the measures need to be practiced for best results and coordinated with the partner/coach. The nurse provides support and encouragement for the woman and her partner using nonpharmacologic methods. Although women can't consciously direct the labor contractions, they can control how they respond to them, thereby enhancing their feelings of control.

Continuous Labor Support

Continuous labor support involves offering a sustained presence to the laboring woman by providing emotional support, comfort measures, advocacy, information and advice, and support for the partner (Gagnon, Meier, & Waghorn, 2007). A woman's family, a midwife, a nurse, a doula, or anyone else close to the woman can provide this continuous presence. A support person can assist the woman to ambulate, reposition herself, and use breathing techniques. A support person can also aid with the use of acupressure, massage, music therapy, or therapeutic touch. During the natural course of childbirth, a laboring woman's functional ability is limited secondary to pain, and she often has trouble making decisions. The support person can help make them based on his or her knowledge of the woman's birth plan and personal wishes.

Research has validated the value of continuous labor support versus intermittent support in terms of lower operative deliveries, cesarean births, and requests for pain medication (Armstrong & Feldman, 2007).

▶ *Take* NOTE!

The human presence is of immeasurable value to make the laboring woman feel secure.

Hydrotherapy

Hydrotherapy is a nonpharmacologic measure in which the woman immerses herself in warm water for relaxation and relief of discomfort. When the woman enters the warm water, the warmth and buoyancy help to release muscle tension and can impart a sense of well-being (Koenig, 2007). Warm water provides soothing stimulation of nerves in the skin, promoting vasodilatation, reversal of sympathetic nervous response, and a reduction in catecholamines (Blackburn, 2007). Contractions are usually less painful in warm water because the warmth and buoyancy of the water have a relaxing effect.

There are a wide range of hydrotherapy options available, from ordinary bathtubs to whirlpool baths and showers, combined with low lighting and music. Many hospitals provide showers and whirlpool baths for laboring women for pain relief. However, hydrotherapy is more commonly practiced in birthing centers managed by midwives. The recommendation for initiating hydrotherapy is that the woman be in active labor (more than 5 cm dilated) to prevent the slowing of labor contractions secondary to muscular relaxation. The woman's membranes can be intact or ruptured. Women are encouraged to stay in the bath or shower as long as they feel they are comfortable. The water temperature should not exceed body temperature, and the bath time typically is limited to 1 to 2 hours (Koenig, 2007).

Hydrotherapy is an effective pain-management option for many women. Women who are experiencing a healthy pregnancy can be offered this option, but the potential benefits or risks to the woman are still not known (Fink, Irwin, & Mitchell, 2007).

Ambulation and Position Changes

Ambulation and position changes during labor are another extremely useful comfort measure. Historically, women adopted a variety of positions during labor, rarely using the recumbent position until recently. The medical profession has favored recumbent positions during labor, but without evidence to demonstrate their appropriateness (Sleutel, Schultz, & Wyble, 2007).

Changing position frequently (every 30 minutes or so)—sitting, walking, kneeling, standing, lying down, getting on hands and knees, and using a birthing ball—helps relieve pain (Fig. 14.9). Position changes also may help to speed labor by adding the benefits of gravity and changing the shape of the pelvis. Research has found that the position that the woman assumes and the frequency of position changes have a profound effect on uterine activity and efficiency. Allowing the woman to obtain a position of comfort frequently facilitates a favorable fetal rotation by altering the alignment of the presenting part with the pelvis. As the mother continues to change position based on comfort, the optimal presentation is afforded (Gilbert, 2007). Supine and sitting positions should be avoided, since they may interfere with labor progress and can cause compression of the vena cava and decrease blood return to the heart.

Swaying from side to side, rocking, or other rhythmic movements may also be comforting. If labor is progressing

slowly, ambulating may speed it up again. Upright positions such as walking, kneeling forward, or doing the lunge on the birthing ball give most women a greater sense of control and active movement than just lying down. Table 14.2 highlights some of the more common positions that can be used during labor and birth.

Acupuncture and Acupressure

Acupuncture and acupressure can be used to relieve pain during labor. Although controlled research studies of these methods are limited, there is adequate evidence that both are useful in relieving pain associated with labor and birth. However, both methods require a trained, certified clinician, and such a person is not available in many birth facilities (Hantoushzadeh, Alhusseini, & Lebaschi, 2007).

Acupuncture involves stimulating key trigger points with needles. This form of Chinese medicine has been practiced for approximately 3,000 years. Classical Chinese teaching holds that throughout the body there are meridians or channels of energy (*qi*) that when in balance regulate body functions. Pain reflects an imbalance or obstruction of the flow of energy. The purpose of acupuncture is to restore *qi*, thus diminishing pain (Koenig, 2007). Stimulating the trigger points causes the release of endorphins, reducing the perception of pain.

Acupressure involves the application of a firm finger or massage at the same trigger points to reduce the pain sensation. The amount of pressure is important. The intensity of the pressure is determined by the needs of the woman. Holding and squeezing the hand of a woman in labor may trigger the point most commonly used for both techniques. Some acupressure points are found along the spine, neck, shoulder, toes, and soles of the feet (Armstrong & Feldman, 2007). A Cochrane Collaboration review found that acupuncture may indeed reduce labor pain, but the number of women studied has been small (Smith et al., 2006).

Attention Focusing and Imagery

Attention focusing and imagery uses many of the senses and the mind to focus on stimuli. The woman can focus on tactile stimuli such as touch, massage, or stroking. She may focus on auditory stimuli such as music, humming, or verbal encouragement. Visual stimuli might be any object in the room, or the woman can imagine the beach, a mountaintop, a happy memory, or even the contractions of the uterine muscle pulling the cervix open and the fetus pressing downward to open the cervix. Some women focus on a particular mental activity such as a song, a chant, counting backwards, or a Bible verse. Breathing, relaxation, positive thinking, and positive visualization work well for mothers in labor. The use of these techniques keeps the sensory input perceived during the contraction from reaching the pain center in the cortex of the brain (Armstrong & Feldman, 2007).

FIGURE 14.9 Various positions for use during labor. (**A**) Ambulation. (**B**) Leaning forward. (**C**) Sitting in a chair. (**D**) Using a birthing ball.

Therapeutic Touch and Massage

Therapeutic touch and massage use the sense of touch to promote relaxation and pain relief. Massage works as a form of pain relief by increasing the production of endorphins in the body. Endorphins reduce the transmission of signals between nerve cells and thus lower the perception of pain (Blackburn, 2007). In addition, touching and massage distract the woman from discomfort.

Therapeutic touch is based on the premises that the body contains energy fields that lead to either good or ill health and that the hands can be used to redirect the energy fields that lead to pain (Arenson & Drake, 2007). To be done correctly, this technique must be learned and

practiced. Some women prefer a light touch, while others find a firmer touch more soothing. Massage of the neck, shoulders, back, thighs, feet, and hands can be very comforting. The use of firm counterpressure in the lower back or sacrum is especially helpful for back pain during contractions (Fig. 14.10). Contraindications for massage include skin rashes, varicose veins, bruises, or infections (Leonard, 2007).

Effleurage is a light, stroking, superficial touch of the abdomen, in rhythm with breathing during contractions. It is used as a relaxation and distraction technique from discomfort. The external fetal monitor belts may interfere with the ability to accomplish this.

TABLE 14.2 COMMON POSITIONS FOR USE DURING LABOR AND BIRTH

Standing	• Takes advantage of gravity during and between contractions • Makes contractions feel less painful and be more productive • Helps fetus line up with angle of maternal pelvis • Helps to increase urge to push in second stage of labor
Walking	• Has the same advantages as standing • Causes changes in the pelvic joints, helping the fetus move through the birth canal
Standing and leaning forward on partner, bed, birthing ball	• Has the same advantages as standing • Is a good position for a backrub • May feel more restful than standing • Can be used with electronic fetal monitor
Slow dancing (standing with woman's arms around partner's neck, head resting on his chest or shoulder, with his hands rubbing woman's lower back; sway to music and breathe in rhythm if it helps)	• Has the same advantages as walking • Back pressure helps relieve back pain • Rhythm and music help woman relax and provide comfort
The lunge (standing facing a straight chair with one foot on the seat with knee and foot to the side; bending raised knee and hip, and lunging sideways repeatedly during a contraction, holding each lunge for 5 seconds; partner holds chair and helps with balance)	• Widens one side of the pelvis (the side toward lunge) • Encourages rotation of baby • Can also be done in a kneeling position
Sitting upright	• Helps promote rest • Has more gravity advantage than lying down • Can be used with electronic fetal monitor
Semi-sitting (setting the head of the bed at a 45-degree angle with pillows used for support)	• Has the same advantages as sitting upright • Is an easy position if on a bed
Sitting on toilet or commode	• Has the same advantages as sitting upright • May help relax the perineum for effective bearing down
Rocking in a chair	• Has the same advantages as sitting upright • May help speed labor (rocking movement)
Sitting, leaning forward with support	• Has the same advantages as sitting upright • Is a good position for a backrub
On all fours, on hands and knees	• Helps relieve backache • Assists rotation of baby in posterior position • Allows for pelvic rocking and body movement • Relieves pressure on hemorrhoids • Allows for vaginal examinations • Is sometimes preferred as a pushing position by women with back labor
Kneeling, leaning forward with support on a chair seat, the raised head of the bed, or on a birthing ball	• Has the same advantages as all-fours position • Puts less strain on wrists and hands
Side-lying	• Is a very good position for resting and convenient for many kinds of medical interventions • Helps lower elevated blood pressure • May promote progress of labor when alternated with walking • Is useful to slow a very rapid second stage • Takes pressure off hemorrhoids • Facilitates relaxation between contractions

(continued)

TABLE 14.2 COMMON POSITIONS FOR USE DURING LABOR AND BIRTH (continued)

Squatting	• May relieve backache • Takes advantage of gravity • Requires less bearing-down effort • Widens pelvic outlet • May help fetus turn and move down in a difficult birth • Helps if the woman feels no urge to push • Allows freedom to shift weight for comfort • Offers an advantage when pushing, since upper trunk presses on the top of the uterus
Supported squat (leaning back against partner, who supports woman under the arms and takes the entire woman's weight; standing up between contractions)	• Requires great strength in partner • Lengthens trunk, allowing more room for fetus to maneuver into position • Lets gravity help
Dangle (partner sitting high on bed or counter with feet supported on chairs or footrests and thighs spread; woman leaning back between partner's legs, placing flexed arms over partner's thighs; partner gripping sides with his thighs; woman lowering herself and allowing partner to support her full weight; standing up between contractions)	• Has the same advantages of a supported squat • Requires less physical strength from the partner

Sources: Albers, 2007; Armstrong & Feldman, 2007; Koenig, 2007; Walsh, 2007.

EVIDENCE-BASED PRACTICE 14.1
The Effects of Complementary and Alternative Therapies for Pain Management in Labor on Maternal and Perinatal Morbidity

● Study

The pain of labor can be intense, with tension, anxiety, and fear making it worse. Many women would like to labor without using drugs and turn to alternatives to manage pain. These alternative methods include acupuncture, mind-body techniques, massage, reflexology, herbal medicines or homoeopathy, hypnosis, and music. This review examined currently available evidence supporting the use of alternative and complementary therapies for pain management in labor. Fourteen trials were included in the review, with data reporting on 1,537 women using different modalities of pain management; 1,448 women were included in the meta-analysis.

▲ Findings

Acupuncture and hypnosis may help relieve labor pain. There is insufficient evidence about the benefits of music, massage, relaxation, white noise, acupressure, and aromatherapy, and no evidence about the effectiveness of massage or other complementary therapies. In summary, acupuncture and hypnosis may be beneficial for the management of pain during labor; however, the number of women studied has been small. Few other complementary therapies have been subjected to proper scientific study.

■ Nursing Implications

Although this study didn't offer conclusive evidence that alternative therapies for pain management work better than pharmacologic or invasive methods, they should not be discounted. Many women wish to avoid artificial means to control the discomfort of labor. The nurse should be supportive and open-minded about a woman's efforts to meet her pain management goals.

Smith, C. A., Collins, C. T., Cyna, A. M., & Crowther, C. A. (2006). Complementary and alternative therapies for pain management in labor. *Cochrane Database of Systematic Reviews* 2006, Issue 4. Art. No.: CD003521. DOI: 10.1002/14651858.CD003521.pub2.

FIGURE 14.10 Nurse massaging the client's back during a contraction while she ambulates during labor.

Breathing Techniques

Breathing techniques are effective in producing relaxation and pain relief through the use of distraction. If the woman is concentrating on slow-paced rhythmic breathing, she isn't likely to fully focus on contraction pain. Breathing techniques are often taught in childbirth education classes (see Chapter 12 for additional information).

Breathing techniques use controlled breathing to reduce the pain experienced through a stimulus–response conditioning. The woman selects a focal point within her environment to stare at during the first sign of a contraction. This focus creates a visual stimulus that goes directly to her brain. The woman takes a deep cleansing breath, which is followed by rhythmic breathing. Verbal commands from her partner supply an ongoing auditory stimulus to her brain. Effleurage can be combined with the breathing to provide a tactile stimulus, all blocking pain sensations to her brain.

Benefits of practicing patterned breathing include:

- Breathing becomes an automatic response to pain.
- Breathing increases relaxation and can be used for deal with life's everyday stresses.
- The steady rhythm of breathing is calming during labor.
- Breathing provides a sense of well-being and a measure of control.
- Breathing brings purpose to each contraction, making them more productive.
- Breathing provides more oxygen for the mother and fetus (American Pregnancy Association, 2007).

Many couples learn patterned-paced breathing during their childbirth education classes. Three levels may be taught, each beginning and ending with a cleansing breath. In the first pattern, also known as slow-paced breathing, the woman inhales slowly through her nose and exhales through pursed lips. The breathing rate is typically 6 to 9 bpm. In the second pattern, also called shallow or modified-paced breathing, the woman inhales and exhales through her mouth at a rate of 4 breaths every 5 seconds. The rate can be accelerated to 2 breaths per second to assist her to relax. The third pattern, pattern paced breathing, is similar to modified-paced breathing except that the breathing is punctuated every few breaths by a forceful exhalation through pursed lips. All breaths are kept equal and rhythmic and can increase as contractions increase in intensity (Lyon, 2007).

Many childbirth educators do not recommend specific breathing techniques or try to teach parents to breathe the "right" way during labor and birth. Couples are encouraged to find breathing styles that enhance their relaxation and use them. There are numerous benefits to controlled and rhythmic breathing in childbirth (outlined above), and many women choose these techniques to manage their discomfort during labor.

Pharmacologic Measures

With varying degrees of success, generations of women have sought ways to relieve the pain of childbirth. Pharmacologic pain relief during labor includes systemic analgesia and regional or local anesthesia. Women have seen dramatic changes in pharmacologic pain management options over the years. Methods have evolved from biting down on a stick to a more complex pharmacologic approach such as epidural/intrathecal analgesia. Systemic analgesia and regional analgesia/anesthesia have become less common, while newer neuraxial analgesia/anesthesia techniques involving minimal motor blockade have become more popular. **Neuraxial analgesia/anesthesia** is the administration of analgesic (opioids) or anesthetic (medication capable of producing a loss of sensation in an area of the body) agents, either continuously or intermittently, into the epidural or intrathecal space to relieve pain. Low-dose and ultra-low-dose epidural analgesia, spinal analgesia, and combined spinal-epidural analgesia have replaced the traditional epidural for labor (Kuczkowski, 2007). This shift in pain management allows a woman to be an active participant in labor.

▶ *Take* NOTE!

Regardless of which approach is used during labor, the woman has the right to choose the methods of pain control that will best suit her and meet her needs.

► *Consider THIS!*

When I was expecting my first child, I was determined to put my best foot forward and do everything right. I was an experienced OB nurse, and in my mind doing everything right was expected behavior. I was already 2 weeks past my calculated due date and I was becoming increasingly worried. That particular day I went to work with a backache but felt no contractions.

I managed to finish my shift but felt completely wiped out. As I walked to my car outside the hospital, my water broke and I felt the warm fluid run down my legs. I went back inside to be admitted for this much-awaited event.

Although I had helped thousands of women go through their childbirth experience, I was now the one in the bed and not standing alongside it. My husband and I had practiced our breathing techniques to cope with the discomfort of labor, but this "discomfort" in my mind was more than I could tolerate. So despite my best intentions of doing everything right, within an hour I begged for a painkiller to ease the pain. While the medication took the edge off my pain, I still felt every contraction and truly now appreciate the meaning of the word "labor." Although I wanted to use natural childbirth without any medication, I know that I was a full participant in my son's birthing experience, and that is what "doing everything right" was for me!

Thoughts: Doing what is right varies for each individual, and as nurses we need to support whatever that is. Having a positive outcome from the childbirth experience is the goal; the means it takes to achieve it is less important. How can nurses support women in making their personal choices to achieve a healthy outcome? Are any women "failures" if they ask for pain medication to tolerate labor? How can nurses help women overcome this stigma of being a "wimp"?

Systemic Analgesia

Systemic analgesia involves the use of one or more drugs administered orally, intramuscularly, or intravenously; they become distributed throughout the body via the circulatory system. Depending on which administration method is used, the therapeutic effect of pain relief can occur within minutes and last for several hours. The most important complication associated with the use of this class of drugs is respiratory depression. Therefore, women given these drugs require careful monitoring. Opioids given close to the time of birth can cause central nervous system depression in the newborn, necessitating the administration of naloxone (Narcan) to reverse the depressant effects of the opioids.

Several drug categories may be used for systemic analgesia:

- Opioids, such as butorphanol (Stadol), nalbuphine (Nubain), meperidine (Demerol), or fentanyl (Sublimaze)
- Ataractics, such as hydroxyzine (Vistaril) or promethazine (Phenergan)
- Benzodiazepines, such as diazepam (Valium) or midazolam (Versed)
- Barbiturates, such as secobarbital (Seconal) or pentobarbital (Nembutal)

Drug Guide 14.1 highlights some of the major drugs used for systemic analgesia.

Systemic analgesics are typically administered parenterally, usually through an existing intravenous (IV) line. Nearly all medications given during labor cross the placenta and have a depressant effect on the fetus; therefore, it is important for the woman to receive the least amount of systemic medication that relieves her discomfort so that it does not cause any harm to the fetus (Cheng & Caughey, 2007). Historically opioids have been administered by nurses, but in the past decade there has been increasing use of client-controlled intravenous analgesia (patient-controlled analgesia [PCA]). With this system, the woman is given a button connected to a computerized pump on the IV line. When the woman desires analgesia, she presses the button and the pump delivers a preset amount of medication. This system provides the woman with a sense of control over her own pain management and active participation in the childbirth process.

Opioids

Opioids are morphine-like medications that are most effective for the relief of moderate to severe pain. Opioids typically are administered IV. Of all of the synthetic opioids (butorphanol [Stadol], nalbuphine [Nubain], fentanyl [Sublimaze], and meperidine [Demerol]), meperidine is the most commonly used opioid for the management of pain during labor. Opioids are associated with newborn respiratory depression, decreased alertness, inhibited sucking, and a delay in effective feeding (Bagwell, 2007).

Opioids decrease the transmission of pain impulses by binding to receptor site pathways that transmit the pain signals to the brain. The effect is increased tolerance to pain and respiratory depression related to a decrease in sensitivity to carbon dioxide (Skidmore-Roth, 2007).

All opioids are considered good analgesics. However, respiratory depression can occur in the mother and fetus depending on the dose given. They may also cause a decrease in FHR variability identified on the fetal monitor strip. This FHR pattern change is usually transient. Other systemic side effects include nausea, vomiting, pruritus, delayed gastric emptying, drowsiness, hypoventilation, and newborn depression. To reduce the incidence of new-

DRUG GUIDE 14.1 COMMON AGENTS USED FOR SYSTEMIC ANALGESIA

Type	Drug	Comments
Opioids	Morphine 2–5 mg IV	May be given IV, intrathecally, or epidurally Rapidly crosses the placenta Can cause maternal and neonatal CNS depression Decreases uterine contractions
	Meperidine (Demerol) 25–50 mg IV	May be given IV or epidurally with maximal fetal uptake 2–3 hours after administration Can cause CNS depression Decreases fetal variability
	Butorphanol (Stadol) 1 mg IV q3–4h	Is given IV Is rapidly transferred across the placenta Causes neonatal respiratory depression
	Nalbuphine (Nubain) 10 mg IV	Is given IV Causes less maternal nausea and vomiting Causes decreased FHR variability, fetal bradycardia and respiratory depression
	Fentanyl (Sublimaze) 25–50 mcg IV	Is given IV or epidurally Can cause maternal hypotension, maternal and fetal respiratory depression Rapidly crosses placenta
Ataractics	Hydroxyzine (Vistaril) 50 mg IM	Does not relieve pain but reduces anxiety and potentiates opioid analgesic effects Is used to decrease nausea and vomiting
	Promethazine (Phenergan) 25 mg IV	Is used for antiemetic effect when combined with opioids Causes sedation and reduces apprehension May contribute to maternal hypotension and neonatal depression
Benzodiazepines	Diazepam (Valium) 2–5 mg IV	Is given to enhance pain relief of opioid and cause sedation May be used to stop eclamptic seizures Decreases nausea and vomiting Can cause newborn depression; therefore, lowest possible dose should be used
	Midazolam (Versed) 1–5 mg IV	Is not used for analgesic but amnesia effect Is used as adjunct for anesthesia Is excreted in breast milk
Barbiturates	Secobarbital (Seconal) 100 mg PO/IM	Causes sedation Is used in very early labor to alter a dysfunctional pattern
	Pentobarbital (Nembutal) 100 mg PO/IM	Is not used for pain relief in active labor Crosses placenta and is secreted in breast milk

Sources: Cheng & Caughey, 2007; Edmonds, 2007; Evron & Ezri, 2007; Skidmore-Roth, 2007; Wood, 2007.

born depression, birth should occur within 1 hour or after 4 hours of administration to prevent the fetus from receiving the peak concentration (Cheng & Caughey, 2007).

Opioid antagonists such as naloxone (Narcan) are given to reverse the effects of the central nervous system depression, including respiratory depression, caused by opioids. Opioid antagonists also are used to reverse the side effects of neuraxial opioids, such as pruritus, urinary retention, nausea, and vomiting, without significantly decreasing analgesia (Skidmore-Roth, 2007). Consult a current drug guide for more specifics on these drug categories.

Ataractics

The ataractic group of medications is used in combination with an opioid to decrease nausea and vomiting and lessen anxiety. These adjunct drugs potentiate the effectiveness of the opioid so that a lesser dose can be given. They may also be used to increase sedation. Promethazine (Phenergan) can be given IV, but hydroxyzine (Vistaril) must be given by mouth or by intramuscular injection into a large muscle mass. Neither drug affects the progress of labor, but either may cause a decrease in FHR variability and possible newborn depression (Albers, 2007).

Benzodiazepines

Benzodiazepines are used for minor tranquilizing and sedative effects. Diazepam (Valium) also is given IV to stop seizures due to pregnancy-induced hypertension. However, it is not used during labor itself. It can be administered to calm a woman who is out of control, thereby enabling her to relax enough so that she can participate effectively during her labor process rather than fighting against it. Lorazepam (Ativan) can also be used for its tranquilizing effect, but increased sedation is experienced with this medication (Skidmore-Roth, 2007). Midazolam (Versed), also given IV, produces good amnesia but no analgesia. It is most commonly used as an adjunct for anesthesia. Diazepam and midazolam cause central nervous system depression for both the woman and the newborn.

Barbiturates

The barbiturate drug group is used only in early labor or in a prolonged latent phase that produces enough discomfort that the woman cannot sleep. Barbiturates are given orally or intramuscularly to produce a light sleep to alter a dysfunctional labor pattern or to calm a very anxious woman in early labor. The goal in giving a barbiturate is to promote therapeutic rest for a few hours to enhance the woman's ability to cope with active labor. These drugs cross the placenta and cause central nervous system depression in the newborn (Skidmore-Roth, 2007).

Regional Analgesia/Anesthesia

Regional analgesia/anesthesia provides pain relief without loss of consciousness. It involves the use of local anesthetic agents, with or without added opioids, to bring about pain relief or numbness through the drug's effects on the spinal cord and nerve roots. Obstetric regional analgesia generally refers to a partial or complete loss of pain sensation below the T8 to T10 level of the spinal cord (Edmonds, 2007).

The routes for regional pain relief include epidural block, combined spinal–epidural block, local infiltration, pudendal block, and intrathecal (spinal) analgesia/anesthesia. Local and pudendal routes are used during birth for episiotomies; epidural and intrathecal routes are used for pain relief during active labor and birth. The major advantage of regional pain-management techniques is that the woman can participate in the birthing process and still have good pain control.

Epidural Block

Approximately 60% of laboring women in the United States receive an epidural block for pain relief during labor. In urban areas, many hospitals approach 90% use of epidurals (Kuczkowski, 2007).

An epidural block involves the injection of a drug into the epidural space, which is located outside the dura mater between the dura and the spinal canal. The epidural space is typically entered through the third and fourth lum-

bar vertebrae with a needle, and a catheter is threaded into the epidural space. The needle is removed and the catheter is left in place to allow for continuous infusion or intermittent injections of medicine (Fig. 14.11). An epidural block provides analgesia and anesthesia and can be used for both vaginal and cesarean births. It has evolved from a regional block producing total loss of sensation to analgesia with minimal blockade. The effectiveness of epidural analgesia depends on the technique and medications used. It is usually started after labor is well established, typically when cervical dilation is greater than 5 cm.

Theoretically, epidural local anesthetics could block all labor pain if used in large volumes and high concentrations. However, pain relief is balanced against other goals such as walking during the first stage of labor, pushing effectively in the second stage, and minimizing maternal and fetal side effects.

An epidural is contraindicated for women with a previous history of spinal surgery or spinal abnormalities, coagulation defects, infections, and hypovolemia. It also is contraindicated for the woman who is receiving anticoagulation therapy.

Complications include nausea and vomiting, hypotension, fever, pruritus, intravascular injection, and respiratory depression. Effects on the fetus during labor include fetal distress secondary to maternal hypotension (Bagwell, 2007). Ensuring that the woman avoids a supine position after an epidural catheter has been placed will help to minimize hypotension.

Changes in epidural drugs and techniques have been made to optimize pain control while minimizing side effects. Today most women receive a continuous lumbar epidural infusion of a local anesthetic, typically a drug whose name ends in "caine," and an opioid. To decrease motor blockade, bupivacaine (Sensorcaine) and ropivacaine (Naropin) have replaced lidocaine (Xylocaine), and drug concentrations have been lowered (Kuczkowski, 2007).

The addition of opioids, such as fentanyl or morphine, to the local anesthetic helps decrease the amount of motor block obtained. Continuous infusion pumps are used to administer the epidural analgesia, allowing the woman to be in control and administer a bolus dose on demand (Smiley & Stephenson, 2007).

Combined Spinal–Epidural Analgesia

Another epidural technique is combined spinal–epidural (CSE) analgesia. This technique involves inserting the epidural needle into the epidural space and subsequently inserting a small-gauge spinal needle through the epidural needle into the subarachnoid space. An opioid, without a local anesthetic, is injected into this space. The spinal needle is then removed and an epidural catheter is inserted for later use.

CSE is advantageous because of its rapid onset of pain relief (within 3 to 5 minutes) that can last up to 3 hours. It also allows the woman's motor function to remain active.

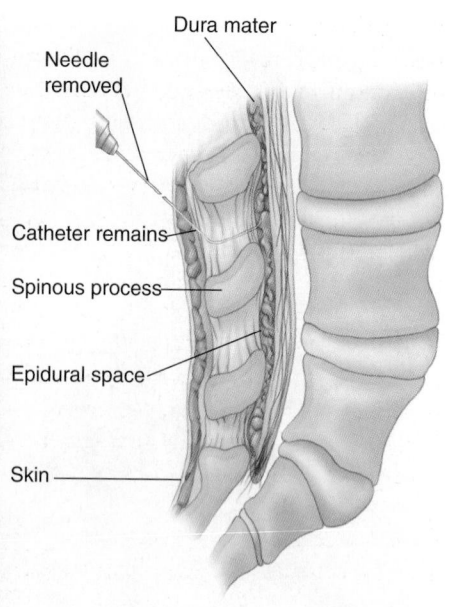

FIGURE 14.11 Epidural catheter insertion. (**A**) A needle is inserted into the epidural space. (**B**) A catheter is threaded into the epidural space; the needle is then removed. The catheter allows medication to be administered intermittently or continuously to relieve pain during labor and childbirth.

Her ability to bear down during the second stage of labor is preserved because the pushing reflex is not lost, and her motor power remains intact. The CSE technique provides greater flexibility and reliability for labor than either spinal or epidural analgesia alone (Kuczkowski, 2007). When compared with traditional epidural or spinal analgesia, which often keeps the woman lying in bed, CSE allows her to ambulate ("walking epidural") (Kuczkowski, 2007). Ambulating during labor provides several benefits: it may help control pain better, shorten the first stage of labor, increase the intensity of the contractions, and decrease the possibility of an operative vaginal or cesarean birth.

Although women can walk with CSE, they often choose not to because of sedation and fatigue. Often health care providers don't encourage or assist women to ambulate for fear of injury (Ros et al., 2007). Currently, anesthesiologists are performing walking epidurals using continuous infusion techniques as well as CSE and patient-controlled epidural analgesia (Smiley & Stephenson, 2007).

Complications include maternal hypotension, intravascular injection, accidental intrathecal blockade, postdural puncture headache, inadequate or failed block, and pruritus. Hypotension and associated FHR changes are managed with maternal positioning (semi-Fowler's position), intravenous hydration, and supplemental oxygen (Kuczkowski, 2007).

Patient-Controlled Epidural Analgesia

Patient-controlled epidural analgesia (PCEA) involves the use of an indwelling epidural catheter with an infusion of medication and a programmed pump that allows the woman to control the dosing. This method allows the woman to have a sense of control over her pain and reach her own individually acceptable analgesia level. When compared with the traditional epidural analgesia, PCEA provides equivalent analgesia with lower anesthetic use, lower rates of supplementation, and higher client satisfaction (Smiley & Stephenson, 2007).

With PCEA, the woman uses a hand-held device connected to an analgesic agent that is attached to an epidural catheter. When she pushes the button, a bolus dose of agent is administered via the catheter to reduce her pain. This method allows her to manage her pain at will without having to ask a staff member to provide pain relief.

Local Infiltration

Local infiltration involves the injection of a local anesthetic, such as lidocaine, into the superficial perineal nerves to numb the perineal area. This technique is done by the physician or midwife just before performing an episiotomy (surgical incision into the perineum to facilitate birth) or before suturing a laceration. Local infiltration does not alter the pain of uterine contractions, but it does numb the immediate area of the episiotomy or laceration. Local infiltration does not cause side effects for the woman or her newborn.

Pudendal Nerve Block

A pudendal nerve block refers to the injection of a local anesthetic agent (e.g., bupivacaine, ropivacaine) into the

FIGURE 14.12 Pudendal nerve block.

pudendal nerves near each ischial spine. It provides pain relief in the lower vagina, vulva, and perineum (Fig. 14.12).

A pudendal block is used for the second stage of labor, an episiotomy, or an operative vaginal birth with outlet forceps or vacuum extractor. It must be administered about 15 minutes before it would be needed to ensure its full effect. A transvaginal approach is generally used to inject an anesthetic agent at or near the pudendal nerve branch. Neither maternal nor fetal complications are common.

Spinal (Intrathecal) Analgesia/Anesthesia

The spinal (intrathecal) pain-management technique involves injection of an anesthetic "caine" agent, with or without opioids, into the subarachnoid space to provide pain relief during labor or cesarean birth. The contraindications are similar to those for the epidural block. Adverse reactions for the woman include hypotension and spinal headache.

The subarachnoid injection of opioids alone, a technique termed intrathecal narcotics, has been gaining popularity since it was introduced in the 1980s. A narcotic is injected into the subarachnoid space, providing rapid pain relief while still maintaining motor function and sensation (Edmonds, 2007). An intrathecal narcotic is given during the active phase (more than 5 cm dilation) of labor. Compared with epidural blocks, intrathecal narcotics are easy to administer, provide rapid-onset pain relief, are less

likely to cause newborn respiratory depression, and do not cause motor blockade (Edmonds, 2007). Although pain relief is rapid with this technique, it is limited by the narcotic's duration of action, which may be only a few hours and not last through the labor. Additional pain measures may be needed to sustain pain management.

General Anesthesia

General anesthesia is typically reserved for emergency cesarean births when there is not enough time to provide spinal or epidural anesthesia or if the woman has a contraindication to the use of regional anesthesia. It can be started quickly and causes a rapid loss of consciousness. General anesthesia can be administered by IV injection, inhalation of anesthetic agents, or both. Commonly, thiopental, a short-acting barbiturate, is given IV to produce unconsciousness. This is followed by administration of a muscle relaxant. After the woman is intubated, nitrous oxide and oxygen are administered. A volatile halogenated agent may also be administered to produce amnesia (Cheng & Caughey, 2007).

All anesthetic agents cross the placenta and affect the fetus. The primary complication with general anesthesia is fetal depression, along with uterine relaxation and potential maternal vomiting and aspiration.

Although the anesthesiologist or nurse anesthetist administers the various general anesthesia agents, the nurse needs to be knowledgeable about the pharmacologic aspects of the drugs used and must be aware of airway management. Ensure that the woman is NPO and has a patent IV. In addition, administer a non-particulate (clear) oral antacid (e.g., Bicitra or sodium citrate) or a proton pump inhibitor (Protonix) as ordered to reduce gastric acidity. Assist with placement of a wedge under the woman's right hip to displace the gravid uterus and prevent vena cava compression in the supine position. Once the newborn has been removed from the uterus, assist the perinatal team in providing supportive care.

Nursing Care During Labor and Birth

WATCH & LEARN

Childbirth, a physiologic process that is fundamental to all human existence, is one of the most significant cultural, psychological, spiritual, and behavioral events in a woman's life. Although the act of giving birth is a universal phenomenon, it is a unique experience for each woman. Continuous evaluation and appropriate intervention for women during labor are key to promoting a positive outcome for the family.

The nurse's role in childbirth is to ensure a safe environment for the mother and her newborn. Nurses begin evaluating the mother and fetus during the admission procedures at the health care agency and continue to do so throughout labor. It is critical to provide anticipatory guidance and explain each procedure (fetal monitoring, intravenous therapy, medications given, and expected reactions) and what will happen next. This will prepare the woman for the upcoming physical and emotional challenges, thereby helping to reduce her anxiety. Acknowledging her support systems (family or partner) helps allay their fears and concerns, thereby assisting them in carrying out their supportive role. Knowing how and when to evaluate a woman during the various stages of labor is essential for all labor and birth nurses to ensure a positive maternal experience and a healthy newborn.

A major focus of care for the woman during labor and birth is assisting her with maintaining control over her pain, emotions, and actions while being an active participant. Nurses can help and support women to be actively involved in their childbirth experience by allowing time for discussion, offering companionship, listening to worries and concerns, paying attention to the woman's emotional needs, and offering information to help her understand what is happening in each stage of labor.

Nursing Care During the First Stage of Labor

Depending on how far advanced the woman's labor is when she arrives at the facility, the nurse will determine assessment parameters of maternal–fetal status and plan care accordingly. The nurse will provide high-touch, low-tech supportive nursing care during the first stage of labor when admitting the woman and orienting her to the labor and birth suite. Nursing care during this stage will include taking an admission history (reviewing the prenatal record); checking the results of routine laboratory tests and any special tests such as chorionic villi sampling, amniocentesis, genetic studies, and biophysical profile done during pregnancy; asking the woman about her childbirth preparation (birth plan, classes taken, coping skills); and completing a physical assessment of the woman to establish a baseline of values for future comparison.

Key nursing interventions include:

- Identifying the estimated date of birth from the client and the prenatal chart
- Validating the client's prenatal history to determine fetal risk status
- Determining fundal height to validate dates and fetal growth
- Performing Leopold's maneuvers to determine fetal position, lie, and presentation
- Checking FHR
- Performing a vaginal examination (as appropriate) to evaluate effacement and dilation progress
- Instructing the client and her partner about monitoring techniques and equipment
- Assessing fetal response and FHR to contractions and recovery time

- Interpreting fetal monitoring strips
- Checking FHR baseline for accelerations, variability, and decelerations
- Repositioning the client to obtain an optimal FHR pattern
- Recognizing FHR problems and initiating corrective measures
- Checking amniotic fluid for meconium staining, odor, and amount
- Comforting client throughout testing period and labor
- Supporting client's decisions regarding intervention or avoidance of intervention
- Assessing client's support system and coping status frequently

In addition to these interventions to promote optimal outcomes for the mother and fetus, the nurse must document care accurately and in a timely fashion. Accurate and timely documentation helps to decrease professional liability exposure and minimize the risk of preventable injuries to women and infants during labor and birth (Walsh, 2007). Guidelines for recording care include documenting:

- All care rendered, to prove that standards were met
- Conversations with all providers, including notification times
- Nursing interventions before and after notifying provider
- Use of the chain of command and response at each level
- All flow sheets and forms, to validate care given
- All education given to client and response to it
- Facts, not personal opinions
- Initial nursing assessment, all encounters, and discharge plan
- All telephone conversations (Hamilton & Wright, 2007)

This standard of documentation is needed to prevent or defend against litigation, which is prevalent in the childbirth arena.

Assessing the Woman upon Admission

The nurse usually first comes in contact with the woman either by phone or in person. It is important to ascertain whether the woman is in true or false labor and whether she should be admitted or sent home. Upon admission to the labor and birth suite, the highest priorities include assessing FHR, assessing cervical dilation/effacement, and determining whether membranes have ruptured or are intact. These assessment data will guide the critical thinking in planning care for the patient.

If the initial contact is by phone, establish a therapeutic relationship with the woman. Speaking in a calm, caring tone facilitates this. When completing a phone assessment, include questions about the following:

- Estimated date of birth, to determine if term or preterm
- Fetal movement (frequency in the past few days)

- Other premonitory signs of labor experienced
- Parity, gravida, and previous childbirth experiences
- Time from start of labor to birth in previous labors
- Characteristics of contractions, including frequency, duration, and intensity
- Appearance of any vaginal bloody show
- Membrane status (ruptured or intact)
- Presence of supportive adult in household or if she is alone

When speaking with the woman over the telephone, review the signs and symptoms that denote true versus false labor, and suggest various positions she can assume to provide comfort and increase placental perfusion. Also suggest walking, massage, and taking a warm shower to promote relaxation. Outline what foods and fluids are appropriate for oral intake in early labor. Throughout the phone call, listen to the woman's concerns and answer any questions clearly.

Reducing the risk of liability exposure and avoiding preventable injuries to mothers and fetuses during labor and birth can be accomplished by adhering to two basic tenets of clinical practice: (1) use applicable evidence and/or published standards and guidelines as the foundation of care, and (2) whenever a clinical choice is presented, chose client safety (Collins, 2006). With these two tenets in mind, advise the woman on the phone to contact her health care provider for further instructions or to come to the facility to be evaluated, since ruling out true labor and possible maternal–fetal complications cannot be done accurately over the phone.

Additional nursing responsibilities associated with a phone assessment include:

- Consulting the woman's prenatal record for parity status, estimated date of birth, and untoward events
- Calling the health care provider to inform him or her of the woman's status
- Preparing for admission to the perinatal unit to ensure adequate staff assignment
- Notifying the admissions office of a pending admission

If the nurse's first encounter with the woman is in person, an assessment is completed to determine whether she should be admitted to the perinatal unit or sent home until her labor advances. Entering a facility is often an intimidating and stressful event for women since it is an unfamiliar environment. Giving birth for the first time is a pivotal event in the lives of most women. Therefore, demonstrate respect when addressing the client; listen carefully and express interest and concern. Nurses must value and respect women and promote their self-worth and sense of control by allowing them to participate in making decisions (Hackley, Kriebs, & Rousseau, 2007).

An admission assessment includes maternal health history, physical assessment, fetal assessment, laboratory studies, and assessment of psychological status. Usually the facility has a form that can be used throughout labor and birth to document assessment findings (Fig. 14.13).

Maternal Health History

A maternal health history should include typical biographical data such as the woman's name and age and the name of the delivering health care provider. Other information that is collected includes the prenatal record data, including the estimated date of birth, a history of the current pregnancy, and the results of any laboratory and diagnostic tests, such as blood type, Rh status, and group B streptococcal status; past pregnancy and obstetric history; past health history and family history; prenatal education; list of medications; risk factors such as diabetes, hypertension, and use of tobacco, alcohol, or illicit drugs; reason for admission, such as labor, cesarean birth, or observation for a complication; history of potential domestic violence; history of previous preterm births; allergies; time of last food ingestion; method chosen for infant feeding; name of birth attendant and pediatrician; and pain management plan.

Ascertaining this information is important so that an individualized plan of care can be developed for the woman. If, for example, the woman's due date is still 2 months away, it is important to establish this information so interventions can be initiated to arrest the labor immediately or notify the intensive perinatal team to be available. In addition, if the woman is a diabetic, it is critical to monitor her glucose levels during labor, to prepare for a surgical birth if dystocia of labor occurs, and to alert the newborn nursery of potential hypoglycemia in the newborn after birth. By collecting important information about each woman they care for, nurses can help improve the outcomes for all concerned.

Be sure to observe the woman's emotions, support system, verbal interaction, body language and posture, perceptual acuity, and energy level. Also note her cultural background and language spoken. This psychosocial information provides cues about the woman's emotional state, culture, and communication systems. For example, if the woman arrives at the labor and birth suite extremely anxious, alone, and unable to communicate in English, how can the nurse meet her needs and plan her care appropriately? It is only by assessing each woman physically and psychosocially that the nurse can make astute decisions regarding proper care. In this case, an interpreter would be needed to assist in the communication process between the staff and the woman to initiate proper care.

It is important to acknowledge and try to understand the cultural differences in women with cultural backgrounds different from that of the nurse. Attitudes toward childbirth are heavily influenced by the culture in which the woman has been raised. As a result, within every society, specific attitudes and values shape the woman's childbearing behaviors. Be aware of what these are. When carrying out a cultural assessment during the admission

ADMISSION ASSESSMENT OBSTETRICS

▲ PATIENT IDENTIFICATION ▲

ADMISSION DATA

Date	Time	Via
		☐ Ambulatory ☐ Wheelchair ☐ Stretcher

Grav.	Term	Pre-term	Ab.	Living	EDC	LMP	GA

Prev. adm. date _____ Reason _____

Obstetrician _____ Pediatrician _____

Ht. _____ Wt. _____ Wt. gain _____

Allergies (meds/food) ☐ None _____ ☐ Hx latex sensitivity

BP _____ T _____ P _____ R _____

FHR _____ Vag exam _____

Reason for Admission

☐ Labor / SROM ☐ Induction _____

☐ Primary C/S _____ ☐ Repeat C/S

☐ Observation _____

☐ OB / Medical complication _____

Onset of labor: ☐ Not in labor

Date _____ Time _____

Membranes: ☐ Intact

☐ Ruptured / Date _____ Time _____

☐ Clear ☐ Meconium ☐ Bloody ☐ Foul

Vaginal bleeding: ☐ None

☐ Normal show ☐ _____

Current Pregnancy Labs   ☐ NPC

☐ POL ☐ PPROM ☐ Cerclage

☐ PIH ☐ Chr. HTN ☐ Other _____

☐ Diabetes _____ Diet _____

☐ Insulin _____

☐ Amniocentesis _____ Results _____

Bld type / RH ____ Date Rhogam ____

Antibody screen ☐ Neg ☐ Pos

Rubella ☐ Non-immune ☐ Immune

Diabetic screen ☐ Normal ☐ Abnormal

Recent exposure to chick pox ☐

Current meds: _____

_____

	Pos	Neg	Tested
Hepatitis B	☐	☐	☐ No
HIV	☐	☐	☐ No
Group B strep	☐	☐	☐ No
GC	☐	☐	☐ No
Chlamydia	☐	☐	☐ No
RPR	☐	☐	☐ No

Previous OB History

☐ POL ☐ Multiple gestation

☐ Prev C/S type _____ Reason _____

☐ PIH ☐ Chronic HTN ☐ Diabetes _____

☐ Stillbirth/demise ☐ Neodeath ☐ Anomalies

☐ Precipitous labor (<3 H) ☐ Macrosomia

☐ PP Hemorrhage

☐ Hx Transfusion reaction ☐ Yes ☐ No

☐ Other _____

Latest risk assessment ☐ None

1. _____ 3. _____

2. _____ 4. _____

Date _____

Signature _____ Time _____

NEUROLOGICAL

☐ WNL

Variance: ☐ HA

☐ Scotoma / visual changes

Reflexes ☐ < 2 + ☐ > 2 +

☐ Clonus ____ bts

☐ Numbness ☐ Tingling

☐ Hx Seizures

☐ _____

RESPIRATORY

☐ WNL

Variance: ☐ Hx Asthma ☐ URI

Respirations: ☐ < 12 ☐ > 24

Effort: ☐ SOB

☐ Shallow ☐ Labored

Auscultation:

☐ Diminished ☐ Crackles

☐ Wheezes ☐ Rhonchi

	No	Yes
Cough for greater than 2 weeks?	☐	☐
Is the cough productive?	☐	☐
Blood in the sputum?	☐	☐
Experiencing any fever or night sweats?	☐	☐
Ever had TB in the past?	☐	☐
Recent exposure to TB?	☐	☐
Weight loss in last 3 weeks?	☐	☐

If the patient answers yes to any three of the above questions implement policy and procedure # 5725-0704.

GASTROINTESTINAL

☐ WNL

Variance: ☐ Heartburn

☐ Epigastric pain   Nausea

☐ Vomiting ☐ Diarrhea

☐ Constipation ☐ Pain

☐ Wt. Gain < 2lbs / month**

☐ Recent change in appetite of < 50% of usual intake for > 5 days

☐ _____

INTEGUMENTARY

☐ WNL

Variance: ☐ Rash ☐ Lacerations

☐ Abrasion ☐ Swelling

☐ Uticaria ☐ Bruising

☐ Diaphoretic/hot

☐ Clammy/cold

☐ Scars

FETAL ASSESSMENT

☐ WNL

Variance:

☐ NRFS

FHR ☐ < 110 ☐ > 160

LTV ☐ Absent ☐ Minimal

☐ Increased

STV Absent

Decelerations: _____

☐ Decreased fetal movement

☐ IUGR

☐ _____

CARDIOVASCULAR

☐ WNL

Variance:

☐ MVP

Heart rate: ☐ < 60 ☐ > 100

B/P: Systolic: ☐ < 90 ☐ > 140

Diastolic: ☐ < 50 ☐ > 90

☐ Edema _____

☐ Chest pain / palpitations

☐ _____

MUSCULOSKELETAL

☐ WNL

Variance:

☐ Numbness ☐ Tingling

☐ Paralysis ☐ Deformity

☐ Scoliosis

☐ _____

GENITOURINARY

☐ WNL

Variance: ☐ Albumin _____

Output: ☐ < 30 cc/Hr.

☐ UTI ☐ Rx ☐ Frequency

☐ Dysuria ☐ Hematuria

☐ CVA Tenderness

☐ Hx STD

☐ Vag. discharge _____

☐ Rash ☐ Blisters

☐ Warts ☐ Lesions

☐ _____

EARS, NOSE, THROAT, AND EYES

☐ WNL

Variance:

☐ Sore throat ☐ Eyeglasses

☐ Runny nose ☐ Contact lenses

☐ Nasal congestion

☐ _____

PSYCHOSOCIAL

☐ WNL

Variance: ☐ Hx depression

☐ Yes ☐ No

☐ Emotional behavioral care

Affect: ☐ Flat ☐ Anxious

☐ Uncooperative ☐ Combative

Living will ☐ Yes ☐ No

☐ On chart

Healthcare surrogate ☐ Yes ☐ No

☐ On chart

Are you being hurt, hit, frightened by anyone at home or in your life? ☐ Yes ☐ No

Religious preference _____

Tobacco use	☐ Denies ☐ Yes	Amt _____
Alcohol use	☐ Denies ☐ Yes	Amt _____
Drug use	☐ Denies ☐ Yes	Amt type _____
Primary language	☐ English ☐ Spanish	

PAIN ASSESSMENT

	No	Yes
1. Do you have any ongoing pain problems?	☐	☐
2. Do you have any pain now?	☐	☐

3. If any of the above questions are answered yes, the patient has a positive pain screening.

4. *Patient to be given pain management education material.*
   Complete pain / symptom assessment on flowsheet.

5. *Please proceed to complete pain assessment.*

FIGURE 14.13 Sample documentation form used for admission to the perinatal unit. (Used with permission. Briggs Corporation, 2001.)

> ### BOX 14.2 Questions for Providing Culturally Competent Care During Labor and Birth
>
> - Where were you born? How long have you lived in the Untied States?
> - What languages do you speak and read?
> - Who are your major support people?
> - What are your religious practices?
> - How do you view childbearing?
> - Are there any special precautions or restrictions that are important?
> - Is birth considered a private or a social experience?
> - How would you like to manage your labor discomfort?
> - Who will provide your labor support?
>
> Sources: Bowers (2007); D'Avanzo (2008); Giger & Davidhizar (2007).

process, ask questions (Box 14.2) to help plan culturally competent care during labor and birth.

Physical Examination

The physical examination typically includes a generalized assessment of the woman's body systems, including hydration status, vital signs, auscultation of heart and lung sounds, and measurement of height and weight. The physical examination also includes the following assessments:

- Fundal height measurement
- Uterine activity, including contraction frequency, duration, and intensity
- Status of membranes (intact or ruptured)
- Cervical dilatation and degree of effacement
- Fetal status, including heart rate, position, and station
- Pain level

These assessment parameters form a baseline against which the nurse can compare all future values throughout labor. The findings should be similar to those of the woman's prepregnancy and pregnancy findings, with the exception of her pulse rate, which might be elevated secondary to her anxious state with beginning labor.

Laboratory Studies

On admission, laboratory studies typically are done to establish a baseline. Although the exact tests may vary among facilities, they usually include a urinalysis via clean-catch urine specimen and complete blood count (CBC). Blood typing and Rh factor analysis may be necessary if the results of these are unknown or unavailable. In addition, if the following test results are not included in the maternal prenatal history, it may be necessary to perform them at this time. They include syphilis screening, hepatitis B (HbsAg) screening, group B streptococcus, HIV testing

(if woman gives consent), and possible drug screening if the history is positive.

Group B streptococcus (GBS) is a gram-positive organism that is present in 10% to 30% of all healthy women (Kenner & Lott, 2007). These women are asymptomatic carriers but can cause GBS disease of the newborn through vertical transmission. The mortality rate of infected newborns varies according to time of onset (early or late). Risk factors for GBS include maternal intrapartum fever, prolonged ruptured membranes, previous birth of an infected newborn, and GBS bacteriuria in the present pregnancy.

In 2002 ACOG and the American Academy of Pediatrics (AAP) issued guidelines that advised universal screening of pregnant women at 35 to 37 weeks' gestation for GBS and intrapartum antibiotic therapy for GBS carriers (Reingold et al., 2007). Maternal infections associated with GBS include acute chorioamnionitis, endometritis, and urinary tract infection. Neonatal clinical manifestations include pneumonia and sepsis. Identified GBS carriers receive IV antibiotic prophylaxis (penicillin G or ampicillin) at the onset of labor or ruptured membranes.

If her HIV status is not documented, the woman being admitted to the labor and birth suite should have rapid HIV testing done. To reduce perinatal transmission, HIV-positive women are given zidovudine (2 mg/kg IV over an hour, and then a maintenance infusion of 1 mg/kg per hour until birth) or a single 200-mg oral dose of nevirapine at the onset of labor; the newborn is given 2 mg/kg orally between 48 and 72 hours of life (Kenner & Lott, 2007). To further reduce the risk of perinatal transmission, ACOG and the U.S. Public Health Service recommend that HIV-infected women with plasma viral loads of more than 1,000 copies per milliliter be counseled regarding the benefits of elective cesarean birth (Jamieson et al., 2007). Additional interventions to reduce the transmission risk would include avoiding use of scalp electrode for fetal monitoring or doing a scalp blood sampling for fetal pH, delaying amniotomy, and avoiding invasive procedures such as forceps or vacuum-assisted devices. The nurse stresses the importance of all interventions and the goal to reduce transmission of HIV to the newborn.

Continuing Assessment During the First Stage of Labor

After the admission assessment is complete, assessment continues for changes that would indicate that labor is progressing as expected. Assess the woman's knowledge, experience, and expectations of labor. Typically, blood pressure, pulse, and respirations are assessed every hour during the latent phase of labor unless the clinical situation dictates that vital signs be taken more frequently. During the active and transition phases, they are assessed every 30 minutes. The temperature is taken every 4 hours throughout the first stage of labor unless the clinical situation dictates more frequent measurement (maternal fever).

Vaginal examinations are performed periodically to track labor progress. This assessment information is shared with the woman to reinforce that she is making progress toward the goal of birth. Uterine contractions are monitored for frequency, duration, and intensity every 30 to 60 minutes during the latent phase, every 15 to 30 minutes during the active phase, and every 15 minutes during transition. Note the changes in the character of the contractions as labor progresses, and inform the woman of her progress. Continually determine the woman's level of pain and her ability to cope and use relaxation techniques effectively.

When the fetal membranes rupture, spontaneously or artificially, assess the FHR and check the amniotic fluid for color, odor, and amount. Assess the FHR intermittently or continuously via electronic monitoring. During the latent phase of labor, assess the FHR every 30 to 60 minutes; in the active phase, assess FHR at least every 15 to 30 minutes. Also, be sure to assess the FHR before ambulation, prior to any procedure, and prior to administering analgesia or anesthesia to the mother. Table 14.3 summarizes assessments for the first stage of labor.

*R*emember Sheila from the chapter-opening scenario? *What is the nurse's role with Sheila in active labor? What additional comfort measures can the labor nurse offer Sheila?*

Nursing Interventions

Nursing interventions during the admission process should include:

- Asking about the client's expectations of the birthing process
- Providing information about labor, birth, pain-management options, and relaxation techniques
- Presenting information about fetal monitoring equipment and the procedures needed
- Monitoring FHR and identifying patterns that need further intervention
- Monitoring the mother's vital signs to obtain a baseline for later comparison
- Reassuring the client that her labor progress will be monitored closely and nursing care will focus on ensuring fetal and maternal well-being throughout

As the woman progresses through the first stage of labor, nursing interventions include:

- Encouraging the woman's partner to participate
- Keeping the woman and her partner up to date on the progress of the labor
- Orienting the woman and her partner to the labor and birth unit and explaining all of the birthing procedures
- Providing clear fluids (e.g., ice chips) as needed or requested
- Maintaining the woman's parenteral fluid intake at the prescribed rate if she has an IV

TABLE 14.3 **SUMMARY OF ASSESSMENTS DURING THE FIRST STAGE OF LABOR**

Assessments*	Latent Phase (0–3 cm)	Active Phase (4–7 cm)	Transition (8–10 cm)
Vital signs (BP, pulse, respirations)	Every 30–60 min	Every 30 min	Every 15–30 min
Temperature	Every 4 hours	Every 4 hours	Every 4 hours
Contractions (frequency, duration, intensity)	Every 30–60 min by palpation or continuously if EFM	Every 15–30 min by palpation or continuously if EFM	Every 15 min by palpation or continuously if EFM
Fetal heart rate	Every hour by Doppler or continuously by EFM	Every 30 min by Doppler or continuously by EFM	Every 15–30 min by Doppler or continuously by EFM
Vaginal examination	Initially on admission to determine phase and as needed based on maternal cues to document labor progression	As needed to monitor labor progression	As needed to monitor labor progression
Behavior/psychosocial	With every client encounter: talkative, excited, anxious	With every client encounter: self-absorbed in labor; intense and quiet now	With every client encounter: discouraged, irritable, feels out of control, declining coping ability

*The frequency of assessments is dictated by the health status of the woman and fetus and can be altered if either one of their conditions changes.
EFM, electronic fetal monitoring.

- Initiating or encouraging comfort measures, such as backrubs, cool cloths to the forehead, frequent position changes, ambulation, showers, slow dancing, leaning over a birth ball, side-lying, or counterpressure on lower back (Teaching Guidelines 14.1)
- Encouraging the partner's involvement with breathing techniques
- Assisting the woman and her partner to focus on breathing techniques
- Informing the woman that the discomfort will be intermittent and of limited duration; urging her to rest between contractions to preserve her strength; and encouraging her to use distracting activities to lessen the focus on contractions
- Changing bed linens and gown as needed
- Keeping the perineal area clean and dry

TEACHING GUIDELINES 14.1

Positioning During the First Stage of Labor

- Walking with support from your partner (adds the force of gravity to contractions to promote fetal descent)
- Slow-dancing position with your partner holding you (adds the force of gravity to contractions and promotes support from and active participation of your partner)
- Side-lying with pillows between the knees for comfort (offers a restful position and improves oxygen flow to the uterus)
- Semi-sitting in bed or on a couch leaning against the partner (reduces back pain because fetus falls forward, away from the sacrum)
- Sitting in a chair with one foot on the floor and one on the chair (changes pelvic shape)
- Leaning forward by straddling a chair, a table, or a bed or kneeling over a birth ball (reduces back pain, adds the force of gravity to promote descent; possible pain relief if partner can apply sacral pressure)
- Sitting in a rocking chair or on a birth ball and shifting weight back and forth (provides comfort because rocking motion is soothing; uses the force of gravity to help fetal descent)
- Lunge by rocking weight back and forth with foot up on chair during contraction (uses force of gravity by being upright; enhances rotation of fetus through rocking)
- Open knee–chest position (helps to relieve back discomfort) (Armstrong & Feldman, 2007)

- Supporting the woman's decisions about pain management
- Monitoring maternal vital signs frequently and reporting any abnormal values
- Ensuring that the woman takes deep cleansing breaths before and after each contraction to enhance gas exchange and oxygen to the fetus
- Educating the woman and her partner about the need for rest and helping them plan strategies to conserve strength
- Monitoring FHR for baseline, accelerations, variability, and decelerations
- Checking on bladder status and encouraging voiding at least every 2 hours to make room for birth
- Repositioning the woman as needed to obtain optimal heart rate pattern
- Communicating requests from the woman to appropriate personnel
- Respecting the woman's sense of privacy by covering her when appropriate
- Offering human presence by being present with the woman, not leaving her alone for long periods
- Being patient with the natural labor pattern to allow time for change
- Reporting any deviations from normal to the health care professional so that interventions can be initiated early to be effective (Sauls, 2007)

See Nursing Care Plan 14.1.

Remember Sheila, who was admitted in active labor? She has progressed to the transition phase (8 cm dilated) and is becoming increasingly more uncomfortable. She is using a patterned-paced breathing pattern now but thrashing around in the hospital bed.

Nursing Management During the Second Stage of Labor

Nursing care during the second stage of labor focuses on supporting the woman and her partner in making active decisions about her care and labor management, implementing strategies to prolong the early passive phase of fetal descent, supporting involuntary bearing-down efforts, providing instruction and assistance, and using maternal positions that can enhance descent and reduce pain (Sleutel, Schultz, & Wyble, 2007). Research suggests that strong pushing during the second stage may be accompanied by a significant decline in fetal pH and may cause maternal muscle and nerve damage if done too early (Sauls, 2007). Shortening the phase of active pushing and lengthening the early phase of passive descent can be achieved by encouraging the woman not to push until she has a strong desire to do so and until the descent and rotation of the fetal head are well advanced. Effective

Nursing Care Plan 14.1

OVERVIEW OF THE WOMAN IN THE ACTIVE PHASE OF THE FIRST STAGE OF LABOR

Candice, a 23-year-old gravida 1, para 0 (G1,P0) is admitted to the labor and birth suite at 39 weeks' gestation having contractions of moderate intensity every 5 to 6 minutes. A vaginal examination reveals her cervix is 80% effaced and 5 cm dilated. The presenting part (vertex) is at 0 station and her membranes ruptured spontaneously 4 hours ago at home. She is admitted and an IV is started for hydration and vascular access. An external fetal monitor is applied. FHR is 140 bpm and regular. Her partner is present at her bedside. Candice is now in the active phase of the first stage of labor, and her assessment findings are as follows: cervix dilated 7 cm, 80% effaced; moderate to strong contractions occurring regularly, every 3 to 5 minutes, lasting 45 to 60 seconds; at 0 station on pelvic examination; FHR auscultated loudest below umbilicus at 140 bpm; vaginal show—pink or bloody vaginal mucus; currently apprehensive, inwardly focused, with increased dependency; voicing concern about ability to cope with pain; limited ability to follow directions.

NURSING DIAGNOSIS: Anxiety related to labor and birth process and fear of the unknown related to client's first experience

Outcome Identification and Evaluation
Client will remain calm and in control as evidenced by ability to make decisions and use positive coping strategies.

Interventions: Promoting Positive Coping Strategies
- Provide instruction regarding the labor process to allay anxiety.
- Reorient the woman to the physical environment and equipment as necessary to keep her informed of events.
- Encourage verbalization of feelings and concerns to reduce anxiety.
- Listen attentively to woman and partner to demonstrate interest and concern.
- Inform woman and partner of standard procedures/processes to ensure adequate understanding of events and procedures.
- Frequently update woman of progress and labor status to provide positive reinforcement for actions.
- Reinforce relaxation techniques and provide instruction if needed to aid in coping.
- Encourage participation of the partner in the coaching role; role-model to facilitate partner participation in labor process to provide support and encouragement to the client.
- Provide a presence and remain with woman as much as possible to provide comfort and support.

NURSING DIAGNOSIS: Pain related to effects of contractions and cervical dilatation and events of labor

Outcome Identification and Evaluation
Client will maintain a tolerable level of pain and discomfort as evidenced by statements of pain relief, pain rating of 2 or less on pain rating scale, and absence of adverse effects in client and fetus from analgesia or anesthesia.

Interventions: Providing Pain Relief
- Monitor vital signs, observe for signs of pain, and have client rate pain on a scale of 0 to 10 to provide baseline for comparison.
- Encourage client to void every 1 to 2 hours to decrease pressure from a full bladder.
- Assist woman to change positions frequently to increase comfort and promote labor progress.
- Encourage use of distraction to reduce focus on contraction pain.
- Suggest pelvic rocking, massage, or back counterpressure to reduce pain.
- Assist with use of relaxation and breathing techniques to promote relaxation.
- Use touch appropriately (backrub) when desired by the woman to promote comfort.
- Integrate use of nonpharmacologic measures for pain relief, such as warm water, birthing ball, or other techniques to facilitate pain relief.
- Administer pharmacologic agents as ordered when requested to control pain.
- Provide reassurance and encouragement between contractions to foster self-esteem and continued participation in labor process.

(continued)

Nursing Care Plan 14.1 (continued)

NURSING DIAGNOSIS: Risk of infection related to vaginal examinations following rupture of membranes

Outcome Identification and Evaluation
Client will remain free of infection as evidenced by absence of signs and symptoms of infection, vital signs and FHR within acceptable parameters, lab test results within normal limits, and clear amniotic fluid without odor.

Interventions: Preventing Infection
- Monitor vital signs (every 1 to 2 hours after ROM) and FHR frequently as per protocol to allow for early detection of problems; report fetal tachycardia (early sign of maternal infection) to ensure prompt treatment.
- Provide frequent perineal care and pad changes to maintain good perineal hygiene.
- Change linens and woman's gown as needed to maintain cleanliness.
- Ensure that vaginal examinations are performed only when needed to prevent introducing pathogens into the vaginal vault.
- Monitor lab test results such as white blood cell count to assess for elevations indicating infection.
- Use aseptic technique for all invasive procedures to prevent infection transmission.
- Carry out good handwashing techniques before and after procedures and use standard precautions as appropriate to minimize risk of infection transmission.
- Document amniotic fluid characteristics—color, odor—to establish baseline for comparison.

---

pushing can be achieved by assisting the woman to assume a more upright or squatting position (Hanson, 2006).

Perineal lacerations or tears can occur during the second stage when the fetal head emerges through the vaginal introitus. The extent of the laceration is defined by depth: a first-degree laceration extends through the skin; a second-degree laceration extends through the muscles of the perineal body; a third-degree laceration continues through the anal sphincter muscle; and a fourth-degree laceration also involves the anterior rectal wall. Special attention needs to be paid to third- and fourth-degree lacerations to prevent fecal incontinence (Lowder et al., 2007). The primary care provider should repair any lacerations during the third stage of labor.

An **episiotomy** is an incision made in the perineum to enlarge the vaginal outlet and theoretically to shorten the second stage of labor. Alternative measures such as warm compresses and continual massage with oil have been successful in stretching the perineal area to prevent cutting it. Certified nurse midwives (CNMs) can cut and repair episiotomies, but they frequently use alternative measures if possible.

▶ *Take NOTE!*

Further research needs to be done to validate the efficacy of natural measures versus the episiotomy.

The midline episiotomy is the most commonly used one in the United States because it can be easily repaired and causes the least amount of pain (Albers & Borders, 2007). Figure 14.14 shows episiotomy locations.

Assessment
Assessment is continuous during the second stage of labor. Hospital policies dictate the specific type and timing of assessments, as well as the way in which they are documented. Assessment involves identifying the signs typical of the second stage of labor, including:

- Increase in apprehension or irritability
- Spontaneous rupture of membranes
- Sudden appearance of sweat on upper lip
- Increase in blood-tinged show
- Low grunting sounds from the woman
- Complaints of rectal and perineal pressure
- Beginning of involuntary bearing-down efforts

Other ongoing assessments include the contraction frequency, duration, and intensity; maternal vital signs every 5 to 15 minutes; fetal response to labor as indicated by FHR monitor strips; amniotic fluid for color, odor, and amount when membranes are ruptured; and the woman and her partner's coping status (Table 14.4).

Assessment also focuses on determining the progress of labor. Associated signs include bulging of the perineum, labial separation, advancing and retreating of the newborn's head during and between bearing-down efforts,

FIGURE 14.14 Location of an episiotomy. (**A**) Midline episiotomy. (**B**) Right and left mediolateral episiotomies.

and **crowning** (fetal head is visible at vaginal opening; Fig. 14.15).

A vaginal examination is completed to determine if it is appropriate for the woman to push. Pushing is appropriate if the cervix has fully dilated to 10 cm and the woman feels the urge to do so.

Nursing Interventions

Nursing interventions during this stage focus on motivating the woman, encouraging her to put all her efforts to pushing this newborn to the outside world, and giving her feedback on her progress. If the woman is pushing and not making progress, suggest that she keep her eyes open

TABLE 14.4   SUMMARY OF ASSESSMENTS DURING THE SECOND, THIRD, AND FOURTH STAGES OF LABOR

Assessments*	Second Stage of Labor (Birth of Neonate)	Third Stage of Labor (Placenta Expulsion)	Fourth Stage of Labor (Recovery)
Vital signs (BP, pulse, respirations)	Every 5–15 min	Every 15 min	Every 15 min
Fetal heart rate	Every 5–15 min by Doppler or continuously by EFM	Apgar scoring at 1 and 5 min	Newborn—complete head-to-toe assessment; vital signs every 15 min until stable
Contractions/uterus	Palpate every one	Observe for placental separation	Palpating for firmness and position every 15 min for first hour
Bearing down/pushing	Assist with every effort	None	None
Vaginal discharge	Observe for signs of descent—bulging of perineum, crowning	Assess bleeding after expulsion	Assess every 15 min with fundus firmness
Behavior/psychosocial	Observe every 15 min: cooperative, focus is on work of pushing newborn out	Observe every 15 min: often feelings of relief after hearing newborn crying; calmer	Observe every 15 min: usually excited, talkative, awake; needs to hold newborn, be close, and inspect body

*The frequency of assessments is dictated by the health status of the woman and fetus and can be altered if either one of their conditions changes.
EFM, electronic fetal monitoring.

FIGURE 14.15 Crowning.

during the contractions and look toward where the infant is coming out. Changing positions every 20 to 30 minutes will also help in making progress. Positioning a mirror so the woman can visualize the birthing process and how successful her pushing efforts are can help motivate her.

During the second stage of labor, an ideal position would be one that opens the pelvic outlet as wide as possible, provides a smooth pathway for the fetus to descend through the birth canal, takes advantage of gravity to assist the fetus to descend, and gives the mother a sense of being safe and in control of the labor process (Hanson, 2006). Some suggestions for positions in the second stage include:

- Lithotomy with feet up in stirrups: most convenient position for caregivers
- Semi-sitting with pillows underneath knees, arms, and back
- Lateral/side-lying with curved back and upper leg supported by partner
- Sitting on birthing stool: opens pelvis, enhances the pull of gravity, and helps with pushing
- Squatting/supported squatting: gives the woman a sense of control
- Kneeling with hands on bed and knees comfortably apart

Other important nursing interventions during the second stage include:

- Providing continuous comfort measures such as mouth care, position changes, changing bed linen and underpads, and providing a quiet, focused environment
- Instructing the woman on the following bearing-down positions and techniques:

- Pushing only when she feels an urge to do so
- Using abdominal muscles when bearing down
- Using short pushes of 6 to 7 seconds
- Focusing attention on the perineal area to visualize the newborn
- Relaxing and conserving energy between contractions
- Pushing several times with each contraction
- Pushing with an open glottis and slight exhalation (Roberts, Gonzalez, & Sampselle, 2007)
- Continuing to monitor contraction and FHR patterns to identify problems
- Providing brief, explicit directions throughout this stage
- Continuing to provide psychosocial support by reassuring and coaching
- Facilitating the upright position to encourage the fetus to descend
- Continuing to assess blood pressure, pulse, respirations, uterine contractions, bearing-down efforts, FHR, coping status of the client and her partner
- Providing pain management if needed
- Providing a continuous nursing presence
- Offering praise for the client's efforts
- Preparing for and assisting with delivery by:
  - Notifying the health care provider of the estimated time frame for birth
  - Preparing the delivery bed and positioning client
  - Preparing the perineal area according to the facility's protocol
  - Offering a mirror and adjusting it so the woman can watch the birth
  - Explaining all procedures and equipment to the client and her partner
  - Setting up delivery instruments needed while maintaining sterility
  - Receiving newborn and transporting him or her to a warming environment, or covering the newborn with a warmed blanket on the woman's abdomen
  - Providing initial care and assessment of the newborn (see the Birth section that follows)

Sheila is completely dilated now and experiencing the urge to push. How can the nurse help Sheila with her pushing efforts? What additional interventions can the labor nurse offer Sheila now?

Birth

The second stage of labor ends with the birth of the newborn. The maternal position for birth varies from the standard lithotomy position to side-lying to squatting to standing or kneeling, depending on the birthing location, the woman's preference, and standard protocols. Once the woman is positioned for birth, cleanse the vulva and perineal areas. The primary health care provider then takes charge after donning protective eyewear, masks, gowns, and gloves and performing hand hygiene.

Once the fetal head has emerged, the primary care provider explores the fetal neck to see if the umbilical cord is wrapped around it. If it is, the cord is slipped over the head to facilitate delivery. As soon as the head emerges, the health care provider suctions the newborn's mouth first (because the newborn is an obligate nose breather) and then the nares with a bulb syringe to prevent aspiration of mucus, amniotic fluid, or meconium (Fig. 14.16). The umbilical cord is double-clamped and cut between the clamps. With the first cries of the newborn, the second stage of labor ends.

In addition to encouraging Sheila to rest between pushing and offering praise for her efforts, what is the nurse's role during the birthing process?

Immediate Care of the Newborn

Once the infant is born, place him or her under the radiant warmer, dry him or her, assess him or her, wrap him or her in warmed blankets, and place him or her on the woman's abdomen for warmth and closeness. In some health care facilities, the newborn is placed on the woman's abdomen immediately after birth and covered with a warmed blanket. In either scenario, the stability of the

FIGURE 14.16 Suctioning the newborn immediately after birth.

newborn dictates the location of aftercare. The nurse can also assist the mother with breastfeeding her newborn for the first time.

Assessment of the newborn begins at the moment of birth and continues until the newborn is discharged. Drying the newborn and providing warmth to prevent heat loss by evaporation is essential to help support thermoregulation and provide stimulation. Placing the newborn under a radiant heat source and putting on a stockinet cap will further reduce heat loss after drying.

Assess the newborn by assigning an Apgar score at 1 and 5 minutes. The Apgar score assesses five parameters—heart rate (absent, slow, or fast), respiratory effort (absent, weak cry, or good strong yell), muscle tone (limp, or lively and active), response to irritation stimulus, and color—that evaluate a newborn's cardiorespiratory adaptation after birth. The parameters are arranged from the most important (heart rate) to the least important (color). The newborn is assigned a score of 0 to 2 in each of the five parameters. The purpose of the Apgar assessment is to evaluate the physiologic status of the newborn; see Chapter 18 for additional information on Apgar scoring.

Secure two identification bands on the newborn's wrist and ankle that match the band on the mother's wrist to ensure the newborn's identity. This identification process is completed in the birthing suite before anyone leaves the room. Some health care agencies also take an early photo of the newborn for identification in the event of abduction (Healthcare Risk Management, 2007).

Other types of newborn security systems can also be used to prevent abduction. Some systems have sensors that are attached to the newborn's identification bracelet or cord clamp. An alarm is set off if the bracelet or clamp activates receivers near exits. Others have an alarm that is activated when the sensor is removed from the newborn (Fig. 14.17). Even with the use of electronic sensors, the parents, nursing staff, and security personnel are responsible for prevention strategies and ensuring the safety and protection of all newborns (Healthcare Risk Management, 2007).

Sheila gave birth to a healthy 7-pound, 7-ounce baby girl. She is eager to hold and nurse her newborn. What is the initial care of the newborn? How can the nurse meet the needs of both the newborn and Sheila, who is exhausted but eager to bond with her newborn?

Nursing Management During the Third Stage of Labor

During the third stage of labor, strong uterine contractions continue at regular intervals under the continuing influence of oxytocin. The uterine muscle fibers shorten, or retract, with each contraction, leading to a gradual decrease in the

FIGURE 14.17 An example of a security sensor applied to a newborn's arm.

size of the uterus, which helps shear the placenta away from its attachment site. The third stage is complete when the placenta is delivered. Nursing care during the third stage of labor primarily focuses on immediate newborn care and assessment and being available to assist with the delivery of the placenta and inspecting it for intactness.

Three hormones play important roles in the third stage. During this stage the woman experiences peak levels of oxytocin and endorphins, while the high adrenaline levels that occurred during the second stage of labor to aid with pushing begin falling. The hormone oxytocin causes uterine contractions and helps the woman to enact instinctive mothering behaviors such as holding the newborn close to her body and cuddling the baby.

Skin-to-skin contact immediately after birth and the newborn's first attempt at breastfeeding further augment maternal oxytocin levels, strengthening the uterine contractions that will help the placenta to separate and the uterus to contract to prevent hemorrhage. Endorphins,

the body's natural opiates, produce an altered state of consciousness and aid in blocking out pain. In addition, the drop in adrenaline level from the second stage, which had kept the mother and baby alert at first contact, causes most women to shiver and feel cold shortly after giving birth.

▶ **Take** NOTE!

A crucial role for nurses during this time is to protect the natural hormonal process by ensuring unhurried and uninterrupted contact between mother and newborn after birth, providing warmed blankets to prevent shivering, and allowing skin-to-skin contact and breastfeeding.

Assessment

Assessment during the third stage of labor includes:

- Monitoring placental separation by looking for the following signs:
  - Firmly contracting uterus
  - Change in uterine shape from discoid to globular ovoid
  - Sudden gush of dark blood from vaginal opening
  - Lengthening of umbilical cord protruding from vagina
- Examining placenta and fetal membranes for intactness the second time (the health care provider assesses the placenta for intactness the first time) (Fig. 14.18)
- Assessing for any perineal trauma, such as the following, before allowing the birth attendant to leave:
  - Firm fundus with bright-red blood trickling: laceration
  - Boggy fundus with red blood flowing: uterine atony
  - Boggy fundus with dark blood and clots: retained placenta

FIGURE 14.18 Placenta. (**A**) Fetal side. (**B**) Maternal side.

- Inspecting the perineum for condition of episiotomy, if performed
- Assessing for perineal lacerations and ensuring repair by birth attendant

Nursing Interventions

Interventions during the third stage of labor include:

- Describing the process of placental separation to the couple
- Instructing the woman to push when signs of separation are apparent
- Administering an oxytocic if ordered and indicated after placental expulsion
- Providing support and information about episiotomy and/or laceration
- Cleaning and assisting client into a comfortable position after birth, making sure to lift both legs out of stirrups (if used) simultaneously to prevent strain
- Repositioning the birthing bed to serve as a recovery bed if applicable
- Assisting with transfer to the recovery area if applicable
- Providing warmth by replacing warmed blankets over the woman
- Applying an ice pack to the perineal area to provide comfort to episiotomy if indicated
- Explaining what assessments will be carried out over the next hour and offering positive reinforcement for actions
- Ascertaining any needs
- Monitoring maternal physical status by assessing:
  - Vaginal bleeding: amount, consistency, and color
  - Vital signs: blood pressure, pulse, and respirations taken every 15 minutes
  - Uterine fundus, which should be firm, in the midline, and at the level of the umbilicus
- Recording all birthing statistics and securing primary caregiver's signature
- Documenting birthing event in the birth book (official record of the facility that outlines every birth event), detailing any deviations

Nursing Management During the Fourth Stage of Labor

The fourth stage of labor begins after the placenta is expelled and lasts up to 4 hours after birth, during which time recovery takes place. This recovery period may take place in the same room where the woman gave birth, in a separate recovery area, or in her postpartum room. During this stage, the woman's body is beginning to undergo the many physiologic and psychological changes that occur after birth. The focus of nursing management during the fourth stage of labor involves frequent close observation for hemorrhage, provision of comfort measures, and promotion of family attachment.

Assessment

Assessments during the fourth stage center on the woman's vital signs, status of the uterine fundus and perineal area, comfort level, lochia amount, and bladder status. During the first hour after birth, vital signs are taken every 15 minutes, then every 30 minutes for the next hour if needed. The woman's blood pressure should remain stable and within normal range after giving birth. A decrease may indicate uterine hemorrhage; an elevation might suggest preeclampsia.

The pulse usually is typically slower (60 to 70 bpm) than during labor. This may be associated with a decrease in blood volume following placental separation. An elevated pulse rate may be an early sign of blood loss. The blood pressure usually returns to its prepregnancy level and therefore is not a reliable early indicator of shock. Fever is indicative of dehydration (less than 100.4°F or 38°C) or infection (above 101°F), which may involve the genitourinary tract. Respiratory rate is usually between 16 and 24 breaths per minute and regular. Respirations should be unlabored unless there is an underlying pre-existing respiratory condition.

Assess fundal height, position, and firmness every 15 minutes during the first hour following birth. The fundus needs to remain firm to prevent excessive postpartum bleeding. The fundus should be firm (feels like the size and consistency of a grapefruit), located in the midline and below the umbilicus. If it is not firm (boggy), gently massage it until it is firm (see Nursing Procedure 22.1 for more information). Once firmness is obtained, stop massaging.

 ▶ *Take* NOTE!

If the fundus is displaced to the right of the midline, suspect a full bladder as the cause.

The vagina and perineal areas are quite stretched and edematous following a vaginal birth. Assess the perineum, including the episiotomy if present, for possible hematoma formation. Suspect a hematoma if the woman reports excruciating pain or cannot void or if a mass is noted in the perineal area. Also assess for hemorrhoids, which can cause discomfort.

Assess the woman's comfort level frequently to determine the need for analgesia. Ask the woman to rate her pain on a scale of 1 to 10; it should be less than 3. If it is higher, further evaluation is needed to make sure there aren't any deviations contributing to her discomfort.

Assess vaginal discharge (lochia) every 15 minutes for the first hour and every 30 minutes for the next hour. Palpate the fundus at the same time to ascertain its firmness and help to estimate the amount of vaginal discharge. In addition, palpate the bladder for fullness, since many women receiving an epidural block experience limited sensation in the bladder region. Voiding should produce large amounts of urine (diuresis) each time. Palpation of the woman's bladder after each voiding helps to ensure complete emptying. A full bladder will displace the uterus to either side of the midline and potentiate uterine hemorrhage secondary to bogginess.

Nursing Interventions

Nursing interventions during the fourth stage might include:

- Providing support and information to the woman regarding episiotomy repair and related pain-relief and self-care measures
- Applying an ice pack to the perineum to promote comfort and reduce swelling
- Assisting with hygiene and perineal care; teaching the woman how to use the perineal bottle after each pad change and voiding; helping the woman into a new gown
- Monitoring for return of sensation and ability to void (if regional anesthesia was used)
- Encouraging the woman to void by ambulating to bathroom, listening to running water, or pouring warm water over the perineal area with the peribottle
- Monitoring vital signs and fundal and lochia status every 15 minutes and documenting them
- Promoting comfort by offering analgesia for afterpains and warm blankets to reduce chilling
- Offering fluids and nourishment if desired
- Encouraging parent–infant attachment by providing privacy for the family
- Being knowledgeable about and sensitive to typical cultural practices after birth
- Assisting the mother to nurse, if she chooses, during the recovery period to promote uterine firmness (the release of oxytocin from the posterior pituitary gland stimulates uterine contractions)
- Teaching the woman how to assess her fundus for firmness periodically and to massage it if it is boggy
- Describing the lochia flow and normal parameters to observe for postpartum
- Teaching safety techniques to prevent newborn abduction
- Demonstrating the use of the portable sitz bath as a comfort measure for her perineum if she had a laceration or an episiotomy repair
- Explain comfort/hygiene measures and when to use them
- Assisting with ambulation when getting out of bed for the first time
- Providing information about the routine on the mother–baby unit or nursery for her stay
- Observing for signs of early parent–infant attachment: fingertip touch to palm touch to enfolding of the infant (Leonard, 2007)

▪▪▪ Key Concepts

- A nurse provides physical and emotional support during the labor and birth process to assist a woman to achieve her goals.
- When a woman is admitted to the labor and birth area, the admitting nurse must assess and evaluate the risk status of the pregnancy and initiate appropriate interventions to provide optimal care for the client.
- Completing an admission assessment includes taking a maternal health history; performing physical assessment on the woman and fetus, including her emotional and psychosocial status; and obtaining the necessary laboratory studies.
- The nurse's role in fetal assessment for labor and birth includes determining fetal well-being and interpreting signs and symptoms of possible compromise. Determining the fetal heart rate (FHR) pattern and assessing amniotic fluid characteristics are key.
- FHR can be assessed intermittently or continuously. Although the intermittent method allows the client to move about during labor, the information obtained intermittently does not provide a complete picture of fetal well-being from moment to moment.
- Assessment parameters of the FHR are classified as baseline rate, baseline variability (long-term and short-term), and periodic changes in the rate (accelerations and decelerations).
- The nurse monitoring the laboring client needs to be knowledgeable about which parameters are reassuring, nonreassuring, and ominous so that appropriate interventions can be instituted.
- For a nonreassuring FHR pattern, the nurse should notify the health care provider about the pattern and obtain further orders, making sure to document all interventions and their effects on the FHR pattern.
- In addition to interpreting assessment findings and initiating appropriate inventions for the laboring client, accurate and timely documentation must be carried out continuously.
- Today's women have many safe nonpharmacologic and pharmacologic choices for the management of pain during childbirth. They may be used individually or in combination to complement one another.
- Nursing management for the woman during labor and birth includes comfort measures, emotional support, information and instruction, advocacy, and support for the partner.
- Nursing care during the first stage of labor includes taking an admission history (reviewing the prenatal record), checking the results of routine laboratory work and special tests done during pregnancy, asking the woman about her childbirth preparation (birth plan, classes taken, coping skills), and completing a physical assessment of the woman to establish a baseline of values for future comparison.

- Nursing care during the second stage of labor focuses on supporting the woman and her partner in making decisions about her care and labor management, implementing strategies to prolong the early passive phase of fetal descent, supporting involuntary bearing-down efforts, providing instruction and assistance, and encouraging the use of maternal positions that can enhance descent and reduce the pain.

- Nursing care during the third stage of labor primarily focuses on immediate newborn care and assessment and being available to assist with the delivery of the placenta and inspecting it for intactness.

- The focus of nursing management during the fourth stage of labor involves frequently observing the mother for hemorrhage, providing comfort measures, and promoting family attachment.

REFERENCES

Albers, L. L. (2007). The evidence for physiologic management of the active phase of the first stage of labor. *Journal of Midwifery & Women's Health, 52*(3), 207–215.

Albers, L. L., & Borders, N. (2007). Minimizing genital tract trauma and related pain following spontaneous vaginal birth. *Journal of Midwifery & Women's Health, 52*(3), 246–253.

American College of Obstetricians and Gynecologists (ACOG). (2005). *Fetal heart rate patterns: Monitoring, interpretation, and management* (Practice Bulletin Number 62). Washington, DC: Author.

American Hospital Association (AHA). (2007). *Hospital statistics.* Chicago: Author.

American Pregnancy Association. (2007). *Patterned breathing during labor.* Available at: http://www.americanpregnancy.org/labornbirth/patternedbreathing.htm.

Arenson, J., & Drake, P. (2007). *Maternal and newborn health.* Sudbury, MA: Jones and Bartlett Publishers.

Armstrong, P., & Feldman, S. (2007). *A wise birth: Bringing together the best of natural childbirth and modern medicine.* London, UK: Pinter and Martin Limited.

Association of Women's Health, Obstetric and Neonatal Nurses (AWHONN). (2006). *Fetal assessment* (Clinical Position Statement). Washington, DC: Author.

Bagwell, G. A. (2007). Resuscitation and stabilization of the newborn and infant. In C. Kenner & J. W. Lott (Eds.), *Comprehensive neonatal care: An interdisciplinary approach* (Chapter 38, pp. 666–676). St. Louis, MO: Saunders Elsevier.

Bakker, P. C., Kurver, P. H., Kuik, D. J., & Van Grijn, H. P. (2007). Elevated uterine activity increases the risk of fetal acidosis at birth. *American Journal of Obstetrics and Gynecology, 196*(4), 313–319.

Blackburn, S. T. (2007) *Maternal, fetal, and neonatal physiology: A clinical perspective* (3rd ed.). St. Louis, MO: Saunders Elsevier.

Bowers, P. (2007). Cultural perspectives in childbearing. *Nursing Spectrum.* Available at: http://www.nurse.com/ce/course.html?CCID=3245.

Cheng, Y. W., & Caughey, A. B. (2007). Normal labor and delivery. *eMedicine.* Available at: http://www.emedicine.com/med/topic3239.htm

Collins, D. (2006). Legally speaking: Risk management in obstetrics and gynecology. *Contemporary OB/GYN, 51*(11), 38–42.

D'Avanzo, C. E. (2008). *Cultural health assessment* (4th ed.). St. Louis: Mosby Elsevier.

Dillon, P. M. (2007). *Nursing health assessment: A critical thinking, case studies approach* (2nd ed.). Philadelphia: F. A. Davis Company.

Edmonds, K. (2007). *Dewhurst's textbook of obstetrics and gynecology* (7th ed.). Oxford, UK: Blackwell Publishers Limited

Evron, S., & Ezri, T. (2007). Options for systemic labor analgesia. *Current Opinions in Anesthesiology, 20*(3), 181–185.

Fink, J. L., Irwin, G., & Mitchell, R. (2007). Clinical tips. *RN, 70*(2), 44–45.

Frieden, F. J., & Chan, Y. (2007). Antepartum care. In R. E. Rakel & E. T. Bope (Eds.), *Conn's current therapy 2007* (Section 16, pp. 1168–1175). Philadelphia: Saunders Elsevier.

Gagnon, A. J., Meier, K. M., & Waghorn, K. (2007). Continuity of nursing care and its link to cesarean birth rate. *Birth: Issues in Perinatal Care, 34*(1), 26–31.

Giger, J. N., & Davidhizar, R. E. (2007). *Transcultural nursing* (5th ed.). St. Louis: Mosby.

Gilbert, E. S. (2007). *Manual of high risk pregnancy and delivery* (4th ed.). St. Louis, MO: Mosby.

Grimes-Dennis, J., & Berghella, V. (2007). Cervical length and prediction of preterm delivery. *Current Opinion in Obstetrics & Gynecology, 19*(2), 191–195.

Hackley, B., Kriebs, J. M., & Rousseau, M. E. (2007) *Primary care of women: A guide for midwives and women's health providers.* Sudbury, MA: Jones and Bartlett Publishers.

Hale, R. (2007). Monitoring fetal and maternal wellbeing. *British Journal of Midwifery, 15*(2), 107–110.

Hamilton, E., & Wright, E. (2007). Labor pains: Unraveling the complexity of OB decision making. *Critical Care Nursing Quarterly, 29*(4), 342–353.

Hanson, L. (2006). Pushing for change. *Journal of Perinatal & Neonatal Nursing, 20*(4), 282–285.

Hantoushzadeh, S., Alhusseini, N., & Lebaschi, A. H. (2007). The effects of acupuncture during labor on nulliparous women: A randomized controlled trial. *Australian & New Zealand Journal of Obstetrics & Gynecology, 47*(1), 26–30.

Healthcare Risk Management. (2007). Infant abduction raises questions about health care security and vigilance. *Healthcare Risk Management, 29*(5), 49–52.

Herbst, A., & Nilsson, C. (2006). Diagnosis of early preterm labor. *British Journal of Obstetrics & Gynecology,* Supplement 2, 113, 60–67.

Institute for Clinical Systems Improvement (ICSI). (2007). *ICSI Health Care Guidelines: Management of labor* (2nd ed.). Available at: http://www.icsi.org/labor/labor__management_of__full_version__2.html.

Jamieson, D. J., Read, J. S., Kourtis, A., et al. (2007). Cesarean delivery for HIV-infected women: Recommendations and controversies. *American Journal of Obstetrics and Gynecology, 197*(3 Suppl), S96–100.

Kenner, C., & Lott, J. W. (2007). *Comprehensive neonatal care: An interdisciplinary approach* (4th ed.). St. Louis, MO: Saunders Elsevier.

Koenig, D. (2007). Special delivery. *Natural Health, 37*(4), 51–58.

Kuczkowski, K. M. (2007). Labor pain and its management with the combined spinal-epidural analgesia: What does an obstetrician need to know? *Archives of Gynecology & Obstetrics, 275*(3), 183–185.

Leonard, P. (2007). Childbirth education: A handbook for nurses. *Nursing Spectrum.* Available at: http://nsweb/nursingspectrum.com/ce/m350c.htm.

Lockwood, C. (2007). Intrapartum EFM: How can we better identify the at-risk fetus? *Contemporary OB/GYN, 52*(1), 15–16.

Lowder, J. L., Burrows, L. J., Krohn, M. A., & Weber, A. M. (2007). Risk factors for primary and subsequent anal sphincter lacerations: A comparison of cohorts by parity and prior mode of delivery. *American Journal of Obstetrics & Gynecology, 196*(4), 344–349.

Lyon, E. (2007). *Big book of birth.* New York: Penguin Group (USA).

Menihan, C. A., & Kopel, E. (2008). *Electronic fetal monitoring: Concepts and applications* (2nd ed.). Philadelphia: Lippincott Williams & Wilkins.

Miller, K. E. (2007). Maternal oxygen affects nonreassuring FHR patterns. *American Family Physician, 75*(1), 111–114.

Moses, S. (2007). Fetal scalp blood sampling. *Family Practice Notebook.* Available at: http://www.fpnotebook.com/OB76.htm.

Murray, M. L. (2007). *Antepartal and intrapartal fetal monitoring* (3rd ed.). New York: Springer Publishing Company, Inc.

National Institute of Child Health and Human Development (NICHD). (2006). *NICHD terminology for fetal heart rate characteristics.* Available at: http://www.nichd.nih.gov/search.cfm? search_string=electronic+fetal+monitoring.

Peek, M. J., Condous, G. S., & Nanan, R. K. (2007). Fetal pulse oximetry and cesarean delivery. *New England Journal of Medicine, 356*(13), 1337–1340.

Reingold, A., Gershman, K., Petit, S., et al. (2007). Perinatal group B streptococcal disease after universal screening recommendations. *Journal of the American Medical Association, 298*(12), 1390–1392.

Roberts, J. M., Gonzalez, C. B., & Sampselle, C. (2007). Why do supportive birth attendants become directive of maternal bearing-down efforts in second-stage labor? *Journal of Midwifery & Women's Health, 52*(2), 134–141.

Ros, A., Felberbaum, R., Jahnke, I., Diedrich, K., Schmucker, P., & Huppe, M. (2007). Epidural anesthesia for labor: Does it influence the mode of delivery? *Archives of Gynecology & Obstetrics, 275*(4), 269–274.

Sauls, D. (2007). Nurses' attitudes toward provision of care and related health outcomes. *Nursing Research, 56*(2), 117–123.

Skidmore-Roth, L. (2007). *Mosby's 2007 nursing drug reference* (20th ed.). St. Louis, MO: Mosby Elsevier.

Sleutel, M., Schultz, S., & Wyble, K. (2007). Nurses' views of factors that help and hinder their intrapartum care. *Journal of Obstetric, Gynecologic & Neonatal Nursing, 36*(3), 203–211.

Smiley, R. M., & Stephenson, L. (2007). Patient-controlled analgesia for labor. *International Anesthesiology Clinics, 45*(1), 83–98.

Smith, C. A., Collins, C. T., Cyna, A. M., & Crowther, C. A. (2006). Complementary and alternative therapies for pain management in labor. *Cochrane Library.* 2006(4), CD003521; 2009358378.

Society of Obstetricians and Gynecologists of Canada (SOGC). (2006). Fetal health surveillance in labor (SOGC Clinical Practice Guidelines). *Journal of Obstetrics and Gynecology in Canada.* Available at: http://www.sogc.org/.

U.S. Department of Health and Human Services (USDHHS). (2000). *Healthy people 2010: Understanding and improving health* (2nd ed.). Chapter 16: Maternal, Infant, and Child Health. (DHHS Publication 017-001-00550-9). Washington, DC: Author.

Walsh, D. (2007). *Evidence-based care for normal labor and birth.* Andover, UK: Taylor & Francis, Inc.

Wood, S. (2007). Coping with labor pain. *March of Dimes.* Available at: http://www.marchofdimes.com/pnhec/240_12936.asp.

WEBSITES

Academy for Guided Imagery, Inc.: www.interactiveimagery.com
American College of Obstetricians and Gynecologists: www.acog.org
American Public Health Association: www.apha.org
Association of Labor Assistants and Childbirth Educators: www.alace.org
Association of Women's Health, Obstetric and Neonatal Nurses (AWHONN): www.awhonn.org
Birthworks: www.birthworks.org
Evidence-Based Nursing: www.evidencebasednursing.com
Child Find: www.childfind.org
Department of Health and Human Services: www.4women.gov
Diversity Rx: www.diversityrx.org
Doulas of North America: www.dona.org
Ethnomed: http://ethnomed.org
HypnoBirthing Institute: www.hypnobirthing.com
International Childbirth Education Association: www.icea.org
Lamaze International: www.lamaze-childbirth.com
National Center for Missing and Exploited Children: www.missingkids.com
Transcultural Health Links: www.iun.edu/~libemb/trannurs/trannurs.htm

CHAPTER WORKSHEET

MULTIPLE CHOICE QUESTIONS

1. When a client in labor is fully dilated, which instruction would be most effective to assist her in encouraging effective pushing?

   a. Hold your breath and push through entire contraction.

   b. Use chest-breathing with the contraction.

   c. Pant and blow during each contraction.

   d. Push for 6 to 7 seconds several times during each contraction.

2. During the fourth stage of labor, the nurse palpates the uterus on the right side and sees a saturated perineal pad. What is the nurse's first action?

   a. Massage the uterus vigorously.

   b. Have the client void and reassess her.

   c. Notify the primary care provider.

   d. Document as a normal finding.

3. When managing a client's pain during labor, nurses should:

   a. Make sure the agents given don't prolong labor.

   b. Know that all pain-relief measures are similar.

   c. Support the client's decisions and requests.

   d. Not recommend nonpharmacologic methods.

4. When caring for a client during the active phase of labor without continuous electronic fetal monitoring, the nurse would intermittently assess FHR every:

   a. 15 minutes

   b. 5 minutes

   c. 30 minutes

   d. 60 minutes

5. The nurse notes the presence of transient fetal accelerations on the fetal monitoring strip. Which intervention would be most appropriate?

   a. Reposition the client on the left side.

   b. Begin 100% oxygen via face mask.

   c. Document this reassuring pattern.

   d. Call the health care provider immediately.

CRITICAL THINKING EXERCISES

1. Carrie, a 20-year-old primigravida at term, comes to the birthing center in active labor (dilation 5 cm and 80% effaced, −1 station) with ruptured membranes. She states she wants an "all-natural" birth without medication. Her partner is with her and appears anxious but supportive. On the admission assessment, Carrie's prenatal history is unremarkable; vital signs are within normal limits; FHR via Doppler ranges between 140 and 144 bpm and is regular.

   a. Based on your assessment data and the woman's request not to have medication, what nonpharmacologic interventions could you offer her?

   b. What positions might be suggested to facilitate fetal descent?

2. Several hours later, Carrie complains of nausea and turns to her partner and angrily tells him to not touch her and to go away.

   a. What assessment needs to be done to determine what is happening?

   b. What explanation can you offer Carrie's partner regarding her change in behavior?

STUDY ACTIVITIES

1. Share experiences within a post-clinical conference group regarding the pain management interventions of the patients to which you were assigned. Compare and evaluate the effectiveness of different methods used, maternal behavior observed, and neonatal outcome in terms of Apgar scores.

2. On the fetal heart monitor, the nurse notices an elevation of the fetal baseline with the onset of contractions. This elevation would describe _____.

3. Compare and contrast a local birthing center to a community hospital's birthing suite in terms of the pain-management techniques and fetal monitoring used.

4. Select a childbirth website for expectant parents and critique the information provided in terms of its educational level and amount of advertising.

UNIT FIVE

POSTPARTUM PERIOD

POSTPARTUM ADAPTATIONS

KEY TERMS

engorgement
engrossment
involution
lactation

letting-go phase
lochia
puerperium

taking-hold phase
taking-in phase
uterine atony

LEARNING OBJECTIVES

Upon completion of the chapter, the learner will be able to:

1. Define the key terms used in this chapter.
2. Explain the systemic physiologic changes occurring in the woman after childbirth.
3. Identify the phases of maternal role adjustment as described by Reva Rubin.
4. Analyze the psychological adaptations occurring in the mother's partner after childbirth.

B̃etsy had been home only 3 days when she called the OB unit where she had given birth and asked to speak to the lactation consultant. She reported pain in both breasts. Her nipples were tender due to frequent breastfeeding and she described her breasts as heavy, hard, and swollen.

Wow

A new mother's expectations are seen through rose-colored glasses, and at times her fantasy is better than the reality.

The postpartum period is a critical transitional time for a woman, her newborn, and her family on physiologic and psychological levels. The **puerperium** period begins after the delivery of the placenta and lasts approximately 6 weeks. During this period the woman's body begins to return to its prepregnant state, and these changes generally resolve by the sixth week after giving birth. However, the postpartum period can also be defined to include the changes in all aspects of the mother's life that occur during the first year after a child is born. Some believe that the postpartum adjustment period lasts well into the first year, making the fourth phase of labor the longest. Keeping this in mind, the true postpartum period may last between 9 and 12 months as the mother works to lose the weight she gained while pregnant, adjusts psychologically to the changes in her life, and takes on the new role of mother.

This chapter describes the major physiologic and psychological changes that occur in a woman after childbirth. Various systemic adaptations take place throughout the woman's body. In addition, the mother and the family adjust to the new addition psychologically. The birth of a child changes the family structure and the roles of the family members. The adaptations are dynamic and continue to evolve as physical changes occur and new roles emerge.

Maternal Physiologic Adaptations

During pregnancy, the woman's entire body changed to accommodate the needs of the growing fetus. After birth, the woman's body once again undergoes significant changes in all body systems to return her body to its prepregnant state.

Reproductive System Adaptations

The reproductive system goes through tremendous adaptations to return to the prepregnancy state. All organs and tissues of the reproductive system are involved. The female reproductive system is unique in its capacity to remodel throughout the woman's reproductive life. The events after birth, with the shedding of the placenta and subsequent uterine involution, involve substantial tissue destruction and subsequent repair and remodeling. For example, the woman's menstrual cycle, interrupted during pregnancy, will begin to return several weeks after childbirth. The uterus, which has undergone tremendous expansion during pregnancy to accommodate progressive fetal growth, will return to its prepregnant size over several weeks. The mother's breasts have grown to prepare for lactation and do not return to their prepregnant size as the uterus does.

Uterus

The uterus returns to its normal size through a gradual process of **involution**, which involves retrogressive changes

that return it to its nonpregnant size and condition. Involution involves three retrogressive processes:

1. Contraction of muscle fibers to reduce those previously stretched during pregnancy
2. Catabolism, which reduces enlarged, individual myometrial cells
3. Regeneration of uterine epithelium from the lower layer of the decidua after the upper layers have been sloughed off and shed during lochial discharge (Blackburn, 2007)

The uterus, which weighs approximately 1,000 g (2.2 lb) soon after birth, undergoes physiologic involution as it returns to its nonpregnant state. Approximately 1 week after birth, the uterus shrinks in size by 50% and weighs about 500 g (1 lb); at the end of 6 weeks, it weighs approximately 60 g (2 oz), about the weight before the pregnancy (Arenson & Drake, 2007; Blackburn, 2007; Fig. 15.1). During the first few days after birth, the uterus typically descends from the level of the umbilicus at a rate of 1 cm (1 fingerbreadth) per day. By 3 days, the fundus lies 2 to 3 fingerbreadths below the umbilicus (or slightly higher in multiparous women). By the end of 10 days, the fundus usually cannot be palpated because it has descended into the true pelvis.

If these retrogressive changes do not occur as a result of retained placental fragments or infection, subinvolution results. Subinvolution is generally responsive to early diagnosis and treatment. Factors that facilitate uterine involution include complete expulsion of amniotic membranes and placenta at birth, a complication-free labor and birth process, breastfeeding, and early ambulation.

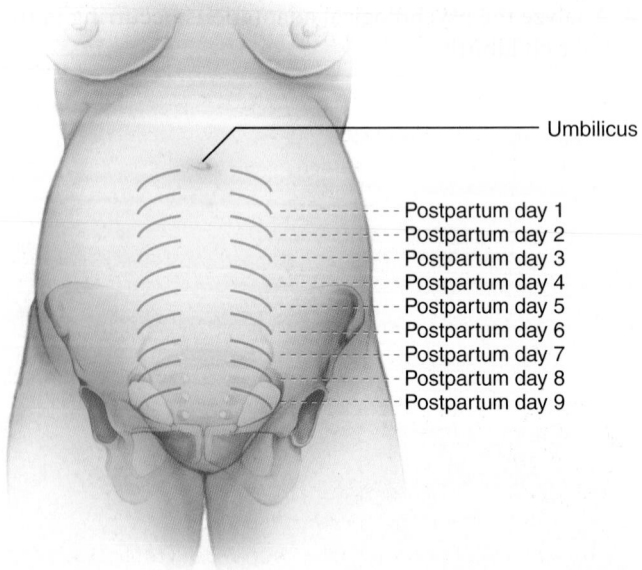

FIGURE 15.1 Uterine involution.

Factors that inhibit involution include a prolonged labor and difficult birth, incomplete expulsion of amniotic membranes and placenta, uterine infection, overdistention of uterine muscles (such as by multiple gestation, hydramnios, or a large singleton fetus), a full bladder (which displaces the uterus and interferes with contractions), anesthesia (which relaxes uterine muscles), and close childbirth spacing (frequent and repeated distention decreases tone and causes muscular relaxation).

Lochia

Lochia is the vaginal discharge that occurs after birth. It results from involution, during which the superficial layer of the decidua basalis becomes necrotic and is sloughed off. Immediately after childbirth, lochia is bright red and consists mainly of blood, fibrinous products, decidual cells, and red and white blood cells. The lochia from the uterus is alkaline but becomes acidic as it passes through the vagina. It is roughly equal to the amount occurring during a heavy menstrual period. The average amount of lochial discharge is 240 to 270 mL (8 to 9 oz) (Nash, 2007).

Women who have had cesarean births tend to have less flow because the uterine debris is removed manually along with delivery of the placenta. Lochia is present in most women for at least 3 weeks after childbirth, but it persists in some women for as long as 6 weeks.

Lochia passes through three stages: lochia rubra, lochia serosa, and lochia alba:

- Lochia rubra is a deep-red mixture of mucus, tissue debris, and blood that occurs for the first 3 to 4 days after birth. As uterine bleeding subsides, it becomes paler and more serous.
- Lochia serosa is the second stage. It is pinkish brown and is expelled 3 to 10 days postpartum. Lochia serosa primarily contains leukocytes, decidual tissue, red blood cells, and serous fluid.
- Lochia alba is the final stage. The discharge is creamy white or light brown and consists of leukocytes, decidual tissue, and reduced fluid content. It occurs from days 10 to 14 but can last 3 to 6 weeks postpartum in some women and still be considered normal.

Lochia at any stage should have a fleshy smell; an offensive odor usually indicates an infection, such as endometritis.

> ▶ **Take** NOTE!
>
> *A danger sign is the reappearance of bright-red blood after lochia rubra has stopped. Reevaluation by the health care professional is essential if this occurs.*

Afterpains

Part of the involution process involves uterine contractions. Subsequently, many women are frequently bothered by painful uterine contractions termed afterpains. All women experience afterpains, but they are more acute in multiparous women secondary to repeated stretching of the uterine muscles. This repeated stretching reduces muscle tone, allowing for alternate uterine contraction and relaxation. The uterus of a primiparous woman tends to remain contracted after giving birth unless she is breastfeeding; had a prolonged, difficult labor and birth; or had an overdistended uterus secondary to multiple gestation, hydramnios, or retained blood clots or placental fragments.

> ▶ **Take** NOTE!
>
> *Afterpains are usually stronger during breastfeeding because oxytocin released by the sucking reflex strengthens the contractions. Mild analgesics can reduce this discomfort.*

Cervix

The cervix typically returns to its prepregnant state by week 6 of the postpartum period. The cervix gradually closes but never regains its prepregnant appearance. Immediately after childbirth, the cervix is shapeless and edematous and is easily distensible for several days. The cervical os gradually closes and returns to normal by 2 weeks, whereas the external os widens and never appears the same after childbirth. The external cervical os is no longer shaped like a circle, but instead appears as a jagged slit-like opening, often described as a "fish mouth" (Fig. 15.2).

Vagina

Shortly after birth, the vaginal mucosa is edematous and thin, with few rugae. As ovarian function returns and estrogen production resumes, the mucosa thickens and rugae return in approximately 3 weeks. The vagina gapes at the

A   B

FIGURE 15.2 Appearance of the cervical os. (**A**) Before the first pregnancy. (**B**) After pregnancy.

opening and is generally lax. The vagina returns to its approximate prepregnant size by 6 to 8 weeks postpartum but will always remain a bit larger than it had been before pregnancy.

Normal mucus production and thickening of the vaginal mucosa usually return with ovulation (Edmonds, 2007). Ovulation can return as early as a month after childbirth in women who are not breastfeeding, with a mean time frame of 3 months. The mean time to ovulation in breastfeeding women is approximately 6 months, but this can vary greatly depending on breast-feeding patterns (Walsh, 2007). Localized dryness and coital discomfort (dyspareunia) usually plague most women until menstruation returns. Water-soluble lubricants can reduce discomfort during intercourse. Box 15.1 lists some commonly available water-soluble lubricants.

Perineum

The perineum is often edematous and bruised for the first day or two after birth. If the birth involved an episiotomy or laceration, complete healing may take as long as 4 to 6 months in the absence of complications at the site, such as hematoma or infection (Blackburn, 2007). Perineal lacerations may extend into the anus and cause considerable discomfort for the mother when she is attempting to defecate or ambulate. The presence of swollen hemorrhoids may also heighten discomfort. Local comfort measures such as ice packs, pouring warm water over the area via a peribottle, witch hazel pads, anesthetic sprays, and sitz baths can relieve pain. See Evidence-Based Practice 15.1.

Supportive tissues of the pelvic floor are stretched during the childbirth process, and restoring their tone may take up to 6 months. Pelvic relaxation can occur in any woman experiencing a vaginal birth. Nurses should encourage all women to practice Kegel exercises to improve pelvic floor tone, strengthen the perineal muscles, and promote healing.

> ▶ *Take* NOTE!
>
> *Failure to maintain and restore perineal muscular tone leads to urinary incontinence later in life for many women.*

Cardiovascular System Adaptations

The cardiovascular system undergoes dramatic changes after birth. During pregnancy, the heart is displaced slightly upward and to the left. This reverses as the uterus undergoes involution. Cardiac output remains high for the first few days postpartum and then gradually declines to nonpregnant values within 3 months of birth.

Blood volume, which increased substantially during pregnancy, drops rapidly after birth and returns to normal within 4 weeks postpartum (Arenson & Drake, 2007). The decrease in both cardiac output and blood volume reflects the birth-related blood loss (an average of 500 mL with a vaginal birth and 1,000 mL with a cesarean birth). Blood plasma volume is further reduced through diuresis, which occurs during the early postpartum period (Cheng & Caughey, 2007). Despite the decrease in blood volume, the hematocrit level remains relatively stable and may even increase, reflecting the predominant loss of plasma. Thus, an acute decrease in hematocrit is not an expected finding and may indicate hemorrhage.

Pulse and Blood Pressure

The increase in cardiac output during pregnancy begins to diminish after birth. This decrease in cardiac output is reflected in bradycardia (50 to 70 bpm) for the first 2 weeks postpartum. This slowing of the heart rate is related to the increased blood that flows back to the heart and to the central circulation after it is no longer perfusing the placenta. This increase in central circulation brings about an increased stroke volume and allows a slower heart rate to provide ample maternal circulation. Gradually, cardiac output returns to prepregnant levels by 3 months after childbirth (Blackburn, 2007).

Tachycardia (heart rate above 100 bpm) in the postpartum woman warrants further investigation. It may indicate hypovolemia, dehydration, or hemorrhage. However, because of the increased blood volume during pregnancy, a considerable loss may be well tolerated and not cause a compensatory cardiovascular response such as tachycardia. In most instances of postpartum hemorrhage, blood pressure and cardiac output remain increased because of the compensatory increase in heart rate. Thus, a decrease

---

BOX 15.1 **Water-Soluble Lubricants**

- Astroglide
- Aqua Lube Personal
- Devine No. 9
- Emerita
- Eros
- ID Glide sensual lubricant
- JO water-based lubricant
- K-Y personal lubricant
- Life Styles personal lubricant
- Liquid Silk
- Nature's Dew
- Pre-Seed Intimate
- Replens
- Slippery Stuff

EVIDENCE-BASED PRACTICE 15.1
Rectal Analgesia for Pain From Perineal Trauma Following Childbirth

● Study
Perineal pain from a tear and/or surgical cut (episiotomy) is a common problem following vaginal birth. Strategies to reduce perineal trauma and the appropriate repair of any perineal damage sustained are important for avoiding and alleviating pain. Numerous pain-relief treatments are used in clinical practice, such as local anesthetics, oral analgesics, therapeutic ultrasound, antiseptics, and nonpharmacologic applications such as ice packs and baths. This review assesses the evidence for using rectal analgesia for pain relief following perineal trauma caused by childbirth.

▲ Findings
This review of trials found that NSAID rectal suppositories are associated with less pain up to 24 hours after birth, and less additional analgesia is required. More research is required to assess the longer-term outcomes, maternal satisfaction, and effects, if any, on breast milk, mother–baby bonding, and sexual functioning.

■ Nursing Implications
According to the study, NSAID rectal suppositories were helpful in relieving postpartum pain. Nurses can offer this intervention to their patients and explain the evidence-based practice behind it.

Hedayati, H., Parsons, J., & Crowther, C. A. (2003). Rectal analgesia for pain from perineal trauma following childbirth. *Cochrane Database of Systematic Reviews* 2003, Issue 3. Art. No.: CD003931. DOI: 10.1002/14651858.CD003931.

in blood pressure and cardiac output are not expected changes during the postpartum period. Early identification is essential to ensure prompt intervention.

Blood pressure values should be similar to those obtained during the labor process. In some women there may be a slight transient increase lasting for about a week after childbirth (Edmonds, 2007). A significant increase accompanied by headache might indicate preeclampsia and requires further investigation. A decreased blood pressure may suggest orthostatic hypotension or uterine hemorrhage.

Coagulation
Clotting factors that increased during pregnancy tend to remain elevated during the early postpartum period. Giving birth stimulates this hypercoagulability state further. As a result, these coagulation factors remain elevated for 2 to 3 weeks postpartum (Hackley, Kriebs, & Rousseau, 2007). This hypercoagulable state, combined with vessel damage during birth and immobility, places the woman at risk for thromboembolism (blood clots) in the lower extremities and the lungs.

Blood Cellular Components
Red blood cell production ceases early in the puerperium, causing mean hemoglobin and hematocrit levels to decrease slightly in the first 24 hours. Over the next 2 weeks, both levels rise slowly. The white blood count, which increases in labor, remains elevated for first 4 to 6 days after birth but then falls to 6,000 to 10,000/mm³. This white blood cell elevation can complicate a diagnosis of infection in the immediate postpartum period.

Urinary System Adaptations

Pregnancy and birth can have profound effects on the urinary system. During pregnancy, the glomerular filtration rate and renal plasma flow increase significantly. Both usually return to normal by 6 weeks after birth.

Many women have difficulty feeling the sensation to void after giving birth if they received an anesthetic block during labor (which inhibits neural functioning of the bladder) or if they received oxytocin to induce or augment their labor (antidiuretic effect). These women will be at risk for incomplete emptying, bladder distention, difficulty voiding, and urinary retention. In addition, urination may be impeded by:

- Perineal lacerations
- Generalized swelling and bruising of the perineum and tissues surrounding the urinary meatus
- Hematomas
- Decreased bladder tone as a result of regional anesthesia
- Diminished sensation of bladder pressure as a result of swelling, poor bladder tone, and numbing effects of regional anesthesia used during labor (Nash, 2007)

Difficulty voiding can lead to urinary retention, bladder distention, and ultimately urinary tract infection (UTI). Urinary retention and bladder distention can cause displacement of the uterus from the midline to the right and can inhibit the uterus from contracting properly, which increases the risk of postpartum hemorrhage. Urinary retention is a major cause of **uterine atony**, which allows excessive bleeding. Frequent voiding of small amounts (less than 150 mL) suggests urinary retention with overflow, and catheterization may be necessary to empty the bladder to restore tone.

Postpartum diuresis occurs as a result of several mechanisms: the large amounts of intravenous fluids given during labor, a decreasing antidiuretic effect of oxytocin as its level declines, the buildup and retention of extra fluids during pregnancy, and a decreasing production of aldosterone—the hormone that decreases sodium retention and increases urine production (Blackburn, 2007). All these factors contribute to rapid filling of the bladder within 12 hours of birth. Diuresis begins within 12 hours after childbirth and continues throughout the first week postpartum. Normal function returns within a month after birth (Edmonds, 2007).

▶ **Consider** THIS!

Have you ever felt like a real idiot by not being able to complete a simple task in life? I had a beautiful baby boy after only 6 hours of labor. My epidural worked well and I actually felt very little discomfort throughout my labor. Because it was in the middle of the night when they brought me to my postpartum room, I felt a few hours of sleep would be all I needed to be back to normal. During an assessment early the next morning, the nurse found my uterus had shifted to the right from my midline, and I was instructed to empty my bladder. I didn't understand why the nurse was concerned about where my uterus was located and, besides, I didn't feel any sensation of a full bladder. But I did get up anyway and tried to comply. Despite all the nurse's tricks of running the faucet for sound effects, in addition to having warm water poured over my thighs via the peri-bottle, I was unable to urinate. How could I not accomplish one of life's simplest tasks?

Thoughts: Women who receive regional anesthesia frequently experience reduced sensation to their perineal area and do not feel a full bladder. The nursing assessment revealed a displaced uterus secondary to a full bladder. What additional "tricks" can be used to assist this woman to void? What explanation should be offered to her regarding why she is having difficulty urinating?

Gastrointestinal System Adaptations

The GI system quickly returns to normal because the gravid uterus is no longer filling the abdominal cavity and producing pressure on the abdominal organs. Progesterone levels, which caused relaxation of smooth muscle during pregnancy and diminished bowel tone, also are declining.

Regardless of the type of delivery, most women experience decreased bowel tone and sluggish bowels for several days after birth. Decreased peristalsis occurs in response to analgesics, surgery, diminished intraabdominal pressure, low-fiber diet and insufficient fluid intake,

and diminished muscle tone. In addition, women with an episiotomy, perineal laceration, or hemorrhoids may fear pain or damage to the perineum with their first bowel movement and may attempt to delay it. Subsequently, constipation is a common problem during the postpartum period. A stool softener can be prescribed for this reason.

Most women are hungry and thirsty after childbirth, commonly related to NPO restrictions and the energy expended during labor. Their appetite returns to normal immediately after giving birth.

▶ **Take** NOTE!

Anticipate the woman's need to replenish her body with food and fluids, and provide both soon after she gives birth.

Musculoskeletal System Adaptations

The effects of pregnancy on the muscles and joints vary widely. During pregnancy, the hormones relaxin, estrogen, and progesterone relax the joints. After birth, levels of these hormones decline, resulting in a return of all joints to their prepregnant state, with the exception of the woman's feet. Parous women will note a permanent increase in their shoe size (Hackley, Kriebs, & Rousseau, 2007).

Woman commonly experience fatigue and activity intolerance and have a distorted body image for weeks after birth secondary to declining relaxin and progesterone levels, which cause hip and joint pain that interferes with ambulation and exercise. Good body mechanics and correct position are important during this time to prevent low back pain and injury to the joints. Within 6 to 8 weeks after delivery, joints are completely stabilized and return to normal.

During pregnancy, stretching of the abdominal wall muscles occurs to accommodate the enlarging uterus. This stretching leads to a loss in muscle tone and possibly separation of the longitudinal muscles (rectus abdominis muscles) of the abdomen. Separation of the rectus abdominis muscles, called diastasis recti, is more common in women who have poor abdominal muscle tone before pregnancy. After birth, muscle tone is diminished and the abdominal muscles are soft and flabby. Specific exercises are necessary to help the woman regain muscle tone. Fortunately, diastasis responds well to exercise, and abdominal muscle tone can be improved (see Chapter 16 for more information about exercises to improve muscle tone).

▶ **Take** NOTE!

If rectus muscle tone is not regained through exercise, support may not be adequate during future pregnancies.

Integumentary System Adaptations

Another system that experiences lasting effects of pregnancy is the integumentary system. As estrogen and progesterone levels decrease, the darkened pigmentation on the abdomen (linea nigra), face (melasma), and nipples gradually fades. Some women experience hair loss during pregnancy and the postpartum periods. Approximately 90% of hairs are growing at any one time, with the other 10% entering a resting phase. Because of the high estrogen levels present during pregnancy, an increased number of hairs go into the resting phase, which is part of the normal hair loss cycle. The most common period for hair loss is within 3 months after birth, when estrogen returns to normal levels and more hairs are allowed to fall out. This hair loss is temporary, and regrowth generally returns to normal levels in 6 to 12 months (Lyon, 2007).

Striae gravidarum (stretch marks) that developed during pregnancy on the breasts, abdomen, and hips gradually fade to silvery lines. However, these lines do not disappear completely. Although many products on the market claim to make stretch marks disappear, their effectiveness is highly questionable.

The profuse diaphoresis (sweating) that is common during the early postpartum period is one of the most noticeable adaptations in the integumentary system. Many women will wake up drenched with perspiration during the puerperium. This postpartal diaphoresis is a mechanism to reduce the amount of fluids retained during pregnancy and restore prepregnant body fluid levels. It can be profuse at times. It is common, especially at night during the first week after birth. Reassure the client that this is normal and encourage her to change her gown to prevent chilling.

Respiratory System Adaptations

Respirations usually remain within the normal adult range of 16 to 24 breaths per minute. As the abdominal organs resume their nonpregnant position, the diaphragm returns to its usual position. Anatomic changes in the thoracic cavity and rib cage caused by increasing uterine growth resolve quickly. As a result, discomforts such as shortness of breath and rib aches are relieved. Tidal volume, minute volume, vital capacity, and functional residual capacity return to prepregnant values, typically within 1 to 3 weeks of birth (Blackburn, 2007).

Endocrine System Adaptations

The endocrine system undergoes several changes rapidly after birth. Levels of circulating estrogen and progesterone drop quickly with delivery of the placenta. Decreased estrogen levels are associated with breast engorgement and with the diuresis of excess extracellular fluid accumulated during pregnancy (Edmonds, 2007). Estrogen is at its lowest level a week after birth. For the woman who is not breastfeeding, estrogen levels begin to increase by 2 weeks after birth. For the breastfeeding woman, estrogen levels remain low until breastfeeding frequency decreases.

Other placental hormones (hCG, hPL, progesterone) decline rapidly after birth. hCG levels are nonexistent at the end of the first postpartum week and hPL is undetectable within 1 day after birth (Blackburn, 2007). Progesterone levels are undetectable by 3 days after childbirth, and production is reestablished with the first menses. Prolactin levels decline within 2 weeks for the woman who is not breastfeeding and remain elevated for the lactating woman (Blackburn, 2007).

Think back to Betsy, the woman experiencing painful changes in her breasts. What is Betsy describing to the lactation consultant? Why has the condition of her breasts changed compared to when she was in the hospital?

Lactation

Lactation is the secretion of milk by the breasts. It is thought to be brought about by the interaction of progesterone, estrogen, prolactin, and oxytocin. Breast milk typically appears 3 days after childbirth.

During pregnancy, the breasts increase in size and functional ability in preparation for breastfeeding. Within the first month of gestation, the ducts of the mammary glands grow branches, forming more lobules and alveoli. These structural changes make the breasts larger, more tender, and heavy. Each breast gains nearly 1 lb in weight by term, the glandular cells fill with secretions, blood vessels increase in number, and there are increased amounts of connective tissue and fat cells (Blackburn, 2007).

Prolactin from the anterior pituitary gland, secreted in increasing levels throughout pregnancy, triggers the synthesis and secretion of milk after the woman gives birth. During pregnancy, prolactin, estrogen, and progesterone cause synthesis and secretion of colostrum, which contains protein and carbohydrate but no milk fat. It is only after birth takes place, when the high levels of estrogen and progesterone are abruptly withdrawn, that prolactin is able to stimulate the glandular cells to secrete milk instead of colostrum. This takes place within 2 to 3 days after giving birth. Oxytocin acts so that milk can be ejected from the alveoli to the nipple. Therefore, sucking by the newborn will release milk. Prolactin levels increase in response to nipple stimulation during feedings. Prolactin and oxytocin result in milk production if stimulated by sucking (Walsh, 2007) (Fig. 15.3). If the stimulus (sucking) is not present, as with a woman who is not breastfeeding, breast engorgement and milk production will subside within 2 to 3 days postpartum.

Typically, during the first 2 days after birth, the breasts are soft and nontender. The woman also may report a tingling sensation in both breasts. After this time, breast changes depend on whether the mother is breastfeeding or taking measures to prevent lactation.

FIGURE 15.3 Physiology of lactation.

Engorgement is the process of swelling of the breast tissue as a result of an increase in blood and lymph supply as a precursor to lactation (Bainbridge, 2007). Breasts increase in vascularity and swell in response to prolactin 2 to 4 days after birth. If engorged, the breasts will be hard and tender to touch. They are temporarily full, tender, and very uncomfortable until the milk supply is ready. Frequent emptying of the breasts helps to minimize discomfort and resolve engorgement. Standing in a warm shower or applying warm compresses immediately before feedings will help to soften the breasts and nipples in order to allow the newborn to latch on easier. These measures will also enhance the letdown reflex. Between feedings, applying cold compresses to the breasts helps to reduce swelling. To maintain milk supply, the breasts need to be stimulated by a nursing infant, a breast pump, or manual expression of the milk (Fig. 15.4).

*R*emember Betsy, with the breast discomfort? The *lactation consultant explained that she was experiencing normal breast engorgement and offered several suggestions to help her. What relief measures might they be? What reassurance can be given to Betsy at this time?*

FIGURE 15.4 Mother using breast pumps to stimulate milk production.

If the woman is not breastfeeding, relief measures include wearing a tight, supportive bra 24 hours daily, applying ice to her breasts for approximately 15 to 20 minutes every other hour, and not stimulating the breasts by squeezing or manually expressing milk from the nipples. In addition, avoiding exposing the breasts to warmth (e.g., a hot shower) will help relieve breast engorgement. In women who are not breastfeeding, engorgement typically subsides within 2 to 3 days with these measures.

Ovulation and Return of Menstruation

Changing hormone levels constantly interact with one another to produce bodily changes. Four major hormones are influential during the postpartum period: estrogen, progesterone, prolactin, and oxytocin. Estrogen is the major female hormone during pregnancy, but levels drop profoundly at birth and reach their lowest level a week into the postpartum period. Progesterone quiets the uterus to prevent a preterm birth during pregnancy, and its increasing levels during pregnancy prevent lactation from starting before birth takes place. As with estrogen, progesterone levels decrease dramatically after birth and are undetectable 72 hours after birth. Progesterone levels are reestablished with the first menstrual cycle (Blackburn, 2007).

During the postpartum period, oxytocin stimulates the uterus to contract during the breastfeeding session and for as long as 20 minutes after each feeding. Oxytocin also acts on the breast by eliciting the milk letdown reflex during breastfeeding. Prolactin is also associated with the breastfeeding process by stimulating milk production. In women who breastfeed, prolactin levels remain elevated into the sixth week after birth (Nash, 2007). The levels of the hormone increase and decrease in proportion to nipple stimulation. Prolactin levels decrease in nonlactating women, reaching prepregnant levels by the third postpartum week (Edmonds, 2007). High levels of prolactin have been found to delay ovulation by inhibiting ovarian response to FSH (Edmonds, 2007).

The timing of first menses and ovulation after birth differs between women who are and are not breastfeeding. For nonlactating women, menstruation usually resumes 7 to 9 weeks after giving birth, with the first cycle being anovulatory (Walsh, 2007). The return of menses in the lactating woman depends on breastfeeding frequency and duration. It can return anytime from 2 to 18 months after childbirth, depending on whether the woman is exclusively breastfeeding or supplementing with formula. The first postpartum menstrual period may be heavier than prepregnant ones and is frequently anovulatory (Hackley, Kriebs, & Rousseau, 2007).

> ▶ **Take** NOTE!
>
> *Ovulation may occur before menstruation; therefore, breastfeeding is not a reliable method of contraception. Other methods of family planning must be used to control fertility (Alexander et al., 2007).*

Betsy tries several of the measures the lactation consultant suggested to relieve her breast discomfort but is still having heaviness and pain. She feels discouraged and tells the nurse she is thinking of reducing her breastfeeding and using formula to feed her newborn. Is that a good choice? Why or why not? What interventions will help Betsy get through this difficult time?

Psychological Adaptations

Mothers' and fathers' experiences of pregnancy are necessarily different, and this difference continues after childbirth as they both adjust to their new parenting roles. Parenting involves caring for infants physically and emotionally to foster the growth and development of responsible, caring adults. During the early months of parenthood, mothers experience more life changes and get more satisfaction from their new roles than fathers. However, fathers interact with their newborns much like mothers (Thorpe, 2007). Early parent–infant contact after birth improves attachment behaviors. Other members of the newborn's family, such as siblings and grandparents, also

experience changes related to the birth of the newborn. Chapter 16 describes these changes.

Maternal Psychological Adaptations

Postpartum depression affects the transition to the maternal role for many mothers. Between 50% and 80% of new mothers suffer from the short-lived postpartum mood disorder termed "baby blues." In addition, each year in the United States, up to 28% of new mothers or more than 400,000 new mothers suffer debilitating postpartum depression, a prevalence that continues unabated (AWHONN, 2007). Postpartum depression can lead to alienation from loved ones, daily dysfunction secondary to overwhelming sorrow and disorientation, and, at its most extreme, personal terror resulting in dangerous thoughts and violent actions. For additional information, see Chapter 22.

The woman experiences a variety of responses as she adjusts to a new family member, postpartum discomforts, changes in her body image, and the reality of change in her life. In the early 1960s, Reva Rubin identified three phases that a mother goes through to adjust to her new maternal role. Rubin's maternal role framework can be used to monitor the client's progress as she "tries on" her new role as a mother. Absence of these processes or inability to progress through the phases satisfactorily may impede the appropriate development of the maternal role (Rubin, 1984). Although Rubin's maternal role development theories are of value, some of her observations regarding the length of each phase may not be completely relevant for the contemporary woman of the 21st century. Today, many women know their infant's gender, have "seen" their fetus in utero through four-dimensional ultrasound, and have a working knowledge of childbirth and child care. They are less passive than in years past and progress through the phases of attaining the maternal role at a much faster pace than Rubin would have imagined. Still, Rubin's framework is timeless for assessing and monitoring expected role behaviors when planning care and appropriate interventions.

Taking–In Phase

The **taking-in phase** is the time immediately after birth when the client needs sleep, depends on others to meet her needs, and relives the events surrounding the birth process. This phase is characterized by dependent behavior. During the first 24 to 48 hours after giving birth, mothers often assume a very passive role in meeting their own basic needs for food, fluids, and rest, allowing the nurse to make decisions for them concerning activities and care. They spend time recounting their labor experience to anyone who will listen. Such actions help the mother integrate the birth experience into reality—that is, the pregnancy is over and the newborn is now a unique individual, separate from herself. When interacting with the newborn, new mothers spend time claiming the newborn and touching him or her, commonly identifying specific features in the newborn, such as "he has my nose" or "his fingers are long like his father's" (Fig. 15.5).

▶ **Take** NOTE!

The taking-in phase typically lasts 1 to 2 days and may be the only phase observed by nurses in the hospital setting because of the shortened postpartum stays that are the norm today.

Taking-Hold Phase

The **taking-hold phase**, the second phase of maternal adaptation, is characterized by dependent and independent maternal behavior. This phase typically starts on the second to third day postpartum and may last several weeks.

As the client regains control over her bodily functions during the next few days, she will be taking hold and becoming preoccupied with the present. She will be particularly concerned about her health, the infant's condition, and her ability to care for him or her. She demonstrates increased autonomy and mastery of her own body's functioning, and a desire to take charge with support and help from others. She will show independence by caring for herself and learning to care for her newborn, but she still requires assurance that she is doing well as a mother. She expresses a strong interest in caring for the infant by herself.

Letting-Go Phase

In the **letting-go phase**, the third phase of maternal adaptation, the woman reestablishes relationships with other people. She adapts to parenthood through her new role as a mother. She assumes the responsibility and care for the newborn with a bit more confidence now (Arenson & Drake, 2007). The focus of this phase is to move forward by assuming the parental role and to separate herself from the symbiotic relationship that she and her newborn had during pregnancy. She establishes a lifestyle that includes the infant. The mother relinquishes the fantasy infant and accepts the real one.

Partner Psychological Adaptations

For partners, whether they are husbands, significant others, boyfriends, same-sex life partners, or just friends, becoming a parent or just sharing the childbirth experience can be a perplexing time as well as a time of great change. This transition is influenced by many factors, including participation in childbirth, relationships with significant others, competence in child care, the family role organization, the individual's cultural background, and the method of infant feeding.

▶ **Take** NOTE!

Most research findings stress the importance of early contact between the father or significant other and the newborn, as well as participation in infant care activities, to foster the relationship (Thorpe, 2007).

Infants have a powerful effect on their fathers and others, who become intensely involved with them (Fig. 15.6). The father's or significant other's developing bond with the newborn—a time of intense absorption, preoccupation, and interest—is called engrossment.

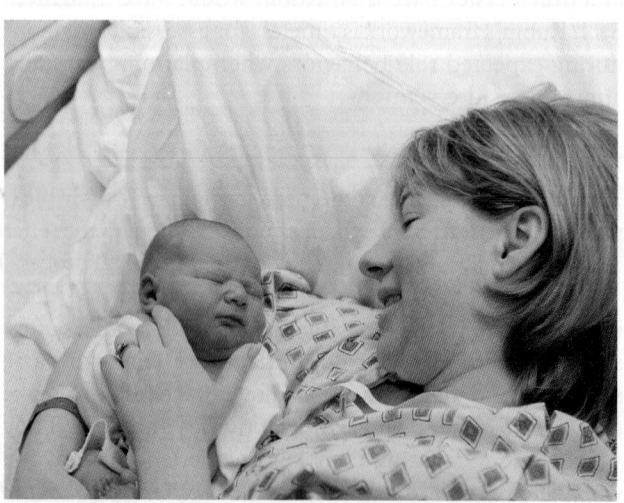

FIGURE 15.5 Mother bonding with newborn during the taking-in phase.

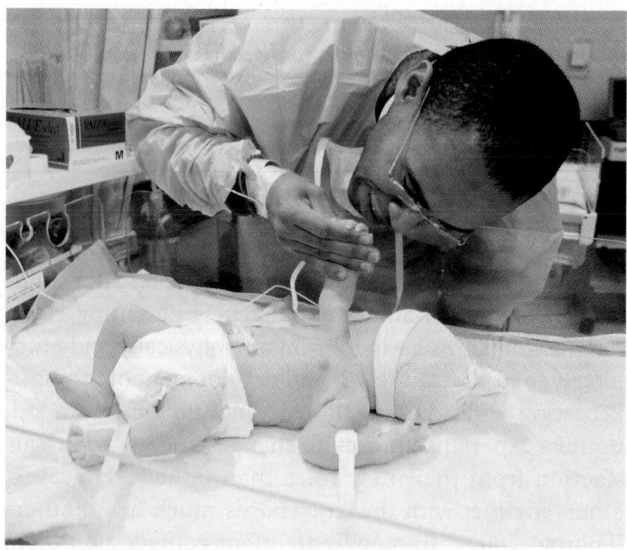

FIGURE 15.6 Engrossment of the father and his newborn.

Engrossment

Engrossment is characterized by seven behaviors:

1. Visual awareness of the newborn—the father or partner perceives the newborn as attractive, pretty, or beautiful
2. Tactile awareness of the newborn—the father or partner has a desire to touch or hold the newborn and considers this activity to be pleasurable
3. Perception of the newborn as perfect—the father or partner does not "see" any imperfections
4. Strong attraction to the newborn—the father or partner focuses all attention on the newborn when he is in the room
5. Awareness of distinct features of the newborn—the father or partner can distinguish his newborn from others in the nursery
6. Extreme elation—the father or partner feels a "high" after the birth of his child
7. Increased sense of self-esteem—the father or partner feels proud, "bigger," more mature, and older after the birth of his child (Sears & Sears, 2006)

Frequently, fathers or partners are portrayed as well-meaning but bumbling when caring for newborns. However, they have their own unique way of relating to their newborns and can become as nurturing as mothers. A father or partner's nurturing responses may be less automatic and slower to unfold than a mother's, but they are capable of a strong bonding attachment to their newborns (Sears & Sears, 2006). Encouraging fathers or partners to express their feelings by seeing, touching, and holding their son or daughter and by cuddling, talking to, and feeding him or her will help to cement this new relationship. Reinforcement of this engrossing behavior helps fathers or partners to make a positive attachment during this critical period.

Three-Stage Role Development Process

Similar to mothers, fathers or partners also go through a predictable three-stage process during the first 3 weeks as they too "try on" their roles as parents. The three stages are expectations, reality, and transition to mastery (Sears & Sears, 2006).

Stage 1: Expectations

New fathers or partners pass through stage 1 (expectations) with preconceptions about what home life will be like with a newborn. Many men may be unaware of the dramatic changes that can occur when this newborn comes home to live with them. For some, it is an eye-opening experience.

Stage 2: Reality

Stage 2 (reality) occurs when fathers or partners realize that their expectations in stage 1 are not realistic. Their feelings change from elation to sadness, ambivalence, jealousy, and frustration. Many wish to be more involved in the newborn's care and yet do not feel prepared to do so. Some find parenting fun but at the same time do not feel fully prepared to take on that role.

Stage 3: Transition to Mastery

In stage 3 (transition to mastery), the father or partner makes a conscious decision to take control and be at the center of his newborn's life regardless of his preparedness. This adjustment period is similar to that of the mother's letting-go phase, when she incorporates the newest member into the family.

■■■ Key Concepts

- The puerperium period refers to the first 6 weeks after delivery. During this period, the mother experiences many physiologic and psychological adaptations to return her to the prepregnant state.
- Involution involves three processes: contraction of muscle fibers to reduce stretched ones, catabolism (which reduces enlarged, individual cells), and regeneration of uterine epithelium from the lower layer of the decidua after the upper layers have been sloughed off and shed in lochia.
- Lochia passes through three stages: lochia rubra, lochia serosa, and lochia alba during the postpartal period.
- Maternal blood plasma volume decreases rapidly after birth and returns to normal within 4 weeks postpartum.
- Reva Rubin (1984) identified three phases the mother goes through to adjust to her new maternal role. The phases of maternal postpartum adjustment are taking in, taking hold, and letting go.
- The transition to fatherhood is influenced by many factors, including participation in childbirth, relationships with significant others, competence in child care, the family role organization, the father's cultural background, and the method of infant feeding.
- Like mothers, men go through a predictable three-stage process during the first 3 weeks as they too "try on" their roles as fathers or partners. The three stages include expectations, reality, and transition to mastery.

REFERENCES

Alexander, L. L., LaRosa, J. H., Bader, H., & Garfield, S. (2007). *New dimensions in women's health* (4th ed.). Sudbury, MA: Jones and Bartlett Publishers.

Arenson, J., & Drake, P. (2007). *Maternal and newborn health.* Sudbury, MA: Jones and Bartlett Publishers.

AWHONN. (2007). Conquering postpartum depression. *Nursing for Women's Health, 11*(4), 422–423.

Bainbridge, J. (2007). Dealing with breast and nipple soreness when breastfeeding. *British Journal of Midwifery, 13*(9), 552–556.

Blackburn, S. T. (2007). *Maternal, fetal, and neonatal physiology* (3rd ed.). Philadelphia: Saunders Elsevier.

Cheng, Y. W., & Caughey, A. B. (2007) Normal labor and delivery. *eMedicine.* Available at: http://www.emedicine.com/MED/topic3239.htm.

Edmonds, K. (2007). *Dewhurst's textbook of obstetrics and gynecology* (7th ed.). Oxford, UK: Blackwell Publishing Limited.

Hackley, B., Kriebs, J. M., & Rousseau, M. E. (2007). *Primary care of women: A guide for midwives and women's health providers.* Sudbury, MA: Jones & Bartlett Publishers.

Lyon, E. (2007). *Big book of birth.* New York: Penguin Group (USA).

Nash, L. R. (2007). Postpartum care. In R. E. Rachel & E. T. Bope (Eds.), *Conn's current therapy 2007* (Section 16, pp. 1190–1193). Philadelphia: Saunders Elsevier.

Rubin, R. (1984). *Maternal identity and the maternal experience.* New York: Springer.

Sears, R. W., & Sears, J. M. (2006). *Fathers' first steps: 25 things every dad should know.* Boston, MA: Harvard Common Press.

Thorpe, K. (2007). Child health nurses supporting parents. *Australian Nursing Journal, 14*(8), 32–35.

Walsh, D. (2007). *Evidence-based care for normal labor and birth: A guide for midwives.* Andover, UK: Taylor & Francis, Inc.

WEBSITES

American College of Nurse-Midwives: www.midwife.org
Association for Perinatal Psychology and Health: www.birthpsychology.com
Association of Maternal & Child Health Programs: www.amchpl.org
Center for Postpartum Health: www.postpartumhealth.com
Depression after Delivery: www.depressionafterdelivery.com
Home-Based Working Moms: www.hbwm.com
International Lactation Consultants Association: www.ilca.org
La Leche League: www.lalecheleague.org
Midwifery Today, Inc.: www.midwiferytoday.com
National Center for Fathering: www.fathers.com
National Parenting Center: www.tnpc.com
National Women's Health Information Center: www.4women.gov
Parenthood Web: www.parenthoodweb.com
Parenting Q & A: www.parenting-qa.com
Parents Anonymous, Inc.: www.parentsanonymous.org
Parents Helping Parents: www.php.com
Postpartum Support International: www.chss.iup.edu/postpartum/

CHAPTER WORKSHEET

MULTIPLE CHOICE QUESTIONS

1. Postpartal breast engorgement occurs 48 to 72 hours after giving birth. What physiologic change influences breast engorgement?

   a. An increase in blood and lymph supply to the breasts

   b. A decrease in estrogen and progesterone levels

   c. Colostrum production increases dramatically

   d. Fluid retention in the breasts due to the intravenous fluids given during labor

2. In the taking-in maternal role phase described by Rubin (1984), the nurse would expect the woman's behavior to be characterized as which of the following?

   a. Gaining self-confidence

   b. Adjusting to her new relationships

   c. Being passive and dependent

   d. Resuming control over her life

3. The nurse is explaining to a postpartal woman that the afterpains she is experiencing can be the result of which of the following?

   a. Manipulation of the uterus during labor

   b. A large infant weighing more than 8 lb

   c. Pregnancies that were too closely spaced

   d. Contractions of the uterus after birth

4. The nurse would expect a postpartal woman to demonstrate lochia in which sequence?

   a. Rubra, alba, serosa

   b. Rubra, serosa, alba

   c. Serosa, alba, rubra

   d. Alba, rubra, serosa

5. The nurse is assessing Ms. Smith, who gave birth to her first child 5 days ago. What findings by the nurse would be expected?

   a. Cream-colored lochia; uterus above the umbilicus

   b. Bright-red lochia with clots; uterus 2 finger-breadths below umbilicus

   c. Light pink or brown lochia; uterus 4 to 5 finger-breadths below umbilicus

   d. Yellow, mucousy lochia; uterus at the level of the umbilicus

6. Prioritize the postpartum mother's needs 4 hours after giving birth by placing a number 1, 2, 3, or 4 in the blank before each need.

   _____ Learn how to hold and cuddle the infant

   _____ Watch a baby bath demonstration given by the nurse

   _____ Sleep and rest without being disturbed for a few hours

   _____ Interaction time with the infant to facilitate bonding

CRITICAL THINKING EXERCISES

1. A new nurse assigned to the postpartum mother–baby unit makes a comment to the oncoming shift that Ms. Griffin, a 25-year-old primipara, seems lazy and shows no initiative in taking care of herself or her baby. The nurse reported that Ms. Griffin talks excessively about her labor and birth experience and seems preoccupied with herself and her needs, not her newborn's care. She wonders if something is wrong with this mother because she seems so self-centered and has to be directed to do everything.

   a. Is there something "wrong" with Ms. Griffin's behavior? Why or why not?

   b. What maternal role phase is being described by the new nurse?

   c. What role can the nurse play to support the mother through this phase?

2. Mrs. Lenhart, a primipara, gave birth to a healthy baby boy yesterday. Her husband John seemed elated at the birth, calling his friends and family on his cell phone minutes after the birth. He passed out cigars and praised his wife for her efforts. Today, when the nurse walked into their room, Mr. Lenhart seemed very anxious around his new son and called for the nurse whenever the baby cried or needed a diaper change. He seemed standoffish when asked to hold his son, and he spent time talking to other fathers in the waiting room, leaving his wife alone in the room.

   a. Would you consider Mr. Lenhart's paternal behavior to be normal at this time?

   b. What might Mr. Lenhart be feeling at this time?

   c. How can the nurse help this new father adjust to his new role?

STUDY ACTIVITIES

1. Find an Internet resource that discusses general postpartum care for new mothers who might have questions after discharge. Evaluate the website's information as to how credible, accurate, and current it is.

2. Prepare a teaching plan for new mothers, outlining the various physiologic changes that will take place after discharge.

3. The term that describes the return of the uterus to its prepregnant state is _____.

4. A deviated fundus to the right side of the abdomen would indicate a _____.

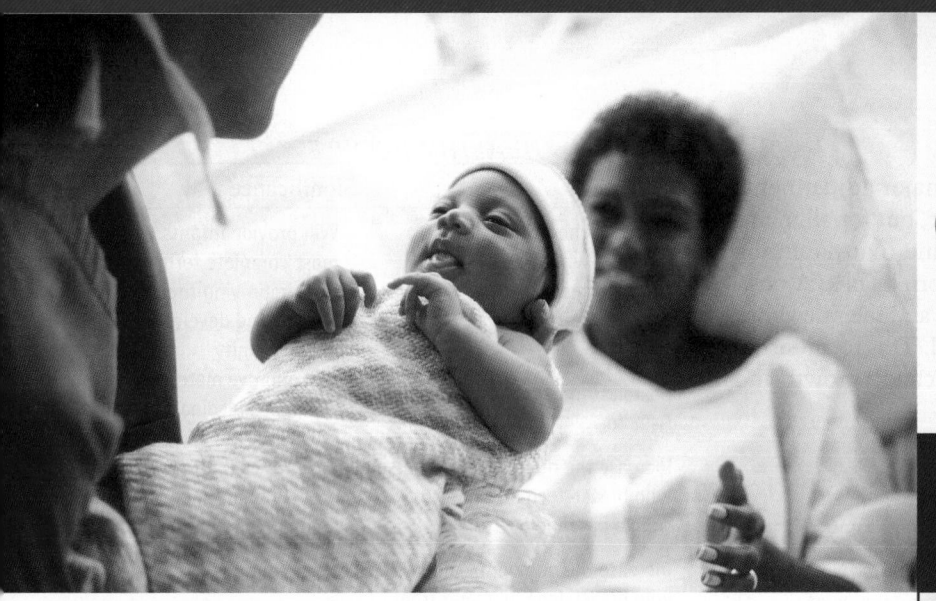

NURSING MANAGEMENT DURING THE POSTPARTUM PERIOD

KEY TERMS

attachment
bonding
en face position

Kegel exercises
mastitis
peribottle

postpartum blues
sitz bath

LEARNING OBJECTIVES

Upon completion of the chapter, the learner will be able to:

1. Define the key terms.
2. List the parameters that need to be assessed during the postpartum period.
3. Compare the bonding and attachment process.
4. Identify behaviors that enhance or inhibit the attachment process.
5. Outline nursing management for the woman and her family during the postpartum period.
6. Discuss the role of the nurse in promoting successful breast-feeding.
7. List areas of health education needed for discharge planning, home care, and follow-up.

*R*aina is a 24-year-old Muslim primipara who has just been admitted to the postpartum unit. Her husband sits at the bedside but doesn't seem to give her any physical or emotional support after her lengthy labor and difficult birth.

Wow *Parenting is an intimate, interactive, continuous, lifelong process.*

The postpartum period is a time of major adjustments and adaptations not just for the mother, but for all members of the family. It is during this time that parenting starts and a relationship with the newborn begins. A positive, loving relationship between parents and their newborn promotes the emotional well-being of all. This relationship endures and has profound effects on the child's growth and development.

▶ *Take* NOTE!

Parenting is a skill that is often learned by trial and error, with varying degrees of success. Successful parenting, a continuous and complex interactive process, requires the parents to learn new skills and to integrate the new member into the family.

Once the infant is born, each system in the mother's body takes several weeks to return to its nonpregnant state. The physiologic changes in women during the postpartum period are dramatic. Nurses should be aware of these changes and should be able to make observations and assessments to validate normal occurrences and detect any deviations.

In addition to physical assessment and care of the woman in the postpartum period, strong social support is vital to help her integrate the baby into the family. In today's mobile society, extended families may live far away and may be unable to help care for the new family. As a result, many new parents turn to health care professionals for information as well as physical and emotional support during this adjustment period. Nurses can be an invaluable resource by serving as mentors, teaching about self-care measures and baby care basics, and providing emotional support. Nurses can "mother" the new mother by offering physical care, emotional support, and information and practical help. The nurse's support and care through this critical time can increase the new parents' confidence, giving them a sense of accomplishment in their parenting skills.

One important intervention during the postpartum period is promotion of breast-feeding. *Healthy People 2010* includes breast-feeding as a goal for maternal, infant, and child health.

As in all nursing care, nurses should provide culturally competent care during the postpartum period. The nurse should engage in ongoing cultural self-assessment and overcome any stereotypes that perpetuate prejudice or discrimination against any cultural group (Bowers, 2007). Providing culturally competent nursing care during the postpartum period requires time, open-mindedness, and patience. To promote positive outcomes, the nurse should

HEALTHY PEOPLE 2010

Objective	Significance
Increase the proportion of mothers who breast-feed their babies.	• Will provide infants with the most complete form of nutrition, improving their health, growth and development, and immunity
Increase the number of mothers who breast-feed during early postpartum from a baseline of 64% to 75%.	• Will improve maternal health via breast-feeding's beneficial effects
Increase the number of mothers who breast-feed at 6 months from a baseline of 29% to 50%.	• Will increase the rate of breast-feeding, particularly among low-income and certain racial and ethnic populations who are less likely to begin breast-feeding in the hospital or to sustain it through the infant's first year
Increase the number of mothers who breast-feed at 1 year from a baseline of 16% to 25%.	

be sensitive to the woman's and family's culture, religion, and ethnic influences (see "Providing Optimal Cultural Care" in the Nursing Interventions section).

Remember the couple introduced at the beginning of the chapter? When the postpartum nurse comes to examine Raina, her husband quickly leaves the room and returns a short time later after the examination is complete. How do you interpret his behavior toward his wife? What might you communicate to this couple?

This chapter describes the nursing management of the woman and her family during the postpartum period. It outlines physical assessment parameters for new mothers and newborns. It also focuses on bonding and attachment behaviors; nurses need to be aware of these behaviors so they can perform appropriate interventions. Steps to address physiologic needs such as comfort, self-care, nutrition, and contraception are described. Ways to help the woman and her family adapt to the birth of the newborn are also discussed (Fig. 16.1).

Nursing management during the postpartum period focuses on assessing the woman's ability to adapt to the physiologic and psychological changes occurring at this time (see Chap. 15 for a detailed discussion of these adaptations). Family members are also assessed to determine how well they are making the transition to this new stage. Based on assessment findings, the nurse plans and implements care to address the family's needs. Because of today's shortened lengths of stay, the nurse may be able to focus only on priority needs and may need to arrange for follow-up in the home to ensure that all the family's needs are met.

FIGURE 16.1 Parents and grandmother interacting with the newborn.

Assessment

Comprehensive nursing assessment begins within an hour after the woman gives birth and continues through discharge.

▶ *Take* NOTE!

Nurses need a firm grasp of normal findings so that they can recognize abnormal findings and intervene appropriately.

This assessment includes vital signs and physical and psychosocial assessments. Although the exact protocol may vary among facilities, postpartum assessment typically is performed as follows:

- During the first hour: every 15 minutes
- During the second hour: every 30 minutes
- During the first 24 hours: every 4 hours
- After 24 hours: every 8 hours (Simpkin & James, 2006)

During each assessment, keep in mind risk factors that may lead to complications, such as infection or hemorrhage, during the recovery period (Box 16.1). Early identification is critical to ensure prompt intervention.

As with any assessment, always review the woman's medical record for information about her pregnancy, labor, and birth. Note any preexisting conditions, any complications that occurred during pregnancy, labor, birth, and immediately afterward, and any treatments provided.

Postpartum assessment of the mother typically includes vital signs, pain level, and a systematic head-to-toe review of body systems. The acronym BUBBLE-EE—breasts, uterus, bladder, bowels, lochia, episiotomy/perineum, extremities, and emotional status—can be used as a guide for this head-to-toe review (Blackburn, 2007).

BOX 16.1 **Factors Increasing the Woman's Risk for Postpartum Complications**

Risk Factors for Postpartum Infection
- Operative procedure (forceps, cesarean birth, vacuum extraction)
- History of diabetes, including gestational-onset diabetes
- Prolonged labor (more than 24 hours)
- Use of indwelling urinary catheter
- Anemia (hemoglobin less than 10.5 mg/dL)
- Multiple vaginal examinations during labor
- Prolonged rupture of membranes (more than 24 hours)
- Manual extraction of placenta
- Compromised immune system (HIV positive)

Risk Factors for Postpartum Hemorrhage
- Precipitous labor (less than 3 hours)
- Uterine atony
- Placenta previa or abruptio placentae
- Labor induction or augmentation
- Operative procedures (vacuum extraction, forceps, cesarean birth)
- Retained placental fragments
- Prolonged third stage of labor (more than 30 minutes)
- Multiparity, more than three births closely spaced
- Uterine overdistention (large infant, twins, hydramnios)

While assessing the woman and her family during the postpartum period, be alert for danger signs (Box 16.2). Notify the primary health care provider immediately if any are noted.

Postpartum assessment also includes assessing the parents and other family members, such as siblings and grandparents, for attachment and bonding with the newborn.

BOX 16.2 **Postpartum Danger Signs**

- Fever more than 38°C (100.4°F)
- Foul-smelling lochia or an unexpected change in color or amount
- Visual changes, such as blurred vision or spots, or headaches
- Calf pain with dorsiflexion of the foot
- Swelling, redness, or discharge at the episiotomy site
- Dysuria, burning, or incomplete emptying of the bladder
- Shortness of breath or difficulty breathing
- Depression or extreme mood swings

Vital Signs

Obtain vital signs and compare them with the previous values, noting and reporting any deviations. Vital sign changes can be an early indicator of complications.

Temperature

Use a consistent measurement technique (oral, axillary, or tympanic) to get the most accurate readings. Typically, the new mother's temperature during the first 24 hours postpartum is within the normal range. Some women experience a slight fever, up to 38°C (100.4°F), during the first 24 hours. This elevation may be the result of dehydration because of fluid loss during labor. Temperature should be normal after 24 hours with replacement of fluids lost during labor and birth (Arenson & Drake, 2007). A temperature above 38°C (100.4°F) at any time or an abnormal temperature after the first 24 hours may indicate infection and must be reported. Abnormal temperature readings warrant continued monitoring until an infection can be ruled out through cultures or blood studies.

Pulse

Because of the changes in blood volume and cardiac output after delivery, relative bradycardia may be noted. The woman's pulse rate may range from 50 to 70 bpm. Pulse usually stabilizes to prepregnancy levels within 10 days (Blackburn, 2007).

Tachycardia in the postpartum woman can suggest anxiety, excitement, fatigue, pain, excessive blood loss, infection, or underlying cardiac problems. Further investigation is warranted to rule out complications.

Respirations

Respiratory rates in the postpartum woman should be within the normal range of 16 to 20 breaths per minute. Any change in respiratory rate out of the normal range might indicate pulmonary edema, atelectasis, or pulmonary embolism and must be reported. Lungs should be clear on auscultation.

Blood Pressure

Assess the woman's blood pressure and compare it with her usual range. Report any deviation from this range. Elevations in blood pressure from baseline might suggest pregnancy-induced hypertension; decreases may suggest dehydration or excessive blood loss.

Blood pressure also may vary based on the woman's position, so assess blood pressure with the woman in the same position every time. Be alert for orthostatic hypotension, which can occur when the woman moves rapidly from a lying or sitting position to a standing one.

Pain

Pain, the fifth vital sign, is assessed along with the other four parameters. Question the woman about the type of pain and its location and severity. Have the woman rate the pain using a numeric scale from 0 to 10 points.

Many postpartum orders will have the nurse premedicate the woman routinely for afterbirth pains rather than wait for her to experience them first. The goal of pain management is to have the woman's pain scale rating maintained between 0 to 2 points at all times, especially after breast-feeding. This can be accomplished by assessing the woman's pain level frequently and preventing pain by administering analgesics. If the woman has severe pain in the perineal region despite use of physical comfort measures, check for a hematoma by inspecting and palpating the area. If one is found, notify the health care provider immediately.

Breasts

Inspect the breasts for size, contour, asymmetry, engorgement, or erythema. Check the nipples for cracks, redness, fissures, or bleeding, and note whether they are erect, flat, or inverted. Flat or inverted nipples can make breast-feeding challenging for both mother and infant. Cracked, blistered, fissured, bruised, or bleeding nipples in the breast-feeding woman are generally indications that the baby is improperly positioned on the breast. Palpate the breasts lightly to ascertain if they are soft, filling, or engorged, and document your findings. For women who are not breast-feeding, use a gentle, light touch to avoid breast stimulation, which would exacerbate engorgement. As milk is starting to come in, the breasts become firmer; this is charted as "filling." Engorged breasts are hard, tender, and taut. Ask the woman if she is having any nipple discomfort. Palpate the breasts for any nodules, masses, or areas of warmth, which may indicate a plugged duct that may progress to **mastitis** if not treated promptly. Any discharge from the nipple should be described and documented if it is not colostrum (creamy yellow) or foremilk (bluish white).

Uterus

Assess the fundus (top portion of the uterus) to determine the degree of uterine involution. If possible, have the woman empty her bladder before assessing the fundus. If the patient has had a cesarean birth and has a PCA pump, instruct her to self-medicate prior to fundal assessment to decrease her discomfort. Using a two-handed approach with the woman in the supine position and the bed in a flat position or as low as possible, palpate the abdomen gently, feeling for the top of the uterus while the other hand is placed on the lower segment of the uterus to stabilize it (Fig. 16.2).

The fundus should be midline and should feel firm. A boggy or relaxed uterus is a sign of uterine atony. This can be the result of bladder distention, which displaces the uterus upward and to the right, or retained placental fragments. Either situation predisposes the woman to hemorrhage.

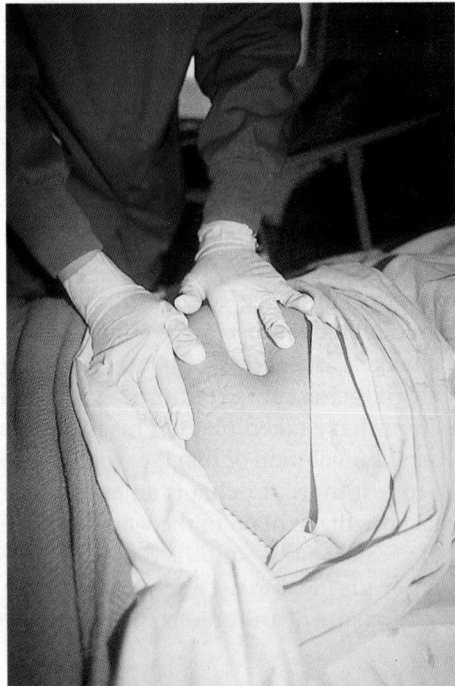

FIGURE **16.2** Palpating the fundus.

Once the fundus is located, place your index finger on the fundus and count the number of fingerbreadths between the fundus and the umbilicus (1 fingerbreadth is approximately equal to 1 cm). One to 2 hours after birth, the fundus typically is between the umbilicus and the symphysis pubis. Approximately 6 to 12 hours after birth, the fundus usually is at the level of the umbilicus.

Normally, the fundus progresses downward at a rate of one fingerbreadth (or 1 cm) per day after childbirth (Cunningham et al., 2005). On the first postpartum day, the top of the fundus is located 1 cm below the umbilicus and is recorded as U-1. Similarly, on the second postpartum day, the fundus would be 2 cm below the umbilicus and should be recorded as U-2, and so on. If the fundus is not firm, gently massage the uterus using a circular motion until it becomes firm.

Bladder

Considerable diuresis—as much as 3,000 mL—may follow for several days after childbirth, decreasing by the third day (Blackburn, 2007). However, many postpartum women do not sense the need to void even if their bladder is full. Women who received regional anesthesia during labor are at risk for bladder distention and for difficulty voiding until sensation returns within several hours after birth.

Assess for voiding problems by asking the woman the following questions:

- Have you (passed your water, urinated, gone to the bathroom) yet?
- Have you noticed any burning or discomfort with urination?
- Do you have any difficulty passing your urine?
- Do you feel that your bladder is empty when you finish urinating?
- Do you have any signs of infection such as urgency, frequency, or pain?
- Are you able to control the flow of urine by squeezing your muscles?
- Have you noticed any leakage of urine when you cough, laugh, or sneeze?

Assess the bladder for distention and adequate emptying after efforts to void. Palpate the area over the symphysis pubis. If empty, the bladder is not palpable. Palpation of a rounded mass suggests bladder distention. Also percuss the area: a full bladder is dull to percussion. If the bladder is full, lochia drainage will be more than normal because the uterus cannot contract to suppress the bleeding.

▶ **Take** NOTE!

Note the location and condition of the fundus; a full bladder tends to displace the uterus up and to the right.

After the woman voids, palpate and percuss the area again to determine adequate emptying of the bladder. If the bladder remains distended, the woman may be retaining urine in her bladder, and measures to initiate voiding should be instituted. Be alert for signs of infection, including infrequent or insufficient voiding (less than 200 mL), discomfort, burning, urgency, or foul-smelling urine (Simpkin & James, 2006). Document urine output.

Bowels

Spontaneous bowel movements may not occur for 2 to 3 days after giving birth because of a decrease in muscle tone in the intestines during labor. Normal patterns of bowel elimination usually return within 8 to 14 days after birth (Blackburn, 2007).

Inspect the woman's abdomen for distention, auscultate for bowel sounds in all four quadrants, and palpate for tenderness. The abdomen typically is soft, nontender, and nondistended. Bowel sounds are present in all four quadrants. Ask the woman if she has had a bowel movement or has passed gas since giving birth, because constipation is a common problem during the postpartum period and most women do not offer this information unless asked about it. Normal assessment findings are active bowel sounds, passing gas, and a nondistended abdomen.

Lochia

Assess lochia in terms of amount, color, odor, and change with activity and time. To assess how much a woman is bleeding, ask her how many perineal pads she has used in the past 1 to 2 hours and how much drainage was on each pad. For example, did she saturate the pad completely, or was only half of the pad covered with drainage? Ask about the color of the drainage, odor, and the presence of any clots. Lochia has a definite musky scent, with an odor similar to that of menstrual flow without any large clots. Foul-smelling lochia suggests an infection, and large clots suggest poor uterine involution, necessitating additional intervention.

To determine the amount of lochia, observe the amount of lochia saturation on the perineal pad and relate it to time (Fig. 16.3). Lochia flow will increase when the woman gets out of bed (lochia pools in the vagina and the uterus while she is lying down) and when she breastfeeds (oxytocin release causes uterine contractions). A woman who saturates a perineal pad within 30 to 60 minutes is bleeding much more than one who saturates a pad in 2 hours. Typically, the amount of lochia is described as follows:

• Scant: a 1- to 2-inch lochia stain on the perineal pad or approximately a 10-mL loss
• Light or small: an approximately 4-inch stain or a 10- to 25-mL loss
• Moderate: a 4- to 6-inch stain with an estimated loss of 25 to 50 mL
• Large or heavy: a pad is saturated within 1 hour after changing it (Nash, 2007)

The total volume of lochia is approximately 240 to 270 mL (8 to 9 oz), and the amount decreases daily (Blackburn, 2007). Check under the woman to make sure there isn't additional blood hidden and not absorbed on her perineal pad.

Report any abnormal findings, such as heavy, bright-red lochia with large tissue fragments or a foul odor. If excessive bleeding occurs, the first step would be to mas-

sage the boggy fundus until it is firm to reduce the flow of blood. Document all findings.

Women who had a cesarean birth will have less lochia discharge than those who had a vaginal birth, but stages and color changes remain the same. Although the woman's abdomen will be tender after surgery, the nurse must palpate the fundus and assess the lochia to make sure they are within the normal range and that there is no excessive bleeding.

Anticipatory guidance to give the woman at discharge should include information about lochia and the expected changes. Urge the woman to notify her health care provider if lochia rubra returns after the serosa and alba transitions have taken place. This is abnormal and may indicate subinvolution or that the woman is too active and needs to rest more. Lochia is an excellent medium for bacterial growth. Explain to the woman that frequent changing of perineal pads, continued use of her peribottle for rinsing her perineal area, and handwashing before and after pad changes are important infection control measures.

Episiotomy and Perineum

To assess the episiotomy and perineal area, position the woman on her side with her top leg flexed upward at the knee and drawn up toward her waist. If necessary, use a penlight to provide adequate lighting during the assessment. Wearing gloves and standing at the woman's side with her back to you, gently lift the upper buttock to expose the perineum and anus (Fig. 16.4). Inspect the episiotomy for irritation, ecchymosis, tenderness, or hematomas. Assess for hemorrhoids and their condition.

During the early postpartum period, the perineal tissue surrounding the episiotomy is typically edematous and slightly bruised. The normal episiotomy site should not have redness, discharge, or edema. The majority of healing takes place within the first 2 weeks, but it may take 4 to 6 months for the episiotomy to heal completely (Blackburn, 2007).

FIGURE 16.3 Assessing lochia.

FIGURE 16.4 Inspecting the perineum.

Lacerations to the perineal area sustained during the birthing process that were identified and repaired also need to be assessed to determine their healing status. Lacerations are classified based on their severity and tissue involvement:

- First-degree laceration—involves only skin and superficial structures above muscle
- Second-degree laceration—extends through perineal muscles
- Third-degree laceration—extends through the anal sphincter muscle
- Fourth-degree laceration—continues through anterior rectal wall

Assess the episiotomy and any lacerations at least every 8 hours to detect hematomas or signs of infection. Large areas of swollen, bluish skin with complaints of severe pain in the perineal area indicate pelvic or vulvar hematomas. Redness, swelling, increasing discomfort, or purulent drainage may indicate infection. Both findings need to be reported immediately.

A white line the length of the episiotomy is a sign of infection, as is swelling or discharge. Severe, intractable pain, perineal discoloration, and ecchymosis indicate a perineal hematoma, a potentially dangerous condition. Report any unusual findings. Ice can be applied to relieve discomfort and reduce edema; sitz baths also can promote comfort and perineal healing (see "Promoting Comfort" in the Nursing Interventions section).

Extremities

During pregnancy, the state of hypercoagulability protects the mother against excessive blood loss during childbirth and placental separation. However, this hypercoagulable state can increase the risk of thromboembolic disorders during pregnancy and postpartum. Three factors predispose women to thromboembolic disorders during pregnancy: stasis (compression of the large veins because of the gravid uterus), altered coagulation (state of pregnancy), and localized vascular damage (may occur during birthing process). All of these increase the risk of clot formation.

> ▶ *Take* NOTE!
>
> *Pulmonary embolism occurs in 1 in 2,000 pregnancies and is a major cause of maternal mortality (Moses, 2007).*

Pulmonary emboli typically result from dislodged deep vein thrombi in the lower extremities. Risk factors associated with thromboembolic conditions include:

- Anemia
- Diabetes mellitus
- Cigarette smoking
- Obesity
- Preeclampsia secondary to exaggeration of hypercoagulable state
- Hypertension
- Varicose veins
- Pregnancy
- Oral contraceptive use
- Cesarean birth
- Previous thromboembolic disease
- Multiparity
- Inactivity
- Advanced maternal age (Hackley, Kriebs, & Rousseau, 2007)

Because of the subtle presentation of thromboembolic disorders, the physical examination may not be enough to detect them. The woman may report lower extremity tightness or aching when ambulating that is relieved with rest and elevation of the leg. Edema in the affected leg (typically the left), along with warmth and tenderness, may also be noted. A duplex ultrasound (two-dimensional ultrasound and Doppler ultrasound that compresses the vein to assess for changes in venous flow) in conjunction with the physical findings frequently is needed for a conclusive diagnosis (Kuntz, Cheesman, & Powers, 2006).

Women with an increased risk for this condition during the postpartum period should wear antiembolism stockings or use sequential compression devices to reduce their risk of thrombophlebitis. Encouraging the client to ambulate after childbirth reduces the incidence of thrombophlebitis.

Emotional Status

Assess the woman's emotional status by observing how she interacts with her family, her level of independence, energy levels, eye contact with her infant (within a cultural context), posture and comfort level while holding the newborn, and sleep and rest patterns. Be alert for mood swings, irritability, or crying episodes.

Remember Raina and her "quiet" husband, the Muslim couple? The postpartum nurse informs Raina that her doctor, Nancy Schultz, has been called away for emergency surgery and won't be available the rest of the day. The nurse explains that Dr. Robert Nappo will be making rounds for her. Raina and her husband become upset. Why? Is culturally competent care being provided to this couple?

Bonding and Attachment

Nurses can be instrumental in promoting attachment by assessing attachment behaviors (positive and negative) and intervening appropriately if needed. Nurses must be able to identify any family discord that might interfere with the attachment process. Remember, however, that mothers from different cultures may behave differently from what is expected in your own culture. For example, Native American mothers tend to handle their newborns less often and use cradle boards to carry them. Native American mothers and many Asian-American mothers delay breast-feeding until their milk comes in, because colostrum is considered harmful for the newborn (Bowers, 2007). Don't assume that different behavior is wrong.

Meeting the newborn for the first time after birth can be an exhilarating experience for parents. Although the mother has spent many hours dreaming of her unborn and how he or she will look, it is not until after birth that they meet face to face. They both need to get to know one another and to develop feelings for one another.

Bonding is the close emotional attraction to a newborn by the parents that develops during the first 30 to 60 minutes after birth. It is unidirectional, from parent to infant. It is thought that optimal bonding of the parents to a newborn requires a period of close contact within the first few minutes to a few hours after birth (Mercer, 2006). The mother initiates bonding when she caresses her infant and exhibits certain behaviors typical of a mother tending her child. The infant's responses to this, such as body and eye movements, are a necessary part of the process. During this initial period, the infant is in a quiet, alert state, looking directly at the holder.

> ▶ *Take* NOTE!
>
> *The length of time necessary for bonding depends on the health of the infant and mother, as well as the circumstances surrounding the labor and birth (Fowles & Horowitz, 2006).*

Attachment is the development of strong affection between an infant and a significant other (mother, father, sibling, and caretaker) (Grossman, Grossman, & Waters, 2006). This tie between two people is psychological rather than biological, and it does not occur overnight. The process of attachment follows a progressive or developmental course that changes over time. Attachment is an individualized and multifactorial process that differs based on the health of the infant, the mother, environmental circumstances, and the quality of care the infant receives (Wilson et al., 2007). It occurs through mutually satisfying experiences. Maternal attachment begins during pregnancy as the result of fetal movement and maternal fantasies about the infant and continues through the birth and postpartum periods. Attachment behaviors include seeking, staying close to, and exchanging gratifying experiences with the infant (Grossman, Grossman,

& Waters, 2006). In a high-risk pregnancy, the attachment process may be complicated by premature birth (lack of time to develop a relationship with the unborn baby) and by parental stress due to the fetal and/or maternal vulnerability.

Bonding is a vital component of the attachment process and is necessary in establishing parent–infant attachment and a healthy, loving relationship. During this early period of acquaintance, mothers touch their infants in a very characteristic manner. Mothers visually and physically "explore" their infants, initially using their fingertips on the infant's face and extremities and progressing to massaging and stroking the infant with their fingers. This is followed by palm contact on the trunk. Eventually, mothers draw their infant toward them and hold the infant. Mothers also interact with their infants through eye-to-eye contact in the *en face* **position** (Mercer, 2006) (Fig. 16.5).

Generally, research on attachment has found that the process is similar for fathers as for mothers, but the pace may be different. Like mothers, fathers manifest attachment behaviors during pregnancy; indeed, Grossman et al. (2006) found that the best predictor of early postnatal attachment for fathers is fetal attachment. Becoming a father requires a man to build on the experiences he has had throughout childhood and adolescence. Fathers develop an emotional tie with their infants in a variety of ways. They seek and maintain closeness with the infant and can recognize characteristics of the infant. They feel a sense of responsibility for the infant's growth and development (Wilson et al., 2007).

Attachment is a process; it does not occur instantaneously, even though many parents believe in a romanticized version of attachment, which happens right after birth. A delay in the attachment process can occur if a mother's physical and emotional states are adversely affected by exhaustion, pain, the absence of a support system, anesthesia, or an unwanted outcome (Feldman, 2007).

FIGURE 16.5 *En face* position.

> ▶ *Take* NOTE!
>
> *Many midwives teach fathers to massage their partners, which has been proven to have a positive effect on the pregnancy, labor, bonding and attachment, and perhaps on family dynamics (Whitehouse, 2006).*

The developmental task for the infant is learning to differentiate between trust and mistrust. If the mother or caretaker is consistently responsive to the infant's care, meeting the baby's physical and psychological needs, the infant will likely learn to trust the caretaker, view the world as a safe place, and grow up to be secure, self-reliant, trusting, cooperative, and helpful. However, if the infant's needs are not met, the child is more likely to face developmental delays, neglect, and child abuse (Logsdon, Wisner, & Pinto-Foltz, 2006).

"Becoming" a parent may take 4 to 6 months. The transition to parenthood, according to Mercer (2006), involves four stages:

1. Commitment, attachment, and preparation for an infant during pregnancy
2. Acquaintance with and increasing attachment to the infant, learning how to care for the infant, and physical restoration during the first weeks after birth
3. Moving toward a new normal routine in the first 4 months after birth
4. Achievement of a parenthood role around 4 months

The stages overlap, and the timing of each is affected by variables such as the environment, family dynamics, and the partners (Mercer, 2006).

Factors Affecting Attachment

Attachment behaviors are influenced by three major factors:

1. Parents' background (includes the care that the parents received when growing up, cultural practices, relationship within the family, experience with previous pregnancies and planning and course of events during pregnancy, postpartum depression)
2. Infant (includes the infant's temperament and health at birth)
3. Care practices (the behaviors of physicians, midwives, nurses, and hospital personnel, care and support during labor, first day of life in separation of mother and infant, and rules of the hospital or birthing center) (Grossman, Grossman, & Waters 2006)

Attachment occurs more readily with the infant whose temperament, health, appearance, and gender fit the par-

ent's expectations. If the infant does not meet these expectations, attachment can be delayed (Wilson et al., 2007).

Factors associated with the health care facility or birthing unit can also hinder attachment. These include:

• Separation of infant and parents immediately after birth and for long periods during the day
• Policies that discourage unwrapping and exploring the infant
• Intensive care environment, restrictive visiting policies
• Staff indifference or lack of support for parent's caretaking attempts and abilities

Critical Attributes of Attachment

The terms "bonding" and "attachment" are often used interchangeably, even though they involve different time frames and interactions. Attachment stages include proximity, reciprocity, and commitment.

Proximity refers to the physical and psychological experience of the parents being close to their infant. This attribute has three dimensions:

1. Contact—The sensory experiences of touching, holding, and gazing at the infant are part of proximity-seeking behavior.
2. Emotional state—The emotional state emerges from the affective experience of the new parents toward their infant and their parental role.
3. Individualization—Parents are aware of the need to differentiate the infant's needs from themselves and to recognize and respond to them appropriately, making the attachment process also, in some way, one of detachment.

Reciprocity is the process by which the infant's abilities and behaviors elicit parental response. Reciprocity is described by two dimensions: complementary behavior and sensitivity. Complementary behavior involves taking turns and stopping when the other is not interested or becomes tired. An infant can coo and stare at the parent to elicit a similar parental response to complement his or her behavior. Parents who are sensitive and responsive to their infant's cues will promote their development and growth. Parents who become skilled at recognizing the ways their infant communicates will respond appropriately by smiling, vocalizing, touching, and kissing.

Commitment refers to the enduring nature of the relationship. The components of this are twofold: centrality and parent role exploration. In centrality, parents place the infant at the center of their lives. They acknowledge and accept their responsibility to promote the infant's safety, growth, and development. Parent role exploration is the parents' ability to find their own way and integrate the parental identity into themselves (Grossman, Grossman, & Waters, 2006).

TABLE 16.1 POSITIVE AND NEGATIVE ATTACHMENT BEHAVIORS

	Positive Behaviors	Negative Behaviors
Infant	Smiles; is alert; demonstrates strong grasp reflex to hold parent's finger; sucks well, feeds easily; enjoys being held close; makes eye-to-eye contact; follows parent's face; appears facially appealing; is consolable when crying	Feeds poorly, regurgitates often; cries for long periods, colicky and inconsolable; shows flat affect, rarely smiles even when prompted; resists holding and closeness; sleeps with eyes closed most of time; stiffens body when held; is unresponsive to parents; doesn't pay attention to parents' faces
Parent	Makes direct eye contact; assumes *en face* position when holding infant; claims infant as family member, pointing out common features; expresses pride in infant; assigns meaning to infant's actions; smiles and gazes at infant; touches infant, progressing from fingertips to holding; names infant; requests to be close to infant as much as allowed; speaks positively about infant	Expresses disappointment or displeasure in infant; fails to "explore" infant visually or physically; fails to claim infant as part of family; avoids caring for infant; finds excuses not to hold infant close; has negative self-concept; appears uninterested in having infant in room; frequently asks to have infant taken back to nursery to be cared for; assigns negative attributes to infant and calls infant inappropriate, negative names (e.g., frog, monkey, tadpole)

Sources: Grossman, Grossman, & Waters, 2007; Nash, 2007; Oppenheim & Goldsmith, 2007.

Positive and Negative Attachment Behaviors

Positive bonding behaviors include maintaining close physical contact, making eye-to-eye contact, speaking in soft, high-pitched tones, and touching and exploring the infant. Table 16.1 highlights typical positive and negative behaviors of attachment.

Nursing Interventions

In terms of postpartum hospital stays today, "less is more." If the woman had a vaginal delivery, she may be discharged within 48 hours. If she had a cesarean birth, she may remain hospitalized from 72 to 96 hours. This shortened stay leaves little time for nurses to prepare the woman and her family for the many changes that will occur when she returns home. Nurses need to use this limited time to address the following topics: pain and discomfort, immunizations, nutrition, activity and exercise, lactation, discharge teaching, sexuality and contraception, and follow-up (see Nursing Care Plan 16.1).

▶ **Take** NOTE!

Always adhere to standard precautions when providing direct care to reduce the risk of disease transmission.

Providing Optimal Cultural Care

As the face of America is becoming more diverse, nurses must be prepared to care for childbearing families from various cultures. In many cultures, women and their families are cared for and nurtured by their community for weeks and even months after the birth of a new family member. Box 16.3 highlights some of the major cultural variants during the postpartum period.

Nurses need to remember that childbearing practices and beliefs vary in different cultures. To provide appropriate nursing care, the nurse should determine the patient's preferences before intervening. Cultural practices may include dietary restrictions, certain clothes, taboos, activities for maintaining mental health, and the use of silence, prayer, or meditation. Restoring health may involve taking folk medicines or conferring with a tribal healer (Srivastava, 2007).

*R*aina and her husband are upset at the thought of having a male doctor care for her because Muslim women are very modest and prefer having a same-sex care provider. What should the nurse do in this situation?

Promoting Comfort

The postpartum woman may have discomfort and pain from a variety of sources, such as an episiotomy, perineal lacerations, an edematous perineum, inflamed hemorrhoids, engorged breasts, afterbirth pains secondary to uterine contractions in breast-feeding and multiparous mothers, and sore nipples if breast-feeding. Nonpharmacologic and pharmacologic measures can be used to decrease pain and discomfort.

Applications of Cold and Heat

Commonly, an ice pack is the first measure used after a vaginal birth to relieve perineal discomfort from edema, an

Nursing Care Plan 16.1

OVERVIEW OF THE POSTPARTUM WOMAN

Belinda, a 26-year-old G2P2, is a patient on the mother–baby unit after giving birth to a term 8-lb, 12-oz baby boy yesterday. The night nurse reports that she has an episiotomy, complains of a pain rating of 7 points on a scale of 1 to 10, is having difficulty breast-feeding, and had heavy lochia most of the night. The nurse also reports that the patient seems focused on her own needs and not on her infant. Assessment this morning reveals the following:

B: Breasts are soft with colostrum leaking; nipples cracked
U: Uterus is one fingerbreadth below the umbilicus; deviated to right
B: Bladder is palpable; patient states she hasn't been up to void yet
B: Bowels have not moved; bowel sounds present; passing flatus
L: Lochia is moderate; peripad soaked from night accumulation
E: Episiotomy site intact; swollen, bruised; hemorrhoids present
—
E: Extremities; no edema over tibia, no warmth or tenderness in calf
E: Emotional status is "distressed" as a result of discomfort and fatigue

NURSING DIAGNOSIS: Impaired tissue integrity related to episiotomy

Outcome Identification and Evaluation
The woman remains free of infection, without any signs and symptoms of infection, and exhibits evidence of progressive healing as demonstrated by clean, dry, intact episiotomy site.

Interventions: Promoting Tissue Integrity
- Monitor episiotomy site for redness, edema, and signs of infection.
- Assess vital signs at least every 4 hours *to identify changes suggesting infection.*
- Apply ice pack to episiotomy site *to reduce swelling.*
- Instruct patient on use of sitz bath *to promote healing, hygiene, and comfort.*
- Encourage frequent perineal care and peripad changes *to prevent infection.*
- Recommend ambulation *to improve circulation and promote healing.*
- Instruct patient on positioning *to relieve pressure on perineal area.*
- Demonstrate use of anesthetic sprays *to numb perineal area.*

NURSING DIAGNOSIS: Pain related to episiotomy, sore nipples, and hemorrhoids

Outcome Identification and Evaluation
The woman experiences a decrease in pain, reporting that her pain has diminished to a tolerable level, rating it as 2 points or less.

Interventions: Providing Pain Relief
- Thoroughly inspect perineum *to rule out hematoma as cause of pain.*
- Administer analgesic medication as ordered as needed *to promote comfort.*
- Carry out comfort measures to episiotomy as outlined earlier *to reduce pain.*
- Explain discomforts and reassure the client that they are time-limited to assist in coping with pain.
- Apply Tucks pads to swollen hemorrhoids *to induce shrinkage and reduce pain.*
- Suggest frequent use of sitz bath *to reduce hemorrhoid pain.*
- Administer stool softener and laxative *to prevent straining with first bowel movement.*
- Observe positioning and latching-on technique while breast-feeding. Offer suggestions based on observations to correct positioning/latching on *to minimize trauma to the breast.*
- Suggest air-drying of nipples after breast-feeding and use of plain water *to prevent nipple cracking.*
- Teach relaxation techniques when breast-feeding *to reduce anxiety and discomfort.*

(continued)

Nursing Care Plan 16.1 (continued)

NURSING DIAGNOSIS: Risk for ineffective coping related to mood alteration and pain

Outcome Identification and Evaluation

The woman copes with mood alterations, as evidenced by positive statements about newborn and participation in newborn care.

Interventions: Promoting Effective Coping

- Provide a supportive, nurturing environment and encourage the mother to vent her feelings and frustrations to relieve anxiety.
- Provide opportunities for the mother to rest and sleep *to combat fatigue.*
- Encourage the mother to eat a well-balanced diet *to increase her energy level.*
- Provide reassurance and explanations that mood alterations are common after birth secondary to waning hormones after pregnancy *to increase the mother's knowledge.*
- Allow the mother relief from newborn care *to afford opportunity for self-care.*
- Discuss with partner expected behavior from mother and how additional support and help are needed during this stressful time *to promote partner's participation in care.*
- Make appropriate community referrals for mother–infant support *to ensure continuity of care.*
- Encourage frequent skin-to-skin contact and closeness between mother and infant *to facilitate bonding and attachment behaviors.*
- Encourage client to participate in infant care and provide instructions as needed *to foster a sense of independence and self-esteem.*
- Offer praise and reinforcement of positive mother–infant interactions *to enhance self-confidence in care.*

episiotomy, or laceration. It is applied during the fourth stage of labor and can be used for the first 24 hours to reduce perineal edema and to prevent hematoma formation, thus reducing pain and promoting healing. Ice packs are wrapped in a disposable covering or clean washcloth and are applied to the perineal area. Usually the ice pack is applied for 20 minutes and removed for 10 minutes. Many commercially prepared ice packs are available, but a latex glove filled with crushed ice and covered can also be used if the mother is not allergic to latex. Ensure that the ice pack is changed frequently to promote good hygiene and to allow for periodic assessments.

The **peribottle** is a plastic squeeze bottle filled with warm tap water that is sprayed over the perineal area after each voiding and before applying a new perineal pad. Usually the peribottle is introduced to the woman when she is assisted to the bathroom to freshen up and void for the first time—in most instances, once vital signs are stable after the first hour. Provide the woman with instructions on how and when to use the peribottle. Reinforce this practice each time she changes her pad, voids, or defecates, making sure that she understands to direct the flow of water from front to back. The woman can take the peribottle home and use it over the next several weeks until her lochia discharge stops. The peribottle can be used by women who had either vaginal or cesarean births to provide comfort and hygiene to the perineal area.

After the first 24 hours, a **sitz bath** with warm water may be prescribed and substituted for the ice pack to reduce local swelling and promote comfort for an episiotomy, perineal trauma, or inflamed hemorrhoids. The change from cold to warm therapy enhances vascular circulation and healing (Steen, Briggs, & King, 2006). Before using a sitz bath, the woman should cleanse the perineum with a peribottle or take a shower using mild soap.

Most health care agencies use plastic disposable sitz baths that women can take home. The plastic sitz bath consists of a basin that fits on the commode; a bag filled with warm water is hung on a hook and connected via a tube onto the front of the basin (Fig. 16.6). Teaching Guidelines 16.1 highlights the steps in using a sitz bath.

Advise the woman to use the sitz bath several times daily to provide hygiene and comfort to the perineal area. Encourage her to continue this measure after discharge.

Some facilities have hygienic sitz baths called Suri-Gators in the bathroom that spray an antiseptic, water, or both onto the perineum. The woman sits on the toilet with legs apart so that the nozzle spray reaches her perineal area.

Keep in mind that tremendous hemodynamic changes are taking place within the mother during this early postpartum period, and her safety must be a priority. Fatigue, blood loss, the effects of medications, and lack of food may cause her to feel weak when she stands up. Assisting the woman to the bathroom to instruct her on how to use the peribottle and sitz bath is necessary to ensure her safety. Many women become lightheaded or dizzy when they get out of bed and need direct physical assistance. Staying in the woman's room, ensuring that the emer-

BOX 16.3 Cultural Influences During the Postpartum Period

African-American
- Mother may share care of the infant with extended family members.
- Experiences of older women within the family influence infant care.
- Mothers may protect their newborns from strangers for several weeks.
- Mothers may not bathe their newborns for the first week. Oils are applied to skin and hair to prevent dryness and cradle cap.
- Silver dollars may be taped over the infant's umbilicus in an attempt to flatten the slightly protruding umbilical stump.
- Sleeping with parents is a common practice (Bowers, 2007).

Amish
- Women consider childbearing their primary role in society.
- They generally oppose birth control.
- Pregnancy and childbirth are considered a private matter; they may conceal it from public knowledge.
- Women typically do not respond favorably when hurried to complete a self-care task. Nurses need to take cues from women indicating their readiness to complete morning self-care activities (Bowers, 2007).

Appalachian
- Infant colic is treated by passing the newborn through a leather horse's collar or administering weak catnip tea.
- An asafetida bag (a gum resin with a strong odor) is tied around the infant's neck to ward off disease.
- Women may avoid eye contact with nurses and health care providers.
- Women typically avoid asking questions even though they do not understand directions.
- The grandmother may rear the infant for the mother (Armstrong & Feldman, 2007).

Filipino-American
- Grandparents often assist in the care of their grandchildren.
- Breast-feeding is encouraged, and some mothers breast-feed their children for up to 2 years.
- Women have difficulty discussing birth control and sexual matters.
- Strong religious beliefs prevail and bedside prayer is common.
- Families are very close-knit and numerous visitors can be expected to the hospital after childbirth (Srivastava, 2007).

Japanese-American
- Cleanliness and protection from cold are essential components of newborn care. Nurses should give the daily bath to the infant.

- Newborns routinely are not taken outside the home because it is believed that they should not be exposed to outside or cold air. Infants should be kept in a quiet, clean, warm place for the first month of life.
- Breast-feeding is the primary method of feeding.
- Many women stay in their parents' home for 1 to 2 months after birth.
- Bathing the infant can be the center of family activity at home (Bowers, 2007).

Mexican-American
- The newborn's grandmother lives with the mother for several weeks after birth to help with housekeeping and child care.
- Most women will breast-feed more than 1 year. The infant is carried in a *rebozo* (shawl) that allows easy access for breast-feeding.
- Women may avoid eye contact and may not feel comfortable being touched by a stranger. Nurses need to respect this feeling.
- Some women may bring religious icons to the hospital and may want to display them in their room (Srivastava, 2007).

Muslim
- Modesty is a primary concern; nurses need to protect the client's modesty.
- Muslims are not permitted to eat pork; check all food items before serving.
- Muslims prefer a same-sex health care provider; male–female touching is prohibited except in an emergency situation.
- A Muslim woman stays in the house for 40 days after birth, being cared for by the female members of her family.
- Most women will breast-feed, but religious events call for periods of fasting, which may increase the risk of dehydration or malnutrition.
- Women are exempt from obligatory five-times-daily prayers as long as lochia is present.
- Extended family is likely to be present throughout much of the woman's hospital stay. They will need an empty room to perform their prayers without having to leave the hospital (Cassar, 2006).

Native American
- Women are secretive about pregnancies and do not reveal them early.
- Touching is not a typical female behavior and eye contact is brief.
- They resent being hurried and need time for sitting and talking.
- Most mothers breast-feed and practice birth control (Srivastava, 2007).

FIGURE 16.6 Sitz bath set-up.

TEACHING GUIDELINES 16.1

Using a Sitz Bath

1. Close clamp on tubing before filling bag with water to prevent leakage.
2. Fill sitz bath basin and plastic bag with warm water (comfortable to touch).
3. Place the filled basin on the toilet with the seat raised and the overflow opening facing toward the back of the toilet.
4. Hang the filled plastic bag on a hook close to the toilet or an IV pole.
5. Attach the tubing to the opening on the basin.
6. Sit on the basin positioned on the toilet seat and release the clamp to allow warm water to irrigate the perineum.
7. Remain sitting on the basin for approximately 15 to 20 minutes.
8. Stand up and pat the perineum area dry. Apply a clean peripad.
9. Tip the basin to remove any remaining water and flush the toilet.
10. Wash the basin with warm water and soap and dry it in the sink.
11. Store basin and tubing in a clean, dry area until the next use.
12. Wash hands with soap and water.

gency call light is readily available, and being available if needed during this early period will ensure safety and prevent accidents and falls.

Topical Preparations

Several treatments may be applied topically for temporary relief of pain and discomfort. One such treatment is a local anesthetic spray such as Dermoplast or Americaine. These agents numb the perineal area and are used after cleansing the area with water via the peribottle and/or a sitz bath.

For hemorrhoid discomfort, cool witch hazel pads, such as Tucks Pads, can be used. The pads are placed at the rectal area, between the hemorrhoids and the perineal pad. These pads cool the area, help relieve swelling, and minimize itching.

Analgesics

Analgesics such as acetaminophen (Tylenol) and oral nonsteroidal anti-inflammatory drugs (NSAIDs) such as ibuprofen (Motrin) are prescribed to relieve mild postpartum discomfort. For moderate to severe pain, a narcotic analgesic such as codeine or oxycodone in conjunction with aspirin or acetaminophen may be prescribed. Instruct the woman about adverse effects of any medication prescribed. Common adverse effects of oral analgesics include dizziness, lightheadedness, nausea and vomiting, constipation, and sedation (Skidmore-Roth, 2007).

Also inform the woman that the drugs are secreted in breast milk. Nearly all medications that the mother takes are passed into her breast milk; however, the mild analgesics (e.g., acetaminophen or ibuprofen) are considered relatively safe for breast-feeding mothers (Tomasulo, 2007). Administering a mild analgesic approximately an hour before breast-feeding will usually relieve afterpains and/or perineal discomfort.

Assisting With Elimination

The bladder is edematous, hypotonic, and congested immediately postpartum. Consequently, bladder distention, incomplete emptying, and inability to void are common. A full bladder interferes with uterine contraction and may lead to hemorrhage, because it will displace the uterus out of the midline. Encourage the woman to void. Often, assisting her to assume the normal voiding position on the commode facilitates this. If the woman has difficulty voiding, pouring warm water over the perineal area, hearing the sound of running tap water, blowing bubbles through a straw, taking a warm shower, drinking fluids, or placing her hand in a basin of warm water may stimulate voiding. If these actions do not stimulate urination within 4 to 6 hours after giving birth, catheterization may be needed. Palpate the bladder for distention and ask the woman if she is voiding in small amounts (less than 100 mL) frequently (retention with overflow). If catheterization is necessary, use sterile technique to reduce the risk of infection.

EVIDENCE-BASED PRACTICE 16.1
Topically Applied Anesthetics for Treating Perineal Pain After Childbirth

● **Study**

The perineum (the area between the vagina and rectum) may be traumatized during childbirth following a tear or a surgical cut (episiotomy). Perineal trauma after childbirth affects millions of women around the world each year. The degree of perineal pain and discomfort associated with perineal trauma is often underestimated. Pain often interferes with basic daily activities such as walking, sitting, and passing urine and also detracts from the experience of motherhood. Local anesthetics are easy to use and inexpensive, but their effectiveness needs to be assessed. A study was performed to assess the effects of topically applied anesthetics to relieve perineal pain after childbirth while the mother was still in the hospital and after discharge. This review of trials found eight studies using a variety of anesthetics.

▲ **Findings**

Data were insufficient to show that the topical anesthetics helped relieve perineal pain, and long-term effects were not assessed. More research is required to assess the effectiveness of topical anesthetics on pain, longer-term outcomes, women's relationships, and quality of life, as well as the effectiveness of different topical anesthetics.

■ **Nursing Implications**

Although this study could not validate topical anesthetics' effectiveness in relieving perineal pain, they do provide relief to many postpartum women. The nurse should assess each woman individually and offer other comfort alternatives such as warm sitz baths, ice packs, and ambulation. Further research will be needed to offer proof that topical anesthetics are an effective pain relief measure.

Hedayati, H., Parsons, J., & Crowther, C. A. (2006). Topically applied anesthetics for treating perineal pain after childbirth. *Cochrane Database of Systematic Reviews* 2006, Issue 2. Art. No.: CD004223. DOI: 10.1002/14651858.CD004223.pub2.

Decreased bowel motility during labor, high iron content in prenatal vitamins, postpartum fluid loss, and the adverse effects of pain medications and/or anesthesia may predispose the postpartum woman to constipation. In addition, the woman may fear that bowel movements will cause pain or injury, especially if she had an episiotomy or a laceration that was repaired with sutures.

Usually a stool softener, such as docusate (Colace), with or without a laxative might be helpful if the client has difficulty with bowel elimination. Other measures, such as ambulating and increasing fluid and fiber intake, may also help. Nutritional instruction might include increasing fruits and vegetables in the diet; drinking plenty of fluids (8 to 12 cups) to keep the stool soft; drinking small amounts of prune juice and/or hot liquids to stimulate peristalsis; eating high-fiber foods such as bran cereals, whole grains, dried fruits, fresh fruits, and raw vegetables; and walking daily.

Promoting Activity, Rest, and Exercise

The postpartum period is an ideal time for nurses to promote the importance of physical fitness, help women incorporate exercise into their lifestyle, and encourage them to overcome barriers to exercise. The lifestyle changes that occur postpartum may affect a woman's health for decades. Early ambulation is encouraged to reduce the risk of thromboembolism and to improve strengthening.

Many changes occur postpartum, and caring for a newborn alters the woman's eating and sleeping habits, work schedules, and time allocation. Postpartum fatigue is common during the early days after childbirth, and it may continue for weeks or months (Runquist, 2007). It affects the mother's relationships with significant others and her ability to fulfill household and child care responsibilities. Be sure that the mother recognizes her need for rest and sleep and is realistic about her expectations. Some suggestions include the following:

• Nap when the infant is sleeping, because getting uninterrupted sleep at night is difficult.
• Reduce participation in outside activities and limit the number of visitors.
• Determine the infant's sleep–wake cycles and attempt to increase wakeful periods during the day so the baby sleeps for longer periods at night.
• Eat a balanced diet to promote healing and to increase energy levels.
• Share household tasks to conserve your energy.
• Ask the father or other family members to provide infant care during the night periodically so that you can get an uninterrupted night of sleep.
• Review your family's daily routine and see if you can "cluster" activities to conserve energy and promote rest.

The demands of parenthood may reduce or prevent exercise in even the most committed person. A targeted exercise program and proper body mechanics can help new mothers deal with the physical challenges of motherhood. Emphasize the benefits of a regular exercise program, which include:

• Helps the woman to lose pregnancy weight
• Increases energy level so the woman can cope with her new responsibilities

- Speeds the return to prepregnant size and shape
- Provides an outlet for stress (Druxman & Petersen, 2006)

More than one third of American women are overweight (CDC, Office of Women's Health, 2007). Although the average gestational weight gain is small (approximately 25 to 35 lb), excess weight gain and failure to lose weight after pregnancy are important predictors of long-term obesity. Breast-feeding and exercise may help to control weight in the long term (AAP, 2005).

▶ **Take** NOTE!

Women who have not returned to their prepregnant weight by 6 months are likely to retain the extra weight (Hackley, Kriebs, & Rousseau, 2007). Encourage women to lose their pregnancy weight by 6 months postpartum, and refer those who don't to community weight-loss programs.

The postpartum woman may face some obstacles to exercising, including physical changes (ligament laxity), competing demands (newborn care), lack of information about weight retention (inactivity equates to weight gain), and stress incontinence (leaking of urine during activity).

A healthy woman with an uncomplicated vaginal birth can resume exercise in the immediate postpartum period. Advise the woman to start slowly and increase the level of exercise over a period of several weeks as tolerated. Jogging strollers may be an option for some women, allowing them to exercise with their newborns. Also, exercise videos and home exercise equipment allow mothers to work out while the newborn naps.

Exercising after giving birth promotes feelings of well-being and restores muscle tone lost during pregnancy. Routine exercise should be resumed gradually, beginning with Kegel exercises on the first postpartum day and, by the second week, progressing to abdominal, buttock, and thigh-toning exercises (Druxman & Petersen, 2006). Walking is an excellent form of early exercise as long as the woman avoids jarring and bouncing movements, because joints do not stabilize until 6 to 8 weeks postpartum. Exercising too much too soon can cause the woman to bleed more and her lochia may return to bright red.

Recommended exercises for the first few weeks postpartum include abdominal breathing, head lifts, modified sit-ups, double knee roll, and pelvic tilt (Teaching Guidelines 16.2). The number of exercises and their duration is gradually increased as the woman gains strength.

Remember that cultures have different attitudes toward exercise. Some cultures (e.g., Haitian, Arab-

TEACHING GUIDELINES 16.2

Exercising

Abdominal Breathing

1. While lying on a flat surface (floor or bed), take a deep breath through your nose and expand your abdominal muscles (they will rise up from your midsection).
2. Slowly exhale and tighten your abdominal muscles for 3 to 5 seconds.
3. Repeat this several times.

Head Lift

1. Lie on a flat surface with knees flexed and feet flat on the surface.
2. Lift your head off the flat surface, tuck it onto your chest, and hold for 3 to 5 seconds.
3. Relax your head and return to the starting position.
4. Repeat this several times.

Modified Sit-Ups

1. Lie on a flat surface and raise your head and shoulders 6 to 8 inches so that your outstretched hands reach your knees.
2. Keep your waist on the flat surface.

3. Slowly return to the starting position.
4. Repeat, increasing in frequency as your comfort level allows.

Double Knee Roll

1. Lie on a flat surface with your knees bent.
2. While keeping your shoulders flat, slowly roll your knees to your right side to touch the flat surface (floor or bed).
3. Roll your knees back over your body to the left side until they touch the opposite side of the flat surface.
4. Return to the starting position on your back and rest.
5. Repeat this exercise several times.

Pelvic Tilt

1. Lie on your back on a flat surface with your knees bent and your arms at your side.
2. Slowly contract your abdominal muscles while lifting your pelvis up toward the ceiling.
3. Hold for 3 to 5 seconds and slowly return to your starting position.
4. Repeat several times..

American, and Mexican) expect new mothers to observe a specific period of bed rest or activity restriction; thus, it would be inappropriate to recommend active exercise during the early postpartum period (Bowers, 2007).

Preventing Stress Incontinence

Fifty percent of all parous women develop some degree of pelvic prolapse in their lifetime that is associated with stress incontinence (Thomason & DeLancey, 2007). The more vaginal deliveries a woman has had, the more likely she is to have stress incontinence. Stress incontinence can occur with any activity that causes an increase in intra-abdominal pressure. Postpartum women might consider low-impact activities such as walking, biking, swimming, or low-impact aerobics so they can resume physical activity while strengthening the pelvic floor.

Suggestions to prevent stress incontinence are:

- Start a regular program of Kegel exercises after childbirth.
- Lose weight if necessary; obesity is associated with stress incontinence.
- Avoid smoking; limit intake of alcohol and caffeinated beverages, which irritate the bladder.

Kegel exercises help to strengthen the pelvic floor muscles if done properly and regularly (Lemarck, 2007). Kegel exercises were originally developed by Dr. Arnold Kegel as a method of controlling incontinence in women after childbirth. The principle behind these exercises is that strengthening the muscles of the pelvic floor improves urethral sphincter function.

While providing postpartum care, instruct women on primary prevention of stress incontinence by discussing the value and purpose of Kegel exercises. Approach the subject sensitively, avoiding the term "incontinent." The terms "leakage," "loss of urine," or "bladder control issues" are more acceptable to most women.

▶ **Take** NOTE!

When properly performed, Kegel exercises have been effective in preventing or improving urinary continence (Lemack, 2007).

Women can perform Kegel exercises, doing ten 5-second contractions, whenever they change diapers, talk on the phone, or watch TV. Teach the woman to perform Kegel exercises properly; help her to identify the correct muscles by trying to stop and start the flow of urine when sitting on the toilet (Teaching Guidelines 16.3). Kegel exercises can be done without anyone knowing.

Assisting With Self-Care Measures

Demonstrate and discuss with the woman ways to prevent infection during the postpartum period. Because she

---

TEACHING GUIDELINES 16.3

Performing Kegel Exercises

1. Identify the correct pelvic floor muscles by contracting them to stop the flow of urine while sitting on the toilet.
2. Repeat this contraction several times to become familiar with it.
3. Start the exercises by emptying the bladder.
4. Tighten the pelvic floor muscles and hold for 10 seconds.
5. Relax the muscle completely for 10 seconds.
6. Perform 10 exercises at least three times daily. Progressively increase the number that you perform.
7. Perform the exercises in different positions, such as standing, lying, and sitting.
8. Keep breathing during the exercises.
9. Don't contract your abdominal, thigh, leg, or buttocks muscles during these exercises.
10. Relax while doing Kegel exercises and concentrate on isolating the right muscles.
11. Attempt to tighten your pelvic muscles before sneezing, jumping, or laughing.
12. Remember that you can perform Kegel exercises anywhere without anyone noticing.

---

may experience lochia drainage for as long as a month after childbirth, describe practices to promote well-being and healing. These measures include:

- Frequently change perineal pads, applying and removing them from front to back to prevent spreading contamination from the rectal area to the genital area.
- Avoid using tampons after giving birth to decrease the risk of infection.
- Shower once or twice daily using a mild soap. Avoid using soap on nipples.
- Use a sitz bath after every bowel movement to cleanse the rectal area and relieve enlarged hemorrhoids.
- Use the peribottle filled with warm water after urinating and before applying a new perineal pad.
- Avoid tub baths for 4 to 6 weeks, until joints and balance are restored, to prevent falls.
- Wash your hands before changing perineal pads, after disposing of soiled pads, and after voiding (Brown, 2006).

To reduce the risk of infection at the episiotomy site, reinforce proper perineal care with the client, showing her how to rinse her perineum with the peribottle after she voids or defecates. Stress the importance of always patting gently from front to back and washing her hands thoroughly before and after perineal care. For hemorrhoids, have the client apply witch hazel-soaked pads

(Tucks Pads), ice packs to relieve swelling, or hemorrhoidal cream or ointment if ordered.

Ensuring Safety

One of the safety concerns during the postpartum period is orthostatic hypotension. When the woman moves from a lying or sitting position to a standing one rapidly, her blood pressure can suddenly drop, causing her pulse rate to increase. She may become dizzy and faint. Be aware of this problem and initiate the following safeguards:

- Check blood pressure first before ambulating the client.
- Elevate the head of the bed for a few minutes before ambulating the client.
- Have the client sit on the side of the bed for a few moments before getting up.
- Help the client to stand up, and stay with her.
- Ambulate alongside the client and provide support if needed.
- Frequently ask the client how her head feels.
- Stay close by to assist if she feels lightheaded.

Additional topics to address concern infant safety. Instruct the woman to place the newborn back in the crib on his or her back if she is feeling sleepy. If the woman falls asleep while holding the infant, she might drop him or her. Also, instruct mothers to keep the door to their room closed when their infant is in their room with them. They should check the identification of anyone who enters their room or who wants to take the infant out of the room. This will prevent infant abduction.

Counseling About Sexuality and Contraception

Sexuality is an important part of every woman's life. Women want to get back to "normal" as soon as possible after giving birth, but the couple's sexual relationship cannot be isolated from the psychological and psychosocial adjustments that both partners are going through.

Postpartum women may hesitate to resume sexual relations for a number of reasons. Many postpartum women have fatigue, weakness, vaginal bleeding, perineal discomfort, hemorrhoids, sore breasts, decreased vaginal lubrication resulting from low estrogen levels, and dyspareunia. Fatigue, the physical demands made by the infant, and the stress of new roles and responsibilities may stress the emotional reserves of couples. New parents may not get much privacy or rest, both of which are necessary for sexual pleasure (Pastore, Owens, & Raymond, 2007).

Men may feel they now have a secondary role within the family, and they may not understand their partner's daily routine. These issues, combined with the woman's increased investment in the mothering role, can strain the couple's sexual relationship.

Although couples are reluctant to ask, they often want to know when they can safely resume sexual intercourse after childbirth. Typically, sexual intercourse can be resumed once bright-red bleeding has stopped and the perineum is healed from an episiotomy or lacerations. This is usually by the third to the sixth week postpartum. However, there is not a set, prescribed time to resume sexual intercourse after childbirth. Each couple must set their own time frame when they feel it is appropriate to resume sexual intercourse.

When counseling the couple about sexuality, determine what knowledge and concerns the couple have about their sexual relationship. Inform the couple that fluctuations in sexual interest are normal. Also inform the couple about what to expect when resuming sexual intercourse and how to prevent discomfort. Precoital vaginal lubrication may be impaired during the postpartum period, especially in women who are breast-feeding. Use of water-based gel lubricants (KY jelly, Astroglide) can help. Pelvic floor exercises, in addition to preventing stress incontinence, can also enhance sensation.

Contraceptive options should be included in the discussions with the couple so that they can make an informed decision before resuming sexual activity. Many couples are overwhelmed with the amount of new information given to them during their brief hospitalization, so many are not ready for a lengthy discussion about contraceptives. Presenting a brief overview of the options, along with literature, may be appropriate. It may be suitable to ask them to think about contraceptive needs and preferences and advise them to use a barrier method (condom with spermicidal gel or foam) until they choose another form of contraceptive. This advice is especially important if the follow-up appointment will not occur for 4 to 6 weeks after childbirth, as many couples will resume sexual activity before this time. Some postpartum women ovulate before their menstrual period returns and thus need contraceptive protection to prevent another pregnancy.

Open and effective communication is necessary for effective contraceptive counseling so that information is clearly understood. Provide clear, consistent information appropriate to the woman and her partner's language, culture, and educational level. This will help them select the best contraceptive method (Engin-Ustun et al., 2007).

Promoting Nutrition

The postpartum period can be a stressful one for myriad reasons, such as fatigue, the physical stress of pregnancy and birth, and the nonstop work required to take care of the newborn and to meet the needs of other family members. As a result, the new mother may ignore her own nutrition needs. Whether she is breast-feeding or bottle-feeding, encourage the new mother to take good care of herself and eat a healthy diet so that the nutrients lost during pregnancy can be replaced and she can return to a healthy weight. In general, nutrition recommendations for the postpartum woman include the following:

- Eat a wide variety of foods with high nutrient density.
- Eat meals that require little or no preparation.

- Avoid high-fat fast foods.
- Drink plenty of fluids daily—at least 2,500 mL (approximately 84 oz).
- Avoid fad weight-reduction diets and harmful substances such as alcohol, tobacco, and drugs.
- Avoid excessive intake of fat, salt, sugar, and caffeine.
- Eat the recommended daily servings from each food group (Box 16.4).

The breast-feeding mother's nutritional needs are higher than they were during pregnancy. The mother's diet and nutritional status influence the quantity and quality of breast milk. To meet the needs for milk production, the woman's nutritional needs increase as follows:

- Calories: +500 cal/day for the first and second 6 months of lactation
- Protein: +20 g/day, adding an extra 2 cups of skim milk
- Calcium: +400 mg daily—consumption of four or more servings of milk
- Fluid: +2 to 3 quarts of fluids daily (milk, juice or water); no sodas

Certain foods (usually gaseous or strong-flavored ones) eaten by the mother may affect the flavor of the breast milk or cause gastrointestinal problems for the infant. Not all infants are affected by the same foods. If the particular food item seems to cause a problem, urge the mother to eliminate that food for a few days to see if the problem disappears.

BOX 16.4 **Nutritional Recommendations for Nutrition During the Postpartum Period**

Recommendations for the Lactating Woman From the Food Guide Pyramid
- Fruits: 4 servings
- Vegetables: 4 servings
- Milk: 4 to 5 servings
- Bread, cereal, pasta: 12 or more servings
- Meat, poultry, fish, eggs: 7 servings
- Fats, oils, and sweets: 5 servings (Dudek, 2006)

General Dietary Guidelines for Americans from the Food Guide Pyramid (for the Non-lactating Woman)
- Fruits: 2 to 4 servings
- Vegetables: 3 to 5 servings
- Milk: 2 to 3 servings
- Breads, grains, and cereals: 6 to 11 servings
- Meat, poultry, fish, eggs: 2 to 3 servings
- Fats, oils, and sweets: use sparingly (USDA & USDHHS, 2005)

▶ *Take NOTE!*

During the woman's brief stay in the health care facility, she may demonstrate a healthy appetite and eat well. Nutritional problems usually start at home when the mother needs to make her own food selections and prepare her own meals. This is a crucial area to address during follow-up.

Supporting the Woman's Choice of Feeding Method

While there is considerable evidence that breast-feeding has numerous health benefits, many mothers choose to feed their infants formula for the first year of life. Nurses must be able to deliver sound, evidence-based information to help the new mother choose the best way to feed her infant and must support her in her decision (Lawson, 2007).

Many factors affect a woman's choice of feeding method, such as culture, employment demands, support from significant others and family, and knowledge base. Although breast-feeding is encouraged, be sure that couples have the information they need to make an informed decision. Whether a couple chooses to breast-feed or bottle-feed the newborn, support and respect their choice.

Certain women should not breast-feed. Drugs such as antithyroid drugs, antineoplastic drugs, alcohol, or street drugs (amphetamines, cocaine, PCP, marijuana) enter the breast milk and would harm the infant, so women taking these substances should not breast-feed. To prevent HIV transmission to the newborn, women who are HIV positive should not breast-feed. Other contraindications to breast-feeding include a newborn with an inborn error of metabolism such as galactosemia or PKU, a current pregnancy, or a serious mental health disorder that would prevent the mother from remembering to feed the infant consistently.

Providing Assistance With Breast-Feeding and Bottle-Feeding

First-time mothers often have many questions about feeding, and even women who have had experience with feeding may have questions. Regardless of whether the postpartum woman is breast-feeding or bottle-feeding her newborn, she can benefit from instruction.

Providing Assistance with Breast-Feeding

WATCH LEARN

The American Academy of Pediatrics (AAP, 2005) recommends breast-feeding for all full-term newborns. Exclusive breast-feeding is sufficient to support optimal growth and development for approximately the first 6 months of life. Breast-feeding should be continued for at least the first year of life and beyond for as long as mutually desired by mother and child. Educating a mother about breast-feeding will increase the likelihood of a successful breast-feeding experience.

At birth, all newborns should be quickly dried, assessed, and, if stable, placed immediately in uninterrupted skin-to-skin contact (kangaroo care) with their mother. This is good practice whether the mother is going to breast-feed or bottle-feed her infant. Kangaroo care provides the newborn with optimal physiologic stability, warmth, and opportunities for the first feed (Kenner & Lott, 2007).

The benefits of breast-feeding are clear (see Chap. 18). To promote breast-feeding, the Baby-Friendly Hospital Initiative, an international program of the World Health Organization and the United Nations Children's Fund, was started in 1991. As part of this program, the hospital or birth center should take the following 10 steps to provide "an optimal environment for the promotion, protection, and support of breast-feeding":

1. Have a written breast-feeding policy that is communicated to all staff.
2. Educate all staff to implement this written policy.
3. Inform all women about the benefits and management of breast-feeding.
4. Show all mothers how to initiate breast-feeding within 30 minutes of birth.
5. Give no food or drink other than breast milk to all newborns.
6. Demonstrate to all mothers how to initiate and maintain breast-feeding.
7. Encourage breast-feeding on demand.
8. Allow no pacifiers to be given to breast-feeding infants.
9. Establish breast-feeding support groups and refer mothers to them.
10. Practice rooming-in 24 hours daily (UNICEF, 2007).

The nurse is responsible for encouraging breast-feeding when appropriate. For the woman who chooses to breast-feed her infant, the nurse or lactation consultant will need to spend time instructing her how to do so successfully. Many women have the impression that breast-feeding is simple. Although it is a natural process, women may experience some difficulty in breast-feeding their newborns. Nurses can assist mothers in smoothing out this transition. Assist and provide one-to-one instruction to breast-feeding mothers, especially first-time breast-feeding mothers, to ensure correct technique. Suggestions are highlighted in Teaching Guidelines 16.4.

▶ **Take** NOTE!

Some newborns "latch on and catch on" right away, and others take more time and patience. Inform new mothers about this to reduce their frustration and uncertainty about their ability to breast-feed.

Tell mothers that they need to believe in themselves and their ability to accomplish this task. They should not panic if breast-feeding does not go smoothly at first; it takes time and practice. Additional suggestions to help mothers relax and feel more comfortable breast-feeding, especially when they return home, include the following:

• Select a quiet corner or room where you won't be disturbed.
• Use a rocking chair to soothe both you and your infant.
• Take long, slow deep breaths to relax before nursing.
• Drink while breast-feeding to replenish body fluids.
• Listen to soothing music while breast-feeding.
• Cuddle and caress the infant while feeding.
• Set out extra cloth diapers within reach to use as burping cloths.
• Allow sufficient time to enjoy each other in an unhurried atmosphere.
• Involve other family members in all aspects of the infant's care from the start.

Providing Assistance With Bottle-Feeding

If the mother or couple has chosen to bottle-feed their newborn, the nurse should respect and support their decision. Discuss with the parents what type of formula they will use. Commercial formulas are classified as cow's milk-based (Enfamil, Similac), soy protein-based (Isomil, Prosobee, Nursoy), or specialized or therapeutic formulas for infants with protein allergies (Nutramigen, Pregestimil, Alimentum). Commercial formulas can also be purchased in various forms: powdered (must be mixed with water), condensed liquid (must be diluted with equal amounts of water), ready to use (poured directly into bottles), and prepackaged (ready to use in disposable bottles).

Newborns need about 108 cal/kg or approximately 650 cal/day (Dudek, 2006). Therefore, explain to parents that a newborn will need to 2 to 4 ounces to feel satisfied at each feeding. Until about age 4 months, most bottle-fed infants need six feedings a day. After this time, the number of feedings declines to accommodate other foods in the diet, such as fruits, cereals, and vegetables (Escott-Stump, 2007). For more information on newborn nutrition and bottle feeding, see Chapter 18.

When teaching the mother about bottle-feeding, provide the following guidelines:

• Make feeding a relaxing time, a time to provide both food and comfort to your newborn.
• Use the feeding period to promote bonding by smiling, singing, making eye contact, and talking to the infant.
• Always hold the newborn when feeding. Never prop the bottle.
• Use a comfortable position when feeding the newborn. Place the newborn in your dominant arm, which is supported by a pillow. Or have the newborn in a semi-upright position supported in the crook of your arm (this position reduces choking and the flow of milk into the middle ear).

TEACHING GUIDELINES 16.4

Breast-Feeding Suggestions

- Explain that breast-feeding is a learned skill for both parties.
- Offer a thorough explanation about the procedure.
- Instruct the mother to wash her hands before starting.
- Inform her that her afterpains will increase during breast-feeding.
- Make sure the mother is comfortable (pain-free) and not hungry.
- Tell the mother to start the feeding with an awake and alert infant showing hunger signs.
- Assist the mother to position herself correctly for comfort.
- Urge the mother to relax to encourage the let-down reflex.
- Guide the mother's hand to form a "C" to access the nipple.
- Have the mother lightly tickle the infant's upper lip with her nipple to stimulate the infant to open the mouth wide.
- Help her to latch on by bringing the infant rapidly to the breast with a wide-open mouth.
- Show her how to check that the newborn's mouth position is correct, and tell her to listen for a sucking noise.
- Demonstrate correct removal from the breast, using her finger to break the suction.
- Instruct the mother on how to burp the infant between breasts.
- Show her different positions, such as cradle and football holds and side-lying positions (see Chap. 18).
- Reinforce and praise the mother for her efforts.
- Allow ample time to answer questions and address concerns.
- Refer the mother to support groups and community resources.

- Tilt the bottle so that the nipple and the neck of the bottle are always filled with formula. This prevents the infant from taking in too much air.
- Stimulate the sucking reflex by touching the nipple to the infant's lips.
- Refrigerate any powdered formula that has been combined with tap water.
- Discard any formula not taken; do not keep it for future feedings.
- Burp the infant frequently, and place the baby on his or her back or side for sleeping.
- Use only iron-fortified infant formula for first year (Lawson, 2007).

Teaching About Breast Care

Regardless of whether or not the mother is breast-feeding her newborn, urge her to wear a very supportive, snug bra 24 hours a day to support enlarged breasts and promote comfort. A woman who is breast-feeding should wear a supportive bra throughout the lactation period. A woman who is not nursing should wear it until engorgement ceases, and then should wear a less restrictive one. The bra should fit snugly while still allowing the mother to breathe without restriction. All new mothers should use plain water to clean their breasts, especially the nipple area; soap is drying and should be avoided.

Assessing the Breasts

Instruct the mother how to examine her breasts daily. Daily assessment includes the milk supply (breasts will feel full as they are filling), the condition of the nipples (red, bruised, fissured, or bleeding), and the success of breast-feeding. The fullness of the breasts may progress to engorgement in the breast-feeding mother if feedings are delayed or breast-feeding is ineffective. Palpating both breasts will help identify whether the breasts are soft, filling, or engorged. A similar assessment of the breasts should be completed on the nonlactating mother to identify any problems, such as engorgement or mastitis.

Alleviating Breast Engorgement

Breast engorgement usually occurs during the first week postpartum. It is a common response of the breasts to the sudden change in hormones and the presence of an increased amount of milk. Reassure the woman that this condition is temporary and usually resolves within 72 hours.

Alleviating Breast Engorgement in the Breastfeeding Woman

If the mother is breast-feeding, encourage frequent feedings, at least every 2 to 3 hours, using manual expression just before feeding to soften the breast so the newborn can latch on more effectively. Advise the mother to allow the newborn to feed on the first breast until it softens before switching to the other side. See Chapter 18 for more information on alleviating breast engorgement and other common breast-feeding concerns.

Alleviating Breast Engorgement and Suppressing Lactation in the Bottle-Feeding Woman

If the woman is bottle-feeding, explain that breast engorgement is a self-limiting phenomenon that disappears as increasing estrogen levels suppress milk formation (i.e., lactation suppression). Encourage the woman to use ice packs, to wear a snug, supportive bra 24 hours a day, and to take mild analgesics such as acetaminophen. Encourage her to avoid any stimulation to the breasts that might foster milk production, such as warm showers or pumping or massaging the breasts. Medication is no longer given to hasten lactation suppression. Teaching Guidelines 16.5 provides tips on lactation suppression.

Promoting Family Adjustment and Well-Being

The postpartum period involves extraordinary physiologic, psychological, and sociocultural changes in the life of a woman and her family. Adapting to the role of a parent is not an easy process. The postpartum period is a "getting-to-know-you" time when parents begin to integrate the newborn into their lives as they reconcile the fantasy child with the real one. This can be a very challenging

TEACHING GUIDELINES 16.5

Suppressing Lactation

1. Wear a supportive, snugly fitting bra 24 hours daily, but not one that binds the breasts too tightly or interferes with your breathing.
2. Suppression may take 5 to 7 days to accomplish.
3. Take mild analgesics to reduce breast discomfort.
4. Let shower water flow over your back rather than your breasts.
5. Avoid any breast stimulation in the form of sucking or massage.
6. Drink to quench your thirst. Restricting your fluid intake will not dry up your milk.
7. Reduce your salt intake to decrease fluid retention.
8. Use ice packs or cool compresses (e.g., cool cabbage leaves) inside the bra to decrease local pain and swelling; change them every 30 minutes (Arenson & Drake, 2007).

period for families. Nurses play a major role in assisting families to adapt to the changes, promoting a smooth transition into parenthood. Appropriate and timely interventions can help parents adjust to the role changes and promote attachment to the newborn.

For couples who already have children, the addition of a new member may bring role conflict and challenges. The nurse should provide anticipatory guidance about siblings' responses to the new baby, increased emotional tension, child development, and meeting the multiple needs of the expanding family. Although the multiparous woman has had experience with newborns, do not assume that her knowledge is current and accurate, especially if some time has elapsed since her previous child was born. Reinforcing information is important for all families.

Promoting Parental Roles

Parents' roles develop and grow when they interact with their newborn (see Chap. 15 for information on maternal and paternal adaptation). The pleasure they derive from this interaction stimulates and reinforces this behavior. With repeated, continued contact with the newborn, parents learn to recognize cues and understand the newborn's behavior. This positive interaction contributes to family harmony.

Nurses need to know the stages parents go through as they make their new parenting roles fit into their life experience. Assess the parents for attachment behaviors (normal and deviant), adjustment to the new parental role, family member adjustment, social support system, and educational needs. To promote parental role adaptation and parent–newborn attachment, include the following nursing interventions:

- Provide as much opportunity as possible for parents to interact with their newborn. Encourage exploration, holding, and providing care.
- Model behaviors by holding the newborn close and speaking positively.
- Always refer to the newborn by name in front of the parents.
- Speak directly to the newborn in a calm voice.
- Encourage both parents to pick up and hold the newborn.
- Point out the newborn's response to parental stimulation.
- Point out the positive physical features of the newborn.
- Involve both parents in the newborn's care and praise them for their efforts.
- Evaluate the family's strengths and weaknesses and readiness for parenting.
- Assess for risk factors such as lack of social support and the presence of stressors.
- Observe the effect of culture on the family interaction to determine whether it is appropriate.
- Monitor parental attachment behaviors to determine whether alterations require referral. Positive behaviors include holding the newborn closely or in an *en face* position, talking to or admiring the newborn, or demonstrating closeness. Negative behaviors include avoiding contact with the newborn, calling it names, or showing a lack of interest in caring for the newborn (see Table 16.1).
- Monitor the parents' coping behaviors to determine alterations that need intervention. Positive coping behaviors include positive conversations between the partners, both parents wanting to be involved with newborn care, and lack of arguments between the parents. Negative behaviors include not visiting, limited conversations or periods of silence, and heated arguments or conflict.
- Identify the support systems available to the new family and encourage them to ask for help. Ask direct questions about home or community support. Make referrals to community resources to meet the family's needs.
- Arrange for community home visits in high-risk families to provide positive reinforcement of parenting skills and nurturing behaviors with the newborn.
- Provide anticipatory guidance about the following before discharge to reduce the new parents' frustration:
  - Newborn sleep–wake cycles (they may be reversed)
  - Variations in newborn appearance
  - Infant developmental milestones (growth spurts)
  - How to interpret crying cues (hunger, wet, discomfort)
  - Techniques to quiet a crying infant (car ride)
  - Sensory enrichment/stimulation (colorful mobile)
  - Signs and symptoms of illness and how to assess for fever
  - Important phone numbers, follow-up care, and needed immunizations

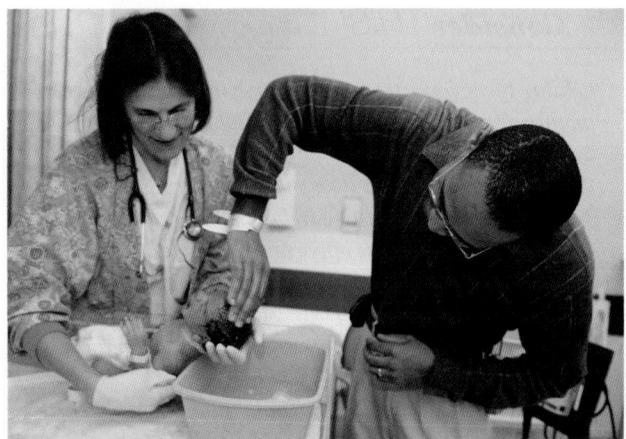

FIGURE 16.7 Father participating in newborn care.

- Physical and emotional changes associated with the postpartum period
- Need to integrate siblings into care of the newborn; stress that sibling rivalry is normal and offer ways to reduce it
- Ways to make time together for the couple
- Appropriate community referral resources

In addition, nurses can help fathers to feel more competent in assuming their parental role by teaching and providing information (Fig. 16.7). Education can dispel any unrealistic expectations they may have, helping them to cope more successfully with the demands of fatherhood and thereby fostering a nurturing family relationship.

Explaining Sibling Roles

It can be overwhelming to a young child to have another family member introduced into his or her small, stable world. Although most parents try to prepare siblings for the arrival of their new little brother or sister, many young children experience stress. They may view the new infant as competition, or fear that they will be replaced in the parents' affection. All siblings need extra attention from their parents and reassurance that they are loved and important.

▶ *Consider* THIS!

Katie and Molly have been excited about having a new baby sister since they were told about their mother's pregnancy. The 6-year-old twins are eagerly looking out the front window, waiting for their parents to bring their new sister, Jessica, home. The girls are big enough to help their mother care for their new sibling, and for the past few months they have been fixing up the new nursery and selecting baby clothes. They practiced diapering their dolls—their mother was specific about not using any powder or lotion on Jessica's bottom—and

(continued)

▶ *Consider* THIS! (continued)

holding them correctly to feed them bottles. Finally, their mother arrives home from the hospital with Jessica in her arms!

The girls notice that their mother is very protective of Jessica and watches them carefully when they care for her. They fight over the opportunity to hold her or feed her. What is special to both of them is the time they spend alone with their parents. Although a new family member has been added, the twins still feel special and loved by their parents.

Thoughts: Bringing a new baby into an established family can cause conflict and jealousy. What preparation did the older siblings have before Jessica arrived? Why is it important for parents to spend time with each sibling separately?

Many parents need reassurance that sibling rivalry is normal. Suggest the following to help parents minimize sibling rivalry:

- Expect and tolerate some regression (thumb sucking, bedwetting).
- Explain childbirth in an appropriate way for the child's age.
- Encourage discussion about the new infant during relaxed family times.
- Encourage the sibling(s) to participate in decisions, such as the baby's name and toys to buy.
- Take the sibling on the tour of the maternity suite.
- Buy a T-shirt that says "I'm the [big brother or big sister]."
- Spend "special time" with the child.
- Read with the child. Some suggested title include *Things to Do with A New Baby* (Ormerod, 1984); *Betsy's Baby Brother* (Wolde, 1975); *The Berenstain Bears' New Baby* (Berenstain, 1974); and *Mommy's Lap* (Horowitz & Sorensen, 1993).
- Plan time for each child throughout the day.
- Role-play safe handling of a newborn, using a doll. Give the preschooler or school-age child a doll to care for.
- Encourage older children to verbalize emotions about the newborn.
- Purchase a gift that the child can give to the newborn.
- Purchase a gift that can be given to the child by the newborn.
- Arrange for the child to come to the hospital to see the newborn (Fig. 16.8).
- Move the sibling from his or her crib to a youth bed months in advance of the birth of the newborn.
- Encourage grandparents to pay attention to the older child when visiting (Rector, 2007).

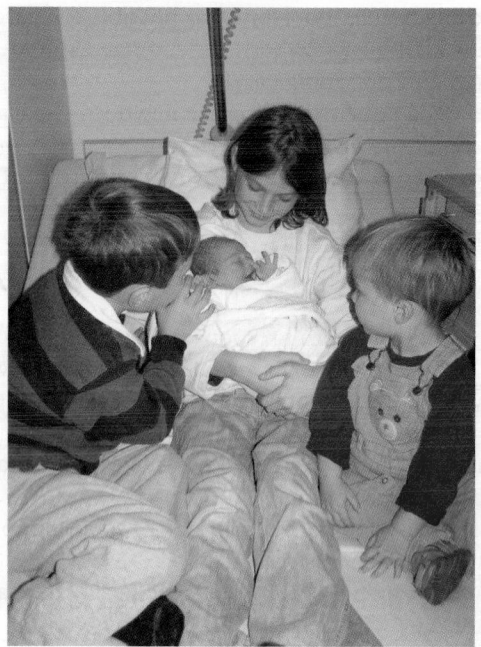

FIGURE 16.8 Sibling visitation.

Discussing Grandparents' Role

Grandparents can be a source of support and comfort to the postpartum family if effective communication skills are used and roles are defined. The grandparents' role and involvement will depend on how close they live to the family, their willingness to become involved, and cultural expectations of their role. Just as parents and siblings go through developmental changes, so too do grandparents. These changes can have a positive or negative effect on the relationship.

Newborn care, feeding, and childrearing practices have changed since the grandparents raised the parents. New parents may lack parenting skills but nonetheless want their parents' support without criticism. A grandparent's "take-charge approach" may not be welcome by new parents who are testing their own parenting roles, and family conflict may ensue. However, many grandparents respect their adult children's wishes for autonomy and remain "resource people" for them when requested.

▶ *Take* NOTE!

Grandparents' involvement can enrich the lives of the entire family if accepted in the right context and dose by the family.

Nurses can assist in the grandparents' role transition by assessing their communication skills, role expectations, and support skills during the prenatal period. Find out whether the grandparents are included in the couple's social support network and whether their support is wanted or helpful. If they are, and it is, then encourage the grandparents to learn about the parenting, feeding, and childrearing skills their children have learned in childbirth classes. This information is commonly found in "grandparenting" classes, which introduce new parenting concepts and bring the grandparents up to date on childbirth practices today.

Teaching About Postpartum Blues

The postpartum period is typically a happy yet stressful time, because the birth of an infant is accompanied by enormous physical, social, and emotional changes. The postpartum woman may report feelings of emotional lability, such as crying one minute and laughing the next. **Postpartum blues** are transient emotional disturbances beginning in the first week after childbirth and are characterized by anxiety, irritability, insomnia, crying, loss of appetite, and sadness (Fooladi, 2006). These symptoms typically begin 3 to 4 days after childbirth and resolve by day 10 (Bennett, 2007). These mood swings may be confusing to new mothers but usually are self-limiting.

Postpartum blues are thought to affect up to 75% of all new mothers; this condition is the mildest form of emotional disturbance associated with childbearing (March of Dimes, 2007). The mother maintains contact with reality consistently and symptoms tend to resolve spontaneously without therapy within 1 to 2 weeks.

> ▶ **Take** NOTE!
>
> *Postpartum blues have been regarded as brief, benign, and without clinical significance, but several studies have proposed a link between blues and subsequent depression in the 6 months following childbirth (Vaughn, 2006).*

Postpartum blues requires no formal treatment other than support and reassurance because it does not usually interfere with the woman's ability to function and care for her infant. Further evaluation is necessary, however, if symptoms persist more than 2 weeks (Ey, 2007). Nurses can ease a mother's distress by encouraging her to vent her feelings and by demonstrating patience and understanding with her and her family. Suggest that getting outside help with housework and infant care might help her to feel less overwhelmed until the blues ease. Provide telephone numbers she can call when she feels down during the day. Making women aware of this disorder while they are pregnant will increase their knowledge about this mood disturbance, which may lessen their embarrassment and increase their willingness to ask for and accept help if it does occur.

The postpartum woman also is at risk for postpartum depression and postpartum psychosis; these conditions are discussed in Chapter 22.

Preparing for Discharge

The AAP and the American College of Obstetricians and Gynecologists (ACOG) state that the length of stay in the health care facility should be individualized for each mother and baby. A shortened hospital stay may be indicated if the following criteria are met:

- Mother is afebrile and vital signs are within normal range.
- Lochia is appropriate amount and color for stage of recovery.
- Hemoglobin and hematocrit values are within normal range.
- Uterine fundus is firm; urinary output is adequate.
- ABO blood groups and RhD status are known and, if indicated, anti-D immunoglobulin has been administered.
- Surgical wounds are healing and no signs of infection are present.
- Mother is able to ambulate without difficulty.
- Food and fluids are taken without difficulty.
- Self-care and infant care are understood and demonstrated.
- Family or other support system is available to care for both.
- Mother is aware of possible complications (AAP & ACOG, 2007).

Providing Immunizations

Prior to discharge, check the immunity status for rubella for all mothers and give a subcutaneous injection of rubella vaccine if they are not serologically immune (titer less than 1:10). Be sure that the client signs a consent form to receive the vaccine. Nursing mothers can be vaccinated because the live, attenuated rubella virus is not communicable. Inform all mothers receiving immunization about adverse effects (rash, joint symptoms, and a low-grade fever 5 to 21 days later) and the need to avoid pregnancy for at least 3 months after being vaccinated because of the risk of teratogenic effects (CDC, 2007).

If the client is Rh negative, check the Rh status of the newborn. Verify that the woman is Rh negative and has not been sensitized, that the Coombs' test is negative, and that the newborn is Rh positive. Mothers who are Rh negative and have given birth to an infant who is Rh positive should receive an injection of Rh immunoglobulin within 72 hours after birth to prevent a sensitization reaction in the Rh-negative woman who received Rh-positive blood cells during the birthing process. The usual protocol for the Rh-negative woman is to receive two doses of Rh immunoglobulin (RhoGAM), one at 28 weeks' gestation and the second dose within 72 hours after childbirth. A signed consent form is needed after a thorough explanation is provided about the procedure, including its purpose, possible adverse effects, and effect on future pregnancies.

Ensuring Follow-Up Care

New mothers and their families need to be attended to over an extended period of time by nurses knowledgeable about mother care, infant feeding (breast-feeding and bottle-feeding), infant care, and nutrition. Although continuous nursing care stops on discharge from the hospital or birthing center, extended episodic nursing care needs to be provided at home. Some of the challenges faced by the current families after discharge are described in Box 16.5.

Many new mothers are reluctant to "cut the cord" after their brief stay in the health care facility and need expanded community services. Women who are discharged too early from the hospital run the risk of uterine subinvolution, discomfort at an episiotomy or cesarean site, infection, fatigue, and maladjustment to their new role. Postpartum nursing care should include a range of family-focused care, including telephone calls, outpatient clinics, and home visits. Typically, public health nurses, community and home health nurses, and the health care provider's office staff will provide postpartum care after hospital discharge.

Providing Telephone Follow-Up

Telephone follow-up typically occurs during the first week after discharge to check on how things are going at home. Calls can be made by perinatal nurses within the agency as part of follow-up care or by the local health department nurses. A disadvantage to a phone call assessment is that the nurse cannot see the client and thus must rely on the mother or the family's observations. The experienced nurse needs to be able to recognize distress and give appropriate advice and referral information if needed.

BOX 16.5 Challenges Facing Families After Discharge

- Lack of role models for breast-feeding and infant care
- Lack of support from the new mother's own mother if she did not breast-feed
- Increased mobility of society, which means that extended family may live far away and cannot help care for the newborn and support the new family
- Feelings of isolation and limited community ties for women who work full time
- Shortened hospital stays: parents may be overwhelmed by all the information they are given in the brief hospital stay
- Prenatal classes usually focus on the birth itself rather than on skills needed to care for themselves and the newborn during the postpartum period
- Limited access to education and support systems for families from diverse cultures

---

Source: Nash, 2007.

Providing Outpatient Follow-Up

For mothers with established health care providers such as private pediatricians and obstetricians, visits to the office are arranged soon after discharge. For the woman with an uncomplicated vaginal birth, an office visit is usually scheduled for 4 to 6 weeks after childbirth. A woman who had a cesarean birth frequently is seen within 2 weeks after hospital discharge. Hospital discharge orders will specify when these visits should be made. Newborn examinations and further diagnostic laboratory studies are scheduled within the first week.

▶ **Take** NOTE!

Infants discharged before they are 48 hours old should be seen by a pediatrician or health care provider by the time they are 96 hours old; those discharged after they are 48 hours old should be seen by the time they are 120 hours old (Langan, 2006).

Outpatient clinics are available in many communities. If family members run into a problem, the local clinic is available to provide assessment and treatment. Clinic visits can replace or supplement home visits. Although these clinics are open during daytime hours only and the staff members are unfamiliar with the family, they can be a valuable resource for the new family with a problem or concern.

Providing Home Visit Follow-Up

Home visits are usually made within the first week after discharge to assess the mother and newborn. During the home visit, the nurse assesses for and manages common physical and psychosocial problems. In addition, the home nurse can help the new parents adjust to the change in their lives. The postpartum home visit usually includes the following:

- Maternal assessment: general well-being, vital signs, breast health and care, abdominal and musculoskeletal status, voiding status, fundus and lochia status, psychological and coping status, family relationships, proper feeding technique, environmental safety check, newborn care knowledge and health teaching needed (Fig. 16.9 shows sample assessment forms)
- Infant assessment: physical examination, general appearance, vital signs, home safety check, child development status, any education needed to improve parents' skills

The home care nurse must be prepared to support and educate the woman and her family in the following areas:

- Breast-feeding or bottle-feeding technique and procedures

(text continues on page 472)

Maternal Assessment
Maternal/Newborn Record System

Page 1 of 2

PATIENT IDENTIFICATION

Record No. _____

Name _____

Home
address _____
STREET

CITY   STATE   ZIP

Date __MO_/_DAY_/_YR__ Time begin: _____ Date of delivery __MO_/_DAY_/_YR__
                        Time end: _____

Medication allergy   ☐ None Identify_____
Significant health history ☐ None Identify_____

PHYSICAL

TEMP.	PULSE	RESP.	BP	/

Breasts   ☐ Nursing   ☐ Non-nursing
Color   ☐ Normal   ☐ Reddened
Condition   ☐ Soft   ☐ Firm   ☐ Engorged   ☐ Blocked ducts
Secretion   ☐ Colostrum   ☐ Milk   ☐ Other _____
Support bra   ☐ No   ☐ Yes, fit ☐ Appropriate
                                            ☐ Inappropriate

Nipples (If nursing) ☐ Erect ☐ Flat ☐ Inverted
   Condition ☐ Intact   ☐ Bruised   ☐ Blistered
             ☐ Fissured   ☐ Bleeding ☐ Scabbed
   Care   ☐ Water only ☐ Soap   ☐ Air dry
             ☐ Topical agent (type/frequency) _____

             ☐ Other _____
Self-exam   ☐ Accurate ☐ Inaccurate/instructed

Abdomen

Diastasis recti ☐ Absent   ☐ Present_____cm
                 ☐ Exercise taught
Incision   ☐ None
   Type   ☐ Transverse ☐ Vertical ☐ Umbilical
   Closure   ☐ Staples   ☐ Sutures   ☐ Steri-strips
   Condition   ☐ Approximated   ☐ Open _____cm
                 ☐ Redness _____
                 ☐ Swelling _____
                 ☐ Discharge _____
                 ☐ Other _____

Reproductive Tract

Uterus   ☐ Firm   ☐ Firm with massage   ☐ Boggy
         Height_____ ☐ Midline   ☐ Displaced L R
         ☐ Non tender   ☐ Tender   ☐ With touch ☐ Constant
Lochia   ☐ Rubra   ☐ Serosa   ☐ Alba
         ☐ Clots (describe)_____
         ☐ Fleshy odor   ☐ Foul odor
         Pads   Type_____   Number/day_____

         Saturation %├────┼────┼────┼────┤
                     0   25   50   75   100

Perineum ☐ Intact   ☐ Laceration
          ☐ Episiotormy   Type_____ Extension_____
Condition ☐ Redness _____
          ☐ Edema _____
          ☐ Eccymosis _____
          ☐ Discharge _____
          ☐ Approximation _____
Care   ☐ Front-to-back cleansing   ☐ Peri-bottle
          ☐ Soap/water
          ☐ Ice ☐ Sitz bath ☐ Warm ☐ Cool
          ☐ Topical agent (type/frequency) _____

          ☐ Other _____

Elimination

Urinary tract
   Voiding pattern   ☐ Normal   ☐ Incontinence
                      ☐ Bladder distention ☐ Catheter (type) _____
   Signs of infection ☐ None/reviewed ☐ Urgency ☐ Frequency
                      ☐ Dysuria ☐ CVA tenderness L R
Gastrointestinal tract
   Bowel pattern   ☐ Normal ☐ No BM
                      ☐ Constipation ☐ Diarrhea
                      ☐ Meds/treatments (type, frequency, effect) _____

   Hemorrhoids   ☐ No ☐ Yes (describe) _____
                      ☐ Meds/treatments (type, frequency, effect) _____

Lower Extremities

Edema   ☐ None   ☐ Pedal   ☐ Ankle   ☐ Pretibial   ☐ Thigh
         ☐ Pitting (describe) _____
Signs of thrombophlebitis   ☐ None

	L	R		L	R
Homan's sign	☐	☐	Redness	☐	☐
Pain	☐	☐	Warmth	☐	☐
Swelling	☐	☐			

Pain	**No**	**Yes**	
		Managed	Problematic
Abdominal incision	☐	☐	☐
Back	☐	☐	☐
Breasts	☐	☐	☐
Headache	☐	☐	☐
Hemorrhoid	☐	☐	☐
Nipple	☐	☐	☐
Perineum	☐	☐	☐
Uterine cramping	☐	☐	☐
Other _____	☐	☐	☐

Analgesic ☐ No
           ☐ Yes (type/dose/frequency) _____

Reportable danger signs ☐ Aware   ☐ Unaware/instructed

TESTS ☐ None
           ☐ Urinalysis
           ☐ CBC
           ☐ _____

IDENTIFIED NEEDS

_____
_____
_____
_____
_____
_____
_____
_____
_____

Signature _____

A

FIGURE **16.9** Sample postpartum home visit assessment form. (**A**) Maternal
assessment. (*continued*)

Maternal Assessment
Maternal/Newborn Record System

Page 2 of 2

ACTIVITIES OF DAILY LIVING - 24 HOUR HISTORY

Date __MO__ / __DAY__ / __YR__

Nutrition

Appetite   ☐ Good   ☐ Fair   ☐ Poor
Usual pattern   ☐ Yes ☐ No
Special diet   ☐ No   ☐ Yes _____
Food intolerance/allergy   ☐ No   ☐ Yes _____
Vitamin/mineral supplement ☐ No   ☐ Yes _____
Fluid intake (type/amount) _____

BREAKFAST	LUNCH	DINNER	SNACKS

General Hygiene   ☐ Adequate   ☐ Inadequate (describe)

Sleep/Activity

Amount of Activity
Night, uninterrupted _____ hrs

Naps ☐ No ☐ Yes _____ hrs

Fatigue ☐ None ☐ Minimal ☐ Moderate
        ☐ Exhausted

Activities
Limitations ☐ None   Identify _____

	Appropriate	Inappropriate/instructed
☐ Self-care	☐ Infant care	
Stair climbing	☐	☐
Lifting	☐	☐
Household tasks	☐	☐
Outside home	☐	☐
Other _____		

Exercise
☐ None

	Accurate	Inaccurate/instructed
Kegel	☐	☐
Postpartum	☐	☐
Other _____		

PSYCHOLOGICAL

Review of Labor and Birth

Missing pieces   ☐ No   ☐ Yes
Unmet expectations   ☐ No   ☐ Yes
Unresolved feelings   ☐ No   ☐ Yes
Pertinent data _____

Emotional Status   ☐ Happy ☐ Ambivalent ☐ Anxious
                       ☐ Sad ☐ Other _____
Postpartum-depression (Key on reverse side)
☐ 0 ☐ 1 ☐ 2 ☐ 3 ☐ 4
☐ Signs/Symptoms Reviewed

General Comments   (body image, role changes, concerns) _____
_____
_____

Postpartum Timetable   (Key on reverse side)
☐ Taking in ☐ Taking hold ☐ Letting go

SEXUALITY

	Aware	Unaware/instructed
Relationship with partner		
Adjustment	☐	☐
Expressions of affection	☐	☐
Resuming Intercourse		
Timing (lack of lochia, comfort)	☐	☐
Vaginal dryness	☐	☐
Milk ejection (if lactating)	☐	☐
Position variation	☐	☐
Libidinal changes	☐	☐
Return of Menses	☐	☐

Contraceptive Method
☐ None   ☐ Undecided/aware of options
☐ Natural family planning
☐ Cervical cap
☐ Condom
☐ Diaphragm
☐ Hormones ☐ Pill ☐ Injection ☐ Implant
☐ IUD
☐ Spermicide
☐ Sterilization ☐ Female ☐ Male
☐ Other _____

Accurate use ☐ Yes ☐ No/instructed

IDENTIFIED NEEDS
_____
_____
_____
_____

Signature _____

FIGURE 16.9 (continued)

PATIENT IDENTIFICATION

Record No. _____

Maternal Assessment
Maternal/Newborn Record System

Name _____
Home
address _____
STREET
CITY   STATE   ZIP

Date MO / DAY / YR Time begin: _____ Date of Birth MO / DAY / YR
                    Time end: _____
Significant history ☐ None Identify _____

PHYSICAL

Temp _____ Pulse (rate/rhythm) _____ Resp _____
Weight _____ Birth weight _____ % Change _____
Length _____ Head _____ Chest _____

HEAD/NECK

	Level	Bulging	Depressed
1. Fontanels			
Anterior	☐	☐	☐
Posterior	☐	☐	☐

Sutures ☐ Open ☐ Closed ☐ Overriding
2. Variations ☐ Molding ☐ Caput ☐ Cephalhematoma

	NORMAL	ABNORMAL	DETAIL VARIATIONS/ ABNORMAL FINDINGS
3. Face (symmetry)	☐	☐	
4. Eyes (symmetry, conjunctiva, sciera, eyelids, PERL)	☐	☐	
5. Ears (shape, position, auditory response)	☐	☐	
6. Nose (patency)	☐	☐	
7. Mouth (lip, mucous membranes, tongue, palate)	☐	☐	
8. Neck (ROM, symmetry)	☐	☐	
Chest			
9. Appearance (shape, breasts, nipples)	☐	☐	
10. Breath sounds	☐	☐	
11. Clavicles	☐	☐	
Cardiovascular			
12. Heart sounds	☐	☐	
13. Brachial/femoral pulses (compare strength, equality)	☐	☐	
Abdomen			
14. Appearance (shape, size)	☐	☐	
15. Cord (condition)	☐	☐	
16. Liver (less than or equal to 3 cm ↓ ®costal margin)	☐	☐	
Genitalia			
17. Female (labia, introitus, discharge	☐	☐	
18. Male (meatus, scrotum, testes)	☐	☐	
19. Circumcision ☐ No ☐ Yes	☐	☐	
Musculoskeletal			
20. Muscle tone	☐	☐	
21. Extremities (symmetry, digits, ROM)	☐	☐	
22. Hips (symmetry, ROM)	☐	☐	
23. Spine (alignment, integrity)	☐	☐	
Neurologic			
24. Reflexes (presence, symmetry)			
Moro	☐	☐	
Grasp	☐	☐	
Babinski	☐	☐	
25. Cry (presence, quality)	☐	☐	

PHYSICAL (CONT'D)
Skin
Turgor ☐ Good ☐ Poor
Condition ☐ Smooth ☐ Dry, cracked ☐ Peeling
Color ☐ Pink ☐ Ruddy ☐ Cyanotic ☐ Pale
☐ Jaundice (note levels)
☐ Head (3 mg/dl)
☐ Head and upper chest (6 mg/dl)
☐ Head and entire chest (9 mg/dl)
☐ Head, chest and abdomen to umbilicus (12 mg/dl)
☐ Head, chest and entire abdomen (15 mg/dl)
☐ Head, chest, abdomen, legs and feet (18 mg/dl)
Variations (Rashes, lesions, birthmarks). _____

NUTRITION
Feeding
Reflexes ☐ Root ☐ Suck ☐ Swallow
Hunger cues identified ☐ Yes ☐ No/instructed

BREAST	FORMULA
Frequency ___ times in ___ hours	Type _____
Time per breast ___ min ___ min	Amount _____ oz.
Positioning ☐ Correct	Frequency _____
☐ Incorrect _____	Preparation ☐ Correct
Latch ☐ Correct	☐ Incorrect _____
☐ Incorrect _____	
Appropriate audible swallows	☐ Correct
☐ Yes ☐ No _____	☐ _____

Satiation demonstrated ☐ Yes
☐ No (describe) _____
Regurgitation ☐ No ☐ Yes (describe) _____
Pacifier use ☐ No ☐ Yes (type/pattern) _____

Stool (number/day, color, consistency) _____
Urine (number/day, color) _____

BEHAVIOR
Sleep/Activity Pattern (24 hours)
Sleep (16–20 hrs) ☐ Yes ☐ No (describe) _____

Awake-alert (2–3 hrs) ☐ Yes ☐ No (describe) _____

Awake-crying (2–4 hrs) ☐ Yes ☐ No (describe) _____

Consolability (Key on reverse) ☐ 0 ☐ 1 ☐ 2 ☐ 3 ☐ 4

TESTS ☐ None   Time
☐ Metabolic screen kit no. _____ _____
☐ Bilirubin   _____
☐ Hematocrit   _____
☐ _____   _____
☐ _____   _____

INENTIFIED NEEDS _____
_____
_____
_____

Signature _____

B

FIGURE 16.9 (continued) (B) Newborn assessment. (Used with permission: Copyright Briggs Corporation. Professional Nurse Associates.)

- Appropriate parenting behavior and problem solving
- Maternal/newborn physical, psychosocial, and culture–environmental needs
- Emotional needs of the new family
- Warning signs of problems and how to prevent or eliminate them
- Sexuality issues, including contraceptive use
- Immunization needs for both mother and infant
- Family dynamics for smooth transition
- Links to health care providers and community resources

■■■ Key Concepts

■ The transitional adjustment period between birth and parenthood includes education about baby care basics, the role of the new family, emotional support, breast-feeding or bottle-feeding support, and maternal mentoring.

■ Sensitivity to how childbearing practices and beliefs vary for multicultural families and how best to provide appropriate nursing care to meet their needs are important during the postpartum period.

■ A thorough postpartum assessment is key to preventing complications as is frequent handwashing by the nurse, especially between handling mothers and infants.

■ The postpartum assessment using the acronym BUBBLE-EE (breasts, uterus, bowel, bladder, lochia, episiotomy/perineum, extremities, and emotions) is a helpful guide in performing a systematic head-to-toe postpartum assessment.

■ Lochia is assessed according to its amount, color, and change with activity and time. It proceeds from lochia rubra to serosa to alba.

■ Because of shortened agency stays, nurses must use this brief time with the client to address areas of comfort, elimination, activity, rest and exercise, self-care, sexuality and contraception, nutrition, family adaptation, discharge, and follow-up.

■ The AAP advocates breast-feeding for all full-term newborns, maintaining that, ideally, breast milk should be the sole nutrient for the first 6 months and continued with foods until 12 months of life or longer.

■ Successful parenting is a continuous and complex interactive process that requires the acquisition of new skills and the integration of the new member into the existing family unit.

■ Bonding is a vital component of the attachment process and is necessary in establishing parent–infant attachment and a healthy, loving relationship; attachment behaviors include seeking and maintaining close proximity to, and exchanging gratifying experiences with, the infant.

■ Nurses can be instrumental in facilitating attachment by first understanding attachment behaviors (positive and negative) of newborns and parents, and intervening appropriately to promote and enhance attachment.

■ New mothers and their families need to be attended to over an extended period of time by nurses knowledgeable about mother care, newborn feeding (breast-feeding and bottle-feeding), newborn care, and nutrition.

REFERENCES

American Academy of Pediatrics (AAP) & American College of Obstetricians & Gynecologists (ACOG). (2007). *Pediatric clinical practice guidelines and policies* (7th ed.). Washington, DC: American Academy of Pediatrics.

American Academy of Pediatrics (AAP). (2005). Policy Statement: Breastfeeding and the use of human milk. *Pediatrics, 115*(2), 496–507.

Arenson, J., & Drake, P. (2007). *Maternal and newborn health.* Sudbury, MA: Jones and Bartlett Publishers.

Armstrong, P., & Feldman, S. (2007). *A wise birth: Bringing together the best of natural childbirth and modern medicine.* London: Pinter & Martin Limited.

Bennett, S. S. (2007). *Postpartum depression for dummies.* Indianapolis: John Wiley & Sons, Inc.

Blackburn, S. T. (2007). *Maternal, fetal, and neonatal physiology* (3rd ed.). Philadelphia: Saunders Elsevier.

Bowers, P. (2007). *Cultural perspectives in childbearing.* Available at: http://www.nurse.com/ce/course.html?CCID=3245.

Brown, S. H. E. (2006). Tender Beginnings program: An educational continuum for the maternity patient. *Journal of Perinatal & Neonatal Nursing, 20*(3), 210–219.

Cassar, L. (2006). Cultural expectations of Muslims and Orthodox Jews in regard to pregnancy and the postpartum period: A study in comparison and contrast. *International Journal of Childbirth Education, 21*(2), 27–30.

Center for Disease Control and Prevention, Office of Women's Health. (2007). *Overweight and obesity among U.S. adults.* Available at: www.cdc.gov/od/spotlight/nwhw/pubs/overwght.htm.

Centers for Disease Control and Prevention (CDC). (2007). *Adult immunizations.* Available at: http://www.cdc.gov/nip/publications/VIS/vis-mmr.pdf.

Cunningham, F. G., Gant, N. F., Leveno, K. J., Gilstrap, L. C., Hauth, J. C., & Wenstrom, K. D. (2005). *Williams' obstetrics* (22nd ed.). New York: Lippincott Williams & Wilkins.

Druxman, L., & Peterson, C. (2006). Postpartum exercise. *IDEA Fitness Journal, 3*(10), 34–37.

Dudek, S. G. (2006). *Nutrition essentials for nursing practice* (5th ed.). Philadelphia: Lippincott Williams & Wilkins.

Engin-Ustun, Y., Ustun, Y., Cetin, F., Meydanli, M., Kafkasli, A., & Sezgin, B. (2007). Effect of postpartum counseling on postpartum contraceptive use. *Archives of Gynecology & Obstetrics, 275*(6), 429–432.

Escott-Stump, S. (2007). *Nutrition and diagnosis-related care* (6th ed.). Philadelphia: Lippincott Williams & Wilkins.

Ey, J. L. (2007). Postpartum depression. *Clinical Pediatrics, 46*(3), 290–291.

Feldman, R. (2007). Parent-infant synchrony and the construct of shared timing; physiologic precursors, developmental outcomes, and risk conditions. *Journal of Child Psychology & Psychiatry, 48*(3/4), 329–354.

Fooladi, M. M. (2006). Therapeutic tears and postpartum blues. *Holistic Nursing Practice, 20*(4), 204–211.

Fowles, E. R., & Horowitz, A. (2006). Clinical assessment of mothering during infancy. *JOGNN, 35*(5), 662–670.

Grossman, K. E., Grossman, K., & Waters, E. (2006). *Attachment from infancy to adulthood.* New York: Guilford Publications, Inc.

Hackley, B., Kriebs, J. M., & Rousseau, M. E. (2007). *Primary care of women: A guide for midwives and women's health providers.* Sudbury, MA: Jones and Bartlett Publishers.

Insel, P., Ross, D., & Turner, E. (2007). *Nutrition* (3rd ed.) Sudbury, MA: Jones and Bartlett.

Kenner, C., & Lott, J. W. (2007). *Comprehensive neonatal care: An interdisciplinary approach* (4th ed.). St. Louis: Saunders Elsevier.

Kersey-Matusiak, G., Gerace, L. M., Bowers, P., & Salimbene, S. (2007). Cultural competence for the global nurse. *Nursing Spectrum.* Available at: http://www.nurse.com/ce/course.html?CCID=3687.

Kuntz, J. G., Cheesman, J. D., & Powers, R. D. (2006). Acute thrombotic disorders. *American Journal of Emergency Medicine, 24*(4), 460–467.

Langan, R. C. (2006). Discharge procedures for healthy newborns. *American Family Physician, 73*(5), 849–853.

Lawson, M. (2007). Contemporary aspects in infant feeding. *Pediatric Nursing, 19*(2), 39–44.

Lemack, G. E. (2007). Incontinence: Helping women stay in control. *Cortlandt Forum, 20*(1), 53–54.

Logsdon, M. C., Wisner, K. L., & Pinto-Foltz, M. D. (2006). The impact of postpartum depression on mothering. *JOGNN, 35*(5), 652–658.

March of Dimes. (2007). *The postpartum blues.* Available at: http://www.marchofdimes.com/pnhec/188_15754.asp.

Mercer, R. T. (2006). Nursing support of the process of becoming a mother. *JOGNN, 35*(5), 649–651.

Moses, S. (2007). Pulmonary embolism in pregnancy. *Family Practice Notebook.* Available at: http://www.fpnotebook.com/ LUN117.htm.

Nash, L. R. (2007). Postpartum care. In R. E. Rakel & E. T. Bope (Eds.), *Conn's current therapy 2007* (Section 16, pp. 1190–1193). Philadelphia: Saunders Elsevier.

Oppenheim, D., & Goldsmith, D. F. (2007). *Attachment theory in clinical work with children: Bridging the gap between research and practice.* New York: Guilford Publications, Inc.

Pastore, L., Owens, A., & Raymond, C. (2007). Postpartum sexuality concerns among first-time parents from one U.S. academic hospital. *Journal of Sexual Medicine, 4*(1), 115–123.

Rector, L. (2007). *Supporting siblings and their families during intensive baby care.* Baltimore: Paul H. Brookes Publishing.

Runquist, J. (2007). Persevering through postpartum fatigue. *JOGNN, 36*(1), 28–37.

Simpkin, K. R., & James, D. C. (2006). Postpartum care. *Nursing Spectrum.* Available at: http://www.nurse.com/ce/syllabus.html? CCID=3455.

Skidmore-Roth, L. (2007). *Mosby's 2007 nursing drug reference* (20th ed.). St. Louis: Mosby Elsevier.

Srivastava, R. (2007). *The healthcare professional's guide to clinical cultural competence.* Philadelphia: Elsevier Health Sciences.

Steen, M., Briggs, M., & King, D. (2006). Alleviating postnatal perineal trauma: To cool or not to cool? *British Journal of Midwifery, 14*(5), 304–308.

Thomason, A., & DeLancey, J. (2007). Urinary incontinence symptoms during and after pregnancy in continent and incontinent primiparas. *International Urogynecology Journal & Pelvic Floor Dysfunction, 18*(2), 147–151.

Tomasulo, P. (2007). LactMed-New NLM Database on drugs and lactation. *Medical Reference Services Quarterly, 26*(1), 51–58.

United States Department of Agriculture (USDA), United States Department of Health and Human Services (USDHHS). (2005). *Healthy eating pyramid.* Center for Nutrition Policy and Promotion. Available at: www.cnpp.usda.gov/pyramid-update/ index.html.

United States Department of Health and Human Resources (USDHHS), Public Health Department. (2000). *Healthy people 2010.* Available at: www.healthypeople.gov/document/HTML/Volume2/ 16MICH.htm.

United Nations International Children's Emergency Fund (UNICEF). (2007). *The Baby-Friendly Hospital Initiative.* Available at: http://www.unicef.org/programme/breastfeeding/baby.htm#10.

Vaughn, J. E. (2006). Behavioral health. When it's not postpartum blues: Recognizing postpartum depression. *Case Management, 12*(3), 8–9.

Whitehouse, K. (2006). That loving touch. *Practicing Midwife, 9*(3), 22–25.

Wilson, C. L., Rholes, W. S., Simpson, J. A., & Tran, S. (2007). Labor, delivery, and early parenthood: An attachment theory perspective. *Personality and Social Psychology Bulletin, 33*(4), 505–518.

WEBSITES

American College of Nurse-Midwives: www.midwife.org
Association for Perinatal Psychology and Health: www.birthpsychology.com
Association of Maternal & Child Health Programs: www.amchpl.org
Baby-Friendly USA: www.babyfriendlyusa.org
Center for Postpartum Health, www.postpartumhealth.com
Depression after Delivery: www.depressionafterdelivery.com
Home-Based Working Moms: www.hbwm.com
International Lactation Consultants Association: www.ilca.org
La Leche League International: www.lalecheleague.org
Midwifery Today, Inc.: www.midwiferytoday.com
National Alliance for Breast-feeding Advocacy: www.naba-breast-feeding.org
National Center for Fathering: www.fathers.com
National Parenting Center: www.tnpc.com
National Women's Health Information Center: www.4women.gov
Parenthood Web: www.parenthoodweb.com
Parenting Q & A: www.parenting-qa.com
Parents Anonymous, Inc.: www.parentsanonymous.org
Parents Helping Parents: www.php.com

CHAPTER WORKSHEET

MULTIPLE CHOICE QUESTIONS

1. When assessing a postpartum woman, which of the following would lead the nurse to suspect postpartum blues?

   a. Panic attacks and suicidal thoughts

   b. Anger toward self and infant

   c. Periodic crying and insomnia

   d. Obsessive thoughts and hallucinations

2. Which of these activities would best help the postpartum nurse to provide culturally sensitive care for the childbearing family?

   a. Taking a transcultural course

   b. Caring for only families of his or her cultural origin

   c. Teaching Western beliefs to culturally diverse families

   d. Educating himself or herself about diverse cultural practices

3. Which of the following suggestions would be most appropriate to include in the teaching plan for a postpartum woman who needs to lose weight?

   a. Increase fluid intake and acid-producing foods in her diet.

   b. Avoid empty-calorie foods and increase exercise.

   c. Start a high-protein diet and restrict fluids.

   d. Eat no snacks or carbohydrates.

4. After teaching a group of breast-feeding women about nutritional needs, the nurse determines that the teaching was successful when the women state that they need to increase their intake of which nutrients?

   a. Carbohydrates and fiber

   b. Fats and vitamins

   c. Calories and protein

   d. Iron-rich foods and minerals

5. Which of the following would lead the nurse to suspect that a postpartum woman was developing a complication?

   a. Fatigue and irritability

   b. Perineal discomfort and pink discharge

   c. Pulse rate of 60 bpm

   d. Swollen, tender, hot area on breast

6. Which of the following would the nurse assess as indicating positive bonding between the parents and their newborn?

   a. Holding the infant close to the body

   b. Having visitors hold the infant

   c. Buying expensive infant clothes

   d. Requesting that the nurses care for the infant

7. Which activity would the nurse include in the teaching plan for parents with a newborn and an older child to reduce sibling rivalry when the newborn is brought home?

   a. Punishing the older child for bedwetting behavior

   b. Sending the sibling to the grandparents' house

   c. Planning a special time daily for the older sibling

   d. Allowing the sibling to share a room with the infant

8. The major purpose of the first postpartum homecare visit is to:

   a. Identify complications that require interventions

   b. Obtain a blood specimen for PKU testing

   c. Complete the official birth certificate

   d. Support the new parents in their parenting roles

CRITICAL THINKING EXERCISES

1. As a nurse working on a postpartum unit, you enter the room of Ms. Jones, a 22-year-old primipara, and find her chatting on the phone while her newborn is crying loudly in the bassinette, which has been pushed into the bathroom. You pick up and comfort the newborn. While holding the baby, you ask the client if she was aware her newborn was crying. She replies, "That's about all that monkey does since she was born!" You hand the newborn to her and she places the newborn on the bed away from her and continues her phone conversation.

   a. What is your nursing assessment of this encounter?

   b. What nursing interventions would be appropriate?

   c. What specific discharge interventions may be needed?

2. Jennifer Adamson, a 34-year-old single primipara, left the hospital after a 36-hour stay with her newborn son. She lives alone in a one-bedroom walk-up apartment. As the postpartum home health nurse visiting her 2 days later, you find the following:

- Tearful client pacing the floor holding her crying son

- Home cluttered and in disarray

- Fundus firm and displaced to right of midline

- Moderate lochia rubra; episiotomy site clean, dry, and intact

- Vital signs within normal range; pain rating less than 3 points on scale of 1 to 10

- Breasts engorged slightly; supportive bra on

- Newborn assessment within normal limits

- Distended bladder upon palpation; reporting urinary frequency

a. Which of these assessment findings warrants further investigation?

b. What interventions are appropriate at this time, and why?

c. What health teaching is needed before you leave this home?

3. The nurse walks into the room of Lisa Drew, a 24-year-old primigravida. She asks the nurse to hand her the bottle sitting on the bedside table, stating, "I'm going to finish it off because my baby only ate half of it 3 hours ago when I fed him."

a. What response by the nurse would be appropriate at this time?

b. What action should the nurse take?

c. What health teaching is needed for Lisa prior to discharge?

STUDY ACTIVITIES

1. Identify three questions that a nurse would ask a postpartum woman to assess for postpartum blues.

2. Find a website that offers advice to new parents about breast-feeding. Critique the site, the author's credentials, and the accuracy of the content.

3. Outline instructions you would give to a new mother on how to use her peribottle.

4. Breast tissue swelling secondary to vascular congestion after childbirth and preceding lactation describes _____.

5. Listen to the postpartum story of one of your assigned patients and share it with your peers in class or as part of online discussion.

UNIT SIX

THE NEWBORN

NEWBORN ADAPTATION

KEY TERMS

cold stress
jaundice
meconium
neonatal period

neurobehavioral response
neutral thermal
    environment (NTE)

periodic breathing
reflex
thermoregulation

LEARNING OBJECTIVES

Upon completion of the chapter, the learner will be able to:

1. Define the key terms used in this chapter.
2. Identify the major changes in body systems that occur as the newborn adapts to extrauterine life.
3. List the primary challenges faced by the newborn during the adaptation to extrauterine life.
4. Explain the three behavioral patterns of newborn behavioral adaptation.
5. Discuss the five typical behavioral responses of the newborn.

The Healthy Start home care nurse reviewed the patient's file in her car before she got out: 18-year-old primipara, 1 week postpartum with a term newborn girl weighing 7 pounds. The new mother, Maria, greeted the nurse at the door and let her inside the house. After performing a postpartum assessment on Maria and an assessment of her newborn daughter, the nurse asked Maria if she had any questions or concerns. Maria's eyes welled up with tears: she is worried that her daughter can't see.

Wow

Newborns can't always be judged by their outer wrapping; rather, we should focus on the awesome gift inside.

When a child is born, the exhaustion and stress of labor are over for the parents, but now the newborn must begin the work of physiologically and behaviorally adapting to the new environment. The first 24 hours of life can be the most precarious (Blackburn, 2007).

The **neonatal period** is defined as the first 28 days of life. After birth, the newborn is exposed to a whole new world of sounds, colors, smells, and sensations. The newborn, previously confined to the warm, dark, wet intrauterine environment, is now thrust into an environment that is much brighter and cooler. As the newborn adapts to life after birth, numerous physiologic changes occur (Table 17.1).

Awareness of the adaptations that are occurring forms the foundation for providing support to the newborn during this crucial time. Physiologic and behavioral changes occur quickly during this transition period. Being aware of any deviations from the norm is crucial to ensure early identification and prompt intervention.

This chapter describes the physiologic changes of the newborn's major body systems. It also discusses the behavioral adaptations, including behavioral patterns and the newborn's behavioral responses, that occur during this transition period.

Physiologic Adaptations

The mechanics of birth require a change in the newborn for survival outside the uterus. Immediately, respiratory gas exchange, along with circulatory modifications, must occur to sustain extrauterine life. During this time, as newborns strive to attain homeostasis, they also experience complex changes in major organ systems. Although the transition usually takes place within the first 6 to 10 hours of life, many adaptations take weeks to attain full maturity.

Cardiovascular System Adaptations

During fetal life, the heart relies on certain unique structures that assist it in providing adequate perfusion of vital body parts. The umbilical vein carries oxygenated blood from the placenta to the fetus. The ductus venosus allows the majority of the umbilical vein blood to bypass the liver and merge with blood moving through the vena cava, bringing it to the heart sooner. The foramen ovale allows more than half the blood entering the right atrium to cross immediately to the left atrium, thereby passing the pulmonary circulation. The ductus arteriosus connects the pulmonary artery to the aorta, which allows bypassing of the pulmonary circuit. Only a small portion of blood passes through the pulmonary circuit for the main purpose of perfusion of the structure, rather than for oxygenation. The fetus depends on the placenta to provide oxygen and nutrients and to remove waste products.

At birth, the circulatory system must switch from fetal to newborn circulation and from placental to pulmonary gas exchange. The physical forces of the contractions of labor and birth, mild asphyxia, increased intracranial pressure as a result of cord compression and uterine contractions, as well as cold stress immediately experienced after birth lead to an increased release in catecholamines that is critical for the changes involved in the transition to

TABLE 17.1 ANATOMIC AND PHYSIOLOGIC COMPARISON OF THE FETUS AND NEWBORN

Comparison	Fetus	Newborn
Respiratory system	Fluid-filled, high-pressure system causes blood to be shunted from the lungs through the ductus arteriosus to the rest of the body.	Air-filled, low-pressure system encourages blood flow through the lungs for gas exchange; increased oxygen content of blood in the lungs contributes to the closing of the ductus arteriosus (becomes a ligament).
Site of gas exchange	Placenta	Lungs
Circulation through the heart	Pressures in the right atrium are greater than in the left, encouraging blood flow through the foreman ovale.	Pressures in the left atrium are greater than in the right, causing the foreman ovale to close.
Hepatic portal circulation	Ductus venosus bypasses; maternal liver performs filtering functions	Ductus venosus closes (becomes a ligament); hepatic portal circulation begins.
Thermoregulation	Body temperature is maintained by maternal body temperature and the warmth of the intrauterine environment.	Body temperature is maintained through a flexed posture and brown fat.

Source: Klossner, N. J., & Hatfield, N. (2006). *Introductory maternity and pediatric nursing*. Philadelphia: Lippincott Williams & Wilkins.

extrauterine life. The increased levels of epinephrine and norepinephrine stimulate increased cardiac output and contractility, surfactant release, and promotion of pulmonary fluid clearance (Kenner & Lott, 2007).

Fetal Structures

Changes in circulation occur immediately at birth as the fetus separates from the placenta (Fig. 17.1). When the umbilical cord is clamped, the first breath is taken and the lungs begin to function. As a result, systemic vascular resistance increases and blood return to the heart via the inferior vena cava decreases. Concurrently with these changes, there is a rapid decrease in pulmonary vascular resistance and an increase in pulmonary blood flow (Blackburn, 2007). The foramen ovale functionally closes with a decrease in pulmonary vascular resistance, which leads to a decrease in right-sided heart pressures. An increase in systemic pressure, after clamping of the cord, leads to an increase in left-sided heart pressures. Ductus arteriosus, ductus venosus, and umbilical vessels that were vital during fetal life are no longer needed. Over a period of months these fetal vessels form nonfunctional ligaments.

Before birth, the foramen ovale allowed most of the oxygenated blood entering the right atrium from the inferior vena cava to pass into the left atrium of the heart. With the newborn's first breath, air pushes into the lungs, triggering an increase in pulmonary blood flow and pulmonary venous return to the left side of the heart. As a result, the

pressure in the left atrium becomes higher than in the right atrium. The increased left atrial pressure causes the foramen ovale to close, thus allowing the output from the right ventricle to flow entirely to the lungs. With closure of this fetal shunt, oxygenated blood is now separated from nonoxygenated blood. The subsequent increase in tissue oxygenation further promotes the increase in systemic blood pressure and continuing blood flow to the lungs. The foramen ovale normally closes functionally at birth when left atrial pressure increases and right atrial pressure decreases. Permanent anatomic closure, though, really occurs throughout the next several weeks.

During fetal life, the ductus arteriosus, located between the aorta and the pulmonary artery, protected the lungs against circulatory overload by shunting blood (right to left) into the descending aorta, bypassing the pulmonary circulation. Its patency during fetal life is promoted by continual production of prostaglandin E2 (PGE2) by the ductus arteriosus (T. W. Hansen, 2007). The ductus arteriosus becomes functionally closed within the first few hours after birth. Oxygen is the most important factor in controlling its closure. Closure depends on the high oxygen content of the aortic blood resulting from aeration of the lungs at birth. At birth, pulmonary vascular resistance decreases, allowing pulmonary blood flow to increase and oxygen exchange to occur in the lungs. It occurs secondary to an increase in PO_2 coincident with the first breath and umbilical cord occlusion when it is clamped.

FIGURE 17.1 Cardiovascular adaptations of the newborn. Note the changes in oxygenation between (**A**) prenatal circulation and (**B**) postnatal (pulmonary) circulation.

The ductus venosus shunted blood from the left umbilical vein to the inferior vena cava during intrauterine life. It closes within a few days after birth, because this shunting is no longer needed as a result of activation of the liver. The activated liver now takes over the functions of the placenta (which was expelled at birth). The ductus venosus becomes a ligament in extrauterine life.

The two umbilical arteries and one umbilical vein begin to constrict at birth, because with placental expulsion, blood flow ceases. In addition, peripheral circulation increases. Thus, the vessels are no longer needed and they too become ligaments.

Heart Rate

During the first few minutes after birth, the newborn's heart rate is approximately 120 to 180 bpm. Thereafter, it begins to decrease to an average of 120 to 130 bpm (Arenson & Drake, 2007). The newborn is highly dependent on heart rate for maintenance of cardiac output and blood pressure. Although the blood pressure is not taken routinely in the healthy term newborn, it is usually highest after birth and reaches a plateau within a week after birth.

> ▶ **Take** NOTE!
>
> *Transient functional cardiac murmurs may be heard during the neonatal period as a result of the changing dynamics of the cardiovascular system at birth (Wheeler & McCaffrey, 2007).*

The fluctuations in both the heart rate and blood pressure tend to follow the changes in the newborn's behavioral state. An increase in activity, such as wakefulness, movement, or crying, corresponds to an increase in heart rate and blood pressure. In contrast, the compromised newborn demonstrates markedly less physiologic variability overall. Tachycardia may be found with volume depletion, cardiorespiratory disease, drug withdrawal, and hyperthyroidism. Bradycardia is often associated with apnea and is often seen with hypoxia.

Blood Volume

The blood volume of the newborn depends on the amount of blood transferred from the placenta at birth. It is usually estimated to be 80 to 85 mL/kg of body weight in the term infant (Blackburn, 2007). However, the volume may vary as much as 25% to 40%, depending on when clamping of the umbilical cord occurs. Early (before 30 to 40 seconds) or late (after 3 minutes) clamping of the umbilical cord changes circulatory dynamics during transition. Recent studies show the benefits of delayed cord clamping as improving the newborn's cardiopulmonary adaptation, preventing childhood anemia without increasing hypervolemia-related risks, increasing blood pressure, improving oxygen transport, and increasing red blood cell flow. Although a tailored approach is required in the case of cord clamping, the balance of available data suggests that delayed cord clamping should be the method of choice (Levy & Blickstein, 2006; Mercer et al., 2007). Further research is needed to explain the relationship among oxygen transport, red blood cell volume, and initiation of breathing, thereby indicating whether early or delayed cord clamping is beneficial.

Blood Components

Fetal red blood cells are large, but few in number. After birth, the red cell count gradually increases as the cell size decreases, because they live in an environment with much higher PO_2. A newborn's red cells have a life span of 80 to 100 days, compared to 120 days in adults.

Hemoglobin initially declines as a result of a decrease in neonatal red cell mass (physiologic anemia of infancy). Leukocytosis (elevated white blood cells) is present as a result of birth trauma soon after birth. The newborn's platelet count and aggregation ability are the same as adults.

The newborn's hematologic values are affected by the site of the blood sample (capillary blood has higher levels of hemoglobin and hematocrit compared with venous blood), placental transfusion (delayed cord clamping and normal shift of plasma to extravascular spaces, which causes higher levels of hemoglobin and hematocrit), and gestational age (increased age is associated with increased numbers of red cells and hemoglobin) (Blackburn, 2007). Table 17.2 lists normal newborn blood values.

Respiratory System Adaptations

The first breath of life is a gasp that generates an increase in transpulmonary pressure and results in diaphragmatic descent. Hypercapnia, hypoxia, and acidosis resulting from normal labor become stimuli for initiating respirations. Inspiration of air and expansion of the lungs allow for an increase in tidal volume (amount of air brought into the lungs). Surfactant is a surface tension-reducing lipoprotein found in the newborn's lungs that prevents alveolar collapse at the end of expiration and loss of lung volume. It lines the alveoli to enhance aeration of gas-free lungs, thus reducing surface tension and lowering the pressure required to open the alveoli. Normal lung function is dependent upon surfactant, which permits a decrease in

TABLE 17.2 **NORMAL NEWBORN BLOOD VALUES**

Lab Data	Normal Range
Hemoglobin	17–20 g/dL
Hematocrit	52%–63%
Platelets	100,000–300,000/µL
Red blood cells	5.1–5.8 (1,000,000/µL)
White blood cells	10–30,000/mm³

surface tension at end-expiration (to prevent atelectasis) and an increase in surface tension during lung expansion (to facilitate elastic recoil on inspiration). Surfactant provides the lung stability needed for gas exchange. The newborn's first breath, in conjunction with surfactant, overcomes the surface forces to permit aeration of the lungs. The chest wall of the newborn is floppy because of the high cartilage content and poorly developed musculature. Thus, accessory muscles to help in breathing are ineffective.

One of the most crucial adaptations that the newborn makes at birth is adjusting from a fluid-filled intrauterine environment to a gaseous extrauterine environment. During fetal life, the lungs are expanded with an ultrafiltrate of the amniotic fluid. During and after birth, this fluid must be removed and replaced with air. Passage through the birth canal allows intermittent compression of the thorax, which helps eliminate the fluid in the lungs. Pulmonary capillaries and the lymphatics remove the remaining fluid.

If fluid is removed too slowly or incompletely (e.g., with decreased thoracic squeezing during birth or diminished respiratory effort), transient tachypnea (respiratory rate above 60 bpm) of the newborn occurs. Examples of situations involving decreased thoracic compression and diminished respiratory effort include cesarean birth and sedation in newborns (Kenner & Lott, 2007).

▶ **Take** NOTE!

A baby born by cesarean delivery does not have the same benefit of the birth canal squeeze as does the newborn born by vaginal delivery. Closely observe the respirations of the newborn after cesarean delivery.

Lungs

Before the newborn's lungs can maintain respiratory function, the following events must occur:

- Initiation of respiratory movement
- Expansion of the lungs
- Establishment of functional residual capacity (ability to retain some air in the lungs on expiration)
- Increased pulmonary blood flow
- Redistribution of cardiac output (McLenan, 2007)

Initial breathing is probably the result of a reflex triggered by pressure changes, noise, light, chilling, compression of the fetal chest during delivery, and high carbon dioxide and low oxygen concentrations of the newborn's blood. Many theories address the initiation of respiration in the newborn, but most are based on speculation from observations rather than on empirical research (Wheeler & McCaffrey, 2007). Research continues to search for answers to these questions.

Respirations

After respirations are established in the newborn, they are shallow and irregular, ranging from 30 to 60 breaths per minute, with short periods of apnea (less than 15 seconds). The newborn's respiratory rate varies according to his or her activity; the more active the newborn, the higher the respiratory rate, on average. Signs of respiratory distress to observe for include cyanosis, tachypnea, expiratory grunting, sternal retractions, and nasal flaring. Respirations should not be labored, and the chest movements should be symmetric. In some cases, **periodic breathing** may occur, which is the cessation of breathing that lasts 5 to 10 seconds without changes in color or heart rate (Arenson & Drake, 2007). Periodic breathing may be observed in newborns within the first few days of life and requires close monitoring.

▶ **Take** NOTE!

Apneic periods lasting more than 15 seconds with cyanosis and heart rate changes require further evaluation (Kenner & Lott, 2007).

Body Temperature Regulation

Newborns are dependent on their environment for the maintenance of body temperature, much more so immediately after birth than later in life. One of the most important elements in a newborn's survival is obtaining a stable body temperature to promote an optimal transition to extrauterine life. On average, a newborn's temperature ranges from 36.5° to 37.5°C (97.9° to 99.7°F).

Thermoregulation is the process of maintaining the balance between heat loss and heat production. It is a critical physiologic function that is closely related to the transition and survival of the newborn. An appropriate thermal environment is essential for maintaining a normal body temperature. Compared with adults, newborns tolerate a narrower range of environmental temperatures and are extremely vulnerable to both under- and overheating. Nurses play a key role in providing an appropriate environment to help newborns maintain thermal stability.

▶ **Consider** THIS!

When I look down at my little miracle of life in my arms, I can't help but beam with pride at this great accomplishment. She seems so vulnerable and defenseless, and yet is equipped with everything she needs to survive at birth. When the nurse brought my daughter in for the first time after birth, I wanted to see and feel every part of her. Much to my dismay, she was

(continued)

▶ *Consider* THIS! *(continued)*

wrapped up like a mummy in a blanket and she had a pink knit cap on her head. I asked the nurse why all the babies had to look like they were bound for the North Pole with all these layers on. Wasn't she aware it was summertime and probably at least 80 degrees outside?

The nurse explained that newborns lose body heat easily and need to be kept warm until their temperature stabilizes. Even though I wanted to get up close and personal with my baby, I decided to keep the pink polar bear outfit on her.

Thoughts: Newborns may be born with "everything they need to survive" on the outside, but they still experience temperature instability and lose heat through radiation, evaporation, convection, and conduction. Because the newborn's head is the largest body part, a great deal of heat can be lost if a cap is not kept on the head. What guidance can be given to this mother before discharge to stabilize her daughter's temperature while at home? What simple examples can be used to demonstrate your point?

Heat Loss

Newborns have several characteristics that predispose them to heat loss:

- Thin skin with blood vessels close to the surface
- Lack of shivering ability to produce heat involuntarily
- Limited stores of metabolic substrates (glucose, glycogen, fat)
- Limited use of voluntary muscle activity or movement to produce heat
- Large body surface area relative to body weight
- Lack of subcutaneous fat, which provides insulation
- Little ability to conserve heat by changing posture (fetal position)
- No ability to adjust their own clothing or blankets to achieve warmth
- Inability to communicate that they are too cold or too warm

Every newborn struggles to maintain body temperature from the moment of birth, when the newborn's wet body is exposed to the much cooler environment of the birthing room. The amniotic fluid covering the newborn cools as it evaporates rapidly in the low humidity and air-conditioning of the room. The newborn's temperature may decrease 3 to 5 degrees within minutes after leaving the warmth of the mother's uterus (99.6°F) (Mercer et al., 2007).

The transfer of heat depends on the temperature of the environment, air speed, and water vapor pressure or humidity. Heat exchange between the environment and the newborn involves the same mechanisms as those with any physical object and its environment. These mechanisms are conduction, convection, evaporation, and radiation. Prevention of heat loss is a key nursing intervention (Fig. 17.2).

Conduction

Conduction involves the transfer of heat from one object to another when the two objects are in direct contact with each other. Conduction refers to heat fluctuation between the newborn's body surface when in contact with other solid surfaces, such as a cold mattress, scale, or circumcision restraining board. Heat loss by conduction can also occur when touching a newborn with cold hands or when the newborn has direct contact with a colder object such as a metal scale. Using a warmed cloth diaper or blanket to cover any cold surface touching a newborn directly helps to prevent heat loss through conduction.

Convection

Convection involves the flow of heat from the body surface to cooler surrounding air or to air circulating over a body surface. An example of convection-related heat loss would be a cool breeze that flows over the newborn. To prevent heat loss by this mechanism, keep the newborn out of direct cool drafts (open doors, windows, fans, air conditioners) in the environment, work inside an isolette as much as possible and minimize opening portholes that allow cold air to flow inside, and warm any oxygen or humidified air that comes in contact with the newborn. Using clothing and blankets in isolettes is an effective means of reducing the newborn's exposed surface area and providing external insulation. Also, transporting the newborn to the nursery in a warmed isolette, rather than carrying him or her, helps to maintain warmth and reduce exposure to the cool air.

Evaporation

Evaporation involves the loss of heat when a liquid is converted to a vapor. Evaporative loss may be insensible (such as from skin and respiration) or sensible (such as from sweating). Insensible loss occurs, but the individual isn't aware of it. Sensible loss is objective and can be noticed. It depends on air speed and the absolute humidity of the air. For example, when the baby is born, the body is covered with amniotic fluid. The fluid evaporates into the air, leading to heat loss. Heat loss via evaporation also occurs when bathing a newborn. Drying newborns immediately after birth with warmed blankets and placing a cap on their head will help to prevent heat loss through evaporation. In addition, drying the newborn after bathing will help prevent heat loss through evaporation. Promptly changing wet linens, clothes, or diapers will also reduce heat loss and prevent chilling.

A. Conduction

B. Convection

C. Evaporation

D. Radiation

FIGURE 17.2 The four mechanisms of heat loss in the newborn. (**A**) Conduction.
(**B**) Convection. (**C**) Evaporation. (**D**) Radiation.

Radiation

Radiation involves loss of body heat to cooler, solid surfaces in close proximity but not in direct contact with the newborn. The amount of heat loss depends on the size of the cold surface area, the surface temperature of the body, as well as the temperature of the receiving surface area. For example, when a newborn is placed in a single-wall isolette next to a cold window, heat loss from radiation occurs. Newborns will become cold even though they are in a heated isolette. To reduce heat loss by radiation, keep cribs and isolettes away from outside walls, cold windows, and air conditioners. Also, using radiant warmers for transporting newborns and when performing procedures that may expose the newborn to the cooler environment will help reduce heat loss.

A warmed transporter is an enclosed isolette on wheels. A radiant warmer is an open bed with a radiant heat source above. This type of environment allows health care professionals to reach the newborn to carry out procedures and treatments (see Evidence-Based Practice 17.1).

Overheating

The newborn is also prone to overheating. Limited insulation and limited sweating ability can predispose any newborn to overheating. Control of body temperature is achieved via a complex negative feedback system that creates a balance between heat production, heat gain, and heat loss. The primary heat regulator is located in the hypothalamus and the central nervous system. The immaturity of the newborn's central nervous system makes it difficult to create and maintain this balance. Therefore, the newborn can become overheated easily. For example, an isolette that is too warm or one that is left too close to a sunny window may lead to hyperthermia. Although heat production can substantially increase in response to a cool environment, basal metabolic rate and the resultant heat produced cannot be reduced. Over-heating increases fluid loss, the respiratory rate, and the metabolic rate considerably.

Thermoregulation

Thermoregulation, the balance between heat loss and heat production, is related to the newborn's rate of metabolism and oxygen consumption. The newborn attempts to conserve heat and increase heat production in the following ways: increasing the metabolic rate, increasing muscular activity through movement, increasing peripheral vasoconstriction, and assuming a fetal position to hold in heat and minimize exposed body surface area.

An environment in which body temperature is maintained without an increase in metabolic rate or oxygen use is called a **neutral thermal environment (NTE)**. Within an NTE, the rates of oxygen consumption and metabolism are minimal, and internal body temperature is maintained because of thermal balance. It promotes growth and stability and minimizes heat (energy) and water loss (McLenan, 2007). Because newborns have difficulty maintaining their body heat through shivering or other mechanisms, they need a higher environmental temperature to maintain an NTE. If the environmental temperature decreases, the newborn responds by consuming more oxygen. The respiratory rate increases (tachypnea) in re-

---

EVIDENCE-BASED PRACTICE 17.1
Radiant Warmers Versus Incubators for Regulating Body Temperature in Newborns

● Study
Providing a thermoneutral environment is an essential component of the immediate and longer-term care of newborn. The methods currently used include incubators and open-care systems, with or without modifications such as heat shields and plastic wrap. The system used must allow ready access to the infant while minimizing alterations in the immediate environment.

This study was performed to assess the effects of radiant warmers versus incubators on neonatal fluid and electrolyte balance, morbidity, and mortality. Eight studies were included in this review.

▲ Findings
Compared with incubators, radiant warmers caused a statistically significant increase in insensible water loss and a trend toward increased oxygen consumption that was not statistically significant. Due to small numbers, effects on important clinical outcomes could not be adequately assessed. A comparison of radiant warmers with heat shields versus incubators without heat shields showed a trend for increased insensible water loss in the radiant warmer group, but the difference was not statistically significant. No difference was shown in terms of oxygen consumption.

Further randomized controlled trials are required to assess the effects of radiant warmers versus incubators in neonatal care on important short- and long-term outcomes.

■ Nursing Implications
Preventing cold stress in newborns is essential in assisting them to make the physiologic transition to extrauterine life. This study compared two heat sources but failed to reach a clear consensus as to which was better. Nurses can apply these results in caring for newborns by making sure that fluid intake is sufficient to make up for insensible water loss when the baby is under either heat source. In addition, they can assist in future research about heat sources that support thermoregulation in the newborn.

Flenady, V. J., & Woodgate, P. G. (2007). Radiant warmers versus incubators for regulating body temperature in newborn infants. *Cochrane Database of Systematic Reviews,* 00075320-100000000-00251, Issue 4, 2007.

sponse to the increased need for oxygen. As a result, the newborn's metabolic rate increases.

The newborn's primary method of heat production is through nonshivering thermogenesis, a process in which brown fat (adipose tissue) is oxidized in response to cold exposure. Brown fat is a special kind of highly vascular fat found only in newborns. The brown coloring is derived from the fat's rich supply of blood vessels and nerve endings. These fat deposits, which are capable of intense metabolic activity—and thus generate a great deal of heat—are found between the scapulae, at the nape of the neck, in the mediastinum, and in areas surrounding the kidneys and adrenal glands. Brown fat makes up about 2% to 6% of body weight in the full-term newborn (Blackburn, 2007). When the newborn experiences a cold environment, the release of norepinephrine increases, which in turn stimulates brown fat metabolism by the breakdown of triglycerides. Cardiac output increases, increasing blood flow through the brown fat tissue. Subsequently, this blood becomes warmed as a result of the increased metabolic activity of the brown fat.

Newborns can experience heat loss through all four mechanisms, ultimately resulting in cold stress. **Cold stress** is excessive heat loss that requires a newborn to use compensatory mechanisms (such as nonshivering thermogenesis and tachypnea) to maintain core body temperature (Cinar & Filiz, 2006). The consequences of cold stress can be quite severe. As the body temperature decreases, the newborn becomes less active, lethargic, hypotonic, and weaker. All newborns are at risk for cold stress, particularly within the first 12 hours of life. However, preterm newborns are at the greatest risk for cold stress and experience more profound effects than full-term newborns because they have less fat stores, poorer vasomotor responses, and less insulation to cope with a hypothermic event.

Cold stress in the newborn can lead to the following problems if not reversed: depleted brown fat stores, increased oxygen needs, respiratory distress, increased glucose consumption leading to hypoglycemia, metabolic acidosis, jaundice, hypoxia, and decreased surfactant production (McLenan, 2007).

> ▶ *Take NOTE!*
>
> *Nurses must be aware of the thermoregulatory needs of the newborn and must ensure that these needs are met to provide the newborn with the best start possible.*

To minimize the effects of cold stress and maintain an NTE, the following interventions are helpful:

• Prewarming blankets and hats to reduce heat loss through conduction
• Keeping the infant transporter (warmed isolette) fully charged and heated at all times
• Drying the newborn completely after birth to prevent heat loss from evaporation
• Encouraging skin-to-skin contact with the mother if the newborn is stable
• Promoting early breastfeeding to provide fuels for nonshivering thermogenesis
• Using heated and humidified oxygen
• Always using radiant warmers and double-wall isolettes to prevent heat loss from radiation
• Deferring bathing until the newborn is medically stable, and using a radiant heat source while bathing (Fig. 17.3)
• Avoiding the placement of a skin temperature probe over a bony area or one with brown fat, because it does not give an accurate assessment of the whole body temperature (most temperature probes are placed over the liver when the newborn is supine or side-lying)

Hepatic System Function

At birth, the newborn's liver assumes the functions that the placenta handled during fetal life. These functions include

FIGURE 17.3 Bathing a newborn under a radiant warmer to prevent heat loss.

iron storage, carbohydrate metabolism, blood coagulation, and conjugation of bilirubin.

Iron Storage

As red blood cells are destroyed after birth, the iron is released and is stored by the liver until new red cells need to be produced. Newborn iron stores are determined by total body hemoglobin content and length of gestation. At birth, the term newborn has iron stores sufficient to last approximately 4 to 6 months (Garfunkel, Kaczorowski, & Christy, 2007).

Carbohydrate Metabolism

When the placenta is lost at birth, the maternal glucose supply is cut off. Initially, the newborn's serum glucose levels decline. Usually, a term newborn's blood glucose level is 70% to 80% of the maternal blood glucose level (Kenner & Lott, 2007).

Glucose is the main source of energy for the first several hours after birth. With the newborn's increased energy needs after birth, the liver releases glucose from glycogen stores for the first 24 hours. Initiating feedings helps to stabilize the newborn's blood glucose levels. Typically a newborn's blood glucose levels are assessed using a heel stick sample of blood on admission to the nursery and again at approximately 4 hours of age.

Bilirubin Conjugation

The liver is also responsible for the conjugation of bilirubin—a yellow to orange bile pigment produced by the breakdown of red blood cells. In utero, elimination of bilirubin in the blood is handled by the placenta and the mother's liver. However, once the cord is cut, the newborn must now assume this function.

Bilirubin normally circulates in plasma, is taken up by liver cells, and is changed to a water-soluble pigment that is excreted in the bile. This conjugated form of bilirubin is excreted from liver cells as a constituent of bile.

The principal source of bilirubin in the newborn is the hemolysis of erythrocytes. This is a normal occurrence after birth, when fewer red blood cells are needed to maintain extrauterine life.

When red blood cells die after approximately 80 days of life, the heme in their hemoglobin is converted to bilirubin. Bilirubin is released in an unconjugated form called indirect bilirubin, which is fat-soluble. Enzymes, proteins, and different cells in the reticuloendothelial system and liver process the unconjugated bilirubin into conjugated bilirubin or direct bilirubin. This form is water-soluble and now enters the gastrointestinal system via the bile and is eventually excreted through feces. The kidneys also excrete a small amount.

Newborns produce bilirubin at a rate of approximately 6 to 8 mg/kg/day. This is more than twice the production rate in adults, primarily because of relative polycythemia and increased red blood cell turnover. Bilirubin produc-

tion typically declines to the adult level within 10 to 14 days after birth (Maisels, 2006). In addition, the metabolic pathways of the liver are relatively immature and thus cannot conjugate bilirubin as quickly as needed.

Failure of the liver cells to break down and excrete bilirubin can cause an increased amount of bilirubin in the bloodstream, leading to jaundice (Stokowski, 2006). Bilirubin is toxic to the body and must be excreted. Blood tests ordered to determine bilirubin levels measure bilirubin in the serum. Total bilirubin is a combination of indirect (unconjugated) and direct (conjugated) bilirubin.

When unconjugated bilirubin pigment is deposited in the skin and mucous membranes, jaundice typically results. **Jaundice**, also known as icterus, refers to the yellowing of the skin, sclera, and mucous membranes that results from increased bilirubin blood levels. Visible jaundice as a result of increased blood bilirubin levels occurs in more than half of all healthy newborns. Even in healthy term newborns, extremely elevated blood levels of bilirubin during the first week of life can cause kernicterus, a permanent and devastating form of brain damage (W. R. Hansen, 2007).

Common risk factors for the development of jaundice include fetal–maternal blood group incompatibility, prematurity, breastfeeding, drugs (such as diazepam [Valium], oxytocin [Pitocin], sulfisoxazole/erythromycin [Pediazole], and chloramphenicol [Chloromycetin]), maternal gestational diabetes, infrequent feedings, male gender, trauma during birth resulting in cephalhematoma, cutaneous bruising, polycythemia, previous sibling with hyperbilirubinemia, infections such as TORCH (toxoplasmosis, other viruses, rubella, cytomegalovirus, herpes simplex viruses), and ethnicity such as Asian or Native American (W. R. Hansen, 2007).

The causes of newborn jaundice can be classified into three groups based on the mechanism of accumulation:

1. Bilirubin overproduction, such as from blood incompatibility (Rh or ABO), drugs, trauma at birth, polycythemia, delayed cord clamping, and breast milk jaundice
2. Decreased bilirubin conjugation, as seen in physiologic jaundice, hypothyroidism, and breastfeeding
3. Impaired bilirubin excretion, as seen in biliary obstruction (biliary atresia, gallstones, neoplasm), sepsis, chromosomal abnormality (Turner syndrome, trisomy 18 and 21), and drugs (aspirin, acetaminophen, sulfa, alcohol, steroids, antibiotics) (Stokowski, 2006)

Jaundice in the newborn is discussed in more detail in Chapter 24.

Gastrointestinal System Adaptations

The full-term newborn has the capacity to swallow, digest, metabolize, and absorb food taken in soon after birth. At birth, the pH of the stomach contents is mildly acidic, reflecting the pH of the amniotic fluid. The once-sterile gut changes rapidly, depending on what feeding is received.

Mucosal Barrier Protection

An important adaptation of the gastrointestinal system is the development of a mucosal barrier to prevent the penetration of harmful substances (bacteria, toxins, and antigens) present within the intestinal lumen. At birth, the newborn must be prepared to deal with bacterial colonization of the gut. Colonization is dependent on oral intake. It usually occurs within 24 hours of age and is required for the production of vitamin K (Kenner & Lott, 2007). If harmful substances are allowed to penetrate the mucosal epithelial barrier under pathologic conditions, they can cause inflammatory and allergic reactions (Blackburn, 2007).

▶ **Take** NOTE!

Human breast milk provides a passive mechanism to protect the newborn against the dangers of a deficient intestinal defense system. It contains antibodies, viable leukocytes, and many other substances that can interfere with bacterial colonization and prevent harmful penetration.

Stomach and Digestion

The stomach of the newborn has a capacity ranging from 30 to 90 mL, with a variable emptying time of 2 to 4 hours. The cardiac sphincter and nervous control of the stomach is immature, which may lead to uncoordinated peristaltic activity and frequent regurgitation. Immaturity of the pharyngoesophageal sphincter and absence of lower esophageal peristaltic waves also contribute to the reflux of gastric contents. Avoiding overfeeding and stimulating frequent burping may minimize regurgitation. Most digestive enzymes are available at birth, allowing newborns to digest simple carbohydrates and protein. However, they have limited ability to digest complex carbohydrates and fats, because amylase and lipase levels are low at birth. As a result, newborns excrete a fair amount of lipids, resulting in fatty stools.

Adequate digestion and absorption are essential for newborn growth and development. Normally, term newborns lose 5% to 10% of their birthweight as a result of insufficient caloric intake within the first week after birth, shifting of intracellular water to extracellular space, and insensible water loss. To gain weight, the term newborn requires an intake of 108 kcal/kg/day from birth to 6 months of age (Begany & Mascarenhas, 2007).

Bowel Elimination

The frequency, consistency, and type of stool passed by newborns vary widely. The evolution of a stool pattern begins with a newborn's first stool, which is meconium. **Meconium** is composed of amniotic fluid, shed mucosal cells, intestinal secretions, and blood. It is greenish black, has a tarry consistency, and is usually passed within 12 to 24 hours of birth. The first meconium stool passed is sterile, but this changes rapidly with ingestion of bacteria through feedings. After feedings are initiated, a transitional stool develops, which is greenish brown to yellowish brown, thinner in consistency, and seedy in appearance.

▶ **Take** NOTE!

Newborns who are fed early pass stools sooner, which helps to reduce bilirubin buildup.

The last development in the stool pattern is the milk stool. The characteristics differ in breast-fed and formula-fed newborns. The stools of the breast-fed newborn are yellow-gold, loose and stringy to pasty in consistency, and typically sour-smelling. The stools of the formula-fed newborn vary depending on the type of formula ingested. They may be yellow, yellow-green, or greenish and loose, pasty, or formed in consistency, and they have an unpleasant odor.

Renal System Changes

The majority of term newborns void immediately after birth, indicating adequate renal function. Although the newborn's kidneys can produce urine, they are limited in their ability to concentrate it until about 3 months of age, when the kidneys mature. Until that time, a newborn voids frequently and the urine has a low specific gravity (1.001 to 1.020). About six to eight voidings daily is average for most newborns; this indicates adequate fluid intake (Arenson & Drake, 2007).

The renal cortex is relatively underdeveloped at birth and does not reach maturity until 12 to 18 months of age. At birth, the glomerular filtration rate (GFR) is approximately 30% of normal adult values, reaching approximately 50% of normal adult values by the 10th day of life and full adult values by the first year of life (Blackburn, 2007). The low GFR and the limited excretion and conservation capability of the kidney affect the newborn's ability to excrete salt, water loads, and drugs.

▶ **Take** NOTE!

The possibility of fluid overload is increased in newborns; keep this in mind when administering intravenous therapy to a newborn.

Immune System Adaptations

Essential to the newborn's survival is the ability to respond effectively to hostile environmental forces. The newborn's immune system begins working early in gestation, but many of the responses do not function adequately during the early neonatal period. The intrauterine environment usually protects the fetus from harmful microorganisms and the need for defensive immunologic responses. With exposure to a wide variety of microorganisms at birth, the newborn must develop a balance between its host defenses and the hostile environmental organisms to ensure a safe transition to the outside world.

Responses of the immune system serve three purposes: defense (protection from invading organisms), homeostasis (elimination of worn-out host cells), and surveillance (recognition and removal of enemy cells). The newborn's immune system response involves recognition of the pathogen or other foreign material, followed by activation of mechanisms to react against and eliminate it. All immune responses primarily involve leukocytes (white blood cells).

The immune system's responses can be divided into two categories: natural and acquired immunity. These mechanisms are interrelated and interdependent; both are required for immunocompetency.

Natural Immunity

Natural immunity includes responses or mechanisms that do not require previous exposure to the microorganism or antigen to operate efficiently. Physical barriers (such as intact skin and mucous membranes), chemical barriers (such as gastric acids and digestive enzymes), and resident nonpathologic organisms make up the newborn's natural immune system. Natural immunity involves the most basic host defense responses: ingestion and killing of microorganisms by phagocytic cells.

Acquired Immunity

Acquired immunity involves two primary processes: (1) the development of circulating antibodies or immunoglobulins capable of targeting specific invading agents (antigens) for destruction and (2) formation of activated lymphocytes designed to destroy foreign invaders. Acquired immunity is absent until after the first invasion by a foreign organism or toxin.

Immunoglobulins are subdivided into five classes: IgA, IgD, IgE, IgG, and IgM. The newborn depends largely on three immunoglobulins for defense mechanisms: IgG, IgA, and IgM.

IgG is the major immunoglobulin and the most abundant, making up about 80% of all circulating antibodies (Blackburn, 2007). It is found in serum and interstitial fluid. It is the only class able to cross the placenta, with active placental transfer beginning at approximately 20 to 22 weeks' gestation. IgG produces antibodies against bacteria, bacterial toxins, and viral agents.

IgA is the second most abundant immunoglobulin in the serum. IgA does not cross the placenta, and maximum levels are reached during childhood. This immunoglobulin is believed to protect mucous membranes from viruses and bacteria. IgA is predominantly found in the gastrointestinal and respiratory tracts, tears, saliva, colostrum, and breast milk.

▶ **Take** NOTE!

A major source of IgA is human breast milk, so breastfeeding is believed to have significant immunologic advantages over formula feeding (Blackburn, 2007).

IgM is found in blood and lymph fluid and is the first immunoglobulin to respond to infection. It does not cross the placenta, and levels are generally low at birth unless there is a congenital intrauterine infection. IgM offers a major source of protection from blood-borne infections. The predominant antibodies formed during neonatal or intrauterine infection are of this class.

Integumentary System Adaptations

The most important function of the skin is to provide a protective barrier between the body and the environment. It limits the loss of water, prevents absorption of harmful agents, protects thermoregulation and fat storage, and protects against physical trauma. The epidermal barrier begins to develop during mid-gestation and is fully formed by about 32 weeks' gestation. Although the neonatal epidermis is similar to the adult epidermis in thickness and lipid composition, skin development is not complete at birth (Hale, 2007). Although the basic structure is the same as that of an adult, the less mature the newborn, the less mature the skin functions. Fewer fibrils connect the dermis and epidermis in the newborn compared with the adult. Also in a newborn, the risk of injury producing a break in the skin from tape, monitors, and handling is greater than for an adult. In addition, sweat glands are present at birth, but full adult functioning is not present until the second or third year of life (Blackburn, 2007). Exposure to air after birth accelerates epidermal development in all newborns (Hale, 2007).

Newborns vary greatly in appearance. Many of the variations are temporary and reflect the physiologic adaptations that the newborn is experiencing. Skin coloring varies, depending on the newborn's age, race or ethnic group, temperature, and whether he or she is crying. Skin color changes with both the environment and health status. At birth, the newborn's skin is dark red to purple. As the newborn begins to breathe air, the skin color changes to red. This redness normally begins to fade the first day.

Neurologic System Adaptations

The nervous system consists of the brain, spinal cord, 12 cranial nerves, and a variety of spinal nerves that come from the spinal cord. Neurologic development follows cephalocaudal (head to toe) and proximal–distal (center to outside) patterns. Myelin develops early on in sensory impulse transmitters. Thus, the newborn has an acute sense of hearing, smell, and taste. The newborn's sensory capabilities include:

- Hearing—well developed at birth, responds to noise by turning to sound
- Taste—ability to distinguish between sweet and sour by 72 hours old
- Smell—ability to distinguish between mother's breast milk and breast milk from others
- Touch—sensitivity to pain, responds to tactile stimuli
- Vision—ability to focus on objects only in close proximity (7–12 inches away); tracks objects in midline or beyond (90 inches); this is the least mature sense at birth (McLenan, 2007)

Remember Maria, the new mother who is worried that her daughter can't see? What might the new mother notice about her daughter's behavior? What might be the new mother's expectations?

Successful adaptations demonstrated by the respiratory, circulatory, thermoregulatory, and musculoskeletal systems indirectly indicate the central nervous system's successful transition from fetal to extrauterine life, because it plays a major role in all these adaptations. In the newborn, congenital reflexes are the hallmarks of maturity of the central nervous system, viability, and adaptation to extrauterine life.

The presence and strength of a reflex is an important indication of neurologic development and function. A **reflex** is an involuntary muscular response to a sensory stimulus. It is built into the nervous system and does not need the intervention of conscious thought to take effect (Arenson & Drake, 2007). Many neonatal reflexes disappear with maturation, although some remain throughout adulthood.

The arcs of these reflexes end at different levels of the spine and brain stem, reflecting the function of the cranial nerves and motor systems. The way newborns blink, move their limbs, focus on a caretaker's face, turn toward sound, suck, swallow, and respond to the environment are all indications of their neurologic abilities. Congenital defects within the central nervous system are frequently not overt but may be revealed in abnormalities in tone, posture, or behavior (Kenner & Lott, 2007). Damage to the nervous system (birth trauma, perinatal hypoxia) during the birthing process can cause delays in the normal growth, development, and functioning of the newborn. Early identification may help to identify the cause and to start early intervention to decrease long-term complications or permanent sequelae.

Newborn reflexes are assessed to evaluate neurologic function and development. Absent or abnormal reflexes in a newborn, persistence of a reflex past the age when it is normally lost, or redevelopment of an infantile reflex in an older child or adult may indicate neurologic pathology. (See Chapter 18 for a description of newborn reflex assessment.)

The Healthy Start nurse explained to Maria that all newborns are born with some degree of myopia (can't see distances) and that 20/20 vision isn't generally achieved until 2 years of age. What developmental information should the nurse discuss with Maria?

Behavioral Adaptations

In addition to adapting physiologically, the newborn also adapts behaviorally. All newborns progress through a specific pattern of events after birth, regardless of their gestational age or the type of birth they experienced.

Behavioral Patterns

The newborn usually demonstrates a predictable pattern of behavior during the first several hours after birth, characterized by two periods of reactivity separated by a sleep phase. Behavioral adaptation is a defined progression of events triggered by stimuli from the extrauterine environment after birth.

First Period of Reactivity

The first period of reactivity begins at birth and lasts for 30 minutes. The newborn is alert and moving and may appear hungry. This period is characterized by myoclonic movements of the eyes, spontaneous Moro reflexes, sucking motions, chewing, rooting, and fine tremors of the extremities (Dabrowski, 2007). Respiration and heart rate are elevated but gradually begin to slow as the next period begins.

This period of alertness allows parents to interact with their newborn and to enjoy close contact with their new baby (Fig. 17.4). The appearance of sucking and rooting behaviors provides a good opportunity for initiating breastfeeding. Many newborns latch on the nipple and suck well at this first experience.

FIGURE 17.4 The first period of reactivity is an optimal time for interaction.

FIGURE 17.5 Newborn during the second period of reactivity. Note the newborn's wide-eyed interest.

Period of Deceased Responsiveness

At 30 to 120 minutes of age, the newborn enters the second stage of transition—that of sleep or a decrease in activity. This phase is referred to as a period of decreased responsiveness. Movements are less jerky and less frequent. Heart and respiratory rates decline as the newborn enters the sleep phase. The muscles become relaxed, and responsiveness to outside stimuli diminishes. During this phase, it is difficult to arouse or interact with the newborn. No interest in sucking is shown. This quiet time can be used for both mother and newborn to remain close and rest together after labor and the birthing experience.

Second Period of Reactivity

The second period of reactivity begins as the newborn awakens and shows an interest in environmental stimuli. This period lasts 2 to 8 hours in the normal newborn (Vandenberg, 2007). Heart and respiratory rates increase. Peristalsis also increases. Thus, it is not uncommon for the newborn to pass meconium during this period. In addition, motor activity and muscle tone increase in conjunction with an increase in muscular coordination (Fig. 17.5).

Interaction between the mother and the newborn during this second period of reactivity is encouraged if the mother has rested and desires it. This period also provides a good opportunity for the parents to examine their newborn and ask questions.

▶ *Take* NOTE!

Teaching about feeding, positioning for feeding, and diaper-changing techniques can be reinforced during this time.

Newborn Behavioral Responses

Newborns demonstrate several predictable responses when interacting with their environment. How they react to the world around them is termed a **neurobehavioral response**. It comprises predictable periods that are probably triggered by external stimuli.

Expected newborn behaviors include orientation, habituation, motor maturity, self-quieting ability, and social behaviors. Any deviation in behavioral responses requires further assessment, because it may indicate a complex neurobehavioral problem.

Orientation

The response of newborns to stimuli is called orientation. They become more alert when they sense a new stimulus in their environment. Orientation reflects newborns' response to auditory and visual stimuli, demonstrated by their movement of head and eyes to focus on that stimulus. Newborns prefer the human face and bright shiny objects. As the face or object comes into their line of vision, newborns respond by staring at the object intently. Newborns use this sensory capacity to become familiar with people and objects in their surroundings.

Remember Maria, who was concerned about her newborn daughter's vision? She told the nurse that her daughter didn't show any interest in her pastel-colored homemade mobile she had hung across the room from her crib. What suggestions can the nurse make to Maria regarding the placement of the mobile and the types and colors of objects used to promote orientation in her newborn daughter?

Habituation

Habituation is the newborn's ability to process and respond to visual and auditory stimuli—that is, how well and appropriately he or she responds to the environment. Habituation is the ability to block out external stimuli after the newborn has become accustomed to the activity. During the first 24 hours after birth, newborns should increase their ability to habituate to environmental stimuli and sleep. Habituation provides a useful indicator of their neurobehavioral intactness.

Motor Maturity

Motor maturity depends on gestational age and involves evaluation of posture, tone, coordination, and movements. These activities enable newborns to control and coordinate movement. When stimulated, newborns with good motor organization demonstrate movements that are rhythmic and spontaneous. Bringing the hand up to the mouth is an example of good motor organization. As newborns adapt to their new environment, smoother movements should be observed. Such motor behavior is a good indicator of the newborn's ability to respond and adapt accordingly—that is, process stimuli appropriately by the central nervous system.

Self-Quieting Ability

Self-quieting ability refers to newborns' ability to quiet and comfort themselves. Newborns vary in their ability to console themselves or to be consoled. "Consolability" is how newborns are able to change from the crying state to an active alert, quiet alert, drowsy, or sleep state. They console themselves by hand-to-mouth movements and sucking, alerting to external stimuli and motor activity (Arenson & Drake, 2007). Assisting parents to identify consoling behaviors to quiet their newborn if the newborn is not able to self-quiet is important. These behaviors include rocking, holding, gently patting, and softly singing to them.

Social Behaviors

Social behaviors include cuddling and snuggling into the arms of the parent when the newborn is held. Usually newborns are very sensitive to being touched, cuddled, and held. Cuddliness is very important to parents, because they frequently gauge their ability to care for their newborn by the newborn's acceptance or positive response to their actions. This can be assessed by the degree to which the newborn nestles into the contours of the holder's arms. Most newborns cuddle, but some will resist. Assisting parents to assume comforting behaviors (e.g., by cooing while holding their newborn) and praising them for their efforts can help foster cuddling behaviors.

■■■ Key Concepts

- The neonatal period is defined as the first 28 days of life. As the newborn adapts to life after birth, numerous physiologic changes occur.

- At birth, the cardiopulmonary system must switch from fetal to neonatal circulation and from placental to pulmonary gas exchange.
- One of the most crucial adaptations that the newborn makes at birth is the adjustment of a fluid medium exchange from the placenta to the lungs and that of a gaseous environment.
- Neonatal RBCs have a life span of 80 to 100 days in comparison with the adult RBC life span of 120 days, which causes several adjustment problems.
- Thermoregulation is the maintenance of balance between heat loss and heat production. It is a critical physiologic function that is closely related to the transition and survival of the newborn.
- The newborn's primary method of heat production is through nonshivering thermogenesis, a process in which brown fat (adipose tissue) is oxidized in response to cold exposure. Brown fat is a special kind of highly vascular fat found only in newborns.
- Heat loss in the newborn is the result of four mechanisms: conduction, convection, evaporation, and radiation.
- Responses of the immune system serve three purposes: defense (protection from invading organisms), homeostasis (elimination of worn-out host cells), and surveillance (recognition and removal of enemy cells).
- In the newborn, congenital reflexes are the hallmarks of maturity of the central nervous system, viability, and adaptation to extrauterine life.
- The newborn usually demonstrates a predictable pattern of behavior during the first several hours after birth, characterized by two periods of reactivity separated by a sleep phase.

REFERENCES

Arenson, J., & Drake, P. (2007). *Maternal and newborn health.* Sudbury, MA: Jones and Bartlett Publishers.

Begany, M., & Mascarenhas, M. (2007). Normal infant feeding. In R. E. Rakel & E. T. Bope (Eds.), *Conn's current therapy 2007* (Section 16, pp. 1210–1214). Philadelphia: Saunders Elsevier.

Blackburn, S. T. (2007). *Maternal fetal and neonatal physiology: A clinical perspective.* (3rd ed.). Philadelphia: Saunders Elsevier.

Cinar, N. D., & Filiz, T. M. (2006). Neonatal thermoregulation. *Journal of Neonatal Nursing, 12*(2), 69–74.

Dabrowski, G. A. (2007). Skin-to-skin contact: Giving birth back to mothers and babies. *AWHONN Lifelines, 11*(1), 64–71.

Garfunkel, L. C., Kaczorowski, J., & Christy, C. (2007). *Pediatric clinical advisor: Instant diagnosis and treatment* (2nd ed.). St. Louis, MO: Mosby Elsevier Health Sciences.

Hale, R. (2007). Protecting neonates' delicate skin. *British Journal of Midwifery, 15*(4), 231–235.

Hansen, T. W. (2007). Patency of the ductus arteriosus in the newborn—now you want it, now you don't. *Pediatric Critical Care Medicine, 8*(3), 302–303.

Hansen, W. R. (2007). Neonatal jaundice. *eMedicine.* Available at: http://www.emedicine.com/ped/topic1061.htm.

Kenner, C., & Lott, J. W. (2007). *Comprehensive neonatal care: An interdisciplinary approach* (4th ed.). St. Louis, MO: Saunders Elsevier.

Levy, T., & Blickstein, I. (2006). Timing of cord clamping revisited. *Journal of Perinatal Medicine, 34*(4), 293–297.

Maisels, M. J. (2006). Neonatal jaundice. *Pediatrics in Review, 27*(12), 443–454.

McLenan, D. (2007). Care of the high-risk neonate. In R. E. Rakel & E. T. Bope (Eds.), *Conn's current therapy 2007* (Section 16, pp. 1200–1210). Philadelphia: Saunders Elsevier.

Mercer, J. S., Erickson-Owens, D. A., Graves, B., & Haley, M. M. (2007). Evidence-based practices for the fetal to newborn transition. *Journal of Midwifery & Women's Health, 52*(3), 262–272.

Stokowski, L. A. (2006). Foundations in newborn care: Fundamentals of phototherapy for neonatal jaundice. *Advances in Neonatal Care, 6*(6), 303–312.

Vandenberg, K. A. (2007). State systems development in high-risk newborns in the neonatal intensive care unit: Identification and management of sleep, alertness, and crying. *Journal of Perinatal & Neonatal Nursing, 21*(2), 130–139.

Wheeler, D. S., & McCaffrey, M. J. (2007). Resuscitation of the newborn. In R. E. Rakel & E. T. Bope (Eds.), *Conn's current therapy 2007* (Section 16, pp. 1193–1200). Philadelphia: Saunders Elsevier.

WEBSITES

Academy of Neonatal Nursing: www.academyonline.org
American Academy of Pediatrics: www.aap.org
National Association of Neonatal Nurses: www.nann.org
Neonatal Network: www.neonatalnetwork.com

CHAPTER WORKSHEET

MULTIPLE CHOICE QUESTIONS

1. When assessing the term newborn, the following are observed: newborn is alert, heart and respiratory rates have stabilized, and meconium has been passed. The nurse determines that the newborn is exhibiting behaviors indicating:

   a. Initial period of reactivity

   b. Second period of reactivity

   c. Decreased responsiveness period

   d. Period of sleep

2. When caring for a newborn, the nurse ensures that the doors of the nursery are closed and minimizes opening of the isolette portholes to prevent heat loss via which mechanism?

   a. Conduction

   b. Evaporation

   c. Convection

   d. Radiation

3. After teaching a group of nursing students about thermoregulation and appropriate measures to prevent heat loss by evaporation, which of the following student behaviors would indicate successful teaching?

   a. Transporting the newborn in an isolette

   b. Maintaining a warm room temperature

   c. Placing the newborn on a warmed surface

   d. Drying the newborn immediately after birth

4. After birth, the nurse would expect which fetal structure to close as a result of increases in the pressure gradients on the left side of the heart?

   a. Foramen ovale

   b. Ductus arteriosus

   c. Ductus venosus

   d. Umbilical vein

5. Which of the following newborns could be described as breathing normally?

   a. Newborn A is breathing deeply, with a regular rhythm, at a rate of 20 bpm

   b. Newborn B is breathing diaphragmatically with sternal retractions, at a rate of 70 bpm

   c. Newborn C is breathing shallowly, with 40-second periods of apnea and cyanosis

   d. Newborn D is breathing shallowly, at a rate of 36 bpm, with short periods of apnea

6. When assessing a term newborn (6 hours old), the nurse auscultates bowel sounds and documents recent passing of meconium. These findings would indicate:

   a. Abnormal gastrointestinal newborn transition and need to be reported

   b. An intestinal anomaly that needs immediate surgery

   c. A patent anus with no bowel obstruction and normal peristalsis

   d. A malabsorption syndrome resulting in fatty stools

CRITICAL THINKING EXERCISES

1. As the nurse manager, you have been orienting a new nurse in the nursery for the past few weeks. Although she has been demonstrating adequacy with most procedures, today you observe her bathing several newborns without covering them, weighing them on the scale without a cover, leaving the storage door open with the transporter nearby, and leaving the newborns' head covers and blankets off after showing them to family members through the nursery observation window.

   a. What is your impression of this behavior?

   b. What principles concerning thermoregulation need to be reinforced?

   c. How will you evaluate whether your instructions have been effective?

2. The most important adaptations for the newborn to make after birth are to establish respirations, make cardiovascular adjustments, and establish thermoregulation. Nursing care focuses on monitoring and supporting adjustments to extrauterine adaptation. Write appropriate nursing intervention to help achieve the following newborn adaptations:

   a. Respiratory adaptation

   b. Safety, including prevention of infection

   c. Thermoregulation

STUDY ACTIVITIES

1. While in the nursery clinical setting, identify the period of behavioral reactivity (first, inactivity, or second period) for two newborns born at different times. Share your findings in post-conference that clinical day.

2. Obtain a set of vital signs (temperature, pulse, respiration) of a newborn on admission to the nursery. Repeat this procedure and compare changes in the values several hours later. Discuss what changes in the vital signs you would expect during this transitional period.

3. Find two websites about transition to extrauterine life that can be shared with other nursing students as well as nursery nurses. Critique the information presented in terms of how accurate and current it is.

4. The most common mechanism of heat loss in the newborn is _____.

NURSING MANAGEMENT OF THE NEWBORN

KEY TERMS

acrocyanosis
Apgar score
caput succedaneum
cephalhematoma
circumcision
Epstein's pearls
erythema toxicum

gestational age
harlequin sign
infant abduction
immunizations
milia
molding
Mongolian spots

nevus flammeus
nevus vasculosus
ophthalmia neonatorum
phototherapy
pseudomenstruation
stork bites
vernix caseosa

LEARNING OBJECTIVES

Upon completion of the chapter, the learner will be able to:

1. Define the key terms.
2. Discuss the assessments performed during the immediate newborn period.
3. Select interventions that meet the immediate needs of the term newborn.
4. List the components of a typical physical examination of a newborn.
5. Identify common variations that can be noted during a newborn's physical examination.
6. List common concerns in the newborn and appropriate interventions.
7. Compare the importance of the newborn screening tests.
8. Explain common interventions that are appropriate during the early newborn period.
9. Discuss the nurse's role in meeting the newborn's nutritional needs.
10. Outline discharge planning content and education needed for the family with a newborn.

*K*elly, a 16-year-old first-time mother, calls the hospital maternity unit 3 days after being discharged home. She tells the nurse that her newborn son "looks like a canary" and "isn't nursing well." She wonders what is wrong.

Wow

You can send a more powerful message with your actions and behavior than with words alone.

Immediately after the birth of a newborn, all parents are faced with the task of learning and understanding as much as possible about caring for this new family member, even if the parents already have other children. In their new or expanded role as parents, they will face many demands and challenges. For most, this is a wonderful, exciting time filled with many discoveries and much information.

Parents learn as they watch the nurse interacting with their newborn. Nurses play a major role in teaching parents about normal newborn characteristics and about ways to foster optimal growth and development. This role is even more important today because of limited hospital stays.

The newborn has come from a dark, small, enclosed space in the mother's uterus into the bright, cold extrauterine environment. Nurses can easily forget that they are caring for a small human being who is experiencing his or her first taste of human interaction outside the uterus. The newborn period is an extremely important one, and two National Health Goals have been developed to address this critical period.

HEALTHY PEOPLE 2010

Objective	Significance
Increase the proportion of mothers who breast-feed their babies during the early postpartum period from a baseline of 64% to 75%. Increase the proportion of mothers who breast-feed at 6 months from a baseline of 29% to 50%. Increase the proportion of mothers who breast-feed at 1 year from a baseline of 16% to 25%. Ensure appropriate newborn bloodspot screening, newborn hearing screening, follow-up testing, and referral services. Ensure that all newborns are screened at birth for conditions mandated by their state-sponsored newborn screening programs. Ensure that follow-up diagnostic testing for screening positives is performed within an appropriate time period.	• Will emphasize the importance of breast milk as the most complete form of nutrition for infants • Will help to promote infant health, growth, immunity, and development throughout the newborn and infant periods • Will help to foster early detection and prompt treatment for conditions, thereby lessening the incidence of illness, disability, and death associated with these conditions and their overall effects on the newborn, infant, and family

Source: U.S. DHHS, 2000.

It is also easy to overlook the intensity with which parents and visitors observe the actions of nurses as they care for the new family member. Nurses need to serve as a model for giving nurturing care to newborns.

This chapter provides information about assessment and interventions in the period immediately following the birth of a newborn and during the early newborn period.

Nursing Management During the Immediate Newborn Period

The period of transition from intrauterine to extrauterine life occurs during the first several hours after birth. During this time, the newborn is undergoing numerous adaptations, many of which are occurring simultaneously (see Chap. 17 for more information on the newborn's adaptation). The neonate's temperature, respiration, and cardiovascular dynamics stabilize during this period. Close observation of the newborn's status is essential. Careful examination of the newborn at birth can detect anomalies, birth injuries, and disorders that can compromise adaptation to extrauterine life. Problems that occur during this critical time can have a lifelong impact.

Assessment

The initial newborn assessment is completed in the birthing area to determine whether the newborn is stable enough to stay with the parents or whether resuscitation or immediate interventions are necessary. A second assessment is done within the first 2 to 4 hours, when the newborn is admitted to the nursery. A third assessment is completed before discharge. The purpose of these assessments is to determine whether the baby is normal, to provide information to the parents, and to identify apparent physical abnormalities (Arenson & Drake, 2007).

During the initial newborn assessment, look for signs that might indicate a problem, including:

• Nasal flaring
• Chest retractions
• Grunting on exhalation
• Labored breathing
• Generalized cyanosis
• Abnormal breath sounds: rhonchi, crackles (rales), wheezing, stridor
• Abnormal respiratory rates (tachypnea, more than 60 breaths/minute; bradypnea, less than 25 breaths/minute)
• Flaccid body posture
• Abnormal heart rates (tachycardia, more than 160 bpm; bradycardia, less than 100 bpm)
• Abnormal newborn size: small or large for gestational age

If any of these findings are noted, medical intervention may be necessary.

Apgar Scoring

The **Apgar score**, introduced in 1952 by Dr. Virginia Apgar, is used to evaluate newborns at 1 minute and 5 minutes after birth. An additional Apgar assessment is done at 10 minutes if the 5-minute score is less than 7 points (Keenan, 2006). Assessment of the newborn at 1 minute provides data about the newborn's initial adaptation to extrauterine life. Assessment at 5 minutes provides a clearer indication of the newborn's overall central nervous system status.

Five parameters are assessed with Apgar scoring. A quick way to remember the parameters of Apgar scoring is as follows:

- A = appearance (color)
- P = pulse (heart rate)
- G = grimace (reflex irritability)
- A = activity (muscle tone)
- R = respiratory (respiratory effort)

Each parameter is assigned a score ranging from 0 to 2 points. A score of 0 points indicates an absent or poor response; a score of 2 points indicates a normal response (Table 18.1). A normal newborn's score should be 8 to 10 points. The higher the score, the better the condition of the newborn. If the Apgar score is 8 points or higher, no intervention is needed other than supporting normal respiratory efforts and maintaining thermoregulation. Scores of 4 to 7 points signify moderate difficulty and scores of 0 to 3 points represent severe distress in adjusting to extrauterine life. The Apgar score is influenced by the presence of infection, congenital anomalies, physiologic immaturity, maternal sedation via medications, and neuromuscular disorders (Keenan, 2006).

When the newborn experiences physiologic depression, the Apgar score characteristics disappear in a predictable manner: first the pink coloration is lost, next the respiratory effort, and then the tone, followed by reflex irritability and finally heart rate (Kenner & Lott, 2007).

▶ *Take* NOTE!

Although Apgar scoring is done at 1 and 5 minutes, it also can be used as a guide during the immediate newborn period to evaluate the newborn's status for any changes because it focuses on critical parameters that must be assessed throughout the early transition period.

Length and Weight

Parents are eager to know their newborn's length and weight. These measurements are taken soon after birth. A disposable tape measure or a built-in measurement board located on the side of the scale can be used. Length is measured from the head of the newborn to the heel with the newborn unclothed (Fig. 18.1). Because of the flexed position of the newborn after birth, place the newborn in a supine position and extend the leg completely when measuring the length. The expected length of a full-term newborn is usually 48 to 53 cm (19 to 21 inches). Molding can affect measurement (Dillon, 2007).

TABLE 18.1 **APGAR SCORING FOR NEWBORNS**

Parameter (Assessment Technique)	0 Point	1 Point	2 Points
Heart rate (auscultation of apical heart rate for 1 full minute)	Absent	Slow (<100 bpm)	>100 bpm
Respiratory effort (observation of the volume and vigor of the newborn's cry; auscultation of depth and rate of respirations)	Apneic	Slow, irregular, shallow	Regular respirations (usually 30–60 breaths/minute), strong, good cry
Muscle tone (observation of extent of flexion in the newborn's extremities and newborn's resistance when the extremities are pulled away from the body)	Limp, flaccid	Some flexion, limited resistance to extension	Tight flexion, good resistance to extension with quick return to flexed position after extension
Reflex irritability (flicking of the soles of the feet or suctioning of the nose with a bulb syringe)	No response	Grimace or frown when irritated	Sneeze, cough, or vigorous cry
Skin color (inspection of trunk and extremities with the appropriate color for ethnicity appearing within minutes after birth)	Cyanotic or pale	Appropriate body color; blue extremities (acrocyanosis)	Completely appropriate color (pink on both trunk and extremities)

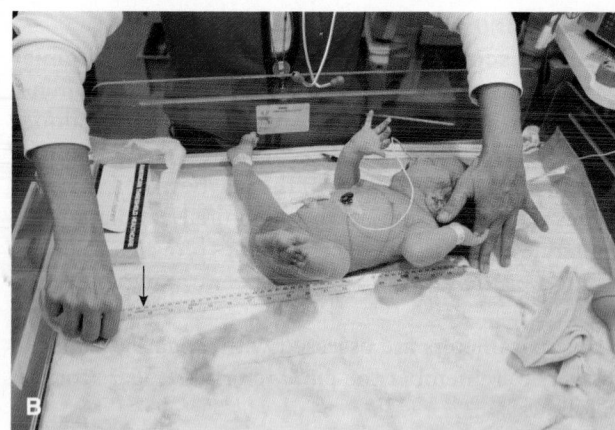

FIGURE 18.1 Measuring a newborn's length. (**A**) The nurse extends the newborn's leg and marks the pad at the heel. (**B**) The nurse measures from the newborn's head to the heel mark.

Most often, newborns are weighed using a digital scale that reads the weight in grams. Typically, the term newborn weighs 2,700 to 4,000 g (6 to 9 lb; Fig. 18.2). Birthweights less than 10% or more than 90% on a growth chart are outside the normal range and need further investigation. Weights taken at later times are compared with previous weights and are documented with regard to gain or loss on a nursing flow sheet. Newborns typically lose approximately 10% of their initial birth weight by 3 to 4 days of age secondary to loss of meconium, extracellular fluid, and

FIGURE 18.2 Weighing a newborn. Note how the nurse guards the newborn from above to prevent injury.

limited food intake. This weight loss is usually regained by the 10th day of life (Kliegman et al., 2007).

Newborns can be classified by their birthweight regardless of their gestational age (AAP, 2007a) as follows:

- Low birthweight: <2,500 g (<5.5 lb)
- Very low birthweight: <1,500 g (<3.5 lb)
- Extremely low birthweight: <1,000 g (<2.5 lb)

Vital Signs

Heart rate and respiratory rate are assessed immediately after birth with Apgar scoring. Heart rate, obtained by taking an apical pulse for 1 full minute, typically is 120 to 160 bpm. Newborns' respirations are assessed when they are quiet or sleeping. Place a stethoscope on the right side of the chest and count the breaths for 1 full minute to identify any irregularities. The newborn respiratory rate is 30 to 60 breaths/minute with symmetric chest movement. Heart and respiratory rates are assessed every 30 minutes until stable for 2 hours after birth. Once stable, the heart rate and respiratory rates are checked every 8 hours (Kenner & Lott, 2007).

Axillary temperature is typically assessed not immediately after birth but on admission to the nursery or when the initial newborn assessment is carried out (e.g., the LDR room). The normal axillary temperature for a term newborn is 36.5° to 37.5°C (97.9° to 99.7°F). Rectal temperatures are no longer taken because of the risk of perforation (Blackburn, 2007). The thermometer or temperature probe is held in the midaxillary space according to manufacturer's directions and hospital protocol. Temperature is reassessed every 30 minutes until it has been stable for 2 hours, then every 8 hours until discharge (Kliegman et al., 2007).

Blood pressure is not usually assessed as part of a normal newborn examination unless there is a clinical indication or low Apgar scores. If assessed, an oscillometer (Dinamap) is used. The typical range is 50 to 75 mmHg

TABLE 18.2 NEWBORN VITAL SIGNS

Newborn Vital Signs	Ranges of values
Temperature	36.5° to 37.5°C (97.9° to 99.7°F)
Heart rate (pulse)	120 to 160 bpm; can increase to 180 during crying
Respirations	30 to 60 breaths/minute at rest; will increase with crying
Blood pressure	50 to 75 mmHg systolic, 30 to 45 mmHg diastolic

(systolic) and 30 to 45 mmHg (diastolic). Crying, moving, and late clamping of the umbilical cord will increase systolic pressure (Dillon, 2007).

Typical values for newborn vital signs are provided in Table 18.2.

Gestational Age Assessment

To determine a newborn's **gestational age** (the stage of maturity), physical signs and neurologic characteristics are assessed. Typically, gestational age is determined by using a tool such as the Dubowitz/Ballard or New Ballard Score system (Fig. 18.3). This scoring system provides an objective estimate of gestational age by scoring the specific parameters of physical and neuromuscular maturity. Points are given for each assessment parameter, with a low score of −1 point or −2 points for extreme immaturity to 4 or 5 points for postmaturity. The scores from each section are added together to correspond to a specific gestational age in weeks.

The physical maturity section of the examination is done during the first 2 hours after birth. The physical maturity assessment section of the Ballard examination evaluates physical characteristics that appear different at different stages depending on a newborn's gestational maturity. Newborns who are physically mature have higher scores than those who are not. The areas assessed on the physical maturity examination include:

• Skin texture—typically ranges from sticky and transparent to smooth, with varying degrees of peeling and cracking, to parchment-like or leathery with significant cracking and wrinkling
• Lanugo—soft downy hair on the newborn's body, which is absent in preterm newborns, appears with maturity, and then disappears again with postmaturity
• Plantar creases—creases on the soles of the feet, which range from absent to covering the entire foot, depending on maturity (the greater the number of creases, the greater the newborn's maturity)
• Breast tissue—the thickness and size of breast tissue and areola (the darkened ring around each nipple), which range from being imperceptible to full and budding

• Eyes and ears—eyelids can be fused or open and ear cartilage and stiffness determine the degree of maturity (the greater the amount of ear cartilage with stiffness, the greater the newborn's maturity)
• Genitals—in males, evidence of testicular descent and appearance of scrotum (which can range from smooth to covered with rugae) determine maturity; in females, appearance and size of clitoris and labia determine maturity (a prominent clitoris with flat labia suggests prematurity, whereas a clitoris covered by labia suggests greater maturity)

The neuromuscular maturity section typically is completed within 24 hours after birth. Six activities or maneuvers that the newborn performs with various body parts are evaluated to determine the newborn's degree of maturity:

1. Posture—How does the newborn hold his or her extremities in relation to the trunk? The greater the degree of flexion, the greater the maturity. For example, extension of arms and legs is scored as 0 point and full flexion of arms and legs is scored as 4 points.
2. Square window—How far can the newborn's hands be flexed toward the wrist? The angle is measured and scored from more than 90 degrees to 0 degrees to determine the maturity rating. As the angle decreases, the newborn's maturity increases. For example, an angle of more than 90 degrees is scored as −1 point and an angle of 0 degrees is scored as 4 points.
3. Arm recoil—How far do the newborn's arms "spring back" to a flexed position? This measure evaluates the degree of arm flexion and the strength of recoil. The reaction of the arm is then scored from 0 to 4 points based on the degree of flexion as the arms are returned to their normal flexed position. The higher the points assigned, the greater the neuromuscular maturity (for example, recoil less than a 90-degree angle is scored as 4 points).
4. Popliteal angle—How far will the newborn's knees extend? The angle created when the knee is extended is measured. An angle less than 90 degrees indicates greater maturity. For example, an angle of 180 degrees is scored as −1 point and an angle of less than 90 degrees is scored as 5 points.
5. Scarf sign—How far can the elbows be moved across the newborn's chest? An elbow that does not reach midline indicates greater maturity. For example, if the elbow reaches or nears the level of the opposite shoulder, this is scored as −1 point; if the elbow does not cross the proximate axillary line, it is scored as 4 points.
6. Heel to ear—How close can the newborn's feet be moved to the ears? This maneuver assesses hip flexibility: the lesser the flexibility, the greater the newborn's maturity. The heel-to-ear assessment is scored in the same manner as the scarf sign.

NEUROMUSCULAR MATURITY

NEUROMUSCULAR MATURITY SIGN	SCORE							RECORD SCORE HERE
	−1	0	1	2	3	4	5	
POSTURE								
SQUARE WINDOW (Wrist)	>90°	90°	60°	45°	30°	0°		
ARM RECOIL		180°	140°–180°	110°–140°	90°–110°	<90°		
POPLITEAL ANGLE	180°	160°	140°	120°	100°	90°	<90°	
SCARF SIGN								
HEEL TO EAR								
						TOTAL NEUROMUSCULAR MATURITY SCORE		

SCORE

Neuromuscular ——
Physical ——
Total ——

MATURITY RATING

Score	Weeks
−10	20
−5	22
0	24
5	26
10	28
15	30
20	32
25	34
30	36
35	38
40	40
45	42
50	44

PHYSICAL MATURITY

PHYSICAL MATURITY SIGN	SCORE							RECORD SCORE HERE
	−1	0	1	2	3	4	5	
SKIN	sticky, friable, transparent	gelatinous, red, translucent	smooth, pink, visible veins	superficial peeling and/or rash, few veins	cracking pale areas, rare veins	parchment, deep cracking, no vessels	leathery, cracked, wrinkled	
LANUGO	none	sparse	abundant	thinning	bald areas	mostly bald		
PLANTAR SURFACE	heel-toe 40–50 mm: −1 <40 mm: −2	>50 mm no crease	faint red marks	anterior transverse crease only	creases ant. 2/3	creases over entire sole		
BREAST	imperceptible	barely perceptible	flat areola no bud	stippled areola 1–2 mm bud	raised areola 3–4 mm bud	full areola 5–10 mm bud		
EYE-EAR	lids fused loosely: −1 tightly: −2	lids open pinna flat stays folded	sl. curved pinna; soft; slow recoil	well-curved pinna; soft but ready recoil	formed and firm instant recoil	thick cartilage, ear stiff		
GENITALS (Male)	scrotum flat, smooth	scrotum empty, faint rugae	testes in upper canal, rare rugae	testes descending, few rugae	testes down, good rugae	testes pendulous, deep rugae		
GENITALS (Female)	clitoris prominent and labia flat	prominent clitoris and small labia minora	prominent clitoris and enlarging minora	majora and minora equally prominent	majora large, minora small	majora cover clitoris and minora		
						TOTAL PHYSICAL MATURITY SCORE		

FIGURE 18.3 Gestational age assessment tool. (Ballard, J. L., Khoury, J. C., Wedig, K., et al. [1991]. New Ballard Score, expanded to include extremely premature infants. *Journal of Pediatrics, 119*[3], 417–423.)

After the scoring is completed, the 12 scores are totaled and then compared with standardized values to determine the appropriate gestational age in weeks. Scores range from very low in preterm newborns to very high for mature and postmature newborns.

Typically newborns are also classified according to gestational age as:

- Preterm or premature—born before 37 weeks' gestation, regardless of birthweight
- Term—born between 38 and 42 weeks' gestation
- Postterm or postdates—born after completion of week 42 of gestation
- Postmature—born after 42 weeks and demonstrating signs of placental aging

Using the information about gestational age and then considering birthweight, newborns can also be classified as follows:

- Small for gestational age (SGA)—weight less than the 10th percentile on standard growth charts (usually <5.5 lb)
- Appropriate for gestational age (AGA)—weight between 10th and 90th percentiles
- Large for gestational age (LGA)—weight more than the 90th percentile on standard growth charts (usually >9 lb)

Chapter 23 describes these variations in birthweight and gestational age in greater detail.

> ▶ *Take* NOTE!
>
> *Gestational age assessment is important because it allows the nurse to plot growth parameters and to anticipate problems related to prematurity, postmaturity, and growth abnormalities.*

Nursing Interventions

During the immediate newborn period, care focuses on helping the newborn to make the transition to extrauterine life. The nursing interventions include maintaining airway patency, ensuring proper identification, administering prescribed medications, and maintaining thermoregulation.

Maintaining Airway Patency

Immediately after birth, a newborn is suctioned to remove fluids and mucus from the mouth and nose. Typically, the newborn's mouth is suctioned first with a bulb syringe to remove debris and then the nose is suctioned. Suctioning in this manner helps to prevent aspiration of fluid into the lungs by an unexpected gasp.

When suctioning a newborn with a bulb syringe, compress the bulb before placing it into the oral or nasal cavity. Release bulb compression slowly, making sure the tip is placed away from the mucous membranes to draw up the excess secretions. Remove the bulb syringe from the mouth or nose, and then, while holding the bulb syringe tip over an emesis basin lined with paper towel or tissue, compress the bulb to expel the secretions. Repeat the procedure several times until all secretions are removed.

> ▶ *Take* NOTE!
>
> *Always keep a bulb syringe near the newborn in case he or she develops sudden choking or a blockage in the nose.*

Ensuring Proper Identification

Before the newborn and family leave the birthing area, be sure that agency policy about identification is followed. Typically, the mother and newborn, and possibly the father, receive matching identification bracelets. The newborn commonly receives two ID bracelets, one on a wrist and one on an ankle. The mother receives a matching one, usually on her wrist. The ID bands usually state name, gender, date and time of birth, and identification number. The same identification number is on the bracelets of all the family members.

These ID bracelets provide for the safety of the newborn and must be secured before the mother and newborn leave the birthing area. The ID bracelets are checked by all nurses to validate that the correct newborn is brought to the right mother if they are separated for any period of time (Fig. 18.4). They also serve as the official newborn identification and are checked before initiating any procedure on that newborn and on discharge from the unit (AAP, 2007). Taking the newborn's picture within 2 hours after birth with a color camera or color video/digital image also helps prevent mix-ups and abduction. Some facilities use electronic devices that sound an alarm if the newborn is removed from the area.

Newborns' footprints may also be taken, using a form that includes the mother's fingerprint, name, and date and time of the birth. Some states require footprints of the newborn, although many studies point out that birthing room staff members do not take consistently legible footprints suitable for identification purposes (Kenner & Lott, 2007). Many states have stopped requiring newborn footprints, and thus other means of identification are needed, such as collecting cord blood at the time of birth for DNA testing and live scans to capture digital forensic-quality prints that are suitable for identification purposes (Cohen, 2007).

Administering Prescribed Medications

During the immediate newborn period, two medications are commonly ordered: vitamin K and eye prophylaxis with

FIGURE 18.4 The nurse checks the newborn's identification band against the mother's.

either erythromycin or tetracycline ophthalmic ointment (Drug Guide 18.1).

Vitamin K

Vitamin K, a fat-soluble vitamin, promotes blood clotting by increasing the synthesis of prothrombin by the liver. A deficiency of this vitamin would delay clotting and might lead to hemorrhage.

Generally, the bacteria of the intestine produce vitamin K in adequate quantities. However, the newborn's bowel is sterile, so vitamin K is not produced in the intestine until after microorganisms are introduced, such as with the first feeding. Usually it takes about a week for the newborn to produce enough vitamin K to prevent vitamin K deficiency bleeding (Wasee, 2006).

The efficacy of vitamin K in preventing early vitamin K deficiency bleeding is firmly established and has been the standard of care since the AAP recommended it in the early 1960s. They recommend that vitamin K be administered to all newborns soon after birth in a single intramuscular dose of 0.5 to 1 mg (AAP, 2007) (Fig. 18.5). They suggest that additional research is needed to validate the efficacy and safety of oral forms of vitamin K, which have been used in many parts of the world but currently are not recommended in the United States.

Eye Prophylaxis

All newborns in the United States, whether delivered vaginally or by cesarean birth, must receive an instillation of a prophylactic agent in their eyes within an hour or two of birth. This is mandated in all 50 states to pre-

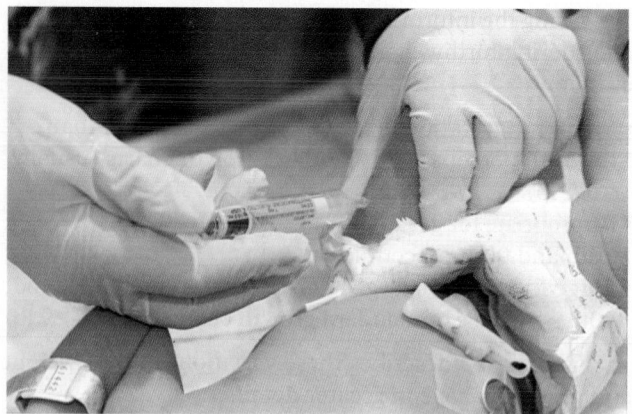

FIGURE 18.5 The nurse administers vitamin K IM to the newborn.

vent **ophthalmia neonatorum**, which can cause neonatal blindness (CDC, 2007). Ophthalmia neonatorum is a hyperacute purulent conjunctivitis occurring during the first 10 days of life. It is usually contracted during birth when the baby comes in contact with infected vaginal discharge of the mother (CDC, 2007). Most often both eyelids become swollen and red with purulent discharge.

Prophylactic agents that are currently recommended include erythromycin 0.5% ophthalmic ointment or tetracycline 1% ophthalmic ointment in a single application. Silver nitrate solution was formerly used but has little efficacy in preventing chlamydial eye disease (CDC, 2007).

Regardless of which agent is used, instillation should be done as soon as possible after birth (Fig. 18.6). If

DRUG GUIDE 18.1 Drugs for the Newborn

Drug	Action/Indication	Nursing Implications
Phytonadione (vitamin K [Aqua-MEPHYTON, Konakion, Mephyton])	Provides the newborn with vitamin K (necessary for production of adequate clotting factors II, VII, IX, and X by the liver) during the first week of birth until newborn can manufacture it Prevents vitamin K deficiency bleeding (VKDB) of the newborn	• Administer within 1 to 2 hours after birth. • Give as an IM injection at a 90-degree angle into the middle third of the vastus lateralis muscle. • Use a 25-gauge, 5/8-in needle for injection. • Hold the leg firmly and inject medication slowly after aspirating. • Adhere to standard precautions. • Assess for bleeding at injection site after administration.
Erythromycin ophthalmic ointment 0.5% or tetracycline ophthalmic ointment 1%	Provides bactericidal and bacteriostatic actions to prevent *Neisseria gonorrhoeae* and *Chlamydia trachomatis* conjunctivitis Prevents ophthalmia neonatorum	• Be alert for chemical conjunctivitis for 1–2 days. • Wear gloves, and open eyes by placing thumb and finger above and below the eye. • Gently squeeze the tube or ampoule to apply medication into the conjunctival sac from the inner canthus to the outer canthus of each eye. • Do not touch the tip to the eye. • Close the eye to make sure the medication permeates. • Wipe off excess ointment after 1 minute.

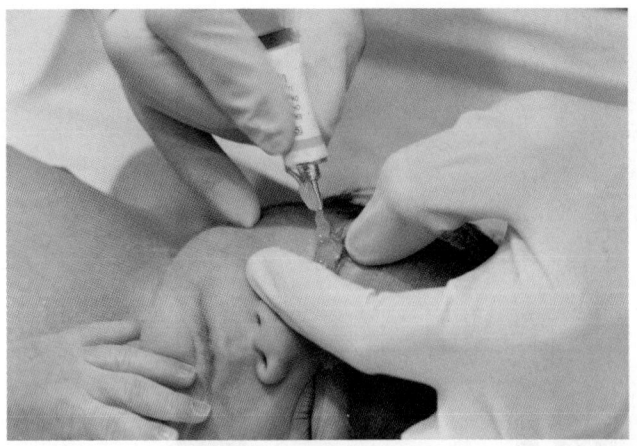

FIGURE 18.6 The nurse administers eye prophylaxis.

instillation is delayed to allow visualization and bonding, the nursery staff should make sure the agent is administered when the newborn reaches the nursery for observation and assessment.

Inform all parents about the eye treatment, including why it is recommended, what problems may arise if the treatment is not given, and possible adverse effects of the treatment.

▶ **Take** NOTE!

Parents have the right to refuse this treatment, but if they received adequate teaching about the treatment and understand its importance, they usually will consent to it.

Maintaining Thermoregulation

Newborns have trouble regulating their temperature, especially during the first few hours after birth (see Chap. 17 for a complete discussion). Therefore, maintaining body temperature is crucial.

Assess body temperature frequently during the immediate newborn period. The baby's temperature should be taken every 30 minutes for the first 2 hours or until the temperature has stabilized, and then every 8 hours until discharge (AAP, 2007).

Commonly a thermistor probe (automatic sensor) is attached to the newborn to record body temperature on a monitoring device. The probe is taped to the newborn's abdomen, usually in the right upper quadrant, which allows for position changes without having to readjust the probe. The other end of the thermistor probe is inserted into the radiant heat control panel. Temperature parameters are set on an alarm system connected to the heat panel that will sound if the newborn's temperature falls out of the set range. Check the probe connection period-

ically to make sure that it remains secure. Remember the potential for heat loss in newborns, and perform all nursing interventions in a way that minimizes heat loss and prevents hypothermia.

Axillary temperatures can also be used to assess the newborn's body temperature. At one time, rectal thermometers were routinely used to monitor body temperature, but their use is no longer recommended because of the risk of traumatizing the rectal lining (Blackburn, 2007). A newborn's temperature typically is maintained at 36.5° to 37.5°C (97.7° to 99.7°F) (Kenner & Lott, 2007).

Nursing interventions to help maintain body temperature include:

- Dry the newborn immediately after birth to prevent heat loss through evaporation.
- Wrap the baby in warmed blankets to reduce heat loss via convection.
- Use a warmed cover on the scale to weigh the unclothed newborn.
- Warm stethoscopes and hands before examining the baby or providing care.
- Avoid placing newborns in drafts or near air vents to prevent heat loss through convection.
- Delay the initial bath until the baby's temperature has stabilized to prevent heat loss through evaporation.
- Avoid placing cribs near cold outer walls to prevent heat loss through radiation.
- Put a cap on the newborn's head after it is thoroughly dried after birth.
- Place the newborn under a temperature-controlled radiant warmer (Fig. 18.7).

Nursing Management During the Early Newborn Period

The early newborn period is a time of great adjustment for both the mother and the newborn, both of whom are adapting to many physiologic and psychological changes. In the past, mothers and newborns remained in the health care facility while these dramatic changes were taking place, with nurses and doctors readily available. However, today shorter hospital stays are the norm, and new mothers can easily be overwhelmed by having to go through all of these changes in such a short time: the woman gives birth, experiences marked physiologic and psychological changes, and must adapt to her newborn and learn the skills needed to care for herself and the baby, all within 24 to 48 hours.

The nurse's role is to assist the mother and her newborn through this dramatic transition period. The newborn needs continued health assessment, and the mother needs to be taught to care for the new baby. At discharge, the new mother may panic and feel insecure about her role as primary caretaker. Nurses play a major role in promoting the newborn's transition by providing ongoing assessment and

FIGURE 18.7 Maintaining thermoregulation. (**A**) Radiant warmer. (**B**) Isolette.

care and in promoting the woman's confidence by serving as a role model and teaching about proper newborn care.

Assessment

The newborn requires ongoing assessment after leaving the birthing area to ensure that his or her transition to extrauterine life is progressing without problems. The nurse uses the data gathered during the initial assessment as a baseline for comparison.

Perinatal History

Pertinent maternal and fetal data are vital to formulate a plan of care for the mother and her newborn. Historical information is obtained from the medical record and from interviewing the mother. Review the maternal history because it provides pertinent information, such as the presence of certain risk factors that could affect the newborn. Keep in mind that a comprehensive maternal history may not be available, especially if the mother has had limited or no prenatal care.

Historical information usually includes the following:

- Mother's name, medical record number, blood type, serology result, rubella and hepatitis status, and history of substance abuse
- Other maternal tests that are relevant to the newborn and care, such as HIV and group B streptococcus status
- Intrapartum maternal antibiotic therapy (type, dose, and duration)
- Maternal illness that can affect the pregnancy, evidence of chorioamnionitis, maternal use of medications such as steroids
- Prenatal care, including timing of first visit and subsequent visits

- Risk for blood group incompatibility, including Rh status and blood type
- Fetal distress or any nonreassuring fetal heart rate patterns during labor
- Known inherited conditions such as sickle cell anemia and phenylketonuria (PKU)
- Birthweights of previous live-born children, along with identification of any newborn problems
- Social history, including tobacco, alcohol, and recreational drug use
- History of depression or domestic violence
- Cultural factors, including primary language and educational level
- Pregnancy complications associated with abnormal fetal growth, fetal anomalies, or abnormal results from tests of fetal well-being
- Information on the progress of labor, birth, labor complications, duration of ruptured membranes, and presence of meconium in the amniotic fluid
- Medications given during labor, at birth, and immediately after birth
- Time and method of delivery, including presentation and the use of forceps or a vacuum extractor
- Status of the newborn at birth, including Apgar scores at 1 and 5 minutes, the need for suctioning, weight, gestational age, vital signs, and umbilical cord status
- Medications administered to the newborn
- Postbirth maternal information, including placental findings, positive cultures, and presence of fever

Newborn Physical Examination

The initial newborn physical examination, which may demonstrate subtle differences related to the newborn's age, is carried out within the first 24 hours after birth. For example, a newborn who is 30 minutes old has not yet completed the normal transition from intrauterine to extrauterine life, and thus variability may exist in vital signs and in respiratory, neurologic, gastrointestinal, skin, and cardiovascular systems. Therefore, a comprehensive examination should be delayed until after the newborn has completed the transition.

In a quiet newborn, begin the examination with the least invasive and noxious elements of the examination (auscultation of heart and lungs). Then examine the areas most likely to irritate the newborn (e.g., examining the hips and eliciting the Moro reflex). A general visual assessment provides an enormous amount of information about the well-being of a newborn. Initial observation gives an impression of a healthy (stable) versus an ill newborn and a term versus a preterm newborn.

A typical physical examination of a newborn includes a general survey of skin color, posture, state of alertness, head size, overall behavioral state, respiratory status, gender, and any obvious congenital anomalies. Check the overall appearance for anything unusual. Then complete the examination in a systematic fashion.

*R*emember Kelly, who called the home health nurse and said her newborn son "looks like a canary"? What additional information is needed about the baby? What might be causing his yellow color?

Anthropometric Measurements

Shortly after birth, after the gender of the child is revealed, most parents want to know the "vital statistics" of their newborn—length and weight—to report to their family and friends. Additional measurements, including head and chest circumference, are also taken and recorded. Abdominal measurements are not routinely obtained unless there is a suspicion of pathology that causes abdominal distention. The newborn's progress from that point on will be validated based on these early measurements. These measurements will be compared with future serial measurements to determine growth patterns, which are plotted on growth charts to evaluate normalcy. Therefore, accuracy is key.

Length

The average length of most newborns is 50 cm (20 in), but it can range from 45 to 55 cm (18 to 22 in). Measure length with the unclothed newborn lying on a warmed blanket placed on a flat surface with the knees held in an extended position. Then run a tape measure down the length of the newborn—from the head to the soles of the feet—and record this measurement in the newborn's record (see Fig. 18.1).

Weight

At birth the average newborn weighs 3,400 g (7.5 lb), but normal birthweights can range from 2,500 to 4,000 g (5 lb, 8 oz to 8 lb, 14 oz). Newborns are weighed immediately after birth and then daily. Newborns usually lose up to 10% of their birthweight within the first few days of life, but regain it in approximately 10 days. Newborns are weighed on admission to the nursery or are taken to a digital scale to be weighed and returned to the mother's room.

First, balance the scale if it is not balanced. Place a warmed protective cloth or paper as a barrier on the scale to prevent heat loss by conduction; recalibrate the scale to zero after applying the barrier. Next, place the unclothed newborn in the center of the scale. Keep a hand above the newborn for safety (see Fig. 18.2).

Weight is affected by racial origin, maternal age, size of the parents, maternal nutrition, and placental perfusion (Lawrence, 2006). Weight should be correlated with gestational age. A newborn who weighs more than normal might be LGA or an infant of a diabetic mother (IDM); a newborn who weighs less than normal might be SGA or preterm or might have a genetic syndrome. It is important to identify the cause for the deviation in size and to monitor the newborn for complications common to that etiology.

Head Circumference

The average newborn head circumference is 32 to 38 cm (13 to 15 in). Measure the circumference at the head's widest diameter (the occipitofrontal circumference). Wrap a flexible or paper measuring tape snugly around the newborn's head and record the measurement (Fig. 18.8A).

> ▶ **Take** NOTE!
>
> *Head circumference may need to be remeasured at a later time if the shape of the head is altered from birth.*

The head circumference should be approximately one fourth of the newborn's length (Lawrence, 2006). A small head might indicate microcephaly caused by rubella, toxoplasmosis, or SGA status; an enlarged head might indicate hydrocephalus or increased intracranial pressure. Both need to be documented and reported for further investigation.

Chest Circumference

The average chest circumference is 30 to 36 cm (12 to 14 in). It is generally equal to or about 2 to 3 cm less than the head circumference (Burns et al., 2009). Place a flexible or paper tape measure around the unclothed newborn's chest at the nipple line without pulling it taut (see Fig. 18.8B).

> ▶ **Take** NOTE!
>
> *The head and chest circumferences are usually equal by about 1 year of age.*

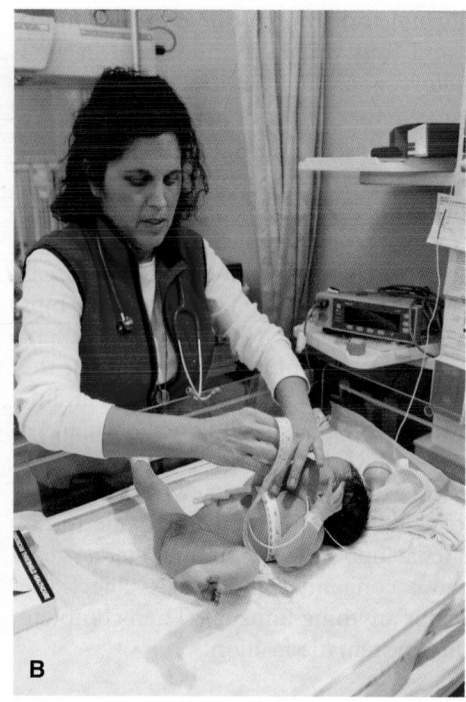

FIGURE 18.8 (**A**) Measuring head circumference. (**B**) Measuring chest circumference.

Vital Signs

In the newborn, temperature, pulse, and respirations are monitored frequently and compared with baseline data obtained immediately after birth. Generally, vital signs (excluding blood pressure) are taken:

- On admission to the nursery or in the LDR room after the parents are allowed to hold and bond with the newborn
- Once every 30 minutes until the newborn has been stable for 2 hours
- Then once every 4 to 8 hours until discharge (AAP, 2007)

Blood pressure is not routinely assessed in a normal newborn unless the baby's clinical condition warrants it. This schedule can change depending on the baby's health status.

Obtain a newborn's temperature by placing an electronic temperature probe in the midaxillary area or by monitoring the electronic thermistor probe that has been taped to the abdominal skin (applied when the newborn was placed under a radiant heat source).

Monitor the newborn's temperature hourly for changes until it stabilizes. On average, a newborn's temperature is 36.5° to 37.5°C (97.9° to 99.7°F). If the temperature is higher, adjust the environment, such as removing some clothing or blankets. If the temperature is lower, check the radiant warmer setting or add a warmed blanket. Report any abnormalities to the primary health care provider if simple adjustments to the environment do not change the baby's temperature.

Obtain an apical pulse by placing the stethoscope over the fourth intercostal space on the chest. Listen for a full minute, noting rate, rhythm, and abnormal sounds such as murmurs. In the typical newborn, the heart rate is 120 to 160 bpm, with wide fluctuations with activity and sleep. Sinus arrhythmia is a normal finding. Murmurs detected during the newborn period do not necessarily indicate congenital heart disease, but they need to be assessed frequently over the next several months to see if they persist.

Also palpate the apical, femoral, and brachial pulses for presence and equality (Fig. 18.9). Report any abnormalities to the primary health care provider for evaluation.

Assess respirations by observing the rise and fall of the chest for 1 full minute. Respirations should be symmetric, slightly irregular, shallow, and unlabored at a rate of 30 to 60 breaths/minute. The newborn's respirations are predominantly diaphragmatic, but they are synchronous with abdominal movements. Also auscultate breath sounds. Note any abnormalities, such as tachypnea, bradypnea, grunting, gasping, periods of apnea lasting longer than 20 seconds, asymmetry or decreased chest expansion, abnormal breath sounds (rhonchi, crackles), or sternal retractions. Some variations might exist early after birth, but if the abnormal pattern persists, notify the primary health care provider.

Skin

Observe the overall appearance of the skin, including color, texture, turgor, and integrity. The newborn's skin should be smooth and flexible, and the color should be consistent with genetic background.

FIGURE **18.9** Assessing the newborn's vital signs. (**A**) Assessing the apical pulse. (**B**) Palpating the femoral pulse. (**C**) Palpating the brachial pulse.

Skin Condition and Color

Check skin turgor by pinching a small area of skin over the chest or abdomen and note how quickly it returns to its original position. In a well-hydrated newborn, the skin should return to its normal position immediately. Skin that remains "tented" after being pinched indicates dehydration. A small amount of lanugo (fine downy hair) may be observed over the shoulders and on the sides of the face and upper back. There may be some cracking and peeling of the skin. The skin should be warm to the touch and intact.

The newborn's skin often appears blotchy or mottled, especially in the extremities. Persistent cyanosis of fingers, hands, toes, and feet with mottled blue or red discoloration and coldness is called **acrocyanosis**. It may be seen in newborns during the first few weeks of life in response to exposure to cold. Acrocyanosis is normal and intermittent.

Newborn Skin Variations

While assessing the skin, note any rashes, ecchymoses or petechiae, nevi, or dark pigmentation. Skin lesions can be congenital or transient; they may be a result of infection or may result from the mode of birth. If any are present, observe the anatomic location, arrangement, type, and color. Bruising may result from the use of devices such as a vacuum extractor during delivery. Petechiae may be the result of pressure on the skin during the birth process. Forceps marks may be observed over the cheeks and ears. A small puncture mark may be seen if internal fetal scalp electrode monitoring was used during labor.

Common skin variations include vernix caseosa, stork bites or salmon patches, milia, Mongolian spots, erythema toxicum, harlequin sign, nevus flammeus, and nevus vasculosus (Fig. 18.10).

Vernix caseosa is a thick white substance that protects the skin of the fetus. It is formed by secretions from the fetus's oil glands and is found during the first 2 or 3 days after birth in body creases and the hair. It does not need to be removed because it will be absorbed into the skin.

Stork bites or salmon patches are superficial vascular areas found on the nape of the neck, on the eyelids, and between the eyes and upper lip (see Fig. 18.10A). The name comes from the marks on the back of the neck where, as myth goes, a stork may have picked up the baby. They are caused by a concentration of immature blood vessels and are most visible when the newborn is crying. They are considered a normal variant, and most fade and disappear completely within the first year.

Milia are unopened sebaceous glands frequently found on a newborn's nose. They may also appear on the chin and forehead (see Fig. 18.10B). They form from oil glands and disappear on their own within 2 to 4 weeks. When they occur in a newborn's mouth and gums, they are termed **Epstein's pearls**. They occur in approximately 60% of newborns (AAP, 2007b).

Mongolian spots are blue or purple splotches that appear on the lower back and buttocks of newborns (see Fig. 18.10C). They tend to occur in African-American, Asian, and Indian newborns but can occur in dark-skinned newborns of all races. The spots are caused by a concentration of pigmented cells and usually disappear within the first 4 years of life (Kliegman et al., 2007).

Erythema toxicum (newborn rash) is a benign, idiopathic, generalized, transient rash that occurs in up to 70% of all newborns during the first week of life. It consists of small papules or pustules on the skin resembling flea bites. The rash is common on the face, chest, and back (see Fig. 18.10D). One of the chief characteristics

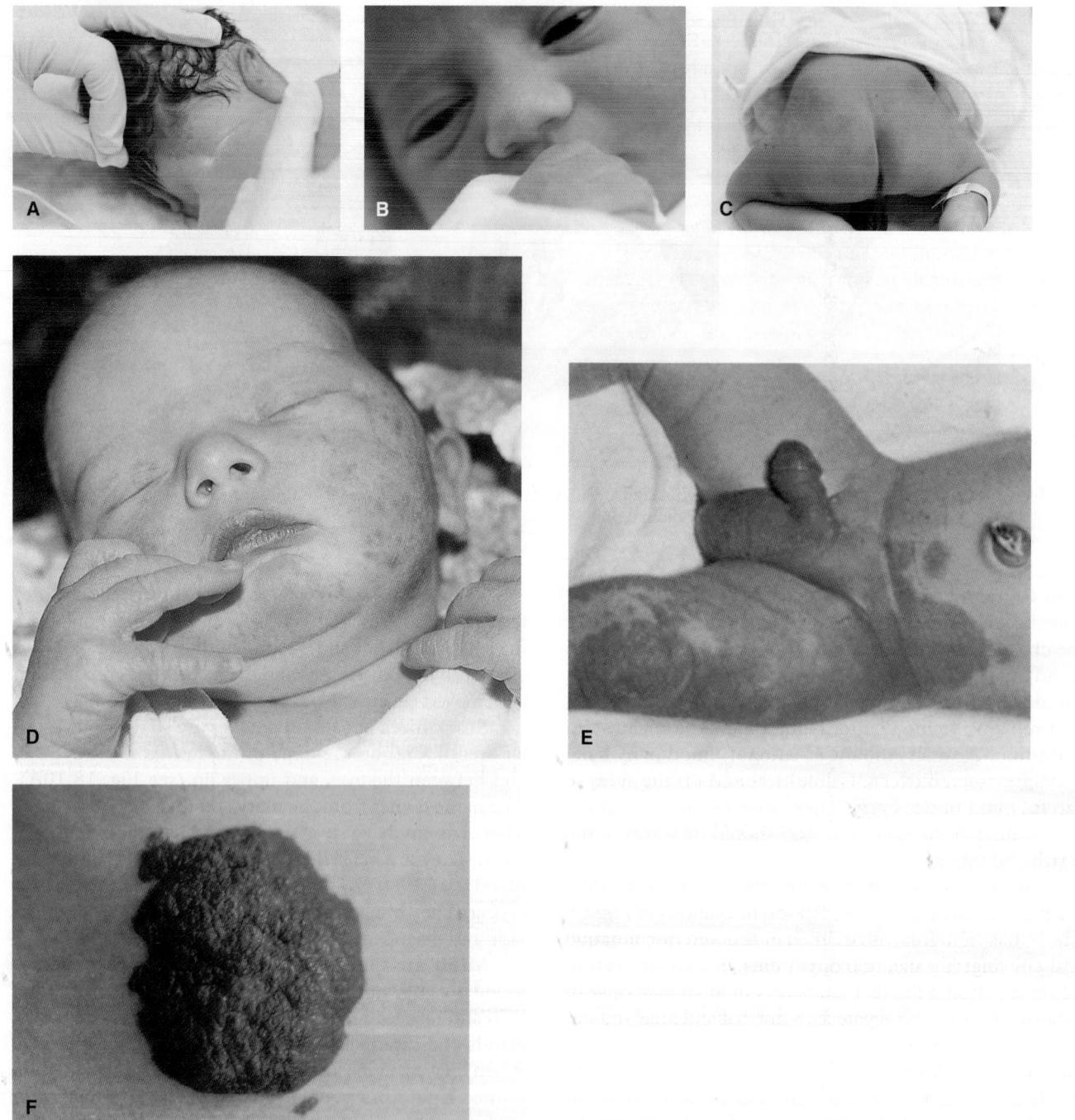

FIGURE 18.10 Common skin variations. (**A**) Stork bite. (**B**) Milia. (**C**) Mongolian spots. (**D**) Erythema toxicum. (**E**) Nevus flammeus (port-wine stain). (**F**) Strawberry hemangioma.

of this rash is its lack of pattern. It is caused by the newborn's eosinophils reacting to the environment as the immune system matures (AAP, 2007b). It does not require any treatment and disappears in a few days.

Harlequin sign refers to the dilation of blood vessels on only one side of the body, giving the newborn the appearance of wearing a clown suit. It gives a distinct midline demarcation, which is described as pale on the nondependent side and red on the opposite, dependent side. It results from immature autoregulation of blood flow and is commonly seen in low-birthweight newborns when there is a positional change (Dillon, 2007). It is transient, lasting as long as 20 minutes, and no intervention is needed.

Nevus flammeus, also called a port wine stain, commonly appears on the newborn's face or other body areas (see Fig. 18.10E). It is a capillary angioma located directly below the dermis. It is flat with sharp demarcations and is purple–red. This skin lesion is made up of mature capillaries that are congested and dilated. It ranges in size from a few millimeters to large, occasionally involving as much as half the body surface. Although it does not grow in area or size, it is permanent and will not fade. Port wine stains may be associated with structural malformations, bony or muscular overgrowth, and certain cancers. Recent studies have noted an association between port wine birthmarks and childhood cancer, so newborns with these lesions should be monitored with periodic eye examinations, neurologic imaging, and extremity measurements (Johnson et al., 2007). Pulsed dye laser surgery has been used to remove larger lesions with some success (AAP, 2007b).

Nevus vasculosus, also called a strawberry mark or strawberry hemangioma, is a benign capillary hemangioma in the dermal and subdermal layers. It is raised, rough, dark red, and sharply demarcated (see Fig. 18.10F). It is commonly found in the head region within a few weeks after birth and can increase in size or number. Commonly seen in premature infants weighing less than 1,500 g (Kenner & Lott, 2007), these hemangiomas tend to resolve by age 3 without any treatment.

Head

Head size varies with age, gender, and ethnicity and has a general correlation with body size. Inspect a newborn's head from all angles. The head should appear symmetric and round. As many as 90% of the congenital malformations present at birth are visible on the head and neck, so careful assessment is very important (AAP, 2007a).

The newborn has two fontanels at the juncture of the cranial bones. The anterior fontanel is diamond-shaped and closes by 18 to 24 months. Typically it measures 4 to 6 cm at the largest diameter (bone to bone). The posterior one is triangular, smaller than the anterior fontanel (usually fingertip size or 0.5 to 1 cm), and closes by 6 to 12 weeks. Palpate both fontanels, which should be soft, flat, and open. Then palpate the skull. It should feel smooth and fused, except at the area of the fontanels. Also assess the size of the head and the anterior and posterior fontanels, and compare them with appropriate standards.

Variations in Head Size and Appearance

During inspection and palpation, be alert for common variations that may cause asymmetry. These include caput succedaneum, cephalhematoma, and molding.

Molding is the elongated shaping of the fetal head to accommodate passage through the birth canal (Fig. 18.11). It occurs with a vaginal birth from a vertex position in which elongation of the fetal head occurs with prominence of the occiput and overriding sagittal suture line. It typically resolves within a week after birth without intervention.

Caput succedaneum describes localized edema on the scalp that occurs from the pressure of the birth process. It is commonly observed after prolonged labor. Clinically,

FIGURE 18.11 Molding in a newborn's head.

it appears as a poorly demarcated soft tissue swelling that crosses suture lines. Pitting edema and overlying petechiae and ecchymosis are noted (Fig. 18.12A). The swelling will gradually dissipate in about 3 days without any treatment. Newborns who were delivered via vacuum extraction usually have a caput in the area where the cup was used.

Cephalhematoma is a localized effusion of blood beneath the periosteum of the skull. This condition is due to disruption of the vessels during birth. It occurs after prolonged labor and use of obstetric interventions such as low forceps or vacuum extraction. The clinical features include a well-demarcated, often fluctuant swelling with no overlying skin discoloration. The swelling does not cross suture lines and is firmer to the touch than an edematous area (see Fig. 18.12B). Cephalhematoma usually appears on the second or third day after birth and disappears within weeks or months (Simonson et al., 2007).

Common Abnormalities in Head or Fontanel Size

Common abnormalities in head or fontanel size that may indicate a problem include:

• Microcephaly—a head circumference more than 2 standard deviations below average or less than 10% of normal parameters for gestational age, caused by failure of brain development (Cohen, 2007). It can be familial, with autosomal dominant or recessive inheritance, and it may be associated with infections (cytomegalovirus) and syndromes such as trisomy 13 and 18, and fetal alcohol syndrome (Kenner & Lott, 2007).

FIGURE 18.12 (**A**) Caput succedaneum involves the collection of serous fluid and often crosses the suture line. (**B**) Cephalhematoma involves the collection of blood and does not cross the suture line.

- Macrocephaly—a head circumference more than 90% of normal, typically related to hydrocephalus (Dillon, 2007). It is often familial (with autosomal dominant inheritance) and can be either an isolated anomaly or a manifestation of other anomalies, including hydrocephalus and skeletal disorders (achondroplasia).
- Large fontanels—more than 6 cm in the anterior diameter bone to bone or more than a 1-cm diameter in the posterior fontanel; possibly associated with malnutrition, hydrocephaly, congenital hypothyroidism, trisomies 13, 18, and 21, and various bone disorders such as osteogenesis imperfecta
- Small or closed fontanels—smaller-than-normal anterior and posterior diameters or fontanels that are closed at birth; associated with microcephaly or premature synostosis (union of two bones by osseous material) (Blackburn, 2007)

Face

Observe the newborn's face for fullness and symmetry. The face should have full cheeks and should be symmetric when the baby is resting and crying. If forceps were used during birth, the newborn may have bruising and reddened areas over both cheeks and parietal bones secondary to the pressure of the forceps blades. Reassure the parents that this resolves without treatment, and point out improvement each day.

Problems with the face can also involve facial nerve paralysis caused by trauma from the use of forceps. Paralysis is usually apparent on the first or second day of life. Typically, the newborn will demonstrate asymmetry of the face with the inability to close the eye and move the lips on the affected side. Newborns with facial nerve paralysis have difficulty making a seal around the nipple, and con-

sequently milk or formula drools from the paralyzed side of the mouth. Most facial nerve palsies resolve spontaneously within days, although full recovery may require weeks to months. Attempt to determine the cause from the newborn's history.

Nose

Inspect the nose for size, symmetry, position, and lesions. The newborn's nose is small and narrow. The nose should have a midline placement, patent nares, and an intact septum. The nostrils should be of equal size and should be patent. A slight mucus discharge may be present, but there should be no actual drainage. The newborn is a preferential nose breather and will use sneezing to clear the nose if needed. The newborn can smell after the nasal passages are cleared of amniotic fluid and mucus (AAP, 2007a).

Mouth

Inspect the newborn's mouth, lips, and interior structures. The lips should be intact with symmetric movement and positioned in the midline; there should not be any lesions. Inspect the lips for pink color, moisture, and cracking. The lips should encircle the examiner's finger to form a vacuum. Variations involving the lip might include cleft upper lip (separation extending up to the nose) or thin upper lip associated with fetal alcohol syndrome.

Assess the inside of the mouth for alignment of the mandible, intact soft and hard palate, sucking pads inside the cheeks, a midline uvula, a free-moving tongue, and working gag, swallow, and sucking reflexes. The mucous membranes lining the oral cavity should be pink and moist, with minimal saliva present.

Normal variations might include Epstein's pearls (small, white epidermal cysts on the gums and hard palate that disappear in weeks), erupted precocious teeth that may need to be removed to prevent aspiration, and thrush (white plaque inside the mouth caused by exposure to *Candida albicans* during birth), which cannot be wiped away with a cotton-tipped applicator.

Eyes

Inspect the external eye structures, including the eyelids, lashes, conjunctiva, sclera, iris, and pupils, for position, color, size, and movement. There may be marked edema of the eyelids and subconjunctival hemorrhages due to pressure during birth. The eyes should be clear and symmetrically placed. Test the blink reflex by bringing an object close to the eye; the newborn should respond quickly by blinking. Also test the newborn's pupillary reflex: pupils should be equal, round, and reactive to light bilaterally. Assess the newborn's gaze: he or she should be able to track objects to the midline. Movement may be uncoordinated during the first few weeks of life. Many newborns have transient strabismus (deviation or wandering of eyes independently) and searching nystagmus (involuntary repetitive eye movement), which is caused by immature muscular control. These are normal for the first 3 to 6 months of age.

Examine the internal eye structures. A red reflex (luminous red appearance seen on the retina) should be seen bilaterally on retinoscopy. The red reflex normally shows no dullness or irregularities.

Chemical conjunctivitis commonly occurs within 24 hours of instillation of eye prophylaxis after birth. There is lid edema with sterile discharge from both eyes. Usually it resolves within 48 hours without treatment.

Ears

Inspect the ears for size, shape, skin condition, placement, amount of cartilage, and patency of the auditory canal. The ears should be soft and pliable and should recoil quickly and easily when folded and released. Ears should be aligned with the outer canthi of the eyes. Low-set ears are characteristic of many syndromes and genetic abnormalities, such as trisomy 13 and 18, and internal organ abnormalities involving the renal system.

An otoscopic examination is not typically done because the newborn's ear canals are filled with amniotic fluid and vernix caseosa, which would make visualization of the tympanic membrane difficult.

Newborn hearing screening is required by law in most states (discussed later in the chapter). Hearing loss is the most common birth defect in the United States: One in 1,000 newborns is profoundly deaf and 2 to 3 in 1,000 have partial hearing loss (Wrightson, 2007). Delays in identification and intervention may affect the child's cognitive, verbal, behavioral, and emotional development. Screening at birth has reduced the age at which newborns with hearing loss are identified and has improved early intervention rates dramatically (AAP, 2007b). Prior to universal newborn screening, children were usually older than 2 years

before significant congenital hearing loss was detected; by this time it had already affected their speech and language skills (USPSTF, 2006).

Causes of hearing loss can be conductive, sensorineural, or central. Risk factors for congenital hearing loss include cytomegalovirus infection and preterm birth necessitating a stay in the neonatal intensive care unit.

To assess for hearing ability generally, observe the newborn's response to noises and conversations. The newborn typically turns toward these noises and startles with loud ones.

Neck

Inspect the newborn's neck for movement and ability to support the head. The newborn's neck will appear almost nonexistent because it is so short. Creases are usually noted. The neck should move freely in all directions and should be capable of holding the head in a midline position. The newborn should have enough head control to be able to hold it up briefly without support. Report any deviations such as restricted neck movement or absence of head control.

Also inspect the clavicles, which should be straight and intact. The clavicles are the bones mostly commonly broken in infants, especially large ones. In most cases, the fractured clavicle is asymptomatic, but decreased or absent movement and pain or tenderness on movement of the arm on the affected side may be noted (Kenner & Lott, 2007). Treatment involves immobilization and minimizing pain.

Chest

Inspect the newborn's chest for size, shape, and symmetry. The newborn's chest should be round, symmetric, and 2 to 3 cm smaller than the head circumference. The xiphoid process may be prominent at birth, but it usually becomes less apparent when adipose tissue accumulates. Nipples may be engorged and may secrete a white discharge. This discharge, which occurs in both boys and girls, is a result of exposure to high levels of maternal estrogen while in utero. This enlargement and milky discharge usually dissipates within a few weeks. Some newborns may have extra nipples, called supernumerary nipples. They are typically small, raised, pigmented areas vertical to the main nipple line, 5 to 6 cm below the normal nipple (AAP, 2007a). They tend to be familial and do not contain glandular tissue. Reassure parents that these extra small nipples are harmless.

The newborn chest is usually barrel-shaped with equal anteroposterior and lateral diameters, and symmetric. Auscultate the lungs bilaterally for equal breath sounds. Normal breath sounds should be heard, with little difference between inspiration and expiration. Fine crackles can be heard on inspiration soon after birth as a result of clearing amniotic fluid from the lungs. Diminished breath sounds might indicate atelectasis, effusion, or poor respiratory effort (Dillon, 2007).

Listen to the heart when the newborn is quiet or sleeping. S1 and S2 heart sounds are accentuated at birth. The point of maximal impulse (PMI) is a lateral to midclavicular line located at the fourth intercostal space. A displaced PMI may indicate tension pneumothorax or cardiomegaly. Murmurs are often heard and are usually benign, but if present after the first 12 hours of life should be evaluated to rule out a cardiac disorder (Kliegman et al., 2007).

Abdomen

Inspect the abdomen for shape and movement. Typically the newborn's abdomen is protuberant but not distended. This contour is a result of the immaturity of the abdominal muscles. Abdominal movements are synchronous with respirations because newborns are, at times, abdominal breathers.

Auscultate bowel sounds in all four quadrants and then palpate the abdomen for consistency, masses, and tenderness. Perform auscultation and palpation systematically in a clockwise fashion until all four quadrants have been assessed. Palpate gently to feel the liver, the kidneys, and any masses. The liver is normally palpable 1 to 3 cm below the costal margin in the midclavicular line. The kidneys are 1 to 2 cm above and to both sides of the umbilicus. Normal findings would include bowel sounds in all four quadrants and no masses or tenderness on palpation. Absent or hyperactive bowel sounds might indicate an intestinal obstruction. Abdominal distention might indicate ascites, obstruction, infection, masses, or an enlarged abdominal organ (Cohen, 2007).

Inspect the umbilical cord area for the correct amount of blood vessels (two arteries and one vein). The umbilical vein is larger than the two umbilical arteries. Evidence of only a single umbilical artery is associated with renal and gastrointestinal anomalies. Also inspect the umbilical area for signs of bleeding, infection, granuloma, or abnormal communication with the intra-abdominal organs (Walsh, 2007).

Genitalia

Inspect the penis and scrotum in the male. In the circumcised male newborn, the glans should be smooth, with the meatus centered at the tip of the penis. It will appear reddened until it heals. For the uncircumcised male, the foreskin should cover the glans. Check the position of the urinary meatus: it should be in the midline at the glans tip. If it is on the ventral surface of the penis, hypospadias is present; if it is on the dorsal surface of the penis, it is termed epispadias. In either case, circumcision should be avoided until further evaluation.

Inspect the scrotum for size, symmetry, color, presence of rugae, and location of testes. The scrotum usually appears relatively large and should be pink in white neonates and dark brown in neonates of color. Rugae should be well formed and should cover the scrotal sac. There should not be bulging, edema, or discoloration (Fig. 18.13A).

FIGURE 18.13 Newborn genitalia. (**A**) Male genitalia. Note the darkened color of the scrotum. (**B**) Female genitalia.

Palpate the scrotum for evidence of the testes, which should be in the scrotal sac. The testes should feel firm and smooth and should be of equal size on both sides of the scrotal sac in the term newborn. Undescended testes (cryptorchidism) might be palpated in the inguinal canal in preterm infants; they can be unilateral or bilateral. If the testes are not palpable within the scrotal sac, further investigation is needed.

In the female newborn, inspect the external genitalia. The urethral meatus is located below the clitoris in the midline (Dillon, 2007). In contrast to the male genitalia, the female genitalia will be engorged: the labia majora and minora may both be edematous. The labia majora is large and covers the labia minora. The clitoris is large and the hymen is thick. These findings are due to the maternal hormones estrogen and progesterone (see Fig. 18.13B). A vaginal discharge composed of mucus mixed with blood may also be present during the first few weeks of life. This discharge, called **pseudomenstruation**, requires no treatment. Explain this phenomenon to the parents.

Variations in female newborns may include a labial bulge, which might indicate an inguinal hernia; ambiguous genitalia; a rectovaginal fistula with feces present in the vagina; and an imperforate hymen.

Inspect the anus in both male and female newborns for position and patency. Passage of meconium indicates patency. If meconium is not passed, a lubricated rectal thermometer can be inserted or a digital examination can be performed to determine patency. Abnormal findings would include anal fissures or fistulas and no meconium passed within 24 hours after birth.

Extremities and Back

Inspect the newborn's upper extremities for appearance and movement. Inspect the hands for shape, number, and position of fingers and presence of palmar creases. The newborn's arms and hands should be symmetric and should move through range of motion without hesitation. Observe for spontaneous movement of the extremities. Each hand should have five digits. Note any extra digits (polydactyly) or fusing of two or more digits (syndactyly). Most newborns have three palmar creases on the hand. A single palmar crease, called a simian line, is frequently associated with Down syndrome.

A brachial plexus injury can occur during a difficult birth involving shoulder dystocia. Erb's palsy is an injury resulting from damage to the upper plexus during labor and birth. The affected arm hangs limp alongside the body, and the affected shoulder and arm are adducted, extended, and internally rotated with a pronated wrist. The Moro reflex is absent on the affected side in brachial palsy. Complete recovery may take 3 to 6 months (Adegbehingbe et al., 2007).

Assess the lower extremities in the same manner. They should of equal length, with symmetric skin folds. Inspect the feet for clubfoot (a turning-inward position), which is secondary to intrauterine positioning. This may be positional or structural. Perform the Ortolani and Barlow maneuvers to identify congenital hip dislocation, commonly termed developmental dysplasia of the hip (DDH). Nursing Procedure 18.1 highlights the steps for performing these maneuvers.

Inspect the back. The spine should appear straight and flat and should be easily flexed when the baby is held in a prone position. Observe for the presence of a tuft of

---

Nursing Procedure 18.1

PERFORMING ORTOLANI AND BARLOW MANEUVERS

Purpose: To Detect Congenital Developmental Dysplasia of the Hip

Ortolani Maneuver

1. Place the newborn in the supine position and flex the hips and knees to 90 degrees at the hip.
2. Grasp the inner aspect of the thighs and abduct the hips (usually to approximately 180 degrees) while applying upward pressure.

A

3. Listen for any sounds during the maneuver. There should be no "cluck" or "click" heard when the legs are abducted. Such a sound indicates the femoral head hitting the acetabulum as the head re-enters the area. This suggests developmental hip dysplasia.

Barlow Maneuver

1. With the newborn still lying supine and grasping the inner aspect of the thighs (as just mentioned), adduct the thighs while applying outward and downward pressure to the thighs.

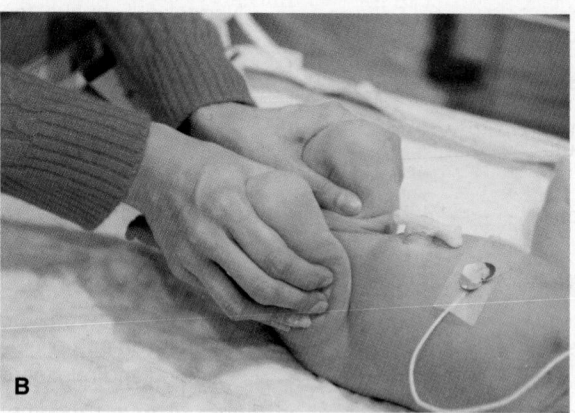

B

2. Feel for the femoral head slipping out of the acetabulum; also listen for a click (Dillon, 2007).

hair, a pilonidal dimple in the midline, a cyst, or a mass along the spine. These abnormal findings should be documented and reported to the primary health care provider.

Table 18.3 summarizes the newborn assessment.

Neurologic Status
Assess the newborn's state of alertness, posture, muscle tone, and reflexes.

Newborn Alertness, Posture, and Muscle Tone
The newborn should be alert and not persistently lethargic. The normal posture is hips abducted and partially flexed, with knees flexed. Arms are adducted and flexed at the elbow. Fists are often clenched, with fingers covering the thumb.

To assess for muscle tone, support the newborn with one hand under the chest. Observe how the neck muscles hold the head. The neck extensors should be able to hold the head in line briefly. There should be only slight head lag when pulling the newborn from a supine position to a sitting one.

Newborn Reflexes
Assess the newborn's reflexes to evaluate neurologic function and development. Absent or abnormal reflexes in a newborn, persistence of a reflex past the age when the reflex is normally lost, or return of an infantile reflex in an older child or adult may indicate neurologic pathology (Table 18.4). Reflexes commonly assessed in the newborn include sucking, Moro, stepping, tonic neck, root-

TABLE 18.3 NEWBORN ASSESSMENT SUMMARY

Assessment	Usual Findings	Variations and Common Problems
Anthropometric measurements	Head circumference: 33–37 cm (13–14 in) Chest circumference: 30–33 cm (12–13 in) Weight: 2,500–4,000 g (5.5–8.5 lb) Length: 45–55 cm (19–21 in)	SGA, LGA, preterm, postterm
Vital signs	Temperature: 36.5°–37.5°C (97°–99°F) Apical pulse: 120–160 bpm Respirations: 30–60 breaths/minute	
Skin	Normal: smooth, flexible, good skin turgor, warm	Jaundice, acrocyanosis, milia, Mongolian spots, stork bites
Head	Normal: varies with age, gender, ethnicity	Microcephaly, macrocephaly, enlarged fontanels
Face	Normal: full cheeks, facial features symmetric	Facial nerve paralysis, nevus flammeus, nevus vasculosus
Nose	Normal: small, placement in the midline and narrow, ability to smell	Malformation or blockage
Mouth	Normal: aligned in midline, symmetric, intact soft and hard palate	Epstein's pearls, erupted precocious teeth, thrush
Neck	Normal: short, creased, moves freely, baby holds head in midline	Restricted movement, clavicular fractures
Eyes	Normal: clear and symmetrically placed on face	Chemical conjunctivitis, subconjunctival hemorrhages
Ears	Normal: soft and pliable with quick recoil when folded and released	Low-set ears, hearing loss
Chest	Normal: round, symmetric, smaller than head	Nipple engorgement, whitish discharge
Abdomen	Normal: protuberant contour, soft, three vessels in umbilical cord	Distended, only two vessels in umbilical cord
Genitals	Normal male: smooth glans, meatus centered at tip of penis Normal female: swollen female genitals as a result of maternal estrogen	Edematous scrotum in males, vaginal discharge in females
Extremities and spine	Normal: extremities symmetric with free movement	Congenital hip dislocation; tuft or dimple on spine

TABLE 18.4 **NEWBORN REFLEXES: APPEARANCE AND DISAPPEARANCE**

Reflex	Appearance	Disappearance
Blinking	Newborn	Persists into adulthood
Moro	Newborn	3–6 mo
Grasp	Newborn	3–4 mo
Stepping	Birth	1–2 mo
Tonic neck	Newborn	3–4 mo
Sneeze	Newborn	Persists into adulthood
Rooting	Birth	4–6 mo
Gag reflex	Newborn	Persists into adulthood
Cough reflex	Newborn	Persists into adulthood
Babinski sign	Newborn	12 mo

ing, Babinski, and palmar grasp reflex. Spinal reflexes tested include truncal incurvation (Galant reflex) and anocutaneous reflex (anal wink).

The sucking reflex is elicited by gently stimulating the newborn's lips by touching them. The newborn will typically open the mouth and begin a sucking motion. Placing a gloved finger in the newborn's mouth will also elicit a sucking motion (Fig. 18.14A).

The Moro reflex, also called the embrace reflex, occurs when the neonate is startled. To elicit this reflex, place the newborn on his or her back. Support the upper body weight of the supine newborn by the arms, using a lifting motion, without lifting the newborn off the surface. Then release the arms suddenly. The newborn will throw the arms outward and flex the knees; the arms then return to the chest. The fingers also spread to form a C. The newborn initially appears startled and then relaxes to a normal resting position (see Fig. 18.14B).

Assess the stepping reflex by holding the newborn upright and inclined forward with the soles of the feet touching a flat surface. The baby should make a stepping motion or walking, alternating flexion and extension with the soles of the feet (see Fig. 18.14C).

The tonic neck reflex resembles the stance of a fencer and is often called the fencing reflex. Test this reflex by having the newborn lie on the back. Turn the baby's head to one side. The arm toward which the baby is facing should extend straight away from the body with the hand partially open, whereas the arm on the side away from the face is flexed and the fist is clenched tightly. Reversing the direction to which the face is turned reverses the position (see Fig. 18.14D).

Elicit the rooting reflex by stroking the newborn's cheek. The newborn should turn toward the side that was stroked and should begin to make sucking movements (see Fig. 18.14E).

The Babinski reflex should be present at birth and disappears at approximately 1 year of age. It is elicited by stroking the lateral sole of the newborn's foot from the heel toward and across the ball of the foot. The toes should fan out. A diminished response indicates a neurologic problem and needs follow-up (see Fig. 18.14F).

The newborn exhibits two grasp reflexes: palmar grasp and plantar grasp. Elicit the palmar grasp reflex by placing a finger on the newborn's open palm. The baby's hand will close around the finger. Attempting to remove the finger causes the grip to tighten. Newborns have strong

FIGURE 18.14 Newborn reflexes. (**A**) Sucking reflex. (**B**) Moro reflex. *(continued)*

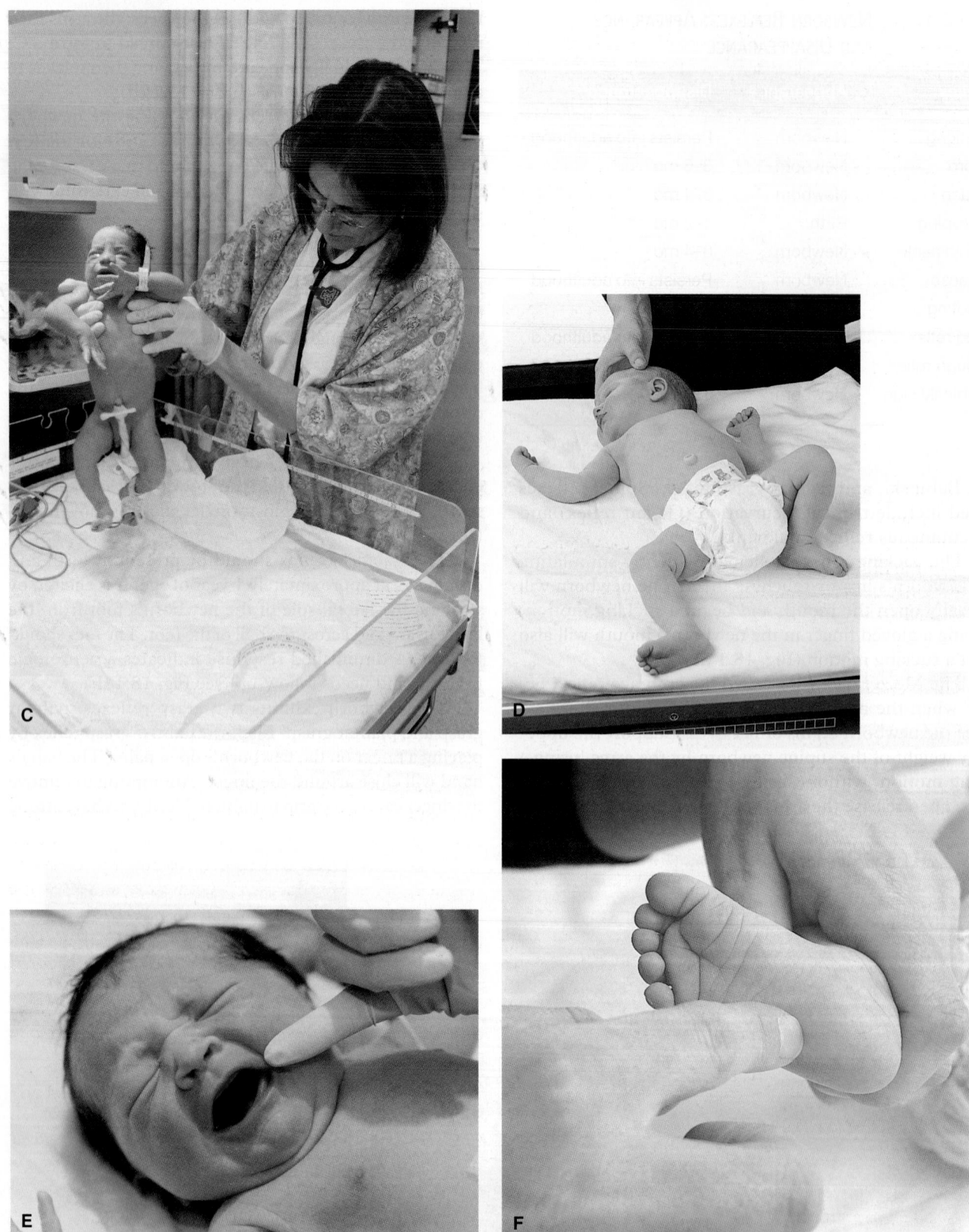

FIGURE 18.14 (continued) (**C**) Stepping reflex. (**D**) Tonic neck reflex. (**E**) Rooting reflex. (**F**) Babinski reflex. *(continued)*

FIGURE 18.14   (continued) (**G**) Palmar grasp. (**H**) Plantar grasp.

grasps and can almost be lifted from a flat surface if both hands are used. The grasp should be equal bilaterally (see Fig. 18.14G).

The plantar grasp is similar to the palmar grasp. Place a finger just below the newborn's toes. The toes typically curl over the finger (see Fig. 18.14H).

Blinking, sneezing, gagging, and coughing are all protective reflexes and are elicited when an object or light is brought close to the eye (blinking), something irritating is swallowed or a bulb syringe is used for suctioning (gagging and coughing), or an irritant is brought close to the nose (sneezing).

The truncal incurvation reflex (Galant reflex) is present at birth and disappears in a few days to 4 weeks. With the newborn in a prone position or held in ventral suspension, apply firm pressure and run a finger down either side of the spine. This stroking will cause the pelvis to flex toward the stimulated side. This indicates T2–S1 innervation. Lack of response indicates a neurologic or spinal cord problem.

The anocutaneous reflex (anal wink) is elicited by stimulating the perianal skin close to the anus. The external sphincter will constrict (wink) immediately with stimulation. This indicates S4–5 innervation (Kenner & Lott, 2007).

Nursing Interventions

Developing confidence to care for their newborn is challenging for most couples. It takes time and patience and a great deal of instruction provided by the nurse. "Showing and telling" parents about their newborn and all the procedures (e.g., feeding, bathing, changing, handling) involved in daily care are key nursing interventions.

Providing General Newborn Care

Generally, newborn care involves bathing and hygiene, diaper care, cord care, circumcision care, use of appropriate clothing, environmental safety measures, and pre-

vention of infection. Nurses should teach these skills to parents and should serve as role models for appropriate and consistent interaction with newborns. Demonstrating respect for the newborn and family helps foster a positive atmosphere to promote the newborn's growth and development.

Bathing and Hygiene

Immediately after birth, drying the newborn and removing blood may minimize the risk of infection caused by hepatitis B, herpesvirus, and HIV, but the specific benefits of this practice remain unclear. Until the newborn has been thoroughly bathed, standard precautions should be used when handling the newborn.

Newborns are bathed primarily for aesthetic reasons, and bathing is postponed until thermal and cardiorespiratory stability is ensured. Traditional reasons why nurses bathe the newborn are so they can conduct a physical assessment, reduce the effect of hypothermia, and allow the mother to rest (Cohen, 2007). However, recent research suggests that nurses do not need to give the newborn an initial bath to reduce heat loss; rather, the parents could be given this opportunity, supported by nurses. A study found that the amount of heat loss was similar in newborns bathed by parents versus newborns who were bathed by nurses (Walsh, 2007).

Wear gloves, because of potential exposure to maternal blood on the newborn, and perform the bath quickly, drying the baby thoroughly to prevent heat loss by evaporation. Move from the "cleanest" area (the eyes) to the most soiled area (the diaper area) to prevent cross-contamination.

Use plain warm water on the face and eyes, adding a mild soap (e.g., Dove) to cleanse the remainder of the body. Instruct the parents to wash the face and neck gently after each feeding to prevent rashes and to prevent the odor that can develop when milk accumulates in the neck creases.

Wash the hair using running water so that the scalp can be thoroughly rinsed. A mild shampoo or soap can be used. Wash both fontanel areas. Frequently parents avoid these "soft spots" because they fear that they will "hurt the baby's brain" if they rub too hard. Reassure parents that there is a strong membrane providing protection. Urge the parents to clean and rinse these areas well. If the anterior fontanel is not rinsed well after shampooing, cradle cap (dry flakes on the scalp) can develop. In Figure 18.15, the nurse is showing the father how to bathe his newborn.

After bathing, place the newborn under the radiant warmer and wrap him or her securely in blankets to prevent chilling. Check the baby's temperature within an hour to make sure it is within normal limits. If it is low, place the newborn under a radiant heat source again.

The literature suggests that tub bathing for the first bath, as opposed to sponge bathing, can be done without significantly lowering the newborn's temperature or increasing rates of cord infection in healthy term newborns (AAP, 2007c).

After the initial bath, the newborn may not receive another full one during the stay in the birthing unit. The diaper area will be cleansed at each diaper change, and any milk spilled will be cleaned. Clear water and a mild soap are appropriate to cleanse the diaper area. The use of lotions, baby oil, and powders is not encouraged because oils and lotions can lead to skin irritation and can cause rashes. Powders should not be used because they can be inhaled, causing respiratory distress. If the parents want to use oils and lotions, have them apply a small amount onto their hand first, away from the newborn; this warms the lotion. Then the parents should apply the lotion or oil sparingly.

Instruct parents that a bath two or three times weekly is sufficient for the first year; more frequent bathing may dry the skin. Parents should not fully immerse the newborn into water until the umbilical cord area is healed—up to 2 weeks after birth. Encourage parents to give the

infant a sponge bath until the umbilical cord falls off and the navel area is healed completely. If the newborn has been circumcised, advise parents to wait until that area has also healed (usually 1 to 2 weeks). Until then, clean the penis with mild soap and water and apply a small amount of Vaseline to the tip to prevent the diaper from adhering to the penis. Instruct parents to apply the diaper loosely and place the newly circumcised male infant on his side or back to prevent pressure and irritation on the penis.

Encourage the parents to gather all items needed before starting the bath: a soft, clean washcloth; two cotton balls to clean the eyes; mild, unscented soap and shampoo; towels or blankets; a tub or basin with warm water; a clean diaper; and a change of clothes. Other guidelines for bathing newborns are given in Teaching Guidelines 18.1.

Elimination and Diaper Area Care

Newborn elimination patterns are highly individualized. Usually the urine is light amber in color. Soaking 6 to 12 diapers a day indicates adequate hydration. Stools can

---

TEACHING GUIDELINES 18.1

Bathing a Newborn

- Select a warm room with a flat surface at a comfortable working height.
- Before the bath, gather all supplies needed so they will be within reach.
- Never leave the newborn alone or unattended at any time during the bath.
- Undress the newborn down to shirt and diaper.
- Always support the newborn's head and neck when moving or positioning him or her.
- Place a blanket or towel underneath the newborn for warmth and comfort.
- In this order, progressing from the cleanest to the dirtiest areas:
  - Wipe eyes with plain water, using either cotton balls or a washcloth. Wipe from the inner corner of the eyes to the outer with separate wipes.
  - Wash the rest of the face, including ears, with plain water.
  - Using baby shampoo, gently wash the hair and rinse with water.
  - Pay special attention to body creases, and dry thoroughly.
  - Wash extremities, trunk, and back. Wash, rinse, dry, cover.
  - Wash diaper area last, using soap and water, and dry; observe for rash.
- Put on a clean diaper and clean clothes after the bath.

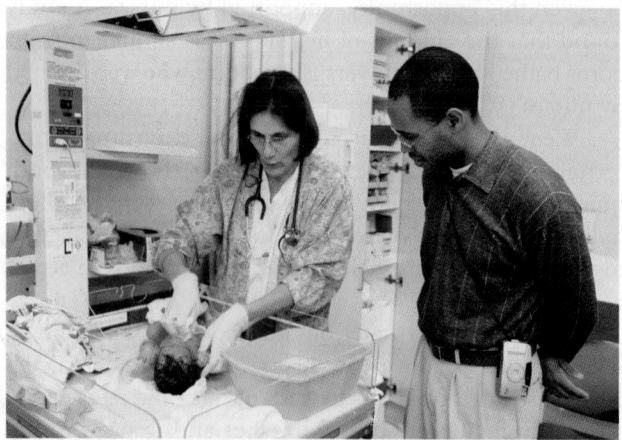

FIGURE 18.15 The nurse demonstrates bathing a newborn while the father watches.

change in color, texture, and frequency without signaling a problem. Meconium is passed for the first 48 hours after birth; the stools appear thick, tarry, sticky, and dark green. Transitional stools (thin, brown to green, less sticky than meconium) typically appear by day 3 after initiation of feeding. The stool characteristics after transitional stool depend on whether the newborn is breast-fed or bottle-fed. Breast-fed newborns typically pass mustard-colored, soft stool with a seedy consistency; formula-fed newborns pass yellow to brown, formed stool with a pasty consistency. As long as the newborn seems content, is eating normally, and shows no signs of illness, minor changes in bowel movements should not be a concern.

The newborn needs to be checked frequently to see whether a diaper change is needed, especially after feeding. Adhere to standard precautions when providing diaper area care. Instruct parents to keep the top edge of the diaper below the umbilical cord area to prevent irritation and to allow air to help dry the cord.

Meconium can be difficult to remove from the skin. Use plain water or special cleansing wipes if necessary to clean the area. Teach parents how to clean the diaper area properly and how to prevent skin irritation. Encourage them to avoid products such as powder and fragranced items, which could be irritating.

Discuss the pros and cons of using cloth diapers versus disposable diapers so that the parents can make informed decisions. Regardless of the type of diapers used, up to 10 diapers a day, or about 70 a week, will be needed.

Additional information about diapering might include:

- Before diapering, make sure all supplies are within reach, including clean diaper, cleaning agent or wipes, and ointment.
- Lay the newborn on a changing table and remove the dirty diaper.
- Use water and mild soap or wipes to gently wipe the genital area clean; wipe from front to back for girls to avoid urinary tract infections.
- Wash your hands thoroughly before and after changing diapers.

While performing diaper area care, parents should observe the area closely for irritation or rash. Tips for preventing or healing a diaper rash include:

- Change diapers frequently, especially after bowel movements.
- Apply a "barrier" cream, such as A & D ointment, after cleaning with mild soap and water.
- Use dye- and fragrance-free detergents to wash cloth diapers.
- Avoid the use of plastic pants, because they tend to hold in moisture.
- Expose the newborn's bottom to air several times a day.
- Place the newborn's buttocks in warm water after he or she had a diaper on all night.

▶ **Take** NOTE!

Advise parents that a rash that persists for more than 3 days may be fungal in origin and may require additional treatment. Encourage the parents to notify the health care provider.

Cord Care

The umbilical cord begins drying within hours after birth and is shriveled and blackened by the second or third day. Within 7 to 10 days, it sloughs off and the umbilicus heals. During this transition, frequent assessments of the area are necessary to detect any bleeding or signs of infection. Cord bleeding is abnormal and may occur if the cord clamp is loosened. Any cord drainage is also abnormal and is generally caused by infection, which requires immediate treatment.

To protect the cord area during each diaper change, apply the appropriate agent (e.g., triple dye, alcohol, or an antimicrobial agent), according to facility policy, to the cord stump to prevent any ascending infections. Single-use agents for cleaning are recommended to prevent cross-contamination with other newborns. Expect to remove the cord clamp approximately 24 hours after birth by using a cord-cutting clamp. However, if the cord is still moist, keep the clamp in place and ensure a referral to home health care so that the home care nurse can remove it after discharge. Always adhere to agency policies regarding cord care; changes in policy may be necessary based on new research findings.

Many parents avoid contact with the cord site to make sure they don't "bother" it. Teach them how to care for the cord site when they go home to prevent complications (Teaching Guidelines 18.2).

Circumcision Care

Circumcision is the surgical removal of all or part of the foreskin (prepuce) of the penis (AAP, 2007c). This has been traditionally done for hygiene and medical reasons and is the oldest known religious rite. In the Jewish faith, circumcision is a ritual that is performed by a *mohel* (ordained circumciser) on the eighth day after birth if possible. The circumcision is followed by a religious ceremony during which the newborn is named.

There are three commonly used methods of circumcision: the Gomco clamp, the Plastibell device, and the Mogen clamp. During the circumcision procedure, part of the foreskin is removed by clamping and cutting with a scalpel (Gomco or Mogen clamp) or by using a Plastibell. The Plastibell is fitted over the glans, and the excess foreskin is pulled over the plastic ring. A suture is tied around the rim to apply pressure to the blood vessels, creating hemostasis. The excess foreskin is cut away. The plastic rim remains in place until healing occurs.

TEACHING GUIDELINES 18.2

Umbilical Cord Care

- Observe for bleeding, redness, drainage, or foul odor from the cord stump and report it to your newborn's primary care provider immediately.
- Avoid tub baths until the cord has fallen off and the area has healed.
- Expose the cord stump to the air as much as possible throughout the day.
- Fold diapers below the level of the cord to prevent contamination of the site and to promote air-drying of the cord.
- Observe the cord stump, which will change color from yellow to brown to black. This is normal.
- Never pull the cord or attempt to loosen it; it will fall off naturally.

The plastic ring typically loosens and falls off in approximately 1 week (Kenner & Lott, 2007) (Fig. 18.16).

The debate over routine newborn circumcision continues in the United States. For many years, the purported benefits and harms of circumcision have been debated in the medical literature and society at large, with no clear consensus to date. Despite the controversy, circumcision is the most common surgical procedure performed on newborns, and almost two thirds of American male newborns are circumcised (Cunningham et al., 2005).

A policy statement by the AAP indicates that newborn circumcision has potential disadvantages and risks as well as medical benefits and advantages. Risks to the newborn include infection, hemorrhage, skin dehiscence, adhesions, urethral fistula, and pain. Benefits to the newborn include the following:

- Urinary tract infections are slightly less common in circumcised boys; however, rates are low in both circumcised and uncircumcised boys and are easily treated without long-term sequelae.
- Sexually transmitted infections are less common in circumcised males, but the risk is believed to be related more to behavioral factors than to circumcision status. However, circumcised males have a 50% lower risk of acquiring HIV infection (Ridings & Amaya, 2007).
- There appears to be a slightly lower rate of penile cancer in circumcised males; however, penile cancer is rare and risk factors such as genital warts, infection with human papillomavirus (HPV), multiple sex partners, and cigarette smoking seem to play a much larger role in causing penile cancer than circumcision status (Kliegman et al., 2007).

The new AAP recommendations state that if parents decide to circumcise their newborn, pain relief must be provided. Research has found that newborns circumcised without analgesia experience pain and stress, indicated by changes in heart rate, blood pressure, oxygen saturation, and cortisol levels (Ridings & Amaya, 2007). Analgesic methods may include EMLA cream (a topical mixture of local anesthetics), a dorsal penile nerve block with buffered lidocaine, acetaminophen, a sucrose pacifier, and swaddling (Cunningham et al., 2005).

The AAP recommends that parents be given accurate and unbiased information about the risks and benefits of circumcision. As with other newborn procedures, research continues. Nurses must keep informed about current medical research to allow parents to make informed decisions. The absence of compelling medical evidence in favor of or against newborn circumcision makes informed consent of parents of paramount importance. The circumcision discussion involves cultural, religious, medical, and emotional considerations. Nurses may have difficulty remaining unbiased and unemotional as they present the facts to parents. Circumcision is a very personal decision for parents, and the nurse's major responsibility is to inform the parents of the risks and benefits of the pro-

FIGURE 18.16 Circumcision. (**A**) Before the procedure. (**B**) Clamp applied and foreskin removed. (**C**) Appearance after circumcision.

cedure and to address concerns so that the parents can reach a fully informed decision.

> ▶ *Take* NOTE!
>
> *The decision to circumcise the male newborn is often a social one, with the strongest factor being whether the newborn's father is himself circumcised (AAP, 2007).*

Immediately after circumcision, the tip of the penis is usually covered with petroleum jelly–coated gauze to keep the wound from sticking to the diaper. Continued care of this site includes:

- Assess for bleeding every 30 minutes for at least 2 hours.
- Document the first voiding to evaluate for urinary obstruction or edema.
- Squeeze soapy water over the area daily and then rinse with warm water. Pat dry.
- Apply a small amount of petroleum jelly with every diaper change if the Plastibell was used; clean with mild soap and water if other techniques were used.
- Fasten the diaper loosely over the penis and avoiding placing the newborn on his abdomen to prevent friction.

If a Plastibell has been used, it will fall off by itself in about a week. Inform parents of this and advise them not to pull it off sooner. Also instruct the parents to check daily for any foul-smelling drainage, bleeding, or unusual swelling.

If the newborn is uncircumcised, wash the penis with mild soap and water after each diaper change and do not force the foreskin back; it will retract normally over time.

Safety

Newborns are completely dependent on those around them to ensure their safety. Their safety must be ensured while in the health care facility and after they are discharged. Parental education is key, especially as the newborn grows and develops and begins to respond to and explore his or her surroundings (Teaching Guidelines 18.3).

Environmental Safety

People who enter a health care facility for treatment expect to be safe there until they return home, but ensuring a safe environment can be a daunting challenge to a health care facility.

Consider this scenario: A woman dressed in nurse's clothing entered the hospital room of a new mother soon after she had given birth. This "nurse" told the mother she needed to take her newborn to the nursery to have him weighed. Sometime later, a staff nurse making her routine rounds realized something was wrong when she

---

TEACHING GUIDELINES 18.3

General Newborn Safety

- Have emergency telephone numbers readily available, such as those for emergency medical assistance and the poison control center.
- Keep small or sharp objects out of reach to prevent them from being aspirated.
- Put safety plugs in wall sockets within the child's reach to prevent electrocution.
- Do not leave the infant alone in any room without a portable intercom on.
- Always supervise the newborn in the tub: a newborn can drown in 2 inches of water.
- Make sure the crib or changing table is sturdy, without any loose hardware, and is painted with lead-free paint.
- Avoid placing the crib or changing table near blinds or curtain cords.
- Provide a smoke-free environment for all infants.
- Place all infants on their backs to sleep to prevent sudden infant death syndrome.
- To prevent falls, do not leave the newborn alone on any elevated surface.
- Use sun shields on strollers and hats to avoid overexposing the newborn to the sun.
- To prevent infection, thoroughly wash your hands before preparing formula.
- Thoroughly investigate any infant care facility before using it.

Source: AAP, 2007b.

---

saw that the newborn's bassinet in the mother's room was empty and the mother was sound asleep in her bed. The staff nurse called security immediately because she suspected that a newborn abduction had taken place.

This is a typical abduction scenario that is repeated many times throughout the United States each year. In **infant abduction**, someone who is not a family member takes a child less than 1 year old (Cohen, 2007). Infant abductions are traumatic for the parents, the community, and the health care facility. The facility may also face huge financial liability if a lawsuit is filed by the parents.

Abductions typically occur during the day and are usually carried out by women who are not criminally sophisticated. Many of these women experienced a pregnancy loss in the past; they are often emotionally immature and compulsive, with low self-esteem. Most female abductors can play the role of a hospital employee convincingly (Healthcare Risk Management, 2007).

Health care agencies are challenged to prevent infant abduction by instituting sound security practices and systems (AWHONN Lifelines, 2007). Such measures include the following:

- All newborns must be transported in cribs and not carried.
- Nurses must respond immediately to any security alarm that sounds on the unit.
- Newborns must never be unattended at any time, especially in hallways.
- All staff must wear appropriate identification at all times.
- Scrubs should not be worn by nursing staff on the postpartum unit.
- Personnel should be wary of visitors who do not seem to be visiting a specific mother.
- The electronic security system should be checked to make sure it works.
- Proper functioning and placement of any electronic sensors used on newborns should be ensured.
- Parents should be taught what infant abduction is; why infant security is important; the schedule of nursery, feeding, and visiting hours; rules about visitor access; the facility's security policies and procedures; what parents can do to protect their infant in the hospital; which staff members are allowed to handle the newborn; and what a proper ID looks like.

Providing a safe and secure environment is a shared responsibility of the facility, staff, and parents. Preventing abductions requires everyone to learn and follow the rules and policies.

Car Safety

Every state requires the use of car seats for infants and children, because motor vehicle accidents are still the leading cause of unintentional injury and death in children under age 5 (AAP, 2007d). In more than half of these deaths, the child was unrestrained.

Despite evidence that the use of car seats can reduce the morbidity and mortality of motor vehicle crashes, parents who lack knowledge about them may underuse or misuse them (AAP, 2007d). Make sure that both parents understand the importance of safely transporting their newborn in a federally approved safety car seat every time the infant rides in a car. Do not release any newborn unless the parents have a car seat in place for their newborn's ride home (Fig. 18.17). If they cannot afford one, many community organizations will provide one for them. According to the AAP, no one car seat is considered to be the "safest" or the "best," but rather consistent and proper use is the key to preventing injuries and deaths. Instruct parents in the following:

- Select a car seat that is appropriate for the child's size and weight.
- Use the car seat correctly, every time the child is in the car.
- Use rear-facing car seats for infants until they are at least 1 year old and weigh 20 lb.

FIGURE 18.17 Newborn in a properly secured car seat.

- Make sure the harness (most seats have a three- to five-point harness) is in the slots at or below the shoulders.

Infection Prevention

The nurse plays a major role in preventing infection in the newborn environment. Ways to control infection are as follows:

- Minimize exposure of newborns to organisms.
- Wash your hands before and after providing care, and insist that all personnel wash their hands before handling any newborn.
- Do not allow ill staff or visitors to visit or handle newborns.
- Monitoring the umbilical cord stump and circumcision site for signs of infection.
- Providing eye prophylaxis by instilling prescribed medication soon after birth.
- Educate parents about appropriate home measures that will prevent infections, such as practicing good hand washing before and after diaper changes, keeping the newborn well hydrated, avoiding bringing the infant into crowds (which may expose him or her to colds and flu viruses), observing for early signs of infection (fever, vomiting, loss of appetite, lethargy, labored breathing, green watery stools, drainage from umbilical cord site or eyes), and keeping pediatrician appointments for routine immunizations.

Promoting Sleep

Although many parents feel their newborns need them every minute of the day, babies actually need to sleep much of the day initially. Usually newborns sleep up to 15 hours daily. They sleep for 2 to 4 hours at a time but do not sleep through the night because their stomach capacity is too small to go long periods without nourishment.

► *Take* NOTE!

All newborns develop their own sleep patterns and cycles, but it may take several months before the newborn sleeps through the night.

Parents should place the newborn on his or her back to sleep. To prevent suffocation, all fluffy bedding, quilts, sheepskins, stuffed animals, and pillows should be removed from the crib.

Parents should be informed that the practice of "co-sleeping" (sharing a bed) is not safe: for example, infants who sleep in adult beds are up to 40 times more likely to suffocate than those who sleep in cribs (Buswell & Spatz 2007). Suffocation can occur when the infant gets entangled in bedding or caught under pillows, or slips between the bed and the wall or the headboard and mattress. The parent may accidentally roll against or on top of the baby. The safest place for a newborn to sleep is in a crib, without any movable objects close by.

Teach parents to avoid other unsafe conditions, such as placing the newborn in the prone position, using a crib that does not meet federal safety guidelines, allowing window cords to hang loose and in close proximity to the crib, or setting the room temperature too high (can cause overheating) (Adler, Hyderi, & Hamilton, 2006).

Enhancing Bonding

Encourage and enhance parent–newborn interaction by involving both parents with the baby and demonstrating appropriate nurturing behaviors:

- Say "hello" and introduce yourself to the newborn.
- Ask the parents permission to care for and hold their newborn. This helps parents to realize that they are responsible for their child and reminds nurses of their role.
- Show parents the power of a soothing voice to calm the newborn.
- Provide care to the newborn in the least stressful way.
- Demonstrate ways to wake the newborn up gently to feed better.
- Tell parents what you are doing, why you are doing it, and how they can duplicate what you are doing at home.
- Offer the opportunity for parents to perform care while you observe them. Support their efforts to soothe the newborn throughout the care process.
- Help parents to interpret the communication cues the newborn uses.
- Point out the efforts the newborn is making to connect with the parents (e.g., alerting to the familiar voice, following the parents while they are speaking, quieting when held securely).

One of the most pleasurable aspects of newborn care is being close to them. Bonding begins soon after birth when parents cradle their newborn and gently stroke him or her with their fingers. Provide parents with opportunities for "skin-to-skin" contact with the newborn, holding the baby against their own skin when feeding or cradling. Many newborns respond very positively to gentle massage. If necessary, recommend books and videos that cover the subject.

For newborns, crying is their only way to communicate that something is wrong. Try to find out the reason why: Is the diaper wet? Is the room too hot or too cold? Is the baby uncomfortable (e.g., diaper rash or tight clothing)? Suggest the following ways in which parents can soothe an upset newborn:

- Try feeding or burping to relieve air or stomach gas.
- Lightly rub the newborn's back and speak softly to him or her.
- Gently sway side to side, or rock back and forth in a rocking chair.
- Talk with the newborn while making eye contact.
- Take the newborn for a walk in a stroller or carriage to get fresh air.
- Change the baby's position from back to side or vice versa.
- Try singing, reciting poetry and nursery rhymes, or reading to the baby.
- Turn on a musical mobile above the newborn's head.
- Give more physical contact by walking, rocking, or patting the newborn.
- Swaddle the newborn to provide a sense of security and comfort. To do this:
  - Spread out a receiving blanket, with one corner folded slightly.
  - Lay the newborn face up with head at the folded corner.
  - Wrap the left corner over the baby's body and tuck it beneath the baby.
  - Bring the bottom corner over the baby's feet.
  - Wrap the right corner around the baby, leaving only the head exposed.

Assisting With Screening Tests

Screening newborns for problems is important because some potentially life-threatening metabolic diseases may not be obvious at birth. Newborn screening tests that are required in most states before discharge are used to check for certain genetic and inborn errors of metabolism and hearing. Early identification and initiation of treatment can prevent significant complications and can minimize the negative effects of untreated disease.

Genetic and Inborn Errors of Metabolism Screening

Although each state mandates which conditions must be tested, the most common screening tests are for PKU, hypothyroidism, galactosemia, and sickle cell disease (Table 18.5).

TABLE 18.5 SELECTED CONDITIONS SCREENED FOR IN THE NEWBORN

Condition	Description	Clinical Picture/ Effect If Not Treated	Treatment	Timing of Screening
PKU	Autosomal recessive inherited deficiency in one of the enzymes necessary for the metabolism of phenylalanine to tyrosine—essential amino acids found in most foods	Irritability, vomiting of protein feedings, and a musty odor to the skin or body secretions of the newborn; if not treated, mental and motor retardation, seizures, microcephaly, and poor growth and development	Lifetime diet of foods low in phenylalanine (low protein) and monitoring of blood levels (Lawson, 2007); special newborn formulas available: Phenex and Lofenalac	Universally screened for in the United States; testing is done 24–48 hours after protein feeding (PKU)
Congenital hypothyroidism	Deficiency of thyroid hormone necessary for normal brain growth, calorie metabolism, and development; may result from maternal hypothyroidism	Increased risk in newborns with birthweight <2,000 g or >4,500 g, and those of Hispanic and Asian ethnic groups; feeding problems, growth and breathing problems; if not treated, irreversible brain damage and mental retardation	Lifelong thyroid replacement therapy (Dudek, 2006)	Testing (measures thyroxin [T4] and TSH) is done between days 4 and 6 of life.
Galactosemia	Absence of the enzyme needed for the conversion of the milk sugar galactose to glucose	Poor weight gain, vomiting, jaundice, mood changes, loss of eyesight, seizures, and mental retardation; if untreated, galactose buildup causing permanent damage to the brain, eyes, and liver, and eventually death	Eliminate milk from diet; substitute soy milk	First test done on discharge from the hospital with a follow-up test within 1 month
Sickle cell anemia	Recessively inherited abnormality in hemoglobin structure, most commonly found in African-American newborns	Anemia developing shortly after birth; increased risk for infection, growth restriction, vaso-occlusive crisis	Maintenance of hydration and hemodilution, rest, electrolyte replacement, pain management, blood replacement, and antibiotics	Bloodspot obtained at same time of other newborn screening tests or prior to 3 months of age

The trend toward early discharge of newborns can affect the timing of screening and the accuracy of some test results. For example, the newborn needs to ingest enough breast milk or formula to elevate phenylalanine levels for the screening test to identify PKU accurately,

so newborn screening for PKU testing should not be performed before 24 hours of age.

Screening tests for genetic and inborn errors of metabolism require a few drops of blood taken from the newborn's heel (Fig. 18.18). These tests are usually per-

FIGURE 18.18 Screening for PKU. (**A**) Performing a heel stick. (**B**) Applying the blood specimen to the card for screening.

formed shortly before discharge. Newborns who are discharged before 24 hours of age need to have repeat tests done within a week in an outpatient facility.

Be aware of which conditions your state regularly screens for at birth to ensure that the parents are taught about the tests and the importance of early treatment. Also be familiar with the optimal time frame for screening and conditions that could affect the results. Ensure that a satisfactory specimen has been obtained at the appropriate time and that circumstances that could cause false results have been minimized. Send out specimens and completed forms within 24 hours of collection to the appropriate laboratory (Kenner & Lott, 2007).

Hearing Screening

Hearing loss is the most common birth disorder in the United States: approximately three to five newborns out of every 1,000 have some degree of hearing loss. Unlike a physical deformity, hearing loss is not clinically detectable at birth and thus remains difficult to assess (Wrightson, 2007). Factors associated with an increased risk of hearing loss include:

• Family history of childhood sensory hearing loss
• Congenital infections such as cytomegalovirus, rubella, toxoplasmosis, herpes

• Craniofacial anomalies involving the pinna or ear canal
• Low birthweight (less than 1,500 g)
• Postnatal infections such as bacterial meningitis
• Head trauma
• Hyperbilirubinemia requiring an exchange transfusion
• Exposure to ototoxic drugs, especially aminoglycosides
• Perinatal asphyxia (USPSTF, 2006)

Delays in identification and intervention may affect the child's language development, academic performance, and cognitive development. Detection before 3 months greatly improves outcomes. Because of this, auditory screening programs for all newborns are recommended by the AAP and are mandated by law in over 30 states. Screening only infants with risk factors is not enough, because as many as 50% of infants born with hearing loss have no known risk factors (AAP, 2007b). Early identification and intervention can prevent severe psychosocial, educational, and language development delays.

The current goals of *Healthy People 2010* (see the Healthy People 2010 display earlier in this chapter) are to screen all infants by 1 month of age, confirm hearing loss with an audiologic examination by 3 months of age, and treat with comprehensive early intervention services before 6 months of age (USDHHS, Volume II, Objective 16-20).

All newborns should be screened prior to discharge to ensure that any newborn with a hearing loss is not missed. Those with suspected hearing loss should be referred for follow-up assessment (Box 18.1 discusses screening methods). In addition, nurses should ensure that testing is accurate to facilitate early diagnosis and intervention services and to optimize the newborn's developmental potential.

BOX 18.1 **Newborn Hearing Screening Methods**

A newborn's hearing can be screened in one of two ways: otoacoustic emission (OAE) or automated auditory brain stem response (ABR). In OAE, an earphone is placed in the infant's ear canal and the sounds produced by the newborn's inner ear are measured in response to certain tones or clicks presented through the earphone. Preset parameters in the equipment decide whether the OAEs are sufficient for the newborn to pass or whether a referral is necessary for further evaluation.

In ABR, an earphone is placed in the ear canal or an earmuff is placed over the newborn's ear, and a soft, rapid tapping noise is presented. Electrodes placed around the newborn's head, neck, and shoulders record neural activity from the infant's brain stem in response to the tapping noises. The ABR tests how well the ear and the nerves leading to the brain work. Like OAEs, automated ABR screening is sensitive to more than mild degrees of hearing loss, but a "pass" does not guarantee normal hearing.

Source: AAP, 2007a.

EVIDENCE-BASED PRACTICE 18.1
Universal Neonatal Hearing Screening Versus Selective Screening as Part of the Management of Childhood Deafness

● **Study**

The principal factors that determine how deafness affects a child's development are the degree of hearing impairment and the age at which it is diagnosed. A number of factors are thought to increase the risk of hearing impairment, such as low birthweight, prematurity, and perinatal hypoxia and jaundice. The high incidence of deafness in children without risk factors and the introduction of simple new screening tests with high sensitivity and specificity have led many prestigious bodies to recommend universal early detection programs for deafness rather than screening that targets high-risk groups. A study was performed to compare the long-term effectiveness of a universal neonatal screening and early treatment program for hearing impairment versus screening and treatment of high-risk neonates only.

▲ **Findings**

This review found no randomized trials that compared the long-term results of these screening programs. Controlled trials and before-and-after studies are needed to address this issue.

■ **Nursing Implications**

Although additional research is needed, nurses should encourage all parents to have their newborns screened. The AAP recommends hearing screening for all newborns so that early interventions can be provided to prevent speech, language, and cognitive development impairments. This information should be stressed during discharge planning activities and follow-up tests if warranted.

Puig, T., Municio, A., & Medà, C. (2006). Universal neonatal hearing screening versus selective screening as part of the management of childhood deafness. *Cochrane Database of Systematic Reviews* 2006, Issue 2. Art. No.: CD003731. DOI: 10.1002/14651858.CD003731.pub2

Dealing With Common Concerns

During the newborn period of transition, certain conditions can develop that require intervention. These conditions, although not typically life-threatening, can be a source of anxiety for the parents. Common concerns include transient tachypnea of the newborn, physiologic jaundice, and hypoglycemia.

Transient Tachypnea of the Newborn

Transient tachypnea of the newborn appears soon after birth. It is accompanied by retractions, expiratory grunting, or cyanosis and is relieved by low-dose oxygen therapy. Mild or moderate respiratory distress typically is present at birth or within 6 hours of birth. This condition usually resolves within 3 days.

Transient tachypnea of the newborn occurs when the fetal liquid in the lungs is removed slowly or incompletely. This can be due to the lack of thoracic squeezing that occurs during a cesarean birth, or diminished respiratory effort if the mother received central nervous system depressant medication. Prolonged labor, macrosomia of the fetus, and maternal asthma also have been associated with this condition (Asenjo, 2007).

Nursing interventions include providing supportive care (giving oxygen, ensuring warmth, observing respiratory status frequently, and allowing time for the pulmonary capillaries and the lymphatics to remove the remaining fluid). The clinical course is relatively benign, but any newborn respiratory issue can be very frightening to the parents. Provide a thorough explanation and reassure them that the condition will resolve over time.

Physiologic Jaundice

Physiologic jaundice is very common in newborns, with the majority demonstrating yellowish skin, mucous membranes, and sclera within the first 3 days of life. In any given year, approximately 60% of the newborns in the United States will experience clinical jaundice (Deshpande & Ramer, 2007). Jaundice is the visible manifestation of hyperbilirubinemia. It typically results from the deposition of unconjugated bilirubin pigment in the skin and mucous membranes.

Factors that contribute to the development of physiologic jaundice in the newborn include an increased bilirubin load because of relative polycythemia, a shortened erythrocyte life span (80 days compared with the adult 120 days), and immature hepatic uptake and conjugation processes (Deshpande & Ramer, 2007). Normally the liver removes bilirubin from the blood and changes it to a form in which it can be excreted. As the red blood cell breakdown continues at a fast pace, the newborn's liver cannot keep up with bilirubin removal. Thus, bilirubin accumulates in the blood, causing a yellowish discoloration on the skin.

The AAP has recently released guidelines for the prevention and management of hyperbilirubinemia in newborns. These include:

• Promotion and support of successful breast-feeding practices to make sure the newborn is well hydrated and stooling frequently to promote elimination of bilirubin
• Completion of a systematic assessment before discharge for the risk of severe hyperbilirubinemia

- Early and focused follow-up based on the risk assessment
- When indicated, treatment of newborns with phototherapy or exchange transfusion to prevent kernicterus (AAP, 2006b)

Assess for jaundice in all newborns by pressing gently with a fingertip on the bridge of the nose, sternum, or forehead. If jaundice is present, the blanched area will appear yellow before the capillary refill (Kenner & Lott, 2007).

Measures that parents can take to reduce the risk of jaundice include exposing the newborn to natural sunlight for short periods of time throughout the day to help oxidize the bilirubin deposits on the skin, provide breastfeeding on demand to promote elimination of bilirubin through urine and stooling, and avoiding glucose water supplementation, which hinders elimination.

If or when the levels of unconjugated serum bilirubin increase and do not return to normal levels with increased hydration, phototherapy is used. The serum level of bilirubin at which phototherapy is initiated is a matter of clinical judgment by the physician, but it is often begun when bilirubin levels reach 12 to 15 mg/dL in the first 48 hours of life in a term newborn (Arenson & Drake, 2007). **Phototherapy** involves exposing the newborn to ultraviolet light, which converts unconjugated bilirubin into products that can be excreted through feces and urine.

> ► **Take** NOTE!
>
> Exposure of newborns to sunlight represents the first documented use of phototherapy in the medical literature. Sister J. Ward, a charge nurse in Essex, England, in 1956 recognized that when jaundiced newborns were exposed to the sun they became less yellow. This observation changed the entire treatment of jaundice in newborns (Maisels, 2006).

Phototherapy reduces bilirubin levels in the blood by breaking down unconjugated bilirubin into colorless compounds. These compounds can then be excreted in the bile. Phototherapy aims to curtail the increase in bilirubin blood levels, thereby preventing kernicterus, a condition in which unconjugated bilirubin enters the brain. If not treated, kernicterus can lead to brain damage and death.

During the past several decades, phototherapy has generally been administered with either banks of fluorescent lights or spotlights. Factors that determine the dose of phototherapy include spectrum of light emitted, irradiance of light source, design of light unit, surface area of newborn exposed to the light, and distance of the newborn from the light source (Cohen, 2006). For phototherapy to be effective, the rays must penetrate as much

of the skin as possible. Thus, the newborn must be naked and turned frequently to ensure maximum exposure of the skin. Several side effects of standard phototherapy have been identified: frequent loose stools, increased insensible water loss, transient rash, and potential retinal damage if the newborn's eyes are not covered sufficiently.

Recently, fiberoptic pads (Biliblanket or Bilivest) have been developed that can be wrapped around the newborn or on which the newborn can lie. The light is delivered from a tungsten–halogen bulb through a fiberoptic cable and is emitted from the sides and ends of the fibers inside a plastic pad (Cohen, 2006). These products work on the premise that phototherapy can be improved by delivering higher-intensity therapeutic light to decrease bilirubin levels. The pads do not produce appreciable heat like the banks of lights or spotlights do, so insensible water loss is not increased. Eye patches also are not needed; thus, parents can feed and hold their newborns continuously to promote bonding.

When caring for newborns receiving phototherapy for jaundice, nurses must do the following:

- Closely monitor body temperature and fluid and electrolyte balance.
- Observe skin integrity (as a result of exposure to diarrhea and phototherapy lights).
- Provide eye protection to prevent corneal injury related to phototherapy exposure.
- Encourage parents to participate in their newborn's care to prevent parent–infant separation.

See Chapter 24 for a more detailed discussion of hyperbilirubinemia.

The home health nurse made a postpartum visit to Kelly to assess the situation. Kelly's son was slightly jaundiced when the home health nurse pressed gently over his sternum, but Kelly said he was nursing better compared with the previous 2 days. What home suggestions can the nurse make to Kelly to reduce the jaundice? What specific education about physiologic jaundice is needed?

Hypoglycemia

Hypoglycemia affects as many as 40% of all full-term newborns (Kenner & Lott, 2007). It is defined as a blood glucose level of less than 35 mg/dL or a plasma concentration of less than 40 mg/dL (Kenner & Lott, 2007). In newborns, blood glucose levels fall to a low point during the first few hours of life because the source of maternal glucose is removed when the placenta is expelled. This period of transition is usually smooth, but certain newborns are at greater risk for hypoglycemia: infants of diabetic mothers, preterm newborns, and newborns with IUGR, inadequate caloric intake, sepsis, asphyxia, hypothermia, polycythemia, glycogen storage disorders, and endocrine deficiencies (Kliegman et al., 2007).

Most newborns experience transient hypoglycemia and are asymptomatic. The symptoms, when present, are nonspecific and include jitteriness, lethargy, cyanosis, apnea, seizures, high-pitched or weak cry, and poor feeding. If hypoglycemia is prolonged or is left untreated, serious, long-term adverse neurologic sequelae such as learning disabilities and mental retardation can occur (Cohen, 2007). Subsequently, early diagnosis and appropriate intervention are essential for all newborns.

Nursing care of the hypoglycemic newborn includes monitoring for signs of hypoglycemia or identifying high-risk newborns prone to this disorder based on their perinatal history, physical examination, body measurements, and gestational age. Check the blood glucose level of all newborns within the first few hours after birth and every 4 hours thereafter. More frequent monitoring and early feeding may be necessary for newborns considered to be high risk. Prevent hypoglycemia in newborns at risk by initiating early feedings with breast milk or formula. If hypoglycemia persists despite feeding, notify the primary health care provider for orders such as intravenous therapy with dextrose solutions. Anticipate hypoglycemia in certain high-risk newborns and begin assessments immediately on nursery admission.

Promoting Nutrition

Several physiologic changes dictate the type and method of feeding throughout the newborn's first year. Some of these changes include the following:

- Stomach capacity is limited to about 90 mL at birth. The emptying time is short (2 to 3 hours) and peristalsis is rapid. Therefore, small, frequent feedings are needed at first, with amounts progressively increasing with maturity.
- The immune system is immature at birth, so the baby is at a high risk for food allergies during the first 4 to 6 months of life. Introducing solid foods prior to this time increases the risk of developing food allergies.
- Pancreatic enzymes and bile to assist in digestion of fat and starch are in limited supply until about 3 to 6 months of age. Infants cannot digest cereal prior to this time.
- The kidneys are immature and unable to concentrate urine until about 4 to 6 weeks of age. Excess protein and mineral intake can place a strain on kidney function and can lead to dehydration. Infants need to consume more water per unit of body weight than adults do as a result of their high body weight from water.
- Immature muscular control at birth changes over time to assist in the feeding process by improving head and neck control, hand–eye coordination, swallowing, and ability to sit, grasp, and chew. At about 4 to 6 months, inborn reflexes disappear, head control develops, and the infant can sit to be fed, making spoon-feeding possible (Dudek, 2006).

Newborn Nutritional Needs

As newborns grow, their energy and nutrient requirements change to meet their body's changing needs. During infancy, energy, protein, vitamin, and mineral requirements per pound of body weight are higher than at any other time of life. These high levels are needed to fuel the rapid growth and development during this stage of life. Generally, an infant's birthweight doubles in the first 4 to 6 months of life and triples within the first year (Dillon, 2007).

A newborn's caloric needs range from 80 to 120 cal/kg body weight. For the first 3 months, the infant needs 110 cal/kg/day; this decreases to 100 cal/kg/day from 3 to 6 months (Begany & Mascarenhas, 2007). Breast milk and formulas contain approximately 20 cal/oz, so the caloric needs of young infants can be met if several feedings are given throughout the day.

Fluid requirements for the newborn and infant range from 100 to 150 mL/kg daily. This requirement can be met through breast or bottle feedings. Additional water supplementation is not necessary. Adequate carbohydrates, fats, protein, and vitamins are achieved through consumption of breast milk or formula. The AAP recommends that bottle-fed infants be given iron supplementation, because iron levels are low in all types of formula milk. This can be achieved by giving iron-fortified formula from birth. The breast-fed infant draws on iron reserves for the first 6 months and then needs iron-rich foods or supplementation added at 6 months of age. The AAP (2007c) also has recommended that all infants (breast- and bottle-fed) receive a daily supplement of vitamin D starting within the first 2 months of life to prevent rickets and vitamin D deficiency. It is also recommended that fluoride supplementation be given to infants not receiving fluoridated water after the age of 6 months (AAP, 2007c).

Supporting the Choice of Feeding Method

Parents typically decide about the method of feeding well before the infant is born. Prenatal and childbirth classes present information about breast-feeding versus bottle feeding and allow the parents to make up their minds about which method is best for them. Various factors can influence their decision, including socioeconomic status, culture, employment, social support available, level of education, range of care interventions provided during pregnancy, childbirth, and the early postpartum period, and especially partner support (Pryor & Huggins, 2007). Nurses can provide evidence-based information to assist the couple in making their decision. Regardless of which method is chosen, the nurse needs to respect and support the couple.

Feeding the Newborn

The newborn can be fed at any time during the transition period if assessments are normal and a desire is demonstrated. Before the newborn can be fed, determine his or her ability to suck and swallow. Clear any mucus in the nares or mouth with a bulb syringe before initiating feeding. Auscultate bowel sounds, check for abdominal distention, and inspect the anus for patency. If these parameters are within normal limits, newborn feeding may be started. Most newborns are on demand feeding schedules and are allowed to feed when they awaken. When they go home, mothers are encouraged to feed their newborns every 2 to 4 hours during the day and only when the newborn awakens during the night for the first few days after birth.

Parents often have many questions about feeding. Generally, newborns should be fed on demand whenever they seem hungry. Most newborns will give clues about their hunger status by crying, placing their fingers or fist in their mouth, rooting around, and sucking.

Newborns differ in their feeding needs and preferences, but most breast-fed ones need to be fed every 2 to 3 hours, nursing for 10 to 20 minutes on each breast. The length of feedings is up to the mother and newborn. Encourage the mother to respond to cues from her infant and not feed according to a standard or preset schedule.

Formula-fed newborns usually feed every 3 to 4 hours, finishing a bottle in 30 minutes or less. Bottle-fed infants consume about 2 to 4 fluid ounces at first and double their intake within a few weeks of age (Begany & Mascarenhas, 2007). If the newborn seems satisfied, wets 6 to 10 diapers daily, produces several stools a day, sleeps well, and is gaining weight regularly, then he or she is probably receiving sufficient breast milk or formula.

Newborns swallow air during feedings, which causes discomfort and fussiness. Parents can prevent this by burping them frequently throughout the feeding. Tips about burping include:

- Hold the newborn upright with his or her head on the parent's shoulder (Fig. 18.19A).
- Support the head and neck while the parent gently pats or rubs the newborn's back (Fig.18.19B).
- Have the newborn sit on the parent's lap, while supporting the baby's chest and head. Gently rub the newborn's back with the other hand.
- Lay the newborn on the parent's lap with the baby's back facing up.
- Support the newborn's head in the crook of the parent's arm and gently pat or rub the back.

▶ **Take** NOTE!

It is the upright position, not the strength of the patting or rubbing, that allows the newborn to release air accumulated in the stomach.

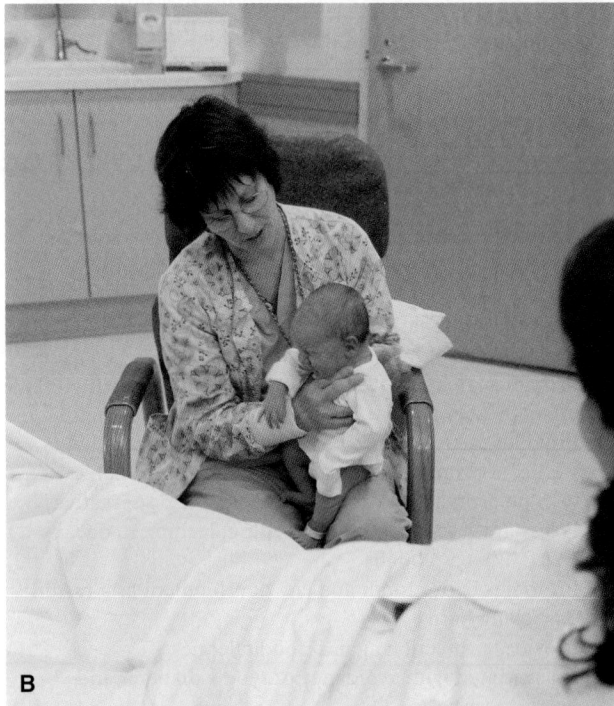

FIGURE 18.19 The nurse demonstrates holding the newborn upright over the shoulder (**A**) and sitting the newborn upright, supporting the neck and chin (**B**).

Stress to parents that feeding time is more than an opportunity to get nutrients into their newborn; it is also a time for closeness and sharing. Feedings are as much for the baby's emotional pleasure as his or her physical well-being. Encourage parents to maintain eye contact with the newborn during the feeding, hold him or her comfortably close to them, and talk softly during the feeding to promote closeness and security.

Breast-Feeding

There is consensus in the medical community that breast-feeding is optimal for all newborns. The AAP and the American Dietetic Association recommend breast-feeding exclusively for the first 6 months of life, continuing it in conjunction with other food at least until the newborn's first birthday (AAP, 2007c). Box 18.2 highlights the advantages of breast-feeding for the mother and newborn.

Mothers should continue to breast-feed during mild illnesses such as colds or the flu. However, in the United States mothers with HIV are advised not to breast-feed.

The composition of breast milk changes over time from colostrum, to transitional milk, and finally to mature milk. Colostrum is a thick, yellowish substance secreted during the first few days after birth. It is high in protein, minerals, and fat-soluble vitamins. It is rich in immunoglobulins (IgA), which help protect the newborn's gastrointestinal tract against infections. It is a natural laxative that helps rid the intestinal tract of meconium quickly (Pryor & Huggins, 2007).

BOX 18.2 Advantages of Breast-Feeding

Advantages for the Newborn
- Contributes to the development of a strong immune system
- Stimulates growth of positive bacteria in digestive tract
- Reduces incidence of stomach upset, diarrhea, and colic
- Begins the immunization process at birth by providing passive immunity
- Promotes optimal mother–infant bonding
- Reduces risk of newborn constipation
- Promotes greater developmental gains in preterm infants (AAP, 2006a, 2006b)
- Provides easily tolerated and digestible formula that is sterile, at proper temperature, and readily available with no artificial colorings, flavorings, or preservatives
- Is less likely to result in overfeeding, leading to obesity (AAP, 2006a, 2006b)
- Promotes better tooth and jaw development as a result of sucking hard
- Provides protection against food allergies
- Is associated with avoidance of type 1 diabetes and heart disease

Advantages for the Mother
- Can facilitate postpartum weight loss
- Stimulates uterine contractions to control bleeding
- Promotes uterine involution as a result of release of oxytocin
- Lowers risk of breast cancer and osteoporosis
- Affords some protection against conception, although it is not a reliable contraceptive method (Pryor & Huggins, 2007)

Transitional milk occurs between colostrum and mature milk and contains all the nutrients in colostrum, but it is thinner and less yellow than colostrum. This transitional milk is replaced by true or mature milk around day 10 after birth. Mature milk appears bluish and is not as thick as colostrum. It provides 20 cal/oz and contains:

- Protein—Although the content is lower than formula, it is ideal to support growth and development for the newborn. The majority of protein is whey, which is easy to digest.
- Fat—Approximately 58% of total calories are fat, but they are easy to digest. Essential fatty acid content is high, as is the level of cholesterol, which helps develop enzyme systems capable of handling cholesterol later in life.
- Carbohydrate—Approximately 35% to 40% of total calories are in the form of lactose, which stimulates the growth of natural defense bacteria in the gastrointestinal system and promotes calcium absorption.
- Water—Water, the major nutrient in breast milk, makes up 85% to 95% of the total volume. Total milk volume varies with the age of the infant and demand.
- Minerals—Breast milk contains calcium, phosphorus, chlorine, potassium, and sodium, with trace amounts of iron, copper, and manganese. Iron absorption is about 50%, compared with about 4% for iron-fortified formulas.
- Vitamins—All vitamins are present in breast milk; vitamin D is the lowest in amount. Debate about the need for vitamin D supplementation is ongoing.
- Enzymes—Lipase and amylase are found in breast milk to assist with digestion (Dudek, 2006).

Breast-Feeding Assistance

Breast-feeding can be initiated immediately after birth. If the newborn is healthy and stable, wipe the newborn from head to toe with a dry cloth and place him or her skin-to-skin on the mother's abdomen. Then cover the newborn and mother with another warmed blanket to hold in the warmth. Immediate mother–newborn contact takes advantage of the newborn's natural alertness after a vaginal birth and fosters bonding. This immediate contact also reduces maternal bleeding and stabilizes the newborn's temperature, blood glucose level, and respiratory rate (AAP, 2007c).

Left alone on the mother's abdomen, a healthy newborn scoots upward, pushing with the feet, pulling with the arms, and bobbing the head until finding and latching on to the mother's nipple. A newborn's sense of smell is highly developed, which also helps in finding the nipple. As the newborn moves to the nipple, the mother produces high levels of oxytocin, which contracts the uterus, thereby minimizing bleeding. Oxytocin also causes the breasts to release colostrum when the newborn sucks on the nipple. Colostrum is rich in antibodies and thus provides the newborn with her "first immunization" against infection.

Keys to successful breast-feeding include:

- Initiating breast-feeding within the first hour of life if the newborn is stable
- Following the newborn's feeding schedule—8 to 12 times in 24 hours
- Providing unrestricted periods of breast-feeding
- Offering no supplement unless medically indicated
- Having a lactation consultant observe a feeding session
- Avoiding artificial nipples and pacifiers except during a painful procedure
- Feeding from both breasts over each 24-hour period
- Watching for indicators of sufficient intake from infant:
  - Six to ten wet diapers daily
  - Waking up hungry 8 to 12 times in 24 hours
  - Acting content and falling asleep after feeding
- Keeping the newborn with the mother throughout the hospital stay

Help position the newborn so that latching-on is effective and is not painful for the mother. Placing pillows or a folded blanket under the mother's head may help, or rolling her to one side and tucking the newborn next to her. Assess both the mother and newborn during this initial session to determine needs for assistance and education. One tool used frequently in this assessment is the LATCH scoring tool (Table 18.6). The higher the score, the less nursing intervention is needed by the mother and baby.

Breast-Feeding Positioning

The mother and infant must be in comfortable positions to ensure breast-feeding success. The four most common positions for breast-feeding are the football, cradle, across-the-lap, and side-lying holds. Each mother, on experimentation, can decide which positions feel most comfortable for her (Fig. 18.20).

In the football hold, the mother holds the infant's back and shoulders in her palm and tucks the infant under her arm. Remind the mother to keep the infant's ear, shoulder, and hip in a straight line. The mother supports the breast with her hand and brings it to the infant's lips to latch on. She continues to support the breast until the infant begins to nurse. This position allows the mother to see the infant's mouth as she guides her infant to the nipple. This is a good choice for mothers who have had a cesarean birth because it avoids pressure on the incision.

The cradling position is the one most commonly used. The mother holds the baby in the crook of her arm, with the infant facing the mother. The mother supports the breast with her opposite hand.

In the across-the-lap position, the mother places a pillow across her lap, with the infant facing the mother. The mother supports the infant's back and shoulders with her palm and supports her breast from underneath. After the infant is in position, the infant is pulled forward to latch on.

In the side-lying position, the mother lies on her side with a pillow supporting her back and another pillow supporting the newborn in the front. To start, the mother props herself up on an elbow and supports the newborn with that arm, while holding her breast with the opposite hand. Once nursing is started, the mother lies down in a comfortable position.

To promote latching-on, instruct the mother to make a C or a V with her fingers. In the C hold, the mother places her thumb well above the areola and the other four fingers

TABLE 18.6 THE LATCH SCORING TOOL

Parameters	0 Point	1 Point	2 Points
L: Latch	Sleepy infant, no sustained latch achieved	Must hold nipple in infant's mouth to sustain latch and suck; must stimulate infant to continue to suck	Grasps nipple; tongue down; rhythmic sucking
A: Audible swallowing	None	A few observed with stimulation	Spontaneous and intermittent both <24 hours old and afterward
T: type of nipple	Inverted (drawn inward into breast tissue)	Flat (not protruding)	Everted or protruding out after stimulation
C: comfort of nipple	Engorged, cracked bleeding; severe discomfort	Filling; reddened, small blisters or bruises; mild to moderate discomfort	Soft, nontender
H: hold (positioning)	Nurse must hold infant to breast	Minimal assistance; help with positioning, then mother takes over	No assistance needed by nurse

Sources: AAP (2006a, 2006b, 2007); Pryor & Huggins (2007).

FIGURE 18.20 Breast-feeding positions.

below the areola and under the breast. In the V hold, the mother places her index finger above the areola and her other three fingers below the areola and under the breast. Either method can be used as long as the mother's hand is well away from the nipple so the infant can latch on.

Breast-Feeding Education

Breast-feeding is not an innate skill in human mothers. Almost all women have the potential to breast-feed successfully, but many fail because of inadequate knowledge. Nursing Care Plan 18.1 gives typical nursing diagnoses, outcomes, and interventions. For many mothers and newborns, breast-feeding goes smoothly from the start, but for others it is a struggle. Nurses can help throughout the experience by demonstrating techniques and offering encouragement and praise for success. Nurse should emphasize that the key to successful breast-feeding is correct positioning and latching-on.

Teaching by nurses has been shown to have a significant effect on both the ability to breast-feed successfully and the duration of lactation (Dudek, 2006). During the first few breast-feeding sessions, mothers want to know how often they should be nursing, whether breast-feeding is going well, if the newborn is getting enough nourishment, and what problems may ensue and how to cope with them. Education for the breast-feeding mother is highlighted in Teaching Guidelines 18.4.

*R*emember Kelly, who was concerned about jaundice in her newborn son? At her son's 2-week well-baby checkup at the clinic, his bilirubin level came back within normal limits. Kelly still felt he was not getting enough to eat and stated that she might switch to formula-feeding her son. What information can the nurse present to promote and reinforce breast-feeding? Should the nurse make a referral to the lactation consultant?

Breast Milk Storage and Expression

If the breast-feeding mother becomes separated from the newborn for any reason (e.g., work, travel, illness), she needs instruction on how to express and store milk safely. Expressing milk can be done manually (hand compression of breast) or by using a breast pump. Manual or hand pumps are inexpensive and can be used by mothers who occasionally need an extra bottle if they are going out. Electric breast pumps are used for mothers who experience a lengthy separation from their infants and need to pump their breasts regularly (Fig. 18.21).

To ensure the safety of expressed breast milk, instruct the mother in the following:

• Wash your hands before expressing milk or handling breast milk.
• Use clean containers to store expressed milk.
• Use sealed and chilled milk within 24 hours.
• Discard any milk that has been refrigerated more than 72 hours.
• Use any frozen expressed milk within 3 months.
• Do not use microwave ovens to warm chilled milk.
• Discard any used milk; never refreeze it.
• Store milk in quantities to be used for each feeding (2 to 4 oz).
• Thaw milk in warm water before using (AAP, 2007b).

Nursing Care Plan 18.1

OVERVIEW OF THE MOTHER AND NEWBORN HAVING DIFFICULTY WITH BREAST-FEEDING

Baby boy James, weight 7 lb, 4 oz, was born a few hours ago. His mother, Jane, is a 19-year-old gravida 1, para 1. His Apgar scores were 9 points at both 1 and 5 minutes. Labor and birth were unremarkable, and James was admitted to the nursery for assessment. After stabilization, James was brought to his mother, who had said she wished to breast-feed. The postpartum nurse assisted Jane with positioning and latching-on and left the room for a few minutes. On returning, Jane was upset, James was crying, and Jane stated she wanted a bottle of formula to feed him since she didn't have milk and her nipples hurt.

Assessment reveals a young, inexperienced mother placed in an uncomfortable situation with limited knowledge of breast-feeding. Anxiety from the mother transferred to James, resulting in crying. The mother, apprehensive about breast-feeding, needs additional help.

NURSING DIAGNOSIS: Knowledge deficit related to breast-feeding skills

Outcome Identification and Evaluation
Mother will demonstrate understanding of breast-feeding skills as evidenced by use of correct positioning and technique, and verbalization of appropriate information related to breast-feeding.

Interventions: Providing Education
- Instruct mother on proper positioning for breast-feeding; suggest use of football hold, side-lying position, modified cradle, and across-the-lap position to ensure comfort and *to promote ease in breast-feeding.*
- Review breast anatomy and milk letdown reflex *to enhance mother's understanding of lactation.*
- Observe newborn's ability to suck and latch on to the nipple *to assess whether newborn has adequate ability.*
- Monitor sucking and newborn swallowing for several minutes *to ensure adequate latching on and to assess intake.*
- Reinforce nipple care with water and exposure to air *to maintain nipple integrity.*

NURSING DIAGNOSIS: Anxiety related to breast-feeding ability and irritable, crying newborn

Outcome Identification and Evaluation
Mother will verbalize increased comfort with breast-feeding as evidenced by positive statements related to breast-feeding and verbalization of desire to continue to breast-feed newborn.

Interventions: Reducing Anxiety
- Ensure that the environment is calm and soothing without distractions *to promote maternal and newborn relaxation.*
- Show mother correct latching-on technique *to promote breast-feeding.*
- Assist in calming newborn by holding and talking *to ensure that the newborn is relaxed prior to latching on.*
- Reassure mother she can be successful at breast-feeding *to enhance her self-esteem and confidence.*
- Encourage frequent trials and attempts *to enhance confidence.*
- Encourage the mother to verbalize her anxiety/fears *to reduce anxiety.*

NURSING DIAGNOSIS: Pain related to breast-feeding and incorrect latching-on technique

Outcome Identification and Evaluation
Mother will experience a decrease in pain during breast-feeding as evidenced by statements of less nipple pain.

Interventions: Reducing Pain
- Suggest several alternate positions for breast-feeding *to increase comfort.*
- Demonstrate how to break suction before removing infant from breast *to minimize trauma to nipple.*
- Inspect nipple area *to promote early identification of trauma.*
- Reinforce correct latching-on technique *to prevent nipple trauma.*
- Administer pain medication if indicated *to relieve pain.*
- Instruct about nipple care between feedings *to maintain nipple integrity.*

TEACHING GUIDELINES 18.4

Breast-Feeding

- Set aside a quiet place where you can be relaxed and won't be disturbed. Relaxation promotes milk letdown.
- Sit in a comfortable chair or rocking chair or lie on a bed. Try to make each feeding calm, quiet, and leisurely. Avoid distractions.
- Listen to soothing music and sip a nutritious drink during feedings.
- Initially, nurse the newborn every few hours to stimulate milk production. Remember that the supply of milk is equal to the demand—the more sucking, the more milk.
- Watch for signals from the infant to indicate that he or she is hungry, such as:
  - Nuzzling against the mother's breasts
  - Demonstrating the rooting reflex by making sucking motions
  - Placing fist or hands in mouth to suck on
  - Crying and squirming
  - Smacking of the lips
- Stimulate the rooting reflex by touching the newborn's cheek to initiate sucking.
- Look for signs indicating that the newborn has latched on correctly: wide-open mouth with the nipple and much of the areola in the mouth, lips rolled outward, and tongue over lower gum, visible jaw movement drawing milk out, rhythmic sucking with an audible swallowing (soft "ka" or "ah" sound indicates the infant is swallowing milk).
- Hold the newborn closely, facing the breast, with the newborn's ear, shoulder, and hip in direct alignment.
- Nurse the infant on demand, not on a rigid schedule. Feed every 2 to 3 hours within a 24-hour period for a total of 8 to 12 feedings.
- Alternate the breast you offer first; identify with a safety pin on bra.
- Vary your position for each feeding to empty breasts and reduce soreness.
- Look for signs that the newborn is getting enough milk:
  - At least six wet diapers and two to five loose yellow stools daily
  - Steady weight gain after the first week of age
  - Pale-yellow urine, not deep yellow or orange
  - Sleeping well, yet looks alert and healthy when awake (AAP, 2007a)
- Wake up the newborn if he or she has nursed less than 5 minutes by unwrapping him or her.
- Before removing the baby from the breast, break the infant's suction by inserting a finger.
- Burp the infant to release air when changing breasts and at the end of the breast-feeding session.
- Avoid supplemental formula feedings to prevent "nipple confusion" (Pryor & Huggins, 2007)
- Do not take drugs or medications unless approved by the health care provider.
- Avoid drinking alcohol or caffeinated drinks because they pass through milk.
- Do not smoke while breast-feeding; it increases the risk of sudden infant death syndrome.
- Always wash your hands before expressing or handling milk to store.
- Wear nursing bras and clothes that are easy to undo.

Common Breast-Feeding Concerns

Breast-feeding women may experience problems such as cracked nipples, engorgement, or mastitis. Breast-feeding should not be painful for the mother. If she has sore, cracked nipples, the first step is to find the cause. Incorrect positioning or latching-on, removing the infant from the breast without first breaking the suction, or wearing a bra that is too tight can cause cracked or sore nipples. Cracked nipples can increase the risk of mastitis because a break in the skin may allow *Staphylococcus aureus* or other organisms to enter the body.

Sore nipples usually are caused by improper infant attachment, which traumatizes the tissue. The nurse should review techniques for proper positioning and latching-on. Recommend the following to the mother:

- Use only water, not soap, to clean the nipples to prevent dryness.
- Express some milk before feeding to stimulate the milk ejection reflex.
- Avoid using breast pads with plastic liners, and change pads when they are wet.
- Wear a comfortable bra that is not too tight.
- Apply a few drops of breast milk to the nipples after feeding.
- Rotate positions when feeding the infant to promote complete breast emptying.
- Leave the nursing bra flaps down after feeding to allow nipples to air-dry.
- Inspect the nipples daily for redness or cracks (Arenson & Drake, 2007).

To ease nipple pain and trauma, reinforce appropriate latching-on and remind the woman about the need to break the suction at the breast before removing the newborn from the breast. Additional measures may include

FIGURE 18.21 Hand-held breast pump.

applying cold compresses over the area and massaging breast milk onto the nipple after feeding.

Engorgement may occur as the milk comes in around day 3 or 4 after birth of the newborn. Explain to the mother that engorgement, though uncomfortable, is self-limited and will resolve as the newborn continues to nurse. The mother should continue to nurse during engorgement to avoid a plugged milk duct, which could lead to mastitis. Provide the following tips for relieving engorgement:

• Take warm to hot showers to encourage milk release.
• Express some milk manually before breast-feeding.
• Wear a supportive nursing bra 24 hours a day to provide support.
• Feed the newborn in a variety of positions—sitting up and then lying down.
• Massage the breasts from under the axillary area down toward the nipple.
• Increase the frequency of feedings.
• Apply warm compresses to the breasts prior to nursing.
• Stay relaxed while breast-feeding.
• Use a breast pump if nursing or manual expression is not effective.
• Remember that this condition is temporary and resolves quickly.

Mastitis, or inflammation of the breast, causes flu-like symptoms, chills, fever, and malaise. These symptoms may occur before the development of soreness, aching, swelling, and redness in the breast (usually the upper outer quadrant). This condition usually occurs in just one breast when a milk duct becomes blocked, causing inflammation, or through a cracked or damaged nipple, allowing bacteria to infect a portion of the breast. Treatment con-

sists of rest, warm compresses, antibiotics, breast support, and continued breast-feeding (the infection will not pass into the breast milk). Explain to the mother that it is important to keep the milk flowing in the infected breast, whether it is through nursing or manual expression or with a breast pump.

Formula Feeding

Despite the general acknowledgment that breast-feeding is the most desirable means of feeding infants, about 40% of mothers choose formula feeding and need education about this procedure. Formula-fed infants grow more rapidly than breast-fed infants not only in weight but also in length (Begany & Mascarenhas, 2007).

Formula feeding requires more than just opening, pouring, and feeding. Parents need information about the types of formula available, preparation and storage of formula, equipment, feeding positions, and the amount to feed their newborn. The mother also needs to know how to prevent lactation (see Chap. 16 for more information).

Commercially prepared formulas are regulated by the Food and Drug Administration (FDA) and are manufactured by Meade Johnson (Enfamil) or Ross Laboratories (Similac) in the United States. Normal full-term infants usually receive conventional cow's milk-based formula, but this decision is made by the health care provider. If the infant shows signs of a reaction or lactose intolerance, a switch to another formula type is recommended. The general recommendation is for all infants to receive iron-fortified formula until the age of 1 year. The latest generation of infant formulas includes some fortification with docosahexaenoic acid (DHA) and arachidonic acid (ARA), two natural components of breast milk. Researchers have found that formulas with DHA and ARA can enhance visual and cognitive development in children (Lawson, 2007).

Commercial formulas come in three forms: powder, concentrate, and easy to feed or ready to use. All are similar in terms of nutritional content but differ in expense. Powdered formula is the least expensive, with concentrated formula the next most expensive. Both must be mixed with water before using. Ready-to-feed formula is the most expensive; it can be opened and poured into a bottle and fed directly to the infant.

Parents need information about the equipment needed for formula feeding. Basic supplies are 4 to 6 4-oz bottles, 8 to 10 8-oz bottles, 8 to 10 nipple units, a bottle brush, and a nipple brush. A key area of instruction is assessing for flow of formula through the nipple and checking for any nipple damage. When the bottle is filled and turned upside down, the flow from the nipple should be approximately one drop per second. If the parents are using bottles with disposable bags, instruct them to make sure they have a tight-fitting nipple to prevent leaks. Frequent observation of the flow rate from the nipple and the condition of the nipple will prevent choking and aspiration associated with too fast a rate of delivery. Ask the parents to fill a bottle with formula and then turn it upside down and observe the rate at which the formula drips from the bottle. If it is too fast (more than one drop/second), then the nipple should be replaced.

Correct formula preparation is critical to the newborn's health and development. Mistakes in dilution may result if the parents do not understand how to prepare the formula or make measurement errors. The safety of the water supply should be considered. If well water is used, parents should sterilize the water by boiling it or should use bottled water. Many health care providers still recommend that all water used in formula preparation be brought to a rolling boil for 1 to 2 minutes and should be cooled to room temperature before use.

Opened cans of ready-made or concentrated formula should be covered and refrigerated after being prepared for the day (24 hours). Instruct parents to discard any unused portions after 48 hours.

> ▶ *Take* NOTE!
>
> *Any formula left in the bottle after feeding should also be discarded, because the infant's saliva has been mixed with it.*

To warm refrigerated formula, advise the parents to place the bottle in a pan of hot water and test the temperature by letting a few drops fall on the inside of the wrist. If it is comfortably warm to the mother, it is the correct temperature.

Formula-Feeding Assistance

The process of feeding a newborn formula from a bottle should mirror breast-feeding as closely as possible. Although nutrition is important, so are the emotional and interactive components of feeding. Encourage parents to cuddle their newborn closely and position him or her so that the head is in a comfortable position, not too far back or turned, which makes swallowing difficult. Also urge parents to communicate with their newborn during the feedings by talking and singing to him or her.

Although it may seem that bottle feeding is not a difficult task, many new parents find it awkward. At first glance, holding an infant and a bottle appears simple enough, but both the position of the baby and the angle of the bottle must be correct.

Formula-Feeding Positions

Advise mothers to feed their newborns in a relaxed and quiet setting to create a sense of calm for themselves and the baby. Make sure that comfort is a priority for both mother and newborn. The mother can sit in a comfortable chair, using a pillow to support the arm in which she is holding the baby. The mother can cradle the newborn in a semi-upright position, supporting the newborn's head in the crook of her arm. Holding the newborn close during feeding provides stimulation and helps prevent choking. Holding the newborn's head raised slightly will help prevent formula from washing backward into the eustachian tubes in the ears, which can lead to an ear infection.

Formula-Feeding Education

Parents require teaching about the correct preparation and storage of formula as well as the techniques for feeding. See Teaching Guidelines 18.5.

Proper positioning makes bottle feeding easier and more enjoyable for both mother and newborn. As in breast-feeding, frequent burping is key. Advise the parents to hold the bottle so that formula fills the nipple, thus allowing less air to enter. Infants get fussy when they swallow air during feedings and need to be relieved of it every 2 to 3 oz.

TEACHING GUIDELINES 18.5

Formula-Feeding

- Wash your hands with soap and water before preparing formula.
- Mix the formula and water amounts exactly as the label specifies.
- Always hold the newborn and bottle during feedings; never prop the bottle.
- Never freeze formula or warm it in the microwave.
- Place refrigerated formula in a pan of hot water for a few minutes to warm.
- Test the temperature of the formula by shaking a few drops on the wrist.
- Hold the bottle like a pencil, keeping it tipped to prevent air from entering. Position the bottle so that the nipple remains filled with milk.
- Burp the infant after every few ounces to allow air swallowed to escape.
- Move the nipple around in the infant's mouth to stimulate sucking.
- Always keep a bulb syringe close by to use if choking occurs.
- Avoid putting the infant to bed with a bottle to prevent "baby bottle tooth decay."
- Feed the newborn approximately every 3 to 4 hours.
- Use an iron-fortified formula for the first year.
- Prepare enough formula for the next 24 hours.
- Check nipples regularly and discard any that are sticky, cracked, or leaking.
- Store unmixed, open liquid formula in the refrigerator for up to 48 hours.
- Throw away any formula left in the bottle after each feeding.

Emphasize to parents that an electrolyte imbalance can occur in infants who are fed formula that has been incorrectly mixed. Hypernatremia can result from formula that is mixed too thickly; the high concentration of sodium is too much for the baby's immature kidneys to handle. As a result, sodium is excreted along with water, leading to dehydration. Mixing the formula with too much water in an effort to save money can lead to failure to thrive and lack of weight gain (AAP, 2007b).

Weaning and Introduction of Solid Foods

Eventually, breast-feeding or formula feeding ends. Weaning involves the transition from breast to bottle, from breast or bottle to cup, or from liquids to solids. Weaning from breast-feeding to cup has several advantages over weaning to a bottle because it eliminates the step of weaning first to a bottle and then to a cup. Another advantage is that the bottle does not become a security object for the infant.

Weaning can be done because the mother is returning to work and cannot keep breast-feeding, or because the infant is losing interest in breast-feeding and showing signs of independence. There is no "right" time to wean; it depends on the desires of the mother and infant. Weaning represents a significant change in the way the mother and infant interact, and each mother must decide for herself when she and her infant are ready to take that step. Either one can start the weaning process, but usually it occurs between 6 months and 1 year of age.

To begin weaning from the breast, instruct mothers to substitute breast-feeding with a cup or bottle. Often the midday feeding is the easiest feeding to replace. A trainer cup with two handles and a snap-on lid with a spout is appropriate and minimizes spilling. Because weaning is a gradual process, it may take months. Instruct parents to proceed slowly and let the infant's willingness and interest guide them.

Weaning from the bottle to the cup also needs to be timed appropriately for mother and infant. Typically, the night bottle is the last to be given up, with cup drinking substituted throughout the day. Slowly diluting the formula with water over a week can help in this process; the final result is an all-water bottle. To prevent the baby from sucking on the bottle during the night, remove it from the crib after the infant falls asleep.

When infants double their birthweight and weigh at least 13 lb, it is time to consider introducing solid foods. Readiness cues include:

- Consumption of 32 oz of formula or breast milk daily (estimated)
- Ability to sit up with minimal support and turn head away to indicate fullness
- Reduction of protrusion reflex so cereal can be propelled to back of throat
- Demonstration of interest in food others around them are eating

- Ability to open mouth automatically when food approaches it

When introducing solid foods, certain principles apply:

- Only one new single-ingredient food (e.g., rice cereal or carrots) should be introduced at a time to watch for allergies.
- Infants should be allowed to set the pace regarding how much they wish to eat.
- New foods should not be introduced more frequently than every 3 to 5 days.
- Fruits are added after cereals; then vegetables and meats are introduced; eggs are introduced last.
- A relaxed, unhurried, calm atmosphere for meals is important.
- A variety of foods are provided to ensure a balanced diet.
- Infants should never be force-fed (Lawson, 2007).

Nurses can promote good feeding practices by actively listening to new mothers, helping them clarify their feelings and discussing solutions. A warm, sincere manner and tone of voice will put an anxious mother at ease. Giving accurate information, making suggestions, and presenting options will enable the mother to decide what is best for her and her infant. Nurses should be sensitive to the individual, family, and economic and cultural differences among mothers before offering suggestions for feeding practices that may not be appropriate.

Preparing for Discharge

Preparing the parents for discharge is an essential task for the nurse. Because of today's shorter hospital stays, the nurse must identify the major teaching topics that need to be covered. Nurses should assess the parents' baseline knowledge and learning needs and plan how to meet them. Using the following principles fosters a learner-centered approach:

- Make the environment conducive to learning. Encourage the parents to feel comfortable during this intense time by using support and praise.
- Allow the parents to provide input about the content and the process of learning. What do they want and need to learn?
- Build the parents' self-esteem by confirming that their responses to the entire birthing process and aftercare are legitimate, and others have felt the same way.
- Ensure that what the parents learn is relevant to their day-to-day home situation.
- Encourage responsibility by reinforcing that their emotional and physical responses are within the normal range.
- Respect cultural beliefs and practices that are important to the family by taking into account their heritage and health beliefs regarding newborn care. Examples include placing a bellyband over the newborn's navel

(Hispanics and African-Americans), delaying naming the newborn (Asian-Americans and Haitians), and delaying breast-feeding (Native Americans; they regard colostrum as "bad") (Bowers, 2007).

While in the hospital, women have ready access to support and hands-on instruction regarding feeding and newborn care. When the new mother is discharged, this close supervision and support by nurses should not end abruptly. Providing the new parents with the phone number of the mother–baby unit will help them through this stressful transitional period. Giving the new family information and offering backup support via the telephone will increase parenting success.

► *Consider* THIS!

I have always prided myself on being very organized and in control in most situations, but survival at home after childbirth wasn't one of them. I left the hospital 24 hours after giving birth to my son because my doctor said I could. The postpartum nurse encouraged me to stay longer, but wanting to be in control and sleeping in my own bed again won out. I thought my baby would be sleeping while I sent out birth announcements to my friends and family—wrong! What happened instead was my son didn't sleep as I imagined and my nipples became sore after breast-feeding every few hours. I was weary and tired and wanted to sleep, but I couldn't. Somehow I thought I would be getting a full night's sleep because I was up throughout the day, but that was a fantasy too. At 2 o'clock in the morning when you are up feeding your baby, you feel you are the only one in the world up at that time and feel very much alone. My feelings of being organized and in control all the time have changed dramatically since I left the hospital. I have learned to yield to the important needs of my son and derive satisfaction from being able to bring comfort to him and to let go of my control.

Thoughts: It is interesting to see how a newborn changed this woman's need to organize and control her environment. What "tips of survival" could the nurse offer this woman to help in her transition to home with her newborn? How can friends and family help when women arrive home from the hospital with their newborns?

Ensuring Follow-Up Care

Most newborns are scheduled for their first health follow-up appointment within 2 to 4 days after discharge so they can have additional laboratory work done as part of the newborn screening series, especially if they were discharged within 48 hours. After this first visit, the typical schedule of health care visits is as follows: 2 to 4 weeks of age; 2, 4, and 6 months of age for checkups and vaccines; 9 months of age for a checkup; 12 months for a checkup and tuberculosis testing; 15 and 18 months for checkups and vaccines; and 2 years of age for a checkup. These appointments provide an opportunity for parents to ask questions and receive anticipatory guidance as their newborn grows and develops.

In addition to encouraging parents to keep follow-up appointments, advise parents to call their health care provider if they notice signs of illness in their newborn. They should know which over-the-counter medicines should be kept on hand. Review the following warning signs of illness with parents:

- Temperature of 38.3°C (101°F) or higher
- Forceful, persistent vomiting, not just spitting up
- Refusal to take feedings
- Two or more green, watery diarrheal stools
- Infrequent wet diapers and change in bowel movements from normal pattern
- Lethargy or excessive sleepiness
- Inconsolable crying and extreme fussiness
- Abdominal distention
- Difficult or labored breathing

Providing Immunization Information

Parents also need instructions about immunizations for their newborn. **Immunization** is the process of rendering an individual immune or of becoming immune to certain communicable diseases (AAP, 2007). The purpose of the immune system is to identify unknown (non-self) substances in the body and develop a defense against these invaders. Disease prevention by immunization is a public health priority and is one of the leading health indicators as part of *Healthy People 2010*. Despite many advances in vaccine delivery, the goal of universal immunization has not been reached (AAP, 2007). Nurses can help to meet this national goal by educating new parents about the importance of disease prevention through immunizations.

Immunity can be provided either passively or actively. Passive immunity is protection transferred via already formed antibodies from one person to another. Passive immunity includes transplacental passage of antibodies from a mother to her newborn, immunity passed through breast milk, and immunity from immunoglobulins. Passive immunity provides limited protection and decreases over a period of weeks or months (Blackburn, 2007). Active immunity is protection produced by an individual's own immune system. It can be obtained by having the actual disease or by receiving a vaccine that produces an immunologic response by that person's body. Active immunity may be lifelong either way.

Young infants and children are susceptible to various illnesses because their immune systems are not yet mature. Many of these illnesses can be prevented by following the recommended schedule of childhood immunizations; Figure 18.22 shows the 2008 Childhood Immunization

Recommended Immunization Schedule for Persons Aged 0–6 Years—UNITED STATES • 2008
For those who fall behind or start late, see the catch-up schedule

Vaccine ▼ Age ►	Birth	1 month	2 months	4 months	6 months	12 months	15 months	18 months	19–23 months	2–3 years	4–6 years
Hepatitis B[1]	HepB	HepB		see footnote1	HepB						
Rotavirus[2]			Rota	Rota	Rota						
Diphtheria, Tetanus, Pertussis[3]			DTaP	DTaP	DTaP	see footnote3	DTaP				DTaP
Haemophilus influenzae type b[4]			Hib	Hib	Hib[4]	Hib					
Pneumococcal[5]			PCV	PCV	PCV	PCV				PPV	
Inactivated Poliovirus			IPV	IPV	IPV						IPV
Influenza[6]						Influenza (Yearly)					
Measles, Mumps, Rubella[7]						MMR					MMR
Varicella[8]						Varicella					Varicella
Hepatitis A[9]						HepA (2 doses)				HepA Series	
Meningococcal[10]										MCV4	

Range of recommended ages

Certain high-risk groups

This schedule indicates the recommended ages for routine administration of currently licensed childhood vaccines, as of December 1, 2007, for children aged 0 through 6 years. Additional information is available at www.cdc.gov/vaccines/recs/schedules. Any dose not administered at the recommended age should be administered at any subsequent visit, when indicated and feasible. Additional vaccines may be licensed and recommended during the year. Licensed combination vaccines may be used whenever any components of the combination are indicated and other components of the vaccine are not contraindicated and if approved by the Food and Drug Administration for that dose of the series. Providers should consult the respective Advisory Committee on Immunization Practices statement for detailed recommendations, including for **high-risk conditions:** http://www.cdc.gov/vaccines/pubs/ACIP-list.htm. Clinically significant adverse events that follow immunization should be reported to the Vaccine Adverse Event Reporting System (VAERS). Guidance about how to obtain and complete a VAERS form is available at www.vaers.hhs.gov or by telephone, 800-822-7967.

1. Hepatitis B vaccine (HepB). *(Minimum age: birth)*
At birth:
• Administer monovalent HepB to all newborns prior to hospital discharge.
• If mother is hepatitis B surface antigen (HBsAg) positive, administer HepB and 0.5 mL of hepatitis B immune globulin (HBIG) within 12 hours of birth.
• If mother's HBsAg status is unknown, administer HepB within 12 hours of birth. Determine the HBsAg status as soon as possible and if HBsAg positive, administer HBIG (no later than age 1 week).
• If mother is HBsAg negative, the birth dose can be delayed, in rare cases, with a provider's order and a copy of the mother's negative HBsAg laboratory report in the infant's medical record.
After the birth dose:
• The HepB series should be completed with either monovalent HepB or a combination vaccine containing HepB. The second dose should be administered at age 1–2 months. The final dose should be administered no earlier than age 24 weeks. Infants born to HBsAg-positive mothers should be tested for HBsAg and antibody to HBsAg after completion of at least 3 doses of a licensed HepB series, at age 9–18 months (generally at the next well-child visit).
4-month dose:
• It is permissible to administer 4 doses of HepB when combination vaccines are administered after the birth dose. If monovalent HepB is used for doses after the birth dose, a dose at age 4 months is not needed.

2. Rotavirus vaccine (Rota). *(Minimum age: 6 weeks)*
• Administer the first dose at age 6–12 weeks.
• Do not start the series later than age 12 weeks.
• Administer the final dose in the series by age 32 weeks. Do not administer any dose later than age 32 weeks.
• Data on safety and efficacy outside of these age ranges are insufficient.

3. Diphtheria and tetanus toxoids and acellular pertussis vaccine (DTaP). *(Minimum age: 6 weeks)*
• The fourth dose of DTaP may be administered as early as age 12 months, provided 6 months have elapsed since the third dose.
• Administer the final dose in the series at age 4–6 years.

4. Haemophilus influenzae type b conjugate vaccine (Hib). *(Minimum age: 6 weeks)*
• If PRP-OMP (PedvaxHIB® or ComVax® [Merck]) is administered at ages 2 and 4 months, a dose at age 6 months is not required.
• TriHIBit® (DTaP/Hib) combination products should not be used for primary immunization but can be used as boosters following any Hib vaccine in children age 12 months or older.

5. Pneumococcal vaccine. *(Minimum age: 6 weeks for pneumococcal conjugate vaccine [PCV]; 2 years for pneumococcal polysaccharide vaccine [PPV])*
• Administer one dose of PCV to all healthy children aged 24–59 months having any incomplete schedule.
• Administer PPV to children aged 2 years and older with underlying medical conditions.

6. Influenza vaccine. *(Minimum age: 6 months for trivalent inactivated influenza vaccine [TIV]; 2 years for live, attenuated influenza vaccine [LAIV])*
• Administer annually to children aged 6–59 months and to all eligible close contacts of children aged 0–59 months.
• Administer annually to children 5 years of age and older with certain risk factors, to other persons (including household members) in close contact with persons in groups at higher risk, and to any child whose parents request vaccination.
• For healthy persons (those who do not have underlying medical conditions that predispose them to influenza complications) ages 2–49 years, either LAIV or TIV may be used.
• Children receiving TIV should receive 0.25 mL if age 6–35 months or 0.5 mL if age 3 years or older.
• Administer 2 doses (separated by 4 weeks or longer) to children younger than 9 years who are receiving influenza vaccine for the first time or who were vaccinated for the first time last season but only received one dose.

7. Measles, mumps, and rubella vaccine (MMR). *(Minimum age: 12 months)*
• Administer the second dose of MMR at age 4–6 years. MMR may be administered before age 4–6 years, provided 4 weeks or more have elapsed since the first dose.

8. Varicella vaccine. *(Minimum age: 12 months)*
• Administer second dose at age 4–6 years; may be administered 3 months or more after first dose.
• Do not repeat second dose if administered 28 days or more after first dose.

9. Hepatitis A vaccine (HepA). *(Minimum age: 12 months)*
• Administer to all children aged 1 year (i.e., aged 12–23 months). Administer the 2 doses in the series at least 6 months apart.
• Children not fully vaccinated by age 2 years can be vaccinated at subsequent visits.
• HepA is recommended for certain other groups of children, including in areas where vaccination programs target older children.

10. Meningococcal vaccine. *(Minimum age: 2 years for meningococcal conjugate vaccine (MCV4) and for meningococcal polysaccharide vaccine (MPSV4))*
• Administer MCV4 to children aged 2–10 years with terminal complement deficiencies or anatomic or functional asplenia and certain other high-risk groups. MPSV4 is also acceptable.
• Administer MCV4 to persons who received MPSV4 3 or more years previously and remain at increased risk for meningococcal disease.

FIGURE 18.22 Recommended childhood immunization schedule.

Schedule. Readers can view the latest CDC immunization schedule by visiting www.cdc.gov/nip. The schedule for immunizations should be reviewed with parents, stressing the importance of continued follow-up health care to preserve their infant's health.

The newborn's first immunization (hepatitis B) is received in the hospital soon after birth. The first dose can also be given by age 2 months if the mother is HbsAg negative. If the mother is HbsAg positive, then the newborn should receive hepatitis B vaccine and hepatitis B immunoglobulin within 12 hours of birth (Cunningham et al., 2005).

Education for the parents should include the risks and benefits for each vaccine and possible adverse effects. Federal law requires a consent form to be signed before administering a vaccine. Parents have the right to refuse immunizations based on their religious beliefs and can sign a waiver noting their decision. The nurse administering the vaccine must document the date and time it was given, name and manufacturer, lot number and expiration date of the vaccine given, site and route of administration, and the name and title of the nurse who administered the vaccine.

■■■ Key Concepts

- The period of transition from intrauterine to extrauterine life occurs during the first several hours after birth. It is a time of stabilization for the newborn's temperature, respiration, and cardiovascular dynamics.
- The newborn's bowel is sterile at birth. It usually takes about a week for the newborn to produce vitamin K in sufficient quantities to prevent VKDB.
- It is recommended that all newborns in the United States receive an instillation of a prophylactic agent (erythromycin or tetracycline ophthalmic ointment) in their eyes within an hour or two of being born.
- Nursing measures to maintain newborns' body temperature include drying them immediately after birth to prevent heat loss through evaporation, wrapping them in prewarmed blankets, putting a hat on their head, and placing them under a temperature-controlled radiant warmer.
- The specific components of a typical newborn examination include a general survey of skin color, posture, state of alertness, head size, overall behavioral state, respiratory status, gender, and any obvious congenital anomalies.
- Gestational age assessment is pertinent because it allows the nurse to plot growth parameters and to anticipate potential problems related to prematurity/postmaturity and growth abnormalities such as SGA/LGA.
- After the newborn has passed the transitional period and stabilized, the nurse needs to complete ongoing assessments, vital signs, weight and measurements, cord care, hygiene measures, newborn screening tests, and

various other tasks until the newborn is discharged home from the birthing unit.
- Important topics about which to educate parents include environmental safety, newborn characteristics, feeding and bathing, circumcision and cord care, sleep and elimination patterns of newborns, safe infant car seats, holding/positioning, and follow-up care.
- Newborn screening tests consist of hearing and certain genetic and inborn errors of metabolism tests required in most states for newborns before discharge from the birth facility.
- The AAP and the American Dietetic Association recommend breast-feeding exclusively for the first 6 months of life and that it continue along with other food at least until the first birthday.
- Parents who choose not to breast-feed need to know what types of formula are available, preparation and storage of formula, equipment, feeding positions, and how much to feed their infant.
- Common problems associated with the newborn include transient tachypnea, physiologic jaundice, and hypoglycemia.
- Transient tachypnea of the newborn appears soon after birth; is accompanied by retractions, expiratory grunting, or cyanosis; and is relieved by low-dose oxygen.
- Physiologic jaundice is a very common condition in newborns, with the majority demonstrating yellowish skin, mucous membranes, and sclera within the first 3 days of life. Newborns undergoing phototherapy in the treatment of jaundice require close monitoring of their body temperature, fluid, and electrolyte balance; observation of skin integrity; eye protection; and parental participation in their care.
- The newborn with hypoglycemia requires close monitoring for signs and symptoms of hypoglycemia if present. In addition, newborns at high risk need to be identified based on their perinatal history, physical examination, body measurements, and gestational age. Blood glucose levels of all newborns are checked within the first few hours after birth and every 4 hours thereafter.
- The schedule for immunizations should be reviewed with parents, stressing the importance of continual follow-up health care to preserve their infant's health.

REFERENCES

Adegbehingbe, O., Owa, J. A., Kuti, O., & Oginni, L. M. (2007). Orthopedic birth trauma: A reflection of current perinatal care. *Internet Journal of Gynecology and Obstetrics, 6*(2), 8–20.

Adler, M. R., Hyderi, A., & Hamilton, A. (2006). What are the safe sleeping arrangements for infants? *Journal of Family Practice, 55*(12), 1083–1087.

American Academy of Pediatrics (AAP). (2006a). *A woman's guide to breast-feeding.* Available at www.aap.org/family/brstguid.htm.

American Academy of Pediatrics (AAP). (2006b). Breast-feeding and the use of human milk. AAP policy statement. *Pediatrics, 115,* 496–506.

American Academy of Pediatrics (AAP). (2007a). *Bright futures guidelines for health supervision of infants, children, and adolescents.* Washington, DC: AAP.

American Academy of Pediatrics (AAP). (2007b). *Heading home with your newborn: From birth to reality.* Washington, DC: AAP.

American Academy of Pediatrics (AAP). (2007c). *Pediatric clinical practice guidelines and policies: A compendium of evidence-based research for pediatric practice* (7th ed.). Washington, DC: AAP.

American Academy of Pediatrics (AAP). (2007d). *Car safety seats: A guide for families 2007.* Available at www.aap.org/family/carseatguide.htm.

Arenson, J., & Drake, P. (2007). *Maternal and newborn health.* Sudbury, MA: Jones and Bartlett Publishers.

Asenjo, M. (2007). Transient tachypnea of the newborn. *eMedicine.* Available at www.emedicine.com/radio/topic710.htm.

AWHONN Lifelines. (2007). Preventing infant abduction: A parent's guide. *AWHONN Lifelines, 10*(6), 521–522.

Begany, M., & Mascarenhas, M. (2007). Normal infant feeding. In R. E. Rakel & E. T. Bope (Eds.), *Conn's current therapy 2007* (Section 16, pp. 1210–1214). Philadelphia: Saunders Elsevier.

Blackburn, S. T. (2007). *Maternal, fetal, and neonatal physiology: A clinical perspective* (3rd ed.). St. Louis: Saunders Elsevier.

Bowers, P. (2007). Cultural aspects of childbearing. *Nursing Spectrum.* Available at http://www.nurse.com/ce/syllabus.html?CCID=3245.

Burns, C. E., Dunn, A. M., Brady, M. A., Starr, N. B., & Blosser, C. G. (2009). *Pediatric primary care* (4th ed.). St. Louis: Saunders Elsevier.

Buswell, S. D., & Spatz, D. L. (2007). Parent-infant co-sleeping and its relationship to breastfeeding. *Journal of Pediatric Health Care, 21*(1), 22–28.

Centers for Disease Control and Prevention (CDC). (2007). *Sexually transmitted diseases treatment guidelines.* Available at: www.cdc.gov/STD/treatment.

Cohen, S. (2007). *Critical thinking in the pediatric unit: Skills to assess, analyze and act.* Marblehead, MA: HCPro, Inc.

Cohen, S. M. (2006). Jaundice in the full-term newborn. *Pediatric Nursing, 32*(3), 202–208.

Cunningham, F. G., Leveno, K. J., Bloom, S. L., Hauth, J. C., Gilstrap, L. C., & Wenstrom, K. D. (2005). *Williams obstetrics* (22nd ed.). New York: McGraw-Hill Medical Publishing Division.

Deshpande, P. G., & Ramer, T. (2007). Breast milk jaundice. *eMedicine.* Available at: http://www.emedicine.com/ped/topic282.htm.

Dillon, P. M. (2007). *Nursing health assessment: A critical thinking, case studies approach.* Philadelphia: F. A. Davis.

Dudek, S. G. (2006). *Nutrition essentials for nursing practice* (5th ed.). Philadelphia: Lippincott Williams & Wilkins.

Healthcare Risk Management. (2007). Infant abduction raises questions about health care security and vigilance. *Healthcare Risk Management, 29*(5), 49–60.

Johnson, K. J., Spector, L. G., Klebanoff, M. A., & Ross, J. A. (2007). Childhood cancer and birthmarks in the collaborative perinatal project. *Pediatrics, 119*(5), 1088–1093.

Keenan, W. (2006). Apgar score—How consistent is it? *Pediatric Alert, 31*(19), 113–114.

Kenner, C., & Lott, J. W. (2007). *Comprehensive neonatal care: An interdisciplinary approach* (4th ed.). St. Louis: Saunders Elsevier.

Kliegman, R. M., Behrman, R. E., Jenson, H. B., & Stanton, B. F. (2007). *Nelson's textbook of pediatrics* (18th ed.). St. Louis: Saunders Elsevier.

Lawrence, E. J. (2006). Focus on the physical. Part 1: A matter of size. *Advances in Neonatal Care, 6*(6), 313–322.

Lawson, M. (2007). Contemporary aspects of infant feeding. *Pediatric Nursing, 19*(2), 39–45.

Maisels, M. J. (2006). What's in a name? Physiologic and pathologic jaundice: The conundrum of defining normal bilirubin levels in the newborn. *Pediatrics, 118*(2), 805–807.

Mukherjee, S. (2007). Hyperbilirubinemia, unconjugated. *eMedicine.* Available at: http://www.emedicine.com/med/topic1066.htm.

Pryor, G., & Huggins, K. (2007). *Nursing mother, working mother: The essential guide to breastfeeding your baby before and after you return to work* (2nd ed.). Harvard, MA: The Harvard Common Press.

Ridings, H., & Amaya, M. (2007). Male neonatal circumcision: An evidence-based review. *Journal of the American Academy of Physician Assistants, 20*(2), 32–36.

Simonson, C., Barlow, P., Dehennin, N., Sphel, M., Toppet, V., Murillo, D., & Rozenberg, S. (2007). Neonatal complications of vacuum-assisted delivery. *Obstetrics and Gynecology, 109*(3), 626–633.

U.S. Department of Health and Human Services (USDHHS). (2000). *Healthy people 2010: Understanding and improving health* (2nd ed.). DHHS publication 017-001-00550-9. Washington, DC: Author.

U.S. Prevention Services Task Force (USPSTF). (2006). *The guide to clinical prevention services.* Agency for Healthcare Research and Quality. Washington, DC: AHRQ Pub.No. 06-0588.

Walsh, D. (2007). *Evidence-based care for normal labor and birth: A guide for midwives.* London: Taylor and Francis, Inc.

Wasee, M. (2006). Vitamin K and hemorrhagic disease of newborns. *Southern Medical Journal, 99*(11), 1199–1200.

Wrightson, A. S. (2007) Universal newborn hearing screening. *American Family Physician, 75*(9), 1349–1352.

WEBSITES

American Academy of Pediatrics, Newborn Screening Facts Sheets: www.aap.org/policy/01565.html
American Academy of Pediatrics, Breast-feeding and use of human milk: www.aap.org/policy/re9729.html
American Social Health Association: www.vaccines.ashastd.org
Baby Trend: www.babytrend.com
Breast-feeding information: www.breastfeeding.com
Bright Future Lactation Resource Center: www.bflrc.com
CDC's National Immunization Program: www.cdc.gov/nip
Graco/Century: www.gracobaby.com
Immunization Action Coalition: www.immunize.org
La Leche League International: www.lalecheleague.org
March of Dimes, newborn screening tests: www.marchofdimes.com/professionals/681–1200.asp
National Center for Missing and Exploited Children: www.missingkids.com
National Healthy Mothers, Healthy Babies Coalition: www.hmhb.org
National Institute of Child Health and Human Development: www.nih.gov
National Newborn Screening and Genetics Resource Center: http://genes-r-us.uthscsa.edu/resources/newborn/screestatus.htm
Neonatal Network: www.neonatalnetwork.com
Safeline Corporation: www.safelinekids.com
Vaccine Education Center: www.vaccine.chop.edu

CHAPTER WORKSHEET

MULTIPLE CHOICE QUESTIONS

1. At birth, a newborn's assessment reveals the following: heart rate of 140 bpm, loud crying, some flexion of extremities, crying when bulb syringe is introduced into the nares, and a pink body with blue extremities. The nurse would document the newborn's Apgar score as:

   a. 5 points

   b. 6 points

   c. 7 points

   d. 8 points

2. The nurse is explaining phototherapy to the parents of a newborn. The nurse would include which of the following as the purpose?

   a. Increase surfactant levels

   b. Stabilize the newborn's temperature

   c. Destroy Rh-negative antibodies

   d. Oxidize bilirubin on the skin

3. The nurse administers a single dose of vitamin K intramuscularly to a newborn after birth to promote:

   a. Conjugation of bilirubin

   b. Blood clotting

   c. Foreman ovale closure

   d. Digestion of complex proteins

4. A prophylactic agent is instilled in both eyes of all newborns to prevent which of the following conditions?

   a. Gonorrhea and chlamydia

   b. Thrush and Enterobacter

   c. *Staphylococcus* and syphilis

   d. Hepatitis B and herpes

5. The AAP recommends that all newborns be placed on their backs to sleep to reduce the risk of:

   a. Respiratory distress syndrome

   b. Bottle mouth syndrome

   c. Sudden infant death syndrome

   d. GI regurgitation syndrome

6. Which of the following immunizations is received by newborns before hospital discharge?

   a. Pneumococcus

   b. Varicella

   c. Hepatitis A

   d. Hepatitis B

7. Which condition would be missed if newborns are screened before they have tolerated protein feedings for at least 48 hours?

   a. Hypothyroidism

   b. Cystic fibrosis

   c. Phenylketonuria

   d. Sickle cell disease

CRITICAL THINKING EXERCISES

1. Linda Scott, an African-American mother who delivered her first baby and is on the mother–baby unit, calls the nursery nurse into her room and expresses concern about how her daughter looks. Ms. Scott tells the nurse that her baby's head looks like a "banana" and is mushy to the touch, and she has "white spots" all over her nose. In addition, there appear to be "big bluish bruises" all over her baby's buttocks. She wants to know what is wrong with her baby and whether these problems will go away.

   a. How should the nurse respond to Ms. Scott's questions?

   b. What additional newborn instruction might be appropriate at this time?

   c. What reassurance can be given to Ms. Scott regarding her daughter's appearance?

2. At approximately 12:30 a.m. on a Friday, a woman enters a hospital through a busy emergency room. She is wearing a white uniform and a lab coat with a stethoscope around her neck. She identifies herself as a new nurse coming back to check on something she had left on the unit on an earlier shift. She enters a postpartum client's room containing the mother's newborn, pushes the open crib down a hallway, and escapes through an exit. The security cameras aren't working. The infant isn't discovered missing until the 2 a.m. check by the nurse.

a. What impact does an infant abduction have on the family and the hospital?

b. What security measure was the weak link in the chain of security?

c. What can hospitals do to prevent infant abduction?

STUDY ACTIVITIES

1. Interview a new mother on the postpartum unit on her second day about the changes she has noticed in her newborn's appearance and behavior within the past 24 hours. Discuss your interview findings at post conference.

2. Demonstrate a newborn bath to a new mother in her room, using the principle of bathing from the cleanest to the dirtiest body part. Discuss the questions asked by the mother and her reaction to the demonstration in post conference.

3. Go to the La Leche League website (www. lalecheleague.org). Review the information it provides on breast-feeding. How helpful would it be to a new mother?

4. Debate the risks and benefits of neonatal circumcision within your nursing group at post conference. Did either side present a stronger position? What is your opinion, and why?

CHILDBEARING AT RISK

NURSING MANAGEMENT OF PREGNANCY AT RISK: PREGNANCY-RELATED COMPLICATIONS

KEY TERMS

abortion
abruptio placentae
ectopic pregnancy
gestational hypertension
gestational trophoblastic
    disease (GTD)

high-risk pregnancy
hyperemesis gravidarum
multiple gestation
oligohydramnios
polyhydramnios
placenta previa

premature rupture of
    membranes (PROM)
preterm premature
    rupture of membranes
    (PPROM)

LEARNING OBJECTIVES

Upon completion of the chapter, the learner will be able to:

1. Define the term "high-risk pregnancy."
2. Explain common factors that might place a pregnancy at high risk.
3. Identify the causes of vaginal bleeding during early and late pregnancy.
4. Outline nursing assessment and management for the pregnant woman experiencing vaginal bleeding.
5. Develop a plan of care for the woman experiencing preeclampsia, eclampsia, and HELLP syndrome.
6. Explain the pathophysiology of polyhydramnios and subsequent management.
7. Select factors in a woman's prenatal history that place her at risk for premature rupture of membranes (PROM).
8. Formulate a teaching plan for maintaining the health of pregnant women experiencing a high-risk pregnancy.

*H*elen, a 35-year-old G5 P4, presented to the labor and birth suite with severe abdominal pain. She reports that the pain began suddenly about an hour ago while she was resting. She has had two prior cesarean births and thus far has had an uneventful past 32 weeks. Helen appears distressed and is moaning. What additional assessments do you need to care for Helen? What might be your immediate nursing action?

WOW

Detours and bumps along the road of life can be managed, but many cannot be entirely cured.

Most people view pregnancy as a natural process with a positive outcome—the birth of a healthy newborn. Unfortunately, conditions can occur that may result in negative outcomes for the fetus, mother, or both. A **high-risk pregnancy** is one in which a condition exists that jeopardizes the health of the mother, her fetus, or both. The condition may result from the pregnancy, or it may be a condition that was present before the woman became pregnant.

Approximately one in four pregnant women is considered to be at high risk or diagnosed with complications (Jung & Erogul, 2007). Women who are considered to be at high risk have a higher morbidity and mortality compared with mothers in the general population. The risk status of a woman and her fetus can change during the pregnancy, with a number of problems occurring during labor, birth, or afterward, even in women without any known previous antepartal risk. Examples of high-risk conditions include gestational diabetes and ectopic pregnancy. These conditions are specifically addressed in *Healthy People 2010.* Early identification of the woman at risk is essential to ensure that appropriate interventions are instituted promptly, increasing the opportunity to change the course of events and provide a positive outcome.

The term "risk" may mean different things to different groups. For example, health care professionals may focus on the disease processes and treatments to prevent complications. Nurses may focus on nursing care and on the psychosocial impact on the woman and her family. Insurance companies may concentrate on the economic issues related to the high-risk status. The woman's attention may be focused on her own needs and those of her family. Together, working as a collaborative team, the ultimate goal of care is to ensure the best possible outcome for the woman, her fetus, and her family.

Risk assessment begins at the first antepartal visit and continues with each subsequent visit because factors may be identified in later visits that were not apparent during earlier visits. For example, as the nurse and client develop a trusting relationship, previously unidentified or unsuspected factors (such as drug abuse or intimate partner violence) may be revealed. Through education and support, the nurse can encourage the client to inform her health care provider of these concerns, and necessary interventions or referrals can be made.

Various factors must be considered when determining a woman's risk for adverse pregnancy outcomes (Britt, Eden, & Evans, 2006), and a comprehensive approach to high-risk pregnancy is needed. For example, prenatal stress and distress have been shown to have significant consequences for the mother, child, and family (Price et al., 2007). Risks are grouped into broad categories based on threats to health and pregnancy outcome. Current categories of risk are biophysical, psychosocial, sociodemographic, and environmental (Gilbert, 2007) (Box 19.1).

This chapter describes the major conditions directly related to the pregnancy that can complicate a pregnancy, possibly affecting maternal and fetal outcomes. These include bleeding during pregnancy (spontaneous abortion, ectopic pregnancy, gestational trophoblastic disease, cervical insufficiency, placenta previa, and abruptio placentae), hyperemesis gravidarum, gestational hypertension, HELLP syndrome, gestational diabetes, blood incompatibility, amniotic fluid imbalances (hydramnios and oligohydramnios), multiple gestation, and premature rupture of membranes. Chapter 20 addresses preexisting conditions that can complicate a woman's pregnancy as well as populations that are considered to be at high risk.

Bleeding During Pregnancy

Bleeding at any time during pregnancy is potentially life-threatening. Bleeding can occur early or late in the pregnancy and may result from numerous conditions. Conditions commonly associated with early bleeding (first half of pregnancy) include spontaneous abortion, ectopic pregnancy, gestational trophoblastic disease, and conditions associated with midtrimester bleeding, such as cervical insufficiency. Conditions associated with late bleeding include placenta previa and abruptio placentae, which usually occur after the 20th week of gestation.

HEALTHY PEOPLE 2010

Objective	Significance
Decrease the proportion of pregnant women with gestational diabetes	• Will help to promote proper prepregnant and pregnancy glycemic control; foster careful perinatal obstetric monitoring, thereby helping to reduce perinatal death and congenital abnormalities • Will help to reinforce the importance of good nutrition during pregnancy as paramount in increasing better pregnancy outcomes
Reduce ectopic pregnancies	• Will help to focus attention on the need for initiating prenatal care early and for continued monitoring throughout pregnancy, thus helping to decrease maternal mortality related to ectopic pregnancies through early detection

Source: U.S. DHHS, 2000.

BOX 19.1 Factors Placing a Woman at Risk During Pregnancy

Biophysical Factors
- Genetic conditions
- Chromosomal abnormalities
- Multiple pregnancy
- Defective genes
- Inherited disorders
- ABO incompatibility
- Large fetal size
- Medical and obstetric conditions
- Preterm labor and birth
- Cardiovascular disease
- Chronic hypertension
- Incompetent cervix
- Placental abnormalities
- Infection
- Diabetes
- Maternal collagen diseases
- Pregnancy-induced hypertension
- Asthma
- Postterm pregnancy
- Hemoglobinopathies
- Nutritional status
- Inadequate dietary intake
- Food fads
- Excessive food intake
- Under- or overweight status
- Hematocrit value less than 33%
- Eating disorder

Psychosocial Factors
- Smoking
- Caffeine
- Alcohol
- Drugs
- Inadequate support system
- Situational crisis
- History of violence
- Emotional distress
- Unsafe cultural practices

Sociodemographic Factors
- Poverty status
- Lack of prenatal care
- Age younger than 15 years or older than 35 years
- Parity—all first pregnancies and more than five pregnancies
- Marital status—increased risk for unmarried
- Accessibility to health care
- Ethnicity—increased risk in nonwhite women

Environmental Factors
- Infections
- Radiation
- Pesticides
- Illicit drugs
- Industrial pollutants
- Second-hand cigarette smoke
- Personal stress (Gilbert, 2007; Blackburn, 2007)

Source: Blackburn, 2007; Gilbert, 2007.

▶ SPONTANEOUS ABORTION

An **abortion** is the loss of an early pregnancy, usually before week 20 of gestation. Abortion can be spontaneous or induced. A spontaneous abortion refers to the loss of a fetus resulting from natural causes—that is, not elective or therapeutically induced by a procedure. The term *miscarriage* is often used by nonmedical people to denote an abortion that has occurred spontaneously. A miscarriage can occur during early pregnancy, and many women who miscarry may not even be aware that they are pregnant. About 80% of spontaneous abortions occur within the first trimester.

The overall rate for spontaneous abortion in the United States is reported to be 15% to 20% of recognized pregnancies in the United States. However, with the development of highly sensitive assays for human chorionic gonadotropin (hCG) levels that detect pregnancies prior to the expected next menses, the incidence of pregnancy loss increases significantly—to about 60% to 70% (Puscheck & Pradhan, 2007).

Pathophysiology

The causes of spontaneous abortion are varied and often unknown. The most common cause for first-trimester abortions is fetal genetic abnormalities, usually unrelated to the mother. Those occurring during the second trimester are more likely related to maternal conditions, such as incompetent cervix, congenital or acquired anomaly of the uterine cavity, hypothyroidism, diabetes mellitus, chronic nephritis, use of crack cocaine, inherited and acquired thrombophilias, lupus, and acute infection such as rubella virus, cytomegalovirus, herpes simplex virus, bacterial vaginosis, and toxoplasmosis (Simpson, 2007).

Nursing Assessment

When a pregnant woman calls and reports vaginal bleeding, she must be seen as soon as possible by a health care professional to ascertain the etiology. Varying degrees of vaginal bleeding, low back pain, abdominal cramping, and passage of products of conception tissue may be reported.

Ask the woman about the color of the vaginal bleeding (bright red is significant) and the amount—for example, question her about the frequency with which she is changing her peripads (saturation of one peripad hourly is significant) and the passage of any clots or tissue. Instruct her to save any tissue or clots passed and bring them with her to the health care facility. Also, obtain a description of any other signs and symptoms the woman may be experiencing, along with a description of their severity and duration. It is important to remain calm and listen to the woman's description.

When the woman arrives at the health care facility, assess her vital signs and observe the amount, color, and characteristics of the bleeding. Ask her to rate her current pain level, using an appropriate pain assessment tool. Also, evaluate the amount and intensity of the woman's abdominal cramping or contractions, and assess the woman's level of understanding about what is happening to her. A thorough assessment helps in determining the type of spontaneous abortion, such as threatened abortion, inevitable abortion, incomplete abortion, complete abortion, missed abortion, and habitual abortion, that the woman may be experiencing (Table 19.1).

Nursing Management

Nursing management of the woman with a spontaneous abortion focuses on providing continued monitoring and psychological support, for the family is experiencing acute loss and grief. An important component of this support is reassuring the woman that spontaneous abortions usually result from an abnormality and that her actions did not cause the abortion.

Providing Continued Monitoring

Continued monitoring and ongoing assessments are essential for the woman experiencing a spontaneous abortion. Monitor the amount of vaginal bleeding through pad counts and observe for passage of products of conception tissue. Assess the woman's pain and provide appropriate pain management to address the cramping discomfort.

Assist in preparing the woman for procedures and treatments such as surgery to evacuate the uterus or medications such as misoprostol or PGE2. If the woman is Rh negative and not sensitized, expect to administer RhoGAM within 72 hours after the abortion is complete. Drug Guide 19.1 gives more information about these medications.

Providing Support

A woman's emotional reaction may vary depending on her desire for this pregnancy and her available support network. Provide both physical and emotional support. In addition, prepare the woman and her family for the assessment process, and answer their questions about what is happening.

Explaining some of the causes of spontaneous abortions can help the woman to understand what is happening and may allay her fears and guilt that she did something to cause this pregnancy loss. Most women experience an acute sense of loss and go through a grieving process with a spontaneous abortion. Providing sensitive listening, counseling, and anticipatory guidance to the woman and her family will allow them to verbalize their feelings and ask questions about future pregnancies.

The grieving period may last as long as 2 years after a pregnancy loss, with each person grieving in his or her own way. Encourage friends and family to be supportive but give the couple space and time to work through their loss. Referral to a community support group for parents who have experienced a miscarriage can be very helpful during this grief process.

▶ ECTOPIC PREGNANCY

An **ectopic pregnancy** is any pregnancy in which the fertilized ovum implants outside the uterine cavity. Ectopic pregnancies occur in from 1 in every 40 to 1 in every 100 pregnancies in the United States (March of Dimes, 2007). Their incidence has increased dramatically in the past few decades as a result of improved diagnostic techniques, such as more sensitive beta-hCG assays and the availability of transvaginal ultrasound (Silver, 2007).

With an ectopic pregnancy, rupture and hemorrhage may occur due to the growth of the embryo. A ruptured ectopic pregnancy is a medical emergency. It is a potentially life-threatening condition and involves pregnancy loss. It is the leading cause of maternal mortality in the first trimester and accounts for 10% to 15% of all pregnancy-related deaths (Lipscomb, 2007).

Pathophysiology

Normally, the fertilized ovum implants in the uterus. With an ectopic pregnancy, the ovum implants outside the uterus. The most common site for implantation is the fallopian tubes, but some ova may implant in the cornua of the uterus, the ovary, the cervix, or the abdominal cavity (Fig. 19.1) (Sepilian & Wood, 2007). None of these anatomic sites can accommodate placental attachment or a growing embryo.

Ectopic pregnancies usually result from conditions that obstruct or slow the passage of the fertilized ovum through the fallopian tube to the uterus. This may be a physical blockage in the tube, or failure of the tubal epithelium to move the zygote (the cell formed after the egg is fertilized) down the tube into the uterus. In the general population, most cases are the result of tubal scarring secondary to pelvic inflammatory disease. Organisms such

TABLE 19.1 CATEGORIES OF ABORTION

Category	Assessment Findings	Diagnosis	Therapeutic Management
Threatened abortion	Vaginal bleeding (often slight) early in a pregnancy No cervical dilation or change in cervical consistency Mild abdominal cramping Closed cervical os No passage of fetal tissue	Vaginal ultrasound to confirm if sac is empty Declining maternal serum hCG and progesterone levels to provide additional information about viability of pregnancy	Conservative supportive treatment Possible reduction in activity in conjunction with nutritious diet and adequate hydration
Inevitable abortion	Vaginal bleeding (greater than that associated with threatened abortion) Rupture of membranes Cervical dilation Strong abdominal cramping Possible passage of products of conception	Ultrasound and hCG levels to indicate pregnancy loss	Vacuum curettage if products of conception are not passed, to reduce risk of excessive bleeding and infection Prostaglandin analogs such as misoprostol to empty uterus of retained tissue (only used if fragments are not completely passed)
Incomplete abortion (passage of some of the products of conception)	Intense abdominal cramping Heavy vaginal bleeding Cervical dilation	Ultrasound confirmation that products of conception still in uterus	Client stabilization Evacuation of uterus via dilation and curettage (D&C) or prostaglandin analog
Complete abortion (passage of all products of conception)	History of vaginal bleeding and abdominal pain Passage of tissue with subsequent decrease in pain and significant decrease in vaginal bleeding	Ultrasound demonstrating an empty uterus	No medical or surgical intervention necessary Follow-up appointment to discuss family planning
Missed abortion (nonviable embryo retained in utero for at least 6 weeks)	Absent uterine contractions Irregular spotting Possible progression to inevitable abortion	Ultrasound to identify products of conception in uterus	Evacuation of uterus (if inevitable abortion does not occur): suction curettage during first trimester, dilation and evacuation during second trimester Induction of labor with intravaginal PGE2 suppository to empty uterus without surgical intervention
Habitual abortion	History of three or more consecutive spontaneous abortions Not carrying the pregnancy to viability or term	Validation via client's history	Identification and treatment of underlying cause (possible causes such as genetic or chromosomal abnormalities, reproductive tract abnormalities, chronic diseases or immunologic problems) Cervical cerclage in second trimester if incompetent cervix is the cause

DRUG GUIDE 19.1 MEDICATIONS USED WITH SPONTANEOUS ABORTIONS

Medication	Action/Indications	Nursing Implications
Misoprostol (Cytotec)	Stimulates uterine contractions to terminate a pregnancy; to evacuate the uterus after abortion to ensure passage of all the products of conception	• Monitor for side effects such as diarrhea, abdominal pain, nausea, vomiting, dyspepsia. • Assess vaginal bleeding and report any increased bleeding, pain, or fever. • Monitor for signs and symptoms of shock, such as tachycardia, hypotension, and anxiety.
Mifepristone (RU-486)	Acts as progesterone antagonist, allowing prostaglandins to stimulate uterine contractions; causes the endometrium to slough; may be followed by administration of misoprostol within 48 hours	• Monitor for headache, vomiting, diarrhea, and heavy bleeding. • Anticipate administration of antiemetic prior to use to reduce nausea and vomiting. • Encourage client to use acetaminophen to reduce discomfort from cramping.
PGE2, dinoprostone (Cervidil, Prepidil Gel, Prostin E2)	Stimulates uterine contractions, causing expulsion of uterine contents; to expel uterine contents in fetal death or missed abortion during second trimester, or to efface and dilate the cervix in pregnancy at term	• Bring gel to room temperature before administering. • Avoid contact with skin. • Use sterile technique to administer. • Keep client supine 30 minutes after administering. • Document time of insertion and dosing intervals. • Remove insert with retrieval system after 12 hours or at the onset of labor. • Explain purpose and expected response to client.
Rh(D) immunoglobulin (Gamulin, HydroRho-D, RhoGAM)	Suppresses immune response of nonsensitized Rh-negative patients who are exposed to Rh-positive blood; to prevent isoimmunization in Rh-negative women exposed to Rh-positive blood after abortions, miscarriages, and pregnancies	• Administer intramuscularly in deltoid area. • Give only MICRhoGAM for abortions and miscarriages <12 weeks unless fetus or father is Rh negative (unless patient is Rh positive, Rh antibodies are present). • Educate woman that she will need this after subsequent deliveries if newborns are Rh positive; also check lab study results prior to administering the drug.

as *Neisseria gonorrhoeae* and *Chlamydia trachomatis* preferentially attack the fallopian tubes, producing silent infections. A recent study reported a twofold increased risk for ectopic pregnancy in women with a history of a chlamydia infection (Bakken, Skjeldestad, & Nordbo, 2007). Even with early treatment, tubal damage can occur.

Therapeutic Management

The therapeutic management of ectopic pregnancy depends on whether the tube is intact or has ruptured. Historically, the treatment of ectopic pregnancy was limited to surgery, but medical therapy is currently available.

If the fallopian tube is still intact, medical management becomes an option. To be eligible for medical therapy, the client must be hemodynamically stable, with no signs of active bleeding in the peritoneal cavity, and the mass (which must measure less than 4 cm as determined by ultrasound) must be unruptured (Lipscomb, 2007). The potential advantages include avoidance of surgery, the preservation of tubal patency and function, and a lower

cost. Methotrexate, prostaglandins, misoprostol, and actinomycin have all been used in the medical (nonsurgical) management of ectopic pregnancy, with a reported success rate of approximately 90% (Lipscomb, 2007).

Methotrexate, the agent most commonly used, is a folic acid antagonist that inhibits cell division in the developing embryo. It typically has been used as a chemotherapeutic agent in the treatment of leukemias, lymphomas, and carcinomas. It has been shown to produce results similar to that for surgical therapy in terms of high success rate, low complication rate, and good reproductive potential (Vitthala, Cheema, & Misra, 2007). Adverse effects associated with methotrexate include nausea, vomiting, stomatitis, diarrhea, gastric upset, increased abdominal pain, and dizziness. Prior to receiving the single-dose intramuscular injection to treat unruptured pregnancies, the woman needs to be counseled on the risks, benefits, adverse effects, and the possibility of failure of medical therapy, which would result in tubal rupture, necessitating surgery (Selway, 2006). The woman

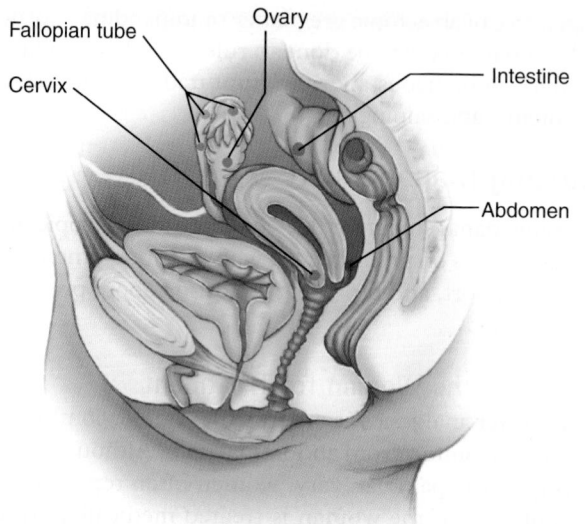

FIGURE 19.1 Possible sites for implantation with an ectopic pregnancy.

is then instructed to return weekly for follow-up laboratory studies for the next several weeks until beta-hCG titers decrease.

Surgical management for the unruptured fallopian tube might involve a linear salpingostomy to preserve the tube—an important consideration for the woman wanting to preserve her future fertility.

With a ruptured ectopic pregnancy, surgery is necessary as a result of possible uncontrolled hemorrhage. A laparotomy with a removal of the tube (salpingectomy) may be necessary. With earlier diagnosis and medical management, the focus has changed from preventing maternal death to facilitating rapid recovery and preserving fertility.

Regardless of the treatment approach (medical or surgical), the woman's beta-hCG level is monitored until it is undetectable to ensure that any residual trophoblastic tissue that forms the placenta is gone. Also, all Rh-negative unsensitized clients are given Rh immunoglobulin to prevent isoimmunization in future pregnancies.

Nursing Assessment

Nursing assessment focuses on determining the existence of an ectopic pregnancy and whether or not it has ruptured.

Health History and Physical Examination

Assess the client thoroughly for signs and symptoms that may suggest an ectopic pregnancy. The onset of signs and symptoms varies, but they usually begin at about the seventh or eighth week of gestation. A missed menstrual period, adnexal fullness, and tenderness may indicate an unruptured tubal pregnancy. As the tube stretches, the pain

EVIDENCE-BASED PRACTICE 19.1
Ectopic Pregnancy: Selecting the Best Intervention

● **Study**

The incidence of ectopic pregnancy, which involves implantation of the fertilized ovum outside the uterine cavity, has increased over the past several decades due to advances in diagnostic methods. The most common site for implantation is in the fallopian tube (thus the name tubal pregnancy). If left untreated, tubal rupture and hemorrhage can occur. At one time, surgery was the only available treatment option. However, treatment today may involve expectant care, medication therapy, or surgery (laparoscopic or open approach). Questions have arisen as to the effectiveness and safety of these treatments.

A study was conducted to evaluate the effectiveness of major types of treatment for ectopic pregnancy. Data were collected from 35 randomized controlled trials that compared the treatments for ectopic pregnancies.

▲ **Findings**

The open approach to surgery was significantly more effective in removing the ectopic pregnancy than the laparoscopic approach, but the laparoscopic approach was more cost-effective. Medication therapy involving fixed multiple doses of methotrexate was effective in women who had low pregnancy hormone levels without any evidence of bleeding. Expectant management was less successful than drug therapy, but the information on this treatment option was inadequate.

■ **Nursing Implications**

This study identified three important treatment options available to a woman with an ectopic pregnancy. Nurses can use this information in their practice as a basis for formulating a teaching plan about treatment options. Nurses can use the information from this study when reviewing the health care provider's recommendations for treatment. As a result, women can make a more informed decision. Nurses also can advocate for medication therapy for women who have low pregnancy hormone levels and no bleeding.

Hajenius, P. J., Mol, F., Mol, B. W. J., Bossuyt, P. M. M., Ankum, W. M., & van der Veen, F. (2007). Interventions for tubal ectopic pregnancy. *Cochrane Database of Systematic Reviews* 2007. Issue 1. Art. No.: CD000324.DOI: 10.1002/14651858.CD000324.pub2.

increases. Pain may be unilateral, bilateral, or diffuse over the abdomen.

> ▶ *Take* NOTE!
>
> *The hallmark of ectopic pregnancy is abdominal pain with spotting within 6 to 8 weeks after a missed menstrual period. Although this is the classic triad, all three of these signs and symptoms occur in only about 50% of cases. Many women have symptoms typical of early pregnancy, such as breast tenderness, nausea, fatigue, shoulder pain, and low back pain.*

In addition, review the client's history for possible contributing factors. These may include:

- Previous ectopic pregnancy
- History of sexually transmitted infections (STIs)
- Fallopian tube scarring from pelvic inflammatory disease
- In utero exposure to diethylstilbestrol
- Endometriosis
- Previous tubal or pelvic surgery
- Infertility and infertility treatments, including use of fertility drugs
- Uterine abnormalities such as fibroids
- Presence of intrauterine contraception
- Use of progestin-only mini-pill (slows ovum transport)
- Postpartum or post-abortion infection
- Increasing age (older than 35 years)
- Cigarette smoking (Brown-Guttovz, 2006)

If rupture or hemorrhage occurs before treatment begins, symptoms may worsen and include severe, sharp, and sudden pain in the lower abdomen as the tube tears open and the embryo is expelled into the pelvic cavity; feelings of faintness; referred pain to the shoulder area, indicating bleeding into the abdomen, caused by phrenic nerve irritation; hypotension; marked abdominal tenderness with distention; and hypovolemic shock.

Laboratory and Diagnostic Testing

The use of transvaginal ultrasound to visualize the misplaced pregnancy and low levels of serum beta-hCG assist in diagnosing an ectopic pregnancy. The ultrasound determines whether the pregnancy is intrauterine, assesses the size of the uterus, and provides evidence of fetal viability. The visualization of an adnexal mass and the absence of an intrauterine gestational sac are diagnostic of ectopic pregnancy (Condous, 2006). In a normal intrauterine pregnancy, beta-hCG levels typically double every 2 to 4 days until peak values are reached 60 to 90 days after conception. Concentrations of hCG decrease after 10 to 11 weeks and reach a plateau at low levels by 100 to 130 days (Blackburn, 2007). Therefore, low beta-hCG levels are suggestive of an ectopic pregnancy or impending abortion. Additional tests may be done to rule out other conditions such as spontaneous abortion, ruptured ovarian cyst, appendicitis, and salpingitis.

Nursing Management

Nursing management for the woman with an ectopic pregnancy focuses on preparing the woman for treatment, providing support, and providing education about preventive measures.

Preparing the Woman for Treatment

Administer analgesics as ordered to promote comfort and relieve discomfort from abdominal pain. Although the intensity of the pain can vary, women often report a great deal of pain. If the woman is treated medically, explain the medication that will be used and what she can expect. Also review signs and symptoms of possible adverse effects. If treatment will occur on an outpatient basis, outline the signs and symptoms of ectopic rupture (severe, sharp, stabbing, unilateral abdominal pain; vertigo/fainting; hypotension; and increased pulse) and advise the woman to seek medical help immediately if they occur.

If surgery is needed, close assessment and monitoring of the client's vital signs, bleeding (peritoneal or vaginal), and pain status are critical to identify hypovolemic shock, which may occur with tubal rupture. Prepare the client physiologically and psychologically for surgery or any procedure. Provide a clear explanation of the expected outcome. Astute vigilance and early referral will help reduce short- and long-term morbidity.

Providing Emotional Support

The woman with an ectopic pregnancy requires support throughout diagnosis, treatment, and aftercare. A woman's psychological reaction to an ectopic pregnancy is unpredictable. However, it is important to recognize she has experienced a pregnancy loss in addition to undergoing treatment for a potentially life-threatening condition. The woman may find it difficult to comprehend what has happened to her because events occur so quickly. In the woman's mind, she had just started a pregnancy and now it has ended abruptly. Help her to make this experience "more real" by encouraging her and her family to express their feelings and concerns openly, and validating that this is a loss of pregnancy and it is okay to grieve over the loss.

Provide emotional support, spiritual care, client education, and information about community support groups available (such as Resolve through Sharing) as the client grieves for the loss of her unborn child and comes to terms with the medical complications of the situation. Acknowledge the client's pregnancy and allow her to discuss her feelings about what the pregnancy means. Also, stress the need for follow-up blood testing for several weeks to monitor hCG titers until they return to zero, indicating resolution of the ectopic pregnancy. Ask about her feelings and concerns about her future fertility, and provide teaching about the need to use contraceptives for at least three menstrual cycles to allow her reproductive tract to heal and the tissue to be repaired. Include the woman's partner in this discussion to make sure both parties understand what has happened, what intervention is needed, and what the future holds regarding childbearing.

Educating the Client

Preventing ectopic pregnancies through screening and client education is essential. Many can be prevented by avoiding conditions that might cause scarring of the fallopian tubes. In addition, a contributing factor to the development of ectopic pregnancy is a previous ectopic pregnancy. Therefore, educating the woman is crucial.

Prevention education may include the following:

- Reduce risk factors such as sexual intercourse with multiple partners or intercourse without a condom.
- Avoid contracting STIs that lead to pelvic inflammatory disease (PID).
- Obtain early diagnosis and adequate treatment of STIs.
- Avoid the use of intrauterine contraceptive methods to reduce the risk of repeat ascending infections, which can be responsible for tubal scarring.
- Use condoms to decrease the risk of infections that cause tubal scarring.
- Seek prenatal care early to confirm the location of pregnancy.

▶ GESTATIONAL TROPHOBLASTIC DISEASE (GTD)

Gestational trophoblastic disease (GTD) comprises a spectrum of neoplastic disorders that originate in the placenta. Gestational tissue is present, but the pregnancy is not viable. The incidence is about 1 in 1,000 pregnancies in the United States; in Asian countries, the rate is as much as 15 times higher (Moore & Ware, 2007). The two most common types of GTD are hydatidiform mole (partial and complete) and choriocarcinoma.

Pathophysiology

Hydatidiform mole is a benign neoplasm of the chorion in which the chorionic villi degenerate and become transparent vesicles containing clear, viscid fluid. Hydatiform mole is classified as complete or partial, distinguished by differences in clinical presentation, pathology, genetics, and epidemiology (Garner et al., 2007). The complete mole contains no fetal tissue and develops from an "empty egg," which is fertilized by a normal sperm (the paternal chromosomes replicate, resulting in 46 all-paternal chromosomes). The embryo is not viable and dies. No circu-

FIGURE 19.2 Complete hydatiform mole. The chorionic villi degenerate and become filled with a viscid fluid, forming transparent vesicles.

lation is established, and no embryonic tissue is found. The complete mole is associated with the development of choriocarcinoma. The partial mole has a triploid karyotype (69 chromosomes), because two sperm have provided a double contribution by fertilizing the ovum (Fig. 19.2).

▶ *Consider THIS!*

We had lived across the dorm hall from each other during nursing school but really didn't get to know each other except for a casual hello in passing. When we graduated, Rose went to work in the emergency room and I in OB. We saw each other occasionally in the employee cafeteria, but a quick hello was all that we usually exchanged. I heard she married one of the paramedics who worked in the ER and was soon pregnant. I finally got to say more than hello when she was admitted to the OB unit bleeding during her fourth month of pregnancy. What was discovered was gestational trophoblastic disease and not a normal pregnancy. I remember holding her in my arms as she wept. She was told she had a complete molar pregnancy after surgery, and she would need extensive follow-up for the next year. I lost track of her that summer as my life became busier. Around Thanksgiving time, I heard she had died from choriocarcinoma. I attended her funeral, finally, to get the time to say a final hello and good-bye, but this time with sadness and tears.

Thoughts: Rose was only 26 years old when she succumbed to this very virulent cancer. I think back

(continued)

> ▶ *Consider* THIS! *(continued)*
>
> *and realize I missed knowing this brave young woman and wished that I had taken the time to say more than hello. Could her outcome have been different? Why wasn't it recognized earlier? Did she not follow up after her diagnosis? I can only speculate regarding the whom, what, and where. She lived a short but purposeful life, and hopefully continued research will change other women's outcomes in the future.*

The exact cause of molar pregnancy is unknown, but researchers are looking into a genetic basis. Studies have revealed some remarkable features about molar pregnancies, including:

- Ability to invade into the wall of the uterus
- Tendency to recur in subsequent pregnancies
- Possible development into choriocarcinoma, a virulent cancer with metastasis to other organs
- Influence of nutritional factors, such as protein deficiency
- Tendency to affect older women more often than younger women

Having a molar pregnancy (partial or complete) results in the loss of the pregnancy and the possibility of developing choriocarcinoma, a chorionic malignancy from the trophoblastic tissue. The most frequent sites of metastases are the lungs, lower genital tract, brain, liver, kidney and gastrointestinal tract (Hernandez, 2007).

Therapeutic Management

Treatment consists of immediate evacuation of the uterine contents as soon as the diagnosis is made and long-term follow-up of the client to detect any remaining trophoblastic tissue that might become malignant. Dilation and suction curettage (D&C) are used to empty the uterus. The tissue obtained is sent to the laboratory for analysis to evaluate for choriocarcinoma. Serial levels of hCG are used to detect residual trophoblastic tissue for 1 year. If any tissue remains, hCG levels will not regress. In 80% of women with a benign hydatidiform mole, serum hCG titers steadily drop to normal within 8 to 12 weeks after evacuation of the molar pregnancy. In the other 20% of women with a malignant hydatidiform mole, serum hCG levels begin to rise (Hernandez, 2007).

Due to the increased risk for cancer, the client is advised to receive extensive follow-up therapy for the next 12 months. The follow-up protocol may include:

- Baseline hCG level, chest radiograph, and pelvic ultrasound
- Weekly serum hCG level until it drops to zero and remains at that level for 3 consecutive weeks, then

monthly for 6 months, then every 2 months for the remainder of the year
- Chest radiograph every 6 months to detect pulmonary metastasis
- Regular pelvic examinations to assess uterine and ovarian regression
- Systemic assessments for symptoms indicative of lung, brain, liver, or vaginal metastasis
- Strong recommendation to avoid pregnancy for 1 year because the pregnancy can interfere with the monitoring of hCG levels
- Use of a reliable contraceptive for at least 1 year (Gilbert, 2007)

Nursing Assessment

The nurse plays a crucial role in identifying and bringing this condition to the attention of the health care provider based on sound knowledge of the typical clinical manifestations and through astute antepartal assessments.

Clinical manifestations of GTD are very similar to those of spontaneous abortion at about 12 weeks of pregnancy. Assess the woman for potential clinical manifestations at each antepartal visit. Be alert for the following:

- Report of early signs of pregnancy, such as amenorrhea, breast tenderness, fatigue
- Brownish vaginal bleeding/spotting
- Anemia
- Severe morning sickness (due to high hCG levels)
- Fluid retention and swelling
- Uterine size larger than expected for pregnancy dates
- Extremely high hCG levels present; no single value considered diagnostic
- Early development of preeclampsia (usually not present until after 24 weeks)
- Absence of fetal heart rate or fetal activity
- Expulsion of grapelike vesicles (possible in some women)

The diagnosis is made by high hCG levels and the characteristic appearance of the vesicular molar pattern in the uterus via transvaginal ultrasound.

Nursing Management

Nursing management of the woman with GTD focuses on preparing her for a D&C, providing emotional support to deal with the loss and potential risks, and educating her about the risk that cancer may develop after a molar pregnancy and the strict adherence needed with the follow-up program. The woman must understand the need for the continued follow-up care regimen to improve her chances of future pregnancies and to ensure her continued quality of life.

Preparing the Client

Upon diagnosis, the client will need an immediate evacuation of the uterus. Perform preoperative care, preparing the client physically and psychologically for the procedure.

Providing Emotional Support

To aid the client and her family in coping with the loss of the pregnancy and the possibility of a cancer diagnosis, use the following interventions:

- Listen to their concerns and fears.
- Allow them time to grieve for the pregnancy loss.
- Acknowledge their loss and sad feelings (say you are sorry for their loss).
- Encourage them to express their grief; allow them to cry.
- Provide them with as much factual information as possible to help them make sense of what is happening.
- Enlist support from additional family and friends as appropriate and with the client's permission.

Educating the Client

After GTD is diagnosed, teach the client about the condition and appropriate interventions that may be necessary to save her life. Explain each phase of treatment accurately and provide support for the woman and her family as they go through the grieving process.

As with any facet of health care, be aware of the latest research and new therapies. Inform the client about her follow-up care, which will probably involve close clinical surveillance for approximately 1 year, and reinforce its importance in monitoring the client's condition. Tell the client that serial serum beta-hCG levels are used to detect residual trophoblastic tissue. Continued high or increasing hCG titers are abnormal and need further evaluation.

Inform the client about the possible use of chemotherapy, such as methotrexate, which may be started as prophylaxis. Strongly urge the client to use a reliable contraceptive to prevent pregnancy for 1 year, as a pregnancy would interfere with tracking the serial beta-hCG levels used to identify a potential malignancy. Stress the need for the client to cooperate and adhere to the plan of therapy throughout this year-long follow-up.

▶ CERVICAL INSUFFICIENCY

Cervical insufficiency, also called premature dilatation of the cervix, describes a weak, structurally defective cervix that spontaneously dilates in the absence of contractions in the second trimester, resulting in the loss of the pregnancy. The incidence of cervical insufficiency is less than 1%; estimates range from 1 in 500 to 1 in 2,000 pregnancies, accounting for approximately 20% to 25% of midtrimester losses (Fox & Chervenak, 2008).

Pathophysiology

The exact mechanism contributing to cervical insufficiency is not known. The incompetent cervix may have less elastin, less collagen, and greater amounts of smooth muscle than the normal cervix (Evans, 2007). Several theories have been proposed that focus on damage to the cervix as a key component.

Cervical insufficiency is likely to be the clinical endpoint of many pathologic processes, such as congenital cervical hypoplasia, in utero diethylstilbestrol (DES) exposure that caused cervical hypoplasia, trauma to the cervix (conization, amputation, obstetric laceration, or forced cervical dilatation [may occur during elective pregnancy termination]). Other conditions such as previous precipitous birth, a prolonged second stage of labor, or increased uterine volume (multiple gestation, hydramnios) are associated with cervical insufficiency (Vyas et al., 2006). However, the exact etiology of cervical insufficiency is not known.

Cervical length also has been associated with cervical insufficiency and subsequently preterm birth. Recent studies have examined the association between a short cervical length and the risk of preterm birth. Some have demonstrated a continuum of risk between a shorter cervix on ultrasound and a higher risk of preterm birth, leading to the hypothetical argument that women with a short cervix on ultrasound might benefit from cervical cerclage, but there have been conflicting results (Lotgering, 2007; Vidaeff & Ramin, 2007).

Therapeutic Management

Cervical insufficiency may be treated in a variety of ways: bed rest; pelvic rest; avoidance of heavy lifting; or surgically, via a procedure of a cervical cerclage in the second trimester. Cervical cerclage involves using a heavy purse-string suture to secure and reinforce the internal os of the cervix (Fig. 19.3).

According to the American College of Obstetricians & Gynecologists (ACOG) (2003), if a short cervix is identified at or after 20 weeks and no infection (chorioamnionitis) is present, the decision to proceed with cerclage should be made with caution. There have been limited numbers of well-designed randomized studies to support its efficacy. Suture displacement, rupture of membranes, and chorioamnionitis are the most common complications associated with cerclage placement, and their incidence varies widely in relation to the timing and indications for

FIGURE 19.3 Cervical cerclage.

the cerclage (Ressel, 2004). The optimal timing for cerclage removal is unclear, according to ACOG (2003).

Nursing Assessment

Nursing assessment focuses on obtaining a thorough history to determine any risk factors that might have a bearing on this pregnancy—previous cervical trauma, preterm labor, fetal loss in the second trimester, or previous surgeries or procedures involving the cervix. History may reveal a previous loss of pregnancy around 20 weeks.

Also be alert for complaints of vaginal discharge or pelvic pressure. Commonly with cervical insufficiency the woman will report a pink-tinged vaginal discharge or an increase in pelvic pressure. Cervical dilation also occurs. If this continues, rupture of the membranes, release of amniotic fluid, and uterine contractions occur, subsequently resulting in delivery of the fetus, often before it is viable.

> ▶ *Take* NOTE!
>
> *The diagnosis of cervical insufficiency remains difficult in many circumstances. The cornerstone of diagnosis is a history of midtrimester pregnancy loss associated with painless cervical dilatation without evidence of uterine activity.*

Transvaginal ultrasound typically is done around 20 weeks' gestation to determine cervical length and evaluate for shortening. Cervical shortening occurs from the internal os outward and can be viewed on ultrasound as funneling. The amount of funneling can be determined by dividing funnel length by cervical length. The most common time at which a short cervix or funneling develops is 18 to 22 weeks, so ultrasound screening should be performed during this interval (Fox & Chervenak, 2008). A cervical length less than 25 mm is abnormal between 14 weeks and 24 weeks and may increase the risk of preterm labor.

Expect the woman (particularly a woman with pelvic pressure, backache, or increased mucoid discharge) to undergo serial transvaginal ultrasound evaluations every few days to avoid missing rapid changes in cervical dilation or until the trend in cervical length can be characterized (Bernasko et al., 2006).

Nursing Management

Nursing management focuses on monitoring the woman very closely for signs of preterm labor: backache, increase in vaginal discharge, rupture of membranes, and uterine contractions. Provide emotional support and education to allay the couple's anxiety about the well-being of their fetus. Provide preoperative care and teaching as indicated

if the woman will be undergoing cerclage. Teach the client and her family about the signs and symptoms of preterm labor and the need to report any changes immediately. Also reinforce the need for activity restrictions (if appropriate) and continued regular follow-up. Continuing surveillance throughout the pregnancy is important to promote a positive outcome for the family.

▶ PLACENTA PREVIA

Placenta previa is a bleeding condition that occurs during the last two trimesters of pregnancy. In placenta previa (literally, "afterbirth first"), the placenta implants over the cervical os. It may cause serious morbidity and mortality to the fetus and mother. It complicates approximately 5 of 1,000 births or 1 in every 200 pregnancies and is associated with potentially serious consequences from hemorrhage, abruption (separation) of the placenta, or emergency cesarean birth (Joy & Lyon, 2007).

Pathophysiology

The exact cause of placenta previa is unknown. It is initiated by implantation of the embryo in the lower uterus. With placental attachment and growth, the cervical os may become covered by the developing placenta. Placental vascularization is defective, allowing the placenta to attach directly to the myometrium (accreta), invade the myometrium (increta), or penetrate the myometrium (percreta).

Placenta previa is generally classified according to the degree of coverage or proximity to the internal os, as follows (Fig. 19.4):

- Total placenta previa: the internal cervical os is completely covered by the placenta
- Partial placenta previa: the internal os is partially covered by the placenta
- Marginal placenta previa: the placenta is at the margin or edge of the internal os
- Low-lying placenta previa: the placenta is implanted in the lower uterine segment and is near the internal os but does not reach it

Therapeutic Management

Therapeutic management depends on the extent of bleeding, the amount of placenta over the cervical os, whether the fetus is developed enough to survive outside the uterus, the position of the fetus, the mother's parity, and the presence or absence of labor (Zeltzer, 2007).

If the mother and fetus are both stable, therapeutic management may involve expectant ("wait-and-see") care. This care can be carried out at home or on an antepartal unit in the health care facility. If there is no active bleeding and the client has readily available access to reliable

FIGURE 19.4 Classification of placenta previa. (**A**) Marginal. (**B**) Partial. (**C**) Complete.

Marginal   Partial   Complete

transportation, can maintain bed rest at home, and can comprehend instructions, expectant care at home is appropriate. However, if the client requires continuous care and monitoring and cannot meet the home care requirements, the antepartal unit is the best environment.

Nursing Assessment

Nursing assessment involves a thorough history, including possible risk factors, and physical examination. Evaluate the client closely for these risk factors:

• Advancing maternal age (more than 35 years)
• Previous cesarean birth
• Multiparity
• Uterine insult or injury
• Cocaine use
• Prior placenta previa
• Infertility treatment
• Asian ethnic background (incidence is increased in Asian cultural groups)
• Multiple gestations
• Previous induced surgical abortion
• Smoking
• Previous myomectomy to remove fibroids
• Smoking (Ko & Yoon, 2007)

Health History and Physical Examination

Ask the client if she has any problems associated with bleeding, now or in the recent past. The classical clinical presentation is painless, bright-red vaginal bleeding occurring during the second or third trimester. The initial bleeding usually is not profuse and it ceases spontaneously, only to recur again. The first episode of bleeding occurs (on average) at 27 to 32 weeks' gestation. The bleeding is thought to arise secondary to the thinning of the lower uterine segment in preparation for the onset of labor. When the bleeding occurs at the implantation site in the lower uterus, the uterus cannot contract adequately and stop the flow of blood from the open vessels. Typically with

normal placental implantation in the upper uterus, minor disruptive placental attachment is not a problem, because there is a larger volume of myometrial tissue able to contract and constrict bleeding vessels.

Assess the client for uterine contractions, which may or may not occur with the bleeding. Palpate the uterus; typically it is soft and nontender on examination. Auscultate the fetal heart rate; it commonly is within normal parameters. Fetal distress is usually absent but may occur when cord problems arise, such as umbilical cord prolapse or cord compression, or when the client has experienced blood loss to the extent that maternal shock or placental abruption has occurred (Oppenheimer, 2007).

Laboratory and Diagnostic Testing

To validate the position of the placenta, a transvaginal ultrasound is done. In addition, magnetic resonance imaging may be ordered when preparing for delivery because it allows identification of placenta accreta (placenta abnormally adherent to the myometrium), increta (placenta accreta with penetration of the myometrium), or percreta (placenta accreta with invasion of the myometrium to the peritoneal covering, causing rupture of the uterus) in addition to placenta previa. These placental abnormalities, although rare, carry a very high morbidity and mortality rate, possibly necessitating a hysterectomy at delivery.

Nursing Management

Whether the care setting is in the client's home or in the health care facility, the nurse focuses on monitoring the maternal–fetal status, including assessing for signs and symptoms of vaginal bleeding and fetal distress, and providing support and education to the client and her family, including what events and diagnostic studies are being performed. For the majority of women, a cesarean birth will be planned. Nursing Care Plan 19.1 discusses the nursing process for the woman with placenta previa.

Nursing Care Plan 19.1

OVERVIEW OF THE WOMAN WITH PLACENTA PREVIA

Sandy, a 39-year-old G5, P4, multigravida client at 32 weeks' gestation, was admitted to the labor and birth suite with sudden vaginal bleeding. Sandy had no further active bleeding and did not complain of any abdominal discomfort or tenderness. She did complain of occasional "tightening" in her stomach. Her abdomen palpated soft. Fetal heart rates were in the 140s with accelerations with movement. She was placed on bed rest with bathroom privileges. Ultrasound identified a low-lying placenta with a viable, normal-growth fetus. She was diagnosed with placenta previa and admitted for observation and surveillance of fetal well-being. Her history revealed two previous cesarean births, smoking half a pack of cigarettes per day, and endometritis infection after birth of her last newborn. Additional assessment findings included painless, bright-red vaginal bleeding with initial bleeding ceasing spontaneously; irregular, mild, and sporadic uterine contractions; fetal heart rate and maternal vital signs within normal range; fetus in transverse lie; anxiety related to the outcome of pregnancy; and expression of feelings of helplessness.

NURSING DIAGNOSIS: Ineffective tissue perfusion (fetal and maternal) related to blood loss

Outcome Identification and Evaluation
Client will maintain adequate tissue perfusion as evidenced by stable vital signs, decreased blood loss, few or no uterine contractions, normal fetal heart rate patterns and variability, and positive fetal movement

Interventions: Maintaining Adequate Tissue Perfusion
- Establish IV access *to allow for administration of fluids, blood, and medications as necessary.*
- Obtain type and cross-match for at least 2 U blood products *to ensure availability should bleeding continue.*
- Obtain specimens as ordered for blood studies, such as CBC and clotting studies *to establish a baseline and use for future comparison.*
- Monitor output *to evaluate adequacy of renal perfusion.*
- Administer IV fluid replacement therapy as ordered *to maintain blood pressure and blood volume.*
- Palpate for abdominal tenderness and rigidity *to determine bleeding and evidence of uterine contractions.*
- Institute bed rest *to reduce oxygen demands.*
- Assess for rupture of membranes *to evaluate for possible onset of labor.*
- Avoid vaginal examinations *to prevent further bleeding episodes.*
- Complete an Rh titer *to identify need for RhoGAM.*
- Avoid nipple stimulation *to prevent uterine contractions.*
- Continuously monitor for contractions or PROM *to allow for prompt intervention.*
- Administer tocolytic agents as ordered *to stall preterm labor.*
- Monitor vital signs frequently *to identify possible hypovolemia and infection.*
- Assess frequently for active vaginal bleeding *to minimize risk of hemorrhage.*
- Continuously monitor fetal heart rate with electronic fetal monitor *to evaluate fetal status.*
- Assist with fetal surveillance tests as ordered *to aid in determining fetal well-being.*
- Observe for abnormal fetal heart rate patterns, such as loss of variability, decelerations, tachycardia, *to identify fetal distress.*
- Position patient in side-lying position with wedge for support *to maximize placental perfusion.*
- Assess fetal movement *to evaluate for possible fetal hypoxia.*
- Teach woman to monitor fetal movement *to evaluate well-being.*
- Administer oxygen as ordered *to increase oxygenation to mother and fetus.*

Nursing Care Plan 19.1 (continued)

NURSING DIAGNOSIS: Anxiety related to threats to self and fetus

Outcome Identification and Evaluation
Client will experience a decrease in anxiety as evidenced by verbal reports of less anxiety, use of effective coping measures, and calm demeanor

Interventions: Minimizing Anxiety
- Provide factual information about diagnosis and treatment, and explain interventions and the rationale behind them *to provide client with understanding of her condition.*
- Answer questions about health status honestly *to establish a trusting relationship.*
- Speak calmly to patient and family members *to minimize environmental stress.*
- Encourage the use of past effective techniques for coping *to promote relaxation and feelings of control.*
- Acknowledge and facilitate the woman's spiritual needs *to promote effective coping.*
- Involve the woman and family in the decision-making process *to foster self-confidence and control over situation.*
- Maintain a presence during stressful periods *to allay anxiety.*
- Use the sense of touch if appropriate *to convey caring and concern.*
- Encourage talking as a means *to release tension.*

Monitoring Maternal–Fetal Status

Assess the degree of vaginal bleeding; inspect the perineal area for blood that may be pooled underneath the woman. Estimate and document the amount of bleeding. Perform a peripad count on an ongoing basis, making sure to report any changes in amount or frequency to the health care provider. If the woman is experiencing active bleeding, prepare for blood typing and cross-matching in the event a blood transfusion is needed.

▶ **Take** NOTE!

Avoid doing vaginal examinations in the woman with placenta previa. They may disrupt the placenta and cause hemorrhage.

Monitor maternal vital signs and uterine contractility frequently for changes. Have the client rate her level of pain using an appropriate pain rating scale.

Assess fetal heart rates via Doppler or electronic monitoring to detect fetal distress. Monitor the woman's cardiopulmonary status, reporting any difficulties in respirations, changes in skin color, or complaints of difficulty breathing. Have oxygen equipment readily available should fetal or maternal distress develop. Encourage the client to lie on her side to enhance placental perfusion.

If the woman has an intravenous (IV) line inserted, inspect the IV site frequently. Alternately, anticipate the insertion of an intermittent IV access device such as a saline lock, which can be used if quick access is needed for fluid restoration and infusion of blood products. Obtain laboratory tests as ordered, including complete blood count (CBC), coagulation studies, and Rh status if appropriate.

Administer pharmacologic agents as necessary. Give Rh immunoglobulin if the client is Rh negative at 28 weeks' gestation. Monitor tocolytic medication if prevention of preterm labor is needed.

Providing Support and Education

Determine the woman's level of understanding about placenta previa and the associated procedures and treatment plan. Doing so is important to prevent confusion and gain her cooperation. Provide information about the condition and make sure that all information related is consistent with information from the primary care provider. Explain all assessments and treatment measures as needed. Act as a client advocate in obtaining information for the family.

Teach the woman how to perform and record daily fetal movement. This action serves two purposes. One, it provides valuable information about the fetus. Two, it is an activity that the client can participate in, thereby fostering some feeling of control over the situation.

If the woman will require prolonged hospitalization or home bed rest, assess the physical and emotional impact that this may have on her. Evaluate her coping mechanisms to help determine how well she will be able to adjust to and cooperate with the treatment plan. Allow the client to verbalize her feelings and fears and provide emotional support. Also, provide opportunities for distraction—educational videos, arts and crafts, computer games, reading books— and evaluate the client's response.

In addition to the emotional impact of prolonged bed rest, thoroughly assess the woman's skin to prevent skin breakdown and to help alleviate her discomfort secondary to limited physical activity. Instruct the woman in appropriate skin care measures. Encourage her to eat a balanced diet with adequate fluid intake to ensure adequate nutrition and hydration and prevent complications associated with urinary and bowel elimination secondary to bed rest.

Teach the client and family about any signs and symptoms that should be reported immediately. In addition, prepare the woman for the possibility of a cesarean birth. The woman must notify her health care provider about any bleeding episodes or backaches (may indicate preterm labor contractions) and must adhere to the prescribed bed rest regimen. To ensure compliance and a positive outcome, she needs to be aware of the purpose of all of the observations that need to be made.

ABRUPTIO PLACENTAE

Abruptio placentae is the separation of a normally located placenta after the 20th week of gestation and prior to birth that leads to hemorrhage. It is a significant cause of third-trimester bleeding, with a high mortality rate. It occurs in about 1% of all pregnancies throughout the world (Gaufberg, 2007), or 1 in 120 pregnancies. The overall fetal mortality rate for placental abruption is 20% to 40%, depending on the extent of the abruption. Maternal mortality is approximately 6% in abruptio placentae and is related to cesarean birth and/or hemorrhage/coagulopathy (Deering & Satin, 2007).

Pathophysiology

The etiology of this condition is unknown; however, it has been proposed that abruption starts with degenerative changes in the small maternal arterioles, resulting in thrombosis, degeneration of the decidua, and possible rupture of a vessel. Bleeding from the vessel forms a retroplacental clot. The bleeding causes increased pressure behind the placenta and results in separation (Collins, 2007).

Fetal blood supply is compromised and fetal distress develops in proportion to the degree of placental separation. This is caused by the insult of the abruption itself and by issues related to prematurity when early birth is required to alleviate maternal or fetal distress.

Abruptio placentae is classified according to the extent of separation and the amount of blood loss from the maternal circulation. Classifications include:

- Mild (grade 1): minimal bleeding (less than 500 mL), marginal separation (10% to 20%), tender uterus, no coagulopathy, no signs of shock, no fetal distress
- Moderate (grade 2): moderate bleeding (1,000 to 1,500 mL), moderate separation (20% to 50%), continuous abdominal pain, mild shock
- Severe (grade 3): absent to moderate bleeding (more than 1,500 mL), severe separation (more than 50%), profound shock, agonizing abdominal pain, and development of disseminated intravascular coagulopathy (DIC) (Gilbert, 2007)

Abruptio placentae also may be classified as partial or complete, depending on the degree of separation. Alternately, it can be classified as concealed or apparent, by the type of bleeding (Fig. 19.5).

Remember Helen, the pregnant woman with severe abdominal pain? Electronic fetal monitoring revealed uterine hypertonicity with absent fetal heart sounds. Palpation of her abdomen revealed rigidity and extreme tenderness in all four quadrants. Her vital signs were as follows—temperature, afebrile; pulse 94; respirations 22; blood pressure 130/90 mm Hg. What might you suspect as the cause of Helen's abdominal pain? What course of action would you anticipate for Helen?

Therapeutic Management

Treatment of abruptio placentae is designed to assess, control, and restore the amount of blood lost; to provide a positive outcome for both mother and newborn; and to prevent coagulation disorders, such as DIC (Box 19.2). Emergency measures include starting two large-bore IV lines with normal saline or lactated Ringer's solution to combat hypovolemia, obtaining blood specimens for evaluating hemodynamic status values and for typing and cross-matching, and frequently monitoring fetal and maternal well-being. After the severity of abruption is determined and appropriate blood and fluid replacement is given, cesarean birth is done immediately if fetal distress is evident. If the fetus is not in distress, close monitoring continues, with delivery planned at the earliest signs of fetal distress. Because of the possibility of fetal blood loss through the placenta, a neonatal intensive care team should be available during the birth process to assess and treat the newborn immediately for shock, blood loss, and hypoxia.

If the woman develops DIC, treatment focuses on determining the underlying cause of DIC and correcting it. Replacement therapy of the coagulation factors is achieved by transfusion of fresh-frozen plasma along with cryoprecipitate to maintain the circulating volume and provide oxygen to the cells of the body. Anticoagulant therapy (low-molecular-weight heparin), packed red cells, platelet concentrates, antithrombin concentrates, and nonclotting protein-containing volume expanders, such as plasma protein fraction or albumin, are also used to combat this serious condition (Bick, 2007). Prompt identification and early intervention are essential for a woman with acute DIC associated with abruptio placentae to treat DIC and possibly save her life.

Nursing Assessment

Abruptio placentae is a medical emergency. The nurse plays a critical role in assessing the pregnant woman presenting with abdominal pain and/or experiencing vaginal bleeding, especially in a concealed hemorrhage, in which

FIGURE 19.5 Classifications of abruptio placentae. (**A**) Partial abruption with concealed hemorrhage. (**B**) Partial abruption with apparent hemorrhage. (**C**) Complete abruption with concealed hemorrhage.

A Partial abruption, concealed hemorrhage

B Partial abruption, apparent hemorrhage

C Complete abruption, concealed hemorrhage

the extent of bleeding is not recognized. Rapid assessment is essential to ensure prompt, effective interventions to prevent maternal and fetal morbidity and mortality. Comparison Chart 19.1 compares placenta previa with abruptio placentae.

BOX 19.2 Disseminated Intravascular Coagulation (DIC)

DIC is a bleeding disorder characterized by an abnormal reduction in the elements involved in blood clotting resulting from their widespread intravascular clotting (Gilbert, 2007). This disorder can occur secondary to abruptio placentae.

Simply put, the clinical and pathologic manifestations of DIC can be described as a loss of balance between the clot-forming activity of thrombin and the clot-lysing activity of plasmin. Therefore, too much thrombin tips the balance toward the prothrombic state and the client develops clots. Alternately, too much clot lysis (fibrinolysis) results from plasmin formation and the client hemorrhages. Small clots form throughout the body, and eventually the blood-clotting factors are used up, rendering them unavailable to form clots at sites of tissue injury. Clot-dissolving mechanisms are also increased, which result in bleeding (possibly severe).

DIC can be stimulated by many factors, including sepsis, malignancy, and obstetric conditions such as placental abruption, missed abortion or retained dead fetus, amniotic fluid embolism, and eclampsia.

Laboratory studies that assist in the diagnosis include:
• Decreased fibrinogen and platelets
• Prolonged PT and aPTT
• Positive D-dimer tests and fibrin (split) degradation products (objective evidence of the simultaneous formation of thrombin and plasmin) (Furlong & Furlong, 2007)

Health History and Physical Examination

Begin the health history by assessing the woman for risk factors that may predispose her to abruptio placentae, such as maternal smoking, advanced maternal age (over 35 years old), poor nutrition, multiple gestation, excessive intrauterine pressure caused by hydramnios, hypertension, severe trauma (e.g., auto accident, intimate partner violence), cocaine use, alcohol ingestion, and multiparity (Norwitz & Schorge, 2006; Zeltzer, 2007). Ask the woman about her previous pregnancies to determine if she has experienced a prior abruption. In addition, be alert for other notable risk factors, such as male fetal gender, chorioamnionitis, prolonged premature ruptured membranes (more than 24 hours), oligohydramnios, preeclampsia, and low socioeconomic status (Deering & Satin, 2007).

Assess the woman for bleeding. As the placenta separates from the uterus, hemorrhage ensues. It can be apparent, appearing as vaginal bleeding, or it can be concealed. Vaginal bleeding is present in 80% of women diagnosed with abruptio placentae and may be significant enough to jeopardize both maternal and fetal health within a short time frame. The remaining 20% of abruptions are associated with a concealed hemorrhage and the absence of vaginal bleeding. Monitor the woman's level of consciousness, noting any signs or symptoms that may suggest shock.

▶ *Take NOTE!*

Vital signs can be within normal range, even with significant blood loss, because a pregnant woman can lose up to 40% of her total blood volume without showing signs of shock (Gilbert, 2007).

Assess the woman for complaints of pain, including the type, onset, and location. Ask if she has had any contractions. Palpate the abdomen, noting any contractions,

COMPARISON CHART 19.1 PLACENTA PREVIA VERSUS ABRUPTIO PLACENTAE

Manifestation	Placenta Previa	Abruptio Placentae
Onset	Insidious	Sudden
Type of bleeding	Always visible; slight, then more profuse	Can be concealed or visible
Blood description	Bright red	Dark
Discomfort/Pain	None (painless)	Constant; uterine tenderness on palpation
Uterine tone	Soft and relaxed	Firm to rigid
Fetal heart rate	Usually in normal range	Fetal distress or absent
Fetal presentation	May be breech or transverse lie; engagement is absent	No relationship

uterine tenderness, tenseness, or rigidity. Ask if she has noticed any changes in fetal movement and activity. Decreased fetal movement may be the presenting complaint, resulting from fetal jeopardy or fetal death (Oyelese & Ananth, 2006). Assess fetal heart rate and continue to monitor it electronically.

▶ **Take** NOTE!

Classic manifestations of abruptio placentae include painful, dark-red vaginal bleeding (port wine color) because the bleeding comes from the clot that was formed behind the placenta; "knife-like" abdominal pain; uterine tenderness; contractions; and decreased fetal movement. Rapid assessment is essential to ensure prompt, effective interventions to prevent maternal and fetal morbidity and mortality.

Laboratory and Diagnostic Testing

Laboratory and diagnostic tests may be helpful in diagnosing the condition and guiding management. These studies may include:

- CBC—determines the current hemodynamic status; however, it is not reliable for estimating acute blood loss
- Fibrinogen levels—typically are increased in pregnancy (hyperfibrinogenemia); thus, a moderate dip in fibrinogen levels might suggest coagulopathy (DIC) and, if profuse bleeding occurs, the clotting cascade might be compromised
- Prothrombin time (PT)/activated partial thromboplastin time (aPTT)—determines the client's coagulation status, especially if surgery is planned
- Type and cross-match—determines blood type if a transfusion is needed
- Kleihauer–Betke test—detects fetal red blood cells in the maternal circulation, determines the degree of fetal–maternal hemorrhage, and helps calculate the

appropriate dosage of RhoGAM to give to Rh-negative clients
- Nonstress test—demonstrates findings of fetal jeopardy manifested by late decelerations or bradycardia
- Biophysical profile—aids in evaluating clients with chronic abruption; a low score (less than 6 points) suggests possible fetal compromise (Collins, 2007)

Ultrasound is not useful for making a definitive diagnosis because the clot is sonographically visible in less than 50% of the cases (Zeltzer, 2007).

Nursing Management

Nursing management of the woman with abruptio placentae warrants immediate care to provide the best outcome for both mother and fetus.

Ensuring Adequate Tissue Perfusion

Upon arrival to the facility, place the woman on strict bed rest and in a left lateral position to prevent pressure on the vena cava. This position provides uninterrupted perfusion to the fetus. Expect to administer oxygen therapy via nasal cannula to ensure adequate tissue perfusion. Monitor oxygen saturation levels via pulse oximetry to evaluate the effectiveness of interventions.

Obtain maternal vital signs frequently, as often as every 15 minutes as indicated, depending on the woman's status and amount of blood loss. Observe for changes in vital signs suggesting hypovolemic shock and report them immediately. Also expect to insert an indwelling urinary (Foley) catheter to assess hourly urine output and initiate an IV infusion for fluid replacement using a large-bore catheter.

Assess fundal height for changes. An increase in size would indicate bleeding. Monitor the amount and characteristics of any vaginal bleeding as frequently as every 15 to 30 minutes. Be alert for signs and symptoms of DIC, such as bleeding gums, tachycardia, oozing from the IV insertion site, and petechiae, and administer blood products as ordered if DIC occurs.

Institute continuous electronic fetal monitoring. Assess uterine contractions and report any increased uterine tenseness or rigidity. Also observe the tracing for tetanic uterine contractions or changes in fetal heart rate patterns suggesting fetal compromise.

Providing Support and Education

A woman diagnosed with abruptio placentae may be filled with a sense of heightened anxiety and apprehension, for her own health as well as that of her fetus. Communicate empathy and understanding of the client's experience, and provide emotional support throughout this frightening time. Remain with the couple, acknowledge their emotions and fears, and address their spiritual and cultural needs. Answer their questions about the status of their fetus openly and honestly, being sure to explain indicators of fetal well-being. Provide information about the various diagnostic tests, treatments, and procedures that may be done, including the possible need for a cesarean birth.

Depending on the client's status, extent of bleeding, and length of gestation, the fetus may not survive. If the fetus does survive, he or she most likely will require neonatal intensive care. Assist the client and family to deal with the loss or with the birth of a newborn in the neonatal intensive care unit.

Although abruptio placentae is not a preventable condition, client education is important to help reduce the risk for a recurrence of this condition. Encourage the woman to avoid drinking, smoking, or using drugs during pregnancy. Urge her to seek early and continuous prenatal care and to receive prompt health care if any signs and symptoms occur in future pregnancies.

Think back to Helen, the pregnant woman described at the beginning of the chapter. She was diagnosed with abruptio placentae and was prepared for an emergency cesarean birth. On exploration, there was almost a 75% abruption, with approximately 800 mL of concealed blood between the uterus and the placenta. In addition, she lost an additional 500 mL during surgery. What in Helen's history may have placed her at increased risk for abruption? What assessments and interventions would be essential during her postpartum recovery secondary to her large blood loss? What psychosocial interventions would be necessary due to her fetal loss?

Hyperemesis Gravidarum

At least 80% of women experience nausea and vomiting during their pregnancy (Lane, 2007). The term *morning sickness* is often used to describe this condition when symptoms are relatively mild. Such symptoms usually disappear after the first trimester. This mild form mostly affects the quality of life of the woman and her family, whereas the severe form—hyperemesis gravidarum—results in dehydration, electrolyte imbalance, and the need for hospitalization (Wilcox & Edelman, 2007).

Unlike morning sickness, **hyperemesis gravidarum** is a complication of pregnancy characterized by persistent, uncontrollable nausea and vomiting that persists beyond the 20th week of pregnancy, causing weight loss of more than 5% of prepregnancy body weight, dehydration, metabolic acidosis from starvation, alkalosis from loss of hydrochloric acid, and hypokalemia (Lamondy, 2007).

Hyperemesis is estimated to occur in approximately 5 per 1,000 pregnancies. The prevalence increases in molar pregnancies and multiple gestations. Its peak incidence occurs between 8 and 12 weeks of pregnancy, and it usually resolves by week 16 (Ogunyemi, 2007).

▶ **Take** NOTE!

Every pregnant woman needs to be instructed to report any episodes of severe nausea and vomiting or episodes that extend beyond the first trimester.

Pathophysiology

Although the exact cause of nausea and vomiting is unknown, its effects—decreased placental blood flow, decreased maternal blood flow, and acidosis—can threaten the health of the mother and fetus. Dehydration can also lead to preterm labor (Lane, 2007). Numerous theories abound, but few studies have produced scientific evidence to identify the etiology of this condition. It is likely that multiple factors contribute to it.

Elevated levels of hCG are present in all pregnant women during early pregnancy, usually declining after 12 weeks. This corresponds to the usual duration of morning sickness. In hyperemesis gravidarum, the hCG levels are often higher and extend beyond the first trimester. Symptoms exacerbate the disease. Decreased fluid intake and prolonged vomiting cause dehydration; dehydration increases the serum concentration of hCG, which in turn exacerbates the nausea and vomiting—a vicious cycle. A few other theories that have been proposed to explain its etiology include:

- Endocrine theory—high levels of hCG and estrogen during pregnancy
- Metabolic theory—vitamin B6 deficiency
- Psychological theory—psychological stress increases the symptoms

Therapeutic Management

Conservative management in the home is the first line of treatment for the woman with hyperemesis gravidarum. This usually focuses on dietary and lifestyle changes.

If conservative management fails to alleviate the client's symptoms and nausea and vomiting continue, hospitalization is necessary to reverse the effects of severe nausea and vomiting.

On admission to the hospital, blood tests are ordered to assess the severity of the client's dehydration, electrolyte imbalance, ketosis, and malnutrition. Parenteral fluids and drugs are ordered to rehydrate the woman and reduce the symptoms. The first choice for fluid replacement is generally 5% dextrose in lactated Ringer's solution with vitamins (pyridoxine [B6]) and electrolytes added. Oral food and fluids are withheld for the first 24 to 36 hours to allow the GI tract to rest. Antiemetics may be administered rectally or intravenously to control the nausea and vomiting initially because the woman is considered NPO. Once her condition stabilizes and she is allowed oral intake, medications may be administered orally.

If the client does not improve after several days of bed rest, "gut rest," IV fluids, and antiemetics, total parenteral nutrition or feeding through a percutaneous endoscopic gastrostomy tube is instituted to prevent malnutrition.

The FDA has not approved any drugs for the treatment of nausea and vomiting in pregnancy, but the risk of administration must be balanced against the sequelae of prolonged starvation and dehydration. Finding a drug that works for any given client is largely a matter of trial and error. If one drug is ineffective, another class of drugs with a different mechanism of action may help. Promethazine (Phenergan) and prochlorperazine (Compazine) are among the older preparations usually tried first. If they fail to relieve symptoms, newer drugs such as on-

dansetron (Zofran) may be tried. Most drugs are given parenterally or rectally (Lane, 2007) (Drug Guide 19.2).

Few women receive complete relief of symptoms from any one therapy. Complementary and alternative medicine therapies appeal to many to help supplement traditional ones. Some popular therapies include acupressure, massage, therapeutic touch, ginger, and the wearing of Sea-bands to prevent nausea and vomiting. Recent research has reported a positive effect of using acupressure over the Neiguan point on the wrist by Sea-bands to control nausea and vomiting associated with pregnancy (Lane, 2007).

Nursing Assessment

Nursing assessment of the woman with hyperemesis gravidarum requires a thorough history and physical examination to identify signs and symptoms associated with this disorder. The client is extremely uncomfortable. She may experience many hours of lost work productivity and sleep, and hyperemesis may damage family relationships. If hyperemesis progresses untreated, it may cause neurologic disturbances, renal damage, retinal hemorrhage, or death (Lane, 2007). Laboratory and diagnostic tests aid in determining the severity of the disorder.

Health History and Physical Examination
Begin the history by asking the client about the onset, duration, and course of her nausea and vomiting. Ask her about any medications or treatments she used and how effective they were in relieving her nausea and vomiting. Obtain a diet history from the client, including a dietary

DRUG GUIDE 19.2 MEDICATIONS USED FOR HYPEREMESIS GRAVIDARUM

Medication	Action/Indications	Nursing Implications
Promethazine (Phenergan)	Diminishes vestibular stimulation and acts on the chemoreceptor trigger zone (CTZ) Symptomatic relief of nausea and vomiting, and motion sickness	Be alert for urinary retention, dizziness, hypotension, and involuntary movements. Institute safety measures to prevent injury secondary to sedative effects Offer hard candy and frequent rinsing of mouth for dryness.
Prochlorperazine (Compazine)	Acts centrally to inhibit dopamine receptors in the CTZ and peripherally to block vagus nerve stimulation in the GI tract Controls severe nausea and vomiting	Be alert for abnormal movements and for neuroleptic malignant syndrome such as seizures, hyper-/hypotension, tachycardia, and dyspnea. Assess mental status, intake/output Caution patient not to drive as a result of drowsiness or dizziness Advise to change position slowly to minimize effects of orthostatic hypotension.
Odansetron (Zofran)	Blocks serotonin peripherally, centrally, and in the small intestine Prevents nausea and vomiting	Monitor for possible side effects such as diarrhea, constipation, abdominal pain, headache, dizziness, drowsiness, and fatigue. Monitor liver function studies as ordered.

Sources: Hodgson & Kizior, 2007; Lilley et al., 2007.

recall for the past week. Note the client's knowledge of nutrition and need for appropriate nutritional intake. Be alert for patterns that may contribute to or trigger her distress. Also ask about any complaints of ptyalism (excessive salivation), anorexia, indigestion, and abdominal pain or distention. Ask if she has noticed any blood or mucus in her stool.

Review the client's history for possible risk factors, such as young age, nausea and vomiting with previous pregnancy, history of intolerance of oral contraceptives, nulliparity, trophoblastic disease, multiple gestation, emotional or psychological stress, gastroesophageal reflux disease, primigravida status, obesity, hyperthyroidism, and *Helicobacter pylori* seropositivity (Ogunyemi, 2007). Weigh the client and compare this weight to her weight before she began experiencing symptoms and to her prepregnancy weight to estimate the degree of loss. With hyperemesis, weight loss usually exceeds 5% of body mass.

Inspect the mucous membranes for dryness and check skin turgor for evidence of fluid loss and dehydration. Assess blood pressure for changes, such as hypotension, that may suggest a fluid volume deficit. Also note any complaints of weakness, fatigue, activity intolerance, dizziness, or sleep disturbances.

Assess the client's perception of the situation. Note any evidence of depression, anxiety, irritability, mood changes, and decreased ability to concentrate, which can add to her emotional distress (Lamondy, 2007). Determine the woman's support systems that are available for help.

Laboratory and Diagnostic Testing

The results of laboratory and diagnostic tests may provide clues to the severity or etiology of the disorder: These may include:

- Liver enzymes—elevations of aspartate aminotransferase (AST) and alanine aminotransferase (ALT) are usually present
- CBC—elevated levels of red blood cells and hematocrit, indicating dehydration
- Urine ketones—positive when the body breaks down fat to provide energy in the absence of inadequate intake
- Blood urea nitrogen (BUN)—increased in the presence of salt and water depletion
- Urine specific gravity—greater than 1.025, possibly indicating concentrated urine linked to inadequate fluid intake or excessive fluid loss
- Serum electrolytes—decreased levels of potassium, sodium, and chloride resulting from excessive vomiting and loss of hydrochloric acid in stomach
- Ultrasound—evaluation for molar pregnancy or multiple gestation (Wilcox & Edelman, 2007)

Nursing Management

Nursing management for the client with hyperemesis gravidarum focuses on promoting comfort by controlling the client's nausea and vomiting and promoting adequate nutrition. In addition, the nurse plays a major role in supporting and educating the client and her family.

Promoting Comfort and Nutrition

During the initial period, expect to withhold all oral food and fluids, maintaining NPO status to allow the GI tract to rest. In addition, administer prescribed antiemetics to relieve the nausea and vomiting and IV fluids to replace fluid losses. Monitor the rate of infusion to prevent overload and assess the IV insertion site to prevent infiltration or infection. Also administer electrolyte replacement therapy as ordered to correct any imbalances, and periodically check serum electrolyte levels to evaluate the effectiveness of therapy.

Provide physical comfort measures such as hygiene measures and oral care. Pay special attention to the environment, making sure to keep the area free of pungent odors. As the client's nausea and vomiting subside, gradually introduce oral fluids and foods in small amounts. Monitor intake and output and assess the client's tolerance to the increase in intake.

Providing Support and Education

Women with hyperemesis gravidarum commonly are fatigued physically and emotionally. Many are exhausted, frustrated, and anxious. Offer reassurance that all interventions are directed toward promoting positive pregnancy outcomes for both the woman and her fetus. Providing information about the expected plan of care may help to alleviate the client's anxiety. Listen to her concerns and feelings, answering all questions honestly. Educate the woman and her family about the condition and its treatment options (Teaching Guidelines 19.1). Teach the client about therapeutic lifestyle changes, such as avoiding stressors and fatigue that may trigger nausea and vomiting. Offer ongoing support and encouragement and promote active participation in care decisions, thereby empowering the client and her family. Attempting to provide the client with a sense of control may help her overcome the feeling that she has lost control. If necessary, refer the client to a spiritual advisor or counseling. Also suggest possible local or national support groups that the client may contact for additional information.

Arrange for possible home care follow-up for the client and reinforce discharge instructions to promote understanding. Collaborate with community resources to ensure continuity of care.

Gestational Hypertension

Gestational hypertension is characterized by hypertension without proteinuria after 20 weeks of gestation and a return of the blood pressure to normal postpartum. Previously, gestational hypertension was known as pregnancy-induced hypertension or toxemia of pregnancy, but these terms are no longer used. Gestational hypertension is clin-

TEACHING GUIDELINES 19.1

Teaching to Minimize Nausea and Vomiting

- Avoid noxious stimuli—such as strong flavors, perfumes, or strong odors such as frying bacon—that might trigger nausea and vomiting.
- Avoid tight waistbands to minimize pressure on abdomen.
- Eat small, frequent meals throughout the day—six small meals.
- Separate fluids from solids by consuming fluids in between meals.
- Avoid lying down or reclining for at least 2 hours after eating.
- Use high-protein supplement drinks.
- Avoid foods high in fat.
- Increase your intake of carbonated beverages.
- Increase your exposure to fresh air to improve symptoms.
- Eat when you are hungry, regardless of normal mealtimes.
- Drink herbal teas containing peppermint or ginger.
- Avoid fatigue and learn how to mange stress in life.
- Schedule daily rest periods to avoid becoming overtired.
- Eat foods that settle the stomach, such as dry crackers, toast, or soda.

ically characterized by a blood pressure of 140/90 mm Hg or more on two occasions at least 6 hours apart (Gibson & Carson, 2007). Gestational hypertension can be differentiated from chronic hypertension, which appears before the 20th week of gestation; or hypertension before the current pregnancy, which continues after the woman gives birth.

Gestational hypertension is the second leading cause of maternal death in the United States after thromboembolism, accounting for almost 15% of such deaths, and the most common complication reported during pregnancy. Hypertension complicates 12% to 20% of pregnancies and the rate has increased steadily, approximately 30% to 40% since 1990, for all ages, races, and ethnic groups. The highest rates are in women younger than 20 or older than 40 (Weismiller, 2007).

ACOG (2007a) and the National High Blood Pressure Education Program (2000) have identified a classification system for hypertensive disorders. Hypertension may be a preexisting condition (chronic hypertension) or it may present for the first time during pregnancy (gestational hypertension). Regardless of its onset, hypertension jeopardizes the well-being of the mother as well as the fetus.

The classification of hypertensive disorders in pregnancy currently consists of four categories:

- Gestational hypertension: blood pressure elevation (140/90 mm Hg) identified after midpregnancy without proteinuria
- Chronic hypertension: hypertension prior to the pregnancy or diagnosed before week 20 of gestation
- Transient hypertension: hypertension without preeclampsia at the time of birth, during labor, or within 24 hours postpartum; resolution within 12 weeks postpartum to normotensive blood pressure levels
- Chronic hypertension with preeclampsia: chronic hypertension with new proteinuria or exacerbation of previously controlled blood pressure, or proteinuria, thrombocytopenia, or elevated liver enzymes (ACOG, 2007; Blackburn, 2007).

Gestational hypertension can be classified as preeclampsia or eclampsia. Each is associated with specific criteria. Preeclampsia is further categorized as mild or severe. Comparison Chart 19.2 highlights these classifications.

Pathophysiology

Gestational hypertension remains an enigma. The condition can be devastating to both the mother and fetus, and yet the etiology still remains a mystery to medical science despite decades of research. Many theories exist, but none have truly explained the widespread pathologic changes that result in pulmonary edema, oliguria, seizures, thrombocytopenia, and abnormal liver enzymes (Podymow & August, 2007). Despite the results of several research studies, the use of aspirin or supplementation with calcium, magnesium, zinc, or antioxidant therapy (vitamin C and E), salt restriction, diuretic therapy, or fish oils has not proved to prevent this destructive condition.

The underlying mechanisms involved with this disorder are vasospasm and hypoperfusion. In addition, endothelial injury occurs, leading to platelet adherence, fibrin deposition, and the presence of schistocytes (fragment of an erythrocyte).

Generalized vasospasm results in elevation of blood pressure and reduced blood flow to the brain, liver, kidneys, placenta, and lungs. Decreased liver perfusion leads to impaired liver function and subcapsular hemorrhage. This is demonstrated by epigastric pain and elevated liver enzymes in the maternal serum. Decreased brain perfusion leads to small cerebral hemorrhages and symptoms of arterial vasospasm such as headaches, visual disturbances, blurred vision, and hyperactive deep tendon reflexes (DTRs). A thromboxane/prostacyclin imbalance leads to increased thromboxane (potent vasoconstrictor and stimulator of platelet aggregation) and decreased prostacyclin (potent vasodilator and inhibitor of platelet aggregation), which contribute to the hypertensive state. Decreased kidney perfusion reduces the glomerular filtra-

COMPARISON CHART 19.2 PREECLAMPSIA VERSUS ECLAMPSIA

	Mild Preeclampsia	Severe Preeclampsia	Eclampsia
Blood pressure	>140/90 mm Hg after 20 weeks' gestation	>160/110 mm Hg	Same as severe preeclampsia
Proteinuria	300 mg/24 h or greater than 1+ protein on a random dipstick urine sample	>500 mg/24 hours; greater than 3+ on random dipstick urine sample	Marked proteinuria
Seizures/coma	No	No	Yes
Hyperreflexia	No	Yes	Yes
Other signs and symptoms	Mild facial or hand edema Weight gain	Headache Oliguria Blurred vision, scotomata (blind spots) Pulmonary edema Thrombocytopenia (platelet count <100,000 platelets/mm^3) Cerebral disturbances Epigastric or RUQ pain HELLP	Severe headache Generalized edema RUQ or epigastric pain Visual disturbances Cerebral hemorrhage Renal failure HELLP

tion rate (GFR), resulting in decreased urine output and increased serum levels of sodium, BUN, uric acid, and creatinine, further increasing extracellular fluid and edema. Increased capillary permeability in the kidneys allows albumin to escape, which reduces plasma colloid osmotic pressure and moves more fluid into extracellular spaces; this leads to pulmonary edema and generalized edema. Poor placental perfusion resulting from prolonged vasoconstriction helps to contribute to intrauterine growth restriction, premature separation of the placenta (abruptio placentae), persistent fetal hypoxia, and acidosis. In addition, hemoconcentration (resulting from decreased intravascular volume) causes increased blood viscosity and elevated hematocrit (ACOG, 2007a).

Therapeutic Management

Management of the woman with gestational hypertension varies depending on the severity of her condition and its effects on the fetus. Typically the woman is managed conservatively if she is experiencing mild symptoms. However, if the condition progresses, management becomes more aggressive.

Management for Mild Preeclampsia

Conservative strategies for mild preeclampsia are used if the woman exhibits no signs of renal or hepatic dysfunction or coagulopathy. A woman with mild elevations in blood pressure may be placed on bed rest at home. She is encouraged to rest as much as possible in the lateral recumbent position to improve uteroplacental blood flow, reduce her blood pressure, and promote diuresis. In addition, antepartal visits and diagnostic testing—such as CBC, clotting studies, liver enzymes, and platelet levels—

increase in frequency. The woman will be asked to monitor her blood pressure daily (every 4 to 6 hours while awake) and report any increased readings; she will also measure the amount of protein found in urine using a dipstick and will weigh herself for any weight gain. Daily fetal movement counts also are implemented. If there is any decrease in movement, the woman needs to be evaluated by her health care provider that day. A balanced, nutritional diet with no sodium restriction is advised. In addition, she is encouraged to drink six to eight 8-oz glasses of water daily.

If home management fails to reduce the blood pressure, admission to the hospital is warranted and the treatment strategy is individualized based on the severity of the condition and the gestational age at the time of diagnosis. During the hospitalization, the woman with mild preeclampsia is monitored closely for signs and symptoms of severe preeclampsia or impending eclampsia (e.g., persistent headache, hyperreflexia). Blood pressure measurements are frequently recorded along with daily weights to detect excessive weight gain resulting from edema. Fetal surveillance is instituted in the form of daily fetal movement counts, nonstress testing, and serial ultrasounds to evaluate fetal growth and amniotic fluid volume to confirm fetal well-being. Expectant management usually continues until the pregnancy reaches term, fetal lung maturity is documented, or complications develop that warrant immediate birth (Mundy, 2006).

Prevention of disease progression is the focus of treatment during labor. Blood pressure is monitored frequently and a quiet environment is important to minimize the risk of stimulation and to promote rest. IV magnesium sulfate is infused to prevent any seizure activity, along with antihypertensives if blood pressure values begin to rise. Calcium gluconate is kept at the bedside in case the magnesium level becomes toxic. Continued close monitoring of neurologic status is warranted to detect any signs or symptoms of hypoxemia, impending seizure activity, or increased intracranial pressure. An indwelling urinary (Foley) catheter usually is inserted to allow for accurate measurement of urine output.

Management for Severe Preeclampsia

Severe preeclampsia may develop suddenly and bring with it high blood pressure of more than 160/110 mmHg, proteinuria of more than 5 g in 24 hours, oliguria of less than 400 mL in 24 hours, cerebral and visual symptoms, and rapid weight gain. This clinical picture signals severe preeclampsia, and immediate hospitalization is needed.

Treatment is highly individualized and based on disease severity and fetal age. Birth of the infant is the only cure, because preeclampsia depends on the presence of trophoblastic tissue. Therefore, the exact age of the fetus is assessed to determine viability.

Severe preeclampsia is treated aggressively because hypertension poses a serious threat to mother and fetus. The goal of care is to stabilize the mother–fetus dyad and prepare for birth. Therapy focuses on controlling hypertension, preventing seizures, preventing long-term morbidity, and preventing maternal, fetal, or newborn death (Weismiller, 2007). Intense maternal and fetal surveillance starts when the mother enters the hospital and continues throughout her stay.

The woman in labor with severe preeclampsia typically receives oxytocin to stimulate uterine contractions and magnesium sulfate to prevent seizure activity. Oxytocin and magnesium sulfate can be given simultaneously via infusion pumps to ensure both are administered at the prescribed rate. The client is evaluated closely for magnesium toxicity. If at all possible, a vaginal delivery is preferable to a cesarean birth. PGE2 gel may be used to ripen the cervix. A cesarean birth may be performed if the client is seriously ill. A pediatrician/neonatologist must be available in the birthing room to care for the newborn. A newborn whose mother received high doses of magnesium sulfate needs to be monitored for respiratory depression, hypocalcemia, and hypotonia (Blackburn, 2007).

Management of Eclampsia

In the woman who develops an eclamptic seizure, the convulsive activity begins with facial twitching, followed by generalized muscle rigidity. Respirations cease for the duration of the seizure, resulting from muscle spasms, thus compromising fetal oxygenation. Coma usually follows the seizure activity, with respiration resuming. Eclamptic seizures are life-threatening emergencies and require immediate treatment to decrease maternal morbidity and mortality.

As with any seizure, the initial management is to clear the airway and administer adequate oxygen. Positioning the woman on her left side and protecting her from injury during the seizure are key. Suction equipment must be readily available to remove secretions from her mouth after the seizure is over. IV fluids are administered after the seizure at a rate to replace urine output and additional insensible losses. Fetal heart rate is monitored closely. Magnesium sulfate is administered IV to prevent further seizures. Hypertension is controlled with antihypertensive medications. After the seizures are controlled, the woman's stability is assessed and birth via induction or cesarean birth is performed (Blincoe, 2007).

If the woman's condition remains stable, she will be transferred to the postpartum unit for care. If she becomes unstable after giving birth, she may be transferred to the critical care unit for closer observation.

Nursing Assessment

Preventing complications related to hypertension during pregnancy requires the use of assessment, advocacy, and counseling skills. Assessment begins with the accurate measurement of the client's blood pressure at each encounter. In addition, nurses need to assess for subjective complaints that may indicate progression of the disease—visual changes, severe headaches, unusual bleeding or bruising, or epigastric pain (Blincoe, 2007). The significant signs of gestational hypertension—proteinuria and hypertension—occur without the woman's awareness. Unfortunately, by the time symptoms are noticed, gestational hypertension can be severe.

▶ *Take* NOTE!

The absolute blood pressure (value that validates elevation) of 140/90 mmHg should be obtained on two occasions 6 hours apart to be diagnostic of gestational hypertension. Proteinuria is defined as 300 mg or more of urinary protein per 24 hours or more than 1+ protein by chemical reagent strip or dipstick of at least two random urine samples collected at least 6 hours apart with no evidence of UTI (ACOG, 2007a).

Health History and Physical Examination

Take a thorough history during the first antepartal visit to identify whether the woman is at risk for preeclampsia. Risk factors include:

• Primigravida status
• Chromosomal abnormalities
• Structural congenital anomalies
• Multifetal pregnancy
• History of preeclampsia in a previous pregnancy
• Excessive placental tissue, as is seen in women with GTD

- Chronic stress
- Family history of preeclampsia (mother or sister)
- Lower socioeconomic group
- History of diabetes, hypertension, or renal disease
- Poor nutrition
- African-American ethnicity
- Age extremes (younger than 20 or older than 40)
- Obesity (Weismiller, 2007)

In addition, complete a nutritional assessment that includes the woman's usual intake of protein, calcium, daily calories, and fluids.

Women at risk for preeclampsia require more frequent prenatal visits throughout their pregnancy, and they require teaching about problems so that they can report them promptly.

Blood pressure must be measured carefully and consistently. Obtain all measurements with the woman in the same position (blood pressure is highest in the sitting position and lowest in the side-lying position) and by using the same technique (automated vs. manual). This standardization in position and technique will yield the most accurate readings (Weismiller, 2007).

Obtain the client's weight (noting gain since last visit), and assess for amount and location of edema. Asking questions such as, "Do your rings still fit on your fingers?" or "Is your face puffy when you get up in the morning?" will help to determine whether fluid retention is present or if the woman's status has changed since her last visit.

▶ *Take* NOTE!

Although edema is not a cardinal sign of preeclampsia, weight should be monitored frequently to identify sudden gains in a short time span. Current research relies less on the classic triad of symptoms (hypertension, proteinuria, and edema or weight gain) and more on decreased organ perfusion, endothelial dysfunction (capillary leaking and proteinuria), and elevated blood pressure as key indicators (Gibson & Carson, 2007).

If edema is present, assess the distribution, degree, and pitting. Document your findings and identify whether the edema is dependent or pitting. Dependent edema is present on the lower half of the body if the client is ambulatory, where hydrostatic pressure is greatest. It is usually observed in the feet and ankles or in the sacral area if the client is on bed rest.

Pitting edema is edema that leaves a small depression or pit after finger pressure is applied to a swollen area (Gibson & Carson, 2007). Record the depth of pitting demonstrated when pressure is applied. Although subjective, the following is used to record relative degrees:

- 1+ pitting edema = 2-mm depression into skin; disappears rapidly
- 2+ pitting edema = 4-mm skin depression; disappears in 10 to 15 seconds
- 3+ pitting edema = 6-mm depression into skin; lasts more than 1 minute
- 4+ pitting edema = 8-mm depression into skin; lasts 2 to 3 minutes

At every antepartal visit, assess the fetal heart rate with a Doppler device. Also check a clean-catch urine specimen for protein using a dipstick.

Laboratory and Diagnostic Testing

Various laboratory tests may be performed to evaluate the woman's status. Typically these include a CBC, serum electrolytes, BUN, creatinine, and hepatic enzyme levels. Urine specimens are checked for protein; if levels are 1-2+ or greater, a 24-hour urine collection is completed.

Nursing Management

Nursing management of the woman with gestational hypertension focuses on close monitoring of blood pressure and ongoing assessment for evidence of disease progression. Throughout the client's pregnancy, fetal surveillance is key.

Intervening With Preeclampsia

The woman with mild preeclampsia requires frequent monitoring to detect changes because preeclampsia can progress rapidly. Instruct all women in the signs and symptoms of preeclampsia and urge them to contact their health care professional for immediate evaluation should any occur.

Typically women with mild preeclampsia can be managed at home if they have a good understanding of the disease process, are stable, have no abnormal laboratory test results, and demonstrate good fetal movement (Teaching Guidelines 19.2). The home care nurse makes frequent visits and follow-up phone calls to assess the woman's condition, to assist with scheduling periodic evaluations of the fetus (such as nonstress tests), and to evaluate any changes that might suggest a worsening of the woman's condition.

Early detection and management of mild preeclampsia is associated with the greatest success in reducing progression of this condition. As long as the client carries out the guidelines of care as outlined by the health care provider and she remains stable, home care can continue to maintain the pregnancy until the fetus is mature. If disease progression occurs, hospitalization is required.

Intervening With Severe Preeclampsia

The woman with severe preeclampsia requires hospitalization. Maintain the client on complete bed rest in the left lateral lying position. Ensure that the room is dark

TEACHING GUIDELINES 19.2

Teaching for the Woman With Mild Preeclampsia

- Rest in a quiet environment to prevent cerebral disturbances.
- Drink 8 to 10 glasses of water daily.
- Consume a balanced, high-protein diet including high-fiber foods.
- Obtain intermittent bed rest to improve circulation to the heart and uterus.
- Limit your physical activity to promote urination and subsequent decrease in blood pressure.
- Enlist the aid of your family so that you can obtain appropriate rest time.
- Perform self-monitoring as instructed, including
  - Taking your own blood pressure twice daily
  - Checking and recording weight daily
  - Performing urine dipstick twice daily
  - Recording the number of fetal kicks daily
- Contact the home health nurse if any of the following occurs:
  - Increase in blood pressure
  - Protein present in urine
  - Gain of more than 1 lb in 1 week
  - Burning or frequency when urinating
  - Decrease in fetal activity or movement
  - Headache (forehead or posterior neck region)
  - Dizziness or visual disturbances
  - Increase in swelling in hands, feet, legs, and face
  - Stomach pain, excessive heartburn, or epigastric pain
  - Decreased or infrequent urination
  - Contractions or low back pain
  - Easy or excessive bruising
  - Sudden onset of abdominal pain
  - Nausea and vomiting

and quiet to reduce stimulation. Give sedatives as ordered to encourage quiet bed rest. The client is at risk for seizures if the condition progresses. Therefore, institute and maintain seizure precautions, such as padding the side rails and having oxygen, suction equipment, and call light readily available to protect the client from injury.

> ▶ *Take NOTE!*
>
> *Preeclampsia increases the risk of placental abruption, preterm birth, intrauterine growth restriction, and fetal distress during childbirth. Be prepared!*

Closely monitor the client's blood pressure. Administer antihypertensives as ordered to reduce blood pressure (Drug Guide 19.3). Assess the client's vision and level of consciousness. Report any changes and any complaints of headache or visual disturbances. Offer a high-protein diet with 8 to 10 glasses of water daily. Monitor the client's intake and output every hour and administer fluid and electrolyte replacements as ordered. Assess the woman for signs and symptoms of pulmonary edema, such as crackles and wheezing heard on auscultation, dyspnea, decreased oxygen saturation levels, cough, neck vein distention, anxiety, and restlessness (Blincoe, 2007).

To achieve a safe outcome for the fetus, prepare the woman for possible testing to evaluate fetal status as preeclampsia progresses. These may include the nonstress test, serial ultrasounds to track fetal growth, amniocentesis to determine fetal lung maturity, Doppler velocimetry to screen for fetal compromise, and biophysical profile to evaluate ongoing fetal well-being (Jung & Erogul, 2007).

Other laboratory tests may be performed to monitor the disease process and to determine if it is progressing into HELLP syndrome. These include liver enzymes such as lactic dehydrogenase (LDH), ALT, and AST; chemistry panel, such as creatinine, BUN, uric acid, and glucose; CBC, including platelet count; coagulation studies, such as PT, PTT, fibrinogen, and bleeding time; and a 24-hour urine collection for protein and creatinine clearance.

Administer parenteral magnesium sulfate as ordered to prevent seizures. Assess deep tendon reflexes (DTRs) to evaluate the effectiveness of therapy. Clients with preeclampsia commonly present with hyperreflexia. Severe preeclampsia causes changes in the cortex, which disrupts the equilibrium of impulses between the cerebral cortex and the spinal cord. Brisk reflexes (hyperreflexia) are the result of an irritable cortex and indicate central nervous system involvement (Warden & Euerle, 2007).

Diminished or absent reflexes occur when the client develops magnesium toxicity. Because magnesium is a potent neuromuscular blockade, the afferent and efferent nerve pathways do not relay messages properly and hyporeflexia develops. Common sites used to assess DTRs are biceps reflex, triceps reflex, patellar reflex, Achilles reflex, and plantar reflex. Nursing Procedure 19.1 highlights the steps for assessing the patellar reflex.

The National Institute of Neurological Disorders and Stroke (NINDS), a division of the National Institutes of Health, published a scale in the early 1990s that, although subjective, is used widely today. It grades reflexes from 0 to 4+. Grades 2+ and 3+ are considered normal, whereas grades 0 and 4 may indicate pathology (Table 19.2). Because these are subjective assessments, to improve communication of reflex results, condensed descriptor categories such as absent, average, brisk, or clonus should be used rather than numeric codes (Gilbert, 2007).

Clonus is the presence of rhythmic involuntary contractions, most often at the foot or ankle. Sustained clonus

DRUG GUIDE 19.3 MEDICATIONS USED WITH PREECLAMPSIA AND ECLAMPSIA

Medication	Action/Indications	Nursing Implications
Magnesium sulfate	Blockage of neuromuscular transmission, vasodilation Prevention and treatment of eclamptic seizures.	Administer IV loading dose of 4–6 g over 30 minutes, continue maintenance infusion of 2–4 g/hour as ordered. Monitor serum magnesium levels closely. Assess DTRs and check for ankle clonus. Have calcium gluconate readily available in case of toxicity. Monitor for signs and symptoms of toxicity, such as flushing, sweating, hypotension, and cardiac and central nervous system depression.
Hydralazine hydrochloride (Apresoline)	Vascular smooth muscle relaxant, thus improving perfusion to renal, uterine, and cerebral areas Reduction in blood pressure	Administer 5–10 mg by slow IV bolus every 20 minutes. Use parenteral form immediately after opening ampule. Withdraw drug slowly to prevent possible rebound hypertension. Monitor for adverse effects such as palpitations, headache, tachycardia, anorexia, nausea, vomiting, and diarrhea.
Labetalol hydrochloride (Normodyne)	Alpha 1 and beta blocker Reduction in blood pressure	Be aware that drug lowers blood pressure without decreasing maternal heart rate or cardiac output. Administer IV bolus dose of 10–20 mg and then administer IV infusion of 2 mg/minute until desired blood pressure value achieved. Monitor for possible adverse effects such as gastric pain, flatulence, constipation, dizziness, vertigo, and fatigue.
Nifedipine (Procardia)	Calcium channel blocker/dilation of coronary arteries, arterioles, and peripheral arterioles Reduction in blood pressure, stoppage of preterm labor	Administer 10 mg orally for three doses and then every 4–8 hours. Monitor for possible adverse effects such as dizziness, peripheral edema, angina, diarrhea, nasal congestions, cough.
Sodium nitroprusside	Rapid vasodilation (arterial and venous) Severe hypertension requiring rapid reduction in blood pressure	Administer via continuous IV infusion with dose titrated according to blood pressure levels. Wrap IV infusion solution in foil or opaque material to protect from light. Monitor for possible adverse effects, such as apprehension, restlessness, retrosternal pressure, palpitations, diaphoresis, abdominal pain.
Furosemide (Lasix)	Diuretic action, inhibiting the reabsorption of sodium and chloride from the ascending loop of Henle Pulmonary edema (used only if condition is present)	Administer via slow IV bolus at a dose of 10–40 mg over 1–2 minutes. Monitor urine output hourly. Assess for possible adverse effects such as dizziness, vertigo, orthostatic hypotension, anorexia, vomiting, electrolyte imbalances, muscle cramps, and muscle spasms.

Sources: Hodgson & Kizior, 2007; Lilley et al., 2007.

Nursing Procedure 19.1

ASSESSING THE PATELLAR REFLEX

Purpose: To Evaluate for Nervous System Irritability Related to Preeclampsia

1. Place the woman in the supine position (or sitting upright with the legs dangling freely over the side of the bed or examination table).
2. If lying supine, have the woman flex her knee slightly.
3. Place a hand under the knee to support the leg and locate the patellar tendon. It should be midline just below the knee cap.
4. Using a reflex hammer or the side of your hand, strike the area of the patellar tendon firmly and quickly.
5. Note the movement of the leg and foot. A patellar reflex occurs when the leg and foot move (documented as 2+).
6. Repeat the procedure on the opposite leg.

confirms central nervous system involvement. Nursing Procedure 19.2 highlights the steps when testing for ankle clonus.

With magnesium sulfate administration, the client is at risk for magnesium toxicity. Closely assess the client for signs of toxicity, which include a respiratory rate of

TABLE 19.2   GRADING DEEP TENDON REFLEXES

Description of Finding	Grade
Reflex absent, no response detected	0
Hypoactive response, diminished	1
Reflex in lower half of normal range	2
Reflex in upper half of normal range	3
Hyperactive, brisk, clonus present	4

Sources: Arenson & Drake, 2007; Weber, 2007.

Nursing Procedure 19.2

TESTING FOR ANKLE CLONUS

Purpose: To Evaluate for Nervous System Irritability Related to Preeclampsia

1. Place the woman in the supine position.
2. Have the client slightly bend her knee and place a hand under the knee to support it.
3. Dorsiflex the foot briskly and then quickly release it.
4. Watch for the foot to rebound smoothly against your hand. If the movement is smooth without any rapid contractions of the ankle or calf muscle, then clonus is not present; if the movement is jerky and rapid, clonus is present.
5. Repeat on the opposite side.

less than 12 breaths per minute, absence of deep tendon reflexes, and a decrease in urinary output, below 30 mL per hour. Also monitor serum magnesium levels. Although exact levels may vary among agencies, serum magnesium levels ranging from 4 to 7 mEq/L are considered therapeutic, whereas levels more than 8 mEq/dL are generally considered toxic. As levels increase, the woman is at risk for severe problems:

- 10 mEq/L: possible loss of DTRs
- 15 mEq/L: possible respiratory depression
- 25 mEq/L: possible cardiac arrest (Podymow & August, 2007)

If signs and symptoms of magnesium toxicity develop, expect to administer calcium gluconate as the antidote.

Throughout the client's stay, closely monitor her for signs and symptoms of labor. Perform continuous electronic fetal monitoring to assess fetal well-being. Note trends in baseline rate and presence or absence of accelerations or decelerations. Also observe for signs of fetal distress and report them immediately. Administer glucocorticoid treatment as ordered to enhance fetal lung maturity and prepare for labor induction if the mother's condition warrants.

Keep the client and family informed of the woman's condition and educate them about the course of treatment. Provide emotional support for the client and family. Severe preeclampsia is very frightening for the client and her family, and most expectant mothers are very anxious about their own health as well as that of the fetus. To allay anxiety, use light touch to comfort and reassure her that the necessary actions are being taken. Actively listening to her concerns and fears and communicating them to the health care provider is important in keeping lines of communication open. Offering praise for small accomplishments can provide positive reinforcement for behaviors that should be continued.

Intervening for Eclampsia

The onset of seizure activity identifies eclampsia. Typically, eclamptic seizures are generalized and start with facial twitching. The body then becomes rigid, in a state of tonic muscular contraction. The clonic phase of the seizure involves alternating contraction and relaxation of all body muscles. Respirations stop during seizure activity and resume shortly after it ends. Client safety is the primary concern during eclamptic seizures. If possible, turn the client to her side and remain with her. Make sure that the side rails are up and padded. Dim the lights and keep the room quiet.

Document the time and sequence of events as soon as possible. After the seizure activity has ceased, suction the nasopharynx as necessary and administer oxygen. Continue the magnesium sulfate infusion to prevent further seizures. Ensure continuous electronic fetal monitoring, evaluating fetal status for changes. Also assess the client for uterine contractions. After the client is stabilized, prepare her for the birthing process as soon as possible to reduce the risk of perinatal mortality.

Providing Follow-Up Care

After delivery of the newborn, continue to monitor the client for signs and symptoms of preeclampsia/eclampsia for at least 48 hours. Expect to continue to administer magnesium sulfate infusion for 24 hours to prevent seizure activity, and monitor serum magnesium levels for toxicity.

Assess vital signs at least every 4 hours, along with routine postpartum assessments—fundus, lochia, breasts, bladder, bowels, and emotional state attention when performing the fundal assessment and assessing lochia. Monitor urine output closely. Diuresis is a positive sign that, along with a decrease in proteinuria, signals resolution of the disease.

HELLP

HELLP is an acronym for hemolysis, elevated liver enzymes, and low platelets. HELLP syndrome occurs in about 20% of pregnant women diagnosed with severe preeclampsia. Although it has been reported as early as 17 weeks' gestation, most of the time it is diagnosed between 22 and 36 weeks' gestation (White, 2006). HELLP syndrome leads to an increased maternal risk for developing liver hematoma or rupture, stroke, cardiac arrest, seizure, pulmonary edema, DIC, subendocardial hemorrhage, adult respiratory distress syndrome, renal damage, sepsis, hypoxic encephalopathy, and maternal or fetal death (White, 2006).

Pathophysiology

The hemolysis that occurs is termed microangiopathic hemolytic anemia. It is thought to happen when red blood cells become fragmented as they pass through small, damaged blood vessels. Elevated liver enzymes are the result of reduced blood flow to the liver secondary to obstruction from fibrin deposits. Hyperbilirubinemia and jaundice result from liver impairment. Low platelets result from vascular damage, the result of vasospasm, and platelets aggregate at sites of damage, resulting in thrombocytopenia in multiple sites (Basama & Granger, 2007).

Therapeutic Management

The treatment for HELLP syndrome is based on the severity of the disease, the gestational age of the fetus, and the condition of the mother and fetus. The client should be admitted or transferred to a tertiary center with a neonatal intensive care unit. Additional treatments include magnesium sulfate, antihypertensives, and correction of the coagulopathies that accompany HELLP syndrome. After this syndrome is diagnosed and the woman's condition is stable, birth of the infant is indicated.

Magnesium sulfate is used prophylactically to prevent seizures. Antihypertensives such as hydralazine or labetalol are given to control blood pressure. Blood component therapy—such as fresh-frozen plasma, packed red cells, or platelets—is transfused to address the microangiopathic hemolytic anemia. Birth may be delayed up to 96 hours so that betamethasone or dexamethasone can be given to stimulate lung maturation in the preterm fetus.

Nursing Assessment

Nursing assessment of the woman with HELLP is similar to that for the woman with severe preeclampsia. Be alert for complaints of nausea (with or without vomiting), malaise, epigastric or right upper quadrant pain, and demonstrable edema. Perform systematic assessments frequently, as indicated by the woman's condition and response to therapy.

A diagnosis of HELLP syndrome is made based on laboratory test results, including:

- Low hematocrit that is not explained by any blood loss
- Elevated LDH (liver impairment)
- Elevated AST (liver impairment)
- Elevated ALT (liver impairment)

- Elevated BUN
- Elevated bilirubin level
- Elevated uric acid and creatinine levels (renal involvement)
- Low platelet count (less than 100,000 cells/mm³)

Nursing Management

Nursing management of the woman diagnosed with HELLP syndrome is the same as that for the woman with severe preeclampsia. Closely monitor the client for changes and provide ongoing support throughout this experience.

Gestational Diabetes

Gestational diabetes is a condition involving glucose intolerance that occurs during pregnancy. It is discussed in greater detail in Chapter 20.

Blood Incompatibility

Blood incompatibility most commonly involves blood type or the Rh factor. Blood type incompatibility, also known as ABO incompatibility, is not as severe a condition as Rh incompatibility. ABO incompatibility rarely causes significant hemolysis, and antepartum treatment is not warranted. Rh sensitization occurs in approximately 1 in 1,000 births to Rh-negative women (Salem, 2007).

According to the CDC (2007), Rh disease affected 16,000 newborns in the United States annually before RhoGAM administration was used to prevent it. Despite prevention measures, there still are approximately 4,000 infants annually affected with Rh disease.

Pathophysiology

Hemolysis associated with ABO incompatibility is limited to type O mothers with fetuses who have type A or B blood. In mothers with type A and B blood, naturally occurring antibodies are of IgM class, which do not cross the placenta, whereas in type O mothers, the antibodies are predominantly IgG in nature. Because A and B antigens are widely expressed in a variety of tissues besides red blood cells, only a small portion of antibodies crossing the placenta are available to bind to fetal red cells. In addition, fetal red cells appear to have less surface expression of A or B antigen, resulting in few reactive sites—hence the low incidence of significant hemolysis in affected neonates.

With ABO incompatibility, usually the mother is blood type O, with anti-A and anti-B antibodies in her serum; the infant is blood type A, B, or AB. The incompatibility arises as a result of the interaction of antibodies present in maternal serum and the antigen sites on the fetal red cells.

Rh incompatibility is a condition that develops when a woman with Rh-negative blood type is exposed to Rh-positive blood cells and subsequently develops circulating titers of Rh antibodies. Individuals with Rh-positive blood type have the D antigen present on their red cells, whereas individuals with an Rh-negative blood type do not. The presence or absence of the Rh antigen on the red blood cell membrane is genetically controlled.

In the United States, 15% of the population lack the Rh surface antigen on the erythrocyte and are considered Rh negative. The vast majority (85%) of individuals are considered Rh positive (Alan, 2007).

Rh incompatibility most commonly arises with exposure of an Rh-negative mother to Rh-positive fetal blood during pregnancy or birth, during which time erythrocytes from the fetal circulation leak into the maternal circulation. After a significant exposure, alloimmunization or sensitization occurs. As a result, maternal antibodies are produced against the foreign Rh antigen.

Theoretically, fetal and maternal blood does not mix during pregnancy. In reality, however, small placental accidents (transplacental bleeds secondary to minor separation), abortions, ectopic pregnancy, abdominal trauma, trophoblastic disease, amniocentesis, placenta previa, and abruptio placentae allow fetal blood to enter the maternal circulation and initiate the production of antibodies to destroy Rh-positive blood. The amount of fetal blood necessary to produce Rh incompatibility varies. In one study, less than 1 mL of Rh-positive blood was shown to result in sensitization of women who are Rh negative (Salem, 2007).

Once sensitized, it takes approximately a month for Rh antibodies in the maternal circulation to cross over into the fetal circulation. In 90% of cases, sensitization occurs during delivery (Blackburn, 2007). Thus, most firstborn infants with Rh-positive blood type are not affected because the short period from first exposure of Rh-positive fetal erythrocytes to the birth of the infant is insufficient to produce a significant maternal IgG antibody response.

The risk and severity of alloimmune response increase with each subsequent pregnancy involving a fetus with Rh-positive blood. A second pregnancy with an Rh-positive fetus often produces a mildly anemic infant, whereas succeeding pregnancies produce infants with more serious hemolytic anemia.

Nursing Assessment

At the first prenatal visit, determine the woman's blood type and Rh status. Also obtain a thorough health history, noting any reports of previous events involving hemorrhage to delineate the risk for prior sensitization. When the client's history reveals an Rh-negative mother who may be pregnant with an Rh-positive fetus, prepare the client for an antibody screen (indirect Coombs test) to determine whether she has developed isoimmunity to the Rh antigen. This test detects unexpected circulating antibodies in a woman's serum that could be harmful to the fetus (Gilbert, 2007).

Nursing Management

If the indirect Coombs test is negative (meaning no antibodies are present), then the woman is a candidate for RhoGAM. If the test is positive, RhoGAM is of no value because isoimmunization has occurred. In this case, the fetus is carefully monitored for hemolytic disease.

The incidence of isoimmunization has declined dramatically as a result of prenatal and postnatal RhoGAM administration after any event in which blood transfer may occur. The standard dose is 300 μg, which is effective for 30 mL of fetal blood. Rh immunoglobulin helps to destroy any fetal cells in the maternal circulation before sensitization occurs, thus inhibiting maternal antibody production. This provides temporary passive immunity, thereby preventing maternal sensitization.

The current recommendation is that every Rh-negative nonimmunized woman receives RhoGAM at 28 weeks' gestation and again within 72 hours after giving birth. Other indications for RhoGAM include:

• Ectopic pregnancy
• Chorionic villus sampling
• Amniocentesis
• Prenatal hemorrhage
• Molar pregnancy
• Maternal trauma
• Percutaneous umbilical sampling
• Therapeutic or spontaneous abortion
• Fetal death
• Fetal surgery (Blackburn, 2007)

Despite the availability of RhoGAM and laboratory tests to identify women and newborns at risk, isoimmunization remains a serious clinical reality that continues to contribute to perinatal and neonatal mortality. Nurses, as client advocates, are in a unique position to make sure test results are brought to the health care provider's attention so appropriate interventions can be initiated. In addition, nurses must stay abreast of current literature and research regarding isoimmunization and its management. Stress to all women that early prenatal care can help identify and prevent this condition. Since Rh incompatibility is preventable with the use of RhoGAM, prevention remains the best treatment. Nurses can make a tremendous impact to ensure positive outcomes for the greatest possible number of pregnancies through education.

Amniotic Fluid Imbalances

Amniotic fluid develops from several maternal and fetal structures, including the amnion, chorion, maternal blood, fetal lungs, GI tract, kidneys, and skin. Any alteration in one or more of the various sources will alter the amount of amniotic fluid. Polyhydramnios and oligohydramnios are two imbalances associated with amniotic fluid.

▶ POLYHYDRAMNIOS

Polyhydramnios, also called hydramnios, is a condition in which there is too much amniotic fluid (more than 2,000 mL) surrounding the fetus between 32 and 36 weeks. It occurs in approximately 3% of all pregnancies and is associated with fetal anomalies of development (Rajiah & Banerjee, 2007). It is associated with poor fetal outcomes because of the increased incidence of preterm births, fetal malpresentation, and cord prolapse.

There are several causes of polyhydramnios. Generally, too much fluid is being produced, there is a problem with the fluid being taken up, or both. It can be associated with maternal disease and fetal anomalies, but it can also be idiopathic in nature.

Therapeutic Management

Treatment may include close monitoring and frequent follow-up visits with the health care provider if the hydramnios is mild to moderate. In severe cases in which the woman is in pain and experiencing shortness of breath, an amniocentesis or artificial rupture of the membranes is done to reduce the fluid and the pressure. Removal of fluid by amniocentesis is only transiently effective. A noninvasive treatment may involve the use of a prostaglandin synthesis inhibitor (indomethacin) to decrease amniotic fluid volume by decreasing fetal urinary output, but this may cause premature closure of the fetal ductus arteriosus (Boyd & Carter, 2007).

Nursing Assessment

Begin the assessment with a thorough history, being alert to risk factors such as maternal diabetes or multiple gestation. Review the maternal history for information about possible fetal anomalies, including fetal esophageal or intestinal atresia, neural tube defects, chromosomal deviations, fetal hydrops, central nervous system or cardiovascular anomalies, and hydrocephaly.

Determine the gestational age of the fetus and measure the woman's fundal height. With hydramnios, there is a discrepancy between fundal height and gestational age, or a rapid growth of the uterus is noted. Assess the woman for complaints of discomfort in her abdomen, such as being severely stretched and tight. Also note any reports of uterine contractions, which may result from overstretching of the uterus. Assess for shortness of breath resulting from pressure on her diaphragm and inspect her lower extremities for edema, which results from increased pressure on the vena cava.

Palpate the abdomen and obtain fetal heart rate. Often the fetal parts and heart rate are difficult to obtain because of the excess fluid present.

Prepare the woman for possible diagnostic testing to evaluate for the presence of possible fetal anomalies. An ultrasound usually is done to measure the pockets of amniotic fluid to estimate the total volume. In some cases, ultrasound also is helpful in finding the etiology of polyhydramnios, such as multiple pregnancy or a fetal structural anomaly.

Nursing Management

Nursing management of the woman with polyhydramnios focuses on ongoing assessment and monitoring for symptoms of abdominal pain, dyspnea, uterine contractions, and edema of the lower extremities. Explain to the woman and her family that this condition can cause her uterus to become overdistended and may lead to preterm labor and preterm rupture of membranes. Outline the signs and symptoms of both conditions and instruct the woman to contact her health care provider if they do occur. If a therapeutic amniocentesis is performed, assist the health care provider and monitor maternal and fetal status throughout for any changes.

▶ OLIGOHYDRAMNIOS

Oligohydramnios is a decreased amount of amniotic fluid (less than 500 mL) between 32 weeks and 36 weeks' gestation. It occurs in 5% to 8% of all pregnancies. Oligohydramnios may result from any condition that prevents the fetus from making urine or blocks it from going into the amniotic sac.

This condition puts the fetus at an increased risk of perinatal morbidity and mortality (Blackburn, 2007). Reduction in amniotic fluid reduces the ability of the fetus to move freely without risk of cord compression, which increases the risk for fetal death and intrapartal hypoxia.

Therapeutic Management

The woman with oligohydramnios can be managed on an outpatient basis with serial ultrasounds and fetal surveillance through nonstress testing and biophysical profiles. As long as fetal well-being is demonstrated with frequent testing, no intervention is necessary. If fetal well-being is compromised, however, birth is planned along with amnioinfusion (the transvaginal infusion of crystalloid fluid to compensate for the lost amniotic fluid). The fluid is introduced into the uterus through an intrauterine pressure catheter. The infusion is administered in a controlled fashion to prevent overdistention of the uterus. Amnioinfusion is thought to improve abnormal fetal heart rate patterns, decrease cesarean births, and possibly minimize the risk of neonatal meconium aspiration syndrome (Norwitz & Schorge, 2006).

Nursing Assessment

Review the maternal history for factors associated with oligohydramnios, including:

- Uteroplacental insufficiency
- Premature rupture of membranes prior to labor onset
- Hypertension of pregnancy
- Maternal diabetes
- Intrauterine growth restriction
- Postterm pregnancy
- Fetal renal agenesis
- Polycystic kidneys
- Urinary tract obstructions

Assess the client for complaints of fluid leaking from the vagina. Leaking of amniotic fluid from the vagina occurs with rupture of the amniotic sac. Leaking in conjunction with a uterus that is small for expected dates of gestation also suggests oligohydramnios. Unfortunately, the woman may not present with any symptoms. Typically, the reduced volume of amniotic fluid is identified on ultrasound.

Nursing Management

Nursing management of the woman with oligohydramnios involves continuous monitoring of fetal well-being during nonstress testing or during labor and birth by identifying nonreassuring patterns on the fetal monitor. Variable decelerations indicating cord compression are common. Changing the woman's position might be therapeutic in altering this fetal heart rate pattern. After the birth, evaluate the newborn for signs of postmaturity, congenital anomalies, and respiratory difficulty.

Assist with amnioinfusion as indicated and continue to assess the woman's vital signs, contraction status, and fetal heart rate throughout the procedure. Provide comfort measures such as changing the bed linens and the woman's bed clothes frequently because of the constant leakage of fluid from the vagina. Also provide frequent perineal care during the infusion.

Multiple Gestation

Multiple gestation is defined as more than one fetus being born to a pregnant woman. This includes twins, triplets, and higher-order multiples such as quadruplets on up. In the past two decades, the number of multiple gestations in the United States has jumped dramatically because of the widespread use of fertility drugs, older women having babies, and assisted reproductive technologies to treat infertility. About one third of live births from assisted reproductive technology result in more than one infant, and twins represent 85% of those multiple-birth children (Grainger, Frazier, & Rowland, 2006). In the United States, the overall prevalence of twins is approximately 12 per 1,000, and two thirds are dizygotic (Zach & Pramanik, 2007). The increasing number of multiple gestations is a concern because women who are expecting more than one infant are at high risk for preterm labor, hydramnios, hyperemesis gravidarum, anemia, preeclampsia, and antepartum hemorrhage. Fetal/newborn risks or complications include prematurity, respiratory distress syndrome, birth asphyxia/perinatal depression, congenital anomalies (central nervous system, cardiovascular, and GI defects), twin-to-twin transfusion syndrome (transfusion of blood from one twin [i.e., donor] to the other twin [i.e., recipient]), intrauterine growth restriction, and becoming conjoined twins (Zach & Pramanik, 2007).

The two types of twins are monozygotic and dizygotic (Fig. 19.6). Monozygotic twins develop when a single, fertilized ovum splits during the first 2 weeks after conception. Monozygotic twins also are called identical twins. Two sperm fertilizing two ova produce dizygotic twins, which are called fraternal twins. Separate amnions, chorions, and placentas are formed in dizygotic twins. Triplets can be monozygotic, dizygotic, or trizygotic.

Therapeutic Management

When a multiple gestation is confirmed, the woman is followed with serial ultrasounds to assess fetal growth patterns and development. Biophysical profiles along with nonstress tests are ordered to determine fetal well-being. Many women are hospitalized in late pregnancy to prevent preterm labor and receive closer surveillance. During the intrapartum period the woman is closely monitored, with a perinatal team available to assist after birth. Operative delivery is frequently needed due to fetal malpresentation.

Nursing Assessment

Obtain a health history and physical examination. Be alert for complaints of fatigue and severe nausea and vomiting. Assess the woman's abdomen and fundal height. Typically with a multiple gestation the uterus is larger than expected based on the estimated date of birth. Laboratory test results may reveal anemia. Prepare the woman for ultrasound, which typically confirms the diagnosis of a multiple gestation.

Nursing Management

During the prenatal period, care focuses on providing education and support for the woman in areas of nutrition, increased rest periods, and close observation for pregnancy complications—anemia, excessive weight gain, proteinuria, edema, vaginal bleeding, and hypertension. Instruct the woman to be alert for and report immediately any signs and symptoms of preterm labor—contractions, uterine cramping, low back ache, increase in vaginal discharge, loss of mucus plug, pelvic pain, and pressure.

With the onset of labor, expect to monitor fetal heart rates continuously. Prepare the woman for an ultrasound to assess the presentation of each fetus to determine the best delivery approach. Ensure that extra nursing staff and the perinatal team are available for any birth or newborn complications.

After the babies are born, closely assess the woman for hemorrhage by frequently assessing uterine involution. Palpate the uterine fundus and monitor the amount and characteristics of lochia.

Throughout the entire pregnancy, birth, and hospital stay, inform and support the woman and her family. Encourage them to ask questions and verbalize any fears and concerns.

Premature Rupture of Membranes

Premature rupture of membranes (PROM) is the rupture of the bag of waters before the onset of true labor. There are a number of associated conditions and complications, such as infection, prolapsed cord, abruptio placentae, and preterm labor. This is the single most common diagnosis associated with preterm births (Gilbert, 2007).

PROM occurs in approximately 12% of all births (ACOG, 2007b). If prolonged (greater than 24 hours), the woman's risk for infection (chorioamnionitis, endometritis, sepsis, and neonatal infections) increases and

FIGURE 19.6 Multiple gestation with twins. (**A**) Dizygotic twins, where each fetus has its own placenta, amnion, and chorion. (**B**) Monozygotic twins, where the fetuses share one placenta, two amnions, and one chorion.

this risk continues to increase as the duration of rupture time increases. The time interval from rupture of membranes to the onset of regular contractions is termed the latent period.

The terminology pertaining to PROM can be confusing. PROM is rupture of the membranes prior to the onset of labor and is used appropriately when referring to a woman who is beyond 37 weeks' gestation, has presented with spontaneous rupture of the membranes, and is not in labor. Related terms include **preterm premature rupture of membranes (PPROM)**, which is defined as rupture of membranes prior to the onset of labor in a woman who is *less* than 37 weeks of gestation. Perinatal risks associated with PPROM may stem from immaturity, including respiratory distress syndrome, intraventricular hemorrhage, patent ductus arteriosus, and necrotizing enterocolitis.

The exact cause of PROM is not known. In many cases, PROM occurs spontaneously.

Therapeutic Management

Treatment of PROM typically depends on the gestational age. Under no circumstances is an unsterile digital cervical examination done until the woman enters active labor, to minimize infection exposure. If the fetal lungs are mature, induction of labor is initiated. PROM is not a lone indicator for surgical birth. If the fetal lungs are immature, expectant management is carried out with adequate hydration, reduced physical activity, pelvic rest, and close observation for possible infection, such as with frequent monitoring of vital signs and laboratory test results (e.g., the white blood cell count). Corticosteroids may be given to enhance fetal lung maturity if lungs are immature, although this remains controversial. Recent studies have shown clear benefits of antibiotics to decrease neonatal morbidity associated with PPROM (ACOG, 2007b).

Nursing Assessment

Nursing assessment focuses on obtaining a complete health history and performing a physical examination to determine maternal and fetal status. An accurate assessment of the gestational age and knowledge of the maternal, fetal, and neonatal risks are essential to appropriate evaluation, counseling, and management of women with PROM and PPROM.

Health History and Physical Examination

Review the maternal history for risk factors such as infection, increased uterine size (hydramnios, macrosomia, multifetal gestation), uterine and fetal anomalies, lower socioeconomic status, STIs, cervical insufficiency, vaginal bleeding, and cigarette smoking during pregnancy. Ask about any history or current symptoms of UTI (frequency, urgency, dysuria, or flank pain) or pelvic or vaginal infection (pain or vaginal discharge).

Assess for signs and symptoms of labor, such as cramping, pelvic pressure, or back pain. Also assess her vital signs, noting any signs indicative of infection such as fever and elevated white blood cell count (more than 18,000 cells/mm^3) (Jazayeri & Galan, 2007).

Institute continuous electronic fetal heart rate monitoring to evaluate fetal well-being. Conduct a vaginal examination to ascertain the cervical status in PROM. If PPROM exists, a sterile speculum examination (where the examiner inspects the cervix but does not palpate it) is done rather than a digital cervical examination because it may diminish latency (period of time from rupture of membranes to birth) and increase newborn morbidity (Cunningham et al., 2005).

Observe the characteristics of the amniotic fluid. Note any evidence of meconium, or a foul odor. When meconium is present in the amniotic fluid, it typically indicates fetal distress related to hypoxia. Meconium stains the fluid yellow to greenish brown, depending on the amount present. A foul odor of amniotic fluid indicates infection. Also observe the amount of fluid. A decreased amount of amniotic fluid reduces the cushioning effect, thereby making cord compression a possibility. Key assessments are summarized in Box 19.3.

Laboratory and Diagnostic Testing

To diagnose PROM or PPROM, several procedures may be used: the Nitrazine test, fern test, or ultrasound. After the insertion of a sterile speculum, a sample of the fluid

---

BOX 19.3 **Key Assessments With Premature Rupture of Membranes**

For the woman with PROM, the following assessments are essential:

- Determining the date, time, and duration of membrane rupture by client interview
- Ascertaining gestational age of the fetus based on date of mother's LMP, fundal height, and ultrasound dating
- Questioning the woman about possible history of or recent UTI or vaginal infection that might have contributed to PROM
- Assessing for any associated labor symptoms, such as back pain or pelvic pressure
- Assisting with or performing diagnostic tests to validate leakage of fluid, such as Nitrazine test, "ferning" on slide, and ultrasound
- Continually assessing for signs of infection including
  - Elevation of maternal temperature and pulse rate
  - Abdominal/uterine tenderness
  - Fetal tachycardia more than 160 bpm
  - Elevated white blood cell count and C-reactive protein
  - Cloudy, foul-smelling amniotic fluid

in the vaginal area is obtained. With a Nitrazine test, pH of the fluid is tested; amniotic fluid is more basic (7.0) than normal vaginal secretions (4.5). Nitrazine paper turns blue in the presence of amniotic fluid. However, false-positive results can occur if blood, urine, semen, or antiseptic chemicals are also present; all will increase the pH.

For the fern test, a sample of vaginal fluid is place on a slide to be viewed directly under a microscope. Amniotic fluid will develop a fern-like pattern when it dries because of sodium chloride crystallization. If both of these tests are inconclusive, a transvaginal ultrasound can also be used to determine whether membranes have ruptured by demonstrating a decreased amount of amniotic fluid (oligohydramnios) in the uterus (Jazayeri & Galan, 2007).

Other laboratory and diagnostic tests that may be used include:

- Urinalysis and urine culture for UTI or asymptomatic bacteriuria
- Cervical test or culture for chlamydia or gonorrhea
- Vaginal culture for bacterial vaginosis and trichomoniasis
- Vaginal introital/rectal culture for group B streptococcus

Nursing Management

Nursing management for the woman with PROM or PPROM focuses on preventing infection and identifying uterine contractions. The risk for infection is great because of the break in the amniotic fluid membrane and its close proximity to vaginal bacteria. Therefore, monitor maternal vital signs closely. Be alert for a temperature elevation or an increase in pulse, which could indicate infection. Also monitor the fetal heart rate continuously, reporting any fetal tachycardia (which could indicate a maternal infection) or variable decelerations (suggesting cord compression). If variable decelerations are present, anticipate amnioinfusion based on agency policy. Evaluate the results of laboratory tests such as a CBC. An elevation in white blood cells would suggest infection. Administer antibiotics if ordered.

Encourage the woman and her partner to verbalize their feelings and concerns. Educate them about the purpose of the protective membranes and the implications of early rupture. Keep them informed about planned interventions, including potential complications and required therapy. As appropriate, prepare the woman for induction or augmentation of labor as appropriate if she is near term.

If labor doesn't start within 48 hours, the woman with PPROM may be discharged home on expectant management, which may include:

- Antibiotics if cervicovaginal cultures are positive
- Activity restrictions
- Education about signs and symptoms of infection and when to call with problems or concerns (Teaching Guidelines 19.3)

TEACHING GUIDELINES 19.3

Teaching for the Woman With PPROM

- Monitor your baby's activity by performing fetal kick counts daily.
- Check your temperature daily and report any temperature increases to your health care provider.
- Watch for signs related to the beginning of labor. Report any tightening of the abdomen or contractions.
- Avoid any touching or manipulating of your breasts, which could stimulate labor.
- Do not insert anything into your vagina or vaginal area.
- Maintain any specific activity restrictions as recommended.
- Wash your hands thoroughly after using the bathroom and make sure to wipe from front to back each time.
- Keep your perineal area clean and dry.
- Take your antibiotics as directed if your health care provider has prescribed them.
- Call your health care provider with changes in your condition, including fever, uterine tenderness, feeling like your heart is racing, and foul-smelling vaginal discharge.

- Frequent fetal testing for well-being
- Ultrasound every 3 to 4 weeks to assess amniotic fluid levels
- Possible corticosteroid treatment depending on gestational age
- Daily kick counts to assess fetal well-being

■■■ Key Concepts

- Identifying risk factors early on and ongoing throughout the pregnancy is important to ensure the best outcome for every pregnancy. Risk assessment should start with the first prenatal visit and continue with subsequent visits.
- The three most common causes of hemorrhage early in pregnancy (first half of pregnancy) are spontaneous abortion, ectopic pregnancy, and GTD.
- Ectopic pregnancies occur in about 1 in 50 pregnancies and have increased dramatically during the past few decades.
- Having a molar pregnancy results in the loss of the pregnancy and the possibility of developing choriocarcinoma, a chronic malignancy from the trophoblastic tissue.
- The classic clinical picture presentation for placenta previa is painless, bright-red vaginal bleeding occurring during the third trimester.

- Treatment of abruptio placentae is designed to assess, control, and restore the amount of blood lost; to provide a positive outcome for both mother and infant; and to prevent coagulation disorders.

- DIC can be described in simplest terms as a loss of balance between the clot-forming activity of thrombin and the clot-lysing activity of plasmin.

- Hyperemesis gravidarum is a complication of pregnancy characterized by persistent, uncontrollable nausea and vomiting before the 20th week of gestation.

- Gestational hypertension is the leading cause of maternal death in the United States and the most common complication reported during pregnancy.

- HELLP is an acronym for hemolysis, elevated liver enzymes, and low platelets.

- Rh incompatibility is a condition that develops when a woman of Rh-negative blood type is exposed to Rh-positive fetal blood cells and subsequently develops circulating titers of Rh antibodies.

- Hydramnios occurs in approximately 3 to 4% of all pregnancies and is associated with fetal anomalies of development.

- Nursing care related to the woman with oligohydramnios involves continuous monitoring of fetal well-being during nonstress testing or during labor and birth by identifying nonreassuring patterns on the fetal monitor.

- The increasing number of multiple gestations is a concern because women who are expecting more than one infant are at high risk for preterm labor, hydramnios, hyperemesis gravidarum, anemia, preeclampsia, and antepartum hemorrhage.

- Nursing care related to PROM centers on infection prevention and identification of preterm labor contractions.

- Early identification of preterm labor would allow for appropriate interventions that may prolong the pregnancy, such as transferring the woman to a facility with a neonatal intensive care unit for prenatal care, administering glucocorticoids to the mother to promote fetal lung maturity, and giving appropriate antibiotics to treat infections to arrest the labor process.

- It is essential that nurses teach all pregnant women how to detect the early symptoms of preterm labor and what to do if they experience contractions or cramping that does not go away.

REFERENCES

Alan, R. (2007). *Rh incompatibility and isoimmunization.* March of Dimes. Available at: http://healthlibrary.epnet.com/GetContent.aspx?token=8482e079-8512-47c2-960c-a403c77a5e4c&chunkiid=11595.

American Academy of Pediatrics, American College of Obstetricians and Gynecologists. (2003). *Guidelines for perinatal care* (5th ed.). Washington, DC: Author.

American College of Obstetricians and Gynecologists (ACOG). (2003). ACOG practice bulletin: Cervical insufficiency. *Obstetrics and Gynecology, 102,* 1091–1099.

American College of Obstetricians and Gynecologists (ACOG). (2007a). *ACOG practice bulletin: Diagnosis and management of preeclampsia and eclampsia updated.* Number 33. Washington, DC: Author.

American College of Obstetricians and Gynecologists (ACOG). (2007b). ACOG Practice Bulletin No. 80: Premature rupture of membranes. *Obstetrics and Gynecology, 109*(4), 1007–1020.

Arenson, J., & Drake, P. (2007). *Maternal and newborn health.* Sudbury, MA: Jones and Bartlett Publishers.

Bakken, I. J., Skjeldestad, F. E., & Nordbo, S. A. (2007). *Chlamydia trachomatis* infections increase the risk for ectopic pregnancy: A population-based, nested case-control study. *Sexually Transmitted Diseases, 34*(3), 166–169.

Basama, F. M., & Granger, K. (2007). Case report: Postpartum class 1 HELLP syndrome. *Archives of Gynecology & Obstetrics, 275*(3), 187–189.

Bernasko, J., Lee, R., Pagano, M., & Kohn, N. (2006). Is routine prophylactic cervical cerclage associated with significant prolongation of triplet gestation? *Journal of Maternal-Fetal & Neonatal Medicine, 19*(9), 575–578.

Bick, R. L. (2007). Disseminated intravascular coagulation. In R. E. Rakel & E. T. Bope (Eds.), *Conn's current therapy 2007* (Section 6, pp. 502–505). Philadelphia: Saunders Elsevier.

Blackburn, S. (2007). *Maternal, fetal, and neonatal physiology: A clinical perspective* (3rd ed.). St. Louis: W. B. Saunders.

Blincoe, A. J. (2007). Hypertension in pregnancy: The importance of monitoring. *British Journal of Midwifery, 15*(1), 47–50.

Boyd, R. L., & Carter, B. S. (2007). Polyhydramnios and oligohydramnios. *eMedicine.* Available at: http://www.emedicine.com/ped/topic1854.htm.

Britt, D. W., Eden, R. D., & Evans, M. I. (2006). Matching risk and resources in high-risk pregnancies. *Journal of Maternal-Fetal and Neonatal Medicine, 19*(10), 645–650.

Brown-Guttovz, H. (2006). Myths and facts about ectopic pregnancy. *Nursing, 36*(8), 70.

Centers for Disease Control and Prevention (CDC). (2007). *Rh disease fact sheet.* Available at: http://www.marchofdimes.com/professionals/14332_1220.asp

Collins, N. J. (2007). Abruptio placentae. *Wild Iris Medical Education.* Available at: http://www.nursingceu.com/courses/81/index_nceu.html.

Condous, G. (2006). Ectopic pregnancy: Risk factors and diagnosis. *Australian Family Physician, 35*(11), 854–857.

Cunningham, F. G., Gant, N. F., Leveno, K. J., Gilstrap, L. C., Hauth, J. C., & Wenstrom, K. D. (2005). *Williams' obstetrics* (22nd ed.). New York: McGraw-Hill.

Deering, S. H., & Satin, A. (2007). Abruptio placentae. *eMedicine.* Available at www.emedicine.com/med/topic6.htm.

Evans, A. T. (2007). *Manual of Obstetrics* (7th ed.). Philadelphia: Lippincott Williams & Wilkins.

Fox, N. S., & Chervenak, F. A. (2008). Cervical cerclage: A review of the evidence. *Obstetrical & Gynecological Survey, 63*(1), 58–65.

Furlong, M. A., & Furlong, B. R. (2007). Disseminated intravascular coagulation. *eMedicine.* Available at: http://www.emedicine.com/emerg/topic150.htm.

Garner, E. I., Goldstein, D. P., Feltmate, C. M., & Berkowitz, R. S. (2007). Gestational trophoblastic disease. *Clinical Obstetrics & Gynecology, 50*(1), 112–122.

Gaufberg, S. V. (2007). Abruptio placentae. *eMedicine.* Available at www.emedicine.com/emerg/topic12.htm.

Gibson, P., & Carson, M. (2007). Hypertension and pregnancy. *eMedicine.* Available at: http://www.emedicine.com/med/topic3250.htm.

Gilbert, E. (2007). *Manual of high-risk pregnancy and delivery* (4th ed.). St. Louis: Mosby, Inc.

Grainger, D. A., Frazier, L. M., & Rowland, C. A. (2006). Preconception care and treatment with assisted reproductive technologies. *Maternal & Child Health Journal, 10*(5), Supplement: S161–164.

Hajenius, P. J., Mol, F., Mol, B. W. J., Bossuyt, P. M. M., Ankum, W. M., & van der Veen, F. (2007). Interventions for tubal ectopic pregnancy. *Cochrane Database of Systematic Reviews* 2007. Issue 1. Art. No.: CD000324.DOI: 10.1002/14651858.CD000324.pub2.

Hernandez, E. (2007). Gestational trophoblastic neoplasia. *eMedicine.* Available at: http://www.emedicine.com/med/topic866.htm.

Hodgson, B. B., & Kizior, R. J. (2007). *Saunders nursing drug handbook.* Philadelphia: Elsevier Health Sciences.

Jazayeri, A., & Galan, H. (2007). Premature rupture of membranes. *eMedicine*. Available at: http://www.emedicine.com/med/topic3256.htm.

Joy, S., & Lyon, D. (2007). Placenta previa. *eMedicine*. Available at: www.emedicine.com/med/topics3271/htm.

Jung, D. C., & Erogul, M. (2007). Pregnancy, preeclampsia. *eMedicine*. Available at: http://www.emedicine.com/emerg/topic480.htm.

Ko, P., & Yoon, Y. (2007). Placenta previa. *eMedicine*. Available at: www.emedicine.com/emerg/topic427.htm.

Lamondy, A. M. (2007). Managing hyperemesis gravidarum. *Nursing, 37*(2), 66–68.

Lane, C. A. (2007). Nausea and vomiting of pregnancy: A tailored approach treatment. *Clinical Obstetrics & Gynecology, 50*(1), 100–111.

Lilley, L. L., Harrington, S., & Snyder, J. S. (2007). *Pharmacology and the nursing process* (5th ed.). Philadelphia: Elsevier Health Sciences.

Lipscomb, G. H. (2007). Ectopic pregnancy. In R. E. Rakel & E. T. Bope (Eds.), *Conn's current therapy 2007* (Section 16, pp. 1175–1178). Philadelphia: Saunders Elsevier.

Lotgering, F. K. (2007). Clinical aspects of cervical insufficiency. *BMC Pregnancy and Childbirth, 7*(1), 17–20.

March of Dimes (2007). *Ectopic pregnancy.* Available at: http://www.marchofdimes.com/pnhec/188_851.asp.

Moore, L. E., & Ware, L. E. (2007). Hydatidiform mole. *eMedicine*. Available at: http://www.emedicine.com/med/topic1047.htm.

Mundy, D. C. (2006). *Diagnosis and management of preeclampsia/eclampsia.* Available at: www.acog.org/acog_sections/download/MOPreeclampsia20061016.ppt- 2007-03-14.

National High Blood Pressure Education Program. (2000). Working Group in High Blood Pressure in Pregnancy report. *American Journal of Obstetrics and Gynecology, 183*, S1–S22.

Norwitz, E. R., & Schorge, J. O. (2006). *Obstetrics and gynecology at a glance* (2nd ed.). Malden, MA: Blackwell Publishing Ltd.

O'Brien, J. M. (2006). Management of cervical insufficiency and bulging fetal membranes. *Obstetrics & Gynecology, 107*(6), 1421–1422.

Ogunyemi, D. A. (2007). Hyperemesis gravidarum. *eMedicine*. Available at: http://www.emedicine.com/med/topic1075.htm.

Oppenheimer, L. (2007). Diagnosis and management of placenta previa. *Journal of Obstetrics & Gynecology Canada, 29*(3), 261–266.

Oyelese, Y., & Ananth, C. V. (2006). Placental abruption. *Obstetrics and Gynecology, 108*(4), 1005–1016.

Podymow, T., & August, P. (2007). Hypertension in pregnancy. *Advances in Chronic Kidney Disease, 14*(2), 178–190.

Price, S., Lake, M., Breen, G., Carson, G., Quinn, C., & O'Connor, T. (2007). The spiritual experience of high risk pregnancy. *JOGNN, 36*(1), 63–70.

Puscheck, E., & Pradhan, A. (2007). First-trimester pregnancy loss. *eMedicine*. Available at: http://www.emedicine.com/med/topic3310.htm.

Rajiah, P., & Banerjee, B. (2007). Polyhydramnios. *eMedicine*. Available at: http://www.emedicine.com/radio/topic566.htm.

Ressel, G. W. (2004). Practice guidelines: ACOG releases bulletin on managing cervical insufficiency. *American Family Physician*. Available at www.aafp.org/afp/20040115/practice.html.

Salem, L. (2007). Rh incompatibility. *eMedicine*. Available at www.emedicine.com/emerg/topic507.htm.

Selway, J. (2006). The challenge of ectopic pregnancy. *Journal for Nurse Practitioners, 2*(9), 583–592.

Sepilian, V., & Wood, E. (2007). Ectopic pregnancy. *eMedicine*. Available at www.emedicine.com/med/topic3212.htm.

Silver, R. M. (2007). Fetal death. *Obstetrics & Gynecology, 109*(1), 153–167.

Simpson, J. L. (2007). Causes of fetal wastage. *Clinical Obstetrics & Gynecology, 50*(1), 10–30.

U.S. Department of Health and Human Services. (2000). *Healthy people 2010* (conference edition, in two volumes). Washington, DC: Author.

Vidaeff, A. C., & Ramin, S. M. (2007). From concept to practice: The recent history of preterm delivery prevention: cervical competence. *American Journal of Perinatology, 23*(1), 3–13.

Vitthala, S., Cheema, M. K., & Misra, P. K. (2007). Medical management of ectopic pregnancy using methotrexate. *Internet Journal of Gynecology & Obstetrics, 6*(2), 4–10.

Vyas, N. A., Vink, J. S., Ghidini, A., Pezzullo, J. C., Korker, V., Landy, H. J., & Poggi, S. H. (2006). Risk factors for cervical insufficiency after term delivery. *American Journal of Obstetrics & Gynecology, 195*(3), 787–791.

Warden, M., & Euerle, B. (2007). Preeclampsia. *eMedicine*. Available at: http://www.emedicine.com/med/topic1905.htm.

Weber, J. R. (2007). *Nurses' handbook of health assessment* (6th ed.). Philadelphia: Lippincott Williams & Wilkins.

Weismiller, D. G. (2007). Hypertension disorders of pregnancy. In R. E. Rakel & E. T. Bope (Eds.), *Conn's current therapy 2007* (Section 16, pp. 1180–1189). Philadelphia: Saunders Elsevier.

White, A. (2006). Emergency care for patients with HELLP syndrome. *Advanced Emergency Nursing Journal, 28*(4), 338–345.

Wilcox, S. R., & Edelman, A. (2007). Pregnancy, hyperemesis gravidarum. *eMedicine*. Available at www.emedicine.com/emerg/topic479.htm.

Zach, T., & Pramanik, A. (2007). Multiple births. *eMedicine*. Available at www.emedicine.com/ped/topic2599.htm.

Zeltzer, J. S. (2007). Vaginal bleeding in late pregnancy. In R. E. Rakel & E. T. Bope (Eds.), *Conn's current therapy 2007* (Section 16, pp. 1178–1180). Philadelphia: Saunders Elsevier.

WEBSITES

American Academy of Pediatrics: www.aap.org

American College of Obstetricians and Gynecologists: www.acog.org

Association of Women's Health, Obstetric & Neonatal Nurses: www.awhonn.org

March of Dimes: www.modimes.org

Resolve through Sharing: www.ectopicpregnancy.com

Sidelines High-Risk Pregnancy Support Office: www.sidelines.org

CHAPTER WORKSHEET

MULTIPLE CHOICE QUESTIONS

1. A woman diagnosed with preeclampsia is to receive magnesium sulfate. The rationale for this drug is to:

   a. Reduce CNS irritability to prevent seizures

   b. Provide supplementation of an important mineral she needs

   c. Prevent constipation during and after the birthing process

   d. Decrease musculoskeletal tone to augment labor

2. A woman is suspected of having abruptio placentae. Which of the following would the nurse expect to assess as a classic symptom?

   a. Painless, bright-red bleeding

   b. "Knife-like" abdominal pain

   c. Excessive nausea and vomiting

   d. Hypertension and headache

3. RhoGAM is given to Rh-negative women to prevent maternal sensitization. In addition to pregnancy, Rh-negative women would also receive this medication after which of the following?

   a. Therapeutic or spontaneous abortion

   b. Head injury from a car accident

   c. Blood transfusion after a hemorrhage

   d. Unsuccessful artificial insemination procedure

4. After teaching a woman about hyperemesis gravidarum and how it differs from the typical nausea and vomiting of pregnancy, which statement by the woman indicates that the teaching was successful?

   a. "I can expect the nausea to last through my second trimester."

   b. "I should drink fluids with my meals instead of in between them."

   c. "I need to avoid strong odors, perfumes, or flavors."

   d. "I should lie down after I eat for about 2 hours."

5. A pregnant woman, approximately 12 weeks' gestation, comes to the emergency department after calling her health care provider's office and reporting moderate vaginal bleeding. Assessment reveals cervical dilation and moderately strong abdominal cramps. She reports that she has passed some tissue with the bleeding. The nurse interprets these findings to suggest which of the following?

   a. Threatened abortion

   b. Inevitable abortion

   c. Incomplete abortion

   d. Missed abortion

CRITICAL THINKING EXERCISES

1. Suzanne, a 16-year-old primigravida, presents to the maternity clinic complaining of continual nausea and vomiting for the past 3 days. She states she is approximately 15 weeks pregnant and has been unable to hold anything down or take any fluids in without throwing up for the past 3 days. She reports she is dizzy and weak. On examination, Suzanne appears pale and anxious. Her mucous membranes are dry, skin turgor is poor, and her lips are dry and cracked.

   a. What is your impression of this condition?

   b. What risk factors does Suzanne have?

   c. What intervention is appropriate for this woman?

2. Gloria is an obese 39-year-old primigravida of African-American descent who is diagnosed with gestational hypertension. Her history reveals that her sister developed preeclampsia during her pregnancy. When describing her diet to the nurse, Gloria mentions that she tends to eat a lot of fast food.

   a. What risk factors does Gloria have that increase her risk for gestational hypertension?

   b. When assessing Gloria, what assessment findings would lead the nurse to suspect that Gloria has developed severe preeclampsia?

STUDY ACTIVITIES

1. Ask a community health maternity nurse how the signs and symptoms of gestational hypertension (including preeclampsia and eclampsia) are taught, and how effective efforts have been to reduce the incidence in the area.

2. Find a website designed to help parents who have suffered a pregnancy loss secondary to a spontaneous abortion. What is its audience level? Is the information up to date?

3. A pregnancy in which the blastocyst implants outside the uterus is an _____ pregnancy.

4. The most serious complication of hydatidiform mole is the development of _____ afterward.

5. Discuss various activities a woman with a multiple gestation could engage in to help pass the time when ordered to be on bed rest at home for 2 months.

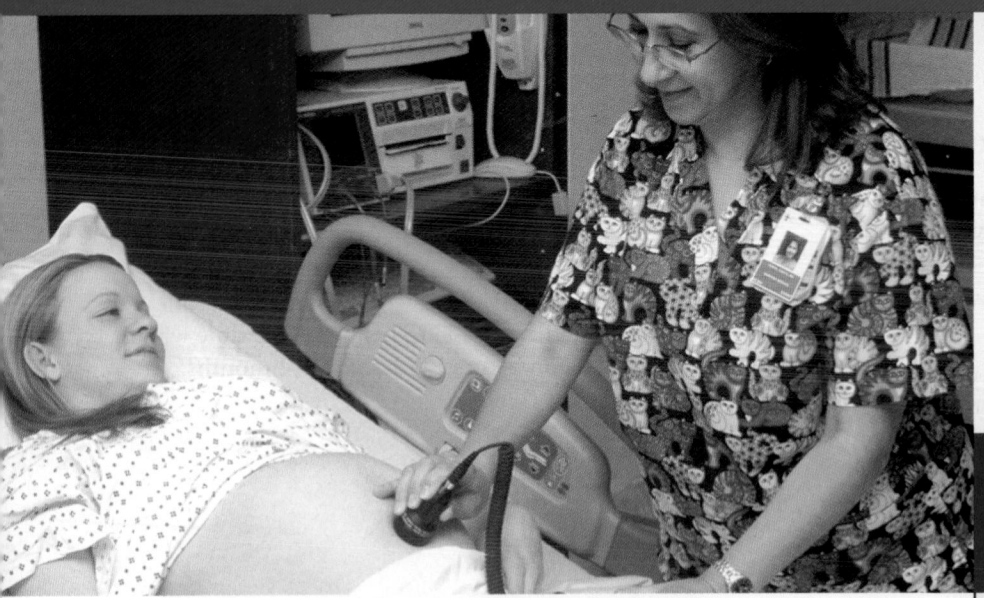

NURSING MANAGEMENT OF THE PREGNANCY AT RISK: SELECTED HEALTH CONDITIONS AND VULNERABLE POPULATIONS

KEY TERMS

acquired immunodeficiency syndrome (AIDS)
adolescence
anemia
fetal alcohol spectrum disorder (FASD)
gestational diabetes mellitus

glycosylated hemoglobin (HbA1C) level
human immunodeficiency virus (HIV)
impaired fasting glucose
impaired glucose tolerance
neonatal abstinence syndrome

perinatal drug abuse
pica
pregestational diabetes
teratogen
type 1 diabetes
type 2 diabetes

LEARNING OBJECTIVES

Upon completion of the chapter, the learner will be able to:

1. Identify at least two conditions present before pregnancy that can have a negative effect on a pregnancy.
2. Explain how a condition present before pregnancy can affect the woman physiologically and psychologically when she becomes pregnant.
3. Differentiate the nursing assessment and management for a pregnant woman with diabetes from that of a pregnant woman without diabetes.
4. Explore how congenital and acquired heart conditions can affect a woman's pregnancy.
5. Describe the nursing assessment and management of a pregnant woman with cardiovascular disorders and respiratory conditions.
6. Differentiate among the types of anemia affecting pregnant women in terms of prevention and management.
7. Describe the most common infections that can jeopardize a pregnancy, and propose possible preventive strategies.
8. Explain the nurse's role in the prevention and management of adolescent pregnancy.

Rose, a thin 16-year-old appearing very pregnant, came into the clinic wheezing and having difficulty catching her breath. She had missed several previous prenatal visits but arrived at the clinic today in distress. Rose has a history of asthma since she was 5 years old. How might Rose's current condition affect her pregnancy? Is this picture typical of the pregnant asthmatic?

Wow

As the sun sets each day, nurses should make sure they have done something for others, and should try to be understanding even under the most difficult of conditions.

LEARNING OBJECTIVES (continued)

9. Identify the impact of pregnancy on a woman over the age of 35.
10. Develop a plan of care for the pregnant woman who is HIV positive.
11. Examine the effects of substance abuse during pregnancy.

Pregnancy and childbirth are exciting yet complex facets within the continuum of women's health. Ideally the pregnant woman is free of any conditions that can affect a pregnancy, but in reality many women enter pregnancy with a multitude of health-related or psychosocial issues that can have a negative impact on the outcome.

Many pregnant women express the wish, "I hope my baby is born healthy." Nurses can play a major role in helping this become a reality by educating women before they become pregnant. Conditions such as diabetes, cardiac and respiratory disorders, anemias, and specific infections frequently can be controlled through close prenatal management so that their impact on pregnancy is minimized. Nurses can provide pregnancy-prevention strategies when counseling teenagers. Meeting the developmental needs of pregnant adolescents is a challenge. Finally, lifestyle choices can place many women at risk during pregnancy, and nurses need to remain nonjudgmental in working with these special populations. Lifestyle choices such as use of alcohol, nicotine, and illicit substances during pregnancy are addressed in a National Health goal.

Chapter 19 described pregnancy-related conditions that place the woman at risk. This chapter addresses common conditions that can have a negative impact on the pregnancy and special populations at risk, outlining appropriate nursing assessment and management for each condition or situation. The unique skills of nurses, in conjunction with the other members of the health care team, can increase the potential for a positive outcome in many high-risk pregnancies.

Diabetes Mellitus

Diabetes mellitus is a chronic disease characterized by a relative lack of insulin or absence of the hormone, which is necessary for glucose metabolism. The chronic hyperglycemia of diabetes is associated with long-term damage, dysfunction, and failure of the eyes, kidneys, nerves, heart, and blood vessels. The prevalence of diabetes in the United States is increasing at an alarming rate, already reaching epidemic proportions. A contributing factor to these increasing rates is the incidence of obesity. Diabetes is a common endocrine disorder, affecting up to 14% of all pregnancies (American Diabetes Association [ADA], 2007a).

Diabetes commonly is classified based on disease etiology (ADA, 2007a). These groups include:

- **Type 1 diabetes**: absolute insulin deficiency (due to an autoimmune process); usually appears before the age of 30 years; approximately 10% of those diagnosed have type 1 diabetes
- **Type 2 diabetes**: insulin resistance or deficiency (related to obesity, sedentary lifestyle); diagnosed primarily in adults older than 30 years of age but is now being seen in children; accounts for 90% of all diagnosed cases.
- **Impaired fasting glucose** and **impaired glucose tolerance**: characterized by hyperglycemia at a level lower than what qualifies as a diagnosis of diabetes (fasting blood glucose level between 100 and 125 mg/dL; blood glucose level between 140 and 199 mg/dL after a 2-hour glucose tolerance test, respectively); symptoms of diabetes are absent; newborns are at risk for being large for gestational age (LGA)
- **Gestational diabetes mellitus**: glucose intolerance with its onset during pregnancy or first detected in pregnancy

During pregnancy, diabetes typically is categorized into two groups: **pregestational diabetes** (alteration in carbohydrate metabolism identified before conception), which includes women with type 1 or type 2 disease; and gestational diabetes, which develops during pregnancy.

HEALTHY PEOPLE 2010	
Objective	Significance
Increase abstinence from alcohol, cigarettes, and illicit drugs among pregnant women Increase in reported abstinence in the past month from substances by pregnant women Alcohol from a baseline of 86% to 94% Binge drinking from a baseline of 99% to 100% Cigarette smoking from abaseline of 87% to 99% Illicit drugs from a baseline of 98% to 100%	Will help to focus attention on measures for reducing substance exposure and use, thereby minimizing the effects of these substances on the fetus and newborn

USDHHS, 2000.

Pregestational diabetes complicates 0.2% to 0.3% of all pregnancies and affects more than 15,000 women annually. Gestational diabetes occurs in approximately 8% of all pregnant women, and those rates are higher among women of color. It is associated with either neonatal complications such as macrosomia, hypoglycemia, and birth trauma or maternal complications such as preeclampsia and cesarean birth. Gestational diabetes complicates more than 200,000 pregnancies annually in the United States and accounts for 90% of diabetic pregnancies (ADA, 2007a).

Before the discovery of insulin in 1922, most women with diabetes were infertile or experienced spontaneous abortion (March of Dimes, 2007b). Over the past several decades, great strides have been made in improving the outcomes of pregnancy in women with diabetes, but this chronic metabolic disorder remains a high-risk condition during pregnancy. A favorable outcome requires commitment on the woman's part to comply with frequent prenatal visits, dietary restrictions, self-monitoring of blood glucose levels, frequent laboratory tests, intensive fetal surveillance, and perhaps hospitalization.

Pathophysiology

With diabetes, there is a deficiency of or resistance to insulin. This alteration interferes with the body's ability to obtain essential nutrients for fuel and storage. If a pregnant woman has pregestational diabetes or develops gestational diabetes, the profound metabolic alterations that occur during pregnancy and that are necessary to support the growth and development of fetus can be affected.

▶ *Consider* THIS!

Scott and I had been busy all day setting up the new crib and nursery, and we finally sat down to rest. I was due any day, and we had been putting this off until we had a long weekend to complete the task. I was excited to think about all the frilly pinks that decorated her room. I was sure that my new daughter would love it as much as I loved her already. A few days later I barely noticed any fetal movement, but I thought that she must be as tired as I was by this point.

That night I went into labor and kept looking at the worried faces of the nurses and the midwife in attendance. I had been diagnosed with gestational diabetes a few months ago and had tried to follow the instructions regarding diet and exercise, but old habits are hard to change when you are 38 years old. I was finally told after a short time in the labor unit that they couldn't pick up a fetal heartbeat and an ultrasound was to be done—still no heartbeat was detected. Scott and I were finally told that our daughter was a stillborn. All I could think about was that she would never get to see all the pink colors in the nursery. . .

Maternal metabolism is directed toward supplying adequate nutrition for the fetus. In pregnancy, placental hormones cause insulin resistance at a level that tends to parallel the growth of the fetoplacental unit. As the placenta grows, more placental hormones are secreted. Human placental lactogen (hPL) and growth hormone (somatotropin) increase in direct correlation with the growth of placental tissue, rising throughout the last 20 weeks of pregnancy and causing insulin resistance. Subsequently, insulin secretion increases to overcome the resistance of these two hormones. In the nondiabetic pregnant woman, the pancreas can respond to the demands for increased insulin production to maintain normal glucose levels throughout the pregnancy (Cypryk et al., 2007). However, the woman with glucose intolerance or diabetes during pregnancy cannot cope with changes in metabolism resulting from insufficient insulin to meet the needs during gestation.

Over the course of pregnancy, insulin resistance changes. It peaks in the last trimester to provide more nutrients to the fetus. The insulin resistance typically results in postprandial hyperglycemia, although some women also have an elevated fasting blood glucose level (Homko & Reece, 2006). With this increased demand on the pancreas in late pregnancy, women with diabetes or glucose intolerance cannot accommodate the increased insulin demand; glucose levels rise as a result of insulin deficiency, leading to hyperglycemia. Subsequently, the mother and her fetus can experience major problems (Table 20.1).

Therapeutic Management

Preconception counseling is key for the woman with pregestational diabetes (the alteration in carbohydrate metabolism is identified before conception) to ensure that her disease state is stable. The goals of preconception care are to:

- Integrate the woman into the management of her diabetes
- Achieve the lowest glycosylated hemoglobin A1C test results without excessive hypoglycemia
- Ensure effective contraception until stable glycemia is achieved
- Identify and evaluate long-term diabetic complications such as retinopathy, nephropathy, neuropathy, cardiovascular disease, and hypertension (ADA, 2007b)

Excellent control of blood glucose, as evidenced by normal fasting blood glucose levels and a **glycosylated hemoglobin (HbA1C) level** (a measurement of the average glucose levels over the past 100 to 120 days), is crucial to achieve the best pregnancy outcome. A glycosylated hemoglobin level of less than 7% indicates good control; a value of more than 8% indicates poor control and warrants intervention (ADA, 2007b).

Preconception counseling also is important in helping to reduce the risk of congenital malformation. The most common malformations associated with diabetes occur in the renal, cardiac, skeletal, and central nervous systems. Since these defects occur by the eighth week of gestation, preconception counseling is critical. The rate

TABLE 20.1 DIABETES AND PREGNANCY: EFFECTS ON THE MOTHER AND FETUS

Effects on the Mother	Effects on the Fetus/Neonate
• Polyhydramnios due to fetal diuresis caused by hyperglycemia • Gestational hypertension of unknown etiology • Ketoacidosis due to uncontrolled hyperglycemia • Preterm labor secondary to premature membrane rupture • Stillbirth in pregnancies complicated by ketoacidosis and poor glucose control • Hypoglycemia as glucose is diverted to the fetus (occurring in first trimester) • Urinary tract infections resulting from excess glucose in the urine (glucosuria), which promotes bacterial growth • Chronic monilial vaginitis due to glucosuria, which promotes growth of yeast • Difficult labor, cesarean birth, postpartum hemorrhage secondary to an overdistended uterus to accommodate a macrosomic infant	• Cord prolapse secondary to polyhydramnios and abnormal fetal presentation • Congenital anomaly due to hyperglycemia in the first trimester (cardiac problems, neural tube defects, skeletal deformities, and genitourinary problems) • Macrosomia resulting from hyperinsulinemia stimulated by fetal hyperglycemia • Birth trauma due to increased size of fetus, which complicates the birthing process (shoulder dystocia) • Preterm birth secondary to hydramnios and an aging placenta, which places the fetus in jeopardy if the pregnancy continues • Fetal asphyxia secondary to fetal hyperglycemia and hyperinsulinemia • Intrauterine growth restriction (IUGR) secondary to maternal vascular impairment and decreased placental perfusion, which restricts growth • Perinatal death due to poor placental perfusion and hypoxia • Respiratory distress syndrome (RDS) resulting from poor surfactant production secondary to hyperinsulinemia inhibiting the production of phospholipids, which make up surfactant • Polycythemia due to excessive red blood cell (RBC) production in response to hypoxia • Hyperbilirubinemia due to excessive RBC breakdown from hypoxia and an immature liver unable to break down bilirubin • Neonatal hypoglycemia resulting from ongoing hyperinsulinemia after the placenta is removed • Subsequent childhood obesity and carbohydrate intolerance

Sources: March of Dimes, 2007b; Gilbert, 2007; Blackburn, 2007.

of congenital anomalies in women with pregestational diabetes can be reduced if excellent glycemic control is achieved at the time of conception (Varughese et al., 2007). This information needs to be stressed with all diabetic women contemplating a pregnancy.

In addition, the woman with pregestational diabetes needs to be evaluated for complications of diabetes. This evaluation should be part of baseline screening and continuing assessment during pregnancy.

Therapeutic management for the woman with gestational diabetes mellitus (defined as glucose intolerance with its onset during pregnancy or first detected during pregnancy) focuses on tight glucose control. The ADA (2007b) recommends maintaining a fasting blood glucose level below 95 mg/dL, with postprandial levels below 140 mg/dL and 2-hour postprandial levels below 120 mg/dL. In comparison, for pregnant women without diabetes, near-normal glucose values include a fasting value between 60 to 90 mg/dL, a 1-hour postprandial value of 100 to 120 mg/dL, and a 2-hour postprandial value of 60 to 120 mg/dL. Such tight control has been advocated because it is associated with a reduction in macrosomia (Scollan-Koliopoulos, Guadagno, & Walker, 2006).

Women with diabetes need comprehensive prenatal care. The primary goals of care are to maintain glycemic control and minimize the risks of the disease on the fetus.

Key aspects of treatment include nutritional management, insulin regimens, and close maternal and fetal surveillance.

Nutritional management focuses on maintaining balanced glucose levels and providing enough energy and nutrients for the pregnant woman, while avoiding ketosis, and minimizing the risk of hypoglycemia in women treated with insulin (Edelstein & Herbold, 2007). Women who receive dietary instruction and follow it have been shown to have a better pregnancy outcome than those who don't receive dietary advice (Henriksen, 2006). For the woman with gestational diabetes, nutritional management may be all that is necessary.

Insulin, which doesn't cross the placenta, historically has been the medication of choice for treating hyperglycemia in pregnancy. Recent studies have examined the use of oral hypoglycemic medications in pregnancy. Several studies have used glyburide (Diabeta) with promising results. When oral agents are prescribed, additional treatment with insulin may be necessary as the pregnancy advances (Scollan-Koliopoulos, Guadagno, & Walker, 2006). More research is indicated to establish the drug's safety and efficacy in managing diabetes in pregnancy before it can be considered an evidence-based practice (Homko & Reece, 2006; Rochon et al., 2006).

The ADA recommends that women diagnosed with gestational diabetes by a 3-hour glucose tolerance test receive nutritional counseling from a registered dietitian. The ADA also recommends insulin therapy if diet is unsuccessful in achieving a fasting glucose level below 105 mg/dL, a 1-hour postprandial level below 155 mg/dL, or 2-hour postprandial level below 130 mg/dL (ADA, 2007b).

The American College of Obstetricians and Gynecologists (ACOG) recommends the use of diet or insulin to achieve a 1-hour postprandial blood glucose level of 130 mg/dL. Both ADA and ACOG believe that further studies are needed to establish the safety of oral antidiabetic agents. Glycemic control—regardless of whether it involves diet, insulin, or oral agents—leads to fewer cases of shoulder dystocia, hyperbilirubinemia requiring phototherapy, nerve palsy, bone fracture, large for gestational age status, and fetal macrosomia (ADA, 2008).

Insulin remains the medication of choice for glycemic control in pregnant and lactating women with any type of diabetes (Ekpebegh et al., 2007). Generally, insulin doses are reduced in the first trimester to prevent hypoglycemia resulting from increased insulin sensitivity as well as from nausea and vomiting. Newer short-acting insulins such as lispo (Humalog) and aspart (Novolog), which do not cross the placenta, may help reduce postprandial hyperglycemia, episodes of hypoglycemia between meals (Hackley, Kriebs, & Rousseau, 2007). Target fasting glucose values of 60 to 90 mg/dL and 1-hour postprandial values less than 120 mg/dL are necessary to provide good glycemic control and good pregnancy outcomes (Frieden & Chan, 2007). Changes in diet and activity level add to the need for changes in insulin dosages throughout pregnancy.

Insulin regimens vary, and controversy remains over the best strategy for insulin delivery in pregnancy. Many health care providers use a split-dose therapy ($\frac{2}{3}$ of the daily dose in the morning and the remaining $\frac{1}{3}$ in the evening). Others advocate the use of an insulin pump to deliver a continuous subcutaneous insulin infusion. Regardless of which protocol is used, frequent blood glucose measurements are necessary, and the insulin dosage is adjusted on the basis of daily glucose levels.

EVIDENCE-BASED PRACTICE 20.1
Selecting Methods of Insulin Administration for Pregnant Women With Diabetes

● Study

A woman who has diabetes and becomes pregnant is at risk for various problems, both for herself and her fetus. The goal during pregnancy is to maintain optimal glucose control. For these women, insulin is the mainstay of treatment. Unfortunately blood glucose levels are not static and insulin requirements change throughout pregnancy.

Insulin typically is administered subcutaneously, commonly in multiple doses throughout the day. However, it also may be administered via a continuous subcutaneous infusion. The question arises as to which method of insulin administration affords the best control of blood glucose levels. The belief is that the continuous infusions would provide better blood glucose control and thus reduce the risks of problems for the mother and fetus.

A study was conducted comparing the effects of continuous subcutaneous insulin infusions with multiple daily doses of insulin therapy. The study involved a search of randomized controlled trials comparing these two methods of administration and their effect on neonatal birthweight, perinatal mortality, fetal anomalies, and maternal hypo- and hyperglycemia. Two studies consisting of 60 women were reviewed and a meta-analysis was performed.

▲ Findings

Women receiving continuous insulin infusions experienced an increase in birthweight of their infants compared to mothers receiving multiple daily doses of insulin. However, the researchers did not identify this difference as clinically significant. The researchers found no significant differences in perinatal mortality, fetal anomalies, or maternal hypo- and hyperglycemia between the two groups. The researchers attributed this to the small number of trials reviewed and the limited sample size of participants in the study. They concluded that there was insufficient evidence to support one method being better than the other. The researchers recommended additional research using a more vigorous approach and larger samples of women.

■ Nursing Implications

This study, although inconclusive, does underscore the need for glucose control in women with pregestational diabetes. Nurses need to be aware of these findings so that they can integrate knowledge of adequate blood glucose control when teaching pregnant women with diabetes about its potential effects, regardless of the method for insulin administration. Nurses also need to be cognizant of the various methods for insulin administration so that they can incorporate the information from this study to provide individualized care to the pregnant woman with diabetes, thereby promoting the best possible outcomes for the mother and her fetus.

Farrar, D., Tuffnell, D. J., & West, J. Continuous subcutaneous insulin infusion versus multiple daily injections of insulin for pregnant women with diabetes. *Cochrane Database of Systematic Reviews* 2007. Issue 3. Art. No.: CD005542.DOI: 10.1002/14651858.CD005542.pub2.

Close maternal and fetal surveillance is also essential. Frequent laboratory tests are done during pregnancy to monitor the woman's status and glucose control. Fetal surveillance via diagnostic testing aids in evaluating fetal well-being and assisting in determining the best time for birth.

For the laboring woman with diabetes, intravenous saline is given and blood glucose levels are monitored every 1 to 2 hours. Glucose levels are maintained below 110 mg/dL throughout labor to reduce the likelihood of neonatal hypoglycemia. If necessary, an infusion of regular insulin may be given to maintain this level (ADA, 2007b). If the woman was receiving insulin during her pregnancy, adjustments in dosage may be necessary after birth since glucose diversion across the placenta to supply the growing fetus is no longer present and insulin resistance is now removed. Frequently, the woman with gestational diabetes can remain controlled through diet and weight management; the woman with type 1 diabetes usually returns to prepregnant levels of insulin administration (Modder, 2008).

Nursing Assessment

Nursing assessment begins at the first prenatal visit. A thorough history and physical examination in conjunction with specific laboratory and diagnostic testing aids in developing an individualized plan of care for the woman with diabetes.

Health History and Physical Examination

For the woman with pregestational diabetes, obtain a thorough history of the preexisting diabetic condition. Ask about her duration of disease, management of glucose levels (insulin injections, insulin pump, or oral hypoglycemic agents), dietary adjustments, presence of vascular complications and current vascular status, current insulin regimen, and technique used for glucose testing. Review any information that she may have received as part of her preconception counseling and measures that were implemented during this time.

Be knowledgeable about the woman's nutritional requirements and assess the adequacy and pattern of her dietary intake. Assess her blood glucose self-monitoring in terms of technique, frequency, and her ability to adjust the insulin dose based on the changing patterns. Ask about the frequency of episodes of hypoglycemia or hyperglycemia to ascertain the woman's ability to recognize and treat them. Continue to assess her for signs and symptoms of hypo- and hyperglycemia.

During antepartum visits, assess the client's knowledge about her disease, including the signs and symptoms of hypoglycemia, hyperglycemia, and diabetic ketoacidosis, insulin administration techniques, and the impact of pregnancy on her chronic condition. If possible have the woman demonstrate her technique for blood glucose monitoring and insulin administration if appropriate. Although the client may have had diabetes for some time,

do not assume that she has a firm knowledge base about her disease process or management of it (Fig. 20.1).

Assess the woman's risk for gestational diabetes at the first prenatal visit. The ADA (2007b) recommends assessing all women for risk factors and then determining the need for additional testing in the high-risk group only. Factors that place a woman at high risk include:

- Previous infant with congenital anomaly (skeletal, renal, central nervous system, cardiac)
- History of gestational diabetes or hydramnios in a previous pregnancy
- Family history of diabetes
- Age 35 or older
- Previous infant weighing more than 9 pounds (4,000 g)
- Previous unexplained fetal demise or neonatal death
- Maternal obesity (Body Mass Index [BMI] > 30)
- Hypertension
- Hispanic, Native American, or African-American ethnicity
- Recurrent monilia infections that don't respond to treatment
- Signs and symptoms of glucose intolerance (polyuria, polyphagia, polydipsia, fatigue)
- Presence of glycosuria or proteinuria (Hackley, Kriebs, & Rousseau, 2007)

Women with clinical characteristics consistent with a high risk for gestational diabetes should undergo glucose testing as soon as feasible.

Provide close ongoing assessment throughout the antepartal period. Women with gestational diabetes mellitus are at increased risk for preeclampsia and glucose control-related complications such as hypoglycemia, hyperglycemia, and ketoacidosis. Gestational diabetes of any severity increases the risk of fetal macrosomia. It is also associated with an increased frequency of maternal hypertensive disorders and operative births. This may be the result of fetal growth disorders (ADA, 2007b).

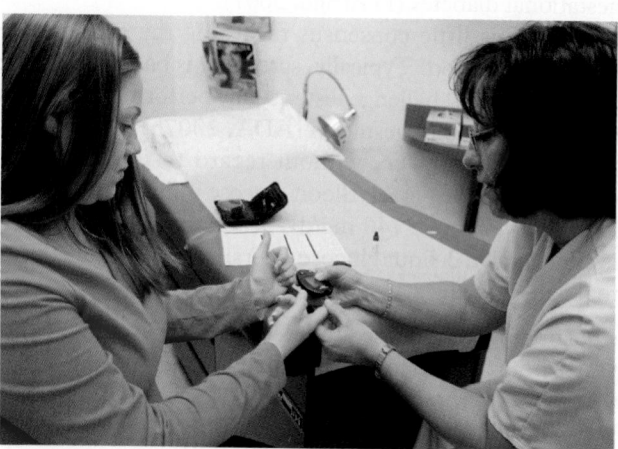

FIGURE 20.1 The nurse is demonstrating the technique for self-blood glucose monitoring with a pregnant client.

Even though gestational diabetes is diagnosed during pregnancy, the woman may have had glucose intolerance before the pregnancy. Therefore, monitor the woman closely for signs and symptoms of possible complications.

Also assess the woman's psychosocial adaptation to her condition. This assessment is critical to gain her co-operation for a change in regimen or the addition of a new regimen throughout pregnancy. Identify her support systems and note any financial constraints, as she will need more intense monitoring and frequent fetal surveillance.

Laboratory and Diagnostic Testing

The results of laboratory and diagnostic tests provide valuable information about maternal and fetal well-being. Women with pregestational diabetes and those discovered to have gestational diabetes require ongoing maternal and fetal surveillance to promote the best outcome.

Screening

ACOG and ADA currently recommend a risk analysis of all pregnant women at their first prenatal visit and additional screening of all high-risk pregnant women again at 24 to 28 weeks, or earlier if risk factors are present. If the initial screening risk assessment is low, additional screening may not be necessary. Pregnant women who fulfill all of the following criteria need not be screened:

• No history of glucose intolerance
• Less than 25 years old
• Normal body weight
• No family history (first-degree relative) of diabetes
• No history of poor obstetric outcome
• Not from an ethnic/racial group with a high prevalence of diabetes (ADA, 2007b)

If the initial risk assessment is high, rescreening should take place between 24 and 28 weeks. A woman with abnormal early results may have had diabetes before the pregnancy, and her fetus is a great risk for congenital anomalies. An elevated glycosylated hemoglobin supports the likelihood of gestational diabetes (D'Arrigo, 2007).

There is little consensus regarding the appropriate screening method. Typically, screening is based on a 50-g 1-hour glucose challenge test, usually performed between week 24 and 28 of gestation (ADA, 2007b). A 50-g oral glucose load is given, without regard to the timing or content of the last meal. Blood glucose is measured 1 hour later; a level above 140 mg/dL is abnormal. If the result is abnormal, a 3-hour glucose tolerance test is done. Normal values are:

• Fasting blood glucose level: less than 105 mg/dL
• At 1 hour: less than 190 mg/dL
• At 2 hours: less than 165 mg/dL
• At 3 hours: less than 145 mg/dL

A diagnosis of gestational diabetes can be made only after an abnormal result is obtained on the glucose toler-ance test. Two or more abnormal values confirm a diagnosis of gestational diabetes (ADA, 2007a).

Surveillance

Maternal surveillance may include the following:

• Urine check for protein (may indicate the need for further evaluation for preeclampsia) and for nitrates and leukocyte esterase (may indicate a urinary tract infection)
• Urine check for ketones (may indicate the need for evaluation of eating habits)
• Kidney function evaluation every trimester for creatinine clearance and protein levels
• Eye examination in the first trimester to evaluate the retina for vascular changes
• HbA1c every 4 to 6 weeks to monitor glucose trends (Hackley, Kriebs, & Rousseau, 2007)

Fetal surveillance may include ultrasound to provide information about fetal growth, activity, and amniotic fluid volume and to validate gestational age. Alpha-fetoprotein levels may be obtained to detect congenital anomalies such as an open neural tube or ventral wall defects of omphalo-cele or gastroschisis, and a fetal echocardiogram may be necessary to rule out cardiac anomalies. A biophysical profile helps to monitor fetal well-being and uteroplacental profusion, and nonstress tests commonly are performed weekly after 28 weeks' gestation to evaluate fetal well-being. As the pregnancy progresses, an amniocentesis may be done to determine the lecithin/sphingomyelin (L/S) ratio and the presence of phosphatidyl glycerol (PG) to evaluate whether the fetal lung is mature enough for birth (Frieden & Chan, 2007).

Nursing Management

The ideal outcome of every pregnancy is a healthy newborn and mother. Nurses can be pivotal in realizing this positive outcome for women with pregestational or gestational diabetes by implementing measures to minimize risks and complications. Since the woman with diabetes is considered to be at high risk, antepartal visits occur more frequently (every 2 weeks up to 28 weeks and then twice a week until birth), providing the nurse with numerous opportunities for ongoing assessment, education, and counseling (Nursing Care Plan 20.1).

Promoting Optimal Glucose Control

At each visit, review the mother's blood glucose levels, including any laboratory tests and self-monitoring results. Reinforce with the woman the need to perform blood glucose monitoring (usually four times a day, before meals and at bedtime) and to keep a record of the results. If appropriate, obtain a fingerstick blood glucose level to evaluate the accuracy of self-monitoring results. Also assess the woman's techniques for monitoring blood glucose levels and for administering insulin if ordered, and offer support and guidance. If the woman is receiving insulin

Nursing Care Plan 20.1

OVERVIEW OF THE PREGNANT WOMAN WITH TYPE 1 DIABETES

Donna, a 30-year-old woman with type 1 diabetes, presents to the maternity clinic for preconception care. She has been a diabetic for 8 years and takes insulin twice daily by injection. She does blood glucose self-monitoring four times daily. She reports that her disease is fairly well controlled, but "I'm worried about how my diabetes will affect a pregnancy and my baby. Will I need to make changes in my routine? Will my baby be normal?" She reports that she recently had a foot infection and needed to go to the emergency room because it led to an episode of ketoacidosis. She states that her last glycosylated hemoglobin A1c test results were abnormal.

NURSING DIAGNOSIS: Deficient knowledge related to type 1 diabetes, blood glucose control, and effects of condition on pregnancy as evidenced by questions about effect on pregnancy, possible changes in regimen, and pregnancy outcome

Outcome Identification and Evaluation

Client will demonstrate increased knowledge of type 1 diabetes and effects on pregnancy *as evidenced by proper techniques for blood glucose monitoring and insulin administration, ability to modify insulin doses and dietary intake to achieve control, and verbalization of need for glycemic control prior to pregnancy, with blood glucose levels remaining within normal range.*

Interventions: Providing Client Teaching

- Assess client's knowledge of diabetes and pregnancy *to establish a baseline from which to develop an individualized teaching plan.*
- Review the underlying problems associated with diabetes and how pregnancy affects glucose control *to provide client with a firm knowledge base for decision making.*
- Review signs and symptoms of hypoglycemia and hyperglycemia and prevention and management measures *to ensure client can deal with them should they occur.*
- Provide written materials describing diabetes and care needed for control *to provide opportunity for client's review and promote retention of learning.*
- Observe client administering insulin and self-glucose testing for technique and offer suggestions for improvement if needed *to ensure adequate self-care ability.*
- Discuss proper foot care *to prevent future infections.*
- Teach home treatment for symptomatic hypoglycemia *to minimize risk to client and fetus.*
- Outline acute and chronic diabetic complications *to reinforce the importance of glucose control.*
- Discuss use of contraceptives until blood glucose levels can be optimized before conception occurs *to promote best possible health status before conception.*
- Explain the rationale for good glucose control and the importance of achieving excellent glycemic control before pregnancy *to promote a positive pregnancy outcome.*
- Review self-care practices (blood glucose monitoring and frequency of testing; insulin administration; adjustment of insulin dosages based on blood glucose levels) *to foster independence in self-care and feelings of control over the situation.*
- Refer client for dietary counseling *to ensure optimal diet for glycemic control.*
- Outline obstetric management and fetal surveillance needed for pregnancy *to provide client with information on what to expect.*
- Discuss strategies for maintaining optimal glycemic control during pregnancy *to minimize risks to client and fetus.*

Nursing Care Plan 20.1 (continued)

NURSING DIAGNOSIS: Anxiety related to future pregnancy and its outcome secondary to underlying diabetes as evidenced by questions about her condition's effect on the baby and baby being normal

Outcome Identification and Evaluation
Client will openly express her feelings related to her diabetes and pregnancy *as evidenced by statements of feeling better about her pre-existing condition and pregnancy outlook, and statements of understanding related to future childbearing by linking good glucose control with positive outcomes for both herself and offspring.*

Interventions: Minimizing Anxiety
* Review the need for a physical examination *to evaluate for any effects of diabetes on the client's health status.*
* Explain the rationale for assessing client's blood pressure, vision, and peripheral pulses at each visit *to provide information related to possible effects of diabetes on health status.*
* Identify any alterations in present diabetic condition that need intervention *to aid in minimizing risks that may increase client's anxiety level.*
* Review potential effects of diabetes on pregnancy *to promote client understanding of risks and ways to control or minimize them.*
* Encourage active participation in decision making and planning pregnancy *to promote feelings of control over the situation and foster self-confidence.*
* Discuss feelings about future childbearing and managing pregnancy *to help reduce anxiety related to uncertainties.*
* Encourage client to ask questions or voice concerns *to help decrease anxiety related to the unknown.*
* Emphasize the use of frequent and continued surveillance of client and fetal status during pregnancy *to reduce the risk of complications and aid in alleviating anxieties related to the unknown.*
* Provide positive reinforcement for healthy behaviors and actions *to foster continued use and enhancement of self-esteem.*

---

therapy, assist with any changes needed if glucose levels are not controlled.

Obtain a urine specimen and check for glucose, protein, and ketones. Ask the woman if she has had any episodes of hypoglycemia and what she did to alleviate them.

Discuss dietary measures related to blood glucose control (Fig. 20.2). In addition, recommend the following:

• Avoid weight loss and dieting during pregnancy.
• Ensure that food intake is adequate to prevent ketone formation and promote weight gain.
• Eat three meals a day plus three snacks to promote glycemic control.
  –40% of calories from good-quality complex carbohydrates
  –35% of calories from protein sources
  –25% of calories from unsaturated fats (ADA, 2007b)

▶ *Take* NOTE!

Nutrient requirements and recommendations for weight gain for the pregnant woman with diabetes are the same as those for the pregnant nondiabetic woman.

If necessary, arrange for consultation with a dietitian or nutritionist to individualize the dietary plan. Also encourage the women to participate in an exercise program that includes at least three sessions lasting longer than 15 min-

utes per week. Exercise may lessen the need for insulin or dosage adjustments.

When caring for the laboring woman with pregestational or gestational diabetes, adjust the intravenous flow rate and the rate of supplemental regular insulin based on

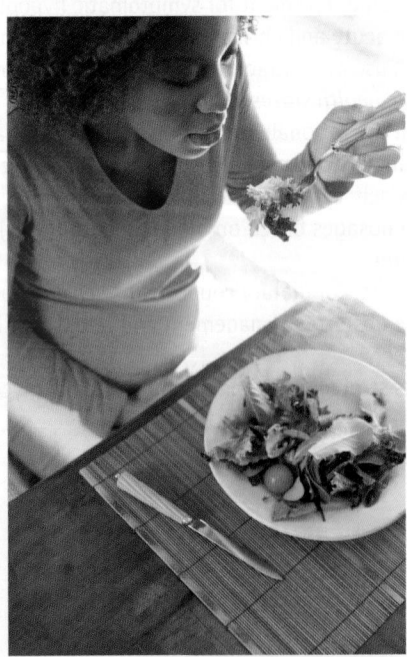

FIGURE 20.2 The pregnant client eating a nutritious meal to ensure adequate glucose control.

the blood glucose levels as ordered. Monitor blood glucose levels every 1 to 2 hours or more frequently if necessary. Keep a syringe with 50% dextrose solution available at the bedside to treat profound hypoglycemia. Monitor fetal heart rate patterns throughout labor to detect nonreassuring patterns. Assess maternal vital signs every hour, in addition to assessing the woman's urinary output with an indwelling catheter. If a cesarean birth is scheduled, monitor the woman's blood glucose levels hourly and administer short-acting insulin or glucose based on the blood glucose levels as ordered.

After birth, monitor blood glucose levels every 2 to 4 hours and continue intravenous fluid administration as ordered. Encourage breastfeeding to assist in maintaining good glucose control. For the woman with pregestational diabetes and type 1 or 2 diabetes, expect insulin needs to decrease rapidly after birth: they may be reduced by half of the antepartum dose as meals are started (Hackley, Kriebs, & Rousseau, 2007). Some women may return to their prepregnancy insulin dosage.

The therapy plan after childbirth is individualized for each woman. If recommended dietary modifications are carried out along with weight loss, the woman with gestational diabetes may return to her normal glucose levels. This is also true for the woman with pregestational diabetes, except that she will return to her prepregnancy insulin administration levels. This provides the nurse with a wonderful opportunity to reinforce healthy lifestyle interventions on the postpartum unit. Nurses can also become involved with community-based education to continue to offer their expertise.

Preventing Complications

Assess the woman closely for signs and symptoms of complications at each visit. Anticipate possible complications and plan appropriate interventions or referrals. Check the woman's blood pressure for changes and evaluate for proteinuria when obtaining a urine specimen. These might suggest the development of preeclampsia. Measure fundal height and review gestational age. Note any discrepancies between fundal height and gestational age or a sudden increase in uterine growth. These may suggest hydramnios.

Encourage the woman to perform daily fetal movement counts to monitor fetal well-being. Tell her specifically when she should notify her health care provider. Also prepare the woman for the need for frequent laboratory and diagnostic testing to evaluate fetal status. Assist with serial ultrasounds to monitor fetal growth and with nonstress tests and biophysical profiles to assess fetal well-being.

Providing Client Education and Counseling

The pregnant woman with diabetes requires counseling and education about the need for strict glucose monitoring, diet and exercise, and signs and symptoms of complications. Encourage the client and her family to make any

lifestyle changes needed to optimize the pregnancy outcome. Providing dietary education and lifestyle advice that extends beyond pregnancy may lower the risk that the woman will have gestational diabetes in subsequent pregnancies as well as type 2 diabetes (Scollan-Koliopoulos, Guadagno, & Walker, 2006). At each visit stress the importance of performing blood glucose screening and documenting the results. With proper instruction, the client and her family will be able to cope with all the changes in her body during pregnancy (Teaching Guidelines 20.1).

Review discussions about the timing of birth and the rationale. Counsel the client about the possibility of cesarean birth for an LGA infant, or inform the woman who will be giving birth vaginally about the possible need for augmentation with oxytocin (Pitocin).

> ▶ *Take* NOTE!
>
> *In the woman with well-controlled diabetes, birth is typically not induced before term unless there are complications, such as preeclampsia or fetal compromise. An early delivery date might be set for the woman with poorly controlled diabetes who is having complications.*

Instruct the client about the benefits of breastfeeding related to blood glucose control. Breastfeeding helps to normalize blood glucose levels. Therefore, encourage the woman to breastfeed her newborn. Also teach the woman receiving insulin for her diabetes that her insulin needs after birth will drastically decrease. Inform her that she will need a repeat glucose challenge test at a postpartum visit (ADA, 2007b).

For the woman with gestational diabetes, the focus is on lifestyle education. Women with gestational diabetes have a greater than 50% increased risk of developing type 2 diabetes (ADA, 2007a). Inform the woman that screening most likely will be done at the postpartum follow-up appointment in 6 weeks. Women with normal results at that visit typically are screened every 3 years thereafter (ADA, 2007a). Teach her how to maintain an optimal weight to reduce her risk of developing diabetes. If necessary, refer the woman to a dietitian to help outline a balanced nutritious diet.

Cardiovascular Disorders

Every minute, an American woman dies of cardiovascular disease (American Heart Association [AHA], 2007). Cardiovascular disease is the leading cause of death for men and women in the United States. It kills nearly 500,000 women each year. Despite the prominent reduction in cardiovascular mortality among men, the rate has not declined for women. Cardiovascular disease has killed more women then men since 1984 (AHA, 2007). In addition to being the number-one killer of women, at

TEACHING GUIDELINES 20.1

Teaching for the Pregnant Woman With Diabetes

- Be sure to keep your appointments for frequent prenatal visits and tests for fetal well-being.
- Perform blood glucose self-monitoring as directed, usually before each meal and at bedtime. Keep a record of your results and call your healthcare provider with any levels outside the established range. Bring your results to each prenatal visit.
- Perform daily "fetal kick counts." Document them and report any decrease in activity.
- Drink 8 to 10 8-ounce glasses of water each day to prevent bladder infections and maintain hydration.
- Wear proper, well-fitted footwear when walking to prevent injury.
- Engage in a regular exercise program such as walking to aid in glucose control, but avoid exercising in temperature extremes.
- Consider breastfeeding your infant to lower your blood glucose levels.
- If you are taking insulin:
  - Administer the correct dose of insulin at the correct time every day.
  - Eat breakfast within 30 minutes after injecting regular insulin to prevent a reaction.
  - Plan meals at a fixed time and snacks to prevent extremes in glucose levels.
- Avoid simple sugars (cake, candy, cookies), which raise blood glucose levels.
- Know the signs and symptoms of hypoglycemia and treatment needed:
  - Sweating, tremors, cold, clammy skin, headache
  - Feeling hungry, blurred vision, disorientation, irritability
  - Treatment: Drink 8 ounces of milk and eat two crackers or glucose tablets
- Carry "glucose boosters" (such as Life Savers) to prevent hypoglycemia.
- Know the signs and symptoms of hyperglycemia and treatment needed:
  - Dry mouth, frequent urination, excessive thirst, rapid breathing
  - Feeling tired, flushed, hot skin, headache, drowsiness
  - Treatment: Notify health care provider, since hospitalization may be needed
- Wear a diabetic identification bracelet at all times.
- Wash your hands frequently to prevent infections.
- Report any signs and symptoms of illness, infection, and dehydration to your health care provider, because these can affect blood glucose control.

the time of diagnosis women have both a poorer overall prognosis and a higher risk of death than men diagnosed with heart disease (Peddicord, 2005). More women die of heart disease, stroke, and other cardiovascular diseases than men, yet many women do not realize they are at risk. These diseases kill more women each year than the next five causes of death combined (AHA, 2007).

Approximately 3% of pregnant women have cardiac disease, which is responsible for 10% to 25% of maternal deaths (Cunningham et al., 2005). The prevalence of cardiac disease is increasing as a result of lifestyle patterns, including cigarette smoking, diabetes, and stress. As women are delaying childbearing, the incidence of cardiac disease in pregnancy will continue to increase. Rheumatic heart disease used to represent the majority of cardiac conditions during pregnancy, but congenital heart disease now constitutes nearly half of all cases of heart disease encountered during pregnancy. Classic symptoms of heart disease mimic common symptoms of late pregnancy, such as palpitations, shortness of breath with exertion, and occasional chest pain. Few women with heart disease die during pregnancy, but they are at risk for other complications, such as heart failure, arrhythmias, and stroke. Their offspring are also at risk of complications, such as premature birth, low birthweight for gestational age, respiratory distress syndrome, intraventricular hemorrhage, and death (Abdin, 2006).

CONGENITAL AND ACQUIRED HEART DISEASE

Congenital heart disease often involves structural defects that are present at birth but may not be discovered at that time (Table 20.2). Until recently women with congenital heart disease didn't live long enough to bear children. Today, due to new surgical techniques to correct these defects, many of these women can complete a successful pregnancy at relatively low risk when appropriate counseling and optimal care are provided. Increasing numbers of women with complex congenital heart disease are reaching childbearing age. Complications such as growth restriction and preterm and premature birth and fetal and neonatal mortality are more common among children of women with congenital heart disease. The risk of complications is determined by the severity of the cardiac lesion, the presence of cyanosis, the maternal functional class, and the use of anticoagulation (Karamermer & Roos-Hesselink, 2007).

Women with certain congenital conditions should avoid pregnancy. These include uncorrected tetralogy of Fallot or transposition of the great arteries, and Eisenmenger's syndrome, a defect with both cyanosis and pulmonary hypertension (Karamermer & Roos-Hesselink, 2007).

TABLE 20.2 SELECTED HEART CONDITIONS AFFECTING PREGNANCY

Condition	Description	Management
Tetralogy of Fallot	Congenital defect involving four structural anomalies: obstruction to pulmonary flow; ventricular septal defect (abnormal opening between the right and left ventricles); dextroposition of the aorta (aortic opening overriding the septum and receiving blood from both ventricles); and right ventricular hypertrophy (increase in volume of the myocardium of the right ventricle) (O'Toole, 2005)	Hospitalization and bed rest possible after the 20th week with hemodynamic monitoring via a pulmonary artery catheter to monitor volume status Oxygen therapy may be necessary during labor and birth.
Atrial septal defect (ASD)	Congenital heart defect involving a communication or opening between the atria with left-to-right shunting due to greater left-sided pressure Arrhythmias present in some women	Treatment with atrioventricular nodal blocking agents, and at times with electrical cardioversion (Gilbert & Harmon, 2006)
Ventricular septal defect (VSD)	Congenital heart defect involving an opening in the ventricular septum, permitting blood flow from the left to the right ventricle. Complications include arrhythmias, heart failure, and pulmonary hypertension (McMahon, 2007).	Rest with limited activity if symptomatic
Patent ductus arteriosus	Abnormal persistence of an open lumen in the ductus arteriosus between the aorta and the pulmonary artery after birth; results in increased pulmonary blood flow and redistribution of flow to other organs (Hermes-DeSantis & Clyman, 2006)	Surgical ligation of the open ductus during infancy; subsequent problems minimal after surgical correction
Mitral valve prolapse	Very common in the general population, occurring most often in younger women Leaflets of the mitral valve prolapse into the left atrium during ventricular contraction. The most common cause of mitral valve regurgitation if present during pregnancy (Wooley & Boudoulas, 2007) Usually improvement in mitral valve function due to increased blood volume and decreased systemic vascular resistance of pregnancy; most women are able to tolerate pregnancy well.	Most women are asymptomatic; diagnosis is made incidentally. Occasional palpations, chest pain, or arrhythmias in some women, possibly requiring beta-blockers Usually no special precautions are necessary during pregnancy.
Mitral valve stenosis	Most common chronic rheumatic valvular lesion in pregnancy Causes obstruction of blood flow from the atria to the ventricle, thereby decreasing ventricular filling and causing a fixed cardiac output Resultant pulmonary edema, pulmonary hypertension, and right ventricular failure (Barker et al., 2006) Most pregnant women with this condition can be managed medically.	General symptomatic improvement with medical management involving diuretics, beta-blockers, and anticoagulant therapy Activity restriction, reduction in sodium, and potentially bed rest if condition severe

(continued)

TABLE 20.2 SELECTED HEART CONDITIONS AFFECTING PREGNANCY (continued)

Condition	Description	Management
Aortic stenosis	Narrowing of the opening of the aortic valve, leading to an obstruction to left ventricular ejection (Balentine & Eisenhart, 2008). Women with mild disease can tolerate hypervolemia of pregnancy; with progressive narrowing of the opening, cardiac output becomes fixed. Diagnosis can be confirmed with echocardiography. Most women can be managed with medical therapy, bed rest, and close monitoring.	Diagnosis confirmed with echocardiography Pharmacologic treatment with beta-blockers and/or antiarrhythmic agents to reduce risk of heart failure and/or dysrhythmias Bed rest/limited activity and close monitoring
Peripartum cardiomyopathy	Rare congestive cardiomyopathy that may arise during pregnancy. Multiparity, age, multiple fetuses, hypertension, an infectious agent, autoimmune disease, or cocaine use may contribute to its presence (Mooney, 2007). Development of heart failure in the last month of pregnancy or within 5 months of giving birth without any preexisting heart disease or any identifiable cause	Preload reduction with diuretic therapy Afterload reduction with vasodilators Improvement in contractility with inotropic agents Nonpharmacologic approaches include salt restriction and daily exercise such as walking or biking. The question of whether another pregnancy should be attempted is controversial due to the high risk of repeat complications.
Myocardial infarction	Rare during pregnancy but incidence is expected to increase as older women are becoming pregnant and the risk factors for coronary artery disease become more prevalent Factors contributing to MI include family history, stress, smoking, age, obesity, multiple fetuses, hypercholesterolemia, and cocaine use (Gibson & Carson, 2007). Increased plasma volume and cardiac output during pregnancy increase the cardiac workload as well as the myocardial oxygen demands; imbalance in supply and demand may contribute to myocardial ischemia.	Usual treatment modalities for any acute MI along with consideration for the fetus Anticoagulant therapy, rest, and lifestyle changes to preserve the health of both parties

Sources: Balentine & Eisenhart, 2008; Gibson & Carson, 2007; McMahon, 2007; Mooney, 2007; O'Toole, 2005.

Acquired heart disease is typically rheumatic in origin (see Table 20.2). The incidence of rheumatic heart disease has declined dramatically in the past several decades because of prompt identification of streptococcal throat infections and treatment with antibiotics. When the heart is involved, valvular lesions such as mitral stenosis, prolapse, or aortic stenosis are common.

Many women are postponing childbearing until the fourth or fifth decade of life. With advancing maternal age, underlying medical conditions such as hypertension, diabetes, and hypercholesterolemia contributing to ischemic heart disease become more common and increase the incidence of acquired heart disease complicating pregnancy. Coronary artery disease and myocardial infarction may result.

A woman's ability to function during the pregnancy is often more important than the actual diagnosis of the cardiac condition. The following is a functional classification system developed by the Criteria Committee of the New York Heart Association (1994) based on past and present disability and physical signs:

- Class I: asymptomatic with no limitation of physical activity
- Class II: symptomatic (dyspnea, chest pain) with increased activity
- Class III: symptomatic (fatigue, palpitations) with normal activity
- Class IV: symptomatic at rest or with any physical activity

The classification may change as the pregnancy progresses and the woman's body must cope with the increasing stress on the cardiovascular system resulting from the numerous physiologic changes taking place. Typically, a woman with class I or II cardiac disease can go through a pregnancy without major complications. A woman with class III disease usually has to maintain bed rest during pregnancy. A woman with class IV disease should avoid pregnancy (McCann, 2007). Women with cardiac disease may benefit from preconception counseling so that they know the risks before deciding to become pregnant.

Maternal mortality varies directly with the functional class at pregnancy onset. ACOG has adopted a three-tiered classification according to the risk of death during pregnancy (Box 20.1).

BOX 20.1 **Classification of Maternal Mortality Risk**

Group I (minimal risk) has a mortality rate of 1% and comprises women with:
- Patent ductus arteriosus
- Tetralogy of Fallot, corrected
- Atrial septal defect
- Ventricular septal defect
- Mitral stenosis, class I and II

Group II (moderate risk) has a mortality rate of 5% to 15% and comprises women with:
- Tetralogy of Fallot, uncorrected
- Mitral stenosis with atrial fibrillation
- Aortic stenosis, class III and IV
- Aortic coarctation without valvular involvement
- Artificial valve replacement

Group III (major risk) has a 25% to 50% mortality rate and comprises women with:
- Pulmonary hypertension
- Complicated aortic coarctation
- Previous myocardial infarction

Sources: Gilbert & Harmon, 2006; Gilbert, 2007; Blackburn, 2007.

Pathophysiology

Numerous hemodynamic changes occur in all pregnant women. These normal physiologic changes can overstress the woman's cardiovascular system, increasing her risk for problems. Increased cardiac workload and greater myocardial oxygen demand during pregnancy place the woman's cardiovascular system at high risk for morbidity and mortality.

> ▶ **Take** NOTE!
>
> Uterine blood flow increases by at least 1 liter per minute, requiring the body to produce more blood during pregnancy. This results in a 25% increase in red blood cells, a 50% expansion of plasma volume during pregnancy, and an overall hemodilution. In addition, the increase in total red blood cellular volume includes an increase in clotting factors and platelets, defining the hypercoagulable state of pregnancy (Dobbenga-Rhodes & Prive, 2006). These changes start as early as the second month of gestation.

Similarly, cardiac output increases steadily during pregnancy by 30% to 50% over prepregnancy levels: stroke volume increases 20% to 30% from prepregnant levels, and the maternal heart rate increases by 10 to 20 beats per minute. The increase is due to both the expansion in blood volume and the augmentation of stroke volume and heart rate. Other hemodynamic changes associated with pregnancy include a decrease in both the systemic vascular resistance and pulmonary vascular resistance, thereby lowering the systolic and diastolic blood pressure. In addition, the hypercoagulability associated with pregnancy might increase the risk of arterial thrombosis and embolization. These normal physiologic changes are important for a successful adaptation to pregnancy but create unique physiologic challenges for the woman with cardiac disease (Comparison Chart 20.1).

Therapeutic Management

Ideally, a woman with a history of congenital or acquired heart disease should consult her health care provider before becoming pregnant and should undergo a risk assessment. This risk assessment must consider the woman's functional capacity, exercise tolerance, degree of cyanosis, medication needs, and history of arrhythmias. Data needed for risk assessment can be acquired from a thorough cardiovascular history and examination, a 12-lead electrocardiogram (ECG), and evaluation of oxygen saturation levels by pulse oximetry. The impact of heart disease on a woman's childbearing potential needs to be clearly explained, and information on how pregnancy may affect her and the fetus is important. This allows women to make an informed choice

COMPARISON CHART 20.1   CARDIOVASCULAR CHANGES: PREPREGNANCY VS PREGNANCY

Measurement	Prepregnancy	Pregnancy
Heart rate	72 (±10 bpm)	+10–20%
Cardiac output	4.3 (±0.9 L/min)	+30% to 50%
Blood volume	5 L	+20% to 50%
Stroke volume	73.3 (±9 mL)	+30%
Systemic vascular resistance	1,530 (±520 dyne/cm/sec)	–20%
Oxygen consumption	250 mL/minute	+20–30%

Sources: Blincoe, 2007; Blackburn, 2007; Harvey, 2007.

whether they wish to accept the risks associated with pregnancy. When possible, any surgical procedures, such as valve replacement, should be done before pregnancy to improve fetal and maternal outcomes (Uebing et al., 2006).

If the woman presents for care after she has become pregnant, prenatal counseling focuses on the impact of the hemodynamic changes of pregnancy, the signs and symptoms of cardiac compromise, and dietary and lifestyle changes needed. More frequent prenatal visits (every 2 weeks until the last month and then weekly) are usually needed to ensure the health and safety of the mother and fetus.

Nursing Assessment

Frequent and thorough assessments are crucial during the antepartum period to ensure early detection of and prompt intervention for problems. Assess the woman's vital signs, noting any changes. Auscultate the apical heart rate and heart sounds, being especially alert for abnormalities, including irregularities in rhythm or murmurs. Check the client's weight and compare to baseline and weights obtained on previous visits. Report any weight gain outside recommended parameters. Inspect the extremities for edema and note any pitting.

Question the woman about fetal activity, and ask if she has noticed any changes. Report any changes such as a decrease in fetal movements. Ask the woman about any symptoms of preterm labor, such as low back pain, uterine contractions, and increased pelvic pressure and vaginal discharge, and report them immediately. Assess the fetal heart rate and review serial ultrasound results to monitor fetal growth.

Assess the client's lifestyle and her ability to cope with the changes of pregnancy and its effect on her cardiac status and ability to function. Evaluate the client's understanding of her condition and what restrictions and lifestyle changes may be needed to provide the best outcome for her and her fetus. A healthy infant and mother at the end of pregnancy is the ultimate goal. As the client's pregnancy advances, expect her functional class to be revised based on her level of disability. Suggest realistic modifications.

The nurse plays a major role in recognizing the signs and symptoms of cardiac decompensation. Decompensation refers to the heart's inability to maintain adequate circulation. As a result, tissue perfusion in the mother and the fetus is impaired. The pregnant woman is most vulnerable for this complication from 28 to 32 weeks of gestation and in the first 48 hours postpartum (Witcher & Harvey, 2006). Assess the woman for the following signs and symptoms:

- Shortness of breath on exertion, dyspnea
- Cyanosis of lips and nail beds
- Swelling of face, hands, and feet
- Jugular vein engorgement
- Rapid respirations
- Abnormal heartbeats, reports of heart racing or palpitations
- Chest pain with effort or emotion
- Syncope with exertion
- Increasing fatigue
- Moist, frequent cough

 ▶ *Take NOTE!*

Assessing the pregnant woman with heart disease for cardiac decompensation is vital because the mother's hemodynamic status determines the health of the fetus.

Nursing Management

Nursing management of the pregnant woman with heart disease focuses on assisting with measures to stabilize the mother's hemodynamic status, because a decrease in maternal blood pressure or volume will cause blood to be shunted away from the uterus, thus reducing placental perfusion. Pregnant women with cardiac disease also need assistance in reducing risks that would lead to complications or further cardiac compromise. Therefore, education and counseling are critical. Collaboration between the cardiologist, obstetrician, perinatologist, and nurse is needed to promote the best possible outcome.

Encourage the woman to continue taking her cardiac medications as prescribed. Review the indications, actions, and potential side effects of the medications. Reinforce the importance of frequent antepartal visits and close medical supervision throughout the pregnancy.

Discuss the need to conserve energy. Help the client to prioritize household chores and childcare to allow rest periods. Encourage the client to rest in the side-lying position, which enhances placental perfusion.

Encourage the client to eat nutritious foods and consume a high-fiber diet to prevent straining and constipation. Discuss limiting sodium intake if indicated to reduce fluid retention. Contact a dietitian to assist the woman in planning nutritionally appropriate meals.

Assist the woman in preparing for diagnostic tests to evaluate fetal well-being. Describe the tests that may be done, such as ECG and echocardiogram, and explain the need for serial nonstress testing, usually beginning at approximately 32 weeks.

Instruct the woman in how to monitor fetal activity and movements. Urge her to do this daily and report any changes in activity immediately.

Although the morbidity and mortality rates of pregnant women with cardiac disease have decreased greatly, congestive heart failure, cardiac arrhythmia, thromboembolism, angina, hypoxemia, and infective endocarditis can occur (Witcher & Harvey, 2006). Explain the signs and symptoms of these complications and review the sign and symptoms of cardiac decompensation, encouraging the woman to notify her health care provider if any occur.

Provide support and encouragement throughout the antepartal period. Assess the support systems available to the client and her family, and encourage her to use them. If necessary, assist with referrals to community services for additional support.

During labor, anticipate the need for invasive hemodynamic monitoring, and make sure the woman has been prepared for this beforehand. Monitor her fluid volume carefully to prevent overload. Anticipate the use of epidural anesthesia if a vaginal birth is planned. After birth, assess the client for fluid overload as peripheral fluids mobilize. This fluid shift from the periphery to the central circulation taxes the heart, and signs of heart failure such as cough, progressive dyspnea, edema, palpitations, and crackles in the lung bases may ensue before postpartum diuresis begins. Because hemodynamics do not return to baseline for several days after childbirth, women at intermediate or high risk require monitoring for at least 48 hours postpartum (Barker et al., 2006).

▶ CHRONIC HYPERTENSION

Chronic hypertension exists when the woman has high blood pressure before pregnancy or before the 20th week of gestation, or when hypertension persists for more than 12 weeks postpartum. The Seventh Report of the Joint National Committee on Prevention, Detection, Evaluation, and Treatment of High Blood Pressure (JNC, 2003) has classified blood pressure as follows:

• Normal: systolic less than 120 mmHg, diastolic less than 80 mmHg
• Prehypertension: systolic 120 to 139 mmHg, diastolic 80 to 89 mmHg
• Mild hypertension: systolic 140 to 159 mmHg, diastolic 90 to 99 mmHg
• Severe hypertension: systolic 160 mm Hg or higher, diastolic 100 mm Hg or higher

Chronic hypertension occurs in up to 22% of women of childbearing age, with the prevalence varying according to age, race, and BMI. It complicates at least 5% of pregnancies, with 1 in 4 women developing preeclampsia during pregnancy (Blincoe, 2007). Chronic hypertension is typically seen in older, obese women with glucose intolerance. The most common complication is preeclampsia, which is seen in approximately 25% of women who enter the pregnancy with hypertension (Podymow & August, 2007; Tihtonen et al., 2007). (See Chapter 19 for more information about preeclampsia.)

Therapeutic Management

Preconception counseling is important in fostering positive outcomes. Typically, it involves lifestyle changes such as diet, exercise, weight loss, and smoking cessation.

Treatment for women with chronic hypertension focuses on maintaining normal blood pressure, preventing superimposed preeclampsia/eclampsia, and ensuring normal fetal development. Once the woman is pregnant, antihypertensive agents are typically reserved for severe hypertension (150 to 160 mmHg/100 to 110 mmHg). Methyldopa (Aldomet) is commonly prescribed because of its safety record during pregnancy. This slow-acting antihypertensive agent helps to improve uterine perfusion. Other antihypertensive agents that can be used include labetalol (Transdate), atenolol (Tenorium), and nifedipine (Procardia) (Gibson & Carson, 2007).

Lifestyle changes are needed and should continue throughout gestation. The woman with chronic hypertension will be seen more frequently (every 2 weeks until 28 weeks and then weekly until birth) to monitor her blood pressure and to assess for any signs of preeclampsia. At approximately 24 weeks' gestation, the woman will be instructed to document fetal movement. At this same time, serial ultrasounds will be ordered to monitor fetal growth and amniotic fluid volume. Additional tests will be included if the client's status changes.

Nursing Assessment

Nursing assessment of the woman with chronic hypertension involves a thorough history and physical examination. Review the woman's history closely for risk factors. The pathogenesis of hypertension is multifactorial and includes many modifiable risk factors such as smoking, obesity, caffeine intake, excessive alcohol intake, excessive salt intake, and use of nonsteroidal anti-inflammatory drugs. Also be alert for nonmodifiable risk factors such as increasing age and African-American race (Sharp, 2006). Ask if the woman has received any preconceptual counseling and what measures have been used to prevent or control hypertension.

Assess the woman's vital signs, in particular her blood pressure. Evaluate her blood pressure in all three positions (sitting, lying, and standing) and note any major differences in the readings. Assess her for orthostatic hypertension when she changes her position from sitting to standing. Document your findings.

· Ask the woman if she monitors her blood pressure at home; if so, inquire about the typical readings. Ask the woman if she uses any medications for blood pressure control, including the drug, dosage, and frequency of administration, as well as any side effects. Ask the woman about lifestyle modifications that she has used to address any modifiable risk factors, and their effectiveness.

Hypertension during pregnancy decreases uteroplacental perfusion. Therefore, fetal well-being must be assessed and closely monitored. Anticipate serial ultrasounds to assess fetal growth and amniotic fluid volume. Question the woman about fetal movement and evaluate her report of daily "kick counts." Assess fetal heart rate at every visit.

Nursing Management

Preconception counseling is the ideal time to discuss lifestyle changes to prevent or control hypertension. One area to cover during this visit would be the Dietary Approaches to Stop Hypertension (DASH) diet, which contains an adequate intake of potassium, magnesium, and calcium. Sodium is usually limited to 2.4 g. Suggest aerobic exercise, although the woman should cease it once the pregnancy is confirmed. Encourage smoking cessation and avoidance of alcohol. If the woman is overweight, encourage her to lose weight before becoming pregnant, not during the pregnancy (Dudek, 2006). Stressing the positive benefits of a healthy lifestyle might help motivate the woman to make the modifications and change unhealthy habits.

Assist the woman in scheduling appointments for antepartum visits every 2 weeks until 28 weeks' gestation and then weekly. Prepare the woman for frequent fetal assessments. Explaining the rationale for the need to monitor fetal growth is important to gain the woman's cooperation. Carefully monitor the woman for signs and symptoms of abruptio placentae (abdominal pain, rigid abdomen, vaginal bleeding), as well as superimposed preeclampsia (elevation in blood pressure, weight gain, edema, proteinuria). Alerting the woman to these risks allows early identification and prompt intervention.

Stress the importance of daily periods of rest (1 hour) in the left lateral recumbent position to maximize placental perfusion. Encourage women with chronic hypertension to use home blood pressure monitoring devices. Urge the woman to report any elevations. As necessary, instruct the woman and her family how to take and record a daily blood pressure, and reinforce the need for her to take her medications as prescribed to control her blood pressure and to ensure the well-being of her unborn child. Praising her for her efforts at each prenatal visit may motivate her to continue the regimen throughout her pregnancy.

The close monitoring of the woman with chronic hypertension continues during labor and birth and during the postpartum period to prevent or identify the onset of preeclampsia. Accurate and frequent blood pressure readings and careful administration of antihypertensive medications, if prescribed, are essential components of care. Stressing the need for continued medical supervision after childbirth is vital to motivate the woman to maintain or initiate lifestyle changes and dietary habits and stay compliant with her medication regimen.

Respiratory Conditions

During pregnancy, the respiratory system is affected by hormonal changes, mechanical changes, and prior respiratory conditions. These changes can cause a woman with a history of compromised respiration to decompensate during pregnancy. While upper respiratory infections are typically self-limiting, chronic respiratory conditions, such as asthma or tuberculosis, can have a negative effect on the growing fetus when alterations in oxygenation occur in the mother. The outcome of pregnancy in a woman with a respiratory condition depends on the severity of the oxygen alteration as well as the degree and duration of hypoxia on the fetus.

▶ ASTHMA

Asthma affects approximately 1% to 4% of pregnancies. It affects 20 million Americans and is one of the most common and potentially serious medical conditions to complicate pregnancy (Arenson & Drake, 2007). Maternal asthma is associated with an increased risk of infant death, preeclampsia, intrauterine growth retardation (IUGR), preterm birth, and low birthweight. These risks are linked to the severity of asthma: more severe asthma increases the risk (National Asthma Education Prevention Program [NAEPP], 2007).

Remember Rose, the pregnant teenager with asthma in acute distress described at the beginning of the chapter? What therapies might be offered to control her symptoms? Should she be treated differently than someone who is not pregnant? Why or why not?

Pathophysiology

Asthma, an allergic-type inflammatory response of the respiratory tract to various stimuli, is also known as reactive airway disease because the bronchioles constrict in response to allergens, irritants, and infections. In addition to bronchoconstriction, inflammation of the airways produces thick mucus that further limits the movement of air and makes breathing difficult.

The normal physiologic changes of pregnancy affect the respiratory system. While the respiratory rate does not change, hyperventilation increases at term by 48% due to high progesterone levels. Diaphragmatic elevation and a decrease in functional lung residual capacity occur late in pregnancy, which may reduce the woman's ability to inspire deeply to take in more oxygen. Oxygen consumption and the metabolic rate both increase, placing additional stress on the woman's respiratory system (American Academy of Allergy, Asthma, and Immunology [AAAAI], 2007).

Both the woman and her fetus are at risk if asthma is not well managed during pregnancy. When a pregnant woman has trouble breathing, her fetus also has trouble getting the oxygen it needs for adequate growth and development. Severe persistent asthma has been linked to the development of maternal hypertension, preeclampsia, placenta previa, uterine hemorrhage, and oligohydramnios. Women whose asthma is poorly controlled during pregnancy are at increased risk of preterm birth, low birthweight, and stillbirth (Hackley, Kriebs, & Rousseau, 2007).

The severity of the condition improves in one third of pregnant women, remains unchanged in one third, and worsens in one third (Hackley, Kriebs, & Rousseau, 2007). However, the effect of pregnancy on asthma is unpredictable. The greatest increase in asthma attacks usually occurs between 24 and 36 weeks' gestation; flare-ups are rare during the last 4 weeks of pregnancy and during labor (AAAAI, 2007).

Therapeutic Management

Asthma should be treated as aggressively in pregnant women as in nonpregnant women because the benefits of averting an asthma attack outweigh the risks of medications. The goals of treatment are to prevent hospitalization, emergency room visits, work loss, and chronic disability. NAEPP recommends three specific drugs to be used during pregnancy to control asthma:

- Budesonide (inhaled-corticosteroid)
- Albuterol (short-acting beta2 agonist)
- Salmeterol (long-acting beta2 agonist)

Oral corticosteroids are not recommended for the treatment of asthma during pregnancy, but they can be used to treat severe asthma attacks during pregnancy (AAAAI, 2007).

Nursing Assessment

Obtain a thorough history of the disease, including the woman's usual therapy and control measures. Question the woman about asthma triggers and strategies used to reduce exposure to them (Box 20.2). Review the client's medication therapy regimen.

Auscultate the lungs and assess respiratory and heart rates. Include the rate, rhythm, and depth of respirations; skin color; blood pressure and pulse rate; and signs of fatigue. Patients with an acute asthma attack often present with wheezing, chest tightness, tachypnea, nonproductive coughing, shortness of breath, and dyspnea. Lung auscultation findings might include diffuse wheezes and rhonchi, bronchovesicular sounds, and a more prominent expiratory phase of respiration compared to the inspiratory phase (More, 2007). If the pregnancy is far enough along, the fetal heart rate is measured and routine prenatal assessments (weight, blood pressure, fundal height, urine for protein) are completed.

Laboratory studies usually include a complete blood count with differential (to assess the degree of nonspecific inflammation and identify anemia) and pulmonary function tests (to assess the severity of an attack and to provide a baseline to evaluate the client's response to treatment).

Nursing Management

Nursing management focuses on client education about the condition and the skills necessary to manage it: self-monitoring, correct use of inhalers, identifying and limiting exposure to asthma triggers, and following a long-term plan for managing asthma and for promptly handling signs and symptoms of worsening asthma. Client education fosters adherence to the treatment regimen, thereby promoting an optimal environment for fetal growth and development.

Ensure that the woman understands drug actions and interactions, the uses and potential abuses of asthma

---

BOX 20.2 Common Asthma Triggers

- Smoke and chemical irritants
- Air pollution
- Dust mites
- Animal dander
- Seasonal changes with pollen, molds, and spores
- Upper respiratory infections
- Esophageal reflux
- Medications, such as aspirin and nonsteroidal anti-inflammatory drugs (NSAIDs)
- Exercise
- Cold air
- Emotional stress

Sources: AAAAI, 2007; Little & Sinert, 2008; Gilbert, 2007.

medications, and the signs and symptoms that require medical evaluation. Reviewing potential perinatal complications with the woman is helpful in motivating her to adhere to the prescribed regimen. At each antepartum visit, reassess the efficacy of the treatment plan to determine whether adjustments are needed.

Taking control of asthma in pregnancy is the responsibility of the client along with her health care team. Providing the client with the knowledge and tools to monitor her condition, control triggers and her environment (Teaching Guidelines 20.2), and use medications to prevent acute exacerbations assist the client in taking control. Facilitating a partnership with the woman will improve perinatal outcomes.

When teaching the pregnant woman with asthma, cover the following topics:

• Signs and symptoms of asthma progression and exacerbation
• Importance and safety of medication to the fetus and to herself
• Warning signs that indicate the need to contact the health care provider
• Potential harm to the fetus and to herself by undertreatment or delay in seeking help
• Prevention and avoidance of known triggers
• Home use of metered-dose inhalers
• Adverse effects of medications

During labor, monitor the client's oxygenation saturation by pulse oximetry and provide pain management

TEACHING GUIDELINES 20.2

Teaching to Control Environmental Triggers

• Remove any carpeting in the house, especially the bedroom, to reduce dust mites.
• Use allergen-proof encasing on the mattress, box spring, and pillows.
• Wash all bedding in hot water.
• Remove dust collectors in house, such as stuffed animals, books, knick-knacks.
• Avoid pets in the house to reduce exposure to pet dander.
• Use a high-efficiency particulate air-filtering system in the bedroom.
• Do not smoke, and avoid places where you can be exposed to passive cigarette smoke from others.
• Stay indoors and use air conditioning when the pollen or mold count is high or air quality is poor.
• Wear a covering over your nose and mouth when going outside in the cold weather.
• Avoid exposure to persons with colds, flu, or viruses.

through epidural analgesia to reduce stress, which may trigger an acute attack. Continuously monitor the fetus for distress during labor and assess fetal heart rate patterns for hypoxia. Assess the newborn for signs and symptoms of hypoxia.

▶ *Take NOTE!*

Successful asthma management can reduce adverse perinatal outcomes: preeclampsia, preterm birth, and low birthweight.

Rose, the pregnant teenager described earlier, is concerned about passing her asthma on to her baby. What should the nurse discuss with her? What questions should the nurse ask to help in identifying triggers in Rose's environment to prevent future asthma attacks?

▶ TUBERCULOSIS

Tuberculosis (TB) is a disease that has been around for years but never seems to go away completely. Globally, TB is second only to HIV/AIDS as a cause of illness and death in adults, accounting for over 9 million cases of active disease and 2 million deaths each year. Someone in the world is newly infected with TB every second. Overall, one third of the world's population is currently infected with TB (World Health Organization [WHO], 2007). Although it is not prevalent in the United States, a resurgence was noted starting in the mid-1980s secondary to the AIDS epidemic and immigration. Left undiagnosed and untreated, each person with active TB will infect on average between 10 and 15 people each year (WHO, 2007). With the large numbers of immigrants coming to the United States, all nurses must be skilled in screening for and managing this condition.

A person becomes infected by inhaling the infectious organism, *Mycobacterium tuberculosis*, which is carried on a droplet nuclei and spread by airborne transmission. The lung is the major site of involvement, but the lymph glands, meninges, bones, joints, and kidneys can become infected. Women can remain asymptomatic for long periods of time as the organism may lie dormant. Pregnant women with untreated TB are more likely to have preeclampsia, miscarriage, preterm labor, an underweight infant, an infant with a low Apgar score, and perinatal death (Bothamley, 2006). The newborn is at risk of postnatally acquired TB if the mother still has active TB at the time of birth. Therefore, prenatal diagnosis and effective treatment of the mother are essential.

Therapeutic Management

Therapeutic management of TB during pregnancy is essentially the same as that for the general population. Medications are the cornerstone of treatment to prevent infection from progressing. The medical therapy for pregnant women is a combination of medications such as isoniazid, rifampin, and ethambutol, taken daily for up to 9 months. These anti-TB agents appear to have minimal teratogenic risks and may be started as soon as the diagnosis of TB is made. However, extensive research has not been done to determine the definitive safety of these drugs (Herchline & Amorosa, 2007).

Nursing Assessment

Review the woman's history for risk factors such as immunocompromised status, recent immigration status, homelessness or overcrowded living conditions, and injectable drug use. Women emigrating from developing countries such as Latin America, Asia, the Indian subcontinent, Eastern Europe, Russia, China, Mexico, Haiti, and Africa with high rates of TB also are at risk.

At antepartum visits, be alert for clinical manifestations of TB, including fatigue, fever or night sweats, nonproductive cough, slow weight loss, anemia, hemoptysis, and anorexia (Noyes & Popay, 2007). If TB is suspected or the woman is at risk for developing TB, anticipate screening with purified protein derivative (PPD) administered by intradermal injection. If the client has been exposed to TB, a reddened induration will appear within 72 hours. If the test is positive, anticipate a follow-up chest x-ray with lead shielding over the abdomen and sputum cultures to confirm the diagnosis.

Nursing Management

Compliance with the multidrug therapy is critical to protect the woman and her fetus from progression of TB. Provide education about the disease process, the mode of transmission, prevention, potential complications, and the importance of adhering to the treatment regimen.

Stressing the importance of health-promotion activities throughout the pregnancy is important. Some suggestions might include avoiding crowded living conditions, avoiding sick people, maintaining adequate hydration, eating a nutritious, well-balanced diet, keeping all prenatal appointments to evaluate fetal growth and well-being, and getting plenty of fresh air by going outside frequently. Determining the woman's understanding of her condition and treatment plan is important for compliance. A language interpreter may be needed to validate and reinforce her understanding if she does not speak English.

Breastfeeding is not contraindicated during the medication regimen and should in fact be encouraged. Management of the newborn of a mother with TB involves preventing transmission by teaching the parents not to cough, sneeze, or talk directly into the newborn's face. Nurses need to stay current about new therapies and screening techniques to treat this centuries-old disease.

Hematologic Conditions

Anemia, a reduction in red blood cell volume, is measured by hematocrit (Hct) or a decrease in the concentration of hemoglobin (Hgb) in the peripheral blood. This results in reduced capacity of the blood to carry oxygen to the vital organs of the mother and fetus. Anemia is a sign of an underlying problem but does not indicate its origin.

▶ IRON DEFICIENCY ANEMIA

Iron deficiency anemia affects one in four pregnancies and is usually related to an inadequate dietary intake of iron (McCann, 2007). It is a very common state in pregnant women. Anemia during the early part of pregnancy can increase the likelihood of preterm birth, low birthweight, and perinatal mortality (Blackburn, 2007). With significant maternal iron depletion, the fetus will attempt to store iron, but at the cost to the mother. Anemia at term increases the perinatal risk for both the mother and newborn. The risks of hemorrhage (impaired platelet function) and infection during and after birth also are increased.

Therapeutic Management

The goals of treatment for iron deficiency anemia in pregnancy are to eliminate symptoms, correct the deficiency, and replenish iron stores. The CDC recommends routine iron supplementation for all pregnant women at a low dose of 30 mg/day beginning at the first prenatal visit. Attempting to meet maternal iron requirements solely through diet in the face of diminished iron stores is difficult.

Nursing Assessment

Review the mother's history for factors that may contribute to the development of iron deficiency anemia, including poor nutrition, hemolysis, **pica** (consuming non-food substances), multiple gestation, limited intervals between pregnancies, and blood loss. Assess the woman's dietary intake as well as the quantity and timing of ingestion of substances that interfere with iron absorption, such as tea, coffee, chocolate, and high-fiber foods. Ask the woman if she has fatigue, weakness, malaise, anorexia, or increased susceptibility to infection, such as frequent colds. Inspect the skin and mucous membranes, noting any pallor. Obtain vital signs and report any tachycardia.

Prepare the woman for laboratory testing. Laboratory tests usually reveal low Hgb (<11 g/dL), low Hct (<35%), low serum iron (<30 ug/dL), microcytic and hypochromic cells, and low serum ferritin (<100 mg/dL).

▶ *Take* NOTE!

Hemoglobin and hematocrit decrease normally during pregnancy in response to an increase in blood plasma in comparison to red blood cells. This hemodilution can lead to physiologic anemia of pregnancy, which is expected in the second trimester of pregnancy. This hemodilution phenomenon should not be confused with an iron deficiency anemia, in which the Hgb would be below 11 g/100 mL and Hct below 35%.

Nursing Management

Nursing management of the woman with iron deficiency anemia focuses on encouraging compliance with drug therapy and providing dietary instruction about the intake of foods high in iron. Although iron constitutes a minimal percentage of the body's total weight, it has several major roles: it assists in the transport of oxygen and carbon dioxide throughout the body, it aids in the production of red blood cells, and it plays a role in the body's immune response.

Stress the importance of taking the prenatal vitamin and iron supplement consistently. Encourage the woman to take the iron supplement with vitamin C-containing fluids such as orange juice, which will promote absorption, rather than milk, which can inhibit iron absorption. Taking iron on an empty stomach improves its absorption, but many women cannot tolerate the gastrointestinal discomfort it causes. In such cases, advise the woman to take it with meals. Instruct the woman about adverse effects, which are predominantly gastrointestinal and include gastric discomfort, nausea, vomiting, anorexia, diarrhea, metallic taste, and constipation. Suggest that the woman take the iron supplement with meals and increase her intake of fiber and fluids to help overcome the most common side effects.

Provide dietary counseling. Recommend foods high in iron, such as dried fruits, whole grains, green leafy vegetables, meats, peanut butter, and iron-fortified cereals (Dudek, 2006). Anticipate the need for a referral to a dietitian. Teaching Guidelines 20.3 highlights instructions for the pregnant woman with iron deficiency anemia.

▶ THALASSEMIA

Thalassemia is a group of hereditary anemias in which synthesis of one or both chains of the hemoglobin molecule (alpha and beta) is defective. A low Hgb and a microcytic, hypochromic anemia result. The prevalence and severity of thalassemia depend on the woman's racial

---

TEACHING GUIDELINES 20.3

Teaching for the Woman With Iron Deficiency Anemia

- Take your prenatal vitamin daily; if you miss a dose, take it as soon as you remember.
- For best absorption, take iron supplement between meals.
- Avoid taking iron supplement with coffee, tea, chocolate, and high-fiber food.
- Eat foods rich in iron, such as:
  - Meats, green leafy vegetables, legumes, dried fruits, whole grains
  - Peanut butter, bean dip, whole-wheat fortified breads and cereals
- For best iron absorption from foods, consume the food along with a food high in vitamin C.
- Increase your exercise, fluids, and high-fiber foods to reduce constipation.
- Plan frequent rest periods during the day.

background: persons of Mediterranean, Asian, Italian, or Greek heritage and African-Americans are most frequently affected. Beta-thalassemia is the most common form found in the United States (Curran & Poggi, 2007).

Thalassemia occurs in two forms: alpha-thalassemia and beta-thalassemia. Alpha-thalassemia (minor), the heterozygous form, results from the inheritance of one abnormal gene from either parent, placing the offspring in a carrier trait state. These women have little or no hematologic disease and are clinically asymptomatic (silent carrier state). Beta-thalassemia (major) is the form involving inheritance of the gene from both parents. Beta-thalassemia major can be very severe. Genetic counseling might be necessary when decisions about childbearing are being made.

Thalassemia minor has little effect on the pregnancy, although the woman will have mild, persistent anemia. This anemia does not respond to iron therapy, and iron supplements should not be prescribed. Women with thalassemia major do not usually become pregnant because of lifelong severe hemolysis, anemia, and premature death (Hackley, Kriebs, & Rousseau, 2007).

Management of thalassemia during pregnancy depends on the severity of the disease. Identification and screening are important to plan care. The woman's ethnic background, medical history, and blood studies are analyzed. If the woman is determined to be a carrier, screening of the father of the child is indicated. Knowledge of the carrier state of each parent provides the genetic counselor with knowledge about the risk that the fetus will be a carrier or will have the disease (Curran & Poggi, 2007).

CHAPTER 20 NURSING MANAGEMENT OF THE PREGNANCY AT RISK: SELECTED HEALTH CONDITIONS AND VULNERABLE POPULATIONS **609**

Mild anemia may be present, and instructions to rest and avoid infections are helpful. Nurses should provide supportive care and expectant management throughout the pregnancy.

SICKLE CELL ANEMIA

Sickle cell anemia is an autosomal recessive inherited condition that results from a defective hemoglobin molecule (hemoglobin S). It is found most commonly in African-Americans, Southeast Asians, and Middle Eastern populations. About 1 in 10 African-Americans are carriers of the trait, while approximately 3 in 800 are affected with the disease (McCann, 2007). People with only one gene for the trait (heterozygous) will have sickle cell trait without obvious symptoms of the disease and with little effect on the pregnancy.

Pathophysiology

In the human body, the hemoglobin molecule serves as the oxygen-carrying component of the red blood cells. Most people have several types of circulating hemoglobin (HbA and HbA2) that make up the majority of their circulatory system. In sickle cell disease, the abnormal hemoglobin S (HbS) replaces HbA and HbA2. This abnormal hemoglobin (HbS) becomes sickle-shaped as a result of any stress or trauma such as infection, fever, acidosis, dehydration, physical exertion, excessive cold exposure, or hypoxia. Significant anemia results. (See Chapter 46 for more information about sickle cell disease.)

Sickle cell anemia during pregnancy is associated with more severe anemia and frequent vaso-occlusive crises, with increased maternal and perinatal morbidity and mortality. In pregnant women with sickle cell anemia, complications can occur at any time during gestation, labor and birth, or postpartum. This is believed to be secondary to hormonal modifications, hypercoagulable state, and increased susceptibility to infection. Microvascular sickling in the placental circulation is associated with miscarriages, placental abruption, preeclampsia, preterm labor, intrauterine growth restriction, and low birthweight (El-sayegh & Shapiro, 2007).

Therapeutic Management

Ideally, women with hemoglobinopathies are screened before conception and are made aware of the risks of sickle cell anemia to themselves and to the fetus. A blood hemoglobin electrophoresis is done for all women from high-risk ancestry at their first prenatal visit to determine the types and percentages of hemoglobin present. This information should help them in making reproductive decisions.

Treatment depends on the health status of the woman. During pregnancy, only supportive therapy is used: blood transfusions for severe anemia, analgesics for pain, and antibiotics for infection.

Nursing Assessment

Assess the woman for signs and symptoms of sickle cell anemia. Ask the woman if she has anorexia, dyspnea, or malaise. Inspect the color of the skin and mucous membranes, noting any pallor. Be alert for indicators of sickle cell crisis, including severe abdominal pain, muscle spasms, leg pains, joint pain, fever, stiff neck, nausea and vomiting, and seizures (McCann, 2007).

Nursing Management

Clients require emotional support, education, and follow-up care to deal with this chronic condition, which can have a great impact on the woman and her family. Monitor vital signs, fetal heart rate, weight gain, and fetal growth. Assess hydration status at each visit and urge the client to drink 8 to 10 glasses of fluid daily to prevent dehydration. Teach the client about the need to avoid infections (including meticulous handwashing), cigarette smoking, alcohol consumption, and temperature extremes.

Assist the woman in scheduling frequent fetal well-being assessments, such as biophysical profiles, nonstress tests, and contraction stress tests, and monitor laboratory test results for changes. Throughout the antepartal period, be alert for early signs and symptoms of crisis.

During labor, encourage rest and provide pain management. Oxygen supplementation is typically used throughout labor, along with intravenous fluids to maintain hydration. The fetal heart rate is monitored closely. After giving birth, the woman is fitted with antiembolism stockings to prevent blood clot formation. Before discharge from the facility after birth of the newborn, discuss family planning options.

Infections

A wide variety of infections can affect the progression of pregnancy, possibly having a negative impact on the outcome. The effect of the infection depends on the timing and severity of the infection and the body systems involved. Common viral infections include cytomegalovirus (CMV), rubella, herpes simplex, hepatitis B, varicella, parvovirus B19, and several sexually transmitted infections (Table 20.3). Toxoplasmosis and group B streptococcus are common nonviral infections. Only the most common infections will be discussed here.

CYTOMEGALOVIRUS

Cytomegalovirus (CMV) is the most common congenital and perinatal viral infection in the world, possibly affecting up to 3% of all newborns (Ross, Jones, & Lynch,

TABLE 20.3 SEXUALLY TRANSMITTED INFECTIONS AFFECTING PREGNANCY

Infection/Organism	Effect on Pregnancy and Fetus/Newborn	Implications
Syphilis (*Treponema pallidum*)	Maternal infection increases risk of premature labor and birth. Newborn may be born with congenital syphilis—jaundice, rhinitis, anemia, IUGR, and CNS involvement.	All pregnant women should be screened for this STI and treated with benzathine penicillin G 2.4 million units IM to prevent placental transmission.
Gonorrhea (*Neisseria gonorrhoeae*)	Majority of women are asymptomatic. It causes ophthalmia neonatorum in the newborn from birth through infected birth canal.	All pregnant women should be screened at first prenatal visit, with repeat screening in the third trimester. All newborns receive mandatory eye prophylaxis with tetracycline or erythromycin within the first hour of life. Mother is treated with ceftriaxone (Rocephin) 125 mg IM in single dose before going home.
Chlamydia (*Chlamydia trachomatis*)	Majority of women are asymptomatic. Infection is associated with infertility and ectopic pregnancy, spontaneous abortions, preterm labor, premature rupture of membranes, low birthweight, stillbirth, and neonatal mortality. Infection is transmitted to newborn through vaginal birth. Neonate may develop conjunctivitis or pneumonia.	All pregnant women should be screened at first prenatal visit and treated with erythromycin.
Human papillomavirus (HPV)	Infection causes warts in the anogenital area, known as condylomata acuminata. These warts may grow large enough to block a vaginal birth. Fetal exposure to HPV during birth is associated with laryngeal papillomas.	Warts are treated with trichlorocetic acid, liquid nitrogen, or laser therapy under colposcopy. A quadrivalent HPV vaccine (Gardasil) against the viral types most likely to cause cervical cancer (types 16 and 18) and genital warts (types 6 and 11) has been licensed in the United States for girls and women 9 to 26 years old. The vaccine is 95% to 100% effective (Zimmerman, 2007). It is hoped that this vaccine will reduce the number of HPV-positive pregnant women in the future.
Trichomonas (*Trichomonas vaginalis*)	Infection produces itching and burning, dysuria, strawberry patches on cervix, and vaginal discharge. Infection is associated with premature rupture of membranes and preterm birth.	Treatment is with a single 2-g dose of metronidazole (Flagyl).

Sources: CDC STD Treatment Guidelines, 2006; Moore & Saybold, 2007.

2006). Pregnant women acquire active disease primarily from sexual contact, blood transfusions, kissing, and contact with children in daycare centers. The virus can be found in virtually all body fluids. Prevalence rates in women in the United States range from 50% to 85% (Hoerst & Samson, 2007). The incidence of primary CMV infection in pregnant women in the United States ranges from 1% to 3% (Hoerst & Samson, 2007). CMV infection during pregnancy may result in abortion, stillbirth, low birthweight, IUGR, microcephaly, deafness, blindness, mental retardation, jaundice, or congenital or neonatal infection. The first or primary infection, if it occurs during pregnancy, is the most dangerous to the fetus: the fetus has a 40% to 50% chance of being infected.

Most women are asymptomatic and don't know they have been exposed to CMV. Symptoms of CMV in the fetus and newborn, known as cytomegalovirus inclusion disease (CID), include hepatomegaly, thrombocytopenia, IUGR, jaundice, microcephaly, hearing loss, chorioretinitis, and mental retardation (Hoerst & Samson, 2007). Since there is no therapy that prevents or treats CMV infections, nurses are responsible for educating and supporting childbearing-age women at risk for CMV infection. Stressing the importance of good handwashing and use of sound hygiene practices can help to reduce transmission of the virus.

▶ RUBELLA

Rubella, commonly called German measles, is spread by droplets or through direct contact with a contaminated object. The risk of a pregnant woman transmitting this virus through the placenta to her fetus increases with earlier exposure to the virus. When infection occurs within the first month after conception, 50% of fetuses show signs of infection; in the second month following conception, 25% of fetuses will be infected; and in the third month, 10% of fetuses will be affected (Santis et al., 2006).

Education for primary prevention is key. Ideally, all women have been vaccinated and have adequate immunity against rubella. However, all women are still screened at their first prenatal visit to determine their status. A rubella antibody titer 1:8 or greater proves evidence of immunity. Women who are not immune should be vaccinated during the immediate postpartum period so they will be immune before becoming pregnant again (CDC, 2007c). Nurses need to check the rubella immune status of all new mothers and should make sure all mothers with a titer of less than 1:8 are immunized prior to discharge after birth of the newborn.

▶ HERPES SIMPLEX VIRUS

Approximately 50 million people are infected with genital herpes in the United States, and 500,000 new cases are diagnosed annually. Despite strategies designed to prevent perinatal transmission, the number of cases of newborn herpes simplex virus (HSV) infection continues to rise, mirroring the rising prevalence of genital herpes infection in women of childbearing age (Fischer, 2007).

HSV is a DNA virus with two subtypes: HSV-1 and HSV-2. HSV-1 infections were traditionally associated with oral lesions (fever blisters), whereas HSV-2 infections occurred in the genital region. Currently, either type can be found in either location (Fischer, 2007).

Infection occurs by direct contact of the skin or mucous membranes with an active lesion through such activities as kissing, sexual (vaginal, oral, anal) contact, or routine skin-to-skin contact. HSV is associated with infections of the genital tract that when acquired during pregnancy can result in severe systemic symptoms in the mother and significant morbidity and mortality in the newborn (Baker, 2007). Once the virus enters the body, it never leaves.

Infants born to mothers with a primary HSV infection have a 30% to 50% risk of acquiring the infection via perinatal transmission near or during birth. Recurrent genital herpes simplex infections carry a 1% to 3% risk of neonatal infection if the recurrence occurs around the time of vaginal birth (Xu et al., 2007).

The greatest risk of transmission is when the mother develops a primary infection near term and it is not recognized. Most neonatal infections are acquired at or around the time of birth through either ascending infection after ruptured membranes or contact with the virus at the time of birth. The method and timing of birth in a woman with genital herpes are controversial. The CDC recommends that in the absence of active lesions, a vaginal birth is acceptable, but if the woman has active herpetic lesions near or at term, a cesarean birth should be planned (CDC, 2008).

Management for the woman with genital herpes during pregnancy involves caring for her as well as reducing the risk of newborn herpes. Since the majority of newborn herpes cases result from perinatal transmission of the virus during vaginal birth, and because transmission can result in severe neurologic impairment or death, treatment of the mother with an antiviral agent such as acyclovir must be started as soon as the culture comes back positive. Universal screening for herpes is not economically sound, so nurses need to remain knowledgeable about current practice to provide accurate and sensitive care to all women.

▶ HEPATITIS B VIRUS

Hepatitis B virus (HBV) is one of the most prevalent chronic diseases in the world. HBV can be transmitted through contaminated blood, illicit drug use, and sexual contact. The virus is 100 times more infectious than HIV and, unlike HIV, it can live outside the body in dried blood for more than a week (Hoerst & Samson, 2007).

Sexual transmission accounts for most adult HBV infections in the United States. Acutely infected women develop hepatitis with anorexia, nausea, vomiting, fever, abdominal pain, and jaundice. In women with acute hepatitis B, vertical transmission occurs in approximately 10% of newborns when infection occurs in the first trimester and in 80% to 90% of newborns when acute infection occurs in the third trimester. Without intervention, 70% to 90% of infants born to women who are positive for hepatitis B will have chronic hepatitis B by 6 months of age (Kripke, 2007).

In addition, hepatitis B infection during pregnancy is associated with an increased risk of preterm birth, low birthweight, and neonatal death. Newborns infected with HBV are likely to become chronic carriers of the virus, becoming reservoirs for continued infection in the population (CDC, 2007e). The fetus is at particular risk during birth because of the possible contact with contaminated blood at this time.

Nursing Assessment

Review the woman's history for factors placing her at high risk:

• History of sexually transmitted infections
• Household contacts with HBV-infected persons
• Employment as a health care worker
• Abuse of intravenous drugs
• Sex worker (prostitute)
• Foreign born
• Multiple sexual partners
• Chinese, Southeast Asian, or African heritage
• Sexual partners who are HBV infected (CDC, 2007e)

At the first prenatal visit, all pregnant women should be screened for hepatitis B surface antigen (HbsAg) via blood studies. Expect to repeat this screening later in pregnancy for women in high-risk groups (Hoerst & Samson, 2007).

Nursing Management

If a woman tests positive for HBV, expect to administer HBV immune globulin (HBIG, Hep-B-Gammagee). The newborn receives HBV vaccine (Recombivax-HB, Engerix-B) within 12 hours of birth. The second and third doses of the vaccine are given at 1 month and 6 months of age (CDC, 2007e). The CDC recommends routine vaccination of all newborns.

Women who are HbsAg-negative may be vaccinated safely during pregnancy. No current research supports the use of surgical births to reduce vertical transmission of HBV. Breastfeeding by mothers with chronic HBV infection does not increase the risk of viral transmission to their newborns (Pyrsopoulos & Reddy, 2007).

Client education related to prevention of HBV is essential. Teach the woman about safer sex practices, good handwashing techniques, and the use of standard precautions (Teaching Guidelines 20.4). Protection can be afforded with the highly effective hepatitis B vaccine.

Permanent remission of the disease even with treatment rarely occurs. Therefore, therapy is directed at long-term suppression of viral replication and prevention of end-stage liver disease. Urge the woman to consume a

TEACHING GUIDELINES 20.4

Teaching to Prevent Hepatitis B Virus

• Abstain from alcohol.
• Avoid intravenous drug exposure or sharing of needles.
• Encourage all household contacts and sexual partners to be vaccinated.
• Receive immediate treatment for any sexually transmitted infection.
• Know that your newborn will receive the hepatitis B vaccine soon after birth.
• Use good handwashing techniques at all times.
• Avoid contact with blood or body fluids.
• Use barrier methods such as condoms during sexual intercourse.
• Avoid sharing any personal items, such as razors, toothbrushes, or eating utensils.

high-protein diet and avoid fatigue. A healthy lifestyle can help delay disease progression. Initiate an open discussion about the modes of transmission and use of condoms to prevent spread.

▶ VARICELLA ZOSTER VIRUS

Varicella zoster virus (VZV), a member of the herpesvirus family, is the virus that causes both varicella (chickenpox) and herpes zoster (shingles). Pregnant women are at risk for developing varicella when they come in close contact with children who have active infection. Maternal varicella can be transmitted to the fetus through the placenta, leading to congenital varicella syndrome, if the mother is infected during the first half of pregnancy, via an ascending infection during birth, or by direct contact with infectious lesions, leading to infection after birth. Varicella occurs in approximately 1 to 7 of 10,000 pregnancies (Anderson & Safdar, 2007).

Congenital varicella syndrome can occur in newborns of mothers infected during early pregnancy. It is characterized by low birthweight, skin lesions in a dermatomal distribution, spontaneous abortion, chorioretinitis, cataracts, cutaneous scarring, limb hypoplasia, microcephaly, ocular abnormalities, mental retardation, and early death (Laartz & Gompf, 2007).

Preconception counseling is important for preventing this condition. A major component of counseling involves determining the woman's varicella immunity. The vaccine is administered if needed. Provide education to women who work in occupations that increase the risk of exposure to the virus, such as daycare workers, teachers of young children, and staff caring for children in institutional settings.

Varicella during pregnancy can be associated with severe illnesses for both the mother and her newborn. If contracted in the first half of pregnancy, some pregnant women are at risk for developing varicella pneumonia, which may put them at risk of life-threatening ventilatory compromise and death (Sauerbrei & Wutzler, 2007). If the mother develops varicella rashes close to her due date, generalized neonatal varicella leading to death in about 20% of cases can be expected (Gardella & Brown, 2007). Maternal infection is preventable by preconception vaccination.

▶ PARVOVIRUS B19

Parvovirus B19 infection occurs worldwide. The incidence of acute B19 infection in pregnancy is about 3% (Malee, 2007). Parvovirus B19 is a common, self-limiting benign childhood virus that causes erythema infectiosum, also known as fifth disease (referring to its "fifth place" in a list of common childhood infections). Approximately 50% to 65% of women of reproductive age have developed immunity to parvovirus B19 (Broliden, Tolfvenstam, & Norbeck, 2006).

Pathophysiology

The infection is spread transplacentally, by the oropharyngeal route in casual contact, and through infected blood. Infection of the fetus occurs through transplacental passage of the virus. Acute infection in pregnancy can cause B19 infection in the fetus, leading to nonimmune fetal hydrops secondary to severe anemia or fetal loss, depending on the gestational age at the time of infection. The risk to the fetus is greatest when the woman is exposed and infected within the first 20 weeks of gestation. In addition to hydrops, other fetal effects of parvovirus include spontaneous abortion, congenital anomalies (central nervous system, craniofacial, and eye), and long-term effects such as hepatic insufficiency, myocarditis, and learning disabilities (Cunningham & Rennels, 2006).

Therapeutic Management

Generally, diagnosis of parvovirus is based on clinical symptoms and serologic antibody testing for parvovirus immunoglobulin G and parvovirus immunoglobulin M (IgM). Parvovirus B19 infection is followed by lifelong immunity, which is shown by positive serum B19 IgG. Pregnant women who have been exposed to or who develop symptoms of parvovirus B19 require assessment to determine whether they are susceptible to infection (nonimmune). If the woman is immune, she can be reassured

that she will not develop infection and that the virus will not adversely affect her pregnancy. If she is nonimmune, then referral to a perinatologist is recommended and counseling regarding the risks of fetal transmission, fetal loss, and hydrops is necessary. Knowledge of how best to manage it during pregnancy lags behind our understanding of the potential adverse consequences.

Intrauterine B19 infection is a cause of fetal anemia, hydrops, and demise, and perhaps also of congenital anomalies. The best strategy for surveillance of the infected pregnant woman is serial ultrasounds for detection of hydropic changes and fetal anemia, and treatment for severe fetal anemia. Serial ultrasounds are advocated because the rates of fetal death and complications peak 4 to 6 weeks after exposure, but they can occur as late as 3 months following onset of symptoms (Elbaz et al., 2007).

The infected newborn is assessed for any anomaly and followed for up to 6 years to identify any sequelae (Cunningham & Rennels, 2006).

Nursing Assessment

Review the mother's history for any risk factors. Schoolteachers, daycare workers, and women living with school-aged children are at highest risk for being seropositive for parvovirus B19, especially if a recent outbreak has occurred in those settings. Also assess the woman for specific signs and symptoms. The characteristic rash starts on the face with a "slapped-cheeks" appearance and is followed by a generalized maculopapular rash. Fever, arthralgia, and generalized malaise are usually present in the mother. Prepare the mother for antibody testing.

Nursing Management

Prevention is the best strategy. Stress the need for handwashing after handling children; cleaning toys and surfaces that children have been in contact with; and avoiding the sharing of food and drinks. Screening for parvovirus B19 during early pregnancy may help in early diagnosis, but the cost-effectiveness of a national screening program has not been accepted to date. The nurse can provide information regarding risk factors and potential complications if exposed and support the parent's decision.

▶ GROUP B STREPTOCOCCUS

Group B streptococcus (GBS) is a naturally occurring bacterium found in 10% to 35% of healthy adults. Women who test positive for the GBS bacteria are considered carriers. Carrier status is transient and doesn't indicate illness. Approximately 25% of pregnant women carry GBS in the rectum or vagina, thus introducing the risk of colonization of the fetus during birth. GBS affects about 1 in every 2,000 newborns in the United States

(March of Dimes, 2007d). Approximately 1 out of every 100 to 200 newborns born to mothers who carry GBS will develop signs and symptoms of GBS disease. Although GBS is rarely serious in adults, it can be life-threatening to newborns. GBS is the most common cause of sepsis and meningitis in newborns and is a frequent cause of newborn pneumonia (Moos, 2006). Newborns with early-onset (within a week after birth) GBS infections may have pneumonia or sepsis, whereas late-onset (after the first week) infections often manifest with meningitis (CDC, 2007b).

Genital tract colonization poses the most threat to the newborn because of exposure during birth and to the mother because of ascending infection after the membranes rupture. GBS colonization in the mother is thought to cause chorioamnionitis, endometritis, and postpartum wound infection.

Therapeutic Management

Antibiotic therapy usually is effective in treating women with GBS infections of the urinary tract or uterus, or chorioamnionitis without any sequelae. According to the 2002 CDC guidelines, all pregnant women should be screened for GBS at 35 to 37 weeks' gestation. Vaginal and rectal specimens are cultured for the presence of the bacterium. If positive, the woman should be treated with intravenous antibiotics during labor.

Penicillin G is the treatment of choice for GBS infection because of its narrow spectrum. Alternative antibiotics can be prescribed for clients with a penicillin allergy. The drug is usually administered intravenously at least 4 hours before birth so that it can reach adequate levels in the serum and amniotic fluid to reduce the risk of newborn colonization. Close monitoring is required during the administration of intravenous antibiotics because severe allergic reactions can occur rapidly.

Nursing Assessment

Review the woman's prenatal history, asking about any previous infection. Determine if the woman's membranes have ruptured and the time of rupture. Rupture of amniotic membranes greater than 18 hours increases the risk for infection. Monitor the mother's vital signs, reporting any maternal fever greater than 100.4°F. Assess the woman for other risk factors for perinatal transmission of GBS, including previous colonization with GBS, low socioeconomic status, African-American race, age less than 20 years, positive colonization at 35 to 37 weeks' gestation, GBS in urine sample, previous birth of GBS-positive newborn, preterm birth, and use of invasive obstetric procedures (March of Dimes, 2007d). Document this information to help prevent vertical transmission to the newborn.

Many women with GBS infection are asymptomatic, but they may have urinary tract infections, uterine infections, and chorioamnionitis.

Nursing Management

Nurses play major roles as educators and advocates for all women and newborns to reduce the incidence of GBS infections. Ensure that pregnant women between 35 and 37 weeks' gestation are screened for GBS infection during a prenatal visit. Record the results and notify the birth attendant if the woman has tested positive for GBS. During labor, be prepared to administer intravenous antibiotics to all women who are GBS positive.

▶ TOXOPLASMOSIS

Toxoplasmosis is a relatively widespread parasitic infection caused by a one-celled organism, *Toxoplasma gondii.* When a pregnant woman is exposed to this protozoan, the infection can pose serious risks to her fetus. Between 1 in 1,000 and 8,000 newborns are born infected with toxoplasmosis in the United States (Hokelek & Safdar, 2006). It is transferred by hand to mouth after touching cat feces while changing the cat litter box or through gardening in contaminated soil. Consuming undercooked meat, such as pork, lamb, or venison, can also transmit this organism.

A pregnant woman who contracts toxoplasmosis for the first time has approximately a 40% chance of passing the infection to her fetus (March of Dimes, 2007e). Although the woman typically remains asymptomatic, transmission to her fetus can occur throughout pregnancy. A fetus that contracts congenital toxoplasmosis typically has a low birthweight, enlarged liver and spleen, chorioretinitis, jaundice, neurologic damage, and anemia (Peyron et al., 2006).

Treatment of the woman during pregnancy to reduce the risk of congenital infection is a combination of pyrimethamine and sulfadiazine. Treatment with sulfonamides during pregnancy has been shown to reduce the risk of congenital infection.

Prevention is the key to managing this infection. Nurses play a key role in educating the woman about measures to prevent toxoplasmosis (Teaching Guidelines 20.5).

Vulnerable Populations

Every year there are an estimated 220 million pregnancies worldwide, with about 6 million of them in the United States (Alan Guttmacher Institute, 2007). Each pregnancy runs the risk of an adverse outcome for the mother and the baby, but risks are dramatically increased for certain vulnerable populations: adolescents, women over the age of 35, women who are HIV positive, and women who abuse substances. While risks cannot be totally eliminated once pregnancy has begun, they can be reduced through appropriate and timely interventions.

TEACHING GUIDELINES 20.5

Teaching to Prevent Toxoplasmosis

- Avoid eating raw or undercooked meat, especially lamb or pork. Cook all meat to an internal temperature of 160°F throughout.
- Clean cutting boards, work surfaces, and utensils with hot soapy water after contact with raw meat or unwashed fruits and vegetables.
- Peel or thoroughly wash all raw fruits and vegetables before eating them.
- Wash hands thoroughly with warm water and soap after handling raw meat.
- Avoid feeding the cat raw or undercooked meats.
- Avoid emptying or cleaning the cat's litter box. Have someone else do it daily.
- Keep the cat indoors to prevent it from hunting and eating birds or rodents.
- Avoid uncooked eggs and unpasteurized milk.
- Wear gardening gloves when in contact with outdoor soil.
- Avoid contact with children's sandboxes, because cats can use them as litter boxes.

Every woman's experience with pregnancy is unique and personal. The circumstances each one faces and what pregnancy means to her involve emotions and experiences that belong solely to her. Many women in these special population groups go through this experience in confusion and isolation, feeling desperately in need of help but not knowing where to go. Although all pregnant women experience these emotions to a certain extent, but they are heightened in women who have numerous psychosocial issues. Pregnancy is a stressful time. Pregnant women face wide-ranging changes in their lives, relationships, and bodies as they move toward parenthood. These changes can be challenging for a woman without any additional stresses but are even more so in the face of age extremes, illness, or substance abuse.

Skilled nursing interventions are essential to promote the best outcome for the client and her baby. Timely support and appropriate interventions during the perinatal period can have long-standing implications for the mother and her newborn, ultimately with the goal of stability and integration of the family as a unit.

▶ PREGNANT ADOLESCENT

Adolescence lasts from the onset of puberty to the cessation of physical growth, roughly from 11 to 19 years of age. Adolescents vacillate between being children and being adults. They need to adjust to the physiologic changes their bodies are undergoing and establish a sexual identity during this time. They search for personal identity and desire freedom and independence of thought and action. However, they continue to have a strong dependence on their parents (O'Toole, 2005).

Each year in the United States, approximately 1 million adolescents, or 10% of girls between the ages of 15 to 19 years, become pregnant. These pregnancies, which account for 11% of all births, are typically unintended and occur outside of marriage (Alan Guttmacher Institute, 2006). In addition, about half of all teen pregnancies occur within 6 months of first having sexual intercourse. Of girls who become pregnant, one in six will have a repeat pregnancy within 1 year. Most of these girls are unmarried, and many are not ready for the emotional, psychological, and financial responsibilities of parenthood (March of Dimes, 2007a). Adolescent pregnancy is further complicated by the adolescent's lack of financial resources: the income of teen mothers is half that of women who have given birth in their 20s (March of Dimes, 2007a).

Although the incidence of teenage pregnancy has steadily declined since the early 1990s, it continues to be higher in the United States than in any other industrialized country (Alan Guttmacher Institute, 2006). Even this reduced incidence represents what is considered an unacceptably high level of pregnancy in an age group that is likely to suffer the social consequences of early pregnancy most. Subsequently, adolescent pregnancy is considered a major health problem and is addressed in Healthy People 2010.

Impact of Pregnancy in Adolescence

Adolescents are a unique group with special needs related to their stage of development. Adolescent pregnancy can be an emotionally charged situation, laden with ethical dilemmas and decisions. Topics such as abstinence, safer sex, abortion, and the decision to have a child are sensitive issues.

HEALTHY PEOPLE 2010

Objective	Significance
Reduce pregnancy among adolescent females from a baseline of 68 pregnancies per 1,000 adolescent girls to 43 pregnancies per 1,000 adolescent girls	Will help to foster a continued decline in adolescent pregnancy rates by focusing on interventions related to pregnancy prevention, including safe sex practices and teaching about the complications associated with adolescent pregnancy

USDHHS, 2000.

Adolescent pregnancy is an area when a nurse's moral convictions may influence the care that he or she provides to clients. Nurses need to examine their own beliefs about teen sexuality to identify personal assumptions. Putting aside one's moral convictions may be difficult, but it is necessary when working with pregnant adolescents. To be effective, health care providers must be able to communicate with adolescents in a manner they can understand and respect them as individuals.

Developmental Issues

An adolescent must accomplish certain developmental tasks to advance to the next stage of maturity. These developmental tasks include:

- Seeking economic and social stability
- Developing a personal value system
- Building meaningful relationships with others (Fig. 20.3)
- Becoming comfortable with their changing bodies
- Working to become independent from their parents
- Learning to verbalize conceptually (Zarrett & Eccles, 2006)

Adolescents have special needs when working to accomplish their developmental tasks and making a smooth transition to young adulthood. One of the biggest areas of need is sexual health. Adolescents commonly lack the information, skills, and services necessary to make informed choices related to their sexual and reproductive health. Developmentally, adolescents are trying to figure out who they are and how they fit into society. As adolescents mature, their parents become less influential and peers become more influential. Peer pressure can lead adolescents to participate in sexual activity, as can the typical adolescent's belief that "it won't happen to me" (Box 20.3).

As a result, unplanned pregnancies occur. Work on the developmental tasks of adolescence, especially identity, can be interrupted as the adolescent attempts to integrate the tasks of pregnancy, bonding, and preparing to

FIGURE 20.3 Adolescent girls sharing time together.

BOX 20.3 Possible Factors Contributing to Adolescent Pregnancy

- Early menarche
- Peer pressure to become sexually active
- Sexual or other abuse as a child
- Lack of accurate contraceptive information
- Fear of telling parents about sexual activity
- Feelings of invulnerability
- Poverty (85% of births occur in poor families)
- Culture or ethnicity (high incidence in Hispanic and African-American girls)
- Unprotected sex
- Low self-esteem and inability to negotiate
- Lack of appropriate role models
- Strong need for someone to love
- Drug use, truancy from school, or other behavioral problems
- Wish to escape a bad home situation
- Early dating without supervision

Sources: March of Dimes, 2008; Langille, 2007.

---

care for another with the tasks of developing self-identity and independence. A pregnant adolescent must try to meet her own needs along with those of her fetus. The process of learning how to separate from the parents while learning how to bond and attach to a newborn brings conflict and stress. A pregnancy can exacerbate an adolescent's feeling of loss of control (Secco et al., 2007).

Health and Social Issues

Adolescent pregnancy has a negative impact in terms of both health and social consequences. For example, seven out of ten adolescents will drop out of school. More than 75% will receive public assistance within 5 years of having their first child. In addition, children of adolescent mothers are at greater risk of preterm birth, low birthweight, child abuse, neglect, poverty, and death (As-Sanie, Gantt, & Rosenthal, 2004). The younger the adolescent is at the time of the first pregnancy, the more likely it is that she will have another pregnancy during her teens (Holub et al., 2007).

The psychosocial risks associated with early childbearing often have an even greater impact on mothers, families, and society than the obstetric or medical risks (Zeck et al., 2007). Pregnant adolescents experience higher rates of domestic violence and substance abuse. Those experiencing abuse are more likely to abuse substances, receive inadequate prenatal care, and have lower pregnancy weight compared with those who are not (Magill & Wilcox, 2007). Moreover, substance abuse (cigarettes, alcohol, or illicit drugs) can contribute to low birthweight, IUGR, preterm births, newborn addiction, and sepsis (March of Dimes, 2007a).

Although early childbearing (12 to 19 years of age) occurs in all socioeconomic groups, it is more prevalent among poor women and those from minority backgrounds, who face more obstetric and newborn risks than their more affluent counterparts (March of Dimes, 2007a). Poverty often contributes to delayed prenatal care and medical complications related to poor nutrition, such as anemia.

The financial burden of adolescent pregnancy is high and costs taxpayers an estimated $7 billion to $15 billion annually in the United States (Alan Guttmacher Institute, 2007). Much of the expense stems from Medicaid, food stamps, state health department maternity clinics, Aid to Families and Children, and direct payments to health care providers. However, this amount does not address the costs to society in terms of the loss of human resources and the far-reaching intergenerational effects of adolescent parenting.

For some adolescents, pregnancy may be seen as a hopeless situation: a grim story of poverty and lost dreams, of being trapped in a life that was never wanted. Health-related behaviors, such as smoking, diet, sexual behavior, and help-seeking behaviors, that are developed during adolescence often endure into later life (Goodman et al., 2007). The consequences associated with an adolescent's less-than-optimal health status at this age due to pregnancy can ultimately affect her long-term health and that of her children.

However, some adolescents can create a happy, stable life for themselves and their children by facing their challenges and working hard to beat the odds.

Recall Rose, the pregnant teenager with asthma. What issues would be important for the nurse to discuss with her related to her pregnancy, her asthma, and her age?

Nursing Assessment

Assessment of the pregnant adolescent is the same as that for any pregnant woman. However, when dealing with pregnant teens, the nurse also needs to ask:

• How does the girl see herself in the future?
• Are realistic role models available to her?
• How much does she know about child development?
• What financial resources are available to her?
• Does she work? Does she go to school?
• What emotional support is available to her?
• Can she resolve conflicts and manage anger?
• What does she know about health and nutrition for herself and her child?
• Will she need help dealing with the challenges of the new parenting role?
• Does she need information about community resources?

Having an honest regard for adolescents requires getting to know them and being able to appreciate the important aspects of their life. Doing so forms a basis for the nurse's clinical judgment and promotes care that takes into account the concerns and practical circumstances of the teen and her family. Skillful practice includes knowing how and when to advise a teen and when to listen and refrain from giving advice. Giving advice can be misinterpreted as "preaching," and the adolescent will probably ignore the information. The nurse must be perceptive, flexible, and sensitive and must work to establish a therapeutic relationship.

Nursing Management

For adolescents, as for all women, pregnancy can be a physically, emotionally, and socially stressful time. The pregnancy is often both the result of and cause of social problems and stressors that can be overwhelming to them. Nurses must support adolescents during the transition from childhood into adulthood, which is complicated by their emergence into motherhood. Assist the adolescent in identifying family and friends who want to be involved and provide support throughout the pregnancy.

Help the adolescent identify the options for this pregnancy, such as abortion, self-parenting of the child, temporary foster care for the baby or herself, or placement of the child for adoption. Explore with the adolescent why she became pregnant. Becoming aware of why she decided to have a child is necessary to help with the development of the adolescent and her ability to parent. Identify barriers to seeking prenatal care, such as lack of transportation, too many problems at home, financial concerns, the long wait for an appointment, and lack of sensitivity on the part of the health care system. Encourage the girl to set goals and work toward them. Assist her in returning to school and furthering her education. As appropriate, initiate a referral for career or job counseling.

Stress that the girl's physical well-being is important for both her and her developing fetus, which depends on her for its own health-related needs. Assist with arrangements for care, including stress management and self-care.

Having a healthy newborn eases the transition to motherhood somewhat, rather than having to deal with the added stress of caring for an unhealthy baby (Secco et al., 2007). Monitor weight gain, sleep and rest patterns, and nutritional status to promote positive outcomes for both. Stress the importance of attending prenatal education classes. Provide appropriate teaching based on the adolescent's developmental level and emphasize the importance of continued prenatal and follow-up care. Monitor maternal and fetal well-being throughout pregnancy and labor (Fig. 20.4).

FIGURE 20.4 A pregnant adolescent receiving care during labor.

Nurses can also play a major role in preventing adolescent pregnancies, perhaps by volunteering to talk to teen groups. Box 20.4 highlights the key areas for teaching adolescents about pregnancy prevention.

Tackling the many issues surrounding adolescent pregnancy is difficult. Making connections with clients is crucial regardless of how complex their situation is. The future challenges nurses to find solutions to teenage pregnancies. Nurses must take proactive positions while working with adolescents, parents, schools, and communities to reduce the problems associated with early childbearing.

BOX 20.4 **Topics for Teaching Adolescents to Prevent Pregnancy**

- High-risk behaviors that lead to pregnancy
- Involvement in programs such as Free Teens, Teen Advisors, or Postponing Sexual Involvement
- Planning and goal setting to visualize their futures in terms of career, college, travel, and education
- Choice of abstinence or taking a step back to become a "second-time virgin"
- Discussions about sexuality with a wiser adult—someone they respect can help put things in perspective
- Protection against sexually transmitted infections and pregnancy if they choose to remain sexually active
- Critical observation and review of peers and friends to make sure they are creating the right atmosphere for friendship
- Empowerment to make choices that will shape their life for years to come, including getting control of their own lives now
- Appropriate use of recreational time, such as sports, drama, volunteer work, music, jobs, church activities, and school clubs

---

Sources: March of Dimes, 2007a; King-Jones, 2008; Lesesne et al., 2008.

▶ THE PREGNANT WOMAN OVER AGE 35

The term "elderly primip" is used to describe women ages 35 or older who are pregnant for the first time. A few decades ago, a woman having a baby after the age of 35 probably was giving birth to the last of several children, but today she may be having her first. With advances in technology and the tendency of women to seek career advancement prior to childbearing, the dramatic increase in women having first pregnancies after the age of 35 will likely continue.

Impact of Pregnancy on the Older Woman

Whether childbearing is delayed by choice or by chance, starting a family at age 35 is different and not without risks. Women in this age group may already have chronic health conditions that may put the pregnancy at risk. In addition, numerous studies have shown that increasing maternal age is a risk factor for infertility and spontaneous abortions, gestational diabetes, chronic hypertension, preeclampsia, preterm labor and birth, multiple pregnancy, genetic disorders and chromosomal abnormalities, placenta previa, IUGR, low Apgar scores, and surgical births (Hilton, 2006). However, even though increased age implies increased complications, most women today who become pregnant after age 35 have healthy pregnancies and healthy newborns (March of Dimes, 2007c).

Nursing Assessment

Nursing assessment of the pregnant woman over age 35 is the same as that for any pregnant woman. For a woman of this age, a preconception visit is important to identify chronic health problems that might affect the pregnancy and also to address lifestyle issues that may take time to modify. Encourage the older woman to plan for the pregnancy by seeing her health care provider before getting pregnant to discuss preexisting medical conditions, medications, and lifestyle choices. Assess the woman for risk factors such as cigarette smoking, poor nutrition, overweight or underweight, alcohol use, or illicit drug use.

A preconception visit also provides the opportunity to educate the woman about risk factors and provide information on how to modify her lifestyle habits to improve the pregnancy outcome. Assist the woman with lifestyle changes so that she can begin pregnancy in an optimal state of health. For example, if the woman is overweight, educate her about weight loss so that she can start the pregnancy at a healthy weight. If the woman smokes, encourage smoking cessation to reduce the effects of nicotine on herself and her fetus.

Prepare the woman for laboratory and diagnostic testing to establish a baseline for future comparisons. The risk of having a baby with Down syndrome increases with age, especially over age 35. Amniocentesis is routinely offered to all older women to allow the early detection of numerous chromosomal abnormalities, including Down syndrome. Additionally, a quadruple blood test screen (alpha fetoprotein [AFP], human chorionic gonadotropin [hCG], unconjugated estriol [UE], and inhibin A [placental hormone]) drawn between 15 and 20 weeks of pregnancy can be helpful in screening for Down syndrome and neural tube defects.

Nursing Management

During routine prenatal visits, the nurse can play a key role in promoting a healthy pregnancy. Consider social, genetic, and environmental factors that are unique to the older pregnant women and prepare to address these factors when providing care. Although research has shown increases in preterm labor and births, low-birthweight newborns, and operative interventions for older women, many carry their pregnancies to term without incident (Tough et al., 2007).

Assess the woman's knowledge about risk factors and measures to reduce them. Educate her about measures to promote a positive outcome. Encourage her to get early and regular prenatal care. Advise her to eat a variety of nutritious foods, especially fortified cereals, enriched grain products, and fresh fruits and vegetables, and drink at least six to eight glasses of water daily and to take the prescribed vitamin containing 400 micrograms of folic acid daily. Also stress the need for her to avoid alcohol intake during pregnancy, avoid exposure to second-hand smoke, and take no drugs unless they are prescribed. Provide continued surveillance of the mother and fetus throughout the pregnancy.

▶ WOMEN WHO ARE HIV POSITIVE

Human immunodeficiency virus (HIV) is a retrovirus that is transmitted by blood and body fluids. The number of people living with HIV infection in 2006 was estimated at nearly 40 million, including approximately 20 million women of childbearing age and 2.5 million children, most of whom acquired HIV from mother-to-child transmission (CDC, 2007a).

Despite the revolutionary strides that have been made in treatment and detection and recent clinical advances and cautious optimism associated with combination therapies and vaccines, the number of individuals who are HIV positive continues to climb worldwide. Intensive efforts notwithstanding, there still remains no real "cure" on the horizon (Lampe, 2006).

Historically, HIV/AIDS was associated with the male homosexual community and intravenous drug users, but currently the prevalence of HIV/AIDS is now increasing more rapidly among women than men. Women are the fastest-growing segment of persons becoming infected with HIV; transmission in women occurs most frequently from sexual contact (64%) and from intravenous drug use (33%) (CDC, 2007a). Most women, a large number of whom are mothers, have acquired the disease through heterosexual contact. The risk of acquiring HIV through heterosexual contact is greater for women due to exposure to the higher viral concentration in semen. In addition, sexual intercourse may cause breaks in the vaginal lining, increasing the chances that the virus will enter the woman's body. Fifty percent of all the HIV/AIDS cases worldwide occur in women. AIDS is the third leading cause of death among all U.S. women aged 25 to 44 years and the leading cause of death among African-American women in this age group (CDC, 2007a).

Pathophysiology

The three recognized modes of HIV transmission are unprotected sexual intercourse with an infected partner, contact with infected blood or blood products, and perinatal transmission.

> ▶ ***Take*** NOTE!
>
> *HIV is not transmitted by doorknobs, faucets, toilets, dirty dishes, mosquitoes, wet towels, coughing or sneezing, shaking hands, or being hugged or by any other indirect method.*

The virus attacks the T4 cells, decreases the CD4 cell count, and disables the immune system. The HIV condition can progress to a severe immunosuppressed state termed **acquired immunodeficiency syndrome (AIDS)**. AIDS is a progressive, debilitating disease that suppresses cellular immunity, predisposing the infected person to opportunistic infections and malignancies. The CDC defines AIDS as an HIV-infected person with a specific opportunistic infection or a CD4 count of less than 200. Eventually, death occurs. The time from infection with HIV to development of AIDS is a median of 11 years but varies depending on whether the patient is taking current antiretroviral therapy (Johnsen, 2007). Research indicates that pregnancy does not accelerate the progression of HIV to AIDS or death (Cressey & Lallemant, 2007).

Once infected with HIV, the woman develops antibodies that can be detected with the enzyme-linked immunosorbent assay (ELISA) and confirmed with the Western blot test. Antibodies develop within 6 to 12 weeks after exposure, although this latent period is much longer in some women. Table 20.4 highlights the four stages of HIV infection according to the CDC (2007a).

Impact of HIV on Pregnancy

When a woman who is infected with HIV becomes pregnant, the risks to herself, her fetus, and the newborn are great. The risks are compounded by problems such as drug abuse, lack of access to prenatal care, poverty, poor nutrition, and high-risk behaviors such as unsafe sex practices and multiple sex partners, which can predispose the woman to additional sexually transmitted infections such as herpes, syphilis, or human papillomavirus (HPV). Additional risk factors to assess for include women who exchange sex for money or drugs or have sex partners who do; women whose past or present sex partners were HIV infected; and women who had a blood transfusion between 1978 and 1985 (U.S. Preventive Services Task Force [USPSTF], 2006b). Subsequently, pregnant women who are HIV positive are at risk for preterm delivery, premature rupture of membranes, intrapartal or postpartum hemorrhage, postpartum infection, poor wound healing, and genitourinary tract infections (CDC, 2007a).

Perinatal transmission of HIV (from the mother to the fetus or child) also can occur. However, such cases have decreased in the past several years in the United States, primarily due to the use of zidovudine (ZDV) therapy in pregnant women infected with HIV. This has not been the case in poor countries without similar resources. The Joint United Nations programs on HIV/AIDS (UN-AIDS) estimates that over 600,000 new infections due to mother-to-child transmission occur annually. This number is expected to increase rapidly as the prevalence rises in Southeast Asia (Johnsen, 2007). Perinatal transmission rates are as high as 35% when there is no intervention (antiretroviral therapy) and below 5% when antiretroviral treatment and appropriate care are available.

With perinatal transmission, approximately 25% to 50% of children manifest AIDS within the first year of life, and about 80% have clinical symptoms of the disease within 3 to 5 years (Johnsen, 2007). Breastfeeding is a major contributing factor for mother-to-child transmission, and the infected mother must be informed about this (Dao et al., 2007). The U.S. Public Health Service recommends that women who are HIV positive should avoid breastfeeding to prevent HIV transmission to the newborn. Given the devastating effects of HIV infection on children, preventing its transmission is critical (Lampe, 2006).

In addition to perinatal transmission, the fetus and newborn also are at risk for prematurity, IUGR, low birthweight, and infection. Prompt treatment with antiretroviral medications for the HIV-infected infant may slow the progression of the disease.

Therapeutic Management

Women who are seropositive for HIV require counseling about the risk of perinatal transmission and the potential for obstetric complications. The risk of perinatal transmission directly correlates with the viral load (Johnsen, 2007). A discussion of the options on continuing the pregnancy, medication therapy, risks, perinatal outcomes, and treatment is warranted. Women who elect to continue with the pregnancy should be treated with antiretroviral therapy regardless of their CD4 count or viral load.

Drug therapy is the mainstay of treatment for pregnant women infected with HIV. The standard treatment is

TABLE 20.4 STAGES OF HIV INFECTION OUTLINED BY THE CDC

Stages	Description	Clinical Picture
I	Acute infection	Early stage with pervasive viral production Flu-like symptoms 2–4 weeks after exposure Signs and symptoms: weight loss, low-grade fever, fatigue, sore throat, night sweats, and myalgia
II	Asymptomatic infection	Viral replication continues within lymphatics Usually free of symptoms; lymphadenopathy
III	Persistent generalized lymphadenopathy	Possibly remaining in this stage for years; AIDS develops in most within 7–10 years Opportunistic infections occur
IV	End-stage disease (AIDS)	Severe immune deficiency High viral load and low CD4 counts Signs and symptoms: bacterial, viral, or fungal opportunistic infections, fever, wasting syndrome, fatigue, neoplasms, and cognitive changes

oral antiretroviral drugs given twice daily from 14 weeks' gestation until giving birth, intravenous administration during labor, and oral syrup for the newborn in the first 6 weeks of life (Hackley, Kriebs, & Rousseau, 2007). The goal of therapy is to reduce the viral load as much as possible, which reduces the risk of transmission to the fetus.

Decisions about the birthing method to be used are made on an individual basis based on several factors involving the woman's health. Some reports suggest that cesarean birth may reduce the risk of HIV infection (Johnsen, 2007). Efforts to reduce instrumentation, such as avoiding the use of an episiotomy, fetal scalp electrodes, and fetal scalp sampling, will reduce the newborn's exposure to bodily fluids.

With appropriate therapies, the prognosis for pregnant women with HIV infection has improved significantly. In addition, the newborns of women with HIV infection who have received treatment usually do not become infected. Unfortunately, therapy is complicated and medications are expensive. Moreover, the medications are associated with numerous adverse effects and possible toxic reactions. These therapies offer a dual purpose: reduce the likelihood of mother-to-infant transmission and provide optimal suppression of the viral load in the mother. The core goal of all medical therapy is to bring the client's viral load to an undetectable level, thus minimizing the risk of transmission to the fetus and newborn.

Nursing Assessment

Nursing assessment begins with a thorough history and physical examination. In addition, the woman is offered screening for HIV antibodies.

Health History and Physical Examination

Review the woman's history for risk factors, such as unsafe sex practices, multiple sex partners, and injectable drug use. Also have the woman complete a risk assessment survey. In addition, question the woman about any flu-like symptoms such as a low-grade fever, fatigue, sore throat, night sweats, diarrhea, cough, skin lesions, or muscle pain.

Perform a complete physical examination. Obtain the woman's weight and determine if she has lost weight recently. Assess for signs and symptoms of sexually transmitted infections (STIs), such as vulvovaginal candidiasis, bacterial vaginosis, HSV, chancroid, CMV, or chlamydia because of the increased risk for STIs.

▶ **Take** NOTE!

Women who request an HIV test despite reporting no individual risk factors should be considered at risk, since many are not likely to disclose their high-risk behaviors.

Laboratory and Diagnostic Testing

The U.S. Public Health Service recommends that all pregnant women be offered HIV antibody testing, regardless of their risk of infection, and that testing be done during the initial prenatal evaluation (Lampe, 2006). Testing is essential because treatments are available that can reduce the likelihood of perinatal transmission and maintain the health of the woman.

▶ **Take** NOTE!

Screening only women who are identified as high risk based on their histories is inadequate due to the prolonged latency period that can exist after exposure. Also, research indicating that treatment with antiretroviral agents could reduce vertical transmission from the infected mother to the newborn has dramatically increased the importance of HIV antibody screening in pregnancy.

Offer all women who are pregnant or planning a pregnancy HIV testing using ELISA. Prepare the woman with a reactive screening test for an additional test, such as the Western blot or an immunofluorescence assay. The Western blot is the confirmatory diagnostic test. A positive antibody test confirmed by a supplemental test indicates that the woman has been infected with HIV and can pass it on to others. HIV antibodies are detectable in at least 95% of women within 3 months after infection (Cressey & Lallemant, 2007).

In addition to the usual screening tests done in normal pregnancy, additional testing for STIs may be necessary. Women infected with HIV have high rates of STIs, especially HPV, vulvovaginal candidiasis, bacterial vaginosis, syphilis, HSV, chancroid, CMV, gonorrhea, chlamydia, and hepatitis B (Hackley, Kriebs, & Rousseau, 2007).

Nursing Management

Women infected with HIV should have comprehensive prenatal care, which starts with pretest and posttest counseling. In pretest counseling, the client completes a risk assessment survey and the nurse explains the meaning of positive versus negative test results, obtains informed consent for HIV testing, and educates the woman on how to prevent HIV infection by changing lifestyle behaviors if needed. Posttest counseling includes informing the client of the test results, reviewing the meaning of the results again, and reinforcing safer sex guidelines. All pretest and posttest counseling should be documented in the client's chart.

Educating the Client

Pregnant clients are dealing with many issues at their first prenatal visit. The confirmation of pregnancy may be accompanied by feelings of joy, anxiety, depression, or other emotions. Simultaneously, the client is given many pamphlets and receives advice and counseling about many important health issues (e.g., nutrition, prenatal development, appointment schedules). This health teaching may be done while the woman feels excited, tired, and anxious. To expect women to understand detailed explanations of a complex disease entity (HIV/AIDS) too may be unrealistic. Determine the client's readiness for this discussion.

Identify the client's individual needs for teaching, emotional support, and physical care. Approach education and counseling of HIV-positive pregnant women in a caring, sensitive manner. Address the following information:

- Infection control issues at home
- Safer sex precautions
- Stages of the HIV disease process and treatment for each stage
- Symptoms of opportunistic infections
- Preventive drug therapies for her unborn infant
- Avoidance of breastfeeding
- Referrals to community support, counseling, and financial aid
- Client's support system and potential caretaker
- Importance of continual prenatal care
- Need for a well-balanced diet
- Measures to reduce exposure to infections

Be knowledgeable about HIV infection and how HIV is transmitted and share this knowledge with all women. Nurses also can work to influence legislators, public health officials, and the entire health establishment toward policies to address the HIV epidemic. Research toward treatment and cure is tremendously important, but the major key to prevention of the spread of the virus is education. Nurses play a major role in this education.

Supporting the Client

Be aware of the psychosocial sequelae of HIV/AIDS. A diagnosis of HIV can put a woman into an emotional tailspin, where she is worried about her own health and that of her unborn infant. She may experience grief, fear, or anxiety about the future of her children. Along with the medications that are so important to her health maintenance, address the woman's mental health needs, family dynamics, capacity to work, and social concerns and provide appropriate support and guidance.

Be aware of your personal beliefs and attitudes toward women who are HIV positive or have AIDS. Incorporate this awareness in your actions as you help the woman face the reality of the diagnosis and treatment options. Empathy, understanding, caring, and assistance are key to helping the client and her family.

Preparing for Labor, Birth, and Afterward

Current evidence suggests that cesarean birth performed before the onset of labor and before the rupture of mem-

branes significantly reduces the rate of perinatal transmission. ACOG recommends that HIV-positive women be offered elective cesarean birth to reduce the rate of transmission beyond that which may be achieved through antiretroviral therapy. They further suggest that operative births be performed at 38 weeks' gestation and that amniocentesis be avoided to prevent contamination of the amniotic fluid with maternal blood. Decisions concerning the method of delivery should be based on the woman's viral load, the duration of ruptured membranes, the progress of labor, and other pertinent clinical factors (USPHSTF, 2006b).

Prepare the woman physically and emotionally for the possibility of cesarean birth and assist as necessary. Ensure that she understands the rationale for the surgical birth.

After the birth of the newborn, the motivation for taking antiretroviral medications may be lower, thus affecting the woman's compliance with therapy. Encourage the woman to continue therapy for her own sake as well as that of the newborn. Nurses can make a difference in helping women to adhere to their complex drug regimens.

Reinforce family planning methods during this time, incorporating a realistic view of her disease status. The use of oral contraceptives with concurrent use of condoms is recommended (Lampe, 2006). Advise the woman that breastfeeding is not recommended. Instruct the HIV-positive woman in self-care measures, including the proper method for disposing of perineal pads to reduce the risk of exposing others to infected body fluids. Finally, teach the HIV-positive woman the signs and symptoms of infection in newborns and infants, encouraging her to report any to the health care provider.

▶ *Take* NOTE!

When providing direct care, **ALWAYS** *follow standard precautions.*

▶ THE PREGNANT WOMAN WITH SUBSTANCE ABUSE

Perinatal drug abuse is the use of alcohol and other drugs by pregnant women. The incidence of substance abuse during pregnancy is highly variable because most pregnant women are reluctant to reveal the extent of their use. The National Institute on Drug Abuse estimates that 6% of the women in the United States have used illicit drugs while pregnant. These include cocaine, marijuana, heroin, and psychotherapeutic drugs that were not prescribed by a health care professional. More than 18% used alcohol and 21% smoked cigarettes during their pregnancy (National Institute on Drug Abuse [NIDA], 2007a).

Impact of Substance Abuse on Pregnancy

The use of drugs, legal or not, increases the risk of medical complications in the mother and poor birth outcomes in the newborn. The placenta acts as an active transport mechanism, not as a barrier, and substances pass from a mother to her fetus through the placenta. Thus, the fetus as well as the mother experiences substance use, abuse, and addiction. Additionally, fetal vulnerability to drugs is much greater because the fetus has not developed the enzymatic system needed to metabolize drugs (Hackley, Kriebs, & Rousseau, 2007).

A woman who claims to have taken no drugs while pregnant may be unaware that substances such as hair dye, diet cola, paint, or over-the-counter (OTC) medications for colds or headaches are still considered drugs. Thus, it is very difficult to get a true picture of the real use of drugs by pregnant women.

Many drugs are considered to have a teratogenic effect on growing fetuses. A **teratogen** is any environmental substance that can cause physical defects in the developing embryo and fetus. Pregnant women with substance abuse commonly present with polysubstance abuse, which is likely to be more damaging than the use of any single substance. Thus, it is inherently difficult to ascribe a specific perinatal effect to any one substance (Rassool & Villar-Luis, 2006).

Effects of Addiction

Addiction is a multifaceted process that is affected by environmental, psychological, family, and physical factors. Women who use drugs, alcohol, or tobacco come from all socioeconomic backgrounds, cultures, and lifestyles. Factors associated with substance abuse during a pregnancy may include low self-esteem, inadequate support systems, low self-expectations, high levels of anxiety, socioeconomic barriers, involvement in abusive relationships, chaotic familial and social systems, and a history of psychiatric illness or depression. Women often become substance abusers to relieve their anxieties, depression, and feelings of worthlessness (Jones, 2006).

Societal attitudes regarding women and substance abuse may prohibit them from admitting the problem and seeking treatment. Society sanctions women for failing to live up to expectations of how a pregnant woman "should" behave, thereby possibly driving them further away from the treatment they so desperately need. For many reasons, pregnant women who abuse substances feel unwelcome in prenatal clinics or medical settings. Often they seek prenatal care late or not at all. They may fear being shamed or reported to legal or child protection authorities. A nonjudgmental atmosphere and unbiased teaching to all pregnant women regardless of their lifestyle is crucial. A caring, concerned manner is critical to help these women feel safe and respond honestly to assessment questions.

Pregnancy can be a motivator for some who want to try treatment. The goal of therapy is to help the client deal with pregnancy by developing a trusting relationship. Providing a full spectrum of medical, social, and emotional care is needed.

Effects of Commonly Abused Substances

Substance abuse during pregnancy, particularly in the first trimester, has a negative effect on the health of the mother and the growth and development of the fetus. The fetus experiences the same systemic effects as the mother, but often more severely. The fetus cannot metabolize drugs as efficiently as the expectant mother and will experience the effects long after the drugs have left the women's system. Substance abuse during pregnancy is associated with preterm labor, abortion, IUGR, abruptio placentae, low birthweight, neurobehavioral abnormalities, and long-term childhood developmental consequences (Rassool & Villar-Luis, 2006). Table 20.5 summarizes the effects of selected drugs during pregnancy.

TABLE 20.5   EFFECTS OF SELECTED DRUGS ON PREGNANCY

Substance	Effect on Pregnancy
Alcohol	Spontaneous abortion, inadequate weight gain, IUGR, fetal alcohol spectrum disorder, the leading cause of mental retardation
Caffeine	Vasoconstriction and mild diuresis in mother; fetal stimulation, but teratogenic effects not documented via research
Nicotine	Vasoconstriction, reduced uteroplacental blood flow, decreased birthweight, abortion, prematurity, abruptio placentae, fetal demise
Cocaine	Vasoconstriction, gestational hypertension, abruptio placentae, abortion, "snow baby syndrome," CNS defects, IUGR
Marijuana	Anemia, inadequate weight gain, "amotivational syndrome," hyperactive startle reflex, newborn tremors, prematurity, IUGR
Narcotics	Maternal and fetal withdrawal, abruptio placentae, preterm labor, premature rupture of membranes, perinatal asphyxia, newborn sepsis and death, intellectual impairment, malnutrition
Sedatives	CNS depression, newborn withdrawal, maternal seizures in labor, newborn abstinence syndrome, delayed lung maturity

Sources: CDC, 2007d; Gilbert & Harmon, 2006; Jones, 2006.

Alcohol

Alcohol abuse is a major public health issue in the United States. Alcohol is a teratogen, a substance known to be toxic to human development. Approximately 10% of pregnant women report alcohol consumption (CDC, 2007d). Theoretically, no mother would give a glass of wine, beer, or hard liquor to her newborn, but when she drinks, her embryo or fetus is exposed to the same blood alcohol concentration as she is. The teratogenic effects of heavy maternal drinking have been recognized since 1973, when fetal alcohol syndrome was first described. Fetal alcohol syndrome is now a classification under the broader term of **fetal alcohol spectrum disorder (FASD)**; this disorder includes the full range of birth defects, such as structural anomalies and behavioral and neurocognitive disabilities caused by prenatal exposure to alcohol (Green, 2007). The incidence of FASD in the United States is estimated to be one or two cases per 1,000 live births (National Organization on Fetal Alcohol Syndrome [NoFAS], 2007). It is the leading cause of mental retardation (CDC, 2007d).

Not every woman who drinks during pregnancy will give birth to an affected child. Based on the best research available, the following is known about alcohol consumption during pregnancy:

- Intake increases the risk of alcohol-related birth defects, including growth deficiencies, facial abnormalities, central nervous system impairment, behavioral disorders, and intellectual development.
- No amount of alcohol consumption is considered safe during pregnancy.
- Damage to the fetus can occur at any stage of pregnancy, even before a woman knows she is pregnant.
- Cognitive defects and behavioral problems resulting from prenatal exposure are lifelong.
- Alcohol-related birth defects are completely preventable (U.S. Department of Health and Human Services [USDHHS], 2007).

Risk factors for giving birth to an alcohol-affected newborn include maternal age, socioeconomic status, ethnicity, genetic factors, poor nutrition, depression, family disorganization, unplanned pregnancy, and late prenatal care (Hackley, Kriebs, & Rousseau, 2007). Identification of risk factors strongly associated with alcohol-related birth outcomes could help identify high-risk pregnancies requiring intervention.

Characteristics of FASD include craniofacial dysmorphia (thin upper lip, small head circumference, and small eyes), IUGR, microcephaly, and congenital anomalies such as limb abnormalities and cardiac defects. Long-term sequelae include postnatal growth restriction, attention deficits, delayed reaction time, and poor scholastic performance (NoFAS, 2007). The complex neurobehavioral problems typically manifest themselves insidiously. Children with prenatal alcohol exposure struggle with cognitive, academic, social, emotional, and behavioral challenges.

BOX 20.5 Common Cognitive and Behavioral Problems Associated With FASD

- Attention-deficit/hyperactivity disorder (ADHD)
- Inability to foresee consequences
- Inability to learn from previous experience
- Lack of organization
- Learning difficulties
- Poor abstract thinking
- Poor impulse control
- Speech and language problems
- Poor judgment

These challenges reduce the child's ability to learn and function successfully in many structured environments (Green, 2007). Common cognitive and behavioral problems are listed in Box 20.5, and Figure 20.5 illustrates the characteristic facial features. See Chapter 24 for a more detailed discussion of the newborn with FASD.

One of the biggest challenges in determining the true prevalence of FASD is how to recognize the syndrome, which depends in part on the age and physical features of the person being assessed. Difficulty in identifying alcohol abuse is due to the client's denial of alcohol use, unwillingness to report alcohol consumption, underreporting, and limited ability to recollect the frequency, quantity, and type of alcohol consumed. This makes it difficult to identify women who are drinking during pregnancy, institute preventive measures, or refer them for treatment.

Women who drink excessively while pregnant are at high risk for giving birth to children with birth defects. To prevent these defects, women should stop drinking during

FIGURE 20.5 Typical facial characteristics of a newborn with FASD.

all phases of a pregnancy. Unfortunately, many women continue to drink during their pregnancy despite warnings from professionals.

Currently, it is not known whether there is a minimal amount of alcohol safe to drink during pregnancy; an occasional glass of wine might be harmless or might not be. Therefore, eliminating alcohol consumption during pregnancy is the ultimate goal to prevent FASD. Most women know they shouldn't drink during pregnancy, but the "window of vulnerability"—the time lag between conception and the discovery of pregnancy—may put substantial numbers of children at risk. Additionally, traditional alcohol-screening questionnaires, such as the Michigan Alcoholism Screening Test (MAST) and the CAGE Questionnaire, are not sensitive enough to detect low levels of alcohol consumption among women.

Several challenges remain in preventing birth defects due to alcohol consumption:

• Ways to improve clinical recognition of high-risk women who drink alcohol
• Ways to intervene more effectively to modify drinking behaviors
• In utero approaches to prevent or minimize fetal injury
• Strategies to address the neurodevelopmental problems of children affected by maternal alcohol ingestion

Caffeine

Caffeine, a CNS stimulant, is present in varying amounts in such common products as coffee, tea, colas, and chocolate. It is also in cold remedies and analgesics. Birth defects have not been linked to caffeine consumption, but maternal coffee consumption decreases iron absorption and may increase the risk of anemia during pregnancy. The FDA recommends that pregnant women eliminate or limit their consumption of caffeine to less than 300 mg/day, or the equivalent of three cups of coffee or cola (Hoffman & Brown, 2006).

Nicotine

Nicotine, found in cigarettes, is another substance that is harmful to the pregnant women and her fetus. Nicotine, which causes vasoconstriction, transfers across the placenta and reduces blood flow to the fetus, contributing to fetal hypoxia. When compared with alcohol, marijuana, and other illicit drug use, tobacco use is less likely to decline as the pregnancy progresses (Wang, 2007). Smoking is associated with adverse pregnancy outcomes. However, these adverse outcomes can be avoided if the woman stops smoking before becoming pregnant.

Smoking increases the risk of spontaneous abortion, preterm labor and birth, maternal hypertension, placenta previa, and abruptio placentae. The perinatal death rate among infants of smoking mothers is 20% to 35% higher (Raatikainen, Huurinainen, & Heinonen, 2007).

Smoking has also been considered an important risk factor for low birthweight, sudden infant death syndrome (SIDS), and cognitive deficits, especially in language, reading, and vocabulary, as well as poorer performances on tests of reasoning and memory. Researchers have also reported behavior problems, such as increased activity, inattention, impulsivity, opposition, and aggression (Wang, 2007).

Women who smoke during the pregnancy also continue to smoke after giving birth, and thus the infant will be exposed to nicotine after birth. This environmental or passive exposure affects the child's development and increases the risk of childhood respiratory disorders.

Cocaine

Cocaine use is second only to marijuana in women who abuse drugs during pregnancy. The incidence of cocaine exposure in utero is 1 to 10 per 1,000 live births (Weekes & Lee, 2006).

Cocaine is a psychoactive drug derived from the leaves of the coca plant, which grows in the Andes Mountains of Peru, Ecuador, and Bolivia. The freebase form, called "crack" because of the cracking or popping noise made in its preparation, is less expensive, easily made, and smokable. Cocaine is a powerful vasoconstrictor. When sniffed into the mucous membranes of the nose, it produces an intense "rush" that some have compared to an orgasmic experience. Smoked crack is absorbed rapidly by the pulmonary vasculature and reaches the brain's circulation in 6 to 8 seconds (NIDA, 2007b).

Cocaine use produces vasoconstriction, tachycardia, and hypertension in both the mother and the fetus (Weekes & Lee, 2006). Uteroplacental insufficiency may result from reduced blood flow and placental perfusion. Chronic use can result in low birthweight, the most common effect of cocaine use in pregnancy (NIDA, 2007b).

Studies suggest that perinatal cocaine use increases the risk of preterm labor, abortion, abruptio placentae, IUGR, intrauterine fetal distress and demise, seizures, withdrawal, and cerebral infarcts. Cocaine may increase the risk of uterine rupture and congenital anomalies (NIDA, 2007b). Fetal anomalies associated with cocaine use in early pregnancy involve neurologic problems such as neural tube defects and microcephaly; cardiovascular anomalies such as congenital heart defects; genitourinary conditions such as prune belly syndrome, hydronephrosis, and ambiguous genitalia; and gastrointestinal system problems such as necrotizing enterocolitis (Jones, 2006). Some infants exposed to cocaine in utero show increased irritability and are difficult to calm and soothe to sleep.

Marijuana

Marijuana is the most commonly used illicit drug in America, with over 90 million people having tried it at least once. It is often called pot, reefer, herb, widow, hash, grass, weed, Mary Jane, or MJ (NIDA, 2007c). Marijuana is a preparation of the leaves and flowering tops of *Cannabis sativa,* the hemp plant, which contains a number of pharmacologically active agents. Tetrahydrocannabinol (THC) is the most active ingredient of marijuana. With heavy smoking, THC narrows the bronchi and bronchioles and produces inflammation of the mucous membranes. Smoking marijuana causes tachycardia and a reduction in blood pressure, resulting in orthostatic hypotension.

The effects of marijuana smoking on pregnancy are not yet fully understood because there are very few studies on its long-term effects on child development. One can speculate that the effects of marijuana on the immature nervous system may be subtle and not detected until more complex functions are required, usually in a formal educational setting. There is some evidence that marijuana increases the risk of spontaneous abortion and preterm delivery (Barros et al., 2006). Although marijuana is not considered teratogenic, many newborns display altered responses to visual stimuli, increased tremulousness, and a high-pitched cry, which might indicate CNS insults (Wang, 2007). A strong correlation exists between the use of marijuana and the use of alcohol and cigarettes.

Opiates and Narcotics

Opiates and narcotics include opium, heroin (known as horse, junk, smack, downtown), morphine, codeine, hydromorphone (Dilaudid; little D), oxycodone (Percodan, perkies), meperidine (Demerol, demise), and methadone (meth, dollies). These drugs are central nervous system depressants that soothe and lull. They may be used medically for pain, but all have a high potential for abuse. Most cause an intense addiction in both mother and newborn.

Narcotic dependence is particularly problematic in pregnant women. It leads to medical, nutritional, and social neglect by the woman due to the long-term risks of physical dependence, malnutrition, compromised immunity, hepatitis, and fatal overdose (Alexander et al., 2007). Taking opiates or narcotics during pregnancy places the woman at increased risk for preterm labor, IUGR, and preeclampsia (Wang, 2007).

Heroin is the most common illicitly used opioid. It is derived from the seeds of the poppy plant and can be sniffed, smoked, or injected. It crosses the placenta via simple diffusion within 1 hour of maternal consumption (Dodge, Brady, & Maguire, 2007). Use of heroin during pregnancy is believed to affect the developing brain of the fetus and may cause behavioral abnormalities in childhood (Alexander et al., 2007).

The most common harmful effect of heroin and other narcotics on newborns is withdrawal, or **neonatal abstinence syndrome** (see Chapter 24). This collection of symptoms may include irritability, hypertonicity, a high-pitched cry, vomiting, diarrhea, respiratory distress, disturbed sleeping, sneezing, diaphoresis, fever, poor sucking, tremors, and seizures (Ebner et al., 2007).

Withdrawal from opiates during pregnancy is extremely dangerous for the fetus, so a prescribed oral methadone maintenance program combined with psychotherapy is recommended for the pregnant woman. This closely supervised treatment program reduces withdrawal symptoms in the newborn, reduces drug cravings, and blocks the euphoric effects of narcotic drugs in order to reduce illicit drug use. Methadone maintenance provides a steady state of opiate levels, thus reducing the risk of withdrawal to the fetus and exposure to HIV and other STIs because the mother is no longer injecting drugs. However, methadone has the same withdrawal consequences for women and newborns as heroin does (Burns et al., 2007).

Sedatives

Sedatives relax the central nervous system and are used medically for inducing relaxation and sleep, relieving tension, and treating seizures. Sedatives easily cross the placenta and can cause birth defects and behavioral problems. Infants born to mothers who abuse sedatives during pregnancy may be physically dependent on the drugs themselves and are more prone to respiratory problems, feeding difficulties, disturbed sleep, sweating, irritability, and fever (Alexander et al., 2007).

Methamphetamines

Methamphetamine use among pregnant women has increased rapidly in the United States. This highly addictive stimulant is commonly known as speed, meth, or chalk. In its smoked form, it is often referred to as ice, crystal, crank, and glass. It is a white, odorless, bittertasting powder that was developed from its parent drug, amphetamine, and was used originally in nasal decongestants and bronchial inhalers. The maternal effects include increased energy and alertness, an intense rush, decreased appetite, tachycardia, and tachypnea. Chronic use can lead to psychosis, including paranoia, hallucinations, memory loss, and aggressive or violent behavior (Derlet & Albertson, 2006). Few studies have been done on the effects of methamphetamine abuse during pregnancy, but the few done indicate an increased risk for preterm births, placental abruption, fetal growth restriction, and congenital anomalies (NIDA, 2007d). These findings are hard to interpret, however, due to small sample size and polydrug use of the participants.

Nursing Assessment

Complete a thorough history and physical examination to evaluate a client for substance use and abuse. Substance abuse screening in pregnancy is done to detect the use of any substance known or suspected to exert a deleterious effect on the client or her fetus. Routinely ask about substance abuse with all women of childbearing age, inform them of the risks involved, and advise them against continuing. Screening questionnaires are helpful in identifying potential users, may reduce the stigma of asking clients about substance abuse, and result in a more accurate and consistent evaluation. The questions in Box 20.6 may be helpful in assessing a client who is at risk for substance abuse during pregnancy. Using "accepting" terminology may encourage the woman to give honest answers without fear of reproach.

A urine toxicology screen may also be helpful in determining drug use, although a urine screen identifies only recent or heavy use of drugs. The length of time a drug is present in urine is as follows:

- Cocaine: 24 to 48 hours in an adult, 72 to 96 hours in an infant
- Heroin: 24 hours in an adult, 24 to 48 hours in an infant
- Marijuana: 1 week to 1 month in an adult, up to a month or longer in an infant
- Methadone: up to 10 days in an infant (Wang, 2007)

Nursing Management

If the woman's drug screen is positive, use this as an opportunity to discuss prenatal exposure to substances that may be harmful. The discussion may lead the nurse to refer the client for a diagnostic assessment or identify an intervention such as counseling that may be helpful. Being nonjudgmental is a key to success; a client is more apt to

trust and reveal patterns of abuse if the nurse does not judge her and her lifestyle choices.

A positive drug screen in a newborn warrants an investigation by the state protection agency. In the interim, institute measures to reduce stress and stimuli to promote the newborn's comfort (see Chapter 24 for a more in-depth discussion).

Be proactive, supportive, and accepting when caring for the client. Assure women with substance abuse problems that sharing information of a confidential nature with health care providers will not render them liable to criminal prosecution. Provide counseling and education, emphasizing the following:

- Effects of substance exposure on the fetus
- Interventions to improve mother–child attachment and improve parenting
- Psychosocial support if treatment is needed to reduce substance abuse
- Referral to outreach programs to improve access to treatment facilities
- Hazardous legal substances to avoid during pregnancy
- Follow-up of children born to substance-dependent mothers
- Dietary counseling to improve the pregnancy outcome for both mother and child
- Drug screening to identify all drugs a client is using
- More frequent prenatal visits to monitor fetal well-being
- Maternal and fetal benefits of remaining drug-free
- Cultural sensitivity
- Coping skills, support systems, and vocational assistance

Substance abuse is a complex problem that requires sensitivity to each woman's unique situation and contributing factors. Be sure to address individual psychological and sociocultural factors to help the woman to regain control of her life. Treatment must combine different approaches and provide ongoing support for women learning to live drug-free. Developing personal strengths, such as communication skills and assertiveness, and self-confidence will help the woman in resisting the drug use. Encourage the use of appropriate coping skills. Enhancing self-esteem also helps provides a foundation to avoid drugs.

■■■ Key Concepts

- Preconception counseling for the woman with diabetes is helpful in promoting blood glucose control to prevent congenital anomalies.
- The classification system for diabetes commonly used is based on disease etiology and not pharmacology management; the classification includes type 1 diabetes, type 2 diabetes, gestational diabetes, and impaired fasting glucose and impaired glucose tolerance.
- A functional classification for heart disease during pregnancy is based on past and present disability: class I,

---

BOX 20.6   **Sample Questions for Assessing Substance Use**

- Have you ever used recreational drugs? If so, when and what?
- Have you ever taken a prescription drug other than as intended?
- What are your feelings about drug use during pregnancy?
- How often do you smoke cigarettes? How many per day?
- How often do you drink alcohol?

If the assessment reveals substance use, obtain additional information by using the RAFFT questions, which are a sensitive screening instrument for identifying substance abuse (Weekes & Lee, 2006):

R: Do you drink or take drugs to **R**elax, improve your self-image, or fit in?

A: Do you ever drink or take drugs while **A**lone?

F: Do you have any close **F**riends who drink or take drugs?

F: Does a close **F**amily member have a problem with alcohol or drugs?

T: Have you ever gotten in **T**rouble from drinking or taking drugs?

asymptomatic with no limitation of physical activity; class II, symptomatic (dyspnea, chest pain) with increased activity; class III, symptomatic (fatigue, palpitation) with normal activity; and class IV, symptomatic at rest or with any physical activity.

■ Chronic hypertension exists when the woman has a blood pressure of 140/90 mm Hg or higher before pregnancy or before the 20th week of gestation or when hypertension persists for more than 12 weeks postpartum.

■ Successful management of asthma in pregnancy involves elimination of environmental triggers, drug therapy, and client education.

■ Ideally, women with hematologic conditions are screened before conception and are made aware of the risks to themselves and to a pregnancy.

■ A wide variety of infections, such as rubella, herpes simplex, hepatitis B, varicella, parvovirus B19, and many sexually transmitted infections can affect the pregnancy, having a negative impact on its outcome.

■ The younger the adolescent is at the time of the first pregnancy, the more likely it is that she will have another pregnancy during her teens. About 1 million teenagers between the ages of 15 and 19 become pregnant each year; about half give birth and keep their infants.

■ The nurse's role in caring for the pregnant adolescent is to assist her in identifying the options for this pregnancy, including abortion, self-parenting of the child, temporary foster care for the baby or herself, or placement for adoption.

■ The prevalence of HIV/AIDS is increasing more rapidly among women then men: half of all the HIV/AIDS cases worldwide now occur in women. There are only three recognized modes of HIV transmission: unprotected sexual intercourse with an infected partner, contact with infected blood or blood products, and perinatal transmission. Breastfeeding is a major contributing factor in mother-to-child transmission of HIV.

■ Cases of perinatal AIDS have decreased in the past several years in the United States, primarily because of the use of zidovudine (ZDV) therapy in pregnant women with HIV. The U.S. Public Health Service recommends that all pregnant women should be offered HIV antibody testing regardless of their risk of infection, and that testing should be done during the initial prenatal evaluation.

■ Pregnant women with substance abuse problems commonly abuse several substance, making it difficult to ascribe a specific perinatal effect to any one substance. Societal attitudes regarding pregnant women and substance abuse may prohibit them from admitting the problem and seeking treatment.

■ Substance abuse during pregnancy is associated with preterm labor, abortion, low birthweight, CNS and fetal anomalies, and long-term childhood developmental consequences.

■ Fetal alcohol spectrum disorder is a lifelong yet completely preventable set of physical, mental, and neurobehavioral birth defects; it is the leading cause of mental retardation in the United States.

■ Nursing management for the woman with substance abuse focuses on screening and preventing substance abuse to reduce the high incidence of obstetric and medical complications as well as the morbidity and mortality among passively addicted newborns.

REFERENCES

Abdin, S. (2006). Care of pregnant women with heart disease: A multidisciplinary approach. *British Journal of Midwifery, 14*(10), 592–595.

Alan Guttmacher Institute. (2006). *U.S. teenager pregnancy statistics: National and state trends and trends by race and ethnicity.* New York: Author, 1–56.

Alan Guttmacher Institute. (2007). *In the know about pregnancy, contraception and abortion.* Available at: http://www.guttmacher.org/in-the-know/pregnancy.html.

Alexander, L. L., LaRosa, J. H., Bader, H., & Garfield, S. (2007). *New dimensions in women's health* (4th ed.). Sudbury: Jones & Bartlett Publishers.

American Academy of Allergy, Asthma & Immunology (AAAAI). (2007). *Managing asthma during pregnancy.* The National Asthma Education Prevention Program. Available at: http://www.aaaai.org/patients/topicofthemonth/0506/.

American Diabetes Association (ADA). (2008). Standards of medical care in diabetes in 2008. *Diabetes Care,* Supplement 1, S12–54.

American Diabetes Association (ADA). (2007a). Diagnosis and classification of diabetes mellitus. *Diabetes Care, 30*(Supplement 1), S42–47.

American Diabetes Association (ADA). (2007b). Standards of medical care in diabetes—2007. *Diabetes Care, 30*(Supplement 1), S4–S41.

American Heart Association (AHA). (2007). *Women and heart disease facts.* Available at: http://www.americanheart.org/presenter.jhtml?identifier=3039318.

Anderson, W. E., & Safdar, A. (2007). Varicella-zoster virus. *eMedicine.* Available at: http://emedicine.com/med/topic2361.htm.

Arenson, J., & Drake, P. (2007). *Maternal and newborn health.* Sudbury, MA: Jones and Bartlett Publishers.

As-Sanie, S., Gantt, A., & Rosenthal, M. S. (2004). Pregnancy prevention in adolescents. *American Family Physician, 70*(8), 1517–1524.

Baker, D. A. (2007). Consequences of herpes simplex virus in pregnancy and their prevention. *Current Opinion in Infectious Diseases, 20*(1), 73–76.

Balentine, J. & Eisenhart, A. (2008). Aortic stenosis. *eMedicine* [Online]. Available at: http://www.emedicine.com/EMERG/topic40.htm.

Barker, D., Lewis, N., Mason, G., & Tan, L. (2006). Maternal cardiovascular medicine: Toward better care for pregnant women with heart disease. *British Journal of Cardiology, 13*(6), 399–402.

Barros, M. C., Guinburg, R., Peres, C., Mitsuhiro, S., Chalem, E., & Laranjeira, R. R. (2006). Exposure to marijuana during pregnancy alters neurobehavior in the early neonatal period. *Journal of Pediatrics, 149,* 781–787.

Blackburn, S. T. (2007). *Maternal, fetal, & neonatal physiology: A clinical perspective* (3rd ed.). Philadelphia: Saunders.

Blincoe, A. J. (2007). Hypertension in pregnancy: The importance of monitoring. *British Journal of Midwifery, 15*(1), 50–53.

Bothamley, J. (2006). Tuberculosis in pregnancy: The role for midwives in diagnosis and treatment. *British Journal of Midwifery, 14*(4), 182–185.

Broliden, K., Tolfvenstam, T., & Norbeck, O. (2006). Clinical aspects of parvovirus B19 infection. *Journal of Internal Medicine, 260,* 285–304.

Burns, L., Mattick, R. P., Lim, K., & Wallace, C. (2007). Methadone in pregnancy: Treatment, retention and neonatal outcomes. *Addiction, 102*(2), 264–270.

CDC. (2006). *STD treatment guidelines.* Available at: http://www.cdc.gov/std/treatment/2006/toc.htm.

CDC. (2007a). *HIV/AIDS among women.* Available at: http://www.cdc.gov/hiv/topics/women/resources/factsheets/print/women.htm.

CDC. (2007b). *Prevention of perinatal group B streptococcal disease: revised guidelines from CDC.* Available at: http://www.cdc.gov/groupbstrep/hospitals/hospitals_guidelines_summary.htm.

CDC. (2007c). *Rubella.* Available at: www.cdc.gov/nip/publications/pink/rubella.pdf.

CDC (2007d). Fact sheet: Alcohol consumption among women who are pregnant. *Morbidity and Mortality Weekly Report, 54*(9), 229–230.

CDC (2007e). *Fact sheet: Viral hepatitis B.* Available at: http://www.cdc.gov/ncidod/diseases/hepatitis/b/fact.htm.

CDC. (2008). *Genital herpes: CDC fact sheet* [Online]. Available at: http:www.cdc.gov/std/herpes/STDFact-herpes.htm.

Cressey, T. R., & Lallemant, M. (2007). Pharmacogenetics of anti-retroviral drugs for the treatment of HIV-infected patients: An update. *Infection, Genetics & Evolution, 7*(2), 333–342.

Criteria Committee of the New York Heart Association. (1994). *Nomenclature and criteria for diagnosis of diseases of the heart and great vessels* (9th ed.). Dallas: American Heart Association.

Cunningham, D., & Rennels, M. B. (2006). Parvovirus B19 infection. *eMedicine.* Available at: http://www.emedicine.com/ped/topic192.htm.

Cunningham, F. G., Gant, N. F., Leveno, K. J., et al. (2005). *Williams' obstetrics* (22nd ed.). New York: McGraw-Hill.

Curran, D., & Poggi, S. H. (2007). Hematologic disease and pregnancy. *eMedicine.* Available at: http://www.emedicine.com/med/topic3254.htm.

Cypryk, K., Vilsboll, T., Nadel, I., Smyczynska, J., Holst J., & Lewinski, A. (2007). Normal secretion of the incretin hormones glucose-dependent insulinotropic polypeptide and glucagon-like peptide-1 during gestational diabetes mellitus. *Gynecologic Endocrinology, 23*(1), 58–62.

Dao, H., Mofenson, L. M., Ekpini, R., Gilks, C. F., Barnhart, M., Bolu, O., & Shaffer, N. (2007). International recommendations on antiretroviral drugs for treatment of HIV-infected women and prevention of mother-to-child HIV transmission in resource-limited settings. *American Journal of Obstetrics & Gynecology, 197*(3), S42–S55.

D'Arrigo, T. (2007). Pre-pregnant care cuts risks. *Diabetes Forecast, 60*(2), 16–17.

Derlet, R., & Albertson, T. (2006). Methamphetamine. *eMedicine.* Available at: http://www.emedicine.com/EMERG/topic859.htm.

Dobbenga-Rhodes, Y. A., & Prive, A. M. (2006). Assessment and evaluation of the woman with cardiac disease during pregnancy. *Journal of Perinatal & Neonatal Nursing, 20*(4), 295–233.

Dodge, P., Brady, M., & Maguire, B. (2007). Initiation of a nurse-developed interdisciplinary plan of care for opiate addiction in pregnant women and their infants. *International Journal of Childbirth Education, 21*(2), 21–24.

Dudek, S. G. (2006). *Nutrition essentials for nursing practice* (5th ed.). Philadelphia: Lippincott Williams & Wilkins.

Ebner, N., Rohrmeister, K., Winklbaur, B., Baewert, A., Jagsch, R., Peternell, A., Thau, K., & Fischer, G. (2007). Management of neonatal abstinence syndrome in neonates born to opioid maintained women. *Drug and Alcohol Dependence, 87*(2/3), 131–138.

Edelstein, S., & Herbold, N. (2007). *Nurse's pocket guide to nutrition.* Sudbury, MA: Jones and Bartlett Publishers.

Ekpebegh, C. O., Coetzee, E. J., van der Merwe, L., & Levitt, N. S. (2007). A 10-year retrospective analysis of pregnancy outcome in pregestational type 2 diabetes: Comparison of insulin and oral glucose-lowering agents. *Diabetic Medicine, 24*(3), 253–258.

Elbaz, W. F., Coyle, P., Hunter, A., & Farrag, S. (2007). Erythrovirus B19 as a potential cause of fetal hydrops: Assessing awareness. *British Journal of Midwifery, 15*(7), 440–444.

Elsayegh, D., & Shapiro, J. M. (2007). Sickle cell vasoocclusive crisis and acute chest syndrome at term pregnancy. *Southern Medical Journal, 100*(1), 77–79.

Farrar, D., Tuffnell, D. J., & West, J. Continuous subcutaneous insulin infusion versus multiple daily injections of insulin for pregnant women with diabetes. *Cochrane Database of Systematic Reviews* 2007. Issue 3. Art. No.: CD005542.DOI: 10.1002/14651858.CD005542.pub2.

Fischer, R. (2007). Genital herpes in pregnancy. *eMedicine.* Available at: http://www.emedicine.com/med/topic3554.htm.

Frieden, F. J., & Chan, Y. (2007). Diabetes mellitus in pregnancy. In R. E. Rakel & E. T. Bope (Eds.), *Conn's current therapy 2007* (pp. 1169–1271). Philadelphia: Saunders Elsevier.

Gardella, C., & Brown, Z. A. (2007). Managing varicella zoster infection in pregnancy. *Cleveland Clinic Journal of Medicine, 74*(4), 290–296.

Gibson, P., & Carson, M. (2007). Hypertension and pregnancy. *eMedicine* Available at: http://emedicine.com/med/topic3250.htm.

Gilbert, E., & Harmon, J. (2006). *Manual of high-risk pregnancy and delivery* (4th ed.). St. Louis: Mosby.

Gilbert, E. S. (2007). *Manual of high risk pregnancy and delivery* (4th ed.). St. Louis: Mosby Elsevier.

Goodman, D., Klerman, L., Johnson, K., Chang, C., & Marth, N. (2007). Geographic access to family planning facilities and the risk of unintended and teenage pregnancy. *Maternal & Child Health Journal, 11*(2), 145–152.

Green, J. H. (2007). Fetal alcohol spectrum disorders: Understanding the effects of prenatal alcohol exposure and supporting students. *Journal of School Health, 77*(3), 103–108.

Hackley, B., Kriebs, J. M., & Rousseau, M. E. (2007). *Primary care of women: A guide for midwives and women's health providers.* Sudbury, MA: Jones and Bartlett Publishers.

Harner, H. M. (2004). Domestic violence and trauma care in teenage pregnancy: does paternal age make a difference? *JOGNN, 33*(3), 312–319.

Harvey, E. A. (2007). Hypertensive disorders or pregnancy. *Nursing Spectrum.* Available at: http://nsweb.nursingspectrum.com/ce/m23c-1.htm.

Henriksen, T. (2006). Nutrition and pregnancy outcome. *Nutrition Reviews, 64*(5), 19–23.

Herchline, T., & Amorosa, J. K. (2007). Tuberculosis. *Emedicine.* Available at: http://www.emedicine.com/MED/topic2324.htm.

Hermes-DeSantis, E. R., & Clyman, R. I. (2006). Patent ductus arteriosus: Pathophysiology and management. *Journal of Perinatology,* Supplement, 26, S14–S18.

Hilton, L. (2006). Pregnancy after 40: What's the risk? *Nursing Spectrum, 18A*(20), 19, 31.

Hoerst, B., & Samson, L. (2007). Perinatal infections. *Nursing Spectrum.* Available at: http://www.nurse.com/ce/course.html?CCID=2803.

Hoffman, D. J., & Brown, G. D. (2006). Neonatal abstinence syndrome secondary to in-utero caffeine exposure. *Neonatal Intensive Care, 19*(6), 24–25.

Hokelek, M., & Safdar, A. (2006). Toxoplasmosis. *eMedicine.* Available at: http://www.emedicine.com/med/topic2294.htm.

Holub, C., Kershaw, T., Ethier, K., Lewis, J., Milan, S., & Ickovics, J. (2007). Prenatal and parenting stress on adolescent maternal adjustment: Identifying a high-risk subgroup. *Maternal & Child Health Journal, 11*(2), 153–159.

Homko, C. J., & Reece, E. A. (2006). Insulins and oral hypoglycemic agents in pregnancy. *Journal of Maternal-Fetal and Neonatal Medicine, 19*(11), 679–686.

Johnsen, C. (2007). Preventing perinatal HIV transmission. *Nursing Spectrum.* Available at: http://www.nurse.com/ce/course.html?CCID=3239.

Joint National Committee (JNC). (2003). *Seventh Report of the Joint National Committee on Prevention, Detection, Evaluation, and Treatment of High Blood Pressure.* National Institutes of Health (NIH), National Heart, Lung, and Blood Institute. NIH Publication No. 035233. Washington, DC: NIH.

Jones, H. E. (2006). Drug addiction during pregnancy: Advances in maternal treatment and understanding child outcomes. *Current Directions in Psychological Science, 15*(3), 126–130.

Karamermer, Y., & Roos-Hesselink, J. W. (2007). Pregnancy and adult congenital heart disease. *Expert Review of Cardiovascular Therapy, 5*(5), 859–869.

King-Jones, T. C. (2008). Caring for pregnant adolescents: Perils and pearls of communication. *Nursing for Women's Health, 12*(2), 114–119.

Kripke, C. (2007). Hepatitis B vaccine for infants of HbsAg-positive mothers. *American Family Physician, 75*(1), 49–50.

Laartz, B., & Gompf, S. G. (2007). Viral infections and pregnancy. *EMedicine.* Available at: http://www.emedicine.com/med/topic3270.htm.

Lampe, M. A. (2006). Human immunodeficiency virus-1 and pre-conceptual care. *Maternal & Child Health Journal,* Supplement 10, 195–197.

Langille, D. B. (2007). Teenage pregnancy: Trends, contributing factors and the physicians' role. *Canadian Medical Association Journal, 176*(11), 1601–1602.

Lesesne, C. A., Lewis, K. M., White, C. P., Green, D. C., Duffy, J. L., & Wandersman, A. (2008). Promoting science-based approaches to teen pregnancy prevention: Proactively engaging the three systems of interactive systems framework. *American Journal of Community Psychology, 41*(3/4), 379–392.

Little, M. & Sinert, R. (2008). Pregnancy, asthma. *eMedicine* [Online]. Available at: http://www.emedicine.com/emerg/TOPIC476.HTM.

Magill, M. K., & Wilcox, R. (2007). Adolescent pregnancy and associated risks: Not just a result of maternal age. *American Family Physician, 75*(9), 1310–1311.

Malee, M. P. (2007). Parvovirus B19 infection. *Contemporary OB/GYN, 52*(5), 70–74.

March of Dimes. (2007a). *Teenage pregnancy.* Available at: http://www.marchofdimes.com/professionals/681_1159.asp.

March of Dimes. (2007b). *Diabetes in pregnancy.* Available at: http://marchofdimes.com/professionals/14332_1197.asp.

March of Dimes. (2007c). *Pregnancy after 35: Quick reference and fact sheet.* Available at: http://www.modimes.org/professionals/681_1155.asp.

March of Dimes. (2007d). *Group B strep infection.* Available at: http://www.marchofdimes.com/professionals/681_1205.asp.

March of Dimes. (2007e). *Toxoplasmosis.* Available at: http://www.marchofdimes.com/printableArticles/681_1228.asp?printable=true.

McCann, J. A. S. (2007). *Maternal-neonatal nursing made incredibly easy* (2nd ed.). Philadelphia: Lippincott Williams & Wilkins.

McMahon, W. S. (2007). Congenital heart disease. In R. E. Rakel & E. T. Bope (Eds.), *Conn's current therapy 2007* (Section 5, pp. 378–379). Philadelphia: Saunders Elsevier.

Menato, G., Bo, S., Signorile, A., Gallo, M., Cotrino, I., Poala, C., & Massobrio, M. (2008). Current management of gestational diabetes mellitus. *Expert Review of Obstetrics Gynecology, 3*(1), 73–91.

Modder, J. (2008). Diabetes in pregnancy: Can we make a difference? *International Journal of Obstetrics & Gynecology, 115*(4), 419–420.

Mooney, M. (2007). Managing cardiac disease in pregnancy. *British Journal of Midwifery, 15*(2), 76–78.

Moore, S. L., & Seybold, V. K. (2007). HPV vaccine. *Clinical Reviews, 17*(1), 36–41.

Moos, M. K. (2006) Group B strep: A prevention success story. *AWHONN Lifelines, 9*(6), 484–486.

More, D. (2007). Asthma in pregnancy. *About allergies.* Available at: http://allergies.about.com/od/allergiesandpregnancy/a/asthmapregnancy.htm.

National Asthma Education and Prevention Program (NAEPP). (2007). NAEPP Expert Panel Report: Managing asthma during pregnancy. *Journal of Allergy & Clinical Immunology, 115,* 36–46.

National Institute on Drug Abuse (NIDA). (2007a). *Drug use during pregnancy.* Available at: http://search2.google.cit.nih.gov/search?q=pregnancy&site=NIDA&client=NIDA_frontnd&proxystylesheet=NIDA_frontend&output=xml_no_dtd&filter=0&getfields=*&btnG.x=16&btnG.y=11.

National Institute on Drug Abuse (NIDA). (2007b). *Cocaine abuse and addiction.* Available at: http://www.nida.nih.gov/ResearchReports/Cocaine/cocaine4.html#maternal.

National Institute on Drug Abuse (NIDA). (2007c). *Marijuana.* Available at: http://www.drugabuse.gov/Infofacts/marijuana.html.

National Institute on Drug Abuse (NIDA). (2007d). *Methamphetamine abuse and addiction.* Available at: http://www.drugabuse.gov/ResearchReports/methamph/methamph5.html.

National Organization on Fetal Alcohol Syndrome (NoFAS). (2007). *What is fetal alcohol syndrome?* Available at: http://www.nofas.org/main/what_is_FAS.htm.

Noyes, J., & Popay, J. (2007). Directly observed therapy and tuberculosis: How can a systemic review of qualitative research contribute to improving services? A qualitative meta-synthesis. *Journal of Advanced Nursing, 57*(3), 227–243.

O'Toole, M. T. (2005). *Encyclopedia and dictionary of medicine, nursing, and allied health* (7th ed.). Philadelphia: Saunders.

Peddicord, K. (2005). Healthy hearts for women. *AWHONN Lifelines, 9*(1), 35–38.

Peyron, F., Wallon, M., Liou, C., & Garner, P. (2006). Treatments for toxoplasmosis in pregnancy. *Cochrane Library* (4), CD001684.

Podymow, T., & August, P. (2007). Hypertension in pregnancy. *Advances in Chronic Kidney Disease, 14*(2), 178–190.

Pyrsopoulos, N. T., & Reddy, K. R. (2007). Hepatitis B. *eMedicine.* Available at: http://www.emedicine.com/med/topic992.htm.

Raatikainen, K., Huurinainen, P., & Heinonen, S. (2007). Smoking in early gestation or through pregnancy: A decision crucial to pregnancy outcome. *Preventive Medicine, 44*(1), 59–63.

Rassool, G. H., & Villar-Luis, M. (2006). Reproductive risks of alcohol and illicit drugs: An overview. *Journal of Addictions Nursing, 17,* 211–213.

Rochon, M., Rand, L., Roth, L., & Gaddipati, S. (2006). Glyburide for the management of gestational diabetes: Risk factors predictive of failure associated pregnancy outcomes. *American Journal of Obstetrics and Gynecology, 195*(4), 1090–1094.

Ross, D. S., Jones, J. L., & Lynch, M. F. (2006). Toxoplasmosis, cytomegalovirus, listeriosis, and preconception care. *Maternal & Child Health Journal, 10*(5), Supplement: S187–S191.

Samson, L., Ferguson, H. W., & Scanlon, R. M. (2007). Chronic medical conditions and pregnancy, part I. *Nursing Spectrum.* Available at: http://nsweb.nursingspectrum.com/ce/m23ac.htm.

Santis, M., Cavaliere, A. F., Straface, G., & Caruso, A. (2006). Rubella infection in pregnancy. *Reproductive Toxicology, 21*(4), 390–398.

Sauerbrei, A., & Wutzler, P. (2007). Varicella-zoster virus infection during pregnancy: Current concepts of prevention, diagnosis and therapy. *Medical Microbiology & Immunology, 196*(2), 95–102.

Scollan-Koliopoulos, M., Guadagno, S., & Walker, E. A. (2006). Gestational diabetes management: Guidelines to a healthy pregnancy. *Nurse Practitioner, 31*(6), 14–25.

Secco, M. L., Profit, S., Kennedy, E., Walsh, A., Letourneau, N., & Stewart, M. (2007). Factors affecting postpartum depressive symptoms of adolescent mothers. *JOGNN, 36*(1), 47–54.

Sharp, K. (2006). Hypertension: Just the facts. *Clinical Journal of Oncology Nursing, 10*(6), 727–730.

Tihtonen, K., Koobi, T., Huhtala, H., & Uotila, J. (2007). Hemodynamic adaptation during pregnancy in chronic hypertension. *Hypertension in Pregnancy, 26*(3), 315–328.

Tough, S., Benzies, K., Fraser-Lee, N., & Newburn-Cook, C. (2007). Factors influencing childbearing decisions and knowledge of perinatal risks among Canadian men and women. *Maternal & Child Health Journal, 11*(2), 189–198.

Uebing, A., Steer, P. J., Yentis, S. M., & Gatzoulis, M. A. (2006). Pregnancy and congenital heart disease. *British Medical Journal, 332,* 401–406.

U.S. Department of Health and Human Services (USDHHS). (2000). *Healthy people 2010* (Conference Edition, vol. 1). Washington, DC.

U.S. Department of Health and Human Services (USDHHS). (2007). *U.S. Surgeon General releases advisory on alcohol use in pregnancy.* HHS Office of the Surgeon General. Available at: http://hhs.gov/surgeongeneral/pressreleases/sg02222007.html.

U.S. Preventive Services Task Force (USPSTF). (2006a). *The guide to clinical preventive services 2006.* USDHHS: AHRQ Pub. No. 06-0588.

U.S. Preventive Services Task Force (USPSTF). (2006b). *Updated USPHSTF recommendations for the use of antiretroviral drugs in pregnant HIV-1-infected women for maternal health and interventions to reduce perinatal HIV-1 transmission in the United States.* Available at: http://aidsinfo.nih.gov.

Varughese, G. I., Chowdhury, S. R., Warner, D. P., & Barton, D. M. (2007). Preconception care of women attending adult general diabetes clinics—Are we doing enough? *Diabetes Research & Clinical Practice, 76*(1), 142–145.

Wang, M. (2007). Perinatal drug abuse and neonatal withdrawal. *eMedicine.* Available at: http://www.emedicine.com/ped/topic2631.htm.

Weekes, A. J., & Lee, D. S. (2006). Substance abuse: Cocaine. *eMedicine*. Available at: http://www.emedicine.com/ped/topic2666.htm.

Witcher, P. M., & Harvey, C. J. (2006). Modifying labor routines for the woman with cardiac disease. *Journal of Perinatal & Neonatal Nursing, 20*(4), 303–311.

Wooley, C. F., & Boudoulas, H. (2007). Mitral valve prolapse: The floppy mitral valve, mitral valve prolapse, and mitral valvular regurgitation. In R. E. Rakel & E. T. Bope (Eds.), *Conn's current therapy 2007* (Section 5, pp. 386–390). Philadelphia: Saunders Elsevier.

World Health Organization (WHO). (2007). *Tuberculosis*. Available at: http://www.who.int/mediacentre/factsheets/fs104/en/.

Xu, F., Markowitz, L. E., Gottlieb, S. L., & Berman, S. M. (2007). Seroprevalence of herpes simplex virus types 1 and 2 in pregnant women in the United States. *American Journal of Obstetrics & Gynecology, 196*(1), 43–46.

Zarrett, N., & Eccles, J. (2006). The passage to adulthood: Challenges of late adolescence. *New Directions for Youth Development*, Fall (111), 13–28.

Zeck, W., Bjelic-Radisic, V., Haas, J., & Greimel, E. (2007). Impact of adolescent pregnancy on the future life of young mothers in terms of social, familial, and educational changes. *Journal of Adolescent Health, 41*(4), 380–388.

WEBSITES

Alan Guttmacher Institute: www.agi-usa.org

Alcoholics Anonymous: www.alcoholics-anonymous.org

American Academy of Pediatrics: www.aap.org

American College of Obstetricians and Gynecologists: www.acog.org

American Diabetes Association: www.diabetes.org

American Lung Association: www.lungusa.org

American Medical Association HIV/AIDS Resource Center: www.ama-assn.org/special/hiv

American Society of Addiction Medicine: www.asam.org

Association of Nurses in AIDS Care: www.anacnet.org

Association of Women's Health, Obstetric & Neonatal Nurses: www.awhonn.org

Asthma and Allergy Foundation of America: www.aafa.org

Allergy & Asthma Network of Mothers of Asthmatics: www.breatherville.org

CDC National Prevention Information Network: 1-800-458-5231, www.cdcnpin.org

HIV websites: www.hivinsite.ucsf.edu, www.hivatis.org

International Nurses Society on Addictions: www.intnsa.org

March of Dimes: www.modimes.org

Narcotics Anonymous: www.na.org

National Campaign to Prevent Teen Pregnancy: www.teenpregnancy.org

National Clearinghouse for Alcohol and Drug Abuse Information: www.health.org

National Heart, Lung and Blood Institute of NIH: www.nhlbi.nih.gov

National Institute on Drug Abuse: www.nida.nih.gov

National Organization for Fetal Alcohol Syndrome: www.nofas.org

Planned Parenthood: www.plannedparenthood.org

Sex Information and Education Council of United States: www.siecus.org

Sidelines High Risk Pregnancy Support Office: www.sidelines.org

Tobacco Information and Prevention Source (TIPS): www.cdc.gov/tobacco

Women for Sobriety Support Group: www.womenforsobriety.org

CHAPTER WORKSHEET

MULTIPLE CHOICE QUESTIONS

1. Which of the following would the nurse include when teaching a pregnant woman about the pathophysiologic mechanisms associated with gestational diabetes?

   a. Pregnancy fosters the development of carbohydrate cravings.

   b. There is progressive resistance to the effects of insulin.

   c. Hypoinsulinemia develops early in the first trimester.

   d. Glucose levels decrease to accommodate fetal growth.

2. When providing prenatal education to a pregnant woman with asthma, which of the following would be important for the nurse to do?

   a. Explain that she should avoid steroids during her pregnancy.

   b. Demonstrate how to assess her blood glucose levels.

   c. Teach correct administration of subcutaneous bronchodilators.

   d. Ensure she seeks treatment for any acute exacerbation.

3. Which of the following conditions would most likely cause a pregnant woman with type 1 diabetes the greatest difficulty during her pregnancy?

   a. Placenta previa

   b. Hyperemesis gravidarum

   c. Abruptio placentae

   d. Rh incompatibility

4. Women who drink alcohol during pregnancy:

   a. Often produce more alcohol dehydrogenase

   b. Usually become intoxicated faster than before

   c. Can give birth to an infant with fetal alcohol spectrum disorder

   d. Gain fewer pounds throughout the gestation

5. When explaining to a pregnant woman about HIV infection and transmission, which of the following would the nurse include?

   a. It primarily occurs when there is a large viral load in the blood.

   b. HIV is most commonly transmitted via sexual contact.

   c. It affects the majority of infants of mothers with HIV infection.

   d. Nurses are most frequently affected due to needle sticks.

CRITICAL THINKING EXERCISES

1. A client at 26 weeks' gestation came to the clinic to follow up on her previous 1-hour glucose screening. Her results had come back outside the accepted screening range, and a 3-hour glucose tolerance test (GTT) had been ordered. It resulted in three abnormal values, confirming a diagnosis of gestational diabetes. As the nurse in the prenatal clinic you are seeing her for the first time.

   a. What additional information will you need to provide care for her?

   b. What education will she need to address this new diagnosis?

   c. How will you evaluate the effectiveness of your interventions?

2. A 14-year-old girl comes to the public health clinic with her mother. The mother tells you that her daughter has been "out messing around and has gotten herself pregnant." The girl is crying quietly in the corner and avoids eye contact with you. The mother reports that her daughter "must be following in my footsteps" because she became pregnant when she was only 15 years old. The client's mother goes back out into the waiting room and leaves the client with you.

   a. What is your first approach with the client to gain her trust?

   b. List the client's educational needs during this pregnancy.

   c. What prevention strategies are needed to prevent a second pregnancy?

3. Linda, a 27-year-old G3P2, is admitted to the labor and birth suite because of preterm rupture of membranes at an estimated 35 weeks' gestation. She has received no prenatal care and reports this was an unplanned pregnancy. Linda appears distracted and very thin. She reports that her two previous children have been in foster care since birth because the child welfare authorities "didn't think I was an adequate mother." She denies any recent use of alcohol or

drugs, but you smell alcohol on her breath. She has a spontaneous vaginal birth a few hours later, producing a 4-lb baby boy with Apgar scores of 8 at 1 minute and 9 at 5 minutes.

a. What aspects of this woman's history may lead the nurse to suspect that this infant may be at risk for fetal alcohol spectrum disorder?

b. What additional screening or laboratory tests might validate your suspicion?

c. What physical and neurodevelopmental deficits might present later in life if the infant has fetal alcohol spectrum disorder?

STUDY ACTIVITIES

1. In the maternity clinic or hospital setting, interview a pregnant woman with a preexisting medical condition (e.g., diabetes, asthma, sickle cell anemia) and find out how this condition affects her life and this pregnancy, especially her lifestyle choices.

2. You have a close friend who has a problem with alcohol but denies it. She now admits to you that she thinks she is pregnant because she missed her period. What specific information and advice should you give her concerning alcohol use during pregnancy?

3. Should marijuana be legalized in the United States? What impact might your view (pro or con) have on pregnant women and their offspring?

4. Outline a discussion you might have with an HIV-positive pregnant woman who doesn't see the need to take antiretroviral agents to prevent perinatal transmission.

5. The nurse is preparing a teaching session about breastfeeding for a group of pregnant women who have various infections listed below. The nurse would include women with which of the following conditions? Select all that apply.

a. Hepatitis B

b. Parvovirus B19

c. Herpesvirus type 2

d. HIV-positive status

e. Cytomegalovirus

f. Varicella-zoster virus

NURSING MANAGEMENT OF LABOR AND BIRTH AT RISK

Jennifer, a 29 year-old G1P0, is at 41 weeks' gestation. Her health care provider has recommended that she come in for induction. She is very anxious about doing this since she has heard "horror stories" about the "hard painful contractions" that can result. What can the nurse do to calm her fears?

KEY TERMS

amnioinfusion
cesarean birth
dystocia
forceps
hypertonic uterine
   dysfunction
hypotonic uterine
   dysfunction

labor induction
macrosomia
postterm pregnancy
precipitous labor
preterm labor
shoulder dystocia

tocolytic
umbilical cord prolapse
vacuum extractor
vaginal birth after
   cesarean (VBAC)

LEARNING OBJECTIVES

Upon completion of the chapter, the learner will be able to:

1. Define dystocia.
2. Identify the four major abnormalities or problems associated with dysfunctional labor patterns, giving examples of each problem.
3. Describe the nursing management for the woman with dysfunctional labor experiencing a problem with the powers, passenger, passageway, and psyche.
4. Develop a plan of care for the woman experiencing preterm labor.
5. Discuss the nursing assessment and management of the woman experiencing a postterm pregnancy.
6. Explain four obstetric emergencies that can complicate labor and birth, including appropriate management for each.
7. Compare and contrast the nursing management for the woman undergoing labor induction or augmentation, forceps- and vacuum-assisted birth.
8. Summarize the plan of care for a woman who is to undergo a cesarean birth.
9. Discuss the key areas to be addressed when caring for a woman who is to undergo vaginal birth after cesarean (VBAC).

Wow

In face of a crisis or a potentially bad outcome, add a mixture of warmth and serenity to your technical abilities.

Most women describe pregnancy as an exciting time in their life, but the development of an unexpected problem can suddenly change this description dramatically. Consider the woman who has had a problem-free pregnancy and then suddenly develops a condition during labor, changing a routine situation into a possible crisis. Many complications occur with little or no warning and present challenges for the perinatal health care team as well as the family. The nurse plays a major role in identifying the problem quickly and coordinating immediate intervention, ultimately achieving a positive outcome.

National Health Goals address maternal and newborn outcomes involving complications of labor and birth and cesarean birth (USDHHS, 2000). These goals are highlighted in Healthy People 2010 21.1.

This chapter will address several conditions occurring during labor and birth that may increase the risk of an adverse outcome for the mother and fetus. It also describes birth-related procedures that may be necessary for the woman who develops a condition that increases her risk or that may be needed to reduce the woman's risk for developing a condition, thus promoting optimal maternal and fetal outcomes. Nursing management of the woman and her family focuses on professional support and compassionate care.

Dystocia

Dystocia, defined as abnormal or difficult labor, can be influenced by a vast number of maternal and fetal factors. Dystocia is said to exist when the progress of labor deviates from normal; it is characterized by a slow and abnormal progression of labor. It occurs in approximately 8% to 11% of all labors and is the leading indicator for primary cesarean birth in the United States (Joy & Lyon, 2007).

To characterize a labor as abnormal, a basic understanding of normal labor is essential. Normal labor starts with regular uterine contractions that are strong enough to result in cervical effacement and dilation. Early in labor, uterine contractions are irregular and cervical effacement and dilation occur gradually. When cervical dilation reaches 4 cm and uterine contractions become more powerful, the active phase of labor begins. It is usually during the active phase that dystocia becomes apparent. Because dystocia cannot be predicted or diagnosed with certainty, the term "failure to progress" is often used. This term includes lack of progressive cervical dilation, lack of descent of the fetal head, or both. An adequate trial of labor is needed to declare with confidence that dystocia or "failure to progress" exists.

Early identification of and prompt interventions for dystocia are essential to minimize risk to the woman and fetus. According to American College of Obstetrics and Gynecology (ACOG, 2003a), factors associated with an increased risk for dystocia include epidural analgesia, excessive analgesia, multiple gestation, hydramnios, maternal exhaustion, ineffective maternal pushing technique, occiput posterior position, longer first stage of labor, nulliparity, short maternal stature (less than 5 feet tall), fetal birth weight (more than 8.8 lb), shoulder dystocia, abnormal fetal presentation or position (breech), fetal anomalies (hydrocephalus), maternal age older than 35 years, gestational age more than 41 weeks, chorioamnionitis, ineffective uterine contractions, and high fetal station at complete cervical dilation.

Dystocia can result from problems or abnormalities involving the expulsive forces (known as the "powers"); presentation, position, and fetal development (the "passenger"); the maternal bony pelvis or birth canal (the "passageway"); and maternal stress (the "psyche"). Table 21.1 summarizes the diagnosis, therapeutic management, and nursing management of the common problems associated with dystocia.

▶ PROBLEMS WITH THE POWERS

When the expulsive forces of the uterus become dysfunctional, the uterus may either never fully relax (hypertonic contractions), placing the fetus in jeopardy, or relax too much (hypotonic contractions), causing ineffective contractions. Still another dysfunction can occur when the uterus contracts so frequently and with such intensity that a very rapid birth will take place (precipitous labor).

(text continues on page 643)

HEALTHY PEOPLE 2010	
Objective	**Significance**
Reduce maternal illness and complications due to pregnancy	• Will help to focus attention on the need for close antepartum surveillance and identification of risk factors for maternal illness and complications, particularly those most likely to be associated with maternal death
Reduce maternal complications during hospitalized labor and delivery from a baseline of 31.2/100 deliveries to a target of 24/100 deliveries	
Reduce cesarean births among low-risk (full term, singleton, vertex presentation) women	• Will help to promote development of specific guidelines for trials of labor and labor management, continual labor support, and practice patterns, while helping to ensure positive maternal and newborn outcomes
Reduce the number of cesarean births in women giving birth for the first time from a baseline of 18% to 15%	
Reduce the number of cesarean births in women with prior cesarean birth from 72% to 63%	

USDHHS, 2000.

TABLE 21.1 DIAGNOSIS AND MANAGEMENT OF COMMON PROBLEMS ASSOCIATED WITH DYSTOCIA

	Description	Diagnosis	Therapeutic Management	Nursing Management
Problems with the powers				
Hypertonic uterine dysfunction *more than 15mmHg*	Occurring in the latent phase of the first stage of labor (cervical dilation of <4 cm); uncoordinated. Force of contraction typically in the midsection of uterus at the junction of the active upper and passive lower segments of the uterus rather than in the fundus. Loss of downward pressure to push the presenting part against the cervix (Gilbert & Harmon, 2007). Woman commonly becomes discouraged due to lack of progress; also has increased pain secondary to uterine anoxia.	Characteristic hypertonicity of the contractions and the lack of labor progress	Therapeutic rest with the use of sedatives to promote relaxation and stop the abnormal activity of the uterus. Identification and intervention of any contributing factors. Ruling out abruptio placentae (also associated with high resting tone and persistent pain). Onset of a normal labor pattern occurs in many women after a 4- to 6-hour rest period (Gilbert, 2007).	Institute bed rest and sedation to promote relaxation and reduce pain. Assist with measures to rule out fetopelvic disproportion and fetal malpresentation. Evaluate fetal tolerance to labor pattern, such as monitoring of FHR patterns. Assess for signs of maternal infection. Promote adequate hydration through IV therapy. Provide pain management via epidural or IV analgesics. Assist with amniotomy to augment labor. Explain to woman and family about dysfunctional pattern. Plan for operative birth if normal labor pattern is not achieved.
Hypotonic uterine dysfunction *less than 10mmHg*	Often termed secondary uterine inertia because the labor begins normally and then the frequency and intensity of contractions decrease (Joy & Lyon, 2007). Possible contributing factors: overdistended uterus with multifetal pregnancy or large single fetus, too much pain medicine given too early in labor, fetal malposition, and regional anesthesia (Bonilla & Forouzan, 2007).	Evaluation of the woman's labor to confirm that she is having hypotonic active labor rather than a long latent phase. Evaluation of maternal pelvis and fetal presentation and position to ensure that they are not contributing to the prolonged labor without noticeable progress.	Identification of possible cause of inefficient uterine action (a malpositioned fetus, a too small maternal pelvis, overdistention of the uterus with fluid or a macrosomic fetus), Rupture of amniotic sac (amniotomy) if all causes ruled out. Possible augmentation with oxytocin (Pitocin) to stimulate effective uterine contractions. Cesarean birth if amniotomy and augmentation ineffective.	Administer oxytocin as ordered once fetopelvic disproportion is ruled out. Assist with amniotomy if membranes are intact. Provide continuous electronic fetal monitoring. Monitor vital signs, contractions, and cervix continually. Assess for signs of maternal and fetal infection. Explain to woman and family about dysfunctional pattern. Plan for surgical birth if normal labor pattern is not achieved or fetal distress occurs. *check for CPD*

Precipitous labor	Abrupt onset of higher-intensity contractions occurring in a shorter period of time instead of the more gradual increase in frequency, duration, and intensity that typifies most spontaneous labors	Identification based on the rapidity of progress through the stages of labor	Vaginal delivery if maternal pelvis is adequate	Closely monitor woman with previous history. Anticipate use of scheduled induction to control labor rate. Administer pharmacologic agents, such as tocolytics, to slow labor. Stay in constant attendance to monitor progress.
Problems with the passenger				
Persistent occiput posterior position	Engagement of fetal head in the left or right occipito-transverse position with the occiput rotating posteriorly rather than into the more favorable occiput anterior position (fetus born facing upward instead of the normal downward position) (Bonilla & Forouzan, 2007). Labor usually much longer and more uncomfortable (causing increased back pain during labor) if fetus remains in this position. Possible extensive caput succedaneum and molding from the sustained occiput posterior position.	Leopold maneuvers and vaginal examination to determine position of fetal head in conjunction with the mother's complaints of severe back pain (back of fetal head pressing on mother's sacrum and coccyx).	Labor to proceed, preparing the woman for a long labor (spontaneous resolution possible). Comfort measures and maternal positioning to help promote fetal head rotation.	Assess for complaints of intense back pain in first stage of labor. Anticipate possible use of forceps to rotate to anterior position at birth or manual rotation to anterior position at end of second stage. Assess for prolonged second stage of labor with arrest of descent (common with this malposition). Encourage maternal position changes to promote fetal head rotation: hands and knees and rocking pelvis back and forth; side-lying position; side lunges during contractions; sitting, kneeling, or standing while leaning forward; squatting position to give birth and enlarge pelvic outlet. Prepare for possible cesarean birth if rotation is not achieved. Administer agents as ordered for pain relief (effective pain relief crucial to help the woman to tolerate the back discomfort). Apply low back counterpressure during contractions to ease the discomfort. Use other

(continued)

TABLE 21.1 DIAGNOSIS AND MANAGEMENT OF COMMON PROBLEMS ASSOCIATED WITH DYSTOCIA (continued)

Description	Diagnosis	Therapeutic Management	Nursing Management
			helpful measures to attempt to rotate the fetal head, including lateral abdominal stroking in the direction that the fetal head should rotate, assisting the client into a hands-and-knees position (all fours); and squatting, pelvic rocking, stair climbing, assuming a side-lying position toward the side that the fetus should rotate, and side lunges (WHO, 2007). Provide measures to reduce anxiety. Continuously reinforce the woman's progress. Teach woman about measures to facilitate fetal head rotation.
Face and brow presentation	Face presentation with complete extension of the fetal head. Brow presentation: fetal head between full extension and full flexion so that the largest fetal skull diameter presents to the pelvis.	Diagnosis only once labor is well established via vaginal examination; palpation of facial features as the presenting part rather than the fetal head	Vaginal birth possible with face presentation with an adequate maternal pelvis and fetal head rotation; cesarean birth if head rotates backward. Cesarean birth for brow presentation unless head flexes.	Assist with evaluating for fetopelvic disproportion. Anticipate cesarean birth if vertex position is not achieved. Explain fetal malposition to the woman and her partner. Provide close observation for any signs of fetal hypoxia, as evidenced by late decelerations on the fetal monitor.
Breech presentation	Fetal buttocks, or breech, presenting first rather than the head. 1. Frank breech: buttock as the presenting part, with hips flexed and legs and knees extended upward 2. Complete breech (or full breech): buttock as presenting part, with hips flexed and knees flexed in a "cannonball" position	Vaginal examination to determine breech presentation. Ideally, ultrasound to confirm a clinically suspected presentation and to identify any fetal anomalies.	The optimal method of birth is controversial: cesarean birth by some providers unless the fetus is small and the mother has a large pelvis; vaginal birth by others with each occurrence treated individually and labor monitored very closely.	Assess for associated conditions such as placenta previa, hydramnios, fetal anomalies, and multiple gestation. Arrange for ultrasound to confirm fetal presentation. Assist with external cephalic version possible after 36 weeks and administer tocolytics to assist with external cephalic version.

3. Footling or incomplete breech: One or two feet as the presenting part, with one or both hips extended

Regardless of the birth method selected, the risk for trauma is high. Breech vaginal births are not recommended by ACOG and come with a higher risk to the mother and infant than a planned surgical birth (ACOG, 2001). Vaginal delivery: fetus allowed to spontaneously deliver up to the umbilicus; then maneuvers to assist in the delivery of the remainder of the body, arms, and head; fetal membranes left intact as long as possible to act as a dilating wedge and to prevent cord prolapse; anesthesiologist and pediatrician present.

Caesarean birth; Use of external cephalic version to reduce the chance of breech presentation at birth; attempted after the 36th week of gestation but before the start of labor (some fetuses spontaneously turn to a cephalic presentation on their own toward term, and some will return to the breech presentation if external cephalic version is attempted too early [Fischer, 2007]); variable success rates, with risk for fractured bones, ruptured viscera, abruptio placentae, fetomaternal hemorrhage, and umbilical cord

Anticipate trial labor for 4 to 6 hours to evaluate progress if version is unsuccessful. Plan for cesarean birth if no progress is seen or fetal distress occurs.
After external cephalic version, administer RhoGAM to the Rh-negative woman to prevent a sensitization reaction if trauma has occurred and the potential for mixing of blood exists (Gilbert, 2007).

(continued)

TABLE 21.1 DIAGNOSIS AND MANAGEMENT OF COMMON PROBLEMS ASSOCIATED WITH DYSTOCIA (continued)

	Description	Diagnosis	Therapeutic Management	Nursing Management
			entanglement (Fischer, 2007). Tocolytic drugs to relax the uterus, as well as other methods, to facilitate external cephalic version at term (Jenis, 2007). Individual evaluation of each woman for all factors before any interventions are initiated.	Intervene immediately due to cord compression.
Shoulder dystocia	Delivery of fetal head with neck not appearing; retraction of chin against the perineum; shoulders remaining wedged behind the mother's pubic bone, causing a difficult birth with potential for injury to both mother and baby. If shoulders still above the brim at this stage, no advancement. Newborn's chest trapped within the vaginal vault; chest unable to expand with respiration (although nose and mouth are outside). Risk of umbilical cord compression between the fetal body and the maternal pelvis.	Emergency, often unexpected complication. Diagnosis made when newborn's head delivers without delivery of neck and remaining body structures. Primary risk factors, including suspected infant macrosomia (weight >4,500 g), maternal diabetes mellitus, excessive maternal weight gain, abnormal maternal pelvic anatomy, maternal obesity, postdates pregnancy, short stature, a history of previous shoulder dystocia, and use of epidural analgesia (Gurewitsch et al., 2006).	If anticipated, preparatory tasks instituted: alerting of key personnel; education of woman and family regarding steps to be taken in the event of a difficult birth; emptying of woman's bladder to allow additional room for possible maneuvers needed for the birth. McRobert's maneuver. Suprapubic pressure (not fundal) (see Fig. 21.1). Combination of maneuvers effective in more than 50% of cases of shoulder dystocia (Abenhaim et al., 2007). Newborn resuscitation team readily available.	Perform McRobert's maneuver and application of suprapubic pressure. Assist with positioning the woman in squatting position, hands-and-knees position, or lateral recumbent position for birth to free shoulder. Anticipate cesarean birth if no success in dislodging shoulders. Clear room of unnecessary clutter to make room for additional personnel and equipment (Anderson, 2007). After the birth, assess newborn for crepitus, deformity, Erb's palsy, or bruising, which might suggest neurologic damage or a fracture (Arenson & Drake, 2007).
Multiple gestation	More than one fetus, leading to uterine overdistention and possibly resulting in hypotonic contractions and abnormal presentations of the fetuses. Fetal hypoxia during labor a significant threat due to placenta providing oxygen and nutrients to more than one fetus.	Nearly all multiples are now diagnosed early by ultrasound. Most women go into labor before 37 weeks.	Admission to facility with specialized care unit if woman goes into labor. Spontaneous progression of labor if woman has no complicating factors and first fetus is in longitudinal lie. Separate monitoring of each fetal heart rate during labor and birth.	Assess for hypotonic labor pattern due to overdistention. Evaluate for fetal presentation, maternal pelvic size, and gestational age to determine mode of delivery. Ensure presence of neonatal team for birth of multiples. Anticipate need for cesarean birth, which is common in multiple gestations.

Variation	Effects on labor	Diagnostic findings	Medical management	Nursing management
(continued from previous page)			After birth of first fetus, clamping of cord and lie of the second twin assessed. Possible external cephalic version necessary to assist in providing a longitudinal lie. Second and subsequent fetuses at greater risk for birth-related complications, such as umbilical cord prolapse, malpresentation, and abruptio placentae (Zach & Pramanik, 2007). Cesarean birth if risk factors high.	
Excessive fetal size and abnormalities	Macrosomia leading to fetopelvic disproportion (fetus unable to fit through the maternal pelvis to be born vaginally). Reduced contraction strength due to overdistention by large fetus leading to a prolonged labor and the potential for birth injury and trauma. Fetal abnormalities possibly interfering with fetal descent, leading to prolonged labor and difficult birth.	A diagnosis of fetal macrosomia can be confirmed by measuring the birthweight after birth. Suspicion of macrosomia based on the findings of an ultrasound examination before onset of labor (if suspected due to conditions such as maternal diabetes or obesity, estimation of fetal weight via ultrasound). Leopold's maneuvers to estimate fetal weight and position on admission to labor and birth unit.	Scheduled cesarean birth if diagnosis is made before the onset of labor to reduce the risk of injury to both the newborn and the mother. If identified by Leopold's maneuvers, possible trial of labor to evaluate progress; however, providers usually opt to proceed with a cesarean birth in a primigravida with a macrosomic fetus (Catalano, 2007).	Assess for inability of fetus to descend. Anticipate need for vacuum and forceps-assisted births (common). Plan for cesarean birth if maternal parameters are inadequate to give birth to large fetus.
Problems with the passageway	Contraction of one or more of the three planes of the pelvis. Poorer prognosis for vaginal birth in women with android and platypelloid types of pelvis. Contracted pelvis involving reduction in one or more of the pelvic diameters interfering with progress	Shortest A-P diameter <10 cm or greatest transverse diameter <12 cm. (Approximation of A-P diameter via measurement of diagonal conjugate, which in the contracted pelvis is <11.5 cm). X-ray pelvimetry to determine the smallest A-P diameter	Focus on allowing natural forces of labor contractions to push the largest diameter (biparietal) of the fetal head beyond the obstruction or narrow passage. Possible forceps and vacuum extraction to assist navigation through this passageway.	Assess for poor contractions, slow dilation, prolonged labor. Evaluate bowel and bladder status to reduce soft tissue obstruction and allow increased pelvic space. Anticipate trial of labor; if no labor progression after an adequate trial, plan for cesarean birth.

(continued)

TABLE 21.1 DIAGNOSIS AND MANAGEMENT OF COMMON PROBLEMS ASSOCIATED WITH DYSTOCIA (continued)

	Description	Diagnosis	Therapeutic Management	Nursing Management
	of labor: inlet, midpelvis, and outlet contracture. Obstruction in the birth canal, such as placenta previa that partially or completely obstructs the internal os of the cervix, fibroids in the lower uterine segment, a full bladder or rectum, an edematous cervix caused by premature bearing-down efforts, and human papillomavirus (HPV) warts.	through which the fetal head must pass. Interischial tuberous diameter of <8 cm possibly compromising outlet contracture (outlet and midpelvic contractures frequently occur together).		
Problems with the psyche	Release of stress-related hormones (catecholamines, cortisol, epinephrine, beta-endorphin), which act on smooth muscle (uterus) and reduce uterine contractility. Excessive release of catecholamines and other stress-related hormones not therapeutic. Release also results in decreased uteroplacental perfusion and increased risk for poor newborn adjustment (Gilbert, 2007).	Ruling out of other possible causes of dystocia	Treatment dependent on woman's responses such as anxiety, fear, anger, frustration, or denial (highly variable due to woman's understanding of the condition itself, past experiences, previous coping mechanisms, and the amount of family and nursing support received). Appropriate medical or surgical interventions depending on the underlying condition.	Provide comfortable environment—dim lighting, music. Encourage partner to participate. Provide pain management to reduce anxiety and stress. Ensure continuous presence of staff to allay anxiety. Provide frequent updates concerning fetal status and progress. Provide ongoing encouragement to minimize the woman's stress and help her to cope with labor and to promote a positive, timely outcome. Assist in relaxation and comfort measures to help her body work more effectively with the forces of labor. Engage the woman in conversation about her emotional well-being; offer anticipatory guidance and reassurance to increase her self-esteem and ability to cope, decrease frustration, and encourage cooperation.

Hypertonic uterine dysfunction occurs when the uterus never fully relaxes between contractions. Subsequently, contractions are erratic and poorly coordinated because more than one uterine pacemaker is sending signals for contraction. Placental perfusion becomes compromised, thereby reducing oxygen to the fetus. These hypertonic contractions exhaust the mother, who is experiencing frequent, intense, and painful contractions with little progression. This dysfunctional pattern occurs in early labor and affects nulliparous women more than multiparous women (Cheng & Caughey, 2007).

Hypotonic uterine dysfunction occurs during active labor (dilation more than 4 cm) when contractions become poor in quality and lack sufficient intensity to dilate and efface the cervix. The major risk with this complication is hemorrhage after giving birth because the uterus cannot contract effectively to compress blood vessels.

Precipitous labor is one that is completed in less than 3 hours. Women experiencing precipitous labor typically have soft perineal tissues that stretch readily, permitting the fetus to pass through the pelvis quickly and easily. Maternal complications are rare if the maternal pelvis is adequate and the soft tissues yield to a fast fetal descent. Potential fetal complications may include head trauma, such as intracranial hemorrhage or nerve damage, and hypoxia due to the rapid progression of labor (Sharf et al., 2007).

▶ PROBLEMS WITH THE PASSENGER

Any presentation other than occiput anterior or a slight variation of the fetal position or size increases the probability of dystocia. These variations can affect the contractions or fetal descent through the maternal pelvis. Common problems involving the fetus include occiput posterior position, breech presentation, multifetal pregnancy, excessive size (macrosomia) as it relates to cephalopelvic disproportion (CPD), and structural anomalies.

Persistent occiput posterior is the most common malposition, occurring in about 15% of laboring women. The reasons for this malposition are often unclear. This position presents slightly larger diameters to the maternal pelvis, thus slowing fetal descent. A fetal head that is poorly flexed may be responsible. In addition, poor uterine contractions may not push the fetal head down into the pelvic floor to the extent that the fetal occiput sinks into it rather than being pushed to rotate in an anterior direction.

Face and brow presentations are rare and are associated with fetal abnormalities (anencephaly), pelvic contractures, high parity, placenta previa, hydramnios, low birthweight, or a large fetus (WHO, 2007).

Breech presentation, which occurs in 3% to 4% of labors, is frequently associated with multifetal pregnancies, grand multiparity (more than five births), advanced mater-

nal age, placenta previa, hydramnios, preterm births, and fetal anomalies such as hydrocephaly (Lee, El-Sayed, & Gould, 2007). In a persistent breech presentation, an increased frequency of prolapsed cord, placenta previa, low birthweight from preterm birth, fetal or uterine anomalies, and perinatal morbidity and mortality from a difficult birth may occur (Cunningham et al., 2005). Perinatal mortality is increased two- to four-fold with a breech presentation, regardless of the mode of delivery (Lee, El-Sayed, & Gould, 2007).

Shoulder dystocia is defined as the obstruction of fetal descent and birth by the axis of the fetal shoulders after the fetal head has been delivered. The incidence of shoulder dystocia is increasing due to increasing birthweight, with reports of it in up to 2% of vaginal births. It is one of the most anxiety-provoking emergencies encountered in labor. Failure of the shoulders to deliver spontaneously places both the woman and the fetus at risk for injury. Postpartum hemorrhage, secondary to uterine atony or vaginal lacerations, is the major complication to the mother. Transient Erb's or Duchenne's brachial plexus palsies and clavicular or humeral fractures are the most common fetal injuries encountered with shoulder dystocia (WHO, 2007). Newborns experiencing shoulder dystocia typically have greater shoulder-to-head and chest-to-head disproportions compared with those delivered without dystocia (Cunningham et al., 2005). Prompt recognition and appropriate management, such as with McRobert's maneuver or suprapubic pressure, can reduce the severity of injuries to the mother and newborn (Fig. 21.1).

▶ **Take** NOTE!

Prompt recognition and appropriate management of shoulder dystocia can reduce the severity of injuries to the mother and infant. Immediately assess the infant for signs of trauma such as a fractured clavicle, Erb's palsy, or neonatal asphyxia. Assess the mother for excessive vaginal bleeding and blood in the urine from bladder trauma.

Multiple gestation refers to twins, triplets, or more infants within a single pregnancy (Box 21.1). The incidence is increasing, primarily as a result of infertility treatment (both ovarian stimulation and in vitro fertilization) and an increased number of women giving birth at older ages (March of Dimes, 2007b). The incidence of twins is approximately 1 in 30 conceptions, with about two thirds of them due to the fertilization of two ova (dizygotic or fraternal) and about one third occurring from the splitting of one fertilized ovum (monozygotic or identical twins). One in approximately 8,100 pregnancies results in triplets (March of Dimes, 2007b). The most

A   B

FIGURE 21.1 Maneuvers to relieve shoulder dystocia. (**A**) McRobert's maneuver. The mother's thighs are flexed and abducted as much as possible to straighten the pelvic curve. (**B**) Suprapubic pressure. Pressure is applied just above the pubic bone, pushing the fetal anterior shoulder downward to displace it from above the mother's symphysis pubis. The newborn's head is depressed toward the mother's anus while suprapubic pressure is applied.

BOX 21.1 Multiple Gestation

As the name implies, multiple gestation involves more than one fetus. These fetuses can result from fertilization of a single ovum or multiple ova. Twin pregnancies that are single-ovum conceptions (monozygotic twins) share one chorion (membrane closest to the uterus), and each twin has his or her own amnion (membrane surrounding the amniotic fluid). One fertilized ovum splits into two separate individuals who are said to be natural clones. They have separate amniotic sacs and placentas, are identical in appearance, and are always the same gender. Twin pregnancies that are multiple-ova conceptions (dizygotic twins) result from two ova fertilized by two sperm. Genetically, dizygotic twins are as alike (or unlike) as any other pair or siblings.

The fetuses of a twin gestation, whether monozygotic or dizygotic, are slightly "squashed" because two fetuses develop in a space usually occupied by one. This compression is reflected in the slowing of weight gain in both twins compared to that for singletons (Zach & Pramanik, 2007).

Multiple births other than twins can be of the identical type, the fraternal type, or combinations of the two. Triplets can occur from the division of one zygote into two, with one dividing again, producing identical triplets, or they can come from two zygotes, one dividing into a set of identical twins, and the second zygote developing as a single fraternal sibling, or from three separate zygotes. Triplets are said to occur once in 7,000 births and quadruplets once in 660,000 births (March of Dimes, 2007b). In recent years, fertility drugs used to induce ovulation have resulted in a greater frequency of quadruplets, quintuplets, sextuplets, and even octuplets.

---

common maternal complication is postpartum hemorrhage resulting from uterine atony.

Excessive fetal size and abnormalities can also contribute to labor and birth dysfunctions. **Macrosomia**, in which a newborn weighs 4,000 to 4,500 g (8.13 to 9.15 lb) or more at birth, complicates approximately 10% of all pregnancies (Jazayeri & Contreras, 2007). Fetal abnormalities may include hydrocephalus, ascites, or a large mass on the neck or head. Complications associated with dystocia related to excessive fetal size and anomalies include an increased risk for postpartum hemorrhage, dysfunctional labor, fetopelvic disproportion, soft tissue laceration during vaginal birth, fetal injuries or fractures, and asphyxia (Joy & Lyon, 2007).

▶ PROBLEMS WITH THE PASSAGEWAY

Problems with the passageway (pelvis and birth canal) are related to a contraction of one or more of the three planes of the maternal pelvis: inlet, midpelvis, and outlet. The female pelvis can be classified into four types based on the shape of the pelvic inlet, which is bounded anteriorly by the posterior border of the symphysis pubis, posteriorly by the sacral promontory, and laterally by the linea terminalis. The four basic types are gynecoid, anthropoid, android, and platypelloid (see Chapter 12 for additional information). Contraction of the midpelvis is more common than inlet contraction and typically causes an arrest of fetal descent. Obstructions in the maternal birth canal, such as swelling of the soft maternal tissue and cervix, termed soft tissue dystocia, also can hamper fetal descent and impede labor progression outside the maternal bony pelvis.

PROBLEMS WITH THE PSYCHE

Many women experience an array of emotions during labor, which may include fear, anxiety, helplessness, being alone, and weariness. These emotions can lead to psychological stress, which indirectly can cause dystocia.

Nursing Assessment

Begin the assessment by reviewing the client's history to look for risk factors for dystocia. Include in the assessment the mother's frame of mind to identify fear, anxiety, stress, lack of support, and pain, which can interfere with uterine contractions and impede labor progress. Helping the woman to relax will promote normal labor progress.

Assess the woman's vital signs. Note any elevation in temperature (might suggest an infection) or changes in heart rate or blood pressure (might signal hypovolemia). Evaluate the uterine contractions for frequency and intensity. Question the woman about any changes in her contraction pattern, such as a decrease or increase in frequency or intensity, and report these. Assess fetal heart rate and pattern, reporting any abnormal patterns immediately.

Assess fetal position via Leopold's maneuvers to identify any deviations in presentation or position, and report any deviations. Assist with or perform a vaginal examination to determine cervical dilation, effacement, and engagement of the fetal presenting part. Evaluate for evidence of membrane rupture. Report any malodorous fluid.

Nursing Management

Nursing management of the woman with dystocia, regardless of the etiology, requires patience. The nurse should provide physical and emotional support to the client and her family. The final outcome of any labor depends on the size and shape of the maternal pelvis, the quality of the uterine contractions, and the size, presentation, and position of the fetus. Thus, dystocia is diagnosed not at the start of labor but rather after it has progressed for a time.

Promoting the Progress of Labor

The nurse plays a major role in determining the progress of labor. Continue to assess the woman, frequently monitoring cervical dilation and effacement, uterine contractions, and fetal descent, and document that all assessed parameters are progressing. Evaluate progress in active labor by using the simple rule of 1 cm/hour for cervical dilation. When the woman's membranes rupture, if they have not already ruptured, observe for visible cord prolapse.

> ▶ *Take* NOTE!
>
> *If a dysfunctional labor occurs, contractions will slow or fail to advance in frequency, duration, or intensity; the cervix will fail to respond to uterine contractions by dilating and effacing; and the fetus will fail to descend.*

Throughout labor, assess the woman's fluid balance status. Check skin turgor and mucous membranes. Monitor intake and output. Also monitor the client's bladder for distention at least every 2 hours and encourage her to empty her bladder often. In addition, monitor her bowel status. A full bladder or rectum can impede descent.

Continue to monitor fetal well-being. If the fetus is in the breech position, be especially observant for visible cord prolapse and note any variable decelerations in heart rate. If either occurs, report it immediately.

Be prepared to administer a labor stimulant such as oxytocin (Pitocin) if ordered to treat hypotonic labor contractions. Anticipate the need to assist with manipulations if shoulder dystocia is diagnosed. Prepare the woman and her family for the possibility of a cesarean birth if labor does not progress.

Providing Physical and Emotional Comfort

Employ physical comfort measures to promote relaxation and reduce stress. Offer blankets for warmth and a backrub, if the client wishes, to reduce muscle tension. Provide an environment conducive to rest so the woman can conserve her energy. Lower the lights and reduce external noise by closing the hallway door. Offer a warm shower to promote relaxation (if not contraindicated). Use pillows to support the woman in a comfortable position, changing her position every 30 minutes to reduce tension and to enhance uterine activity and efficiency. Offer her fluids/food as appropriate to moisten her mouth and replenish her energy (Fig. 21.2).

Assist with providing counterpressure along with backrubs if the fetus is in the occiput posterior position. Encourage the woman to assume different positions to promote fetal rotation. Upright positions are helpful in facilitating fetal rotation and descent. Also encourage the woman to visualize the descent and birth of the fetus.

Assess the woman's level of pain and degree of distress. Administer analgesics as ordered or according to the facility's protocol.

Evaluate the mother's level of fatigue throughout labor, such as verbal expressions of feeling exhausted, inability to cope in early labor, or inability to rest or calm down between contractions. Praise the woman and her partner for their efforts. Provide empathetic listening to increase the client's coping ability, and remain with the client to demonstrate caring.

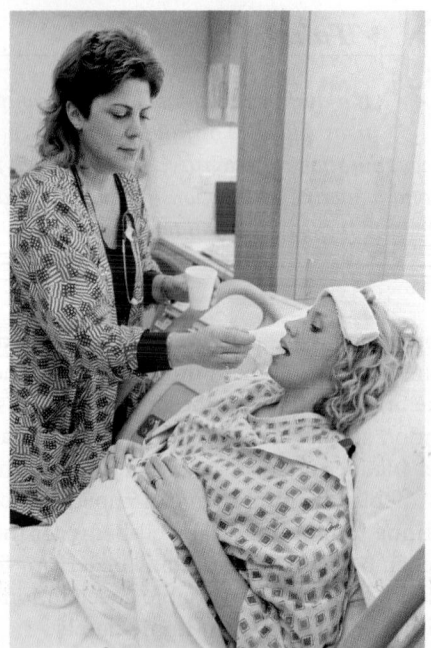

FIGURE 21.2 The nurse applies a cool, moist washcloth to the client's forehead and offers her ice chips to combat thirst and provide comfort for the woman experiencing dystocia.

Promoting Empowerment

Educate the client and family about dysfunctional labor and its causes and therapies. Explain therapeutic interventions that may be needed to assist with the labor process. Encourage the client and her partner to participate in decision making about interventions.

Assist the woman and partner in expressing their fears and anxieties. Provide encouragement to help them to maintain control. Support the client and her partner in their coping efforts. Keep the woman and her partner informed of progress and advocate for them.

Preterm Labor

Preterm labor is defined as the occurrence of regular uterine contractions accompanied by cervical effacement and dilation before the end of the 37th week of gestation. If not halted, it leads to preterm birth.

Preterm births remain one of the biggest contributors to perinatal morbidity and mortality in the world. According to the March of Dimes (2007c, 2007d, 2007e), about 12% of births (one in eight infants) in the United States are premature.

Preterm birth is one of the most common obstetric complications, and its sequelae have a profound effect on the survival and health of the newborn. The rate of preterm births in the United States has increased 35% in the past 20 years. Preterm births account for 75% of neurodevelopmental disorders and other serious morbidities,

as well as behavioral and social problems. They account for 85% of all perinatal morbidity and mortality. In addition, up to $30 billion is spent on maternal and infant care related to prematurity (March of Dimes, 2007c). Infants born prematurely also are at risk for serious sequelae such as respiratory distress syndrome, infections, congenital heart defects, thermoregulation problems that can lead to acidosis and weight loss, intraventricular hemorrhage, feeding difficulties resulting from diminished stomach capacity and an underdeveloped suck reflex, and neurologic disorders related to hypoxia and trauma at birth (Gray, 2006). Although great strides have been made in neonatal intensive care, prematurity remains the leading cause of death within the first month of life and is the second leading cause of all infant deaths (March of Dimes, 2007c).

The exact cause of preterm labor is not known. Currently, prevention is the goal.

Therapeutic Management

Predicting the risk of preterm labor is valuable only if there is an available intervention that is likely to improve the situation. According to ACOG, many factors must be considered before selecting an intervention. Many factors influence the decision to intervene when women present with symptoms of preterm labor, including the probability of progressive labor, gestational age, and the risks of treatment. ACOG (2003b) recommends the following as guidelines:

• There are no clear first-line **tocolytic** drugs (drugs that promote uterine relaxation by interfering with uterine contractions) to manage preterm labor. Clinical circumstances and the health care provider's preference should dictate treatment.
• Antibiotics do not appear to prolong gestation and should be reserved for group B streptococcal prophylaxis in women in whom birth is imminent.
• Tocolytic drugs may prolong pregnancy for 2 to 7 days; during this time, steroids can be given to improve fetal lung maturity and the woman can be transported to a tertiary care center.

Despite these recommendations, health care providers continue to prescribe pharmacologic treatment for preterm labor at home and in the hospital setting. This treatment often includes oral or intravenous tocolytics and varying degrees of activity restriction (Fig. 21.3). Antibiotics may also be prescribed to treat presumed or confirmed infections. Steroids may be given to enhance fetal lung maturity between 24 weeks and 34 weeks' gestation.

Tocolytic Therapy

The decision to stop preterm labor is individualized based on risk factors, extent of cervical dilation, membrane status, fetal gestational age, and presence or absence of infection. Tocolytic therapy is most likely ordered if preterm

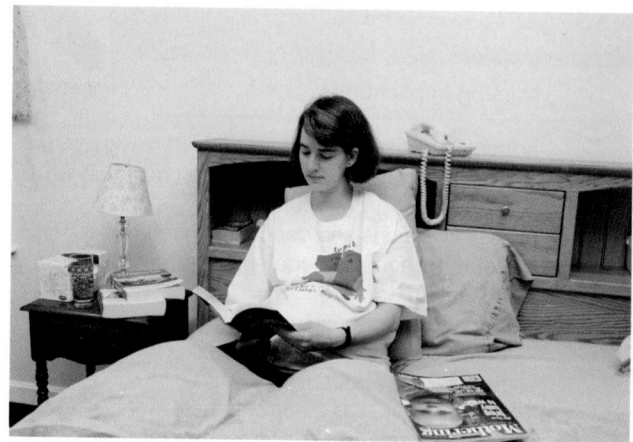

FIGURE 21.3 The mother with preterm labor resting in bed at home.

labor occurs before the 34th week of gestation in an attempt to delay birth and thereby to reduce the severity of respiratory distress syndrome and other complications associated with prematurity. Tocolytic therapy does not typically prevent preterm birth, but it may delay it. It is contraindicated for abruptio placentae, acute fetal distress or death, eclampsia or severe preeclampsia, active vaginal bleeding, dilation of more than 6 cm, chorioamnionitis, and maternal hemodynamic instability (Griffin, 2007).

Medications most commonly used for tocolysis include magnesium sulfate (which reduces the muscle's ability to contract), terbutaline (Brethine, a beta-adrenergic), indomethacin (Indocin, a prostaglandin synthetase inhibitor), and nifedipine (Procardia, a calcium channel blocker). These drugs are used "off label": this means they are effective for this purpose but have not been officially tested and developed for this purpose by the FDA (Tan et al., 2006). All these medications have serious side effects, and the woman needs close supervision when they are being administered (Drug Guide 21.1).

Corticosteroids

Corticosteroids given to the mother in preterm labor can help prevent or reduce the frequency and severity of respiratory distress syndrome in premature infants delivered between 24 weeks and 34 weeks' gestation. The beneficial effects of corticosteroids on fetal lung maturation have been reported within 48 hours of initial administration (Blackburn, 2007). These drugs require at least 24 hours to become effective, so timely administration is crucial.

Nursing Assessment

The preterm birth rate cannot be reduced until there are ways to predict the risk for preterm birth. Because the etiology is often multifactorial, an individualized approach is needed.

Health History and Physical Examination

The signs of preterm labor are subtle and may be overlooked by the client as well as the health care professional. Obtain a thorough health history and be alert for risk factors associated with preterm labor and birth (Box 21.2).

Frequently, women are unaware that uterine contractions, effacement, and dilation are occurring, thus making early intervention ineffective in arresting preterm labor and preventing the birth of a premature newborn. Ask the woman about any complaints, being alert for the subtle symptoms of preterm labor, which may include:

- Change or increase in vaginal discharge
- Pelvic pressure (pushing-down sensation)
- Low, dull backache
- Menstrual-like cramps
- Heaviness or aching in the thighs
- Uterine contractions, with or without pain
- Intestinal cramping, with or without diarrhea (Gilbert, 2007; Gray, 2006)

Assess the pattern of the contractions: the contractions must be persistent, such that four contractions occur every 20 minutes or eight contractions occur in 1 hour. Evaluate cervical dilation and effacement: cervical effacement is 80% or greater and cervical dilation is greater than 1 cm (AAP & ACOG, 2003). On examination, engagement of the fetal presenting part will be noted.

Laboratory and Diagnostic Testing

Commonly used diagnostic testing for preterm labor risk assessment includes a complete blood count to detect infection, which may be a contributing factor to preterm labor; urinalysis to detect bacteria and nitrites, which are indicative of a urinary tract infection; and an amniotic fluid analysis to determine fetal lung maturity and the presence of subclinical chorioamnionitis.

Four other tests may be used for preterm labor prediction: fetal fibronectin testing, cervical length evaluation by transvaginal ultrasound, salivary estriol, and home monitoring of uterine activity to recognize preterm contractions. Fetal fibronectin and cervical length examinations have a high negative predictive value and are thus better at predicting which pregnant women are unlikely to have a preterm birth as opposed to predicting those who will (Grimes-Dennis & Berghella, 2007).

Fetal Fibronectin

Fetal fibronectin, a glycoprotein produced by the chorion, is found at the junction of the chorion and decidua (fetal membranes and uterus). It is present in cervicovaginal fluid prior to delivery, regardless of gestational age. It is not found in vaginal secretions unless there has been a disruption between the chorion and decidua. The test is a useful marker for impending membrane rupture within 7 to 14 days if the level increases to greater than 0.05 ug/mL. Conversely, if fetal fibronectin is not present, there is a

DRUG GUIDE 21.1 MEDICATIONS USED WITH PRETERM LABOR

Drug	Action/Indication	Nursing Implications
Magnesium sulfate	Relaxes uterine muscles to stop irritability and contractions, to arrest uterine contractions for preterm labor (off-label use). Has been used in seizure prophylaxis and treatment of seizures in preeclamptic and eclamptic patients for almost 100 years (Lilley, Harrington, & Snyder, 2007).	Administer IV with a loading dose of 4–6 g over 15–30 minutes initially, and then maintain infusion at 1–4 g per hour. Assess vital signs and deep tendon reflexes (DTRs) hourly; report any hypotension or depressed or absent DTRs. Monitor level of consciousness; report any headache, blurred vision, dizziness, or altered level of consciousness. Perform continuous electronic fetal monitoring; report any decreased fetal heart rate variability, hypotonia, or respiratory depression. Monitor intake and output hourly; report any decrease in output (<30 mL/hour). Assess respiratory rate; report respiratory rate <12 breaths/minute; auscultate lung sounds for evidence of pulmonary edema. Monitor for common maternal side effects, including flushing, nausea and vomiting, dry mouth, lethargy, blurred vision, and headache. Assess for nausea, vomiting, transient hypotension, lethargy. Assess for signs and symptoms of magnesium toxicity, such as decreased level of consciousness, depressed respirations and DTRs, slurred speech, weakness, and respiratory and/or cardiac arrest. Have calcium gluconate readily available at the bedside to reverse magnesium toxicity.
Terbutaline sulfate (Brethine)	Relaxes smooth muscles to calm uterus, inhibits uterine activity to arrest preterm labor	This drug is usually effective in delaying birth for up to 48 hours (Tan et al., 2006). Monitor the mother for adverse effects such as tachycardia, hypotension, palpitations, tremors, chest pain, hypokalemia, water retention, nausea, vomiting, diarrhea, hyperglycemia, decreased urinary output, and nervousness. Monitor fetal well-being, noting any adverse effects such as tachycardia or heart failure. Adverse effects are dose-related and will increase as dose is increased. Perform cardiac assessment of woman to rule out preexisting cardiac disease and diabetes. Institute continuous fetal monitoring. Assess vital signs frequently for changes. Discontinue drug for the following: maternal tachycardia >120 bpm, hypotension <90/60 mmHg, fetal heart rate >180 bpm, signs of maternal pulmonary edema. Have propranolol (Inderal) available to reverse cardiac adverse effects.
Indomethacin (Indocin)	Inhibits prostaglandins, which stimulate contractions; inhibits uterine activity to arrest preterm labor	Continuously assess vital signs, uterine activity, and fetal heart rate. Administer oral form with food to reduce GI irritation.

(handwritten annotation on left side:)
loading dose
4g over 20 min
maintain
2g/hr increasing 1g an hr
until contraction stop
then titrate down

(handwritten annotation under Terbutaline:)
beta adrenergic

Drug	Action/Indication	Nursing Implications
		Do not give to women with peptic ulcer disease. Schedule ultrasound to assess amniotic fluid volume and function of ductus arteriosus before initiating therapy; monitor for signs of maternal hemorrhage. Be alert for maternal adverse effects such as nausea, vomiting, heartburn, rash, prolonged bleeding time, oligohydramnios, and hypertension. Monitor for neonatal adverse effects, including constriction of ductus arteriosus, premature ductus closure, necrotizing enterocolitis, oligohydramnios, and pulmonary hypertension.
Nifedipine (Procardia)	Blocks calcium movement into muscle cells, inhibits uterine activity to arrest preterm labor	Use caution if giving this drug with magnesium sulfate because of increased risk for hypotension. Monitor blood pressure hourly if giving with magnesium sulfate; report a pulse rate >110 bpm. Monitor for fetal effects such as decreased uteroplacental blood flow manifested by fetal bradycardia, which can lead to fetal hypoxia. Monitor for adverse effects, such as flushing of the skin, headache, transient tachycardia, palpitations, postural hypertension, peripheral edema, and transient fetal tachycardia.
Betamethasone (Celestone)	Promotes fetal lung maturity by stimulating surfactant production, prevents or reduces risk of respiratory distress syndrome and intraventricular hemorrhage in the preterm neonate less than 34 weeks' gestation	Administer two doses intramuscularly 24 hours apart. ~12 mg doses~ Monitor for maternal infection or pulmonary edema. ← especially w/ mag sulfate Educate parents about potential benefits of drug to preterm infant. Assess maternal lung sounds and monitor for signs of infection.

[handwritten notes: watch glucose; Dexamethasone 4 doses 12 hrs apart; Penicillin for Group B Strep]

98% chance that the woman will not go into preterm labor (Incerti et al., 2007).

A sterile applicator is used to collect a cervicovaginal sample during a speculum examination. The result is either positive (fetal fibronectin is present) or negative (fetal fibronectin is not present). Interpretation of fetal fibronectin results must always be viewed in conjunction with the clinical findings; it is not used as a lone indicator for predicting preterm labor.

Transvaginal Ultrasound

Transvaginal ultrasound of the cervix has been used as a tool to predict preterm labor in high-risk pregnancies and to differentiate between true and false preterm labor. Three parameters are evaluated during the transvaginal ultrasound: cervical length and width, funnel width and length, and percentage of funneling. Measurement of the closed portion of the cervix visualized during the transvaginal ultrasound is the single most reliable parameter

for prediction of preterm delivery in high-risk women (Blackburn, 2007).

Cervical length varies during pregnancy and can be measured fairly reliably after 16 weeks' gestation using an ultrasound probe inserted in the vagina. A cervical length of 3 cm or more indicates that delivery within 14 days is unlikely. Women with a short cervical length of 2.5 cm during the mid-trimester have a substantially greater risk of preterm birth prior to 35 weeks' gestation. As with fetal fibronectin testing, negative results can be reassuring and prevent unnecessary interventions (Grimes-Dennis & Berghella, 2007).

Home Uterine Activity Monitoring

Home monitoring of uterine activity can identify women in preterm labor at an early stage to reduce the rate of preterm birth (Gilbert, 2007). Home uterine activity monitoring does not prevent preterm labor or birth; rather, it provides supplemental client education and

BOX 21.2 **Risk Factors Associated With Preterm Labor and Birth**

- African-American race (double the risk)
- Maternal age extremes less than 16 years and more than 40 years old
- Low socioeconomic status
- Alcohol or other drug use, especially cocaine
- Poor maternal nutrition
- Maternal periodontal disease
- Cigarette smoking
- Low level of education
- History of prior preterm birth (triples the risk)
- Uterine abnormalities, such as fibroids
- Low pregnancy weight for height
- Preexisting diabetes or hypertension
- Multiple gestation
- PROM
- Late or no prenatal care
- Short cervical length
- STIs: gonorrhea, *Chlamydia*, trichomoniasis
- Bacterial vaginosis (50% increased risk) (Pretorius et al., 2007)
- Chorioamnionitis
- Hydramnios
- Gestational hypertension
- Cervical insufficiency
- Short interpregnancy interval: less than 1 year between births
- Placental problems, such as placenta previa and abruption placenta
- Maternal anemia
- UTI
- Domestic violence
- Stress, acute and chronic (March of Dimes, 2007c)

clinical data for the health care provider in an effort to prolong gestation and maximize pregnancy outcomes through timely clinical interventions. It involves client education, daily client assessment, data collection, and data interpretation (Gray, 2007).

The woman is asked to wear an ambulatory tocodynamometer and transmit data to the nurse or health care provider daily via telephone lines. Uterine and fetal activity data are transmitted to perinatal nurses who are available around the clock for detection of uterine contractions, in addition to picking up the fetal heart rate. Women are also asked to record uterine activity (uterine pressure, back pain, or cramps) they experience for an hour twice a day and then speak to a perinatal nurse, who analyzes the results.

If the number of contractions exceeds a predetermined threshold, the woman drinks 8 to 12 oz of water, rests, empties her bladder, and then repeats uterine monitoring. The effectiveness of this type of screening remains controversial (Morrison & Chauhan, 2003).

Nursing Management

Nurses play a key role in reducing preterm labor and births to improve pregnancy outcomes for both mothers and their infants. Early detection of preterm labor is currently the best strategy to improve outcomes. Because of the numerous factors associated with preterm labor, it is challenging to identify and address all of them, especially when women experiencing contractions are frequently falsely reassured and not assessed thoroughly to determine the cause. This delay impedes initiation of interventions to reduce infant death and morbidity.

Preterm birth prevention programs for women at high risk have used self-monitoring of symptoms and patterns, weekly cervical examinations, telephone monitoring, home visiting, and home uterine activity monitoring, alone or in combination, with mixed results (Gray, 2006).

Nursing management of the woman with preterm labor involves administering tocolytic therapy if indicated, thoroughly educating the client, and providing psychological support during the process.

Administering Tocolytic Therapy

A firm diagnosis of preterm labor is necessary before treatment is considered. Diagnosis requires the presence of both uterine contractions and cervical change (or an initial cervical examination of more than 2 cm and/or more than 80% effacement in a nulliparous client). A cause for preterm labor should always be sought. Absolute contraindications to tocolytic agents include intrauterine infection, fetal distress, vaginal bleeding, prolonged premature rupture of the membranes, and intrauterine demise (Norwitz & Schorge, 2006). Bed rest and hydration are commonly recommended, but without proven efficacy.

Short-term pharmacologic therapy remains the cornerstone of management. However, there are no studies to suggest that any tocolytic agent can delay birth for longer than 48 hours (Stein, 2007). No single agent has a clear therapeutic advantage.

Magnesium sulfate may be ordered. This agent acts as a physiologic calcium antagonist and a general inhibitor of neurotransmission. Expect to administer it intravenously. Monitor the woman for nausea, vomiting, headache, weakness, hypotension, and cardiopulmonary arrest. Assess the fetus for decreased fetal heart rate variability, drowsiness, and hypotonia. Magnesium has a wide margin of safety and is commonly used as a first choice.

Although calcium channel blockers may be prescribed to manage preterm labor, available literature provides little evidence that they have better efficacy in treating preterm labor than magnesium sulfate (ACOG, 2003b). Administer calcium channel blockers (nifedipine) orally or sublingually every 4 to 8 hours as ordered. Monitor the woman for hypotension, reflex tachycardia, headache, nausea, and facial flushing.

If beta-adrenergic agonists (terbutaline) are ordered, expect to administer the agent intravenously during the initial period and then switch to the oral route for maintenance therapy. Closely assess the woman for side effects, including jitteriness, anxiety, restlessness, nausea, and tachycardia. Assess the fetus for tachycardia, hypotension, and hypoglycemia.

Supportive nursing care is needed for the woman in preterm labor whether the contractions are stopped with tocolytic therapy or not. Nursing tasks include monitoring vital signs, measuring intake and output, encouraging bed rest on the woman's left side to enhance placental perfusion, monitoring the fetal heart rate via an external monitor continuously, limiting vaginal examinations to prevent an ascending infection, and monitoring the mother and fetus closely for any adverse effects from the tocolytic agents. Offering the couple ongoing explanations will help prepare them for the birth.

Educating the Client

Ensure that every pregnant woman receives basic education about preterm labor, including information about harmful lifestyles, the signs of genitourinary infections and preterm labor, and the appropriate response to these symptoms. Teach the client how to palpate for and time uterine contractions. Provide written materials to support this education at a level and in a language appropriate for the client. Also educate clients about the importance of prenatal care, risk reduction, and recognizing the signs and symptoms of preterm labor. Teaching Guidelines 21.1 highlights important instructions related to preventing preterm labor.

Explaining to the couple what is happening in terms of labor progress, the treatment regimen, and the status of the fetus is important to reduce the anxiety associated with the risk of giving birth to a preterm infant. Educate them about the importance of promotion of fetal lung maturity with corticosteroids. Include supportive family members in all education. Allow time for the woman and her family to express their concerns about the possible outcome for the infant and the possible side effects of the tocolytic therapy. Encourage them to vent any feelings, fears, and anger they may experience. Provide the woman and her family with an honest appraisal of the situation and plan of treatment throughout her care.

Providing Psychological Support

Preterm labor and birth present multifactorial challenges for everyone involved. If the woman's activities are restricted, additional stresses may be placed on the family, contributing to the crisis. Assess the stress levels of the client and family, and make appropriate referrals. Emphasize the need for more frequent supervision and office visits, and encourage clients to talk to their health care provider for reassurance.

Every case of spontaneous preterm labor is unique. Care must take into account the clinical circumstances, and the full and informed consent of the woman and her

TEACHING GUIDELINES 21.1

Teaching to Prevent Preterm Labor

- Avoid traveling for long distances in cars, trains, planes, or buses.
- Avoid lifting heavy objects, such as laundry, groceries, or a young child.
- Avoid performing hard, physical work, such as yard work, moving of furniture, or construction.
- Visit a dentist in early pregnancy to evaluate and treat periodontal disease.
- Enroll in a smoking cessation program if you are unable to quit on your own.
- Curtail sexual activity until after 37 weeks if experiencing preterm labor symptoms.
- Consume a well-balanced nutritional diet to gain appropriate weight.
- Avoid the use of substances such as marijuana, cocaine, and heroin.
- Identify factors and areas of stress in your life, and use stress management techniques to reduce them.
- If you are experiencing intimate partner violence, seek resources to modify the situation.

Recognize the signs and symptoms of preterm labor and notify your birth attendant if any occur:

- Uterine contractions, cramping, or low back pain
- Feeling of pelvic pressure or fullness
- Increase in vaginal discharge
- Nausea, vomiting, and diarrhea
- Leaking of fluid from vagina

If you are experiencing any of these signs or symptoms, do the following:

- Stop what you are doing and rest for 1 hour.
- Empty your bladder.
- Lie down on your side. *left side*
- Drink two to three glasses of water.
- Feel your abdomen and make note of the hardness of the contraction. Call your health care provider and describe the contraction as
  - Mild if it feels like the tip of the nose
  - Moderate if it feels like the tip of the chin
  - Strong if it feels like your forehead (Simhan & Caritis, 2007)

partner is needed. Half of all women who ultimately give birth prematurely have no identifiable risk factors. Nurses should be sensitive to any complaint and should provide appropriate assessment, information, and follow-up. Sensitivity to the subtle differences between normal pregnancy sensations and the prodromal symptoms of preterm labor is a key factor in ensuring timely care. Offer clarification and validation of the woman's symptoms.

If tocolytic therapy isn't successful in stopping uterine contractions, support the couple through this stressful period to prepare them for the birth. Keep them informed of all progress and changes; for example, continuously monitor maternal and fetal vital signs, especially the maternal temperature to detect signs of early infection. Offer one-on-one contact and be available throughout this difficult and anxiety-producing period.

Postterm Labor

A term pregnancy usually lasts 38 to 42 weeks. A **postterm pregnancy** is one that continues past the end of the 42nd week of gestation, or 294 days from the first day of the last menstrual period. Postterm pregnancies account for about 3% to 12% of births (Butler & Wilkes, 2007). Incorrect dates account for the majority of these cases: many women have irregular menses and thus cannot identify the date of their last menstrual period accurately.

Recall Jennifer described at the beginning of the chapter, who was at 41 weeks' gestation. What information would be most important to determine on admission to the facility? What interventions might the nurse anticipate when she arrives?

The exact etiology of a postterm pregnancy is unknown because the mechanism for the initiation of labor is not completely understood. Theories suggest there may be a deficiency of estrogen and continued secretion of progesterone that prohibits the uterus from contracting, but no evidence has validated this. A woman who has one postterm pregnancy is at greater risk for another in subsequent pregnancies.

Postterm pregnancies may adversely affect both the mother and fetus or newborn. Maternal risk is related to the large size of the fetus at birth, which increases the chances that a cesarean birth will be needed. Other issues might include dystocia, birth trauma, postpartum hemorrhage, and infection. Mechanical or artificial interventions such as forceps or vacuum-assisted birth and labor induction with oxytocin may be necessary. In addition, maternal exhaustion and feelings of despair over this prolonged gestation can add to the woman's anxiety level and reduce her coping ability.

Fetal risks associated with a postterm pregnancy include macrosomia, shoulder dystocia, brachial plexus injuries, and cephalopelvic disproportion. All of these conditions predispose this fetus to birth trauma or a surgical birth. The perinatal mortality rate at more than 42 weeks of gestation is twice that at term and increases six-fold and higher at 43 weeks of gestation and beyond. Uteroplacental insufficiency, meconium aspiration, and intrauterine infection contribute to the increased rate of perinatal deaths (Heimstad et al., 2006). As the placenta ages, its perfusion decreases and it becomes less efficient at delivering oxygen and nutrients to the fetus. Amniotic fluid volume also begins to decline by 40 weeks of gestation, possibly leading to oligohydramnios, subsequently resulting in fetal hypoxia and an increased risk of cord compression because the cushioning effect offered by adequate fluid is no longer present. Hypoxia and oligohydramnios predispose the fetus to aspiration of meconium, which is released by the fetus in response to a hypoxic insult (Gümezoglu, Crowther, & Middleton, 2006). All of these issues can compromise fetal well-being and lead to fetal distress.

Nursing Assessment

Obtain a thorough history to determine the estimated date of birth. Many women are unsure of the date of their last menstrual period, so the date given may be unreliable. Despite numerous methods used to date pregnancies, many are still misdated. Accurate gestational dating via ultrasound is essential.

Antepartum assessment for a postterm pregnancy typically includes daily fetal movement counts done by the woman, nonstress tests done twice weekly, amniotic fluid assessments as part of the biophysical profile, and weekly cervical examinations to evaluate for ripening. In addition, assess the following:

- Client's understanding of the various fetal well-being tests
- Client's stress and anxiety concerning her lateness
- Client's coping ability and support network

Nursing Management

Once the dates are established and postdate status is confirmed, monitoring fetal well-being becomes critical. When determining the plan of care for a woman with a postterm pregnancy, the first decision is whether to deliver the baby or wait. If the decision is to wait, then fetal surveillance is key. If the decision is to have the woman deliver, labor induction is initiated. Both decisions remain controversial, and there is no clear answer about which option is more appropriate. Therefore, the plan must be individualized.

Think back to Jennifer, who is scheduled for labor induction. What ongoing nursing assessments would be important when providing care for her?

Providing Support

The intense surveillance is time-consuming and intrusive, adding to the anxiety and worry already being experienced by the woman about her overdue status. Be alert to the woman's anxiety and allow her to discuss her feelings. Provide reassurance about the expected time range for birth

EVIDENCE-BASED PRACTICE 21.1
Labor Induction and Outcomes for Women Beyond Term

● **Study**

Postterm pregnancies may adversely affect both the mother and fetus or newborn. Placental perfusion decreases as the placenta ages and becomes less efficient at delivering oxygen and nutrients to the fetus. Amniotic fluid volume also begins to decline by 40 weeks of gestation, increasing the fetus's risk for oligohydramnios, meconium aspiration, and cord compression. However, questions arise: What is the best time for inducing labor in a postterm pregnancy? Does labor induction improve maternal and fetal outcomes, or would it be better to wait for spontaneous labor to begin? A study was conducted to compare the effects of inducing labor in women at or beyond term with those of waiting for spontaneous labor to begin. A search was conducted for randomized controlled trials that compared labor induction with waiting for spontaneous labor to begin in women who were at term or postterm. Two review authors collected the data and analyzed the trials. A total of 19 trials involving almost 8,000 women were evaluated.

▲ **Findings**

Based on the trials analyzed, fewer perinatal deaths occurred in women who underwent labor induction at 41 completed weeks of gestation or later. Fewer newborns experienced meconium aspiration syndrome with induction at 41 weeks or more. Women at 37 to 40 weeks' gestation who received expectant management were more likely to undergo a cesarean birth compared to those in the same gestational week range who received induction. Statistical analysis, however, showed that these differences were not significant.

■ **Nursing Implications**

Although the study did not reveal results that were statistically significant, nurses need to be aware of the potential benefits and limitations associated with labor induction so that they can provide women and their families with the most appropriate information about options for a postterm pregnancy. Nurses can integrate information from this study in their teaching about the risks associated with postterm pregnancy. They can also use this information to help answer the couple's questions about induction and its effectiveness as well as provide anticipatory guidance about the procedure. Doing so fosters empowerment of the woman and her family, promoting optimal informed decision making.

Gülmezoglu, A. M., Crowther, C. A., & Middleton, P. (2006). Induction of labour for improving birth outcomes for women at or beyond term. *Cochrane Database of Systematic Reviews* 2006. Issue 4. Art. No.: CD004945.DOI:10.1002/14651858.CD004945.pub2.

and the well-being of the fetus based on the assessment tests. Validating the woman's stressful state due to the prolonged pregnancy provides an opportunity for her to verbalize her feelings openly.

Educating the Woman and Her Partner

Teach the woman and her partner about the testing required and the reasons for each test. Also describe the methods that may be used for cervical ripening if indicated. Explain about the possibility of induction if the woman's labor isn't spontaneous or if a dysfunctional labor pattern occurs. Also prepare the woman for the possibility of a surgical delivery if fetal distress occurs.

Providing Care During the Intrapartum Period

During the intrapartum period, continuously assess and monitor fetal heart rate (FHR) to identify potential fetal distress early (e.g., late or variable decelerations) so that interventions can be initiated. Also monitor the woman's hydration status to ensure maximal placental perfusion. When the membranes rupture, assess amniotic fluid characteristics (color, amount, and odor) to identify previous fetal hypoxia and prepare for prevention of meconium aspiration. Report meconium-stained amniotic fluid imme-

diately when the membranes rupture. Anticipate the need for amnioinfusion to minimize the risk of meconium aspiration by diluting the meconium in the amniotic fluid expelled by the hypoxic fetus. In addition, monitor the woman's labor pattern closely because dysfunctional patterns are common (Gilbert, 2007).

Encourage the woman to verbalize her feelings and concerns, and answer all her questions. Provide support, presence, information, and encouragement throughout this time.

Women Requiring Labor Induction and Augmentation

Ideally, all pregnancies go to term, with labor beginning spontaneously. However, many women need help to initiate or sustain the labor process. **Labor induction** involves the stimulation of uterine contractions by medical or surgical means to produce delivery before the onset of spontaneous labor. The labor induction rate is at an all-time high in the United States. The widespread use of artificial induction of labor for convenience has contributed to the recent increase in the number of cesarean births.

Evidence is compelling that elective induction of labor significantly increases the risk of cesarean birth, instrumented delivery, use of epidural analgesia, and neonatal intensive care unit admission, especially for nulliparous women (Crane, 2006).

Labor induction is not an isolated event: it brings about a cascade of other interventions that may or may not produce a favorable outcome. Labor induction also involves intravenous therapy, bed rest, continuous electronic fetal monitoring, significant discomfort from stimulating uterine contractions, epidural analgesia/anesthesia, and a prolonged stay on the labor unit (Wing, 2006).

Labor augmentation enhances ineffective contractions after labor has begun. Continuous electronic FHR monitoring is necessary.

There are multiple medical and obstetric reasons for inducing labor, the most common being postterm gestation. Other indications for inductions include prolonged premature rupture of membranes, gestational hypertension, renal disease, chorioamnionitis, dystocia, intrauterine fetal demise, isoimmunization, and diabetes (Bueno et al., 2007). Contraindications to labor induction include complete placenta previa, abruptio placentae, transverse fetal lie, prolapsed umbilical cord, a prior classic uterine incision that entered the uterine cavity, pelvic structure abnormality, previous myomectomy, vaginal bleeding with unknown cause, invasive cervical cancer, active genital herpes infection, and abnormal FHR patterns (ACOG, 2004b). In general, labor induction is indicated when the benefits of birth outweigh the risks to the mother or fetus for continuing the pregnancy. However, the balance between risk and benefit remains controversial.

▶ **Take** NOTE!

Before labor induction is started, fetal maturity (dating, ultrasound, amniotic fluid studies) and cervical readiness (vaginal examination, Bishop scoring) must be assessed. Both need to be favorable for a successful induction.

Therapeutic Management

The decision to induce labor is based on a thorough evaluation of maternal and fetal status. Typically, this includes an ultrasound to evaluate fetal size, position, and gestational age and to locate the placenta; pelvimetry to rule out fetopelvic disproportion; a nonstress test to evaluate fetal well-being; a phosphatidylglycerol (PG) level to assess fetal lung maturity; Nitrazine paper and/or fern test to confirm ruptured membranes; complete blood count and urinalysis to rule out infection; and a vaginal examination to evaluate the cervix for inducibility (ACOG, 2004). Accurate dating of the pregnancy also is essential before cervical ripening and induction are initiated to prevent a preterm birth.

Cervical Ripening

There has been increasing awareness that if the cervix is unfavorable or unripe, a successful vaginal birth is unlikely. Cervical ripeness is an important variable when labor induction is being considered. A ripe cervix is shortened, centered (anterior), softened, and partially dilated. An unripe cervix is long, closed, posterior, and firm. Cervical ripening usually begins prior to the onset of labor contractions and is necessary for cervical dilatation and the passage of the fetus.

Various scoring systems to assess cervical ripeness have been introduced, but the Bishop score is most commonly used today. The Bishop score helps identify women who would be most likely to achieve a successful induction (Table 21.2). The duration of labor is inversely correlated with the Bishop score: a score over 8 indicates a successful vaginal birth. Bishop scores of less than 6 usually indicate that a cervical ripening method should be used prior to induction (Rai & Schreiber, 2007).

Nonpharmacologic Methods

Nonpharmacologic methods for cervical ripening are less frequently used today, but nurses need to be aware of them and question clients about their use. Methods may include herbal agents such as evening primrose oil, black haw, black and blue cohosh, and red raspberry leaves. In

TABLE 21.2 **BISHOP SCORING SYSTEM**

Score	Dilation (cm)	Effacement (%)	Station	Cervical Consistency	Position of Cervix
0	Closed	0–30%	–3	Firm	Posterior
1	1–2 cm	40–50%	–2	Medium	Midposition
2	3–4 cm	60–70%	–1 or 0	Soft	Anterior
3	5–6 cm	80%	+1 or +2	Very soft	Anterior

Modified from Bishop, E. H. (1964). Pelvic scoring for elective induction. *Obstetrics & Gynecology, 24*(2), 267.

addition, castor oil, hot baths, and enemas are used for cervical ripening and labor induction. The risks and benefits of these agents are unknown.

Another nonpharmacologic method suggested for labor induction is sexual intercourse along with breast stimulation. This promotes the release of oxytocin, which stimulates uterine contractions. In addition, human semen is a biological source of prostaglandins used for cervical ripening. According to a Cochrane Review, sexual intercourse with breast stimulation would appear beneficial, but safety issues have not been fully evaluated, nor can this activity be standardized (Kavanagh, Kelly, & Thomas, 2007). Therefore, its use as a method for labor induction is not validated by research.

Mechanical Methods

Mechanical methods are used to open the cervix and stimulate the progression of labor. All share a similar mechanism of action—application of local pressure stimulates the release of prostaglandins to ripen the cervix. Potential advantages of mechanical methods, compared with pharmacologic methods, may include simplicity or preservation of the cervical tissue or structure, lower cost, and fewer side effects. The risks associated with these methods include infection, bleeding, membrane rupture, and placental disruption (Boulvain et al., 2007).

For example, an indwelling (Foley) catheter (e.g., 26 French) can be inserted into the endocervical canal to ripen and dilate the cervix. The catheter is placed in the uterus, and the balloon is filled. Direct pressure is then applied to the lower segment of the uterus and the cervix. This direct pressure causes stress in the lower uterine segment and probably the local production of prostaglandins (Rai & Schreiber, 2007).

Hygroscopic dilators absorb endocervical and local tissue fluids; as they enlarge, they expand the endocervix and provide controlled mechanical pressure. The products available include natural osmotic dilators (laminaria, a type of dried seaweed) and synthetic dilators containing magnesium sulfate (Lamicel, Dilapan). Hygroscopic dilators are advantageous because they can be inserted on an outpatient basis and no fetal monitoring is needed. As many dilators are inserted in the cervix as will fit, and they expand over 12 to 24 hours as they absorb water. Absorption of water leads to expansion of the dilators and opening of the cervix. They are a reliable alternative when prostaglandins are contraindicated or unavailable (Gelber, 2006).

Surgical Methods

Surgical methods used to ripen the cervix and induce labor include stripping of the membranes and performing an amniotomy. Stripping of the membranes is accomplished by inserting a finger through the internal cervical os and moving it in a circular direction. This motion causes the membranes to detach. Manual separation of the amniotic membranes from the cervix is thought to induce cervical ripening and the onset of labor (Rai & Schreiber, 2007).

An amniotomy involves inserting a cervical hook (Amniohook) through the cervical os to deliberately rupture the membranes. This promotes pressure of the presenting part on the cervix and stimulates an increase in the activity of prostaglandins locally. Risks associated with these procedures include umbilical cord prolapse or compression, maternal or neonatal infection, FHR deceleration, bleeding, and client discomfort (Shobeiri, Tehranian, & Nazari, 2007).

When either of these techniques is used, amniotic fluid characteristics (such as whether it is clear or bloody, or meconium is present) and the FHR pattern must be monitored closely.

Pharmacologic Agents

The use of pharmacologic agents has revolutionized cervical ripening. The use of prostaglandins to attain cervical ripening has been found to be highly effective in producing cervical changes independent of uterine contractions (Sifakis et al., 2007). In some cases, women will go into labor, requiring no additional stimulants for induction. Induction of labor with prostaglandins offers the advantage of promoting both cervical ripening and uterine contractility. A drawback of prostaglandins is their ability to induce excessive uterine contractions, which can increase maternal and perinatal morbidity (Hofmeyr & Gulmezoglu, 2007). Prostaglandin analogs commonly used for cervical ripening include dinoprostone gel (Prepidil), dinoprostone inserts (Cervidil), and misoprostol (Cytotec). Misoprostol (Cytotec), a synthetic PGE1 analog, is a gastric cytoprotective agent used in the treatment and prevention of peptic ulcers. It can be administered intravaginally or orally to ripen the cervix or induce labor. It is available in 100-mcg or 200-mcg tablets, but doses of 25 to 50 mcg are typically used. However, it is not approved by the FDA for cervical ripening since several reports found higher levels of uterine rupture associated with its use (USFDA, 2007) (Drug Guide 21.2). Furthermore, it is contraindicated for women with prior uterine scars and therefore should not be used for cervical ripening in women attempting a VBAC.

Oxytocin

Oxytocin is a potent endogenous uterotonic agent used for both artificial induction and augmentation of labor. It is produced naturally by the posterior pituitary gland and stimulates contractions of the uterus. For women with low Bishop scores, cervical ripening is typically initiated before oxytocin is used. Once the cervix is ripe, oxytocin is the most popular pharmacologic agent used for inducing or augmenting labor. Frequently a woman with an unfavorable cervix is admitted the evening before induc-

DRUG GUIDE 21.2 DRUGS USED FOR CERVICAL RIPENING AND LABOR INDUCTION

Drug	Action/Indication	Nursing Implications
Dinoprostone (Cervidil insert; Prepidil gel)	Directly softens and dilates the cervix/to ripen cervix and induce labor	Provide emotional support. Administer pain medications as needed. Frequently assess degree of effacement and dilation. Monitor uterine contractions for frequency, duration, and strength. Assess maternal vital signs and FHR pattern frequently. Monitor woman for possible adverse effects such as headache, nausea and vomiting, and diarrhea.
Misoprostol (Cytotec)	Ripens cervix/to induce labor	Instruct client about purpose and possible adverse effects of medication. Ensure informed consent is signed per hospital policy. Assess vital signs and FHR patterns frequently. Monitor client's reaction to drug. Initiate oxytocin for labor induction at least 4 hours after last dose was administered. Monitor for possible adverse effects such as nausea and vomiting, diarrhea, uterine hyperstimulation, and non-reassuring FHR pattern.
Oxytocin (Pitocin)	Acts on uterine myofibrils to contract/to initiate or reinforce labor	Administer as an IV infusion via pump, increasing dose based on protocol until adequate labor progress is achieved. Assess baseline vital signs and FHR and then frequently after initiating oxytocin infusion. Determine frequency, duration, and strength of contractions frequently. Notify health care provider of any uterine hypertonicity or abnormal FHR patterns. Maintain careful I & O, being alert for water intoxication. Keep client informed of labor progress. Monitor for possible adverse effects such as hyperstimulation of the uterus, impaired uterine blood flow leading to fetal hypoxia, rapid labor leading to cervical lacerations or uterine rupture, water intoxication (if oxytocin is given in electrolyte-free solution or at a rate exceeding 20 mU/min), and hypotension.

[handwritten annotations:]
max: 20-40 mu/min
stop → late decelerations
variable decelerations
FHR brady

tion to ripen her cervix with one of the prostaglandin agents. Then induction begins with oxytocin the next morning if she has not already gone into labor. Doing so markedly enhances the success of induction.

Response to oxytocin varies widely: some women are very sensitive to even small amounts. The most common adverse effect of oxytocin is uterine hyperstimulation, leading to fetal compromise and impaired oxygenation (Smith & Merrill, 2006). The response of the uterus to the drug is closely monitored throughout labor so that the oxytocin infusion can be titrated appropriately. In addition, oxytocin has an antidiuretic effect, resulting in decreased urine flow that may lead to water intoxication. Symptoms to watch for include headache and vomiting.

Oxytocin is administered via an intravenous infusion pump piggybacked into the main intravenous line at the port most proximal to the insertion site. Usually 10 units of oxytocin is added to 1 L of isotonic solution to achieve an infusion rate of 1 mU/min = 6 mL/hr. The dose is titrated according to protocol to achieve stable contractions every 2 to 3 minutes lasting 40 to 60 seconds (Briggs & Wan, 2006). The uterus should relax between contractions. If the resting uterine tone remains above 20 mmHg, uteroplacental insufficiency and fetal hypoxia can result. This underscores the importance of continuous FHR monitoring.

Oxytocin has many advantages: it is potent and easy to titrate, it has a short half-life (1 to 5 minutes), and it is generally well tolerated. Induction using oxytocin has side effects (water intoxication, hypotension, and uterine hypertonicity), but because the drug does not cross the placental barrier, no direct fetal problems have been observed (Khan, Khan, & Ashraf, 2007) (Fig. 21.4).

[handwritten annotations at bottom:]
water intoxication → nausea/vomiting,
hypotension, tachycardia

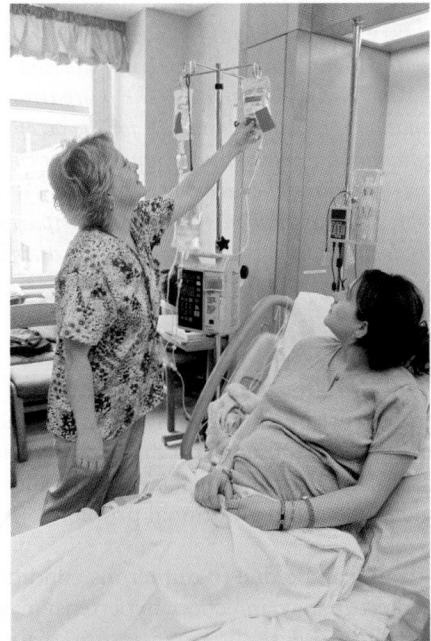

FIGURE 21.4 The nurse monitors an intravenous infusion of oxytocin being administered to a woman in labor.

*R*emember Jennifer, the young woman described at the beginning of the chapter? After her cervix is ripened, an oxytocin infusion is started and her progress is slow. What encouragement can the nurse offer? After a few hours, her contractions begin to increase in intensity and frequency. What typical pain management measures can the nurse implement, and how would the nurse evaluate the effectiveness of these measures?

Nursing Assessment

Nursing assessment of the woman who is undergoing labor induction or augmentation involves a thorough history and physical examination. Review the woman's history for relative indications for induction or augmentation, such as diabetes, hypertension, postterm status, dysfunctional labor pattern, prolonged ruptured membranes, and maternal or fetal infection, and for contraindications such as placenta previa, overdistended uterus, active genital herpes, fetopelvic disproportion, fetal malposition, or severe fetal distress.

Assist with determining the gestational age of the fetus to prevent a preterm birth. Assess fetal well-being to validate the client's and fetus's ability to withstand labor contractions. Evaluate the woman's cervical status, including cervical dilatation and effacement, and station via vaginal examination as appropriate before cervical ripening or induction is started. Determine the Bishop score to determine the probable success of induction.

> ▶ *Take* NOTE!
>
> *Nurses working with women in labor play an important role acting as the "eyes" and "ears" for the birth attendant because they remain at the client's bedside throughout the entire experience. Close, frequent assessment and follow-up interventions are essential to ensure the safety of the mother and her unborn child during cervical ripening and labor induction or augmentation.*

Nursing Management

Explain to the woman and her partner about the induction or augmentation procedure clearly, using simple terms (Teaching Guidelines 21.2). Ensure that an informed consent has been signed after the client and her

TEACHING GUIDELINES 21.2

Teaching in Preparation for Labor Induction

- Your health care provider may recommend that you have your labor induced. This may be necessary for a variety of reasons, such as elevated blood pressure, a medical condition, prolonged pregnancy over 41 weeks, or problems with fetal heart rate patterns or fetal growth.
- Your health care provider may use one or more methods to induce labor, such as stripping the membranes, breaking the amniotic sac to release the fluid, administering medication close to or in the cervix to soften it, or administering a medication called oxytocin (Pitocin) to stimulate contractions.
- Labor induction is associated with some risks and disadvantages, such as overactivity of the uterus; nausea, vomiting, or diarrhea; and changes in fetal heart rate.
- Prior to inducing your labor, your health care provider may perform a procedure to ripen your cervix to help ensure a successful induction.
- Medication may be placed around cervix the day before you are scheduled to be induced.
- During the induction, your contractions may feel stronger than normal. However, the length of your labor may be reduced with induction.
- Medications for pain relief and comfort measures will be readily available.
- Health care staff will be present throughout labor.

partner have received complete information about the procedure, including its advantages, disadvantages, and potential risks. Ensure that the Bishop score has been determined before proceeding. Nursing Care Plan 21.1 presents an overview of the nursing care for a woman undergoing labor induction.

Administering Oxytocin

If not already done, prepare the oxytocin infusion by diluting 10 units of oxytocin in 1,000 mL of lactated Ringer's solution. Use an infusion pump on a secondary line connected to the primary infusion. Start the oxytocin infusion in mU/min or milliliters per hour as ordered. Typically, the initial dose is 0.5 to 1 mU/min; anticipate increasing the rate in increments of 1 to 2 mU/min every 30 to 60 minutes. Maintain the rate once the desired contraction frequency has been reached. To ensure adequate maternal and fetal surveillance during induction or augmentation, the nurse-to-client ratio should not exceed 1:2 (Briggs & Wan, 2006).

During induction or augmentation, monitoring of the maternal and fetal status is essential. Apply an external electronic fetal monitor or assist with placement of an internal device. Obtain the mother's vital signs and the FHR every 15 minutes during the first stage. Evaluate the contractions (frequency, duration, and intensity) and resting tone, and adjust the oxytocin infusion rate accordingly. Monitor the FHR, including baseline rate, baseline variability, and decelerations, to determine whether the oxytocin rate needs adjustment. Discontinue the oxytocin and notify the birth attendant if uterine hyperstimulation or a nonreassuring FHR pattern occurs. Perform or assist with periodic vaginal examinations to determine cervical dilation and fetal descent: cervical dilation of 1 cm/hour typically indicates satisfactory progress.

Continue to monitor the FHR continuously and document it every 15 minutes during the active phase of labor and every 5 minutes during the second stage. Assist with pushing efforts during the second stage.

Measure and record intake and output to prevent excess fluid volume. Encourage the client to empty her bladder every 2 hours to prevent soft tissue obstruction.

Providing Pain Relief and Support

Assess the woman's level of pain. Ask her frequently to rate her pain and provide pain management as needed. Offer position changes and other non-pharmacologic measures. Note her reaction to any medication given, and document its effect. Monitor her need for comfort measures as contractions increase.

Throughout induction and augmentation, frequently reassure the woman and her partner about the fetal status and labor progress. Provide them with frequent updates on the condition of the woman and the fetus. Assess the woman's ability to cope with stronger contractions (Kuczkowski, 2007). Provide support and encouragement as indicated.

After a very long day, Jennifer gives birth to a healthy baby boy with Apgar scores of 9 at 1 minute and 10 at 5 minutes. When transferring her to the postpartum unit, what information is essential to include for the accepting nurse? What specific nursing information should be given to the nursery nurse regarding the laboring experience? With such a lengthy labor, what assessments might the postpartum nurse be especially focused on for the first few hours after birth?

Intrauterine Fetal Demise

When an unborn life suddenly ends with fetal loss, the family members are profoundly affected. The sudden loss of an expected child is tragic and the family's grief can be very intense: it can last for years and can cause extreme psychological stress and emotional problems (Lindsey & Azad, 2007).

Fetal death can be due to numerous conditions, such as prolonged pregnancy, infection, hypertension, advanced maternal age, Rh disease, uterine rupture, diabetes, congenital anomalies, cord accident, abruption, premature rupture of membranes, or hemorrhage; it may go unexplained (Gilbert, 2007). Early pregnancy loss may be through a spontaneous abortion (miscarriage), an induced abortion (therapeutic abortion), or a ruptured ectopic pregnancy. A wide spectrum of feelings may be expressed, from relief to sadness and despair. A stillbirth can occur at any gestational age, and typically there is little or no warning other than reduced fetal movement.

The period following a fetal death is extremely difficult for the family. For many women, emotional healing takes much longer than physical healing. The feelings of loss can be intense. The grief response in some women may be so great that their relationships become strained, and healing can become hampered unless appropriate interventions and support are provided.

Fetal death also affects the health care staff. Despite the trauma that the loss of a fetus causes, some staff members avoid dealing with the bereaved family, never talking about or acknowledging their grief. This seems to imply that not discussing the problem will allow the grief to dissolve and vanish. As a result, the family's needs go unrecognized. Failing to keep the lines of communication open with a bereaved client and her family closes off some of the channels to recovery and healing that may be desperately needed. Subsequently, the bereaved family members may feel isolated.

Nursing Assessment

History and physical examination are of limited value in the diagnosis of fetal death, since the only history tends to be recent absence of fetal movement. An inability to obtain fetal heart sounds on examination suggests fetal demise, but an ultrasound is necessary to confirm the absence of fetal cardiac activity. Once fetal demise is confirmed, induction of labor is indicated.

Nursing Care Plan 21.1

OVERVIEW OF THE WOMAN UNDERGOING LABOR INDUCTION

Rose, a 29-year-old primipara, is admitted to the labor and birth suite at 40 weeks' gestation for induction of labor. Assessment reveals that her cervix is ripe and 80% effaced, and dilated to 2 cm. Rose says, "I'm a bit nervous about being induced. I've never been through labor before and I'm afraid that I'll have a lot of pain from the medicine used to start the contractions." She consents to being induced but wants reassurance that this procedure won't harm the baby. Upon examination, the fetus is engaged and in a cephalic presentation, with the vertex as the presenting part. Her partner is at her side. Induction is initiated with oxytocin. Rose reports that contractions have started and are beginning to get stronger.

NURSING DIAGNOSIS: Anxiety related to induction of labor and lack of experience with labor *as evidenced by statements about being nervous, not having gone through labor before and fear of pain*

Outcome Identification and Evaluation
Client will experience decrease in anxiety as evidenced by ability to verbalize understanding of procedures involved and use of positive coping skills to reduce anxious state.

Interventions: Minimizing Anxiety
- Provide a clear explanation of the labor induction process *to provide client and partner with a knowledge base.*
- Maintain continuous physical presence *to provide physical and emotional support and demonstrate concern for maternal and fetal well-being.*
- Explain each procedure before carrying it out and answer questions *to promote understanding of procedure and rationale for use and decrease fears of the unknown.*
- Review with client measures used in the past to deal with stressful situations *to determine effectiveness;* encourage use of past effective coping strategies *to aid in controlling anxiety.*
- Instruct client's partner in helpful measures to assist client in coping and encourage their use *to foster joint participation in the process and feelings of being in control and to provide support to the client.*
- Offer frequent reassurance of fetal status and labor progress *to help alleviate client's concerns and foster continued participation in the labor process.*

NURSING DIAGNOSIS: Risk for injury (maternal or fetal) related to induction procedure *as evidenced by client's concerns about fetal well-being and possible adverse effects of oxytocin administration*

Outcome Identification and Evaluation
Client will remain free of complications associated with induction *as evidenced by progression of labor as expected, delivery of healthy newborn, and absence of signs and symptoms of maternal and fetal adverse effects.*

Interventions: Promoting Maternal and Fetal Safety
- Follow agency's protocol for medication use and infusion rate *to ensure accurate, safe drug administration.*
- Set up oxytocin IV infusion to piggyback into the primary IV infusion line *to allow for prompt discontinuation should adverse effects occur.*
- Use an infusion pump *to deliver accurate dose as ordered.*
- Gradually increase oxytocin dose in increments of 1 to 2 mU/min every 30 to 60 minutes based on assessment findings and protocol *to promote effective uterine contractions.*
- Maintain oxytocin rate once desired frequency of contractions has been reached *to ensure continued progress in labor.*
- Accurately monitor contractions for frequency, duration, and intensity and resting tone *to prevent development of hypertonic contractions.*
- Maintain a nurse–client ratio of 1:2 *to ensure maternal and fetal safety.*
- Monitor FHR via electronic fetal monitoring during induction and continuously observe the FHR response to titrated medication rate *to ensure fetal well-being and identify adverse effects immediately.*
- Obtain maternal vital signs every 1 to 2 hours or as indicated by agency's protocol, reporting any deviations, *to promote maternal well-being and allow for prompt detection of problems.*
- Communicate with birth attendant frequently concerning progress *to ensure continuity of care.*

(continued)

Nursing Care Plan 21.1 (continued)

- Discontinue oxytocin infusion if tetanic contractions (>90 seconds), uterine hyperstimulation (<2 minutes apart), elevated uterine resting tone, or a nonreassuring FHR pattern occurs *to minimize risk of drug's adverse effects.*
- Provide client with frequent reassurance of maternal and fetal status *to minimize anxiety.*

NURSING DIAGNOSIS: Pain related to uterine contractions *as evidenced by client's statements about contractions increasing in intensity and expected effect of oxytocin administration*

Outcome Identification and Evaluation
Client will report a decrease in pain as evidenced by statements of increased comfort and pain rating of 3 or less on numeric pain rating scale.

Interventions: Promoting Comfort and Pain Relief
- Explain to the client that she will experience discomfort sooner than with naturally occurring labor *to promote client's awareness of events and prepare client for the experience.*
- Frequently assess client's pain using a pain rating scale *to quantify client's level of pain and evaluate effectiveness of pain-relief measures.*
- Provide comfort measures, such as hygiene, backrubs, music, and distraction, and encourage the use of breathing and relaxation techniques *to help promote relaxation.*
- Provide support for her partner *to aid in alleviating stress and concerns.*
- Employ nonpharmacologic methods, such as position changes, birthing ball, hydrotherapy, visual imagery, and effleurage, *to help in managing pain and foster feelings of control over situation.*
- Administer pharmacologic agents such as analgesia or anesthesia as appropriate and as ordered *to control pain.*
- Continuously reassess client's pain level *to evaluate effectiveness of pain management techniques used.*

Nursing Management

The nurse can play a major role in assisting the grieving family. With skillful intervention, the bereaved family may be better prepared to resolve their grief and move forward. To assist families in the grieving process, include the following measures:

- Provide accurate, understandable information to the family.
- Encourage discussion of the loss and venting of feelings of grief and guilt.
- Provide the family with baby mementos and pictures to validate the reality of death.
- Allow unlimited time with the stillborn infant after birth to validate the death; provide time for the family members to be together and grieve; offer the family the opportunity to see, touch, and hold the infant.
- Use appropriate touch, such as holding a hand or touching a shoulder.
- Inform the chaplain or the religious leader of the family's denomination about the death and request his or her presence.
- Assist the parents with the funeral arrangements or disposition of the body.
- Provide the parents with brochures offering advice about how to talk to other siblings about the loss.
- Refer the family to the support group SHARE Pregnancy and Infant Loss Support, Inc., which is designed for those who have lost an infant through abortion, miscarriage, fetal death, stillbirth, or other tragic circumstances.

- Make community referrals to promote a continuum of care after discharge.

Women Experiencing an Obstetric Emergency

Obstetric emergencies are challenging to all labor and birth personnel because of the increased risk of adverse outcomes for the mother and fetus. Quick clinical judgment and good critical decision making will increase the odds of a positive outcome for both mother and fetus. This chapter will discuss a few of these emergencies: umbilical cord prolapse, placental abruption, uterine rupture, and amniotic fluid embolism.

▶ UMBILICAL CORD PROLAPSE

An **umbilical cord prolapse** is the protrusion of the umbilical cord alongside (occult) or ahead of the presenting part of the fetus (Fig. 21.5). This condition occurs in 1 out of every 300 births and requires prompt recognition and intervention for a positive outcome (March of Dimes, 2007f). Cord prolapse occurs in 3% of deliveries when the fetus is in the vertex position and in 3.7% of deliveries when the fetus is in the breech position. The risk is increased further when the presenting part does not fill the lower uterine segment, as is the case with incomplete

FIGURE 21.5 Prolapsed cord.
(**A**) Prolapse within the uterus.
(**B**) Prolapse with the cord visible
at the vulva.   **A**   **B**

breech presentations (5% to 10%), premature infants, and multiparous women (Morgan & Ross, 2007). With a 50% perinatal mortality rate, it is one of the most catastrophic events in the intrapartum period (Enakpene, Omigbodun, & Arowojolu, 2006).

Pathophysiology

Prolapse usually leads to total or partial occlusion of the cord. Since this is the fetus's only lifeline, fetal perfusion deteriorates rapidly. Complete occlusion renders the fetus helpless and oxygen-deprived. The fetus will die if the cord compression is not relieved.

Nursing Assessment

Prevention is the key to managing cord prolapse by identifying clients at risk for this condition. Carefully assess each client to help predict her risk status. Be aware that cord prolapse is more common in pregnancies involving malpresentation, growth restriction, prematurity, ruptured membranes with a fetus at a high station, hydramnios, grandmultiparity, and multifetal gestation (Dilbaz et al., 2006). Continuously assess the client and fetus to detect changes and to evaluate the effectiveness of any interventions performed.

▶ *Take* NOTE!

When the presenting part does not fully occupy the pelvic inlet, prolapse is more likely to occur.

Nursing Management

Prompt recognition of a prolapsed cord is essential to reduce the risk of fetal hypoxia resulting from prolonged cord compression. When membranes are artificially ruptured, assist with verifying that the presenting part is well applied to the cervix and engaged into the pelvis. If pressure or compression of the cord occurs, assist with measures to relieve the compression. Typically, the examiner places a sterile gloved hand into the vagina and holds the presenting part off the umbilical cord until delivery. Changing the woman's position to a modified Sims, Trendelenburg, or knee–chest position also helps relieve cord pressure. Monitor fetal heart rate, maintain bedrest, and administer oxygen if ordered. Provide emotional support and explanations as to what is going on to allay the woman's fears and anxiety. If the mother's cervix is not fully dilated, prepare the woman for an emergency cesarean birth to save the fetus's life.

▶ PLACENTAL ABRUPTION

Placental abruption refers to premature separation of a normally implanted placenta from the maternal myometrium. Abruptio placentae occurs in about 1% of all pregnancies throughout the world (March of Dimes, 2007a). Risk factors include preeclampsia, gestational hypertension, seizure activity, uterine rupture, trauma, smoking, cocaine use, coagulation defects, previous history of abruption, domestic violence, and placental pathology. These conditions may force blood into the underlayer of the placenta and cause it to detach (Deering & Satin, 2007).

Management of placental abruption depends on the gestational age, the extent of the hemorrhage, and maternal–fetal oxygenation perfusion/reserve status (see Chapter 19 for additional information on abruptio placentae). Treatment is based on the circumstances. Typically once the diagnosis is established, the focus is on maintaining the cardiovascular status of the mother and developing a plan to deliver the fetus quickly. A cesarean birth takes place if the fetus is still alive. A vaginal birth may take place if there is fetal demise.

▶ UTERINE RUPTURE

Uterine rupture is a catastrophic tearing of the uterus at the site of a previous scar into the abdominal cavity. Its onset is often marked only by sudden fetal bradycardia, and treatment requires rapid surgery for good outcomes. From the time of diagnosis to delivery, only 10 to 30 minutes are available before clinically significant fetal morbidity occurs. Fetal morbidity occurs secondary to catastrophic hemorrhage, fetal anoxia, or both.

Nursing Assessment

Review the mother's history for risk conditions such as uterine scars, prior cesarean births, prior rupture, trauma, prior invasive molar pregnancy, history of placenta percreta or increta, malpresentation, labor induction with excessive uterine stimulation, and crack cocaine use (Nahum & Pham, 2007). Reviewing a client's history for risk factors might prove to be life-saving for both mother and fetus.

Generally, the first and most reliable symptom of uterine rupture is sudden fetal distress. Other signs may include acute and continuous abdominal pain with or without an epidural, vaginal bleeding, hematuria, irregular abdominal wall contour, loss of station in the fetal presenting part, and hypovolemic shock in the woman, fetus, or both (Nahum & Pham, 2007).

Timely management of uterine rupture depends on prompt detection. Because many women desire a trial of labor after a previous cesarean birth, the nurse must be familiar with the signs and symptoms of uterine rupture. It is difficult to prevent uterine rupture or to predict which women will experience rupture, so constant preparedness is necessary.

Screening all women with previous uterine surgical scars is important, and continuous electronic fetal monitoring should be used during labor because this may provide the only indication of an impending rupture.

Nursing Management

Because the presenting signs may be nonspecific, the initial management will be the same as that for any other cause of acute fetal distress. Urgent delivery by cesarean birth is usually indicated. Monitor maternal vital signs and observe for hypotension and tachycardia, which might indicate hypovolemic shock. Assist in preparing for an emergency cesarean birth by alerting the operating room staff, anesthesia provider, and neonatal team. Insert an indwelling urinary (Foley) catheter if one is not in place already. Inform the woman of the seriousness of this event and remind her that the health care staff will be working quickly to ensure her health and that of her fetus. Remain calm and provide reassurance that everything is being done to ensure a safe outcome for both.

The life-threatening nature of uterine rupture is underscored by the fact that the maternal circulatory system delivers approximately 500 mL of blood to the term uterus every minute (Kennare et al., 2007). Maternal death is a real possibility without rapid intervention. Newborn outcome after rupture depends largely on the speed with which surgical rescue is carried out.

> ▶ **Take** NOTE!
>
> *When excessive bleeding occurs during the childbirth process and it persists or signs such as bruising or petechiae appear, disseminated intravascular coagulation (DIC) should be suspected.*

▶ AMNIOTIC FLUID EMBOLISM

Amniotic fluid embolism is a rare and often fatal event characterized by the sudden onset of hypotension, hypoxia, and coagulopathy. Amniotic fluid containing particles of debris (e.g., hair, skin, vernix, or meconium) enters the maternal circulation and obstructs the pulmonary vessels, causing respiratory distress and circulatory collapse (O'Shea & Eappen, 2007). The incidence is approximately 1 case per 8,000 to 80,000 pregnancies and carries a maternal mortality rate as high as 80% (Schoening, 2007).

Pathophysiology

Normally, amniotic fluid does not enter the maternal circulation because it is contained within the uterus, sealed off by the amniotic sac. An embolus occurs when the barrier between the maternal circulation and the amniotic fluid is broken and amniotic fluid enters the maternal venous system via the endocervical veins, the placental site (if the placenta is separated), or a site of uterine trauma. This condition has a high mortality rate: as many as 50% of women die within the first hour after the onset of symptoms, and about 85% of survivors have permanent hypoxia-induced neurologic damage (Moore, 2006).

Although medical science has supplied many answers to questions about this condition, health care providers remain largely unable to predict or prevent an amniotic fluid embolism or to decrease its mortality rate.

Nursing Assessment

No test can diagnose an amniotic fluid embolism. Therefore, the nurse's assessment skills are critical. Immediate recognition and diagnosis of this condition are essential to improve maternal and fetal outcomes. Until recently, the diagnosis could be made only after an autopsy of the mother revealed squamous cells, lanugo hair, or other fetal and amniotic material in the pulmonary arterial vasculature (Gilbert, 2007).

The clinical appearance is varied, but most women report difficulty breathing. Other symptoms include hypotension, cyanosis, seizures, tachycardia, coagulation failure, disseminated intravascular coagulation, pulmonary edema, uterine atony with subsequent hemorrhage, adult respiratory distress syndrome, and cardiac arrest (Moore & Ware, 2007).

▶ *Take* NOTE!

Amniotic fluid embolism should be suspected in any pregnant women with an acute onset of dyspnea, hypotension, and disseminated intravascular coagulation. By knowing how to intervene, the nurse can promote a better chance of survival for both the mother and her newborn.

Nursing Management

Upon recognizing the signs and symptoms, institute supportive measures: oxygenation (resuscitation and 100% oxygen), circulation (intravenous fluids, inotropic agents to maintain cardiac output and blood pressure), control of hemorrhage and coagulopathy (oxytocic agents to control uterine atony and bleeding), seizure precautions, and administration of steroids to control the inflammatory response (Schoening, 2007).

Care is largely supportive and aimed at maintaining oxygenation and hemodynamic function and correcting coagulopathy. There is no specific therapy that is life-saving once this condition starts. Adequate oxygenation is necessary, with endotracheal intubation and mechanical ventilation for most women. Vasopressors are used to maintain hemodynamic stability. Management of disseminated intravascular coagulation may involve replacement with packed red blood cells or fresh-frozen plasma as necessary. Oxytocin infusions and prostaglandin analogs can be used to address uterine atony.

Explain to the client and family what is happening and what therapies are being instituted. The woman is usually transferred to a critical care unit for intensive observation and care. Assist the family to express their feelings and provide support as needed.

▶ WOMEN REQUIRING BIRTH-RELATED PROCEDURES

Most women can give birth without the need for operative obstetric interventions. Most will expect to have a "natural" birth experience and don't anticipate the need for medical intervention. However, in some situations interventions are necessary to safeguard the health of the mother and fetus. The most common birth-related procedures are amnioinfusion, episiotomy (see Chapter 14), forceps-assisted or vacuum-assisted birth, cesarean birth,

and vaginal birth following a previous cesarean birth. Nurses play a major role in helping the couple to cope with any unanticipated procedures by offering thorough explanations of the procedure, its anticipated benefits and risks, and any other options available.

▶ AMNIOINFUSION

Amnioinfusion is a technique in which a volume of warmed, sterile, normal saline or Ringer's lactate solution is introduced into the uterus through an intrauterine pressure catheter to increase the volume of fluid when oligohydramnios is present (Boyd & Carter, 2008). It is used to change the relationship of the uterus, placenta, cord, and fetus to improve placental and fetal oxygenation. Instilling an isotonic glucose-free solution into the uterus helps to cushion the umbilical cord or dilute thick meconium (Xu et al., 2007).

This procedure is commonly indicated for severe variable decelerations due to cord compression, oligohydramnios due to placental insufficiency, postmaturity or rupture of membranes, preterm labor with premature rupture of membranes, and thick meconium fluid. However, it does not prevent meconium aspiration syndrome (ACOG, 2006). Contraindications to amnioinfusion include vaginal bleeding of unknown origin, umbilical cord prolapse, amnionitis, uterine hypertonicity, and severe fetal distress (ACOG, 2006).

There is no standard protocol for amnioinfusion. After obtaining informed consent, a vaginal examination is performed to evaluate for cord prolapse, establish dilation, and confirm presentation. Next, 250 to 500 mL of warmed normal saline or lactated Ringer's solution is administered using an infusion pump over 20 to 30 minutes. Overdistention of the uterus is a risk, so the amount of fluid infused must be monitored closely (Boyd & Carter, 2008).

When caring for the woman who is receiving an amnioinfusion, include the following:

- Explain the need for the procedure, what it involves, and how it may solve the problem.
- Inform the mother that she will need to remain on bed rest during the procedure.
- Assess the mother's vital signs and associated discomfort level.
- Maintain intake and output records.
- Assess the duration and intensity of uterine contractions frequently to identify overdistention or increased uterine tone.
- Monitor the FHR pattern to determine whether the amnioinfusion is improving the fetal status.
- Prepare the mother for a possible cesarean birth if the FHR does not improve after the amnioinfusion.

FIGURE 21.6 Forceps delivery. (**A**) Example of forceps. (**B**) Forceps being applied to the fetus.

▶ FORCEPS- OR VACUUM- ASSISTED BIRTH

Forceps or a vacuum extractor may be used to apply traction to the fetal head or to provide a method of rotating the fetal head during birth. **Forceps** are stainless-steel instruments, similar to tongs, with rounded edges that fit around the fetus's head. Some forceps have open blades and some have solid blades. Outlet forceps are used when the fetal head is crowning and low forceps are used when the fetal head is at a +2 station or lower but not yet crowning. The forceps are applied to the sides of the fetal head. The type of forceps used is determined by the birth attendant. All forceps have a locking mechanism that prevents the blades from compressing the fetal skull (Fig. 21.6).

A **vacuum extractor** is a cup-shaped instrument attached to a suction pump used for extraction of the fetal head (Fig. 21.7). The suction cup is placed against the occiput of the fetal head. The pump is used to create negative pressure (suction) of approximately 50 to 60 mmHg. The birth attendant then applies traction until the fetal head emerges from the vagina.

The indications for the use of either method are similar and include a prolonged second stage of labor, a nonreassuring FHR pattern, failure of the presenting part to fully rotate and descend in the pelvis, limited sensation and inability to push effectively due to the effects of regional anesthesia, presumed fetal jeopardy or fetal distress, maternal heart disease, acute pulmonary edema, intrapartum infection, maternal fatigue, or infection (Pope & O'Grady, 2006).

The use of forceps or a vacuum extractor poses the risk of tissue trauma to the mother and the newborn. Maternal trauma may include lacerations of the cervix, vagina,

FIGURE 21.7 Vacuum extractor for delivery. (**A**) Example of a vacuum extractor. (**B**) Vacuum extractor applied to the fetal head to assist in delivery.

or perineum; hematoma; extension of the episiotomy incision into the anus; hemorrhage; and infection. Potential newborn trauma includes ecchymoses, facial and scalp lacerations, facial nerve injury, cephalhematoma, and caput succedaneum (Cunningham et al., 2005).

Prevention is key to reducing the use of these techniques. Preventive measures include frequently changing the client's position, encouraging ambulation if permitted, frequently reminding the client to empty her bladder to allow maximum space for birth, and providing adequate hydration throughout labor. Additional measures include assessing maternal vital signs, the contraction pattern, the fetal status, and the maternal response to the procedure. Provide a thorough explanation of the procedure and the rationale for its use. Reassure the mother that any marks or swelling on the newborn's head or face will disappear without treatment within 2 to 3 days. Alert the postpartum nursing staff about the use of the technique so that they can observe for any bleeding or infection related to genital lacerations.

CESAREAN BIRTH

WATCH&LEARN

A **cesarean birth** is the delivery of the fetus through an incision in the abdomen and uterus. A classic (vertical) or low transverse incision may be used; today, the low transverse incision is more common (Fig. 21.8).

High cesarean birth rates are an international concern. The number of cesarean births has steadily risen in the United States: today approximately 29% or one in three births occur this way (ACOG, 2008). Although there has been some decline in rates since the 1980s, the United States still has a way to go to reduce its surgical birth rates (USDHHS, 2000).

Several factors may explain this increased incidence of cesarean deliveries: the use of electronic fetal monitoring, which identifies fetal distress early; the reduced number of forceps-assisted births; older maternal age and reduced parity, with more nulliparous women having infants; convenience to the client and doctor; and a increase in malpractice suits (Katz, 2006).

Cesarean birth is a major surgical procedure with increased risks compared to a vaginal birth. The client is at risk for complications such as infection, hemorrhage, aspiration, pulmonary embolism, urinary tract trauma, thrombophlebitis, paralytic ileus, and atelectasis. Fetal injury and transient tachypnea of the newborn also may occur (Gagnon, Meir, & Waghorn, 2007).

Spinal, epidural, or general anesthesia is used for cesarean births. Epidural anesthesia is most commonly used today because it is associated with less risk and most women wish to be awake and aware of the birth experience.

Nursing Assessment

Review the woman's history for indications associated with cesarean birth and complete a physical examination. Any condition that prevents the safe passage of the fetus through the birth canal or that seriously compromises maternal or fetal well-being may be an indication for a cesarean birth. Examples include active genital herpes, fetal macrosomia, fetopelvic disproportion, prolapsed umbilical cord, placental abnormality (placenta previa or abruptio placentae), previous classic uterine incision or scar, gestational hypertension, diabetes, positive HIV status, and dystocia. Fetal indications include malpresentation (nonvertex presentation), congenital anomalies (fetal neural tube defects, hydrocephalus, abdominal wall defects), and fetal distress (Humenick, 2006).

Nursing Management

Once the decision has been made to proceed with a cesarean birth, assess the woman's knowledge of the procedure and necessary preparation. Assist with obtaining diagnostic tests as ordered. These tests are usually ordered to ensure the well-being of both parties and may include a complete blood count; urinalysis to rule out infection; blood type and cross-match so that blood is available for transfusion if needed; an ultrasound to determine fetal position and placental location; and an amniocentesis to determine fetal lung maturity if needed.

Although the nurse's role in a cesarean birth can be very technical and skill-oriented at times, the focus must remain on the woman, not the equipment surrounding the bed. Care should be centered on the family, not the surgery. Provide education and minimize separation of the mother, father, and newborn. Remember that the client is anxious and concerned about her welfare as well as that of

FIGURE 21.8 Low transverse incision for cesarean birth.

her child. Use touch, eye contact, therapeutic communication, and genuine caring to provide couples with a positive birth experience, regardless of the type of delivery.

Providing Preoperative Care

Client preparation varies depending on whether the cesarean birth is planned or unplanned. The major difference is the time allotted for preparation and teaching. In an unplanned cesarean birth, institute measures quickly to ensure the best outcomes for the mother and fetus. Ensure that the woman has signed an informed consent, and allow for discussion of fears and expectations. Provide essential teaching and explanations to reduce the woman's fears and anxieties.

Ascertain the client's and family's understanding of the surgical procedure. Reinforce the reasons for surgery given by the surgeon. Outline the procedure and expectations of the surgical experience. Ensure that all diagnostic tests ordered have been completed, and evaluate the results. Explain to the woman and her family about what to expect postoperatively. Reassure the woman that pain management will be provided throughout the procedure and afterward. Encourage the woman to report any pain.

Ask the woman about the time she last had anything to eat or drink. Document the time and what was consumed. Throughout the preparations, assess maternal and fetal status frequently.

Provide preoperative teaching to reduce the risk of postoperative complications. Demonstrate the use of the incentive spirometer and deep-breathing and leg exercises. Instruct the woman on how to splint her incision.

Complete the preoperative procedures, which may include:

- Preparing the surgical site as ordered
- Starting an intravenous infusion for fluid replacement therapy as ordered
- Inserting an indwelling (Foley) catheter and informing the client about how long it will remain in place (usually 24 hours)
- Administering any preoperative medications as ordered; documenting the time administered and the client's reaction

Maintain a calm, confident manner in all interactions with the client and family. Help transport the client and her partner to the operative area.

Providing Postoperative Care

Postoperative care for the mother who has had a cesarean delivery is similar to that for one who has had a vaginal birth, with a few additional measures. Assess vital signs and lochia flow every 15 minutes for the first hour, then every 30 minutes for the next hour, and then every 4 hours if stable. Assist with perineal care and instruct the client in the same. Inspect the abdominal dressing and document

description, including any evidence of drainage. Assess uterine tone to determine fundal firmness. Check the patency of the intravenous line, making sure the infusion is flowing at the correct rate. Inspect the infusion site frequently for redness.

Assess the woman's level of consciousness if sedative drugs were administered. Institute safety precautions until the woman is fully alert and responsive. If a regional anesthetic was used, monitor for the return of sensation to the legs.

Assess for evidence of abdominal distention and auscultate bowel sounds. Assist with early ambulation to prevent respiratory and cardiovascular problems and to promote peristalsis. Monitor intake and output at least every 4 hours initially and then every 8 hours as indicated.

Encourage the woman to cough, perform deep-breathing exercises, and use the incentive spirometer every 2 hours. Administer analgesics as ordered and provide comfort measures, such as splinting the incision and pillows for positioning. Assist the client to move in bed and turn side to side to improve circulation. Also encourage the woman to ambulate to promote venous return from the extremities.

Encourage early touching and holding of the newborn to promote bonding. Assist with breastfeeding initiation and offer continued support. Suggest alternate positioning techniques to reduce incisional discomfort while breastfeeding.

Review with the couple their perception of the surgical birth experience. Allow them to verbalize their feelings and assist them in positive coping measures. Prior to discharge, teach the woman about the need for adequate rest, activity restrictions such as lifting, and signs and symptoms of infection.

▶ VAGINAL BIRTH AFTER CESAREAN

Vaginal birth after cesarean (VBAC) describes a woman who gives birth vaginally after having at least one previous cesarean birth. Despite evidence that some women who have had a cesarean birth are candidates for vaginal birth, most women who have had a cesarean birth once undergo another for subsequent pregnancies (Caughey, 2006).

The choice of a vaginal or a repeat cesarean birth can be offered to women who had a lower abdominal incision. However, controversy remains. The argument against VBAC focuses on the risk of uterine rupture and hemorrhage. Although the risk of uterine rupture is relatively low, the rate of fetal mortality in the event of a uterine rupture is extremely high.

Contraindications to VBAC include a prior classic uterine incision, prior transfundal uterine surgery (myomectomy), uterine scar other than low-transverse cesarean scar, contracted pelvis, and inadequate staff or facility if an emergency cesarean birth in the event of uterine rupture is required (Caughey, 2006). Most women go through a trial of labor to see how they progress, but this must be performed in an environment capable of handling the emergency of uterine rupture. The use of cervical ripening agents increases the risk of uterine rupture and thus is contraindicated in VBAC clients. The woman considering induction of labor after a previous cesarean birth needs to be informed of the increased risk of uterine rupture with an induction than with spontaneous labor (Meddings et al., 2007).

Women are the primary decision makers about the choice of birth method, but they need education about VBAC during their prenatal course. Management is similar for any women experiencing labor, but certain areas require special focus:

• Consent: Fully informed consent is essential for the woman who wants to have a trial of labor after cesarean birth. The client must be advised about the risks as well as the benefits. She must understand the ramifications of uterine rupture, even though the risk is small.
• Documentation: Recordkeeping is an important component of safe client care. If and when an emergency occurs, it is imperative to take care of the client, but also to keep track of the plan of care, interventions and their timing, and the client's response. Events and activities can be written right on the fetal monitoring tracing to correlate with the change in fetal status.
• Surveillance: A nonreassuring fetal monitor tracing in a woman undergoing a trial of labor after a cesarean birth should alert the nurse to the possibility of uterine rupture. Terminal bradycardia must be considered an emergency situation, and the nurse should prepare the team for an emergency delivery.
• Readiness for emergency: According to ACOG criteria for a safe trial of labor for a woman who has had a previous cesarean birth, the physician, anesthesia provider, and operating room team must be immediately available. Anything less would place the women and fetus at risk (ACOG, 2004a).

Nurses must act as advocates, giving input on the appropriate selection of women who wish to undergo VBAC. Nurses also need to become experts at reading fetal monitoring tracings to identify a nonreassuring pattern and set in motion an emergency delivery. Including all these nursing strategies will make VBAC safer for all.

■■■ Key Concepts

■ Risk factors for dystocia include epidural analgesia, occiput posterior position, longer first stage of labor, nulliparity, short maternal stature (<5 feet tall), high birth weight, maternal age older than 35 years, gestational age more than 41 weeks, chorioamnionitis, pelvic contractions, macrosomia, and high station at complete cervical dilation.
■ Dystocia may result from problems in the powers, passenger, passageway, or psyche.
■ Problems involving the powers that lead to dystocia include hypertonic uterine dysfunction, hypotonic uterine dysfunction, and precipitous labor.
■ Management of hypertonic labor pattern involves therapeutic rest with the use of sedatives to promote relaxation and stop the abnormal activity of the uterus.
■ Any presentation other than occiput or a slight variation of the fetal position or size increases the probability of dystocia.
■ Multiple gestation may result in dysfunctional labor due to uterine overdistention, which may lead to hypotonic dystocia, and abnormal presentations of the fetuses.
■ During labor, evaluation of fetal descent, cervical effacement and dilation, and characteristics of uterine contractions are paramount to determine progress or lack thereof.
■ Antepartum assessment for a postterm pregnancy typically includes daily fetal movement counts done by the woman, nonstress tests done twice weekly, amniotic fluid assessments as part of the biophysical profile, and weekly cervical examinations to check for ripening for induction.
■ Once the cervix is ripe, oxytocin is the most popular pharmacologic agent used for inducing or augmenting labor.
■ Generally, the first and most reliable symptom of uterine rupture is fetal distress.
■ Amniotic fluid embolism is a rare but often fatal event characterized by the sudden onset of hypotension, hypoxia, and coagulopathy.
■ Cesarean births have steadily risen in the United States; today, approximately one in five births occurs this way. Cesarean birth is a major surgical procedure and has increased risks over vaginal birth.

REFERENCES

Abenhaim, H., Kinch, R., Morin, L., Benjamin, A., & Usher, R. (2007). Effect of prepregnancy body mass index categories on obstetrical and neonatal outcomes. *Archives of Gynecology and Obstetrics, 275*(1), 39–43.
American Academy of Pediatrics (AAP) and American College of Obstetricians and Gynecologists (ACOG). (2003). *Guidelines for perinatal care* (5th ed.). Washington, DC: Author.
ACOG. (2001). ACOG committee opinion: Number 256. Mode of term single breech delivery. *International Journal of Gynecology and Obstetrics, 77*(1), 65–66.
ACOG. (2003a). *Dystocia and augmentation of labor. Clinical management guidelines for obstetricians-gynecologists.* ACOG Practice Bulletin No. 49. Washington, DC: Author.
ACOG. (2003b). ACOG practice bulletin: Management of preterm labor. *Obstetrics and Gynecology, 101*, 1039–1047.
ACOG. (2004a). Guidelines for VBAC. *American Family Physician, 70*(7), 1397–1399.

ACOG. (2004b). Management of postterm pregnancy (Practice Bulletin #55). *Obstetrics and Gynecology, 194,* 639–646.

ACOG. (2006). Amnioinfusion does not prevent meconium aspiration syndrome. ACOG Committee on Obstetric Practice, number 346. *Obstetrics & Gynecology, 108*(4), 1053–1055.

ACOG. (2008). Rising cesarean birth rates in U.S. tied to obesity, ACOG's 54th annual meeting. [online] Available at: http://www.medpagetoday.com/MeetingCoverage/ACOG/tb/3268.

Anderson, T. (2007). Cochrane made simple: Can midwives prevent shoulder dystocia? *Practicing Midwife, 10*(1), 36–37.

Arenson, J., & Drake, P. (2007). *Maternal and newborn health.* Sudbury, MA: Jones and Bartlett Publishers.

Blackburn, S. (2007). *Maternal, fetal, and neonatal physiology: A clinical perspective* (3rd ed.). St. Louis: W. B. Saunders.

Bonilla, M. M., & Forouzan, I. (2007). Dystocia. *eMedicine.* Available at: http://www.eMedicine.com/med/topic3280.htm.

Boulvain, M., Kelly, A., Lohse, C., Stan, C., & Irion, O. (2007). Mechanical methods for induction of labor. *Cochrane Database of Systematic Reviews 2007* Issue 1: DOI: 10.1002/14651858.CD001233.

Boyd, R. L., & Carter, B. S. (2008). Polyhydramnios and oligohydramnios. *eMedicine.* Available at: http://www.emedicine.com/ped/topic 1854.htm.

Briggs, G. G., & Wan, S. R. (2006). Drug therapy during labor and delivery. *American Journal of Health-System Pharmacists, 63*(12), 1131–1139.

Bueno, B., San-Frutos, L., Perez-Medina, T., Barbancho, C., & Bajo, J. (2007). The labor induction: Integrated clinical and sonographic variables that predict the outcome. *Journal of Perinatology, 27*(1), 4–8.

Butler, J. R., & Wilkes, P. T. (2007). Postterm pregnancy. *eMedicine.* Available at: http://www.emedicine.com/med/topic3248.htm.

Catalano, P. M. (2007). Management of obesity in pregnancy. *Obstetrics and Gynecology, 109*(2), 419–433.

Caughey, A. B. (2006). Vaginal birth after cesarean delivery. *eMedicine.* Available at: http://www.emedicine.com/med/topic3434.htm.

Cheng, Y. W., & Caughey, A. B. (2007). Normal labor and delivery. *eMedicine.* Available at: http://www.emedicine.com/med/topic 3239.htm.

Crane, J. M. (2006). Factors predicting labor induction success: A critical analysis. *Clinical Obstetrics & Gynecology, 49*(3), 573–584.

Cunningham, F. G., Leveno, K. J., Bloom, S. L., Hauth, J. C., Gilstrap, L., & Wenstrom, K. D. (2005). *Williams' obstetrics* (22nd ed.). New York: McGraw-Hill.

Deering, S. H., & Satin, A. (2007). Abruptio placentae. *eMedicine.* Available at: http://www.emedicine.com/med/topic6.htm.

Dilbaz, B., Ozturkoglu, E., Dilbaz, S., Ozturk, N., Sivaslioglu, A., & Haberal, A. (2006). Risk factors and perinatal outcomes associated with umbilical cord prolapse. *Archives of Gynecology & Obstetrics, 274*(2), 104–107.

Ecker, J., & Frigoletto, F. D. (2007). Cesarean delivery and the risk-benefit calculus. *New England Journal of Medicine, 356*(9), 885–888.

Enakpene, C. A., Omigbodun, A. O., & Arowojolu, A. O. (2006). Perinatal mortality following umbilical cord prolapse. *International Journal of Gynecology & Obstetrics, 95*(1), 44–45.

Fischer, R. (2007). Breech presentation. *eMedicine.* Available at: http://www.emedicine.com/med/topic3272.htm.

Gagnon, A. J., Meier, K. M., & Waghorn, K. (2007). Continuity of nursing care and its link to cesarean birth rate. *Birth: Issues in Perinatal Care, 34*(1), 26–31.

Gelber, S. (2006). Mechanical methods of cervical ripening and labor induction. *Clinical Obstetrics & Gynecology, 49*(3), 642–657.

Gilbert, E. (2007). *Manual of high-risk pregnancy and delivery* (4th ed.). St. Louis: Mosby.

Gray, B. A. (2006). How nurses can identify, treat and prevent preterm labor. *AWHONN Lifelines, 10*(5), 380–389.

Griffin, G. (2007). Are oral beta-mimetics effective maintenance therapies after threatened preterm labor? *American Family Physician, 75*(5), 648–649.

Grimes-Dennis, J., & Berghella, V. (2007). Cervical length and prediction of preterm delivery. *Current Opinion in Obstetrics & Gynecology, 19*(2), 191–195.

Gülmezoglu, A. M., Crowther, C. A., & Middleton, P. (2006). Induction of labour for improving birth outcomes for women at or beyond term. *Cochrane Database of Systematic Reviews* 2006. Issue 4. Art. No.: CD004945.DOI:10.1002/14651858.CD004945.pub2.

Gurewitsch, E. D., Johnson, E., Hamzehzadeh, S., & Allen, R. H. (2006). Risk factors for brachial plexus injury with and without shoulder dystocia. *American Journal of Obstetrics and Gynecology, 194,* 486–492.

Heimstad, R., Romundstad, P. R., Eik-Nes, S. H., & Salvesen, K. A. (2006). Outcomes of pregnancy beyond 37 weeks of gestation. *Obstetrics and Gynecology, 108*(3), 500–508.

Hofmeyr, G. J., & Gulmezoglu, A. M. (2007). Vaginal misoprostol for cervical ripening and induction of labor. *Cochrane Database of Systematic Reviews 2007* Issue 1. Art. No.: CD000941. DOI: 10.1002/14651858.CD000941.

Humenick, S. (2006). NIH weighs in on cesarean birth. *Journal of Perinatal Education, 15*(1), 3.

Incerti, M., Ghidini, A., Korker, V., & Pezzullo, J. (2007). Performance of cervicovaginal fetal fibronectin in a community hospital setting. *Archives of Gynecology & Obstetrics, 275*(5), 347–351.

Jazayeri, A., & Contreras, D. (2007). Macrosomia. *eMedicine.* Available at: http://emedicine.com/med/topic3279.htm.

Jenis, A. (2007). Pregnancy, breech delivery. *eMedicine.* Available at: http://www.emedicine.com/emerg/topic868.htm.

Joy, S., & Lyon, D. (2007). Diagnosis of abnormal labor. *eMedicine.* Available at: http://www.emedicine.com/med/topic3488.html.

Katz, V. L. (2006). Cesarean birth. *Obstetrics & Gynecology, 108*(1), 2–3.

Kavanagh, J., Kelly, A., & Thomas, J. (2007). Sexual intercourse for cervical ripening and induction of labor. *Cochrane Database of Systematic Reviews* 2007 Issue 1: CD003093. DOI: 10.1002/14651858. CD003093.

Kennare, R., Tucker, G., Heard, A., & Chan, A. (2007). Risks of adverse outcomes in the next birth after a first cesarean delivery. *Obstetrics & Gynecology, 109*(2), 270–276.

Khan, R. A., Khan, Z. E., & Ashraf, O. (2007). Concurrent versus sequential methods for labor induction at term. *International Journal of Gynecology & Obstetrics, 96*(2), 94–97.

Kuczkowski, K. M. (2007). Labor pain and its management with the combined spinal-epidural analgesia: What does an obstetrician need to know? *Archives of Gynecology & Obstetrics, 275*(3), 183–185.

Lee, H. C., El-Sayed, Y. Y., & Gould, J. B. (2007). Delivery mode by race for breech presentation in the U.S. *Journal of Perinatology, 27*(3), 147–153.

Lilley, L. L., Harrington, S., & Snyder, J. S. (2007). *Pharmacology and the nursing process* (5th ed.). St. Louis: Elsevier Health Sciences.

Lindsey, J. L., & Azad, S. (2007). Evaluation of fetal death. *eMedicine.* Available at: http://www.emedicine.com/med/topic3235.htm.

March of Dimes. (2007a). *Placental abruption.* Available at: http://www.marchofdimes.com/pnhec/188_1135.asp.

March of Dimes. (2007b). *Multiples: Twins, triplets and beyond.* Available at: http://www.marchofdimes.com/professionals/681_4545.asp.

March of Dimes. (2007c). *Preterm labor and birth: A serious pregnancy complication.* Available at: http://www.marchofdimes.com/printable Articles/240_1080.asp?printable=true.

March of Dimes. (2007d). *Preterm birth.* Available at: http://www.marchofdimes.com/prematurity/5196_5799.asp.

March of Dimes. (2007e). *Preterm labor.* Available at: http://www.marchofdimes.com/pnhec/188_1080.asp.

March of Dimes. (2007f). *Umbilical cord abnormalities.* Available at: http://www.marchofdimes.com/professionals/681_4546.asp.

Meddings, F., Phipps, F. M., Haith-Cooper, M., & Haigh, J. (2007). Vaginal birth after cesarean section (VBAC): exploring women's perceptions. *Journal of Clinical Nursing, 16*(1), 160–167.

Moore, J. (2006). Amniotic fluid embolism: On the trail of an elusive diagnosis. *Lancet, 368*(9545), 1399–1401.

Moore, L. E., & Ware, D. (2007). Amniotic fluid embolism. *eMedicine.* Available at: http://emedicine.com/med/topic122.htm.

Morgan, B. L. G., & Ross, M. G. (2007). Umbilical cord complications. *eMedicine.* Available at: http://www.emedicine.com/med/topic3276.htm.

Morrison, J. C., & Chauhan, S. P. (2003). Current status of home uterine activity monitoring. *Clinics in Perinatology, 30*(4), 757–801.

Nahum, G. G., & Pham, K. Q. (2007). Uterine rupture in pregnancy. *eMedicine.* Available at: http://www.emedicine.com/med/topic3746.htm.

Norwitz, E. R., & Schorge, J. O. (2006). *Obstetrics and gynecology at a glance* (2nd ed.). Malden, MA: Blackwell Publishing, Ltd.

O'Shea, A., & Eappen, S. (2007). Amniotic fluid embolism. *International Anesthesiology Clinics, 45*(1), 17–28.

Pope, C. S., & O'Grady, J. P. (2006). Vacuum extraction. *eMedicine.* Available at: http://www.emedicine.com/med/topic3389.htm.

Pretorius, C., Jagatt, A., & Lamont, R. (2007). The relationship between periodontal disease, bacterial vaginosis, and preterm birth. *Journal of Perinatal Medicine, 35*(2), 93–99.

Rai, J., & Schreiber, J. R. (2007). Cervical ripening. *eMedicine.* Available at: http://www.emedicine.com/med/topic3282.htm.

Schoening, A. M. (2007). Amniotic fluid embolism: Recognizing trouble. *Nursing 2007, 37*(1), 64–67.

Sharf, Y., Farine, D., Batzalel, M., Megel, Y., Shenhav, M., Jaffa, A., & Barnea, O. (2007). Continuous monitoring of cervical dilatation and fetal head station during labor. *Medical Engineering & Physics, 29*(1), 61–71.

Shobeiri, F., Tehranian, N., & Nazari, M. (2007). Amniotomy in labor. *International Journal of Gynecology & Obstetrics, 96*(3), 197–198.

Sifakis, S., Angelakis, E., Avgoustinakis, E., Fragouli, Y., Mantas, N., Koukoura, O., Vardaki, E., & Koumantakis, E. (2007). A randomized comparison between intravaginal misoprostol and prostaglandin E2 for labor induction. *Archives of Gynecology and Obstetrics, 275*(4), 263–267.

Simhan, H., & Caritis, S. (2007). Prevention of preterm delivery. *New England Journal of Medicine, 357*(5), 477–487.

Smith, J. G., & Merrill, D. C. (2006). Oxytocin in induction of labor. *Clinical Obstetrics & Gynecology, 49*(3), 594–608.

Stein, A. M. (2007). *Maternity and women's health nursing.* Clifton Park, NY: Thomson Delmar Learning.

Tan, T. C., Devendra, K., Tan, L. K., & Tan, H. K. (2006). Tocolytic treatment for the management of preterm labor: A systematic review. *Singapore Medical Journal, 47*(5), 361–366.

U.S. Department of Health and Human Services (USDHHS), Public Health Service. (2000). *Healthy People 2010* (conference edition, in two volumes). U.S. Department of Health and Human Services. Washington, DC: U.S. Government Printing Office.

U.S. Food and Drug Administration (USFDA). (2007). *Misoprostol (marketed as Cytotec) information. FDA Alert—Risks of use in labor and delivery.* Available at: http://www.fda.gov/CDER/Drug/infopage/misoprostol/default.htm.

Wing, D. A. (2006). Symposium on cervical ripening and labor induction. *Clinical Obstetrics & Gynecology, 49*(3), 549–550.

World Health Organization (WHO). (2007). Malpositions and malpresentations: A guide for midwives and doctors. Available at: http://www.who.int/reproductive-health/impac/Symptoms/Malpositions__malpresetations_S69_S81.html.

Xu, H., Hofmeyr, J., Roy, C., & Fraser, W. D. (2007). Intrapartum amnioinfusion for meconium-stained amniotic fluid: A systematic review of randomized controlled trials. *International Journal of Obstetrics & Gynecology, 114*(4), 383–390.

Zach, T., & Pramanik, A. K. (2007). Multiple births. *eMedicine.* Available at: http://www.emedicine.com/ped/topic2599.htm.

WEBSITES

American Academy of Pediatrics: www.app.org
American College of Obstetricians and Gynecologists: www.acog.org
American Society of Reproductive Medicine: www.asrm.org
Association of Women's Health, Obstetric and Neonatal Nurses: www.awhonn.org
Birthrites: Healing after Cesarean, Inc.: www.birthrites.org
Department of Health and Human Services: www.4women.gov
International Cesarean Awareness Network: www.ican-online.org
March of Dimes: www.modimes.org
Mothers of Super Twins: www.mostonline.org
National Perinatal Association: www.nationalperinatal.org
SHARE Parents Support Group: www.nationalshareoffice.com/
Sidelines: High Risk Pregnancy Support Group: www.sidelines.org
Smoke-free Families: www.smokefreefamilies.org
VBAC: www.vbac.com

CHAPTER WORKSHEET

MULTIPLE CHOICE QUESTIONS

1. When reviewing the medical record of a client, the nurse notes that the woman has a condition in which the fetus cannot physically pass through the maternal pelvis. The nurse interprets this as:

   a. Cervical insufficiency

   b. Contracted pelvis

   c. Maternal disproportion

   d. Fetopelvic disproportion

2. The nurse would anticipate a cesarean birth for a client who has which active infection present at the onset of labor?

   a. Hepatitis

   b. Herpes simplex virus

   c. Toxoplasmosis

   d. Human papillomavirus

3. After a vaginal examination, the nurse determines that the client's fetus is in an occiput posterior position. The nurse would anticipate that the client will have:

   a. Intense back pain

   b. Frequent leg cramps

   c. Nausea and vomiting

   d. A precipitous birth

4. When assessing the following women, which would the nurse identify as being at the greatest risk for preterm labor?

   a. Woman who had twins in a previous pregnancy

   b. Client living in a large city

   c. Woman working full-time as a computer programmer

   d. Client with a history of a previous preterm birth

5. The rationale for using a prostaglandin gel for a client prior to the induction of labor is to:

   a. Stimulate uterine contractions

   b. Numb cervical pain receptors

   c. Prevent cervical lacerations

   d. Soften and efface the cervix

6. A client who was in active labor and whose cervix had dilated to 4 cm experiences a weakening in the intensity and frequency of her contractions and exhibits no further progress in labor. The nurse interprets this as a sign of:

   a. Hypertonic labor

   b. Precipitous labor

   c. Hypotonic labor

   d. Dysfunctional labor

CRITICAL THINKING EXERCISES

1. Marsha, a 26-year-old multipara, is admitted to the labor and birth suite in active labor. After a few hours, the nurse notices a change in her contraction pattern—poor contraction intensity and no progression of cervical dilatation beyond 5 cm. Marsha keeps asking about her labor progress and appears anxious about "how long this labor is taking."

   a. Based on the nurse's findings, what might you suspect is going on?

   b. How can the nurse address Marsha's anxiety?

   c. What are the appropriate interventions to change this labor pattern?

2. Marsha activates her call light and states, "I feel increased wetness down below."

   a. What might be occurring?

   b. How will the nurse confirm the suspicions?

   c. What interventions are appropriate for this finding?

STUDY ACTIVITIES

1. Visit the SHARE Pregnancy and Infant Loss Support, Inc. website (http://www.nationalshareoffice.com/) and assess its helpfulness to parents.

2. Outline the fetal and maternal risks associated with a postterm pregnancy.

3. An abnormal or difficult labor describes

   _____.

NURSING MANAGEMENT OF THE POSTPARTUM WOMAN AT RISK

KEY TERMS

mastitis

metritis

postpartum depression

postpartum hemorrhage

subinvolution

thrombophlebitis

uterine atony

uterine inversion

LEARNING OBJECTIVES

Upon completion of the chapter, the learner will be able to:

1. Define the major conditions that place the postpartum woman at risk.
2. Explain the risk factors, assessment, preventive measures, and nursing management of common postpartum complications.
3. Differentiate the causes of postpartum hemorrhage based on the underlying pathophysiologic mechanisms.
4. Outline the nurse's role in assessing and managing the care of a woman with a thromboembolic condition.
5. Discuss the nursing management of a woman who develops a postpartum infection.
6. Identify at least two affective disorders that can occur in women after birth, describing specific therapeutic management for each.

*J*oan gave birth about an hour ago to her fifth baby boy, who weighed 10 pounds, and she is resting in bed when the nurse comes in to assess her. She tells the nurse that she feels like there is "something really wet" between her legs. She also feels a bit lightheaded. What would the nurse suspect is happening? What findings would support the nurse's suspicion? What should the nurse do first?

Wow

After holding their breath during the childbirth experience, nurses shouldn't let it out fully and relax until the woman and baby are discharged.

Typically, recovery from childbirth proceeds normally both physiologically and psychologically. It is a time filled with many changes and wide-ranging emotions, and the new mother commonly experiences a great sense of accomplishment. However, the woman can experience deviations from the norm, developing a postpartum condition that places her at risk. These high-risk conditions or complications can become life-threatening. Healthy People 2010 addresses these risks in two National Health Goals.

This chapter will address the nursing management of the most common conditions that place the postpartum woman at risk: hemorrhage, infection, thromboembolic disease, and postpartum affective disorders.

Postpartum Hemorrhage

Postpartum hemorrhage is a potentially life-threatening complication that can occur after both vaginal and cesarean births. It is the leading cause of maternal mortality worldwide: it is estimated that worldwide, 150,000 women die of postpartum hemorrhage annually—one every four minutes (American College of Obstetricians & Gynecologists [ACOG], 2006). More than half of all maternal deaths occur within 24 hours of giving birth, most commonly from excessive bleeding.

Postpartum hemorrhage is defined as a blood loss greater than 500 mL after vaginal birth or more than 1,000 mL after a cesarean birth. Blood loss that occurs within 24 hours of birth is termed *early postpartum hemorrhage;* blood loss that occurs 24 hours to 6 weeks after birth is termed *late postpartum hemorrhage.* However, this definition is arbitrary, because estimates of blood loss at birth are subjective and generally inaccurate. Studies have suggested that health care providers consistently underestimate actual blood loss (Smith & Brennan, 2007). A more objective definition of postpartum hemorrhage would be any amount of bleeding that places the mother in hemodynamic jeopardy.

Pathophysiology

Excessive bleeding can occur at any time between the separation of the placenta and its expulsion or removal. The most common cause of postpartum hemorrhage is **uterine atony**, failure of the uterus to contract and retract after birth. The uterus must remain contracted after birth to control bleeding from the placental site. Any factor that causes the uterus to relax after birth will cause bleeding—even a full bladder that displaces the uterus.

Over the course of a pregnancy, maternal blood volume increases by approximately 50% (from 4 to 6 L). The plasma volume increases twice as much in comparison to the total red blood cell volume. As a result, hemoglobin and hematocrit fall. The increase in blood volume meets the perfusion demands of the low-resistance uteroplacental unit and provides a reserve for the blood loss that occurs at delivery (Cunningham et al., 2005). Given this increase, the typical signs of hemorrhage (e.g., falling blood pressure, increasing pulse rate, and decreasing urinary output) do not appear until as much as 1,800 to 2,100 mL of blood has been lost (Gilbert and Harmon, 2007). In addition, accurate determination of actual blood loss is difficult because of blood pooling inside the uterus, on peripads, mattresses, and the floor. Since no universal clinical standard exists, nurses must remain vigilant, assessing for risk factors and checking clients carefully before the birth attendant leaves the birthing area.

Other causes of postpartum hemorrhage include lacerations of the genital tract, episiotomy, retained placental fragments, uterine inversion, coagulation disorders, and hematomas of the vulva, vagina, or subperitoneal areas (ACOG, 2006). A helpful way to remember the causes of postpartum hemorrhage is by using the "4 Ts": tone, tissue, trauma, and thrombosis (Anderson & Etches, 2007).

Tone

Altered uterine muscle tone most commonly results from overdistention of the uterus. Overdistention can be caused by multifetal gestation, fetal macrosomia, polyhydramnios, fetal abnormality, or placental fragments. Other causes might include prolonged or rapid, forceful labor, especially if stimulated; bacterial toxins (e.g., chorioamnionitis, endomyometritis, septicemia); use of anesthesia, especially halothane; and magnesium sulfate used in the treatment of preeclampsia (Nash, 2007). Overdistention of the uterus is a major risk factor for uterine atony, the most common cause of early postpartum hemorrhage, which can lead to hypovolemic shock.

HEALTHY PEOPLE *2010*	
Objective	Significance
Reduce maternal deaths from a baseline of 7.1 maternal deaths per 100,000 live births to 3.3 maternal deaths per 100,000 live births.	Will help foster the need for early identification of problems and prompt intervention to reduce the potential negative outcomes of pregnancy and birth
Reduce maternal illness and complications due to pregnancy	Will help to contribute to lower rates of rehospitalization, morbidity, and mortality by focusing on thorough assessments in the postpartum period
Related to postpartum complications, including postpartum depression	Will help to minimize the devastating effects of complications during the postpartum period and the woman's ability to care for her newborn

DHHS, 2000.

Tissue

Uterine contraction and retraction lead to detachment and expulsion of the placenta after birth. Classic signs of placental separation include a small gush of blood with lengthening of the umbilical cord and a slight rise of the uterus in the pelvis. Complete detachment and expulsion of the placenta permit continued contraction and optimal occlusion of blood vessels. Failure of complete placental separation and expulsion leads to retained fragments, which occupy space and prevent the uterus from contracting fully to clamp down on blood vessels; this can lead to hemorrhage. After the placenta is expelled, a thorough inspection is necessary to confirm its intactness; tears or fragments left inside may indicate an accessory lobe or placenta accreta (an uncommon condition in which the chorionic villi adhere to the myometrium, causing the placenta to adhere abnormally to the uterus and not separate and deliver spontaneously). Profuse hemorrhage results because the uterus cannot contract fully.

A prolapse of the uterine fundus to or through the cervix so that the uterus is turned inside out after birth is called **uterine inversion**. This condition is associated with grand multiparity, abnormal adherence of the placenta, excessive traction on the umbilical cord, vigorous fundal pressure, precipitous labor, or vigorous manual removal of the placenta. Acute postpartum uterine inversion is rare, with an estimated incidence of 1 in 2,000 births (Pope & O'Grady, 2006). Prompt recognition and rapid treatment to replace the inverted uterus will avoid morbidity and mortality for this serious complication (Smith & Brennan, 2006).

Subinvolution refers to incomplete involution of the uterus or failure to return to its normal size and condition after birth (Dorland, 2007). Complications of subinvolution include hemorrhage, pelvic peritonitis, salpingitis, and abscess formation (Weydert & Benda, 2006). Causes of subinvolution include retained placental fragments, distended bladder, uterine myoma, and infection. All of these conditions contribute to delayed postpartum bleeding. The clinical picture includes a postpartum fundal height that is higher than expected, with a boggy uterus; the lochia fails to change colors from red to serosa to alba within a few weeks. This condition is usually identified at the woman's postpartum examination 4 to 6 weeks after birth with a bimanual vaginal examination or ultrasound. Treatment is directed toward stimulating the uterus to expel fragments with a uterine stimulant, and antibiotics are given to prevent infection.

Trauma

Damage to the genital tract may occur spontaneously or through the manipulations used during birth. Lacerations and hematomas resulting from birth trauma can cause significant blood loss. Hematomas can present as pain or as a change in vital signs disproportionate to the amount of blood loss. Uterine inversion can occur secondary to pressure or pulling on the umbilical cord when the placenta is still firmly attached to the fundus after the infant has been born. Additionally, uterine rupture can cause damage to the genital tract and is more common in women with previous cesarean incisions or those who had undergone any procedure resulting in disruption of the uterine wall, including myomectomy, perforation of the uterus during a dilation and curettage (D&C), biopsy, or intrauterine device (IUD) insertion (Smith & Brennan, 2006).

Trauma can also occur after prolonged or vigorous labor, especially if the uterus has been stimulated with oxytocin or prostaglandins. Trauma can also occur after extrauterine or intrauterine manipulation of the fetus.

Cervical lacerations commonly occur during a forceps delivery or in mothers who have not been able to resist bearing down before the cervix is fully dilated. Vaginal sidewall lacerations are associated with operative vaginal births but may occur spontaneously, especially if the fetal hand presents with the head. Lacerations can arise during manipulations to resolve shoulder dystocia. Lacerations should always be suspected in the face of a contracted uterus with bright-red blood continuing to trickle out of the vagina.

Thrombosis

Thrombosis (blood clots) helps to prevent postpartum hemorrhage immediately after birth by providing hemostasis. Fibrin deposits and clots in supplying vessels play a significant role in the hours and days after birth. Disorders that interfere with the clot formation can lead to postpartum hemorrhage. Medication used to prevent hemorrhage by stimulating uterine contractions may delay the appearance of coagulation disorders. Coagulopathies should be suspected when postpartum bleeding persists without any identifiable cause (ACOG, 2006).

Ideally, the client's coagulation status is determined during pregnancy. However, if she received no prenatal care, coagulation studies should be ordered immediately to determine her status. Abnormal results typically include decreased platelet and fibrinogen levels, increased prothrombin time, partial thromboplastin time, and fibrin degradation products, and a prolonged bleeding time (Anderson & Etches, 2007). Conditions associated with coagulopathies in the postpartum client include idiopathic thrombocytopenic purpura, von Willebrand disease, and disseminated intravascular coagulation.

Idiopathic Thrombocytopenia Purpura

Idiopathic thrombocytopenia purpura (ITP) is a disorder of increased platelet destruction caused by the development of autoantibodies to platelet-membrane antigens. The incidence of ITP in adults is approximately 66 cases per 1 million per year (Silverman, 2007). Thrombocytopenia, capillary fragility, and increased bleeding time define the disorder, commonly manifested by easy bruising, bleeding from mucous membranes, menorrhagia, epistaxis, bleeding gums, hematomas, and severe hemorrhage after a cesarean birth or lacerations (Sood & Abrams, 2007). Glucocorticoids and immune globulin are the mainstays of medical therapy.

von Willebrand Disease

von Willebrand disease (vWD) is a congenital bleeding disorder, inherited as an autosomal dominant trait. It is characterized by a prolonged bleeding time, a deficiency of von Willebrand factor, and impairment of platelet adhesion (Dorland, 2007). In the United States, it is estimated to affect fewer than 3% of the population (Geil, 2007). Most cases remain undiagnosed due to lack of awareness, difficulty in diagnosis, a tendency to attribute bleeding to other causes, and variable symptoms (Kadir et al., 2007). The disorder is characterized by excessive bruising, prolonged nosebleeds, and prolonged oozing from wounds after surgery and after childbirth. The goal of therapy is to correct the defect in platelet adhesiveness by raising the level of von Willebrand factor with medications (Franchini & Lippi, 2007).

Disseminated Intravascular Coagulation

Disseminated intravascular coagulation (DIC) is a life-threatening, acquired pathologic process in which the clotting system is abnormally activated, resulting in widespread clot formation in the small vessels throughout the body (Levi & Schmaier, 2007). It can cause postpartum hemorrhage by altering the blood clotting mechanism. DIC is always a secondary diagnosis that occurs as a complication of abruptio placentae, amniotic fluid embolism, intrauterine fetal death with prolonged retention of the fetus, severe preeclampsia, septicemia, and hemorrhage. Clinical features include petechiae, ecchymoses, bleeding gums, fever, hypotension, acidosis, hematomas, tachycardia, proteinuria, uncontrolled bleeding during birth, and acute renal failure (Bick, 2007). Treatment goals are to maintain tissue perfusion through aggressive administration of fluid therapy, oxygen, heparin, and blood products.

Therapeutic Management

Therapeutic management focuses on the underlying cause of the hemorrhage. For example, uterine massage is used to treat uterine atony. If retained placental fragments are the cause, the fragments are usually manually separated and removed and a uterine stimulant is given to promote the uterus to expel fragments. Antibiotics are administered to prevent infection. Lacerations are sutured or repaired. Glucocorticoids and intravenous immunoglobulin, intravenous anti-RhoD, and platelet transfusions may be given. A splenectomy may be necessary if the bleeding tissues do not respond to medical management.

In vWD, there is a decrease in von Willebrand factor, which is necessary for platelet adhesion and aggregation. It binds to and stabilizes factor VIII of the coagulation cascade (Franchini & Lippi, 2007). Desmopressin, a synthetic form of vasopressin (antidiuretic hormone), may be used to treat vWD. This drug stimulates the release of stored factor VIII and von Willebrand factor from the lining of blood vessels, which increases platelet adhesiveness and shortens bleeding time. Other treatments that may be ordered include clotting factor concentrates, replacement of von Willebrand factor and factor VIII (Alphanate, Humate-P); antifibrinolytics (Amicar); and nonsteroidal anti-inflammatory drugs (NSAIDs) that do not cause platelet dysfunction (Geil, 2007).

Nursing Assessment

Pregnancy and childbirth involve significant health risks, even for women with no preexisting health problems. There are an estimated 14 million cases of pregnancy-related hemorrhage every year, with some of these women bleeding to death. Most of these deaths occur within 4 hours of giving birth and are a result of problems during the third stage of labor (ACOG, 2006). The period after the birth and the first hours postpartum are crucial times for the prevention, assessment, and management of bleeding. Compared with other maternal risks such as infection, bleeding can rapidly become life-threatening, and nurses, along with other health care providers, need to identify this condition quickly and intervene appropriately.

Begin by reviewing the mother's history, including labor and birth history, for risk factors associated with postpartum hemorrhage (Box 22.1).

Since the most common cause of immediate severe postpartum hemorrhage is uterine atony (failure of the

---

BOX 22.1 **Factors Placing a Woman at Risk for Postpartum Hemorrhage**

- Prolonged first, second, or third stage of labor
- Previous history of postpartum hemorrhage
- Multiple gestation
- Fetal macrosomia
- Uterine infection
- Manual extraction of placenta
- Arrest of descent
- Maternal exhaustion, malnutrition, or anemia
- Mediolateral episiotomy
- Preeclampsia
- Precipitous birth
- Maternal hypotension
- Previous placenta previa
- Coagulation abnormalities
- Birth canal lacerations
- Operative birth (forceps or vacuum)
- Augmented labor with medication
- Coagulation abnormalities
- Grand multiparity
- Polyhydramnios (Anderson & Etches, 2007)

uterus to contract properly after birth), assess uterine tone after birth by palpating the fundus for firmness and location. A soft, boggy fundus indicates uterine atony.

> ▶ *Take* NOTE!
>
> *A soft, boggy uterus that deviates from the midline suggests that a full bladder is interfering with uterine involution. If the uterus is not in correct position (midline), it will not be able to contract to control bleeding.*

Assess the amount of bleeding. If bleeding continues even though there are no lacerations, suspect retained placental fragments. The uterus remains large with painless, dark-red bleeding mixed with clots. This cause of hemorrhage can be prevented by carefully inspecting the placenta for intactness.

If trauma is suspected, attempt to identify the source and document it. Typically, the uterus will be firm with a steady stream or trickle of unclotted bright-red blood noted in the perineum. Most deaths from postpartum hemorrhage are not due to gross bleeding, but rather to inadequate management of slow, steady blood loss (Anderson & Etches, 2007).

Assess for hematoma. The uterus would be firm, with bright-red bleeding. Observe for a localized bluish bulging area just under the skin surface in the perineal area (Fig. 22.1). Often the woman will report severe perineal or pelvic pain and will have difficulty voiding. In addition, she may exhibit hypotension, tachycardia, and anemia (Gilbert & Harmon, 2007).

FIGURE 22.1 Perineal hematoma. Note the bulging swollen mass.

Inspect the skin and mucous membranes for gingival bleeding or petechiae and ecchymoses. Check venipuncture sites for oozing or prolonged bleeding. These findings might suggest a coagulopathy as a cause of postpartum hemorrhage. Also assess the amount of lochia, which would be much greater than usual. Urinary output would be diminished, with signs of acute renal failure. Vital signs would show an increased pulse rate and a decreased level of consciousness. However, signs of shock do not appear until hemorrhage is far advanced due to the increased fluid and blood volume of pregnancy.

Nursing Management

Massage the uterus if uterine atony is noted. The uterine muscles are sensitive to touch; massage stimulates the muscle fibers to contract. Massage the boggy uterus to stimulate contractions and expression of any accumulated blood clots while supporting the lower uterine segment. As blood pools in the vagina, stasis of blood causes clots to form; they need to be expelled as pressure is placed on the fundus. Overly forceful massage can tire the uterine muscles, resulting in further uterine atony and increased pain. See Nursing Procedure 22.1 for the steps in massaging the fundus.

If repeated fundal massage and expression of clots fail, medication is probably needed to cause the uterus to contract in order to control bleeding from the placental site. The injection of an uterotonic drug immediately after birth is an important intervention used to prevent postpartum hemorrhage. Oxytocin (Pitocin); methylergonovine maleate (Methergine); a synthetic analog of prostaglandin E1, misoprostol (Cytotec); and a derivative of prostaglandin (PGF2a), carboprost (Hemabate), are drugs used to manage postpartum hemorrhage (Drug Guide 22.1). However, misoprostol is not approved by the U.S. Food and Drug Association for this purpose. The choice of which uterotonic drug to use for management of bleeding depends on the judgment of the health care provider, the availability of drugs, and the risks and benefits of the drug.

*R*emember Joan, the woman described at the beginning of the chapter? The nurse assesses her and finds that her uterus is boggy. What would the nurse do next? What additional nursing measures might be used if Joan's fundus remains boggy? When should the health care provider be notified?

Maintain the primary IV infusion and be prepared to start a second infusion at another site if blood transfusions are necessary. Draw blood for type and cross-match and send it to the laboratory. Administer oxytocics as ordered, correlating and titrating the infusion rate to assessment findings of uterine firmness and lochia. Assess for visible vaginal bleeding, and count or weigh perineal pads.

Nursing Procedure 22.1

MASSAGING THE FUNDUS

Purpose: To Promote Uterine Contraction

1. After explaining the procedure to the woman, place one gloved hand (usually the dominant hand) on the fundus.
2. Place the other gloved hand on the area above the symphysis pubis (this helps to support the lower uterine segment).
3. With the hand on the fundus, gently massage the fundus in a circular manner. Be careful not to overmassage the fundus, which could lead to muscle fatigue and uterine relaxation.
4. Assess for uterine firmness (uterine tissue responds quickly to touch).
5. If firm, apply gentle yet firm pressure in a downward motion toward the vagina to express any clots that may have accumulated.
6. Do not attempt to express clots until the fundus is firm because the application of firm pressure on an uncontracted uterus could cause uterine inversion, leading to massive hemorrhage.
7. Assist the woman with perineal care and applying a new perineal pad.
8. Remove gloves and wash hands.

▶ *Take* NOTE!

When weighing perineal pads to determine blood loss, remember that 1 g of pad weight is equivalent to 1 mL of blood loss (Cohen, 2006).

Check vital signs every 15 to 30 minutes, depending on the acuity of the mother's health status. Monitor her complete blood count to identify any deficit or assess the adequacy of replacement. Assess the woman's level of consciousness to determine changes that may result from inadequate cerebral perfusion.

If a full bladder is present, assist the woman to empty her bladder to reduce displacement of the uterus. If the woman cannot void, anticipate the need to catheterize her to relieve bladder distention.

Prepare the woman for removal of retained placental fragments. These usually are manually separated and removed by the health care provider. Be sure that the health care provider remains long enough after birth to assess the bleeding status of the woman and determine the etiology. Assist the health care provider with suturing any lacerations immediately to control hemorrhage and repair the tissue.

Continually assess the woman for signs and symptoms of hemorrhagic shock, a condition in which inadequate perfusion of organs results in insufficient availability of oxygen to satisfy the metabolic needs of the tissues (Dorland, 2007). Subsequently a catabolic state develops, leading to inflammation, endothelial dysfunction, and disruption of normal metabolic processes in vital organs. Once these events become established, the process of shock is often irreversible, even if volume and red blood cell deficits are corrected (Cohen, 2006).

Monitor the woman's blood pressure, pulse, capillary refill, mental status, and urinary output. These assessments allow estimation of the severity of blood loss and help direct treatment. If the woman develops hemorrhagic shock, interventions focus on controlling the source of blood loss; restoring adequate oxygen-carrying capacity; and maintaining adequate tissue perfusion. Successful treatment depends on efficient collaboration among all health care team members to meet the woman's specific needs.

For the woman with ITP, expect to administer glucocorticoids, IV immunoglobulin, IV anti-RhoD, and platelet transfusions. Prepare the woman for a splenectomy if the bleeding tissues do not respond to medical management.

Be alert for women with abnormal bleeding tendencies, ensuring that they receive proper diagnosis and treatment. Teach them how to prevent severe hemorrhage by

DRUG GUIDE 22.1 DRUGS USED TO CONTROL POSTPARTUM HEMORRHAGE

Drug	Action/Indication	Nursing Implications
Oxytocin (Pitocin)	Stimulates the uterus to contract/to contract the uterus to control bleeding from the placental site	Assess fundus for evidence of contraction and compare amount of bleeding every 15 minutes or according to orders. Monitor vital signs every 15 minutes. Monitor uterine tone to prevent hyperstimulation. Reassure client about the need for uterine contraction and administer analgesics for comfort. Offer explanation to client and family about what is happening and the purpose of the medication. Provide nonpharmacologic comfort measures to assist with pain management. Set up the IV infusion to be piggybacked into a primary IV line. This ensures that the medication can be discontinued readily if hyperstimulation or adverse effects occur while maintaining the IV site and primary infusion.
Methylergonovine maleate (Methergine)	Stimulates the uterus/to prevent and treat postpartum hemorrhage due to atony or subinvolution	Assess baseline bleeding, uterine tone, and vital signs every 15 minutes or according to protocol. Offer explanation to client and family about what is happening and the purpose of the medication. Monitor for possible adverse effects, such as hypertension, seizures, uterine cramping, nausea, vomiting, and palpitations. Report any complaints of chest pain promptly.
Prostaglandin (PGF-2α, Carboprost, Hemabate)	Stimulates uterine contractions/to treat postpartum hemorrhage due to uterine atony when not controlled by other methods	Assess vital signs, uterine contractions, client's comfort level, and bleeding status as per protocol. Offer explanation to client and family about what is happening and the purpose of the medication. Monitor for possible adverse effects, such as fever, chills, headache, nausea, vomiting, diarrhea, flushing, and bronchospasm.

learning how to feel for and massage their fundus when boggy, assisting the nurse to keep track of the number of and amount of bleeding on perineal pads, and avoiding any medications with antiplatelet activity such as aspirin, antihistamines, or NSAIDs.

If the woman develops DIC, institute emergency measures to control bleeding and impending shock and prepare to transfer her to the intensive care unit. Identification of the underlying condition and elimination of the causative factor are essential to correct the coagulation problem. Be ready to replace fluid volume, administer blood component therapy, and optimize the mother's oxygenation and perfusion status to ensure adequate cardiac output and end-organ perfusion. Continually reassess the woman's coagulation status via laboratory studies.

Monitor vital signs closely, being alert for changes that signal an increase in bleeding or impending shock. Observe for signs of bleeding, including spontaneous bleeding from gums or nose, petechiae, excessive bleeding from the cesarean incision site, hematuria, and blood in the stool. These findings correlate with decreased blood volume, decreased organ and peripheral tissue perfusion, and clots in the microcirculation (Bick, 2007).

▶ **Take** NOTE!

Always remember the four causes of postpartum hemorrhage and the appropriate intervention for each: 1. Uterine atony—massage and oxytocics; 2. Retained placental tissue—evacuation and oxytocics; 3. Lacerations or hematoma—surgical repair; 4. Thrombosis (bleeding disorders)—blood products.

Institute measures to avoid tissue trauma or injury, such as giving injections and drawing blood. Also provide emotional support to the client and her family throughout this critical time by being readily available and providing explanations and reassurance.

An IV oxytocin infusion is started for Joan. What assessments will need to be done frequently to make sure Joan is not losing too much blood? What discharge instructions need to be reinforced with Joan?

Thromboembolic Conditions

A thrombosis (blood clot within a blood vessel) can cause an inflammation of the blood vessel lining (**thrombophlebitis**), which in turn can lead to a thromboembolism (obstruction of a blood vessel by a blood clot carried by the circulation from the site of origin). Thrombi can involve the superficial or deep veins in the legs or pelvis. Superficial venous thrombosis usually involves the saphenous venous system and is confined to the lower leg. Superficial thrombophlebitis may be caused by the use of the lithotomy position during birth. Deep venous thrombosis can involve deep veins from the foot to the calf, to the thighs, or pelvis. In both locations, thrombi can dislodge and migrate to the lungs, causing a pulmonary embolism.

The three most common thromboembolic conditions occurring during the postpartum period are superficial venous thrombosis, deep venous thrombosis, and pulmonary embolism. Although thromboembolic disorders occur in less than 1% of all postpartum women, pulmonary embolus can be fatal if a clot obstructs the lung circulation; thus, early identification and treatment are paramount.

Pathophysiology

Thrombus (blood clot) formation results typically results from venous stasis, injury to the innermost layer of the blood vessel, and hypercoagulation. Venous stasis and hypercoagulation are both common in the postpartum period.

If a clot dislodges and travels to the pulmonary circulation, pulmonary embolism can occur. Pulmonary embolism is a potentially fatal condition that occurs when the pulmonary artery is blocked by a blood clot that has traveled from another vein into the lungs, causing an obstruction and infarction. When the clot is large enough to block one or more of the pulmonary vessels that supply the lungs, it can result in sudden death. Pulmonary embolism is the leading cause of pregnancy-related death in the United States, occurring in 2 out of 100,000 live births (Shaughnessy, 2007).

Nursing Assessment

Assess the woman closely for risk factors and signs and symptoms of thrombophlebitis. Look for risk factors in the woman's history such as use of oral contraceptives before the pregnancy, smoking, employment that necessitates prolonged standing, history of thrombosis, thrombophlebitis, or endometritis, or evidence of current varicosities. Also look for other factors that can increase a woman's risk, such as prolonged bed rest, diabetes, obesity, cesarean birth, progesterone-induced distensibility of the veins of the lower legs during pregnancy, severe anemia, varicose veins, advanced maternal age (older than 35), and multiparity (Feied & Handler, 2007).

Ask the woman if she has pain or tenderness in the lower extremities. Suspect superficial venous thrombosis in a woman with varicose veins who reports tenderness and discomfort over the site of the thrombosis, most commonly in the calf area. The area appears reddened along the vein and is warm to the touch. The woman will report increased pain in the affected leg when she ambulates and bears weight.

Manifestations of deep venous thrombosis are often absent and diffuse. If they are present, they are caused by an inflammatory process and obstruction of venous return. Calf swelling, erythema, warmth, tenderness, and pedal edema may be noted. A positive Homans' sign (pain in the calf upon dorsiflexion) is not a definitive diagnostic sign and is no longer recommended as an indicator of deep vein thrombosis because calf pain can also be caused by a strained muscle or contusion (Feied & Handler, 2007).

Be alert for signs and symptoms of pulmonary embolism, including unexplained sudden onset of shortness of breath and severe chest pain. The woman may be apprehensive and diaphoretic. Additional manifestations may include tachypnea, tachycardia, hypotension, syncope, distention of the jugular vein, decreased oxygen saturation (shown by pulse oximetry), cardiac arrhythmias, hemoptysis, and a sudden change in mental status as a result of hypoxemia (Shaughnessy, 2007). Prepare the woman for a lung scan to confirm the diagnosis.

Nursing Management

Nursing management focuses on preventing thrombotic conditions, promoting adequate circulation if thrombosis occurs, and educating the client about preventive measures, anticoagulant therapy, and danger signs.

Preventing Thrombotic Conditions

Prevention of thrombotic conditions is an essential aspect of nursing management and can be achieved with the routine use of simple measures:

- Developing public awareness about risk factors, symptoms, and preventive measures
- Preventing venous stasis by encouraging activity that causes leg muscles to contract and promotes venous return (leg exercises and walking)
- Using intermittent sequential compression devices to produce passive leg muscle contractions until the woman is ambulatory
- Elevating the woman's legs above her heart level to promote venous return
- Stopping smoking to reduce or prevent vascular vasoconstriction
- Applying compression stockings and removing them daily for inspection of legs
- Performing passive range-of-motion exercises while in bed
- Using postoperative deep-breathing exercises to improve venous return by relieving the negative thoracic pressure on leg veins

- Reducing hypercoagulability with the use of warfarin, aspirin, and heparin
- Preventing venous pooling by avoiding pillows under knees, not crossing legs for long periods, and not leaving legs up in stirrups for long periods
- Padding stirrups to reduce pressure against the popliteal angle
- Avoiding sitting or standing in one position for prolonged periods
- Using a bed cradle to keep linens and blankets off extremities
- Avoiding trauma to legs to prevent injury to the vein wall
- Increasing fluid intake to prevent dehydration
- Avoiding the use of oral contraceptives

In women at risk, early ambulation is the easiest and most cost-effective method. Use of elastic compression stockings (TED hose or Jobst stockings) decrease distal calf vein thrombosis by decreasing venous stasis and augmenting venous return (Comerota & Chahwan, 2007). Women who are at a high risk for thromboembolic disease based on risk factors or a previous history of deep vein thrombosis or pulmonary embolism may be placed on prophylactic heparin therapy during pregnancy. Standard heparin or a low-molecular-weight heparin such as enoxaparin (Lovenox) can be given, since neither drug crosses the placenta. It is typically discontinued during labor and birth and then restarted during the postpartum period.

Promoting Adequate Circulation

For the woman with superficial venous thrombosis, administer NSAIDs for analgesia, provide for rest and elevation of the affected leg, apply warm compresses to the affected area to promote healing, and use antiembolism stockings to promote circulation to the extremities.

Implement bed rest and elevation of the affected extremity for the woman with deep vein thrombosis. These actions help to reduce interstitial swelling and promote venous return from that leg. Apply antiembolism stockings to both extremities as ordered. Fit the stockings correctly to avoid excess pressure and constriction and urge the woman to wear them at all times. Sequential compression devices can also be used for women with varicose veins, a history of thrombophlebitis, or a surgical birth.

Anticoagulant therapy using a continuous IV infusion of heparin usually is initiated to prolong the clotting time and prevent extension of the thrombosis. Monitor the woman's coagulation studies closely; these might include activated partial thromboplastin time (aPTT), whole blood partial thromboplastin time, and platelet levels. A therapeutic aPTT value typically ranges from 35 to 45 seconds, depending on which standard values are used (Pagana & Pagana, 2007). Also apply warm moist compresses to the affected leg and administer analgesics as ordered to decrease the discomfort.

After several days of IV heparin therapy, expect to begin oral anticoagulant therapy with warfarin (Coumadin)

as ordered and monitor coagulation studies. In most cases, the woman will continue to take this medication for several months after discharge.

For the woman who develops a pulmonary embolism, institute emergency measures immediately. The objectives of treatment are to prevent growth or multiplication of thrombi in the lower extremities, prevent more thrombi from traveling to the pulmonary vascular system, and provide cardiopulmonary support if needed. Administer oxygen via mask or cannula as ordered and initiate IV heparin therapy titrated according to the results of the coagulation studies. Maintain the client on bed rest, and administer analgesics as ordered for pain relief. Be prepared to assist with administering thrombolytic agents, such as alteplase (tPA), which might be used to dissolve pulmonary emboli and the source of the thrombus in the pelvis or deep leg veins, thus reducing the potential for a recurrence.

Educating the Client

Provide teaching about the use of anticoagulant therapy and danger signs that should be reported (Teaching Guidelines 22.1). Provide anticipatory guidance, support, and education about associated signs of complications and risks. Focus teaching on the following issues:

- Elimination of modifiable risk factors for deep vein thrombosis (smoking, use of oral contraceptives, a sedentary lifestyle, and obesity)
- Importance of using compression stockings
- Avoidance of constrictive clothing and prolonged standing or sitting in a motionless, leg-dependent position
- Danger signs and symptoms (sudden onset of chest pain, dyspnea, and tachypnea) to report to the health care provider

Postpartum Infection

Infection during the postpartum period is a common cause of maternal morbidity and mortality. Overall, postpartum infection is estimated to occur in up to 8% of all births. There is a higher occurrence in cesarean births than in vaginal births (Gilbert & Harmon, 2007).

Postpartum infection is defined as a fever of 38°C or 100.4°F or higher after the first 24 hours after childbirth, occurring on at least 2 of the first 10 days after birth, exclusive of the first 24 hours (Dorland, 2007).

Infections can easily enter the female genital tract externally and ascend through the internal genital structures. In addition, the normal physiologic changes of childbirth increase the risk of infection by decreasing the vaginal acidity due to the presence of amniotic fluid, blood, and lochia, all of which are alkaline. An alkaline environment encourages the growth of bacteria.

Postpartum infections usually arise from organisms that constitute the normal vaginal flora, typically a mix of aerobic and anaerobic species. Generally, they are polymicrobial and involve the following microorganisms: *Staphylococcus aureus, Escherichia coli*, Klebsiella, *Gardnerella*

TEACHING GUIDELINES 22.1

Teaching to Prevent Bleeding Related to Anticoagulant Therapy

• Watch for possible signs of bleeding and notify your health care provider if any occur:
  • Nosebleeds
  • Bleeding from the gums or mouth
  • Black tarry stools
  • Brown "coffee ground" vomitus
  • Red to brown speckled mucus from a cough
  • Oozing at incision, episiotomy site, cut, or scrape
  • Pink, red, or brown-tinged urine
  • Bruises, "black and blue marks"
  • Increased lochia discharge (from present level)
• Practice measures to reduce your risk of bleeding:
  • Brush your teeth gently using a soft toothbrush.
  • Use an electric razor for shaving.
  • Avoid activities that could lead to injury, scrapes, bruising, or cuts.
  • Do not use any over-the-counter products containing aspirin or aspirin-like derivatives.
  • Avoid consuming alcohol.
  • Inform other health care providers about the use of anticoagulants, especially dentists.
• Be sure to comply with follow-up laboratory testing as scheduled.
• If you accidentally cut or scrape yourself, apply firm direct pressure to the site for 5 to 10 minutes. Do the same after receiving any injections or having blood specimens drawn.
• Wear an identification bracelet or band that indicates that you are taking an anticoagulant.

vaginalis, gonococci, coliform bacteria, group A or B hemolytic streptococci, *Chlamydia trachomatis,* and the anaerobes that are common to bacterial vaginosis (Kennedy, 2007). Common postpartum infections include metritis, wound infections, urinary tract infections, and mastitis.

▶ METRITIS

Although usually referred to clinically as endometritis, postpartum uterine infections typically involve more than just the endometrial lining. **Metritis** is an infectious condition that involves the endometrium, decidua, and adjacent myometrium of the uterus. Extension of metritis can result in parametritis, which involves the broad ligament and possibly the ovaries and fallopian tubes, or septic pelvic thrombophlebitis, which results when the infection

spreads along venous routes into the pelvis (Simmons & Bammel, 2007).

The uterine cavity is sterile until rupture of the amniotic sac. As a consequence of labor, birth, and associated manipulations, anaerobic and aerobic bacteria can contaminate the uterus. In most cases, the bacteria responsible for pelvic infections are those that normally reside in the bowel, vagina, perineum, and cervix, such as *E. coli, Klebsiella pneumoniae,* or *G. vaginalis.*

The risk of metritis increases dramatically after a cesarean birth; it complicates from 10% to 20% of cesarean births. This is typically an extension of chorioamnionitis that was present before birth (indeed, that may have been why the cesarean birth was performed). In addition, trauma to the tissues and a break in the skin (incision) provide entrances for bacteria to enter the body and multiply (Kennedy, 2007).

▶ WOUND INFECTIONS

Any break in the skin or mucous membranes provides a portal for bacteria. In the postpartum woman, sites of wound infection include cesarean surgical incisions, the episiotomy site in the perineum, and genital tract lacerations (Fig. 22.2). Wound infections are usually not identified until the woman has been discharged from the hospital because symptoms may not show up until 24 to 48 hours after birth.

▶ URINARY TRACT INFECTIONS

Urinary tract infections are most commonly caused by bacteria often found in bowel flora, including *E. coli,* Klebsiella, Proteus, and Enterobacter species. Invasive manipulation of the urethra (e.g., urinary catheterization), frequent vaginal examinations, and genital trauma increase the likelihood of a urinary tract infection.

▶ MASTITIS

A common problem that may occur within the first 2 weeks postpartum is an inflammation of the breast, termed **mastitis**. It can result from any event that creates milk stasis: insufficient drainage of the breast, rapid weaning, oversupply of milk, pressure on the breast from a poorly fitting bra, a blocked duct, missed feedings, and breakdown of the nipple via fissures, cracks, or blisters (Betzold, 2007). The most common infecting organism is *S. aureus,* which comes from the breastfeeding infant's mouth or throat (Kennedy,

FIGURE 22.2 Postpartum wound infections. (**A**) Infected episiotomy site. (**B**) Infected cesarean birth incision.

A   **B**

2007). Infection can be transmitted from the lactiferous ducts to a secreting lobule, from a nipple fissure to periductal lymphatics, or by circulation (Gilbert & Harmon, 2007) (Fig. 22.3). A breast abscess may develop if mastitis is not treated adequately.

Therapeutic Management

When metritis occurs, broad-spectrum antibiotics are used to treat the infection. Management also includes measures to restore and promote fluid and electrolyte balance, provide analgesia, and provide emotional support. In most treated women, fever drops and symptoms cease within 48 to 72 hours after the start of antibiotic therapy.

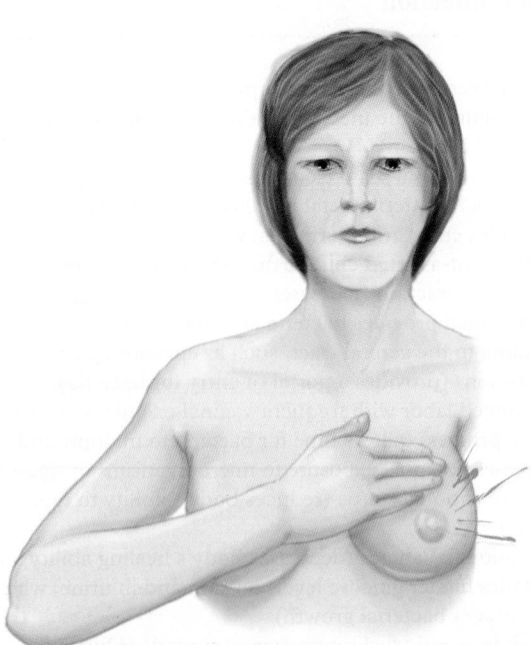

FIGURE 22.3 With mastitis, an area on one breast is tender, hot, red, and painful.

Management for wound infections involves recognition of the infection, followed by opening of the wound to allow drainage. Aseptic wound management with sterile gloves and frequent dressing changes if applicable, good handwashing, frequent perineal pad changes, hydration, and ambulation to prevent venous stasis and improve circulation are initiated to prevent development of a more serious infection or spread of the infection to adjacent structures. Parenteral antibiotics are the mainstay of treatment. Analgesics are also important, because women often experience discomfort at the wound site.

If the woman develops a urinary tract infection, fluids are used to treat dehydration. Antibiotics may be ordered if appropriate.

Treatment of mastitis focuses on two areas: emptying the breasts and controlling the infection. The breast can be emptied either by the infant sucking or by manual expression. Increasing the frequency of nursing is advised. Lactation need not be suppressed. Control of infection is achieved with antibiotics. In addition, ice or warm packs and analgesics may be needed.

▶ *Take* NOTE!

Regardless of the etiology of mastitis, the focus is on reversing milk stasis, maintaining milk supply, and continuing breastfeeding, along with providing maternal comfort and preventing recurrence.

Nursing Assessment

Perinatal nurses are the primary caregivers for postpartum women and have a unique opportunity to identify subtle changes that place women at risk for infection.

Nurses play a key role in identifying signs and symptoms that suggest a postpartum infection. Today women are commonly discharged 24 to 48 hours after giving birth. Therefore, nurses must assess new mothers for risk factors and identify early, subtle signs and symptoms of an infectious process. Factors that place a woman at risk for a postpartum infection are highlighted in Box 22.2.

Review the client's history and physical examination and labor and birth record for factors that might increase her risk for developing an infection. Then complete the assessment (using the "BUBBLE-HE" parameters discussed in Chapter 16), paying particular attention to areas such as the abdomen and fundus, breasts, urinary tract, episiotomy, lacerations, or incisions, being alert for signs and symptoms of infection (Table 22.1).

> ▶ *Take* NOTE!
>
> *A postpartum infection is commonly associated with an elevated temperature, as mentioned previously. Other generalized signs and symptoms may include chills, foul-smelling vaginal discharge, headache, malaise, restlessness, anxiety, and tachycardia. In addition, the woman may have specific signs and symptoms based on the type and location of the infection.*

When assessing the episiotomy site, use the acronym "REEDA" (redness, ecchymosis, edema, drainage or discharge, and approximation of wound edges) to ensure complete evaluation of the site (Arenson & Drake, 2007). Monitor the woman's vital signs, especially her temperature, for changes that may signal an infection.

Nursing Management

Nursing management focuses on preventing postpartum infections. Use the following guidelines to reduce the incidence of postpartum infections:

- Maintain aseptic technique when performing invasive procedures such as urinary catheterization, when changing dressings, and during all surgical procedures.
- Use good handwashing technique before and after each client care activity.
- Reinforce measures for maintaining good perineal hygiene.
- Use adequate lighting and turn the client to side to assess the episiotomy site.
- Screen all visitors for any signs of active infections to reduce the client's risk of exposure.
- Review the client's history for preexisting infections or chronic conditions.
- Monitor vital signs and laboratory results for any abnormal values.
- Monitor the frequency of vaginal examinations and length of labor.

BOX 22.2 **Factors Placing a Woman at Risk for Postpartum Infection**

- Prolonged (>18 to 24 hours) premature rupture of membranes (removes the barrier of amniotic fluid so bacteria can ascend)
- Cesarean birth (allows bacterial entry due to break in protective skin barrier)
- Urinary catheterization (could allow entry of bacteria into bladder due to break in aseptic technique)
- Regional anesthesia that decreases perception to void (causes urinary stasis and increases risk of urinary tract infection)
- Staff attending to woman are ill (promotes droplet infection from personnel)
- Compromised health status, such as anemia, obesity, smoking, drug abuse (reduces the body's immune system and decreases ability to fight infection)
- Preexisting colonization of lower genital tract with bacterial vaginosis, *Chlamydia trachomatis,* group B streptococci, *Staphylococcus aureus,* and *Escherichia coli* (allows microbes to ascend)
- Retained placental fragments (provides medium for bacterial growth)

- Manual removal of a retained placenta (causes trauma to the lining of the uterus and thus opens up sites for bacterial invasion)
- Insertion of fetal scalp electrode or intrauterine pressure catheters for internal fetal monitoring during labor (provides entry into uterine cavity)
- Instrument-assisted childbirth, such as forceps or vacuum extraction (increases risk of trauma to genital tract, which provides bacteria access to grow)
- Trauma to the genital tract, such as episiotomy or lacerations (provides a portal of entry for bacteria)
- Prolonged labor with frequent vaginal examinations to check progress (allows time for bacteria to multiply and increases potential exposure to microorganisms or trauma)
- Poor nutritional status (reduces body's ability to repair tissue)
- Gestational diabetes (decreases body's healing ability and provides higher glucose levels on skin and in urine, which encourages bacterial growth)
- Break in aseptic technique during surgery or birthing process (allows entry of bacteria)

TABLE 22.1   SIGNS AND SYMPTOMS OF POSTPARTUM INFECTIONS

Postpartum Infection	Signs and Symptoms
Metritis	Lower abdominal tenderness or pain on one or both sides
	Temperature elevation (>38°C)
	Foul-smelling lochia
	Anorexia
	Nausea
	Fatigue and lethargy
	Leukocytosis and elevated sedimentation rate
Wound infection	Weeping serosanguineous or purulent drainage
	Separation of or unapproximated wound edges
	Edema
	Erythema
	Tenderness
	Discomfort at the site
	Maternal fever
	Elevated white blood cell count
Urinary tract infection	Urgency
	Frequency
	Dysuria
	Flank pain
	Low-grade fever
	Urinary retention
	Hematuria
	Urine positive for nitrates
	Cloudy urine with strong odor
Mastitis	Flulike symptoms, including malaise, fever, and chills
	Tender, hot, red, painful area on one breast
	Inflammation of breast area
	Breast tenderness
	Cracking of skin or around nipple or areola
	Breast distention with milk

- Assess frequently for early signs of infection, especially fever and the appearance of lochia.
- Inspect wounds frequently for inflammation and drainage.
- Encourage rest, adequate hydration, and healthy eating habits.
- Reinforce preventive measures during any interaction with the client.

If the woman develops an infection, review treatment measures, such as antibiotic therapy if ordered, and any special care measures, such as dressing changes, that might be needed (Nursing Care Plan 22.1).

Client teaching is a priority due to today's short lengths of stay after delivery. Some infections may not manifest until after discharge. Review the signs and symptoms of infection, emphasizing the danger signs that need to be reported to the health care provider. Most importantly, stress proper handwashing, especially after perineal care and before and after breastfeeding. Also reinforce measures to promote breastfeeding, including proper breast care (see Chapter 16). Teaching Guidelines 22.2 highlights the major teaching points for a woman with a postpartum infection.

Postpartum Affective Disorders

The postpartum period involves extraordinary physiologic, psychological, and sociocultural changes in the life

Nursing Care Plan 22.1

OVERVIEW OF THE WOMAN WITH A POSTPARTUM COMPLICATION

Jennifer, a 16-year-old G1P1, gave birth to a boy 3 days ago. It was a cesarean birth due to cephalopelvic disproportion following 25 hours of labor with ruptured membranes. Her temperature is 102.6° F (39.2° C). She is complaining of chills and malaise and says, "My incision really hurts." Jennifer rates her pain as 7 to 8 out of 10. The incision site is red, swollen, and very warm to the touch. A 5-cm area of purulent drainage is noted on the dressing; a 3-cm area of the incision is slightly opened, with the wound edges separated. Jennifer's lochia is scant and dark red, with a strong odor. She asks the nurse to take her baby back to the nursery because she doesn't feel well enough to care for him.

NURSING DIAGNOSIS: Ineffective thermoregulation related to bacterial invasion *as evidenced by fever, complaints of chills and malaise, and statement of not feeling well*

Outcome Identification and Evaluation
Jennifer will exhibit a return to normothermia *as evidenced by a body temperature being maintained below 99° F, reports of a decrease in chills and malaise, and statements of feeling better.*

Interventions: Promoting Fever Reduction
- Assess vital signs every 2 to 4 hours and record results *to monitor progress of infection.*
- Administer antipyretics as ordered *to reduce temperature and help combat infection.*
- Encourage fluid intake *to promote fluid balance.*
- Document intake and output *to assess hydration status.*
- Offer cool bed bath or shower *to reduce temperature.*
- Place cool cloth on forehead and/or back of neck *for comfort.*
- Change bed linen and gown when damp from diaphoresis *to provide comfort and hygiene.*

NURSING DIAGNOSIS: Impaired skin integrity related to wound infection as *evidenced by purulent drainage, redness, swelling, and separation of wound edges*

Outcome Identification and Evaluation
Jennifer will experience a resolution of wound infection as *evidenced by a reduction in redness, swelling, and drainage from wound, absence of purulent drainage, and beginning signs and symptoms of wound healing.*

Interventions: Promoting Wound Healing
- Administer antibiotic therapy as ordered *to treat infection.*
- Perform frequent dressing changes and wound care as ordered *to promote wound healing;* monitor dressing for drainage, including amount, color, and characteristics, *to evaluate for resolution of infection.*
- Use aseptic technique *to prevent spread of infection.*
- Encourage fluid intake *to maintain fluid balance;* encourage adequate dietary intake, including protein, *to promote healing.*

NURSING DIAGNOSIS: Acute pain related to infectious process

Outcome Identification and Evaluation
Client reports a decrease in pain *as evidenced by pain rating of 0 or 1 on pain scale; verbalization of relief with pain management, and statements of feeling better and ability to rest comfortably.*

Interventions: Relieving Pain
- Place client in semi-Fowler's position *to facilitate drainage and relieve pressure.*
- Assess pain level on pain scale of 0 to 10 *to quantify pain level;* reassess pain level after intervening *to determine effectiveness of intervention.*
- Assess fundus gently *to ensure appropriate involution.*
- Administer analgesics as needed and on time as ordered *to maintain pain relief.*
- Provide for rest periods *to allow for healing.*
- Assist with positioning in bed with pillows *to promote comfort.*
- Offer nonpharmacologic pain measures such as a backrub *to ease aches and discomfort if desired and enhance effectiveness of analgesics.*

Nursing Care Plan 22.1 (continued)

NURSING DIAGNOSIS: Risk for impaired parent–infant attachment related to effects of postpartum infection *as evidenced by mother's request to take baby back to the nursery*

Outcome Identification and Evaluation

Jennifer begins to bond with newborn appropriately with each exposure *as evidenced by desire to spend time with newborn, expression of positive feelings toward newborn when holding him, increasing participation in care of newborn as client's condition improves, and statements about help and support at home to care for self and newborn.*

Interventions: Promoting Mother–Newborn Interaction

- Promote adequate rest and sleep *to ensure adequate energy for interaction and wound healing.*
- Bring newborn to mother after she is rested and had an analgesic *to allow mother to focus her energies on the child.*
- Progressively allow the client to care for her infant or comfort him as her energy level and pain level improve *to promote self-confidence in caring for the newborn.*
- Offer praise and positive reinforcement for caretaking tasks; stress positive attributes of newborn to mother while caring for him *to facilitate bonding and attachment.*
- Contact family members to participate in care of the newborn *to allow mother to rest and recover from infection.*
- Encourage mother to care for herself first and then the newborn *to ensure adequate energy for newborn's care.*
- Arrange for assistance and support after discharge from hospital *to provide necessary backup.*
- Refer to community health nurse for follow-up care of mother and newborn at home *to foster continued development of maternal–infant relationship.*

---

of a woman and her family. It is an exhilarating time for most women, but for others it may not be what they had expected. Women have varied reactions to their childbearing experiences, exhibiting a wide range of emotions. Typically, the delivery of a newborn is associated with positive feelings such as happiness, joy, and gratitude for the birth of a healthy infant. However, women may also feel weepy, overwhelmed, or unsure of what is happening to them. They may experience fear about loss of control; they may feel scared, alone, or guilty, or as if they have somehow failed.

Postpartum affective disorders have been documented for years, but only recently have they received medical attention. Plummeting levels of estrogen and progesterone immediately after birth can contribute to postpartum mood disorders. It is believed that the greater the change in these hormone levels between pregnancy and postpartum, the greater the chance for developing a mood disorder (Edler, Jones, & Venis, 2007).

Many types of affective disorders occur in the postpartum period. Although their description and classification may be controversial, the disorders are commonly classified on the basis of their severity as postpartum or baby blues, postpartum depression, and postpartum psychosis.

▶ POSTPARTUM OR BABY BLUES

Many postpartum women (approximately 50% to 90%) experience the "baby blues" (ACOG, 2007). The woman exhibits mild depressive symptoms of anxiety, irritability, mood swings, tearfulness, increased sensitivity, feelings of being overwhelmed, and fatigue (Edler, Jones, & Venis, 2007). The "blues" typically peak on postpartum days 4 and 5 and usually resolve by postpartum day 10. Although the woman's symptoms may be distressing, they do not reflect psychopathology and usually do not affect the mother's ability to function and care for her infant.

Baby blues are usually self-limiting and require no formal treatment other than reassurance and validation of the woman's experience, as well as assistance in caring for herself and the newborn. However, follow-up of women with postpartum blues is important, because up to 20% go on to develop postpartum depression (Alexander et al., 2007).

▶ POSTPARTUM DEPRESSION

Depression is more prevalent in women than in men, which may be related to biological, hormonal, and psychosocial factors. If the symptoms of postpartum blues last beyond 6 weeks and seem to get worse, the mother may be experiencing **postpartum depression**, a major depressive episode associated with childbirth (Edler, Jones, & Venis, 2007). As many as 20% of all mothers develop postpartum depression (ACOG, 2007). It affects approximately 500,000 mothers in the United States each year, and about half of these women receive no mental health evaluation or treatment (ACOG, 2007). Unlike the postpartum blues, women with postpartum depression feel

TEACHING GUIDELINES 22.2

Teaching for the Woman With a Postpartum Infection

- Continue your antibiotic therapy as prescribed.
  - Take the medication exactly as ordered and continue with the medication until it is finished.
  - Do not stop taking the medication even when you are feeling better.
- Check your temperature every day and call your health care provider if it is above 100.4°F (38°C).
- Watch for other signs and symptoms of infection, such as chills, increased abdominal pain, change in the color or odor of your lochia, or increased redness, warmth, swelling, or drainage from a wound site such as your cesarean incision or episiotomy. Report any of these to your health care provider immediately.
- Practice good infection prevention:
  - Always wash your hands thoroughly before and after eating, using the bathroom, touching your perineal area, or providing care for your newborn.
  - Wipe from front to back after using the bathroom.
  - Remove your perineal pad using a front-to-back motion. Fold the pad in half so that the inner sides of the pad that were touching your body are against each other. Wrap in toilet tissue or place in a plastic bag and discard.
  - Wash your hands before applying a new pad.
  - Apply a new perineal pad using a front-to-back motion. Handle the pad by the edges (top and bottom or sides) and avoid touching the inner aspect of the pad that will be against your body.
  - When performing perineal care with the peribottle, angle the spray of water to that it flows from front to back.
  - Drink plenty of fluids each day and eat a variety of foods that are high in vitamins, iron, and protein.
  - Be sure to get adequate rest at night and periodically throughout the day.

worse over time, and changes in mood and behavior do not go away on their own.

Postpartum depression affects not only the woman but also the entire family. Identifying depression early can substantially improve the client and family outcomes. Postpartum depression usually has a more gradual onset and becomes evident within the first 6 weeks postpartum.

Postpartum depression may lend itself to prophylactic intervention because its onset is predictable, the risk period for illness is well defined, and women at high risk potentially could be identified using a screening tool. This is not the case for all women, however (see Evidence-Based

▶ *Consider* THIS!

As an assertive practicing attorney in her thirties, my first pregnancy was filled with nagging feelings of doubt about this upcoming event in my life. Throughout my pregnancy I was so busy with trial work that I never had time to really evaluate my feelings. I was always reading about the bodily changes that were taking place, and on one level I was feeling excited, but on another level I was emotionally drained. Shortly after the birth of my daughter, those suppressed nagging feelings of doubt surfaced big time and practically immobilized me. I felt exhausted all the time and was only too glad to have someone else care for my daughter. I didn't breastfeed because I thought it would tie me down too much. Although at the time I thought this "low mood" was normal for all new mothers, I have since found out it was postpartum depression. How could any woman be depressed about this wondrous event?

Thoughts: Now that postpartum depression has been "taken out of the closet" and recognized as a real emotional disorder, it can be treated. This woman showed tendencies during her pregnancy but was able to suppress the feelings and go forward. Her description of her depression is very typical of many women who suffer in silence, hoping to get over these feelings in time. What can nurses do to promote awareness of this disorder? Can it be prevented?

Practice 22.1). Prophylaxis starts with a prenatal risk assessment and education. Based on the woman's history of prior depression, prophylactic antidepressant therapy may be needed during the third trimester or immediately after giving birth. Management mirrors that of any major depression—a combination of antidepressant medication, antianxiety medication, and psychotherapy in an outpatient or inpatient setting (Jung et al., 2007). Marital counseling may be necessary if marital problems are contributing to the woman's depressive symptoms.

▶ POSTPARTUM PSYCHOSIS

At the severe end of the continuum of postpartum emotional disorders is postpartum psychosis, which occurs in one or two women per 1,000 births (Edler, Jones, & Venis, 2007). It generally surfaces within 3 weeks of giving birth and is manifested by sleep disturbances, fatigue, depression, and hypomania. The mother will be tearful, confused, and preoccupied with feelings of guilt and worthlessness. Early symptoms resemble those of depression, but they may escalate to delirium, hallucinations, anger toward her-

EVIDENCE-BASED PRACTICE 22.1
Preventing Postpartum Depression Using Psychosocial Interventions

● Study

Postpartum depression can be a devastating condition for women and their families. There is a lack of knowledge about its cause, and women receive limited education about the possibility of depression after birth. Research has shown the effectiveness of treatment strategies that integrate psychosocial and psychological variables. The question then arises that if management addressing these variables is effective, would psychosocial interventions provided during pregnancy and the early postpartum period be effective in preventing postpartum depression?

Two reviewers searched multiple databases and contacted experts in the field. They also scanned secondary references and contacted several trial researchers for additional information. Both reviewers were involved in evaluating the methodology of the study and in extracting data. Information was gathered from all published and unpublished randomized controlled trials that compared psychosocial or psychological interventions with typical care during the antepartal, intrapartal, and postpartal periods. The researchers used relative risk for categorical data and weighted mean difference for continuous data. The study included 15 trials involving over 7,600 women.

▲ Findings

Women who received some type of psychosocial intervention had the same risk for developing postpartum depression as the women who received routine care; thus, the psychosocial intervention was not effective in preventing postpartum depression. However, statistical analysis found that intensive psychosocial support from public health nurses or midwives in the postpartum period was beneficial. The use of psychosocial interventions primarily during the postpartum period also was more effective than when these interventions were also used in the prenatal period. Interventions focusing on women at risk appear to be more effective than those geared to the overall maternal population. Individualized interventions were found to be more effective than those designed for groups. However, the risk for developing postpartum depression for either group did not differ significantly.

■ Nursing Implications

Although the study failed to identify effective measures for preventing postpartum depression, it did provide some useful information for nurses to incorporate when providing care to pregnant women throughout the perinatal period. Nurses need to remain alert for risk factors associated with postpartum depression so they can initiate appropriate interventions for these at-risk women. Nurses can implement psychosocial interventions during the prenatal period, keeping in mind that these interventions need to be continued throughout the postpartum period. They can also advocate for their clients upon discharge to ensure appropriate follow-up and support in the community.

Dennis, C.-L., & Creedy, D. (2004). Psychosocial and psychological interventions for preventing postpartum depression. *Cochrane Database of Systematic Reviews 2004,* Issue 4. Art. No.: CD001134. DOI:10.1002/14651858.CD001134.pub2.

self and her infant, bizarre behavior, manifestations of mania, and thoughts of hurting herself and the infant. The mother frequently loses touch with reality and experiences a severe regressive breakdown, associated with a high risk of suicide or infanticide (Johnson, 2007).

Most women with postpartum psychosis are hospitalized for up to several months. Psychotropic drugs are almost always part of treatment, along with individual psychotherapy and support group therapy.

> ▶ *Take NOTE!*
>
> *The greatest hazard of postpartum psychosis is suicide. Infanticide and child abuse are also risks if the woman is left alone with her infant. Early recognition and prompt treatment of this disorder are imperative.*

Nursing Assessment

Postpartum affective disorders are often overlooked and go unrecognized despite the large percentage of women who experience them. The postpartum period is a time of increased vulnerability, but few women receive education about the possibility of depression after birth. In addition, many women may feel ashamed of having negative emotions at a time when they "should" be happy; thus, they don't seek professional help. Nurses can play a major role in providing guidance about postpartum affective disorders, detecting manifestations, and assisting women to obtain appropriate care.

Begin the assessment by reviewing the history to identify general risk factors that could predispose a woman to depression:

• Poor coping skills
• Low self-esteem
• Numerous life stressors

- Mood swings and emotional stress
- Previous psychological problems or a family history of psychiatric disorders
- Substance abuse
- Limited or lack of social support network

Also review the history for specific pregnancy and birth factors that may increase the woman's risk for depression. These may include a history of postpartum depression, evidence of depression during the pregnancy, prenatal anxiety, a difficult or complicated pregnancy, traumatic birth experience, or birth of a high-risk or special-needs infant (Johnson, 2007).

Be alert for physical findings. Assess the woman's activity level, including her level of fatigue. Ask about her sleeping habits, noting any problems with insomnia. When interacting with the woman, observe for verbal and nonverbal indicators of anxiety as well as her ability to concentrate during the interaction. Difficulty concentrating and anxious behaviors suggest a problem. Also assess her nutritional intake: weight loss due to poor food intake may be seen. Assessment can identify women with a high-risk profile for depression, and the nurse can educate them and make referrals for individual or family counseling if needed. Some common assessment findings associated with postpartum depression are listed in Box 22.3.

Nursing Management

Nursing management focuses on assisting any postpartum woman to cope with the changes of this period. Encourage the client to verbalize what she is going through and emphasize the importance of keeping her expectations realistic. Assist the woman in structuring her day to regain a sense of control over the situation. Encourage her to seek help if necessary, using available support systems. Also reinforce the need for good nutrition and adequate exercise and sleep (Linter & Gray, 2006).

The nurse can play an important role in assisting women and their partners with postpartum adjustment. Providing facts about the enormous changes that occur during the postpartum period is critical. This information would include changes in the woman's body. Review the signs and symptoms of all three affective disorders. This information is typically included as part of prenatal visits and childbirth education classes. Know the risk factors associated with these disorders and review the history of clients and their families. Use specific, nonthreatening questions to aid in early detection, such as, "Have you felt down, depressed, or hopeless lately? Have you felt little interest or pleasure in doing things recently?"

Discuss factors that may increase a woman's vulnerability to stress during the postpartum period, such as sleep deprivation and unrealistic expectations, so couples can understand and respond to those problems if they occur. Stress that many women need help after childbirth and that help is available from many sources, including people they already know. Assisting women to learn how to ask for help is important so they can gain the support they need. Also provide educational materials about postpartum emotional disorders. Have available referral sources for psychotherapy and support groups appropriate for women experiencing postpartum adjustment difficulties.

■■■ Key Concepts

- Postpartum hemorrhage is a potentially life-threatening complication of both vaginal and cesarean births. It is the leading cause of maternal mortality in the United States.
- A good way to remember the causes of postpartum hemorrhage is the "4 Ts": tone, tissue, trauma, and thrombosis.
- Uterine atony is the most common cause of early postpartum hemorrhage, which can lead to hypovolemic shock.
- Oxytocin (Pitocin), methylergonovine maleate (Methergine), and prostaglandin PGF2a (Hemabate) are drugs used to manage postpartum hemorrhage.
- Failure of the placenta to separate completely and be expelled interferes with the ability of the uterus to contract fully, thereby leading to hemorrhage.
- Causes of subinvolution include retained placental fragments, distended bladder, uterine myoma, and infection.
- Lacerations should always be suspected when the uterus is contracted and bright-red blood continues to trickle out of the vagina.
- Conditions that cause coagulopathies may include idiopathic thrombocytopenic purpura (ITP), von Willebrand disease (vWD), and disseminated intravascular coagulation (DIC).

BOX 22.3 **Common Assessment Findings Associated With Postpartum Depression**

- Loss of pleasure or interest in life
- Low mood, sadness, tearfulness
- Exhaustion that is not relieved by sleep
- Feelings of guilt
- Irritability
- Inability to concentrate
- Anxiety
- Despair
- Compulsive thoughts
- Loss of libido
- Loss of confidence
- Sleep difficulties (insomnia)
- Loss of appetite
- Feelings of failure as a mother (Litner & Gray, 2006)

- Pulmonary embolism is a potentially fatal condition that occurs when the pulmonary artery is obstructed by a blood clot that has traveled from another vein into the lungs, causing obstruction and infarction.
- The major causes of a thrombus formation (blood clot) are venous stasis and hypercoagulation, both common in the postpartum period.
- Postpartum infection is defined as a fever of 38° C (100.4° F) or higher after the first 24 hours after childbirth, occurring on at least 2 of the first 10 days exclusive of the first 24 hours.
- Common postpartum infections include metritis, wound infections, urinary tract infections, and mastitis.
- Postpartum emotional disorders are commonly classified on the basis of their severity: "baby blues," postpartum depression, and postpartum psychosis.
- Management of postpartum depression mirrors the treatment of any major depression—a combination of antidepressant medication, antianxiety medication, and psychotherapy in an outpatient or inpatient setting.

REFERENCES

Alexander, L. L., LaRosa, J. H., Bader, H., & Garfield, S. (2007). *New dimensions in women's health* (4th ed.). Sudbury, MA: Jones and Bartlett Publishers.

American College of Obstetricians and Gynecologists (ACOG). (2006). Clinical management guidelines: Postpartum hemorrhage. ACOG Practice Bulletin Number 76. *Obstetrics and Gynecology, 108*(4), 1039–1047.

American College of Obstetricians and Gynecologists (ACOG). (2007). *Spotlight on postpartum depression.* ACOG News Release. Available at: http://www.acog.org/from_home/publications/press_releases/nr02-30-07-2.cfm.

Anderson, J. M., & Etches, D. (2007). Prevention and management of postpartum hemorrhage. *American Family Physician, 75*(6), 875–882.

Arenson, J., & Drake, P. (2007). *Maternal and newborn health.* Sudbury, MA: Jones and Bartlett Publishers.

Betzold, C. M. (2007). An update on the recognition and management of lactational breast inflammation. *Journal of Midwifery & Women's Health, 52*(6), 595–605.

Bick, R. L. (2007). Disseminated intravascular coagulation. In R. E. Rakel & E. T. Bope (Eds.), *Conn's current therapy 2007* (Section 6, pp. 502–505). Philadelphia: Saunders Elsevier.

Cohen, W. R. (2006). Hemorrhagic shock in obstetrics. *Journal of Perinatal Medicine, 34*(4), 271–280.

Comerota, A. J., & Chahwan, S. (2007). Venous thrombosis. In R. E. Rakel & E. T. Bope (Eds.), *Conn's current therapy 2007* (Section 5, pp. 435–445). Philadelphia: Saunders Elsevier.

Cunningham, F. G., Gant, N. F., & Leveno, K. J. (2005). Conduct of normal labor and delivery. In: *Williams' obstetrics* (22nd ed., pp. 320–325). New York: McGraw-Hill.

Dennis, C. L., & Creedy, D. (2004). Psychosocial and psychological interventions for preventing postpartum depression. *Cochrane Database of Systematic Reviews 2004,* Issue 4. Art. No.: CD001134. DOI:10.1002/14651858.CD001134.pub2.

Dorland, W. A. N. (2007). *Dorland's illustrated medical dictionary* (30th ed.). St. Louis, MO: Saunders Elsevier.

Edler, C. R., Jones, H. W., & Venis, J. A. (2007). Beyond the baby blues: Postpartum depression. *Nursing Spectrum.* Available at: http://nsweb.nursingspectrum.com/ce/ce72d.htm.

Feied, C., & Handler, J. A. (2007). Thrombophlebitis. *eMedicine.* Available at: http://www.emedicine.com/emerg/topic582.htm.

Franchini, M., & Lippi, G. (2007). The role of von Willebrand factor in hemorrhagic and thrombotic disorders. *Critical Reviews in Clinical Laboratory Sciences, 44*(2), 115–149.

Geil, J. D. (2007). Von Willebrand disease. *eMedicine.* Available at: http://emedicine.com/ped/topic2419.htm.

Gilbert, E. S., & Harmon, J. S. (2007). *Manual of high-risk pregnancy and delivery* (4th ed.). St. Louis, MO: Mosby Elsevier.

Johnson, R. (2007). Mental illness in primary women's health care. In B. Hackley, J. M. Kriebs, & M. E. Rousseau (Eds.), *Primary care of women: A guide for midwives and women's health providers* (Chapter 9, pp. 249–312). Sudbury, MA: Jones and Bartlett Publishers.

Jung, V., Short, R., Letourneau, N., & Andrews, D. (2007). Interventions with depressed mothers and their infants: Modifying interactive behaviors. *Journal of Affective Disorders, 98*(3), 199–205.

Kadir, R. A., Kingman, C. E., Chi, C., Lee, C. A., & Economides, D. L. (2007). Is primary postpartum hemorrhage a good predictor of inherited bleeding disorders? *Hemophilia, 13*(2), 178–181.

Kennedy, E. (2007). Postpartum infections. *eMedicine.* Available at: http://www.emedicine.com/emerg/topic482.htm.

Levi, M., & Schmaier, A. H. (2007). Disseminated intravascular coagulation. *eMedicine.* Available at: http://www.emedicine.com/med/topic577.htm.

Lintner, N. C., & Gray, B. A. (2006). Childbearing and depression. *AWHONN Lifelines, 10*(1), 50–57.

MacMullen, N. J., Dulski, L. A., & Meagher, B. (2005). Red alert: Perinatal hemorrhage. *MCN, 30*(1), 46–51.

Nash, L. R. (2007). Postpartum care. In R. E. Rakel & E. T. Bope (Eds.), *Conn's current therapy 2007* (Section 16, pp. 1190–1193). Philadelphia: Saunders Elsevier.

Pagana, K. D., & Pagana, T. J. (2007). *Mosby's diagnostic and laboratory test reference* (8th ed.). St. Louis, MO: Mosby Elsevier.

Pope, C. S., & O'Grady, J. P. (2006). Malposition of the uterus. *eMedicine.* Available at: http://www.emedicine.com/med/topic3473.htm.

Shaughnessy, K. (2007). Massive pulmonary embolism. *Critical Care Nurse, 27*(1), 39–50.

Silverman, M. A. (2007). Idiopathic thrombocytopenic purpura. *eMedicine.* Available at: http://www.emedicine.com/emerg/topic282.htm.

Simmons, G. T., & Bammel, B. M. (2007). Endometritis. *eMedicine.* Available at: http://www.emedicine.com/MED/topic676.htm.

Smith, J. R., & Brennan, B. G. (2006). Management of the third stage of labor. *eMedicine.* Available at: http://www.emedicine.com/med/topic3569.htm.

Smith, J. R., & Brennan, B. G. (2007). Postpartum hemorrhage. *eMedicine.* Available at: http://emedicine.com/med/topic3568.htm.

Sood, S., & Abrams, C. S. (2007). Platelet-mediated bleeding disorders. In R. E. Rakel & E. T. Bope (Eds.), *Conn's current therapy 2007* (Section 6, pp. 499–501). Philadelphia: Saunders Elsevier.

U.S. Department of Health and Human Services (USDHHS), Public Health Service. (2000). *Healthy People 2010* (conference edition, in two volumes). U.S. Department of Health and Human Services. Washington, DC: U.S. Government Printing Office.

Weydert, J. A., & Benda, J. A. (2006). Subinvolution of the placental site as an anatomic cause of postpartum uterine bleeding. *Archives of Pathology & Laboratory Medicine, 130*(10), 1538–1542.

WEBSITES

A Place to Remember: www.aplacetoremember.com
Center for Postpartum Health: http://www.postpartumhealth.com
Depression: www.nimh.nih.gov/publicat/depwomenknows.cfm
Depression After Delivery, Inc. (D.A.D.): www.depressionafterdelivery.com
International Childbirth Educator's Association: www.icea.org
LaLeche League & Breastfeeding Resource Center: www.lalecheleague.org
Learning about von Willebrand Disease: www.allaboutbleeding.com
National Hemophilia Foundation: www.hemophilia.org
National Institute of Mental Health: www.nimh.nih.gov
National Women's Health Information Center: www.4women.gov
Parents Helping Parents: www.php.com
Postpartum Support International: www.postpartum.net
World Federation of Hemophilia: www.wfh.org

CHAPTER WORKSHEET

MULTIPLE CHOICE QUESTIONS

1. A postpartum mother appears very pale and states she is bleeding heavily. The nurse should first:

   a. Call the client's health care provider immediately.

   b. Immediately set up an intravenous infusion of magnesium sulfate.

   c. Assess the fundus and ask her about her voiding status.

   d. Reassure the mother that this is a normal finding after childbirth.

2. A postpartum woman reports hearing voices and says, "The voices are telling me to do bad things." The nurse interprets these findings as suggesting:

   a. Postpartum psychosis

   b. Postpartum anxiety disorder

   c. Postpartum depression

   d. Postpartum blues

3. When implementing the plan of care for a postpartum woman who gave birth just a few hours ago, the nurse vigilantly monitors the client for which complication?

   a. Deep vein thrombosis

   b. Postpartum psychosis

   c. Uterine infection

   d. Postpartum hemorrhage

4. Which of the following would the nurse expect to include in the plan of care for a woman with mastitis who is receiving antibiotic therapy?

   a. Stop breastfeeding and apply lanolin.

   b. Administer analgesics and bind both breasts.

   c. Apply warm or cold compresses and administer analgesics.

   d. Remove the nursing bra and expose the breast to fresh air.

5. While assessing a postpartum multiparous woman, the nurse detects a boggy uterus midline 2 cm above the umbilicus. Which intervention would be the priority?

   a. Assessing vital signs immediately

   b. Measuring her next urinary output

   c. Massaging her fundus

   d. Notifying the woman's obstetrician

6. Methergine has been ordered for a postpartum woman because of excessive bleeding. The nurse should question this order if which of the following is present?

   a. Minimal lochia flow

   b. Tender inflamed breasts

   c. Pulse rate of 68 beats per minute

   d. Blood pressure of 158/96 mm Hg

CRITICAL THINKING EXERCISES

1. Mrs. Griffin had a 22-hour labor before a cesarean birth. Her membranes ruptured 20 hours before she came to the hospital. Her fetus showed signs of fetal distress, so internal electronic fetal monitoring was used. Her most recent test results indicate she is anemic.

   a. What postpartum complication is this new mother at highest risk for? Why?

   b. What assessments need to be done to detect this complication?

   c. What nursing measures will the nurse use to prevent this complication?

2. Tammy, a 32-year-old G9P9, had a spontaneous vaginal birth 2 hours ago. Tammy has been having a baby each year for the past 9 years. Her lochia has been heavy, with some clots. She hasn't been up to void since she had epidural anesthesia and has decreased sensation to her legs.

   a. What factors place Tammy at risk for postpartum hemorrhage?

   b. What assessments are needed before planning interventions?

   c. What nursing actions are needed to prevent a postpartum hemorrhage?

3. Lucy, a 25-year-old G2P2, gave birth 2 days ago and is expected to be discharged today. She had severe postpartum depression 2 years ago with her first child. Lucy has not been out of bed for the past 24 hours, is not eating, and provides no care for herself or her newborn. Lucy states she already has a boy at home and not having a girl this time is disappointing.

   a. What factors/behaviors place Lucy at risk for an affective disorder?

   b. Which interventions might be appropriate at this time?

   c. What education does the family need prior to discharge?

Study Activities

1. Compare and contrast postpartum blues, postpartum depression, and postpartum psychosis in terms of their features and medical management.

2. Select a website from the ones listed at the end of the chapter. Critique it regarding its helpfulness to parents, the correctness of the information, and when it was last updated.

3. Interview a woman who has given birth and ask if she had any complications and what was most helpful to her during the experience.

4. The number-one cause of postpartum hemorrhage is _____.

5. When giving report to the nurse who will be caring for a woman and her newborn in the postpartum period, what information should the labor nurse convey?

THE NEWBORN AT RISK

NURSING CARE OF THE NEWBORN WITH SPECIAL NEEDS

KEY TERMS

appropriate for
   gestational age
asphyxia
extremely low birthweight
large for gestational age

late preterm newborn
low birthweight
postterm newborn
preterm newborn

retinopathy of prematurity
small for gestational age
term newborn
very low birthweight

LEARNING OBJECTIVES

Upon completion of the chapter, the learner will be able to:

1. Explain factors that assist in identifying a newborn at risk due to variations in birthweight and gestational age.
2. Select contributing factors and common complications associated with dysmature infants and their management.
3. Compare and contrast a small-for-gestational-age newborn and a large-for-gestational-age newborn; a postterm and preterm newborn.
4. Discuss associated conditions that affect the newborn with variations in birthweight and gestational age, including appropriate management.
5. Outline the nurse's role in helping parents experiencing perinatal grief or loss.
6. Integrate knowledge of the risks associated with late preterm births into nursing interventions, discharge planning, and parent education.

nna and her husband were stunned when she went into labor at 7 months' gestation. They couldn't understand what would cause her to give birth early, but it happened. When they approached the NICU, Anna took a deep breath and looked down at her tiny baby with tubes coming from everywhere. What feelings might they be experiencing at this moment? Do you think that guilt would be one of those feelings? If so, why?

Wow

Guiding a parent's hand to touch a frail or ill newborn demonstrates courage and compassion under very difficult circumstances and is a powerful tool in helping to deal with the newborn's special needs.

Most newborns are born between 38 and 40 weeks' gestation and weigh 6 to 8 lb, but variations in birthweight or gestational age can occur, and newborns with these variations have special needs. Gestational age at birth is inversely correlated with the risk that the infant will experience physical, neurologic, or developmental sequelae (March of Dimes, 2007b, 2007c). Some newborns are born very ill and need special advanced care to survive.

When a woman gives birth to a newborn with problems involving immaturity or birthweight, especially one who is considered high risk, she may go through a grieving process in which she mourns the loss of the healthy full-term newborn she had expected. Through this process she learns to come to terms with the experience she now faces.

The development of new technologies and regionalized care centers for the care of newborns with special needs has resulted in significant improvements. Nurses need to have a sound knowledge base to identify the newborn with special needs and to provide coordinated care.

The key to identifying a newborn with special needs related to birthweight or gestational age variation is an awareness of the factors that could place a newborn at risk. These factors are similar to those that would suggest a high-risk pregnancy and include:

- Maternal nutrition (malnutrition or overweight)
- Substandard living conditions
- Low socioeconomic status
- Maternal age of less than 20 or more than 35 years old
- Substance abuse
- Failure to seek prenatal care
- Smoking or exposure to passive smoke
- Periodontal disease
- Multiple gestation
- Extreme maternal stress
- Abuse and violence
- Placental complications (placenta previa or abruptio placentae)
- History of previous preterm birth
- Maternal disease (e.g., hypertension or diabetes)
- Maternal infection (e.g., urinary tract infection or chorioamnionitis)
- Exposure to occupational hazards (Gilbert, 2007)

Being able to anticipate the birth of a newborn at risk allows the birth to take place at a health care facility equipped with the resources to meet the mother's and newborn's needs. This is important in reducing mortality and morbidity.

Healthy People 2010 identifies preterm births and low birthweight as important national health goals (U.S. Department of Health and Human Services [USDHHS], 2000).

This chapter discusses the nursing management of newborns with special needs related to variations in birth-

HEALTHY PEOPLE 2010

Objective	Significance
Increase the proportion of very low birthweight (VLBW) infants born at level III hospitals or subspecialty perinatal centers	• Will help to promote the delivery of high-risk infants in settings that have the technological capacity to care for them, ultimately reducing the morbidity and mortality rates for these infants
Reduce low birthweight (LBW) from a baseline of 7.6% to a target of 5%; reduce very low birthweight (VLBW) from a baseline of 1.4% to 0.9%	• Will help to emphasize the issue of LBW as a risk factor associated with newborn death, helping to promote measures to reduce this risk factor and thus contributing to significant reductions in infant mortality
Reduce the total number of preterm births from a baseline of 11.6% to 7.6% Reduce the number of live births at 32 to 36 weeks' gestation from a baseline of 9.6% to 6.4% Reduce the number of live births at less than 32 weeks' gestation from a baseline of 2% to 1.1%	• Will help to emphasize the role of preterm birth as the leading cause of newborn deaths unrelated to birth defects • Will aid in promoting an overall reduction in infant illness, disability, and death

USDHHS, 2000.

weight and gestational age. It also describes selected associated conditions affecting these newborns. Due to the frailty of these newborns, the care of the family experiencing perinatal loss and the role of the nurse in helping the family cope also are addressed.

Birthweight Variations

Fetal growth is influenced by maternal nutrition, genetics, placental function, environment, and a multitude of other factors. Assigning size to a newborn is a way to measure and monitor the growth and development of the newborn at birth. Newborns can be classified according to their weight and weeks of gestation, and knowing the group into which a newborn fits is important.

Appropriate for gestational age (AGA) characterizes approximately 80% of newborns and describes a newborn with a normal height, weight, head circumference, and body mass index (BMI; Dorland, 2007). Being in the AGA group confers the lowest risk for any problems. These infants have lower morbidity and mortality than other groups.

Small-for-gestational-age (SGA) newborns typically weigh less than 2,500 g (5 lb 8 oz) at term due to less

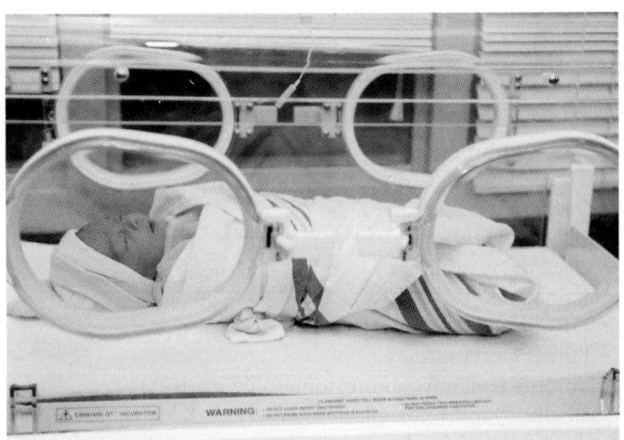

FIGURE 23.1 A low birthweight newborn in an isolette.

growth in utero than expected. A newborn is also classified as SGA if his or her birthweight is at or below the 10th percentile as correlated with the number of weeks of gestation on a growth chart.

Large-for-gestational-age (LGA) describes newborns whose birthweight is above the 90th percentile on a growth chart and who weigh more than 4,000 g (8 lb 13 oz) at term due to accelerated growth for length of gestation (Herranz et al., 2007).

The following terms describe other newborns with marginal weights at birth and of any gestational age:

- **Low birthweight**: less than 2,500 g (5.5 lb) (Fig. 23.1)
- **Very low birthweight**: less than 1,500 g (3 lb 5 oz)
- **Extremely low birthweight**: less than 1,000 g (2 lb 3 oz)

▶ SMALL-FOR-GESTATIONAL-AGE NEWBORNS

Newborns are considered SGA when they weigh less than two standard deviations for gestational age or fall below the 10th percentile on a growth chart for gestational age. These infants can be preterm, term, or postterm.

In some SGA newborns, the rate of growth does not meet the expected growth pattern. Termed intrauterine growth restriction (IUGR), these newborns also are considered at risk, with the perinatal morbidity and mortality rate increased substantially compared to that of the appropriate-for-age newborn (Cunningham et al., 2005). IUGR is the pathologic counterpart of SGA. However, an important distinction to make between SGA and IUGR newborns is that not all who are SGA have IUGR. The converse also is true: not all newborns who have IUGR are SGA. Some SGA newborns are constitutionally small: they are statistically small but otherwise healthy.

Conditions altering fetal growth produce insults that affect all organ systems and are known to produce two patterns of growth that depend on the timing of the insult to the developing embryo or fetus. An early insult (typically occurring before 28 weeks) results in overall growth restriction, with all organs being small. These SGA infants never catch up in size when compared with normal children. An insult later in gestation (after 28 weeks) results in intrauterine malnutrition, but optimal postnatal nutrition generally restores normal growth potential and carries a better prognosis than earlier insults (Kenner & Lott, 2007).

Historically, IUGR has been categorized as symmetric or asymmetric. Symmetric IUGR refers to fetuses with equally poor growth rates of the head, the abdomen, and the long bones. Asymmetric IUGR refers to infants whose head and long bones are spared compared to their abdomen and internal organs. The current belief is that in most cases IUGR is a continuum from asymmetry (early stages) to symmetry (late stages) (Harper & Lam, 2007).

Fetal growth is dependent on genetic, placental, and maternal factors. Cognitive and motor development during infancy forms the basis for children's subsequent development. Newborns who experience nutritional deficiencies in utero and are born SGA are at risk for cognitive deficits that can undermine their academic performance throughout their lives (Kristensen et al., 2007).

The fetus is thought to have an inherent growth potential that, under normal circumstances, yields a healthy newborn of appropriate size. The maternal–placental–fetal units act in harmony to meet the needs of the fetus during gestation. However, growth potential in the fetus can be limited, and this is analogous to failure to thrive in the infant. The causes of both can be intrinsic or environmental. Factors that can contribute to the birth of an SGA newborn are highlighted in Box 23.1.

Nursing Assessment

Assessment of the SGA infant begins by reviewing the maternal history to identify risk factors such as smoking, drug abuse, chronic maternal illness, hypertension, multiple gestation, or genetic disorders. This information allows the nurse to anticipate a possible problem and to be prepared to intervene quickly should one occur. At birth, perform a thorough physical examination, closely observing the newborn for typical characteristics, including:

- Head disproportionately large compared to rest of body
- Wasted appearance of extremities
- Reduced subcutaneous fat stores
- Decreased amount of breast tissue
- Scaphoid abdomen (sunken appearance)
- Wide skull sutures secondary to inadequate bone growth
- Poor muscle tone over buttocks and cheeks
- Loose and dry skin that appears oversized
- Thin umbilical cord

BOX 23.1 **Factors Contributing to the Birth of SGA Newborns**

- Maternal causes
  - Chronic hypertension
  - Diabetes mellitus with vascular disease
  - Autoimmune diseases
  - Living at a high altitude (hypoxia)
  - Smoking
  - Substance abuse (heroin, cocaine, methamphetamines)
  - Hemoglobinopathies (sickle cell anemia)
  - Preeclampsia
  - Chronic renal disease
  - Malnutrition
  - TORCH group infections
- Placental factors
  - Abnormal cord insertion

- Chronic abruption
- Decreased surface area, infarction
- Decreased placental weight
- Placenta previa
- Placental insufficiency
- Fetal factors
  - Trisomy 13, 18, and 21
  - Turner's syndrome
  - Chronic fetal infection (cytomegalovirus [CMV], rubella, syphilis, toxoplasmosis)
  - Congenital anomalies (heart, diaphragmatic hernia, tracheoesophageal fistula)
  - Radiation exposure
  - Multiple gestation

Sources: Harper & Lam, 2007; Kenner & Lott, 2007; and Neonatal Handbook, 2007e

---

Also assess the SGA newborn for any congenital malformations, neurologic insults, or indications of infection. SGA newborns commonly face problems after birth because of the decrease in placental function during gestation. Table 23.1 highlights some of the common problems associated with SGA newborns and others experiencing a variation in birthweight or gestational age. Anticipate the need for and provide resuscitation as indicated by the newborn's condition.

Nursing Management

Interventions for the SGA infant may include obtaining weight, length, and head circumference, comparing them to standards, and documenting the findings. Perform frequent serial blood glucose measurements as ordered and monitor vital signs, being particularly alert for changes in respiratory status that might indicate respiratory distress. Institute measures to maintain a neutral thermal environment to prevent cold stress and acidosis.

Initiate early and frequent oral feedings unless contraindicated. At birth the newborn's glucose level is 70% of the mother's serum glucose (Aylott, 2006a). Any newborn stressed at birth uses up available glucose stores with resulting hypoglycemia, a plasma glucose concentration at or below 40 mg/dL (Stanley, 2006). With the loss of the placenta at birth, the newborn now must assume control of glucose homeostasis through intermittent oral feedings. If oral feedings are not accepted, an intravenous infusion with 10% dextrose in water may be needed to maintain the glucose level above 40 mg/dL. Weigh the newborn daily and ensure that he or she has adequate rest periods to decrease metabolic requirements.

Observe for clinical signs of polycythemia and monitor blood results. Asymptomatic newborns with a hematocrit between 60% and 70% may simply be supported with fluids, close observation, and a repeat hematocrit

level in 4 to 6 hours (Kates & Kates, 2007). If the newborn is symptomatic, partial exchange transfusion may be used, but this treatment is considered controversial.

Provide anticipatory guidance to parents about any treatments and procedures that are being done. Emphasize the need for close follow-up and careful monitoring of the infant's growth in length, weight, and head circumference and feeding patterns throughout the first year of life to confirm any "catch-up" growth taking place.

▶ LARGE-FOR-GESTATIONAL-AGE NEWBORNS

A newborn whose weight is above the 90th percentile on growth charts or two standard deviations above the mean weight for gestational age is defined as LGA. The range of weight is 4,000 to 5,000 g, or more than 9 lb. LGA infants may be preterm, term, or postterm. Based on these definitions, up to 10% of all births involve an LGA newborn (March of Dimes, 2007a).

Because of the newborn's large size, vaginal birth may be difficult and occasionally results in birth injury. In addition, shoulder dystocia, clavicular fractures, and facial palsies are common. The incidence of cesarean births is very high with LGA newborns to avoid arrested labor and birth trauma.

▶ *Take* NOTE!

Diabetes is commonly associated with LGA newborns. However, due to poor placental perfusion, the newborn may experience IUGR and be SGA.

TABLE 23.1   COMMON PROBLEMS ASSOCIATED WITH NEWBORNS EXPERIENCING A VARIATION IN BIRTHWEIGHT OR GESTATIONAL AGE

Problem	Occurrence	Etiology/Pathophysiology	Assessment Findings	Nursing Implications
Perinatal asphyxia	SGA newborns (common)	Poor tolerance to stress of labor, frequently leading to acidosis and hypoxia Living in hypoxic environment prior to birth, leaving little to no oxygen reserves available to withstand stress of labor: —Uterine contractions increase hypoxic stress —Possible depletion of glycogen stores due to chronic hypoxic state, leading to fetal distress —Impaired uteroplacental circulation due to maternal and uterine conditions predisposing to perinatal depression Compromised newborn at birth experiencing difficulty adjusting to extrauterine environment	Fetal distress (bradycardia, decelerations) during labor Low Apgar scores (Deshpande, 2007)	Anticipate possible problem; assess for maternal risk factors. Initiate resuscitation measures immediately at birth.
	Postterm newborns	Placental deprivation or oligohydramnios, leading to cord compression and subsequent reduction in perfusion to fetus		
	Preterm newborns (common)	Surfactant deficiency Unstable chest wall Immaturity of respiratory control centers in the CNS Small respiratory passages, increasing risk for obstruction Inability to clear mucus from airways		
Difficulty with thermoregulation	SGA newborns (common)	Less muscle mass, less brown fat, less heat-preserving subcutaneous fat, and limited ability to control skin capillaries (Aylott, 2006b) Associated with depleted glycogen stores, poor subcutaneous fat stores, and disturbances in CNS thermoregulation due to hypoxia (Kenner & Lott, 2007)	Temperature <36.4° C; temperature instability; skin cool to touch; cyanosis of hands and feet Bradypnea (<25 bpm) and tachypnea (>60 breaths/min)	Maintain a neutral thermal environment to promote stabilization of newborn's temperature. Assess skin temperature and respiration characteristics. Monitor arterial blood gases and blood glucose levels.

(continued)

TABLE 23.1 COMMON PROBLEMS ASSOCIATED WITH NEWBORNS EXPERIENCING A VARIATION IN BIRTHWEIGHT OR GESTATIONAL AGE (continued)

Problem	Occurrence	Etiology/Pathophysiology	Assessment Findings	Nursing Implications
	Postterm newborns	Increased risk for acidosis and hypoglycemia secondary to metabolic stress (Neonatal Handbook, 2007j) Loss of subcutaneous fat second to placental insufficiency Use of stored nutrients for nutrition due to lost ability of placenta to nourish fetus Subsequent wasting of subcutaneous fat, muscle, or both (Aylott, 2006b) Loss of natural insulation (subcutaneous fat) important in temperature regulation	Tremors, irritability Wheezing, crackles, retractions Restlessness, lethargy Hypotonia Weak or high-pitched cry Seizures Poor feeding Grunting (Galligan, 2006) Acidosis	Eliminate sources of heat loss: —Dry newborn thoroughly. —Wrap in warmed blanket with stockinette cap on head. —Use radiant heat source.
	Preterm newborns (common) Late preterm infant (common)	Immaturity of CNS (temperature-regulating center) interferes with ability to regulate body temperature Inadequate amounts of subcutaneous fat Lack of muscle tone and flexion to conserve heat Inadequate brown fat to generate heat Limited muscle mass activity, reducing ability to produce own heat Inability to shiver to generate heat		
Hypoglycemia	SGA newborns (common) LGA newborns (common)	Increased metabolic rate and lack of adequate glycogen stores to meet newborn's metabolic needs Commonly associated with infants of diabetic mothers Abrupt cessation of high-glucose maternal blood supply with birth and continued insulin production by the newborn Limited ability to release glucagons and catecholamines, which normally stimulate glucagon breakdown and glucose release	Often subtle Lethargy, tachycardia Respiratory distress Jitteriness Drowsiness Poor feeding, feeble sucking Hypothermia, temperature instability Diaphoresis Weak cry Seizures Hypotonia	Monitor blood glucose levels, initially on arrival to nursery and hourly thereafter. Maintain fluid and electrolyte balance. Watch for subtle changes. Initiate early oral feedings if possible; if not, administer IV infusion with 10% dextrose in water.

Problem	Occurrence	Etiology/Pathophysiology	Assessment Findings	Nursing Implications
	Postterm newborns	Hypoxia secondary to depleted glycogen reserves Placental insufficiency secondary to placental aging contributing to chronic fetal nutritional deficiency further depleting glycogen stores	Blood glucose levels <40 mg/dL for term newborns, <20 mg/dL for preterm newborns (Kenner & Lott, 2007)	
	Preterm newborns Late preterm infants	Immature sucking and swallowing leading to insufficient intake Perinatal hypoxia Increased energy expenditure Decreased subcutaneous and brown fat with little to no glycogen stores		
Polycythemia	SGA newborns	Chronic mild hypoxia secondary to placental insufficiency Stimulation of erythropoietin release, leading to increased RBC production	Venous hematocrit >65% Plethora (ruddy appearance) Weak sucking reflex	Ensure adequate hydration (orally or IV). Monitor hematocrit levels (goal is ~60%). Administer partial exchange transfusion, albumin or normal saline IV to reduce RBC volume and increase fluid volume (controversial).
	LGA newborns	Secondary to fetal hypoxia, trauma with bleeding, increased erythropoietin production, or delayed cord clamping (Lessaris, 2007)	Tachypnea Jaundice Lethargy Jitteriness Hypotonia Irritability Feeding difficulties Difficulty in arousing Seizures	
	Postterm newborns	Intrauterine hypoxia triggers increased RBC cell production to compensate for lower oxygen levels.		
Meconium aspiration	SGA newborns	Release of meconium into amniotic fluid prior to birth Inhalation of meconium-containing amniotic fluid by the newborn, leading to aspiration	Green amniotic fluid with rupture of membranes during labor Green staining of the umbilical cord or fingernails Difficulty initiating respirations	Initiate resuscitation measures as necessary. Suction airways and support ventilation (see Chapter 24 for more information).
	Postterm newborns	Commonly associated with chronic intrauterine hypoxia Struggling by fetus making respiratory efforts and bearing down with abdominal muscles, leading to expulsion of meconium into amniotic fluid Normal sucking and swallowing by fetus leads to meconium filling airways.		

(continued)

TABLE 23.1 COMMON PROBLEMS ASSOCIATED WITH NEWBORNS EXPERIENCING A VARIATION IN BIRTHWEIGHT OR GESTATIONAL AGE (continued)

Problem	Occurrence	Etiology/Pathophysiology	Assessment Findings	Nursing Implications
Hyperbilirubinemia	LGA newborns (common)	Associated with polycythemia and RBC breakdown Inability to tolerate feedings in the first few days of life, leading to increased enterohepatic circulation of bilirubin Excessive bruising secondary to birth trauma, leading to higher-than-normal bilirubin levels	Elevated serum bilirubin levels Jaundice Tea-colored urine Clay-colored stools	Ensure adequate hydration. Institute early feedings if possible. Administer phototherapy (see Chapter 24 for more information).
	Preterm newborns Late preterm infants	Increased breakdown of RBCs and immature liver function to handle excess load		
Birth trauma	LGA newborns	Large size requiring use of operative birth procedure	Obvious deformities Bruising Edema Asymmetrical movement	Perform complete physical and neurologic assessment of the newborn. Note symmetry of structure and function. Assist parents in understanding situation (see Chapter 24 for more information).

Nursing Assessment

Assessment of the LGA newborn begins with a review of the maternal history, which can provide clues as to whether the woman has an increased risk of giving birth to an LGA newborn. Maternal factors that increase the chance of bearing an LGA newborn include maternal diabetes mellitus or glucose intolerance, multiparity, prior history of a macrosomic infant, postdates gestation, maternal obesity, male fetus, and genetics (Jazayeri, 2007).

At birth, assess the newborn for common characteristics. The typical LGA newborn has a large body and appears plump and full-faced. The increase in body size is proportional. However, the head circumference and body length are in the upper limits of intrauterine growth. These newborns have poor motor skills and have difficulty in regulating behavioral states. LGA newborns are more difficult to arouse to a quiet alert state (Neonatal Handbook, 2007f).

Thoroughly assess the LGA newborn at birth to identify traumatic birth injuries such as fractured clavicles, brachial palsy, facial paralysis, phrenic nerve palsy,

skull fractures, or hematomas. Perform a neurologic examination to identify any nerve palsies, looking for abnormalities such as immobility of the upper arm. Observe and document any injuries discovered to allow for early intervention and improved outcomes.

Obtain frequent blood glucose levels as ordered to evaluate for hypoglycemia. The clinical signs are often subtle and include lethargy, apathy, drowsiness, irritability, tachypnea, weak cry, temperature instability, jitteriness, seizures, apnea, bradycardia, cyanosis or pallor, feeble suck and poor feeding, hypotonia, and coma. Other disorders, including septicemia, severe respiratory distress, and congenital heart disease, may present with similar findings. In addition, be alert for other common problems, such as polycythemia and hyperbilirubinemia (see Table 23.1 earlier in this chapter).

Nursing Management

Assist in stabilizing the LGA newborn. Monitor blood glucose levels within 30 minutes of birth and repeat the screening every hour. Recheck levels before feedings and also immediately in any infant suspected of having or showing clinical signs of hypoglycemia, regardless of age (Aylott, 2006a). To help prevent hypoglycemia, initiate feedings, which can be formula or breast milk, with intravenous glucose supplementation as needed.

If the newborn's blood glucose level is below 25 mg/dL, institute immediate treatment with intravenous glucose, regardless of clinical symptoms (Aylott, 2006a). Monitor and record intake and output and obtain daily weights to aid in evaluating nutritional intake.

Observe for signs of polycythemia and hyperbilirubinemia and report any immediately to the health care provider so that early interventions can be taken to prevent poor long-term neurologic development outcomes. Polycythemia and hyperviscosity are associated with fine and gross motor delays, speech delays, and neurologic sequelae (Neonatal Handbook, 2007g). Increasing fluid volume aids in decreasing blood viscosity. Partial exchange transfusion with plasma or normal saline may be used to lower hematocrit and decrease blood viscosity, but this treatment remains controversial. Hydration, early feedings, and phototherapy are used to treat hyperbilirubinemia (see Chapter 24 for more information about hyperbilirubinemia). Provide parental guidance about the treatments and procedures being done and about the need for follow-up care for any abnormalities identified.

Gestational Age Variations

The mean duration of pregnancy, calculated from the first day of the last normal menstrual period, is approximately 280 days, or 40 weeks. Gestational age is typically measured in weeks: a newborn born before completion of 37 weeks is classified as a **preterm newborn** and one born after completion of 42 weeks is classified as a **postterm newborn**. An infant born from the first day of 38th week through 42 weeks is classified as a **term newborn**. As of 2006, a new classification has been added, the **late preterm newborn**—one who is born between 34 weeks and 36 weeks, 6 days of gestation.

Precise knowledge of a newborn's gestational age is imperative for effective postnatal management. Determination of gestational age by the nurse assists in planning appropriate care for the newborn and provides important information regarding potential problems that need interventions. See Chapter 18 for more information on assessing gestational age.

▶ *Take* NOTE!

Although preterm and postterm newborns may appear to be at opposite ends of the gestational age spectrum and are very different in size and appearance, both are at high risk and need special care.

▶ POSTTERM NEWBORN

A pregnancy that extends beyond 42 weeks' gestation produces a postterm newborn. Other terms used to describe these late births include postmature, prolonged pregnancy, or postdates pregnancy. Postterm newborns may be LGA, SGA, or dysmature (newborn weighs less than established normal parameters for estimated gestational age [IUGR]), depending on placental function.

The reason why some pregnancies last longer than others is not completely understood. What is known is that women who experience one postterm pregnancy are at increased risk in subsequent pregnancies. The incidence of prolonged pregnancy is approximately 10% (Gilbert, 2007).

The ability of the placenta to provide adequate oxygen and nutrients to the fetus after 42 weeks' gestation is thought to be compromised, leading to perinatal mortality and morbidity. As the placenta loses its ability to nourish the fetus, the fetus uses stored nutrients to stay alive, and wasting occurs. This wasted appearance at birth is secondary to the loss of muscle mass and subcutaneous fat.

▶ *Consider* THIS!

I had been waiting for this baby my whole married life and now I was told to wait even longer. I was into my third week past my due date and was just told that if I didn't go into labor on my own, the doctor would induce me on Monday. As I waddled out of his office into the hot summer sun, I thought about all the comments that would await me at the office: "You're not still pregnant, are you?" "Weren't you due last month?" "You look as big as a house." "Are you sure you aren't expecting triplets?" I started to get into my car when I felt warm fluid slide down my legs. Although I was embarrassed at my wetness, I was thrilled I wouldn't have to go back to the office and drove myself to the hospital. Within hours my wait was finally over with the birth of my son, a postterm infant with peeling skin and a thick head of hair. He was certainly worth the wait!

Thoughts: Although most due dates are within plus or minus 2 weeks, we can't "go to the bank with it" because so many factors influence the start of labor. This woman was anxious about her overdue status, but nature prevailed. The old adage "when the fruit is ripe, it will fall" doesn't always bring a good outcome: many women need a little push to bring a healthy newborn forth. What happens when the fetus stays inside the uterus too long? What other features are typical of postterm infants?

Nursing Assessment

A thorough assessment of the postterm newborn upon admission to the nursery provides a baseline from which to identify changes in clinical status. Review the maternal history for any risk factors associated with postterm birth. Also be aware of the common physical characteristics and be able to identify any deviation from the expected. Postterm newborns typically exhibit the following characteristics:

• Dry, cracked, wrinkled skin
• Long, thin extremities
• Creases that cover the entire soles of the feet
• Wide-eyed, alert expression
• Abundant hair on scalp
• Thin umbilical cord
• Limited vernix and lanugo
• Meconium-stained skin
• Long nails (Kenner & Lott, 2007)

Assess the newborn's gestational age and complete a physical examination to identify any abnormalities. Review the medical record to determine the color of the amniotic fluid when membranes ruptured and observe for a meconium-stained umbilical cord and fingernails to assess for possible meconium aspiration. Careful suctioning at the time of birth and afterwards, if the condition dictates it, reduces the incidence of meconium aspiration. Also be alert for other typical complications associated with a postterm newborn, such as perinatal asphyxia, hypoglycemia, hypothermia, and polycythemia, and be prepared to initiate early interventions (see Table 23.1 earlier in the chapter).

Nursing Management

The birth of a postterm newborn creates a crisis for the mother and her family. In most situations, birth of a newborn requiring special care was not anticipated. Postterm newborns are susceptible to several birth challenges secondary to placental dysfunction that place them at risk for asphyxia, hypoglycemia, and respiratory distress. The nurse must be vigilant for complications when managing these newborns.

The postterm newborn is at high risk for perinatal asphyxia, which is usually attributed to placental deprivation or oligohydramnios that leads to cord compression, thereby reducing perfusion to the fetus. Anticipating the need for newborn resuscitation is a priority. The newborn resuscitation team needs to be available in the birthing suite for immediate backup. The newborn may require transport to the neonatal intensive care unit (NICU) for continuous assessment, monitoring, and treatment, depending on his or her status after resuscitation.

Monitor and maintain the postterm newborn's blood glucose levels once stabilized. Intravenous dextrose 10% and/or early initiation of feedings will help stabilize the blood glucose levels to prevent central nervous system sequelae.

Also monitor the postterm newborn's skin temperature, respiration characteristics, results of blood studies, such as arterial blood gases (ABGs) and serum bilirubin levels, and neurologic status. Institute measures to prevent or reduce the risk of hypothermia by eliminating sources of heat loss: thoroughly dry the newborn at birth, wrap him or her in a warmed blanket, and place a stockinet cap on the newborn's head. Providing environmental warmth via a radiant heat source will help stabilize the newborn's temperature.

Closely assess all postterm newborns for polycythemia. Providing adequate hydration helps to reduce the viscosity of the newborn's blood to prevent thrombosis. Be alert to the early, often subtle signs to promote early identification and prompt treatment to prevent any neurodevelopmental delays.

▶ PRETERM NEWBORN

A preterm newborn is one who is born before the completion of 37 weeks of gestation. Although the national birth rate has been declining since the 1990s, the preterm birth rate has been climbing rapidly. Approximately one in eight babies, or 12%, is born before the 37th week of gestation (March of Dimes, 2007c). Prematurity is now the leading cause of death within the first month of life and the second leading cause of all infant deaths.

The etiology of half of all preterm births is unknown (March of Dimes, 2007b, 2007c). Preterm births take an enormous financial toll, estimated to be in the billions of dollars. They also take an emotional toll on those involved.

Changes in perinatal care practices, including regional care, have reduced newborn mortality rates. Transporting high-risk pregnant women to a tertiary center for birth rather than transferring the neonate after birth is associated with a reduction in neonatal mortality and morbidity (Vargo & Trotter, 2007). Despite increasing survival rates, preterm infants continue to be at high risk for neurodevelopmental disorders such as cerebral palsy or mental retardation, intraventricular hemorrhage, congenital anomalies, neurosensory impairment, behavioral problems, and chronic lung disease (Kipiani, Tatishvili, & Sirbiladze, 2007). Making sure that all pregnant women receive quality prenatal care throughout pregnancy is a major method for preventing preterm births.

Effects of Prematurity on Body Systems

Since the preterm newborn did not remain in utero long enough, every body system may be immature, affecting the newborn's transition from intrauterine to extrauterine life and placing him or her at risk for complications.

Without full development, organ systems are not capable of functioning at the level needed to maintain extrauterine homeostasis (March of Dimes, 2007b, 2007c).

*R*ecall Anna, who was described at the beginning of the chapter; she gave birth to a newborn at 7 months' gestation. What problems would you anticipate that her newborn might have?

Respiratory System

The respiratory system is one of the last body systems to mature. Therefore, the preterm newborn is at great risk for respiratory complications. A few of the problems that affect the preterm newborn's breathing ability and adjustment to extrauterine life include:

- Surfactant deficiency, leading to the development of respiratory distress syndrome
- Unstable chest wall, leading to atelectasis
- Immature respiratory control centers, leading to apnea
- Smaller respiratory passages, leading to an increased risk for obstruction
- Inability to clear fluid from passages, leading to transient tachypnea

Cardiovascular System

The preterm newborn has great difficulty in making the transition from intrauterine to extrauterine life in terms of changing from a fetal to a newborn circulation pattern. Higher oxygen levels in the circulation once air breathing begins spur this transition. If the oxygen levels remain low secondary to perinatal asphyxia, the fetal pattern of circulation may persist, causing blood flow to bypass the lungs. Another problem affecting the cardiovascular system is the increased incidence of congenital anomalies associated with continued fetal circulation—patent ductus arteriosus and an open foramen ovale. In addition, impaired regulation of blood pressure in preterm newborns may cause fluctuations throughout the circulatory system. One of special note is cerebral blood flow, which may predispose the fragile blood vessels in the brain to rupture, causing intracranial hemorrhage (Lissauer & Weindling, 2006).

Gastrointestinal System

Preterm newborns usually lack the neuromuscular coordination required to maintain the suck, swallow, and breathing regimen necessary for sufficient calorie and fluid intake to support growth. Perinatal hypoxia causes shunting of blood from the gut to more important organs such as the heart and brain. Subsequently, ischemia and damage to the intestinal wall can occur. This combination of shunting, ischemia, damage to the intestinal wall, and poor sucking ability places the preterm infant at risk for malnutrition and weight loss.

In addition, preterm newborns have a small stomach capacity, weak abdominal muscles, compromised metabolic function, limited ability to digest proteins and absorb nutrients, and weak or absent suck and gag reflexes. All of these limitations place the preterm newborn at risk for nutritional deficiency and subsequent growth and development delays (Neonatal Handbook, 2007h).

Currently, minimal enteral feeding is used to prepare the preterm newborn's gut to overcome the many feeding difficulties associated with gastrointestinal immaturity. It involves the introduction of small amounts, usually 0.5 to 1 mL/kg/h, of enteral feeding to induce surges in gut hormones that enhance maturation of the intestine. This minute amount of breast milk or formula given via gavage feeding prepares the gut to absorb future introduction of nutrients. It builds mucosal bulk, stimulates development of enzymes, enhances pancreatic function, stimulates maturation of gastrointestinal hormones, reduces gastrointestinal distention and malabsorption, and enhances transition to oral feedings (Blackburn, 2007).

Renal System

The renal system of the preterm newborn is immature, reducing the baby's ability to concentrate urine and slowing the glomerular filtration rate. As a result, the risk for fluid retention, with subsequent fluid and electrolyte disturbances, increases. In addition, preterm newborns have limited ability to clear drugs from their systems, thereby increasing the risk of drug toxicity. Close monitoring of the preterm newborn's acid–base and electrolyte balance is critical to identify metabolic inconsistencies. Prescribed medications require strict evaluation to prevent overwhelming the preterm baby's immature renal system.

Immune System

The preterm newborn's immune system is very immature, increasing his or her susceptibility to infections. A deficiency of IgG may occur because transplacental transfer does not occur until after 34 weeks' gestation. This protection is lacking if the baby was born before this time. In addition, preterm newborns have an impaired ability to manufacture antibodies to fight infection if they were exposed to pathogens during the birth process. Moreover, the preterm newborn's thin skin and fragile blood vessels provide a limited protective barrier, adding to the increased risk for infection. Thus, anticipating and preventing infections is the goal; preventing infections has a better outcome than treating them.

Central Nervous System

The preterm newborn is susceptible to injury and insult to the central nervous system (CNS), increasing the potential for long-term disability into adulthood. Like all newborns, preterm newborns have difficulty in temperature regulation and maintaining stability. However, their risk for heat loss is compounded by inadequate amounts of insulating subcutaneous fat; lack of muscle tone and flexion to conserve heat; inadequate brown fat to generate heat; limited muscle mass activity, reducing the possibility of producing their own heat; inability to shiver to generate heat; and an immature temperature-regulating center in the brain (Blackburn, 2007). Preventing cold stress, which would increase the newborn's metabolic and oxygen needs, is crucial. The goal is to create a neutral thermal environment in which oxygen consumption is minimal but body temperature is maintained (Kenner & Lott, 2007).

In addition, the preterm newborn is especially susceptible to hypoglycemia due to immature glucose control mechanisms, decreased glucose stores, and a reduced availability of alternative fuels such as ketone bodies.

▶ *Take* NOTE!

Glucose is needed by the brain and CNS to maintain and support numerous body system functions.

Nursing Assessment

Preterm newborns are at high risk for numerous problems and require special care. When preterm labor develops and cannot be stopped by medical interventions, plans for appropriate management of the mother and the preterm newborn are necessary, such as transporting them to a regional center with facilities to care for preterm newborns or notifying the facility's NICU. Depending on the degree of prematurity, the preterm newborn may be kept in the NICU for months.

A thorough assessment of the preterm newborn upon admission to the nursery provides a baseline from which to identify changes in clinical status. Be aware of the common physical characteristics and be able to identify any deviation from the expected (Fig. 23.2). Common physical characteristics of preterm infants may include:

• Birthweight of less than 5.5 lb
• Scrawny appearance
• Head disproportionately larger than chest circumference
• Poor muscle tone
• Minimal subcutaneous fat
• Undescended testes
• Plentiful lanugo (soft, downy hair), especially over the face and back
• Poorly formed ear pinna, with soft, pliable cartilage
• Fused eyelids
• Soft and spongy skull bones, especially along suture lines
• Matted scalp hair, wooly in appearance
• Absent to a few creases in the soles and palms
• Minimal scrotal rugae in male infants; prominent labia and clitoris in female infants

• Thin, transparent skin with visible veins
• Breast and nipples not clearly delineated
• Abundant vernix caseosa (Kenner & Lott, 2007)

Be alert for evidence that might suggest that the preterm newborn is developing a complication (see Table 23.1 earlier in the chapter).

Review the maternal history to identify risk factors for preterm birth and check antepartum and intrapartum records for maternal infections to anticipate the need for treatment. Maternal risk factors associated with preterm birth include a previous preterm delivery, low socioeconomic status, preeclampsia, hypertension, poor maternal nutrition, smoking, multiple gestation, infection, advanced maternal age, and substance abuse.

Assess the newborn's gestational age and assess for IUGR if appropriate. Inspect the newborn's skin closely, especially skin color. Assess vital signs, including temperature via skin probe to identify hypothermia or fever, and heart rate for tachycardia or bradycardia. Evaluate the newborn's respiratory effort and respiratory rate. Observe for periods of apnea lasting longer than 20 seconds. Monitor oxygen saturation levels by pulse oximetry to validate perfusion status. Note and report any signs of respiratory distress. Auscultate lung and heart sounds, being especially alert for possible murmur, which would indicate the presence of patent ductus arteriosus in a preterm newborn.

Assess neurologic status by observing the newborn's behavior. Note any restlessness, hypotonia, or weak cry or sucking effort and report unusual findings.

Monitor laboratory studies such as hemoglobin and hematocrit for signs of polycythemia. Screen for hypoglycemia upon admission and then hourly, always observing for nonspecific signs of hypoglycemia such as lethargy, poor feeding, and seizures. Evaluate serum bilirubin concentrations.

Also assess the mother and family members. Identify family strengths and coping mechanisms to establish a basis for intervention.

Nursing Management

The birth of a preterm newborn creates a crisis for the mother and family. Multiple studies have found that hospitalization for preterm newborns is often followed by negative mental health/behavioral outcomes, anxiety and depressive disorders, and developmental problems (Melnyk, Feinstein, & Fairbanks, 2006). Preterm newborns present with immaturity of all organ systems, abundant physiologic challenges, and significant morbidity and mortality (Kenner & Lott, 2007). The nurse must be vigilant for complications when managing preterm newborns (Fig. 23.3 and Nursing Care Plan 23.1).

Promoting Oxygenation

Newborns normally start to breathe without assistance and often cry after birth, being stimulated by a change in pres-

FIGURE 23.2 Characteristics of a preterm newborn. (**A**) Few plantar creases. (**B**) Soft, pliable ear cartilage, matted hair, and fused eyelids. (**C**) Lax posture with poor muscle tone. (**D**) Breast and nipple area barely visible. (**E**) Male genitalia with minimal rugae on scrotum. (**F**) Female genitalia with prominent labia and clitoris.

sure gradients and environmental temperature. The work of taking that first breath is primarily due to overcoming the surface tension of the walls of the terminal lung units at the gas–tissue interface. Subsequent breaths require less inspiratory pressure since there is an increase in functional capacity and air retained. By 1 minute of age, most new-

borns are breathing well. A newborn who fails to establish adequate, sustained respiration after birth is said to have **asphyxia**. On a physiologic level, it is defined as an impairment in gas exchange resulting in a decrease in oxygen in the blood (hypoxemia) and an excess of carbon dioxide or hypercapnia that leads to acidosis. Asphyxia is the most

FIGURE 23.3 The physical condition of a preterm newborn demands skilled assessment and nursing care.

common clinical insult in the perinatal period that results in brain injury, which may lead to mental retardation, cerebral palsy, or seizures (Blackburn, 2007).

The preterm infant lacks surfactant. Surfactant lowers surface tension in the alveoli and stabilizes them to prevent their collapse. Even if preterm newborns can initiate respirations, they have a limited ability to retain air due to insufficient surfactant. Therefore, preterm newborns develop atelectasis quickly without alveoli stabilization. The inability to initiate and establish respirations leads to hypoxemia and ultimately hypoxia (decreased oxygen), acidosis (decreased pH), and hypercarbia (increased carbon dioxide). This change in the newborn's biochemical environment may inhibit the transition to extrauterine circulation, thus allowing fetal circulation patterns to persist.

Failure to initiate extrauterine breathing or failure to breathe well after birth leads to hypoxia (too little oxygen in the cells of the body). As a result, the heart rate falls, cyanosis develops, and the newborn becomes hypotonic and unresponsive. Although this can happen with any newborn, the risk is higher in preterm newborns.

Prevention and early identification of newborns at risk are key. Prenatal risk factors that can help identify the newborn who may need resuscitation at birth secondary to asphyxia include:

- History of substance abuse
- Gestational hypertension
- Fetal distress due to hypoxia before birth
- Chronic maternal diseases such as diabetes or a heart or renal condition
- Maternal or perinatal infection

- Placental problems (placenta previa or abruptio placentae)
- Umbilical cord problems (nuchal or prolapsed)
- Difficult or traumatic birth
- Multiple births
- Congenital heart disease
- Maternal anesthesia or recent analgesia
- Preterm or postterm birth (Neonatal Handbook, 2007i)

Note the newborn's Apgar score at 1 and 5 minutes. If the score is below 7 at either time, resuscitation efforts are needed. Several diagnostic studies may be done to identify underlying etiologies. For example, a chest x-ray helps to identify structural abnormalities that might interfere with respirations. Blood studies may be done, such as cultures to rule out an infectious process, a toxicology screen to detect any maternal drugs in the newborn, and a metabolic screen to identify any metabolic conditions (Lissauer & Weindling, 2007). Monitor vital signs continuously, check blood glucose levels for hypoglycemia secondary to stress, and maintain a neutral thermal environment to promote energy conservation and minimize oxygen consumption.

Resuscitating the Newborn

Any newborn can be born with asphyxia without warning. Approximately 10% of newborns require some assistance to begin breathing at birth. Anticipation, adequate preparation, accurate evaluation, and prompt initiation of support are critical for successful newborn resuscitation. Have all basic equipment immediately available and in working order. Ensure that the equipment is evaluated daily, and document its condition and any needed repairs. Box 23.2 lists the equipment needed for basic newborn resuscitation.

Determine the need for resuscitation by performing a rapid assessment using the following four questions:

- What is the gestational age of this newborn?
- Was the amniotic fluid clear of meconium or cloudy (infection present)?
- Is the newborn breathing or crying now?
- Does the newborn have good muscle tone?

If the answers are "yes" to all questions, then routine care is initiated: provide warmth, clear the airway, dry the newborn, and assess color. If the answer to any of these questions is "no," the newborn should receive one or more of the following actions, according to this sequence:

1. Stabilization—Dry the newborn thoroughly with a warm towel; provide warmth by placing him or her under a radiant heater to prevent rapid heat loss through evaporation; position the head in a neutral position to open the airway; clear the airway with a bulb syringe or suction catheter; stimulate breathing. At times, handling and rubbing the newborn with a dry towel may be all that is needed to stimulate respirations.

Nursing Care Plan 23.1

OVERVIEW OF THE CARE OF A PRETERM NEWBORN

Alice, an 18-year-old, felt she had done everything right during her first pregnancy and certainly didn't anticipate giving birth to a preterm newborn at 32 weeks' gestation. When Mary Kaye was born, she had respiratory distress and hypoglycemia and couldn't stabilize her temperature. Assessment revealed the following: newborn described as scrawny in appearance; skin thin and transparent with prominent veins over abdomen; hypotonia with lax, extended positioning; weak sucking reflex when nipple offered; respiratory distress with tachypnea (70 breaths/min), nasal flaring, and sternal retractions; low blood glucose level suggested by lethargy, tachycardia, jitteriness; axillary temperature of 36° C (96.8° F) despite warmed blanket; weight 2,146 g (4.73 lb); length 45 cm (17.72 inches).

NURSING DIAGNOSIS: Ineffective breathing pattern related to immature respiratory system and respiratory distress as evidenced by tachypnea, nasal flaring, and sternal retractions

Outcome Identification and Evaluation
Newborn's respiratory status returns to adequate level of functioning as evidenced by rate remaining within 30 to 60 breaths/min, maintenance of acceptable oxygen saturation levels, and minimal to absent signs of respiratory distress.

Interventions: Promoting Optimal Breathing Pattern
- Assess gestational age and risk factors for respiratory distress *to allow early detection.*
- Anticipate need for bag and mask setup and wall suction *to allow for prompt intervention should respiratory status continue to worsen.*
- Assess respiratory effort (rate, character, effort) *to identify changes.*
- Assess heart rate for tachycardia and auscultate heart sounds *to determine worsening of condition.*
- Observe for cues (grunting, shallow respirations, tachypnea, apnea, tachycardia, central cyanosis, hypotonia, increased effort) *to identify need for additional oxygen.*
- Maintain slight head elevation *to prevent upper airway obstruction.*
- Assess skin color *to evaluate tissue perfusion.*
- Monitor oxygen saturation level via pulse oximetry *to provide objective indication of perfusion status.*
- Provide supplemental oxygen as indicated and ordered *to ensure adequate tissue oxygenation.*
- Assist with any ordered diagnostic tests, such as chest x-ray and arterial blood gases, *to determine effectiveness of treatments.*
- Cluster nursing activities *to reduce oxygen consumption.*
- Maintain a neutral thermal environment *to reduce oxygen consumption.*
- Monitor hydration status *to prevent fluid volume deficit or overload.*
- Explain all events and procedures to the parents *to help alleviate anxiety and promote understanding of the newborn's condition.*

NURSING DIAGNOSIS: Ineffective thermoregulation related to lack of fat stores and hypotonia as evidenced by extended positioning, low axillary temperature despite warmed blanket, respiratory distress, and lethargy

Outcome Identification and Evaluation
Newborn will demonstrate ability to regulate temperature as evidenced by temperature remaining in normal range (36.5° to 37.5° C) and absent signs of cold stress.

Interventions: Promoting Thermoregulation
- Assess the axillary temperature every hour or use a thermistor probe *to monitor for changes.*
- Review maternal history *to identify risk factors contributing to problem.*
- Monitor vital signs, including heart rate and respiratory rate, every hour *to identify deviations.*
- Check radiant heat source or isolette *to ensure maintenance of appropriate temperature of the environment.*
- Assess environment for sources of heat loss or gain through evaporation, conduction, convection, or radiation *to minimize risk of heat loss.*
- Avoid bathing and exposing newborn *to prevent cold stress.*
- Warm all blankets and equipment that come in contact with newborn; place warmed cap on the newborn's head and keep it on *to minimize heat loss.*

(continued)

Nursing Care Plan 23.1 (continued)

- Encourage kangaroo care (mother or father holds preterm infant underneath clothing skin-to-skin and upright between breasts) *to provide warmth.*
- Educate parents on how to maintain a neutral thermal environment, including importance of keeping the newborn warm with a cap and double-wrapping with blankets and changing them frequently to keep dry *to promote newborn's adjustment.*
- Demonstrate ways to safeguard warmth and prevent heat loss.

NURSING DIAGNOSIS: Risk for imbalanced nutrition: less than body requirements related to poor sucking and lack of glycogen stores necessary to meet the newborn's increased metabolic demands as evidenced by weak sucking reflex, low birthweight, and signs and symptoms of hypoglycemia, including lethargy, tachycardia, and jitteriness

Outcome Identification and Evaluation

Newborn will demonstrate adequate nutritional intake, remaining free of signs of hypoglycemia as evidenced by blood glucose levels being maintained above 45 mg/dL, enhanced sucking ability, and appropriate weight gain.

Interventions: Promoting Optimal Nutrition

- Identify newborn at risk based on behavioral characteristics, body measurements, and gestational age *to establish a baseline and allow for early detection.*
- Assess blood glucose levels as ordered *to determine status and establish a baseline for interventions.*
- Obtain blood glucose measurements upon admission to nursery and every 1 to 2 hours as indicated *to evaluate for changes.*
- Observe behavior for signs of low blood glucose *to allow early identification.*
- Initiate early oral feedings or gavage feedings *to maintain blood glucose levels.*
- If oral or gavage feedings aren't tolerated, initiate an IV glucose infusion *to aid in stabilizing blood glucose levels.*
- Assess skin for pallor and sweating *to identify signs of hypoglycemia.*
- Assess neurologic status for tremors, seizures, jitteriness, and lethargy *to identify further drops in blood glucose levels.*
- Monitor weight daily for changes *to determine effectiveness of feedings.*
- Maintain temperature using warmed blankets, radiant warmer, or warmed isolette *to prevent heat loss and possible cold stress and reduce energy demands.*
- Monitor temperature *to prevent cold stress resulting in decreased blood glucose levels.*
- Offer opportunities for non-nutritive sucking on premature-size pacifier *to satisfy sucking needs.*
- Monitor for tolerance of oral feedings, including intake and output, *to determine effectiveness.*
- Administer IV dextrose if newborn is symptomatic *to raise blood glucose levels quickly.*
- Decrease energy requirements, including clustering care activities and providing rest periods, *to conserve glucose and glycogen stores.*
- Inform parents about procedures and treatments, including rationale for frequent blood glucose levels, *to help reduce their anxiety.*

---

2. Ventilation
3. Chest compressions
4. Administration of epinephrine and/or volume expansion (AHA/AAP, 2006).

The decision to progress from one set of actions to the next and the need for further resuscitative efforts is determined by the assessment of respirations, heart rate, and color (AHA/AAP, 2006).

When performing newborn resuscitation, use the mnemonic "ABCDs" (airway, breathing, circulation, and drugs) to remember the sequence of steps (Box 23.3).

Resuscitation measures are continued until the newborn has a pulse above 100 bpm, a good cry, or good breathing efforts and a pink tongue. This last sign indicates a good oxygen supply to the brain (AHA/AAP, 2006).

Throughout the resuscitation period, keep the parents informed of what is happening to their newborn and what is being done and why. Provide support through this initial crisis. Once the newborn is stabilized, encourage bonding by having them stroke, touch, and when appropriate hold the newborn.

Administering Oxygen

Oxygen administration is a common therapy in newborn nurseries. Although it has been used in newborns for over 75 years, there is no universal agreement on the most ap-

---

BOX 23.2 **Basic Equipment for Newborn Resuscitation**

- A wall vacuum suction apparatus
- A wall source or tank source of 100% oxygen with a flow meter
- A neonatal self-inflating ventilation bag with correct-sized face masks
- A selection of endotracheal tubes (2.5, 3.0, or 3.5 mm) with introducers
- A laryngoscope with a small, straight blade and spare batteries and bulbs
- Ampules of naloxone (Narcan) with syringes and needles
- A wall clock to document timing of activities and events
- A supply of disposable gloves in a variety of sizes for staff to use

---

BOX 23.3 **ABCDs of Newborn Resuscitation**

- **Airway**
  - Place infant's head in "sniffing" position.
  - Suction mouth, then nose.
  - Suction trachea if meconium-stained and newborn is NOT vigorous (strong respiratory effort, good muscle tone, and heart rate > 100 bpm).
- **Breathing**
  - Use positive-pressure ventilation (PPV) for apnea, grasping, or pulse <100 bpm.
  - Ventilate at rate of 40 to 60 breaths/minute.
  - Listen for raising heart rate, audible breath sounds.
  - Look for slight chest movement with each breath.
  - Use carbon dioxide detector after intubation.
- **Circulation**
  - Start compressions if heart rate is <60 after 30 seconds of effective PPV.
  - Give 3 compressions: 1 breath every 2 seconds.
  - Compress one third of the anterior-posterior diameter of the chest.
- **Drugs**
  - Give epinephrine if heart rate is <60 after 30 seconds of compressions and ventilation.
  - *Caution:* Epinephrine dosage is different for endotracheal and IV routes!
    - Epinephrine: 1:10,000 concentration
      - 0.1 to 0.3 mL/kg IV
      - 0.3 to 1 ml/kg via endotracheal tube (AHA/AAP, 2006)

---

propriate range at which oxygen levels should be maintained for newborns experiencing hypoxia, nor is there a standard time frame for oxygen to be administered (Neonatal Handbook, 2007d). While this uncertainty continues, nurses will experience a wide variation in practice in terms of modes of administration, monitoring, blood levels, and target ranges for both short- and long-term oxygen therapy.

A guiding principle, though, is that oxygen therapy should be targeted to levels appropriate to the condition, gestational age, and postnatal age of the newborn. Oxygen therapy must be used judiciously to prevent **retinopathy of prematurity (ROP)**, a major cause of blindness in preterm newborns in the past. ROP is a potentially blinding eye disorder that occurs when abnormal blood vessels grow and spread through the retina, eventually leading to retinal detachment. The incidence of ROP is inversely proportional to the preterm baby's birthweight. Approximately 400 to 600 children become blind because of ROP in the United States annually (Lyon & Warren, 2006).

Although the role of oxygen in the pathogenesis of ROP is unclear, current evidence suggests that it is linked to the duration of oxygen use rather than the concentration. Thus, the use of 100% oxygen to resuscitate a newborn should not pose a problem (National Eye Institute, 2007). However, an ophthalmology consult for follow-up after discharge is essential for preterm infants who have received extensive oxygen therapy. See Chapter 38 for a more in-depth discussion of this condition.

Respiratory distress in preterm infants is commonly caused by a deficiency of surfactant, retained fluid in the lungs (wet lung syndrome), meconium aspiration, pneumonia, hypothermia, or anemia. The principles of care are the same regardless of the cause of respiratory distress. First, keep the newborn warm, preferably in a warmed iso-lette or with an overhead radiant warmer, to conserve the baby's energy and prevent cold stress. Handle the newborn as little as possible, because stimulation often increases the oxygen requirement. Provide energy through calories via intravenous dextrose or gavage or continuous tube feedings to prevent hypoglycemia. Treat cyanosis with an oxygen hood or blow-by oxygen placed near the newborn's face if respiratory distress is mild and short-term therapy is needed. Record the following important observations every hour or more frequently if indicated, and document any deterioration or changes in respiratory status:

- Respiratory rate, quality of respirations, and respiratory effort
- Airway patency, including removal of secretions per facility policy
- Skin color, including any changes to duskiness, blueness, or pallor
- Lung sounds on auscultation to differentiate breath sounds in upper and lower fields
- Equipment required for oxygen delivery, such as:
  - Blow-by oxygen delivered via mask or tube for short-term therapy

FIGURE 23.4 **(A)** A preterm newborn receiving oxygen therapy via a nasal cannula. The newborn also has an enteral feeding tube inserted for nutrition. **(B)** A preterm newborn receiving mechanical ventilation.

- Oxygen hood (oxygen is delivered via a plastic hood placed over the newborn's head)
- Nasal cannula (oxygen is delivered directly through the nares) (Fig. 23.4A)
- Continuous positive airway pressure (CPAP), which prevents collapse of unstable alveoli and delivers high levels of inspired oxygen into the lungs
- Mechanical ventilation, which delivers consistent assisted ventilation and oxygen therapy, reducing the work of breathing for the fatigued infant (see Fig. 23.4B)
- Correct placement of endotracheal tube (if present)
- Heart rate, including any changes
- Oxygen saturation levels via pulse oximetry to evaluate need for therapy modifications based on hemoglobin
- Maintenance of oxygen saturation level from 87% to 95% (Aylott, 2006b)
- Nutritional intake, including calories provided, to prevent hypoglycemia and method of feeding, such as gavage, intravenous, or continuous enteral feedings
- Hydration status, including any signs and symptoms of fluid overload
- Laboratory tests, including ABGs, to determine effectiveness of oxygen therapy
- Administration of medication, such as exogenous surfactant

If the newborn shows worsening cyanosis or if oxygen saturation levels fall below 87%, prepare to give additional oxygen as ordered. Throughout care, strict asepsis, including handwashing, is vital to reduce the risk of infection.

Maintaining Thermal Regulation

Immediately after birth, dry the newborn with a warmed towel and then place him or her in a second warm, dry towel before performing the assessment. This drying prevents rapid heat loss secondary to evaporation. Newborns who are active, breathing well, and crying are stable and can be placed on their mother's chest ("kangaroo care") to promote warmth and prevent hypothermia. Preterm newborns who are not considered stable may be placed under a radiant warmer or in a warmed isolette after they are dried with a warmed towel.

Typically newborns use nonshivering thermogenesis for heat production by metabolizing their own brown adipose tissue. However, the preterm newborn has an inadequate supply of brown fat because he or she left the uterus before it was adequate. The preterm newborn also has decreased muscle tone and thus cannot assume the flexed fetal position, which reduces the amount of skin exposed to a cooler environment. In addition, preterm newborns have large body surface areas compared to weight. This allows an increased transfer of heat from their bodies to the environment.

Typically, a preterm newborn who is having problems with thermal regulation is cool to cold to the touch. The hands, feet, and tongue may appear cyanotic. Respirations are shallow or slow, or signs of respiratory distress are present. The newborn is lethargic and hypotonic, feeds poorly, and has a feeble cry. Blood glucose levels are probably low, leading to hypoglycemia, due to the energy expended to keep warm.

When promoting thermal regulation for the preterm newborn:

- Remember the four mechanisms for heat transfer and ways to prevent loss:
  - Convection: heat loss through air currents (avoid drafts near the newborn)
  - Conduction: heat loss through direct contact (warm everything the newborn comes in contact with, such as blankets, mattress, stethoscope)
  - Radiation: heat loss without direct contact (keep isolettes away from cold sources and provide insulation to prevent heat transfer)
  - Evaporation: heat loss by conversion of liquid into vapor (keep the newborn dry and delay the first bath until the baby's temperature is stable)

- Frequently assess the temperature of the isolette or radiant warmer, adjusting the temperature as necessary to prevent hypo- or hyperthermia.
- Assess the newborn's temperature every hour until stable.
- Observe for clinical signs of cold stress, such as respiratory distress, central cyanosis, hypoglycemia, lethargy, weak cry, abdominal distention, apnea, bradycardia, and acidosis.
- Remember the complications of hypothermia and frequently assess the newborn for signs:
  - Metabolic acidosis secondary to anaerobic metabolism used for heat production, which results in the production of lactic acid
  - Hypoglycemia due to depleted glycogen stores
  - Pulmonary hypertension secondary to pulmonary vasoconstriction
- Monitor the newborn for signs of hyperthermia such as tachycardia, tachypnea, apnea, warm to touch, flushed skin, lethargy, weak or absent cry, and CNS depression; adjust the environmental temperature appropriately.
- Explain to the parents the need to maintain the newborn's temperature, including the measures used; demonstrate ways to safeguard warmth and prevent heat loss.

Promoting Nutrition and Fluid Balance

Providing nutrition is challenging for preterm newborns because their needs are great but their ability to take in optimal amounts of energy/calories is reduced due to their compromised health status. Individual nutritional needs are highly variable.

Depending on their gestational age, preterm newborns receive nutrition orally, enterally, or parenterally via infusion. Several different methods can be used to provide nutrition: parenteral feedings administered through a percutaneous central venous catheter for long-term venous access with delivery of total parenteral nutrition (TPN), or enteral feedings, which can include oral feedings (formula or breast milk), continuous nasogastric tube feedings, or intermittent gavage tube feedings. Gavage feedings are commonly used for compromised newborns to allow them to rest during the feeding process. Many have a weak suck and become fatigued and thus cannot consume enough calories to meet their needs.

Most newborns born after 34 weeks' gestation without significant complications can feed orally. Those born before 34 weeks' gestation typically start with parenteral nutrition within the first 24 hours of life. Then enteral nutrition is introduced and advanced based on the degree of maturity and clinical condition. Ultimately, enteral nutrition methods replace parenteral nutrition.

To promote nutrition and fluid balance in the preterm newborn:

- Measure daily weight and plot it on a growth curve.
- Monitor intake; calculate fluid and caloric intake daily.
- Assess fluid status by monitoring weight; urinary output; urine specific gravity; laboratory test results such as serum electrolyte levels, blood urea nitrogen, creatinine, and hematocrit; skin turgor; and fontanels (Kenner & Lott, 2007). Be alert for signs of dehydration, such as a decrease in urinary output, sunken fontanels, temperature elevation, lethargy, and tachypnea.
- Continually assess for enteral feeding intolerance; measure abdominal girth, auscultate bowel sounds, and measure gastric residuals before the next tube feeding.
- Encourage and support breastfeeding by facilitating maternal breast pumping.
- Encourage nuzzling at the breast in conjunction with kangaroo care if the newborn is stable.

▶ **Take** NOTE!

When assessing the fluid status of a preterm newborn, palpate the fontanels. Sunken fontanels suggest dehydration; bulging fontanels suggest overhydration.

Preventing Infection

Prevention of infection is critical when caring for preterm newborns. Infections are the most common cause of morbidity and mortality in the NICU population (Kenner & Lott, 2007). Nursing assessment and early identification of problems are imperative to improve outcomes.

Preterm newborns are at risk for infection because their early birth deprived them of maternal antibodies needed for passive protection. Preterm newborns also are susceptible to infection because of their limited ability to produce antibodies, asphyxia at birth, and thin, friable skin that is easily traumatized, providing an entry portal for microorganisms.

Early detection is crucial. The clinical manifestations can be nonspecific and subtle: apnea, diminished activity, poor feeding, temperature instability, respiratory distress, seizures, tachycardia, hypotonia, irritability, pallor, jaundice, and hypoglycemia. Report any of these to the primary care provider immediately so that treatment can be instituted.

Include the following interventions when caring for a preterm or postterm newborn to prevent infection:

- Assess for risk factors in maternal history that place the newborn at increased risk.
- Monitor for changes in vital signs such as temperature instability, tachycardia, or tachypnea.
- Assess oxygen saturation levels and initiate oxygen therapy as ordered if oxygen saturation levels fall below acceptable parameters.
- Assess feeding tolerance, typically an early sign of infection.

- Monitor laboratory test results for changes.
- Avoid using tape on the newborn's skin to prevent tearing.
- Use equipment that can be thrown away after use.
- Adhere to standard precautions; use clean gloves to handle dirty diapers and dispose of them properly.
- Use sterile gloves when assisting with any invasive procedure; attempt to minimize the use of invasive procedures.
- Remove all jewelry on your hands prior to washing hands; wash hands upon entering the nursery and in between caring for newborns.
- Avoid coming to work when ill, and screen all visitors for contagious infections.

Preventing Complications

Preterm newborns face a myriad of possible complications as a result of their fragile health status or the procedures and treatments used. Some of the more common complications in preterm newborns include respiratory distress syndrome, periventricular-intraventricular hemorrhage, bronchopulmonary dysplasia, ROP, hyperbilirubinemia, anemia, necrotizing enterocolitis, hypoglycemia, infection or septicemia, delayed growth and development, and mental or motor delays (March of Dimes, 2007b). Several of these complications are described in Chapter 24.

Remember Anna, who was in a state of shock when she entered the NICU to see her preterm baby for the first time? How could the nurse have prepared her for this event? What information needs to be given at the isolette to reduce her anxiety and fear now?

Providing Appropriate Stimulation

Newborn stimulation involves a series of activities to encourage normal development. Research on developmental interventions shows that when preterm newborns, in particular, receive sensorimotor interventions such as rocking, skin-to-skin contact with parents, containment (swaddling and surrounded by blanket rolls), music, non-nutritive sucking, breastfeeding, massage, holding, or sleeping on waterbeds, they gain weight faster, progress in feeding abilities more quickly, and show improved interactive behavior compared to preterm newborns who were not stimulated (Field et al., 2006). Conversely, overstimulation may have negative effects by reducing oxygenation and causing stress. A newborn reacts to stress by flaying the hands or bringing an arm up to cover the face. When overstimulated, such as by noise, lights, excessive handling, alarms, and procedures, and stressed, heart and respiratory rates decrease and periods of apnea or bradycardia may follow (Blackburn, 2007).

Appropriate developmental stimulation that would not overtax the compromised newborn might include

FIGURE 23.5 A preterm newborn receiving non-nutritive sucking.

kangaroo (skin-to-skin) holding, rocking, soft singing or music, cuddling, gentle stroking of the infant's skin, colorful mobiles, gentle massage, waterbed mattresses, and non-nutritive sucking opportunities (Fig. 23.5) or providing sucrose if tolerated.

The NICU environment can be altered to provide periods of calm and rest for the newborn by dimming the lights, lowering the volume and tone of conversations, closing doors gently, setting the telephone ringer to the lowest volume possible, clustering nursing activities, and covering the isolette with a blanket to act as a light shield to promote rest at night.

Encourage parents to hold and interact with their newborn. Doing so helps to acquaint the parents with their newborn, promotes self-confidence, and fosters parent–newborn attachment (Fig. 23.6).

Think back to Anna, the woman who gave birth to a preterm newborn at 7 months' gestation. Anna will be discharged but her newborn will be staying in the NICU for a while. What interventions would be appropriate to facilitate bonding despite their separation? What support can be provided specifically to her family?

Managing Pain

Pain is an unpleasant sensory and emotional experience felt by all humans. Newborns feel pain and require the same level of pain assessment and management as adults. Common indicators of pain in the newborn who is unable

FIGURE 23.6 A mother bonding with her preterm newborn.

BOX 23.4 **Newborn Pain Prevention and Management Guidelines**

• Newborn pain frequently goes unrecognized and undertreated.
• Pain assessment is an essential activity prior to pain management.
• Newborns experience pain, and analgesics should be given.
• A procedure considered painful for an adult should also be considered painful for a newborn.
• Developmental maturity and health status must be considered when assessing for pain in newborns.
• Newborns may be more sensitive to pain than adults.
• Pain behavior is frequently mistaken for irritability and agitation.
• Newborns are more susceptible to the long-term effects of pain.
• Adequate pain management may reduce complications and mortality.
• Nonpharmacologic measures can prevent, reduce, or eliminate newborn pain.
• Sedation does not provide pain relief and may mask pain responses.
• A newborn's response to both pharmacologic and nonpharmacologic pain therapy should be assessed within 30 minutes of administration or intervention.
• Health care professionals are responsible for pain assessment and treatment.
• Written guidelines are needed on each newborn unit.

Source: Kenner & Lott, 2007.

to vocalize include facial expressions, body movements, and physiologic changes (Kenner & Lott, 2007). Untreated pain in newborns may result in increased morbidity and length of stay in the NICU, exaggerated responses to pain in later life, and altered psychosocial development (Koeppel, 2007). Parents commonly expect that health care providers will use appropriate measure to prevent pain in their newborns, but there are gaps in knowledge about the most effective way to accomplish this.

Assessment of pain in the newborn remains a contentious and vexing problem. Newborns in the NICU are subjected to repeated procedures that cause them pain. Newborns, whether preterm, full term, or postterm, do experience pain, but the pain is difficult to validate with consistent behaviors. Considering that ill newborns undergo multiple noxious stimuli from invasive procedures, such as lumbar punctures, heel sticks, venipuncture, line insertions, chest tube placement, specimen collections, endotracheal intubation and suctioning, and mechanical ventilation, common sense would suggest that newborns experience pain from these many activities and interventions. However, pain management in infants was not addressed formally until various professional and accrediting organizations issued position statements and clinical recommendations in an effort to promote effective pain management (AAP, 2006a, 2006b). An international consortium established principles of newborn pain prevention and management that all nurses must be familiar with and apply (Box 23.4).

Several psychometric tools are available to assess pain in the newborn. Examples include the Pain Assessment Tool (PAT), which evaluates respirations, heart rate, oxy-

gen saturation, and blood pressure; the Premature Infant Pain Profile (PIPP), which assesses heart rate and oxygen saturation; the CRIES tool (cry, requires oxygen, increased vital signs, expression and sleeplessness); and the Neonatal Infant Pain Scale (NIPS), which evaluates respiratory patterns. Most are based on facial expressions, crying patterns, change in vital signs, and body movements (AAP, 2006a). See Chapter 35 for a more in-depth discussion of pain assessment and management.

Nurses play a key role in assessing a newborn's pain level. Assess the newborn frequently. Pain is considered the "fifth vital sign" and should be assessed as frequently as the other four vital signs. Differentiate pain from agitation by observing for changes in vital signs, behavior, facial expression, and body movement. Suspect pain if the newborn exhibits the following:

• Sudden high-pitched cry
• Facial grimace with furrowing of brow and quivering chin
• Increased muscle tone
• Oxygen desaturation

- Body posturing, such as squirming, kicking, arching
- Limb withdrawal and thrashing movements
- Increase in heart rate, blood pressure, pulse, and respirations
- Fussiness and irritability (Arenson & Drake, 2007)

The goals of pain management are to minimize the amount, duration, and severity of pain and to assist the newborn in coping. Effective pain management strategies for newborns include preventing, limiting, or avoiding noxious stimuli; using nonpharmacologic techniques to reduce pain; and administering pharmacologic agents when appropriate. Box 23.5 lists some of the more commonly used nonpharmacologic pain management techniques for the preterm newborn.

The number of analgesics available for use with preterm newborns is limited. Morphine and fentanyl, usually administered intravenously, are the most commonly used opioids for moderate to severe pain. Acetaminophen is effective for mild pain. Benzodiazepines are used as sedatives during painful procedures and can be combined with opioids for more effectiveness. Local or topical anesthetics (e.g., EMLA cream) also may be used before procedures such as venipuncture, lumbar puncture, and intravenous catheter insertion (AAP, 2006b).

Be vigilant in assessing for adverse effects (respiratory depression or hypotension) when administering pharmacologic agents for pain management, especially in preterm newborns with neurologic impairment. These negative effects are usually dose- and route-related, so be knowledgeable about the pharmacokinetics and therapeutic dosing of any drug administered.

Promoting Growth and Development

In the late 1970s, researchers evaluated the NICU environment in terms of light and sound levels, caregiving activities, and handling of newborns. As a result of this research, many environmental modifications were made to reduce the stress and overstimulation of the NICU, and the concept of developmentally supportive care was introduced. Developmentally supportive care is defined as care of a newborn or infant to support positive growth and development. Developmental care focuses on what newborns or infants can do at that stage of development; it uses therapeutic interventions only to the point that they are beneficial; and it provides for the development of the newborn–family unit (Neonatal Handbook, 2007b).

Developmental care is a philosophy of care that requires rethinking the relationships between newborns, families, and health care providers. It includes a variety of activities designed to manage the environment and individualize the care of the preterm or high-risk ill newborn based on behavioral observations (see Evidence-Based Practice 23.1). The goal is to promote a stable, well-organized newborn who can conserve energy for growth and development (Hendricks-Munoz & Prendergast, 2007).

Developmental care includes these strategies:

- Clustering care to promote rest and conserve the infant's energy
- Flexed positioning to simulate in utero positioning
- Environmental management to reduce noise and visual stimulation
- Kangaroo care to promote skin-to-skin sensation
- Placement of twins in the same isolette or open crib to reduce stress
- Activities to promote self-regulation and state regulation:
  - Surrounding the newborn with nesting rolls/devices
  - Swaddling with a blanket to maintain the flexed position
  - Providing sheepskin or a waterbed to simulate the uterine environment
  - Providing non-nutritive sucking (calms the infant)
  - Providing objects to grasp (comforts the newborn)
- Promotion of parent–infant bonding by making parents feel welcome in the NICU
- Open, honest communication with parents and staff
- Collaboration with the parents in planning the infant's care (Davidson et al., 2007)

Developmental care can be fostered by clustering the lights in one area so that no lights are shining directly on newborns, installing visual alarm systems and limiting overhead pages to minimize noise, and monitoring continuous and peak noise levels. Nurses can play an active role

---

BOX 23.5 **Nonpharmacologic Techniques to Reduce Pain in the Preterm Newborn**

- Gentle handling, rocking, caressing, cuddling, and massaging
- Rest periods before and after painful procedures
- Kangaroo care (skin-to-skin contact) during procedure
- Breastfeeding, if able, to reduce pain from minor procedures
- Use of a facilitated tuck (holding arms and legs in a flexed position)
- Application of topical anesthetics prior to venipuncture or lumbar puncture
- Swaddling and positioning to establish physical boundaries
- Non-nutritive sucking (pacifier dipped in sucrose) prior to procedure
- Minimal use of tape, with gentle removal to avoid skin tears
- Warm blankets for wrapping to facilitate relaxation
- Reduction of environmental stimuli by removing or turning down noxious stimuli such as noise from alarms, beepers, loud conversations, and bright lights
- Distraction, such as with colored objects or mobiles (AAP, 2006a, 2006b)

EVIDENCE-BASED PRACTICE 23.1
Promoting Development and Preventing Morbidity in Preterm Infants

● Study

Preterm newborns are at risk due to their immature body systems. This is compounded by the newborn's increased risk for complications and illnesses and his or her exposure to numerous stimuli in the NICU environment. Together, these stressors can interfere with the newborn's growth and development. Developmental care is a philosophy that includes a wide range of activities to manage the environment and individualize care. The belief is that it can reduce the effects of these stressors. Activities typically associated with developmental care include controlling external stimuli, clustering care activities, and positioning and swaddling the preterm newborn.

A study was done to examine the effects of developmental care on preterm newborns. The study evaluated relevant outcomes such as neurodevelopment, weight gain, length of hospital stay, duration of mechanical ventilation, and physiologic stress. A computerized search of all articles, controlled trials, and conference and symposia proceedings was done. Two independent experts identified the data from all relevant randomized trials that compared the elements of developmental care to routine nursery care for newborns less than 37 weeks' gestation. The researchers identified 36 controlled trials.

▲ Findings

Assessing the benefits of developmental care was difficult because most of the studies reviewed included multiple interventions and many of the trials had small sample sizes. Therefore, the authors could not determine whether any one intervention was more effective than another. Overall, they reported that developmental care had limited benefits and no major harmful effects. It had a limited benefit on decreasing moderate to severe chronic lung disease, decreasing the incidence of necrotizing colitis, and improving family outcomes. Evidence was also limited related to the long-term positive effect on behavior and movement at 5 years corrected age. However, individualized developmental care activities showed some positive effects in improving neurodevelopmental outcomes.

■ Nursing Implications

Although the study found that developmental care for preterm newborns was of limited benefit, it emphasized that this type of care had no major harmful effects. Nurses can integrate these findings into their care for preterm newborns with the understanding that they are beneficial but that the effect may be limited. Nurses can advocate for individualizing the activities involved in developmental care based on the newborn's needs. They also can play a key role in fostering research to help determine which stressors seem to be the most troublesome and which specific activities are of the greatest benefit. In addition, nurses can assist in identifying appropriate short- and long-term outcome measures.

Symington, A., & Pinelli, J. (2006). Developmental care for promoting development and preventing morbidity in preterm infants. *Cochrane Database of Systematic Reviews* 2006. Issue 2. Art. No.: CD001814. DOI: 10.1002/14651858.CD001814.pub2.

by serving on committees that address these issues. In addition, nurses can provide direct developmentally supportive care. Doing so involves careful planning of nursing activities to provide the ideal environment for the newborn's development. For example:

- Dim the lights and cover isolettes at night to simulate nighttime.
- Support early extubation from mechanical ventilation.
- Encourage early and consistent feedings with breast milk.
- Administer prescribed antibiotics judiciously.
- Position the newborn as if he or she was still in utero (a nesting fetal position).
- Promote kangaroo care by encouraging parents to hold the newborn against the chest for extended periods each day.
- Coordinate care to respect sleep and awake states.

Throughout the newborn's stay, work with the parents, developing a collaborative partnership so they feel comfortable caring for their newborn. Be prepared to make referrals to community support groups to enhance coping (McGrath, 2006).

Promoting Parental Coping

Generally, pregnancy and the birth of a newborn are exciting times, but when the newborn has serious, perhaps life-threatening problems, the exciting experience suddenly changes to one of anxiety, fear, guilt, loss, and grief.

Parents are typically unprepared for the birth of a preterm newborn and commonly experience an array of emotions, including disappointment, fear for the survival of the newborn, and anxiety due to the separation from their newborn immediately after birth (Mok & Sui, 2006). Early interruptions in the bonding process and concern about the newborn's survival can create extreme anxiety and interfere with attachment (Mercer & Walker, 2006).

Nursing interventions aimed at reducing parental anxiety include:

- Reviewing with them the events that have occurred since birth
- Providing simple relaxation and calming techniques (visual imagery, breathing)
- Exploring their perception of the newborn's condition and offering explanations
- Validating their anxiety and behaviors as normal reactions to stress and trauma
- Providing a physical presence and support during emotional outbursts
- Exploring the coping strategies they used successfully in the past and encouraging their use now
- Encouraging frequent visits to the NICU
- Addressing their reactions to the NICU environment and explaining all equipment used
- Identifying family and community resources available to them (Franklin, 2006)

Preparing for Discharge

Discharge planning typically begins with evidence that recovery of the newborn is certain. However, the exact date of discharge may not be predictable. The goal of the discharge plan is to make a successful transition to home care. Essential elements for discharge are a physiologically stable infant, a family who can provide the necessary care with appropriate support services in place in the community, and a primary care physician available for ongoing care.

The care of each high-risk newborn after discharge requires careful coordination to provide ongoing multidisciplinary support for the family. The discharge planning team typically includes the parents, primary care physician, neonatologists, neonatal nurses, and a social worker. Other professionals, such as surgical specialists and pediatric subspecialists, occupational, physical, speech, and respiratory therapists, nutritionists, home health care nurses, and a case manager, may be included as needed. Critical components of discharge planning are summarized in Box 23.6.

Nurses involved in the discharge process are instrumental in bridging the gap between the hospital and home. Interventions typically include:

- Assessing the physical status of the mother and the newborn
- Discussing the early signs of complications and what to do if they occur
- Reinforcing instructions for infant care and safety
- Stressing the importance of proper car seat use
- Providing instructions for medication administration
- Reinforcing instructions for equipment operation, maintenance, and troubleshooting
- Teaching infant cardiopulmonary resuscitation and emergency care

BOX 23.6 Critical Components of Discharge Planning

- Parental education—involvement and support in newborn care during NICU stay will ensure their readiness to care for the infant at home
- Evaluation of unresolved medical problems—review of the active problem list and determination of what home care and follow-up is needed
- Implementation of primary care—completion of newborn screening tests, immunizations, examinations such as funduscopic exam for ROP, and hematologic status evaluation
- Development of home care plan, including assessment of:
  - Equipment and supplies needed for care
  - In-home caregiver's preparation and ability to care for infant
  - Adequacy of the physical facilities in the home
  - An emergency care and transport plan if needed
  - Financial resources for home care costs
  - Family needs and coping skills
  - Community resources, including how they can be accessed

- Demonstrating techniques for special care procedures such as dressings, ostomy care, artificial airway maintenance, chest physiotherapy, suctioning, and infant stimulation
- Providing breastfeeding support or instruction on gavage feedings
- Assisting with defining roles in the adjustment period at home
- Assessing the parents' emotional stability and coping status
- Providing support and reassurance to the family
- Reporting abnormal findings to the health care team for intervention
- Following up with parents to assure them that they have a "lifeline"

Dealing With Perinatal Loss

Perinatal loss is a profound experience for the family. It engenders a unique kind of mourning since the infant is so much a part of the parents' identity. Instead of celebrating a new life as they expected, parents are mourning the loss of dreams and hopes and the loss of an extension of themselves. NICU nurses face a difficult situation when caring for newborns who may not survive. Newborn death is incomprehensible to most parents. This makes the grieving process more difficult because what is happening "can't be real." Deciding whether to see, touch, or hold the dying newborn is extremely difficult for many parents. Nurses play a major role in assisting parents to make their dying newborn "real" to them by providing them with as many memories as possible and encouraging them to see, hold, touch, dress, and take care of the infant and take photographs. These actions help to validate the parents' sense of loss, relive the experience, and attach significance to the meaning of loss. A lock of hair, a name card, or an identification bracelet may serve as important mementoes that can ease the grieving process. The memories created by these interventions can be useful allies in the grieving process and in resolving grief (Callister, 2006).

Parent–newborn interaction is vital to the normal processes of attachment and bonding. The detachment process involved in a newborn's death is equally important for parents. Nurses can aid in this process by helping parents to see their newborn through the maze of equipment, explaining the various procedures and equipment, encouraging them to express their feelings about the newborn's status, and providing time for them to be with their dying newborn (Kavanaugh & Moro, 2006).

A common reaction by many people when learning that a newborn is not going to survive is one of avoidance. Nurses are no exception. It is difficult to initiate a conver-

sation about such a sensitive issue without knowing how the parents are going to react and cope with the impending loss. One way to begin a conversation with the parents is to convey concern and acknowledge their loss. Active listening can give parents a safe place to begin the healing process. The relationship that the nurse establishes with the parents is a unique one, providing an opportunity for both the nurse and the parents to share their feelings.

Be aware of personal feelings about loss and how these feelings are part of one's own life and personal belief system. Actively listen to the parents when they are talking about their experiences. Communicate empathy (understanding and feeling what another person is feeling), respect their feelings, and respond to them in helpful and supportive ways (Kavanaugh & Moro, 2006). Table 23.2 highlights appropriate interventions for a family experiencing a perinatal loss before and after a newborn dies.

In a time of crisis or loss, individuals are often more sensitive to other people's reactions. For example, the parents may be extremely aware of the nurse's facial expressions, choice of words, and tone of voice. Talking quickly,

TABLE 23.2 ASSISTING PARENTS TO COPE WITH PERINATAL LOSS

Before the newborn's death	Respect variations in the family's spiritual needs and readiness. Assess cultural beliefs and practices that may bring comfort; respect culturally appropriate requests for truth telling and informed refusal. Initiate spiritual comfort by calling the hospital clergy if appropriate; offer to pray with the family if appropriate. Encourage the parents to take photographs, make memory boxes, and record their thoughts in a journal. Explore with family members how they dealt with previous losses. Discuss techniques to reduce stress, such as meditation and relaxation. Recommend that family members maintain a healthy diet and get adequate rest and exercise to preserve their health. Participate in early and repeated care conferencing to reduce family stress. Allow family to be present at both medical rounds and resuscitation; provide explanations of all procedures, treatments, and findings; answer questions honestly and as completely as possible. Provide opportunities for the family to hold the newborn if they choose to. Assess the family's support network. Provide suggestions as to how friends can be helpful to the family.
After the newborn's death	Help the family to accept the reality of death by using the word "died." Acknowledge their grief and the fact that their newborn has died. Help the family to work through their grief by validating and listening. Provide the family with realistic information about the causes of death. Offer condolences to the family in a sincere manner. Encourage the father to cry and grieve with his partner. Provide opportunities for the family to hold the newborn if they desire.
At the time of the release of the newborn's body	Reassure the family that their feelings and grieving responses are normal. Encourage the parents to have a funeral or memorial service to bring closure. Suggest that the parents plant a tree or flowers to remember the infant. Address attachment issues concerning subsequent pregnancies. Provide information about local support groups. Provide anticipatory guidance regarding the grieving process. Present information about any impact on future childbearing, and refer the parents to appropriate specialists or genetic resources.

Sources: Callister, 2006; Cote-Arsenault & Donato, 2007; Kobler, Limbo, & Kavanaugh, 2007.

in a businesslike fashion, or ignoring the loss may inhibit parents from discussing their pain or how they are coping with it. Parents may need to vent their frustrations and anger, and the nurse may become the target. Validate their feelings and attempt to reframe or refocus the anger toward the real issue of loss. An example would be to say, "I understand your frustration and anger about this situation. You have experienced a tremendous loss and it must be difficult not to have an explanation for it at this time." Doing so helps to defuse the anger while allowing them to express their feelings.

When assisting bereaved parents, start where the parents are in the grief process to avoid imposing your own agenda on them. You may feel uncomfortable at not being able to change the situation or take the pain away. The nurse's role is to provide immediate emotional support and facilitate the grieving process. Supporting and strengthening the family bond in the face of perinatal loss is essential.

▶ LATE PRETERM NEWBORN

A late preterm newborn is an infant born between 34 weeks and 36 weeks, 6 days of gestation. In recent years, the subject of late preterm birth has received much attention, since this population of preterm newborns represents more than 70% of all preterm births in the United States and has increased by 30% in the past 20 years (National Center for Health Statistics, 2006). With the sharp rise in the number of cesarean births performed, the incidence of late preterm newborns will also rise. Perinatal nurses need to understand the risks of late preterm births and the unique needs of this population to facilitate timely assessment and intervention to improve outcomes.

Some of the challenges facing the late preterm newborn include respiratory distress (secondary to cesarean births, maternal gestational diabetes, chorioamnionitis, premature rupture of membranes, and fetal distress); thermoregulation issues related to limited ability to flex the trunk and extremities to decrease exposed surface area; hypoglycemia related to the first two challenges (respiratory distress and cold stress); jaundice and hyperbilirubinemia related to a gestational age of 36 weeks or less; and feeding challenges related to immature suck and swallowing reflexes (Askin et al., 2007). These challenges are similar to those facing the preterm newborn and require similar management. Nurses and parents must be aware of the risks associated with late preterm births to optimize care and outcomes for this group of newborns.

■■■ Key Concepts

■ Variations in birthweight and gestational age can place a newborn at risk for problems that require special care.

■ Variations in birthweight include the following categories: small for gestational age, appropriate for gestational age, and large for gestational age. Newborns who are small or large for gestational age have special needs.

■ The small-for-gestational-age newborn faces problems related to a decrease in placental function in utero; these problems may include perinatal asphyxia, hypothermia, hypoglycemia, polycythemia, and meconium aspiration.

■ Risk factors for the birth of a large-for-gestational-age infant include maternal diabetes mellitus or glucose intolerance, multiparity, prior history of a macrosomic infant, postdates gestation, maternal obesity, male fetus, and genetics. Large-for-gestational-age newborns face problems such as birth trauma due to cephalopelvic disproportion, hypoglycemia, and jaundice secondary to hyperbilirubinemia.

■ Variations in gestational age include postterm and preterm newborns. Postterm newborns may be large or small for gestational age or dysmature, depending on placental function.

■ The postterm newborn may develop several complications after birth, including fetal hypoxia, hypoglycemia, hypothermia, polycythemia, and meconium aspiration.

■ Preterm birth is the leading cause of death within the first month of life and the second leading cause of all infant deaths.

■ The preterm newborn is at risk for complications because his or her organ systems are immature, thereby impeding the transition from intrauterine life to extrauterine life.

■ Newborns can experience pain, but their pain is difficult to validate with consistent behaviors.

■ Newborns with gestational age variations, primarily preterm newborns, benefit from developmental care, which includes a variety of activities designed to manage the environment and individualize the care based on behavioral observations.

■ Nurses play a key role in assisting the parents and family of a newborn with special needs to cope with this crisis situation, including dealing with the possibility that the newborn may not survive. Nurses working with parents experiencing a perinatal loss can help by actively listening, understanding the parents' experiences, and communicating empathy.

■ The goal of discharge planning is to make a successful transition to home care.

REFERENCES

American Academy of Pediatrics (AAP). (2006a). *Guidelines for neonatal resuscitation: Translating evidence-based guidelines for NRP.* Available at: http://www.aap.org/nrp/nrpmain.html.

American Academy of Pediatrics (AAP). (2006b). Prevention and management of pain in the neonate: An update. *Pediatrics, 118*(5), 2231–2241.

American Heart Association (AHA) and American Academy of Pediatrics (AAP). (2006). Neonatal resuscitation program (NRP). *Neonatal Network, 25*(2), 145–151.

Arenson, J., & Drake, P. (2007). *Maternal and newborn health.* Sudbury, MA: Jones and Bartlett Publishers.

Askin, D. F., Bakewell-Sachs, S., Medoff-Cooper, B., Rosenberg, S., & Santa-Donato, A. (2007). Late preterm infant assessment guide. *AWHONN,* Washington, DC.

Aylott, M. (2006a). The neonatal energy triangle. Part 1: Metabolic adaptation. *Pediatric Nursing, 18*(6), 38–42.

Aylott, M. (2006b). The neonatal energy triangle. Part 2: Thermoregulation and respiratory adaptation. *Pediatric Nursing, 18*(7), 38–42.

Blackburn, S. (2007). *Maternal, fetal and neonatal physiology: A clinical perspective* (3rd ed.). Philadelphia: Saunders Elsevier.

Callister, L. C. (2006). Perinatal loss. *Journal of Perinatal & Neonatal Nursing, 20*(3), 227–234.

Clark, D. A., & Clark, M. B. (2007). Meconium aspiration syndrome. *eMedicine.* Available at: www.emedicine.com/ped/topic768.htm.

Côté-Arsenault, D., & Donato, K. (2007). Restrained expectations in late pregnancy following loss. *JOGNN: Journal of Obstetric, Gynecologic, & Neonatal Nursing, 36*(6), 550–557.

Cunningham, F. G., Leveno, K. J., Bloom, S. L., Hauth, J. C., Gilstrap, L. C., & Wenstrom, K. D. (2005). *Williams obstetrics* (22nd ed.). New York: McGraw-Hill.

Davidson, J. E., Powers, K., Hedayat, K. M., et al. (2007). Clinical practice guidelines for support of the family in the patient-centered intensive care unit: American College of Critical Care Medicine Task Force. *Critical Care Medicine, 35*(2), 605–622.

Deshpande, S. (2007). Early postnatal blood lactate predicts short-term outcome in infants with perinatal asphyxia. *Early Human Development, 83*(2), 128–129.

Dorland, W. A. N. (2007). *Dorland's illustrated medical dictionary* (30th ed.). St. Louis: Saunders Elsevier.

Field, T., Hernandez-Reif, M., Feijo, L., & Freedman, J. (2006). Prenatal, perinatal and neonatal stimulation: A survey of neonatal nurseries. *Infant Behavior & Development, 29*(1), 24–31.

Franklin, C. (2006). The neonatal nurse's role in parental attachment in the NICU. *Critical Care Nursing Quarterly, 29*(1), 81–85.

Galligan, M. (2006). Proposed guidelines for skin-to-skin treatment of neonatal hypothermia. *MCN, 31*(5), 298–306.

Gilbert, E. S. (2007). *Manual of high-risk pregnancy and delivery* (4th ed.). St. Louis: Mosby.

Harper, T., & Lam, G. (2007). Fetal growth restriction. *eMedicine.* Available at: www.emedicine.com/med/topic3247.htm.

Hendricks-Munoz, K. D., & Prendergast, C. C. (2007). Barriers to provision of developmental care in the NICU: Neonatal nursing perceptions. *American Journal of Perinatology, 24*(2), 71–77.

Herranz, L., Pallardo, L., Hillman, N., et al. (2007). Maternal third trimester hyperglycemic excursions predict large-for-gestational-age infants in type 1 diabetic pregnancy. *Diabetes Research & Clinical Practice, 75*(1), 42–46.

Jazayeri, A. (2007). Macrosomia. *eMedicine.* Available at: http://www.emedicine.com/med/topic3279.htm.

Kates, E. H., & Kates, J. S. (2007). Anemia and polycythemia in the newborn. *Pediatrics in Review, 28*(1), 33–35.

Kavanaugh, K., & Morro, T. (2006). Supporting parents after stillbirth or newborn death. *AJN, 106*(9), 74–79.

Kenner, C., & Lott, J. W. (2007). *Comprehensive neonatal care: An interdisciplinary approach* (4th ed.). St. Louis: Saunders.

Kipiani, T., Tatisvili, N., & Sirbiladze, T. (2007). Long-term neurological developments of the preterm newborns. *Georgian Medical News, 142,* 42–45.

Kobler, K., Limbo, R., & Kavanaugh, K. (2007). Meaningful moments: The use of ritual in perinatal and pediatric death. *MCN: The American Journal of Maternal Child Nursing, 32*(5), 288–297.

Koeppel, R. (2007). Assessment and management of acute pain in the newborn. *AWHONN.* Available at: http://www.awhonn.org.

Kristensen, S., Salihu, H., Keith, L., et al. (2007). SGA subtypes and mortality risk among singleton births. *Early Human Development, 83*(2), 99–105.

Laroia, N. (2006). Birth trauma. *eMedicine.* Available at: www.emedicine.com/ped/topic2836.htm.

Lessaris, K. J. (2007). Polycythemia of the newborn. *eMedicine.* Available at: www.emedicine.com/ped/topic2479.htm.

Leu, M., & Diament, MJ. (2006). Meconium aspiration. *eMedicine.* Available at: www.emedicine.com/radio/topic426.htm.

Lissauer, T., & Weindling, A. (2006). *Neonatology at a glance.* Ames, IA: Blackwell Publishers.

Lyon, D. W., & Warren, D. F. (2006). A clinical guide to retinopathy of prematurity. *Review of Optometry, 143*(12), 53–61.

March of Dimes. (2007a). *Diabetes in pregnancy.* Available at: http://www.marchofdimes.com/professionals/14332_1197.asp.

March of Dimes. (2007b). *Complications of preterm birth.* Available at: www.marchofdimes.com/prematurity/5512.asp.

March of Dimes. (2007c). *Prematurity.* Available at: www.marchofdimes.com/prematurity/5408_5576.asp.

McGrath, J. M. (2006). Family-centered developmental care begins before birth. *Journal of Perinatal & Neonatal Nursing, 20*(3), 195–196.

Melnyk, B. M., Feinstein, N., & Fairbanks, E. (2006). Two decades of evidence to support implementation of the COPE program as standard practice with parents of young children unexpectedly hospitalized/critically ill children and premature infants. *Pediatric Nursing, 32*(5), 475–481.

Mercer, R. T., & Walker, L. O. (2006). A review of nursing interventions to foster becoming a mother. *JOGNN, 35*(5), 568–582.

Mok, E., & Sui, L. (2006). Nurses as providers of support for mothers of premature infants. *Journal of Clinical Nursing, 15*(6), 726–734.

National Center for Health Statistics (NCHS). (2006). Percent distribution of preterm births in the United States. *National Vital Statistics Reports, 55*(1), 22.

National Eye Institute. (2007). *Retinopathy of prematurity (ROP).* U.S. National Institutes of Health Resource Guide. Available at: http://nei.nih.gov/health/rop/index.asp.

Neonatal Handbook. (2007a). *Breastfeeding issues.* Available at: http://www.netsvic.org.au/nets/handbook/?doc_id=907.

Neonatal Handbook. (2007b). *Developmental care.* Available at: http://www.netsvic.org.au/nets/handbook/?doc_id=719.

Neonatal Handbook. (2007c). *Jaundice in the first two weeks of life.* Available at: http://www.netsvic.org.au/nets/handbook/?doc_id=458.

Neonatal Handbook. (2007d). *Respiratory distress syndrome.* Available at: http://www.rwh.org.au/nets/handbook/index.cfm?doc_id=603.

Neonatal Handbook. (2007e). *Small-for-gestational-age infants.* Available at: http://www.netsvic.org.au/nets/handbook/?doc_id=821.

Neonatal Handbook. (2007f). *Infant of a diabetic mother.* Available at: http://www.netsvic.org.au/nets/handbook/?doc_id=889.

Neonatal Handbook. (2007g). *Polycythemia.* Available at: http://www.netsvic.org.au/nets/handbook/?doc_id=636.

Neonatal Handbook. (2007h). *Nutrition of the preterm infant.* Available at: http://www.rch.org.au/nets/handbook/index.cfm?doc_id=909.

Neonatal Handbook. (2007i). *Perinatal asphyxia.* Available at: http://www.rch.org.au/nets/handbook/index.cfm?doc_id=11236.

Neonatal Handbook. (2007j). *Metabolic diseases.* Available at: http://www.rch.org.au/nets/handbook/index.cfm?doc_id=895.

Stanley, C. A. (2006). Hypoglycemia in the neonate. *Pediatric Endocrinology Reviews, 4*(1), 76–81.

U.S. Department of Health and Human Services (USDHHS), Public Health Service. (2000). *Healthy People 2010* (conference edition, in two volumes). Washington, DC.: U.S. Government Printing Office.

Vargo, L. E., & Trotter, C. W. (2007). The premature infant: Nursing assessment and management. *March of Dimes Nursing Modules* (2nd ed.). #33-1995-05.

WEBSITES

March of Dimes: www.marchofdimes.com

National Association of Neonatal Nurses: www.nann.org

Neonatal Network: www.neonatalnetwork.com

Parental Guide for Developmentally Supportive Care: www.comeunity.com/premature/baby/supportive-care.html

Physical and Developmental Environment of the High-Risk Infant: www.med.usf.edu/tsinger

Premature Infant: www.premature-infant.com

CHAPTER WORKSHEET

MULTIPLE CHOICE QUESTIONS

1. The nurse documents that a newborn is postterm based on the understanding that he was born after:

   a. 38 weeks' gestation

   b. 40 weeks' gestation

   c. 42 weeks' gestation

   d. 44 weeks' gestation

2. SGA and LGA newborns have an excessive number of red blood cells because of:

   a. Hypoxia

   b. Hypoglycemia

   c. Hypocalcemia

   d. Hypothermia

3. Because subcutaneous and brown fat stores were used for survival in utero, the nurse would assess an SGA newborn for which of the following?

   a. Hyperbilirubinemia

   b. Hypothermia

   c. Polycythemia

   d. Hypoglycemia

4. In assessing a preterm newborn, which of the following findings would be of greatest concern?

   a. Milia over the bridge of the nose

   b. Thin transparent skin

   c. Poor muscle tone

   d. Heart murmur

5. In dealing with parents experiencing a perinatal loss, which of the following nursing interventions would be most appropriate?

   a. Sheltering the parents from the bad news

   b. Making all the decisions regarding care

   c. Encouraging them to participate in the newborn's care

   d. Leaving them by themselves to allow time to grieve

6. The nurse is providing care to several newborns with variations in gestational age and birthweight. When developing the plan of care for these newborns, the nurse focuses on energy conservation to promote growth and development. Which measures would the nurse include in the nursing plans of care? Select all that apply.

   a. Keeping the handling of the newborn to a minimum

   b. Maintaining a neutral thermal environment

   c. Decreasing environmental stimuli

   d. Initiating early oral feedings

   e. Using thermal warmers in all cribs

7. Which of the following concepts would the nurse incorporate into the plan of care when assessing pain in a newborn with special needs?

   a. Newborns experience pain primarily with surgical procedures.

   b. Preterm newborns in the NICU are at least risk for pain.

   c. Pain assessment needs to be comprehensive and frequent.

   d. A newborn's facial expression is the primary indicator of pain.

CRITICAL THINKING EXERCISES

1. After fetal distress was noted on the monitor, a postterm newborn was delivered via a difficult vacuum extraction. The newborn had low Apgar scores and had to be resuscitated before being transferred to the nursery. Once admitted, the nurse observed the following behaviors: jitteriness, tremors, hypotonia, lethargy, and rapid respirations.

   a. What might these behaviors indicate?

   b. For what other conditions might this newborn be at high risk?

   c. What intervention is needed to address this newborn's condition?

2. A preterm newborn was born at 35 weeks following an abruptio placentae due to a car accident. He was transported to the NICU at a nearby regional medical center. After being stabilized, he was placed in an isolette close to the door and placed on a cardiac monitor. A short time later, the nurse notices that he is cool to the touch and lethargic, has a weak cry, and has an axillary temperature of 36°C.

   a. What might have contributed to this newborn's hypothermic condition?

b. What transfer mechanism may have been a factor?

c. What intervention would be appropriate for the nurse to initiate?

3. A term SGA newborn weighing 4 lb was brought to the nursery for admission a short time after birth. The labor and birth nurse reports the mother was a heavy smoker and a cocaine addict and experienced physical abuse throughout her pregnancy. After stabilizing the newborn and correcting the hypoglycemia with oral feedings, the nurse observes the following: acrocyanosis, ruddy color, poor circulation to the extremities, tachypnea, and irritability.

a. What complication might this SGA newborn be manifesting?

b. What factors may have contributed to this complication?

c. What would be an appropriate intervention to manage this condition?

STUDY ACTIVITIES

1. At a community health department maternity clinic, secure permission to interview the parents of a special needs child. Ask about their feelings throughout the experience. How are they managing and coping now?

2. Visit the March of Dimes website and review this group's national campaign to reduce the incidence of prematurity. Are their strategies workable or not? Explain your reasoning.

3. A common metabolic disorder present in both SGA and LGA newborns after birth is

_____.

4. A 10-lb LGA newborn is brought to the nursery after a difficult vaginal birth. The nursery nurse should focus on detecting birth injuries such as

_____.

NURSING MANAGEMENT OF THE NEWBORN AT RISK: ACQUIRED AND CONGENITAL NEWBORN CONDITIONS

KEY TERMS

alcohol–related birth
    defects
asphyxia
caput succedaneum
cephalhematoma
fetal alcohol spectrum
    disorder

fetal alcohol syndrome
gastrochisis
hyperbilirubinemia
infant of a diabetic mother
kernicterus
meconium aspiration
    syndrome

neonatal abstinence
    syndrome
neonatal sepsis
omphalocele
respiratory distress
    syndrome

Kelly, a 27-year-old G2P1, comes to the labor and birth area in active labor. She tells you she is overdue and relieved to finally be giving birth. Her membranes rupture on admission, revealing meconium-stained fluid. What additional nursing assessments need to be carried out now? What risk factors need to be considered in when developing Kelly's plan of care?

LEARNING OBJECTIVES

After completion of the chapter, the learner will be able to:

1. Identify the most common acquired conditions affecting the newborn.
2. Describe the nursing management of a newborn experiencing respiratory distress syndrome.
3. Outline the birthing room preparation and procedures necessary to prevent meconium aspiration syndrome in the newborn at birth.
4. Differentiate risk factors for the development of necrotizing enterocolitis.
5. Explain the impact of maternal diabetes on the newborn and the care needed.
6. Describe the assessment and intervention for a newborn experiencing substance withdrawal after birth.
7. Identify assessment and nursing management for newborns sustaining trauma and birth injuries.
8. Outline the assessment, interventions, prevention, and management of hyperbilirubinemia in newborns.
9. Summarize the interventions appropriate for a newborn with neonatal sepsis.
10. Describe four gastrointestinal system congenital anomalies that can occur in a newborn.

Wow

Courage and faith in oneself project onto others, giving them the strength to persevere.

LEARNING OBJECTIVES (continued)

11. Formulate a plan of care for a newborn with an acquired or congenital condition.
12. Discuss the importance of parental participation in care of the newborn with a congenital or acquired condition, including the nurse's role in facilitating parental involvement.

Advances in prenatal and neonatal medical and nursing care throughout the industrialized world have led to a marked increase in the number of newborns who have survived a high-risk pregnancy but experience acquired or congenital conditions. These newborns are considered at risk: that is, they are susceptible to morbidity and mortality because of the acquired or congenital disorder. Several National Health Goals address the issues of acquired and congenital conditions in newborns (Healthy People 2010 24.1).

Technological and pharmacologic advances, in conjunction with standardized policies and procedures, over the past several decades have significantly improved survival rates for at-risk newborns. However, morbidity remains an important sequela. For example, some of these newborns are at risk for continuing health problems that require long-term technological support. Other newborns remain at risk for physical and developmental problems into the school years and beyond. Providing the complex care needed to maintain the child's health and well-being will have a tremendous emotional and economic impact on the family. Nurses are challenged to provide support to mothers and their families when neonatal well-being is threatened.

Acquired disorders typically occur at or soon after birth. They may result from problems or conditions experienced by the woman during her pregnancy or at birth, such as diabetes, maternal infection, or substance abuse, or conditions associated with labor and birth, such as prolonged rupture of membranes or fetal distress. However, there may be no identifiable cause for the disorder.

Congenital disorders are disorders present at birth, usually due to some type of malformation that occurred during the antepartal period. Congenital disorders, which typically involve a problem with inheritance, include structural anomalies (commonly referred to as birth defects), chromosomal disorders, and inborn errors of metabolism. Most congenital disorders have a complex etiology, involving many interacting genes, gene products, and social and environmental factors during organogenesis. Some alterations can be prevented or compensated for with pharmacologic, nutritional, or other types of interventions, while others cannot be changed. Only through a better understanding of the complex interplay of genetic, environmental, social, and cultural factors can these

HEALTHY PEOPLE 2010	
Objective	**Significance**

1. Reduce fetal and infant deaths
  Decrease the number of all infant deaths (within 1 year) from a baseline of 7.2/ 1,000 live births to 4.5/ 1,000 live births.
  Decrease the number of neonatal deaths (within the first 28 days of life) from a baseline of 4.8 to 2.9 deaths/ 1,000 live births.
  Decrease the number of post-neonatal deaths from a baseline of 2.4 to 1.2 deaths/ 1,000 live births.
  Reduce the number of deaths related to all birth defects from a baseline of 1.6 to 1.1 deaths/1,000 live births.
	Will foster early and consistent prenatal care, including education to place infants on their backs for naps and sleeping to prevent SIDS and avoidance of exposing the newborn to cigarette smoke

2. Reduce the occurrence of developmental disabilities
  Reduce the number of children with mental retardation from a baseline of 131 to 124 children/10,000.
  Reduce the number of children with cerebral palsy from a baseline of 32.2 to 31.5 children/ 10,000.
  Reduce the number of children with autism spectrum disorder.
	Will promote measures for close antepartal and intrapartal monitoring of women at risk, subsequently reducing the incidence of disabilities, leading to a reduction in long-term effects and costs of care

3. Reduce the occurrence of fetal alcohol syndrome	Will foster programs for at-risk groups, including adolescents, about the effects of substance abuse, especially alcohol, during pregnancy

DHHS, 2000; available online at www.healthypeople.gov

devastating and life-changing outcomes be prevented (Arenson & Drake, 2007).

This chapter addresses selected acquired and congenital newborn conditions. In addition, it describes the nurse's role in assessment and management, emphasizing parental education and support. Nurses play a key role in helping the parents cope with the stress of having an ill newborn.

Acquired Disorders

▶ NEONATAL ASPHYXIA

As the newborn makes the transition to life outside the fluid-filled intrauterine environment, dramatic changes must occur to facilitate newborn respirations. Newborns normally start to breathe with routine warming, drying, airway suctioning, and mild stimulation. Most newborns make this transition such that by 1 minute of age, they are breathing well on their own. A newborn who fails to establish adequate, sustained respiration after birth is said to have **asphyxia**. Physiologically, asphyxia can be defined as impairment in gas exchange resulting in a decrease in blood oxygen levels (hypoxemia) and an excess of carbon dioxide or hypercapnia that leads to acidosis.

Asphyxia is the most common clinical insult in the perinatal period. As many as 10% of newborns require some degree of active resuscitation to stimulate breathing (Cunningham et al., 2005). According to the World Health Organization, 4 to 9 million cases of neonatal asphyxia occur annually worldwide, accounting for approximately 20% of all newborn deaths. More than a million newborns who survive asphyxia at birth develop long-term problems such as cerebral palsy, mental retardation, and speaking, hearing, visual, and learning disabilities (Maternal and Neonatal Health [MNH], 2007).

Pathophysiology

Asphyxia occurs when oxygen delivery is insufficient to meet metabolic demands, resulting in hypoxia, hypercarbia, and metabolic acidosis. Any condition that reduces oxygen delivery to the fetus can result in asphyxia. These conditions may include maternal hypoxia, such as from cardiac or respiratory disease, anemia, or postural hypotension; maternal vascular disease that leads to placental insufficiency, such as diabetes or hypertension; cord problems such as compression or prolapse; and postterm pregnancies, which may trigger meconium release into the amniotic fluid.

Initially, the newborn uses compensatory mechanisms including tachycardia and vasoconstriction to help bring oxygen to the vital organs for a time. However, without intervention, these mechanisms fail, leading to hypotension, bradycardia, and eventually cardiopulmonary arrest.

With failure to breathe well after birth, the newborn will develop hypoxia (too little oxygen in the cells of the body). As a result, the heart rate falls, cyanosis develops, and the newborn becomes hypotonic and unresponsive.

Think back to Kelly, described at the beginning of the chapter. She gives birth to a son weighing approximately 2,500 g; he appears postterm and small for gestational age. His skin is stained yellow-green and he is limp, cyanotic, and apneic at birth. The initial assessment once the newborn is under the radiant warmer indicates that resuscitation and tracheal suctioning are needed. What is the nurse's role during resuscitation? What assessments will be needed during this procedure?

Nursing Assessment

The key to successful treatment of newborn asphyxia is early identification and recognition of newborns who may be at risk. Review the perinatal history for risk factors, including:

• Trauma: injury to the central or peripheral nervous system secondary to a long or difficult labor, a precipitous birth, multiple gestation, abnormal presentation, cephalopelvic disproportion, shoulder dystocia, or extraction by forceps or vacuum
• Intrauterine asphyxia: for example, fetal hypoxia secondary to maternal hypoxia, diabetes, hypertension, anemia, cord compression, or meconium aspiration
• Sepsis: acquired bacterial or viral organisms from infected amniotic fluid, maternal infection, or direct contact while passing through the birth canal
• Malformation: congenital anomalies including facial or upper airway deformities, renal anomalies, pulmonary hypoplasia, neuromuscular disorders, esophageal atresia, or neural tube defects
• Hypovolemic shock: secondary to abruptio placentae, placenta previa, or cord rupture resulting in blood loss to the fetus
• Medication: drugs given to mother during labor that can affect the fetus by causing placental hypoperfusion and hypotension; use of hypnotics, analgesics, anesthetics, narcotics, oxytocin, and street drugs during pregnancy

At birth, assess the newborn immediately. Observe the infant's color, noting any pallor or cyanosis. Assess the work of breathing. Be alert for apnea, tachypnea, gasping respirations, grunting, nasal flaring, or retractions. Evaluate heart rate and note bradycardia. Assess the newborn's temperature, noting hypothermia. Determine the Apgar score at 1 and 5 minutes; an Apgar score below 7 at either time indicates that resuscitation is needed.

Anticipate diagnostic testing to identify etiologies for the newborn's asphyxia. For example, a chest x-ray may identify structural abnormalities that might interfere with respiration. A blood culture may identify an infectious process. A blood toxicology screen may detect any maternal drugs in the newborn (Kenner & Lott, 2007).

Nursing Management

Management of the newborn experiencing asphyxia includes immediate resuscitation. Ensure that the equipment needed for resuscitation is readily available and in working order. Essential equipment includes a wall suction apparatus, an oxygen source, a newborn ventilation bag, endotracheal tubes (2 to 3 mm), a laryngoscope, and ampules of naloxone (Narcan) with syringes and needles for administration (see Chapter 23 for a more detailed discussion of resuscitation).

Dry the newborn quickly with a warm towel and then place him or her under a radiant heater to prevent rapid heat loss through evaporation. Handling and rubbing the newborn with a dry towel may be all that is needed to stimulate the onset of breathing. If the newborn fails to respond to stimulation, then active resuscitation is needed.

The procedure for newborn resuscitation is easily remembered by the "ABCDs"—airway, breathing, circulation, and drugs (see Chapter 23, Box 23.3). Continue resuscitation until the newborn has a pulse above 100 bpm, a good cry, or good breathing efforts and a pink tongue. This last sign indicates a good oxygen supply to the brain (Brodsky & Ouellette, 2007).

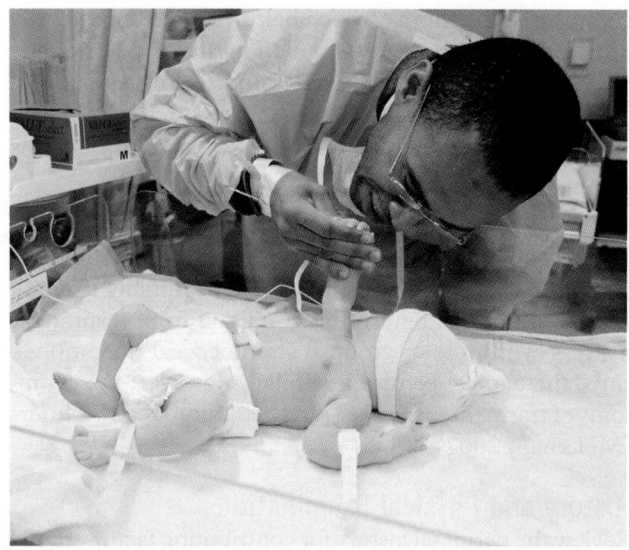

FIGURE 24.1 A father interacting with his newborn once the newborn's condition has stabilized.

> ▶ **Take** NOTE!
>
> *According to the American Heart Association and American Academy of Pediatrics Emergency Care Guidelines for Neonatal Resuscitation, resuscitation efforts may be stopped if the newborn exhibits no heart beat and no respiratory effort after 10 minutes of continuous and adequate resuscitation (AHA/AAP, 2005; Zaichkin, 2006).*

Provide continued observation and assessment of the newborn who has been successfully resuscitated. Monitor the newborn's vital signs and oxygen saturation levels closely for changes. Maintain a neutral thermal environment to prevent hypothermia, which would increase the newborn's metabolic and oxygen demands. Check the blood glucose level and observe for signs of hypoglycemia; if this develops, it can further stress the newborn.

The need for resuscitative measures can be extremely upsetting for the parents. Explain to them the initial resuscitation activities being performed and offer ongoing explanations about any procedures being done, equipment being used, or medications given. Provide physical and emotional support to the parents through the initial crisis and throughout the newborn's stay. When the newborn is stable, allow parents to spend time with their newborn to promote bonding (Fig. 24.1). Point out the newborn's positive attributes and give frequent updates on his or her status. Role-model techniques for holding, interacting with, and caring for the newborn to decrease the parents' anxiety.

*R*emember Kelly, the young woman described at the beginning of the chapter? Her son is intubated and tracheal suctioning is performed. Positive-pressure ventilation is also started with a self-inflating bag and 50% oxygen. Ventilation is continued for 1 minute and then gradually discontinued. The heart rate is now 120 bpm, and spontaneous respirations are noted. When free-flow oxygen is administered, the newborn begins to cry and turn pink. What continued care is needed in the special care nursery? What explanation should be offered to Kelly regarding her son?

▶ TRANSIENT TACHYPNEA OF THE NEWBORN

Transient tachypnea of the newborn (TTN) is a condition involving a mild degree of respiratory distress. It is described as the retention of lung fluid or transient pulmonary edema (McLenan, 2007). It usually occurs within a few hours of birth and resolves by 72 hours of age. TTN occurs in approximately 11 per 1,000 live births (Asenjo, 2007).

Pathophysiology

Most newborns make the transition from fetal to newborn life without incident. During fetal life, the lungs are filled with a serous fluid because the placenta, not the lungs, is used for nutrient and gas exchange. During and after birth, this fluid must be removed and replaced with air. Passage through the birth canal during a vaginal birth compresses the thorax, which helps remove the majority of this fluid. Pulmonary circulation and the lymphatic drainage remove the remaining fluid shortly after birth. TTN occurs when the liquid in the lung is removed slowly or incompletely.

Nursing Assessment

Astutely observe the newborn with respiratory distress because TTN is a diagnosis of exclusion. Initially it might be difficult to distinguish this condition from respiratory distress syndrome or group B streptococcal pneumonia, since the clinical picture is similar. However, the symptoms of transient tachypnea rarely last more than 72 hours (McLenan, 2007).

History and Physical Examination

Review the perinatal history for contributing factors. TTN is commonly seen in newborns who are sedated or have been born via cesarean birth. Also check the history for evidence of a prolonged labor, fetal macrosomia, and maternal asthma and smoking. These factors are associated with a higher incidence of TTN (Rodriguez, 2006).

Closely assess the newborn for signs of TTN. Within the first few hours of birth, observe for tachypnea, expiratory grunting, retractions, labored breathing, nasal flaring, and mild cyanosis (Asenjo, 2007). Mild to moderate respiratory distress is present by 6 hours of age, with respiratory rates as high as 100 to 140 breaths per minute (Kenner & Lott, 2007). Also inspect the newborn's chest for hyperextension or a barrel shape. Auscultate breath sounds, which may be slightly diminished secondary to reduced air entry.

Laboratory and Diagnostic Testing

To aid in the diagnosis, a chest x-ray may be done. It usually reveals mild symmetric lung overaeration and prominent perihilar interstitial markings and streaking. These findings correlate with lymphatic engorgement of retained fetal fluid (Asenjo, 2007).

Nursing Management

Nursing management focuses on providing adequate oxygenation and determining whether the newborn's respiratory manifestations appear to be resolving or persisting. Provide supportive care while the retained lung fluid is reabsorbed. Administer intravenous (IV) fluids and/or gavage feedings until the respiratory rate decreases enough to allow safe oral feeding. Provide supplemental oxygen via a nasal cannula or oxygen hood to maintain adequate oxygen saturation. Maintain a neutral thermal environment with minimal stimulation to minimize oxygen demand.

Provide ongoing assessment of the newborn's respiratory status. As TTN resolves, the newborn's respiratory rate declines to 60 breaths per minute or less, the oxygen requirement decreases, and the chest x-ray shows resolution of the perihilar streaking. Provide reassurance and progress reports to the parents to help them cope with this crisis.

▶ RESPIRATORY DISTRESS SYNDROME

Despite improved survival rates and advances in perinatal care, many high-risk newborns are at risk for respiratory problems, particularly **respiratory distress syndrome** (RDS), a breathing disorder resulting from lung immaturity and lack of alveolar surfactant. Since the link between RDS and surfactant deficiency was discovered more than 30 years ago, tremendous strides have been made in understanding the pathophysiology and treatment of this disorder. The introduction of prenatal steroids to accelerate lung maturity and the development of synthetic surfactant can be credited with the dramatic improvements in the outcome of newborns with RDS (Rodriguez, 2006).

RDS affects an estimated 25,000 infants born alive in the United States annually. The incidence declines with degree of maturity at birth. It occurs in 60% of preterm newborns of less than 28 weeks' gestation, 30% of those born at 28 to 34 weeks, and less than 5% of those born after 34 weeks (American Lung Association [ALA], 2007). Intensive respiratory care, usually with mechanical ventilation, is necessary.

Pathophysiology

Lung immaturity and surfactant deficiency contribute to the development of RDS. Surfactant is a complex mixture of phospholipids and proteins that adheres to the alveolar surface of the lungs. Surfactant forms a coating over the inner surface of the alveoli, reducing the surface tension and preventing alveolar collapse at the end of expiration. In the affected newborn, surfactant is deficient or lacking, and this deficit results in stiff lungs and alveoli that tend to collapse, leading to diffuse atelectasis. The work of breathing is increased because increased pressure similar to that required to initiate the first breath is needed to inflate the lungs with each successive breath. Hypoxemia and acidemia result, leading to vasoconstriction of the pulmonary vasculature. Right-to-left shunting occurs and alveolar capillary circulation is limited, further inhibiting surfactant production. As the disease progresses, fluid and fibrin leak from the pulmonary capillaries, causing hyaline membranes to form in the bronchioles, alveolar ducts, and alveoli. These membranes further decrease gas exchange. A vicious cycle is created, compounding the problem (Blackburn, 2007).

Nursing Assessment

Nursing assessment focuses on keen observation to identify the signs and symptoms of respiratory distress. In addition, assessment aids in differentiating RDS from other respiratory conditions, such as TTN or group B streptococcal pneumonia.

History and Physical Examination

Review the history for risk factors associated with RDS; these include perinatal asphyxia regardless of gestational age, cesarean birth in the absence of preceding labor (related to the lack of thoracic squeezing), male gender, and maternal diabetes. It is believed that each of these conditions has an impact on surfactant production, thus resulting in RDS in the term infant (Stoll & Kliegman, 2004).

▶ *Take* NOTE!

Prolonged rupture of membranes, intrauterine growth restriction (IUGR), gestational hypertension, maternal heroin addiction, and use of prenatal corticosteroids reduce the newborn's risk for RDS because of the physiologic stress imposed on the fetus. Chronic stress experienced by the fetus in utero accelerates the production of surfactant before the 35th week of gestation and thus reduces the incidence of RDS at birth.

The newborn with RDS usually demonstrates signs at birth or within a few hours of birth. Observe the infant for expiratory grunting, nasal flaring, chest wall retractions, see-saw respirations, and generalized cyanosis. Auscultate the heart and lungs, noting tachycardia (rates above 150 to 180), fine inspiratory crackles, and tachypnea (rates above 60 breaths per minute). Use the Silverman-Anderson index assessment tool to determine the degree of respiratory distress. The index involves observation of five features, each of which is scored as 0, 1, or 2 (Fig. 24.2). The higher the score, the greater the respiratory distress. A score over 7 suggests severe respiratory distress.

Laboratory and Diagnostic Testing

The diagnosis of RDS is based on the clinical picture and x-ray findings. A chest x-ray reveals hypoaeration, underexpansion, and a "ground glass" pattern (Brodsky & Ouellette, 2007; Mattson & Smith, 2004).

Nursing Management

If untreated, RDS will worsen. However, it appears to be a self-limiting disease, with respiratory symptoms declining after 72 hours. This decline parallels the production of surfactant in the alveoli (McLenan, 2007). The newborn needs supportive care until surfactant is produced. Effective therapies for established RDS include conventional mechanical ventilation, continuous positive airway pressure (CPAP), or positive end-expiratory pressure (PEEP) to prevent volume loss during expiration, and surfactant therapy. The use of exogenous surfactant replacement

therapy to stabilize the newborn's lungs until postnatal surfactant synthesis matures has become a life-saver.

Care of the newborn with RDS is primarily supportive and requires a multidisciplinary approach to obtain the best outcomes. Therapy focuses on improving oxygenation and maintaining optimal lung volumes. Expect to transfer the newborn to the neonatal intensive care unit (NICU) soon after birth. Apply the basic principles of newborn care, such as thermoregulation, cardiovascular and nutritional support, normal glucose level maintenance, and infection prevention, to achieve the therapeutic goals of reducing mortality and minimizing lung trauma.

Anticipate the administration of surfactant replacement therapy, prophylactically or as a rescue approach. With prophylactic administration, surfactant is given within minutes after birth, thus providing replacement surfactant before severe RDS develops. Rescue treatment is indicated for newborns with established RDS who require mechanical ventilation and supplemental oxygen. The earlier the surfactant is administered, the better the effect on gas exchange (Kenner & Lott, 2007).

Administer the prescribed oxygen concentration via nasal cannula. Anticipate the need for ventilator therapy, which has greatly improved in the past several years, with significant advances in conventional and high-frequency ventilation therapies (Fig. 24.3). Recent studies show no difference in outcomes for newborns who received early treatment with high-frequency oscillatory ventilation compared with those receiving conventional mechanical ventilation (Blackburn, 2007). Although mechanical ventilation has increased survival rates, it is also a contributing factor to bronchopulmonary dysplasia, pulmonary hypertension, and retinopathy of prematurity (Cunningham et al., 2005).

In addition, support the newborn with RDS using the following interventions:

- Continuously monitor the infant's cardiopulmonary status via invasive or noninvasive means (e.g., arterial lines or auscultation, respectively).
- Monitor oxygen saturation levels continuously; assess pulse oximeter values to determine oxygen saturation levels.
- Closely monitor vital signs, acid–base status, and arterial blood gases.
- Administer broad-spectrum antibiotics if blood cultures are positive.
- Administer sodium bicarbonate or acetate as ordered to correct metabolic acidosis.
- Provide fluids and vasopressor agents as needed to prevent or treat hypotension.
- Test blood glucose levels and administer dextrose as ordered for prevention or treatment of hypoglycemia.
- Cluster caretaking activities to avoid overtaxing and compromising the newborn.
- Place the newborn in the prone position to optimize respiratory status and reduce stress.

Score

Feature observed	0	1	2
Chest movement	Synchronized respirations	Lag on respirations	Seesaw respirations
Intercostal retraction	None	Just visible	Marked
Xiphoid retraction	None	Just visible	Marked
Nares dilation	None	Minimal	Marked
Expiratory grunt	None	Audible by stethoscope	Audible by unaided ear

FIGURE 24.2 Assessing the degree of respiratory distress. (Used with permission from Silverman, W. A., & Anderson, D. H. [1956]. A controlled clinical trial of effects of water mist on obstructive respiratory signs, death rate, and necroscopy findings among premature infants. *Pediatrics, 17*[4], 1–9.)

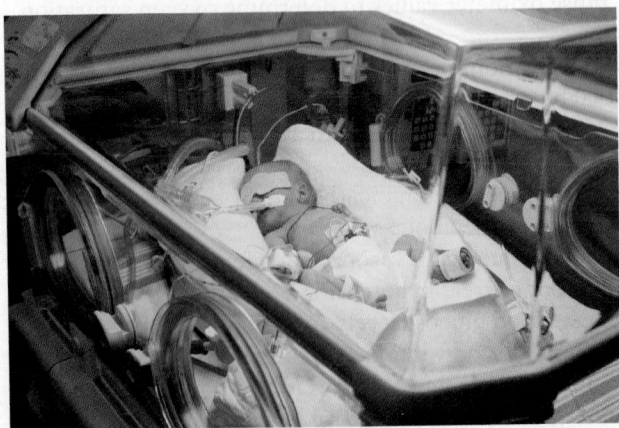

FIGURE 24.3 A newborn with RDS receiving mechanical ventilation.

- Perform gentle suctioning to remove secretions and maintain a patent airway.
- Assess level of consciousness to identify intraventricular hemorrhage.
- Provide sufficient calories via gavage and IV feedings.
- Maintain adequate hydration and assess for signs of fluid overload.
- Provide information to the parents about treatment modalities; give thorough but simple explanations about the rationales for interventions.
- Encourage the parents to participate in care (Blackburn, 2007).

Provide ongoing assessment and be alert for complications. These may include air leak syndrome, bronchopulmonary dysplasia (chronic lung disease), patent ductus arteriosus, congestive heart failure, intraventricular hemorrhage, retinopathy of prematurity, necrotizing enterocolitis, complications resulting from intravenous catheter use (infection, thrombus formation), and developmental delay or disability (Stoll & Kliegman, 2004).

MECONIUM ASPIRATION SYNDROME

Meconium is a viscous green substance composed primarily of water and other gastrointestinal secretions that can be noted in the fetal gastrointestinal tract as early as 10 to 16 weeks' gestation (Clark & Clark, 2007). It is expelled as the newborn's first stool after birth. **Meconium aspiration syndrome** occurs when the newborn inhales particulate meconium mixed with amniotic fluid into the lungs while still in utero or on taking the first breath after birth. It is a common cause of newborn respiratory distress and can lead to severe illness. Meconium staining of the amniotic fluid, with the possibility of aspiration, occurs in approximately 20% of pregnancies at term (Cunningham et al., 2005). Aspiration induces airway obstruction, surfactant dysfunction, hypoxia, and chemical pneumonitis with inflammation of pulmonary tissues. In severe cases, it progresses to persistent pulmonary hypertension and death (Cunningham et al., 2005). About 3% to 5% of infants with meconium aspiration syndrome die (Wiswell, Tin, & Ohler, 2007).

Pathophysiology

Meconium may be passed in utero secondary to hypoxic stress. Hypoxia induces the fetus to gasp or attempt to breathe. The fetus may bear down and pass meconium into the amniotic fluid or he or she may experience a vagal reflex that causes relaxation of the anal sphincter, allowing meconium to be passed into the amniotic fluid. The fetus then sucks or swallows this amniotic fluid in utero, or the infant may aspirate meconium with the first breath after birth as air rushes into the lungs.

Although the etiology is not well understood, the effects of meconium can be harmful to the fetus. Meconium alters the amniotic fluid by reducing antibacterial activity and subsequently increasing the risk of perinatal bacterial infection. Additionally, meconium is very irritating because it contains enzymes from the fetal pancreas.

When aspirated into the lungs, meconium blocks the bronchioles, causing an inflammatory reaction as well as a decrease in surfactant production. Gas exchange is impaired and atelectasis occurs. A ball–valve effect occurs when air is inspired into the alveoli but cannot be fully expired secondary to reduced airway diameter. Significant respiratory distress is followed by persistent pulmonary hypertension, right-to-left shunting of blood, and patent ductus arteriosus. Conventional mechanical ventilation, extracorporeal membrane oxygenation (ECMO), nitric oxide, high-frequency ventilation, or liquid ventilation may be necessary.

Nursing Assessment

Review prenatal and birth records to identify newborns who may be at high risk for meconium aspiration. Predisposing factors for meconium aspiration syndrome include postterm pregnancy; breech, forceps, or vacuum extraction births; prolonged or difficult labor associated with fetal distress in a term or postterm newborn; maternal hypertension or diabetes; oligohydramnios; IUGR; prolapsed cord; or acute or chronic placental insufficiency (Kenner & Lott, 2007).

Assess the amniotic fluid for meconium staining when the maternal membranes rupture. Green-stained amniotic fluid suggests the presence of meconium in the amniotic fluid and should be reported immediately. After birth, note any yellowish-green staining of the umbilical cord and nails and skin. This staining indicates that meconium has been present for some time.

Consider Kelly, the 27-year-old woman who gave birth to a son who required resuscitation. What findings would lead the nurse to suspect that her son aspirated meconium? What risk factors in Kelly's history would support the diagnosis of meconium aspiration syndrome?

▶ ***Take** NOTE!*

Recent evidence suggests that newborns with meconium staining do not routinely require intrapartum suctioning (before the birth of the shoulders). Tracheal suctioning is warranted if the newborn does not exhibit a strong respiratory effort, good muscle tone, and a heart rate greater than 100 beats per minute (AHA/AAP, 2005).

Observe the newborn for a barrel-shaped chest with an increased anterior-posterior (AP) chest diameter (similar to that found in a patient with chronic obstructive pulmonary disease), prolonged tachypnea, progression from mild to severe respiratory distress, intercostal retractions, end-expiratory grunting, and cyanosis (Clark & Clark, 2007). Auscultate the lungs, noting coarse crackles and rhonchi.

Chest x-rays show patchy, fluffy infiltrates unevenly distributed throughout the lungs and marked hyperaeration mixed with areas of atelectasis. Arterial blood gas analysis will indicate metabolic acidosis with a low blood pH, decreased PaO_2, and increased $PaCO_2$ (Wiswell,

Tin, & Ohler, 2007). Direct visualization of the vocal cords for meconium staining using a laryngoscope can confirm the presence of meconium below the larynx.

Nursing Management

Nursing management focuses on ensuring adequate tissue perfusion and minimizing oxygen demand and energy expenditure. Caring for the newborn with meconium aspiration begins in the birthing unit when the birth attendant identifies meconium-stained amniotic fluid with membrane rupture during labor. Upon delivery of the newborn's head, before the newborn takes the first breath, the nasal cavity and then the posterior pharynx are gently suctioned to decrease the potential for aspiration. If the newborn is significantly depressed at birth, secondary clearing of the lower airways by direct tracheal suctioning may be necessary. Repeated suctioning and stimulation are limited to prevent overstimulation and further depression (Clark & Clark, 2007). Usually the newborn is transferred to the NICU for close monitoring.

Maintain a neutral thermal environment, including placing the newborn under a radiant warmer or in a warmed isolette, to prevent hypothermia. In addition, minimize handling to reduce energy expenditure and oxygen consumption that could lead to further hypoxemia and acidosis.

Administer oxygen therapy as ordered via nasal cannula or with positive-pressure ventilation. Monitor oxygen saturation levels via pulse oximetry to evaluate the newborn's response to treatment and to detect changes. Increased pulmonary pressures associated with meconium aspiration may cause blood to be shunted away from the lungs. The newborn may exhibit uneven pulmonary ventilation, with hyperinflation in some areas and atelectasis in others. This leads to poor perfusion and subsequent hypoxemia, which in turn may increase pulmonary vasoconstriction, resulting in a worsening of hypoxemia and acidosis.

Expect to administer hyperoxygenation to dilate the pulmonary vasculature and close the ductus arteriosus or nitric oxide inhalation to decrease pulmonary vascular resistance, or to use high-frequency oscillatory ventilation to increase the chance of air trapping (Clark & Clark, 2007). In addition, administer vasopressors and pulmonary vasodilators as prescribed and administer surfactant as ordered to counteract inactivation by meconium. Monitor arterial blood gas results for changes and assist with measures to correct acid–base imbalances to facilitate perfusion of tissues and prevent pulmonary hypertension (Cunningham et al., 2005). If these measures are ineffective, be prepared to assist with the use of ECMO, a modified type of heart–lung machine.

In addition, perform the following interventions:

- Cluster newborn care to minimize oxygen demand.
- Administer broad-spectrum antibiotics to treat bacterial pneumonia.

- Administer sedation to reduce oxygen consumption and energy expenditure.
- Continuously monitor the newborn's condition.
- Reassure and support the parents throughout the experience (McLenan, 2007).

► PERSISTENT PULMONARY HYPERTENSION OF THE NEWBORN

Persistent pulmonary hypertension of the newborn, previously referred to as persistent fetal circulation, is a cardiopulmonary disorder characterized by marked pulmonary hypertension that causes right-to-left extrapulmonary shunting of blood and hypoxemia. Persistent pulmonary hypertension can occur idiopathically or as a complication of perinatal asphyxia, meconium aspiration syndrome, pneumonia, congenital heart defects, metabolic disorders such as hypoglycemia, hypothermia, hypovolemia, hyperviscosity, acute hypoxia with delayed resuscitation, sepsis, and RDS. It occurs in 2 to 6 newborns per 1,000 live births of term, near-term, or postterm infants (Steinhorn, 2007).

Pathophysiology

Normally, pulmonary artery pressure decreases when the newborn takes the first breath. However, interference with this ability to breathe allows pulmonary pressures to remain increased. Hypoxemia and acidosis also occur, leading to vasoconstriction of the pulmonary artery. These events cause an elevation in pulmonary vascular resistance. Normally, the decrease in pulmonary artery pressure and pulmonary vascular resistance with breathing leads to the closure of the ductus arteriosus and foramen ovale. However, with persistent pulmonary hypertension, pulmonary vascular resistance is elevated to the point that venous blood is diverted to some degree through fetal structures, such as the ductus arteriosus or foramen ovale, causing them to remain open, leading to a right-to-left shunting of blood into the systemic circulation. This diversion of blood bypasses the lungs, resulting in systemic arterial hypoxemia.

Nursing Assessment

Assess the newborn's status closely. A newborn with persistent pulmonary hypertension demonstrates tachypnea within 12 hours after birth. Observe for marked cyanosis, grunting, and retractions. Auscultate the heart, noting a systolic ejection murmur, and measure blood pressure for hypotension resulting from both heart failure and persistent hypoxemia (Kenner & Lott, 2007). Measure oxygen saturation via pulse oximetry and report low values. Prepare the newborn for an echocardiogram, which will reveal right-to-left shunting of blood that confirms the diagnosis.

Nursing Management

When caring for the newborn with persistent pulmonary hypertension, pay meticulous attention to detail, with continuous monitoring of the newborn's oxygenation and perfusion status and blood pressure. The goals of therapy include improving alveolar oxygenation, inducing metabolic alkalosis by administering sodium bicarbonate, correcting hypovolemia and hypotension with the administration of volume replacement and vasopressors, and anticipating use of ECMO when support has failed to maintain acceptable oxygenation (Steinhorn, 2007).

Provide immediate resuscitation after birth and administer oxygen therapy as ordered. Early and effective resuscitation and correction of acidosis and hypoxia are helpful in preventing persistent pulmonary hypertension. Monitor arterial blood gases frequently to evaluate the effectiveness of oxygen therapy. Provide respiratory support, which frequently necessitates the use of mechanical ventilation. Administer prescribed medications, monitor cardiopulmonary status, cluster care to reduce stimulation, and provide support and education to the parents.

> ▶ **Take** NOTE!
>
> *Almost any procedure, such as suctioning, weighing, changing diapers, or positioning, can precipitate severe hypoxemia due to the instability of the pulmonary vasculature. Therefore, minimize the newborn's exposure to stimulation as much as possible.*

▶ PERIVENTRICULAR–INTRAVENTRICULAR HEMORRHAGE

Periventricular–intraventricular hemorrhage is defined as bleeding that usually originates in the subependymal germinal matrix region of the brain, with extension into the ventricular system (Brodsky & Ouellette, 2007). It is a common problem in preterm infants, especially in those born before 32 weeks. A significant number of these newborns will incur brain injury, leading to complications that may include hydrocephalus, seizure disorders, periventricular leukomalacia (an ischemic injury resulting from inadequate perfusion of the white matter adjacent to the ventricles), cerebral palsy, learning disabilities, vision or hearing deficits, and mental retardation. Identifying preventive strategies to reduce the incidence of these brain insults is a national public health priority (McLenan, 2007).

The incidence of ventricular hemorrhage depends on the gestational age at birth. Up to 50% of newborns weighing 1,500 g or less or born at 30 weeks' gestation or

less will have evidence of hemorrhage. Only about 4% of term newborns show evidence of ventricular hemorrhage. Very-low-birthweight infants have the earliest onset of hemorrhage and the highest mortality rate (Brodsky & Ouellette, 2007).

Pathophysiology

The preterm newborn is at greatest risk for periventricular–intraventricular hemorrhage because cerebral vascular development is immature, making it more vulnerable to injury. The earlier the newborn is, the greater the likelihood for brain damage. While all areas of the brain can be injured, the periventricular area is the most vulnerable.

Each ventricular area contains a rich network of capillaries that are very thin and fragile and can rupture easily. The causes of rupture vary and include fluctuations in systemic and cerebral blood flow, increases in cerebral blood flow from hypertension, IV infusions, seizure activity, increases in cerebral venous pressure due to vaginal delivery, hypoxia, and respiratory distress. With a preterm birth, the fetus is suddenly transported from a well-controlled uterine environment into a highly stimulating one. This tremendous physiologic stress and shock may contribute to the rupture of periventricular capillaries and subsequent hemorrhage. Most hemorrhages occur in the first 72 hours after birth (Cunningham et al., 2005).

Periventricular–intraventricular hemorrhage is classified according to a grading system of I to V (least severe to most severe) (Blackburn, 2007). The prognosis is guarded, depending on the grade and severity of the hemorrhage. Generally, newborns with mild hemorrhage (grades I and II) have a much better developmental outcome than those with severe hemorrhage (grades III and IV).

Nursing Assessment

The signs of periventricular–intraventricular hemorrhage vary significantly; no clinical signs may be evident. Closely monitor newborns who are at an increased risk, such as those who are preterm or of low birthweight. Also assess for risk factors such as acidosis, asphyxia, unstable blood pressure, meningitis, seizures, acute blood loss, hypovolemia, respiratory distress with mechanical ventilation, intubation, apnea, hypoxia, suctioning, use of hyperosmolar solutions, rapid volume expansion, and activities that involve handling.

Evaluate the newborn for an unexplained drop in hematocrit, pallor, and poor perfusion as evidenced by respiratory distress and oxygen desaturation. Note seizures, lethargy or other changes in level of consciousness, weak suck, high-pitched cry, or hypotonia. Palpate the anterior fontanel for tenseness. Assess vital signs, noting bradycardia and hypotension. Evaluate laboratory data for changes indicating metabolic acidosis or glucose instability (Annibale & Hill, 2007). Frequently a bleed can progress rapidly and result in shock and death. Prepare the newborn for cranial ultrasonography, the diagnostic tool of choice to detect hemorrhage.

Nursing Management

Prevention of preterm birth is essential in preventing periventricular–intraventricular hemorrhage. Promote community awareness of factors that may contribute to periventricular–intraventricular hemorrhage, such as a lack of prenatal care, maternal infection, alcohol consumption, and smoking (Kenner & Lott, 2007). Identify risk factors that can lead to hemorrhage, and focus care on interventions to decrease the risk of hemorrhage. For example, institute measures to prevent perinatal asphyxia and birth trauma and provide developmental care in the NICU. If a preterm birth is expected, having the mother deliver at a tertiary care facility with a NICU would be most appropriate.

Care of the newborn with periventricular-intraventricular hemorrhage is primarily supportive. Correct anemia, acidosis, and hypotension with fluids and medications. Administer fluids slowly to prevent fluctuations in blood pressure. Avoid rapid volume expansion to minimize changes in cerebral blood flow. Keep the newborn in a flexed, contained position with the head elevated to prevent or minimize fluctuations in intracranial pressure. Continuously monitor the newborn for signs of hemorrhage, such as changes in the level of consciousness, bulging fontanel, seizures, apnea, and reduced activity level. Also, measure head circumference daily.

Minimize handling of the newborn by clustering nursing care, and limit stimulation in the newborn's environment to reduce stress. Also reduce the newborn's exposure to noxious stimuli to avoid a fluctuation in blood pressure and energy expenditure. Provide adequate oxygenation to promote tissue perfusion but controlled ventilation to decrease the risk of pneumothorax.

Support for the parents to cope with the diagnosis and potential long-term sequelae is essential. The long-term neurodevelopmental outcome is determined by the severity of the bleed. Provide education and emotional support for the parents throughout the newborn's stay. Discuss expectations for short-term and long-term care needs with the parents and assist them in obtaining the necessary support from appropriate community resources.

▶ NECROTIZING ENTEROCOLITIS

Necrotizing enterocolitis (NEC) is a serious gastrointestinal disease occurring in newborns. It is the most common and most serious acquired gastrointestinal disorder among hospitalized preterm neonates and is associated with significant acute and chronic morbidity and mortality (Stoll & Kliegman, 2007). NEC occurs in 1 to 3 cases per 1,000 live births, affecting 1% to 5% of all newborns in intensive care units (Stoll & Kliegman, 2007). Attempts to improve gastrointestinal function and reduce the risk of NEC include enteral antibiotics, judicious administration of parenteral fluids, human milk feedings, antenatal corticosteroids, enteral probiotics (*Lactobacillus acidophilus*), and slow continuous drip feedings (Neu, 2007).

Pathophysiology

The pathophysiology of NEC is not clearly understood and is thought to be multifactorial in nature. Current research points to three major pathologic mechanisms that lead to NEC: bowel ischemia, bacterial flora, and the effect of feeding (Neu, 2007).

During perinatal or postnatal stress, oxygen is shunted away from the gut to more important organs such as the heart and brain. Ischemia and intestinal wall damage occur, allowing bacteria to invade. High-solute feedings allow bacteria to flourish. Mucosal or transmucosal necrosis of part of the intestine occurs (Wood, 2007). Although any region of the bowel can be affected, the distal ileum and proximal colon are the regions most commonly involved. NEC usually occurs between 3 and 12 days of life, but it can occur weeks later in some newborns.

Nursing Assessment

NEC can be devastating, and astute assessment is crucial. Assessing the newborn for the development of NEC includes the health history and physical examination as well as laboratory and diagnostic testing.

Health History and Physical Examination

Assess the newborn's history for risk factors associated with NEC. In addition to preterm birth, prenatal and postnatal predisposing risk factors are highlighted in Box 24.1.

Also observe the newborn for common signs and symptoms, which may include:

- Abdominal distention and tenderness
- Bloody stools
- Feeding intolerance, characterized by bilious vomiting
- Signs of sepsis
- Lethargy
- Apnea
- Shock

Always keep the possibility of NEC in mind when dealing with preterm newborns, especially when enteral feedings are being administered. Note respiratory distress, cyanosis, lethargy, decreased activity level, temperature instability, feeding intolerance, diarrhea, bile-stained emesis, or grossly bloody stools. Assess blood pressure, noting hypotension. Evaluate the neonate's abdomen for distention, tenderness, and visible loops of bowel (Verklan & Walden, 2004). Measure the abdominal circumference,

BOX 24.1 Predisposing Factors for the Development of Necrotizing Enterocolitis

Prenatal Factors
- Preterm labor
- Prolonged rupture of membranes
- Preeclampsia
- Maternal sepsis
- Amnionitis
- Uterine hypoxia

Postnatal Factors
- Respiratory distress syndrome
- Patent ductus arteriosus
- Congenital heart disease
- Exchange transfusion
- Low birthweight
- Low Apgar scores
- Umbilical catheterization
- Hypothermia
- Gastrointestinal infection
- Hypoglycemia
- Asphyxia

noting an increase. Determine residual gastric volume prior to feeding; when it is elevated, be suspicious for NEC.

Laboratory and Diagnostic Testing

Common laboratory and diagnostic tests ordered for assessment of NEC include:

- Kidney, ureter, and bladder (KUB) of the abdomen x-ray: confirms the presence of pneumatosis intestinalis (air in the bowel wall) and persistently dilated loops of bowel (Verklan & Walden, 2004; Wood, 2007)
- Blood values: may demonstrate metabolic acidosis, increased white blood cells, thrombocytopenia, neutropenia, electrolyte imbalance or disseminated intravascular coagulation (DIC)

Nursing Management

Nursing management of the newborn with NEC focuses on maintaining fluid and nutritional status, providing supportive care, and teaching the family about the condition and prognosis. Therapeutic management initially consists of bowel rest and antibiotic therapy. Serial KUB x-rays are used to assess the resolution or progression of NEC. If medical treatment fails to stabilize the newborn or if free air is present on a left lateral decubitus film, surgical intervention will be necessary to resect the portion of necrotic bowel. Surgery for NEC usually requires the placement of a proximal enterostomy until the anastomosis site is ready for reconnection.

Maintaining Fluid and Nutritional Status

If NEC is suspected, immediately stop enteral feedings until a diagnosis is made. Administer IV fluids initially to restore proper fluid balance. If ordered, administer total parenteral nutrition (TPN) to keep the newborn supported nutritionally. Give prescribed IV antibiotics to prevent sepsis from the necrotic bowel (if surgery is required, antibiotics may be needed for an extended period of time). Institute gastric decompression as ordered with an orogastric tube attached to low intermittent suction. Carefully monitor intake and output. Restart enteral feedings once the disease has resolved (normal abdominal examination and KUB negative for pneumatosis) or as determined postoperatively by the surgeon.

Providing Supportive Care

Manage pain by administering analgesics as ordered. Infection control is important, with an emphasis on careful handwashing. In addition, implement these interventions in an ongoing manner:

- Check stools for evidence of blood and report any positive findings.
- Measure the abdominal girth.
- Palpate the abdomen for tenderness and rigidity.
- Auscultate for normal bowel sounds.
- Observe the abdomen for redness or shininess, which indicates peritonitis.

Teaching the Family

The diagnosis of NEC may cause significant family anxiety. Listen to the family's worries and fears. Answer their questions honestly. Inform the family that medically treated NEC is usually limited to a short period and resolves within 48 hours of stopping oral feedings. Explain that surgically treated NEC, however, can be a much lengthier process. The amount of bowel that has necrosed, as determined during the bowel resection, significantly increases the likelihood of long-term medical problems. Short bowel syndrome may result from a large resection (short bowel syndrome is discussed in Chapter 41). Reassure the family that although some infants have more involved cases of NEC, the improved parenteral nutrition formulations have improved the outcomes for these infants. Provide education about ostomy care if surgery is required (refer to page 1335 for a discussion of ostomy care). Promote interaction with their newborn.

▶ INFANTS OF DIABETIC MOTHERS

An **infant of a diabetic mother** is one born to a woman with pregestational or gestational diabetes (see Chapter 20 for additional information). The newborn of a diabetic woman is at high risk for numerous health-related complications, especially hypoglycemia. In light of the increasing incidence of type 2 diabetes among women of childbearing age due to obesity, it is important to educate women about the potential impact of poor glycemic control on their offspring.

Impact of Diabetes on the Newborn

For more than a century, it has been known that diabetes during pregnancy can have severe adverse effects on fetal and newborn outcomes. Infants of diabetic mothers have increased morbidity and mortality in the perinatal period. The incidence of major congenital anomalies is much greater for these newborns than for other newborns. Poor glycemic control in the first trimester, during organogenesis, is thought to be a major reason for congenital malformations. The most common types of malformations in infants of diabetic mothers involve the cardiovascular, skeletal, central nervous, gastrointestinal, and genitourinary systems. Cardiac anomalies are the most common (Kwik et al., 2007).

Infants of diabetic mothers are longer and weigh more than newborns of similar gestational age. They also have increased organ weights (organomegaly) and excessive fat deposits on the shoulders and trunk, contributing to the increased overall body weight and predisposing them to shoulder dystocia. These newborns are macrosomic (an infant whose birthweight exceeds 4,500 g). These oversized newborns frequently require cesarean births for cephalopelvic disproportion and are often hypoglycemic in the first few hours after birth.

Despite their increased size and weight, they may be remarkably frail, showing behaviors similar to those of a preterm newborn. Thus, birthweight may not be a reliable criterion of maturity. Newborns of women with diabetes but without vascular complications often tend to be large for gestational age (LGA), whereas those of women with diabetes and vascular disease are usually small for gestational age (SGA).

Pathophysiology

The large size of the infant born to a diabetic mother occurs secondary to exposure to high levels of maternal glucose crossing the placenta into the fetal circulation. Maternal hyperglycemia acts as a fuel to stimulate increased production of fetal insulin, which in turn promotes somatic growth within the fetus. The fetus responds to these high levels by producing more insulin, which acts as a growth factor in the fetus (Blackburn, 2007). How the fetus will be affected and the problems that the newborn experiences depend on the severity, duration, and control of the diabetes in the mother. Table 24.1 summarizes the common problems that may occur in infants of diabetic mothers.

Nursing Assessment

Assessment begins in the prenatal period by identifying women with diabetes and taking measures to control maternal glucose levels (see Chapter 20 for information on management of the pregnant woman with diabetes).

Physical Examination
At birth, inspect the newborn for these characteristic features:

- Full rosy cheeks with a ruddy skin color
- Short neck (some describe "no-neck" appearance)
- Buffalo hump over the nape of the neck
- Massive shoulders with a full intrascapular area
- Distended upper abdomen due to organ overgrowth
- Excessive subcutaneous fat tissue, producing fat extremities (Fig. 24.4)

Be alert for hypoglycemia, which may occur immediately after birth or within an hour. Assess blood glucose levels, which should remain above 40 mg/dL. Closely assess the newborn for signs of hypoglycemia, including listlessness, hypotonia, apathy, poor feeding, apneic episodes with a drop in oxygen saturation, cyanosis, temperature instability, pallor and sweating, tremors, irritability, and seizures.

Assess the newborn for signs of birth trauma involving the head (tense, bulging fontanels, cephalhematoma, skull fractures, and facial nerve paralysis), shoulders and extremities (posturing, paralysis), and skin (bruising). Inspect the newborn for compromised oxygenation by examining the skin for cyanosis, pallor, mottling, and sluggish capillary refill. Take the newborn's temperature frequently and provide a neutral thermal environment to prevent cold stress, which would increase the glucose utilization and contribute to the hypoglycemic state.

Laboratory and Diagnostic Testing
Determine baseline serum calcium, magnesium, and bilirubin levels and monitor them frequently for changes (Table 24.2). Hypocalcemia is typically manifested in the first 2 to 3 days of life as a result of birth injury or a prolonged delay in parathyroid hormone production. Hypomagnesemia parallels calcium levels and is suspected only when hypocalcemia does not respond to calcium replacement therapy. Red blood cell breakdown leads to increased hematocrit and polycythemia. In addition, hyperbilirubinemia may be caused by slightly decreased extracellular fluid volume, hepatic immaturity, and birth trauma forming enclosed hemorrhages. It can appear within the first 24 hours of life (pathologic) or after 24 hours of life (physiologic).

Nursing Management

The focus of care for these infants is early detection and initiation of therapy to address potential problems (Nursing

TABLE 24.1 COMMON PROBLEMS OF INFANTS OF DIABETIC MOTHERS

Condition	Description	Effects
Macrosomia	Newborn with an excessive birthweight; arbitrarily defined as a birthweight >4,000 g (8 lb 13 oz) to 4,500 g (9 lb 15 oz) or >90% for gestational age Complication in 10% of all pregnancies in the United States	Increased risk for shoulder dystocia, traumatic birth injury, birth asphyxia Risks for newborn hypoglycemia and hypomagnesemia, polycythemia, and electrolyte disturbances Increased maternal risk for surgical birth, postpartum hemorrhage and infection, and birth canal lacerations Increased risk of developing type 2 diabetes later in life for both Higher weight and accumulation of fat in childhood and a higher rate of obesity in adults
Respiratory distress syndrome (RDS)	Cortisol-induced stimulation of lecithin/sphingomyelin (phospholipids) necessary for lung maturation is antagonized due to the high insulin environment within the fetus due to mother's hyperglycemia. Less mature lung development than expected for gestational age Decrease in the phospholipid phosphatidylglycerol (PG), which stabilizes surfactant, compounding risk	Most commonly, breathing normally at birth but developing labored, grunting respiration with cough and a hoarse complaining cry within a few hours with chest retractions and varying degrees of cyanosis IDMs with vascular disease seldom develop RDS because the chronic stress of poor intrauterine perfusion leads to increased production of steroids, which accelerates lung maturation.
Hypoglycemia	Glucose is the major source of energy for organ function. Typical characteristics: – Poor feedings – Jitteriness – Lethargy – High-pitched or weak cry – Apnea – Cyanosis and seizures Some newborns asymptomatic.	Low blood glucose levels are problematic during early post-birth period due to abrupt cessation of high-glucose maternal blood supply and the continuation of insulin production by the newborn. Limited ability to release glucagon and catecholamines, which normally stimulate glucagon breakdown and glucose release Prolonged and untreated hypoglycemia leads to serious, long-term adverse neurologic sequelae such as learning disabilities and mental retardation.
Hypocalcemia and hypomagnesemia	Hypocalcemia (drop in calcium levels) manifested by tremors, hypotonia, apnea, high-pitched cry, and seizures due to abrupt cessation of maternal transfer of calcium to fetus primarily in third trimester and experiencing birth asphyxia Associated hypomagnesemia directly related to the maternal level before birth About half of IDMs affected	Newborn is at risk for a prolonged delay in parathyroid hormone production and cardiac dysrhythmias.
Polycythemia	Venous hematocrit of >65% in the newborn Increased oxygen consumption by IDM secondary to fetal hyperglycemia and hyperinsulinemia Increased fetal erythropoiesis secondary to intrauterine hypoxia due to placental insufficiency from maternal diabetes Hypoxic stimulation of increased red blood cell (RBC) production as compensatory mechanism	Increased viscosity, resulting in poor blood flow predisposing newborn to decreased tissue oxygenation and development of microthrombi

(continued)

TABLE 24.1   COMMON PROBLEMS OF INFANTS OF DIABETIC MOTHERS (continued)

Condition	Description	Effects
Hyperbilirubinemia	Usually seen within the first few days after birth, manifested by a yellow appearance of the sclera and skin Excessive red cell hemolysis necessary to break down increased RBCs in circulation due to polycythemia Resultant elevated bilirubin levels Excessive bruising secondary to birth trauma of macrosomic infants, further adding to high bilirubin levels	If untreated, high levels of unconjugated bilirubin may lead to kernicterus (neurologic syndrome that results in irreversible damage) with long-term sequelae that include cerebral palsy, sensorineural hearing loss, and mental retardation.
Congenital anomalies	Occur in up to 10% of IDMs, accounting for 30% to 50% of perinatal deaths Incidence is greatest among SGA newborns. Overall, approximately three times the usual incidence of congenital anomalies compared to newborns from the non-diabetic general population.	Most common anomalies: – Coarctation of the aorta – Atrial and ventricular septal defects – Transposition of the great vessels – Sacral agenesis – Hip and joint malformations – Anencephaly – Spina bifida – Caudal dysplasia – Hydrocephalus

Sources: Arenson & Drake, 2007; Blackburn, 2007; Kenner & Lott, 2007; McLenan, 2007.

Rosy cheeks

Wide shoulders

Poor feeding

Excessive subcutaneous fat on extremities

Distended abdomen

FIGURE 24.4 Characteristics of an infant of a diabetic mother.

Care Plan 24.1). Perform a head-to-toe physical assessment to identify congenital anomalies. Institute measures to correct hypoglycemia, hypocalcemia, hypomagnesemia, dehydration, and jaundice. Provide oxygenation and ventilatory support as necessary.

Preventing Hypoglycemia

Prevent hypoglycemia by providing early oral feedings with formula or breast milk at frequent intervals (every 2 to 3 hours). Feedings help to control glucose levels, reduce hematocrit, and promote bilirubin excretion. Maintain a neutral thermal environment to avoid cold stress, which may stimulate the metabolic rate, thereby increasing the demand for glucose. Provide rest periods to decrease energy demand and expenditure.

Monitor blood glucose levels via heel stick every hour for the first 4 hours of life and then every 3 to 4 hours

TABLE 24.2   CRITICAL LABORATORY VALUES FOR INFANTS OF DIABETIC MOTHERS

Hypoglycemia	<40 mg/dL
Hypocalcemia	<7 mg/dL
Hypomagnesemia	<1.5 mg/dL
Hyperbilirubinemia	>12 mg/dL (term infant)
Polycythemia	>65% (venous hematocrit)

OVERVIEW OF AN INFANT OF A DIABETIC MOTHER

Jamie, a 38-year-old Hispanic woman, gave birth to a term large-for-gestational-age newborn weighing 10 lb. She had a history of gestational diabetes but had not received any prenatal care. She arrived at the hospital in active labor. Despite macrosomia, the newborn's Apgar scores were 8 and 9 at 1 and 5 minutes respectively. No resuscitative measures were needed.

One hour after birth, assessment revealed a pale, irritable newborn with sweating and several episodes of apnea. A glucose level obtained at this time via a heel stick was 35 mg/dL. Two hours later, the newborn begins exhibiting signs of respiratory distress—grunting, nasal flaring, retractions, tachypnea (respiratory rate 72 breaths/minute), and tachycardia (heart rate 176 bpm).

NURSING DIAGNOSIS: Risk for unstable glucose level related to hypoglycemia secondary to intrauterine hyperinsulin state resulting from maternal gestational diabetes as evidenced by low blood glucose level, irritability, pallor, sweating, and apnea

Outcome Identification and Evaluation
The newborn will exhibit adequate glucose control *as evidenced by maintaining blood glucose levels above 40 mg/dL and an absence of clinical signs of hypoglycemia.*

Interventions: Promoting Glucose Control
- Monitor blood glucose levels hourly for the first 4 hours and then every 3 to 4 hours or as necessary *to detect hypoglycemia, which would be <40 mg/dL.*
- Continue to observe for manifestations of hypoglycemia, such as pallor, tremors, jitteriness, lethargy, and poor feeding, *to allow for early detection and prompt intervention, thereby minimizing the risk of complications associated with hypoglycemia.*
- Monitor temperature frequently and institute measures to maintain a neutral thermal environment *to prevent cold stress, which would increase metabolic demands and further deplete glycogen stores.*
- Initiate early feedings every 2 to 3 hours or as appropriate or administer glucose supplements as ordered *to prevent hypoglycemia caused by the newborn's hyperinsulin state.* Administer IV glucose infusions as ordered *to correct hypoglycemia if glucose levels do not stabilize with feeding.*
- Cluster infant care activities and provide for rest periods *to conserve the newborn's energy and reduce use of glucose and glycogen stores.*
- Reduce environmental stimuli by dimming lights and speaking softly *to reduce energy demands and further utilization of glucose.*
- Explain all events and procedures to the mother *to help alleviate anxiety and promote understanding of the newborn's condition.*

NURSING DIAGNOSIS: Impaired gas exchange related to respiratory distress secondary to delayed lung maturity resulting from inhibition of pulmonary surfactant production due to fetal hyperinsulinemia as evidenced by grunting, nasal flaring, retractions, tachypnea, and tachycardia

Outcome Identification and Evaluation
Newborn will demonstrate signs of adequate oxygenation without respiratory distress *as evidenced by respiratory rate and vital signs within acceptable parameters, absence of nasal flaring, retractions, and grunting, and oxygen saturation and arterial blood gas levels within acceptable parameters.*

Interventions: Promoting Oxygenation
- Monitor newborn's vital signs *to establish a baseline and evaluate for changes.*
- Assess airway patency and perform gentle suctioning as ordered *to ensure patency and allow for adequate oxygen intake.*
- Position the newborn prone *to optimize respiratory status and reduce stress.*
- Assess lung sounds for changes *to allow early detection of change in status.*
- Continuously monitor oxygen saturation levels via pulse oximetry *to determine adequacy of tissue perfusion.*
- Assess arterial blood gas results *to detect changes indicating acidosis, hypoxemia, or hypercarbia, which would suggest hypoxia.* Administer medications as ordered *to correct acidosis.*
- Administer oxygen as ordered *to promote adequate tissue perfusion.*
- Assess newborn's skin to identify cyanosis, pallor, and mottling *to detect changes indicating compromised oxygenation.*
- Administer surfactant replacement therapy as ordered *to aid in stabilizing the newborn's lungs until postnatal surfactant synthesis improves.*
- Institute measures to maintain normal blood glucose levels and a neutral thermal environment, cluster care activities, and reduce excessive stimuli *to reduce oxygen demand and consumption.*

until stable. Document the results. Report unstable glucose values if oral feedings do not maintain and stabilize the newborn's blood glucose levels. If glucose levels are not stabilized, initiate IV glucose infusions as ordered and monitor that the infusions are flowing at the prescribed rate.

Maintaining Fluid and Electrolyte Balance

Monitor serum calcium levels for changes indicating the need for supplementation, such as with oral or IV calcium gluconate. Assess the newborn for signs of hypocalcemia, such as tremors, jitteriness, twitching, seizures, and high-pitched cry.

Also administer fluid therapy as ordered to maintain adequate hydration. Monitor serum bilirubin levels and institute phototherapy if the newborn is over 24 hours old.

Providing Parental Support

Assist the parents and family in understanding the newborn's condition and need for frequent monitoring. Offer support and information to the parents and family. They may erroneously interpret the newborn's large size as an indication that the newborn is free of problems. Encourage open communication and listen with empathy to the family's fears and concerns. Provide frequent opportunities for the parents to interact with their newborn. Make appropriate referrals to social services and community resources as necessary to help the family cope.

▶ BIRTH TRAUMA

Injuries to the newborn from the forces of labor and birth are categorized as birth trauma. In the past, numerous injuries were associated with difficult births requiring external or internal version or mid- or high forceps deliveries. Today, however, cesarean births have contributed to the decline in birth trauma.

Significant birth trauma accounts for fewer than 2% of neonatal deaths and stillbirths in the United States (Kenner & Lott, 2007). Improved prenatal diagnosis and monitoring during labor have helped to reduce the incidence of birth injuries today.

Pathophysiology

The process of birth is a blend of compression, contractions, torques, and traction. Birth traumas are injuries sustained by the newborn during the birthing process. When fetal size, presentation, or neurologic immunity complicates this process, the forces of labor and birth may lead to tissue damage, edema, hemorrhage, or fracture in the newborn. For example, birth trauma may result from the pressure of birth, especially in a prolonged or abrupt

labor, abnormal or difficult presentation, cephalopelvic disproportion, or mechanical forces, such as forceps or vacuum used during delivery. Table 24.3 summarizes the most common types of birth trauma.

Nursing Assessment

Recognition of trauma and birth injuries is imperative so that early treatment can be initiated. Review the labor and birth history for risk factors, such as a prolonged or abrupt labor, abnormal or difficult presentation, cephalopelvic disproportion, or mechanical forces, such as forceps or vacuum used during delivery. Also review the history for multiple fetus deliveries, large-for-date infants, extreme prematurity, large fetal head, or newborns with congenital anomalies.

Complete a careful physical and neurologic assessment of every newborn admitted to the nursery to establish whether injuries exist. Inspect the head for lumps, bumps, or bruises. Note if swelling or bruising crosses the suture line. Assess the eyes and face for facial paralysis, observing for asymmetry of the face with crying or appearance of the mouth being drawn to the unaffected side. Ensure that the newborn spontaneously moves all extremities. Note any absence of or decrease in deep tendon reflexes or abnormal positioning of extremities.

Assess and document symmetry of structure and function. Be prepared to assist with scheduling diagnostic studies to confirm trauma or injuries, which will be important in determining treatment modalities.

Nursing Management

Nursing management is primarily supportive and focuses on assessing for resolution of the trauma or any associated complications along with providing support and education to the parents. Provide the parents with explanations and reassurance that these injuries usually resolve with minimal or no treatment. Parents are alarmed when their newborn is unable to move an extremity or demonstrates asymmetric facial movements. Provide parents with a realistic picture of the situation to gain their understanding and trust. Be readily available to answer questions and teach them how to care for the newborn, including any modifications that might be necessary. Allow parents adequate time to understand the implications of the birth trauma or injury and what treatment modalities are needed, if any. Provide them with information about the length of time until the injury will resolve and when and if they need to seek further medical attention for the condition. Spending time with the parents and providing them with support, information, and teaching are important to allow them to make decisions and care for their newborn. Anticipate the need for community referral for ongoing follow-up and care, if necessary.

TABLE 24.3 COMMON TYPES OF BIRTH TRAUMA

Type	Description	Findings	Treatment
Fractures	Most often occur during breech births or shoulder dystocia in newborns with macrosomia Mid-clavicular fractures are the most common type of fracture, secondary to shoulder dystocia. Long bone fractures of humerus or femur, usually mid-shaft, also can occur.	Mid-clavicular fractures: The newborn presents with irritability and does not move the arm on the affected side either spontaneously or when the Moro reflex is elicited. Femoral or humeral long bone fractures: The newborn shows loss of spontaneous leg or arm motion respectively; usually swelling and pain accompany the limited movement. X-rays confirm the fracture.	Mid-clavicular fractures typically heal rapidly and uneventfully; arm motion may be limited by pinning the newborn's sleeve to the shirt. Femoral and humeral shaft fractures are treated with splinting. Healing and complete recovery are expected within 2 to 4 weeks without incident (Laroia, 2007). Explanation to the parents and reassurance are needed.
Brachial plexus injury	Primarily in large babies, babies with shoulder dystocia, or breech delivery Results from stretching, hemorrhage within a nerve, or tearing of the nerve or the roots associated with cervical cord injury Associated traumatic injuries include fracture of the clavicle or humerus or subluxations of the shoulder or cervical spine. Erb's palsy is an upper brachial plexus injury. Klumpke's palsy is an injury to the lower brachial plexus (lower brachial injuries are less common).	In Erb's palsy, the involved extremity usually presents adducted, prone, and internally rotated; shoulder movement is absent; Moro, bicep, and radial reflexes are absent, but the grasp reflex is usually present. Klumpke's palsy is manifested by weakness in the hand and wrist; grasp reflex is absent.	Erb's palsy usually involves immobilization of the upper arm across the upper abdomen/chest to protect the shoulder from excessive motion for the first week; then gentle passive range-of-motion exercises are performed daily to prevent contractures. There is usually no associated sensory loss, and this condition usually improves rapidly. Treatment for Klumpke's palsy involves placing the hand in a neutral position and using passive range-of-motion exercises. In some cases deficits may persist, requiring continuing observation.
Cranial nerve trauma	Most common is facial nerve palsy. Frequently attributed to pressure resulting from forceps May also result from pressure on the nerve in utero, related to fetal positioning such as the head lying against the shoulder	Physical findings include asymmetry of the face when crying; mouth may be drawn towards the unaffected side; wrinkles are deeper on the unaffected side. The paralyzed side may be smooth, with a swollen appearance. Eye is persistently open on the affected side.	Most infants begin to recover in the first week, but full resolution may take up to several months; parents need reassurance about this. In most cases, treatment is not necessary, only observation. If the eye is affected and unable to close, protection with patches and synthetic tears may be necessary. Parents need instruction about how to feed the newborn, since he or she cannot close the lips around the nipple without having milk seep out.

(continued)

TABLE 24.3 COMMON TYPES OF BIRTH TRAUMA (continued)

Type	Description	Findings	Treatment
Head trauma	Mild trauma can cause soft tissue injuries such as cephalhematoma and caput succedaneum; greater trauma can cause depressed skull fractures. **Cephalhematoma** (subperiosteal collection of blood secondary to the rupture of blood vessels between the skull and periosteum) occurs in 2.5% of all births and typically appears within hours after birth (Cunningham et al., 2005). **Caput succedaneum** (soft tissue swelling) is caused by edema of the head against the dilating cervix during the birth process. Subarachnoid hemorrhage (one of the most common types of intracranial trauma) may be due to hypoxia/ischemia, variations in blood pressure, and the pressure exerted on the head during labor. Bleeding is of venous origin, and underlying contusions also may occur (Laroia, 2007). Subdural hemorrhage (hematomas) occurs less often today because of improved obstetric techniques. Typically, tears of the major veins or venous sinuses overlying the cerebral hemispheres or cerebellum (most common in newborns of primaparas and large newborns, or after an instrumented birth) are the cause. Increased pressure on the blood vessels inside the skull leads to tears. Depressed skull fractures (rare) may result from the pressure of a forceps delivery; can also occur during spontaneous or cesarean births and may be associated with other head trauma causing subdural bleeding, subarachnoid hemorrhage, or brain trauma (Laroia, 2007).	In cephalhematoma, suture lines delineate its extent; usually located on one side, over the parietal bone. In caput succedaneum, swelling is not limited by suture lines: it extends across the midline and is associated with head molding. It does not usually cause complications other than a misshapen head. Swelling is maximal at birth and then rapidly decreases in size. In subarachnoid hemorrhage, some RBCs may appear in the CSF of full-term newborns. Newborns may present with apnea, seizures, lethargy, or abnormal findings on a neurologic examination (Rodriguez, 2007). Subdural hemorrhage can be asymptomatic, or the neonate can exhibit seizures, enlarging head size, decreased level of consciousness, or abnormal findings on a neurologic examination, with hypotonia, a poor Moro reflex, or extensive retinal hemorrhages. Depressed skull fractures can be observed and palpated as depressions. Confirmation by x-ray is necessary.	Cephalhematoma resolves gradually over 2 to 3 weeks without treatment (see Chapter 18). Caput succedaneum usually resolves over the first few days without treatment (see Chapter 18). Subarachnoid hemorrhage requires minimal handling to reduce stress. Subdural hematoma requires aspiration; can be life-threatening if it is in an inaccessible location and cannot be aspirated (Laroia, 2007). Depressed skull fractures typically require a neurosurgical consultation.

▶ NEWBORNS OF SUBSTANCE-ABUSING MOTHERS

It is generally assumed that all pregnant women want to provide a healthy environment for their unborn child and know how to avoid harm. However, for women who use substances such as drugs or alcohol, this may not be the case. Substance use during pregnancy exposes the fetus to the possibility of IUGR, prematurity, neurobehavioral and neurophysiologic dysfunction, birth defects, infections, and long-term developmental sequelae (Kenner & Lott, 2007).

It is difficult to establish the true prevalence of substance use in pregnant women; many women deny taking any nonprescribed substance because of the associated social stigma and legal implications. The National Institute on Drug Abuse (NIDA) suggests that approximately 1 in 10 newborns are exposed to one or more mood-altering drugs in utero (NIDA, 2007f). Drug exposure may go unrecognized in these newborns, and they may be discharged from the newborn nursery at risk for medical and social problems, including abuse and neglect.

Tobacco, alcohol, and marijuana are the substances most commonly abused during pregnancy. Other drugs may include opioids such as morphine, codeine, methadone, meperidine, and heroin; CNS stimulants such as amphetamines and cocaine; CNS depressants such as barbiturates, diazepam (Valium), and sedative–hypnotics; and hallucinogens, such as LSD, inhalants, glue, paint thinner, nail polish remover, and nitrous oxide (NIDA, 2007f). Table 24.4 highlights commonly used substances and their effects on the fetus and newborn.

▶ *Consider* THIS!

I admit, I had led a reckless life since I was a teen. I rebelled against my mother's authority and started smoking and doing drugs just to "check out" of my painful world. It was one big blast after another with a high and then a low. I never considered the consequences of my behavior then and never thought it would hurt anyone until I learned I was about 4 months pregnant. I convinced myself that if I cut back, everything would be fine.

Now, as I stand here in the NICU watching my tiny son struggle for air and tremble all over, I am not so convinced that I didn't hurt anyone except myself. As I witness my son fight against MY nicotine and drug addiction, my heart is heavy with guilt. I wonder how I could have thought that my troubles wouldn't become another's plight sooner or later. What must I have been thinking to isolate my addiction and not

(continued)

▶ *Consider* THIS! *(continued)*

consider the impact that it would have on my mother and my son?

Thoughts: This woman honestly regrets what her addiction has done to her son as she stands watching him go through withdrawal. Her lifestyle choices do affect others, despite her previous denial. One problem with addiction is the difficulty in getting help after deciding to finally quit. There aren't enough rehab centers to deal with the large numbers needing their services and it can be difficult to get into one. What can be offered to pregnant women who abuse substances? How can nurses increase community awareness about the impact of this problem, especially during pregnancy?

Substance abuse during pregnancy is the subject of much controversy. The timing of drug ingestion usually determines the type and severity of damage to the fetus. Frequently, the woman uses more than one substance, which compounds the problem. Nurses must be knowledgeable about the issues of substance abuse and must be alert for opportunities to identify, prevent, manage, and educate women and families about this key public health issue.

Fetal Alcohol Syndrome

The adverse effects of alcohol consumption have been recognized for centuries, but the associated pattern of fetal anomalies was not labeled until the early 1970s. The distinctive pattern identified three specific findings: growth restriction (prenatal and postnatal), craniofacial structural anomalies, and CNS dysfunction. These distinctive findings were called **fetal alcohol syndrome**, characterized by physical and mental disorders that appear at birth and remain problematic throughout the child's life. However, there are also circumstances in which the effects of prenatal alcohol exposure are apparent, but the newborn does not meet all of the criteria. In an attempt to include those who do not meet the strict criteria, the terms "fetal alcohol effects," "alcohol-related birth defects," and "alcohol-related neurologic defects" are used to describe children with a variety of problems thought to be related to alcohol consumption during pregnancy. The Institutes of Medicine coined the term **fetal alcohol spectrum disorder** as a way of describing the broader effects of prenatal alcohol exposure. Children with fetal alcohol syndrome are at the severe end of the spectrum (Manning & Hoyne, 2007). Newborns with some but not all of the symptoms of fetal alcohol syndrome are described as having **alcohol-related birth defects**. Fetal alcohol effects may include

(text continues on page 747)

TABLE 24.4 SUBSTANCES AND THEIR EFFECTS ON THE FETUS AND NEWBORN

Substance	Description	Effects on Fetus and Newborn	Nursing Implications
Alcohol	Consumption is pervasive and widely accepted, with use, abuse, and addiction affecting all levels of society. It is a common misconception that a substance sold to the public without restriction is safe.	Fetal alcohol syndrome (one of the most common known causes of mental retardation) Fetal alcohol spectrum disorders Alcohol-related birth defects	Provide education that decreasing or eliminating alcohol consumption during pregnancy is the only way to prevent fetal alcohol syndrome and fetal alcohol effects. Assist pregnant woman in finding a treatment program if possible. Inform all women who are pregnant or planning to become pregnant about the detrimental effects of alcohol during pregnancy. Educate women using a nonjudgmental, culturally connected approach. Warn women that there is no safe time to drink or amount of alcohol they can consume.
Tobacco/nicotine	Nicotine is an addictive substance. It causes epinephrine release from adrenal cortex, leading to initial stimulation followed by depression and fatigue, causing the user to seek more nicotine. Increased numbers of women are smoking (at least 11% smoke during pregnancy; March of Dimes, 2007c). Over 2,500 chemicals are found in cigarette smoke, including nicotine, tar, carbon monoxide, and cyanide. It is unknown which are harmful, but nicotine and carbon monoxide are believed to play a role in causing adverse pregnancy outcomes.	Impaired oxygenation of mother and fetus due to nicotine crossing placenta and carbon monoxide combining with hemoglobin Increased risk for low birthweight (risk almost doubled), small for gestational age, and preterm birth Increased risk for sudden infant death syndrome (SIDS) and chronic respiratory illness (MNH, 2007)	Provide teaching to women about healthy behaviors. Provide support for smoking cessation. Individualize counseling based on factors associated with the woman's smoking and challenges faced (why woman smokes, stressors in life, and social support network). Suggest options such as group smoking cessation programs, relaxation techniques, individual counseling, hypnosis, and partner-support counseling.
Marijuana	Most widely used illicit psychoactive substance in Western world and most commonly used illicit drug in the United States (NIDA, 2007d) Derived from *Cannabis sativa* plant	Not shown to have teratogenic effects on fetus; no consistent types of malformations identified Intrauterine growth restriction (IUGR) is common due to delivery of carbon monoxide to fetus (NIDA, 2007d). Increased risk for small for gestational age	Provide teaching to women about healthy behaviors. Provide support for cessation of marijuana use.

Substance	Description	Effects on Fetus and Newborn	Nursing Implications
		Altered responses to visual stimuli, sleep-pattern abnormalities, photophobia, lack of motor control, hyperirritability, increased tremulousness, and high-pitched cry noted in infants of mothers who smoked marijuana Research related to long-term effects is continuing (NIDA, 2007d).	
Methamphetamines	Addictive stimulant; use releases high levels of dopamine, which stimulates brain cells, enhancing mood and body movement High potential for abuse and addiction; can be inhaled, injected, smoked, or taken orally Many street names, such as speed, meth, ice, and chalk Primary effects include accelerated heart and respiratory rate, elevated blood pressure, papillary dilation; secondary effects include loss of appetite. Used medically as treatment for obesity and narcolepsy in adults and hyperactivity in children	Little research on use during pregnancy because its use is less common than cocaine or narcotics Fetal effects similar to cocaine (suggesting vasoconstriction as possible underlying mechanism) Possible maternal malnutrition, leading to problems with fetal growth and development Increased risk for preterm birth and low-birthweight newborns Infants may have withdrawal symptoms, including dysphoria, agitation, jitteriness, poor weight gain, abnormal sleep patterns, poor feeding, frantic fist sucking, high-pitched cry, respiratory distress soon after birth, frequent infections, and significant lassitude (Arenson & Drake, 2007). Long-term effects are not known.	Provide teaching to women about healthy behaviors. Provide support for cessation of methamphetamine use. Monitor the woman for weight changes; emphasize the need for adequate nutritional intake to support fetal growth and development.
Cocaine	Strong CNS stimulant that interferes with reabsorption of dopamine Physical effects: vasoconstriction; pupillary dilation; increased temperature, heart rate, and blood pressure Taken orally, sublingually, intranasally, intravenously, and via inhalation Estimated that 30% to 40% of cocaine addicts are female Maternal cocaine use during pregnancy is a significant health problem (March of Dimes, 2007b). Increased potential for use of multiple drugs if mother using cocaine	Preterm birth and lower birthweight Unclear impact on later development Speculation that cocaine interferes with infant's cognitive development, leading to learning and memory difficulties later in life (Kenner & Lott, 2007) Associated congenital anomalies: GU, cardiac, and CNS defects, and prune belly syndrome Other typical newborn characteristics: smaller head circumference, piercing cry, limb defects, ambiguous genitalia, poor feeding, poor visual and auditory responses, poor sleep patterns, decreased impulse control, stiff, hyperextended positioning, irritability and hypersensitivity, inability to respond to caretaker (Blackburn, 2007)	Educate the woman about the effects of cocaine use on the fetus and newborn. Assess for use of other substances. Provide teaching to women about healthy behaviors. Provide support and guidance for cessation of cocaine and other substance use.

(continued)

TABLE 24.4   SUBSTANCES AND THEIR EFFECTS ON THE FETUS AND NEWBORN (continued)

Substance	Description	Effects on Fetus and Newborn	Nursing Implications
Heroin	Illegal, highly addictive opiate derived from morphine that can be sniffed, smoked, or injected Possible consequences include HIV infection, tuberculosis, crime, violence, and family disruption. Severe physical addiction; CNS depressant producing mental dullness and drowsiness	Newborns of heroin-addicted mothers are born dependent on heroin. Increased risk for transmission of hepatitis B and C and HIV to newborns when mothers share needles Significantly increased rates of stillbirth, IUGR, preterm birth, and newborn mortality (3 to 7 times greater; NIDA, 2007b, 2007c) Small-for-gestational age newborns, meconium aspiration, high incidence of SIDS, and delayed effects from subacute withdrawal (restlessness, continual crying, agitation, sneezing, vomiting, fever, diarrhea, seizures, irritability, and poor socialization [possibly persisting for 4 to 6 months]; March of Dimes, 2007b) Intrauterine death or preterm birth is possible with abrupt cessation of heroin use.	Educate the woman about the effects of heroin use on the fetus and newborn. Assess for use of other substances. Provide teaching to women about healthy behaviors. Warn the woman not to abruptly stop heroin use. Encourage her to enroll in a methadone maintenance program.
Methadone	Synthetic opiate narcotic used primarily as maintenance therapy for heroin addiction	Improvement in many of the detrimental fetal effects associated with heroin use Withdrawal symptoms are common in newborns. Possible low birthweight due to symmetric fetal growth restriction Increased severity and longer period of withdrawal (due to methadone's longer half-life) Seizures (commonly severe) do not usually occur until 2 to 3 weeks of age, when the newborn is at home. Increased rate of SIDS (3 to 4 times higher; Goff & O'Connor, 2007)	Methadone maintenance programs are the standard of care for women with narcotic addiction. Inform the woman about the benefits and risks of methadone use vs. heroin use. Advantages include improved fetal and newborn growth, reduced risk of fetal death, and reduced risk of HIV infections. Advise the woman that she will need to return consistently to receive the prescribed methadone dose. Reinforce the need for continued prenatal care. Inform the woman that she can breastfeed her newborn while receiving methadone. Teach mother and caregivers about signs and symptoms of methadone withdrawal.

such problems as low birthweight, developmental delays, and hyperactivity. Box 24.2 summarizes the manifestations of fetal alcohol syndrome.

Worldwide, the incidence of fetal alcohol syndrome is 1 to 3 cases per 1,000 live births, and that of fetal alcohol effects is 3 to 5 per 1,000 live births (March of Dimes, 2007a). Current estimates indicate that approximately 13% of women of childbearing age are either problem drinkers or alcoholics; therefore, the number of fetuses exposed to alcohol during utero increases dramatically (March of Dimes, 2007a).

Fetal alcohol syndrome is one of the most common known causes of mental retardation, and it is the only cause that is entirely preventable. The effects last a lifetime. Children with this syndrome have varying degrees of psycholog-

ical and behavioral problems and often find it difficult to hold a job and live independently (CDC, 2007b).

Decreasing or eliminating alcohol consumption during pregnancy is the only way to prevent fetal alcohol syndrome and fetal alcohol effects. Unfortunately, few treatment programs address the needs of pregnant women, so many newborns are exposed to alcohol in utero.

Neonatal Abstinence Syndrome

Newborns of women who abuse tobacco, illicit substances, caffeine, and alcohol can exhibit withdrawal behavior. Withdrawal symptoms occur in 60% of all newborns exposed to drugs (Arenson & Drake, 2007). Drug dependency acquired in utero is manifested by a constellation of neurologic and physical behaviors and is known as **neonatal abstinence syndrome**. Although often treated as a single entity, neonatal abstinence syndrome is not a single pathologic condition. The manifestations of withdrawal are a function of the drug's half-life, the specific drug or combination of drugs used, dosage, route of administration, timing of drug exposure, and length of drug exposure (Kuschel, 2007). Typical newborn behaviors include CNS hypersensitivity, autonomic dysfunction, and gastrointestinal disturbances (Marcellus, 2007). Neonatal abstinence syndrome has both medical and developmental consequences for the newborn.

Nursing Assessment

Several assessment tools can be used to assess a drug-exposed newborn. Figure 24.5 shows an example. Regardless of the tool used for assessment, address these key areas:

- Maternal history to identify risk behaviors for substance abuse:
  - Previous unexplained fetal demise
  - Lack of prenatal care
  - History of missed prenatal appointments
  - Severe mood swings
  - Precipitous labor
  - Poor nutritional status
  - Abruptio placentae
  - Hypertensive episodes
  - History of drug abuse
- Laboratory test results (toxicology) to identify substances in mother and newborn
- Signs of neonatal abstinence syndrome (use the "WITHDRAWAL" acronym; see description below)
- Evidence of seizure activity and need for protective environment

The newborn's behavior often prompts the health care provider or nurse to suspect intrauterine drug exposure (Box 24.3). The newborn physical examination may also reveal low birthweight for gestational age or drug- or alcohol-related birth defects and dysfunction.

> ### BOX 24.2 Clinical Picture of Fetal Alcohol Syndrome
>
> - Microcephaly (head circumference <10th percentile)★
> - Small palpebral (eyelid) fissures★
> - Abnormally small eyes
> - Intrauterine growth restriction
> - Maxillary hypoplasia (flattened or absent)
> - Epicanthal folds (folds of skin of the upper eyelid over the eye)
> - Thin upper lip★
> - Missing vertical groove in median portion of upper lip★
> - Short upturned nose
> - Short birth length and low birthweight
> - Joint and limb defects
> - Altered palmar crease pattern
> - Prenatal or postnatal growth ≤10th percentile★
> - Congenital cardiac defects (septal defects)
> - Delayed fine and gross motor development
> - Poor eye–hand coordination
> - Clinically significant brain abnormalities★
> - Mental retardation
> - Narrow forehead
> - Performance substantially below expected level in cognitive or developmental functioning, executive or motor functioning, and attention or hyperactivity; social or language skills★
> - Inadequate sucking reflex and poor appetite
>
> ---
>
> ★Diagnosis of fetal alcohol syndrome requires the presence of three findings:
> 1. Documentation of all three facial abnormalities
> 2. Documentation of growth deficits (height, weight or both below 10th percentile)
> 3. Documentation of CNS abnormalities (structural, neurologic, or functional)
>
> Source: National Center on Birth Defects and Developmental Disabilities (NCBDDD) (2004). Fetal alcohol syndrome: guidelines for referral and diagnosis (p. 20). Atlanta: Centers for Disease Control and Prevention (CDC), Department of Health and Human Services (DHHS)

CENTRAL NERVOUS SYSTEM DISTURBANCES

SIGNS AND SYMPTOMS	SCORE	AM							PM			
Excessive high-pitched cry	2											
Continuous high-pitched cry	3											
Sleeps <1 hour after feeding	3											
Sleeps <2 hours after feeding	2											
Sleeps <3 hours after feeding	1											
Hyperactive Moro reflex	2											
Markedly hyperactive Moro refex	3											
Mild tremors disturbed	1											
Moderate–severe tremors disturbed	2											
Mild tremors undisturbed	1											
Moderate–severe tremors undisturbed	4											
Increased muscle tone	2											
Excoloration (specify area)	1											
Myoclonic jerks	3											
Generalized convulsions	5											

METABOLIC / VASOMOTOR/RESPIRATORY DISTURBANCES

Sweating												
Fever <101 (99–100.8°F/37.2–38.2°C)	1											
Fever >101 (38.2°C and higher)	2											
Frequent yawning (>3– 4 times/interval)	1											
Mottling	1											
Nasal stuffiness	1											
Sneezing (>3–4 times/interval)	1											
Nasal flaring	2											
Respiratory rate >60 / min	1											
Respiratory rate >60 / min, with retractions	2											

GASTROINTESTINAL DISTURBANCES

Excessive sucking	1											
Poor feeding	2											
Regurgitation	2											
Projectile vomiting	3											
Loose stools	2											
Watery stools	3											
TOTAL SCORE												

FIGURE 24.5 Neonatal abstinence scoring system (From Cloherty, J. P., & Stark, A. P. [1998]. *Manual of neonatal care* [4th ed., pp. 26–27]. Boston: Little, Brown.)

BOX 24.3 Manifestations of Neonatal Abstinence Syndrome

CNS Dysfunction
- Tremors
- Generalized seizures
- Hyperactive reflexes
- Restlessness
- Hypertonic muscle tone, constant movement
- Shrill, high-pitched cry
- Disturbed sleep patterns

Metabolic, Vasomotor, and Respiratory Disturbances
- Fever
- Frequent yawning
- Mottling of the skin
- Sweating
- Frequent sneezing
- Nasal flaring
- Tachypnea >60 bpm
- Apnea

Gastrointestinal Dysfunction
- Poor feeding
- Frantic sucking or rooting
- Loose or watery stools
- Regurgitation or projectile vomiting (Belik & Hawes, 2007; Kuschel, 2007; Marcellus, 2007)

Labels on figure: Irritability; Disturbed sleep patterns; Frequent sneezing; Shrill, high-pitched cry; Vomiting; Constant movement; Tachypnea; Tremors; Diarrhea; Hyperreflexia, clonus

---

▶ **Take** NOTE!

Cocaine-exposed newborns are typically fussy, irritable, and inconsolable at times. Cocaine-exposed infants demonstrate poor coordination of sucking and swallowing, making feeding time frustrating for the newborn and caregiver alike.

Assess the newborn for signs of neonatal abstinence syndrome. Use the acronym WITHDRAWAL to focus the assessment:

W = Wakefulness: sleep duration less than 1 to 3 hours after feeding
I = Irritability
T = Temperature variation, tachycardia, tremors
H = Hyperactivity, high-pitched persistent cry, hyperreflexia, hypertonus
D = Diarrhea, diaphoresis, disorganized suck
R = Respiratory distress, rub marks, rhinorrhea
A = Apneic attacks, autonomic dysfunction
W = Weight loss or failure to gain weight
A = Alkalosis (respiratory)
L = Lacrimation (Belik & Hawes, 2007)

Assist with obtaining diagnostic studies to identify the severity of withdrawal. Toxicology screening of the newborn's blood, urine, and meconium identifies the substances to which the newborn has been exposed.

In general, a urine screen signifies only recent newborn exposure to maternal use of drugs. It can detect marijuana use up to a month earlier, cocaine use up to 96 hours earlier, heroin use 24 to 48 hours earlier, and methadone use up to 10 days earlier (Belik & Hawes, 2007).

Nursing Management

The needs of the substance-exposed newborn are multiple, complex, and costly, both to the health care system and to society. Substance abuse takes place among people of all colors, sizes, shapes, incomes, types, and conditions. Most pregnant women are unaware of the adverse impact their substance abuse can have on the newborn.

Nurses are in a unique position to help because they interact with high-risk mothers and newborns in many settings, including the community, health care facilities, and family agencies. It is the responsibility of all nurses to identify, educate, counsel, and refer pregnant women with substance-abusing problems. For example, nurses can be instrumental in increasing the number of pregnant women who make a serious attempt to quit smoking by using the "5 A's" approach:

- Ask: Ask all women if they smoke and would like to quit.
- Advise: Encourage the use of clinically proven treatment plans.
- Assess: Provide motivation by discussing the "5 R's":
  - Relevance of quitting to the woman
  - Risk of continued smoking to the fetus
  - Rewards of quitting for both
  - Roadblocks to quitting
  - Repeat at every visit
- Assist: Help the woman to protect her fetus and newborn from the negative effects of smoking.
- Arrange: Schedule follow-up visits to reinforce the woman's commitment to quit.

Although this approach is geared to smoking cessation, nurses can adapt it to focus on cessation for any substance use. Early, supportive, ongoing nursing care is critical to the well-being of the mother and her newborn.

Caring for a substance-exposed newborn remains a major challenge to health care professionals. The major goals include providing comfort to the newborn by relieving symptoms, improving feeding and weight gain, preventing seizures, promoting mother–newborn interactions, and reducing the incidence of newborn mortality and abnormal development (Belik & Hawes, 2007).

Promoting Comfort

Keep environmental stimuli to a minimum. For example, decrease stimuli by dimming the lights in the nursery, and swaddle the newborn tightly to decrease irritability behaviors. Other techniques such as gentle rocking, using a flexed position, and offering a pacifier can help manage CNS irritability. A pacifier also helps satisfy the newborn's need for nonnutritive sucking. Use a calm, gentle approach when handling the newborn and plan activities to avoid overstimulating the newborn, allowing time for rest periods.

Meeting Nutritional Needs

When feeding the newborn, use small amounts and position the newborn upright to prevent aspiration and to facilitate rhythmic sucking and swallowing. Breastfeeding is encouraged unless the mother is still using drugs. Monitor the newborn's weight daily to evaluate the success of food intake. Assess hydration; check skin turgor and fontanels. Assess the frequency and characteristics of bowel movements and monitor the newborn's fluid and electrolyte and acid–base status.

Preventing Complications

Pharmacologic treatment is warranted if conservative measures, such as swaddling and decreased environmental stimulation, are not adequate. The AAP recommends that for newborns with confirmed drug exposure, drug therapy is indicated if the newborn has seizures, diarrhea and vomiting resulting in excessive weight loss and dehydration, poor feeding, inability to sleep, and fever unrelated to infection (AAP Committee on Substance Abuse, 2005). Common medications used in the management of newborn withdrawal include morphine, paregoric, phenobarbital, tincture of opium, methadone, clonidine, chlorpromazine, and diazepam (Marcellus, 2007). Administer the prescribed medications and document the newborn's behavioral responses.

The newborn is at risk for skin breakdown. Weight loss, diarrhea, dehydration, and irritability can contribute to this risk. Provide meticulous skin care and protect the newborn's elbows and knees against friction and abrasions.

Promoting Parent–Newborn Interaction

For a mother who abuses substances, the birth of a drug-exposed newborn is both a crisis and an opportunity. The mother may feel guilty about the newborn's condition. Many of these newborns are unresponsive and have disorganized sleeping and feeding patterns. When awake, they can be easily overstimulated and irritated. Such characteristics make parent–newborn interactions difficult and frustrating, leading to possible detachment and avoidance (Burd, 2007). In addition, the mother may be single and a victim of physical and sexual abuse and may have a limited support system. Many of these mothers may have had poor parenting themselves, lack information about characteristic infant behaviors, and have unrealistic expectations about the newborn's abilities (Goff & O'Connor, 2007). Instruct the mother or caretaker how to care for the newborn, including what to do after the newborn goes home (Teaching Guidelines 24.1).

On the other hand, the newborn may be a powerful motivator for the mother to undergo treatment and seek recovery. Refer the mother to community agencies to address addiction and the infant's developmental needs (Gilbert, 2006). The nurse can play a pivotal role in assisting her to abstain from drug use and to promote effective parenting skills.

▶ HYPERBILIRUBINEMIA

Hyperbilirubinemia is a total serum bilirubin level above 5 mg/dL resulting from unconjugated bilirubin being deposited in the skin and mucous membranes (Blackburn, 2007). Hyperbilirubinemia is exhibited as jaundice (yellowing of the body tissues and fluids). Newborn jaundice is one of the most common reasons for hospital readmission. It occurs in 60% to 80% of term

TEACHING GUIDELINES 24.1

Caring for Your Newborn at Home

- Position your newborn with the head elevated to prevent choking.
- To aid your newborn's sucking and swallowing during feeding, position the chin downward and support it with your hand.
- Place your newborn on his or her back to sleep or nap, never on the stomach.
- Keep a bulb syringe close by to suction your newborn's mouth in case of choking.
- Cluster newborn care (bathing, feeding, dressing) to prevent overstimulation.
- If your newborn is fussy or crying, try these measures to help calm him or her:
  - Wrap your newborn snugly in a blanket and gently rock in rocking chair.
  - Take the baby for a ride in the car (using a newborn car seat).
  - Play soothing music and "dance" with the newborn.
  - Use a wind-up swing with music.
- To help your newborn get to sleep, try these measures:
  - Schedule a bath with a gentle massage prior to bedtime.
  - Change diaper and clothes to make the baby comfortable.
  - Feed the baby just prior to bedtime.
  - If the newborn cries when put in crib and all needs are met, allow him or her to cry.
  - Use a rocking chair to feed and sing a soft lullaby.
- Call your primary care provider if you observe withdrawal behaviors such as:
  - Slight tremors (shaking) of hands and legs
  - Stiff posture when held in your arms
  - Irritability and frequent fussiness
  - High-pitched cry, excessive sucking motions
  - Erratic sleep pattern
  - Frequent yawning, nasal stuffiness, sweating
  - Prolonged time needed to feed
  - Frequent vomiting after feeding

newborns in the first week of life and in virtually all preterm newborns (Rodriguez et al., 2008).

Pathophysiology

Newborn jaundice results from an imbalance in the rate of bilirubin production and bilirubin elimination. This imbalance determines the pattern and degree of newborn hyperbilirubinemia (Blackburn, 2007).

During the newborn period, a rapid transition from the intrauterine to the extrauterine pattern of bilirubin physiology occurs. Fetal unconjugated bilirubin is normally cleared by the placenta and the mother's liver in utero, so total bilirubin at birth is low. After the umbilical cord is cut, the newborn must conjugate bilirubin (convert a lipid-soluble pigment into a water-soluble pigment) in the liver on his or her own. The rate and amount of bilirubin conjugation depend on the rate of red blood cell breakdown, the bilirubin load, the maturity of the liver, and the number of albumin-binding sites (Kenner & Lott, 2007). Bilirubin production increases after birth mainly because of a shortened red blood cell lifespan (70 days in the newborn vs. 90 days in the adult) combined with an increased red blood cell mass. Therefore, the amount of bilirubin the newborn must deal with is large compared to that of an adult.

Bilirubin has two forms—unconjugated or indirect, which is fat-soluble and toxic to body tissues, and conjugated or direct, which is water-soluble and nontoxic. Elevated serum bilirubin levels are manifested as jaundice in the newborn. Typically the total serum bilirubin level rises over the first 3 to 5 days and then declines.

Physiologic Jaundice

Physiologic jaundice is the manifestation of the normal hyperbilirubinemia seen in newborns, appearing during the third to fourth days of life, due to the limitations and abnormalities of bilirubin metabolism. It occurs in 60% of term infants and up to 80% of preterm infants (Blackburn, 2007). Serum bilirubin levels reach up to 10 mg/dL and then decline rapidly over the first week after birth (Cunningham et al., 2005). Most newborns have been discharged by the time this jaundice peaks (at about 72 hours).

Physiologic jaundice may result from an increased bilirubin load because of relative polycythemia, a shortened red blood cell lifespan, immature hepatic uptake and conjugation process, and increased enterohepatic circulation (McLenan, 2007). Newborns with delayed passage of meconium are more likely to develop physiologic jaundice (Blackburn, 2007).

Physiologic jaundice differs between breastfed and bottle-fed newborns in relation to the onset of symptoms. Breastfed newborns typically have peak bilirubin levels on the fourth day of life; levels for bottle-fed newborns usually peak on the third day of life. The rate of bilirubin decline is less rapid in breastfed newborns compared to bottle-fed newborns because bottle-fed newborns tend to have more frequent bowel movements. Jaundice associated with breastfeeding presents in two distinct patterns: early-onset breastfeeding jaundice and late-onset breast milk jaundice.

Early-Onset Breastfeeding Jaundice

Early-onset breastfeeding jaundice is probably associated with ineffective breastfeeding practices because of relative caloric deprivation in the first few days of life. Decreased volume and frequency of feedings may result in mild dehydration and the delayed passage of meconium. This delayed defecation allows enterohepatic circulation reuptake of bilirubin and an increase in the serum level of unconjugated bilirubin. To prevent this, strategies to promote early effective breastfeeding are important. The AAP guidelines recommend early and frequent breastfeeding without supplemental water or dextrose-water unless medically indicated (AAP, 2005). Early frequent feedings can provide the newborn with adequate calories and fluid volume (via colostrum) to stimulate peristalsis and passage of meconium to eliminate bilirubin.

Late-Onset Breastfeeding Jaundice

Late-onset breastfeeding jaundice occurs later in the newborn period, with the bilirubin level usually peaking in the 6th to 14th day of life. Total serum bilirubin levels may be 12 to 20 mg/dL, but the levels are not considered pathologic (Simpson, 2007). The specific cause of late-onset breast milk jaundice is not entirely understood, but it may be related to a change in the milk composition resulting in enhanced enterohepatic circulation. Additional research is needed to determine the cause. Interrupting breastfeeding is not recommended unless bilirubin levels reach dangerous levels; if this occurs, breastfeeding is stopped for only 1 or 2 days. Substituting formula during this short break usually results in a prompt decline of bilirubin levels.

Pathologic Jaundice

Pathologic jaundice is manifested within the first 24 hours of life when total bilirubin levels increase by more than 5 mg/dL/day and the total serum bilirubin level is higher than 17 mg/dL in a full-term infant (Ozen & Mukherjee, 2007). Conditions that alter the production, transport, uptake, metabolism, excretion, or reabsorption of bilirubin can cause pathologic jaundice in the newborn. A few conditions that contribute to red blood cell breakdown and thus higher bilirubin levels include polycythemia, blood incompatibilities, and systemic acidosis. These altered conditions can lead to high levels of unconjugated bilirubin, possibly reaching toxic levels and resulting in a severe condition called kernicterus.

Kernicterus (yellow nucleus) or bilirubin encephalopathy is a preventable neurologic disorder characterized by encephalopathy, motor abnormalities, hearing and vision loss, and death (Maisels & Newman, 2007). Neurotoxicity develops because unconjugated bilirubin has a high affinity for brain tissue, and bilirubin not bound to albumin is free to cross the blood–brain barrier and damage cells of the CNS.

In the acute stage, the newborn becomes lethargic, irritable, and hypotonic and sucks poorly. If the hyperbilirubinemia is not treated, the newborn becomes hypertonic, with arching and seizures. A high-pitched cry may

be noted. These changes can occur rapidly, so all newborns must be assessed for jaundice and tested if indicated so that treatment can be initiated.

The most common condition associated with pathologic jaundice is hemolytic disease of the newborn secondary to incompatibility of blood groups of the mother and the newborn. The most frequent conditions are Rh factor and ABO incompatibilities.

> ▶ *Take* NOTE!
>
> *Significant jaundice in the newborn less than 24 hours of age should be immediately reported to the physician, as it may indicate a pathologic process.*

Rh Isoimmunization

Rh incompatibility or isoimmunization develops when an Rh-negative woman who has experienced Rh isoimmunization subsequently becomes pregnant with an Rh-positive fetus. The maternal antibodies cross the placenta into the fetal circulation and begin to break down the red blood cells (Fig. 24.6). Destruction of the fetal red blood cells leads to fetal anemia and hemolytic disease of the newborn. The severity of the fetal hemolytic process depends on the level and effectiveness of anti-D antibodies and the capacity of the fetal system to remove antibody-coated cells.

Intrauterine transfusions with Rh-negative, type O blood may be life-saving if done in time. The widespread administration of Rh immune globulin (RhoGAM), combined with aggressive fetal surveillance and transfusion, has reduced the incidence of hemolytic disease of the newborn.

Immune hydrops, also called hydrops fetalis, is a severe form of hemolytic disease of the newborn that occurs when pathologic changes develop in the organs of the fetus secondary to severe anemia. Hydrops fetalis results from fetal hypoxia, anemia, congestive heart failure, and hypoproteinemia secondary to hepatic dysfunction. ABO and Rh incompatibilities can both cause hydrops fetalis, but Rh disease is the more common cause. Typically, hydrops is not observed until the hemoglobin drops below approximately 4 g/dL (hematocrit <15%) (Huang et al., 2007). Fetuses with hydrops may die in utero from profound anemia and circulatory failure. The placenta is very enlarged and edematous. One sign of severe anemia and impending death is the sinusoidal fetal heart rate pattern (Cunningham et al., 2005).

ABO Incompatibility

ABO incompatibility is an immune reaction that occurs when the mother has type O blood and the fetus has type A, B, or AB blood. Although it occurs more frequently

Subsequent Rh⊕fetus

FIGURE 24.6 Rh isoimmunization.
(**A**) The Rh-negative mother is
exposed to Rh-positive antigens.
(**B**) Maternal antibodies form.
(**C**) Rh antibodies are transferred
to the fetus.

A   B   C

than Rh incompatibilities, it causes less severe problems and rarely results in hemolytic disease severe enough to be clinically diagnosed and treated. Enlargement of the spleen and liver may be found in newborns with ABO incompatibility, but hydrops fetalis is rare (Kenner & Lott, 2007). Because the antibodies resulting in ABO incompatibility occur naturally, it is impossible to eliminate this type of incompatibility.

Women with type O blood develop anti-A or anti-B antibodies throughout their life through foods they eat and exposure to infections. Most species of anti-A and anti-B antibodies are immunoglobin M (IgM), which cannot cross the placenta and thus cannot gain access to the fetal red blood cells. Some anti-A and anti-B antibodies from the mother may cross the placenta to the fetus during the first pregnancy and can cause hemolysis of fetal blood cells.

Nursing Assessment

Nurses play an important role in early detection and identification of jaundice in the newborn. Keen observation skills are essential.

Health History and Physical Examination

Review the medical record for factors that might predispose the newborn to hyperbilirubinemia, such as:

- Polycythemia
- Significant bruising or cephalhematoma, which increases bilirubin production
- Infections such as TORCH (toxoplasmosis, hepatitis B, rubella, cytomegalovirus, herpes simplex virus)
- Use of drugs during labor and birth such as diazepam (Valium) or oxytocin (Pitocin)
- Prematurity
- Gestational age of 34 to 36 weeks
- Hemolysis due to ABO incompatibility or Rh isoimmunization
- Macrosomic infant of a diabetic mother

- Delayed cord clamping, which increases the erythrocyte volume
- Decreased albumin binding sites to transport unconjugated bilirubin to the liver because of acidosis
- Delayed meconium passage, which increases the amount of bilirubin that returns to the unconjugated state and can be absorbed by the intestinal mucosa
- Siblings who had significant jaundice
- Inadequate breastfeeding leading to dehydration, decreased caloric intake, weight loss, and delayed passage of meconium
- Ethnicity, such as Asian-American, Mediterranean, or Native American
- Male gender (Kenner & Lott, 2007)

Perform a complete physical examination. Assess the skin, mucous membranes, sclerae, and bodily fluids (tears, urine) for a yellow color. Detect jaundice by observing the infant in a well-lit room and blanching the skin with digital pressure over a bony prominence. Typically, jaundice begins on the head and gradually progresses to the abdomen and extremities. Also inspect for pallor (anemia), excessive bruising (bleeding), and dehydration (sluggish circulation), which may contribute to the development of jaundice and the risk for kernicterus.

Assess the newborn for Rh incompatibility. Be alert for clinical manifestations such as ascites, congestive heart failure, edema, pallor, jaundice, hepatosplenomegaly, hydramnios, thick placenta, and dilation of the umbilical vein (Blackburn, 2007).

The hydropic newborn appears pale, edematous, and limp at birth and typically requires resuscitation. The newborn with immune hydrops exhibits severe generalized edema, organ hypertrophy and enlargement, and effusion of fluid into body cavities.

Laboratory and Diagnostic Testing

Determine maternal and fetal blood types, checking for incompatibilities (Comparison Chart 24.1). Assess lab-

COMPARISON CHART 24.1 RH VS. ABO
INCOMPATIBILITY

Clinical Picture	Rh Incompatibility	ABO Incompatibility
First-born	Rare	Common
Later pregnancies	More severe	No increase in severity
Jaundice	Moderate to severe	Mild
Hydrops fetalis	Frequent	Rare
Anemia	Frequently severe	Rare
Ascites	Frequent	Rare
Hepatosplenomegaly	Frequent	Common

oratory values for bilirubin (both unconjugated and conjugated). Bilirubin levels establish the diagnosis of hyperbilirubinemia. The newborn with Rh incompatibility demonstrates a rapidly rising unconjugated bilirubin level at birth or in the first 24 hours. Also expect to obtain alkaline phosphatase, liver enzymes, and prothrombin time and partial thromboplastin time, as well as:

• Direct Coombs test—to identify hemolytic disease of the newborn; positive results indicate that the newborn's red blood cells have been coated with antibodies and thus are sensitized
• Hemoglobin concentration—for evidence of anemia
• Blood type—to determine Rh status and any incompatibility of the newborn
• Total serum protein—to detect reduced binding capacity of albumin
• Reticulocyte count—to identify an elevated level indicating increased hemolysis

Assist with obtaining blood specimens. Use cord blood for hemoglobin concentration measurements; use a heel stick for direct Coombs testing and bilirubin levels. Prepare the parents and newborn for radiologic evaluation if necessary to determine abnormalities that may be causing the jaundice.

Nursing Management

Nursing management of a newborn with hyperbilirubinemia requires a comprehensive approach. As members of the health care team, nurses share in the responsibility for early detection and identification, family education, management, and follow-up of the mother and newborn. Documentation of the timing of onset of jaundice is essential to differentiate between physiologic (>24 hours) and pathologic jaundice (<24 hours).

Nurses can improve care by offering their presence and support.

Reducing Bilirubin Levels

Encourage early initiation of feedings to prevent hypoglycemia and provide protein to maintain the albumin levels to transport bilirubin to the liver. Ensure newborn feedings (breast milk or formula) every 2 to 3 hours to promote prompt emptying of bilirubin from the bowel. Encourage the mother to breastfeed (8 to 12 feedings per day) to prevent inadequate intake and thus dehydration. Supplement breast milk with formula to supply protein if bilirubin levels continue to increase with breastfeeding only. Monitor serum bilirubin levels frequently to reduce the risk of severe hyperbilirubinemia.

Phototherapy

For the newborn with jaundice, regardless of its etiology, phototherapy is used to convert unconjugated bilirubin to the less toxic water-soluble form that can be excreted. Phototherapy, via special lights placed above the newborn or a fiber-optic blanket placed under the newborn and wrapped around him or her, involves blue wavelengths of light to alter unconjugated bilirubin in the skin. For the newborn receiving phototherapy, place the newborn under the lights or on the fiberoptic blanket, exposing as much skin as possible. Cover the newborn's genitals and shield the eyes to protect these areas from becoming irritated or burned when using direct lights. Assess the intensity of the light source to prevent burns and excoriation (Fig. 24.7).

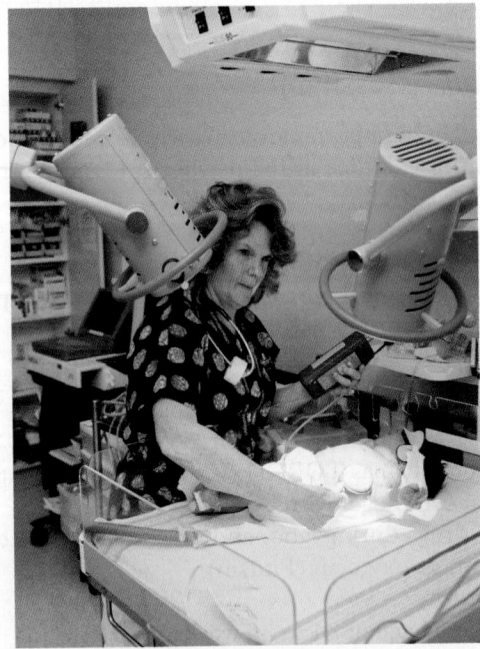

FIGURE 24.7 A newborn receiving phototherapy. Here the nurse is checking the intensity of the lights with a meter.

Turn the newborn every 2 hours to maximize the area of exposure, removing the newborn from the lights only for feedings. Maintain a neutral thermal environment to decrease energy expenditure, and assess the newborn's neurologic status frequently.

Assess the newborn's temperature every 3 to 4 hours as indicated. Monitor fluid intake and output closely and assess daily weights for gains or losses. Check skin turgor for dehydration.

With feedings, remove the newborn from the lights and remove the eye shields to allow interaction with the newborn. Encourage breast or bottle feedings every 2 to 3 hours. Follow agency policy about removing the eye shields periodically to assess the eyes for discharge or corneal irritation secondary to eye shield pressure. Typically, the eyes are assessed and eye shields removed once a shift.

Monitor stool for consistency and frequency. Unconjugated bilirubin excreted in the feces will produce a greenish appearance, and typically stools are loose. Lack of frequent green stools is a cause for concern.

Provide meticulous skin care. Assess skin surfaces frequently for dryness and irritation secondary to the dehydrating effects of phototherapy and irritation from highly acidic stool to prevent excoriation and skin breakdown (Simpson, 2007). Monitor the newborn's skin turgor.

Exchange Transfusion

If the total serum bilirubin level remains elevated after intensive phototherapy, an exchange transfusion, the quickest method for lowering serum bilirubin levels, may be necessary (Springer & Annibale, 2007). In the presence of hemolytic disease, severe anemia, or a rapid rise in the total serum bilirubin level, an exchange transfusion is recommended. An exchange transfusion removes the newborn's blood and replaces it with nonhemolyzed red blood cells from a donor. During the transfusion, monitor the newborn's cardiovascular status continuously because serious complications can arise, such as acid–base imbalances, infection, hypovolemia, and fluid and electrolyte imbalances. Exchange transfusion is used only as a second-line therapy after phototherapy has failed to yield results. Intensive nursing care is needed.

Assist the physician with an exchange transfusion if necessary. Monitor the newborn's status closely for changes, especially in vital signs and heart rate and rhythm, before, during, and after the procedure.

Providing Parent Teaching and Support

Nurses can help the parents to understand the diagnostic tests and treatment modalities by offering individualized teaching. Explore with the family their understanding of jaundice and treatment modalities to reduce anxiety and gain their cooperation in monitoring the infant. Teach the parents about jaundice and its potential risk using written and verbal material. Also show the parents how to identify newborn behaviors that might indicate rising bilirubin

levels. Emphasize the need to seek treatment from their pediatrician should any of the following occur:

• Lethargy, sleepiness, poor muscle tone, floppiness
• Poor sucking, lack of interest in feeding
• High-pitched cry

Teach the parents how to assess their newborn for signs of jaundice because physiologic jaundice may not occur until after the newborn is discharged. Reinforce the need for appropriate follow-up with the primary care provider within 48 to 72 hours after discharge to assess jaundice status (Keren & Bhutani, 2007).

The need for phototherapy can be anxiety-producing for the parents. Explain the rationale for the procedure and demonstrate techniques that the parents can use to interact with their newborn. Additional education about phototherapy may be necessary when home phototherapy is used (Teaching Guidelines 24.2).

▶ NEWBORN INFECTIONS

Newborns are susceptible to infections because their immune system is immature and slow to react. The antibodies that newborns received from their mother during pregnancy and from breast milk help protect them from invading organisms. However, these need time to reach optimal levels.

Bacterial infections of the newborn affect approximately 4 out of every 1,000 live births (McLenan, 2007). Making the diagnosis of sepsis in newborns is difficult due to its nonspecific symptoms. The mortality rate from newborn sepsis may be as high as 50% if untreated. Infection is a major cause of death during the first month of life, contributing to 13% to 15% of all neonatal deaths (Anderson-Berry & Bellig, 2007).

Pathophysiology

When a pathologic organism overcomes the newborn's defenses, infection and sepsis results. **Neonatal sepsis** is the presence of bacterial, fungal, or viral microorganisms or their toxins in blood or other tissues. Infections that have an onset within the first month of life are termed newborn infections. Exposure to a pathogenic organism, whether a virus, fungus, or bacteria, occurs, and it enters the newborn's body and begins to multiply.

Newborn infections are usually grouped into three classes according to their time of onset: congenital infection, acquired in utero (intrauterine infections) by vertical transmission with onset before birth; early-onset infections, acquired by vertical transmission in the perinatal period, either shortly before or during birth; and late-onset infections, acquired by horizontal transmission in the nursery. As many as 80% to 90% of neonatal infections have

TEACHING GUIDELINES 24.2

Caring for Your Newborn Receiving Home Phototherapy

- Inspect your newborn's skin, eyes, and mucous membranes for a yellow color.
- Remember that a home health nurse will come to visit and help you set up the light system.
- Keep the lights about 12 to 30 inches above your newborn.
- Cover your newborn's eyes with patches or cotton balls and gauze to protect them.
- Keep the newborn undressed except for the diaper area; fold the diaper down below the newborn's navel in the front and as far as possible in the back to expose as much skin area as possible.
- Turn your newborn every 2 hours so that all areas of the body are exposed.
- Remove the newborn from the lights only for feeding.
- Remove the eye patches during feedings so that you can interact with your newborn.
- Record your newborn's temperature, weight, and fluid intake daily.
- Document the frequency, color, and consistency of all stools; the stools should be loose and green as the bilirubin is broken down.
- Keep the skin clean and dry to prevent irritation.
- Feed your newborn frequently, including supplemental glucose water if allowed to provide added fluid, protein, and calories.
- Rock, cuddle, or hold the newborn to promote bonding when out of the lights.
- Contact your pediatrician or home health care agency with any questions or changes, including refusing feedings, fewer than five wet diapers in one day, vomiting of complete amounts of feeding, or elevated temperature.
- Keep appointments for follow-up laboratory testing to monitor bilirubin levels.

their onset in the first 2 days of life (CDC, 2007). Comparison Chart 24.2 compares the three classes of newborn infections.

Nursing Assessment

Nursing assessment focuses on early identification of a newborn at risk for infection to allow for prompt treatment, thus reducing mortality and morbidity. Be aware of the myriad risk factors associated with newborn sepsis. Among the factors that contribute to the newborn's overall vulnerability to infection are poor skin integrity, invasive procedures, exposure to numerous caregivers, and an

environment conducive to bacterial colonization (Kenner & Lott, 2007).

Few newborn infections are easy to recognize because manifestations usually are nonspecific. Early symptoms can be vague because of the newborn's inability to mount an inflammatory response. Often, the observation is that the newborn does not "look right." Assess the newborn for common nonspecific signs of infection, including:

- Hypothermia
- Pallor or duskiness
- Hypotonia
- Cyanosis
- Poor weight gain
- Irritability
- Seizures
- Jaundice
- Grunting
- Nasal flaring
- Apnea and bradycardia
- Lethargy
- Hypoglycemia
- Poor feeding (lack of interest in feeding)
- Abdominal distention (Anderson-Berry & Bellig, 2007)

Since infection can be confused with other newborn conditions, laboratory and radiographic tests are needed to confirm the presence of infection. Be prepared to coordinate the timing of the various tests and assist as necessary.

Evaluate the complete blood count with a differential to identify anemia, leukocytosis, or leukopenia. Elevated C-reactive protein levels may indicate inflammation. As ordered, obtain x-rays of the chest and abdomen, which may reveal infectious processes located there. Blood, cerebrospinal fluid, and urine cultures are indicated to identify the location and type of infection present. Positive cultures confirm that the newborn has an infection.

Nursing Management

To enhance the newborn's chance of survival, early recognition and diagnosis are key. Often the diagnosis of sepsis is based on a suspicious clinical picture. Antibiotic therapy is usually started before the laboratory results identify the infecting pathogen (see Evidence-Based Practice). Along with antibiotic therapy, circulatory, respiratory, nutritional, and developmental support is important. Antibiotic therapy is continued for 7 to 21 days if cultures are positive, or it is discontinued within 72 hours if cultures are negative. With the use of antibiotics along with early recognition and supportive care, mortality and morbidity rates have been reduced greatly.

Nurses possess the education and assessment tools to decrease the incidence of and reduce the impact of infections on women (see Chapter 20 for additional information) and their newborns. Implement measures for prevention and early recognition, including:

COMPARISON CHART 24.2   INTRAUTERINE VS. EARLY-ONSET VS. LATE-ONSET NEWBORN INFECTIONS

	Intrauterine (Congenital)	Early-Onset Infections	Late-Onset Infections
Risk factors	-Immature immune system IgM, IgA, and T lymphocytes -Decreased gastric acid, which is needed to reduce organisms	-Prolonged rupture of membranes -Urinary tract infections -Preterm labor -Prolonged or difficult labor -Maternal fever -Colonization with group B streptococci -Maternal infections	-Low birthweight -Prematurity -Meconium staining -Need for resuscitation -Birth asphyxia -Improper handwashing
Common causative organisms	-Cytomegalovirus -Rubella -Toxoplasmosis -Syphilis	-*Escherichia coli* -Group B streptococci -*Klebsiella pneumoniae* -*Listeria monocytogenes* -Other enteric gram-negative bacilli	-*Candida albicans* -Coagulase-negative staphylococci -*Staphylococcus aureus* -*E. coli* -Enterobacter -Klebsiella -Serratia -Pseudomonas -Group B streptococci
Mechanism of infection	-Organism crossing placenta into fetal circulatory system; organism residing in amniotic fluid -Ascent of organism via the vagina, ultimately infecting membranes and causing rupture and leading to respiratory and gastrointestinal tract infections	Most occur during birthing process when newborn comes into contact with infected birth canal (newborn cannot defend against host organisms). -Newborn susceptibility to infection by exogenous organisms possibly due to inadequacy of physical barriers (thin, friable skin with little subcutaneous tissue) -Lack of gastric acidity, possibly resulting in easy colonization by environmental organisms -Aspiration of microorganisms during birth with development of pneumonia	More common in newborns undergoing invasive procedures such as endotracheal intubation or catheter insertion; break in skin or mucosal protection barrier.

Sources: Blackburn (2007); Brousseau & Sharieff (2007), Kenner & Lott (2007).

- Formulating a sepsis prevention plan that includes education of all members of the health care team on identification and treatment of sepsis
- Screening all newborns daily for signs of sepsis
- Monitoring sepsis cases and outcomes to reinforce continued quality-improvement measures or to modify current practices
- Outlining and carrying out measures to prevent nosocomial infections, such as:
  - Thorough handwashing hygiene for all staff
  - Frequent oral care and inspections of mucous membranes

- Proper positioning and turning to prevent skin breakdown
- Use of strict aseptic technique for all wound care
- Frequent monitoring of invasive catheter sites for signs of infection
- Identifying newborns at risk for sepsis by reviewing risk factors
- Monitoring vital sign changes and observing for subtle signs of infection
- Monitoring for signs of organ system dysfunction:
  - Cardiovascular compromise—tachycardia and hypotension

EVIDENCE-BASED PRACTICE 24.1
Treating Neonatal Sepsis With Gentamicin Given as a Once-Daily Dose or as Multiple Doses per Day

● **Study**

Sepsis in a newborn can be fatal, and the signs and symptoms can be vague. Antibiotic therapy is usually initiated before the infection is confirmed by cultures. Gentamicin is a common antibiotic used to treat neonatal sepsis because of its effectiveness against gram-negative pathogens. However, gentamicin, like other aminoglycosides, can have adverse effects on hearing and kidney function, leading to questions about the most effective dosing regimen. Studies have shown that once-a-day dosing is most effective in older children and adults, but these studies do not address the neonatal population.

A study involving neonates with confirmed or suspected sepsis was completed to evaluate the effectiveness and safety of two types of dosing regimens: once-a-day dosing and multiple-doses-per-day dosing. All randomized or quasi-randomized controlled trials involving a comparison of one daily dose with multiple doses per day of gentamicin to newborns less than 28 days of age were selected. Information about clinical effectiveness, pharmacokinetic effectiveness, ototoxicity, and nephrotoxicity was collected. Of the 24 studies initially selected, 11 were evaluated. Most of the studies used intravenous infusion of gentamicin as the method of administration.

One study used a bolus dose of gentamicin administered over 1 minute; two other studies used intramuscular administration.

▲ **Findings**

Regardless of the dosing regimen, gentamicin was shown to be effective in treating the sepsis. The once-daily dosing regimen appeared to be more effective: appropriate peak and trough levels of the drug were obtained more frequently when compared to the multiple dosing regimen. The studies found no evidence of ototoxicity or nephrotoxicity with either regimen.

■ **Nursing Implications**

The study confirmed the effectiveness of gentamicin in the treatment of neonatal sepsis, but it did not determine whether a once-daily dose was more effective than multiple doses per day in treating sepsis. Nurses can integrate the findings of this study into their practice when caring for newborns who are at risk for or have developed sepsis. Regardless of the regimen ordered, nurses can be diligent in ensuring that peak and trough drug levels are monitored. Although the study showed no evidence of hearing and kidney adverse effects, nurses still need to monitor the newborns for this possibility.

Rao, S. C., Ahmed, M., & Hagan, R. (2006). One dose per day compared to multiple doses per day of gentamicin for treatment of suspected or proven sepsis in neonates. *Cochrane Database of Systematic Reviews* 2006. Issue 1. Art. No.: CD005091.

- Respiratory compromise—respiratory distress and tachypnea
- Renal compromise—oliguria or anuria
- Systemic compromise—abnormal blood values
- Providing comprehensive sepsis treatment:
  - Circulatory support with fluids and vasopressors
  - Supplemental oxygen and mechanical ventilation
  - Obtaining culture samples as requested
  - Antibiotic administration as ordered, observing for side effects
  - Promoting newborn comfort
  - Assessing the family's educational needs and providing instructions as necessary

Perinatal infections continue to be a public health problem, with severe consequences for those affected. By promoting a better understanding of newborn infections and appropriate use of therapies, nurses can lower the mortality rates associated with severe sepsis, especially with appropriate timing of interventions. The potential for nursing interventions to identify, prevent, and minimize the risk for sepsis is significant. Primary disease prevention must be a major focus for nurses. Family education plays a key role in the prevention of perinatal infections, in addition to following accepted practices in immunization.

Congenital Conditions

Congenital conditions can arise from many etiologies, including single-gene disorders, chromosome aberrations, exposure to teratogens, and many sporadic conditions of unknown cause. Congenital conditions may be inherited or sporadic, isolated or multiple, apparent or hidden, gross or microscopic. They cause nearly half of all deaths in term newborns and cause long-term sequelae for many. The incidence varies according to the type of defect. When a serious anomaly is identified prenatally, the parents can decide whether or not to continue the pregnancy. When an anomaly is identified at or after birth, parents need to be informed promptly and given a realistic appraisal of the severity of the condition, the prognosis, and treatment options so that they can participate in all decisions pertaining to their child.

Congenital conditions can affect virtually any body system. This chapter describes those congenital conditions that require immediate treatment or affect the newborn in the period immediately after birth. Other congenital conditions, such as congenital heart disease or CNS defects, are discussed in later chapters due to their long-term nature and ongoing effects.

▶ ESOPHAGEAL ATRESIA AND TRACHEOESOPHAGEAL FISTULA

Esophageal atresia and tracheoesophageal fistula are gastrointestinal anomalies in which the esophagus and trachea do not separate normally during embryonic development.

Esophageal atresia refers to a congenitally interrupted esophagus where the proximal and distal ends do not communicate; the upper esophageal segment ends in a blind pouch and the lower segment ends a variable distance above the diaphragm (Fig. 24.8).

Tracheoesophageal fistula is an abnormal communication between the trachea and esophagus. When associated with esophageal atresia, the fistula most commonly occurs between the distal esophageal segment and the trachea. The incidence of esophageal atresia is 1 per 3,000 to 4,000 live births (Blackburn, 2007).

Pathophysiology

Several types of esophageal atresia exist, but the most common anomaly is a fistula between the distal esopha-

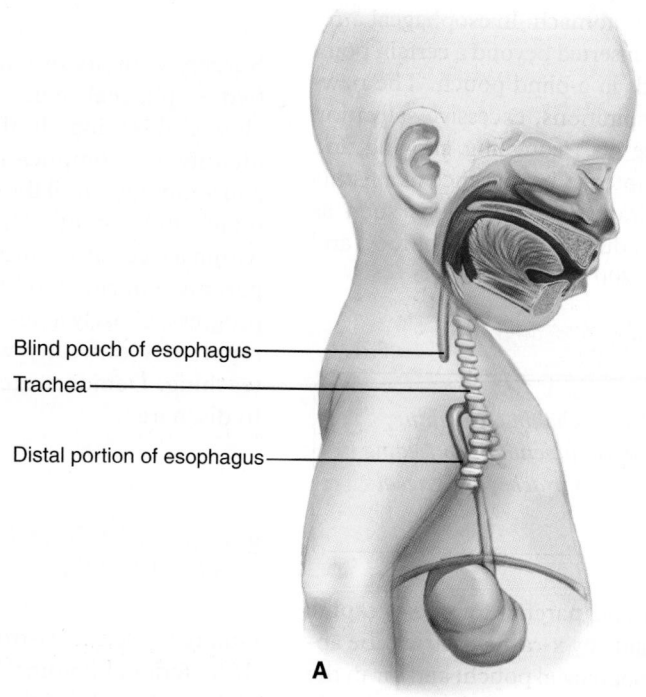

Blind pouch of esophagus —————

Trachea —————

Distal portion of esophagus —————

A

FIGURE 24.8 Esophageal atresia and tracheoesophageal fistula. (**A**) The most common type of esophageal atresia, in which the esophagus ends in a blind pouch and a fistula connects the trachea with the distal portion of the esophagus. (**B**) The upper and distal portions of the esophagus end in a blind pouch. (**C**) The esophagus is one segment, but a portion of it is narrowed. (**D**) The upper portion of the esophagus connects to the trachea via a fistula.

B   **C**   **D**

gus and the trachea, which occurs in 86% of newborns with an esophageal defect. Esophageal atresia and tracheoesophageal fistula are thought to be the result of incomplete separation of the lung bed from the foregut during early fetal development. A large percentage of these newborns have other congenital anomalies involving the vertebra, kidneys, heart, and musculoskeletal and gastrointestinal systems (Rodriguez, 2006); most have several anomalies.

Nursing Assessment

Review the maternal history for polyhydramnios. Often this is the first sign of esophageal atresia because the fetus cannot swallow and absorb amniotic fluid in utero, leading to accumulation. Soon after birth, the newborn may exhibit copious, frothy bubbles of mucus in the mouth and nose, accompanied by drooling. Abdominal distention develops as air builds up in the stomach. In esophageal atresia, a gastric tube cannot be inserted beyond a certain point because the esophagus ends in a blind pouch. The newborn may have rattling respirations, excessive salivation and drooling, and "the three C's" (coughing, choking, and cyanosis) if feeding is attempted. The presence of a fistula increases the risk of respiratory complications such as pneumonitis and atelectasis due to aspiration of food and secretions (Kenner & Lott, 2007).

> ▶ **Take** NOTE!
>
> The "three C's" of choking, coughing, and cyanosis in conjunction with feeding are considered the classic signs of tracheoesophageal fistula and atresia.

Prepare the newborn and parents for radiographic evaluation. Diagnosis is made by x-ray: a gastric tube appears coiled in the upper esophageal pouch, and air in the gastrointestinal tract indicates the presence of a fistula (Kenner & Lott, 2007). Once a diagnosis of esophageal atresia is established, begin preparations for surgery if the newborn is stable.

Nursing Management

Nursing management focuses on preparing the newborn and parents for surgery and providing meticulous postoperative care.

Providing Preoperative Care
Preoperative nursing interventions include the following measures:

- Initiate nothing by mouth (NPO) status.
- Elevate the head of the bed 30 to 45 degrees to prevent reflux and aspiration.

- Monitor hydration status and fluid and electrolyte balance; administer and monitor parenteral IV fluid infusions.
- Assess and maintain the patency of the orogastric tube; monitor the functioning of the tube, which is attached to low continuous suction; and avoid irrigation of the tube to prevent aspiration.
- Have oxygen and suctioning equipment readily available should the newborn experience respiratory distress.
- Assist with diagnostic studies to rule out other anomalies.
- Use comfort measures to minimize crying and prevent respiratory distress; provide nonnutritive sucking.
- Inform the parents about the rationales for the aspiration prevention measures.
- Document frequent observations of the newborn's condition (Kenner & Lott, 2007).

Providing Postoperative Care
Surgery consists of closing the fistula and joining the two esophageal segments. Postoperative care involves closely observing all of the newborn's body systems to identify any complications. Expect to administer TPN and antibiotics until the esophageal anastomosis is proven intact and patent. Then begin oral feedings, usually within a week after surgery (Blackburn, 2007). Keep the parents informed of their newborn's condition and progress. Closely assess the newborn during feeding and report any difficulty with swallowing. Provide parent teaching. Demonstrate and reinforce all teaching prior to discharge.

▶ OMPHALOCELE AND GASTROSCHISIS

Omphalocele and gastroschisis are congenital anomalies of the anterior abdominal wall. An **omphalocele** is a defect of the umbilical ring that allows evisceration of the abdominal contents into an external peritoneal sac. Defects vary in size; they may be limited to bowel loops or may include the entire gastrointestinal tract and liver (Fig. 24.9). Bowel malrotation is common, but the displaced organs are usually normal. Omphaloceles are associated with other anomalies in more than 70% of the cases. This anomaly is usually detected during routine prenatal ultrasound of the fetus or during investigation of an increased alpha-fetoprotein level (Glasser, 2006).

Gastroschisis is a herniation of the abdominal contents through an abdominal wall defect, usually to the left or right of the umbilicus (McLenan, 2007). Gastroschisis differs from omphalocele in that there is no peritoneal sac protecting the herniated organs, and thus exposure to amniotic fluid makes them thickened, edematous, and inflamed (Rodriguez, 2006). Gastroschisis is associated

FIGURE 24.9 Omphalocele in a newborn. Note the large, protruding sac.

with significant newborn mortality and morbidity rates. Despite surgical correction, feeding intolerance, failure to thrive, and prolonged hospital stays occur in nearly all newborns with this anomaly (Glasser, 2006).

Each of these diagnoses requires that a pediatric surgeon be available at delivery to determine the extent of the defect and complications.

Nursing Assessment

Review the maternal history for factors associated with high-risk pregnancies, such as maternal illness and infection, drug use, smoking, and genetic abnormalities. These factors are also associated with omphalocele and gastroschisis. They contribute to placental insufficiency and the birth of a small-for-gestational-age or preterm newborn, the populations in which both of these abdominal defects most commonly occur. The combined incidence of both congenital abdominal wall anomalies is 1 in 2,000 births (Glasser, 2006).

Omphalocele and gastroschisis are readily observed. Note the appearance of the protrusion on the abdomen and evidence of a sac. Inspect the sac closely for the presence of organs, most commonly the intestines but sometimes the liver. Also inspect the contents for any twisting of the intestines. Note the color of the organs within the sac and measure the size of the omphalocele.

Also perform a complete physical examination of the newborn. Typically these congenital conditions are associated with other congenital anomalies, such as those involving the cardiovascular, genitourinary, and central nervous systems.

Nursing Management

Nursing management of newborns with omphalocele or gastroschisis focuses on preventing hypothermia, maintaining perfusion to the eviscerated abdominal contents by minimizing fluid loss, and protecting the exposed ab-

dominal contents from trauma and infection. These objectives can be accomplished by placing the infant in a sterile drawstring bowel bag that maintains a sterile environment for the exposed contents, allows visualization, reduces heat and moisture loss, and allows heat from radiant warmers to reach the newborn. The newborn is placed feet-first into the bag and the drawstring is secured around the torso (McLenan, 2007). Strict sterile technique is necessary to prevent contamination of the exposed abdominal contents.

An orogastric tube attached to low suction is used to prevent intestinal distention. IV therapy is administered to maintain fluid and electrolyte balance and provide a route for antibiotic therapy. Monitor the newborn's fluid status frequently. Closely observe the exposed bowel for vascular compromise, such as changes in color or a decrease in temperature, and report these immediately.

Providing Postoperative Care

Surgical repair of both defects occurs after initial stabilization and comprehensive evaluation for any other anomalies. It may have to occur in stages, depending on the defect (Box 24.4).

Postoperative care involves providing pain management, monitoring respiratory and cardiac status, monitoring intake and output, assessing for vascular compromise, maintaining the orogastric tube to suction, documenting the amount and color of drainage, and administering ordered medications and treatments (Lund, Bauer, & Berrios, 2007). Also be alert for complications, such as short bowel syndrome (see Chapter 41 for additional information).

BOX 24.4 **Surgery to Repair Omphalocele and Gastroschisis**

Surgical repair of gastroschisis is an emergency due to the high risk of intestinal atresia, resulting in obstruction. Primary repair of gastroschisis is usually performed without incident, unless the contents are unable to fit into the abdominal cavity. This occurs more often with a large omphalocele, requiring the surgeon to do a staged closure. This involves covering the defect with a synthetic material that is sequentially squeezed like toothpaste to reduce the defect into the abdominal cavity. After enough of the defect is in the abdominal cavity, a surgical repair is then performed (Islam, 2008). If damage to the exposed organs occurs, such as necrosis, then the necrotic sections are removed during the repair. If a significant amount of small intestine is lost, then the complication of short bowel syndrome may occur.

Promoting Parent–Newborn Interaction

The parents need continued support and progress reports on their newborn. They may be distraught at the sight of the anomaly, and they may be frightened to touch their newborn. Encourage the parents to touch the newborn and participate in care as much as possible. Because of the nature of this defect, bonding opportunities will be limited initially. However, strongly encourage frequent visiting. In addition, provide information to the parents about the defect, treatment modalities, and prognosis. After surgery, instruct the parents in care measures and provide them with home care instructions. Anticipate the need for a referral to a home health care agency and community resources for support.

◗ IMPERFORATE ANUS

An imperforate anus is a gastrointestinal system malformation of the anorectal area that may occur in several forms. The rectum may end in a blind pouch that does not connect to the colon, or it may have fistulas (openings) between the rectum and the perineum, the vagina in girls or the urethra in boys (Fig. 24.10). The malformations occur during early fetal development and are associated with anomalies in other body systems.

Imperforate anus occurs in about 1 of every 5,000 live births (March of Dimes, 2006). The defect can be further classified as a high or low type, depending on its level. The level significantly influences the outcome in terms of fecal continence as well as management (Blackburn, 2007).

Surgical intervention is needed for both high and low types of imperforate anus. Surgery for a high type of defect involves a colostomy in the newborn period, with corrective surgery performed in stages to allow for growth. Surgery for the low type of anomaly, which frequently in-

cludes a fistula, involves closure of the fistula, creation of an anal opening, and repositioning of the rectal pouch into the anal opening. A major challenge for either type of surgical repair is finding, using, or creating adequate nerve and muscle structures around the rectum to provide for normal evacuation.

Nursing Assessment

In the newborn, observe for an appropriate anal opening. If the anal opening exists, observe for passage of meconium stool within the first 24 hours of life. Assess urine output to identify genitourinary problems. For the newborn with an imperforate anus, inspection of the perineal area would reveal absence of the usual opening. In addition, meconium generally is not passed or present within 24 hours of birth.

In the infant with suspected imperforate anus, assess for common signs of intestinal obstruction, which may occur as a result of the malformation. These include abdominal distention and bilious vomiting.

Prepare the newborn and family for radiographic studies that may be ordered to assess for complications associated with imperforate anus.

Nursing Management

Nursing management focuses on preparing the newborn and parent for surgery and providing postoperative care. Preoperatively, maintain the newborn's NPO status and provide gastric decompression. Administer IV therapy and antibiotic therapy as ordered and monitor the newborn's hydration status. Provide a full explanation of the defect, surgical options, potential complications, typical postoperative course, and long-term care needed to the parents. Make sure they are aware of the available treatment modalities. Prepare them for the possibility that the newborn may require an ostomy. Provide support to the parents and family.

Postoperative care includes ensuring adequate pain relief, maintaining NPO status and gastric decompression until normal bowel function is restored, and providing colostomy care if applicable.

◗ BLADDER EXSTROPHY

In bladder exstrophy, the bladder protrudes onto the abdominal wall because the abdominal wall failed to close during embryonic development. Wide separation of the rectus muscles and the symphysis pubis accompanies this defect. Virtually all affected male infants have associated epispadias. The upper urinary tract is usually normal. The incidence is approximately 1 in 24,000 to 40,000 live births (Kenner & Lott, 2007). Initial bladder closure is completed within 48 hours after birth. Further surgical re-

FIGURE 24.10 Imperforate anus, in which the rectum ends in a blind pouch.

construction is performed in several stages at about 2 to 3 years of age. (See Chapter 42 for more information.)

■■■ Key Concepts

■ Asphyxia, the most common clinical insult in the perinatal period, results in brain injury and may lead to mental retardation, cerebral palsy, or seizures.

■ Transient tachypnea of the newborn occurs when the liquid in the lung is removed slowly or incompletely.

■ Common risk factors for respiratory distress syndrome (RDS) include young gestational age, perinatal asphyxia regardless of gestational age, cesarean birth in the absence of labor (related to the lack of thoracic squeeze), male gender, and maternal diabetes.

■ Meconium aspiration has three major pulmonary effects: airway obstruction, surfactant dysfunction, and chemical pneumonitis.

■ The management of persistent pulmonary hypertension of the newborn requires meticulous attention to detail, with continuous monitoring of oxygenation, blood pressure, and perfusion.

■ Periventricular/intraventricular hemorrhage is bleeding that usually originates in the subependymal germinal matrix region of the brain with extension into the ventricular system.

■ Necrotizing enterocolitis (NEC) is a serious gastrointestinal disease of unknown etiology in newborns that can result in necrosis of a segment of the bowel.

■ Infants of diabetic mothers are at risk for malformations most frequently involving the cardiovascular, skeletal, central nervous, gastrointestinal, and genitourinary systems; cardiac anomalies are the most common.

■ Factors that place the newborn at risk for birth trauma include cephalopelvic disproportion, maternal pelvic anomalies, oligohydramnios, prolonged or rapid labor, abnormal presentation, fetal prematurity, fetal macrosomia, and fetal abnormalities.

■ Women who use drugs during their pregnancy expose their unborn child to the possibility of intrauterine growth restriction, prematurity, neurobehavioral and neurophysiologic dysfunction, birth defects, infections, and long-term developmental sequelae.

■ Newborns of women who abuse tobacco, illicit substances, caffeine, and alcohol can exhibit withdrawal behavior.

■ Physiologic jaundice is a common, normal newborn phenomenon that appears during the second or third day of life and then declines over the first week after birth. Pathologic jaundice is manifested within the first 24 hours of life when total bilirubin levels increase by more than 5 mg/dL/day and the total serum bilirubin level is higher than 17 mg/dL in a full-term infant.

■ Newborn infections are usually classified according to the time of onset and grouped into three categories: congenital infection, acquired in utero by vertical trans-

mission with onset before birth; early-onset neonatal infections, acquired by vertical transmission in the perinatal period, either shortly before or during birth; and late-onset neonatal infections, acquired by horizontal transmission in the nursery.

■ Congenital conditions can arise from many etiologies including single-gene disorders, chromosome aberrations, exposure to teratogens, and many sporadic conditions of unknown cause. Congenital structural anomalies may be inherited or sporadic, isolated or multiple, apparent or hidden, and gross or microscopic.

■ Esophageal atresia refers to a congenitally interrupted esophagus where the proximal and distal ends do not communicate; the upper esophageal segment ends in a blind pouch and the lower segment ends a variable distance above the diaphragm. Tracheoesophageal fistula is an abnormal communication between the trachea and esophagus.

■ Omphalocele and gastroschisis are congenital anomalies of the anterior abdominal wall. An omphalocele is a defect of the umbilical ring that allows evisceration of abdominal contents into an external peritoneal sac. Gastroschisis is a herniation of abdominal contents through an abdominal wall defect, usually to the left or right of the umbilicus.

REFERENCES

American Academy of Pediatrics (AAP). (2005). AAP policy statement of breastfeeding and the use of human milk. *Pediatrics, 115*(2), 496–506.

American Academy of Pediatrics (AAP) Committee on Substance Abuse. (2005). Tobacco, alcohol, and other drugs: The role of the pediatrician in prevention, identification, and management of substance abuse. *Pediatrics, 115*(3), 816–821.

American Diabetes Association (ADA). (2007a). *Diabetic statistics for women.* Available at: http://www.diabetes.org/diabetes-statistics/women.jsp.

American Diabetes Association (ADA). (2007b). *Gestational diabetes.* Available at: http://www.diabetes.org/gestational-diabetes.jsp.

American Heart Association and American Academy of Pediatrics. (2005). *Summary of major changes in the 2005 AAP/AHA Emergency Cardiovascular Care Guidelines for Neonatal Resuscitation: translating evidence-based guidelines to the NRP.* Available at: http://www.aap.org/nrp/nrpmain.html.

American Lung Association (ALA). (2007). *Respiratory distress syndrome of the newborn fact sheet.* Lung Disease Data and Minority Lung Disease Data. Available at: http://www.lungusa.org/site/pp.asp?c=dvLUK9O0E&b=35693.

Anderson-Berry, A. L., & Bellig, L. L. (2007). Neonatal sepsis. *eMedicine.* Available at: http://www.emedicine.com/ped/topic2630.htm.

Annibale, D. J., & Hill, J. (2007). Periventricular hemorrhage-intraventricular hemorrhage. *eMedicine.* Available at: http://www.emedicine.com/ped/topic2595.htm.

Arenson, J., & Drake, P. (2007). *Maternal and newborn health.* Sudbury, MA: Jones and Bartlett Publishers.

Asenjo, M. (2007). Transient tachypnea of the newborn. *eMedicine.* Available at: http://www.emedicine.com/radio/topic710.htm.

Belik, J., & Hawes, J. (2007). Neonatal abstinence syndrome. *eMedicine.* Available at: http://emedicine.com/ped/topic2760.htm.

Blackburn, S. T. (2007). *Maternal, fetal and neonatal physiology: A clinical perspective* (3rd ed.). St. Louis: Saunders Elsevier.

Brodsky, D., & Ouellette, M. A. (2007). *Primary care of the premature infant.* Philadelphia: Elsevier Health Sciences.

Brousseau, T. J., & Sharieff, G. Q. (2007). Neonatal emergencies. *WebMD.* Available at: http://www.medscape.com/viewprogram/7232_pnt.

Burd, L. J. (2007). Interventions in FASD: We must do better. *Child: Care, Health & Development, 33*(4), 398–400.

Centers for Disease Control and Prevention (CDC). (2007a). *Surgeon General's report: Women and smoking fact sheet: tobacco use and reproductive outcomes.* Available at: http://www.cdc.gov/tobacco/sgr/sgr_forwomen/factsheet_outcomes.htm.

Centers for Disease Control and Prevention (CDC). (2007b). *Fetal alcohol syndrome: Guidelines for referral and diagnosis.* National Task Force on FAS/FAE. Atlanta: Centers for Disease Control and Prevention.

Clark, D. A., & Clark, M. B. (2007). Meconium aspiration syndrome. *eMedicine.* Available at: http://www.emedicine.com/ped/topic768.htm.

Cunningham, F. G., Leveno, K. J., Bloom, S. L., Gilstrap, L. C., Hauth, J. C., & Wenstrom, K. D. (2005). *Williams' obstetrics* (22nd ed.). New York: McGraw-Hill.

Gilbert, E. S. (2006). *Manual of high-risk pregnancy and delivery* (3rd ed.). St. Louis: Mosby.

Glasser, J. G. (2007). Omphalocele and gastroschisis. *eMedicine.* Available at: http://www.emedicine.com/ped/topic1642.htm.

Goff, M., & O'Connor, M. (2007). Perinatal care of women maintained on methadone. *Journal of Midwifery & Women's Health, 52*(3), 23–26.

Huang, H. R., Tsay, P. K., Chiang, M. C., Lien, R., & Chou, Y. H. (2007). Prognostic factors and clinical features in liveborn neonates with hydrops fetalis. *American Journal of Perinatology, 24*(1), 33–38.

Islam, S. (2008). Clinical care outcomes in abdominal wall defects. *Current Opinions in Pediatrics, 20*(3), 305–310.

Kenner, C., & Lott, J. W. (2007). *Comprehensive neonatal care: An interdisciplinary approach* (4th ed.). St. Louis: Saunders Elsevier.

Keren, R., & Bhutani, V. K. (2007). Predischarge risk assessment for severe neonatal hyperbilirubinemia. *NeoReviews, 8*(2), 68–75.

Kuschel, C. (2007). Managing drug withdrawal in the newborn infant. *Seminars in Fetal & Neonatal Medicine, 12*(2), 127–133.

Kwik, M., Seeho, S. K. M., Smith, C., McElduff, A., & Morris, J. M. (2007). Outcomes of pregnancies affected by impaired glucose tolerance. *Diabetes Research & Clinical Practice, 77*(2), 263–268.

Laroia, N. (2007). Birth trauma. *eMedicine.* Available at http://www.emedicine.com/ped/topic2836.htm.

Lund, C. H., Bauer, K., & Berrios, M. (2007). Gastroschisis. *Journal of Perinatal & Neonatal Nursing, 21*(1), 63–68.

Maisels, M. J., & Newman, T. B. (2007). Kernicterus and evidence-based medicine. *Pediatrics, 119*(5), 1038–1039.

Manning, M. A., & Hoyme, E. H. (2007). Fetal alcohol spectrum disorders: A practical clinical approach to diagnosis. *Neuroscience & Behavioral Reviews, 31*(2), 230–238.

Marcellus, L. (2007). Neonatal abstinence syndrome: Reconstructing the evidence. *Neonatal Network, 26*(1), 33–40.

March of Dimes. (2006). *Birth defects.* Available at: http://search.marchofdimes.com/cgi-bin/MsmGo.exe?grab_id=0&page_id=713&query=congenital%20defects&hiword=DEFECT%20DEFECTIVE%20DEFECTOS%20congenital%20defects%20.

March of Dimes. (2007a). *Drinking alcohol during pregnancy.* March of Dimes Fact Sheets. Available at: http://www.marchofdimes.com/professionals/681_1170.asp.

March of Dimes. (2007b). *Illicit drug use during pregnancy.* MOD Quick Reference: Fact Sheets. Available at: http://www.marchofdimes.com/professionals/14332_1169.asp.

March of Dimes. (2007c). *Smoking during pregnancy.* March of Dimes Fact Sheets. Available at: http://www.marchofdimes.com/professionals/14332_1171.asp.

Maternal & Neonatal Health (MNH). (2007). *Best practices: Detecting and treating newborn asphyxia.* MNH Program. Available at: http://www.mnh.jhpiego.org/best/detasphyxia.asp.

McLenan, D. (2007). Care of the high-risk neonate. In R. E. Rakel & E. T. Bope (Eds.), *Conn's current therapy 2007* (Section 16, pp. 1200–1210). Philadelphia: Saunders Elsevier.

Mercer, J. S., Erickson-Owens, D. A., Graves, B., & Haley, M. M. (2007). Evidence-based practices for the fetal to newborn transition. *Journal of Midwifery & Women's Health, 52*(3), 262–272.

National Center on Birth Defects and Developmental Disabilities (NCBDDD). (2004). *Fetal alcohol syndrome: Guidelines for referral and diagnosis* (p. 20). Atlanta: Centers for Disease Control and Prevention (CDC), Department of Health and Human Services (DHHS).

National Institute on Drug Abuse (NIDA). (2007a). *NIDA InfoFacts: crack and cocaine.* National Institutes of Health. Available at: http://www.drugabuse.gov/infofacts/cocaine.html.

National Institute on Drug Abuse (NIDA). (2007b). *NIDA InfoFacts: Heroin.* National Institutes of Health. Available at: http://www.nida.nih.gov/Infofacts/heroin.html.

National Institute on Drug Abuse (NIDA). (2007c). *NIDA Research Report: Heroin abuse and addiction.* NIH Publication Number 05–4165. Available at: http://www.drugabuse.gov/ResearchReports/Heroin/heroin4.html.

National Institute on Drug Abuse (NIDA). (2007d). *NIDA InfoFacts: Marijuana.* National Institutes of Health. Available at: http://www.nida.nih.gov/Infofacts/marijuana.html.

National Institute on Drug Abuse (NIDA). (2007e). *NIDA InfoFacts: Methamphetamine.* National Institutes of Health. Available at: http://www.drugabuse.gov/infofacts/methamphetamine.html.

National Institute on Drug Abuse (NIDA). (2007f). *NIDA InfoFacts: Pregnancy and drug use trends.* National Institutes of Health. Available at: http://www.drugabuse.gov/Infofacts/pregnancytrends.html.

Neu, J. (2007). Gastrointestinal development and meeting the nutritional needs of premature infants. *American Journal of Clinical Nutrition, 85*(2), 629S–634S.

Ozen, N., & Mukherjee, S. (2007). Hyperbilirubinemia, unconjugated. *eMedicine.* Available at: http://www.emedicine.com/med/topic1066.htm.

Rao, S. C., Ahmed, M., & Hagan, R. (2006). One dose per day compared to multiple doses per day of gentamicin for treatment of suspected or proven sepsis in neonates. *Cochrane Database of Systematic Reviews* 2006. Issue 1. Art. No.: CD005091.DOI: 10.1002/14651858.CD005091.pub2.

Rodriguez, R., Fanaroff, A., & Lissauer, T. (2008). *Neonatology at a glance.* Malden, MA: John Wiley.

Simpson, K. R. (2007). Kernicterus prevention. *MCN, 32*(2), 132.

Springer, S. C., & Annibale, D. J. (2007). Kernicterus. *eMedicine.* Available at: http://www.emedicine.com/ped/topic1247.htm.

Steinhorn, R. H. (2007). Pulmonary hypertension, persistent-newborn. *eMedicine.* Available at: http://www.emedicine.com/ped/topic2530.htm.

Stoll, B. J., & Kliegman, P. M. (2007). Neonatal necrotizing enterocolitis (NEC). In R. E. Behrman, R. M. Kliegman, & H. B. Jenson (Eds.), *Nelson textbook of pediatrics* (18th ed.). Philadelphia: W. B. Saunders.

U.S. Department of Health and Human Services (USDHHS). (2000). *Healthy people 2010:* Volumes 1 and 2 (conference ed.). Washington, DC: U.S. Government Printing Office.

Verklan, M. T., & Walden, M. (2004). *Core curriculum for neonatal intensive care nursing* (3rd ed.). St. Louis: Elsevier Saunders.

Wheeler, D. S., & McCaffrey, M. J. (2007). Resuscitation of the newborn. In R. E. Rakel & E. T. Bope (Eds.), *Conn's current therapy 2007* (Section 16, pp. 1193–1200). Philadelphia: Saunders Elsevier.

Wiswell, T. E., Tin, W., & Ohler, K. (2007), Evidence-based use of adjunctive therapies to ventilation. *Clinics in Perinatology, 34*(1), 191–204.

Wood, B. P. (2007). Necrotizing enterocolitis. *eMedicine.* Available at: http://www.emedicine.com/radio/topic469.htm.

Woods, D. (2007). *Neonatal resuscitation.* International Association for Maternal and Neonatal Health (IAMANEH). Available at: http://www.gfmer.ch/Medical_education_En/PGC_RH_2004/Neonatal_asphyxia.htm.

Zaichkin, J. (2006). NPR 2006: What you should know. *Neonatal Network, 25*(2), 145–151.

WEBSITES

AHRQ's Tobacco Pathfinder: www.ahrq.gov
American Diabetes Association: www.diabetes.org
Birth Defects for Children: www.birthdefects.org

Centers for Disease Control and Prevention: www.cdc.gov

Esophageal Atresia/Tracheoesophageal Fistula Family Support Connection: www.eatef.org

March of Dimes Birth Defects Foundation: www.marchofdimes.com

Narcotics Anonymous: www.na.org

National Center on Birth Defects and Developmental Disabilities: www.cdc.gov/ncbddd/fas

National Clearinghouse for Alcohol and Drug Abuse Information: www.health.org

National Institute on Alcohol Abuse and Alcoholism: www.niaaa.nih.gov

National Organization on Fetal Alcohol Syndrome: www.nofas.org

National Women's Health Information Center: www.4woman.gov

Neonatal Network: www.neonatalnetwork.com

Parental Guide for Developmentally Supportive Care: www.comeunity.com/premature/baby/supportive-care.html

Partnership for a Drug-Free America: www.drugfreeamerica.org

Physical and Developmental Environment of the High-Risk Infant: www.med.usf.edu/~tsinger

Safe Motherhood Initiative: www.safemotherhood.org

SHARE Pregnancy & Infant Loss Support, Inc.: www.nationalshareoffice.com

Substance Abuse & Mental Health Services: www.findtreatment.samhsa.gov

CHAPTER WORKSHEET

MULTIPLE CHOICE QUESTIONS

1. Which finding would lead the nurse to suspect that a newborn is experiencing respiratory distress syndrome?

   a. Abdominal distention

   b. Acrocyanosis

   c. Depressed fontanels

   d. Nasal flaring

2. When assessing the substance-exposed newborn, which finding would the nurse expect?

   a. Calm facial appearance

   b. Daily weight gain

   c. Increasing irritability

   d. Feeding and sleeping well

3. A newborn with tracheoesophageal fistula is likely to present with which assessment finding?

   a. Subnormal temperature

   b. Absent Moro reflex

   c. Inability to swallow

   d. Drooling from mouth

4. The nurse would be most alert for the development of transient tachypnea in a newborn who:

   a. Was born by cesarean birth

   b. Received no sedation

   c. Has a mother with heart disease

   d. Is small for gestational age

CRITICAL THINKING EXERCISES

1. As the nursery nurse, you receive a newborn from the labor and birth suite and place him under the radiant warmer. The nurse who gives you the report states that the mother couldn't remember when her membranes broke before labor and that she ran a fever during labor for the past few hours. The Apgar scores were good, but the newborn seemed lethargic. As you begin your assessment, you note that he is pale and floppy and has a subnormal temperature; heart rate is 180 bpm and respiratory rate is 70 breaths per minute.

   a. What in the mother's history should raise a red flag to the nurse?

   b. What condition is this newborn at high risk for?

   c. What interventions are appropriate for this condition?

2. Terry, a day-old baby girl, is very fretful, and calming measures don't seem to work. As the nursery nurse you notice that she is losing weight and her formula intake is poor, even though she is manifesting hungry behavior. The mother received no prenatal care and denied drug use, but her drug screen was positive for heroin.

   a. What additional information do you need to obtain from the mother?

   b. What additional laboratory work might be needed for Terry?

   c. What specific measures need to be made for her ongoing care?

3. Baby boy Sims, a term newborn, was brought to the nursery. His mother received no prenatal care, but the newborn's Apgar scores were fine. As the nurse carried out her newborn assessment, she noted an imperforate anus and palpated no testicles in the scrotal sac.

   a. What additional assessments should the nurse complete?

   b. Are anorectal agenesis and genitourinary tract anomalies common?

   c. What diagnostic tests might be ordered? What might be included in the treatment plan for this newborn?

STUDY ACTIVITIES

1. Arrange for a tour of a regional NICU to see the nurse's role in caring for sick neonates. Ask the nurse to give a quick history of each newborn's condition. Was the nurse's role like you imagined? What was your impression of the NICU, and how would you describe it to expectant parents?

2. Select a website from the list at the end of the chapter. What kind of information is given? How helpful would it be for parents with an infant diagnosed with a specific condition?

3. A herniation of a newborn's abdominal contents present at birth describes _____.

UNIT NINE

HEALTH PROMOTION FOR THE GROWING CHILD AND FAMILY

GROWTH AND DEVELOPMENT OF THE NEWBORN AND INFANT

KEY TERMS

anticipatory guidance
binocularity
cephalocaudal
colic
development

discipline
growth
maturation
object permanence
proximodistal

solitary play
stranger anxiety
temperament

LEARNING OBJECTIVES

Upon completion of the chapter, the learner will be able to:

1. Identify normal developmental changes occurring in the newborn and infant.
2. Identify the gross and fine motor milestones of the newborn and infant.
3. Express an understanding of language development in the first year of life.
4. Describe nutritional requirements of the newborn and infant.
5. Develop a nutritional plan for the first year of life.
6. Identify common issues related to growth and development in infancy.
7. Demonstrate knowledge of appropriate anticipatory guidance for common developmental issues.

Allison Johnson is a 6-month-old girl brought to the clinic by her mother and father for her 6-month check-up. As new parents, they have a list of questions and concerns. On assessment you find that Allison's weight is 16 pounds, length 25¾ inches, and head circumference 17 inches. As the nurse caring for her, assess Allison's growth and development, and then teach the parents what changes to expect in Allison over the next few months.

Wow

Of all the joys that lighten our hearts, what joy is welcomed like a newborn child?

The newborn or neonatal period of infancy is defined as the period from birth until 28 days of age. Infancy is defined as the period from birth to 12 months of age. Growth and development are interrelated, ongoing processes in infancy and childhood. **Growth** refers to an increase in physical size. **Development** is the sequential process by which infants and children gain various skills and functions. Heredity influences growth and development by determining the child's potential, while environment contributes to the degree of achievement. **Maturation** refers to an increase in functionality of various body systems or developmental skills.

Growth and Development Overview

Growth and developmental changes in the first year of life are numerous and dramatic. Physical growth, maturation of body systems, and gross and fine motor skills progress in an orderly and sequential fashion. Though timing may vary from infant to infant, the order in which developmental skills are acquired is consistent. Infants also exhibit vast amounts of learning in the psychosocial and cognitive, language and communication, and social/ emotional domains. Adequate growth and development are indicative of health in the infant or young child. Nurses must be familiar with normal developmental milestones so that they can accurately assess the infant's development as well as provide age-appropriate anticipatory guidance to the parents.

Achievement of developmental milestones may be assessed in a variety of ways. While obtaining the health history, the nurse may ask the parent or caregiver if the skill is present and when it was attained. The infant may also demonstrate the skill during the interview or examination, or the nurse may elicit the skill from the infant. A number of screening tools are also used to assess development, such as the Denver II Developmental Screening Test (see Appendix B), Prescreening Developmental Questionnaire (PDQ II), Ages and Stages Questionnaire (ASQ), Infant Toddler Checklist for Language and Communication, and Infant Development Inventory.

Ill or premature infants may exhibit delayed acquisition of physical growth and developmental skills. When as- sessing the growth and development of a premature infant, use the infant's adjusted age to determine expected outcomes. To determine adjusted age, subtract the number of weeks that the infant was premature from the infant's chronological age. Plot growth parameters and assess developmental milestones based on adjusted age. For example, a 6-month-old boy who was born at 28 weeks' gestation was born 12 weeks early (3 months), so subtract 3 months from his chronological age of 6 months to obtain an adjusted age of 3 months. This infant would demonstrate healthy growth if he were the size of a 3-month-old, and he should be expected to achieve the developmental milestones of a 3-month-old rather than a 6-month-old.

▶ PHYSICAL GROWTH

Ongoing assessments of growth are important so that too-rapid or inadequate growth can be identified early. With early identification, the cause can be diagnosed and the potential for further appropriate growth maximized. Infants grow very rapidly over the first 12 months of life. Weight, length, and head and chest circumference are all indicators of physical growth in the newborn and infant (Table 25.1).

Weight

The average newborn weighs 7 lb 8 oz (3,400 g) at birth. Newborns lose up to 10% of their body weight over the first 5 days of life. The average newborn then gains about 20 to 30 g per day and regains his or her birthweight by 10 to 14 days of age. Most infants double their birthweight by 4 to 6 months of age and triple their birthweight by the time they are 1 year old.

Height

The average newborn is 19 to 21 inches (48 to 53 cm) long at birth. During the first 6 months, length increases by 1 inch (2.5 cm) per month, then by about a half-inch per month in the second 6 months.

Head and Chest Circumference

Average head circumference of the full-term newborn is 13 to 14 inches (33 to 35 cm). The head circumference

TABLE 25.1 AVERAGE MEASUREMENTS OF INFANTS AT BIRTH AND 6 AND 12 MONTHS

Age	Weight	Length	Head Circumference
Birth	7.5 lb (3,400 g)	19–21 in (48–53 cm)	13–14 in (33–35 cm)
6 months	15 lb (6.8 kg)	25–27 in (63.5–68.5 cm)	16.5–17.5 in (42–44.5 cm)
12 months	23 lb (10.5 kg)	28–30 in (71–76 cm)	17.7–18.7 in (45–47.5 cm)

is about 1 inch (2 to 3 cm) greater than the chest circumference, which averages 12 to 13 inches (30.5 to 33 cm). The head circumference increases rapidly during the first 6 months; the average increase is about 0.6 inch (1.5 cm) per month. From 6 to 12 months of age, the head circumference increases an average of 0.2 inch (0.5 cm) monthly. The chest circumference is not routinely measured after the newborn period but does increase in size as the child grows.

ORGAN SYSTEM MATURATION

The newborn and infant's organ systems undergo significant changes as the infant grows. Systems that undergo significant change include the neurologic system, the cardiovascular system, the respiratory system, the gastrointestinal (digestive) system, the renal system, the hematopoietic system, the immunologic system, and the integumentary system.

Neurologic System

The infant experiences tremendous changes in the neurologic system over the first year of life. Critical brain growth and continued myelinization of the spinal cord are occurring. Involuntary movement progresses to voluntary control, and immature vocalizations and crying progress to the ability to speak as a result of maturational changes of the neurologic system.

States of Consciousness

The normal term newborn's ability to move sequentially through states of consciousness reassures parents and health care providers that the neurologic system, though immature, is intact. A normal newborn will ordinarily move through six states of consciousness:

1. Deep sleep: The infant lies quietly without movement.
2. Light sleep: The infant may move a little while sleeping and may startle to noises.
3. Drowsiness: Eyes may close; the infant may be dozing.
4. Quiet alert state: The infant's eyes are open wide and the body is calm.
5. Active alert state: The infant's face and body move actively.
6. Crying: The infant cries or screams and the body moves in a disorganized fashion.

Newborns usually progress through these states slowly, rather than going from deep sleep immediately into outright crying.

Brain Growth

The nervous system continues to mature throughout infancy, and the increase in head circumference is indicative of brain growth. The brain undergoes tremendous growth during the first 2 years of life. By 6 months of age the infant's brain weighs half that of the adult brain. At age 12 months, the brain has grown considerably, weighing 2½ times what it did at birth. Usually, the anterior fontanel remains open until 12 to 18 months of age to accommodate this rapid brain growth. However, the fontanel may close as early as 9 months of age, and this is not of concern in the infant with age-appropriate growth and development.

In general, the neurologic system matures a significant amount over the first year of life. Myelination of the spinal cord and nerves continues over the first 2 years. Maturation of the nervous system and continued myelination are necessary for the tremendous developmental skills that are achieved in the first 12 months. During the first few months of life, reflexive behavior is replaced with purposeful action.

Reflexes

Primitive reflexes are subcortical and involve a whole-body response. Selected primitive reflexes present at birth include Moro, root, suck, asymmetric tonic neck, plantar and palmar grasp, step, and Babinski. Except for the Babinski, which disappears around 1 year of age, these primitive reflexes diminish over the first few months of life, giving way to protective reflexes. Protective reflexes (also termed postural responses or reflexes) are motor responses related to maintenance of equilibrium. These responses are prerequisites for appropriate motor development and remain throughout life once they are established. The protective reflexes include the righting and parachute reactions. Appropriate presence and disappearance of primitive reflexes, as well as development of protective reflexes, are indicative of a healthy neurologic system. Persistence of primitive reflexes beyond the usual age of disappearance may indicate an abnormality of the neurologic system and should be investigated.

Table 25.2 gives descriptions and illustrations of several primitive and protective reflexes, as well as the timing of appearance and disappearance of these reflexes.

Respiratory System

The respiratory system continues to mature over the first year of life. The respiratory rate slows from an average of 30 to 60 breaths in the newborn to about 20 to 30 in the 12-month-old. The newborn breathes irregularly, with periodic pauses. As the infant matures, the respiratory pattern becomes more regular and rhythmic.

In comparison with the adult, in the infant:

• The nasal passages are narrower.
• The trachea and chest wall are more compliant.
• The bronchi and bronchioles are shorter and narrower.
• The larynx is more funnel-shaped.
• The tongue is larger.
• There are significantly fewer alveoli.

(text continues on page 775)

TABLE 25.2 SELECTED PRIMITIVE AND PROTECTIVE REFLEXES IN INFANCY

	Description	Age Reflex Appears	Age Reflex Disappears
Primitive Reflexes			
Root	When infant's cheek is stroked, the infant turns to that side, searching with mouth.	Birth	3 months
Suck	Reflexive sucking when nipple or finger is placed in infant's mouth	Birth	2–5 months
Moro	With sudden extension of the head, the arms abduct and move upward and the hands form a "C."	Birth	4 months

	Description	Age Reflex Appears	Age Reflex Disappears
Asymmetric tonic neck	While lying supine, extremities are extended on the side of the body to which the head is turned and opposite extremities are flexed (also called the "fencing" position).	Birth	4 months
Palmar grasp	Infant reflexively grasps when palm is touched.	Birth	4–6 months
Plantar grasp	Infant reflexively grasps with bottom of foot when pressure is applied to plantar surface.	Birth	9 months

(continued)

TABLE 25.2   SELECTED PRIMITIVE AND PROTECTIVE REFLEXES IN INFANCY (continued)

	Description	Age Reflex Appears	Age Reflex Disappears
Babinski	Stroking along the lateral aspect of the sole and across the plantar surface results in fanning and hyperextension of the toes.	Birth	12 months

	Description	Age Reflex Appears	Age Reflex Disappears
Step	With one foot on a flat surface, the infant puts the other foot down as if to "step."	Birth	4–8 weeks

Protective Reflexes

	Description	Age Reflex Appears	Age Reflex Disappears
Neck righting	Neck keeps head in upright position when body is tilted.	4–6 months	Persists
Parachute (sideways)	Protective extension with the arms when tilted to the side in a supported sitting position	6 months	Persists
Parachute (forward)	Protective extension with the arms when held up in the air and moved forward. The infant reflexively reaches forward to catch himself.	6–7 months	Persists

	Description	Age Reflex Appears	Age Reflex Disappears
Parachute (backward)	Protective extension with the arms when tilted backward	9–10 months	Persists

These anatomic differences place the infant at higher risk for respiratory compromise. The respiratory system does not reach adult levels of maturity until about 7 years of age. The lack of IgA in the mucosal lining of the upper respiratory tract also contributes to the frequent infections that occur in infancy.

Cardiovascular System

The heart doubles in size over the first year of life. As the cardiovascular system matures, the average pulse rate decreases from 120 to 140 in the newborn to about 100 in the 1-year-old. Blood pressure steadily increases over the first 12 months of life, from an average of 60/40 in the newborn to 100/50 in the 12-month-old. The peripheral capillaries are closer to the surface of the skin, thus making the newborn and young infant more susceptible to heat loss. Over the first year of life, thermoregulation (the body's ability to stabilize body temperature) becomes more effective: the peripheral capillaries constrict in response to a cold environment and dilate in response to heat.

Gastrointestinal System

Teeth

Occasionally, an infant is born with one or more teeth (termed natal teeth) or develops teeth in the first 28 days of life (termed neonatal teeth). The presence of natal or neonatal teeth may be associated with other birth anomalies. The vast majority of newborns do not have teeth at birth, nor do they develop them in the first month of life. On average, the first primary teeth begin to erupt between the ages of 6 and 8 months. The primary teeth (also termed deciduous teeth) are lost later in childhood and will be replaced by the permanent teeth. The gums around the emerging tooth often swell. The lower central incisors are usually the first to appear, followed by the upper central incisors (Fig. 25.1). The average 12-month-old has four to eight teeth.

Digestion

The newborn's digestive system is not developed fully. Small amounts of saliva are present for the first 3 months of life and ptyalin is present only in small amounts in the saliva. Gastric digestion occurs as a result of the presence of hydrochloric acid and rennin. The small intestine is about 250 cm long and grows to the adult length over the first few years of life. The stomach capacity is relatively small at birth, holding about one-half to 1 ounce. However, by 1 year of age the stomach can accommodate three full meals and several snacks per day. In the duodenum, three enzymes in particular are important for digestion. Trypsin is available in sufficient quantities for protein digestion after birth. Amylase (needed for complex carbohydrate digestion) and lipase (essential for appropriate fat digestion) are both deficient in the infant and do not reach adult levels until about 5 months of age.

FIGURE 25.1 Sequence and average age of tooth eruption.

The liver is also immature at birth. The ability to conjugate bilirubin and secrete bile is present after about 2 weeks of age. Conjugation of medications may remain immature over the first year of life. Other functions of the liver, including gluconeogenesis, vitamin storage, and protein metabolism, remain immature during the first year of life.

Stools

The consistency and frequency of stools change over the first year of life. The newborn's first stools (meconium) are the result of digestion of amniotic fluid swallowed *in utero*. They are dark green to black and sticky (Fig. 25.2). In the first few days of life the stools become yellowish or tan. Generally the formula-fed infant has stools the consistency of peanut butter. Breastfed infants' stools are usually looser in texture and appear seedy. Newborns may have as many as eight to ten stools per day or as few as one stool every day or two. After the newborn period, the number of stools may decrease, and some infants do not have a bowel movement for several days. Infrequent stooling is considered normal if the bowel movement remains soft. Due to the immaturity of the gastrointestinal system, newborns and young infants often grunt, strain, or cry while attempting to have a bowel movement. This is not of concern unless the stool is hard and dry. Stool color and texture may change depending on the foods

FIGURE 25.2 (**A**) Meconium stool. (**B**) Typical stool after the first few days. Note the yellowish, seedy stool of a breastfed infant.

that the infant is ingesting. Iron supplements may cause the stool to appear black or very dark green.

> ▶ **Take** NOTE!
>
> *Parents should call the primary care provider if the infant's stools are red, white, or black; mucus-like; frequent and watery; frothy or foul-smelling; hard, dry, formed, or pellet-like; or if the baby is vomiting.*

Genitourinary System

In the infant, extracellular fluid (lymph, interstitial fluid, and blood plasma) accounts for about 35% of body weight and intracellular fluid accounts for 40%, compared with the adult quantities of 20% and 40% respectively. Thus, the infant is more susceptible to dehydration. Infants urinate frequently and the urine has a relatively low specific gravity. The renal structures are immature and the glomerular filtration rate, tubular secretion, and reabsorption as well as renal perfusion are all reduced compared with the adult. The glomeruli reach full maturity by 2 years of age.

Integumentary System

In utero the infant is covered with vernix caseosa, which protects the developing infant's skin. At birth, the infant may be covered with vernix (earlier gestational age) or vernix may be found in the folds of the skin, axilla, and groin areas (later gestational age). Production of vernix

ceases at birth. Fine downy hair (lanugo) covers the body of many newborns. Often this hair is lost over time and is not replaced. Darker-skinned races tend to have more lanugo present at birth than those with light skin.

Acrocyanosis (blueness of the hands and feet) is normal in the newborn; it decreases over the first few days of life (Fig. 25.3). Newborns often experience mottling of the skin (a pink-and-white marbled appearance) because of their immature circulatory system. Mottling decreases over the first few months of life.

The newborn and young infant's skin is relatively thinner than that of the adult, with the peripheral capillaries being closer to the surface. This may cause increased absorption of topical medications.

Hematopoietic System

Significant changes in the hematopoietic system occur over the first year of life. At birth, fetal hemoglobin (HgbF) is present in large amounts. After birth the production of fetal hemoglobin nearly ceases, and adult hemoglobin (HgbA) is produced in steadily increasing amounts throughout the first 6 months. Since HgbF has a shorter lifespan than HgbA, infants may experience physiologic anemia at age 2 to 3 months. During the last 3 months of gestation, maternal iron stores are transferred to the fetus. The newborn typically has 0.3 to 0.5 g of iron stores available. As the high hemoglobin concentration of the newborn decreases over the first 2 to 3 months, iron is reclaimed and stored. These stores may be sufficient for the first 6 to 9 months of life but will become depleted if iron supplementation does not occur. Ongoing iron intake is required throughout the first 15 years of life in order to reach the adult level of 5 g.

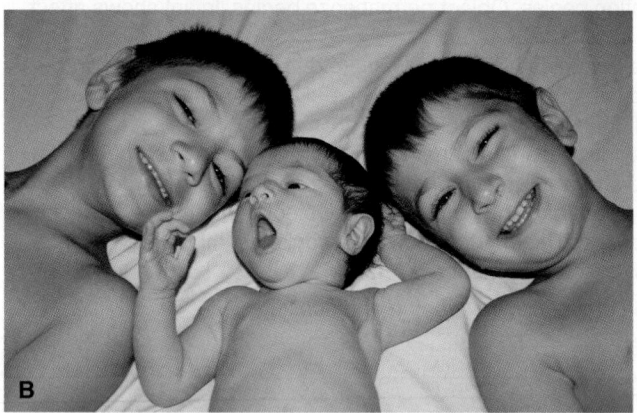

FIGURE 25.3 (**A**) Acrocyanosis. Note blueness of the hands. (**B**) Mottling of the skin in a young infant.

> ▶ *Take* NOTE!
>
> *Maternal iron stores are transferred to the fetus throughout the last trimester of pregnancy. Infants born prematurely miss all or at least a portion of this iron store transfer, placing them at increased risk for iron deficiency anemia compared with term infants.*

Immunologic System

Newborns receive large amounts of immunoglobulin G (IgG) through the placenta from their mothers. This confers immunity during the first 3 to 6 months of life for antigens to which the mother was previously exposed. Infants then synthesize their own IgG, reaching approximately 40% of adult levels at age 12 months. Immunoglobulin M (IgM) is produced in significant amounts after birth, reaching adult levels by 9 months of age. Immunoglobulin A (IgA), immunoglobulin D (IgD), and immunoglobulin E (IgE) production increases very gradually, maturing in early childhood.

▶ PSYCHOSOCIAL DEVELOPMENT

Erik Erikson (1963) identifies the psychosocial crisis of infancy as Trust versus Mistrust. Development of a sense of trust is crucial in the first year, as it serves as the foundation for later psychosocial tasks. The parent or primary caregiver can have a significant impact on the infant's development of a sense of trust. When the infant's needs are consistently met, the infant develops this sense of trust. But if the parent or caregiver is inconsistent in meeting the infant's needs in a timely manner, then the infant develops a sense of mistrust. Table 25.3 lists activities that promote a sense of trust in infancy.

▶ COGNITIVE DEVELOPMENT

The first stage of Jean Piaget's theory of cognitive development is referred to as the sensorimotor stage (birth to 2 years) (Piaget, 1969). Infants learn about themselves and the world through their developing sensory and motor capacities. Infants' development from birth to 1 year of age can be divided into four substages within the sensorimotor stage: reflexes, primary circular reaction, secondary circular reaction, and coordination of secondary schemes. Cause and effect guides most of the cognitive development seen in infancy (see Table 25.3).

The concept of **object permanence** begins to develop between 4 and 7 months of age and is solidified by about 8 months of age. If an object is hidden from the infant's sight, he or she will search for it in the last place it was seen, knowing it still exists. This development of object permanence is essential for the development of self-image. By age 12 months the infant knows he or she is separate from the parent or caregiver. Self-image is also promoted through the use of mirrors. By 12 months of age, infants can see themselves in the mirror. The 12-month-old will explore objects in different ways, such as throwing, banging, dropping, and shaking. He or she may imitate gestures and knows how to use certain objects correctly (e.g., puts phone to ear, turns up cup to drink, attempts to comb hair).

▶ MOTOR SKILL DEVELOPMENT

Infants exhibit phenomenal increases in their gross and fine motor skills over the first 12 months of life.

Gross Motor Skills

The term "gross motor skills" refers to those that use the large muscles (e.g., head control, rolling, sitting, and walking). Gross motor skills develop in a **cephalocaudal**

TABLE 25.3 DEVELOPMENTAL THEORIES

Theorist	Stage	Activities
Erikson	Trust vs. Mistrust (birth to 1 year)	Caregivers respond to the infant's basic needs by feeding, changing diapers, and cleaning, touching, holding, and talking to the infant. This creates a sense of trust in the infant.
		As the nervous system matures, infants realize they are separate beings from their caregivers. Over time the infant learns to tolerate small amounts of frustration and trusts that although gratification may be delayed, it will eventually be provided.
Piaget	Sensorimotor (birth to 2 years)	Infant uses senses and motor skills to learn about the world.
	Substage 1: use of reflexes (birth to 1 month)	Reflexive sucking brings the pleasure of ingesting nutrition. Infant begins to gain control over reflexes; recognizes familiar objects, odors, and sounds.
	Substage 2: primary circular reactions (1 to 4 months)	Thumb-sucking may occur by chance; then the infant repeats it on purpose to bring pleasure. Imitation begins. Object permanence begins. Infant shows affect.
	Substage 3: secondary circular reactions (4 to 8 months)	Infant repeats actions to achieve wanted results (e.g., shakes rattle to hear the noise it makes). The infant's actions are purposeful but the infant does not always have an end goal in mind.
	Substage 4: coordination of secondary schemes (8 to 12 months)	Infants coordinate previously learned schemes with previously learned behaviors. They may grasp and shake a rattle intentionally or crawl across the room to reach a desired toy. Infant can anticipate events. Object permanence is present at about 8 months of age. The infant begins to associate symbols with events (e.g., waving goodbye means someone is leaving)
Freud	Oral stage (birth to 1 year)	Pleasure is focused on oral activities: feeding and sucking.

fashion (from the head to the tail) (Fig. 25.4). In other words, the baby learns to lift the head before learning to roll over and sit. At birth, babies have poor head control and need to have their necks supported when being held. They can lift their heads only slightly while in a prone position. Over the next several months the infant's motor skills progress at a dramatic rate. First the infant achieves head control, then the ability to roll over, sit, crawl, pull to stand, and, usually around a year of age, to walk independently. Table 25.4 gives details on when the infant develops each specific gross motor skill. Progression of gross motor skills is illustrated in Figures 25.5 through 25.7.

▶ *Take NOTE!*

Warning signs that may indicate problems with motor development include the following: arms and legs are stiff or floppy; child cannot support head at 3 to 4 months of age; child reaches with one hand only; child cannot sit with assistance at 6 months of age; child does not crawl by 12 months of age; child cannot stand supported by 12 months of age.

FIGURE 25.4 Gross motor skills develop in a cephalocaudal direction, fine motor skills in a proximodistal fashion.

TABLE 25.4   DEVELOPMENT OF GROSS MOTOR SKILLS
IN INFANCY

Age	Gross Motor Skills
1 month	Lifts and turns head to side in prone position Head lag when pulled to sit Rounded back in sitting
2 months	Raises head and chest, holds position Improving head control
3 months	Raises head to 45 degrees in prone Slight head lag in pull to sit
4 months	Lifts head and looks around Rolls from prone to supine Head leads body when pulled to sit
5 months	Rolls from supine to prone and back again Sits with back upright when supported
6 months	Tripod sits
7 months	Sits alone with some use of hands for support
8 months	Sits unsupported
9 months	Crawls, abdomen off floor
10 months	Pulls to stand Cruises
12 months	Sits from standing position Walks independently

FIGURE 25.5 When pulled to sit, an infant shows (**A**) significant head lag (newborn; 2 or 3 weeks old), (**B**) improving head control (2 months old), and (**C**) no head lag (4 months old).

Fine Motor Skills

Fine motor development includes the maturation of hand and finger use. Fine motor skills develop in a **proximodistal** fashion (from the center to the periphery) (see Fig. 25.4). In other words, the infant first bats with the whole hand, eventually progressing to gross grasping, before being capable of fine fingertip grasping (Fig. 25.8). The newborn's hand movements are involuntary in nature, whereas the 12-month-old is capable of feeding himself or herself with a cup and spoon. By 12 months of age the infant should be able to eat with his or her fingers and assist with dressing (e.g., pushing an arm through the sleeve). Table 25.5 gives details on when the infant develops each specific fine motor skill.

▶ SENSORY DEVELOPMENT

Though hearing should be fully developed at birth, the other senses continue to develop as the infant matures. Though they mature at different rates, sight, smell, taste, and touch all continue to develop after birth.

Sight

The newborn is nearsighted, preferring to view objects at a distance of 8 to 15 inches. Newborns prefer the human face to other objects and may even imitate the facial expressions made by those caring for them. In addition to human faces, newborns show a preference for certain objects, particularly those with contrasts such as black-and-white stripes. The

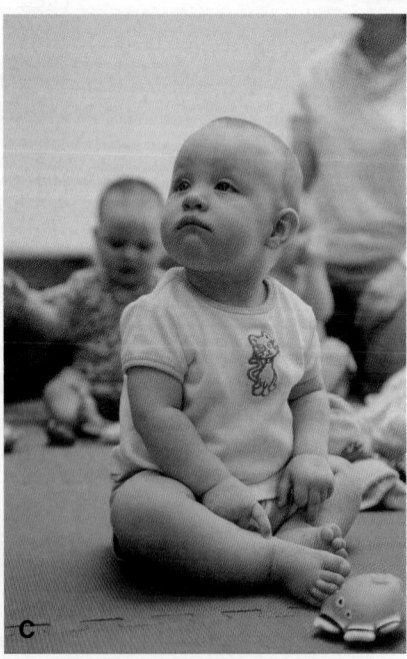

FIGURE 25.6 Development of sitting. (**A**) At 4 months, the infant requires significant support. (**B**) The 6-month-old infant sits in tripod fashion. (**C**) The 8-month-old sits alone.

newborn's eyes wander and occasionally cross. At 1 month of age the infant can recognize by sight the people he or she knows best. The infant will study objects within his or her visual range closely. The ability to fuse two ocular images into one cerebral picture (**binocularity**) begins to develop at 6 weeks of age and is well established by 4 months of age. Full color vision develops by 7 months of age, as do distance vision and the ability to track objects.

Hearing

The newborn's hearing is intact at birth and as acute as that of an adult. Newborns prefer the sound of human voices to nonhuman sounds. By 1 month of age the infant can recognize the sounds of those he or she knows best.

Smell and Taste

The sense of smell develops rapidly: the 7-day-old infant can differentiate the smell of his or her mother's breast milk from that of another woman and will preferentially turn toward the mother's smell. Newborns prefer sweet tastes to all others. This persists for several months, and eventually the infant will accept non-sweet flavors.

Touch

The sense of touch is perhaps the most important of all the senses for newborn communication. Even the most immature infant responds to soothing stroking. The infant prefers soft sensations to coarse sensations. The infant dislikes rough handling and may cry. Holding, stroking, rocking, and cuddling calms infants when they are upset and makes them more alert when they are drowsy. Infants learn to understand their caregiver's moods by the way they touch them.

▶ ***Take*** NOTE!

Warning signs that may indicate problems with sensory development include the following: young infant does not respond to loud noises; child does not focus on a near object; infant does not start to make sounds or babble by 4 months of age; infant does not turn to locate sound at age 4 months; infant crosses eyes most of the time at age 6 months.

▶ COMMUNICATION AND LANGUAGE DEVELOPMENT

For several months, crying is the only means of communication for the newborn and infant. The basic reason for crying is unmet needs. The 1- to 3-month-old baby coos, makes other vocalizations, and demonstrates differentiated crying. At 4 to 5 months of age, the infant makes simple vowel sounds, laughs aloud, performs "raspberries," and vocalizes in response to voices. The infant also responds

FIGURE 25.7 Development of locomotion. (**A**) At 4 months the infant pushes up from a prone position. (**B**) At 8 months, the infant crawls with the abdomen off the floor. (**C**) The infant pulls to stand by 10 months of age. (**D**) The infant cruises along furniture or (**E**) takes steps with assistance at 10 to 11 months of age. (**F**) The infant independently stands from a crouched position and walks around 12 months of age (plus or minus 3 months).

FIGURE 25.8 Development of the pincer grasp. Note the gross (whole-hand) approach to grasping a small object (**A**), compared with the fine (thumb-to-finger) ability (**B**).

to his or her own name and begins to respond to "no." Between 4 and 7 months the infant begins to distinguish emotions based on tone of voice. Squealing and yelling begin around 6 months of age; these may be used to express joy or displeasure. At age 7 to 10 months, babbling begins and progresses to strings (e.g., mamama, dadada) without meaning. The infant at this age is also able to respond to simple commands. At 9 to 12 months of age the infant begins to attach meaning to "mama" and "dada" and starts to imitate other speech sounds. The average 12-month-old uses two or three recognizable words with meaning, recognizes objects by name, and starts to imitate animal sounds. At this age, the infant pays increasing

attention to speech and tries to imitate words; he or she may also say, "uh-oh." The 12-month-old also babbles with inflection (this babbling has the rhythm and timing of spoken language, but few of the "words" make sense).

It is very important for the parent or caregiver to talk to the infant in order for the infant to learn communication skills. Sometimes regression in language development occurs briefly when the child is focusing energy on other skills, such as crawling or walking. As long as the infant's hearing is normal, language acquisition should continue to progress. Infants in bilingual families may "language mix" (uses some words from each language). This is considered to be a normal progression in language development for these children, but it makes it more difficult for the health care provider to determine delays in communication skills (Goldstein, 2006).

TABLE 25.5 DEVELOPMENT OF FINE MOTOR SKILLS IN INFANCY

Age	Fine Motor Skills
1 month	Fists mostly clenched Involuntary hand movements
3 months	Holds hand in front of face, hands open
4 months	Bats at objects
5 months	Grasps rattle
6 months	Releases object in hand to take another
7 months	Transfers object from one hand to the other
8 months	Gross pincer grasp (rakes)
9 months	Bangs objects together
10 months	Fine pincer grasp Puts objects into container and takes them out
11 months	Offers objects to others and releases them
12 months	Feeds self with cup and spoon Makes simple mark on paper Pokes with index finger

▶ **Take** NOTE!

Warning signs that may indicate problems in language development are as follows: infant does not make sounds at 4 months of age; infant does not laugh or squeal by 6 months of age; infant does not babble by 8 months of age; infant does not use single words with meaning at 12 months of age (mama, dada).

▶ SOCIAL AND EMOTIONAL DEVELOPMENT

The newborn spends much of the time sleeping, but by 2 months of age the infant is ready to start socializing. The infant exhibits a first real smile at age 2 months. He or she spends a great deal of time while awake watching and observing what is going on around him or her. By about 3 months of age the infant will start an interaction with a caregiver by smiling widely and possibly gurgling.

This prompts the caregiver to smile back and talk to the infant. The infant responds with more smiling, cooing, and gurgles as well as moving the arms and legs. The 3- to 4-month-old will also mimic the parent's facial movements, such as widening the eyes and sticking out the tongue. The baby may hesitate at first, but once the other person responds pleasantly to the infant, the infant engages and gets into the interaction. The infant may cry when the pleasant interaction stops. At 6 to 8 months of age the infant may enjoy socially interactive games such as patty-cake and peek-a-boo.

Stranger Anxiety

Around the age of 8 months the infant may develop **stranger anxiety**. The previously happy and very friendly infant may become clingy and whiny when approached by strangers or people not well known. Stranger anxiety is an indicator that the infant is recognizing himself or herself as separate from others. As the infant becomes more aware of new people and new places, he or she may view an interaction with a stranger as threatening and may start crying, even if the parent is right there. Family members whom the child sees infrequently, as well as others the child does not spend a lot of time with, should approach the infant calmly and slowly, with the parent in sight. Sometimes this will prevent a sudden crying spell.

Separation Anxiety

Separation anxiety may also start in the last few months of infancy. The infant becomes quite distressed when the parent leaves. The infant will eventually calm down and become engaged with the current caregiver. It is not until the infant is older that cognition and memory are sufficient for him or her to understand that the parent will come back.

> ▶ *Take* NOTE!
>
> *Warning signs of possible problems with social/emotional development include the following: child does not smile at people at 3 months of age; child refuses to cuddle; child does not seem to enjoy people; child shows no interest in peek-a-boo at 8 months of age.*

Temperament

Temperament is an individual's nature; it is referred to as the "how" of behavior (Zolten & Long, 2006). Temperament ranges from low or moderately active, regular, and predictable to highly active, more intense, and less adaptable. These are all considered normal along a continuum. An infant's innate temperament affects the way he or she responds to the environment. As parents take note of their infant's usual activity level, how intensely he or she reacts with others and the environment, and how stimulated the baby becomes with interactions, they start to learn about their infant's temperament. The parent should note how adaptable and flexible the infant is as well as how predictable and persistent the baby is.

When parents are familiar with how the baby approaches life on a routine basis, they will be better able to recognize when the baby is not acting like himself or herself. Nurses can help parents interpret observations about their infant's temperament and recommend ways to support the infant's individual behavior. Some infants are slower to warm up than others; those infants should be approached slowly and calmly. Some infants exhibit increased levels of activity compared to quieter, more passive babies; those infants generally require more direct play with the parent or caregiver and will be the type of older infant who is in constant motion. Some infants are loud and some are not. The quiet infant may become overwhelmed with excessive stimulation, whereas the very active baby may need additional stimulation to be satisfied. Becoming familiar with the infant's temperament also helps the parents describe the best approach to the infant by others (e.g., child care workers or health care professionals).

▶ CULTURAL INFLUENCES ON GROWTH AND DEVELOPMENT

Many cultural differences have an impact on growth and development. For instance, certain ethnic groups tend to be shorter than others because of their genetic makeup. These children will not grow to be as tall as those of another ethnic background. Cultural feeding practices in some cultures may lead to overweight in some children. Some cultures and certain religions advocate vegetarianism; those children need nutritional assessment to ensure they are getting enough protein intake for adequate growth.

Parenting styles and health promotion behaviors can also be significantly influenced by culture. Parents and extended family are the most significant influences in an infant's life in most cultures. Certain cultures place a high value upon independence and may encourage their infants to develop quickly, while other cultures "baby" their infants for longer periods. In most cultures the mother takes primary responsibility for caring for the child, but in some cultures, major health-related decisions may be deferred to the father or grandparents.

Health beliefs are often strongly influenced by an individual's religious or spiritual background. Sometimes this creates conflict in the health care setting when the health providers have a different value system than that of the infant's family.

In some cultures infants and children share a bed with their parents. When an infant or child is hospitalized and is accustomed to sleeping with the parents, it may be difficult and distressing for him or her to try to sleep alone.

The nurse should explore the family's cultural practices related to growth and development. Usually these practices are not harmful and can be supported by the health care team, but safety must always be considered.

The nurse should not make assumptions about a family's cultural practices based on their skin color, accent, or name; rather, the nurse should perform an adequate assessment.

> ▶ *Take* NOTE!
>
> *Many communities now include people from a variety of cultures, so it is important for nurses to practice transcultural nursing (nursing care that is directed by cultural aspects and that respects the individual's differences). Many nurse researchers are exploring the cultural aspects of health care and the impact that cultural diversity has upon health.*

Refer back to Allison Johnson, who was introduced at the beginning of the chapter. What developmental milestones would you expect Allison to have reached by this age? How would this be different if Allison had been born 6 weeks premature?

The Nurse's Role in Newborn and Infant Growth and Development

WATCH&LEARN

Growth and development affect every aspect of the infant's life. As infants progress through various stages of development, they do so in a predictable fashion. Growth and development are sequential and orderly, though some children develop at faster rates than others. It is important for the nurse to understand growth and development. Health care visits through infancy often focus primarily on **anticipatory guidance** (educating parents and caregivers about what to expect in the next phase of development). The purpose of anticipatory guidance is to give parents the tools they need to support their infant's development in a safe fashion.

Hospital nurses also need to use their knowledge of growth and development when caring for ill infants. Hospitalization often requires the infant to be confined to the crib or the hospital room. Nurses must support growth and development within the constraints imposed by the child's illness.

▶ NURSING PROCESS OVERVIEW

After the infant's current growth and development status has been assessed, problems related to growth and development may be identified. The nurse may then identify one or more nursing diagnoses, including:

- Ineffective breastfeeding
- Risk for disproportionate growth
- Imbalanced nutrition, less than body requirements
- Risk for impaired parent/infant attachment
- Delayed growth and development
- Risk for caregiver role strain

Nursing care planning for the infant with growth and development issues should be individualized based on the infant's and family's needs. The Nursing Care Plan Overview can be used as a guide in planning nursing care for the infant with a growth and development problem. The nurse may choose the appropriate nursing diagnoses from the plan and individualize them as needed. The nursing care plan is intended to serve as a guide, not as an all-inclusive growth and development care plan.

▶ PROMOTING HEALTHY GROWTH AND DEVELOPMENT

Adding a new person to the family produces both excitement and anxiety. Newborns are completely reliant upon their parents or caregivers to fill every need. It is quite a burden and precious responsibility that new parents are taking on. Many parents read the latest books about caring for newborns, while others rely on information received from family and friends. Newborns and their mothers spend only a short time in the hospital after delivery, so it is very important that parents can care for their newborn and know when to call the primary care provider with concerns.

Periodic screening for adequate growth and development is recommended by the American Academy of Pediatrics (AAP) for all infants and children. The prevention of devastating disease is another priority for infants and children. The AAP and the Advisory Committee on Immunization Practices (ACIP) have made recommendations for immunization schedules. Immunizations are a very important part of the newborn and infant's health visits. Nurses caring for newborns and infants should be familiar with the recommended infant/child periodic screenings (check-ups) as well as the current immunization schedule (see Chapter 30, for further information on immunizations).

Promoting Growth and Development Through Play

Experts in child development and behavior have said repeatedly that play is the work of children. Infants practice their gross and fine motor skills and language through play. Play is a natural way for infants and children to learn. Play is critical to infant development, as it gives infants the opportunity to explore their environment, practice new skills, and solve problems. The newborn prefers

(text continues on page 787)

Nursing Care Plan 25.1

GROWTH AND DEVELOPMENT ISSUES IN THE NEWBORN AND INFANT

NURSING DIAGNOSIS: Breastfeeding, ineffective, related to lack of exposure, misconceptions, or knowledge deficit as evidenced by first baby, mother's verbalization, or nursing observations

Outcome Identification and Evaluation

Mother/infant dyad will experience successful breastfeeding: *infant will latch on, suck and swallow at the breast; mother will not experience sore nipples.*

Interventions: Promoting Effective Breastfeeding

- Educate mother on recognition of and response to infant hunger cues *to promote on-cue breastfeeding, which will establish milk supply.*
- Educate mother on appropriate diet and fluid intake *to ensure ability to manufacture adequate supply of breast milk.*
- Demonstrate breastfeeding positions with infant at the breast *(appropriate positioning increases probability of successful latch).*
- Assess infant's latch technique, sucking motion, and audible swallowing *(an appropriately latched infant will take most of the areola in the mouth, suck in spurts, and demonstrate audible swallowing).*
- Assess infant voiding/stool patterns: *at least six voids per day and passage of stool ranging from one or more per day to one every several days is a normal pattern for breastfed infants.*
- Assess infant weight gain: *gain of 15 to 30 g per day after the second week of life indicates infant is receiving appropriate nutrition.*
- Assess mother's nipples for redness or soreness; *if infant appropriately latches on, nipples will not become sore.*

NURSING DIAGNOSIS: Risk for altered growth pattern (risk factors: caregiver knowledge deficit, first infant, premature infant, or maladaptive feeding behaviors)

Outcome Identification and Evaluation

Infant will demonstrate adequate growth and appropriate feeding behaviors: *steady increases in weight, length, and head circumference; infant feeds appropriately for age.*

Interventions: Promoting Adequate Growth

- Observe mother/infant dyad breastfeeding or bottle-feeding *to determine need for further education or identify infant difficulties with feeding.*
- Educate mother about appropriate breastfeeding or bottle-feeding *so that mother is aware of what to expect in normal feeding pattern.*
- When infant is old enough, provide education about addition of solid foods, spoon and cup feeding: *after 6 months of age breast milk or formula needs to be supplemented with a variety of foods.*
- Determine need for additional caloric intake if necessary *(premature infants and infants with chronic illnesses or metabolic disorders often need adjustments in caloric intake to demonstrate adequate or catch-up growth).*
- Obtain daily weights (if hospitalized, weekly if outpatient) and weekly length and head circumference *to determine whether feeding pattern is sufficient to promote adequate growth.*

(continued)

Nursing Care Plan 25.1 (continued)

NURSING DIAGNOSIS: Nutrition, altered, less than body requirements, related to possible ineffective feeding pattern or inadequate caloric intake as evidenced by failure to gain weight or by inadequate increases in weight, length, and head circumference over time

Outcome Identification and Evaluation

Infant will take in adequate nutrients using effective feeding pattern: *infant will demonstrate adequate weight gain (15 to 30 g per day) and steady increases in length and head circumference.*

Interventions: Promoting Adequate Nutritional Intake

- Assess current feeding pattern and daily intake *to determine areas of concern.*
- Increase frequency of breastfeeding or volume of bottle feeding *if needed to meet caloric needs.*
- Introduce solid foods on age-appropriate schedule: *introducing solids at the right time improves the chances that the child will learn to take solid foods.*
- Limit juice intake or discontinue altogether *(juice has little nutritive value and displaces nutrients from breast milk or formula).*
- Use human milk fortifier (if ordered) *to increase caloric density of breast milk.*
- Increase caloric density of formula (if ordered) by mixing to a more concentrated level or with additives (fats or carbohydrates) *to provide increased calories needed to support adequate growth.*
- If infant is taking solids already, choose higher-calorie foods *to maximize nutrient intake.*

NURSING DIAGNOSIS: Parent/infant attachment, altered, risk for (risk factors: premature infant, parental knowledge deficit about normal newborn activity and care, infant with difficult temperament or medical problems)

Outcome Identification and Evaluation

Parent and infant will demonstrate appropriate attachment via *eye contact, parental response to infant cues, parental verbalization of caring for infant, infant response to parent's caretaking behaviors.*

Interventions: Encouraging Appropriate Parent–Infant Attachment

- Assess parent's response to infant cues *to determine degree of attachment and level of parent's knowledge about infant care.*
- Assess infant's response to parent's caretaking behaviors *to determine degree of attachment.*
- Determine infant's temperament *to counsel parent effectively about responses appropriate for that type of temperament.*
- Encourage *en face* positioning for holding or feeding the young infant *to encourage give-and-take response between infant and parent.*
- Encourage parent to meet infant's needs promptly and with affection *to promote sense of trust in the infant.*
- Reinforce parent's attempts at improving attachment with infant *(positive reinforcement naturally encourages appropriate behaviors).*

NURSING DIAGNOSIS: Growth and development, altered, related to speech, motor, psychosocial, or cognitive concerns as evidenced by delay in meeting expected milestones

Outcome Identification and Evaluation

Development will be maximized: *infant will make continued progress toward attainment of developmental milestones.*

Interventions: Maximizing Development

- Perform developmental evaluation of the infant *to determine infant's current level of functioning.*
- Offer age-appropriate play, activities, and toys *to encourage further development.*
- Carry out interventions as prescribed by developmental specialist, physical therapist, occupational therapist, or speech therapist *(repeated exposure to the activities or exercises is needed to make developmental progress).*
- Provide support to parents of infants with developmental concerns, *as developmental progress can be slow and it is difficult for families to stay motivated and maintain hope.*

Nursing Care Plan 25.1 (continued)

NURSING DIAGNOSIS: Caregiver role strain, risk for (risk factors: first baby, knowledge deficit about infant care, lack of prior exposure, fatigue if premature, ill, or developmentally delayed infant)

Outcome Identification and Evaluation
Parent will experience competence in role: *will demonstrate appropriate caretaking behaviors and verbalize comfort in new role.*

Interventions: Preventing Caregiver Role Strain
- Assess parent's knowledge of newborn/infant care and the issues that arise as a part of normal development *to determine parent's needs.*
- Provide education on normal newborn/infant care *so that parents have the knowledge they need to appropriately care for their new baby.*
- Provide anticipatory guidance related to normal infant development *to prepare parents for what to expect next and how to intervene.*
- Encourage respite for parents *(even a few hours away from the demands of an infant's care can rejuvenate the parents).*

NURSING DIAGNOSIS: Injury, risk for (risk factors: developmental age, infant curiosity, rapidly progressing motor abilities)

Outcome Identification and Evaluation
Infant safety will be maintained: *infant will remain free from injury.*

Interventions: Preventing Injury
- Encourage car seat safety *to decrease risk of injury related to motor vehicles.*
- Childproof home: *as infant becomes more mobile, he or she will want to explore everything, increasing risk of injury.*
- Parents should have the Poison Control Center phone number available: *should an accidental ingestion occur, Poison Control can give parents the best advice for appropriate intervention.*
- Never leave an infant unattended in the sink, bathtub, or swimming pool *to prevent drowning.*
- Teach parents first aid measures and infant CPR *to minimize consequences of injury should it occur.*
- Parents should watch the infant at all times *(no amount of childproofing can replace the watchful eye of a caring parent).*

---

interacting with the parent to toys. Parents can talk to and sing to their newborns while participating in the daily activities that infants need, such as feeding, bathing, and changing diapers. Newborns and young infants love to watch people's faces and often appear to mimic the expressions they see.

As infants become older, toys may be geared toward the motor skills or language skills that the child is developing. Parents can promote fine motor development in infants by providing age-appropriate toys. For example, a rattle that a young infant can hold promotes reaching and attaining. The older infant builds fine motor skills by stacking cups or placing smaller toys inside of larger ones. Gross motor skills are reinforced and practiced over and over again when the infant wants to reach something he or she is interested in.

When playing with toys, the infant usually engages in **solitary play**; he or she does not share with other infants or directly play with other infants. A wide variety of toys are available for infants, but infants often enjoy the most basic ones, such as plastic containers of various shapes and sizes, soft balls, and wooden or plastic spoons.

Books are also very important toys for infants. Reading to all ages of infants is appropriate, and the older infant develops fine motor skills by learning to turn book pages.

Table 25.6 lists age-appropriate toys.

Promoting Early Learning

Research has shown that reading aloud and sharing books during early infancy are critical to the development of neural networks that are important in the later tasks of reading and word recognition. Reading books increases listening comprehension. Infants demonstrate their excitement about picture books by kicking and waving their arms and babbling when looking at them. At 6 to 12 months, the infant reaches for books and brings them to the mouth. Over time, reading leads to acquisition of language skills. Reading picture books and simple stories to infants starts a good habit that should be continued throughout childhood.

Promoting Safety

The most common cause of death in infants between the ages of 6 and 12 months is injury. As infants become more mobile, they risk injury from falls down stairs and off chairs, tables, and other structures. Curiosity leads the

TABLE 25.6 APPROPRIATE TOYS FOR NEWBORNS AND INFANTS

Age	Appropriate Toys
Newborn to 1 month	• Mobile with contrasting colors or patterns • Unbreakable mirror • Soft music via tape or music box • Soft, brightly colored toys
1 to 4 months	• Bright mobile • Unbreakable mirror • Rattles • Singing by parent or caregiver, varied music • High-contrast patterns in books or images
4 to 7 months	• Fabric or board books • Different types of music • Easy-to-hold toys that do things or make noise (fancy rattles) • Floating, squirting bath toys • Soft dolls or animals
8 to 12 months	• Plastic cups, bowls, buckets • Unbreakable mirror • Large building blocks • Stacking toys • Busy boxes (with buttons or knobs that make things happen) • Balls • Dolls • Board books with large pictures • Toy telephone • Push–pull toys (older infants)

infant to explore potentially dangerous items, such as electrical outlets, hot stove or furnace vents, mop buckets, and toilets. Since infants explore so much with their mouths, small objects or hard foods pose a choking hazard. The infant will invariably pick up any accessible object and bring it to the mouth. With increasing dexterity, poisoning from medications, household cleaning products, or other substances also becomes a problem.

Safety in the Car

Motor vehicle accidents are one source of injury, particularly if the infant is improperly restrained. Infants should never be transported in a motor vehicle without proper restraint. Infant car seats should face the rear of the car until the infant is 12 months of age and weighs 20 pounds. The car seat should be secured tightly in the center of the back seat. The infant should never be placed in a front seat that is equipped with an airbag.

Infants should never be left unattended in a motor vehicle. The temperature rises very quickly inside a closed vehicle, and an infant can suffocate from heat in a closed vehicle in the summer. Even during cooler weather, the heat generated within a closed vehicle can reach three to five times the exterior temperature. Kidnapping is also a concern if the baby is left unattended in a vehicle.

Additional information on car safety can be found on www.childsafety.org, www.safekids.org, and www.carseat.org and through the National Highway Traffic Safety Administration at www.nhtsadot.gov.

Safety in the Home

The baby's crib should have a firm mattress that fits snugly in the crib on a secure support. The distance between crib slats should be 2⅜ inches or less to prevent injury. All crib edges should be smooth. Only well-fitting crib sheets should be used, not sheets intended for large beds. Crib side rails should always be raised when the parent is not right next to the crib. Additional information about crib and playpen safety can be found at www.safekids.org.

Even before the infant can roll over, he or she wiggles and pushes with the feet. The infant can easily fall from a changing table, sofa, or crib with the side rails down, so the infant should never be left unattended on any surface. If infant seats, bouncy seats, or swings are used, the infant should always be restrained in the seat with the appropriate straps.

The AAP does not recommend the use of infant walkers, because the walker may tip over and the baby fall out of it or the infant may fall down the stairs in it. Walkers allow infants access to things they may not otherwise be capable of reaching until they are able to walk alone, such as hot stoves and items on the edge of the countertop.

As the infant becomes more mobile, learning to crawl and walk, new safety issues arise. Safety gates should be used at the tops and bottoms of stairways. Gates may also be used to block curious infants from rooms that may pose physical danger to them because of sharp-edged furniture or decorative objects. Electrical outlets should be covered with approved safety covers. Cabinets and drawers should be secured with child safety latches. Medications, household cleaning supplies, and other potentially hazardous substances should be stored completely out of reach of infants.

Choking is a risk because infants immediately bring small items to the mouth for exploration. To avoid choking, recommend the following to parents:

• Use only toys recommended for children 0 to 12 months of age.
• Avoid stuffed animals with eyes or buttons that can be dislodged by the persistent infant.
• Keep the floor free of small items (accidentally dropped coins, paper clips, straight pins).
• Avoid feeding popcorn, nuts, carrot slices, grapes, and hot dog pieces to infants.

Suffocation is also a risk for infants. Cribs should not have pillows, comforters, stuffed animals, or other soft items in them. Keep plastic bags of any size away from infants. Avoid the risk of strangulation by keeping window blind and drapery cords out of the infant's reach.

Though no safety measure is as effective as close supervision by a watchful parent or caregiver, the above safety measures can be critical to the infant's well-being.

Safety in the Water

Infants can drown in a very small amount of water. Never leave an infant unattended in the sink, a baby bathtub or standard bathtub, a swimming or wading pool, or any other body of water, even if it is quite shallow. The bathroom door should be kept closed and the toilet lid down. Water should be emptied from tubs, pails, or buckets immediately after use. If the family has a swimming pool, a locked fence or locked screen enclosure should surround it. Exterior doors should be kept locked to prevent the older infant from wandering out to the pool. The AAP recommends that parents use caution when enrolling their infant in an aquatic or swim program. The program should be geared toward water survival skills rather than swimming skills, as the infant is not developmentally ready for formal swimming lessons. Completing an aquatic program does not decrease the risk of drowning; vigilant supervision is still always required.

*R*emember *Allison Johnson, the infant described in the beginning of the chapter? What anticipatory guidance related to safety would you provide to Allison's parents?*

Promoting Nutrition

Adequate nutrition is essential for growth and development. Breastfeeding and bottle-feeding of infant formula are both acceptable means of nutrition in the newborn and infant. Breast milk or formula supplies all of the infant's daily nutritional requirements until 4 to 6 months of age, at which time solid foods may be introduced.

Cultural Factors

Many dietary practices are affected by culture, both in the types of food eaten and in the approach to progression of infant feeding. Some ethnic groups tend to be lactose-intolerant (particularly blacks, Native Americans, and Asians); therefore, alternative sources of calcium must be offered. Explore the cultural practices of the family related to infant feeding so that you can support the family's cultural values.

Nutritional Needs

Newborns and infants are experiencing tremendous growth and need diets that support these rapid changes. Table 25.7 compares fluid and caloric needs in the newborn and infant.

Breastfeeding

The National Association of Pediatric Nurse Practitioners (NAPNAP), the AAP, the American College of Obstetrics and Gynecology, the American Dietetic Association, and the U.S. Breastfeeding Committee of the Department of Health and Human Services all recommend breastfeeding as the natural and preferred method of newborn and infant feeding. In their position statement on breastfeeding (2001), NAPNAP identifies "human milk as superior to all substitute feeding methods." Breast milk provides complete infant nutrition.

Breastfeeding or feeding of expressed human milk is recommended for all infants, including sick or premature newborns (with rare exceptions). The exceptions include infants with galactosemia, maternal use of illicit drugs and a few prescription medications, maternal untreated active tuberculosis, and maternal human immunodeficiency virus (HIV) infection in developed countries.

Data from *Healthy People 2010* (2000) indicate that in 1998 64% of U.S. women breastfed in the early postpartum period, 29% of infants were breastfeeding at 6 months of age, and only 16% were still breastfeeding at 1 year of age. Even partial breastfeeding is helpful and offers some of the health benefits of breastfeeding. Pediatric nurses in the community and the hospital are in an excellent position to promote and support breastfeeding, thereby contributing to the *Healthy People 2010* goal of increasing the proportion of mothers who breastfeed their babies.

Breastfeeding Technique

Breastfeeding mothers may not have established adequate breastfeeding prior to leaving the hospital after birth of the newborn. The pediatric nurse may encounter an infant-mother dyad experiencing difficulty with breastfeeding for

TABLE 25.7 NUTRITIONAL REQUIREMENTS

Nutritional Requirements	Newborn	Infant
Fluid	140–160 mL/kg/day	100 mL/kg/day for first 10 kg, 50 mL/kg/day for next 10 kg
Calories	105–108 kcal/kg/day	1 to 6 months: 108 kcal/kg 6 to 12 months: 98 kcal/kg

a variety of reasons. Thus the pediatric nurse must be competent in counseling the breastfeeding mother. Refer to Chapter 18 for complete information related to breastfeeding positions and technique.

The breastfeeding infant does not need supplementation with water or formula even in the first few days of life as long as the newborn continues to wet 6 to 8 diapers per day. After several days of age, the mother's milk supply should be well established. Adequate urine output and bowel movements, as well as continued weight gain in the infant, indicate the adequacy of breastfeeding. Working mothers in particular may need additional support from the nurse in order to continue breastfeeding if they desire to do so. Common problems occurring with breastfeeding are addressed in Teaching Guidelines 25.1. Additional reliable resources for mothers who desire to breastfeed may be found on the following websites: www.aap.org/healthtopics/breastfeeding.cfm, www.breastfeeding.com, www.lalecheleague.org, www.medela.com, and www.promom.org.

Bottle Feeding

For the mother who does not desire to, or cannot, breastfeed, commercially prepared formulas are available for bottle-feeding. These formulas are designed to imitate human milk. Standard infant formulas based on cow's milk provide 20 kcal/ounce and use lactose as a source for carbohydrates. Vegetable oil is used as the source of fat; whey or casein provides protein. Newer cow's milk–based formulas contain long-chain polyunsaturated fatty acids that are thought to improve brain development. Ordinary cow's milk is not recommended for the first year of life.

> ▶ *Take* NOTE!
>
> *Cow's milk does not provide an adequate balance of nutrients for the growing infant, especially iron. It may also overload the infant's renal system with inappropriate amounts of protein, sodium, and minerals.*

TEACHING GUIDELINES 25.1

Promoting Breastfeeding

Problem	Solutions
Sore nipples	Prevention: encourage appropriate latch on from the beginning. Expose nipples to air between feedings. Allow breast milk to dry on nipples. Aloe vera or vitamin E may help to heal sore nipples. Medical-grade lanolin or preservative-free lanolin (Lansinoh) may be helpful.
Engorgement	Apply warm compresses or encourage the mother to take a warm shower prior to having the baby latch on. Warmth encourages some of the milk to be released, allowing the breast to soften and making it easier for the infant to latch on.
Poor sucking	Feed on cue, not on a schedule. Encourage the sleepy infant by stroking the feet, undressing, and rubbing the head.
Inadequate milk supply	Decrease maternal stress. Encourage adequate maternal diet and fluid intake. Mothers who return to work must pump in order to keep up milk supply when away from infant.
Father feels left out	Encourage father to participate in other aspects of care.
Mother worries about adequacy of breast milk	If infant is voiding six times per day and gaining weight, then he or she is receiving enough milk and appropriate nutrition.

Only formulas that are fortified with iron should be used. Iron stores that the infant received prenatally are depleted by 4 to 6 months of age. To prevent iron-deficiency anemia, poor growth patterns, and impaired development, iron-fortified formulas must be used. The AAP recommends that commercial formulas provide 10 to 12 mg of iron per liter (AAP, Committee on Nutrition, 1999). Commercial formulas also provide an adequate blend of essential vitamins and minerals.

Feeding Patterns

Infant feeding is an opportune time to establish good eating behaviors. The infant should always be held while being bottle-fed. Cradling in a semi-upright position allows for additional bonding time, as the infant can see the caregiver's face while feeding (Fig. 25.9). Talking or singing during feeding time also increases bonding. As with breastfed infants, the bottle-fed infant should be fed on cue. Overfeeding with the bottle increases the incidence of gastroesophageal reflux, so families need to learn their baby's cues to hunger and satiety.

It is important to feed the baby when he or she displays signs of hunger. Crying is a late sign of hunger; earlier signs include making sucking motions, sucking on hands, or putting the fist to the chin. The infant should be burped two or three times per feeding, when he or she slows feeding or stops sucking. Newborns may only take a half-ounce to 1 ounce per feeding initially, working up to 2 to 3 ounces in the first few days. They need to feed about six to ten times per day. The infant will gradually be able to ingest more formula per feeding. By 3 to 4 months of age, babies feed four or five times per day and take 6 to 7 ounces per feeding. Most infants will not require specific amounts per feeding; the infant should be fed until full. To prevent overfeeding, healthy bottle-fed infants should be allowed to self-regulate the amount of formula ingested per feeding. When the baby is satiated, he or she might fall asleep, spit out the nipple or formula, play with the nipple, or lie quietly, only sucking once in a while.

Types of Formulas and Bottles

Parents may choose to use commercial formulas that are ready-to-feed or available as a concentrate or as a powder. Parents should follow the instructions for mixing the concentrate or powder to avoid dehydration or fluid and electrolyte imbalances. Ready-to-feed formula should be used as is and never diluted.

A wide variety of baby bottle and nipple types are available for formula feeding, and the choice is purely individual. Few infants require special nipples or bottles. Box 25.1 gives guidelines on preparation and storage of formula and care of bottles.

Special Formulas

Special formulas may be needed for the infant who is allergic to a particular component of standard formula or has a renal, hepatic, metabolic, or intestinal disorder. For example, lactose-free cow's milk formulas are available for the lactose-intolerant child. Formulas using soy as the base ingredient instead of whey or casein are also available. Soy formulas are necessary for infants with a milk allergy, and they may be appealing to the vegetarian family.

These special formulas are designed to meet the nutritional needs of infants, depending on the disorder. Infants who fail to gain weight may be placed on standard infant formula prepared to deliver a higher caloric density per

FIGURE 25.9 Technique for bottle-feeding the infant.

BOX 25.1   Preparation and Storage of Bottles and Formula

- Wash nipples and bottles in hot soapy water and rinse well OR
- Run nipples and bottles through the dishwasher.
- Store tightly covered ready-to-feed formula can after opening in refrigerator for up to 48 hours.
- After mixing concentrate or powdered formula, store tightly covered in refrigerator for up to 48 hours.
- Do not reheat and reuse partially used bottles. Throw away the unused portion after each feeding.
- Do not add cereal to the formula in the bottle.
- Do not sweeten formula with honey.
- Warm formula by placing bottle in a container of hot water.
- Do not microwave formula.

ounce. Preterm infants (those born at less than 36 weeks' gestation) need adequate nutrition to exhibit catch-up growth. Good catch-up growth (quadrupling or even quintupling the birth weight) in the first year or so of life is critical for adequate head growth and avoidance of neuro-developmental consequences. Premature infant follow-up formulas are designed to provide additional calories, protein, and a particular calcium-to-phosphorus ratio as well as the vitamins and minerals needed for adequate catch-up growth.

Progressing to Solid Foods

After 6 months of age, infants usually require the nutrients available in solid foods in addition to their breast milk or formula. Progressing to feeding solid foods can be exciting and trying. Before solid foods are attempted, the infant should be assessed for readiness to progress. Parents need instruction in choosing appropriate solid foods and support in the progression process.

Assessing Infant Readiness

Several factors contribute to the appropriate timing of solid food introduction. The tongue extrusion reflex is necessary for sucking to be an automatic reaction—that is, when a nipple or other item is placed in the mouth, the tongue extrudes and sucking begins. This reflex disappears at about 4 to 6 months of age. Introducing solid food with a spoon prior to 4 to 6 months of age will result in extrusion of the tongue. The parent may think that the infant does not want the food and is spitting it out intentionally, but this is not the case; the infant simply must be mature enough to eat with a spoon (absence of extrusion reflex).

The ability to swallow solid food does not become completely functional until 4 to 6 months of age. Enzymes to appropriately digest food other than breast milk and formula are also not present in sufficient quantities until the age of 4 to 6 months.

Before the introduction of solid foods and the cup, the infant should be able to sit supported in a high chair. Solids should be fed with a spoon, with the infant in an upright position.

Choosing Appropriate Solid Foods

Iron-fortified rice cereal mixed with a small amount of breast milk or formula is a good choice for the first solid food. The cereal is easily digested and its taste is generally well accepted. The cereal should be quite thin at first; it can be mixed to a thicker consistency as the infant gets older. Once the feeding of cereal with a spoon is successful, other single foods may be introduced. The foods should be puréed to a smooth consistency, whether prepackaged "baby food" or puréed at home.

The introduction of one new food every 4 to 7 days is recommended. This allows for identification of food allergies (Box 25.2). No salt, sugar, or other seasoning should be added to these first foods.

BOX 25.2 Foods to Avoid in Infancy

- Honey
- Egg yolks and meats (until 10 months of age)
- Excessive amounts of fruit juice
- Foods likely to cause choking
  - Peanuts
  - Popcorn
  - Other small hard foods (e.g., raw carrot chunks)
  - Grapes and hot dog slices (must be cut in smaller pieces)
- Foods likely to result in allergic reaction
  - Citrus
  - Strawberries
  - Wheat
  - Cow's milk
  - Egg whites
  - Peanut butter

Generally, by 8 months of age the infant is ready for more texture in his or her foods. Soft, smashed table food without large chunks is appropriate. Finger foods such as Cheerios, soft green bean pieces, or soft peas may also be offered. Avoid hard foods that the infant may choke on. Strained, puréed, or mashed meats may be introduced at 10 to 12 months of age.

The cup should be introduced at 6 to 8 months of age. One ounce of breast milk or formula should be placed in the cup while the infant is learning. This will decrease the amount of mess should the cup be spilled. Old-fashioned sippy cups are generally acceptable for use, though older infants quickly learn to drink from an ordinary cup with assistance when they are thirsty. Newer "no-spill" sippy cups are not recommended for general home use. They require sucking much like a bottle and do not really encourage the child to learn cup drinking. They should be reserved for use on long trips in the car or other instances in which spills should be avoided (Bailey, 2007).

Fruit juice is unnecessary and should not be introduced until 6 months of age. If juice is given, it should be limited to 2 to 4 ounces per day. Fruit itself is much more nutritious than fruit juice. If infants are allowed to consume larger quantities of juice, it can displace important nutrients from breast milk or formula.

Promoting Healthy Eating Habits

Infants and children learn about food within a social context, so the family plays an important role in creating healthy eating habits. Families "model" eating behaviors; infants and children learn about eating through watching others. Lifelong eating patterns are often established in childhood, so it is important to emphasize healthy eating practices beginning in infancy (Savage et al., 2007). Parents should not let infants eat whatever they want (permissive feeding style); this will lead to fights over eating in the future. Infants may require as many as 20 exposures to a new food before it is accepted. On the other hand, infants should not be coerced into eating all that is provided (authoritarian feeding style). Forcing an infant to eat when he or she is full sets the child up for overeating in the future and may lead to more power struggles. Parents need to find a balance between the permissive and authoritarian feeding styles to establish lifelong healthy eating patterns in their children. By providing education about appropriate diet and feeding behaviors, the nurse can help the family to accomplish this goal.

Think back to Allison Johnson. What questions should you ask Allison's parents related to her nutritional intake? What anticipatory guidance related to nutrition would be appropriate?

Promoting Healthy Sleep and Rest

Newborns sleep about 20 hours a day, waking frequently to feed and quickly returning to sleep. By 3 months of age, most infants sleep 7 to 8 hours per night without waking. They will continue to take about three naps a day. By 4 months of age the infant is more active and alert and may have more trouble going to sleep in the evening. Night waking may occur, but the infant should be capable of sleeping through the night and does not require a night feeding. By 12 months of age infants sleep 8 to 12 hours per night and take two naps per day.

Discuss safe sleeping practices with parents of newborns and infants; the baby should sleep on a firm mattress without pillows or comforters. The baby's bed should be placed away from air conditioner vents, open windows, and open heaters. Sudden infant death syndrome (SIDS) has been associated with prone positioning of newborns and infants, so the infant should be placed to sleep on the back. See Healthy People 2010.

▶ *Take NOTE!*

The AAP has determined that side sleeping is not as safe as supine sleeping.

In the newborn period, the primary caregiver should try to sleep when the baby is sleeping. Since newborns need to be fed every 1½ to 3 hours around the clock, parents may become exhausted quickly and are often eager for the infant to sleep through the night. Adding rice cereal to the evening bottle has not been proven to discour-

HEALTHY PEOPLE 2010	
Objective	Significance
Increase the percentage of healthy full-term infants who are put down to sleep on their backs.	• Begin teaching about "back to sleep" at prenatal or newborn visit. • Use each encounter with the young infant as an opportunity to reinforce the supine position for sleep.

age night waking and is not recommended. Provide support to parents of newborns and educate them on infant sleeping patterns.

It is important to establish a bedtime routine around 4 months of age due to the infant's increased alertness and activity level. The baby who is 4 months or older needs a time of calming and relaxation before going to sleep. A consistent bedtime routine should be established, perhaps a bath followed by rocking, singing, or reading. The infant should fall asleep in his or her own crib rather than being rocked to sleep or held until sleeping and then put in the crib. After 4 months of age, infants must learn to soothe themselves back to sleep following night waking. Older infants may exhibit head banging as a form of self-soothing and use it to fall asleep at night. Night feedings are unnecessary at this age and will create a routine of further night waking that will be difficult to break. Parents should minimize attention and stimulation provided during a night waking. Briefly checking on the infant to ascertain his or her safety, followed by placing the infant back in a lying position and telling him or her good night, is all that is needed. This may have to be repeated several times before the infant falls back to sleep. It is important to keep interactions brief during the night waking so that the infant learns to fall back to sleep on his or her own. Continued issues with night waking should be discussed with the infant's primary care provider.

What anticipatory guidance should you provide to Allison's parents in relation to sleep?

Promoting Healthy Teeth and Gums

Healthy teeth and gums require proper oral hygiene and appropriate fluoride supplementation. Children over 6 months of age whose drinking water source contains less than 0.3 parts per million may require fluoride supplementation. Excess fluoride ingestion can result in discoloration of the teeth (fluorosis). Early childhood dental caries can result from pooling of milk or juice around teeth and gums.

Before tooth eruption, parents should clean the child's gums after feeding with a damp washcloth. After teeth have erupted, parents can continue to use a soft cloth for tooth cleaning and then eventually use a small soft-bristled toothbrush. Toothpaste is unnecessary in infancy. Infants should not be allowed to take milk or juice bottles to bed, as the high sugar content of the fluid in contact with the teeth all night leads to dental caries (see section on baby bottle mouth below). Weaning from the bottle at age 12 to 15 months may help prevent dental caries. No-spill sippy cups have also been implicated in the development of dental caries and should be avoided. The American Academy of Pediatric Dentistry recommends that infants receive their first dental visit by the age of 1 year.

Promoting Appropriate Discipline

Parenting requires ever-changing adaptations to the developing infant's needs. Unconditional love, patience, and compassion must be balanced with the parents' needs. **Discipline** helps build self-esteem in children as well as sets standards for social interactions. The primary goal of discipline is to teach an infant limits. Discipline should be used to help the infant solve problems. The infant's activities are based on the basic needs of food, security, warmth, love, and comfort. Misbehavior is the result of an unmet need, and the parents should respond accordingly.

As the infant is undergoing rapid changes in motor skills, safety needs increase. Nurses should encourage the parents to "childproof" their home so that the infant can develop physical skills without being at risk. In a childproof home, fewer restrictions need to be placed on the infant's behavior, and he or she can explore.

Physical punishment or spanking should never be used in infancy. Infants are at increased risk for physical injury from spanking and cannot make the connection between the spanking and the undesirable behavior (Brazelton & Sparrow, 2006). Providing a safe environment, redirection away from undesirable behaviors, and saying "no" in appropriate instances are far more effective. For example, when the infant is in potential danger (e.g., inserting a key into an electrical outlet, attempting to ingest a poisonous substance, or reaching into the toilet), the parent must use a firm but calm and brisk approach. If the infant knows the parent is serious, he or she will usually comply more quickly.

Remaining calm, firm, and consistent is necessary. Immediacy is also an important component of appropriate discipline. The infant cannot make the connection between a subsequent punishment or discussion of behavior with the earlier event itself. Positive reinforcement should be used to support good behavior.

Addressing Child Care Needs

Many mothers work outside the home, there are many single-parent families, and many families live a distance away from relatives. In all of these circumstances, infants may need to be cared for outside the home, often in child care settings or home day care centers.

Parents contemplating child care must consider a number of factors. Do they want a sitter to come to their home? Will they use a traditional day care center or a home care situation with fewer children? How much can they afford? If families choose to use a freestanding day care center or a home-based day care center, they should make sure that the provider is appropriately licensed. Parents should feel comfortable with the caregiver-to-child ratio. Are the caregivers trained in infant CPR and first aid? Families may need to visit or interview several facilities before finding one that meets their requirements.

When an older infant is attending a child care situation for the first time, it may be helpful to visit the center once or twice beforehand so that the infant can get used to the caregivers from the comfort and security of the parent's lap. Warn parents that separation anxiety in late infancy can cause a disturbing crying episode when the parent leaves. Reassure parents that the infant will not suffer harm due to the separation.

► ADDRESSING COMMON DEVELOPMENTAL CONCERNS

Parents commonly have multiple concerns during normal infant growth and development. Although most of these issues are not actual disease states or behavior problems, nurses must be aware of these issues to recognize them and to intervene appropriately.

Colic

Healthy 6-week-old infants cry for a total of about 3 hours every day. Crying and fussing are more prevalent in the evenings. By age 12 weeks, the total amount of crying is about 1 hour per day, and infants are better able to soothe themselves by this age. **Colic** is defined as inconsolable crying that lasts 3 hours or longer per day and for which there is no physical cause. It typically resolves by 3 months of age, coinciding with the age at which infants are better able to soothe themselves (e.g., by finger sucking). The cause of colic is thought to be problems in the gastrointestinal or neurologic system (probably system immaturity), temperament, or parenting style of the mother or father (Lobo et al., 2004). Some parents are overly anxious or overly attentive or, at the other extreme, may not give the infant the attention he or she needs. Any of these may contribute to a baby's fussing and crying.

Prolonged crying leads to increased stress among caregivers. Failure to stop the crying leads to frustration, and crying that prevents the parents from sleeping contributes to the exhaustion they are already experiencing.

Educate parents that normal crying increases by the time the infant is 6 weeks old and diminishes by about 12 weeks. When faced with a colicky baby, parents should develop a stepwise approach to checking that all of the infant's basic needs are met. When these needs are met, attempts at soothing the infant may be used. Reducing stimulation may decrease the length of crying. Carrying the infant more may also be helpful. Some infants respond to the motion of an infant swing or a car ride. Vibration, white noise, or swaddling may also help to decrease fussing in some infants. Pacifiers can be soothing to babies who need additional non-nutritive sucking. Parents should try one intervention at a time, taking care not to stimulate the infant excessively in the process of searching for solutions. Nurses should provide ongoing support to the parents of a colicky infant and reassure them that this is a temporary condition that will resolve in time.

Spitting Up

Spitting up (regurgitating small amounts of stomach contents) occurs in all infants, and a significant number of normal infants spit up excessively (Barr, 2003). Although spitting up after feeding is normal, it can be a cause of great concern to parents. Overfed babies who feed based on a parent-designed schedule and those who burp poorly are more likely to spit up. For some infants, the amount and frequency of spitting up are significant, and it may indicate gastroesophageal reflux.

Teach parents that feeding smaller amounts on a more frequent basis may help to decrease spitting-up episodes. Always burp the baby at least two or three times per feeding. Keep the baby upright for 30 minutes after feeding and do not lay the infant prone after feeding. Avoid bouncing or excess activity immediately after feeding. Positioning in an infant seat compresses the stomach and is not recommended. When placing the baby in bed, position him or her on the side with the head of the bed slightly elevated.

Reassure parents that if the infant is wetting at least six diapers per 24 hours and gaining weight, the spitting up is normal. If the infant vomits one third or more of most feedings, chokes when vomiting, or experiences forceful emesis, the primary care provider should be notified.

Thumb Sucking, Pacifiers, and Security Items

Infants demonstrate a clear need for non-nutritive sucking: even fetuses can be observed sucking their thumbs or fingers *in utero*. Thumb sucking is a healthy self-comforting activity. Infants who suck their thumbs or pacifiers often are better able to soothe themselves than those who do not. Studies have not shown that sucking either thumbs or pacifiers leads to the need for orthodontic braces unless the sucking continues well beyond the early school-age period. However, pacifier use has been associated with the increased incidence of otitis media (Comina et al., 2006), and hygiene is always a concern as pacifiers often fall on the floor.

Infants may also become attached to a doll, stuffed animal, or blanket. Just like thumb sucking, the attachment item gives the infant the security to self-soothe when he or she is uncomfortable.

Families need to explore their feelings and cultural preferences about sucking habits and security items. Parents should not try to break the habit during a stressful time for the infant. When the infant is intensely trying to master a new skill such as sitting or walking, he or she may need the sucking or security item to self-soothe. Pacifiers and security items can be physically taken away at some point, but the thumb is attached. The infant who has become attached to thumb sucking should not have additional attention drawn to the issue, as that may prolong thumb sucking.

Families of infants who use pacifiers may want to wean the infant from the pacifier when the child is 6 to 9 months of age. This is the time when the need for additional sucking naturally decreases. Attempts to wean the child from a security blanket or toy should probably be reserved for after infancy (see Evidence-Based Practice).

Teething

Discomfort is common as the tooth breaks through the periodontal membrane. Infants may drool, bite on hard objects, or increase finger sucking. Some infants may become very irritable, refuse to eat, and not sleep well. Fever, vomiting, and diarrhea are generally not considered a sign of teething but rather of illness.

Teething pain results from inflammation. Teach parents that application of cold may be soothing to the gums. The infant may chew on a frozen teething ring, or parents can rub an ice cube wrapped in a washcloth on the gums. Over-the-counter topical anesthetics such as baby Orajel may also be helpful. Parents should apply the ointment correctly to the gums, avoiding the lips, as these ointments cause numbing. Occasionally, oral acetaminophen or ibuprofen may be given to relieve pain.

Refer back to 6-month-old Allison Johnson. List some common developmental concerns of 6-month-old infants. What anticipatory guidance related to these concerns would you provide to her parents?

■■■ Key Concepts

- Infancy encompasses the period from birth to age 12 months.
- The infant exhibits tremendous growth, doubling the birthweight by 6 months of age and tripling it by 12 months of age.
- Most organ systems are immature at birth and develop and mature over the first year of life.

EVIDENCE-BASED PRACTICE 25.1
Benefits and Risks of Pacifier Use

● **Study**

The authors review the history of pacifier use and several recent research studies that attempted to determine the risks and benefits of pacifier use. The majority of the studies were performed within the early part of the 21st century.

▲ **Findings**

Upon analysis of the various research studies, the authors reached several conclusions. Pacifier use has been shown to lower the risk of Sudden Infant Death Syndrome (SIDS) when used at the time of sleep. Additional benefits include assistance in development of neurologic maturity in preterm infants and not shortening breastfeeding duration in preterm or term infants older than 1 month of age. Potential risks include shortening of breastfeeding duration if

a pacifier is used before 1 month of age, increased incidence of otitis media when used after 1 year of age, and development of dental misalignment.

■ **Nursing Implications**

In light of the potential risks and benefits of pacifier use, nurses must be prepared to provide parents with accurate information related to the use of pacifiers. Educate parents to avoid introduction of the pacifier until breastfeeding is well established (4 weeks of age), to use pacifiers only during periods of sleep, and to never force a pacifier on an infant or replace a pacifier in a sleeping infant's mouth. Additionally, parents should begin to wean the infant from the pacifier in late infancy so that it is not used past 1 year of age.

Marter, A., & Agruss, J. C. (2007). Pacifiers: An update on use and misuse. *Journal for Specialists in Pediatric Nursing, 12*(4), 278–285.

■ Child development is orderly, sequential, and predictable, progressing in a cephalocaudal and proximodistal fashion.

■ The infant is mastering the psychosocial task of Trust versus Mistrust.

■ Cognitive development in infancy is sensorimotor; infants use their senses and progressing motor skills to master their environment.

■ The 12-month-old babbles expressively and uses two or three words with meaning.

■ Promotion of safety is of key importance throughout infancy.

■ Breastfeeding is the natural and preferred method for infant feeding.

■ Breastfed and bottle-fed infants should both be fed on cue rather than on a parent-designed schedule.

■ Solid foods should be introduced at age 4 to 6 months. A spoon should be used to feed the infant, and rice cereal should be the first food. New foods should be introduced no more frequently than every 4 to 7 days.

■ The cup may be introduced at 6 months of age. No-spill sippy cups are generally not recommended.

■ Spitting up and colic are parts of normal development in the otherwise thriving infant and do not require medical intervention.

REFERENCES

American Academy of Pediatric Dentistry. (2007). Policy on use of fluoride. Retrieved August 28, 2007 from http://www.aapd.org/media/Policies_Guidelines/P_FluorideUse.pdf.

American Academy of Pediatrics. (2001). Policy statement: The use and misuse of fruit juice in pediatrics (RE0047). *Pediatrics, 107*(5), 1201–1213.

American Academy of Pediatrics. (2004a). *Guidance for effective discipline.* Retrieved August 28, 2007 from http://aappolicy.aappublications.org/cgi/content/full/pediatrics;101/4/723.

American Academy of Pediatrics. (2004b). *Policy statement: Swimming programs for infants and toddlers.* Retrieved August 28, 2007 from http://aappolicy.aappublications.org/cgi/content/full/pediatrics;105/4/868.

American Academy of Pediatrics. (2005a). Policy statement, breastfeeding and the use of human milk. *Pediatrics, 115*(2), 496–506.

American Academy of Pediatrics. (2005b). Policy statement, the changing concept of sudden infant death syndrome: diagnostic coding shifts, controversies regarding the sleeping environment, and new variable to consider in reducing risk. *Pediatrics, 116*(5), 1245–1255.

American Academy of Pediatrics. (2007a). *Car safety seats: A guide for families 2007.* Retrieved August 28, 2007 from http://www.aap.org/family/carseatguide.htm.

American Academy of Pediatrics. (2007b). *Policy use: The use and misuse of fruit juice in pediatrics.* Retrieved August 28, 2007 from http://aappolicy.aappublications.org/cgi/content/full/pediatrics;107/5/1210.

American Academy of Pediatrics, Committee on Nutrition. (1999). Policy statement: Iron fortification of infant formulas (RE9865). *Pediatrics, 104*(1), 119–123.

American Academy of Pediatrics, The Injury Prevention Program. (2007a). Age-related safety sheets, birth to 6 months. Retrieved August 28, 2007 from http://www.aap.org/family/birthto6.htm.

American Academy of Pediatrics, The Injury Prevention Program. (2007b). Age-related safety sheets, 6 to 12 months. Retrieved August 28, 2007 from http://www.aap.org/family/6to12mo.htm.

American Dietetic Association. (2005). Promoting and supporting breastfeeding. *Journal of the American Dietetic Association, 105*(5), 810–818.

Barr, R. G. (2003). Crying and colic. In Rudolph, C. D., Rudolph, A. M., Hostetter, M. K., Lister, G., & Siegel, N. J. (Eds.), *Rudolph's pediatrics, 21st ed.* New York: McGraw-Hill.

Bailey, E. (2007). *Proper dental care is critical to child's health.* Retrieved August 28, 2007 from http://www.gloucestertimes.com/pulife/local_story_236093935.

Brazelton, T. B., & Sparrow, J. D. (2006). *Touchpoints, birth to 3.* Cambridge, MA: Da Capo Press.

Bright Horizons. (2006). *A guide for quality care for your baby.* Retrieved August 28, 2007 from http://www.brighthorizons.com/Site/pages/infant_web_checklist.pdf.

Center for Prevention and Early Intervention Policy. (2005). *Literacy, bonding, and school readiness.* Tallahassee, FL: Florida State University.

Comina, E., Marion, K., Renaud, F. N. R., Dore, J., Bergeron, E., & Freney, J. (2006). Pacifiers: A microbial reservoir. *Nursing & Health Sciences, 8*(4), 216–223.

Erikson, E. H. (1963). *Childhood and society* (2nd ed.). New York: W. W. Norton and Company.

Gabbard, G. O. (2000). Psychoanalysis. In B. J. Sadock & V. A. Sadock (Eds.), *Kaplan and Sadock's comprehensive textbook of psychiatry* (7th ed.). Philadelphia: Lippincott Williams & Wilkins.

Gilger, M. A. (2006). Normal gastrointestinal function. In J. A. McMillan (Ed.), *Oski's pediatrics: Principles and practice* (4th ed.). Philadelphia: Lippincott Williams & Wilkins.

Goldenring, J. M. (2007). What to tell parents before they leave the hospital. *Contemporary Pediatrics, 24*(4), 52–79.

Goldstein, B. A. (2006). Clinical implications of research on language development and disorders in bilingual children. *Seminars in Speech and Language, 26*(4), 305–321.

Green, M., & Palfrey, J. S. (Eds). (2002). *Bright futures: Guidelines for health supervision of infants, children, and adolescents* (2nd ed., rev.). Arlington, VA: National Center for Education in Maternal and Child Health.

Johannes, B., & Menei, L. (2007). Happy babies, happy parents: Calming techniques ease moms' minds. *2007 Pediatrics Specialty Guide,* 20–21.

Leininger, M. M., & MacFarland, M. R. (2005). *Culture, care, diversity and universality: A worldwide nursing theory* (2nd ed.). Sudbury, MA: Jones & Bartlett.

Lobo, M. L., Kotzer, A. M., Keefe, M. R., Brady, E., Deloian, B., Froese-Fretz, A., & Barbosa, G. (2004). Current beliefs and management strategies for treating infant colic. *Journal of Pediatric Health Care, 18*(3), 115–122.

National Association of Pediatric Nurse Practitioners. (2006). *Guide to common breastfeeding problems.* Cherry Hill, N.J.: Author.

National Association of Pediatric Nurse Practitioners. (2006). *Healthy eating and activity together (HEAT) clinical practice guideline: Identifying and preventing overweight in childhood.* Cherry Hill, NJ: Author.

National Association of Pediatric Nurse Practitioners. (2007). NAP-NAP position statement on breastfeeding. *Journal of Pediatric Health Care, 21,* 39A–40A.

National Association of Pediatric Nurse Practitioners. (2007b). *Successful bottlefeeding.* Retrieved August 28, 2007 from http://napnap.org/Docs/bottle_eng.pdf.

National Association of Pediatric Nurse Practitioners. (2007c). *The scoop on babies' poop.* Retrieved August 28, 2007 from http://napnap.org/Docs/poop_eng.pdf.

National Association for Sport & Physical Education. (2007). *Active start: A statement of physical activity guidelines for children birth to five years.* Retrieved August 28, 2007 from http://www.aahperd.org/naspe/template.cfm?template=ns_active.html.

National Heart Lung and Blood Institute. (2007). *How can iron-deficiency anemia be prevented?* Retrieved August 28, 2007 from http://www.nhlbi.nih.gov/health/dci/Diseases/ida/ida_prevention.html.

Palmer, F. B., & Capute, A. J. (2006). Streams of development: The keys to developmental assessment. In J. A. McMillan (Ed.), *Oski's pediatrics: Principles and practice* (4th ed.). Philadelphia: Lippincott Williams & Wilkins.

Piaget, J. (1969). *The theory of stages in cognitive development.* New York: McGraw-Hill.

Safe Kids USA. (2007a). *Safety tips: Car.* Retrieved August 28, 2007 from http://www.usa.safekids.org/tier2_rl.cfm?folder_id=170.

Safe Kids USA. (2007b). *Safety tips: Baby, crib safety checklist.* Retrieved August 28, 2007 from http://www.usa.safekids.org/tier3_cd.cfm?folder_id=167&content_item_id=1290.

Savage, J. S., Fisher, J. O., & Birch, L. L. (2007). Parental influence on eating behavior: Conception to adolescence. *The Journal of Law, Medicine & Ethics, 35*(1), 22–34.

Schuman, A. T. (2007). The ABCs of toy safety: More than just child's play. *Contemporary Pediatrics, 24*(7), 49–57, 64.

Shelov, S. P., Trubo, R., & Hannemann, R. E. (Eds.) (2004). *Caring for your baby and young child: Birth to age 5* (4th ed.). New York: Bantam Books.

Small, L., Melnyk, B. M., & Strasser, A. (2007). Preventing obesity in young children. *Advance for Nurse Practitioners, 15*(3), 35–40.

Southall, J. (2007). Well-child visits should serve as a time to approach patients holistically. *Infectious Diseases in Children, 20*(6), 39–40.

Storey, M., Holt, K., & Sotfka, D. (Eds.). (2002). *Bright futures in practice: Nutrition* (2nd ed.). Arlington, VA: National Center for Education in Maternal and Child Health.

Zolten, K., & Long, N. (2006). *Center for effective parenting: Infant temperament.* Retrieved August 28, 2007 from http://www.parenting-ed.org/handouts/infant%20temperament.pdf.

WEBSITES

Georgia Department of Public Health–Growth and Development: health.state.ga.us/publications/growthdev/months.asp

American Academy of Pediatrics: www.aap.org

Online community for new fathers: www.brandnewdad.com

Nemours Center for Children's Health Media: www.kidshealth.com

Parent-supported group for children's health, growth, and development: www.kidsource.com

American Academy of Pediatric Dentistry: www.aapd.org

University of Washington-Nursing Child Assessment Satellite Training: www.ncast.org

Teething information from Del Pharmaceuticals: www.orajel.com

Johnson & Johnson Pediatric Institute: www.pediatricinstitute.com

Safe Kids USA: www.usa.safekids.org/

The Zero to Three: National Center for Infants, Toddlers and Families: www.zerotothree.org

CHAPTER WORKSHEET

MULTIPLE CHOICE QUESTIONS

1. The mother of a 3-month-old boy asks the nurse about starting solid foods. What is the most appropriate response by the nurse?

   a. "It's okay to start puréed solids at this age if fed via the bottle."

   b. "Infants don't require solid food until 12 months of age."

   c. "Solid foods should be delayed until age 6 months, when the infant can handle a spoon on his own."

   d. "The tongue extrusion reflex disappears at age 4 to 6 months, making it a good time to start solid foods."

2. The father of a 2-month-old girl is expressing concern that his infant may be getting spoiled. The nurse's best response is:

   a. "She just needs love and attention. Don't worry; she's too young to spoil."

   b. "Consistently meeting the infant's needs helps promote a sense of trust."

   c. "Infants need to be fed and cleaned; if you're sure those needs are met, just let her cry."

   d. "Consistency in meeting needs is important, but you're right, holding her too much will spoil her."

3. Parents of an 8-month-old girl express concern that she cries when left with the babysitter. How does the nurse best explain this behavior?

   a. Crying when left with the sitter may indicate difficulty with building trust.

   b. Stranger anxiety should not occur until toddlerhood; this concern should be investigated.

   c. Separation anxiety is normal at this age; the infant recognizes parents as separate beings.

   d. Perhaps the sitter doesn't meet the infant's needs; choose a different sitter.

4. The nurse is providing anticipatory guidance to the mother of a 6-month-old-infant. What is the best instruction by the nurse in relation to the infant's oral health?

   a. "Start brushing her teeth after all the baby teeth come in."

   b. "Use a washcloth with toothpaste to clean her mouth."

   c. "Clean your baby's gums, then new teeth, with a washcloth."

   d. "Rinse your baby's mouth with water after every feeding."

5. A 9-month-old infant's mother is questioning why cow's milk is not recommended in the first year of life as it is much cheaper than formula. What rationale does the nurse include in her response?

   a. It is permissible to substitute cow's milk for formula at this age as he is so close to 1 year old.

   b. Cow's milk is iron poor and does not provide the proper balance of nutrients for the infant.

   c. As long as the mother provides whole milk, rather than skim, she can start cow's milk in infancy.

   d. If the mother cannot afford the infant formula, she should dilute it to make it last longer.

CRITICAL THINKING EXERCISES

1. The mother of an 11-month-old boy who was born at 24 weeks' gestation is concerned about his size and motor skills. What information should the nurse provide?

2. An infant's mother thinks there may be something wrong with him because "he spits up so much." What further information should the nurse obtain?

3. If you determine that the infant in the question above is experiencing normal spitting up associated with his developmental age, develop a brief teaching plan to review with the mother.

STUDY ACTIVITIES

1. A mother brings her 9-month-old boy to the clinic for a well-child check-up. She has questions about feeding, speech, and walking. Develop a teaching plan of anticipatory guidance for the 9-month-old infant.

2. Develop a safety plan for the 12-month-old infant.

3. In the clinical setting, observe two infants of the same age, one who is developing appropriately for his or her age and one who is delayed. Note the similarities and differences between the two infants.

CHAPTER 26

GROWTH AND DEVELOPMENT OF THE TODDLER

KEY TERMS

animism
echolalia
egocentrism
expressive language
food jag

individuation
parallel play
physiologic anorexia
receptive language
regression

ritualism
separation
separation anxiety
sibling rivalry
telegraphic speech

LEARNING OBJECTIVES

Upon completion of the chapter, the learner will be able to:

1. Explain normal physiologic, psychosocial, and cognitive changes occurring in the toddler.
2. Identify the gross and fine motor milestones of the toddler.
3. Demonstrate an understanding of language development in the toddler years.
4. Discuss sensory development of the toddler.
5. Demonstrate an understanding of emotional/social development and moral/spiritual development during toddlerhood.
6. Implement a nursing care plan to address common issues related to growth and development in toddlerhood.
7. Encourage growth and learning through play.
8. Develop a teaching plan for safety promotion in the toddler period.
9. Demonstrate an understanding of toddler needs related to sleep and rest, as well as dental health.
10. Develop a nutritional plan for the toddler based on average nutritional requirements.
11. Provide appropriate anticipatory guidance for common developmental issues that arise in the toddler period.
12. Demonstrate an understanding of appropriate methods of discipline for use during the toddler years.
13. Identify the role of the parent in the toddler's life and determine ways to support, encourage, and educate the parents about toddler growth, development, and concerns during this period.

J̄ose Gonzales is a 2-year-old boy brought to the clinic by his mother and father for his 2-year-old check-up. During your assessment, you find that his weight is 30 pounds, height 33 inches, and head circumference 19.5 inches. As the nurse caring for him, assess Jose's growth and development, and then provide appropriate anticipatory guidance to the parents.

Wow

Toddlers will take risks and make many mistakes, but remember that both are an essential part of their growth.

The toddler period encompasses the second 2 years of life, from age 1 year to age 3 years. This period is a time of significant advancement in growth and development for the child. It can also be quite a challenging time for parents. The theme during the toddler years is one of holding on and letting go. Having learned that parents are predictable and reliable, the toddler is now learning that his or her behavior has a predictable, reliable effect on others. The challenge is to encourage independence and autonomy while keeping the curious toddler safe.

▶ *Take* NOTE!

As more grandparents are assuming the primary caregiver role for their grandchildren, nurses should be alert to the possibility of increased stress that is placed upon the older caregiver, particularly during the active and sometimes trying years of toddlerhood.

Growth and Development Overview

Infancy is a time of intense growth and development. Both physical growth and acquisition of new motor skills slow somewhat during the toddler years. Refinement of motor skills, continued cognitive growth, and acquisition of appropriate language skills are of prime importance during toddlerhood. The nurse uses the knowledge of normal toddler development as a roadmap for behavioral assessment of the 1- to 3-year-old child.

▶ PHYSICAL GROWTH

The toddler's height and weight continue to increase steadily, though the increase occurs at a slower velocity compared to infancy. Toddler gains in height and weight tend to occur in spurts, rather than in a linear fashion (Fig. 26.1). The average toddler weight gain is 3 to 5 pounds per year. Length/height increases by an average of 3 inches per year. Toddlers generally reach about half of their adult height by 2 years of age. Head circumference increases about 1 inch from when the child is between 1 and 2 years of age, then increases an average of a half-inch per year until age 5. The anterior fontanel should be closed by the time the child is 18 months old. Head size becomes more proportional to the rest of the body near the age of 3 years.

FIGURE 26.1 The typical toddler appearance is that of a rounded abdomen, a slight swayback, and a wide-based stance.

▶ ORGAN SYSTEM MATURATION

Though not as pronounced as the changes occurring during infancy, the toddler's organ systems continue to grow and mature in their functioning. Significant functional changes occur within the neurologic, gastrointestinal, and genitourinary systems. The respiratory and cardiovascular systems undergo changes as well.

Neurologic System

Brain growth continues through toddlerhood, and the brain reaches about 90% of its adult size by 2 years of age. Myelinization of the brain and spinal cord continues to progress and is complete around 24 months of age. Myelinization results in improved coordination and equilibrium as well as the ability to exercise sphincter control, which is important for bowel and bladder mastery. Integration of the primitive reflexes occurs in infancy, allowing for the emergence of the protective reflexes near the end of infancy or early in toddlerhood. The forward or downward parachute reflex is particularly helpful when the child starts to toddle. Rapid increase in language skills is evidence of continued progression of cognitive development.

Respiratory System

The respiratory structures continue to grow and mature throughout toddlerhood. The alveoli continue to increase in number, not reaching the adult number until about 7 years of age. The trachea and lower airways continue to grow but remain small compared with the adult. The tongue is relatively large in comparison to the size of the mouth. Tonsils and adenoids are large and the Eustachian tubes are relatively short and straight.

Cardiovascular System

The heart rate decreases and blood pressure increases in toddlerhood. Blood vessels are close to the skin surface and so are compressed easily when palpated.

Gastrointestinal System

The stomach continues to increase in size, allowing the toddler to consume three regular meals per day. Pepsin production matures by 2 years of age. The small intestine continues to grow in length, though it does not reach the maximum length of 2 to 3 meters until adulthood. Stool passage decreases in frequency to one or two per day, with as many as 25% of toddlers having a bowel movement every other day. The color of the stool may change (yellow, orange, brown, or green) depending upon the toddler's diet. Since the toddler's intestines remain somewhat immature, the toddler often passes whole pieces of difficult-to-digest food such as corn kernels. Bowel control is generally achieved by the end of the toddler period.

Genitourinary System

Bladder and kidney function reach adult levels by 16 to 24 months of age. The bladder capacity increases, allowing the toddler to retain urine for increased periods of times. Urine output should be about 1 mL/kg/hour. The urethra remains short in both the male and female toddler, making them more susceptible to urinary tract infections compared to adults.

Musculoskeletal System

During toddlerhood, the bones increase in length and the muscles mature and become stronger. The abdominal musculature is weak in early toddlerhood, resulting in a pot-bellied appearance. The toddler appears to have a swayback along with the potbelly. Around 3 years of age, the musculature strengthens and the abdomen is flatter in appearance.

▶ PSYCHOSOCIAL DEVELOPMENT

Erikson defines the toddler period as a time of autonomy versus shame and doubt. It is a time of exerting indepen-

dence. Since the toddler developed a sense of trust in infancy, he or she is ready to give up dependence and to assert his or her sense of control and autonomy (Erikson, 1963). The toddler is struggling for self-mastery, to learn to do for himself or herself what others have been doing for him or her. Toddlers often experience ambivalence about the move from dependence to autonomy, and this results in emotional lability. The toddler may quickly change from happy and pleasant to crying and screaming. Exertion of independence also results in the toddler's favorite response, "no." The toddler will often answer "no" even when he or she really means "yes."

This negativism—always saying "no"—is a normal part of healthy development and is occurring as a result of the toddler's attempt to assert his or her independence. Table 26.1 gives further information related to developing a sense of autonomy.

Cognitive Development

According to Jean Piaget (1969), toddlers move through the last two substages of the first stage of cognitive development, the sensorimotor stage, between 12 and 24 months of age. Young toddlers engage in tertiary circular reactions and progress to mental combinations. Rather than just repeating a behavior, the toddler is able to experiment with a behavior to see what happens. By 2 years of age, toddlers are capable of using symbols to allow for imitation. With increasing cognitive abilities, toddlers may now engage in delayed imitation. For example, they may imitate a household task that they observed a parent doing several days ago.

Piaget identified the second stage of cognitive development as the preoperational stage. It occurs in children between ages 2 and 7 years. During this stage toddlers begin to become more sophisticated with symbolic thought. The thinking of the older toddler is far more advanced than that of the infant or young toddler, who views the world as a series of objects. During the preoperational stage, objects begin to have characteristics that make them unique from one another. Objects are considered large or small, a particular color or shape, or a unique texture. This moves beyond the connection of sensory information and physical action. Words and images allow the toddler to begin this process of developing symbolic thought by providing a label for the objects' characteristics.

Toddlers also use symbols in dramatic play. First they imitate life with appropriate toy objects, and then they are able to substitute objects in their play. A bowl may be used to pretend to eat from, but then later it can be used upside down on the head as a hat (Fig. 26.2). Human feelings and characteristics may also be attributed to objects (**animism**). See Table 26.1 for further explanation of cognitive development in toddlerhood.

TABLE 26.1 DEVELOPMENTAL THEORIES

Theorist	Stage	Activities
Erikson	Autonomy vs. Shame & Doubt Age 1–3 years	Achieves autonomy and self-control Separates from parent/caregiver Withstands delayed gratification Negativism abounds Imitates adults and playmates Spontaneously shows affection Increasingly enthusiastic about playmates Cannot take turns in games until age 3 years

Piaget	Sensorimotor
	  Substage 5: Tertiary
	    Circular Reactions
	  Age: 12–18 months
	
	  Substage 6:
	    Mental Combinations
	  Age: 18–24 months
		Differentiating self from objects
		Increased object permanence (knows that objects that are out of sight still
		    exist [e.g., cookies in the cabinet])
		Uses ALL senses to explore environment
		Places items in and out of containers
		Imitates domestic chores (domestic mimicry)
		Imitation is more symbolic
		Starting to think before acting
		Understands requests and is capable of following simple directions
		Has a sense of ownership (my, mine)

	Preoperational Age: 2–7 years	Time, space, and causality understanding is increasing Uses mental trial and error rather than physical Makes mechanical toys work Plays make-believe with dolls, animals, and people Increased use of language for mental representation Understands concept of "two" Starting to make connections between an experience in the past and a new one that is currently occurring Sorts objects by shape and color Completes puzzles with four pieces Play becomes more complex
Freud	Anal Stage Age: 1–3 years	Focus is on achieving anal sphincter control. Satisfaction and/or frustration may occur as the toddler learns to withhold and expel stool.

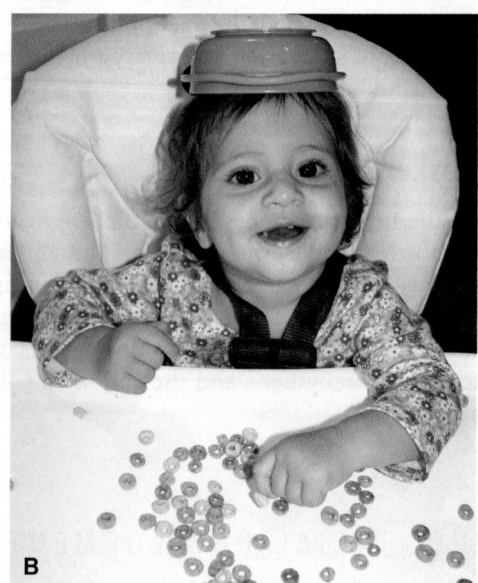

FIGURE 26.2 The toddler will (**A**) pretend with items in the way they are intended to be used as well as (**B**) find other creative uses for them.

▶ MOTOR SKILL DEVELOPMENT

Toddlers continue to gain new motor skills as well as refine others. Walking progresses to running, climbing, and jumping. Pushing or pulling a toy, throwing a ball, and pedaling a tricycle are accomplished in toddlerhood. Fine motor skills progress from holding and pinching to the ability to manage utensils, hold a crayon, string a bead, and use a computer. Development of eye–hand coordination is necessary for the refinement of fine motor skills. These increased abilities of mobility and manipulation help the curious toddler explore and learn more about his or her environment (Fig. 26.3). As the toddler masters a new task, he or she has confidence to conquer the next challenge. Thus, mastery in motor skill development contributes to the toddler's growing sense of self-esteem. The toddler who is eager to face challenges will likely develop more quickly than one who is reluctant. The senses of sight, hearing, and touch are useful in helping to coordinate gross and fine motor movement.

Gross Motor Skills

As gross motor skills are mastered and then used repeatedly, the large muscle groups in the toddler are strength-ened. The "toddler gait" is characteristic of new walkers. The toddler does not walk smoothly and maturely. Instead, the legs are planted widely apart, toes are pointed forward, and the toddler seems to sway from side to side while moving forward (Fig. 26.4). Often the toddler seems to speed along, pitching forward, appearing ready to topple over at any moment. The toddler may fall often, but will use outstretched arms to catch himself or herself (parachute reflex). After about 6 months of practice walking, the toddler's gait is smoother and the feet are closer together. By 3 years of age, the toddler walks in a heel-to-toe fashion similar to that of adults. Toddlers often use physical actions such as running, jumping, and hitting to express their emotions because they are only just learning to express their thoughts and feelings verbally. Table 26.2 lists motor skill expectations in relation to age.

Fine Motor Skills

Fine motor skills in the toddler period are improved and perfected. Holding utensils requires some control and agility, but even more is needed for buttoning and zipping. Adequate vision is necessary for the refinement of fine motor skills because eye–hand coordination is crucial for directing the fingers, hand, and wrist to accomplish small muscle tasks such as fitting a puzzle piece or stringing a bead. See Table 26.2 for age expectations for various motor skills.

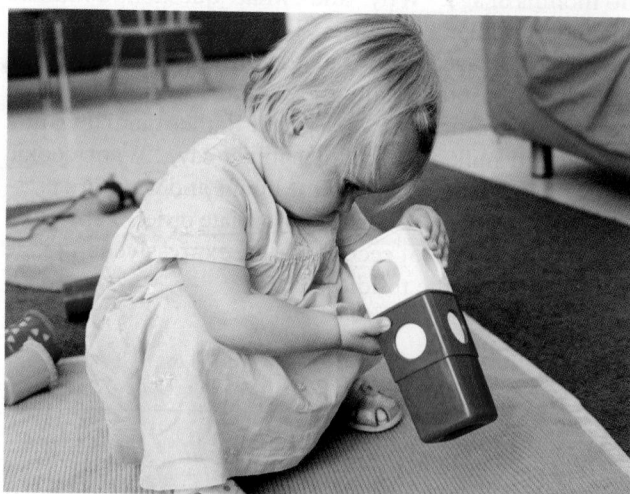

FIGURE 26.3 The toddler's curiosity about the world increases, as does her ability to explore it.

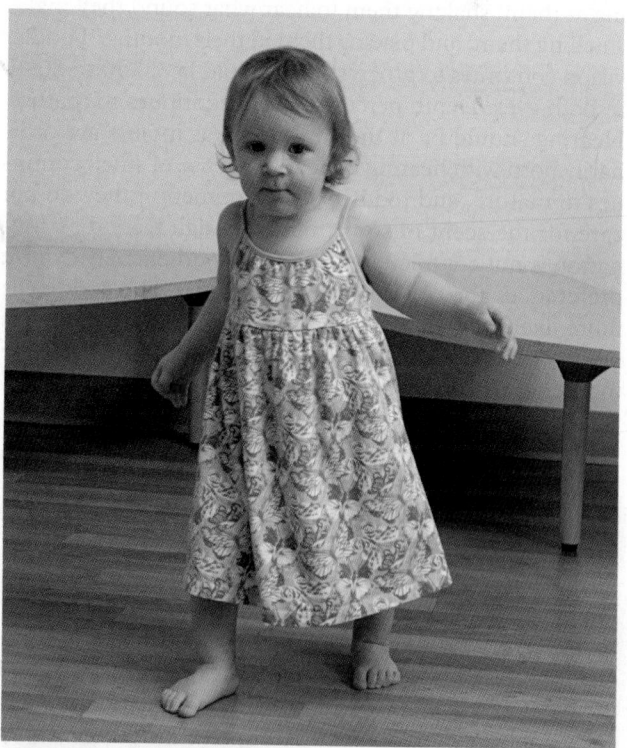

FIGURE 26.4 The young toddler (early walker) walks with a wide-based stance, feet pointing forward and arms akimbo.

TABLE 26.2   MOTOR SKILL DEVELOPMENT

Age	Expected Gross Motor Skill	Expected Fine Motor Skills
12–15 months	Walks independently	Feeds self finger foods Uses index finger to point
18 months	Climbs stairs with assistance Pulls toys while walking	Masters reaching, grasping, and releasing: stacks blocks, puts things in slots Turns book pages (singly with board book, multiple if paper) Removes shoes and socks Stacks four cubes
24 months	Runs Kicks ball Can stand on tiptoe Carries several toys, or a large toy while walking Climbs onto and down from furniture without assistance	Builds tower of six or seven cubes Right- or left-handed Imitates circular and vertical strokes Scribbles and paints Starting to turn knobs Puts round pegs into holes
36 months	Climbs well Pedals tricycle Runs easily Walks up and down stairs with alternate feet Bends over easily without falling	Undresses self Copies circle Builds tower of nine or ten cubes Holds a pencil in writing position Screws/unscrews lids, nuts, bolts Turns book pages one at a time

▶ SENSORY DEVELOPMENT

Toddlers use all of their senses to explore the world around them. Toddlers examine new items by feeling them, looking at them, shaking them to hear what sound they make, smelling them, and placing them in their mouths. Toddler vision continues to progress and should be 20/50 to 20/40 in both eyes. Depth perception also continues to mature. Hearing should be at the adult level, as infants are ordinarily born with hearing intact. The sense of smell continues to mature, and toddlers may comment if they do not care for the scent of something. Though taste discrimination is not completely developed, toddlers may exhibit preferences for certain flavors of foods. The toddler is more likely to try a new food if its appearance or smell is familiar. Lack of complete taste discrimination places the toddler at risk of accidental ingestion.

▶ COMMUNICATION AND LANGUAGE DEVELOPMENT

Language development occurs rapidly during the toddler years. The acquisition of language is a dynamic and complex process. The child's age and social interactions and the types of language to which he has been exposed influence language development. **Receptive language** development (the ability to understand what is being said or asked) is typically far more advanced than **expressive language** development (the ability to communicate one's desires and feelings). In other words, the toddler understands language and is able to follow commands far sooner than he or she can actually use the words themselves. Language is a very important part of the toddler's ability to organize his or her world and actually make sense of it. Thoughtfully planned use of language can provide behavior guidance and contribute to the avoidance of power struggles. In regard to expressive language development, the young toddler begins to use short sentences and will progress to a vocabulary of 50 words by 2 years of age. **Echolalia** (repetition of words and phrases without understanding) normally occurs in toddlers less than 30 months of age. "Why" and "what" questions dominate the older toddler's language. Telegraphic speech is common in the 3-year-old. **Telegraphic speech** refers to speech that contains only the essential words to get the point across, much like a telegram. Rather than "I want a cookie and milk," the toddler might say, "Want cookie milk." In telegraphic speech the nouns and verbs are present and are verbalized in the appropriate order. Table 26.3 gives an overview of receptive and expressive language development in the toddler.

▶ *Take* NOTE!

Stuttering usually has its onset at between 2 and 4 years of age. It occurs more often in boys than in girls. About 75% of all cases of stuttering resolve within 1 to 2 years after they start.

TABLE 26.3 LANGUAGE DEVELOPMENT IN TODDLERS

Age	Receptive Language	Expressive Language
12 months	Understands common words independent of context Follows a one-step command accompanied by gesture	Uses a finger to point to things Imitates or uses gestures such as waving goodbye Communicates desires with word and gesture combinations Vocal imitation First word
15 months	Looks at adult when communicating Follows a one-step command without gesture Understands 100–150 words	Repeats words that he or she hears Babbles in what sound like sentences
18 months	Understands the word "no" Comprehends 200 words Sometimes answers the question, "What's this?"	Uses at least 5–20 words Uses names of familiar object
24 months	Points to named body parts Points to pictures in books Enjoys listening to simple stories Names a variety of objects in the environment Beginning to use "my" or "mine"	Vocabulary of 40–50 words Sentences of two or three words (me up, want cookie) Asks questions (what that?) Uses simple phrases Uses descriptive words (hungry, hot) Two thirds of what child says should be understandable Repeats overheard words
30 months	Follows a series of two independent commands	Vocabulary of 150–300 words
36 months	Understands most sentences Understands physical relationships (on, in, under) Participates in short conversations May follow a three-part command	Speech usually understood by those who know the child, about half understood by those outside family Asks "why?" Three- to four-word sentences Talks about something that happened in the past Vocabulary of 1,000 words Can say name, age, and gender Uses pronouns and plurals

Early identification and referral of children with potential speech delays is critical. If a delay is identified, early intervention may increase the child's potential to acquire age-appropriate receptive and expressive language skills.

▶ **Take** NOTE!

Children with preexisting conditions such as genetic syndromes that are known to have an effect on language development should be referred to a speech–language pathologist as soon as the condition is recognized rather than waiting until the child exhibits a delay.

Of special concern in the toddler years is the development of speech and language in potentially bilingual children. At the age of 1 to 2 years, the potentially bilingual child may blend two languages—that is, parts of the word in both languages are blended into one word. At age 2 to 3 years, the potentially bilingual toddler may mix languages within a sentence. Thus, the assessment of adequate language development is more complicated in bilingual children. Parents of potentially bilingual children may find support and resources at the website www.nethelp.no/cindy/biling-fam.html.

▶ **Take** NOTE!

Bilingual children often mix languages, and thus speech delay may be more difficult to assess in this population. The bilingual child should have command of 20 words (between both languages) by 20 months of age and should be making word combinations. If this is not the case, further investigation may be warranted.

▶ EMOTIONAL AND SOCIAL DEVELOPMENT

Emotional development in the toddler years is focused on **separation** and **individuation**. Seeing oneself as separate from the parent or primary caregiver is accompanied by forming a sense of self and learning to exert control over one's environment. As this need to feel in control of his or her world emerges, the toddler displays **egocentrism** (focus on self). This need for control results in emotional lability: very happy and pleasant one moment, then over-reacting to limit setting with a temper tantrum in the next moment. As toddlers identify the boundaries between themselves and the parent or primary caregiver, they learn to negotiate a balance between attachment and independence. Toddlers initially rely on the parents' communication and signals in order to initiate appropriate behavior or inhibit undesirable behavior. They have a difficult time choosing between sets of behaviors as they occur in different situations. Power struggles often occur in this age group, and it is important for parents and caregivers to thoughtfully and intentionally develop the rituals and routines that will provide stability and security for the toddler. Many toddlers rely upon a security item (blanket, doll, or bear) to comfort themselves in stressful situations (Fig. 26.5). This ability to self-soothe is a function of autonomy and is viewed as a sign of a nurturing environment, rather than, as one might suspect, one of neglect.

Children also begin to learn about gender differences in the toddler years. They observe the differences between male and female body parts if they are exposed to them. Toddlers may question parents about these differences and may begin to explore their own genitals. Toddlers also begin to understand and mimic social gender differences. They make observations about gender-specific behavior dependent upon what they are exposed to.

Aggressive behaviors are typically displayed during the toddler years. Toddlers may hit, bite, or push other children and grab toys. Adults can assist the toddler in building empathy by pointing out when someone is hurt and explaining what happened. Toddlers should not be blamed for their impulsive behavior; rather, they should be guided toward socially acceptable actions in order to foster development of appropriate social judgment. It is particularly important for the parent or caregiver to serve as a role model for appropriate behavior, rather than losing his or her own temper, in order for the toddler to be able to learn how to acceptably handle frustrations. Offering limited choices is one way of allowing toddlers some control over their environment and helping them to establish a sense of mastery. Since toddlers naturally have a short attention span, they tend to dawdle. As the toddlers become more self-aware, they start to develop emotions of self-consciousness such as embarrassment and shame.

Though toddlers are becoming more self-aware, they still do not have clear body boundaries. They do not clearly understand the body's functions, though they are beginning to make appropriate connections. Feces may be viewed as a part of the child, and the toddler may become upset at seeing it disappear in the toilet. The toddler will protect his or her body by resisting intrusive procedures such as temperature or blood pressure measurement.

Separation Anxiety

As toddlers become increasingly skilled at mobility, they realize that if they have the capability of leaving, then so does the parent. As self-awareness develops and conflicts over closeness versus exploration occur, **separation anxiety** may reemerge in the 18- to 24-month period. Power struggles may escalate and distress at separating from the parent may increase. Again, a predictable routine with appropriate limit setting may help toddlers to feel safer and more secure during this period. From the age of 24 to 36 months, separation anxiety again eases. The older toddler begins to have a concept of object constancy: he or she has an internal representation of the parent or caregiver and is better able to tolerate separation, knowing that a reunion will occur.

Temperament

Temperament is the biological basis for personality. It is our emotional and motivational core, around which the personality develops over time. Temperament affects how the toddler interacts with the environment. The easygoing toddler may adapt more easily and not mind changes in routine as much as other toddlers. The easygoing toddler usually sleeps and eats well and has more predictable and regular behaviors. However, the toddler may still express

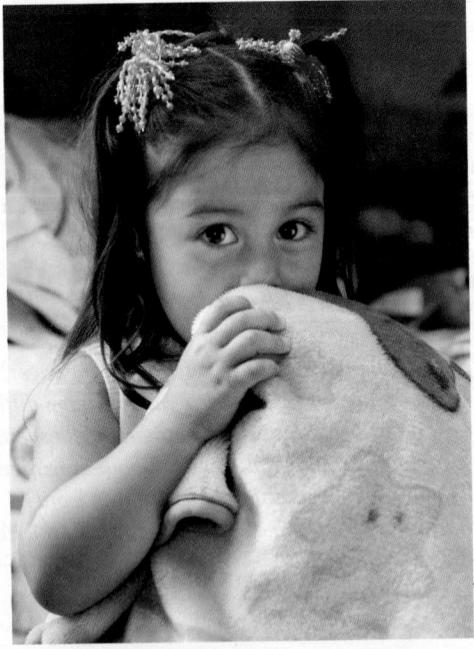

FIGURE 26.5 The toddler may be able to self-soothe and produce a sense of comfort during this stage of establishing autonomy by relying upon a security item such as a doll, bear, or blanket.

frustration by having a temper tantrum. The "difficult" toddler is more likely to have intense reactions, negative or positive, with temper tantrums being more likely, more frequent, and more intense than in other toddlers. The structure and routine that toddlers need to feel secure are essential for the difficult toddler; otherwise, the child feels insecure and as a result is more likely to behave inappropriately. The difficult toddler is also the most active of the three temperament types. The slow-to-warm-up toddler is more of a loner and may be very shy. He or she may experience more difficulty with separation anxiety. The behavior of the slow-to-warm-up toddler is more passive; the toddler may be very watchful and withdrawn and may take longer to mature. Changes in routine usually do not result in as much upset, since the toddler's natural reaction is one of passivity.

Based on the toddler's temperament, make suggestions to the parents for interacting with the toddler in various situations. For example, to avoid temper tantrums in the difficult toddler, suggest that the parent should be especially diligent about maintaining structure and routine as well as avoiding tantrum triggers such as fatigue and hunger. Explain to parents that they may need to exercise additional patience with new activities to which the slow-to-warm-up toddler may need extra time becoming accustomed.

Fears

Common fears of toddlers include loss of parents (which contributes to separation anxiety) and fear of strangers. Some toddlers may be very slow to warm up to people they do not know. The nurse caring for a toddler in the outpatient or hospital setting should take the time to establish a relationship with the toddler in order to allay the toddler's fears. Toddlers may be afraid of loud noises and large or unfamiliar animals. Going to sleep may be a scary time for toddlers as they may be afraid of the dark. A nightlight in the toddler's room may be very helpful.

▶ MORAL AND SPIRITUAL DEVELOPMENT

During the toddler years, children may feel comfort from the routine of praying, but they do not understand religious beliefs because of their limited cognitive abilities. Reading simple Bible stories can lay a foundation for later religious teachings. Kohlberg's (1984) description of moral development places the older toddler in the preconventional level. The toddler is only just beginning to learn right from wrong and does not understand the larger concept of morality. The toddler will base his or her actions on the avoidance of punishment and the attainment of pleasure. Older toddlers begin to feel empathy for others.

▶ CULTURAL INFLUENCES ON GROWTH AND DEVELOPMENT

Homelessness or poverty may directly influence the toddler's ability to grow adequately, as resources for the purchase and preparation of appropriate food may be lacking. Appropriate toys (safe ones) may also not be available in those situations. Food customs continue to have an impact on the child's diet and ability to ingest appropriate nutrients. Individual families' value systems have an impact on the toddler's development as well. Some parents desire to keep their child a "baby" for a longer period, thus delaying weaning or continuing to feed the child baby food or puréed food for a longer period. Other families may highly value independence and encourage the toddler to walk everywhere on his or her own rather than carrying the child.

Culture may also affect emotional development. Some families start at a very young age to discourage crying in boys, encouraging them to "act like a big boy" or "be a man." Ridicule for crying at this age may hurt the toddler's self-concept. Educating families about normal growth and development while continuing to value and support cultural practices is important.

Remember Jose Gonzales, whom you met at the beginning of the chapter? What developmental milestones would you expect him to have reached at his age?

The Nurse's Role in Toddler Growth and Development

WATCH & LEARN

The toddler's growth and development affects his or her everyday life as well as the family's. Though some toddlers may grow more quickly or reach developmental milestones sooner than others, growth and development remains orderly and sequential. Health care visits throughout toddlerhood continue to focus on growth and development. The nurse must have a good understanding of the changes that occur during the toddler years in order to provide appropriate anticipatory guidance and support to the family.

When the toddler is hospitalized, growth and development may be altered. The toddler's primary task is establishing autonomy, and the toddler's focus is mobility and language development. Hospitalization removes most opportunities for the toddler to learn through exploration of the environment. Isolation for contagious illness further constrains the toddler's ability to find some control over the environment. The nurse caring for the hospitalized toddler must use knowledge of normal growth and development to be successful in interactions with the toddler, promote continued development, and recognize delays (see Chapter 32) (Fig. 26.6).

▶ NURSING PROCESS OVERVIEW

Upon completion of assessment of the toddler's current growth and development status, problems or issues related to growth and development may be identified. The nurse may then identify one or more nursing diagnoses, including but not limited to:

- Delayed growth and development
- Imbalanced nutrition, less than body requirements
- Interrupted family processes
- Readiness for enhanced parenting
- Risk for caregiver role strain
- Risk for delayed development
- Risk for disproportionate growth
- Risk for injury

Nursing care planning for the toddler with growth and development issues should be individualized based on the toddler's and family's needs. The nursing care plan may be used as a guide in planning nursing care for the toddler with a growth or developmental concern. The nurse may choose the appropriate nursing diagnoses from the following plan and individualize them as needed. The nursing care plan is intended to serve as a guide only and is not intended to be an inclusive growth and development plan.

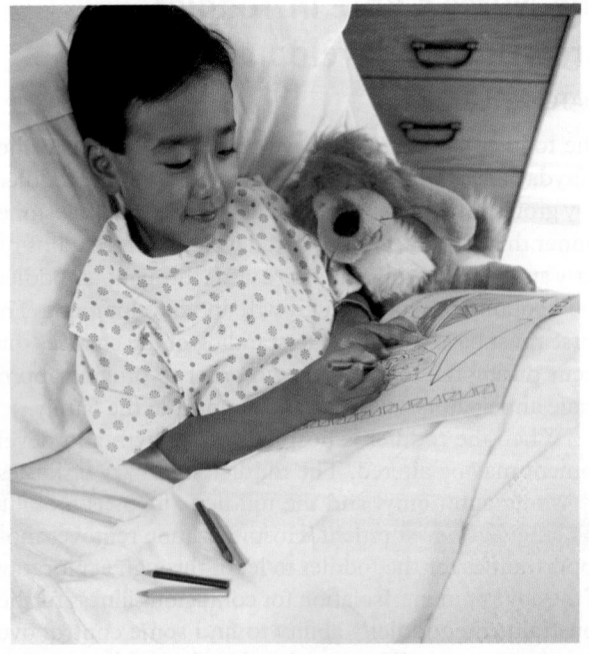

FIGURE 26.6 The hospitalized toddler continues to enjoy developmental tasks appropriate for his or her age, such as coloring.

▶ PROMOTING HEALTHY GROWTH AND DEVELOPMENT

Parents who give their toddler love and respect regardless of the child's gender, behavior, or capabilities are helping to lay the foundation for self-esteem. Self-esteem is also built through familiarity with the daily routine. Routine and ritual help toddlers develop a conscience. Making expectations known through everyday routines helps to avoid confrontations. If the toddler knows the routine, he or she knows what to expect and how he or she is expected to act. When routine and limits are absent, the toddler develops feelings of uncertainty and anxiety. Limit setting (and remaining consistent with those limits) helps toddlers master their behavior, develop self-esteem, and become successful participants in the family. Children then are able to learn about cooperation throughout the predictable flow of daily life. Nurses need to be aware of normal developmental expectations in order to determine whether the toddler is progressing appropriately. Table 26.4 lists potential signs of developmental delay. Any toddler with one or more of these concerns should be referred for further developmental evaluation.

Promoting Growth and Development Through Play

Play is the major socializing medium for toddlers. Parents should limit television viewing and encourage creative and physical play instead. Toddlers typically play alongside another child (**parallel play**) rather than cooperatively (Fig. 26.7). The short attention span of the toddler will make him or her often change toys and types of play. It is important to provide a variety of safe toys to allow the toddler many different opportunities for exploring the environment. Toddlers do not need expensive toys; in fact, regular household items sometimes make the most enjoyable toys. Toddlers are egocentric, a normal part of their development. This makes it difficult for them to share. As they are developing a sense of self (who they are as a person), they may see their toys as an extension of themselves. Learning to share occurs in later toddlerhood. Toddlers also like dramatic play and play that recreates familiar activities in the home. Toddlers like to listen to music of all kinds and will often dance to whatever they hear on the radio. Toddlers enjoy drums, xylophones, cymbals, and toy pianos. Musical instruments made at home are also enjoyed. A few pebbles or coins inside an empty water bottle with the top tightly secured is a great music maker; an empty butter tub with a lid and a pair of wooden spoons makes a nice drum.

Adequate physical activity is necessary for the development and refinement of movement skills. Toddlers need

(text continues on page 811)

Nursing Care Plan 26.1

GROWTH AND DEVELOPMENT ISSUES IN THE TODDLER

NURSING DIAGNOSIS: Risk for injury related to curiosity, increased mobility, and developmental immaturity

Outcome Identification and Evaluation
Toddler safety will be maintained: *Toddler will remain free from injury.*

Interventions: Preventing Injury
- Teach and encourage appropriate use of forward facing car seat *to decrease risk of toddler injury related to motor vehicles.*
- Teach toddlers to stay away from the street and provide constant supervision *to prevent pedestrian injury.*
- Require bicycle helmet use while riding any wheeled toy *to prevent head injury and form habit of helmet use.*
- Childproof the home *to provide a developmentally safe environment for the curious and increasingly mobile toddler.*
- Post poison control center phone number *in case of accidental ingestion.*
- Never leave a toddler unattended in a tub or pool or near any body of water *to prevent drowning.*
- Teach parents first-aid measures and child CPR *to minimize consequences of injury should it occur.*
- Provide close observation and keep side rails up on crib/bed in hospital *because toddlers are at particularly high risk for falling or becoming entangled in tubing as they attempt mobility.*

NURSING DIAGNOSIS: Imbalanced nutrition, less than body requirements, related to inappropriate nutritional intake to sustain growth needs (excess juice or milk intake, inadequate food variety intake) as evidenced by failure to attain adequate increases in height and weight over time

Outcome Identification and Evaluation
Toddler will consume adequate nutrients while using an appropriate feeding pattern: *Toddler will demonstrate weight gain and increases in height.*

Interventions: Promoting Appropriate Nutrition
- Assess current feeding schedule and usual intake, as well as methods used to feed, *to determine areas of adequacy versus inadequacy.*
- Determine toddler's ability to drink from cup, finger feed, swallow, and consume textures *to determine if additional exposure is needed or if further interventions such as speech or occupational therapy are required.*
- Weigh toddler daily on same scale if hospitalized, weekly on same scale if at home, and plot growth patterns weekly or monthly as appropriate on standardized growth charts *to determine if growth is improving.*
- Wean from bottle by 15 months of age *to discourage excess milk or juice intake in toddler who can carry bottle around.*
- Limit juice to 4 to 6 ounces per day and milk to 16 to 24 ounces per day *to discourage sense of fullness achieved with excess milk or juice intake, thereby increasing appetite for solid foods.*
- Provide three nutrient-dense meals and at least two healthy snacks per day *to encourage adequate nutrient consumption.*
- Feed toddler on a similar schedule daily, without distractions and with the family: *toddlers respond well to routine and structure and may eat better in the social context of meals, and they become distracted easily (TV should be off).*

NURSING DIAGNOSIS: Delayed growth and development related to motor, cognitive, language, or psychosocial concerns as evidenced by delay in meeting expected milestones

Outcome Identification and Evaluation
Development will be enhanced: *Toddler will make continued progress toward realization of expected developmental milestones.*

Interventions: Enhancing Growth and Development
- Screen for developmental capabilities *to determine toddler's current level of functioning.*
- Offer age-appropriate toys, play, and activities (including gross motor) *to encourage further development.*
- Perform interventions as prescribed by physical, occupational, or speech therapist: *participation in those activities helps to promote function and accomplish acquisition of developmental skills.*
- Provide support to families of toddlers with developmental delay *(progress in achieving developmental milestones can be slow and ongoing motivation is needed).*
- Reinforce positive attributes in the toddler *to maintain motivation.*
- Model age-appropriate communication skills *to illustrate suitable means for parenting the toddler.*

(continued)

Nursing Care Plan 26.1 (continued)

NURSING DIAGNOSIS: Risk for disproportionate growth related to excess milk or juice intake, late bottle weaning, and consumption of inappropriate foods or in excess amounts

Outcome Identification and Evaluation
Toddler will grow appropriately and not become overweight or obese: *Toddler will achieve weight and height within the 5th to 85th percentiles on standardized growth charts.*

Interventions: Promoting Proportionate Growth
- Wean from bottle and discourage use of no-spill sippy cups by 15 months of age *(will keep mobile toddler from carrying around and continually drinking from cup or bottle).*
- Provide juice (4–6 ounces per day) and milk (16–24 ounces per day) from a cup at meal and snack time *to encourage appropriate cup drinking and limit intake of nutrient-poor, high-calorie fluids.*
- Provide only nutrient-rich foods without high sugar content for meals and snacks; *even if the toddler won't eat, it is inappropriate to provide high-calorie junk food just so the toddler eats something.*
- Ensure adequate physical activity *to stimulate development of motor skills and provide appropriate caloric expenditure. This also sets the stage for forming life-long habit of appropriate physical activity.*

NURSING DIAGNOSIS: Interrupted family processes related to issues with toddler development, hospitalization, or situational crisis as evidenced by decreased parental visitation in hospital, parental verbalization of difficulty with current situation, possible crisis related to health of family member other than the toddler

Outcome Identification and Evaluation
Family will demonstrate adequate functioning: *Family will display coping and psychosocial adjustment.*

Interventions: Enhancing Family Functioning
- Assess the family's level of stress and ability to cope *to determine family's ability to cope with multiple stressors.*
- Engage in family-centered care *to provide a holistic approach to care of the toddler and family.*
- Encourage the family to verbalize feelings *(verbalization is one method of decreasing anxiety levels),* and acknowledge feelings and emotions.
- Encourage family visitation and provide for sleeping arrangements for a parent or caregiver to stay in the hospital with the toddler *(contributes to family's sense of control of situation).*
- Involve family members in toddler's care, *giving them a feeling of control and connectedness.*

NURSING DIAGNOSIS: Readiness for enhanced parenting related to parental desire for increased skills and success with toddler as evidenced by current healthy relationships and verbalization of desire for improved skills

Outcome Identification and Evaluation
Parent will provide safe and nurturing environment for the toddler.

Interventions: Increasing Parenting Skill Set
- Use family-centered care *to provide holistic approach.*
- Educate parent about normal toddler development *to provide basis for understanding the parenting skills needed in this time period.*
- Acknowledge and encourage parent's verbalization of feelings related to chronic illness of child or difficulty with normal toddler behavior *to validate the normalcy of the parent's feelings.*
- Encourage positive parenting with respect to toddlers and their normal development *(helps parents develop approaches to toddlers that can be used in place of anger and frustration).*
- Acknowledge and admire positive parenting skills already present *to contribute to parents' confidence in their abilities to parent.*
- Role model appropriate parenting behaviors related to communicating with and disciplining the toddler *(role modeling actually shows rather than just telling the parent what to do).*

TABLE 26.4 SIGNS OF DEVELOPMENTAL DELAY

Age or Time Frame	Concern
After independent walking for several months	• Persistent tiptoe walking • Failure to develop a mature walking pattern
By 18 months	• Not walking • Not speaking 15 words • Does not understand function of common household items
By 2 years	• Does not use two-word sentences • Does not imitate actions • Does not follow basic instructions • Cannot push a toy with wheels
By 3 years	• Difficulty with stairs • Frequent falling • Cannot build tower of more than four blocks • Difficulty manipulating small objects • Extreme difficulty in separation from parent or caregiver • Cannot copy a circle • Does not engage in make-believe play • Cannot communicate in short phrases • Does not understand simple instructions • Little interest in other children • Unclear speech, persistent drooling

at least 30 minutes of structured physical activity and anywhere from 1 to several hours of unstructured physical activity per day. Indoor and outdoor play areas should encourage play activities that use the large muscle groups. The activity must occur within a safe environment. Outdoor play structures should be positioned over surfaces that are soft enough to absorb a fall, such as sand, wood chips, or sawdust (Fig. 26.8). Box 26.1 lists recommended age-appropriate toys.

Promoting Early Learning

The parent–child relationship and the interactions between parent and child form the context for the toddler's early learning.

Promoting Language Development

Talking and singing to the toddler during routine activities such as feeding and dressing provides an environment

FIGURE 26.7 Parallel play. The toddler usually plays alongside another child rather than cooperatively.

FIGURE 26.8 Toddlers love outdoor physical play, such as climbing on playground equipment. An adult should always supervise toddlers when they are playing outdoors.

BOX 26.1   Appropriate Toys for Toddlers

- Familiar household items such as plastic bowls and cups of various sizes, large plastic serving utensils, pots and pans, wooden spoons, cardboard boxes and tubes (from paper towel rolls), old magazines, baskets, purses, hats
- Child-size household item toys (kitchen, broom, vacuum cleaner, lawnmower, telephone, and so on)
- Blocks, cars and trucks, plastic animals, trains, plastic figures (family, community helpers), simple dolls, stuffed animals, balls, doll beds and carriages
- Manipulative toys with knobs, wind-ups and buttons that make things happen; putting large pegs or shapes into matching holes, stringing large beads on shoelaces, blocks and containers that stack, jigsaw puzzles with large pieces, toys that can be taken apart and put back together again
- Gross motor toys: play gym, push and pull toys, wagons, tricycle or other ride-on toys, tunnels
- Tape or CD players for music, various musical instruments
- Chalk, large crayons, finger paint, Play-Doh, washable markers
- Bucket, plastic shovel and other containers for sand and water play
- Squeaking, floating, squirting toys for the bath

that encourages conversation. Frequent, repetitive naming helps the toddler learn appropriate words for objects. The parent or caregiver should be attentive to what the toddler is saying as well as to his or her moods. Using clarification validates the toddler's emotions and ideas. Parents should listen to and answer the toddler's questions. They should sit down quietly with the toddler and gently repeat what the toddler is saying. Encouragement and elaboration convey confidence and interest to the toddler. The toddler needs time to complete his or her thoughts without being interrupted or rushed because he or she is just starting to be able to make the connections necessary to transfer thoughts and feelings into language.

Parents should not overreact to the child's use of the word "no." They can give the toddler opportunities to use the word "no" appropriately by asking silly questions such as, "Can a cat drive a car?" or "Is a banana purple?" When promoting language development, the parent or primary caregiver should teach the toddler appropriate words for body parts and objects and should help the toddler choose appropriate words to label feelings and emotions. Toddlers' receptive language and interpretation of body language and subtle signs far surpass their expressive language, especially at a younger age.

Parents should avoid discussing scary or serious topics in the presence of the toddler, since the toddler is very adept at reading emotions.

If the parents speak a foreign language in addition to English, both languages should be used in the home.

Encouraging Reading

Reading to the toddler every day is one of the best ways to promote language and cognitive development (Fig. 26.9). Toddlers particularly enjoy homemade or purchased books about feelings, family, friends, everyday life, animals and nature, and fun and fantasy. Board books have thick pages that are easier for young toddlers to turn; older toddlers can turn paper pages one at a time. The toddler may also enjoy "reading" the story to the parent. Reach Out and Read, a program designed to promote early literacy, offers tips for reading with young children (see Teaching Guidelines 26.1).

Choosing a Preschool

The older toddler may benefit from the structure and socialization provided by attending preschool. Attending preschool will help the toddler become more mature and independent and give the toddler a different source for a sense of accomplishment. At this age, toddlers need supervised play with some direction that fosters their cognitive development. A strict curriculum is not necessary in this age group. When choosing a preschool, the parent or caregiver should look for an environment that has the following qualities:

- Goals and an overall philosophy with which the parents agree (promotion of independence and self-confidence through structured and free play)
- Teachers and assistants trained in early childhood development as well as child cardiopulmonary resuscitation (CPR)
- Small class sizes and an adult-to-child ratio with which the parent feels comfortable
- Disciplinary procedures consistent with the parents' values
- Parents can visit at any time

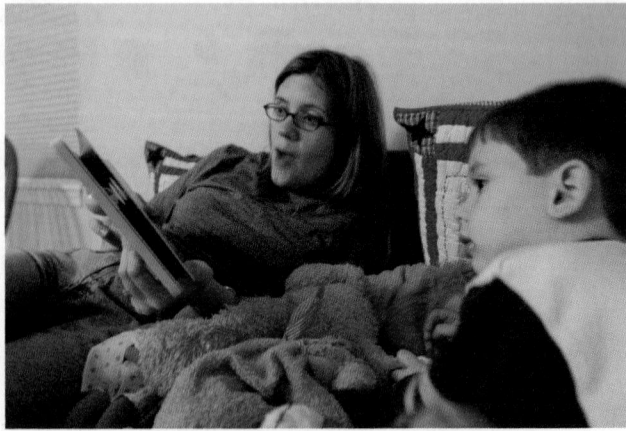

FIGURE 26.9 Reading to a toddler daily is one of the best ways to promote language development and school readiness.

TEACHING GUIDELINES 26.1

Tips for Reading with Young Children

- Make reading part of every day: Read at bedtime or on the bus.
- Have fun: Children who love books learn to read. Books can be part of special time with your child.
- A few minutes is OK: Young children can sit for only a few minutes for a story, but as they grow they will sit longer.
- Talk about the pictures: You do not have to read the book to tell a story.
- Let your child turn the pages: Babies need board books and help to turn pages, but your 3-year-old can do it alone.
- Show your child the cover page: Explain what the story is about.
- Show your child the words: Run your finger along the words as you read them.
- Make the story come alive: Create voices for the story characters and use your body to tell the story.
- Ask questions about the story: What do you think will happen next? What is this?
- Let your child ask questions about the story: Use the story as an opportunity to engage in conversation and to talk about familiar activities and objects.
- Let your child tell the story: Children as young as 3 years old can memorize a story, and many children love an opportunity to express their creativity. (Reach Out and Read, 2006)

- School is childproofed inside and out
- Appropriate hygiene procedures, including prohibiting sick children from attending

Teach the parents how to ease the toddler's transition to attending preschool. Encourage parents to talk about going to preschool and visit the school a couple of times. On the first day, parents should calmly and in a matter-of-fact tone tell the toddler that they will return to pick him or her up. If the toddler expresses separation anxiety, the parent should remain calm and follow through with the plan for school attendance. After a few days of attendance, the toddler will be accustomed to the new routine and crying when parting from the parent should be minimal.

Promoting Safety

Safety is of prime concern throughout the toddler period. Curiosity, mobility, and lack of impulse control all contribute to the incidence of unintentional injury in toddlerhood. Even the most watchful and caring parents have toddlers who run into the street, otherwise disappear from parents, and fall down the stairs. Toddlers require direct

observation and cannot be trusted to be left alone. A childproof environment provides a safe place for the toddler to explore and learn. Motor vehicle accidents, drowning, choking, burns, falls, and poisoning are the most common injuries suffered by toddlers. Safety and injury prevention focuses on these categories.

Safety in the Car

The safest place for the toddler to ride is in the back seat of the car. Parents should use the appropriate size and style of car seat for the child's weight and age as required by the state. At a minimum, all children over 20 pounds and up to 40 pounds should be in a forward-facing car seat with harness straps and a clip. A toddler riding in a pickup truck should never ride in the cargo area or truck bed. A full rear seat in the truck is the preferred placement for the toddler car seat. If an appropriate rear seat is unavailable, the air bag should be disarmed and the forward-facing car seat should be secured appropriately in the truck seat. The top tether is additionally required for all forward-facing car seats (Fig. 26.10). Drivers should avoid using the cell phone or attempting to intervene with the children while they are driving. Excellent resources about car seat safety appropriate for both parents and professionals can be found at www.bucklebear.com, www.nhtsa.dot.gov, www.usa.safekids.org, and www.seatcheck.org.

Safety in the Home

Key areas of concern for keeping toddlers safe in the home include avoiding exposure to tobacco smoke, preventing injury, and preventing poisoning.

Avoiding Exposure to Tobacco Smoke

Environmental exposure to tobacco smoke has been associated with increased risk of respiratory disease and infection, decreased lung function, and increased incidence of middle ear effusion and recurrent otitis media. It may also hinder neurodevelopment and may be associated with behavior problems (World Health Organization, 2007). Parents should avoid cigarette smoking entirely to best protect their children. Even smoking outside of the home is suboptimal because smoke lingers on parents' clothing and children who are often carried (such as younger toddlers) face more exposure. Counsel parents to stop smoking (optimal), but if they continue smoking never to smoke inside the home or car with children present.

Preventing Injury

The toddler is able to open drawers and doors, unlock deadbolts, and climb anywhere he or she wants to go. Toddlers have a limited concept of body boundaries and essentially no fear of danger. Toddlers may fall from any height to which they can climb (e.g., play structures, tables, counters). They may also fall from wheeled toys such as tricycles. As toddlers gain additional height and hand dexterity they are able to reach potentially dangerous items

FIGURE 26.10 The top tether further secures the forward-facing car seat. This tether has been a requirement on all forward-facing car seats manufactured since 1999, and most vehicles manufactured after 1999 have a specific attachment for the top tether. (U.S. Department of Transportation, National Highway Traffic Safety Administration.)

on the counter or stove, leading to an accidental ingestion, burn, or cut.

To prevent injury in the home, stress the following to parents:

- Never leave a toddler unsupervised out of doors.
- Lock doors to dangerous rooms.
- Install safety gates at the top and bottom of staircases.
- Ensure that window locks are operable; if windows are left opened, then secure all window screens.
- Keep pot handles on the stove turned inward, out of an inquisitive toddler's reach.
- Teach the toddler to avoid the oven, stove, and iron.
- Keep electrical equipment, cords, and matches out of reach.
- Remove firearms from the home, or keep them in a locked cabinet out of the toddler's reach.
- Always require the child to wear a helmet approved by the Consumer Products Safety Commission (CSPC) when riding a wheeled toy. This starts the habit of helmet wearing early, so it can be more easily carried over to the bicycle-riding years of the future.
- Begin teaching the toddler about watching for cars when crossing the street, but always carry or hold the hand of the toddler when crossing the street.
- Teach the toddler to avoid unknown animals.

▶ *Take* NOTE!

"Bernie Burn," by Sarah Cruz, RN, is a book designed to educate parents and their toddlers about burn prevention while entertaining them. It is endorsed by the American Journal of Nursing and is available from www.littleboots publishing.com.

Preventing Poisoning

As toddlers become more mobile, they are increasingly able to explore their environment and more easily and efficiently gain access to materials that may be unsafe for them to handle. Their natural curiosity leads them into situations that may place them in danger. Poor taste discrimination in this age group allows for ingestion of chemicals or other materials that older children would find too unpleasant to swallow. Box 26.2 lists most potentially dangerous ingested poisons. Discuss poison prevention in the home at each well-child visit (see Healthy People 2010). The American Academy of Pediatrics recommends that potentially poisonous substances (e.g., medications, cleaners, hair care products, car care products) be stored out of the toddler's teach, out of the toddler's sight, and in a childproof, locked cabinet.

Encourage all families to:

- Store all substances in original containers only.
- Never store any liquid other than soda in a soda pop bottle.
- Do not allow toddlers access to baby powder, lotion, cream, or other toddler hygiene products.

BOX 26.2 **Most Dangerous Potential Poisons**

- Medicines (especially iron)
- Cleaning products
- Antifreeze, windshield washer solution
- Alcohol
- Pesticides
- Gasoline, kerosene, lamp oil, furniture polish
- Wild mushrooms

American Association of Poison Control Centers, 2004

HEALTHY PEOPLE 2010

Objective	Significance
Reduce nonfatal poisonings	• Use every encounter with the toddler's family as an opportunity to educate about preventing poisonings.

- Ensure all medications have child-safety caps.
- Do not leave within the toddler's reach medications such as lozenges or samples that are not packaged in safety bottles.
- Be very careful with medications that are provided in transdermal patch form.
- Do not refer to medicines as candy, as the toddler may mistake pills for candy and ingest them.
- Do not expose toddlers to hazardous vapors such as paints, cleaners, tobacco smoke, and especially street drugs such as crack and marijuana.
- Keep "button" batteries secured and away from a toddler's reach.
- Keep house plants off the floor, remove them from the home, or hang them or place them on a high shelf.

> ▶ *Take* NOTE!
>
> *The American Academy of Pediatrics (AAP, 2007b) recommends that all families post the Poison Control Center number in a readily accessible place in the home: (800) 222-1222. The AAP discourages the use of syrup of ipecac in the home to induce vomiting after an accidental ingestion.*

Safety in the Water

Drowning is the leading cause of unintentional injury and death in U.S. children, with the highest rate of drowning occurring in 1- to 2-year-olds (AAP, 2003, 2004b). Drowning may occur in very small volumes of water such as a toilet, bucket, or bathtub, as well as the obvious sites such as swimming pools and other bodies of water. Toddlers' large heads in relation to their body size place them at risk for toppling over into a body of water that they are inquisitive about. Toddlers should be supervised at all times when in or around the water. In general, most children do not have the physical and cognitive capabilities necessary to truly learn how to swim until 4 years of age. Parents who want to enroll a toddler in a swimming class should be aware that a water safety skills class would be most appropriate. However, even toddlers who have completed a swimming program still need *constant* supervision in the water. Box 26.3 gives recommendations for the prevention of drowning.

BOX 26.3 Preventing Drowning

- Pools should be fenced with locked gates or screened with locked doors.
- Interior doors should be kept locked.
- Young children should never be left unattended in or near water.
- Water wings or "floaties" are not a substitute for adult supervision or for personal flotation devices.
- U.S. Coast Guard-approved life preservers or personal flotation devices should be available when a young child is in or near a body of water.
- Parents and caregivers should be trained in child cardiopulmonary resuscitation (CPR).

Remember Jose Gonzales, the 2-year-old introduced at the beginning of the chapter? What anticipatory guidance related to safety should you provide to his parents?

Promoting Nutrition

The toddler's ability to chew and swallow is improving, and he or she learns to use utensils effectively to feed himself or herself. The early years lay a foundation for the future, and a great deal of parental and societal interest is focused upon nutrition and eating. Forming healthy eating habits has its foundation early in life, and diet has significant influence upon the child's future health status. By establishing healthier food choice patterns early in life, the child is better able to continue these healthy choices later in life. The child less than 2 years of age should not have his or her fat intake restricted, but this does not mean that unhealthy foods such as sweets should be eaten liberally. A diet high in nutrient-rich foods and low in nutrient-poor high-calorie foods such as sweets is appropriate for children of all ages. See Healthy People 2010.

Weaning

The timing of weaning from breastfeeding is influenced by a number of factors such as cultural beliefs, local and regional ethnic beliefs, the mother's work schedule, desired child spacing, or societal feelings about the nature

HEALTHY PEOPLE 2010

Objective	Significance
Reduce growth retardation among low-income children under age 5 years.	• Counsel families about the appropriate toddler diet. • Refer eligible families to WIC for grocery supplementation and nutritional counseling.

of the mother–infant relationship. The extent and duration of breastfeeding are inversely related to the development of obesity later in life: children who breastfeed longer are less likely to become obese than those who breastfeed for shorter periods of time. Thus, extending breastfeeding into toddlerhood is believed to be beneficial to the child. Extended breastfeeding provides nutritional, immunologic, and emotional benefits to the child. Contrary to popular belief, it is biologically possible to become pregnant while breastfeeding. Breastfeeding a newborn appropriately can occur while continuing to nurse its older sibling.

Weaning from breastfeeding tends to occur earlier in the United States than in countries around the world, despite recommendations on length of breastfeeding by a number of organizations. Most professional organizations recommend breastfeeding for at least 1 year.

Weaning is a highly individualized decision. Educate the mother about the benefits of extended breastfeeding and support her in her decision to wean at a given time.

Weaning from the bottle should occur by 12 to 15 months of age. Prolonged bottle-feeding is associated with the development of dental caries. No-spill "sippy cups" contain a valve that requires sucking by the toddler in order to obtain fluid, thus functioning similar to a baby bottle. Hence, no-spill sippy cups can also be associated with dental caries and are not recommended. Cups with spouts that do not contain valves are acceptable. The 12- to 15-month-old is developmentally capable of consuming adequate fluid amounts using a cup.

Teaching About Nutritional Needs

Adequate calcium intake and appropriate exercise lay the foundation for proper bone mineralization. The toddler requires an average intake of 500 mg calcium per day. Dairy products are considered the primary sources of dietary calcium. One cup of low-fat or whole milk, 8 ounces of low-fat yogurt, and 1½ ounces of cheddar cheese each provide 300 mg of calcium. Broccoli, oranges, sweet potatoes, tofu, and dried beans or legumes are also good sources of calcium (35 to 120 mg calcium per serving).

> ▶ **Take** NOTE!
>
> Though a half-cup of cooked spinach contains 120 mg of calcium, it is essentially non-bioavailable, making spinach a poor source of calcium.

Iron-deficiency anemia in the first 2 years of life may be associated with developmental and psychomotor delays. Although it is important for toddlers to consume adequate amounts of iron, they tend to have the lowest daily iron intake of any age group. When breast-

feeding or formula feeding ends (most often at 1 year of age), it is often replaced with iron-poor cow's milk. Limiting milk intake to 16 ounces per day, as well as limiting juice intake, can be helpful. Encourage the parents to provide iron-fortified cereals and other foods rich in iron and vitamin C.

> ▶ **Take** NOTE!
>
> Toddlers who consume a strictly vegan diet (no food from animal sources) are at risk for deficiencies in vitamin D, vitamin B12, and iron. Supplementation with these nutrients should occur to promote adequate nutrition and growth.

Fat or cholesterol intake should not be restricted in children under age 2 years. The first 2 years of life require high energy intake because they are a time of very rapid growth and development. To promote healthy cholesterol levels, children over age 2 years should consume a diet with a total fat content between 20% and 30% of total calories. Saturated fats should account for less than 10% of total calories. Due to daily variations and the pickiness of the toddler, fat intake should be evaluated over a period of several days. The daily recommended intake of fiber for a 1- to 3-year-old is 19 grams. Figure 26.11 gives guidance on serving sizes and daily nutritional needs. Box 26.4 lists common sources of several nutrients.

Parents should encourage toddlers to drink water. Juice intake should be limited to 4 to 6 ounces per day. Milk intake should be limited to 16 to 24 ounces per day. Juice and milk should be served along with meals or snacks. Water should be offered for between-meal drinking. Toddlers should drink from a cup.

Advancing Solid Foods

Parents should offer three full meals and two snacks daily. Portion sizes for toddlers are about one-quarter the size of adult portions. Large portions of a new or different food on the toddler's plate may intimidate the toddler. Normal toddler behaviors of mouthing, handling, tasting, extruding the food from the mouth, and then resampling the food often occur. These behaviors are distasteful to some parents but are a normal part of toddler development. Parents need to understand and tolerate these behaviors rather than scolding the toddler for them. Toddlers are often afraid to try new things anyway, so the parent or caregiver should be flexible with the toddler's acceptance or rejection of new foods. If the toddler refuses healthy food choices at meal or snack time, parents should not substitute high-fat, high-sugar, processed food "just to make sure he's eating something." This sets the stage for future power struggles. The parent decides which foods will be served or

Food Guide Pyramid For Your Young Child

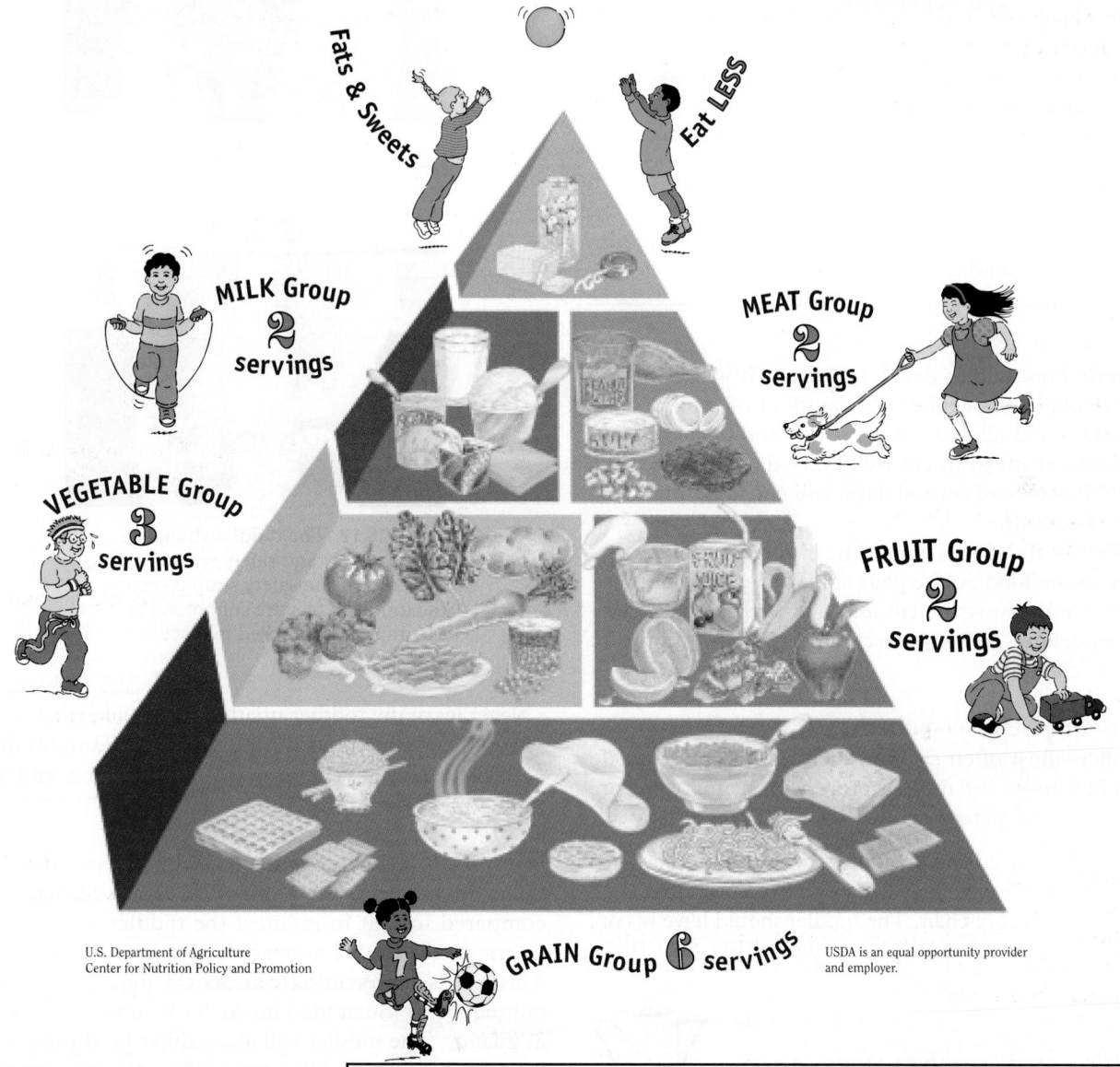

U.S. Department of Agriculture
Center for Nutrition Policy and Promotion

USDA is an equal opportunity provider and employer.

FOOD IS FUN and learning about food is fun, too. Eating foods from the Food Guide Pyramid and being physically active will help you grow healthy and strong.

What Counts As One Serving?

Grain Group
1 slice of bread
½ cup of cooked rice or pasta
½ cup of cooked cereal
1 ounce of ready-to-eat cereal

Vegetable Group
½ cup of chopped raw or cooked vegetables
1 cup of raw leafy vegetables

Fruit Group
1 piece of fruit or melon wedge
¾ cup of juice
½ cup of canned fruit
¼ cup of dried fruit

Milk Group
1 cup of milk or yogurt
2 ounces of cheese

Meat Group
2 to 3 ounces of cooked lean meat, poultry, or fish

½ cup of cooked dry beans, or 1 egg counts as 1 ounce of lean meat.
2 tablespoons of peanut butter count as 1 ounce of meat

Fats and Sweets
Limit calories from these.

**Four- to 6-year-olds can eat these serving sizes. Offer 2- to 3-year-olds less, except for milk.
Two- to 6-year-old children need a total of 2 servings from the milk group each day.**

Provided by _____

NIBBLES FOR HEALTH 2 Nutrition Newsletters for Parents of Young Children, USDA, Food and Nutrition Service

FIGURE 26.11 The U.S. Department of Agriculture's Young Child Food Pyramid provides a guide for parents and caregivers for determining adequate nutritional intake. (USDA, http://www.fns.usda.gov/tn/Resources/Nibbles/fgp_nibbles.pdf.)

BOX 26.4 **Key Nutrients Provided by Fruits and Vegetables**

Dietary fiber: applesauce, carrots, corn, green beans, mangos, pears

Folate: avocados, broccoli, green peas, oranges, spinach and dark greens, strawberries

Vitamin A: apricots, cantaloupe, carrots, mangos, spinach and dark greens, sweet potatoes

Vitamin C: broccoli, cantaloupe, green peas, oranges, potatoes, strawberries, tomatoes

FIGURE 26.12 The toddler should be appropriately and safely seated in the high chair. The safety strap is secure, the toddler's feet are supported, and the tray table is locked in place.

offered. The toddler decides how much will be eaten. The toddler self-regulates the amount of food needed to sustain and allow further growth and development. The toddler may not eat well every day but generally, over the course of several days, will consume the foods he or she needs.

Foods should be served near room temperature. Some of the food on the plate should be soft and moist. Food should always be cut into bite-size pieces. Teaching Guidelines 26.2 gives recommendations on ways to prevent choking.

Promoting Self-Feeding

Toddlers most often eat with their fingers, but they do need to learn to use utensils properly. The following are suggestions for parents:

• Use a child-sized spoon and fork with dull tines.
• Seat the toddler in a high chair or at a comfortable height in a secure chair. The toddler should have his or her feet supported rather than dangling (Fig. 26.12).

TEACHING GUIDELINES 26.2

Avoiding Choking

• Slowly add foods that are more difficult to chew as the toddler becomes more adept at chewing.
• Cut all foods into bite-sized pieces.
• Avoid foods that are hard to chew and may become lodged in the airway, such as:
  • Nuts
  • Gumdrops or other chewy candies
  • Raw carrots
  • Peanut butter (by itself)
  • Popcorn
• Cut hotdogs and grapes into quarters. Cook carrots until soft; if serving raw, then grate them.
• Always supervise the toddler while he or she is eating.

• Never leave the toddler unattended while eating.
• Minimize distractions during mealtime. Turn off the television and serve food to the toddler along with the other members of the family.

Promoting Healthy Eating Habits

Since the toddler's rate of growth has slowed somewhat compared to that in infancy, the toddler requires less caloric intake for his or her size compared to the infant. This results in **physiologic anorexia**: toddlers simply do not require as much food intake for their size as they did in infancy. The toddler will also exhibit **food jags**. During a food jag, the toddler may prefer only one particular food for several days, then not want it for weeks. Again, it is important for the parent to continue to offer healthy food choices during a food jag and not give in by allowing the toddler to eat junk food.

The normal developmental issue of testing limits will also occur for the toddler at mealtime. Since toddlers still have limited ability to express their emotions with words, they use nonverbal behaviors to do so. While eating, the toddler may dislike the taste of a particular food or experience a feeling of fullness but will communicate that feeling by screaming or throwing food. When the child exhibits these behaviors, the parent must remain calm and remove the toddler from the situation. Meals should be eaten in a calm and pleasant environment. Parents should serve as role models for appropriate eating habits, but toddlers may also be willing to try more foods if they are exposed to other children who eat those foods. Praise the child for trying a new food, and never punish the toddler for refusing to try something new. A new food may need to be offered many times in a row before the toddler chooses to try it. Parents should be sure to include foods the child is familiar with and likes to eat at the same meal that the new food is being introduced. Teaching Guidelines 26.3 lists alternative foods that meet nutritional needs and a list of books for parents of the picky eater.

Preventing Overweight and Obesity

In the child younger than 3 years of age, the greatest risk factor for the development of overweight or obesity is having an obese parent. The nurse can screen for overweight in the child over 2 years of age by calculating the body mass index (BMI) and plotting the BMI on the standardized age- and gender-appropriate growth charts (see Appendix A for growth charts, and refer to Chapter 31 for BMI calculation instructions). Trends over time may be predictive of the development of overweight or obesity.

TEACHING GUIDELINES 26.3

Meeting Nutritional Needs of the Picky Eater

Alternative Food Choices for the Picky Eater
- Won't drink milk? Obtain calcium through yogurt (frozen or regular), cheese, pudding, and hot cocoa.
- Poor meat intake? Obtain iron through unsweetened iron-fortified cereals or breakfast bars, raisins; cook with an iron skillet.
- Loves processed white bread? Encourage fiber intake with fresh fruits and vegetables, bran muffins, beans or peas (can be in soup).
- Refuses vegetables? Encourage vitamin A intake with apricots, sweet potatoes, and vegetable juices.

Books for Parents of the Picky Eater
- *Coping with a Picky Eater: A Guide for the Perplexed Parent* by W. Wilkoff. New York: Simon & Schuster, 1998.
- *First Foods* by M. Stoddard. New York: Dorling-Kindersley Publishing, Inc., 1998.
- *How to Get Your Kid to Eat . . . but not too much* by E. Satter. Boulder, CO: Bull Publishing Co., 1987.
- *The "Everything" Baby's First Food Book* by J. Tarlou. Holbrook, MA: Adams Media Corp., 2001.
- *The Family Nutrition Book* by W. Sears & M. Sears. Boston: Little Brown & Co., 1999.
- *The Healthy Baby Meal Planner* by A. Karmel. New York: Simon & Schuster, 2001.

Another factor in development of obesity in young children is juice intake. Since most young children like the sweet taste of juice, they may drink excessive amounts of it. Toddlers who drink excess fruit juice and eat well may develop overweight or obesity because of the high sugar content in the juice. On the other end of the spectrum, some children may actually feel full from juice consumption and decrease their intake of solid foods. These children are at risk for malnutrition. Fruit juice intake should be limited to 4 to 6 ounces per day.

▶ *Take* NOTE!

Young children should consume only pasteurized juice, as unpasteurized juice consumption places the toddler at increased risk of Escherichia coli, Salmonella, *and* Cryptosporidium *infection.*

Refer back to Jose Gonzales. What questions should you ask his parents related to his nutritional intake? What anticipatory guidance related to nutrition would be appropriate?

Promoting Healthy Sleep and Rest

The 18-month-old requires 13.5 hours of sleep per day, the 24-month-old 13 hours, and the 3-year-old 12 hours. A typical toddler should sleep through the night and take one daytime nap. Most children discontinue daytime napping at around 3 years of age. The toddler who slept in a crib as an infant will need to move to a youth or toddler bed or even a full-size bed usually sometime in the toddler period. When the crib becomes unsafe (that is, when the toddler becomes physically capable of climbing over the rails), then he or she must make the transition to a bed.

Consistent bedtime rituals help the toddler prepare for sleep. Choose a bedtime and stick to it as much as possible. The nightly routine might include a bath followed by reading a story. The routine should be a calm period with minimal outside distractions. Toddlers often require a security item to help them get to sleep. Older toddlers may be afraid of the dark, so a nightlight is often helpful.

Night waking is a problem for some toddlers. This may occur as a result of change in routine or as a desire for nighttime attention. Attention during night waking should be minimized so that the toddler receives no reward for being awake at night. The book, "Solve Your Child's Sleep Problems," by Dr. Richard Ferber (2006, New York: Fireside Publishing), is an excellent resource for the family with a toddler who resists bedtime or is a persistent night waker. For some toddlers, night waking is caused by nightmares. As the imagination and capacity for make-believe grow, the toddler may not be able to distinguish between reality and pretend. The parent should hold and comfort the toddler after a nightmare. Limiting television viewing (especially shortly before bedtime) may be helpful in limiting nightmares.

Some families practice "co-sleeping" (when children sleep in the parents' bed). Although some professionals believe that co-sleeping may interfere with the toddler's struggle for independence, this theory has not been proven. The nurse should support the family's choice for sleep arrangements unless the co-sleeping is unsafe either physically or psychologically. Refer to safebedsharing.org for bedsharing safety guidelines.

Provide anticipatory guidance to Jose Gonzales' parents in relation to his sleep.

Promoting Healthy Teeth and Gums

By 30 months of age, the toddler should have a full set of primary ("baby") teeth. Parents may not be aware of the importance of preventing cavities in primary teeth since they will eventually be replaced by the permanent teeth. Poor oral hygiene, prolonged use of a bottle or no-spill sippy cup, lack of fluoride intake, and delayed or absent professional dental care may all contribute to the development of dental caries. Cleaning of the toddler's teeth should progress from brushing with simply water to using a very small amount (pea-sized) of fluoridated toothpaste with brushing beginning at 2 years of age (Fig. 26.13). Weaning from the bottle no later than 15 months of age and severely restricting use of a no-spill sippy cup (the kind that requires sucking for fluid delivery) is recommended.

At age 1 year, the toddler should have his or her first dentist visit to establish current health of the teeth and gums. Eating should be limited to meal and snack times, as "grazing" throughout the day exposes the teeth to food throughout the day. Carbohydrate-containing foods combined with oral bacteria create a decreased oral pH level that is optimal for the development of dental caries (cavities). See Healthy People 2010.

Public water fluoridation is a public health initiative that ensures that most children receive adequate fluoride intake to prevent dental caries. Table 26.5 gives recommendations regarding fluoride supplementation. If the water supply contains adequate fluoride, no other supplementation is necessary other than brushing with a small amount of fluoride-containing toothpaste after age 2 years. Excess fluoride ingestion should be avoided, as it contributes to the development of fluorosis (mottling of the

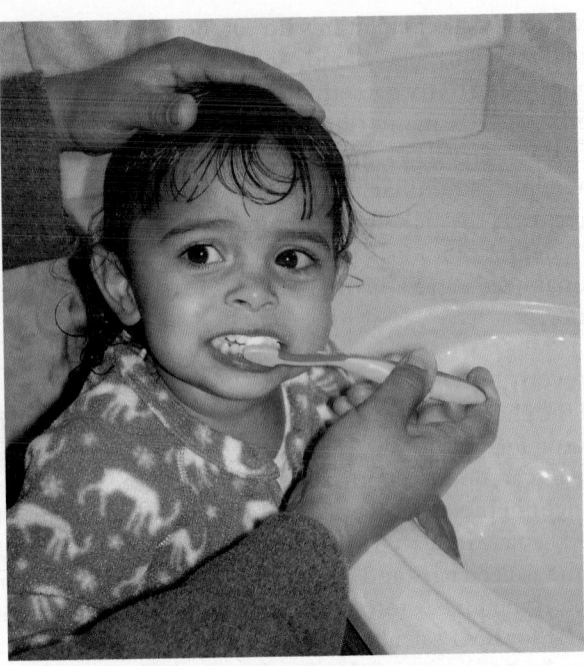

FIGURE 26.13 The parent should brush the toddler's teeth to ensure proper cleaning of the teeth, gums, and tongue. Use only water for brushing before 2 years of age and a pea-sized amount of fluoride-containing toothpaste after age 2 years.

enamel). Fluorosis occurs most often in the toddler years. Risk factors for fluorosis development include:

- High fluoride levels in the local water supply
- Use of fluoride-containing toothpaste prior to age 2 years
- Excessive ingestion of fluoride either in toothpaste or foods
  - Fluoride-containing foods: tea, ready-to-eat infant foods containing chicken, white or purple grape juice, and beverages, processed foods and cereals that were manufactured with fluoride-containing water

Promoting Appropriate Discipline

Discipline is a common concern during toddlerhood. The toddler's intense personality and extreme emotional re-

HEALTHY PEOPLE 2010	
Objective	Significance
Reduce the proportion of children with untreated dental decay.	• Encourage weaning from bottle by 15 months of age. • Discourage use of no-spill sippy cups. • Refer any toddler with potential or existing caries to pediatric dentist.

TABLE 26.5 RECOMMENDATIONS FOR FLUORIDE SUPPLEMENTATION

	Fluoride Ion Level in Drinking Water (ppm)		
Age	<0.3 ppm	0.3–0.6 ppm	>0.6 ppm
Birth to 6 months	None	None	None
6 months to 3 years	0.25 mg/day	None	None
3–6 years	0.50 mg/day	0.25 mg/day	None
6–16 years	1.0 mg/day	0.50 mg/day	None

ppm: parts per million is equivalent to 1 mg/liter

These recommendations are public domain at www.ada.org and were approved by the American Dental Association, the American Academy of Pediatrics, and the American Academy of Pediatric Dentistry.

actions can be difficult for parents to understand and cope with. The toddler needs firm, gentle guidance to learn what the expectations are and how to meet them. The parent's love and respect for the toddler teach the toddler to care about himself or herself and for others. Affection is as important as the guidance aspect of discipline. Having realistic expectations of what the toddler is capable of learning and understanding can help the parent in the disciplinary process. The toddler's intense push for autonomy can often test a parent's limits. The easygoing infant usually becomes more challenging in toddlerhood. The toddler's continual quest for new experiences often places the toddler at risk, and his or her negativism very often taxes the parent's patience.

In an effort to prevent the toddler from experiencing harm and in response to his or her continual testing of limits, parents often resort to spanking. Though commonly accepted, the American Academy of Pediatrics and the National Association of Pediatric Nurse Practitioners recommend against corporal or physical punishment (AAP 2004a; NAPNAP, 2006b). Recent research points out the dangers inherent in the use of corporal punishment as well as the possibilities for negative effects on the child's future behavior (Box 26.5). Spanking or other forms of corporal punishment lead to a pro-violence attitude, create resentment and anger in some children, and contribute to the cycle of violence (NAPNAP, 2006). See Evidence-Based Practice 26.1.

▶ **Take** NOTE!

Toddlers less than 18 months of age should NEVER be spanked, as there is an increased possibility of physical injury in this age group. Also, the infant/young toddler is not capable of linking the spanking with the undesired behavior.

Normal toddler development includes natural curiosity, and this curiosity often results in dangerous or problematic activities for the toddler. Toddlers have a difficult time learning the rules and in general do not behave badly intentionally. Providing a childproof environment will allow the toddler to participate in safe exploration, which will meet his or her developmental needs and decrease the frequency of intervention needed on the part of the parents.

BOX 26.5 Negative Impact of Physical Punishment

- Spanking is less effective than time-out or other discipline measures to reduce undesired behavior in children.
- The toddler less than 18 months of age:
  - Is not capable of making the appropriate connections between spanking and the undesired behavior
  - Is at increased risk for physical injury from spanking than older children
- Physical punishment:
  - May lead to a pro-violence attitude
  - May create resentment in the toddler
  - Is a poor model for learning effective problem solving
  - May be correlated with antisocial and criminal behavior later in life
  - Leads to increased aggression in preschoolers, school-aged children, and adults
  - When used frequently, may weaken the parent–child relationship
- Childhood corporal punishment increases the probability of depression and substance abuse in adulthood.
- Spanking may lead to more severe forms of punishment and to actual child abuse and maltreatment.
- The more frequently children are hit or spanked, the more likely they are to hit their own children and to be involved in spouse abuse as adults.

AAP, 2004a; NAPNAP, 2006b

EVIDENCE-BASED PRACTICE 26.1
Corporal Punishment and Behavior Problems in Early Childhood

● Study

A large volume of research indicates that there are few, if any, positive developmental outcomes associated with the use of corporal punishment (spanking). In order to determine if negative consequences resulted, the authors used data from a large longitudinal ongoing multicenter study, the National Institute of Child Health and Human Development Study of Early Child Care and Youth Development. They reviewed the data from over 100 children, performing analyses that specifically controlled for contextual and parenting variables as well as for partial child effects. The Home Observation for the Measurement of the Environment (HOME) was administered when the children were 15, 36, and 54 months of age. The HOME measurement determined the use of corporal punishment. To determine the presence of behavior problems, the Child Behavior Checklist was administered at 36 months of age and again when the child was in the first grade.

▲ Findings

Multiple regression analysis was performed on the data sets, controlling for variables such as the child's gender, ethnicity, and temperament as well as maternal sensitivity and depression. The results established a causal link between the use of corporal punishment and child adjustment, particularly an increase in behavior problems during toddlerhood.

■ Nursing Implications

Targeted interventions may have a positive impact on decreasing the use of corporal punishment in young children. Advise parents about the risks associated with corporal punishment. Provide them with education about appropriate alternative methods of discipline, including limit-setting with consistent follow-through, extinction, and time-out. Support parents' efforts to use alternative methods of discipline.

Mulvaney, M. K., & Mebert, C. J. (2007). Parental corporal punishment predicts behavior problems in early childhood. *Journal of Family Psychology, 21*(3), 389–397.

Discipline should focus on limit setting, negotiation, and techniques to assist the toddler to learn problem solving. Parents should provide consistency and commit to the limits that are set.

Offering realistic choices helps give the toddler a sense of mastery. Rules should be simple and limited in number. Maintaining the toddler's schedule of meals and rest/sleep will help to prevent conflicts that occur as a result of hunger or fatigue. Toddlers should not be made to share, as this is a concept they do not understand. Parents should encourage simple activities enjoyed by the children involved and avoid confrontation over toys. Parents should offer toddlers appropriate choices to help them develop autonomy, but should not offer a choice when none exists.

Positive reinforcement should be used as much as possible. "Catching" a child being good helps to reinforce appropriate or desirable behaviors. When the toddler is displaying appropriate behavior, the parent should reward the child consistently with praise and physical affection.

"Time out" can be used effectively at around 2.5 to 3 years of age (refer to Chapter 6 for details). "Extinction" is a particularly useful technique with 2- and 3-year-olds. Extinction involves systematic ignoring of the undesired behavior. Parents sometimes unknowingly contribute to the occurrence of an unwanted behavior simply by the attention they give the toddler (even if is negative in nature, it is still attention). Parents who want to extinguish an annoying (non-dangerous) behavior should resolve to ignore

it every time it occurs. When the child withholds the behavior or performs the opposite (appropriate) behavior, they should use compliments and praise. It may be difficult to ignore a difficult behavior, but the results are well worth the effort. Teaching Guidelines 26.4 provides tips on avoiding power struggles and offering appropriate guidance to toddlers.

► ADDRESSING COMMON DEVELOPMENTAL CONCERNS

Common developmental concerns of the toddler period are toilet teaching, temper tantrums, thumb sucking or pacifier use, sibling rivalry, and regression. An understanding of the normalcy of negativism, temper tantrums, and sibling rivalry will help the family cope with these issues. Prepare parents for these developmental events by giving appropriate anticipatory guidance.

Toilet Teaching

When myelinization of the spinal cord is achieved around age 2 years, the toddler is capable of exercising voluntary control over the sphincters. Girls may be ready for toilet teaching earlier than boys. Toddlers are ready for toilet teaching when:

• Bowel movements occur on a fairly regular schedule.

TEACHING GUIDELINES 26.4

Providing Toddlers with Guidance

- When giving the toddler instructions, tell the child what to do, NOT what not to do. This allows for a positive focus. If you must say "no," "don't," or "stop," then follow with a direction of what to do instead.
- Offer limited choices, when a choice is truly available. Say, "Do you want to wear your blue hat or your red hat?" NOT "Do you want to put on your hat?" This gives the toddler some, but not all, control.
- Role model appropriate communication, but don't feel like you have to speak nicely all the time. If the situation warrants, use a firm and even tone to get the point across. Avoid yelling.
- Pay attention to the inflection in your voice. A statement or direction should not end in a questioning tone or with "Okay?" Be clear. Statements should sound like statements, and only questions should end in a questioning tone.
- When a toddler behaves aggressively, label the child's feelings calmly, but be firm and consistent with the expectation. For example, "I know you're mad at your friend, but it is not okay to hit."

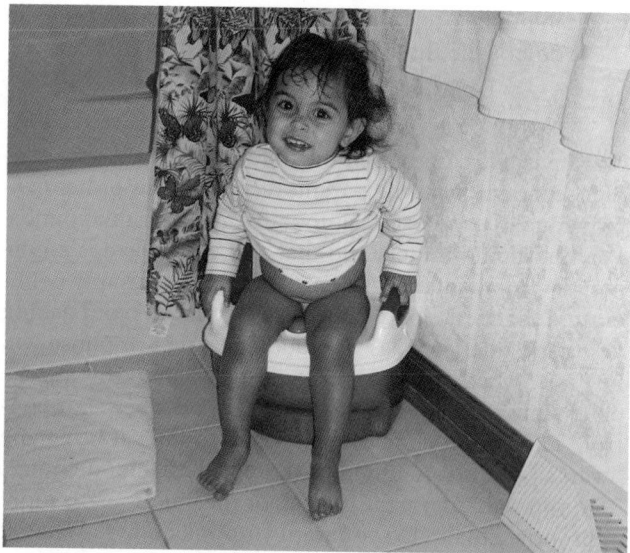

FIGURE 26.14 The toddler will feel most comfortable with a potty chair that sits on the floor.

- The toddler expresses knowledge of the need to defecate or urinate. This may be through verbalization, change in activity, or gestures such as:
  - Looks into or grabs diaper
  - Squats
  - Crosses legs
  - Grimaces and/or grunts
  - Hides behind a door or the couch when defecating
- The diaper is not always wet (this indicates the ability to hold the urine for a period of time).
- The toddler is willing to follow instructions.
- The toddler walks well alone and is able to pull down his or her pants.
- The toddler follows caregivers to the bathroom.
- The toddler climbs onto the potty chair or toilet.

Parents should approach toilet teaching with a calm, positive, and nonthreatening manner. Initially it may be helpful to allow the toddler to observe a same-sex family member using the toilet. Start with the toddler fully clothed on the potty chair or toilet while the parent or caregiver talks about what the toilet is used for and when. The toddler will feel most comfortable with a toddler potty chair that sits on the floor (Fig. 26.14). If a potty chair is unavailable, facing toward the toilet tank may make the toddler feel more secure, as the buttocks remain on the

front of the seat rather than sinking through the toilet seat opening. After a week or longer, remove a dirty diaper and place the contents in the toilet. Next try having the toddler sit on the potty chair or toilet without pants or diaper on. The toddler may benefit from watching a caregiver or friend use the toilet. It may also be beneficial to demonstrate using the potty chair with a baby doll that wets.

Parents should always use gentle praise and no reproaches. Usually the best time to achieve success with defecation on the toilet is following a meal. When the toddler has achieved success with bowel control, bladder control will come next. It may be many months before nighttime bladder control is achieved, and the toddler may still require a diaper at night. Parents should use appropriate words for body parts, urination, and defecation, then use those words consistently so the toddler understands what to say and do.

After a couple of weeks of successful toileting, the toddler may start wearing training pants. When toddlers have an accident and don't make it to the toilet, gently remind them about toileting and let them help clean up. Toddlers should never be punished for bowel or bladder "accidents."

With so much attention focused on the genitalia during toilet teaching and the frequency of being without a diaper, it is natural for toddlers to become more focused on their own genitalia. Boys and girls both will explore their genitalia and discover the resulting pleasurable sensation. Masturbation in the toddler often causes a great deal of discomfort in the parent. The parent should not draw attention to the activity, as that may increase its frequency. The parent should calmly explain to the toddler that this is an activity that may only be done in private. If the toddler is masturbating excessively or refuses to stop when in public, then there may be additional stressors in the toddler's life that should be explored.

Negativism

Negativism is common in the toddler period. As the toddler separates from the parent, recognizes his or her own individuality, and exerts autonomy, negativism abounds. Parents should understand that this negativism is a normal developmental occurrence and not necessarily deliberate defiance (though that also occurs). Avoid asking yes-or-no questions, as the toddler's usual response will be "no," whether he or she means it or not. Offering the child simple choices will give the toddler a sense of control. The parent should not ask the toddler if he or she "wants" to do something, if there is actually no choice. "Do you want to use the red cup or the blue cup?" is more appropriate than "Do you want your milk now?" When it is time to go outside, don't ask, "Do you want to put your shoes on?" Instead, state in a matter-of-fact tone that shoes must be worn outside, and give the toddler a choice of type of shoe or color of socks. If the child continues with negative answers, then the parent should remain calm and make the decision for the child.

Temper Tantrums

Even children who displayed an easygoing personality as infants may lose their temper frequently during the toddler years (Fig. 26.15). A toddler who was more intense as an infant may have more temper tantrums. Temper tantrums are a natural result of the frustration that toddlers experience. Toddlers are eager to explore new things, but their efforts are often thwarted (usually for safety reasons). Tod-

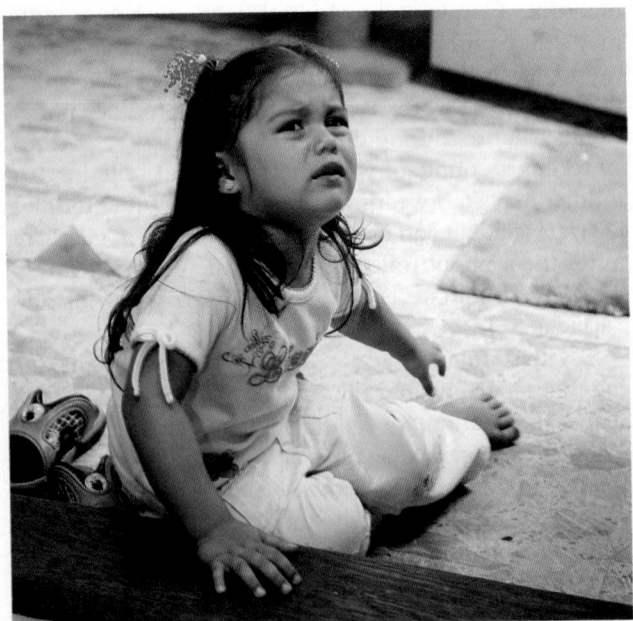

FIGURE 26.15 Tantrums are a normal component of toddler development.

dlers do not behave badly on purpose. They need time and maturity to learn the rules and regulations. Some of their frustration may come from lack of language skills to express themselves. Toddlers are just starting to learn how to verbalize feelings and to use alternative actions rather than just "pitching a fit." The temper tantrum may be manifested as a screaming and crying fit or a full-blown episode in which the toddler throws himself or herself on the floor kicking, screaming, and pounding, perhaps even holding the breath. Fatigue or hunger may limit the toddler's coping abilities and promote negative behavior and temper tantrums.

Although tantrums are annoying to parents and caregivers, they are a normal part of the toddler's quest for independence. As toddlers mature, they become better able to express themselves and to understand their environment.

Parents need to learn their toddler's behavioral cues in order to limit activity that is frustrating. When the parent notes the beginnings of frustration, a friendly warning might be given. Intervening early with an activity change might prevent a tantrum. Use distraction, refocusing, or removal from the situation.

When a temper tantrum does occur, the best course of action is to ignore the behavior and ensure that the child is safe during the tantrum. Physical punishment will probably just prolong the tantrum and in fact produce more intense negative behavior. If the tantrum occurs in public, it may be necessary for the parent to immobilize the child with a big bear hug and use a calm voice to soothe the toddler. It is very important for parents to model self-control. Since toddlers' tantrums most often result from frustration, the role-modeled behavior of self-control helps to teach toddlers to control their temper when they can't get what they want.

Thumb Sucking and Pacifiers

Infants bring their hands to their mouths and begin thumb sucking as a form of self-soothing. This habit may continue into the toddler years and beyond. The pacifier is used for the same reason. Toddlers may calm themselves in a stressful situation by thumb sucking or sucking on a pacifier. Opinions about thumb and finger sucking and pacifier use are significantly affected by family history and culture. For most children there is no need to worry about a sucking habit until it is time for the permanent teeth to erupt. Prolonged and frequent sucking in the withdrawn child is more likely to yield changes to the tooth and jaw structure than sucking that is primarily used for self-soothing. Parents must sort through their own feelings about thumb sucking and pacifier use and then decide how they want to handle the habit.

To ensure safety with pacifier use:

- Use only one-piece pacifiers.
- Replace worn pacifiers with new ones.
- Never tie a pacifier around a toddler's neck.

Parents may want to limit thumb sucking and pacifier use to bedtime, in the car, and in stressful situations. The parent should calmly discuss these limits with the toddler and then remain consistent about enforcing them.

Sibling Rivalry

Many families have subsequent children when their first child is a toddler. The toddler has been accustomed to being the baby and receiving a great deal of attention, both at home and with the extended family. Since toddlers are normally egocentric, bringing a new baby into the home may be quite disruptive. To minimize issues with **sibling rivalry**, parents should attempt to keep the toddler's routine as close to normal as possible. Spend individual time with the toddler on a daily basis. Involve the toddler in the care of the baby. The toddler is capable of fetching a diaper or T-shirt, entertaining the baby with a toy, or helping sing a song to calm the baby. "Helping" the parent care for the baby gives the toddler a sense of importance (Fig. 26.16). The toddler will need significant support while holding the baby.

Regression

Some toddlers experience **regression** during a stressful event (e.g., the birth of a sibling, hospitalization). Stress in a toddler's life affects his or her ability to master new developmental tasks. During regression, the toddler may want to go back to an earlier stage. He or she may desire a bottle or pacifier long ago forgotten. The toddler may stop displaying previously achieved language or motor skills. A significant stress in the toddler's life may also disrupt the toilet teaching process (toilet teaching may not be achieved near the time a sibling is born). When regression occurs, parents should ignore the regressive behavior and offer praise for age-appropriate behavior or attainment of skills.

*R*efer to Jose Gonzales, the 2-year-old in the case study. List common developmental concerns of the toddler. What anticipatory guidance related to these concerns would the nurse provide to Jose's parents?

■■■ Key Concepts

- The toddler's organ systems are continuing to mature, and growth slows during this period as compared with infancy.
- The psychosocial task of the toddler years is to attain a sense of autonomy and to experience separation and individuation.
- Cognitive development in toddlerhood progresses from sensorimotor in nature to preoperational.
- The toddler refines gross motor skills after learning to walk and builds fine motor skills through the use of utensils and various manipulative toys.
- The toddler progresses from limited expressive language capabilities to a vocabulary of 900 by age 3 years.
- Toddlers use all of their senses to explore and learn about their environment.
- Visual acuity progresses to at least 20/50 in the toddler period.
- Negativism abounds in toddlers as they attempt to exert their independence.
- Very ritualistic, toddlers feel safer and more secure when clear limits are enforced and a structured routine is followed.
- The toddler is starting to learn right from wrong and bases actions on punishment avoidance.
- Toddler development may be promoted through active gross motor play, books, music, and block building.
- Safety is a primary concern in the toddler years as the child is more mobile, very curious, and experimenting with autonomy.
- Poisoning in the toddler period may be prevented through proper storage of medications and other potentially poisonous substances and appropriate supervision.
- Consistent bedtime rituals help ease the toddler's transition to sleep.
- All primary teeth are erupted by 30 months of age and may be kept healthy with appropriate tooth brushing and fluoride supplementation.
- The toddler may experience a decrease in appetite as growth slows, yet he or she still needs appropriate nutritional intake for continued development.

FIGURE 26.16 The toddler may be more likely to accept the new baby in a positive manner if she feels that this is "our baby," not just "mommy's baby." This toddler is meeting her new brother for the first time.

- Toilet teaching can be achieved after myelinization of the spinal cord is complete, usually around 2 years of age.

- Thumb sucking, pacifier use, security items, and temper tantrums are expected issues in the toddler years.

- Toddler discipline should focus on clear limits and consistency. It should not involve spanking. It should be balanced with a caring and nurturing environment along with frequent praise for appropriate behavior.

- Parental role modeling of appropriate behavior, especially related to dealing with frustration, is beneficial to toddlers.

- Parents play an important role in toddler development, not only by providing a loving environment but also by role modeling appropriate behavior in most areas of daily life.

REFERENCES

Ackley, B., & Ladwig, G. (2006). *Nursing diagnosis handbook: A guide to planning care* (7th ed.). St. Louis: Mosby.

American Academy of Pediatric Dentistry. (2007). *Policy on use of fluoride.* Retrieved August 28, 2007 from http://www.aapd.org/media/Policies_Guidelines/P_FluorideUse.pdf.

American Academy of Pediatrics. (2003). Policy Statement: Prevention of drowning in infants, children and adolescents. *Pediatrics, 112*(2), 437–439.

American Academy of Pediatrics. (2004a). *Guidance for effective discipline.* Retrieved August 28, 2007 from http://aappolicy.aappublications.org/cgi/content/full/pediatrics;101/4/723.

American Academy of Pediatrics. (2004b). *Policy statement: Swimming programs for infants and toddlers.* Retrieved August 26, 2007 from http://aappolicy.aappublications.org/cgi/content/full/pediatrics;105/4/868.

American Academy of Pediatrics. (2007a). *Car safety seats: A guide for families 2007.* Retrieved August 28, 2007 from http://www.aap.org/family/carseatguide.htm.

American Academy of Pediatrics. (2007b). *Poison prevention and treatment tips.* Retrieved August 28, 2007 from http://www.aap.org/advocacy/releases/poisonpreventiontips.htm.

American Academy of Pediatrics. (2007c). *Policy statement: Poison treatment in the home.* Retrieved August 28, 2007 from http://aappolicy.aappublications.org/cgi/content/full/pediatrics;112/5/1182#SEC2.

American Academy of Pediatrics. (2007d). *Policy use: The use and misuse of fruit juice in pediatrics.* Retrieved August 28, 2007 from http://aappolicy.aappublications.org/cgi/content/full/pediatrics;107/5/1210.

American Academy of Pediatrics, Committee on Nutrition. (2003). Prevention of pediatric overweight and obesity. *Pediatrics, 104*(5), 1152–1157.

American Academy of Pediatrics, The Injury Prevention Program. (2007a). *Age-related safety sheets: 1 to 2 years.* Retrieved August 28, 2007 from http://www.aap.org/family/1to2yrs.htm.

American Academy of Pediatrics, The Injury Prevention Program. (2007b). *Age-related safety sheets: 2 to 4 years.* Retrieved August 28, 2007 from http://www.aap.org/family/2to4yrs.htm.

American Dietetic Association. (2002). *5 a day for young children up to 2 years of age.* Accessed 12/11/03 at http://www.webdietitians.org/Public/NutritionInformation/92_nfs0302.cfm

Brazelton, T. B., & Sparrow, J. D. (2006). *Touchpoints, birth to 3.* Cambridge, MA: Da Capo Press.

Butler, F. R., & Zakari, N. (2005). Grandparents parenting grandchildren: Assessing health status, parental stress and social supports. *Journal of Gerontological Nursing, 31*(3), 43–54.

Cathey, M., & Gaylord, N. (2004). Picky eating: A toddler's approach to mealtime. *Pediatric Nursing, 30*(2), 101–109.

Cincinnati Children's Hospital Medical Center. (2006). *Toddler nutrition.* Retrieved August 28, 2007 from http://www.cincinnatichildrens.org/health/info/nutrition/eat/toddler-nutrition.htm.

Erikson, E. H. (1963). *Childhood and society* (2nd ed.). New York: W.W. Norton and Company.

Gilger, M. A. (2006). Normal gastrointestinal function. In J. A. McMillan (Ed.), *Oski's pediatrics: Principles and practice* (4th ed.). Philadelphia: Lippincott Williams & Wilkins.

Goldstein, B. A. (2006). Clinical implications of research on language development and disorders in bilingual children. *Seminars in Speech and Language, 26*(4), 305–321.

Green, M., & Palfrey, J. S. (Eds.). (2002). *Bright futures: Guidelines for health supervision of infants, children, and adolescents* (2nd ed., rev.). Arlington, VA: National Center for Education in Maternal and Child Health.

Kohlberg, L. (1984). *Moral development.* New York: Harper & Row.

Lumeng, J. (2005). Is the picky eater a cause for concern? *Contemporary Pediatrics, 22*(3), 71–82.

Mandleco, B. (2004). *Growth and development handbook: Newborn through adolescence.* Clifton Park, NY: Delmar Learning.

National Association of Pediatric Nurse Practitioners. (2006a). *Healthy eating and activity together (HEAT) clinical practice guideline: Identifying and preventing overweight in childhood.* Cherry Hill, NJ: Author.

National Association of Pediatric Nurse Practitioners. (2006b). NAPNAP position statement on corporal punishment. *Journal of Pediatric Health Care, 20*(6), A43–A44.

National Association of Pediatric Nurse Practitioners. (2007a). *Building blocks to help toddlers eat well.* Retrieved August 28, 2007 from http://napnap.org/Docs/hungry_eng.pdf.

National Association of Pediatric Nurse Practitioners. (2007b). NAPNAP position statement on breastfeeding. *Journal of Pediatric Health Care, 21,* 39A–40A.

National Association for Sport & Physical Education. (2007). *Active start: A statement of physical activity guidelines for children birth to five years.* Retrieved August 28, 2007 from http://www.aahperd.org/naspe/template.cfm?template=ns_active.html.

Nelms, B. C. (2006). Discipline: Parents need our help. *Journal of Pediatric Health Care, 19*(4), 195–196.

Palmer, F. B., & Capute, A. J. (2006). Streams of development: The keys to developmental assessment. In J. A. McMillan (Ed.), *Oski's pediatrics: Principles and practice* (4th ed.). Philadelphia: Lippincott Williams & Wilkins.

Papalia, D. E., Olds, S. W., & Feldman, F. D. (2006). *Human development* (10th ed.). New York: McGraw-Hill.

Piaget, J. (1969). *The theory of stages in cognitive development.* New York: McGraw-Hill.

Reach Out and Read. (2006). *Reading tips.* Retrieved August 28, 2007 from http://www.reachoutandread.org/FileRepository/ReadingTips.pdf.

Safe Bed Sharing.org (2007). *Keep it safe.* Retrieved August 28, 2007 from http://www.safebedsharing.org/safetyguidelines.html.

Safe Kids USA. (2007). *Safety tips: Car.* Retrieved August 28, 2007 from http://www.usa.safekids.org/tier2_rl.cfm?folder_id=170.

Safe Kids Worldwide. (2007). *Preventing injury to children in motor vehicle crashes.* Retrieved August 28, 2007 from http://www.usa.safekids.org/content_documents/MVO_tips.pdf.

Savage, J. S., Fisher, J. O., & Birch, L. L. (2007). Parental influence on eating behavior: Conception to adolescence. *The Journal of Law, Medicine & Ethics, 35*(1), 22–34.

Schmitt, B. D. (2004). Toilet training problems: Underachievers, refusers, and stool holders. *Contemporary Pediatrics, 21*(4), 71–82.

Schuman, A. T. (2007). The ABCs of toy safety: More than just child's play. *Contemporary Pediatrics, 24*(7), 49–57, 64.

Shelov, S. P., Trubo, R., & Hannemann, R. E. (Eds.) (2004). *Caring for your baby and young child: Birth to age 5* (4th ed.). New York: Bantam Books.

Small, L., Melnyk, B. M., & Strasser, A. (2007). Preventing obesity in young children. *Advance for Nurse Practitioners, 15*(3), 35–40.

Storey, M., Holt, K., & Sotfka, D. (Eds.). (2002). *Bright futures in practice: Nutrition* (2nd ed.). Arlington, VA: National Center for Education in Maternal and Child Health.

Wilson, M. H., & Levin-Goodman, R. (2006). Injury prevention and control. In J. A. McMillan (Ed.), *Oski's pediatrics: Principles and practice* (4th ed.). Philadelphia: Lippincott Williams & Wilkins.

World Health Organization. (2007). *Passive smoking*. Retrieved August 28, 2007 from http://www.who.int/tobacco/en/atlas10.pdf.

Zebrowski, P. M. (2003). Developmental stuttering. *Pediatric Annals, 32*(7), 453–465.

WEBSITES

American Academy of Pediatrics: www.aap.org
American Academy of Pediatric Dentistry: www.aapd.org
Information on child passenger safety: www.bucklebear.com
American Dietetic Association: www.eatright.org
Produce for Better Health Foundation: www.5aday.com
Infant and toddler nutrition: www.gerber.com
Nemours Center for Children's Health Media: www.kidshealth.com

Parent-supported group for children's health, growth, and development: www.kidsource.com
Source for burn prevention book "Bernie Burn": www.littleboots publishing.com
Bilingual families webpage: www.nethelp.no/cindy/biling-fam.html
National Highway Traffic Safety Administration: www.nhtsa.dot.gov
Johnson & Johnson Pediatric Institute: www.pediatricinstitute.com
Early literacy promotion: www.reachoutandread.org
Car seat inspection and seat recalls: www.seatcheck.org
Safe Kids USA: www.usa.safekids.org/
United States Department of Agriculture; information on young child food guide pyramid: www.usda.gov/wps/portal/usdahome
Zero to Three: National Center for Infants, Toddlers and Families: www.zerotothree.org

CHAPTER WORKSHEET

MULTIPLE CHOICE QUESTIONS

1. The nurse is caring for a hospitalized 30-month-old who is resistant to care, angry, and yells "no" all the time. The nurse identifies this toddler's behavior as

   a. Problematic, as it interferes with needed nursing care

   b. Normal for this stage of growth and development

   c. Normal because the child is hospitalized and out of his routine

2. The mother of a 15-month-old is concerned about a speech delay. She describes her toddler as being able to understand what she says, sometimes following commands, but using only one or two words with any consistency. What is the nurse's best response to this information?

   a. The toddler should have a developmental evaluation as soon as possible.

   b. If the mother would read to the child, then speech would develop faster.

   c. Receptive language normally develops earlier than expressive language.

   d. The mother should ask her pediatrician for a speech therapy evaluation.

3. A 2-year-old is having a temper tantrum. What advice should the nurse give the mother?

   a. For safety reasons, the toddler should be restrained during the tantrum.

   b. Punishment should be initiated, as tantrums should be controlled.

   c. The mother should promise the toddler a reward if the tantrum stops.

   d. The tantrum should be ignored as long as the toddler is safe.

4. What is the best advice about nutrition for the toddler?

   a. Encourage cup drinking and give water between meals and snacks.

   b. Encourage unlimited milk intake, because toddlers need the protein for growth.

   c. Avoid sugar-sweetened fruit drinks and allow as much natural fruit juice as desired.

   d. Allow the toddler unlimited access to the sippy cup to ensure adequate hydration.

5. To gain cooperation from a toddler, what is the best approach by the nurse?

   a. Immediately pick the toddler up from the mother's lap.

   b. Kneel in front of the toddler while he or she is on the mother's lap.

   c. Do the nursing tasks quickly so the toddler can play.

   d. Ask the toddler if it is okay if you begin the needed task.

CRITICAL THINKING EXERCISES

1. Develop a teaching plan about safety to present to a toddler-age preschool class.

2. Construct a 3-day menu for a 2-year-old, one that is realistic and will provide the nutrients needed.

3. Develop a plan for educating the parent of a 34-month-old who has been resistant to toilet teaching. Include assessments the nurse will make as well as the plan for teaching.

STUDY ACTIVITIES

1. Visit a preschool that provides care for special-needs toddlers as well as typical toddlers. Perform a developmental assessment on a typical toddler and one with special needs (both the same age). Compare and contrast your findings.

2. Care for two average 2-year-olds in the clinical setting. Describe each toddler's behavior, response to the parent, and response to the nurse and list strategies used to gain compliance and minimize stress to the toddler.

3. Observe in the toddler classroom of a typical preschool. Choose two toddlers the same age with different temperaments. Record the toddlers' differences and similarities in response to structure and authority, interactions with classmates, attention levels, and language and activity levels.

GROWTH AND DEVELOPMENT OF THE PRESCHOOLER

KEY TERMS

animism
empathy
imaginary friend

magical thinking
preoperational thought
school readiness

telegraphic speech
transduction

LEARNING OBJECTIVES

Upon completion of the chapter, the learner will be able to:

1. Identify normal physiologic, cognitive, and psychosocial changes occurring in the preschool-aged child.
2. Express an understanding of language development in the preschool years.
3. Implement a nursing care plan that addresses common concerns or delays in the preschooler's development.
4. Integrate knowledge of preschool growth and development with nursing care and health promotion of the preschool-aged child.
5. Develop a nutrition plan for the preschool-aged child.
6. Identify common issues related to growth and development during the preschool years.
7. Demonstrate knowledge of appropriate anticipatory guidance for common developmental issues that arise in the preschool period.

Nila Patel is a 4-year-old girl brought to the clinic by her mother and father for her school check-up. During your assessment you measure her weight to be 44 pounds and her height 40 inches. As the nurse caring for her, assess Nila's growth and development, and then provide appropriate anticipatory guidance to her parents.

Wow

Quality parenting is achieved only by example.

The preschool period is the period between 3 and 6 years of age. This is a time of continued growth and development. Physical growth continues much more slowly compared to earlier years. Gains in cognitive, language, and psychosocial development are substantial throughout the preschool period. Many tasks that began during the toddler years are mastered and perfected during the preschool years. The child has learned to tolerate separation from parents, has a longer attention span, and continues to learn skills that will lead to later success in the school-age period. Preparation for success in school occurs during the preschool period because most children enter elementary school by the end of the preschool period.

Growth and Development Overview

The healthy preschooler is slender and agile, with an upright posture. The formerly clumsy toddler becomes more graceful, demonstrating the ability to run more smoothly. Athletic abilities may begin to develop. Major development occurs in the area of fine motor coordination. Psychosocial development is focused on the accomplishment of initiative. Preconceptual thought and intuitiveness dominate cognitive development. The preschooler is an inquisitive learner and absorbs new concepts like a sponge absorbs water.

▶ PHYSICAL GROWTH

The average preschool age child will grow 2.5 to 3 inches (6.5–7.8 cm) per year. The average 3-year-old is 37 inches tall (96.2 cm), the average 4-year-old is 40.5 inches tall (103.7 cm), and the average 5-year-old is 43 inches tall (118.5 cm). Average weight gain during this time period is about 5 pounds (2.3 kg) per year. The average weight of a 3-year-old is 32 pounds (14.5 kg), increasing to an average weight of 41 pounds (18.6 kg) by age 5. The loss of baby fat and the growth of muscle during the preschool years give the child a stronger and more mature appearance (Fig. 27.1). The length of the skull also increases slightly, with the lower jaw becoming more pronounced. The upper jaw widens through the preschool years in preparation for the emergence of permanent teeth, usually starting around age 6.

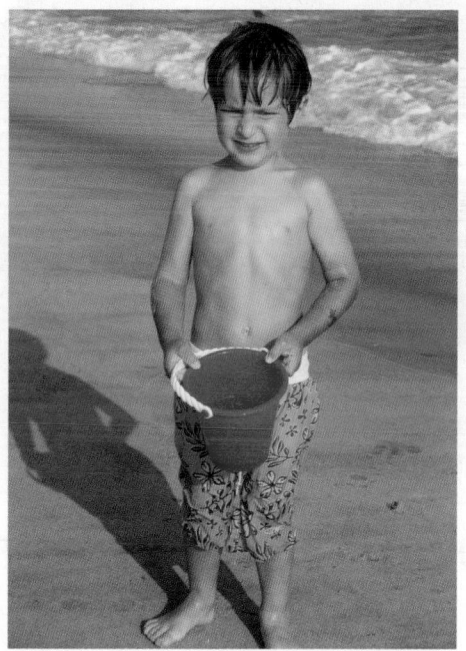

FIGURE 27.1 The preschool child has a more slender appearance and erect posture than the toddler.

3 years. The respiratory structures are continuing to grow in size, and the number of alveoli continues to increase, reaching the adult number at about 7 years of age. The eustachian tubes remain relatively short and straight. Heart rate decreases and blood pressure increases slightly during the preschool years. An innocent heart murmur may be heard upon auscultation, and splitting of the second heart sound may become evident. The preschooler should have 20 deciduous teeth present.

The small intestine is continuing to grow in length. Stool passage usually occurs once or twice per day in the average preschooler. The 4-year-old generally has adequate bowel control. The urethra remains short in both boys and girls, making them more susceptible to urinary tract infections than adults. Bladder control is usually present in the 4- and 5-year-old child, but an occasional accident may occur, particularly in stressful situations or when the child is absorbed in an interesting activity.

The bones continue to increase in length and the muscles continue to strengthen and mature. However, the musculoskeletal system is still not fully mature, making the preschooler susceptible to injury, particularly with overexertion or excess activity.

▶ ORGAN SYSTEM MATURATION

Most of the body systems have matured by the preschool years. Myelination of the spinal cord allows for bowel and bladder control to be complete in most children by age

▶ PSYCHOSOCIAL DEVELOPMENT

According to Erik Erikson, the psychosocial task of the preschool years is establishing a sense of initiative versus guilt (Erikson, 1963). The preschooler is an inquisitive

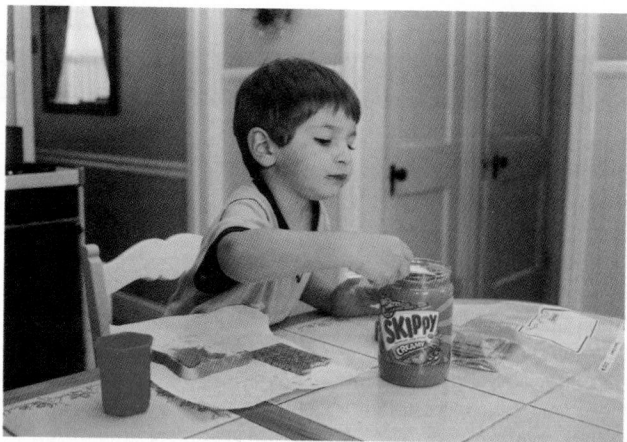

FIGURE 27.2 Allowing the preschooler to assist with simple household tasks such as preparing a sandwich encourages the development of initiative.

The child in the intuitive phase can count 10 or more objects, correctly name at least four colors, and better understand the concept of time, and he or she knows about things that are used in everyday life, such as appliances, money, and food. The preschooler uses **transduction** when reasoning: he or she extrapolates from a particular situation to another, even though the events may be unrelated. The preschooler also attributes lifelike qualities to inanimate objects (**animism**). Table 27.1 gives further examples illustrating this developmental stage.

The acquisition of language skills in the toddler period is enhanced in the preschool period. The expansion of vocabulary enables the preschooler to progress further with symbolic thought. At this age, children do not completely understand the concept of death or its permanence: they may ask when their grandparent or pet who died is returning.

learner, very enthusiastic about learning new things. Preschoolers feel a sense of accomplishment when succeeding in activities (Fig. 27.2), and feeling pride in one's accomplishment helps the child to use initiative. However, when the child extends himself or herself further than current capabilities allow, he or she may feel a sense of guilt. The superego or conscience development is completed during the preschool period, and this is the basis for moral development (understanding right and wrong). Table 27.1 gives examples illustrating the stage of initiative versus guilt.

COGNITIVE DEVELOPMENT

According to Jean Piaget's theory, the preschool-age child continues in the preoperational stage. Preoperational thought dominates during this stage and is based on a self-centered understanding of the world. In the preconceptual phase of preoperational thought, the child remains egocentric and is able to approach a problem from a single point of view only. The young preschooler may understand the concept of counting and begins to engage in fantasy play.

Magical thinking is a normal part of preschool development. The preschooler believes that his or her thoughts are all-powerful. The fantasy experienced through magical thinking allows the preschooler to make room in his or her world for the actual or the real. Through make-believe and magical thinking, preschool children satisfy their curiosity about differences in the world around them.

The preschooler often has an **imaginary friend** as well. This friend serves as a creative way for the preschooler to sample different activities and behaviors and practice conversational skills. Despite this imagination, the preschooler is able to switch easily between fantasy and reality throughout the day.

MORAL AND SPIRITUAL DEVELOPMENT

The preschool child can understand the concepts of right and wrong and is developing a conscience. That inner voice that warns or threatens is developing in the preschool years. Kohlberg identified this stage (between 4 and 10 years) as the preconventional stage, which is characterized by a punishment-and-obedience orientation. Preschool children see morality as external to themselves; they defer to power (that of the adult). The child's moral standards are those of their parents or other adults who influence them, not necessarily their own. Preschoolers adhere to those standards to gain rewards or avoid punishment. Since the preschool child is facing the psychosocial task of initiative versus guilt, it is natural for the child to experience guilt when something goes wrong. The child may have a strong belief that if someone is ill or dying, then he or she may be at fault and the illness or death is punishment.

As the child's moral development progresses, he or she learns how to deal with angry feelings. Sometimes the way the child chooses to deal with those feelings may be inappropriate, such as fighting and biting. Preschoolers are so involved in imagination and fantasy that lying begins to occur at this age. Preschoolers also use their limited life experiences to make sense of and help them cope with crisis. They need to learn the socially acceptable limits of behavior and are also learning the rewards of manners. The preschool child begins to help out in the family and begins to understand the concept of give-and-take in relationships.

During the preoperational phase of cognitive development, the preschooler's concept of faith is intuitive and projective in nature (Fosarelli, 2003). The preschool child's imagination allows for anything to be possible, so he or she does not have a logical view of the world (as adults

TABLE 27.1 **DEVELOPMENTAL THEORIES**

Theorist	Stage	Activities
Erikson	Initiative vs. Guilt Age 3–6 years	Likes to please parents Begins to plan activities, make up games Initiates activities with others Acts out the roles of other people (real and imaginary) Develops sexual identity Develops conscience May take frustrations out on siblings Likes exploring new things Enjoys sports, shopping, cooking, working Feels remorse when makes wrong choice or behaves badly Cooperates with other children Negotiates solutions to conflicts
Piaget	Preoperational substage: Preconceptual phase Age: 2–4 years	Exhibits egocentric thinking, which lessens as the child approaches age 4 Short attention span Learns through observing and imitating Displays animism Forms concepts that are not as complete or as logical as the adult's Able to make simple classifications By age 4 understands the concept of opposites (hot/cold, soft/hard) Reasoning is that of specific to specific Has an active imagination
	Preoperational substage: Intuitive phase Age 4–7 years	Able to classify and relate objects Has intuitive thought processes; knows if something is right or wrong, though cannot state why Tolerates others' differences but doesn't understand them Very curious about facts Knows acceptable cultural rules Uses words appropriately but often without true understanding of their meaning Has a more realistic sense of causality May begin to question parents' values
Kohlberg	Punishment–obedience orientation Age 2–4 years (preconventional morality)	Determines good vs. bad dependent upon associated punishment Children may learn inappropriate behavior at this stage if parental intervention does not occur (if the child hits, bites, or is verbally disrespectful but is not punished for these activities, the child will view those behaviors as good and continue to participate in them)
Freud	Phallic stage Age 3–7 years	Child's pleasure centers on genitalia and masturbation. Superego is developing and conscience is emerging. Oedipal stage occurs: jealousy and rivalry toward same-sex parent, with love of the opposite-sex parent. This usually resolves by the end of the preschool years, when the child develops a strong identification with the same-sex parent.

do). Preschool children have limited life experiences, so they may project a feeling onto a new person or situation. They may use this projection to help them understand what is going on around them. Preschoolers may project their parents' or caregiver's feelings or characteristics onto "God": if mommy gets angry, then God is probably also angry.

The family's religious beliefs may affect the child's diet, the mode of discipline that parents use, and even how the parents view their children. Knowing about a family's practices of prayer or meditation is helpful to the pediatric nurse, who can help continue the ritual when the child is ill or hospitalized (Fig. 27.3).

MOTOR SKILL DEVELOPMENT

As the preschooler's musculoskeletal system continues to mature, existing motor skills become refined and new ones develop. The preschooler has more voluntary control over his or her movements and is less clumsy than the toddler.

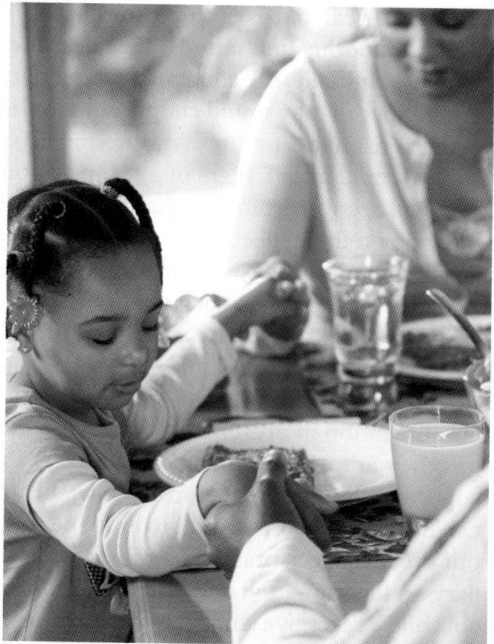

FIGURE 27.3 The preschool child may participate in religious rituals without having full understanding of their meaning.

FIGURE 27.4 The older toddler runs well, can hold a ball, and can balance on one foot.

Significant refinement in fine motor skills occurs during the preschool period (Table 27.2).

Gross Motor Skills

The preschooler is agile while standing, walking, running, and jumping (Fig. 27.4). He or she can go up and down stairs and walk forward and backward easily. Standing on tiptoes or on one foot still requires extra concentration. The preschooler seems to be in constant motion. He or she also uses the body to understand new concepts (such as using the arms in a "chug-chug" motion when describing how the train wheels work).

Fine Motor Skills

The 3-year-old can move each finger independently and is capable of grasping utensils and crayons in adult fashion,

TABLE 27.2 MOTOR SKILL DEVELOPMENT

Age	Expected Gross Motor Skills	Expected Fine Motor Skills
4 years	• Throws ball overhand • Kicks ball forward • Catches bounced ball • Hops on one foot • Stands on one foot up to 5 seconds • Alternates feet going up and down steps • Moves backward and forward with agility	• Uses scissors successfully • Copies capital letters • Draws circles and squares • Traces a cross or diamond • Draws a person with two to four body parts • Laces shoes
5 years	• Stands on one foot 10 seconds or longer • Swings and climbs well • May skip • Somersaults • May learn to skate and swim	• Prints some letters • Draws person with body and at least six parts • Dresses/undresses without assistance • Can learn to tie laces • Uses fork, spoon, and knife (supervised) well • Copies triangle and other geometric patterns • Mostly cares for own toileting needs

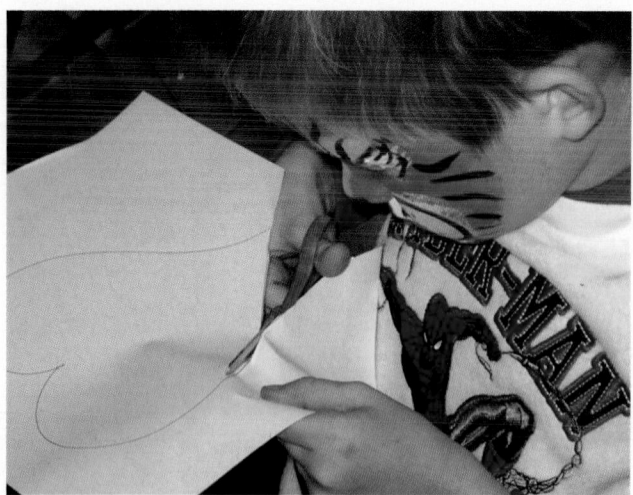

FIGURE 27.5 The 5-year-old has the fine motor dexterity to cut well with scissors.

with the thumb on one side and the fingers on the other. He or she can also scribble freely, copy a circle, trace a square, and feed himself or herself without spilling much. These skills become refined over the next 2 years, and by 5 years of age the child can write letters, cut with scissors more accurately, and tie shoelaces (Fig. 27.5).

▶ SENSORY DEVELOPMENT

Hearing is intact at birth and should remain so throughout the preschool years. The senses of smell and touch continue to develop throughout the preschool years. The young preschooler may have a less discriminating sense of taste than the older child, putting him or her at increased risk for accidental ingestion. Visual acuity continues to progress and should be equal bilaterally. The typical 5-year-old has visual acuity of 20/40 or 20/30. Color vision is intact at this age.

▶ COMMUNICATION AND LANGUAGE DEVELOPMENT

The acquisition of language allows the preschool child to express thoughts and creativity. The preschool years are a time of refinement of language skills. The 3-year-old exhibits **telegraphic speech**, using short sentences that contain only the essential information. Vocabulary at 3 years comprises about 900 words. The preschool child may acquire as many as 10 to 20 new words per day and at age 5 usually has a vocabulary of 2,100 words. By the end of the preschool period, the child is using sentences that are adult-like in structure (Table 27.3).

The 3- to 6-year-old is starting to develop fluency (the ability to smoothly link sounds, syllables, and words when speaking). Initially, the child may exhibit dysfluency or stuttering. Speech may sound choppy, or the child may say repeated consonants or "um." Stuttering usually has its onset between 2 and 4 years of age, and about 75% of children will recover from it without therapy. Parents should slow down their speech and should give the child time to speak without rushing or interrupting. Some sounds remain difficult for the preschooler to enunciate properly: "f," "v," "s," and "z" sounds are usually mastered by age 5 years, but some children do not master the sounds of "sh," "l," "th," and "r" until age 6 or later.

Communication in preschool children is concrete in nature, as they are not yet capable of abstract thought. Despite its concrete nature, the preschooler's communication can be quite elaborate and involved; he or she may talk about dreams and fantasies. In addition to acquiring vocabulary and learning the correct use of grammar, the preschool child's receptive language skills are also becoming refined.

The preschooler is very much in tune with the parent's moods and easily picks up on negative emotions in conversations. If the preschooler hears parents discussing things that are frightening to the child, the preschooler's imagination may fuel the development of fears and lead to misinterpretation of what the child has heard.

In the potentially bilingual child, by 4 years of age the child will cease the language mixing exhibited during the toddler years and should be able to use each language as a separate system.

▶ EMOTIONAL AND SOCIAL DEVELOPMENT

By the time a child enters kindergarten, he or she should have developed a useful set of social skills that will help him or her have successful experiences in the school setting as well as in life in general. These skills include cooperation, sharing (of things and feelings), kindness, generosity, affection display, conversation, expression of feelings, helping others, and making friends.

Preschoolers tend to have strong emotions. They can be very excited, happy, and giddy in one moment, then extremely disappointed in the next. The preschool child has a vivid imagination, and fears are very real to preschoolers. Most children this age have learned to control their behaviors. They should be able to name the feelings they are having rather than acting on them. Strong feelings may be expressed through outlets such as clay or Play-Doh, water play, drawing or painting, or through dramatic play such as with puppets.

Preschoolers are developing a sense of identity. They recognize that they are boys or girls. They know that they belong to a particular family, community, or culture.

TABLE 27.3 COMMUNICATION SKILLS IN THE PRESCHOOL CHILD

Age	Communication Abilities
4 years	• Speaks in complete sentences using adult-like grammar • Tells a story that is easy to follow • 75% of speech understood by others outside of family • Asks questions with "who," "how," "how many" • Stays on topic in a conversation • Understands the concepts of "same" and "different" • Asks many questions • Knows names of familiar animals • Names common objects in books and magazines • Knows at least one color • Uses language to engage in make-believe • Follows a three-part command • Can count a few numbers • Vocabulary of 1,500 words
5 years	• Persons outside of the family can understand most of the child's speech • Explains how an item is used • Participates in long, detailed conversations • Talks about past, future, and imaginary events • Answers questions that use "why" and "when" • Can count to 10 • Recalls part of a story • Speech should be completely intelligible, even if the child has articulation difficulties • Speech is generally grammatically correct • Vocabulary of 2,100 words • Says name and address

They take pride in using self-control rather than giving in to their impulses. The preschool child is capable of helping others and being involved in routines and transitions.

Parents can encourage and assist preschool children with developing the social and emotional skills that will be needed when the child enters school. Preschool children thrive on one-to-one communication with a parent. During interactive communication, children learn to express their feelings and ideas. Interactive communication fosters not only emotional and moral development but also self-esteem and cognitive development. Asking the preschool child questions requires the child to think out his or her own intention or motivation and encourages vocabulary development. Parents may use individual communication as a time to explore right and wrong, thus further contributing to moral development. Being listened to while answering parents' questions gives preschoolers a sense that they are valued, that what they think and have to say matters.

Establishing a few simple rules and enforcing them consistently gives preschoolers the structure and security they need while promoting moral development. Parents or caregivers can help the child give a name to the emotion that is being experienced. Fears are very real to preschoolers because of their active imaginations and may result in a

variety of emotions. Parents should validate the feeling or emotion, then discuss with the child alternatives for dealing with the emotion.

Preschoolers are developing their sense of identity, and parents should encourage preschoolers to do simple things for themselves, like dressing and washing their hands and face (Fig. 27.6). Parents should give the child the time he or she needs to complete the task. This helps to establish a sense of accomplishment.

At this age, the child may begin to show an interest in basic sexuality. The preschooler may want to know why boys' and girls' bodies are different, how the reproductive organs function, and where babies come from. The parent should answer the child honestly and directly, using the correct anatomic terms. Long explanations are not necessary, just simple answers. This curiosity is a normal function of the preschool years, and the curiosity may also involve playing with the genitals (see the section on masturbation later in this chapter).

Friendships

Preschoolers need interactions with friends as well. Learning how to make and keep a friend is an important part of social development. Friends may be other children in the neighborhood or those at preschool or day care. A special

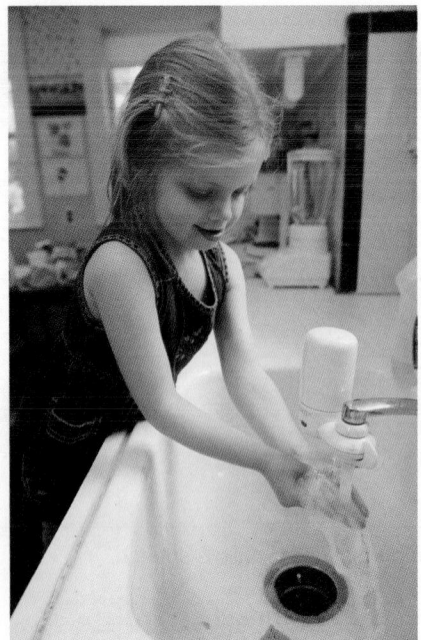

FIGURE 27.6 Encouraging the preschooler to complete simple tasks by himself or herself helps to build self-esteem.

friend is someone the preschooler can care about, talk to, and play with (Fig. 27.7). The preschooler is more likely to agree to rules and wants to please friends and be like them. The preschooler loves to sing, dance, and act and will enjoy these activities with friends. Disagreements may occur, but the parent can encourage the children to express their views, discuss and resolve conflicts, and continue being friends.

Temperament

By the time children are 3 years old, they recognize that what they do actually matters. It is helpful for the parent to view the child as an active participant in the parent–child relationship. The child's temperament has become a reliable indicator of how a parent might expect the child to react in a certain situation. When the parent is in tune with the preschooler's temperament, it is easier to find ways to ease transitions and changes for that child. In the area of task orientation, temperament may range from the highly attentive and persistent to the more distractible and active.

A child's social flexibility is also evident by this age. A child who is quite adaptable will handle stimuli from the outside world in an approaching rather than a withdrawing manner. Temperament also determines the extent of reactivity (the child's sensory threshold of responsiveness, high versus low). This determines the quality of the child's mood and the intensity of reactions to stimuli, change, or situations. When the parents are familiar with the child's task orientation, social flexibility, and reactivity, they can better structure activities and situations for the child.

The 4-year-old is better at learning self-control and can use setbacks in appropriate behavior as opportunities for growth. Temper tantrums should ease off by this age as the child's language skills are more capable of keeping up with complex ideas. The 4-year-old is able to see the rewards of growing up. This awareness of self-power may, however, lead to additional fears. The 5-year-old who has a more vulnerable type of temperament, as opposed to a confident temperament, may be more apt to experience fears.

Fears

With their vivid imaginations, preschoolers experience a variety of fears. Preschoolers may be scared of loud noises such as fire engine sirens or barking dogs. Imaginary monsters may scare the child. Preschoolers are often afraid of people they do not know as well as strange people (Santa Claus or people who look or dress very differently from what they are accustomed to). Many preschoolers are afraid of the dark. Preschoolers may also fear insects as well as animals they are not familiar with. The preschooler's memory is long enough that he or she may fear returning to the doctor's office when a painful procedure occurred during the prior visit.

Parents should acknowledge fears rather than minimizing them. They can then collaborate with the child on strategies for dealing with the fear.

FIGURE 27.7 The preschool child begins to develop friendships.

▶ CULTURAL INFLUENCES ON GROWTH AND DEVELOPMENT

Children may learn prejudice or bias at home before entering school or day care. The ways that families view other races or cultures may be subtly or overtly demonstrated in routine daily activities. The preschool child is developing a conscience, so attitudes of tolerance or bias may influence the child's values. As in the toddler period, the value that the family places on independence will affect the child's development of a healthy self-concept.

Some cultures value reading and education more than others. If reading is not valued in the home, the preschool child's first experience with books may not occur until he or she is in school.

Food served in the home is often very specific to the family's ethnic background. As the preschool child is exposed to persons of other cultures in school, he may or may not like the food that is served. Exploring customs or cultural practices that the family participates in is important so that these practices may be safely incorporated into the child's plan of care.

*R*efer back to Nila, who was introduced in the beginning of the chapter. What developmental milestones would you expect Nila to have reached at this age? Nila's mother expresses concerns about her child's imaginary friend, Sasha. How would you respond?

The Nurse's Role in Preschool Growth and Development

WATCH & LEARN

Growth and development in the preschool child remains orderly and sequential. Some preschoolers grow faster than others or reach various developmental milestones sooner than others. Nurses must be aware of the usual growth and development patterns for this age group so that they can assess preschool children appropriately and provide guidance to their families. The changes that the preschool child is experiencing affect not only the child but also the family. Health care visits throughout the preschool period continue to focus on expected growth and development and anticipatory guidance. An additional concern is the preparation for school entry (school readiness).

If the preschooler is hospitalized, growth and development may be altered. Hospitalization hinders the preschool child's ability to explore the environment and engage in make-believe play and thus presents a challenge for the curious and inquisitive child. If the child must be isolated for a contagious illness, the opportunities for exploration and experimentation are further restricted. In addition, a sick preschooler may feel a sense of guilt, worrying that maybe he or she caused the illness by negative thoughts or behaviors.

When caring for the hospitalized preschooler, the nurse must use knowledge of normal growth and development to recognize potential delays, promote continued appro-

priate growth and development, and interact successfully with the preschooler.

▶ NURSING PROCESS OVERVIEW

Upon completion of assessment of the preschool child's growth and development status, problems or issues related to growth and development may be identified. The nurse may then identify one or more nursing diagnoses, including but not limited to:

• Delayed growth and development
• Imbalanced nutrition, less than body requirements
• Interrupted family processes
• Readiness for enhanced parenting
• Risk for caregiver role strain
• Risk for delayed development
• Risk for disproportionate growth
• Risk for injury

Planning nursing care for the preschool child with growth and development issues should take into account the preschooler's and family's individual needs. The nursing care plan may be used as a guide in planning nursing care for the preschooler with a growth or developmental concern. The nurse may choose the appropriate nursing diagnoses from the following plan and individualize them as needed. The nursing care plan is intended to serve as a guide only and is not intended to be an inclusive growth and development plan.

▶ PROMOTING HEALTHY GROWTH AND DEVELOPMENT

The building of self-esteem continues throughout the preschool period. It is of particular importance during these years, as the preschooler's developmental task is focused on the development of initiative rather than guilt. A sense of guilt will contribute to low self-esteem, whereas a child who is rewarded for his or her initiative will have increased self-confidence. The parent who provides a loving and nurturing environment for the preschooler builds upon the earlier foundation.

Routine and ritual continue to be important throughout the preschool years, as they help the child to develop a sense of time as well as provide the structure for the child to feel safe and secure. Daily routine continues to assist with the development of conscience in the preschooler. As in toddlerhood, making expectations known through everyday routines helps to avoid confrontations. The preschooler is developing the maturity to know how to behave in various situations and is capable of learning manners.

(text continues on page 840)

Nursing Care Plan 27.1

GROWTH AND DEVELOPMENT ISSUES IN THE PRESCHOOL CHILD

NURSING DIAGNOSIS: Risk for injury related to developmental age, environment, and motor vehicle travel

Outcome Identification and Evaluation
Child's safety will be maintained: *Child will remain free from injury.*

Interventions: Preventing Injury
- Teach and encourage appropriate use of forward-facing car seat or booster seat if greater than 40 pounds *to decrease risk of injury related to motor vehicles.*
- Teach preschoolers to stay away from street and to cross the street only when holding the hand of an adult *to prevent pedestrian injury.*
- Require bicycle helmet use while riding any wheeled toy *to prevent head injury and form habit of helmet use.*
- Teach the preschooler appropriate safety rules in the home (avoiding electric outlets, etc.): *the preschooler is able to follow simple directions and carry out directives. Limits help him or her to organize the environment.*
- Post poison control center phone number *(in case of accidental ingestion; the preschool child is very curious).*
- Never leave a preschool child unattended in a tub or pool or near any body of water *to prevent drowning.*
- Provide swimming lessons for children age 4 or 5 *to encourage water safety, but not as a replacement for adult supervision.*
- Teach parents first-aid measures and child CPR *to minimize consequences of injury should it occur.*
- Provide close observation and keep side rails up on bed in hospital *because the preschool child continues to be at risk for falling or injuring self on equipment or tubing (because of curiosity).*

NURSING DIAGNOSIS: Imbalanced nutrition, less than body requirements, related to inappropriate nutritional intake to sustain growth needs (excess juice or milk intake, inadequate food variety intake) as evidenced by failure to attain adequate increases in height and weight over time

Outcome Identification and Evaluation
Child will consume adequate nutrients: *Child will demonstrate weight gain and increases in height.*

Interventions: Promoting Appropriate Nutrition
- Assess current feeding schedule and usual intake, as well as methods used to feed, *to determine areas of adequacy versus inadequacy.*
- Determine if the preschooler is unable to drink from a cup or does not finger feed or use utensils properly, or if the child has difficulty swallowing or tolerating certain textures of foods *to determine if further interventions such as speech or occupational therapy are required.*
- Weigh child daily on same scale if hospitalized, weekly on same scale if at home, and plot growth patterns weekly or monthly as appropriate on standardized growth charts *to determine if growth is improving.*
- Limit juice to 4 to 6 ounces per day, milk to 16 to 24 ounces per day, *to discourage sense of fullness achieved with excess milk or juice intake, thereby increasing appetite for appropriate solid foods.*
- Provide three nutrient-dense meals and at least two healthy snacks per day *to encourage adequate nutrient consumption.*
- Feed child on a similar schedule daily, without distractions and with the family: *preschool children continue to respond well to routine and structure. They are more interested in the social context of meals and are still apt to become distracted easily, so the TV should be off at mealtimes.*

Nursing Care Plan 27.1 (continued)

NURSING DIAGNOSIS: Delayed growth and development related to motor, cognitive, language, or psychosocial concerns as evidenced by delay in meeting expected milestones

Outcome Identification and Evaluation
Development will be enhanced: *Child will make continued progress toward realization of expected developmental milestones.*

Interventions: Enhancing Growth and Development
- Screen for developmental capabilities *to determine child's current level of functioning.*
- Offer age-appropriate toys, play, and activities (including gross motor) *to encourage further development.*
- Perform interventions as prescribed by physical, occupational, or speech therapist: *participation in those activities helps to promote function and accomplish acquisition of developmental skills.*
- Provide support to families of preschoolers with developmental delay *(progress in achieving developmental milestones can be slow and ongoing motivation is needed).*
- Reinforce positive attributes in the child *to maintain motivation.*
- Model age-appropriate communication skills *to illustrate suitable means for parenting the preschooler.*

NURSING DIAGNOSIS: Risk for disproportionate growth related to excess milk or juice intake, consumption of inappropriate foods or in excess amounts

Outcome Identification and Evaluation
Child will grow appropriately and not become overweight or obese: *Child will achieve weight and height within the 5th to 85th percentiles on standardized growth charts.*

Interventions:
- Discourage use of no-spill sippy cups *(they contribute to dental caries and allow unlimited access to fluids, possibly decreasing appetite for appropriate solid foods).*
- Provide juice (4–6 ounces per day) and milk (16–24 ounces per day) from a cup at meal and snack time and water in between *to avoid having the child drink excessive juice or milk.*
- Provide only nutrient-rich foods without high sugar content for meals and snacks; *even if the preschooler is a picky eater, it is inappropriate to provide high-calorie junk food just so the child eats something.*
- Teach parents to role model appropriate eating (nutrient-rich, varied diet) *to encourage child to try/accept new foods, as well as become familiar with a variety of food.*
- Severely limit the intake of fast foods and foods with high sugar and fat content *to decrease intake of nutrient-poor, high-calorie foods.*
- Ensure adequate physical activity *to stimulate development of motor skills and provide appropriate caloric expenditure. This also sets the stage for forming lifelong habit of appropriate physical activity.*
- Teach parents to limit television viewing to 1 to 2 hours per day *to encourage participation in physical activities.*

NURSING DIAGNOSIS: Interrupted family processes related to issues with preschool child's development, hospitalization, or situational crisis as evidenced by decreased parental visitation in hospital, parental verbalization of difficulty with current situation, possible crisis related to health of family member other than the preschool child

Outcome Identification and Evaluation
Family will demonstrate adequate functioning: *Family will display coping and psychosocial adjustment.*

Interventions: Enhancing Family Functioning
- Assess the family's level of stress and ability to cope *to determine family's ability to cope with multiple stressors.*
- Engage in family-centered care *to provide a holistic approach to care of the preschooler and family.*
- Encourage the family to verbalize feelings *(verbalization is one method of decreasing anxiety levels)* and acknowledge feelings and emotions.
- Use puppets or dramatic play with the child *to elicit the preschooler's feelings about the current situation.*
- Encourage family visitation and provide for sleeping arrangements for a parent or caregiver to stay in the hospital with the preschooler; *this contributes to family's sense of control in situation.*
- Involve family members in preschooler's care, *giving them a feeling of control and connectedness.*

(continued)

Nursing Care Plan 27.1 (continued)

NURSING DIAGNOSIS: Readiness for enhanced parenting related to parental desire for increased skill level and success with preschool child as evidenced by current healthy relationships and verbalization of desire for improved skills

Outcome Identification and Evaluation

Parent will provide safe and nurturing environment for the preschool child: *Parents will verbalize new skills they will employ in the family.*

Interventions: Increasing Parenting Skill Set

- Use family-centered care *to provide holistic approach.*
- Educate parent about normal preschool development *to provide basis of understanding for parenting skills needed in this time period.*
- Acknowledge and encourage parents' verbalization of feelings related to chronic illness of child or difficulty with normal preschool behavior; *this validates the normalcy of parents' feelings.*
- Encourage positive parenting and respect for preschooler and his/her normal development *(helps parents develop approaches to preschoolers that can be used in place of anger and frustration).*
- Acknowledge and admire positive parenting skills already present *to contribute to parents' confidence in their abilities to parent.*
- Role model appropriate parenting behaviors related to communicating with and disciplining the child *(role modeling actually demonstrates rather than just verbalizes what the parent should strive for).*

Setting limits (and remaining consistent with those limits) continues to be important in the preschool period. Consistent limits provide the preschooler with expectation and guidance. As the preschooler increasingly participates in fantasy and imagination, the limits of routine and structure help guide his or her behavior and ability to distinguish reality.

Nurses caring for preschoolers should have knowledge of normal developmental expectations so they can determine whether the preschool child is progressing appropriately. Table 27.4 lists potential signs of developmental delay. A preschool child with one or more of these concerns should be referred for further developmental evaluation.

Promoting Growth and Development Through Play

Providing sincere encouragement for the preschool child's efforts and accomplishments helps him or her develop a sense of initiative. Giving children opportunities to decide how and with whom they want to play also helps them develop initiative. Preschool children like to write, color, draw, paint with a brush or their fingers, and trace or copy patterns (Fig. 27.8). They may start small collections that may be sorted. They like using toys for their intended purpose as well as for whatever invented purpose they can imagine.

Preschoolers begin to play cooperatively with one another. Play may be focused around a distinct theme. They define roles, make up rules, and assign jobs. They are able to work together toward a common goal such as building a house or fort with discarded boxes. Cooperative play encourages the preschool child to learn to share, take turns and compromise, listen to others' opinions, consider the feelings of others, and use self-control and overcome fears.

Preschoolers have incredible imaginations and love to play "make-believe" (Fig. 27.9). Encouraging pretend play and providing props for dress-up stimulates curiosity and creativity. Fantasy play is usually cooperative in nature. It encourages the preschooler to develop social skills such as taking turns, communication, paying attention, and responding to one another's words and actions. Fantasy play also allows preschoolers to explore complex social ideas such as power, compassion, and cruelty. Through role playing, children begin to develop their sexual identity as well.

Since preschool children have vivid imaginations, it is important to be careful about what television they watch. The preschooler should be limited to 1 to 2 hours per day of quality television. The violence in some television programs may scare the preschool child or inspire him or her to act out violent behavior.

Most preschoolers also engage in dramatic play, fueled by their innate curiosity and vivid imaginations. Three-year-olds may not realize that they are pretending. They run from scary creatures, make plans, and pack their backpacks (never intending to actually leave). Four-year-olds are more sophisticated with dramatic or pretend play: they know they are pretending, and they use dress-up clothes and props to act out more complex roles and scenarios (Fig. 27.10). Five-year-olds are capable of quite complex scenarios. They pretend they are real or fantasy characters.

TABLE 27.4 SIGNS OF DEVELOPMENTAL DELAY

Age	Concern
4 years	• Cannot jump in place or ride a tricycle • Cannot stack four blocks • Cannot throw ball overhand • Does not grasp crayon with thumb and fingers • Difficulty with scribbling • Cannot copy a circle • Does not use sentences with three or more words • Cannot use the words "me" and "you" appropriately • Ignores other children or does not show interest in interactive games • Will not respond to people outside the family; still clings or cries if parents leave • Resists using toilet, dressing, sleeping • Does not engage in fantasy play
By 5 years	• Unhappy or sad often • Little interest in playing with other children • Unable to separate from parent without major protest • Is extremely aggressive • Is extremely fearful or timid, or unusually passive • Cannot build tower of six to eight blocks • Easily distracted; cannot concentrate on single activity for 5 minutes • Rarely engages in fantasy play • Trouble with eating, sleeping, or using the toilet • Cannot use plurals or past tense • Cannot brush teeth, wash and dry hands, or undress efficiently

They often use dramatic play to express anxiety, try out negative feelings, or conquer their fears. For example, a child who is afraid of getting a shot at the doctor's office may work through that feeling with pretend play.

Parents should encourage physical activity in the preschool child. Regular physical activity improves gross motor skills, may enhance the child's self-confidence, and allows the child to expend excess energy. Establishing the habit of daily physical activity in the early years is important in the long-term goal of avoiding obesity. The main goal of organized sports at this age should be fun and enjoyment, although of course safety must remain a priority.

Beware of sophisticated toys that claim to teach the young child. These toys are often very expensive and are not necessary. Box 27.1 lists appropriate playthings for the preschool child.

FIGURE 27.8 The preschool child loves to create things, so coloring and molding clay are ideal activities for children this age.

FIGURE 27.9 Preschool children enjoy imitative play.

Promoting Early Learning

The family is the foundation for the child's early growth and development. Parents serve as role models for behavior related to education and learning, as well as instilling values in their children. School readiness is a topic that has received a significant amount of national attention in recent years. To succeed in school, children need a safe, responsive home environment that allows them to learn and explore, as well as structure and limits that allow them to learn the socially acceptable behaviors that they will need in school. Language development is critical to the ability to succeed in school and can be encouraged through books and reading. Each of these components is important in readying the child for education in a more formal setting. Promoting language development, choosing a preschool,

FIGURE 27.10 Preschool children love to dress up and pretend.

BOX 27.1 **Appropriate Toys for Preschoolers**

- Blocks, simple jigsaw puzzles (four to six large pieces), pegboards, wooden bead with string
- Supplies for creativity: chalk, large crayons, finger paint, Play-Doh or clay, washable markers, paper, paint and paintbrush, scissors, paste, or glue
- Puppets, dress-up clothes and props for dramatic play
- Bucket, plastic shovel and other containers for sand and water play
- Play kitchen with accessories and pretend food (empty food boxes can be recycled for kitchen play)
- Squeaking, floating, squirting toys for the bath
- Sandbox with shovel and various toys for building
- Dolls that can be dressed and undressed (large buttons, zippers, and snaps), doll care accessories (diapers, bottles, carriage, crib)
- Gross motor toys: tricycle or big wheel (with helmet), jungle gym or swing set (with supervision), hula hoop, tunnel, wagon
- Blocks, Legos, cars and trucks, plastic animals, trains, plastic figures (family, community helpers), stuffed animals, balls, sewing cards
- Tape or CD players for music, various musical instruments
- Simple card and board games (older preschooler)
- Dollhouse with furniture and accessories, people and animals

and making the transition to kindergarten are discussed in more detail below.

Promoting Language Development

The parent serves as the child's first teacher. The interactions between parent and child in relation to books and other play activities model the types of interactions that the child will later have in school. Asking open-ended questions stimulates the development of thinking as well as language in the preschool child. The preschooler is a great imitator, so the parent should serve as a role model for appropriate language. Parents should avoid swearing, as the child is sure to repeat "bad words" even if he or she does not understand what they mean. Allowing children to pursue interests at their own pace will help them to develop the literacy and numeric skills that will enable them to later focus on academic skills.

Preschoolers enjoy books with pictures that tell stories (Fig. 27.11). Stories with repeated phrases help to keep the child's attention. Children like stories that describe experiences similar to their own. The preschool child demonstrates early literacy skills by reciting stories or portions of books. He or she also may retell the story from the book, pretend to read books, and ask questions about the story. The preschool child has enough focus and expanded atten-

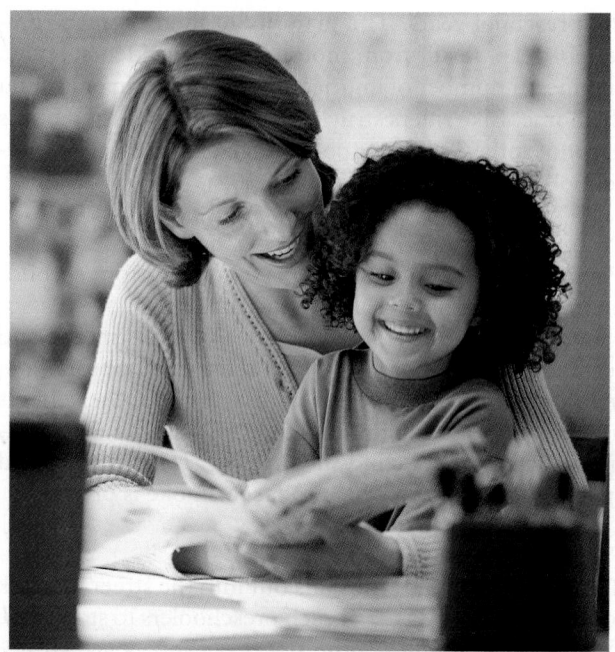

FIGURE 27.11 Preschool children enjoy being read to and looking at the pictures that go along with the story.

tion to notice when a page is skipped during reading and will call it to the parent's attention.

> ▶ **Take** NOTE!
>
> *Risk factors for lack of social and emotional readiness for school include insecure attachment in the early years, maternal depression, parental substance abuse, and low socioeconomic status. Nurses should screen for these factors and make referrals if appropriate.*

Choosing a Preschool/Starting Kindergarten

Many parents choose to enroll their child in preschool. Preschool should be used primarily as an opportunity to foster the child's social skills and accustom him or her to the group environment. When selecting a preschool the parent may want to consider the accreditation of the school, the teachers' qualifications, and recommendations of other parents. The focus of the school environment is also important: What is the daily schedule of activities? Is the school very structured, or does it have a looser environment? The parents must decide how focused on curriculum they want the school to be. The parent should observe the classroom, evaluating the environment, noise level, and sanitary practices as well as how the children interact with each other and how the teachers interact with the children.

The type of discipline used in the school is also an important factor. Parents should not choose a preschool

that uses corporal punishment. The American Academy of Pediatrics discourages the use of corporal punishment in the school setting. Corporal punishment may hurt a child's self-esteem as well as his or her ability to achieve in school. It may also lead to disruptive and violent behavior in the classroom. As preschool is the foundation for later education, the child should have the opportunity to build self-esteem and the skills needed for the more formal setting of elementary school.

Whether or not the child attended preschool, kindergarten will be the next big step. Kindergarten hours may be longer than preschool hours, and kindergarten is usually held 5 days per week. This may be a significant change for some children. For most children, the setting and personnel in kindergarten will be new to the child. Rules and expectations are often very different as well. When discussing starting kindergarten with the preschool child, parents should do so in an enthusiastic fashion, keeping the conversation light and positive. Parents should meet with the child's teacher prior to the start of school, if possible, to discuss particular needs or concerns. Parents may want to schedule a tour of the school for the preschooler or attend the school's open house with the child to ease the transition. Practicing the new daily routine prior to the start of school will also be helpful.

Most states require up-to-date immunizations and a health screening of the child before he or she enters kindergarten, so advise parents to plan ahead and schedule these in a timely fashion so that school entrance is not delayed.

Promoting Safety

In the United States, accidental injury remains the leading cause of death for children between the ages of 1 and 14 years. Preschoolers are at an ideal age to be taught about safety and safe behaviors. They are cognitively able to absorb concrete information and they desire to master the situations they are in, but they continue to display poor judgment related to safety issues. Their engagement in fantasy is so strong that it makes it difficult for them to master complicated cause-and-effect relationships. The preschool child is capable of learning safe behaviors but may not always be able to transfer those behaviors to a different situation. Parents must continue to closely supervise preschool children to avoid accidental injury during this period.

Safety in the Car

The young preschooler who weighs less than 40 pounds should use a forward-facing car seat with harness and top tether. The preschooler who weighs between 40 and 80 pounds should ride in a booster seat that uses both the lap and shoulder belts (Fig. 27.12). When the child is large enough to sit up straight with the knees bent at the front edge of the seat, he or she may sit directly on the seat of the car with the lap/shoulder belt securely and appropriately

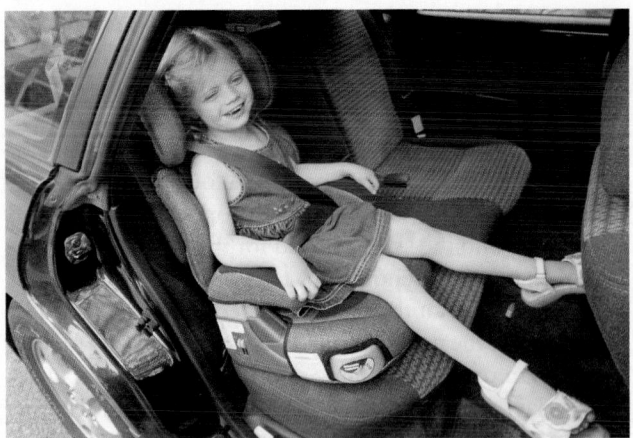

FIGURE 27.12 The preschool child who weighs more than 40 pounds should be appropriately secured in an approved booster seat.

attached. The lap belt should sit low over the hips and upper thighs and the shoulder belt should stay on the shoulder and close to the chest. The back seat of the car is always the safest place for a child to ride. If a child under 12 years of age must sit in the front seat because there are not enough rear seats available, then the front passenger seat air bag should be deactivated. Children should never ride in the cargo area of a pickup truck. See Healthy People 2010 (see Evidence-Based Practice 27.1).

> ▶ **Take** NOTE!
>
> *Although motor vehicle accidents remain a major cause of injury and death in the preschool age group, many families do not use appropriate car seat/seat belt safety with their children. Child passenger safety technicians are available to provide proper installation of car seats. To find one in your area, visit www.nhtsa.dot.gov/people/injury/childps/contacts or www.seatcheck.org. The NHTSA Auto Safety Hot Line may be reached at (888) 327-4236.*

Safety in the Home

Handguns, matches, bodies of water, bicycle riding, and poisons continue to be sources of potential injury during

the preschool years. The majority of injuries in the preschool years result from motor vehicle accidents, with a significant number of injuries also occurring in or around the home. Bike riders struck by motor vehicles and burns account for a significant percentage of deaths in the preschool age group (Dowd et al., 2002).

Preventing Exposure to Tobacco Smoke

Parents should protect their preschoolers from secondhand tobacco smoke. Exposure to tobacco smoke is associated with an increased incidence of otitis media and respiratory infections, as well as increased symptoms and medication use in children with asthma. Other effects include decreased lung function and behavioral difficulties. The preschool child should never be in an enclosed space (such as a car) where tobacco smoke is present.

Preventing Injury

The preschool child who runs out into the street is at risk for being struck by a car. Teach preschoolers to stop at the curb and never go into the street without a grown-up. The preschooler may learn to ride a bicycle (with or without training wheels). The child must wear an approved bicycle helmet any time he or she rides the bicycle, even if it is just in the driveway. Requiring helmet use in the early years will lead to the habit of helmet use as the child gets older. Allowing the preschooler to choose his or her own helmet may encourage the child to use the helmet.

Bicycles should be safe for this age group. The size must be correct; the balls of the feet should reach both pedals while the child is sitting on the seat and has both hands on the handlebars. Children under 5 years of age have difficulty learning to use hand-operated brakes, so traditional pedal-back brakes are recommended in this age group. Preschoolers are not mature enough to ride a bicycle in the street even if they are riding with adults, so they should always ride on the sidewalk.

It is important to make the inside of the home safe for the preschool child. Parents should install and maintain smoke alarms in the home. Increased physical dexterity and refinement of motor skills enable the preschooler to strike matches or use a lighter and start a fire. The preschool child is capable of washing his or her hands independently, so the water heater should be set at 120°F or below to prevent scalding.

The preschooler's active imagination and desire to play make-believe may result in a firearm injury. The average preschooler is physically capable of handling and firing a gun, particularly a handgun, which is smaller and lighter. If present in the home, firearms should be kept in a locked cabinet with the ammunition stored elsewhere.

Preventing Poisoning

Though it is continuing to develop, preschoolers still have unrefined taste discrimination, placing them at risk for accidental ingestion. Parents should never try to coax a child to take a vitamin supplement, tablet, or pill by calling

EVIDENCE-BASED PRACTICE 27.1
Interventions Directed Toward Acquiring and Using Booster Seats for Children 4 to 8 Years Old

● Study

Children outgrow toddler car seats around the age of 4 years or when they weigh 40 pounds. Regular seat belts do not fit children properly. The purpose of booster seats for the 4- to 8-year-old child is to raise him or her higher on the seat of the car, in order for the adult seat belt to secure the child properly. Booster seats provide increased comfort and safety for this age group. Booster seat use in this age group has been shown to decrease injury and death via motor vehicle accident by nearly 60%. The authors reviewed five studies involving 3,070 subjects and performed a meta-analysis of the study results. Each of the randomized controlled trials reviewed assessed the efficacy of interventions directed toward increasing booster seat use.

▲ Findings

The authors' meta-analysis of the studies revealed that interventions directed toward improving booster seat use can make a difference. Enforcement of booster seat law was the weakest intervention. More successful interventions all included education of parents about the importance and appropriate use of booster seats. Providing a free booster seat upon completion of the training or an incentive coupon to receive a discount upon purchase were the most helpful interventions.

■ Nursing Implications

Parents want to protect their children from injury when riding in motor vehicles, but many may lack the knowledge or financial resources to do so. Nurses are in a unique position to provide ongoing, repeated education about the importance of booster seat use for the preschooler to families wherever they encounter them. Nurses can also seek out resources in their individual communities to provide financial incentives to assist families with obtaining a booster seat. Nurses should always praise preschoolers for complying with booster seat use while riding in vehicles.

Ehiri, J. E., Ejere, H. O. D., Magnussen, L., Emusu, D., King, W., & Osberg, J. S. (2007). Interventions for promoting booster seat use in four to eight year olds traveling in motor vehicles. *The Cochrane Library 2007, 4.*

---

it "candy." Dangerous fluids should be stored in their original containers and should be kept out of reach of preschoolers; they should not be poured into containers that look like ordinary drinking glasses or cups. Potentially dangerous cleaning or personal health and beauty products, gardening and pool chemicals, as well as automotive materials should be kept out of reach of preschoolers and in a locked cabinet if possible. Medications should have childproof caps and should be kept in a locked cabinet. The poison control telephone number should be posted on or near the home phone (1-800-222-1222).

Safety in the Water

Five years of age is an appropriate time for a child to learn to swim. Children at this age are physically capable of this activity and have the cognitive maturity to accomplish the task of swimming and basic water safety. Swimming programs should focus on appropriate swim techniques as well as safety measures. Parents and caregivers should be trained in infant/child CPR. Homes with swimming pools should have lifesaving devices readily accessible. Preschoolers should be taught never to dive into water until an adult has verified its depth. Preschoolers are still too young to be left unattended around any body of water, even if they know how to swim. Preschoolers should never be allowed to swim in a canal or any fast-moving water. Preschoolers who are riding in boats or fishing off riverbanks should wear a personal flotation device. Parents should also be cautioned about close supervision of young children walking, skating, or riding near thin or weak ice. See Healthy People 2010.

▶ *Take* NOTE!

The American Academy of Pediatrics recommends that all swimming pools be secured by a fence that is at least 5 feet high and has a self-latching gate to protect young children from entering a pool area unattended (AAP, 2003).

HEALTHY PEOPLE 2010

Objective	Nursing Significance
Reduce drownings.	• Never leave a young child unattended in or near the water. • Educate families about water safety. • Remind families that the preschooler's ability to swim does not replace the need for constant supervision while in the pool or other body of water.

*R*ecall Nila Patel, the 4-year-old presented at the beginning of the chapter. What anticipatory guidance related to safety should you provide to her parents?

Promoting Nutrition

The preschool child has a full set of primary teeth, is able to chew and swallow competently, and has learned to use utensils fairly effectively to feed himself or herself (Fig. 27.13). As in the toddler years, it is important for the preschool child to continue to learn and build upon healthy eating habits. These habits will last throughout the child's life. A diet high in nutrient-rich foods such as whole grains, vegetables, fruits, appropriate dairy foods, and lean meats is appropriate for the preschooler. Nutrient-poor, high-calorie foods such as sweets and typical fast foods should be offered only in limited amounts.

Nutritional Needs

The 3- to 5-year-old requires 500 to 800 mg calcium and 10 mg iron daily. The 3-year-old should consume 19 mg dietary fiber daily, while the 4- to 8-year-old requires 25 mg dietary fiber per day. Box 27.2 lists good calcium and iron sources. The typical preschooler requires about 85 kcal/kg of body weight. Saturated fats should account for less than 10% of total calories. Preschool children's diets should include a daily total fat intake of no less than 20% and not more than 30% of total calories to promote and maintain healthy cholesterol levels.

▶ *Take* NOTE!

Drinking excess amounts of milk may lead to iron deficiency, as the calcium in milk blocks iron absorption.

FIGURE 27.13 The preschool child has the manual dexterity to handle utensils appropriately and feed himself or herself independently.

BOX 27.2 **Daily Calcium and Iron Recommendations for Preschool Children**

Calcium: 500 mg (3-year-old), 800 mg (4- to 8-year-old)   **Iron: 10 mg**

Calcium in foods:
- 8 oz low-fat or whole milk: 300 mg
- 8 oz low-fat yogurt: 300 mg
- 1½ oz cheddar cheese: 300 mg
- 1 oz dried white beans (cooked): 160 mg
- ¼ cup tofu: 125 mg
- 1 medium orange: 50 mg
- ½ cup mashed sweet potatoes: 44 mg
- ½ cup cooked or 1½ cup raw broccoli: 35 mg

Iron in foods:
- ¾ cup 100% fortified prepared cereal: 18 mg
- ¾ cup 50% fortified prepared cereal: 9 mg
- 3 oz beef: 3 mg
- 3 oz chicken leg: 3 mg
- ½ cup cooked lentils: 3 mg
- 3 oz chicken breast: 2 mg
- ¼ cup fresh cooked spinach: 1.6 mg
- ¼ cup tofu: 0.9 mg
- 1 slice enriched bread: 0.8 to 0.9 mg
- ¼ cup frozen spinach, cooked: 0.7 mg

Promoting Healthy Eating Habits

Preschool children may be picky eaters. They may eat only a limited variety of foods or foods prepared in certain ways and may not be very willing to try new things. The 3- or 4-year-old may exhibit "food fads," eating only certain foods over a several-day period. As the child gets older, pickiness lessens. By 5 years of age the child is more focused on the social context of eating: table conversation and manners. The 5-year-old is generally more willing to at least try new foods and may like to help with meal preparation and clean-up as appropriate.

If the preschooler is growing well, then the pickiness is not a cause for concern. A larger concern may be the negative relationship that can develop between the parent and child relating to mealtime. The more the parent coaxes, cajoles, bribes, and threatens, the less likely the child is to try new foods or even eat the ones he or she likes that are served. The parent must maintain a positive and patient demeanor at mealtime. The child should be offered a healthy diet, with foods from all groups over the course of the day as recommended by the USDA. The "Food Guide Pyramid for Your Young Child" (from the United States Department of Agriculture) may be used to plan the preschool child's daily diet. See Figure 26.9 in Chapter 26, and note the explanation of serving sizes at the bottom of the chart.

The parent should maintain a matter-of-fact approach, offer the meal or snack, and then allow the child to decide

HEALTHY PEOPLE 2010

Objective	Nursing Significance
Increase the proportion of persons aged 2 years and older who meet dietary recommendations for calcium.	• Screen preschoolers for appropriate dietary intake of calcium. • Educate families about calcium content in foods. • Assist families with choosing a diet that meets calcium needs and is appealing to the young child.

how much of the food, if any, he or she is going to eat. High-fat, nutrient-poor snacks should not be substituted for healthy foods just to coax the child to "eat something." See Healthy People 2010.

Preventing the Development of Overweight and Obesity

Worldwide, over 22 million children under 5 years old are obese. In the past 30 years, the number of U.S. children and adolescents who are overweight has doubled. According to the National Health and Nutrition Examination Survey, 21% of all 2- to 5-year-olds are either overweight or at risk of overweight (NAPNAP, 2006a). Overweight and obese children are at risk for hypertension, hyperlipidemia, and the development of insulin resistance. Children whose weight is at or above the 95th percentile when 3 to 6 years old have a 50% chance of being obese as adults (Krebs et al., 2004). The risk is increased if one or both parents are overweight.

Parents are in an opportune position to exert a positive influence on their preschooler's nutritional intake and activity level. The habits learned in early childhood will likely carry over into the school-age, adolescent, and adult years. Children whose parents take an authoritarian approach to mealtime may learn to overeat, as they are encouraged to finish the entire meal ("Clean your plate!"). If they are offered appropriate, healthy food choices and access to high-calorie, nutrient-poor food is limited, preschoolers will learn to self-regulate (eat only until full). Food should not be used as either reward or punishment.

Parents should remain positive and patient at mealtime. Mealtimes should continue to be structured. Unstructured meals lead to an increase in fat and calorie consumption. Increased amount of calories as fat has been linked to a higher body mass index (BMI) in preschool children. To limit the chance that overeating will occur, preschoolers should be offered a variety of healthy foods at each meal. This may include one each of a protein source, grain, vegetable, and fruit. The preschool child's serving size is usually one third to one half of the recommended size of an adult serving. The preschool child may imitate the other eaters at the table. Parents have a prime chance to be good role models, setting an example of eating vegetables and fruits.

As with toddlers, fruit juice should be limited to 4 to 6 ounces per day, as excess consumption can lead to excess weight gain. Preschoolers should be encouraged to drink water.

Limiting television viewing and encouraging physical activity are also important strategies for the prevention of overweight and obesity.

Refer back to Nila Patel, the 4-year-old introduced at the beginning of the chapter. What questions should you ask Nila's parents related to nutritional intake? What anticipatory guidance related to nutrition would be appropriate? Nila's mother expresses concerns regarding obesity. How would you address these?

Promoting Healthy Sleep and Rest

The preschool child needs about 12 hours of sleep each day. Some preschool children continue to take a nap during the day. Unless very tired, many preschool children will resist going to bed from time to time. Bedtime rituals continue to be reassuring to children, and it is important to continue them in the preschool years. Having a time of relaxation with a decrease in stimulation will allow the child to fall asleep more easily. Some children continue to need a security item at bedtime or naptime. A nightlight in the bedroom may be necessary, as many children this age are afraid of the dark. Teaching Guidelines 27.1

TEACHING GUIDELINES 27.1

Bedtime Routines

• Establish a bedtime as well as morning wake-up time, and enforce them consistently.
• Avoid sugar or caffeine consumption in the evening.
• Avoid stimulating activities such as roughhousing before bedtime.
• Do not allow television watching in bed.
• Make the child's bedroom an inviting and comfortable area of the home.
• Provide a nightlight in the child's bedroom if he or she is afraid of the dark.
• Conform to a nightly routine:
  • Television off at a certain time
  • Bath
  • Quiet game or story reading/telling
  • Bedtime prayer or song
• Maintain quiet in the bedroom and nearby to increase the child's ability to fall asleep.

gives information about assisting parents to establish a bedtime routine.

Nightmares often occur in preschool children as a result of the child's struggle to distinguish what is real from what is not. When a child awakens from a nightmare, he or she is often crying and may be able to recount what the dream was about. Parents should validate the child's fear rather than discounting it. Saying, "Yes, I agree, monsters are scary; it's a good thing they aren't real" is more appropriate than, "Don't be silly: monsters aren't real." Sometimes children benefit from reading stories about dreams. Recommended books include:

• *Bedtime for Frances* by Russell Hoban
• *Ben's Dream* by Chris van Allsberg
• *In the Night Kitchen* by Maurice Sendak
• *There's a Nightmare in My Closet* by Mercer Mayer

Nightmares should not be confused with night terrors. After a nightmare, the child is aroused and interactive, but night terrors are different: a short time after falling asleep, the child seems to awaken and is screaming. The child usually does not respond much to the parent's soothing, but he or she eventually stops screaming and goes back to sleep. Night terrors are often frightening for parents because the child does not seem to be responding to them. One technique that may help to decrease the incidence of night terrors is to wake the child about 30 to 45 minutes into the sleep cycle. If continued nightly for about a week, the cycle of night terrors may be broken. See Comparison Chart 27.1.

Think back to Nila Patel. What anticipatory guidance would you provide to her parents in relation to sleep during the preschool years?

Promoting Healthy Teeth and Gums

Dental caries prevention continues to be important and can be achieved through daily brushing and flossing. Parents should use only a pea-sized amount of toothpaste to prevent excess fluoride consumption, which can contribute to fluorosis. The preschooler may brush his or her own teeth, but the parent must continue to supervise to ensure adequate brushing. Parents must perform flossing because the preschool child cannot perform this task adequately.

Cariogenic foods should be avoided. If sugary foods are consumed, the mouth should be rinsed with water if it is not possible to brush the teeth immediately. The preschool child should visit the dentist every 6 months.

▶ *Take* NOTE!

Dental caries prevention is important in the primary teeth, because loss of these teeth to caries may affect the proper formation of permanent teeth as well as the width of the dental arch.

Promoting Appropriate Discipline

Successful discipline results from a loving and nurturing environment in which the preschooler's self-esteem is fostered and where limits are well chosen and enforced consistently. Spanking (striking with the open hand) is the least effective discipline practice and is discouraged by the American Academy of Pediatrics and the National Association of Pediatric Nurse Practitioners. Belts, switches, paddles, or other items should never be used to strike a

COMPARISON CHART 27.1 NIGHTMARES VERSUS NIGHT TERRORS

	Nightmare	Night Terror
Definition	Scary or bad dream followed by awakening	Partial arousal from deep sleep
When parents become aware	Child awakens parent after episode is over	Screaming and thrashing during the episode awakens the parent
Timing	Usually in the second half of the night	Usually about an hour after falling asleep
Behavior	Crying, may be scared after awakening	Sits up, thrashes, cries, screams, talks, looks wild-eyed. Sweats, may have racing heartbeat.
Responsiveness	Responsive to parent's soothing and reassurances	Child unaware of parent's presence, may scream and thrash more if restrained
Return to sleep	Difficulty going back to sleep if afraid	Rapidly returns to sleep without full awakening
Memory of occurrence	May remember the dream and talk about it later	No memory of event

Information from Ferber, R. (2006). *Solve your child's sleep problems*. New York: Fireside.

child. The use of physical punishment has been associated with a number of additional problems in adulthood, such as antisocial and criminal behaviors (see Chapter 26).

If parents are consistent with discipline while encouraging the preschooler's normal growth and development of imagination and make-believe, the child will learn to accept that certain things are not allowed. The sense of initiative can be preserved and guilt avoided if the rules are clear and enforced consistently.

> ▶ *Take* NOTE!
>
> *The more frequently children are hit in the preschool years, the more anger they report as adults (AAP, 2004a).*

Minimize the occurrence of misbehavior by anticipating conditions likely to lead to the undesired or risky action. When the situation becomes difficult, parents should use distraction to changes the preschooler's focus. When discussing the misbehavior, be certain to label the behavior and not the child. This helps to preserve the preschooler's self-esteem. When teaching preschoolers about undesired behavior, be sure they also understand the reason why it is wrong or unacceptable to do it. This helps to encourage the child to use internal controls over behavior. Parents should serve as role models for self-control, including choice of words, the tone they are delivered in, and the actions that accompany them.

Children work harder to obtain praise than to receive punishment, so always reward positive behaviors. Preschool children are becoming capable of understanding the concept of right and wrong. They start to understand each other's feelings (**empathy**) and are cognitively capable of remembering basic rules.

Time-out or time away from the situation can be very effective in this age group. The punishment should be used only for intentional misbehavior (knowing something is forbidden but doing it anyway). It is particularly helpful with dangerous or destructive behavior. The preschooler is given a warning that time-out will occur if the behavior does not stop. The preschooler is removed from the situation and must stay in time-out for a specified period of time. A particular time-out area is helpful; a boring corner of the room without distractions available is a good location. The generally recommended period of time is to require 1 minute of time-out per year of age; thus, a 4-year-old would be in time-out for 4 minutes. Set the timer so the child will know when the time-out is over. If the child gets up before the prescribed time, replace the child in time-out and restart the timer. Time-out works best if used each and every time the undesirable behavior occurs. Also, praise the child when he or she follows the rules and behaves appropriately.

A simple and clear explanation of the misbehavior should be given to the child; parents should also talk about acceptable alternative strategies that the child can use in the future instead of the undesired behavior. Removal of a privilege such as playing with a favorite toy can be as effective as time-out.

Books and other media that are available to help educate parents about appropriate discipline and to help the child learn self-control are listed in Box 27.3.

BOX 27.3 **Selected Resources for Parent and Preschoolers**

Books for Parents (about discipline)
- *How to Talk so Kids will Listen and Listen so Kids will Talk* by A. Faber & E. Mazlish (Harper Resource)
- *Kids are Worth It: Giving Your Children the Gift of Inner Discipline* by B. Colorosos (Harper Collins Publishers)
- *Positive Discipline A to Z: 1001 Solutions to Everyday Parenting Problems* by J. Nelson, L. Lott, & S. G. Glenn (Three Rivers Press)
- *Setting Limits with Your Strong-willed Child: Eliminating Conflict by Establishing Clear, Firm and Respectful Boundaries* by R. MacKenzie (Three Rivers Press)
- *The Case Against Spanking: How to Discipline Children without Hitting* by I. A. Hyman (Jossey-Bass)
- *The Nurturing Parent: How to Raise Creative, Loving, Responsible Children* by J. S. Dacey & A. J. Packer (Fireside)
- *Without Spanking or Spoiling: a Practical Approach to Toddler and Preschool Guidance* by E. Crary (Parenting Press)

Books for Preschoolers (about dealing with feelings and learning how to behave):
- *Hands are Not for Hitting* by M. Agassi (Free Spirit Publishing)
- *I Can't Wait* by E. Crary (Parenting Press)
- *I Want It* by E. Crary (Parenting Press)
- *I Want to Play* by E. Crary (Parenting Press)
- *I Was so Mad* by M. Mayer (Golden Books)
- *I Was so Mad* by N. Simon & D. Leder (Albert Whitman & Company)
- *I'm Excited* by E. Crary (Parenting Press)
- *I'm Frustrated* by E. Crary (Parenting Press)
- *I'm Mad* by E. Crary (Parenting Press)
- *I'm Scared* by E. Crary (Parenting Press)
- *Feet are not for Kicking* by E. Verdick (Free Spirit Publishing)
- *Teeth are not for Biting* by E. Verdick (Free Spirit Publishing)
- *When Sophie gets Angry . . . Really, Really Angry* by M. Bang (Blue Sky Press)
- *Words are not for Hurting* by E. Verdick (Free Spirit Publishing)

▶ ADDRESSING COMMON
DEVELOPMENTAL CONCERNS

Common developmental concerns of the preschool period include lying, sex education, and masturbation. Parents often express difficulty in dealing with these issues with their preschool children. Offering appropriate anticipatory guidance may give the parents the support and confidence they need to deal with these issues.

Lying

Lying is common in preschool children. It may occur because the child fears punishment, has gotten carried away with imagination, or is imitating what he or she sees the parent do. The parent should ascertain the reason for the lie before punishing the child. If the child has broken a rule and fears punishment, then the parent must determine the truth. The child needs to learn that lying is usually far worse than the misbehavior itself. The punishment for the misbehavior should be lessened if the child admits the truth. The parent should remain calm and serve as a role model of an even temper. The next time the misbehavior occurs, the child will be more apt to simply tell the truth.

If the child's lying is really just his or her imagination getting carried away, then the parent should guide the child in distinguishing between myth and reality. The preschooler's imagination is very vivid, and the child needs direction in the use of that faculty. Parents should serve as role models of appropriate behavior for their children to learn it. Children who lie because they hear their parents do it simply must not see or hear their parents do it.

Sex Education

Preschoolers are keen observers but are still not able to interpret all that they see correctly. The child may recognize, but not understand, sexual activity. Preschoolers are very inquisitive and want to learn about everything around them; therefore, they are very likely to ask questions about sex and where babies come from. Before attempting to answer questions, parents should try to find out first what the child is really asking and what the child already thinks about that subject. Then they should provide a simple, direct, and honest answer. The child needs only the information that he or she is requesting. Additional questions will occur in the future and should be addressed as they arise.

Masturbation

The normal curiosity of the preschool years often leads children to explore their own genitals. This behavior may be upsetting to some parents, but masturbation is a healthy and natural part of normal preschool development if it occurs in moderation. If the parent overreacts to this behavior, then it may occur more frequently. Masturbation should be treated in a matter-of-fact way by the parent. The child needs to learn certain rules about this activity: nudity and masturbation are not acceptable in public. The child should also be taught safety: no other person can touch the private parts unless it is the parent, doctor, or nurse checking to see when something is wrong.

*T*hink back to Nila Patel. What are some developmental concerns that are common during the preschool years? What anticipatory guidance related to these concerns would you provide to Nila's parents?

■■■ Key Concepts

■ The preschool child grows at a slower rate and takes on a more slender and upright appearance than the toddler.

■ The primary psychosocial task of the preschool period is developing a sense of initiative.

■ Cognitive development moves from an egocentric approach to the world toward a more empathetic understanding of what happens outside of the self.

■ The preschooler gains additional motor skills and displays significant refinement of fine motor abilities.

■ Cognitive and language skills that develop in the preschool years help prepare the child for success in school.

■ Dysfluency or hesitancy in speech is a normal finding in the preschool period and occurs as a result of the fast pace with which the preschooler is gaining language skills and vocabulary.

■ The vocabulary of a preschooler increases to about 2,100 words, and the child speaks in full sentences with appropriate use of tense and prepositions.

■ Appropriate growth and development should be maintained in the ill or hospitalized child.

■ Recognizing concerns or delays in growth and development is essential so that the appropriate referrals may be made and intervention can begin.

■ The preschool child requires a well-balanced diet with fat content between 20 and 30 percent of calories consumed.

■ Adequate physical activity and provision of a nutrient-dense diet (rather than foods high in fat and sugar) are the foundation for obesity prevention in the preschool child.

■ Adequate dental care is important for the health of the primary teeth.

■ Preschoolers need about 12 hours of sleep per day and benefit from a structured bedtime routine.

■ Due to the active imagination of the preschooler, nightmares and night terrors may begin during this period.

■ Safety and injury prevention remain a focus in the preschool years.

■ Structure, appropriate limit setting, and consistency are the keys for effective discipline in the preschool period.

■ Time-out is an effective disciplinary measure for pre-schoolers.

■ Masturbation may occur as the preschooler discovers his or her body. If not excessive, it is considered a normal part of growth and development.

REFERENCES

American Academy of Pediatric Dentistry. (2007). *Policy on use of fluoride.* Retrieved August 28, 2007 from http://www.aapd.org/media/Policies_Guidelines/P_FluorideUse.pdf.

American Academy of Pediatrics. (2003). Policy statement: Prevention of drowning in infants, children and adolescents. *Pediatrics, 112*(2), 437–439.

American Academy of Pediatrics. (2004a). *Guidance for effective discipline.* Retrieved August 28, 2007 from http://aappolicy.aappublications.org/cgi/content/full/pediatrics;101/4/723.

American Academy of Pediatrics. (2004b). *Policy statement: Swimming programs for infants and toddlers.* Retrieved August 28, 2007 from http://aappolicy.aappublications.org/cgi/content/full/pediatrics;105/4/868.

American Academy of Pediatrics. (2006). *Corporal punishment in schools.* Retrieved August 28, 2007 from http://aappolicy.aappublications.org/cgi/content/full/pediatrics;106/2/343.

American Academy of Pediatrics. (2007a). *Car safety seats: A guide for families 2007.* Retrieved August 28, 2007 from http://www.aap.org/family/carseatguide.htm.

American Academy of Pediatrics. (2007b). *Poison prevention and treatment tips.* Retrieved August 28, 2007 from http://www.aap.org/advocacy/releases/poisonpreventiontips.htm.

American Academy of Pediatrics. (2007c). *Policy statement: Poison treatment in the home.* Retrieved August 28, 2007 from http://aappolicy.aappublications.org/cgi/content/full/pediatrics;112/5/1182.

American Academy of Pediatrics. (2007d). *Policy statement: The uses and misuse of fruit juice in pediatrics.* Retrieved August 28, 2007 from http://aappolicy.aappublications.org/cgi/content/full/pediatrics;107/5/1210.

American Academy of Pediatrics, The Injury Prevention Program. (2007a). *Age-related safety sheets: 2 to 4 years.* Retrieved August 28, 2007 from http://www.aap.org/family/2to4yrs.htm.

American Academy of Pediatrics, The Injury Prevention Program. (2007b). *Age-related safety sheets: 5 years.* Retrieved August 28, 2007 from http://www.aap.org/family/5years.htm.

Bautista, S. R., & Flynn, J. R. (2006). Trauma prevention in children. *Pediatric Annals, 35*(2), 85–90.

Brazelton, T. B. (2001). *Touchpoints three to six: Your child's emotional and behavioral development.* Cambridge, MA: Perseus Publishing Company.

Christakis, D. A., & Zimmerman, F. J. (2007). Children & television: A primer for pediatricians. *Contemporary Pediatrics, 24*(3), 31–42.

Erikson, E. H. (1963). *Childhood and society* (2nd ed.). New York: W. W. Norton and Company.

Ferber, R. (2006). *Solve your child's sleep problems* (2nd ed.). New York: Fireside.

Fosarelli, P. (2003). Children and the development of faith: Implications for pediatric practice. *Contemporary Pediatrics, 20*(1), 85–98.

Green, M., & Palfrey, J. S. (Eds.). (2002). *Bright futures: Guidelines for health supervision of infants, children, and adolescents* (2nd ed., rev.). Arlington, VA: National Center for Education in Maternal and Child Health.

Krebs, N. F., Collins, J., & Johnson, S. L. (2004). Screen for and treat overweight in 2-to 5-year-olds? Yes! *Contemporary Pediatrics.* [Electronic version] Available at: www.contemporarypediatrics.com

Meadows-Oliver, M. (2007). Using our heads: What PNPs need to know about helmets. *Journal of Pediatric Health Care, 21*(4), 265–267.

National Association of Pediatric Nurse Practitioners. (2006a). *Healthy eating and activity together (HEAT) clinical practice guideline: identifying and preventing overweight in childhood.* Cherry Hill, NJ: Author.

National Association of Pediatric Nurse Practitioners. (2006b). NAPNAP position statement on corporal punishment. *Journal of Pediatric Health Care, 20*(6), A43–A44.

National Association for Sport & Physical Education. (2007). *Active start: A statement of physical activity guidelines for children birth to five years.* Retrieved August 28, 2007 from http://www.aahperd.org/NASPE/ns_active.html.

Papalia, D. E., Olds, S. W., & Feldman, F. D. (2006). *Human development* (10th ed.). New York: McGraw-Hill.

Passehl, B., McCarroll, C., Buechner, J., Gearring, C., Smith, A. E., & Trowbridge, F. (2004). Preventing childhood obesity: Establishing healthy lifestyle habits in the preschool years. *Journal of Pediatric Healthcare, 18*(6), 315–319.

Piaget, J. (1969). *The theory of stages in cognitive development.* New York: McGraw-Hill.

Reach Out and Read. (2006). *Reading tips.* Retrieved August 28, 2007 from http://www.reachoutandread.org/FileRepository/ReadingTips.pdf.

Safe Kids USA. (2007). *Safety tips: Car.* Retrieved August 28, 2007 from http://www.usa.safekids.org/tier2_rl.cfm?folder_id=170.

Safe Kids Worldwide. (2007). *Preventing injury to children in motor vehicle crashes.* Retrieved August 28, 2007 from http://www.usa.safekids.org/content_documents/MVO_tips.pdf.

Savage, J. S., Fisher, J. O., & Birch, L. L. (2007). Parental influence on eating behavior: Conception to adolescence. *The Journal of Law, Medicine & Ethics, 35*(1), 22–34.

Schuman, A. J. (2007). The ABCs of toy safety: More than just child's play. *Contemporary Pediatrics, 24*(7), 49–57, 64.

Shelov, S. P., Trubo, R., Hannemann, R. E. (Eds.). (2004). *Caring for your baby and young child: Birth to age 5* (4th ed.). New York: Bantam Books.

Small, L., Melnyk, B. M., & Strasser, A. (2007). Preventing obesity in young children. *Advance for Nurse Practitioners, 15*(3), 35–40.

Smith, J., & McSherry, W. (2004). Spirituality and child development: A concept analysis. *Journal of Advanced Nursing, 42*(3), 307–315.

Storey, M., Holt, K., & Sotfka, D. (Eds.). (2002). *Bright futures in practice: Nutrition* (2nd ed.). Arlington, VA: National Center for Education in Maternal and Child Health.

World Health Organization. (2007). *Passive smoking.* Retrieved August 28, 2007 from http://www.who.int/tobacco/en/atlas10.pdf.

Yuma, P. J., & Maldonado, M. (2006). Booster seats: Protecting the forgotten child. *Journal of Pediatric Health Care, 20*(2), 137–140.

Zebrowski, P. M. (2003). Developmental stuttering. *Pediatric Annals, 32*(7), 453–458.

WEBSITES

American Academy of Pediatrics: www.aap.org

Children's Nutrition Research Center at Baylor College of Medicine in cooperation with U.S. Department of Agriculture: www.bcm.tmc.edu/cnrc

Child nutrition and health section of the Food and Nutrition Information Center: www.fnic.nal.usda.gov

Early language intervention programs: www.hanen.org

Nemours Center for Children's Health Media: www.kidshealth.com

Bilingual families webpage: www.nethelp.no/cindy/biling-fam.html

National Highway Traffic Safety Administration: www.nhtsa.dot.gov

Promotion of nutritional health of children and adolescents: www.nutritionforkids.com

Safe Kids USA: www.usa.safekids.org/

CHAPTER WORKSHEET

MULTIPLE CHOICE QUESTIONS

1. The nurse is caring for a hospitalized 4-year-old who insists on having the nurse perform every assessment and intervention on her imaginary friend first. She then agrees to have the assessment or intervention done to herself. The nurse identifies this preschooler's behavior as:

   a. Problematic; the child is old enough to begin to have a basis in reality.

   b. Normal, because the child is hospitalized and out of her routine.

   c. Normal for this stage of growth and development.

   d. Problematic, as it interferes with needed nursing care.

2. The mother of a 3-year-old is concerned about her child's speech. She describes her preschooler as hesitating at the beginning of sentences and repeating consonant sounds. What is the nurse's best response?

   a. Hesitancy and dysfluency are normal during this period of development.

   b. Reading to the child will help model appropriate speech.

   c. Expressive language concerns warrant a developmental evaluation.

   d. The mother should ask her pediatrician for a speech therapy evaluation.

3. The mother of a 4-year-old asks for advice on using time-out for discipline with her child. What advice should the nurse give the mother?

   a. If spanking is not working, then time-out is not likely to be helpful either.

   b. Place the child in time-out for 4 minutes.

   c. Use time-out only if removing privileges is unsuccessful.

   d. The child should stay in time-out until crying ceases.

4. A 5-year-old child is not gaining weight appropriately. Organic problems have been ruled out. What is the priority action by the nurse?

   a. Allow the child unlimited access to the sippy cup to ensure adequate hydration.

   b. Encourage sweets for the extra caloric content.

   c. Teach the mother about nutritional needs of the preschooler.

   d. Assess the child's usual intake pattern at home.

CRITICAL THINKING EXERCISES

1. Teach a preschool class about bicycle and street safety. Be certain to design the content at an appropriate developmental level.

2. Construct a 3-day menu for a picky 4-year-old. Include three daily meals and two snacks. Follow the nutritional guidelines recommended by the USDA.

3. Color or draw with a preschool child. Analyze the drawings and interactions or discussions you have with the child, relating them to psychosocial and cognitive development expected at this age.

STUDY ACTIVITIES

1. Care for two average 3-, 4-, or 5-year-old children in the clinical setting (make sure both are the same age). Describe each child's development level, response to hospitalization, and family dynamics.

2. Visit a preschool that provides care for special needs children as well as typically developing children. Perform a development assessment on a typical child and one with special needs (both the same age). Compare and contrast your findings.

3. Observe in a 3-, 4- or 5-year-old classroom of a typical preschool. Choose two children who are the same age with different temperaments. Record the differences and similarities in their response to structure and authority, interactions with classmates, attention levels, and language and activity levels.

GROWTH AND DEVELOPMENT OF THE SCHOOL-AGE CHILD

CHAPTER *28*

KEY TERMS

bruxism
caries
industry
inferiority
malocclusion

prepubescence
principle of
    conservation
school-age child
school refusal

secondary sexual
    characteristics
self-esteem

LEARNING OBJECTIVES

Upon completion of the chapter, the learner will be able to:

1. Identify normal physiologic, cognitive, and moral changes occurring in the school-age child.
2. Describe the role of peers and schools in the development and socialization of the school-age child.
3. Identify the developmental milestones of the school-age child.
4. Identify the role of the nurse in promoting safety for the school-age child.
5. Demonstrate knowledge of the nutritional requirements of the school-age child.
6. Identify common developmental concerns in the school-age child.
7. Demonstrate knowledge of the appropriate nursing guidance for common developmental concerns.

*L*awrence Jones is a 10-year-old boy brought to the clinic by his mother for his annual school check-up. During your assessment you measure his weight at 62 pounds and his height at 54 inches. As the nurse caring for him, assess Lawrence's growth and development, and then provide appropriate anticipatory guidance to his mother.

WOW

Always give a hundred percent, and you will never doubt your ability to succeed.

853

School-age children, between the ages of 6 and 12 years, are experiencing a time of slow progressive physical growth, while their social and developmental growth accelerates and increases in complexity. The focus of their world expands from family to teachers, peers, and other outside influences (e.g., coaches, media). The child at this stage becomes increasingly more independent while participating in activities outside the home.

Growth and Development Overview

The school-age years are a time of continued maturation of the child's physical, social, and psychological characteristics. It is during this time that children move toward abstract thinking and seek approval of peers, teachers, and parents. Their eye–hand–muscle coordination allows them to participate in organized sports in school or the community. The **school-age child** values school attendance and school activities. The nurse uses knowledge of normal growth and development of the school-age child to assist the child with coping with disruptions and changes during this time period.

▶ PHYSICAL GROWTH

From 6 to 12 years of age, children grow an average of 2 inches (5 centimeters) per year, increasing their height by at least 1 foot. An increase of 4 to 6 pounds (2 to 3 kilograms) per year in weight is expected. In the early school-age years, girls and boys are similar in height and weight and appear thinner and more graceful than in previous years. In later school-age years, most girls begin to surpass boys in both height and weight. (See Appendix A for growth charts.)

Preadolescent boys and girls do not want to be different from peers of the same sex or the opposite sex, although there are differences in physical and physiologic growth during the school-age years. These differences, especially **secondary sexual characteristics**, are concerning and often a source of embarrassment for both sexes.

The differences between girls and boys are more apparent at the end of the middle-school years and may become extreme and a source of emotional problems. These differences in height and weight relationships, and changes in growth patterns, should be explained to parents and children (Fig. 28.1). Physical maturity is not necessarily associated with emotional and social maturity. An 8-year-old who is the size of an 11-year-old will think and act like an 8-year-old. Many times, the expectations placed on these children are unrealistic and can impact the self-esteem and competence of the child. This can work in reverse, to similar effect, for an 11-year-old who is the size of an 8-year-old and is therefore treated as such.

▶ ORGAN SYSTEMS MATURATION

Maturation of organs may differ with age or gender. Maturation of organs remains fairly consistent until late school age. In the late school-age years (10- to 12-year-olds), boys experience a slowed growth in height and increased weight gain, which may lead to obesity. During this time,

FIGURE 28.1 The different growth rates of school-age children are depicted by these same-age school-age children.

girls may begin to have changes in the body that soften body lines. Preadolescence is a period of rapid growth, especially for girls.

Neurologic System

The brain and skull grow very slowly during the school-age years. Brain growth is complete by the time the child is 10 years of age. The shape of the head is longer and the growth of the facial bones changes facial proportions.

Respiratory System

The respiratory system continues to mature with the development of the lungs and alveoli, resulting in fewer respiratory infections. Respiratory rates decrease, abdominal breathing disappears, and respirations become diaphragmatic in nature. The frontal sinuses are developed by 7 years of age. Tonsils decrease in size from the preschool years, but they remain larger than adolescents'. The adenoids and tonsils may appear large normally, even in the absence of infection.

Cardiovascular System

The school-age child's blood pressure increases and the pulse rate decreases. The heart grows more slowly during the middle years and is smaller in size in relation to the rest of the body than at any other development stage.

Gastrointestinal System

During the school-age years, all 20 primary deciduous teeth are lost, replaced by 28 of 32 permanent teeth, with the exception of the third molars. The school-age child experiences fewer gastrointestinal upsets compared with earlier years. Stomach capacity increases, which permits retention of food for longer periods of time. In addition, the caloric needs of the school-age child are lower than in the earlier years.

Genitourinary System

Bladder capacity increases, but varies among individual children. Girls generally have a greater bladder capacity than boys. Urination patterns vary with the amount of fluids ingested, the time they were ingested, and the stress level of the child. The formula for bladder capacity is age in years plus 2 ounces. Therefore, the bladder capacity of the 7-year-old would be 9 ounces. The larger capacity of the bladder allows for the child to experience longer periods between voiding.

Prepubescence

The late school-age years are also referred to as *preadolescence* (the time between middle childhood and the 13th birthday). During preadolescence, **prepubescence** occurs. Prepubescence typically occurs in the 2 years before the beginning of puberty and is characterized by the development of secondary sexual characteristics, a period of rapid growth for girls, and a period of continued growth for boys. There is approximately 2 years' difference in the onset of prepubescence between boys and girls. Sexual development in both boys and girls can lead to a negative perception of physical appearance and lowered self-esteem. Early development in girls can lead to embarrassment, concern over physical appearance, and low self-esteem. Delayed development in boys can lead to a negative self-concept, resulting in substance abuse or reckless use of non-automobile vehicles. Early development may lead to risk-taking behaviors in both boys and girls. It is important for the nurse and parents to educate the late school-age child about body changes to decrease anxiety and promote comfort with these body changes.

Musculoskeletal System

Musculoskeletal growth leads to greater coordination and strength, yet the muscles are still immature and can be injured easily. Bones continue to ossify throughout childhood, but mineralization is not complete until maturity.

Immune System

Lymphatic tissues continue to grow until the child is 9 years old; immunoglobulins A and G (IgA and IgG) reach adult levels at around 10 years of age. Due to the lymphatic system becoming more competent in localizing infections and producing antibody–antigen responses, school-age children may have fewer infections. They may experience more infections during the first 1 to 2 years of school due to exposure to other children who may have infections.

▶ PSYCHOSOCIAL DEVELOPMENT

Erikson (1963) describes the task of the school-age years to be a sense of **industry** vs. **inferiority**. During this time, the child is developing his sense of self-worth by becoming involved in multiple activities at home, school, and in the community, which develops his cognitive and social skills. He is very interested in learning how things are made and work. The school-age child's satisfaction from achieving success in developing new skills leads him to an increased sense of self-worth and level of competence. It is the role of the parents, teachers, coaches, and nurses of the school-age child to identify areas of competency and to build on the child's successful experiences to promote mastery, success, and self-esteem. If the expectations of adults are set too high, the child will develop a sense of inferiority and incompetence that can affect all aspects of his life. See Table 28.1 for a further explanation of psychosocial development in school-age children.

TABLE 28.1 DEVELOPMENTAL THEORIES

Theorist	Stage	Activities
Erikson	Industry vs. inferiority	Interested in how things are made and run Success in personal and social tasks Increased activities outside home—clubs, sports Increased interactions with peers Increased interest in knowledge Needs support and encouragement from important people in child's life Needs support when child is not successful Inferiority occurs with repeated failures with little support or trust from those who are important to the child
Piaget	Concrete operational	Learns by manipulating concrete objects Lacks ability to think abstractly Learns that certain characteristics of objects remain constant Understands concepts of time Engages in serial ordering, addition, subtraction Classifies or groups objects by their common elements Understands relationships among objects Starts collections of items Can reverse thought process

Kohlberg	Conventional
	  Stage 3: interpersonal conforming, "good child, bad child"
	  Age 7–10 years
	  Stage 4: "law and order"
	  Age 10–12 years
		An act is wrong because it brings punishment
		Behavior is completely wrong or right
		Does not understand the reason behind rules
		If child and adult differ in opinions, the adult is right
		Can put self in another person's position
		Begins to exercise the "golden rule"
		Acts are judged in terms of intention, not just punishment

Freud	Latency	A time of tranquility between the Oedipal phase of early childhood and adolescence—focuses on activities that develop social and cognitive skills Develops social skills in relating to same-sex friends through joining clubs like Brownies, Girl Scouts, Boy Scouts

◗ COGNITIVE DEVELOPMENT

Piaget's stage of cognitive development for the 7- to 11-year-old is the period of concrete operational thoughts. In developing concrete operations, the child is able to assimilate and coordinate information about her world from different dimensions. She is able to see things from another person's point of view and think through an action, anticipating its consequences and the possibility of having to re-think the action. She is able to use stored memories of past experiences to evaluate and interpret present situations. The school-age child also develops the ability to classify or divide things into different sets and to identify their relationships to each other. The school-age child is able to classify members of four generations on a family tree vertically and horizontally, and at the same time see that one person can be a father, son, uncle, and grandson. It is at this time that the school-age child develops an interest in collecting objects. She starts out collecting multiple objects and becomes more selective as she gets older. Also, during concrete operational thinking, the school-age child develops an

understanding of the **principle of conservation**—that matter does not change when its form changes. For example, if the child pours a half-cup of water into a short, wide glass and into a tall, thin glass, she still only has a half-cup of water despite the fact that it looks like the tall, thin glass has more (Fig. 28.2). She learns about conserving matter in a sequence ranging from the simplest to the more complex. See Table 28.1 for further information about cognitive development of school-age children.

◗ MORAL AND SPIRITUAL DEVELOPMENT

During the school-age years, the child's sense of morality is constantly being developed. According to Kohlberg, the school-age child is at the conventional stage of moral development. The 7- to 10-year-old usually follows rules out of a sense of being a "good" person. He wants to be a good person to his parents, friends, and teachers and to

FIGURE **28.2** School-age children understand the theory of conservation (**A**). If you pour an equal amount of liquid into two glasses of unequal shape (**B**), the amount of water you have remains the same despite the unequal appearance in the two glasses (**C**).   **A**   **B**   **C**

himself. The adult is viewed as being right. This is stage 3: interpersonal conformity (good child, bad child), according to Kohlberg. Ten- to 12-year-olds progress to stage 4: the "law and order" stage. At this stage, the child can determine if an action is good or bad based upon the reason for the action, not just on the possible consequences of the action. The older school-age child's behavior is guided by the child's desire to cooperate and by his respect for others. This leads to the school-age child's ability to understand and incorporate into his behavior the concept of the "golden rule." See Table 28.1 for additional information about the moral development of school-age children.

It is during school age that children develop an interest in religion. They are still concrete thinkers and are guided by their family's religious and cultural beliefs. They are comforted by the rituals of their religion, but are just beginning to understand the differences between natural and supernatural. Incorporating religious practices in their lives can assist school-age children in coping with different stressors.

impulses of exploration. Children between 8 and 10 years of age are less restless, but their energy level continues to be high with activities more subdued and directed. These children exhibit greater rhythm and gracefulness of muscular movements, allowing them to participate in physical activities that require longer and more concentrated attention and effort, such as baseball or soccer.

Between the ages of 10 and 12 years of age (the pubescent years for girls), energy levels remain high but are more controlled and focused. Physical skills in this age group are similar to adults', with strength and endurance increasing during adolescence.

All school-age children should be encouraged to engage in physical activities and learn physical skills that contribute to their health for the rest of their lives. Cardiovascular fitness, weight control, emotional tension release, and development of leadership and following skills are enhanced through physical activity and team sports.

▶ MOTOR SKILL DEVELOPMENT

Gross and fine motor skills continue to mature throughout the school-age years. Refinement of motor skills occurs, and speed and accuracy increase. To assess the motor skills of school-age children, ask questions about participation in sports and after-school activities, band membership, constructing models, and writing skills.

Gross Motor Skills

During the school-age years, coordination, balance, and rhythm improve, facilitating the opportunity to ride a two-wheel bike, jump rope, dance, and participate in a variety of other sports (Fig. 28.3). Older school-age children may become awkward due to their bodies growing faster than their ability to compensate.

School-age children between the ages of 6 and 8 enjoy gross motor activities such as bicycling, skating, and swimming. They are enthralled with the world and are in constant motion. Sometimes fear is limited due to the strong

FIGURE **28.3** Jumping rope is an example of the increased development of gross motor skills of the school-age child.

Fine Motor Skills

Myelinization of the central nervous system is reflected by refinement of fine motor skills. Eye–hand coordination and balance improve with maturity and practice. Hand usage improves, becoming steadier and independent and granting an ease and precision that allows these children to write, print words, sew, or build models or other crafts. The child between 10 and 12 years of age begins to exhibit manipulative skills comparable to adults. School-age children take pride in activities that require dexterity and fine motor skills such as playing musical instruments (Fig. 28.4). Talent and practice become the keys to proficiency.

▶ SENSORY DEVELOPMENT

All senses are mature early in the school-age years. The typical school-age child has 20/20 visual acuity. In addition, ocular muscular control, peripheral vision, and color discrimination are fully developed by the time the child is 7 years of age. Good vision is essential to the physical development and educational progression of school-age children. Vision screening programs conducted by school nurses identify problems with vision and result in appropriate referrals when warranted. Some problems frequently identified include amblyopia, uncorrected refractive errors or other eye defects, and malalignment of the eyes (called *strabismus*). If untreated by age 9 years of age, amblyopia can cause irreversible visual loss. This condition is correctable prior to this time with glasses or patching. Proper screening and referral, as well as notification to parents of the existing condition, are essential to the education and socialization of the school-age child (www.aao.org).

Hearing deficits that are severe are usually diagnosed in infancy, but the less severe may not be diagnosed until the child enters school and has difficulty learning or with speech. It is important to screen children for hearing deficits to ensure proper educational and social progression. With loud music heard over long periods of time each day, there are concerns about these environmental noises affecting hearing in the school-age and adolescent populations.

The sense of smell is mature and can be tested in the school-age child by using scents that children are familiar with, such as chocolate or other familiar odors. In addition, the school-age child may be tested for the sense of touch with objects to discriminate cold from hot, soft from hard, and blunt from sharp.

▶ COMMUNICATION AND LANGUAGE DEVELOPMENT

Language skills continue to accelerate during the school-age years. Vocabulary expands to 8,000 to 14,000 words. Culturally specific words are used, with bilingual children speaking English in school and a second language at home. The school-age child learns to read and reading efficiency improves language skills. Reading skills are improved with increased reading exposure. School-age children begin to use more complex grammatical forms such as plurals and pronouns. Also, they develop metalinguistic awareness—an ability to think about language and comment on its properties. This enables them to enjoy jokes and riddles due to their understanding of double meanings, and play on words and sounds. They are also beginning to understand metaphors such as "a stitch in time saves nine." School-age children may experiment with profanity and dirty jokes if exposed. This age group tends to imitate parents, family members, or others. Therefore, role modeling is very important.

▶ EMOTIONAL AND SOCIAL DEVELOPMENT

Patterns of temperamental traits identified in infancy may continue to influence behavior in the school-age child. Analyzing past situations may provide clues to the way a child may react to new or different situations. Children may react differently over time due to their experiences and abilities. Self-esteem is the child's view of their individual worth. This view is impacted by feedback from family, teachers, and other authority figures.

Temperament

Temperament has been described as the way individuals behave. Some descriptions of temperament are that the

FIGURE 28.4 School-age children improve their fine motor skills so they can play musical instruments well.

child is *easy, slow to warm,* or *difficult.* These behaviors vary from the child who is easy (even-tempered and predictable) to the child labeled as difficult (due to high activity levels, irritability, and moodiness). The child who is easy may adapt to school entry and other experiences smoothly and with little or no stress. The slow-to-warm child may be slow to adapt to changes. The slow-to-warm school-age child may exhibit discomfort when placed in different or new situations such as school. This child may need time to adjust to the new place or situation, and may demonstrate frustration with tears or somatic complaints. The slow-to-warm child should be allowed time to adjust to new situations and people (such as teachers) within his or her own time frame. All of these factors may impact the younger school-age child upon entering the school environment, with changes in authority and the introduction of many peers. The difficult or easily distracted child may benefit from an introduction to the new experience and people by role-playing, by visiting the site and being introduced to the teachers, and by hearing stories or participating in conversations about the upcoming school experience. These children require patience, firmness, and understanding to make the transition into a new situation or experience such as school. The Behavioral Style Questionnaire (BSQ) (McDevitt & Carey, 1978) is a temperament questionnaire for children 3 to 7 years old; the Middle Childhood Temperament Questionnaire is another tool for children 8 to 12 years of age (Hegvik, McDevitt, & Carey, 1982). These tools may be useful for determining type of temperament and guiding interventions.

Self-Esteem Development

Self-esteem mirrors the child's individual self-worth and consists of both positive and negative qualities. Children strive to achieve internalized goals of attainment, although they continually receive feedback from individuals they perceive as authorities (parent or teacher). By the school-age years, children have received feedback related to their performance or tasks. The direction of this feedback influences the child's opinion of self-worth, which influences self-esteem and self-evaluation.

Children face the process of self-evaluation from a framework of either self-confidence or self-doubt. Children who have mastered the earlier developmental task of autonomy and initiative face the world with feelings of pride rather than shame.

If school-age children regard themselves as worthwhile, they have a positive self-concept and high self-esteem. Significant adults in school-age children's lives can manipulate the environment to facilitate success. This success impacts the self-esteem of the child.

Body Image

Body image is how the school-ager perceives his or her body. School-age children are knowledgeable about the human body but may have different perceptions about body parts. School-age children are very interested in peers' views and acceptances of their body, body changes, and clothing. This age group may model themselves after parents, peers, and persons in movies or on television. It is important for late school-agers to feel accepted by peers. If they feel different and are teased, there may be lifelong effects.

School-Age Fears

School-age children are less fearful of harm to their body than in their preschool years, but fear being kidnapped or undergoing surgery. They continue to fear the dark and worry about their past behaviors. They fear death and are fascinated by death and dying. They are less fearful of dogs and noises. The school-age child needs reassurance that his or her fears are normal for this developmental age. Parents, teachers, and other caretakers should discuss the fears and answer questions posed by the child (Child Development Institute, 2007).

Peer Relationships

The child's concept of self is shaped by relationships with others. Peer relationships influence children's independence from parents. Peers play an important role in the approval and critiquing of skills of school-age children. Previously, only adults such as parents and teachers have been authorities; now, peers influence school-age children's perceptions of themselves. Peer relationships help to support the school-age child by providing enough security to risk the parental conflict brought about when establishing independence. School-age children associate with peers of the same sex most of the time. Although games and other activities are shared by both boys and girls, the child's concept of the appropriate sex role is influenced by his or her relationship with peers.

Continuous peer relationships provide the most important social interaction for school-age children. Valuable lessons are learned from interactions with children their own age. Children learn to respect differing points of view that are represented in their groups (Fig. 28.5). Peer groups establish norms and standards that signify acceptance or rejection. Children may modify behavior to gain acceptance. A characteristic of school-age children is their formation of groups with rules and values. Peer and peer-group identification are essential to the socialization of the school-age child.

Teacher and School Influences

School serves as a means to transmit values of society and to establish peer relationships. Secondary only to the family, school exerts a profound influence on the social development of the child. Often school requires changes for the child and parent. The child enters an environment that requires conforming to group activities that are structured

FIGURE 28.5 School-age children like to join clubs. These children, in the acting club at school, are rehearsing for a play.

and directed by an adult other than the parent. The parent's attitude and support influences the child's transition into the school setting. Parents that are positive and supportive promote a smooth entry into school. Parents that encourage clinging behaviors may delay a successful transition into school.

To facilitate the transition from home to school, the teacher must have the personality and knowledge of development that will allow him or her to meet the needs of young children. Even though the teacher's responsibilities are primarily to stimulate and guide intellectual development, they must share in shaping the child's attitudes and values. The system of awards and punishment administered by teachers affects the self-concept of children and influences their response to school. Teachers and school are important in shaping the socialization, self-concept, and intellectual development of children.

Family Influences

The school-age years are a time for peer relationships, questioning of parents, and the potential for parental conflict but continued respect for family values. School-age years are the beginning of the time of peer-group influence, with testing of parental and family values. Although the peer group is influential, the family's values usually predominate when parental and peer-group values come into conflict. Even though the school-age child may question the parents' values, the child will usually incorporate the values from parents into his or her values.

Many times in the late school-age and preadolescent period, the child may prefer to be in the company of peers and show a decreased interest in family functions. This may require an adjustment for parents. Parents' awareness of this developmental trend and their continuing support for the child is important while they continue to enforce restrictions and control of behaviors. The school-ager is beginning to strive for independence, but parental au-

thority and controls continue to impact choices and values. School-age children continue to need parenting. They do not need parents as pals.

▶ CULTURAL INFLUENCES ON GROWTH AND DEVELOPMENT

Culture influences habits, beliefs, language, and values. School-age children thrive on learning the music, language, traditions, holidays, games, values, gender roles, and other aspects of culture. Nurses must be aware of the effects on children of various groups' family structures and traditional values. The school-age child's cultural and ethnic backgrounds must be considered when assessing growth and development, including differences in growth in children of different racial and cultural backgrounds. Cultural implications must be considered for all children and families in order to provide appropriate care.

*R*efer back to Lawrence Jones, who was introduced at the beginning of this chapter. What developmental milestones would you expect him to have reached by this age?

The Nurse's Role in School-Age Growth and Development

WATCH & LEARN

The nurse's role in school-age growth and development includes assessing growth and development, promoting healthy growth and development, and addressing common developmental concerns. The nursing process overview would include an assessment of the individual child and identification of nursing diagnoses needing intervention or referral. The nurse promotes healthy growth and development through anticipatory guidance and goal attainment.

▶ NURSING PROCESS OVERVIEW

Upon completion of assessment of the school-age child's current growth and development status, problems or issues related to growth and development may be identified. The nurse may then identify one or more nursing diagnoses, including:

• Risk for disproportionate growth
• Imbalanced nutrition: more than body requirements
• Delayed growth and development

• Risk for caregiver role strain
• Risk for injury

Nursing care planning for the school-age child with growth and development issues should be individualized based on the school-age child's and family's needs. The nursing care plan can be used as a guide in planning nursing care for the school-age child with a growth and development concern. The nurse may choose the appropriate nursing diagnoses from Nursing Care Plan 28.1 and individualize them as needed. The nursing care plan is intended to serve as a guide, not to be an all-inclusive growth and development care plan.

▶ PROMOTING HEALTHY GROWTH AND DEVELOPMENT

The family plays a critical role in promoting healthy growth and development of the school-age child. Respectful interchange of communication between the parent and child will foster self-esteem and self-confidence. This respect will give the child confidence in achieving personal, educational, and social goals appropriate for his or her age. The nurse should study interactions between parents and school-age children to observe for this respect or lack of respect ("putting the child down"). The nurse can model appropriate behaviors by listening to the child and making appropriate responses. The nurse can be a resource for parents and an advocate for the child in promoting healthy growth and development.

Promoting Growth and Development Through Play

Cooperative play is exhibited by the school-age child. Play for the school-age child includes both organized cooperative activities (such as team sports) and solitary activities. School-age children have the coordination and intellect to participate with other children their age in sports such as soccer, baseball, football, and tennis. The school-age child comprehends that his or her cooperation with others will lead to a unified whole for the team. Additionally, the child learns rules and the value of playing by the rules.

School-age children also enjoy solitary activities including board, card, video, and computer games, and dollhouse and other small-figure play (Fig. 28.6). Many schoolagers start collections of stamps, cars, or other valuable or not-so-valuable items. During the school-age years, children may also begin a scrapbook or keep a diary. They may participate in activities such as dance or karate. Girls and boys may join clubs, gangs, or special interest groups.

Active play has decreased in recent years as television viewing and computer games have increased. This trend has resulted in health risks such as obesity, type 2 diabetes, and cardiovascular problems.

Promoting Learning

School attendance and learning are very important to the school-age child. Parent–child, child–teacher, and child–peer relationships and activities influence the school-age child's learning.

Formal Education

Most children are excited about starting school and making new friends. They like the notion of getting books, having book bags, and having homework assignments. The reality of the work involved with school and homework may decrease the enthusiasm about school.

Peers are very important within this age group. Both peers and teachers influence children. Attending school may be their first experience interacting with a large number of children their own age. Through this interaction, children learn cooperation, competition, and the importance of following the rules. Peer approval and influences grow as the child matures. Teachers have significant influences on children. They help to guide the child's intellectual development by rewarding successes and helping the child deal with failures. The student–teacher relationship is a key to success. Teachers play a role in fostering feelings of industry and preventing feelings of inferiority (Fig. 28.7). School-age children also learn skills, rules, values, and other ways to work with peers and other authority figures.

Parental support is important for school adjustment and achievement. Parents must collaborate with teachers and school personnel to ensure that the child is fulfilling the expectations and requirements for this age group in school. Parents must monitor the child's homework assignments and friends, and observe for any changes in behavior that would indicate school or behavioral problems.

Reading

Encouraging reading is an excellent way to promote learning in the school-age child. Trips to the library and purchasing books help to promote a love of reading. School-age children enjoy being read to as well as reading on their own. Younger school-age children (6 to 8 years) enjoy books that are simple to read with few words on a page, such as the Dr. Seuss books. They enjoy books about animals and trains and simple mysteries. Children 8 to 10 years of age have more advanced reading skills and enjoy those books from early childhood, plus more classic novels and adventures such as the Harry Potter series. Older children enjoy horror stories, mysteries, romances, and adventure stories as well as classic novels. School-age children of all ages benefit from books on topics related to things they may be experiencing, such as a visit to the hospital for a surgical procedure. See Box 28.1 for ideas for parents to promote reading in the school-age child.

Nursing Care Plan 28.1

GROWTH AND DEVELOPMENT ISSUES OF THE SCHOOL-AGE CHILD

NURSING DIAGNOSIS: Risk for disproportionate growth (risk factors: caregiver knowledge deficit, frequent illnesses)

Outcome Identification and Evaluation

School-age child will demonstrate adequate growth: *appropriate weight gain for age and gender*

Interventions: Promoting Proportionate Growth

- Assess parent's knowledge of nutritional needs of school-age children *to determine need for further education.*
- Plot out height, weight, and body mass index (BMI) *to detect possible pattern.*
- Determine need for additional caloric intake if necessary *(if very active in sports, if have a chronic illness).*
- Educate mother about appropriate serving sizes and foods *so that mother is aware of what to expect for school-age children.*

NURSING DIAGNOSIS: Imbalanced nutrition, more than body requirements, related to lack of exercise, increased caloric intake, poor food choices

Outcome Identification and Evaluation

School-age child will lose weight at an appropriate rate: *increase amount of exercise, make appropriate eating choices, decrease caloric intake to appropriate amount for age and gender*

Interventions: Promoting Nutrition

- Assess knowledge of parents and child about nutritional needs of school-age children *to determine deficits in knowledge.*
- Have child keep food and exercise diary for 1 week *to determine current patterns of eating and exercise.*
- Interview parents in relationship to their eating habits and exercise habits *to determine where adjustments might need to be made.*
- Analyze preceding data, and base recommendations for changes on these data.
- Discuss ways to decrease temptation to overeat and to make good meal choices (see Teaching Guideline 28.2).
- Have child assist in meal planning and grocery shopping *to allow him some sense of control in process.*
- Incorporate increase in daily exercise, which will stress sense of self-improvement *to increase caloric expenditure and self-esteem.*
- Decrease TV/computer time *to increase caloric expenditure.*
- Develop reward system *to increase self-esteem.*
- Investigate joining weight-loss program for school-age children *to increase self-esteem and to increase awareness that other children have the same problem.*

NURSING DIAGNOSIS: Growth and development, delayed related to speech, motor, psychosocial, or cognitive concerns as evidenced by delay in meeting expected school performances

Outcome Identification and Evaluation

Development will be maximized: School-age child will make continued progress toward attainment of expected school performances.

Interventions: Promoting Growth and Development

- Perform scheduled evaluation of the school-age child by school and health care provider *to determine current functioning.*
- Develop realistic multidisciplinary plan *to ensure maximizing resources.*
- Carry out interventions as prescribed by developmental specialist, physical therapist, occupational therapist, or speech therapist at home and at school *to maximize benefit of interventions.*
- Have scheduled evaluation meetings to be able *to adapt interventions as soon as possible.*

Nursing Care Plan 28.1 (continued)

NURSING DIAGNOSIS: Caregiver role strain, risk for (risk factors: new sibling in household, knowledge deficit about school-age issues, lack of prior exposure, fatigue, ill or developmentally delayed child)

Outcome Identification and Evaluation
Parent will experience competence in role: *will demonstrate appropriate caretaking behaviors and verbalize comfort in caring for a school-age child*

Interventions: Preventing Caregiver Role Strain
- Assess parent's knowledge of school-age children and the issues that arise as a part of normal development *to determine parent's needs.*
- Provide education on normal issues of school-age children so that parents are armed with the knowledge they need *to appropriately care for their school-age child.*
- Provide anticipatory guidance related to upcoming expected issues related to school-age development *to prepare parents for what to expect next and how to intervene.*

NURSING DIAGNOSIS: Injury, risk for (risk factors: curiosity, increasing cognitive skills and motor abilities)

Outcome Identification and Evaluation
School-age child's safety will be maintained: *will remain free from injury*

Interventions: Preventing Injury
- Discuss safety measures needed for the following: bikes, scooters, guns, skateboards, cars, water, and playground *to decrease risk of injury related to those areas.*
- Discuss and develop a fire safety plan *to decrease risk of injury related to fire.*
- Discuss appropriate safety equipment needed for each sport *to decrease risk of injury.*
- Discuss appropriate sports to participate in depending upon age, sex, and maturity of child *to prevent possible injury and to promote child's self-esteem.*
- Parents should have the poison control center phone number available *(in the event of accidental ingestion, poison control can give parents the best advice for appropriate intervention).*
- Teach parents and child first-aid measures and child cardiopulmonary resuscitation (CPR) *to minimize consequences of injury should it occur.*
- Discuss influence of peers on actions of school-age children *to prevent possible injury due to mimicking behavior.*

FIGURE 28.6 This school-age girl enjoys solitary play with her dollhouse and dolls.

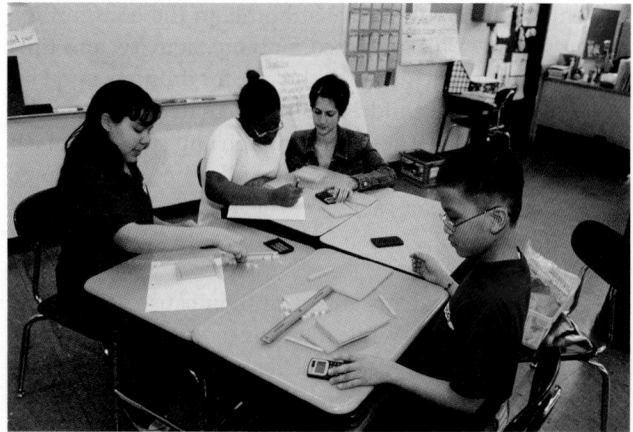

FIGURE 28.7 School is important to the school-age child.

BOX 28.1 **Promotion of Reading in School-Age Children**

- Parents, read to and with your children.
- Ask teachers and librarians for advice on books appropriate for your child.
- Choose stories that the child can relate to if the child has difficulty reading.
- Choose books with movement if the child has a short attention span.
- Take advantage of all reading opportunities (cereal boxes, road signs).
- Provide choices for the child to select a book of interest.
- Talk about the text and ask questions to improve understanding.
- Keep a record of what the child is reading.
- Visit a library, get a library card, and check out books.
- Parents, demonstrate role modeling through reading books.

Promoting Safety

School-age children become more independent with age. This independence leads to an increased self-confidence and decreased fears, which may contribute to accidents and injuries. School age is a time that the child may walk to school with peers who may influence his or her behavior. Increased independence may also increase exposure to dangerous situations such as the approach of strangers or unsafe streets. Promotion of safe habits during the school-age years is important for parents and nurses. See Teaching Guidelines 28.1 for additional information on safety education for nurses and parents.

Unintentional injuries are the leading cause of death in children between 1 and 21 years of age (CDC, 2007a). Each year, 20 million children sustain an injury sufficiently severe to seek medical attention (CDC, 2007b). School-age children are very active at home, in the community, and at school. This increased mobility, activity, and time away from parents increases the risk for unintentional injuries. School-age children continue to need supervision and guidance. They need information and rules about car safety, pedestrian safety, bicycle and other sport safety, fire safety, and water safety.

Car Safety

Motor vehicle accidents are a common cause of injury in the school-age child. While traveling in the car, school-age children should always sit in the rear seat. The front seat is dangerous because of passenger-side airbags in most new-model cars. The school-age child should use a three-point restraint system in the rear seat of the car with the shoulder strap and lap belt fitted snugly. In addition, a school-age child over 40 pounds (generally 4 to 8 years of age) should use a belt-positioning, forward-facing booster seat using both lap and shoulder belts. School-age children who outgrow the convertible restraint can sit in a booster seat until their head is higher than the vehicle seat back (usually 4'9" and taller). Children under 12 years of age should not ride in the front seat of a vehicle with an airbag.

Pedestrian Safety

Children between the ages of 5 and 9 have the highest incidence of pedestrian-related injuries. Young school-age children between 6 and 8 years of age should walk to school or the bus with an older friend, sibling, or parent. Darting out into the street without looking both ways or from between cars is a common occurrence in the school-age years. Teach children safe street and pedestrian practices.

Bicycle and Sport Safety

Bicycling, riding scooters, skateboarding, and inline skating or rollerskating are common activities of school-age children. Laws in most states require helmets for riding bicycles and scooters. In addition, when skating or skateboarding, school-age children should wear a helmet, kneepads, and elbow pads.

Research has shown that head injuries due to bicycle accidents have been reduced by 85% by wearing a well-fitting helmet. National estimates of bicycle helmet ownership in school-age children are 50%, and only approximately 50% of those wear helmets each time they ride their bicycles (see Healthy People 2010). It is important for children to wear helmets that fit and that do not obstruct their vision or hearing. Because school-age children have completed most of their skull growth, a helmet can be worn into adolescence. It is important for the child to have a bicycle that is appropriate for his or her size and age. The child should be able to plant both feet on the ground when sitting on the seat of the bike (Fig. 28.8). It is important to stress to parents the importance of appropriate size and not to get a bike for the child to "grow into." If older school-agers are using the bike for transportation on busy streets, they should be taught to use bike lanes and to give appropriate hand signals for turning. Non-motorized and motorized scooters also place children at risk for injury, so counsel families about the use of protective gear.

Fire Safety

School-age children are eager to help parents with cooking and ironing. They are curious about fire and are drawn to play with fire, matches, and fireworks. Serious burns can occur from any exposure to fire. Educate children about the hazards of fire. In addition, teach children proper behavior around fires at home and outdoors. Always supervise children in the use of matches. In the home setting, parents should develop a fire safety plan with their children, teach children what to do if their clothes catch on fire, and practice evacuating the house in the event of a fire.

TEACHING GUIDELINES 28.1

Safety Issues and Interventions of the School-Age Child

Safety Issue	Interventions
Car safety	• Should wear seat belt or be in age- and weight-appropriate booster seat at all times. • Fasten seat belt before car is started. • Children under 12 years must sit in back seat. • Utilize childproof locks in back seat. • Establish rules of conduct in car.
Pedestrian safety	• Child should look right, left, then right again before crossing the street. • Cross only at safe crossings. • Older children and adults should provide supervision of younger children. • Should only walk on sidewalks. • Should not dart out between parked cars. • In parking lots, should watch for cars backing up. • If children are playing outside, drivers should be aware of their presence before backing up.
Bike safety: general	• Have a well-maintained and appropriate-size bike for child. • Parents should orient the child to the bike. • Child should demonstrate his or her ability to ride bike safely before being allowed to ride on street. • Safe areas for bike riding should be established as well as routes to and from area of activities. • Should not ride bike barefoot, with someone else on bike, or with clothing that might get entangled in the bike. • Should wear sturdy, well-fitting shoes. • Should wear ANSI-approved helmets. • Bike should be inspected often to ensure it is in proper working order. • A basket should be used to carry heavy objects.
Bike safety in traffic	• All traffic signs and signals must be observed. • If riding at night, the bike should have lights and reflectors and the rider should wear light-colored clothes. • Should ride on the side of the road traveling with traffic. • Should keep close to the side of the road and in single file. • Should watch and listen for cars. • Should not wear headphones while riding a bike. • Never hitch a ride on any vehicles.
Sports safety	• Match sport to child's ability and desire. • Sports program should have warm-up procedure. • Coaches should be trained in cardiopulmonary resuscitation (CPR) and first aid. • Child should wear appropriate protection devices for individual sport.
Skateboarding and inline skating safety	• Should wear helmet, and protective padding on knees, elbows, and wrists • Should not skate in traffic or on streets or highways. • Skating on homemade ramps could be dangerous—should assess ramps for any hazards before skating.
All-terrain vehicle safety	• Should not be operated by children less than 16 years of age. • Should wear helmet and protective coverings. • No nighttime riding. • Should not be used on public roads. • Should not stand up in the vehicle or ride in a person's lap.

(continued)

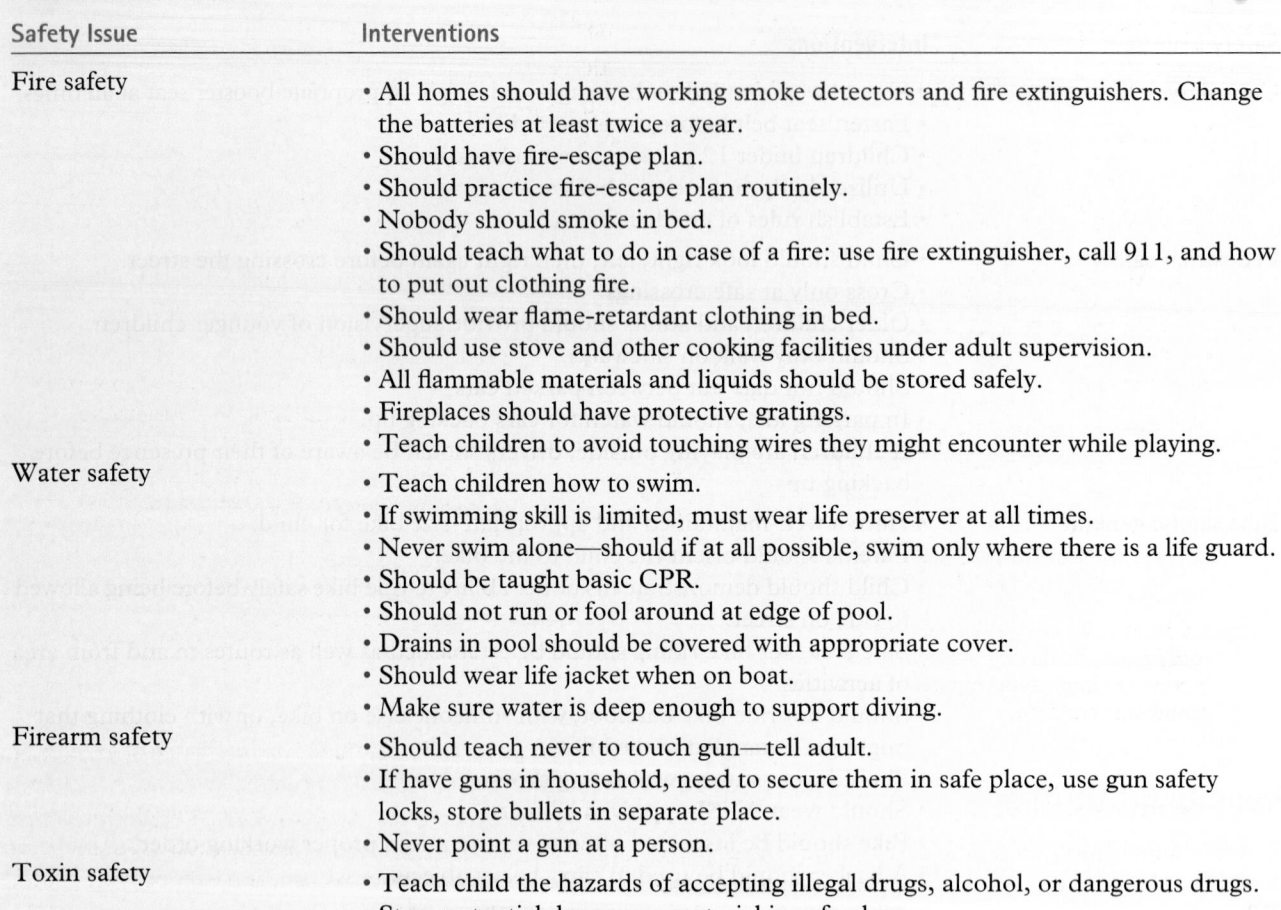

TEACHING GUIDELINES 28.1 (continued)

Safety Issues and Interventions of the School-Age Child

Safety Issue	Interventions
Fire safety	• All homes should have working smoke detectors and fire extinguishers. Change the batteries at least twice a year. • Should have fire-escape plan. • Should practice fire-escape plan routinely. • Nobody should smoke in bed. • Should teach what to do in case of a fire: use fire extinguisher, call 911, and how to put out clothing fire. • Should wear flame-retardant clothing in bed. • Should use stove and other cooking facilities under adult supervision. • All flammable materials and liquids should be stored safely. • Fireplaces should have protective gratings. • Teach children to avoid touching wires they might encounter while playing.
Water safety	• Teach children how to swim. • If swimming skill is limited, must wear life preserver at all times. • Never swim alone—should if at all possible, swim only where there is a life guard. • Should be taught basic CPR. • Should not run or fool around at edge of pool. • Drains in pool should be covered with appropriate cover. • Should wear life jacket when on boat. • Make sure water is deep enough to support diving.
Firearm safety	• Should teach never to touch gun—tell adult. • If have guns in household, need to secure them in safe place, use gun safety locks, store bullets in separate place. • Never point a gun at a person.
Toxin safety	• Teach child the hazards of accepting illegal drugs, alcohol, or dangerous drugs. • Store potential dangerous material in safe place.

In the school setting, children should be aware of the appropriate response to fire drills and fire drills should be conducted on a regular basis.

Water Safety

Teach school-age children swim and water safety. An adult should always supervise children when they are swimming to prevent water-related accidents.

HEALTHY PEOPLE 2010

Objective	Nursing Significance
Increase use of helmets by bicyclists.	• Provide education to children and their parents about avoiding head injury through helmet use. • Encourage child to choose a helmet that appeals to him or her (one that looks "cool").

Abuse in Children

Child abuse, including physical abuse and sexual abuse, are common crimes of violence against children. Three million reports of child abuse are made annually, but the true incidence may be triple that figure (ChildHelp, 2006). In 2002, more than 88,000 children were victims of sexual abuse (Kellogg & Committee on Child Abuse and Neglect, 2005). The abusers of children are family, friends, and strangers. It is important for parents to teach children the concept of "good touch" vs. "bad touch" prior to school-age years. Whenever the school-age child's behavior yields suspicion of physical or sexual abuse, the nurse should report to the appropriate authorities in his or her state. These topics will be discussed in more depth in Chapter 51.

Remember Lawrence Jones, the 10-year-old presented in the case study? What anticipatory guidance related to safety should you provide to his mother?

FIGURE 28.8 Wearing the appropriate safety equipment and having an appropriately sized bicycle are important to prevent injuries in school-age children.

Promoting Nutrition

Growth, body composition, and body shape remain constant during late school-age years. Needed calories decrease while the appetite increases. In preparation for adolescence, the body fat composition of school-age children increases. This tendency toward increased body fat occurs earlier in girls than in boys, with the amount of increase greater in girls. Boys have more lean body mass per inch of height than girls.

Diet preferences established in the preschool years continue during the school-age period. As the child grows older, influences of family, media, and peers can impact the eating habits of this age group. Some of these influences are parents' work schedule, outside activities, and exercise level of the child. Decreased exercise levels and poor nutritional choices lead to the mounting problem of obesity seen in this age group. See Box 28.2 for appropriate questions to ask the child and parent regarding nutritional status. Healthy People 2010 provides objectives and actions to improve the nutritional health of children.

Nutritional Needs

School-age children with an average body weight of 20 to 35 kilograms need approximately 70 calories per kilogram daily (1,400 to 2,100 calories per day). The average water requirement per 24 hours ranges from 1,800 to 2,200 milliliters per day. The child needs 28 grams of protein and

---

BOX 28.2 Dietary Questions

Questions for the Child
- How often do you eat together as a family?
- What are the usual mealtimes?
- How often does the family eat out?
- Do you eat breakfast regularly?
- Where do you eat lunch?
- What do you drink/how much?
- What foods do you eat most often?
- What is your favorite food?
- How often do you eat fast foods?
- What type of exercise do you do?

Questions for the Parents
- How would you describe your child's usual appetite?
- Do you have any special cultural/religious practices regarding food?
- Has your child gained or lost weight recently?
- Do you have any concerns about his or her eating behaviors?
- How does your child exercise? Your family?
- Is there a family history of cancer, hypertension, diabetes, obesity, or heart disease?

---

800 milligrams of calcium for maintenance of growth and good nutrition. Calcium is needed for the development of strong bones and teeth. Milk, yogurt, and cheese provide protein, vitamins, and minerals and are an excellent source of calcium. Meats, poultry, fish, and eggs provide protein, vitamins, and minerals.

HEALTHY PEOPLE 2010

Objective	Nursing Significance
Increase the proportion of persons age 2 years and older who consume at least two daily servings of fruit; three daily servings of vegetables, with at least one-third being dark-green or deep-yellow vegetables; and six daily servings of grain products, with at least three being whole grain. Increase the proportion of persons age 2 years and older who consume less than 10% of calories from saturated fat, and who consume no more than 30% of calories from fat.	• Educate families about the importance of whole grains, fruits, and vegetables in the diet. • Encourage the child to choose fruits and vegetables that appeal to him or her. • Provide creative suggestions for vegetable preparation to make them more appealing to children. • Educate families about saturated fat–containing foods. • Offer suggestions for alternate sources of protein and fats (chicken or fish, olive oil).

Nutritional Guidelines

School-age children should choose culturally appropriate foods and snacks from the Food Guide Pyramid. School-age children need to limit intake of fat and processed sugars. A prudent diet limits the use of fatty meats, high-fat dairy products, eggs, and hydrogenated shortenings and promotes the consumption of fish and the substitution of polyunsaturated vegetable oils and margarines. The American Heart Association has endorsed a diet for school-age children that includes the recommendations listed in Box 28.3.

Regarding Lawrence Jones, what questions should you ask Lawrence's mother related to nutritional intake? What anticipatory guidance related to nutrition would be appropriate?

Promoting Healthy Sleep and Rest

The number of hours of sleep required for growth and development decreases with age. Children between the ages of 6 and 8 years require about 12 hours of sleep per night. Children between 8 and 10 years of age require 10 to 12 hours of sleep per night, and children between 10 and 12 years of age need 9 to 10 hours of sleep per night. Young school-age children may need an occasional brief nap for an energy boost after being in school for most of the day. Bedtime rituals and consistent schedules continue to be important throughout the school-age years. Parents must facilitate the bedtime schedule and quiet time before bed. Bedtime is a special time for parents and children to read together, listen to stories or soothing music, share events of the day, and exchange expressions of affection. Children should have bedtime expectations as well as wake-up times and methods for waking up (alarm, calling by parent, and so forth).

BOX 28.3 **American Heart Association's Diet Recommendations for School-Age Children**

- A high-quality protein with every meal
- Milk with added vitamin D and other low-fat dairy products
- Vegetables high in vitamin A
- Fruits high in vitamin C
- Whole-grain or enriched breads or cereals
- Vegetable oils high in polyunsaturated fats
- Meats (4 servings per week of 4 ounces each)
- Fish (1–2 times per week)
- Poultry (1–2 times per week)
- Dark green, leafy, or deep yellow vegetables (at least 4 times per week)
- Eggs (4 times per week)

Night terrors or sleepwalking may occur in 6- to 8-year-olds but should be resolved between the ages of 8 and 10 years. In the older school-age child (11 to 12 years), encourage parents to allow a variation in the sleep schedule on the weekends and a regular schedule on weekdays.

Provide anticipatory guidance to Lawrence Jones's mother in relation to proper sleep for her 10-year-old son.

Promoting Healthy Teeth and Gums

Dental **caries** remains the leading disease in the United States, even though the incidence has been reduced since the introduction of fluoride (www.dentalcare.com). Dental care with emphasis on prevention of caries is important in this age group. Sometimes dental care is not considered to be important by parents of young children because the primary teeth will be replaced by permanent teeth. This perception leads to complications of permanent teeth such as **malocclusion** (see Healthy People 2010).

Proper alignment of teeth is important to tooth formation, speech development, and physical appearance. Many school-age children need braces or other orthodontic devices to correct malocclusion, a condition in which the teeth are crowded, crooked, or misaligned. **Bruxism** or teeth grinding while asleep may continue in the school-age years. Bruxism may result in grinding away of tooth enamel. Teeth grinding may be due to malalignment. A dental evaluation should be scheduled if consistent teeth grinding occurs.

School-age children need to brush their teeth two to three times per day for 3 minutes each time (Fig. 28.9). Parents should replace the toothbrush (soft) every 3 to 4 months. Flossing the teeth at least once daily is recommended by the American Dental Association. Parents must monitor teeth brushing, observe for abnormal alignment of their child's teeth, and schedule regular dental examinations every 6 months to ensure good dental health and prevent dental problems. Children may need help with brushing teeth until they are between 7 and 10 years of age. Dental sealants are recommended for all school-age children. The sealant is a plastic coating applied to biting surfaces to seal out tooth decay on permanent back teeth.

HEALTHY PEOPLE 2010

Objective	Nursing Significance
Reduce the proportion of children and adolescents who have dental caries in their primary or permanent teeth. Increase the proportion of children who have received dental sealants to their molar teeth.	• Encourage appropriate toothbrushing and flossing. • Educate child and family about fluoride use. • Refer school-age children to dentist for molar sealants. • Assist families lacking dental insurance to find resources for the provision of dental care.

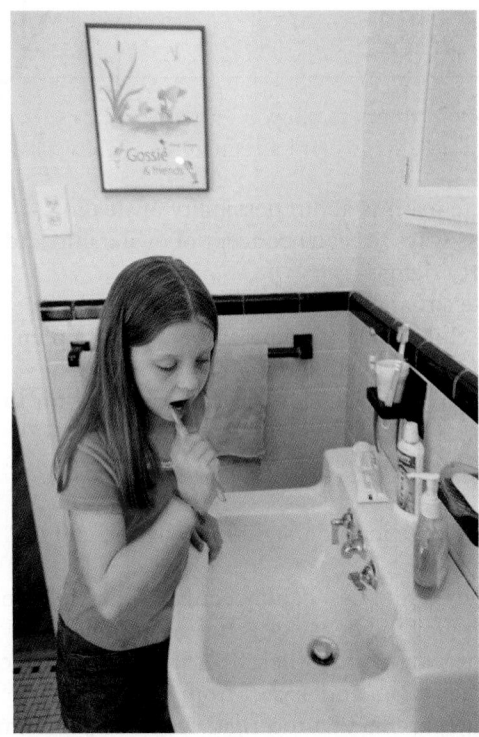

FIGURE 28.9 Using correct technique to brush the teeth is important in the prevention of cavities.

In addition, parents should give a fluoride supplement (as directed by the dentist) to their children if fluoride is not in the town's water supply.

Children wearing braces are more prone to cavities; encourage them to brush their teeth after meals and snacks. School nurses can assist these children with brushing after lunch. In addition, the school nurse should promote dental health through education on dental care and gum problems that result from lack of proper dental care. Diet can play a part in dental health. Limiting sticky, high-sugar, and high-carbohydrate foods will decrease the possibility of cavities.

Promoting Appropriate Discipline

Because of the increasing ability of the school-age child to view situations from different angles, the school-age child should be able to see how his actions affect others. Children between 6 and 8 years old are beginning to see the effects of behaviors on others. They are also beginning to realize that their behaviors can have consequences. Children between 8 and 12 years of age are fully aware of the cause and effect of their behaviors. They should be able to express emotions without using violence. Discipline techniques with consequences have both *natural* and *logical* consequences. Natural consequences allow the child to learn the results of their actions. For example, if the child throws a toy out of the window, then he cannot play with the toy anymore. In logical consequences, if the child does not put away her bike, she does not get to ride the bike for the rest of the day.

In disciplining children, parents should teach children the rules established by the family, values, and social rules of conduct. Rules should provide the school-age child with guidelines about behavior that is acceptable and unacceptable. School-age children look to their parents for guidance and as role models. Parents should role model appropriate expressions of feelings and emotions and allow the child to express emotions and feelings. Discuss the effects of the child's temperament on his or her behavior, as well as what constitutes age-appropriate behavior. Include how the parents' temperament can influence the child's temperament.

Effective guidance and discipline focus on the development of the child. They can preserve the child's self-esteem and dignity. Discuss with parents guidelines regarding discipline. Explain to parents that they should never belittle the child. Children may view parents and caretakers negatively if they are consistently belittled or insulted. These negative actions can inhibit learning and teach the child to react unkindly to others. Instead, parents should discipline with praise. Positive acknowledgements of progress are likely to encourage healthy development and appropriate behavior (AAP, 2004). Discuss with parents how to be realistic when planning activities so as to not overwhelm the child, resulting in misbehavior. Encourage parents to say "no" only when they mean it, to avoid a negative atmosphere in the home, and to avoid inconsistency.

When misbehaviors occur, the type and amount of discipline is based upon different factors:

- Developmental level of both the child and the parents
- Severity of the misbehavior
- Established rules of the family
- Temperament of the child
- Response of the child to rewards

Keep in mind that school-age children should participate in developing a plan of action for their misbehavior. Whatever methods of discipline are chosen, it is important that parents are consistent in providing discipline in a nurturing environment.

▶ ADDRESSING COMMON DEVELOPMENTAL CONCERNS

The developmental task (according to Erikson) of the school-age child is industry. The school-age child is busy learning, achieving, and exploring. As the school-age child becomes more independent, forces other than the family such as television, video games, and peers influence them. Some of these influences are positive and others are negative. Some of the common developmental concerns for the school-age child are discussed in the following sections. Guidelines to assist the parents and nurses when encountering these concerns are included in Teaching Guidelines 28.2.

TEACHING GUIDELINES 28.2

Addressing Common Developmental Concerns

Television and Video Games

- Limit television watching and video-game playing to 2 hours per day.
- Monitor television programs.
- Prohibit television or video games with violence.
- Do not put television or video games in children's bedrooms.
- Provide a schedule of accepted television programs for viewing each week.
- Co-view television and video games with the child.
- Encourage sports, interactive play, and reading.

Obesity

- Provide healthy meals and snacks.
- Schedule and encourage daily exercise.
- Encourage involvement in sports.
- Restrict TV and computer-game use.
- Limit the amount of fast-food intake.
- Provide education about healthy nutrition.
- Never use food as a reward.
- Be a good role model.

School Phobia

- Return child to school.
- Investigate cause of the fear.
- Support child.
- Collaborate with teachers.
- Praise success in school attendance.

Latchkey Kids

- Provide rules to follow and expectations, such as
  - Not answering the door or phone
  - No friends in the house when parents are not home
  - No playing with fire
- Teach child to call a trusted neighbor when help is needed and 911 in the event of emergency.
- Post all resource numbers, including after-school help lines if available, in a clearly viewable spot.
- Purchase caller ID for the phone system.
- Enroll the child in an after-school program if available.
- Discuss limitations of outside play.
- Discuss limitations of television viewing and video-game use.
- Make sure the child knows how to contact the parent.
- Set clear homework expectations.
- DO NOT keep guns in the home.

Stealing

- Educate parents about possibility of stealing.
- Discuss ways to teach concept of ownership and property rights.
- Handle situation openly.
- Assist child in developing and enacting a plan to return what was stolen.
- Make sure the punishment is appropriate for the action.

Lying

- Help parents in understanding why the child is lying.
- When the child lies, calmly confront the child and explain why the behavior is not acceptable.
- Educate parents that their behavior should reflect what they teach and expect from their child.
- Educate parents that too-rigid or severe punishments can decrease the child's sense of worth.
- Seek professional help if lying persists in the older school-age child, to rule out underlying problems.

Cheating

- Educate parents that the child must be mature enough to understand the concept of rules.
- Handle cheating situations openly.
- Help parents to understand why their child is cheating and to modify the trigger.
- Develop appropriate punishment; inappropriate punishment could undermine the child.
- Educate parents that their behavior should reflect what they expect from their child.
- Seek professional help if cheating persists in the older school-age child, to rule out underlying problems.

Bullying

The Bullied Child

- Educate parents whose children are at risk for being bullied
  - Children who appear different from the majority
  - Children who act different from the majority
  - Children who have low self-esteem
  - Children with a mental or psychological problem
- Teach parents to role play different scenarios the child may face at school; show the child different ways to react to being bullied.

TEACHING GUIDELINES 28.2 (continued)

Addressing Common Developmental Concerns

- Impress upon the child that he or she did not cause the bullying.
- Develop ways to increase the child's self-esteem at home.
- Discuss the situation with the teacher and develop a plan of care.

The Bullying Child

- Educate parents on reasons why it is important to correct the behavior.
- Discuss ways the child can appropriately show his or her anger and feelings.
- Have parents help the child to see how it feels to be bullied.
- Do not allow fighting at home.
- Reward settling of conflicts without violence.

Tobacco and Alcohol Education

- Inquire about tobacco and alcohol use.
- Discuss the physical and social dangers of tobacco and alcohol use.
- Urge parents to be good role models.
- Limit reading and media materials about alcohol and tobacco use.
- Discuss the influences of tobacco and alcohol use by peers.
- Educate the child on spit tobacco. Let them know it is just as dangerous as smoking tobacco.
- Advocate for a smoke-free environment in the home and other places frequented.
- Avoid having tobacco and alcohol products readily available in the home.

Television and Video Games

The influence of television and video games upon the school-age child is a growing concern for parents and child specialists. Children in the United States spend about 4 hours a day either watching TV or playing video games. During that time, a child will see 8,000 murders by the end of grade school and 40,000 commercials a year. Although a school-age child can determine what is real from what is fantasy, research has shown that this amount of time in front of the TV—watching it or playing video games— can lead to aggressive behavior, less physical activity, and altered body image (see Healthy People 2010).

Although some television shows and video games can have positive influences on children, teach parents guidelines on the use of TV and video games. Parents should set limits on how much TV watching the child can have. The American Academy of Pediatrics recommends 2 hours or less of television viewing per day. The parent should establish guidelines on when the child can watch TV, for example, after homework or when chores are completed. Television watching should not be used as a reward. The parents should be aware of what the child is watching.

Watch the programs together and use that opportunity to discuss the subject matter with the child. There should be no TV during dinner and no TV in the child's room. The parents need to set an example for the child. Read instead of watching TV or do a physical activity together as a family. If the TV causes fights or arguments, it should be turned off for a period of time.

Obesity

The National Health and Nutrition Examination Survey (NHANES) found that more and more children are overweight. Over the past three decades the number of overweight children and adolescents more than tripled. Thirty percent of 6- to 11-year-olds are overweight or at risk for overweight (NAPNAP, 2006). Overweight is classified as a body mass index (BMI) greater than 85% and obese is classified as a BMI greater than 95% (see Healthy People 2010).

Obesity occurs when the intake of calories and food exceeds the expenditures. Some factors linked to causing

HEALTHY PEOPLE 2010

Objective	Nursing Significance
Increase the proportion of children and adolescents who view television 2 or fewer hours per day.	• Assist families to identify activities other than television for the child to participate in. • Praise craft, music, and sports participation.

HEALTHY PEOPLE 2010

Objective	Nursing Significance
Reduce the proportion of children and adolescents who are overweight or obese.	• Screen all children for the development of overweight as indicated by an increasing body mass index (BMI) for their age. • Provide accurate diet counseling. • Encourage daily physical activity. • Counsel parents to limit television/computer time daily.

obesity include family role modeling, lack of exercise, and unstructured meals as well as cultural, genetic, environmental, and socioeconomic factors. Some factors that influence lack of exercise include the decreased number of days that school systems offer physical education programs and recess. Also, some children live in unsafe neighborhoods and have no safe place to play outside; therefore they spend time in sedentary activities such as watching TV. Children with low metabolic rates and increased numbers of fat cells tend to gain more weight. Obese children are at risk for cardiovascular diseases, type 2 (non–insulin dependent) diabetes, and orthopedic problems. Also, psychosocial problems and eating disorders are prevalent. When parents do not have knowledge of nutrition, do not monitor snacks or meals, and have unstructured meals, habits are established that lead to obesity. A lack of exercise also contributes to obesity.

Preventing obesity in childhood is important because the fat cells of childhood are carried into adulthood obesity and contribute to disease. Due to the risk of obesity, encourage parents to never use food as a reward. To prevent obesity, establish regular mealtimes and offer healthy foods and snacks. Encourage parents to praise their child's good food choices and to role model appropriate eating and exercise.

School Phobia

School refusal (also called *school phobia* or *school avoidance*) has been defined as frequent absences, dropping out of school, or academic disengagement or disruption (Kearney, 2006). School phobia needs to be defined both symptomatically and operationally as the cause for the anxiety. School avoidance occurs in approximately 5% of school-age children. These children may refuse to attend school or create reasons why they cannot go to school.

Some of the fears expressed by school-refusing children include tests, bullying, teacher reprimands, anxieties over toileting in a public bathroom, physical harm, or undressing in the locker room. Due to the emotional distress caused in these children when attending school, they are frequently classified as having school phobia. Young children may complain of stomachache or headache and older children may complain of palpitations or feeling faint.

It is important to investigate specific causes of school refusal/school phobia and take appropriate actions. The physician or nurse practitioner should conduct a physical examination of the child to rule out any physical illness. After these measures are taken, the parent, teacher, school counselor, and school administrator may devise a plan to assist the student to overcome a specific fear. In uncomplicated cases, parents must return the child to school as soon as possible. There may be altered schedules (partial days or decreased hours) to help promote a successful transition back to school. Another idea to help desensitize the child may be to have him or her spend part of the day in the counselor's or school nurse's office.

Latchkey Children

With both parents in the workforce, many children return home alone without adult supervision for a number of hours. These "latchkey kids" are more prone to misbehave and to take risks. The American Academy of Pediatrics recommends that a child come home to a parent, another adult, or a responsible adolescent (www.aap.org).

Most young children are not capable of handling stress or making decisions on their own before 11 or 12 years of age. However, some school-age children are more mature and can be left alone by 8 to 10 years of age; maturity is the key, not the age. Despite the level of maturity, children who are unsupervised are more likely to use alcohol and illegal drugs. In addition, latchkey children may feel isolated from friends because friends may be prohibited from entering the home when parents are not present (American Academy of Child and Adolescent Psychiatry, 2004).

If children come home to no supervision, they should know the names, addresses, and phone numbers of parents and a neighbor, as well as emergency numbers. They should be given rules about answering the door and the phone. They should tell anyone who comes to the door or who calls that mom is home but busy at this time. Directions as to the handling of the house key and fire safety should be taught and demonstrated (see Teaching Guidelines 28.2).

Stealing, Lying, and Cheating

It is during the school-age years that antisocial behaviors can emerge. Children who were previously well behaved may now exhibit behaviors of stealing, lying, and cheating. Parents are usually disturbed by this change in behavior. In turn, they have difficulty in addressing these issues and need help in providing appropriate interventions.

Children between 6 and 8 years old do not fully understand the concept of ownership and property rights. These children may steal things because they like the look of the item. Stealing in the 8- to 10-year-old may occur because the child desires the item or to impress the child's peers. The 10- to 12-year-old child may steal for the same reasons as children between 8 and 10 years of age. In addition, these older children may steal to supplement their perceived inadequate income.

Lying is more common in children between 6 and 8 years old. It is acceptable for these children to tell tall tales, but they should know what truth is and what make-believe is. These younger children typically lie to avoid punishment. However, they do not like others to lie and will tell on them if they lie. Children between 8 and 12 years old typically lie because they are unable to meet expectations of family and peers. They also lie to impress others. If lying persists in older school-age children, parents should discuss the matter with a health care provider because the lying may be evidence of underlying problems.

The concept of cheating is not well understood until the child is 7 years old. Before this age, the desire to "win"

EVIDENCE-BASED PRACTICE 28.1
Benefits of Bully-Prevention Education

● **Study**

Child conduct problems continue to pose a problem in elementary schools. In addition to the behavioral disruption that occurs as a result of bullying and victimization, prior research has demonstrated that child bullies and victims are at increased risk for mental health problems and antisocial behavior. This study was performed over a 2-year period utilizing fourth-grade classrooms at 28 public elementary schools. The group-randomized trial assigned classrooms to receive a program aimed at bullying and aggression prevention or to receive no treatment at all. Self-reported bullying and victimization were then analyzed after the 2-year trial.

▲ **Findings**

Upon analysis of the findings, the researchers reported a mild decrease in bullying and a greater decrease in bullying victimization. It appears that bullying-prevention programs in elementary schools may be effective in decreasing aggression and violence in the school-age group.

■ **Nursing Implications**

Nurses should continue to educate parents and teachers about bullying. Encourage children to be involved in peer groups. Become actively involved in the local elementary school bullying-prevention program. When bullies are identified, refer them for education in alternative means of emotional expression such as social skills training.

Jensen, J. M., & Dieterich, W. A. (2007). Effects of a skills-based prevention program on bullying and bully victimization among elementary school children. *Prevention Science, 8,* 285–296.

is most important and rigid rules are hard to understand. In children between 8 and 12 years old, the concept of cheating is fully understood. It is usually done because of peer pressure, strong pressure placed on the child to succeed by parents, and a sense of low self-esteem. If cheating persists in older school-age children, parents should discuss the matter with a health care provider because the behavior may indicate underlying problems.

In dealing with children who exhibit stealing, lying, or cheating behaviors, parents must first realize the importance of their own behaviors in those areas. Parents are role models to the school-age child. Therefore, when the child sees or hears that parents lie, steal, or cheat (e.g., parents bragging about cheating on their taxes), they think it is all right to mimic those behaviors. Secondly, parents must directly confront any stealing, lying, or cheating behaviors and discuss (and follow through consistently with) the consequences of such behaviors (see Teaching Guideline 28.2).

Bullying

Bullying, defined as inflicting verbal, emotional, or physical abuse upon others, is on the increase during the school-age years. Bullied children are those who report themselves as being lonely and having difficulty in forming friendships. The children who perform the bullying are those children who are reported to have low self-esteem, poor grades, and poor interpersonal skills.

In general, about 10% of all children attending school are frightened and afraid most of the day. Most of the bullying occurs at school. Both boys and girls are bullied; boys usually bully boys and use force more often. Girls can be bullied by both sexes using mainly social alienation and intimidation. Both girls and boys can bully. Girls are usually the bullies in grades 1 through 3, and boys are typically the bullies in grades 4 and above.

Being bullied can have negative results on children throughout life. These children often have increased episodes of common childhood illnesses of headaches, stomachaches, and sleep problems. After the problem of either being bullied or being the bully has been identified, parents must work with the child, the school, and the health care provider to solve the problem (see Teaching Guidelines 28.2 and Evidence-Based Practice).

Tobacco and Alcohol Education

School-age children are eager to grow up and be independent. Peers and acceptance are very important at this time. School-age children may be exposed to messages that are in conflict with their parents' values regarding smoking and alcohol. Peers often exert pressure for children to experiment with tobacco and alcohol (see Healthy People 2010).

School-age children are ready to absorb information that deals with drugs and alcohol. Information from parents or other adults who are major influences in the child's life is essential at this time to set clear rules and model

HEALTHY PEOPLE 2010

Objective	Nursing Significance
Reduce initiation of tobacco use among children and adolescents.	• Educate children and families about the dangers of tobacco use.

behaviors for children to embrace. Discussions with children need to be based on facts and focused on the present. Some topics for discussion include:

- What alcohol and drugs are like and how they harm you
- Differences in medical use vs. illegal use of drugs
- How to think critically to interpret messages seen in advertising, media, sports, and entertainment personalities

See Teaching Guidelines 28.2.

Recall Lawrence Jones, the 10-year-old presented at the beginning of the chapter. List potential developmental problems he may experience. What anticipatory guidance related to these concerns should you provide to his mother?

■■■ Key Concepts

- Physical growth is slow and steady, with social and cognitive development progressing rapidly, during the school-age years of 6 to 12. Height increases approximately 2 inches per year and weight gain is 1½ to 3 kilograms (3 to 6 pounds) per year. Boys are taller and heavier than girls during this time period.
- With the entrance into the school system, school-age children have the influences of peers and teachers.
- With the development of gross motor skills and involvement in sports at school and in the community, safety education and practices are required. Also, with the participation in cooperative sports, injuries occur.
- Visual acuity is reaching maturation and 20/20 vision is expected by 7 years of age.
- Increased independence leads to increased exposure to safety hazards.
- The school-age child develops the cognitive ability to classify objects and to identify relationships among objects.
- Dental care is very important to prevent dental caries, malocclusion, and other problems. In early school age, the first primary teeth will be lost.
- The onset of puberty may occur by the later school-age years.
- Erikson's developmental task for the age group is the development of a sense of industry.
- Peers are very important, especially peers of the same sex. School-age children usually have a best friend and belong to clubs. They have collections of nonvaluable items such as rocks, clips, and so forth.
- School-age children are capable of concrete operations, solving problems, and making decisions. They continue to need guidance, rules, and directions from parents.
- The school-age child develops a conscience and knows cultural and social values. He can understand and obey rules.

- The school-age child incorporates religious practices into her life, which may be a source of comfort during stressful times.
- The nurse's role includes educating parents and school-age children in promoting health and safety.
- Nurses should inform the school-age child about expected developmental changes in the body to promote self-esteem and self-confidence.

REFERENCES

Alba-Fisch, M. (2007). *Temperament: Miss or match.* Retrieved August 28, 2007 from http://www.taconicnet.com/articles/temperament.php.

American Academy of Child & Adolescent Psychiatry. (2004). *Home alone children.* Retrieved August 28, 2007 from http://aacap.org/page.ww?name=Home+Alone+Children&section=Facts+for+Families.

American Academy of Pediatric Dentistry. (2007). *Policy on use of fluoride.* Retrieved August 28, 2007 from http://www.aapd.org/media/Policies_Guidelines/P_FluorideUse.pdf.

American Academy of Pediatrics. (2003). Policy statement: Prevention of drowning in infants, children and adolescents. *Pediatrics, 112*(2), 437–439.

American Academy of Pediatrics. (2004). *Guidance for effective discipline.* Retrieved August 28, 2007 from http://aappolicy.aappublications.org/cgi/content/full/pediatrics;101/4/723.

American Academy of Pediatrics. (2006). Active healthy living: Prevention of childhood obesity through increased physical activity. *Pediatrics, 117*, 1834–1842.

American Academy of Pediatrics. (2006). *Corporal punishment in schools.* Retrieved August 28, 2007 from http://aappolicy.aappublications.org/cgi/content/full/pediatrics;106/2/343.

American Academy of Pediatrics, The Injury Prevention Program. (2007a). *Age-related safety sheets: 6 years.* Retrieved August 28, 2007 from http://www.aap.org/family/6years.htm.

American Academy of Pediatrics, The Injury Prevention Program. (2007a). *Age-related safety sheets: 8 years.* Retrieved August 28, 2007 from http://www.aap.org/family/8years.htm.

American Academy of Pediatrics, The Injury Prevention Program. (2007a). *Age-related safety sheets: 10 years.* Retrieved August 28, 2007 from http://www.aap.org/family/10years.htm.

American Heart Association, Gidding, S. S., Dennison, B. A., Birch, L. L., Daniels, S. R., Gilman, M. W., Lichtenstien, A. H., Rattay, K. T., Steinberger, J., Stettler, N., & Van Horn, L. (2006). Dietary recommendations for children and adolescents: A guide for practitioners. *Pediatrics, 117*(2), 544–559.

Barakat, I. S., & Clark, J. A. (2005). *Positive discipline and child guidance.* Retrieved July 9, 2006 from http://muextension.missouri.edu/xplor/hesguide/humanrel/gh6119.htm.

Bautista, S. R., & Flynn, J. R. (2006). Trauma prevention in children. *Pediatric Annals, 35*(2), 85–90.

Bindler, R. M., & Bruya, M. A. (2007). Evidence for identifying children at risk for being overweight, cardiovascular disease, and type 2 diabetes in primary care. *Journal of Pediatric Health Care, 20*(2), 82–87.

Centers for Disease Control. (2007a). *10 leading causes of death, United States, 2004, all races, both sexes.* Retrieved August 28, 2007 from http://webappa.cdc.gov/cgi-bin/broker.exe.

Centers for Disease Control. (2007b). *The injury pyramid.* Retrieved August 28, 2007 from http://www.cdc.gov/HealthyYouth/injury/slides/injury_guidelines.ppt#4.

ChildHelp. (2006). *Child abuse statistics.* Retrieved August 28, 2007 from http://www.childhelp.org/resources/learning-center/statistics.

Child Development Institute. (2007). *Helping your child deal with fears and phobias.* Retrieved August 28, 2007 from http://www.childdevelopmentinfo.com/disorders/fears.htm.

Christakis, D. A., & Zimmerman, F. J. (2007). Children and television: A primer for pediatricians. *Contemporary Pediatrics, 24*(3), 31–42.

Desantis-Moniaci, D., & Altshuler, L. (2007). Comprehensive behavioral treatment of overweight and the pediatric practice. *Pediatrics Annals, 36*(2), 102–108.

Edelman, C. L., & Mandle, C. L. (2006). *Health promotion throughout the life span* (6th ed.). St. Louis: Mosby.

Erikson, E. (1963). *Childhood and society* (2nd ed.). New York: Norton.

Green, M., & Palfrey, J. S. (Eds.). (2002). *Bright futures: Guidelines for health supervision of infants, children, and adolescents* (2nd ed., rev.). Arlington, VA: National Center for Education in Maternal and Child Health.

Gunturu, S. D., & Ten, S. (2007). Complications of obesity in childhood. *Pediatric Annals, 36*(2), 96–101.

Hegvik, R., McDevitt, S., & Carey, W. (1982). The middle childhood temperament questionnaire/develop. *Journal of Developmental and Behavioral Pediatrics, 3*(4), 197–200.

Heyman, R. B. (2007). Combating underage drinking with the 6 g's. *Contemporary Pediatrics, 24*(6), 63–75.

Hockenberry, M., Wilson, D., Winkelstein, M. L., & Kline, N. (2003). *Wong's infant care of infants and children* (7th ed.). St. Louis, MO: Mosby.

Kearney, C. (2006). Dealing with school refusal behavior, a primer for family physicians: Workable solutions for unhappy youth and frustrated parents. *Journal of Family Practice, 55*(8), 685–692.

Kellogg, N., & Committee on Child Abuse and Neglect. (2005). The evaluation of sexual abuse in children. *Pediatrics, 116*(2), 506–512.

McDevitt, S., & Carey, W. (1978). The measurement of temperament in 3–7 year old children. *Journal of Child Psychology and Psychiatry, 19*, 245–253.

Meadows-Oliver, M. (2007). Using our heads: What PNPs need to know about helmets. *Journal of Pediatric Health Care, 21*(4), 265–267.

National Association for Sport & Physical Education. (2007). *Active start: A statement of physical activity guidelines for children birth to five years.* Retrieved August 28, 2007 from http://www.aahperd.org/NASPE/ns_active.html.

National Association of Pediatric Nurse Practitioners. (2006a). *Healthy eating and activity together (HEAT) clinical practice guideline: Identifying and preventing overweight in childhood.* Cherry Hill, NJ: Author.

National Association of Pediatric Nurse Practitioners. (2006b). NAPNAP position statement on corporal punishment. *Journal of Pediatric Health Care, 20*(6), A43–A44.

Nield, L. S., Stenger, J. P., & Kamat, D. (2007). Dental disease: pearls about those pearly whites. *Consultant for Pediatricians, 6*(8), 449–454.

Papalia, D. E., Olds, S. W., & Feldman, R. D. (2006). *Human development.* New York: McGraw-Hill.

Rosenbaum, M. (2007). Epidemiology of pediatric obesity. *Pediatric Annals, 26*(2), 89–95.

Safe Kids USA. (2007). *Safety tips: Car.* Retrieved August 28, 2007 from http://www.usa.safekids.org/tier2_rl.cfm?folder_id=170.

Safe Kids Worldwide. (2007). *Preventing injury to children in motor vehicle crashes.* Retrieved August 28, 2007 from http://www.usa.safekids.org/content_documents/MVO_tips.pdf.

Savage, J. S., Fisher, J. O. & Birch, L. L. (2007). Parental influence on eating behavior: Conception to adolescence. *The Journal of Law, Medicine & Ethics, 35*(1), 22–34.

Schuman, A. J. (2007). The ABCs of toy safety: More than just child's play. *Contemporary Pediatrics, 24*(7), 49–57, 64.

Storey, M., Holt, K., & Sotfka, D. (Eds.). (2002). *Bright futures in practice: Nutrition* (2nd ed.). Arlington, VA: National Center for Education in Maternal and Child Health.

World Health Organization. (2007). *Passive smoking.* Retrieved August 26, 2007 from http://www.who.int/tobacco/en/atlas10.pdf.

Yuma, P. J., & Maldonado, M. (2006). Booster seats: Protecting the forgotten child. *Journal of Pediatric Health Care, 20*(2), 137–140.

WEBSITES

Sports Illustrated for Kids (online): sikids.com/

American Academy of Pediatrics: www.aap.org

American Association of Pediatric Dentistry: www.aapd.org

American Academy of Ophthalmology: www.aao.org

Dental care information: www.dentalcare.com/drn.htm

American Dietetic Association: www.eatright.org

Healthy People 2010: www.healthypeople.gov/

Healthy Schools.org is a nonprofit organization devoted to decreasing environmental exposures in schools: www.healthyschools.org

Kids' website of the U.S. Department of Health and Human Services: www.hhs.gov/kids/

Nemours Center for Children's Health Media: www.kidshealth.org/

Sutter Health Institute website for preteens: www.pamf.org/preteen/mybody/

Center for Sports Parenting: www.sportsparenting.org/csp/

Safe Kids USA: www.usa.safekids.org/

CHAPTER WORKSHEET

MULTIPLE CHOICE QUESTIONS

1. The successful resolution of developmental tasks for the school-age child, according to Erikson, would be identified by:

    a. Learning from repeating tasks.

    b. Developing a sense of worth and competence.

    c. Using fantasy and magical thinking to cope with problems.

    d. Developing a sense of trust.

2. Which of the following are reasons that stealing occurs in school-age children? (Choose all that apply)

    a. To escape punishment

    b. High self-esteem

    c. Low expectations of family/peers

    d. Lack of sense of propriety

    e. Strong desire to own something

3. Which activities will promote weight loss in an obese school-age child? (Choose all that apply)

    a. Unlimited computer and TV time

    b. Role modeling by family

    c. Becoming active in sports

    d. Eating unstructured meals

    e. Involving child in meal planning and grocery shopping

    f. Drinking three glasses of water per day

4. As the school nurse conducting screening for vision in a 6-year-old child, you would refer the child to a specialist if the visual acuity in both eyes is:

    a. 20/20

    b. 20/25

    c. 20/30

    d. 20/50

5. The mother of two sons, ages 6 and 9, states they want to play on the same baseball team. As the school nurse, what advice would you give their mother?

    a. Having the boys on the same team will make it more convenient for the mother.

    b. Levels of coordination and concentration differ, so the boys need to be on different teams.

    c. Put the boys on the same team because they are both school-age children.

    d. It is best to avoid putting the boys on the same team to prevent sibling rivalry.

CRITICAL THINKING EXERCISES

1. Ms. Sams brings her 8-year-old son (Frank) to the pediatrician's office for his annual exam. She states that she is concerned about his recent behavior. He went to the grocery store with his friend and his friend's mother and he came home with a Matchbox car. The friend's mother stated she had not purchased the car.

    a. What would be your response to Ms. Sams?

    b. Ms. Sams said she still has the car. What would you advise Ms. Sams to do to make Frank aware of consequences of his actions?

2. Sally's mother is asking the nurse advice about purchasing a 2-wheeled bike for her 7-year-old. What guidance should the nurse offer this parent?

3. Ms. Shaw brings in her 11-year-old daughter for a well-child check. The schoolager says to the nurse, "I look different from my friends. I do not wear bras and my friends are already wearing bras." What would be an appropriate response to this schoolager?

4. Johnny is a 9-year-old whose mother and father both work during the day. He returns home after school. How should the parents prepare Johnny for this experience? What safety rules would be included in the education for Johnny?

STUDY ACTIVITIES

1. Attend a sporting event (such as soccer or baseball) with school-age teams. Describe the coordination and gross motor functioning of this group.

2. Attend a first-grade class. Observe the behaviors exhibited by the school-age children in this class. How do these behaviors compare with normal values for this age group?

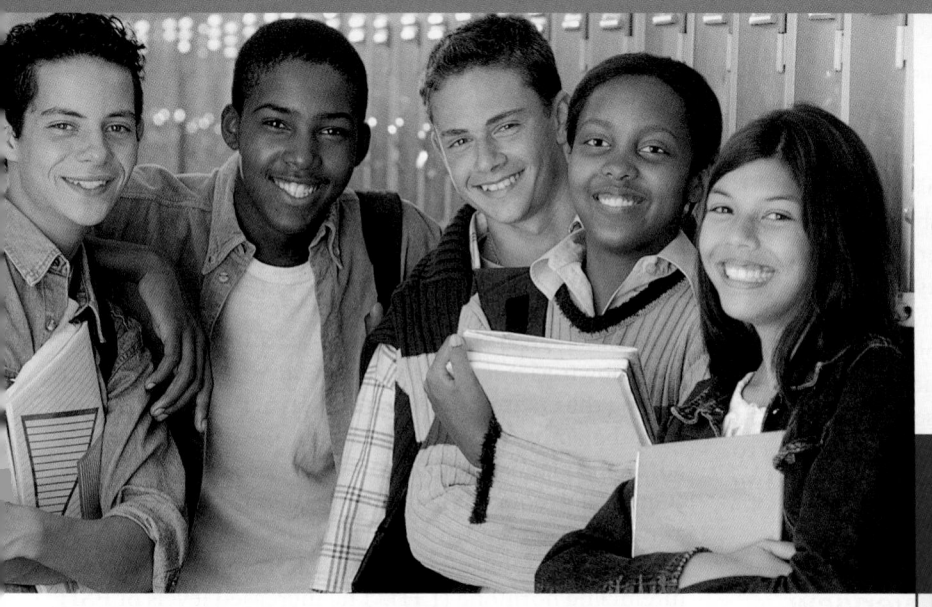

GROWTH AND DEVELOPMENT OF THE ADOLESCENT

KEY TERMS

adolescence
adolescent egocentrism
invincibility

menarche
peer groups
puberty

risk-taking behaviors
sexuality

LEARNING OBJECTIVES

Upon completion of the chapter, the learner will be able to:

1. Identify normal physiologic changes, including puberty, occurring in the adolescent.
2. Discuss psychosocial, cognitive, and moral changes occurring in the adolescent.
3. Identify changes in relationships with peers, family, teachers, and community during adolescence.
4. Describe interventions to promote safety during adolescence.
5. Demonstrate knowledge of the nutritional requirements of the adolescent.
6. Demonstrate knowledge of the development of sexuality and its influence on dating during adolescence.
7. Identify common developmental concerns of the adolescent.
8. Demonstrate knowledge of the appropriate nursing guidance for common developmental concerns.

Cho Chung is a 15-year-old girl brought to the clinic by her mother for her annual school check-up. During your assessment you measure Cho's weight at 110 pounds and her height at 60 inches. As the nurse caring for her, assess Cho's growth and development, and then provide appropriate anticipatory guidance to her and her mother.

WOW
The only way to grow is to let go...

Adolescence spans the years of transition from childhood to adulthood, which is usually between the ages of 11 and 20 years. There is some overlap between late school age and adolescence. The adolescent experiences drastic changes in the physical, cognitive, psychosocial, and psychosexual areas. With this rapid growth during adolescence, the development of secondary sexual characteristics, and interest in the opposite sex, the adolescent needs the support and guidance of parents and nurses to facilitate healthy lifestyles and to reduce **risk-taking behaviors**.

Growth and Development Overview

Adolescence is a time of rapid growth with dramatic changes in body size and proportions. The magnitude of these changes is second only to the growth in infancy. During this time sexual characteristics develop and reproductive maturity is achieved. The age of onset and the duration of the physiologic changes vary from individual to individual. Generally girls enter **puberty** earlier (at 9 to 10 years of age) than boys (at 10 to 11 years). Adolescents will represent varying levels of identity formation and will offer unique challenges to the nurse (Table 29.1).

▶ PHYSIOLOGIC CHANGES ASSOCIATED WITH PUBERTY

The secretion of estrogen in girls and testosterone in boys stimulates the development of breast tissue in girls, pubic hair in both sexes, and changes in male genitalia. These biological changes that occur during adolescence are known as *puberty*. Puberty is the result of triggers among the environment, the central nervous system, the hypothalamus, the pituitary gland, the gonads, and the adrenal glands. Gonadotropin-releasing hormone (GnRH), produced by the hypothalamus, travels to the anterior pituitary gland to stimulate the production and secretion of follicle-stimulating hormone (FSH) and luteinizing hormone (LH). The increased levels of FSH and LH stimulate the gonadal response. LH stimulates ovulation in girls and acts on testicular Leydig cells in boys, prompting maturation of the testicles and testosterone production. FSH with LH stimulates sperm production. Estrogen, progesterone, and testosterone and other androgens are released from the gonads and affect biological changes and changes in various organs, including alterations in muscles, bones, skin, and hair follicles.

Adolescents experience physical development, hormonal changes, and sexual maturation during puberty

TABLE 29.1 **PHYSIOLOGIC CHANGES OF ADOLESCENCE**

Stage of Adolescence	Changes in Females	Changes in Males
Early adolescence (11–14 years)	Pubic hair begins to curl and spread over mons pubis; genitalia pigmentation increases. Breast bud and areola continue to enlarge; no separation of breast. First menstrual period (average 12.8 years)	Pubic hair spreads laterally, begins to curl; pigmentation increases. Growth and enlargement of testes in scrotum (scrotum reddish in color) and continued lengthening of penis. Leggy look due to extremities growing faster than the trunk
Middle adolescence (14–16 years)	Pubic hair becomes coarse in texture and continues to curl; amount of hair increases. Areola and papilla separate from the contour of the breast to form a secondary mound.	Pubic hair becomes coarser in texture and takes on adult distribution. Testes and scrotum continue to grow; scrotal skin darkens; penis grows in width, and glans penis develops. May experience breast enlargement. Voice changes; more masculine due to rapid enlargement of the larynx and pharynx as well as lung changes
Late adolescence (17–20 years)	Mature pubic hair distribution and coarseness	Mature pubic hair distribution and coarseness. Breast enlargement disappears. Adult size and shape of testes, scrotum, and penis; scrotal skin darkening

that correlate to Freud's genital stage of psychosexual development. The genital stage begins with the production of sex hormones and maturation of the reproductive system.

Girls reach physical maturity before boys and menstruation usually begins between the ages of 9 and 15 years (average 12.8 years). Breast budding (thelarche) occurs at approximately age 9 to 11 years and is followed by the growth of pubic hair. African-American girls reach **menarche** slightly earlier than Caucasian girls (Burns et al., 2004).

The first sign of pubertal changes in boys is testicular enlargement in response to testosterone secretion, usually occurring in Tanner stage 2. As testosterone levels increase, the penis and scrotum enlarge, hair distribution increases, and scrotal skin texture changes. During late puberty, boys will typically experience their first ejaculation, which may occur while they are sleeping (nocturnal emissions). Nurses should provide anticipatory guidance to adolescent males regarding involuntary nocturnal emissions (wet dreams) to assure them that this is a normal occurrence.

Tanner stages 3 to 5 usually occur during adolescence. Refer to Figures 31.28, 31.34, and 31.36 for an illustration of the increase in breast tissue and pubic hair distribution in girls, and scrotal and penile changes as well as hair distribution changes in boys. The nurse should provide guidance to adolescents about the normalcy of the sexual feelings and evolving body changes that occur during puberty.

▶ PHYSICAL GROWTH

Diet, exercise, and hereditary factors influence the height, weight, and body build of the adolescent. Over the past three decades, adolescents have become taller and heavier than their ancestors and the beginning of puberty is earlier. During the early adolescent period, there is an increase in the percentage of body fat and the head, neck, and hands reach adult proportions.

The rapid growth during adolescence is secondary only to that of the infant years and is a direct result of the hormonal changes of puberty. Both girls and boys experience changes in appearance and size. Height in girls increases rapidly after menarche and usually ceases 2 to 2½ years after menarche. Boys' growth spurt occurs later than girls' and usually begins between the ages of 10½ and 16 years and ends sometime between the ages of 13½ and 17½ years. Peak height velocity (PHV) occurs at approximately 12 years of age in girls or at about 6 to 12 months after menarche. Boys reach PHV at about 14 years of age. Peak weight velocity (PWV) occurs about 6 months after menarche in girls and at about 14 years of age in boys. Muscle mass increases in boys and fat deposits increase in girls (Fig. 29.1).

During early adolescence growth is rapid, but it decreases in middle and late adolescence. Height for adolescent boys who are between the 50th and 95th percentile ranges from 52½ inches (132 centimeters) to 69½ inches (176.8 centimeters). Weight of boys in these percentiles ranges from 77¼ pounds (35.3 kilograms) to 211 pounds

FIGURE 29.1 These adolescents reflect the differences in sizes and shapes seen in adolescents of the same age.

(95.76 kilograms). On average, boys will gain 10 to 30 centimeters (4 to 12 inches) in height and 7 to 30 kilograms (15 to 65 pounds) in weight.

Height for girls who are between the 50th and 95th percentile ranges from 57 inches (144.8 centimeters) to 68½ inches (173.6 centimeters), with weight ranging from 60 pounds (27.24 kilograms) to 181 pounds (82.47 kilograms). On average, girls will gain 5 to 20 centimeters (2 to 8 inches) in height and 7 to 25 kg (15 to 55 pounds) in weight during adolescence. See Appendix A for growth charts for this age group. Refer to Chapter 31 for instructions for calculating body mass index (BMI).

▶ ORGAN SYSTEM MATURATION

Adolescence is a time of metabolic slowing and of increasing size of some organs. The basal metabolic rate (BMR) reaches the adult level during late adolescence.

Neurologic System

During adolescence there is continued brain growth although the size of the brain does not increase significantly. Neurons do not increase in number, but growth of the myelin sheath enables faster neural processing.

Respiratory System

The adolescent years see an increase in diameter and length of the lungs. Respiratory rate decreases and reaches the adult rate of 15 to 20 breaths per minute. Respiratory volume and vital capacity increase. Volume and capacity are greater in boys than girls, which may be associated with increased chest and shoulder size in boys. The growth of the laryngeal cartilage, larynx, and vocal cords produces the voice changes experienced in adolescence. Deepening of both male and female voices occurs but is more pronounced in boys (Edelman & Mandle, 2006).

Cardiovascular System

There is an increase in size and strength of the heart. Systolic blood pressure increases and heart rate decreases. Blood volume reaches higher levels in boys than girls, which may be due to boys' greater muscle mass.

Gastrointestinal System

The adolescent has a full set of permanent teeth with the exception of the last four molars (permanent teeth) which may erupt at age 17 to 20 years. The liver, spleen, kidneys, and digestive tract enlarge during the growth spurt in early adolescence, but do not change in function. These systems are mature in early school age.

Musculoskeletal System

The ossification of the skeletal system is incomplete until late adolescence in boys. Ossification is more advanced in girls and occurs at an earlier age. During the growth spurt, muscle mass and strength increase. At similar stages of development, muscle development is generally greater in boys. Estrogen, progesterone, and testosterone (sex steroids) and other androgens are released from the gonads and affect changes in the muscles and bones. Low estrogen levels tend to stimulate skeletal growth, while higher levels inhibit growth. During middle adolescence, shoulder, chest, and hip breadth increase.

Integumentary System

During adolescence the skin becomes thick and tough. Under the influence of androgens, the sebaceous glands become more active, particularly on the face, back, and genitals. Due to the increased levels of testosterone during Tanner stages 4 and 5 in both boys and girls, both sexes may have increased sebum production, which may lead to the development of acne and oily hair.

The exocrine and apocrine sweat glands function at adult levels during adolescence. The exocrine glands are all over the body and they produce sweat that helps to eliminate body heat through evaporation. The apocrine glands are found in the axillae, genital, and anal areas, and around the breasts. The apocrine sweat glands produce sweat in response to hair follicles. This sweat is produced continuously and is stored and released in response to emotional stimuli.

▶ PSYCHOSOCIAL DEVELOPMENT

According to Erikson, it is during adolescence that teenagers achieve a sense of identity. As the adolescent is trying out many different roles in regard to his relationships with peers, family, community, and society, he is developing his own individual sense of self. If he is not successful in forming his own sense of self, he develops a sense of role confusion or diffusion. The adolescent culture becomes very important to the teenager. It is through his involvement with teenage groups that the adolescent finds support and help with developing his own identity.

Erikson believed that during the task of developing his own sense of identity, the adolescent revisits each of the previous stages of development. The sense of trust is encountered as the adolescent strives to find out whom and what ideals he can have faith in. In revisiting the stage of autonomy, the adolescent is seeking out ways to express his individuality in an effective manner. He would avoid behaviors that would "shame" or ridicule him in front of his peers. The sense of initiative is revisited as the adolescent develops his vision for what he might become. And the sense of industry is again encountered as the adolescent makes his choice to participate in different activities at school, in the community, at church, and in the work force.

The ability of the adolescent to successfully form a sense of self is dependent upon how well the adolescent successfully completed the former stages of development. Erikson believed that if the adolescent has been successful, he could develop resources during adolescence to overcome any gaps in previous developmental stages. If the adolescent believes that he cannot express himself in any manner due to societal restrictions, he will develop role confusion. See Table 29.2 for additional information.

TABLE 29.2 DEVELOPMENTAL THEORIES

Theories	Stages	Activities
Erikson (psychosocial)	Identity vs. role confusion or diffusion Early (11–14 years)	Focuses on bodily changes Experiences frequent mood changes Importance placed upon conformity to peer norms and peer acceptance Strives to master skills within peer groups Defining boundaries with parents and authority figures Early stage of emancipation—struggles to separate from parents while still desiring dependence upon them Identifies with same-sex peers Takes more responsibility for own behaviors
	Middle (14–16 years)	Continues to adjust to changed body image Tries out different roles within peer groups Need for acceptance by peer group at the highest level Interested in attracting opposite gender Time of greatest conflict with parents/authority figures Able to understand implications of behavior and decisions
	Late (17–20 years)	Roles within peer groups established Feels secure with body image Has matured sexual identity Has idealistic career goals Importance of individual friendships emerges Process of emancipation from family almost complete
Piaget (cognitive)	Formal Operations Early (11–14 years)	Limited abstract thought process Egocentrically thinking Eager to apply limited abstract process to different situations and to peer groups
	Middle (14–17 years)	Increased ability to think abstractly or in more idealistic terms Able to solve verbal and mental problems using scientific methods Thinks he or she is invincible—risky behaviors increase Likes making independent decisions Becomes involved/concerned with society, politics
	Late (17–20 years)	Abstract thinking is established Develops critical thinking skills—tests different solutions to problems Less risky behaviors Develops realistic goals and career plans
Kohlberg	Postconventional Level III Early (11–14 years)	Morals based upon peer, family, church, and societal morals Asks broad, usually unanswerable questions about life
	Middle (14–17 years)	Developing own set of morals—evaluates individual morals in relation to peer, family, and societal morals
	Late (17–20 years)	Internalizes own morals and values Continues to compare own morals and values to those of society Evaluates morals of others

◆ COGNITIVE DEVELOPMENT

According to Piaget, the adolescent progresses from a concrete framework of thinking to an abstract one. It is the formal operational period. During this period, the adolescent develops the ability to think outside of the present; that is, he or she can incorporate into thinking concepts that do exist as well as concepts that might exist. Her thinking becomes logical, organized, and consistent. She is able to think about a problem from all points of view, ranking the possible solutions while solving the problem. Not all adolescents achieve formal operational reasoning at the same time.

In the early stages of formal operational reasoning, the adolescent's thinking is egocentric. She is very idealistic, constantly challenging the way things are and wondering why things cannot change. These activities lead to the adolescent's feeling of being omnipotent. The adolescent must undergo this way of thinking, even though it can frustrate adults, in her quest to reach formal operational reasoning. As the teenager progresses towards middle adolescence, her thinking becomes very introspective. She assumes others are just as interested in what interests her, which leads her to feel unique, special, and exceptional. That feeling of "being exceptional" leads to the risk-taking behaviors of which teenagers are well known. Also, the teenager feels very committed to her viewpoints. She tries very hard to convince others of her viewpoints and embraces strongly those causes that support her opinions. This idealism can cause the adolescent to reject her family, her culture, her church, and her community beliefs, which can cause conflict with her family, culture, church, and community. See Table 29.2 for additional information.

◆ MORAL AND SPIRITUAL DEVELOPMENT

It is during the adolescent years that teenagers develop their own set of values and morals. According to Kohlberg, adolescents are experiencing the postconventional stage of moral development. It is only because adolescents are developing their formal operational way of thinking that they can experience the postconventional stage of moral development. At the beginning of this stage, teenagers begin to question the status quo. The majority of their choices are based upon emotions while they are questioning societal standards. As they progress to developing their own set of morals, adolescents realize that moral decisions are based upon rights, values, and principles that are agreeable to a given society. They also realize that those rights, values, and principles can be in conflict with the laws of the given society, but they are able to reconcile the differences. Because adolescents undergo the process of developing their own set of morals at different rates, they might find that their friends view a situation differently. This dif-

ference can lead to conflicts and the forming of different friendships. See Table 29.2 for additional information.

Adolescents also begin to question their formal religious practices. As they progress through adolescence, teenagers become more interested in the spiritualism of their religion than in the actual practices of their religion. As teenagers become older, organized religion becomes less important in their lives; rather, their religious beliefs become more personalized.

Referring back to Cho Chung, identify the stage of psychosocial development that she should be in according to Erikson. What approaches for assessment and teaching would be most effective based on the stage you identified?

◆ MOTOR SKILL DEVELOPMENT

During adolescence, the teenager refines and continues to develop his or her gross and fine motor skills. Because of this period of rapid growth spurts, teenagers may experience times of decreased coordination and have a diminished ability to perform previously learned skills, which can be worrisome for the teenager.

Gross Motor Skills

It is usually during early adolescence that teenagers begin to develop endurance. Their concentration has increased so they can follow complicated instructions. Coordination can be a problem because of the uneven growth spurts. During middle adolescence, speed and accuracy increase while coordination also improves. Teenagers become more competitive with each other (Fig. 29.2). During late adolescence, the teenager usually

FIGURE 29.2 Adolescents become involved in competitive sports, which draw upon their gross motor skills.

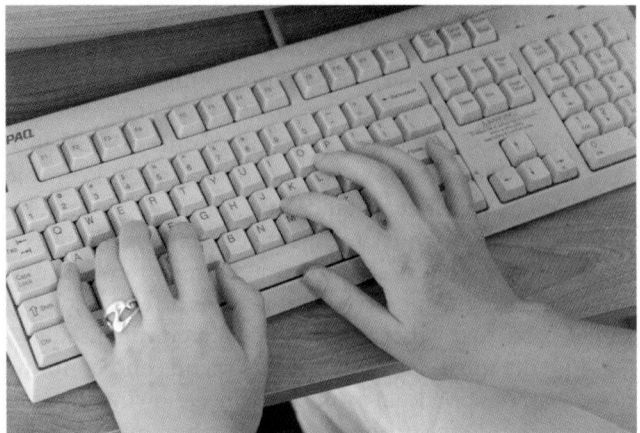

FIGURE 29.3 Using computers has increased the fine motor skills of adolescents.

narrows his or her areas of interest and concentrates on the needed relevant skills.

Fine Motor Skills

The use of computers has greatly increased the fine motor skills of teenagers (Fig. 29.3). In the early adolescent years, the teenager increases his ability to manipulate objects. His handwriting is neat and he increases his finger dexterity. The middle adolescent years see the teenager refining his dexterity skills. By late adolescence, the teenager has developed precise eye–hand coordination and finger dexterity.

▶ COMMUNICATION AND LANGUAGE DEVELOPMENT

Language skills continue to develop and be refined during adolescence. During early adolescence, verbal vocabulary is close to 8,000 words and reading vocabulary is over 50,000 words. Adolescents have improved communication skills, using correct grammar and parts of speech. Vocabulary and communication skills continue to develop during middle adolescence. However, the usage of colloquial speech (slang) increases, causing communication with people other then peers to be difficult at times. By late adolescence, language skills are comparable to those of adults.

▶ EMOTIONAL AND SOCIAL DEVELOPMENT

Adolescents undergo a great deal of change in the areas of emotional and social development as they grow and mature into adults. Areas that are affected include the

adolescent's relationship with parents; self-concept and body image; importance of peers; and **sexuality** and dating.

Relationship With Parents

Families and parents of adolescents experience changes and conflict that require adjustments and the understanding of adolescent development. The adolescent is striving for self-identity and increased independence. He or she spends more time with peers and less time with family and attending family functions. Parents sense that they have less influence on the adolescent as the teen questions family values and becomes more mobile. This may lead to a family crisis, and the parents may respond by setting stricter limits or asking questions about the teen's activities and friends. Other parents may drop all rules and assume that the adolescent can manage herself. Both of these responses increase tension in the family.

With the adolescent attempting to establish some level of independence—and the family learning to let go while focusing on aging parents, their marriage, and other children—a state of disequilibrium occurs. The family may experience more stress than at any other time.

Some families have better outcomes with their adolescents than others. Families who listen to and continue to demonstrate affection for and acceptance of their adolescent have a more positive outcome. This does not mean that the family accepts all of the teen's ideas or actions, but they are willing to listen and attempt to negotiate some limits. For tips to improve communication with teenagers, see Box 29.1.

Siblings experience changes in the relationship with the adolescent brother or sister; the older sibling may attempt to parent and the younger sibling may regress in an attempt to avoid the family conflict. Understanding the

BOX 29.1 Ways to Improve Communication with Teens

- Set aside appropriate amount of time to discuss subject matter without interruptions.
- Talk face to face. Be aware of body language.
- Ask questions to see why he feels that way.
- Ask her to be patient as you tell your thoughts.
- Choose words carefully so he understands you.
- Tell her exactly what you mean.
- Give praise and approval to your teenager often.
- Speak to him as an equal—don't talk down to him.
- Be aware of your tone of voice and body language.
- Don't pretend you know all the answers.
- Admit that you do make mistakes.
- Rules and limits should be set fairly.

status of the adolescent–family relationship is essential for the nurse.

Self-Concept and Body Image

Self-concept and self-esteem are tied to body image many times. Adolescents who perceive their body as being different than peers or as less than ideal may view themselves negatively. Adolescent girls often are influenced by peers and the media and want to weigh less and have smaller hips, waist, or thighs. Boys tend to view themselves as being too thin or not muscular enough.

Sexual characteristics are important to the adolescent's self-concept and body image. Boys are concerned about the size of their penis and facial hair while girls are concerned about breast size and the onset of menstruation. Larger breasts are considered more feminine and menstruation is considered the right of passage into adulthood. All of these body changes are important to the adolescent's self-concept.

Importance of Peers

Peer groups play an essential role in the identity of the adolescent. Adolescent peer relationships are very important in providing opportunities to learn about negotiating differences; for recreation, companionship, and someone to share problems with; for learning peer loyalty; and for creating stability during transitions or times of stress. Learning to work out differences with peers is a skill that is important throughout life. Peers serve as someone safe to discuss family issues with, as the teen emotionally moves away from the family while trying to find his or her identity. Due to changes that have taken place within family systems in society, peer groups play a significant role in the socialization of adolescents (Fig. 29.4).

Peers serve as credible sources of information, role model social behaviors, and act as sources of social reinforcement. Friends provide an opportunity for fun and excitement. Peers impact teens' appearance, dress, social behavior, and language. Peers also can have positive influences on each other, such as promoting college attendance, or negative influences such as involvement with alcohol, drugs, or gangs. Early and middle adolescence are periods when teens are prone to join gangs. Peer role modeling and peer acceptance may lead to the formation of a gang that provides a collective identity and gives a sense of belonging. Peer pressure, companionship, and protection are the most frequent reasons given for joining gangs, particularly those associated with criminal activity.

Parents must know their teen's friends and continue to be aware of potential problems while allowing the teen the independence to become his or her own person. Nurses must remind parents of the importance of peers and the impact they have on the teen's decisions and life choices. The transition to greater peer involvement requires guidance and support. Adolescents who do not have parental or adult supervision and opportunities for conversation with adults may be more susceptible to peer influences and at higher risk for poor peer selections.

Sexuality and Dating

Adolescence is a critical time in the development of sexuality. Sexuality includes the thoughts, feelings, and behaviors related to the adolescent's sexual identity. Adolescents usually begin experimentation with heterosexual and homosexual behaviors, although these behaviors may occur earlier in some cultures.

An interest in the opposite sex occurs during adolescence (Fig. 29.5). Some of the reasons cited for this devel-

FIGURE 29.5 Dating becomes an important aspect of the teenager's life.

FIGURE 29.4 Peers play an important role in shaping the adolescent's identity.

oping interest are physical development and body changes, peer-group pressure, and curiosity. During the past several decades, the age of beginning to date in the United States has dropped. Girls are between 14 and 15 years old, and boys are 15 to 16 years old. Teen dating can range from group dating to single dating to serious relationships. Most early adolescents spend more time in activities with mixed-sex groups, such as dances and parties, than they do dating as a couple. Popular dating activities today include going out to dinner or the movies, "hanging out" at the mall, or visiting each other's home. During early adolescence, teens tend to date for fun and recreation. Also, they may see dating as a way to upgrade social standing by being seen with a popular boy or an attractive girl.

Middle and late adolescents have group and single dates. Most teens have been involved in at least one romantic relationship by middle adolescence (O'Sulliven et al., 2007). Dating or spending time with a potential romantic partner is viewed as a major developmental marker for teens and is one of the most challenging adjustments. Teens who date frequently report more depression and lower levels of autonomy, and experience a higher level of parental conflict even though they have been found to have higher levels of self-esteem and are classified as more popular.

Trends in dating are changing, but dating remains a developmental milestone for the adolescent.

Adolescents may experiment with homosexual behavior, though homosexual behavior as a teen does not necessarily indicate that the adolescent will maintain a homosexual orientation. Gay and lesbian adolescents face many challenges due to society's nonacceptance and peer insensitivity. Teens who self-declare as homosexual during high school are at increased risk for such problems as suicide, victimization, risky sexual behaviors, and substance abuse.

Of greatest concern to parents during the adolescent period of developing sexuality and dating are unwanted pregnancy, sexually transmitted infections (STIs), and teen feelings of despair over failed relationships. Many times adolescents are not worried about negative consequences of sexual activity and believe "it will not happen to me."

Cho Chung's mother states that she is concerned about the changes that have occurred in her and Cho's relationship over the past year. Cho seems much more self-centered, always wants to be with her friends, is very critical of her mother and father and seems to be constantly in conflict with them. Based on what you know about this stage of development, what guidance, including approaches and techniques, can you discuss with Mrs. Chung to address her concerns?

CULTURAL INFLUENCES ON GROWTH AND DEVELOPMENT

Although the adolescent's culture continues to influence the teenager, the desire to be in harmony with peers becomes paramount. That desire can cause conflict with his family and culture. Today's adolescents live in a rapidly changing, increasingly culturally diverse world. They are exposed to many different cultures and ethnic groups. In 2006, over 40% of children and adolescents in the United States will be minorities (Federal Interagency Forum on Child and Family Statistics, 2007).

Attitudes regarding adolescence vary among different cultures. Certain cultures may have more permissive attitudes toward issues facing adolescents, while others are more conservative, for example towards sexuality. Experiencing a rite of passage ceremony to signal the adolescent's movement to adult status varies among cultures. The American culture does not universally have a rite of passage for teenagers. Some religious and social groups do have ceremonies that signal a movement toward the maturity of adulthood, for example, the Jewish bar or bat mitzvah, the Catholic confirmation, and social debuts. In many parts of the world, separate "youth cultures" have developed in an attempt to blend traditional and modern worlds for the adolescent.

It is important for the nurse to recognize the ethnic background of each client. Research has shown that certain ethnic groups are at higher risk for certain diseases. For example, adolescent African-Americans are at higher risk for developing hypertension. But the major barrier to the adolescent's health and successful achievement of the tasks of adolescence is socioeconomic status. Adolescents at a lower socioeconomic level are at higher risk for developing health care problems and risk-taking behaviors; this may be due to their inability to access health care and to obtain needed services. In caring for adolescents, recognize the influence of their culture, ethnicity, and socioeconomic level upon them.

The Nurse's Role in Adolescent Growth and Development

During adolescence, the teenager faces many challenges. His or her fluctuating relationships with parents and other adult figures may limit the teen from seeking assistance in dealing with the common issues of adolescence. In dealing with adolescents, be aware that they behave unpredictably, are inconsistent with their need for independence, have sensitive feelings, may interpret situations differently from what they are, think friends are extremely important, and have a strong desire to belong. The following Nursing Process Overview will address promoting healthy growth and development and dealing with common developmental concerns.

NURSING PROCESS OVERVIEW

Upon completion of assessment of the adolescent's current growth and development status, problems or issues related to growth and development may be identified. The nurse may then identify one or more nursing diagnoses, including:

- Risk for disproportionate growth
- Imbalanced nutrition: more than body requirements
- Delayed growth and development
- Risk for caregiver role strain
- Risk for injury
- Ineffective coping

Nursing care planning for the adolescent with growth and development issues should be individualized based on the adolescent's and family's needs. Nursing Care Plan 29.1 can be used as a guide in planning nursing care for the adolescent with a growth and development concern. The nurse may choose the appropriate nursing diagnoses from this plan and individualize them as needed. The nursing care plan is intended to serve as a guide, not to be an all-inclusive growth and development care plan.

▶ PROMOTING HEALTHY GROWTH AND DEVELOPMENT

WATCH▸LEARN

It takes multiple groups who address multiple issues to promote healthy growth and development in the adolescent. Some of these groups include sports teams in the school or the community, peers, teachers, band and choir members, and so forth. Also, the family's support and love will influence growth and development.

Promoting Growth and Development Through Sports and Physical Fitness

Many adolescents are involved in team sports that provide avenues for exercise. High levels of physical activity may reduce cardiovascular disease risk factors during adolescence. Adolescents probably spend more time and energy participating in sports than any other age group. Participation in sports contributes to the adolescent's development, educational process, and better health. Sports and games provide an opportunity to interact with peers while enjoying socially accepted stimulation and conflict. Competition in sports activities helps the teenager in processing self-appraisal and in developing self-respect and concern for others.

Every sport has some potential for injury. Rapidly growing bones, muscles, joints, and tendons are more vulnerable to unusual strains and fractures (see Evidence-Based Practice 29.1). The American Academy of Pediatrics (2006) encourages sports participation by young persons and encourages parents and coaches to be aware of early warning signs of fatigue, dehydration, and injury. See Chapter 44 for a discussion of sports injuries.

In relation to youth sports, the role of the nurse is to educate to prevent injuries (Fig. 29.6). This education should include discouraging participation when the teen is tired or has an existing injury.

Additionally, adolescence is a good time to develop an exercise program, with aerobic exercise at least 30 minutes per day, four times per week. Nurses should encourage all adolescents to be physically active daily or at least four times per week.

Promoting Learning

School, teachers, family, and peers influence education and learning for the adolescent. Also, activities such as athletics and club membership enhance learning through interactions with peers, coaches, club leaders, and others.

School

School plays an essential part in preparing adolescents for the future. Completing school prepares the adolescent for college or employment to make an adequate income. Schools in the United States may not meet the developmental needs of all adolescents. Minority students may not be at the appropriate grade level and the dropout rate may be higher than in nonminority students. Dropout rates are highest among Hispanic and American Indian students. Another influencing factor is a lack of parental involvement. Due to single parent families and both parents being in the work force, parents have less time to devote to involvement in their child's school activities.

There is evidence that the transition from elementary school to middle school at age 12 or 13, and then the transition to high school, both occur at the time of physical changes, which may have a negative effect on teens. It is important to observe for transition problems into middle or high school, which may be exhibited by failing grades or behavior problems. Also, students who experience difficulties in school, resulting in negative evaluations and failing grades, may feel alienated from school. Students with failing grades and those repeating grades exhibit more emotional behavior and are more likely to engage in risky behaviors such as tobacco and alcohol use. In 2003, 9% of adolescent boys and 3% of adolescent girls reported carrying a weapon to school (CDC, 2004b). Schools that support peer-group relationships, promote health and fitness, encourage parental involvement, and strengthen community relationships have better student outcomes. Parents, teachers, and health care providers should provide guidance and support.

Nursing Care Plan 29.1

GROWTH AND DEVELOPMENT OF THE ADOLESCENT

NURSING DIAGNOSIS: Risk for disproportionate growth (risk factors: caregiver and adolescent knowledge deficit, low self-esteem, frequent illnesses)

Outcome Identification and Evaluation

Adolescent will demonstrate adequate growth: *appropriate weight gain for age and sex*

Intervention: Promoting Appropriate Physical Growth

- Assess parents' and adolescent's knowledge of nutritional needs of adolescents *to determine need for further education.*
- Educate parents and adolescent about appropriate serving sizes and foods *so that they are aware of what to expect for adolescents.*
- Determine need for additional caloric intake if necessary *(if very active in sports, if have a chronic illness).*
- Plot out height, weight, and body mass index (BMI) *to detect possible pattern.*
- Assess for risk factors for developing eating disorder *to refer to if needed and plan interventions.*

NURSING DIAGNOSIS: Nutrition, more than body requirements, imbalanced, related to lack of exercise, increased caloric intake, poor food choices, and stresses of adolescence

Outcome Identification and Evaluation

Adolescent will lose weight at an appropriate rate: *increase amount of exercise, make appropriate eating choices, decrease caloric intake to appropriate amount for age and sex*

Intervention: Promoting Appropriate Nutrition

- Assess knowledge of parents and adolescent about nutritional needs of teenagers *to determine deficits in knowledge.*
- Have adolescent keep a detailed food and exercise diary for 1 week *to determine current patterns of eating and exercise.*
- Interview family in relationship to their eating habits and exercise habits *to determine where adjustments might need to be made.*
- Discuss changes in a positive manner—talk about developing healthy eating habits instead of dieting *to promote compliance.*
- Analyze preceding data, and base recommendations for changes on these data *to promote compliance and to prioritize recommendations.*
- Discuss ways to decrease temptation to overeat, for example, eat slowly, put down the fork between bites, serve food on smaller plates, and count mouthfuls *to allow time to realize that you are full.*
- Have adolescent create meal plans and grocery shop *to allow him or her some sense of control and decision-making.*
- Incorporate increase in daily exercise, which will stress sense of self-improvement to *increase caloric expenditure and self-esteem.*
- Decrease TV/computer time *to increase caloric expenditure.*
- Encourage peer exercise activities *to increase peer interactions and to help teen to realize that others are like him or her.*
- Develop reward system *to increase self-esteem.*
- Investigate joining weight loss program for adolescents *to increase self-esteem and encourage weight loss.*

NURSING DIAGNOSIS: Growth and development, delayed, related to speech, motor, psychosocial, or cognitive concerns as evidenced by delay in meeting expected school performances

Outcome Identification and Evaluation

Development will be maximized: Adolescent will make continued progress toward attainment of expected school performance.

Interventions: Promoting Growth and Development

- Perform scheduled evaluation of the adolescent by school and health care provider *to determine current functioning.*
- Develop realistic multidisciplinary plan *to ensure maximizing resources.*
- Carry out interventions as prescribed by developmental specialist, physical therapist, occupational therapist, or speech therapist at home and at school *to maximize benefit of interventions.*
- Have scheduled evaluation meetings *to be able to adapt interventions as soon as possible.*

(continued)

Nursing Care Plan 29.1 (continued)

NURSING DIAGNOSIS: Caregiver role strain, risk for (risk factors: knowledge deficit about adolescent issues, lack of prior exposure, fatigue, ill or developmentally delayed child)

Outcome Identification and Evaluation
Parent will experience competence in role: *will demonstrate appropriate caretaking behaviors and verbalize comfort in caring for an adolescent*

Interventions: Preventing Caregiver Role Strain
* Assess parent's knowledge of adolescents and the issues that arise as a part of normal development *to determine parent's needs.*
* Provide education on normal issues of adolescence *so that parents are armed with the knowledge they need to appropriately care for their adolescents.*
* Provide anticipatory guidance related to upcoming expected issues related to adolescent development *to prepare parents for what to expect next and how to intervene in an appropriate manner.*

NURSING DIAGNOSIS: Injury, risk for (risk factors: increased motor and cognitive skills and feeling of invincibility)

Outcome Identification and Evaluation
Adolescent's safety will be maintained: *will remain free from injury*

Interventions: Preventing Injury
* Discuss safety measures needed for the following: bikes, scooters, guns, skateboards, cars, and water *to decrease risk of injury related to those areas.*
* Discuss and develop a fire safety plan *to decrease risk of injury related to fire.*
* Discuss appropriate safety equipment needed for each sport *to decrease risk of injury.*
* Discuss appropriate sports to participate in depending upon age, sex, and maturity of adolescent *to prevent possible injury.*
* Teach parents and adolescent first-aid measures and cardiopulmonary resuscitation (CPR) *to minimize consequences of injury should it occur.*
* Discuss influence of peers upon actions of adolescents *to prevent possible injury due to mimicking behavior.*

NURSING DIAGNOSIS: Coping, ineffective, risk for (risk factors: low self-esteem, poor relationship with parents and peers, participating in risk-taking behaviors)

Outcome Identification and Evaluation
Adolescent will demonstrate adequate coping abilities *as evidenced by management of stress of adolescence and no evidence of participating in risk-taking behaviors.*

Interventions: Promoting Effective Coping
* Assess adolescent's knowledge of normal stress facing teenagers *to determine current knowledge.*
* Assess adolescent's present coping skills *to determine areas for improvement/support.*
* Encourage parents to accept teenager as a unique individual.
* Discuss with parents and adolescent normal developmental issues facing teens *to give them knowledge needed to cope.*
* Provide different situations the teen might be faced with and encourage teen to develop different solutions.
* Allow for increasing independence and opportunities to solve own problems *to improve coping skills.*
* Encourage parents to provide unconditional love *to improve self-esteem.*
* Assess for any evidence of any risk-taking behaviors (drugs, smoking, suicide) *to identify need for early interventions.*

Other Activities
Adolescents are involved in many other activities that influence learning. Some of these activities include: (1) school activities such as band, choir, or clubs requiring high achievement; (2) athletic activities in the school and community and sometimes in the state or region; (3) art, sewing, and building classes; and (4) work activities when the late adolescent may have a part-time job.

Promoting Safety
Unintentional and intentional injuries are the leading causes of death in persons in the United States under 35 years of age (Minoño, Heron, & Smith, 2006). "At least one adolescent (10 to 19 years of age) dies of an injury every hour of every day," resulting in about 15,000 such deaths each year. Injuries kill more adolescents than

FIGURE 29.6 Stretching before exercise is an important part of exercise.

HEALTHY PEOPLE 2010

Objective	Significance
Increase high-school completion.	• Encourage school attendance and completion when encountering teens for well-child or sick visits. • Refer children who have difficulty concentrating or learning for further evaluation. • Praise school accomplishments.

all diseases combined. Unintentional injury accounts for about 60% of adolescent injury deaths, while violence (homicide and suicide) accounts for the remaining 40%. Males are more likely than females to die of any type of injury (CDC, 2004b).

Influencing factors related to the prevalence of adolescent injuries include increased physical growth; insufficient psychomotor coordination for the task; abundance of energy; impulsivity; peer pressure; and inexperience. Impulsivity, inexperience, and peer pressure may place the teen in a vulnerable situation between knowing what

is right and wanting to impress peers. On the other hand, teens have a feeling of invulnerability, which may contribute to negative outcomes. Alcohol and other drugs are contributing factors in automobile and firearm accidents among adolescents. Most of the serious or fatal injuries in adolescents are preventable (Fig. 29.7). Nurses must educate parents and adolescents on car, gun, and water safety to prevent unintentional injuries. See Teaching Guideline 29.1 for information on promoting safety.

Motor Vehicle Safety

The largest numbers of adolescent injuries are due to motor vehicle crashes. When the adolescent passes his or her driving test, he or she is able to drive legally. However, driving is complex and requires judgments that the teen is often incapable of exhibiting. Also, the typical adolescent

EVIDENCE-BASED PRACTICE 29.1
Interventions Directed Toward Prevention of Ankle Ligament Injury or Sprain

● **Study**

Adolescents are increasingly involved in organized sports that put them at risk for injury. Soccer and basketball, in particular, result in a very high incidence of ankle injuries, and ankle sprains are very commonly treated in acute care. Inversion of the plantar-flexed foot is the most common mechanism of ankle injury resulting in damage to the lateral ligament complex. The authors analyzed 14 randomized or quasi-randomized trials that included data for a total of 8,279 participants. The intervention evaluated included use of modified footwear (high-top athletic shoes), external ankle supports, coordination training, and health education. The study evaluated the occurrence as well as the recurrence of ankle sprains.

▲ **Findings**

Ankle coordination and strength training may be beneficial in the prevention of ankle sprains, but the results from the

included studies were not powerful. However, the review provided sufficient evidence that the use of semi-rigid orthoses reduces the risk of ankle sprain in the young athlete and adult. Use of these devices was shown to be particularly helpful in preventing reinjury of the ankle.

■ **Nursing Implications**

Nurses should recommend the use of semi-rigid ankle orthoses to adolescent athletes participating in sports such as soccer and basketball. Although physical conditioning of the ankle was not decisively proved to decrease the risk of ankle injury, it was not proved to be harmful so it should still be encouraged in student athletes. Exercises designed to improve coordination and proprioception should be included. At a minimum, adolescent athletes participating in high-risk sports should wear high-top athletic shoes in order to provide some protection against the occurrence of ankle injury.

Handoll, H. H. G., Rowe, B. H., Quinn, K. M., & de Bie, R. (2007). Interventions for preventing ankle ligament injuries. *The Cochrane Library 2007, 4.*

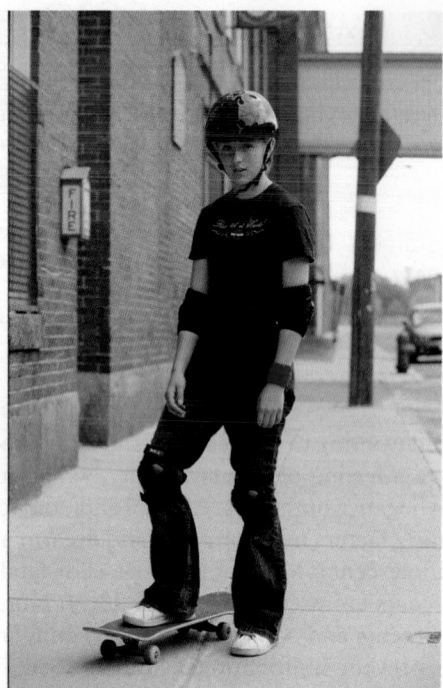

FIGURE 29.7 Wearing appropriate safety equipment can prevent injuries.

is opposed to authority and is interested in showing peers and others his or her independence. The Youth Risk Behavior Surveillance Survey of high school students found that 16.4% had rarely worn seat belts, and over 33% had ridden with a driver who was drinking alcohol. Adolescents who drive after drinking are more likely than adults to have a crash. Adolescents are also vulnerable to crashes at night. Adolescents do most of their driving at night and have over 50% of their accidents then. Adolescents also cause a disproportionate number of deaths among other passengers and pedestrians (National Highway Traffic Safety Association, n.d.).

It is essential to promote driver education, to teach about the importance of wearing seat belts, and to explain laws about teen driving and curfews (Fig. 29.8). See Teaching Guidelines 29.1 for additional information.

Firearm Safety

The risk of dying from a firearm injury among 15- to 19-year-olds has increased by 77% since 1985. In this age group, a firearm causes one in four deaths. Provide education about gun safety. Guns in the home must be kept and locked in a safe location, with ammunition kept separately. Parents must teach adolescents about the dangers

---

TEACHING GUIDELINES 29.1

Promoting Safety

Safety Issue	Activity
Motor vehicle	• Wear seat belt at all times.
	• Do not drive with someone who is impaired.
	• Take driver-education course.
	• Establish driving rules between parent and adolescent prior to getting license.
	• Have all passengers wear seat belts.
	• Do not use cell phone while driving, drink and drive, or drive when tired.
	• Maintain car in good condition.
	• Drive with adult supervision for period of time after receiving license.
Bike: General	• Have a well-maintained and appropriate-size bike for adolescent.
	• Adolescent should demonstrate his or her ability to ride bike safely before being allowed to ride on street.
	• Safe areas for bike riding should be established as well as routes to and from area of activities.
	• Should not ride bike barefoot, with someone else on bike, or with clothing that might get entangled in the bike.
	• Should wear sturdy, well-fitting shoes and ANSI-approved helmets.
	• Bike should be inspected often to ensure it is in proper working order.
	• A basket should be used to carry heavy objects.
Bike: in traffic	• All traffic signs and signals must be observed.
	• If riding at night, the bike should have lights and reflectors and the rider should wear light-colored clothes.
	• Should ride on the side of the road traveling with traffic and keep close to the side of the road in single file.
	• Should watch and listen for cars and never hitch a ride on any vehicle.
	• Should not wear headphones while riding a bike.

Promoting Safety

Safety Issue	Activity
All-terrain vehicles	• Should not be operated by adolescent less than 16 years of age. • Helmet and protective coverings required. • No nighttime riding. • Not for use on public roads or if teen has been drinking or using drugs. • Do not stand up in the vehicle or ride in a person's lap.
Skateboards/Skates	• Wear helmet, and protective padding on knees, elbows, and wrists. • Do not skate in traffic or on streets or highways. • Skating on homemade ramps could be dangerous—assess ramps for any hazards before skating.
Water safety	• Learn how to swim; if swimming skill is limited, must wear life preserver at all times. • Never swim alone—should, if at all possible, swim only where there is a life guard. • Learn basic cardiopulmonary resuscitation (CPR). • Do not run or fool around at edge of pool. • Drains in pool should be covered with appropriate cover. • Wear life jacket when on boat. • Make sure there is enough water to support diving. • Do not swim if drinking alcohol or using drugs.
Firearms	• If guns are in household, should take firearm safety class, secure guns in safe place, use gun safety locks, store bullets in separate place. • Never point a gun at a person.
Fire safety	• All homes should have working smoke detectors and fire extinguishers. Change the batteries at least twice a year. • Have fire-escape plan and practice the plan routinely. • No smoking in bed. • Teach what to do in case of a fire: use fire extinguisher, call 911, and how to put out clothing fire. • All flammable materials and liquids should be stored safely. • Fireplaces should have protective gratings. • Avoid touching any downed power lines.
Machinery	• Use safety devices. • Receive training on how to use equipment. • Do not use when alone.
Sports	• Match sport to adolescent's ability and desire. • Sports program should have warm-up procedure and hydration policy. • Undergo sports physical before start of activity. • Coaches should be trained in CPR and first aid. • Wear appropriate protection devices for individual sport.
Sun	• Use sunscreen with both ultraviolet A (UVA) and ultraviolet B (UVB) protection. • Apply sunscreen prior to going out and reapply sunscreen often. • Limit sun exposure, especially between 10 a.m. and 2 p.m. • Wear hat and sunglasses while outside.
Personal safety	• Never go with a stranger. • Do not enter a car when the driver has been drinking. • Notify adult where you are when out after dark. • Keep cell phone fully charged. • Never give out personal information over the Internet. • Say "no" to drugs, alcohol, smoking, or to being touched when you do not want to be touched.
Toxins	• Teach the hazards of accepting illegal drugs, alcohol, dangerous drugs. • Store potential dangerous material in safe place.

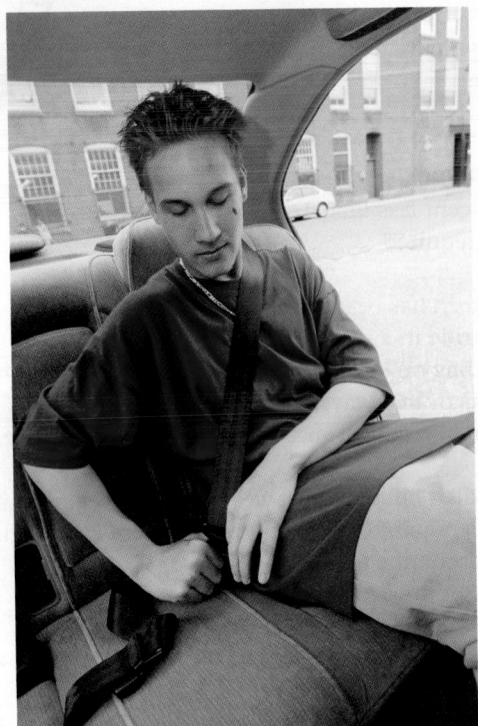

FIGURE 29.8 The use of seat belts has led to fewer fatal injuries in car accidents.

of playing with firearms. See Teaching Guidelines 29.1 for additional information on gun safety.

Water Safety

Drowning is a needless cause of death in adolescents. Many drownings are a result of risk-taking behaviors. With the independence of the adolescent, many times adult supervision is not prevalent and the teen takes a dare that results in drowning. Provide water safety education and proper supervision to decrease the incidence of risk taking. Teach about swimming lessons for nonswimmers. See Teaching Guidelines 29.1 for additional information.

Remember Cho Chung, the 15-year-old presented at the beginning of the chapter? What anticipatory guidance related to safety should you provide to Cho and her mother?

Promoting Nutrition

Nutritional needs are increased during adolescence due to accelerated growth and sexual maturation. Adolescents may appear to be hungry constantly and need regular meals and snacks with adequate nutrients to meet the body's anaerobic requirements. Multiple factors influence the adolescent's diet and eating habits (Box 29.2). According to Centers for Disease Control and Prevention (CDC) data, 67% of children between 6 and 19 years of age ex-

---

BOX 29.2 Factors Influencing the Adolescent's Diet

- Peer pressure
- Busy schedules
- Concern about weight control
- Convenience of fast food

---

ceed the dietary guidelines recommended for fat intake; 72% exceed recommendations for saturated fat; and only 21% of high school students eat the five recommended daily servings of fruits and vegetables. Due to this, over 9 million children and adolescents are overweight. In 6- to 11-year-olds, the number of children who are overweight has doubled in the past 20 years. In 12- to 19-year-olds, the obesity rate has tripled over the same period of time.

Nutritional Needs

Teenagers have a need for increased calories, zinc, calcium, and iron for growth. However, the number of calories needed for adolescence depends on the teen's age and activity level as well as growth patterns. Teenage girls who are active require about 2,200 calories per day. Teenage boys who are active require between 2,500 and 3,000 calories per day. Adolescents require about 1,200 to 1,500 milligrams of calcium each day. Adolescents should be made aware of foods high in calcium, including milk, white beans, broccoli, cheese, and yogurt. Adolescent males require 12 milligrams of iron each day and females require 15 milligrams each day. Advise adolescents about foods high in iron (see Box 29.3 and Healthy People 2010). Protein requirements for adolescent girls are 46 grams per day, and 45 to 59 grams for boys. Some foods high in protein are meats, fish, poultry, beans, and dairy products.

BOX 29.3 Foods High in Iron

- Beef, chicken, fish
- Liver
- Peanut butter
- Nuts and seeds
- Green peas, lima beans
- Spinach
- Strawberries
- Tomato juice
- Whole-grain bread
- Raisins
- Watermelon

Objective	Significance
Reduce iron deficiency among young children and females of childbearing age.	• Educate parents and teens about iron-containing foods. • Encourage adolescent females to consume a diet high in iron-rich foods.

Nutritional Assessment

The nurse must understand normal growth and development of the adolescent in order to provide guidance that fits the quest for independence and the need for teens to make their own choices. Assess the eating habits and diet preferences of the adolescent. The assessment should include an evaluation of foods from the different food groups that the adolescent eats each day. Also, assess the number of times that fast foods, snacks, and other junk food are eaten per week. This assessment will help the nurse to guide the adolescent in making better food choices at home and in fast-food establishments. Many fast-food restaurants offer baked chicken sandwiches and salads with fewer calories and less fat. Adolescents may be guided in alternating hamburger and fries with more nutritious choices. Remember that planning should always include the adolescent.

Nutritional Guidelines

The official U.S. dietary guidelines are based on the Food Guide Pyramid (see Appendix H). This pyramid, designed by the U.S. Department of Agriculture, illustrates a healthy, balanced diet with recommendations for eating foods from the main food groups each day with the exception of fats, oils, and sweets. Table 29.3 outlines daily serving recommendations based on caloric requirements (lower, moderate, or higher). Nurses may use the information in Table 29.3 to help teens plan a healthy diet for themselves. Active teenage girls should eat the number of servings recommended in the "Moderate" column of Table 29.3. Active teenage boys should eat the number of servings recommended in the "Higher" column. Adoles-

cents who are overweight and dieting should base their daily intake on the serving recommendations in the "Lower" column.

What questions should you ask Cho Chung and her mother related to nutritional intake? What anticipatory guidance related to nutrition would be appropriate?

Promoting Healthy Sleep and Rest

The average number of hours of sleep that teens require per night is 8. On the weekends, they may sleep 10 to 12 hours per night. In this independence-seeking phase of adolescence, the teen may stay up later to do homework or to complete projects and may have difficulty awakening in the morning. Rapid growth and increased activities may produce fatigue and the need for more rest. Parents may relate that the teen sleeps all the time and never has the time or energy to help with household chores. Explain to parents the need to discourage late hours on school nights because they may affect school performance. Provide advice to teens and parents about having realistic expectations; encourage them to agree on a level of normalcy and adequate rest for the teen so that he or she can still fulfill responsibilities in the home.

Provide anticipatory guidance to Cho Chung and her mother in relation to sleep during the adolescent years.

Promoting Healthy Teeth and Gums

Most permanent teeth have erupted with the possible exception of the third molars (wisdom teeth). These molars may become impacted and require surgical removal. The rate of cavities decreases but the need for routine dental visits every 6 months and brushing two to three times per day is very important. Some of the conditions that occur during adolescence include malocclusion, gingivitis, and tooth avulsion. Malocclusion occurs in approximately 50% of adolescents, resulting from facial and mandibular bone growth. The treatment includes braces and other

TABLE 29.3 **SAMPLE DIET FOR THREE CALORIC LEVELS**

Calories for Three Caloric Levels	Lower (About 1,600 Calories)	Moderate (About 2,200 Calories)	Higher (About 2,800 Calories)
Grain group servings	6	9	11
Vegetable group servings	3	4	5
Fruit group servings	2	3	4
Milk group servings	2–3	2–3	2–3
Meat group (ounces)	5	6	7

dental devices. Teach the adolescent to brush the teeth more frequently if he or she has braces or other dental devices. Gingivitis is inflammation of the gums and breakdown of gingival epithelium due to diet and hormonal changes. The use of dental devices/braces makes cleaning more difficult and contributes to gingivitis. Tooth avulsion (knocked-out teeth) may occur during sports and other activities such as falls. The avulsed tooth should be reimplanted as soon as possible. The nurse may see the teen first so it is important that nurses know the proper procedure, which is to reinsert the tooth into its socket if possible or to store it in cool milk or normal saline for transport to the dentist.

Promoting Personal Care

Promotion of personal care during adolescence is an important topic to cover with the adolescent and his or her parents. Topics to discuss include general hygiene tips, caring for body piercings and tattoos, preventing suntanning, and promoting a healthy sexual identity.

General Hygiene Tips

Adolescents find that frequent baths and deodorant use are important due to apocrine sweat gland secretory activity. Also, to decrease oily skin due to sexual steroids and hormones, teach the adolescent to wash his or her face two to three times per day with plain unscented soap. Vigorous scrubbing should be discouraged because it could irritate the skin and lead to follicular rupture. The hair should be shampooed daily to remove excess oil from the hair and scalp. Many over-the-counter medications are available for beginning acne or acne with a few lesions. These preparations may cause drying or redness. Discourage adolescents from squeezing acne lesions to prevent further irritation and permanent scarring. If the adolescent has severe acne, encourage him or her to ask a parent to make an appointment with a dermatologist.

Caring for Body Piercings and Tattoos

Today, body piercing on the tongue, lip, eyebrow, navel, and nipple is common (Fig. 29.9). Other sites such as the genitals, chin cleft, knuckles, and even the uvula have been used. Generally, body piercing is harmless, but nurses should caution teens about performing these procedures under nonsterile conditions and should educate them about complications. Qualified personnel using sterile needles should perform the procedure. Teach the adolescent to cleanse the pierced area twice a day and more often at some sites.

The complications of body piercing vary by site. Infections from body piercing usually result from unclean tools of the trade. Some of the infections that may occur as a result of unclean tools include hepatitis, tetanus, tuberculosis, and human immunodeficiency virus (HIV). Also, keloid formation and allergies to metal may occur. The

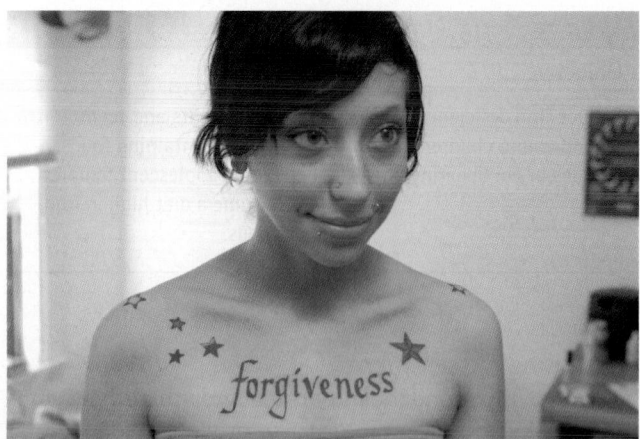

FIGURE 29.9 Having multiple piercings and tattoos can lead to certain health risks.

navel is an area prone to infection because it is a moist area that endures friction from clothing. After a navel infection occurs, it may take up to a year to heal. Pierced ear cartilage also heals slowly and is prone to infection. Tongue piercings heal very quickly, usually within 4 weeks, probably due to the antiseptic effects of saliva. Other concerns with tongue piercing include tooth damage from biting on the jewelry or partial paralysis if the jewelry pierces a nerve.

Tattoos are becoming more popular among adolescents and are not necessarily a mark of gang membership. Tattoos serve to define one's identity (see Fig. 29.9). Because of the invasiveness of the tattooing procedure, it should be considered a health-risk situation. Like piercings, tattoos are open wounds predisposing to infection.

Little regulation exists in the tattoo business, and nurses should educate adolescents about the risk of blood-borne infections, skin infections, and allergic reactions to dyes used in the tattoo process. Teach teens to cleanse tattoos with an antibacterial soap and water several times a day and to keep the area moist with an ointment to prevent scab formation. Refer to Box 29.4 for additional information about tattoos.

BOX 29.4 **What Adolescents Need to Know About Tattooing**

- Infections occur as a result of nonsterile equipment used in the procedure.
- Tattoos are open wounds predisposing to infection; sites require proper care with antibacterial soap and water several times per day and application of ointment.
- For most people a tattoo is permanent; new procedures for removal are painful and expensive.

Preventing Suntanning

Suntanning is popular among adolescents and is influenced by the media, which promotes a link between tan skin and beauty. There is no such thing as a good tan. Most exposure to ultraviolet rays occurs during childhood and adolescence, thereby putting people at risk for the development of skin cancer. However, it is difficult to convince adolescents that tanning is harmful to their skin and puts them at risk for skin cancer later in life (see Healthy People 2010).

Educate teens about the benefits and effects of different sun protection products. Explain to them that sun damage and skin cancers can be prevented if sunscreens are used as directed on a regular basis. Encourage sunscreen or sunblock use for water sports, beach activities, and participation in outdoor sports. Also, make adolescents aware of allergies to some sunscreen products. See Teaching Guideline 29.1 for additional information.

Promoting a Healthy Sexual Identity

Encourage parents and teens to have sexuality discussions. In addition, nurses should ensure that adolescents have the knowledge, skills, and opportunities that enable them to make responsible decisions regarding sexual behaviors and sexual orientation. Education for the adolescent should include a discussion about media influences and the use of sexuality to promote products. This discussion should make the adolescent aware of the motives of the media and the need to be an individual and not be influenced by television, magazines, and other forms of advertisement. Encourage parents to be aware of who their adolescents are dating and where they go on their dates. Refer to Teaching Guidelines 29.2 for information on counseling related to adolescent sexuality.

Promoting Appropriate Discipline

Adolescents naturally misbehave or do not follow the rules of the house, and parents must determine how to respond.

TEACHING GUIDELINES 29.2

Adolescent Sexuality

- It should be your choice to engage in sexual relations. Do not be influenced by peers. When you say "no," be firm and clear about your position.
- Pregnancy, sexually transmitted infections, and human immunodeficiency virus (HIV) infection can occur with any sexual encounter without the use of barrier methods of contraception. Use appropriate contraception if sexually active. Discuss abstinence as a contraceptive method.
- Sexual activity in a mature relationships should be pleasurable to both parties. If your sexual partner is not interested in your pleasure, you need to reconsider the relationship.

Adolescents need to know the rules and expectations. After rules are established, parents must explain to the adolescent the consequences of breaking the rules.

Offer guidance to parents related to disciplining teens. The parent and the teen should collaborate on what the consequences will be if the rules are broken. Parents must acknowledge and offer reinforcement and support when the teen follows the rules. Consistency and predictability are the cornerstones of discipline, and praise is the most powerful reinforcer of learning.

► ADDRESSING COMMON DEVELOPMENTAL CONCERNS

Adolescence is a time of rapid growth and development with maturation of sexuality. The adolescent period begins with a child and ends with the expectation of adulthood. There are many developmental concerns that present during this period, including obesity, violence, suicide, and homicide. The following is an overview of some of these concerns.

Obesity

Over 9 million children and adolescents in the United States are overweight. Over a 20-year time period, from 1980 to 2000, the number of overweight adolescents tripled from 5% to 15%. Although obesity has increased in all segments of the U.S. population, there are differences specific to race, ethnicity, and socioeconomic status. The prevalence of obesity is highest in Hispanic and African-American teens between the ages of 12 and 19 years. Obesity rates are higher in females and in adolescents of lower socioeconomic status.

HEALTHY PEOPLE 2010

Objective	Significance
Increase the proportion of persons who use at least one of the following protective measures that may reduce the risk of skin cancer: avoid the sun between 10 a.m. and 4 p.m., wear sun-protective clothing when exposed to sunlight, use sunscreen with a sun protection factor (SPF) of 15 or higher, and avoid artificial sources of ultraviolet light.	• Encourage female teens to use sunscreen-containing makeup. • Discourage teen use of tanning beds. • Remind students to use sunscreen during outdoor organized-sports practice. • Educate teens and families about the risks associated with sun exposure.

This increase in obesity in adolescents has led to increases in hypertension, heart disease, and type 2 diabetes. Influential factors causing obesity include food choices, eating practices, and lack of exercise. One study indicated that only 75% to 78% of adolescents ages 11 to 19 eat breakfast. Also, less than 40% of adolescents ages 12 to 19 meet the daily dietary requirement of vegetables and fruits while exceeding the recommendation for saturated fats. Adolescents are busy and eat on the run with many meals from fast-food facilities. In addition, many schools have decreased or discontinued physical education, which has resulted in a more sedentary lifestyle leading to weight gain. Interest in computer games and television watching at home has decreased physical activity and exercise and further contributed to weight gain and obesity (see Healthy People 2010).

Nurses must make parents and adolescents aware of factors leading to obesity. Nurses should recommend:

- Proper nutrition and healthy food choices
- Good eating habits
- Decreased fast-food intake
- Exercising for 30 minutes at least four times per week
- Parents/adolescents exercising more at home
- Decreased computer use and television watching

Violence

The CDC's Injury Center defines violence as threatened or actual physical force or power initiated by an individual that results in physical or psychological injury or death. More than 877,700 adolescents and young adults between 10 and 24 years of age were injured as a result of violence in 2002. Approximately 1 in 13 of these injuries resulted in hospitalization (CDC, 2007f). The issue of youth violence is a growing concern in America's communities. The health and well-being of adolescents and society are threatened by this violence. See Box 29.5 for factors contributing to adolescent violence.

BOX 29.5 **Factors Contributing to Adolescent Violence**

- Crowded conditions/housing
- Low socioeconomic status
- Limited parental supervision
- Single parent families/both parents in workforce
- Access to guns or cars
- Drug or alcohol use
- Low self-esteem
- Racism
- Peer or gang pressure
- Aggression

Homicide

Homicide is the fourth leading cause of death in children between 10 and 14 years old, and the second leading cause of death in 15- to 19-year-olds. Most young homicide victims are killed with guns. In 2003, 82% of homicide victims age 10 to 24 years were killed with firearms (CDC, 2006b). Refer to Box 29.5 for factors that contribute to violence among adolescents. In a nationwide survey conducted in 2004, 17% of students reported carrying a weapon on one or more days within the past 30 days (CDC, 2006b) (see Healthy People 2010).

Suicide

Suicide is the third leading cause of death in adolescents 15 to 19 years of age. In a CDC study in 2001, 19.3% of adolescents surveyed related that they had seriously considered suicide within the past 12 months. The rate of suicide among teens between 15 and 19 years old increased by 11% from 1980 to 1997, and by 10% in 10- to 14-year-olds in the same time period. In 1999, more teenagers and young adults died from suicide than from cancer, heart disease, acquired immunodeficiency syndrome (AIDS),

---

HEALTHY PEOPLE 2010	
Objective	**Significance**
Increase the proportion of adolescents who engage in moderate physical activity for at least 30 minutes on 5 or more of the previous 7 days, and vigorous physical activity that promotes cardiorespiratory fitness 3 or more days per week for 20 or more minutes per occasion.	• For the nonexercising teen, advise to start slowly by walking. • Work with the teen to identify physical activities that interest the teen. • Praise efforts to participate in a routine exercise plan. • Identify an athletic individual that the teen identifies with and encourage similar activities in the teen.

HEALTHY PEOPLE 2010	
Objective	**Significance**
Reduce homicides, physical fighting among adolescents, weapon carrying by adolescents on school property, rate of suicide attempts by adolescents.	• Screen teens at all encounters for indications of violent behaviors. • Provide education related to decreasing school violence at middle and high schools. • Encourage alternate, appropriate methods for dispelling anger. • Screen teens at all encounters for indications of depression.

birth defects, stroke, and chronic lung disease combined (CDC, 2007c). Among adolescents ages 15 to 19, firearm-related suicides accounted for more than 60% of the increase in the overall suicide rate from 1980 to 1997 (see Healthy People 2010).

Dating Violence

Violent behavior that takes place in a context of dating or courtship is not a rare event. Thirty percent of teens state that either they or someone they know has experienced dating violence. Females are victims of dating violence more often than males and suffer more injuries than males. Dating violence in the teen years is a risk factor for continued violence exposure in adulthood. Risk factors for dating violence include living in a broken home or rural area, inadequate parental supervision, condoning violence, substance use, prior victimization, dropping out of high school, and risky sexual practices (Mars & Valdez, 2007).

Gangs

Much of youth violence is a result of the behavior of adolescent gangs. Nationwide there are an estimated 23,388 gangs with 664,906 members; approximately 3% are female. In one study, the risk factors for gang involvement were family, friends, neighborhood, and interpersonal issues. Peers are ranked as being most influential in female gang involvement, followed by neighborhood, family, and self. Gang membership may aid in the formation of identity by providing status and a sense of belonging. Gang membership occurs in cities and in suburban areas, but may differ in composition. The gangs in rural or suburban areas are more diverse racially and include both males and females. All socioeconomic groups are represented in gang membership. Gangs threaten and intimidate with violent behaviors and guns (Archer & Grascia, 2005).

Nursing Interventions to Decrease Youth Violence

Nurses working with adolescents should include violence prevention in anticipatory guidance. Violence is a learned behavior. It is often reinforced by the media, television, music, and personal example. Explain to parents, teachers, and peers the importance of being good role models because violence is a learned behavior. Parents should monitor video games, music, television, and other media to decrease exposure to violence. Parents need to know who their adolescent's friends are and monitor for negative behaviors and actions.

The identification of adolescents at risk for suicide is a very important task for the nurse, parents, peers, and counselors. See Box 29.6 for signs of risk factors. The National Center for Injury Prevention and Control (NCIPC) is working to create awareness of suicide as a serious public health problem and is developing strategies to reduce injuries and deaths due to suicide.

BOX 29.6 Risk Factors for Suicide in Adolescents

- Depression
- Mental health changes
- Poor school performance
- Family disorganization
- Substance abuse
- Homosexuality
- Giving away valued possessions
- Being a loner/having no close friends
- Changes in behavior

Substance Use

Agents commonly abused by children and adolescents include alcohol, hallucinogens, sedatives, analgesics, anxiolytics, steroids, inhalants, and stimulants. The substance abused is related to its availability and cost. Two common substances that are more accessible and have the highest incidence of use are tobacco and alcohol. Each day, approximately 4,000 young people under the age of 18 try their first cigarette; 80% of adult smokers started smoking before age 18. It is estimated that 90% of adolescents have tried alcohol by the time they reach adulthood. Research consistently supports the hypothesis that drug use progresses from beer or wine to cigarettes or hard liquor and then to marijuana, followed by illicit drugs.

Some of the long-term effects and consequences of drug and alcohol use include: possibility of overdose and death; unintentional injuries; irrational behaviors; inability to think clearly; unsafe driving and legal consequences; problems with relationships with family and friends; sexual activity and STIs; and health problems such as liver problems (hepatitis) and cardiac problems (sudden death with cocaine). Refer to Table 29.4 for commonly abused drugs and behaviors exhibited (see Healthy People 2010).

Tobacco

Tobacco use remains the leading preventable cause of death in the United States, causing more than 440,000 deaths each year. Long-term consequences of youth smoking are reinforced by the fact that most young people who smoke regularly continue to smoke throughout adulthood. Each day in the United States, about 4,000 12- to 17-year-olds take their first cigarette. More than 6.4 million people will die prematurely because of smoking as adolescents. Although the overall rate of smoking has declined since 1999, rates still remain high: 22% of high-school students report current cigarette use. Seven percent of high-school students use smokeless tobacco (CDC, 2004a). Teens who smoke are three times more

TABLE 29.4 DRUGS COMMONLY ABUSED

Drug	Manifestations	Considerations
Marijuana	Red eyes, dry mouth, euphoria, relaxation, decreased motivation, loss of inhibition	Considered a gateway drug
Cocaine	Weight loss, euphoria, elation, agitation, pressured speech, tachycardia, hypertension, anorexia, insomnia	Psychotic behavior with large doses; if combined with other drugs can be fatal
Opiates	Elation, euphoria, detachment, drowsiness, constricted pupils, slurred speech, impaired judgment	Self-neglect with malnutrition and dehydration; criminal behaviors to get drugs; infections at injection sites
Amphetamines	Euphoria, agitation, weight loss, insomnia, tachycardia, hypertension	Possible paradoxical effect of depression in children
Hallucinogens	Hallucinations, illusions, depersonalization, heightened awareness, dilated pupils, hypertension, increased salivation, distorted perceptions	Panic flashbacks long after use of drugs; psychotic behaviors
Phencyclidine hydrochloride (PCP)	Euphoria, distorted perceptions, agitation, violence, antisocial behaviors, hypertension, increased salivation, increased pain response	Irrational behaviors, panic, psychosis
Barbiturates	Euphoria followed by depression or hostility; impaired judgment; decreased inhibitions; slurred speech; incoordination	Often used with stimulants; may have a paradoxical effect of hyperactivity in children

likely than nonsmokers to use alcohol, eight times more likely to use marijuana, and 22 times more likely to use cocaine. Smoking is associated with a host of other risky behaviors, including fighting and engaging in unprotected sex (Focus Adolescent Services, 2007). The short-term health effects of smoking include damage to the respiratory system, addiction to nicotine, and the associated risk of other drug use. Smoking negatively impacts physical fitness and lung growth and increases the potential for addiction in adolescents. Smokeless tobacco may also cause many problems. It can lead to bleeding gums and

sores in the mouth that never heal. Smokeless tobacco use leads to discoloration of the teeth and eventually may lead to cancer.

Alcohol

The Youth Risk Behavior Survey found that about 75% of adolescents under the age of 18 have consumed alcohol, although the legal drinking age is 21. Forty-three percent of teens reported current alcohol use, and 25% admitted to episodic binge drinking (CDC, 2006b). The findings revealed that there were no substantial differences among various sociodemographic subgroups with respect to drinking rates, although alcohol use is lowest in African-Americans and highest in whites. The incidence of alcohol use increases throughout adolescence. Almost two thirds of 12th graders who report consuming alcohol also reported at least one alcohol-related problem. Alcohol use as an adolescent can lead to prevailing alcohol use as an adult and contribute to physical health problems. It may also precede other drug abuse.

Illicit Drugs

Adolescents may also experiment with or abuse illicit drugs. Substance abuse remains a widespread problem among American adolescents. Although experimentation with marijuana has decreased between 1991 and 2003 among the adolescent population, it still remains the most widely used illicit drug (Eaton et al., 2006). The Youth Risk Behavior Survey revealed that almost 8% of teens

HEALTHY PEOPLE 2010

Objective	Significance
Reduce the proportion of adolescents who report that they rode, during the previous 30 days, with a driver who had been drinking alcohol. Reduce steroid use among adolescents. Increase the proportion of adolescents who disapprove of substance abuse and smoking.	• Provide education in the office, hospital, or school related to adverse effects of tobacco, alcohol, and illicit substance use. • Educate families, teens, and coaches about the negative effects of anabolic steroids. • Praise teens for abstaining from the above substances and rising above peer pressure.

had used cocaine, 12.5% had tried inhalants, and 4% had used illegal steroids (CDC, 2006b).

Data reveal that illicit drug usage for individual drugs reflects rapidly changing determinants specific to that drug. Influencing factors include the psychoactive potential and benefits reported, how risky the drug is to use, how acceptable is it to peer groups, and the accessibility of the drug (Johnston et al., 2006).

Nursing Interventions to Decrease Substance Use Among Teens

Educate the adolescent on the problems related to alcohol use and abuse. Topics that should be discussed include:

- Short- and long-term effects of alcohol, tobacco, and drugs on health
- Risk factors and implications for unintentional injuries and sexual activity
- Short- and long-term effects of alcohol, tobacco, and drugs on relationships and school performance and progression
- The how and why of chemical dependency
- Impact of substance abuse on society
- Importance of maintaining a healthy lifestyle
- Importance of resisting peer pressure to use drugs and alcohol
- Importance of having confidence in his or her own judgement
- Providing the teen with accurate and up-to-date information (Children of Alcoholics Foundation, n.d.)

Think back to Cho, who was introduced at the beginning of the chapter. List common developmental concerns of the adolescent. What anticipatory guidance related to these concerns would you provide?

■■■ Key Concepts

- Adolescence is a period of rapid and variable growth in the areas of physical, psychosocial, cognitive, and moral development.
- The adolescent is developing his own identity, becoming an abstract thinker, and developing his own set of morals and values. Inability to successfully develop an individual identity leads to poor preparation for the challenges of adulthood.
- Relationships with parents fluctuate widely during adolescence. The teenager eventually becomes emancipated from her parents.
- Peers become most important—guiding mainly the early and middle adolescent in his decisions, while the late adolescent can usually formulate his own decisions.
- Adolescence is a critical time in the development of sexuality. Sexuality includes the thoughts, feelings, and behaviors surrounding the adolescent's sexual identity.

- The egocentric and invincible thought processes of the adolescent can lead to injuries. Health care providers must emphasis safety regarding cars, bikes, water, firearms, and fire.
- Motor vehicle accidents are the number one cause of death in adolescents.
- Nutritional habits of the adolescent lead to deficiency in vitamins and minerals needed for the rapid growth during this period.
- Obesity in adolescents is a growing health concern. Health care providers are facing increased numbers of adolescents with hypertension, type 2 diabetes, and hyperlipidemia.
- Substance abuse and experimentation is common during adolescence; it is associated with other risk-taking behaviors such as injuries and sexual activity.
- Health care providers must work collaboratively with the adolescent in the development of interventions to promote health.

REFERENCES

Advocates for Youth. (2007). *Gay, lesbian, bisexual, transgender, and questioning (GLBTQ) youth.* Retrieved November 9, 2007 from http://www.advocatesforyouth.org/glbtq.htm.
Alba-Fisch, M. *Temperament: miss or match.* Retrieved November 9, 2007 from http://www.taconicnet.com/articles.php.
American Academy of Pediatric Dentistry. (2007). *Policy on use of fluoride.* Retrieved August 28, 2007 from http://www.aapd.org/media/Policies_Guidelines/P_FluorideUse.pdf.
American Academy of Pediatrics. (2003). Policy statement: Prevention of drowning in infants, children and adolescents. *Pediatrics, 112*(2), 437–439.
American Academy of Pediatrics. (2004a). *Guidance for effective discipline.* Retrieved August 28, 2007 from http://aappolicy.aappublications.org/cgi/content/full/pediatrics;101/4/723.
American Academy of Pediatrics. (2006). Active healthy living: Prevention of childhood obesity through increased physical activity. *Pediatrics, 117*, 1834–1842.
American Academy of Pediatrics. (2006). *Corporal punishment in schools.* Retrieved August 28, 2007 from http://aappolicy.aappublications.org/cgi/content/full/pediatrics;106/2/343.
American Academy of Pediatrics. (2006). The teen driver. *Pediatrics, 118*, 2570–2581.
American Academy of Pediatrics, Council on Sports Medicine and Fitness and Council on School Health. (2006). Active health living: prevention of childhood obesity through increased physical activity. *Pediatrics, 117*, 1834–1842.
American Academy of Pediatrics, The Injury Prevention Program. (2007a). *Age-related safety sheets: 2 to 4 years.* Retrieved August 28, 2007 from http://www.aap.org/family/2to4yrs.htm.
Barakat, I.S., & Clark, J.A. (2005). *Positive discipline and child guidance.* Retrieved July 9, 2006 from http://muextension.missouri.edu/xplor/hesguide/humanrel/gh6119.htm.
Bautista, S.R., & Flynn, J.R. (2006). Trauma prevention in children. *Pediatric Annals, 35*(2), 85–90.
Biaglioli, F.E., Chesnutt, J.C., Paladine, H.L., Powers, E.C., & Eiff, M.P. (2007). Managing overweight adolescents. *Contemporary Pediatrics, 24*(6), 37–59.
Bindler, R.M., & Bruya, M.A. (2007). Evidence for identifying children at risk for being overweight, cardiovascular disease, and type 2 diabetes in primary care. *Journal of Pediatric Health Care, 20*(2), 82–87.
Centers for Disease Control and Prevention. (2004a). Cigarette use among high school students: United States 1991-2003. *Morbidity and Mortality Weekly Report, 53*(52), 499-502.

Centers for Disease Control and Prevention. (2004b). Violence-related behaviors among high school students: United States, 1991-2003. *Morbidity and Mortality Weekly, 53*(29), 651-655.

Centers for Disease Control and Prevention. (2007). *10 leading causes of death, United States, 2004, all races, both sexes.* Retrieved August 28, 2007 from http://webappa.cdc.gov/cgi-bin/broker.exe.

Centers for Disease Control and Prevention. (2007). *The injury pyramid.* Retrieved August 28, 2007 from http://www.cdc.gov/HealthyYouth/injury/slides/injury_guidelines.ppt#4.

Centers for Disease Control and Prevention. (2007b). *Physical activity and the health of young people.* Retrieved November 9, 2007 from http://www.cdc.gov/HealthyYouth/PhysicalActivity/.

Centers for Disease Control and Prevention. (2006). *CDC's position on tattooing and HCV infection.* Retrieved November 9, 2007 from http://www.cdc.gov/ncidod/diseases/hepatitis/c/tattoo.htm.

Centers for Disease Control and Prevention. (2007a). *Overweight and obesity: Health consequences.* Retrieved November 9, 2007 from http://www.cdc.gov/nccdphp/dnpa/obesity/consequences.htm.

Centers for Disease Control and Prevention. (2007f). *Tobacco use.* Retrieved November 9, 2007 from http://www.cdc.gov/HealthyYouth/tobacco/index.htm.

Centers for Disease Control and Prevention. (2006b). Youth risk behavior surveillance—United States, 2005. *Morbidity and Mortality Weekly Report, 55* (SS-5).

Centers for Disease Control and Prevention, National Center for Injury Prevention and Control. (2007). *Youth violence: Fact sheet.* Retrieved November 9, 2007 from http://www.cdc.gov/ncipc/factsheets/yvfacts.htm.

ChildHelp. (2006). *Child abuse statistics.* Retrieved August 28, 2007 from http://www.childhelp.org/resources/learning-center/statistics.

Child Trends. (2006). *Dating.* Retrieved November 9, 2007 from http://www.childtrendsdatabank.org/indicators/73dating.cfm.

Christakis, D. A., & Zimmerman, F.J. (2007). Children and television: A primer for pediatricians. *Contemporary Pediatrics, 24*(3), 31–42.

Cool Nurse. (2007). *Dating.* Retrieved November 9, 2007 from http://www.coolnurse.com/dating.htm.

Desantis-Moniaci, D., & Altshuler, L. (2007). Comprehensive behavioral treatment of overweight and the pediatric practice. *Pediatrics Annals, 36*(2), 102–108.

Eaton, D.K., Kann, L., Kinchen, S., Ross, J., et al. (2006). Youth risk behavior surveillance: United States, 2005. *Morbidity and Mortality Weekly, 55* (SS05), 1-108.

Erikson, E. (1963). *Childhood and society* (2nd ed.). New York: Norton.

Green, M., & Palfrey, J.S. (eds). (2002). *Bright futures: Guidelines for health supervision of infants, children, and adolescents* (2nd ed., rev.). Arlington, VA: National Center for Education in Maternal and Child Health.

Gunturu, S.D., & Ten, S. (2007). Complications of obesity in childhood. *Pediatrics Annals, 36*(2), 96–101.

Heyman, R.B. (2007). Combating underage drinking with the 6 g's. *Contemporary Pediatrics, 24*(6), 63–75.

Hickman, L.J., Jaycox, L.H. & Aronoff, J. (2004). Dating violence among adolescents: Prevalence, gender distribution, and prevention program effectiveness. *Trauma, Violence & Abuse, 5*(2), 1223-1242.

Kohlberg, L. (1984). *Essays on moral development.* San Francisco: Harper & Row.

Meadows-Oliver, M. (2007). Using our heads: What PNPs need to know about helmets. *Journal of Pediatric Health Care, 21*(4), 265–267.

National Association for Sport & Physical Education. (2007). *Active start: A statement of physical activity guidelines for children birth to five years.* Retrieved August 28, 2007 from http://www.aahperd.org/NASPE/ns_active.html.

National Association of Pediatric Nurse Practitioners. (2006a). *Healthy eating and activity together (HEAT) clinical practice guide-line: Identifying and preventing overweight in childhood.* Cherry Hill, NJ: Author.

National Association of Pediatric Nurse Practitioners. (2006b). NAP-NAP position statement on corporal punishment. *Journal of Pediatric Health Care, 20*(6), A43–A44.

National Highway Traffic Safety Association. (n.d.). *Teen Safety.* Retrieved July 9, 2006 from http://www.nhtsa.dot.gov/people/outreach/safesobr/19qp/sect2/page3.html.

Nield, L.S., Stenger, J.P., & Kamat, D. (2007). Dental disease: Pearls about those pearly whites. *Consultant for Pediatricians, 6*(8), 449–454.

Piaget, J. (1969). *The theory of stages in cognitive development.* New York: McGraw-Hill.

Rosenbaum, M. (2007). Epidemiology of pediatric obesity. *Pediatric Annals, 26*(2), 89–95.

Safe Kids USA. (2007). *Safety tips: Car.* Retrieved August 28, 2007 from http://www.usa.safekids.org/tier2_rl.cfm?folder_id=170.

Safe Kids Worldwide. (2007). *Preventing injury to children in motor vehicle crashes.* Retrieved August 28, 2007 from http://www.usa.safekids.org/content_documents/MVO_tips.pdf.

Shelov, S.P., Trubo, R., Hannemann, R.E. (Eds.). (2004). *Caring for your baby and young child: Birth to age 5* (4th ed.). New York: Bantam Books.

Storey, M., Holt, K., & Sotfka, D. (Eds.). (2002). *Bright futures in practice: Nutrition* (2nd ed.). Arlington, VA: National Center for Education in Maternal and Child Health.

Savage, J.S., Fisher, J.O., & Birch, L.L. (2007). Parental influence on eating behavior: Conception to adolescence. *The Journal of Law, Medicine & Ethics, 35*(1), 22–34.

Tanner, J. (1962). *Growth at adolescence* (2nd ed.). Oxford, England: Blackwell Scientific Publications.

United States Department of Health and Human Services. (2000). *Healthy people 2010* (2nd ed., 2 vols.). Washington, DC: U.S. Government Printing Office.

World Health Organization. (2007). *Passive smoking.* Retrieved August 26, 2007 from http://www.who.int/tobacco/en/atlas10.pdf.

WEBSITES

American Academy of Pediatrics: www.aap.org

American Academy of Pediatric Dentistry: www.aapd.org

American Heart Association: www.americanheart.org/

Centers for Disease Control and Prevention: www.cdc.gov/

Growth chart information from the CDC: www.cdc.gov/growthcharts/

Powerful Bones. Powerful Girls. The National Bone Health Campaign: www.cdc.gov/powerfulbones/

CDC's Tobacco Information and Prevention Source (TIPS): www.cdc.gov/tobacco/

Teen health website (Canada): www.chebucto.ns.ca/health/TeenHealth/

Sexuality and sexual health information for adolescents: www.coolnurse.com/sex_stuff.htm

Dental care information from Proctor & Gamble: www.dentalcare.com/drn.htm

American Dietetic Association: www.eatright.org

Internet clearinghouse of information, resources and support for helping teens: www.focusas.com/

Information on a healthy school environment: www.healthyschools.org

Information on adolescent nutrition: www.keepkidshealthy.com/adolescent/adolescentnutrition.html

Teen's homepage on Nemours Foundation Kids' Health website: www.kidshealth.org/teen/

American Obesity Association: www.obesity.org

Internet safety for kids: www.safekids.com

Sports Illustrated for Kids: www.sikids.com/

CHAPTER WORKSHEET

MULTIPLE CHOICE QUESTIONS

1. When giving parents guidance for the adolescent years, the nurse would advise the parents to: (Choose all that apply)

   a. Accept the adolescent as a unique individual.

   b. Provide strict, inflexible rules.

   c. Listen and try to be open to the adolescent's views.

   d. Screen all of his or her friends.

   e. Respect the adolescent's privacy.

   f. Provide unconditional love.

2. In developing a weight-loss plan for an adolescent, which would the nurse include? (Choose all that apply)

   a. Have parents make all of the meal plans.

   b. Eat slowly and place the fork down between each bite.

   c. Have the family exercise together.

   d. Refer to an adolescent weight-loss program.

   e. Keep a food and exercise diary.

3. Which is associated with early adolescence? (Choose all that apply)

   a. Uses scientific reasoning to solve problems

   b. Still at times wants to be dependent upon parents

   c. Incorporates own set of morals and values

   d. Is influenced by peers and values memberships in cliques

4. What has the most influence in deterring an adolescent from beginning to drink alcohol?

   a. Drinking habits of parents

   b. Drinking habits of peers

   c. Drinking philosophy of adolescent's culture

   d. Drinking philosophy of adolescent's religion

CRITICAL THINKING EXERCISES

1. During a sports physical examination, Susan, a 16-year-old, tells her health care provider that she is overweight. What additional information would the health care provider obtain?

2. The parents of Joe, a 14-year-old, talk to the school nurse about Joe's behavior at home. He is moody, fights with his younger siblings, only wants to be on his computer, and does not want to go on the family vacation. What advice would the nurse give the parents?

3. Jane tells the school nurse that she might be homosexual. What additional information would the nurse obtain?

4. Alicia's parents are worried because all of Alicia's friends wear heavy makeup and have multiple piercings and hair colors. What advice would the nurse give Alicia's parents?

STUDY ACTIVITIES

1. Talk to an early, middle, and late adolescent. Compare and contrast their interactions with you. Identify what psychosocial, cognitive, and moral stage they are in, using examples from their conversations with you.

2. Have an adolescent keep a food and exercise diary for one week. Analyze the information. Develop with the adolescent any interventions needed to promote healthy eating and exercise habits.

3. Plan a class on the dangers of smoking for 15-year-olds.

4. Plan a class for parents on how to keep the lines of communication open for adolescents.

UNIT TEN

FOUNDATIONS OF PEDIATRIC NURSING

HEALTH SUPERVISION

KEY TERMS

active immunity
developmental screenings
developmental
    surveillance

immunity
medical home
passive immunity
risk assessment

screening tests
selective screening
universal screening

LEARNING OBJECTIVES

Upon completion of the chapter, the learner will be able to:

1. Describe the principles of health supervision.
2. List the three components of a health supervision visit.
3. Use instruments appropriately for developmental and functional testing of children.
4. Demonstrate knowledge of the principles of immunization.
5. Identify barriers to immunization.
6. Identify challenges to health supervision for children with chronic illnesses.

Three-year-old Maya Randall and 9-month-old Evan Randall are brought to the clinic by their father. Maya was last seen in the clinic when she was 1 year old, and Evan has never been seen. The father says that they have both been healthy so they did not need to come to the clinic before this. Maya is complaining of a sore throat, which is what prompted today's visit.

Wow
It is never too late to start prevention. It begins with a genuine desire for health improvement.

Principles of Health Supervision

Health supervision involves providing services proactively, with the goal of optimizing the child's level of functioning. This chapter is organized around the three components of health supervision: developmental surveillance and screening; injury and disease prevention; and health promotion. Health supervision begins at birth and continues through adolescence. Health supervision is vital to every child and is most effective when the child has a centralized source of health care. Any place publicly accessible by children and families can be an appropriate setting for health supervision services—private physicians' offices, community health departments, sliding-scale clinics, homeless shelters, daycare centers, and schools. The framework for the health supervision visit is developed from national guidelines available through the U.S. Department of Health and Human Services (DHHS), the American Medical Association (AMA), and the American Academy of Pediatrics (AAP). These organizations also provide guidelines for children with chronic health problems and services and information regarding unique situations such as the internationally adopted child.

Wellness

The focus of pediatric health supervision is wellness. The health supervision visit provides an opportunity to maximize health promotion for the child, family, and community. Nurses have the ability to promote optimal health during these encounters. Health supervision visits must be viewed as part of a continuum of care, not as the accomplishment of isolated tasks.

Medical Home

A **medical home** is the primary health care provider who has a long-term and comprehensive relationship with the family. This continuing relationship promotes trust between the provider and the family and leads to comprehensive, coordinated, and cost-effective care. The medical home is the setting that allows the highest level of health supervision. To be effective, the medical home must be accessible, family-centered, and community-based. It must be integrated into the child's world, not adjacent to it. Characteristics of a medical home are displayed in Box 30.1.

Partnerships

The child is the focus of the health supervision visit. However, the child's health is linked to the needs and resources of his or her family and community. For instance, if the family is in turmoil because of divorce, drug abuse, or parental health problems, the child is less likely to receive the attention and energy that he or she needs

---

BOX 30.1   Characteristics of a Medical Home

- Preventive care activities
- Ambulatory and inpatient care available 24 hours a day
- Continuity of care from infancy through adolescence
- Availability of subspecialty consultation and referrals
- Interactive relationships with school and community agencies
- A centralized database containing all pertinent information

Green, M., & Palfrey, J. (Eds.) (2002). *Bright futures: Guidelines for health supervision of infants, children, and adolescents* (2nd ed.). Arlington, VA: National Center for Education in Maternal and Child Health.

---

to thrive. Likewise, a community with high levels of poverty, poor infrastructure, and lack of resources will not be able to provide the support services needed to allow children to reach their full potential. To be effective, the nurse must offer commitment and develop an ongoing partnership with the child, family, and community. These partnerships allow for mutual goal setting, marshalling of resources, and development of optimal health practices.

The partnership between the child and the health supervision team develops over time. In infancy the family is the surrogate for the child in the partnership. The child's participation in the partnership increases at a rate that is developmentally appropriate. The child's increasing influence in the partnership allows the nurse to tailor health supervision to the child's needs. The partnership allows the child to take increasing responsibility for his or her personal health and optimizes health promotion.

Nurses must validate and enhance the role of family members as they influence and inform the child's concept of wellness. The health care community must involve the family to have a significant impact on a child's health. The family wants the best possible outcome for their child, and health care decisions are based on the knowledge they possess. The nurse can greatly facilitate trust by acknowledging that the family has unique insights to offer on their child's health. Nurses can also strengthen the partnership between the family and the health care community by recognizing the family's healthy practices, addressing their health issues, and strengthening their skills. By contributing to the partnership, both the nurse and the family enhance the chance of success for health care plans, but families are the ones who must implement any health care strategy and know what expected outcomes are reasonable. Their feedback is invaluable to formulating an effective long-term health supervision plan that optimizes their child's wellness.

> ▶ *Take* NOTE!
>
> *Observe the parent–child interaction during the health supervision visit. The nurse can learn much about the family dynamic by observing the family for behavioral clues:*
>
> - *Does the parent make eye contact with the infant?*
> - *Does the parent anticipate and respond to the infant's needs?*
> - *Are parents effective when dealing with a toddler's temper tantrum?*
> - *Do the parents' comments increase the school-age child's sense of self-worth?*
>
> *Behavioral observations are crucial to the proper assessment of the family's needs and issues.*

Partnerships between the community and the health promotion team benefit the community as well as individual clients. When nurses develop partnerships with community agencies such as schools, churches, and ancillary health facilities, barriers to care can be overcome. The nurse becomes aware of available resources in the community that can benefit an individual family. With input from community partners, the nurse can perform an assessment of the community's needs. The assessment then provides the foundation for the development of community-based health promotion programs. These programs expand the resources of the community, which in turn enhances the health of its members.

Special Issues in Health Supervision

Special issues in health supervision include cultural influences, community influences, health supervision and the chronically ill child, and health supervision and the internationally adopted child.

Cultural Influences on Health Supervision

A person's definition of health is influenced by his or her culture. Successful interactions result when the nurse is aware of the beliefs and interactive styles that are often present in members of a specific culture. If the goals of the health care plan are not consistent with the health belief system of the family, the plan has little chance for success. Optimal wellness for the child requires the nurse and the family to negotiate a mutually acceptable plan of care. A plan must balance the cultural beliefs and practices of the family with those of the health care establish-

ment. The nurse must possess cultural competence and sensitivity for the partnership to be successful.

Most health promotion and disease prevention strategies in the United States have a future-based orientation and view the client as an active and controlling agent in his or her own health. This reflects the dominant culture; however, the challenge to the nurse is to develop strategies that are meaningful to clients from other cultures. Significant numbers of clients belong to cultures with a present-based orientation. For these clients, health promotion activities need shorter-term goals and outcomes to be useful. Clients with a fatalistic worldview will see any actions on their part as ineffective. They may feel that a god figure or supernatural forces control their fate and that health is a gift to be appreciated, not a goal to be pursued. Certain cultures believe health is the result of being in harmony within oneself and the larger universe. From this viewpoint, taking a medication or receiving a treatment is not an effective way to restore health because it does not address the problem of being "out of harmony."

However, just because an individual belongs to a certain culture does not guarantee that he or she subscribes to all of its values. The nurse should explore each client's specific beliefs during the health interview.

Community Influences on Health Supervision

The child is a member of a community as well as a family and a culture. Each community has unique strengths, weaknesses, and values. A community can be a contributor to a child's health or be the cause of his or her illnesses. The child's health cannot be totally separated from the health of the surrounding community.

Ideally the child's medical home is within the family's community. If home and access to medical care are close, barriers such as lack of transportation, expense of travel, and time away from the parents' workplace are reduced. Having the medical home within the community facilitates bonds between the health team and schools, churches, and support services and agencies. Community support and resources are necessary for children with significant problems. A close working relationship between the child's health care provider and community agencies is an enormous benefit to the child (see the earlier section on partnerships).

The community assessment may reveal problems that are causing or contributing to the child's health problems. A deteriorating infrastructure can contribute to decreased access to care and increased risk of injury or illness. Poverty has been linked to low birthweight and premature birth, among other health problems. Substandard housing can be directly related to lead poisoning and asthma. Children from communities suffering the large-scale breakdown of family relationships and loss of support systems will be at increased risk for depression, violence and abuse, substance abuse, and human immunodeficiency virus (HIV) infection. A thorough knowledge of the family's community is needed before a health surveillance program can be effective.

Health Supervision and the Child With Chronic Illness

Effective health supervision must be responsive to the individual child's situation. The child with a chronic illness needs to be assessed repeatedly to determine his or her health maintenance needs. These assessments determine the frequency of visits and types of interventions needed. The impact of the illness on the child's functional health patterns determines whether standard health supervision visits need to be augmented.

An effective partnership among the child's medical home, family, and community is vital for a child with a chronic illness. Coordination of specialty care, community agencies, and family support networks enhances the quality of life and health of these children. Access to care and services minimizes the risk of injury from the illness. Support groups and community-based resources optimize the family's adaptation to the stressors of chronic illness.

Comprehensive health supervision includes frequent psychosocial assessments. Issues to be covered include:

• Health insurance coverage
• Transportation to health care facilities
• Financial stressors
• Family coping
• School's response to the chronic illness

These are often stressful and emotionally charged issues. The nurse with a trusting and ongoing relationship with the child and family is in the best position to help with these issues. The nurse can assist the family to find financial and medical assistance programs, take advantage of community resources, and participate in support groups. The nurse can also educate school personnel about the child's illness and assist them in maximizing the child's potential for academic success.

Health Supervision and the Child Adopted Internationally

Health supervision of the internationally adopted child must include comprehensive screening for infectious disease. In 2000, nearly 20,000 children were adopted from countries outside the United States, many from areas with a high prevalence of infectious diseases. China and Russia typically supply 50% of all international adoptees. Korea, Guatemala, Romania, Vietnam, and the Ukraine account for 32% of internationally adopted children. Proper screening is important not only to the child's health but also to the

adopting family and the larger community. Screening is recommended within the first few weeks of the child's arrival into the United States.

Intestinal parasites are a common problem: approximately 25% of international adoptees have one or more pathogens. *Giardia lamblia,* the most common pathogen, is found in 19% of these children. Infected children are frequently symptom-free, so universal screening is recommended.

Latent tuberculosis is also common, affecting up to 19% of this population. Though active tuberculosis infection has been rarely reported, an extensive outbreak of tuberculosis occurred in a North Dakota community in 1998. The index case was an internationally adopted child from the Marshall Islands. Universal screening is recommended for this high-risk population.

Universal screening for hepatitis B, HIV, and syphilis infections is recommended. Due to lack of resources in the home country, screening and treatment for these diseases are sporadic and ineffective. If testing is documented, it is likely to be unreliable. Testing supplies may have been outdated or improperly stored. Also, the test may have been performed before the child's seroconversion occurred.

Components of Health Supervision

Developmental surveillance and screening, injury and disease prevention, and health promotion are the critical components of health supervision for children. Disease prevention and health promotion are concepts well established in adult health supervision. Injury prevention and developmental surveillance/screening are additional components of pediatric health supervision visits that help every child achieve his or her optimal state of wellness.

Developmental Surveillance and Screening

Developmental surveillance is an ongoing collection of skilled observations made over time during health care visits. Components include:

• Noting and addressing parental concerns
• Obtaining a developmental history
• Making accurate observations
• Consulting with relevant professionals

Developmental screenings are brief assessment procedures that identify children who warrant more intensive assessment and testing. Developmental screening assessments may be observational or by caregiver report (Fig. 30.1).

Development, or the emergence of the child's abilities, is a longitudinal process. Within the trust and security of the medical home, family and health care providers

FIGURE 30.1 Developmental screening provides the opportunity for the nurse to identify problems in the child's development.

can share observations and concerns. In collaboration, the family and the health care provider observe the child's accomplishments or milestones over time. Data collection for developmental surveillance of infants and young children is performed through developmental questionnaires, health care provider observations, and a thorough physical examination. School records and test results can provide academic performance data for the older child. Input from teachers, coaches, and other adults involved with the child can give insight into the child's emotional and social development.

When developmental delay is suspected, frequent developmental surveillance is warranted. Reemphasizing parental roles and responsibilities fosters cooperation and compliance. It is therefore crucial that parents understand the need for frequent assessments. A pattern of developmental delays warrants a formal evaluation.

The pediatric nurse must understand normal growth and development and become proficient at screening for problems related to development. The historical information obtained from the parent or primary caregiver about developmental milestones may indicate warning signs or identify risks for developmental delay (Table 30.1). Factors placing the infant or toddler at risk for developmental problems include:

- Birthweight less than 1,500 g
- Gestational age less than 33 weeks
- Central nervous system abnormality
- Hypoxic ischemic encephalopathy
- Maternal prenatal alcohol or drug abuse
- Hypertonia
- Hypotonia
- Hyperbilirubinemia requiring exchange transfusion
- Kernicterus
- Congenital malformations
- Symmetric intrauterine growth deficiency

TABLE 30.1 INFANT/TODDLER DEVELOPMENTAL WARNING SIGNS

Age	Warning Sign	Possible Developmental Concern
Any age	No response to environmental stimulus	Sensory deficit
Any age	Persistently up on toes (longer than 30 seconds) in supported standing position	Cerebral palsy
Before 3 months	Rolls over	Hypertonia
After 2–3 months	Persistent fisting	Neurologic dysfunction
After 4 months	Persistent head lag	Hypotonia
5 months	Not reaching for toys	Motor, visual, or cognitive deficit
6 months	Lack of tripod sitting	Hypotonia
6 months	Not smiling	Visual deficit, attachment issue
6 months	Primitive reflex persistence	Neurologic dysfunction
6 months	Not babbling	Hearing deficit
9 months	No reciprocal vocalizations or facial expressions	Autism spectrum disorders
12 months	No spoon or crayon use	Fine motor delay
15–18 months	Not walking	Gross motor delay
18 months	No imitative play	Autism spectrum disorders
Prior to 18 months	Hand dominance present	Hemiplegia in opposite upper extremity
18 months	No first word	Hearing deficit, expressive language deficit
24 months	Echolalia (repetitive speech) or inability to follow simple commands	Social delay or autism spectrum disorders

- Perinatal or congenital infection
- Suspected sensory impairment
- Chronic (more than 3 months) otitis media with effusion
- Inborn error of metabolism
- HIV infection
- Lead level above 19 mg/dL
- Parental concern about developmental issues
- Parent with less than high school education
- Single parent
- Sibling with developmental problems
- Parent with developmental disability or mental illness

Infants or children with any of these risk factors should be carefully screened for developmental delays. This screening should occur in a prospective manner, with screenings occurring at frequent intervals to identify concerns early.

> ▶ **Take** NOTE!
>
> *Any child who "loses" a developmental milestone—for example, the child able to sit without support who now cannot—needs an immediate full evaluation, since this indicates a significant neurologic problem.*

A number of developmental screening tools are available to guide the nurse in assessing development (Table 30.2). The Denver II is a frequently used tool (see Appendix G). The Denver II should be used for diagnostic purposes only when administered by specifically trained personnel. Nurses not trained in the use of the Denver II should use screening tools based on the Denver II. Many screening methods assist the nurse in identifying infants and children who may have developmental delays, thus allowing for prompt identification and referral for evaluation. Additional data can be used to determine a school-age child's developmental level, include handwriting samples, ability to draw, school performance, and social skills.

Injury and Disease Prevention

Disease prevention is defined as interventions performed to protect clients from a disease or to identify it at an early stage and lessen its consequences. These interventions are determined by the results of the nurse's assessment, nationally accepted practice guidelines, and the family's goals. Components of disease prevention include screening tests and immunizations.

Injury prevention is primarily accomplished through education, anticipatory guidance, and physical changes in the environment. Injuries can be unintentional (poisoning, falls, or drowning) or intentional (child abuse, homi-

cide, or suicide). The types of injuries a child is most likely to encounter vary greatly among age groups. Although aggressive public health initiatives have decreased mortality rates of childhood injuries significantly in the past 50 years, continued vigilance and innovation are needed. The nurse, in partnership with the family and the community, can have an enormous impact on child safety. Specific interventions are discussed in Chapters 4 through 8.

Screening Tests

Screening tests are procedures or laboratory analyses used to identify clients with a certain condition. These tests are done to ensure that no person with the disorder is missed. They have a high sensitivity (a high false-positive rate) and a low specificity (a low false-negative rate). If a screening test is positive, follow-up tests with higher specificity are performed. A **risk assessment** is performed by the health care professional in conjunction with the client and includes objective as well as subjective data to determine the likelihood that the client will develop a condition.

In **universal screening**, an entire population is screened regardless of the client's individual risk. This type of screening is performed when a reliable risk assessment procedure is not available. In contrast, **selective screening** is done when a risk assessment indicates the client has one or more risk factors for the disorder.

> ▶ **Take** NOTE!
>
> *To increase cooperation from young children during screenings, set up a reward system. Easy-to-do rewards include:*
>
> - *Stamping the back of the child's hand with a "smiley face"*
> - *Making an eye cover by placing two stickers back to back over a tongue blade and letting the child keep the cover after the screening*
> - *Copying a design onto a sheet of paper and letting the child take it home to color*
> - *Letting the child play with a simple device such as a penlight or stethoscope*

Metabolic Screening

State law determines which metabolic screening tests are mandatory in that state. In some states, mandatory screening is limited to as few as four diseases. In addition to screening for hearing loss, the March of Dimes currently recommends universal newborn metabolic screening tests for 28 disorders for which effective treatment is available:

- Amino acid metabolism disorders: phenylketonuria, maple syrup urine disease, homocystinuria, citrullinemia, argininosuccinic acidemia, tyrosinemia type I

TABLE 30.2 DEVELOPMENTAL SCREENING TOOLS

Age	Screening Tool	Definition	Nursing Implications
Birth–6 years	Denver II	Assesses personal–social, fine motor–adaptive, language, and gross motor skills	Administered by nurse. Requires props (e.g., ball, crayon, doll), available in the Denver II kit. Simple to learn to administer.
Birth–6 years	Denver PRQ	Assesses personal–social, fine motor–adaptive, language, and gross motor skills	Parental report of all items on the Denver II
Birth–6 years	Child Development Inventory (CDI)	Simple questions about infant, toddler, or preschooler behaviors. Measures social, self-help, gross motor, fine motor, expressive language, language comprehension, letters, numbers, and general development as appropriate.	A parental-report screening tool
Birth–6 years	Ages and Stages Questionnaire (ASQ)	Assesses communication, gross motor, fine motor, personal–social, and problem-solving skills	A parental-report screening tool, scored by the nurse after completion to determine child's progress in each of the developmental areas
Birth–8 years	Parents' Evaluation of Developmental Status (PEDS)	Screens for a wide range of developmental, behavioral, and family issues	A parental-report screening tool that can also be used in nurse interview format. Also available in Spanish.
12–96 months	Batelle Developmental Inventory Screening Test	Assesses fine and gross motor, adaptive, personal–social, receptive and expressive language, and cognitive skills	Direct elicitation, parental description, and examiner observation. Requires special training.
1–42 months	Bayley Scales of Infant Development II	Provides a mental and motor scale for assessment of cognitive, language, personal–social, and fine and gross motor development. A behavior rating scale is obtained during the testing.	Direct elicitation. Thorough. Requires special training.
Birth–3 years	Early Language Milestone Scale	Screens for auditory expressive and receptive, visual components of speech	Requires standardized kit
2½–7 years	Denver Articulation Screening	Screens for articulation disorders	5 minutes to administer. Does not evaluate language ability.
5–17 years	Goodenough-Harris Drawing Test	A nonverbal screen for mental ability (intelligence)	Child draws a person, which is analyzed for body parts, clothing, proportion, and perspective.

- Organic acid metabolism disorders: isovaleric acidemia, glutaric acidemia type I, hydroxymethyl-glutaric aciduria, multiple carboxylase deficiency, methylmalonic acidemia due to mutase deficiency, methylmalonic acidemia cblA and cblB forms, 3-methylcrotonyl-CoA carboxylase deficiency, propionic acidemia, beta-ketothiolase deficiency
- Fatty acid oxidation disorders: medium-chain acyl-CoA dehydrogenase deficiency, very-long-chain acyl-CoA dehydrogenase deficiency, long-chain 3-OH acyl-CoA dehydrogenase deficiency, trifunctional protein deficiency, carnitine uptake defect
- Hemoglobinopathies: sickle cell anemia, HbS/beta-thalassemia, HbS/C disease

• Others: congenital hypothyroidism, biotinidase deficiency, congenital adrenal hyperplasia, classical galactosemia, cystic fibrosis

During the initial health supervision visit, the nurse should confirm that newborn metabolic screening was performed prior to discharge from the birthing unit. If the test was not performed or was performed at less than 48 hours of age, the screening should be performed at that visit. The metabolic screening results need to be noted in the child's permanent record at the medical home.

Hearing Screening

The AAP recommends hearing screening of all infants. Hearing loss is a common condition in newborns, and even mild hearing loss can cause serious delays in social and emotional development, language acquisition, and cognitive function. Identification of hearing loss by 3 months of age is crucial to reduce the impact on the child's development. Targeted screening based on risk factors will identify only 50% of infants with hearing loss. Screening should be done before discharge from the birthing unit; if not, the newborn needs to be screened before 1 month of age. Behavioral observations of the infant's response to sounds, such as a ringing bell, are not sensitive enough to preclude mild to moderate hearing loss. Accepted methodologies for screening newborn hearing are displayed in Table 30.3.

Screening for hearing loss in older children begins with a history from the primary caregivers. If any problems are noted, audiometry should be performed. When the child is capable of following simple commands reliably, the nurse can perform some basic procedures to screen for hearing loss. The whisper test is easy to perform but to be valid requires a quiet room that is away from distractions. The Weber and Rinne tests can be used to screen for sensorineural or conductive hearing loss (Fig. 30.2).

Universal hearing screening with objective testing is recommended at ages 4, 5, 6, 8, 10, 12, 15, and 18 years. More frequent screening is recommended if there is any behavior that indicates the child's hearing may be impaired. Repeated hearing screenings are recommended if a child has risk factors for acquired hearing loss such as those listed in Box 30.2.

Vision Screening

Newborns with ocular structural abnormalities are at high risk for vision impairment. Vision screening is performed at every scheduled health supervision visit. The screening procedures for children younger than 3 years of age or for nonverbal children involve evaluating the child's ability to fixate on and follow objects. The neonate should be able to fixate on an object 10 to 12 inches from the face. After fixation, the infant should be able to follow the object to the midline. By 2 months of age, the infant

should be able to follow the object 180 degrees. The technique of photoscreening can help identify problems such as ocular malalignment, refractive error, and lens and retinal problems.

> ▶ **Take** NOTE!
>
> *Use objects with black and white patterns when performing vision screening on an infant less than 6 months of age. The infant's vision at this age is more attuned to high-contrast patterns than to colors. Try checkerboard patterns or concentric circles. Animal figures like pandas and dalmatians also work well.*

After the age of 3 years, a variety of standardized age-appropriate vision screening charts are available. These charts include the "tumbling E" and Allen figures (Fig. 30.3A, B). These charts allow for a more precise vision assessment and aid the nurse in identifying preschool children with visual acuity problems. By age 5 or 6, most children know the alphabet well enough to use the traditional Snellen chart for vision screening (see Fig. 30.3C). Table 30.4 gives further information about vision screening tools.

Screenings should be performed when children are alert, as fatigue and lack of interest can mimic poor vision. When using any vision screening chart, several simple steps need to be followed:

• Place the chart at the child's eye level.
• Place a mark on the floor 20 feet from the chart.
• Align the child's heels on the mark.
• Have the child read each line with one eye covered and then with the other eye covered (Fig. 30.4).
• Have the child read each line with both eyes.

In addition to visual acuity screening, children should also be screened for color discrimination.

Any child with eye abnormalities or who has failed visual screening needs to be evaluated by a specialist appropriately trained to treat children.

Iron Deficiency Anemia Screening

Iron deficiency is the leading nutritional deficiency in the United States. The increased incidence of iron deficiency anemia is directly associated with periods of diminished iron stores, rapid growth, and high metabolic demands. At 6 months of age, the in utero iron stores of a full-term infant are almost depleted. The adolescent growth spurt warrants constant iron replacement. Pregnant adolescents are at even higher risk for iron deficiency due to the demands of the mother's growth spurt and the needs of the developing fetus.

TABLE 30.3 HEARING SCREENING METHODS

Test Name	Age Group	Characteristics	Nursing Implications
Auditory brain stem response (ABR)	Newborn–6 months	Measures electroencephalographic waves Test results may be affected by ear debris	Infant must be quiet (sedation may be needed).
Evoked otoacoustic emissions (EOAE)	Newborn–6 months or developmentally delayed children at the infant's level of functioning	The machine produces clicks that stimulate cilia in the cochlea and measures the response.	Infant must be quiet. Test results may be inaccurate in first 24 hours of life.
Visual reinforcement audiometry (VRA)	6 months–2 years	Visual reward is linked to a tone signal. Child looks to the visual reward in response to the tone. Reward is activated, reinforcing the response.	Child must be alert and happy for best results. Schedule for after sleep/rest period. Allow child to sit in parent's lap.
Tympanometry	Over 7 months	Measures tympanic membrane mobility and determines middle ear pressure	The probe must form a seal with the canal. The child must remain still to obtain a valid result.
Conditioned play audiometry (CPA)	2–4 years	Similar to VRA except uses "listening games" Child does listening game at the tone and receives social reward. May be used when developmental age is 2 years	See Nursing Implications for VRA.
Pure-tone (conventional) audiometry	4 years and older	Measures hearing acuity through a range of frequencies and intensities Child must wear earphones. Performed in a soundproof room if possible	Teach the child the desired motor response before screening. Administer conditioning trials. Offer two presentations of stimulus to ensure reliability. At a minimum, screen 1,000-, 2,000-, and 4,000-hertz levels at 20 decibels.
Whisper test	4 years and older	One ear is occluded. Examiner stands behind the child and whispers a word. The child must accurately repeat the whispered word.	The child must be in a quiet room and away from distractions. The child should be alert and well rested for accurate results. Consider a reward system to increase compliance.
Weber test	6 years and older	Place a vibrating tuning fork in the middle of the top of the head. Ask if the sound is in one ear or both ears. The sound should be heard in both ears.	The child must understand the instructions and be able to cooperate.
Rinne test	6 years and older	Place a vibrating tuning fork on the mastoid process to assess bone conduction. The child signals when the sound is gone. Next place a vibrating tuning fork outside the ear to test air conduction. The child signals when the sound is gone. For a passing test, air conduction time should be twice as long as bone conduction time.	The child must understand the instructions and be able to cooperate.

FIGURE 30.2 (**A**) The Weber test screens for hearing by assessing sound conducted via bone. (**B**) The Rinne test screens for hearing by comparing sound conduction via bone to sound conduction via air.

Guidelines for universal iron deficiency anemia screening vary. The Centers for Disease Control and Prevention (CDC) recommend universal screening of high-risk children at various age intervals. The AAP recommends universal screening of all infants at 9 to 12 months, boys at 12 to 18 years, and adolescent girls during all routine physical examinations. Both the CDC and the AAP have similar recommendations for selective screening (Boxes 30.3 and 30.4).

Lead Screening

Elevated blood lead levels (10 mcg/dL or higher) remain a preventable environmental health threat. Although the prevalence of elevated lead levels has declined over the past two decades, certain communities still possess a high level of lead exposure. In 1997 the CDC released guidelines to aid state and local health authorities in determining which children are at risk for elevated blood lead levels. These children are likely to benefit from lead screening. Federal Medicaid policy requires that all participating children be screened for blood lead levels.

The CDC recommends universal screening for children living in areas where more than 27% of the houses were constructed before 1950. It also recommends universal screening of children if more than 12% of the 1- and 2-year-olds in a specific population have elevated blood lead levels. Targeted screening based on risk assessment is

BOX 30.2 Risk Factors for Hearing Impairment

• Family history of hearing loss
• Prenatal infection
• Anomalies of the head, face, or ears
• Low birthweight (<1,500 g)
• Hyperbilirubinemia requiring exchange transfusion
• Ototoxic medications
• Low Apgar scores: 4 or less at 1 minute, or 6 or less at 5 minutes
• Mechanical ventilation lasting 5 days
• Syndrome associated with hearing loss
• Bacterial meningitis
• Neurodegenerative disorders
• Persistent pulmonary hypertension
• Otitis media with effusion for 3 months

HEALTHY PEOPLE 2010

Objective	Significance
Increase the proportion of newborns who are screened for hearing loss by age 1 month, have audiologic evaluation by age 3 months, and are enrolled in appropriate intervention services by age 6 months.	• Determine results of newborn hearing screening at first newborn checkup. • Refer any infant with possible hearing deficit for further evaluation. • Ensure infants with hearing impairment receive appropriate augmentation (hearing aids).
Increase the proportion of persons who have had a hearing examination on schedule.	• Ensure all children and adolescents receive hearing screenings with well-child checkups as appropriate.

Source: USDHHS, 2007.

FIGURE 30.3 (**A**) The "tumbling E" chart is appropriate for children who do not yet know the alphabet but who can follow instructions to indicate the direction that the arms of the "E" are pointing. (**B**) A picture chart similar to the Allen object recognition chart is appropriate for vision screening in the preschool-age child. (**C**) The Snellen eye chart may be used for children age 6 or older who know the alphabet.

recommended for other children. In addition to assessing risk by location and population, an individual assessment needs to be performed. A community-specific questionnaire or the three-question personal risk questionnaire from the AAP (Box 30.5) should be used.

Hypertension Screening

Systemic hypertension occurs in 1% to 3% of children. Universal hypertension screening for children beginning at 3 years of age is recommended. If the child has risk factors for systemic hypertension, such as preterm birth or congenital heart disease, then screening begins when the risk factor becomes apparent.

The guidelines for determining hypertension in children and adolescents mirror the adult guidelines (Box 30.6). Preadolescents whose blood pressure is in the 90th to 95th percentile are considered to have prehypertension. Adolescents whose blood pressure is 120/80 mmHg are considered prehypertensive, even if their ranking is below the 90th percentile. Anticipatory guidance on diet and lifestyle changes is appropriate for any child with prehypertension. Refer to Chapter 40 for additional information on hypertension.

Hyperlipidemia Screening

Atherosclerosis has been documented in children, and a link exists between high lipid levels and the development of these lesions. Selectively screening children at high risk for hyperlipidemia can reduce their lifelong risk of coronary artery disease.

TABLE 30.4 VISION SCREENING TOOLS

Screening Tool	Age	Nursing Implications
Snellen letters or numbers	School-age	The child must know his or her letters or numbers for the test to be valid.
"Tumbling E"	Preschool	The child points in the direction that the "E" is facing.
LEA symbols or Allen figures	Preschool	The child should first identify the pictures with both eyes at a comfortable distance prior to monocular testing to ensure validity of the test.
Ishihara	School-age	Screens for color discrimination (numbers composed of dots, hidden within other dots)
Color Vision Testing Made Easy (CVTME)	Preschool	Uses dot pictures like the Ishihara, but instead of numbers has easily identified shapes imbedded in the dots

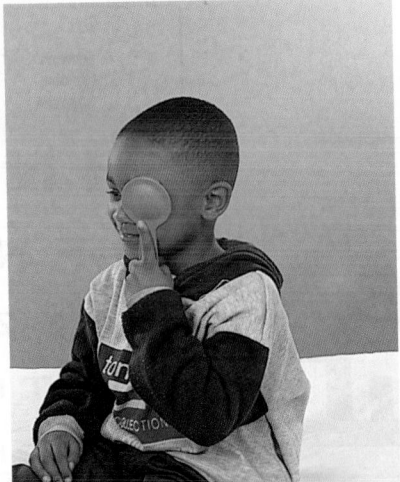

FIGURE 30.4 One eye must be covered while the other is tested in order to detect discrepancies in visual acuity between the two eyes and identify amblyopia early.

The risk assessment focuses on the child's family history. Children whose parents or grandparents had premature cardiovascular disease (before 55 years of age) or who have a parent with hypercholesterolemia are screened. If the child's family history is not available, screening is done at the discretion of the health care provider. The nurse also assesses for factors that may contribute to hyperlipidemia, such as sedentary lifestyle, cigarette smoking, obesity, and high-fat dietary intake. Children with diseases such as diabetes and hypertension are also candidates for hyperlipidemia screening. Box 30.7 gives details.

Remember Maya and Evan, the children introduced at the beginning of the chapter? How would you assess their growth and development? Which screening tests are warranted for them, and why? What further information would you need to determine which tests should be performed?

HEALTHY PEOPLE 2010

Objective	Significance
Increase the proportion of preschool children age 5 years and under who receive vision screening.	• Use preschool-appropriate vision screening tool to assess vision. • Ensure screening begins at age 3.

Source: USDHHS, 2007.

BOX 30.3 Comparing Iron Deficiency Anemia Screening Guidelines

CDC Recommendations

Universal Screening
• High-risk children only:
  • Ages 9–12 months
  • Repeat 6 months later
  • Ages 2–5 years annually
• Girls ages 12–18 years: once every 5–10 years

Selective Screening
Assess infants and children for risk factors at:
• 9–12 months
• 15–18 months
• 2–18 years annually
Screen clients with risk factors.

AAP Recommendations

Universal Screening
• Screen all infants at 9–12 months.
• Screen boys ages 12–18 years at routine physical examinations during their peak growth period.
• Screen adolescent girls during all routine physical examinations.

Selective Screening
Assess infants and children for risk factors at:
• 9–12 months
• 15–18 months
• 2–18 years annually
Screen clients with risk factors.

Immunizations

Immunization is the key disease prevention activity during childhood health supervision visits. The development of effective vaccines, beginning in the 1940s, revolutionized children's health care. Immunization allowed the focus to shift from disease treatment to disease prevention. The nurse needs to understand the principles of immunizations, the proper use of vaccines, and barriers to immunization. Armed with this knowledge, the nurse can partner with families to provide the highest level of disease protection to children (Fig. 30.5).

Principles of Immunization

The immune system has the ability to recognize materials present in the body as "self" or "non-self." Foreign materials (non-self) are called antigens. When an antigen is recognized by the immune system, the immune system responds by producing antibodies (immunoglobulins) or directing special cells to destroy and remove the antigen.

Immunity is the ability to destroy and remove a specific antigen from the body. The acquisition of immunity

BOX 30.4 Risk Factors for Iron Deficiency Anemia

- Periods of rapid growth
- Low-birthweight or preterm infants
- Low dietary intake of meat, fish, poultry, and ascorbic acid
- Macrobiotic diets
- Inappropriate consumption of cow's milk
- Use of infant formula not fortified with iron
- Exclusive breastfeeding after age 6 months without iron-fortified supplemental foods
- Meal skipping, frequent dieting
- Pregnancy or recent pregnancy
- Intensive physical training
- Recent blood loss, heavy/lengthy menstrual periods
- Chronic use of aspirin or nonsteroidal anti-inflammatory drugs
- Parasitic infections

Children at High Risk for Iron Deficiency Anemia
- Low-income families
- Those eligible for the Special Supplemental Nutrition Program for Women, Infants, and Children (WIC)
- Migrants or recently arrived refugees

BOX 30.5 A Basic Personal-Risk Questionnaire for Lead Exposure in Children

1. Does your child live in or regularly visit a house or childcare facility that was built before 1950?
2. Does your child live in or regularly visit a house or childcare facility built before 1978 that is being or has recently been renovated or remodeled (within the past 6 months)?
3. Does your child have a sibling or playmate who has or did have lead poisoning?

Reproduced with permission from *Pediatrics, 101,* 1072–1078. Copyright ©1998 American Academy of Pediatrics.

HEALTHY PEOPLE 2010

Objective	Significance
Eliminate elevated blood lead levels in children.	• Screen for lead exposure. • Ensure that high-risk children have blood lead levels measured.

Source: USDHHS, 2007.

BOX 30.6 Preadolescent Childhood Hypertension Guidelines

Optimal	<90th percentile
Prehypertension	90th to 95th percentile
Stage I	>95th percentile up to 5 mmHg above 99th percentile
Stage II	5 mmHg above 99th percentile, or higher

can be active or passive. **Passive immunity** is produced when the immunoglobulins of one person are transferred to another. This immunity lasts only weeks or months. Passive immunity can be obtained by injection of exogenous immunoglobulins. It can also be transferred from mothers to infants via colostrum or the placenta. **Active immunity** is acquired when a person's own immune system generates the immune response. Active immunity lasts for many years or for a lifetime. This long-term protection is the result of immunologic memory. After the initial immune response, specialized cells for that antigen continue to exist. When an antigen returns, these memory cells very rapidly produce a fresh supply of antibodies to reestablish protection. This immunity can occur after exposure to natural pathogens or after exposure to vaccines. Vaccines mimic the characteristics of the natural antigen. The immune system mounts a response and establishes an immunologic memory as it would for an infection.

BOX 30.7 Hyperlipidemia Screening

Screen if parents or grandparents, at <55 years of age, have/had documented:
- Coronary atherosclerosis
- Myocardial infarction
- Angina pectoris
- Peripheral vascular disease
- Cerebrovascular disease
- Sudden cardiac death

Screen if a parent's blood cholesterol level is 240 mg/dL or higher. Screen at health care provider's discretion:
- Parental history is unobtainable.
- Child has diabetes or hypertension.
- Child has lifestyle risk factors:
  - Cigarette smoking
  - Obesity
  - Sedentary lifestyle
  - High-fat dietary intake

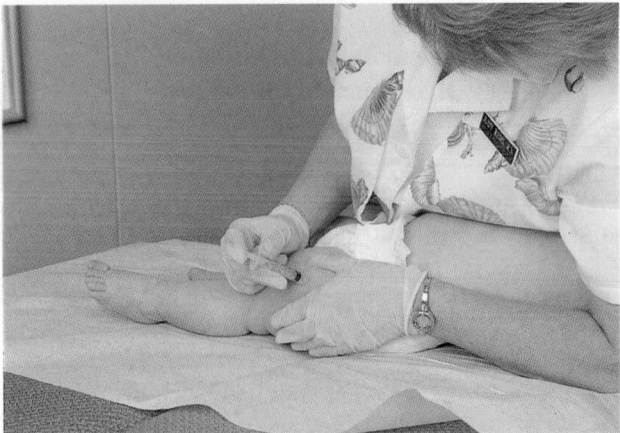

FIGURE 30.5 Nurse restraining infant for intramuscular injection into the vastus lateralis.

The classification of vaccines is based on the characteristics of the antigen present. The antigen may be viral or bacterial. It may be live attenuated (weakened) or killed. It may be the whole antigen or a portion of it (fractional).

- Live attenuated vaccines are modified living organisms that are weakened. The organism can produce an immune response but does not produce the complications of the illness.
- Killed vaccines contain whole dead organisms; they are incapable of reproducing but are capable of producing an immune response.
- Toxoid vaccines contain protein products produced by bacteria called toxins. The toxin is heat-treated to weaken its effect, but it retains its ability to produce an immune response.
- Conjugate vaccines are the result of chemically linking the bacterial cell wall polysaccharide (sugar-based) portions with proteins. This dramatically increases the immune response compared to presenting the polysaccharide portion alone.
- Recombinant vaccines use genetically engineered organisms. For example, the hepatitis B vaccine is produced by splicing a gene portion of the virus into a gene of a yeast cell. The yeast cell is then able to produce hepatitis B surface antigen to use for vaccine production.

HEALTHY PEOPLE 2010

Objective	Significance
Increase the proportion of young children who receive all vaccines that have been recommended for universal administration for at least 5 years.	• Immunize at every opportunity. If a child is due or past due for vaccinations, provide them at a sick visit if not contraindicated. • Educate families about the benefits and risks of immunization.

Source: USDHHS, 2007.

The safety and efficacy of existing vaccines are constantly being reviewed, and research to improve vaccines is ongoing. The goal is to refine vaccines so that a maximum immune response is produced with the least amount of risk for the client.

Immunization Management

The Advisory Committee on Immunization Practices (ACIP), a branch of the CDC, reviews the recommended immunization schedules at least yearly and updates the schedule to ensure that it reflects current best practices (Tables 30.5 and 30.6). In addition to the recommended schedule, the ACIP publishes a "catch-up" schedule for children who have not been adequately immunized (Table 30.7). The child's immunization record must be compared with the latest edition of these schedules when assessing the need for immunization.

> ▶ *Take* NOTE!
>
> *When obtaining an immunization history from the parent, ask, "When and where did your child receive his (or her) last immunization?" The answer will provide more information than simply asking, "Are your child's immunizations up to date?" The nurse can compare this information with that on the immunization record; discover in what settings the child is getting health care; and use the information as a starting point in a discussion of any reactions to previous immunizations.*

Vaccine storage and administration affect the efficacy of a vaccine. Improperly stored or reconstituted vaccines can be ineffective. The vaccine must be given by the correct route; not all vaccines are given intramuscularly (Box 30.8; Table 30.8). The manufacturer's package insert is the best reference source for any vaccine.

> ▶ *Take* NOTE!
>
> *Proper vaccine storage is critical to vaccine efficacy. If you suspect that a vaccine was not maintained at the proper storage temperature, do not use it! An ineffective vaccine is of no use in preventing disease.*

The Public Health Service Act outlines standards of practice for immunization programs. The act requires that Vaccine Information Statements (VIS; Fig. 30.6) be provided to parents before an immunization is given. In accordance with the concept of partnership with the

(text continues on page 922)

TABLE 30.5 CDC RECOMMENDED IMMUNIZATION SCHEDULE FOR PERSONS AGED 0–6 YEARS—UNITED STATES, 2008

For those who fall behind or start late, see the catch-up schedule

Vaccine ▼ Age ▶	Birth	1 month	2 months	4 months	6 months	12 months	15 months	18 months	19–23 months	2–3 years	4–6 years
Hepatitis B[1]	HepB	HepB		see footnote 1		HepB					
Rotavirus[2]			Rota	Rota	Rota						
Diphtheria, Tetanus, Pertussis[3]			DTaP	DTaP	DTaP	see footnote 3	DTaP				DTaP
Haemophilus influenzae type b[4]			Hib	Hib	*Hib*[4]	Hib					
Pneumococcal[5]			PCV	PCV	PCV	PCV				PPV	
Inactivated Poliovirus			IPV	IPV		IPV					IPV
Influenza[6]						Influenza (Yearly)					
Measles, Mumps, Rubella[7]						MMR					MMR
Varicella[8]						Varicella					Varicella
Hepatitis A[9]						HepA (2 doses)				HepA Series	
Meningococcal[10]										MCV4	

Range of recommended ages

Certain high-risk groups

This schedule indicates the recommended ages for routine administration of currently licensed childhood vaccines, as of December 1, 2007, for children aged 0 through 6 years. Additional information is available at www.cdc.gov/vaccines/recs/schedules. Any dose not administered at the recommended age should be administered at any subsequent visit, when indicated and feasible. Additional vaccines may be licensed and recommended during the year. Licensed combination vaccines may be used whenever any components of the combination are indicated and other components of the vaccine are not contraindicated and if approved by the Food and Drug Administration for that dose of the series. Providers should consult the respective Advisory Committee on Immunization Practices statement for detailed recommendations, including for **high-risk conditions:** http://www.cdc.gov/vaccines/pubs/ACIP-list.htm. Clinically significant adverse events that follow immunization should be reported to the Vaccine Adverse Event Reporting System (VAERS). Guidance about how to obtain and complete a VAERS form is available at www.vaers.hhs.gov or by telephone, 800-822-7967.

1. Hepatitis B vaccine (HepB). *(Minimum age: birth)*
At birth:
 • Administer monovalent HepB to all newborns prior to hospital discharge.
 • If mother is hepatitis B surface antigen (HBsAg) positive, administer HepB and 0.5 mL of hepatitis B immune globulin (HBIG) within 12 hours of birth.
 • If mother's HBsAg status is unknown, administer HepB within 12 hours of birth. Determine the HBsAg status as soon as possible and if HBsAg positive, administer HBIG (no later than age 1 week).
 • If mother is HBsAg negative, the birth dose can be delayed, in rare cases, with a provider's order and a copy of the mother's negative HBsAg laboratory report in the infant's medical record.
After the birth dose:
 • The HepB series should be completed with either monovalent HepB or a combination vaccine containing HepB. The second dose should be administered at age 1–2 months. The final dose should be administered no earlier than age 24 weeks. Infants born to HBsAg-positive mothers should be tested for HBsAg and antibody to HBsAg after completion of at least 3 doses of a licensed HepB series, at age 9–18 months (generally at the next well-child visit).
4-month dose:
 • It is permissible to administer 4 doses of HepB when combination vaccines are administered after the birth dose. If monovalent HepB is used for doses after the birth dose, a dose at age 4 months is not needed.

2. Rotavirus vaccine (Rota). *(Minimum age: 6 weeks)*
 • Administer the first dose at age 6–12 weeks.
 • Do not start the series later than age 12 weeks.
 • Administer the final dose in the series by age 32 weeks. Do not administer any dose later than age 32 weeks.
 • Data on safety and efficacy outside of these age ranges are insufficient.

3. Diphtheria and tetanus toxoids and acellular pertussis vaccine (DTaP). *(Minimum age: 6 weeks)*
 • The fourth dose of DTaP may be administered as early as age 12 months, provided 6 months have elapsed since the third dose.
 • Administer the final dose in the series at age 4–6 years.

4. *Haemophilus influenzae* type b conjugate vaccine (Hib). *(Minimum age: 6 weeks)*
 • If PRP-OMP (PedvaxHIB® or ComVax® [Merck]) is administered at ages 2 and 4 months, a dose at age 6 months is not required.
 • TriHIBit® (DTaP/Hib) combination products should not be used for primary immunization but can be used as boosters following any Hib vaccine in children age 12 months or older.

5. Pneumococcal vaccine. *(Minimum age: 6 weeks for pneumococcal conjugate vaccine [PCV]; 2 years for pneumococcal polysaccharide vaccine [PPV])*
 • Administer one dose of PCV to all healthy children aged 24–59 months having any incomplete schedule.
 • Administer PPV to children aged 2 years and older with underlying medical conditions.

6. Influenza vaccine. *(Minimum age: 6 months for trivalent inactivated influenza vaccine [TIV]; 2 years for live, attenuated influenza vaccine [LAIV])*
 • Administer annually to children aged 6–59 months and to all eligible close contacts of children aged 0–59 months.
 • Administer annually to children 5 years of age and older with certain risk factors, to other persons (including household members) in close contact with persons in groups at higher risk, and to any child whose parents request vaccination.
 • For healthy persons (those who do not have underlying medical conditions that predispose them to influenza complications) ages 2–49 years, either LAIV or TIV may be used.
 • Children receiving TIV should receive 0.25 mL if age 6–35 months or 0.5 mL if age 3 years or older.
 • Administer 2 doses (separated by 4 weeks or longer) to children younger than 9 years who are receiving influenza vaccine for the first time or who were vaccinated for the first time last season but only received one dose.

7. Measles, mumps, and rubella vaccine (MMR). *(Minimum age: 12 months)*
 • Administer the second dose of MMR at age 4–6 years. MMR may be administered before age 4–6 years, provided 4 weeks or more have elapsed since the first dose.

8. Varicella vaccine. *(Minimum age: 12 months)*
 • Administer second dose at age 4–6 years; may be administered 3 months or more after first dose.
 • Do not repeat second dose if administered 28 days or more after first dose.

9. Hepatitis A vaccine (HepA). *(Minimum age: 12 months)*
 • Administer to all children aged 1 year (i.e., aged 12–23 months). Administer the 2 doses in the series at least 6 months apart.
 • Children not fully vaccinated by age 2 years can be vaccinated at subsequent visits.
 • HepA is recommended for certain other groups of children, including in areas where vaccination programs target older children.

10. Meningococcal vaccine. *(Minimum age: 2 years for meningococcal conjugate vaccine (MCV4) and for meningococcal polysaccharide vaccine (MPSV4))*
 • Administer MCV4 to children aged 2–10 years with terminal complement deficiencies or anatomic or functional asplenia and certain other high-risk groups. MPSV4 is also acceptable.
 • Administer MCV4 to persons who received MPSV4 3 or more years previously and remain at increased risk for meningococcal disease.

TABLE 30.6 CDC RECOMMENDED IMMUNIZATION SCHEDULE FOR PERSONS AGED 7–18 YEARS—
UNITED STATES, 2008

For those who fall behind or start late, see the green bars and the catch-up schedule

Vaccine ▼ Age ▶	7–10 years	11–12 years	13–18 years
Diphtheria, Tetanus, Pertussis[1]	*see footnote 1*	Tdap	Tdap
Human Papillomavirus[2]	*see footnote 2*	HPV (3 doses)	HPV Series
Meningococcal[3]	MCV4	MCV4	MCV4
Pneumococcal[4]	PPV		
Influenza[5]	Influenza (Yearly)		
Hepatitis A[6]	HepA Series		
Hepatitis B[7]	HepB Series		
Inactivated Poliovirus[8]	IPV Series		
Measles, Mumps, Rubella[9]	MMR Series		
Varicella[10]	Varicella Series		

Range of recommended ages

Catch-up immunization

Certain high-risk groups

This schedule indicates the recommended ages for routine administration of currently licensed childhood vaccines, as of December 1, 2007, for children aged 7–18 years. Additional information is available at www.cdc.gov/vaccines/recs/schedules. Any dose not administered at the recommended age should be administered at any subsequent visit, when indicated and feasible. Additional vaccines may be licensed and recommended during the year. Licensed combination vaccines may be used whenever any components of the combination are indicated and other components of the vaccine are not contraindicated and if approved by the Food and Drug Administration for that dose of the series. Providers should consult the respective Advisory Committee on Immunization Practices statement for detailed recommendations, including for **high risk conditions:** http://www.cdc.gov/vaccines/pubs/ACIP-list.htm. Clinically significant adverse events that follow immunization should be reported to the Vaccine Adverse Event Reporting System (VAERS). Guidance about how to obtain and complete a VAERS form is available at www.vaers.hhs.gov or by telephone, 800-822-7967.

1. Tetanus and diphtheria toxoids and acellular pertussis vaccine (Tdap). *(Minimum age: 10 years for BOOSTRIX® and 11 years for ADACEL™)*
- Administer at age 11–12 years for those who have completed the recommended childhood DTP/DTaP vaccination series and have not received a tetanus and diphtheria toxoids (Td) booster dose.
- 13–18-year-olds who missed the 11–12 year Tdap or received Td only are encouraged to receive one dose of Tdap 5 years after the last Td/DTaP dose.

2. Human papillomavirus vaccine (HPV). *(Minimum age: 9 years)*
- Administer the first dose of the HPV vaccine series to females at age 11–12 years.
- Administer the second dose 2 months after the first dose and the third dose 6 months after the first dose.
- Administer the HPV vaccine series to females at age 13–18 years if not previously vaccinated.

3. Meningococcal vaccine.
- Administer MCV4 at age 11–12 years and at age 13–18 years if not previously vaccinated. MPSV4 is an acceptable alternative.
- Administer MCV4 to previously unvaccinated college freshmen living in dormitories.
- MCV4 is recommended for children aged 2–10 years with terminal complement deficiencies or anatomic or functional asplenia and certain other high-risk groups.
- Persons who received MPSV4 3 or more years previously and remain at increased risk for meningococcal disease should be vaccinated with MCV4.

4. Pneumococcal polysaccharide vaccine (PPV).
- Administer PPV to certain high-risk groups.

5. Influenza vaccine.
- Administer annually to all close contacts of children aged 0–59 months.
- Administer annually to persons with certain risk factors, health-care workers, and other persons (including household members) in close contact with persons in groups at higher risk.

- Administer 2 doses (separated by 4 weeks or longer) to children younger than 9 years who are receiving influenza vaccine for the first time or who were vaccinated for the first time last season but only received one dose.
- For healthy nonpregnant persons (those who do not have underlying medical conditions that predispose them to influenza complications) ages 2–49 years, either LAIV or TIV may be used.

6. Hepatitis A vaccine (HepA).
- Administer the 2 doses in the series at least 6 months apart.
- HepA is recommended for certain other groups of children, including in areas where vaccination programs target older children.

7. Hepatitis B vaccine (HepB).
- Administer the 3-dose series to those who were not previously vaccinated.
- A 2-dose series of Recombivax HB® is licensed for children aged 11–15 years.

8. Inactivated poliovirus vaccine (IPV).
- For children who received an all-IPV or all-oral poliovirus (OPV) series, a fourth dose is not necessary if the third dose was administered at age 4 years or older.
- If both OPV and IPV were administered as part of a series, a total of 4 doses should be administered, regardless of the child's current age.

9. Measles, mumps, and rubella vaccine (MMR).
- If not previously vaccinated, administer 2 doses of MMR during any visit, with 4 or more weeks between the doses.

10. Varicella vaccine.
- Administer 2 doses of varicella vaccine to persons younger than 13 years of age at least 3 months apart. Do not repeat the second dose if administered 28 or more days following the first dose.
- Administer 2 doses of varicella vaccine to persons aged 13 years or older at least 4 weeks apart.

TABLE 30.7 CATCH-UP IMMUNIZATION SCHEDULE FOR PERSONS AGED 4 MONTHS–18 YEARS WHO START LATE OR WHO ARE ≥1 MONTH BEHIND—UNITED STATES, 2008

The table below provides catch-up schedules and minimum intervals between doses for children whose vaccinations have been delayed. A vaccine series does not need to be restarted, regardless of the time that has elapsed between doses. Use the section appropriate for the child's age.

CATCH-UP SCHEDULE FOR PERSONS AGED 4 MONTHS–6 YEARS					
Vaccine	**Minimum Age for Dose 1**	**Minimum Interval Between Doses**			
		Dose 1 to Dose 2	**Dose 2 to Dose 3**	**Dose 3 to Dose 4**	**Dose 4 to Dose 5**
Hepatitis B[1]	Birth	4 weeks	8 weeks (and 16 weeks after first dose)		
Rotavirus[2]	6 wks	4 weeks	4 weeks		
Diphtheria, Tetanus, Pertussis[3]	6 wks	4 weeks	4 weeks	6 months	6 months[3]
Haemophilus influenzae type b[4]	6 wks	**4 weeks** if first dose administered at younger than 12 months of age **8 weeks (as final dose)** if first dose administered at age 12-14 months **No further doses needed** if first dose administered at 15 months of age or older	**4 weeks**[4] if current age is younger than 12 months **8 weeks (as final dose)**[4] if current age is 12 months or older and second dose administered at younger than 15 months of age **No further doses needed** if previous dose administered at age 15 months or older	**8 weeks (as final dose)** This dose only necessary for children aged 12 months–5 years who received 3 doses before age 12 months	
Pneumococcal[5]	6 wks	**4 weeks** if first dose administered at younger than 12 months of age **8 weeks (as final dose)** if first dose administered at age 12 months or older or current age 24–59 months **No further doses needed** for healthy children if first dose administered at age 24 months or older	**4 weeks** if current age is younger than 12 months **8 weeks (as final dose)** if current age is 12 months or older **No further doses needed** for healthy children if previous dose administered at age 24 months or older	**8 weeks (as final dose)** This dose only necessary for children aged 12 months–5 years who received 3 doses before age 12 months	
Inactivated Poliovirus[6]	6 wks	4 weeks	4 weeks	4 weeks[6]	
Measles, Mumps, Rubella[7]	12 mos	4 weeks			
Varicella[8]	12 mos	3 months			
Hepatitis A[9]	12 mos	6 months			
CATCH-UP SCHEDULE FOR PERSONS AGED 7–18 YEARS					
Tetanus, Diphtheria/ Tetanus, Diphtheria, Pertussis[10]	7 yrs[10]	4 weeks	**4 weeks** if first dose administered at younger than 12 months of age **6 months** if first dose administered at age 12 months or older	**6 months** if first dose administered at younger than 12 months of age	
Human Papillomavirus[11]	9 yrs	4 weeks	12 weeks (and 24 weeks after the first dose)		
Hepatitis A[9]	12 mos	6 months			
Hepatitis B[1]	Birth	4 weeks	8 weeks (and 16 weeks after first dose)		
Inactivated Poliovirus[6]	6 wks	4 weeks	4 weeks	4 weeks[6]	
Measles, Mumps, Rubella[7]	12 mos	4 weeks			
Varicella[8]	12 mos	**4 weeks** if first dose administered at age 13 years or older **3 months** if first dose administered at younger than 13 years of age			

1. Hepatitis B vaccine (HepB).
- Administer the 3-dose series to those who were not previously vaccinated.
- A 2-dose series of Recombivax HB® is licensed for children aged 11–15 years.

2. Rotavirus vaccine (Rota).
- Do not start the series later than age 12 weeks.
- Administer the final dose in the series by age 32 weeks.
- Do not administer a dose later than age 32 weeks.
- Data on safety and efficacy outside of these age ranges are insufficient.

3. Diphtheria and tetanus toxoids and acellular pertussis vaccine (DTaP).
- The fifth dose is not necessary if the fourth dose was administered at age 4 years or older.
- DTaP is not indicated for persons aged 7 years or older.

4. *Haemophilus influenzae* type b conjugate vaccine (Hib).
- Vaccine is not generally recommended for children aged 5 years or older.
- If current age is younger than 12 months and the first 2 doses were PRP-OMP (PedvaxHIB® or ComVax® [Merck]), the third (and final) dose should be administered at age 12–15 months and at least 8 weeks after the second dose.
- If first dose was administered at age 7–11 months, administer 2 doses separated by 4 weeks plus a booster at age 12–15 months.

5. Pneumococcal conjugate vaccine (PCV).
- Administer one dose of PCV to all healthy children aged 24–59 months having any incomplete schedule.
- For children with underlying medical conditions, administer 2 doses of PCV at least 8 weeks apart if previously received less than 3 doses, or 1 dose of PCV if previously received 3 doses.

6. Inactivated poliovirus vaccine (IPV).
- For children who received an all-IPV or all-oral poliovirus (OPV) series, a fourth dose is not necessary if third dose was administered at age 4 years or older.

- If both OPV and IPV were administered as part of a series, a total of 4 doses should be administered, regardless of the child's current age.
- IPV is not routinely recommended for persons aged 18 years and older.

7. Measles, mumps, and rubella vaccine (MMR).
- The second dose of MMR is recommended routinely at age 4–6 years but may be administered earlier if desired.
- If not previously vaccinated, administer 2 doses of MMR during any visit with 4 or more weeks between the doses.

8. Varicella vaccine.
- The second dose of varicella vaccine is recommended routinely at age 4–6 years but may be administered earlier if desired.
- Do not repeat the second dose in persons younger than 13 years of age if administered 28 or more days after the first dose.

9. Hepatitis A vaccine (HepA).
- HepA is recommended for certain groups of children, including in areas where vaccination programs target older children. See *MMWR* 2006;55(No. RR-7):1–23.

10. Tetanus and diphtheria toxoids vaccine (Td) and tetanus and diphtheria toxoids and acellular pertussis vaccine (Tdap).
- Tdap should be substituted for a single dose of Td in the primary catch-up series or as a booster if age appropriate; use Td for other doses.
- A 5-year interval from the last Td dose is encouraged when Tdap is used as a booster dose. A booster (fourth) dose is needed if any of the previous doses were administered at younger than 12 months of age. Refer to ACIP recommendations for further information. See *MMWR* 2006;55(No. RR-3).

11. Human papillomavirus vaccine (HPV).
- Administer the HPV vaccine series to females at age 13–18 years if not previously vaccinated.

BOX 30.8 **Vaccine Administration Routes**

Intramuscular	Subcutaneous
DTaP, DT, Tdap	IPV
Hepatitis A, hepatitis B	MMR
Hib	Varicella
Influenza (trivalent)	MPSV4
Pneumococcal	
HPV	
MCV4	

Modified from Immunization Action Coalition (2007). *Administering vaccines: dose, route, site, and needle size.* Available at http://www.immunize.org/catg.d/p3085.pdf.

---

parents, allow ample time for them to read the VIS and to discuss their concerns. If the parents do not understand the information presented, they should feel comfortable asking questions. If the parents are illiterate, present the information orally and verify that the parents understand it. If the information in the VIS is not in the parent's native language, have a translator present the information.

At this time, ask the parents about the child's reactions to previous immunizations, and screen for precautions and contraindications for each vaccine to be administered. Before the vaccine is given, the parents must sign consent forms.

Any clinically significant adverse event that occurs after an immunization should be reported to the Vaccine Adverse Event Reporting System (VAERS). For assistance in obtaining and completing a VAERS form, call 800-822-7967 or visit www.vaers.hhs.gov.

Documentation in the child's permanent record includes the following:

- Date the vaccine was administered
- Name of vaccine (commonly used abbreviation is acceptable)
- Lot number and expiration date of vaccine
- Manufacturer's name
- Site and route by which vaccine was administered (e.g., left deltoid, IM)
- Edition date of VIS given to the parents
- Name and address of the facility administering the vaccine (where the permanent record will be kept)
- Name of the person administering the immunization

Families should be provided with a copy of the child's immunizations. This reinforces the importance of the procedure and reminds the parents to keep the child's immunizations up to date.

Figure 30.7 shows a typical vaccine administration record.

Vaccine Descriptions

This section reviews the most commonly used vaccines. These immunizations are recommended by the ACIP and the AAP. Each state has laws that determine which immunizations are required for school admittance. These requirements can be waived if a contraindication or precaution to the vaccine exists. *Contraindications* are conditions that justify withholding an immunization either permanently or temporarily. There are only two permanent contraindications: (1) an anaphylactic or systemic allergic reaction to a vaccine component or (2) with pertussis immunization, encephalopathy without an identified cause within 7 days of the immunization. Temporarily postponing vaccinations is recommended if the child has a severe illness with a high fever or immunosuppression or has recently received blood products. Vaccination should not be postponed because of a minor respiratory illness or a low-grade fever. *Precautions* are conditions

---

TABLE 30.8 **VACCINE ADMINISTRATION: NEEDLE AND SITE SELECTION**

Client	Needle Size	Needle Length (Inches)	Site
Intramuscular			
Birth–28 days	25 gauge	⅝	Anterolateral thigh
1–12 months	23–25 gauge	1	Anterolateral thigh
1–2 years	23–25 gauge	1 to 1.25 ⅝ to 1	Anterolateral thigh Deltoid
3–18 years	22–25 gauge	1 to 1.25 ⅝ to 1	Anterolateral thigh Deltoid
Subcutaneous			
1–12 months	23–25 gauge	⅝	Fat of anterolateral thigh
>12 months	23–25 gauge	⅝	Fatty tissue over triceps

Immunization Action Coalition (2007). *Administering vaccines: dose, route, site, and needle size.* Available at http://www.immunize.org/catg.d/p3085.pdf.

DIPHTHERIA TETANUS & PERTUSSIS VACCINES

W H A T   Y O U   N E E D   T O   K N O W

1 | Why get vaccinated?

Diphtheria, tetanus, and pertussis are serious diseases caused by bacteria. Diphtheria and pertussis are spread from person to person. Tetanus enters the body through cuts or wounds.

DIPHTHERIA causes a thick covering in the back of the throat.
- It can lead to breathing problems, paralysis, heart failure, and even death.

TETANUS (Lockjaw) causes painful tightening of the muscles, usually all over the body.
- It can lead to "locking" of the jaw so the victim cannot open his mouth or swallow. Tetanus leads to death in up to 2 out of 10 cases.

PERTUSSIS (Whooping Cough) causes coughing spells so bad that it is hard for infants to eat, drink, or breathe. These spells can last for weeks.
- It can lead to pneumonia, seizures (jerking and staring spells), brain damage, and death.

Diphtheria, tetanus, and pertussis vaccine (DTaP) can help prevent these diseases. Most children who are vaccinated with DTaP will be protected throughout childhood. Many more children would get these diseases if we stopped vaccinating.

DTaP is a safer version of an older vaccine called DTP. DTP is no longer used in the United States.

2 | Who should get DTaP vaccine and when?

Children should get 5 doses of DTaP vaccine, one dose at each of the following ages:
- ✓ 2 months
- ✓ 4 months
- ✓ 6 months
- ✓15-18 months
- ✓ 4-6 years

DTaP may be given at the same time as other vaccines.

3 | Some children should not get DTaP vaccine or should wait

- Children with minor illnesses, such as a cold, may be vaccinated. But children who are moderately or severely ill should usually wait until they recover before getting DTaP vaccine.

- Any child who had a life-threatening allergic reaction after a dose of DTaP should not get another dose.

- Any child who suffered a brain or nervous system disease within 7 days after a dose of DTaP should not get another dose.

- Talk with your doctor if your child:
  - had a seizure or collapsed after a dose of DTaP,
  - cried non-stop for 3 hours or more after a dose of DTaP,
  - had a fever over 105°F after a dose of DTaP.

Ask your health care provider for more information. Some of these children should not get another dose of pertussis vaccine, but may get a vaccine without pertussis, called **DT**.

4 | Older children and adults

DTaP is not licensed for adolescents, adults, or children 7 years of age and older.

But older people still need protection. A vaccine called **Tdap** is similar to DTaP. A single dose of Tdap is recommended for people 11 through 64 years of age. Another vaccine, called **Td**, protects against tetanus and diphtheria, but not pertussis. It is recommended every 10 years. There are separate Vaccine Information Statements for these vaccines.

| Diphtheria/Tetanus/Pertussis | 5/17/2007 |

FIGURE 30.6 Federal law mandates the use of Vaccine Information Statements (VIS). These should be given to the parent or primary caregiver for each vaccine the child receives.

5 | What are the risks from DTaP vaccine?

Getting diphtheria, tetanus, or pertussis disease is much riskier than getting DTaP vaccine.

However, a vaccine, like any medicine, is capable of causing serious problems, such as severe allergic reactions. The risk of DTaP vaccine causing serious harm, or death, is extremely small.

Mild Problems (Common)

- Fever (up to about 1 child in 4)
- Redness or swelling where the shot was given (up to about 1 child in 4)
- Soreness or tenderness where the shot was given (up to about 1 child in 4)

These problems occur more often after the 4th and 5th doses of the DTaP series than after earlier doses. Sometimes the 4th or 5th dose of DTaP vaccine is followed by swelling of the entire arm or leg in which the shot was given, lasting 1-7 days (up to about 1 child in 30).

Other mild problems include:

- Fussiness (up to about 1 child in 3)
- Tiredness or poor appetite (up to about 1 child in 10)
- Vomiting (up to about 1 child in 50)

These problems generally occur 1-3 days after the shot.

Moderate Problems (Uncommon)

- Seizure (jerking or staring) (about 1 child out of 14,000)
- Non-stop crying, for 3 hours or more (up to about 1 child out of 1,000)
- High fever, over 105°F (about 1 child out of 16,000)

Severe Problems (Very Rare)

- Serious allergic reaction (less than 1 out of a million doses)
- Several other severe problems have been reported after DTaP vaccine. These include:
  - Long-term seizures, coma, or lowered consciousness
  - Permanent brain damage.
  These are so rare it is hard to tell if they are caused by the vaccine.

Controlling fever is especially important for children who have had seizures, for any reason. It is also important if another family member has had seizures. You can reduce fever and pain by giving your child an *aspirin-free* pain reliever when the shot is given, and for the next 24 hours, following the package instructions.

6 | What if there is a moderate or severe reaction?

What should I look for?

Any unusual conditions, such as a serious allergic reaction, high fever or unusual behavior. Serious allergic reactions are extremely rare with any vaccine. If one were to occur, it would most likely be within a few minutes to a few hours after the shot. Signs can include difficulty breathing, hoarseness or wheezing, hives, paleness, weakness, a fast heart beat or dizziness. If a high fever or seizure were to occur, it would usually be within a week after the shot.

What should I do?

- **Call** a doctor, or get the person to a doctor right away.
- **Tell** your doctor what happened, the date and time it happened, and when the vaccination was given.
- **Ask** your doctor, nurse, or health department toreport the reaction by filing a Vaccine Adverse Event Reporting System (VAERS) form.

Or you can file this report through the VAERS web site at **www.vaers.hhs.gov**, or by calling **1-800-822-7967**. *VAERS does not provide medical advice*

7 | The National Vaccine Injury Compensation Program

In the rare event that you or your child has a serious reaction to a vaccine, a federal program has been created to help pay for the care of those who have been harmed.

For details about the National Vaccine Injury Compensation Program, call **1-800-338-2382** or visit the program's website at **www.hrsa.gov/vaccinecompensation.**

8 | How can I learn more?

- Ask your health care provider. They can give you the vaccine package insert or suggest other sources of information.

- Call your local or state health department's immunization program.

- Contact the Centers for Disease Control and Prevention (CDC):
  - Call **1-800-232-4636 (1-800-CDC-INFO)**
  - Visit the National Immunization Program's website at **www.cdc.gov/nip**

U.S. DEPARTMENT OF HEALTH & HUMAN SERVICES
Centers for Disease Control and Prevention

Vaccine Information Statement	
DTaP (5/17/07)	42 U.S.C. § 300aa-26

FIGURE 30.6 (continued)

EVIDENCE-BASED PRACTICE 30.1
Which Intramuscular Thigh Vaccination Technique Results in the Fewest Adverse Reactions in Infants and Toddlers?

● **Study**

The incidence of vaccine-preventable diseases is decreasing, yet concern remains about adverse reactions following intramuscular immunizations. This single-center study, comprising 375 subjects age 2, 4, 6, or 18 months, used a blinded randomized controlled design to evaluate three techniques of intramuscular thigh injection: (1) the World Health Organization (WHO) recommendation—a 25-gauge, 16-mm (⅝-inch) needle inserted at a 90-degree angle to the long axis of the femur with the skin compressed between the thumb and index finger; (2) the Australian method—a 23-gauge, 25-mm (1-inch) needle inserted at the junction of the upper and middle thirds of the vastus lateralis at a 45- to 60-degree angle, pointing towards the knee; and (3) the U.S. technique—a 23-gauge, 25-mm (1-inch) needle inserted into the upper lateral quadrant at a 45-degree angle to the long axis of the femur and posterior at a 45-degree angle to the table top, with the thigh muscle bunched and the baby supine.

▲ **Findings**

Overall, the WHO technique resulted in less irritability and bruising than the other two techniques.

■ **Nursing Implications**

Parents often have concerns about adverse reactions associated with immunization. The 90-degree WHO technique is easier than the angled injection recommended in the Australian and U.S. techniques and reduces the risk of hitting bone with the longer needle. The amount of muscle varies with the size of the infant and toddler, so the nurse must ensure that the needle is long enough to place the medication intramuscularly. If a 1-inch-long needle is deemed necessary, the 90-degree angle technique may still be used to decrease the incidence of adverse reactions.

Diggle, L. (2006). The WHO technique for intramuscular thigh vaccination in infants and toddlers had fewer adverse reactions than two other techniques. *Evidence-Based Nursing, 9,* 9.

---

that increase the risk of an adverse reaction or may impair the child's ability to acquire immunity from the vaccine. On an individualized basis, providers must weigh the benefits of immunization against the likelihood of an adverse event. A summary of precautions and contraindications is presented in Table 30.9.

Diphtheria, Tetanus, and Pertussis Vaccines

Immunization against diphtheria, tetanus, and pertussis diseases is given via a combination vaccine. The vaccine currently used for children under age 7 is diphtheria, tetanus, acellular pertussis (DTaP). It contains diphtheria and tetanus toxoids and pertussis cell wall proteins. The older version of this vaccine—diphtheria, tetanus, pertussis (DPT)—contained killed whole cells of pertussis bacteria and caused more frequent and severe adverse reactions than DTaP. Diphtheria and tetanus (DT) vaccine is used for children under age 7 who have contraindications to pertussis immunization. Full-strength diphtheria toxoid causes significant adverse reactions in people over the age of 7 years. For this group, the TdaP adolescent preparation vaccine is used: it contains tetanus toxoid, reduced diphtheria toxoid, and acellular pertussis vaccine. The lowercase "d" is used to designate the lower dose of diphtheria toxoid. The ACIP recommends that TdaP be used for all tetanus boosters in older children (11 to 12 years) and adolescents, because TdaP provides a boost to diphtheria and pertussis immunization.

▶ *Take* NOTE!

Pertussis cases have steadily risen since the 1970s, with 34% of cases occurring in adolescents. This increase prompted the AAP's recommendation to change the tetanus booster for older children and adolescents from Td to TdaP beginning in 2006, to provide continuing protection against pertussis infection.

Haemophilus influenzae Type B Vaccines

Haemophilus influenzae type B is a bacterium that causes several life-threatening illnesses in children under 5 years of age. These infections include meningitis, epiglottitis, and septic arthritis. *Haemophilus influenzae* type B conjugate vaccines (Hib) have been extremely effective in cutting the rates of these diseases in children. There are several different types of Hib conjugate vaccines. HibTITER (HbOC) and ActHib (PRP-T) require three doses for the primary infant series, while PedvaxHIB and Comvax (PRP-OMP) require two doses. These vaccines are interchangeable, but if different brands are administered to a child, then a total of three doses is necessary to complete the primary series in infants. Hib vaccine is not given to children 5 years of age or older.

(text continues on page 928)

Vaccine Administration Record
for Children and Teens

Patient name: _____

Birthdate: _____

Chart number: _____

Vaccine	Type of Vaccine[1] (generic abbreviation)	Date given (mo/day/yr)	Source (F,S,P)[2]	Site[3]	Vaccine		Vaccine Information Statement		Signature/ initials of vaccinator
					Lot #	Mfr.	Date on VIS[4]	Date given[4]	
Hepatitis B[5] (e.g., HepB, Hib-HepB, DTaP-HepB-IPV) Give IM.									
Diphtheria, Tetanus, Pertussis[5] (e.g., DTaP, DTaP-Hib, DTaP-HepB-IPV, DT, Tdap, Td) Give IM.									
Haemophilus influenzae type b[5] (e.g., Hib, Hib-HepB, DTaP-Hib) Give IM.									
Polio[5] (e.g., IPV, DTaP-HepB-IPV) Give IPV SC or IM. Give DTaP-HepB-IPV IM.									
Pneumococcal (e.g., PCV, conjugate; PPV, polysaccharide) Give PCV IM. Give PPV SC or IM.									
Rotavirus (Rv) Give oral (po).									
Measles, Mumps, Rubella[5] (e.g., MMR, MMRV) Give SC.									
Varicella[5] (e.g., Var, MMRV) Give SC.									
Hepatitis A (HepA) Give IM.									
Meningococcal (e.g., MCV4; MPSV4) Give MCV4 IM and MPSV4 SC.									
Human papillomavirus (e.g., HPV) Give IM.									
Influenza[5] (e.g., TIV, inactivated; LAIV, live attenuated) Give TIV IM. Give LAIV IN.									
Other									

1. Record the generic abbreviation for the type of vaccine given (e.g., DTaP-Hib, PCV), *not* the trade name.
2. Record the source of the vaccine given as either F (Federally-supported), S (State-supported), or P (supported by Private insurance or other Private funds).
3. Record the site where vaccine was administered as either RA (Right Arm), LA (Left Arm), RT (Right Thigh), LT (Left Thigh), IN (Intranasal), or O (Oral).
4. Record the publication date of each VIS as well as the date it is given to the patient.
5. For combination vaccines, fill in a row for each separate antigen in the combination.

Technical content reviewed by the Centers for Disease Control and Prevention, Nov. 2006.

www.immunize.org/catg.d/p2022b.pdf • Item #P2022 (11/06)

Immunization Action Coalition • 1573 Selby Ave. • St. Paul, MN 55104 • (651) 647-9009 • www.immunize.org • www.vaccineinformation.org

FIGURE 30.7 Sample of a vaccine administration record.

TABLE 30.9 CONTRAINDICATIONS AND PRECAUTIONS FOR COMMONLY USED VACCINES

Vaccine	Contraindications	Precautions
Hepatitis A (HepA)	• Standard contraindications* • Infants <12 months of age	Moderate or severe illness
Hepatitis B (HepB)	Standard contraindications*	• Moderate or severe illness with or without acute fever • Infants <2,000 g if mother is HBsAg negative
Diphtheria, tetanus, acellular pertussis (DTaP) Tetanus, diphtheria, acellular pertussis (TdaP)	• Standard contraindications* • Previous encephalopathy within 7 days after diphtheria, tetanus, pertussis (DTP) vaccine or DTaP	• Temperature 105° F (40.5° C) within 48 hours after previous dose • Continuous crying lasting 3 hours within 48 hours after previous dose • Previous convulsion within 3 days after immunization • Pale or limp episode or collapse within 48 hours after previous dose • Unstable progressive neurologic problem • History of Guillain-Barré syndrome within 6 weeks
Diphtheria, tetanus (DT)	Standard contraindications*	
Measles, mumps, rubella (MMR)	• Standard contraindications*† • Pregnancy or possibility of pregnancy within 4 weeks • Blood products within the past 5 months • Immunocompromised status • If not given same day as varicella and/or yellow fever, hold until spaced 28 days apart	Thrombocytopenia or history of thrombocytopenic purpura
Varicella	• Standard contraindications*† • Pregnancy or possibility of pregnancy within 4 weeks • Blood products received within the past 5 months • Immunocompromised status • If not given same day as MMR and/or yellow fever, hold until spaced 28 days apart	• Do not give within 24 hours of antiviral medications. • Family history of congenital or hereditary immunodeficiency
Inactivated poliovirus (IPV)	Standard contraindications*‡	• Moderate or severe acute illness • Pregnancy
Haemophilus influenzae type B (Hib)	Standard contraindications*	• Moderate or severe acute illness
Trivalent inactivated influenza vaccine (TIV)	Standard contraindications*	• History of Guillain-Barré syndrome within 6 weeks
Live attenuated influenza vaccine (LAIV)	• Standard contraindications* • Client <5 years old • Client 5 or more years old with chronic illnesses • Client with close contact with severely immunosuppressed persons	Do not give within 48 hours of antiviral medications.
Pneumococcal conjugate vaccine (PCV7)	Standard contraindications*	Moderate or severe acute illness
Pneumococcal polysaccharide vaccine (PPV23)		

*1. Do not administer if client has had an anaphylactic reaction to prior dose of vaccine or any of its components. 2. Do not administer if client has a moderate to severe acute illness. Minor illnesses are not a reason to postpone immunization.

†Inquire about neomycin or gelatin allergies.

‡Inquire about neomycin, streptomycin, or polymyxin B allergies.

Polio Vaccine

Inactivated polio vaccine (IPV) is the only polio vaccine currently recommended in the United States. It is a killed virus vaccine that poses no risk for vaccine-acquired disease. Oral polio vaccine (OPV), a live attenuated virus vaccine, was the preferred polio vaccine until 2000. At that time it became apparent that the only victims of poliomyelitis were people who had acquired it from OPV. The ACIP determined that in this country the risks of OPV outweighed the benefits and withdrew its recommendation of OPV.

Measles, Mumps, and Rubella Vaccines

Measles, mumps, and rubella (MMR) is a live attenuated virus combination vaccine. It is the one most commonly used in childhood immunizations. MMR can be given the same day as other live attenuated virus vaccines such as varicella vaccine. However, if not given on the same day, the immunizations should be spaced at least 28 days apart. Anaphylactic reactions are believed to be associated with the neomycin or gelatin components of the vaccine rather than the egg component. The vaccine is not prepared from the allergenic albumen portion of the egg, so egg allergy is no longer a contraindication for measles vaccine. Pregnancy in a child's mother is not a contraindication to the vaccination of the child. Individual measles, mumps, and rubella vaccines are available if needed.

Hepatitis A Vaccine

Hepatitis A vaccine (HepA) is an inactivated whole virus vaccine. The vaccine has been demonstrated to be about 94% effective in preventing hepatitis A infection. Hepatitis A is spread through close physical contact and by eating or drinking contaminated food or water. It is one of the most frequently reported vaccine-preventable diseases in the United States. Young children are particularly susceptible to hepatitis A because of their close contact with other children, inadequate hygiene practices, and their tendency to place everything in their mouth. Hepatitis A vaccine is recommended to be given to all children at age 12 months, followed by a repeat dose in 6 to 12 months.

Hepatitis B Vaccine

Hepatitis B vaccine (HepB) is a recombinant vaccine. The vaccine is 80% to 90% effective in preventing hepatitis B infection. For infants, the mother's HBsAg status determines when immunization for hepatitis B begins. If the mother's status is positive or unknown, the neonate is immunized within the first 12 hours of life, at 1 to 2 months of age, and at 6 months of age. This is vital, because up to 90% of infected neonates develop chronic carrier status and will be predisposed to cirrhosis and hepatic cancer. If the mother's status is negative, immunizations are given routinely at 2, 4, and 6 months of age. Because hepatitis B is a sexually transmitted infection, it is important to verify the immunization status of all adolescents.

Varicella Vaccine

Varicella vaccine (Var) is a live attenuated virus vaccine. All children age 12 to 15 months who have not had varicella (chickenpox) should be immunized. A second dose is recommended at age 4 to 6 years. The vaccine provides effective postexposure prophylaxis if administered within 3 to 5 days after exposure. Varicella vaccine may be given the same day as other live attenuated virus vaccines. However, if not given on the same day, the immunizations should be spaced at least 28 days apart. Pregnancy in a child's mother is not a contraindication to the vaccination of the child.

Pneumococcal Vaccines

Streptococcus pneumoniae (pneumococcus) is the most common cause of pneumonia, sepsis, and meningitis in children under 2 years of age. The two available pneumococcal vaccines are pneumococcal conjugate vaccine (PCV) and pneumococcal polysaccharide vaccine (PPV). PCV contains seven strains of Streptococcus pneumoniae. It stimulates an immune response in infants and is given at 2 months of age as part of the initial immunization series. PPV contains 23 strains of Streptococcus pneumoniae. It does not provoke an immune response in children under 2 years of age. PPV is given to children over 2 years old who are at high risk for pneumococcal sepsis. This group includes children with anatomic/functional asplenia; sickle cell disease; chronic cardiac, pulmonary, or renal disease; diabetes mellitus; HIV infection; or immunosuppression.

Influenza Vaccines

Influenza immunization is recommended yearly for children between the ages of 6 and 59 months. Children 2 years old or older should be vaccinated if they have chronic health problems. Caregivers and household contacts of these children should also be immunized. The vaccine can also be given to anyone wishing to have immunity.

There are two influenza vaccines available, the trivalent inactivated influenza vaccine (TIV) and the live attenuated influenza vaccine (LAIV). LAIV is given intranasally and is indicated for healthy persons between the ages of 5 and 49 years. The virus in LAIV can replicate, and a person who has received LAIV can shed virus for a week. LAIV should not be given to anyone who will be in contact with an immunosuppressed person requiring a protected environment. TIV is suitable for any eligible person age 6 months or older. TIV is not capable of causing disease and is given by intramuscular injection.

Rotavirus Vaccine

Rotavirus is the most common cause of severe gastroenteritis among young children. The virus is shed in the stool and easily spreads via the fecal–oral route. Rotavirus accounts for about 50% of annual hospitalizations for gastroenteritis in children. Severe, watery, crampy diarrhea quickly leads to dehydration in the infected child. The most severe disease occurs in children ages 3 to 35 months.

The rotavirus vaccine is a live vaccine targeting five strains of rotavirus and is given via the oral route to infants less than 32 weeks of age.

Human Papillomavirus Vaccine

Human papillomavirus (HPV) is a DNA tumor virus transmitted through direct skin-to-skin contact. HPV is contracted most often during vaginal or anal penetrative sexual acts. HPV infection is most common in adolescents and young adults aged 15 to 24 years who are sexually active. HPV causes genital warts and is responsible for the development of cervical cancer. For these reasons, the ACIP and AAP have recommended that HPV vaccination occur in preadolescent girls. The three-vaccine series should begin at age 11 to 12 years. The vaccine is anticipated to prevent most cases of genital warts and cervical cancer.

Meningococcal Vaccine

Meningococcal disease may manifest as meningitis or as a deadly blood infection (meningococcemia). It is caused by the bacterium *Neisseria meningitiditis*, which is spread through direct contact or by air droplets. Since the 1990s, the incidence of meningococcal disease among adolescents and young adults has increased about 60%. About 10% to 12% of infected persons die; of the remaining victims, about 20% suffer severe long-term consequences (National Meningitis Association, 2007). For these reasons, the meningococcal vaccine is now recommended for all previously unvaccinated children at age 11 to 12 years. These children should receive the meningococcal conjugated vaccine (MCV4). Certain high-risk groups may be vaccinated at 2 years of age (through age 10) with the meningococcal polysaccharide vaccine (MPSV4).

Recall the Randall children, introduced at the beginning of the chapter. What immunizations would be appropriate for them to receive? Explain how you would administer the injections, and discuss any contraindications or precautions.

Barriers to Immunization

A fully immunized child is protected from the discomforts and complications of many infectious diseases. Disease prevention spares the family the emotional and financial burdens that serious illnesses can cause. Immunization programs prevent devastating epidemics in a community. Health care dollars not spent treating preventable diseases can be used for other urgent issues. Despite the numerous advantages of immunization, many children in this country are not fully immunized.

Many factors lead to children not being fully immunized. Parental concerns about vaccine safety are a significant cause of inadequate immunization. Misconceptions of what constitutes a contraindication to vaccination and having more than one health care provider are major contributors to inadequate immunization status. The more children in a family, the less likely the children are to be fully vaccinated. The costs for vaccines can also deter families from obtaining immunizations. Parents may want to postpone some of the scheduled immunizations because they are concerned about the effects of multiple injections on their child. Postponing a portion of the immunizations puts the child at risk for contracting disease. Disrupting the optimal spacing of the immunizations can decrease the efficacy of vaccine, further putting the child at risk.

Overcoming Barriers to Immunization

The AAP recommends the use of a manufacturer-produced combination vaccine whenever it will reduce the number of injections at a visit. These combination vaccines have been studied and approved by the U.S. Food and Drug Administration (FDA). The nurse should never mix separate vaccines in the same syringe unless expressly permitted in the product insert for all vaccines involved. Examples of combination vaccines are:

- DTaP: diphtheria, tetanus, acellular pertussis
- MMR: measles, mumps, rubella
- HepB-Hib: hepatitis B virus and *Haemophilus influenzae* type B

The Vaccines for Children (VFC) program was implemented in 1994. Prior to this program, free vaccines were available only through public health agencies. By providing free vaccines to low-income and uninsured families through their private health care providers, immunization rates have increased tremendously. Additional information on the VFC program is available at http://www.cdc.gov/vaccines/programs/vfc/default.htm.

Establishing a medical home for every child will alleviate many of the factors associated with lack of immunization. Parents who have a long-term, trusting relationship with a health care provider are more likely to have their concerns about vaccine safety discussed and removed. Missed opportunities for immunizations can be reduced by:

- Maintaining a centralized immunization record
- Verifying immunization status at every visit, not just health supervision visits
- Verifying the status of siblings accompanying the child to the appointment
- Providing parents with up-to-date information on vaccines geared to their concerns and needs

Two excellent resources for vaccination recommendations in the United States are the CDC's Vaccines and Immunizations website (http://www.cdc.gov/vaccines/default.htm) and the National Immunization Hotline (800-235-2522).

Discuss potential barriers to the Randall children being fully immunized. As a nurse, how can you help overcome these barriers?

Health Promotion

Health promotion focuses on maintaining or enhancing the physical and mental health of clients. The principal components of health promotion are identifying risk factors for a disease, facilitating lifestyle changes to eliminate or reduce those risk factors, and empowering clients at the individual and community level to develop resources to optimize their health. The nurse implements health promotion through education and anticipatory guidance.

Partnership development is the key strategy for success when implementing a health promotion activity. Identifying key stakeholders from the community allows problems to be solved and provides additional venues for disseminating information. Health promotion messages can be reinforced at schools, daycare centers, community agencies, and churches. If families have difficulty getting to health care facilities, the community arenas may be the primary source of health promotion.

Providing Anticipatory Guidance

Anticipatory guidance is primary prevention. The nurse partners with the parents to create a "road map" to optimal health for the child. *Healthy People 2010* provides a framework for determining health promotion goals. *Bright Futures: Guidelines for Health Supervision of Infants, Children, and Adolescents* (Green & Palfrey, 2002) is another valuable resource.

The "skeleton" of the guidance provided involves common childhood health problems. The nurse fleshes out that information using the results of risk assessments and screening tests, health concerns unique to the child, and the interests and concerns of the parents. Age-related anticipatory guidance information is provided in Chapters 4 through 8.

Provide appropriate anticipatory guidance for 3-year-old Maya and 9-month-old Evan.

Promoting Oral Health Care

Effective oral health practices are essential to the overall health of children and adolescents. Dental care is the most prevalent unmet health need among children in the United States. Poor oral health can have significant negative effects on systemic health. Children who suffer from dental caries have an increased incidence of pain, a decreased appetite, and sleep pattern disturbances. They are at increased risk for abscesses and systemic infections.

Optimal oral health is not limited to the prevention and treatment of dental caries. It includes anticipatory guidance about non-nutritive sucking habits, injury prevention, oral cancer prevention, and tongue and lip piercing. Preventing and treating malocclusion can have a significant benefit for children. Comprehensive health care is not possible if oral health is not a priority in the health delivery system.

Optimizing oral health can benefit the community as well as the individual client. There has been a 60% reduc-

tion in early childhood caries over the past 50 years since community water supplies were fluoridated at optimal levels. The cost of pediatric oral health care could be reduced 50% with the proper use of fluoride treatments coupled with other preventive measures. These health care dollar savings will enhance community resources.

Having a dental home enhances the likelihood that the child will obtain appropriate preventive and routine care. The American Academy of Pediatric Dentistry (AAPD) adopted the policy of the dental home in 2001. It is modeled on the AAP medical home policy. The dental home provides the same benefits to the child as the medical home. Characteristics of a dental home are listed in Box 30.9. The AAPD recommends that the dental home be established by the infant's first birthday.

Promoting Healthy Weight

Childhood obesity is a growing problem. The number of overweight children has doubled since 1980; the rate for teens has tripled. The principal causes of this increase in obesity are unhealthy eating habits and decreased physical activity. Research has demonstrated that weight is best managed with a combination of diet and exercise. Nurses can have the maximum effect in promoting healthy weight in children by encouraging activities that address both healthy eating patterns and physical fitness. Children, parents, and communities are all targets for healthy weight promotion by nurses.

The focus of healthy weight promotion should be health-centered, not weight-centered. Emphasizing the

HEALTHY PEOPLE 2010

Objective	Significance
Reduce the proportion of children and adolescents who have dental caries in their primary or permanent teeth.	• Teach children and adolescents appropriate toothbrushing and flossing techniques. • Encourage use of fluoride-containing toothpastes. • Encourage routine dental visits.

Source: USDHHS, 2007.

BOX 30.9 Characteristics of the Dental Home

- Preventive health program based on risk assessment
- Anticipatory guidance on oral health developmental issues
- Plans for emergency dental trauma
- Anticipatory guidance on oral hygiene
- Comprehensive dental care
- Referral to specialists for care not available at the dental home

benefits of health through an active lifestyle and nutritious eating creates a nurturing environment for the child. This allows the child to maintain his or her self-esteem. Linking success to numbers on a scale increases the possibility of developing eating disorders, nutritional deficiencies, and body hatred. A health-centered orientation also allows the family to develop a lifestyle that incorporates its cultural food patterns and traditions.

The nurse can stress the benefits of the mother's healthy nutritional habits on the fetus at prenatal visits. Parents who have a healthy eating pattern are likely to maintain and encourage those patterns in their children. The nurse provides parents with anticipatory guidance about age-related eating patterns during each health supervision visit. Parents with toddlers and preschoolers may need training in ways to cope with the child's growing autonomy while providing a variety of nutritious options.

The nurse can begin directly advising children on healthy foods starting at age 3. Information and teaching modalities need to be age-appropriate. With colorful posters and games, the nurse can teach the preschool child the difference between healthy and unhealthy food choices. As children enter school, group and peer-led activities can be very effective. The nurse must gear material toward the teen's growing autonomy in making self-care decisions.

Before providing education to school-age and teenage children, it is important to obtain nutritional histories directly from them because increasingly they are eating meals away from the family table. As they spend more time away from their parents, they need to develop the ability to make nutritious choices. The goal is to help older children develop strategies for making healthy choices as part of their increasingly independent lifestyle. Detailed anticipatory guidance is provided in Teaching Guidelines 30.1 and in Chapters 28 through 32.

TEACHING GUIDELINES 30.1

Healthy Eating

Breakfast

1. Don't skip breakfast. You will not have enough energy to play well later in the day. Skipping breakfast can also lower your grades in school.
2. Avoid eating high-sugar foods at breakfast. They will make you sleepy during the day.
3. Start your breakfast with some fruit. A small glass of juice, berries on your cereal, or a banana is a good choice.
4. Protein is important at breakfast. Milk, either in a glass or on cereal, is a good source of protein; so is yogurt or peanut butter.

Lunch

1. Check the quality of school-provided lunches. If they are high in fat or sugar, bring your lunch. Many schools publish their daily menus in advance. Check the newspaper or ask the school for a copy.
2. Add a variety of healthy alternatives to your lunches.
   a. Try different types of breads. Pitas, wraps, bagels, and taco shells can be a good change of pace in the sandwich routine.
   b. Freeze fruits before putting them in the lunch box. This will keep the lunch items cool and the fruit fresh-tasting. Canned pineapple and grapes freeze well; so do bananas.
   c. Try alternatives to high-fat chips. Dried fruits, baked pretzels, and animal crackers are a few examples of tasty, healthy treats.
   d. Low-fat chocolate milk is more nutritious than prepackaged juice boxes, which have high sugar concentrations.

Snacks

1. Limit snacks to after school and bedtime. Light snacks such as yogurt or fruit provide good hunger management. A very hungry child will tend to overeat at meals.
2. Children need to learn to eat only when they are hungry. Children often eat out of boredom. Discourage nonstop grazing by planning activities to occupy the child.

Dinner

1. Plan your menu a week ahead. Planning ahead reduces the likelihood of eating out or getting take-out food. Restaurant foods are more likely to be high in fats and carbohydrates.
2. Prepare homemade healthy versions of take-out favorites. Top prepared pizza crust with cooked chicken, vegetables, mushrooms, and cheese. Serve the pizza with a salad for a complete and healthy meal. "Make your own tacos" nights, using lean hamburger and low-fat sour cream, can be a lot of fun for children.
3. Don't turn dinner into a battle zone. Forcing children to eat foods they do not like will only deepen their dislike of them. Give them the healthy foods they do enjoy and eventually they will explore more options.
4. Lead by example. Children eventually adopt the eating patterns of their parents. If they see their parents eat vegetables, they will eventually try them.

Healthy physical activity can take many forms. During the preschool years, nurses should encourage parents to provide a wide variety of physical activities. This exposure to multiple types of exercise allows the child to find the one that is most enjoyable and increases the chances that he or she will maintain an active lifestyle. The focus should be on noncompetitive, fun activities. When the child enters school, the lure of television and computers can significantly diminish the amount of time spent in physical activity. Parents can encourage their children to stay physically active in several ways. They can limit the amount of time spent in sedentary activities and actively encourage the child to pursue any exercise that he or she enjoys. In addition to verbal encouragement, parents can promote exercise by participating in exercise with the child. A simple family walk can increase physical fitness while providing time for interaction between parent and child. Teaching Guidelines 30.2 gives additional suggestions for promoting physical activity.

TEACHING GUIDELINES 30.2

Healthy Activity

1. Plan physical activities that your family can do as a group.
2. Write exercise activities on your family's daily schedule.
3. Look for activities that appeal to your child's interest, such as dance, team sports, or swimming.
4. Place value on noncompetitive as well as competitive activities.
5. Show your child you believe exercise is important. Exercise daily yourself.
6. Encourage the community to develop safe areas for spontaneous games and activities.

Promoting Personal Hygiene

Handwashing is the first personal hygiene topic that needs to be introduced to children. Handwashing prevents disease by limiting a child's exposure to pathogens. The nurse can introduce the topic to preschool children using cartoons and games. Have the child sing "Twinkle, Twinkle Little Star" while washing his or her hands; this encourages adequate cleansing time. Use soap containers and towels with colorful characters to make the experience more fun. The school-age child can understand the concepts of germs and disease. Slogans such as "Let's drown a germ" can serve as a reminder of the importance of handwashing. The "Glo Germ" program (www.glogerm.com) is very effective in this age group. A nontoxic substance that shines under a black light is placed on the children's hands. The children can follow how germs travel from object to object. After washing their hands, the children can see if they did a good job.

In response to peer pressure, teenagers are usually stringent about personal hygiene. Young teens may need guidance in dealing with pubescent body changes such as body odor, fungal infections such as tinea pedis (athlete's foot), and acne.

Promoting Safe Sun Exposure

Skin cancer is a significant health problem in the United States. Blistering sunburns in children substantially increase the risk of melanoma and other skin cancers. People with fair skin are at highest risk for skin cancers, but anyone can become sunburned and develop skin cancer. When teaching clients about safe sun exposure, remind them that harmful ultraviolet (UV) rays can reflect off water, snow, sand, and concrete, so being in the shade or under an awning does not guarantee protection. Adequate sun protection requires using sunscreen, avoiding peak sun hours, and wearing proper clothing. Teaching Guidelines 30.3 gives more detailed instruc-

TEACHING GUIDELINES 30.3

Safe Sun Exposure

Sunscreen

1. Use sunscreen lotions every day. Harmful ultraviolet (UV) rays penetrate clouds and cause damaging sunburns.
2. Use sunscreens with a sun protection factor (SPF) of 15 or higher. An adequate amount for an average-sized child is half an ounce.
3. Apply sunscreens half an hour before sun exposure.
4. Reapply every hour if the child is perspiring heavily.
5. Reapply immediately after swimming.
6. Infants 6 months old or younger should not use sunscreens. Take steps to avoid sun exposure completely with this age group.

Clothing

1. Wear hats. The brim of the hat should be 4 inches or more and should shade the ears. Straw hats need to have a sunproof liner to be effective. Children introduced to hats as infants usually accept hats as part of the "outfit."
2. Wear UV-blocking sunglasses. The eye is the second most common site for melanoma.

3. Wear long, loose, and lightweight clothing for maximum sun protection.

Lifestyle

1. Avoid sun exposure between 10 a.m. and 4 p.m. This is when UV rays are strongest.
2. Ask your health care provider if your medication will increase your sensitivity to UV rays. If the answer is yes, take extra precautions to reduce sun exposure.
3. Avoid tanning parlors. The devices emit UV rays just like the sun and can cause damage.
4. Check the UV index before going out. The higher the index, the more precautions you should take. UV index figures are available in newspapers, TV, and radio weather reports and on the Internet.
5. Advocate for safe-sun scheduling of recreational activities. Talk to others about scheduling outdoor activities before 10 a.m., after 4 p.m., or in the shade.
6. Consider UV-blocking plastic film for your house and car windows.

---

tions. With proper sun protection starting in infancy, 80% of skin cancers could be prevented.

▶ *Take* NOTE!

Give children the following physical reference when doing health promotion on safe sun exposure. Tell the child, "Play outside only when your shadow is taller than you are." The child's shadow will be "taller" before 10 a.m. and after 2 p.m. The nurse can demonstrate this concept by placing a ruler on end and shining a bright light over it. As the nurse moves the light, the child will see the ruler's shadow lengthen.

■■■ Key Concepts

- Health supervision for children is a dynamic process. Optimal wellness for the child can only occur if the nurse forms meaningful partnerships with the child, the family, and the community. These partnerships allow for free exchange of information and the establishment of mutually agreed upon goals. The medical home exists when there is a single primary care provider for the

child. The medical home establishes a trusting long-term relationship with the child and family. This relationship leads to comprehensive, coordinated, and cost-effective care for the child.

- Health supervision has three components: developmental surveillance and screening; injury and disease prevention; and health promotion.
- Developmental surveillance is an ongoing process requiring a skilled observer and interviewer. To be effective, the nurse must understand normal growth and development expectations and be proficient at developmental screening procedures and techniques. Caregivers are most likely to reveal risk factors or warning signs for developmental delay when the nurse has a long-term and trusting relationship with the family.
- Screening tests are part of injury and disease prevention. They are modalities that identify treatable disease in an early or asymptomatic state and allow for cure or lessening of the disease's injury.
- Vision and hearing screening are functional testing modalities that the nurse must be proficient in administering in order for the child's results to be valid.
- Immunizations are a cornerstone of pediatric disease prevention. The nurse increases the effectiveness of immunization by understanding the principles of immunization and applying them to the client's individ-

ual circumstances. Adhering to good immunization management practices, as outlined by the ACIP and the AAP, enhances the benefits and reduces the risks of immunization.

- Barriers to full immunization include fragmentation of health care, concerns about vaccine safety, financial constraints, and lack of knowledge. The nurse can be pivotal in assuring that children and adolescents are fully immunized by serving as client educator and advocate.

- Children with chronic illnesses have a critical need for comprehensive and coordinated health supervision. Children with chronic illnesses require more frequent health supervision assessments. These children must have a medical home. The location of that medical home may be with a knowledgeable primary health care provider or at a multidisciplinary specialty facility. The location is determined by the child's needs and the family's preferences.

- The nurse incorporates frequent assessments of the many psychosocial stressors faced by families of children with chronic illnesses when establishing health care plans for them.

REFERENCES

American Academy of Pediatric Dentistry. (2004). *Policy on the dental home.* Retrieved July 24, 2007, from http://www.aapd.org/media/Policies_Guidelines/P_DentalHome.pdf.

American Academy of Pediatric Dentistry. (2007a). *Guideline on periodicity of examination, preventive dental services, anticipatory guidance and oral treatment for children.* Retrieved September 14, 2007, from http://www.aapd.org/media/Policies_Guidelines/G_Periodicity.pdf.

American Academy of Pediatric Dentistry. (2007b). *Policy on use of fluoride.* Retrieved September 14, 2007, from http://www.aapd.org/media/Policies_Guidelines/P_FluorideUse.pdf.

American Academy of Pediatrics. (2004). Ensuring culturally effective pediatric care: Implications for education and health policy. *Pediatrics, 114*(6), 1677–1685.

American Academy of Pediatrics. (2005a). Lead exposure in children: Prevention, detection, and management. *Pediatrics, 116*(4), 1036–1046.

American Academy of Pediatrics. (2005b). *Preschool vision screening for healthcare professionals.* Elk Grove Village, IL: Author.

American Academy of Pediatrics. (2006a). Active healthy living: Prevention of childhood obesity through increased physical activity. *Pediatrics, 117*, 1834–1842.

American Academy of Pediatrics. (2006b). Identifying infants and young children with developmental disorders in the medical home: An algorithm for developmental surveillance and screening. *Pediatrics, 118*(1), 405–420.

American Academy of Pediatrics. (2007a). *Eye examination in infants, children, and young adults by pediatricians.* Retrieved September 14, 2007, from http://aappolicy.aappublications.org/cgi/content/full/pediatrics%3b111/4/902.

American Academy of Pediatrics. (2007b). *Protecting your child from the sun.* Retrieved September 14, 2007, from http://www.aap.org/family/protectsun.htm.

American Academy of Pediatrics, Committee on Infectious Diseases. (2007c). Recommended immunization schedules for children and adolescents—United States, 2007. *Pediatrics, 119*(1), 207–208.

American Heart Association: Gidding, S. S., Dennison, B. A., Birch, L. L., Daniels, S. R., Gilman, M. W., Lichtenstein, A. H., Rattay, K. T., Steinberger, J., Stettler, N., & Van Horn, L. (2006). Dietary recommendations for children and adolescents: A guide for practitioners. *Pediatrics, 117*(2), 544–559.

Atkinson, W., Hamborsky, J., McIntyre, L., & Wolfe, S. (Eds.) (2007). *Epidemiology and prevention of vaccine-preventable diseases* (10th ed.). Washington, DC: Public Health Foundation.

Centers for Disease Control and Prevention. (2003). Surveillance for elevated blood lead levels among children—United States, 1997–2001. *Morbidity and Mortality Weekly Report, 52*(SS10), 1–21.

Centers for Disease Control and Prevention. (2005). *Preventing lead poisoning in young children.* Atlanta: Author.

Centers for Disease Control and Prevention. (2007a). Prevention of varicella. *Morbidity and Mortality Weekly Report, 56*(RR-4), 1–40.

Centers for Disease Control and Prevention. (2007b). Recommended immunization schedules for persons aged 0–18 years—United States, 2007. *Morbidity and Mortality Weekly Report, 55*(51 & 52), Q1–Q4.

Centers for Disease Control and Prevention. (2008). Recommended immunization schedules for person age 0–18 years—United States. *MMWR Weekly, 57*(01), Q1–Q4.

Cincinnati Children's Hospital Medical Center. (2007). *Healthy foods and snacking.* Retrieved September 14, 2007, from http://www.cincinnatichildrens.org/health/info/nutrition/eat/food.htm.

De Michele, A. M., & Ruth, R. A. (2005). Newborn hearing screening. *eMedicine.* Retrieved September 14, 2007, from http://www.emedicine.com/ent/topic576.htm#section~prevalence_of_hearing_loss.

Glo-germ program. (n.d.). Retrieved September 14, 2007, from http://www.glogerm.com.

Green, M., & Palfrey, J. (Eds.) (2002). *Bright futures: Guidelines for health supervision of infants, children, and adolescents* (2nd ed., rev.). Arlington, VA: National Center for Education in Maternal and Child Health. Retrieved September 14, 2007, from www.brightfutures.org/bf2/pdf/index.html.

Immunization Action Coalition. (2007). *Administering vaccines: Dose, route, site, and needle size.* Retrieved September 14, 2007, from http://www.immunize.org/catg.d/p3085.pdf.

March of Dimes. (2007). *Recommended newborn screening tests: 29 disorders.* Retrieved September 14, 2007, from http://www.marchofdimes.com/professionals/14332_15455.asp.

National Association of Pediatric Nurse Practitioners. (2006a). *Healthy Eating and Activity Together (HEAT) clinical practice guideline: Identifying and preventing overweight in childhood.* Cherry Hill, NJ: Author.

National Heart, Lung, and Blood Institute. (2005). *The fourth report on the diagnosis, evaluation and treatment of high blood pressure in children and adolescents* (NIH Publication No. 05-5267). Washington, DC: U.S. Department of Health and Human Services.

National Meningitis Association. (2007). *About meningococcal disease.* Retrieved September 14, 2007, from http://www.nmaus.org/about_meningitis/.

Pickering, L. K. (Ed.) (2006). *Red book: 2006 report of the committee on infectious diseases* (27th ed.). Elk Grove Village, IL: American Academy of Pediatrics.

Staat, M. (2002). Infectious disease issues in internationally adopted children. *Pediatric Infectious Disease Journal, 21*, 257–258.

Story, M., Holt, K., & Sofka, D. (2002). *Bright futures in practice: Nutrition* (2nd ed.). Arlington, VA: National Center for Education in Maternal and Child Health.

U.S. Department of Health and Human Services. (2000). *Healthy People 2010.* Retrieved September 14, 2007, from http://www.healthypeople.gov.

U.S. Preventive Services Task Force. (2006). Screening for iron deficiency anemia, including iron supplementations for children and pregnant women: Recommendation statement. *American Family Physician, 74*(3), 461–464.

Weber, J., & Kelly, J. (2006). *Health assessment in nursing* (3rd ed.). Philadelphia: Lippincott Williams & Wilkins.

Wrightson, A. S. (2007). Universal newborn hearing screening. *American Family Physician, 75*(9), 1349–1352.

WEBSITES

American Academy of Pediatrics: www.aap.org

American Association of Pediatric Ophthalmology and Strabismus: www.aapos.org

American Optometric Association: www.aoa.org

Bright Futures: www.brightfutures.org

Centers for Disease Control and Prevention/National Center on Birth Defects and Developmental Disabilities: childdevelopmentwww.cdc.gov/ncbddd/child/screen_provider.htm

Healthy People 2010 National Health Goals: www.healthypeople.gov

Immunization Action Coalition: www.immunize.org

Institute for Vaccine Safety at Johns Hopkins University of Public Health: www.vaccinesafety.edu

International Hearing Society: www.ihsinfo.org

National Network for Immunization Information: www.immunizationinfo.org

Prevent Blindness America: www.preventblindness.org

Vaccine Adverse Event Reporting System: vaers.hhs.gov

Vaccine and immunization information from the Centers for Disease Control and Prevention: www.cdc.gov/vaccines/default.htm

Vision 2020, The Right to Sight: www.v2020.org

CHAPTER WORKSHEET

MULTIPLE CHOICE QUESTIONS

1. During the health interview, the mother of a 4-month-old says, "I'm not sure my baby is doing what he should be." What is the nurse's best response?

   a. "I'll be able to tell you more after I do his physical."

   b. "Fill out this developmental screening questionnaire and then I can let you know."

   c. "Tell me more about your concerns."

   d. "All mothers worry about their babies. I'm sure he's doing well."

2. An infant boy is at your facility for his initial health supervision visit. He is 2 weeks old and responds to a bell during his examination. You review all his birth records and find no documentation that a newborn hearing screening was performed. What is the best action by the nurse?

   a. Do nothing; responding to the bell proves the infant does not have a hearing deficit.

   b. Schedule the infant immediately for newborn hearing screening.

   c. Ask the mother to observe for signs that the infant is not hearing well.

   d. Screen again with the bell at the infant's 2-month health supervision visit.

3. A 15-month-old girl is having her first health supervision visit at your facility. Her mother has not brought a copy of the child's immunization record but believes she is fully immunized: "She had immunizations 3 months ago at the local health department." Which would be the best action by the nurse?

   a. Ask the mother to bring the records to the 18-month health supervision visit.

   b. Start the "catch-up" schedule because there are no immunization records.

   c. Keep the child at the facility while the mother returns home for the records.

   d. Call the local health department and verify the child's immunization status.

4. A 4-year-old child is having a vision screening performed. Which screening chart would be best for determining the child's visual acuity?

   a. Snellen

   b. Ishihara

   c. Allen figures

   d. CVTME

5. Which facility fulfills the characteristics of a medical home?

   a. An urgent care center

   b. A primary care pediatric practice

   c. A mobile outreach immunization program

   d. A dermatology practice

6. When should the child's first examination by a dentist occur?

   a. By the first birthday

   b. By the second birthday

   c. By entry into kindergarten

   d. By entry into first grade

CRITICAL THINKING EXERCISES

1. During a health supervision visit for a 5-year-old boy, the mother tells you she is worried about his hearing. Your facility has been his medical home since birth. He was the product of a normal pregnancy and delivery. He has had frequent ear infections since the age of 8 months. Six months ago he had a ruptured appendix. He was treated with an aminoglycoside. He has been fully recovered for 4 months.

   a. During the health interview, what information should the nurse elicit from the mother?

   b. What information should the nurse verify from the permanent medical record?

   c. What risk factors for hearing loss does this child have?

   d. What is the best course of action at this time?

2. The nurse is examining a 4-year-old to determine his readiness for school. Describe the developmental, vision, and hearing screening tools that will help the nurse to identify any problems.

STUDY ACTIVITIES

1. Develop an immunization plan for the following well children: a 2-month-old, an 18-month-old who has never been immunized, and a 5-year-old who was current with all immunizations at age 2.

2. This is the first health supervision visit, since arriving in this country 1 week ago, for a 3-year-old international adoptee from Russia. Develop a plan for this visit.

3. Develop a healthy weight program for the following: a preschool class, a family in which the parents and the two school-age children are mildly overweight, and a teenage girl who is of normal weight but fears "getting fat."

HEALTH ASSESSMENT OF CHILDREN

KEY TERMS

accommodation
acrocyanosis
auscultation
body mass index (BMI)
cerumen
chief complaint

fontanel
inspection
lanugo
obligate nose breathing
palpation
PERRLA

point of maximal impulse
  (PMI)
stadiometer
Tanner stages
tympanometer

LEARNING OBJECTIVES

Upon completion of the chapter, the learner will be able to:

1. Demonstrate an understanding of the appropriate health history to obtain from the child and the parent or primary caregiver.
2. Individualize elements of the health history depending upon the age of the child.
3. Discuss important concepts related to health assessment in children.
4. Describe the appropriate sequence of the physical examination in the context of the child's developmental stage.
5. Perform a health assessment using approaches that relate to the age and developmental stage of the child.
6. Distinguish normal variations in the physical examination from differences that may indicate serious alterations in health status.
7. Determine the sexual maturity of females and males based upon evaluation of the secondary sex characteristics.

Elliot Simmons, 3 years old, is brought to the clinic for his annual examination. His mother states that he is very fearful and anxious about this visit.

WOW

Growth and development is a journey, on which many children venture without a map.

Assessment of the child's health status involves many components: the health interview and history; observation of the parent–child interaction; physical examination; and the child's emotional, physiological, cognitive, and social development. The nurse's skills are vital to the success of the assessment process. The nurse must (Mandleco, 2005):

- Establish rapport and trust
- Demonstrate respect for the child and the parent or caregiver
- Communicate effectively by actively listening, demonstrating empathy, and providing feedback
- Observe systematically
- Obtain accurate data
- Validate and interpret data accurately

The focus of the assessment process depends on the purpose of the visit and the needs of the patient. Assessment is an ongoing process and is repeated to varying degrees at every encounter. Expert nurses are constantly evaluating all of those in their care, whether directly or indirectly as part of conversation and play. Indeed, some of the subtlest developmental signs may express themselves only during relaxed and casual interaction with a child. You can observe gait while watching a child run down the hall; assess fine motor skills and social adaptation while playing a board game; or observe balance and coordination when bouncing a ball. Playful activities such as tickling a child can give the nurse feedback related to upper body strength when the child attempts to push the nurse's arms away. Nurses must also learn to perform a comprehensive and thorough examination of a child in an efficient manner.

A thorough and thoughtful assessment of a child is the foundation upon which a nurse determines the needs of and plan of care for the patient. Nothing can replace it for giving the nurse a snapshot of the life and health of the child. A comprehensive history, a thorough examination, and developmental or cognitive testing as appropriate will provide practical information about the health of a child and guide the nurse's plan of care. The history and physical examination also provide a time for health education, teaching about expected growth and development, and discussing healthy lifestyle choices. The nurse uses critical thinking skills to analyze the data and establish priorities for nursing intervention or follow-up.

The health assessment may be documented using a number of formats. The information should be easily retrievable and available to all members of the child's health care team.

Health History

The health history provides the nurse with an overall picture of what the child has experienced, highlighting areas of concern such as recurrent upper respiratory infections or headaches. This not only helps the nurse to assess those specific areas more comprehensively but also provides the opportunity to ask focused questions and identify areas where education may be needed. The time used to obtain the health history also gives the nurse an opportunity to interact with the child in a nonthreatening manner, while the child watches the interactions between the nurse and the primary caregiver.

▶ PREPARING FOR THE HEALTH HISTORY

Appropriate materials and a suitable environment are needed when performing a thorough health history. Take into account family roles and values. Consider the age and developmental stage of the child so that you can approach the child appropriately and possibly involve him or her in the health history. Observe the child–parent interaction. Determine the extent of the health history that is needed in a given situation. Being well organized and staying flexible will help ensure success.

Gathering Materials and Preparing Yourself for the Health History

Before you begin, make sure you have materials to record your history data (either a computer or chart paper and a pen), a private space with adequate lighting, chairs for adults and the nurse, and a bed or examination table for the child. The space should be safe for your patient's developmental stage and allow you uninterrupted time for your examination. Sit down for as much of the history taking as possible to demonstrate a relaxed and welcoming manner.

Approaching the Parent or Caregiver

Greet the parent or caregiver by name. While interviewing the parent, provide toys or books to occupy the child, allowing the parent to concentrate on your questions. Use open-ended questions and avoid making judgmental comments. Show respect by remaining approachable. Remember that the structure of the family and its roles and dynamics will affect how the family communicates and how they make decisions about health care. Demonstrate patience and help the parent stay on track when there are several children in the family. Throughout the interview, refer to the child by name and use the correct gender when referring to the child, demonstrating interest and competence.

Approaching the Child

Show a professional demeanor while still being warm and friendly to the caregivers and child. A white examination coat or all-white uniform may be frightening to children, who may associate the uniform with painful experiences or find it too unfamiliar. The nurse can wear a variety of professional-looking outfits, whether colorful uniform tops, aprons, or smocks worn over white uniforms, or everyday clothing, depending on the setting of the nurse's practice. Make eye contact if possible and address the child by name. Use slow deliberate gestures rather than very quick or grand ones, which may be frightening to shy children.

Some young children will warm up when given time to be invisible in the room, such as hiding behind a parent before they tentatively appear. Make physical contact with the child in a nonthreatening way at first. Briefly cuddling a newborn before returning it to the caregiver, warmly shaking the hand of older children and teens, and laying your hand on the head or arm of toddlers and preschoolers will convey a gentle demeanor. A joke, a puppet, a silly story, or even a simple magic trick may coax the child into warming up. Being at the same eye level as the child can also be more reassuring than standing over the child. This may require having extra seating for the nurse at the same level as the child and parent/caregiver. Aim to be seen as a trustworthy adult who is the child's partner in feeling better and staying healthy.

Elicit the child's cooperation by allowing him or her control over the pace, the order, or anything else that the child can control while still allowing you to obtain the information you need. All of this establishes a personal relationship with the child and helps gain his or her cooperation.

Communicating With the Child During the Health History

The child should be given opportunities to actively participate in the health history and assessment process. For young children, such as toddlers and preschoolers, ask them to point to where it hurts and allow them to answer questions. Validation of the information by the parent/caregiver is essential because of the limited comprehension and language use of children at these ages. The school-aged child can be more accurate because of his or her increased language skills and maturity level.

Initially, address the child and obtain as much information from him or her as possible. School-aged children should be able to answer questions about interactions with friends and siblings and school and activities they enjoy or are involved in. Ask the parent/caregiver if any additional information or observations should be included.

Adolescents may not feel comfortable addressing health issues, answering questions, or being examined in the presence of the parent/caregiver. The nurse must establish a trusting relationship with the adolescent to provide him or her with optimal health care. Ask adolescents whether they would be more comfortable answering questions alone in the examination area or whether they prefer for their parents to be present. Either way, the parent/caregiver will have an opportunity to talk with the nurse after the health history and assessment are completed.

Demonstrate an interest in the teen by asking questions about school, work, hobbies or activities, and friendships. Begin with these topics to make the teen feel comfortable in communicating with you. Communicate honestly with the adolescent and explain the rationale for various aspects of the health history. Teens are very sensitive to nonverbal communication, so be very aware of your gestures and expressions. Once a rapport has been established, move on to more emotionally charged questions that relate to sexuality, substance use, depression, and suicide.

Always assure the teen that complete confidentiality will be maintained to the extent possible. Current state law will determine the types of information that may be withheld from parents. If the information that the nurse receives indicates that the teen may be in danger, then the nurse must inform the teen that the information will be shared with other providers and/or the parents.

Observing the Parent–Child Interaction

Observation of the parent–child interaction begins during the focused conversation of the health interview and continues throughout the physical examination. Explore the family dynamics, not only through questions but also by observing the family for behavioral clues. Does the parent make eye contact with the infant? Does the parent anticipate and respond to the infant's needs? Are the parents ineffective when dealing with a toddler's temper tantrum? The plan of care may need to be adjusted to teach appropriate responses to the infant's needs or toddler's behavior. Do the parents' comments increase the school-age child's sense of self-worth? Behavioral observations are crucial to proper assessment of the family's needs.

Does the parent seem to be coping with the health issue or does he or she appear overwhelmed? Is the parent's/caregiver's behavior appropriate? Does the child look at the parent/caregiver before answering? Does the child seem relaxed and happy with the parent/caregiver, or is the child tense? The infant will appear calm and relaxed if his or her needs are generally met. Crying may occur when the baby is ill or frightened but may also indicate discomfort with the parent or caregiver. Use a calm and comforting voice with the infant. Infants respond well to higher-pitched and soothing voices.

When observing the relationship between the adolescent and the parent/caregiver, does the parent/caregiver allow the adolescent to speak, or does he or she frequently interrupt? Does the parent/caregiver contradict what is being said? Observe the body language of the adolescent. Does the adolescent seem relaxed or tense? Since adolescents are between childhood and adulthood, they have unique needs. They are in a time of multiple physical and emotional changes, many of which they cannot control. They need to know that the nurse is interested in what they have to say. The use of open-ended questions allows the adolescent to talk. "Tell me about your. . . ." or "What have you noticed about. . . ." are comfortable phrases to use to elicit the information needed.

Be aware of your reactions to the adolescent's questions or behaviors, such as your nonverbal and facial expressions. Talk with the adolescent using accurate language that is developmentally and age-appropriate.

Determining the Type of History Needed

The purpose of the examination will determine how comprehensive the history must be. If the health care provider rarely sees the child or if the child is critically ill, a complete and detailed history is in order, no matter what the setting. The child who has received routine health care and presents with a mild illness may need only a problem-focused history. In critical situations, some of the history taking must be delayed until after the child's condition is stabilized. Evaluate the situation to determine the best timing and the extent of the history. Also, be sensitive to repetitive interviews in hospital situations, and collaborate with physicians or other members of the health care team to ensure that a family already under stress does not need to undergo prolonged or repetitive questioning.

*R*emember Elliot, the 3-year-old being seen for his annual examination? When you enter the room, he is hiding behind his mother's legs. Considering his age and developmental level, how will you proceed with obtaining a health history?

▶ PERFORMING A HEALTH HISTORY

The health interview is the foundation of an accurate health assessment. Information about the child's health will come not only from a physical examination, but also from a careful conversation or interview with the child and/or the caregiver. Depending on the intent of the health assessment, many of the questions will be direct, and many will require the caregiver or child to answer simply "yes" or "no." In other than emergency situations, though, asking open-ended questions offers an excellent opportunity to learn more about the patient's life. For example, "Are you happy at school?" may elicit a brief nod of the head, whereas "Tell me what it's like on your school playground" may result in a story about the child's friends, the kind of activities they enjoy, any bullying that goes on, and so forth. These stories will provide the nurse with clues to the child's stage of physical, emotional, and moral development as well as his or her functional status.

Establish a therapeutic relationship with the child and family. Without the trust that comes from this therapeutic relationship, the family may not reveal vital information due to fear, embarrassment, or mistrust. Use therapeutic communication techniques such as active listening, open-ended questions, and eliminating barriers to communication. Establishing a "medical home" where ongoing health supervision occurs encourages the formation of trust through continuity of care and the family's continuing relationships with health care providers (see Chapter 30).

Components of the Health Interview

The structure of the health interview is determined by the nature of the visit. At an initial visit, large amounts of historical data are collected. Having the family fill out a questionnaire can save time, but a questionnaire is not a substitute for the health interview. The questionnaire may serve as a springboard to begin structured conversations between the family and the nurse. At subsequent visits the health interview can focus on the pertinent issues of that visit as well as any health issues that are being monitored.

The health history includes demographics, chief complaint and history of present illness, past health history, review of systems, family health history, developmental history, functional history, and family composition, resources, and home environment.

> ▶ **Take** NOTE!
>
> *Any questionnaires used in the health care setting must be appropriate to the reading level and primary language of the person filling them out.*

Demographics

Questions should start with simple and nonintrusive ones; once a rapport between the nurse and patient has started, sensitive questions can be asked. First obtain data such as the child's name, nickname, birth date, and gender. Determine the child's race or ethnicity, the language the child understands, and the language the child speaks. Record the child's address and home telephone number and the parent's or caregiver's work telephone number. Identify who the historian is (the child or the parent or caregiver), and note how reliable you consider this source of information to be. Do not assume that an adult with the child is the child's parent. Establish the relationship of the adult to the child, and ask who cares for the child if that person does not. Determine the composition of the household, including other children and other family members or other persons who live there.

Chief Complaint and History of Present Illness

Next, ask about the **chief complaint** (reason for the visit). The reason may not always be apparent to you. A question such as, "What can I help you with today?" or "What did you notice in your baby/child that you wanted to have checked today?" is very welcoming. The response from the child or parent may be a functional problem, a developmental concern, or a disease.

Record the chief complaint in the child's or parent's own words.

Next address the history related to the present illness. For each concern, determine its onset, duration, characteristics and course (location, signs, symptoms, exposures, and so on), previous episodes in patient or family, previous testing or therapies, what makes it better and what makes it worse, and what the concern means to the child and family. Inquire about any exposure to infectious agents.

Past Health History

Ask about the prenatal history (any problems with pregnancy), perinatal history (any problems with labor and delivery), past illnesses, or any other health or developmental problems. Document the child's prior history of illnesses (recurrent, chronic, or serious) and any accidents or injuries in the past. Inquire about any operations or hospitalizations the child has had. Document the child's diet. Note the child's allergies to foods, medications, animals, environmental or contact agents, or latex products. Determine the child's reaction to the allergen as well as its severity. Determine the child's immunization status (refer to Chapter 30 for further information on immunizations). Record any medications the child is taking, the dosage and schedule, as well as when the last dose was given. In preadolescent and adolescent females, determine menstrual history.

Family Health History

Obtaining information about the family's health is a key part of a health interview. Perform a three-generation family health history. This information may be documented in a genogram (Fig. 31.1). Asking about the age and health status of mother, father, siblings, and other family members helps to identify trends and specific health issues. For example, do the grandparents have early-onset coronary artery disease? If they do, the child may benefit from additional health screening. Siblings may exhibit a genetic disease or carry a trait for the disease. This family health information helps to guide future health planning.

Review of Systems

Inquire about current or past history of problems related to:

• Growth and development
• Skin

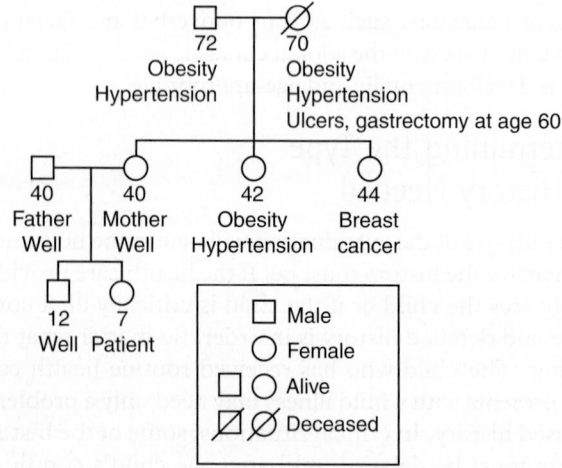

FIGURE 31.1 Genogram.

- Head and neck
- Eyes and vision
- Ears and hearing
- Mouth, teeth, and throat
- Respiratory system and breasts
- Cardiovascular system
- Gastrointestinal system
- Genitourinary system
- Musculoskeletal system
- Neurologic system
- Endocrine system
- Hematologic system

Table 31.1 provides specific questions related to each of these systems.

Developmental History

Determine the age when landmarks in gross motor control were achieved, such as sitting, standing, walking, pedaling, and so on. Ask whether the child has attained fine motor skills such as grasping, releasing, pincer grasp, crayon or utensil use, and handwriting skills. Note the child's age and extent of language acquisition. Document speech problems such as a lisp or stuttering. The rate of developmental skill acquisition may vary from child to child, but the sequence of skill attainment should remain the same. Inquire about self-care ability (e.g., tying shoes, dressing, brushing teeth) and, in the younger child, how toilet training is progressing. Assess feeding skills, including how well the child drinks from a cup and uses utensils or whether the

TABLE 31.1 QUESTIONS FOR THE REVIEW OF SYSTEMS

Systems	Has the Child Experienced:
Growth and development	Weight loss or gain, appropriate energy and activity levels, fatigue, behavioral changes such as irritability, nervousness, anger, or increased crying
Skin	Easy bruising or bleeding, rash, lesion, skin disease, pruritus, birthmarks, or change in mole, pigment, hair, or nails
Head and neck	Head injury, headache, dizziness, syncope
Eyes and vision	Pain, redness, discharge, diplopia, strabismus, cataracts, vision changes, reading difficulties, need to sit close to the board at school or close to the TV at home
Ears and hearing	Earache, recurrent ear infection, tubes in eardrums, discharge, difficulty hearing, ringing, excess cerumen
Mouth, teeth, and throat	Swollen gums, pain with teething, caries, tooth loss, toothache, sores, difficulty with chewing or swallowing, hoarseness, sore throat, mouth breathing, change in voice
Respiratory system and breasts	Nasal congestion or discharge, cough, wheeze, noisy breathing, snoring, shortness of breath or other difficulty breathing, problems with or changes in breasts
Cardiovascular system	Murmur, color change (cyanosis), exertional dyspnea, activity intolerance, palpitations, extremity coldness, high blood pressure, high cholesterol
Gastrointestinal system	Nausea, vomiting, abdominal pain, cramping, diarrhea, constipation, stool-holding, anal pain or itching
Genitourinary system	Dysuria; polyuria; oliguria; narrow urine stream; dark, cloudy, or discolored urine; difficulty with toilet training; bedwetting *Boys:* undescended testicles, pain in penis or scrotum, sores or lesions, discharge, scrotal swelling when crying, changes in scrotum or penis size, addition of pubic hair *Girls:* vaginal discharge, itching rash, problems with menstruation or menstrual cycle, development of pubic hair
Musculoskeletal system	Joint or bone pain, stiffness, swelling, injury (e.g., broken bones or sprains), movement limitation, decreased strength, altered gait, changes in coordination, back pain, posture changes or spinal curvature
Neurologic system	Numbness, tingling, difficulty learning, altered mood or ability to stay alert, tremors, tics, seizures
Endocrine system	Increased thirst, excessive appetite, delayed or early pubertal changes, problems with growth
Hematologic system	Swelling of lymph nodes, pale color, excessive bruising

Data from Burns, C., Dunn, A., Brady, M., Starr, N., & Blosser, C. (2004). *Pediatric primary care: A handbook for nurse practitioners.* Philadelphia: W. B. Saunders; Jarvis, C. (2008). *Physical examination and health assessment* (5th ed.). St. Louis: Saunders; Weber, J., & Kelley, J. (2005). *Health assessment in nursing* (3rd ed.). Philadelphia: Lippincott Williams & Wilkins.

child has any special requirements. Inquire about social skills and comfort articles (e.g., blankets, stuffed animals). Note whether the child has a habit of thumb or finger sucking or using a pacifier. Document daycare attendance and preschool or school adjustment and achievements.

Functional History

The functional history should contain information about the child's daily routine. Inquire about:

- Safety measures (e.g., car seats and their placement, use of seat belts, smoke detectors, bike helmets)
- Routine health care and dental care (including dates of dental care and what was done)
- Nutrition, including a 24-hour dietary recall or week-long food diary, use of supplements and vitamins, feeding pattern and satisfaction with diet, amount of "junk food" consumed, food likes and dislikes, and the parent's perception of the child's nutrition (refer to Chapters 25 through 29 for nutritional needs at various ages)
- Physical activity and organized sports, play, and recreation
- Television and computer habits
- Sleep behavior and bedtime
- Elimination patterns and any concerns
- Hearing or vision problems (dates of last screenings and results)
- Relationships with other family members and friends, coping and temperament, discipline strategies, attention or school behavior problems
- Religious involvement and other spiritual practices
- Use of adaptive and assistive devices such as eyeglasses or contact lenses, hearing aids, walker, braces, wheelchair
- Sexual practices

Family Composition, Resources, and Home Environment

Determine the marital status of the parents. Does the child live with the parents, a stepparent, or other family member? Is the child adopted or in foster care? Are the parents the primary caretakers for the child? If not, the primary caretaker should be included in the interview process if possible. Parents may not know some of the child's routines if the child spends much of the time being cared for by someone else. Working parents may learn about a health or behavior issue only after being alerted by the child's daycare center or babysitter. It may be helpful to expand the family history to include the grandparents and their interaction with the child.

Determine the employment status of the parents and their occupations, as this could affect the child's overall well-being; for example, the parents' work schedule may not allow them to spend much time with the child. Assess family income and financial resources, including health insurance and food stamps or other governmental supplemental income. Major family changes can also affect how the parents and child interact, so evaluate for relationship problems or changes.

Ask about the family's home and its age and the home environment. Is there a safe outdoor play area? If there is a pool, are safety features in place? Determine whether the home has electricity and an indoor water supply. Also determine whether the home has heating, air conditioning, and refrigeration. What pets does the family have? How are they housed? Are there infestations of insects or rodents in the home?

> ▶ **Take** NOTE!
>
> *Homes or apartments built prior to 1978 may contain lead-based paint, and children who live there are at an increased risk for the development of lead poisoning.*

Performing a Physical Examination

After the history comes the physical examination. It should focus on the chief complaint or any of the systems that engaged the nurse's critical thinking while taking the history. The examination will reflect the nurse's general practice style, the developmental stage and age of the child, the temperament of the child and caregiver, and the health status of the child. A very ill child will not waste energy protesting the examination, so the nurse can move quickly in that situation. A healthy child, however, will express his or her normal developmental stage and will show varying degrees of resistance to the examination.

▶ PREPARING FOR THE PHYSICAL EXAMINATION

When performing the physical examination, being prepared and organized ensures that you will obtain the needed information. The appropriate methods to use and ways to approach the child depend on the child's developmental stage.

Gathering Materials and Preparing for the Examination

The examination area should include an exam table or the child's hospital crib or bed. Appropriate lighting is necessary for adequate observation and inspection. Gather the equipment necessary for the examination such as clean gloves, stethoscope, thermometer, sphygmomanometer, tape measure, reflex hammer, penlight, otoscope/ophthalmoscope, tongue depressor, and cotton ball. An infant or adult scale is needed, as well as a **stadiometer** for children capable of standing independently. Young children may be frightened by seeing a large amount of equipment, so take out one piece of equipment at a time. Some children can be very resistant to what they see as a threat or an invasion of their privacy, so it may help to have washable toys in the examination area to use as distractions during the assessment.

Children and their parents may be able to sense any frustration or anxiety on the part of the examiner, so display a confident and matter-of-fact approach. If the child is not cooperative, do not become discouraged; more time and explanation will usually do the trick.

Regardless of the child's age, if the examination room is cold, the child will be uncomfortable and possibly less cooperative. Provide appropriate covers to ensure the child's comfort, or have the child remain dressed until the time of the examination.

Approaching the Child

Approach the child according to his or her developmental age and stage. Table 31.2 outlines a general approach to the physical examination in each broad developmental category.

If several children are to be seen at the same time, begin with the child who will be most cooperative. If the other children do not see anything scary and realize that their sibling was examined without a problem, it sets the stage for better cooperation from the younger ones.

Newborns and Infants

If the infant is asleep, auscultate the heart, lungs, and abdomen first while the baby is quiet. Count the heart rate and respiratory rate before undressing the baby. Completely undress newborns and infants down to their diaper, removing it just at the end to examine the genitalia, anus, spine, and hips. It is best to examine the infant 1 to 2 hours before a feeding. Having the parent or caregiver hold the child during the examination can help to alleviate fears and anxieties (Fig. 31.2). Allow the parent or caregiver to be a nurturer rather than assisting with painful procedures, unless there are no other choices available.

Perform the assessment in a head-to-toe manner, leaving the most traumatic procedures, such as examination of the ears, nose, mouth, and throat, until last. Also delay eliciting the Moro reflex until the end of the examination, as the startling sensation may make the infant cry. Use firm, gentle handling while examining the infant. Make sure your hands and the stethoscope are warm. Perform the assessment as quickly and completely as possible. Use a soft and crooning voice, smile, and engage the infant in eye contact. If the baby is crying, a pacifier may be useful and brightly colored objects may help distract him or her.

▶ *Take* NOTE!

Many older infants demonstrate stranger anxiety as a normal part of development. If the infant is not being held by the parent, make sure the parent is within the infant's view; this will increase the baby's comfort and cooperation.

Toddlers and Preschoolers

Toddlers and preschoolers usually prefer to remove their clothing one item at a time as needed for the examination. After one area is examined, the child may feel more comfortable replacing that item of clothing before removing another one. An examination gown is usually not necessary before school age. Again, make certain the room temperature is comfortable.

When the nurse enters the room, a child of this age is often sitting or standing by the parent. Incorporate play as appropriate during the health assessment. Remember your own facial expressions and tone. Use little touch at the beginning of the encounter with the child and the caregiver.

Introduce the equipment to be used slowly, explaining briefly what is going to happen. Let the child touch and hold the equipment whenever possible, even taking a parent's temperature or putting the blood pressure cuff on a teddy bear (Fig. 31.3). The toddler will prefer to sit on the caregiver's lap. When the toddler must be supine for the abdominal examination, sit in your chair knee-to-knee with the caregiver so the toddler may lie back on the caregiver's and your laps.

Praise the child for being cooperative during the examination. "You did such a good job holding still while I listened to your chest" and similar phrases give positive feedback to the child.

If the child is uncooperative, assess as thoroughly as possible and move on to the next area to be assessed. The caregiver may need to place an arm around the toddler's body to provide restraint for invasive procedures. Use short phrases to tell the toddler what you are going to do, rather than asking if it is OK.

▶ *Take* NOTE!

Toddlers are egocentric. Telling a toddler how well another child behaved probably will not be helpful in gaining the young child's cooperation.

The preschooler may fear body invasion and mutilation and will withdraw from any procedure or assessment that is viewed as intrusive. Otherwise, the sense of initiative often leads the preschooler to be cooperative. The

TABLE 31.2 DEVELOPMENTAL CONSIDERATIONS FOR EXAMINATION

	Newborn	Infant	Toddler	Preschool	School-age	Early Teen	Late Teen
Place to perform examination	May lie on examination table or in caregiver's lap.	In caregiver's lap or on exam table with caregiver right beside infant.	Allow some freedom of movement where possible; child may stand between sitting caregiver's legs or sit on the lap.	Some may be willing to sit on exam table with caregiver standing close by with hand on the leg.	Sitting on examination table where they still have eye contact with caregiver.	Some may be willing to have their caregiver wait outside the exam room.	Explain to the caregiver that the teen needs privacy and that he or she should wait outside the exam room.
Examination direction	Keep up a running dialog with the caregiver, explaining each step as you do it.	Continue to explain each step to the caregiver; address child by name. Perform most invasive parts last.	Introduce yourself to caregiver and child; explain most steps to the child and all steps to caregiver; allow child to handle instruments. Perform most invasive parts last.	Allow child to decide the order of the examination; explain what the instruments do and let the child try them; speak to the caregiver before and after the examination.	Include the child in all parts of the examination; use head-to-toe approach with genital exam last. Speak to the caregiver before and after the examination.	Speak to the child using mature language; appeal to his or her desire for self-care. Use a head-to-toe approach, with genital exam last.	Explain confidentiality to caregiver and teen; allow time talking with them together and separately. Use a head-to-toe approach, with genital exam last.

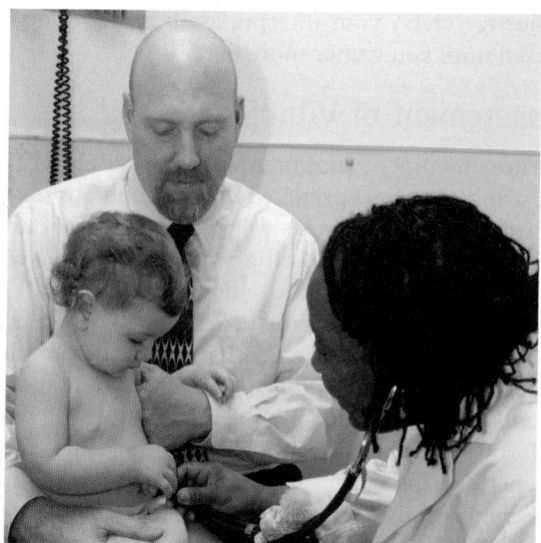

FIGURE 31.2 The infant or toddler may feel more comfortable and secure being examined while sitting in the parent or caregiver's lap.

preschooler may be willing to undress completely, leaving just the underpants on. Use simple explanations to inform the child about each step of the examination, offering reassurance as appropriate. Allow him or her to "help" by holding the stethoscope or penlight. If choices are available, offer them to the child. Again, always compliment the child on his or her cooperation.

▶ ***Take*** NOTE!

Preschoolers like to play games. To encourage deep breathing during lung auscultation, hold up a finger or a lit penlight and instruct the child to "blow it out."

FIGURE 31.3 The preschooler enjoys listening to her mother's heart first.

School-Age Children

The school-age child's thinking is still very concrete, but he or she can be objective and realistic. Avoid using medical jargon and words that may have a double meaning to a young child. Instead of "take your temperature," "take your blood pressure," "hit your knee," or "test," say, "Let's see how warm you are," "I want to listen to you breathe," and other phrases that describe, in words the child can understand, what you are preparing to do. The school-age child may be very interested in how things work and why certain things need to be done and will be responsive to truthful and simple explanations. Instruments that are colorful or look like toys are very helpful until adolescence, when teens are put off by childish things.

Always respect a child's desire to avoid pain and insult. Allow children to wear their underpants under the examination gown to provide a sense of security until the genitalia need to be examined. Allow the child to replace his or her clothing as soon as possible. Privacy and respect for the child's feelings are important to children of this age.

▶ ***Take*** NOTE!

Describing and commenting on your findings during the physical examination is interesting to the school-age child, as children of this age like to learn about how the body works.

Adolescents

Provide privacy while the adolescent is undressing and putting on a gown. Demonstrate an attitude of respect. Perform the assessment in a head-to-toe manner, exposing only the area to be examined. Provide information about physical changes in a matter-of-fact way, such as, "the hair on your legs is what is expected at this time." This provides information related to sensitive areas that the teen may be reluctant to ask about. It also provides the adolescent with information about the sexual development that is normal and expected. Allow opportunities for the teen to ask questions without the caregiver being present. Assure the adolescent that there are no "dumb questions" about the changes being experienced. Teenage girls should remove their bra so that you can do a breast examination, teach breast self-examination, and check for scoliosis. If the nurse is a male and the patient is an adolescent female, it is appropriate for a female staff member to be present during the breast and genital examination.

Steps of the Physical Examination

The physical examination of children, just as for adults, begins with a systematic **inspection**: checking color, warmth, characteristics, and texture visually and smelling for any odor. **Palpation** follows inspection to validate your observations. Percussion is a useful tool for determining the location, size, and density of organs or masses. Tapping with the reflex hammer elicits deep tendon reflexes. The stethoscope is used to auscultate the heart, lungs, and abdomen.

Performing a Physical Examination

A complete examination includes assessment of the general appearance, vital signs, body measurements, pain assessment, as well as examination of the head, neck, eyes, ears, nose, mouth and throat, skin, thorax and lungs, breasts, heart and peripheral perfusion, abdomen, genitalia and rectum, musculoskeletal system, and neurologic system. The nurse in most settings will not be assessing the breasts, genitalia, or eyes or ears in detail. Be aware of the role of the nurse in different settings and how the nurse can facilitate the assessment process.

General Appearance

Never discount first impressions. As you become more comfortable performing physical examinations, you will develop an ability to describe what you see and hear. Does the child give an impression of being ill or well? What is the child's expression and energy level? Note lethargy, listlessness, excessive activity, or inappropriate attention span for the child's age. Observe the child's state of alertness and whether he or she is responding appropriately to the stress of the situation. Note the child's posture and positioning:

- The newborn's posture is flexed, with arms and legs tucked in.
- The older infant should have improving head and then trunk control.
- The toddler demonstrates lordosis (swayback) and bowlegs, with a relatively large head and protuberant belly.
- The preschooler is more slender and upright in appearance.
- The school-age child and adolescent should demonstrate an upright, straight, and well-balanced posture.

Note whether the child's development appears appropriate. Observing the child initially may yield a wealth of information about the child's development. Is the child active, moving about the room? Does the child's speech seem appropriate for his or her age? Notice whether the family interacts appropriately with one another and the child. Does the child appear clean and well cared for? Does the child appear well nourished or small for age or obese? Do you smell tobacco or alcohol on the family's clothing? Does the child have a toy or transitional object? Is there a baby bottle or pacifier nearby? Do the siblings appear equally well cared for? Is there tension in the room between adults or adolescents? This initial quick assessment of general appearance will serve the nurse well if it is objective; delay your interpretation of what you have assessed until you gather more data.

Measurement of Vital Signs

Measure, document, and interpret the vital signs of children using age-appropriate equipment and approaches. The child's age and size, as well as knowledge of underlying health conditions, will affect your analysis of the vital signs. Vital signs are the temperature, pulse rate, respiratory rate, and blood pressure. In terms of vital signs, there is greater fluctuation in what is considered normal in children compared to adults. Therefore, count the heart rate and respiratory rate for a full minute (this will require comforting an infant or distracting a young child). If possible, perform these measurements when the child is quiet; if the child is crying or otherwise active during the assessment, document this. Many acute care settings require continuous measurement of vital signs using specific monitoring equipment. Also assess the child's pain level when assessing the vital signs.

Temperature

Temperature is measured as it is in adults. Thermometers are available in glass, electronic, and digital types. Use the same type of equipment consistently to allow reliable comparisons to be made and to permit tracking of temperatures during the course of illness. No matter which type of thermometer is used, ensure accuracy by carefully following the manufacturer's instructions.

The routes for taking the child's temperature are tympanic, temporal, oral, axillary, and rectal. Evidence is conflicting as to which method actually correlates best with the child's core, bladder, or arterial temperature, but recent studies support the use of a tympanic temperature as the most accurate, if it is appropriately obtained (El Radhi & Patel, 2006; Nimah et al., 2006). Take the child's temperature using the least invasive method that is best accepted by the child, parent, and health care provider.

▶ **Take** NOTE!

Glass thermometers are rarely used today due to the federal safety recommendations related to glass and mercury.

Choosing a method of measuring temperature depends on what is available at the facility and the child's age and physical condition. Tympanic thermometers measure the temperature within seconds, so this route is ideal for most children. Tympanic temperature reflects the pulmonary artery temperature. Tympanic thermometers are now available with smaller speculums, more appropriate for the infant or young child's ear canal. The accuracy of a tympanic temperature reading depends on the user's technique (Nursing Procedure 31.1). The tympanic method is not affected by the presence of ear wax, but it may be affected by vernix in the newborn's ear.

Temporal scanning is a newer method of temperature measurement that uses infrared scanning on the skin over the temporal artery combined with a mathematical computation to determine the child's arterial temperature. The arterial temperature is considered the most accurate reflection of body temperature. Measure temperature on the exposed side of the head (not the side that has been lying on a pillow or covered by a hat). Slide the sensor tip externally in a horizontal line across the child's forehead, midway between the eyebrows and hairline and ending at the temporal artery (Fig. 31.4). Hold it there until the device registers the temperature reading, which usually requires 1 second. Accuracy may be affected by excessive sweating.

Oral temperature is highly reliable if the child can cooperate. By 4 years of age, the child can hold an electronic oral thermometer in the mouth well enough to obtain a reading. Place the probe under the tongue. The child's mouth remains closed until the device registers the temperature. Have the child sit or lie quietly while the temperature is being taken. Electronic devices provide a temperature reading in as little as 4 seconds, but again the length of time varies with manufacturer. Oral intake, oxygen administration, and nebulized medications or treatments may affect oral temperature.

The axillary method works well for children who are uncooperative, neurologically impaired, or immunosuppressed or have injuries or surgery to the oral cavity. Place the tip of the electronic or digital thermometer in the axilla to obtain the reading. Make sure the tip is

FIGURE 31.4 Temporal artery thermometers are noninvasive and well tolerated by young children. For an accurate reading, move hair to expose forehead and hairline.

indeed in the axilla and not just between the arm and the child's side. Hold the thermometer parallel rather than perpendicular to the child's side to obtain the most accurate reading. Keep the child's arm pressed down to the side until the thermometer registers, which will be as little as 10 seconds with certain electronic models but 2 or 3 minutes with digital models commonly used at home.

Though long considered to reflect core temperature, the rectal route is invasive, not well accepted by children or parents, and probably unnecessary with the modern alternative methods now available. In addition to its intrusiveness, obtaining the rectal temperature runs the risks of damaging the rectal mucosa and inducing bradycardia in young infants. To take the rectal temper-

Nursing Procedure 31.1

TYMPANIC TEMPERATURE

1. Note age of child. If younger than 3 years, pull the earlobe back and down.
2. Insert the tympanic thermometer gently into the ear canal with the infrared sensor beam directed toward the center of the tympanic membrane rather than the sides of the ear canal.
3. Push the button to take the temperature and hold until a reading is obtained. The length of time required for the temperature to register varies per manufacturer but is only a few seconds at most.

ature, position the young infant supine with legs flexed. The older infant or child should be prone or side-lying. Small children may lie across the parent's lap for additional comfort. Apply a water-soluble jelly to the covered probe, insert the thermometer past the anal sphincter no more than 1 inch (2.5 cm), and hold it there until the temperature registers (as little as 15 seconds with certain electronic models but longer with digital models). See Evidence-Based Practice 31.1.

▶ *Take NOTE!*

Avoid the rectal route of temperature measurement in the neonate and the immunosuppressed child, as well as the child who has diarrhea, a bleeding disorder, or a history of rectal surgery.

Pulse

Assess the heart rate while the child is resting or sleeping. The heart rate in infants is much faster than in adults. It also varies in infants and children who are anxious, fearful, or crying. As the child grows, the heart rate slows and the range of normal values narrows. Table 31.3 lists heart rate ranges according to the child's age. The radial pulse is difficult to palpate accurately in children less than 2 years of age because the blood vessels lie close to the skin surface and are easily obliterated. For children younger than 2 years of age, auscultate the apical pulse with the stethoscope for a full minute. The **point of maximum intensity (PMI)**, the point on the chest wall where the heartbeat is heard most distinctly, is just above and outside the left nipple of the infant at the third or fourth intercostal space. The PMI moves to a more medial and slightly lower area until 7 years of age, when it is heard best at the fourth or fifth interspace at the midclavicular line (see the section below on chest examination for more information). Apical pulse rate should also be taken if the child has a cardiac problem such as an irregular heart rate or a congenital heart defect, as well as before administration of certain medications such as digoxin. During this procedure with children, allow the young child to examine or handle the stethoscope to become familiar with the equipment. In older children, palpate the radial pulse for a full minute (Fig. 31.5). Note any irregularities in strength or rhythm.

Finally, document the method used to obtain pulse measurement as well as any activity of the child during the assessment and any action taken.

▶ *Take NOTE!*

In the infant and young child, the heart rate is often quite elevated due to fear or anxiety when the stethoscope is placed on the chest initially. For an accurate heart rate, wait several seconds until the rate slows, then count for 1 full minute.

EVIDENCE–BASED PRACTICE 31.1
Pacifier Thermometers

● Study

Nurses and parents are concerned with being able to measure temperature accurately with the least invasive method possible. Research trials on pacifier thermometry in the past have been limited. The researchers utilized a convenience sample of children aged 7 days to 24 months in a prospective, cross-sectional study. Subjects were limited to those without gastrointestinal illness or contraindication to either the sublingual or rectal method of temperature measurement. Each child underwent pacifier temperature measurement with recordings at 3 and 6 minutes. The result was adjusted upward .5° F. as recommended by the thermometer manufacturer. Rectal temperature was then taken.

▲ Findings

Analysis of the pairs of recorded temperatures for each subject revealed close agreement between the rectal temperature and the adjusted 6-minute pacifier temperatures.

Differences between the two were not statistically significant. Variations between measurements are certain to occur when temperature is measured at different sites, so the researcher does not recommend replacing rectal thermometers with pacifier thermometers when a rectal temperature is indicated. Rather, it is the researcher's recommendation to use the pacifier thermometer as a screening tool.

■ Nursing Implications

Pacifier thermometers are an acceptable tool for temperature screening in children 7 days to 24 months of age. Nurses must use the thermometer properly, as well as instruct parents in its appropriate use if it is to be used at home. Consistent use of one particular method is important for tracking trends in temperature management over time. The mathematical upward adjustment of .5° F. must be included in the reporting of temperatures measured by pacifier thermometry.

Braun, C. A. (2006). Accuracy of pacifier thermometers in young children. *Pediatric Nursing, 32*(5), 413–418.

TABLE 31.3 **HEART RATE AND RESPIRATORY RATE RANGES BY AGE GROUP**

	Infant	Toddler	Preschooler	School-age	Adolescent
Heart rate	80–150	80–140	80–130	75–120	70–100
Respiratory rate	20–40	20–40	20–30	16–22	15–20

Respiratory Rate

Assess respirations when the child is resting or sitting quietly, since respiratory rate often changes when infants or young children cry, feed, or become more active. They also tend to breathe faster when they are anxious or scared. The most accurate respiratory rate is obtained before disturbing the infant or child. This can often be done easily when the parent/caregiver is holding the child before any clothing is removed. Count the respiratory rate for a full minute to ensure accuracy. Infants' respirations are primarily diaphragmatic, so count the abdominal movements. After 1 year of age, count the thoracic movements. Table 31.3 lists ranges of respiratory rate according to the child's age. Document the rate, activity of the child, any deviations from normal, and any action taken.

▶ **Take** NOTE!

Infants normally display an uneven or irregular breathing pattern, with short pauses between some breaths. This may be accentuated when they are ill.

Measuring Oxygen Saturation

Since the incidence of respiratory dysfunction is high in children who are ill, pulse oximetry is often routinely included in the vital signs assessment. This method is reliable and noninvasive. Pulse oximetry determines the oxygen saturation (SaO_2) in blood by using a sensor that measures the absorption of light waves as they pass through highly perfused areas of the body. The pulse rate on the oximeter should coincide with the apical pulse rate to ensure that the oxygen saturation reading is accurate. Nursing Procedure 31.2 details how to use the pulse oximeter. Identify whether pulse oximetry monitoring will be continuous or intermittent (as with vital signs).

A few guidelines to follow when using pulse oximetry are as follows:

• The probe may be placed on the finger, toe, ear, or foot. Avoid placing the probe on the same extremity with a blood pressure cuff or an intravenous or other type of line.
• Use the physician's orders or health care agency guidelines to set parameters for high and low pulse rate as well as high and low oxygen saturation. Never turn off the alarm settings.
• Ensure that the probe is not applied too tightly, as this will prevent venous flow and cause inaccurate readings.

Potential sources of errors in pulse oximeter readings include abnormal hemoglobin value, hypotension, hypothermia, ambient light interference, motion artifact, and skin breakdown. Falsely low readings may be associated with a nonsecure connection (movement of child's foot or hand), cold extremities/hypothermia, and hypovolemia. Falsely high readings may be associated with carbon monoxide poisoning and anemia.

Blood Pressure

The National Heart, Lung, and Blood Institute (NHLBI) recommends that children over 3 years of age have their blood pressure measured at least once during every health care episode. Children under 3 years old should have blood pressure measured if they have one of the following risk factors:

• History of prematurity, very low birthweight, or other neonatal intensive care complication
• Congenital heart disease
• Recurrent urinary tract infections, hematuria, proteinuria, known renal disease or urologic malformations, family history of congenital renal disease

FIGURE 31.5 Assessing the radial pulse of a young child.

Nursing Procedure 31.2

PULSE OXIMETRY MONITORING

1. Explain the procedure to the child and family (use a penlight to show how the sensor "looks through the skin").
2. Attach the probe to the child and connect to the monitor.
3. Set the parameters for the alarm if monitoring pulse oximetry continuously.
4. Observe and record pulse rate and oxygen saturation.
5. Record the activity level of the child and the percentage of oxygen in use.
6. Check skin condition and rotate sensor position every few hours.

Types of probes
a. infant continuous

b. finger continuous

c. finger intermittent

- Malignancy, bone marrow transplant or solid organ transplant
- Treatment with medications that raise BP
- Systemic illnesses associated with hypertension such as neurofibromatosis and tuberous sclerosis
- Increased intracranial pressure (NHLBI, 2005)

In the hospital or outpatient setting when a child is ill or undergoing surgery or a procedure, the frequency of blood pressure measurement will depend on the child's physical status. Measurement of blood pressure can be frightening to a young child, so include an age-appropriate explanation and perform the procedure after obtaining the pulse rate and respirations (Fig. 31.6). Accuracy of blood pressure measurement depends on the cuff size, as well as the operator's skill and accurate calibration of an electronic

FIGURE 31.6 Allowing children to handle the equipment gives them some control over the situation.

device. The National Heart, Lung, and Blood Institute (NHLBI) recommends that the cuff bladder width be at least 40% of the circumference of the upper arm at its midpoint. The cuff bladder length should cover 80% to 100% of the circumference of the upper arm. Various pediatric and infant cuffs are available, as well as larger thigh cuffs that may be used on an arm in an obese adolescent.

> ▶ *Take* NOTE!
>
> *Using an accurate cuff size is important: a wider cuff yields a lower reading and a narrower cuff yields a higher reading.*

Measure blood pressure in the upper arm, lower arm, thigh, or calf/ankle. The size of the cuff should match the extremity used. The measurement should be taken in the same limb, at the same place, and in the same position with each subsequent measurement to ensure consistency in tracking the blood pressure. To measure blood pressure using the upper arm, place the limb at the level of the heart, place the cuff around the upper arm, and auscultate at the brachial artery. When obtaining blood pressure in the lower arm, again, position the limb at the level of the heart, place the cuff above the wrist, and auscultate the radial artery. For measurement in the thigh, place the cuff above the knee and auscultate the popliteal artery. To obtain blood pressure on the calf or ankle, place the cuff above the malleoli or at the midcalf and auscultate the posterior tibial or dorsal pedal artery. Figure 31.7 shows appropriate cuff placement and auscultation points for the various sites.

The NHLBI recommends auscultation as the preferred method of obtaining blood pressure readings in children (Fig. 31.8). Systolic pressure in children is read at the moment the first Korotkoff sound is heard as the manometer pressure is lowered. The point at which the sound disappears is the diastolic pressure. The systolic blood pressure sometimes can be heard to a measurement of zero, so document the reading as systolic pressure over "P" for pulse.

Due to the small arm vessels in infants and young children, it may be very difficult to hear the Korotkoff sounds by auscultation. Alternative methods for obtaining blood pressure measurements in children include the use of Doppler or oscillometric (Dinamap) devices. The Doppler ultrasound method uses high-frequency sound waves that bounce off body parts to obtain blood pressure. Apply the gel to the Doppler end and listen with the Doppler device where you would ordinarily auscultate.

With either the Doppler method or auscultation, inflate the cuff 20 mm Hg past the point where the distal pulse disappears. Oscillometric equipment measures the mean arterial pulse and then calculates the systolic and diastolic readings. The accuracy of this method depends heavily on ongoing validation and calibration. Also, the cuff inflates to a preset value often far higher than the infant or child's blood pressure, resulting in a tight, uncomfortable cuff being in place for a longer period of time.

> ▶ *Take* NOTE!
>
> *If the oscillometric device yields a blood pressure greater than the 90th percentile for gender and height, repeat the reading using auscultation.*

In children older than 1 year, the systolic pressure in the thigh tends to be 10 to 40 mm Hg higher than in the arm; the diastolic pressure remains the same. Refer to Appendix I for the NHLBI blood pressure levels based on gender and height. Systolic blood pressure increases

A B C D

Brachial artery

Radial artery

Popliteal artery

Dorsalis pedis artery

Posterior tibial artery

FIGURE 31.7 Various positions of cuff placement and auscultation area for obtaining blood pressure. (**A**) Upper arm. (**B**) Lower arm. (**C**) Thigh. (**D**) Calf/ankle.

FIGURE 31.8 Auscultation is the preferred method for measuring blood pressure in children.

if the child is crying or anxious, so measure the blood pressure with the child quiet and relaxed. If the reading is lower in the leg than in the arm, always consider co-arctation of the aorta or interference with circulation to the lower extremities. Also pay attention to the pulse pressure (the difference between the systolic and diastolic readings): unusually wide (more than 50 mm Hg) or narrow (less than 10 mm Hg) pulse pressure readings suggest a congenital heart defect.

Infants and children presenting with cardiac complaints should have blood pressures assessed in all four extremities and also in the sitting, lying, and standing positions.

Document the method and site used, the activity of the child, any changes that may have occurred, and any actions or interventions performed.

Pain Assessment

Pain is considered to be the "fifth vital sign." Use the FLACC pain scale to measure pain in children who are too young to verbally or conceptually quantify their pain, or when there is a language barrier. The FLACC pain scale consists of a possible 10 points, with 0, 1, or 2 points given for each of five clinical signs (see Table 35.7 in Chapter 35).

Children who are older and can express that pain is worsening or improving should use the Pain Faces Scale (see Fig. 35.3 in Chapter 35). Explain that each face represents a person who is happy or sad, depending on how much or how little pain he has: 0 is for a person who is "very happy because he doesn't hurt at all"; 1 means "it hurts just a little bit"; 2, "it hurts a little more"; 3, "it hurts even more"; 4, "it hurts a whole lot"; and 5, "it hurts as much as you can imagine—but you don't have to be crying to feel this bad." Then ask the child to point to the face that best describes the amount of pain being felt.

For additional information related to pain assessment, refer to Chapter 35.

Body Measurements

Appropriate growth in children is usually an indicator of good health. A child who is not growing well may be in poor health, have inappropriate or inadequate dietary intake, or have a chronic disease. Accurate assessment of growth is a critical skill for the pediatric nurse and one that is rarely needed when caring for adults.

Determine the child's height or length, weight, and weight for length or **body mass index (BMI)**. Measure the head circumference for healthy children under age 3. Plot these measurements on a graph so they can be compared with earlier measurements and those of the child's peers. Additional anthropometric measurements used in children may include the chest circumference, mid-upper arm circumference, and skinfold measurement at the triceps, abdomen, or subscapular regions, but these are not performed routinely and are usually used only when a nutritionist consultation is necessary.

The growth chart is a screening tool for nutritional problems as well as a useful screen for chronic illness. Record each measurement in ink with a small dot at the correct location for the child's age and the date of the measurement written above it. Then use a plastic straight-edge to connect the previous measurement to the most current one. Children grow at variable rates; in infancy and pre-puberty, the growth velocity is normally more rapid. The growth chart allows the nurse to compare the patient to other children of the same age and gender while allowing for normal genetic variation. When measurements fall close to the same percentiles over time, growth is normal for that child. Children whose measurements fall within the 5th and 95th percentiles are generally considered within the normal growth range.

Sudden or sustained changes in percentile may indicate a chronic disorder, emotional difficulty, or nutritional intake problem. These findings require further assessment of the physical status of the child as well as other types of evaluations such as dietary intake or serum laboratory measurements.

Appendix F provides growth charts for boys and girls, ages birth to 36 months and 2 to 20 years. Special growth charts are available for children with Down syndrome, Turner syndrome, and ethnic groups that are typically smaller in stature as adults. Children may be as much as 10% above or below the predicted measurement and still be normal. Look for a trend over time of healthy growth that is neither too fast nor too slow.

▶ *Take NOTE!*

The most valid and reliable growth charts are those supplied by epidemiologists at the Centers for Disease Control and Prevention.

Length or Height

Calculate the length of the infant and toddler in a lying position until the age of 24 months. Use a measuring board (Fig. 31.9) or a cloth or paper measuring tape. Stretch out the legs to get a full extension of the body. Marking the examination paper at the child's head and extended foot is an option. Make sure that the growth chart where the measurement is plotted is marked for length and not height, as the two measurements differ. Document the length in centimeters and inches.

Once the child can cooperate and stand independently, begin measuring the standing height. Using a stadiometer is best (Fig. 31.10), but a cloth or paper tape can be used. Ask the child to remove his or her shoes and check that the back, shoulders, buttocks, and heels are against the wall, with the pelvis tucked as much as possible to correct for lordosis. The chin should be parallel to the floor. Plot this measurement on a growth chart marked for height rather than length. Record the height in centimeters as well as feet and inches.

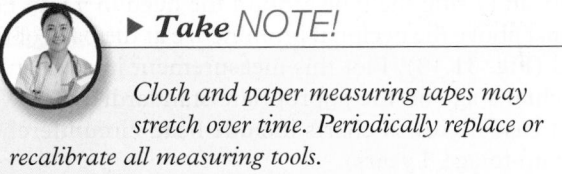

► **Take** NOTE!

Cloth and paper measuring tapes may stretch over time. Periodically replace or recalibrate all measuring tools.

Weight

Measure weight on a scale that is calibrated between every measurement. Just before placing the child on the electronic scale, press the "zero" or "tare" button and make sure the reading is 0. Calibrate the balance-type scale by setting the weight at zero, observing the beam balance, and making adjustments as necessary. Infants

FIGURE 31.10 Standing height is most accurately measured with the stadiometer.

and toddlers should be weighed on a platform-type electronic or balance scale, with examination paper placed between the child and the scale surface. Calibrate the scale with the examination paper in place. Remove the infant's diaper immediately before placing him or her on the scale. Toddlers may sit on the scale with the nurse or caregiver nearby to avoid falls (Fig. 31.11). Weigh older children and adolescents on a standing scale (Fig. 31.12). They may keep their underpants on and wear a lightweight examination gown.

An alternate method for obtaining weight, though much less accurate, is to weigh the caregiver initially and then weigh the caregiver holding the child. The difference between the two weights is the child's weight.

Regardless of the method used, weigh the infant to the nearest 10 g (or half-ounce) and the toddler and older child to the nearest 100 g (or quarter-pound). Record the weight in kilograms and in pounds.

Weight for Length

For children between the ages of newborn and 36 months, plot weight on the growth chart in comparison to the child's length. This allows the nurse to determine whether the child is a healthy weight for how long he or she is. Children placing less than the 5th percentile on the weight-for-length chart are considered underweight. Those placing greater than the 95th percentile are considered to be overweight.

Body Mass Index

With the recent increase in obesity in children, BMI is becoming an important measurement. BMI is a measure of

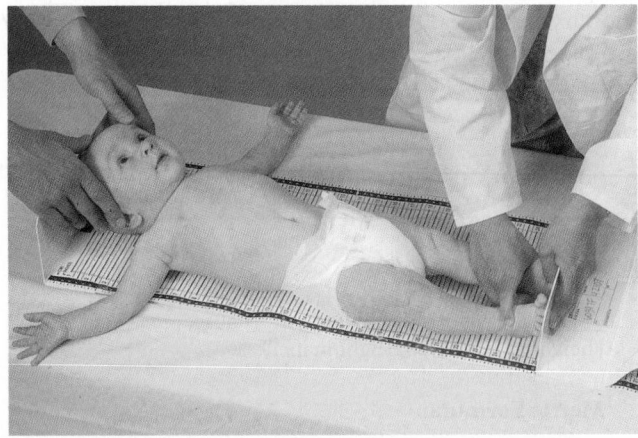

FIGURE 31.9 The recumbent measuring board is the most accurate method for obtaining a length measurement in infants and very young children.

FIGURE 31.11 A nurse or caregiver should remain nearby while weighing the infant or toddler.

FIGURE 31.12 Children who can stand independently can be weighed on a regular standing balance scale.

body fat and is determined by comparing the child's height and weight. Calculate the BMI using the child's weight and height by either the English or metric method. Box 31.1 provides BMI calculation formulas. BMI is included on the charts for children ages 2 to 20 years. Plot the BMI on the growth chart according to the child's age. A child whose BMI for age plots at less than the 5th percentile is considered to be underweight. BMI between the 85th and 95th percentiles indicates risk for overweight. BMI greater than the 95th percentile indicates the child is overweight.

The growth chart can indicate when a child is not growing adequately and can also be used to predict the development of overweight and obesity.

Head Circumference

Measure head circumference at well-child visits and upon hospital admission until the third birthday. Then measure it at the annual well-child visit until 6 years old if there are problems such as microcephaly or macrocephaly present at age 3. Measure the largest point across the skull, not including the ears, with a non-stretching cloth or paper tape. Begin at the forehead just above the eyebrows and bring the tape around the head in a taut circle just above the occipital prominence at the back of the head (Fig. 31.13). Plot this measurement in relation to the child's age on the appropriate standardized growth chart (usual growth charts include head circumference only up to age 3 years).

Monitoring Equipment

Sometimes children in acute care settings require continuous monitoring of vital signs. This monitoring could be via an apnea monitor or a cardiopulmonary monitor. The apnea monitor measures abnormal or irregular breathing in infants. The cardiopulmonary monitor generally measures heart rate and respiratory rate. Additional equipment on this monitor also allows for blood pressure and temperature monitoring. Set high and low alarm limits according to the health care facility's policies. Figure 31.14 indicates the placement of electrodes for the apnea and cardiopulmonary monitors. Assess the skin where the electrodes are placed to ensure there is no skin breakdown. If the

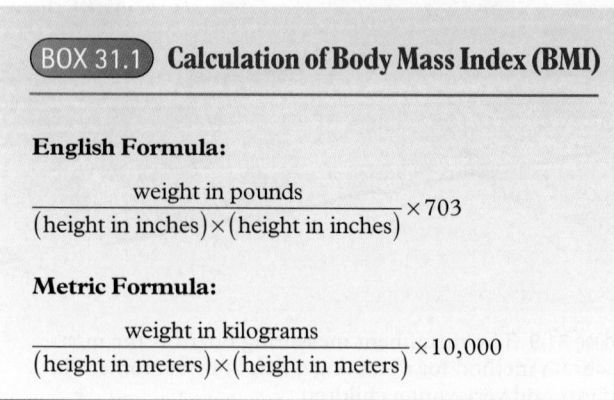

BOX 31.1 **Calculation of Body Mass Index (BMI)**

English Formula:

$$\frac{\text{weight in pounds}}{(\text{height in inches}) \times (\text{height in inches})} \times 703$$

Metric Formula:

$$\frac{\text{weight in kilograms}}{(\text{height in meters}) \times (\text{height in meters})} \times 10,000$$

Objective	Significance
Reduce the proportion of children and adolescents who are overweight or obese.	• Screen for overweight in all children by plotting weight for length of children less than 36 months and BMI for age for children age 2–20 years. • Assess dietary intake and activity level in all children at risk for or overweight. • Provide diet and activity recommendations to attain a healthy weight or BMI. • Refer significantly overweight children to a pediatric endocrinologist.

alarm sounds, immediately check the child to ensure the leads are not disconnected or the child is not in distress.

Skin

The skin is the body's largest organ and reveals information about a child's nutrition, respiratory, cardiac, endocrine, and hydration status all at a glance. A careful skin examination provides an invaluable understanding of a child's health.

Inspection

Inspect the color of the skin. The color should be appropriate to the child's racial or ethnic background, with the nail beds, conjunctivae, soles of the feet, and palms of the hands appearing pink. Normal variations include the following:

• Blueness of the hands and feet, known as **acrocyanosis**, is normal in babies up to several days of age and results from an immature circulatory system

FIGURE 31.13 Measure occipito-frontal head circumference at the largest point.

FIGURE 31.14 Placement of cardiac apnea monitor leads: white on the right upper chest, black on the left upper chest, red on the abdomen (not over bone).

completing the switch from fetal to extrauterine life (see Fig. 25.3 in Chapter 25).

• Cooling or warming the newborn and young infant may produce a vasomotor response that causes a mottling of the skin over the trunk and extremities (see Fig. 25.3).

• Babies of darkly pigmented Native American, African, and Asian parents will be paler than their parents for many months until the melanocytes in the epidermis begin production.

• Dark-skinned infants commonly have hyperpigmented areolas, genitals, and linea nigra.

Other variations related to skin color are discussed in Box 31.2.

Inspect the skin for the presence of **lanugo**. All infants display some degree of lanugo (soft, downy hair on the body, particularly the face and back). Lanugo is more

---

BOX 31.2 **Variations in Skin Color and Their Causes**

• **Pallor** (defined as decreased pinkness in light-skinned patients, ashy-gray in dark-skinned) is caused by anemia, shock, fever, or syncope.

• **Peripheral cyanosis** (blue discoloration) occurs in nails, soles, and palms and may be caused by anxiety or cold; also associated with central cyanosis.

• **Central cyanosis** (blueness of the lips, tongue, oral mucosa, trunk) is caused by hypoxia or circulatory collapse.

• Overall yellow color (**jaundice**) may be physiologic in the newborn or related to liver or hematopoietic disease in any age child.

• **Yellowing** of nose, palms, and soles may result from excess intake of yellow vegetables.

• **Redness** of the skin results from blushing, exposure to cold, hyperthermia, inflammation (localized), or alcohol ingestion.

• **Lack of color** in skin, hair, and eyes is related to albinism.

abundant in infants of Hispanic descent and in premature infants and recedes over the first few weeks of life.

Inspect the entire body for nevi and vascular and other lesions. Note their location, size, distribution, characteristics, and color. Pigmented nevi (also termed birthmarks) are indicated by a darker patch of skin and generally do not fade over time. Note the presence of hyperpigmented nevi (formerly called Mongolian spots), which appear as blue or gray, variably and irregularly shaped macules (Fig. 31.15). These are a common finding in dark-skinned infants. These nevi fade over months to years as the child's skin pigment darkens. Do not mistake hyperpigmented nevi for bruises. Inspect the skin for vascular lesions. Table 31.4 describes vascular lesions and their significance.

Rashes are common in children and are often associated with communicable diseases. Describe the rash in detail, noting types of lesions, distribution, drying, scabbing, and any drainage. The newborn and young infant may display milia (small white papules) on the forehead, chin, nose, and cheeks. These recede spontaneously. In adolescents the skin examination may reveal open or closed comedones (pimples or blackheads) across the face, chest, and back. Teens may sport tattoos, brandings, or various body piercings; inspect these areas for signs of infection such as erythema or drainage (Fig. 31.16).

Document the presence of any lacerations, abrasions, or burns. Note the distribution of the injury and whether it seems consistent with the mechanism described in the health history. Be alert to the possibility of child abuse if the type or number of burns, lacerations, or bruises seems unusual for the situation.

▶ **Take** NOTE!

Petechiae or ecchymosis may be found over areas traumatized by the birth process; these may take a few weeks to resolve. Certain cultures use "cupping" or "coining" when a child is ill, and these practices may yield bruises or mild burns.

FIGURE 31.15 Transient hyperpigmentation most often occurs in darker-skinned infants.

Palpation

Palpate the skin for temperature, moisture, texture, turgor, and edema. Use the back of your hand to assess the skin's temperature, comparing the right side of the body to the left and the upper body to the lower. The skin should feel uniformly warm. Cool extremities are associated with environmentally cool temperatures as well as impending circulatory collapse and shock. Warm skin may be associated with fever or sunburn, or locally a burn or infectious process. The skin should feel fairly dry, occasionally moister in the creases. Dry, flaking skin may occur in the young infant, particularly if born postmaturely. Overall skin dryness in the well-hydrated child may occur with excess sun exposure, poor nutrition, or

TABLE 31.4 VASCULAR LESIONS AND THEIR SIGNIFICANCE

Description	Significance
Salmon nevi: light pink macule usually on eyelids, nasal bridge, back of neck ("stork bite")	Usually fade over time, but may never go away completely. No complications.
Strawberry nevus: raised reddish papule made of blood vessels (hemangiomas)	Present at or develop after birth; recede over time, usually by age 9 years. Usually no complications.
Nevus flammeus: dark purple-red flat patch, grows with the child ("port-wine stain")	May be associated with Sturge-Weber syndrome. May be disfiguring; may be removed with laser therapy.
Ecchymosis: purplish discoloration, changing to blue, brown, black (bruise)	Common on lower extremities in young children. Should correlate with the injury.
Petechiae: pinpoint reddish purple macules that do not blanch when pressed	Broken tiny blood vessels; occur with coughing, bleeding disorders, meningococcemia
Purpura: larger purple macules	Bleeding under the skin; occur with bleeding disorders, meningococcemia

FIGURE 31.16 Adolescent with multiple piercings.

overbathing. Moist skin occurs with perspiration, fever resolution, and shock. The infant's and young child's skin is very soft ordinarily. Older children should continue to have a smooth and even skin texture. The preadolescent and adolescent may have oily-feeling skin on the face, shoulders, or back.

Assess skin turgor by elevating the skin on the abdomen in the infant or on the back of hand in the older child or teen. The "pinched-up" skin should quickly return to place. Skin that remains tented is strongly suggestive of moderate to severe dehydration. When edema is present, palpate the edematous area to determine its extent. Palpate any lumps or protrusions to determine firmness or tenderness. Palpate lesions or rashes with a gloved hand to document the size and extent of the lesions.

Hair and Nails

Inspect the hair and scalp, noting distribution of hair as well as color, texture, amount, and quality. The young infant's hair may be absent entirely or quite thick; it will be replaced by hair that is of a texture and color closer to what the child will have throughout childhood. Coarse, dry hair at any age may indicate a thyroid disorder or nutritional deficiency. Inspect the scalp thoroughly; it should be free from lesions and infestations. Note the presence of a greasy, scaly plaque on the scalp of infants; termed seborrheic dermatitis or cradle cap, it is benign and easily treated.

Inspect the nails for color, shape, and condition. Full-term infants may have long, papery fingernails that can scratch their skin if not trimmed. Children should have healthy nails. Dry, brittle nails may indicate a nutritional deficiency. Inspect the skin around the nails to ensure that it is intact and without signs of infection. Many children (especially school-age children) have a nervous habit of nail biting or hangnail biting or pulling.

Inspect the school-age child's or adolescent's toenails to ensure they are trimmed in a horizontal fashion. Self-trimming of toenails either too low or in a curved fashion places the child at risk for the development of ingrown

nails. Clubbing of the nails indicates chronic hypoxemia related to respiratory or cardiac disease. Nails that curve inward or outward may be hereditary or linked with injury, infection, or iron deficiency anemia.

Head

Examining the head is critical in the newborn and infant periods but should not be overlooked in older children as an opportunity to check for diseases of the scalp and functional and developmental problems that are reflected in poor hygiene of the head and scalp. Note hair distribution and any bald or thinning areas. Use of gloves may be indicated, depending on the overall scalp cleanliness and chance of infestation by head lice (seen as small grayish specks near the base of hair shafts).

Inspection

Examine the head and face for shape and symmetry. In newborns, the head may be temporarily misshapen from uterine positioning or a long vaginal delivery. Some infants have a slight flattening of the back of the head since the recommended sleeping position is supine. Note any irregularities or asymmetry. Observe the infant's head shape by looking down on it from above. Observe whether the head appears centered on the neck or tilts to one side. After 4 months of age, the infant should have achieved enough head control to hold the head erect and in midline when placed in a vertical position. Pull the infant from the supine position into sitting to determine the extent of head lag. To determine the extent of head control in older infants and children, ask the child to turn the head in different directions, either by simple commands or by following a colorful object.

Observe the infant's face when crying, smiling, or babbling for symmetry of muscle movement. In children who are old enough to follow directions, a game of "Simon Says" is a playful way to determine facial symmetry and strength; ask them to puff out their cheeks, make kisses, look surprised, stick out their tongue, and so on (effectively testing function of cranial nerve VII [facial]).

▶ *Take* NOTE!

When you note a flattened occiput in an infant, encourage the parent or caregiver to allow the infant "tummy time" while awake and observed and to change the infant's head position frequently when upright in an infant seat.

Palpation

Gently palpate the anterior and posterior **fontanels** (Fig. 31.17), which remain open in infancy to allow for rapid brain growth in the first months of life. Note the size of the fontanels. The anterior fontanel is about the

FIGURE 31.17 Note location and size of the fontanels. The anterior fontanel is diamond-shaped and closes between the ages of 9 and 18 months.

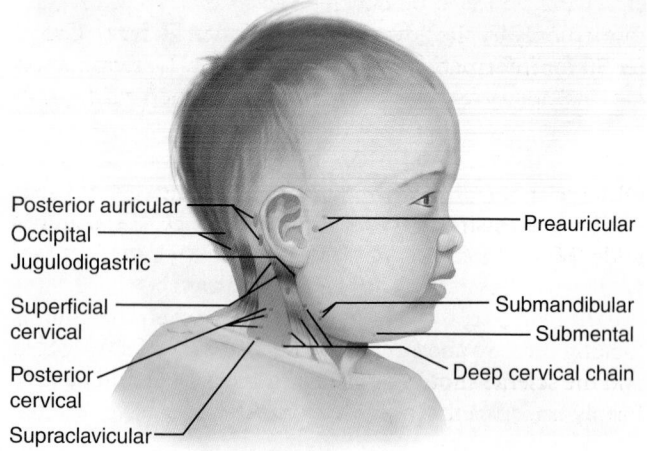

FIGURE 31.18 Location of lymph nodes.

size of a quarter at birth and slowly gets smaller until it can no longer be felt when it is closed by the age of 9 to 18 months. The posterior fontanel is much smaller and may close any time between shortly after birth and approximately 2 months of age. The fontanel should be neither depressed nor taut and bulging, though it is not uncommon to see it pulsate or briefly bulge if the baby cries. In an acutely ill infant, assess the fontanels while obtaining the vital signs. Dehydration can cause the fontanels to be sunken; increased intracranial pressure and overhydration can cause them to bulge. Palpate the skull for asymmetry, overriding or open sutures, and lumps or other deformities. Palpate the jaw joints as the child bites down to assess cranial nerve V (trigeminal). Use the fingertips to palpate for occipital, postauricular, preauricular, submental, and submandibular lymph nodes, noting their size, mobility, and consistency (Fig. 31.18).

> ▶ **Take** NOTE!
>
> *Large fontanels may be associated with Down syndrome or congenital hypothyroidism. A fontanel that becomes larger over time rather than smaller may indicate the development of hydrocephalus, especially if accompanied by an accelerated increase in head circumference.*

Neck

Inspect the neck for symmetry. The infant's neck is short, but by 4 years of age the child's neck should be similar in appearance to the adult's. Webbing or excessive neck skin folds may be associated with Turner syndrome, and lax neck skin may occur with Down syndrome. Assess the flexibility of the neck through a full range of motion. Take younger children through a passive range of motion. Older

children will be able to look in all directions on command and stretch their chins to the chests themselves. Test cranial nerve XI (accessory) in the older child by having the child attempt to turn the head against resistance. Assessment of neck mobility is particularly important when infections of the central nervous system are suspected. Pain or resistance to range of motion may indicate meningeal irritation. Do not assess neck mobility in the trauma victim.

Palpate the neck for masses and lymph nodes. Palpate the cervical and clavicular lymph nodes with the distal part of the fingers using gentle but firm pressure in a circular motion. Tilt the child's head upward slightly to allow better access. Assess the lymph nodes for swelling, mobility, temperature, and tenderness. In healthy infants and adolescents, the cervical lymph nodes are usually not palpable, whereas they are often found to be small, nontender, and mobile in healthy children from the ages of 1 year through 11 years (see Fig. 31.18 for locations of lymph nodes). Enlarged cervical lymph nodes frequently occur in association with upper respiratory infections and otitis media. Significant enlargement should be reported to the physician or nurse practitioner. Palpate the trachea; the thyroid is usually palpable only in older children.

> ▶ **Take** NOTE!
>
> *The infant or child who has experienced trauma should have the cervical spine maintained completely immobile until a radiologist has determined that the spinal cord is not damaged.*

Eyes

Assessment of the eyes includes evaluation of the external and internal structures as well as screening for visual acuity. Any nurse caring for a child should be adept at examining the external structures. Assessment of the internal structures will also be covered below but is usually performed only by the advanced practitioner. Refer to Chapter 30 for information on vision screening. Determination of visual acuity tests the function of cranial nerve II (optic).

External Structures

Observe the eyes for symmetry and spacing, even distribution of eyelashes and eyelids, and presence of epicanthal folds. Note the child's ability to blink, reporting inability to do so. The eyes should look symmetrical and both should be facing forward in the midline when the child is looking directly ahead. The iris should be perfectly round and the sclerae should be clear. The cornea should be uniformly transparent. Inspect the corners of the eye (medial and lateral canthus) and the conjunctiva (lining of the eyelids). They should be free of discharge, inflammation, or swelling. Epicanthal folds may be present in children of Asian descent, children with genetic abnormalities, or those with fetal alcohol spectrum disorder. Using a small penlight or ophthalmoscope, inspect the function and clarity of the pupil by putting your non-dominant hand on the child's forehead and moving the light toward and away from each eye. This will elicit the blink reflex. Next observe whether the pupil contracts with the light and expands when the light is removed. Make the same motion with a small toy or object and direct the child to look at it. The eyes demonstrate **accommodation,** or focusing at different distances, if the pupil constricts as the object moves closer. If normal findings are present, report **PERRLA** (pupils are equal, round, reactive to light and accommodation) (Fig. 31.19). This is a particularly important assessment in head and eye injuries, as well as when other neurologic concerns are present. Absence of pupillary reflexive action after age 3 weeks may indicate blindness.

FIGURE 31.19 The pupils should be equal, round and reactive to light and accommodation (PERRLA).

(Fig. 31.20). The cover test also assesses eye muscle strength. Cover one of the child's eyes and instruct the child to focus on an interesting object. The eye should not waver. While the child is still focusing with the first eye, remove the cover from the second. Observe the uncovered eye for movement. Report any movement or drift.

To test peripheral vision, have the child focus on a specific point or object directly in front. Bring a finger or a small object from beyond the range of vision into the area of the peripheral vision. When the child sees the ob-

> ▶ *Take* NOTE!
>
> *The normal infant may exhibit intermittent strabismus (crossing of the eyes) until about 3 months of age. However, persistent strabismus at any age or intermittent strabismus after 3 months of age should be evaluated by a pediatric ophthalmologist.*

Check extraocular muscle motility and function of cranial nerves III and IV (oculomotor and abducens) by instructing the child to follow the light through the six cardinal positions of gaze. Infants and very young children will follow an interesting object. This tests cranial nerve III (oculomotor). Instruct the older child to look downward and inward (testing cranial nerve IV [trochlear]). Assess eye muscle strength using two tests. Using the Hirschberg test, bring the penlight to the middle of your face and direct the child to look at it. The small dot of reflected light seen in the iris should be symmetrically placed in each eye

FIGURE 31.20 Note reflected light falling symmetrically on each pupil with the Hirschberg test.

ject from the side, while still focusing on the object or point in front, the child should say "stop." This also tests cranial nerve II (optic).

Internal Structures

Assessment of the internal structures of the eye is best accomplished by an advanced practitioner with experience in this type of assessment. An adequate assessment requires that the child cooperate. Restraint for eye examination does not usually prove fruitful, as movement and tearing of the eyes interfere with the accuracy of the examination. Use the ophthalmoscope to inspect the internal eye structures. Observe the glow of the pupil, which appears red (creamy-colored in children with very dark eye color). Inspect the optic disk, macula, fovea, and blood vessels. Refer any child with blurring or bulging of the optic disk or hemorrhage of vessels to a pediatric ophthalmologist for further evaluation.

> ▶ **Take** NOTE!
>
> *Immediately report absence of the red reflex in one or both eyes, as this may indicate the presence of cataracts.*

Ears

Assessment of the ears includes evaluation of the external and internal structures as well as screening for hearing. Any nurse caring for a child should be adept at examining the external structures. Assessment of the internal structures will also be covered below but is usually performed only by the advanced practitioner. Refer to Chapter 30 for information on hearing screening. Testing of hearing also tests the function of cranial nerve VIII (acoustic).

External Structures

Assess the placement of the external ears on the head. They should be symmetrical and placed no lower than the eyes. The pinna should deviate no more than 10 degrees from an imaginary line that is perpendicular to a line drawn between the outer canthus of the eye and the top of the ear. Low-set ears may be associated with genetic abnormalities or syndromes (Fig. 31.21). Note protrusion or flattening of the ears, which may be normal for that child or may indicate inflammation (protrusion) or persistent side-lying (flattening). Note the presence of pits or skin tags in the preauricular area. Observe the exterior ear canal. A waxy **cerumen** that is soft and an orangish-brown color is normally found lubricating and protecting the external ear canal and should be left in place or washed gently away when bathing. Note drainage from the ear canal, which is always considered abnormal. Pull on the auricle and palpate the mastoid process, neither of which should result in pain in the healthy child.

FIGURE 31.21 Low-set ears may be associated with chromosomal or other genetic anomalies.

> ▶ **Take** NOTE!
>
> *Impacted and dry cerumen can be softened with a few drops of mineral or cooking oil and then gently irrigated from the canal with an ear syringe and warm water.*

Internal Structures

Use a **tympanometer** to assess the mobility of the eardrum (tympanic membrane). Gently pull down on the earlobe of infants and toddlers and up on the outer edge of the pinna in older children to straighten the ear canal, and press the tip of the tympanometer over the external canal. A reading of air pressure is recorded by the instrument, and this is useful to assess middle ear disease. Many tympanometers record a wave pattern that may be printed to include in the child's chart.

A nurse practitioner or physician generally performs inspection of the ear canal and tympanic membrane with an otoscope (Fig. 31.22). The otoscopic examina-

FIGURE 31.22 Otoscopic examination allows visualization of the internal structures of the ear.

tion is usually performed near the end of the physical assessment for infants and young children, as they are often quite resistant to this intrusive procedure. The infant or toddler may require restraint in the parent's lap for the otoscopic evaluation. The preschooler may cooperate if the nurse uses a game such as looking for pretend puppies or potatoes in the child's ear. As with the tympanometer, gently pull down on the earlobe of the infant or toddler and up on the outer edge of the pinna in older children to straighten the ear canal. Use an otoscopic speculum appropriate to the size of the child's ear canal. Insert the speculum into the ear canal to visualize the canal and the tympanic membrane. The canal should be pink, should have tiny hairs, and should be free from scratches, drainage, foreign bodies, and edema. The tympanic membrane should appear pearly pink or gray and should be translucent, allowing visualization of the bony landmarks. It may be red if the child has been crying recently. Compress the pneumatic insufflator bulb to provide a puff of air; this causes motion of the tympanic membrane when the middle ear is healthy. Note abnormalities such as a fluid level, bubble or pus behind the tympanic membrane, tympanic membrane immobility, holes or perforations in the tympanic membrane, and the presence of tympanostomy tubes, scarring, or vesicles.

▶ *Take* NOTE!

Never attempt to flush a foreign object out with water until it has been identified, because small pieces of sponge, clay, or vegetative material like peas or beans swell with water, further obstructing the ear canal.

Nose and Sinuses

The nose, as with all facial features in a child, should be symmetrical, but it can be displaced temporarily by birth trauma in newborns. Children of Asian or African descent often display a flattened nasal bridge as a normal variation. Ensure that the nares provide unobstructed airflow by alternately occluding one nostril at a time and observing for air movement through the other nostril. If the child is breathing comfortably, there should be little nostril movement visible. Adolescents may have pierced their nose or nasal septum; ensure that the site is free from infection or loose jewelry that could migrate into the sinuses. Ideally the nose should not be draining, though clear mucus may be present if the child has been crying. Assess the amount, color, thickness, and presence of any odor if drainage is present. Inspect the interior of the nose by tilting the child's head backward and pushing the tip of the nose upward. Direct the beam of a penlight in the nostril. The nasal mucosa should be uniformly firm, pink, and free from edema, excoriation, or masses. Test the older child's sense of smell by having the child close the eyes and identify a familiar scent such as peppermint or coffee (cranial nerve I [olfactory]). Palpate the sinuses for tenderness.

▶ *Take* NOTE!

*Infants up to 3 to 6 months of age have traditionally been thought to be **obligate nose breathers** because of their long soft palate and relatively large tongue, which allows for swallowing without aspiration during breast or artificial nipple feeding. This lessens with age and as the infant becomes better able to breathe through the mouth when necessary.*

Mouth and Throat

Wear a powder-free glove to examine the mouth, teeth, and throat. Inspection of the exterior of the mouth may be done at any point in the examination. Infants and young children may find assessment of the mouth and particularly the pharynx and uvula to be quite intrusive, so delay that part of the assessment until the end of the examination, after otoscopic evaluation. Assess the character and quality of the child's voice and the infant's cry. It should be neither too hoarse nor too shrill.

Inspection of the Mouth

Observe the lips for color, symmetry, and absence of inflammation or edema. Salivation in infants begins at about 3 months of age; drooling occurs because the infant does not learn to swallow saliva until several months later. Next, inspect the interior of the mouth. The mouth is the first part of the digestive system, and a pink, moist, healthy mucosal lining is indicative of a healthy gastrointestinal tract. In infants, the tongue should lie within the mouth at rest and should be capable of extending over the lower gum line to help the baby feed. The tongue extrusion reflex is normal in infants up until the age of 6 months and allows the infant to suckle easily from birth. Observe movement of the tongue when the infant or young child babbles or cries. Ask the older child to touch the tongue to the roof of the mouth and then stick out the tongue and move it from side to side (testing cranial nerve XII [hypoglossal]). Full movement should be present and the tongue should be free from lesions or exudate. Visualize the hard and soft palate (which should be intact) or palpate with the gloved finger.

Most infants have no teeth before the fifth to sixth month. When the teeth begin to erupt, they usually erupt symmetrically at the rate of about one a month, until toddlers have 20 teeth by 30 months of age. The infant may drool for several months before teething. During teething the gums will be swollen at the location of the impending tooth. In older children, the secondary teeth replace the primary teeth much more slowly and with little discomfort from the 5th to the 20th year. Figure 31.23 shows the usual permanent tooth eruption pattern.

Look for dental caries or alignment problems and inspect the gums for signs of infection. Test cranial nerve IX (glossopharyngeal) by having the child identify taste with the posterior portion of the tongue.

▶ **Take** NOTE!

Natal (present at birth) or neonatal (erupting by 30 days of age) teeth should be evaluated by a pediatric dentist for potential extraction, as they may pose an aspiration risk.

Inspection of the Throat

Inspect the tonsils, uvula, and oropharynx. Assess the infant's throat during a yawn or cry, as any forcible attempt to depress the tongue with a tongue depressor produces a strong reflex elevation of the base of the tongue that completely blocks the view of the pharynx. The young child will require restraint so that the nurse can depress the tongue and visualize the back of the mouth without injuring the child (Fig. 31.24). Asking the older child to open wide, stick out the tongue, and say "aaaah" simultaneously will allow for a quick look at the tonsils and pharynx without the need to use a tongue depressor, but the nurse must be very quick because the tongue rises rapidly after those maneuvers are performed.

Upper Teeth	Erupt
Central incisor	7-8 yrs.
Lateral incisor	8-9 yrs.
Canine (cuspid)	11-12 yrs.
First premolar (first bicuspid)	10-11 yrs.
Second premolar (second bicuspid)	10-12 yrs.
First molar	6-7 yrs.
Second molar	12-13 yrs.
Third molar (wisdom tooth)	17-21 yrs.
Lower Teeth	**Erupt**
Third molar (wisdom tooth)	17-21 yrs.
Second molar	11-13 yrs.
First molar	6-7 yrs.
Second premolar (second bicuspid)	11-12 yrs.
First premolar (first bicuspid)	10-12 yrs.
Canine (cuspid)	9-10 yrs.
Lateral incisor	7-8 yrs.
Central incisor	6-7 yrs.

Figure 31.23 Usual sequence of permanent tooth eruption.

FIGURE 31.24 The young child may need to be restrained so that the throat examination can be done safely.

Tonsils usually cannot be seen in the infant. As the child becomes a toddler, the tonsils become dramatically larger and then begin to decrease in size again by the ninth year. The tonsils should be pink and often have crypts on their surfaces, which are sometimes filled with debris. Is the uvula at midline? Does it rise if the gag reflex is elicited (cranial nerve X [vagus])? Inspect the oropharynx, which should be pink and free from exudate.

▶ *Take* NOTE!

If a gag reflex is inadvertently elicited in the very ill child, the airway may become compromised. Therefore, the pharynx should be examined by asking the child to say "aaah" rather than by depressing the tongue with a tongue depressor.

Thorax and Lungs

Assessment of the thorax and lungs begins by observing the shape and contour of the thorax and determining work of breathing. Accurate auscultation of the lungs is essential, since children often have respiratory infections and disorders and may exhibit alterations in respiratory effort and breath sounds. Note the child's color, which should be pink; cyanosis indicates hypoxia. Listen for audible stridor (inspiratory high-pitched sound), expiratory grunting or snoring, audible wheezing (heard with the naked ear), or cough. Document type and extent of cough. Observe the nail beds for clubbing, which occurs with diseases inducing chronic hypoxic states.

Thorax

Examine the chest with the head in a midline position to determine size and shape as well as symmetry, movement, and bony landmarks. The newborn's chest should be smooth and round, with the transverse diameter nearly equal to the anterior-posterior diameter. The shape of the chest progresses to that of the adult by age 5 to 6 years. At that time the anterior-posterior diameter is about half the transverse diameter (Fig. 31.25). At the point where the xiphoid process and the right and left costal margins meet, the costal angle should measure 90 degrees or less. Inspect for structural deformity such as pectus excavatum (depressed sternum) or pectus carinatum (protuberant sternum) (Fig. 31.26). Note symmetric movement of the chest wall with respiration. Infants and younger children are primarily diaphragmatic breathers, so the abdomen and chest will rise and fall together. Older children, particularly adolescent females, demonstrate thoracic breathing, yet the abdomen and chest should continue to rise and fall together. Asymmetry of chest wall movement is an abnormal finding.

A

B

FIGURE 31.25 (**A**) The newborn's chest is round. (**B**) The adult chest has an anterior-posterior diameter about twice the transverse diameter.

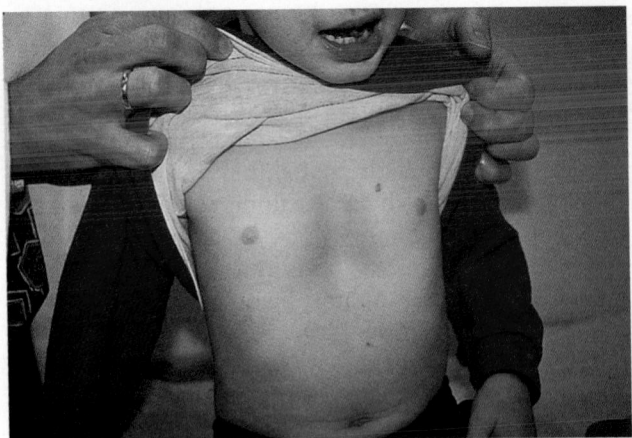

FIGURE 31.26 Pectus excavatum: note depression in xiphoid area.

Observe the depth and regularity of respirations, noting the length of the inspiratory and expiratory phases in relation to each other. The newborn and young infant demonstrate an irregular respiratory pattern. Older infants and children should have a more regular respiratory pattern.

Assess the child's respiratory effort by first observing for nasal flaring, which indicates labored breathing. Observe the chest wall and shoulders for accessory muscle use, which normally is not present. If retractions are present, note their location and severity. Typical locations for retraction include the intercostal, subcostal, substernal, suprasternal, and clavicular regions (Fig. 31.27). Pay attention to the position the child naturally assumes to breathe comfortably: children in respiratory distress often sit forward and are uncomfortable lying down or talking.

Lungs

Experienced examiners may palpate and percuss the lungs before using **auscultation** to evaluate the breath sounds. Palpate for symmetric respiratory excursion by placing the thumbs and fingers together along the costal margin on

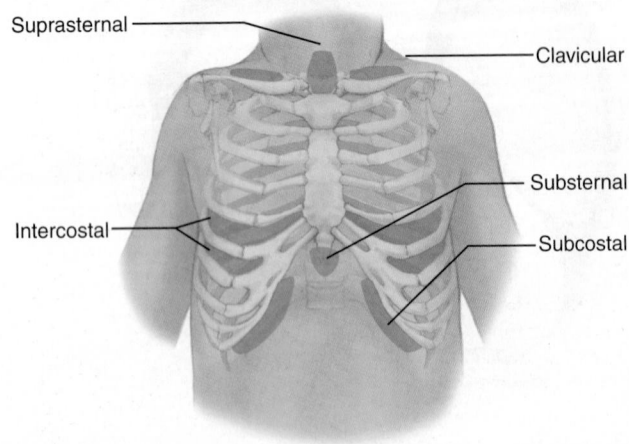

FIGURE 31.27 Location of retractions.

the chest or back. Movement should be symmetric with each breath. Palpate for the normal presence of tactile fremitus with the palms or fingertips while the infant is crying or the older child says "99." Indirectly percuss the lungs of older children, noting resonance over lung fields. Hyperresonance may be present in conditions resulting in hyperaeration of the lungs, such as asthma.

Auscultation

Use the bell of the stethoscope or switch to a small diaphragm to auscultate lung sounds in the infant or child. The adult-sized diaphragm may be used for the adolescent. Auscultate the lung fields with the infant or child in a sitting position, even if that requires propping the infant in a parent's lap. Infants and young children have loud breath sounds because of their thin chest walls. Breath sounds should be clear with adequate aeration throughout all lung fields. Listen to a full inspiration and expiration at the apices of the lungs as well as symmetrically across the entire lung field, systematically comparing the right to the left side. Listen on the anterior chest, posterior chest, and in the axillary regions.

Playing games may encourage younger children to cooperate with deep breathing during lung assessment. The child can blow a cotton ball up in the air, blow a pinwheel, or "blow out" the light of the penlight. Older children are capable of deep breathing when instructed to do so.

The child who has a respiratory disorder or who is experiencing respiratory distress may exhibit diminished breath sounds, most often in the lung bases. Diminished breath sounds are softer and quieter than lung sounds demonstrating adequate aeration. In the healthy infant or child, no adventitious sounds should be heard. If noisy breath sounds are heard in the infant or young child, particularly over all lung fields, compare the sound to the noises heard over the trachea or within the nose. Infants and young children with secretions in the nasopharyngeal area may have those sounds transmitted over the lung fields. These sounds usually clear with coughing or airway suctioning; they are not true adventitious sounds. Note adventitious breath sounds such as wheezes or crackles, documenting their location and whether they are present on inspiration, expiration, or both. It is most important to describe the abnormal breath sounds being heard rather than attempting to classify the sounds. Adventitious lung sounds are associated with a variety of disorders, and extensive experience is required to appropriately classify lung sounds. Adventitious breath sounds should be reported for further evaluation.

Breasts

Assess the breasts of children of all ages and both genders. Note the size of the breasts in relation to the age of the child. Palpate the axillary lymph nodes during the breast assessment.

Inspection

Observe the breasts for position, shape, size, symmetry, and color. Newborns of both genders may have swollen nipples from the influence of maternal estrogen, but by several weeks of age the nipples should be flat and should continue to be so in all prepubertal children. In children the nipples are located lateral to the midclavicular line, usually between the fourth and fifth rib. The areola becomes darker in color as the child approaches puberty. Overweight children may appear to have enlarged breasts due to adipose tissue. Note the location of additional (supernumerary) nipples if present (usually located along the mammary ridge); they may appear as darkly pigmented elevated or nipple-like spots. These are usually of no concern as they do not change over time, but they may be associated with renal disorders.

Inspect the breasts for the current stage of development: widening of the areola, elevation of the nipple, and increase in breast size. Female breast development may begin as early as age 8 but starts by age 13 in most girls. Breast development then continues in a characteristic pattern but usually is asymmetric, with one breast larger than the other throughout the lifespan. The sexual maturity rating scale developed by Tanner in 1962 is used to describe breast development (**Tanner stages**; Fig. 31.28). Adolescent boys may develop gynecomastia (enlargement of the breast tissue) due to hormonal pubertal changes. When the hormone levels stabilize, male adolescents then have flat nipples. Occasionally gynecomastia is caused by marijuana use, anabolic steroids, or hormonal dysfunction.

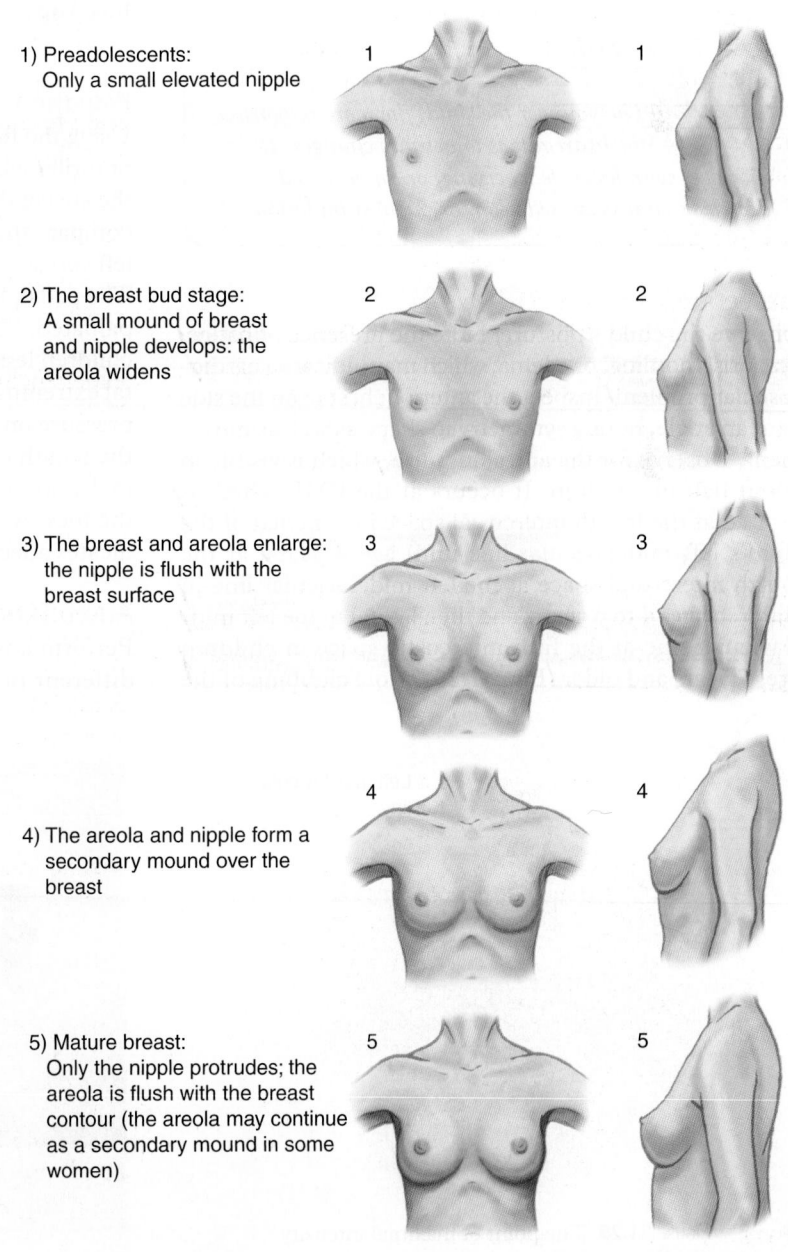

1) Preadolescents:
   Only a small elevated nipple

2) The breast bud stage:
   A small mound of breast and nipple develops: the areola widens

3) The breast and areola enlarge: the nipple is flush with the breast surface

4) The areola and nipple form a secondary mound over the breast

5) Mature breast:
   Only the nipple protrudes; the areola is flush with the breast contour (the areola may continue as a secondary mound in some women)

FIGURE 31.28 Tanner sexual maturity rating for breast development.

Palpation

Palpate the breasts in a systematic fashion. A tender nodule palpated just under the nipple confirms pubertal changes. This change may be difficult to assess in girls with excessive adipose tissue. Normal breast tissue should feel smooth, firm, and elastic. Note masses or nodules if present. Palpate for axillary lymph nodes with the child's arms relaxed at the side but slightly abducted. Note size and texture of nodes if present.

Heart and Peripheral Perfusion

The examination of the heart in children is identical to that of adults except for the focus of the examiner's attention. Congenital heart defects are the most common cause of heart problems in children, and children with these defects present differently than adults with heart disease.

> ▶ *Take* NOTE!
>
> *The younger the child, the more responsive the heart rate is to activity changes. It increases with fever, fear, crying, or anxiety and decreases with sleep, sedation, or vagal stimulation.*

Inspection

Observe the child's posture. Note the presence of pallor, cyanosis, mottling, or edema, which may indicate a cardiovascular problem. Inspect the anterior chest from the side or at an angle, noting symmetry in shape as well as movement. Observe for the apical impulse, which is visible in about half of children. It occurs at the PMI, which is located at the fourth intercostal space just medial of the child's left midclavicular line until age 4 years, at the fourth intercostal space at the left midclavicular line in children ages 4 to 6 years, and then lateral to the left midclavicular line at the fifth intercostal space in children ages 7 years and older (Fig. 31.29). Note clubbing of the

FIGURE 31.30 It is important to assess brachial and femoral pulses simultaneously to determine equality or differences in strength and intensity.

fingertips or distention of neck veins, both of which may be associated with congenital heart disease.

Palpation

Using the fingertips, palpate the chest for lifts and heaves or thrills, which are not normal. Palpate the apical pulse in the area of the PMI (see Fig. 31.29). Check the pulses and compare the upper body to lower body pulses, as well as left versus right, noting strength and quality (Fig. 31.30). The pedal, brachial, and femoral pulses are usually easily palpated. The radial pulse is very difficult to palpate in children less than 2 years of age. Note warmth of the distal extremities. To assess capillary refill time, place slight pressure on the nail beds and quickly release it. Observe the length of time required for refill and return to original color. Compare capillary refill time of the fingers to the toes. A capillary refill time of less than 3 seconds indicates adequacy of perfusion.

Auscultation

Perform auscultation of the heart with the child in two different positions, upright and reclined (Fig. 31.31).

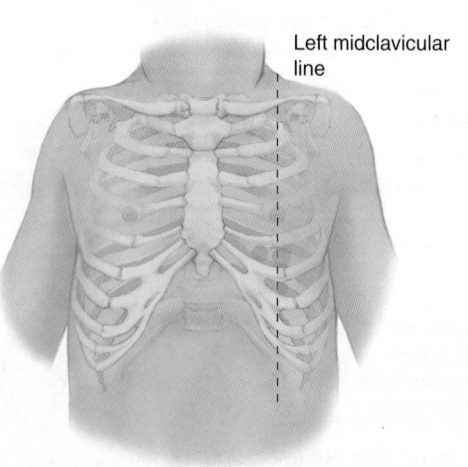

FIGURE 31.29 The point of maximal intensity (PMI) or apical impulse.

Left midclavicular line

FIGURE 31.31 Auscultating the child's heart.

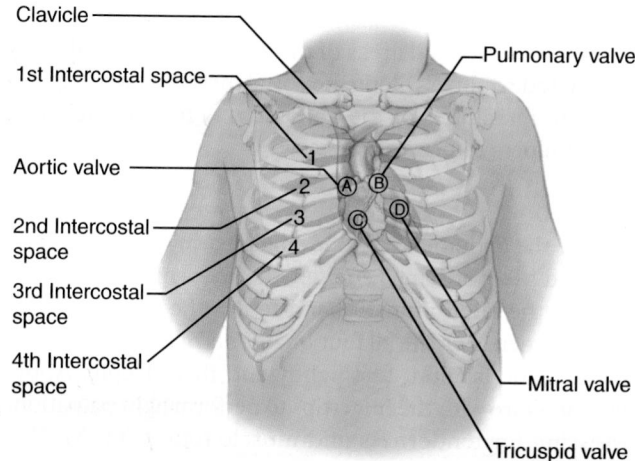

Clavicle

1st Intercostal space

Aortic valve

2nd Intercostal space

3rd Intercostal space

4th Intercostal space

Pulmonary valve

Mitral valve

Tricuspid valve

FIGURE 31.32 Areas where the sounds of heart valves radiate. A: Aortic valve—second intercostal space, just right of sternum. P: Pulmonic valve—second intercostal space, just left of sternum. T: Tricuspid valve—fourth intercostal space, just right of sternum. M: Mitral valve—fourth intercostal space at left midclavicular line.

occurs in many infants and young children. S3 may be heard in many healthy children and is considered normal, though the child with a chronic cardiac condition may develop an S3 when congestive heart failure is present. S4 is usually considered abnormal, most often occurring with cardiac disease.

Sinus arrhythmia is a common and normal finding in children and adolescents. It results in an irregular heart rhythm: the heart rate increases with inhalation and decreases with exhalation. If the child holds his or her breath, the rhythm becomes regular.

▶ **Take** NOTE!

S1 should not vary in intensity at a particular point. If it does, this may indicate a cardiac arrhythmia and the child should be referred for further evaluation.

Auscultate the heart rate in the area of the PMI (see Fig. 31.29). As you begin auscultation, listen first for respirations and note their timing so as not to confuse the heart sounds with the lung sounds. A crying infant may help by briefly holding his or her breath between cries. Once you are confident that you are listening to the heart, be sure to listen for 1 to 3 minutes because of the irregularity of rhythms in some children. Count the heart rate, which should be consistent with the palpated pulse (either radial or brachial).

Develop a systematic approach to auscultation of the heart. Listen over all four valvular areas anteriorly (Fig. 31.32). In the infant or younger child, also auscultate the heart in the axillary region and posteriorly (certain murmurs radiate to these areas). Note S1, S2, extra heart sounds, or murmurs. S1 is usually loudest at the mitral and tricuspid areas and increases in intensity with fever, exercise, and anemia. S2 is usually most intense at the aortic and pulmonic areas. A split S2 heard at the apex

Auscultate for murmurs. Note the location (where it is heard best or loudest) and timing of the murmur. A systolic murmur occurs in association with S1 (closure of the atrioventricular valves), a diastolic murmur in association with S2 (closure of the semilunar valves). Also note the duration of murmur. Does it occur early or late in diastole or systole? Does it occur all the way across systole (holosystolic)? Note the intensity of the murmur. Table 31.5 discusses grading of murmur intensity.

Innocent murmurs occur frequently in children because of the child's more dynamic circulation, thin chest wall, and angulated vessels. An innocent murmur is most often heard at the second or fourth intercostal space, and its timing is systolic. The innocent murmur is usually medium-pitched and musical. Often an innocent murmur disappears when the child changes position. A venous hum that is heard in the supraclavicular area and possibly radiating down the chest is considered an innocent murmur. Refer any child with a murmur to an experienced practitioner for further evaluation.

TABLE 31.5   GRADING HEART MURMURS IN CHILDREN

Grade	Sound
1	Barely audible; sometimes heard, sometimes not. Usually heard only with intense concentration
2	Quiet, soft; heard each time the chest is auscultated
3	Audible, intermediate intensity
4	Audible, with a palpable thrill
5	Loud, audible with edge of the stethoscope lifted off the chest
6	Very loud, audible with the stethoscope placed near but not touching the chest

Abdomen

The abdomen contains organs related to the genitourinary and lymphatic systems, in addition to the gastrointestinal system. These structures lie within the abdomen in approximately the same location as they do in adults. Dividing the abdomen into quadrants simplifies the description of normal organ location and the reporting of abnormalities. Draw an imaginary vertical line from the xiphoid process to the symphysis pubis. Cross this with an imaginary perpendicular line through the umbilicus. The sequence of physical examination is altered for the abdominal assessment: auscultation is done before percussion and palpation because manipulation of the lower abdomen may affect the bowel sounds.

Inspection

Inspect the abdomen for size, shape, and symmetry. The abdomen in the infant and toddler is rounded and protuberant until the abdominal musculature becomes well developed. Though rounded, the abdomen should not be distended (at any age). By adolescence, the stature is more erect and the abdomen begins to appear flat when standing and concave when supine. The thin skin of a young child may allow the visualization of superficial venous circulation across the abdomen. Inspect the abdomen for movement. At eye level with the abdomen, note abdomen and thorax movement occurring simultaneously. Visible peristaltic waves are abnormal and should be reported immediately.

Inspect the newborn's umbilicus for color, bleeding, odor, and drainage. The umbilical stump should slowly dry, become black and hard, and fall away from the cutaneous navel by the end of the second week of life. Note drainage or granulation at the umbilical site indicating delayed drying of the umbilical stump. Inspect the umbilicus in older infants and young children for the presence of umbilical hernia. Because the umbilicus divides the rectus abdominis muscle, it is not uncommon to see an umbilical hernia protrude through and become larger when the infant or toddler strains or cries. This is a benign finding and will usually disappear as the abdomen becomes stronger. Adolescents may have jewelry piercing the umbilicus.

Auscultation

Auscultate the abdomen using the diaphragm or the bell of the stethoscope pressed firmly against the abdomen. Count the bowel sounds in each of the four quadrants for a full minute. Bowel sounds should be present by a few hours after birth and should remain active throughout life. Note whether bowel sounds are normally active, hyperactive, hypoactive, or absent. Normal bowel sounds can be described as growls, gurgles and clicking sounds. Hypoactive bowel sounds may occur postoperatively. Hyperactive bowels sounds are common with diarrhea. Classify bowel sounds as absent after listening for 5 full minutes in each area. Absent bowel sounds may indicate ileus or peritonitis.

Percussion

Indirectly percuss all areas of the abdomen. Normal findings include dullness along the costal margins and tympany over the remainder of the abdomen. A full bladder may yield dullness to percussion.

Palpation

Palpate the abdomen with the child in a supine position. If the child's legs are small enough, the knees may be brought up with the nondominant hand to flex the hips and relax the abdomen. Palpate all four quadrants of the abdomen in a systematic fashion, first lightly and then deeply. Apply light pressure with the fingertips to perform light palpation, assessing for tenderness and muscle tone (Fig. 31.33). Note skin turgor by gently elevating a piece of skin and allowing it to fall back into place. Perform deep palpation to assess the organs and any masses. Place one hand on top of the other and palpate from the lower quadrants to the upper (see Fig. 31.33). The edge of the liver may be felt at the right costal margin, and the tip of the spleen can be felt at the left costal margin. The descending colon may be felt in the left lower quadrant as a small column and the blad-

FIGURE 31.33 (**A**) Light and (**B**) deep palpation of the abdomen.

der as a soft balloon below the umbilicus. The kidneys are rarely palpable. The abdomen should be soft and nontender to palpation. Report firmness, tenderness, or masses. Palpate the inguinal area for the presence of hernia or enlarged lymph nodes.

> ▶ **Take** NOTE!
>
> *To decrease ticklishness with abdominal palpation, place a flat, warm, still hand on the abdomen while distracting the child before palpation begins. An alternate technique is to first palpate with the child's hand under the examiner's hand.*

Genitalia and Anus

Examination of the genitals should immediately follow the abdominal assessment in the younger child and should be reserved for the end of the assessment in the adolescent. Though the anus is part of the gastrointestinal tract, it is best assessed during the genital examination. Ensure privacy for the older child and adolescent. Keep the child covered as much as possible. Use a casual, matter-of-fact approach to place the child or teen at ease. During the genital examination, teach the child or adolescent about normal variations and changes with puberty, as well as issues related to health promotion.

Male

Inspect the penis and scrotum for size, color, skin integrity, and obvious masses. The obese boy's penis may appear small because of additional skin folds. Penis size should correlate with pubertal stage (Fig. 31.34). The penis may have a foreskin that covers the glans, protecting and lubricating it. If present, do not forcibly retract the foreskin. In circumcised males the urinary meatus is exposed and should be at the tip of the glans. Assess the meatus for absence of discharge. If possible, observe the stream of urine for strength of flow and patency of the urethral orifice. Skin lesions may indicate sexually transmitted infection. A foreskin that cannot be retracted in a boy over 3 years of age may indicate phimosis. Report abnormal findings.

> ▶ **Take** NOTE!
>
> *When you first remove a male infant's diaper, this is the ideal time to assess the force of the urine stream and the erection reflex, as the cool air may make the infant void and briefly experience an erection.*

From top to bottom:

1) No pubic hair and scrotum size and proportion the same as during childhood

2) Few straight hairs at base of penis, little or no penis enlargement, testes/scrotum begin to enlarge

3) Sparse pubic hair growth over entire pubis, penis begins to lengthen, scrotum continues to enlarge

4) Thick pubic hair growth but not on thighs, penis grows in length and diameter, testes almost full grown

5) Pubic hair growth spread over medial thighs, penis and scrotum are adult size and shape

FIGURE 31.34 Tanner male sexual maturity rating for genitalia and pubic hair.

Assess the presence and distribution of pubic hair. Inspect the scrotum for size, slight asymmetry, color, and absence of edema. The scrotum may initially be swollen from birth trauma or maternal hormones, but this swelling should decrease in the first few days of life. The scrotum is ordinarily more deeply pigmented than the rest of the boy's skin. Figure 31.34 illustrates scrotal changes that occur with puberty. Assess the testicles by placing one finger over the inguinal canal and palpating the scrotum with the other. This prevents the retractile testes in a young child from slipping back up the inguinal canal. The testicles should be smooth, of similar sizes, and freely move-

FIGURE 31.35 Placing a digit over the inguinal canal during testicular palpation prevents retraction of the testis into the canal.

Stage 1 Preadolescents.
No pubic hair. Mons and labia covered with fine vellus hair as on abdomen.

Stage 2 Growth sparse and mostly on labia. Long, downy hair, slightly pigmented, straight or only slightly curly.

Stage 3 Growth sparse and spreading over mons pubis. Hair darker, coarser, curlier.

Stage 4 Hair is adult in type but over smaller area; none on medial thigh.

Stage 5 Adult in type and pattern; inverse triangle. Also on medial thigh surface.

FIGURE 31.36 Tanner female sexual maturity rating for pubic hair.

able. The infant's testicles may be palpated in the scrotum or in the inguinal canal, where they can be easily moved into the scrotum with gentle pressure from the examiner's nondominant hand (Fig. 31.35). Beyond infancy, allow the boy to sit cross-legged to reduce the cremasteric reflex that retracts the testicles during palpation. An adolescent boy may need to stand for the nurse to fully palpate the scrotum. Document the presence of both testicles in the scrotal sac, if they are retractile, or if they are absent. Report undescended testicle or other abnormal findings.

Female

In most cases, the female genitalia examination is limited to assessment of the external genitalia. Internal examination is not routinely performed before maturity unless the adolescent anticipates becoming or is sexually active or requests birth control or if pathology is suspected. If an internal examination is needed, refer the child or adolescent to the appropriate advanced practitioner or physician.

Position the infant in the parent's lap or on the examination table or crib. The toddler or preschooler should be examined in the parent's lap, in a frog-legged position. The school-age or adolescent girl should lie on the examination table or bed. Provide for privacy by keeping the genital area covered until it is time for the examination.

Perform the assessment of the external genitalia in a systematic fashion. First, determine the presence and distribution of pubic hair. Infants and young girls (particular those of dark-skinned races) may have a small amount of downy pubic hair. Otherwise, the appearance of pubic hair indicates the onset of pubertal changes, sometimes prior to breast changes. Pubic hair generally begins to appear by age 11 years, with age 13 being the latest. Figure 31.36 illustrates the development of pubic hair through puberty in girls.

Inspect the labia majora and minora for size, color, and skin integrity. The newborn's labia minora are swollen from the effects of maternal estrogen but will decrease in size and be hidden by the labia majora within the first weeks of life. Redness or swelling of the labia may occur with infection, sexual abuse, or masturbation. Lesions on the external genitalia may indicate sexually transmitted infection. Gently spread the labia to inspect the clitoris, urethral meatus, and vaginal opening. Some girls may prefer to spread the labia themselves. The urinary meatus and vaginal orifice should be visible and not occluded by the hymen. It is not uncommon to see a hymenal tag. Note clitoral size. Inspect the urinary meatus and vaginal opening for edema or redness, which should not be present. Observe for any vaginal discharge. A small amount of blood-tinged or mucoid discharge may be noted in the first few weeks of life as a result of maternal hormone exposure. A small amount of clear mucus-like discharge is normal in all females. If present, document labial adhesion or other abnormal findings.

Anus

Inspect the anal area for fissures, rash, hemorrhoids, prolapse, or skin tags. Examine the infant's anal area while examining the genitalia. The younger child may lie back in the parent's lap and flex the knees to the chest. The older child or adolescent may be prone or in a side-lying position. If the adolescent boy is already standing for the scrotal assessment, have him bend forward so that you can assess the anal area. The anus should appear moist and hairless. Gently stroke the anal area to elicit the anal reflex (quick contraction). If indicated, inspect anal sphincter tone by inserting a gloved finger lubricated with water-soluble jelly just inside the anal sphincter.

Musculoskeletal

Assessment of the musculoskeletal system includes examination of the clavicles and shoulders, spine, extremities, joints, and hips. Determining the child's ability to move all extremities through the full range of motion is also important.

Clavicles and Shoulders

Palpate the clavicles. In the newborn, tenderness or crepitus reveals a fracture sustained at birth. In the older infant or child, a bump indicates callus formation with clavicle fracture. Test shoulder strength and the function of cranial nerve XI in the older child by requesting that the child shrug the shoulders while you apply downward pressure.

Spine

Observe the child's resting posture and alignment of the trunk. The newborn's position will look like the position the baby preferred *in utero* and is one of general flexion. The older infant moves more and can sit unassisted in the second half of the first year. Toddlers stand with a wide-based gait, a slightly swayed back, and the abdomen slightly protruding. The posture straightens in the preschool and school-age years. Adolescents often demonstrate kyphosis as the skeleton and muscles are both growing rapidly (Fig. 31.37).

Inspect the child's spine. The newborn's spine has a single C-shaped curve and remains rounded for the first 3 months of life. The cervical curve begins to develop around 3 to 4 months of age as the baby gains head control. By 12 to 18 months of age, the lumbar curve develops, which corresponds to the onset of walking. The S-shaped spine in older children and adolescents is similar to that of the adult's. The spine should be flexible, with good muscle tone and no rigidity. Assess the back, and hip and shoulder heights for symmetry.

Examine the preadolescent and adolescent for the development of scoliosis. Refer to Chapter 44 for information about scoliosis screening. Scoliosis screening is

FIGURE 31.37 The teen's posture often demonstrates kyphosis.

generally performed during well-child examinations by the physician or nurse practitioner or by the middle or high school nurse on a particular day of the school year.

Note mobility of the vertebral column by having the child bend forward and side to side. Flex the neck and move it from side to side. No resistance or pain should occur. Inspect the back for discoloration, tufts of hair, or dimples. A normal pilonidal dimple is sometimes seen at the base of the spine, but there should be no tuft of hair or nevi along the spine. Document and report abnormal findings.

Extremities

All children, even newborns, should be able to move all extremities spontaneously. Screen the infant younger than 6 months of age for developmental dysplasia of the hip by performing the Ortolani and Barlow maneuvers (refer to Chapter 44 for additional information). These maneuvers are usually best performed by a proficient examiner. Inspect and palpate the child's upper and lower extremities. Assess for symmetry in size, contour, movement, warmth, and color of the extremities. The infant's feet and legs appear bowed secondary to *in utero* positioning but can be straightened through passive range of motion. Observe the child in a standing position. Bowing of the lower legs (internal tibial torsion) lessens as the toddler begins to bear weight and usually resolves in the second or third year of life as the strength of the muscles and bones increases. When it persists past that time, it is termed genu varum (bow legs). Genu valgum (knock knee) is usually present until the child is 7 years old. Observe the child walking, noting any difficulty with leg position or balance.

If the child is reluctant to walk, use play as a way to elicit the behavior. The school-age child should have gait and leg appearance similar to that of the adult.

Note the normal flat foot in the toddler and young child. The arch develops as the child grows and the muscles become less lax, though some children may continue with flexible flat feet; this is considered a normal variation.

Perform passive range of motion of the young infant's extremities. Inability to straighten the foot to midline may indicate clubfoot. Count the fingers and toes, noting abnormalities such as polydactyly (increased number of digits) or syndactyly (webbing of the digits). Palpate the joints for warmth or tenderness. Check the mobility of the joints of the upper and lower extremities by performing range of motion. Determine lower extremity muscle strength by having the child push against the examiner's hands with the soles of the forefoot. Assess upper extremity strength by having the child squeeze the examiner's crossed fingers and/or push up or down against the examiner's outstretched hands.

► *Take* NOTE!

Slight tremors may be noticed in the infant's extremities in the first month of life.

Neurologic

The neurologic examination should include level of consciousness, balance and coordination, sensory function, and reflexes. Motor function is assessed within the musculoskeletal section. Cranial nerve function is generally tested within other portions of the physical assessment as it applies to that section.

Level of Consciousness

Note the state of alertness and attentiveness to parents and the environment in the newborn and infant. Older infants become interactive with other people, as do toddlers and preschoolers. Younger children demonstrate orientation by positive interaction with family members and by crying or fussing when they feel threatened. By school age, the child should be oriented to name and place and a few years later should be able to state the date as well (even if only the day of the week).

Balance and Coordination

Balance and coordination are controlled by the cerebellum. Observe the child's gait to assess balance and coordination. Observe toddlers and older children rising and walking from a seated and supine position. They should be able to stand and balance without straining or holding

on to objects. Continue to test cerebellar function by having the younger child skip or hop and requesting that the older child or adolescent walk heel to toe. Further tests of cerebellar function responsible for balance and coordination are discussed in Box 31.3. Demonstrate each test and make sure the child understands your instructions.

Sensory Testing

Portions of sensory testing related to most of the cranial nerves, vision, hearing, taste, and smell have already been incorporated into other sections as appropriate within the physical assessment. Test cranial nerve V (trigeminal) by lightly touching the child's cheek with a cotton ball. The young infant will root toward the side that is touched. With the child's eyes closed, ask the child to identify other locations where he or she is lightly touched (several different ones) to assess sensation. Ask the child to tell you when he or she is touched. Make a game of this activity to encourage cooperation in younger children. In the older child who knows the definition of sharp and dull, test for these sensations with the child's eyes closed. Use the rounded end of a tongue blade for dull and the broken edge of a tongue blade for the sharp sensation. The child should be able to discriminate the sensations of sharp and dull.

BOX 31.3 **Cerebellar Function Testing**

- **Romberg:** Ask the school-age or older child to stand still with eyes closed and arms down by the sides. Observe the child for leaning (stand close in case this does occur). This is considered a positive Romberg test, indicating cerebellar dysfunction.

For the following tests, the child should demonstrate accuracy and smoothness:
- **Heel-to-shin:** Have the child lie in a supine position, place one heel on the opposite knee, and run it down the shin.
- **Rapid alternating movements:** The child pats the thighs with the hands, lifts them, turns them over, pats the thighs with the back of the hands, and repeats the process multiple times. An alternate test is for the child to touch the thumb to each finger of the same hand starting at the index finger, then reverse the direction and repeat.
- **Finger-to-finger:** The child's eyes are open. The child touches the examiner's outstretched finger with the index finger, then touches his or her own nose. The examiner moves the finger to a different spot and the child repeats this process several times.
- **Finger-to-nose:** The child's eyes are closed. The child stretches the arm with the index finger extended, then touches his or her nose with that finger, keeping the eyes closed.

Reflexes

Assess the infant's primitive and protective reflexes. The primitive reflexes involve a whole-body response and are subcortical in nature. Selected primitive reflexes present at birth include Moro, root, suck, asymmetric tonic neck, plantar and palmar grasp, step, and Babinski. Most of the primitive reflexes diminish over the first few months of life, giving way to protective or postural reflexes. Protective reflexes are motor responses related to maintenance of equilibrium. They are necessary for appropriate motor development and remain throughout life once they are established. The protective reflexes include the righting and parachute reactions.

Place one finger in each of the infant's hands to elicit the palmar grasp reflex (usually disappears by age 3 to 4 months). Touch the thumb to the ball of the infant's foot to elicit the plantar grasp reflex. The infant's toes will curl down (this reflex disappears by 8 to 10 months). Refer to Table 25.2 and Figures 25.1 through 25.6 in Chapter 25 for additional explanation of the other reflexes. Appropriate presence and disappearance of primitive reflexes, as well as development of protective reflexes, is indicative of a healthy neurologic system. Primitive reflexes that persist beyond the usual age of disappearance may indicate an abnormality of the neurologic system and should be further investigated.

Assess deep tendon reflexes in all infants and children. Appropriate responses indicate that the reflex arc is intact. Use the reflex hammer in all ages or the curved tips of the two first fingers to elicit the responses in infants. The limb must be relaxed and the muscle partly stretched. Use a snapping motion of the wrist to tap with the fingertips or the reflex hammer. Test the biceps, triceps, patellar, and Achilles reflexes as you would in the adult. It may help to place a finger under the infant's knee to encourage relaxation. Young children who tense up when their reflexes are being tested may relax the area if you have them focus on another area, so have the child clasp the hands while testing the Achilles and patellar reflexes. As the child focuses on the hands, the lower extremities relax. Distraction may also be helpful.

Grade the strength of the response using the standard scale from 0 to 4+:

• 0: no response
• 1+: diminished or sluggish
• 2+: average
• 3+: brisker than average
• 4+: very brisk, may involve clonus

The newborn's deep tendon reflexes are normally brisk (3+). They decrease to average (2+), usually by 4 months of age. Healthy children should have reflexes of 2+ if the reflex has been elicited properly. Absent, sluggish, or hyperreactive responses usually indicate disease.

Refer back to Elliot, the 3-year-old from the beginning of the chapter. What are some important considerations when performing his physical examination?

▪▪▪ Key Concepts

■ The health history in children includes more than just the chief complaint, history of present illness, and past medical history; it is important to include the perinatal history and developmental milestones.

■ Allow the chief complaint to determine which parts of the history require more in-depth investigation.

■ The developmental history will warrant more attention in the younger child, while school performance and adjustment will be more important in the school-age child and adolescent.

■ Though the parent will provide most of the health history for the infant and young child, allow the young verbal child to answer questions during the health history as appropriate.

■ Direct health history questions to the school-age child and adolescent, seeking clarification from the parents as needed.

■ Provide confidentiality and privacy for the adolescent during the health history.

■ Weight and length or height should be assessed at each well-child visit to determine adequacy of growth.

■ Measure head circumference until age 3 years to monitor brain growth.

■ Perform hearing and vision screenings for children of all ages.

■ BMI can be used to identify children who are overweight or at risk for being overweight.

■ The normal range of vital signs varies based on the child's age.

■ The sequence of the physical examination in children should be based on the child's developmental age, his or her level of cooperation, and the severity of the illness.

■ Obtain heart rate and respiratory rate and auscultate the heart and lungs while the infant or young child is quiet.

■ Perform intrusive procedures such as examination of the ears, mouth, and throat last in the infant or young child.

■ Perform the health assessment in a head-to-toe fashion in the school-age child or adolescent, reserving the genitalia and anus examination for last.

■ Plan the health assessment in such a way as to minimize trauma to the child or adolescent.

■ Use age-appropriate measurement tools to assess pain in children.

■ Allow the infant or young child to remain in the parent's lap for as much of the assessment as possible so that the child feels secure.

- Use age-appropriate games during the health assessment to gain cooperation in the younger child.

- Having the young boy sit cross-legged for a testicular examination may reduce the cremasteric reflex.

- The newborn may exhibit a wide variety of normal skin variations.

- The infant's fontanels should be soft and flat; report a bulging fontanel immediately.

- Jaundice (outside of the newborn period), pallor, cyanosis, and poor skin turgor indicate illness and may need immediate intervention.

- Heart murmurs should be assessed for intensity, location, and duration. They may be innocent or may indicate a congenital heart defect.

- The infant's chest wall is relatively thin, allowing upper airway sounds to be transmitted throughout the lung fields.

- Substernal or xiphoid retractions indicate that the child is laboring to breathe, whereas a fixed, depressed sternum (pectus excavatum) is a structural abnormality.

- The Tanner stages of sexual maturity provide a basis for assessing pubertal development in boys and girls. Use the breast and pubic hair charts for girls and the pubic hair and penis and scrotum size chart for boys.

REFERENCES

American Academy for Pediatric Ophthalmology and Strabismus. (2005). *Vision screening for infants and children.* Retrieved October 6, 2007 from http://www.aapos.org/displaycommon.cfm?an=1&subarticlenbr=54.

American Academy of Pediatrics. (2000). Clinical practice guideline: Early detection of developmental dysplasia of the hip (AC0001). *Pediatrics, 105*(4), 896–905.

American Academy of Pediatrics. (2007). Year 2007 position statement: Principles and guidelines for early hearing detection and intervention programs. *Pediatrics, 120*, 898–921.

Anonymous. (n.d.). Points on the pediatric physical exam. Columbia University College of Physicians and Surgeons, Pediatric Clerkship. Available at http://www.columbia.edu/itc/hs/medical/clerkships/peds/Student_Information/Reference_Materials/Pediatric_PE.html#PhysicalExam.

Barnes, K. (2004). *Paediatrics: A clinical guide for nurse practitioners.* New York: Elsevier.

Barton, S. J., Gaffney, R., Chase, T., Rayens, M. K., & Piyabanditkul, L. (2003). Pediatric temperature measurement and child/parent/nurse preference using three temperature measurement instruments. *Journal of Pediatric Nursing, 18*(1), 314–320.

Benjamin, J. T. (2004). *The continuity clinic notebook: An unfinished story (Department of Pediatrics, Medical College of Georgia).* Retrieved April 20, 2006, from http://www.mcg.edu/pediatrics/CCNotebook/index.htm.

Burns, C., Dunn, A., Brady, M., Starr, N., & Blosser, C. (2004). *Pediatric primary care: A handbook for nurse practitioners.* Philadelphia: W. B. Saunders.

Centers for Disease Control and Prevention. (2007). *Using the BMI-for-age growth charts.* Retrieved October 6, 2007, from http://www.cdc.gov/nccdphp/dnpa/growthcharts/training/modules/module1/text/page1a.htm

Centers for Disease Control and Prevention. (2007). *CDC growth charts: United States.* Retrieved October 6, 2007, from http://www.cdc.gov/nchs/about/major/nhanes/growthcharts/background.htm.

Centers for Disease Control and Prevention. (2007). *Clinical growth charts.* Retrieved October 6, 2007, from http://www.cdc.gov/nchs/about/major/nhanes/growthcharts/clinical_charts.htm.

DeMeulenaere, S. (2007). Pulse oximetry: Uses and limitations. *The Journal for Nurse Practitioners, 3*(5), 312–317.

El Radhi, A. S., & Barry, W. (2006). Thermometry in paediatric practice. *Archives of Disease in Childhood, 91*, 351–356.

El Radhi, A. S., & Patel, S. (2006). An evaluation of tympanic thermometry in a paediatric emergency department. *Emergency Medicine Journal, 23*(1), 40–41.

Engel, J. K. (2006). *Mosby's pocket guide to pediatric assessment* (5th ed.). St. Louis: Elsevier.

Erickson, B. A. (2003). *Heart sounds and murmurs across the lifespan, with audiotape* (4th ed.). St. Louis: Elsevier.

Exergen Corporation. (2005). *Temporal artery thermometer consumer information center.* Available at http://www.exergen.com/medical/TAT/tatconsumerpage.htm.

Hebbar, K., Fortenberry, J. D., Merritt, R., & Easley, K. (2005). Comparison of temporal artery thermometer to standard temperature measurements in pediatric intensive care unit patients. *Pediatric Critical Care Medicine, 6*(5), 557–561.

Jarvis, C. (2008). *Physical examination and health assessment* (5th ed.). St. Louis: Saunders.

Kelley, P. E., Friedman, N. R., Johnson, C. E., & Yoon, P. J. (2007). Ear, nose, & throat. In Hay, W. W., Levin, M. J., Sondheimer, J. M., & Deterding, R. R., *Current pediatric diagnosis and treatment* (18th ed.). New York: McGraw-Hill.

Mandleco, B. (2004). *Growth and development handbook: Newborn through adolescence.* Clifton Park, NY: Delmar Learning.

Mandleco, B. (2005). *Pediatric nursing skills and procedures.* Clifton Park, NY: Thomson Delmar.

Mansson, M. E., & Dykes, A. K. (2004). Practices for preparing children for clinical examinations and procedures in Swedish pediatric wards. *Pediatric Nursing, 30*(3), 182–187, 229.

Manworren, R., & Hynan, L. (2003). Clinical validation of FLACC: Preverbal patient pain scale. *Pediatric Nursing, 29*(2), 140–146.

Mau, M. K., Yamasato, K. S., & Yamamoto, L. G. (2005). Normal oxygen saturation values in pediatric patients. *Hawaii Medical Journal, 64*(2), 42, 44–45.

Miller, S. (n.d.). *Introduction to the pediatric physical exam (video).* Columbia University College of Physicians and Surgeons, Pediatric Clerkship. Available at http://www.columbia.edu/itc/hs/medical/clerkships/peds/Student_Information/Reference_Materials/Pediatric_PE.html.

Musumba, C. O., Griffiths, K. L., Ross, A., & Newton, C. R. J. C. (2005). Comparison of axillary, rectal and tympanic temperature measurements in children admitted with malaria. *Journal of Tropical Pediatrics, 51*(4), 242–244.

Nellcor Puritan Bennett, Inc. (2007). *Clinician's guide to Nellcor sensors.* Retrieved October 6, 2007 from http://www.nellcor.com/_Catalog/PDF/Product/CliniciansSensorGuide.pdf.

Nimah, M. M., Bshesh, K., Callahan, J. D., & Jacobs, B. R. (2006). Infrared tympanic thermometry in comparison with other temperature measurement techniques in febrile children. *Pediatric Critical Care Medicine, 7*(1), 48–55.

Ottar-Pfeifer, W. (2005). When should children have their eyes checked? *Insight: The Journal of the American Society of Ophthalmic Registered Nurses, 30*(2), 17–22.

Popovich, D. M., Richiuso, N., & Gale, D. (2004). Pediatric health care providers' knowledge of pulse oximetry. *Pediatric Nursing, 30*(1), 14–20.

Salyer, J. W. (2003). Neonatal and pediatric pulse oximetry. *Respiratory Care, 48*(4), 386–396.

Sands, R., & Drack, A. (2007). Eye. In Hay, W. W., Levin, M. J., Sondheimer, J. M., & Deterding, R. R., *Current pediatric diagnosis & treatment* (18th ed.). New York: McGraw-Hill.

Siberry, G. K., Diener-West, M., Schappell, E., & Karron, R. A. (2005). Comparison of temple temperatures with rectal temperatures in children under two years of age. *Clinical Pediatrics, 41*(6), 405–414.

Sondheimer, H. M., Yetman, A. T., & Miyamoto, S. D. (2007). Cardiovascular diseases. In Hay, W. W., Levin, M. J., Sondheimer, J. M., & Deterding, R. R., *Current pediatric diagnosis & treatment* (18th ed.). New York: McGraw-Hill.

Tanner, J. M. (1962). *Growth at adolescence.* Oxford, England: Blackwell Scientific Publications.

Thilo, E. H. & Rosenberg, A. A. (2007). The newborn infant. In Hay, W. W., Levin, M. J., Sondheimer, J. M., & Deterding, R. R., *Current pediatric diagnosis & treatment* (18th ed.). New York: McGraw-Hill.

U.S. Department of Health and Human Services, National Institutes of Health, National Heart, Lung, and Blood Institute. (2005). *The fourth report on the diagnosis, evaluation, and treatment of high blood pressure in children and adolescents* (NIH Publication No. 05-5267). Washington, D.C.: U.S. Department of Health and Human Services.

U.S. Department of Health and Human Services, Substance Abuse and Mental Health Services Administration. (2006). *Fetal alcohol spectrum disorder (FASD): The basics.* Retrieved October 6, 2007, from http://fascenter.samhsa.gov/educationTraining/fasdBasics.cfm.

Weber, J., & Kelley, J. (2006). *Health assessment in nursing* (3rd ed.). Philadelphia: Lippincott Williams & Wilkins.

Willis, M., Merkel, S., Voepel-Lewis, T., & Malviya, S. (2003). FLACC behavioral pain assessment scale: A comparison with the child's self-report. *Pediatric Nursing, 29*(3), 95–198.

Wong, D., & Baker, C. (1988). Pain in children: Comparison of assessment scales. *Pediatric Nursing, 14*, 9–17.

WEBSITES

American Academy of Pediatrics: www.aap.org

Kids' Health for Kids—Nemours Foundation: kidshealth.org/kid

Maternal and Child Health Bureau: mchb.hrsa.gov

Agency for Healthcare Research and Quality, Child and Adolescent Health: www.ahrq.gov/child

Bright Futures at Georgetown University: www.brightfutures.org

Centers for Disease Control: www.cdc.gov/

Child Trends Data Bank: www.childtrendsdatabank.org

U.S. Food and Drug Administration's Kids' Home Page: www.fda.gov/oc/opacom/kids/default.htm

Healthy People 2010: www.healthypeople.gov

HHS for Kids (U.S. Department of Health and Human Services): www.hhs.gov/kids

National Association of Pediatric Nurse Practitioners: www.napnap.org

Society of Pediatric Nurses: www.pedsnurses.org

Chapter Worksheet

Multiple Choice Questions

1. A 5-year-old boy visits the physician's office with an upper respiratory infection. Which approach would give the nurse the most information about the child's developmental level?

   a. Playing a game with the child.

   b. Talking with the child about the teddy bear next to him.

   c. Using a screening tool during a follow-up office visit.

   d. Asking the 10-year-old sibling about the child.

2. Which statement indicates the best sequence for the nurse to conduct an assessment in a non-emergency situation?

   a. Introduce yourself, ask about any problems, take a history, do the physical examination.

   b. Perform the physical examination and then ask the family if there are any problems in the child's life.

   c. Do the physical examination while at the same time asking about the child's previous illnesses; then talk about the family's concerns.

   d. Get a complete history of the family's health beliefs and practices, then assess the child.

3. What approach by the nurse would most likely encourage a child to cooperate with an assessment of physical and developmental health?

   a. Explain to the child what's going to happen when the child asks questions.

   b. Explain what is going to happen in words the child can understand.

   c. Force them to cooperate by having a parent hold them down.

   d. Give the child a sticker before beginning the examination.

4. A sleeping 5-month-old girl is being held by the mother when the nurse comes in to do a physical examination. What assessment should be done initially?

   a. Listening to the bowel sounds.

   b. Counting the heart rate.

   c. Checking the temperature.

   d. Looking in the ears.

5. Which assessment finding is considered normal in children?

   a. Irregular respiratory rate and rhythm.

   b. Split S2 and sinus arrhythmia.

   c. Decreased heart rate with crying.

   d. Genu varum past the age of 5 years.

Critical Thinking Exercises

1. A soft and muffled heart murmur is heard in a 4-year-old patient. The mother states that she has never heard that the child has a murmur. What should the nurse do?

2. A nurse is helping a new mother breastfeed her 4-day-old baby. The mother notices that the baby has a bluish cast to the skin on his hands and that sometimes the infant has a tremor. She asks the nurse if the baby is cold, though the baby is swaddled and comfortably resting against the mother's skin. How might the nurse help teach this mother?

3. Devise a plan for encouraging cooperation of the toddler or preschooler during various parts of the physical examination.

Study Activities

1. In the clinical setting, obtain a health history on an infant, child, or adolescent.

2. In the clinical setting, compare the approach you use for the physical examination of a toddler versus a school-aged child or adolescent.

3. No matter how thoughtfully and appropriately you plan your assessment, odds are good that you will have difficulty assessing a 2-year-old. Discuss with your classmates the strategies that you have used for success and brainstorm with them about their ideas for assessing a crying or resistant young child.

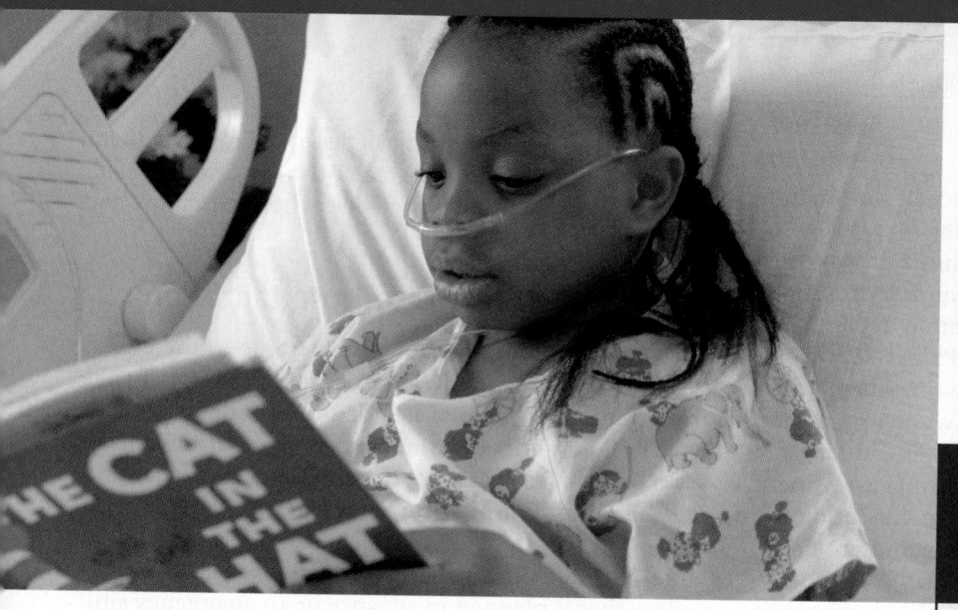

Chapter number "32" appears at top right with image.

CHAPTER 32

NURSING CARE OF CHILDREN DURING ILLNESS AND HOSPITALIZATION

KEY TERMS

child life specialist
denial
magical thinking

regression
sensory deprivation
sensory overload

separation anxiety
therapeutic hugging
therapeutic play

LEARNING OBJECTIVES

Upon completion of the chapter, the learner will be able to:

1. Identify the major impact and stressors of illness and hospitalization for children in the various developmental stages.
2. Identify the reactions and responses of children and their families during illness and hospitalization.
3. Explain the factors that influence the reactions and responses of children and their families during illness and hospitalization
4. Describe the nursing care that minimizes stressors for children who are ill or hospitalized.
5. Discuss the major components of admission for children to the hospital.
6. Outline the nursing interventions required for children in specific units or situations in the hospital.
7. Discuss appropriate safety measures to use when caring for children of all ages.
8. Describe basic care procedures for children in various health care settings.
9. Review the major components and nursing responsibilities related to client education and discharge from the hospital.

Jake Jorgenson, 8 years old, was brought to the clinic with a history of headaches, vomiting not related to feeding, and changes in his gait. Initial testing leads to a suspected brain tumor. Jake is to be admitted to the neurologic service at a pediatric hospital for further testing and treatment. Up until this point he has been a healthy child with no previous hospitalizations. He lives at home with his parents and two siblings, Jenny, age 11, and Joshua, age 5. As a nurse on this unit, how can you help prepare Jake and his family for this hospitalization?

WOW

Sick children need love, hope, faith, and most of all a positive attitude from their nurse.

Illness, with the occasional consequence of hospitalization, affects children and their families in a variety of ways. Hospitalization is often confusing, complex, and overwhelming for children and their families. Reactions and responses to illness and hospitalization depend on a number of factors, including the child's developmental stage. Nursing strategies are needed to prepare children and their families for this experience while minimizing negative effects. These strategies include identifying the needs of children and families through astute assessment of nonverbal and verbal behaviors, then validating the information with accurate interpretation and providing appropriate responses and interventions.

Although the nurse implements these strategies throughout the interaction with the child and family, a critical time to ensure the best outcome for the child and family is during the admission process. The nurse assesses the learning needs and abilities of the child and family. For the interventions to be successful, the nurse must communicate and teach in the most effective method for the individual child and family. The nurse also evaluates the child's and family's competence in performing specific activities prior to discharge.

Hospitalization in Childhood

In today's health care environment, children receive much of their care for illnesses in community health settings such as physician's offices, urgent care settings, or day surgery centers. As a result of this trend, fewer children may actually be admitted to a hospital unit, and those who are hospitalized are generally acutely ill. In addition, hospital stays are often shorter due to economic trends in the health care environment, such as the delivery system of managed care and other factors that attempt to control costs. Acute conditions, trauma, or chronic diseases or illnesses requiring surgical intervention lead to hospitalization for children.

According to Child Health USA 2005, diseases of the respiratory system account for the majority of hospitalizations in children under 5 years of age, while diseases of the respiratory system, mental health problems, injuries, and gastrointestinal disorders lead to more hospitalizations in older children. Adolescents between 15 and 19 years of age are often hospitalized because of problems related to pregnancy, childbearing, and mental health (U.S. Department of Health and Human Services, 2005).

Other health problems begin before birth or immediately following birth, such as congenital heart disease or gastrointestinal atresia. Just when they are getting used to the idea of having a new child, the family must also deal with illness and possibly extended hospitalizations. Specific genetic or environmental factors also predispose the child to disease and injury, such as the genetic disorder of hemophilia or the environmental sit-

uation of homelessness. Many of these factors or situations put the child and family at greater risk for chronic health conditions and long periods of illness, hospitalization, and even death.

Children's Reactions to Hospitalization

In general, children are more vulnerable to the effects of illness and hospitalization because this is a change from their usual state of health and routine. They also have limited understanding and coping mechanisms to assist them in resolving the stressors that might occur during this time. Hospitalization creates a series of traumatic and stressful events in a climate of uncertainty for children and their families, whether it is an elective procedure that is planned in advance or an emergency situation resulting from trauma. The stressors that children experience in relation to hospitalization may result in various reactions. Children react to the stresses of hospitalization before admission, during hospitalization, and after discharge.

Besides the physiologic effects of the health problem, the effects of illness and hospitalization on a child include anxiety and fear related to the overall process and the potential for bodily injury, physical harm, and pain. In addition, children are separated from their homes, families, friends, and what is familiar to them, which may result in **separation anxiety** (distress related to removal from family and familiar surroundings). There is a general loss of control over their lives and sometimes their emotions and behaviors. The result may be feeling of anger and guilt, **regression** (return to a previous stage of development), acting out, and other types of defense mechanisms to cope with these effects. Children's typical coping strategies are tested during this experience.

Fear and Anxiety

For many children entering the hospital is like entering a foreign world. The result is fear and anxiety. Often anxiety stems from the rapid onset of the illness or injury, particularly when the child has limited experiences with disease or injury. The child becomes distressed about the unfamiliar environment, procedures, and situations, such as the strange words being used, ominous-looking equipment, strangers in unusual attire (e.g., surgical caps, masks, gowns), unfamiliar and frightening noises and smells, or the sounds of other children crying. Overall, hospitalization is a difficult experience for children.

Normal fears of childhood include the fear of separation, loss of control, and bodily injury, mutilation, or harm. Children's fears are similar to adult fears of the unknown, including fear of unfamiliar environments and losing control. In the hospital, children may be exposed to people, situations, and procedures that may be new to them and cause them pain (Fig. 32.1).

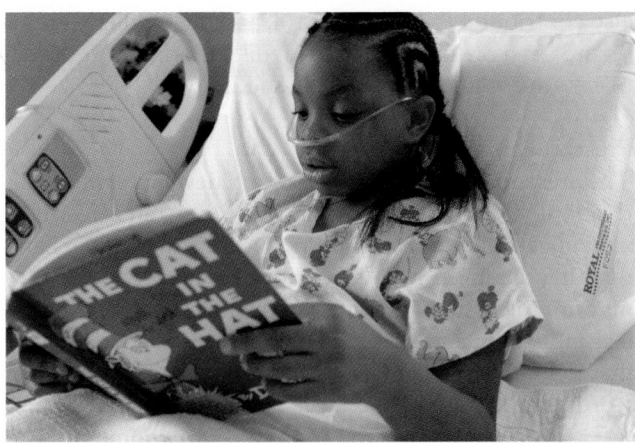

FIGURE 32.1 The presence of familiar objects and home routines normalizes the environment and helps the child cope with hospitalization. Reading a favorite bedtime story can be comforting.

▶ *Take* NOTE!

Wollin et al. (2004) interviewed 120 children between the ages of 5 and 12 and their parents to assess preoperative anxiety and fear. Needles, postoperative pain, the unknown, and the presence of many unrecognizable people in the room increased anxiety for children.

Separation Anxiety

Separation anxiety is a major stressor for children of certain ages. It occurs most frequently in children from middle infancy throughout the preschool years, with the peak incidence occurring between the ages of 6 and 30 months.

Separation anxiety consists of three stages. The first phase, protest, occurs when the child is separated from the parents or primary caretaker. This phase may last from a few hours to several days. The child reacts aggressively to this separation and exhibits great distress by crying, expressing agitation, and rejecting others who attempt to offer comfort. The child may also display anger and inconsolable grief.

If the parents do not return within a short time, the child exhibits the second phase, despair. The child displays hopelessness by withdrawing from others, becoming quiet without crying, and exhibiting apathy, depression, lack of interest in play and food, and overall feelings of sadness.

Detachment (also known as **denial**) is the third and final phase of separation anxiety. During this phase the child forms coping mechanisms to protect against further emotional pain. This occurs more often in long-term separations. During this stage, the child shows interest in the environment, starts to play again, and forms superficial relationships with the nurses and other children. If the

parents return, the child ignores them. A child in this phase of separation anxiety exhibits resignation, not contentment. It is more difficult to reverse this stage, and developmental delays may occur.

Today, health care providers primarily observe the first and second stages because of the shorter hospital stays and the more common use of a family-centered approach to care.

Loss of Control

When hospitalized, children experience a significant loss of control. This loss of control increases the perception of threat and affects their coping skills. They lose control over routine self-care and their usual tasks and play as well as decisions related to the care of their own bodies. In the hospital, the child's usual routine is disrupted. He or she cannot choose what to do and at what time. The child can no longer accomplish simple tasks independently as he or she does at home or school. Confinement to the bed or crib worsens this loss of control. For example, if connected to tubes or intravenous lines, the child may not even be able to visit the bathroom alone.

Hospitalization also affects the child's control over decisions related to his or her own body. Many of the procedures and treatments that occur in the hospital are invasive or are at least disturbing to children, and much of the time they do not have the option to refuse to undergo them. Adults are presumed to be competent to make health care decisions, but generally children are not. Though the parents and nurses of hospitalized children have the children's best interest in mind, children often feel powerless when in the hospital, not having their feelings and wishes respected and having minimal control over events.

▶ *Take* NOTE!

When advocating for a child, make sure to include the child's voice. Do not assume what his or her wishes may be; ask about them directly.

Reactions Based on Developmental Level

Children's responses to the stressors of fear, separation anxiety, and loss of control vary depending on their age and developmental level. Although children are increasingly able to adapt as they grow older, lack of understanding about the need for hospitalization can make adaptation difficult. Moreover, hospitals threaten the sense of control that children are striving for as they develop (Romino et al., 2005).

Infants

Newborns and infants are adapting to life outside the womb with rapid growth and development and establishment of a healthy attachment to parents or primary care-givers. They are dependent on others for nurturance and protection. They gain a sense of trust in the world through rhythmic and reciprocal patterns of contact and feeding, resulting in bonding to the primary caregiver. They need a secure pattern of restful sleep, satisfaction of oral and nutritional needs, relaxation of body systems, and spontaneous response to communication and gentle stimuli. The caregiver–infant attachment is critical for psychological health, especially during periods of illness and hospitalization.

Unfortunately, during illness and hospitalization, these critical patterns of feeding, contact, comfort, sleeping, elimination, and stimulation are disrupted, resulting in fear, separation anxiety, and loss of control. By 5 to 6 months of age, infants have developed an awareness of self as separate from mother. As a result, infants of this age are acutely aware of the absence of their primary caregiver and become fearful of unfamiliar persons. Infants may be separated from their parents when hospitalized if the parents cannot room-in because of hospital policy or if they must work or care for other children. This results in separation anxiety.

The infant's oral needs, the basic source of infant satisfaction, are often not met in the hospital due to the condition of the child or the procedures that must be performed. The infant is accustomed to having his or her basic needs met by the parent when he or she cries or gestures. The constraints of hospitalization result in loss of control over the environment, leading to additional anxiety in the infant.

Toddlers

Toddlers are more aware of self and can communicate their desires. Because their autonomy is developing, toddlers need to master accomplishments to minimize the development of shame and doubt. Control becomes an issue for toddlers. Toddlers also need opportunities to explore, and they need consistent routines. In addition, toddlers are aware of the need for care and protection from others, so they need familiarity and closeness to the primary caregiver. When the toddler is hospitalized, disruption occurs in this development of autonomy.

Toddlers are often fearful of strangers and can recall traumatic events. Simply walking toward the treatment room where a traumatic procedure previously occurred may upset the toddler. Ordinarily a resurgence in separation anxiety occurs during the toddler years. When the toddler is separated from his or her parents or caregivers in an unfamiliar environment, separation anxiety is compounded. In response to this anxiety, toddlers may demonstrate behaviors such as pleading for the parents to stay, physically trying to go after the parents, throwing temper tantrums, and refusing to comply with usual routines. Restrictions related to mobility and new skill acquisition result in loss of control. Disruption in usual routines

also contributes to loss of control, and the toddler feels insecure. As a result, regression in toilet training and refusal to eat are common reactions in toddlers.

Preschoolers

The preschooler has better verbal and developmental skills to adapt to various situations, but illness and hospitalization can still be stressful. Preschoolers may understand that they are in the hospital because they are sick, but they may not understand the cause of their illness. Preschoolers fear mutilation and are afraid of intrusive procedures since they do not understand the body's integrity. They interpret words literally and have an active imagination. Therefore, when the nurse says, "I need to take some blood," preschoolers' fantasies may run wild. They may not understand the concept of blood and may think everything will come out of their body. They may think that blood is "taken" the same way a child picks up a toy to take it out of the room. Preschoolers' thinking is egocentric; they believe that some personal deed or thought caused their illness, which can lead to guilt and shame. These feelings may be internalized. Overall, preschoolers' concrete, egocentric, and **magical thinking** (type of thinking that allows for fantasies and creativity) limits their ability to understand, so communication and interventions must be on their level.

Separation anxiety may not be as much of an issue as it is for toddlers since preschoolers may already be spending time away from parents in preschool. They are, however, still acutely aware of the comfort and security that their family provides for them, so disruptions in these relationships lead to challenges. The preschooler may constantly ask for his or her parents or ask to call the parents. He or she may quietly cry, refuse to eat or take medication, or generally be uncooperative.

In addition, the hospitalized preschooler loses control over the environment. The preschooler is naturally curious about his or her surroundings and learns best by observing and working with objects. This might be limited during hospitalization. Because the preschooler cannot participate in typical activities and explore the environment as usual, the child's normal creative, curious nature may give rise to a variety of fantasies that may present challenges.

School-Age

School-age children generally are hospitalized because of long-term illnesses or trauma. The general task of their development stage, to develop confidence through a sense of industry, can be disrupted during hospitalization. Even at this time, they generally want to continue to learn and maintain their skills and abilities. The stress of illness or anxiety related to diagnostic tests and therapeutic interventions may lead to inward or outward expressions of distress. If they have learned various coping skills, this distress may be minimized. After 11 years of age there is an increased awareness of physiologic, psychological, and behavioral causes of illness and injury. Typically, the school-age child has a more realistic understanding of the reasons for the illness and can better comprehend explanations. School-age children are concerned about disability and death, and they fear injury and pain. They want to know why procedures and tests are being performed. They can understand cause and effect and how it relates to their illness. They are uncomfortable with any type of sexual examination.

Separation anxiety is not as much of an issue for school-age children. They are accustomed to periods of separation and may already be experiencing some separation anxiety related to being in school. At the same time, they may be missing school and friends as they try to adjust to the unfamiliar environment. They may feel that friends will forget them if they remain in the hospital for a long time. Some school-age children may regress and become needy, demanding their parents' attention or playing with special "comfort toys" they used at a younger age.

Since school-age children are accustomed to controlling self-care and typically are highly social, they like being involved. They are used to making choices about meals and activities. Hospitalization presents loss of control by limiting their activities, making them feel helpless and dependent. This may result in feelings of loneliness, boredom, isolation, and depression. The key is to give them opportunities to maintain independence, retain a sense of control, enhance self-esteem, and continue to work toward achieving a sense of industry.

Adolescents

Adolescents fear injury and pain. Since appearance is important to them, they are concerned with how the illness or injury will affect their body image. Anything that changes their perceptions of themselves has a major impact on their response. Typically, adolescents do not like to be different; they like "being cool," which means being in control and not showing how afraid they really are. They also may feel ambivalent about wanting their parents. Adolescents typically do not experience separation anxiety from being away from their parents; instead, their anxiety comes from being separated from friends.

Loss of control is a key factor affecting the behavior of adolescents who are hospitalized. Anger, withdrawal, or general lack of cooperation may occur due to the feelings of loss of control. In addition, their desire to appear confident may led them to question everything that is being done or that they are asked to do. Their feelings of invincibility may cause them to take risks and be noncompliant with treatment. Overall, adolescents strive for independence, self-assertion, and liberation while developing their identity.

Factors Affecting Children's Reaction to Hospitalization

Various factors have a great impact on the ability of children to handle illness and hospitalization. These factors may increase or diminish the fears of the child who is ill and hospitalized. Each child responds differently and will perceive the hospital experience differently. Box 32.1 lists the various factors affecting a child's response to illness and hospitalization.

Developmental Abilities and Perceptions

The child's age, cognitive level, and developmental level will affect his or her perceptions of actual events, and this in turn will affect his or her reaction to illness and hospitalization. Younger children, with their limited life experience and immature intellectual capacities, have a more difficult time comprehending what is happening to them. This can be particularly true for toddlers and preschoolers, who perceive the intactness of their bodies to be exposed during physical intrusions. In addition, they frequently interpret illness as punishment for wrongdoing or hospital procedures as hostile, mutilating acts. Thus, children younger than 5 are more vulnerable to emotional distress from hospitalization.

Previous Experiences

In general, children's lack of understanding and experience of illness, hospitalization, and hospital procedures contributes to their anxiety level. However, previous experience with hospitalization and other health-related experiences can either facilitate preparation or impair it if the experiences were perceived as negative. For example, the child who associates the hospital with the birth of a sibling may view this experience as positive. However, the child who associates the hospital with the serious illness or death of a relative or close friend will probably view the experience as negative.

BOX 32.1 **Factors Affecting a Child's Response to Illness and Hospitalization**

- Amount of separation from parent/caregiver
- Age
- Developmental level
- Cognitive level
- Previous experience with illness and hospitalization
- Recent life stresses and changes
- Type and amount of preparation
- Temperament
- Innate and acquired coping skills
- Seriousness of the diagnosis/onset of illness or injury (e.g., acute or chronic)
- Support systems available, including the family and health care professionals
- Cultural background
- Parents' reaction to illness and hospitalization

The type of experience may contribute to increased anxiety and fear if the child must be admitted to the hospital. If children have had previous experiences, how the experience unfolded and their response to it will determine many of their reactions to hospitalization. Older children may cling to their parents, kick, or create a scene because of their previous experience. One research study compared the psychological responses of children hospitalized in a pediatric intensive care unit with those hospitalized on a general unit. Results showed that children who were younger, more severely ill, and who endured more invasive procedures had significantly more medical fears, a lower sense of control over their health, and ongoing posttraumatic stress responses for 6 months after discharge (Zengerle-Levy, 2006).

Recent Stresses and Changes and Individual Coping Skills

The effects of hospitalization on children are influenced by the nature and severity of the health problem, the condition of the child, and the degree to which activities and routines differ from those of everyday life. A lack of sensory stimulation in the hospital environment produces listlessness, indifference, unhappiness, and even appetite changes. When the child's motor activity is restricted, anger and hyperactivity may result. Play, recreation, and educational opportunities can provide an outlet to distract the child from the illness, provide pleasant experiences, and help the child understand his or her condition.

The child's ability to work through a situation will also affect his or her responses to illness and hospitalization. This ability depends on the age of the child, his or her perceptions of the event, previous encounters with health care personnel, and support from significant others. Table 32.1 lists various coping skills used by children and suggestions for promoting positive coping.

Parents' Response to Child's Hospitalization

Children take in their parents' anxiety and concern. Even whispers can set off children's imaginations. For example, preschoolers may invent elaborate stories to explain what is happening to them. Parents who do not tell children the truth or do not answer their questions confuse and frighten them and may weaken the child's trust in the parents. It is important for children to believe that someone is in control and that the person can be trusted. Some parents, however, have their own fears and insecurities. Thus, a child's reaction often is related to the parents' reaction to the illness and hospitalization.

The relationship between the family and the hospital staff may either add to or ease the child's stress. This relationship can contribute significantly to the quality of the environment. Hospital personnel must assume responsibility for the care of hospitalized children by maintaining good partnerships with families.

*R*emember Jake, the 8-year-old with a suspected brain tumor? What responses to hospitalization might you see in him and his family?

The Hospitalized Child's Family

Whether planned or unplanned, hospitalization increases the family's stress and anxiety level. The illness or serious injury of one family member affects all members of the family because the process disrupts the family's usual routines and may alter family roles. Parents and siblings have their own reactions to this experience.

Reactions of Parents

Watching a child in pain is difficult, especially when the parent is assisting with the procedure by holding the child. The parent may feel guilty for not seeking care sooner. Parents may also exhibit other feelings such as denial, anger, depression, and confusion. Parents may deny that the child is ill. They may express anger, especially directed at the nursing staff, another family member, or a higher power because of their loss of control in caring for the child. Depression may occur because of exhaustion and the psychological and physical requirements of spending long hours in a hospital caring for a child. Confusion may develop because of dealing with an unfamiliar environment or the loss of a parental role. Finally, the parents'

TABLE 32.1 CHILDREN AND COPING

Behavior/Methods for Coping	Suggestions to Promote Coping
Ignore or negate the problem Stoicism, passive acceptance Acting out—yelling, kicking, screaming, crying Anger, withdrawal, rejection Intellectualizing	Breathing techniques such as blowing bubbles, pinwheels, or party noise-makers Distraction with books or games Imagery with tapes or scenarios Music Teaching before events or procedures

marriage may be strained because of dual roles, long separation, and increased stress.

A recent study indicates that parents have experiences in four categories: facing boundaries, attempting to understand, coping with uncertainty, and seeking reassurance from caregivers (Stratton, 2004). First, parents feel helpless when they play a passive role in their child's care, such as when a medical procedure is required that hurts the child. Then parents attempt to understand by becoming informed and understanding the procedures. Next, they deal with the fear of uncertainty and attempt to promote a sense of comfort by interacting with the hospital staff. Finally, they seek reassurance from the caregivers.

Reactions of Siblings

Siblings of children who are hospitalized may experience jealousy, insecurity, resentment, confusion, and anxiety. They may have difficulty understanding why their sibling is ill or getting all the attention, leaving little for them. They may wonder if their sibling is going to die or ever return home. They may worry that their sibling's illness is going to happen to them. Certain age groups, such as preschoolers, may feel that they caused the illness. Their magical and egocentric thinking, combined with little information, contributes to their fears that they may have caused the illness or injury by their thoughts, wishes, or behaviors (Winch, 2001). If the family roles or routines change significantly, the siblings may feel insecure or anxious. They may develop changes in behavior or in school performance.

> ▶ *Take* NOTE!
>
> *Research supports the need to provide support and information to the siblings to decrease their stress, anxiety, and confusion.*

Factors Influencing Family Reactions

The parenting style and the family–child relationship can influence the hospital experience as well as the family members' coping skills. Cultural, ethnic, and religious variations, values, and practices related to illness, general response to stress, and attitudes about the care of a sick child have a significant influence on the family's response. For example, religious beliefs can raise problems or can be a source of strength to the family and child. Families already in crisis or without support systems have a more difficult time dealing with the added stress of hospitalization. Chapter 2 gives further explanations of some of these influences on children and their families.

*J*ake's parents are very upset that he has to be hospitalized. His mother says to you, "I'm worried how Jake is going to react to all of this. What can we do to help him?" How would you address his mother's concerns?

The Nurse's Role in Caring for the Hospitalized Child

In most instances, the nurse is the primary person involved in the care of a hospitalized child. The nurse is probably the first one to see the child and family and will spend more time with them than other health care providers. Nurses are part of a medical community that makes decisions in the child's best interest, but the nurse needs to bear in mind the child's rights and must try to minimize the child's distress so that the hospital stay will be as pleasant an experience as possible. When establishing strategies to care for children in the hospital, nurses should examine the general effects of hospitalization on children in each developmental stage and should strive to understand the factors affecting hospitalization as well as the reactions of the child and family. Nursing Care Plan 32.1 summarizes the nursing care associated with a hospitalized child.

The initial contact with children and their families establishes the foundation for a trusting relationship. Each institution has its own criteria for admission and transfer of pediatric clients, formulated in light of its mission, abilities, and limitations. Use favorite toys and common television shows to establish rapport. Allow the child to participate in the conversation without the pressure of having to comply with requests or undergo any procedures. A trusting relationship can be built by using appropriate language, games, and play such as singing a song during a procedure, preparing the child adequately for procedures, and providing explanations and encouragement. Get down to the child's level and play on his or her terms.

The next two phases involve making judgments and providing feedback. Decisions must be made that will affect the trust the child has developed. For example, it is imperative to decide how much control the child will have during treatment, how much information to share with the child about upcoming events, and whether parents should participate. Reinforce the child's use of coping strategies that lead to healthy outcomes by providing options whenever it is safe to do so. Finally, the comfort and reassurance phase uses techniques such as praising the child and providing opportunities to cuddle with a favorite toy.

Preparing Children and Families for Hospitalization

When preparing children for hospitalization, be aware of the situations that may create distress in a child and try

(text continues on page 989)

Nursing Care Plan 32.1

OVERVIEW FOR THE HOSPITALIZED CHILD AND FAMILY

NURSING DIAGNOSIS: Anxiety related to hospital situation, fear of injury or bodily mutilation, separation from family or friends, changes in routine, painful procedures and treatments, and unfamiliar events and surroundings as evidenced by crying, fussing, withdrawal, or resistance

Outcome Identification and Evaluation

Child and family will exhibit a decrease in anxiety level as evidenced by positive coping strategies, verbalization or playing out of feelings, appropriate behaviors, positive interactions with staff, child and parent cooperation and participation, and absence of signs and symptoms of increasing anxiety and fear.

Interventions: Minimizing Anxiety

- Orient child and family to the unit and the child's room *to familiarize them with the facility.*
- Assess for signs and symptoms of anxiety and fear *to establish a baseline and assess effectiveness of interventions.*
- Place the child in a room with another child of a similar age, developmental level, and condition severity *to promote sharing.*
- Provide atraumatic care *to minimize exposure to distress, which would increase anxiety.*
- Explain all events, treatments, procedures, and activities to the parents and child (at a level the child can understand) in a calm, relaxed manner *to help the child prepare for what is to come and decrease fear of the unknown. A calm, relaxed manner helps to establish rapport and instill trust.*
- Encourage parents to room-in if possible *to provide the child with support;* if parents cannot stay, encourage them to call *to reduce child's fear of being alone.*
- Urge parents to inform the child when they will be leaving and when they are expected to return *to help child cope with their absence and promote trust.*
- Assess child's usual routine at home and attempt to incorporate aspects of usual routine into hospital routine *to ease the transition to the hospital and promote the child's participation in routine.*
- Offer comfort measures such as holding, stroking, and rocking *to relieve distress.*
- Encourage the child to play (unstructured and therapeutic play as necessary) *to allow for expression of feelings and fears and promote energy expenditure.*
- Suggest that parents bring in a special toy or object from home *to promote feelings of security.*
- Provide positive reinforcement for participation in care activities *to foster self-esteem.*
- Assess for regression behaviors and inform parents that such behaviors are common *to alleviate their concerns about this behavior.*
- Provide consistency with care measures *to facilitate trust and acceptance.*

NURSING DIAGNOSIS: Risk for powerlessness related to lack of control over procedures, treatments, and care, and changes in usual routine

Outcome Identification and Evaluation

Child and family will demonstrate an increase in control over the situation as evidenced by participation in care activities, identification of needs and choices, and incorporation of appropriate aspects of child's usual routine with that of the hospital.

Interventions: Promoting Control

- Encourage child and parents to identify areas of concern *to help determine priority needs.*
- Encourage parent and child to participate in care activities *to promote feelings of control.*
- Incorporate aspects of child's routine at home and use terms similar to those used at home *to foster a sense of normalcy.*
- Offer child choices as much as possible, such as options for foods, drinks, hygiene, activities, or clothing (if appropriate) *to promote feelings of individuality and control.*
- Allow child opportunities for being out of bed or room within limitations as appropriate *to foster independence.*
- Work with child, as age and development allow, and family to set up a schedule to *promote structure and routine.*

Nursing Care Plan 32.1 (continued)

NURSING DIAGNOSIS: Deficient diversional activity related to confinement in bed or health care facility, limited mobility, activity restrictions, or equipment as evidenced by verbalization of boredom, lack of participation in play, reading, or schoolwork

Outcome Identification and Evaluation
Child will participate in diversional activities as evidenced by engagement in unstructured and therapeutic play that is developmentally appropriate and interaction with family, staff, and other children.

Interventions: Promoting Adequate Diversional Activities
- Question child and family about favorite types of activities *to establish a baseline for developing appropriate choices during hospitalization.*
- Assist with planning activities within the limits of the child's condition *to maintain muscle tone and strength without overexerting the child.*
- Spend time with the child *to provide stimulation and foster trust.*
- Enlist the aid of a child life specialist *to provide suggestions for appropriate activities.*
- Encourage interaction with other children *to promote sharing and avoid loneliness.*
- Provide developmentally appropriate opportunities for unstructured and therapeutic play *to facilitate expression of feelings.*
- Encourage short trips to the playroom or activity room *to provide a change of scenery and sensory stimulation.*
- Integrate play activities with nursing care *to achieve therapeutic effect.*

NURSING DIAGNOSIS: Interrupted family processes related to separation from child due to hospitalization, increased demands of caring for an ill child, changes in role function, and effect of hospitalization on other family members such as siblings, as evidenced by parental verbalization of issues, parental presence in hospital, or child's hospitalization requiring parent to miss work

Outcome Identification and Evaluation
Family will demonstrate positive coping strategies as evidenced by visiting frequently and staying with the child as necessary, sharing of family responsibilities, obtaining assistance for relief or respite, and visiting by other members of the child's family and friends.

Interventions: Maximizing Family Functioning
- Encourage parents and family members to verbalize concerns about child's illness, diagnosis, and prognosis *to promote family-centered care and identify areas where intervention may be needed.*
- Explain therapies, procedures, child's behaviors, and plan of care to parents to *promote understanding of the child's status and plan of care, which helps to decrease anxiety.*
- Encourage parental involvement in care *to promote feelings of the parents being needed and valued, providing them with a sense of control over their child's health.*
- Identify support system for family and child *to identify resources available for coping.*
- Educate family and child on additional resources available *to promote a wider base of support to deal with the situation.*
- Suggest ways that parents can divide time between child and other siblings *to prevent feelings of guilt.*
- Provide support and positive reinforcement *to promote family coping and foster family strength.*
- Encourage frequent visits by family members, including siblings as appropriate, *to promote ongoing family functioning.*
- Stress the need for adequate rest, sleep, exercise, and nutrition for family members *to promote family health and minimize stress of hospitalization on family.*
- Assist with referrals for resources and help from additional family members and friends as necessary *to allow for respite or relief of care responsibilities.*
- Encourage family to maintain usual routine as much as possible *to minimize the effects of hospitalization on family functioning.*

(continued)

Nursing Care Plan 32.1 (continued)

NURSING DIAGNOSIS: Self-care deficit related to immobility, activity restrictions, regression, or use of equipment, devices, or prescribed treatments as evidenced by inability to feed, bathe, or dress self or accomplish other activities of daily living

Outcome Identification and Evaluation
Child will participate in self-care within limitations of condition as evidenced by assisting with bathing and hygiene, feeding, toileting, and dressing and grooming.

Interventions: Promoting Self-Care
- Assess child's usual routine for self-care and self-care abilities *to provide a baseline for individualizing interventions.*
- Provide child-sized equipment and devices *to promote child's ability to complete the self-care task.*
- Encourage parents and child to do as much self-care as possible, within limitations of the child's condition and developmental level, *to promote feelings of independence and foster growth and development.*
- Offer praise and encouragement for activities performed *to foster self-esteem, confidence, and competence.*
- Ensure adequate rest periods *to minimize energy expenditure associated with self-care activities.*

NURSING DIAGNOSIS: Risk for delayed growth and development related to stressors associated with hospitalization, current condition or illness, separation from family, and sensory overload or sensory deprivation

Outcome Identification and Evaluation
Child will demonstrate developmentally appropriate milestones as evidenced by age-appropriate behaviors and activities.

Interventions: Promoting Growth and Development
- Assess child's developmental stage *to establish a baseline and determine appropriate strategies.*
- Use unstructured and therapeutic play and adaptive toys *to promote developmental functioning.*
- Provide stimulating environment when possible *to maximize potential for growth and development.*
- Praise accomplishments and emphasize child's abilities *to foster self-esteem and encourage feelings of confidence and competence.*
- Include parents in techniques to foster growth and development *to promote feelings of control in their child's care.*

NURSING DIAGNOSIS: Deficient knowledge related to hospitalization, surgery, treatments, procedures, required care, and follow-up as evidenced by questioning and verbalization, lack of prior exposure

Outcome Identification and Evaluation
Child and family will demonstrate understanding of all aspects of child's current situation as evidenced by identification of child's and family's needs, verbal statements of understanding and/or need for additional information, return demonstration of procedures and treatments, and verbalization of instructions for follow-up and continued care.

Interventions: Providing Child and Family Teaching
- Assess child's and family's willingness to learn *to ensure effective teaching.*
- Provide family with time to adjust to diagnosis *to facilitate their ability to learn and participate in the child's care.*
- Repeat information *to promote multiple opportunities for child and family to learn.*
- Teach in short sessions *to prevent overloading the child and parents with information.*
- Gear teaching to appropriate level of understanding for the child and the family (depends on age of child, physical condition, memory) *to promote learning.*
- Provide reinforcement and rewards *to facilitate the teaching/learning process.*
- Use multiple modes of learning, such as written information, verbal instruction, demonstrations, and media, when possible *to facilitate learning and retention of information.*
- Provide the child and family with written step-by-step instructions for procedures or care *to provide a reference if needed at a later date.*
- Have child and family provide return demonstrations of care procedures *to ensure effectiveness of teaching.*
- Arrange for trial home care during hospitalization and after discharge as appropriate *to ensure understanding and provide opportunities for additional teaching and learning.*

to minimize or eliminate them. Even the most minor situations may be frightening to young children. New experiences, unfamiliar sights and sounds, disruption of sleep patterns, and pain associated with procedures and treatments are major causes of stress for the hospitalized child and family (Zengerle-Levy, 2006). Table 32.2 presents some hospital activities that may seem scary or stressful to a child and gives suggestions for preparing the child and family. Thoughtful preparation for these situations may relieve the stress. Educate children about what to expect so they can cope with their imagination and distin-

guish reality from fantasy. Describe the intervention and the sequence of steps that will occur, and include sensory information such as how the child will feel.

Good preparation can reduce the child's fears and increase his or her ability to cope with the hospital experience. Preparation should include exploring the child's perceptions, reviewing previous experiences, and identifying coping strategies. Useful techniques include the following:

• Perform nursing care on stuffed animals or dolls and allow the child to do the same.

TABLE 32.2 STRATEGIES TO REDUCE FEAR OF COMMON HOSPITALIZATION SITUATIONS

Situation	Strategies to Reduce Fear
Procedure involving intrusion into the body or use of equipment or technology	Describe the procedure and equipment in terms the child can understand. Review the steps of the procedure or steps involved with the use of the equipment. Explain what the child's role will be and what is or isn't allowed. If appropriate, have the child rehearse with the equipment or role play.
Darkness, such as with radiologic examinations or at night	Keep a light on in the examination area. Use a night light in the child's room. If possible, allow the child to hold the caregiver's or nurse's hand or a favorite toy.
Transport to other areas of the hospital	Allow caregiver to accompany child if possible. Inform the child of where he or she is going, about how long he or she will be there, and approximately when he or she will return. Introduce the child to the person who will be transporting the child.
Numerous personnel in and out of child's room	Identify all staff members working with the child (each shift and each day). Place a small board in the child's room with the name of the nurse caring for the child that shift or day. Inform the child how long the nurse will be caring for the child (adapt this information according to the child's cognitive level; for example, instead of saying that you'll be there for 8 hours, say, "I'll be your nurse until just before dinnertime" or "I'll be your nurse until you go for your test"). Say good-bye to the child when leaving for the day; tell the child about his or her new nurse; inform the child of when you will return.

- Avoid the use of medical terms.
- Allow the child to handle some equipment.
- Teach the child the steps of the procedure or inform him or her exactly what will happen during the hospital stay.
- Show the child the room where he or she will be staying.
- Introduce the child to the health care personnel with whom he or she will come in contact.
- Explain the sounds the child may hear.
- Let the child sample the food that will be served.

All techniques used to prepare the child for hospitalization should emphasize the philosophy of atraumatic care. "The main goal of preparation is for the child to participate in a dialogue and a demonstration of the coming procedure so he or she can better understand the situation" (Mansson & Dykes, 2004). Adapt all information to the cognitive and developmental level of the child. Identify what role the child will play in the situation: it is always helpful for children to have something to do, since it shows them that they are included. A rehearsal of what will occur in the hospital allows the child to become comfortable with the situation. If time permits, provide pamphlets that describe the procedure and suggest preparation activities for the child at home before admission.

The child and family may be able to take a tour of the hospital unit or the surgical facility. Videotapes or DVDs, photographs, and books on hospitalization and surgery can serve as resources for the family and child. Many institutions offer programs to familiarize children and families with the hospital experience. For example, one institution uses a "train ride" to help them understand what to expect (Herron, 2005). During the ride, opportunities are provided for role playing, and during stops along the way the child can see, touch, and feel the equipment that may be used (Fig. 32.2).

The American Society of Anesthesiologists has prepared a coloring book entitled "My Trip to the Hospital." This book is designed to alleviate some of the fears that younger children may have related to the hospital experience. It describes the process from admission (whether it be to the hospital or ambulatory surgery center) through discharge and includes information about preoperative testing, anesthesia, and recovery. The book also includes information for parents. The book is available online at http://www.asahq.org/patientEducation/mytrip.htm.

Parents are instrumental in preparing children by reviewing the materials that are given, answering questions, and being truthful and supportive. Teaching Guidelines 32.1 provides suggestions for parents in preparing their child for hospitalization. Table 32.3 discusses strategies for preoperative teaching.

Admitting the Child to the Facility

Admitting the child to the facility involves preparing him or her for admission and introducing the child to the unit where he or she will be staying. Use the appropriate hospital forms. Chapter 2 gives general information about communicating with and teaching children and families.

In today's health care environment, the admission process occurs quickly, with little time for extensive preparation; this is why preparation before admission is so important. Of course, the urgency of the child's medical condition also may limit the amount of preparation that can be done in advance.

Types of Admissions and Nursing Care

The hospital units to which a child may be admitted include:

- General inpatient unit
- Emergency and urgent care department

FIGURE 32.2 A child is being prepared for hospitalization by becoming familiar with some of the equipment that might be used.

TEACHING GUIDELINES 32.1

Preparing Your Child for Hospitalization

- Read stories about experiences with hospital or surgery.
- Talk about going to the hospital and what it will be like coming home.
- Be honest and encourage the child to ask questions.
- Visit the hospital and go through the preadmission tour if time permits.
- Provide support to the child via your presence, telephone calls, and special items brought from home.
- Encourage the child to draw pictures to express how he or she is feeling.
- Include siblings in the preparation.

TABLE 32.3 STRATEGIES FOR PREOPERATIVE TEACHING

Developmental Level	Implications for Teaching
Infants and toddlers	Encourage parents to use a soft tone of voice and stroking and secure, comfortable holding positions to promote calm.
	Remind parents to use positive facial expressions.
	Encourage the parent or caregiver to stay with the child as much as possible.
	Use terms that the child and parents can understand.
	For toddlers, provide information as close to the day of surgery as possible to prevent undue anxiety.
Preschoolers and school-age children	Provide factual explanations using terms the child and parents can understand.
	Incorporate pictures and other visual aids in explanation.
	Tailor the timing of education to meet the child's learning needs, allowing enough time for the child to ask questions. Some recommend that information be provided no more than 1 week beforehand for school-age children. (Justus et al., 2006).
Adolescents	Provide detailed explanations of the procedure at least 7 to 10 days beforehand.
	Answer questions honestly, ensuring privacy at all times.
	Remain available for questions or concerns arising before or after surgery.

- Pediatric intensive care unit
- Outpatient or special procedures unit
- Rehabilitation unit or hospital

Regardless of the site of care, nursing care must begin by establishing a trusting, caring relationship with the child and family. Smile, introduce yourself, and give your title. Let the child and family know what will happen and what is expected of them. Ask the family and child what names they prefer to be called by. Maintain eye contact at the appropriate level. With a younger child, start with the family first so the child can see that the family trusts you. Communicate with children at age-appropriate levels.

The next step, as the child's medical condition allows, involves an orientation to the hospital unit. Briefly explain policies and routines and the personnel who will be involved in the care of the child.

During the nursing interview that follows, obtain information about the child's history, routines, and reason for admission. Obtain baseline vital signs, height and

weight, and perform a physical assessment. Each health care setting has its own policies and procedures for this. Recognize the needs of the family and child during this process. If some of this information already exists, do not ask for it again, except to confirm vital information such as allergies, medications taken at home, and history of the illness. Typically, the information is collected immediately if the child's condition is urgent; otherwise, the information is collected within 8 hours, except for the information that is required for safe care.

General Inpatient Unit Stays

Today, general inpatient unit stays for children are shorter and involve more acute conditions, resulting in little time for admission preparation. Many times the admission procedure and treatment actually occur simultaneously. Sometimes the stay is in a special 23-hour observation unit so the child is in the setting for less than 24 hours. General hospital stays may be in a pediatric hospital, a pediatric unit in a general hospital, or a general unit that occasionally admits children. General units often lack child-oriented services, such as play areas, child-size equipment, and staff familiar with caring for children.

> ▶ *Take* NOTE!
>
> *When a child is admitted to a general unit, take extra time to orient and explain the routines and procedures to the child and family. Emphasize that the parents can stay with the child (if institutional policy permits). If possible, place the child in a room close to the nurses' station and order food appropriate for the child's age and developmental level.*

Emergency and Urgent Care Departments

The number-one reason for illness and hospitalization in children is injuries from accidents. Many times a family's first experience with the acute care setting is the urgent care or emergency department. Due to the situation, the child and family may experience increased anxiety, and it may become overwhelming as uncertainties develop and critical decisions must be made. The family may be frightened, insecure, and in a state of shock.

Procedures and tests are performed quickly, with minimal time for preparation. The family is often ill prepared for the visit, having little money or clothing with them. Siblings may be present if the parents did not have time to get a sitter.

Due to the fast pace of the emergency department, the family may be hesitant to ask questions, so keep the family and child well informed. Allow the family to stay with the child, provide support, and allow the family, and when appropriate the child, to participate in decisions.

Families may have a strong fear of the unknown and may be terrified that the child will die or be permanently disabled. Help the family to identify their concerns and their support systems. Prepare them for what they will experience. Provide comfort such as holding, touching, talking softly, and other appropriate interventions according to age and developmental level.

Pediatric Intensive Care Units

The pediatric intensive care unit (PICU) specializes in caring for children in crisis. The same principles and concepts of general care of children apply to this setting, but everything is intensified. Families will be faced with an unfamiliar, high-tech environment and a large number of staff.

Families must deal with the critical situation that brought them to the PICU. The child will likely experience pain, unusual noises, and increased stimulation and will probably undergo uncomfortable procedures. Parents may

face the possibility of losing their child. Sometimes the child cannot talk, eat, or display other appropriate developmental behaviors. **Sensory overload** (increased stimulation) or **sensory deprivation** (lack of stimulation) can affect both child and family.

Welcome families (if institutional policy permits) and encourage them to stay with the child and participate in care. Explain everything to the parents and, when appropriate, to the child. Frequently touch the child and encourage the parents to comfort him or her. Listen for clues about what the child and family need during the PICU stay.

Outpatient or Special Procedure Units

Outpatient or special procedure units are used to keep hospital stays short and decrease the cost of hospitalization. These units may be a part of a general hospital or a freestanding facility. Typically, the child and family arrive in the morning; the child has the procedure, test, or surgery and then goes home later that same day. Examples of procedures performed in outpatient settings include tympanostomy tube placement, hernia repair, tonsillectomy, cystoscopy, bronchoscopy, and chemotherapy.

This setting minimizes separation of the child from the family. In addition, there is minimal disruption of the family pattern, a decreased risk of infection, and decreased cost. However, these units do not have the equipment for overnight stays, so if complications develop, the child will need to be transported to another facility or another area of the hospital.

Rehabilitation Units

The rehabilitation unit provides care for children beyond the initial period of illness or injury. The care involves an interdisciplinary approach that assists the child to reach his or her potential and achieve developmental skills. For example, rehabilitation units help children regain abilities lost due to neurologic injuries or serious burns. The facilities often resemble a home environment, with special services to help children to relearn activities of daily living and to help them deal with the physical or mental challenges associated with the original illness or injury. Typically, families are encouraged to participate and are given support for their child's eventual return home. There is a balance of nurturing and firm discipline while the child reclaims independence.

Isolation Rooms

Isolation rooms are used for situations involving the risk for infection. When a child is admitted with an infectious disease, or to rule out an infectious disease, or if the child has impaired immune function, isolation will be instituted. Children in this setting may experience sensory deprivation due to the limited contact with others and the use of personal protective equipment such as gloves, masks, and gowns.

Encourage the family to visit often, and help them to understand the reason for the isolation and any special procedures that are required. Introduce yourself before entering the room and allow the child to view your face before applying a mask. Continue to have contact with the child and hold or touch the child often, especially if the parents are not present.

Addressing the Effects of Hospitalization Developmentally

When addressing the fears, separation anxiety, and loss of control that occur in hospitalized children, the nurse should consider the child's age and cognitive or developmental level. Interventions are then based on how the child experiences these stressors at that age or developmental level. The content, timing, setting, and method of preparation are also based on the child's age and cognitive or developmental level. General guidelines for addressing fear and anxiety, separation anxiety, and loss of control are provided in Box 32.2.

Newborns and Infants

Assess the development or lack of development that is occurring in the infant, and assess the baby's attachment to the parents or primary caregivers. The infant's facial expression is the most consistent indicator of pain or bodily injury. To decrease fear and minimize separation anxiety, avoid separation from the primary caregiver if possible; this will also promote healthy attachment. If the parent or primary caregiver cannot stay with the infant, arrange for volunteers to provide consistent comfort to the baby. Maintaining the infant's home routine related to sleep and feeding helps decrease feelings of loss of control. Weigh the infant daily, at the same time, on the same scale. Monitor intake and output closely. Be alert to signs of discomfort other than crying, such as a furrowed brow or tense body posture. Additional nursing goals related to promoting growth and development of the infant are presented in Table 32.4.

Toddlers

Key nursing concerns when caring for toddlers are separation anxiety, growth and development, and autonomy. Establishing a trusting relationship with the toddler through nonthreatening play may decrease the amount of fear the toddler feels. Be alert to subtle, nonverbal indicators of grief or discontent.

Encourage the parent or primary caregiver to stay with the toddler in the hospital to decrease separation anxiety. Maintaining the home routine related to meals and sleep or a nap provides structure and may help decrease the toddler's feelings of loss of control. If indicated, weigh the toddler daily. Closely monitor intake and output. Refer to Table 32.4 for additional nursing considerations related to promoting growth and development in the hospitalized toddler.

BOX 32.2 **Guidelines to Address the General Effects of Hospitalization**

Minimizing Fear and Anxiety
- Consider the effects of magical thinking.
- Explain everything to children and their families before it occurs (see Chapter 35).
- Use age-appropriate communication techniques. Include the family in this process so they can help the child cope with fears.
- Allow time for children to play out their fears and concerns.
- Talk to the child and parents using a soft, comforting tone of voice, with the parent or caregiver holding the child.

Addressing/Minimizing Separation Anxiety
- Know the stages of separation anxiety and be able to recognize them.
- Remember that behaviors demonstrated during the first stage do not indicate that the child is "bad."
- Encourage the family to stay with the child.
- Help the child cope, and intervene before the behaviors of detachment occur.
- Try guided imagery, using the child's imagination and enjoyment of play, to help the child relax (Bricher, 2000).

Addressing Loss of Control
- Minimize physical restrictions, altered routines and rituals, and dependency issues, because they produce loss of control.
- Allow as much independence as possible within the constraints of the diagnosis.
- Recognize the child's inherent powerlessness in the hospital setting and explore strategies that give children an opportunity to participate in their own health care decisions (Bricher, 2000).

Preschoolers

Nursing care for hospitalized preschoolers focuses on their special needs, fears, and fantasies. When working with preschoolers, remember that they use magical thinking and fantasy. Be honest and specific, providing information just prior to the intervention to allay the child's fears. As with toddlers, encouraging parental involvement may decrease the amount of separation anxiety the preschooler experiences while in the hospital. Allowing the preschooler to make simple decisions such as which color bandage to use or whether to take medicine from a cup or syringe helps the child to feel some sense of control. Table 32.4 gives specific nursing considerations related to promoting growth and development for the preschooler in the hospital.

TABLE 32.4   NURSING CONSIDERATIONS FOR PROVIDING SAFE, DEVELOPMENTALLY APPROPRIATE CARE

	Ensuring Safety	Promoting Healthy Growth and Development
Infants	• Maintain close supervision of the infant. • Keep one hand on the infant when crib sides are down. • Keep crib rails up all the way when the infant is in the crib. • Avoid leaving small objects that are harmful or that can be swallowed in the crib. • Provide safe and appropriate toys for the infant. • Place infants in rooms close to the nurses' station. • Encourage a family member to stay with the infant at all times.	• Use the *en face* position when holding newborns. • Smile and talk to the infant during bathing, feeding, and other interactions. • Minimize the number of painful or uncomfortable procedures. • Provide comfort during and after procedures by holding or talking, using soothing tones and movements. • When handling the infant, use smooth, continuous movements. • Use gentle stroking and holding, which may reduce stress. • Serve as a role model for first-time parents. • Encourage the family to maintain home routines while in hospital, planning nursing care around the usual feeding and sleep times. • Use the pacifier between feedings to satisfy nonnutritive sucking needs.
Toddlers	• Keep crib side rails up with overhead crib protection intact when the toddler is in the crib. • Never leave a toddler alone in the room unless secured in the crib. • Use a bed only for the older toddler who has an adult present in the room at all times. • Avoid leaving small objects than can be swallowed or are harmful in the crib or bed. • Place crib out of reach of cords, equipment, and electrical outlets. • Provide safe and appropriate toys for the toddler. • Always have someone with the toddler when ambulating.	• Encourage the parent to stay with the toddler to decrease separation anxiety. • To promote autonomy, allow the toddler to make appropriate choices, such as which juice to take the medicine with. • Encourage active play in the playroom or with push/pull toys in the hallway (accompanied by an adult). • Expect and plan for regression in areas of toilet training, eating, and other behaviors. • Expect increased temper tantrums in general and intense reactions to intrusive procedures. • Maintain home routine while in hospital, planning nursing care around the usual feeding and sleep times. • Give simple directions with choices appropriate to the hospital situation. • Place toddlers in rooms close to the nurses' station. • Provide close supervision while encouraging independence.
Preschoolers	• Keep bed in low position with the side rails up when the preschooler is in the bed. • Instruct the child to call the nurse or caregiver for help getting out of bed. • Keep harmful objects out of reach of the child.	• Encourage parents to stay with the preschooler in the room as well as other areas of the hospital. • Encourage the preschooler to be involved in care by providing choices and opportunities for the child to help. • Use play as an opportunity to work through the preschooler's fears. • Explain activities in simple, concrete terms, being cautious with the words you use because of the preschooler's fantasies and magical thinking. • Expect reactions to pain and bodily injury to be verbally aggressive and specific. • Try to maintain home routines while the child is in the hospital, working them into the plan of care when possible.

	Ensuring Safety	Promoting Healthy Growth and Development
School-age children	• Keep the bed in the low position with the side rails up while the child is in the bed, explaining that this is a hospital rule, not a punishment.	• Provide opportunities for the child to be involved in care. • Allow children to select their meals, assist with treatments, and keep their rooms neat. • Allow visits with other children if condition allows. • Encourage parents to tell the child when they will return. • Plan care around the child's usual home routines (meals, sleep). • Encourage the child to do schoolwork.
Adolescents	• Be aware of the adolescent's whereabouts. The teen may not wish to stay in the room but may become confused about where the room or unit is located in the hospital.	• Allow teens to interact with others. • Alter hospital routines as possible to allow the teen to sleep in or stay up later at night. • Provide others close to their age as roommates. • Encourage visits from friends. • Provide emotional support for feelings of being alone or away from friends; be alert for regression, which may result in the teen becoming emotional. • Answer questions honestly and with appropriate information. • Give the teen a sense of control by allowing choices. • Be sensitive to concerns about being "different."

School-Age Children

Provide honest information using concrete, meaningful words to the school-age child to minimize fear of the unknown. School-age children are still very attached to their parents, so encouraging parental involvement or rooming-in decreases separation anxiety. Involve the child in making simple decisions and planning the schedule as appropriate to give him or her a sense of control. Nursing considerations when caring for hospitalized school-age children include ensuring safety and promoting growth and development (see Table 32.4).

Adolescents

The adolescent may or may not express fears. Educate the teen honestly: younger teens require more concrete explanations, while older teens can process more abstract concepts. Respect the teen's need for privacy. Encourage visits from the adolescent's friends to minimize anxiety related to separation. Prepare a mutually agreeable schedule with the teen, as appropriate, that includes the teen's preferences while incorporating the required nursing care. Collaborating with the adolescent will provide the teen with increased control. Refer to Table 32.4 for additional nursing considerations related to care of the adolescent in the hospital.

Think back to Jake, the 8-year-old from the beginning of the chapter. Discuss nursing care you could provide that will help minimize stressors.

Preparing the Child and Family for Surgery

If the child is to undergo a surgical procedure, whether in the hospital or an outpatient setting, special interventions are necessary. The parents should be allowed to stay with the child until surgery begins. Parents should also be allowed to be with the child when he or she wakes up in the post-anesthesia recovery area. Good preparation provides reassurance and comfort to the child and allows him or her to know what will happen and what is expected of him or her.

Preoperative Care

Preoperative care for the child who is to undergo surgery is similar to that for an adult. The major difference is that the preparation and teaching must be geared to the child's age and developmental level. Many facilities offer special programs to help prepare children and families for the surgical experience. Presurgical preparation programs allow children and their families to experience a "trial run" in a supportive environment to reduce anxiety, increase knowledge, and enhance coping skills (Justus et al., 2006). Books, including the one cited earlier by the American Society of Anesthesiologists, are helpful in preparing the child and family.

Child and family teaching is essential. Like any intervention, adapt the teaching to the child's developmental level. For example, when teaching a toddler or preschooler about breathing exercises, have the child blow a pinwheel or cotton balls across the table through a straw.

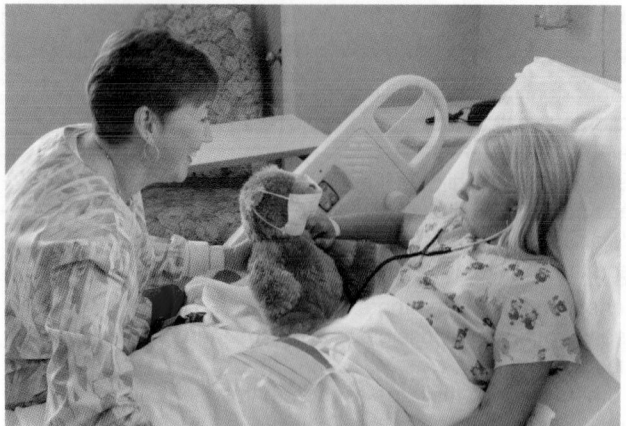

FIGURE 32.3 Using a stuffed animal to explain a surgical procedure to the child.

FIGURE 32.4 Safety is an essential aspect of pediatric nursing. A clear plastic cover over the crib prevents the older infant or toddler from climbing out and falling.

The child will enjoy the activity while also reaping the respiratory benefits of the activity.

In preparation for surgery, use items such as stuffed animals or dolls to help children understand what is going to happen to them (Fig. 32.3). Allow the child to role-play various experiences with dolls. Dolls designed to simulate surgical experiences have been developed. For example, Shadow Buddies (www.shadowbuddies.org) are custom-made dolls that have the same illness or surgery as the child; the doll may have an ostomy, scar, or catheter. The dolls were developed to help children cope with their illness or disease and send the message that it is okay to be different. These dolls also provide the child with a companion to talk to.

> ▶ *Take* NOTE!
>
> *The presence of parents during anesthesia induction reduces child and parent anxiety as well as the incidence of adverse effects (Romino et al., 2005).*

Maintaining Safety During Hospitalization

Safety is a critical aspect of care of the child in the hospital. Due to their age and developmental level, children are vulnerable to harm. Ensure the child has an identification band in place at all times. Sometimes in implementing interventions an armband is removed, so make sure it is attached to another extremity. Monitor children closely to avoid accidents such as a child pushing the wrong knob, picking up a piece of equipment or supplies left in the bed or room, or climbing out of bed (Fig. 32.4). Table 32.4 provides nursing goals for ensuring safe, developmentally appropriate care for the hospitalized child.

Use of Restraints

When caring for children, some type of restriction may be necessary. The restriction, often referred to as a restraint, may be needed to ensure the child's safety, allow a therapeutic or diagnostic procedure to be done, immobilize a body part or limit movement, or prevent disruption of prescribed therapy. However, restraints can be overused and can cause harm. As a result, the Joint Commission on Accreditation of Healthcare Organizations (JCAHO, 2005) issued standards related to the use of restraints designed to safeguard clients' physical safety and psychological well-being.

According to these standards, hospitals are required to have a policy in place that specifies the following:

- Reason for the restraint
- Client assessment parameters identifying the need for the restraint
- Use of at least one alternative method for restriction before using a restraint
- Use of the least restrictive type of restraint for the purpose after the decision is made that a restraint is necessary
- Need for a written order by a licensed independent practitioner (LIP) within 1 hour of application of the restraint
- Need for evaluation by LIP within 1 hour of application of the restraint

In addition, the JCAHO standards also identify the need for specific staff training and frequent assessment and appropriate discontinuation of use.

> ▶ *Take* NOTE!
>
> *When deciding whether it is necessary to restrain a child, consider the child's age, developmental level, mental status, and threat to others and self.*

EVIDENCE-BASED PRACTICE 32.1
Preventing Falls in the Hospitalized Child

Hospitals are increasingly emphasizing the importance of client safety. Due to developmental issues, children are at a high risk of falls. Pediatric and adult clients fall for different reasons. Can adult fall risk factor scales assist in predicting falls in children? What variables increase the risk of falling for the pediatric client?

● Study
A descriptive study was done to identify risk factors in hospitalized children based on two adult fall risk factor scales, the Morse Fall Scale and the Hendrich II Fall Risk Model. A retrospective chart audit was performed to identify 100 hospitalized children who had fallen. Each client who had fallen was matched according to chronological age and year of hospitalization with a child who had not fallen. Analysis was performed to describe sample demographics, length of stay, and environmental fall characteristics. Further analysis was done to determine statistically significant differences in children who fell and those who did not fall based on the risk factor scales.

▲ Findings
A statistically significant difference was found using the Morse Fall Scale between fallers and non-fallers for

history of falls, impaired gait, and mental status. However, the tools used to assess fall risk in adults do not appear to be applicable to children, as several items defined on adult fall scales do not apply to children. The authors determined that a valid and reliable pediatric fall rating scale needs to be developed. The study also showed that having a caregiver in attendance did not provide adequate protection against falls. Visits to the bathroom and entry and exit from a bed were associated with increased fall risk.

■ Nursing Implications
Factors such as an unfamiliar environment, impaired gait, and disorientation contribute to falls in hospitalized children. Nurses should educate caregivers about the risk of falls, providing appropriate guidance for assisting their child when getting into and out of bed or using the bathroom. Orient the child to the environment, repeatedly if necessary. Continue close supervision and monitor disoriented children and those with an impaired gait very frequently.

Razmus, I., Wilson, D., Smith, R., & Newman, E. (2006). Falls in hospitalized children. *Pediatric Nursing, 32*(6), 568–572.

Restraints can promote physical distress in a child. Children also may view restraints as punishment. Before a restraint is used, other measures need to be tried. Explain why the child should not touch the intravenous site or should maintain a certain position so that he or she has a basic understanding of what is necessary. This may be all that is necessary for an older child.

Therapeutic hugging (a holding position that promotes close physical contact between the child and a parent or caregiver) may be used for certain procedures or treatments where the child must remain still. For example, the parent can hold the child in his or her lap snugly to prevent the child from moving during an injection or venipuncture. This technique may be used to position a child for intravenous access, injections, an otoscopic examination, or a lumbar puncture. When using this technique, make sure the parent understands his or her role and knows which body parts to hold still in a safe manner.

Alternatively, distraction or stimulation (such as with a toy) can help to gain the child's cooperation. One-to-one supervision and behavior modification techniques may be other alternatives to the use of restraints.

If it is determined that a restraint is needed, select the most appropriate, least restrictive type of restraint. For example, if the child has an intravenous catheter in the antecubital space that stops flowing when the child bends

the arm, an elbow restraint or arm board, rather than a soft wrist restraint or four-point extremity restraint, would be appropriate. Table 32.5 lists the types of restraints and the major issues associated with the use of restraints in children.

> ▶ ***Take*** NOTE!
>
> *When selecting a restraint, the nurse must choose the least restrictive type and apply it for the shortest time necessary.*

Before applying a restraint, explain the reason for the restraint to the child and the parents. Emphasize that the rationale is to maintain the child's safety; the restraint is not punishment. Having the child and parents state the reason for the restraint demonstrates their understanding.

A written order for the restraint and an evaluation of the child by a LIP must occur within 1 hour of applying the restraint. In addition, the nurse must do the following:

• Ensure that the restraint fits properly.
• Secure the restraints with ties to the bed or crib frame, not the side rails.

TABLE 32.5 TYPES OF RESTRAINTS AND ASSOCIATED SAFETY CONCERNS

Type of Restraint	Purpose	Safety Concerns
Soft limb restraint	Wrist or ankle restraint to prevent range of motion of extremities	Check wrist or ankle for any sign of circulatory, integumentary, or neurologic compromise.
Elbow restraint	Prevents child from flexing and reaching face, head, IV and other tubes	Position the restraint so it does not rub against axilla. Check pulse, temperature, and capillary refill of the extremity.
Mummy restraint	Body restraint using a sheet folded in a square appropriate to size of infant or young child to secure the whole body of the child or every extremity except for one	Ensure that all extremities are secured within the sheet.

Type of Restraint	Purpose	Safety Concerns
Jacket (vest) restraint	Jacket worn by child with ties attached to the child's back and to side of bed. Used to keep children flat in bed, such as after surgery, or safe in chair.	Ensure the child can turn head to side and that the head of the bed is elevated. Place ties in back so child cannot manipulate them.
Crib top bubble restraint	Clear plastic cover over the bed to prevent older infant or young child from falling and climbing out of bed	Ensure that there are no tears or loose plastic.

- Use a clove-hitch type of knot to secure the restraints with ties (this allows for quick, easy access and release of the restraint).
- Check restraints 15 minutes following initial placement and then every hour for proper placement.
- Assess the temperature of the affected extremities, pulses, and capillary refill, initially after 15 minutes and then every hour after placement.
- Remove the restraint every 2 hours to allow for range of motion and repositioning, with documentation of this process and any findings.
- Encourage parent participation, providing continuous explanations about the reasons for the restraints and tentative time frame for use.
- Offer positive reinforcement to the child and parents.
- Review the criteria for removing the restraints; document removal and continued assessment.

Transport of the Child

Children may need to be transported to other units for diagnostic tests or surgery, to different areas in the same unit, such as the playroom or treatment room, or for discharge. When the child is transported to other areas, specific guidelines need to address safety issues, the age and developmental level of the child, the child's physical condition, and the destination. These factors need to be considered before transport so that the appropriate method can be used with the least amount of risk for the child. Various methods to transport children include carrying the infant and using strollers, wagons, or rolling beds (Fig. 32.5). If possible, the parents should accompany the child to offer support and comfort.

When carrying an infant, good support of the back and head is vital. Rails should be up on all beds and wagons. Use safety belts with strollers and wheelchairs.

▶ **Take** NOTE!

Never leave a child unattended during transport. Keep the child visible at all times during the transport.

Providing Basic Care for the Hospitalized Child

Basic care involves general hygiene measures, including bathing, hair care, oral care, and nutritional care. Young children are dependent on an adult for most, if not all, of their self-care needs. If parents are present, allow them to provide care for the child to decrease the child's stress. Older children may perform hygiene measures themselves but may need some assistance from the nurse.

General Hygiene Measures

General hygiene measures help to maintain healthy skin, hair, and teeth. Skin is a complex structure; its primary function is to protect the tissues that it encloses and to protect itself. Injury to the child's skin may occur when inserting and maintaining an intravenous line, removing a dressing, positioning a child in bed, changing a diaper, using and removing electrode patches, and maintaining restraints. Risk factors for problems include impaired mobility, protein malnutrition, edema, incontinence, sensory loss, anemia, and infection. A good time to assess the skin is during bath time.

Bathing

Bathing infants and children is a common daily hygiene measure in the health care environment. Although the parents or primary caregiver often does this in today's family-centered environment, the nurse is still responsible for ensuring that bathing is done safely and hygienically. Adhere to safety principles to prevent falls, burns, and aspiration of water. Never leave a child alone in a bathtub. Use a gentle, pH-balanced soap with moisturizer if there is a need to rehydrate the skin. Note any condition that might require special considerations or further assessment, such as paralysis, loss of sensation, surgical incisions, skin traction/cast, external lines (intravenous lines, urinary catheters, or feeding tubes), or other alterations in skin integrity. Pay close attention to the ears, between skinfolds, the neck, the back, and the genital area for alterations in skin integrity. Table 32.6 highlights specific developmental considerations for bathing.

Before bathing and performing other hygiene measures, assess the family's preferences and home practices for the child, such as time of day, rituals, special equipment, and allergies to products. This is a good time to assess the amount of assistance that might be required by the parents and to address learning needs related to hygiene. Follow general guidelines in bathing any client with regard to equipment, room temperature, privacy, and use of products such as deodorant and lotion.

Hair Care

Lying in bed can make the hair matted and tangled. Avoid pulling on the child's hair when combing or brushing it. If necessary, use commercial detangling solutions to ease combing.

If the hair requires washing, this is often done during the daily bath for infants. Typically, shampooing once or twice a week is sufficient for younger children. Adolescents may need more frequent shampooing due to the increase in sebaceous gland secretion. The frequency of shampooing also varies based on the child's condition; for example, if the child has experienced diaphoresis, more frequent shampooing may be indicated.

Shampooing may be done at the bedside with specially adapted equipment, at a readily accessible sink while the

A

B

C

D

FIGURE 32.5 Methods for transporting the infant or child. (**A**) Cradle method for carrying infants up to 3 months of age. One hand grasps the infant's thighs; the other arm supports the infant's head and back. (**B**) Football method for carrying infants up to 2 months of age. The forearm and hand support the body and head of the infant. (**C**) The "over-the-shoulder" method for carrying infants up to 7 months of age. Support the head if the infant does not have head control. (**D**) A wagon with rails and padding is used to transport small children.

child is sitting in a chair or lying on a stretcher, or in a tub or shower. Commercial no-rinse shampoos may be available for use. With these products, the shampoo is applied to the hair and then brushed or combed out.

If the child uses a tub or shower for hair care, monitor the child's safety throughout to ensure that the child does not slip and fall due to the slippery surface or is burned because of improper water temperature.

The child's ethnicity may require special measures for hair care. For example, a child of African-American descent may use a broad-toothed comb for hair care. Ask the child's parents to bring one from home if one is not available. Also ask the child and parents about any products used on the hair to make it easier to handle; the parents can bring some from home. Encourage the parents to help with braiding or plaiting of the hair if desired.

▶ **Take** NOTE!

The hair of African-Americans typically is easier to comb when wet, so if possible comb the child's hair soon after shampooing.

Oral Hygiene

Oral hygiene is an important part of basic care. Wipe the infant's gums with a wet cloth after each feeding. Assist children in brushing and flossing their teeth after each feeding or meal and before bedtime. The child who is immunosuppressed needs special attention to oral hygiene, such as using soft toothbrushes and moistened gauze sponges to prevent bleeding and careful inspection of the oral cavity for areas of breakdown.

TABLE 32.6   DEVELOPMENTAL CONSIDERATIONS
             FOR BATHING

Age of Child	Special Considerations
Infants	Use a sponge bath or tub bath to bathe young infants who cannot sit unaided. Support the infant's body at all times. Ensure appropriate water temperature. Avoid use of talcum powder.
Toddlers	Bathe older infants and toddlers at the bedside or in a regular bathtub, depending on their health condition.
School-age children and adolescents	Older children may prefer a shower if available and acceptable for their health condition. Assess whether a shower would be safe. Provide privacy.

Nutritional Care

Adequate nutrition is necessary for growth and development and tissue repair, so it is an essential component of care for the ill or hospitalized child.

Frequently, the ill or hospitalized child experiences a loss of appetite, which can affect the child's nutritional status. This may be compounded by other problems such as nausea and vomiting and NPO restrictions for testing or surgery.

▶ *Take* NOTE!

Never attempt to force a child to eat. This can exacerbate nausea and vomiting and can lead to an aversion to food that extends past the hospital stay (Hockenberry, 2005).

If possible, schedule procedures or treatments away from mealtimes. In younger children, refusing to eat may be related to the child's feeling of separation; in others, refusing to eat may reflect the child's attempt to control the situation. Encourage parents to use gentle persuasion instead of force to assist with intake. They should give the child choices about what to eat; this reinforces the child's sense of control. Remind parents that the child's appetite will probably improve as his or her condition improves. Teaching Guidelines 32.2 provides tips for promoting

TEACHING GUIDELINES 32.2

**Promoting Nutrition
for Your Hospitalized Child**

- Check with the nurse about any restrictions related to your child's diet. Find out if intake and output are being monitored.
- Encourage your child to eat his or her favorite foods.
- Assist your child with eating or drinking as necessary; be present at mealtimes to promote socialization.
- Frequently offer small cups of fluid and finger foods; avoid giving large quantities at one time.
- Try offering fluids at different temperatures at different times for variety.
- Remember that children can ingest greater amounts of thin liquids (e.g., gelatin or carbonated drinks) than thicker liquids (e.g., cream soups or milkshakes).
- Include ice chips as fluid intake. Ice is approximately equivalent to half the same amount of water (e.g., 1 cup of ice equals a half-cup of water).
- Use straws (unless not allowed) and brightly colored utensils, cups, or dishes to provide contrast and stimulation.
- Offer the child choices; allow the child to choose what he or she wants from the menu.
- Avoid spicy or highly seasoned foods.
- Talk with the dietitian to see if any special preferences can be addressed.
- Offer praise to your child for what he or she eats or drinks.
- Never punish the child for not eating or drinking.
- Encourage the older child to help keep track of what he or she eats and drinks.

nutrition in the hospitalized child. Although geared to parents, nurses also can incorporate these guidelines into the child's plan of care.

Providing Play, Activities, and Recreation for the Hospitalized Child

Play is an important component in the child's plan of care. Today many health care settings providing care for children have playrooms with age-appropriate toys, equipment, and other creative activities (Fig. 32.6). If the facility is large enough, there may even be a separate area for teens where they can listen to music, play video games, and visit with peers. Obviously, some children will not be able to use these facilities if their activity level is restricted or if isolation is necessary. Children may also play in their rooms. Ensure that opportunities for unstructured play are provided to all children who can engage in play.

FIGURE 32.6 Children occupied in a hospital playroom. It is important to provide age-appropriate activities for younger and older children alike.

Therapeutic play may be used to teach children about their health status or to allow them to work through issues in their lives.

> ▶ *Take* NOTE!
>
> *Avoid using the term "playroom" when caring for older school-aged children and adolescents. Instead, call it the "activity room" or "social room." Doing so promotes a greater feeling of maturity and makes it more likely that they will use the area.*

Child Life Specialist

The **child life specialist** (CLS) is a specially trained individual who provides programs that prepare children for hospitalization, surgery, and other procedures that could be painful (Child Life Council, 2008). The CLS is a member of the multidisciplinary team and works in conjunction with the health care providers and parents to foster an atmosphere that promotes the child's well-being. Services provided by a CLS include:

- Nonmedical preparation for tests, surgeries, and other medical procedures
- Support during medical procedures
- Therapeutic play
- Activities to support normal growth and development
- Sibling support
- Grief and bereavement support
- Emergency room interventions for children and families
- Hospital preadmission tours and information programs
- Outpatient consultation with families (Child Life Council, 2007a)

> ▶ *Take* NOTE!
>
> *Keep the bed or crib and playroom as "safe" places. Perform invasive procedures such as venipunctures in the treatment room if possible. Never perform any nursing interventions in the playroom, no matter how nonthreatening they may appear to the nurse.*

Unstructured Play

Unstructured play allows children to control events, ideas, and relationships. Encourage parents to bring small toys and favorite stuffed animals from home to make the child feel more comfortable in the strange environment of the hospital. Children also enjoy receiving small new toys as surprises when they are hospitalized. Many children enjoy diversional activities such as playing board games or electronic games, reading books, and watching TV, videos, or DVDs. Quiet activities appropriate to the child's developmental level provide the opportunity for play and encourage the use and development of fine motor skills even if the child is confined to bed. Infants and toddlers enjoy manipulating blocks and playing with stacking toys. The preschooler may enjoy coloring, dollhouses, or playing with plastic building blocks such as Legos. School-age children and adolescents may enjoy playing video games or building a model geared toward their developmental level.

Play as Part of Nursing Care

Play is also an important part of nursing care. Use play as appropriate while providing routine nursing care to the child. An example of the use of play in nursing care involves the school-age child's love of competition and games. To increase range of motion in a school-age child who is hospitalized for traction due to a fracture, have the child throw a soft sponge ball or beanbag ball into a hoop, and compete against the child. To increase deep breathing, encourage the child to blow bubbles or blow a whistle. To increase intake of fluids, help the child create a graph to chart the number of glasses of fluids he or she drinks over a period of time. Award the child a sticker, baseball card, special pencil, or other small item if he or she reaches a certain level.

When using play as part of nursing care, it is important to evaluate the outcome of play. Play used in the manner described above should enhance the child's outcome. For example, for the child blowing bubbles, determine whether this activity enhanced coughing and deep breathing.

Therapeutic Play

WATCH & LEARN

Another important aspect of play is **therapeutic play**. Health care professionals use therapeutic play to help the child deal with the physical and psychological challenges of illness and hospitalization. Therapeutic play is nondirected and focuses on helping the child cope with feelings and fears. Supervised play with medical equipment in the hospital environment can help children work thorough their feelings about what has happened to them (Fig. 32.7). In a large hospital or a children's hospital, the CLS typically coordinates these activities. Goals include maintaining normal living patterns, minimizing psychological trauma, and promoting optimal development of the child. If a CLS is not available, the nurse provides this type of activity. There is a greater emphasis on the developmental and psychosocial implications of illness and hospitalization and validation of the child's voice.

In emotional outlet play or traumatic play, the child acts out or dramatizes real-life stressors. For example, using a wooden hammer and pegs, a soft sponge ball, or boxing gloves can allow the child to express anger over separation from family and friends. Commercial toys such as anatomically correct dolls and puppets have removable parts so children can see various organs of the

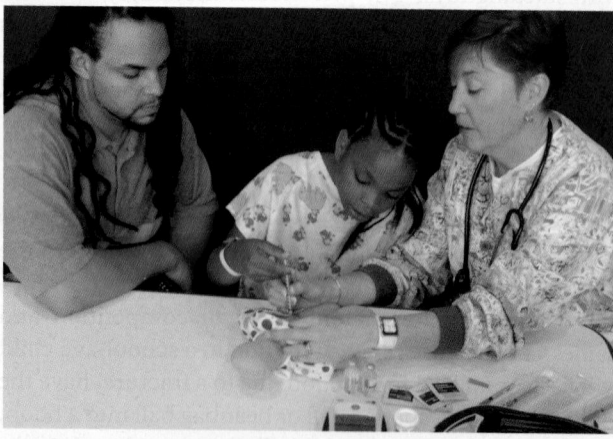

FIGURE 32.7 The nurse supervises play with medical equipment to help the child work through her feelings about being hospitalized.

body. Sometimes younger children "talk" to puppets and dolls, allowing them to express their feelings to a nonthreatening "person" about a specific situation or what they want from the health care provider. For example, the Shadow Buddies dolls mentioned earlier in the chapter provide a way of coping with a specific condition. The company creates an ostomy buddy who has a stoma, a cancer buddy with thinning hair and a chest catheter for chemotherapy treatments, and a heart buddy who has a chest incision and a repaired heart. If the child has a dressing, the doll can also get one.

Other types of therapeutic play include drawing and supervised "needle play." Drawing is a way for the child to express his or her thoughts and feelings. Supervised "needle play" assists children who must undergo frequent blood work, injections, or intravenous procedures. A doll can receive an injection as the child works out his or her anger and anxiety. Keep in mind safety and the child's growth and development level before planning this type of directed play; an adult must always be present.

Promoting Schoolwork and Education During Hospitalization

Promote schoolwork and the child's typical activities while he or she is in the hospital. Determine the amount of this schoolwork by assessing the child's condition, the availability of teachers, and the family situation. Many children's hospitals have teachers at the hospitals; there may be classrooms too. These teachers work closely with the child's neighborhood school to continue schoolwork as the child's condition permits. Hospitals without the educational staff will rely on parents to coordinate with the child's school. Parents may bring in schoolbooks and the child's homework for completion while in the hospital. This connection to the child's school as well as interactions with peers helps maintain normalcy for the child and minimizes the disruption of everyday life.

Addressing the Needs of Family Members

Assess the factors that may influence the family's reaction to the child's hospitalization and plan the care of the child to accommodate some of these issues. Encourage families to have support systems in place before, during, and after hospitalization. Using good communication and tailoring nursing actions to the family's needs and preferences increase the parents' satisfaction with the health care setting (Marino & Marino, 2000).

Parents and Caregivers
As stated previously, the anxiety level of caregivers greatly affects the anxiety level of the child. Thus, it is important to help the family members work through their feelings. Common sources of parental anger when a child is hospi-

talized include visiting restrictions, an unexpected change in the child's health status, confusion resulting from conflicting or insufficient information provided by the hospital staff, and feeling undervalued in the care of their child (Griffin, 2003).

The importance of family involvement to the well-being of the child is reflected in the philosophies, policies, procedures, and physical environments where care is delivered. The philosophy of family-centered care places the family at the core of care. The family is the primary and continuing provider of care for the child. Encourage parents to room-in with the child throughout the hospital stay, if possible. Facilities can be designed to welcome family participation. For example, having computer ports and fax machines available and providing extra meals and beds for the parents can encourage parents to participate in care. View the parents as vital members of the health care team and partners in the care of the ill child.

Siblings

Family-centered care recognizes the need to treat the child in context of the family, including siblings. Important questions that will affect how siblings deal with the hospitalization of their brother or sister include:

- Was the admission an emergency?
- Were there previous admissions, and how did the siblings perceive those hospitalizations?
- How serious is the illness or trauma?
- Is the prognosis known?

Address the sibling's possible feelings of guilt. Use educational materials, allow time for visits, send photographs back and forth between siblings, and allow siblings to talk on the phone.

Providing Client Teaching

Not all experiences with hospitalization are negative: in fact, the experience may enhance the child's and family's coping skills, bolster self-esteem, and provide new socialization experiences. It may allow the child to master self-care skills and provides an opportunity for the child and family to learn new information. Parents may learn more about their child's growth and development skills as well as additional parenting or caregiving skills, resulting in improved parenting abilities. In addition, the child's overall health may be improved because of the hospital stay if the child receives current immunizations and the parents learn more about health care practices.

The overall goals of client and family teaching are to minimize the child's and family's stress, educate them about treatment and nursing care in the hospital, and ensure the family can provide appropriate care at home upon discharge. Providing support before, during, and after hospitalization may minimize stress.

Preadmission programs can introduce the child and family to the setting. During the hospital stay, forming partnerships with the child and family, using strategies to promote coping, and providing appropriate preparation for procedures, tests, and surgery serve to decrease stress.

Assess the child's and family's knowledge of the illness and hospital experience. This provides a baseline for teaching. Include hospital rules in child and family teaching. Behavioral changes in hospitalized children often disturb parents or caregivers. Determine the child's usual patterns of behavior and explain to the parents about the child's reaction to hospitalization. Encourage the family to maintain consistent discipline even while in the hospital to provide structure for the child as well as to prevent discipline issues after discharge. Also discuss how siblings may react to the hospitalization, and provide appropriate teaching to the siblings. Every interaction the nurse has with the child or family provides an opportunity for teaching. Explain the purpose of even simple procedures such as vital signs assessment to the child and family. Provide ongoing information about the child's illness or trauma, treatment plan, and expected outcomes. Chapter 2 provides general principles related to teaching children and their families.

Preparing the Child and Family for Discharge

Discharge planning actually begins upon admission. The nurse assesses the family's resources and knowledge level to determine what education and referrals they may need. Upon discharge, children and their parents or caregivers receive written instructions about home care, and a copy is retained in the medical record. These instructions are individualized for the child. Generally, discharge instructions should include:

- Follow-up appointment information
- Guidelines about when to contact the physician or nurse practitioner (e.g., new or worsening symptoms or indications that the child is not improving)
- Diet
- Activity level allowed
- Medications, including dose, times to be given, route, adverse effects, and special instructions; any prescriptions should be included
- Information on additional treatments the child requires at home
- Specific dates for when the child may return to school or daycare
- Names and phone numbers of agencies the family has been referred to, such as durable medical equipment providers

Provide and review educational booklets that give basic health information or general care for a child with a

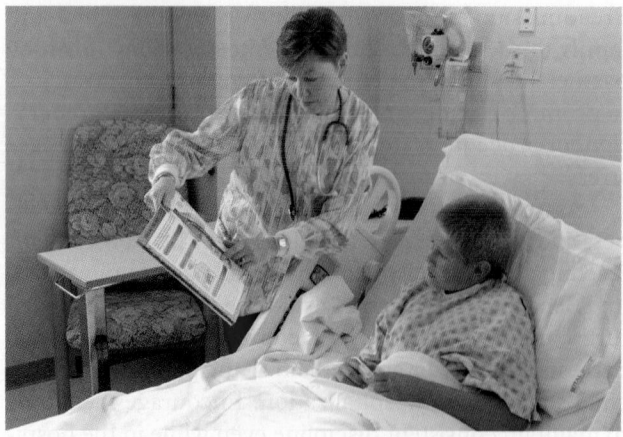

FIGURE 32.8 The nurse uses charts with pictures to perform client teaching before the child goes home.

particular disease (Fig. 32.8). Videotapes, DVDs, or CD-ROMs may also be used if available. The ability to watch a procedure over and over is helpful to some families. Explain, demonstrate, and request a return demonstration of any treatments or procedures to be done at home. Provide a written schedule if the child is to receive multiple medications, tube feedings, or other medical treatments. For complicated cases, a written teaching plan may be used to provide continuity of child/family education between various nurses. As the family attempts to perform each task, document whether the caregiver continues to require assistance or prompting with the task or whether he or she can perform the task independently.

Parents of children with multiple medical needs may benefit from a trial period of home care. This occurs while the child is still in the hospital, but the parents or caregivers provide all of the care that the child requires. Support the family and praise their accomplishments during this trial period.

■■■ Key Concepts

■ Stressors associated with hospitalization include separation from family and routines; fear of an unknown environment; potential for pain, bodily injury, or mutilation; and loss of control.

■ Responses of children to the general stressors of hospitalization include anxiety, fear, anger, guilt, and regression.

■ Parents may experience anger or guilt related to the hospitalization of their child.

■ The responses of children and families to hospitalization can be influenced by the age and developmental level of the child, their perceptions of the situation, previous experiences, separation from family and peers, coping skills, and the preparation and support provided by the family, facility, and health care providers.

■ Whatever the reason for admission, preparation for admission is vital.

■ Upon admission to the hospital or outpatient unit, orient the child and family to the unit, discuss unit rules, and begin patient/family teaching.

■ Since due to their age and developmental level children may be vulnerable to harm, the nurse must use appropriate safety measures in caring for children (e.g., identification of children, use of restraints and transportation, basic hygiene measures).

■ Nursing care is directed toward meeting the child's needs related to self-care, separation anxiety, growth and development, diversion, family, control, teaching, pain relief, and coping.

■ Play, including therapeutic play, is an important strategy to prepare children for hospitalization and to help them adapt to the effects of illness and hospitalization. It provides an emotional outlet, opportunities for teaching and learning, and the ability to become familiar with a situation and improve physiologic abilities. A child life specialist is a specially trained individual who is a member of the child's multidisciplinary team. He or she works in conjunction with the child's health care providers and parents to foster an atmosphere that promotes the child's well-being.

■ Family-centered care and atraumatic care are philosophies that pay special attention to the concerns of the family and child during hospitalization.

■ Providing support to hospitalized children and their families is critical for minimizing stress.

■ Discharge planning begins upon admission. Each interaction with the family is an opportunity for patient teaching.

REFERENCES

Bricher, G. (2000). Children in the hospital: Issues of power and vulnerability. *Pediatric Nursing, 26*(3), 277–282.
Child Life Council. (1998–2003). What is a child life specialist? Available at: http://www.childlife.org/About/what_is_specialist.htm.
Child Life Council. (2007). *How a child life specialist can help you.* Retrieved May 16, 2008 from http://www.childlife.org/The%20Child%20Life%20Professional/HowaChildLifeSpecialistCanHelpYou.cfm.
Child Life Council. (2008). *Child life: Empowering children and families to cope with life's challenges.* Retrieved May 16, 2008 from http://www.childlife.org/files/AboutChildLife2008.pdf.
Griffin, T. (2003). Facing challenges to family-centered care, II: Anger in the clinical setting. *Pediatric Nursing, 29*(3), 212–214.
Herron, R. (2005). Young patients learn "on tour" with Pediatric Express. *Advance for Nurses, 3*(24), 10.
Hockenberry, M. (2005). *Wong's essentials of pediatric nursing.* St. Louis: Mosby.
Joint Commission on Accreditation of Healthcare Organizations. (2005). *Setting the standard: The Joint Commission and health care safety and quality.* Oakbrook Terrace, IL: JCAHO.
Justus, R., Wyles, D., Wilson, J., Rode, D., Walther, V., & Lim-Sulit, N. (2006). Preparing children and families for surgery: Mount Sinai's multidisciplinary perspective. *Pediatric Nursing, 31*(1), 35–43.

Mansson, M. E., & Dykes, A. (2004). Practices for preparing children for clinical examination and procedures in Swedish pediatric wards. *Pediatric Nursing, 30*(3), 182.

Marino, B. L., & Marino, E. K. (2000). Practice applications of research. Parents' report of children's hospital care: What it means for your practice. *Pediatric Nursing, 26*(2), 195–198.

Romino, S. L., Keatley, V. M., Secrest, J., & Good, K. (2005). Parental presence during anesthesia induction in children. *AORN Journal, 81*(4), 779–792.

Stratton, K. M. (2004). Parents' experiences of their child's care during hospitalization. *Journal of Cultural Diversity, 11*(1), 4.

U.S. Department of Health and Human Services, Health Resources and Services Administration, Maternal and Child Health Bureau (2005). *Child health USA 2005.* U.S. Department of Health and Human Services.

Winch, A. (2001). Role play: A nurse's role in helping well children cope with a parent's serious illness and/or hospitalization. *Journal of the Society of Pediatric Nurses, 6*(1), 42–46.

Wollin, S. R., Plummer, J. L., Owen, H., et al. (2004). Anxiety in children having elective surgery. *Journal of Pediatric Nursing, 19*(2), 128–132.

Zengerle-Levy, K. (2006). Nursing the child who is alone in the hospital. *Pediatric Nursing, 32*(3), 226–231.

WEBSITES

American Academy of Pediatrics: www.aap.org
Institute for Family-Centered Care: www.familycentercare.org
Starbright Foundation: www.starbright.org

CHAPTER WORKSHEET

MULTIPLE CHOICE QUESTIONS

1. The nurse would most likely assess separation anxiety in which of these children?

   a. A 2-month-old infant

   b. A 15-month-old toddler

   c. A 4-year-old preschooler

   d. An 11-year-old child

2. When developing the preoperative plan of care for an adolescent, the nurse plans interventions to address the adolescent's anxieties and fears related to:

   a. Separation from parents

   b. Punishment for wrongdoing

   c. Changes in body image

   d. Magical thinking

3. The nurse is preparing a 5-year-old boy for surgery on his lower leg. His mother is helping him into the hospital gown and the boy fights removal of his underwear. What is the most appropriate nursing action?

   a. Allow the mother to remove the underwear.

   b. Tell the boy he is acting childishly.

   c. Notify the OR that the underwear is on.

   d. Allow the boy to keep his underwear on.

4. A 6-month-old infant requires restraint to prevent removal of his nasogastric tube. What is the priority nursing intervention?

   a. Tie the restraint loosely to prevent skin breakdown.

   b. Leave the baby unrestrained when directly observed.

   c. Position the restrained infant prone to prevent aspiration.

   d. Place the infant in a room near the nurses' station.

5. A 10-year-old child on a regular diet refuses to eat the food on her meal tray. She requests chicken nuggets, French fries, and ice cream. What is the best nursing action?

   a. Ask that the child's desired foods be sent up from the kitchen.

   b. Negotiate with the child to eat at least part of the food on the tray.

   c. Remove a privilege.

   d. Offer the child cereal and milk from stock on the nursing unit.

CRITICAL THINKING EXERCISES

1. Becky, an 8-year-old, is admitted to the pediatric unit for an emergency surgery. She is in third grade and very active in after-school programs. Her mother is with her during the admission process but will have to return to work shortly after Becky returns from surgery to the pediatric unit. Would the nurse expect Becky to show separation anxiety? What are the three top nursing diagnoses for Becky?

2. A 6-year-old is admitted to the general pediatric unit after spending several hours in the emergency department with an acute asthma attack. Her mother and two younger siblings are present, but the mother plans to leave shortly to take the siblings home. The father will visit in about 2 hours, after work. What is the overall goal for this child's care? What could the nurse say to promote coping in this child? What would be the best answer if the mother asks if she should stay?

STUDY ACTIVITIES

1. Shadow a child life specialist in a hospital. Identify his or her role and how he or she works with the nursing staff.

2. Follow a child and family during the admission process, from preadmission to initial time on the unit, to identify the procedures and tasks involved. Examine the response of the child and family and how the nursing staff responds to their needs.

3. Spend a day in radiology or the emergency room to learn about the strategies used to prepare children for various procedures.

4. Develop a teaching plan to orient a toddler or preschooler and his or her family to a nursing unit. Include the resources, personnel, and techniques to include in the teaching plan.

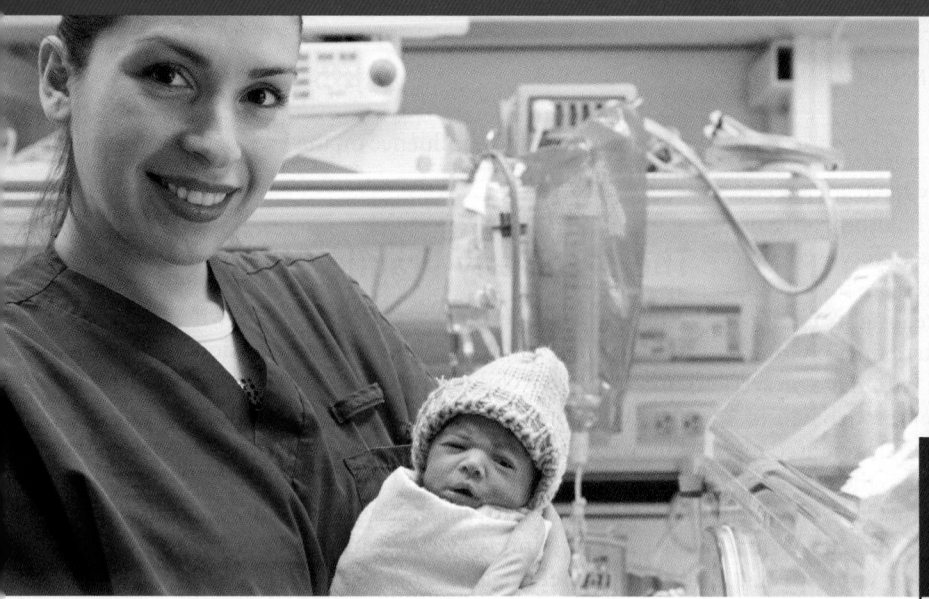

NURSING CARE OF THE CHILD WITH SPECIAL NEEDS

KEY TERMS

chronic illness
developmental delay

developmental disability
palliative care

respite care
terminal illness

LEARNING OBJECTIVES

Upon completion of the chapter, the learner will be able to:

1. Analyze the impact that being a child with special needs has on the child and family.
2. Describe ways that nurses assist children with special needs and their families to obtain optimal functioning.
3. Identify anticipated times when the child and family will require additional support.
4. Plan for transition of the special needs child from the inpatient facility to the home, and from pediatric to adult medical care.
5. Discuss early intervention and public school education for the special needs child.
6. Differentiate developmental responses to death and appropriate interventions.
7. Discuss key elements related to pediatric end-of-life care.

Preet Singh, a 2-year-old boy who was born at 27 weeks' gestation, is seen in your clinic for the first time. He has a history of hydrocephalus and developmental delay. During the examination, his mother states, "I'm concerned about finding a good, affordable preschool for Preet. His older brother attends public school, but I can't imagine Preet there." After further discussion with Preet's mother, you realize he has not been involved in an early intervention program.

WOW

The touch of a mother's hand and the sound of her voice bring comfort to her special child, and when you bring comfort, you strengthen both of them.

As medicine and scientific technology have advanced, the number of children surviving with health problems that require long-term interventions has increased significantly (Hewitt-Taylor, 2005). Children are now living with conditions that require high-tech treatments for survival. The Maternal Child Health Bureau defines children with special health care needs as those who have or are at risk for a chronic physical, developmental, behavioral, or emotional condition beyond needs generally required by children (Jackson Allen, 2004). According to the National Survey of Children with Special Health Care Needs, about 12.8% of children in the United States have special health care needs. Of those children with special needs, almost 25% are reported as having conditions that affect their activities usually, always, or a great deal of the time (U.S. Department of Health and Human Services, 2004).

In addition to the direct effects of their special needs, these children and their families are often inadequately insured, have financial needs, have unmet family support needs, or have difficulty obtaining the specialty care that the child requires. Nationwide, 11% report not having a personal doctor or nurse ("medical home") (U.S. Department of Health and Human Services, 2004). Children with special health care needs generally require more intensive and diverse health services, as well as coordination of those services, than do typical children (Child and Adolescent Health Measurement Initiative, 2006). It can be challenging for the family of a child with special needs to navigate the system and obtain all of the services their child requires.

Another difficult situation that families may encounter is losing a child to the disease process. A child's chronic illness may progress to the point of becoming terminal. Despite the increased survival rates for children with cancer as a result of improved treatment options and protocols, cancer remains the leading cause of death from disease in all children over the age of 1 year. Less frequently, other diseases also lead to **terminal illness** in children, with congenital defects and traumatic injuries being the more common causes. Caring for the dying child is a family-centered, multidisciplinary process. Nurses must respond to the child's and family's physiologic, emotional, and spiritual needs during this difficult time. Children display differing responses to the dying process and impending death depending on their developmental level. Children and their families need significant amounts of support throughout the process of dying.

For children with special needs, the pediatric nurse fills the critical role of child and family advocate and case manager. When a child is dying, nurses provide physical care of the child and also strive to meet the emotional needs of the child and family. Nurses are in a unique position, both in the inpatient and outpatient setting, to have a significant and positive influence on the lives of these children and their families.

The Medically Fragile Child

When an infant is born very prematurely, when a child is injured and requires long-term rehabilitation and special care, or when a child is diagnosed with a complex chronic health condition, the parents are often devastated initially. The parents of medically fragile children may feel they must adapt to the risk and protect their child. They are interested in preserving their family while compensating for the past, and they cautiously look to the future and become hopeful again. While the infant or child is still in the hospital, nurses can help parents build on their strengths, empowering them to care for their medically fragile infant or special needs child. Education is paramount and should begin as early in the hospitalization as possible. In many situations, particular discharge needs are known early in the course of the infant's or child's hospitalization. Nurses should provide anticipatory guidance about the course of treatment and the expected outcome.

Most children with **chronic illness**, or those who are dependent on technology, progress through stages of growth and development just as typical children do, though possibly at a slower pace. The exception is the child with significant psychomotor retardation, though some developmental progression may occur. Children with special health care needs desire to be treated as normal (Wang & Barnard, 2004), and they want to experience the same events that other children do.

Of particular concern is a growing subset of children with emotional, behavioral, and developmental problems. Children with these needs have even greater difficulty receiving the care and services they require. Many children with emotional, behavioral, or developmental problems also have health problems. Often, these children's problems are not diagnosed early and treatment is difficult. Ongoing counseling and therapy is very difficult for some families to obtain (CDC, 2005). Ultimately, this has a negative impact on the child's physical and mental health and may result in decreased achievement and productivity as the child matures. See Healthy People 2010.

HEALTHY PEOPLE 2010

Objective	Nursing Significance
Reduce the proportion of children and adolescents with disabilities who are reported to be sad, unhappy, or depressed.	Screen children with special health care needs for depression or sadness. Refer children and their families to mental health providers as needed.

Effect of Special Needs on the Child and Family

The child with special needs and his or her family are both affected by the child's condition and way of living. Each member of the family experiences effects related to the child's special needs. Family members' experiences and their responses to the child's illness influence each other directly. They also affect the coping ability of the child with special needs. Children's ability to cope is significantly affected by the family's response to stressors.

Effects on the Child

Children with special health care needs experience differing effects of the chronic illness or disability based on their developmental level, which naturally changes over time for most children.

Infants may fail to develop a sense of trust or attach appropriately with the parents because of frequent hospitalizations, often with multiple caregivers involved, lack of consistency in nurturing, or parental detachment or grieving over the child's condition. The infant's ability to learn through sensorimotor exploration may be impaired due to lack of appropriate stimulation, confinement to a crib, or increased contact with painful experiences.

The toddler may experience difficulty developing autonomy because of increased dependency on the parent or overinvolvement by the parent. Motor and language skill development may be delayed if the toddler is not given adequate opportunities to test his or her limits and abilities.

Limited opportunity also reduces the preschooler's development of a sense of initiative. The preschooler may experience limited opportunities for socialization, causing him or her to withdraw or to feel criticized. Body image development may be hindered due to painful exposures and anxiety. In preschoolers, magical thinking may lead to feelings of guilt for having caused their own disease or condition.

The school-age child may have limited opportunities to achieve a sense of industry because of school absence and inability to participate in activities or competitive events. Lack of socialization limits the school-age child's ability to form peer relationships. The ability to learn via concrete operations is affected by the child's physical limitations or possibly the treatments required.

Adolescents may feel as though they are different from their peers because of their lack of skills/abilities or their appearance. This may hinder the teen's ability to form a sense of personal identity. Since the teen with special health care needs often requires significant amounts of support from the parents, it may be difficult for the adolescent to achieve independence. If the earlier stages of cognitive development have been delayed, then reaching the level of abstract thinking may be blocked.

The child with special health care needs may be able to focus on the positive experiences in his or her life as a method of coping, leading to as much independence as possible. Other children may always feel different from their peers (in a negative sense) and withdraw. Irritability and acting out may also occur. Some children may be compliant and/or seek support for themselves. The child's coping pattern may change over time or with certain situations, such as relapse or worsening of the condition. Children with overprotective parents may display marked dependence and may be very fearful. Children whose parents have been overly indulgent may be more independent and defiant. The nurse must assess the child's individual response to the current health care status and intervene as appropriate.

Effects on the Parents

Raising a child with special needs is generally not the life parents expected to have. Some parents may adapt over time and ultimately accept the child's illness or disability. Others may adapt but do not accept the child's condition and experience the continual fading and re-emergence of chronic sorrow. Denial of their child's problem may prevent parents from progressing through grief, but it also allows them to have hope (Rolland & Walsh, 2006).

Caring for the special needs child at home (rather than having the child in a facility) may decrease the parents' feelings of anxiety and helplessness (Fig. 33.1). As with typically developing children, parents enjoy witnessing the emotional and social growth of the child (Wang & Barnard, 2004). Parents of special needs children experience a multitude of emotions and changes in their lives; they report that they "live worried" (Coffey, 2006). They feel helpless and overwhelmed at discharge from the hospital. Though willing to carry the burden, they may experience fear, anger,

FIGURE 33.1 The special needs child often requires a significant amount of care at home.

sadness, guilt, frustration, or resentment. Many parents experience grief as a result of losing the "perfect child" they dreamed of.

Stressors of Daily Living

Families with a child who has special health care needs experience life differently than other families. They may have to change their housing situation to accommodate the child's needs. Their sleep is affected. Constant supervision of the technology-dependent child makes it difficult to carry out other basic household activities. In addition to basic childcare and running of the household, medical and technical care must be incorporated into daily life. The family's identity and the parents' employment may be altered radically. Holidays and vacations are affected, as it is difficult to plan activities. Nursing and other health care professional visits are disruptive to family life.

Mothers appear to carry the larger burden of care, though fathers are not unaffected. Somehow, parents eventually take charge, and though they fear failure, they display vigilance, can negotiate and seek information, and become advocates for their child and experts on his or her care. Though parents may feel trapped, isolated, and experience a loss of freedom, their need to survive as a family continues to motivate them. Parents may feel a need to be with their child at all times and experience stress related to coping with the heavy load of caregiving (Case-Smith, 2004).

The extended burden of caregiving can also have adverse health effects on caregivers: only a small percentage of parents of children with special health care needs report that they routinely participate in health-promoting activities for themselves (Kuster et al., 2004). Additionally, parents of children with special health care needs are at increased risk for the development of depression (Wang & Barnard, 2004).

In addition to the caregiving burden, parents experience role conflicts, financial burdens, and the struggle between independence in providing care and the isolation associated with it. It is very difficult to enjoy spontaneous events outside the home because so much planning is necessary (Case-Smith, 2004).

The possibility of independence revolves around mobility issues, education, and assistive technology. Though education for all children is federally mandated, parents have anxiety about educational decisions and also find it difficult to obtain the support and educational services the child needs.

Additional stress is associated with transition times in the care of a special needs child. These transition times include:

- Initial diagnosis or change in prognosis
- Increased symptoms
- When the child moves to a new setting (hospital, school)
- During a parent's absence
- During periods of developmental change

Vulnerable Child Syndrome

"Vulnerable child syndrome" is a clinical state in which the parents' reactions to a serious illness or event in the child's past continue to have long-term psychologically harmful effects on the child and parents for many years. The parents view the child as being at higher risk for medical, developmental, or behavioral problems (Kerruish et al., 2005). Parents exhibit excessive unwarranted concerns and seek health care for their child very frequently. Risk factors for the development of vulnerable child syndrome include preterm birth, congenital anomaly, newborn jaundice, handicapping condition, an accident or illness that the child was not expected to recover from, or crying or feeding problems in the first 5 years of life (Pearson & Boyce, 2004). The parent has difficulty separating from the child, and the child senses that anxiety and then develops symptoms that reinforce the parent's fears. Alternatively (or additionally), the parents may to try to retain control, particularly at times of increasing independence, and fear disciplining the child as they do not want to "upset" the child (Pearson & Boyce, 2004).

Effects on Siblings

The siblings of children with special health care needs are also affected dramatically. Their relationship with their parents is different than it would have been if they had a typical brother or sister. Parents often need to spend more time with the child with special needs and have less time with their healthy children. Children exhibit emotional and psychological responses to their sibling's long-term needs. Knowledge about the sibling's illness, attitude toward and adjustment to it, the sibling's own self-esteem, how socially supported the sibling is, and the parents' awareness of sibling's feelings are all related to how well the sibling adjusts (Hewitt-Taylor, 2005).

Nursing Management of the Medically Fragile Child

Family-centered care provides the optimal framework for caring for medically fragile children and their families. Family-centered care minimizes the impact of chronic illness and maximizes the child's developmental potential. To provide the best nursing care for these children and the families, the nurse must first develop a trusting relationship with the family.

To ensure optimal functioning, children with special health care needs require comprehensive and coordinated services from multiple professionals. These professionals should work collaboratively to address the child's health, educational, psychological, and social service needs (Farmer, 2005). In addition to case management and advocacy, nursing management focuses on screening and ongoing assessment of the child, provision of home care, care of the technology-dependent child, education and support of the child and family, and referral for resources.

Developing a Therapeutic Relationship

Raising children is always challenging, but for the parent of a special needs child it is often overwhelming and exhausting. The parents' needs change continuously, so it is best if the family has a permanent relationship with a health care provider. This promotes trust and a more efficient two-way flow of information (Nuutila & Salanterä, 2006).

Respect the parents' range of emotions and work with them as a team to manage the child's care. Parents need to be recognized for complying with the treatment plan or for other small gains that are made (Jackson Allen, 2004). Empowering the family strengthens them and gives them self-confidence (Lindblad et al., 2005). Feeling supported and invigorated gives parents strength, energy, and hope. Box 33.1 lists principles related to family involvement.

Screening and Ongoing Assessment

Nurses should perform screening to identify children with unmet health care needs (Jackson Allen, 2004). A screening tool developed by the Child and Adolescent Health Measurement Initiative (Fig. 33.2) may help to identify children with special health care needs. Additional information related to the screening tool is available at http://www.cahmi.org/pages/Sections.aspx?Section=10.

Children with special health care needs may attain developmental milestones more slowly than typically developing children. If the Denver II is used for ongoing developmental surveillance of the young child, then the results should be compared from visit to visit to determine progress rather than using it as a screening tool. Assess special needs children and their families for vulnerable child syndrome.

Promoting Home Care

Home is the most developmentally appropriate environment for all children, even those who are technology dependent. The child's home provides an emotionally nurturing and socially stimulating environment. Children desire to be cared for at home, and those who are cared for at home display an improved physical, emotional, psychological, and social status (Wang & Barnard, 2004).

Technology-dependent children may require supplemental oxygen, assisted ventilation, tracheostomy care, assisted enteral or parenteral feeding, or parenteral medication administration. Traditionally, hospitalization would have been required for these children—in fact, intensive care would have been necessary for children who need assisted ventilation—but with advances in technology, today even children with extensive medical and developmental needs may be cared for at home. Early discharge planning is important, and parents will need detailed instructions and support in caring for the technology-dependent child at home.

Early Discharge Planning

Early discharge planning and ongoing inclusion and education of the family facilitates continuity of care (Swartz, 2005). Box 33.2 provides information about preparing the medically fragile child for discharge.

Caring for the Technology-Dependent Child at Home

Home care nurses are often involved in the care of technology-dependent children. Caring for a technology-dependent child at home is a complex process, yet children thrive in the home care setting with appropriate intervention and care. Many parents feel that rearing a technology-dependent child is different only because of the presence of the equipment. Nurses may tend to think that parents treat the technology-dependent child differently than the other children, while parents value normalization and want to raise and provide discipline to all of their children in the same manner. Parents should tell nurses about their child-rearing expectations, and nurses need to respect the parents' wishes.

Improved collaboration between parents and home care nurses may decrease the parents' stress and maximize opportunities for appropriate growth and development in the technology-dependent child. Thus, a strong relationship, good communication, and negotiation skills are assets to the family and child.

Help the family to incorporate the medical regimen into daily life to minimize the child's self-perception of being "different" (Green & Ray, 2006). Teach families about the technical issues, such as home and travel oxygen therapy, use of the ventilator, suctioning, chest percussion and postural drainage, tube feedings and care of the feeding tube, and medications. Assist parents with the planning and management of routine care, respiratory treatments, nutritional support, and developmental interventions. Reinforce exercises and techniques as prescribed by developmental therapists (Romanko, 2005). Refer to Chapter 2 for additional information about home care nursing.

BOX 33.1 **Principles Related to Family Involvement**

Families:
- Define who they are and their culture
- Need to have their basic needs met
- Need to have access to information and training
- Deserve to receive culturally competent care
- Can identify priorities and concerns that lead to policy change
- Know their strengths, limitations, and fears
- Share decision-making power and responsibility for outcomes

Adapted from Federation of Families for Children's Mental Health. (2007). *FFCMH principles for family involvement.*

(text continues on page 1016)

CAHMI Children with Special Health Care Needs (CSHCN) Screening Tool
(mail or telephone)

1. Does your child currently need or use **medicine prescribed by a doctor** (other than vitamins)?
   - ☐ Yes ⇐ Go to Question 1a
   - ☐ No ⇐ Go to Question 2

    1a. Is this because of ANY medical, behavioral or other health condition?
   - ☐ Yes ⇐ Go to Question 1b
   - ☐ No ⇐ Go to Question 2

    1b. Is this a condition that has lasted or is expected to last for _at least_ 12 months?
   - ☐ Yes
   - ☐ No

2. Does your child need or use more **medical care, mental health or educational services** than is usual for most children of the same age?
   - ☐ Yes ⇐ Go to Question 2a
   - ☐ No ⇐ Go to Question 3

    2a. Is this because of ANY medical, behavioral or other health condition?
   - ☐ Yes ⇐ Go to Question 2b
   - ☐ No ⇐ Go to Question 3

    2b. Is this a condition that has lasted or is expected to last for _at least_ 12 months?
   - ☐ Yes
   - ☐ No

3. Is your child **limited or prevented** in any way in his or her ability to do the things most children of the same age can do?
   - ☐ Yes ⇐ Go to Question 3a
   - ☐ No ⇐ Go to Question 4

    3a. Is this because of ANY medical, behavioral or other heath condition?
   - ☐ Yes ⇐ Go to Question 3b
   - ☐ No ⇐ Go to Question 4

    3b. Is this a condition that has lasted or is expected to last for _at least_ 12 months?
   - ☐ Yes
   - ☐ No

4. Does your child need or get **special therapy**, such as physical, occupational or speech therapy?
   - ☐ Yes ⇐ Go to Question 4a
   - ☐ No ⇐ Go to Question 5

    4a. Is this because of ANY medical, behavioral or other health condition?
   - ☐ Yes ⇐ Go to Question 4b
   - ☐ No ⇐ Go to Question 5

    4b. Is this a condition that has lasted or is expected to last for _at least_ 12 months?
   - ☐ Yes
   - ☐ No

5. Does your child have any kind of emotional, developmental or behavioral problem for which he or she needs or gets **treatment or counseling**?
   - ☐ Yes ⇐ Go to Question 5a
   - ☐ No

    5a. Has this problem lasted or is it expected to last for _at least_ 12 months?
   - ☐ Yes
   - ☐ No

FIGURE 33.2 The CSHCN Screener. (Reprinted with permission from the Child and Adolescent Health Management Initiative.)

Scoring the Children with Special Health Care Needs (CSHCN©) Screening Tool

Conceptual background

The CSHCN Screener uses consequences-based criteria to screen for children with chronic or special health needs. To qualify as having chronic or special health needs, the following set of conditions must be met:

       a) The child currently experiences a specific consequence.

       b) The consequence is due to a medical or other health condition.

       c) The duration or expected duration of the condition is 12 months or longer.

The first part of each screener question asks whether a child experiences one of five different health consequences:

       1) Use or need of prescription medication

       2) Above-average use or need of medical, mental health or educational services

       3) Functional limitations compared with others of same age

       4) Use or need of specialized therapies (OT, PT, speech, etc.)

       5) Treatment or counseling for emotional or developmental problems

The second and third parts* of each screener question ask those responding "yes" to the first part of the question whether the consequence is due to any kind of health condition and if so, whether that condition has lasted or is expected to last for at least 12 months.

     *NOTE: CSHCN screener question 5 is a two-part question. Both parts must be answered "yes" to qualify.

All three parts of at least one screener question (or in the case of question 5, the two parts) must be answered "yes" in order for a child to meet CSHCN Screener criteria for having a chronic condition or special health care need.

The CSHCH Screener has three "definitional domains." These are:

       1) Dependency on prescription medications

       2) Service use above that considered usual or routine

       3) Functional limitations

The definitional domains are not mutually exclusive categories. A child meeting the CSHCN Screener© criteria for having a chronic condition may qualify for one or more definitional domains (see diagram below).

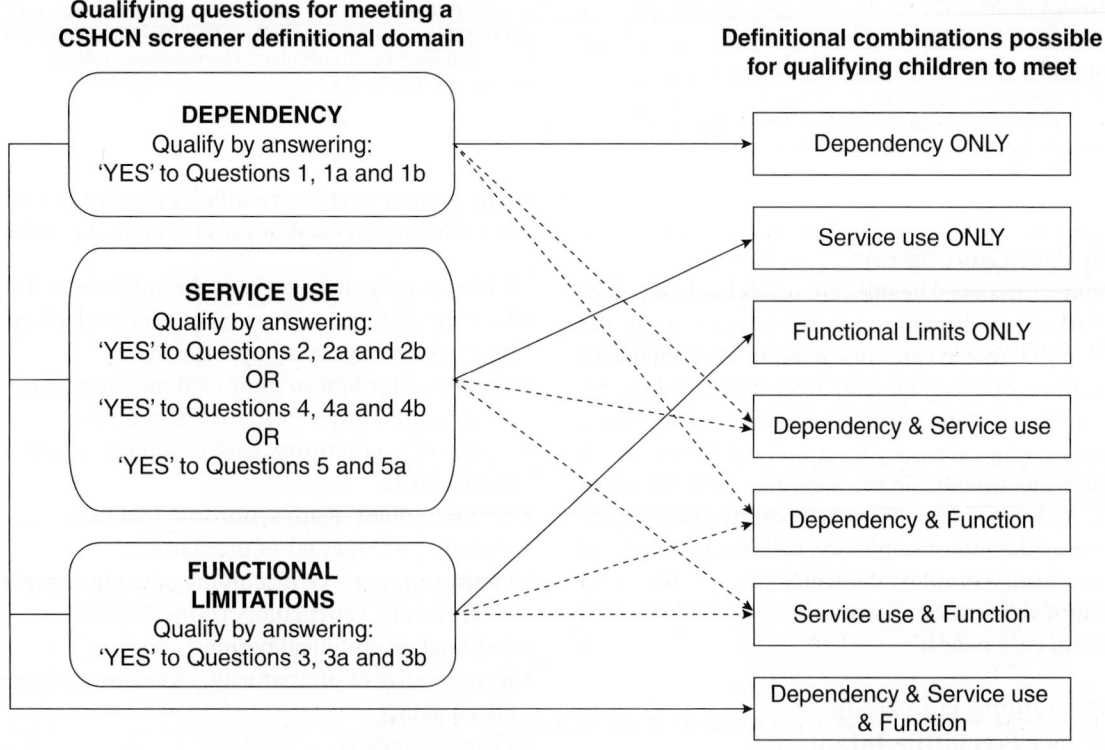

FIGURE 33.2 (continued)

BOX 33.2 **Preparing for Home Care Before Discharge**

• Promote liaison with community resources. Develop communication between various services. Plan appointments. Set up home nursing care (either private duty or visits).
• Teach skills, encouraging active caregiving in the hospital setting to increase the parents' self-confidence
• Discuss psychological and emotional issues with parents.
• Obtain/organize equipment and supplies (running out of supplies may cause significant stress on families).
• Refer the family for necessary financial resources.
• Ensure the family's home environment is adequate (enough room for equipment, electricity on, air conditioner for warm weather, heater for cold weather, and refrigeration for food).
• For the baby being discharged from the NICU:
  • Teach the parents about the infant's cues and behaviors and the preemie's different sleep–wake patterns.
  • Encourage kangaroo care and infant massage while in the NICU (as the infant's condition allows).
  • Educate the parents about possible effects on short- and long-term neurodevelopment.
  • Refer to local early intervention program.
  • Assist the family with finding a primary care provider who is experienced in the ongoing follow-up of high-risk infants.

Data from Bakewell-Sachs, S., & Genarro, S. (2004). Parenting the post-NICU premature infant. *MCN, 29*(6), 398–403; and Hewitt-Taylor, J. (2005). Caring for children with complex and continuing health needs. *Nursing Standard, 19*(42), 41–47.

Providing Care Coordination

Once a child with special health care needs has been identified and has been discharged to the home setting, the nurse plays a vital role in care coordination. Any child with special health care needs benefits from a medical home. The nurse in the medical home is a critical team member, providing ongoing care coordination and follow-up. If such services are available in the local area, refer the child and family with special needs to an integrated health program that provides interdisciplinary, collaborative care for children requiring complex, coordinated care. Box 33.3 lists nursing interventions for families of children with special health care needs.

Providing Ongoing Follow-Up of the Former Premature Infant

Many former premature infants experience a myriad of medical and developmental problems throughout infancy, early childhood, and beyond. Upon or following discharge,

---

BOX 33.3 **Nursing Interventions for Families of Children with Special Health Care Needs**

• Flag the special needs child's chart.
• Develop written health plans.
• Provide care coordination and collaboration with specialists in other disciplines, early intervention, schools and public agencies.
• Address needs for prior authorization for treatments, medication or specialist referrals; retain copies in the child's chart of authorization forms and approvals.
• Modify office routines to promote family and child comfort.
• Assist parents with childcare decisions. Help parents to understand the child's limits and abilities and the potential health issues (e.g., infections and injuries) associated with childcare.
• Know community resources available to children with special health care needs.
• When the child is hospitalized, encourage high levels of parental participation (if desired by the parent).
• Provide care coordination across multiple health settings.
• Educate childcare providers on child health needs.
• Help parents get involved with parent support networks.

Data from Jackson Allen, P. L. (2004). Children with special health care needs: National survey of prevalence and health care needs. *Pediatric Nursing, 30*(4), 307–314; and Onufer, C. N. (2006). New momentum on building a medical home for the child with a chronic health problem. *Contemporary Pediatrics, 23*(10), 65–66, 66–70, 72–73.

---

many former premature infants display one or many of the following medical or developmental problems:

• Chronic lung disease (bronchopulmonary dysplasia)
• Cardiac changes such as right ventricular hypertrophy and pulmonary artery hypertension
• Growth retardation, poor feeding, anemia of prematurity, other nutrient deficiencies
• Apnea of prematurity, gastroesophageal reflux disease, bradycardia
• Sudden infant death syndrome (SIDS)
• Rickets (osteopenia) of prematurity
• Hydrocephalus, ventriculomegaly, abnormal head MRI results, ventriculoperitoneal shunt
• Inguinal or umbilical hernias
• Retinopathy of prematurity, strabismus, decreased visual acuity
• Hearing deficits
• Delayed dentition
• Gross motor, fine motor, and language delay, sensory integration issues

Over the long term, former premature infants are at higher risk than typical infants of developing cognitive delay, cerebral palsy, attention-deficit disorder, learning disabilities, difficulties with socialization, and vulnerable child syndrome. Additionally, many former premature infants display alterations in muscle tone at or shortly after discharge from the neonatal intensive care unit (NICU) that require physical therapy intervention.

For these reasons, high-risk infants require special attention and thorough, appropriate assessment to discern subtle changes that may affect their long-term physical, cognitive, emotional, and social outcome. The pediatric nurse should have an understanding of the special concerns that former premature infants and children as well as their families may face.

From the beginning, encourage families to keep a binder that includes all of the infant's pertinent check-up, insurance, and medical and developmental information; this will serve as a resource for the parents, and they will be able to supply complete information when visiting various providers (Kelly, 2006c).

Providing Routine Well-Child Care of the Former Premature Infant

Former premature infants require similar well-child care as typical infants do, with additional visits for management of multiple complex medical issues and developmental screening/intervention. Teach families routine newborn care, including bathing, dressing, and avoidance of passive cigarette smoke. All visits for primary care follow-up will be scheduled based on the infant's chronological age.

Prior to discharge from the NICU, the infant will be tested for oxygen desaturation while seated in the car seat. Clearance will be obtained prior to the infant's discharge. Former preemies require car seat use just as other infants do. Help the parents to find methods of padding the car seat or adding an additional semi-firm cushion inside the seat for the infant to ride in the car safely. Some infants may need to continue cardiac/apnea monitoring while in the car seat.

Since the former premature infant is at increased risk for SIDS compared to the general population, it is critical to teach parents to put the infant on his or her back to sleep (although this is contraindicated with gastroesophageal disease).

Give immunizations according to the current CDC-recommended immunization schedule, based on the infant's chronological age (Kelly, 2006a). All former preemies should receive the flu vaccine as recommended after 6 months chronological age. Respiratory syncytial virus (RSV) prophylaxis is critical for certain groups of premature infants. Administer palivizumab (Synagis) vaccine according to the recommended schedule (refer to Chapter 39 for additional information about RSV prophylaxis) (Kelly, 2006b; Romanko, 2005).

Assessing Growth and Development of the Former Premature Infant

When assessing growth and development of the infant or child who was born prematurely, determine the child's adjusted or corrected age so that you can perform an accurate assessment. The corrected or adjusted age should be used for evaluating progression in growth as well as development. For example, if a 6-month-old infant was born at 28 weeks' gestation (12 weeks or 3 months early), his growth and development expectations are those of a 3-month-old (corrected age). Continue to correct age for growth and development until the child is 3 years old.

Many former premature infants require special diets to foster catch-up growth. Extra calories are needed for increased growth needs. Additional calcium and phosphorus are required for bone mineralization. For these reasons, former preemies should be fed breast milk fortified with additional nutrients or a commercially prepared formula specific for premature infants. When former preemies demonstrate consistent adequate growth (usually by 6 months corrected age), they may be switched to a "term infant formula" such as Similac or Enfamil, concentrated to higher caloric density if needed. Assess the infant's ability to suck efficiently and refer him or her to occupational or speech therapy if the infant is a slow feeder or has difficulty feeding.

All anticipatory guidance related to nutrition is based on the child's corrected age. In other words, begin solids at 6 months corrected age, not chronologic age, and delay the addition of whole milk until 12 months corrected age, rather than 1 year chronologic age. Signs that the former premature infant may be ready to attempt spoon feeding include interest in feeding, decrease in tongue thrust, and adequate head control (Kelly, 2006a).

Early screening and intervention for issues related to development are critical to the attainment of optimal development in the former preemie. The comorbidities that ex-preemies exhibit in the form of prior and current medical problems place these infants at high risk for **developmental delay** (Kelly, 2006b). Even mild developmental delays warrant evaluation and intervention. The Denver II may be used as a screening tool for developmental concerns in the ex-preemie, though it does not always identify children at risk. Parent-report questionnaires demonstrate fairly accurate estimations of developmental problems, and their use is recommended by the American Academy of Pediatrics (AAP, 2006). Most importantly, assess the child's development based on corrected age until the child is 3 years old. Refer infants and children early if developmental concerns are suspected.

Identifying and Managing Failure to Thrive and Feeding Disorders in Children With Special Needs

Failure to thrive (FTT) is a term used to describe inadequate growth in infants and children. The child fails to demonstrate appropriate weight gain over a prolonged period of time. Length or height velocity and head circumference growth may also be affected. Typical children may experience FTT, but it is much more common in the child with special needs. Adequate nutrition is critical for appropriate brain growth in the first 2 years of life and obviously for growth in general throughout childhood and adolescence. **Developmental disability** may contribute to FTT, as the child's ability to consume adequate nutrition is impaired because of sensory or motor delays, such as with cerebral palsy. Other organic causes of failure to thrive include inability to suck and/or swallow correctly, malabsorption, diarrhea, vomiting, or alterations in metabolism and caloric/nutrient needs associated with a variety of chronic illnesses. Infants and children with cardiac or metabolic disease, chronic lung disease (bronchopulmonary dysplasia), cleft palate, or gastroesophageal reflux disease are at particular risk. Feeding disorders or food refusal may occur in infants or children who have required prolonged mechanical ventilation, long-term enteral tube feedings, or an unpleasant event such as a choking episode. Inorganic causes of FTT include neglect, abuse, behavioral problems, lack of appropriate maternal interaction, poor feeding techniques, lack of parental knowledge, or parental mental illness. Poverty is the single greatest contributing risk factor (Block et al., 2005).

The two categories of causes are not mutually exclusive. Organic causes of FTT may lead to behavioral problems that potentiate problems with adequate growth; hence FTT is thought of as a multifactorial problem.

Screen all children for FTT to identify them early (Locklin, 2005). In addition to poor growth, the infant or child with FTT may present with a history of developmental delay or loss of acquired milestones. Infants or children with feeding problems may display nipple, spoon, or food refusal; difficulty sucking; disinterest in feeding; or difficulty progressing from liquid to puréed to textured food. Perform a detailed dietary history and instruct the parents to complete a 3-day food diary to identify what the child actually eats and drinks. Assess the parent–child interaction, with particular attention to the parent's ability to read and respond to the infant's or child's cues. Observe feeding, noting the child's oral interest or aversion, oral–motor coordination, and swallowing ability, as well as parent–child interactions before, during, and after the feeding (Block et al., 2005). Further aversion to eating may occur as the parent's anxiety over the thought of the child not eating or losing weight leads to attempts to force-feed the child.

Significant FTT may require hospitalization for evaluation and management. Sometimes enteral tube feedings are necessary in order for children with FTT or feeding disorders to demonstrate adequate growth. Box 33.4 lists nursing interventions for the hospitalized child with FTT.

BOX 33.4 **Nursing Interventions During Hospitalization for Failure to Thrive**

- Observe parent/child interactions, especially during feedings.
- Develop an appropriate feeding schedule.
- Provide feedings as prescribed (usually 120 kcal/kg/day is needed to demonstrate proper weight gain).
- Weigh the child daily and maintain strict records of intake and output.
- Educate parents about proper feeding techniques and volumes.
- Provide extensive support to alleviate parental anxiety related to the child's inability to gain weight.

▶ **Take** NOTE!

Infants with FTT related to maternal neglect may be less interactive than other infants and avoid eye contact.

Promoting Growth and Development

When caring for the infant with special health care needs in the hospital, provide consistent caregivers to encourage the infant to develop a sense of trust. Allow and encourage the parent to stay with the infant, providing a comfortable place for the parent to sleep. To promote attachment, emphasize the baby's positive qualities. Encourage developmentally appropriate skills and allow the infant to have pleasurable experiences through all of the senses.

For the toddler, begin developmentally appropriate limit-setting and discipline. Encourage independence as the toddler is able. Modify gross motor and sensory activities to accommodate the toddler's limitations. To encourage a sense of control, offer the toddler simple choices. As the preschooler develops, encourage mastery of self-help skills as the child is able. Encourage socialization with same-age peers to develop a sense of friendship. Reinforce to the child that the illness or disability is not a punishment for wrongdoing or the child's fault in any way.

Encourage the school-age child to attend school and make up work that must be missed for medical treatments or appointments. Provide education to the school staff and other students about the child's special needs. Promote involvement in appropriate sports activities; music, drama, or art activities; and clubs such as Boy Scouts or Girl Scouts. Educate the child about the illness or disability and the course of treatment.

Inform parents of teens that those with chronic illness often participate in the same activities as typical teens, such

EVIDENCE-BASED PRACTICE 33.1
Life Skills Intervention for Children With Cystic Fibrosis and Effects of Intervention on Psychosocial Adjustment, Functional Health Status, and Physiological Status Over Time

● **Study**

Improved survival and an altered course for cystic fibrosis have led to a need to balance psychosocial and developmental needs in affected children. The authors performed a blinded, randomized controlled trial at four university cystic fibrosis (CF) centers. One hundred and sixteen children were participants in the study over a 9-month period of time. The intervention performed consisted of a home visit to assess each child's knowledge and management of CF. Information was provided using an educational problem-solving approach. Subsequent focus groups were held and the children discussed how to deal with peer issues.

▲ **Findings**

Children who participated in the intervention group had greater improvements in loneliness, global self-worth, and

perceived illness experience. The intervention did not demonstrate an impact upon physical or functional health status but did improve psychosocial status.

■ **Nursing Implications**

In addition to CF, many chronic and debilitating conditions affect children's quality of life. Any school-age or older child with a chronic condition that impairs physical functioning would benefit from interventions similar to those performed in this study. In particular, nurses who work in settings that allow them to have long-term relationships with these children have the potential to positively influence their lives. Nurses should help children learn communication and problem-solving skills that could lessen the impact of their chronic condition.

Christian, B. J., & D'Auria, J. P. (2006). Building life skills for children with cystic fibrosis: Effectiveness of an intervention. *Nursing Research, 55,* 300–307.

as risk-taking, rebelling, and trying out different identities. Assist the teen with coping and interpersonal skills. Promote involvement in activities with other teens with special needs as well as typical adolescents. Ensure that the teen participates in rites of passage as able, such as attending the prom or obtaining a driver's license. Discuss future plans with the teen, such as college or vocation, as well as transition to an adult health care provider. See Evidence-Based Practice 33.1.

Providing Resources to the Child and Family

Nurses should be familiar with community resources available to children with special health care needs. Educational opportunities for children with special health care needs include early intervention programs and programs offered through the public school system. Financial resources, respite care, and complementary therapies are other areas the nurse should become familiar with.

Educational Opportunities for the Special Needs Child

The foundation for health and development in children is laid during the first years of life. Children with special health care needs often require multiple developmental interventions and special education in the early years in order to reach their developmental potential later in childhood. Children learn best when they are at the stage of maximal readiness, and the early years must not be

missed as an opportunity for development. See Healthy People 2010.

Early intervention programs are intended to enhance the development of infants and toddlers with, or at risk for, disabilities, thereby minimizing educational costs and special education. Early intervention is also directed toward enhancing the capacity of families to meet their child's needs as well as to maximize the likelihood of independent living.

The Individuals with Disabilities Education Improvement Act (IDEA) of 2004 (formerly called Public Law 99-457) mandates government-funded care coordination and special education for children up to 3 years of age. This early intervention program is administered through each state. Federal law allows each state to define

HEALTHY PEOPLE 2010

Objective	Nursing Significance
Increase the proportion of children and youth with disabilities who spend at least 80 percent of their time in regular education programs.	Ensure that children under age 3 years who may qualify are referred to the local early intervention program. Encourage families to advocate for their child's needs on the individualized education plan.

"developmental disability" differently, but in general an evaluation of the child's physical, language, emotional, and social capabilities is performed by qualified personnel to determine eligibility. The law guarantees that eligible children will obtain access to services that will enhance their development. Children who qualify for services receive care coordination, and an individualized family service plan is developed by the service coordinator in conjunction with the family. The service coordinator manages the developmental services and special education that the child requires.

The intent of the program is that the child receives services in a "natural environment," so most services occur in the home or daycare center. Home visits by the service coordinator and maintenance of regular contact with the family ensure the success of the program.

Refer children suspected of developmental delay to the local early intervention program. For children receiving these services, collaborate with the service coordinator on an ongoing basis, with particular involvement at hospital discharge and when transition of services occurs at age 3 years.

Think back to Preet, the 2-year-old boy with a history of hydrocephalus and developmental delay, from the beginning of the chapter. Discuss with his mother the educational opportunities that are available for Preet. Explain what early intervention is and why it is important for Preet.

Schools may have a profound impact on the child's overall health and development. Some children with special needs do not require additional services to succeed in school. For these children, the nurse's role is to assess for school success or failure and determine the effect of the school environment on the child's health. The Individuals with Disabilities Education Act, reauthorized in 2004, provides for the education of children with special needs through the public school system, from age 3 to 21 years. These services are provided within the public school system.

According to the law, each special needs student is entitled to an individualized education program (IEP), which is a written plan designed to meet the preschool, primary, or secondary school student's individual needs. A committee consisting of the child's parent, a regular teacher, a special education teacher, and various other specialists develops the IEP. Nurses may be called to serve upon this committee. The IEP must include measurable short- and long-term goals. Parents are informed of the student's progress routinely and the IEP is reviewed at least annually.

Preschool special education through the local public school system is provided from age 3 to 5 years; access to the curriculum is ensured for all children. A child is eligible for special needs preschool when a significant delay is present in the cognitive, language, adaptive, social-emotional, or motor development domains to the extent that it adversely affects the child's learning ability. The child receives (in the school setting) developmental therapy as needed to augment his or her ability to participate in the education process. The least restrictive environment is preferred, with special needs children participating in classes containing age-appropriate typical peers whenever possible. Special needs preschool services are often offered in the elementary school setting.

Financial and Insurance Resources

Many special needs children whose families demonstrate financial need may be eligible for Supplemental Security Income (SSI). This program was created in 1972 through Public Law 92-603. SSI is a cash assistance program, and monthly benefits vary per individual. SSI qualification also qualifies the child for state-administered Medicaid. Medicaid benefits vary slightly from state to state but generally cover medical visits, medication, hospitalization, and limited adjuvant therapies. The State Children's Health Insurance Program (SCHIP) provides low-cost health insurance to eligible children. Eligibility and the extent of benefits provided by SCHIP vary by state.

Public Law 94-566 provides for state-administered Title V programs under the Maternal and Child Health Bureau Block Grant program. State Title V programs provide community-based, comprehensive service coordination for children with special needs (USA.gov, 2007).

Internet Resource for Special Children (www.irsc.org) is an online directory providing a wealth of links to resources for special needs children. Additional online resources include www.childrensdisabilities.info and www.specialchild.com.

Respite Care

Primary caregivers of children with special health care needs must be dedicated, skillful, vigilant, and knowledgeable. Constant care is a stress on the primary caregiver, who needs temporary relief from the daily caregiving demands. **Respite care** provides an opportunity for families to take a break from the daily intensive caregiving responsibilities. Respite care should meet the child's health care needs and offer the child developmental opportunities. Finding and using respite care that the family is comfortable with and trusts may decrease the family's stress and lead to an enhanced quality of life for special needs children and their families. Nurses can facilitate access to respite care, educate respite providers, and ensure quality respite care practices through involvement in community agencies.

Complementary Therapies

Adjuvant therapies are often used by families of children with special health care needs. These may include, among others, homeopathic and herbal medicine, pet therapy,

hippotherapy, music, and massage. Many families desire to blend natural or Eastern medicine with traditional allopathic medicine for their special needs child in search of palliation or a cure. When obtaining the health history, ask specifically about homeopathy or herbal medications the child may be taking.

Pet therapy may be used to decrease stress or as a component of psychotherapy.

Hippotherapy is also referred to as horseback riding for the handicapped, therapeutic horseback riding, or equine-facilitated psychotherapy. Individuals with almost any cognitive, physical, or emotional disability may benefit from therapeutic riding or other supervised interaction with horses. The unique movement of the horse under the child helps the child with physical disabilities to achieve increased flexibility, balance, and muscle strength. Children with mental or emotional disabilities may experience increased self-esteem, confidence, and patience as a result of the unique relationship with the horse. A physical therapist or psychotherapist (depending on the situation) generally works very closely with specially trained equine staff. Box 33.5 lists chronic medical conditions for which hippotherapy may be beneficial. Additional information may be obtained through the North American Riding for the Handicapped Association (www.narha.org) or the American Hippotherapy Association (www.american hippotherapyassociation.org).

Music may be used to induce positive behavioral changes or various other positive effects (Gasalberti, 2006).

Massage therapy may be beneficial to a wide variety of children. It may be used to reduce pain, promote relaxation, or demonstrate a specific positive effect related to the child's particular medical condition (Gasalberti, 2006).

> ▶ *Take* NOTE!

Become familiar with the risks and benefits of homeopathic and herbal medications, as many families use these treatments in an effort to improve their child's quality of life or outcome.

Providing Support and Education

At the time of initial diagnosis, allow and encourage the family to express their feelings. Parents of children with special health care needs require emotional, practical, economic, and social support. Encourage parents to obtain help with daily routines. Encourage stress reduction for the parents through exercise and allowing time for themselves. Be a supportive and encouraging listener, making sure to nurture the whole child, not just his or her special condition (Jackson Allen, 2004).

Parents value peer support groups, sometimes feeling that only other parents of disabled or chronically ill children could understand the heartache, fear, and other emotions they often experience. Pediatric nurses should be proactive in helping families find support systems (Coffey, 2006).

Fathers have the same concerns about their children as mothers do, but they may show this concern differently. It is important for nurses to involve them in the child's care. Teach skills to both parents, and actively involve fathers by asking about their observations and opinions (Ahmann, 2006).

Parents become the experts on their child's needs and care and they should be recognized as such. Parents want to be taken seriously and do not like being ignored (Lindblad et al., 2005). They should be viewed as having reliable and valuable information about their children. By being an active and reflective listener, the nurse can demonstrate to the parents that their opinion is valued, in addition to finding out what the child really needs. Some parents may hesitate to volunteer information, unsure about which information the nurse needs. Show respect for the parents' knowledge of their child's needs by seeking advice on the child's daily care, medical/physical needs, and current developmental level, no matter what the site of care is (Bowie, 2004). See Healthy People 2010.

BOX 33.5 Conditions Benefiting from Hippotheraphy

- Muscular dystrophy
- Cerebral palsy
- Visual impairment
- Down syndrome
- Mental retardation
- Autism
- Multiple sclerosis
- Emotional disabilities
- Brain injury
- Myelomeningocele
- Spinal cord injury
- Amputation
- Attention-deficit disorder
- Learning disabilities
- Deafness
- Cerebrovascular accident (stroke)

HEALTHY PEOPLE 2010

Objective	Nursing Significance
(Developmental) Increase the proportion of children with special health care needs who have access to a medical home.	In the primary care setting, build a relationship with the family to establish a medical home. If available, refer families to multidisciplinary programs for medically complex children.

Families may need additional support from the nurse at times of transition (discussed previously). As the equipment or treatment needs change, adjust the teaching plan. Educate the child and family about the use of adaptive equipment. Ensure that families understand how specific activities must be modified to accommodate the child's needs. Provide anticipatory guidance related to expected developmental changes, including resources and laws related to education. Act as a liaison between the family and the daycare center or school. As the child grows and matures, encourage parents to relinquish caregiving tasks to the child as appropriate to encourage independence and promote self-esteem.

Assisting the Adolescent With Special Health Needs Making the Transition to Adulthood

Adolescence is a time of physical changes, psychosocial challenges, and initiation of independence from parents. The adolescent with a chronic illness or one who is technology dependent may experience this period differently than other teens. Puberty is often affected by chronic illness (either delayed or earlier). Chronic illness may lead to isolation from peers at a time when peer interaction is the core of psychosocial development. Teens may struggle to fit in with their peers by hiding their illness or health care needs (ignoring them), complying poorly with treatment regimens, or participating in risky behaviors. At a time when the child should be developing independence from the parents, he or she may be experiencing significant dependence related to the special health condition. Adolescents with chronic health disorders demonstrate mental illness at a rate three to four times higher than normally developing adolescents (Burns et al., 2006). For these reasons, the adolescent with special health care needs may require increased amounts of support from the nurse.

With the tremendous increase in technology and health care, over 85% of all children with chronic illness or special health care needs live into adulthood (Yeo & Sawyer, 2005). Making the transition to adult care for a child with special health care needs can be difficult. A written plan for transition to adult care should be initiated in mid-adolescence. Advance planning leads to a smoother transition to adult care. Have ongoing conversations with the teen about this transition. Issues to be resolved prior to the transition include financial resources for medical care, college or vocational school attendance, living arrangements, and caretaking arrangements.

The Adolescent Health Transition Project (AHTP) recommends the following schedule:

• By age 14, ensure that a transition plan is initiated and that the IEP reflects post–high school plans.
• By age 17, explore health care financing for young adults. If needed, notify the local division of vocational rehabilitation by the autumn before the teen is to graduate from high school of the impending transition. Initiate guardianship procedures if appropriate.

• Notify the teen that all rights transfer to him or her at the age of majority. Check the teen's eligibility for SSI the month the child turns 18. Determine if the child is eligible for SSI work incentives.
• If the youth is attending college, contact the college's campus student disability service program.
• By age 21, ensure that the young adult has registered with the Division of Developmental Disabilities for adult services if applicable.

Prior to moving to adult care (with an adult medical specialist), ensure that the adolescent understands the treatment rationale, symptoms of worsening condition, and especially danger signs. Teach the adolescent about when to seek help from a health professional. Introduce the teen to the medical insurance process. At transition, coordinate a seamless transfer by providing a detailed written plan to the care coordinator or advanced practice nurse (after verbal collaboration).

After the transition, serve as a consultant to the adult office in relation to the teen's needs. Consult with a transition services coordinator or other service agency as available in the local community (AHTP, 2007).

The Dying Child

The idea that a child may die is simply unimaginable to most people, yet children die daily. Each year, about 50,000 children die in the U.S. (Himelstein, 2006), and about 28,000 children who die each year are infants (Mellichamp, 2007). Pediatric nurses will inevitably encounter situations in which a child dies. These situations are extremely difficult for all persons involved, and the nurse plays a key role in caring for the dying child and his or her family.

Grieving

Anticipatory grief may be experienced by the family when the diagnosis of terminal illness is made. Families may deny the prognosis, become angry at the health care system or a higher power, or may experience depression. Acute grief is an intense process that occurs around the time of the actual death. Family members may feel short of breath or as though the throat is tight. They may verbalize that the situation is unreal to them or search for reasons why the death was not prevented. Families may also display hostility or restlessness. Each individual will express grief in his or her own manner. Mourning the death of a loved one takes a long time, and families should be supported throughout the process.

Palliative Care of the Dying Child

Appropriate **palliative care** is essential for any child with a life-threatening or progressive incurable condition. Whether palliative care is provided in the home, hospital, or hospice setting, the goal is to provide the best quality of life possible at the end of life while alleviating physical, psychological, emotional, and spiritual suffering. The Last Acts Palliative Care Task Force has established principles on which palliative care of children should be based. These include:

- Respecting patients' goals, preferences, and choices
- Comprehensive caring
- Using the strengths of interdisciplinary resources
- Acknowledging and addressing caregivers' concerns
- Building systems and mechanisms of support (Association of Pediatric Oncology Nurses, 2003)

Hospice Care

Hospice allows for family-centered care in the child's home or a hospice facility. As with adult hospice care, the comfort of the entire family is important. The goals of pediatric hospice care are enhancement of quality of life for the child and family through an individualized plan of care (Children's Hospice International, 2007). The recommended standards for pediatric hospice care do not preclude involvement in ongoing treatment (this is in contrast to adult hospice), but certain eligibility criteria must be met. Parents are educated on ways to comfort and interact with their dying child, such as massage, movement, or singing. Spiritual support is available through a chaplain, social worker, or the family's minister. The nurse not only educates the family about the dying process but also assists them with providing basic care and pain management. The decision to withhold nutrition or hydration may be made in certain instances. Pain management is of utmost importance for the terminally ill child. Ongoing bereavement care is also provided to the family by the hospice after the child's death.

Nursing Management of the Dying Child

Though interdisciplinary care is essential for quality care at the end of life, it is the nurse who plays the key role of child/family advocate and who is usually the constant presence throughout the dying process. Nursing management of the dying child focuses on end-of-life decision making, meeting the child's and family's needs, and assisting the family after the child's death. Throughout the process, focus on the family as the unit of care (Malloy et al., 2006).

Assisting the Family With End-of-Life Decision Making

Parents are obligated not only to protect their children from harm but also to do as much good for them as possible, both from an ethical and legal standpoint (Rushton, 2004). When the time comes for end-of-life decision making, parents are often torn about the "right" course of action. Parents may be asked to make decisions about stopping treatment, withdrawing treatment, providing palliative care, or consenting to do not resuscitate (DNR) orders. Patients, parents, and health care providers are generally in agreement that continued suffering is not desired for any child with a terminal illness. When all possible curative attempts have been made, then survival is no longer possible.

Nurses involved in this process must examine their own values related to dying and consider the American Nurses Association's code of ethics for nurses as well. The family's feelings must also be acknowledged. During the process of end-of-life decision making, health care providers must assure families that the focus of care is changing and that the child is not being abandoned (Rushton, 2004). Emphasize to parents that no matter what their decision is, the health care team is dedicated to the comfort and expert care of their child.

Ensure that communication is family-centered. Quality of life must be taken into consideration when making decisions to continue or withhold treatment (Jacobs, 2005). Provide parents facing end-of-life decisions with honest information and education from the time of the diagnosis/prognosis forward. Anticipate that parents may vacillate in the decision-making process. Clarify information for them and allow them private time to discuss the options. Do not make judgments about or question the parents' decision. Be sensitive to any ethnic, spiritual, or cultural preferences during the terminal stage of the illness. Encourage parents to interact with other parents who have a child with a terminal illness.

Allowing Natural Death

The decision to institute a DNR order is one of the most difficult decisions a family may ever have to make. DNR refers to withholding cardiopulmonary resuscitation should the child's heart stop beating. Parents may initially feel like this means they are giving up on their child. Nurses must educate families that resuscitation may be inappropriate and lead to more suffering than if death were allowed to occur naturally. The parents need to understand that when a palliative care route is chosen, rather than continuing a curative or treatment route, the focus of the child's care is changing but that the child and family are not being abandoned. Families may wish to specify a certain extent of resuscitation that they feel more comfortable with (e.g., allowing supplemental oxygen but not providing chest compressions). Some institutions are now replacing the DNR terminology with "allow natural death" (AND), which may be more acceptable to families facing the decision to withhold resuscitation (Knox & Lenehan, 2005).

Involving the Dying Child in the Decision-Making Process

End-of-life decision making often involves ethical dilemmas for the patient, family, and health care team. This is particularly true when the parents' wishes conflict with the child's or adolescent's desires. Children should be involved in decision making to the extent that they are able. Discuss intervention within the context of the child's condition and wishes. Children over the age of 7 may "assent" to the continuation or withdrawal of treatment (Kon, 2006). Be available to the older child or adolescent to provide support and information if he or she desires. Talk with the child or adolescent with the parents present, as well as in private. Maintain the child's comfort and dignity. Encourage the child to spend time with other children with a terminal illness. Assure the child that everything will be done to make him or her comfortable.

Consult parents about the timing and depth of end-of-life discussions. Just as parents do, the terminally ill child may vacillate in the decision-making process. Remain sensitive, and respect the child's decisions.

Organ or Tissue Donation

With large numbers of organ transplant candidates on waiting lists and the shortage of viable organs, pediatric organ and tissue donation is a priority. For many families, knowing that a child's organs or tissues may save another child's life provides a way to help others despite their own loss. A healthy child who dies unexpectedly is an excellent candidate for organ donation. Many chronic illnesses in children preclude the option of organ or tissue donation, though individual determinations of eligibility should be made.

The discussion of organ donation should be separated from the discussion of impending death or brain death notification. Written consent is necessary for organ donation, so the family must be appropriately informed and educated. Many families who never thought about it before may consider the option of donation if adequately educated about the process. All expenses for organ procurement are borne by the recipient's family, not the donor's. Ask whether the dying child ever expressed a wish to donate organs and whether the parents have considered it.

Families need to know that procurement of the organs does not mar the child's appearance, so that an open casket at the child's funeral is still possible if the family desires. The donating child will not suffer further because of organ donation. The organs or tissues will be harvested in a timely fashion after the declaration of death, so the family need not worry about delay of the wake or funeral. The family's cultural and religious beliefs must be considered, and the team discussing organ donation with the family must do so in a sensitive and ethical manner.

Managing Pain and Discomfort

Pain management is an essential component of care for the child with a terminal illness. Providing for comfort enhances the child's quality of life and minimizes suffering. Assess pain using a developmentally appropriate tool (see Chapter 35 for further information). Provide pain medication around the clock rather than on an "as needed" basis to prevent recurrence or escalation of pain. Determine the child's preferred comfort measures and use them to provide additional relief. Change the child's position frequently but gently to minimize discomfort. Limit nursing care to comfort measures that ease the child's discomfort. Maintain a calm environment, minimizing noise and light.

Easing Anxiety or Fears

Involve the parents and other family members in all phases of the child's care. Explain all aspects of care to the child to minimize anxiety related to nursing interventions. Answer the child's questions honestly. Involve the child in decision making whenever possible. Limit interventions to those related to palliation, rather than treatment, advocating for the child as needed. Remain with the child when a parent or family member is not in the room so the child will not fear dying alone.

Providing Nutrition

Since the body naturally requires less nutrition as the child is dying, do not excessively coax the child to eat or drink. Offer frequent small meals or snacks of the child's choosing. Soups and shakes require less energy to eat and so may be desirable. If the child desires a different food, provide that one. Keep strong odors away from the child to decrease nausea. Administer antiemetics as needed. Provide mouth care and keep the lips lubricated to keep the mouth feeling clean and prevent the discomfort associated with chapped lips. Make sure the environment is a pleasant one for eating.

Supporting the Dying Child and Family

To foster a holistic connection with the child and family, be attuned to the entire family's needs and emotions. Nurses provide physical care through specific tasks and interventions for the dying child, but they also need to be fully present with the child and family. In general, people are uncomfortable with the concept of a dying child. Nurses should work through their own feelings about the situation to be able to be "in the moment" with the child and family. Ask yourself: Can I be fully present with this family? If not, then what can I change to be so?

Families and dying children benefit from the presence of the nurse, not just the interventions he or she performs. Families report that the simple of act of being present with the family is very healing (Mellichamp, 2007). Listen to the child and family; be still and silent for a time to accomplish this. Foster respect for the whole child by attending to him or her as such.

Respect the parents of the dying child by helping them honor the commitments they have made to their child. Acknowledge that parents have diverse needs for information and participation in decision making. Allow and encourage family customs or rituals in relation to death and dying. Families may desire the pastor or priest to be present when the child's death is imminent. Certain rituals may be desired, depending on the family's religious or spiritual background. Ensure that these important events occur, and alter nursing care routines as needed to accommodate them. Respect the family's need to participate in these rituals and customs.

Work collaboratively with the family and health care team to provide for the needs of the child and family (Rushton, 2005). Resources for families of a dying child are listed in Box 33.6. The Make-a-Wish Foundation (www.wish.org) works to grant the wishes of terminally ill children, giving the child and family an experience of hope, strength, and love.

Meeting the Dying Child's Needs According to Developmental Stage

It is important to provide the type of support and education that the dying child needs according to his or her developmental stage. For the infant, unconditional love and trust are of utmost importance. Ensure that the infant's family is available to the child. The toddler, 1 to 3 years old, thrives on familiarity and routine. Maximize the toddler's time with parents, be consistent, provide favorite toys, and ensure physical comfort. Spirituality in the preschool years focuses on the concept of right versus wrong. The 3- to 5-year-old may see death as punishment for wrongdoing; correct this misunderstanding. Use honest and precise language. Help the parents to teach the child that though the family will miss the child, it will continue to function without him or her.

BOX 33.6 Resources for Families of a Dying Child

Websites
- www.joyandhope.org: Project Joy and Hope
- www.chionline.org: Children's Hospice International
- www.compassionatefriends.org: Compassionate Friends

Books
- *Gentle Willow: A Story for Children about Dying* by Joyce Mills
- *35 Ways to Help a Grieving Child* by the Dougy Center for Grieving Children
- *Sad Isn't Bad* by Michaeline Mundy
- *A Child Asks. . . . What Does Dying Mean?* by Lake Pylant Monhollon
- *Talking with Children and Young People about Death and Dying: a Workbook* by Mary Turner
- *The Worst Loss: How Families Heal from the Death of a Child* by Barbara Rosof
- *I Have No Intention of Saying Goodbye: Parents Share Their Stories of Hope and Healing After a Child's Death* by Sandy Fox
- *Stars in the Deepest Night: After the Death of a Child* by Genesse Gentry
- *The Bereaved Parent* by Harriet Schiff
- *You are Special* by Max Lucado

The school-age child has a concrete understanding of death. Children who are 5 to 10 years old need specific, honest details (as desired). Encourage the child to help make decisions, and help the child to establish a sense of control.

The young adolescent (10 to 14 years old) will benefit from reinforcement of self-esteem, self-respect, and a sense of worth. Respect the child's need for privacy and time alone as well as time requested with peers. Support the need for independence and encourage the child to participate in decision making. The older teen (14 to 18 years of age) has a more adult-like understanding of death and will need further support through honest, detailed explanations and will want to feel truly involved and listened to.

■■■ Key Concepts

- Children with special health care needs are those who have, or are at risk for, a chronic physical, developmental, behavioral, or emotional condition that generally requires more intensive and diverse health services, as well as coordination of those services, than do typical children.
- Most children with chronic illnesses or who are dependent on technology progress through stages of growth and development just as typical children do, though possibly at a slower pace, and desire to be treated as normal children.
- Parents of special needs children experience a multitude of emotions and changes in their lives, often carrying a heavy caregiving burden. They become the experts on their child's care and should be empowered and supported in their efforts.
- Children with special health care needs are at increased risk for the development of vulnerable child syndrome, which may have psychologically harmful effects on the child and parents for many years.
- Home is the most developmentally appropriate environment for children with special health care needs and those who are technology dependent. Children display an improved physical, emotional, psychological, and social status when they are cared for at home.
- Family-centered care provides the optimal framework for caring for children and families with special needs. Empowering the family strengthens them. A medical home or permanent relationship with the health care provider benefits the family, as care coordination and advocacy are provided.
- Use adjusted (or corrected) age when assessing growth and development of the infant or child who was born prematurely. Provide early screening and intervention for issues related to development to maximize the former preemie's potential for growth and development.
- Become familiar with the risks and benefits of adjuvant therapies used by some families of children with special health care needs.

■ Screen children with special health care needs for failure to thrive or a feeding disorder.

■ Screening helps to identify children with unmet health needs early so that intervention may begin.

■ The child and family with special needs may require additional support during times of transition, such as at initial diagnosis or change in prognosis, when symptoms increase, when the child moves to new setting (hospital, school), during periods of developmental change, or during a parent's absence.

■ Early discharge planning and ongoing inclusion and education of the family facilitate continuity of care. During mid-adolescence, initiate a written plan to help the special needs child make the transition to adult care.

■ Early intervention provides care coordination (developmental services and special education), as well as an individualized family service plan for qualifying children and their families.

■ Each special needs student is entitled to an individualized education program (IEP), which is a written plan that is designed to meet the preschool, primary, or secondary school student's needs.

■ Younger children who are dying generally need for their families to be close and to trust their needs will be provided for. Older children require honest explanations given at a level appropriate for the child's age or developmental stage.

■ Support the dying child and the family throughout the end-of-life decision-making process, providing facts as desired about palliative care, hospice, and organ donation.

REFERENCES

Books and Journals

108th Congress of the United States. (2004). *Individuals with Disabilities Education Improvement Act of 2004.* Retrieved September 3, 2006, from http://frwebgate.access.gpo.gov/cgi-bin/getdoc.cgi?dbname=108_cong_public_laws&docid=f:publ446.108.

Adolescent Health Transition Project. (2007). *A resource for adolescents with special health care needs, chronic illnesses, physical or developmental disabilities.* Retrieved November 17, 2007 from http://depts.washington.edu/healthtr/.

Ahmann, E. (2006). Supporting fathers' involvement in children's health care. *Pediatric Nursing, 32*(1), 88–90.

American Academy of Pediatrics, Committee on Children with Disabilities. (2001). Counseling families who choose complementary and alternative medicine for their child with chronic illness or disability. *Pediatrics, 107*(3), 598–601.

American Academy of Pediatrics, Council on Children with Disabilities. (2005). Policy statement, care coordination in the medical home: Integrating health and related systems of care for children with special health care needs. *Pediatrics, 116*(5), 1238–1244.

American Academy of Pediatrics, Council on Children with Disabilities. (2006). Policy statement: Identifying infants and young children with developmental disorders in the medical home, an algorithm for developmental surveillance and screening. *Pediatrics, 116*(1), 405–420.

American Academy of Pediatrics, Medical Home Initiatives for Children with Special Needs Project Advisory Committee. (2002). Policy statement: The medical home. *Pediatrics, 110*(1), 184–186.

American Nurses Association. (2001). *Code of ethics for nurses with interpretive statements.* Washington, DC: American Nurses Association.

Association of Pediatric Oncology Nurses. (2003). *Precepts of palliative care for children, adolescents and their families.* Retrieved November 17, 2007, from http://www.apon.org/files/public/last_acts_precepts.pdf.

Ayoob, K. T., & Barresi, I. (2007). Feeding disorders in children: Taking an interdisciplinary approach. *Pediatric Annals, 36*(8), 478–483.

Bakewell-Sachs, S., & Genarro, S. (2004). Parenting the post-NICU premature infant. *MCN, 29*(6), 398–403.

Baum, L. S. (2004). Internet parent support groups for primary caregivers of a child with special health care needs. *Pediatric Nursing, 30*(5), 381–401.

Blann, L. E. (2005). Early intervention for children and families with special needs. *MCN, 30*(4), 263–268.

Block, R. W., Krebs, N. F., the Committee on Child Abuse and Neglect, and the Committee on Nutrition. (2005). Failure to thrive as a manifestation of child neglect. *Pediatrics, 116*(5), 1234–1237.

Bowie, H. (2004). Mommy first. *Pediatric Nursing, 30*(3), 203–206.

Bratton, S. L., Kolovos, N. S., Roach, E. S., et al. (2006). Pediatric organ transplantation needs: organ donation best practices. *Archives of Pediatrics and Adolescent Medicine, 160*(5), 468–472.

Burns, J. J., Sadof, M., & Kamat, D. (2006). The adolescent with a chronic illness. *Pediatric Annals, 35*(3), 207–216.

Case-Smith, J. (2004). Parenting a child with a chronic medical condition. *American Journal of Occupational Therapy, 58*, 551–560.

Centers for Disease Control and Prevention. (2005). Mental health in the United States: Health care and well being of children with chronic emotional, behavioral, or developmental problems—United States 2001. *Morbidity and Mortality Weekly Report (54)*, 985–989.

Child and Adolescent Health Measurement Initiative. (n.d.). *The children with special health care needs (CSHCN) screener©.* Retrieved November 17, 2007 from http://cahmi.org/ViewDocument.aspx?DocumentID=115.

Children's Hospice International. (2007). *About children's hospice, palliative and end-of-life care.* Retrieved November 17, 2007, from http://www.chionline.org/resources/about.php.

Coffey, J. S. (2006). Parenting a child with chronic illness: A metasynthesis. *Pediatric Nursing, 32*(1), 51–59.

Farmer, J. E. (2005). Comprehensive primary care for children with special health care needs in rural areas. *Pediatrics, 116*(3), 649–656.

Federation of Families for Children's Mental Health. (2007). *FFCMH principles for family involvement.* Retrieved November 17, 2007, from http://www.ffcmh.org/publication_pdfs/PrinciplesFamilyInvolve.pdf.

Gance-Cleveland, B. (2006). Family-centered care: Decreasing health disparities. *Journal for Specialists in Pediatric Nursing, 11*(1), 72–76.

Gasalberti, D. (2006). Alternative therapies for children and youth with special health care needs. *Journal of Pediatric Health Care, 20*(2), 133–136.

Green, A., & Ray, T. (2006). Attention to child development: A key piece of family-centered care for cardiac transplant recipients. *Journal for Specialists in Pediatric Nursing, 11*(2), 143–148.

Heilferty, C. M. (2004). Spiritual development and the dying child: the pediatric nurse practitioner's role. *Journal of Pediatric Health Care, 18*, 271–275.

Hewitt-Taylor, J. (2005). Caring for children with complex and continuing health needs. *Nursing Standard, 19*(42), 41–47.

Higgins, S. S., & Tong, E. (2003). Transitioning adolescents with congenital heart disease into adult health care. *Progress in Cardiovascular Nursing, 18*(2), 93–98.

Himelstein, B. P. (2006). Palliative care for infants, children, adolescents, and their families. *Journal of Palliative Medicine, 9*(1), 162–181.

Inkelas, M., & Garro, N. (2005). A picture of needs for children with special health-care needs: What we are learning from the national survey. *Journal of Pediatric Nursing, 20*(3), 207–210.

Jackson Allen, P. L. (2004). Children with special health care needs: National survey of prevalence and health care needs. *Pediatric Nursing, 30*(4), 307–314.

Jacobs, H. H. (2005). Ethics in pediatric end-of-life care: A nursing perspective. *Journal of Pediatric Nursing, 20*(5), 360–369.

Johnson, C. P., Kastner, T. A., & the Committee/Section on Children with Disabilities of the American Academy of Pediatrics. (2005). Helping families raise children with special health care needs at home. *Pediatrics, 115*(2), 507–511.

Kelly, M. M. (2006a). Primary care issues for the healthy premature infant. *Journal of Pediatric Health Care, 20*(5), 293–299.

Kelly, M. M. (2006b). The basics of prematurity. *Journal of Pediatric Health Care, 20*(4), 238–244.

Kelly, M. M. (2006c). The medically complex premature infant in primary care. *Journal of Pediatric Health Care, 20*(6), 367–373.

Kerruish, N. J., Settle, K., Campbell-Stokes, P., & Taylor, B. J. (2005). Vulnerable Baby Scale: Development and piloting of a questionnaire to measure maternal perceptions of their baby's vulnerability. *Journal of Paediatrics and Child Health, 41*(8), 419–423.

Knox, C., & Lenehan, G. P. (2005). Allow natural death: A more humane approach to discussing end-of-life directives. *Journal of Emergency Nursing, 31*(6), 560–561.

Kon, A. A. (2006). Assent in pediatric research. *Pediatrics, 117*(5), 1806–1810.

Kornhaber, L., Ridgway, E., & Kathirithamby, R. (2007). Occupational and physical therapy approaches to sensory and motor issues. *Pediatric Annals, 36*(8), 484–494.

Kuster, P. A., Badr, L. K., Chang, B. L., et al. (2004). Factors influencing health-promoting activities of mothers caring for ventilator-assisted children. *Journal of Pediatric Nursing, 19*(4), 276–287.

Lewis, M. (2007). Discharge management for children with complex needs. *Paediatric Nursing, 19*(4), 26–30.

Lindblad, B., Rasmussen, B. H., & Sandman, P. (2005). Being invigorated in parenthood: Parents' experiences of being supported by professionals when having a disabled child. *Journal of Pediatric Nursing, 20*(4), 288–297.

Lobar, S. L., Youngblut, J. M., & Brooten, D. (2006). Cross-cultural beliefs, ceremonies, and rituals surrounding death of a loved one. *Pediatric Nursing, 32*(1), 44–50.

Locklin, M. (2005). The redefinition of failure to thrive from a case study perspective. *Pediatric Nursing, 31*(6), 474–479.

Malloy, P., Ferrell, B., Virani, R., et al. (2006). Palliative care education for pediatric nurses. *Pediatric Nursing, 32*(6), 555–561.

Mellichamp, P. (2007). End-of-life care for infants. *Home Healthcare Nurse, 25*(1), 41–44.

Nuutila, L., & Salanterä, S. (2006). Children with a long-term illness: parents' experiences of care. *Journal of Pediatric Nursing, 21*(2), 153–160.

Onufer, C. N. (2006). New momentum on building a medical home for the child with a chronic health problem. *Contemporary Pediatrics, 23*(10), 65–66, 69–70, 72–73.

Pearson, S. R., & Boyce, W. T. (2004). The vulnerable child syndrome. *Pediatrics in Review, 25*(10), 345–349.

Rolland, J. S., & Walsh, F. (2006). Facilitating family resilience with childhood illness and disability. *Current Opinion in Pediatrics, 18*(5), 527–538.

Romanko, E. A. (2005). Caring for children with bronchopulmonary dysplasia in the home setting. *Home Healthcare Nurse, 23*(2), 95–102.

Romesberg, T. (2004). Understanding grief: A component of neonatal palliative care. *Journal of Hospice and Palliative Nursing, 6*(3), 161–170.

Rushton, C. H. (2004). Ethics and palliative care in pediatrics: When should parents agree to withdraw life-sustaining therapy for children? *AJN, 104*(4), 54–63.

Rushton, C. H. (2005). A framework for integrated pediatric palliative care: Being with dying. *Journal of Pediatric Nursing, 20*(5), 311–325.

Schulman, L. H., Meringolo, D., & Scott, G. (2007). Early intervention: A crash course for pediatricians. *Pediatric Annals, 36*(8), 463–469.

Stille, C. J., & Antonelli, R. C. (2004). Coordination of care for children with special health care needs. *Current Opinion in Pediatrics, 16*(6), 700–705.

Sullivan-Bolyai, S., Sadler, L., Knafl, K. A., & Gilliss, C. L. (2004). Great expectations: A position description for parents as caregivers: Part II. *Pediatric Nursing, 30*(1), 52–56.

Swartz, M. K. (2005). Parenting preterm infants: A meta-synthesis. *MCN, 30*(2), 115–120.

USA.gov. (2007). *Title V–maternal and child health services block grant.* Retrieved November 17, 2007 from http://www.ssa.gov/OP_Home/ssact/title05/0500.htm.

U.S. Department of Health and Human Services, Health Resources and Services Administration, Maternal and Child Health Bureau. (2004). *The national survey of children with special health care needs chartbook 2001.* Rockville, MD: U.S. Department of Health and Human Services.

Wang, K. K., & Barnard, A. (2004). Technology-dependent children and their families: A review. *Journal of Advanced Nursing, 45*(1), 36–46.

Yeo, M., & Sawyer, S. (2005). Chronic illness and disability. *BMJ, 330*, 721–723.

WEBSITES

Adolescent Health Transition Project: http://depts.washington.edu/healthtr/

National Newborn Screening and Genetics Resource Center: http://genes-r-us.uthscsa.edu

Building the Legacy: IDEA 2004: http://idea.ed.gov/

End-of-life Nursing Education Consortium: www.aacn.nche.edu/elnec

American Academy of Pediatrics: www.aap.org

American Hippotherapy Association: www.americanhippotherapyassociation.org

National Center on Birth Defects and Developmental Disabilities, promoting optimal fetal, infant, and child development; preventing birth defects and developmental disabilities; enhancing quality of life for those with disabilities: www.cdc.gov/ncbddd

Articles and resources for families of children with disabilities: www.childrensdisabilities.info/

Children's Hospice International: www.chionline.org

Division of Early Childhood, promoting support of families and optimal development of young children with or at risk for developmental delays and disabilities: www.dec-sped.org

Voice for health care consumers, dedicated to achieving high-quality, affordable health care for all Americans: www.familiesusa.org

Institute for Family-Centered Care: www.familycenteredcare.org/

A national clearinghouse for information and education related to the health care of children with special health needs: www.familyvoices.org

Federation for Children with Special Needs: www.fcsn.org

Federation of Families for Children's Mental Health: www.ffcmh.org

Kids as Self-Advocates: www.fvkasa.org/

National Center for Hearing Assessment and Management: www.infanthearing.org

Initiative for Pediatric Palliative Care: www.ippcweb.org

Internet Resource for Special Children: www.irsc.org

American Academy of Pediatrics, National Center of Medical Home Initiatives for Children with Special Needs: www.medicalhomeinfo.org

March of Dimes Resource Center, addressing personal and complex problems related to pregnancy and birth defects: www.marchofdimes.com

North American Riding for the Handicapped Association: www.narha.org

National Early Childhood Technical Assistance Center: www.nectas.unc.edu

National Dissemination Center for Children with Disabilities: www.nichcy.org/

Parents of Premature Babies, Inc., a nonprofit foundation supporting parents of preterm infants: www.preemie-l.org

Preemies.Org; helps parents of premature infants find other parents using various Internet resources: www.preemies.org

Resources for parents and caregivers of children with special needs: www.specialchild.com

Social Security Administration: www.ssa.gov

Make-a-Wish Foundation: www.wish.org

Zero to Three, supporting healthy development and well-being of infants and toddlers and their families: www.zerotothree.org

CHAPTER WORKSHEET

MULTIPLE CHOICE QUESTIONS

1. The parents of a 5-year-old with special health care needs talk to the parents of a 10-year-old with a similar condition for quite a while each day. What is the nurse's interpretation of this behavior?

   a. The nurse has not provided enough emotional support for the parents.

   b. This relationship between the children's parents is potentially unhealthy.

   c. Support between parents of special children is extremely valuable.

   d. Confidentiality is a pressing issue in this particular situation.

2. The nurse is caring for a child who has received all possible medical care for cancer, yet continues to experience relapse and metastasis. It is time to make the transition from curative care attempts to palliative care. What is the most important nursing consideration at this time?

   a. The health care professionals should make the decision about the child's care.

   b. The family may lose a sense of hope, so cancer treatments should continue.

   c. Involve the family in the decision-making process about the shift to palliative care.

   d. Palliative care can take place only at home, so the child should be discharged.

3. The nurse is caring for a 3-year-old with a gastrostomy tube and tracheostomy who is on supplemental oxygen and multiple medications. The mother is rooming in during this hospitalization. What is the priority nursing action?

   a. Incorporate the mother's assistance in care when convenient.

   b. Recognize the mother as the expert on her child's needs and care.

   c. Recommend that the mother go home to get some rest.

   d. Provide family-centered care since the mother is there.

4. The nurse is caring for a child with a developmental disability who is starting kindergarten this year. The mother is tearful and doesn't want the child to go to school. What is the best response by the nurse?

   a. "Do you need some time alone to collect yourself?"

   b. "You've known for a while this time would come."

   c. "Can I call your husband or a friend for you?"

   d. "It is normal to feel stressed or sad at this time."

5. The parents of a child with a developmental disability ask the nurse for advice about disciplining their child. What is the best response by the nurse?

   a. "You should choose methods that are most congruent with your values about discipline."

   b. "Children like this really can't follow directions, so they may be very hard to discipline."

   c. "Punish your child only for socially unacceptable or offending behaviors."

   d. "Spanking works well for this type of child, as they really don't like pain."

CRITICAL THINKING EXERCISES

1. A 15-year-old boy is dying of cancer after all medical care options have been exhausted. Describe the plan of care for this child and his family. What strategies should the nurse use to support the child and his family through this difficult process?

2. A 5-month-old infant who was born at 24 weeks' gestation is ready to be discharged from the NICU. She will be going home on oxygen, gastrostomy tube feedings, and eight medications. Develop a teaching plan for the family.

STUDY ACTIVITIES

1. In the clinical setting, care for a child with a terminal illness. Reflect in your clinical journal about the feelings you had during the care of the child, as well as the feelings and behaviors that you noticed in the child, siblings, parents, and nursing staff.

2. Visit a preschool that provides care for developmentally delayed and typical children. Choose two same-age children, one with a disability or impairment and the other a typical healthy child. Perform a Denver developmental screening or development assessment on each of the two children. Compare and contrast your findings.

3. Spend the day with a home care nurse providing care for a technology-dependent child. What obstacles has the family overcome to have this child at home? What adjustments does the nurse make to provide family-centered care in the home (as compared to the hospital setting)?

MEDICATION ADMINISTRATION, INTRAVENOUS THERAPY, AND NUTRITIONAL SUPPORT

KEY TERMS

biotransformation
bolus feeding
enteral nutrition
gastrostomy

gavage feedings
infiltration
parenteral nutrition
pharmacodynamics

pharmacokinetics
residual
total parenteral nutrition

LEARNING OBJECTIVES

Upon completion of this chapter, the learner will be able to:

1. Describe atraumatic methods for preparing children for procedures.
2. Describe the "eight rights" of pediatric medication administration.
3. Explain the physiologic differences in children affecting a medication's pharmacodynamic and pharmacokinetic properties.
4. Accurately determine recommended pediatric medication doses.
5. Demonstrate the proper technique for administering medication to children via the oral, rectal, ophthalmic, otic, intravenous, intramuscular, and subcutaneous routes.
6. Integrate the concepts of atraumatic care in medication administration for children.
7. Identify the preferred sites for peripheral and central intravenous medication administration.
8. Describe nursing management related to maintenance of intravenous infusions in children, as well as prevention of complications.
9. Explain nursing care related to enteral tube feedings.
10. Describe nursing management of the child receiving total parenteral nutrition.

*L*ily Kline, a 9-month-old, is admitted to your unit for failure to thrive. The physician has ordered insertion of a nasogastric tube to begin gavage feedings. The parents are very nervous and upset about this. They ask, "What will this tube do for Lily? It sounds very uncomfortable. What do you have to do to insert it? Will it have to stay in all the time? Won't it move?" How would you address their concerns?

WOW

Quality technical skills delivered by a caring hand are a vital part of good nursing care

The ill child often requires medications, intravenous (IV) therapy, or enteral nutrition to restore health. These procedures occur most often in the inpatient setting, but with today's advanced technology many children may receive treatment in the home, daycare center, school, physician's office, or other community setting.

This chapter begins with an overview of the important aspects of caring for a child who is to undergo a procedure. The key elements of and guidelines for care related to medication administration, IV therapy, and nutritional support in children will be discussed. Child and parent education is emphasized. The chapter will focus on adapting and modifying nursing procedures based on the child's growth and development and providing these treatments using a family-centered, atraumatic approach.

Children and Procedures

Children undergo numerous diagnostic and therapeutic procedures in a wide range of settings during their development. Medication administration, IV therapy, and nutritional support are just three examples. These procedures may be performed in the community or outpatient setting or in a care facility. Regardless of the procedure to be performed and the setting, children, like adults, need thorough preparation before the procedure and support during and after the procedure to promote the best outcome.

Before the Procedure

Appropriate preparation for procedures helps to decrease the child's and family's anxiety level, promote the child's cooperation, and support the child's and family's coping skills. Adequate preparation also helps to foster the child's feeling of mastery over a potentially stressful event, as undergoing invasive procedures in particular is extremely distressing for children.

Preparation may include psychological preparation (including explanation and education) as well as preparing the child physically. Employ the concept of atraumatic care when preparing children for a procedure. General guidelines for preparation include the following:

- Provide a description of and the reason for the procedure using age-appropriate language ("the doctor will look at your blood to see why you are sick").
- Describe where the procedure will occur ("the x-ray department has big machines that won't hurt you; it's a little cold there too").
- Introduce strange equipment the child may see ("you will lie on a special bed that moves in the big machine, but you can still see out").
- Describe how long the procedure will last ("you will be in the x-ray department until lunchtime").
- Identify unusual sensations that may occur during the procedure ("you may smell something different" [e.g., alcohol smell], "the MRI machine makes loud noises").
- Inform the child if any pain is involved.
- Identify any special care required after the procedure ("you will need to lie quietly for 15 minutes afterward").

> ▶ *Take* NOTE!
>
> *In the hospital, perform all invasive procedures in the treatment room or a room other than the child's room. The child's room should remain a safe and secure area.*

A major aspect of preparation involves play. In general, young children respond better to play materials and older children benefit more from viewing peer modeling films. However, consider the child's temperament, coping strategies, and previous experiences as well as developmental needs and cognitive abilities. First, gain trust and provide support. Include the child's parents, because parents are usually the greatest source of comfort for the child. Be short, simple, and appropriate in explaining situations at the child's level of development. Explain what is to be done and what is expected of the child. Avoid terms that have double meanings or might be confusing. Table 34.1 lists alternative words or phrases to use for terms that may be confusing or misunderstood.

During the Procedure

Use a firm, positive, confident approach that provides the child with a sense of security. Encourage cooperation by involving the child in decision making and allowing the child to select from a list or group of appropriate choices. Allow the child to express feelings of anger, anxiety, fear, frustration, or any other emotions. Often this is how a child communicates and copes with the situation. Tell the child that it is okay to scream or cry, but that it is very important to hold still. Use distraction methods such as those listed in Box 34.1.

Toddlers and preschoolers often resist procedures despite preparation for them. Being held down or restrained is often more traumatizing to the young child than the procedure itself. Use alternative methods (positions that provide comfort for the child) to keep the child still during the procedure (Fig. 34.1). The older child can be held while using a book or story for distraction.

After the Procedure

After the procedure, hold and comfort the child. Cuddle and soothe infants. Encourage children to express their feelings through play, such as dramatic play or use of puppets. Gross motor activities such as pounding or throwing are also helpful for children to discharge pent-up feelings and energy. School-age children and adolescents may not outwardly demonstrate behavior indicating the need for

TABLE 34.1 ALTERNATIVES FOR CONFUSING OR MISUNDERSTOOD TERMS

Term to Avoid	How Children Might Interpret It	Use These Terms Instead
Catheter	Too technical	Tube
Deaden	Kill?	Make sleepy
Dye	"Die"	Special medicine to help the doctor see _____ (part of the body) better
Electrodes	Too technical	Stickers, ticklers, snaps
ICU	"I see you"	Special room with your own nurse
Incision, cut open, make a hole	Too explicit	Special or small opening
Monitor	Too technical	TV screen
Organ	Like a piano?	Special place in the body
Pain	May be too explicit	Child's word for hurt; "boo-boo"
Put to sleep, anesthesia	May confuse with putting a pet to sleep	Special kind of sleep
Shot	Children are scared of shots	Medication under the skin
Stool	Like you sit on?	"Poop" or child's word for it
Stretcher or gurney	"Stretch her"	Rolling bed or special bed on wheels
Take your temperature/BP	Where are you going to "take" them?	See how warm you are/hug your arm
Test	Like at school? (the child will need to perform)	See how your heart is working
Tourniquet	Too technical	Special kind of rubber band
Urine	"You're in?"	"Pee" or child's word for it
X-ray	Don't understand	Picture or big camera to take pictures of the inside of your body

Partially adapted from Florida Children's Hospital, *Suggested vocabulary to use with children.*

comforting; however, provide them with opportunities to express their feelings and be comforted. Remember to praise children for appropriate behavior during the procedure and after all interventions are completed.

Medication Administration

WATCH & LEARN

At one time or another, every child will need to receive medication. As with adults, pediatric medication administration is a critical component of safe and effective nursing care. However, the incidence of potentially harmful medication errors may be three times as high in pediatrics compared to adults (Ghaleb et al., 2006). Therefore, the need for safety takes on even greater importance due to the physiologic, psychological, and cognitive differences inherent in children. The pediatric nurse must adapt administration principles and techniques to meet the child's needs. Medication administration, regardless of the route, requires a solid knowledge base about the drug and its action.

As with medication administration to any patient, the nurse must adhere to the "rights" of medication administration (Box 34.2). Confirming the child's identity and double-checking the dosage before administration of any medication are two critical safeguards that play a major role in preventing medication errors.

BOX 34.1   Distraction Methods

- Have the child point toes inward and wiggle them.
- Ask the child to squeeze your hand.
- Encourage the child to count aloud.
- Sing a song and have the child sing along.
- Point out the pictures on the ceiling.
- Have the child blow bubbles.
- Play music appealing to the child.

▶ *Take* NOTE!

If a parent, caregiver, or patient questions whether a medication should be given, listen attentively, answer their questions, and double check the order.

FIGURE 34.1 Positioning a child for comfort during a painful procedure. (**A**) Sitting on the parent's lap while undergoing allergy testing provides this toddler with a sense of comfort. (**B**) Position the infant cuddled over the parent's (preferable) or the nurse's shoulder when obtaining a heelstick. (**C**) Use "therapeutic hugging" to maintain a child's position when the child is receiving an IM injection. (**D**) Use "therapeutic hugging" to position a child while the child is having an IV line inserted.

Differences in Pharmacodynamics and Pharmacokinetics

Although a drug's mechanism of action is the same in any individual, the physiologic immaturity of some body systems in a child can affect a drug's **pharmacodynamics** (behavior of the medication at the cellular level). As a result, the body may not respond to the drug as intended. The intended effect may be enhanced or diminished, necessitating a change in the dosage to ensure optimal effectiveness without increasing the child's risk for toxicity.

The child's age, weight, body surface area, and body composition also can affect the drug's **pharmacokinetics** (movement of drugs throughout the body via absorption, distribution, metabolism, and excretion). Drugs are administered to children via many of the same routes that are used for adults. However, this similarity ends once the drug is administered.

During the absorption process, drugs move from the administration site into the bloodstream. In infants and young children, the absorption of orally administered medications is affected by slower gastric emptying, increased

BOX 34.2 **Eight Rights of Pediatric Medication Administration**

Right Medication
- Check order and expiration dates.
- Know action of medication and potential side effects (use pharmacy, drug formulary).
- Ensure that the medication provided is the medication that is ordered.

Right Patient
- Confirm patient identity since children may deny their identity in attempt to avoid an unpleasant situation, play in another child's bed, or remove ID bracelet.
- Confirm identity each time medication is given.
- Verify child's name with caregiver to provide additional verification.

Right Time
- Give within 20 to 30 minutes of the ordered time.
- For a medication given on an as-needed (PRN) basis, know when it was last given and how much was given during the past 24 hours.

Right Route of Administration
- Check ordered route and ensure this is the most effective and safe route for this child; clarify any order that is confusing or unclear.
- Give the medication by the route ordered. If there is a need to change route, always check with prescriber (e.g., if a child is vomiting and has an order for an oral

medication, the medication may need to be given via the IV or rectal route).

Right Dose
- Calculate the recommended dose according to child's weight and double-check your calculations.
- Always question the pharmacist and/or prescriber if the ordered dose falls outside the recommended dose range.
- Unusually large or small volumes or dosages should always be verified.

Right Documentation
- Record administration of the medication on the appropriate paper or computerized form according to agency policy.
- Ensure that all medications administered and refused are documented.

Right to Be Educated
- Provide simple explanations to the child based on his or her level of understanding.
- Explain to the parents or caregiver about the medication to be given and what to expect from it.
- Use a positive, firm approach with the child.

Right to Refuse
- Provide explanations to the child and parents to clarify any misconceptions or relieve fears.
- Reinforce the rationale for medication use.
- Respect the child's or parents' option to refuse.

---

intestinal motility, a proportionately larger small intestine surface area, higher gastric pH, and decreased lipase and amylase secretion compared with adults. Intramuscular absorption in infants and young children is affected by amount of muscle mass, muscle tone and perfusion, as well as vasomotor instability. Similarly, decreased perfusion alters subcutaneous absorption. Absorption by these routes is erratic and may be decreased. In contrast, topical absorption of medications is increased in infants and young children because the stratum corneum is thinner and well hydrated (Lilley et al., 2005; Woo, 2004).

The distribution (movement of a drug from the blood to interstitial spaces and then into cells) of medications is also altered in infants and young children. Medication distribution in children is affected by:

- Higher percentage of body water than adults
- More rapid extracellular fluid exchange
- Decreased body fat
- Liver immaturity, altering first-pass elimination
- Decreased amounts of plasma proteins available for drug binding
- Immature blood–brain barrier, allowing permeation by certain medications (Lilley et al., 2005; Pickar, 2004; Woo, 2004)

Metabolism of medications in children is altered because of differences in hepatic enzyme production and the child's increased metabolic rate. **Biotransformation** (the alteration of chemical structures from their original form, which allows for the eventual excretion of the substance) is affected by the same variations affecting distribution in children. In addition, the immaturity of the kidneys until the age of 1 to 2 years affects renal blood flow, glomerular filtration, and active tubular secretion. This results in a longer half-life and increases the potential for toxicity of drugs primarily excreted by the kidneys (Lilley et al., 2005; Woo, 2004).

Developmental Issues and Concerns

Children are constantly growing and developing. The specific psychosocial, cognitive, physical, and motor developmental levels of children are important. Nurses need a solid understanding of growth and development to ensure safe administration of medications to children. Table 34.2 details some growth and development issues related to administering medications to children. Always give developmentally appropriate, truthful explanations before administering medications to children. Include why the drug is needed, what the child will experience,

TABLE 34.2 GROWTH AND DEVELOPMENT ISSUES RELATED TO PEDIATRIC MEDICATION ADMINISTRATION

Stage of Development	Issue/Concern	Nursing Interventions
Infant	Development of trust, which is fostered by consistent care; development of stranger anxiety later in infancy	Involve parents in medication administration to reduce stress for infant. Ensure that parents hold and comfort infant during intervention.
Toddler	Development of autonomy with displays of negativism; rituals, routines, and choices necessary to maintain some sense of control	Follow routines and rituals from home in giving medications if these are safe and positive approaches. Involve parents in medication administration. Offer simple choices (e.g., "Do you want Mom or me to give you your medicine?"). Allow child to touch or handle equipment as appropriate.
Preschooler	Development of initiative, which is fostered when they sense they are helping	Provide an opportunity to play with the equipment and respond positively to explanations and comforting. Provide choices that are possible and keep them simple (e.g., "Do you want juice or water with your medication?" or "Which medication do you want to take first?"). Do not ask, "Will you take your medicine now?" Involve parents in medication administration. Be aware that giving suppositories is particularly upsetting to this age group because of their fears of bodily intrusion and mutilation.
School-aged child	Development of industry, benefiting from being a part of their care; generally very cooperative	Explain to child in simple terms the purpose of the medication. Seek their assistance, such as putting pills in cup or opening the packet, and allow a broader range of choices. Establish a reward system to enhance their cooperation if necessary.
Adolescent	Development of identity, benefiting from much more control over their care	Approach in same manner as adults, with respect and sensitivity to their needs. Maintain the adolescent's privacy as much as possible.

what is expected of the child, and how the parents can participate and support their child. Refer to Chapters 25 through 29 for further information about growth and developmental issues.

The child's past experiences with taking medications and the approaches that may have been used will often affect how the child reacts. Always approach children positively; let your manner convey the belief that they can accomplish this needed behavior. Never label the child as "bad" if he or she did not fully cooperate in taking medication. When medications must be administered with a needle (intramuscularly or subcutaneously), assure the child that this method is not a consequence of the child's behavior. Help parents to work through the feelings of frustration that may result from the child's re-

fusal to cooperate with medication administration. Provide parents with facts about growth and developmental issues and children's fears and anxiety related to medication administration. Model alternative ways for the parents to deal with undesirable behavior.

▶ **Take** NOTE!

Always administer medications promptly, assist the child in holding still using a comforting position for the child, and reward positive behavior.

Determination of Correct Dose

Administering the correct dose is a key component of medication administration. Incorrect dosing is the most commonly reported medication error in the pediatric population (Ghaleb et al., 2006). Many drug references list recommended pediatric dosages, and nurses are responsible for checking doses to ensure that they are appropriate for the child. Two common methods for determining pediatric doses are based on the unit of drug per kilogram of body weight or body surface area (BSA).

Dose Determination by Body Weight

The most common method for calculating pediatric medication doses is based on body weight. The recommended dosage is usually expressed as the amount of drug to be given over a 24-hour period (mg/kg/day) or as a single dose (mg/kg/dose). Differentiate between the 24-hour dosage and the single dose. Use these guidelines to determine the correct dose by body weight:

1. Weigh the child.
2. If the child's weight is in pounds, convert it to kilograms (divide the child's weight in pounds by 2.2).
3. Check a drug reference for the safe dose range (for example, 10 to 20 mg/kg of body weight).
4. Calculate the low safe dose (Box 34.3).
5. Calculate the high safe dose.
6. Determine if the dose ordered is within this range.

BOX 34.3 Dosage Calculation Using Body Weight

After converting the child's weight in pounds to kilograms and checking the safe dose range:
- Calculate the low safe dose range (e.g., 10 to 20 mg/kg and the child weighs 30 kg):
  - Set up a proportion using the low safe dose range
    $10 \text{ mg}/1 \text{ kg} = x \text{ mg}/30 \text{ kg}$
  - Solve for x by cross-multiplying:
    $1 \times x = 10 \times 30$
    $x = 300 \text{ mg}$
- Calculate the high safe dose range:
  - Set up a proportion using the high safe dose range
    $20 \text{ mg}/1 \text{ kg} = x \text{ mg}/30 \text{ kg}$
  - Solve for x by cross-multiplying:
    $1 \times x = 20 \times 30$
    $x = 600$
- Compare the safe dose range (for this example, 300 to 600 mg) with the ordered dose. If the dose falls within the range, the dose is safe. If the dose falls outside the range, notify the prescriber.

The pediatric dosage should not exceed the minimum recommended adult dosage. Generally, once a child or adolescent weighs 50 kg or greater, the adult dose is frequently prescribed. However, always verify that the dose does not exceed the recommended adult dose (Pickar, 2004).

Dose Determination by Body Surface Area

Calculating the dosage based on BSA takes into account the child's metabolic rate and growth. It is commonly used for chemotherapeutic agents. Some recommended medication doses may read "mg/BSA/dose." To determine the dose using BSA, you will need to know the child's height and weight, which will be plotted on a nomogram (Fig. 34.2). A nomogram is a graph divided into three columns: height (left column), surface area (middle column), and weight (right column). Use these guidelines to determine BSA:

1. Measure the child's height.
2. Determine the child's weight.
3. Using the nomogram, draw a line to connect the height measurement in the left column and the weight measurement in the right column.
4. Determine the point where this line intersects the line in the surface area column. This is the BSA, expressed in meters squared (m^2).

FIGURE 34.2 A nomogram to determine body surface area.

Once you have determined the BSA, use the recommended dosage range to calculate the safe dosage.

Oral Administration

Medications to be given via the oral route are supplied in many forms, such as liquids (elixirs, syrups, or suspensions), powders, tablets, and capsules. Generally, children under the age of 5 to 6 are at risk for aspiration because they have difficulty swallowing tablets or capsules. Therefore, if a tablet or capsule is the only oral form available, it needs to be crushed or opened and mixed with a pleasant-tasting liquid or a small amount (generally no more than a tablespoon) of a nonessential food such as applesauce. However, never crush or open an enteric-coated or time-release tablet or capsule. The crushed tablet or inside of a capsule may taste bitter, so never mix it with formula or other essential foods. Otherwise, the child may associate the bitter taste with the food and later refuse to eat it.

▶ *Take* NOTE!

Certain drug formulations should not be crushed. Before crushing a pill or opening a capsule, always check that this will not alter the intended effects of the drug.

Liquid medications, primarily suspensions, may be less concentrated at the top of the bottle than at the bottom of the bottle. Always shake the liquid to ensure even drug distribution. The key to administering liquid forms of oral medications is to use calibrated equipment such as a medicine cup, spoon, plastic oral syringe, or dropper (Fig. 34.3). If a dropper is packaged with a certain medication, never use it to administer another medication, since the drop size may vary from one dropper to another. If using a syringe for oral administration, only use the type intended for oral medications, not one designed for parenteral administration. When using a dropper or oral syringe (without a needle) for infants or young children, direct the liquid toward the posterior side of the mouth. Give the drug slowly in small amounts (0.2 to 0.5 mL) and allow the child to swallow before more medication is placed in the mouth (Fig. 34.4). A nipple without the bottle attached is sometimes used to administer medication to infants. Place the medication directly in the nipple and keep the nipple filled with medication as the infant sucks so no air is taken in while the infant takes the medication. Always place the infant or young child upright (at least a 45-degree angle) to avoid aspiration. The toddler or young preschooler may enjoy using the oral syringe to squirt the medicine into his or her mouth. Older children can take oral medication from a medicine cup or measured medicine spoon.

As children adapt to swallowing tablets or capsules, administration is similar to that of adults. When helping the younger child learn how to swallow medication, the tablet or capsule can be placed at the back of the tongue or

FIGURE 34.3 Devices used to administer oral medications to children.

FIGURE 34.4 Position the infant or young child for safe medication administration.

in a small amount of food such as ice cream or applesauce. Always tell children if there is medicine in the food; otherwise they may not trust you.

> ▶ *Take* NOTE!
>
> *Use the medicine cup or syringe with proper calibration instead of household cups or measuring spoons, since they are not calibrated and may deliver an incorrect dose of medication.*

When the child has a nasogastric, orogastric, nasojejunal, nasoduodenal, **gastrostomy** (opening into the stomach), or jejunostomy tube, oral medications may be given via these devices. The tube allows for the medication to be placed directly into the stomach or small intestine area. Be aware that not all medications can be placed directly into the duodenum or jejunum. Medication for administration via a tube must be supplied in a liquid form, or a crushed tablet or opened capsule can be mixed with a liquid (Box 34.4). Always check tube placement prior to administering the medication. After administration, flush the tube to maintain patency.

> ▶ *Take* NOTE!
>
> *Never force an oral medication into a child's mouth or pinch the child's nose. Doing so increases the risk for aspiration and interferes with the development of a trusting relationship.*

BOX 34.4 **Guidelines for Administering Medications via Gastrostomy or Jejunostomy Tubes**

- Give liquid medications directly into the tube.
- Mix powdered medications well with warm water first.
- Crush tablets and mix with warm water to prevent tube occlusion.
- Open up capsules and mix the contents with warm water to dissolve the contents and prevent tube occlusion.
- Flush the tube with water after administering medications to ensure that the entire amount of medication has been given and to prevent tube occlusion.

Adapted from Children's Healthcare of Atlanta. (2004). *Gastrostomy tube home care manual.*

Rectal Administration

The rectal route is not a preferred route for medication administration in children. The drug's absorption may be erratic and unpredictable. The method is invasive and can be extremely upsetting to the toddler and preschooler because of age-related fears and may be embarrassing to the school-age child or adolescent. However, the rectal route may be used when the child is vomiting or receiving nothing by mouth (NPO). Use age-appropriate explanations and reassurance. Helping the child to maintain the correct position may be necessary to ensure proper insertion and safety.

Lubricate the suppository well with a water-soluble lubricant. With the child in the side-lying position, insert the suppository into the rectum quickly but gently. Wear gloves or use a finger cot to insert the suppository. Insert the suppository above the anal sphincter. For an infant or child under the age of 3, use the fifth finger for insertion. For an older child, use the index finger. To prevent expulsion of the suppository, hold the buttocks together for several minutes or until the child loses the urge to defecate. If the child has a bowel movement within 10 to 30 minutes after administration of the medication, examine the stool for the presence of the suppository. If it is observed, notify the health care provider to determine if the drug needs to be administered again.

Ophthalmic Administration

Many children have a fear of having anything placed in their eyes. Provide older children with an age-appropriate explanation to gain their cooperation. Ophthalmic medications are typically supplied in the form of drops or ointment. Ensure that the medication is at room temperature, as chilled medication may be uncomfortable to the child. Proper positioning of the child is necessary to control the child's head, keep the child's hands from interfering, and prevent injury to the eye. Attempt to administer the medication when the child is not crying to ensure that the medication reaches its intended target area.

Wash hands thoroughly and don gloves. Place the child in the supine position, slightly hyperextending the neck with the head lower than the body so the medication will be dispersed over the cornea. Rest the heel of your hand on the child's forehead to stabilize it. Retract the lower eyelid and place the medication in the conjunctival sac; maintain sterile technique by being careful not to touch the tip of the tube or dropper to the sac. For eye drops, place the prescribed number of drops into the lower conjunctival sac (Fig. 34.5). For ointment, apply the medication in a thin ribbon from the inner canthus outward without touching the eye or eyelashes. If the child is old enough to cooperate, instruct the child to gently close the eyes to allow the medication to be dispersed.

FIGURE 34.5 Administering eye drops: gently press the lower lid down and have the child look up as the medication is instilled into the lower conjunctival sac.

If a child is uncooperative, he or she may need to be immobilized in order to administer the eye drops. Alternatively, one or two drops on the inner canthus of the closed eye can be administered while the child is lying supine (Myers, Wallace, & Johnson, 2005). When the child opens his or her eye, the drop enters the eye. Always ensure that excess medication is wiped from the skin to prevent systemic absorption. Punctal occlusion after application is also important to slow systemic absorption and ensure the medicine stays in the eye.

Children often require ophthalmic medications at home. Parents or caregivers need instruction about how to administer this type of medication. Teaching Guidelines 34.1 provides information on administering eye drops and eye ointments.

Otic Administration

Medications for otic administration are typically in the form of ear drops. This route of administration can be

TEACHING GUIDELINES 34.1

Applying Eye Medications

• Wash your hands with soap and water. Dry them thoroughly using paper towels or a clean cloth.
• Allow the eye drops or ointment to come to room temperature (if the medication was stored in the refrigerator). If necessary, warm the eye drops or ointment tube in the palm of your hand. Keep the cap on to avoid any spillage.
• Remove the cap, placing it on a dry, clean surface.
• For young children (3 years or less), obtain assistance to keep their arms and fingers away during the procedure. If doing this procedure alone, wrap the child in a towel or blanket, keeping the arms inside.
• If you are applying eye drops, it may be easiest if you are standing or sitting behind the child, looking over the back of the child's head as he or she reclines. If you are applying an eye ointment, it may be easiest to face the child directly.
• Using one hand, hold the child's forehead in place while raising the eyelid with your thumb.
• With your other hand, hold the eye drop bottle or ointment tube above the eye, using an extended finger against the child's cheek, forehead, or nose to steady your hand.

• Gently squeeze the eye drop bottle, dispensing the proper number of drops, or gently squeeze the ointment tube, dispensing a small trail (about 2 cm) of ointment into the gap between the lower portion of the eye and bottom eyelid.
• Make sure the tip of the bottle or tube does not make contact with the eye or any other surface.
• For eye drops, gently press your finger against the inside corner where the eye meets the nose for about 1 minute, blocking the tears and medication from exiting through the tear duct. This will help the eye retain more of the medication. If your child is old enough, he or she may be able to do this unassisted.
• For ointment, have the child close his or her eye and not rub the area.
• Ask the child not to blink or squeeze the eye shut more than normal, as this may wash away the medication prematurely.
• Gently dab away any tears or medication on the face with a clean tissue.
• If necessary, clean the tip of the bottle or tube with a clean tissue and recap.
• Wash your hands again and dry them thoroughly.

Source: The Pediatric Glaucoma and Cataract Family Association; http://www.pgcfa.org/drops.htm, http://www.pgcfa.org/ointment.htm)

upsetting to the child because he or she cannot see what is happening. The child often receives otic drugs for an earache, and he or she may fear that the ear drops will increase the pain. Explain the procedure to the younger child in terms that he or she can understand to help allay these fears. Gain the older child's cooperation by explaining the purpose of the medication and the procedure for administration.

Reinforce the need for the child to keep the head still. Younger children may require assistance to do so. Be sure that the ear drops are at room temperature. If necessary, roll the container between the palms of your hands to help warm the drops. Using cold ear drops can cause pain and possibly vertigo when they reach the eardrum.

Place the child in a supine or side-lying position with the affected ear exposed (Fig. 34.6). Pull the pinna downward and back in children under the age of 3 and upward and back in older children. Instill the medication using a dropper. Then have the child remain in the same position for several minutes to ensure that the medication stays in the ear canal. Massage the area anterior to the affected ear to promote passage of the medication into the ear canal. If necessary, place a piece of cotton or a cotton ball loosely in the ear canal to prevent the medication from leaking.

Nasal Administration

Nasally administered medications are typically drops and sprays. Administering nose drops to infants and young children may be difficult, and additional help may be needed to help maintain the child's position. For nose drops, position the child supine with the head hyperextended to ensure that the drops will flow back into the nares. A pillow or folded towel can be used to facilitate this hyperextension. Place the tip of the dropper just at or inside the nasal opening, taking care not to touch the nares with the dropper (Fig. 34.7). Doing so might stimulate the child to sneeze. Although the nasal membranes are not sterile, the drop solution is, and sneezing would contaminate the dropper, leading to contamination of the drop solution when the dropper is returned to the bottle. Once the drops are instilled, maintain the child's head in hyperextension for at least 1 minute to ensure that the drops have come in contact with the nasal membranes.

For nasal sprays, position the child upright and place the tip of the spray bottle just inside the nasal opening and tilted toward the back. Squeeze the container, providing just enough force for the spray to be expelled from the container. Using too great a force can push the spray solution and secretions into the sinuses or eustachian tube.

FIGURE 34.6 Administering ear drops. (**A**) For a child over age 3 years, the nurse pulls the pinna of the affected ear up and back. (**B**) For the child less than 3 years of age, the nurse pulls the pinna of the ear down and back.

FIGURE 34.7 Administering nose drops. Tilt the head down and back to instill nose drops.

▶ *Take* NOTE!

In young infants, instill the medication in one naris at a time, since they are obligate nose breathers.

Intramuscular Administration

Intramuscular (IM) administration delivers medication to the muscle. In children, this method of medication administration is used infrequently because it is painful and children often lack adequate muscle mass for medication absorption. However, IM administration is used to administer certain medications, such as many immunizations.

Muscle development and the amount of fluid to be injected determine IM injection sites in children. Needle size (gauge and length) is determined by the size of the muscle and the viscosity of the medication. For example, more viscous medications often require a larger-gauge needle. In addition, the needle must be long enough to ensure that the medication reaches the muscle.

The preferred injection site for infants is the vastus lateralis muscle. An alternative site is the rectus femoris muscle. The dorsogluteal site, often used in adults, is not used in children until the child has been walking for at least a year. The muscle has not fully developed and the sciatic nerve occupies a larger portion of this area in the young child. The deltoid muscle is used as an IM injection site in children after the age of 4 to 5 years of age due to the small muscle mass. Figure 34.8 illustrates IM injection sites.

Select the needle size and gauge based on the size of the child's muscle. The goal is to use the smallest length and gauge that will deposit the medication in the muscle. Table 34.3 provides general guidelines for solution amount, needle size, and needle gauge when administering IM medications.

Insert the needle into the skin at a 90-degree angle. If the child is a very small infant or has a small muscle mass, use a 45-degree angle.

Subcutaneous and Intradermal Administration

Subcutaneous (SC) administration distributes medication into the fatty layers of the body. It is used primarily for insulin administration. Subcutaneous layers differ among individuals. The preferred sites for SC administration include the anterior thigh, buttocks, upper arms, and abdomen. Use a 3/8- or 5/8-inch needle. Spread the skin tightly or pinch up the skin with the nondominant hand to isolate the tissue from the muscle. Insert the needle at a 45- to 90-degree angle, release the skin if pinched, and inject the medication slowly.

Intradermal (ID) administration deposits medication just under the epidermis. The forearm is the usual site for administration. ID administration is used primarily for tuberculosis screening and allergy testing. A 1-mL syringe with a 5/8-inch, 25- or 27-gauge needle is commonly used to administer the medication. Insert the needle beneath the skin at a 5- to 15-degree angle.

Intravenous Administration

Intravenous (IV) medication administration is commonly used with children, especially when a rapid response to a drug is desired or when absorption via other routes is difficult due to the child's illness or condition. In some cases, the IV route is the only effective method for administering a medication. Use of the IV route requires that the child have an IV device inserted, peripherally or centrally. Although insertion of this device is invasive and traumatic for the child, IV medication administration is considered to be less traumatic when compared to the trauma associated with multiple injections. Unfortunately, the veins of a child are small and easily irritated.

Most medications given by the IV route must be given at a specified rate and diluted properly to prevent overdose or toxicity due to the rapid onset of action that occurs with this route. Therefore, administering medications via the IV route requires knowledge of the drug, the amount of drug to be administered, the minimum dilution of the drug, the type of solution for dilution or infusion, the length of time for infusion, the rate of infusion, the IV tubing volume capacity, and the compatibility of various solutions and medications (Algren & Arnow, 2005). Careful maintenance of the IV site is required to prevent complications.

The primary method for IV medication administration is a syringe pump. This method provides a highly precise rate of infusion. Nursing Procedure 34.1 gives the steps for administering medication via a syringe pump.

If a pump is unavailable, the medication may be administered via a volume control device. The medication is added to the device with a specified amount of compatible fluid and then infused at the ordered rate.

Direct IV push medication typically is reserved for emergency situations and when therapeutic blood levels must be reached quickly to achieve the desired effect (Weinstein, 2006). Direct IV push administration requires that the drug be diluted appropriately and given at a specified rate, such as over 2 to 3 minutes. Care must be taken to prevent fluid overload, which may occur due to flushing needed to maintain IV patency and prevent drug incompatibilities, and from the administration of multiple drug therapies.

Providing Atraumatic Care

When administering any medication, including oral medications, use the principles of atraumatic care (see Chapters 2 and 35 for more information). Children can

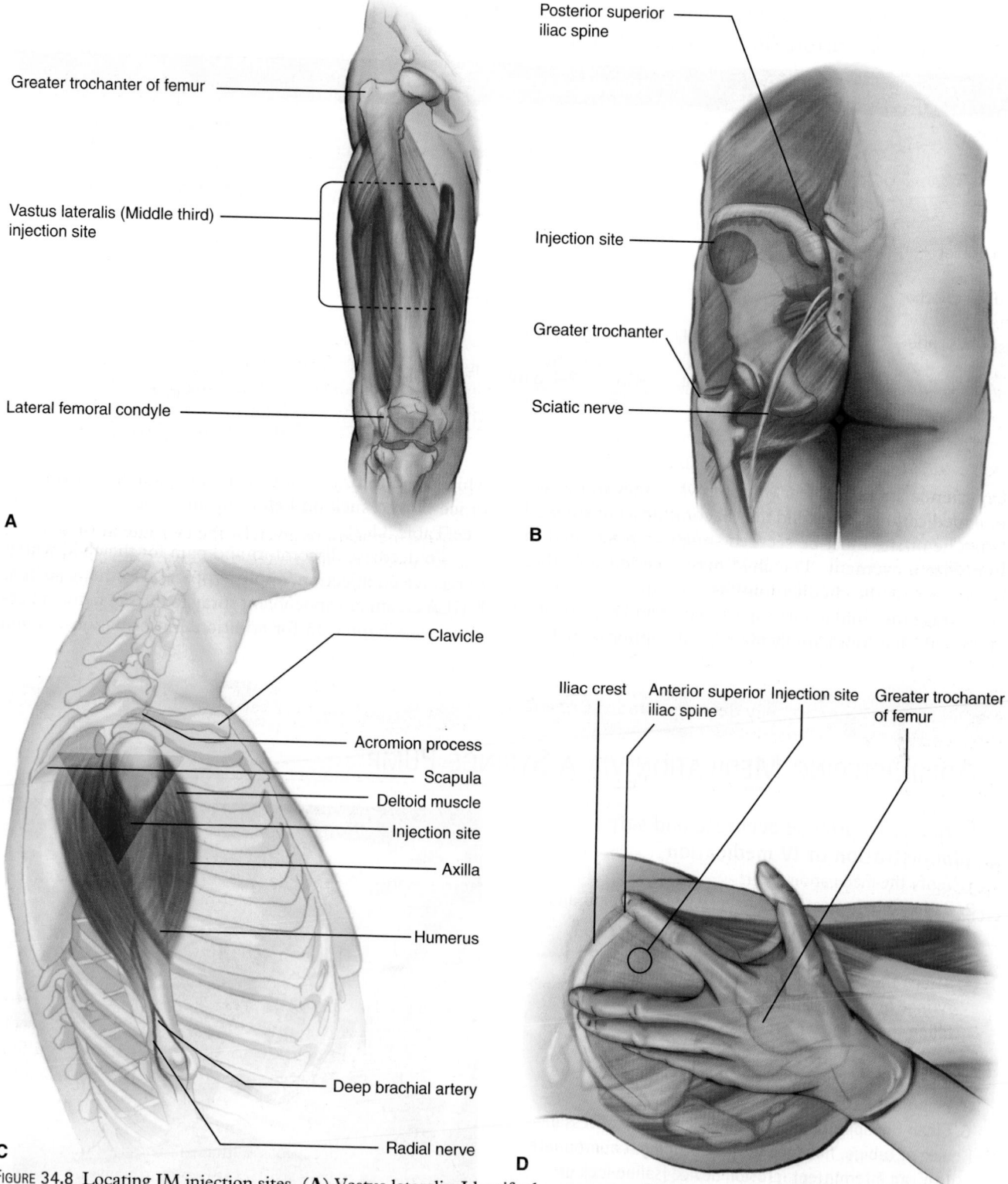

FIGURE 34.8 Locating IM injection sites. (**A**) Vastus lateralis: Identify the greater trochanter and the lateral femoral condyle; inject in middle third and anterior lateral aspect. (**B**) Dorso-gluteal: Place hand on iliac crest and locate the posterosuperior iliac spine; inject in the outer quadrant formed when an imaginary line is drawn between the trochanter and the iliac spine. (**C**) Deltoid: Locate the lateral side of the humerus, one to two fingerwidths below the acromion process. Inject into upper third of muscle. (**D**) Ventrogluteal: Place palm of left hand on right greater trochanter so index finger points toward anterosuperior iliac spine, spread middle finger to form a V, and inject in the middle of the V.

TABLE 34.3   GUIDELINES FOR SOLUTION AMOUNT, NEEDLE LENGTH, AND NEEDLE GAUGE FOR IM INJECTIONS

	Solution Amount					
	Vastus Lateralis	Dorsogluteal	Ventrogluteal	Deltoid	Needle Length	Needle Gauge
Infant	0.5–1 mL	Not recommended	Not recommended	Not recommended	⅝ inch	25–27
Toddler	1 mL	Not recommended	1 mL	0.5 mL	⅝ to 1 inch	22–23
Preschooler	1.5 mL	1.5 mL	1.5 mL	0.5 mL	⅝ to 1 inch	22–23
School age	1.5–2 mL	1.5–2 mL	1.5–2 mL	0.5 mL	⅝ to 1.5 inch	22–23
Adolescent	2–2.5 mL	2–2.5 mL	2–2.5 mL	1 mL	⅝ to 1.5 inch	22–23

experience stress and fear or upset when they must take oral medications. The child may become upset or stressed when he or she must be secured snugly or positioned to minimize movement. The child may experience further discomfort if the medication has an unpleasant taste. Encourage the child to participate in care and provide the child with developmentally appropriate options, such as which fluid to drink with the medication or which flavor of ice pop to suck on before or after the administration (see Table 34.2).

To decrease discomfort and pain for the child who is to receive an injection, apply a topical anesthetic such as EMLA cream or vapocoolant spray to the site before injection (see Chapter 35 for additional information). When

Nursing Procedure 34.1

ADMINISTERING MEDICATION VIA A SYRINGE PUMP

Purpose: To provide accurate and safe administration of IV medication

1. Verify the medication order.
2. Gather the medication and necessary equipment and supplies.
3. Wash hands and put on gloves.
4. Attach the syringe pump tubing to the medication syringe and purge air from the tubing by gently filling the tubing with medication from the syringe.
5. Insert the syringe into the pump according to the manufacturer's directions.
6. Clean the appropriate port on the child's IV access device or tubing, flush the device or tubing if appropriate (e.g., an intermittent infusion device [saline lock or heparin lock]), and attach the syringe tubing to the IV tubing or device.
7. Set the infusion rate on the pump as ordered.
8. When the medication infusion is completed, flush the syringe pump tubing to deliver any medication remaining in the tubing, according to institution protocol.
9. Document the procedure and the child's response to it.

preparing the site for injection, clean it with alcohol or an antiseptic solution and allow this solution to dry.

Ensuring that the child doesn't move is essential to prevent injury. When administering an injection to a young child, at least two adults should hold him or her; this may also be necessary to help an older child to remain still. Use positions that are comforting to the child, such as those in Figure 34.1. After administration, encourage the parents or caregivers to hold and cuddle the child and offer praise.

Educating the Child and Parents

Teaching the child and parents or caregivers about medication administration is a key component of patient education. Many medications are given in the home, making the parents or caregivers the persons responsible for administration. They need to know what medications they are giving and why, how to give them, and what to expect from the drug, including adverse effects. If the medication is to be given via injection, parents and caregivers need to learn how to administer the injection properly.

Parents and caregivers commonly need suggestions about the best ways to administer the medication to their child. Provide them with tips for administration, such as mixing unpleasant-tasting medications with applesauce or yogurt or offering a favorite liquid as a chaser. Also teach the parents how to measure the amount of drug to be given. Encourage them to use a calibrated device and not a typical household spoon, which can vary in the amount that it holds. Teaching Guidelines 34.2 gives pointers about oral medication administration.

Intravenous Therapy

IV access provides a route for the administration of medications and fluids. It is commonly used for children because it is the quickest, and often the most effective, method of administration. As with adults, numerous sites and various devices and equipment may be used to provide IV therapy over a short or long period of time. When administering IV therapy, safety is crucial. The nurse must have a solid knowledge base about the fluids or medications to be given as well as a thorough understanding of the child's physical and emotional development. Venipuncture can be a terrifying and painful experience for children and their families. Nurses play a crucial role in providing support and education to the child and family before, during, and after the procedure (refer to Chap. 2 for additional information related to provision of atraumatic care with procedures).

Sites

IV therapy may be administered via a peripheral vein or a central vein. Peripheral IV therapy sites commonly include the hands, feet, and forearms (Fig. 34.9). In infants up to about the age of 9 months, the scalp veins may be used. The scalp veins are easily visualized, being covered only by

TEACHING GUIDELINES 34.2

Administering Oral Medications

- Be firm when telling your child that it is time for his or her medication. State, "It's time for your medicine" instead of asking, "Will you take your medicine?" or "Can you take your medicine for me?"
- Allow your child to choose an appropriate liquid to help swallow the medication or drink after taking it. Limit the choices to two or three.
- Never bribe or threaten your child to take his or her medication.
- Never refer to the medication as "candy."
- Be honest about the taste of the medication. If necessary, mix it with another food such as applesauce, yogurt, or syrup to help mask the taste.
- If the medication's taste cannot be masked or disguised, have your child hold his or her nose while taking the medication (taste and smell are closely related).
- Do not mix the medication with formula or baby food.
- Always check with your health care provider and pharmacy about opening capsules or crushing tablets and mixing them with food. Some medications should not be opened or crushed.
- If you are giving a liquid using an oral syringe or dropper, place the medication slowly along the inside of the cheek. Never squirt the medication forcibly to the back of the child's throat. It may cause the child to gag and spit out the medication or aspirate it into his or her lungs.
- Always praise the child after taking the medication and provide comfort and cuddling.

a thin layer of subcutaneous tissue. These veins do not have valves, so the device may be inserted in either direction, although the preference would be in the direction of blood flow. However, use of a scalp vein requires that that area of the infant's head be cleared of hair to enhance visualization. They also can be frightening to parents who may think the fluid is infusing into the infant's brain. Thus, scalp veins are usually used only if attempts at other sites have been unsuccessful. When used, ensure appropriate education of the parents prior to insertion.

▶ **Take** NOTE!

When selecting an IV site in an extremity, always choose the most distal site. Doing so prevents injury to the veins superior to the site and allows additional access sites should complications develop in the most distal site.

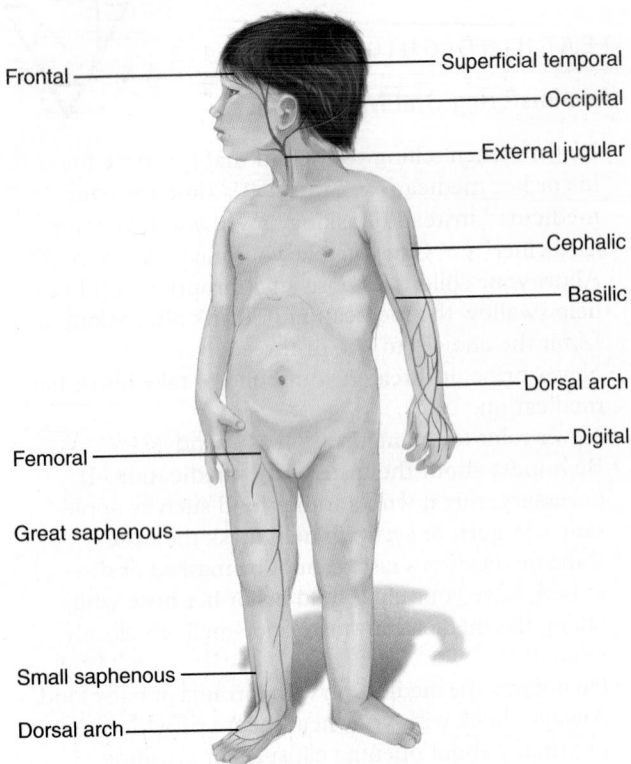

Frontal
Superficial temporal
Occipital
External jugular
Cephalic
Basilic
Dorsal arch
Digital
Femoral
Great saphenous
Small saphenous
Dorsal arch

FIGURE 34.9 Preferred peripheral sites for IV insertion.

Central IV therapy usually is administered through a large vein, such as the subclavian, femoral, or jugular vein or the vena cava. The tip of the device lies in the superior vena cava just at the entrance to the right atrium. The device is inserted surgically or percutaneously and exits the body typically in the chest area, just below the clavicle. A device can be inserted via a peripheral vein, such as the median, cephalic, or basilic vein, and then threaded into the superior vena cava.

Equipment

The choice of equipment is determined by the solution or medication to be administered, the duration of the therapy, the age and developmental level of the child, the child's status, and the condition of his or her veins. Various types of IV devices are commercially available. In addition, different types of tubing and infusion control devices may be necessary.

Peripheral Access Devices

Devices used for peripheral venous access in a child include over-the-needle catheters or winged-infusion sets, commonly referred to as "butterflies" or scalp vein needles. These devices are inserted into the vein and then connected to the IV solution via tubing to provide a continuous infusion of fluid. These devices can also be inserted for intermittent use if the child does not require a continuous fluid infusion. Typically, the hub of the device is capped or plugged to allow intermittent access, such as for administering medications or obtaining blood specimens. When used in this manner, these devices are termed peripheral intermittent infusion devices or saline or heparin locks.

Needle size on the device also varies. Typically, the needle ranges from 21 to 25 gauge, depending on the child's size. The rule of thumb is to use the smallest-gauge catheter with the shortest length possible to prevent traumatizing the child's fragile veins. Typically, peripheral IV devices are used for short-term therapy, usually averaging 3 to 5 days. Midline catheters are also available. These catheters are longer than peripheral catheters and can stay in for 2 to 4 weeks. They are seated deep in the cephalic or basilic veins, but the tip does not extend past the axilla.

Central Access Devices

Numerous devices for central venous access are available. The type chosen depends on several factors, including the duration of the therapy, the child's diagnosis, the risks to the child from insertion, and the ability of the child and family to care for the device. The device may have one or multiple lumens. Although central venous access devices can be used short term, the majority are used for moderate-to long-term therapy.

Central venous access devices are indicated when the child lacks suitable peripheral access, requires IV fluid or medication for more than 3 to 5 days, or is to receive specific treatments, such as the administration of highly concentrated solutions or irritating drugs that require rapid dilution. Patient preference is also a consideration. Central venous access is advantageous because it provides vascular access without the need for multiple IV starts, thus decreasing discomfort and fear. However, central venous access devices are associated with complications such as thrombosis due to partial occlusion of the vessel and infection at the site as well as in the blood due to the direct access to the central circulation (de Jonge et al., 2005). Typically, a chest x-ray is performed after a central venous access device is inserted to verify proper placement. No fluids are administered until correct placement is confirmed. Table 34.4 describes the major types of central venous access devices.

Infusion Control Devices

Infants and young children are at increased risk for fluid volume overload compared with adults. Also, malfunction at the IV insertion site, such as infiltration, may result in much greater injury than a similar incident would cause in an adult. Therefore, IV fluids must be carefully administered and monitored. To ensure accurate fluid administration, infusion control devices such as infusion pumps, syringe pumps, and volume control sets may be used.

TABLE 34.4 TYPES OF CENTRAL VENOUS ACCESS DEVICES

Device	Description
Nontunneled central venous catheter (CVC)	Usually used short term One or more lumens Surgical or percutaneous insertion most commonly via the subclavian, internal jugular, or femoral vein with the tip of the catheter at the top of the superior vena cava just above the right atrium Useful for emergency situations Catheter sutured in place at the exit site
Peripherally inserted central catheters (PICC)	Short- to moderate-term therapy Insertion via a peripheral vein such as antecubital, basilic, cephalic, or medial antecubital vein Catheter typically threaded into superior vena cava; distal tip terminates in the superior vena cava, inferior vena cava, or proximal right atrium Insertion via saphenous vein with tip terminating in inferior vena cava above the diaphragm for infants Single or multiple lumens PICC insertion requires additional training and advanced skill.
Tunneled central venous catheter (e.g., Groshong, Hickman/Broviac)	Usually for long-term use Catheter inserted by a physician via small incision in jugular or subclavian vein and tunneled in the subcutaneous tissue under the skin Initially sutured in place to stabilize position; sutures removed after approximately 1 to 2 weeks when cuff on catheter attaches to subcutaneous tissue Single or multiple lumens Some have valves that prevent backflow of blood and air entrance.
Implanted ports (e.g., Port-a-Cath, Infus-a-Port, Mediport)	Surgically inserted by a physician Stainless-steel port with a polyurethane or silicone catheter attached Catheter tip lying in subclavian or jugular vein; port implanted under skin in a subcutaneous pocket, usually on the upper chest wall Port covered completely by skin and visible only as a slight bulging on the chest; possibly more appealing to the older child and adolescent because there are no visible parts or dressings Access to port via a specially angled, non-coring needle (Huber needle) Site preparation and pain relief measures necessary before accessing the port

Infusion pumps used for children are similar to those used for adults. Typically, the IV solution bag is attached to a calibrated volume control set that has been filled with a specified amount of IV solution (Fig. 34.10). The fluid chamber holds a maximum of 100 to 150 mL of fluid that can be infused over a specified period of time as ordered. Usually, a maximum of a 2-hour infusion amount in the chamber avoids accidental fluid overload in the pediatric population. This chamber can be filled every 1 to 2 hours so only small amounts of ordered quantities of fluid can infuse and the child is protected from receiving too much fluid volume.

In addition, syringe pumps may be used to deliver fluid and medications to children. These pumps can be programmed to deliver minute amounts of fluid over controlled periods of time (see discussion on p. 000 for additional information about syringe pumps).

Fluid Administration

Administering IV fluids to an infant or child requires close attention to the child's fluid status. Typically, the amount of fluid to be administered in a day (24 hours) is determined by the child's weight (in kg) using the following formula:

100 mL per kg of body weight for the first 10 kg
50 mL per kg of body weight for the next 10 kg
20 mL per kg of body weight for the remainder of body weight in kg

Table 34.5 gives examples of calculating a child's fluid requirements using body weight. Once the 24-hour total fluid requirement is determined, this amount is divided by 24 hours to arrive at the correct hourly rate of infusion.

Figure 34.10 Volume control infusion device.

Inserting Peripheral IV Access Devices

Peripheral IV devices are used for most IV therapies. Prior to insertion, review the child's diagnosis and medical history for information that may affect therapy, such as site selection or insertion. For example, a child who has a history of chronic illness may have heightened fears and anxieties related to insertion due to his or her previous experiences or difficulty in accessing IV sites. Typically, the nondominant extremity should be used for insertion, but this may not be possible if a right-handed child has a cast on his left arm.

Check the orders for the prescribed therapy. Determine the purpose and length of the IV therapy and the type of fluid or medication that is to be administered. This information aids in selecting the best device and insertion site. For example, the device needs to be of an adequate gauge to allow the solution or medication to infuse into the vein while at the same time allowing enough blood flow around the device to promote dilution of the infusion.

Establish rapport with the child and parents. Inform them about IV therapy and what to expect. Be honest with the child. Explain that the venipuncture will hurt but only for a short time. Provide the child with a time frame that he or she can understand, such as the time it takes to brush his or her teeth or eat a snack. If possible, use therapeutic play to assist the child in coping (see Chapter 32 for more information).

Insertion of an IV therapy device is traumatic. Follow the principles of atraumatic care, including the following:

• Gather all equipment needed before approaching the child.
• If possible, select a site using hand veins rather than wrist or upper arm veins to reduce the risk of phlebitis. Avoid using lower extremity veins if possible because these are associated with an increased risk of thrombophlebitis and other complications (Cook, 2007)
• Ensure adequate pain relief using pharmacologic and nonpharmacologic methods prior to insertion of the device (see Chapter 35 for more information about management of pain related to procedures).
• Allow the antiseptic used to prepare the site to dry completely before attempting insertion.
• Use a barrier such as a gauze or washcloth or the sleeve of the child's gown under the tourniquet to avoid pinching or damaging the skin.

TABLE 34.5 INTRAVENOUS MAINTENANCE FLUID CALCULATIONS BY BODY WEIGHT

<10 kg in weight	100 mL per kg of weight = # mL for 24 hours Example: A child weighs 7.4 kg. 7.4 × 100 = 740 mL (daily requirement) 740/24 = 30.8 or 31 mL/hour
11–20 kg in weight	100 mL per kg of weight for the first 10 kg + 50 mL/kg for the next 10 kg = # mL for 24 hours Example: A child weighs 16 kg. (10 × 100 = 1,000) plus (6 × 50 = 300) Total = 1,300 mL (daily requirement) 1,300/24 = 54 mL/hour
>20 kg in weight	100 mL/kg for the first 10 kg + 50 mL/kg for the next 10 kg + 20 mL/kg for each kg > 20 kg = # mL for 24 hours Example: A child weighs 30 kg. (10 × 100 = 1,000) plus (10 × 50 = 500) plus (10 × 20 = 200) Total = 1,700 mL (daily requirement) 1,700/24 = 70.8 or 71 mL/hr

- If the child's veins are difficult to locate, use a device to transilluminate the vein (shows the vein's size and direction of travel).
- Make only two attempts to gain access; if you are unsuccessful after two attempts, allow another individual two attempts to access a site. If still unsuccessful, evaluate the need for insertion of another device.
- Encourage parental participation as appropriate in helping to position the child or to provide comfort positioning, such as therapeutic hugging.
- Coordinate care with other departments such as the laboratory for blood specimen collection to minimize the number of venipunctures for the child.
- Secure the IV line using a minimal amount of tape or transparent dressing.
- Protect the site from bumping by using a security device such as the I.V. House dressing (Fig. 34.11).

Maintaining IV Fluid Therapy

Throughout the course of therapy, monitor the fluid infusion rate and volume closely, as often as every hour. If a volume control set is used to administer the IV infusion, fill the device with the allotted amount of fluid that the child is to receive in 1 hour. Doing so prevents inadvertent administration of too much fluid. Never assume that just because an infusion pump is in use, the infusion is being administered without problems. Pumps can malfunction. The tubing can become blocked, or the IV device can move out of the vein lumen. Not enough fluid, fluid overload, or infiltration of the solution into the tissues can occur.

In addition to monitoring the fluid infusion, closely monitor the child's output. Expected urine output for children and adolescents is 1.0 to 2.0 mL/kg/hour (Weinstein, 2006).

> ▶ **Take** NOTE!
>
> *When measuring the output of an infant or child who is not toilet-trained or who is incontinent, weigh the diaper to determine the output. Remember that 1 gram of weight is equal to 1 mL of fluid.*

Historically, padded armboards and footboards were used to prevent movement of the IV device, but today these are considered mechanical restraints and as such should be used only as a last resort when no less restrictive method is available or effective. Padded boards also can interfere with inspection of the insertion site. They also restrict movement, increasing the risk of contractures; they may be uncomfortable; and they can irritate the underlying tissue, leading to excoriation and infection. Moreover, research has failed to demonstrate that the use of armboards promotes patency of the IV line (Algren & Arnow, 2005).

Flushing the IV line when the device is used intermittently may be necessary to maintain patency, such as before and/or after medication is administered and after obtaining blood specimens. However, there is much debate as to how often flushing should be done and the best flush solution to use, heparin or saline. Saline has been found to be more compatible with the numerous solutions and medications administered intravenously and less expensive and less irritating to the vein; also, the incidence of pain and phlebitis is less. Heparin is expensive and incompatible with numerous medications and solutions, and it can affect clotting time, depending on the concentration of the flush solution used. Evidence appears to support the use of normal saline flush with catheters larger than 24 gauge, but more studies are needed to determine the effectiveness of normal saline flushes with catheters smaller than 24 gauge. Additional research is also needed to determine the specific frequency interval for flushing and the volume and concentration of the flush solution to

FIGURE 34.11 (A) IV House over the IV site on a child's hand. (B) IV House over the site on an infant's foot.

use (Knue et al., 2006). Always follow your agency's policy for flushing IV lines.

If the child is receiving IV therapy via a central venous access device, provide site care using sterile technique and flush the device according to agency policy. Note the exit site for the device and inspect it frequently for signs of infection. If the device has multiple lumens, label each lumen with its use (i.e., blood specimen, medication, or fluid). Always check the compatibilities of solutions and medications being given simultaneously.

> ▶ **Take** NOTE!
>
> *When flushing or administering medications through a peripherally inserted central catheter (PICC) line, use a 5-mL syringe or larger, because PICC lines are fragile. Using a larger-volume syringe exerts less pressure on the PICC, thereby reducing the risk of complications.*

Preventing Complications

IV therapy is an invasive procedure that is associated with numerous complications. Strict aseptic technique is necessary when inserting the device and caring for the site. Adherence to standard precautions is key. Inspect the insertion site every 1 to 2 hours for inflammation or **infiltration** (inadvertent infusion of a nonirritant solution or medication into the surrounding tissue) (Weinstein, 2006). Note signs of inflammation such as warmth, redness, induration, or tender skin. Check closely for signs of infiltration such as cool, blanched, or puffy skin. Use of a transparent dressing or IV House dressing provides easy access for assessing the IV insertion site. These types of dressings also help to prevent movement of the catheter hub, thus minimizing the risk of mechanical irritation and complications such as phlebitis or infection.

Typically, an IV site is changed every 72 hours and at any time when the integrity of the system has been compromised or contamination is suspected (Weinstein, 2006). However, with children, the 72-hour time frame may need to be adjusted to minimize the child's exposure to the repeated trauma of insertion. Follow the agency's policies and procedures related to site changes. Consider an alternative route for fluid and medication administration or the insertion of an alternative IV device, such as a PICC line. The majority of catheter-related bloodstream infections occur with the use of central venous lines. These infections result in increased morbidity, mortality, and health care costs. Prevention is paramount. Nurses need to practice proper hand hygiene, use maximal barrier protection during insertion, assess the site frequently, provide proper site care using strict sterile technique, and ensure the patient's CVC is removed as soon as it is no longer needed.

Discontinuing the IV Device

Prepare the child for removal of the IV device in much the same manner as for insertion. Many children may fear the removal of the device to the same extent that they feared its insertion. Explain what is to occur and enlist the child's help in the removal. If appropriate, allow the child to assist in removing the tape or dressing. This gives the child a sense of control over the situation and also encourages his or her cooperation. In addition, practice atraumatic care by doing the following:

- Use water or adhesive remover to help loosen the tape.
- If a transparent dressing is in place, gently lift off the dressing by pulling up opposite corners using a motion parallel to the skin surface.
- Avoid using scissors to cut the tape, but if cutting the tape is necessary, be sure that the child's fingers are clear of the tape and scissors.
- Turn off the infusion solution and pump.
- Once all tape and dressings are removed, gently slide the IV device out using a motion opposite to that used for the insertion.
- Apply pressure to the site with a dry gauze dressing and then cover with a small adhesive bandage. If possible, allow the child to choose the bandage.

> ▶ **Take** NOTE!
>
> *If the IV site was in the arm at or near the antecubital space, do not have the child bend his or her arm after removal of the device. Doing so increases the risk of hematoma formation.*

Nutritional Support

Adequate nutrition is important for all individuals but especially for children. The quality of a child's nutrition during the growing years has a major effect on his or her overall health and development (Klossner & Hatfield, 2006). The presence of a chronic illness, disease, or trauma can increase the child's nutritional demands; if the child cannot meet these even with oral supplementation, other measures may be necessary to provide nutritional support. Such measures may include **enteral nutrition** (delivery of nutrition into the gastrointestinal tract via a tube) and **parenteral nutrition** (IV delivery of nutritional substances). The nutritional plan is determined by the child's age, developmental level, and health status.

Enteral Nutrition

Enteral nutrition, commonly called tube feedings, involves the insertion of a tube so that feedings can be delivered directly into the child's gastrointestinal tract. The tube may be inserted via the nose or mouth or through an opening in the abdominal area, with the tube ending in the stomach or small intestine. Nasogastric or orogastric through tube feedings, a tube from the nose to the stomach or from the mouth to the stomach, respectively, are commonly referred to as **gavage feedings**. Nasoduodenal or nasojejunal feedings involve a tube that is inserted through the nose and ends in either the duodenum or jejunum. Gastrostomy feedings involve the insertion of a gastrostomy tube through an opening in the abdominal wall and into the stomach. Jejunostomy feedings are similar to gastrostomy feedings except that the tube lies in the jejunum.

Enteral nutrition is indicated for children who have a functioning gastrointestinal tract but cannot ingest enough nutrients orally. The child may be unconscious or have a severely debilitating condition that interferes with his or her ability to consume adequate food and fluids. Other conditions that may warrant the use of enteral nutrition include:

• Failure to thrive
• Inability to suck or tiring easily during sucking
• Abnormalities of the throat or esophagus
• Swallowing difficulties or risk for aspiration
• Respiratory distress
• Metabolic conditions
• Severe gastroesophageal reflux disease (GERD)
• Surgery
• Severe trauma

Enteral feedings may be given via nasogastric, orogastric, nasojejunal, nasoduodenal, gastrostomy, or jejunostomy tubes (Fig. 34.12). Table 34.6 provides additional

FIGURE 34.12 (**A**) Gastrostomy tube. (**B**) Low-profile (button) gastrostomy tube. The filled balloon keeps the tube in place inside the stomach.

information about these types of feeding tubes. Enteral feedings are less costly than parenteral feedings; they are considered a safer alternative for nutritional support and are associated with improved outcomes (Westhus, 2004). Tube misplacement is a serious complication of enteral feeding.

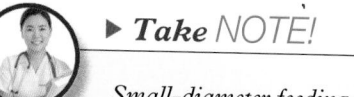

▶ *Take* NOTE!

Small-diameter feeding tubes, though more comfortable, may easily become dislodged if the child coughs vigorously.

Inserting a Nasogastric or Orogastric Feeding Tube

Tubes for gavage feeding can be inserted via the nose or mouth. For infants, who are obligate nose breathers, insertion via the mouth may be appropriate. Oral insertion also promotes sucking in the infant. For the older child, nasal insertion is usually the preferred method. If the tube is to remain in place, the nose also is considered to be more comfortable. Nursing Procedure 34.2 gives the steps for inserting a gavage feeding tube.

Once the gavage feeding tube is inserted, checking for placement is essential. Tube placement must be confirmed each time the tube is inserted and prior to each use. Radiologic confirmation of tube placement is considered the most accurate method, but the risks associated with repeated radiation exposure to verify tube placement prohibit its use (Westhus, 2004). Several methods have been proposed as reliable for checking tube placement; but no single method has been shown to be consistently accurate for continually assessing tube placement. Refer to Box 34.5 for methods to verify feeding tube placement.

Even with these methods, tube malpositioning can occur. Research also has suggested using measurements of bilirubin, trypsin, and pepsin levels to enhance assessment of tube placement, but no methods are available for bedside testing of these levels (Huffman et al., 2004). Therefore, nurses need to be vigilant in checking for tube placement using the recommended methods and be cautious and proactive if there is any suspicion that the tube may be misplaced.

If the gavage feeding tube is to remain in place, secure it to the child's cheek. Do not tape the tube to the child's forehead because this could lead to irritation and pressure on and possible breakdown of the nasal mucosa. Also measure the length of the tube extending from the nose or mouth to the end and record this information. Double-check this measurement before administering each intermittent tube feeding to verify that the feeding tube is in the proper position. Once the position of the gavage feeding tube is confirmed, the feeding solution or medication can be administered.

TABLE 34.6   TYPES OF ENTERAL FEEDING TUBES

Type of Tube	Indication	Nursing Implications
Nasogastric (inserted via the nose into the stomach) Orogastric (inserted via the mouth into the stomach)	Short-term enteral feeding. Orogastric usually limited to young infants only.	• Long-term use or repeated insertion causes irritation and discomfort. • Silicone and polyurethane tubes are very flexible and more comfortable; they require a stylet or guidewire for insertion. • Length of long-term use varies according to the type of tube used and the institution protocol. Periodically a nasogastric tube is removed and reinserted via the opposite nostril to prevent pressure on the nasal mucosa. • Maintaining orogastric placement between feedings can be difficult due to oral secretions.
Nasoduodenal (inserted via the nose to the duodenum) or nasojejunal (inserted via the nose to the jejunum)	Short-term enteral feeding. Indicated if child has trouble digesting food, cannot use his or her gastrointestinal tract secondary to congenital anomalies or surgery, or is at risk for or has a history of severe reflux or aspiration.	• Silicone and polyurethane tubes with weighted tip allow tube to pass from pylorus into small intestines. • Agency may require special training in order to place at bedside; may also be performed in radiology. • Length of use same as nasogastric or orogastric tubes.
Gastrostomy (surgically inserted through the abdominal wall into the stomach) Jejunostomy (surgically inserted through the abdominal wall into the jejunum)	Long-term enteral feeding or when esophageal atresia or stricture is present. Jejunostomy tubes are indicated when gastric feeding is not tolerated.	• The inner section of the tube is below the skin surface with the tip located in the stomach or jejunum (may be balloon, winged, or mushroom-shaped). The outer section appears above the skin surface at the insertion site and has an opening or feeding port to which the feeding solution is attached. • Low-profile gastrostomy device (gastrostomy button) is flush with the abdominal surface. The flip-top opening is anchored by a dome that fits against the stomach wall. Less conspicuous, it allows the child to be more active and mobile. • After initial insertion, the tube length is measured from the insertion site to the far end of the tube and recorded. This measurement is checked at least daily to ensure that the tube has not moved. • For any gastrostomy or jejunostomy tube, the type and size of tube inserted as well as the amount required to fill the balloon if present should be known.

▶ **Take** NOTE!

Instilling air into the tube and then auscultating for the sound is no longer considered a viable method for checking tube placement. Air instilled into a tube that is positioned above the gastroesophageal sphincter can still be auscultated as air in the stomach, thereby giving a false-positive result.

Remember Lily, the 9-month-old infant diagnosed with failure to thrive who is to receive gavage feedings with a nasogastric tube? What equipment will be needed, and what steps will you take to complete the procedure?

Administering Enteral Feedings

Enteral feedings can be given continuously or intermittently, regardless of the type of tube used. Intermittent

INSERTING A GAVAGE FEEDING TUBE

Purpose: To provide a means for delivering nutrition to the child's functioning gastrointestinal tract

1. Verify the order for gavage feeding.
2. Explain the procedure to the child and parents using appropriate language geared to the child's development level.
3. Gather the necessary equipment; remove formula for feeding from refrigerator if appropriate and allow it to come to room temperature.
4. Wash hands and put on gloves.
5. Inspect the child's nose and mouth for deformities that may interfere with passage of the tube.
6. Position the infant supine with the head slightly elevated and with the neck slightly hyperextended so that the nose is pointed upward. If necessary, place a rolled towel or blanket under the neck to help in maintaining this position. Assist the older child to a sitting position if appropriate. Alternatively, have the parent or another person hold the child to promote comfort and reassurance. Enlist the aid of additional persons, such as a parent or other health care team member, to assist in maintaining the child's position.
7. Determine the tubing length for insertion: measure from the tip of the nose to the earlobe to the middle of the area between the xiphoid process and umbilicus. Mark this measurement on the tube with an indelible pen or with a piece of tape.

8. Lubricate the tube with a generous amount of sterile water or water-soluble lubricant to promote passage of the tube and minimize trauma to the child's mucosa.
9. Insert the tube into one of the nares or the mouth. Direct a nasally inserted tube straight back toward the occiput; direct an orally inserted tube toward the back of the throat.
10. Advance the tube slowly to the designated length; encourage the child (if capable) to swallow frequently to assist with advancing the tube.
11. Watch for signs of distress, such as gasping, coughing, or cyanosis, indicating that the tube is in the airway. If these signs develop, withdraw the tube and allow the child to rest before attempting reinsertion.
12. Check for proper placement of the tube by attaching a syringe to the end of the tube and aspirating stomach contents; the pH of the aspirate should be less than 6 (indicating gastric acid) and the color of the aspirate should be clear, tan, or green (indicating gastric secretions); return any aspirated contents to the stomach.
13. Document the type of tube inserted, length of tubing inserted, measurement of external tubing length after insertion, and confirmation of placement.

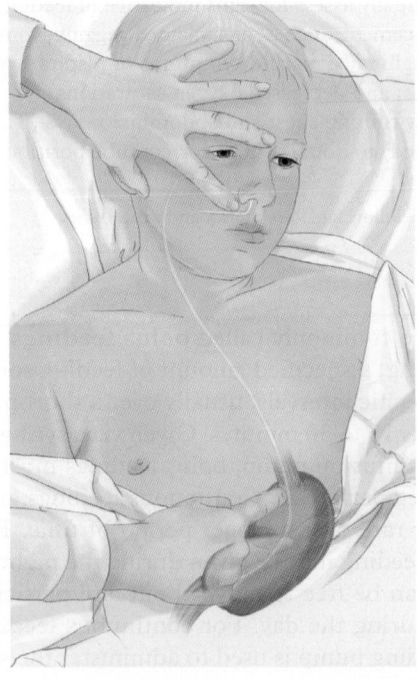

Methods for Verification of Feeding Tube Placement

- Obtain radiographic confirmation of proper tube placement after initial placement.
- After initial confirmation, document pH of aspirate; document insertion distance and external length of tube in the chart. Mark and document the tube's exit site from the nose or mouth.
- Use bedside techniques at regular intervals to determine proper tube positioning.
  - Measuring pH
    - Gastric secretions have a pH < 5. Small intestine secretions will usually have a pH > 6, but this does not reliably predict proper tube placement. A pH > 6 can occur with respiratory or esophageal placement, with proper tube placement (gastric or intestinal) when feedings are given continuously, or if the child is receiving acid-inhibiting medications. Therefore, if the pH is > 5 additional assessment is warranted.
  - Observing appearance of fluid aspirated from tube
    - Gastric secretions are usually grassy green or clear and colorless and can have off-white or tan mucus shreds. It may also be brown-tinged if blood is present.
    - Intestinal secretions are often bile stained, light golden yellow to brownish green. They tend to be thicker and more translucent than gastric secretions.
    - Respiratory secretions can be white, yellow, straw colored, or clear.
  - Check external markings on tube and external tube length to determine if the tube seems to have migrated or been misplaced.
  - Continually assess for signs indicative of feeding tube misplacement, such as unexplained gagging, vomiting, or coughing; signs and symptoms of respiratory distress; and decreased oxygen saturations.
  - Review routine chest and abdominal x-rays (if obtained) to double check correct tube position.

*Note: Always follow agencies' policy and procedures.

feedings are commonly called **bolus feedings**. With a bolus feeding, a specified amount of feeding solution is given at specific intervals, usually over a short period of time such as 15 to 30 minutes. Given via a syringe, feeding bag, or infusion pump, bolus feedings most closely resemble regular meals. Continuous feedings are given at a slower rate over a longer period of time. In some cases, the feeding may be given during the night so that the child can be free to move about and participate in activities during the day. For continuous feedings, an enteral feeding pump is used to administer the solution at a prescribed rate.

Checking for tube placement is a priority before administering any intermittent tube feeding and periodically during continuous tube feedings, regardless of the type of tube being used. (Refer to Table 34.6.) For gastrostomy and jejunostomy tubes, ensure that the calibration, if present, has not changed. Measure the length of the tube daily from the exit site on the stomach to the end of the tube. Aspiration of stomach contents is still recommended in some literature, and checking the pH can assist in verifying proper placement. Once placement is confirmed, the feeding can be given. Also, measure the gastric **residual** (the amount remaining in the stomach; indicates gastric emptying time) by aspirating the gastric contents with a syringe, measuring it, and then replacing the contents. Check the residuals periodically, according to the facility's policy, such as every 4 to 6 hours, and before each intermittent feeding. If the residual volume exceeds the amount specified by the physician's order, hold the feeding and notify the physician.

Begin the feeding by placing the child in a supine position with the head and shoulders elevated approximately 30 degrees so that the feeding will remain in the stomach area. Flush the tube with a small amount of water to clear it and prevent occlusion. This is not necessary for a gavage feeding if the tube is being inserted each time a feeding is given. Ensure that the feeding solution is at room temperature. Administer the feeding as per the facility's policy.

Feeding solutions may be placed into the barrel of a syringe or into a feeding bag attached to the feeding tube and allowed to flow by gravity. The rate of flow for gravity-assisted feedings can be increased or decreased by raising or lowering the feeding solution container, respectively. Typically, intermittent feedings last from 15 to 30 minutes. A feeding bag also may be attached to a pump to control the rate of flow. Monitor the child's tolerance to the feeding.

Once the feeding is complete but before the formula completely empties from the container, flush the tube with water. As the water leaves the syringe or tubing, clamp the tube to prevent air from entering the stomach. Then disconnect the syringe or tube-feeding bag from the tube (Children's Healthcare of Atlanta, 2004).

▶ **Take** NOTE!

If the child vomits during the feeding, stop the feeding immediately and turn him onto his side or sit him up.

If the child has a gastrostomy button, open the cap and connect an adaptor or insert extension tubing through the one-way valve. This allows access to the gastric conduit. The feeding solution container is connected to the extension tubing or adaptor and the feeding is given as de-

EVIDENCE-BASED PRACTICE 34.1
Feeding Tube Aspirates, pH, and Enzyme Content as Accurate Predictors of Proper Feeding Tube Placement in Children

Nutritional support is essential in the care of ill children. Many patients require enteral feedings to obtain proper nutrition during illness. Feeding tube placement errors can have a negative impact. Tubes inadvertently placed in the esophagus or in the stomach when they should have been in the intestines increase the risk for aspiration. Tubes placed in the intestines that were intended to be in the stomach can lead to malabsorption and diarrhea. Tubes placed in the lungs can have catastrophic, even fatal results. Extreme care needs to be taken to ensure correct positioning of a feeding tube prior to use. Radiography is the most accurate way to determine that a feeding tube is in the desired location and not inadvertently in the lung. The risk of repeated exposure to radiation makes it unrealistic to use radiography every time feeding tube placement needs to be confirmed.

● Study

A prospective descriptive clinical study was performed at a university-based children's hospital. A convenience sample of 56 children, from birth to 14 years, who required feeding tubes—nasogastric, orogastric, or nasointestinal—was used. Placement of the feeding tube was checked 30 minutes after radiologic confirmation by aspirating 2.5 mL of fluid. The appearance of the fluid was described, pH was deter-

mined by two methods, and the aspirate was assayed for pepsin and trypsin content.

▲ Findings

Mean gastric pH was significantly lower than mean intestinal pH. Color of the gastric aspirate (clear and colorless, green, off-white, or brown) was significantly different than the intestinal aspirate (yellow or bile stained). Both enzymes, pepsin and trypsin, were statistically significant discriminators between gastric and intestinal tube placement. Aspirating fluids from feeding tubes, visually examining the fluid, and assaying the fluid for aspirate characteristics were found to be adaptable from adults to children.

■ Nursing Implications

Nurses need to utilize accurate assessment skills when verifying feeding tube placement. Nurses can feel more confidence that simple bedside tests, such as pH and visual appearance of aspirate, can provide evidence that a feeding tube is placed properly in the stomach. When pH is > 6 and the aspirate's visual appearance is yellow or bile colored, this may indicate intestinal placement, but further assessment and verification is still warranted. Refer to Box 34.5 for further explanation.

Westhaus, N. (2004). Methods to test feeding tube placement in children. *American Journal of Maternal Child Nursing, 29*(5), 290–291.

scribed previously. After the feeding is completed, the extension tubing or adaptor is flushed with water and the flip-top opening is closed.

Burp the infant during and after any type of tube feeding in the same manner as for an infant who is bottle- or breast-fed. Also, position the child on his or her right side with the head slightly elevated, approximately 30 degrees, for about 1 hour after the feeding to facilitate gastric emptying and reduce the risk of aspiration and regurgitation. Weigh the child daily throughout enteral nutrition therapy to determine the effectiveness of the therapy.

Providing Skin and Insertion Site Care

Skin around the insertion gastrostomy or jejunostomy site may become irritated from movement of the tube, moisture, or leakage of stomach or intestinal contents, or due to the adhesive device holding the tube in place. Keeping the skin clean and dry will help prevent most of these problems (Children's Healthcare of Atlanta, 2004). Routine site care includes gentle cleansing with soap and water followed by rinsing or cleaning with water alone.

> ▶ **Take** NOTE!
>
> *Do not rotate a jejunal tube because it can cause kinking (Cincinnati Children's Hospital Medical Center, 2005).*

The skin around a gastrostomy or jejunostomy tube requires cleaning at least once a day. Ordinary soap and water are sufficient to clean about the tube site to prevent buildup. To clean under an external disc or bumper, a cotton-tipped applicator may be used. Diluted hydrogen peroxide may be necessary to clean crusted drainage (Cincinnati Children's Hospital Medical Center, 2005). During insertion site care, rotate the gastrostomy tube or button a quarter-turn to prevent skin adherence and irritation (Children's Healthcare of Atlanta, 2004). Assess the insertion site and condition of the surrounding skin for signs and symptoms of infection, such as erythema, induration, foul drainage, or pain. A small amount of clear or tan drainage is normal. If any drainage is present, a dressing can be placed. This dressing should be changed when soiled. If no drainage is present, do not place a dressing as it can cause undue pressure.

Preventing movement of the tube also helps reduce skin irritation. Check the volume of the balloon with a balloon-tipped device about once or twice a week and reinflate the balloon to the initial volume if needed. The tube should be able to move slightly in and out of the child's stomach. The plastic disc should be snug against the skin but not tight enough to cause pressure. Tube stabilization methods help prevent the tube from moving around and sliding further into the stomach or jejunum. Stabilize the tube by pulling gently on the tubing and sliding the stabilizer bar or disc snugly against the abdomen. Then, measure and record the length of the tube from the exit site of the abdominal wall to the end of the tube. All future measurements should be the same unless the tube length is changed. For tubes without a stabilizer bar or disc or for additional stabilization needs, several other methods may be used, including nipples, tape, tension loops, and hydroactive dressings (Box 34.6).

Promoting Growth and Development

Some children receive all of their nutritional needs through tube feedings, whereas other children use tube feedings as a supplement to eating by mouth. Feeding time is a special time for infants and children. Occasionally, babies who are fed solely through an enteral feeding tube may forget or lose the desire to eat by mouth. Use a pacifier to help avoid this, allowing the infant to associate the nipple in his or her mouth with a feeding. The sucking motion will also exercise the jaw and promote the flow of the feedings. The saliva produced during sucking aids in digestion. Combined with holding the infant and cuddling, rocking, and talking to him or her, this promotes a more normal feeding time.

Talking with children, playing music, or reading a story promotes an active feeding time. At home, encourage parents to include the feeding as a part of regular family mealtime together to provide socialization for the child. Allow the child to participate in the feedings by gathering supplies and administering the actual feeding so that the child may experience independence and adaptation. If the child also eats food by mouth, feed him or her by mouth first and then administer the tube feeding. During tube feedings in bed, make sure the head of the bed is elevated at least 30 degrees to help prevent vomiting and aspiration.

Children with feeding tubes should be allowed as normal a routine as possible. For example, they can crawl, walk, and jump just like children of the same age and developmental level. However, in some cases, contact sports such as football, hockey, and wrestling should be avoided because of the higher risk of injury. Securing the tubing under the child's clothing will prevent it from becoming accidentally dislodged. Dressing younger children in one-piece outfits helps to prevent them from playing with the gastrostomy or jejunostomy tube and helps to protect the insertion site (Fidanza, 2005).

Educating the Child and Family

Educate children receiving enteral feedings and their parents thoroughly about this method of nutritional support. Reinforce the reason for the therapy and provide the child and parents with opportunities to verbalize their concerns and ask questions. Ensure that the parents understand the risks and benefits of the therapy and the expected duration.

Provide the child, if developmentally appropriate, and parents with opportunities to participate in the feeding sessions. This helps allay some of their fears and anxieties and promotes a sense of control over the situation. They will also gain valuable practice in learning the skill should the feedings be required at home. Teaching Guidelines 34.3 identifies important topics to include in the teaching plan for a child receiving enteral nutrition at home. Education also involves helping the family develop appropriate coping strategies to adapt, solve problems, and negotiate for the support and services they will need after discharge.

*R*emember Lily from the beginning of the chapter? She is to be discharged home after having a gastrostomy tube inserted to continue feedings at home.
    What teaching is needed for her family prior to discharge?

Parenteral Nutrition

Nutritional support can be administered IV through a peripheral or central venous catheter. The concentration and components of the solution determine the type of parenteral nutrition. Parenteral nutrition given via a central venous access is termed **total parenteral nutrition (TPN)**. Comparison Chart 34.1 gives information about peripheral and central parenteral nutrition.

Administering TPN

Typically, the health care provider determines the concentration and components of the TPN solution based on a thorough assessment of the child's status, including the results of laboratory testing. This information is used as a baseline for evaluating the effectiveness of therapy.

The solution is prepared under sterile conditions in the pharmacy. For TPN, a central venous access device is inserted and secured, if one is not already in place. Use specialized tubing with an in-line filter (0.22 μm) to prevent small microparticles from entering the circulation. If total nutrient admixture (TNA) is being administered, the use of a 1.2-μg filter is recommended.

BOX 34.6 Methods to Stabilize a Gastrostomy Tube

Nipple Method

1. Cut a piece of skin protectant (e.g., Stomahesive®) to fit around the G-tube, leaving a small amount of skin showing around the tube.
2. Cut a half-inch from the top of a baby-bottle nipple, just large enough to fit snugly over the tube. Cut three or four holes at the base of the nipple to allow air circulation and site assessment. Slip the nipple over the tube.
3. Secure the tube to the Stomahesive® with four pieces of 1-inch-wide tape around the base of the nipple. Do not cover the holes in the nipple.
4. Gently pull on the tube until slight resistance is felt, anchoring the tube against the stomach or intestinal wall.
5. Place another piece of 1-inch-wide tape where the tube meets the nipple, securing the tube in place.

Taping Methods

1. Cut two pieces of 1-inch-wide tape about 4 to 5 inches long.
2. Fold a tab down on each piece of tape.
3. Tape the pieces to the skin and along opposite sides of the tube, sandwiching them together.

OR

1. Cut two pieces of tape about 6 inches long.
2. Form pieces into two tabs by folding the middle third of each one so it will stick onto itself. Apply these two tabs on either side of the tube directly onto the skin.

3. Cut a third piece of tape about 8 inches long, using it to go from one tab over the G-tube to the other tab and back again, leaving space at the tube insertion point. This forms an H with the two tabs.

Tension Loop Method

1. Fold the middle third of a piece of tape onto itself. Place the tape onto the skin about 2 to 3 inches from the tube insertion site.
2. Fold each end of a second piece of tape onto itself to make two tabs. Fold this around the tube 3 inches away from the tube insertion site.
3. Tape the two pieces together, keeping the tube at a 90-degree angle from the abdomen.

Hydroactive Dressing Method

This method of securing a tube may be used if there is skin breakdown or irritation at the insertion site.

1. Cleanse the skin with soap and water, then rinse. Dry well.
2. Cut a 2-by-3-inch piece of hydroactive dressing material, rounding off the corners. Cut through to the center and then cut a small hole the size of the tube.
3. Remove the paper backing off the hydroactive dressing and apply it to the skin, fitting snugly around the tube.

4. Reapply a new dressing every 3 to 5 days or when it becomes wet.

Adapted from Children's Healthcare of Atlanta. (2004). *Gastrostomy tube home care manual.*

Topics to Be Covered for Home Enteral Nutrition

- Type of nutritional support
- Rationale for therapy
- Expected results from therapy
- Duration of therapy
- Frequency of feedings
- Feeding solution and equipment
- Tube insertion technique (if appropriate)
- Methods to check for correct placement
- Steps for administering the feeding (and medication if ordered)
- Procedure for flushing tube
- Frequency of weighing the child
- Signs and symptoms of complications and when to notify health care provider
- Troubleshooting problems, such as clogging of the tube
- Daily tube care (e.g., cleaning the site, rotating tube)
- Site assessment
- Technique for reinsertion/replacement of tube as appropriate
- Equipment suppliers
- Resources for support
- Follow-up visits and referrals

The infusion of the solution is initiated at a slow rate that is gradually increased as ordered based on how the child tolerates the therapy. TPN solutions are highly concentrated glucose solutions that can cause hyperglycemia if given too rapidly. Use of an infusion pump is essential to control the rate of infusion. TPN solutions may be refrigerated until they are to be used. Once started, a single solution of TPN should hang for no longer than 24 hours. Fat emulsions are administered periodically to meet the child's need for essential fatty acids. These solutions are given as a piggyback solution into the TPN line, but below the in-line filter.

Throughout TPN therapy, be vigilant in monitoring the infusion rate, and report any changes in the infusion rate to the health care provider immediately. Adjustments may be made to the rate, but only as ordered by the provider. The infusion rate should never be adjusted more than 10% higher or lower than the current rate (Weinstein, 2006).

Check blood glucose levels frequently, such as every 4 to 6 hours, initially to evaluate for hyperglycemia. These levels can be obtained with a bedside glucose meter. Minimize the trauma and discomfort associated with frequent invasive procedures by using the principles of atraumatic care. If blood glucose levels are elevated, subcutaneous administration of insulin may be needed. Once the child's glucose levels stabilize, the frequency of blood glucose level determinations decreases, such as every 8 to 12 hours, based on the facility's policy.

▶ *Take* NOTE!

If for any reason the TPN infusion is interrupted or stops, begin an infusion of a 10% dextrose solution at the same infusion rate as the TPN. This helps to prevent rebound hypoglycemia that may occur due to the increased insulin secretion by the child's body in response to the use of the highly concentrated TPN solution.

COMPARISON CHART 34.1   PERIPHERAL PARENTERAL NUTRITION VS. TOTAL PARENTERAL NUTRITION

	Peripheral Parenteral Nutrition	Total Parenteral Nutrition
Indications/use	Primarily supplemental Short-term use to supply additional calories and nutrients	Provides all nutrients to meet child's needs Enough calories supplied to maintain a positive nitrogen balance (Weinstein, 2006)
Route	Peripheral vein	Central venous access to allow rapid dilution of hypertonic solution
Child's status	Nutritional status usually within acceptable parameters Oral intake decreased or absent	Child with a nonfunctioning GI tract, such as a congenital or acquired GI disorder Severe failure to thrive Multisystem trauma or organ involvement Preterm newborns
Components	Fluid, electrolytes, and carbohydrates (dextrose); usually no protein or fats Carbohydrate concentration usually limited to 10% (Weinstein, 2006)	Highly concentrated solution of carbohydrates, electrolytes, vitamins, and minerals Lipid emulsion to supply need for essential fatty acids Total nutrient admixture (TNA) with components of TPN plus lipids and other additives in one container

Perform catheter site care, tubing and filter changes, and dressing changes according to the facility's policy. Inspect the insertion site closely for signs of infection. Also monitor the child's vital signs, daily weights, and intake and output closely for changes. In addition, review laboratory test results, which can aid in early detection of problems, such as infection or electrolyte excesses or deficits.

TPN can be administered continuously over a 24-hour period, or after initiation it may be given on a cyclic basis, such as over a 12-hour period during the night. When administering cycled TPN, the solution is infused at half the prescribed rate for the first and last hour to prevent hyper- and hypoglycemia.

Preventing Complications

Nurses play a key role in minimizing the risk for complications related to use of central venous access devices and TPN. Box 34.7 describes these complications. Key measures to reduce the risk of complications include the following:

- Monitor the child's vital signs closely for changes.
- Adhere to strict aseptic technique when caring for the catheter and administering TPN.

BOX 34.7 Complications that can Occur with Central Venous Access Devices and TPN

- Air embolism from inadvertent entry of air into the system during tubing or cap changes or accidental disconnection
- Cardiac tamponade due to catheter advancement with movement of the arm, neck, or shoulder
- Catheter occlusion from the development of a fibrin sheath or thrombus at the catheter tip, malpositioning or kinking, or the deposition of precipitates or a blood clot
- Venous thrombosis from injury to the vessel wall during insertion or movement of the catheter after insertion or from chemical irritation due to administration of concentrated solutions, vesicants, and other medications through the catheter
- Hyperglycemia, typically with too rapid an infusion of TPN
- Hypoglycemia, which may occur with rapid cessation
- Dehydration as the child's body attempts to rid itself of excess glucose through renal excretion
- Electrolyte imbalance (particularly potassium, sodium, calcium, magnesium, and phosphorus)
- Infection at the skin insertion site, along the catheter pathway, or in the bloodstream. Organisms can arise from the skin, hands of caregivers, or other areas such as wound drainage, droplets from the lungs, or urine. For example, connection sites can be contaminated during tubing or dressing changes.

- Ensure that the system remains a closed system at all times. Secure all connections, use occlusive dressings, and clamp the catheter or have the child perform the Valsalva maneuver during tubing and cap changes.
- Adhere to agency policy for flushing of the catheter and maintaining catheter patency.
- Assess intake and output frequently.
- Monitor blood glucose levels and obtain laboratory tests as ordered to evaluate for changes in fluid and electrolytes.

> ▶ *Take* NOTE!
>
> *Never administer any medication, blood, or other solution through the TPN lumen. Doing so increases the risk for contamination of the system and subsequent infection.*

Promoting Growth and Development

Meals are a time for meeting nutritional needs as well as a time for love, comfort, support, and socialization. TPN meets the child's nutritional needs, but the child's need for love and support also must be met. Implement measures similar to those for children receiving enteral nutrition (see discussion earlier in this chapter). Also provide opportunities for holding and cuddling the child. Allow the older child to participate in activities that can help to occupy the time associated with meals. Encourage the child and parents to participate in the care to promote a sense of independence as well as a sense of control over the situation.

Educating the Child and Family

Children who require long-term TPN therapy may receive TPN in the home. Administering TPN at home requires thorough education of the child and parents. This teaching can occur in the health care agency or in the child's home. The amount of information to be taught can be overwhelming, so ensure that ample time is available. Allow time for questions and concerns. Offer emotional support and guidance whenever necessary.

Provide written and verbal instructions about the care involved. Have the child (if appropriate) and parents demonstrate the care needed, including care of the central venous access device. Review with them the measures for obtaining, storing, and handling the solutions and supplies. Develop plans for troubleshooting problems with devices and equipment, and give instructions on how to recognize and treat complications. Also teach them about danger signs and symptoms that require immediate notification. Be sure they have the name and number of a contact person in case of emergency situations.

Initiate the appropriate referrals for support. Specialized home care infusion services are available for follow-up in the home. In addition, social services can be helpful in providing assistance with finances, health insurance reimbursement, scheduling, transportation, emotional support, and community resources.

■■■ Key Concepts

- Children and families need appropriate explanation and education before a procedure is performed. Preparation may include explaining the procedure as well as physically preparing the child. Appropriate preparation helps to decrease the child's and family's anxiety, promote the child's cooperation, and support the child's and family's coping skills.

- The "eight rights" of pediatric medication administration are the right drug, right dose, right route, right time, right patient, right documentation, right to be educated, and right to refuse.

- The physiologic immaturity of some body systems in children can affect a drug's pharmacodynamics, leading to differences in the body's response to the drug and thus enhancing or diminishing the drug's effects. The child's age, weight, body surface area, and body composition can affect the drug's pharmacokinetics.

- The two most common methods for determining pediatric drug doses involve the use of the child's body weight and body surface area.

- Children under the age of 5 to 6 are at risk for aspiration when receiving tablets or capsules because they have difficulty swallowing them; liquids may be more appropriate. When administering oral medications to children, always tell them whether a medication is being mixed with food.

- Medication administration via the rectal route is not preferred because the drug's absorption may be erratic and unpredictable and children find this route extremely upsetting or embarrassing.

- When administering otic medications, pull the pinna downward and back if the child is under age 3, up and back for older children.

- Intramuscular administration is used infrequently in children because it is painful and children often lack the adequate muscle mass. When used with infants, the preferred site is the vastus lateralis muscle.

- Administration of medication via the IV route is common with children, especially when a rapid response to the drug is desired or when absorption via other routes is difficult or impossible. The primary method for IV medication administration is via a syringe pump.

- Preferred sites for peripheral IV therapy include the veins of the hands, feet, and forearms. The scalp vein may be used in infants but only if attempts at other sites have been unsuccessful. The rule of thumb for insertion of any peripheral devices is to use the smallest-gauge catheter for the shortest length of time possible to prevent trauma to the child's fragile veins.

- Central venous therapy usually is administered through a large vein, such as the subclavian, femoral, or jugular vein or vena cava. The tip of the device lies in the superior vena cava just at the entrance to the right atrium. Devices include single- or multiple-lumen short- and long-term catheters, peripherally inserted central catheters, tunneled catheters, and vascular access ports.

- Monitoring intake and output is important when a child is receiving IV therapy. Site inspection, proper care of the site, and proper dressing changes are key to preventing complications.

- Nutritional support can be administered enterally via a nasogastric or orogastric tube (gavage feeding) or via a gastrostomy or jejunostomy device or administered parenterally through a peripheral or central venous access device.

- Enteral nutrition is indicated for children who have a functioning gastrointestinal tract but cannot consume adequate amounts of nutrients orally.

- Prior to any enteral feeding, placement of the feeding tube must be confirmed. The gold standard for confirming placement is with an x-ray. At the bedside, checking the color and pH of the aspirate is used to confirm placement.

- Children receiving TPN require close monitoring of the infusion rate and volume, intake and output, vital signs, and blood glucose levels. Strict aseptic technique is necessary when caring for the central venous access site and TPN infusion.

REFERENCES

Algren, C., & Arnow, D. (2005). Pediatric variations of nursing interventions. In M. J. Hockenberry, *Wong's essentials of pediatric nursing* (7th ed.). St. Louis: Mosby, Inc.

American Academy of Pediatrics, Committee on Hospital Care and Committee on Drugs. (2003). *Prevention of medication errors in the pediatric inpatient setting.* Retrieved December 6, 2006, from http://www.guideline.gov/summary/summary.aspx?ss=15&doc_id=4253&nbr4253.

American Association of Critical Care Nurses. (2005). Practice Alert: Verification of feeding tube placement. Retrieved on January 6, 2008 at http://www.aacn.org/AACN/practiceAlert.nsf/Files/VOFTP/$file/Verification%20of%20Feeding%20Tube%20Placement%2005–2005.pdf.

Association of Operating Room Nurses. (2006). Pediatric medication safety. *AORN Journal, 83*(1), 111–113.

Centers for Disease Control & Prevention (2002). Guidelines for prevention of intravascular catheter-related infections. *Morbidity and Mortality Weekly Report, 55*(RR10), 1–26.

Centers for Disease Control and Prevention. (2005). Intravascular catheter-associated bloodstream infections. Division of Healthcare Quality Promotion (DHQP). Retrieved on January 3, 2007 from http://www.cdc.gov/ncidad/dhqp/dpac_iv.html.

Children's Healthcare of Atlanta. (2004). *Gastrostomy tube home care manual.* Atlanta: Children's Healthcare of Atlanta.

Cincinnati's Children's Hospital Medical Center. (2005). Gastrostomy-jejunostomy tube care. *Abdominal and Digestive Home Care.* Retrieved January 8, 2008 at http://www.cincinnatichildrens.org/health/info/abdomen/home/.

Cook, L. S. (2007). Choosing the right intravascular catheter. *Home Healthcare Nurse, 25*(8), 523–531.

de Jonge, R. C., Polderman, K. H., & Gemke, R. J. (2005). Central venous catheter use in the pediatric patient: Mechanical and infectious complications. *Pediatric Critical Care Medicine, 6*(3), 329–339.

Ellis, J. A., Sharp, D., Newhook, K. & Cohen, J. (2004). Selling comfort: A survey of interventions for needle procedures in a pediatric hospital. *Pain Management Nursing, 5*(4), 144–152.

Fidanza, S. (2006). *What is a gastrostomy?* Retrieved on January 9, 2008 from http://www.med.umich.edu/1libr/pa/pa_gastcare_hhg.htm.

Florida Children's Hospital, Child Life Department. (n.d.). *Atraumatic care: an age-specific approach.* Orlando, FL: Author.

Florida Children's Hospital, Child Life Department. (n.d.). *Suggested vocabulary to use with children.* Orlando, FL: Author.

Ghaleb, M. A., Barber, N., Franklin, B. D., Yeung, V. WS., Khaki, Z. F., & Wong, I. CK. (2006). Systematic review of medication errors in pediatric patients. *Annals of Pharmacotherapy, 40*(10), 1766–1776.

Goldberg, E., Kaye, R., Yaworski, J., & Liacouras, C. (2005). Gastrostomy tubes: Facts, fallacies, fistulas, and false tracts. *Gastroenterology Nursing, 28*(6), 485–494.

Hadaway, L. C. (2006). Keeping central line infection at bay. *Nursing2006, 36*(4), 58–63. Retrieved on January 10, 2008 at http://www.nursing2004.com/pt/re/nursing/pdfhandler.00152193-200604000-00042.pdf;jsessionid=HGGTWNt39zZJG6LZ2TTT2gTTxJ4gJDbXlw4QLcCD0Ng12JKxjBTJ!-1297386286!181195629!8091!-1.

Huffman, S., Jarczyk, K. S., O'Brien, E., et al. (2004). Methods to confirm feeding tube placement: Application of research in practice. *Pediatric Nursing, 30*(1), 10–13.

Huffman, S., Pieper, P., Jarczyk, K. S., Bayne, A. & O'Brien, E. (2004). Methods to confirm feeding tube placement: Application of research in practice [Electronic Version]. *Pediatric Nursing, 30*(1), 10–12. Retrieved on January 6, 2008 http://www.medscape.com/viewarticle/470693_1.

Hughes, R. G. (2005). Reducing pediatric medication errors: Children are especially at risk for medication errors. *American Journal of Nursing, 10*(5), 79–84.

Hughes, R. G. & Ortiz, E. (2005). Medication errors: Why they happen and how they can be prevented. *AJN(Supplement),* 14–24.

Klossner, N. J., & Hatfield, N. (2006). *Introductory maternity and pediatric nursing.* Philadelphia: Lippincott Williams & Wilkins.

Knue, M., Doellman, D., & Jacobs, B. R. (2006). Peripherally inserted central catheters in children. *Journal of Infusion Nursing, 29*(1).

Lilley, L. L., Harrington, S., Snyder, J. S., & Lake, R. E. (2005). *Pharmacology and the nursing process* (4th ed.). St. Louis: Mosby, Inc.

Mandleco, B. L. (2005). *Pediatric nursing skills and procedures.* Clifton Park, NY: Thomson Delmar Learning.

Myers, T. M., Wallace, D. K., & Johnson, S. M. (2005). Ophthalmic medications in pediatric patients. *Comprehensive Ophthalmology Update, 6*(2), 85–101.

Pediatric Glaucoma & Cataract Family Association. (2006). *How to apply eye drops.* Retrieved February 12, 2007, from http://www.pgcfa.org/drops.htm.

Pediatric Glaucoma & Cataract Family Association. (2006). *How to apply eye ointment.* Retrieved February 12, 2007, from http://www.pgcfa.org/ointment.htm.

Pennsylvania Patient Safety Authority. (2006). Confirming feeding tube placement: Old habits die hard. *Patient Safety Advisory, 3*(4). Retrieved on January 6, 2008 at http://www.psa.state.pa.us/psa/lib/psa/advisories/v3n4december2006/confirming_feeding_tube_placement_-_old_habits_die_hard.pdf.

Phillips, S. K. (2004). Pediatric parenteral nutrition: Differences in practice from adult care. *Journal of Infusion Nursing, 166*(27), 166–170.

Potter, P. A., & Perry, A. G. (2005). *Fundamentals of nursing* (6th ed.). St. Louis: Mosby, Inc.

Rosenthal, K. (2005). Kid's stuff: Starting I.V.s in peds. *Nursing Made Incredibly Easy!, 3*(4), 45–50.

Taylor, C., Lillis, C., & Lemone, P. (2005). *Fundamentals of nursing: The art and science of nursing care.* Philadelphia: Lippincott Williams & Wilkins.

Thomas, D. O. (2005). Lessons learned: Basic evidence-based advice for preventing medication errors in children. *Journal of Emergency Nursing, 31*(5), 490–493.

Tracey, D. L. & Patterson, G. E. (2006). Care of the gastrostomy tube in the home. *Home Healthcare Nurse, 24*(6), 381–386.

U.S. Pharmacopeia. (2006). *Error-avoidance recommendations for medications used in pediatric populations.* Retrieved December 6, 2006, from www.usp.org/patientSafety/resources/pedRecommnds 2003-01-22.html.

Weinstein, S. M. (2006). *Plumer's principles and practice of intravenous therapy* (8th ed.). Philadelphia: Lippincott Williams & Wilkins.

Westhus, N. (2004). Methods to test feeding tube placement in children. *MCN: The American Journal of Maternal Child Nursing, 29*(5), 282–291.

Willock, J., Richardson, J., Brazier, A., et al. (2004). Peripheral venipuncture in infants and children. *Nursing Standard, 18*(27), 43–50, 52, 55.

Woo, T. M. (2004). Pediatric pharmacology update, essentials for prescribing. *Advance for Nurse Practitioners, 12*(6), 22–28.

WEBSITES

American Academy of Pediatrics: http://www.aap.org

Medication administration policies: www.familymanagement.com/childcare/policies/medication.administration.html

G-tube Assisted Nutrition: http://www.g-tube.net/spec.spml

Kids with Tubes: http://www.kidswithtubes.org

CHAPTER WORKSHEET

MULTIPLE CHOICE QUESTIONS

1. A nurse is preparing to administer an intramuscular injection to an infant. What is the most appropriate site for this injection?

   a. Deltoid muscle

   b. Vastus lateralis

   c. Dorsogluteal

   d. Rectus femoris

2. A 3-year-child is to receive a medication that is supplied as an enteric-coated tablet. What is the best nursing action?

   a. Crush the tablet and mix it with applesauce.

   b. Dissolve the medication in the child's milk.

   c. Place a pill in the posterior part of the pharynx and tell the child to swallow.

   d. Check with the prescriber to see if an alternative form can be used.

3. The nurse is caring for an infant who weighs 8.2 kg and is NPO and receiving IV fluid therapy. What rate does the nurse calculate as meeting the child's daily fluid requirements?

   a. 82 mL/hour

   b. 41 mL/hour

   c. 34 mL/hour

   d. 22 mL/hour

4. When administering ear drops to a 2-year-old, which action would be most appropriate?

   a. Tell the child that the drops are to treat his infection.

   b. Pull the pinna of the child's ear down and back.

   c. Have the child turn his head to the opposite side after giving the drops.

   d. Massage the child's forehead to facilitate absorption of the medication.

CRITICAL THINKING EXERCISES

1. When reviewing the medical record of a child, the nurse notes that the ordered dose of medication is different from the recommended dose. How should the nurse proceed?

2. While caring for a 5-year-old child who is receiving IV fluid therapy at a rate of 100 mL/hour, the nurse notes that the infusion is running slowly. The insertion site appears slightly reddened and swollen. What should the nurse do next?

3. A school-aged child is to be discharged, continuing TPN therapy at home. The child lives with his parents and two younger siblings. How would the nurse prepare this child and family for discharge? How could the nurse promote growth and development for this child during TPN therapy?

STUDY ACTIVITIES

1. Review the medical records of several children who are on a pediatric unit in your agency. Note the type of medication, route ordered, and what specific interventions are needed for each child related to the medication administration and developmental age of the child. Compile a list of the most commonly used routes.

2. Interview several parents about their experiences in giving medications to their children. From these interviews, develop a teaching sheet that provides tips to facilitate oral medication administration to children.

3. Create a chart that compares and contrasts the subcutaneous, intramuscular, and intravenous methods of medication administration. Include examples of medications given via these routes, onset of action, appropriate sites, and necessary safety measures for each.

4. An infant is to receive intermittent gavage feedings via a nasogastric tube every 6 hours. The feeding tube was inserted with a previous feeding and remains in place. The nurse is preparing to administer the next scheduled feeding. Place the events in the proper sequence.

   _____ a. Check the placement of the feeding tube.
   _____ b. Position the infant on his right side with the head of the bed slightly elevated.
   _____ c. Allow the feeding to come to room temperature.
   _____ d. Flush the tube with water.
   _____ e. Clamp the tube to prevent air from entering the stomach.
   _____ f. Pour the solution into the barrel of the syringe.

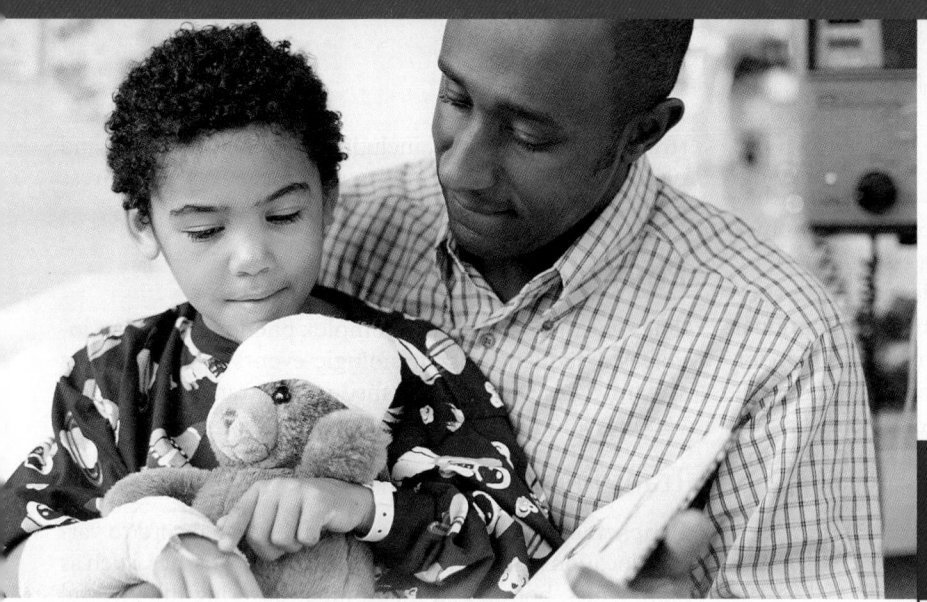

PAIN MANAGEMENT IN CHILDREN

KEY TERMS

acute pain
chronic pain
conscious sedation
drug tolerance
epidural
neuromodulators

neuropathic pain
nociceptive pain
nociceptors
pain
pain threshold

patient-controlled analgesia (PCA)
physical dependence
somatic pain
transduction
visceral pain

LEARNING OBJECTIVES

Upon completion of the chapter, the learner will be able to:

1. Identify the major physiologic events associated with the perception of pain.
2. Discuss the factors that influence the pain response.
3. Identify the developmental considerations of the effects and management of pain in the infant, toddler, preschooler, school-age child, and adolescent.
4. Explain the principles of pain assessment as they relate to children.
5. Understand the use of the various pain rating scales and physiologic monitoring for children.
6. Establish a nursing care plan for children related to management of pain, including pharmacologic and nonpharmacologic techniques and strategies.

Aiden Russell is a 6-year-old on the pediatric unit admitted for a wound infection. He requires BID dressing changes. In report you are told that Aiden cries and fights during the dressing change but otherwise seems to be playing and not experiencing much pain. The nurse reporting off states, "Aiden's mother keeps requesting pain medication for Aiden. She states he's complaining of pain most of the time. I'm not sure if I believe her: when I see Aiden, he's playing Nintendo games or watching television and seems to be fine. I've tried to hold off on his pain medication as long as I can."

WOW

All of our patients in pain deserve as much comfort as we can give.

Pain is a highly individualized, subjective experience that can affect any person of any age. It is a complex phenomenon that involves multiple components and is influenced by a myriad of factors. Pain often has been described as a subjective experience that involves both sensory and emotional factors. **Pain** is defined by the International Association for the Study of Pain as "an unpleasant sensory and emotional experience that is associated with actual or potential tissue damage" (IASP, 2007). The cause of pain is related to the disease process, treatment protocols, surgical interventions, or injury to the child. A definition of pain that is commonly used defines pain as whatever the person says it is, existing whenever the person says it does (McCaffery & Pasero, 1999)—that is, pain is present when the person says that it is. The person experiencing the pain is the only one who can identify pain and know what the pain is like.

Pain is a universal experience. The American Pain Society (1995) has labeled it "the fifth vital sign" to emphasize the importance of assessing pain frequently and providing appropriate treatment. The goal is to encourage health care professionals to assess pain every time that temperature, pulse, respirations, and blood pressure are assessed and to institute measures to manage the pain.

Pain affects adults and children alike, but children may lack the verbal capacity to describe their pain accurately. In addition, many caregivers and health care providers have misconceptions about pain in children, it is difficult to assess the complex nature of the pain experience, and limited resources and research are available related to pain relief strategies for children. All this makes pain management a critical element in the plan of care for children.

Pain is a major source of distress for children and their families as well as health care providers. Pain affects children of all ages, even preterm infants. Various national health associations have issued position papers and guidelines related to the need to treat pain and suffering in children. Effective pain management involves initial pain assessment, therapeutic interventions, and reassessment for all children in any health care setting.

Pain in children can result from numerous causes, including procedures, and can lead to serious physical and emotional consequences, such as increased oxygen consumption and alterations in blood glucose metabolism. In addition, the experience of pain early in life may lead to long-term consequences for the child (Young, 2005). Treating pain reduces anxiety during procedures and decreases the need for physical restraints, reduces anxiety regarding subsequent procedures, and prevents short- and long-term consequences of inadequately treated pain, particularly in newborns.

This chapter describes the pain experience in children, including the types of pain, factors influencing pain, and common fallacies and myths associated with pain in children. The nursing process is applied to provide an overview of the care for a child in pain. Various pain management strategies are described, including nonpharmacologic and pharmacologic interventions and measures to address procedure-related and chronic pain.

Physiology of Pain

The sensation of pain is a complex phenomenon that involves a sequence of physiologic events in the nervous system. These events are transduction, transmission, perception, and modulation.

Transduction

Peripheral nerve fibers extend from the spinal cord to various locations in and throughout the body's tissues, such as skin, joints, bones, and membranes covering the internal organs. At the end of these fibers are specialized receptors, called **nociceptors**, that become activated when they are exposed to noxious stimuli. The noxious stimuli can be mechanical, chemical, or thermal. Mechanical stimuli may include intense pressure to an area, a strong muscular contraction, or extensive pressure due to muscular overstretching. Chemical stimulation may involve the release of mediators, such as histamine, prostaglandins, leukotrienes, or bradykinin, as a response to tissue trauma, ischemia, or inflammation. Thermal stimuli typically involve extremes of heat and cold. This process of nociceptor activation is called **transduction**.

Transmission

When nociceptors are activated by noxious stimuli, the stimuli are converted to electrical impulses that are relayed along the peripheral nerves to the spinal cord and brain. Specialized afferent nerve fibers are responsible for moving the electrical impulse along. Myelinated A-delta fibers are large fibers that conduct the impulse at very rapid rates. The pain transmitted by these fibers is often referred to as fast pain, most commonly associated with mechanical or thermal stimuli (Porth, 2004). Pain also is transmitted by unmyelinated small C fibers. These fibers transmit the impulse slowly and are often activated by chemical stimuli or continued mechanical or thermal stimuli (Porth, 2004). These fibers carry the impulse to the spinal cord via the dorsal horn. Neurotransmitters are released to facilitate the transmission process to the brain.

Several theories have been proposed in an attempt to explain the process of pain transmission. The best known of these is the gate-control theory. According to this theory, the dorsal horn of the spinal cord contains interneuronal or interconnecting fibers. These fibers, when stimulated, close the gate or pathway to the brain, thereby inhibiting or blocking the transmission of the pain impulse. Subsequently, the impulse does not reach the brain where it would be interpreted as pain.

Perception

Once in the dorsal horn of the spinal cord, the nerve fibers divide and then cross to the opposite side and rise upward to the thalamus. The thalamus responds quickly and sends a message to the somatosensory cortex of the brain, where the impulse is interpreted as the physical sensation of pain. The impulses carried by the fast pain A-delta fibers lead to the perception of sharp, stabbing, localized pain that also commonly involves a reflex response to withdraw from the stimulus. The impulses carried by the slow C fibers lead to the perception of diffuse, dull, burning, or aching pain. The point at which the person first feels the lowest intensity of the painful stimulus is termed the **pain threshold** (Fig. 35.1). In addition to sending a message to the cerebral cortex, the thalamus also sends a message to the limbic system, where the sensation is interpreted emotionally, and to the brain stem centers, where autonomic nervous system responses begin.

Modulation

Research has identified substances called **neuromodulators** that appear to modify the pain sensation. These substances have been found to change a person's perception of pain. Examples of these neuromodulators include serotonin, endorphins, enkephalins, and dynorphins.

Pain perception can be modified peripherally or centrally. In the peripheral nerve fibers, chemical substances are released that either stimulate the nerve fibers or sensitize them. Peripheral sensitization allows the nerve fibers to react to a stimulus that is of lower intensity than would be needed to cause pain. As a result, the person perceives more pain. Actions that block or inhibit the release of these substances can lead to a decrease in pain perception.

Modification of pain perception can occur centrally in the spinal cord at the dorsal horn. Substances released by the excited interneurons can potentiate the pain sensation. Other neurochemicals, through their binding to specific receptors, can inhibit the perception of pain.

Types of Pain

Many different systems can be used to classify pain. Most commonly, pain is classified based on its duration, etiology, or source or location.

Classification by Duration

Pain is classified by duration as acute or chronic. **Acute pain** is defined as pain that is associated with a rapid onset of varying intensity. It usually indicates tissue damage and resolves with healing of the injury. Acute pain reflects stimulation of nociceptors and serves a protective function (that is, alerting the person to a problem). Examples of causes of acute pain include trauma, invasive procedures, acute illnesses such as sore throat or appendicitis, and surgery. For example, a child may experience acute pain after operative procedures, trauma, or disease. This type of pain generally last a few days.

FIGURE 35.1 Physiology of pain: (1) Exposure to thermal noxious stimuli results in activation of nociception (transduction). (2) Impulses are relayed along the peripheral nerves to the spinal cord through the dorsal horn (transmission). (3 & 4) This results in the individual feeling the sensation of pain (perception). (5) Neurons in the brain stem send signls back down to the dorsal horn, and these fibers release substances such as endorphins, which can inhibit painful impulses in the dorsal horn. These neurotransmitters are taken back by the body, therefore limiting the analgesic value.

> ▶ **Take** NOTE!
>
> Children often experience pain associated with various procedures done in health care settings. This type of pain is usually short in duration. Preparation of the child and family will help to decrease fears or anxiety. Depending on the type of procedure and the child's age, cognitive level, and temperament, various techniques and methods can be used. Advocating for atraumatic care and adhering to its guidelines will help to minimize procedure-related pain.

Chronic pain is defined as pain that continues past the expected point of healing for injured tissue. It provides no protective function. It may be continuous or intermittent, with and without periods of exacerbation or remission. It often interferes with sleep and performance of activities of daily living, thus impairing a person's ability to function. Environmental and affective factors can exacerbate and perpetuate chronic pain, leading to disability and maladaptive behavior (American Pain Society, 2006). Examples of causes of chronic pain include malignant conditions, arthritis, and fibromyalgia.

Chronic pain may be further classified as malignant pain (also called cancer pain, which is associated with cancer or other potentially life-threatening conditions) and chronic non-cancer pain. Malignant pain may be due to the disease itself or its effects on the body or the procedures and treatments used. Chronic non-cancer pain may be the result of numerous conditions, such as juvenile idiopathic arthritis, multiple sclerosis, chronic pancreatitis, or inflammatory bowel disease.

In children, chronic, recurrent pain is most commonly associated with abdominal pain, headache, limb pain, or chest pain, with only a small percentage of this pain found to have an organic etiology (Behrman, 2004). The signs and symptoms that indicate a possible organic etiology include constant pain, pain that wakes the child from sleep, well-localized pain, and other physical findings such as fever, weight loss, changes in color, consistency, or frequency of stools, and urinary tract symptoms (Behrman, 2004). This type of pain lasts for longer periods of time or comes and goes over a period of time.

Classification by Etiology

Pain can be classified by etiology as nociceptive or neuropathic. **Nociceptive pain** reflects pain due to activation of the A-delta fibers and C fibers by noxious stimuli. The pain perceived often correlates closely with the degree or intensity of the stimulus and the extent of real or possible tissue damage (American Pain Society, 2006). With nociceptive pain, nervous system functioning is intact. Reports of nociceptive pain vary depending on the location of the nociceptors being stimulated, ranging from a sharp or burning, to dull, aching, or cramping, to deep aching or sharp stabbing. Examples of conditions that result in nociceptive pain include chemical burns, sunburn, cuts, appendicitis, and bladder distention.

Neuropathic pain is pain due to malfunctioning of the peripheral or central nervous system. It may be continuous or intermittent and is commonly described as burning, tingling, shooting, squeezing, or spasm-like pain. Examples of neuropathic pain include neuropathies, phantom limb pain, and post-stroke pain.

Classification by Source or Location

Pain also may be classified, by the source or location of the area involved, as somatic pain (superficial and deep) or visceral pain. These classifications typically indicate nociceptive pain. **Somatic pain** refers to pain that develops in the tissues. It can be further divided into two groups: superficial and deep. Superficial somatic pain, often called cutaneous pain, involves stimulation of nociceptors in the skin, subcutaneous tissue, or mucous membranes. Typically the pain is well localized and described as a sharp, pricking, or burning sensation. Superficial somatic pain may be due to external mechanical, chemical, or thermal injury or skin disorders. Tenderness commonly is present. The individual also experiences hyperalgesia (an increased response to noxious stimulus) and allodynia (a painful response to a normally nonpainful or non-noxious stimulus; American Pain Society, 2006).

Deep somatic pain typically involves the muscles, tendons, joints, fasciae, and bones. It can be localized or diffuse and is usually described as dull, aching, or cramping. Deep somatic pain may be due to strain from overuse or direct injury, ischemia, and inflammation. Tenderness and reflex spasm may be present. Additionally, the person may exhibit sympathetic nervous system activation such as tachycardia, hypertension, tachypnea, diaphoresis, pallor, and pupillary dilation.

Visceral pain is pain that develops within organs such as the heart, lungs, gastrointestinal tract, pancreas, liver, gallbladder, kidneys, or bladder. It can be well or poorly localized and is described as a deep ache or sharp stabbing sensation that may be referred to other areas. Visceral pain may be due to distention of the organ, organ muscular spasm or pulling, ischemia, or inflammation. Tenderness, nausea, vomiting, and diaphoresis may be present.

Factors Influencing Pain

Children, like adults, experience neurologic events that result in the perception of pain. However, research has found that environmental and psychological factors may exert a greater influence on the child's perception of pain. Certain factors such as age, gender, cognitive level, temperament, previous pain experiences, and family and cultural background cannot be changed. However, situational factors involving behavioral, cognitive, and emotional aspects can be modified. These situation-specific factors that affect the child's pain experience include "what the child and parents understand, what they and the health care staff do, and how the child and parents feel. Certain situational factors can intensify pain and distress, whereas others can eventually trigger pain episodes, prolong pain-related disability, or maintain the repeated pain episodes in recurrent pain syndrome" (McGrath, 2005).

Age and Gender

Research has demonstrated that the nervous system structures needed for pain impulse transmission and perception are present by the 23rd week of gestation (Blount, Piira, Cohen, & Cheng, 2006). Therefore, children of any age, including preterm newborns, are capable of experiencing pain. Early on, children can interpret pain as an unpleasant sensation, but this interpretation is based on their comparison with other sensations. As they get older, they learn to use words to describe their pain more fully.

Gender also may play a role in a child's perception of pain, but research has failed to yield concrete evidence supporting it.

Cognitive Level

Cognitive level is a key factor affecting a child's pain perception and response and usually goes hand in hand with the child's age. Cognitive level typically increases with age, thereby influencing the child's understanding of the pain and its impact and his or her choices for coping strategies. In addition, as the child's cognitive level increases, his or her ability to communicate information about pain increases. However, this increased understanding and ability to communicate with advancing age may not apply to the child experiencing developmental delays. For example, a developmentally delayed school-aged child or adolescent may have the cognitive level of a toddler or preschooler. Health care providers need to be cognizant of this difference when caring for the child in pain. Numerous research studies have revealed that young children often describe pain in concrete terms, whereas older children use more abstract terms that involve both physical and psychological components (McGrath, 2005).

Temperament

Temperament affects how a child will respond to a situation. Previous experience with a situation or the method used to cope with a new or a threatening or harmful situation along with the child's coping style will affect the child's pain experience. Even mild symptoms of negative mood may affect the perceptions and persistence of pain (Palermo et al., 2005). A child with a "difficult temperament" is more likely to have an increased response to pain.

Previous Pain Experiences

A child identifies pain based on his or her experiences with pain in the past. The number of episodes of pain, the type of pain, the severity or intensity of the previous pain experience, and how the child responded all affect how the child will perceive and respond to the current experience. For example, several research studies have demonstrated that children who had negative experiences with pain involving a routine blood-drawing procedure exhib-

ited an increase in anxiety and stress and greater pain when faced with the procedure again.

Family and Culture

The child's cultural and family background will influence how he or she will express and manage pain. Some cultures transmit the standard of accepting pain stoically; others allow outward expression. The parents have a strong influence on the child's ability to cope. For example, if a parent reacts to the child's pain in a positive manner and offers comfort measures, the child may have an easier time coping. If the parent shows anger or disapproval, the pain experience may be intensified for the child.

Situational Factors

Situational factors involve factors or elements that interact with the child and his or her current situation involving the experience of pain. These factors are highly variable and dependent on the specific situation. Examples of situational factors are highlighted in Table 35.1.

Developmental Considerations

Since children of various developmental ages respond differently to pain and perceive pain in different ways, it is important to review developmental considerations. Refer to Chapters 25 through 29 for a more complete understanding of childhood development. Nurses must understand how children of various ages respond to painful stimuli and what behaviors may be expected based on their developmental level. By understanding these developmental considerations, the nurse can appropriately assess the child's pain and provide effective interventions.

Infants

Research has demonstrated that infants, including preterm infants, experience pain and can distinguish pain from other tactile experiences (McGrath & Hillier, 2003). Much of this research focuses on pain related to invasive procedures, such as heelsticks and intravenous catheter insertion. Research suggests that neonates, especially preterm infants, actually experience pain at a greater intensity than children and adults (Gerik, 2005). The belief is related to the immaturity of the inhibitory mechanisms that develop higher in the central nervous system at a later time during fetal development. These mechanisms are more complex and do not become functional until later in gestation.

In preterm and term newborns, behavioral and physiologic indicators are used for determining pain. Behavioral indicators include facial expression, body movements, and crying. Physiologic indicators include changes in heart rate, respiratory rate, blood pressure, oxygen saturation levels, vagal tone, palmar sweating, and plasma cortisol or

TABLE 35.1 SITUATIONAL FACTORS AFFECTING A CHILD'S PAIN EXPERIENCE

Cognitive	Behavioral	Emotional
Information about condition and pain problem, including cause and prognosis	Distress responses; specific behaviors and actions	Anticipatory anxiety
Knowledge about available therapy	Use of therapies	Heightened distress; feelings about scheduled possibly painful treatments
Expectations about the effectiveness of therapy and about the future	Child's or family's response to pain condition	Fear about undiagnosed condition and continuing pain; impact of pain and illness on family
Ability to identify pain triggers	Resolution of stressful situation	Situation-specific stress such as school, sports
Knowledge about stress reduction	Participation in routine activities	Frustration related to interruption in activities
		Underlying anxiety and depression

Adapted from McGrath, P. A., & Hillier, L. M. (2003). Modifying the psychologic factors that intensify children's pain and prolong disability. In N. L. Schecter, C. B. Berde, & M. Yaster, *Pain in infants, children, and adolescents* (2nd ed., Fig. 6.1, p. 87). Philadelphia: Lippincott Williams & Wilkins.

catecholamine levels (American Academy of Pediatrics and Canadian Paediatric Society, 2006).

In the younger infant, facial expression is the most common response to pain (Fig. 35.2). The brows may be lowered and drawn together, with the eyes tightly closed. The mouth is open, often forming a square. The body may be stiff, and thrashing may be seen. When the area is stimulated, the infant may demonstrate a generalized reflex withdrawal. The infant may exhibit a high-pitched, shrill cry.

The older infant often displays similar behavioral manifestations of pain. The older infant may display an angry facial expression, but the eyes are open. He or she often demonstrates a definite withdrawal response when the area is stimulated. The older infant cries loudly and tries to push away the stimulus that is causing the pain. Other manifestations include irritability, restless sleeping, and poor feeding.

▶ **Take** NOTE!

Although an infant usually exhibits typical behaviors indicating pain, absence of these manifestations does not indicate a lack of a pain; the response to pain is highly variable.

Infants are preverbal, so facial expression, diffuse body movements, and other signs, as indicated above, provide helpful feedback that the infant is in pain.

Infants also demonstrate physiologic responses to pain. These may include:

- Increased heart rate, usually averaging approximately 10 beats per minute; possibly bradycardia in preterm newborns
- Decreased vagal tone
- Decreased oxygen saturation
- Palmar or plantar sweating (as measured by skin conductivity testing); not reliable in infants under 37 weeks' gestation

Research has identified some short- and long-term consequences of inadequately treated pain in newborns (Paediatrics and Child Health Division, 2006). These include hyperalgesia around a wound from such situations

FIGURE 35.2 In the younger infant, facial expression is the most common response to pain.

as repeated heelsticks; an increased risk of developing intraventricular hemorrhage with repeated painful stressors; and a change in the pattern of response to subsequent pain. Children's memories of painful experiences can have long-term consequences for their reaction to later painful events and their acceptance of later health care interventions (von Baeyer et al., 2004). Moreover, preterm infants may be at greater risk for experiencing memories of pain due to the often long hospitalizations involving numerous invasive and painful procedures (Johnston et al., 2003).

Toddlers

Toddlers can react to painless procedures as intensely as painful ones, with intense emotional upset and physical resistance or aggression (Hockenberry et al., 2005). They may bite, hit, scream, or kick. Other behaviors may include being very quiet, pointing to where it hurts, or saying such words as "owww." Facial grimacing and teeth clenching may be noted. They may also react with fear and try to hide or leave the room. They often have limited vocabularies, so it may be difficult for them to express pain. Toddlers may demonstrate regressive behaviors, such as clinging to the parent or crying loudly.

Preschoolers

Since preschoolers may differentiate poorly between their self and the external world, the physical and verbal aggression is more goal-directed. They also may become quiet or try to withdraw and hide: the child may say he or she needs to go to the bathroom or needs to get something from another room. Because of their magical type of thinking, preschoolers may believe pain is a punishment for misbehaving or having bad thoughts. Preschoolers may not verbally report their pain, thinking that pain is something to be expected or that the adults are aware of their pain. They can tell someone where it hurts and can use various tools to describe the severity of pain; however, because they may have limited experience with pain, they may have difficulty distinguishing between types of pain (sharp or dull), describing the intensity of the pain, and determining whether the pain is worse or better.

School-Age Children

School-age children can communicate the type, location, and severity of pain. Children over the age of 8 years can use specific words, such as "sharp as a knife," burning, or pulling, to describe their pain. However, they may deny pain in an attempt to appear brave or to avoid further pain related to a procedure or intervention. They may be more concerned with their fear about the illness and its effects rather than the pain. They also may fear being embarrassed by acting-out behaviors. Thus, a typical response might be to withdraw by staring at the television. Other behaviors may include muscular rigidity, such as clenching the fists, stiffening the body, closing the eyes, wrinkling the forehead, or gritting the teeth.

Adolescents

Adolescents are concerned primarily about body image and fear losing control over their behavior. This may result in denial or refusal of medications. Their mood and what they think is expected of them will also affect their response. Adolescents often ask numerous questions and pay close attention to how others respond to them. Fearing that their behavior may be viewed as juvenile, they may attempt to remain stoic, not exhibiting any emotion. Subtle changes such as increased muscle tension with clenched fists and teeth, rapid breathing, and guarding the affected body part may occur. They may also show lack of interest in everyday activities or a decreased ability to concentrate.

Common Fallacies and Myths About Pain in Children

In general, children respond to pain based on the type of pain, the extent of pain, and their age and developmental level. Table 35.2 highlights some common myths and misconceptions related to pain in children. Because of these myths, children have been medicated less than adults with a similar diagnosis, leading to inadequate pain management.

NURSING PROCESS OVERVIEW FOR THE CHILD IN PAIN

WATCH & LEARN

Nursing care of the child with pain includes nursing assessment, nursing diagnosis, planning, interventions, and evaluation. Each step of this process must be individualized for each patient. A general understanding of the physiology of pain, factors that influence pain, and effective pain management techniques can help to individualize the child's plan of care.

Assessment

Assessment of pain in children consists of both subjective and objective data collection. The acronym **QUESTT** is an excellent way to remember the key principles of pain assessment (Baker & Wong, 1987):

- **Question** the child.
- **Use** a reliable and valid pain scale.
- **Evaluate** the child's behavior and physiologic changes to establish a baseline and determine the effectiveness of the intervention. The child's behavior and motor activity may include irritability and protection as well as withdrawal of the affected painful area.
- **Secure** the parent's involvement.
- **Take** the cause of pain into account when intervening.
- **Take** action.

TABLE 35.2 MYTHS AND MISCONCEPTIONS ABOUT CHILDREN AND PAIN

Myth or Misconception	Fact
Newborns do not feel pain.	Newborns, including preterm newborns, do feel pain. The neurologic and hormonal systems needed for the transmission of painful stimuli are sufficiently developed.
Exposure to pain at an early age has little to no effect on the child. Infants and small children have little memory of pain.	Prolonged or severe pain can lead to increased newborn morbidity. Infants who have experienced pain during the neonatal period respond differently to subsequent painful events (McGrath, 2005). Repeated exposure to painful procedures and events can have long-term consequences. Memories of pain may be stored in the child's nervous system, influencing later reactions to painful stimuli (Johnston et al., 2003).
The intensity of a child's behavioral reaction indicates the intensity of the child's pain.	Numerous factors affect a child's response to pain. Each child is an individual, with his or her own set of responses.
A child who is sleeping or playing is not in pain.	Sleep or play may be a coping strategy for the child in pain. Sleep may reflect exhaustion of the child who is coping with pain.
Children are truthful when they are asked if they are experiencing pain.	Often children deny pain to avoid a painful situation or procedure, embarrassment, or loss of control. Children may assume that others know how they are feeling and thus will not verbalize their complaints.
Children learn to adapt to pain and painful procedures.	Repeated exposure to pain or painful procedures can result in an increase in behavioral manifestations.
Children experience more adverse effects of narcotic analgesics than adults do.	The risk of adverse effects of narcotic analgesics is the same for children as for adults.
Children are more prone to addiction to narcotic analgesics.	Addiction to narcotics when used in children is very rare.

▶ *Take NOTE!*

Children do experience pain, and pain management techniques work just as well with children as they do with adults.

Health History

When assessing pain in children, tailor the assessment to the child's developmental level and ask questions geared to the child's cognitive ability. During the health history, determine the child's previous exposure to pain, if any, and how the child responded. This information will provide clues about how the child copes and his or her current response. Attempt to determine what word the child uses to denote pain. Some children may not understand the term "pain" but do understand terms such as "ouchie" or "boo-boo."

The health history also includes questioning the parents about their cultural beliefs related to pain and their child's usual responses. This information aids in planning developmentally and culturally appropriate family-centered care.

Questioning the Child

When questioning the child, phrase the questions in a manner that the child will be able to understand based

on his or her developmental level. Some input from the child's family may be helpful in determining where best to focus the questions.

Ask the child what pain means to him or her. Use words that the child may comprehend more easily, such as "hurt," "boo-boo," or "ouch," as appropriate. Inquire about similar experiences in the past and how he or she responded. Determine whether the child let others know that he or she was hurting and how this message was conveyed (e.g., crying, acting out, or pointing to the hurting area).

Review the history of the pain and various influences such as cultural aspects, caregiver attitudes or expectations, previous experiences, and any education or teaching related to pain management. Continue to formulate questions to ascertain the following:

- Location, quality, severity, and onset of the pain, as well as the circumstances in which the child experiences the pain. Have the child point to the area where it hurts or identify the location on a diagram or doll.
- Conditions, if any, that preceded the onset of pain and the conditions that followed the onset of pain
- Any associated symptoms, such as weight loss, fever, vomiting, or diarrhea, which may indicate a current illness
- Any recent trauma, including any interventions that were used in an attempt to relieve the pain

Continue the health history by inquiring about what the child wants others, including the nurse, to do when the child hurts. Conversely, ask the child what he or she doesn't want others to do. Finally, question the child about measures that seem to be most effective in relieving the pain. Ask if there is anything special the child wants to tell the nurse, such as a special pain-relief technique or a specific comfort object.

If the child is experiencing chronic or recurrent pain, suggest the child and family record information in a symptom diary. Explain that this will be helpful in identifying the best ways to manage the pain.

Questioning the Parents

Parents play a key role in assessing pain in children. Often it is the parents who provide information about the child's current and past experiences with pain. In addition, parents can provide information about how the child exhibits and responds to pain. Parents may be aware of subtle changes in the child's behavior that may precede the pain, occur with the pain, or indicate relief of pain. Including the parents in this process helps create a positive experience for all involved and promotes feelings of control over the situation.

The questions posed to the parents are similar in focus to those posed to the child. However, more detailed information may be obtained from the parents because they are usually able to describe events more fully or in greater detail due to their higher cognitive level. Parents typically know their child best.

> ▶ *Take* NOTE!
>
> *Parents may assume that nurses have greater expertise when it comes to assessing their child's pain and taking appropriate action. Thus, they may not always report when they notice changes suggesting that their child is uncomfortable. Emphasize the important role that parents play in reporting any changes in their child so that pain relief measures can be instituted as soon as possible.*

When questioning the parents, use the following examples as a guide for assessing the child's pain:

- Has your child ever been in pain before? If so, what was the cause of the pain? How long did he or she have the pain? Where was the pain located?
- How did your child react to the pain? What did you do to lessen the pain?
- Did your child let you know that he or she was in pain? Did he or she tell you or did you notice something?
- Are there any special signs that let you know that your child is hurting? If so, what are they?

- Is there anything that your child does or that you do when he or she is hurting that helps relieve the pain?
- Does one thing work better than another when your child is hurting?
- Is there any special information that you want to tell me about your child?

Using Pain Rating Scales

Various pain assessment or pain rating scales are available. These scales allow the child to report his or her pain, and the pain level is quantified. These standardized rating scales provide a greater alignment between the child's pain and the nurse's assessment of the severity of the pain.

Many health care facilities have specific policies and procedures related to pain assessment, including the frequency of assessment, the rating tool to use, and nursing interventions to be instituted based on the rating. For example, many facilities require assessment of the child using a specific tool with documentation at least once a shift and 30 minutes to 1 hour after a non-pharmacologic or pharmacologic pain-relief intervention. This process provides a more objective method to determine whether the pain is increasing or decreasing and whether pain-relief methods are effective.

> ▶ *Take* NOTE!
>
> *Typically, different pain rating scales are appropriate for different developmental levels. However, children may regress when in pain, so a simpler tool may be needed to make sure that the child understands what is being asked. Regardless of the tool used, nurses need to be consistent in using the same tool so that appropriate comparisons can be made and effective interventions can be planned and implemented. Using the most appropriate tool consistently allows the most accurate assessment of the child's pain.*

FACES Pain Rating Scale. The FACES pain rating scale (Fig. 35.3) is a self-report tool that can be used by children as young as 3 years of age. The scale consists of six illustrations of faces arranged horizontally with expressions ranging from smiling (indicating no hurt) to crying with frowning (indicating hurts worst). Under each face is a short description such as "hurts little bit" and a number. The number scale can be 0, 1, 2, 3, 4, and 5 or 0, 2, 4, 6, 8, and 10. The nurse explains the words associated with each face. Then the child is asked to select the facial expression that best describes how he or she is feeling. The nurse then documents the number corresponding to the word description and face.

Oucher Pain Rating Scale. The Oucher pain rating scale is similar to the FACES scale in that it uses facial expressions to indicate increasing degrees of hurt. However,

Wong-Baker FACES Pain Rating Scale

0	1	2	3	4	5
NO HURT	HURTS LITTLE BIT	HURTS LITTLE MORE	HURTS EVEN MORE	HURTS WHOLE LOT	HURTS WORST

| Alternate coding | 0 | 2 | 4 | 6 | 8 | 10 |

Instructions: Explain to the person that each face is for a person who feels happy because he has no pain (hurt) or sad because he has some or a lot of pain. **Face 0** is very happy because he doesn't hurt at all. **Face 1** hurts just a little bit. **Face 2** hurts a little more. **Face 3** hurts even more. **Face 4** hurts a whole lot. **Face 5** hurts as much as you can imagine, although you don't have to be crying to feel this bad. Ask the person to choose the face that best describes how he is feeling.

FIGURE 35.3 FACES Pain Rating Scale. (From Hockenberry, M. J., Wilson, D., & Winkelstein, M. L. [2005]. *Wong's essentials of pediatric nursing* [7th ed., p. 1259]. St. Louis, MO. Used with permission. Copyright, Mosby.)

FIGURE 35.5 The poker chip tool. Here the nurse asks the child to identify the number of chips that indicate her degree of "hurt."

instead of illustrations, six photographs are used: "no hurt" is placed at the bottom of the arrangement and "most hurt" at the top. Alongside the photos is a scale ranging from 0 to 10 that corresponds to the facial expressions in the photographs (Fig. 35.4). After explaining the photos and numeric scale, the child is asked to point to the number that best describes his or her level of pain.

This scale is useful for self-reporting of pain in children from 3 to 13 years of age. Three different scales have been developed for use with Caucasian, Hispanic, and African-American children.

Poker Chip Tool. The poker chip tool is a self-reporting pain assessment tool that uses four red poker chips to quantify the child's level of pain. The chips are arranged in a horizontal line on a surface in front of the child. Starting with the chip closest to the child's left side, the nurse points to the chip and explains that the first chip means a little hurt, the next chip means more hurt, the third chip means more hurt, and the fourth chip means the worst hurt ever. Then the nurse asks the child how many "pieces of hurt" he or she is having (Fig. 35.5). If the child is not experiencing any pain, typically the child will state that he or she isn't having any. When the child identifies the number of "pieces of hurt," the nurse follows up by asking the child to tell the nurse more about his or her hurt.

The poker chip tool is useful for assessing pain in children who are 4 years of age or older. Children may view this assessment tool as a game since it involves poker chips. However, the nurse needs to ensure that the child has the cognitive ability to distinguish the numbers.

Word-Graphic Rating Scale. The word-graphic rating scale is a self-reporting scale that consists of a line with descriptors underneath: no pain, little pain, medium pain, large pain, and worst possible pain (Fig. 35.6). The nurse explains the line and descriptors to the child. Then

OUCHER!

10 —	
9 —	
8 —	
7 —	
6 —	
5 —	
4 —	
3 —	
2 —	
1 —	
0 —	

FIGURE 35.4 Oucher Pain Rating Scale.

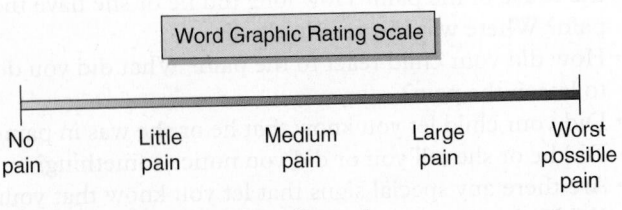

Word Graphic Rating Scale

| No pain | Little pain | Medium pain | Large pain | Worst possible pain |

FIGURE 35.6 Word-graphic rating scale.

the child is asked to make a vertical mark on the horizontal line at the point that best describes the child's level of pain. The nurse uses a ruler to measure the distance from the "no pain" starting point to the area marked by the child. This measurement is recorded as the pain score. The word-graphic rating scale is useful for children 4 to 17 years old.

Visual Analog and Numeric Scales.

Visual analog and numeric scales involve a horizontal or vertical line with marked endpoints. With a visual analog scale, the end points are identified as no pain and worst pain. A numeric scale typically has endpoints of 0 and 10, reflecting no pain and worst pain, respectively (Fig. 35.7). The nurse explains the scale to the child. With the visual analog scale, the child makes a line that best describes the level of pain. The nurse then measures the distance from the "no pain" endpoint to the child's mark and records this as the pain score. With the numeric scale, the nurse asks the child to pick the number that best describes his or her level of pain.

The numeric scale can be used with children as young as 5 years of age, as long as they can count and understand the concepts related to numeric values. Although research has validated use of the visual analog scale with children as young as 4.7 years of age, the preferred minimum age for using this tool is 7 years (Algren, 2005).

Adolescent Pediatric Pain Tool.

The Adolescent Pediatric Pain Tool is a self-report type of tool useful for older children, usually from ages 8 to 17 years. The tool involves three aspects of assessment. In the first assessment the child identifies the location of the pain on two illustrations of the body, front and back views (Fig. 35.8). The child is instructed to color the areas where he or she is hurting. The child is also instructed to color the area as big or as small as how much he or she is hurting. For example, if the hurt is mild or moderate, the child would

color a moderate area of the location; if the pain was severe, he or she would color a much larger area. The second portion of the tool involves a scale that ranges from "no pain" to "worst possible pain"; the child is instructed to identify the severity of his or her pain. The third assessment is a list of words that may be used to describe pain, such as throbbing, pounding, stabbing, or sharp. The child is asked to point to or circle the words that describe the current pain. Children with limited reading skills or vocabulary may have difficulty with some of the words listed to describe pain. Work with the child and encourage the parents to help the child understand the various descriptive words. Parental participation fosters control over the situation and gives the parents some insight into what their child is experiencing.

Physical Examination

Physical examination of the child for pain primarily involves the skills of observation and inspection. These skills are used to assess for physiologic and behavioral changes that indicate pain. Auscultation also may be used to assess for changes in vital signs, specifically heart rate and blood pressure.

Manifestations of Pain

Observe for physical signs and symptoms of pain, keeping in mind the child's developmental level. Look for facial expressions of discomfort, grimacing, or crying. Be alert for movements that may suggest pain. For example, an infant or toddler may pull on the ear when experiencing ear pain. The child may move the head from side to side, suggesting head pain. Typically, children with abdominal pain will lie on one side and draw their knees up to the abdomen. Inspect the child's gait: a limp or avoidance of weight bearing may suggest leg pain. Immobility, guarding of a particular body area, or refusal to move an area may be observed. Inspect the skin for flushing or diaphoresis, possible indicators of pain. Also monitor vital signs for changes. Pulse or heart rate, respiratory rate, and blood pressure may increase. Other physiologic parameters suggesting pain may include elevated intracranial pressure and pulmonary vascular resistance and decreased oxygen saturation levels.

FIGURE 35.7 (A) Visual analog scale. (B) Numeric scale.

▶ *Take* NOTE!

The body responds to acute pain via the sympathetic nervous system, leading to stimulation and subsequently the increase in vital signs. However, if the child has persistent or chronic pain, the body adapts and these changes may be less noticeable; in fact, heart and pulse rate, respiratory rate, and blood pressure may actually decrease.

Right | Left | Left | Right

Sensory

Aching ("pain all over")

Hurting ("pain all over")
Sore ("like a cut")

Beating (procedural pain "spots")

Pounding ("gets on your nerves")

Cutting ("hurts more than a cut")

Like a sharp knife ("stabbing and sharp")

Sharp (no meaning)

Stabbing (no meaning)

Cramping ("everywhere like a plane crash")
Crushing (no meaning)
Pressure ("pushing all over")
Itching ("all over")
Scratching ("helps sometimes")
Shocking (pain "surprises" her)
Splitting ("splitting in half" her body)
Numb ("knows pain is there"/ procedural pain)
Stiff ("cannot move")
Swollen ("meds do not help")
Tight ("cannot move")

Affective

Awful ("cannot do anything")

Crying ("hurts so bad")
Frightening ("scared it won't stop")

Screaming (afraid of "going to the hospital")

Terrifying ("cannot sleep," "really tired," "not going to live")

Dizzy ("don't know where I am")

Evaluative

Annoying ("cannot sleep")

Bad ("cannot stop the hurting")
Miserable ("cannot sleep or do stuff")

Terrible ("don't like it")

Uncomfortable ("can't stay in one spot")

Uncontrollable ("cannot stop it")

Temporal

Always ("pain always there")

Comes and goes ("always pain")
Comes on all of a sudden ("no warning")

Constant ("never goes away")

Continuous ("pain not going away")

Forever ("never will go away")

Once in a while ("in a month sometimes pain; sometimes not")

Sneaks up ("don't know when the pain will happen")
Sometimes ("goes away sometimes; sometimes not")

FIGURE 35.8 Adolescent Pediatric Assessment Tool. (Top) Adolescent Pediatric Pain Tool (APPT): Body Outline (Crandall & Savedra, 2005). (Bottom) Pain Quality: Words chosen and meaning of words (Crandall & Savedra, 2005).

The child also may exhibit behavioral changes indicating pain. Be alert for irritability and restlessness. Watch for clenching of teeth or fists, body stiffening, or increased muscle tension. Note any changes in the child's behavior—for example, a child who previously was talkative and playful who becomes quiet and almost withdrawn. In addition, pay close attention to the child's cultural background and how these beliefs may be affecting the behavioral response to pain.

Each child is an individual with unique responses to pain, so the nurse must ensure that observations of behavior do indeed reflect the child's pain level. To help ensure the accuracy of observations, several physiologic and behavioral assessment tools have been developed to help quantify the observations.

Physiologic and Behavioral Pain Assessment Tools

Use of physiologic and behavioral pain assessment tools allows measurement of specific parameters and changes that would indicate that the child is experiencing pain. These measurements aid in determining the intensity of the pain experience. Along with the self-report pain-rating scales, measurement of these changes allows the nurse to objectively assess pain and the effectiveness of pain management measures.

Neonatal Infant Pain Scale. The Neonatal Infant Pain Scale (NIPS) is a behavioral assessment tool that is useful for measuring pain in preterm and full-term neonates. Six parameters are measured: facial expression, cry, breathing patterns, arms, legs, and state of arousal (Table 35.3). Each parameter except for cry is scored as a 0 or 1; cry is scored as 0, 1, or 2. The scores are totaled; the maximum

score that can be achieved is 7. A higher score indicates increased pain. This tool is not recommended for use in neonates who are too ill to respond or who are receiving paralyzing agents. In these cases, a falsely low score would be produced.

Riley Infant Pain Scale. The Riley Infant Pain Scale (RIPS) is a behavioral assessment tool useful for infants who lack verbal ability. Like NIPS, RIPS measures six parameters: facial expression, body movement, sleep, verbal or vocal ability, consolability, and response to movements and touch (Table 35.4). Each parameter is scored as 0, 1, 2, or 3. The score is totaled; the maximum score that can be achieved is 18. The higher the total score, the more intense the pain.

Pain Observation Scale for Young Children. The Pain Observation Scale for Young Children (POCIS) is a behavioral assessment tool designed for use in children 1 to 4 years of age. This tool measures seven parameters: facial expression, cry, breathing, torso, arms and fingers, legs and toes, and state of arousal (Table 35.5). Each parameter is scored as 0 or 1; the maximum score achievable is 7. The higher the score, the greater the pain being experienced by the child.

CRIES Scale for Neonatal Postoperative Pain Assessment. The CRIES scale is a behavioral assessment tool that also includes measures of physiologic parameters. It was developed to quantify postoperative pain in the newborn. The tool also may be used to monitor the infant's progress over time during recovery or after interventions. The tool assesses five parameters: cry, oxygen required for saturation levels less than 95%, increased vital signs, facial expression, and sleeplessness (Table 35.6).

TABLE 35.3 THE NEONATAL INFANT PAIN SCALE (NIPS)

Parameter	Finding	Score
Facial expression	Relaxed (restful face; neutral expression)	0
	Grimace (tight facial muscles; furrowed brow, chin, or jaw; negative facial expression)	1
Cry	No cry (quiet; not crying)	0
	Whimper (mild intermittent moaning)	1
	Vigorous crying (loud screaming, shrill, continuous)	2
Breathing patterns	Relaxed	0
	Change in breathing (irregular; faster than usual; gagging; breath holding)	1
Arms	Relaxed (no muscular rigidity; occasional random movements of arm)	0
	Flexed/extended (tense, straight, rigid, or rapid flexion or extension)	1
Legs	Relaxed (no muscular rigidity; occasional random movements of leg)	0
	Flexed/extended (tense, straight, rigid, or rapid flexion or extension)	1
State of arousal	Sleeping/awake (quiet, peaceful; settled)	0
	Fussy (alert, restless, thrashing)	1

From Lawrence, J., Alcock, D., McGrath, P., Kay, J., MacMurray, S. B., & Dulberg, C. (1993). The development of a tool to assess neonatal pain. *Neonatal Network, 12*(6), 59–66.

TABLE 35.4   THE RILEY INFANT PAIN SCALE

Parameter	Score
Facial expression	
• Neutral/smiling	0
• Frowning/grimacing	1
• Clenched teeth	2
• Full cry expression	3
Body movement	
• Calm, relaxed	0
• Restless, fidgeting	1
• Moderate agitation or mobility; thrashing, flailing, incessant agitation or strong voluntary mobility	2
• Voluntary immobility	3
Sleep	
• Sleeping quietly with easy respirations	0
• Restless while asleep	1
• Sleeps intermittently (sleep/awake)	2
• Sleeping for prolonged periods of time interrupted by jerky movements or inability to sleep	3
Verbal/vocal	
• No cry	0
• Whimpering, complaining	1
• Pain crying	2
• Screaming, high-pitched cry	3
Consolability	
• Neutral	0
• Easy to console	1
• Not easy to console	2
• Inconsolable	3
Response to movement/touch	
• Moves easily	0
• Winces when touched or moved	1
• Cries out when moved or touched	2
• High-pitched cry or scream when touched or moved	3

From Schade, J. G., Joyce, B. A., Gerkensmeyer, J., & Keck, J. F. (1996). Comparison of three preverbal scales for postoperative pain assessment in a diverse pediatric sample. *Journal of Pain and Symptom Management, 12*(6), 348–359.

Each parameter is scored as 0, 1, or 2 and then totaled. As with other assessment tools, the higher the score, the greater the infant's pain.

FLACC Behavioral Scale for Postoperative Pain in Young Children. The FLACC behavioral scale is a behavioral assessment tool that is useful in assessing a child's pain when the child cannot report accurately his or her level of pain. It has been demonstrated to be a reliable tool for children from age 2 months to 7 years of age. This tool measures five parameters: facial expression, legs, activity, cry, and consolability (Table 35.7). Observe the child with the legs and body uncovered. If the child is awake, observe

TABLE 35.5   THE PAIN OBSERVATION SCALE FOR YOUNG CHILDREN (POCIS)

Parameter	Finding	Score
Facial expression	Neutral	0
	Grimace (negative)	1
Cry	No cry	0
	Moan, scream	1
Breathing	Relaxed and regular	0
	Irregular and indrawn	1
Torso	At rest, inactive	0
	Tense, shivering	1
Arms and fingers	At rest, inactive	0
	Tense, restless	1
Legs and toes	At rest, inactive	0
	Tense, restless	1
State of arousal	Calm, sleepy	0
	Fussy	1

Reprinted with permission of W. J. C. Boelen-van der Loo, Ph.D.

him or her for 2 to 5 minutes; if sleeping, observe the child for 5 minutes or longer. Each parameter is scored as 0, 1, or 2; the scores are totaled, with a maximum achievable score of 10. As with other assessment tools, the higher the score, the greater the pain.

Nursing Diagnoses, Goals, Interventions, and Evaluation

After the assessment is completed, the nurse identifies appropriate nursing diagnoses. The most commonly identified nursing diagnosis would be Acute or Chronic pain. However, the related factors and defining characteristics can vary widely. Nursing diagnoses will focus on the effects of pain on the child—for example, the stress incurred as a result of the pain or the fear or anxiety associated with the pain or events causing the pain. Moreover, pain can affect physiologic functions, such as sleep, nutrition, mobility, and elimination. Examples of common nursing diagnoses may include:

• Acute pain related to repeated need for invasive procedures, surgical experience, recent trauma, or infection
• Chronic pain related to prolonged illness or injury, effects of cancer on surrounding tissues, or treatment-related effects
• Fear related to the unknown, separation from family, anticipation of invasive procedures, or effects of treatment
• Anxiety related to the stress and uncertainty of the situation
• Deficient knowledge related to current condition and appropriate methods for managing pain
• Disturbed sleep pattern related to inability to manage pain effectively

TABLE 35.6 THE CRIES SCALE FOR NEONATAL POSTOPERATIVE PAIN ASSESSMENT

Assessment	0	1	2
Crying	No	High-pitched, but consolable	High-pitched, inconsolable
Oxygen required for saturation above 95%	No	<30%	>30%
Increased vital signs	Heart rate and blood pressure within 10% of preoperative values	Heart rate or blood pressure 11% to 20% higher than preoperative values	Heart rate or blood pressure 21% or more above preoperative values
Expression	No grimace	Grimace	Grimace with grunt
Sleepless	No	Waking at frequent intervals	Constantly awake
Total infant score			

From Krechel, S. W., & Bildner, J. (1995). CRIES: A new neonatal postoperative pain measurement score. Initial testing of validity and reliability. *Paediatric Anaesthesia, 5,* 53–61.

- Impaired mobility related to increased episodes of pain
- Risk for constipation related to potential adverse effects of narcotic analgesic agents

When caring for a child experiencing pain, the ultimate goal is that the child will be free of pain as evidenced by participation in age-appropriate activities of daily living and vital signs within age-appropriate parameters. However, at times, this may be unrealistic, especially if the child is experiencing chronic pain. Therefore, a more appropriate goal would be that the child reports that his or her pain has decreased to a tolerable level. Pain assessment tools can be used to quantify the amount by which the child's pain has decreased. For example, if the child has rated the pain as 7 out of 10, a realistic goal might be that the child reports a pain rating of no more than 4 out of 10. Additional goals

would reflect improvement or resolution of the identified problem. For example, a short-term goal for a child experiencing disturbed sleep due to the pain might be that the child sleeps for a minimum of 4 consecutive hours through the night. A long-term goal might be that the child sleeps for 7 to 8 hours undisturbed through the night.

Various interventions can be used for pain management. These interventions include pharmacologic and nonpharmacologic measures. A guiding principle when caring for the child experiencing pain is the provision of atraumatic care (see Chapters 2 and 34 for more information). For example, apply a topical anesthetic cream to a site early enough before a venipuncture that it becomes effective. Use an intermittent infusion device to obtain multiple blood specimen samples rather than performing repeated venipunctures. Consider the use of sedation

TABLE 35.7 FLACC BEHAVIORAL SCALE

	Scoring		
Category	0	1	2
Face	No particular expression or smile	Occasional grimace or frown, withdrawn, disinterested	Frequent to constant frown, clenched jaw, quivering chin
Legs	Normal position or relaxed	Uneasy, restless, tense	Kicking, or legs drawn up
Activity	Lying quietly, normal position, moves easily	Squirming, shifting back and forth, tense	Arched, rigid, or jerking
Cry	No cry (awake or asleep)	Moans or whimpers, occasional complaint	Crying steadily, screams or sobs, frequent complaints
Consolability	Content, relaxed	Reassured by occasional touching, hugging, or being talked to, distractable	Difficult to console or comfort

Each of the five categories is scored from 0 to 2, which results in a total score between 0 and 10.

for more painful procedures. In addition to pharmacologic measures, cognitive and behavioral approaches are appropriate for pain management, including pain management related to procedures.

Throughout the child's care, be sure to discuss specific goals and interventions with the child and family as appropriate. Include the family in developing appropriate interventions so they can continue to support the child. Education of the child and family about interventions, including various therapies, is key. Play therapy may be helpful in allowing the child to express his or her feelings and adapt to the stressors of the current situation. Ongoing assessment is needed to determine the effectiveness of the pain relief measures in achieving the desired goals.

Nursing Care Plan 35.1 can be used as a guide in planning nursing care for the child experiencing pain. The nursing care plan should be individualized based on the child's symptoms and needs. Specific information related to pain management and the nurse's role will be discussed later in the chapter.

When you enter Aiden's room, he is crying and says his leg hurts. What will be your initial action? What will be your plan of care to manage Aiden's pain (refer to QUESTT assessment)? How would you address the statements made by the nurse in report? What approaches can you use to change staff behavior about pain management?

Management of Pain

Three general principles guide pain management in children:

1. Individualize interventions based on the amount of pain experienced during a procedure and the child's personality.
2. Use nonpharmacologic and pharmacologic approaches to ease or eliminate the pain.
3. Use aggressive pharmacologic treatment with the first procedure.

Strategies for pain management include nonpharmacologic interventions such as distraction, relaxation, and guided imagery and pharmacologic interventions such as analgesics, patient-controlled analgesia, local analgesia, epidural analgesia, and conscious sedation.

Nonpharmacologic Management

Various techniques may be available to assist in managing mild pain in children or augment the effectiveness of medications for moderate or severe pain. Many of these nonpharmacologic techniques assist children in coping with pain and give them an opportunity to feel a sense of mastery or control over the situation. Two types of techniques

are behavior/cognitive strategies and biophysical strategies. With these techniques as well as administration of medications, parents need to be involved in the process.

Behavioral-Cognitive Strategies

Behavioral-cognitive strategies for pain management involve measures that require the child to focus on a specific area rather than the pain. These strategies help to change the interpretation of the painful stimuli, reducing pain perception or making pain more tolerable. In addition, these strategies help to decrease negative attitudes, thoughts, and anxieties, thereby improving the child's coping mechanisms. Typically, these interventions work well with older children, but some younger children also benefit from these techniques if they are adapted to the child's age and developmental level. Common behavioral-cognitive strategies include relaxation, distraction, imagery, biofeedback, thought stopping, and positive self-talk.

Relaxation

Relaxation aids in reducing muscle tension and anxiety. A wide variety of techniques can be used. Relaxation can be as simple as holding an infant or young child closely while stroking the child or speaking in a soft soothing manner, or having the child inhale and exhale slowly using rhythmically controlled deep breathing. It also can involve more sophisticated techniques such as progressive relaxation. With this technique the child is asked to focus on one area of the body and let that body part go limp. Then in an organized fashion, usually working from the toes to the head or vice versa, the child is asked to focus on another body part, making it go limp. Eventually the exercises work through all body areas, leading to relaxation of the entire body.

Distraction

Distraction involves having the child focus on another stimulus, thereby attempting to shield him or her from pain. This technique does not eliminate the pain but does help to make it more tolerable. Various methods can be used for distraction, including:

• Counting
• Repetition of specific phrases or words, such as "ouch"
• Listening to music or singing
• Playing games, including computer games
• Blowing bubbles or blowing pinwheels or party favors
• Listening to favorite stories (Fig. 35.9)
• Watching cartoons, television shows, or movies
• Visiting with friends
• Humor

Humor has been demonstrated to be an effective distracting technique for pain management. However, make sure that the technique is age-appropriate and be sure to determine what or who will make the child laugh. If possible, allow the child and his family to choose the materials that they consider humorous.

Nursing Care Plan 35.1

OVERVIEW FOR THE CHILD IN PAIN

NURSING DIAGNOSIS: Acute pain related to need for invasive procedures, surgery, recent trauma, or infection as evidenced by pain rating scale, facial grimacing, crying, irritability, withdrawal activity, or changes in vital signs

Outcome Identification and Evaluation
Child will achieve adequate comfort level as evidenced by a decrease in rating number (3 or less) on a pain rating scale, quietness, calm resting behaviors, decrease in crying and irritability, and vital signs within acceptable parameters.

Intervention: Promoting Pain Relief
- Assess pain level using a developmentally appropriate pain rating tool *to establish a baseline.*
- Assess for verbal and nonverbal indicators of pain; question parents about child's typical behaviors and previous experiences with pain *to determine factors that may be influencing child's response to pain.*
- Institute nonpharmacologic methods for pain control based on the child's age and cognitive level; encourage parental participation in use of methods *to provide additional support for the child.*
- Administer pharmacologic agents as ordered using the least traumatic route possible *to alter pain impulse transmission and minimize distress while promoting effective pain relief.*
- Explain the action of the drug and what the child should expect from the medication at a level that the child can understand *to promote trust and reduce fear.*
- Give analgesics around the clock if pain is continuous and can be predicted *to maintain steady blood levels of the drug, thereby maximizing the drug's effect.*
- Perform atraumatic care at all times *to minimize the child's exposure to physical and psychological distress.*
- If a procedure is to be done, explain the purpose of the medication before the procedure and what to expect *to help minimize fear of the unknown.*
- Anticipate timing of procedures or situations that may lead to pain and provide appropriate analgesic therapy as ordered *to ensure that therapy is most effective at the time of the procedure.*
- Ensure that the child's environment is quiet and conducive to rest, dim the lights, close the door or curtain *to reduce sensory overload that would increase the child's pain sensation.*
- Encourage the parents to stroke, touch, caress, and hold the child *to promote feelings of security.*
- Reassess child's pain level after use of nonpharmacologic and pharmacologic methods *to determine effectiveness;* anticipate the need to modify or adapt nonpharmacologic methods or adjust analgesic dosage, route, or frequency *to promote maximum pain relief.*
- Perform nursing care activities after administering analgesic *to prevent exacerbating the child's pain.*
- Use diversional activities, distraction, and play appropriate to the child's age and cognitive level *to promote additional pain relief.*

NURSING DIAGNOSIS: Anxiety related to stress and uncertainty of the situation, unknown cause of pain, lack of familiarity with procedures, testing, and health care facility, and painful procedures, as evidenced by crying, irritability, withdrawal, stoic or aggressive behaviors

Outcome Identification and Evaluation
Child and family will demonstrate a decrease in anxiety level as evidenced by age-appropriate positive coping behaviors, verbalization of feelings, playing out of feelings, child and family cooperation with plan of care, and absence of signs and symptoms associated with escalating anxiety.

Intervention: Minimizing Anxiety
- Assess child's and parents' understanding of the situation, including their understanding of what may be causing the pain and the reasons for the procedures and testing, *to provide baseline information about the child's and parents' knowledge and possible clues to anxiety.*
- Spend time with the child and parents discussing what they think might be happening, encouraging child and parents to talk openly about their feelings, *to facilitate continued expressions and communication.* Allow time for questions and answer questions honestly *to establish rapport and build trust.*

(continued)

Nursing Care Plan 35.1 (continued)

- Approach the child and family in a calm, relaxed manner *to foster trust and communication.*
- Allow the child options related to pharmacologic agent administration as much as possible, such as fluid to drink or snack to eat, extremity to use for venipuncture (right or left), color of bandage, or holding tape or dressing, *to foster feelings of control.*
- Provide atraumatic care *to reduce exposure to distress, which would exacerbate the child's anxiety level.*
- Explain any procedures, tests, or activities at a level the child can understand *to reduce fear of the unknown.*
- Incorporate aspects of the child's routine at home as much as possible *to reduce feelings of separation and promote feelings of normalcy.*
- Ensure consistency in care *to facilitate trust and acceptance.*
- Encourage parents in the use of comfort measures such as stroking, cuddling, holding, and rocking *to promote feelings of security and minimize stress.*
- Provide positive reinforcement for choices, participation in activities, and use of appropriate coping methods *to foster self-esteem.*
- Encourage the child's participation in play (unstructured and therapeutic play as needed) *to promote expression of feelings and fears.*

NURSING DIAGNOSIS: Deficient knowledge related to current condition and appropriate methods for managing pain as evidenced by crying, irritability, pushing away, questions and verbalizations about pain and relief methods

Outcome Identification and Evaluation
Child and parents will demonstrate adequate knowledge about the child's current condition and use of pain relief methods as evidenced by statements about the cause of the child's pain, demonstration of chosen nonpharmacologic relief methods, use of pharmacologic agents, and statements related to signs and symptoms of increased and decreased pain.

Intervention: Providing Child and Family Teaching
- Assess child's and parents' knowledge and understanding of child's current condition and current pain level *to establish a baseline for teaching.*
- Provide time for child and parents to ask questions; answer questions honestly and in terms they can understand *to promote learning.*
- Explain in simplified terms how the child's condition is associated with pain or the rationale for procedures needed that may contribute to pain *to promote understanding and foster trust.*
- Teach in short sessions *to prevent overloading the child and parents with information.*
- Provide reinforcement and rewards *to help facilitate the teaching/learning process.*
- Use multiple modes of learning, such as written information, verbal instruction, demonstrations, and media when possible, *to facilitate learning and retention of information.*
- Instruct parents and child as appropriate in nonpharmacologic methods for pain relief; encourage practice and participation by parents in methods chosen *to foster independence and use of method when necessary.*
- Teach child as appropriate and parents about pharmacologic methods for pain relief; review specific information about drug to be used, including action, duration, administration, possible adverse effects, and care necessary when drug is used, *to promote learning*; have child and parents report back information or demonstrate administration *to evaluate effectiveness of teaching.*
- Provide parents with written information about pain relief methods for use at home if indicated *to allow for reference at a later date.*

Nursing Care Plan 35.1 (continued)

NURSING DIAGNOSIS: Disturbed sleep patterns related to inability to manage pain effectively as evidenced by frequent waking by child during night, signs and symptoms of pain including irritability and restlessness, statements about being tired, pain rating scale

Outcome Identification and Evaluation
Child will exhibit increased ability to sleep during night as evidenced by increasing periods of calm and restfulness (initially starting at 2 hours and gradually increasing to 7 to 8 hours), decreased pain level on pain rating scale, and statements of decreased fatigue.

Intervention: Promoting Sleep and Rest
- Assist child in using nonpharmacologic methods of pain relief, such as imagery, distraction, muscle relaxation, *to promote relaxation.*
- Administer pharmacologic pain relief as ordered *to minimize pain interfering with sleep*; anticipate a change in drug therapy if pain relief is inadequate.
- Cluster nursing care activities *to minimize energy expenditure and disruptions in child's ability to rest.*
- Help child with a nighttime routine similar to one he or she uses at home *to promote feelings of security.*
- Offer child back rub, warm bath, or warm liquids, reading a story, or listening to music *to facilitate relaxation*; provide stroking, hugging, cuddling, rocking, and light touch *to promote a sense of security and calm.*
- Dim the lights and close the curtain or door to the room *to provide a quiet, restful environment.*
- Ensure round-the-clock pain relief for the child through the night *to minimize the risk of pain.*

NURSING DIAGNOSIS: Risk for injury related to possible adverse effects of analgesics

Outcome Identification and Evaluation
Child will remain free of any injury related to signs and symptoms of adverse effects of analgesic therapy as evidenced by respiratory rate appropriate for age, no complaints of GI upset, dizziness, or sedation or episodes of constipation, nausea, vomiting, or pruritus.

Intervention: Promoting Safety
- Ensure that the child's call light is within reach *to allow for notification of health care personnel should problems arise.*
- Administer analgesic exactly as prescribed *to reduce the risk of error and development of adverse effects.*
- Assess child's respiratory status closely for changes *to allow for early detection of respiratory depression.*
- If an opioid analgesic is being given, have naloxone readily available *to reverse the action of the narcotic if respiratory depression occurs.*
- Monitor appetite and assess bowel sounds for changes; note any abdominal distention or decreased bowel sounds, *which would suggest decreased peristalsis.*
- Ensure adequate fluid and fiber intake *to reduce risk of constipation.*
- Offer small frequent meals and give medication with food *to minimize risk of GI upset.*
- Assess for nausea and vomiting; if necessary withhold food and fluids *to rest the GI tract* and administer antiemetics until nausea and vomiting resolve.
- Instruct the child to remain in bed after receiving analgesic, raise crib or side rails as appropriate, and instruct the child and parents to have someone accompany the child to the bathroom if allowed *to reduce the risk of falls from sedation.*
- Assess for complaints of itching and observe for rash or reddened areas; if pruritus occurs, urge the child not to scratch and expect to administer antihistamine as ordered *to reduce pruritus.*
- Provide the child with distraction to assist in helping *to reduce effects of pruritus.*

The type of distraction used depends on the age of the child. For example, a younger child may enjoy blowing pinwheels and blowing bubbles. He or she also will enjoy listening to favorite stories or books. Older children may enjoy computer games, listening to favorite music, or visiting with friends.

Imagery
Imagery involves the use of the imagination to create a mental image. This mental image usually is a positive, pleasurable image, but it need not be real. The child is encouraged to include details and sensations that are associated with the image, such as specific descriptions of the image, colors,

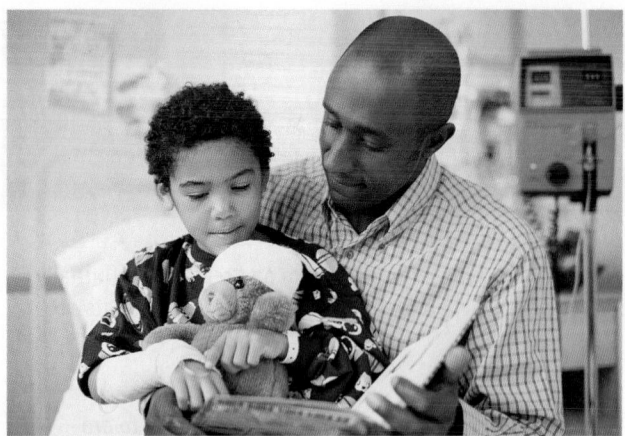

FIGURE 35.9 A child using distraction for pain management.

sounds, feelings, and smells. In some instances, the child may write down or record the image on a tape or compact disc. When pain occurs, the child is encouraged to create the mental image or read or listen to the description.

Biofeedback

Biofeedback involves having the child gain an awareness of his or her body functions and learn ways to modify them voluntarily. The child usually is taught specific skills about how to modify body functions using an apparatus that measures pain-related changes in muscle tone or physio-

logic data, such as blood pressure or pulse rate. This teaching usually is performed by a specialized health care provider and occurs over several sessions, in advance of the pain experience. With practice, the child learns to control the changes without the apparatus. This technique can be used by older children, such as adolescents, who can concentrate for longer periods of time.

Thought Stopping

Thought stopping involves substituting a pleasurable or positive thought for the painful experience. Examples of positive thoughts might be, "It's only for a short time" or "It's important so I get better." The negative component of the pain is not ignored or suppressed; rather, it is transformed into something positive. Thought stopping also can involve the use of short, positive phrases. For example, the child may repeat "quick stick, feel better, go home soon" when he or she anticipates pain or experiences pain.

Thought stopping is a useful method for reducing anxiety before and during events associated with pain. Children can be taught to use this technique anytime they experience anxiety related to a painful experience. Doing so helps to promote the child's sense of control over the situation.

Positive Self-Talk

Positive self-talk is similar to thought stopping in that it involves the use of positive statements. With positive self-

---

EVIDENCE–BASED PRACTICE 35.1

What Are the Effects of Distraction on Pain, Fear, and Distress During Venous Port Access and Venipuncture in Children With Cancer?

Children with cancer undergo multiple procedures, and many describe these procedures as the most distressing part of their disease. Distraction can decrease procedural pain, distress, and fear by redirecting the child from threatening to nonthreatening stimuli, resulting in a therapeutic benefit.

● Study

This study used an intervention-comparison group design in a large university-affiliated pediatric medical center. A convenience sample of 50 children with cancer, from 5 to 18 years old, was randomly assigned to either a comparison or an intervention group. Two oncology nurses performed all port access or venipunctures per institutional guidelines. Both groups received standard care with the intervention group also using a self-selected distracter from a pool of five choices, which were chosen based on recommendations in the literature (*I Spy: Super Challenger* book, bubbles, music, VR glasses that allow the child to watch a video in 3-D and listen to music in stereo sound, and Nintendo Gameboy).

▲ Findings

The pain and fear scores were lower in the intervention group, although the difference was not statistically significant. Fear and distress scores were significantly improved from during to after the procedure in the intervention versus the comparison group. Forty-six percent of those in the intervention group stated the current poke was "better" or "much better" than their last one, compared to 39% in the comparison group. Fifty-nine percent of parents in the intervention group, compared to 16% in the comparison group, felt this venous access or venipuncture was better than the last one. Ninety-one percent of those patients in the intervention group stated that the distracter helped and they would use it again. All of the parents (100%) reported the distracter was effective and they would encourage their child to use it again.

■ Nursing Implications

Nurses need to encourage distraction strategies as they have been shown to positively enhance procedure outcomes. The nurse needs to facilitate and encourage parent participation in the use of distraction strategies.

Windich-Biermeier, A., et al. (2007). Effects of distraction on pain, fear, and distress during venous port access and venipuncture in children and adolescents with cancer. *Journal of Pediatric Oncology Nursing, 24*(1), 8–19.

talk the child is taught to say positive statements when he or she is experiencing pain. For example, the child may be taught to say, "I will feel better and be able to go home and play with my friends."

Biophysical Interventions

Biophysical interventions focus on interfering with the transmission of pain impulses reaching the brain. The interventions involve some type of cutaneous stimulation near the site of the pain. This stimulation decreases the ability of the A-delta and C fibers to transmit pain impulses. Examples of biophysical interventions include application of heat and cold, massage and pressure, and transcutaneous electrical nerve stimulation (TENS).

A particular intervention for infants is nonnutritive sucking, which reduces pain behaviors in neonates undergoing painful procedures (Morash & Fowler, 2004). Infants derive satisfaction from sucking. In addition, they show reduced pain behaviors after ingestion of sucrose or other sweet-tasting solutions such as glucose, since these substances are mediated through the opioid pathways (Morash & Fowler, 2004). Nonnutritive sucking is recommended as a technique for providing atraumatic care, but this method must be used with caution in infants with unstable blood glucose levels.

Heat and Cold Applications

Heat and cold applications alter physiologic mechanisms associated with pain. Cold results in vasoconstriction and alters capillary permeability, leading to a decrease in edema at the site of the injury. Due to vasoconstriction, blood flow is reduced and the release of pain-producing substances such as histamine and serotonin also is decreased. Moreover, transmission of painful stimuli via peripheral nerve fibers is decreased.

Heat results in vasodilation and increases blood flow to the area. It also leads to a decrease in nociceptive stimulation and removal of chemical substances that can stimulate nociceptive fibers. The increase in blood flow alters capillary permeability, leading to a reduction in swelling and pressure on nociceptive nerve fibers. Heat may also trigger the release of endogenous opioids, which mediate the pain response.

Massage and Pressure

Massage and pressure, like other biophysical interventions, are believed to inhibit stimulation of the A-delta and C fibers. These methods are helpful in relaxing muscles and reducing tension. In addition, these techniques can aid in distracting the child. Massage can be as simple as rubbing a body part or pressing on an area such as an injection site for about 10 seconds, or it can be more involved, requiring the use of another person to perform the massage. Lotion or ointment can be used during the massage and may provide a comforting effect. Contralateral pressure or massage (i.e., of the opposite area) may be used, especially if the area of pain cannot be accessed or if the affected area is too painful to touch.

A more formal method of pressure application is acupressure. In acupressure the fingertip, thumb, or a blunt instrument is used to apply gentle, firm pressure to specifically designated sites to control pain. The pressure may be applied in one motion followed by releasing, in a circular motion for several minutes and then releasing, or with a vibrating motion using the fingertips. The motion of applying and then releasing pressure is thought to facilitate the release of endogenous endorphins and enkephalins. The techniques of pressure and massage can be taught to children and parents. The techniques are easy to learn and use.

The Nurse's Role in Nonpharmacologic Pain Intervention

The nurse plays a major role in teaching the child and family about nonpharmacologic pain interventions, helping them choose the most appropriate and most effective methods, and ensuring that the child and parents use

TEACHING GUIDELINES 35.1

Teaching to Manage Pain Without Drugs

- Review the methods available and choose the method(s) that your child and you find best for your situation.
- Learn to identify the ways in which your child shows pain or demonstrates he or she is anxious about the possibility of pain—for example, does he or she get restless, make a face, or get flushed in the face?
- Begin using the technique chosen before your child experiences pain or when your child first indicates he or she is anxious about or beginning to experience pain.
- Practice the technique with your child and encourage the child to use the technique when he or she feels anxious about pain or anticipates that a procedure or experience will be painful.
- Perform the technique with your child; for example, take the deep breath in and out or blow bubbles with him or her; listen to the music or play the computer game with your child.
- Avoid using terms such as "hurt" or "pain" that suggest or cause your child to expect pain.
- Use descriptive terms like pushing, pulling, pinching, or heat.
- Avoid overly descriptive or judgmental statements such as, "this will really hurt a lot" or "this will be terrible."
- Stay with your child as much as possible; speak softly and gently stroke or cuddle your child.
- Offer praise, positive reinforcement, hugs, and support for using the technique even when it was not effective.

the method before pain occurs as well as before the pain increases. Teaching Guidelines 35.1 lists some helpful instructions for the parents and child about nonpharmacologic pain management.

The nurse also assists the child and parents when using the technique, ensuring that they are using the technique correctly and offering suggestions for modifications or adaptations as necessary.

Parents are important components of the pain management program. Give them the option to stay with the child, or let them know that someone else will support the child if they opt not to stay. Offer simple, concrete ways to assist and help the child to manage pain. Many of the nonpharmacologic techniques can be done by parents, and children may respond better if their parents demonstrate the technique and encourage them to use it. Invite parents to participate in decisions as well as act as a coach to their child during procedures. Prepare the parents and explain the most appropriate pain management approaches and strategies. Discuss the type and amount of pain expected as well as the potential complications associated with pain management approaches. Ask how the parent predicts the child will react to a painful situation. Finally, offer techniques and strategies to the parents as they act as the coach during these situations.

> ▶ *Take* NOTE!
>
> *Although parents want to help their children and some are able to act as coaches, the response of the child to pain and stress and to their parents' distraction interventions is highly variable. Some children appear to be soothed by their parents' distraction actions; others appear to become distressed. Be alert to factors that may influence the child's response, including age, sex, diagnosis, ethnicity, previous experience, temperament, anxiety, and coping style. Also be aware of parental factors, including ethnicity, sex, previous experience, belief in the helpfulness of the intervention, parenting style, and parental anxiety (McCarthy & Kleiber, 2006).*

Pharmacologic Management

Pharmacologic interventions involve the administration of drugs for pain relief. Administration may occur using a wide variety of methods. The selection of the method is determined by the drug being administered, the child's status, the type, intensity, and location of the pain, and any factors that may be influencing the child's pain. Research overwhelmingly supports the appropriate use of analgesics to reduce pain perception in children (Broome & Huth, 2003).

Medications Used for Pain Management

Analgesics (medications for pain relief) typically fall into one of two categories: nonopioid analgesics and opioid analgesics. Anesthetics also may be used. Drugs such as sedatives and hypnotics also may be used as adjuvant medications to help minimize anxiety or provide or assist with pain relief when typical analgesics are ineffective.

Nonopioid Analgesics

Nonopioid analgesics include acetaminophen and nonsteroidal anti-inflammatory drugs (NSAIDs) such as ibuprofen, ketorolac, naproxen, indomethacin, diclofenac, and piroxicam (Drug Guide 35.1). These agents may be used to treat mild to moderate pain, often for conditions such as arthritis; joint, bone, and muscle pain; headache; dental pain; and menstrual pain. Acetaminophen, probably the most widely known nonopioid analgesic, also is commonly used to treat fever in children, as is ibuprofen.

> ▶ *Take* NOTE!
>
> *Aspirin should not be used in children for analgesic and antipyretic purposes because of the high risk of Reye's syndrome.*

According to the World Health Organization's pain ladder, acetaminophen and NSAIDs are first-line agents for the treatment of pain (WHO, 2006). Although this ladder was developed for the relief of cancer pain, it can be applied to any patient experiencing pain.

Nonopioid agents are typically administered orally or rectally. In some cases, such as with postoperative pain, they may be administered intravenously as a continuous infusion or as bolus doses (Maunuksela & Olkkola, 2003). Administration via intramuscular injection is not recommended because the injection can cause significant pain and the onset of pain relief is not increased.

Adverse effects commonly associated with these agents include gastrointestinal irritation, blood clotting problems, and renal dysfunction. However, research has demonstrated that children experience only mild gastrointestinal upset and negligible effects on a healthy, well-functioning renal system. Blood clotting problems arise primarily when these agents are given perioperatively before primary hemostasis has occurred (Maunuksela & Olkkola, 2003). Nonopioids are relatively safe, have few incompatibilities with other medications, and do not depress the central nervous system. Unfortunately, they exhibit a ceiling effect for analgesia: after a certain level, they do not provide increasing pain relief even when administered at increased doses. As a result, they may be combined with opioids for more effective pain relief.

Drug	Action/Indication	Nursing Implications
Acetaminophen (Tylenol)	Possible inhibition of cyclooxygenase in the central nervous system. Direct action on hypothalamic heat-regulating center. Mild to moderate pain; arthritis, musculoskeletal pain, headache	• Administer orally or rectally. Do not exceed five doses of drug in 24 hours. • Caution parents to read labels of other over-the-counter (OTC) drugs carefully; some may contain acetaminophen and if given in conjunction may lead to overdose.
Ibuprofen (Motrin, Advil)	Inhibition of prostaglandin synthesis Mild to moderate pain, fever	• Administer orally. • Give with food or after meals if GI upset occurs. • Assess for easy bruising, bleeding gums, or frank or occult blood in urine or stool. • Monitor for nausea, vomiting, GI upset, diarrhea or constipation, dizziness or drowsiness. • Caution parents to read labels of OTC medications closely; some may contain ibuprofen or other NSAIDs and if given in conjunction may lead to overdose.
Other NSAIDs: ketorolac (Toradol), diclofenac (Voltaren), indomethacin (Indocin), naproxen (Naprosyn, Aleve)	Inhibition of prostaglandin synthesis Mild to moderate pain	• Administer oral form with food or after meals if GI upset occurs. • Monitor for headache, dizziness, nausea, vomiting, constipation, or diarrhea. • Assess for signs and symptoms of bleeding, such as bruising, epistaxis, gingival bleeding, or frank or occult blood in urine or stool. • Ketorolac: May also be given IV or IM. In children 2–16 years, recommended as single dose only. • Naproxen: Also available in combination products (caution parents to read OTC labels carefully). • Indomethacin: When administering IV, report oliguria or anuria. • Diclofenac: May also be given rectally.
Opioid agents: morphine, codeine, fentanyl (Sublimaze, Duragesic), hydromorphone (Dilaudid), oxycodone (OxyContin)	Opioid agonist acting primarily at mu-receptor sites (morphine, codeine, fentanyl, hydromorphone, oxycodone) Moderate to severe acute and chronic pain. Morphine: intractable pain, preoperative sedation. Codeine: also suppresses cough reflex. Fentanyl: pain associated with short procedures such as bone marrow aspiration, fracture reductions, suturing.	• Assess respiratory status frequently, noting any decrease in ventilatory rate or changes in breathing patterns; have naloxone readily available in case of respiratory depression (particularly morphine, fentanyl, hydromorphone). • Monitor for sedation dizziness, lethargy, confusion. • Educate parents and child that the drug may make the child sleepy, drowsy, or lightheaded. • Institute safety measures to prevent injury to the child. • Assess bowel sounds for decreased peristalsis; observe for abdominal distention. • Ensure adequate fiber intake and administer stool softeners as prescribed to minimize risk for constipation. • Monitor urine output for changes and report. • Morphine: May cause itching, particularly facial. • Codeine: May cause nausea, vomiting, abdominal pain. IV administration results in apnea and severe hypotension. Most commonly administered orally in combination with acetaminophen. • Fentanyl: Observe for chest wall rigidity, which can occur with rapid IV infusion. • Oxycodone is the opioid component of Tylox and Percocet.

(continued)

DRUG GUIDE 35.1 COMMON DRUGS FOR PAIN MANAGEMENT (continued)

Drug	Action and Indication	Nursing Implications
Mixed opioid agonist–antagonist: pentazocine (Talwin), butorphanol (Stadol), nalbuphine (Nubain)	Pentazocine: antagonist at mu-receptor sites, agonist at kappa-receptor sites. Butorphanol: high affinity for kappa-receptor sites, minimal affinity for sigma-receptor sites. Nalbuphine: partial agonist at kappa-receptor sites, antagonist at mu-receptor sites. Moderate to severe pain. Relief of migraine headache (butorphanol). Preoperative analgesia (nalbuphine).	• Monitor the child for sedation. Educate child and parents that the drug may make the child sleepy, drowsy, or lightheaded. • Institute safety measures to prevent injury to the child. • Pentazocine, butorphanol: Monitor for diaphoresis, dizziness. Assess for tachycardia and hypertension. • Butorphanol is given intranasally for migraine headaches.

Opioid Analgesics

Opioid analgesics are typically used for moderate to severe pain. They are classified as either agonists (when they act as the neurotransmitter at the receptor site) or antagonists (when they block the action at the receptor site). Opioid agents that act as agonists include morphine, codeine, fentanyl, meperidine, hydromorphone, oxycodone, and hydrocodone. Opioids that act as mixed agonists–antagonists include pentazocine, butorphanol, and nalbuphine (see Drug Guide 35.1). Opioids can be administered orally, rectally, intramuscularly, or intravenously. In addition, some agents such as fentanyl can be administered transdermally or transmucosally. Morphine is considered the "gold standard" for all opioid agonists; it is the drug to which all other opioids are compared and is usually the drug of choice for severe pain.

Opioid agonists, such as morphine, are associated with numerous adverse effects, resulting primarily from their depressant action on the central nervous system.

▶ **Take** NOTE!

When administering parenteral or epidural opioids, always have naloxone (Narcan) readily available to reverse the opioid's effects should respiratory depression occur.

Opioids stimulate the chemoreceptor trigger zone (CTZ), leading to nausea and vomiting. Moreover, **drug tolerance** (increased dosage required for the same pain relief previously achieved with a lower dose) and **physical dependence** (need for continued administration of the drug to prevent withdrawal symptoms) are commonly noted when opioids are given repeatedly (Yaster et al., 2003). Drug Guide 35.1 gives additional information related to the opioid analgesics.

▶ **Take** NOTE!

Drug tolerance occurs when increasing doses are required to manage the pain. Physical dependence can occur after as few as 5 days of continuous use of the drug; symptoms of withdrawal begin if it is suddenly stopped. To decrease the risk of withdrawal, the dose can be decreased 10% to 20% per day.

Mixed agonist–antagonists are associated with less respiratory depression than agonists. Unfortunately, like NSAIDs, this group also has a ceiling effect, leading to inadequate effectiveness even with increased dosages. When this occurs, increasing the dosage of the mixed agonist–antagonist or combining it with an agonist provides no additional pain relief.

▶ **Take** NOTE!

Meperidine, an opioid agonist, is not recommended as a first-choice agent for pain relief in children. Meperidine's metabolite, normeperidine, is associated with the development of restlessness, irritability, twitching, agitation, tremors, and most importantly seizures. Normeperidine is a central nervous stimulant and its effects cannot be reversed by an opioid antagonist such as naloxone (American Medical Association, 2006; McCaffrey & Pasero, 1999).

Adjuvant Drugs

Adjuvant drugs are drugs that are used to promote more effective pain relief, either alone or in combination with non-opioids or opioids. Their primary indication is for diagnoses other than pain. These agents are not classified as analgesics but may provide a coanalgesic effect or may treat side effects. Benzodiazepines, such as diazepam and midazolam, help to relieve anxiety. Midazolam also produces amnesia. Anticonvulsants, such as carbamazepine, and tricyclic antidepressants, such as amitriptyline and nortriptyline, are used to treat neuropathic pain.

Local Anesthetics

Local anesthetics are commonly used to provide analgesia for procedures. They are effective in providing successful pain relief with only minimal risk of systemic adverse effects. However, local anesthetics such as lidocaine historically were not used in children because they need to be injected; the belief was that children feared needles and use of a local anesthetic subjected the child to two needle-sticks instead of one. Advances in technology have led to the development of improved methods of delivery such as topical ointments and iontophoresis for administration of local anesthetics, thereby promoting atraumatic care. (For more detailed discussion, see the next section on drug administration methods and later in the chapter on the nurse's role in managing procedure-related pain.)

Drug Administration Methods

With any medication administered for pain management, the timing of administration is vital. Timing depends on the type of pain. For continuous pain, the current recommendation is to administer analgesia around the clock at scheduled intervals to achieve the necessary effect. Scheduled dosing has been associated with decreased pain intensity ratings for children (Paice et al., 2005). As-needed or PRN dosing is not recommended. This method can lead to inadequate pain relief because of the delay before the drug reaches its peak effectiveness, and as a result the child continues to experience pain, possibly necessitating a higher dose of analgesic to achieve relief; this then places the child at risk for overmedication and toxic effects.

For pain that can be predicted or considered temporary, such as with a procedure, analgesia is administered so that the peak action of the drug matches the time of the painful event.

There are various methods for administering pain medications to children. The preferred methods are the oral, rectal, intravenous, topical, or local nerve block routes. Epidural administration and conscious sedation also can be used.

Oral Method

The oral method is often preferred because it is simple, easy, and convenient. The medication may be in the form of a pill, capsule, tablet, syrup, or elixir. Oral administration provides relatively steady blood levels of the drug when administered as a scheduled dose. Effectiveness typically occurs 1 to 2 hours after administration. Higher doses of the medication may be needed to achieve the same ef-

fect when switching the child from a parenteral form to an oral form (Hockenberry et al., 2005).

Rectal Method

The rectal method may be used when the child cannot take the medication orally, such as when he or she has difficulty swallowing or is experiencing nausea and vomiting. It is a viable alternative for drug administration. Some analgesics are available in suppository form; for others that are not, the drug can be compounded into a suppository form. The absorption rate varies with rectal administration, and children may find insertion of a suppository uncomfortable and embarrassing.

Intravenous Method

Intravenous analgesia administration is the method of choice in emergency situations and when pain is severe and quick relief is needed. With intravenous administration, the drug usually takes effect within 5 minutes. Intravenous administration can be accomplished with bolus injections or continuous infusions. Continuous infusions may be preferred over bolus doses because steady blood levels are more easily maintained, thereby enhancing the drug's effect in relieving pain. Typically, opioids such as morphine, hydromorphone, and fentanyl are used due to their short half-life and decreased risk for toxicity.

Patient-Controlled Analgesia

In **patient-controlled analgesia (PCA)**, a computerized pump is programmed to deliver an infusion of analgesics via a catheter inserted intravenously, epidurally, or subcutaneously. The analgesic may be given as a continuous infusion, as a continuous infusion supplemented by patient-delivered bolus doses, or as patient-delivered bolus doses only. Typically the child presses a button to administer a bolus dose. The pump has a lockout function that is preset with the dose and time interval: if the child presses the button before the preset time, he or she will not receive an overdose of medication. By delivering small, frequent doses of opioids, the child can experience pain relief without the effects of oversedation. The child also experiences a sense of control over the pain experience.

PCA has been used successfully in children as young as 5 or 6 years old (D'Arcy, 2007). However, it is essential to assess each child individually and consider his or her developmental level and psychosocial factors in determining appropriate PCA use. The child must have the necessary intellect, manual dexterity, and strength to operate the device. Both the Institute for Safe Medical Practices (ISMP) and the Joint Commission on the Accreditation of Health Care Organizations (JCAHO) have identified infants and young children as not being good candidates for PCA usage (D'Arcy, 2007).

Serious adverse events, such as oversedation, respiratory depression, and even death, can occur when family members, caregivers, or clinicians who are not authorized administer PCA doses "by proxy." The ISMP recommends developing specific criteria in any situation where authorized agent–activated PCA is being used. Proper education and instruction is crucial in any situation where someone other than the patient may be administering PCA doses. To ensure safety with PCA use, each institution must have policies and procedures in place, appropriate education of health care staff, quality-control measures, and quality machines.

PCA has been used to control postoperative pain and the pain associated with trauma, cancer, and sickle cell crisis. It can be used in acute care settings or in the home. Most commonly, morphine, hydromorphone, and fentanyl are the drugs used with PCA. The dosage is based on the child's response. Initial bolus doses commonly range from 0.015 to 0.02 mg/kg. Dosages for infusions depend on the child's age, the opioid used, and the type of pain. A commonly used range for morphine infusion to treat postoperative pain ranges from 0.01 to 0.04 mg/kg/hour. Higher dosage ranges have been used to treat the pain associated with sickle cell crisis and cancer.

Local Anesthetic Application

A local anesthetic may sometimes be used to alleviate the pain associated with procedures such as venipuncture, injections, wound repair, lumbar puncture, or accessing of implanted ports. Local anesthesia is a type of regional analgesia that blocks or numbs specific nerves in a region of the body. Medications called local anesthetics include topical forms, such as creams, agents delivered by iontophoresis, and vapocoolants and skin refrigerants, and injectable forms.

Topical Forms

The first choice for the most effective, painless local anesthesia is EMLA (eutectic mixture of local anesthetics [lidocaine and prilocaine]). It achieves anesthesia to a depth of 2 to 4 mm, so it reduces pain of phlebotomy, venous cannulation, and intramuscular injections for up to 24 hours after the injection. However, it requires a 60-minute application time to intact skin using an occlusive dressing for superficial procedures and up to 2 to 3 hours for deeper, more invasive procedures (Box 35.1). Sometimes EMLA is not used due to the expense and the time needed to allow the drug to act.

> ▶ **Take** NOTE!
> EMLA cream should not be used in those patients with the rare condition of congenital or idiopathic methemoglobinemia and in infants under the age of 12 months who are receiving treatment with methemoglobin-inducing agents, such as sulfonamides.

BOX 35.1 Applying EMLA

Follow these guidelines when applying EMLA:
- Explain the purpose of the medication to the child and parents, reinforcing that it will help the pain go away.
- Check the scheduled time for the procedure; plan to apply the cream 60 minutes before a superficial procedure such as a heelstick or venipuncture or 2 to 3 hours before a deeper procedure such as a lumbar puncture or bone marrow aspiration.
- Place a thick layer of the cream on the skin at the intended site of the procedure, making sure that the area where the cream is being applied is free of any breaks. Do not rub the cream in once it is applied to the skin.
- Use approximately one third to one half of a 5-g tube for an application.
- Cover the site with a transparent dressing such as Tegaderm or Op-site and secure it so that the dressing is occlusive. Alternatively, use plastic film wrap and tape the edges to secure the dressing.
- Instruct the child not to touch the dressing once it is secured. If necessary, cover the occlusive dressing with a protection device or a loosely applied gauze or elastic bandage.
- After the allotted time, remove the occlusive dressing and wipe the cream from the skin. Inspect the skin for a change in color (blanching or redness), which indicates that the medication has penetrated the skin adequately.
- Verify that sensation is absent by lightly tapping or scratching the area. Use this technique also to demonstrate to the child that the anesthetic is effective. If sensation is present, reapply the cream.
- Prepare the child for the procedure. Assess the child's pain after the procedure to evaluate for pain and to differentiate pain from fear and anxiety.

EMLA is available in two forms: a cream and a topical disc. If the disc form is used, an occlusive dressing is not needed. EMLA is approved for use in infants 37 weeks' gestation or older. Maximum dosage and maximum area of application are based on the child's weight. Parents can be taught how to apply the EMLA cream or disc at home in preparation for a procedure (Fig. 35.10).

> ▶ **Take** NOTE!
> EMLA is contraindicated in children who have congenital or idiopathic methemoglobinemia. It must be used cautiously in those under age 12 months who are receiving methemoglobin-inducing agents, such as sulfonamides, phenytoin, phenobarbital, and acetaminophen. Use of these agents in combination with EMLA increases the child's risk for methemoglobinemia, a condition that could lead to cyanosis and hypoxemia.

FIGURE 35.10 A parent applies EMLA cream to the child at home in preparation for a procedure.

TAC (tetracaine, epinephrine, cocaine) and LET (lidocaine, epinephrine, tetracaine) are other examples of topical anesthetics. These are commonly used for lacerations that require suturing. The agent is applied directly to the wound with a cotton ball or swab for 20 to 30 minutes until the area is numb. These methods are not used in patients with known sensitivity to any of these medications.

Researchers have studied LMX4, an over-the-counter topical anesthetic that provides anesthesia to the applied area in 15 to 30 minutes instead of the 60 minutes required by EMLA. The studies showed that an occlusive dressing was not needed when this topical anesthetic was used.

A study published recently in the *Canadian Medical Association Journal* found that a new topical anesthetic containing liposomal lidocaine 4% cream was highly effective in reducing the pain associated with intravenous cannulation. The researchers cited a short onset of action (30 minutes) and minimal vascular effects as benefits. They found that the liposomal encapsulation protects the anesthetic from being metabolized too quickly. Results of this study showed higher intravenous cannulation success rates, less pain, shorter total procedure time, and minor dermal changes among the children (Taddio et al., 2005).

Another choice for local anesthesia is iontophoresis. Iontophoretic lidocaine (Numby Stuff) provides anesthesia to a depth of 8 to 10 mm in approximately 10 minutes and is used over intact skin. A mild electrical current from a small battery-powered generator and two iontophoretic drug-delivery electrodes push drug molecules

(lidocaine HCl 2% with epinephrine 1:100,000) into the skin. This type of local anesthesia is not recommended for use in children who have a history of allergy or sensitivity to these drugs; with children who have electrically sensitive equipment such as a pacemaker; or if damaged skin or scar tissue is present.

Vapocoolant spray, another type of local analgesia, can be sprayed onto the skin or administered using a cotton ball soaked in liquid. The depth of anesthesia is not known, but it appears to provide immediate pain control. It is inexpensive and requires no waiting time. The effect lasts for approximately 1 to 2 minutes.

Injectable Forms

Injectable forms of lidocaine or procaine can be administered subcutaneously or intradermally around the procedural area approximately 5 to 10 minutes before the procedure. Common problems with this form of anesthetic include the pain associated with the subcutaneous injection and some burning associated with lidocaine administration, as well as blanching of the skin.

> ▶ **Take** NOTE!
>
> *The burning that lidocaine causes on injection may be diminished by buffering lidocaine with sodium bicarbonate, using 10 parts lidocaine and 1 part sodium bicarbonate (1 mL of 1% to 2% lidocaine and 0.1 mL of 8.4% sodium bicarbonate). Then inject 0.1 mL or less of the solution intradermally at the site of venipuncture. Anesthetic action is almost immediate. The solution is stable for only approximately 1 week if not refrigerated.*

Epidural Analgesia

For epidural analgesia, a catheter is inserted in the epidural space at L1-2, L3-4, or L4-5. The drug, usually fentanyl or morphine, diffuses into the cerebrospinal fluid and crosses the dura mater to the spinal cord. Then it binds with the opioid receptors located at the dorsal horn. The drugs can be administered as bolus injections (a one-time bolus or on an intermittent schedule), a continuous infusion, or PCA. Usually an opioid, such as morphine, fentanyl, or hydromorphone, is given in conjunction with a long-acting local anesthetic such as bupivacaine.

Epidural analgesia is typically used postoperatively, providing analgesia to the lower body for approximately 12 to 14 hours. The small amount of medication used with this type of analgesia causes less sedation, thereby allowing the child to participate more actively in postoperative care activities. This type of analgesia also is effective for children undergoing upper or lower abdominal surgeries because it controls localized intense pain, somatic pain, and visceral pain.

When epidural analgesia is being administered, additional narcotic analgesics are not given in order to prevent complications such as respiratory depression, pruritus, nausea, vomiting, and urinary retention.

▶ *Take* NOTE!

Respiratory depression, although rare when epidural analgesia is used, is always a possibility. When it does occur, it usually occurs gradually over a period of several hours after the medication is initiated. This allows adequate time for early detection and prompt intervention.

Constant assessment is essential because insertion of an epidural catheter and epidural analgesia can lead to infection at the site of the insertion, epidural hematoma, arachnoiditis, neuritis, or spinal headache (rare) due to a cerebrospinal fluid leak and respiratory depression. Frequent assessment, typically every 1 to 2 hours, of heart rate, respiratory rate, blood pressure, depth of sedation, and pain level is imperative. Assessing for adverse reactions such as nausea and vomiting and pruritus, as well as checking the catheter site and ensuring the occlusive dressing is intact, are all important nursing interventions. The dermatome, which is the area of the body associated with supply by a particular nerve, that innervates the diaphragm can become suppressed during continuous epidural analgesia, resulting in respiratory depression. Therefore the nurse must assess the patient's sensory level frequently. This can be done by using cool water on alcohol pad and bilaterally touching the patient's body every 2 to 3 cm. The level where the patient states he or she feels the temperature change is the level of anesthesia. (Refer to Figure 35.11 for dermatome levels.)

Conscious Sedation

Conscious sedation is a medically controlled state of depressed consciousness that allows protective reflexes to be maintained so the child has the ability to maintain a patent airway and respond to physical or verbal stimulation. This procedure requires adherence to specific protocols as outlined by the Federal Drug Administration Department and Joint Commission on Accreditation of Healthcare Organizations. The depressed state is obtained by using various agents such as morphine, fentanyl, midazolam, or diazepam and other adjuvants such as pentobarbital. Midazolam and fentanyl often are the drugs of choice for conscious sedation because they act quickly, last only a short time, and are available in oral and intravenous formulations (Box 35.2).

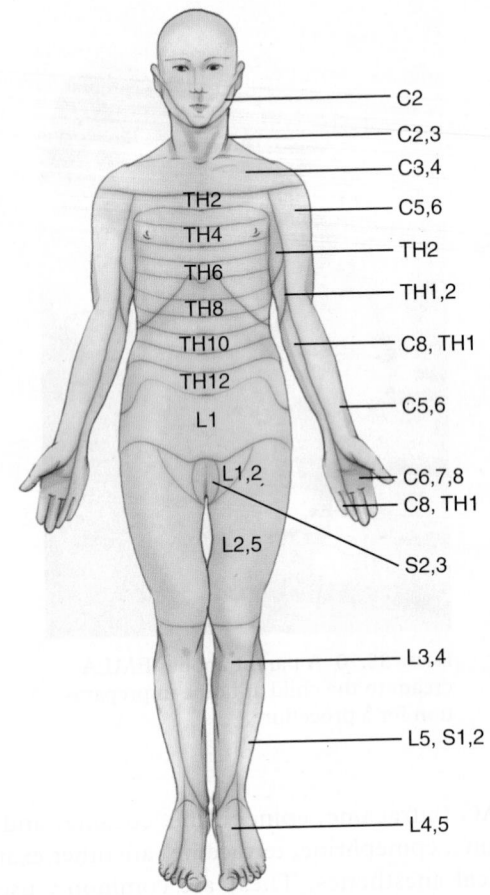

Diagram of Dermatomes

FIGURE 35.11 The level of anesthesia should not go higher than T4, the nipple line, in children.

▶ *Take* NOTE!

The combination of meperidine (Demerol), promethazine (Phenergan), and chlorpromazine (Thorazine), commonly called DPT, is no longer recommended because it has been shown to cause excessive depression of the central nervous system. In addition, chlorpromazine increases the risk of meperidine toxicity, compounding the risk of severe respiratory depression. Promethazine causes extrapyramidal reactions. The combination also must be administered intramuscularly, which causes the child to experience more pain.

Conscious sedation is used for procedures that are painful and stressful. Therefore, the route of administering the medications for sedation should follow the guide-

BOX 35.2 **Oral Forms of Midazolam and Fentanyl**

Two of the most commonly used agents for conscious sedation are midazolam and fentanyl. Each of these is available in an oral form, which promotes atraumatic care.

Oral midazolam syrup
- Clear purplish-red cherry-flavored syrup
- Syrup containing 2 mg/mL
- Recommended dosage: 0.25 to 0.5 mg/kg to a maximum dose of 20 mg
- Action usually within 10 to 20 minutes
- Major adverse effects: respiratory depression and arrest

Fentanyl Oralet
- Oral transmucosal formulation
- Candy-type lozenge on a plastic holder
- Available in 200, 300, and 400 mg
- Recommended dose: 5 to 15 mcg/kg
- Not recommended for use in children weighing less than 15 kg
- Onset of action in about 15 minutes of sucking lozenge; duration of action approximately 1 hour

lines of atraumatic care. Oral, topical, or an existing intravenous route should be used. For example, conscious sedation is suggested instead of restraints, especially for toddlers and preschool children who are undergoing frightening or invasive procedures and who are manifesting extreme anxiety and behavioral upset. Other indications include situations involving:

- Evidence that the child is experiencing a heightened stress reaction—attempting to flee, crying inconsolably, or flailing
- Verbalization by the child that he or she is frightened and does not want to be touched
- Inability to remain immobilized, such as during laceration repair or computed tomography
- Any procedure that is painful and fear-provoking

Personnel administering conscious sedation must be specially trained, and emergency equipment and medications must be readily available.

The Nurse's Role in Pharmacologic Pain Intervention

The nurse plays a major role in providing pharmacologic pain relief. As with any medication, the nurse is responsible for adhering to the five rights of medication administration: right drug, right dose, right route, right time, and right patient. In addition, the nurse also adheres to three additional rights: the right of the child and parents to be educated; the right of the child to refuse the

medication; and the right documentation. The nurse also must have a solid knowledge base about the medications used for pain relief. This knowledge includes information about the drug's pharmacokinetics (absorption, distribution, metabolism, and excretion) and pharmacodynamics (mechanism of action, including adverse effects).

Assessment is crucial when pharmacologic pain interventions are used. An initial assessment of pain provides a baseline from which options for relief can be chosen. Factors that can affect the choice of analgesic, such as the child's age, pain intensity, physiologic status, or previous experiences with pain, also need to be considered. The nurse acts as an advocate for the child and the family to ensure that the most appropriate pharmacologic agent is chosen for the situation.

Assessment is ongoing once the agent is administered. The nurse must monitor physiologic parameters such as level of consciousness, vital signs, oxygen saturation levels, and urinary output for changes that might indicate an adverse reaction to the agent. More intensive monitoring is needed when agents are administered intravenously or epidurally or by conscious sedation. For example, if the child is receiving conscious sedation, interventions include:

- Ensuring that emergency equipment is readily available
- Maintaining a patent airway
- Monitoring the child's level of consciousness and responsiveness
- Assessing the child's vital signs (especially pulse rate, heart rate, blood pressure, and respiratory rate)
- Monitoring oxygen saturation levels

Typically, a specially trained health care provider is specifically designated to perform these activities during the administration of the sedation. Afterwards, the nurse is responsible for ongoing monitoring of the child's status.

Monitor the child closely for evidence of adverse effects. Table 35.8 describes the interventions useful for responding to these adverse effects. Be alert for signs and symptoms of respiratory depression secondary to opioid administration. Have an opioid antagonist such as naloxone (Narcan) and the benzodiazepine antagonist flumazenil (Romazicon) readily available should the child experience respiratory depression.

In addition to assessing physiologic parameters, the nurse must assess the child's and parents' emotional status before and after the agent is administered. For example, increased anxiety and fear may necessitate a change in method of administration, such as topical application instead of an intradermal injection of a local anesthetic. Nonpharmacologic methods may be employed to help lessen anxiety, thereby promoting more effective relief from the drug.

Nurses also are responsible for ensuring that the child and parents are adequately prepared for the use of the pharmacologic agent. The nurse educates the child and

TABLE 35.8 INTERVENTIONS FOR COMMON OPIOID-INDUCED ADVERSE EFFECTS

Adverse Effect	Nursing Interventions
Constipation	Encourage fluid intake unless contraindicated. Ensure intake of high-fiber foods, including fruits, if allowed. Encourage activity, including ambulation if possible. Obtain order for stool softener. Administer laxative as ordered.
Pruritus	Apply cool compresses and lotions. Administer antihistamine as ordered.
Nausea and vomiting	Inform child and parents that these symptoms usually subside in 1 to 2 days. Encourage small frequent meals with bland foods. Administer antiemetic if ordered.

parents about the drug, why it is being used, its intended effects, and possible adverse effects, tailoring the teaching to the child's cognitive level. Provide opportunities for the child and parents to ask questions, offering support and guidance throughout the experience. Provide a demonstration or use visual aids so that the child and parents know exactly what to expect. Encourage the use of play to help the child express fears and anxieties related to the administration.

Management of Procedure-Related Pain

One of the most common causes of pain in children is procedure-related pain. The procedure may be minor, such as an intramuscular injection, heelstick, or venipuncture, or it may be more involved, such as lumbar puncture, bone marrow aspiration, or wound care. Regardless, pain is real for children and painful procedures are often extremely distressing to them. Variables that affect pain include the intensity or length of the procedure and the skill of the health care provider performing the procedure.

The Nurse's Role in Managing Procedure-Related Pain

Through the use of behavioral and pharmacologic approaches, nurses can significantly reduce the pain and distress of procedures. The guiding principle is the provision of atraumatic care to the child, which includes the following:

- Using topical EMLA, iontophoretic lidocaine, vapocoolant spray, or buffered lidocaine at the intended site of a skin or vessel puncture
- Incorporating the use of nonpharmacologic strategies for pain relief in conjunction with pharmacologic methods
- Preparing the child and parents ahead of time about the procedure and then keeping all equipment out of site until it is ready to be used

- Using therapeutic hugging (see Chapter 32) to secure the child
- Using the smallest-gauge needle possible or an automated lancet device to puncture the skin
- Using an intermittent infusion device or peripherally inserted central catheter (PICC) if multiple or repeated blood samples are necessary; coordinating care so that several tests can be performed from one sample if possible
- Opting for venipuncture in newborns instead of heelsticks if the amount of blood needed would require much squeezing
- Using kangaroo care (skin-to-skin contact) for newborns before and after heelstick
- Providing nonnutritive sucking with sucrose solution for newborns several minutes before the procedure (Lefrak, Burch, Caravantes, et al., 2006).

▶ *Take* NOTE!

Individualize interventions based on the painfulness of the procedure and the child's developmental age and personality. Use behavioral-cognitive approaches and pharmacologic interventions. For example, encouraging the school-age child to assist during painful procedures in age-appropriate ways may actually help ease some of the pain related to a heightened state of anxiety, or at least assist the child in coping with the situation. Always use appropriate pharmacologic treatment for the first procedure to provide a painless experience for the child.

Nursing care for the child with procedure-related pain includes the child as well as the parents. Be sure to prepare them for the procedure using an appropriate developmental approach. Promote environmental comfort, too. Ensure that the child's privacy is maintained and that the lighting is adequate for the procedure but not so bright as to cause the child discomfort.

Painful procedures performed in the child's room can lead to an association of pain or fear with the room or bed. Many hospitals have a special treatment room where procedures can be performed. These rooms are usually equipped with many activities, toys, and decorations to help distract the child. The use of a treatment room may not be feasible or desirable in all situations or for all procedures. The ultimate goal is to do what is best for the child; therefore, the nurse needs to consider the needs of the child, the demands of the procedures, and the conditions that would facilitate the best outcome.

Unless contraindicated, encourage the parents to be present before, during, and after the procedure to provide comforting support to the child. Also encourage the child and parents to use nonpharmacologic methods to help maximize pain relief and reduce anxiety. For example, nonpharmacologic methods that are helpful for the toddler and preschooler may include positioning the child on the lap and hugging the child, distracting the child with toys or interactive books, and blowing bubbles.

Play therapy can be useful when preparing children for painful procedures. Encourage children to make decisions about their care related to pain management if their condition or procedure allows. It is also helpful to anticipate and recognize painful situations and provide pain medication before the actual procedure to ensure comfort. Many nonpharmacologic strategies can be enhanced and better implemented with the help of the child life specialist or play therapist, who have specialized training in these techniques.

*R*ecall Aiden from the beginning of the chapter. What are some interventions that may be helpful prior to, during, and after his dressing change?

Management of Chronic Pain

Typically, pain in children is acute pain, but chronic pain is a significant problem in the pediatric population, affecting approximately 15% to 20% of children (American Pain Society, 2006). Historically, chronic pain was defined by the duration of the pain, such as longer than 3 to 6 months. However, research has identified elements associated with chronic pain as occurring much earlier in time. Currently, chronic pain is identified as the complex interplay of biologic, psychological, and environmental factors. According to the American Pain Society, children with chronic pain and their families experience significant emotional and social consequences from the pain and disability; also, the experience of chronic pain in childhood may predispose the individual to chronic pain in adulthood.

The Nurse's Role in Managing Chronic Pain

The nurse's role in managing chronic pain in children is similar to that for the child experiencing acute pain or procedure-related pain. Assessment of the child's pain is key and should include a history of the present problem. Questions should focus on the onset of the pain, its intensity, duration, and location, and any factors that alleviate or exacerbate it. In addition, the nurse needs to question the child and parents about the impact of the pain on the child's daily life, such as sleep, play, eating, school, and interactions with peers, other family members, and friends. Impact on the family's life also is addressed.

Another key area of assessment is determining how the pain affects the child's and family's level of stress. Areas to address include the child's and parents' feelings of hopelessness, anxiety, and depression. Also question the child and parents about what they think has caused the pain and how they have coped with it. In addition, ascertain what methods the child and parents have used to alleviate the pain and the success of these methods. Inquire about any home remedies or alternative therapies that may have been used.

Review past physical examination findings for clues to the underlying problem. Observe the child's overall appearance, gait, and posture. Assess the child's cognitive level and emotional response, especially related to the experience of pain. Expect to complete a neurologic examination and observe for muscle spasms, trigger points, and increased sensitivity to light touch. Abnormal body postures assumed by the child due to chronic pain may result in the development of secondary pain in the muscles and fascia. When children tense their muscles due to fear of examination, somatic pain may occur.

Various nonpharmacologic and pharmacologic strategies are used to manage chronic pain. Often multiple strategies are combined to address pain relief as well as the pain's impact on other areas, such as sleep or school functioning. When pharmacologic agents are used, the oral form is the method of choice. As with any pain management strategy, education of the child and family is paramount. A referral to a pediatric pain specialist may be needed if the child's pain is not controlled effectively.

■■■ Key Concepts

- Pain is a highly individualized subjective experience affecting persons of any age. It is a universal experience and is considered the fifth vital sign.

- Pain management is a critical element in a child's plan of care because children may lack the verbal capacity to describe their pain experience, caregivers and health care providers often have misconceptions about pain, assessment of the complex nature of the pain experience is difficult, and available resources and research related to pain relief strategies in children are limited.

■ The sensation of pain involves a sequence of physiologic events: transduction, transmission, perception, and modulation

■ Pain can be classified by duration as acute or chronic, by etiology as nociceptive or neuropathic, or by source or location as somatic or visceral.

■ Factors influencing a child's perception of pain include age and gender, cognitive level, temperament, previous pain experiences, and family and cultural background, all of which cannot be changed. Situational factors involve behavioral, cognitive, and emotional aspects and can be changed.

■ Infants, including preterm infants, experience pain. Behavioral and physiologic indicators are used to assess pain. Toddlers commonly react with intense emotional upset and physical resistance or aggression. Preschoolers may feel that pain is a punishment for misbehaving or having bad thoughts. School-age children can communicate the type, location, and severity of pain but may deny having pain to appear brave or avoid further pain. Adolescents, with their focus on body image and fear of loss of control, often ask numerous questions and may attempt to remain stoic to avoid being viewed as childish.

■ Assessment of pain in children includes both subjective and objective data. Nurses need to tailor the assessment to the child's developmental level and ask appropriate questions geared to the child's cognitive level. Parental questioning during the health history also is important.

■ Self-report pain rating scales are valuable assessment tools that allow the child's level of pain to be quantified. Examples include the FACES pain rating scale, the Oucher pain rating scale, the poker chip tool, the word-graphic rating scale, visual analog and numeric scales, and the Adolescent Pediatric Pain Tool.

■ Different pain rating scales are appropriate for different developmental levels. However, children may regress when in pain, so a simpler tool may be needed to make sure that the child understands what is being asked. Consistency in using the same tool is essential so that appropriate comparisons can be made and effective interventions can be planned and implemented.

■ Physical examination of the child for pain primarily involves the skills of observation and inspection. These skills are used to assess for physiologic and behavioral changes that indicate pain. Auscultation also may be used to assess for changes in vital signs, specifically heart rate and blood pressure. Physiologic and behavioral pain assessment tools, such as the Neonatal Infant Pain Scale, Riley Infant Pain Scale, Pain Observation Scale for Young Children, the CRIES Scale for Neonatal Postoperative Pain Assessment, and the FLACC Behavioral Scale for Postoperative Pain in Young Children, measure specific parameters and changes that would indicate that the child is in pain.

■ Nonpharmacologic pain management strategies aim to assist children in coping with pain and to give them a sense of mastery or control over the situation. These strategies may be categorized as behavioral-cognitive, in which the child focuses on a specific area or aspect rather than the pain (e.g., relaxation, distraction, imagery, biofeedback, thought stopping, and positive self-talk), or biophysical, in which the focus is on interfering with the transmission of pain impulses reaching the brain (e.g., heat and cold applications, massage and pressure).

■ The nurse plays a major role in teaching the child and family about available nonpharmacologic pain interventions, helping them choose the most appropriate and most effective methods, and ensuring that the child and parents use the method before the pain occurs as well as before it increases.

■ Pharmacologic interventions involve the administration of drugs for pain relief, most commonly nonopioids and opioid analgesics. The selection of the method is determined by the drug being administered, the child's status, the type, intensity, and location of the pain, and any factors that may be influencing the child's pain. The preferred methods for administering analgesics include the oral, rectal, intravenous, or local nerve block routes, epidural administration, and conscious sedation.

■ Nonopioid analgesics used to treat mild to moderate pain include acetaminophen and nonsteroidal anti-inflammatory drugs (NSAIDs) such as ibuprofen, ketorolac, naproxen, and less commonly indomethacin, diclofenac, and piroxicam.

■ Morphine is considered the "gold standard" for all opioid agonists; it is the drug to which all other opioids are compared and is usually the drug of choice for severe pain.

■ Local anesthetics are commonly used to provide analgesia for procedures. They are effective in providing successful pain relief with only minimal risk of systemic adverse effects. The first choice for the most effective, painless local anesthesia is EMLA (eutectic mixture of local anesthetics [lidocaine and prilocaine]). It achieves anesthesia to a depth of 2 to 4 mm, so it reduces pain of phlebotomy, venous cannulation, and intramuscular injections up to 24 hours after injection.

■ Epidural analgesia involves the insertion of a catheter into the epidural space through which drugs can be administered as bolus injections (a one-time bolus or on an intermittent schedule), as a continuous infusion, or as PCA. Usually an opioid, such as morphine, fentanyl, or hydromorphone, is given in conjunction with a long-acting local anesthetic, such as bupivacaine.

■ Conscious sedation is a medically controlled state of depressed consciousness that allows protective reflexes to be maintained so the child has the ability to maintain a patent airway and respond to physical or verbal stimulation.

- When providing pharmacologic pain relief, the nurse must adhere to the five rights of medication administration and have a solid knowledge base about the medications used for pain relief and the drug's pharmacokinetics (absorption, distribution, metabolism, and excretion) and pharmacodynamics (mechanism of action, including adverse effects). Initial and ongoing assessment is crucial.
- The principles of atraumatic care guide nursing interventions for providing pain relief, especially for procedure-related pain.
- Chronic pain in children can significantly affect the child's daily life and activities as well as the family's life.

REFERENCES

Algren, C. (2005). Family-centered care of the child during illness and hospitalization. In M. Hockenberry, *Wong's essentials of pediatric nursing* (7th ed., pp. 637–705). Philadelphia: Elsevier/Mosby.

American Academy of Pediatrics and American Pain Society. (2001). The assessment and management of acute pain in infants, children, and adolescents. *Pediatrics, 108*(3), 793–797.

American Academy of Pediatrics and American Pain Society. (2001). Policy statement: The assessment and management of acute pain in infants, children, and adolescents (0793). *Pediatrics, 105*, 454–461.

American Academy of Pediatrics and Canadian Paediatric Society. (2006). Prevention and management of pain in the Neonate: An update. *Pediatrics, 118*(5), 2231–2240.

American Medical Association. (2006). *AMA pain management: Pediatric pain management (continuing medical education).* Retrieved 9/5/06 from http://www.ama-cmeonline.com/pain_mgmt/module06/01cme/02_01.htm.

American Pain Society. (1995). *Pain: The fifth vital sign.* Los Angeles: American Pain Society.

American Pain Society. (2006). *Pain: Current understanding of assessment, management, and treatments.* APS/National Pharmaceutical Council. Available at http://www.ampainsoc.org/ce/enduring.htm. Accessed 7/6/06.

American Pain Society. (2006). *Pediatric chronic pain. A position statement.* Retrieved on February 3, 2008 at http://www.ampainsoc.org/advocacy/pediatric.htm.

American Society for Pain Management Nursing Position Statement. (2006). Authorized and unauthorized ("PCA by proxy") dosing of analgesic infusion pumps. Retrieved on January 28, 2008 at http://www.aspmn.org/Organization/documents/PCAbyProxy-final-EW_004.pdf.

Baker, C. M. & Wong, D. L. (1987). Q.U.E.S.T.: A process of pain assessment in children. *Orthopaedic Nursing, 6*(1), 11–21.

Beal, J. A. (2005). Evidence for best practices in the neonatal period. *MCN, 30*(6), 397–403.

Behrman, R. E., Kliegman, R. M., & Jenson, H. B. (2004). *Nelson's essentials of pediatrics* (17th ed.). Philadelphia: W. B. Saunders.

Blount, R. L., Piira, T., Cohen, L. L., & Cheng, P. S. (2006). Pediatric procedural pain [Electronic Version]. *Behavior Modification, 30*(1), 24–49.

Boelen-van der Loo, W. J. C., Scheffer, E., de Haan, R. J., & de Groot, C. J. (1999). Clinimetric evaluation of the pain observation scale for young children in children aged between 1 and 4 years after ear, nose, and throat surgery. *Developmental and Behavioral Pediatrics, 20*(4), 222–227.

Britt, R. B. (2005). Using EMLA cream before venipuncture [Electronic Version]. *Nursing2005, 35*(1), 17.

Broome, M. E., & Huth, M. M. (2003). Nursing management of the child in pain. In N. L. Schecter, C. B. Berde, & M. Yaster, *Pain in infants, children, and adolescents* (2d ed., pp. 417–433). Philadelphia: Lippincott Williams & Wilkins.

Byers, J. F., & Thornley, K. (2004). Cueing in to infant pain. *MCN, 29*(2), 84–91.

Cohen, R., & Smetzer, J. (2005). Patient-controlled analgesia safety issues [Electronic version]. *Journal of Pain & Palliative Care Pharmacotherapy, 19*(1), 45–50.

Crandall, M., & Savedra, M. (2005). Multidimensional assessment using the adolescent pediatric pain tool: A case report. *Journal for Specialists in Pediatric Nursing, 10*(3), 115–123.

D'Arcy, Y. (2007). Patient safety issues with patient-controlled analgesia. *Topics in Advanced Practice Nursing eJournal.* Retrieved on January 27, 2008 at http://www.medscape.com/viewarticle/557394_1.

Dlugosz, C. K., Chater, R. W., & Engle, J. P. (2006). Appropriate use of nonprescription analgesics in pediatric patients [Electronic Version]. *Journal of Pediatric Health Care, 20*(5), 316–325.

Gerik, S. M. (2005). Pain management in children: Developmental considerations and mind-body therapies [Electronic Version]. *Southern Medical Journal, 98*(3), 295–302.

Hockenberry, M. J., Wilson, D., & Winkelstein, M. L. (2005). *Wong's essentials of pediatric nursing* (7th ed., p. 1259). St. Louis: Mosby.

Hom, J. & Burg, J. (2008). Pediatrics, sedation. *eMedicine.* Retrieved on January 29, 2008 at http://www.emedicine.com/EMERG/topic403.htm.

International Association for the Study of Pain. (2007). *IASP pain terminology.* Retrieved April 4, 2007 from http://www.iasp-pain.org/AM/Template.cfm?Section=General_Resource_Links&Template=/CM/HTMLDisplay.cfm&ContentID=3058#Pain.

International Association for the Study of Pain. (2005). Why children's pain matters. *Pain Clinical Updates, 13*(4). Retrieved on February 3, 2008 at http://www.iasp-pain.org/AM/Template.cfm?Section=Resources1&Template=/CM/HTMLDisplay.cfm&ContentID=2946.

Johnston, C. C., Stevens, B. J., Boyer, K., & Porter, F. L. (2003). Development of psychologic responses to pain and assessment of pain in infants and toddlers. In N. L. Schecter, C. B. Berde, & M. Yaster, *Pain in infants, children, and adolescents* (2d ed., pp. 105–127). Philadelphia: Lippincott Williams & Wilkins.

Joint Commission on Accreditation of Healthcare Organizations. (2004). Sentinel event alert. Patient controlled analgesia by proxy. Retrieved on January 27, 2008 at www.jointcommission.org/sentinelevents/sentineleventalert.

Krechel, S. W., & Bildner, J. (1995). CRIES: A new neonatal postoperative pain measurement score. Initial testing of validity and reliability. *Paediatric Anaesthesia, 5*, 53–61.

Lawrence, J., Alcock, D., McGrath, P., Kay, J., MacMurray, S. B., & Dulberg, C. (1993). The development of a tool to assess neonatal pain. *Neonatal Network, 12*(6), 59–66.

Lefrak, K., Burch, R., Caravantes, K., Knoerlein, N., DeNolf, J., Duncan, F.; Hampton, C., Johnston, D., Lockey, C. M.-W. RN, et al. (2006). Sucrose analgesia: Identifying potentially better practices [Electronic Version]. *Pediatrics, 118*(Supplement, 2), S197–S202.

Manworren, R. C. B., & Hynan, L. S. (2003). Clinical validation of FLACC: Preverbal patient pain scale. *Pediatric Nursing, 29*(2).

Maunuksela, E., & Olkkola, K. T. (2003). Nonsteroidal anti-inflammatory drugs in pediatric pain management. In N. L. Schecter, C. B. Berde, & M. Yaster, *Pain in infants, children, and adolescents* (2d ed., pp. 171–180). Philadelphia: Lippincott Williams & Wilkins.

McCaffery, M., & Pasero, C. (1999). *Pain: A clinical manual* (2d ed.). St. Louis: Mosby.

McCarthy, A. M., & Kleiber, C. (2006). A conceptual model of factors influencing children's responses to a painful procedure when parents are distraction coaches. *Journal of Pediatric Nursing, 21*(2), 88–98.

McGrath, P. A. (2005). Children—not simply "little adults." In H. Merskey, J. D. Loeser, R. Dubner (Eds.), *The paths of pain 1975–2005* (pp. 433–446). Seattle: IASP Press.

McGrath, P. A., & Hillier, L. M. (2003). Modifying the psychologic factors that intensify children's pain and prolong disability. In N. L. Schecter, C. B. Berde, & M. Yaster, *Pain in infants, children, and adolescents* (2d ed., pp. 85–104). Philadelphia: Lippincott Williams & Wilkins.

Merkel, S. (2006). Use of patient-controlled analgesia in pediatrics. *US Special Populations*, 77–78. Retrieved on January 28, 2008 at http://www.touchbriefings.com/pdf/2032/Merkel.pdf.

Merkel, S. I., Voepel-Lewis, T., Shayevitz, J. R., & Malviya, S. (1997). The FLACC: A behavioral scale for scoring postoperative pain in young children. *Pediatric Nursing, 23*(3), 293–297.

Morash, D., & Fowler, K. (2004). An evidence-based approach to changing practice: Using sucrose for infant analgesia. *Journal of Pediatric Nursing, 19*(5), 366–370.

National Association of Neonatal Nurses. (2006). *Position statement #3019: Pain management in infants.* Retrieved 9/1/06 from http://www.nann.org/i4a/pages/index.cfm?pageid=79

National Library of Medicine. (2006). Table 2, pain assessment tools, the word-graphic rating scale. In *Health services/technology assessment text.* Retrieved 9/10/06 from http://www.ncbi.nlm.nih.gov/books/bv.fcgi?rid=hstat6.section.32536.

O'Rourke, D. (2004). The measurement of pain in infants, children, and adolescents: From policy to practice. *Physical Therapy, 84*(6), 560–570.

Paice, J. A., Noskin, G. A., Vanagunas, A., & Shott, S. (2005). Efficacy and safety of scheduled dosing of opioid analgesic: A quality improvement study. *Journal of Pain, 6*(10), 639–643.

Palermo, T. M. & Kiska, R. (2005). Subjective sleep disturbances in adolescents with chronic pain: Relationship to daily functioning and quality of life. *Journal of Pain, 6*(3), 201–207.

Porth, C. M. (2004). *Pathophysiology: concepts of altered health states* (7th ed.). Philadelphia: Lippincott Williams & Wilkins.

Razmus, I. S., Daltom, M. E., & Wilson, D. (2004). Pain management for newborn circumcision. *Pediatric Nursing, 30*(5), 414–417, 427.

Rogers, T. L. & Ostrow, C. L. (2004). The use of EMLA cream to decrease venipuncture pain in children [Electronic Version]. *Journal of Pediatric Nursing, 19*(1), 33–39.

Schade, J. G., Joyce, B. A., Gerkensmeyer, J., & Keck, J. F. (1996). Comparison of three preverbal scales for postoperative pain assessment in a diverse pediatric sample. *Journal of Pain and Symptom Management, 12*(6), 348–359.

Taddio, A., Soin, H. K., Schuh, S., Koren, G., & Scolnik, D. (2005). Liposomal lidocaine to improve procedural success rates and reduce procedural pain among children: A randomized controlled trial. *Canadian Medical Association Journal, 172*(13), 1691–1695.

Taketokmo, C. K., Hodding, J. H., & Kraus, D. M. (2005). *Lexi-comp's pediatric dosage handbook* (12th ed.). Hudson, OH: Lexi-comp.

Tesler, M. D., Savedra, M. C., Holzemer, W. L., Wilkie, D. J., Ward, J. A., & Paul, S. M. (1991). The word-graphic rating scale as a measure of children's and adolescent's pain intensity. *Research in Nursing and Health, 14*(5), 361–361.

UCLA Pediatric Update. (2006). Multiple modalities relieve chronic pain in children. *Mattel Children's Hospital at UCLA, 13*(1). Retrieved on January 29, 2008 at http://www.uclahealth.org/body.cfm?xyzpdqabc=0&id=122&action=detail&ref=5.1

VanHulle, V. C. (2005). Nurses' knowledge, attitudes, & practices regarding children's pain. *American Journal of Maternal Child Nursing, 30,* 177–183.

von Baeyer, C. L., Marche, T. A., Rocha, E. M., & Salmon, K. (2004). Children's memory for pain: Overview and implications for practice. *Journal of Pain, 5*(5), 241–249.

Willis, M. H. W., Merkel, S. I., Voepel-Lewis, T., & Malviya, S. (2002). FLACC behavioral pain assessment scale: A comparison with the child's self-report. *Pediatric Nursing, 29*(3), 195–198.

Windich-Biermeier, A., Sjoberg, I., Dale, J. C., Eshelman, D., & Guzzetta, C. E. (2007). Effects of distraction on pain, fear, and distress during venous port access and venipuncture in children and adolescents with cancer. *Journal of Pediatric Oncology Nursing, 24*(1), 8–19.

World Health Organization (2006). WHO's pain ladder. Available at: http://www.who.int/cancer/palliative/painladder/en/. Accessed 7/23/06.

Yaster, M., Kost-Byerly, S., & Maxwell, L. G. (2003). Opioid agonists and antagonists. In N. L. Schecter, C. B. Berde, & M. Yaster, *Pain in infants, children, and adolescents* (2d ed., pp. 181–224). Philadelphia: Lippincott Williams & Wilkins.

Young, K. (2005). Pediatric procedural pain. *Annals of Emergency Medicine, 45*(2), 160–171.

WEBSITES

Agency for Healthcare Research and Quality: www.ahrq.gov/clinic/
American Academy of Pediatrics: www.aap.org
American Pain Foundation: www.painfoundation.org
American Pain Society: www.ampainsoc.org
Canadian Pain Society: www.canadianpainsociety.ca
Children's Hospice International: www.chionline.org
City of Hope Pain/Palliative Care Resource Center: http://www.mayday.coh.org
International Association for the Study of Pain (IASP): www.iasp-pain.org
Kids Health: www.kidshealth.org
National Association of Pediatric Nurse Associates and Practitioners: www.napnap.org
National Association of Children's Hospitals and Related Institutions: www.childrenshospitals.net
Society of Pediatric Nurses: www.pedsnurses.org
Virtual Pediatric Hospital: www.virtualpediatrichospital.org
National Association of Neonatal Nurses: www.nann.org

CHAPTER WORKSHEET

MULTIPLE CHOICE QUESTIONS

1. The nurse is preparing to assess the pain of a 3-year-old child who had surgery the day before. Which pain rating scale would be most appropriate for the nurse to use?

    a. FACES Pain Rating Scale

    b. Poker chip tool

    c. Word-graphic rating scale

    d. Visual analog scale

2. When developing the plan of care for a child in pain, the nurse identifies appropriate strategies aimed at modifying which factors influencing pain?

    a. Gender

    b. Cognitive level

    c. Previous pain experiences

    d. Anticipatory anxiety

3. An adolescent who is a competitive swimmer comes to the emergency department complaining of localized aching pain in his shoulder. He states, "I've been practicing really hard and long to get myself ready for my meet this weekend." The area is tender to the touch. The nurse determines that the adolescent is most likely experiencing which type of pain?

    a. Cutaneous pain

    b. Deep somatic pain

    c. Visceral pain

    d. Neuropathic pain

4. After teaching a child's parents about the different methods of distraction that can be used for pain management, which statement by the parents indicates a need for additional teaching?

    a. "We'll have her focus on her hand and count each finger slowly."

    b. "We'll read some of her favorite stories to her."

    c. "We'll have her imagine that she's at the beach this summer."

    d. "She likes to play video games, so we'll bring in some from home."

5. A child is scheduled for a bone marrow aspiration at 4 p.m. The nurse would plan to apply EMLA cream to the intended site at which time?

    a. 1:30 p.m.

    b. 3:00 p.m.

    c. 3:30 p.m.

    d. 4:00 p.m.

CRITICAL THINKING EXERCISES

1. The nurse asks a 12-year-old girl if she is having pain. She denies pain, even though she is lying on her left side holding her abdomen with her knees flexed up to it. What might be some underlying factors leading the child to deny her pain? How would the nurse go about assessing this child's pain?

2. The nurse comes into the room of a 6-year-old who is sleeping. His mother states, "He's asleep, so he's not in pain." How should the nurse respond?

3. A child who is receiving ibuprofen is experiencing increased pain. The dosage of ibuprofen is increased but is no longer effective in providing adequate pain relief. What is occurring? What would be most likely to happen next?

STUDY ACTIVITIES

1. Interview nurses who work on a pediatric unit about their experiences with managing pain in children. Ask them how they assess pain in children and the major methods they use to assist the children in managing their pain.

2. Interview families of children with chronic illnesses who deal with pain. Ask the parents how they assess their children's pain level and what methods they have used in assisting their children in managing pain.

3. Compare and contrast the drugs fentanyl and midazolam when used for conscious sedation in terms of onset of action, duration, primary effects, and antidotes.

4. A child is receiving epidural analgesia with morphine. The nurse would be alert for which of the following adverse effects? Select all that apply.

    _____ a. Respiratory depression

    _____ b. Pruritus

    _____ c. Constipation

    _____ d. Vomiting

    _____ e. Amnesia

    _____ f. Hematoma

UNIT ELEVEN

NURSING CARE OF THE CHILD WITH A HEALTH DISORDER

NURSING CARE OF THE CHILD WITH AN INFECTIOUS OR COMMUNICABLE DISORDER

KEY TERMS

antigen
antibody
chain of infection

communicability
endogenous pyrogens
exanthem

fomite
pathogen
phagocytosis

LEARNING OBJECTIVES

Upon completion of the chapter, the learner will be able to:

1. Discuss anatomic and physiologic differences in children versus adults in relation to the infectious process.
2. Identify nursing interventions related to common laboratory and diagnostic tests used in the diagnosis and management of infectious conditions.
3. Identify appropriate nursing assessments and interventions related to medications and treatments for childhood infectious and communicable disorders.
4. Distinguish various infectious illnesses occurring in childhood.
5. Devise an individualized nursing care plan for the child with an infectious or communicable disorder.
6. Develop client/family teaching plans for the child with an infectious or communicable disorder.

*S*amuel Goldberg, 3 months old, is brought to the clinic by his mother. He presents with a history of fever and nasal congestion. His mother tells you, "He's been very irritable and crying more than usual."

Wow

Complete and lasting freedom from infectious disease remains a dream, but one worth fighting a hard battle for.

Infectious and communicable diseases are the leading cause of death worldwide, and their incidence is increasing in the United States (National Center for Infectious Diseases, 2003). They can lead to serious illness in children and significantly affect the lives of these children and their families. They include bacterial infections (e.g., sepsis), viral infections (e.g., viral exanthems and rabies), and parasitic infections (e.g., roundworm and pediculosis capitis [head lice]). Sexually transmitted infections such as chlamydia and gonorrhea are discussed in Chapter 5.

There has been a dramatic decrease in the incidence and severity of infections and communicable diseases since the advent of vaccines, antibiotics, antiviral drugs, and antitoxins. Some diseases have been effectively controlled, but the vast majority will not be eliminated. New diseases emerge and old diseases are reappearing, sometimes in a drug-resistant form. The Centers for Disease Control & Prevention (CDC) tracks certain infectious diseases. This list of nationally reportable diseases is revised periodically to add new pathogens or remove diseases as their incidence declines. Reporting by the states to the CDC is voluntary, so slight variations exist from state to state. Box 36.1 lists nationally reportable diseases.

Nurses, particularly those working in schools, childcare centers, and outpatient settings, are often the first to see the signs of infectious or communicable diseases in children. These signs are often vague at first, consisting of a sore throat or rash. Therefore, nurses must have accurate assessment skills and be familiar with the signs and symptoms of these common childhood diseases so that they can provide prompt recognition, treatment, and guidance and support to families. Identifying the infectious agent is of primary importance to prevent further spread.

Many infectious diseases can be prevented through simple and inexpensive methods such as handwashing, adequate immunization, proper handling and preparation of food, and judicious antibiotic use. Nurses play a key role in educating parents and the community on ways to prevent infectious and communicable diseases.

Infectious Process

Infection occurs when an organism enters the body and multiplies, causing damage to the tissues and cells. The body's response to this damage due to infection or injury is inflammation. The body delivers fluid, blood, and nutrients to the area of infection or injury and attempts to eliminate the pathogens and repair the tissues. The body does this through vascular and cellular reactions. The vascular response is an initial period of vasoconstriction followed by vasodilatation. This vasodilatation allows for the increase of fluids, blood, and nutrients to the area.

The cellular response involves the arrival of white blood cells (WBCs) to the area. WBCs are the body's

---

BOX 36.1   Nationally Notifiable Diseases

- Chlamydia
- Diphtheria
- Ehrlichiosis
- Gonorrhea
- Lyme disease
- Malaria
- Measles
- Mumps
- Pertussis
- Poliomyelitis, paralytic
- Q fever
- Rabies
- Rocky Mountain spotted fever
- Rubella
- Streptococcal disease, invasive group A
- Syphilis
- Tetanus
- Varicella (morbidity)
- Varicella (deaths only)

For a complete list of nationally notifiable diseases in the United States, go to www.cdc.gov/epo/dphsi/phs/infdis2007r.htm.

HEALTHY PEOPLE 2010

Objective	Significance
Reduce or eliminate indigenous cases of vaccine-preventable diseases. Congenital rubella syndrome (children under age 1 year); diphtheria (persons under age 35 years); *Haemophilus influenzae* type b (children under age 5 years); hepatitis B (persons aged 2 to 18 years); measles (persons of all ages); mumps (persons of all ages); pertussis (children under age 7 years); polio (wild-type virus) (persons of all ages); rubella (persons of all ages); tetanus (persons under age 35); varicella (persons under age 18). Achieve and maintain effective vaccination coverage levels for universally recommended vaccines among young children	• Educate children and their families on the importance of proper immunizations. • Assess immunization status at every healthy encounter. • Provide families with a written record of immunizations given.

TABLE 36.1 FUNCTION OF WHITE BLOOD CELLS BY LEUKOCYTE TYPE

Cell	Cell's Function Is to Combat
Neutrophils (bands and segs)	Pyogenic infection (bacterial)
Eosinophils	Allergic disorders and parasitic infestations
Basophils	Parasitic infections, some allergic disorders
Lymphocytes	Viral infections (measles, rubella, chickenpox, infectious mononucleosis)
Monocytes	Severe infections, by phagocytosis

Source: Fischbach, 2004; adapted from p. 51.

defense against infection or injury. The types of WBCs are neutrophils, lymphocytes, basophils, eosinophils, and monocytes. Elevations in certain portions of the WBC count reflect different processes occurring in the body, such as infection, allergic reaction, or leukemia. Table 36.1 explains the function of each type of WBCs. Each type is generally present in a balanced state; the types are reported as a percentage of the total WBC count or as the number per certain volume of blood.

WBCs use **phagocytosis** to ingest and destroy the **pathogen**. If bacteria escape the action of phagocytosis, they enter the bloodstream and lymph system and the immune system is activated. With activation of the immune system, B lymphocytes (humoral immunity) and T lymphocytes (cell-mediated immunity) are matured and activated. B and T cells recognize and attack infectious pathogens. B cells, which mature in the bone marrow, produce specific antibodies to a specific offending **antigen** (a substance that the body recognizes as foreign). T cells, which mature in the thymus, attack the antigen directly. Once B and T cells have been exposed to an antigen, some cells will remember the antigen: thus, if the particular antigen invades again, the body will act more quickly.

Infection or inflammation caused by bacteria, viruses, or other pathogens stimulates the release of **endogenous pyrogens** (interleukins, tumor necrosis factor, and interferon), resulting in fever. The pyrogens act on the hypothalamus, where they trigger prostaglandin production and increase the body's temperature set point. This triggers the cold response, resulting in shivering, vasoconstriction, and a decrease in peripheral perfusion to help decrease heat loss and allow the body's temperature to rise to the new set point. Fever, defined as a temperature greater than 38°C (100.4°F), then occurs. Box 36.2 gives specific parameters for fever based on the measurement route.

Antipyretics are often used to lower fever and increase client comfort. They decrease the temperature set point by inhibiting the production of prostaglandins, leading to sweating and vasodilation and therefore heat loss and a drop in temperature.

It is important to distinguish between fever and hyperthermia. Hyperthermia occurs when normal thermoregu-

lation fails, resulting in an unregulated rise in core temperature. Hyperthermia may occur if the central nervous system of the child becomes impaired by disease, drugs, and abnormalities of heat production or thermal stressors, such as being left in a hot automobile or exertional heat stroke. In the absence of hyperthermia and in the normally neurologic child, the body does not allow fever to rise to lethal levels. The body actually produces a natural antipyretic, called cryogen. If there is no hyperthermic insult, it is rare to see a child's temperature rise to above 41.4°C (106°F) (Crocetti & Serwint, 2005).

Stages of Infectious Disease

Infectious diseases follow a similar pattern. They progress through certain stages (Table 36.2) in which **communicability** (ability to spread to others) can be predicted. It is important for nurses to understand these stages to help control and manage infectious diseases.

Chain of Infection

The **chain of infection** is the process by which an organism is spread. Behaviors of infants and young children, mainly pertaining to hygiene, increase their risk for infection by promoting the chain of infection. Poor hygiene habits, including lack of handwashing, placing toys and hands in the mouth, drooling, and leaking diapers, all can contribute to the spread of infection and communicable diseases. Table 36.3 reviews the chain of infection and nursing implications related to it.

BOX 36.2 **Definition of Fever by Measurement Route**

- Oral: >37.5°C (99.5°F)
- Rectal: >38°C (100.4°F)
- Axillary: >37.3°C (99.1°F)
- Tympanic: >38°C (100.4°F)

TABLE 36.2 **STAGES OF INFECTIOUS DISEASE**

Stage	Explanation
Incubation	Time from entrance of pathogen into the body to appearance of first symptoms; during this time, pathogens grow and multiply
Prodrome	Time from onset of nonspecific symptoms such as fever, malaise, and fatigue to more specific symptoms
Illness	Time during which client demonstrates signs and symptoms specific to an infection type
Convalescence	Time when acute symptoms of illness disappear

Preventing the Spread of Infection

Nurses play a key role in breaking the chain of infection and preventing the spread of diseases. Nurses must not only follow infection control and prevention practices but also educate parents and children on the measures they can take to prevent the spread of infection.

 ▶ *Take* NOTE!

Frequent handwashing is the most important way to prevent the spread of infection.

Isolation precautions help nurses break the chain of infection and provide strategies to prevent the spread of pathogens among hospitalized clients. Guidelines can be

TABLE 36.3 **CHAIN OF INFECTION**

Chain Link	Explanation	Nursing Implications

Infectious agent	Any agent capable of causing infection; examples: bacteria, viruses, rickettsiae, protozoa, and fungus	• Control or eliminate infectious agents through:
		  • Handwashing
		  • Wearing gloves
		  • Cleaning, disinfection, or sterilization of equipment

Reservoir	A place where the pathogen can thrive and reproduce; examples: human body, animals, insects, food, water, inanimate objects (e.g., stethoscopes)	• Control or eliminate reservoirs. • Control sources of body fluids, drainage, or solutions that may harbor pathogens. • Follow institutional guidelines for disposing of infectious wastes. • Provide proper wound care; change dressings or bandages when soiled. • Assist clients to carry out appropriate skin and oral care. • Keep linens clean and dry.
Portal of exit	A way for the pathogen to exit the reservoir; examples: skin and mucous membranes, respiratory tract, urinary tract, gastrointestinal tract, reproductive tract	• Control portals of exit and educate clients and families. • Cover mouth and nose when sneezing or coughing. • Avoid talking, coughing, or sneezing over open wounds or sterile fields. • Use personal protective equipment.
Modes of transmission	Direct transmission: body-to-body contact Indirect transmission: transferred by **fomite** or vector; spread by droplet or airborne transmission	• Wash hands before and after client contact, invasive procedures, or touching open wounds. • Use personal protective equipment when necessary. • Urge clients and family to wash hands frequently, especially before eating or handling food, after eliminating, and after touching infectious material.
Portal of entry	A way for the pathogen to enter the host; examples: skin and mucous membranes, respiratory tract, urinary tract, gastrointestinal tract, reproductive tract	• Use proper sterile technique during invasive procedures. • Provide appropriate wound care. • Dispose of needles and sharps in puncture-resistant containers. • Provide all clients with their own personal care items.
Susceptible host	Any person who cannot resist the pathogen	• Protect susceptible host by promoting normal body defenses against infection. • Maintain integrity of the client's skin and mucous membranes. • Protect normal defenses by regular bathing and oral care, adequate fluid intake and nutrition, proper immunization.

found on the CDC website (www.cdc.gov/ncidod/dhqp/gl_isolation.html). Additional guidelines are available from various infection control societies and regulatory agencies such as the Occupational Safety and Health Administration. Infection control standards have also been developed by the Joint Commission on Accreditation of Healthcare Organizations. This leads to an array of complex guidelines that all health professionals need to be familiar with.

The Hospital Infection Control Practices Advisory Committee (HICPAC) has presented guidelines for hospitalized clients that include two tiers. Tier 1 is standard precautions, which are designed for the care of all clients in the hospital regardless of their diagnosis. Tier 2 is transmission-based precautions, designed for clients who are known or suspected to be infected with epidemiologically important pathogens. These pathogens can be spread by airborne, droplet, or contact transmission. Box 36.3 gives an overview of standard and transmission-based precautions.

When caring for children, these guidelines may need to be modified. For instance, diaper changing is routine in the pediatric setting. Since it does not usually soil hands, it is not mandatory to wear gloves (except if gloves are required due to transmission-based precautions). According to the standard precaution guidelines, single rooms are required for those who are incontinent and cannot control bodily excretions. Since the majority of young children are incontinent, obviously this guideline is inappropriate in the pediatric setting. Pediatric units often have common rooms, such as playrooms and schoolrooms. Children placed on transmission-based isolation are not allowed to leave their rooms and therefore are not allowed to use these common rooms.

Variations in Pediatric Anatomy and Physiology

Normal immune function is an amazing protective response by the body. It involves complex responses including phagocytosis, humoral immunity, cellular immunity, and activation of the complement system. Blood and lymph are responsible for transporting the agents of the immune system. Due to the immature responses of the immune system, infants and young children are more susceptible to infection. The newborn displays a decreased inflammatory response to invading organisms, contributing to an increased risk for infection. Cellular immunity is generally functional at birth, and humoral immunity occurs when the body encounters and then develops immunity to new diseases. Since the infant has had limited exposure to disease and is losing the passive immunity acquired from maternal antibodies, the risk of infection is higher. Young children continue to have an increased risk for infection and communicable disorders because disease protection from immunizations is not complete. (Refer to Chapter 30 for further details.)

Common Medical Treatments

A variety of medications and other medical treatments are used to treat infectious disorders in children. Most of these treatments will require a physician's order when the child is in the hospital. The most common treatments and medications are listed in Common Medical Treatments 36.1 and Drug Guide 36.1. The nurse caring for the child with an infectious disorder should be familiar with what the procedures are, how they work, and common nursing implications related to use of these modalities.

NURSING PROCESS OVERVIEW FOR THE CHILD WITH A COMMUNICABLE DISORDER

Care of the child with an infectious disorder includes assessment, nursing diagnosis, planning, interventions, and evaluation. There are a number of general concepts related to the nursing process that may be applied to the care of children with infectious disorders. From a general understanding of the care involved for a child with an infectious disorder, the nurse can then individualize the care based on the client's specifics.

Remember Samuel, the 3-month-old with fever, congestion, and irritability? What additional health history and physical examination assessment information should you obtain?

Assessment

Assessment of the child with a communicable or infectious disorder includes health history, physical examination, and laboratory and diagnostic testing.

Health History

The health history comprises past medical history, including the mother's pregnancy history, family history, and history of present illness (when the symptoms started and how they have progressed), as well as treatments used at home. The past medical history might be significant for lack of recommended immunizations, prematurity, maternal infection during pregnancy or labor, prolonged difficult delivery, or immunocompromise. Family history might be significant for lack of immunization or recent infectious or communicable disease. When eliciting the history of the present illness, inquire about the following:

- Any known exposure to infectious or communicable disease
- Immunization history
- History of having any common childhood communicable diseases

(text continues on page 1106)

BOX 36.3 Standard Precautions and Isolation Precautions

Standard Precautions (Tier One)
- Apply to all clients
- Apply to all body fluids, secretions, and excretions except sweat; nonintact skin; and mucous membranes
- Designed to reduce the risk of transmission of microorganisms from recognized and unrecognized sources
- Techniques include:
  - Proper hand hygiene
  - Use of gloves (clean and sterile) when touching blood, body fluids, secretions or excretions, and contaminated items
  - Masks, eye protection, and face shields when client care may include splashing or sprays of blood, body fluid secretions or excretions
  - Fluid-resistant nonsterile gowns, to protect skin and clothing, when client care may include splashing or sprays of blood, body fluid secretions or excretions
  - Client care equipment handled in a manner that prevents skin or mucous membrane exposure and contamination of clothing
  - All used linen is considered contaminated and needs to be handled and disposed of appropriately.
  - Precautions used to prevent injury when using, cleaning, or disposing of needles and sharps
  - Mouthpieces, resuscitation bags, and other ventilation devices should be readily available.

Transmission-Based Precautions (Tier Two)
Designed for clients with known or suspected infection with pathogens for which additional precautions are warranted to interrupt transmission

Airborne
- Designed to reduce the risk of infectious agents transmitted by airborne droplet nuclei or dust particles that may contain the infectious agent
- Examples of such illnesses include measles, varicella, tuberculosis.
- Techniques include standard precautions as well as:
  - Private room (if unavailable, consider cohorting clients with the same disease and consult with an infection control professional)
  - Room with negative air pressure ventilation, with air externally exhausted or high-efficiency particulate air filtered if recirculated
  - If infectious pulmonary tuberculosis is suspected or proven, wear a respiratory protective device, such as N95 respirator, while in the client's room.
  - Susceptible health care personnel should not enter the room of clients with measles or varicella zoster infections. Those with proven immunity to these viruses need not wear a mask.

Droplet
- Designed to reduce the risk of infectious agents transmitted by contact of the conjunctivae or the mucous membranes of the nose or mouth of a susceptible person with large-particle droplets containing pathogens generated from a person (generally through coughing, sneezing, talking, or procedures such as suctioning) who has a clinical disease or who is a carrier of the disease
- Examples of such illnesses include diphtheria, pertussis, streptococcal group A, influenza, mumps, rubella, scarlet fever.
- Techniques include standard precautions as well as:
  - Private room (if unavailable, consider cohorting clients with the same disease. If this is not possible, separation of at least 3 feet between other clients and visitors should be maintained.)
  - Wear a mask if within 3 feet of the client.

Contact
- Most important and most common route of transmission of health care–associated infections
- Designed to reduce the risk of infectious agents transmitted by direct or indirect contact. Direct-contact transmission involves skin-to-skin contact and physical transfer of pathogens between a susceptible host and an infected or colonized person. Examples include client care activities that involve physical contact such as turning and bathing. Direct-contact transmission also can occur between two clients, where one serves as the source of infectious pathogen and the other as a susceptible host. Indirect-contact transmission involves contact of a susceptible host with a contaminated intermediate object, usually inanimate, in the client's environment.
- Examples of such illnesses include diphtheria★, pediculosis, scabies, multidrug-resistant bacteria.
- Techniques include standard precautions as well as:
  - Private room (if unavailable, consider cohorting clients with the same disease)
  - Gloves (clean or sterile) should be used at all times.
  - Proper hand hygiene after glove removal
  - Use gowns, unless the client is continent and contact of clothing with client and client environmental surfaces is not anticipated. Remove gowns before leaving the client's room.

Prevention standards are applied in all health care settings and are modified to meet each setting's unique needs. Health care workers must practice within the specific institution's guidelines.

★Certain infections require more than one precaution.

COMMON MEDICAL TREATMENTS 36.1

Treatment	Explanation	Indications	Nursing Implications
Hydration	Promoting proper fluid balance either orally or intravenously	Child who can't replace insensible loss due to fever, child who is vomiting or has diarrhea	• Encourage oral fluids, if possible. • Offer child preferred fluid; try Popsicles or games to promote fluid intake. • If administering IV fluids, ensure proper fluid and rate per order and assess IV site and fluid intake every hour. • Maintain strict record of intake and output.
Fever reduction	Reducing temperature by use of antipyretics or non-pharmacologic interventions	Febrile child who is uncomfortable or who can't keep up with the increased metabolic demands associated with fever	• Administer antipyretics, such as ibuprofen and acetaminophen. • Avoid aspirin use in children and adolescents. • Use non-pharmacologic interventions such as dressing lightly, removing blankets, use of a fan, tepid bath, and cooling blanket. Make sure that non-pharmacologic measures do not induce shivering or discomfort. If they do, they should be stopped immediately.

DRUG GUIDE 36.1   COMMON DRUGS FOR COMMUNICABLE DISORDERS

Medication	Action/Indication	Nursing Implications
Antibiotics	Kill and prevent the growth of bacteria Used for treatment of bacterial infections such as sepsis	• Check for antibiotic allergies. • Give as prescribed for the length of time prescribed.
Antivirals (e.g., acyclovir)	Kill and prevent the growth of viruses Used for treatment of viral infections such as herpes simplex II	• Observe infusion site for signs of tissue damage. • If administering topically, clean and dry area before application and wear gloves. • Give as prescribed for the length of time prescribed.
Antipyretics (acetaminophen, ibuprofen)	Decrease the temperature set point (only in a child with a raised temperature) by inhibiting the production of prostaglandins, leading to heat loss (through vasodilation and sweating) and resulting in a reduction in fever Used to decrease temperature in the febrile child who is uncomfortable or who can't keep up with the increased metabolic demands associated with fever	• Ensure proper dosing, concentration, and dosing interval. • Avoid aspirin use in children and adolescents. • Avoid ibuprofen use in children with a bleeding disorder. • Assess fever and any related symptoms such as tachycardia, shivering, diaphoresis. • Properly educate caregivers on appropriate dosing, concentration, dosing interval, and use of accurate measuring device.
Antipruritics (usually antihistamines)	Given orally or topically to block the histamine reaction Used to relieve discomfort associated with itching	• When applying topically, wear gloves. • Do not apply to open wounds. • Oral antihistamines may cause drowsiness.

- Fever
- Sore throat
- Lethargy
- Malaise
- Poor feeding or appetite
- Vomiting
- Diarrhea
- Cough
- Rash (in the older child ask for a description of how it feels; is it painful, does it itch?)

▶ *Take* NOTE!

Many childhood infections and communicable diseases involve a rash. Rashes can be difficult to identify; therefore, obtaining a thorough description and history from the caregiver is important.

Physical Examination

Physical examination of the child with an infectious disorder includes inspection, observation, and palpation.

Inspection and Observation

The physical examination should begin with inspection and observation. Assess the child's skin, mouth, throat, and hair for lesions or wounds. Note the color, shape, and distribution of any lesions or wounds. Assess whether there is any exudate from the lesions or wounds. Observe for scratching, restlessness, and avoidance of the use of a body part or guarding of a body part. A thorough and accurate description is important to assist in identifying the rash and causative organism. Observe the child's affect, energy level, and interaction with caregivers. Lethargy can indicate serious infection or sepsis. Observe if there is any discharge from the nose, cough, or respiratory difficulty.

Assess hydration status. Inspect the oral mucosa; dry and pale mucous membranes can indicate dehydration. Observe for other signs of dehydration, such as sunken eyes and no tears with crying.

Assessment of vital signs can provide more information about the child's condition. Elevated temperature can indicate infection. Often tachypnea and tachycardia accompany fever. Hypotension may also occur, but it is usually a late sign with sepsis.

▶ *Take* NOTE!

Neonates may not present with fever; some may be hypothermic.

Palpation

Palpate the skin to assess temperature, moisture, texture, and turgor. In a child with an infectious or communicable disease, the skin may be warm and moist due to fever. Turgor may be decreased secondary to dehydration. In infants, palpate the fontanels; if they are sunken, the infant may be dehydrated. Palpate the rash to determine if it is raised or flat. A thorough picture of the presenting rash can help identify the child's illness. Palpate the lymph nodes and note any that are swollen and tender.

Laboratory and Diagnostic Testing

Common Laboratory and Diagnostic Tests 36.1 discusses the tests used most commonly when communicable disorders are suspected. The tests can assist the physician in diagnosing the disorder and/or be used as guidelines in determining ongoing treatment. Laboratory or non-nursing personnel obtain some of the tests, while the nurse might obtain others. In either instance the nurse should be familiar with how the tests are obtained, what they are used for, and normal versus abnormal results. This knowledge will also be necessary when providing client and family education related to the testing.

Obtaining Blood Specimens

Giving a blood specimen may be very frightening to children because of the fear of needles, pain, and blood loss. Provide atraumatic care when performing venipunctures and other needlesticks in children. Whether the laboratory technician or the nurse is drawing the blood, the procedure should be performed in an area other than the child's bed, such as the treatment room; the child's bed should be kept as a "safe" area. Provide teaching about the procedure based on the child's developmental level and readiness to learn. In infants and younger children, additional assistance with positioning and restraint will be needed in perform the procedure safely and to ensure proper collection. Use a topical anesthetic cream or gel, refrigerant spray, or iontophoresis prior to venipuncture. In young infants, administer oral sucrose beginning 1 to 2 minutes prior to the procedure and throughout the course of the venipuncture. Refer to Chapter 35 for additional information about decreasing venipuncture-related pain in infants and children.

The usual sites for obtaining blood specimens via venipuncture are the superficial veins of the dorsal surface of the hand or the antecubital fossa, although other locations may also be used. In specific situations, the jugular or femoral vein may be used; in this case either the physician or advanced practice nurse will perform the venipuncture.

Capillary puncture of the child's fingertip, the great toe, or the infant's heel may also be used to obtain blood specimens. Fingertip puncture is similar to that in the

COMMON LABORATORY AND DIAGNOSTIC TESTS 36.1

Test	Explanation	Indications	Nursing Implications
Complete blood count (CBC)	Evaluate white blood cell count (particularly the percentage of individual white cells)	Detect the presence of inflammation, infection	• Normal values vary according to age and gender. • White blood cell count differential is helpful in differentiating source of infection. • May be affected by myelo-suppressive drugs
Erythrocyte sedimentation rate (ESR)	Nonspecific test used in conjunction with other tests to determine presence of infection or inflammation	Detect the presence of inflammation, infection	• Send to laboratory immediately; specimens allowed to stand for longer than 3 hours may produce a falsely low result.
C-reactive protein (CRP)	Nonspecific test that measures a type of protein produced in the liver that is present during episodes of acute inflammation or infection Usually used to diagnose bacterial infections; does not consistently rise with viral infections	To detect the presence of infection, CRP is a more sensitive and rapidly responding indicator than ESR.	• Presence of an intrauterine device may cause positive test results because of tissue inflammation. • Exogenous hormones, such as oral contraceptives, may cause increased levels. • Nonsteroidal anti-inflammatories, salicylates, and steroids may cause decreased levels. • Fasting may be required.
Blood culture and sensitivity	Deliberate growing of micro-organism in a solid or liquid medium. Once it has grown, it is tested against various antibiotics to determine which antibiotics will kill it.	Detect the presence of bacteria or yeast, which may have spread from a certain site in the body into the bloodstream Determine which antibiotics the bacteria or yeast is sensitive to	• Follow aseptic technique and hospital protocol to prevent contamination. • Two cultures obtained from two different sites are preferred. • Ideally obtain before administering antibiotics; if client is taking antibiotics, notify laboratory and draw specimen shortly before next dose. • Deliver specimen to laboratory immediately (within 30 minutes).
Stool culture (including stool for ova and parasites [O&P])	To determine if a bacteria or parasite has infected the intestines	Detect pathogens, including parasites or overgrowth of normal flora in the bowel. Indicated for clients with diarrhea, fever, or abdominal pain.	• Stool must be free of urine, water, and toilet paper. • Do not retrieve out of toilet water. • Deliver to laboratory immediately. • Mineral oil, barium, and bismuth interfere with the detection of parasites; specimen collection should be delayed for 7 to 10 days. • Often a minimum of three specimens on 3 separate days are required for adequate examination, since many parasites and worm eggs are shed intermittently.

(continued)

COMMON LABORATORY AND DIAGNOSTIC TESTS 36.1 (continued)

Test	Explanation	Indications	Nursing Implications
Urine culture	Collection of urine to detect the presence of bacteria in the urine	Detect the presence of bacteria in the urine. Indicated for clients with fever of unknown origin, dysuria, frequency or urgency, or if urinalysis suggests infection.	• Should be obtained by midstream clean-catch, catheterization, or suprapubic aspiration. Avoid contamination with stool, vaginal secretions, hands, or clothing. • Placing bags on the perineum is not acceptable due to high chance of contamination. • Obtain before antibiotics are administered. • Deliver to laboratory immediately or refrigerate.
Throat culture	Vigorous swabbing of the tonsillar area and posterior pharynx to detect the presence of invasive organisms	Most reliable method of detecting group A streptococcal pharyngitis Will also detect *Bordatella pertussis, Corynebacterium diphtheriae* May be performed in those with fever of unknown origin	• Ensure specimen is of secretions in the pharyngeal or tonsillar area. • When performing on young children, have adult hold child in lap. • Health care worker needs to stabilize head by placing hand on the child's forehead.

adult, directed to the sides of the fingertip. Great toe puncture is performed in the same way. Capillary heel puncture must be performed in the proper location to avoid striking the medial plantar artery or periosteum (see Nursing Procedure 36.1). Automatic lancet devices can be used to deliver a more precise puncture depth (Folk, 2007). The young infant will benefit from the use of oral sucrose via pacifier before and during the capillary puncture.

Occasionally, blood samples may be obtained from an artery rather than a vein or capillary. Blood gases in particular are usually obtained by arterial puncture. Arterial puncture requires additional training and in many institutions is performed only by the respiratory therapist, physician, or nurse practitioner. Children with indwelling venous access devices may be spared the trauma of puncture for blood specimens. Follow your institution's guidelines for withdrawing blood from peripherally inserted venous catheters or central venous catheters. The initial blood will be discarded to prevent contamination with intravenous fluids or medications such as heparin. The amount discarded depends on the size of the catheter, the weight of the child, and the institution's guidelines. After aspirating the specimen, flush the venous access device with normal saline to prevent clogging. The device may then be reconnected to the intravenous fluid or flushed according to the institution's protocol.

Nursing Diagnoses, Goals, Interventions, and Evaluations

After completing a thorough assessment, the nurse might identify several nursing diagnoses, including:

- Altered Body Temperature: Fever
- Impaired Comfort
- Impaired Skin Integrity
- Risk for Infection
- Fluid Volume Deficit
- Social Isolation
- Knowledge Deficit

After completing an assessment of Samuel, you note the following: rectal temperature of 39°C, poor sucking, and lethargy. Based on these assessment findings, what would your top three nursing diagnoses be for Samuel?

Nursing goals, interventions, and evaluation for the child with a communicable or infectious disorder are based on the nursing diagnoses. Nursing Care Plan Overview 36.1 provides a general guide for planning care for a child with an infectious or communicable disorder. Additional

Nursing Procedure 36.1

CAPILLARY HEEL PUNCTURE

1. Choose the collection site and apply a commercial heel warmer or warm pack for several minutes prior to specimen collection.
2. Assemble equipment:
   - Gloves
   - Automatic lancet
   - Antiseptic wipe
   - Cotton ball or dry gauze
   - Capillary blood collection tube
   - Band-aid
3. Don gloves. Remove the warm pack.
4. Cleanse the site with antiseptic prep pad and allow to dry.
5. Hold the dorsum of the foot with the nondominant hand; with the dominant hand, pierce the heel with the lancet.
6. Wipe away the first drop of blood with the cotton ball or dry gauze.
7. Collect the blood specimen with a capillary specimen collection tube. Avoid squeezing the foot during specimen collection if possible, as it may contribute to hemolysis of the specimen.
8. Hold a dry gauze over the site until bleeding stops, then apply a Band-aid.

---

information about nursing management will be included later in the chapter as it relates to specific disorders.

Managing Fever

Fever is one of the most common reasons parents seek medical attention. Most infections or communicable diseases are accompanied by fever. Many parents have great concerns about fever: they fear febrile seizures, neurologic complications, and a potential serious underlying disease. Many health care providers share these fears. This leads to the common recommendation to intervene and reduce fever. These fears and misconceptions about fever can lead to mismanagement of fever, such as inappropriate dosing of antipyretics or inappropriate use of nonpharmacologic treatments such as sponging the child with alcohol or cold water.

Health care providers need to educate parents that fever is a protective mechanism the body uses to fight infection. Evidence exists that an elevated body temperature actually enhances various components of the immune response. Fever can slow the growth of bacteria and viruses and increase neutrophil production and T-cell proliferation (Crocetti & Serwint, 2005). Studies have shown that the use of antipyretics may prolong illness. Concern also

exists that reducing fever may hide signs of serious bacterial illness.

> ▶ *Take* NOTE!
>
> *Infants less than 3 months of age with a rectal temperature greater than 38°C should be seen by a physician. They are considered at risk for sepsis until proven otherwise due to their immature immune system and inability to localize or handle infection very well.*

In infants over 3 months of age, fever less than 39°C usually does not require treatment (Kliegman et al., 2007). Antipyretics provide symptomatic relief but do not change the course of the infection. The major benefits of decreasing fever are increasing comfort in the child and decreasing fluid requirements, which helps to prevent dehydration. Children with certain underlying conditions, such as cardiovascular disease or pulmonary disease, also benefit from treating fever because such treatment decreases demands on the body.

Home Management of Fever

Fever is typically managed at home, so it is important for nurses to give guidance and instruction at well-child visits; this information should be reviewed at subsequent visits. Written and video materials about fever management may be effective in increasing caregivers' knowledge. Parents can refer to the written instructions when needed (see Teaching Guidelines 36.1).

The use of acetaminophen or ibuprofen to reduce fever in children has been shown to be safe and effective when the appropriate dose is administered at the appropriate interval (Crocetti & Serwint, 2005). Box 36.4 gives dosing recommendations.

> ▶ *Take* NOTE!
>
> *Never give aspirin to children to reduce fever, due to the risk of Reye syndrome.*

Acetaminophen Use

Acetaminophen is widely used and accepted, but toxic reactions can be seen in children. Causes of acetaminophen toxicity include overdosing or incorrect dosing due to failure to read and understand the label instructions, use of an incorrect measuring device or concentration, and co-administration with an over-the-counter fixed-dose combination medication (the parent may not recognize that it has acetaminophen in it). Another factor that may cause acetaminophen toxic-

(text continues on page 1113)

Nursing Care Plan 36.1

OVERVIEW FOR THE CHILD WITH AN INFECTIOUS OR COMMUNICABLE DISORDER

NURSING DIAGNOSIS: Altered body temperature: fever related to infectious disease process as evidenced by rectal temperature greater than 38°C or 100.4°F

Outcome Identification and Evaluation
Child will maintain temperature within adaptive levels and be comfortable and remain hydrated.
Temperature will be 38°C or 100.4°F or less.
Child will verbalize or exhibit signs of comfort during febrile episode; child will demonstrate adequate signs of hydration.

Interventions: Managing Fever
- Assess temperature at least every 4 to 6 hours, 30 to 60 minutes after antipyretic is given and with any change in condition; *recognizing the pattern of fever may help identify source.*
- Use same site and device for temperature measurement *to reflect a more accurate trend in temperature, since different sites can result in significant differences in temperature reading.*
- Administer antipyretics per physician order when the child is experiencing discomfort or cannot keep up with the metabolic demands of the fever. *Fever is a protective response of the body to fight infection. Antipyretics provide symptomatic relief but do not change the course of the infection. The major benefits to decreasing fever are increasing comfort in the child and decreasing fluid requirements, helping to prevent dehydration.*
- Notify physician of temperature per institution or specific order guidelines; *increases in temperature may indicate worsening infection and relevant changes in condition.*
- Assess fluid intake and encourage oral intake or administer intravenous fluids per physician order; *increased metabolic rate and diaphoresis related to fever can cause fluid loss and lead to fluid volume deficit.*
- Keep linens and clothing clean and dry; *diaphoresis can leave clothing and linen soaked, increasing discomfort for the child.*
- Use of non-pharmacologic measures such as tepid bath and removal of clothing and blankets is controversial. If used, discontinue if shivering begins.

NURSING DIAGNOSIS: Impaired comfort related to infectious and/or inflammatory process as evidenced by hyperthermia, pruritus, rash or skin lesions, sore throat, or joint pain

Outcome Identification and Evaluation
Pain or discomfort will be reduced to level acceptable to child.
Child will verbalize absence or decrease of pain using a pain scale (FLACC, faces or linear pain scale), will verbalize decrease in uncomfortable sensations such as itching and aches; infants will exhibit decreased crying and ability to rest quietly.

Interventions: Improving Comfort
- Assess pain and response to interventions frequently with use of pain scales or other pain measurement tools; *provides baseline of pain and allows for evaluation of effectiveness of interventions.*
- Administer analgesics and antipruritics as ordered *to relieve pain via interruption of CNS pathways and to decrease discomfort related to itching.*
- Apply cool compresses to areas of pruritus or provide a cool bath *to decrease inflammation and soothe pruritus.*
- Keep child's fingernails short (use mitts, gloves, or socks over hands if necessary) *to prevent injury to the skin, which leads to increased pain.*
- Encourage child to press on rather than scratch the area of pruritus; *pressing on the area that itches can soothe the itching and prevent scratching, which can lead to skin injury.*
- Provide fluids frequently and offer warm fluids such as soup or cold foods such as Popsicles *to ease the discomfort of a sore throat.*
- Provide cool mist humidification *to ease the discomfort of a sore throat.*
- Dress the child in light clothing; *restrictive clothing and diaphoresis can lead to increased pruritus.*
- Use diversional activities and distraction appropriate to developmental level: *distraction from pain can reduce the need for pharmacologic agents, and distraction for pruritus can minimize scratching.*

Nursing Care Plan 36.1 (continued)

NURSING DIAGNOSIS: Impaired skin integrity related to mechanical trauma secondary to infectious disease process as evidenced by rash, pruritus, and scratching

Outcome Identification and Evaluation

Child will maintain or regain skin integrity.

Child will not demonstrate increased skin breakdown. Child or parent will be able to describe or demonstrate measures to protect and heal skin and proper care for any lesions.

Interventions: Promoting Skin Integrity

- Monitor skin for color changes, temperature, redness, swelling, warmth, pain or signs of infection, changes in rash lesions, distribution, or size *to help identify problems early and allow for prevention of infection; can also provide information regarding the course of the illness.*
- Encourage fluid intake and proper nutrition *to promote wound healing.*
- Keep child's fingernails short (use mitts, gloves, or socks over hands if necessary) *to prevent injury to the skin, which leads to increased pain.*
- Encourage child to press on rather than scratch the area of pruritus; *pressing on the area that itches can soothe the itching and prevent scratching, which can lead to skin injury.*
- Use antipruritics and topical ointments or creams as ordered *to minimize scratching to prevent injury to skin; can aid in healing.*

NURSING DIAGNOSIS: Risk for infection related to insufficient knowledge regarding measures to avoid exposure to pathogens, increased environmental exposure to pathogens, transmission to others secondary to contagious organism or presence of infectious organisms

Outcome Identification and Evaluation

Child will exhibit no signs or symptoms of local or systemic infection. Child will not spread infection to others. *Symptoms of infection will decrease over time; others will remain free of infection. Child and family will demonstrate appropriate hygiene measures using proper technique, such as handwashing, to prevent the spread of infection.*

Interventions: Preventing and Controlling Infection

- Monitor vital signs; *elevation in temperature may indicate infection.*
- Monitor skin lesions for signs of local infection: *redness, warmth, drainage, swelling, and pain at lesions can indicate infection.*
- Maintain aseptic technique and practice good handwashing *to prevent introduction of further infectious agents and prevent transmission to others.*
- Administer antibiotics as prescribed *to prevent or treat bacterial infection.*
- Encourage nutritious diet and proper hydration according to child's preferences and ability to feed orally *to assist body's natural defenses against infection.*
- Isolate child as required based on transmission-based precautions *to prevent nosocomial spread of infection.*
- Teach child and family preventive measures such as good handwashing, covering mouth and nose with cough or sneeze, and proper disposal of used tissues *to prevent nosocomial or community spread of infection.*

(continued)

Nursing Care Plan 36.1 (continued)

NURSING DIAGNOSIS: Fluid volume deficit, risk for, related to increased metabolic demands and insensible loss due to fever, vomiting, poor feeding or intake

Outcome Identification and Evaluation
Fluid volume will be maintained and balanced. *Oral mucosa is moist and pink, skin turgor is elastic, urine output is at least 1 to 2 mL/kg/hr.*

Interventions: Promoting Adequate Fluid Balance
- Administer IV fluids if ordered *to maintain adequate hydration in children who are NPO, unable to tolerate oral intake, or unable to keep up with fluid losses.*
- When oral intake is allowed and tolerated, encourage oral fluids *to promote intake and maintain hydration.*
- Assess for signs of adequate hydration such as pink and moist oral mucosa, elastic skin turgor, adequate urine output *to detect fluid imbalance.*
- Monitor intake and output *to identify fluid imbalance.*
- Assess urine specific gravity, urine and serum electrolytes, blood urea nitrogen, creatinine, and osmolality and daily weights *to monitor fluid status.*

NURSING DIAGNOSIS: Social isolation related to required isolation from peers secondary to transmission-based precautions, as evidenced by disruption in usual play secondary to inability to leave hospital room, activity intolerance, and fatigue

Outcome Identification and Evaluation
Child will participate in stimulating activities. *Child is able to verbalize reason for isolation and length of isolation (if developmentally appropriate); child verbalizes interest in activities.*

Interventions: Preventing Social Isolation
- Explain reasons for transmission-based precautions and length of time; *this helps increase understanding and decrease anxiety about isolation. Children sometimes mistake isolation as punishment. Explaining length of time gives child an endpoint he or she can work toward.*
- Visit child frequently, at least every hour, and try to spend some uninterrupted time to play and allow child time to verbalize feelings about separation from others; *helps establish a therapeutic relationship and demonstrates caring.*
- Let child see caregiver's face before applying mask if appropriate *to help child identify and relate to those caring for him or her and minimize anxiety about strangers and the unknown.*
- Consult child life specialist *to arrange for stimulating activities child enjoys; can help child to understand reasons for isolation.*
- Contact volunteers to spend time with child, if appropriate: *gives child attention and support, which will help child to cope and decrease stress.*

NURSING DIAGNOSIS: Knowledge deficit related to lack of information regarding medical condition, prognosis, and medical needs as evidenced by verbalization, questions, or actions demonstrating lack of understanding regarding child's condition or care

Outcome Identification and Evaluation
Child and family will verbalize accurate information and understanding about condition, prognosis, and medical needs. *Child and family demonstrate knowledge of condition and prognosis and medical needs, including possible causes, contributing factors, and treatment measures.*

Interventions: Providing Client and Family Teaching
- Assess child's and family's willingness to learn: *child and family must be willing to learn in order for teaching to be effective.*
- Provide family with time to adjust to diagnosis *to facilitate adjustment and ability to learn and participate in child's care.*
- Repeat information *to give family and child time to learn and understand.*
- Teach in short sessions; *many short sessions are more helpful than one long session.*
- Gear teaching to level of understanding of the child and family (depends on age of child, physical condition, memory) *to ensure understanding.*
- Provide reinforcement and rewards *to facilitate the teaching/learning process.*
- Use multiple modes of learning involving many senses (provide written, verbal, demonstration, and videos) when possible; *the child and family are more likely to retain information when it is presented in different ways using many senses.*

EVIDENCE-BASED PRACTICE 36.1
The Effect of Physical Methods Such as Sponging on Decreasing Body Temperature in Children

Health care providers commonly recommend physical methods such as sponging to decrease elevated temperature in children.

● Study
The authors reviewed seven randomized and quasi-randomized studies that evaluated the effects of sponging alone or in combination with antipyretic drugs. Study participants included children from the age of 1 month to 15 years.

▲ Findings
Tepid water sponging alone was found to have limited usefulness but may decrease fever in some children if used along with antipyretic drugs. Iced water or alcohol should never be used for sponge bathing as adverse effects such as excess shivering, goose pimples, increased irritability, and febrile seizures occurred more frequently with these types of sponge baths.

■ Nursing Implications
To alleviate some of the concerns that parents have with fever, nurses should educate parents about why fever occurs. Discourage parents from using alcohol baths or ice water to decrease body temperature in children. Counsel parents to administer appropriate doses of antipyretics when fever causes discomfort in the child or if the child is at risk for febrile seizures. Advise parents that tepid bathing in a warm room may safely be used in conjunction with antipyretics to decrease fever in children.

Meremikwu, M., & Oyo-Ita, A. (2007). Physical methods for treating fever in children. *The Cochrane Library 2007, 4.* Indianapolis: John Wiley & Sons.

ity is the controversial but common practice of alternating acetaminophen and ibuprofen to help reduce fever. There is no evidence supporting this practice (Serwint et al., 2007), and it can result in overdose or improper administration. It can be hard for parents to keep track of the time each medication is due. Parents may confuse which medication is given every 4 hours and which is given every 6 hours. They may exceed the recommended daily doses or may confuse the strength or dosage of the medicines.

TEACHING GUIDELINES 36.1

Fever Management

- Fever is a sign of illness, not a disease; it is the body's weapon to fight infection.
- Diurnal variation may allow temperature changes as much as 1°C (1.8°F) over a 24-hour period, peaking in the evening.
- In some children fever can be associated with a seizure or dehydration, but this will not lead to brain damage or death. Discuss the facts about febrile seizures (see Chapter 37 for further information on febrile seizures).
- Watch for the signs and symptoms of dehydration; it is important to provide oral rehydration by increasing fluid intake.
- Dress the child lightly and avoid warm, binding clothing or blankets.
- The use of sponging with tepid water is controversial; if used, encourage the parent to give an antipyretic prior to sponging. Ensure the sponging does not produce shivering (which causes the body to produce heat and maintain the elevated set point), and reinforce the importance of using tepid water, not cold water or alcohol. Instruct the parent to stop if the child experiences discomfort.
- Call the physician for:
  - Any child less than 3 months of age who has a rectal temperature above 38°C (100.4°F)
  - Any child who is lethargic or listless, regardless of temperature
  - Fever lasting more than 3 to 5 days
  - Fever greater than 40.6°C (105°F)
  - Any child who is immunocompromised by illness, such as cancer or HIV, will need further evaluation and treatment.

BOX 36.4 Dose Recommendations for Acetaminophen and Ibuprofen

Acetaminophen, 10 to 15 mg/kg/dose
• No more than every 4 hours
• No more than 5 doses in a 24-hour period
Ibuprofen, 5 to 10 mg/kg/dose
• Only children >6 months of age
• No more than 4 doses in a 24-hour period

▶ *Take* NOTE!

The American Academy of Pediatrics has stated that due to the lack of evidence supporting the safety or efficacy of alternating acetaminophen with ibuprofen for fever management, extreme discretion should be used when considering this therapy.

Managing Skin Rashes

Many infectious or communicable diseases are accompanied by skin rashes. These rashes can be very uncomfortable and irritating for the child. Management often occurs at home, so parents need to be educated on ways to relieve the discomfort and protect and maintain skin integrity. Antipruritics, including oral medications or topical creams or ointments, may be prescribed by the physician (see Drug Guide 36.1). Parents need to be instructed on the importance of maintaining skin integrity to prevent infection or scarring. Teach parents to keep their child's fingernails short and hands clean. Explain the importance of discouraging scratching, and discuss distraction techniques they can use with the child. Cool compresses or cool baths can relieve itching. Encourage the child to press on rather than scratch the itchy area; this can relieve discomfort while maintaining skin integrity. Refer to Chapter 45 for more information on managing skin rashes.

*B*ased on your top three nursing diagnoses for Samuel, describe appropriate nursing interventions.

Sepsis

Sepsis is a systemic overresponse to infection resulting from bacteria (most common), fungi, viruses, or parasites. It can lead to septic shock, which results in hypotension, low blood flow, and multisystem organ failure. Septic shock is a medical emergency and clients are usually admitted to an intensive care unit (see Chapter 52). The cause of sepsis may not be known, but common causative organisms in children include *Neisseria meningitidis*, *Streptococcus pneumoniae*, and *Haemophilus influenzae*. Sepsis can affect any age group but is more common in neonates and young infants. Neonates and young infants have a higher susceptibility due to their immature immune system, inability to localize infections, and lack of IgM immunoglobulin, which is necessary to protect against bacterial infections.

The prognosis for sepsis is variable and depends on the child's age and the cause of the sepsis. The mortality rate may be as high as 40% to 60% for certain types of infections (Kliegman et al., 2007). Neonates are at the highest risk, and 50% of neonatal deaths result from serious bacterial infections in the first month of life (Crawford, 2006). Due to this high mortality rate, when a febrile neonate presents, a full work-up is indicated, and usually admission to the hospital to rule out sepsis is the standard of practice.

Pathophysiology

Sepsis results in the systemic inflammatory response syndrome (SIRS) due to infection. The pathophysiology of sepsis is complex. It results from the effects of circulating bacterial products or toxins, mediated by cytokine release, occurring as a result of sustained bacteremia. The pathogens cause an overproduction of proinflammatory cytokines, previously termed endotoxins, which are responsible for the clinically observable effects of the sepsis. Impaired pulmonary, hepatic, or renal function may result from excessive cytokine release during the septic process.

Therapeutic Management

Therapeutic management of sepsis in infants, especially neonates, is more aggressive than for older children. Neonates and infants with sepsis or even suspected sepsis are treated in the hospital. The infant is admitted for close monitoring along with antibiotic therapy. Intravenous antibiotics are started immediately after the blood, urine, and cerebrospinal fluid cultures have been obtained. The length of therapy and the specific antibiotic used will be determined based on the source of the positive culture and the results of the culture and sensitivity. Common treatment length for positive cultures is 10 to 14 days. If final culture reports are negative and symptoms have subsided, antibiotics may be discontinued (usually after 72 hours of treatment). If the child is not responding to therapy and symptoms worsen, sepsis may be progressing to shock. Management of the child with septic shock is usually done in the intensive care unit.

Nursing Assessment

For a full description of the assessment phase of the nursing process, refer to page 1103. Assessment findings pertinent to sepsis are discussed below.

Health History

Elicit a description of the present illness and chief complaint. Signs of sepsis can vary with each child. Some common signs and symptoms reported during the health history might include:

- Child just does not look or act right
- Crying more than usual, inconsolable
- Fever
- Hypothermia (in neonates and those with severe disease)
- Lethargic and less interactive or playful
- Increased irritability
- Poor feeding or poor suck
- Rash (e.g., petechiae, ecchymosis, diffuse erythema)
- Difficulty breathing
- Nasal congestion
- Diarrhea
- Vomiting
- Decreased urine output
- Hypotonia
- Changes in mental status (confused, anxious, excited)
- Seizures
- Older child may complain of heart racing

Explore the child's current and past medical history for risk factors such as:

- Prematurity
- Lack of immunizations
- Immunocompromise
- Exposure to communicable pathogens

In neonates and young infants, seek pregnancy and labor risk factors such as:

- Premature rupture of membranes or prolonged rupture
- Difficult delivery
- Maternal infection or fever, including sexually transmitted infections
- Resuscitation and other invasive procedures
- Positive maternal group beta-streptococcal vaginosis

Sepsis may occur in the hospitalized child. Assess for risk factors such as:

- Intensive care unit stay
- Presence of central line or other invasive lines or tubes
- Immunosuppression

Physical Examination

Perform a thorough physical examination of the infant or child with proven or suspected sepsis. Specific findings related to inspection and observation are noted below.

Inspection and Observation

Observe the child's general appearance, color, level of arousal, and hydration status. The child with sepsis may appear lethargic and pale and show signs of dehydration. In neonates and infants, observe the quality of their cry

and reaction to parental stimulation, noting weak cry, lack of smile or facial expression, or lack of responsiveness. Inspect the skin for petechiae or other skin lesions. Petechiae may indicate a serious bacterial infection (often *N. meningitidis*), and other skin lesion patterns may help identify the cause of the fever. Observe respiratory effort and rate. The infant or child with sepsis may demonstrate tachypnea and increased work of breathing, such as nasal flaring, grunting, and retractions.

Assess vital signs, noting abnormalities. Note elevation in temperature or hypothermia in the young infant. Note tachypnea or tachycardia in the child or apnea or bradycardia in the infant. Document blood pressure. Hypotension, especially when accompanied by signs of poor perfusion, can be a sign of worsening sepsis with progression to shock (refer to Chapter 52).

> ▶ *Take* NOTE!
>
> Listen to the parents' descriptions of the neonate's or infant's behavior and appearance, as well as changes they have observed. Many times they are the first to notice when their child is not acting right, even before clinical signs of infection are seen.

Laboratory and Diagnostic Tests

Symptoms of sepsis can be vague in infants. Therefore, laboratory tests play a crucial role in confirming or ruling out sepsis. Common laboratory and diagnostic studies ordered for the assessment of sepsis include:

- Complete blood count: WBC levels will be elevated; in severe cases they may be decreased (this is an ominous sign)
- C-reactive protein: elevated
- Blood culture: positive in septicemia, indicating bacteria is present in the blood
- Urine culture: may be positive, indicating presence of bacteria in the urine
- Cerebrospinal fluid analysis: may reveal increased WBCs and protein and low glucose
- Stool culture: may be positive for bacteria or other infectious organisms
- Culture of tubes, catheters, or shunts suspected to be infected: the fluid inside these tubes may be tested for bacteria
- Chest x-ray: may reveal signs of pneumonia such as hyperinflation and patchy areas of atelectasis or infiltration

Nursing Management

Monitor the infant or child closely for changes in condition, especially the development of shock. Administer antibiotics as ordered. Refer to the Nursing Care Plan Overview 36.1

for nursing diagnoses and related interventions. In addition to these interventions, reducing risk for infection and providing education to the child and family should be done.

Preventing Infection

Sepsis is a potentially life-threatening illness, and prevention is important. Handwashing is the most effective intervention against nosocomial infection. Nurses play a key role in minimizing environmental sources by cleaning equipment and disposing of soiled linens and dressings properly and adhering to proper aseptic technique with all invasive procedures. Following your institution's policies and using evidence-based practice guidelines for interventions such as invasive line dressing changes and intravenous tubing changes can reduce the risk of infection. Encourage immunization as recommended. To reduce streptococcus group B infection in neonates, screen pregnant woman; if the results are positive, administer intrapartum antibiotics.

> ▶ *Take* NOTE!
>
> *There has been a dramatic reduction in invasive* Haemophilus influenzae *type B diseases since the widespread use of the Hib vaccine. Meningococcal and pneumococcal vaccines also have decreased the incidence of invasive infection, especially in high-risk children.*

Educating the Child and Family

Early recognition of the signs of sepsis is essential in preventing morbidity and mortality. Educate parents about the importance of fever, especially in neonates and infants less than 3 months old. Instruct parents to contact their health care provider if their infant or neonate has a fever. A health care provider should see any child with a fever accompanied by lethargy, poor responsiveness, or lack of facial expressions. Signs and symptoms of sepsis can be vague and vary from child to child. Parents need to be encouraged to contact their health care provider if they feel their febrile child is "just not acting right."

Bacterial Infections

Bacteria are one-celled organisms that can live, grow, and reproduce. They exist everywhere. Most are completely harmless and some are very useful. Others can lead to disease either because they are in the wrong place in the body or they are designed to invade and cause disease in humans and animals. Children are at a high risk of developing bacterial infections, which can result in life-threatening illness. Fortunately, many bacterial diseases, such as diphtheria, pertussis, and tetanus, can be prevented by immunization (see Chapter 30 for more information on immunizations).

▶ SCARLET FEVER

Scarlet fever is an infection resulting from group A streptococci. The bacteria produce a toxin that causes a rash. Two children may both have a group A streptococcus infection, but both may not get the rash of scarlet fever: only the one who is sensitive to the toxin will develop scarlet fever. It is usually seen in children less than 18 years of age, with the peak incidence between the ages of 4 and 8 years. It is rare in children less than 2 years old. Transmission is airborne and follows contact with respiratory tract secretions. Close contact that occurs in schools and childcare centers facilitates transmission. Foodborne outbreaks have occurred due to human contamination of food. After exposure the incubation period is 2 to 5 days. Communicability is highest during acute infection, and the child is no longer contagious 24 hours after the initiation of appropriate antimicrobial therapy.

There has been a dramatic decrease in the mortality from scarlet fever due to antibiotic use, but complications such as rheumatic fever and glomerulonephritis can still occur.

Nursing Assessment

Symptoms of scarlet fever begin abruptly. The history may reveal a fever greater than 101°F, chills, body aches, loss of appetite, nausea, and vomiting. Inspect the pharynx, which is usually very red and swollen. The tonsils may have yellow or white specks of pus, and cervical lymph nodes may be swollen. Inspect the skin for the most striking symptom of scarlet fever, which is an erythematous rash appearing on the face, trunk, and extremities. The rash is typically absent from the palms and soles of the feet. It looks like a sunburn but feels like sandpaper (Fig. 36.1A). The rash lasts approximately 5 days and is followed by desquamation, typically on the fingers and toes. Early in the illness the tongue develops a thick coat with a strawberry appearance. The tongue will later lose the coating and become bright red (see Fig. 36.1B).

Diagnosis is made by identification of group A streptococcus on throat culture. Several rapid tests for group A streptococcal pharyngitis are available. The accuracy of these tests depends on the quality of the specimen. It is important that the secretions obtained are pharyngeal or tonsillar (see Common Medical Treatments 36.1 for more information on throat cultures).

Nursing Management

Children with scarlet fever are usually cared for at home. Penicillin V is the antibiotic of choice. In those sensitive to penicillin, erythromycin may be used. Educate the family on the importance of taking the antibiotic as directed and finishing all the medicine.

Encourage fluid intake to maintain adequate hydration due to fever. Teach parents ways to provide comfort for the child. A cool mist humidifier can soothe the child's sore

FIGURE 36.1 (**A**) Rash of scarlet fever.
(**B**) Strawberry tongue.

throat. Soft foods, warm liquids like soup, or cold foods like
Popsicles may also be helpful. If the child is hospitalized,
droplet precautions, along with standard precautions, are
necessary.

▶ CAT SCRATCH DISEASE

Cat scratch disease is a relatively common and occasionally
serious disease caused by the bacteria *Bartonella henselae*. It
occurs in both children and adults but is more common in
children under 10 years of age. Cats can carry the bacteria
in their saliva, and in 90% of cases the child has had a recent interaction with cats and often kittens (Pickering,
2006). No evidence exists to support person-to-person
transmission. *B. henselae* is transmitted between cats via the
cat flea. The incubation period is 7 to 12 days, with lymphadenopathy appearing in 5 to 50 days. Therapeutic management is supportive and is aimed at management of
symptoms. The disease itself is usually self-limited, resolving on its own in 2 to 4 months. If lymphadenopathy persists or if the child is immunocompromised, antibiotics may
be needed. Painful, swollen nodes may be treated with needle aspiration to provide symptom relief.

Nursing Assessment

Note history of headaches and fatigue. The history may
also include interaction or rough play with cats or kittens,
resulting in a scratch. Document the temperature, noting
fever. Palpate for enlarged lymph nodes, noting their location. A skin papule may be present or reported. Diagnostic tests are available to detect serum antibodies to
antigens of *Bartonella* species.

Nursing Management

Administer antibiotics if ordered. No transmission-based
isolation is required; standard precautions are sufficient.
Educate the client and family about prevention and control measures. Teach children to avoid rough play with
cats and kittens. Teach parents and children to immediately wash any bites or scratches with soap and running
water. Explain that cats should never lick open wounds
on the child. Control of fleas in cats is important to prevent the spread of *B. henselae*.

▶ DIPHTHERIA

Diphtheria is caused by infection with *Corynebacterium diphtheriae* and may affect the nose, larynx, tonsils, or pharynx.
Tonsillar and pharyngeal infections are the most common
and will be the focus of this discussion. A pseudomembrane
forms over the pharynx, uvula, tonsils, and soft palate
(Fig. 36.2). The neck becomes edematous and lymphadenopathy develops. The pseudomembrane causes airway
obstruction and suffocation. Diphtheria generally occurs
in children less than 15 years old who are unimmunized.
Routine infant immunization can prevent the disease. Therapeutic management involves administration of antibiotics
and antitoxin, as well as airway management.

Nursing Assessment

Children at risk for diphtheria are those who are unimmunized. Note history of sore throat and fever, usually
less than 38.9°C. As the pseudomembrane forms, swallowing becomes difficult and signs of airway obstruction

Figure 36.2 In diphtheria a pseudo-membrane forms over the pharynx, uvula, tonsils, and soft palate.

become apparent. A specimen of the membrane may be cultured for *C. diphtheriae*.

Nursing Management

Close observation of respiratory status is of utmost importance. Administration of antibiotics and the antitoxin is critical to encourage sloughing of the membrane. The child should remain on strict droplet precautions in addition to standard precautions and should maintain bed rest.

▶ PERTUSSIS

Pertussis is an acute respiratory disorder characterized by paroxysmal cough (whooping cough) and copious secretions. It primarily occurs in children 4 years and younger and is most severe in children less than 6 months of age. The disease is caused by *Bordatella pertussis*. The incubation period is 6 to 21 days, usually 7 to 10 days. Pertussis usually starts with 7 to 10 days of cold symptoms. The paroxysmal coughing spells then begin and can last 1 to 4 weeks. Convalescence occurs over the course of several weeks to months. Immunization has decreased the incidence of pertussis, but the increasing numbers of unimmunized children, particularly immigrants, contribute to the incidence of the disease. Complications include seizures, pneumonia, encephalopathy, and death.

Therapeutic Management

Therapeutic management of pertussis focuses on eradicating the bacterial infection and providing respiratory support. CDC guidelines recommend antimicrobial treat-

ment. For infants older than 1 month of age, macrolide drugs, including erythromycin, clarithromycin, and azithromycin, are the drugs of choice. For younger infants, azithromycin should be used and erythromycin and clarithromycin avoided. An alternative to macrolides in children older than 2 months is trimethoprim-sulfamethoxazole (TMP-SMZ).

Nursing Assessment

The most important risk factor for the development of pertussis is lack of immunization. The history may reveal cold and cough symptoms, progressing to paroxysmal coughing spells. During the paroxysms, the child might cough 10 to 30 times in a row, followed by a whooping sound. This might be accompanied by redness in the face, progressive cyanosis, and protrusion of the tongue. Saliva, mucus, and tears flow from the mouth, nose, and eyes. Between the paroxysmal episodes, the child might rest well and appear relatively unaffected. Auscultate the lungs to assess air exchange. The diagnosis may be confirmed by an immunofluorescent assay positive for *B. pertussis*.

Nursing Management

Nursing care will focus on providing a high-humidity environment and frequent suctioning to mobilize secretions. Observe for signs of airway obstruction. Encourage fluids to keep secretions thin and maintain adequate hydration. Offer reassurance to the child and family; the coughing episodes can be very frightening. Droplet precautions along with standard precautions are necessary for the hospitalized child.

▶ TETANUS

Tetanus is an acute, often fatal neurologic disease caused by the toxins produced by *Clostridium tetani*. Tetanus is rare in the United States but continues to be significant worldwide due to lack of routine immunization. It is characterized by increased muscle tone and spasm. *C. tetani* spores can live anywhere but are found most commonly in soil, dust, and feces from humans or animals, such as sheep, cattle, chickens, dogs, cats, and rats. The spores can enter the body through a wound that is contaminated, through a burn, or by injecting contaminated street drugs. Once it enters the body, an anaerobic environment allows it to multiply and a poisonous toxin is released.

There are four forms of tetanus. Neonatal tetanus is the most common worldwide, affecting newborns in the first week of life secondary to an infected umbilical stump or unsterile surgical technique during circumcision. Most women in the United States have been immunized and will pass the immunity to their fetus. Along with proper hygiene during delivery and adequate cord care, this makes this type rare in the United States, but in underdeveloped countries it remains a significant problem. The second form is local tetanus. This rare form is characterized by local muscle spasms within the area of the wound. The third type is cephalic tetanus, which is associated with recurrent otitis media or head trauma. It is also rare and affects the cranial nerves, especially facial nerves. Generalized tetanus is the most common form and results in spasms that progress in a descending fashion beginning at the jaw. The most profoundly affected muscles are those of the neck and back. In the United States the fatality rate associated with tetanus has declined and cases are rare, but 3 out of 10 cases will result in death (Pickering, 2006). The general incubation period is 3 to 21 days; it averages 8 days. Recovery can be long and difficult, and children with tetanus may have to spend several weeks in the hospital in an intensive care setting. It has been suggested that the shorter the incubation period, the higher the risk of more severe illness and poorer prognosis. Complications associated with tetanus include breathing problems, fractures, elevated blood pressure, dysrhythmias, clotting in the blood vessels of the lung, pneumonia, and coma.

Therapeutic management is directed toward supporting respiratory and cardiovascular function. Tetanus immunoglobulin may be given as well as the tetanus vaccine. Removal of the offending organism, by débridement of the wound, may occur, and intravenous antibiotics such as metronidazole may be initiated. In severe cases, the child may require intensive nursing care with mechanical ventilation.

Nursing Assessment

Note history of initial signs such as headache, spasms, crankiness, and cramping of the jaw (lockjaw), which are followed by difficulty swallowing and a stiff neck. Tetanus progresses in a descending fashion to other muscle groups, causing spasms of the neck, arms, legs, and stomach; seizures may result. Document the presence of fever along with an elevated blood pressure and tachycardia. Opisthotonos may be noted due to severe spasms of the neck and back. The spasms or muscle contractions in children may be strong enough to result in fractures. The diagnosis of tetanus is based on the clinical findings of the history and physical examination.

Nursing Management

Nursing management focuses on observing for signs of respiratory distress. Provide a quiet environment with reduced external stimuli to decrease the incidence of spasms. Appropriately manage pain. Encourage adequate nutrition and hydration. Administer sedatives and muscle relaxants as ordered to reduce the pain associated with the muscle spasms and to prevent seizures. Encourage the parents to stay with their child. The child's mental status is unaffected by the disease, and therefore he or she is aware of what is happening. Efforts need to be made to reduce the

child's anxiety and to provide reassuring, sympathetic care to the child and family.

Tetanus is a preventable but potentially fatal disease. Education is essential regarding the importance of receiving this routine immunization (refer to Chapter 30 for immunization schedule) as well as a booster every 10 years. Instructing parents on proper wound care can also help prevent tetanus. All wounds should be cleaned thoroughly and a proper antiseptic used. If a wound is deep and contamination is suspected, the child should be seen by a health care professional. If it has been more than 5 years since the last tetanus dose, a booster may be needed. This can help to neutralize the poison and prevent it from entering the nervous system.

Viral Infections

Viruses are very small particles that infect cells. They cannot multiply on their own and require a living host, such as humans, animals, or plants. They can reproduce only by invading and taking over the host cells. Young children are highly sensitive to viruses, as their resistance is low and exposure is high. Viruses are hard to destroy without damaging or killing the living cells they infect; this is why drugs are not used to control them. Many viral diseases can be prevented by immunization, such as measles, rubella, varicella, mumps, and poliomyelitis (see Chapter 30 for more information on immunizations).

▶ VIRAL EXANTHEMS

Many viral infections of the skin in childhood are called viral exanthems. **Exanthem** means rash or skin eruption. Viral exanthems of childhood often present with a distinct rash pattern that assists in the diagnosis of the virus. Table 36.4 discusses common childhood exanthems. Immunizations have led to a decrease in the incidence of certain viral exanthems, such as measles, rubella, and varicella.

Typically, children with viral exanthems are cared for at home, but there are times when a child may be hospitalized or may develop the disease while being hospitalized. Appropriate transmission-based precautions must be taken. Therapeutic management of the viral exanthems focuses on fever management and relief of discomfort.

Nursing Assessment

Obtain the history of the present illness, noting the onset of rash in relation to the onset of fever. Note accompanying symptoms such as respiratory complaints. Document known exposure to childhood diseases. Note immunization status. Inspect the skin for rash, noting the distribution, type, and extent of lesions. Table 36.4 describes the

(text continues on page 1124)

TABLE 36.4 COMMON VIRAL EXANTHEMS OF CHILDHOOD

Disease	Clinical Manifestations	Management/Complications	Nursing Implications
Rubella (German measles) • Caused by rubella virus • Transmitted by direct or indirect contact with droplets, primarily by nasopharyngeal secretions, but also in blood, stool, and urine. Also transmitted from mother to fetus. • Peak incidence during late winter and early spring • Incubation period: 14 to 23 days (usually 16 to 18) • Communicable 7 days before to 7 days after onset of rash 	• Lymphadenopathy (retroauricular, posterior cervical, postoccipital) 24 hours before the onset of the rash; lasting up to 1 week • Rash begins on face and spreads quickly down the neck, trunk, and extremities; disappears in same order it spread, usually by third day. On the second day the rash may appear pinpoint. Desquamation is minimal. • Mild pruritus. • Polyarthralgia and polyarthritis (rare in children but common in adolescents)	• Usually mild and self-limiting • Treatment is mainly supportive. • Complications: Encephalitis and thrombocytopenia (rare) • Maternal rubella during pregnancy can result in miscarriage, fetal death, or congenital malformations.	• Comfort measures such as antipyretics, antipruritics, and analgesics for joint pain • Contact precautions for the duration of the illness in the hospitalized child • Avoid exposure to pregnant women.
Rubeola (measles) • Caused by measles virus • Transmitted by direct or indirect contact with droplets, primarily by nasopharyngeal secretions, but also blood and urine. Highly contagious. • Incubation period: 10 to 12 days • Communicable 1 to 2 days before the onset of symptoms (3 to 5 days before onset of rash) until 5 days after rash has appeared 	• Prodromal phase: 3 to 5 days, consisting of fever, cough, coryza, conjunctivitis • Followed by Koplik spots • Erythematous maculopapular rash appears 3 to 4 days after the onset of the prodromal phase.	• Treatment is mainly supportive, including antipyretics, bed rest, adequate fluid intake. • Possible vitamin A supplementation in children 6 months to 2 years hospitalized for measles or its complications or those with immunodeficiency (Kliegman et al., 2007) • Complications: otitis media, pneumonia, croup, and diarrhea common in young children; acute encephalitis	• Comfort measures, such as antipyretics and antipruritics • Clean eyes with warm, moist cloth to remove secretions. • Cool mist humidification to alleviate coryza and cough • Droplet precautions until fifth day of rash

Varicella zoster (chickenpox)

- Caused by varicella zoster virus, human herpes virus 3
- Highly contagious. Transmitted by direct contact with infected persons' nasopharyngeal secretions or via airborne spread, to a lesser degree by contact with unscabbed lesions. Also transmitted from mother to fetus.
- Peak incidence late fall, winter, and spring
- Incubation period: 14 to 21 days, usually 14 to 16
- Communicable 1 to 2 days before onset of rash until all vesicles have crusted over (about 3 to 7 days after onset of rash)

- Prodromal symptoms (fever, malaise, anorexia, headache, mild abdominal pain) may be present 24 to 48 hours before the onset of the rash.
- Lesions often appear first on scalp, face, and trunk; initially intensely pruritic erythematous macules that evolve to papules and then form clear, fluid-filled vesicles.
- Vesicles eventually erupt, and then lesions scab and crust. A variety of lesions are present at one time.
- More severe in adolescents and adults than in young children

- Usually self-limiting; treatment is mainly supportive: fever reduction, antipruritics, and skin care to prevent infection of lesions.
- Antiviral therapy and varicella zoster immune globulin may be used in those considered to be at high risk (immunocompromised, pregnant women, and newborns exposed to maternal varicella). Routine antiviral therapy is not recommended for the treatment of uncomplicated varicella infection in otherwise healthy children.
- Complications: bacterial superinfection of skin lesions, thrombocytopenia, arthritis, hepatitis, cerebellar ataxia, encephalitis, meningitis, pneumonia, glomerulonephritis, congenital infection and life-threatening perinatal infection
- Lifelong latent infection occurs; reactivation results in herpes zoster (shingles), uncommon in childhood.

- Comfort measures, such as antipyretics and antipruritics
- Airborne and contact precautions in the hospitalized child for a minimum of 5 days after onset of rash and as long as vesicular lesions are present
- For those with exposure to susceptible persons, airborne and contact precautions, from 8 to 21 days after exposure
- Children may return to school or childcare once lesions have crusted.

(continued)

TABLE 36.4 COMMON VIRAL EXANTHEMS OF CHILDHOOD (continued)

Disease	Clinical Manifestations	Management/Complications	Nursing Implications
Exanthem subitum (roseola infantum or sixth disease) • Caused by human herpes virus 6 (HHV-6); less frequently human herpes virus 7 (HHV-7) • Transmission mode: little is known but suspected to be from saliva of infected person and enters the host through the oral, nasal, or conjunctival mucosa • Peak incidence age 6 to 15 months • Incubation period: 5 to 15 days, average of 10 days • Communicability is unknown, but most likely contagious during febrile stage	• Prodromal phase: usually asymptomatic but may include upper respiratory signs • Clinical illness: high fever ranging from 37.9° to 40°C (101° to 106°F) for 3 to 5 days; resolves abruptly; rash appears 12 to 24 hours later, lasting about 1 to 3 days	• Course is generally benign. • In children who are uncomfortable or irritable or have a history of febrile seizures, antipyretics may be warranted. • Complications: HSV-6 may be responsible for some febrile seizures, encephalitis and meningoencephalitis (rare).	• Comfort measures, such as antipyretics, antipruritics • Standard precautions are sufficient in the hospitalized child.
Erythema infectiosum (fifth disease) • Caused by human parvovirus B19 • Transmitted by large droplet spread from nasopharyngeal viral shedding or percutaneous exposure to blood and blood products. Also transmitted from mother to fetus. • Peak incidence late winter and early spring. • Incubation period: 4 to 21 days, average 16 to 17 days 	• Prodromal phase: mild symptoms, low-grade fever, headache, mild upper respiratory infection • Characteristic rash occurs in three stages: • Begins with erythematous flushing often described as "slapped-cheek" appearance, often with circumoral pallor	• Usually benign and self-limited; supportive treatment is all that is needed. • Blood transfusion may be necessary in children with aplastic crisis. • Complications: arthritis and arthralgia • May result in fetal loss, hydrops fetalis in pregnant woman	• Comfort measures, such as antipyretics, antipruritics • Droplet precautions are required in the hospitalized child. • Inform pregnant women (including health care workers) of the potential risks to the fetus and preventive meas-

- Communicability is uncertain, but most children are no longer infectious by the time the rash appears and diagnosis is made, so isolation or exclusion from school, once child is diagnosed, is unnecessary (those with aplastic crisis may be communicable up to 1 week after onset of symptoms and those who are immunosuppressed with chronic infection and severe anemia may be communicable for months to years).

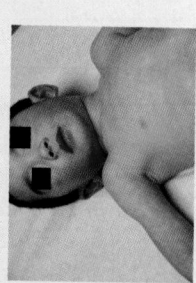

Hand, foot and mouth disease, or herpangina (if only mouth involvement)

- Caused by Coxsackie A viruses (esp. A16). Transmitted by direct contact with infected fecal, oral secretions; spread mostly through saliva.
- Peak incidence during spring and summer, particularly in children who wear diapers (1- to 4-year-olds)
- Most common during spring and summer
- Incubation period: 3 to 6 days
- Communicable from time of infection until fever resolves; virus is shed for several weeks after the infection begins.

- Spreads to trunk
- Moves peripherally, appearing as a maculopapular, lace-like appearance; often pruritic
- Palms and soles are usually spared. Rash fluctuates in intensity and will disappear and reappear with environmental changes such as exposure to sunlight.
- Resolves spontaneously over 1 to 3 weeks
- Children with preexisting anemias may develop aplastic crisis (will have fever, malaise, myalgia, but usually no rash).

- High fever usually occurs first.
- Vesicles on tongue and oral mucosa erode to shallow ulcers; vesicles on hands and feet are football-shaped, with erythematous rims.
- Extensive mouth lesions may lead to anorexia, dehydration, and drooling.

- Usually mild and self-limiting, resolving within 1 week
- Treatment is mainly supportive.
- Complications: dehydration, meningitis, encephalitis, and pulmonary edema

- Contact precautions and good hand hygiene are necessary.
- Encourage oral fluids of preference, Popsicles.
- Provide analgesics as needed.

ures to decrease these risks (strict infection control practices, not caring for those likely to be contagious). The CDC does not recommended routine exclusion from a workplace where an outbreak is occurring.

rash as well as accompanying symptoms for each of the viral exanthems.

Nursing Management

Nursing management of viral exanthems focuses on fever reduction, relief of discomfort, and protection of skin integrity. Encourage hydration. Administer antipyretics and antipruritics as needed (refer to Drug Guide 36.1). Nonpharmacologic interventions to reduce fever, such as tepid sponging and cool compresses, may be used. Refer to Nursing Care Plan 36.1 for additional information; care should be individualized based on the child's and family's response to the illness.

> ▶ *Take* NOTE!
>
> *Trim the child's fingernails or cover hands with mitts, gloves, or socks (which work well with younger infants and children) if the rash itches to help prevent breaks in the skin, which can lead to discomfort and infection.*

▶ MUMPS

Mumps, a contagious disease caused by Paramyxovirus, is characterized by fever and parotitis (inflammation and swelling of the parotid gland). Mumps is spread via contact with infected droplets. Infected individuals are contagious for 1 to 7 days prior to onset of symptoms and for 7 to 9 days after parotid swelling begins. The American Academy of Pediatrics recommends immunization against mumps for all children. Mumps occurs most frequently in unimmunized children between 5 and 19 years of age. About one third of all infected prepubertal boys also develop orchitis (inflammation of the testicle). Complications of mumps include meningoencephalitis with seizures and auditory neuritis, which can result in deafness. Therapeutic management is supportive.

Nursing Assessment

Note history of exposure to infected individuals as well as immunization status. Determine history of low-grade fever and onset and progression of parotid swelling. History may also include malaise, anorexia, headache, and abdominal pain. The parotid swelling is easily observed as swelling of the neck either bilaterally or unilaterally (Fig. 36.3). In boys, note orchitis. The diagnosis is usually based on the history and clinical presentation, but serum may be tested for the presence of mumps immunoglobulin G (IgG) or immunoglobulin M (IgM) **antibody**.

FIGURE 36.3 Parotitis associated with mumps.

Nursing Management

Nursing management of mumps is primarily supportive. Acetaminophen is used for fever management, and occasionally narcotic analgesics are required for pain management. Oral fluids are encouraged to prevent dehydration. If orchitis is present, ice packs to the testicles and gentle testicular support may be helpful. Hospitalized children should be confined to respiratory isolation to prevent spread of the disease. Infected children are considered no longer contagious 9 days following onset of parotid swelling. Current recommendations include first mumps immunization by 15 months of age, followed by a second vaccine between 4 and 6 years of age (see Chapter 30 for information on mumps vaccination).

> ▶ *Take* NOTE!
>
> *In recent years mumps outbreaks have occurred, mainly on college campuses. The mumps vaccine is not 100% effective, and mumps infection can occur in vaccinated individuals. Per the CDC (2006), one dose of MMR prevents 80% of cases and two doses prevent approximately 90% of cases. During an outbreak it is essential to define the population at risk and transmission setting, identify and isolate suspected cases, and identify and vaccinate susceptible individuals (CDC, 2006).*

▶ POLIOMYELITIS

Poliomyelitis is an infection caused by the highly infectious poliovirus, which is an enterovirus. The virus invades the central nervous system and can produce total paralysis. Transmission occurs through direct or indirect contact. The poliovirus is spread most commonly via the fecal-to-oral or oral-to-oral route. Polio most commonly occurs in young children and is also referred to as infantile paralysis. This disease is rare due to effective immunization programs but is still seen in developing countries in the eastern Mediterranean region, India, and Africa.

Nursing Assessment

Initial signs and symptoms include fever, fatigue, headache, vomiting, neck stiffness, and limb pain. Symptoms then progress to tremors of the extremities and possible paralysis. Kernig's sign will be positive and deep tendon reflexes will be hyperactive initially and then diminished. Paralysis is asymmetric and generally affects the legs more than the arms. Respiratory problems can occur if the respiratory center of the brain is involved. The poliovirus can be isolated in feces or the pharynx of infected individuals, and cerebrospinal fluid evaluation generally shows elevated leukocytes and protein.

Nursing Management

Nursing management is aimed at providing supportive care, focusing on maintaining respiratory status and nutritional status until the illness has run its course. Bed rest will usually be ordered, so skin care is a priority. Maintaining self-care and mobility are also important nursing functions. Long-term care providing therapy and bracing to strengthen muscles may be needed during and after hospitalization.

No cure for polio exists, but it can be prevented by the polio vaccine, which is routinely administered in developed countries (refer to the immunization schedule in Chapter 30). Oral polio vaccine (OPV) is a live strain, and thus the virus is shed in the stool for up to 6 weeks after immunization, leading to the risk for vaccine-acquired polio in caregivers. For this reason, OPV has been replaced by inactivated polio vaccine (IPV), an injectable form, in the United States. OPV is still used in developing countries, however, so immigrants or travelers whose children were recently immunized in their home country should take precautions if they are immunocompromised or unvaccinated. Areas where polio is endemic, including Afghanistan, Egypt, India, Niger, Nigeria, and Pakistan, agreed to a massive immunization campaign in 2004 and hope to make polio the first eradicated disease of the 21st century (Stephenson, 2004).

▶ RABIES

Rabies is a preventable viral infection of the central nervous system. It is transmitted to other animals and humans through close contact with the saliva of a rabid animal, usually by a bite. The number of cases of rabies has steadily declined in the United States. It is rare in the United States and Western Europe due to routine vaccination of domestic animals, such as dogs, and the availability of effective postexposure prophylaxis. Now most cases of rabies in these areas are due to wild animals such as raccoons, skunks, bats, and foxes. Rabies continues to be a major health problem in other parts of the world, especially in areas where dogs are not controlled.

Most cases of rabies occur in children less than 15 years of age, and most human deaths occur in developing countries. Children have an increased susceptibility to rabies due to their fearlessness around animals, eagerness to play with animals, shorter stature, and inability to protect themselves. The incubation period for rabies is extremely variable and can range from 20 to 180 days, with the peak at 30 to 60 days (Kliegman et al., 2007). The incubation period tends to be shorter in children. Once symptoms of rabies have developed the prognosis is poor: death usually occurs within days of the onset of symptoms. Prevention is of paramount importance, and eliminating infection in animal vectors is essential. Successful animal vaccination and animal control campaigns in the United States have led to a very low rate of human rabies cases. Rabies among dogs in the United States has been virtually eliminated. Recently, rabies transmitted from other animals, especially bat bites, has become a cause for concern.

The decision to provide postexposure prophylaxis can be complex. The local health department should be contacted. Several factors need to be considered, such as local epidemiology, type of animal involved, availability of the responsible animal for testing or quarantine, and the circumstances of the exposure, such as a provoked versus an unprovoked attack. In the United States, concurrent use of passive and active immunoprophylaxis is recommended. It consists of a regimen of one dose of immune globulin and five doses of human rabies vaccine over a 28-day period. Rabies immune globulin and the first dose of rabies vaccine should be given as soon as possible after exposure, ideally within 24 hours. Additional doses of rabies vaccine should be given on days 3, 7, 14, and 28 after the first vaccination. Rabies immune globulin is infiltrated into and around the wound, with any remaining volume administered intramuscularly at a site distant from the vaccine inoculation. Human rabies vaccine is administered intramuscularly into the anterolateral thigh or deltoid, depending on the age and size of the child. Administration into the gluteus muscle should be avoided, since this site has been associated with vaccine failure (Kliegman et al., 2007).

Nursing Assessment

Note history of an animal bite, especially if it was unprovoked, and exposure to bats. Document history of early symptoms of rabies infection, which are nonspecific and flu-like, such as fever, headache, and general malaise. The child may complain of pain, pruritus, and paresthesia at the bite site. As the virus spreads to the central nervous system, encephalitis develops. The disease will have progressive neurologic manifestations, which may include insomnia, confusion, anxiety, changes in behavior, agitation or excitation, hallucinations, hypersalivation, dysphagia, and hydrophobia, which results from aspiration when swallowing liquid or saliva. In some cases progressive paralysis may be present. The client may have periods of lucidity alternating with these neurologic changes.

Laboratory testing may include hair and saliva specimens from which the virus may be isolated. Serum and cerebrospinal fluid can be tested for antibodies to the rabies virus. Direct fluorescent antibody testing can be done to diagnose rabies in a suspected animal. The test can only be done postmortem and requires brain tissue from the potentially rabid animal.

Nursing Management

Few people survive once symptomatic rabies infection develops. Intensive supportive care is required, but recovery is extremely rare. Therefore, it is vital to educate children and families about the importance of seeking medical care after any animal bite to prevent death from rabies infection. Also, teach children to avoid wild animals, stray animals, and any animal with unusual behavior. Teach children not to provoke or attempt to capture wild or stray animals.

Regardless of whether immunoprophylaxis is initiated, appropriate wound management is necessary in all victims of a bite from a potentially rabid animal. This includes a thorough cleansing of all wounds with soap and water. Irrigation of wounds for at least 10 minutes with a virucidal agent, such as povidone–iodine solution, is recommended (Kliegman et al., 2007).

When caring for a child requiring postexposure prophylaxis, provide support and education to the child and family. Due to the seriousness and urgency surrounding this disease and treatment, the child and family are often very frightened. Consider comfort measures, such as EMLA cream and positioning, when giving immunization.

Vector-Borne Infections

Children are at a particular risk for contracting vector-borne diseases, which are diseases transmitted by ticks, mosquitoes, or other insect vectors (Table 36.5). Young children are unaware of the health risks around them and cannot take protective measures. Their immature immune system leads to a decreased capacity to resist vector-borne diseases. These diseases can be severe and even fatal, though most are treatable if identified early. Many times the child presents initially with nonspecific symptoms. Coupled with the fact that there are few definitive diagnostic tests available, this can lead to difficulty in promptly recognizing and treating these diseases.

Tick-borne diseases are the most common vector-borne illnesses in the United States. Two of the most common will be covered below.

▶ LYME DISEASE

Lyme disease, the most common vector-borne disease in the United States, is caused by the spirochete *Borrelia burgdorferi*. It is transmitted to humans via the bite of an infected blacklegged tick. It has been reported in more than 50 countries and is seen in three distinct regions in the United States. Most cases occur in the Northeast, from southern Maine to northern Virginia. Cases have also been reported in the upper Midwest and the West Coast, especially northern California, but with less frequency. Most cases are seen between April and October. Lyme disease can affect any age group, but the incidence is highest among children 5 to 10 years of age (Kliegman et al., 2007). The prognosis for recovery in children who are treated is excellent.

Therapeutic Management

In most cases Lyme disease can be cured by antibiotics, especially if they are started early in the illness. Doxycycline is the drug of choice for children older than 8 years. Because it can cause permanent discoloration of the teeth, children younger than 8 should be treated with amoxicillin. For clients allergic to penicillin, cefuroxime or erythromycin can be used. Duration of treatment is usually 14 to 21 days.

Nursing Assessment

The clinical signs of Lyme disease are divided into three stages: early localized, early disseminated, and late disease. Untreated clients may progress through the three stages or may present with early disseminated or late disease without having any symptoms of the earlier stages. If children are treated in the early stage, it is uncommon to see them with late disease. Nursing assessment for Lyme disease includes an accurate health history as well as physical examination.

Health History

Explore the health history for a tick bite. Document onset of rash. In early localized disease, the rash usually occurs 7 to 14 days after the tick bite (though it can appear 3 to 32 days after the bite). In early disseminated disease, the

TABLE 36.5 OTHER VECTOR-BORNE ILLNESSES

Disease	Causative Organism	Geographic Distribution	Vector of Transmission	Manifestations
Mediterranean spotted fever (boutonneuse fever)	*Rickettsia conorii*	Africa, Mediterranean region, India, Middle East	Tick bite	• Fever, headache, maculopapular rash • Eschar may be present at tick bite.
Rickettsial pox	*Rickettsia akari*	Northeastern cities in United States, Europe and Asia, mainly urban settings	Mouse mite bite	• Bite becomes a papule, then pustule, then ulcerates and forms eschar at site. • Fever, local adenopathy, headache, myalgia, maculopapular rash that may become vesicular
Epidemic typhus	*Rickettsia prowazekii*	Africa, South America, Central America, Mexico, Asia; occasional cases seen in United States	Louse feces (typically from the body louse) that are rubbed into broken skin or mucous membranes. Cases in United States associated with louse or flea of flying squirrel.	• Abrupt onset of high fever, chills, and myalgia with severe headache and malaise • Rash appears 4 to 7 days after onset of symptoms, beginning on the trunk and spreading to the extremities. • Maculopapular rash becomes petechial or hemorrhagic, then develops brown pigmented areas. • Changes in mental status may occur. • Flying squirrel–related disease typically presents as a milder illness.
Endemic typhus (murine typhus)	*Rickettsia typhi* and *Rickettsia felis*	Worldwide, especially warm coastal ports. In United States, most prevalent in southern Texas and southern California.	Rat flea or cat flea feces	• Headache, myalgia, and chills that slowly worsen • Fever for 10 to 14 days • Rash appears after 3 to 8 days; it is macular or maculopapular with sparse lesions and no hemorrhage.

(continued)

TABLE 36.5 OTHER VECTOR–BORNE ILLNESSES (continued)

Disease	Causative Organism	Geographic Distribution	Vector of Transmission	Manifestations
Scrub typhus	*Orientia tsutsugamushi*	Southern Asia, Japan, Indonesia, Australia, Korea, Asiatic Russia, India, China	Chigger bite	• Possible necrotic eschar at site of bite, fever, headache, myalgia, cough, and gastrointestinal symptoms • Lymphadenopathy, maculopapular rash on trunk and extremities.
Ehrlichioses	3 pathogens: *Ehrlichia chaffeensis*, *Ehrlichia anaplasma*, *Ehrlichia ewimgii*	Mostly in southeastern and south-central United States	Tick	• Fever with clinical signs similar to Rocky Mountain spotted fever. Rash is less commonly associated. • May also present with leukopenia, anemia, and hepatitis
Q fever	*Coxiella burnetii*	Worldwide	Inhalation of infected aerosols, ingestion of contaminated dairy products	• Most cases are initially asymptomatic. Occurs in two forms: • Acute: follows initial exposure and presents with abrupt onset of fever, chills, weakness, headache, and loss of appetite • Chronic: occurs years after initial exposure and may present with endocarditis (in clents with underlying heart disease), hepatitis, or fever of unknown origin
Malaria	*Plasmodium* (four species exist that infect humans: *P. falciparum*, *P. vivax*, *P. ovale*, *P. malariae*)	Endemic in tropical areas of the world. Highest risk in sub-Saharan Africa, Papua New Guinea, the Solomon Islands, and Vanuatu Other areas of risk: Haiti and Indian subcontinent	Bite of *Anopheles* species of mosquito	• High fever with chills, rigors, sweats, and headache, which may be paroxysmal • Nausea, vomiting, diarrhea, cough, arthralgia, abdominal and back pain may also occur. • Anemia and thrombocytopenia with pallor and jaundice may be seen. • May occur in a cyclic pattern, and depending on the species fever may occur every other day or every third day.

rash usually begins 3 to 5 weeks after the tick bite. Note complaints of fever, malaise, mild neck stiffness, headache, fatigue, myalgia, and arthralgia or pain in the joints. In late disease, note recurrent arthritis of the large joints, such as the knees, beginning weeks to months after the tick bite. The child with late disease may or may not have a history of earlier stages of the disease, including erythema migrans.

Physical Examination

Observe for a rash. Early local disease is characterized by a ring-like rash at the site of the tick bite (erythema migrans) (Fig. 36.4). If untreated, the rash gradually expands and will remain for 1 to 2 weeks. Early disseminated disease should be suspected if multiple areas of erythema migrans are found. The multiple lesions are usually smaller than the primary lesions. Note cranial nerve palsies (especially cranial nerve VII), conjunctivitis, or signs of meningeal irritation, which occur in early disseminated disease.

Laboratory and Diagnostic Testing

Immunoglobulin-specific antibody tests may not be positive in the early stage of the disease but may be useful in the later stages. The CDC recommends a two-step test: a sensitive enzyme immunoassay (EIA) or immunofluorescent assay (IFA) followed by a Western immunoblot. If these are negative, no further testing is indicated.

Nursing Management

Administer antibiotics as ordered. In the hospitalized client, no transmission-based precautions are necessary. Educate the client and family on the importance of taking the antibiotic as directed and finishing all the medicine. Another important nursing function is educating the client, family, and community on prevention measures (Box 36.5). For infection to occur, the tick must be attached for 24 to 48 hours, so prompt removal of ticks is essential to the prevention of Lyme disease. Teaching Guidelines 36.2 gives information on tick removal. A vac-

FIGURE 36.4 Erythema migrans, a ring-like rash at the site of the tick bite, occurs in Lyme disease.

> ### BOX 36.5   Prevention of Tick-Borne Illnesses
>
> • Wear appropriate protective clothing when entering tick-infested areas. Clothing should fit tightly around wrists, waists, and ankles. Tuck pants into socks if possible.
> • After leaving the area, check for ticks and remove them promptly.
> • Insect repellent may provide temporary relief but may produce toxicity, especially in children, if used frequently or in large doses.

cine was licensed in 1998 by the U.S. Food and Drug Administration for persons ages 15 to 70, but it has since been withdrawn due to low demand.

▶ ROCKY MOUNTAIN SPOTTED FEVER

Rocky Mountain spotted fever (RMSF) is the most severe and frequently reported rickettsial illness in the United States. A rickettsia is a bacteria of the genus Rickettsiae; these bacteria are carried as a parasite by many ticks, fleas, and lice and cause disease in humans. RMSF is caused by the bacteria *Rickettsia rickettsii*. The American dog tick and Rocky Mountain wood tick are the primary vectors, although others have been implicated. RMSF can be fatal without prompt and appropriate treatment. Most cases occur between April and September.

RMSF occurs throughout the United States; its name is derived from the fact that it was discovered in the Rocky Mountain region, though few cases are found there today. RMSF is more common in the coastal Atlantic states, with

> ### TEACHING GUIDELINES 36.2
>
> **Tick Removal**
>
> • Use fine-tipped tweezers.
> • Protect fingers with a tissue, paper towel, or latex gloves.
> • Grasp tick as close to the skin as possible and pull upward with steady, even pressure.
> • Do not twist or jerk the tick.
> • Once the tick is removed, clean site with soap and water and wash your hands.
> • Save the tick for identification in case the child becomes sick. Place in a sealable plastic bag and put it in your freezer. Write date of bite on the bag.

the highest incidence in North Carolina and Oklahoma. It occurs in all age groups but most frequently in children, with the peak incidence in 5- to 9-year-olds (Kliegman et al., 2007).

Complications of RMSF include noncardiogenic pulmonary edema, cerebral edema, and multiorgan damage. Long-term neurologic involvement, such as partial paralysis of the lower extremities, hearing loss, loss of bladder and bowel control, movement disorders, and language disorders, may be seen, especially in clients with severe illness who require long hospital stays.

Therapeutic Management

The fatality rate from RMSF has decreased with the widespread use of antimicrobial therapy. However, delays in diagnosis and therapy are significant factors associated with severity of disease and death. In most cases RMSF resolves rapidly with appropriate antibiotic therapy, especially if it is started early. Treatments of choice are tetracyclines, such as doxycycline, and chloramphenicol. Chloramphenicol is the preferred drug in children less than 9 years old due to the risk of teeth staining, though some clinicians use doxycycline to treat children less than 9 because tooth discoloration is dose-dependent and children less than 9 are unlikely to need multiple doses (Kliegman et al., 2007). Length of treatment is 5 to 10 days.

Nursing Assessment

Note history of early signs of RMSF, such as sudden onset of fever, headache, malaise, nausea and vomiting, muscle pain, and anorexia. The incubation period varies from 2 to 14 days, with the average being around 7 days after the tick bite. Late signs include a rash, usually seen 2 to 5 days after the onset of the fever, abdominal pain, joint pain, and diarrhea. Inspect the skin for a rash, which starts as small, pink, macular, non-itchy, blanchable spots on the wrists, forearms, and ankles. The rash then spreads rapidly over the entire body, including the soles and palms. After several days the rash will appear red, spotted and petechial, or hemorrhagic (Fig. 36.5). Approximately 10% to 15% of those with RMSF do not have a rash (Kliegman et al., 2007). Laboratory findings may include a low leukocyte count, low or decreasing platelet count, and hyponatremia. Biopsy of the rash with immunofluorescent assay and serologic tests may also be used.

FIGURE 36.5 Rash associated with Rocky Mountain spotted fever.

Nursing Management

Nursing management is similar to that for Lyme disease. Educate the family about completing the antibiotic course, preventing tick bites, and appropriate tick removal (refer to Box 36.5 and Teaching Guidelines 36.2).

Parasitic and Helminthic Infections

Parasites are organisms larger than yeast or bacteria that can cause infection. They live in or on a host. Parasites receive nourishment from the host without benefiting or killing the host. Parasites frequently seen in children are scabies and head lice. A helminth is a parasitic intestinal worm. Helminthic infections seen in children include pinworms, roundworms, and hookworms. Children are at an increased risk for parasitic or helminthic infections due to poor hygiene practices: they are typically more careless about handwashing and they tend to put things in their mouths and share toys and objects with other children.

Nursing Assessment and Management

Parents are often embarrassed when they find out that their child has a parasitic or helminthic infection. Reassure them that these infections can occur in any child. Tables 36.6 and 36.7 give nursing assessment and management information related to specific common parasitic and helminthic infections in children.

(text continues on page 1135)

TABLE 36.6   COMMON PARASITIC INFECTIONS IN CHILDREN

Infection/Causative Organism	Transmission	Clinical Manifestations	Diagnosis/Treatment	Isolation/Control Measures
Pediculosis capitis (head lice) Caused by *Pediculus humanus capitis* (head louse)	Direct contact with hair of infested people, less commonly with personal belongings, such as combs and hats, of those infested. Incubation period from laying of eggs to hatching of nymph is 6 to 10 days; adult lice will appear 2 to 3 weeks later.	Extreme pruritus is the most common symptom. Adult eggs (nits) or lice may be seen, especially behind the ears and at the nape of the neck.	Diagnosis by identification of eggs, nymph, and lice with the naked eye is possible; adult lice are rarely seen. Treatment: Washing hair with a pediculicide such as permethrin, lindane, malathion. Careful instructions on proper use of any product should be given and strict adherence to application instructions encouraged. Detection of living lice 24 hours after treatment suggests incorrect use, a very heavy infestation, reinfestation, or resistance to treatment. Removal of nits after treatment is not necessary to prevent spread but may be done for aesthetic reasons (Pickering, 2006).	Contact precautions Control measures: Household and other close contacts should be examined and if infested treated. Bedmates should be treated prophylactically. Children should not be excluded or sent home from school. Most children can be treated effectively without treating their clothing and bedding. If needed, dry-cleaning clothing or simply sealing it in a plastic bag for 10 days is effective. Disinfection of headgear, pillowcases, and towels by washing in hot water and drying on the hot cycle may be helpful. Soak combs and hairbrushes in pediculicide, shampoo, or hot water (Pickering, 2006). Lice infestation is not a sign of poor hygiene; all socioeconomic groups are affected.
Pediculosis pubis (pubic lice) Caused by *Phthirus pubis*	Transmission usually occurs through sexual contact; also can be through contaminated items such as towels.	Pruritus of anogenital area; other hairy areas of the body, including eyelashes, eyebrows, axilla, beard, can be affected	Diagnosis by identification of eggs, nymph, and lice with the naked eye is possible; adult lice are rarely seen. Same as treatment with pediculicides to treat head lice. Retreat 7 to 10 days later. Use petroleum oil to treat eyelashes and eyebrows.	Contact precautions All sexual contacts should be treated.

TABLE 36.6 COMMON PARASITIC INFECTIONS IN CHILDREN (continued)

Infection/Causative Organism	Transmission	Clinical Manifestations	Diagnosis/Treatment	Isolation/Control Measures
Scabies Caused by *Saracoptes scabiei*	Incubation period from laying of eggs to hatching of nymph is 6 to 10 days; adult lice will appear 2 to 3 weeks later. Transmission usually occurs through prolonged, close personal contact. Incubation period in those without previous exposure is 4 to 6 weeks. People who were previously infested can develop symptoms in 1 to 4 days.	Intense pruritus (especially at night) with presence of erythematous, papular rash with excoriations. The lesions are generally distributed but often are concentrated on the hands and feet and in body folds. May be found on head and neck. In infants and young children and those who are immunocompromised, the rash may include vesicles, pustules, or nodules.	Diagnosis can be made by a history of itching (especially at night), classic rash, and reports of itching in household or sexual contacts. Mites can be seen on microscopic examination of skin scrapings to confirm diagnosis. Treatment: A scabicide, such as permethrin or lindane, should be applied to the entire body below the head. Treatment of infants and young children should include the head, neck, and body. The cream is left on for a specified time (usually 8 to 14 hours) depending on the type of scabicide. Careful instructions on proper use of any product should be given and strict adherence to application instructions should be urged. Itching may not subside for several weeks, even after successful treatment.	Contact precautions. Prophylactic therapy for household members Bedding and clothing worn the 4 days prior to treatment should be laundered in hot water and dried on the hot cycle (mites do not survive more than 3 to 4 days without skin contact). Environmental disinfestation is unnecessary (Pickering, 2006).

TABLE 36.7   COMMON HELMINTHIC INFECTIONS IN CHILDREN

Infection/Causative Organism	Clinical Manifestations	Transmission	Diagnosis/Treatment	Isolation/Control Measures
Roundworm (ascariasis) Caused by *Ascaris lumbricoides*, common in temperate and tropical areas	Loss of appetite, nausea, vomiting, and abdominal pain may be seen. In significant infestation, partial or complete intestinal obstruction may occur. The more worms, the worse the symptoms.	Human feces are the major source of infected eggs. Hand to mouth is the usual route of transmission. The eggs are swallowed due to unclean hands or contaminated food. They pass into the intestine; larvae then hatch, penetrate the intestinal wall, enter the circulatory system, and migrate to any body tissue.	Diagnosis: Once female worms are in the intestine, eggs can be visualized by microscopic evaluation of the stool. Occasionally a worm may be visualized in vomit or stool. Treatment is with mebendazole, albendazole, or pyrantel pamoate.	• Standard precautions are sufficient. • Sanitary disposal of feces • Proper hand hygiene
Hookworm Caused by *Ancylostoma duodenale* (roundworm) (found mainly in Europe, Africa, China, Japan, India, and the Pacific Islands) and *Necator americanus* (roundworm) (found mainly in the Americas, Caribbean, Africa, Asia, and the Pacific)	Most often people are asymptomatic until significant worms are established. May see pruritic erythematous papular rash at entry site (referred to as ground itch) or pulmonary symptoms as the larvae migrate. One of the greatest concerns in chronic infection is anemia (microcytic hypochromic anemia) secondary to blood loss as the worms suck blood and juices from the intestines. This can lead to hypoproteinemia, edema, pica, and wasting. The infection may result in physical or mental retardation in children.	Hookworms are found in soil and enter the host through pores, hair follicles, and even intact skin (hands and feet are major sites of entry). The maturing larvae travel through the circulatory system into the lungs and then up the bron-chial tree and then are swallowed with secretions. They then migrate into the intestinal tract and attach to the wall of the small intestines, where they feed and reproduce. Transmission via ingested soil has been seen with *Ancylostoma duodenale* only.	Diagnosis is made through microscopic examination of feces that reveals hookworm eggs. Treatment: Albendazole, mebendazole, and pyrantel pamoate. In children younger than 2, the World Health Organization recommends half the adult dose of albendazole or mebendazole (Pickering, 2006). Iron supplementation and possible blood transfusion in severe cases	• Standard precautions are sufficient. • Proper sanitation and disposal of feces • Treatment of all known infested people • Screening of high-risk individuals • Encourage the wearing of shoes and avoiding going barefoot.

(continued)

TABLE 36.7 COMMON HELMINTHIC INFECTIONS IN CHILDREN (continued)

Infection/Causative Organism	Clinical Manifestations	Transmission	Diagnosis/Treatment	Isolation/Control Measures
Pinworm Caused by *Enterobius vermicularis* (roundworm)	Some people are asymptomatic. May cause anal itching (pruritus ani), especially at night. Other clinical findings may include teeth grinding at night, weight loss, and enuresis.	Fecal–oral route directly, indirectly, or inadvertently by contaminated hands or shared toys, bedding, clothing, toilet seats Incubation period is 1 to 2 months or longer.	Diagnosis is made when adult worms are visualized in the perianal region; they are best viewed when the child is sleeping. Very few ova are present in stool, so examination of stool is not recommended. Transparent tape pressed to perianal area and then viewed under a microscope may reveal eggs. Three consecutive specimens should be obtained when the child first awakens in the morning. Treatment of choice is mebendazole, pyrantel pamoate, and albendazole, usually single doses and repeated in 2 weeks. All family members should be treated since transmission from person to person is very easy.	Standard precautions are sufficient. Reinfection occurs easily. Infected people should bathe in the morning, which will remove a large portion of the eggs. Frequent changing of underclothes and bedding. Personal hygiene measures such as keeping fingernails short, avoiding scratching of perianal area and nail biting. Good hand hygiene is the most effective preventive measure, especially after using the bathroom and before eating.

▶ *Take* NOTE!

The head louse is becoming increasingly resistant to pediculicides. This may lead parents to resort to home remedies. Parents need to be informed that these remedies are unproven and can be toxic.

As the nurse in a pediatric clinic, you receive a call from a frantic mother. She tells you, "The school sent my daughter home and told me she has lice! We are clean people! I don't understand how this could happen!" How would you address her concerns? Discuss the plan of care for this child. What education and interventions will be necessary to prevent the spread of pediculosis capitis?

■■■ Key Concepts

■ Infants and young children are more susceptible to infection due to their immature immune system. Young children continue to have an increased risk for infections and communicable disorders because disease protection from immunizations is not complete.

■ When obtaining blood cultures, follow aseptic technique and hospital protocol to prevent contamination. Obtain the specimen before administering antibiotics.

■ When administering antipyretics, proper education must be given to caregivers on appropriate dosing, concentration, dosing interval, and use of proper measuring device.

■ Promoting proper fluid balance and reducing temperature in a febrile child are important nursing interventions when caring for a child with an infection or communicable illness.

■ Many childhood infectious and communicable diseases involve a rash. Rashes can be difficult to identify, so a thorough description and history from the caregiver is important.

■ Sepsis, a systemic overresponse to infection resulting from bacteria, fungi, viruses, or parasites, can lead to septic shock. Any infant less than 3 months old with a fever or any child with a fever accompanied by extreme lethargy, unresponsiveness, or lack of facial expressions should be seen by a health care provider.

■ Many bacterial and viral infections, such as diphtheria, tetanus, pertussis, mumps, measles, rubella, varicella, and poliomyelitis, can be prevented by vaccination.

■ Children are at a particular risk for contracting vector-borne diseases, which are disease transmitted by ticks, mosquitoes, or other insect vectors. Two of the most commonly seen are Lyme disease and Rocky Mountain spotted fever.

■ Viral exanthems of childhood often present with a distinct rash pattern that assists in the diagnosis of the virus. Common childhood exanthems include exanthem subitum (roseola infantum), rubella (German measles), rubeola (measles), varicella (chickenpox), and erythema infectiosum (fifth disease).

■ Nurses play a key role in educating the public on the importance of immunizations.

■ Health care providers need to remember and educate parents that fever is a protective mechanism the body uses to fight infection.

REFERENCES

Ackley, B. J., & Ladwig, G. B. (2006). *Nursing diagnosis handbook: A guide to planning care* (7th ed.). St. Louis: Mosby.

Amitai, A., Sinert, R., & Medlin, R. (2006). Tick-borne diseases, Rocky Mountain spotted fever. *eMedicine.* Retrieved 7/22/06 from http://www.emedicine.com/emerg/topic510.htm.

Apolito, K. C. (2006). State of the science: Procedural pain management in the neonate. *Journal of Perinatal and Neonatal Nursing, 20*(1), 56–61.

Atkinson, W., Hamborsky, J., McIntyre, L., & Wolfe, S. (Eds.). (2007). *Epidemiology and prevention of vaccine-preventable diseases* (10th ed.). Washington, DC: Public Health Foundation.

Boyer, K. M., & Severin, P. N. (2006). Sepsis and septic shock. In J. A. McMillan (Ed.), *Oski's pediatrics: Principles and practice* (pp. 918–923). Philadelphia: Lippincott Williams & Wilkins.

Bratton, R. L., & Corey, G. R. (2005). Tick-borne diseases. *American Family Physician, 71*(12), 2323–2330.

Centers for Disease Control and Prevention. (2006). Update: multistate outbreak of mumps—United States, January 1–May 2, 2006. *MMWR Dispatch, 55,* 1–5.

Centers for Disease Control and Prevention. (2007). *Nationally notifiable infectious diseases, United States 2007, revised.* Retrieved September 15, 2007 from http://www.cdc.gov/epo/dphsi/phs/infdis2007r.htm.

Crawford, M. B. (2006). Pediatrics, bacteremia and sepsis. *eMedicine.* Retrieved July 22, 2006 from http://www.emedicine.com/EMERG/topic364.htm#section~author_information.

Crocetti, M. T., & Serwint, J. R. (2005). Fever: Separating fact from fiction. *Contemporary Pediatrics.* Retrieved July 22, 2006 from www.contemporarypediatrics.com/contpeds/content/contentDetail.jsp?id=143315.

Evans, J. C., McCartney, E. M., Lawhon, G., & Galloway, J. (2005). Longitudinal comparison of preterm pain response to repeated heelsticks. *Pediatric Nursing, 31*(3), 216–221.

Fischbach, F. T. (2004). *A manual of laboratory and diagnostic tests* (7th ed.). Philadelphia: Lippincott Williams & Wilkins.

Flinders, D. C., & De Schweinitz, P. (2004). Pediculosis and scabies. *American Family Physician, 69*(2), 341–348.

Folk, L. A. (2007). Guide to capillary heelstick blood sampling in infants. *Advances in Neonatal Care, 7*(4), 171–178.

Goldrick, B. A. (2005). Emerging infections: Pertussis on the rise. *American Journal of Nursing, 105*(1), 69–71.

Hotez, P. J., Brooker, S., Bethony, J. M., Bottazzi, M. E., Loukas, A., & Xiao, S. (2004). Current concepts: Hookworm infection. *New England Journal of Medicine, 351*(8), 799–807.

Kenner, C., & Lott, J. W. (2004). *Neonatal nursing handbook.* St. Louis: Saunders.

Kliegman, R. M., Behrman, R. E., Jenson, H. B., & Stanton, B. F. (2007). *Nelson's textbook of pediatrics* (18th ed.). Philadelphia: Saunders.

Knies, R. C. (2004). Research applied to clinical practice: Sepsis in children. *Emergency Nursing World.* Retrieved 7/22/06 from http://enw.org/Research-SepticKid.htm.

Kucik, C. J., Martin, G. C., & Sortor, B. V. (2004). Common intestinal parasites. *American Family Physician, 69*(5), 1161–1168.

Levin, M. J., & Weinberg, A. (2007). Infections: Viral and rickettsial. In W. W. Hay, M. J. Levin, J. M. Sondheimer, & R. R. Deterding (Eds.), *Current pediatric diagnosis and treatment* (18th ed.) New York: McGraw-Hill.

McMillan, J. A., & Feigin, R. (2006). Diphtheria. In J. A. McMillan (Ed.), *Oski's pediatrics: Principles and practice* (4th ed., pp. 1059–1062). Philadelphia: Lippincott Williams & Wilkins.

Murray, S. S., & McKinnery, E. S. (2006). *Foundations of maternal-newborn nursing* (4th ed.). St. Louis: Saunders.

National Center for Infectious Diseases. (2003). *About the Center.* Retrieved December 19, 2007, from http://www.cdc.gov/ncidod/about.htm

Niederhauser, V. P. (2006). Pediatric primary care. In S. M. Nettina (Ed.), *Lippincott manual of nursing practice* (8th ed., pp. 1350–1381). Philadelphia: Lippincott Williams & Wilkins.

Ogle, J. W., & Anderson, M. S. (2007). Infections: Bacterial and spirochetal. In W. W. Hay, M. J. Levin, J. M. Sondheimer, & R. R. Deterding (Eds.), *Current pediatric diagnosis and treatment* (18th ed.). New York: McGraw-Hill.

Pagana, K. D., & Pagana, T. J. (2006). *Mosby's manual of diagnostic and laboratory tests* (3rd ed.). St. Louis: Mosby.

Pickering, L. K. (Ed.). (2006). *Red book: 2006 report of the committee on infectious diseases* (27th ed.). Elk Grove Village, IL: American Academy of Pediatrics.

Prinzhorn, J., & Churchwell, C. (2004). Fever management in children who are febrile is questionable. *Pediatric Nursing, 30*(4), 322.

Public Health Service, U.S. Department of Health and Human Services, Centers for Disease Control and Prevention, Siegel, J. D.,

Rhinehart, E., Jackson, J., Chiarello, L. & the Healthcare Infection Control Practices Advisory Committee. (2007). *2007 guidelines for isolation precautions: Preventing transmission of infectious agents in health care settings.* Retrieved September 15, 2007 from www.cdc.gov/ncidod/dhqp/gl_isolation.html.

Serwint, J. R., Collier, D. N., & Billings, C. (2007). *Alternating acetaminophen and ibuprofen.* Retrieved September 19, 2007 from http://pedsinreview.aappublications.org/cgi/eletters/28/2/7s.

Stephenson, J. (2004). Polio eradication plan. *JAMA, 291*(77), 813.

Takano-Lee, M., Edman, J. D., Mullens, B. A., & Clark, J. M. (2004). Home remedies to control head lice: Assessment of home remedies to control the human head louse, *Pediculus humanus capitis* (Anoplura: Pediculidae). *Journal of Pediatric Nursing, 19*(6), 393–398.

Weir, E. (2005). Parvovirus B19 infection: Fifth disease and more. *Canadian Medical Association Journal, 172*(6), 743.

WEBSITES

American Social Health Organization: www.ashastd.org

Lyme Disease Foundation: www.lyme.org

Measles Initiative: www.measlesinitiative.org/index3.asp

National Center for Infectious Diseases, Centers for Disease Control and Prevention: www.cdc.gov/ncidod/about.htm

National Foundation for Infectious Diseases: www.nfid.org

National Pediculosis Association: www.headlice.org

CHAPTER WORKSHEET

MULTIPLE CHOICE QUESTIONS

1. Compared with adults, why are infants and children at an increased risk for infection and communicable diseases?

   a. The infant has had limited exposure to disease and is losing the passive immunity acquired from maternal antibodies.

   b. The infant demonstrates an increased inflammatory response.

   c. Cellular immunity is not functional at birth.

   d. Infants have an increased risk for infection until they receive their first set of immunizations.

2. A mother calls the clinic because her 2-year-old daughter has a rectal temperature of 37.8°C (100°F). She wonders how high a fever should be before she should give medications to reduce it. What is the best response by the nurse?

   a. "All fevers should be treated to prevent seizures."

   b. "Antipyretics should be used with any rise in temperature. They can help change the course of the infection."

   c. "Give your child aspirin when her fever is above 38°C (100.4°F)."

   d. "In a normal healthy child, if your child is not uncomfortable, fevers less than 39°C (102.2°F) do not require medication."

3. A neonate should be evaluated by a physician if which signs and symptoms are present?

   a. Acting fussier than normal

   b. Refusing the pacifier

   c. Rectal temperature above 38°C

   d. Mottling that is present during bathing

4. The public health nurse has been asked to provide information to local childcare centers on controlling the spread of infectious diseases. What is the best information the nurse can provide?

   a. The etiology of common infectious diseases

   b. Proper handwashing techniques

   c. The physiology of the immune system

   d. Why children are at a higher risk of infection than adults

CRITICAL THINKING EXERCISES

1. A 12-year-old boy presents with a very sore throat and fever. On assessment you find an erythematous rash on his face that feels like sandpaper. You obtain a throat culture, which is positive for group A streptococcus. What instructions would you give the parents regarding his care at home?

2. A 1-month-old infant is admitted to the hospital to rule out sepsis. What would be your priority nursing interventions?

3. A 4-year-old child presents with a fever and rash. What three of the following items should the nurse obtain during the health history?

   a. Immunization history

   b. Any exposure to communicable or infectious diseases

   c. Whether the child takes a daily vitamin

   d. Thorough description and history of the rash

   e. Mother's immunization history

STUDY ACTIVITIES

1. The 4-year-old presented in question 3 above was diagnosed with varicella zoster virus. Write a nursing care plan for a child with varicella.

2. You are asked to give a presentation to a group of adolescents on sexually transmitted infections, including transmission, symptoms, treatment, and prevention. What information would you include?

3. A child is brought to the school nurse with intense itching. Upon assessment the nurse finds an erythematous, papular rash with excoriations on the child's hands and feet. As suspected, the diagnosis of scabies is confirmed. What teaching is necessary for the parents, family, and classmates of the child?

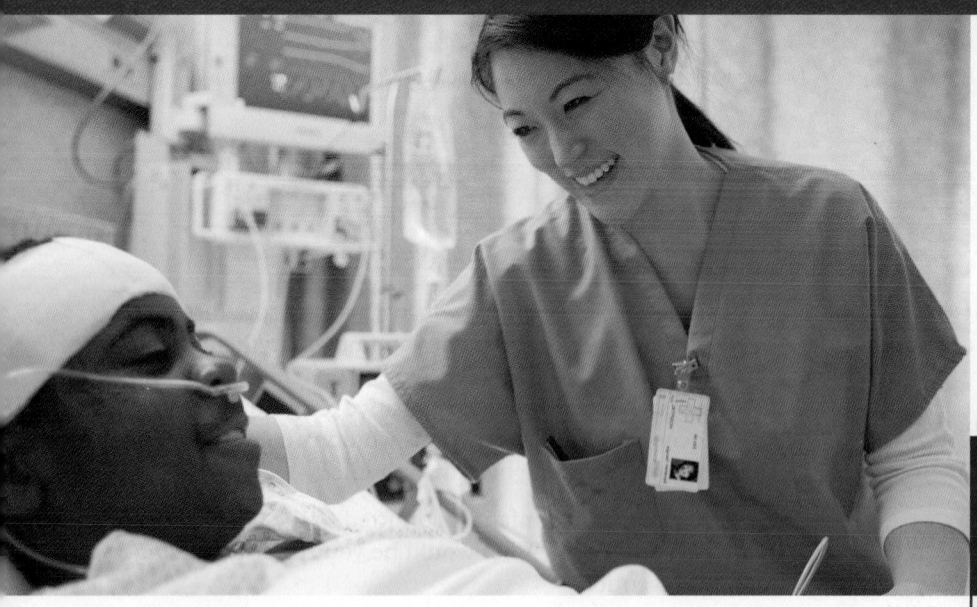

NURSING CARE OF THE CHILD WITH A NEUROLOGIC DISORDER

KEY TERMS

automatism
central nervous system
   (CNS)
cerebrospinal fluid (CSF)
clonic
decorticate posturing

decerebrate posturing
head circumference
intracranial pressure (ICP)
lumbar puncture (LP)
myelinization
myoclonus

neural tube
opisthotonic
postictal
status epilepticus
teratogen
tonic

LEARNING OBJECTIVES

Upon completion of the chapter, the learner will be able to:

1. Compare how the anatomy and physiology of the neurologic system in children differs from adults.
2. Identify various factors associated with neurologic disease in infants and children.
3. Discuss common laboratory and other diagnostic tests useful in the diagnosis of neurologic conditions.
4. Discuss common medications and other treatments used for treatment and palliation of neurologic conditions.
5. Recognize risk factors associated with various neurologic disorders.
6. Distinguish among different neurologic illnesses based on the signs and symptoms associated with them.
7. Discuss nursing interventions commonly used for neurologic illnesses.
8. Devise an individualized nursing care plan for the child with a neurologic disorder.
9. Develop client and family teaching plans for the child with a neurologic disorder.
10. Describe the psychosocial impact of chronic neurologic disorders on children.

Antonio Chapman, 3 months old, has had increased irritability, poor sucking and feeding, and a fever for the past 24 hours. Today he is lethargic with a weak cry and is vomiting his feeds.

WOW

As long as nurses possess inner integrity, they will be able to handle their patient's life's challenges.

Neurologic disorders in children often have a devastating and lasting impact. Neurologic disorders can be divided into several categories, including structural disorders, seizure disorders, infectious disorders, trauma to the neurologic system, blood flow disruption disorders, and chronic disorders.

Nurses must be familiar with neurologic conditions affecting children in order to provide prevention, prompt treatment, guidance, and support to families. Neurologic disorders require acute interventions, but many times have long-lasting implications on the child's health and development. Due to the potentially devastating effects that neurologic disorders can have on children and their families, nurses need to be skilled in assessment and interventions in this area and must be able to provide support throughout the course of the illness and beyond.

Variations in Pediatric Anatomy and Physiology

Neurologic disorders can result from congenital problems as well as from infections or traumas. Certain neurologic conditions occur in children more often than adults and will affect their growth and development. Pediatric clients are at an increased risk for different neurologic problems than adults due to anatomic and physiologic differences.

Brain and Spinal Cord Development

Development of the brain and spinal cord occurs early in gestation, in the first 3 to 4 weeks, from the **neural tube**. Infection, trauma, **teratogens**, and malnutrition during this period can result in malformations in brain and spinal cord development and may affect normal **central nervous system (CNS)** development.

At birth, the cranial bones are not well developed and are unfused. Therefore there is an increased risk for fracture. The brain is highly vascular, leading to an increased risk for hemorrhage. Premature infants are at greater risk for brain damage; the more premature the infant, the greater the risk. The premature infant has more capillaries in the periventricular area, which is the brain tissue that lines the outside of the lateral ventricles. These capillaries are fragile and at greater risk for rupture, leading to intracranial bleeding. Also, because the cranium is very soft in the preterm infant, external pressure can change its shape and cause increased pressure in areas of the brain and possible hemorrhage.

The sutures and fontanels present in the newborn help make the skull more flexible and help to accommodate for brain growth that continues after birth. Closure of the fontanels too early or too late can be indicative of problems with brain growth. The child's spine is very mobile, especially the cervical spine region, resulting in a high risk for cervical spine injury.

Nervous System

The development of the nervous system is complete but immature at birth. The infant is born with all the nerve cells that he or she will have throughout life. However, myelinization of these nerves is incomplete. The speed and accuracy of nerve impulses increases as **myelinization** increases. This process accounts for the acquisition of fine and gross motor movements and coordination in early childhood. Myelinization proceeds in the cephalocaudal direction. For example, infants are able to control the head and neck before the trunk and extremities.

The immaturity of the CNS in preterm infants can result in delayed development of motor skills. Premature newborns may have difficulty coordinating sucking and swallowing, leading to feeding and growth issues. Also, episodes of apnea can be problematic in the preterm newborn due to the underdevelopment of the nervous system.

Head Size

The head of the infant and young child is large in proportion to the body. The head of an infant accounts for a quarter of the body height; in adults it accounts for one eighth of the body height (Fig. 37.1). In addition, the infant's and child's neck muscles are not well developed. Both of these differences lead to an increased incidence of head injury from falls. The head is the fastest growing body part during infancy and continues to grow until the child is 5 years old.

Common Medical Treatments

A variety of interventions, including medical treatments and medications, are used to treat neurologic illness in children. Most of these treatments will require a physician's order when the child is hospitalized. The most common treatments and medications used for neurologic disorders are listed in Common Medical Treatments 37.1 and Drug Guide 37.1.

NURSING PROCESS OVERVIEW FOR THE CHILD WITH A NEUROLOGIC DISORDER

Care of the child with a neurologic disorder includes assessment, nursing diagnosis, planning, interventions, and evaluation. There are a number of general concepts related to the nursing process that can be applied to the management of neurologic disorders. From a general understanding of the care involved for a child with neurologic dysfunction, the nurse can then individualize the care based on client specifics.

Newborn   6 years   25 years

FIGURE 37.1 Proportion of head to body height in the newborn, child, and adult.

*R*emember Antonio, the 3-month-old with lethargy, a weak cry, and vomiting? What additional health history and physical examination assessment information should the nurse obtain?

Assessment

Assessment of neurologic dysfunction in children includes health history, physical examination, and laboratory and diagnostic testing.

▶ **Take** NOTE!

Neurologic assessment should proceed from least invasive to most invasive. The use of toys and familiar objects, as well as incorporating play, will help promote cooperation from the child.

Health History

The health history consists of past medical history, including the mother's pregnancy history, family history, and history of present illness (when the symptoms started and how they have progressed) as well as treatments used at home. The past medical history might be significant for prematurity, difficult birth, infection during preg-

nancy, nausea, vomiting, headaches, changes in gait, falls, visual disturbances, or recent trauma. Family history might be significant for genetic disorders with neurologic manifestations; seizure disorders; or headaches. When eliciting the history of the present illness, inquire about the following:

• Nausea
• Vomiting
• Changes in gait
• Visual disturbances
• Complaints of headaches
• Recent trauma
• Changes in cognition
• Change in consciousness, including any loss of consciousness
• Poor feeding
• Lethargy
• Increased irritability
• Fever
• Neck pain
• Altered muscle tonicity
• Delays in growth and development
• Ingestion or inhalation of neurotoxic substances or chemicals

Physical Examination

Physical examination of the nervous system consists of inspection and observation; palpation; and auscultation.

COMMON MEDICAL TREATMENTS 37.1

Treatment	Explanation	Indications	Nursing Implications
Shunt placement	A catheter is placed in the ventricle to pass the CSF to the peritoneal cavity, atrium of the heart, or pleural spaces. (Ventriculoperitoneal shunts are commonly used.)	Hydrocephalus, increased ICP	Monitor: • For signs and symptoms of increased ICP • Neurologic status closely • Level of consciousness and vital signs • For signs and symptoms of infection
Ventilation	Hyperventilation to decrease $PaCO_2$, which will result in vasoconstriction and therefore decrease ICP Adequate oxygenation to prevent hypoxia and further damage to the brain	Increased ICP	Monitor: • Arterial blood gases • For signs and symptoms of increased ICP • Pulse oximetry
PT/OT/ST	Therapies are used to improve motor function and ability of clients with neurologic disorders.	Head injury, mental retardation	Ensure adequate communication exists within the interdisciplinary team.
External ventricular drainage (EVD)	A catheter is temporarily placed in the ventricle and CSF is drained in a closed system to an external reservoir	Most commonly used with shunt infections until CSF is sterile and shunt can be replaced; treats acute-onset hydrocephalus, meningitis, encephalitis, tumors that cause blockage of CSF, closed head injury, subarachnoid hemorrhage, increased ICP; also can be used to monitor ICP	Monitor: • For signs and symptoms of increased ICP • Neurologic status closely • Level of consciousness and vital signs • For signs and symptoms of infection • Level of collection container when drain is unclamped
Ventricular tap	To reduce accumulation of CSF and decrease ICP	Increased ICP	Monitor: • Level of consciousness • Neurologic status
Vagal nerve stimulator	A nerve stimulator is implanted and a lead wire running under the skin is wrapped around the vagus nerve. The stimulator is programmed to provide the appropriate dose of stimulation at preset intervals; additional stimulation can be administered.	Short- and long-term seizure management in children >12 years of age	Monitor: • For signs and symptoms of infection • For seizure activity
Ketogenic diet	Diet involving high intake of fats, adequate protein, and a very low intake of carbohydrates, resulting in a ketosis state. Child is kept in a mild state of dehydration.	Prevention, control, and reduction of seizures, in particular for children with difficult-to-control seizures	Monitor: • Input and output closely • For seizure activity • Growth and nutritional status The diet is time consuming and many clients find it unpalatable; therefore all families and clients do not accept it.

DRUG GUIDE 37.1

Medication	Action/Indication	Nursing Implications
Antibiotics (oral, parenteral, intrathecal)	Treatment of bacterial meningitis and shunt infections/kill and prevent the growth of bacteria	Check for antibiotic allergies. Monitor serum levels to ensure therapeutic dosing if indicated. Give as prescribed for the length of time prescribed.
Anticonvulsants (oral, parenteral)	Decrease hyperexcitability of nerves Treatment and prevention of seizures	Maintain seizure precautions. Monitor for drug interactions and long-term adverse effects. Monitor and document all seizure activity. Many are used in combination, but need to be aware of interactions and long-term adverse effects. Stopping drug abruptly may precipitate seizures or even status epilepticus.
Benzodiazepines Diazepam (oral, rectal, or parenteral) Lorazepam (parenteral or oral)	Minor sedative that prevents or stops seizures by slowing down the CNS, making abnormal electrical activity unlikely. Treatment for status epilepticus	Diazepam is available in rectal form to stop prolonged seizures in children. Useful for home management; nurses must educate family members on administration and when to call MD. Monitor sedation level and for cessation of seizure activity.
Analgesics (acetaminophen, ibuprofen, ketorolac, morphine)	Blocks pain impulse in response to inhibition of prostaglandin synthesis. Narcotic analgesics (i.e., morphine) act on receptors in the brain to alter perception of pain. Used to treat pain. Used to help avoid increase in ICP.	Monitor for improvements in pain. Monitor sedation and respiratory status with narcotics. Monitor neurologic status closely. Used cautiously because loss of accurate neurologic evaluation can occur
Osmotic diuretics (i.e., mannitol)	Increases plasma osmolality, therefore inducing diffusion back into plasma and extra-vascular space/reduces ICP	Monitor electrolytes. Monitor I/O closely. Monitor vital signs. Monitor for signs and symptoms of increased ICP.
Corticosteroids (i.e., dexamethasone)	Suppresses inflammation and normal immune response/reduces cerebral edema	Give oral doses with food. Dosage must be tapered before discontinuing.

Inspection and Observation

Specific areas to inspect and observe include level of consciousness (LOC); vital signs; head, face, and neck; cranial nerve function; motor function; reflexes; sensory function; and **increased intracranial pressure (ICP)**.

Level of Consciousness (LOC). Begin the physical examination with inspection and observation. Observe the child's LOC, noting a decrease or significant changes. LOC is the earliest indicator of improvement or deterioration of neurologic status. Extreme irritability or lethargy is considered an abnormal finding. Consciousness consists of alertness, which is a wakeful state and includes the ability to respond to stimuli; and cognition, which includes the ability to process stimuli and demonstrate a verbal or motor response. Five different states constitute the levels of consciousness:

1. *Full consciousness* is defined as a state in which the child is awake and alert; is oriented to time, place, and person; and exhibits age-appropriate behaviors.
2. *Confusion* is defined as a state in which disorientation exists. The child may be alert but responds inappropriately to questions.
3. *Obtunded* is defined as a state in which the child has limited responses to the environment and falls asleep unless stimulation is provided.
4. *Stupor* exists when the child only responds to vigorous stimulation.
5. *Coma* defines a state in which the child cannot be aroused, even with painful stimuli.

The Pediatric Glasgow Coma Scale is a popular scale used to standardize degree of consciousness. It consists of three parts: eye opening, verbal response, and motor

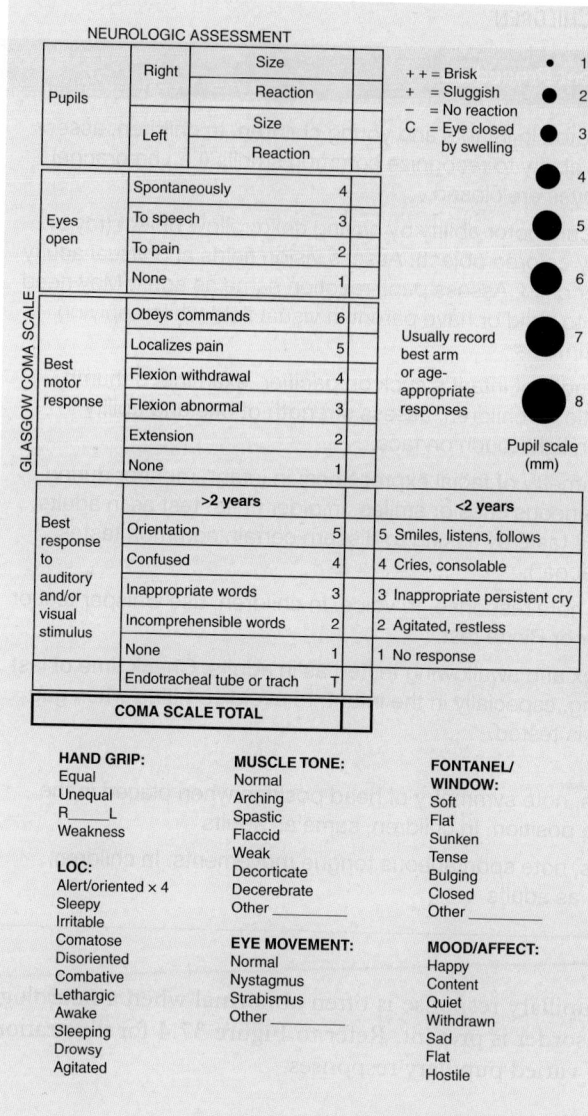

FIGURE 37.2 Pediatric Glasgow Coma Scale (GCS). The Pediatric GCS provides for developmentally appropriate cues to assess level of consciousness (LOC) in infants and children. Numeric values are assigned to the levels of response and the sum provides an overall picture, as well as an objective measure, of the child's LOC. The lower the score, the less responsive the child.

response (Fig. 37.2). When assessing LOC in children, consider that the infant or child may not respond to unfamiliar voices in an unfamiliar environment. Therefore it may be helpful to have a parent present to elicit the response.

▶ *Take* NOTE!

Parents many times will be the first to notice changes in their child's LOC. Listen to parents and respond to their concerns.

▶ *Take* NOTE!

Lack of response to painful stimuli is abnormal and can indicate a life-threatening condition. Report this finding immediately.

Vital Signs. Assessment of vital signs can provide probable underlying causes for altered LOC as well as reveal the adequacy of oxygenation and circulation. Certain neurologic conditions like cerebral infections, increased ICP, coma, brain stem injury, or head injuries can cause alterations in the pediatric client's vital signs.

Head, Face, and Neck. Inspect and observe the head for size and shape. Abnormal skull shape can result from premature closure or widening of sutures. Inspect and observe the face for symmetry. Asymmetry may occur due to paralysis of certain cranial nerves, position *in utero*, or swelling caused by trauma. Assess range of motion of the neck. Alterations in range of motion can indicate CNS infections such as meningitis.

The most dramatic increase in brain volume occurs during the last 3 months of fetal development and the first 2 years of life. The relationship between head and brain growth explains why head circumference is a standard assessment made in children less than 3 years of age. All children less than 3 years old, and any child whose head size is questionable, should have their head circumference measured and plotted on a growth chart (see Appendix F for growth charts). Assessment of the growth trend of the head is important in detecting potential neurologic conditions. Report and investigate any variation in head circumference percentiles over time because variations may indicate abnormal brain or skull growth. A smaller than normal **head circumference** may indicate microcephaly, and a larger than normal head circumference may indicate hydrocephalus.

▶ *Take* NOTE!

Any assessment that involves movement of the head and neck should not be attempted in cases of trauma or suspected trauma until cervical injury is ruled out. Maintain complete immobilization of the cervical spine until that time.

Cranial Nerve Function. Techniques of assessment of cranial nerve function are similar to techniques for adult assessment. The method of obtaining responses may vary based on age and developmental level of the child. Certain elements of the adult assessment may be omitted. Alter-

TABLE 37.1 ASSESSMENT OF CRANIAL NERVES IN INFANTS AND CHILDREN

Cranial Nerve	Function	Assessment Procedure
I (Olfactory)	Sense of smell	Not evaluated in infants and young children. In children, assess child's ability to recognize common smells (i.e., an orange) while eyes are closed.
II (Optic), III (Oculomotor), IV (Trochlear), VI (Abducens)	Vision, motor control and sensation of eye muscles, movement of major eye muscles	Assess oculomotor ability by having child follow object (toy or brightly colored object). Assess vision fields and visual acuity in older child. Assess pupil reaction same as adult. May need to talk to child or have parent in visual field while applying light stimulus
V (Trigeminal)	Mastication muscles and facial sensation	Note strength of infant's suck on pacifier, examiner's thumb, or bottle. In children, assess strength of bite and ability to discern light touch on face.
VII (Facial)	Facial muscles, salivation, and taste	Note symmetry of facial expressions; in infant, monitor during spontaneous cries or smiles. In older child, test as in adults. Assess taste by asking to discern certain common tastes (salt, sugar).
VIII (Acoustic)	Hearing	In infant, note response, to voice. In children, use whisper test or Weber or Rinne test.
IX (Glossopharyngeal), X (Vagus)	Motor impulses to heart and other organs, swallowing, and gag reflex	Gag reflex and swallowing tested as in adults. Check time of last feeding, especially in the infant, to avoid vomiting when gag reflex is tested.
XI (Accessory)	Impulses to muscles of shoulders and pharynx	In infants, note symmetry of head position when placed in the sitting position. In children, same as adults
XII (Hypoglossal)	Motor impulses to tongue and skeletal muscles	In infants, note spontaneous tongue movements. In children, same as adults

ations in cranial nerve function can be the result of compression of a specific nerve, infection, or trauma leading to brain injury. Refer to Table 37.1 for an explanation of cranial nerve assessment in children.

Use the doll's eyes maneuver to evaluate cranial nerves III, IV, and VI. This maneuver can be helpful when assessing an infant, uncooperative child, or comatose client. It examines horizontal and vertical eye movements by turning the head in one direction and assessing if the eyes move symmetrically in the other direction. For example, if you suddenly turn the child's head to the right, the child's eyes should look to the left symmetrically. Assess vertical eye movements in a similar manner by flexing or extending the neck. Absence of expected eye movements may indicate increased ICP.

When assessing oculomotor function, be sure to note nystagmus or sunset appearance of the eyes. Observe for nystagmus by looking for involuntary, rapid, rhythmic eye movements that may be present at rest or with eye movement. Horizontal nystagmus may occur with lesions in the brainstem and can be the result of certain medications (phenytoin in particular). Vertical nystagmus indicates brainstem dysfunction. *Sunsetting* is when the sclera of the eyes is showing over the top of the iris (Fig. 37.3). Sunset eyes may indicate increased ICP as seen in hydrocephalus.

Pupillary response is often abnormal when a neurologic disorder is present. Refer to Figure 37.4 for illustrations of varied pupillary responses.

▶ *Take* NOTE!

Report immediately the sudden presence of fixed and dilated pupils

Motor Function. Alterations in motor function, like changes in gait, muscle tone, or strength, may indicate certain neurologic problems such as increased ICP, head

FIGURE 37.3 Sunsetting of the eyes is a sign of increased intracranial pressure.

FIGURE 37.4 Assessing pupil size and reaction: (**A**) *Pinpoint* is commonly observed in poisonings, brainstem dysfunction, and opiate use. (**B**) *Dilated but reactive* is seen after seizures. *Fixed and dilated* is associated with brainstem herniation secondary to increased intracranial pressure. (**C**) *One dilated but reactive* is associated with intracranial mass.

FIGURE 37.5 (**A**) Decorticate posturing occurs with damage of the cerebral cortex and includes adduction of the arms, flexion at the elbows with arms held over chest, and flexion of the wrists with hands fisted. Lower extremities are adducted and extended. (**B**) Decerebrate posturing occurs with damage to the midbrain and includes extension and pronation of the arms and legs.

injury, and cerebral infections. Observe muscle strength, size, and tone in the infant or child. Assess bilaterally and compare. Observe spontaneous activity, posture, and balance and assess for asymmetrical movements. In the infant, observe resting posture, which will normally be a slightly flexed posture. The infant should be able to extend extremities to a normal stretch. Because cortical control of motor function is lost in certain neurologic disorders, postural reflexes reemerge and are directly related to the area of the brain that is damaged. Therefore, it is important to assess for two distinct types of posturing that may occur. **Decorticate posturing** occurs with damage of the cerebral cortex (Fig. 37.5A). **Decerebrate posturing** occurs with damage at the level of the brainstem (Fig. 37.5B). Both types of posturing are characterized by extremely rigid muscle tone.

Reflexes. Testing of deep-tendon reflexes is part of the neurologic assessment, just as it is in adults. Testing of primitive and protective reflexes in the infant is important because infants cannot perform tasks on command. The Moro, tonic neck, and withdrawal reflexes are important in assessing neurologic health in infants. Refer to Chapter 25

for a further explanation of primitive and protective reflexes in infants (see Chapter 25, Table 25.2). Absence of certain reflexes, persistence of primitive reflexes after age of normal disappearance, or increases in reflexes may be present in specific neurologic conditions.

Sensory Function. When assessing sensory function, the child should be able to distinguish between light touch, pain, vibration, heat, and cold. When assessing an infant, limit the examination to responses to touch or pain. The normal response in a 4-month-old infant will be movement away from the stimulus. In the child, techniques similar to those used in the adult assessment are followed. Make sure to explain what you are doing to the child, especially before the pin-prick test, to gain continued cooperation. Alterations in sensory function can result from brain or spinal cord lesions.

Increased Intracranial Pressure. Increased ICP is a sign that may occur with many neurologic disorders. It may result from head trauma, birth trauma, hydrocephalus, infection, and brain tumors. Observe for signs and symptoms associated with increased ICP while caring for a child with a potential or suspected neurologic disorder. Refer to Comparison Chart 37.1 for early versus late signs and symptoms of increased ICP. As ICP increases, LOC decreases and the signs and symptoms will become more pronounced. It is essential to recognize early signs and symptoms of increased ICP and intervene immediately to prevent long-term damage and possible death.

Palpation

Palpation of the newborn and infant skull and fontanels is an important function of the neurologic examination.

COMPARISON CHART 37.1   EARLY VS. LATE SIGNS OF INCREASED INTRACRANIAL PRESSURE

Early Signs	Late Signs
• Headache	• Lowered level of consciousness
• Vomiting, possibly projectile	• Decreased motor and sensory responses
• Blurred vision, double vision (diplopia)	• Bradycardia
• Dizziness	• Irregular respirations
• Decreased pulse and respirations	• Cheyne-Stokes respirations
• Increased blood pressure or pulse pressure	• Decerebrate or decorticate posturing
• Pupil reaction time decreased and unequal	• Fixed and dilated pupils
• Sunset eyes	
• Changes in level of consciousness, irritability	
• Seizure activity	
• In infant will also see:	
• Bulging, tense fontanel	
• Wide sutures and increased head circumference	
• Dilated scalp veins	
• High-pitched cry	

Changes in size or fullness of the fontanels may exist in certain neurologic conditions and must be noted. A bulging fontanel can be a sign of increased ICP and is seen in such neurologic disorders as hydrocephalus and head traumas. It is normal for the fontanels to be full or bulging during crying; take this into consideration during assessment.

Note any premature closure of fontanels, which can indicate skull deformities such as craniosynostosis. The posterior fontanel normally closes by 2 months of age and the anterior fontanel normally closes by 12 to 18 months of age. In children with hydrocephalus, widening of the fontanels may be noted, along with a tense appearance and a resulting increase in head circumference.

Auscultation

Advanced practitioners may perform auscultation of the skull. Soft, symmetric bruits may be found in children less than 4 years of age or in children with acute febrile illness. A finding of a loud or localized bruit is usually significant and requires immediate further investigation. Increased ICP, resulting from conditions such as hydrocephalus, tumor, or meningitis, frequently produces intracranial bruits. Arterial venous malformations may also produce large bruits.

Laboratory and Diagnostic Testing
Common Laboratory and Diagnostic Tests 37.1 offers an explanation of the most commonly used laboratory and diagnostic tests utilized when considering neurologic disorders. The tests can assist the physician in diagnosing the disorder and/or serve as guidelines in determining ongoing treatment. Laboratory or nonnursing personnel obtain some of the tests, while the nurse might obtain others. In either instance, the nurse should be familiar with how the tests are obtained, what they are used for, and normal versus abnormal results. This knowledge will also be necessary when providing client and family education related to the testing. Many of these tests, such as **lumbar puncture** (LP; see Fig. 37.6), can be frightening to parents and the child. Prepare the family and the child and provide support and reassurance during and after the test or procedure.

After completing an assessment of Antonio, the nurse noted the following: a full anterior fontanel; when being held, Antonio was inconsolable; when lying still, he was calmer and in the opisthotonic position.

Nursing Diagnoses and Related Interventions
Upon completion of a thorough assessment, the nurse might identify several nursing diagnoses, including:

• Decreased intracranial adaptive capacity
• Ineffective tissue perfusion: cerebral
• Risk for injury
• Disturbed sensory perception
• Risk for infection
• Pain
• Self-care deficit
• Impaired physical mobility

(text continues on page 1150)

COMMON LABORATORY AND DIAGNOSTIC TESTS 37.1

Test	Explanation	Indications	Nursing Implications
Lumbar puncture (LP)	Withdrawal of CSF from the subarachnoid space for analysis	To diagnose hemorrhage, infection or obstruction Can obtain measurement of spinal fluid pressure	Assist with proper positioning (see Fig. 37.6). Help child maintain position and remain still. Maintain strict asepsis. Assist with collection and transport of specimen. Encourage fluids after procedure if not contraindicated. Keep child flat for 1 hour if ordered. Apply EMLA cream to puncture site 30–60 min before procedure to reduce pain, if ordered.
Head and neck x-ray	Radiographic image of the head and neck will show skull and spine structures	Detects skull and spinal fractures; shows location and course of ventricular catheters; reveals information about increased intracranial pressure (ICP) and skull defects	Children may be afraid. Allow a parent or family member to accompany the child. If the child is unable or unwilling to stay still for the x-ray, restraint may be necessary. The time of restraint should be limited to the amount of time needed for the x-ray.
Fluoroscopy	Radiographic examination that uses continuous x-rays to show live up-to-date images	Can assess cervical spine for instability during movement	Same as head and neck x-rays. Child will need to cooperate with flexion and extension of neck.
Cerebral angiography	X-ray study of cerebral blood vessels. Involves injection of a contrast medium and use of fluoroscopy	Can assess for vessel defects or space-occupying lesions	Same as head and neck x-rays. Assess for allergy to contrast medium. Push fluids following procedure, if not contraindicated, to help flush out contrast medium.
Ultrasound	Use of sound waves to locate the depth and structure within soft tissues and fluid	Used to assess intracranial hemorrhage in newborns, and ventricular size	Better tolerated by nonsedated children than CT or MRI Can be performed portably at bedside
Computed tomography (CT)	Noninvasive x-ray study that looks at tissue density and structures. Images a "slice" of client's tissue	To diagnose congenital abnormalities, such as neural tube defects, hemorrhage, tumors, fractures	Machine is large and can be frightening to children. Procedure can be lengthy and child must remain still. If unable to do so, sedation may be necessary. Can be performed with or without use of contrast medium; if used, assess for allergy. Encourage fluids postprocedure if not contraindicated.

(continued)

COMMON LABORATORY AND DIAGNOSTIC TESTS 37.1 (continued)

Test	Explanation	Indications	Nursing Implications
Electroencephalogram (EEG)	Measure electrical activity of the brain	To diagnose seizures and brain death	Must remain still. If unable to do so, sedation may be necessary but should be avoided if possible because sedatives can alter the EEG reading. Inform technician of what anticonvulsants the client's taking. Morning anticonvulsants may need to be held.
Magnetic resonance imaging (MRI)	Use of magnetic field to show different tissue compositions	Used to assess tumors and inflammation; used to diagnose congenital abnormalities, such as neural tube defects; shows normal versus abnormal brain tissue	Client may not have any metal devices, internal or external, while undergoing MRI (ensure hospital gown does not have metal snaps). Procedure can be lengthy and child must remain still. Child is placed in long narrow tube and the machine makes a booming noise when it is turned on and off during the procedure; therefore can be difficult to gain cooperation. If the child is unable to remain still, sedation may be necessary. Can be performed with or without use of a contrast medium. If contrast medium is used, assess for allergy. Encourage fluids postprocedure if not contraindicated.
Positron emission tomography (PET)	Similar to CT or MRI but radioisotope is added. Measures physiologic function	Provides information on brain functional development. Can assist in identifying seizure foci. Can assess tumors and brain metabolism.	Procedure can be lengthy and child must remain still. If unable to do so, sedation may be necessary. IV access will be needed for the procedure. Encourage fluids postprocedure if not contraindicated, to help body eliminate radioisotopes.
Intracranial pressure (ICP) monitoring (intraventricular catheter, subarachnoid screw or bolt, epidural sensor, anterior fontanel pressure monitor)	A sensing device is placed in the head that monitors the pressure intracranially.	Used to monitor ICP resulting from hydrocephalus, acute head trauma, and brain tumors. Ventricular catheter also allows for draining of CSF to help reduce ICP.	Usually monitored in critical care setting. Monitor for signs and symptoms of increased ICP. Monitor for infection. Keep head of bed elevated 15–30 degrees. Alarms for monitoring device should remain on at all times. Reduce stimulation and avoid interventions that may cause pain or stress and result in an increased ICP.

Test	Explanation	Indications	Nursing Implications
Video electro-encephalogram (EEG)	Measure electrical activity of the brain continuously along with recorded video of actions and behaviors	Can help determine precise localization of seizure area before surgery. Assists in diagnosis and management of seizures by correlating behaviors with abnormal EEG activity	Ensure that seizure precautions are in place. Parent or caregiver must be with client at all times. Client movements are limited and usually confined to the room. When client changes position, ensure that he or she is still seen by video camera. Boredom can be a problem. Must notify nurse if seizure activity occurs; push the alert button to highlight attack on EEG recoding. Nurse must immediately go to the room, expose as much of the client as possible (remove covers; if at night, turn on light), and avoid blocking the camera. Ask questions (i.e., what is your name, can you raise your left arm, remember the word banana) to help assess responsiveness more accurately. Stay with the client until full recovery has occurred. Ask the client what word you asked them to remember, and document all findings and time of the event.

FIGURE 37.6 Proper positioning for a lumbar puncture. (**A**) The newborn is positioned upright with head flexed forward. (**B**) Child or older infant is positioned on the side with head flexed forward and knees flexed to abdomen.

- Risk for delayed development
- Imbalanced nutrition: less than body requirements
- Risk for deficient fluid volume
- Deficient knowledge
- Interrupted family processes

Nursing goals, interventions, and evaluation for the child with a neurologic disorder are based on the nursing diagnoses.

*B*ased on the assessment findings, what would be your top three prioritized nursing diagnoses for Antonio?

Nursing Care Plan 37.1 may be used as a guide in planning nursing care for the child with a neurologic disorder. It should be individualized based on the client's symptoms and needs. Additional information will be included later in this chapter related to specific disorders.

*B*ased on your top three nursing diagnoses for Antonio, describe appropriate nursing interventions.

Seizure Disorders

Seizures occur in approximately 10% of children (Behrman, Kliegman, & Jenson, 2004). Most seizures are caused by disorders that originate outside of the brain such as a high fever, infection, head trauma, hypoxia, toxins, or cardiac arrhythmias. Less than one third of seizures in children are caused by epilepsy (Behrman et al., 2004). Seizure disorders discussed below include epilepsy, febrile seizures, and neonatal seizures.

▶ EPILEPSY

Epilepsy is a condition in which seizures are triggered recurrently from within the brain. Epilepsy is a common neurologic disorder discovered in childhood, although brain injury or infection can cause epilepsy at any age. Epilepsy is considered present when two or more unprovoked seizures occur more than 24 hours apart. The prognosis for most children with seizures associated with epilepsy is good. Many children will outgrow epilepsy, but some children will have persistent seizures that are difficult to manage and may be unresponsive to pharmacologic interventions. Living with a seizure disorder may have a devastating impact on the quality of life of the child and family.

Pathophysiology

Epilepsy is a complex disorder of the CNS in which brain function is affected. Recurrent or unprovoked seizures are the clinical manifestation of epilepsy and result from a disruption of electrical communication among the neurons of the brain. This disruption results from an imbalance between the excitatory and inhibitory mechanisms in the brain, causing the neurons to either fire when they are not supposed to or not fire when they should. Epilepsy may be acquired and related to brain injury or it may be a familial tendency, but in most cases the cause is unknown.

There are two major categories of seizures: partial and generalized seizures. In partial seizures only one area of the brain is involved, while general seizures involve the entire brain. Partial seizures account for a large portion of childhood seizures and are classified as *simple* or *complex*. Generalized seizures include infantile spasms, absence seizures, tonic-clonic seizures, myoclonic seizures, and atonic seizures. There are many different types of seizures, and the classification of the type of seizure is crucial in assisting with the management and control of seizures. Not all cases are easily classified. The most common seizure types are discussed in Table 37.2.

Therapeutic Management

Management of epilepsy focuses on controlling seizures or reducing their frequency, along with helping the child who has recurrent seizures and his or her family to learn to live with the seizures. The primary mode of treatment is the use of anticonvulsants. There have been significant advances in the treatment of epilepsy due to the many new anticonvulsant medications that have become available in recent years (Table 37.3). Most anticonvulsants are taken orally and are often used in combination. Different medications control different types of seizures, which may be due to individual variation. It can take time to find the right combination to best control an individual's seizures.

If seizures remain uncontrolled, another option for managing them is surgery. Depending on the area of the brain that is affected, it may be possible to remove the area that is responsible for the seizure activity or to interrupt the impulses from spreading and therefore stop or reduce the seizures. The adverse effects range from mild to severe, depending on the area of the brain that is affected. Other nonpharmacologic treatments that may be considered in children with intractable seizures include a ketogenic diet or placement of a vagal nerve stimulator. Refer to Common Medical Treatments 37.1.

Nursing Assessment

For a full description of the assessment phase of the nursing process, refer to page 1140. Assessment findings pertinent to epilepsy are discussed below.

Health History

Elicit a description of the present illness and chief complaint, which will usually involve a seizure episode. Gain information to help characterize the episode as a seizure

(text continues on page 1155)

Nursing Care Plan 37.1

OVERVIEW FOR THE CHILD WITH A NEUROLOGIC DISORDER

NURSING DIAGNOSIS: Decreased intracranial adaptive capacity related to compression of brain tissue due to increased CSF or cerebral edema secondary to increased ICP resulting from brain injury, congenital structural defects, brain tumor, decreased reabsorption of CSF, or shunt malfunction as evidenced by vomiting, headache, complaints of visual disturbances, decreased pulse and respirations, elevated blood pressure or pulse pressure, changes in level of consciousness, increased head circumference, or bulging fontanel

Outcome Identification and Evaluation

Child will remain free of signs and symptoms of increased intracranial pressure as evidenced by *remaining free of headache, vomiting, vision disturbances, vital signs within parameters for age, no signs of altered levels of consciousness, free of excessive irritability or lethargy, head circumference is within parameters for age.*

Interventions: Promoting Adequate Intracranial Adaptive Capacity

- Assess neurologic status closely, monitor for signs and symptoms of increased ICP: *changes in level of consciousness, signs of irritability or lethargy, changes in pupillary reaction can indicate changes in ICP.*
- Monitor vital signs: *decreased pulse and respiratory rate and increased blood pressure or pulse pressure can indicate increased ICP.*
- Measure head circumference in children <3 years of age: *increases in head circumference outside parameters for age can indicate increased ICP.*
- Elevate head of bed 15–30 degrees to *facilitate venous return and can help to reduce ICP.*
- Minimize environmental stimuli and noise, avoid pain-producing procedures if possible: *all can increase ICP.*
- Have emergency equipment ready and available: *increased ICP can result in respiratory or cardiac failure.*
- Notify MD immediately if changes in assessment are noted: *early intervention is critical to prevent neurologic damage and death.*

NURSING DIAGNOSIS: Risk for ineffective (cerebral) tissue perfusion related to increased ICP, alteration in blood flow secondary to hemorrhage, vessel malformation, cerebral edema

Outcome Identification and Evaluation

Child will exhibit adequate cerebral tissue perfusion through course of illness and childhood: *Child will remain alert and oriented with no signs of altered level of consciousness; vital signs will be within parameters for age; motor, sensory, and cognitive function will be within parameters for age; head circumference remains within parameters for age.*

Interventions: Promoting Adequate Tissue Perfusion

- Assess neurologic status closely, monitor for signs and symptoms of increased ICP: *changes in level of consciousness, signs of irritability or lethargy, changes in pupillary reaction can indicate decreased cerebral tissue perfusion.*
- Monitor vital signs: *decreased pulse and respiratory rate and increased blood pressure or pulse pressure can indicate increased ICP, which can lead to decreased cerebral perfusion.*
- Have emergency equipment ready and available: *decreased cerebral perfusion can result in respiratory or cardiac failure.*
- Notify MD immediately if changes in assessment are noted: *early intervention is critical to prevent neurologic damage and death.*

(continued)

Nursing Care Plan 37.1 (continued)

NURSING DIAGNOSIS: Risk for injury related to altered level of consciousness, weakness, dizziness, ataxia, loss of muscle coordination secondary to seizure activity

Outcome Identification and Evaluation

Child will remain free of injury as evidenced by *no signs of aspiration or traumatic injury.*

Interventions: Preventing Injury

- Ensure child has patent airway and adequate oxygenation (have suction, oxygen available at bedside) and place child in side-lying position if possible: *a child with altered level of consciousness may not be able to manage his secretions and is at risk for aspiration and ineffective airway clearance; providing suction and oxygenation can help ensure an open airway and the side-lying position can help secretions drain and prevent obstruction of airway or aspiration.*
- Protect child from hurting self during seizures or changes in level of consciousness by removing environmental obstacles, easing child to lying position, and padding side rails: *helps to keep environment safe.*
- Institute seizure precautions for any child at risk for seizure activity (see Box 37.2): *to help prevent injury that can result from acute seizure activity.*
- With seizure activity do not insert a tongue blade or restrain child: *can lead to injury to caregiver and child.*
- Administer anticonvulsant medications as ordered: *will help to promote cessation and prevention of seizure activity.*
- Assist child with ambulation: *help prevent injury in child with weakness, dizziness, ataxia.*
- Allow for periods of rest: *to prevent fatigue and decrease risk of injury.*

NURSING DIAGNOSIS: Disturbed sensory perception related to presence of neurologic lesion or pressure on sensory or motor nerves secondary to increased ICP, presence of tumor, swelling postoperatively as evidenced by visual disturbances (i.e., reports of double vision), pupillary changes, nystagmus, ataxia, balance disturbances, or loss of response to stimuli

Outcome Identification and Evaluation

Child will be free of changes in sensory perception or will remain at baseline as evidenced by *no complaints of double vision, PERRLA, no disturbances of gait or balance noted, and no increased in loss of responses to stimuli.*

Interventions: Managing Disturbed Sensory Perception

- Assess for changes in sensory perception: *provides baseline data and allows nurse to recognize change in sensory perception early.*
- Monitor child for risk of injury secondary to changes in sensory perception: *visual changes, disturbances of gait or balance increase child's risk for injury.*
- Notify MD of changes in sensory perception: *can indicate increased ICP and medical emergency.*
- Assist child to learn to use adaptive methods to live with permanent changes in sensory perception (i.e., use of eyeglasses) and maximize the use of intact senses: *adaptive devices can enhance sensory input and intact senses can often compensate for impaired senses.*
- Provide familiar sounds (voices, music): *can help relieve anxiety related to changes in sensory perception, especially visual changes.*

Nursing Care Plan 37.1 (continued)

NURSING DIAGNOSIS: Risk for infection related to surgical interventions, presence of foreign body (i.e., shunt), trauma to skull, nutritional deficiencies, stasis of pulmonary secretions and urine, presence of infectious organisms as evidenced by fever, poor feeding, decreased responsiveness and presence of virus or bacteria on laboratory screening

Outcome Identification and Evaluation

Child will exhibit no signs or symptoms of local or systemic infection and will not spread infection to others: *Symptoms of infection will decrease over time; others will remain free of infection.*

Interventions: Preventing Infection

- Monitor vital signs: *elevation in temperature can indicate presence of infection.*
- Monitor incision sites for signs of local infection: *redness, warmth, drainage, swelling, pain at incision site can indicate presence of infection.*
- Maintain aseptic technique—practice good hand washing, use proper technique when managing postoperative incisions and external shunts: *to prevent introduction of further infectious agents.*
- Administer antibiotics as prescribed: *to prevent or treat bacterial infection.*
- Encourage nutritious diet and proper hydration according to child's preferences and ability to feed orally: *to assist body's natural defenses against infection.*
- Isolation of child as required: *to prevent nosocomial spread of infection.*
- Teach child and family preventive measures such as good hand washing, covering mouth and nose upon cough or sneeze, adequate disposal of used tissues: *to prevent nosocomial or community spread of infection.*

NURSING DIAGNOSIS: Self-care deficit related to neuromuscular impairments; cognitive deficits as evidenced by an inability to perform hygiene care and transfer self independently

Outcome Identification and Evaluation

Child will demonstrate ability to care for self within age parameters and limits of disease: *Child is able to feed, dress, manage elimination within limits of disease and age.*

Interventions: Maximizing Self-Care

- Introduce child and family to self-help methods as soon as possible: *promotes independence from the beginning.*
- Encourage family and staff to allow child to do as much as possible: *allows child to gain confidence and independence.*
- Teach specific measures for bowel and urinary elimination as needed: *promotes independence, increases self-care abilities and self-esteem.*
- Collaborate with physical therapy, occupational therapy, and speech therapy departments to provide child and family with appropriate tools to modify environment and methods to promote transferring and self-care: *allows for maximum functioning.*
- Praise accomplishments and emphasize child's abilities: *helps improve self-esteem and encourages feeling of confidence and competence.*
- Balance activity with periods to rest: *to reduce fatigue and increase energy for self-care.*

NURSING DIAGNOSIS: Impaired physical mobility related to muscle weakness, hypertonicity, impaired coordination, loss of muscle function or control as evidenced by an inability to move extremities, to ambulate without assistance, to move without limitations

Outcome Identification and Evaluation

Child will be able to engage in activities within age parameters and limits of disease: *Child is able to move extremities, move about environment, and participate in exercise programs within limits of age and disease.*

Interventions: Maximizing Physical Mobility

- Encourage gross and fine motor activities: *facilitates motor development.*
- Collaborate with physical therapy, occupational therapy, and speech therapy departments to strengthen muscles and promote optimal mobility: *facilitates motor development.*
- Utilize passive and active ROM and teach child and family how to perform: *prevent contractures, facilitate joint mobility and muscle development (active ROM) to help increase mobility.*
- Praise accomplishments and emphasize child's abilities: *helps improve self-esteem and encourages feeling of confidence and competence.*

(continued)

Nursing Care Plan 37.1 (continued)

NURSING DIAGNOSIS: Risk for delayed development related to physical disability, cognitive deficits, activity restrictions

Outcome Identification and Evaluation
Child will demonstrate developmental milestones within age parameters and limits of disease: *Child expresses interest in the environment and people around him or her, and interacts with environment age appropriately.*

Interventions: Maximizing Development
- Use therapeutic play and adaptive toys: *helps facilitate developmental functioning.*
- Provide stimulating environment when possible: *to maximize potential for growth and development.*
- Praise accomplishments and emphasize child's abilities: *helps improve self-esteem and encourages feeling of confidence and competence.*

NURSING DIAGNOSIS: Nutrition, imbalanced: less than body requirements related to vomiting and difficulty feeding secondary to increased ICP; difficulty sucking, swallowing, or chewing; surgical incision pain or difficulty assuming normal feeding position; inability to feed self as evidenced by decreased oral intake, impaired swallowing, weight loss

Outcome Identification and Evaluation
Child will exhibit signs of adequate nutrition as evidenced by: *Weight will remain within parameters for age, skin turgor will be good, I/O will be within normal limits, adequate calories will be ingested, vomiting will cease or decrease.*

Interventions: Promoting Adequate Nutrition
- Monitor height and weight: *insufficient intake will lead to impaired growth and weight gain.*
- Monitor hydration status (moist mucous membranes, elastic skin turgor, adequate urine output): *insufficient intake can lead to dehydration.*
- Use techniques to promote caloric and nutritional intake and teach family (i.e., positioning, modified utensils, soft or blended foods, allow extra time): *these techniques can facilitate intake.*
- Assess respiratory system frequently: *to assess for aspiration.*
- Monitor for nausea and vomiting and medicate if ordered: *to help reduce vomiting and increase intake.*
- Monitor for pain and medicate if ordered: *to help reduce pain related to surgical incisions and trauma, and increase intake.*
- Assist family to assume as normal a feeding position as possible: *to help increase oral intake.*

NURSING DIAGNOSIS: Fluid volume deficit, risk for, related to vomiting, altered level of consciousness, poor feeding or intake, insensible loss due to fever, failure of regulatory mechanisms (as in diabetes insipidus) as evidenced by dry oral mucosa, decreased skin turgor, sudden weight loss, hypotension, and tachycardia

Outcome Identification and Evaluation
Fluid volume will be maintained and balanced: *oral mucosa moist and pink, skin turgor elastic, urine output at least 1–2 cc/kg/hr.*

Interventions: Promoting Adequate Fluid Balance
- Administer IV fluids if ordered: *to maintain adequate hydration in children who are NPO or unable to tolerate oral intake.*
- When oral intake is allowed and tolerated, encourage PO fluids: *to promote intake and maintain hydration.*
- Strict intake and output monitoring: *can help identify fluid imbalance and also detect signs of abnormal pituitary secretions resulting in conditions like syndrome of inappropriate antidiuretic hormone secretion (SIADH) and diabetes insipidus (DI) (see Chapter 48 for further information).*
- Maintain minimum hydration and avoid overhydration in clients where cerebral edema is a concern: *fluid overload can contribute to cerebral edema.*
- Urine specific gravity, urine and serum electrolytes (especially serum sodium), blood urea nitrogen, creatinine and osmolality, and daily weights: *are reliable indicators of fluid status and can also detect signs of abnormal pituitary secretions resulting in conditions like SIADH and DI.*

Nursing Care Plan 37.1 (continued)

NURSING DIAGNOSIS: Knowledge deficit related to lack of information regarding complex medical condition, prognosis, and medical needs as evidenced by verbalization, questions, or actions demonstrating lack of understanding regarding child's condition or care

Outcome Identification and Evaluation
Child and family will verbalize accurate information and understanding about condition, prognosis, and medical needs: *Child and family demonstrate knowledge of condition and prognosis and medical needs including possible causes, contributing factors, and treatment measures.*

Interventions: Providing Client and Family Teaching
- Assess child's and family's willingness to learn: *child and family must be willing to learn for teaching to be effective.*
- Provide family with time to adjust to diagnosis: *will help facilitate adjustment and ability to learn and participate in child's care.*
- Repeat information: *allows family and child time to learn and understand.*
- Teach in short sessions: *many short sessions are found to be more helpful than one long session.*
- Gear teaching to a level of understanding of the child and also the family (depends on age of child, physical condition, memory): *to ensure understanding.*
- Provide reinforcement and rewards: *help facilitate the teaching–learning process.*
- Use multiple modes of learning involving many senses (provide written, verbal, demonstration, and videos) when possible: *child and family more likely to retain information when presented in different ways using many senses.*

NURSING DIAGNOSIS: Family processes, interrupted related to child's illness, hospitalization, diagnosis of chronic illness in child and potential long-term affects of illness as evidenced by family's presence in hospital, missed work, demonstration of inadequate coping

Outcome Identification and Evaluation
Family will maintain functional system of support and demonstrate adequate coping, adaptation of roles and functions, and decreased anxiety: *Parents are involved in child's care, ask appropriate questions, express fears and concerns, and are able to discuss child's care and condition calmly.*

Interventions: Promoting Adequate Family Processes
- Encourage parents and family members to verbalize concerns related to child's illness, diagnosis, and prognosis: *allows the nurse to identify concerns and areas where further education may be needed. Demonstrates family-centered care.*
- Explain therapies, procedures, child's behaviors, and plan of care to parents: *understanding the child's current status and plan of care helps decrease anxiety.*
- Encourage parental involvement in care: *allows parents to feel needed and valued with a sense of control over their child's health.*
- Identify support system for family and child: *helps nurse identify needs and resources available for coping.*
- Educate family and child on additional resources available: *to help them develop a wide base of support.*

---

or as a nonepileptic event (see Box 37.1 for a list of nonepileptic events). It is rare to actually observe the child having a seizure; therefore a complete, accurate, and detailed history from a reliable source is essential. *Questions should include:*

- Where did the event occur—while sleeping, eating, playing, or just after waking?
- Description of child's behavior during the event—what types of movements, progression, length, respiratory status, apnea?
- How did the child act after the event?
- Have the episodes been recurrent? If so, how frequent?

- Any precipitating factors such as a fever, fall, activity, anxiety, infection, or exposure to strong stimuli such as flashing lights or loud noises?

Explore the client's current and past medical history for risk factors such as:

- Family history of seizures or epilepsy
- Any complications during the prenatal, perinatal, or postnatal periods
- Changes in developmental status or delays in developmental milestones
- Any recent illness, fever, trauma, or toxin exposure

TABLE 37.2 COMMON TYPES OF SEIZURES

Type	Description	Characteristics
Infantile spasms	Uncommon type of generalized seizure seen in an epilepsy syndrome of infancy and childhood Usually seen between 3–12 months of age and usually stops by 2–4 years of age	Presents as a sudden jerk followed by stiffening May see: • Head flexed, arms extended, and legs drawn up • Arms flung out, knees are pulled up, and the body bends forward (referred to as "jackknife seizures") • Cry may precede or follow Majority of infants have some brain disorder before seizures begin. The infant seems to stop developing and may lose skills that he or she has already attained after the onset of infantile spasms. Steroid therapy and anticonvulsants are common forms of treatment.
Absence (formerly *petit mal*)	Type of generalized seizure; occurs more frequently in girls than boys Uncommon before age 5	Sudden cessation of motor activity or speech with a blank facial expression or rhythmic twitching of the mouth or blinking of the eyelids Complex absence seizure consists of myoclonic movements of the face, fingers, or extremities and possible loss of body tone. Lasts less than 30 seconds Child may experience countless seizures in a day. Not associated with a post-ictal (after seizure) state May go unrecognized or mistaken for inattentiveness because of subtle change in child's behavior
Tonic-clonic (formerly *grand mal*)	Extremely common generalized seizures. Most dramatic seizure type	Associated with an aura Loss of consciousness occurs and may be preceded by a piercing cry. Presents with entire body experiencing tonic contractions followed by rhythmic clonic contractions alternating with relaxation of all muscle groups Cyanosis may be noted due to apnea. Saliva may collect in the mouth due to inability to swallow. Child may bite tongue. Loss of sphincter control, especially the bladder, is common. Postictal phase: child will be semicomatose or in a deep sleep for approximately 30 minutes to 2 hours; usually responds only to painful stimuli. Child will have no memory of the seizure; may complain of headache and feeling fatigue. Safety of the child is a primary concern. See Teaching Guideline 37.1.
Myoclonic	Type of generalized seizure that involves the motor cortex of the brain. May occur along with other seizure forms.	Sudden, brief, massive muscle jerks that may involve the whole body or one body part Child may or may not lose consciousness.
Atonic	Type of generalized seizure often referred to as "drop attacks." Seen in children with Lennox-Gastaut syndrome	Sudden loss of muscle tone. In children, may only be a sudden drop of the head. Child will regain consciousness within a few seconds to a minute. Can result in injury related to violent fall

Type	Description	Characteristics
Simple partial	Type of partial seizure that occurs in part of the brain. The symptoms seen will depend on which area of the brain is affected.	Motor activity characterized by clonic or tonic movements involving the face, neck, and extremities Can include sensory signs such as numbness, tingling, paresthesia, or pain Usually persists for 10–20 seconds Child remains conscious and may verbalize during the seizure. No post-ictal state
Complex partial	Common type of partial seizure. May begin with a simple partial seizure then progress	May or may not have a preceding aura Consciousness will be impaired. Automatisms and complex purposeful movements are common features in infants and children. Infants will present with behaviors such as lip smacking, chewing, swallowing, and excessive salivation; can be difficult to distinguish from normal infant behavior In older children, will see picking or pulling at bed sheets or clothing, rubbing objects, or running or walking in a nondirective and repetitive fashion These seizures can be difficult to control.
Status epilepticus	Common neurologic emergency in children. Can occur with any seizure activity. Febrile seizures are the most common type. In children with epilepsy, it commonly occurs early in the course of epilepsy. Can be life threatening.	Prolonged or clustered seizures where consciousness does not return between seizures. The age of the child, cause of the seizures, and duration of status epilepticus influence prognosis. Prompt medical intervention is essential to reduce morbidity and mortality. Treatment: • Basic life support—ABCs (airway, breathing, circulation) • Administration of anticonvulsants to cease seizures is crucial. Common medications include benzodiazepines such as lorazepam and diazepam, and fosphenytoin. (See Drug Guide 37.1 and Table 37.3) • Blood glucose levels and electrolytes along with evaluation of the underlying cause should be initiated.

Children known to have epilepsy are often admitted to the hospital for other health-related issues or complications and treatment of their seizure disorder. The health history should include questions related to:

• Age of onset of seizures
• Seizure control—what medications is the child taking and has he or she been able to take them; when was his or her last seizure?
• Description and classification of seizures—does the child lose consciousness; does the child become apneic?
• Precipitating factors that may contribute to onset of seizures
• Adverse effects related to anticonvulsant medications
• Compliance with medication regimen

Physical Examination

Perform a complete neurologic examination. Careful assessment of the child's mental status, language, learning,

behavior, and motor abilities can help provide information about any neurologic deficits. If seizure activity is observed directly, provide a thorough and accurate description of the event. This description needs to include:

• Time of onset and length of seizure activity
• Alterations in behavior such as a cry or changes in facial expression, motor abilities, or sensory alterations prior to the seizure that may indicate an aura
• Precipitating factors such as fever, anxiety, just waking, or eating
• Description of movements and any progression
• Description of respiratory effort and any apnea noted
• Changes in color (pallor or cyanosis) noted
• Position of mouth, any injury to mouth or tongue, inability to swallow, or excessive salivation
• Loss of bladder or bowel control
• State of consciousness during seizure and postictal (after seizure) state—during the seizure the nurse may

TABLE 37.3 COMMON ANTICONVULSANT MEDICATIONS

Medication	Nursing Implications
Phenytoin (IV and PO; IM administration is contraindicated)	Monitor serum levels to ensure therapeutic dosing. Be aware that gingival hyperplasia appears most commonly in children and adolescents. If on prolonged therapy, ensure adequate intake of vitamin D–containing foods. Monitor serum calcium and magnesium levels.
Fosphenytoin (IM or IV only)	Adverse effects are said to be less common than with phenytoin. It does not cause local irritation, but it is a more expensive drug than phenytoin. It is water soluble, therefore allowing faster and easier administration than phenytoin. All dosing is in phenytoin sodium equivalents. It does not precipitate in commonly used IV diluents.
Phenobarbital	Assess for excessive sedation. Monitor serum levels to ensure therapeutic dosing. Monitor for drug interactions. Increase vitamin D–fortified foods or administer supplement if prescribed. Withdrawal symptoms will occur if drug is stopped abruptly. Valproic acid interferes with this drug, causing increased phenobarbital levels.
Felbamate	Monitor for drug interactions, especially if client is taking phenytoin or carbamazepine.
Valproic acid (divalproex sodium, sodium valproate)	Monitor serum levels to ensure therapeutic dosing. Depakote sprinkles are available and useful for children who are unable to tolerate valproate suspension, tablets, or capsules. The contents can be sprinkled on food that does not require chewing.
Carbamazepine	Monitor serum levels to ensure therapeutic dosing; toxicity can occur even with levels slightly above therapeutic range. Plasma concentration decreased by phenytoin, phenobarbital, and valproic acid.
Gabapentin	Do not administer within 2 hours of antacids. Rapidly absorbed in the gastrointestinal tract
Topiramate	Dilantin, tegretol, and valproic acid decrease concentration of topiramate.
Oxcarbazepine	Monitor phenytoin levels if administering concurrently.
Zonisamide	Presence of food will delay absorption. Phenytoin, phenobarbital, and carbamazepine all increase the metabolism of this drug.
Lamotrigine	Valproate inhibits metabolism; therefore, monitor serum blood values and decrease the dose if necessary.
Levetiracetam	Monitor phenytoin levels if administering concurrently. Monitor for difficulty with gait or coordination. B-complex vitamin supplementation can help mange side effects.
Ethosuximide	Give with food GI upset occurs. Monitor closely during periods of dosage adjustment or addition of new medications.

IM, intramuscular; IV, intravenous; PO, by mouth.

BOX 37.1 **Nonepileptic Events**

- Syncope
- Breath holding
- Jitteriness
- Apnea
- Gastroesophageal reflux
- Cardiac conduction abnormalities
- Migraines
- Tics

ask the child to remember a word; after the seizure, assess if child is able to recall it, to help accurately establish current mental state
- Assess: orientation to person, place, and time; motor abilities; speech; behavior; alterations in sensation postictally
- Duration of postictal state

Laboratory and Diagnostic Tests

Laboratory and diagnostic tests are used to evaluate the cause of, and also aid in identifying the type of, seizure activity (refer to Common Laboratory and Diagnostic

Tests 37.1). Common laboratory and diagnostic studies ordered for the diagnosis and assessment of epilepsy include:

- Serum glucose, electrolytes, and calcium—to rule out metabolic causes such as hypoglycemia and hypocalcemia
- Lumbar puncture (LP)—to analyze CSF to rule out meningitis or encephalitis
- Skull x-ray examinations—to evaluate for the presence of fracture or trauma
- Computed tomography (CT) and magnetic resonance imaging (MRI) studies—to identify abnormalities and intracranial bleeds and rule out tumors
- Electroencephalographs (EEGs)—EEG findings may be noted with certain seizure types, but a normal EEG does not rule out epilepsy because seizure activity rarely occurs during the actual testing time. EEGs are useful in evaluating seizure type and assisting in medication selection. They can be useful in differentiating seizures from nonepileptic activity.
- Video EEGs—provide the opportunity to see the child's actual behavior on video, accompanied with EEG changes; can improve the chance of catching a seizure because the monitoring is done over a period of time

Nursing Management

Nursing management focuses on preventing injury during seizures; administering appropriate medication and treatments to prevent or reduce seizures; and providing education and support to the child and family to help them cope with the challenges of living with a chronic seizure disorder. See Box 37.2 for a list of basic seizure precautions. In addition to the nursing diagnoses and related interventions discussed in Nursing Care Plan 37.1, interventions common to epilepsy follow.

Relieving Anxiety

Seizures produce fear and anxiety due to their unpredictable nature along with the uncontrolled, forceful, and at times violent appearance. Instruct parents and family members, along with those in the community who may care for the child, on how to respond in case of a seizure (see Teaching Guidelines 37.1). This will help to empower the parents, family, and other caregivers, and in turn alleviate some of the anxiety that they may feel.

Managing Treatment

Provide child and family teaching and instruction regarding the administration of anticonvulsant therapy and its importance. Included in this discussion should be common adverse effects, the need to continue the medication unless instructed otherwise by the physician, and the need to call the physician if the child is ill and vomiting and unable to take his or her medication. Encourage parents to discuss unwanted adverse effects with the physician so that they can be addressed and noncompliance with the medication regimen can be reduced. The most common cause of breakthrough seizures is noncompliance.

Providing Family Support and Education

Having a child with a chronic seizure disorder can place stress and anxiety on the family that is often due to fears and misconceptions they may have. An important nursing function is to educate not only the child and family but also the community, including the child's teachers and care-

TEACHING GUIDELINES 37.1

How to Respond When Your Child Has a Seizure

Instruct parents and caregivers:
- Remain calm.
- Time seizure episode.
- If child is standing or sitting, ease child to the ground if possible.
- Tight clothing and jewelry around the neck should be loosened if possible.
- Place child on one side and open airway if possible.
- Do not restrain the child.
- Remove hazards in the area.
- Do not forcibly open jaw with a tongue blade or fingers.
- Document length of seizure and movements noted, also cyanosis or loss of bladder or bowel control and any other characteristics.
- Remain with child until fully conscious.
- Call emergency medical services (EMS) if:
  - The child stops breathing
  - Any injury has occurred
  - Seizure lasts for more than 5 minutes
  - This is the child's first seizure
  - Child is unresponsive to painful stimuli after seizure

BOX 37.2   Seizure Precautions

- Padding of side rails and other hard objects
- Side rails raised on bed at all times when child is in bed
- Oxygen and suction at bedside
- Supervision, especially during bathing, ambulation, or other potentially hazardous activities
- Use of a protective helmet during activity may be appropriate.
- Child should wear a medical alert bracelet.

givers, on the reality and facts of the disorder. Encourage parents to be involved in the management of their child's seizures but to allow the child to learn about the disorder and its management as soon as he or she is old enough. Encourage parents to treat the child with epilepsy just as they would a child without this disorder. Children who are brought up no differently than children without epilepsy will be more likely to develop a positive self-image and have increased self-esteem. Any activity restrictions, such as limiting swimming or participation in sports, will be based on the type, frequency, and severity of the seizures the child has. Educate parents and children on any restrictions and encourage parents to place only the necessary restrictions on the child.

The needs of the child and family will change as the child grows and develops. The nurse needs to recognize theses changes and provide appropriate education and support. Referral to support groups is appropriate. The Epilepsy Foundation can be accessed at www.epilepsyfoundation.org. Additional resources can be found at www.paceusa.org and www.epilepsyinstitute.org.

▶ FEBRILE SEIZURES

Febrile seizures are the most common type of seizure seen during childhood. They usually affect children who are less than 5 years of age, with the peak incidence occurring in children between 18 and 24 months old. It is rare to see febrile seizures in children younger than 6 months and older than 7 years of age. This type of seizure is more commonly seen in boys and there is an increased risk for children who have a family history of febrile seizures. Febrile seizures are associated with a fever, usually related to a viral illness. These seizures are usually benign but can be very frightening for both the child and family. The prognosis is generally excellent for febrile seizures. However, febrile seizures may indicate a serious underlying infectious disease, such as meningitis or sepsis. Though rare, complications associated with febrile seizures include status epilepticus, motor coordination deficits, mental retardation, and behavioral problems.

Therapeutic Management

Treatment includes determination of the cause of the fever and interventions to control the fever. The American Academy of Pediatrics does not recommend long-term or intermittent anticonvulsant therapy for the child who has suffered one or more simple febrile seizures (Shinnar & O'Dell, 2004). Rectal diazepam has been shown to be safe and effective in terminating febrile seizures and may be used in children at high risk for febrile seizures or in children whose parents are extremely anxious. Although anticonvulsant prophylaxis is no longer recommended (Behrman et al., 2004), intermittent use of anticonvul-

sants at the time of a fever may be used in select groups of children.

Nursing Assessment

A febrile seizure is usually associated with a core temperature that increases rapidly to 39°C (102.2°F) or higher. The seizure usually presents as a generalized tonic-clonic seizure that lasts a few seconds to 10 minutes and is followed by a brief postictal period of drowsiness. A simple febrile seizure is defined as a generalized seizure lasting less than 15 minutes that occurs once in a 24-hour period and is accompanied by a fever. It is likely to have stopped by the time a child receives medical attention. Diagnosis is made based on a thorough history and physical examination, accompanied by a determination of the source of the fever. In some cases an LP may be performed to rule out meningitis or encephalitis. This will be based on the age and the clinical presentation of the child.

Risk factors for recurrence of a febrile seizure include young age at first febrile seizure and family history of febrile seizures and high fever. Children who experience one or more febrile seizures are at no greater risk of developing epilepsy than the general population. No evidence exists that febrile seizures cause structural damage or cognitive declines.

Nursing Management

Provide parental support and education regarding febrile seizures. Reassure parents of the benign nature of febrile seizures. Counsel parents on controlling fever; discuss how to keep a child safe during a seizure; and provide instruction and demonstration in the administration of rectal diazepam at the onset of a seizure (if applicable). Instruct parents when to call their physician and when to take their child to the emergency room. Reinforce that any recurrent seizure activity will require prompt medical attention.

▶ NEONATAL SEIZURES

The incidence of seizures is higher in the neonatal period than in any other age group. The immature brain is more prone to seizure activity. Neonatal seizures are seizures that occur within the first 4 weeks of life and are most commonly seen within the first 10 days. They are different from those in the child or adult because generalized tonic-clonic seizures tend not to occur during the first month of life. Seizures in newborns are associated with underlying conditions such as hypoxic-ischemic encephalopathy, metabolic disorders (hypoglycemia and hypocalcemia), neonatal infection (meningitis and encephalitis), and intracranial hemorrhage. The prognosis depends mainly on the underlying cause of the seizures and the severity of the insult. There is increasing evidence that neonatal seizures have an adverse effect on neurodevelopment and may predispose the infant to cognitive, behavioral, or epileptic complications later in life.

Therapeutic Management

Acute neonatal seizures should be treated aggressively because repeated seizure activity may result in injury to the brain. Treatment focuses on ensuring adequate ventilation; correcting any underlying metabolic disturbance that may exist, such as hypoglycemia; and possibly administering anticonvulsant therapy. Phenobarbital is often used in the initial management of neonatal seizures but efficacy remains uncertain. The dosage of anticonvulsants may be higher in the neonate because neonates metabolize drugs more rapidly than older infants.

Nursing Assessment

Neonatal seizures may be difficult to recognize clinically and may be accompanied by a normal EEG. Several clinical features may help distinguish seizures from non-epileptic activity, such as tremors or jitteriness, in neonates. Autonomic changes such as tachycardia and elevated blood pressure are common with seizures in neonates, but do not occur with nonepileptic events. Also, nonepileptic movements can be suppressed by gently restraining the limb; in true seizures this is not the case. Ocular deviation may be seen with seizure activity but will not be present with nonepileptic activity. The characteristics of seizures seen in the neonatal period differ from those seen in older children. Five major seizure types have been recognized in the neonatal period. See Table 37.4 for information on types of seizures seen in newborn infants.

Laboratory and diagnostic tests including serum testing (e.g., serum glucose, electrolytes, calcium), LP (to analyze CSF), cranial ultrasound, CT, and MRI may be performed to help determine the cause of the seizures. EEGs and video EEGs may assist in the characterization of neonatal seizures and their medical management.

Nursing Management

Nursing management will focus on carrying out interventions to cease seizure activity; monitoring neurologic status closely; recognizing the seizures; preventing injury during seizure activity; and providing support and education to the parents and family.

Structural Defects

Due to the sensitivity of the development of the neurologic system in the first weeks of embryonic life, there exists a potential for defects to occur. These structural defects include neural tube defects, microcephaly, Arnold-Chiari malformation, hydrocephalus, intracranial arteriovenous malformation, and craniosynostosis.

▶ NEURAL TUBE DEFECTS

Neural tube defects account for the majority of congenital anomalies of the CNS. They affect 0.6 per 1,000 live births in the United States, where there are approximately 3,000 pregnancies annually that are complicated by neural tube defects (Becske & Jallo, 2007; CDC, 2004). They are the second most common major congenital anomaly worldwide, behind cardiac malformations (CDC, 2004). They are serious birth defects of the spine and the brain and include disorders such as spina bifida occulta, myelomeningocele, meningocele, anencephaly, and encephalocele. The neural tube closes between the third and fourth week *in utero*. The cause of neural tube defects is not known but many factors such as drugs, malnutrition, chemicals, and genetics can adversely affect normal CNS development. Strong evidence exists that maternal preconception supplementation of folic acid can decrease the incidence of neural tube defects in pregnancies at risk by 50% (Behrman et al., 2004). In 1992, the United States Public Health Service recommended that all women of childbearing age who are capable of becoming pregnant

TABLE 37.4 TYPES OF SEIZURES SEEN IN NEWBORN INFANTS

Type	Age Affected	Characteristics
Subtle	Preterm and full term	Chewing motions, excessive salivation, alterations in respiratory rate, apnea, blinking, and pedaling movements
Tonic	Preterm	Rigid posturing of the extremities and trunk. May be associated with fixed deviation of the eyes
Focal clonic	Full term	Rhythmic twitching of local muscle groups such as the extremities or face
Multifocal clonic	Full term	Similar to focal clonic, except many muscle groups are involved, frequently simultaneously
Myoclonic	Rare in neonatal period	Brief focal jerks, involving one extremity; or multifocal jerks, involving several body parts

take 0.4 mg (400 mcg) of folic acid daily (Merereau et al., 2004). According to the Centers for Disease Control and Prevention (CDC), the number of pregnancies affected by neural tube defects has decreased from 4,000 (1995–1996) to 3,000 (1999–2000) (Merereau et al., 2004). Prenatal screening of maternal serum for alpha-fetoprotein (AFP) and ultrasound examination at 16 to 18 weeks' gestation can help identify fetuses at risk. Anencephaly and encephalocele are discussed below. Refer to Chapter 43 for information on spina bifida occulta, meningocele, and myelomeningocele.

Anencephaly

Anencephaly is a defect in brain development resulting in small or missing brain hemispheres, skull, and scalp. It occurs when the cephalic or upper end of the neural tube fails to close during the third to fourth week of gestation. These infants are born without both a forebrain and a cerebrum, and the condition is incompatible with life. The remaining brain tissue may be exposed. The incidence of anencephaly is 1 in 1,000 live births (Behrman et al., 2004).

Nursing Assessment

Anencephalic infants have a distinctive appearance, with a large defect noted in the vault of the skull (Fig. 37.7). The mother may have had a difficult labor due to the malformation of the head not allowing it to engage in the cervix. The majority of infants will be stillborn. If not, most anencephalic infants die within hours to several days of

birth. There have been a few cases in which the infant has lived for several months. The infant is usually blind, deaf, unconscious, and unable to feel pain. Some infants born with anencephaly may be born with a brainstem, but the lack of cerebrum rules out the possibility of gaining consciousness. Reflex actions such as respirations, reactions to sound and touch, and ability to suck may be present.

Nursing Management

The prognosis is extremely poor. Nursing management is supportive in nature and focuses on comfort measures for the dying infant. Some parents may have been aware of the diagnosis prenatally due to screening tests such as AFP and ultrasounds. Parents and family will need support and understanding from all health care professionals during this difficult time. Fear of what the child will look like may be overwhelming. Use of an infant cap can be helpful and allow parents to feel more comfortable holding and comforting their infant. Assisting with anticipatory grieving and decision making related to end-of-life care will also be key nursing interventions.

Encephalocele

Encephalocele is a protrusion of the brain and meninges through a skull defect. It results from failure of the anterior portion of the neural tube to close. Infants born with an encephalocele are at risk for visual problems, microcephaly, mental retardation, and seizures. The prognosis, including the extent of complications and cognitive deficits, will depend on the size and location of the encephalocele and involvement of other brain structures. Encephaloceles are often accompanied by craniofacial and other abnormalities such as hydrocephalus, microcephaly, spastic quadriplegia, ataxia, developmental delay, mental and growth retardation, and seizures. Some children who are affected may display normal intelligence.

Treatment consists of surgical repair, including placement of tissues back into the skull and removal of the sac; possible shunt placement to correct associated hydrocephalus; and corrective repair of any craniofacial abnormalities.

Nursing Assessment

Initial assessment postdelivery will reveal a visible external sac protruding from the skull area. It occurs most commonly in the occipital region but can occur elsewhere, such as frontally or nasofrontally. Generally the lesion is covered by skin, but it may also be open. Therefore, assessment to ensure that the sac covering is intact remains important. Assess neurologic status carefully. Before surgical correction, the infant will be thoroughly examined to determine brain tissue involvement or associated anomalies. Diagnostic procedures such as CT, MRI, and ultrasound may be performed.

FIGURE 37.7 Anencephalic infant.

Nursing Management

Nursing management will consist of preoperative and post-operative care, along with symptomatic and supportive care. Preoperative and postoperative care will be similar to that for the child with myelomeningocele, with a focus on preventing rupture of the sac, preventing infection, and providing adequate nutrition and hydration. Infants with an encephalocele are at an increased risk for developing hydrocephalus Therefore, monitor for signs and symptoms of increased ICP and head circumference.

▶ MICROCEPHALY

Microcephaly is defined as a head circumference that is more than three standard deviations below the mean for the age and sex of the infant (Behrman et al., 2004). It may be congenital or it may be acquired and develop in the first few years of life. It generally results in mental retardation due to the lack of functioning brain tissue. There are many causes. Microcephaly can be caused by abnormal development during gestation or follow intrauterine infections such as rubella, toxoplasmosis, and cytomegalovirus. It can also be caused by chromosomal abnormalities or be associated with other syndromes. Acquired microcephaly may occur due to severe malnutrition, perinatal infections, or anoxia in early infancy.

Nursing Assessment

Microcephalic infants will present at birth with a normal or reduced head size. As the child ages, head growth will fail while the face will continue to grow at a normal rate. This results in a small head, a large face, and a loose, often wrinkled scalp. As the child grows older, this smallness of the skull becomes more pronounced. Development of motor functions and speech may be delayed. The degree of mental retardation varies, but it is a common occurrence. Convulsions may be present, and motor deficit ranges from clumsiness to spastic quadriplegia.

Nursing Management

There is no treatment. Nursing care will be supportive and focus on determining the extent of neurologic and cognitive deficits, as well as teaching parents the care of a child with such impairments.

▶ ARNOLD-CHIARI MALFORMATION

Arnold-Chiari malformation consists of two major subgroups—type I and type II. In type I, symptoms are typically seen in adolescence and adulthood. This type is usually not associated with hydrocephalus and is the more benign form. The deformity is a result of the cerebellar tonsils displacing into the upper cervical canal. The client will usually complain of neck pain, recurrent headaches, lower extremity spasticity, and urinary frequency. Type II is the most common and is usually associated with hydrocephalus and myelomeningocele. The deformity results from the cerebellum, the medulla oblongata, and the fourth ventricle displacing into the cervical canal, resulting in an obstruction of the CSF and causing hydrocephalus. The prognosis depends on the extent of the defect. Symptomatic type II Chiari malformation is the leading cause of death in infants and young children with open neural tube defects (Stevenson, 2004). Treatment of the type II Chiari malformation includes surgical decompression.

Nursing Assessment

Approximately 10% of type II Arnold-Chiari malformations result in symptoms in infancy (Behrman et al., 2004). Symptoms consist of weak cry, stridor, and apnea. These symptoms require prompt medical treatment to reduce mortality. Gastrointestinal disturbances along with a history of chronic aspiration, choking, gagging, prolonged feeding times, and weight loss may also be present. Physical signs include coarse upper airway sounds heard on auscultation and diminished or absent gag reflex. In the older child, signs and symptoms seen are subtler and less frequently life threatening. Upper extremity weakness, spasticity, ataxia, and headaches are frequent signs found. Assessment of shunt function is extremely important in the infant and older child presenting with type II Chiari malformation and associated hydrocephalus (refer to "Hydrocephalus" section). An MRI may be performed to help evaluate and diagnose Chiari malformations.

Nursing Management

Nursing management will focus on preoperative and postoperative care; preventing infection; monitoring of blood loss; improvement of preoperative symptoms in the postoperative period; any signs and symptoms of increased ICP; and any resultant CNS injury.

▶ HYDROCEPHALUS

Hydrocephalus is not a specific disease, but results from underlying brain disorders. It is one of the most frequently seen disorders of the nervous system. It results from an imbalance in the production and absorption of CSF. In hydrocephalus, CSF accumulates within the ventricular system and causes the ventricles to enlarge and increases in ICP to occur. Common disorders or illnesses that are associated with hydrocephalus include neural tube defects such as myelomeningocele; intraventricular hemorrhage in premature infants; meningitis; intrauterine viral infections; lesions or malformations of the brain such as posterior fossa brain tumors; Chiari malformations; and nonaccidental injury. Hydrocephalus may be congenital or acquired. Congenital hydrocephalus is present at birth and is often due to environmental influences during fetal development or a genetic disposition. Causes of congenital hydrocephalus include abnormal intrauterine development, as is the case with myelomeningocele, or intrauterine infections. Acquired hydrocephalus develops at the time of birth or at some point after. It can occur at any age and can result from injury or disease. Acquired hydrocephalus can result from trauma, hemorrhage, neoplasms, or infections.

Hydrocephalus is also classified as obstructive or noncommunicating vs. nonobstructive or communicating. Obstructive or noncommunicating hydrocephalus occurs when the flow of CSF is blocked within the ventricular system. Neural tube defects, neonatal meningitis, trauma, tumors, or Chiari malformations usually result in this type of hydrocephalus. One of the most common causes of obstructive or noncommunicating hydrocephalus in children is aqueductal stenosis, which results from the narrowing of the aqueduct of Sylvius (a passageway between the third and fourth ventricles in the middle brain). Nonobstructive or communicating hydrocephalus occurs when the flow of CSF is blocked after it exits from the ventricles. This form of hydrocephalus, in which the CSF can still flow between the ventricles, is most often caused by defective absorption of CSF. Examples include hydrocephalus that results from subarachnoid hemorrhage and intrauterine infections.

Prognosis for the child with hydrocephalus depends mainly on the cause and whether or not brain damage has occurred prior to recognition and treatment. These children are at increased risk for developmental disabilities, visual problems, abnormalities in memory, and reduced intelligence. Long-term follow-up and multidisciplinary care are necessary.

Pathophysiology

CSF is formed primarily in the ventricular system by the choroid plexus. It flows as a result of the pressure gradient that exists between the ventricular system and the venous channels. CSF is absorbed primarily by the arachnoid villi. Hydrocephalus results when there is an obstruction in the ventricular system or obliteration or malfunction of the arachnoid villi. This results in impaired absorption or circulation of the CSF. In rare cases, hydrocephalus can be caused by an overproduction of CSF by the choroid plexus.

Therapeutic Management

Hydrocephalus must be identified early. Treatment needs to be initiated in order to prevent brain tissue damage that can result from the increased ICP that hydrocephalus creates. Specific treatment will depend on the cause. The goals of treatment include relieving hydrocephalus and managing complications associated with the disorder, such as growth and developmental delay. With few exceptions, most cases of hydrocephalus are treated with the surgical placement of an extracranial shunt. Most often a ventriculoperitoneal shunt (VP shunt) is placed. See Figure 37.8

FIGURE 37.8 To treat hydrocephalus, a ventriculoperitoneal (VP) shunt catheter is placed in an enlarged ventricle. The shunt diverts the flow of cerebrospinal fluid (CSF) within the central nervous system to the peritoneum, where CSF is now absorbed across the peritoneal membrane into the body's circulation.

for an illustration of a shunt. The shunt will need to be replaced as the child grows. Therefore, the child will undergo shunt revision surgery at various times during his or her life. It is important for health care professionals and parents to be able to recognize when a shunt needs replacing or when complications are occurring, to decrease the possibility of death or disability that may occur due to increased ICP.

Nursing Assessment

For a full description of the assessment phase of the nursing process, refer to page 1140. Assessment findings pertinent to hydrocephalus are discussed below.

Health History

Explore the pregnancy history and past medical history for:

- Intrauterine infections
- Prematurity with intracranial hemorrhage
- Meningitis
- Mumps encephalitis

Elicit a description of the present illness and chief complaint. Common signs and symptoms reported during the health history of the undiagnosed child might include:

• Irritability
• Lethargy
• Poor feeding
• Vomiting
• Complaints of headache in older children
• Altered, diminished, or changes in LOC

Children known to have hydrocephalus are often admitted to the hospital for shunt malfunctions or other complications of the disease. The health history should include questions related to:

• Neurologic status—have there been changes or decreases in LOC; changes in personality; deterioration in school performance?
• Complaints of headache
• Vomiting
• Visual disturbances
• Any other changes in physical or cognitive state

Physical Examination

Physical examination of the infant or child with hydrocephalus will include inspection and observation; palpation; and percussion.

Inspection and Observation

Observe general appearance and affect. Pay particular attention to the size of the skull and note any asymmetry. Note LOC and motor function. Changes or decreases in LOC may be noted along with brisk reflexes and spasticity of the lower extremities. Symptoms seen vary by age, primarily due to the fact that the infant's skull is able to accommodate the buildup of CSF because the sutures have not closed. In the infant, the most obvious indication is often a rapid increase in head circumference (Fig. 37.9). In the older child, loss of development and changes in personality may be seen. Signs and symptoms associated with increased ICP may be seen (refer to Comparison Chart 37.1).

Palpation

In the infant, palpation of the fontanels may reveal wide-open, bulging fontanels. They will be nonpulsatile and feel tense and very full.

Percussion

Upon percussion of the skull, by advanced practitioners, a positive Macewen's sign may be noted. This is when a "cracked pot" sound is heard during percussion and can indicate separation of the sutures.

Laboratory and Diagnostic Tests

Common laboratory and diagnostic tests ordered for the diagnosis and assessment of hydrocephalus include:

• Skull x-ray studies (may reveal separation of sutures)
• CT
• MRI

CT and MRI are used to evaluate for the presence of hydrocephalus and can also aid in identifying the cause of hydrocephalus. Refer to Common Laboratory and Diagnostic Tests 37.1.

▶ **Consider** *THIS!*

Sandra and Michael Graham have brought their 6-month-old son, Thomas, to the pediatric unit for observation. Thomas's head circumference has increased from the 25th percentile at the 4-month check-up to the 75th percentile at the 6-month check-up. Upon assessment, the nurse notes a bulging anterior fontanel and persistent primitive reflexes.

What do you think is going on?
Identify early signs.
Identify late signs.
Describe nursing care for Thomas.
What teaching will the nurse do with Sandra and Michael?

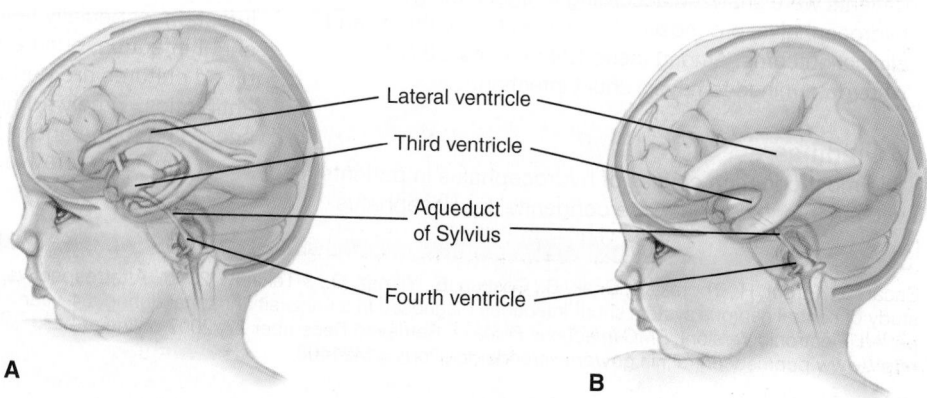

Lateral ventricle
Third ventricle
Aqueduct of Sylvius
Fourth ventricle

FIGURE 37.9 (**A**) Infant without hydrocephalus. (**B**) Infant with hydrocephalus. Note broadening of the forehead and large head size.   **A**   **B**

Nursing Management

Nursing management of the child with hydrocephalus will focus on maintaining cerebral perfusion, minimizing neurologic complications, maintaining adequate nutrition, promoting growth and development, and supporting and educating the child and family. In addition to the nursing diagnoses and related interventions discussed in Nursing Care Plan 37.1, interventions common to hydrocephalus are discussed below.

Preventing and Recognizing Shunt Infection and Malfunction

The major complications associated with shunts are infection and malfunction. Due to the serious nature and potentially devastating affects of shunt infection or malfunction, parents and health professionals need to be aware of the signs and symptoms to provide early recognition and prompt treatment. Signs and symptoms of a shunt infection include elevated vital signs, poor feeding, vomiting, decreased responsiveness, seizure activity, and signs of local inflammation along the shunt tract. Signs and symptoms of shunt malfunction include vomiting, drowsiness, and headache. Signs and symptoms of increased ICP, as listed in Comparison Chart 37.1, can also be in-

dicative of shunt complications. See Evidence-Based Practice 37.1.

Infection can occur at any time but is more common 1 to 2 months after placement. Infection is treated with intravenous antibiotics and, if the infection is persistent, the shunt will be removed and an external ventricular drainage (EVD) system will be put into place until the CSF is sterile (refer to Common Medical Treatments 37.1 and Box 37.3).

> ▶ **Take** NOTE!
>
> *Rapid drainage of CSF, which may occur if the client sits up without the EVD system being clamped, will decrease ICP and can lead to extreme headache, collapse of the ventricles, formation of subdural hematomas, and neurologic deterioration.*

A new shunt will be placed after the infection has cleared. Intrathecal administration of antibiotics may be performed by the physician or advanced practitioner. Keeping the peritoneal surgical incision free of feces and

---

EVIDENCE-BASED PRACTICE 37.1
Clinical Features, Pathogens, and Outcomes of Patients With CSF Shunt Infections

Infection is the most common complication of shunt implantation. Infections of the CNS are a major cause of morbidity and mortality in patients with shunts. Treatment of shunt infections usually results in an increase in hospital stay by 2 or 3 weeks. Many factors have been attributed to increasing the risk of infection, including age, cause of hydrocephalus, type of shunt implanted, and the surgeon's experience.

● Study

A chart review was performed on 124 consecutive patients having a CNS shunt placed over a 4-year period. The patients were analyzed according to age, etiology of hydrocephalus, prognosis, clinical infection features, and clinical outcome. Among these 124 patients, 22 (17.7%) were determined to have a shunt infection.

▲ Findings

The most common causes of hydrocephalus in patients with an infected shunt were congenital hydrocephalus-

myelomeningocele (32%) and meningitis (23%). The most common causative microorganism was *Staphylococcus aureus*. The rate of infection did not differ greatly between type of shunt placed. Children, especially those under 2 years, were more likely than adults to acquire a shunt infection. Fever was the most common symptom noted. Presentation of other manifestations such as nausea, vomiting, malaise, and headache was variable.

■ Nursing Implications

Intraoperative nurses must follow strict aseptic technique during surgical insertion or repair of shunts. Postoperatively, closely monitor the child for signs and symptoms of infection, especially fever. In the child with suspected shunt infection, ensure that CSF examination and blood cultures are performed prior to administration of antibiotics. Timely administration of antibiotic treatment according to the antimicrobial susceptibility and sensitivity is imperative.

Sacar, S., Turgut, H., Toprak, S., Cirak, B., Coskun, E., Yilmaz, O., & Tekin K. (2006). A retrospective study of central nervous system shunt infections diagnosed in a university hospital during a 4-year period [Electronic Version]. *BMC Infectious Disease.* Retrieved December 27, 2007 online at http://www.pubmedcentral.nih.gov/articlerender.fcgi?artid=1421408.

BOX 37.3 Nursing Management of External Ventricular Drainage (EVD) Device

- Ensure all connections are secure and label line as EVD.
- Regularly check that drip chamber of manometer is set at the height prescribed in relation to the client (i.e., zero at clavicle).
- Clamp the drain in the event of client movement or movement anticipated with care. Rezero and open clamps when done.
- Accurately document volume and color of CSF every hour (CSF is normally clear and colorless; cloudiness indicates infection). Notify MD or charge nurse of any significant increase in amount of drainage (if exceeds 10 mL more than previous volumes).
- If minimal or no drainage, check tubing for kinks, blockage, or closed clamps. Check to see if CSF is oscillating in tubing. If blockage is suspected, notify neurosurgery department immediately.
- Entry site into skull should be dressed with a sterile occlusive dressing and should be changed if soiled or nonocclusive.
- Routine CSF samples may be sent for culture and analysis.
- Client may be taking prophylactic antibiotics due to increased risk of infection from the drain.

---

urine can help prevent infection. Additionally, inspect surgical incisions after shunt placement for signs and symptoms of infection and any signs of leaking CSF.

Malfunction of the shunt can occur due to kinking, clogging, or separation of the tubing. Blockage is the most common reported complication. A shunt that has been placed within the past year is at higher risk of malfunction. Early recognition and operative intervention are essential to prevent neurologic deficits or possible death from occurring.

Supporting and Educating the Child and Family

Hydrocephalus is a serious and chronic illness. It will require lifelong follow-up and regular evaluations. It requires early recognition of complications to prevent neurologic damage. Children will require future surgeries and hospitalizations, which can place a strain on the family and its finances. Potential growth and developmental disabilities are an additional strain. The support of the family in establishing realistic goals and helping the child to achieve his or her developmental and educational potential is important.

The family should be involved in the child's care from the time of diagnosis. Initially parents may be frightened because shunt placement involves entering the brain. Provide parents with accurate information regarding the

procedure, and be available to listen to parents' concerns and to answer questions that arise. Ongoing education about the illness and its treatment are important, including signs and symptoms of shunt complications. As the family becomes more comfortable with the diagnosis, treatment, and signs and symptoms of complications, they will become experts on the child's care and will often recognize subtle changes in him or her that may be indicative of shunt complications. Referral to support groups can be helpful for both the family and the child. The National Hydrocephalus Foundation can be accessed at www.nhfonline.org. Additional resources can be found at www.hydroassoc.org and www.hydrocephalus.org.

▶ INTRACRANIAL ARTERIOVENOUS MALFORMATION (AVM)

Intracranial arteriovenous malformation is a rare congenital disorder. It is caused by an abnormal development of blood vessels and can occur in the brain, brainstem, or spinal cord. AVMs that hemorrhage can lead to serious neurologic deficits and even death. However, some cases of AVMs never cause problems. AVMs are the most common cause of hemorrhagic stroke in infants (Molofsky, 2006).

Therapeutic Management

More aggressive treatment strategies are used in children. Treatment options used include surgical excision; endovascular embolization, which involves closing off the vessels of the AVM by injecting glue into them; and radiosurgery, which involves focusing radiation on the AVM. The treatment approach will be based on the age of the client and size and location of the malformation in the brain. The client will usually require at least 24 hours of intensive care monitoring following surgery.

Nursing Assessment

The most common symptoms seen include intracranial hemorrhage (children are more likely to present with hemorrhage than adults), seizures, headaches, and progressive neurologic deficits such as vision problems, loss of speech, problems with memory, and paralysis. In children less than 2 years of age, presentation may include cardiac failure due to arteriovenous shunting in neonates and infants; a large head secondary to hydrocephalus; and seizure activity. Diagnosis is made using diagnostic imaging procedures such as MRI, CT, and arteriography. Due to advances in brain imaging techniques, an increasing number of AVMs are detected before rupture.

Nursing Management

Nursing management for these clients is aimed at supportive care. Monitor for changes in neurologic status, noting any seizure activity, signs or symptoms of increased ICP, or signs and symptoms of intracranial hemorrhage. Hydrocephalus may occur as a result of intracranial hemorrhage secondary to the AVM. An EVD and eventual shunt placement may be necessary (refer to "Hydrocephalus" section).

▶ CRANIOSYNOSTOSIS

Craniosynostosis is premature closure of the cranial sutures (Fig. 37.10). Complete closure of all sutures does not normally occur until late in childhood. Premature closure can inhibit brain growth and a distorted skull appearance will be evident. In cases where only one suture is fused, neurologic impairments are rarely seen. When two or more sutures are fused, neurologic complications such as hydrocephalus with increased ICP are more likely to occur. The incidence of craniosynostosis is approximately 1 in 2,000 births (Behrman et al., 2004). The cause is unknown, but in 10% to 20% of cases a genetic disorder such as Carpenter's syndrome or Apert's, Crouzon's, or Pfeiffer's disease is present (Behrman et al., 2004). There are numerous different types of craniosynostosis; they are listed and illustrated in Table 37.5. The prognosis is good for the majority of infants presenting with craniosynostosis, and normal brain development will occur. Exceptions to this are the infant or child who has associated genetic disorders that involve brain function and development.

Surgical correction may be done and allows for normal expansion of the brain and acceptable appearance of the head and skull. If one suture is fused, the surgical intervention is done mainly for cosmetic reasons. If more than one suture is fused, operative intervention is essential to prevent neurologic complications.

Nursing Assessment

Most cases of craniosynostosis are present at birth. Skull deformity is evident as well as a prominent bony ridge that can be palpated. X-ray studies can confirm fusion of the sutures. It is important that craniosynostosis be detected early if it is not evident at birth because premature closure of the suture lines will inhibit brain development. Therefore, measure head circumference in all children less than 3 years old and compare findings with normal head circumference parameters as well as past measurements of the infant or child.

Nursing Management

Nursing management includes observing hemoglobin and hematocrit levels due to large volumes of blood loss that can occur, and observing for pain, hemorrhage, fever, infection, and swelling. Due to the location of the surgery and incision line, large amounts of facial swelling may be present. This can result in an inability of the child to open his or her eyes for a few days postoperatively. Make sure that parents are aware of this. Encourage the parents to talk to, hold, and comfort their child during this time. Provide support and education to the parents before, during, and after the procedure. Refer families to the Craniosynostosis and Positional Plagiocephaly Support Group, accessible at www.cappskids.org/index.html and 6905 Xanadu Court, Fredericksburg, VA 22407.

▶ POSITIONAL PLAGIOCEPHALY

Since the inception of the "back to sleep" program, which recommends placing all infants supine to sleep to decrease the risk of sudden infant death syndrome (SIDS), there has been a dramatic increase in the incidence of positional plagiocephaly. Positional plagiocephaly refers to asymmetry in head shape without fused sutures. It results from gravitational force exertion on the developing cranium. Plagiocephaly in the infant may lead to torticollis.

Medical treatment for positional plagiocephaly is generally conservative, such as changing the infant's position, encouraging "tummy time," and avoiding excessive use of the car seat for infant seating outside of the automobile. Some infants may benefit from the use of a molding helmet (Fig. 37.11).

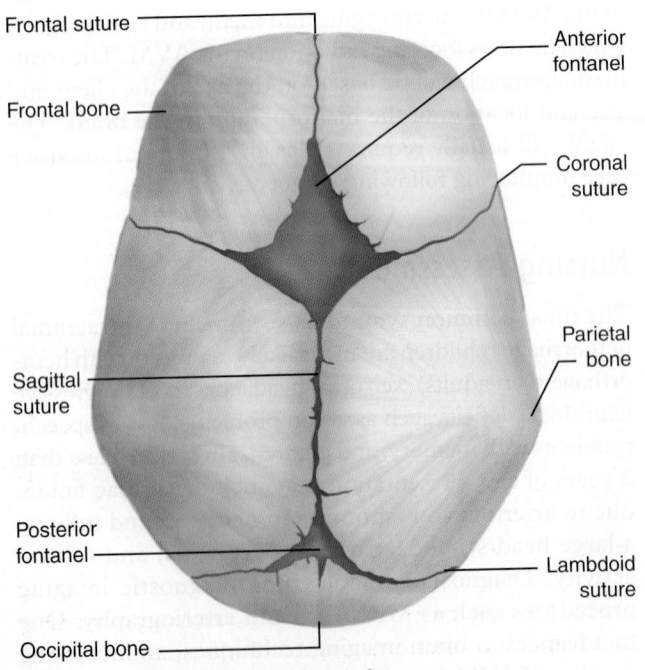

FIGURE 37.10 Skull sutures in the infant.

TABLE 37.5 TYPES OF CRANIOSYNOSTOSIS

Types	Description	
Sagittal synostosis (scaphocephaly)	Sagittal suture is closed. Head grows long and narrow in anterior–posterior direction. Broad forehead and a prominent occiput are present. Most common form	
Metopic synostosis (trigonocephaly)	Metopic suture is closed. Usually a ridge down the forehead can be seen or felt. Triangular-shaped forehead Eyebrows may appear "pinched" on either side. Eyes may also appear close together.	
Unilateral coronal synostosis (anterior plagiocephaly)	Early closure of one side of the coronal suture Forehead and orbital rim (eyebrow) have a flattened appearance on that side.	
Bicoronal synostosis (brachycephaly)	Very flat, recessed forehead Skull is shortened in the anterior–posterior direction. Commonly seen in Apert's and Crouzon's disease	
Lambdoid (posterior plagiocephaly)	Early closure of one lambdoid suture Trapezoid-shaped head in craniosynostosis. Similar to shape found in positional molding or positional plagiocephaly	

Nursing Assessment

View the infant's head from the top, noting asymmetry ranging from flattening on one side posteriorly to posterior flattening associated with anterior bulging (Fig. 37.12). Assess neck range of motion to determine if torticollis is also present. Palpate the cranial sutures, which will not feel overlapped as they do when they are fused. Skull x-ray examination or head CT scan will rule out craniosynostosis by demonstrating evidence of open sutures.

Nursing Management

Nursing management is directed toward repositioning the infant to decrease time spent with the flattened area in the dependent position. Position the infant so that turning

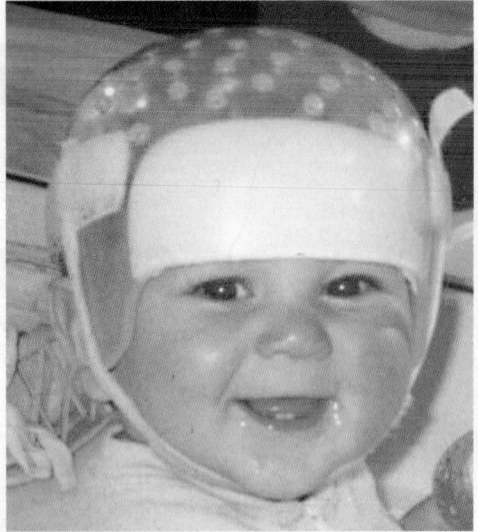

FIGURE 37.11 Molding helmet for positional plagiocephaly.

away from the affected side is necessary for him or her to view objects of interest. Place the infant on the abdomen when awake and supervised. Discourage use of the car seat outside of the automobile. Place a rolled washcloth along the affected side of the head to discourage turning the head in that direction. Following these recommendations may prevent positional plagiocephaly in the infant without congenital torticollis.

FIGURE 37.12 Note flattening of the right posterior parietal and occipital regions of the skull in this infant with positional plagiocephaly.

Infectious Disorders

Infectious disorders of the neurologic system include bacterial meningitis, aseptic meningitis, encephalitis, Reye's syndrome, botulism, and rabies.

▶ BACTERIAL MENINGITIS

Bacterial meningitis is an infection of the meninges, the lining that surrounds the brain and spinal cord. It is a serious illness in children and can lead to brain damage, nerve damage, deafness, stroke, and even death. It requires rapid assessment and treatment. The leading cause of bacterial meningitis in newborns is group B streptococcus and gram-negative enteric bacilli like *Escherichia coli* (Spiro & Spiro, 2004). In children, the leading causative agents are *Neisseria meningitidis* and *Streptococcus pneumoniae* (Spiro & Spiro, 2004). See Table 37.6 for types of meningitis seen in different age groups. In developed countries, disease resulting from *Haemophilus influenzae* type B, once the most common cause of meningitis in children, has decreased dramatically since the introduction of the Hib vaccine. In less developed countries, infection with *H. influenzae* type B still remains a concern. Most cases of bacterial meningitis occur in the winter and early spring, but it can occur year round (Spiro & Spiro, 2004).

Pathophysiology

Bacterial meningitis causes inflammation, swelling, purulent exudates, and tissue damage to the brain. It can occur as a secondary infection to upper respiratory infections, sinus infections, or ear infections, and can also be the result of direct introduction through LP; skull fracture or severe head injury; neurosurgical intervention; congenital structural abnormalities, like spina bifida; or the presence of foreign bodies, like a ventricular shunt or cochlear implants.

TABLE 37.6 **COMMON CAUSES OF MENINGITIS IN DIFFERENT AGE GROUPS**

Causative Organism	Age Affected
Escherichia coli	Newborns and infants
Streptococcus group B	Infants less than 1 month old
Haemophilus influenzae type B	1 month–6 years, typically 6–9 months old
Streptococcus pneumoniae	Children older than 3 months of age and adults
Neisseria meningitidis	Children older than 3 months of age and adults

Therapeutic Management

Bacterial meningitis is a medical emergency and requires prompt hospitalization and treatment. Deterioration may be rapid and occur in less than 24 hours, leading to long-term neurologic damage and even death. Intravenous antibiotics will be started immediately after the LP and blood cultures have been obtained if bacterial meningitis is suspected. The length of therapy and specific antibiotic will be determined based on the analysis and the culture and sensitivity of the CSF. Corticosteroids may be ordered to help reduce the inflammatory process. Specific medical treatment varies based on the suspected causative organism and will be determined by the physician.

Nursing Assessment

For a full description of the assessment phase of the nursing process, refer to page 1140. Assessment findings pertinent to bacterial meningitis are discussed below.

Health History

Elicit a description of the present illness and chief complaint. Common signs and symptoms reported during the health history might include:

- Sudden onset of symptoms
- Preceding respiratory illness or sore throat
- Presence of fever, chills
- Headache
- Vomiting
- Photophobia
- Stiff neck
- Rash
- Irritability
- Drowsiness
- Lethargy
- Muscle rigidity
- Seizures

Symptoms in infants can be more subtle and atypical, but the history may reveal:

- Poor sucking and feeding
- Weak cry
- Lethargy
- Vomiting

Explore the client's current and past medical history for risk factors such as:

- Young age: 1 month to 5 years, with most cases in children less than 1 year of age and young adults 15 to 24 years of age
- Any fever or illness during pregnancy or around delivery (for infants less than 3 months of age)
- Exposure to ill persons
- Exposure to tuberculosis
- Travel history

- History of maternal illness
- Recent neurosurgical procedure or head trauma
- Presence of a foreign body, such as a shunt or a cochlear implant
- Immunocompromised status
- Close-contact living spaces such as dormitories or military bases
- Daycare attendance

Physical Examination

Observe the general appearance of the client. The infant with bacterial meningitis may rest in the **opisthotonic** position (Fig. 37.13), and the older child may complain of neck pain. In the infant a bulging fontanel may be present, which is often a late sign, and the infant may be consolable when lying still as opposed to being held. Presence of positive Kernig's and Brudzinski's signs can indicate irritation of the meninges (Fig. 37.14). Inspect the client for presence of a rash; a petechial, vesicular, or macular rash may be seen.

▶ *Take* NOTE!

Abrupt eruption of a petechial or purplish rash can be indicative of meningococcemia (infection with N. meningitidis*). Immediate medical attention is warranted.*

Laboratory and Diagnostic Tests

Common laboratory and diagnostic studies ordered for the assessment of bacterial meningitis include:

- LP—Fluid pressure will be measured and a sample is obtained for analysis and culture. CSF will reveal increased white blood cells (WBCs) and protein and low glucose (the bacteria present feed on the glucose).
- Complete blood count (CBC)—WBCs will be elevated.
- Blood culture—Performed to rule out sepsis. Blood culture will be positive in cases of septicemia.

FIGURE 37.13 Infant in opisthotonic position: head and neck are hyperextended to relieve discomfort.

FIGURE 37.14 (**A**) Kernig's sign is tested by flexing legs at the hip and knee (**A1**), then extending the knee (**A2**). A positive report of pain along the vertebral column is a positive sign and indicates irritation of meninges. (**B**) Brudzinski's sign is tested by the child lying supine with the neck flexed (**B1**). A positive sign occurs if resistance or pain is met. The child may also passively flex hip and knees in reaction, indicating meningeal irritation (**B2**).

Nursing Management

Quickly initiate supportive measures to ensure proper ventilation, reduce the inflammatory response, and help prevent injury to the brain. Interventions are aimed at reducing ICP and maintaining cerebral perfusion along with treating fluid volume deficit, controlling seizures, and preventing injury that may result from altered LOC or seizure activity. Initiate appropriate isolation precautions. In addition to standard precautions, infants and children diagnosed with bacterial meningitis will be placed on droplet isolation until 24 hours of antibiotics have been received to help prevent transmission to others. Refer to Nursing Care Plan 37.1 for nursing diagnoses and related interventions. In addition to those diagnoses and interventions, reducing fever and preventing bacterial meningitis should be noted.

Reducing Fever

Hyperthermia related to infectious process, increased metabolic rate, and dehydration as evidenced by increased body temperature; warm, flushed skin; and tachycardia may be present. Reducing fever is important to help maintain opti-

mal cerebral perfusion by reducing the metabolic needs of the brain. Administer antipyretics such as acetaminophen and NSAIDS such as ibuprofen, per order. Institute non-pharmacologic measures if needed. Reduction of environmental temperature and the use of cooling blankets, fans, cold compresses, and tepid baths may be helpful in reducing fever. Avoid measures that cause shivering because it increases heat production and is therefore counterproductive as well as uncomfortable for the client.

Preventing Bacterial Meningitis

Bacterial meningitis is a serious illness and prevention is important. It is transmitted by direct close contact with respiratory droplets from the nose or throat. Most at risk are those living with the client or anyone with whom the client played or was in close contact. Postexposure prophylaxis and postexposure immunization may be effective. Control measures should be initiated in environments where risk exists. Disinfect toys and other shared objects to decrease transmission of the microorganisms to others.

To reduce group B streptococcus infection in neonates, screen pregnant women; if the screening results are positive, administer intrapartal antibiotics. Vaccines are available for some specific causative organisms, but complete vaccination prevention is not possible at this time. The Hib vaccine is routine starting at 2 months of age and all children should be immunized to continue the reduction of bacterial meningitis caused by *H. influenzae* type B. The pneumococcal vaccine is also routine for all children starting at 2 months of age and should be considered for preschoolers who are at risk. Children at risk include those with immune deficiency; sickle-cell disease; asplenia; chronic pulmonary, cardiac, or renal disease; diabetes mellitus; cochlear implants; cerebrospinal leaks; and organ transplants.

Since the 1990s, a dramatic increase in the incidence of meningococcal meningitis (and the often fatal blood infection meningococcemia) among adolescents and young adults has occurred. Living in close quarters, sleeping less than usual, and sharing personal items such as drinking glasses and lip balm contribute to the increase in disease. For these reasons, the AAP recommendations advise meningococcal vaccination for all children aged 11 to 12 years; adolescents at high school entry or age 15 (whichever comes first) who have not been previously vaccinated; all college freshmen living in dormitories; and children who are at high risk, such as children with chronic conditions or immune suppression or those who travel to high-risk areas or live in crowded conditions (AAP, 2005). Further information and a resource for families can be obtained through the National Meningitis Association, which can be accessed at www.nmaus.org. (See Healthy People 2010.)

▶ ASEPTIC MENINGITIS

Aseptic meningitis is the most common type of meningitis, and the majority of children affected are less than 5 years of age. If the causative organism can be identified, it is usually a virus. Enteroviruses, like echovirus and coxsackievirus, account for many cases of aseptic meningitis. Less common causes include mumps, herpesvirus, human immunodeficiency virus (HIV), measles, varicella, and polio.

HEALTHY PEOPLE 2010

Objective	Significance
Reduce bacterial meningitis in young children.	• Encourage appropriate immunization as recommended. • Educate families to complete prescribed courses of antibiotics (to avoid progression of minor bacterial infections to meningitis).

Therapeutic Management

Prompt diagnosis and treatment are essential to improve outcomes. The child is treated aggressively as if he or she has bacterial meningitis until the diagnosis is confirmed. Antibiotics are administered and continued until the causative organism is recognized. If the cause is viral, antibiotics may be discontinued and antiviral agents may be started at this time. After diagnosis is confirmed, treatment is mainly supportive in nature and the illness is usually self-limiting, lasting 3 to 10 days.

Nursing Assessment

Elicit a description of the present illness and chief complaint. Common signs and symptoms reported during the health history might include:

• General malaise
• Headache
• Photophobia
• Poor feeding
• Nausea
• Vomiting
• Irritability
• Lethargy
• Neck pain
• Positive Kernig's and Brudzinski's signs

The onset of symptoms may be abrupt or gradual. Assessment is similar to that of the child with bacterial meningitis. Signs and symptoms are similar to those seen in bacterial meningitis, but the child is usually less ill.

Nursing Management

Nursing management is similar to the nursing care of the child with bacterial meningitis and will focus on comfort measures to reduce pain and fever. Aseptic meningitis can be managed successfully at home if the child's neurologic status is stable and he or she is tolerating oral intake.

▶ ENCEPHALITIS

Encephalitis is an inflammation of the brain that may also include an inflammation of the meninges. It is a rare complication and can be caused by protozoan, bacterial, fungal, or viral invasion. In children it is most often associated with a viral illness. Most cases of viral encephalitis in children are of unknown cause. In the United States, common causative organisms include the herpes simplex virus; enteroviruses, such as poliovirus and coxsackievirus; and arthropod-borne viruses. Arthropod-borne viruses (e.g., West Nile and St. Louis encephalitis) are spread by the bites of insects, especially mosquitoes and ticks. Enteroviral infections are usually seen in the late summer and early fall, and arthropod-borne viruses are seen in the summer months.

Recovery from encephalitis can occur in a few days or may be complicated and involve severe neurologic damage with residual effects. Prognosis depends on the age of the child and the causative organism. Prompt diagnosis and treatment are essential. The child suspected of having encephalitis should be hospitalized. Treatment is mainly supportive in nature and focuses on maintaining optimal cerebral perfusion; hydration and nutrition; and injury prevention.

Nursing Assessment

For a full description of the assessment phase of the nursing process, refer to page 1140. Assessment findings pertinent to encephalitis are discussed below.

Health History

Elicit a description of the present illness and chief complaint. Common signs and symptoms reported during the health history might include:

- Fever
- Flu-like symptoms
- Altered LOC
- Headache
- Lethargy
- Drowsiness
- Generalized weakness
- Seizure activity

Explore the client's current history for risk factors such as:

- Recent travel
- Recreational activities, such as hiking and camping
- Animal contacts

Physical Examination

Perform a neurologic examination to distinguish between encephalitis and viral meningitis. In encephalitis, a neurologic examination will reveal changes in sensorium and focal neurologic changes. Neurologic findings vary and reflect the areas of the brain that are involved.

Laboratory and Diagnostic Tests

An LP may be done and the CSF may show an elevated leukocyte count and elevated protein and glucose levels. However, in some cases, levels may be normal. MRI, CT, and EEG procedures may be performed to help identify early changes and provide useful clues in developing a diagnosis.

Nursing Management

Nursing management is similar to nursing care for the child with meningitis. Teach children and their families how to prevent encephalitis. Encephalitis can result from com-plications of childhood illnesses such as measles, mumps, or chickenpox. Explain the importance of keeping children up-to-date in their immunizations. Effective vaccines are available for a few viral pathogens that cause encephalitis (such as rabies virus and Japanese encephalitis virus), but these vaccines are not routine; they are recommended for those at high risk. For example, postexposure rabies vaccines can be administered to a child who was bitten by a suspected rabid animal. Also, those traveling to areas where Japanese encephalitis is endemic, such as India and China, and planning a prolonged stay or extreme outdoor activity should receive the appropriate vaccine. Vector control and avoiding mosquito and tick bites are the best prevention of arthropod-borne infection. Using insect repellent (repellents containing DEET should be used cautiously in children less than 12 years of age and not at all in children less than 1 year of age); wearing clothing that covers the arms and legs; controlling mosquito populations by eliminating areas of standing water where mosquitoes can breed; and using insect traps and public measures such as sprayed insecticides to reduce the mosquito population can all be helpful in reducing the risk of infection with arthropod-borne viruses. Specific antiviral therapy may be used for diseases caused by the herpes simplex virus.

▶ REYE'S SYNDROME

Reye's syndrome is a disease that primarily affects children less than 15 years of age who are recovering from a viral illness. The exact cause of Reye's syndrome is unknown. It has been found that Reye's syndrome is a reaction that is triggered by the use of salicylates or salicylate-containing products to treat a viral infection. This reaction causes brain swelling, liver failure, and death in hours if treatment in not initiated. In the 1980s, the adverse effects of salicylates used to treat viral illnesses began to be publicized and the U.S. Food and Drug Administration (FDA) required warning labels to be placed on all salicylate-containing products, such as aspirin. Since then there has been a dramatic decrease in the occurrence of Reye's syndrome.

Nursing Assessment

Elicit a description of the present illness and chief complaint. Common signs and symptoms reported during the health history might include:

- Severe and continual vomiting
- Changes in mental status
- Lethargy
- Irritability
- Confusion
- Hyperreflexia

Explore the client's current and past medical history for risk factors such as:

- A prodromal viral illness, like chickenpox, croup, flu, or an upper respiratory infection
- Ingestion of salicylate-containing products within 3 weeks of the start of the viral illness

Diagnosis can be confirmed by elevated liver function tests and elevated serum ammonia levels.

Nursing Management

Early recognition and treatment are the most important aspects of managing this illness. Nursing management is aimed at maintaining cerebral perfusion, managing and preventing increased ICP, providing safety measures due to changes in LOC and risk for seizures, and monitoring fluid status to prevent dehydration and overhydration.

Education is an important aspect of preventing this disease. Salicylates are found in many products, including many over-the-counter products such as Alka-Seltzer and Pepto-Bismol. For a complete list, go to www.reyessyndrome.org. Recovery from Reye's syndrome is dependent on the severity of swelling of the brain; some children will make a full recovery, while others may suffer long-term neurologic damage.

▶ BOTULISM

Botulism is a disease that is caused by a toxin produced in the immature intestines of young children resulting from infection with the bacteria *Clostridium botulinum*. It is rare, but can cause serious paralytic illness. Botulism is mainly a food-borne infection but can also be contracted through wound infections or intestinal infections in infants. *C. botulinum* is common in soil and can also be found in a variety of foods, such as improperly preserved home-canned foods. It generally occurs in infants less than 6 months of age. It has been associated with feeding honey and corn syrup to infants; thus these should be avoided in children less than 1 year of age. The disease is not contagious, and the child must ingest the bacterial spores. These spores then multiply in the intestinal tract and produce the toxin, which is absorbed in the immature intestines of the infant. It is generally not a problem for older children because the bacteria do not grow well in mature intestines due to the presence of the normal intestinal flora. Prognosis is good, but if treatment is not initiated, paralysis to the arms, legs, trunk, and respiratory system can develop.

Nursing Assessment

For a full description of the assessment phase of the nursing process, refer to page 1140. Assessment findings pertinent to botulism are discussed below.

Health History

Elicit a description of the present illness and chief complaint. Signs and symptoms usually occur soon after ingestion of the bacteria. Common signs and symptoms in infants reported during the health history might include:

- Constipation
- Poor feeding
- Listlessness
- Generalized weakness
- Weak cry

Common signs and symptoms in older children reported during the health history might include:

- Double vision
- Blurred vision
- Drooping eyelids
- Difficulty swallowing
- Slurred speech
- Muscle weakness

Physical Examination and Laboratory and Diagnostic Tests

Assess for a diminished gag reflex, which is indicative of botulism. Diagnostic tests include culturing of stool and serum. Botulism is a rare disease and is difficult to diagnose because symptoms are similar to those seen in other neurologic diseases. Therefore assessment may include diagnostic tests to help rule out other diseases such as Guillain-Barré syndrome, stroke, and myasthenia gravis.

Nursing Management

Treatment is mainly supportive in nature and focuses on maintaining respiratory status and nutritional status. If ordered, administer botulism toxin early in the course of the disease to reduce the severity and progression of the disease.

Trauma

Trauma or injury is a leading cause of childhood morbidity and mortality in the United States, with the highest rates among minority populations (Morbidity and Mortality Weekly Report, 2007). The child faces significant risk of trauma to his or her developing neurologic system, often leading to neurologic disorders with life-threatening and lasting effects. Neurologic trauma may include head trauma, nonaccidental head trauma, and near drowning.

▶ HEAD TRAUMA

In the United States, injury causes more death in children than disease. Of these injuries, head injury is the most common cause of death and disability in childhood.

Common causes of head trauma in children include falls, motor vehicle accidents, pedestrian and bicycle accidents, and child abuse. Many factors make children more susceptible to head trauma than adults. Larger head size in relation to the body, coupled with a higher center of gravity, causes the child to hit his or her head more readily when involved in motor vehicle accidents, bicycle accidents, and falls. Children are also at risk for injury related to psychosocial factors such as their high activity level, curiosity, incomplete motor development, and their lack of knowledge and judgment skills. Also, their dependence on others to care for them places them at a high risk for injuries caused by child abuse. Children younger than 3 years of age have a very mobile spine, especially in the cervical region, along with immature neck muscles. This places them at a higher risk for injury from acceleration/deceleration injuries, which occur when the head receives a blow or is shaken; the sudden acceleration causes deformation of the skull and movement of the brain, allowing brain contents to strike parts of the skull. Bruising of the brain can occur at the point of impact or at that point distant from the impact where the brain collides with the skull. Another result of brain movement is hemorrhages in the brain, which are caused by the shearing forces that may tear small arteries. The child's thin skull places him or her at increased risk for skull fractures and penetrating injuries resulting from head trauma.

Head trauma is a broad term that can include specific patterns of injury. See Table 37.7 for descriptions of common head injuries seen in children. Head trauma in children is serious because it can cause an immediate threat to the child's life as well as a number of complications that can lead to lifelong impairment of an individual's physical, cognitive, and psychosocial functioning. Prognosis for the child who has suffered a head trauma depends on the extent and severity of the injury as well as any complications (see Healthy People 2010).

Nursing Assessment

For a full description of the assessment phase of the nursing process, refer to page 1140. Assessment findings pertinent to head trauma are discussed below.

Health History
Take a detailed history, including past medical history along with details of the events surrounding the injury such as mental status at the time of the injury, any loss of consciousness, irritability, lethargy, abnormal behavior, vomiting (if so, how many times), any seizure activity, and any complaints of headache, visual changes, or neck pain.

Physical Examination
Perform a thorough physical examination. Initial physical assessment will focus on the ABCs (airway, breath-

ing, and circulation) (refer to Chapter 52 for further information on emergency management). All children who experience head trauma need an assessment of their neurologic function as soon as they are seen. This includes LOC, pupillary response, and any seizure activity. Fixed and dilated pupils, fixed and constricted pupils, or sluggish pupillary reaction to light will warrant prompt intervention.

> ▶ **Take** NOTE!
>
> *A child's spine must remain stabilized after a head injury until spinal cord injury is ruled out.*

Laboratory and Diagnostic Tests
Diagnostic tests that may be utilized include x-ray examinations of the head and neck and CT and MRI scans. These procedures can assist in providing a more definitive diagnosis of the severity and type of trauma.

> ▶ **Take** NOTE!
>
> *If clear liquid fluid is noted draining from the ears or nose, notification of the physician or advanced practitioner is warranted. If the fluid tests positive for glucose, this is indicative of leaking CSF.*

Nursing Management

Nursing management of the child with head trauma depends on the seriousness of the injury. For all head trauma, however, the nurse provides support and education to the family and provides teaching on ways to prevent future head injuries.

Caring for the Child With Mild to Moderate Head Injury
Most children with mild to moderate closed head injury, which refers to brain injury without any penetrating injury to the brain, who suffered no loss of consciousness, no other injury to their head or body, are acting normally after the injury, and were healthy before the injury can be cared for and observed at home. Provide parents and caregivers with clear instructions regarding the care of their child at home. Explain that they must seek medical attention if the child's condition worsens at any time

TABLE 37.7   COMMON HEAD INJURIES SEEN IN CHILDREN

Types	Description	Characteristics
Skull fractures	A break in the bone surrounding the brain	In infants and children less than 2 years old, a great deal of force is needed to produce a skull fracture. Due to the flexibility of the immature skull, it is able to withstand a great degree of deformation before a fracture will occur. Can result in little or no brain damage, but may have serious consequences if the underlying brain tissue is injured
Linear skull fracture	A simple break in the skull that follows a relatively straight line	Most common skull fracture. Can result from minor head injuries such as being struck by a rock, stick, or other object; falls; or motor vehicle accidents. Not usually serious unless there is additional injury to the brain
Depressed skull fractures	The bone is locally broken and pushed inward, causing pressure on the brain.	Can result from forceful impact from a blunt object, such as a hammer or another heavy but fairly small object Surgery is often required to elevate the bony pieces and inspect the brain for evidence of injury.
Diastatic skull fracture	A fracture through the skull sutures	Most commonly occurs in the lamboid sutures (refer to Fig. 37.10 for location of sutures) Usually treatment is not required but observation will be necessary.
Compound skull fracture	A laceration of the skin and splintering of the bone	The fracture can be linear or depressed. Generally is the result of blunt force. Usually requires medical intervention and surgery may be necessary.
Basilar skull fracture	A fracture of the bones that form the base of the skull	Can result from severe blunt head trauma with significant force. Due to the proximity to the brainstem, this is a serious head injury. Findings include CSF rhinorrhea and otorrhea, bleeding from the ear, and orbital or postauricular ecchymosis (bruising behind ear is referred to as Battle's sign), and these children are at increased risk for infection because the fracture may allow a portal of entry into the central nervous system.
Concussion	A mild brain injury that is caused by jarring or shaking and results in disruption or malfunction of the electrical activities of the brain	Most common head injury. Results from a blow or jolt to the head caused by sports injuries, motor vehicle accidents, and falls. Confusion and amnesia after the head injury are seen. Loss of consciousness may or may not occur. Noted symptoms may include increased distractibility, and difficulty with concentration. Treatment includes rest and monitoring for neurologic changes that could indicate a more severe injury, such as increased sleepiness, worsening headache, increased vomiting, worsening confusion, difficulty walking or talking, changes in LOC, and seizures.
Contusion	Bruising of cerebral tissue	Results from a blow to the head from incidents such as a motor vehicle accident, falls, or abuse such as shaken baby syndrome. May cause focal disturbances in vision, strength, and sensation. The signs and symptoms will vary based on the extent of vascular injury and can range from mild weakness to prolonged unconsciousness and paralysis. Treatment includes close monitoring for neurologic changes. Surgery is usually not necessary.

(continued)

TABLE 37.7 COMMON HEAD INJURIES SEEN IN CHILDREN (continued)

Types	Description	Characteristics
Subdural hematoma	Collection of blood between the dura and cerebrum	Low incidence of fracture. Most common in children less than 2 years old, especially infants. Results from birth trauma, falls, bicycle injuries, and abuse such as shaken baby syndrome. Usually consists of venous bleeding. Symptoms may occur within 3 days of trauma or as late as 20 days. Symptoms include vomiting, failure to thrive, changes in LOC, seizures, and retinal hemorrhage. Treatment depends on clinical symptoms, size of clot, and area of the brain involved. In some cases, the bleed may be closely monitored for resolution. In other cases, treatment may include subdural taps in infants and surgical evacuation in older children. Close monitoring of neurologic status and for signs of increased ICP is indicated.
Epidural hematoma	Collection of blood located outside the dura but within the skull	Relatively uncommon. Often results from skull fracture. Seen when head trauma is severe. Usually arterial bleeding, therefore brain compression occurs rapidly and can result in impairment of the brainstem and respiratory or cardiovascular function. Symptoms include vomiting, headache, and lethargy. Treatment depends on clinical symptoms, the size of the clot, and the area of the brain involved. Treatment includes prompt surgical evacuation and cauterization of the artery. The earlier the bleed is recognized and treated, the more favorable the outcome. Close monitoring of neurologic status is indicated.

during the first several days after injury. See Teaching Guidelines 37.2.

Children with mild closed head injury may exhibit some cognitive and behavioral symptoms, such as difficulty paying attention, problems making sense of what has been seen or heard, and forgetting things, in the early days after the injury. The majority make a full recovery. However, some may experience ongoing cognitive and behavioral difficulties, including slow information processing and attention difficulties.

Caring for the Child With Severe Head Injury

Children with more severe head injury may require intensive care initially until stabilized. Focus will be on maintaining the child's airway; monitoring breathing, circulation, and neurologic status closely; preventing and ceasing any seizure activity; and treating any other injuries that may

have occurred as a result of the trauma. Nursing management will continue to focus on evaluation of neurologic status, assessing for changes in LOC and signs and symptoms of increased ICP. Initiate seizure precautions as ordered.

Individualize care to the specific needs of the child. Maintain a quiet environment to help reduce restlessness and irritability. Manage pain and administer sedation as ordered. Observe the level of sedation closely to ensure that LOC will not become altered, which would hinder the ability to assess adequately for neurologic changes. Monitor for the development of complications, which include hemorrhage, infection, cerebral edema, and herniation.

▶ *Take* NOTE!

Parents are extremely helpful resources in evaluating a child's behavior for changes or abnormalities. They can provide insight into whether a behavior seen is normal or abnormal for this child. Examples include the ease at which a child is normally aroused, how much the child normally sleeps during the day, and what is the child's normal visual and hearing acuity.

HEALTHY PEOPLE 2010

Objective	Significance
Increase the number of states and the District of Columbia with laws requiring bicycle helmets for bicycle riders.	• Support legislation locally that calls for bicycle helmet laws. • Participate in local "safe kids" activities to demonstrate support for helmet use

TEACHING GUIDELINES 37.2

Monitoring the Child with Closed Head Injury at Home

Instruct parents and caregivers:

- Stay with the child for the first 24 hours and be ready to take the child to the hospital if necessary.
- Closely observe the child for a few days.
- Wake the child every 2 hours to ensure that he or she moves normally, wakes enough to recognize the caregiver, and responds to the caregiver appropriately.
- Call the medical provider or bring child to the emergency room if the child exhibits any of the following:
  - Constant headache that gets worse
  - Slurred speech
  - Dizziness that does not go away or happens repeatedly
  - Extreme irritability or other abnormal behavior
  - Vomiting more than two times
  - Clumsiness or difficulty walking
  - Oozing blood or watery fluid from ears or nose
  - Difficulty waking up
  - Unequal-sized pupils
  - Unusual paleness that lasts longer than 1 hour
  - Seizures
- Review signs and symptoms of increased intracranial pressure and provide parents with a number they can call if they have questions or concerns.

Head injuries can range from a temporary unconsciousness that resolves quickly to children who may remain in a comatose state for a prolonged time. Nursing management of the comatose child is similar to nursing care of the comatose adult.

Providing Support and Education

Provide support and education for the family of a child who has suffered a head trauma. Encourage involvement in the child's care. The extent of residual neurologic damage and recovery may be unclear for the child with a head injury. This can be frustrating and stressful for parents and family. Encourage verbalization of their feelings and concerns. Rehabilitation of the child with permanent brain damage is an essential component of his or her care. It should begin as soon as possible in the hospital setting and may continue for months to years. This can place a strain on the family and its finances. Families need to be involved in the rehabilitation process. The nurse will be a key member in ensuring the parents and family are involved with the interdisciplinary team.

Preventing Head Injuries

Prevention of head injuries provides the greatest benefit to children and the community. Nurses play a key role in educating the public on topics such as helmet use with certain sports; bicycle and motorcycle safety; seat belt use; and providing adequate supervision of children to help prevent injuries and accidents—and resultant head trauma—from occurring (see Healthy People 2010).

▶ NONACCIDENTAL HEAD TRAUMA

In the United States, inflicted or nonaccidental head trauma is the leading cause of traumatic death and morbidity during infancy (Berger et al., 2006). Causes include violent shaking, referred to as shaken baby syndrome (SBS); blows to the head; and intentional cranial impacts against the wall, furniture, or the floor. The infant's large head size and weak neck muscles place him or her at an increased risk for head trauma due to violent shaking or cranial impacts from adults. The average victim is less than 9 months of age. SBS is a form of child abuse and a significant number of head traumas result from it. It differs from many other forms of child abuse in that frequently there was no intent to harm the child. Shaking happens when the parent or caregiver becomes frustrated or angry because he or she cannot get the baby to stop crying.

The full appearance of neurologic deficits resulting from nonaccidental head trauma may take several years to be identified and recovery can be very slow. Long-term outcomes are not known, but many of these infants and children have poor outcomes and may suffer neurologic defects such as profound mental retardation, spastic quadriplegia, severe motor dysfunction, and blindness. The majority of children with inflicted head injuries have some impairment of motor and cognitive abilities, language, vision, and behavior. These injuries may also contribute to later problems with education and social attainment.

HEALTHY PEOPLE 2010

Objective	Significance
Reduce hospitalization for nonfatal head injuries.	• Educate children and families about safety such as helmet use when inline skating, skateboarding, bicycling, and playing football or other sports that may result in head injury.
	• Encourage appropriate child car seat and seat belt use.
	• Use every encounter with a child and family as an opportunity to provide education related to injury prevention.

Nursing Assessment

The infant who has been a victim of nonaccidental trauma can present in many ways. Symptoms and physical findings may be similar to those seen in children with accidental head trauma or increased ICP related to infection. Therefore many nonaccidental traumas remain unidentified. Nurses are mandatory reporters of abuse (for further information on this, see Chapter 52), and early recognition of suspected child abuse is essential to prevent death and disability from repetitive inflicted head trauma.

Health History

It is important that health care providers review the child's history closely and pay particular attention to the caregivers' explanation of the child's injury. The health care provider should be alert to any discrepancies between the physical injuries and the history of injury given by the parent, if the stories are conflicting, or if the caregivers are unable to give an explanation for the injury. Also, any previous intracranial or skeletal injuries that cannot be explained should be noted.

In less severe cases, common signs and symptoms may include:

- Poor feeding or sucking
- Vomiting
- Lethargy or irritability
- Failure to thrive
- Increased sleeping
- Difficulty arousing

In more severe cases, the symptoms will be more acute and may consist of:

- Seizure activity
- Apnea
- Bradycardia
- Decreased LOC
- Bulging fontanel

Physical Examination

External bruising of the head and face may be evident in some inflicted head traumas. However, no evidence of external trauma, but the presence of intracranial or intraocular hemorrhages, is the classic presentation of SBS. Retinal hemorrhages are seen in the majority of cases, which is a rare finding in accidental or nontraumatic events.

Laboratory and Diagnostic Tests

Diagnostic tests including CT, MRI, ophthalmologic examination to rule out retinal hemorrhages, and skeletal survey x-rays to rule out or confirm other injuries may be performed to help determine the extent and type of injury.

Nursing Management

Treatment and nursing management will be similar to that for the child with accidental head trauma (see earlier section, "Head Trauma"). Prevention of nonaccidental head trauma, including SBS, is a major concern for all health care professionals. Be aware of risk factors related to the potential for SBS to occur. Recognizing these risk factors will allow appropriate intervention and protection of the child to take place. See Box 37.4 for risk factors related to SBS.

Educating parents and caregivers on appropriate ways to handle stress and ways to cope with a crying infant can help to prevent nonaccidental head trauma (see Teaching Guidelines 37.3). Many parents and caregivers may perceive shaking a child as a less violent way to react than other means of enforcing discipline. They need to be aware that shaking a baby, even for only a few seconds, can cause serious brain damage and death. Decreasing mortality and morbidity associated with SBS and nonaccidental injury through early preventive education is an essential nursing concern. Information about the dangers of shaking a baby should be a part of prenatal care and standard discharge teaching on postpartum units. In addition, this information should be provided to the community and in health education classes to reach young potential child care providers.

▶ NEAR DROWNING

Drowning rates have declined, but drowning remains a leading cause of injury-related death in children between the ages of 1 and 19 years (Schnitzer, 2006). Drowning is a preventable problem that is far too prevalent, especially in children. Those at greatest risk of drowning are toddlers and adolescent males.

Near drowning is described as an incident in which a child has suffered a submersion injury and has survived for at least 24 hours. Near-drowning events result in a significant number of injured children and can result in long-term neurologic deficits. In children between the ages of 1 and 4 years, most drowning and near-drowning incidents occur in residential swimming pools (Saluja et al., 2006). Most incidents are accidental and result from inadequately supervising children who are in or near water; lack of use of personal flotation devices while on recreational water apparatus such as boats; and diving accidents.

BOX 37.4 Risk Factors Associated with Shaken Baby Syndrome

- Single parent
- Young parent
- Substance abuse by a parent
- Any external factors present such as financial, social, or physical burdens that place stress on the parent
- Premature or sick infant
- Infant with colic

TEACHING GUIDELINES 37.3

Tips to Calm a Crying Baby

Instruct parents and caregivers
- Try to figure out what is upsetting the baby.
  - Is the baby hungry?
  - Is the baby's diaper dry?
  - Is the baby cold or hot?
  - Is the baby overtired or overstimulated?
  - Is the baby in pain?
  - Is the baby sick or running a fever?
- Try to help the baby relax.
  - Turn down the lights.
  - Swaddle the baby.
  - Walk the baby.
  - Rock the baby.
  - Give the baby a breast, bottle, or pacifier.
  - Shhh, talk to, or sing to the baby.
  - Talk the baby for a stroller or car ride.
- Sometimes the baby may continue to cry after all your efforts. If you feel overwhelmed, frustrated, or angry, focus on keeping the baby safe.
  - Stop what you are doing, take a deep breath, and count to 10.
  - Place the baby in a safe place, such as the crib or playpen.
  - Leave the room and shut the door, and find a quiet place for yourself.
  - Check on the baby every 5–15 minutes.
  - Do not be afraid to call for help; call a friend, relative, or neighbor.

Nursing Assessment

Hypoxia is the primary problem resulting from near drowning. Nursing assessment needs to begin with resuscitative measures. The child may be comatose, hypothermic, lack spontaneous respirations, and present with hypoxia and hypercapnea. Gain information about the site of submersion (was it fresh or salt water), the water temperature, the time of submersion, and how long it was until the child received interventions such as cardiopulmonary resuscitation (CPR) and emergency medical services (EMS).

Nursing Management

Resuscitative measures should be started as soon as the child is pulled from the water, and the child should be transported to a hospital immediately. Management will be based on the degree of cerebral insult that has occurred. The child who has been successfully resuscitated will usually require intensive nursing care and monitoring. Promotion of oxygenation and monitoring for infection related to aspiration of water are primary nursing concerns. Chronic neurologic damage occurs in many near drown-

ings secondary to hypoxia. The child may need rehabilitation and long-term follow-up. Provide parents with support and education relating to their child's condition. Educating children, families, and the community is an important nursing intervention to help prevent drowning (see Teaching Guidelines 37.4).

Blood Flow Disruption

The incidence of pediatric cerebral vascular disorders is estimated to be between 2 and 3 per 100,000 with the highest incidence in the younger child (Molofsky, 2006). Although they occur less often than in adults, they are still an important cause of mortality and chronic morbidity in children. Many children will develop lifelong cognitive and motor impairments. Improvements in imaging techniques have led to an increase in the reported incidence and prevalence of cerebral vascular disorders in children in recent years. Childhood cerebral vascular disorders (stroke) are usually seen after the first month of life. Periventricular/intraventricular (PVH/IVH) hemorrhage is seen in preterm infants and in infants up to 1 month of age (refer to Chapter 24 for further information on PVH/IVH).

▶ CEREBRAL VASCULAR DISORDERS (STROKE)

A cerebral vascular disorder is a sudden disruption of the blood supply to the brain. It affects neurologic functioning, such as movement and speech. Two major types of cerebral vascular disorders are seen in children just as in adults: ischemic stroke and hemorrhagic stroke. Ischemic stroke is more common than hemorrhagic stroke in children. In children, there is a wide array of risk factors and

TEACHING GUIDELINES 37.4

Teaching to Prevent Drowning

Instruct parents and caregivers
- Install proper pool fencing.
- Start water safety training at a young age.
- Never leave an infant or young child without adult supervision in or near water (this includes bathtubs).
- Empty water from all containers, such as 5-gallon buckets, immediately after use.
- Use personal flotation devices at all times when near water.
- Learn cardiopulmonary resuscitation (CPR) and keep emergency numbers handy (make sure babysitters are CPR qualified).
- Know the depth of water before permitting a child to jump or dive.

causes as compared to adults (see Comparison Chart 37.2), but in many cases the cause remains unidentified. The outcomes reported for cerebral vascular disorders in children vary, but many children will develop some neurologic or cognitive deficit.

Nursing Assessment

The clinical presentation will vary according to age, the underlying cause, and the location of the stroke. Signs and symptoms of acute stroke are similar to those seen in the adult and depend on the area of the brain that has been affected. Common signs include:

• Weakness on one side or hemiplegia
• Facial droop
• Slurred speech
• Speech deficits

Strokes in children are diagnosed in the same manner as strokes in adults. However, further tests may need to be run in the child, such as metabolic studies, coagulation tests, echocardiogram, and LP to help identify the cause of the stroke.

Nursing Management

Historically, children have been excluded from adult stroke studies. Therefore, many treatments used in children have had to be adapted from adult studies. Acute treatment is supportive and requires intensive care. The exact treatment will depend on the underlying cause. Nursing man-

agement will be similar to that for the adult client who has suffered a stroke. Care will focus on assessing neurologic status, increasing mobility, providing adequate nutrition and hydration, and encouraging self-care. Rehabilitative care may be initiated, depending on the long-term deficits, to help the child attain optimal function. Parental support and education will be essential in helping them care for a child who has new disabilities..

Chronic Disorders

Chronic disorders in children necessitate multidisciplinary care. Parents and children are in need of a large amount of education and support from the health care team. Chronic neurologic disorders commonly seen in children include headaches and breath holding.

▶ HEADACHES

Acute and chronic headaches, including migraines, are common reasons why children miss school, visit their primary care physicians, and receive subsequent referrals to neurologists. Children with reports or symptoms of headaches need to be examined thoroughly. Headaches may result from sinusitis or eyestrain or can be indicative of more serious conditions such as brain tumors, acute meningitis, or increased ICP. Migraines are a specific

COMPARISON CHART 37.2 RISK FACTORS AND CAUSES OF STROKE IN THE PEDIATRIC CLIENT VS. THE ADULT CLIENT

	Risk Factors and Causes in Children	Risk Factors and Causes in Adults
Ischemic stroke	Cardiac disorders and intracardiac defects (congenital such as ventricular septal defect, atrial septal defect, and aortic stenosis, or acquired such as rheumatic heart disease) Coagulation abnormalities that lead to thrombosis Sickle-cell disease Infection, such as meningitis Arterial dissection Genetic disorders	Cardiac disease, including atherosclerosis Diabetes mellitus Hyperlipidemia Hypercoagulability states Polycythemia Sickle-cell disease Smoking Increased age Male gender Obesity Excessive alcohol consumption
Hemorrhagic stroke	Vascular malformations such as intracranial arteriovenus malformation (AVM) Aneurysms Warfarin therapy Cavernous malformations Malignancy Trauma Coagulation disorders such as hemophilia Thrombocytopenia Liver failure Leukemia Intracranial tumors such as medulloblastomas	Hypertension Aneurysms Use of anticoagulant medications Smoking Increased age Male gender Obesity Excessive alcohol consumption

type of headache. They are benign, recurrent, throbbing headaches often accompanied by nausea, vomiting, and photophobia. Acute migraines can occur in children as young as 3 to 4 years old. The cause of migraine headaches is not well understood.

Therapeutic Management

After other acute or chronic conditions are ruled out, management will focus on treating the child's pain. Pharmacologic measures may be utilized in the treatment of chronic headaches and migraines. Medications used in children to treat and prevent headaches are similar to the medications used to treat adults. Recent attention has been paid to headaches caused by medication overuse. The client may have a primary headache disorder that is exacerbated by the frequent use of medications. Although medication overuse headaches are common in children, they are frequently underrecognized and underdiagnosed.

Nursing Assessment

Elicit a description of the present illness and chief complaint. Important health history information to obtain is onset of the pain, aggravating and alleviating factors, frequency and duration of the pain, time of day the pain usually occurs, location of the pain, and quality and intensity of the pain.

In young children, symptoms of headache may be hard to recognize. However, common signs and symptoms may include:

- Irritability
- Lethargy
- Head holding
- Head banging
- Sensitivity to sound or light

Assessment also includes a thorough physical examination to rule out any life-threatening illness, such as a brain tumor or increased ICP. A detailed neurologic exam is warranted. Neuroimaging may be performed based on the child's history and physical exam, if needed, to rule out a brain tumor or mass as the cause of the headaches.

Nursing Management

Nursing measures will focus on support and education. Reassure the child and family that no serious medical or neurologic disease is present. Because headaches are recurring and the cause may be unknown, pain management can be difficult. Provide education to help the child and parents gain control over the headaches. Teach the child and family to a keep very accurate record of headaches and activities surrounding the headaches to help establish a pattern of occurrence and identify triggering factors. Encourage parents and the child to recognize the triggering factors and to avoid them (Box 37.5). Teach the child and family about pain medications and how to use them. Teach other man-

---

> ### BOX 37.5 Potential Headache Triggers
>
> - Foods, such as chocolate, caffeine, or monosodium glutamate (MSG)-containing foods
> - Changes in hormone levels, around menses and ovulation
> - Changes in:
>   - Weather
>   - Season
>   - Sleep patterns
>   - Meal schedule
> - Stress
> - Intense activity
> - Bright or flickering lights
> - Odors, such as strong perfumes

---

agement techniques, which may include exercise, regular attendance at school, use of biofeedback, stress reduction techniques, and possible psychiatric assessment.

▶ BREATH HOLDING

Breath holding is a benign behavior of childhood, although it is extremely frightening for parents. It is normally seen in children 1 to 3 years old and typically is outgrown by 5 years of age. It is usually triggered by the child becoming angry or stressed after not getting his or her way. It can also occur as a reflexive response to fear, pain, or being startled. The child stops inhaling and exhaling or hyperventilates, the brain becomes anoxic, and the child becomes cyanotic and then passes out. It usually resolves spontaneously. With the loss of consciousness the child will begin breathing on his or her own and will often begin crying, screaming, and trying to catch his or her breath. The spells usually only last 30 to 60 seconds and, as long as the child does not sustain an injury while falling, have no consequences.

Nursing Assessment

The first time a spell occurs, a doctor should evaluate the child because the event could indicate a seizure. Breath holding also has been shown to be aggravated by iron deficiency anemia and, in rare cases, it could indicate a more serious neurologic condition and therefore warrant a full evaluation. Elicit a full description of the episode and events leading up to it. Also, collect a thorough past medical history and perform a complete physical examination.

Nursing Management

If no underlying condition is found, the child needs no therapy. Nursing management should focus on educating and supporting the parents. Breath holding is a scary event and parents will want information on the effects of the behavior and how to prevent the behavior from recurring. Reassure parents that the child will suffer no ill effects from breath holding and that they should not reinforce the breath holding behavior or give in to the child. Encourage parents to maintain a safe environment when an episode is occurring, but to avoid giving extra attention to the child after the event because this could encourage repetition of the behavior.

■■■ Key Concepts

- Development of the brain and spinal cord occurs early in gestation, in the first 3 to 4 weeks. Infection, trauma, teratogens, and malnutrition during this period can result in malformations and may affect normal CNS development.

- The brain of the newborn is highly vascular, leading to an increased risk for hemorrhage.

- The head of the infant and young child is large in proportion to the body and the neck muscles are not well developed, which places the infant at an increased risk of head injury from falls and accidents.

- Neurologic disorders in children can result from congenital problems as well as infections or trauma.

- LP and CSF analysis can be useful in the diagnosis of hemorrhage, infection, or obstruction.

- CT and MRI studies can be useful in diagnosing congenital abnormalities such as neural tube defects, hemorrhage, tumors, fractures, demyelinating, or inflammation.

- EEGs measure the electrical activity of the brain and can be used in diagnosing seizures or brain death.

- Antibiotics are utilized in the treatment of bacterial meningitis and shunt infections.

- Anticonvulsants are used in the treatment and prevention of seizures and are often used in combination.

- Corticosteroids are used to reduce cerebral edema and must be tapered before discontinuing.

- Risk factors associated with neurologic disorders include prematurity, difficult birth, infection during pregnancy, family history of genetic disorders with a neurologic manifestation, seizure disorders, and headaches.

- Alterations in motor function, such as changes in gait or muscle tone or strength, may indicate certain neurologic problems such as increased ICP, head injury, and cerebral infections.

- Increased ICP is a sign that may occur with many neurologic disorders. It may result from head trauma, birth trauma, hydrocephalus, infection, and brain tumors. It is essential that the nurse observes for signs and symptoms associated with increased ICP while caring for a child with a potential or suspected neurologic disorder.

- Sunset eyes may indicate increased ICP as seen in hydrocephalus.

- A bulging fontanel can be a sign of increased ICP and is seen in such neurologic disorders as hydrocephalus and head traumas.

- Cortical control of motor function is lost in certain neurologic disorders; postural reflexes reemerge and are directly related to the area of the brain that is damaged. Decorticate posturing occurs with damage of the cerebral cortex. Decerebrate posturing occurs with damage at the level of the brainstem.

- Hydrocephalus results from an imbalance in the production and absorption of CSF. Key assessment findings include a rapid increase in head circumference seen in the infant, or loss of development and changes in personality in the older child. Signs and symptoms associated with increased ICP may be seen.

- Bacterial meningitis requires rapid assessment and treatment. On assessment, the nurse may find the infant with bacterial meningitis resting in the opisthotonic position, and the older child may complain of neck pain.

- Nursing management of seizures focuses on preventing injury during seizures, instituting seizure precautions, maintaining a patent airway, administering appropriate medication and treatments to prevent or reduce seizures, and providing education and support to the child and family to help them cope with the challenges of living with a chronic seizure disorder.

- Nursing management of the child with hydrocephalus will focus on maintaining cerebral perfusion, minimizing neurologic complications, recognizing and preventing shunt infection and malfunction, maintaining adequate nutrition, promoting growth and development, and supporting and educating the child and family.

- Nursing management of the child with bacterial meningitis will include administration of intravenous antibiotics, reducing ICP, and maintaining cerebral perfusion along with treating fluid volume deficit, controlling seizures, and preventing injury that may result from altered LOC or seizure activity.

- Nurses play a key role in educating the public on topics such as helmet use with certain sports, bicycle and motorcycle safety, seat belt use, and providing adequate supervision of children to help prevent injuries and accidents and resultant head trauma from occurring.

- Many neurologic disorders affect multiple body systems with lifelong deficits that require long-term rehabilitation. Adjusting to the demands this condition places on the child and family is difficult. Parents may need time to accept their child's condition but as soon as possible they should be involved in the child's care.

- Children with neurologic disorders and their families often need large amounts of education and support throughout the child's lifetime. As the child grows, the needs of the family and child will change. The nurse needs to provide ongoing education and support.

- Some neurologic disorders require complete intensive daily care. Adjusting to these demands can be difficult for the family. Encourage respite care and provide meaningful education programs that emphasize independence for the child in the least restrictive educational environment.

Refer caregivers to local resources, including education services and support groups.

REFERENCES

AAP. (2005). *Prevention and control of meningococcal disease: Recommendations for use of meningococcal vaccines in pediatric patients.* Retrieved on December 17, 2007 at http://www.aap.org/advocacy/releases/mengpolicyfinal.pdf.

Atabaki, S. (2007). Pediatric head injury [Electronic Version]. *Pediatrics in Review, 28*(6), 215–224.

Becske, T. & Jallo, G. (2007). Neural tube defects. *eMedicine* (online) Retrieved on December 18, 2007 at http://www.emedicine.com/neuro/topic244.htm

Bechtel, K. & Berger, R. (2006). Inflicted traumatic brain injury: Making the diagnosis in the emergency department [Electronic version]. *Clinical Pediatric Emergency Medicine, 7*(3), 138–142.

Behrman, R. E., Kliegman, R. M., & Jenson, H. B. (2004). *Nelson's textbook of pediatrics* (17th ed.). Philadelphia: Saunders.

Centers for Disease Control and Prevention (CDC). (2004). Use of vitamins containing folic acid among women of childbearing age—United States [electronic version]. *MMWR, 53*(36), 847–850. Retrieved on December 18, 2007 at http://www.cdc.gov/mmwr/preview/mmwrhtml/mm5336a6.htm

Centers for Disease Control and Prevention. (2007). Significant disparities in fatal-injury rates persist between white and minority. *Morbidity and Mortality Weekly Report, 56*(SS05);1–16, retrieved on December 17, 2007 at http://www.medscape.com/viewarticle/556746Children.

Clancy, R. (2006). Summary proceeding from the Neurology Group on Neonatal Seizures [Electronic version]. *Pediatrics, 117*(3), S23-S27.

Fisher, P. G. (2007). First and second seizures: What to know and do. *Contemporary Pediatrics, 24*(4), 80–88.

Freeman, J. M, Kossoff, E. H. & Hartman, A. L. (2007). The ketogenic diet: One decade later [Electronic Version]. *Pediatrics, 119*(3), 535–543.

Hudson, K. (2006). *Hydrocephalus and cerebral spinal fluid drainage.* Retrieved on December 27, 2007 at http://dynamic nursingeducation.com/class.php?class_id=98&pid=10.

Komotar, R. J., Zacharia, B. E., Ellis, J. A., Feldstein, N. A., & Anderson, R. C. E. (2006). Pitfalls for the pediatrician: Positional molding or craniosynostosis. *Pediatric Annals, 35*(5), 365–75.

Kossoff, E. H. & Mankad, D. N. (2006). Medication-overuse headache in children: Is initial preventive therapy necessary? *Journal of Child Neurology, 21*(1), 45–48.

LaRossa, M. M., & Carter, S. L. (2005). *Understanding how the brain develops.* Retrieved July 9, 2006, from www.pediatrics.emory.edu/neonatology/dpc/brain.htm

Lawes, R. (2007). Uncovering the layer of meningitis and encephalitis. *Nursing Made Incredibly Easy!, 5*(4), 26–35.

Leung, A. K. C. & Robson, W. L. M. (2007). Febrile seizures. *Journal of Pediatric healthcare, 21*(4), 250–55.

Marthaler, M. T. (2004). Seizures revisited [Electronic version]. *Critical Care, 35*(4), 71–75. Retrieved July 9, 2006, from Proquest database.

McCaskey, M. S. (2007). Pediatric assessment: The little differences [Electronic Version]. *Home Healthcare Nurse, 25*(1), 20–24.

Milonovich, L. M. (2007). Meningococcemia epidemiology, pathophysiology and management. *Journal of Pediatric Healthcare, 21*(2), 75–80.

Molofsky, W. J. (2006). Managing stroke in children. *Pediatric Annals, 35*(5), 379–84.

Moss, M. (2006). Reye syndrome. *Pediatrics for Parents. 22*(9), 7–9.

Munson, S., Schroth, E. & Ernst, M. (2006). The role of functional neuroimaging in pediatric brain injury [Electronic Version]. *Pediatrics, 117*(4), 1372–1381.

National Institute of Neurological Disorders and Stroke. (2004). Meningitis and encephalitis fact sheet. Retrieved on December 27, 2007 at http://www.ninds.nih.gov/disorders/encephalitis_meningitis/detail_encephalitis_meningitis.htm.

Nield, L. S., Brunner, N. E., Scott, J., & Jaynes, M. (2006). Pediatric stroke: Evaluation, treatment, and follow-up [Electronic Version]. *Applied Neurology.* Retrieved on December 27, 2007 at http://appneurology.com/showArticle.jhtml?articleId=177104315.

Padgett, K., & Boss B. J. (2004). Alterations in neurologic function in children. In S. E. Huether & K. L. Chance (Eds.), *Understanding pathophysiology* (3rd ed., pp. 429–447). St. Louis, MO: Mosby.

Purugganan, D. H. & Adam, A. M. (2006). Abnormalities of head size. *Pediatrics in Review, 27*(12), 473–476.

Roberts, E. G., & Shulkin, B. L. (2004). Technical issues in performing PET studies in pediatric patients [Electronic version]. *Journal of Nuclear Medicine Technology, 32*(1), 5–13. Retrieved July 9, 2006, from Proquest database.

Rubin, D. H., Suecoff, S. A., & Knupp, K. G. (2006). Headaches in children. *Pediatric Annals, 35*(5), 346–353.

Sacar, S., Turgut, H., Toprak, S., Cirak, B., Coskun, E., Yilmaz, O., & Tekin K. (2006). A retrospective study of central nervous system shunt infections diagnosed in a university hospital during a 4-year period [Electronic Version]. *BMC Infectious Disease.* Retrieved December 27, 2007 at http://www.pubmedcentral.nih.gov/articlerender.fcgi?artid=1421408.

Saluja, G., Brenner, R. A., Trumble, A. C., Smith, G. S., et al. (2006). Swimming pool drownings among US residents aged 5–24 years: Understanding racial/ethnic disparities [electronic version]. *American Journal of Public Health, 96*(4), 728–734. Retrieved December 17, 2007 from Proquest database.

Schnitzer, P. G. (2006). Prevention of unintentional childhood injuries [Electronic Version]. *American Family Physician, 74*(11), 1864–70. Retrieved December 17, 2007 from Proquest database.

Shinnar, S., & O'Dell, C. (2004). Febrile seizures. *Pediatric Annals 33*(6), 395–401.

Simpkins, C. J. (2006). Ventriculoperitoneal shunt infections in patients with hydrocephalus [Electronic Version]. *Pediatric Nursing, 31*(6), 457–462.

Sobel, J. (2005). Botulism [Electronic Version]. *Clinical Infectious Diseases, 41*(8), 1167–1174. Retrieved December 17, 2007 from Proquest database.

Spiro, C. S., & Spiro, D. M. (2004). Acute meningitis. *Clinician Reviews, 14*(3), 54–58.

Stevenson, K. L. (2004). Chiari type II malformation: Past, present and future [Electronic version]. *Neurosurgery Focus, 16*(2). Retrieved July 9, 2006 from Proquest database.

Wheeless, J. W. (2004). Treatment of status epilepticus in children. *Pediatric Annals, 33*(6), 377–383.

Wolf, S. M. & McGoldrick, P. E. (2006). Recognition and management of pediatric seizures. *Pediatric Annals, 35*(5), 332–344.

Worrall, K. (2004). Use of the Glasgow Coma Scale in infants. *Paediatric Nursing, 16*(4), 45–50.

Yang, M. (2004). Newborn neurologic examination [Electronic Version]. *Neurology, 62*, E15–E17.

WEBSITES

Brain Injury Association of America: prevention, research, education, and advocacy: www.biausa.org/Pages/splash.html

Craniosynostosis and Positional Plagiocephaly Support, Inc.: resources and education for families: www.cappskids.org/index.html

Children's Hemiplegia and Stroke Association: Support for Children with Hemiplegia, Hemiplegic Cerebral Palsy, Infant Stroke, or Childhood Stroke: www.chasa.org

Epilepsy support group for families: www.geocities.com/epilepsy911

Online support group for children with hemiplegia or hemiplegic cerebral palsy: www.hemikids.org

Hydrocephalus Foundation: www.hydrocephalus.org

Support group for pediatric stroke: www.pediatricstrokenetwork.com/ Pediatric Stroke Network

A childhood stroke support group: www.pediatricstroke.org

National Safe Kids Campaign: www.safekids.org

CHAPTER WORKSHEET

MULTIPLE CHOICE QUESTIONS

1. When compared with adults, why are infants and children at an increased risk of head trauma?

   a. The head of the infant and young child is large in proportion to the body and the neck muscles are not well developed.

   b. The development of the nervous system is complete at birth but remains immature.

   c. The spine is very immobile in infants and young children.

   d. The skull is more flexible due to the presence of sutures and fontanels.

2. At a well-child visit, hydrocephalus may be suspected in an infant if upon assessment the nurse finds:

   a. Narrow sutures

   b. Sunken fontanels

   c. A rapid increase in head circumference

   d. Increase in weight since last visit

3. A 10-year-old child is admitted to the hospital due to history of seizure activity. As his nurse, you are called into the room by his mother who states he is having a seizure. What would be the priority nursing intervention?

   a. Prevention of injury by removing the child from his bed

   b. Prevention of injury by placing a tongue blade in the child's mouth

   c. Prevention of injury by restraining the child

   d. Prevention of injury by placing the child on his side and opening his airway

4. A 6-month-old infant is admitted to the hospital with suspected bacterial meningitis. She is crying, irritable, and lying in the opisthotonic position. The priority nursing intervention would be:

   a. Educate the family on ways to prevent bacterial meningitis.

   b. Initiate appropriate isolation precautions and begin intravenous antibiotics.

   c. Assess the infant's fontanels.

   d. Encourage the mother to hold the infant and feed her.

CRITICAL THINKING EXERCISES

1. A child is seen in the doctor's office after hitting his head while skateboarding. The child suffered no loss of consciousness, and has no external injuries and no significant past medical history. He is acting appropriately at this time. His only complaint is a dull headache. What instructions would you give the parents regarding his care at home? Include when they should seek further medical care.

2. A 10-year-old child is admitted to the pediatric unit after experiencing a seizure. A complete, accurate, and detailed history from a reliable source is essential. What information would you ask for while obtaining the history?

3. A 6-year-old child is admitted to the hospital because of a possible seizure. The child's mother calls the nurse to the room because the child is "jerking all over" and won't respond when she calls the child's name. List appropriate nursing interventions for this child. Prioritize the list of interventions.

4. Describe the impact of cerebral vascular accident in the child as compared with the adult. How does it affect the child's future? How will the nurse provide care differently for the child stroke victim as compared with the adult?

STUDY ACTIVITIES

1. A 4-month-old child with a history of hydrocephalus has undergone surgery for placement of a VP shunt. What information would you include in the teaching plan?

2. Develop an example of a "headache log" that could be used by the family for chronicling the child's headaches, including triggers, relieving factors, and precipitating events. Ensure that the log is developed at a 6th-grade reading level to make it practical for low literacy parents.

3. In the clinical setting, interview the parent of a child who has suffered significant brain trauma or injury (such as head trauma, IVH, or stroke). Talk with the family about the types of care the child requires. Reflect upon this interview in your clinical journal, and compare how the ongoing care for this child compares with that for a typical child.

NURSING CARE OF THE CHILD WITH A DISORDER OF THE EYES OR EARS

CHAPTER 38

KEY TERMS

acuity
amblyopia
blindness
conductive hearing loss
deaf
decibel

hearing impairment
nystagmus
pressure–equalizing tubes
  (PE tubes)
ptosis

sensorineural hearing loss
strabismus
tympanometry
tympanostomy
vision impairment

LEARNING OBJECTIVES

Upon completion of the chapter, the learner will be able to:

1. Differentiate between the anatomic and physiologic differences of the eyes and ears in children as compared with adults.
2. Identify various factors associated with disorders of the eyes and ears in infants and children.
3. Discuss common laboratory and other diagnostic tests useful in the diagnosis of disorders of the eyes and ears.
4. Discuss common medications and other treatments used for treatment and palliation of conditions affecting the eyes and ears.
5. Recognize risk factors associated with various disorders of the eyes and ears.
6. Distinguish between different disorders of the eyes and ears based on the signs and symptoms associated with them.
7. Discuss nursing interventions commonly used in regard to disorders of the eyes and ears.
8. Devise an individualized nursing care plan for the child with a sensory impairment or other disorder of the eyes or ears.
9. Develop patient/family teaching plans for the child with a disorder of the eyes or ears.
10. Describe the psychosocial impact of sensory impairments on children.

Enrique Baxter, a 9-month-old, is brought to the clinic by his mother. His mother tells you, "Enrique has been fussy and not eating or sleeping well for the past 2 days."

Wow

With the help of a nurse's care and healing, the child's senses provide him or her with an antenna to the universe.

C hildren commonly suffer from disorders related to the eyes and ears. Conjunctivitis and otitis media are two very common disorders in childhood. Other inflammatory and infectious conditions also affect the child's eyes or ears. Various alterations such as refractive error, strabismus, and amblyopia affect the development of visual acuity in children. Any alteration in the ear that contributes to hearing loss may have a significant impact on the child's language acquisition. It is important for nurses to be familiar with the most common disorders of the eyes and ears in order to provide appropriate care to these children and to encourage optimal development in all children. In addition, the nurse may be caring for a child with another problem who is also either visually or hearing impaired. The nurse must take these developmental differences into account when planning care for these children.

Variations in Pediatric Anatomy and Physiology

It is important for the nurse to understand the impact of eye and ear disorders on the child's development. Some children may be born with anomalies of the eyes or ears that will have a significant impact on vision and hearing, as well as psychomotor development. On the other hand, disorders affecting the eyes or ears, particularly if chronic or recurrent, can have a significant impact on the development of visual acuity or may cause hearing impairment.

Eyes

Light-skinned children are often born with blue eyes. The iris becomes pigmented over time and eye color is determined by 6 to 12 moths of age. The newborn's sclera may be slightly bluish-tinged but becomes white within weeks. The eyeball of the infant and young child occupies a relatively larger space within the orbit than the adult's does, making it more susceptible to injury (Fig. 38.1).

The spherical shape of the newborn's lens does not allow for distance accommodation, so the newborn sees best at a distance of about 8 to 10 inches. The optic nerve

is not completely myelinated, so color discrimination is incomplete. Visual acuity develops over the first few years of the child's life. At birth, acuity ranges from 20/100 to 20/400. By age 2 to 3 years, the visual acuity of most children is 20/50, with 20/20 achieved by age 6 to 7 years. The rectus muscles are uncoordinated at birth and mature over time so that binocular vision (the ability to focus with both eyes simultaneously) may be achieved by 4 months of age. In the very preterm infant, retinal vascularization is incomplete, so visual acuity may be affected.

Ears

Congenital deformities of the ear are often associated with other body system anomalies and genetic syndromes. The presence of ear anomalies may lead to the search for and subsequent diagnosis of the other anomalies or syndromes. The infant's relatively short, wide, and horizontally placed eustachian tubes allow bacteria and viruses to gain access to the middle ear easily, resulting in increased numbers of ear infections as compared to the adult. As the child matures, the tubes assume a more slanted position, so older children and adults generally have fewer cases of middle ear effusion and infection (Fig. 38.2). Sometimes enlargement of the adenoids contributes to obstruction of the eustachian tubes, leading to infection.

Common Medical Treatments

A variety of interventions are used to treat disorders of the eyes and ears in children. The treatments listed in Common Medical Treatments 38.1 and Drug Guide 38.1 usually require a physician's order when a child is hospitalized.

NURSING PROCESS OVERVIEW FOR THE CHILD WITH A DISORDER OF THE EYES OR EARS

Care of the child with a disorder of the eyes and ears includes assessment, nursing diagnosis, planning, interventions, and evaluation. There are a number of general concepts related to the nursing process that can be applied

FIGURE 38.1 The relatively larger space that the infant's and young child's eyeball occupies within the orbit makes it more susceptible to injury as compared with the adult's eye.

A

Eustachian tube
(adult)

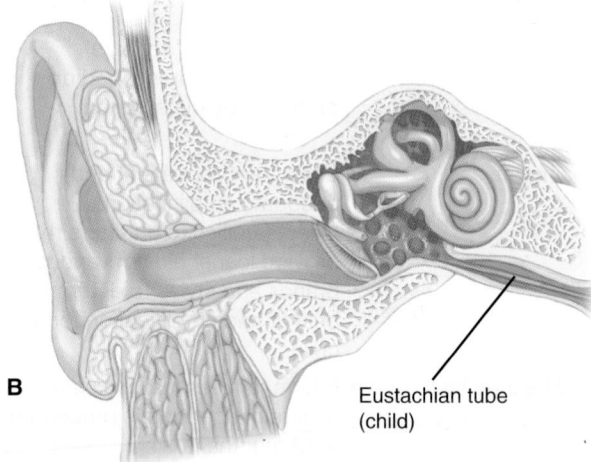

B

Eustachian tube
(child)

FIGURE 38.2 Note the child's relatively shorter, wider eustachian tubes and their horizontal positioning (**B**) as compared with the adult's (**A**).

to disorders of the eyes and ears. From a general understanding of the care involved for a child with alterations in the eyes or ears, the nurse can then individualize the care based on client specifics.

Assessment

Assessment of disorders of the eyes and ears in children includes health history, physical assessment, and laboratory or diagnostic testing.

Remember Enrique, the 9-month-old with fussiness and poor feeding who was not sleeping well? What additional health history and physical examination assessment information should you obtain?

Health History
The health history comprises past medical history, family history, history of present illness, as well as treatments used at home. The past medical history may be significant

for prematurity, genetic defect, eye or ear deformities, visual acuity deficit or blindness, hearing impairment or deafness, recurrent ear infections, or ear surgeries. Family history might be significant for eye or ear deformities or vision or hearing impairment or may reveal contacts for infectious exposure.

When eliciting the history of the present illness, inquire about its onset and progression and the presence of fever, nasal congestion, eye or ear pain, eye rubbing, ear pulling, headache, lethargy, or behavioral changes. Document if the child has corrective lenses or hearing aids prescribed and to what extent these devices are actually used.

Physical Examination
When assessing the eyes and ears, begin with inspection and observation. Additionally, testing of visual activity and hearing may be performed.

Inspection and Observation

The physical examination should begin with inspection and observation. Note whether the child uses eyeglasses, corrective lenses, or a hearing aid. Observe the eyes: note their positioning and symmetry, presence of strabismus, nystagmus, and squinting. The eyelids should open equally (failure to open fully is termed **ptosis**). Note variations in eye slant and the presence of epicanthal folds. Assess the eyes for presence of eyelid edema, sclera color, discharge, tearing, and pupillary equality, as well as size and shape of the pupils. Evert the eyelid to inspect the palpebral conjunctivae for redness. Test for extraocular movements and pupillary light response and accommodation. Note symmetry of corneal light reflex. Note presence of red reflex with an ophthalmoscope. Perform an age-appropriate visual acuity test. Refer to Chapter 30 for more detailed information related to visual acuity testing.

▶ *Take* NOTE!

Attempts to inspect the palpebral conjunctivae may be frightening to children. Ask the older, cooperative child to evert the eyelid himself or herself, while the nurse inspects the conjunctivae.

▶ *Take* NOTE!

Though the sclerae are bluish in newborns, they become white in the first few weeks of life. Blue sclerae that persist beyond a few weeks of life may be an indicator of osteogenesis imperfecta type I, an inherited connective tissue disorder.

COMMON MEDICAL TREATMENTS 38.1

Treatment	Explanation	Indication	Nursing Implications
Warm compress	Warm, moist washcloth	Conjunctivitis	• Use very warm water from the tap (to avoid risk of burning, do not microwave).
Corrective lenses	In eyeglass form or as contact lenses	Correction of astigmatism, refractive error, strabismus	• Use a safety strap to help young children wear their eyeglasses.
Patching	An adhesive patch is applied to the healthier eye for several hours each day.	Strabismus, amblyopia, any other eye condition that results in one eye being weaker than the other	• Inform parents that though difficult to obtain, compliance with patching is critical. • A "pirate patch" may coax preschoolers into compliance.
Eye muscle surgery	Surgical alignment of the eyes	Strabismus	• Protect the operative site with patching. • Use elbow restraints if necessary.
Pressure-equalizing (PE) tubes (tympanostomy tubes)	Tiny plastic tubes inserted in the tympanic membrane	Chronic otitis media with effusion	• Teach parents "dry ears" precautions if prescribed or preferred by the surgeon.
Hearing aids	Amplification device worn in the ear	Hearing impairment	• Ensure appropriate fit and adequate amplification. • Direct families to outfitters that provide loaner aids of various brands and styles to determine best fit and amplification for the child.
Cochlear implants	Surgically inserted electronic prosthetic device	Sensorineural hearing loss	• Inform families that the usual minimum age for this procedure is 12 months.

Inspect the ears: note their size and shape, position, and the presence of skin tags, dimples, or other anomalies (Fig. 38.3). Upon otoscopic examination, note presence of cerumen, discharge, inflammation, or a foreign body in the ear canal. Visualize the tympanic membrane and observe its color, landmarks, and light reflex, as well as presence of perforation, scars, bulging, or retraction. Tympanic membrane mobility may be tested with pneumatic otoscopy. Auditory acuity is tested via the whisper test, audiometry, or other age-appropriate test (refer to

DRUG GUIDE 38.1 COMMON DRUGS FOR EAR AND EYE DISORDERS

Medication	Action	Indication	Nursing Implications
Antibiotics (oral, otic, ophthalmic)	Treatment of bacterial infections of the eyes and ears	Acute otitis media, otitis externa, conjunctivitis	Teach families to complete the entire course as prescribed. Check for drug allergies prior to administration.
Antihistamines	Block histamine reaction	Allergic conjunctivitis	Topical drops used. Oral agents usually prescribed if allergic rhinitis accompanies the conjunctivitis.
Analgesics	Pain relief	Otitis media, otitis externa, after eye or ear surgery	Narcotic analgesics may be necessary in some instances.

FIGURE 38.3 Note the skin tag (**A**) and preauricular pit (**B**) (in front of the ear).

Chapter 30 for a more detailed explanation of hearing testing).

Palpation

Usually, the eyes are not palpated. In the case of injury the upper eyelid may be everted for examination purposes. Palpate the ear for tenderness over the tragus or pinna. Note the presence of tenderness over the mastoid area (tenderness may be present when otitis media progresses to mastoiditis). Palpate for enlarged cervical lymph nodes (this occurs when the eyes or ears are infected).

Laboratory and Diagnostic Testing

The Common Laboratory and Diagnostic Tests display offers an explanation of the laboratory and diagnostic tests most commonly used for disorders of the eyes and ears. These tests can assist the physician in diagnosing the disorder and/or can be used as guidelines in determining ongoing treatment. Laboratory or non-nursing personnel

obtain some of the tests, while the nurse may obtain others. In either instance the nurse should be familiar with how the tests are obtained, what they are used for, and normal versus abnormal results. This knowledge will also be necessary when providing patient and family education related to the testing.

Nursing Diagnoses and Related Interventions

Upon completion of a thorough assessment, the nurse might identify several nursing diagnoses, including:

- Disturbed sensory perception
- Risk for infection
- Pain
- Delayed growth and development
- Impaired verbal communication
- Deficient knowledge
- Interrupted family processes
- Risk for injury

COMMON LABORATORY AND DIAGNOSTIC TESTS 38.1

Test	Explanation	Indication	Nursing Implications
Culture of eye or ear discharge	Fluid draining from the eye or ear is cultured	To determine specific bacteria present and appropriate antibiotic coverage	Easy to collect, relatively pain-free. If drainage must be removed from within the ear canal, more likely to be painful.
Tympanic fluid culture	Culture of fluid aspirated from the middle ear	To determine specific bacteria present and appropriate antibiotic coverage	Painful; usually performed only by specially trained physicians.
Tympanometry	Probe in ear canal measures movement of the eardrum	Determines extent of effusion of the middle ear	Quick and easy to perform (seconds). Requires accurate-sized probe for adequate seal of the ear canal.

After completing an assessment of Enrique, the nurse noted the following: fever, tugging at his ears, and increased crying when lying down. Based on the assessment findings, what would your top three nursing diagnoses be for Enrique?

Nursing goals, interventions, and evaluation for the child with an eye or ear disorder are based on the nursing diagnoses. Nursing Care Plan 38.1 may be used as a guide in planning nursing care for the child with an eye or ear disorder, but it should be individualized based on the patient's symptoms and needs. Refer to Chapter 35 for the nursing care plan for pain management. Additional information will be included later in the chapter as it relates to specific disorders.

Based on your top three nursing diagnoses for Enrique, describe appropriate nursing interventions.

Infectious and Inflammatory Disorders of the Eyes

Infectious and inflammatory disorders of the eyes include conjunctivitis, nasolacrimal duct obstruction, eyelid lesions, and periorbital cellulitis.

▶ CONJUNCTIVITIS

Inflammation of the bulbar or palpebral conjunctiva is referred to as conjunctivitis. It can be infectious, allergic, or chemical in nature. Viruses or bacteria may cause infectious conjunctivitis. Adenoviruses and influenza account for the bulk of cases of viral conjunctivitis. The most common bacterial cause is *Staphylococcus aureus,* but many cases are also caused by *Streptococcus pneumoniae, Haemophilus influenzae,* and other bacteria. In the newborn, *Chlamydia trachomatis* and *Neisseria gonorrhoeae* are more common causes. Infectious conjunctivitis is very contagious, so epidemics are common, particularly in young children. Risk factors for acute infectious conjunctivitis include age less than 2 weeks; daycare, preschool, or school attendance; concomitant viral upper respiratory infection; pharyngitis; or otitis media. Concurrent acute otitis media may occur depending upon the bacterial cause (Cook & Walsh, 2005). Complications from simple infectious conjunctivitis are uncommon. Neonates with chlamydial conjunctivitis may be at risk for the development of chlamydial pneumonia.

Allergic conjunctivitis results from exposure to particular allergens. Allergic conjunctivitis may be a seasonal or year-round complaint. A genetic predisposition to allergic conjunctivitis exists, just as it does for asthma, allergic rhinitis, and atopic dermatitis. Allergic conjunctivitis occurs more frequently in school-age children and adolescents than it does in infants and young children because of repeat exposure to allergens over time. In the case of seasonal allergic conjunctivitis, the severity of symptoms and the number of children affected are directly related to the pollen count in the area.

Therapeutic Management

Therapeutic management of conjunctivitis is prescribed depending upon the cause. Bacterial conjunctivitis is generally treated with an ophthalmic antibiotic preparation (drops or ointment). Viral conjunctivitis is a self-limiting disease and does not require topical medication. Eye drops with an antihistamine or mast cell stabilization effect may be helpful in alleviating symptoms of allergic conjunctivitis. If other allergy signs and symptoms are also present, an oral antihistamine may also be prescribed. Table 38.1 compares bacterial, viral, and allergic conjunctivitis.

Pathophysiology

When bacteria or viruses come in contact with the bulbar or palpebral conjunctiva, they are recognized as foreign antigens and an antigen–antibody immune reaction occurs, resulting in inflammation. Allergic conjunctivitis occurs through a different mechanism. Contact with the allergen results in an allergic response (overreaction of the immune response). The mast cell and histamine mediators are then activated, resulting in inflammation.

Nursing Assessment

Nursing assessment of the child with conjunctivitis, regardless of the cause, is similar. It includes health history, physical examination, and in rare instances laboratory testing.

Health History

Elicit a description of the present illness and chief complaint. Common signs and symptoms reported during the health history might include:

• Redness
• Edema
• Tearing
• Discharge
• Eye pain
• Itching of the eyes (usually with allergic conjunctivitis)

Determine the onset of symptoms and their progression as well as response to treatments used at home. Assess for risk factors for infectious conjunctivitis, such as daycare or school attendance. Note any history of an upper respiratory infection, sore throat, or earache. Question parents about possible infectious exposures. Review the health history for risk factors for allergic conjunctivitis such

Nursing Care Plan 38.1

OVERVIEW FOR THE CHILD WITH A DISORDER OF EYES OR EARS

NURSING DIAGNOSIS: Sensory perception, disturbed (visual) related to visual impairment or blindness as evidenced by lack of reaction to visual stimuli, squinting, holding items close

Outcome Identification and Evaluation

Child will reach maximal vision potential: *Child uses corrective lenses appropriately and is able to participate in play and schoolwork.*

Intervention: Improving Vision

- Encourage corrective lens use *for enhancement of vision.*
- For the severely impaired or blind child, identify yourself via voice and name items in environment for the child *so that the child is aware of his or her surroundings.*
- Support the family's efforts at vision therapy and other habilitation programs *to promote vision enhancement.*
- Engage the parents in bedside caregiving *because the parents' voice and presence are reassuring to the child.*

NURSING DIAGNOSIS: Sensory perception, disturbed (auditory) related to hearing loss as evidenced by lack of reaction to verbal stimuli, delayed attainment of language milestones

Outcome Identification and Evaluation

Child will reach maximal hearing and speech potential: *Child uses aids appropriately and communicates effectively.*

Intervention: Improving Hearing

- Assess hearing ability frequently *because early detection of hearing loss allows for earlier intervention and correction.*
- Assess language development at each visit *to allow for early detection of hearing loss (earlier intervention and correction).*
- Encourage hearing aid use *for amplification of sound.*
- Teach about hearing aid battery safety *to avoid aspiration of battery.*
- Assist child with focusing on sounds in the environment *to encourage listening skills.*
- Refer for and encourage attendance at communication habilitation program *to maximize communication potential.*

NURSING DIAGNOSIS: Risk for infection related to presence of infectious organisms as evidenced by fever, presence of virus or bacteria on laboratory screening.

Outcome Identification and Evaluation

Child will exhibit no signs of secondary infection and will not spread infection to others: *Symptoms of infection decrease over time, and others remain free from infection.*

Intervention: Reducing Infection Risk

- Maintain aseptic technique and practice good hand washing *to prevent introduction of further infectious agents.*
- Limit number of visitors, screening for recent illness, *to prevent further infection.*
- Administer antibiotics if prescribed *to prevent or treat bacterial infection.*
- Encourage nutritious diet according to child's preferences *to assist body's natural infection-fighting mechanisms.*
- Isolate the child as required *to prevent nosocomial spread of infection.*
- Teach child and family preventive measures such as good hand washing, covering mouth and nose when coughing or sneezing, adequate disposal of used tissues, *to prevent nosocomial or community spread of infection.*

(continued)

Nursing Care Plan 38.1 (continued)

NURSING DIAGNOSIS: Growth and development delay, related to sensory impairment as evidenced by delay in attainment of developmental milestones

Outcome Identification and Evaluation
Child will achieve optimum independence for age: *Child participates in age-appropriate developmental activities.*

Intervention: Encouraging Growth and Development
- Encourage attainment of developmental milestones with use of assistive devices as needed *for timely developmental achievements.*
- Foster independence in ADLs *to promote sense of accomplishment.*
- Encourage participation in play with another child or within a group *to promote socialization.*
- Assist family to set limits and apply discipline *because structure and routine provide a secure environment in which the developing child can grow.*
- Encourage friendships with other children with a sensory impairment *to promote socialization and let the child know that he or she is not the only one with these challenges.*

NURSING DIAGNOSIS: Impaired verbal communication related to hearing loss as evidenced by lack of or inarticulate speech, lack of alternate communication channel

Outcome Identification and Evaluation
The child will communicate effectively with the method chosen by the family (this may be sign language, oral/deaf speech, cued speech, or augmentative alternative communication device).

Intervention: Improving Communication
- Encourage choice of and attendance at communication habilitation program *to promote continued learning.*
- Provide consistency between home and hospital in regard to communication style/devices *to promote continued learning.*
- Support the child's efforts at correct speech *to promote speech development through reinforcement and praise.*
- Encourage family to use spoken language and read books at home *to continue to promote appropriate language development.*

NURSING DIAGNOSIS: Deficient knowledge related to sensory impairment (vision or hearing) as evidenced by new diagnosis and parents' questions

Outcome Identification and Evaluation
Parents express understanding of diagnosis and care of child: *Parents verbalize understanding, demonstrate use of assistive devices, or independently perform medical treatments.*

Intervention: Educating the Family
- Review diagnosis and plan of care with the parents *to promote understanding of the disease process.*
- Refer family to resources available for sensory impaired children *to provide further education and support to the parents.*
- Demonstrate medical treatments prescribed or use of assistive devices, requiring a return demonstration, *which shows the parents' ability to provide the prescribed care for the child.*
- Encourage exploration of different communication and learning modes available for the sensory impaired child *to allow the child and family to find the right educational and communication style fit.*

Nursing Care Plan 38.1 (continued)

NURSING DIAGNOSIS: Family processes, interrupted, related to child's sensory impairment as evidenced by parent verbalization, nonverbal communication, altered coping

Outcome Identification and Evaluation

Parents demonstrate adequate coping and decreased anxiety: *Parents are involved in child's care, ask appropriate questions, and are able to discuss child's care and condition calmly.*

Intervention: Encouraging Appropriate Family Interactions

- Encourage parents' verbalization of grief if child is hearing or vision impaired. *Parents must deal with their own feelings of loss to successfully care for the child with an impairment.*
- Encourage parents' verbalization of concerns related to child's illness. *This allows for identification of concerns and demonstrates to the family that the nurse also cares about them, not just the child.*
- Explain therapy, procedures, and child's behavior to parents; *developing an understanding of the child's current status helps decrease anxiety.*
- Encourage parental involvement in care *so that parents may continue to feel needed and valued.*

NURSING DIAGNOSIS: Risk for injury related to vision loss as evidenced by difficulty navigating surroundings

Outcome Identification and Evaluation
The infant or child will remain free from injury.

Intervention: Preventing Injury
- Orient the child to hospital surroundings *because awareness is the first step to preventing injury.*
- Encourage parent to be at bedside *so that the child feels more comfortable.*
- Encourage use of assistive devise *to promote safety.*

---

as a family history and a history of asthma, allergic rhinitis, or atopic dermatitis. Determine seasonality related to the symptoms and whether the symptoms occur after exposure to particular allergens, such as pollen, hay, or animals.

Physical Examination
Observe for eyelid swelling or redness. Inspect the conjunctivae for redness (Fig. 18.4). Note quantity, color, and consistency of discharge. Bacterial infections generally result in a thick, colored discharge, whereas a clear or white discharge is generally seen with viral conjunctivitis. Allergic conjunctivitis often results in a watery discharge, sometimes profuse, which is usually present bilaterally.

Contact with an allergen rubbed into one of the eyes may result in unilateral symptoms. Observe the child for other signs of allergic or atopic disease, and document presence of runny nose or cough as well.

Laboratory and Diagnostic Tests
Cases of bacterial, viral, and allergic conjunctivitis are generally diagnosed based on history and clinical presentation. Cases of viral and allergic conjunctivitis do not warrant laboratory testing. If bacterial conjunctivitis is suspected, then a bacterial culture of the eye drainage may be performed to determine the exact causative organism, thus allowing the most appropriate antibiotic to be prescribed.

TABLE 38.1   TYPES OF CONJUNCTIVITIS

Type of Conjunctivitis	Conjunctivae	Discharge	Additional Findings	Eyelid Edema	Treatment
Bacterial	Inflamed	Purulent, mucoid	Mild pain	Occasional	Antibiotic drops or ointment
Viral	Inflamed	Watery, mucoid	Lymphadenopathy, photophobia, tearing	Usually present	Symptom relief; anti-herpetic agent if cause is herpes
Allergic	Inflamed	Watery or stringy	Itching	Usually present	Antihistamine and/or mast cell stabilizer drops

FIGURE 38.4 (**A**) Bacterial conjunctivitis: note redness of conjunctiva, and eyelid swelling. (**B**) Allergic conjunctivitis: note redness of conjunctiva, clear watery discharge.

Nursing Management

Nursing management of the various types of conjunctivitis focuses on alleviating symptoms and, for infectious causes, preventing spread.

Alleviating Symptoms

Teach parents how to apply eye drops or ointment (antibiotic for bacterial causes and antihistamine or mast cell stabilizer for allergic). Warm compresses may be used to help loosen the crust that accumulates on the eyelids overnight when drainage is copious, particularly with bacterial conjunctivitis.

The child with allergic conjunctivitis may experience perennial or seasonal allergies (or both). Encourage the child to avoid perennial allergens once the offending allergen is determined (refer to Chapter 39 for additional information related to education about perennial allergen avoidance). Seasonal allergies may include tree pollen in the winter or spring, grass pollen in the summer and ragweed, or flower pollen in the fall.

It is impossible to completely eliminate seasonal allergic responses, partly because it is important for children to participate in physical activity outdoors. Teach families to minimize seasonal allergens on the child's skin and hair. Educate families to:

- Encourage the child not to rub or touch the eyes.
- Rinse the child's eyelids periodically with a clean washcloth and cool water.
- When the child comes in from outdoors, wash the child's face and hands.
- Ensure that the child showers and shampoos before bedtime.

▶ **Take** NOTE!

The itching of allergic conjunctivitis may be relieved with cool compresses. An easy way to accomplish this is to have the child hold a tube of yogurt over the affected eye.

Preventing Infectious Spread

Because infectious conjunctivitis is extremely contagious, the parent must wash hands diligently after caring for the child. Teach parents and children about appropriate hand washing, and discourage them from sharing towels and washcloths. Children with viral conjunctivitis may return to school or daycare when symptoms lessen. When mucopurulent drainage is no longer present (usually after 24 to 48 hours of treatment with a topical antibiotic), the child with bacterial conjunctivitis may safely return to daycare or school (Brady, 2005).

▶ **Take** NOTE!

Avoid the use of vasoconstricting eye drops such as Visine to rid the eyes of redness. Rebound vasodilation may occur, and with it the redness returns. This leads to repeated frequent use of the drops to keep the eyes from being red but does not treat the actual cause of the redness.

▶ **Consider** THIS!

Bryn Carle, a 6-year-old, is brought to the clinic by her mother. She presents with redness of the left eye, edema, and drainage. What other assessment information would be helpful? Based on the history and clinical presentation, Bryn is diagnosed with conjunctivitis. What education will be necessary for the family to assist in alleviating symptoms and preventing infectious spread?

▶ NASOLACRIMAL DUCT OBSTRUCTION

Stenosis or simple obstruction of the nasolacrimal duct is a common disorder of infancy, occurring in about 6% to 20% of the general population (Casady et al., 2006). It is unilateral in about 65% of cases. Chronic tearing occurs and build-up in the lacrimal sac causes a mucoid or muco-purulent drainage. Over 90% of all cases resolve spontaneously by 1 year of age (American Association for Pediatric Ophthalmology and Strabismus, 2005). No apparent risk factors exist for the development of nasolacrimal duct obstruction or stenosis. Therapeutic management involves a "wait-and-see" approach. Massage may be prescribed, and if secondary bacterial infection is suspected or confirmed, antibiotic ointment or drops may be ordered. If the obstruction does not resolve by 12 months of age, then the pediatric ophthalmologist may probe the duct to relieve the obstruction (a brief outpatient procedure).

Nursing Assessment

Tearing or discharge from one or both eyes is often first noted at the 2-week checkup. Obtain a thorough history about the eye drainage to distinguish it from neonatal conjunctivitis. Determine the onset and progression of symptoms, as well as the newborn's response to any interventions attempted so far. Upon physical examination, note redness of the lower lid of the affected eye. If drainage is present, note its consistency, color, and quantity. Nasolacrimal duct obstruction is usually a diagnosis based upon clinical presentation, but culture of the eye drainage may be used to rule out conjunctivitis or secondary bacterial infection (Fig. 38.5).

Nursing Management

As previously stated, the majority of cases of nasolacrimal duct stenosis resolve spontaneously by 12 months of age. Nevertheless, the continual tearing and discharge is quite

FIGURE 38.5 Mild eyelid redness and tearing are present in the infant with nasolacrimal duct stenosis. Note the presence of obstruction.

upsetting to the parents. Teach parents to clean the eye area frequently with a moist cloth. In addition, teach parents to massage the nasolacrimal duct, which may change the pressure and cause it to open, allowing drainage to occur. Refer to Teaching Guidelines 38.1 for appropriate nasolacrimal duct massage technique. Ensure that parents are educated about when and how to administer antibiotic eye drops if ordered.

◆ EYELID DISORDERS

Disorders of the eyelid include hordeolum (stye), chalazion, and blepharitis. Hordeolum is a localized infection of the sebaceous gland of the eyelid follicle, usually caused by bacterial invasion. Chalazion is a chronic painless infection of the meibomian gland. Blepharitis refers to chronic scaling and discharge along the eyelid margin. Chalazion may resolve spontaneously. Therapeutic management of hordeolum and blepharitis usually involves the use of antibiotic ointment.

Nursing Assessment

Determine the child's health history, noting onset of symptoms, extent and character of eye discharge, and presence of pain (hordeolum is usually painful). Inspect the eyelids, noting redness along the eyelid margin and presence of eyelid edema (hordeolum, blepharitis). Hordeolum may also be quite visible as an enlarged lesion along the lid margin, with purulent drainage present (Fig. 38.6). Chalazion may be visible as a small nodule on the lid margin. The conjunctivae remain clear with all three of these disorders.

Nursing Management

For hordeolum and blepharitis, instruct parents in the administration of antibiotic ointment. Encourage the use of hot, moist compresses. Inform parents that the stye may require several weeks to resolve completely. Also inform parents that chalazion will usually resolve spontaneously; if it does not, it may require minor surgical drainage.

◆ PERIORBITAL CELLULITIS

Periorbital cellulitis is a bacterial infection of the eyelids and tissue surrounding the eye. The bacteria may gain entry to the skin via an abrasion, laceration, insect bite, foreign body, or impetiginous lesion. Periorbital cellulitis may also result from a nearby bacterial infection, such as sinusitis. *Staphylococcus aureus*, *Streptococcus pyogenes*, and

TEACHING GUIDELINES 38.1

Nasolacrimal Duct Massage

- Using the forefinger or little finger, push on top of the bone (the puncta must be blocked).

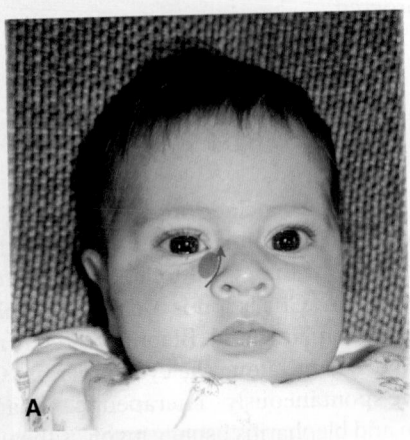

A

- Gently push in and up.

B

- Then gently push downward along the side of the nose.

C

FIGURE 38.6 Hordeolum.

Streptococcus pneumoniae are the most commonly implicated bacteria. The bacteria produce either an enzyme or endotoxins that initiate the inflammatory response. Redness, swelling, and infiltration of the skin by the inflammatory mediators occur.

Therapeutic management of periorbital cellulitis focuses on intravenous antibiotic administration during the acute phase followed by completion of the course with oral antibiotics. Complications of periorbital cellulitis include bacteremia and progression to orbital cellulitis, which is a more extensive infection involving the orbit of the eye.

Nursing Assessment

Note the onset and duration of symptoms, as well as any treatment used so far. Document any history of fever. The child may complain of pain around the eye as well as restricted movement of the eye area. Inspect the eye, noting marked eyelid edema as well as a purplish or red color of the eyelid (Fig. 38.7). Usually the conjunctivae are clear and no discharge is present. If the extent of the edema allows the child to open the eye, assess visual acuity, which should be normal.

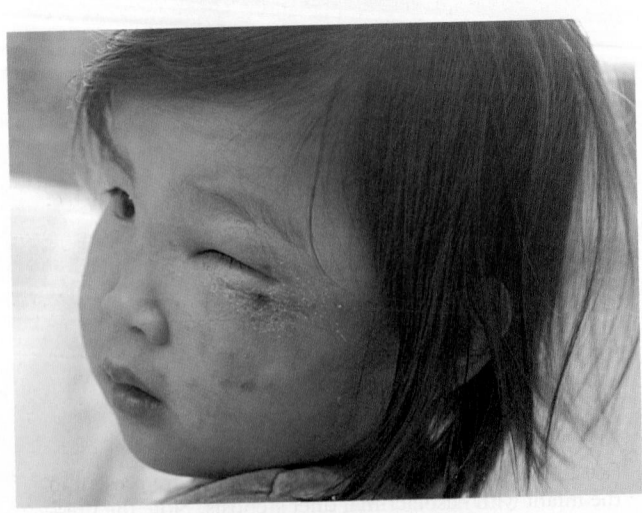

FIGURE 38.7 Periorbital cellulitis.

> ▶ *Take NOTE!*
>
> *Notify the physician immediately if any of these signs of progression to orbital cellulitis occur: conjunctival redness, change in vision, pain with eye movement, eye muscle weakness or paralysis, or proptosis.*

Nursing Management

Apply warm soaks to the eye area for 20 minutes every 2 to 4 hours. Administer intravenous antibiotics as prescribed. Teach families the importance of completing the entire course of oral antibiotic treatment at home. Instruct parents to call the physician or have the child evaluated again if:

- The child is not improving.
- The child reports inability to move the eye.
- Visual acuity changes.
- Proptosis occurs.

Eye Injuries

As mentioned earlier, infants and young children are more susceptible to eye injuries than adults since the eyeball is relatively larger in relation to the space within the orbit. Developmental maturity may also play a part in eye injuries. For example, as infants and toddlers learn to walk and run, they do not have the awareness and maturity to avert disaster. Older children involved in sports and school science experiments are also at risk for eye injuries. A few of the more common eye injuries are eyelid injuries, contusion, scleral hemorrhage, corneal abrasion, a foreign body in the eye, and chemical injury.

Therapeutic management depends on the type of injury. Eyelid lacerations may require suturing. Deep lacerations may result in ptosis at a later date, so these patients should be referred to an ophthalmologist. Simple contusions (black eye) usually need only observation, ice, and analgesics. Scleral hemorrhages resolve gradually without intervention over a few weeks. Corneal abrasions may be allowed to self-heal, or antibiotic ointment may be prescribed. Foreign bodies in the eye require removal to prevent further irritation or abrasion. Chemical injuries require irrigation and vision evaluation.

Nursing Assessment

When a child presents with an eye injury, it is very important to obtain an accurate history related to the injury, followed by a focused physical examination, which consists mostly of inspection and observation. The nurse must determine whether an eye injury is non-emergent or emergent in order to provide rapid and appropriate treatment in the case of an emergency so that vision may be preserved.

Health History

Obtain an accurate history. Determine the mechanism of injury and obtain as much detail about the injury as possible. Questions that should be asked during the health history include:

- When did the injury occur?
- What exactly happened?
- Was an object involved? If so, what type of object, and how fast was it going?
- Was it a splash injury?
- Was the child wearing eye protective gear or eyeglasses when the injury occurred?

Determine the extent of pain if present. Document photosensitivity, sensation of a foreign body in the eye, and blurry or lost vision. Inquire about past medical history, including previous eye injury or surgery or vision problems. Determine the child's immunization status.

Physical Examination

Regardless of the type of eye injury, the examination of the child's eye can be quite difficult. The nurse plays an important role in assisting the child and family to cope with the examination. Children with an eye injury often are in acute pain. The area surrounding the eye swells quickly after blunt trauma. The edema and tearing make the eye examination more difficult. Children are very frightened because of the pain and difficulty seeing. Approach the child in a calm and gentle manner. Soothe and coax the child as the eye is examined. Younger children may need to be restrained briefly in order for the examination to proceed safely.

Note the eyelid placement and look for signs of trauma such as bleeding, edema, and eyelid malformation. Evaluate the child's ability to open the eyes. Use a penlight to evaluate the pupils' response to light and accommodation (in the case of non-emergent eye trauma, the pupils should remain equally round and reactive to light and accommodation [PERRLA]). Note redness or irritation of the sclerae and/or conjunctivae. Observe for excessive tearing. Figure 38.8 shows appropriate technique for eversion and examination of the interior of the eyelid.

In a non-emergent situation, evaluate visual acuity via the use of an age-appropriate vision screening tool (refer to Chapter 30 for additional information related to visual acuity screening). Generally, radiologic testing is used only in emergency situations. Table 38.2 provides assessment information specific to eyelid laceration, simple contusion, scleral hemorrhage, corneal abrasion, and foreign body in the eye.

Twist cotton-tipped swab upward

Look downward

FIGURE 38.8 Eversion of the eyelid for examination. Place a cotton-tipped applicator over the eyelid. Pull the eyelid outward and up over the applicator.

▶ *Take* NOTE!

If pupillary reaction is abnormal, vision is affected (decreased acuity from the child's norm, diplopia, or blurriness), or extraocular movements are affected, the child should be immediately referred to an ophthalmologist for further evaluation.

Nursing Management

Children with urgent or emergent conditions must be referred to an ophthalmologist immediately to preserve vision. Urgent and emergent conditions include:

• Traumatic hyphema
• Blowout fracture
• Ruptured globe

TABLE 38.2   ASSESSMENT OF EYE INJURIES

Description of Injury	Nursing Assessment
Eyelid Injuries: May occur as laceration to the eyelid	• Laceration is noted at any point along the lid • Vision is unaffected
Simple Contusion (Black Eye): Occurs as a result of blunt trauma to the eye area	• Bruising and edema of lids or area surrounding eye • PERRLA • Extraocular movements intact • Visual acuity intact • No diplopia or blurred vision • Pain surrounding eye but not within the eye
Scleral Hemorrhage: Caused by blunt trauma or increased pressure such as with coughing	• Painless • Appears as erythema in the sclera; can be quite large initially • Vision unaffected
Corneal Abrasion: Results from foreign body such as sand, grit, or other small object scratching the cornea	• May have tearing • Eye pain • PERRLA • Vision may be blurry • Photophobia may be present
Foreign Body: May be dirt, glass, or other small particle	• Tearing • Complaint of "something in the eye" • PERRLA • Vision may be blurry

- Thermal injury/corneal flash burn
- Extensive animal bite
- Lid laceration with underlying structural involvement
- Corneal abrasion in which corneal penetration is suspected
- Foreign body embedded in the globe

Managing Non-emergent Eye Injuries

Non-emergent eye injuries usually need only simple management. Assist the physician with positioning and distraction of the child for eyelid laceration suturing. The child may require sedation or pain medication for this procedure.

To decrease edema in the child with a black eye (simple contusion), instruct the parent to apply an ice pack to the area for 20 minutes, then remove it for 20 minutes, and continue to repeat the cycle. Tell the parents and child that bruising of the surrounding eye area may take up to 3 weeks to resolve.

The appearance of a scleral hemorrhage may be frightening. Instruct the parents and child about the benign nature of the hemorrhage and its natural history of resolution without intervention over a period of a few weeks.

If the child with a corneal abrasion has pain, analgesics may be helpful. Tell parents that most corneal abrasions heal on their own. If an antibiotic ointment is prescribed, instruct the parents in appropriate administration of the ointment.

> ▶ **Take** NOTE!
>
> *Patching of the eye with a corneal abrasion is no longer recommended, as children are often able to open the eye under the patch, which causes drying of the eye and further irritation, possibly contributing to prolonged recovery from the abrasion.*

Foreign bodies may be removed from the eye by gently everting the eyelid and wiping the foreign body away with a sterile cotton-tipped applicator. Irrigation with normal saline may also wash the foreign body away.

For chemical injury, irrigate the eye with copious amounts of water. Consult ophthalmology for further evaluation and management.

> ▶ **Take** NOTE!
>
> *Refer the child with a large foreign body in the eye or one that is imbedded in the globe of the eye to the ophthalmologist for appropriate, safe removal.*

Eye injuries can be prevented, and nurses play a vital role in educating the public about prevention of eye injuries and use of appropriate safety equipment. See Healthy People 2010 and Evidence-Based Practice 38.1.

Visual Disorders

Adequate visual development requires appropriate sensory stimulation to both eyes over the first few years of life. When one or both eyes are deprived of this stimulation, visual development does not progress appropriately, and visual impairment or blindness may result. This may occur when the eyes are not aligned properly, visual acuity between the eyes is disparate, or other problems with the eyes exist. If vision disorders are diagnosed at an early age and treatment is begun, then vision may progress normally. However, when these disorders go untreated, the young child's developing vision may be significantly reduced. Children must be appropriately screened for these disorders.

Common visual disorders in childhood include refractive errors, astigmatism, strabismus, amblyopia, nystagmus, glaucoma, and cataracts.

▶ REFRACTIVE ERRORS

The most common cause of visual difficulties in children is refractive errors. When the light that enters the lens does not bend appropriately to allow it to fall directly on the retina, then a refractive error occurs. Young children naturally have hyperopia (farsightedness) because the depth of the eye globe is not fully developed until about age 5 years. These children may have blurriness at close range, but by school age this blurriness usually resolves.

HEALTHY PEOPLE 2010

Objective	Significance
(Developmental) Increase the proportion of public and private schools that require use of appropriate head, face, eye, and mouth protection for students participating in school-sponsored physical activities; increase the use of appropriate personal protective eyewear in recreational activities and hazardous situations around the home	• Educate the family about appropriate use of eye protective equipment during sports, lawn care, chemical use, and other potentially hazardous activities. • Encourage families to provide appropriate supervision of children (particularly young children) to reduce the risk of injury. • Educate families to teach their children safe practices in and around the home (not running with scissors, etc.).

EVIDENCE-BASED PRACTICE 38.1
The Effect of Patching for Corneal Abrasion on Healing and Decreased Pain

● **Study**

Simple corneal abrasions are a common eye complaint. Eye patching with or without antibiotic ointment has often been used despite a lack of evidence for its use. Additionally, patches are difficult to keep on young children and may be associated with corneal erosion. The authors included quasi-randomized and randomized studies evaluating patching versus no patching for treatment of simple corneal abrasion. Eleven trials with a total of 1014 participants were included in the review.

▲ **Findings**

The authors found that patching for simple corneal abrasions did not improve healing on day 1, nor did it decrease the amount of pain experienced. Additionally, binocular vision is lost when one eye is patched. Based on these results, it is not recommended that patching be used for treatment of simple corneal abrasions.

■ **Nursing Implications**

Parents worry significantly when their child experiences even a very mild eye injury. Teach parents about the ability of the cornea to heal quickly from a minor abrasion. Emphasize that non-patched corneal abrasions have been shown to heal more rapidly than those that are patched.

Turner, A. & Rabiu, M. (2007). Patching for corneal abrasion. *The Cochrane Library 2007, 4.*

When the light entering the eye focuses in front of the retina, it results in myopia (nearsightedness). Children who are nearsighted may see well at close range but have difficulty focusing well on the blackboard or other objects at a distance.

The treatment for both hyperopia and myopia is prescription eyeglasses or contact lenses. Generally, a child 12 years of age can demonstrate the responsibility necessary to wear and care for contact lenses. Contact lenses may be used in younger children but are lost or damaged more readily. Because of the continuing refractive development in the child's vision through adolescence, laser surgery for vision correction is not recommended by the American Academy of Ophthalmology until 18 years of age, though it may be done experimentally in some children (AAO, 2007).

Nursing Assessment

Elicit the health history, noting blurred vision, complaints of eye fatigue with reading, or complaints of eye strain (headache, pulling sensation, or eye burning). Note complaints of difficulty concentrating on or maintaining a clear focus on objects up close, avoidance of up-close work, or poor work performance (hyperopia). Note the risk factor of family history of myopia. Observe for squinting when the child looks at objects at a distance. Observe the hyperopic child for the presence of esotropia. Readily observable physical findings are not noted in the myopic child. Test visual acuity using an age-appropriate screening tool (for more information related to visual acuity screening, refer to Chapter 30). Hyperopia is usually not identified with visual acuity screening alone; it usually requires a retinal examination by an ophthalmologist.

Nursing Management

Nursing management of the child with a refractive error focuses on providing education about corrective lens use and monitoring for the need for new eyeglasses or contact lenses.

Educating About Eyeglass Use

Children may or may not be compliant with wearing eyeglasses. Glasses still carry a stigma, and the child may be teased or bullied. However, many children enjoy the improved vision they achieve when wearing their eyeglasses, and this can help them overcome the teasing they might suffer. Encourage the child with newly prescribed eyeglasses to wear them by having the parent spend "special time" with the child doing an activity that requires the glasses (such as reading or drawing). Teach the parent and child to remove eyeglasses with both hands and to lay them on their side (not directly on the lens on any surface). Instruct the child and family about cleaning the glasses daily with mild soap and water or a commercial cleansing agent provided by the optometrist. Use a soft cloth to clean the glasses, not paper towels, tissues, or toilet paper.

Educating About Contact Lens Use

Teach the older child or adolescent how to care for the contact lenses properly, including lens hygiene and lens insertion and removal. Inform the child and parents that protective eyewear should be worn when the child is participating in contact sports. If the eye becomes inflamed, remove the contact lens and wear eyeglasses until the eye is improved. Consult with the child's eye care provider to determine if medications prescribed for an eye problem can be used while the contact lens is in.

Monitoring for Fit and Visual Correction

Encourage the family to complete visual assessments as scheduled. Since the child's vision is continuing to develop and refraction is not stable, the corrective lens prescription may change more frequently than it does in an adult. As the young child in particular is continuing to grow at a rapid rate, the head size is also changing. Eyeglass frames may hurt or pinch the child as the child's head becomes larger. Teach families to check the fit of the glasses monthly. Monitor for signs of ill fit, such as constant removal of the glasses in an older child or rubbing at the glasses or eyes in the very young child. Monitor for squinting, eye fatigue or strain, and complaints of headache or dizziness, which may indicate the need for a change in the lens prescription. See Healthy People 2010.

ASTIGMATISM

In astigmatism the cornea's curvature is uneven, which results in an irregular quality of vision because the light rays are refracted unevenly. Sometimes the lens is irregularly shaped, having the same result.

Nursing Assessment

Explore the health history for symptoms of astigmatism. Children with astigmatism often have blurry vision and difficulty seeing letters as a whole, so their ability to read is affected. They may have headaches or dizziness. Older children may complain of eye fatigue or strain. Children with astigmatism often learn to tilt their heads slightly so that they can focus more effectively. This may lead to "normal" vision screenings, but the headache and dizziness still warrant further examination by an eye specialist. The

diagnosis of astigmatism requires not only a visual acuity test but also a refractive error evaluation by an optometrist or ophthalmologist.

Nursing Management

Corrective lenses can help to, in effect, smooth out the curvature of the cornea, making the light ray refraction occur smoothly. As with refractive errors, encourage the child who requires corrective lenses for astigmatism to wear the eyeglasses or contact lenses regularly.

STRABISMUS

Strabismus refers to misalignment of the eyes. It is common and occurs in about 4% of children (Optometrists Network, 2006). The most common types of strabismus are exotropia and esotropia. In exotropia the eyes turn outward; in esotropia they turn inward. Because of this unequal alignment, visual development in each eye may proceed at different rates. Diplopia (double vision) may result, so vision in one eye may be "turned off" by the brain to avoid diplopia. Many infants have strabismus intermittently, but this usually resolves by 3 months of age. Intermittent strabismus that persists past 3 months of age or constant strabismus at any age warrants referral to an ophthalmologist for further evaluation.

Therapeutic management of strabismus may include patching of the stronger eye or eye muscle surgery. Corrective lenses are also used for strabismus. Complications of strabismus include amblyopia and visual deficits.

Nursing Assessment

Parents may be the first persons to notice that the child's eyes do not face in the same direction. Question parents about the onset of the problem and whether it is continuous or intermittent. If intermittent, does it occur more often when the child is tired? Elicit the health history, noting complaints of blurred vision, tired eyes, squinting or closing one eye in bright sunlight, tilting the head to focus on an object, or a history of bumping into objects (depth perception may be limited).

Observe the child's eyes for obvious exotropia or esotropia. In the absence of an obvious finding, assessment of the symmetry of the corneal light reflex is extremely helpful (Fig. 38.9). The "cover test" is also a useful tool for the identification of strabismus.

True strabismus should not be confused with pseudostrabismus. In pseudostrabismus, the eyes may appear slightly crossed (as in the child with wide nasal bridge and epicanthal folds), but the corneal light reflex remains symmetric.

HEALTHY PEOPLE *2010*	
Objective	**Significance**
(Developmental) Reduce uncorrected visual impairment due to refractive errors; reduce blindness and visual impairment in children and adolescents aged 17 years and under	• Ensure that visual acuity testing begins with an age-appropriate screening tool by 3 years of age and continues yearly throughout childhood and adolescence. • Refer for an eye evaluation any children with complaints of difficulty seeing the front of the classroom or complaints of eye strain or difficulty with close work. • Screen infants and children for asymmetric corneal light reflex for early detection of amblyopia.

FIGURE 38.9 Esotropia. Test for strabismus by observing symmetry of the corneal light reflex. The reflex falls to the left of one pupil and to the right of the other.

Nursing Management

It is extremely important to treat strabismus appropriately in the developing years so that equal visual acuity may be achieved in both eyes. When patching is prescribed, encourage the family to comply with this modality. Encourage eyeglass wearing if prescribed. Provide appropriate postoperative care by protecting the operative site with eye patching.

▶ AMBLYOPIA

Amblyopia refers to poor visual development in the otherwise structurally normal eye. It develops within the first decade of life and if untreated, causes more cases of vision loss than all other conditions together in persons younger than 40 years of age. It occurs in about 2% to 3% of children (Dubowy, 2005). The vision in one eye is reduced because the eye and the brain are not working together properly. While the eyes are fighting to focus differently because of their differences in visual acuity, one eye is stronger than the other. This is why amblyopia is often referred to as "lazy eye."

Amblyopia may be caused by any disorder that affects normal visual development, including strabismus and differences in visual acuity or astigmatism between the two eyes. It may also result from eye trauma, ptosis, or cataract. Children with amblyopia, if untreated, will have worsening of the poorer eye and strain in the better eye, which may also lead to worsening of acuity in that eye. Eventually blindness will result in one or both eyes.

Therapeutic management of amblyopia focuses on strengthening the weaker eye. This may be achieved through patching for several hours per day, using atropine drops in the better eye (once daily), vision therapy, or eye muscle surgery if the cause is strabismus.

Nursing Assessment

One of the most important functions of the nurse is to identify on screening the preschool child with amblyopia. Begin visual acuity testing using an age-appropriate tool

by 3 years of age. Observe for asymmetry of the corneal light reflex in the child of any age. This may be the only sign in the preverbal child.

Nursing Management

It is very important for children with amblyopia to receive appropriate treatment during the early years of visual development. Patching the better eye for several hours each day encourages the eye with poorer vision to be used appropriately and promotes visual development in that eye. The once-daily use of atropine drops in the better eye results in blurring in that eye, similarly encouraging use and development of the weaker eye. Support and encourage children and parents to comply with the patching protocol or atropine drop use.

Promoting eye safety is extremely important for the child with amblyopia; if the better eye suffers a serious injury, both eyes may become blind.

▶ NYSTAGMUS

Nystagmus refers to a very rapid, irregular eye movement. It is described by some as "bouncing" of the eyes. It may occur in children with congenital cataracts, but the most common cause is a neurologic problem. It is difficult for the brain and eyes to communicate when the eyes are in continuous motion; thus, visual development may be affected. Children with nystagmus must receive further evaluation by an ophthalmologist and possibly a neurologist.

▶ INFANTILE GLAUCOMA

Infantile glaucoma is an autosomal recessive disorder that is more common in interrelated marriages or relationships. It is often associated with other genetic disorders. It occurs in about 1 of 10,000 live births (Lighthouse International, 2007). Infantile glaucoma is characterized by obstruction of aqueous humor flow and increased intraocular pressure that results in large, prominent eyes. Vision loss may occur as a result of corneal scarring, optic nerve damage, or, most commonly, amblyopia.

Unlike adult glaucoma, in which medical management is the first step, therapeutic management of infantile glaucoma is focused on surgical intervention. Infantile glaucoma is treated surgically via goniotomy (removal of obstruction of the aqueous humor). Laser surgery is being used as well. Sometimes several surgeries may be necessary to correct the problem. Ongoing medication therapy may also be required.

Nursing Assessment

Note any family history of infantile glaucoma or other genetic disorders. Elicit the health history, noting history of the infant keeping the eyes closed most of the time or rubbing the eyes. Observe the eye for corneal enlargement and clouding; the eye may appear enlarged. Photophobia may occur, so bright light may bother the infant. Tearing or conjunctivitis and eyelid squeezing or spasm may also occur. The pediatric ophthalmologist may use a tonometer to measure the intraocular pressure during the diagnostic phase.

Nursing Management

The main goal of nursing care for the infant with glaucoma is postoperative care. Family education will also be important.

Providing Postoperative Care

Postoperatively the eye will be patched and the child should be maintained on bed rest. Nursing care focuses on protection of the surgical site. Infants and toddlers may require elbow restraints to prevent them from rubbing the affected eye. These children may be quite anxious with one or both eyes patched, since their ability to see will be affected. Use a calm and soothing approach with these children, as well as distraction and developmentally appropriate play activities.

Educating the Family

Instruct parents and children to make sure the child avoids roughhousing and contact sports for at least 2 weeks after surgery. Before the first surgery occurs, prepare parents for the possibility that three or four operations may be necessary. Teach families how to administer postoperative medications. Encourage parents to comply with ongoing recommended visual assessments.

▶ CONGENITAL CATARACT

A congenital cataract is an opacity of the lens of the eye that is present at birth. Sensory amblyopia will result if the infant goes untreated. Complications include visual developmental delay related to amblyopia. In children younger than 5 years of age, congenital cataract causes 16% of the cases of legal blindness (Lighthouse International, 2007). Bilateral cataracts may be associated with metabolic or genetic syndromes. Surgery to remove the opaque lens can be done as early as 2 weeks of age. The infant is then fitted with a contact lens. Intraocular lens implants are also being used (Watkinson & Graham, 2005). The best visual outcomes occur when cataracts are removed prior to 3 months of age. Glaucoma may occur as a complication after cataract surgery.

Nursing Assessment

Note history of lack of visual awareness. Observe the eyes for apparent cloudiness of the cornea (not always visible).

HEALTHY PEOPLE 2010	
Objective	Significance
(Developmental) Reduce visual impairment due to glaucoma (Developmental) Reduce visual impairment due to cataract	• Appropriately screen infants and children for glaucoma or cataract. • Refer suspected cases to a pediatric ophthalmologist for further evaluation.

Upon ophthalmoscopic examination, the red reflex will not be observed in the affected eye.

Nursing Management

Postoperative care focuses on protecting the operative site and providing developmentally appropriate activities. Ensure that the protective eye patch is secure. Elbow restraints may be necessary in the older infant to prevent accidental injury to the operative site. Teach families how to administer antibiotic or corticosteroid ophthalmic drops if prescribed for postoperative use. Once the surgical site is healed, the "good" eye may be patched for several hours a day to promote visual development in the eye with the contact or intraocular lens. Regular visual assessments are critical for determining the adequacy of visual development after cataract removal. Instruct parents about the importance of using sunglasses that block ultraviolet rays in the child who has had a lens removed.

Retinopathy of Prematurity

Retinopathy of prematurity (ROP) is a disorder characterized by rapid growth of retinal blood vessels in the premature infant. In the fetus, retinal vascularization begins at 4 months and progresses until completion at 9 months or shortly after birth. The premature infant is born with incomplete retinal vascularization, yet new vessels continue to grow between the vascularized and nonvascularized retina. Risk factors include low birthweight, early gestational age, sepsis, high light intensity, and hypothermia. Changes in oxygen tension resulting from hypoxia, oxyhemoglobin dissociation curve changes that occur when adult blood is transfused to the premature infant, and the duration/concentration of supplemental oxygen are thought to play an important role in the development of ROP.

Premature infants should have serial examinations by an ophthalmologist until the ROP has regressed and normal vascularization is seen. If ROP continues to progress, laser surgery may be necessary to prevent blindness (Hack & Klein, 2006). Complications of ROP include myopia, glaucoma, and blindness. Strabismus may occur even in cases of regressed (resolved) ROP. Refractive errors and amblyopia may occur as early as 3 months corrected age. In the first year of life, ophthalmologic examinations may occur frequently so that if corrective lenses are needed, they may be prescribed at the earliest possible time. After 1 year corrected age, former premature infants should continue to have yearly ophthalmologic examinations to detect and treat visual deficits early (Verma, Sridhar, & Spitzer, 2003).

Nursing Assessment

Ensure that all former premature infants are routinely screened for visual deficits. Discuss developmental progress with the parents. Observe for the development of strabismus, manifested by an asymmetric corneal light reflex.

Nursing Management

Nursing management of infants with ROP mainly focuses on ensuring that the family is compliant with the ophthalmologist's follow-up recommendations. Recurrent illness or rehospitalization of premature infants may interfere with scheduled eye follow-up appointments. Ensure that these appointments are rescheduled and that the family understands the importance of them. Many children who have regressed ROP or who require cryotherapy have refractive errors, so even when the ROP is considered resolved, these children should still maintain appropriate ophthalmology follow-up.

Visual Impairment

Vision impairment in children refers to acuity of between 20/60 and 20/200 in the better eye on examination. "Legal blindness" is a term used to refer to vision of less than 20/200 or peripheral vision less than 20 degrees. In most cases, vision may be augmented with corrective lenses. Some blind children can differentiate light versus dark, while others live in total darkness.

Visual impairment in children may result from a number of different causes. In the United States, visual impairment and blindness are most often caused by refractive error, astigmatism, strabismus, amblyopia, nystagmus, infantile glaucoma, congenital cataract, retinopathy of prematurity, and retinoblastoma. Factors that increase the risk for developing visual impairment include: prematurity, developmental delay, genetic syndrome, family history of eye disease, African-American heritage, previous serious eye injury, diabetes, HIV, and chronic corticosteroid use. Trauma is also an important cause of blindness in children.

Children with visual impairments often exhibit motor and cognitive delays as well. With one less sense with which to experience their environment, these children may lag behind in developmental milestones. Visual impairments are associated with many other syndromes. For example, many children with fetal alcohol syndrome have visual impairments, and albinism is associated with blindness.

> ▶ *Take* NOTE!
>
> *Laser pointers pose a risk of retinal damage in infants and young children. Damage occurs if the child stares at the red light for longer than 10 seconds. They should not be used as toys.*

Nursing Assessment

Nursing assessment for visual impairment includes a careful health history, physical examination, and visual acuity testing.

Health History

Parents and nurses alike should be alert to signs of potential visual impairment. One of the most important functions of the nurse is to recognize signs of visual impairment as early as possible. These signs may include:

At any age:
• Dull, vacant stare

Infants:
• Does not "fix and follow"
• Does not make eye contact
• Unaffected by bright light
• Does not imitate facial expression

Toddlers and older children:
• Rub, shut, cover eyes
• Squinting
• Frequent blinking
• Holds objects close or sits close to television
• Bumping into objects
• Head tilt, or forward thrust

Physical Examination

Assess for symmetry or asymmetry of corneal light reflex. Perform the "cover test." Use an age-appropriate visual acuity screening tool (refer to Chapter 30 for additional information on visual acuity screening).

Nursing Management

Important nursing functions in relation to visual impairment and blindness are supporting the child and family and promoting socialization, development, and education. In addition, when the child with a visual impairment is hospitalized for any reason, the nurse must plan appropriate care for that child, taking into consideration the child's level of disability. Box 38.1 provides tips on working with the visually impaired child, and these tips should also be taught to families.

Supporting the Child and Family

Provide emotional support to the family with a visually impaired child. Ensure that the child's environment pro-

BOX 38.1 Tips for Interacting With the Visually Impaired Child

- Use the child's name to gain attention.
- Identify yourself and let the child know you are there before you touch the child.
- Encourage the child to be independent while maintaining safety.
- Name and describe people/objects to make the child more aware of what is happening.
- Discuss upcoming activities with the child.
- Explain what other children or individuals are doing.
- Make directions simple and specific.
- Allow the child additional time to think about the response to a question or statement.
- Use touch and tone of voice appropriate to the situation.
- Use parts of the child's body as reference points for the location of items.
- Encourage exploration of objects through touch.
- Describe unfamiliar environments and provide reference points.
- Use the sighted-guide technique when walking with a visually impaired child.

Adapted from the Delta Gamma Center for Children with Visual Impairments.

vides familiarity and security. Encourage activities that stimulate development; these activities will vary from child to child depending upon whether the child also demonstrates impairment in other areas, such as hearing or motor skills. The blind infant will not provide the eye contact that parents are looking for, so educate the parents about other indicators that the infant is acknowledging the parents' presence, such as:

- Increased motor activity
- Eyelid movement
- Changes in breathing pattern
- Making sounds

Encourage the family of a visually impaired child to display affection through touch and tone of voice. Refer families to support networks and other resources for the blind and visually impaired. Box 18.2 lists some on-line resources for families of children who are visually impaired or blind.

Promoting Socialization, Development, and Education

Blind children, since they lack the visual stimulation that children usually receive, may develop self-stimulatory actions in compensation ("blindisms"). Examples of blindisms are eye pressing, rocking, spinning, bouncing,

BOX 38.2 On-line Resources for Families of Children With Visual Impairments

- www.aapos.org: American Association of Pediatric Ophthalmology and Strabismus—Mainly for health care providers, some information and resources for lay persons
- www.acb.org: American Council of the Blind—The nation's leading membership organization of blind and visually impaired people
- www.afb.org: American Foundation for the Blind—Resource for products for people with visual deficits
- www.aoa.org: American Optometric Association—Education and resources for parents
- www.cnib.ca: Canadian National Institute for the Blind—Resources within Canada
- www.helenkeller.org: Helen Keller Services for the Blind—Serves blind, deaf-blind, and visually impaired persons in the New York metropolitan area
- www.icevi.org: International Council for Education of People with Visual Impairment—Promotes equal access to appropriate education for all visually impaired children and youths
- www.lighthouse.org: Lighthouse International—Information on visual disorders, statistics, resources available for families; resource for products for people with visual deficits
- www.nei.nih.gov/: National Eye Institute, a division of the National Institutes of Health—Conducts and
supports vision research; information for the lay person or health care provider for eye examinations and financial resources
- www.nfb.org: National Federation of the Blind—Information, education, and support for the blind
- www.nichcy.org: National Dissemination Center for Children with Disabilities—Provides information, education, and resources for families and educators; also in Spanish
- www.preventblindness.org: Prevent Blindness America—Resources for lay persons
- www.rfbd.org: Recording for the Blind and Dyslexic—Texts and tapes of books
- www.ropard.org: Association for Retinopathy of Prematurity and Related Diseases—Resources for families and health care providers
- www.sightforstudents.org: Sight for Students—Provides vision examinations and glasses to uninsured children across the country
- www.spedex.com/napvi: National Association for Parents of Children with Visual Impairments—Information, referrals, financial resources; also in Spanish
- www.v2020.org: Vision 2020: The Right to Sight—Information, education, goals for prevention and treatment of blindness worldwide

and head banging. These repetitive behaviors may interfere with the child's ability to socialize. Work with the parents to plan a strategy for the development of alternative behaviors specific to the individual child.

Refer the blind or visually impaired child who is younger than 3 years of age to the local district of Early Intervention to establish case management services for the child's developmental needs. After age 3, state laws provide for public education and related services for children with disabilities. An individualized education plan (IEP) should be developed to maximize the child's learning ability. Nurses may be one of the professionals involved in the development of the IEP.

The severely visually impaired or blind child will need to learn to read Braille and will also need to learn to navigate the environment with the use of a cane or via another method.

Otitis Media

Otitis media is defined as inflammation of the middle ear with the presence of fluid. It can be subdivided into two categories. Acute otitis media (AOM) refers to an acute infectious process of the middle ear that may produce a rapid onset of ear pain and possibly fever. Otitis media with effusion (OME) refers to a collection of fluid in the middle ear space without signs and symptoms of infection. Chronic otitis media with effusion (chronic OME) is defined as OME lasting longer than 3 months.

▶ ACUTE OTITIS MEDIA

AOM is a common illness in children, resulting from infection (bacterial or viral) of fluid in the middle ear. AOM has a peak incidence between 3 and 18 months of age (Donaldson, 2006). Increased susceptibility in infants may be partly explained by the short length and horizontal positioning of the eustachian tube, limited response to antigens, and lack of previous exposure to common pathogens. AOM occurs mostly in the fall through spring, with the highest incidence in the winter. AOM often recurs in infants and young children when the fluid in the middle ear becomes reinfected. The most significant risk factors for otitis media are eustachian tube dysfunction and susceptibility to recurrent upper respiratory infections.

Pathophysiology

An upper respiratory infection frequently precedes AOM. Fluid and pathogens travel upward from the nasopharyngeal area, invading the middle ear space. Fluid behind the eardrum has difficulty draining back out toward the nasopharyngeal area because of the horizontal positioning of the eustachian tube. A viral upper respiratory infection may cause AOM or may place the child at risk for bacterial invasion. Pathogens gain access to the eustachian tube, where they proliferate and invade the mucosa. Fever and pain occur acutely. Increased pressure behind the tympanic membrane may result in perforation. This may result in decreased pain and yield drainage in the ear canal. Most perforations heal spontaneously and are completely benign.

AOM is most commonly caused by viral pathogens, *Streptococcus pneumoniae, Haemophilus influenzae,* and *Moraxella catarrhalis*. Viral causes of AOM resolve spontaneously.

After clearance of the infection, fluid remains in the middle ear space behind the tympanic membrane, sometimes for several months (otitis media with effusion). This may occur because of the positioning of the eustachian tubes, resulting in difficulty in draining fluid back to the nasopharyngeal area. OME may also occur because of the high frequency of upper respiratory infections in infants and young children, which again result in back-up of fluid from the nasopharyngeal area.

The most common complications of AOM include:

- Hearing loss
- Expressive speech delay
- Tympanosclerosis (scarring of the tympanic membrane; usually has no effect on hearing)
- Tympanic membrane perforation (acute with resolution or chronic)
- Chronic suppurative otitis media (chronic drainage via perforation or **tympanostomy** tubes)
- Acute mastoiditis (infection of the mastoid process)
- Intracranial infections, including bacterial meningitis and abscesses

Therapeutic Management

Viral causes of AOM usually resolve spontaneously, but bacterial causes may require treatment with an antibiotic. It is unreasonable to obtain a culture of middle ear fluid with every episode of AOM to determine the specific cause. Scientific studies of fluid obtained via tympanostomy in children with AOM have been performed, and clinical decision making is based upon this research. There is great concern in the health care community about the development of antibiotic resistance due to the overuse of antibiotics. For this reason, clinical practice guidelines have been developed for a number of disorders based upon large quantities of research.

Certain diagnosis of AOM is based upon rapid onset of symptoms, signs of fluid in the middle ear, and signs or symptoms of inflammation in the middle ear (complaint of ear pain or visible erythema of the tympanic membrane) (American Academy of Pediatrics & American Academy of Family Physicians, 2004). The choice of antibiotic will depend upon the timing, the child's age, and whether the episode is a first or subsequent infection. The current recommendations by the American Academy of Pediatrics and American Academy of Family Physicians allow for a period of observation or "watchful waiting" in certain children. This allows for natural resolution of AOM related to viral causes and decreases the overuse of antibiotics in the pediatric population.

Recommendations for AOM treatment in previously healthy children are found in Table 18.3. Pain management is also an important component of AOM treatment, as is appropriate follow-up to ensure disease resolution.

Nursing Assessment

Nursing assessment of the child with AOM consists of health history and physical examination.

Health History

Elicit a description of the present illness and chief complaint. Note acute, abrupt onset of signs and symptoms. Common signs and symptoms reported during the health history might include:

- Fever (may be low grade or higher)
- Complaints of otalgia (ear pain)
- Fussiness or irritability
- Crying inconsolably, particularly when lying down
- Batting or tugging at the ears (may also occur with teething or OME, or may be a habit)
- Rolling the head from side to side
- Poor feeding or loss of appetite
- Lethargy
- Difficulty sleeping or awakening crying in the night
- Fluid draining from the ear

Determine the child's response to any treatments used thus far. Explore the child's current and past medical history for risk factors such as:

- Young age
- Daycare attendance
- Previous history of AOM or OME
- Antecedent or concurrent upper respiratory infection
- Other risk factors (Box 38.3)

Physical Examination and Diagnostic Testing

The child may complain of pain when the ear is examined. On otoscopic examination, the tympanic membrane will have a dull or opaque appearance and is bulging and/or red (Fig. 38.10). Sometimes pus (greenish or yellowish) may be visible behind the eardrum. Upon pneumatic otoscopy, the eardrum will be immobile. (A physician or nurse practitioner usually performs otoscopic examination.) If the tympanic membrane has become perforated, drainage may be present in the ear canal, but the canal will otherwise appear normal. Palpate for possible cervical lymphadenopathy. **Tympanometry** is not as useful in the diagnosis of AOM as it is with OME.

Nursing Management

Nursing management of the child with acute otitis media is mainly supportive in nature. It focuses on pain management, family education, and prevention of AOM.

Managing Pain Associated With AOM

Analgesics such as acetaminophen and ibuprofen have been shown to be effective at managing mild to moderate pain associated with AOM. They have the added benefit of reducing fever. Narcotic analgesics such as codeine may be prescribed for severe pain. Application of heat or a cool compress may also be helpful. Instruct the family to have the child lie on the affected side with the heating pad or covered ice pack in place to that ear. Numbing eardrops such as benzocaine (Auralgan) may be helpful in the event of acute, severe pain. They should be used in conjunction with analgesics, though, because of the short duration of action (American Academy of Pediatrics & American Academy of Family Physicians, 2004).

TABLE 38.3 TREATMENT RECOMMENDATIONS FOR **AOM**

Age and Severity of Illness*	Certainty of Diagnosis	Treatment
Less than 6 months old	Certain or possible	Antibiotics
6 months to 2 years	Certain	Antibiotics
6 months to 2 years with severe illness	Possible	Antibiotics
6 months to 2 years with nonsevere illness	Possible	May observe**
Greater than 2 years with severe illness	Certain	Antibiotics
Greater than 2 years with nonsevere illness	Certain	Observe**
Greater than 2 years	Possible	Observe**

*Severe illness is defined as moderate to severe otalgia or fever 39°C or higher. Nonsevere illness is defined as mild otalgia and fever less than 39°C.

**Observation is appropriate only when follow-up can be ensured. If symptoms are persistent or become worse, antibiotics may then be started.

(AAP & AAFP, 2004)

BOX 38.3 **Risk Factors for Acute Otitis Media**

- Eustachian tube dysfunction
- Recurrent upper respiratory infection
- First episode of AOM before 3 months of age
- Daycare attendance (increases exposure to viruses causing upper respiratory infections)
- Previous episodes of AOM
- Family history
- Passive smoking
- Crowding in the home or large family size
- Native American, Inuit, or Australian aborigine ethnicity
- Absence of infant breastfeeding
- Immunocompromise
- Poor nutrition
- Craniofacial anomalies
- Presence of allergies (possibly)

HEALTHY PEOPLE 2010

Objective	Significance
Reduce otitis media in children and adolescents	• Teach children and families the importance of hand washing to avoid the common cold (often a precursor to otitis media). • Teach families the importance of appropriate follow-up for eradication of otitis media. • Educate families about the importance of using antibiotics only for true bacterial infections (in order to decrease the development of resistant organisms, many of which cause otitis media).

Educating the Family

If the treatment selected for AOM is observation or watchful waiting, explain the rationale for this to the family. Ensure that the family understands the importance of returning for re-evaluation if the child is not improving or if the AOM progresses to severe illness. When antibiotics are prescribed, the family must understand the importance of completing the entire course of antibiotics. Families are tempted to stop giving the antibiotic because the child is usually vastly improved after taking the medication for 24 to 48 hours. Follow-up for resolution of AOM is necessary for all children, and the physician or nurse practitioner will determine the timing of that follow-up. Emphasize the importance of follow-up to the parents, educating them about OME and its potential impact on hearing and speech. See Healthy People 2010.

Preventing AOM

Breastfed infants have a lower incidence of AOM than formula-fed infants, and breast milk's immunologic benefits are well known, so encourage mothers to breastfeed for at least 6 to 12 months. Instruct families to avoid excess exposure to individuals with upper respiratory infections to decrease the incidence of these infections in their child. Infants and children should not be exposed to second-hand smoke. Encourage parents to stop smoking. If quitting smoking is not possible, then instruct parents not to smoke inside the house or automobile. Encourage the parents to have the child immunized with Prevnar and, when appropriate, influenza vaccine.

Though not yet clinically or scientifically proven, Xylitol syrup, a sucrose substitute, may also be protective.

A

Pars flaccida

Lateral process

Manubrium

} Malleus

Pars tensa

B

FIGURE 38.10 (A) Normal tympanic membrane. (B) Acute otitis media: note erythema and opacity of the tympanic membrane.

Children who are old enough may chew Xylitol-containing gum. Younger children and infants may be given Xylitol syrup. Care should be taken to avoid excessive dosing, as Xylitol can cause diarrhea.

▶ OTITIS MEDIA WITH EFFUSION

Otitis media with effusion (OME) refers to the presence of fluid within the middle ear space, without signs or symptoms of infection. It may occur independent of AOM or may persist after the infectious process of AOM has resolved. Risk factors for OME include passive smoking, absence of breastfeeding, frequent viral upper respiratory infections, allergy, young age, male sex, adenoid hypertrophy, eustachian tube dysfunction, and certain congenital disorders. Complications of OME include AOM, hearing loss, and deafness.

Nursing Assessment

Nursing assessment of the child with OME includes health history, physical examination, and diagnostic testing.

Health History
Determine the extent of symptoms. Children may be asymptomatic or may experience a popping sensation or fullness behind the eardrum. Explore the health history for risk factors such as passive smoking, absence of breastfeeding, frequent viral upper respiratory infections, allergy, or recent history of AOM.

Physical Examination
Otoscopic examination may reveal a dull, opaque tympanic membrane that may be white, gray, or bluish (Fig. 38.11). If the tympanic membrane is not opaque, a fluid level or air bubble may be visualized. Mobility may be absent or diminished upon pneumatic otoscopy. Tympanometry may be used to confirm the diagnosis of OME.

Nursing Management

OME may take several months to resolve. Nursing management during the resolution phase focuses on education and monitoring for hearing loss.

Educating the Family
Educate the family about the natural history of OME and the anatomical differences in young children that contribute to OME. Inform parents that antihistamines, decongestants, antibiotics, and corticosteroids have not been proven to hasten the resolution of OME and thus are not recommended. OME usually resolves spontaneously, but children should be rechecked every 4 weeks while this resolution is occurring. Teach parents not to feed infants in a supine position and to avoid bottle propping.

Monitoring for Hearing Loss
When OME persists, the primary concern is its effect on hearing. In the infant or toddler who should be experiencing rapid language development, impaired hearing can depress language acquisition significantly. Children with OME who are at risk for speech, language, or learning problems may be referred for evaluation of hearing earlier than a child with OME who isn't at risk (Box 18.4). Children with chronic OME (persistent OME of 3 months' duration or longer) should be referred to a specialist for hearing evaluation. Children who are not already at risk for speech concerns and are not experiencing difficulty with language acquisition may be reassessed every 3 to 6 months as long as hearing loss is not identified. At-risk children may require treatment earlier.

To communicate more effectively with children with OME who have hearing loss:

- Turn off music or television.
- Position yourself within 3 feet of the child before speaking.
- Face the child while speaking.

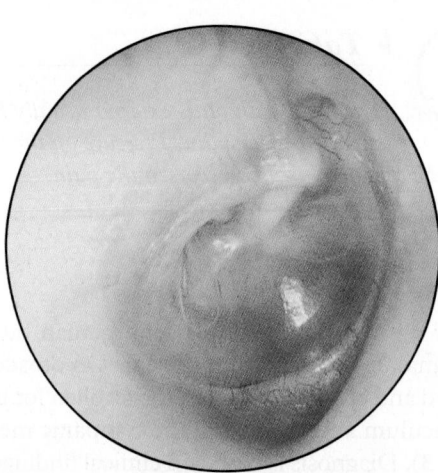

FIGURE **38.11** Otitis media with effusion; note dull white tympanic membrane.

> ### BOX 38.4   Children at Risk for Speech, Language, or Learning Difficulties
>
> - Permanent hearing loss (without OME)
> - Speech/language delay (suspected or diagnosed)
> - Craniofacial disorder that may interfere with speech
> - Any pervasive developmental disorder
> - Genetic disorders or syndromes associated with speech or learning problems
> - Cleft palate
> - Blindness or significant visual impairment

• Use visual cues.
• Increase the volume of your speech only slightly.
• Speak clearly.
• Request preferential classroom seating.

> ▶ *Take* NOTE!
>
> *Evaluation of hearing is recommended when OME lasts 3 months or more if language delay, hearing loss, or a learning problem is suspected.*

Providing Postoperative Care for the Child With Pressure-Equalizing Tubes

The standard treatment for persistent or problematic OME is surgical insertion of **pressure-equalizing (PE) tubes** into the tympanic membrane (via myringotomy). The tubes stay in place for at least several months and generally fall out on their own (Fig. 38.12). The procedure is usually done as an outpatient surgery and the child returns home in the evening. Teach the parents to administer ear drops postoperatively if prescribed. After PE tube placement, the surgeon may recommend avoiding water entry into the ears. If recommended, advise parents to have the child wear earplugs in the bathtub or while swimming.

Placement of the PE tubes allows for adequate hearing, which in turn encourages appropriate speech development. Placement of PE tubes does not prevent middle ear infection. If the middle ear becomes infected with PE tubes in place, the tubes allow infected fluid to drain from the ear. Tell parents to contact their pediatrician if drainage from the ear is noted. After PE tubes are placed, young children often have rapid increases in language acquisition, and parents should observe for this.

FIGURE 38.12 Pressure-equalizing tubes in place in the tympanic membrane.

> ▶ *Take* NOTE!
>
> *Children with PE tubes who swim in a lake must wear earplugs, as lake water is contaminated with bacteria and entry of that water into the middle ear should be avoided.*

▶ OTITIS EXTERNA

Otitis externa is defined as an infection and inflammation of the skin of the external ear canal. *Pseudomonas aeruginosa* and *Staphylococcus aureus* are typical causative agents, though fungi such as *Aspergillus* and other bacteria also may be implicated. Moisture in the canal contributes to pathogen growth. Otitis externa is commonly known as "swimmer's ear" since it occurs more frequently in those who swim often (and thus have wet ear canals). Changing the pH in the ear canal contributes to the inflammatory process (Zoltan, Taylor, & Achar, 2005).

Nursing Assessment

Nursing assessment of the child with otitis externa focuses on the health history and physical examination.

Health History

Elicit a description of the present illness and chief complaint. Note history of ear itching or pain, ear drainage, or a feeling of fullness in the ear canal, with possible difficulty hearing. Note onset and progression of symptoms, as well as the child's response to treatments. Explore the child's current and past medical history for risk factors such as previous episodes of otitis externa or history of recent swimming in a pool, lake, or ocean.

> ▶ *Take* NOTE!
>
> *The child with otitis externa usually has significant ear pain. Pressure on the tragus should be avoided, as it can worsen the pain.*

Physical Examination

Typically a white or colored discharge can be seen in the ear canal or running from the ear. On otoscopy, the canal is red and edematous, often too swollen for insertion of the speculum and viewing of the tympanic membrane (Fig. 38.13). Diagnosis is based on clinical findings. Occasionally the ear drainage is cultured for bacteria or fungus, particularly if otitis externa is not improving with treatment.

FIGURE 38.13 Note edema and erythema of the ear canal as well as purulent discharge in the child with otitis externa.

Nursing Management

The primary goals of nursing management are pain relief, treatment of the infection, and prevention of recurrence.

Managing Pain

Analgesics (often narcotics) may be administered to manage the pain. A warm compress or heating pad to the affected ear is helpful in some children.

Treating the Infection

Antibiotic or antifungal eardrops should be administered as prescribed. In some cases a wick is placed in the ear canal. The wick keeps the antibiotic drops in contact with the skin of the ear canal and promotes healing. Wick insertion can be extremely painful, and younger children will need to be restrained during insertion for their safety.

Preventing Reinfection

Once the infection has resolved, children and their parents should be educated about prevention of further episodes. Since moisture contributes to otitis externa, the ear canals should be kept dry. Encourage the child and parents to use one of the methods described in Teaching Guidelines 38.2 after swimming or showering.

Hearing Loss and Deafness

Infants are ordinarily born with the sense of hearing fully developed. Language development in infancy and early childhood is dependent upon adequate hearing, and even the fluctuating hearing loss associated with intermittent bouts of AOM can hinder language development. Hearing loss may be unilateral (involving one ear) or bilateral (involving both ears). The extent of hearing loss is defined based on the softest intensity of sound that is perceived, described in **decibels** (dB). Levels of hearing loss are:

TEACHING GUIDELINES 38.2

Preventing Otitis Externa

1. Avoid the use of cotton swabs, headphones, and earphones.
2. Wear earplugs when swimming.
3. Promote ear canal dryness and alternate pH. Use one or more of the following methods:
   - Dry the ear canals using a hair dryer set on a lower setting.
   - Administer solutions that have a drying effect on the auditory canal skin and change the pH of the canal to discourage organism growth in susceptible children. The following solutions can be used:
   - A few drops of Domeboro solution can be placed in the canal, and then allowed to run out.
   - A mixture of half rubbing alcohol and half vinegar (squirted into the canal and then allowed to run out). The alcohol solution should be used only when the ear canals are healthy. Using it while the canals are inflamed will cause stinging and increased pain.

- 0 to 20 dB: normal
- 20 to 40 dB: mild loss
- 40 to 60 dB: moderate loss
- 60 to 80 dB: severe loss
- Greater than 80 dB: profound loss (ASHA, 2007)

Hearing loss may be congenital or of delayed onset. Congenital hearing loss affects about 3 infants per 1,000 live births in the United States (NCHAM, 2007b). Most congenital hearing loss is inherited through a recessive gene, with only about 22% of cases resulting from an autosomal dominant trait (Kaye, 2006). Congenital hearing loss accounts for about one half of all the cases of hearing impairment; the remainder are acquired. Premature infants and those with persistent pulmonary hypertension of the newborn are at increased risk for hearing loss compared with other infants (Verma et al., 2003). Hearing loss commonly occurs with a large number of congenital or genetic syndromes, as well as in association with anomalies of the head and face. As of 2005, a variety of newborn universal hearing screening mandates have been passed by legislation in 37 states, thus allowing for earlier identification of infants with congenital hearing loss (NCHAM, 2007a). See Healthy People 2010.

Delayed-onset hearing loss may be conductive, sensorineural, or mixed. **Conductive hearing loss** results when transmission of sound through the middle ear is disrupted, as in the case of OME. When fluid fills the middle ear, the tympanic membrane is unable to move properly, and partial or complete hearing loss occurs. **Sensorineural hearing loss** is caused by damage to the hair cells in the cochlea or along the auditory pathway. This may result from kernicterus, use of ototoxic medication, intrauterine infection with cytomegalovirus or rubella, neonatal or postnatal infection such as meningitis, severe neonatal respiratory depression, or exposure to excess noise. Mixed hearing loss occurs when the cause may be attributed to both conductive and sensorineural problems. See Healthy People 2010.

Regardless of the cause of hearing loss, early intervention can make a difference in the child's ability to communicate. Once the hearing loss has been determined, intervention can begin. Hearing aids, cochlear implants, communication devices, and speech education may enable these children to communicate verbally. Improved communication beginning in infancy and early childhood may also improve the child's school achievement.

> ▶ *Take* NOTE!
>
> *The earplugs or covers used to block ambient noise in premature infants in the NICU may decrease the preemie's risk for hearing loss.*

Nursing Assessment

Nursing assessment of the child with hearing loss or impairment focuses on the health history, physical examination, and hearing testing.

Health History

Common signs and symptoms reported during the health history might include:

Infant:
• Wakes only to touch, not environmental noises
• Does not startle to loud noises
• Does not turn to sound by 4 months of age
• Does not babble at 6 months of age
• Does not progress with speech development

Young child:
• Does not speak by 2 years of age
• Communicates needs through gestures
• Does not speak distinctly, as appropriate for his or her age
• Displays developmental (cognitive) delays
• Prefers solitary play
• Displays immature emotional behavior
• Does not respond to ringing of the telephone or doorbell
• Focuses on facial expressions when communicating

Older child:
• Often asks for statements to be repeated
• Is inattentive or daydreams
• Performs poorly at school
• Displays monotone or other abnormal speech
• Gives inappropriate answers to questions except when able to view face of speaker

At any age:
• Speaks loudly
• Sits very close to TV or radio or turns volume too loud
• Responds only to moderate or loud voices

Signs of hearing loss should be investigated as early as possible in order for appropriate communication intervention to begin.

Explore the child's current and past medical history for risk factors such as congenital anomalies, genetic syndrome, infection, family history, kernicterus, neonatal ventilator use, ototoxic medication, or exposure to excess noise. Note whether newborn hearing screening was done, along with the results.

Physical Examination and Laboratory and Diagnostic Tests

Determine the child's level of interaction with the environment. For preschoolers and older children, administer the whisper test, keeping in mind that this is a gross screening test only. Perform the Weber and Rinne tests (refer to Chapter 30 for further explanation). If further evaluation is needed, the nurse may be responsible for administering an otoacoustic emissions test or auditory brain stem evoked response test, either in the hospital or outpatient office.

Nursing Management

The primary goal of nursing care for the child with a hearing impairment is to provide education and support to the family and child. Individualize care for the child with a hearing impairment and the family based on their specific responses to the hearing impairment.

Augmenting Hearing

Compliance with hearing aids and communication curriculums is critical so that the child can develop hearing and speech. Hearing aids should be cleaned daily with a damp cloth. Batteries are usually changed weekly. When inserting the aid, the volume should be turned down, then adjusted to the appropriate level after insertion. As the infant or child grows, the hearing aid will need to be reassessed for proper fit. Many deaf schools and other organizations provide loaner hearing aids so that the best fit and amplification may be determined prior to purchase. Assist the family to explore this type of option in the local community. See Healthy People 2010.

When cochlear implants are used, the nurse focuses on postoperative care of the incision site and pain management.

Promoting Communication and Education

Families and children need to learn how to communicate effectively with one another. If the child learns American Sign Language, for instance, the parents and siblings should as well. Table 38.4 provides information on communication options for hearing-impaired children and their families. Communication may also be enhanced by the use of text telephone service in the home and closed-caption television. Bells and alarms in the home may use lights rather than sound to alert the child. Provide a sign language

HEALTHY PEOPLE 2010	
Objective	**Significance**
(Developmental) Increase access by persons who have hearing impairments to hearing rehabilitative services and adaptive devices, including hearing aids, cochlear implants, or tactile or other assistive or augmentative devices	• Know resources available in the local area for the deaf and hearing impaired. • Refer children with hearing deficits to these resources and to service providers for augmentative devices.

interpreter for the child at health care visits if the parent is not present for interpretation.

Encouraging Education

Refer the child less than 3 years of age to the local district of Early Intervention for case management of developmental needs. At 3 years of age and beyond, state laws provide for public education and related services for children with disabilities. An IEP should be developed to maximize the child's learning ability. Nurses may be involved in the development of the IEP.

Some children attend schools specifically geared toward deaf students. The choice of school will depend upon the family's preferences and resources.

Providing Support

The diagnosis of a significant disability can be extremely stressful for the family. Encourage families to express their feelings and provide emotional support. Ensure that the needs of any siblings are also attended to. When the family is ready, encourage them to network with other families

TABLE 38.4   **COMPARING COMMUNICATION OPTIONS FOR THE HEARING IMPAIRED**

Spoken Language Oral deaf education (auditory-verbal therapy)	Uses technology to boost auditory potential; teaches children to notice sound and give it meaning. Develops oral speech.
Cued speech	A system using hand signs to clarify lip-reading; gives the person clues about the sounds the speaker is making.
Signed Language American Sign Language (ASL)	Entirely communicated through hand signs, gestures, and facial expressions. Has its own grammar and syntax.
Combination: Total Communication	Combines auditory training and teaching of spoken language with SEE ("signing exact English"; corresponds to the words and syntax of English).
Augmentative and Alternative Communication (AAC) May use gestural communication	Can also include physical devices such as notebooks, communication boards, charts, or computers. Ranges from very low-tech to technologically complex.

BOX 38.5 **On-line Resources for Families of Children With Hearing Impairments**

- www.agbell.org: Alexander Graham Bell Association for the Deaf and Hard of Hearing—Wide range of programs and services, advocating independence through listening and talking
- www.asha.org: American Speech-Language-Hearing Association (ASHA)—Information, education, referrals, and resources for the hearing impaired
- www.audiology.org: American Academy of Audiology (AAA)—Education, referrals for audiologists, resources
- www.chs.ca: Canadian Hearing Society—Resources within Canada
- www.cuedspeech.org: National Cued Speech Association—Promotes and supports the effective use of cued speech
- www.entnet.org: American Academy of Otolaryngology–Head and Neck Surgery—Education and resources
- www.ihsinfo.org: International Hearing Society—Education, referrals, information on hearing aids
- www.jtc.org: John Tracy Clinic—Worldwide free service for families of preschool children with hearing loss
- www.lhh.org: League for the Hard of Hearing—Hearing rehabilitation and human services agency
- www.oraldeafed.org: Oral Deaf Education—Promotes spoken language use in the hearing impaired for effective communication

who have children with similar needs. Educate the family about the child's prescribed plan of care. Refer families to resources and support groups (Box 38.5).

■■■ Key Concepts

- Though hearing is fully developed at birth, visual development continues to progress until about age 7 years.
- The relatively short and horizontally positioned eustachian tubes of infants and young children make them more susceptible to otitis media than adults.
- Binocular vision develops by age 4 months; visual acuity progresses to 20/50 by age 3 years and usually reaches 20/20 by age 7 years.
- To maximize speech and language development, hearing loss should be identified early and intervention begun immediately.
- The corneal light reflex test and cover test are useful tools for identifying strabismus and amblyopia.
- Tympanometry is used to determine the presence of fluid behind the eardrum (such as with otitis media with effusion).
- Topical ophthalmic medications are used to treat certain infectious eye disorders.
- Systemic antibiotics are used for the treatment of periorbital cellulitis and acute otitis media.

- Very premature infants are at high risk of developing visual deficits related to retinopathy of prematurity and are also at increased risk of hearing impairment compared to other infants.
- Children with genetic syndromes or family history are at increased risk of visual and hearing impairments.
- Strabismus, glaucoma, and cataracts may all lead to visual impairment if left untreated.
- Recurrent or constant nasal congestion contributes to otitis media with effusion.
- Asymmetry of the corneal light reflex occurs with true strabismus.
- A cloudy cornea indicates the presence of cataract.
- Eye strain, eye rubbing, and headaches may indicate a visual deficit.
- Delay in language acquisition may occur when hearing loss is present.
- Appropriate hand washing is the single most important factor to reduce the spread of acute viral or bacterial conjunctivitis.
- Otitis externa can be prevented by keeping the ear canal dry and altering canal pH.
- Children with visual disorders should be encouraged to use prescribed corrective lenses.
- The child with hearing loss should receive early intervention with hearing aids or other augmentative devices.
- Hearing and/or vision impairment can significantly hinder developmental progress.
- The fluctuating hearing loss associated with recurrent otitis media and the hearing loss associated with chronic otitis media with effusion can both significantly hinder language development in the infant and toddler.
- Amblyopia must be identified early and treated with patching, corrective lenses, or surgery to prevent visual deterioration and promote appropriate vision development.

REFERENCES

American Academy of Family Physicians, American Academy of Otolaryngology–Head and Neck Surgery, and American Academy of Pediatrics Subcommittee on Otitis Media With Effusion. (2004). Clinical practice guideline: Otitis media with effusion. *Pediatrics, 113,* 1412–1429.

American Academy of Ophthalmology. (2007). *Summary recommendations for LASIK.* Retrieved December 18, 2007 from http://one.aao.org/CE/PracticeGuidelines/ClinicalStatements_Content.aspx?cid=1d8a8b79-4952-4140-9680-50bd53da3f55.

American Academy of Pediatrics. (2002). Use of photoscreening for children's vision screening. *Pediatrics, 109,* 524–525.

American Academy of Pediatrics. (2003). Eye examination in infants, children and young adults by pediatricians. *Pediatrics, 111,* 902–907.

American Academy of Pediatrics. (2006). Screening examination of premature infants for retinopathy of prematurity. *Pediatrics, 117,* 572–576.

American Academy of Pediatrics and American Academy of Family Physicians, Subcommittee on Management of Acute Otitis Media. (2004). Clinical practice guidelines: Diagnosis and management of acute otitis media. *Pediatrics, 113,* 1451–1465.

American Academy of Pediatrics, National Association of Pediatric Nurse Practitioners. (2006). *Universal newborn hearing screening, diagnosis, and intervention guidelines for pediatric medical home providers.* Cherry Hill, N.J.: National Association of Pediatric Nurse Practitioners.

American Association for Pediatric Ophthalmology and Strabismus (AAPOS). (2005). *Congenital nasolacrimal duct obstruction.* [electronic version] available at www.aapos.org.

American Speech-Language-Hearing Association. (2007). *Type, degree and configuration of hearing loss.* Retrieved March 28, 2007 from http://www.asha.org/public/hearing/disorders/types.htm.

Augsburger, J., & Asbury, T. (2008). Ocular and orbital trauma. In Riordan-Eva, P., & Whitcher, J. P., *Vaughan & Asbury's general ophthalmology* (17th ed.). New York: McGraw-Hill.

Block, S. (2005). Diagnosing acute otitis media: It's what you see, not what you hear. *Contemporary Pediatrics, Suppl.,* 3–8.

Bradley, R. (2007). Ear assessment for children and adolescents. *The Journal for Nurse Practitioners, 3*(2), 122–123.

Brady, M. T. (2005). Infectious disease in pediatric out-of-home child care. *American Journal of Infection Control, 33*(5), 276–285.

Brophy, M., Sinclair, S. A., Hostetler, G., & Xiang, H. (2006). Pediatric eye injury-related hospitalizations in the United States. *Pediatrics, 117* (6), 2267.

Brunnell, P. A., Wagner, R. S., Cuming, G. S., Dorfman, M. S., & Murphey, D. K. (2006). Bacterial conjunctivitis in children: Containing the infection. *Infectious Diseases in Children (Suppl.),* 2–19.

Byers, J. F. (2003). Developmental care and the evidence for their use in the NICU. *Maternal Child Nursing, 28*(3), 174–182.

Carlson, L. H. (2005). Otitis media: New information on an old disease. *Nurse Practitioner, 30*(3), 31–41.

Carlson, L. (2007). Inside and out: A review of otitis in children. *Advance for Nurse Practitioners, 15*(5), 51–58.

Casady, D. R., Meyer, D. R., Simon, J. W., Stasior, G. O., & Zobal-Ratner, J. L. (2006). Stepwise treatment paradigm for congenital nasolacrimal duct obstruction. *Ophthalmic Plastic and Reconstructive Surgery, 22*(4), 243–247.

Casey, J. R. (2005). Treatment of AOM post-PCV7: Judicious antibiotic therapy. *Contemporary Pediatrics (Suppl.),* 16–23.

Cook, K. A., & Walsh, M. (2005). *Otitis media.* [electronic version] Available at http://www.emedicine.com/emerg/topic351.htm.

Donaldson, J. D. (2006). Middle ear, acute otitis media, medical treatment. Retrieved December 18, 2007 from http://www.emedicine.com/ent/topic212.htm

Downey, D., & Hurtig, R. (2003). Augmentative and alternative communication. *Pediatric Annals, 32,* 467–474.

Dubowy, S. M. (2005). Vision screening of young children: Taking a second look. *Journal of the American Academy of Physician Assistants, 18*(8), 41–43, 47–49.

Goller, Y. (2006). Cochlear implantation in children: Implications for the primary care provider. *Journal of the American Academy of Nurse Practitioners, 18*(9), 397–408.

Hack, M., & Klein, N. (2006). Young adult attainments of premature infants. *Journal of the American Medical Association, 295*(6), 695–696.

Harrison, C. J. (2004). How will the new guideline for managing otitis media work for your practice? *Contemporary Pediatrics, 21*(6), 24–40.

Harrison, C. J. (2005). The microbiology of acute otitis media: Past, present, and future. *Contemporary Pediatrics (Suppl.),* 8–16.

Joint Committee on Infant Hearing. (2007). Year 2007 position statement: Principles and guidelines for early hearing detection and intervention programs. *Pediatrics, 120*(4), 898–921.

Kaye, C. I. and the Committee on Genetics. (2006). Newborn screening fact sheets. *Pediatrics, 118,* 934–963.

Lighthouse International. (2007). *Causes of blindness.* Retrieved December 18, 2007 from http://www.lighthouse.org/medical/causes-of-blindness/.

Montgomery, D. (2005). A new approach to treating acute otitis media. *Journal of Pediatric Health Care, 19*(1), 50–52.

National Center for Hearing Assessment and Management. (2007a). *EDHI legislation.* Retrieved December 18, 2007 from http://www.infanthearing.org/legislative/index.html.

National Center for Hearing Assessment and Management. (2007b). *Universal newborn hearing screening fact sheet.* Retrieved December 18, 2007 from http://www.infanthearing.org/resources/fact.pdf.

Office of Disease Prevention and Health Promotion. (2000). Chapter 28, vision and hearing. Retrieved December 18, 2007 from http://healthypeople.gov/Document/pdf/Volume2/28Vision.pdf.

Optometrists Network. (2006). *Strabismus.* Retrieved March 28, 2007 from http://www.strabismus.org/.

Randleman, J. B., & Sachdeva, D. (2005). *Chemical eye burns.* Retrieved October 24 2005 from http://www.emedicinehealth.com/chemical_eye_burns/article_em.htm.

Rosenthal, M. (2005). Achieve eradication, rather than clinical cure when treating AOM. *Infectious Diseases in Children, 18*(11), 57–58.

Sadovsky, R. (2003). Distinguishing periorbital from orbital cellulitis. *American Family Physician, 67*(6), 1349, 1353.

Sands, R., & Drack, A. (2007). Eye. In W. W. Hay, M. J. Levin, J. M. Sondheimer, & R. R. Deterding (Eds.), *Current pediatric diagnosis and treatment* (18th ed.) New York: McGraw-Hill.

St. Lukes Cataract and Laser Institute. (2006). *Eye conditions: do you know how to treat a chemical burn?* Retrieved June 24, 2006 from http://www.stlukeseye.com/conditions/chemicalburn.asp.

Wagner, R. S. (2005). Treating pediatric conjunctivitis: A pediatric ophthalmologist's perspective. *Infectious Diseases in Children, 18*(10), 5.

Walling, A. D. (2005). Selecting a topical treatment for seasonal allergic conjunctivitis. *American Family Physician, 71*(7), 1409.

Watkinson, S., & Graham, S. (2005). Visual impairment in children. *Nursing Standard, 19*(51), 58–65.

Westerfeld, C. B., & Kazlas, M. (2007). Pediatric conjunctivitis. *Contemporary Ophthalmology, 6*(3), 1–5.

WEBSITES

American Association of Pediatric Ophthalmology and Strabismus: www.aapos.org

American Council of the Blind (goal is to improve the well-being of all blind and visually impaired people): www.acb.org

Alexander Graham Bell Association for the Deaf and Hard of Hearing: www.agbell.org

American Optometric Association: www.aoa.org

American Speech-Language-Hearing Association (ASHA): www.asha.org

American Academy of Audiology (AAA): www.audiology.com

A division of Helen Keller Worldwide: www.childsight.org

Canadian Hearing Society: www.chs.ca

Canadian National Institute: www.cnib.ca

Marion Downs National Center for Infant Hearing: www.colorado.edu/slhs/mdnc

Delta Gamma Center for Children with Visual Impairments: www.dgckids.org

American Academy of Otolaryngology–Head and Neck Surgery: www.entnet.org

Helen Keller Services for the Blind (helping blind and visually impaired persons to develop independence): www.helenkeller.org

Helen Keller Worldwide: www.hkworld.org

International Council for Education of People with Visual Impairments: www.icevi.org

International Hearing Society: www.ihsinfo.org

National Center for Hearing Assessment and Management: www.infanthearing.org

Jewish Braille International (provides a wide variety of Braille books and magazines): www.jewishbraille.org/

John Tracy Clinic: www.johntracyclinic.org

League for the Hard of Hearing: www.lhh.org

Lighthouse International: www.lighthouse.org

National Eye Institute, a division of the National Institutes of Health: www.nei.nih.gov/

National Federation of the Blind: www.nfb.org

National Information Center for Children and Youth with Disabilities: www.nfb.org

American Nystagmus Network, Inc.: www.nystagmus.org/

Oral Deaf Education: www.oraldeafed.org

Pediatric Glaucoma and Cataract Family Association (Canada): www.pgcfa.org/

Prevent Blindness America: www.preventblindness.org

Association for Retinopathy of Prematurity and Related Diseases: www.ropard.org

Research to Prevent Blindness: www.rpbusa.org

National Association for Parents of Children with Visual Impairments: www.spedex.com.napri

Vision 2020, The Right to Sight: www.v2020.org

CHAPTER WORKSHEET

MULTIPLE CHOICE QUESTIONS

1. Which situation would cause the nurse to become concerned about possible hearing loss?

   a. A 12-month-old who babbles incessantly, making no sense

   b. An 8-month-old who says only "da"

   c. A 3-month-old who startles easily to sound

   d. A 3-year-old who drops the letter "s"

2. A 4-year-old complains of extreme pain when the tragus is touched. Though not diagnostic, this sign is most indicative of which disorder?

   a. Acute otitis media

   b. Acute tympanic effusion

   c. Otitis interna

   d. Otitis externa

3. The nurse is caring for an infant who has undergone surgery for infantile glaucoma. What is the priority nursing intervention?

   a. Place the child prone postoperatively for comfort.

   b. Teach the family use of the contact lens.

   c. Place elbow restraints on the infant.

   d. Provide a mobile for optical stimulation.

4. A 2-year-old has been prescribed eye patching for strabismus 6 hours per day. What teaching does the nurse provide for the mother?

   a. Try to patch 6 hours per day, but if you miss some it is OK.

   b. Patching is necessary to strengthen vision in the weaker eye.

   c. Patching will keep the eye from turning in.

   d. Since the child is so young, patching can be delayed until school age.

CRITICAL THINKING EXERCISES

1. A 16-month-old toddler is being seen for his sixth ear infection. What particular information about his growth and development must the nurse ask about? Be specific about the questions you would ask.

2. How would you distinguish allergic conjunctivitis from acute bacterial conjunctivitis?

3. A 13-month-old has been diagnosed with severe visual impairment. Develop a list of sample nursing diagnoses for this situation.

STUDY ACTIVITIES

1. Develop a sample plan for teaching a low-literacy parent about the etiology, treatment, and complications of recurrent acute otitis media.

2. While in the pediatric clinical setting, compare the play styles of a sighted child with those of a visually impaired child.

3. Research hearing and vision resources in your local community.

NURSING CARE OF THE CHILD WITH A RESPIRATORY DISORDER

KEY TERMS

atelectasis
atopy
clubbing
coryza
cyanosis
expiration
hypoxemia
hypoxia
infiltrate

inspiration
laryngitis
oxygenation
pharyngitis
pulmonary
pulse oximetry
rales
retractions
rhinitis

rhinorrhea
stridor
subglottic stenosis
suctioning
tachypnea
tracheostomy
ventilation
wheeze
work of breathing

LEARNING OBJECTIVES

Upon completion of the chapter, the learner will be able to:

1. Discuss how the anatomy and physiology of the respiratory system in children differs from that of adults.
2. Identify various factors associated with respiratory illness in infants and children.
3. Discuss common laboratory and other diagnostic tests useful in the diagnosis of respiratory conditions.
4. Discuss common medications and other treatments used for treatment and palliation of respiratory conditions.
5. Recognize risk factors associated with various respiratory disorders.
6. Distinguish different respiratory illnesses based on their signs and symptoms.
7. Discuss nursing interventions commonly used for respiratory illnesses.
8. Devise an individualized nursing care plan for the child with a respiratory disorder.
9. Develop client/family teaching plans for the child with a respiratory disorder.
10. Describe the psychosocial impact of chronic respiratory disorders on children.

Alexander Roberts, 4 months old, is brought to the clinic by his mother. He has a cold and has been coughing a great deal for 2 days. Today he has had difficulty taking his bottle and is breathing very quickly. Mrs. Roberts says he seems tired.

Wow

Restoring a full breath allows a child to participate fully in life's adventures.

Respiratory disorders are the most common causes of illness and hospitalization in children. These illnesses range from mild, non-acute disorders (such as the common cold or sore throat) to serious life-threatening conditions (such as epiglottitis). Chronic disorders, such as allergic rhinitis or asthma, can affect quality of life, but frequent acute or recurrent infections also can interfere significantly with the well-being of some children.

Respiratory infections account for the majority of acute illnesses in children. The child's age and living conditions as well as the season of the year can influence the development of respiratory disorders in addition to the course of illness. For example, low-income children have a higher risk for increased severity or increased frequency of disease. Infants and younger children are more likely to deteriorate quickly from a respiratory illness. Certain viruses are more prevalent in the winter, whereas allergen-related respiratory diseases are more prevalent in the spring and fall. Children with chronic illness such as diabetes, congenital heart disease, sickle cell anemia, and cystic fibrosis and children with developmental disorders such as cerebral palsy tend to be more severely affected with respiratory disorders. Parents may have difficulty determining the severity of their child's condition and might either seek care very early in the course of the illness (when it is still very mild) or wait and present to the health care setting when the child is very ill.

Nurses must be familiar with respiratory conditions affecting children so that they can provide guidance and support to families. When children become ill, families often encounter nurses in outpatient settings first. Nurses must be able to ask questions that can help establish the severity of the child's illness and determine whether they must seek care at a health facility. Since respiratory illnesses account for the majority of pediatric admissions to general hospitals, nurses caring for children need to have expert assessment and intervention skills in this area. Detection of worsening respiratory status early in the course of deterioration allows for timely treatment and the chance to prevent a minor problem from becoming a critical illness.

Difficulty with breathing can be very frightening for both the child and parents. The child and the family need the nurse's support throughout a respiratory illness. Nurses are also in the unique position of being able to reduce the burden of respiratory illness in children by identifying these illnesses early, providing education about them, and promoting prevention efforts.

Variations in Pediatric Anatomy and Physiology

Respiratory conditions often affect both the upper and lower respiratory tract, though some affect primarily one or the other. Respiratory dysfunction in children tends to be more severe than in adults, and several differences in

HEALTHY PEOPLE 2010

Objective	Significance
Reduce hospitalization rates for three ambulatory-care-sensitive conditions: pediatric asthma and immunization-preventable pneumonia and influenza.	• Appropriately educate children with asthma and their families about the ongoing management of asthma. • Encourage pneumococcal and influenza vaccinations per recommendations.

the infant's or child's respiratory system account for this increased severity.

Nose

Newborns are obligatory nose breathers until at least 4 weeks of age. The young infant cannot automatically open his or her mouth to breathe if the nose is obstructed. The nares must be patent for breathing to be successful while feeding. Newborns breathe through their mouths only while crying.

The upper respiratory mucus serves as a cleansing agent, yet newborns produce very little mucus, making them more susceptible to infection. However, the newborn and young infant may have very small nasal passages, so when excess mucus is present, airway obstruction is more likely.

Infants are born with maxillary and ethmoid sinuses present. The frontal sinuses (most often associated with sinus infection) and the sphenoid sinuses develop by age 6 to 8 years, so younger children are less apt to acquire sinus infections than are adults.

Throat

The tongue of the infant relative to the oropharynx is larger than in adults. Posterior displacement of the tongue can quickly lead to severe airway obstruction. Through early school age, children tend to have enlarged tonsillar and adenoidal tissue even in the absence of illness. This can contribute to an increased incidence of airway obstruction.

Trachea

The airway lumen is smaller in infants and children than in adults. The infant's trachea is approximately 4 mm wide compared with the adult width of 20 mm. When edema, mucus, or bronchospasm is present, the capacity for air passage is greatly diminished. A small reduction in the diameter of a child's airway can significantly increase resistance to airflow, leading to increased **work of breathing** (Fig. 39.1).

In teenagers and adults the larynx is cylindrical and fairly uniform in width. In infants and children less than 10 years old, the cricoid cartilage is underdeveloped, resulting in laryngeal narrowing. Thus, in infants and children, the larynx is funnel-shaped. When any portion of

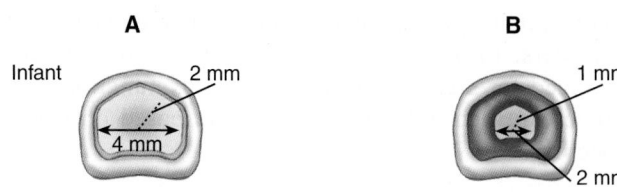

1 mm circumferential edema causes 50% reduction of diameter and radius, increasing pulmonary resistance by a factor of 16.

1 mm circumferential edema causes 20% reduction of diameter and radius, increasing pulmonary resistance by a factor of 2.4.

FIGURE 39.1 (**A**) Note the smaller diameter of the child's airway under normal circumstances. (**B**) With 1 cm of edema present, note the exponential decrease in airway lumen diameter as compared with the adult.

the airway is narrowed, further narrowing from mucus or edema will result in an exponential increase in resistance to airflow and work of breathing. In infants and children, the larynx and glottis are located higher in the neck, increasing the chance of aspiration of foreign material into the lower airways. Congenital laryngomalacia occurs in some infants and results in the laryngeal structure being weaker than normal, yielding greater collapse on **inspiration**. Box 39.1 discusses congenital laryngomalacia.

The child's airway is highly compliant, making it quite susceptible to dynamic collapse in the presence of airway

BOX 39.1 **Congenital Laryngomalacia**

- Inspiratory stridor is present and is intensified with certain positions.
- Suprasternal retractions may be present, but the infant exhibits no other signs of respiratory distress.
- Congenital laryngomalacia is generally a benign condition that improves as the cartilage in the larynx matures. It usually disappears by age 1 year.
- The crowing noise heard with breathing can make parents very anxious. Reassure parents that the condition will improve with time.
- Parents become very familiar with the "normal" sound their infant makes and are often able to identify intensification or change in the stridor. Airway obstruction may occur earlier in infants with this condition, so intensification of stridor or symptoms of respiratory illness should be evaluated early by the primary care provider.

obstruction. The muscles supporting the airway are less functional than those in the adult. Children have a large amount of soft tissue surrounding the trachea, and the mucous membranes lining the airway are less securely attached compared with adults. This increases the risk for airway edema and obstruction. Upper airway obstruction resulting from a foreign body, croup, or epiglottitis can result in tracheal collapse during inspiration.

Lower Respiratory Structures

The bifurcation of the trachea occurs at the level of the third thoracic vertebra in children, compared to the level of the sixth thoracic vertebra in adults. This anatomic difference is important when suctioning children and when endotracheal intubation is required (see Chapter 52 for further discussion). This difference in placement also contributes to risk for aspiration. The bronchi and bronchioles of infants and children are also narrower in diameter than the adult's, placing them at increased risk for lower airway obstruction (see Fig. 39.1). Lower airway obstruction during exhalation often results from bronchiolitis or asthma or is caused by foreign body aspiration into the lower airway.

Alveoli develop at approximately 24 weeks' gestation. Term infants are born with about 50 million alveoli. After birth, alveolar growth slows until 3 months of age and then progresses until the child reaches 7 or 8 years of age, at which time the alveoli reach the adult number of around 300 million. Alveoli make up most of the lung tissue and are the major sites for gas exchange. Oxygen moves from the alveolar air to the blood, while carbon dioxide moves from the blood into the alveolar air. Smaller numbers of alveoli, particularly in the premature and/or young infant, place the child at a higher risk of **hypoxemia** and carbon dioxide retention.

Chest Wall

In older children and adults the ribs and sternum support the lungs and help keep them well expanded. The movement of the diaphragm and intercostal muscles alters volume and pressure within the chest cavity, resulting in air movement into the lungs. Infants' chest walls are highly compliant (pliable) and fail to support the lungs adequately. Functional residual capacity can be greatly reduced if respiratory effort is diminished. This lack of lung support also makes the tidal volume of infants and toddlers almost completely dependent upon movement of the diaphragm. If diaphragm movement is impaired (as in states of hyperinflation such as asthma), the intercostal muscles cannot lift the chest wall and respiration is further compromised.

Metabolic Rate and Oxygen Need

Children have a significantly higher metabolic rate than adults. Their resting respiratory rates are faster and their demand for oxygen is higher. Adult oxygen consumption is 3 to 4 liters per minute, while infants consume 6 to 8 liters per minute. In any situation of respiratory distress, infants and children will develop hypoxemia more rapidly than adults. This may be attributed not only to the child's increased oxygen requirement but also to the effect that certain conditions have on the oxyhemoglobin dissociation curve.

Normal oxygen transport relies upon binding of oxygen to hemoglobin in areas of high pO_2 (pulmonary arterial beds) and release of oxygen from hemoglobin when the partial pressure of oxygen (pO_2) is low (peripheral tissues). Normally, a pO_2 of 95 mm Hg results in an oxygen saturation of 97%. A decrease in oxygen saturation results in a disproportionate (much larger) decrease in pO_2 (Fig. 39.2). Thus, a small decrease in oxygen saturation reflects a larger decrease in pO_2. Conditions such as alkalosis, hypothermia, hypocarbia, anemia, and fetal hemoglobin cause oxygen to become more tightly bound to hemoglobin, resulting in the curve shifting to the left. Common pediatric conditions such as acidosis, hyperthermia, and hypercarbia cause hemoglobin to decrease its affinity for oxygen, further shifting the curve to the right.

Common Medical Treatments

A variety of interventions are used to treat respiratory illness in children. The treatments listed in Common Medical Treatments 39.1 and Drug Guide 39.1 usually require a physician's order when a child is hospitalized.

NURSING PROCESS OVERVIEW FOR THE CHILD WITH A RESPIRATORY DISORDER

Care of the child with a respiratory disorder includes assessment, nursing diagnosis, planning, interventions, and evaluation. There are a number of general concepts related to the nursing process that can be applied to respiratory disorders. From a general understanding of the care involved for a child with respiratory dysfunction, the nurse can then individualize the care based on client specifics.

Assessment

Assessment of respiratory dysfunction in children includes health history, physical examination, and laboratory or diagnostic testing.

*R*emember Alexander, the 4-month-old with the cold, cough, fatigue, feeding difficulty, and fast breathing? What additional health history and physical examination assessment information should the nurse obtain?

Health History

The health history comprises past medical history, family history, and history of present illness (when the symptoms started and how they have progressed) as well as treatments used at home. The past medical history might be significant for recurrent colds or sore throats, **atopy** (such as asthma or atopic dermatitis), prematurity, respiratory dysfunction at birth, poor weight gain, or history of recurrent respiratory illnesses or chronic lung disease. Family history might be significant for chronic respiratory disorders such as asthma or might reveal contacts for infectious exposure. When eliciting the history of the present illness, inquire about onset and progression, fever, nasal congestion, noisy breathing, presence and description of cough, rapid respirations, increased work of breathing, ear, nose, sinus, or throat pain, ear pulling, headache, vomiting with coughing, poor feeding, and lethargy. Also inquire about exposure to second-hand smoke. Children exposed to environmental smoke have an increased incidence of respiratory illnesses such as asthma, bronchitis, and pneumonia (Sheahan & Free, 2005).

Physical Examination

Physical examination of the respiratory system includes inspection and observation, auscultation, percussion, and palpation.

Inspection and Observation

Color. Observe the child's color, noting pallor or cyanosis (circumoral or central). Pallor (pale appearance) occurs as a result of peripheral vasoconstriction in an effort to conserve oxygen for vital functions. **Cyanosis** (a bluish tinge to the skin) occurs as a result of **hypoxia**. It might first present circumorally (just around the mouth) and progress to central cyanosis. Newborns might have blue hands and feet (acrocyanosis), a normal finding. The infant might have pale hands and feet when cold or when ill, as peripheral circulation is not well developed in early

FIGURE 39.2 Normal hemoglobin dissociation curve (*green*), shift to the right (*red*), and shift to the left (*black*).

COMMON MEDICAL TREATMENTS 39.1   RESPIRATORY DISORDERS

Treatment	Explanation	Indications	Nursing Implications
Oxygen	Supplemented via mask, nasal cannula, hood, or tent or via endotracheal or nasotracheal tube	Hypoxemia, respiratory distress	Monitor response via work of breathing and pulse oximetry.
High humidity	Addition of moisture to inspired air	Common cold, croup, tonsillectomy	Infant may require extra blankets with cool mist, and frequent changes of bedclothes under oxygen hood or tent as they become damp.
Suctioning	Removal of secretions via bulb syringe or suction catheter	Excessive airway secretions (common cold, flu, bronchiolitis, pertussis)	Should be done carefully and only as far as recommended for age or tracheostomy tube size, or until cough or gag occurs.
Chest physiotherapy (CPT) and postural drainage	Promotes mucus clearance by mobilizing secretions with the assistance of percussion or vibration accompanied by postural drainage	Bronchiolitis, pneumonia, cystic fibrosis, or other conditions resulting in increased mucus production. Not effective in inflammatory conditions without increased mucus.	May be performed by respiratory therapist in some institutions, by nurses in others. In either case, nurses must be familiar with the technique and able to educate families on its use.
Saline gargles	Relieves throat pain via salt water gargle	Pharyngitis, tonsillitis	Recommended for children old enough to understand the concept of gargling (to avoid choking)
Saline lavage	Normal saline introduced into the airway, followed by suctioning	Common cold, flu, bronchiolitis, any condition resulting in increased mucus production in the upper airway	Very helpful for loosening thick mucus; child may need to be in semi-upright position to avoid aspiration
Chest tube	Insertion of a drainage tube into the pleural cavity to facilitate removal of air or fluid and allow full lung expansion	Pneumothorax, empyema	Should tube become dislodged from container, the chest tube must be clamped immediately to avoid further air entry into the chest cavity.
Bronchoscopy	Introduction of a bronchoscope into the bronchial tree for diagnostic purposes. Also allows for bronchiolar lavage.	Removal of foreign body, cleansing of bronchial tree	Watch for postprocedure airway swelling, complaints of sore throat.

infancy. It is important, then, to note if the cyanosis is central (involving the midline), as this is a true sign of hypoxia. Children with low red blood cell counts might not demonstrate cyanosis as early in the course of hypoxemia as children with normal hemoglobin levels. Therefore, absence of cyanosis or the degree of cyanosis present is not always an accurate indication of the severity of respiratory involvement.

Note the rate and depth of respiration as well as work of breathing. Often the first sign of respiratory illness in infants and children is **tachypnea**.

▶ *Take NOTE!*

A slow or irregular respiratory rate in an acutely ill infant or child is an ominous sign. See Chapter 52.

Nose and Oral Cavity. Inspect the nose and oral cavity. Note nasal drainage and redness or swelling in the nose. Note the color of the pharynx, presence of exudate,

DRUG GUIDE 39.1 COMMON DRUGS FOR RESPIRATORY DISORDERS

Medication	Action/Indications	Nursing Implications
Expectorant (guaifenesin)	Reduces viscosity of thickened secretions by increasing respiratory tract fluid Used for the common cold, pneumonia, and other conditions requiring mobilization and subsequent expectoration of mucus	Encourage deep breathing before coughing in order to mobilize secretions. Maintain adequate fluid intake. Assess breath sounds frequently.
Cough suppressants (dextromethorphan, codeine, hydrocodone)	Relieves irritating, nonproductive cough by direct effect on the cough center in the medulla, which suppresses the cough reflex Used for the common cold, sinusitis, pneumonia, bronchitis	Should be used only with nonproductive coughs in the absence of wheezing
Antihistamines	Treatment of allergic conditions such as allergic rhinitis, asthma	May cause drowsiness or dry mouth
Antibiotics (oral, parenteral)	Treatment of bacterial infections of the respiratory tract such as pharyngitis, tonsillitis, sinusitis, bacterial pneumonia, cystic fibrosis, empyema, abscess, tuberculosis	Check for antibiotic allergies. Should be given as prescribed for the length of time prescribed.
Antibiotics (inhaled)	Treatment of bacterial infections of the respiratory tract in children with cystic fibrosis	Can be given via nebulizer
Beta2-adrenergic agonists (short-acting) (i.e., albuterol, levalbuterol)	Relax airway smooth muscle, resulting in bronchodilation Used for acute and chronic treatment of wheezing and bronchospasm in asthma, bronchiolitis, cystic fibrosis, chronic lung disease. Also used to prevent wheezing in exercise-induced asthma.	May be administered orally or via inhalation Can be used for acute relief of bronchospasm May cause nervousness, tachycardia, and jitteriness Inhaled agents result in fewer systemic side effects.
Beta2-adrenergic agonists (long-acting) (i.e., salmeterol)	Long-acting bronchodilator used in chronic asthma management and for prevention of exercise-induced asthma Long-term control in chronic asthma Prevention of exercise-induced asthma	Administered via inhalation Used only for long-term control or for exercise-induced asthma. Not for relief of bronchospasm in an acute wheezing episode.
Racemic epinephrine	Produces bronchodilation Indicated for croup	Assess lung sounds and work of breathing. Observe for rebound bronchospasm.
Anticholinergic (ipratropium)	Produces bronchodilation in asthma or chronic lung disease	In children, generally used as an adjunct to beta2-adrenergic agonists for treatment of bronchospasm
Antiviral agents (amantadine, rimantadine, zanamivir, oseltamivir)	Treatment and prevention of influenza A	Amantadine, rimantadine: Monitor for confusion, nervousness, and jitteriness. Zanamivir, oseltamivir: Well tolerated but expensive
Virazole (Ribavirin)	Treatment of severe lower respiratory tract infection with RSV, usually reserved for ventilated clients	Administer via aerosol with the small-particle aerosol generator (SPAG). Suction patients on assisted ventilation every 2 hours; monitor pulmonary pressures every 2 to 4 hours. May cause blurred vision and photosensitivity.
Corticosteroids (inhaled)	Exert a potent, locally acting anti-inflammatory effect to decrease the frequency and severity of asthma attacks. May also delay pulmonary damage that occurs with chronic asthma. Also used for chronic lung disease and croup syndromes.	Not for treatment of acute wheezing Rinse mouth after inhalation to decrease incidence of fungal infections, dry mouth, and hoarseness. Minimal systemic absorption makes inhaled steroids the treatment of choice for asthma maintenance program.

Medication	Action/Indications	Nursing Implications
Corticosteroids (oral, parenteral)	Suppress inflammation and normal immune response Used for acute asthma exacerbations, wheezing with chronic lung disease, and severe croup	May cause hyperglycemia May suppress reaction to allergy tests Consult physician if vaccinations are ordered during course of systemic corticosteroid therapy. Short courses of therapy are generally safe. Very effective, but long-term or chronic use can result in peptic ulceration, altered growth, and numerous other side effects. Children on long-term dosing should have growth assessed.
Decongestants (e.g., pseudephedrine)	Treatment of runny or stuffy nose associated with the common cold, sinusitis, or allergic rhinitis in children over age 6	Assess child periodically for nasal congestion. Some children react to decongestants with excessive sleepiness or increased activity.
Leukotriene receptor antagonists (montelukast, zafirlukast, zileuton)	Decrease inflammatory response by antagonizing the effects of leukotrienes to control asthma in children age 1 year and older Montelukast: for allergic rhinitis in children 6 months and older	Given once daily, in the evening Not for relief of bronchospasm during an acute wheezing episode, but may be continued during the episode
Mast-cell stabilizers (cromolyn, nedocromil)	Prevent release of histamine from sensitized mast cells, resulting in decreased frequency and intensity of allergic reactions in children with asthma or chronic lung disease. Also used as pre-exposure treatment for allergens.	Administered via inhalation For prophylactic use, not to relieve bronchospasm during an acute wheezing episode. Can be used 10 to 15 minutes prior to exposure to allergen, to decrease reaction to allergen.
Methylxanthines (theophylline, aminophylline)	To provide for continuous airway relaxation in moderate or severe asthma in order to achieve long-term control Also indicated for apnea of prematurity (see "Caffeine")	Administered orally or intravenously. Sustained-release oral preparation can be used to prevent nocturnal symptoms. Monitor drug levels routinely. Report signs of toxicity immediately: tachycardia, nausea, vomiting, diarrhea, stomach cramps, anorexia, confusion, headache, restlessness, flushing, increased urination, seizures, arrhythmias, insomnia.
Caffeine	Stimulates the respiratory center in infants with apnea of prematurity	See "Methylxanthines."
Pulmozyme (dornase alfa)	Enzyme that hydrolyzes the DNA in sputum, reducing sputum viscosity in children with cystic fibrosis	Administered via nebulizer Monitor for dysphonia and pharyngitis.
Synagis (palivizumab)	Monoclonal antibody used to prevent serious lower respiratory RSV disease in certain high-risk groups of children	Should be administered monthly during the RSV season Given intramuscularly only

HEALTHY PEOPLE 2010	
Objective	**Significance**
Reduce the proportion of children who are regularly exposed to tobacco smoke at home.	• Educate the family about the effects that passive smoking has on children. • Encourage families to join smoking cessation programs.

tonsil size and status, and presence of lesions anywhere in the oral cavity.

Cough and Other Airway Noises. Note the sound of the cough. (Is it wet, productive, dry and hacking, tight? When does the cough occur? Is it only or mainly at night?) If noises associated with breathing are present (grunting, stridor, or audible wheeze) these should also be noted. Grunting occurs on **expiration** and is produced by prema-

FIGURE 39.3 Location of retractions.

Suprasternal notch
(Suprasternal retractions)

Xiphoid area
(Suprasternal retractions)

Ribs
(Intercostal
retractions)

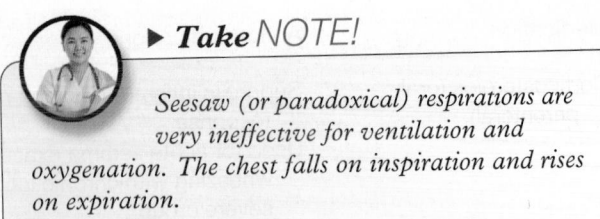

► **Take** NOTE!

Seesaw (or paradoxical) respirations are very ineffective for ventilation and oxygenation. The chest falls on inspiration and rises on expiration.

ture glottic closure. It is an attempt to preserve or increase functional residual capacity. Grunting might occur with alveolar collapse or loss of lung volume, such as in atelectasis, pneumonia, and pulmonary edema. **Stridor**, a high-pitched, readily audible inspiratory noise, is a sign of upper airway obstruction. Sometimes wheezes can be heard with the naked ear; these are referred to as audible wheezes.

Respiratory Effort. Assess respiratory effort for depth and quality. Is breathing labored? Infants and children with significant nasal congestion may have tachypnea, which usually resolves when the nose is cleared of mucus. Mouth breathing also may occur when a large amount of nasal congestion is present. Increased work of breathing, particularly if associated with restlessness and anxiety, usually indicates lower respiratory involvement. Assess for the presence of nasal flaring, retractions, or head bobbing. Nasal flaring can occur early in the course of respiratory illness and is an effort to inhale greater amounts of oxygen.

Retractions (the inward pulling of soft tissues with respiration) can occur in the intercostal, subcostal, substernal, supraclavicular, or suprasternal regions (Fig. 39.3). Document the severity of the retractions: mild, moderate, or severe. Also note the use of accessory neck muscles. Note the presence of paradoxical breathing (lack of simultaneous chest and abdominal rise with the inspiratory phase; Fig. 39.4). Bobbing of the head with each breath is also a sign of increased respiratory effort.

Anxiety and Restlessness. Is the child anxious or restless? Restlessness, irritability, and anxiety result from difficulty in securing adequate oxygen. These might be very early signs of respiratory distress, especially if accompanied by tachypnea. Restlessness might progress to listlessness and lethargy if the respiratory dysfunction is not corrected.

Clubbing. Inspect the fingertips for the presence of **clubbing**, an enlargement of the terminal phalanx of the finger, resulting in a change in the angle of the nail to the fingertip (Fig. 39.5). Clubbing might occur in children with a chronic respiratory illness. It is the result of increased capillary growth as the body attempts to supply more oxygen to distal body cells.

Hydration Status. Note the child's hydration status. The child with a respiratory illness is at risk for dehydration. Pain related to sore throat or mouth lesions may prevent the child from drinking properly. Nasal congestion interferes with the infant's ability to suck effectively at the breast or bottle. Tachypnea and increased work of breathing interfere with the ability to safely ingest fluids.

Assess the oral mucosa for color and moisture. Note skin turgor, presence of tears, and adequacy of urine output.

Auscultation

Assess lung sounds via auscultation. Evaluate breath sounds over the anterior and posterior chest, as well as in the axillary areas. Note the adequacy of aeration. Breath sounds should be equal bilaterally. The intensity and pitch should be equal throughout the lungs; document diminished breath sounds. In the absence of concurrent lower respiratory illness, the breath sounds should be clear throughout all lung fields. During normal respiration, the inspiratory phase is usually softer and longer than the expiratory phase. Prolonged expiration is a sign of bronchial

Synchronized respirations

Lag on respirations

Seesaw respirations

FIGURE 39.4 Seesaw respirations.

FIGURE 39.5 (**A**) Normal fingertip. Early clubbing (**B**) may progress eventually to advanced clubbing (**C**) as a result of chronic hypoxemia.

or bronchiolar obstruction. Bronchiolitis, asthma, pulmonary edema, and an intrathoracic foreign body can cause prolonged expiratory phases.

Infants and young children have thin chest walls. When the upper airway is congested (as in a severe cold), the noise produced in the upper airway might be transmitted throughout the lung fields. When upper airway congestion is transmitted to the lung fields, the congested-sounding noise heard over the trachea is the same type of noise heard over the lungs but is much louder and more intense. To ascertain if these sounds are truly adventitious lung sounds or if they are transmitted from the upper airway, auscultate again after the child coughs or his or her nose has been suctioned. Another way to discern the difference is to compare auscultatory findings over the trachea to the lung fields to determine if the abnormal sound is truly from within the lung or is actually a sound transmitted from the upper airway.

Note adventitious sounds heard on auscultation. Wheezing, a high-pitched sound that usually occurs on expiration, results from obstruction in the lower trachea or bronchioles. Wheezing that clears with coughing is most likely a result of secretions in the lower trachea. Wheezing resulting from obstruction of the bronchioles, as in bronchiolitis, asthma, chronic lung disease, or cystic fibrosis, does not clear with coughing. **Rales** (crackling sounds) result when the alveoli become fluid-filled, such as in pneumonia. Note the location of the adventitious sounds as well as the timing (on inspiration, expiration, or both). Tachycardia might also be present. An increase in heart rate often initially accompanies hypoxemia.

Percussion

When percussing, note sounds that are not resonant in nature. Flat or dull sounds might be percussed over partially consolidated lung tissue, as in pneumonia. Tympany might be percussed with a pneumothorax. Note the presence of hyperresonance (as might be apparent with asthma).

Palpation

Palpate the sinuses for tenderness in the older child. Assess for enlargement or tenderness of the lymph nodes of the head and neck. Document alterations in tactile fremitus detected on palpation. Increased tactile fremitus might occur in a case of pneumonia or pleural effusion. Fremitus might be decreased in the case of barrel chest, as with cystic fibrosis. Absent fremitus might be noted with pneumothorax or atelectasis.

Compare central and peripheral pulses. Note the quality of the pulse as well as the rate. With significant respiratory distress, perfusion often becomes compromised. Poor perfusion might be reflected in weaker peripheral pulses (radial, pedal) when compared to central pulses.

Laboratory and Diagnostic Testing

Common Laboratory and Diagnostic Tests 39.1 explains the laboratory and diagnostic tests most commonly used for a child with a respiratory disorder. The tests can assist the physician in diagnosing the disorder and/or be used as guidelines in determining ongoing treatment. Laboratory or non-nursing personnel obtain some of the tests, while the nurse might obtain others. In either instance the nurse should be familiar with how the tests are obtained, what they are used for, and normal versus abnormal results. This knowledge will also be necessary when providing client and family education related to the testing.

▶ *Take* NOTE!

Ambient light may interfere with pulse oximetry readings. When the pulse oximeter probe is placed on the infant's foot or the young child's toe, covering the probe and foot with a sock may help to ensure an accurate measurement.

Nursing Diagnoses, Goals, Interventions, and Evaluation

Upon completion of a thorough assessment, the nurse might identify several nursing diagnoses, including:

- Ineffective Airway Clearance
- Ineffective Breathing Pattern
- Impaired Gas Exchange
- Risk for Infection
- Pain
- Risk for Fluid Volume Deficit
- Altered Nutrition, less than body requirements
- Activity Intolerance
- Fear
- Altered Family Processes

(text continues on page 1230)

Test	Explanation	Indications	Nursing Implications
Allergy skin testing	Suggested allergen is applied to skin via scratch, pin, or prick. A wheal response indicates allergy to the substance. Carries risk of anaphylaxis. (Nursing note: Antihistamines must be discontinued before testing, as they inhibit the test.)	Allergic rhinitis, asthma	Close observation for anaphylaxis is necessary. Epinephrine and emergency equipment should be readily available. Some children react to the skin test almost immediately; others take several minutes.
Arterial blood gases	Invasive method (requires blood sampling) of measuring arterial pH, partial pressure of oxygen and carbon dioxide, and base excess in blood	Usually reserved for severe illness, the intubated child, or suspected carbon dioxide retention	Hold pressure for several minutes after a peripheral arterial stick to avoid bleeding. Radial arterial sticks are common and can be very painful. Note if the child is crying excessively during the blood draw, as this affects the carbon dioxide level.
Chest x-ray	Radiographic image of the expanded lungs: can show hyperinflation, atelectasis, pneumonia, foreign body, pleural effusion, abnormal heart or lung size	Bronchiolitis, pneumonia, tuberculosis, asthma, cystic fibrosis, bronchopulmonary dysplasia	Children may be afraid of the x-ray equipment. If a parent or familiar adult can accompany the child, often the child is less afraid. If the child is unable or unwilling to hold still for the x-ray, restraint may be necessary. Restraint should be limited to the amount of time needed for the x-ray.
Fluorescent antibody testing	Determines presence of respiratory syncytial virus (RSV), adenovirus, influenza, parainfluenza, or *Chlamydia* in nasopharyngeal secretions	Bronchiolitis, pneumonia	To obtain a nasopharyngeal specimen, instill 1 to 3 mL of sterile normal saline into one nostril, aspirate the contents using a small sterile bulb syringe, place the contents in sterile container, and immediately send them to the lab.
Fluoroscopy	Radiographic examination that uses a fluorescent screen— "real-time" imaging	Identification of masses, abscesses	Requires the child to lie still. Equipment can be frightening. Children may respond to presence of parent or familiar adult.
Gastric washings for AFB	Determines presence of AFB (acid-fast bacilli) in stomach (children often swallow sputum)	Tuberculosis	Nasogastric tube is inserted and saline is instilled and suctioned out of the stomach to obtain the specimen.
Peak expiratory flow	Measures the maximum flow of air (in L/sec) that can be forcefully exhaled in 1 second	Daily use can indicate adequacy of asthma control.	It is important to establish the child's "personal best" by taking twice-daily readings over a 2-week period while well. The average of these is termed "personal best." Charts based on height and age are also available to determine expected peak expiratory flow.

Test	Explanation	Indications	Nursing Implications
Pulmonary function tests	Measure respiratory flow and lung volumes	Asthma, cystic fibrosis, chronic lung disease	Usually performed by a respiratory therapist trained to do the full spectrum of tests. Spirometry can be obtained by the trained nurse in the outpatient setting.
Pulse oximetry	Noninvasive method of continuously (or intermittently) measuring oxygen saturation	Can be useful in any situation in which a child is experiencing respiratory distress	Probe must be applied correctly to finger, toe, foot, hand, or ear in order for the machine to appropriately pick up the pulse and oxygen saturation.
Rapid flu test	Rapid test for detection of influenza A or B	Influenza	Should be done in first 24 hours of illness so that medication administration can begin
Have the child gargle with sterile normal saline and then spit into a sterile container. Send immediately to the lab.
Rapid strep test	Instant test for presence of strep A antibody in pharyngeal secretions	Pharyngitis, tonsillitis	Results in 5 to 10 minutes. Negative tests should be backed up with throat culture.
RAST (radioallergosorbent test)	Measures minute quantities of immunoglobulin E in the blood
Carries no risk of anaphylaxis but is not as sensitive as skin testing	Asthma (food allergies)	Blood test that is usually sent out to a reference laboratory
Sinus x-rays, computed tomography (CT), or magnetic resonance imaging (MRI)	Radiologic tests that may show sinus involvement	Sinusitis, recurrent colds	X-ray results are usually received more quickly than CT or MRI results.
Sputum culture	Bacterial culture of invasive organisms in the sputum	Pneumonia, cystic fibrosis, tuberculosis	Must be true sputum, not mucus from the mouth or nose. Child can deep breathe, cough, and spit, or specimen may be obtained via suctioning of the artificial airway.
Sweat chloride test	Collection of sweat on filter paper after stimulation of skin with pilocarpine
Measures concentration of chloride in the sweat	Cystic fibrosis	May be difficult to obtain sweat in a young infant
Throat culture	Bacterial culture (minimum of 24 to 48 hours required) to determine presence of streptococcus A or other bacteria	Pharyngitis, tonsillitis	Can be obtained on separate swab at same time as rapid strep test to decrease trauma to the child (swab both applicators at once)
Do not perform immediately after the child has had medication or something to eat or drink.
Tuberculin skin test	Mantoux test (intradermal injection of purified protein derivative)	Tuberculosis, chronic cough	Must be given intradermally; not a valid test if injected incorrectly

fter completing an assessment of Alexander, the nurse notes the following: lots of clear secretions in the airway, child appears pale, respiratory rate 68, retractions, nasal flaring, wheezing, and diminished breath sounds. Based on these assessment findings, what would your top three nursing diagnoses be for Alexander?

Nursing goals, interventions, and evaluation for the child with a respiratory disorder are based on the nursing diagnoses. Nursing Care Plan 39.1 can be used as a guide in planning nursing care for the child with a respiratory disorder. The nursing care plan should be individualized based on the client's symptoms and needs; refer to Chapter 35 for detailed information on pain management. Additional information will be included later in the chapter as it relates to specific disorders.

ased on your top three nursing diagnoses for Alexander, describe appropriate nursing interventions.

Oxygen Supplementation

Oxygen may be delivered to the child by a variety of methods (Fig. 39.6). Since oxygen administration is considered a drug, it requires a physician's order, except when following emergency protocols outlined in a health care facility's policies and procedures. Many health care settings develop specific guidelines for oxygen administration that are often coordinated by respiratory therapists, yet the nurse still remains responsible for ensuring that oxygen is administered properly.

Oxygen sources include wall-mounted systems as well as cylinders. The supply of oxygen available from a wall-mounted source is limitless, but use of a wall-mounted source restricts the child to the hospital room. Cylinders are portable oxygen tanks; the D-cylinder holds a little less than 400 liters of oxygen and the E-cylinder holds about 650 liters of oxygen. Cylinders turn on with a gauge attached to the top of the tank. The cylinder is useful for the child on low-flow oxygen because it allows for mobility.

The tank empties relatively quickly if the child requires a high flow of oxygen, so this is not the best oxygen source in an emergency. Respiratory therapists usually maintain the respiratory equipment that is found in the emergency room or hospital. However, in an outpatient setting the nurse may be responsible for maintaining respiratory equipment and checking the level of oxygen in the office's oxygen tanks each day.

▶ **Take** NOTE!

Oxygen is highly flammable, so use safety precautions. Post signs ("Oxygen in Use"); inform the family to avoid matches, lighters, and flammable or volatile materials; and use only facility-approved equipment.

The efficiency of oxygen delivery systems is affected by several variables, including the child's respiratory effort, the liter flow of oxygen delivered, and whether the equipment is being used appropriately. In general, oxygen facemasks come in infant, child, and adult sizes. Select the mask that best fits the child. In addition, ensure that the mask is sealed properly to decrease the amount of oxygen that escapes from the mask. Ensure that the liter flow is set according to the manufacturer's recommendations for use with that particular delivery method. The oxygen flow rate or concentration is usually determined by the physician's order. Whichever method of delivery is used, provide humidification during oxygen delivery to prevent drying of nasal passages and to assist with liquefying secretions. Table 39.1 provides details on oxygen delivery methods.

▶ **Take** NOTE!

Monitor vital signs, color, respiratory effort, pulse oximetry, and level of consciousness before, during, and after oxygen therapy to evaluate its effectiveness.

Acute Infectious Disorders

Acute infectious disorders include the common cold, sinusitis, influenza, pharyngitis, tonsillitis, laryngitis, croup syndromes, respiratory syncytial virus (RSV), pneumonia, and bronchitis.

▶ COMMON COLD

The common cold is also referred to as a viral upper respiratory infection (URI) or nasopharyngitis. Colds can be caused by a number of different viruses, including rhinoviruses, parainfluenza, RSV, enteroviruses, and adenoviruses (National Institute of Allergy and Infectious Diseases, 2007). Recently, human meta-pneumovirus has been identified as an important cause of the common cold (Burke, 2004). Viral particles spread through the air or from person-to-person contact. Colds occur more frequently in winter. They affect children of all ages and have a higher incidence among children who attend daycare and school-age children. It is not unusual for a child to have six to nine colds per year. Spontaneous resolution of the common cold occurs after about 7 to 10 days. Potential complications include secondary bacterial infections of the ears, throat, sinuses, or lungs.

Therapeutic management of the common cold is directed toward symptom relief. Nasal congestion may

(text continues on page 1234)

Nursing Care Plan 39.1

OVERVIEW FOR THE CHILD WITH A RESPIRATORY DISORDER

NURSING DIAGNOSIS: Ineffective airway clearance related to inflammation, increased secretions, mechanical obstruction, or pain as evidenced by presence of secretions, productive cough, tachypnea, and increased work of breathing

Outcome Identification and Evaluation
Child will maintain patent airway, *free from secretions or obstruction, easy work of breathing, respiratory rate within parameters for age.*

Interventions: Maintaining a Patent Airway
- Position with airway open (sniffing position if supine) *to allow adequate ventilation.*
- Humidify oxygen or room air and ensure adequate fluid intake (intravenous or oral) *to liquefy secretions for ease in clearance.*
- Suction with bulb syringe or via nasopharyngeal catheter as needed, particularly prior to bottle-feeding, *to promote clearance of secretions.*
- If tachypneic, maintain NPO status *to avoid aspiration.*
- In older child, encourage expectoration of sputum with coughing *to promote airway clearance.*
- Perform chest physiotherapy if ordered *to mobilize secretions.*
- Ensure emergency equipment is readily available *to avoid delay should airway become unmaintainable.*

NURSING DIAGNOSIS: Ineffective breathing pattern related to inflammatory or infectious process as evidenced by tachypnea, increased work of breathing, nasal flaring, retractions, diminished breath sounds

Outcome Identification and Evaluation
Child will exhibit adequate ventilation: *respiratory rate within parameters for age, easy work of breathing (absence of retractions, accessory muscle use, grunting), clear breath sounds with adequate aeration, oxygen saturation >94% or within prescribed parameters.*

Interventions: Promoting Effective Breathing Patterns
- Assess respiratory rate, breath sounds, and work of breathing frequently *to ensure progress with treatment and so that deterioration can be noted early.*
- Use pulse oximetry to monitor oxygen saturation in the least invasive manner *to note adequacy of oxygenation and ensure early detection of hypoxemia.*
- Position for comfort with open airway and room for lung expansion. Use pillows or padding if necessary to maintain position *to ensure optimal ventilation via maximum lung expansion.*
- Administer supplemental oxygen and/or humidity as ordered *to improve oxygenation.*
- Allow for adequate sleep and rest periods *to conserve energy.*
- Administer antibiotics as ordered: *may be indicated in the case of bacterial respiratory infection.*
- Encourage incentive spirometry and coughing with deep breathing (can be accomplished through play) *to maximize ventilation (play enhances the child's participation).*

NURSING DIAGNOSIS: Gas exchange, impaired, related to airway plugging, hyperinflation, atelectasis, as evidenced by cyanosis, decreased oxygen saturation, and alterations in arterial blood gases

Outcome Identification and Evaluation
Gas exchange will be adequate: *Pulse oximetry reading on room air is within normal parameters for age, blood gases within normal limits, absence of cyanosis.*

Interventions: Promoting Adequate Gas Exchange
- Administer oxygen as ordered *to improve oxygenation.*
- Monitor oxygen saturation via pulse oximetry *to detect alterations in oxygenation.*
- Encourage clearance of secretions via coughing, expectoration, chest physiotherapy, and suctioning *to improve gas exchange.*
- Administer bronchodilators if ordered (albuterol, levalbuterol, and racemic epinephrine) *to treat bronchospasm and improve gas exchange.*
- Provide frequent contact and support to the child and family *to decrease anxiety, which increases the child's oxygen demands.*
- Assess and monitor mental status (confusion, lethargy, restlessness, combativeness): *hypoxemia can lead to changes in mental status.*

(continued)

Nursing Care Plan 39.1 (continued)

NURSING DIAGNOSIS: Risk for infection related to presence of infectious organisms as evidenced by fever or presence of virus or bacteria on laboratory screening

Outcome Identification and Evaluation
Child will exhibit no signs of secondary infection and will not spread infection to others: *symptoms of infection decrease over time; others remain free from infection.*

Interventions: Preventing Infection
- Maintain aseptic technique, practice good handwashing, and use disposable suction catheters *to prevent introduction of further infectious agents.*
- Limit number of visitors and screen them for recent illness *to prevent further infection.*
- Administer antibiotics if prescribed *to prevent or treat bacterial infection.*
- Encourage nutritious diet according to child's preferences and ability to feed orally *to assist body's natural infection-fighting mechanisms.*
- Isolate the child as required *to prevent nosocomial spread of infection.*
- Teach child and family preventive measures such as good handwashing, covering mouth and nose when coughing or sneezing, proper disposal of used tissues *to prevent nosocomial or community spread of infection.*

NURSING DIAGNOSIS: Fluid volume deficit, risk for, related to decreased oral intake, insensible losses via fever, tachypnea, or diaphoresis

Outcome Identification and Evaluation
Fluid volume will be maintained: *Oral mucosa moist and pink, skin turgor elastic, urine output at least 1 to 2 mL/kg/hr.*

Interventions: Maintaining Adequate Fluid Volume
- Administer intravenous fluids if ordered *to maintain adequate hydration in NPO state.*
- When allowed oral intake, encourage oral fluids. Popsicles, favorite fluids, and games can be used *to promote intake.*
- Assess for signs of adequate hydration (elastic skin turgor, moist mucosa, adequate urine output).
- Monitor intake and output *to identify fluid imbalance.*
- Monitor urine specific gravity, urine and serum electrolytes, blood urea nitrogen, creatinine, and osmolality *to determine fluid status.*

NURSING DIAGNOSIS: Nutrition, altered: less than body requirements related to difficulty feeding as evidenced by poor oral intake, tiring with feeding

Outcome Identification and Evaluation
Child will maintain adequate nutritional intake: *Weight is gained or maintained. Child consumes adequate diet for age.*

Interventions: Promoting Adequate Nutritional Intake
- Weigh on same scale at same time daily *so that measurements are consistent.*
- Perform calorie counts over a 3-day period *to determine whether caloric intake is sufficient.*
- Encourage child to choose higher-calorie, protein-rich foods *to optimize growth potential.*
- Coax young children to eat better by playing games and offering favorite foods *to improve intake.*

NURSING DIAGNOSIS: Activity intolerance related to high respiratory demand as evidenced by increased work of breathing and need for frequent rest when playing

Outcome Identification and Evaluation
Child will resume normal activity level: *Activity is tolerated without difficulty breathing. Pulse oximetry readings and vital signs are within parameters for age and activity level.*

Interventions: Increasing Activity Tolerance
- Provide rest periods balanced with periods of activity, and group nursing activities and visits *to allow for sufficient rest.*
- Provide small, frequent meals *to prevent overtiring (energy is expended while eating).*
- Encourage quiet activities that do not require exertion *to prevent boredom.*
- Allow gradual increase in activity as tolerated, keeping pulse oximetry reading within normal parameters, *to minimize risk for further respiratory compromise.*

Nursing Care Plan 39.1 (continued)

NURSING DIAGNOSIS: Fear related to difficulty breathing, unfamiliar personnel, procedures, and environment (hospital), as evidenced by clinging, crying, fussing, verbalization, or lack of cooperation

Outcome Identification and Evaluation

Fear/anxiety will be reduced: *decreased episodes of crying or fussing, happy and playful at times.*

Interventions: Relieving Fear

- Establish trusting relationship with child and family *to decrease anxiety and fear.*
- Explain procedures to child at developmentally appropriate level *to decrease fear of unknown.*
- Provide favorite blanket or bear as well as comfort measures preferred by client such as rocking or music *for added security.*
- Involve parents in care *to give child reassurance and decrease fear.*

NURSING DIAGNOSIS: Family processes, altered, related to child's illness or hospitalization as evidenced by family's presence in hospital, missed work, demonstration of inadequate coping

Outcome Identification and Evaluation

Parents demonstrate adequate coping and decreased anxiety: *Parents are involved in child's care, ask appropriate questions, and are able to discuss child's care and condition calmly.*

Interventions: Promoting Adequate Family Processes

- Encourage parents to discuss their concerns related to child's illness *to identify concerns and show parents that the nurse also cares about them, not just the child.*
- Explain therapy, procedures, and child's behavior to parents *to decrease their anxiety.*
- Encourage parents to be involved in care *so they feel needed and valued.*

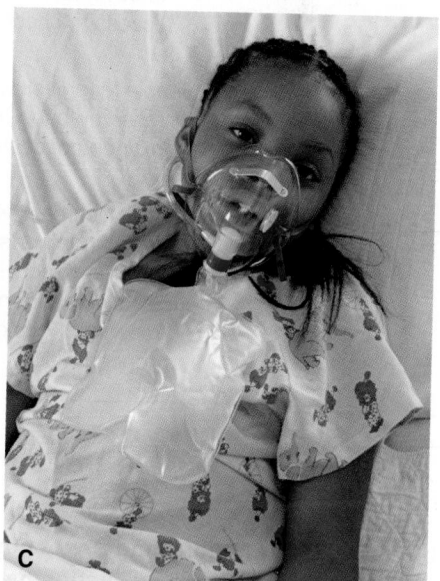

FIGURE 39.6 (**A**) Simple oxygen mask provides about 40% oxygen. (**B**) The nasal cannula provides an additional 4% oxygen per 1 L of oxygen flow (i.e., 1 L will deliver 25% oxygen). (**C**) The nonrebreather mask provides 80% to 100% oxygen.

TABLE 39.1 OXYGEN DELIVERY METHODS

Delivery Method	Description	Nursing Implications
Simple mask	Provides 35% to 60% oxygen with a flow rate of 6 to 10 L/minute. Oxygen delivery percentage is affected by respiratory rate, inspiratory flow, and adequacy of mask fit.	• Must maintain oxygen flow rate of at least 6 L/minute to maintain inspired oxygen concentration and prevent rebreathing of carbon dioxide • Mask must fit snugly to be effective but should not be so tight as to irritate the face.
Venturi mask	Provides 24% to 50% oxygen by using a special gauge at the base of the mask that allows mixing of room air with oxygen flow	• Set oxygen flow rate according to percentage of oxygen desired as indicated on the gauge/dial. • As with simple mask, must fit snugly.
Nasal cannula	Provides low oxygen concentration (22% to 44%)	• Must be used with humidification to prevent drying and irritation of airways • Can provide very small amounts of oxygen (as low as 25 cc/minute) • Maximum recommended liter flow in children is 4 L/minute. • Children can eat or talk while on oxygen. • Inspired oxygen concentration affected by mouth breathing • Requires patent nasal passages
Oxygen tent	Provides high-humidity environment with up to 50% oxygen concentration	• Oxygen level drops when tent is opened. • Must change linen frequently as it becomes damp from the humidity • Secure edges of tent with blankets or by tucking edges under mattress. • Young children may be fearful and resistant. • Mist may interfere with visualization of child inside tent.
Oxygen hood	Provides high concentration (up to 80% to 90%) for infants only. Allows easy access to chest and lower body.	• Liter flow must be set at 10 to 15 L/minute. • Good method for infant but need to remove for feeding • Can and should be humidified
Partial rebreathing mask	Simple facemask with an oxygen reservoir bag. Provides 50% to 60% oxygen concentration.	• Must set liter flow rate at 10 to 12 L/min to prevent rebreathing of carbon dioxide • The reservoir bag does not completely empty when child inspires if flow rate is set properly.
Nonrebreathing mask	Simple facemask with valves at the exhalation ports and an oxygen reservoir bag with a valve to prevent exhaled air from entering the reservoir. Provides 95% oxygen concentration.	• Must set liter flow rate at 10 to 12 L/min to prevent rebreathing of carbon dioxide • The reservoir bag does not completely empty when child inspires if flow rate is set properly.

be relieved via humidity and use of normal saline nasal wash or spray followed by suctioning. Antihistamines are not indicated, as they dry secretions further. Over-the-counter cold preparations are available singly and in combinations. These preparations have not been proven to reduce the length or severity of the cold but may offer symptomatic relief in some children over 6 years of age.

▶ *Take* NOTE!

In October 2007, over-the-counter cold preparations containing decongestants intended for use in infants and young children were removed from the market. Several research studies have not shown the preparations to be effective, and they are known to have potentially serious side effects (AAP, 2007).

EVIDENCE-BASED PRACTICE 39.1
Various Body Positions and Their Effects on Hospitalized Infants and Young Children With Acute Respiratory Distress

● Study

Prone positioning has been found to improve ventilation in some adults with acute respiratory distress and in premature infants with respiratory distress syndrome, but due to the risk of sudden infant death syndrome (SIDS), infants are generally positioned supine. The authors reviewed 21 studies that evaluated the effect of positioning (supine, prone, lateral, elevated, and flat positions) on respiratory function (oxygen saturation, partial pressure of arterial oxygen, oxygenation index, thoraco-abdominal synchrony, and episodes of oxygen desaturation) in infants and young children with acute respiratory distress.

▲ Findings

The only position found to produce a statistically significant improvement in respiratory function was the prone position. The prone position was better in terms of improving ventilation and oxygenation. The other positions did not demonstrate statistically significant differences.

■ Nursing Implications

Nurses should critically consider the result of this review. Certainly, if an alternate position is used, the infant must be closely monitored and the position changed should any level of deterioration occur. If hospitalized infants with acute respiratory distress are placed in the prone position, continuous cardiopulmonary and oxygenation saturation monitoring must be provided because of the risk of SIDS in this age group. Do not encourage families to use the prone position at home when an infant is ill with a respiratory condition.

Wells, D. A., Gillies, D., & Fitzgerald, D. A. (2007). Positioning for acute respiratory distress in hospitalised infants and children. *The Cochrane Library 2007, 4.* Indianapolis: John Wiley & Sons.

Nursing Assessment

The child may have either a stuffy or runny nose. Nasal discharge is usually thin and watery at first but may become thicker and discolored. The color of nasal discharge is not an accurate indicator of viral versus bacterial infection. The child may be hoarse and complain of a sore throat. Cough usually produces very little sputum. Fever, fatigue, watery eyes, and appetite loss may also occur. Symptoms are generally at their worst over the first few days and then decrease over the course of the illness.

Assess for risk factors such as daycare or school attendance. Inspect for edema and vasodilation of the mucosa. Diagnosis is based on clinical presentation rather than laboratory or x-ray studies. Comparison Chart 39.1 differentiates causes of nasal congestion.

Nursing Management

Nursing management of the child with a common cold consists of promoting comfort, providing family education, and preventing spread of the cold.

COMPARISON CHART 39.1 CAUSES OF NASAL CONGESTION

Sign or Symptom	Allergic Rhinitis	Common Cold	Sinusitis
Length of illness	Varies; may have year-round symptoms	10 days or less	Longer than 10 to 14 days
Nasal discharge	Thin, watery, clear	Thick, white, yellow, or green; can be thin	Thick, yellow or green
Nasal congestion	Varies	Present	Present
Sneezing	Varies	Present	Absent
Cough	Varies	Present	Varies
Headache	Varies	Varies	Varies
Fever	Absent	Varies	Varies
Bad breath	Absent	Absent	Varies

Promoting Comfort

Nursing care of the common cold is aimed at supportive measures. Nasal congestion may be relieved with the use of normal saline nose drops, followed by bulb syringe suctioning in infants and toddlers. Older children may use a normal saline nose spray to mobilize secretions. A cool mist humidifier also helps with nasal congestion. Generally, other over-the-counter nose sprays are not recommended for use in children, but they are sometimes prescribed for very short-term use. Promotion of adequate oral fluid intake is important to liquefy secretions.

Educate parents about the use of cold and cough medications. Although they may offer some symptomatic relief, they have not been proven to shorten the length of cold symptoms. Counsel parents to use the appropriate product depending on the symptom relief desired, rather than a combination product. Products containing acetaminophen combined with other "cold symptom" medications may mask a fever in the child who is developing a secondary bacterial infection. As with all viral infections in children, teach parents that aspirin use should be avoided because of its association with Reye syndrome.

Providing Family Education

Currently there are no medications available to treat the viruses that cause the common cold, so symptomatic treatment is all that is necessary. Antibiotics are not indicated unless the child also has a bacterial infection. Explain to parents the importance of reserving antibiotic use for appropriate illnesses. Provide education about the use of normal saline nose drops and bulb suctioning to clear the infant's nose of secretions. Normal saline nasal wash using a bulb syringe to instill the solution is also helpful for children of all ages with nasal congestion. Though normal saline for nasal administration is available commercially, parents can also make it at home (Box 39.2). Teaching Guidelines 39.1 gives instructions on use of the bulb syringe.

Counsel parents about how to recognize complications of the common cold. These include:

- Prolonged fever
- Increased throat pain or enlarged, painful lymph nodes
- Increased or worsening cough, cough lasting longer than 10 days, chest pain, difficulty breathing

- Earache, headache, tooth or sinus pain
- Unusual irritability or lethargy
- Skin rash

If complications do occur, tell parents to notify the health care provider for further instructions or reassessment.

Preventing the Common Cold

Teaching about ways to prevent the common cold is a vital nursing intervention. Explain that frequent handwashing helps to decrease the spread of viruses that cause the common cold. Teach parents and family to avoid second-hand smoke as well as crowded places, especially during the winter. Avoid close contact with individuals known to have a cold. Encourage parents and families to consume a healthy diet and get enough rest.

▶ *Consider THIS!*

> Corey Davis, a 3-year-old, is brought to the clinic by her mother. She presents with a runny nose, congestion, and a nonproductive cough. Her mother says, "She's miserable."
>
> What other assessment information would be helpful?
> Based on the history and clinical presentation, Corey is diagnosed with a common cold. What education would be helpful for this family? Include ways to improve Corey's comfort and ways to prevent the common cold.

▶ SINUSITIS

Sinusitis (also called rhinosinusitis) generally refers to a bacterial infection of the paranasal sinuses. The disease may be either acute or chronic in nature, with the treatment approach varying with chronicity. Approximately 5% of upper respiratory infections are complicated with acute sinusitis. In young children the maxillary and ethmoid sinuses are the main sites of infection. After age 10 years, the frontal sinuses may be more commonly involved. Mucosal swelling, decreased ciliary movement, and thickened nasal discharge all contribute to bacterial invasion of the nose. Nasal polyps also place the child at risk for bacterial sinusitis. Complications include orbital cellulitis and intracranial infections such as subdural empyemas.

Symptoms lasting less than 30 days generally indicate acute sinusitis, whereas symptoms persisting longer than 4 to 6 weeks usually indicate chronic sinusitis. Sinusitis is managed with antibiotic treatment. The course of treatment is a minimum of 10 days. The current American Academy of Pediatrics recommendations state that antibiotics should be continued for 7 days once the child is free from symptoms to eradicate the infection (AAP, 2001).

BOX 39.2 **Homemade Salt Water Nose Drops**

Mix 8 oz distilled water, a half-teaspoon sea salt, and a quarter-teaspoon baking soda. Keeps for 24 hours in the refrigerator, but should be allowed to come to room temperature prior to use.

TEACHING GUIDELINES 39.1

Using the Bulb Syringe to Suction Nasal Secretions

1. Hold the infant on your lap or on the bed with head tilted slightly back.

2. If using saline, instill several drops of saline solution in one of infant's nostrils.

3. Compress the sides of the bulb syringe completely. Use only a rubber-tipped bulb syringe. Place the rubber tip in the infant's nose.

4. Release pressure on the bulb.

5. Remove the syringe and squeeze bulb over tissue or the sink to empty it of secretions.

6. Repeat on other nostril if necessary. Using a bulb syringe prior to bottle-feeding or breastfeeding may relieve congestion enough to allow the infant to suck more efficiently.
7. Clean the bulb syringe thoroughly with warm water after each use and allow to air dry.

Objective	Significance
Reduce the number of courses of antibiotics prescribed for the sole diagnosis of the common cold.	• Appropriately educate families that the cause of the common cold is a number of viruses and that antibiotics are inappropriate for the treatment of viral infections. • Encourage families to use measures such as normal saline nasal washes to decrease symptoms associated with the common cold more quickly.

Naturally, chronic sinusitis requires a longer course of treatment than acute sinusitis. Surgical therapy may be indicated for children with chronic sinusitis, particularly if it is recurrent or if nasal polyps are present.

Nursing Assessment

The most common presentation of sinusitis is persistent signs and symptoms of a cold. Rather than improving after 7 to 10 days, nasal discharge persists. Explore the history for:

• Cough
• Fever
• In preschoolers or older children, halitosis (bad breath)
• Facial pain may or may not be present, so is not a reliable indicator of disease.
• Eyelid edema (in the case of ethmoid sinus involvement)
• Irritability
• Poor appetite

Cold symptoms that are severe and not improving over time may also indicate sinusitis (Leung & Kellner, 2004). Assess for risk factors such as a history of recurrent cold symptoms or a history of nasal polyps.

On physical examination, note eyelid swelling, extent of nasal drainage, and halitosis. Inspect the throat for postnasal drainage. Inspect the nasal mucosa for erythema. Palpate the sinuses, noting pain with mild pressure. The diagnosis may be made based on the history and clinical presentation, augmented by x-ray, computed tomography scan, or magnetic resonance imaging findings in some cases (Leung & Kellner, 2004). (Refer to Comparison Chart 39.1, which differentiates the causes of nasal congestion.)

Nursing Management

Normal saline nose drops or spray, cool mist humidifiers, and adequate oral fluid intake are recommended for children with sinusitis. Teach families the importance of continuing the full course of antibiotics to eradicate the cause of infection. Also educate the family that using decongestants, antihistamines, and intranasal steroids as adjuncts in the treatment of sinusitis has not been shown to be beneficial. Normal saline nose spray or nasal washes may promote drainage (Leung & Kellner, 2004).

▶ INFLUENZA

Influenza viral infection occurs primarily during the winter. "The flu" is spread through inhalation of droplets or contact with fine-particle aerosols. Infected children shed the virus for 1 to 2 days before symptoms begin and may continue increased amounts of viral shedding as compared with adults for as long as 2 weeks. Average annual infection rates in children range from 20% to 50% (Iskander et al., 2007). Influenza viruses primarily affect the upper respiratory epithelium but can cause systemic effects as well. Children with chronic heart or lung conditions, diabetes, chronic renal disease, or immune deficiency are at higher risk than other children for more severe influenza infection.

Bacterial infections of the respiratory system commonly occur as complications of influenza infection, severe pneumococcal pneumonia in particular. Otitis media occurs in 18% to 40% of all influenza cases (Iskander et al., 2007). Less common complications include Reye syndrome and acute myositis. Reye syndrome is an acute encephalopathy that has been associated with aspirin use in the influenza-infected child. Acute myositis is particular to children. A sudden onset of severe pain and tenderness in both calves causes the child to refuse to walk. Due to the potential for complications, a prolonged fever or a fever that returns during convalescence should be investigated.

Nursing Assessment

Children who attend daycare or school are at higher risk for influenza infection than those who are routinely at home. Note the presence of risk factors for severe disease, such as chronic heart or lung disease (such as asthma), diabetes, chronic renal disease, or immune deficiency or children with cancer receiving chemotherapy. School-age children and adolescents experience the illness similarly to adults. Abrupt onset of fever, facial flushing, chills, headache, myalgia, and malaise are accompanied by cough and **coryza.** About half of infected individuals have a dry or sore throat. Ocular symptoms such as photophobia, tearing, burning, and eye pain are common.

Infants and young children exhibit symptoms similar to other respiratory illnesses. Fever greater than 39.5°C is common. Infants may be mildly toxic in appearance and irritable and have a cough, coryza, and pharyngitis. Wheezing may occur, as influenza also can cause bronchiolitis. An erythematous rash may be present, and diarrhea may also occur. The diagnosis may be confirmed by a rapid assay test.

Nursing Management

Nursing management of influenza is mainly supportive. Symptomatic treatment of cough and fever and maintenance of hydration are the focus of care. Amantadine hydrochloride (Symmetrel) and other newer antiviral drugs can reduce the symptoms associated with influenza if started within the first 24 to 48 hours of the illness.

Preventing Influenza Infection

Yearly vaccination against influenza is recommended for high-risk groups. Children 6 months or older are considered high risk if they:

• Have chronic heart or lung conditions
• Have sickle cell anemia or other hemoglobinopathy
• Are under medical care for diabetes, chronic renal disease, or immune deficiency
• Are on long-term aspirin therapy (risk of developing Reye syndrome after the flu)

Among otherwise healthy children, infants and toddlers are at highest risk for developing severe disease. All healthy children between the ages of 6 and 59 months should also be immunized. Refer to Chapter 30 for more information on immunizations.

▶ PHARYNGITIS

Inflammation of the throat mucosa (pharynx) is referred to as **pharyngitis**. A sore throat may accompany nasal congestion and is often viral in nature. A bacterial sore throat most often occurs without nasal symptoms. Group A streptococci account for 15% to 25% of cases, with the remainder being caused by other viruses or bacteria (Martin & Green, 2006).

Suppurative complications of group A streptococcal infection include peritonsillar or retropharyngeal abscess. Peritonsillar abscess may be noted by asymmetric swelling of the tonsils, shifting of the uvula to one side, and palatal edema. Retropharyngeal abscess may progress to the point of airway obstruction, hence requiring careful evaluation and appropriate treatment. Additional complications include acute rheumatic fever (see Chapter 40) and acute glomerulonephritis (see Chapter 42).

Viral pharyngitis is usually self-limited and does not require therapy beyond symptomatic relief. Group A streptococcal pharyngitis requires antibiotic therapy. If either the rapid diagnostic test or throat culture (described below) is positive for group A streptococci, penicillin is generally prescribed. Appropriate alternative antibiotics include amoxicillin and, for those allergic to penicillin, macrolides and cephalosporins (Wong, Blumberg, & Lowe, 2006).

> ▶ **Take** NOTE!
>
> A "strep carrier" is a child who has a positive throat culture for streptococci when asymptomatic. Strep carriers are not at risk for complications from streptococci, as are those who are acutely infected with streptococci and are symptomatic.

Nursing Assessment

Onset of the illness is often quite abrupt. The history may include a fever, sore throat and difficulty swallowing, headache, and abdominal pain, which are quite common. Inquire about recent incidence of viral or strep throat in the family, day care center, or school.

Inspect the pharynx and tonsils, which may demonstrate varying degrees of inflammation (Fig. 39.7). Exudate may be present but is not diagnostic of bacterial infection. Note the presence of petechiae on the palate. Inspect the tongue for a strawberry appearance. Palpate for enlargement and tenderness of the anterior cervical nodes. Inspect the skin for a fine, red, sandpaper-like rash (called scarlatiniform), particularly on the trunk or abdomen, a common finding with streptococcus A infection.

The nurse may obtain a throat swab for rapid diagnostic testing and throat culture. If both tests are being obtained, the applicators may be swabbed simultaneously to decrease perceived trauma to the child. The rapid strep test is a sensitive and reliable measure, rarely resulting in

FIGURE 39.7 Note the redness of the pharynx, tonsillar exudate, and white strawberry tongue coating.

false-positive readings (Farrar-Simpson et al., 2005). If the rapid strep test is negative, the second swab may be sent for a throat culture.

Nursing Management

Nursing management of the child with pharyngitis focuses on promoting comfort and providing family education.

Promoting Comfort

Saline gargles (made with 8 oz of warm water and a half-teaspoon of table salt) are soothing for children old enough to cooperate. Analgesics such as acetaminophen and ibuprofen may ease fever and pain. Sucking on throat lozenges or hard candy may also ease pain. Cool mist humidity helps to keep the mucosa moist in the event of mouth breathing. Encourage the child to ingest Popsicles, cool liquids, and ice chips to maintain hydration.

Providing Family Education

Parents may be accustomed to "sore throats" being treated with antibiotics, but in the case of a viral cause antibiotics will not be necessary and the pharyngitis will resolve in a few days. For the child with streptococcal pharyngitis, urge parents to have the child complete the entire prescribed course of antibiotics (Parmet, 2004). After 24 hours of antibiotic therapy, instruct the parents to discard the child's toothbrush to avoid reinfection. Children may return to daycare or school after they have been receiving antibiotics for 24 hours, as they are considered noncontagious at that point.

▶ TONSILLITIS

Inflammation of the tonsils often occurs with pharyngitis and thus may also be viral or bacterial in nature. Viral infections require only symptomatic treatment. Treatment for bacterial tonsillitis is the same as for bacterial pharyngitis. Occasionally surgical intervention is warranted. Tonsillectomy (surgical removal of the palatine tonsils) may be indicated for the child with recurrent streptococcal tonsillitis, massive tonsillar hypertrophy, or other reasons. When hypertrophied adenoids obstruct breathing, then adenoidectomy (surgical removal of the adenoids) may be indicated.

Nursing Assessment

Note whether fever is present currently or by history. Inquire about the history of recurrent pharyngitis or tonsillitis. Note if the child's voice sounds muffled or hoarse. Inspect the pharynx for redness and enlargement of the tonsils. As the tonsils enlarge, the child may ex-

perience difficulty breathing and swallowing. When tonsils touch at the midline ("kissing tonsils" or 4+ in size), the airway may become obstructed (see Fig. 39.7). Also, if the adenoids are enlarged, the posterior nares become obstructed. The child may breathe through the mouth and may snore. Palpate the anterior cervical nodes for enlargement and tenderness. Rapid test or culture may be positive for streptococcus A.

Nursing Management

Tonsillitis that is medically treated requires the same nursing management as pharyngitis. Nursing care for the child after tonsillectomy is described below.

Promoting Airway Clearance

Until fully awake, place the child in a side-lying or prone position to facilitate safe drainage of secretions. Once alert, he or she may prefer to sit up or have the head of the bed elevated. Suctioning, if necessary, should be done carefully to avoid trauma to the surgical site. Dried blood may be present on the teeth and the nares, with old blood present in emesis. Since the presence of blood can be very frightening to parents, alert them to this possibility.

Maintaining Fluid Volume

Hemorrhage is unusual postoperatively but may occur any time from the immediate postoperative period to as late as 10 days after surgery (Peterson & Losek, 2004). Inspect the throat for bleeding. Mucus tinged with blood may be expected, but fresh blood in the secretions indicates bleeding. Early bleeding may be identified by continuous swallowing of small amounts of blood while awake or sleeping. Other signs of hemorrhage include tachycardia, pallor, restlessness, frequent throat clearing, and emesis of bright red blood.

To avoid trauma to the surgical site, discourage the child from coughing, clearing the throat, blowing the nose, and using straws. Upon discharge, instruct the parents to immediately report any sign of bleeding to the physician. To maintain fluid volume postoperatively, encourage children to take any fluids they desire; Popsicles and ice chips are particularly soothing. Citrus juice and brown or red fluids should be avoided: the acid in citrus juice may irritate the throat, and red or brown fluids may be confused with blood if vomiting occurs.

Relieving Pain

For the first 24 hours after surgery, the throat is very sore. Adequate pain relief is essential to establish adequate oral fluid intake. An ice collar may be prescribed, as well as analgesics with or without narcotics. Counsel parents to maintain pain control upon discharge from the facility, not only for the child's sake but also to enable the child to continue to drink fluids (Louloudes, 2006).

INFECTIOUS MONONUCLEOSIS

Infectious mononucleosis is a self-limited illness caused by the Epstein-Barr virus. It is characterized by fever, malaise, sore throat, and lymphadenopathy. Mononucleosis is commonly called the "kissing disease" since it is transmitted by oropharyngeal secretions. It can occur at any age but is most often diagnosed in adolescents and young adults. Some infected individuals may have concomitant streptococcal pharyngitis. Complications include splenic rupture, Guillain-Barré syndrome, and aseptic meningitis (Jensen, 2004).

Nursing Assessment

Note any history of exposure to infected individuals. Determine history of fever and onset and progression of sore throat, malaise, and other complaints. Observe for periorbital edema. Inspect the pharynx and tonsils for inflammation and patches of gray exudate. Petechiae may be present on the palate. Palpate for bilateral non-tender enlargement of the posterior cervical lymph nodes. After 3 to 5 days of illness, the pharynx may become edematous and the tonsillar exudate more extensive. Lymphadenopathy may progress to include the anterior cervical nodes, which may become tender. Palpate the abdomen for splenomegaly or hepatomegaly. An erythematous maculopapular rash may appear as the illness progresses. Definitive diagnosis may be made by Monospot or Epstein-Barr virus titers.

▶ **Take** NOTE!

The Monospot is usually negative if obtained within the first 7 to 10 days of illness with infectious mononucleosis. Epstein-Barr virus titer is reliable at any point in the illness.

Nursing Management

Nursing management of mononucleosis is primarily symptomatic. The throat may be very sore, so analgesics and salt-water gargles are recommended. Bed rest should be encouraged while the child is febrile. Frequent rest periods may be necessary for several weeks after the onset of illness, as fatigue may persist as long as 6 weeks. During the acute phase, if tonsillar or pharyngeal edema threatens to obstruct the airway, then corticosteroids may be given to decrease the inflammation. In the presence of splenomegaly or hepatomegaly, strenuous activity and contact sports should be avoided. Appearance of rash or jaundice should be reported to the physician.

▶ **Take** NOTE!

Concomitant strep throat in the presence of infectious mononucleosis should be treated with an antibiotic other than ampicillin, as it may cause an allergic-type rash if used in the presence of mononucleosis.

LARYNGITIS

Inflammation of the larynx is termed **laryngitis**. It may occur alone or in conjunction with other respiratory symptoms. It is characterized by a hoarse voice or loss of the voice (so soft as to make it difficult to hear). Oral fluids might offer relief, but resting the voice for 24 hours will allow the inflammation to subside. Laryngitis alone requires no further intervention.

CROUP

Children between 3 months and 3 years of age are the most frequently affected with croup, though croup may affect any child. Croup is also referred to as laryngotracheobronchitis because inflammation and edema of the larynx, trachea, and bronchi occur as a result of viral infection. Parainfluenza is responsible for the majority of cases of croup. Other causes include adenovirus, influenza virus A and B, RSV, and rarely measles virus or *Mycoplasma pneumoniae* (Bjornson et al., 2004). The inflammation and edema obstruct the airway, resulting in symptoms. Mucus production also occurs, further contributing to obstruction of the airway. Narrowing of the subglottic area of the trachea results in audible inspiratory stridor. Edema of the larynx causes hoarseness. Inflammation in the larynx and trachea causes the characteristic barking cough of croup. Symptoms occur most often at night, and croup is usually self-limited, lasting only about 3 to 5 days (Leung et al., 2004).

Croup often presents suddenly at night, with resolution of symptoms in the morning. Complications of croup are rare but may include worsening respiratory distress, hypoxia, or bacterial superinfection (as in the case of bacterial tracheitis). Croup is usually managed on an outpatient basis, with only 1% to 2% of cases requiring hospitalization (Leung et al., 2004).

Corticosteroids (usually a single dose) are used to decrease inflammation, and racemic epinephrine aerosols demonstrate the alpha-adrenergic effect of mucosal vasoconstriction, helping to decrease edema (Bjornson et al., 2004; Schooff, 2005). Children with croup may be hospitalized if they have significant stridor at rest or severe retractions after a several-hour period of observation. Comparison Chart 39.2 compares croup to epiglottitis.

Nursing Assessment

Note the age of the child; children between 3 months and 3 years of age are most likely to present with viral croup (laryngotracheobronchitis). History may reveal a cough that developed during the night (most common presentation) and that sounds like barking (or a seal). Inspect for the presence of mild URI symptoms. Temperature may be normal or elevated mildly. Listen for inspiratory stridor and observe for suprasternal retractions. Auscultate the lungs for adequacy of breath sounds. Various scales are available for scoring croup severity, though these are of limited value in the clinical assessment and treatment of croup (Leung et al., 2004). Croup is usually diagnosed based on history and clinical presentation, but a lateral neck x-ray may be obtained to rule out epiglottitis.

> ▶ **Take** NOTE!
>
> *The child with fever, a toxic appearance, and increasing respiratory distress despite appropriate croup treatment may have bacterial tracheitis (Orenstein, 2004a). Notify the physician of these findings in a child with croup.*

COMPARISON CHART 39.2   CROUP VS. EPIGLOTTITIS

	Spasmodic Croup	Epiglottitis
Preceding illness	None or minimal coryza	None or mild upper respiratory infection
Age group usually affected	3 months to 3 years	1 to 8 years
Onset	Usually sudden, often at night	Rapid (within hours)
Fever	Variable	High
Barking cough, hoarseness	Yes	No
Dysphagia	No	Yes
Toxic appearance	No	Yes
Cause	Viral	*Haemophilus influenzae* type B

TEACHING GUIDELINES 39.2

Home Care of Croup

- Keep the child quiet and discourage crying.
- Allow the child to sit up (in your arms).
- Encourage rest and fluid intake.
- If stridor occurs, take the child into a steamy bathroom for 10 minutes.
- Administer medication (corticosteroid) as directed.
- Watch the child closely. Call the physician if:
  - The child breathes faster, has retractions, or has any other difficulty breathing
  - The nostrils flare or the lips or nails have a bluish tint
  - The cough or stridor does not improve with exposure to moist air
  - Restlessness increases or the child is confused
  - The child begins to drool or cannot swallow

Adapted from Knutson & Aring, 2004.

Nursing Management

If the child's care is being managed at home, advise parents about the symptoms of respiratory distress and instruct them to seek treatment if the child's respiratory condition worsens. Teach parents to expose their child to humidified air (via a cool mist humidifier or steamy bathroom). Though never clinically proven, use of humidified air has long been recommended for alleviating coughing jags and anecdotally has been reported as helpful. Administer dexamethasone if ordered or teach parents about home administration. Explain to parents that the effects of racemic epinephrine last about 2 hours and the child must be observed closely as occasionally a child will worsen again, requiring another aerosol. Teaching Guidelines 39.2 provides information about home care of croup.

▶ EPIGLOTTITIS

Epiglottitis (inflammation and swelling of the epiglottis) is most often caused by *Haemophilus influenzae* type b. Extensive use of the Hib vaccine since the 1980s has resulted in a significant decrease in the incidence of epiglottitis. Epiglottitis usually occurs in children between the ages of 2 and 7 years and can be life-threatening (Leung et al., 2004). Respiratory arrest and death may occur if the airway becomes completely occluded. Additional complications include pneumothorax and pulmonary edema. Therapeutic management focuses on airway maintenance and support. Intravenous antibiotic therapy is necessary.

The child will be managed in the intensive care unit. Comparison Chart 39.2 gives information comparing croup to epiglottitis.

Nursing Assessment

Carefully assess the child with suspected epiglottitis. Note sudden onset of symptoms and high fever. The child has an overall toxic appearance. He or she may refuse to speak or may speak only with a very soft voice. The child may refuse to lie down and may assume the characteristic position, sitting forward with the neck extended. Drooling may be present. Note anxiety or a frightened appearance. Note the child's color. Cough is usually absent. A lateral neck x-ray may be performed to determine whether epiglottitis is present. This is done cautiously, so as not to induce airway obstruction with changes in position of the child's neck (Bjornson et al., 2004).

Nursing Management

Do not leave the child unattended. Keep the child and parents as calm as possible. Allow the child to assume a position of comfort. Do not place the child in a supine position, as airway occlusion may occur. Provide 100% oxygen in the least invasive manner that is acceptable to the child. Do not under any circumstance attempt to visualize the throat: reflex laryngospasm may occur, precipitating immediate airway occlusion. If the child with epiglottitis experiences complete airway occlusion, an emergency tracheostomy may be necessary. Ensure that emergency equipment is available and that personnel trained in intubation of the pediatric occluded airway and percutaneous tracheostomy are notified of the child's presence in the facility (Bjornson et al., 2004).

> ▶ *Take* NOTE!
>
> *Epiglottitis is characterized by dysphagia, drooling, anxiety, irritability, and significant respiratory distress. Prepare for the event of sudden airway occlusion.*

▶ BRONCHIOLITIS (RSV)

Bronchiolitis is an acute inflammatory process of the bronchioles and small bronchi. Nearly always caused by a viral pathogen, RSV accounts for the majority of cases of bronchiolitis, with adenovirus, parainfluenza, and human meta-pneumovirus also being important causative agents. This discussion will focus on RSV bronchiolitis.

The peak incidence of bronchiolitis is in the winter and spring, coinciding with RSV season. RSV season in the United States and Canada generally begins in September or October and continues through April or May. Virtually all children will contract RSV infection within the first few years of life. RSV bronchiolitis occurs most often in infants and toddlers, with a peak incidence around 6 months of age. The severity of disease is related inversely to the age of the child. The frequency and severity of RSV infection decrease with age. Repeated RSV infections occur throughout life but are usually localized to the upper respiratory tract after toddlerhood.

Therapeutic Management

Management of RSV focuses on supportive treatment. Supplemental oxygen, nasal and/or nasopharyngeal suctioning, oral or intravenous hydration, and inhaled bronchodilator therapy are used. Many infants are managed at home with close observation and adequate hydration. Hospitalization is required for children with more severe disease. The infant with tachypnea, significant retractions, poor oral intake, or lethargy can deteriorate quickly, to the point of requiring ventilatory support, and thus warrants hospital admission.

Pathophysiology

RSV is a highly contagious virus and may be contracted through direct contact with respiratory secretions or from particles on objects contaminated with the virus (Lauts, 2005). RSV invades the nasopharynx, where it replicates and then spreads down to the lower airway via aspiration of upper airway secretions. RSV infection causes necrosis of the respiratory epithelium of the small airways, peribronchiolar mononuclear infiltration, and plugging of the lumens with mucus and exudate. The small airways become variably obstructed; this allows adequate inspiratory volume but prevents full expiration. This leads to hyperinflation and atelectasis (Bennett, 2006). Serious alterations in gas exchange occur, with arterial hypoxemia and carbon dioxide retention resulting from mismatching of pulmonary ventilation and perfusion. Hypoventilation occurs secondary to markedly increased work of breathing.

Nursing Assessment

For a full description of the assessment phase of the nursing process, refer to page 1222. Assessment findings pertinent to bronchiolitis are discussed below.

Health History
Elicit a description of the present illness and chief complaint. Common signs and symptoms reported during the health history might include:

• Onset of illness with a clear runny nose (sometimes profuse)
• Pharyngitis

- Low-grade fever
- Development of cough 1 to 3 days into the illness, followed by a wheeze shortly thereafter
- Poor feeding

Explore the child's current and past medical history for risk factors such as:

- Young age (less than 2 years old), more severe disease in a child less than 6 months old
- Prematurity
- Multiple births
- Birth during April to September
- History of chronic lung disease (bronchopulmonary disease)
- Cyanotic or complicated congenital heart disease
- Immunocompromise
- Male gender
- Exposure to passive tobacco smoke
- Crowded living conditions
- Daycare attendance
- School-age siblings
- Low socioeconomic status
- Lack of breastfeeding

Physical Examination
Examination of the child with RSV involves inspection, observation, and auscultation.

Inspection and Observation
Observe the child's general appearance and color (centrally and peripherally). The infant with RSV bronchiolitis might appear air-hungry, exhibiting various degrees of cyanosis and respiratory distress, including tachypnea, retractions, accessory muscle use, grunting, and periods of apnea. Cough and audible wheeze might be heard. The infant might appear listless and uninterested in feeding, surroundings, or parents.

Auscultation
Auscultate the lungs, noting adventitious sounds and determining the quality of aeration of the lung fields. Earlier in the illness, wheezes might be heard scattered throughout the lung fields. In more serious cases, the chest might sound quiet and without wheeze. This is due to significant hyperexpansion with very poor air exchange.

Laboratory and Diagnostic Tests
Common laboratory and diagnostic studies ordered for the assessment of RSV bronchiolitis include:

- Pulse oximetry: oxygen saturation might be significantly decreased
- Chest x-ray: might reveal hyperinflation and patchy areas of atelectasis or infiltration

- Blood gases: might show carbon dioxide retention and hypoxemia
- Nasal-pharyngeal washings: positive identification of RSV can be made via enzyme-linked immunosorbent assay (ELISA) or immunofluorescent antibody (IFA) testing

Nursing Management

RSV infection is usually self-limited, and nursing diagnoses, goals, and interventions for the child with bronchiolitis are aimed at supportive care. Children with less severe disease might require only antipyretics, adequate hydration, and close observation. They can often be successfully managed at home, provided the primary caregiver is reliable and comfortable with close observation. Parents or caregivers should be educated to watch for signs of worsening and must understand the importance of seeking care quickly should the child's condition deteriorate.

Hospitalization is required for children with more severe disease, and children admitted with RSV bronchiolitis warrant close observation. In addition to the nursing diagnoses and related interventions discussed in the Nursing Care Plan for respiratory disorders, interventions common to bronchiolitis follow.

> ▶ *Take* NOTE!
>
> *Currently no safe and effective antiviral drug is available for definitive treatment of RSV. Aerosolized ribavirin is recommended only for the highest-risk, most severely ill patients (Lauts, 2005). Routine antibiotic use is discouraged in RSV bronchiolitis treatment because the secondary bacterial infection rate of the lower airway is very low.*

Maintaining Patent Airway
Infants and young children with RSV tend to have copious secretions. Position the child with the head of the bed elevated to facilitate an open airway. These children often require frequent assessment and suctioning to maintain a patent airway (Lauts, 2005). Use a Yankauer or tonsil-tip suction catheter to suction the mouth or pharynx of older infants or children, rinsing the catheter after each suctioning. Nasal bulb suctioning may be sufficient to clear the airway in some infants, while others will require nasopharyngeal suctioning with a suction catheter. Nursing Procedure 39.1 gives further information. Adjust the pressure ranges for suctioning infants and children between 60 and 100 mm Hg, 40 and 60 mm Hg for premature infants.

Nursing Procedure 39.1

NASOPHARYNGEAL OR ARTIFICIAL AIRWAY SUCTION TECHNIQUE

1. Make sure the suction equipment works properly before starting.
2. After washing your hands, assemble the equipment needed:
   - Appropriate-size sterile suction catheter
   - Sterile gloves
   - Supplemental oxygen
   - Sterile water-based lubricant
   - Sterile normal saline if indicated
3. Don sterile gloves, keeping dominant hand sterile and nondominant hand clean.
4. Preoxygenate the infant or child if indicated.
5. Apply lubricant to the end of the suction catheter.
6. If indicated for loosening of secretions, instill sterile saline.
7. Maintaining sterile technique, insert the suction catheter into the child's nostril or airway.
   - Insert only to the point of gagging if inserting via the nostril.
   - Insert only 0.5 cm further than the length of the artificial airway.
8. Intermittently apply suction for no longer than 10 seconds, while twisting and removing the catheter.
9. Supplement with oxygen after suctioning.

Promoting Adequate Gas Exchange

Infants and children with bronchiolitis might deteriorate quickly as the disease progresses. In the child ill enough to require oxygen, the risk is even greater. Assessment should include work of breathing, respiratory rate, and oxygen saturation. The percentage of inspired oxygen (FiO_2) should be adjusted as needed to maintain oxygen saturation within the desired range. Positioning the infant with the head of the bed elevated may also improve gas exchange. Frequent assessment is necessary for the hospitalized child with bronchiolitis (Steiner, 2004).

▶ Take NOTE!

In the tachypneic infant, slowing of the respiratory rate does not necessarily indicate improvement: often, a slower respiratory rate is an indication of tiring, and carbon dioxide retention may soon be followed by apnea.

Reducing Risk for Infection

Since RSV is easily spread through contact with droplets, inpatients should be isolated according to hospital policy to decrease the risk of nosocomial spread to other clients. Clients with RSV can be safely cohorted. Attention to handwashing is necessary, as droplets might enter the eyes, nose, or mouth via the hands.

Providing Family Education

Educate parents so they can recognize signs of worsening distress. Tell parents to call the physician or nurse practitioner if the child's breathing becomes rapid or more difficult or if the child cannot eat secondary to tachypnea. Children who are less than 1 year of age or who are at higher risk (those who were born prematurely or who have chronic heart or lung conditions) might have a longer course of illness. Instruct parents that cough can persist for several days to weeks after resolution of the disease, but infants usually act well otherwise.

Preventing RSV Disease

Strict adherence to handwashing policies in daycare centers and when exposed to individuals with cold symptoms is important for all groups. Though generally benign in healthy older children, RSV can be devastating in young infants or children with pre-existing risk factors. Palivizumab (Synagis) is a monoclonal antibody that can prevent severe RSV disease in those who are most susceptible. It is given as an intramuscular injection once a month throughout the RSV season. Though quite costly, it is covered by most insurance policies and Medicaid for those who qualify. It is generally indicated for use in certain children less than 2 years of age. Qualifying factors include:

- Prematurity
- Chronic lung disease (bronchopulmonary dysplasia) requiring medication or oxygen
- Certain congenital heart diseases
- Immunocompromise (Bennett, 2006)

Additional information related to Synagis may be found at http://www.synagis.com/.

▶ PNEUMONIA

Pneumonia is an inflammation of the lung parenchyma. It can be caused by a virus, bacteria, *Mycoplasma,* or fungus. It may also result from aspiration of foreign material into the lower respiratory tract (aspiration pneumonia). Pneumonia occurs more often in winter and early spring. It is common in children but is seen most frequently in infants and young toddlers. Viruses are the most common cause of pneumonia in younger children and the least common cause in older children (Table 39.2). Viral pneumonia is usually better tolerated in children of all ages. Children with bacterial pneumonia are more apt to present with a toxic appearance, but they generally recover rapidly if appropriate antibiotic treatment is instituted early.

> ▶ **Take** NOTE!
>
> *Community-acquired pneumonia (CAP) refers to pneumonia in a previously healthy person that is contracted outside of the hospital setting. CAP is a common cause of lower respiratory infection in North America (Ostapchuk et al., 2004).*

Pneumonia is usually a self-limited disease. A child who presents with recurrent pneumonia should be evaluated for chronic lung disease such as asthma or cystic fibrosis. Potential complications of pneumonia include bacteremia, pleural effusion, empyema, lung abscess, and pneumothorax (Nield et al., 2005). Excluding bacteremia, these are often treated with thoracentesis and/or chest tubes as well as antibiotics if appropriate. Pneumatoceles (thin-walled cavities developing in the lung) might occur with certain bacterial pneumonias and usually resolve spontaneously over time.

Therapeutic management of children with less severe disease includes antipyretics, adequate hydration, and close observation. Even bacterial pneumonia can be successfully managed at home if the work of breathing is not severe and oxygen saturation is within normal limits. However, hospitalization is required for children with more severe disease. The child with tachypnea, significant retractions, poor oral intake, or lethargy might require hospital admission for the administration of supplemental oxygen, intravenous hydration, and antibiotics.

TABLE 39.2 **COMMON CAUSES OF PNEUMONIA ACCORDING TO AGE**

Age Group	Most Common Causative Agents
1 to 3 months	RSV, other respiratory viruses (parainfluenza, influenza, adenovirus); *Streptococcus pneumoniae, Chlamydia trachomatis*
4 months to 5 years	Respiratory viruses, *Streptococcus pneumoniae, Chlamydia pneumoniae, Mycoplasma pneumoniae*
5 to 18 years	*Mycoplasma pneumoniae, Chlamydia pneumoniae, Streptococcus pneumoniae*

Sources: Nield et al., 2005; Ostapchuk, 2004.

> ▶ **Take** NOTE!
>
> *Haemophilus influenzae type B has been nearly eliminated as a cause of pneumonia in the United States and other developed countries as a result of universal immunization with Hib vaccine.*

Pathophysiology

Pneumonia occurs as a result of the spread of infectious organisms to the lower respiratory tract from either the upper respiratory tract or the bloodstream. In bacterial pneumonia, mucus stasis occurs as a result of vascular engorgement. Cellular debris (erythrocytes, neutrophils, and fibrin) accumulates in the alveolar space. Relative hyperexpansion with air trapping follows. Inflammation of the alveoli results in **atelectasis** (a collapsed or airless portion of the lung), so gas exchange becomes impaired. The inflammatory response further impairs gas exchange (Nield et al., 2005).

Viral pneumonia usually results in an inflammatory reaction limited to the alveolar wall. Aspiration of food, fluids, or other substances into the bronchial tree can result in aspiration pneumonia. Aspiration is the most common cause of recurrent pneumonia in children and often occurs as a result of gastroesophageal reflux disease. Secondary bacterial infection often occurs following viral or aspiration pneumonia and requires antibiotic treatment.

Nursing Assessment

For a full description of the assessment phase of the nursing process, refer to page 1222. Assessment findings pertinent to pneumonia are discussed below.

Health History

Elicit a description of the present illness and chief complaint. Note onset and progression of symptoms. Common signs and symptoms reported during the health history include:

- Antecedent viral URI
- Fever
- Cough (note type and whether productive or not)
- Increased respiratory rate
- History of lethargy, poor feeding, vomiting, or diarrhea in infants
- Chills, headache, dyspnea, chest pain, abdominal pain, and nausea or vomiting in older children

Explore the child's past and current medical history for risk factors known to be associated with an increase in the severity of pneumonia, such as:

- Prematurity
- Malnutrition

- Passive smoke exposure
- Low socioeconomic status
- Daycare attendance
- Underlying cardiopulmonary, immune, or nervous system disease

Physical Examination

Physical examination consists of inspection, auscultation, percussion, and palpation.

Inspection

Observe the child's general appearance and color (centrally and peripherally). Cyanosis might accompany coughing spells. The child with bacterial pneumonia may appear ill. Assess work of breathing. Children with pneumonia might exhibit substernal, subcostal, or intercostal retractions. Tachypnea and nasal flaring may be present. Describe cough and quality of sputum if produced.

Auscultation

Auscultation of the lungs might reveal wheezes or rales in the younger child. Local or diffuse rales may be present in the older child. Document diminished breath sounds.

Percussion and Palpation

In the older child, percussion might yield local dullness over a consolidated area. Percussion is much less valuable in the infant or younger child. Tactile fremitus felt upon palpation may be increased with pneumonia.

Laboratory and Diagnostic Tests

Common laboratory and diagnostic studies ordered for the assessment of pneumonia include:

- Pulse oximetry: oxygen saturation might be significantly decreased or within normal range
- Chest x-ray: varies according to client age and causative agent. In infants and young children, bilateral air trapping and perihilar **infiltrates** are the most common findings. Patchy areas of consolidation might also be present. In older children, lobar consolidation is seen more frequently.
- Sputum culture: may be useful in determining causative bacteria in older children and adolescents
- White blood cell count: might be elevated in the case of bacterial pneumonia

Nursing Management

Nursing diagnoses, goals, and interventions for the child with pneumonia are primarily aimed at providing supportive care and education about the illness and its treatment. Prevention of pneumococcal infection is also important. Children with more severe disease will require hospitalization. Refer to Nursing Care Plan 39.1 for nursing diagnoses and related interventions. In ad-dition to the interventions listed there, the following should be noted.

Providing Supportive Care

Ensure adequate hydration and assist in thinning of secretions by encouraging oral fluid intake in the child whose respiratory status is stable. In children with increased work of breathing, intravenous fluids may be necessary to maintain hydration. Allow and encourage the child to assume a position of comfort, usually with the head of the bed elevated to promote aeration of the lungs. If pain due to coughing or pneumonia itself is severe, administer analgesics as prescribed. Provide supplemental oxygen to the child with respiratory distress or hypoxia as needed.

Providing Family Education

Educate the family about the importance of adhering to the prescribed antibiotic regimen. Antibiotics may be given intravenously if the child is hospitalized, but upon discharge or if the child is managed on an outpatient basis, oral antibiotics will be used.

Teach the parents of a child with bacterial pneumonia to expect that following resolution of the acute illness, for 1 to 2 weeks the child might continue to tire easily and the infant might continue to need small, frequent feedings. Cough may also persist after the acute recovery period but should lessen over time.

If the child is diagnosed with viral pneumonia, parents might not understand that their child does not require an antibiotic. Pneumonia is often perceived by the public as a bacterial infection, so most parents will need an explanation related to treatment of viral infections. As with bacterial pneumonia, the child may experience a week or two of weakness or fatigue following resolution of the acute illness.

The young child is at risk for the development of aspiration pneumonia. Parents need to understand that the child might be at risk for injury related to his or her age and developmental stage. To prevent recurrent or further aspiration, teach the parents the safety measures in Teaching Guidelines 39.3.

Preventing Pneumococcal Infection

Children at high risk for severe pneumococcal infection should be immunized against it. This includes all children between 0 and 23 months of age, as well as children between 24 and 59 months of age who either never received the vaccine before age 2 or did not receive a booster dose between 12 and 23 months of age. Additionally, children between 24 and 59 months of age with certain conditions such as immune deficiency, sickle cell disease, asplenia, chronic cardiac conditions, chronic lung problems, cerebrospinal fluid leaks, chronic renal insufficiency, diabetes mellitus, and organ transplants, should receive the vaccine. For additional information on immunization, refer to Chapter 30.

TEACHING GUIDELINES 39.3

Preventing Aspiration

- Keep toxic substances such as lighter fluid, solvents, and hydrocarbons out of reach of young children. Toddlers and preschoolers cannot distinguish safe from unsafe fluids due to their developmental stage.
- Avoid oily nose drops and oil-based vitamins or home remedies to avoid lipid aspiration into the lungs.
- Avoid oral feedings if the infant's respiratory rate is 60 or greater to minimize the risk of aspiration of the feeding.
- Discourage parents from "force-feeding" in the event of poor oral intake or severe illness to minimize the risk of aspiration of the feeding.
- Position infants and ill children on their right side after feeding to minimize the risk of aspirating emesis or regurgitated feeding.

► BRONCHITIS

Bronchitis is an inflammation of the trachea and major bronchi. It is often associated with a URI. Bronchitis is usually viral in nature, though *Mycoplasma pneumoniae* is also an important causative agent in children over 6 years of age. Recovery usually occurs within 5 to 10 days. Therapeutic management involves mainly supportive care. Expectorant administration and adequate hydration are important. If *Mycoplasma* is the cause, antibiotics are indicated (Orenstein, 2004b).

Nursing Assessment

The illness might begin with a mild URI. Fever develops, followed by a dry, hacking cough that might become productive in older children. The cough might wake the child at night. Auscultation of the lungs might reveal coarse rales. Respirations remain unlabored. The chest x-ray might show diffuse alveolar hyperinflation and perihilar markings.

HEALTHY PEOPLE 2010

Objective	Significance
Reduce invasive pneumococcal infections.	• Provide accurate information to families about pneumococcal disease. • Encourage pneumococcal immunization per recommendations.

Nursing Management

Nursing management is aimed at providing supportive care. Teach parents that expectorants will help loosen secretions and antipyretics will help reduce the fever, making the child more comfortable. Encourage adequate hydration. Antibiotics are prescribed only in cases believed to be bacterial in nature. Discourage the use of cough suppressants: it is important for accumulated sputum to be raised.

► TUBERCULOSIS

Tuberculosis is a highly contagious disease caused by inhalation of droplets of *Mycobacterium tuberculosis* or *Mycobacterium bovis*. Children usually contract the disease from an immediate household member. Annually about 1,000 U.S. children contract active tuberculosis disease (Reznik & Ozuah, 2005). Nonwhite children and children with chronic illness or malnutrition are more susceptible to infection. After exposure to an infected individual, the incubation period is 2 to 10 weeks. The inhaled tubercle bacilli multiply in the alveoli and alveolar ducts, forming an inflammatory exudate. The bacilli are spread by the bloodstream and lymphatic system to various parts of the body. Though pulmonary tuberculosis is the most common, children may also have infection in other parts of the body, such as the gastrointestinal tract or central nervous system.

In the case of drug-sensitive tuberculosis, the American Academy of Pediatrics recommends a 6-month course of oral therapy. The first 2 months consist of isoniazid,

HEALTHY PEOPLE 2010

Objective	Significance
Reduce tuberculosis. Increase the proportion of all tuberculosis patients who complete curative therapy within 12 months. Increase the proportion of contacts and other high-risk persons with latent tuberculosis infection who complete a course of treatment.	• Assess the health history of all infants, children, and adolescents for risk factors for tuberculosis infection. • Provide tuberculosis screening as recommended. • Refer all tuberculosis infections to the local public health department. • Educate families about the importance of completing medication therapy as prescribed for active and latent tuberculosis, and the need for appropriate follow-up and retesting for tuberculosis infection.

rifampin, and pyrazinamide given daily. This is followed by twice-weekly isoniazid and rifampin; administration must be observed directly (usually by a public health nurse). In the case of multidrug-resistant tuberculosis, ethambutol or streptomycin is given via intramuscular injection (Pickering, 2006).

Nursing Assessment

Routine screening for tuberculosis infection is not recommended for low-risk individuals, but children considered to be at high risk for contracting tuberculosis should be screened using the Mantoux test. Children considered to be at high risk are those who:

• Are infected with HIV
• Are incarcerated or institutionalized
• Have a positive recent history of latent tuberculosis infection
• Are immigrants from or have a history of travel to endemic countries
• Are exposed at home to HIV-infected or homeless persons, illicit drug users, persons recently incarcerated, migrant farm workers, or nursing home residents

Children with chronic illnesses (except HIV infection) are not more likely to become infected with tuberculosis but should receive special consideration and be screened prior to initiation of immunosuppressant therapies (Reznik & Ozuah, 2005).

The presentation of tuberculosis in children is quite varied. Children can be asymptomatic or exhibit a broad range of symptoms. Symptoms may include fever, malaise, weight loss, anorexia, pain and tightness in the chest, and rarely hemoptysis. Cough might or might not be present and usually progresses slowly over several weeks to months. As tuberculosis progresses, the respiratory rate increases and the lung on the affected side is poorly expanded. Dullness to percussion might be present, as well as diminished breath sounds and crackles. Fever persists and pallor, anemia, weakness, and weight loss are present. Diagnosis is confirmed with a positive Mantoux test, positive gastric washings for acid-fast bacillus, and/or a chest x-ray consistent with tuberculosis (Reznik & Ozuah, 2005).

Nursing Management

Hospitalization of children with tuberculosis is necessary only for the most serious cases. Nursing management is aimed at providing supportive care and encouraging adherence to the treatment regimen. Most nursing care for childhood tuberculosis is provided in outpatient clinics, schools, or a public health setting. Supportive care includes ensuring adequate nutrition and adequate rest, providing comfort measures such as fever reduction, preventing exposure to other infectious diseases, and preventing reinfection.

Providing Care for the Child With Latent Tuberculosis Infection

Children who test positive for tuberculosis but who do not have symptoms or radiographic/laboratory evidence of disease are considered to have latent infection. These children should be treated with isoniazid for 9 months to prevent progression to active disease. Follow-up and appropriate monitoring can be achieved via the child's primary care provider or local health department.

Preventing Infection

Tuberculosis infection is prevented by avoiding contact with the tubercle bacillus. Thus, hospitalized children with tuberculosis must be isolated according to hospital policy to prevent nosocomial spread of tuberculosis infection. Promotion of natural resistance through nutrition, rest, and avoidance of serious infections does not prevent infection. Pasteurization of milk has helped to decrease the transmission of *Mycobacterium bovis*. Administration of bacille Calmette-Guérin (BCG) vaccine can provide incomplete protection against tuberculosis, and it is not widely used in the United States.

Acute Noninfectious Disorders

Acute noninfectious disorders include epistaxis, foreign body aspiration, respiratory distress syndrome, acute respiratory distress syndrome, and pneumothorax.

▶ EPISTAXIS

Epistaxis (a nosebleed) occurs most frequently in children before adolescence. Bleeding of the nasal mucosa occurs most often from the anterior portion of the septum. Epistaxis may be recurrent and idiopathic (meaning there is no cause). The majority of cases are benign, but in children with bleeding disorders or other hematologic concerns, epistaxis should be further investigated and treated.

▶ *Take NOTE!*

The child with recurrent epistaxis or epistaxis that is difficult to control should be further evaluated for underlying bleeding or platelet concerns.

Nursing Assessment

Explore the child's history for initiating factors such as local inflammation, mucosal drying, or local trauma (usually nose picking). Inspect the nasal cavity for blood.

Nursing Management

The presence of blood often frightens children and their parents. The nurse and parents should remain calm. The child should sit up and lean forward (lying down may allow aspiration of the blood). Apply continuous pressure to the anterior portion of the nose by pinching it closed. Encourage the child to breathe through the mouth during this portion of the treatment. Ice or a cold cloth applied to the bridge of the nose may also be helpful. The bleeding usually stops within 10 to 15 minutes. Apply petroleum jelly or water-soluble gel to the nasal mucosa with a cotton-tipped applicator to moisten the mucosa and prevent recurrence.

▶ FOREIGN BODY ASPIRATION

Foreign body aspiration occurs when any solid or liquid substance is inhaled into the respiratory tract. It is common in infants and young children and can present in a life-threatening manner. The object may lodge in the upper or lower airway, causing varying degrees of respiratory difficulty. Small, smooth objects such as peanuts are the most frequently aspirated, but any small toy, article, or piece of food smaller than the diameter of the young child's airway can be aspirated.

Foreign body aspiration occurs most frequently in children ages 6 months to 5 years. Children this age are growing and developing rapidly. They tend to explore things with their mouths and can easily aspirate small items.

The child often coughs out foreign bodies from the upper airway. If the foreign body reaches the bronchus, then it may need to be surgically removed via bronchoscopy. Postoperative antibiotics are used if an infection is also present. Complications of foreign body aspiration include pneumonia or abscess formation, hypoxia, respiratory failure, and death (Orenstein, 2004c).

Nursing Assessment

The infant or young child might present with a history of sudden onset of cough, wheeze, or stridor. Stridor suggests that the foreign body is lodged in the upper airway. Sometimes the onset of respiratory symptoms is much more gradual. When the item has traveled down one of the bronchi, then wheezing, rhonchi, and decreased aeration can be heard on the affected side. A chest x-ray will demonstrate the foreign body only if it is radiopaque (Fig. 39.8).

Nursing Management

The most important nursing intervention related to foreign body aspiration is prevention. Anticipatory guidance

FIGURE 39.8 Foreign body is noted in the bronchus on a chest x-ray.

for families with 6-month-olds should include a discussion of aspiration avoidance. This information should be repeated at each subsequent well-child visit through age 5. Tell parents to avoid letting their child play with toys with small parts and to keep coins and other small objects out of the reach of children. Teach parents not to feed peanuts and popcorn to their child until he or she is at least 3 years old. When children progress to table food, teach parents to chop all foods so that they are small enough to pass down the trachea should the child neglect to chew them up thoroughly. Carrots, grapes, and hot dogs should be cut into small pieces. Harmful liquids should be kept out of the reach of children.

▶ *Take* NOTE!

Items smaller than 1.25 inches (3.2 cm) can be aspirated easily. A simple way for parents to estimate the safe size of a small item or toy piece is to gauge its size against a standard toilet paper roll, which is generally about 1.5 inches in diameter.

▶ RESPIRATORY DISTRESS SYNDROME

Respiratory distress syndrome (RDS) is a respiratory disorder that is specific to neonates. It results from lung immaturity and a deficiency in surfactant, so it is seen most often in premature infants. Other infants who might experience RDS include infants of diabetic mothers, those delivered via cesarean section without preceding labor, and those experiencing perinatal asphyxia. It is believed that each of these conditions has an impact on surfactant production, thus resulting in RDS in the term infant (Stoll & Kliegman, 2004).

The administration of surfactant via an endotracheal tube shortly after delivery helps to decrease the incidence and severity of RDS. Management of RDS focuses on intensive respiratory care, usually with mechanical ventilation. Newer techniques for ventilatory support are also available (Table 39.3).

Pathophysiology

The lack of surfactant in the affected newborn's lungs results in stiff, poorly compliant lungs with poor gas exchange. Right-to-left shunting and hypoxemia result. As the disease progresses, fluid and fibrin leak from the pulmonary capillaries, causing a hyaline membrane to form in the bronchioles, alveolar ducts, and alveoli. Presence of the membrane further decreases gas exchange. Complications of RDS include air leak syndrome, bronchopulmonary dysplasia, patent ductus arteriosus and congestive heart failure, intraventricular hemorrhage, retinopathy of prematurity, necrotizing enterocolitis, complications resulting from intravenous catheter use (infection, thrombus formation), and developmental delay or disability (Stoll & Kliegman, 2004).

Nursing Assessment

The onset of RDS is usually within several hours of birth. The newborn exhibits signs of respiratory distress, including tachypnea, retractions, nasal flaring, grunting, and varying degrees of cyanosis. Auscultation reveals fine rales and diminished breath sounds. If untreated,

RDS progresses to seesaw respirations, respiratory failure, and shock.

Nursing Management

Rarely, mucus plugging can occur in the neonate placed on a ventilator after surfactant administration. Therefore, close observation and assessment for adequate lung expansion are critical. In addition to expert respiratory intervention, other crucial nursing goals include maintenance of normothermia, prevention of infection, maintenance of fluid and electrolyte balance, and promotion of adequate nutrition (parenterally or via gavage feeding). Nursing care of the infant with RDS generally occurs in the intensive care unit.

▶ ACUTE RESPIRATORY DISTRESS SYNDROME

Acute respiratory distress syndrome (ARDS) occurs following a primary insult such as sepsis, viral pneumonia, smoke inhalation, or near-drowning. Respiratory distress and hypoxemia occur acutely within 72 hours of the insult in infants and children with previously healthy lungs. The alveolar–capillary membrane becomes more permeable and pulmonary edema develops. Hyaline membrane formation over the alveolar surfaces and decreased surfactant production cause lung stiffness. Mucosal swelling and cellular debris lead to atelectasis. Gas diffusion is impaired significantly. ARDS can progress to respiratory failure and death, though some individuals recover completely or have residual lung disease.

Medical treatment is aimed at improving **oxygenation** and **ventilation**. Mechanical ventilation is used, with special attention to lung volumes and positive end-expiratory

TABLE 39.3 ALTERNATIVES TO TRADITIONAL MECHANICAL VENTILATION

Mode	Description	Additional Information
High-frequency ventilators (high-frequency, oscillating, or jet)	Provide very high respiratory rates (up to 1,200 breaths per minute) and very low tidal volumes	May decrease risk of barotrauma associated with ventilator pressures
Nitric oxide	Causes pulmonary vasodilation, helping to increase blood flow to alveoli	Safe; no long-term developmental risks
Liquid ventilation	Perfluorocarbon liquid acts as a surfactant. Provides an effective medium for gas exchange and increases pulmonary function.	Virtually no reported physiologic sequelae
Extracorporeal membrane oxygenation (ECMO)	Blood is removed from body via catheter, warmed and oxygenated in the ECMO machine, and then returned to infant.	Labor-intensive. Risk of bleeding is great.

pressure (PEEP). Newer treatment modalities show promise for improving outcomes of ARDS.

Nursing Assessment

Tachycardia and tachypnea occur over the first few hours of the illness. Significantly increased work of breathing with nasal flaring and retractions develops. Auscultate for breath sounds, which might range from normal to high-pitched crackles throughout the lung fields. Hypoxemia develops. Bilateral infiltrates can be seen on a chest x-ray.

Nursing Management

Nursing care of the child with ARDS is mainly supportive and occurs in the intensive care unit. Closely monitor respiratory and cardiovascular status. Comfort measures such as hygiene and positioning as well as pain and anxiety management, maintenance of nutrition, and prevention of infection are also key nursing interventions. The acute phase of worsening respiratory distress can be frightening for a child of any age, and the nurse can be instrumental in soothing the child's fears. As the disease worsens and progresses, especially when ventilatory support is required, psychological support of the family as well as education about the intensive care unit procedures will be especially important.

▶ PNEUMOTHORAX

A collection of air in the pleural space is called a pneumothorax. It can occur spontaneously in an otherwise healthy child or as a result of chronic lung disease, cardiopulmonary resuscitation, surgery, or trauma. Trapped air consumes space within the pleural cavity, and the affected lung suffers at least partial collapse. Needle aspiration and/or placement of a chest tube is used to evacuate the air from the chest. Some small pneumothoraces resolve independently, without intervention (Kerby et al., 2007).

Nursing Assessment

Primary pneumothorax (spontaneous) occurs most often in adolescence. The infant or child with a pneumothorax might have a sudden or gradual onset of symptoms. Chest pain might be present as well as signs of respiratory distress such as tachypnea, retractions, nasal flaring, or grunting. Assess risk factors for acquiring a pneumothorax, including chest trauma or surgery, intubation and mechanical ventilation, or a history of chronic lung disease such as cystic fibrosis. Inspect the child for a pale or cyanotic appearance. Auscultate for increased heart rate (tachycardia) and absent or diminished breath sounds on the affected side. The x-ray reveals air within the thoracic cavity (Fig. 39.9).

Nursing Management

The child with a pneumothorax requires frequent respiratory assessments. Pulse oximetry might be used as an adjunct, but clinical evaluation of respiratory status is most useful. In some cases, administration of 100% oxygen hastens the reabsorption of air, but it is generally used only for a few hours. If a chest tube is connected to a dry suction or water seal apparatus, provide care of the drainage apparatus as appropriate (Fig. 39.10). A pair of hemostats should be kept at the bedside to clamp the tube should it become dislodged from the drainage container. The dressing around the chest tube is occlusive and is not routinely changed. If the tube becomes dislodged from the child's chest, apply Vaseline gauze and an occlusive dressing, immediately perform appropriate respiratory assessment, and notify the physician.

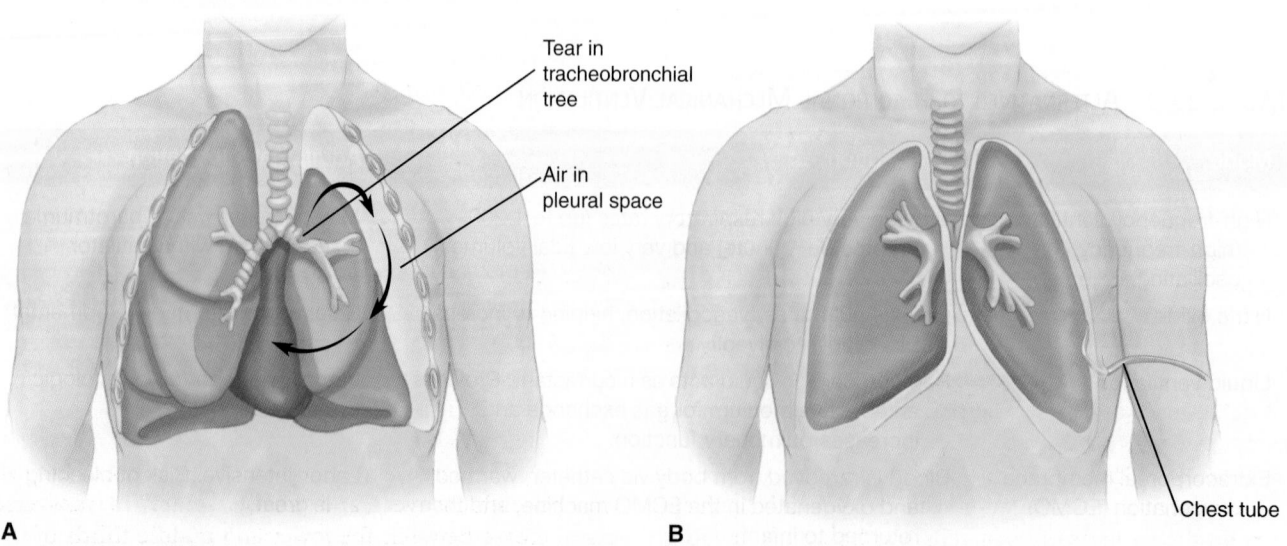

Tear in tracheobronchial tree

Air in pleural space

Chest tube

A   B

FIGURE 39.9 Pneumothorax.

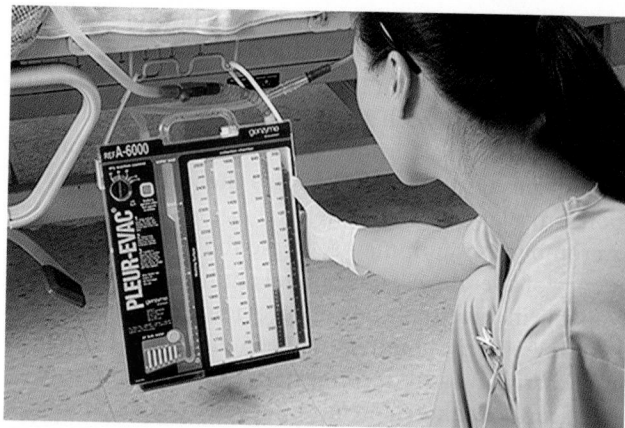

FIGURE 39.10 The chest tube is connected to suction or water seal via a drainage container.

Chronic Diseases

Chronic respiratory disorders include allergic rhinitis, asthma, chronic lung disease (bronchopulmonary dysplasia), cystic fibrosis, and apnea.

▶ ALLERGIC RHINITIS

Allergic **rhinitis** is a common chronic condition in childhood, affecting up to 40% of children (Hagemann, 2005). Allergic rhinitis is associated with atopic dermatitis and asthma, with as many as 60% to 78% of asthmatic children also suffering from allergic rhinitis (Rance, 2007). Perennial allergic rhinitis occurs year-round and is associated with indoor environments. Allergens commonly implicated in perennial allergic rhinitis include dust mites, pet dander, cockroach antigens, and molds. Seasonal allergic rhinitis is caused by elevations in outdoor levels of allergens. It is typically caused by certain pollens, trees, weeds, fungi, and molds. Complications from allergic rhinitis include exacerbation of asthma symptoms, recurrent sinusitis and otitis media, and dental malocclusion.

Pathophysiology

Allergic rhinitis is an intermittent or persistent inflammatory state that is mediated by immunoglobulin E (IgE). In response to contact with an airborne allergen protein, the nasal mucosa mounts an immune response. The antigen (from the allergen) binds to a specific IgE on the surface of mast cells, releasing the chemical mediators of histamine and leukotrienes. The release of mediators results in acute tissue edema and mucus production (Banasiak & Meadows-Oliver, 2005). Late-phase mediators are released and more inflammation results. IgE binds to receptors on the surfaces of mast cells and basophils, creating the sensitization memory that causes the reaction with subsequent allergen exposures. Allergen exposure then results in mast cell degranulation and release of histamine and other chemotactic factors. Histamine and other factors cause nasal vasodilation, watery **rhinorrhea**, and nasal congestion. Irritation of local nerve endings by histamine produces pruritus and sneezing (Hagemann, 2005). Treatment of allergic rhinitis is aimed at decreasing response to these allergic mediators as well as treating inflammation.

Nursing Assessment

For a full description of the assessment phase of the nursing process, refer to page 1222. Assessment findings pertinent to allergic rhinitis are discussed below.

Health History

Elicit a description of the present illness and chief complaint. Common signs and symptoms reported during the health history might include:

- Mild, intermittent to chronic nasal stuffiness
- Thin, runny nasal discharge
- Sneezing
- Itching of nose, eyes, palate
- Mouth breathing and snoring

Determine the seasonality of symptoms. Are they perennial (year-round) or do they occur during certain seasons only? What types of medications or other treatments have been used, and what was the child's response?

Explore the history for the presence of risk factors such as:

- Family history of atopic disease (asthma, allergic rhinitis, or atopic dermatitis)
- Known allergy to dust mites, pet dander, cockroach antigens, pollens, or molds
- Early childhood exposure to indoor allergens
- Early introduction to foods or formula in infancy
- Exposure to tobacco smoke
- Environmental air pollution
- Recurrent viral infections

Nonwhite race and higher socioeconomic status have also been noted as risk factors (Hagemann, 2005).

Physical Examination

Physical examination of the child with allergic rhinitis includes inspection, observation, and auscultation.

Inspection and Observation

Observe the child's facies for red-rimmed eyes or tearing, mild eyelid edema, "allergic shiners" (bluish or grayish cast beneath the eyes), and "allergic salute" (a transverse nasal crease between the lower and middle thirds of the nose that results from repeated nose rubbing) (Fig. 39.11).

Figure 39.11 Allergic shiners beneath the eyes and allergic salute across the nose.

Inspect the nasal cavity. The turbinates may be swollen and gray/blue. Clear mucoid nasal drainage may be observed. Inspect the skin for rash. Listen for nasal phonation with speech.

Auscultation

Auscultate the lungs for adequate aeration and clarity of breath sounds. In the child who also has asthma, exacerbation with wheezing often occurs with allergic rhinitis.

Laboratory and Diagnostic Tests

The initial diagnosis is often made based on the history and clinical findings. Common laboratory and diagnostic studies ordered for the assessment of allergic rhinitis may include:

• Nasal smear (positive for eosinophilia)
• Positive allergy skin test
• Positive RAST

   To distinguish between the causes of nasal congestion, refer to Comparison Chart 39.1.

Nursing Management

In addition to the nursing diagnoses and related interventions discussed in the Nursing Care Plan for disorders of the nose, mouth, and throat, interventions common to allergic rhinitis follow.

Maintaining Patent Airway

The continual nasal obstruction that occurs with allergic rhinitis can be very problematic for some children.

Performing nasal washes with normal saline may keep the nasal mucus from becoming thickened. Thickened, immobile secretions often lead to a secondary bacterial infection. The nasal wash also decongests the nose, allowing for improved nasal airflow. Anti-inflammatory (corticosteroid) nasal sprays can decrease the inflammatory response to allergens. A mast cell stabilizing nasal spray such as cromolyn sodium may decrease the intensity and frequency of allergic responses. Oral antihistamines are now available in once-daily dosing, providing convenience for the family. Some children may benefit from a combined antihistamine/nasal decongestant if nasal congestion is significant. Leukotriene modifiers such as montelukast may also be beneficial for some children (Banasiak & Meadows-Oliver, 2005).

Providing Family Education

One of the most important tools in the treatment of allergic rhinitis is learning to avoid known allergens. Teaching Guidelines 39.4 gives information on educating families about avoidance of allergens. Children may be referred to a specialist for allergen desensitization (allergy shots). Products helpful with control of allergies are available from a number of vendors, such as www.onlineallergyrelief.com.

► ASTHMA

Asthma is a chronic inflammatory airway disorder characterized by airway hyperresponsiveness, airway edema, and mucus production. Airway obstruction resulting from asthma might be partially or completely reversed. Severity ranges from long periods of control with infrequent acute exacerbations in some children to the presence of persistent daily symptoms in others (Kieckhefer & Ratcliffe, 2004). It is the most common chronic illness of childhood and affects about 9 million American children (Kumar et al., 2005). A small percentage of children with asthma account for a large percentage of health care use and expense (Wakefield et al., 2005a, 2005b). Asthma accounts for about 14 million lost school days per year and a significant number of lost workdays on the part of parents (Rhee et al., 2007). The incidence and severity of asthma are increasing; this might be attributed to increased urbanization, increased air pollution, and more accurate diagnosis.

   Severity ranges from symptoms associated only with vigorous activity (exercise-induced bronchospasm) to daily symptoms that interfere with quality of life. Table 39.4 discusses classification of asthma severity. Though uncommon, childhood death related to asthma is also on the rise worldwide. Air pollution, allergens, family history, and viral infections might all play a role in asthma. Many

TEACHING GUIDELINES 39.4

Controlling Exposure to Allergens

Tobacco

- Avoid all exposure to tobacco smoke.
- If parents cannot quit, they must not smoke inside the home or car.

Dust Mites

- Use pillow and mattress covers.
- Wash sheets, pillowcases, and comforters once a week in 130° F water.
- Use blinds rather than curtains in bedroom.
- Remove stuffed animals from bedroom.
- Reduce indoor humidity to <50%.
- Remove carpet from bedroom.
- Clean solid-surface floors with wet mop each week.

Pet Dander

- Remove pets from home permanently.
- If unable to remove them, keep them out of bedroom and off carpet and upholstered furniture.

Cockroaches

- Keep kitchen very clean.
- Avoiding leaving food or drinks out.
- Use pesticides if necessary, but ensure that the asthmatic child is not inside the home when the pesticide is sprayed.

Indoor Molds

- Repair water leaks.
- Use dehumidifier to keep basement dry.
- Reduce indoor humidity to <50%.

Outdoor Molds, Pollen, and Air Pollution

- Avoid going outdoors when mold and pollen counts are high.
- Avoid outdoor activity when pollution levels are high.

TABLE 39.4   ASTHMA SEVERITY CLASSIFICATION IN CHILDREN NOT TAKING LONG-TERM CONTROL MEDICATIONS

Classification	Symptoms	Lung Function	Interference with Normal Activity	Short-Acting Beta2-Agonist Use for Symptom Control
Intermittent	• 1 or 2 times a week • Nighttime symptoms 1 or 2 times a month	FEV 80% or more of predicted	None	1 or 2 days per week
Mild persistent	• Symptoms more than twice a week but less than once a day • Nighttime symptoms 3 or 4 times a month	FEV 80% or more of predicted, variability	Minor limitation	Greater than twice per week, but not more than once a day
Moderate persistent	• Daily symptoms • Nighttime symptoms >1 time a week, but not nightly	FEV 60% to 80% of predicted	Some limitation	Daily
Severe persistent	• Throughout the day • Nighttime symptoms often 7 times per week	FEV less than 60% of predicted	Extremely limited	Several times per day

FEV, forced expiratory volume.
Adapted from National Asthma Education and Prevention Program. (2007). *Expert panel report 3: Guidelines for the diagnosis and management of asthma* (NIH Publication No. 07-4051). Bethesda, MD: National Institutes of Health, National Heart, Lung and Blood Institute.

children with asthma also have gastroesophageal disease, though the relationship between the two diseases is not clearly understood.

A significant long-term complication, chronic airway remodeling, may result from recurrent asthma exacerbation and inflammation. This process involves structural changes such as thickening of the sub-basement membrane, subepithelial fibrosis, airway smooth muscle hypertrophy and hyperplasia, blood vessel proliferation and dilation, and mucous gland hyperplasia and hypersecretion (NAEPP, 2007). In some individuals with poorly controlled asthma, these changes may be permanent, resulting in decreased responsiveness to therapy. Children with asthma are also more susceptible to serious bacterial and viral respiratory infections. Acute complications also include status asthmaticus and respiratory failure.

Pathophysiology

In asthma, the inflammatory process contributes to increased airway activity. Thus, control or prevention of inflammation is the core of asthma management. Asthma results from a complex variety of responses in relation to a trigger. When the process begins, mast cells, T lympho-cytes, macrophages, and epithelial cells are involved in the release of inflammatory mediators. Eosinophils and neutrophils migrate to the airway, causing injury. Chemical mediators such as leukotrienes, bradykinin, histamine, and platelet-activating factor also contribute to the inflammatory response. The presence of leukotrienes contributes to prolonged airway constriction (Banasiak & Meadows-Oliver, 2005). Autonomic neural control of airway tone is affected, airway mucus secretion is increased, mucociliary function changes, and airway smooth muscle responsiveness increases (Kiecheter & Ratcliffe, 2004). As a result, acute bronchoconstriction, airway edema, and mucus plugging occur (Fig. 39.12).

In most children, this process is considered reversible and until recently it was not considered to have long-standing effects on lung function. Current research and scientific thought, however, recognize the concept of airway remodeling. Airway remodeling occurs as a result of chronic inflammation of the airway. Following the acute response to a trigger, continued allergen response results in a chronic phase. During this phase, the epithelial cells are denuded and the influx of inflammatory cells into the airway continues. This results in structural changes of the airway that are irreversible, and further loss of pulmonary function might occur (Kiecheter & Ratcliffe, 2004).

Therapeutic Management

Current goals of medical therapy are avoidance of asthma triggers and reduction or control of inflammatory episodes. The most recent recommendations by the National Asthma Education and Prevention Program (2007) suggest a stepwise approach to medication management as well as control of environmental factors (allergens) and comorbid conditions that affect asthma. The NAEPP guidelines stress periodic assessment of asthma control. Treatment decisions may then be made based on the indi-

Normal airway

Airway with inflammation

Airway with inflammation, bronchospasm, and mucus production

FIGURE 39.12 Note airway edema, mucus production, and bronchospasm occurring with asthma.

vidual's level of asthma control, rather than on the severity at diagnosis.

The stepwise approach to asthma treatment involves increasing medications as the child's condition worsens, then backing off treatment as he or she improves (Table 39.5). Bronchodilators may be used in the acute treatment of bronchoconstriction or in the long-acting form to prevent bronchospasm. Exercise-induced bronchospasm may occur in any child with asthma or as the only symptom in the child with mild intermittent asthma. Most children may avoid exercise-induced bronchospasm by using a longer warm-up period prior to vigorous exercise and, if necessary, inhaling a short-acting bronchodilator just prior to exercise. Long-term prevention usually involves inhaled steroids. Leukotriene modifiers may be used as an alternative but are not preferred for mild persistent asthma (NAEPP, 2007).

TABLE 39.5 STEPWISE APPROACH TO ASTHMA MANAGEMENT

All patients: patient education, environmental control, and management of comorbidities at each step. Consider referral to asthma specialist at step 3. (Step 2 and above are persistent asthma.)

Step 1 (intermittent asthma)
Preferred: short-acting beta2-agonist PRN

Step 2
Preferred: low-dose inhaled corticosteroid
Alternative: cromolyn or leukotriene modifier

Step 3
Preferred: medium-dose inhaled corticosteroid (all ages) OR low-dose inhaled corticosteroid and leukotriene modifier or long-acting beta2-agonist (children over 4 yrs)

Step 4
Preferred: medium-dose inhaled corticosteroids and long-acting beta2-agonist (can use leukotriene modifier in children under 4 yrs)

Step 5
Preferred: high-dose inhaled corticosteroids and long-acting beta2-agonist (or leukotriene modifier or theophylline)

Step 6
Preferred: high-dose inhaled corticosteroids, long-acting beta2-agonist and oral systemic corticosteroids

Adapted from National Asthma Education and Prevention Program. (2007). *Expert panel report 3: Guidelines for the diagnosis and management of asthma* (NIH Publication No. 07-4051). Bethesda, MD: National Institutes of Health, National Heart, Lung and Blood Institute. These recommendations are intended to be used as a guide in individualized asthma care.

HEALTHY PEOPLE 2010

Objective	Significance
Reduce activity limitations among persons with asthma. (Developmental) Reduce the number of school days or workdays missed by persons with asthma. Increase the proportion of persons with asthma who receive formal patient education, including information about community and self-help resources, as an essential part of the management of their condition.	• Encourage appropriate physical activity in children with asthma. • Provide extensive education to children and families about peak flow meter use and its meaning, maintenance and rescue medications, symptoms of asthma exacerbation, and a written plan for how to "step up" and "step down" asthma management. • Refer children and their families to local or Internet resources and support groups. • Refer families to formal classes on asthma education.

▶ *Take* NOTE!

By the end of 2008, all metered-dose inhalers using chlorofluorocarbon (CFC) as the propellant should be off the market. Environmentally friendly formulations of hydrofluoroalkane (HFA) will be used in all metered-dose inhalers by that time (Bederka, 2006).

Nursing Assessment

For a full description of the assessment phase of the nursing process, refer to page 1222. Assessment findings pertinent to asthma are discussed below.

Health History
Elicit a description of the present illness and chief complaint. Common signs and symptoms reported during the health history might include:

• Cough, particularly at night: hacking cough that is initially nonproductive, becoming productive of frothy sputum
• Difficulty breathing: shortness of breath, chest tightness or pain, dyspnea with exercise
• Wheezing

Explore the child's current and past medical history for risk factors such as:

• History of allergic rhinitis or atopic dermatitis
• Family history of atopy (asthma, allergic rhinitis, atopic dermatitis)

• Recurrent episodes diagnosed as wheezing, bronchiolitis, or bronchitis
• Known allergies
• Seasonal response to environmental pollen
• Tobacco smoke exposure
• Poverty

Physical Examination

Physical examination of the child with asthma includes inspection, auscultation, and percussion.

Inspection

Observe the child's general appearance and color. During mild exacerbations, the child's color might remain pink, but as the child worsens, cyanosis might result. Work of breathing is variable. Some children present with mild retractions, while others demonstrate significant accessory muscle use and eventually head-bobbing if not effectively treated. The child may appear anxious and fearful or may be lethargic and irritable. An audible wheeze might be present. Children with persistent severe asthma may have a barrel chest and routinely demonstrate mildly increased work of breathing.

Auscultation and Percussion

A thorough assessment of lung fields is necessary. Wheezing is the hallmark of airway obstruction and might vary throughout the lung fields. Coarseness might also be present. Assess the adequacy of aeration. Breath sounds might be diminished in the bases or throughout. A quiet chest in an asthmatic child can be an ominous sign. With severe airway obstruction, air movement can be so poor that wheezes might not be heard upon auscultation. Percussion may yield hyperresonance.

Laboratory and Diagnostic Tests

Laboratory and diagnostic studies commonly ordered for the assessment of asthma include:

• Pulse oximetry: oxygen saturation may be significantly decreased or normal during a mild exacerbation
• Chest x-ray: usually reveals hyperinflation
• Blood gases: might show carbon dioxide retention and hypoxemia
• Pulmonary function tests (PFTs): can be very useful in determining the degree of disease but are not useful during an acute attack. Children as young as 5 or 6 years might be able to comply with spirometry.
• Peak expiratory flow rate (PEFR): is decreased during an exacerbation
• Allergy testing: skin test or RAST can determine allergic triggers for the asthmatic child

Nursing Management

Initial nursing management of the child with an acute exacerbation of asthma is aimed at restoring a clear airway and effective breathing pattern as well as promoting adequate oxygenation and ventilation (gas exchange). Refer to the Nursing Care Plan. Additional considerations are reviewed below.

Educating the Child and Family

Asthma is a chronic illness and needs to be understood as such. Figure 39.13 displays the "Kids with Asthma Bill of Rights" developed by the American Lung Association. Teach families of children with asthma, and the children themselves, how to care for the disease. Symptom-free periods (often very long) are interspersed with episodes of exacerbation. Parents and children often do not understand the importance of maintenance medications for long-term control. They may view the episodes of exacerbation (sometimes requiring hospitalization or emergency room visits) as an acute illness and are simply relieved when they are over. Frequently during the periods between acute episodes, children are viewed as disease-free and long-term maintenance schedules are abandoned. The prolonged inflammatory process occurring in the absence of symptoms, primarily in children with moderate to severe asthma, can lead to airway remodeling and eventual irreversible disease.

Each child should have a management plan in place to determine when to step up or step down treatment. Figure 39.14 provides an example of a written format that may be helpful to families in the management of asthma. This written action plan should also be kept on file at the child's school, and relief medication should be available to the child at all times. Children who experience exercise-induced bronchospasm may still participate in physical education or athletics but may need to be allowed to use their medicine before the activity. Provide appropriate education to the child and family based on the child's individualized stepwise treatment plan. Stress the concept of maintenance medications for the prevention of future serious disease in addition to controlling or preventing current symptoms.

Educate families and children on the appropriate use of nebulizers, metered-dose inhalers, spacers, dry-powder inhalers, and Diskus, as well as the purposes, functions, and side effects of the medications they deliver. Require return demonstrations of equipment use to ensure that children and families can use the equipment properly (Teaching Guidelines 39.5).

▶ **Take** NOTE!

The NAEPP recommends use of a spacer or holding chamber with metered-dose inhalers to increase the bioavailability of medication in the lungs.

(text continues on page 1263)

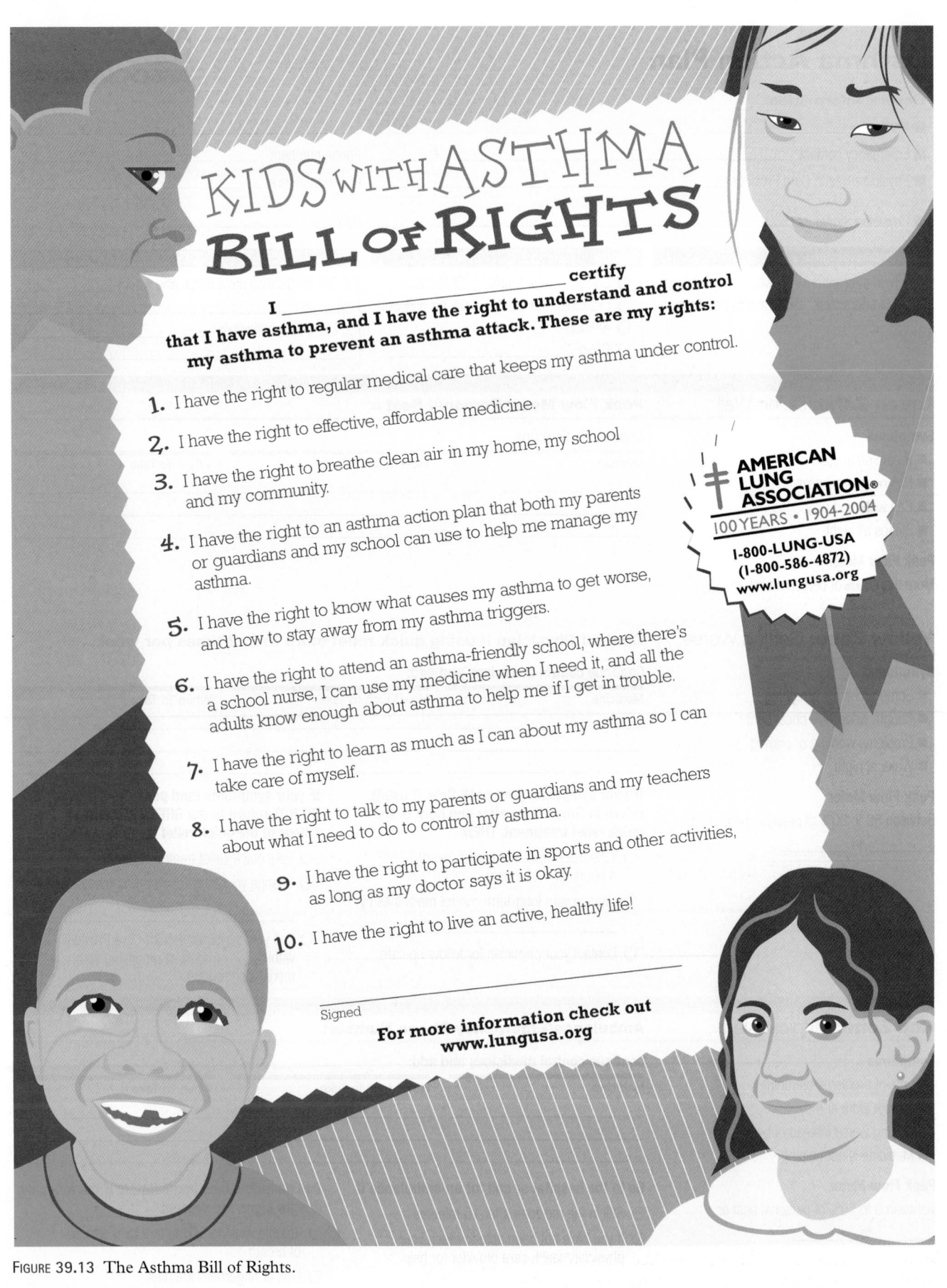

FIGURE 39.13 The Asthma Bill of Rights.

Asthma Action Plan

General Information:

■ Name _____

■ Emergency contact _____   Phone numbers _____

■ Physician/Health Care Provider _____   Phone numbers _____

■ Physician Signature _____   Date _____

Severity Classification	**Triggers**	**Exercise**
○ Mild Intermittent ○ Moderate Persistent ○ Mild Persistent ○ Severe Persistent	○ Colds ○ Smoke ○ Weather ○ Exercise ○ Dust ○ Air pollution ○ Animals ○ Food ○ Other _____	1. Pre-medication (how much and when) _____ 2. Exercise modifications _____

Green Zone: Doing Well   Peak Flow Meter Personal Best = _____

Symptoms

Control Medications

Medicine	How Much to Take	When To Take It
■ Breathing is good		
■ No cough or wheeze		
■ Can work and play		
■ Sleeps all night		

Peak Flow Meter

More than 80% of personal best or _____

Yellow Zone: Getting Worse   Contact Physician if using quick relief more than 2 times per week.

Symptoms

Continue control medicines and add:

Medicine	How Much to Take	When To Take It
■ Some problems breathing		
■ Cough, wheeze or chest tight		
■ Problems working or playing		
■ Wake at night		

Peak Flow Meter

Between 50 to 80% of personal best or
_____ to _____

IF your symptoms (and peak flow, if used) return to Green Zone after one hour of the quick relief treatment, THEN

○ Take quick-relief medication every 4 hours for 1 to 2 days

○ Change your long-term control medicines by

_____

○ Contact your physician for follow-up care

IF your symptoms (and peak flow, if used) DO NOT return to the GREEN ZONE after 1 hour of the quick relief treatment, THEN

○ Take quick-relief treatment again

○ Change your long-term control medicines by

_____

○ Call your physician/Health Care Provider within _____ hours of modifying your medication routine

Red Zone: Medical Alert   Ambulance/Emergency Phone Number: _____

Symptoms

Continue control medicines and add:

Medicine	How Much to Take	When To Take It
■ Lots of problems breathing		
■ Cannot work or play		
■ Getting worse instead of better		
■ Medicine is not helping		

Peak Flow Meter

Between 0 to 50% of personal best or
_____ to _____

Go to the hospital or call for an ambulance if

○ Still in the red zone after 15 minutes

○ If you have not been able to reach your physician/health care provider for help

○ _____

Call an ambulance immediately if the following danger signs are present

○ Trouble walking/talking due to shortness of breath

○ Lips or fingernails are blue

FIGURE 39.14 Asthma action plan.

TEACHING GUIDELINES 39.5

Using Asthma Medication Delivery Devices

Nebulizer

1. Plug in the nebulizer and connect the air compressor tubing.

2. Add the medication to the medicine cup.

3. Attach the mask or the mouthpiece and hose to the medicine cup.

4. Place the mask on the child OR

5. Instruct the child to close the lips around the mouthpiece and breathe through the mouth.

6. After use, wash the mouthpiece and medicine cup with water and allow to air dry.

Metered-Dose Inhaler

1. Shake the inhaler and take off the cap.

(continued)

TEACHING GUIDELINES 39.5 (continued)

Using Asthma Medication Delivery Devices

2. Attach the inhaler to the spacer or holding chamber.

3. Breathe out completely.
4. Put the spacer mouthpiece in the mouth (or place the mask over the child's nose and mouth, ensuring a good seal).

5. Compress the inhaler and inhale slowly and deeply. Hold the breath for a count of 10.

Diskus

1. Hold the Diskus in a horizontal position in one hand and push the thumb grip with the thumb of your other hand away from you until mouthpiece is exposed.

2. Push the lever until it clicks (the dose is now loaded).

3. Breathe out fully.
4. Place your mouth securely around the mouthpiece and breathe in fully and quickly through your mouth.
5. Remove the Diskus, hold the breath for 10 seconds, and then breathe out.

TEACHING GUIDELINES 39.5 (continued)

Using Asthma Medication Delivery Devices

Turbuhaler

1. Hold the Turbuhaler upright. Load the dose by twisting the brown grip fully to the right.

2. Then twist it to the left until you hear it click.

3. Breathe out fully.
4. Holding the Turbuhaler horizontally, place the mouth firmly around the mouthpiece and inhale deeply and forcefully.

5. Remove the Turbuhaler from the mouth and then breathe out.

In children who have more severe asthma, the NAEPP recommends the use of the peak expiratory flow rate (PEFR) to determine daily control. PEFR measurements obtained via a home peak flow meter can be very helpful as long as the meter is used appropriately; Teaching Guidelines 39.6 gives instructions on peak flow meter use. The child's "personal best" is determined collaboratively with the health care practitioner during a symptom-free period. PEFR is measured daily at home using the peak flow meter. The asthma management plan then gives specific instructions based on the PEFR measurement (Table 39.6).

TEACHING GUIDELINES 39.6

Using a Peak Flow Meter

• Slide the arrow down to "zero."
• Stand up straight.
• Take a deep breath and close the lips tightly around the mouthpiece.
• Blow out hard and fast.
• Note the number the arrow moves to.
• Repeat three times and record the highest reading.
• Keep a record of daily readings, being sure to measure peak flow at the same time each day.

Source: Data from the American Lung Association.

▶ *Take NOTE!*

Young children with asthma receiving inhaled medications via a nebulizer should use a snugly fitting mask to ensure accurate deposition of medication to the lungs. "Blow-by" via nebulizer should be discouraged, as medication delivery is variable and unreliable.

Avoidance of allergens is another key component of asthma management. Avoiding known triggers helps to prevent exacerbations as well as long-term inflammatory changes. This can be a difficult task for most families, particularly if the affected child suffers from several allergies.

TABLE 39.6   ASSESSMENT OF PEAK EXPIRATORY FLOW RATE (PEFR)

Zone*	PEFR	Symptoms	Action
Green: Good control	>80% personal best	None	Take usual medications.
Yellow: Caution	50% to 80% personal best	Possibly present	Take short-acting inhaled beta2-agonist right away. Talk to your health care provider.
Red: Medical alert	<50% personal best	Usually present	Take short-acting inhaled beta2-agonist right away. Go to office or emergency department.

*The National Asthma Education and Prevention Program recommended the "traffic light" approach for educating individuals on PEFRs and management plans.

Teaching Guidelines 39.4 outlines strategies for allergen avoidance.

Research has found a lag in parent/child education in relation to asthma management (Horner, 2004). Asthma education is not limited to the hospital or clinic setting. Nurses can become involved in community asthma education: community-centered education in schools, churches, and daycare centers or through peer educators has been shown to be effective. Education should include pathophysiology, asthma triggers, and prevention and treatment strategies. With such a large number of children affected with this chronic disease, community education has the potential to make a broad impact.

School nurses must also become experts in asthma management as well as being committed to ongoing education of the child and family. Resources for schools include:

- Open Airways for Schools: an educational program presented by the American Lung Association or its local chapter, focusing on increasing asthma awareness and compliance with asthma action plans and decreasing asthma emergencies. Contact the local lung association or call 1-800-LUNG-USA.
- Asthma and Allergies at School: a kit available from AANMA at www.breatherville.org/schoolhouse or 1-800-878-4403.
- Healthy School Environments Assessment Tool: http://www.epa.gov/schools/

▶ *Take* NOTE!

Exposure to cigarette smoke increases the need for medications in children with asthma as well as the frequency of asthma exacerbations. Both indoor air quality and environmental pollution contribute to asthma in children.

Promoting the Child's Self-Esteem

Fear of an exacerbation and feeling "different" from other children can harm a child's self-esteem. In qualitative research studies, children have made such statements as "my body shuts down" and "I feel like I'm going to die" (Yoos et al., 2005). The fatigue and fear associated with chronic asthma may reduce the child's confidence and sense of control over his or her body and life. In addition to coping with a chronic illness, the asthmatic child often also has to cope with school-related issues. Moodiness, acting out, and withdrawal correlate with increases in school absence, which can contribute to poor school performance. To live in fear of an exacerbation or to be unable to participate in activities affects the child's self-esteem.

Through education and support, the child can gain a sense of control. Children need to learn to master their disease. Accurate evaluation of asthma symptoms and improvement of self-esteem may help the child to experience less panic with an acute episode. Improved self-esteem might also help the child cope with the disease in general and with being different from his or her peers. The school-age child has the cognitive ability to begin taking responsibility for asthma management, with continued involvement on the part of the parents. Transferring control of asthma care to the child is an important developmental process that will increase the child's feeling of control over the illness (Buford, 2004).

Promoting Family Coping

Parent denial is an issue in many families. The family, through education and encouragement, can become the experts on the child's illness as well as advocates for the child's well-being. The resilient child is better able to cope with the challenges facing him or her, including asthma. Cohesiveness and warmth in the family environment can improve a child's resiliency as well as contribute to family hardiness. Parents need to be allowed to ask questions and voice their concerns. A nurse who understands the family's issues and concerns is better able to plan for support and education. Provide culturally sensitive education and interventions that focus on increasing the family's commitment to and control of asthma management. As the child and parents become confident in their ability to recognize asthma symptoms and cope with asthma and its periodic episodes, the family's ability to cope will improve (Svavarsdottir & Rayens, 2005).

CHRONIC LUNG DISEASE

Chronic lung disease (formerly termed bronchopulmonary dysplasia) is often diagnosed in infants who have experienced RDS and continue to require oxygen at 28 days of age. It is a chronic respiratory condition seen most commonly in premature infants. It results from a variety of factors, including pulmonary immaturity, acute lung injury, barotrauma, inflammatory mediators, and volutrauma. Epithelial stretching, macrophage and polymorphonuclear cell invasion, and airway edema affect the growth and development of lung structures. Cilia loss and airway lining denudation reduce the normal cleansing abilities of the lung. The number of normal alveoli is reduced by one third to one half. Lower birthweights, white race, and male gender pose increased risk for development of chronic lung disease. Complications include pulmonary artery hypertension, cor pulmonale, congestive heart failure, and severe bacterial or viral pneumonia. (Harvey, 2004; Stoll & Kliegman, 2004).

Anti-inflammatory inhaled medications are used for maintenance, and short-acting bronchodilators are used as needed for wheezing episodes. Supplemental long-term oxygen therapy may be required in some infants.

Nursing Assessment

Tachypnea and increased work of breathing are characteristic of chronic lung disease. After discharge from the NICU, these symptoms can continue. Exertion such as activity or oral feeding can cause dyspnea to worsen. Failure to thrive might also be evident. Auscultation might reveal breath sounds that are diminished in the bases. These infants have reactive airway episodes, so wheezing might be present during times of exacerbation. If fluid overload develops, rales may be heard.

Nursing Management

If the infant is oxygen-dependent, provide education to the parents about oxygen tanks, nasal cannula use, pulse oximetry use, and nebulizer treatments. Often these children require increased-calorie formulas to grow adequately. Fluid restrictions and/or diuretics are necessary in some infants. Follow-up echocardiograms might be used to determine resolution of pulmonary artery hypertension prior to weaning from oxygen. Encourage developmentally appropriate activities. It might be difficult for the oxygen-dependent infant or toddler to reach gross motor milestones or explore the environment because the length of the oxygen tubing limits him or her.

Parental support is also a key nursing intervention. After a long and trying period of ups and downs with their newborn in the intensive care unit, parents find themselves exhausted caring for their medically fragile infant at home.

CYSTIC FIBROSIS

Cystic fibrosis is an autosomal recessive disorder that occurs about once in every 3,300 live white births and about once in every 16,000 live black births (Boat, 2004). A deletion occurring on the long arm of chromosome 7 at the cystic fibrosis transmembrane regulator (CFTR) is the responsible gene mutation. DNA testing can be used prenatally and in newborns to identify the presence of the mutation. The American College of Obstetrics and Gynecology currently recommends screening for cystic fibrosis to any person seeking preconception or prenatal care. At present, 11 states include testing for cystic fibrosis as part of newborn screening (Gross et al., 2004).

Cystic fibrosis is the most common debilitating disease of childhood among those of European descent. Medical advances in recent years have greatly increased the length and quality of life for affected children: about 50% now live past the age of 30 years (Boat, 2004), and many live a high-quality life into their 40s (Carpenter & Narsavage, 2004). Complications include hemoptysis, pneumothorax, bacterial colonization, cor pulmonale, volvulus, intussusception, intestinal obstruction, rectal prolapse, gastroesophageal reflux disease, diabetes, portal hypertension, liver failure, gallstones, and decreased fertility.

Therapeutic Management

Therapeutic management of cystic fibrosis is aimed toward minimizing pulmonary complications, maximizing lung function, preventing infection, and facilitating growth. All children with cystic fibrosis who have pulmonary involvement require chest physiotherapy with postural drainage several times daily to mobilize secretions from the lungs. Physical exercise is encouraged. Recombinant human DNase (Pulmozyme) is given daily using a nebulizer to decrease sputum viscosity and help clear secretions. Inhaled bronchodilators and anti-inflammatory agents are prescribed for some children. Aerosolized antibiotics are often prescribed and may be given at home as well as in the hospital. Choice of antibiotic is determined by sputum culture and sensitivity results. Pancreatic enzymes and supplemental fat-soluble vitamins are prescribed to promote adequate digestion and absorption of nutrients and optimize nutritional status. Increased-calorie, high-protein diets are recommended, and sometimes supplemental high-calorie formula, either orally or via feeding tube, is needed. Some children require total parenteral nutrition to maintain or gain weight (McMullen, 2004). Lung transplantation has been successful in some children with cystic fibrosis.

Pathophysiology

In cystic fibrosis, the CFTR mutation causes alterations in epithelial ion transport on mucosal surfaces, resulting in generalized dysfunction of the exocrine glands. The epithelial cells fail to conduct chloride, and water transport abnormalities occur. This results in thickened, tenacious secretions in the sweat glands, gastrointestinal tract, pancreas, respiratory tract, and other exocrine tissues. The increased viscosity of these secretions makes them difficult to clear. The sweat glands produce a larger amount of chloride, leading to a salty taste of the skin and alterations in electrolyte balance and dehydration. The pancreas, in-

trahepatic bile ducts, intestinal glands, gallbladder, and submaxillary glands become obstructed by viscous mucus and eosinophilic material. Pancreatic enzyme activity is lost and malabsorption of fats, proteins, and carbohydrates occurs, resulting in poor growth and large, malodorous stools. Excess mucus is produced by the tracheobronchial glands. Abnormally thick mucus plugs the small airways, and then bronchiolitis and further plugging of the airways occur. Secondary bacterial infection with *Staphylococcus aureus, Pseudomonas aeruginosa,* and *Burkholderia cepacia* often occurs. This contributes to obstruction and inflammation, leading to chronic infection, tissue damage, and respiratory failure. Nasal polyps and recurrent sinusitis are common. Boys have tenacious seminal fluid and experience blocking of the vas deferens, often making them infertile. In girls, thick cervical secretions might limit penetration of sperm (Boat, 2004; Simpson & Ivey, 2005). Table 39.7 gives further details of the pathophysiology

TABLE 39.7 **Pathophysiology of Cystic Fibrosis and Resultant Respiratory and Gastrointestinal Clinical Manifestations**

Defect in the CFTR Gene Affects:	Pathophysiology	Clinical Manifestations
Respiratory tract	• Infection leads to neutrophilic inflammation. • Cleavage of complement receptors and immunoglobin G leads to opsonophagocytosis failure. • Chemoattractant interleukin-8 and elastin degradase contribute to inflammatory response. • Thick, tenacious sputum that is chronically colonized with bacteria results. • Air trapping related to airway obstruction • Pulmonary parenchyma is eventually destroyed.	• Airway obstruction • Difficulty clearing secretions • Respiratory distress and impaired gas exchange • Chronic cough • Barrel-shaped chest • Decreased pulmonary function • Clubbing • Recurrent pneumonia • Hemoptysis • Pneumothorax • Chronic sinusitis • Nasal polyps • Cor pulmonale (right-sided heart failure)
Gastrointestinal tract	• Decreased chloride and water secretion into the intestine (causing dehydration of the intestinal material) and into the bile ducts (causing increased bile viscosity) • Reduced pancreatic bicarbonate secretion • Hypersecretion of gastric acid • Insufficiency of pancreatic enzymes necessary for digestion and absorption • Pancreas secretes thick mucus.	• Meconium ileus • Retention of fecal matter in distal intestine, resulting in vomiting, abdominal distention and cramping, anorexia, right lower quadrant pain • Sludging of intestinal contents may lead to fecal impaction, rectal prolapse, bowel obstruction, intussusception. • Obstructive cirrhosis with esophageal varices, and splenomegaly • Gallstones • Gastroesophageal reflux disease (compounded by postural drainage with chest physiotherapy) • Inadequate protein absorption • Altered absorption of iron and vitamins A, D, E, and K • Failure to thrive • Hyperglycemia and development of diabetes later in life

and resulting respiratory and gastrointestinal clinical manifestations of cystic fibrosis.

Nursing Assessment

For a full description of the assessment phase of the nursing process, refer to page 1222. Assessment findings pertinent to cystic fibrosis are discussed below.

Health History

Elicit a description of the present illness and chief complaint. Common signs and symptoms reported during the health history in the undiagnosed child might include:

• A salty taste to the child's skin (resulting from excess chloride loss via perspiration)
• Meconium ileus or late, difficult passage of meconium stool in the newborn period
• Abdominal pain or difficulty passing stool (infants or toddlers might present with intestinal obstruction or intussusception at the time of diagnosis)
• Bulky, greasy stools
• Poor weight gain and growth despite good appetite
• Chronic or recurrent cough and/or upper or lower respiratory infections

Children known to have cystic fibrosis are often admitted to the hospital for pulmonary exacerbations or other complications of the disease. The health history should include questions related to:

• Respiratory status: has cough, sputum production, or work of breathing increased?
• Appetite and weight gain
• Activity tolerance
• Increased need for pulmonary or pancreatic medications
• Presence of fever
• Presence of bone pain
• Any other changes in physical state or medication regimen

Physical Examination

The physical examination includes inspection, auscultation, percussion, and palpation.

Inspection

Observe the child's general appearance and color. Check the nasal passages for polyps. Note respiratory rate, work of breathing, use of accessory muscles, position of comfort, frequency and severity of cough, and quality and quantity of sputum produced. The child with cystic fibrosis often has a barrel chest (anterior–posterior diameter approximates transverse diameter) (Fig. 39.15). Clubbing of the nail beds might also be present. Note whether rectal prolapse is present. Does the child appear small or thin for his or her age? The child might have a protuberant abdomen and thin extremities, with decreased amounts of subcutaneous fat. Observe for the presence of edema (sign of

Cross section of thorax

A Normal chest   **B** Barrel chest

FIGURE 39.15 (**A**) Normal chest shape—transverse diameter is greater than anterior–posterior diameter. (**B**) Barrel chest—transverse diameter equals anterior–posterior diameter.

cardiac or liver failure). Note distended neck veins or the presence of a heave (signs of cor pulmonale).

Auscultation

Auscultation may reveal a variety of adventitious breath sounds. Fine or coarse crackles and scattered or localized wheezing might be present. With progressive obstructive pulmonary involvement, breath sounds might be diminished. Tachycardia might be present. Note the presence of a gallop (might occur with cor pulmonale). Note the adequacy of bowel sounds.

Percussion

Percussion over the lung fields usually yields hyperresonance due to air trapping. Diaphragmatic excursion might be decreased. Percussion of the abdomen might reveal dullness over an enlarged liver or mass related to intestinal obstruction.

Palpation

Palpation might yield a finding of asymmetric chest excursion if atelectasis is present. Tactile fremitus may be decreased over areas of atelectasis. Note if tenderness is present over the liver (might be an early sign of cor pulmonale).

Laboratory and Diagnostic Tests

Common laboratory and diagnostic studies ordered for the diagnosis and assessment of cystic fibrosis include:

- Sweat chloride test: considered suspicious if the level of chloride in collected sweat is above 50 mEq/L and diagnostic if the level is above 60 mEq/L (Fig. 39.16)
- Pulse oximetry: oxygen saturation might be decreased, particularly during a pulmonary exacerbation
- Chest x-ray: may reveal hyperinflation, bronchial wall thickening, atelectasis, or infiltration
- Pulmonary function tests: might reveal a decrease in forced vital capacity and forced expiratory volume, with increases in residual volume (Boat, 2004; McMullen, 2004)

Nursing Management

Management of cystic fibrosis focuses on minimizing pulmonary complications, promoting growth and development, and facilitating coping and adjustment by the child and family. In addition to the nursing diagnoses and related interventions discussed in the Nursing Care Plan for respiratory disorders, interventions common to cystic fibrosis follow.

Maintaining Patent Airway

Chest physiotherapy is often used as an adjunct therapy in respiratory illnesses, but for children with cystic fibrosis it is a critical intervention. Chest physiotherapy involves percussion, vibration, and postural drainage, and either it or another bronchial hygiene therapy must be performed several times a day to assist with mobilization of secretions. Nursing Procedure 39.2 gives instructions on the chest physiotherapy technique.

For older children and adolescents, the flutter-valve device, positive expiratory pressure therapy, or a high-frequency chest compression vest may also be used. The flutter valve device provides high-frequency oscillation to the airway as the child exhales into a mouthpiece that contains a steel ball. Positive expiratory pressure therapy involves exhaling through a flow resistor, which creates positive expiratory pressure. The cycles of exhalation are repeated until coughing yields expectoration of secretions.

FIGURE 39.16 Sweat chloride test.

The vest airway clearance system provides high-frequency chest wall oscillation to increase airflow velocity to create repetitive cough-like shear forces and to decrease the viscosity of secretions (Chatburn, 2007). Breathing exercises are also helpful in promoting mucus clearance. Encourage physical exercise, as it helps to promote mucus secretion as well as providing cardiopulmonary conditioning. Ensure that Pulmozyme is administered, as well as inhaled bronchodilators and anti-inflammatory agents if prescribed.

Preventing Infection

Vigorous pulmonary hygiene for mobilization of secretions is critical to prevent infection. Aerosolized antibiotics can be given at home as well as in the hospital. Children with frequent or severe respiratory exacerbations might require lengthy courses of intravenous antibiotics.

Maintaining Growth

Pancreatic enzymes must be administered with all meals and snacks to promote adequate digestion and absorption of nutrients. The number of capsules required depends on the extent of pancreatic insufficiency and the amount of food being ingested. The dosage can be adjusted until an adequate growth pattern is established and the number of stools is consistent at one or two per day. Children will need additional enzyme capsules when high-fat foods are being eaten. In the infant or young child, the enzyme capsule can be opened and sprinkled on cereal or applesauce. A well-balanced, high-calorie, high-protein diet is necessary to ensure adequate growth. Some children require up to 1.5 times the recommended daily allowance of calories for children their age. A number of commercially available nutritional formulas and shakes are available for diet supplementation.

In infants, breastfeeding should be continued with enzyme administration. Some infants will require fortification of breast milk or supplementation with high-calorie formulas. Commercially available infant formulas can continue to be used for the formula-fed infant and can be mixed to provide a larger amount of calories if necessary. Supplementation with vitamins A, D, E, and K is necessary. Administer gavage feedings or total parenteral nutrition as prescribed to provide for adequate growth.

Promoting Family Coping

Cystic fibrosis is a serious chronic illness that requires daily interventions. It can be hard to maintain a schedule that requires pulmonary hygiene several times daily as well as close attention to appropriate diet and enzyme supplementation. Adjusting to the demands that the illness places on the child and family is difficult. Continual adjustments within the family must occur. Children are frequently hospitalized, and this may place an additional strain on the family and its finances. Children with cystic fibrosis may express fear or feelings of isolation, and siblings may be worried or jealous (Carpenter & Narsavage, 2004). The

Nursing Procedure 39.2

PERFORMING CHEST PHYSIOTHERAPY

1. Provide percussion via a cupped hand or an infant percussion device. Appropriate percussion yields a hollow sound, not a slapping sound.

2. Percuss each segment of the lung for 1 to 2 minutes.

POSITION #1
UPPER LOBES, Apical segments

POSITION #1, for infants
UPPER LOBES, Apical segments

POSITION #2
UPPER LOBES, Posterior segments

POSITION #3
UPPER LOBES, Anterior segments

POSITION #4
LINGULA

(continued)

Nursing Procedure 39.2 (continued)

POSITION #5
MIDDLE LOBE

POSITION #6
LOWER LOBES, Anterior basal segments

POSITION #7
LOWER LOBES, Posterior basal segments

POSITION #8 & 9
LOWER LOBES, Lateral basal segments

POSITION #10
LOWER LOBES, Superior segments

3. Place the ball of the hand on the lung segment, keeping the arm and shoulder straight. Vibrate by tensing and relaxing your arms during the child's exhalation. Vibrate each lung segment for at least five exhalations.

4. Encourage the child to deep breathe and cough.
5. Change drainage positions and repeat percussion and vibration.

family should be encouraged to lead a normal life through involvement in activities and school attendance during periods of wellness.

> ▶ *Take* NOTE!
>
> *Massage therapy performed by the parent, nurse, or licensed massage therapist may help to decrease anxiety in the child with cystic fibrosis. It may have the added benefit of improving respiratory status, but it does not replace chest physiotherapy (Huth et al., 2005).*

Starting at the time of diagnosis, families often demonstrate significant stress as the severity of the diagnosis and the significance of disease chronicity become real for them. The family should be involved in the child's care from the time of diagnosis, whether in the outpatient setting or in the hospital. Ongoing education about the illness and its treatments is necessary. Once the initial shock of diagnosis has passed and the family has adjusted to initial care, the family usually learns how to manage the requirements of care. Powerlessness gives way to adaptation. As family members become more comfortable with their understanding of the illness and the required treatments, they will eventually become the experts on the child's care. It is important for the nurse to recognize and respect the family's changing needs over time.

Providing daily intense care can be tiring, and noncompliance on the part of the family or child might occur as a result of this fatigue. Overvigilance may also occur as parents attempt to control the difficult situation and protect the child. Families welcome support and encouragement. Most families eventually progress past the stages of fear, guilt, and powerlessness to a way of living that is different than what they anticipated but is something that they can manage.

Refer parents to a local support group for families of children with cystic fibrosis. The Cystic Fibrosis Foundation has chapters throughout the United States (www.cff.org). Additional resources can be found at www.cysticfibrosis.com, www.cfri.org, and www.cfww.org.

Parents of children with a terminal illness might face the death of their child at an earlier age than expected. Assisting with anticipatory grieving and making decisions related to end-of-life care are other important nursing interventions.

Preparing the Child and Family for Adulthood With Cystic Fibrosis

With current technological and medication advances, many more children with cystic fibrosis are surviving to adulthood and into their 30s and 40s. Lung transplantation is now being used in some patients with success, thus prolonging life expectancy (barring transplant complications). Children with cystic fibrosis should have the goal of independent living as an adult, as other children do. Making the transition from a pediatric medical home to an adult medical home should be viewed as a normal part of growing up, similar to completing school or finding a first job (Kennedy et al., 2007). Pediatric clinics are focused on family-centered care that heavily involves the child's parents, but adults with cystic fibrosis need a different focus, one that views them as independent adults.

Clients with cystic fibrosis can make the transition from pediatric to adult care with thoughtful preparation and coordination. They desire and deserve a smooth transition in care that will result in appropriate ongoing medical management of cystic fibrosis in an environment that is geared toward adults rather than children.

Adults with cystic fibrosis are able to find rewarding work and pursue relationships. Most men with cystic fibrosis are capable of sexual intercourse, though unable to reproduce. Females might have difficulty conceiving, and when they do they should be cautioned about the additional respiratory strain that pregnancy causes. All children of parents with cystic fibrosis will be carriers of the gene.

▶ APNEA

Apnea is defined as absence of breathing for longer than 20 seconds; it might be accompanied by bradycardia. Sometimes apnea presents in the form of an acute life-threatening event (ALTE), an event in which the infant or child exhibits some combination of apnea, color change, muscle tone alteration, coughing, or gagging. Apnea may also occur acutely at any age as a result of respiratory distress. This discussion will focus on apnea that is chronic or recurrent in nature or that occurs as part of an ALTE.

Apnea in infants may be central (unrelated to any other cause) or may occur with other illnesses such as sepsis and respiratory infection. Apnea in newborns might be associated with hypothermia, hypoglycemia, infection, or hyperbilirubinemia. Apnea of prematurity occurs secondary to an immature respiratory system. Apnea should not be considered a predecessor to sudden infant death syndrome (SIDS). Current research has not proven this theory, and SIDS generally occurs in otherwise healthy young infants (AAP, Task Force on Sudden Infant Death Syndrome, 2005). Box 39.3 gives more information about SIDS and its prevention.

Therapeutic management of apnea varies depending on the cause. When apnea occurs as a result of another disorder or infection, treatment is directed toward that cause. In the event of apnea, stimulation may trigger the infant to take a breath. If breathing does not resume, rescue breathing or bag-valve-mask ventilation is necessary. Infants and children who have experienced an ALTE or who have chronic apnea may require ongoing cardiac/

BOX 39.3	Sudden Infant Death Syndrome (SIDS)

Definition

Sudden death of a previously healthy infant <1 year of age

Prevention

• Place all infants in the supine position to sleep (even side-lying is not as safe and is not recommended by the AAP).
• Provide a firm sleep surface and avoid soft bedding, excess covers, pillows, and stuffed animals in the crib.
• Avoid maternal prenatal smoking and exposure of the infant to second-hand smoke.
• Ensure the infant sleeps separately from the parents.
• Avoid overbundling or overdressing the infant.
• Encourage pacifier use during naps and at bedtime if the infant is receptive to it (AAP, 2005).

Support and Information

• SIDS Alliance: www.sidsalliance.org
• National Sudden Infant Death Resource Center: www.sidscenter.org
• Association for SIDS and Infant Mortality Program: www.asip1.org
• Sudden Infant Death Syndrome Network, Inc.: ds-network.org/

---

apnea monitoring. Caffeine or theophylline is sometimes administered, primarily in premature infants, to stimulate respirations.

Nursing Assessment

Question the parents about the infant's position and activities preceding the apneic episode. Did the infant experience a color change? Did the infant self-stimulate (breathe again on his or her own), or did he or she require stimulation from the caretaker? Assess risk factors for apnea, which may include prematurity, anemia, and history of metabolic disorders. Apnea may occur in association with cardiac or neurologic disturbances, respiratory infection, sepsis, child abuse, or poisoning.

In the hospitalized infant, note absence of respiration, position, color, and other associated findings, such as emesis on the bedclothes. If an infant who is apneic fails to be stimulated and does not breathe again, pulselessness will result.

Nursing Management

When an infant is noted to be apneic, gently stimulate him or her to take a breath again. If gentle stimulation is unsuccessful, then rescue breathing or bag-valve-mask ventilation must be started.

To avoid apnea in the newborn, maintain a neutral thermal environment. Avoid excessive vagal stimulation and taking rectal temperatures (the vagal response can cause bradycardia, resulting in apnea). Administer caffeine or theophylline if prescribed and teach families about the use of these medications.

Infants with recurrent apnea or ALTE may be discharged on a home apnea monitor (Fig. 39.17). Provide education on use of the monitor, guidance about when to notify the physician or monitor service about alarms, and training in infant CPR. The monitor is usually discontinued after 3 months without a significant event of apnea or bradycardia. In some ways the monitor gives parents peace of mind, but in others it can make them more nervous about the well-being of their child. Also, the alarm on home monitors is extremely loud and parents often go for months with inadequate sleep. Providing appropriate education to the parents about the nature of the child's disorder as well as action to take in the event of apnea may give the family a sense of mastery over the situation, thus decreasing their anxiety. Refer families to local support groups such as those offered by Parent to Parent and Parents Helping Parents.

Tracheostomy

A **tracheostomy** is an artificial opening in the airway; usually a plastic tracheostomy tube is in place to form a patent airway. Tracheostomies are performed to relieve airway obstruction, such as with **subglottic stenosis** (narrowing of the airway sometimes resulting from long-term intubation). They are also used for pulmonary toilet and in the child who requires chronic mechanical ventilation. The tracheostomy facilitates secretion removal, reduces work of breathing, and increases client comfort. In some cases the tracheostomy facilitates mechanical ventilation weaning. It may be permanent or temporary, depending on the indication. The tracheostomy

FIGURE 39.17 The home apnea monitor uses a soft belt with a Velcro attachment to hold two leads in the appropriate position on the chest.

tube varies in size and type depending on the child's airway size and health and the length of time the child will require the tracheostomy. Silastic tracheostomy tubes are soft and flexible; they are available with a single lumen or may have an outer and inner lumen. Both types have an obturator (the guide used during tube changes). Typically, the tubes with inner cannulas are used with older children and in children with increased mucus production. Cuffed tracheostomy tubes are generally used in older children also. The cuff is used to prevent air from leaking around the tube. The funnel-shaped airway in younger children acts a physiological cuff and prevents air leakage. Figure 39.18 shows various types of tracheostomy tubes.

Complications immediately after surgery include hemorrhage, air entry, pulmonary edema, anatomic damage, and respiratory arrest. At any point in time the tracheostomy tube may become occluded and ventilation compromised. Complications of chronic tracheostomy include infection, cellulitis, and formation of granulation tissue around the insertion site (Russell, 2005).

Nursing Assessment

When obtaining the history for a child with a tracheostomy, note the reason for the tracheostomy, as well as the size and type of tracheostomy tube. Inspect the site. The stoma should appear pink and without bleeding or drainage. The tube itself should be clean and free from secretions. The tracheostomy ties should fit securely, allowing one finger to slide beneath the ties (Fig. 39.19). Inspect the skin under the ties for rash or redness. Observe work of breathing.

When caring for the infant or child with a tracheostomy, whether in the intensive care unit, the ward, or the home, a thorough respiratory assessment is necessary. Note presence of secretions and their color, thickness, and amount. Auscultate for breath sounds, which should be clear and equal throughout all lung fields. Pulse oximetry may also be measured. When infection is suspected or secretions are discolored or have a foul odor, a sputum culture may be obtained.

FIGURE 39.19 Properly fitting trach ties. One fingerwidth fits between the ties and the child's neck.

▶ *Take* NOTE!

Keep small toys (risk of aspiration), plastic bibs or bedding (risk of airway occlusion), and talcum powder (risk of inhalation injury) out of reach of the child with a tracheostomy.

Nursing Management

In the immediate postoperative period the infant or child may require restraints to avoid accidental dislodgment of the tracheostomy tube. Infants and children who have had a tracheostomy for a period of time become accustomed to it and usually do not attempt to remove the tube. Since air inspired via the tracheostomy tube bypasses the upper airway, it lacks humidification, and this lack of humidity can lead to a mucus plug in the tracheostomy and hypoxia. Provide humidity to either room air or oxygen via a tracheostomy collar or ventilator, depending on the child's need (Fig. 39.20). Box 39.4 lists the equipment that should be available at the bedside of any child who has a tracheostomy.

Tracheostomies require frequent suctioning to maintain patency. The appropriate length for insertion of the suction catheter depends on the size of the tracheostomy and the child's needs. Place a sign at the head of the child's bed indicating the suction catheter size and the length (in centimeters) that it should be inserted for suctioning. Keep

FIGURE 39.18 Note smaller size and absence of inner cannula on particular brands of pediatric tracheostomy tubes.

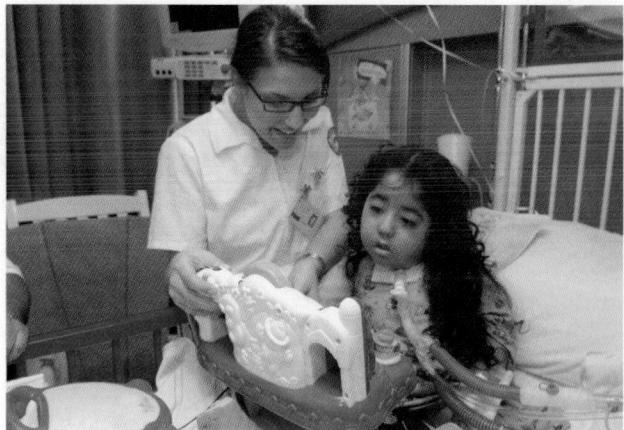

FIGURE 39.20 The trach collar allows for humidification of inspired air or supplemental oxygen.

Nursing Procedure 39.3

TRACHEOSTOMY CARE

1. Gather the necessary equipment:
   - Cleaning solution
   - Gloves
   - Precut gauze pad
   - Cotton-tipped applicators
   - Clean tracheostomy ties
   - Scissors
   - Extra tracheostomy tube in case of accidental dislodgement
2. Position the infant/child supine with a blanket or towel roll to extend the neck.
3. Open all packaging and cut tracheostomy ties to appropriate length if necessary.
4. Cleanse around the tracheostomy site with prescribed solution (half-strength hydrogen peroxide or acetic acid, normal saline or soap and water if at home) and cotton-tipped applicators, working from just around the tracheostomy tube outward.
5. Rinse with sterile water and cotton-tipped applicator in similar fashion.
6. Place the precut sterile gauze under the tracheostomy tube.
7. With the assistant holding the tube in place, cut the ties and remove from the tube.
8. Attach the clean ties to the tube and tie or secure in place with Velcro.

an extra tracheostomy tube of the same size and one size smaller at the bedside in the event of an emergency.

Many pediatric tracheostomy tubes do not have an inner cannula that requires periodic removal and cleaning, so periodic removal and replacement of the chronic tracheostomy tube is required. Clean the removed tracheostomy tube with half-strength hydrogen peroxide and pipe cleaners. Rinse with distilled water and allow it to dry. The tracheostomy tube can be reused many times if adequately cleaned between uses.

Perform tracheostomy care every 8 hours or per institution protocol. Change the tracheostomy tube only as needed or per institution protocol. Nursing Procedure 39.3 gives information about tracheostomy care.

If the older child or teen has a tracheostomy tube with an inner cannula, care of the inner cannula is similar to that of an adult. Involve parents in care of the tracheostomy and begin education about caring for the tracheostomy tube at home as soon as the child is stable. Refer the family to local support groups or to www.tracheostomy.com, which offers many resources for a family whose child has a tracheostomy. The child with a tracheostomy often

qualifies for a Medicaid waiver that will provide a certain amount of home nursing care.

Always change tracheostomy ties with an assistant to avoid accidental dislodgement of the tube.

■■■ Key Concepts

- Respiratory infections account for the majority of acute illnesses in children.
- The upper and lower airways are smaller in children than adults, making them more susceptible to obstruction in the presence of mucus, debris, or edema.
- Newborns are obligatory nose breathers.
- The child's highly compliant airway is quite susceptible to dynamic collapse in the presence of airway obstruction.
- Because they have fewer alveoli, children have a higher risk for hypoxemia than adults.
- Generally, disorders of the nose and throat do not result in increased work of breathing or affect the lungs. Thus, if the lungs are involved, lower respiratory disease must be considered.

BOX 39.4 **Emergency Equipment (Available at Bedside)**

- Two spare tracheostomy tubes (one the same size and one a size smaller)
- Suction equipment
- Stitch cutter (new tracheostomy)
- Spare tracheostomy ties
- Lubricating jelly
- Bag-valve-mask device
- Call bell within child's/parent's reach

■ Wheezing may be associated with a variety of lower respiratory disorders, such as asthma, bronchiolitis, and cystic fibrosis.

■ Pulse oximetry is a useful tool for determining the extent of hypoxia. Findings should be correlated with the child's clinical presentation.

■ Rapid streptococcus and rapid flu tests are very useful for the quick diagnosis of strep throat or influenza so that appropriate treatment may be instituted early in the illness.

■ Supplemental oxygen is often necessary in the child who is hospitalized (particularly with lower respiratory disease). Oxygen should be humidified to prevent drying of secretions.

■ Suctioning, whether with a bulb syringe or suction catheter, is very effective at maintaining airway patency, especially in the younger child or infant.

■ Normal saline nasal wash is an inexpensive, simple, and safe method for decongesting the nose in the case of the common cold, allergic rhinitis, and sinusitis.

■ Infants who were born prematurely, children with a chronic illness such as diabetes, congenital heart disease, sickle cell anemia, or cystic fibrosis, and children with developmental disorders such as cerebral palsy tend to be more severely affected with respiratory disorders.

■ Passive cigarette smoke exposure increases the infant's and child's risk for respiratory disease.

■ Continual swallowing while awake or asleep is an indication of bleeding in the postoperative tonsillectomy patient.

■ Positioning to ease work of breathing and maintaining a patent airway are priorities for the child with a respiratory disorder.

■ To avoid Reye syndrome, aspirin should not be given to treat fever or pain in the infant or child with a viral infection.

■ Infants and children at high risk for serious RSV disease should be immunized with Synagis each RSV season. Children 6 to 23 months of age should be immunized against influenza yearly.

■ Children at high risk for exposure to tuberculosis should be screened for infection.

■ Promoting airway clearance and maintenance, effective breathing patterns, and adequate gas exchange is the priority focus of nursing intervention in pediatric respiratory disease.

■ Children with any degree of respiratory distress require frequent assessment and early intervention to prevent progression to respiratory failure.

■ Avoidance of allergens is critical in the treatment plan for the child with allergic rhinitis.

■ Avoidance of allergic triggers, control of the inflammatory process, and education of the child and family are the focus of asthma management.

■ Chest physiotherapy is extremely useful for mobilizing secretions in any condition resulting in an increase in mucus production and is required in children with cystic fibrosis.

■ Children with chronic respiratory disorders and their families often need large amounts of education and psychosocial support: children often experience fear and isolation, while families must learn to balance care of the chronically ill child with other family life.

REFERENCES

Ackley, B. J., & Ladwig, G. B. (2006). *Nursing diagnosis handbook: A guide to planning care* (7th ed.). St. Louis: Mosby.

American Academy of Pediatrics. (2001). Clinical practice guidelines: Management of sinusitis. *Pediatrics, 108*, 798–808.

American Academy of Pediatrics, Task Force on Sudden Infant Death Syndrome. (2005). Policy Statement: The changing concept of sudden infant death syndrome: Diagnostic coding shifts, controversies regarding the sleeping environment, and new variables to consider in reducing risk. *Pediatrics, 116*(5), 1245–1255.

American Academy of Pediatrics. (2007). *Treating kids' colds without drugs.* Retrieved December 28, 2007, from https://www.aap.org/new/kidcolds.htm.

American Association of Respiratory Care. (2004). AARC clinical practice guideline: Nasotracheal suctioning—2004 revision & update. *Respiratory Care, 49*(9), 1080–1084.

American Heart Association. (2007). *Pediatric advanced life support provider manual.* Dallas: American Heart Association.

Anonymous. (2005). Montelukast sodium for young children. *Nurse Practitioner, 30*(11), 76.

Balinsky, W., & Zhu, C. W. (2004). Pediatric cystic fibrosis: Evaluating costs and genetic testing. *Journal of Pediatric Health Care, 18*, 30–34.

Banasiak, N. C., & Meadows-Oliver, M. (2005). Leukotrienes: Their role in the treatment of asthma and seasonal allergic rhinitis. *Pediatric Nursing, 31*(1), 35–38.

Bederka, M. (2006). Asthma studies you shouldn't miss: A look back at important research developments from 2004–2005. *Advance for Nurse Practitioners.* Available at: http://nurse-practitioners.advanceweb.com/.

Bennett, A. (2006). Respiratory syncytial virus: With treatment choices limited, prevention and education are vital. *Advance for Nurse Practitioners, 14*(10), 71–78.

Bjornson, C. L., Klassen, T. P., Williamson, J., Brant, R., Mitton, C., Plint, A., Bulloch, B., Evered, L., & Johnson, D. W. (2004). A randomized trial of a single dose of oral dexamethasone for mild croup. *New England Journal of Medicine, 351*, 1306–1313.

Boat, T. F. (2004). Cystic fibrosis. In R. E. Behrman, R. M. Kliegman, & H. B. Jenson, *Nelson textbook of pediatrics* (17th ed.). Philadelphia: W. B. Saunders.

Bowden, V. R., & Greenberg, C. S. (2007). *Pediatric nursing procedures.* Philadelphia: Lippincott Williams & Wilkins.

Brunnell, P. (Ed.). (2007). Identifying risk factors for severe RSV infection. *Infectious Diseases in Children, 20*(6-Supplement), 11–16.

Buford, T. A. (2004). Transfer of asthma management responsibility from parents to their school-age children. *Journal of Pediatric Nursing, 19*(1), 3–12.

Burke, M. G. (2004). Human metapneumovirus: Newly recognized villain. *Contemporary Pediatrics.* Available at: www.contemporarypediatrics.com.

Carpenter, D. R., & Narsavage, G. L. (2004). One breath at a time: Living with cystic fibrosis. *Journal of Pediatric Nursing, 19*(1), 25–32.

Celik, S. A., & Kanan, N. (2006). A current conflict: use of isotonic sodium chloride solution on endotracheal suctioning in critically ill patients. *Dimensions of Critical Care Nursing, 25*(1), 11–14.

Chatburn, R. L. (2007). High-frequency assisted airway clearance. *Respiratory Care, 52*(9), 1224–1237.

Cincinnati Children's Hospital Medical Center. (2006). *Evidence-based clinical practice guideline of community-acquired pneumonia in children 60 days to 17 years of age.* Available at: www.guidelines.gov.

DeMeulenaere, S. (2007). Pulse oximetry: Uses and limitations. *Journal for Nurse Practitioners, 3*(5), 312–318.

Edgtton-Winn, M., & Wright, K. (2005). Tracheostomy: A guide to nursing care. *Australian Nursing Journal, 13*(5), S1–S4.

Farrar-Simpson, M. A., Gaffney, K. F., & Deleon, E. E. (2005). School-age girl with sore throat. *Pediatric Nursing, 31*(4), 341–344.

Flume, P. A., Strange, C., Ye, X., Ebeling, M., Hulsey, T., & Clark, L. L. (2005). Pneumothorax in cystic fibrosis. *Chest, 128*(2), 720–728.

Galley, R. (2005). Understanding pulse oximetry. *Clinician Reviews, 15*(10), 32–36.

Gross, S. D., Boyle, C. A., Botkin, J. R., Comeau, A. M., Kharrazi, M., Rosenfeld, M., & Wilfond, B. S. (2004). Newborn screening for cystic fibrosis: Evaluation of benefits and risks and recommendations for state newborn screening programs. *Morbidity and Mortality Weekly Report, 53*(RR12), 1–36.

Grossman, S., & Grossman, L. C. (2005). Pathophysiology of cystic fibrosis: Implications for critical care nurses. *Critical Care Nurse, 25*(4), 46–51.

Hagemann, T. M. (2005). Pediatric allergic rhinitis drug therapy. *Journal of Pediatric Health Care, 19*, 238–244.

Hall, K. L., & Zalman, B. (2005). Evaluation and management of apparent life-threatening events in children. *American Family Physician, 71*(12), 2301–2308.

Harvey, K. (2004). Bronchopulmonary dysplasia. In P. L. Jackson & J. A. Vessey (Eds.), *Primary care of the child with a chronic condition.* St. Louis: Mosby.

Hamilton, C., Steinlechner, B., Gruber, E., Simon, P., & Wollenek, G. (2004). The oxygen dissociation curve: Quantifying the shift. *Perfusion, 19*, 141–144.

Horner, S. D. (2004). Effect of education on school-age children's and parents' asthma management. *Journal for Specialists in Pediatric Nursing, 9*(3), 95–102.

Huth, M. M., Zink, K. A., & Van Horn, N. R. (2005). The effects of massage therapy in improving outcomes for youth with cystic fibrosis: An evidence review. *Pediatric Nursing, 31*(4), 328–332.

Iskander, M., Booy, R., & Lambert, S. (2007). The burden of influenza in children. *Current Opinion in Infectious Diseases, 20*(3), 259–263.

Jensen, H. B. (2004). Epstein-Barr virus. In R. E. Behrman, R. M. Kliegman, & H. B. Jenson (Eds.), *Nelson textbook of pediatrics* (17th ed.). Philadelphia: W. B. Saunders.

Kennedy, A., Sloman, F., Douglass, J. A., & Sawyer, S. M. (2007). Young people with chronic illness: The approach to transition. *Internal Medicine Journal, 37*(8), 555–560.

Kerby, G. S., Accurso, F. J., Deterding, R. R., Balasubramaniam, V., Sagel, S. D., & Cavanaugh, K. L. (2007). Respiratory tract & mediastinum. In W. W. Hay, M. J. Levin, J. M. Sondheimer, & R. R. Detering, *Current pediatric diagnosis and treatment* (18th ed.). New York: McGraw-Hill.

Kieckhefer, G., & Ratcliffe, M. (2004). Asthma. In P. L. Jackson & J. A. Vessey (Eds.), *Primary care of the child with a chronic condition.* St. Louis: Mosby.

Knutson, D., & Aring, A. (2004). Information from your family doctor: What should I know about croup? *American Family Physician, 69*(3), 541–542.

Kumar, C., Edelman, M., & Ficorelli, C. (2005). Children with asthma: A concern for the family. *Maternal Child Nursing, 306*(30), 306–311.

Lauts, N. M. (2005). RSV: Protecting the littlest patients. *RN, 68*(12), 47–51.

Leung, A. K. C., & Kellner, J. D. (2004). Acute sinusitis in children: Diagnosis and management. *Journal of Pediatric Health Care, 18*, 72–76.

Leung, A. K. C., Kellner J. D., & Johnson, D. W. (2004). Viral croup: A current perspective. *Journal of Pediatric Health Care, 18*, 297–301.

Louloudes, A. P. (2006). Pediatric respiratory disorders. In S. M. Nettina (Ed.), *Lippincott manual of nursing practice.* Philadelphia: Lippincott Williams & Wilkins.

Martin, J. M., & Green, M. (2006). Group A streptococcus. *Seminars in Pediatric Infectious Diseases, 17*(3), 140–148.

McCaskey, M. (2007). Pediatric assessment: the little differences. *Home Healthcare Nurse, 25*(1), 20–24.

McCool, F. D., & Rosen, M. J. (2006). Nonpharmacologic airway clearance therapies: AACP evidence-based clinical practice guidelines. *Chest, 129*(1), 250S–259S.

McMillan, J. A., Abramson, J. S., Katz, S. L., & Offit, P. A. (2005). Reducing the risk of influenza: Prevention strategies to help both the young and the old. *Contemporary Pediatrics Supplement, 22*(1), 1–8.

McMullen, A. H. (2004). Cystic fibrosis. In P. L. Jackson & J. A. Vessey (Eds.), *Primary care of the child with a chronic condition* (4th ed.). St. Louis: Mosby.

Myers, T. R. (2005). AARC clinical practice guideline: Selection of an oxygen delivery device for neonatal and pediatric patients. *Respiratory Care, 47*(6), 707–716.

National Asthma Education and Prevention Program. (2007). *Expert panel report 3: Guidelines for the diagnosis and management of asthma* (NIH Publication No. 07-4051). Bethesda, MD: National Institutes of Health, National Heart, Lung and Blood Institute.

National Institute of Allergy and Infectious Diseases. (2007). *Common cold.* Available at: www3.niaid.nih.gov/healthscience/healthtopics/colds/.

Nield, L. S., Mahajan, P., & Kamat, D. M. (2005). Pneumonia: Update on causes and treatment options. *Consultant for Pediatricians, 4*(8), 365–370.

Orenstein, D. M. (2004a). Bacterial tracheitis. In R. E. Behrman, R. M. Kliegman, & H. B. Jenson (Eds.), *Nelson textbook of pediatrics* (17th ed.). Philadelphia: W. B. Saunders.

Orenstein, D. M. (2004b). Bronchitis. In R. E. Behrman, R. M. Kliegman, & H. B. Jenson (Eds.), *Nelson textbook of pediatrics* (17th ed.). Philadelphia: W. B. Saunders.

Orenstein, D. M. (2004c). Foreign bodies in the larynx, trachea and bronchi. In R. E. Behrman, R. M. Kliegman, & H. B. Jenson (Eds.), *Nelson textbook of pediatrics* (17th ed.). Philadelphia: W. B. Saunders.

Ostapchuk, M., Roberts, D. M., & Haddy, R. (2004). Community-acquired pneumonia in infants and children. *American Family Physician, 70*(5), 899–908.

Pagana, K. D., & Pagana, T. J. (2006). *Mosby's manual of diagnostic and laboratory tests* (3rd ed.). St. Louis: Mosby.

Parmet, S. (2004). Sore throat. *Journal of the American Medical Association, 291*(13), 1664.

Pediatric Tuberculosis Collaborative Group. (2004). Targeted tuberculin skin testing and treatment of latent tuberculosis infection in children and adolescents. *Pediatrics, 114*(4 Supplement), 1175–1201.

Peterson, J., & Losek, J. D. (2004). Post-tonsillectomy hemorrhage and pediatric emergency care. *Clinical Pediatrics, 43*, 445–448.

Pickering, L. K. (Ed.). (2006). *AAP Red Book: 2006 report of the committee on infectious diseases.* Elk Grove Village, IL: American Academy of Pediatrics.

Popovich, D. M., Richiuso, N., & Danek, G. (2004). Pediatric health care providers' knowledge of pulse oximetry. *Pediatric Nursing, 30*(1), 14–20.

Prober, C. G. (2004). Pneumonia. In R. E. Behrman, R. M. Kliegman, & H. B. Jenson (Eds.), *Nelson textbook of pediatrics* (17th ed.). Philadelphia: W. B. Saunders.

Rance, K. (2007). The asthma-allergy connection: Complex companions. *Advance for Nurse Practitioners, 15*(4), 31–36.

Reznik, M., & Ozuah, P. O. (2005). A prudent approach to screening for and treating tuberculosis. *Contemporary Pediatrics, 22*(11), 73–88.

Rhee, H., Wenzel, J., & Steeves, R. H. (2007). Adolescents' psychosocial experiences living with asthma: A focus group study. *Journal of Pediatric Health Care, 21*, 99–107.

Robertson, J., & Shilkofski, N. (2005). *The Harriet Lane handbook: A manual for pediatric house officers* (17th ed.). St. Louis: Mosby.

Roman, M. (2005). Tracheostomy care. *MedSurg Nursing, 14*(2), 143–145.

Russell, C. (2005). Providing the nurse with a guide to tracheostomy care and management. *British Journal of Nursing, 14*(8), 428–433.

Schooff, M. (2005). Glucocorticoids for treatment of croup. *American Family Physician, 71*(1), 66.

Selekman, J. (2006). Changes in the screening for tuberculosis in children. *Pediatric Nursing, 32*(1), 73–75.

Sheahan, S. L., & Free, T. A. (2005). Counseling parents to quit smoking. *Pediatric Nursing, 31*(2), 98–109.

Simpson, T., & Ivey, J. (2005). Toddler with a chronic cough. *Pediatric Nursing, 31*(1), 48–49.

Steiner, R. W. P. (2004). Treating acute bronchiolitis associated with RSV. *American Family Physician, 69*(2), 325–330.

Stoll, B. J., & Kliegman, R. M. (2004). Hyaline membrane disease (respiratory distress syndrome). In R. E. Behrman, R. M. Kliegman, & H. B. Jenson (Eds.), *Nelson textbook of pediatrics* (17th ed.). Philadelphia: W. B. Saunders.

Svavarsdottir, E. K., & Rayens, M. K. (2005). Hardiness in families of young children with asthma. *Journal of Advanced Nursing, 50*(4), 381–390.

Taketokmo, C. K., Hodding, J. H., & Kraus, D. M. (2007). *Lexi-comp's pediatric dosage handbook* (14th ed.). Hudson, Ohio: Lexi-comp.

U.S. Department of Health and Human Services. (2000). *Healthy people 2010: Understanding and improving health.* Washington, DC: Department of Health and Human Services.

Wachter, K. (2005). Many children manage own asthma medications. *Pediatric News, 39*(7), 38.

Wakefield, P. L., Sockrider, M. M., & White, L. (2005a). A new approach to wheezing in infants and preschoolers: Shedding light on a difficult diagnosis. *Contemporary Pediatrics, 22*(3), 54–61.

Wakefield, P. L., Sockrider, M. M., & White, L. (2005b). A new approach to wheezing in infants and preschoolers: Toward more effective treatment. *Contemporary Pediatrics, 22*(3), 63–68.

Wong, D. M., Blumberg, D. A., & Lowe, L. G. (2006). Guidelines for the use of antibiotics in acute upper respiratory tract infections. *American Family Physician, 74*(6), 956–969.

Yoos, H. L., Kitzman, H., McMullen, A., Sidora-Arcoleo, K., & Anson, E. (2005). The language of breathlessness: Do families and health care providers speak the same language when describing asthma symptoms? *Journal of Pediatric Health Care, 19*(4), 197–205.

WEBSITES

Aaron's Tracheostomy Site: www.tracheostomy.com

Allergy & Asthma Network Mothers of Asthmatics: www.aanma.org/ (offers extensive resources for families with children who have asthma)

American Academy of Allergy, Asthma, and Immunology: www.aaaai.org

American College of Allergy, Asthma, and Immunology: www.acaai.org/

American Lung Association, section on children and asthma: www.lungusa.org/site/pp.asp?c=dvLUK9O0E&b=22691

Asthma and Allergy Foundation of America: www.aafa.org

Childhood Asthma Foundation: www.childasthma.com

Childhood Asthma Research and Education (CARE) Network: www.asthma-carenet.org/ (founded by the National Heart, Lung and Blood Institute)

Consortium on Children's Asthma Camps: www.asthmacamps.org/asthmacamps/

Cystic Fibrosis Foundation: www.cff.org

Cystic Fibrosis Research, Inc.: www.cfri.org

Cystic Fibrosis Worldwide: www.cfww.org

Education about asthma, section for children, also available in Spanish: www.noattacks.org

Information about asthma and children (supported by AstraZeneca): www.asthmaandchildren.com/

Joint Council of Allergy, Asthma, and Immunology: www.jcaai.org

National Guideline Clearinghouse: www.guideline.gov

National Institute of Allergy and Infectious Disease: www.niaid.nih.gov

Online club for kids with asthma: www.asthmabusters.org/

Support forum for the cystic fibrosis community: www.cysticfibrosis.com

CHAPTER WORKSHEET

MULTIPLE CHOICE QUESTIONS

1. A 5-month-old infant with RSV bronchiolitis is in respiratory distress. The baby has copious secretions, increased work of breathing, cyanosis, and a respiratory rate of 78. What is the most appropriate initial nursing intervention?

   a. Attempt to calm the infant by placing him in his mother's lap and offering him a bottle.

   b. Alert the physician to the situation and ask for an order for a stat chest x-ray.

   c. Suction secretions, provide 100% oxygen via mask, and anticipate respiratory failure.

   d. Bring the emergency equipment to the room and begin bag-valve-mask ventilation.

2. A toddler has moderate respiratory distress, is mildly cyanotic, and has increased work of breathing, with a respiratory rate of 40. What is the priority nursing intervention?

   a. Airway maintenance and 100% oxygen by mask

   b. 100% oxygen and pulse oximetry monitoring

   c. Airway maintenance and continued reassessment

   d. 100% oxygen and provision of comfort

3. The nurse is caring for a child with cystic fibrosis who receives pancreatic enzymes. Which statement by the child's mother indicates an understanding of how to administer the supplemental enzymes?

   a. "I will stop the enzymes if my child is receiving antibiotics."

   b. "I will decrease the dose by half if my child is having frequent, bulky stools."

   c. "Between meals is the best time for me to give the enzymes."

   d. "The enzymes should be given at the beginning of each meal and snack."

4. Which of these factors contributes to infants' and children's increased risk for upper airway obstruction as compared with adults?

   a. Underdeveloped cricoid cartilage and narrow nasal passages

   b. Small tonsils and narrow nasal passages

   c. Cylinder-shaped larynx and underdeveloped sinuses

   d. Underdeveloped cricoid cartilage and smaller tongue

5. Which is the most appropriate treatment for epistaxis?

   a. With the child lying down and breathing through the mouth, apply pressure to the bridge of the nose.

   b. With the child lying down and breathing through the mouth, pinch the lower third of the nose closed.

   c. With the child sitting up and leaning forward, apply pressure to the bridge of the nose.

   d. With the child sitting up and leaning forward, pinch the lower third of the nose closed.

CRITICAL THINKING EXERCISES

1. A 10-month-old girl is admitted to the pediatric unit with a history of recurrent pneumonia and failure to thrive. Her sweat chloride test confirms the diagnosis of cystic fibrosis. She is a frail-appearing infant with thin extremities and a slightly protuberant abdomen. She is tachypneic, has retractions, and coughs frequently. Based on the limited information given here and your knowledge of cystic fibrosis, choose three of the categories below as priorities to focus on when planning her care:

   a. Prevention of bronchospasm

   b. Promotion of adequate nutrition

   c. Education of the child and family

   d. Prevention of pulmonary infection

   e. Balancing fluid and electrolytes

   f. Management of excess weight gain

   g. Prevention of spread of infection

   h. Promoting adequate sleep and rest

2. A boy with asthma is admitted to the pediatric unit for the fourth time this year. The mother expresses frustration that he is getting sick so often. Besides information about onset of symptoms and events leading up to this present episode, what other types of information would you ask for while obtaining the history?

3. The mother of the boy in the previous question tells you that she smokes (but never around the boy), the family has a cat that comes inside sometimes, and she always gives her son the medication prescribed. She gives salmeterol and budesonide as

soon as he starts to cough. When he is not having an episode, she gives him albuterol before his baseball games. Diphenhydramine helps his runny nose in the springtime. Based on this new information, what advice/instructions would you give the mother?

4. A 7-year-old presents with a history of recurrent nasal discharge. He sneezes every time he visits his cousins, who have pets. He lives in an older home that is carpeted. Tobacco smokers live in the home. His mother reports that he snores and is a mouth breather. She says he has symptoms nearly year-round, but they are worse in the fall and the spring. She reports that diphenhydramine is somewhat helpful with his symptoms, but she doesn't like to give it to him on school days because it makes him drowsy. Based on the history above, develop a teaching plan for this child.

5. The nurse is caring for a 4-year-old girl who returned from the recovery room after a tonsillectomy 3 hours ago. She has cried off and on over the past 2 hours and is now sleeping. What areas should the nurse assess and focus on for this patient?

STUDY ACTIVITIES

1. While caring for children in the pediatric setting, compare the signs and symptoms of a child with asthma to those of an infant with bronchiolitis. What are the most notable differences? How does the history of the two children differ?

2. A child with asthma has been prescribed Advair (fluticasone and salmeterol), albuterol, and prednisone. Develop a sample teaching plan for the child and family. Include appropriate use of the devices used to deliver the medications, as well as important information about the medications (uses and adverse effects).

3. While caring for children in the pediatric setting, compare the signs and symptoms and presentation of a child with the common cold to those of a child with either sinusitis or allergic rhinitis.

4. While caring for children in the pediatric setting, review the census of clients and identify those at risk for severe influenza and thus those who would benefit from annual influenza vaccination.

5. Compare the differences in oxygen administration between a young infant and an older child.

NURSING CARE OF THE CHILD WITH A CARDIOVASCULAR DISORDER

Logan Bernstein, 6 weeks old, is brought to the clinic by his mother. He presents with poor feeding. His mother states, "Logan falls asleep while feeding, and he's always very sweaty during feedings."

KEY TERMS

arrhythmia	congenital heart defect	orthotopic
cardiac monitoring	echocardiography	polycythemia
cardiac output	electrocardiogram	sinus bradycardia
cardiomegaly	(ECG, EKG)	sinus tachycardia
clubbing	heart failure	tetralogy of Fallot

LEARNING OBJECTIVES

Upon completion of the chapter, the learner will be able to:

1. Compare anatomic and physiologic differences of the cardiovascular system in infants and children versus adults.
2. Describe nursing care related to common laboratory and diagnostic tests used in the medical diagnosis of pediatric cardiovascular conditions.
3. Distinguish cardiovascular disorders common in infants, children, and adolescents.
4. Identify appropriate nursing assessments and interventions related to medications and treatments for pediatric cardiovascular disorders.
5. Develop an individualized nursing care plan for the child with a cardiovascular disorder.
6. Describe the psychosocial impact of chronic cardiovascular disorders on children.
7. Devise a nutrition plan for the child with cardiovascular disease.
8. Develop patient/family teaching plans for the child with a cardiovascular disorder.

WoW

The heart of the matter is healing the child's heart so he or she can embrace life to its fullest.

Cardiovascular disease is a significant cause of chronic illness and death in children. Typically cardiovascular disorders in children are divided into two major categories: congenital heart disease (CHD) and acquired heart disease. Congenital heart disease is defined as structural anomalies that are present at birth, though they are often not diagnosed until later in life. CHD accounts for the largest percentage of birth defects, and about 40,000 babies are born annually with a **congenital heart defect** (American Heart Association [AHA], 2008c). Acquired heart disease includes disorders that occur after birth. These disorders develop from a wide range of causes, or they can occur as a complication or long-term effect of CHD. Over 100 genes have been identified that may be involved in the development of CHD (Cunningham et al., 2005). Additional noncardiac anomalies occur in about 28% of children with CHD. CHD is also commonly associated with chromosomal abnormalities and occurs at a rate of about 3% in children with first-degree relatives who have CHD (Fixler, 2006). Many congenital heart defects result in heart failure and chronic cyanosis, leading to failure to thrive.

The diagnosis of a cardiovascular disorder in any person can be extremely frightening and overwhelming. This is even truer for the child and his or her parents. Early on, children learn that the heart is necessary for life, so knowing that there is a heart problem can promote feelings of dread. These feelings are compounded by the child's age, the view of the child as being vulnerable and defenseless, and the stressors associated with the disorder itself. The child and parents need much support and reassurance.

Nurses need to have a sound knowledge base about cardiovascular conditions affecting children so that they can provide appropriate assessment, intervention, guidance, and support to the child and family. Cardiovascular disorders require acute interventions that often have long-term implications for the child's health and growth and development. Due to the potentially overwhelming and devastating effects that cardiovascular disorders can have on children and their families, nurses need to be skilled in assessment and interventions in this area and able to provide support throughout the course of the illness and beyond. This chapter describes the nursing management of children with congenital and acquired cardiovascular disorders, highlighting the common procedures used for treatment.

Variations in Pediatric Anatomy and Physiology

The cardiovascular system undergoes numerous changes at birth. Structures that were vital to the fetus are no longer needed. Circulation via the umbilical arteries and vein is replaced with the child's own closed independent circulation. Changes in the size of the heart, pulse rate, and blood pressure also occur.

Circulatory Changes From Gestation to Birth

The fetal heart is developed within the first 21 days of gestation, with the development of the heart rate and fetal blood circulation. The four chambers of the heart and arteries are formed during gestational months 2 through 8. During fetal development, oxygenation of the fetus occurs via the placenta; the lungs, though perfused, do not perform oxygenation and ventilation. The foramen ovale, an opening between the atria, allows blood flow from the right to the left atrium. The ductus arteriosus allows blood flow between the pulmonary artery and the aorta, shunting blood away from the pulmonary circulation (Molczan, 2006; Valente et al., 2006). Figure 40.1 illustrates fetal circulation.

With the first breath, several changes occur in the cardiopulmonary system that enable the newborn to make the transition from fetal circulation to normal circulation. As the newborn breathes for the first time, the lungs inflate, reducing pulmonary vascular resistance to blood flow. As a result, pulmonary artery pressure drops. Subsequently, pressure in the right atrium decreases. Blood flow to the left side of the heart increases the pressure in the left atrium. This change in pressure leads to closure of the foramen ovale. The drop in pressure of the pulmonary artery promotes closure of the ductus arteriosus, which is located between the aorta and pulmonary artery. The ductus venosus, located between the left umbilical vein and the inferior vena cava, closes because of a lack of blood flow and vasoconstriction. The closed ductus arteriosus and ductus venosus eventually become ligaments. With the lack of blood flow to the umbilical arteries and vein, these structures atrophy.

Structural and Functional Differences

The structure and function of the infant's and child's cardiovascular system differ from those of adults, depending on age. In infants and children under 7, the heart lies more horizontally. As a result, the apex lies higher, below the fourth intercostal space. In the infant, the heart lies higher in the chest and occupies over half of the chest width. As the lungs grow over time, the heart is displaced downward. The toddler/preschooler (between 1 and 6 years) has a heart four times the birth size. By school age (between 6 and 12 years) the child's heart is 10 times the size it was at birth. However, the heart is smaller proportionally at this time than at any other stage in life. During the school-age years, the heart grows more vertically within the thoracic cavity. During adolescence, the heart continues to grow in relation to the teen's rapid growth.

At birth, the ventricle walls are similar in thickness, but with time the left ventricular wall thickens. The immature myocytes of the infant's heart are thinner and less compliant than those of the adult. Right ventricular function dominates at birth, and over the first few months of life, left

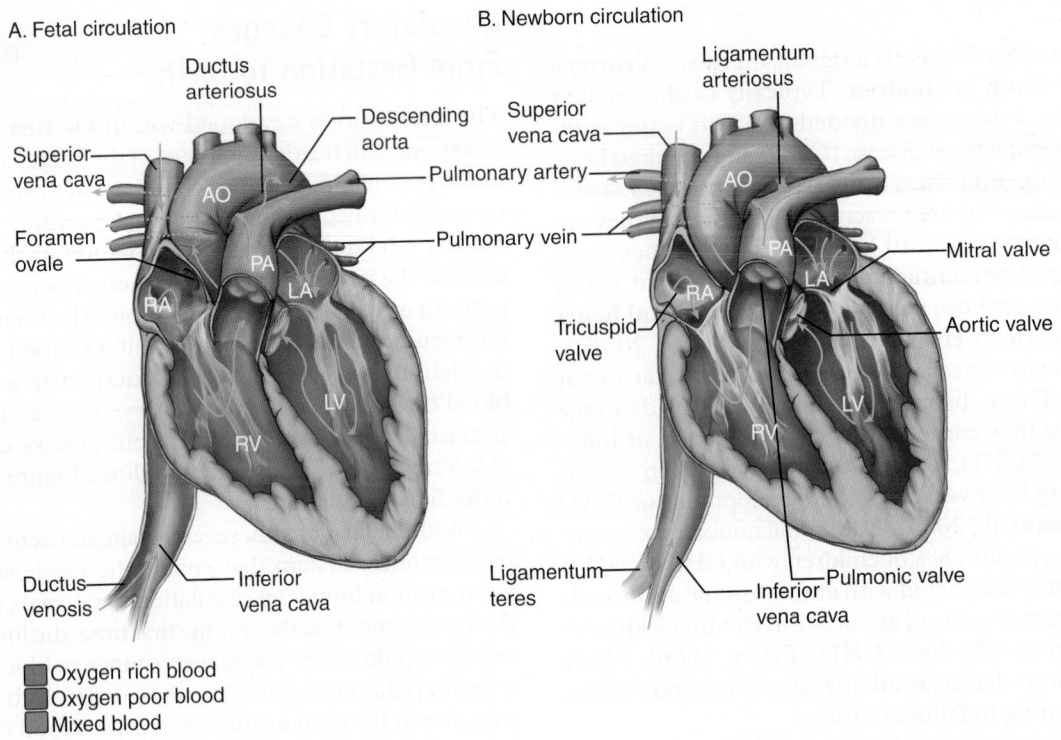

A. Fetal circulation

Ductus arteriosus

Descending aorta

Superior vena cava

Foramen ovale

AO

PA

LA

RA

LV

RV

Ductus venosus

Inferior vena cava

B. Newborn circulation

Ligamentum arteriosus

Superior vena cava

Pulmonary artery

Pulmonary vein

AO

PA

LA

RA

Mitral valve

Tricuspid valve

Aortic valve

LV

RV

Ligamentum teres

Inferior vena cava

Pulmonic valve

Oxygen rich blood
Oxygen poor blood
Mixed blood

FIGURE 40.1 Fetal and newborn circulation.

ventricular function becomes dominant. The infant's heart at rest exhibits a greater resting tension than the adult's, so volume loading or increased stretch may actually lead to decreased **cardiac output**. The infant's sarcoplasmic reticulum is less well organized than the adult's, making the infant dependent on serum calcium for contraction. Inotropic response to calcium in the actin and myosin (contractile proteins) increases with age.

The normal heart rate is higher in infancy than in adulthood, limiting the infant's ability to increase cardiac output by increasing the heart rate. The heart's efficiency increases as the child ages and the heart rate drops over time. The normal infant heart rate averages 120 to 130 beats per minute (bpm), the toddler's or preschooler's is 80 to 105 bpm, the school-age child's is 70 to 80 bpm, and the adolescent's averages 60 to 68 bpm. Innocent murmurs and physiologic splitting of heart sounds may be noted in infancy or childhood. These findings are related to the change in the size of the heart in relation to the thoracic cavity. The infant's and child's blood vessels widen and increase in length over time. The normal infant's blood pressure (BP) is about 80/40 mm Hg. The BP increases over time to the adult level. The toddler or preschooler's BP averages 80 to 100/64 mm Hg, the school-age child's 94 to 112/56 to 60 mm Hg, and the adolescent's 100 to 120/50 to 70 mm Hg (Frietas-Nichols, 2004; Luxner, 2005; Muscari, 2004).

Common Medical Treatments

A variety of medications as well as other medical treatments and surgical procedures are used to treat cardiovascular

problems in children. Most of these treatments will require a physician's order when the child is in the hospital. The most common treatments and medications are listed in Common Medical Treatments 40.1 and Drug Guide 40.1. The nurse caring for the child with a cardiovascular disorder should be familiar with what the procedures and medications are and how they work as well as common nursing implications related to use of these modalities.

▶ **Take** NOTE!

*Give digoxin at regular intervals, every 12 hours, such as at 8 a.m. and 8 p.m., 1 hour before or 2 hours after a feeding. If a digoxin dose is missed and more than 4 hours have elapsed, withhold the dose and give the dose at the regular time; if less than 4 hours have elapsed, give the missed dose. If the child vomits digoxin, **do not** give a second dose. Monitor potassium levels, as a decrease enhances the effects of digitalis, causing toxicity.*

NURSING PROCESS OVERVIEW FOR THE CHILD WITH A CARDIOVASCULAR DISORDER

Care of the child with a cardiovascular disorder includes all of the typical steps of the nursing process: assessment, nursing diagnosis, planning, interventions, and evaluation.

(text continues on page 1285)

COMMON MEDICAL TREATMENTS 40.1

Treatment	Explanation	Indication	Nursing Implications
Oxygen	Supplemented via mask, nasal cannula, hood, tent or via endotracheal/nasotracheal tube	Hypoxemia, respiratory distress, heart failure	Monitor response via work of breathing and pulse oximetry.
Chest physiotherapy (CPT) and postural drainage	Promotes mucus clearance by mobilizing secretions with the assistance of percussion or vibration accompanied by postural drainage (refer to Chapter 39 for additional information related to CPT and postural drainage)	Mobilization of secretions, particularly in postoperative period or with heart failure	May be performed by respiratory therapist in some institutions, by nurses in others. In either case, nurses must be familiar with the technique and able to educate families on its use.
Chest tube	Drainage tube is inserted into the pleural cavity to facilitate removal of air or fluid and allow full lung expansion.	After open heart surgery, pneumothorax	If tube becomes dislodged from container, the chest tube must be clamped immediately to avoid further air entry into the chest cavity.
Pacing	External wiring connected to a small generator used to electrophysiologically correct cardiac arrhythmias or heart block (temporary). Permanent pacing achieved with an implantable internal pacemaker.	Bradyarrhythmias, heart block, cardiomyopathy, sinoatrial or atrioventricular node malfunction	Provide close observation of the child, pacing unit, and ECG. Maintain asepsis at pacing lead insertion site. Explain to child and family that the permanent pacemaker may be felt under the skin. Advise against participation in contact sports.

DRUG GUIDE 40.1

Medication	Action/Indication	Nursing Implications
Alprostadil (Prostin VR: prostaglandin E$_1$)	Direct vasodilation of the ductus arteriosus smooth muscle. Indicated for temporary maintenance of ductus arteriosus patency in infants with ductal-dependent congenital heart defects.	• Apnea occurs in 10% to 20% of neonates within first hour of infusion. • Monitor arterial BP, respiratory rate, heart rate, ECG, temperature, pO$_2$; watch for abdominal distention. • Fresh IV solution required every 24 hours. • Reposition catheter if facial or arm flushing occurs. • Use with caution in neonate with bleeding tendency. • Contraindicated in respiratory distress syndrome or persistent fetal circulation.
Digoxin (Lanoxin)	Increases contractility of the heart muscle by decreasing conduction and increasing force. Used for heart failure, atrial fibrillation, atrial flutter, supraventricular tachycardia.	• Prior to administering each dose, count apical pulse for 1 full minute, noting rate, rhythm, and quality. Withhold if apical pulse is <60 in an adolescent, <90 in an infant. • Avoid giving oral form with meals, as altered absorption may occur. • Monitor serum digoxin levels (therapeutic range: 0.8–2 ng/mL). • Notes signs of toxicity: nausea, vomiting, diarrhea, lethargy, bradycardia. • Ginseng, hawthorn, and licorice intake increases risk for drug toxicity.

(continued)

DRUG GUIDE 40.1 (continued)

Medication	Action/Indication	Nursing Implications
		• Note contraindications (ventricular fibrillation and hypersensitivity to digitalis). • Avoid rapid IV administration, as this may lead to systemic and coronary artery vasoconstriction.
Furosemide (Lasix)	Inhibits resorption of sodium and chloride. Used to manage edema associated with heart failure, and hypertension in combination with antihypertensives.	• Administer with food or milk to decrease GI upset. • Monitor BP, renal function, electrolytes (particularly potassium), and hearing. • May cause photosensitivity.
Heparin	Interferes with conversion of prothrombin to thrombin, preventing clot formation. Indicated for the prophylaxis and treatment of thromboembolic disorders, especially after cardiac surgery.	• Administer SQ, not IM. • Dose is adjusted according to coagulation test results. • Monitor for signs of bleeding, platelet counts. • Ensure that the antidote, protamine sulfate, is available. • Do not administer with uncontrolled bleeding or if subacute bacterial endocarditis is suspected.
Indomethacin (Indocin)	Inhibits prostaglandin synthesis in order to close patent ductus arteriosus.	• Monitor heart rate, BP, ECG, urine output; monitor for murmur. • Monitor serum sodium, glucose, platelet count, BUN, creatinine, potassium, and liver enzymes. • May mask signs of infection. • Note development of edema.
Spironolactone (Aldactone)	Competes with aldosterone to result in increased water and sodium excretion (spares potassium). Used to manage edema due to heart failure and for treatment of hypertension.	• Administer with food. • Monitor serum potassium, sodium, and renal function. • May cause drowsiness, headache, arrhythmia. • May cause false elevations in digitalis level. • Teach patients to avoid high-potassium diets, salt substitutes, and natural licorice. • Contraindicated in hyperkalemia, renal failure, and anuria.
Antibiotics		
Penicillin G benzathine (PCN-G) Penicillin V potassium (Pen-VK)	Inhibits bacterial wall synthesis in susceptible organisms. Indicated in mild to moderate infections, for prophylaxis of endocarditis and rheumatic fever.	• Contraindications include hypersensitivity to penicillins. • Report hypersensitivity reactions (chills, fever, wheezing, pruritus, anaphylaxis) immediately. • PCN-G: administer IM. • Pen-VK: administer orally on empty stomach 1 hour prior to or 2 hours after a meal.
Erythromycin	Inhibits RNA transcription in susceptible organisms. Used in children with penicillin allergy, mild to moderate infections, endocarditis, and for rheumatic fever prophylaxis.	• Contraindicated in preexisting liver disease. • IV administration may result in CV abnormalities. • Abdominal distress common with oral use. • Fever, dizziness, rash may occur.
Antihypertensive Drugs		
Angiotensin-converting enzyme (ACE) inhibitors (captopril [Capoten], enalapril [Vasotec])	Competitive inhibition of ACE for management of hypertension. Heart failure management in conjunction with digitalis and diuretics.	• Monitor BP, renal function, WBC count, serum potassium. • Discontinue if angioedema occurs. • Captopril: administer orally on empty stomach 1 hour before or 2 hours after meals. • Enalapril: may administer orally without regard to food.

Medication	Action/Indication	Nursing Implications
Beta-adrenergic blockers (propranolol [Inderal], atenolol [Tenormin], sotalol [Betapace])	Competitively blocks response to beta-adrenergic stimulation decreasing heart rate and force of contraction. Used for management of hypertension, arrhythmias, and prevention of myocardial infarction.	• Monitor ECG and BP. • Propranolol: administer with food. • Atenolol, sotalol: administer without regard to food. Do not stop drug abruptly. • May result in bradycardia, dizziness, nausea and vomiting, dyspnea, hypoglycemia (propranolol). • Contraindications: heart block, uncompensated heart failure, cardiogenic shock, asthma, or hypersensitivity.
Hydralazine (Apresoline)	Direct vasodilation of arterioles to manage moderate to severe hypertension, heart failure.	• Monitor heart rate, BP. • Closely monitor BP with IV use. • Administer oral dose with food. • May cause palpitations, flushing, tachycardia, dizziness, nausea and vomiting. • Notify physician if flu-like symptoms occur. • Contraindicated in rheumatic valvular disease.

There are a number of general concepts related to the nursing process that may be applied to any child with a cardiovascular disorder. The nurse should be knowledgeable about the procedures, treatments, and medication as well as familiar with the nursing implications related to these interventions. With an understanding of these concepts, the nurse can individualize the care based on the patient's and family's needs.

Remember Logan, the 6-week-old with poor feeding? What additional health history and physical examination assessment information should the nurse obtain?

Assessment

When assessing a child with a cardiovascular disorder, expect to obtain a health history, perform a physical examination, and prepare the child for laboratory and diagnostic testing.

Health History

The health history comprises a history of the present illness, past medical history, and family history. Depending on his or her age, the child should be included in the health history interview; the child's age will determine the degree of involvement and the terminology used. Table 40.1 gives examples of typical questions that can be used when obtaining the child's health history.

History of Present Illness

Elicit the history of the present illness, which addresses when the symptoms started and how they have progressed. Inquire about any treatments and medications used at home. Ask parents about history of orthopnea, dyspnea, easy fatigability, growth delays, squatting, edema, dizziness, and/or frequent occurrences of pneumonia, which can be significant signs of pediatric heart disease (Muscari, 2004). The history of present illness may reveal a history of poor feeding, including fatigue, lethargy, and/or vomiting, or failure to thrive, even with adequate caloric intake. The parents may report diaphoresis, which is often seen in early heart failure. Delays in gross motor development, cyanosis (possibly reported by the parents as more of a gray color than blue), and tachypnea (indicative of heart failure) may also be reported by the parent or caregiver.

Past Medical History

The past medical history includes information about the child as well as the mother's pregnancy history. Assess the child's past medical history for:

• Problems occurring after birth (history of the child's condition after birth may reveal evidence of an associated congenital malformation or other disorder)
• Frequent infections
• Chromosomal abnormalities
• Prematurity
• Autoimmune disorders
• Use of medications, such as corticosteroids

Assess the mother's pregnancy, labor, and delivery history. Be sure to include information about the status of the neonate at birth. Also inquire about maternal use of medications, including illicit or over-the-counter drugs and alcohol; exposure to radiation; presence of hypertension; and maternal viral illnesses such as coxsackievirus, cytomegalovirus, influenza, mumps, or rubella. A history of significant problems related to labor and delivery

TABLE 40.1 EXAMPLES OF QUESTIONS FOR OBTAINING A CHILD'S HEALTH HISTORY

Questions	Provides Information About:
• What types and amounts (dosages) of medications has the child received? What were they used for? • Who prescribed them? • Were they effective? Did the child experience any adverse effects? • To whom does the child go for medical evaluation? How often? Were the visits for regular health check-ups or for situational problems? Were there previous hospitalizations? What for?	• Possible underlying conditions that may be related to the child's current status • Other health care personnel involved in the child's care as well as the parents' health care beliefs and patterns • How the medications may be affecting the child's health • The child's health status and the parents' health care knowledge, practices, and beliefs
• Has the child experienced any growth delay? Does the child have any problems with activity and coordination?	• Problems that may result from impaired cardiac output, adequacy of tissue oxygenation, and concomitant disorders associated with heart disease
• Does the child's skin color change when crying? If so, what color do you see?	• Effectiveness of tissue oxygenation. A blue or gray skin color may be due to cyanosis.
• Does the child stop frequently during play to sit or squat?	• The child's exercise tolerance and tissue oxygenation
• Does the child have feeding difficulty? Does the child tire easily or sleep excessively?	• The child's energy expenditure, ability to tolerate activity, and tissue oxygenation
• Does the child frequently develop strep throat?	• Child's risk for developing rheumatic fever and heart disease

is also important: stress or asphyxia at birth may be related to cardiac dysfunction and pulmonary hypertension in the newborn.

Assess for additional risk factors such as:

• Family history of heart disease or CHD (investigate the history further if heart disease occurred in a first-degree relative)
• Hyperlipidemia
• Diabetes mellitus
• Obesity
• Inactivity
• Stress
• High-cholesterol diet (Freitas-Nichols, 2004; Muscari, 2004)

▶ *Take* NOTE!

Medications taken by pregnant women such as isotretinoin (Accutane) for acne, lithium, and some antiseizure medications may be linked to the development of congenital heart defects. In addition, smoking during pregnancy, febrile illness in the first trimester, rubella infection during pregnancy, exposure of the pregnant woman to strong cleaning products, repeated x-rays, and any harmful or poisonous material can increase the risk of CHD.

Physical Examination

Physical examination of the child with a cardiovascular condition consists of inspection, palpation, and auscultation. In addition, obtain the child's vital signs and measure the child's height and weight. Plot this information on a standard growth chart to evaluate nutritional status and growth. If the child is less than 3 years of age, measure and plot the head circumference also.

Inspection

Assess the child's overall appearance. Inspect the color of the skin, noting cyanosis. Inspect the skin for edema. In infants, peripheral edema occurs first in the face, then the presacral region, and then the extremities. Edema of the lower extremities is characteristic of right ventricular heart failure in older children.

▶ *Take* NOTE!

CHD should be suspected in the cyanotic newborn who does not improve with oxygen administration.

Inspect the fingers and toes for **clubbing**. Clubbing (which usually does not appear until after 1 year of age) implies chronic hypoxia due to severe congenital heart disease. The first sign of clubbing is softening of the nail beds, followed by rounding of the fingernails, followed by shininess and thickening of the nail ends (see Fig. 39.6 in Chapter 39).

Obtain the child's temperature; fever would suggest infection. Assess respirations, including rate, rhythm, and effort. Note location and severity of retractions if present. Inspect the chest configuration, noting any prominence of the precordial chest wall, which is often seen in infants and children with **cardiomegaly**. Note visible pulsations, which may indicate increased heart activity. Also inspect the neck veins for engorgement or abnormal pulsations. Note abdominal distention (Frietas-Nichols, 2004; Muscari, 2004; Valente et al., 2006).

> ▶ *Take* NOTE!
>
> *Children with cardiac conditions resulting in cyanosis will often have baseline oxygen saturations that are relatively low because of the mixing of oxygenated with deoxygenated blood.*

Palpation

Palpate the right and left radial or brachial pulse to assess cardiac rate and rhythm. Throughout infancy and childhood, the rate may vary. Palpate the femoral pulse; it should be readily palpable and equal in amplitude and strength to the brachial or radial pulse. A femoral pulse that is weak or absent in comparison to the brachial pulse is associated with coarctation of the aorta. Significant variations in pulse occur with activity, so the most accurate heart rate may be determined during sleep. In older children, exercise and emotional factors may influence the heart rate. A bounding pulse is characteristic of patent ductus arteriosus or aortic regurgitation. Narrow or thready pulses may occur in children with heart failure or severe aortic stenosis. Note **tachycardia, bradycardia**, irregularities in rhythm, diminished peripheral pulses, or thready pulse. Palpate the child's abdomen for hepatomegaly, a sign of right-sided heart failure in the infant and child.

Auscultation

Auscultate the apical pulse for a full minute to determine heart rate and rhythm. Note irregularities in rhythm, tachycardia or bradycardia. Auscultate the heart for murmurs. Many children have functional or innocent murmurs, but all murmurs must be evaluated on the basis of the following characteristics:

• Location
• Relation to the heart cycle and duration
• Intensity: grade I, soft and hard to hear; grade II, soft and easily heard; grade III, loud without thrill; grade IV,

loud with a precordial thrill; grade IV, loud, audible with a precordial thrill; grade V, loud, audible with a stethoscope; grade VI, very loud, and audible with a stethoscope or with the naked ear
• Quality: harsh, musical, or rough; high, medium, or low pitch
• Variation with position (sitting, lying, standing) (Freitas-Nichols, 2004; Muscari, 2004; Valente et al., 2006)

Auscultate for the character of heart sounds. Note distinct, muffled, or distant heart sounds. Abnormal splitting or intensifying of S2 sounds occurs in children with major heart problems. Ejection clicks, which are high-pitched, are related to problems with dilated vessels and/or valve abnormalities. Heard throughout systole, they can be early, moderate, or late. Clicks on the upper left sternal border are related to the pulmonary area. Aortic clicks are best heard at the apex and can be mitral or aortic in origin. A mild to late ejection click at the apex is typical of a mitral valve prolapse. The S3 heart sound may be heard in children and is associated with cardiac abnormalities. The S4 heart sound is not normally heard and is always associated with cardiac abnormalities (Driscoll, 2006; Muscari, 2004).

Auscultate the BP in the upper extremities and lower extremities and compare the findings; there should be no major differences between the upper and lower extremities. Determine the pulse pressure by subtracting the diastolic pressure from the systolic pressure. The pulse pressure is less than 50 Hg, or less than half the systolic pressure. A widened pulse pressure, which usually is accompanied by a bounding pulse, is associated with patent ductus arteriosus, aortic insufficiency, fever, anemia, or complete heart block. A narrowed pulse pressure is associated with aortic stenosis. Note hypotension or hypertension.

> ▶ *Take* NOTE!
>
> *Children and parents must be alerted if a heart murmur is detected, even if it is benign.*

Laboratory and Diagnostic Testing

Common Laboratory and Diagnostic Tests 40.1 explains the laboratory and diagnostic tests most commonly used when considering cardiovascular disorders in children. The tests can assist the physician in diagnosing the disorder or can be used as guidelines in determining ongoing treatment. Laboratory or non-nursing personnel obtain some of the tests, while the nurse might obtain others. In either instance the nurse should be familiar with how the tests are obtained, what they are used for, and normal versus abnormal results. This knowledge will also be

COMMON LABORATORY AND DIAGNOSTIC TESTS 40.1

Test	Explanation	Indications	Nursing Implications
Arteriogram (angiogram: visualization of arteries or veins)	Radiopaque contrast solution is injected through a catheter and into the circulation. X-rays are then taken to visualize the structure of the heart and blood vessels.	To observe blood flow to parts of body and detect lesions; to confirm a diagnosis. Catheters can be used to remove plaques.	• Make sure the parent signs a consent form. • Administer premedication as ordered. • Obtain child's weight to determine amount of dye needed. • Keep the child NPO before the procedure according to institutional protocol. • After the procedure, maintain the child on bed rest. • Observe the puncture site for bleeding. • Monitor vital signs frequently and check the pulse distal to the site.
Ambulatory electrocardiographic monitoring (Holter)	Monitoring of the heart's electrical patterns for 24 hours using a portable compact unit	To identify and quantify arrhythmias in a 24-hour period during normal daily activities	• Instruct the child and parent to push the "event button" whenever chest pain, syncope, or palpitations occur. • Normal daily activities should be carried out during the testing period. • Having the child wear a snug undershirt over the leads helps to keep them in place.
Chest x-ray	A radiographic film of the chest area; will determine size of the heart and its chambers and pulmonary blood flow	Serves as a baseline for comparison with films taken after surgery; used to identify abnormalities of the lungs, heart, and other structures in the chest	• Instruct patient not to wear jewelry or any metal around neck or on the hospital gown. • Explain to the child and family that no pain or discomfort should result. • If a portable x-ray at bedside is done, remove electrodes temporarily.
Echocardiogram	Noninvasive ultrasound procedure used to assess heart wall thickness, size of heart chambers, motion of valves and septa, and relationship of great vessels to other cardiac structures	Specific diagnosis of structural defects; determines hemodynamics and detects valvular defects	• Assure the child that the echo does not hurt. • Instruct the child about ECG lead placement and use of gel on the scope's wand during the procedure. • Encourage the child to lie still throughout the test.
Electrocardiogram (ECG, EKG)	A graphic record produced by an electrocardiograph (device used to record the electrical activity of the myocardium to detect transmission of the cardiac impulse through the conductive tissues of the muscle). Facilitates evaluation of the heart rate, rhythm, conduction, and musculature.	To detect heart rhythm and chamber overload; also serves as a baseline for measuring postoperative complications	• Assure the child that monitoring is a painless procedure. • Place electrodes in the appropriate location. • The child must lie still during the ECG recording period (usually about 5 minutes). • Wipe electrode paste or jelly off after procedure.

Test	Explanation	Indications	Nursing Implications
Exercise stress test	Monitoring of heart rate, blood pressure, ECG, and oxygen consumption at rest and during exercise	Quantifies exercise tolerance; can be used to provoke symptoms or arrhythmias	• Child should be NPO for 4 hours prior to test. • Obtain baseline ECG and vital signs. • Instruct child to verbalize symptoms during testing. • Usually takes about 45 minutes.
Hemoglobin (Hgb) and hematocrit (Hct)	Measures the total amount of hemoglobin in the blood and indirectly measures the red blood cell number and volume	To detect anemia or polycythemia (may occur with CHD resulting in cyanosis)	• False elevations occur with dehydration. • May be obtained quickly via capillary puncture. • Normal values vary with age.
Partial pressure of oxygen (pO₂)	Measures the amount of oxygen in the blood	To determine the presence and degree of hypoxia	• Most accurate result is with arterial specimen (venous and capillary specimens demonstrate lower levels). • Observe child for cyanosis. • Supplement with oxygen per protocol.

necessary when providing patient and family education related to the testing.

Cardiac Catheterization

Cardiac catheterization is the definitive study for infants and children with cardiac disease and thus deserves special attention in this section on assessment of cardiovascular disorders. Cardiac catheterization has become almost a routine diagnostic procedure and may be performed on an outpatient basis. However, it is highly invasive and not without risks, especially in sick infants and children. Indications for cardiac catheterization include:

• Cardiovascular disease causing cyanosis in infants: these infants need to be catheterized as soon as they are in a reasonably stable condition
• Severe heart failure or progressive problems such as pulmonary edema
• Questionable anatomic or physiologic abnormalities
• Planned cardiac surgery
• Progressive monitoring related to pulmonary hypertension
• Periodic assessment after repair of a cardiac defect
• Therapeutic interventions such as septostomy or balloon valvotomy

Cardiac catheterization may be categorized as diagnostic, interventional, or electrophysiologic. Diagnostic cardiac catheterization typically is used to identify structural defects. Interventional cardiac catheterization is used as a treatment measure to dilate occluded or stenotic structures or vessels or close some defects. Electrophysiologic cardiac catheterization involves the use of electrodes to identify abnormal rhythms and destroy sites of abnormal electrical conduction. The type of catheterization performed varies based on the individual needs of the patient. The procedure lasts from 1 to 3 hours (Driscoll, 2006; Mullins, 2006b; Muscari, 2004).

Performing Cardiac Catheterization

In cardiac catheterization, a radiopaque catheter is inserted into a blood vessel and is then guided through the vessel to the heart with the aid of fluoroscopy. For a right-sided catheterization, the catheter is threaded to the right atrium via a major vein such as the femoral vein. With a left-sided catheterization, the catheter is threaded to the aorta and heart via an artery. Once the tip of the catheter is in the heart, contrast material is injected via the catheter and radiographic images are taken.

While the catheter is in the heart, several procedures can be performed. The blood pressures, changes in cardiac output or stroke volume, and oxygen saturation in each heart chamber and major blood vessels are recorded. With the injection of contrast material, information is revealed about the heart anatomy, ventricular wall motion and ejection fraction, intracardiac pressures and hemodynamic parameters, cardiac valve function, and structural abnormalities. The movement of the contrast material is filmed so that the details of the cardiac procedure are recorded. Samples of heart tissue to evaluate for infection, muscular dysfunction, or rejection after a transplant may also be obtained.

Nursing Management

Although cardiac catheterization may be considered nearly routine, for the child and parents or guardians, the procedure can be a source of much anxiety. Therefore, the nurse needs to educate the parents and, if appropriate for age, the child about all aspects of the procedure. The procedure is commonly performed on an outpatient basis, but some health care providers require the child be admitted for an overnight stay for observation. Nursing management of the child undergoing cardiac catheterization includes preprocedure nursing assessment and preparation of the child and family, postprocedural nursing care, and discharge teaching.

Before the Procedure. A thorough history and physical examination are necessary to establish a baseline. Obtain vital signs. Note fever or other signs and symptoms of infection, which may necessitate rescheduling the procedure. Obtain the child's height and weight to aid in determining medication dosages. Assess the child for any allergies, especially to iodine and shellfish, because some contrast materials contain iodine as a base. Review the child's medications: medications such as anticoagulants are typically withheld for several days or longer prior to the procedure to reduce the child's risk for bleeding. Check the results of any laboratory tests, such as hemoglobin and hematocrit levels.

Perform a complete physical examination. Pay particular attention to assessing the child's peripheral pulses, including pedal pulses. Use an indelible pen to mark the location of the child's pedal pulses so they can be easily assessed after the procedure. Document the location and quality in the child's medical record.

Teach the parents and child, if appropriate, about the procedure, including what the procedure involves, how long it will take, and any special instructions from the health care provider. Use a variety of teaching methods as appropriate, such as videotapes, books, and pamphlets. Adapt these teaching methods to the child's developmental stage. For example, introduce the younger child to equipment through play therapy. For school-age and older children and their parents, offer a tour of the cardiac catheterization laboratory. Mention sounds and sights they may experience during the procedure. Explain the use of intravenous fluid therapy, sedation, and, if ordered, anesthesia to the child and parents. Tell the child that he or she may feel a sensation of the heart racing when the catheter is inserted. Also warn the older child that he or she may experience a feeling of warmth or stinging when the contrast material is injected. Encourage the child to use familiar ways to help him or her relax. If necessary, teach the child simple relaxation measures.

Typically, food and fluid are withheld for 4 to 6 hours before the procedure. Prescribed medications may be taken with a sip of water. On the day of the procedure, check to ensure that a signed informed consent form is on the child's medical record and that all necessary assessment data have been included. Just before the procedure, ask the child to void and administer a sedative, as ordered. If appropriate and permitted, allow the parents to accompany the child to the catheterization area.

Teach the child and family what to expect after the procedure is completed. Inform the parents of the possible complications that might occur, such as bleeding, low-grade fever, loss of pulse in the extremity used for the catheterization, and arrhythmias. Explain to the child that he or she will have a dressing over the catheter site and that he or she will need to keep the leg straight for several hours after the procedure. Teach the child and parent that frequent monitoring will be required after the procedure.

After the Procedure. Throughout the postprocedure period, closely monitor the child for complications of bleeding, **arrhythmia**, hematoma and thrombus formation, and infection. After the procedure, evaluate the child's vital signs, the neurovascular status of the lower extremities, and the pressure dressing over the catheterization site every 15 minutes for the first hour and then every 30 minutes for 1 hour. Vital signs should remain within acceptable parameters. Hypotension may signify hemorrhage due to perforation of the heart muscle or bleeding from the insertion site. Expect to monitor cardiac rhythm and oxygen saturation levels via pulse oximetry for the first few hours after the procedure to help identify possible complications.

Assess the child's distal pulses bilaterally for presence and quality. The pulse of the affected extremity may be slightly less than that of the other extremity in the initial postprocedure period, but it should gradually return to baseline. Also assess the color and temperature of the extremity; pallor or blanching would indicate an obstruction in blood flow. Check capillary refill and sensation to evaluate blood flow to the area.

Maintain bed rest in the immediate postprocedure period. Ensure that the child maintains the extremity in a straight position for approximately 4 to 8 hours, depending on the approach used and the facility's policy. Some facilities require straight positioning for 4 to 6 hours after a right-sided catheterization and for 6 to 8 hours after a left-sided catheterization to ensure healing of the vessel. Inspect the pressure dressing frequently. Check to make sure that it is dry and intact, without evidence of bleeding. Reinforce the dressing as necessary and report any evidence of drainage on the dressing. If there is a risk of the dressing becoming soiled or wet, cover it with plastic.

▶ **Take** NOTE!

If bleeding occurs after a cardiac catheterization, apply pressure 1 inch above the site to create pressure over the vessel, thereby reducing the blood flow to the area.

Monitor the child's intake and output closely to ensure adequate hydration. The contrast material has a diuretic effect, so assess the child for signs and symptoms of dehydration and hypovolemia. Typically, the child resumes oral intake as tolerated, beginning with sips of clear liquids and progressing to his or her preprocedure diet. Continue intravenous fluids as ordered and encourage oral fluid intake as allowed and ordered to promote elimination of the contrast material.

Allow the child to talk about the experience and how and what he or she felt. Provide positive reinforcement for the child's actions.

Provide patient and family education before the child is discharged home (Teaching Guidelines 40.1). Areas to address include site care, signs and symptoms of complications (especially within 24 hours after the catheterization, such as fever, bleeding or bruising at the catheterization site, or changes in color, temperature, or sensation in the extremity used), diet, and activity level.

Nursing Diagnoses and Related Interventions

Upon completion of a thorough assessment, the nurse might identify several nursing diagnoses. These may include but are not limited to:

- Decreased cardiac output
- Ineffective tissue perfusion
- Imbalanced nutrition, less than body requirements
- Risk for delayed growth and development
- Risk for infection
- Excess fluid volume
- Interrupted family process
- Activity intolerance
- Pain

After completing Logan's assessment, the nurse noted the following: poor weight gain, tachypnea with occasional nasal flaring, crackles heard on auscultation, and edema noted in the face, presacral area and extremities. Based on these assessment findings, what would your top three nursing diagnoses be for Logan?

Nursing goals, interventions, and evaluation for the child with a cardiovascular disorder are based on the nursing diagnoses. Nursing Care Plan 40.1 can be used as a guide in planning nursing care for the child with a cardiovascular disorder. The nursing care plan overview should be individualized based on the patient's symptoms and needs. Refer to Chapter 35 for detailed information about pain assessment and management. Additional information will be included later in the chapter as it relates to specific disorders.

Based on your top three nursing diagnoses for Logan, describe appropriate nursing interventions.

TEACHING GUIDELINES 40.1

Providing Care After a Cardiac Catheterization

- Change the pressure dressing on the day after the procedure. Apply a dry sterile dressing or adhesive bandage for the next several days. Keep the dressing dry; cover it with plastic if there is a chance that the dressing could become wet or soiled.
- When changing the dressing, inspect the insertion site for redness, irritation, swelling, drainage, and bleeding. Report any of these to the health care provider.
- Check the temperature, color, sensation, and pulses on the child's extremities and compare. Report any changes to the health care provider.
- Resume the child's usual diet after the procedure; report any nausea or vomiting.
- Check the child's temperature at least once a day for approximately 3 days after the procedure. Report any temperature elevation of 100.4°F or greater.
- Avoid giving the child a tub bath for approximately 3 days after the procedure; use sponge baths or showers instead.
- Discourage strenuous exercise or activity for approximately 3 days after the procedure.
- Watch for changes in the child's appearance, such as changes in skin color, reports of the heart "fluttering" or "skipping a beat," fever, or difficulty breathing.
- Give acetaminophen (Tylenol) or ibuprofen (Motrin) for complaints of pain.
- Schedule a follow-up appointment with the health care provider in the time specified.

Congenital Heart Disease

In North America, more than 1% of newborn infants have CHD resulting from numerous causes. The prevalence of CHD is about 8 per 1,000 live births; premature infants have a higher rate (Fixler, 2006). Many chromosome defects are associated with CHD, including Down syndrome, velocardiofacial syndrome, Turner syndrome, trisomy 13, trisomy 18, Williams syndrome, Prader-Willi syndrome, and cri-du-chat (Marian et al., 2004). About one third of infants with CHD will have disease serious enough to result in death or will require cardiac catheterization or cardiac surgery within the first year of life.

(text continues on page 1295)

Nursing Care Plan 40.1

OVERVIEW FOR THE CHILD WITH A CARDIOVASCULAR DISORDER

NURSING DIAGNOSIS: Decreased cardiac output related to structural defect, congenital anomaly, or ineffective heart pumping as evidenced by arrhythmias, edema, murmur, abnormal heart rate, or abnormal heart sounds

Outcome Identification and Evaluation
Child or infant will demonstrate adequate cardiac output; *will have elastic skin turgor, brisk capillary refill, demonstrate pink color, pulse and blood pressure within normal limits for age, regular heart rhythm, adequate urinary output.*

Interventions: Increasing Cardiac Output
- Monitor vital signs closely, especially BP and heart rate, *to detect increases or decreases.*
- Monitor cardiac rhythm via cardiac monitor *to detect arrhythmias quickly.*
- Observe for signs of hypoxia such as tachypnea, cyanosis, tachycardia, bradycardia, dizziness, and/or restlessness *to identify this change early.*
- Administer oxygen as needed *to correct hypoxia.*
- Place child in knee-to-chest or squatting position as needed *to increase systemic vascular resistance.*
- Administer antiarrhythmics, vasopressors, ACE inhibitors, beta blockers, corticosteroids, or diuretics as prescribed *to improve cardiac output.*
- Monitor for signs of thrombosis such as restlessness, seizure, coma, oliguria, anuria, edema, hematuria, or paralysis *to identify this condition early.*
- Administer adequate hydration *to decrease possibility of thrombosis formation.*
- Cluster nursing care and other activities *to allow adequate periods of rest.*
- Anticipate child's needs *to decrease the child's stress, thereby decreasing oxygen consumption requirement.*

NURSING DIAGNOSIS: Excess fluid volume related to ineffective cardiac muscle function as evidenced by weight gain, edema, jugular vein distention, dyspnea, shortness of breath, abnormal breath sounds, or pulmonary congestion

Outcome Identification and Evaluation
Child will attain appropriate fluid balance, *will lose weight (fluid), edema or bloating will decrease, lung sounds will be clear and heart sounds normal.*

Interventions: Encouraging Fluid Loss
- Weigh daily on same scale in similar amount of clothing; *in children weight is the best indicator of changes in fluid status.*
- Monitor location and extent of edema (measure abdominal girth daily if ascites is present); *decrease in edema indicates positive increase in oncotic pressure.*
- Protect edematous areas from skin breakdown: *edema leads to increased risk for alterations in skin integrity.*
- Auscultate lungs carefully to identify crackles *(indicating pulmonary edema).*
- Assess work of breathing and respiratory rate *(increased work of breathing is associated with pulmonary edema).*
- Assess heart sounds for gallop *(presence of S3 may indicate fluid overload).*
- Maintain fluid restriction as ordered *to decrease intravascular volume and workload on the heart.*
- Strictly monitor intake and output *to quickly note discrepancies and provide intervention.*
- Provide sodium-restricted diet as ordered *(restricting sodium intake allows better renal excretion of extra fluid).*
- Administer diuretics as ordered and monitor for adverse effects. *Diuretics encourage excretion of fluid, elimination of edema, reduce cardiac filling pressures, and increase renal blood flow. Adverse effects include electrolyte imbalance as well as orthostatic hypotension.*

Nursing Care Plan 40.1 (continued)

NURSING DIAGNOSIS: Imbalanced nutrition, less than body requirements, related to increased energy expenditure and fatigue as evidenced by weight loss or height and weight below accepted standards

Outcome Identification and Evaluation
Child will improve nutritional intake resulting in *steady increase in weight and length/height, will feed without tiring easily.*

Interventions: Promoting Adequate Nutrition
• Determine body weight and length/height norm for age *to determine goal to work toward.*
• Assess child for food preferences that fall within dietary restrictions: *child will be more likely to consume adequate amounts of foods that he or she likes.*
• Weigh child daily or weekly (according to physician order or institutional standard) and measure length/height weekly *to monitor for increased growth.*
• Offer highest-calorie meals at the time of day when the child's appetite is the greatest *(to increase likelihood of increased caloric intake).*
• Provide increased-calorie shakes or puddings within diet restriction *(high-calorie foods increase weight gain).*
• Consult with the pediatric dietician *to provide optimal caloric intake within dietary restrictions.*
• Provide small, frequent feedings *to discourage tiring with feeding.*
• Feed infants with special nipple as needed *to decrease amount of energy expended for sucking.*
• Administer vitamin and mineral supplements as prescribed *to attain/maintain vitamin and mineral balance in the body.*

NURSING DIAGNOSIS: Ineffective tissue perfusion related to inadequate cardiac function or cardiac surgery as evidenced by pallor, cyanosis, edema, changes in mental status, prolonged capillary refill, clubbing, or diminished pulses

Outcome Identification and Evaluation
Child will demonstrate adequate tissue perfusion: *Child will be alert, not restless or lethargic, will have pink color, decrease in edema, normal perfusion and strong pulses.*

Interventions: Promoting Tissue Perfusion
• Assess level of consciousness, pulse, BP, peripheral perfusion, and skin color frequently *to determine baseline and ongoing improvement.*
• Administer cardiac glycosides or vasodilators as ordered *to promote cardiac output necessary for proper perfusion.*
• Monitor pulse oximetry and arterial blood gas results *to assess ability to appropriately oxygenate.*
• Supplement oxygen as needed *to provide oxygen to organs for proper functioning.*
• Monitor hemoglobin and hematocrit *to identify blood loss.*
• Strictly assess intake and output *to determine adequacy of renal perfusion.*
• Position with head of bed elevated *to decrease blood volume returning to heart.*
• Change position every 2 to 4 hours *to promote circulation and avoid skin breakdown in areas of poor perfusion.*

NURSING DIAGNOSIS: Risk for delayed growth and development related to effects of cardiac disease and necessary treatments, inadequate nutrition, or frequent separation from caregivers secondary to illness

Outcome Identification and Evaluation
Child will display development appropriate for age, *will display evidence of cognitive and motor function within normal limits (individualized for each child).*

Interventions: Promoting Appropriate Development
• Promote adequate caloric intake *to stimulate growth and provide adequate energy.*
• Provide age-appropriate developmental activities *to stimulate development.*
• Consult with the physical or occupational therapist or child life specialist *to determine activities most appropriate for the child within the constraints of the child's illness.*
• Schedule daily activities to allow for essential rest periods *for energy conservation.*
• Encourage parents, teachers, and playmates to be sensitive to child's self-image, using positive comments, *to improve the child's self-concept.*
• As energy allows, encourage participation in all activities as feasible *to allow the child to feel normal.*

(continued)

Nursing Care Plan 40.1 (continued)

NURSING DIAGNOSIS: Risk for infection related to need for multiple invasive procedures or cardiac surgery as evidenced by break in skin integrity, decreased hemoglobin, or inadequate nutritional intake

Outcome Identification and Evaluation

Child will remain free from infection: *vital signs will be within normal limits, white blood cell count normal, cultures negative. Child will exhibit no signs or symptoms of infection.*

Interventions: Preventing Infection

- Maintain strict hand hygiene *to prevent spread of infectious organisms to the child.*
- Assess temperature *to detect elevation early in course of infection.*
- Avoid contact with persons with known infections *to prevent risk of becoming ill.*
- Ensure appropriate immunization, including pneumococcal and influenza vaccinations, *to prevent development of common childhood illness.*
- Administer prophylactic antibiotics prior to all dental procedures, surgery, and many invasive procedures *to prevent subacute bacterial endocarditis.*
- Encourage good dental hygiene *to reduce the risk of endocarditis.*

NURSING DIAGNOSIS: Interrupted family processes related to crisis associated with heart disease, frequent need for testing and hospitalizations, or stresses associated with care demands, as evidenced by inadequate parental coping, frequent separations of parent and child, or inadequate support

Outcome Identification and Evaluation

Family will maintain functional system of support and will demonstrate adequate coping, adaptation of roles and functions, and decreased anxiety: *Parents are involved in child's care, ask appropriate questions, express fears and concerns, and can discuss child's care and condition calmly.*

Interventions: Promoting Family Processes

- Provide ongoing support to the child and family *to help them cope.*
- Encourage parents and family members to verbalize concerns related to child's illness, diagnosis, and prognosis: *allows the nurse to identify concerns and areas where further education may be needed. Demonstrates family-centered care.*
- Allow families to grieve over the loss of a "perfect" child: *parents must work through those grief feelings so they can be fully "present" for this chronically ill child.*
- Explain therapies, procedures, child's behaviors, and plan of care to parents: *understanding the child's current status and plan of care helps decrease anxiety.*
- Encourage parents to be involved in care: *allows parents to feel needed and valued and gives them a sense of control over their child's health.*
- Identify support system for family and child: *helps nurse identify needs and resources available for coping.*
- Educate family and child on additional resources available *to help them develop a wide base of support.*
- Encourage parents to seek genetic counseling *to provide them with the information required to make an informed decision about having another child.*

Nursing Care Plan 40.1 (continued)

NURSING DIAGNOSIS: Activity intolerance related to ineffective cardiac muscle function, increased energy expenditure, or inability to meet increased oxygen or metabolic demands as evidenced by squatting positions, shortness of breath, cyanosis, or fatigue

Outcome Identification and Evaluation

Child will increase activity level as tolerated: *child participates in play and activities (specify particular activities and level as individualized for each child).*

Interventions: Promoting Activity

- Assess level of fatigue and activity tolerance *to determine baseline for comparison.*
- Note extent of dyspnea, oxygen requirement, or color change with exertion *to provide baseline for comparison.*
- Cluster care activities, allowing rest periods in between, *to conserve child's energy.*
- Work with the parent and child to determine a mutually satisfactory daily schedule *to allow adequate rest and energy conservation.*
- Instruct family and child in prescribed activity restrictions *to prevent fatigue while allowing some activity.*
- In the infant, avoid long periods of crying or prolonged nipple feeding *(expends excessive calories).*
- Provide neutral thermal environment *to avoid increased oxygen and energy needs associated with excessive heat or cold.*

Complications of CHD include heart failure, hypoxemia, growth retardation, developmental delay, and pulmonary vascular disease. As many as 13% of children with CHD experience severe failure to thrive (Chen et al., 2004).

With advances in palliative and corrective surgery in the past 20 years, many more children are now able to survive into adulthood (Fulton & Freed, 2004). As many as 70% to 85% of children with CHD grow to be adults, yet many have problems related to education, insurance, and employment (McDonagh, 2005). Hypothermia and cardiopulmonary bypass required during cardiac surgery for CHD may have a long-term impact on the child's cognitive ability and academic function (Mahle et al., 2006). Due to the potential long-term effects that CHD may have on these children, nurses must be expertly equipped to care for them.

Pathophysiology

The exact cause of CHD is unknown. However, the belief is that it results from an interplay of several factors, including genetics (e.g., chromosomal alterations) and maternal exposure to environmental factors (e.g., toxins, infections, chronic illnesses, and alcohol).

Congenital heart defects result from some interference in the development of the heart structure during fetal life. Subsequently, the septal walls or valves may fail to develop completely, or vessels or valves may be stenotic, narrowed, or transposed. Structures that formed to allow fetal circulation may fail to close after birth, altering the pressures necessary to maintain adequate blood flow.

After birth, with the change from fetal to newborn circulation, pressures within the chambers of the right side of the heart are less than those of the left side and pulmonary vascular resistance is less than that for the systemic circulation. These normal pressure gradients are necessary for adequate circulation to the lungs and the rest of the body. However, these pressure gradients become disrupted if a structure has failed to develop, a fetal structure has failed to close, or a narrowing, stenosis, or transposition of a vessel has occurred. For example, blood typically flows from an area of higher pressure to lower pressure. If the ductus arteriosus fails to close, blood will move from the aorta to the pulmonary artery, ultimately increasing right atrial pressure. With this shunting of blood, highly oxygenated blood can mix with less oxygenated blood, interfering with the amount available to the tissues via the systemic circulation. Some of the defects may result in significant hypoxemia, the sequelae of which include clubbing, polycythemia, exercise intolerance, hypercyanotic spells, brain abscess, and cerebrovascular accident (Fulton & Freed, 2004).

The traditional approach to categorizing CHD has been in terms of whether the child exhibits cyanosis as a clinical manifestation—cyanotic versus acyanotic defects. However, children with acyanotic defects may exhibit cyanosis, and children with cyanotic defects may not demonstrate cyanosis unless they are seriously ill. Many children with congenital heart defects shift between cyanotic and acyanotic states depending on their hemodynamic status (Suddaby, 2001). Therefore, this chapter will categorize the disorders based on hemodynamic characteristics (blood flow patterns in the heart):

- Disorders with decreased pulmonary blood flow: tetralogy of Fallot, tricuspid atresia
- Disorders with increased pulmonary blood flow: patent ductus arteriosus (PDA), atrial septal defect (ASD), ventricular septal defect (VSD)

- Obstructive disorders: coarctation of the aorta, aortic stenosis, pulmonary stenosis
- Mixed disorders: transposition of the great vessels (TGV), total anomalous pulmonary venous return (TAPVR), truncus arteriosus, and hypoplastic left heart syndrome (Suddaby, 2001)

Therapeutic Management

Prenatal education about avoiding certain substances or infection is essential to promote optimal outcomes for the fetus. Parents of children with CHD are encouraged to receive genetic counseling because of the probability of having subsequent children with a congenital heart defect. Children with small septal defects are urged to lead a normal life and often require no medical intervention. Therapeutic management of other forms of CHD focuses on palliative care or a surgical corrective approach necessary for most of the defects. In newborns and very young infants with severe cyanosis (tricuspid atresia, TGV), a prostaglandin infusion will maintain patency of the ductus arteriosus, improving pulmonary blood flow. Definitive correction of structural disorders requires surgical intervention. Table 40.2 describes the surgical procedures used for the various congenital heart defects and the relevant nursing measures. Nursing management for the child with CHD will be provided following the disorders section. See Evidence-Based Practice.

▶ DISORDERS WITH DECREASED PULMONARY BLOOD FLOW

Defects involving decreased pulmonary blood flow occur when there is some obstruction of blood flow to the lungs. As a result of the obstruction, pressure in the right side of the heart increases and becomes greater than that of the left side of the heart. Blood from the higher-pressure right side of the heart then shunts to the lower-pressure left side through a structural defect. Subsequently, deoxygenated blood mixes with oxygenated blood on the left side of the heart. This mixed blood, which is low in oxygen, is pumped via the systemic circulation to the body tissues.

Defects with decreased pulmonary blood flow are characterized by mild to severe oxygen desaturation. Typically, the child exhibits oxygen saturation levels ranging from 50% to 90%, which can produce severe cyanosis. To compensate for low blood oxygen levels, the kidneys produce the hormone erythropoietin to stimulate the bone marrow to produce more red blood cells (RBCs). This increase in RBCs is called **polycythemia**. Polycythemia can lead to an increase in blood volume and possibly blood viscosity, further taxing the workload of the heart. Although the number of RBCs increases, there is no change in the amount of blood that reaches the lungs for oxygenation (Chamberlain, 2006; Driscoll, 2006a).

Disorders within this classification include tetralogy of Fallot and tricuspid atresia.

Tetralogy of Fallot

Tetralogy of Fallot is a congenital heart defect that actually comprises four heart defects: pulmonary stenosis (a narrowing of the pulmonary valve and outflow tract, creating an obstruction of blood flow from the right ventricle to the pulmonary artery), VSD, overriding aorta (enlargement of the aortic valve to the extent that it appears to arise from the right and left ventricles rather than the anatomically correct left ventricle), and right ventricular hypertrophy (the muscle walls of the right ventricle increase in size due to continued overuse as the right ventricle attempts to overcome a high pressure gradient). Surgical intervention is usually required during the first year of life. The rate for survival into adulthood with a good functional long-term result is greater than 90% (Neches et al., 2006a).

Pathophysiology

With pulmonary stenosis, the blood flow from the right ventricle is obstructed and slowed, resulting in a decrease in blood flow to the lungs for oxygenation and a decrease in the amount of oxygenated blood returning to the left atrium from the lungs. The obstructed flow also increases the pressure in the right ventricle. This blood, which is poorly oxygenated, is then shunted across the VSD into the left atrium. Poorly oxygenated blood also travels through the overriding aorta (if it extends to both ventricles). In some cases when the VSD is large, the pressure in the right ventricle may be equal to that of the left ventricle. In this case, the path of blood shunting depends on which circulation is exerting the higher pressure, pulmonary or systemic.

Regardless of which way shunting occurs, a mixing of oxygenated and poorly oxygenated blood occurs, with this blood ultimately being pumped into the systemic circulation. The oxygen saturation of the blood in the systemic circulation is reduced, leading to cyanosis. The degree of cyanosis depends on the extent of the pulmonary stenosis, the size of the VSD, and the vascular resistance of the pulmonary and systemic circulations. In some children, cyanosis is so severe that it leads to severe hypoxia, dysrhythmias, and sudden death (Betz & Sowden, 2005).

Tetralogy of Fallot is usually diagnosed during the first weeks of life due to the presence of a murmur and/or cyanosis. Some newborns may be acutely cyanotic, while others may exhibit only mild cyanosis that gradually becomes more severe, particularly during times of stress as the child grows older. Most often, infants with tetralogy of Fallot have a PDA at birth, providing additional pulmonary blood flow and thereby decreasing the severity of the initial cyanosis. Later, as the ductus arteriosus closes, such as within the first days of life, more severe cyanosis can occur (Fig. 40.2).

(text continues on page 1299)

TABLE 40.2 COMMON SURGICAL PROCEDURES AND NURSING MEASURES FOR CONGENITAL HEART DEFECTS

Disorder	Surgical Procedure	Nursing Measures
Tetralogy of Fallot	Palliation with systemic-to-pulmonary anastomoses: • Blalock-Taussig shunt: an end-to-side anastomosis (or connection with a small Gore-tex tube) of the subclavian artery and the pulmonary artery. • Waterston shunt: anastomosis of the ascending aorta and the pulmonary artery. • Definitive correction involves patch closure of the ventricular septal defect and repair of the pulmonary valve and right ventricular outflow tract.	• Avoid BP measurements and venipunctures in the affected arm after a Blalock-Taussig shunt. Pulse will not be palpable in that arm because of use of the subclavian artery for the shunt. • Monitor for ventricular arrhythmias after corrective repair.
Tricuspid atresia	• Palliation with Blalock-Taussig shunt or pulmonary artery banding may be performed. • At 3 to 6 months of age, the superior vena cava is detached from the heart and connected to the pulmonary artery (Glenn procedure). • By age 2 to 5 years, a modified Fontan procedure may be performed. Systemic venous return is redirected to the pulmonary artery directly.	• Monitor for atrial arrhythmias, left ventricular dysfunction, and protein-losing enteropathy. • Some children may eventually require a pacemaker.
Atrial septal defect	• If small, the defect may be sutured closed. Larger defects may require a patch of pericardium or synthetic material. • Ostium secundum ASD may be repaired percutaneously via cardiac catheterization with an Amplatzer septal occluder (other brands are also available).	• Monitor for atrial arrhythmias (lifelong) after surgical closure. • With the Amplatzer device, strenuous activity should be avoided for 1 month after the procedure.
Ventricular septal defect	• If surgical closure is required, it should be performed before permanent pulmonary vascular changes develop. • Surgical closure may be in the form of suture closure of the VSD, transcatheter placement of a device in the defect, or Dacron patch closure.	• Monitor for ventricular dysrhythmias or AV block. • With the clamshell occluding or Amplatzer device, strenuous activity should be avoided for 1 month after the procedure.
Atrioventricular canal defect	• Pulmonary artery banding as palliation in very young infants. • Surgical correction by 3 to 18 months of age. • Patch closure of the septal defects and suturing of the valve leaflets or valve reconstruction are performed.	• Monitor for complete heart block postoperatively. • Teach parents that mitral regurgitation is a long-term complication and may require valve replacement.
Patent ductus arteriosus	• PDA is closed by coil embolization or device via cardiac catheterization. • May also be surgically ligated.	• Monitor for bleeding and laryngeal nerve damage.
Coarctation of the aorta	• Balloon angioplasty via cardiac catheterization is possible in some children. • Most common surgical repair is resection of the narrowed portion of the aorta, followed by end-to-end reanastomosis.	• Preoperatively, administer prostaglandin medications as ordered to relax the ductal tissue. • Postoperatively, measure and compare BP in all four extremities and quality of upper vs. lower pulses.
Aortic stenosis	• Balloon dilatation is accomplished via the umbilical artery in the newborn or the femoral artery via cardiac catheterization in the older child.	• Provide routine post-catheterization care. • Teach parents that long-term aortic regurgitation requiring valve replacement may occur.

Disorder	Surgical Procedure	Nursing Measures
Pulmonary stenosis	• Balloon dilation valvuloplasty is performed via cardiac catheterization to dilate the valve. This is effective in all but the most severe of cases, which will require surgical valvotomy.	• Provide routine post-catheterization care for balloon dilation. • Explain to parents that prognosis is excellent.
Transposition of the great vessels (arteries)	• Balloon atrial septotomy is usually done as soon as the diagnosis is made. A balloon-tipped catheter is passed through the atrial septum to enlarge the atrial septum. • Surgical correction involves switching the arteries into their normal anatomic positions.	• Administer prostaglandin to maintain the open state of the ductus arteriosus, which will allow the mixing of poorly oxygenated blood with well-oxygenated blood. • Monitor for rapid respirations and cyanosis. • Administer oxygen as needed preoperatively.
Total anomalous pulmonary venous return	The pulmonary vein is repositioned to the back of the left atrium and the ASD is closed.	• Monitor for dysrhythmias, heart block, and persistent heart failure.
Truncus arteriosus	VSD repair, separation of the pulmonary arteries from the aorta, with subsequent connection to the right ventricle with a valve conduit.	• Preoperatively, administer prostaglandin infusion to prevent closing of the ductus arteriosus.
Hypoplastic left heart syndrome	• Heart transplantation is the treatment of choice. • Palliative staged treatment. First: Norwood procedure, reconstruction of the aorta and pulmonary arteries includes a cardiac transplant. Second: bidirectional Glenn procedure, connection of the superior vena cava to the right pulmonary artery to increase the blood flow to the lungs. Third: modified Fontan procedure.	• Preoperatively, administer prostaglandin infusion to prevent closing of the ductus arteriosus. • After palliative repairs, monitor for dysrhythmias or worsening ventricular function.
Valve disorders	• The incompetent valve is replaced with a valve prosthesis.	• Lifelong anticoagulation therapy is necessary with prosthetic valves. • Monitor prothrombin times. • Monitor heart sounds for alterations.

EVIDENCE-BASED PRACTICE 40.1
Effects of Chronic or Intermittent Hypoxia on Cognition in Children

● Study
It is well known that significant hypoxia demonstrates an adverse effect on cognition, yet little is known about the effects of chronic or intermittent hypoxia on cognition in children. Many children with congenital heart disease (CHD) suffer either chronic or intermittent hypoxia. The authors performed a systematic literature review to study this question. Fifty-five studies were included, and a significant proportion of them addressed hypoxia with CHD.

▲ Findings
About 80% of the studies reported adverse effects on cognition in children who suffered chronic or intermittent hypoxia, including developmental and academic achieve-ment. Adverse effects were noted at all childhood age levels except premature infants. The effects were noted even with mild oxygen desaturation.

■ Nursing Implications
It is critical that the developing child be afforded the opportunity to develop optimal cognition. Know the child's normal oxygen saturation so that decreases may be quickly acted upon. Use supplemental oxygen judiciously and within the physician order parameters. Since many children experience improved oxygenation after CHD repair, encourage adequate nutrition so that, in turn, the infant or child will demonstrate growth adequate for safe surgical intervention.

Bass, J. L., Corwin, M., Gozal, D., Moore, C., Nishida, H., Parker, S., Schonwald, A., Wilker, R. E., Stehle, S., & Kinane, T. B. (2004). The effect of chronic or intermittent hypoxia on cognition in childhood: A review of the evidence. *Pediatrics, 114*(3), 805–816.

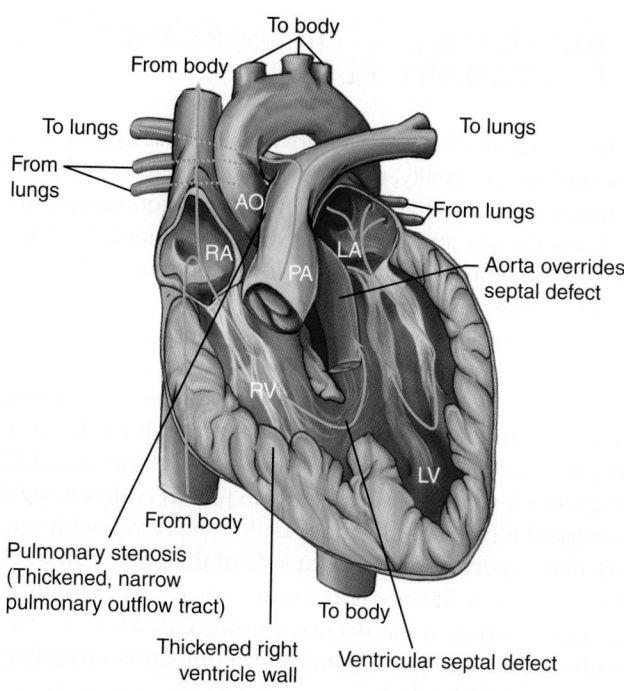

FIGURE 40.2 Tetralogy of Fallot.

To body

From body

To lungs

From lungs

AO

RA

PA

LA

Aorta overrides septal defect

RV

LV

From body

Pulmonary stenosis (Thickened, narrow pulmonary outflow tract)

Thickened right ventricle wall

To body

Ventricular septal defect

■ Oxygen rich blood
■ Oxygen poor blood
■ Mixed blood

Nursing Assessment

Nursing assessment consists of health history, physical examination, and laboratory and diagnostic tests.

Health History and Physical Examination

Obtain the health history, noting a history of color changes associated with feeding, activity, or crying. Determine if the infant or child is demonstrating hypercyanotic spells. Hypercyanosis develops suddenly and is manifested as increased cyanosis, hypoxemia, dyspnea, and agitation. If the infant's oxygen demand is greater than the supply, such as with crying or during feeding, then the spell progresses to anoxia. When the degree of cyanosis is severe and persistent, the infant may become unresponsive. As the infant gets older, he or she may use specific postures, such as bending at the knees or assuming the fetal position, to relieve a hypercyanotic spell. The walking infant or toddler may squat periodically. These positions improve pulmonary blood flow by increasing systemic vascular resistance. Ask the parents if they have noticed any of these unusual positions (Driscoll, 2006a). Note history of irritability, sleepiness, or difficulty breathing.

During the physical examination, observe the skin color and note any evidence of cyanosis. Also observe for changes in skin color with positional changes, and inspect the fingers for clubbing. Note if the child has a hypercyanotic spell during the assessment. Count the child's respiratory rate and observe work of breathing, noting retractions, shortness of breath, or noisy breathing. Docu-

ment oxygen saturation via pulse oximetry; it will likely be decreased. Auscultate the chest for adventitious breath sounds, which may suggest the development of heart failure. Auscultate the heart, noting a loud, harsh murmur characteristic of this disorder.

Laboratory and Diagnostic Tests

Note increased hematocrit, hemoglobin, and RBC count associated with polycythemia. Additional testing may include:

- Echocardiography, possibly revealing right ventricular hypertrophy, decreased pulmonary blood flow, and reduced size of the pulmonary artery
- ECG, indicating right ventricular hypertrophy
- Cardiac catheterization and angiography, which reveal the extent of the structural defects

▶ *Consider* THIS!

Ava Gardener, 2 weeks old, is brought to the clinic by her mother. She presents with trouble feeding. Her mother states, "When Ava eats, she seems to have trouble breathing, and recently I've noticed a bluish color around her lips." What other assessment information would you obtain?

Ava is to be admitted to the hospital secondary to suspected tetralogy of Fallot. What education and interventions may be necessary for this child and family? How can you assist the family to cope?

Tricuspid Atresia

Tricuspid atresia is a congenital heart defect in which the valve between the right atrium and right ventricle fails to develop. As a result, there is no opening to allow blood to flow from the right atrium to the right ventricle and subsequently through the pulmonary artery into the lungs.

Pathophysiology

In tricuspid atresia, blood returning from the systemic circulation to the right atrium cannot directly enter the right ventricle due to agenesis of the tricuspid valve. Subsequently, deoxygenated blood then passes through an opening in the atrial septum (either an ASD or through a patent foramen ovale) into the left atrium, never entering the pulmonary vasculature. Thus, deoxygenated blood mixes with oxygenated blood in the left atrium. The blood then travels to the lungs through a PDA. The foramen ovale and ductus arteriosus must remain open for the newborn to maintain minimally adequate oxygenation (Fig. 40.3).

Nursing Assessment

Nursing assessment consists of health history, physical examination, and laboratory and diagnostic tests.

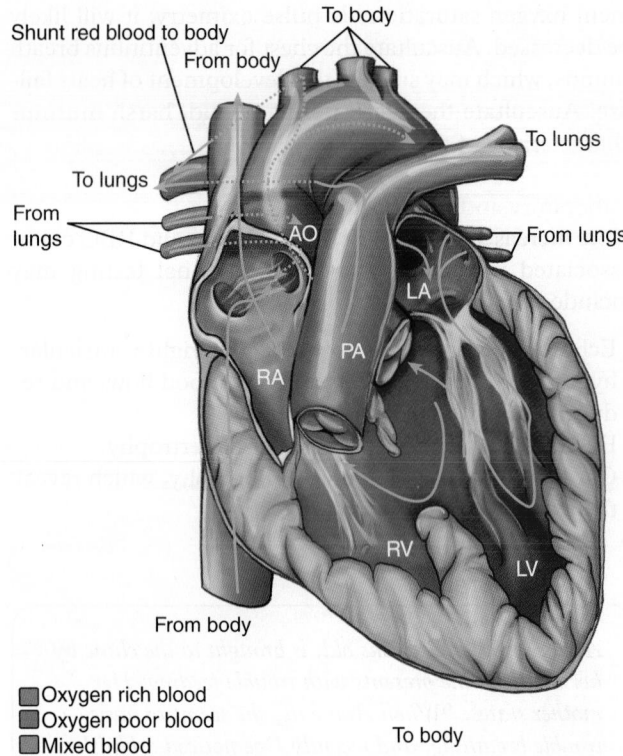

Shunt red blood to body
To body
From body
To lungs
To lungs
From lungs
From lungs
AO
LA
PA
RA
RV
LV
From body

■ Oxygen rich blood
■ Oxygen poor blood
■ Mixed blood
To body

FIGURE 40.3 Tricuspid atresia.

Health History and Physical Examination

Note the infant's history since birth. Document history of cyanosis either at birth or a few days later when the ductus arteriosus closed. Note history of rapid respirations and difficulty with feeding. Inspect the skin for cyanosis or a pale gray color. Observe the apical impulse, noting overactivity. Evaluate the baby's sucking strength (will usually have a weak or poor suck). Count the respiratory rate, noting tachypnea. Note increased work of breathing. Auscultate the lungs, noting crackles or wheezes if heart failure is beginning to develop. Auscultate the heart, noting a murmur. Palpate the skin, noting coolness and clamminess of the extremities. Document the presence of clubbing in the older infant or child.

Laboratory and Diagnostic Testing

Laboratory and diagnostic testing is similar to that for tetralogy of Fallot. A complete blood count (CBC) is needed to assess compensatory increases in hematocrit, hemoglobin, and erythrocyte count (RBC) indicating the development of polycythemia. Oxygen saturation levels (typically reduced) may be determined by pulse oximetry or arterial blood gases. Additional testing may include:

• Echocardiography, revealing absence of tricuspid valve, underdeveloped right ventricle
• ECG, indicating possible heart failure
• Cardiac catheterization and angiography, which reveal the extent of the structural defects

DISORDERS WITH INCREASED PULMONARY FLOW

Most congenital heart defects involve increased pulmonary blood flow. Normally, the left side of the heart has a higher pressure than the right side. Defects with connections involving the left and right sides will shunt blood from the higher-pressure left side to the lower-pressure right side. Even a small pressure gradient such as a 1- to 3-mm difference between the left and right sides will produce a movement of blood from the left to the right. In turn, the increase of blood on the right side of the heart will cause a greater amount of blood to move through the heart. If the amount of blood flowing to the lungs is large, the child may develop **heart failure** early in life. In addition, right ventricular hypertrophy may result. Sometimes with ventricular hypertrophy the right side of the heart pumps so forcefully that left-to-right shunting is reversed to right-to-left shunting. If this occurs, deoxygenated blood mixes with oxygenated blood, thereby lowering the overall blood oxygen saturation level.

Excessive blood flow to the lungs can produce a compensatory response such as tachypnea or tachycardia. Tachypnea increases caloric expenditure; poor cellular nutrition from decreased peripheral blood flow leads to feeding problems. Subsequently, the infant experiences poor weight gain, which retards overall growth and development. Increased pulmonary blood flow results in decreased systemic blood flow, so sodium and fluid retention may occur. Increased pulmonary blood flow also places the child at higher risk for pulmonary infections. As the child grows, the continuous increased pulmonary blood flow will cause vasoconstriction of the pulmonary vessels, actually decreasing the pulmonary blood flow. This may lead to pulmonary hypertension. Therefore, preventing the development of pulmonary disease via early surgical correction is essential.

For children with congenital defects with increased pulmonary blood flow, oxygen supplementation is not helpful. Oxygen acts as a pulmonary vasodilator. If pulmonary dilation occurs, pulmonary blood flow is even greater, causing tachypnea, increasing lung fluid retention, and eventually causing a much greater problem with oxygenation. Over time, continuous increased pulmonary blood flow may cause pulmonary vasoconstriction and pulmonary hypertension. Surgical correction is essential before pulmonary disease develops (Driscoll, 2006a; Gumbiner, 2006; Mullins, 2006a; Vick & Bezold, 2006). Examples of defects with increased pulmonary blood flow are ASD, VSD, atrioventricular canal defect, and PDA.

Atrial Septal Defect

An ASD is a passageway or hole in the wall (septum) that divides the right atrium from the left atrium (Fig. 40.4).

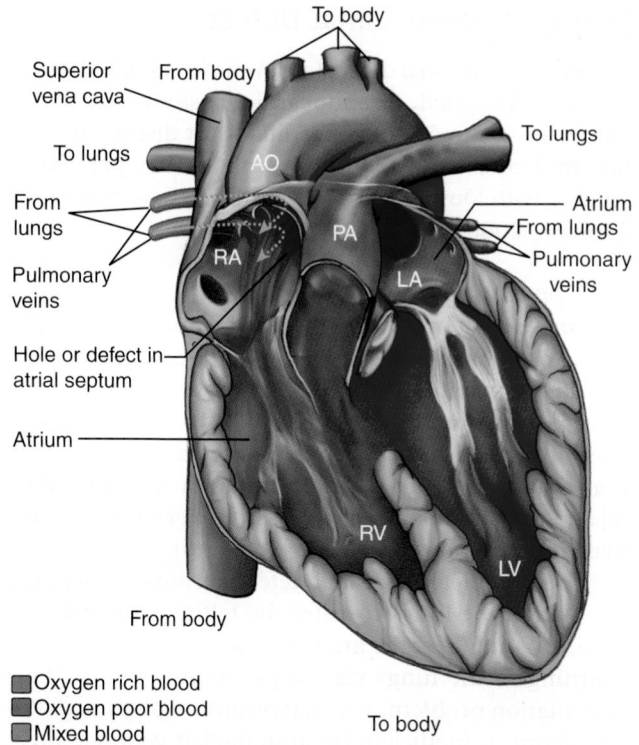

FIGURE 40.4 Atrial septal defect; note the opening between the two atria.

Three types of ASDs are identified based on the location of the opening:

- Ostium primum (ASD1): the opening is at the lower portion of the septum
- Ostium secundum (ASD2): the opening is near the center of the septum
- Sinus venosus defect: the opening is near the junction of the superior vena cava and the right atrium

When the ASD is small, as many as 80% of infants may have a spontaneous closure within the first 18 months of life. If not spontaneously closed by age 3, the child will most likely need corrective surgery.

Pathophysiology

With ASD, blood flows between the opening from the left atrium to the right atrium due to pressure differences. The shunting increases the blood volume entering the right atrium. This, in turn, leads to increased blood flow into the lungs. The defect if untreated can cause problems such as pulmonary hypertension, heart failure, atrial arrhythmias, or stroke (Driscoll, 2006a; Vick & Bezold, 2006).

Nursing Assessment

Most children with ASDs are asymptomatic. However, a very large defect can cause increased blood flow, leading to heart failure, which results in shortness of breath, easy fatigability, or poor growth.

Health History and Physical Examination

Obtain the health history, noting poor feeding as an infant, decreased ability to keep up with peers, or history of difficulty growing. Observe the child's chest, noting a hyperdynamic precordium. Auscultate the heart, noting a fixed split second heart sound and a systolic ejection murmur, best heard in the pulmonic valve area. Palpate along the left sternal border for a right ventricular heave.

Laboratory and Diagnostic Tests

Echocardiography is done to confirm the diagnosis. An **electrocardiogram** may show normal sinus rhythm or prolonged PR intervals. The chest x-ray may show enlargement of the heart and increased vascularity of the lungs.

Ventricular Septal Defect

A VSD is an opening between the right and left ventricular chambers of the heart (Fig. 40.5). It is one of the most common congenital heart defects, with a prevalence of 1.5 to 2.5 per 1,000 live births. VSD accounts for nearly one third of all congenital heart defects (Gumbiner, 2006). Spontaneous closure of the VSD occurs in about 45% of children by age 3 years (most often with smaller defects) (Singh et al., 2004). Long-term outcomes for surgically repaired VSD are good, though the risk of sudden death is increased in those who develop pulmonary hypertension (Roos-Hesselink et al., 2004).

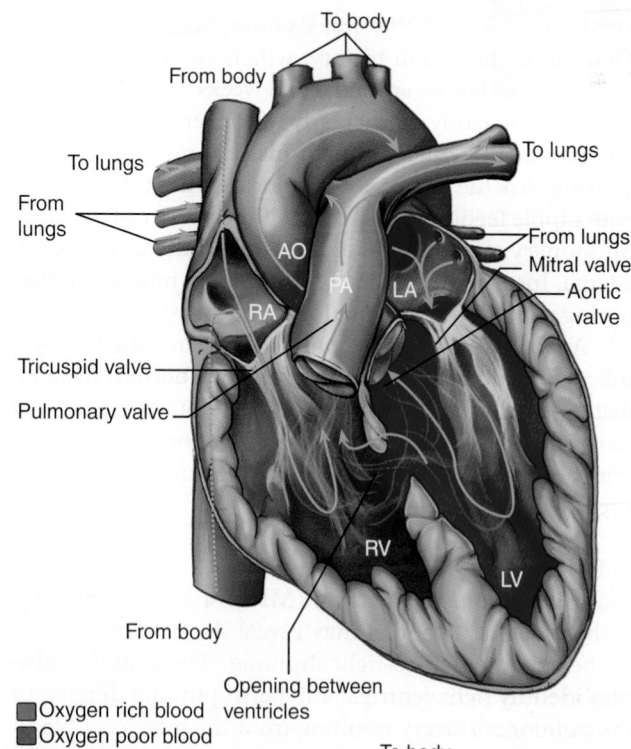

FIGURE 40.5 Ventricular septal defect; note the opening between the ventricles.

Pathophysiology

In VSD, there is an abnormal opening between the right and left ventricles. The opening varies in size, from as small as a pinhole to a complete opening between the ventricles so that the right and left sides are as one. Children with small VSDs may remain asymptomatic. In other children, blood shunts across the opening in the septum. Pulmonary vascular resistance and systemic vascular resistance determine the direction of blood flow. A left-to-right shunt results when pulmonary vascular resistance is low. Increased amounts of blood flowing into the right ventricle are then pumped to the pulmonary circulation, eventually causing an increase in pulmonary vascular resistance. Increased pulmonary vascular resistance leads to increased pulmonary artery pressure (pulmonary hypertension) and right ventricular hypertrophy. When the pulmonary vascular resistance exceeds the systemic vascular resistance, right-to-left shunting of blood across the VSD occurs, resulting in Eisenmenger syndrome (pulmonary hypertension and cyanosis). Heart failure commonly occurs in children with moderate to severe VSD. Children with VSD are also at risk for the development of aortic valve regurgitation as well as infective endocarditis.

Nursing Assessment

Initially, the newborn may not exhibit any signs and symptoms at birth because left-to-right shunting is most likely minimal due to the high pulmonary resistance common after birth.

Health History and Physical Examination

Determine the health history, which commonly reveals signs of heart failure around 4 to 8 weeks of age. Note history of tiring easily, particularly with exertion or feeding. Document the child's growth history, noting difficulty thriving. Ask the parent about color change or diaphoresis with nipple feeding in the infant. Note history of frequent pulmonary infections, shortness of breath, and possibly edema. Inspect the extremities for edema, noting whether pitting is present. Note mild tachypnea.

Auscultate the heart, noting a characteristic holosystolic harsh murmur along the left sternal border. In some instances, a murmur may be noted only with excessive blood flow across the opening. Adventitious lung sounds may be auscultated if the child is experiencing heart failure. Palpate the chest for a thrill.

Laboratory and Diagnostic Tests

Magnetic resonance imaging (MRI) or echocardiogram with color flow Doppler may reveal the opening as well as the extent of left-to-right shunting. These studies also may identify right ventricular hypertrophy and dilation of the pulmonary artery resulting from the increased blood flow. Cardiac catheterization may be used to evaluate the extent of blood flow being pumped to the pulmonary circulation and to evaluate hemodynamic pressures.

Atrioventricular Canal Defect

Atrioventricular canal defect (atrioventricular septal defect [AVSD], AV canal, or endocardial cushion defect) accounts for 4% to 5% of congenital heart disease and occurs in 2 of every 10,000 live births. Forty percent of children with Down syndrome and CHD have this defect (Driscoll, 2006a).

Pathophysiology

AV canal defect occurs as a result of failure of the endocardial cushions to fuse (Fig. 40.6). These cushions are needed to separate the central parts of the heart near the tricuspid and mitral (AV) valves. The complete AV canal defect involves atrial and ventricular septal defects as well as a common AV orifice and a common AV valve. Partial and transitional forms of AV canal defect also occur, involving variations of the complete form.

The complete AV canal defect permits oxygenated blood from the lungs to enter the left atrium and ventricle, crossing over the atrial or ventricular septum and returning to the lungs via the pulmonary artery. This recirculation problem, which typically involves a left-to-right shunt, is inefficient because the left ventricle must pump blood back to the lungs and also meet the body's peripheral demand for oxygenated blood. Subsequently, the left ventricle must pump two to three times more blood than in a normal heart. Therefore, this specific type of cardiac defect causes a large left-to-right shunt; an increased workload of the left ventricle; and high pul-

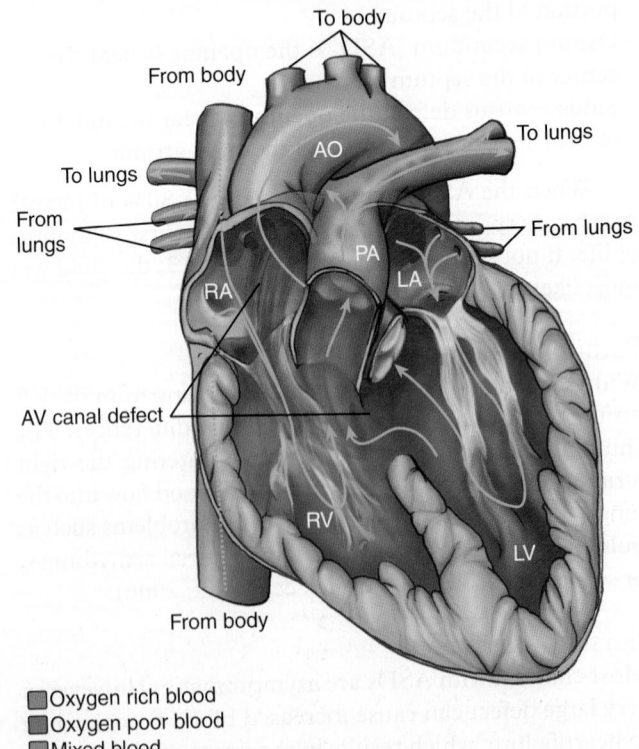

■ Oxygen rich blood
■ Oxygen poor blood
■ Mixed blood

FIGURE 40.6 Atrioventricular canal defect.

monary arterial pressure, resulting in an increased amount of blood in the lungs and causing pulmonary edema (Driscoll, 2006a; Vick & Bezold, 2006).

Nursing Assessment

The infant with a complete AV canal defect commonly exhibits moderate to severe signs and symptoms of heart failure. However, for infants with partial or transitional AV canal defects, the signs and symptoms will be more subtle.

Health History and Physical Examination

Obtain the health history, noting frequent respiratory infections and difficulty gaining weight. Ask the parent if the infant has been experiencing difficulty feeding or increased work of breathing.

Inspect the skin, fingernails, and lips for cyanosis. Observe for retractions, tachypnea, and nasal flaring. Auscultate the lungs and heart, noting rales and a loud murmur. The murmur is commonly noted within the first 2 weeks of life. Infants with partial or transitional AV canal defect may display more subtle signs.

Laboratory and Diagnostic Tests

Echocardiography will reveal the extent of the defect and shunting as well as right ventricular hypertrophy. Electrocardiogram may indicate right ventricular hypertrophy and possible first-degree heart block due to impulse blocking before reaching the AV node.

Patent Ductus Arteriosus

PDA is failure of the ductus arteriosus, a fetal circulatory structure, to close within the first weeks of life (Fig. 40.7). As a result, there is a connection between the aorta and pulmonary artery. PDA is the second most common congenital heart defect and accounts for 10% of CHD cases (Mullins, 2006a). PDA occurs much more frequently in premature than in term infants: 45% of infants less than 1,750 g at birth and 80% of infants less than 1,200 g will display a PDA. PDA occurs 30 times more often in infants born at high altitudes compared with those born at sea level (Driscoll, 2006a). Infants with other congenital heart defects that result in right-to-left shunting of blood and cyanosis may additionally display a PDA. In these infants, the PDA allows for some level of oxygenated blood to reach the systemic circulation.

Pathophysiology

Failure of the ductus arteriosus to close leads to continued blood flow from the aorta to the pulmonary artery. Blood returning to the left atrium passes to the left ventricle, enters the aorta, and then travels to the pulmonary artery via the PDA instead of entering the systemic circulation. This altered blood flow pattern increases the workload of the left side of heart. Pulmonary vascular congestion occurs, causing an increase in pressure. Right

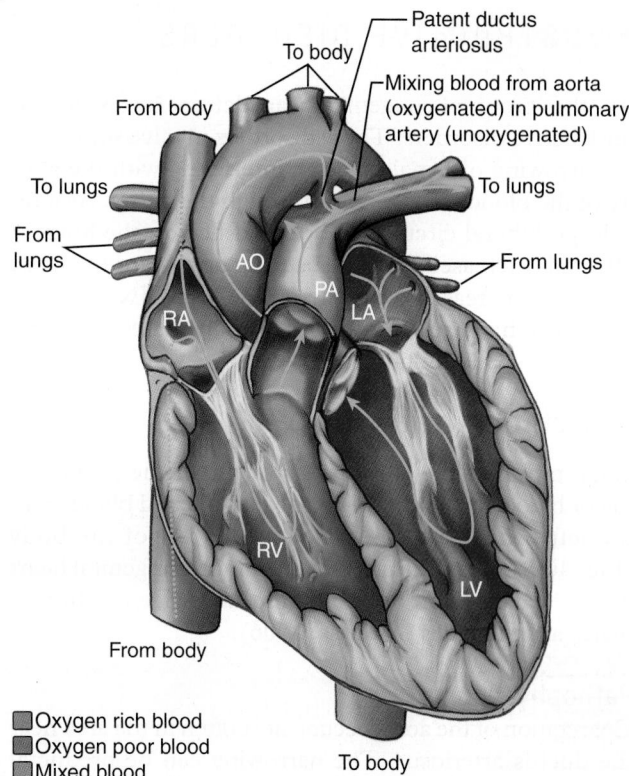

■ Oxygen rich blood
■ Oxygen poor blood
■ Mixed blood

FIGURE 40.7 Patent ductus arteriosus.

ventricular pressure increases in an attempt to overcome this increase in pulmonary pressure. Eventually, right ventricular hypertrophy occurs.

Nursing Assessment

The symptoms of PDA depend on the size of the ductus arteriosus and the amount of blood flow it carries. If it is small, the infant may be asymptomatic. Some infants demonstrate signs and symptoms of heart failure.

Health History and Physical Examination

Determine the health history, which may reveal frequent respiratory infections, fatigue, and poor growth and development. On physical examination, note tachycardia, tachypnea, bounding peripheral pulses, and a widened pulse pressure. The diastolic blood pressure typically is low due to the shunting. Auscultate the lungs and heart, noting rales if heart failure is present. Note a harsh, continuous, machine-like murmur, usually loudest under the left clavicle at the first and second intercostal spaces.

Laboratory and Diagnostic Tests

Echocardiogram reveals the extent of the defective opening and confirms the diagnosis. Electrocardiogram may be normal or it may indicate ventricular hypertrophy, especially if the defect is large. Chest x-ray demonstrates cardiomegaly.

▶ OBSTRUCTIVE DISORDERS

Another group of congenital heart defects is classified as obstructive disorders. These disorders involve some type of narrowing of a major vessel, interfering with the ability of the blood to flow freely through the vessel. As a result, peripheral circulation or blood flow to the lungs is affected. Increased pressure backing up toward the heart causes an increased workload on the heart. Examples of defects in this group include coarctation of the aorta, aortic stenosis, and pulmonic stenosis.

Coarctation of the Aorta

Coarctation of the aorta is narrowing of the aorta, the major blood vessel carrying highly oxygenated blood from the left ventricle of the heart to the rest of the body (Fig. 40.8). It is the third most common congenital heart defect. Coarctation occurs more than twice as often in males as in females (Morriss, 2006).

Pathophysiology

Coarctation of the aorta occurs most often in the area near the ductus arteriosus. The narrowing can be preductal (between the subclavian artery and ductus arteriosus) or postductal (after the ductus arteriosus). As a result of the narrowing, blood flow is impeded, causing pressure to increase in the area proximal to the defect and to decrease in the area distal to it. Thus, blood pressure is increased

in the heart and upper portions of the body and decreased in the lower portions of the body. Left ventricular afterload is increased, and in some children this may lead to heart failure. Collateral circulation also may develop as the body attempts to ensure adequate blood flow to the descending aorta. Due to the elevation in blood pressure, the child is also at risk for aortic rupture, aortic aneurysm, and cerebrovascular accident (CVA).

Nursing Assessment

The extent of the symptoms depends on the severity of the coarctation. Some children with coarctation of the aorta grow well into the school-age years before the defect is discovered.

Health History and Physical Examination

Determine the health history, noting problems with irritability and frequent epistaxis. In older children, there also may be reports of leg pain with activity, dizziness, fainting, and headaches. Assess pulses throughout, noting full, bounding pulses in the upper extremities with weak or absent pulses in the lower extremities. Determine BP in all four extremities. BP in the upper extremities may be 20 mm Hg or higher than that in the lower extremities. Inspect the school-age child's chest, noting notching of the ribs. Auscultate the heart for a soft or moderately loud systolic murmur, most often heard at the base of the heart.

Laboratory and Diagnostic Tests

Diagnosis of coarctation of the aorta is based primarily on the history and physical examination. In addition, an echocardiogram may disclose the extent of narrowing and evidence of collateral circulation. Chest x-ray may reveal left-sided cardiac enlargement and rib notching indicative of collateral arterial enlargement. Other tests, such as electrocardiogram, computed tomography, or MRI, may be done to provide additional evidence about the extent of the coarctation and subsequent effects.

Aortic Stenosis

Aortic stenosis is a condition causing obstruction of the blood flow between the left ventricle and the aorta. The occurrence of aortic stenosis is 4 per 1,000 live births, with 75% of cases occurring in males (Balentine & Eisenhart, 2005).

Pathophysiology

Aortic stenosis can be caused by a muscle obstruction below the aortic valve, an obstruction at the valve itself, or an aortic narrowing just above the valve (Fig. 40.9). The most common type is an obstruction of the valve itself, called aortic valve stenosis. The aortic valve consists of three very pliable leaflets. Normally the leaflets of the aortic valve spread open easily when the left ventricle ejects blood into the aorta. Aortic stenosis occurs when

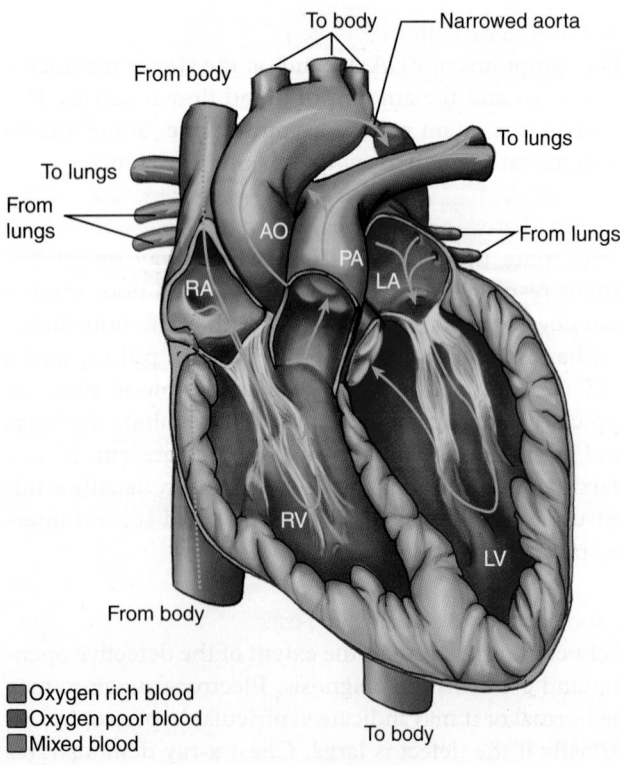

Oxygen rich blood
Oxygen poor blood
Mixed blood

FIGURE 40.8 Coarctation of the aorta.

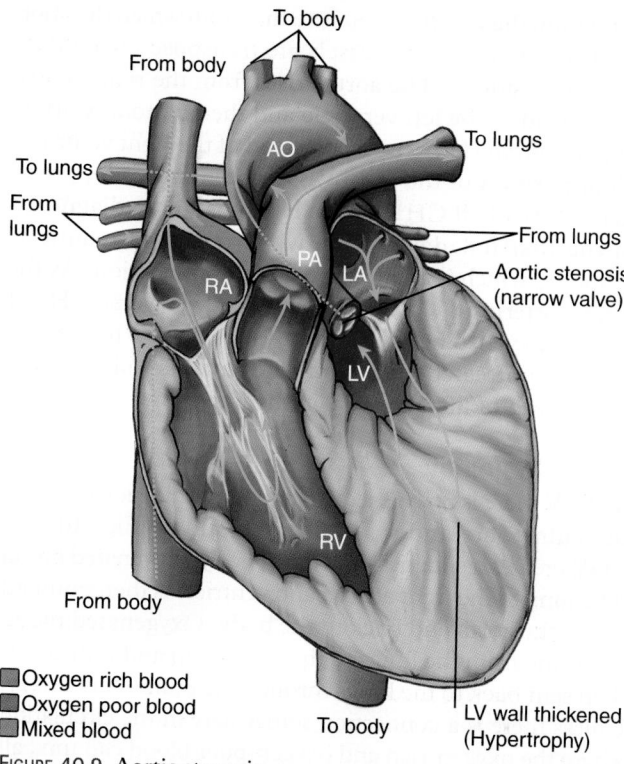

FIGURE 40.9 Aortic stenosis.

the aortic valve narrows, causing an obstruction between the left ventricle and the aorta. As a result, cardiac output decreases. When the aortic valve does not function properly, the left ventricle must work harder to pump blood into the aorta. Because of the increased workload, the left ventricular muscle hypertrophies. If this continues, left ventricular failure can occur, leading to a backup of pressure in the pulmonary circulation and pulmonary edema. Heart failure may occur, but this is more commonly seen in the infant (Driscoll, 2006a).

Nursing Assessment

Typically, the child with aortic stenosis is asymptomatic. However, it is important to obtain an accurate health history and perform a physical examination.

Health History and Physical Examination

Obtain the child's health history, noting easy fatigability or complaints of chest pain similar to anginal pain when active. Dizziness with prolonged standing also may be reported. In the infant, note difficulty with feeding. Palpate the child's pulse; if aortic stenosis is severe, the pulses may be faint. Palpate the child's chest, noting a thrill at the base of the heart. Auscultate the heart, noting a systolic murmur best heard along the left sternal border with radiation to the right upper sternal border.

Laboratory and Diagnostic Tests

The echocardiogram is the most important noninvasive test to identify aortic stenosis. An electrocardiogram may

be normal in children with mild to moderate forms of aortic stenosis. For children with severe aortic stenosis, left ventricular hypertrophy may be determined from the electrocardiogram. For children experiencing easy fatigability and chest pain, an exercise stress test may be done to evaluate the degree of cardiac compromise.

Pulmonary Stenosis

Pulmonary stenosis is a condition that causes an obstruction in blood flow between the right ventricle and the pulmonary arteries. Pulmonary stenosis occurs in 7% to 12% of all cases of CHD (Cheatham, 2006). It is often associated with various genetic syndromes. Children may be asymptomatic, although some children with severe stenosis may exhibit dyspnea and fatigue with exertion (demonstrating hypercyanotic spells similar to those in children with tetralogy of Fallot).

Pathophysiology

Pulmonary stenosis may occur as a muscular obstruction below the pulmonary valve, an obstruction at the valve, or a narrowing of the pulmonary artery above the valve (Fig. 40.10). Valve obstruction is the most common form of pulmonary stenosis. Normally the pulmonary valve is constructed with three thin and pliable valve leaflets; they spread apart easily, allowing the right ventricle to eject blood freely into the pulmonary artery. The most common problem causing pulmonary stenosis is that the pul-

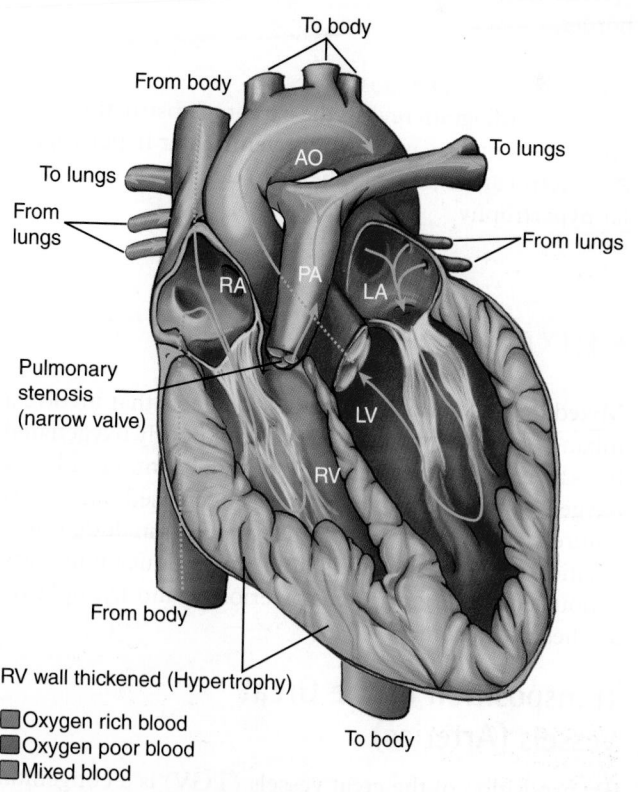

FIGURE 40.10 Pulmonary stenosis.

monary valve leaflets are thickened and fused together along their separation lines, causing the obstruction to blood flow. The right ventricle has an additional workload, causing the muscle to thicken, resulting in right ventricular hypertrophy and decreased pulmonary blood flow. When the pulmonary valve is severely obstructed, the right ventricle cannot eject sufficient blood into the pulmonary artery. As a result, pressure in the right atrium increases, which could lead to a reopening of the foramen ovale. If this occurs, deoxygenated blood would pass through the foramen ovale into the left side of the heart and would then be pumped to the systemic circulation. In some cases, a PDA may be present, thus allowing for some compensation by shunting blood from the aorta to the pulmonary circulation for oxygenation.

Nursing Assessment

The child with pulmonary stenosis may be asymptomatic or may exhibit signs and symptoms of mild heart failure. If the stenosis is severe, the child may demonstrate cyanosis. Therefore, it is important for the nurse to obtain an accurate health history and physical examination.

Health History and Physical Examination

Elicit the health history, noting mild dyspnea or cyanosis with exertion. Document the child's growth history, which is typically normal. Carefully palpate the sternal border for a thrill (not always present). Auscultate the heart, noting a high-pitched click following the second heart sound and a systolic ejection murmur loudest at the upper left sternal border.

Laboratory and Diagnostic Tests

An echocardiogram reveals the extent of obstruction present at the valve, as well as right ventricular hypertrophy. An electrocardiogram also helps to detect right ventricular hypertrophy.

▶ MIXED DEFECTS

Mixed defects are congenital heart defects that involve a mixing of well-oxygenated blood with poorly oxygenated blood. As a result, systemic blood flow contains a lower oxygen content. Cardiac output is decreased, and heart failure occurs. Examples of mixed defects include transposition of the great vessels, total anomalous pulmonary venous connection, truncus arteriosus, and hypoplastic left heart syndrome.

Transposition of the Great Vessels (Arteries)

Transposition of the great vessels (TGV) is a congenital heart defect in which the pulmonary artery and the aorta arise from the ventricle opposite that from which they normally arise. Thus, the vessels are transposed from their normal positions. The aorta arises from the right ventricle instead of the left ventricle and the pulmonary artery arises from the left ventricle instead of the right ventricle. Transposition of the great vessels accounts for approximately 5% of all CHD cases. It is most often diagnosed in the first few days of life when the child manifests cyanosis, which indicates decreased oxygenation. As the ductus arteriosus closes, the symptoms will worsen. Heart failure may also be present in the first weeks to months of life. If untreated, 50% of affected infants will die in the first month of life and 90% in the first year.

Pathophysiology

In TGV there is no connection or communication between the pulmonary and systemic circulations (Fig. 40.11). TGV creates a situation in which poorly oxygenated blood returning to the right atrium and ventricle is then pumped out to the aorta and back to the body. Oxygenated blood returning from the lungs to the left atrium and ventricle is then sent back to the lungs through the pulmonary artery. Unless there is a connection somewhere in the circulation where the oxygen-rich and oxygen-poor blood can mix, all the organs of the body will be poorly oxygenated. Often the ductus arteriosus remains patent, allowing for some mixing of blood. Similarly, if a VSD is also present, mixing of blood may occur and cyanosis will be delayed. However, these associated defects can lead to increased pulmonary blood

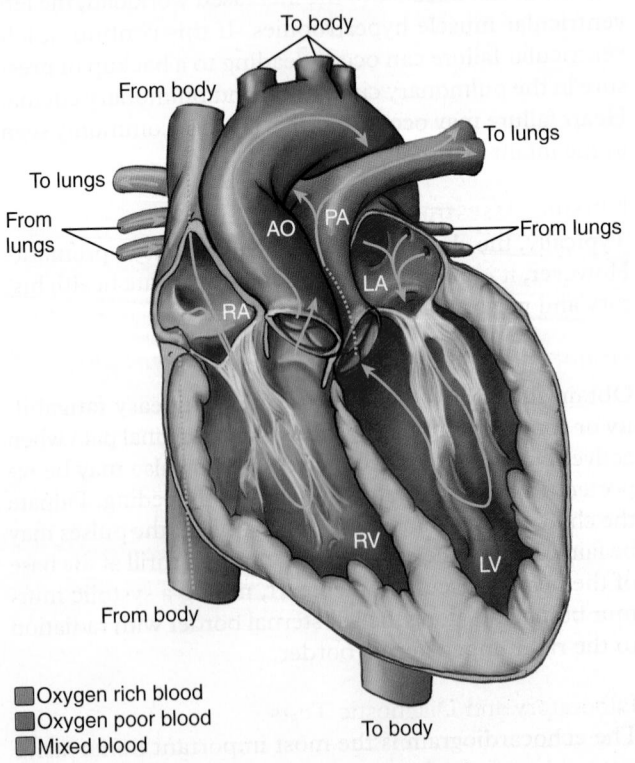

■ Oxygen rich blood
■ Oxygen poor blood
■ Mixed blood

FIGURE 40.11 Transposition of the great vessels.

flow that increases pressure in the pulmonary circulation. This predisposes the child to heart failure.

Nursing Assessment

Significant cyanosis without a murmur in the newborn period is highly indicative of TGV. In about 10% of infants, cyanosis will not develop until several days of age as the PDA closes (Molczan, 2006). In infants with septal defects, cyanosis may be further delayed.

Health History and Physical Examination

Elicit the health history, noting onset of cyanosis with feeding or crying. Observe the infant for cyanosis while active and at rest. Observe the chest, noting a prominent ventricular impulse. Auscultate the heart, noting a loud second heart sound. A murmur may be heard if the ductus remains open or a septal defect is present. If heart failure is present, note edema, tachypnea, and adventitious lung sounds.

Laboratory and Diagnostic Tests

Echocardiography clearly reveals evidence of the transposition. Cardiac catheterization may be performed, determining low oxygen saturation levels due to the mixing of the blood.

Total Anomalous Pulmonary Venous Connection

Total anomalous pulmonary venous connection (TAPVC) is a rare congenital heart defect in which the pulmonary veins do not connect normally to the left atrium; instead, they connect to the right atrium, often by way of the superior vena cava. Males exhibit this disorder three times more often than females (Ward, 2006).

Pathophysiology

Oxygenated blood that would normally enter the left atrium now enters the right atrium and passes to the right ventricle. As a result, the pressure on the right side of the heart increases, leading to hypertrophy. TAPVC is incompatible with life unless there is an associated defect present that allows for shunting of blood from the highly pressured right side of the heart. A patent foramen ovale or an ASD is usually present. Since none of the pulmonary veins connect normally to the left atrium, the only source of blood to the left atrium is blood that is shunted from the right atrium across the defect to the left side of the heart (Fig. 40.12). The highly oxygenated blood from the lungs completely mixes with the poorly oxygenated blood returning from the systemic circulation. This causes an overload of the right atrium and right ventricle. The increased blood volume going into the lungs can lead to pulmonary hypertension and pulmonary edema.

Nursing Assessment

The degree of cyanosis present with TAPVC depends on the extent of the associated defects. For example, if

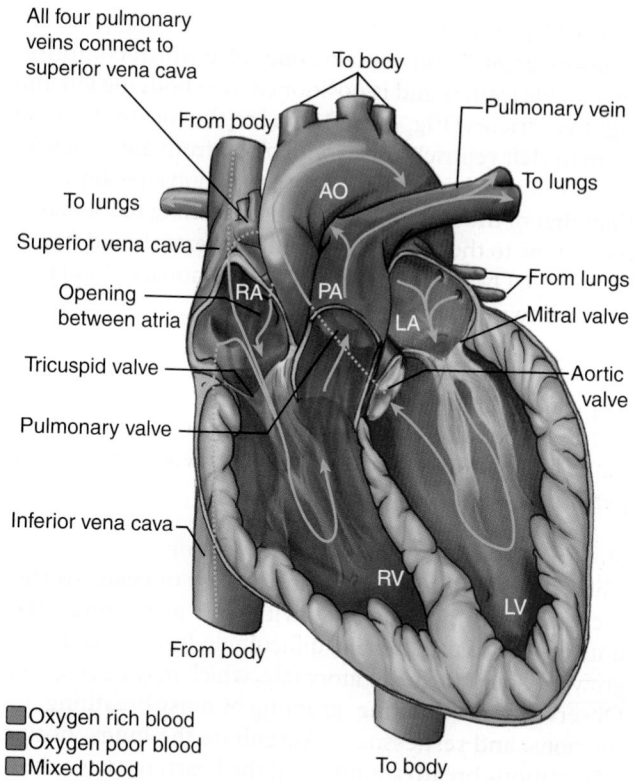

FIGURE 40.12 Total anomalous pulmonary venous connection.

the foramen ovale closes or the ASD is small, significant cyanosis will be present. The physical examination findings will vary depending on the type of TAPVC the infant has, whether obstruction is present, and which other associated cardiac anomalies are present.

Health History and Physical Examination

Note history of cyanosis, tiring easily, and difficulty feeding. Observe the chest for prominence of the right ventricular impulse and retractions with tachypnea. Auscultate the heart, noting fixed splitting of the second heart sound and a murmur. Palpate the abdomen for hepatomegaly.

Laboratory and Diagnostic Tests

An echocardiogram will reveal the abnormal connection of the pulmonary veins, enlargement of the right atrium and right ventricle, and an ASD if present. The chest x-ray will demonstrate an enlarged heart and pulmonary edema. Cardiac catheterization can also be useful to visualize the abnormal connection of the pulmonary veins, particularly if an obstruction is present.

Truncus Arteriosus

Truncus arteriosus is a congenital heart defect in which only one major artery leaves the heart and supplies blood to the pulmonary and systemic circulations. It affects males and females equally and accounts for 1% to 4% of all CHD cases (Slesnick & Kovalchin, 2006). A VSD may also be present.

Pathophysiology

The one great vessel contains one valve which comprises two to five leaflets and is positioned over both the left and right ventricles (Fig. 40.13). Due to the location, blood from the left ventricle mixes with blood from the right ventricle. Pressure in the pulmonary circulation typically is less than that of the systemic circulation, leading to increased blood flow to the lungs. As a result, systemic blood flow is decreased. Over time, the increased pulmonary blood flow can lead to pulmonary vascular disease.

Nursing Assessment

Typically, the infant demonstrates cyanosis in varying degrees depending on the extent of compromise in the systemic circulation. Obtain an accurate health history and perform a physical examination.

Health History and Physical Examination

Elicit the health history, noting history of cyanosis that increases with periods of activity such as feeding. Also note history of tiring easily, difficulty in feeding, and poor growth. Count the respiratory rate, which may be elevated. Observe for nasal flaring, grunting or noisy breathing, retractions, and restlessness. Auscultate the lungs, noting adventitious breath sounds, and the heart, noting a murmur associated with a VSD.

Laboratory and Diagnostic Tests

An echocardiogram will confirm the presence of truncus arteriosus as the anatomy of the great vessels, the single truncal valve, and the VSD will be seen. On rare occasions a cardiac catheterization may be done to determine pressures in the pulmonary arteries.

Hypoplastic Left Heart Syndrome

Hypoplastic left heart syndrome (HLHS) is a congenital heart defect in which all of the structures on the left side of the heart are severely underdeveloped (Fig. 40.14). The mitral and aortic valves are completely closed or very small. The left ventricle is nonfunctional. Thus, the left side of the heart is completely unable to supply blood to the systemic circulation. HLHS is the fourth most common congenital heart defect. It appears to have a multifactorial and autosomal recessive inheritance pattern. Almost 30% of infants with HLHS also have a definable genetic or other congenital anomaly in addition to the heart defect (Eidem, 2006). The options for treatment include palliative care, cardiac transplantation within the first few weeks of life, or palliative reconstructive surgery consisting of three stages, beginning within days to weeks of birth (Kilian, 2006).

Pathophysiology

With HLHS, the right side of the heart is the main working part of the heart. Blood returning from the lungs into the left atrium must pass through an ASD to the right side of the heart. The right ventricle must then pump blood to the lungs and also to the systemic circulation through the PDA. A few days after birth, when the ductus arteriosus

FIGURE 40.13 Truncus arteriosus.

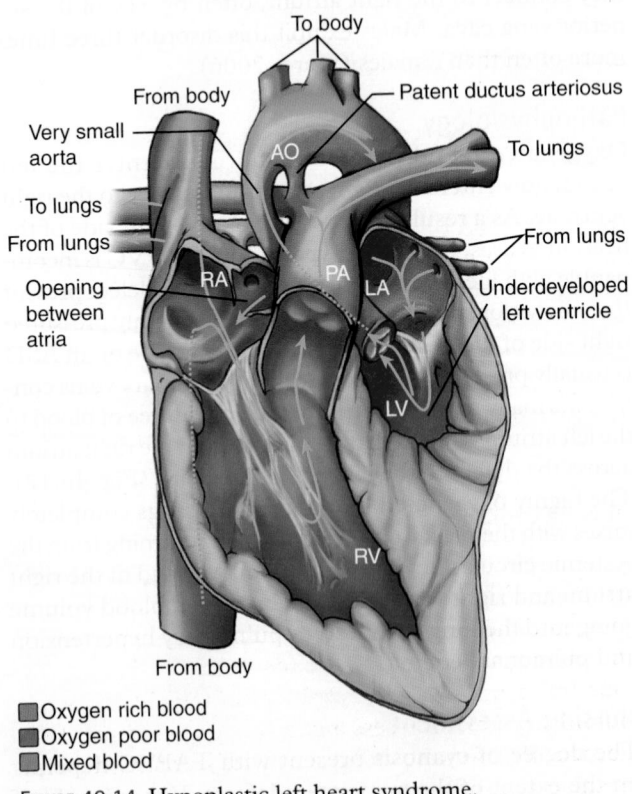

FIGURE 40.14 Hypoplastic left heart syndrome.

closes, the heart cannot pump blood into the systemic circulation, causing poor perfusion of the vital organs and shock. Death will occur rapidly without intervention.

Nursing Assessment

Initially after birth, the newborn may be asymptomatic because the ductus arteriosus is still patent. However, as the ductus begins to close at a few days of age, the newborn will begin to exhibit cyanosis. Some infants may present with circulatory collapse (shock) and must be resuscitated emergently.

Health History and Physical Examination

Obtain the health history, noting onset of cyanosis. Note poor feeding and history of tiring easily. Evaluate the vital signs, noting tachycardia, tachypnea, and hypothermia. Observe for increased work of breathing and gradually increasing cyanosis. Note pallor of the extremities and decreased oxygen saturation via pulse oximetry. Auscultate the heart and lungs. Note adventitious breath sounds, gallop rhythm, single second heart sound, and a soft systolic ejection or holosystolic murmur.

Laboratory and Diagnostic Tests

Prenatally, a fetal echocardiogram can diagnose this syndrome, as can a maternal ultrasound. After birth, the echocardiogram illustrates the defect.

> ▶ NURSING MANAGEMENT OF THE CHILD WITH CONGENITAL HEART DISEASE

The child with a congenital heart defect has multiple needs and requires comprehensive, multidisciplinary care. Nurses play a key role in helping the child and family during this intensely stressful time. Nursing care focuses on improving oxygenation, promoting adequate nutrition, assisting the child and family with coping, providing postoperative nursing care, preventing infection, and providing patient and family education. An important component of education involves preparing the child and parents for discharge. In addition to the nursing management presented below, refer to Nursing Care Plan 40.1 for additional interventions appropriate for the child with CHD. Individualize nursing care specific to the child's needs.

Improving Oxygenation

Due to the hemodynamic changes accompanying the underlying structural defect, oxygenation is key. Provide frequent ongoing assessment of the child's cardiopulmonary status. Assess airway patency and suction as needed. Position the child in Fowler's or semi-Fowler's position to facilitate lung expansion. Monitor vital signs,

especially heart and respiratory rates. Monitor the child's color and oxygen saturation levels closely, using these to guide oxygen administration. Observe for tachypnea and other signs of respiratory distress, such as nasal flaring, grunting, and retractions. Auscultate the lungs for adventitious sounds. Provide humidified supplemental oxygen as ordered, warming it to prevent wide temperature fluctuations. Anticipate the need for assisted ventilation if the child has difficulty maintaining the airway or experiences deterioration in oxygenation capacity. Box 40.1 lists interventions related to relief of hypercyanotic spells.

Promoting Adequate Nutrition

Adequate nutrition is critical to foster growth and development as well as to reduce the risk for infection. Children with congenital heart defects typically have increased nutritional needs due to the increased energy expenditure associated with increased cardiac and respiratory workloads. In addition, many of the defects lead to heart failure, which may affect the child's fluid balance status, further increasing the child's energy expenditure.

Nutrition may be provided orally, enterally, or parenterally. For example, for the newborn or infant, nutrition via breast milk or formula may be provided orally or via gavage feedings. Breastfeeding is usually associated with decreased energy expenditure during the act of feeding, yet some infants in intensive care are not stable enough to breastfeed. Gavage with breast milk is possible, and the use of human milk fortifier (either with breastfeeding or added to the gavage feed) adds additional calories that the infant requires. Formula-fed infants may also require increased-calorie formula, which may be achieved by more concentrated mixing of the formula or through the use of additives such as Polycose or vegetable oil. Consult the nutritionist to determine the individual infant's caloric needs and prescription of appropriate feeding.

Cutting a large hole in the nipple or "cross-cutting" the nipple decreases the work of feeding for some infants. Generally, nipple feedings should be limited to a 20-minute duration, as feeding for longer periods results in excess caloric expenditure. Many infants may feed orally for 20 minutes, receiving the remainder of that feeding via orogastric or nasogastric tube. Offer older children small, frequent feedings to reduce the amount of energy required

---

BOX 40.1 Relieving Hypercyanotic Spells

- Use a calm, comforting approach.
- Place the infant or child in a knee-to-chest position.
- Provide supplemental oxygen.
- Administer morphine sulfate (0.1 mg/kg IV, IM, or SQ).
- Supply IV fluids.
- Administer propranolol (0.1 mg/kg IV).

to feed or eat and to prevent overtiring the child. When needed, administer and monitor total parenteral nutrition as prescribed.

> ▶ *Take* NOTE!
>
> *Breastfeeding a child before and after cardiac surgery may boost the infant's immune system, which can help fight postoperative infection. If breastfeeding is not possible, mothers can pump milk and the breast milk may be given via bottle, dropper, or gavage feeding.*

Assisting the Child and Family to Cope

The diagnosis of CHD is especially overwhelming for the child and the parents. The numerous examinations, diagnostic tests, and procedures are sources of stress for the infant or child regardless of age and for the parents. The parents may fear long-term disability or death or may worry that allowing the child to engage in any activity will worsen his or her status. Thus, the parents may tend to overprotect the child. It is important for the parents to continue parenting the child, even when the child requires extended hospitalizations or intensive care (Fernandes, 2005). Explain all that is happening with the child, using language the parents and child can understand. Allow the parents and child to voice their feelings, concerns, or questions. Provide ample time to address these questions and concerns. Encourage the parents, and the child as developmentally appropriate, to participate in the child's care.

If the child is a newborn or infant, encourage attachment and bonding. Emphasize the child's positive attributes, including the normal aspects of the infant. Help the parents to experience the joy of a new infant, seeing the beauty of the child, no matter how ill the infant is (Fernandes, 2005). Urge the parents to touch, stroke, pat, and talk to the infant. Encourage them to hold the infant close, using kangaroo care as appropriate. If the child is older, offer suggestions as to how the parents can meet the child's emotional needs. For example, encourage them to bring a favorite toy or object from home while the child is hospitalized.

Provide developmentally appropriate explanations to the child. Encourage play therapy to help the child understand what is happening.

Preventing Infection

Teach parents proper hand hygiene. Provide appropriate dental care. Make sure the child receives prophylaxis for infective endocarditis as needed. Ensure that children 24 months or younger who have hemodynamically significant heart defects receive respiratory syncytial virus (RSV) prophylaxis as recommended during RSV season (Ressel, 2004).

Providing Care for the Child Undergoing Cardiac Surgery

Cardiac surgery may be necessary to correct a congenital defect or to provide symptomatic relief. The surgery may be planned as an elective procedure or done as an emergency. Open-heart surgery involves an incision of the heart muscle to repair the internal structures. This may require cardiopulmonary bypass. Closed-heart surgery involves structures related to the heart but not the heart muscle itself and may be performed with or without cardiopulmonary bypass (Kopf & Mello, 2006; Muscari, 2004).

Providing Preoperative Care

The preoperative nursing assessment complements the history and physical examination and provides important baseline information for comparison during the postoperative period. Establish a relationship with the child and parents. Identify problems that may require particular nursing interventions during the postoperative period. Before cardiac surgery, interview the parents and, if age-appropriate, the child. Focus the interview on the history of the present illness, cardiac risk factors, the child's present physical and functional status, additional medical problems, current medications and drug allergies, the child's and family's understanding of the illness and planned procedure, and the family support system.

The preoperative physical assessment includes:

- Temperature and weight measurements
- Examination of extremities for peripheral edema, clubbing, and evaluation of peripheral pulses
- Auscultation of the heart (rate, rhythm, heart sounds, murmurs, clicks, and rubs)
- Respiratory assessment, including respiratory rate, work of breathing, and auscultation of the lungs for breath sounds

Obtain any necessary laboratory and diagnostic tests to establish a baseline. In addition, review the results of any tests done previously. Testing may include CBC, electrolyte levels, clotting studies, urinalysis, cultures of blood and other body secretions, renal and hepatic function tests, chest x-ray, electrocardiogram, echocardiogram, and cardiac catheterization.

In most nonemergent cases, preoperative assessment is performed in an outpatient setting and the patient is admitted to the hospital on the day of surgery. Nursing care during this phase focuses on thorough patient and parent education. If the surgery is an emergency, patient teaching must be done quickly, emphasizing the most important elements of the child's care.

Child and parent education typically includes the following topics:

- Heart anatomy and its function, including what area is involved with the defect that is to be corrected
- Events before surgery, including any testing or preparation such as a skin scrub
- Location of the child after surgery, such as a pediatric intensive care unit, which may include a visit to the unit if appropriate and explanation of the sights and sounds that may be present
- Appearance of the child after surgery (equipment or devices used for monitoring, such as oxygen administration, electrocardiogram leads, pulse oximeter, chest tubes, mechanical ventilation, or intravenous lines)
- Approximate location of the incision and coverage with dressings
- Postoperative activity level, including measures to reduce the risk of complications, such as coughing and deep-breathing exercises, incentive spirometry, early ambulation, and leg exercises
- Nutritional restrictions, such as nothing by mouth for a specified time before surgery and use of intravenous fluids
- Medications, such as anesthesia, sedation, and analgesics as well as medications the child is taking now that need to be continued or withheld

Prepare and educate the child at an age- and developmentally appropriate level. Advise parents to read books with their child about CHD and hospitalization such as:

- "Clifford Visits the Hospital" by N. Bridwell, 2000 (Scholastic Inc.)
- "Franklin Goes to the Hospital" by P. Bourgeois, 2000 (Scholastic Paperbacks)
- "Pump the Bear" by G. O. Whittingon, 2000 (Brown Books)
- "Blue Lewis and Sasha the Great" by C. D. Newell, 2005 (Cally Press)
- "Cardiac Kids: A Book for Families Who Have a Child with Heart Disease" by V. Elder, 1994 (Dayton Area Heart and Cancer Association)
- "When Molly Was in the Hospital: A Book for Brothers and Sisters of Hospitalized Children" by D. Duncan, 1994 (Rayve Productions) (siblings)
- "A Night Without Stars" by J. Howe, 1993 (Camelot) (older children)

Additionally, parents may order "It's My Heart", a parent resource book, free of charge from the Children's Heart Foundation at http://www.childrensheartfoundation.org/its_my_heart.htm.

Parents may also help their child by buying a small thrift-store suitcase, spray-painting it, and allowing the child to decorate it with his or her name, pictures of family, stickers, or favorite story characters. This will be the child's "hospital suitcase" that the child may pack with toys and videos to bring to the hospital. Hospital tours are appropriate for school-age children, and older children and teens may benefit from an intensive care unit tour before surgery.

Instruct parents to stop food and liquids at the designated time, depending on the child's age, and to give all medications as directed. Some medications may be withheld before surgery. If the child's nutritional status is poor or questionable, nutritional supplementation may be ordered for a period of time preoperatively to ensure that the child has the best possible nutritional status before surgery. When it is time for the child to be transported to the surgical area, allow the parents to accompany the child as far as possible, depending on the institution's policy. Also reinforce with the child that the parents will be present at the bedside when he or she awakens from surgery.

Providing Postoperative Care

The child will usually be transported from the operating room to the intensive care unit. Depending on the age, postoperative stability, and type of surgery, the child may stay in the intensive care unit for several hours up to several days. Vigilant nursing care aids in the transition of the child and parents after surgery and reduces the risk of complications.

During the postoperative period the nurse should do the following:

- Assess vital signs frequently, as often as every 1 hour, until stable.
- Assess the color of the skin and mucous membranes, check capillary refill, and palpate peripheral pulses.
- Observe cardiac rate and rhythm via electronic monitoring and auscultate heart rate, rhythm, and sounds frequently.
- Monitor hemodynamic status via arterial and/or central venous lines (left and right atrial, and pulmonary artery pressures, pulmonary artery oxygen saturation).
- Provide site care and tubing changes according to the institution's policy.
- Auscultate lungs for adventitious, diminished, or absent breath sounds.
- Assess oxygen saturation levels via pulse oximetry and arterial blood gases as well as work of breathing and level of consciousness frequently.
- Administer supplemental oxygen as needed.
- Monitor mechanical ventilation and suction as ordered.
- Inspect chest tube functioning, noting amount, color, and character of drainage.
- Inspect the dressing (incision and chest tube) for drainage and intactness. Reinforce or change the dressing as ordered.
- Assess the incision for redness, irritation, drainage, or separation.
- Monitor intake and output hourly.
- Maintain accurate intravenous infusion rate; restrict fluids as ordered to prevent hypervolemia.

- Assess for changes in level of consciousness. Report restlessness, irritability, or seizures.
- Obtain ordered laboratory tests, such as CBC, coagulation studies, cardiac enzyme levels, and electrolyte levels. Report abnormal results.
- Administer medications, such as digoxin or inotropic or vasopressor agents, as ordered, watching the child closely for possible adverse effects.
- Encourage the child to turn, cough, deep breathe, use the incentive spirometer, and splint the incisional area with pillows.
- Assess the child's pain level and administer analgesics as ordered. Allow time for the child to rest and sleep.
- Assist the child to get out of bed as soon as possible and as ordered.
- Assess daily weights.
- Administer small, frequent feedings or meals when oral intake is allowed.
- Position the child in a comfortable position, one that maximizes chest expansion. Change position frequently.
- Assess the child for complications (Box 40.2).
- Provide emotional and physical support to the child and family, making appropriate referrals such as to social services for assistance.
- Prepare the patient and family for discharge (Beke et al., 2005).

▶ *Take* NOTE!

Abrupt cessation of chest tube output accompanied by an increase in heart rate and increased filling pressure (right atrial) may indicate cardiac tamponade (Beke et al., 2005).

BOX 40.2   **Possible Complications After Cardiac Surgery**

- Atelectasis
- Bacterial endocarditis
- Cardiac arrhythmias
- Cardiac tamponade
- Cerebrovascular accident
- Heart failure
- Hemorrhage
- Pleural effusion
- Pneumonia
- Pneumothorax
- Postperfusion syndrome
- Postcardiac surgery syndrome
- Pulmonary edema
- Seizures
- Wound infection

Providing Patient and Family Education

Provide patient and family education throughout the child's stay. Initially, teaching focuses on the underlying defect and measures to treat or control the problem. If the child requires surgery, teaching shifts to preoperative and postoperative events. Emphasize discharge teaching for each admission. Teaching Guidelines 40.2 highlights the major areas to be addressed in patient and family education.

Acquired Cardiovascular Disorders

Acquired cardiovascular disorders occur in children as a result of an underlying cardiovascular problem or may refer to other cardiac disorders that are not congenital. The most common type of acquired cardiovascular disorder in children is heart failure. Other acquired disorders include rheumatic fever, cardiomyopathy, infective endocarditis, hyperlipidemia, hypertension, and Kawasaki disease.

TEACHING GUIDELINES 40.2

Caring for the Child With a Congenital Heart Disease

- Give medications, if ordered, exactly as prescribed.
- Weigh the child at least once a week or as ordered, at approximately the same time of the day with the same scale, and wearing the same amount of clothing.
- Allow the child to engage in activity as directed. Provide time for the child to rest frequently throughout the day to prevent overexertion.
- Provide a nutritious diet, taking into account any restrictions for fluids or foods.
- Use measures to prevent infection, such as frequent handwashing, prophylactic antibiotics, and skin care.
- Adhere to schedule for follow-up diagnostic tests and procedures.
- Support the child's growth and development needs.
- Use available community support services.
- Notify the primary care provider if the child has increasing episodes of respiratory distress, cyanosis, or difficulty breathing; fever; increased edema of the hands, feet, or face; decreased urinary output; weight loss or difficulty eating or drinking; increased fatigue or irritability; decreased level of alertness; or vomiting or diarrhea.

▶ HEART FAILURE

Heart failure occurs most often in children with CHD and is the most common reason for admission to the hospital for children with CHD. Eighty percent of all cases of heart failure in children with CHD occur by the age of 1 year (Freitas-Nichols, 2004). Heart failure also occurs secondary to other conditions such as myocardial dysfunction following surgical intervention for CHD, cardiomyopathy, myocarditis, fluid volume overload, hypertension, anemia, or sepsis or as a toxic effect of certain chemotherapeutic agents used in the treatment of cancer. Heart failure refers to a set of clinical signs and symptoms that reflect the heart's inability to pump effectively to provide adequate blood, oxygen, and nutrients to the body organs and tissues.

The child experiencing heart failure requires a multidisciplinary approach to care. Collaboration is necessary to achieve improved cardiac function, restored fluid balance, decreased cardiac workload, and improved oxygen delivery to the tissues.

Pathophysiology

Cardiac output is controlled by preload (diastolic volume), afterload (ventricular wall tension), myocardial contractility (inotropic state), and heart rate. Protracted alterations in any of these factors may lead to heart failure. In the event of reduced cardiac output, multiple compensatory mechanisms are activated. When the ventricular contraction is impaired (systolic dysfunction), reduced ejection of blood occurs, and therefore cardiac output is reduced. Diminished ability to receive venous return (diastolic dysfunction) occurs when high venous pressures are required to support ventricular function. As a result of decreased cardiac output, the renin-angiotensin-aldosterone system is activated as a compensatory mechanism. Fluid and sodium retention as well as improved contractility and vasoconstriction then occur. Initially blood pressure is supported and organ perfusion is maintained, but increased afterload worsens systolic dysfunction. As the heart chambers dilate, myocardial oxygen consumption increases and cardiac output is limited by excessive wall stretch. Over time, the capacity of the heart to respond to these compensatory mechanisms fails, and cardiac output is further decreased (Francis et al., 2008). Figure 40.15 shows the clinical manifestations that occur related to the mechanisms of heart failure.

Therapeutic Management

Management of heart failure is supportive. Promotion of oxygenation and ventilation is of utmost importance. Digitalis, diuretics, inotropic agents, vasodilators, antiarrhythmics, and antithrombotics have been widely used in children for palliation of symptoms (Rosenthal et al.,

2004). Many children with heart failure require management in the intensive care unit until they are stabilized. Augmenting nutrition and ensuring adequate rest are also key components of management.

Nursing Assessment

For a full description of the assessment phase of the nursing process, refer to page 1285. Specific assessment findings related to heart failure are discussed below.

Health History

When obtaining the health history, elicit a description of the present illness and chief complaint. Common complaints reported during the health history might include:

• Failure to gain weight or rapid weight gain
• Failure to thrive
• Difficulty feeding
• Fatigue
• Dizziness, irritability
• Exercise intolerance
• Shortness of breath
• Sucking and then tiring quickly
• Syncope
• Decreased number of wet diapers

Infants with heart failure often display subtle signs such as difficulty feeding and tiring easily. Pay close attention for reports of these problems from the parents. Also be alert for statements such as "the baby drinks a small amount of breast milk (or formula) and stops, but then wants to eat again very soon afterwards"; "the baby seems to perspire a lot during feedings"; or "the baby seems to be more comfortable when he's sitting up or on my shoulder than when he's lying flat." In addition, the parents may report episodes of rapid breathing and grunting.

The child's current and past medical history also provides additional clues. Question the parents about any history of congenital heart defects and treatments such as surgery to repair the defect. Determine the current medication regimen. Also ask about any recent or past infections, such as streptococcal infections or fever.

Physical Examination

Weigh the child and note recent rapid weight gain or lack of weight gain. Obtain the child's vital signs, noting tachycardia or tachypnea. These findings are often the first indicators of heart failure in an infant or older child. Measure the BP in the upper and lower extremities, comparing the findings for differences. Note decreased BP, which may be due to impaired cardiac muscle function. Inspect the skin color, noting pallor or cyanosis. Also observe for diaphoresis (profuse sweating). Inspect the face, hands, and lower extremities for edema. Observe for increased work of breathing, such as nasal flaring or retractions. Note the presence of a cough, which may be productive with bloody

FIGURE 40.15 Pathophysiology of heart failure. (From Francis et al., 2008).

sputum. Auscultate the apical pulse, noting its location and character. Listen for a murmur, which may suggest a congenital heart defect, a gallop rhythm, or an accentuated third heart sound, suggesting sudden ventricular distention. Auscultate the lungs, noting crackles or wheezes suggestive of pulmonary congestion. Palpate the peripheral pulses, noting weak or thready pulses. Note the temperature and color of the extremities; they may be cool, clammy, and pale.

Assess the child's abdomen, looking for distention indicative of ascites. Gently palpate the abdomen to identify hepatomegaly or splenomegaly.

Laboratory and Diagnostic Tests
The diagnosis of heart failure is based on the child's signs and symptoms and is confirmed with several laboratory and diagnostic tests. These include:

- Chest x-ray, revealing an enlarged heart and/or pulmonary edema
- Electrocardiogram, indicating ventricular hypertrophy
- Echocardiogram, revealing the underlying cause of heart failure, such as a congenital heart defect

Other tests may be done to support the diagnosis. For example, the CBC may show evidence of anemia or infection. Electrolyte levels may reveal hyponatremia secondary to fluid retention and hyperkalemia secondary to tissue destruction or impaired renal function. Arterial blood gas results may demonstrate respiratory alkalosis in mild heart failure or metabolic acidosis. Tissue hypoxia may be evidenced by increased lactic acid and decreased bicarbonate levels.

Nursing Management

Nursing management of the child with heart failure focuses on promoting oxygenation, supporting cardiac function, providing adequate nutrition, and promoting rest.

Promoting Oxygenation
Position the infant or child in a semi-upright position to decrease work of breathing and lessen pulmonary congestion. Suction as needed. Chest physiotherapy and postural drainage may also be beneficial. Administer supplemental oxygen as ordered and monitor oxygen saturation via pulse oximetry. Oxygen also serves the function of vasodilator

and decreases pulmonary vascular resistance. Occasionally, the infant or child with heart failure may require intubation and positive-pressure ventilation to normalize blood gas tension.

> ▶ **Take** NOTE!
>
> *In a child with a large left-to-right shunt, oxygen will decrease pulmonary vascular resistance while increasing the systemic vascular resistance, which leads to increased left-to-right shunting. Monitor the child carefully and use oxygen only as prescribed.*

Supporting Cardiac Function

Administer digitalis, angiotensin-converting enzyme (ACE) inhibitors, and diuretics as prescribed. Digoxin therapy begins with a digitalizing dose divided into several doses (oral or IV) over a 24-hour period to reach maximum cardiac effect. During digitalization, monitor the electrocardiogram for a prolonged PR interval and decreased ventricular rate. Doses are then administered every 12 hours. Monitor the child for signs of digoxin toxicity. Measure BP before and after administration of ACE inhibitors, holding the dose and notifying the physician if the BP falls greater then 15 mm Hg. Observe for signs of hypotension such as lightheadedness, dizziness, or fainting. Weigh the child daily to determine fluid loss. Maintain accurate records of intake and output, restricting fluid intake if ordered. Carefully monitor potassium levels, administering potassium supplements if prescribed. Sodium intake is not usually restricted in the child with heart failure (Rosenthal et al., 2004).

Providing Adequate Nutrition

Due to the increased metabolic rate associated with heart failure, the infant may require as much as 150 calories/kg/day. Older children will also require higher caloric intake than typical children. Offer small, frequent feedings if the child can tolerate them. During the acute phase of heart failure, many infants in particular will require continuous or intermittent gavage feeding to maintain or gain weight. Concentrate infant formula to 24 to 28 calories/ounce as instructed by the nutritionist.

Promoting Rest

Minimize metabolic needs to decrease cardiac demand. The infant or older child with heart failure will usually limit activities based upon energy level. Ensure adequate time for sleep, and attempt to limit disturbing interventions. Provide age-appropriate activities that can be performed quietly or in bed, such as books, drawing, and video or board games. The older child or adolescent with significant heart failure may require home schooling. As the child improves, a rehabilitation program may be helpful for maximizing activity within the child's cardiovascular status limits.

▶ INFECTIVE ENDOCARDITIS

Infective endocarditis is a microbial infection of the endothelial surfaces of the heart's chambers, septum, or valves (most common). Children with congenital heart defects (septum or valve defects) or prosthetic valves are at increased risk of acquiring bacterial endocarditis, which is potentially fatal in these children. Other risk factors for endocarditis include central venous catheters and intravenous drug use. Infective endocarditis occurs when bacteria or fungi gain access to a damaged epithelium. Turbulence in blood flow associated with narrowed or incompetent valves or with a communication between the systemic and pulmonary circulation leads to damage of the endothelium. Thrombi and platelets then adhere to the endothelium, forming vegetations. When a microbe gains access to the bloodstream, it colonizes the vegetation, using the thrombi as a breeding ground. Clumps may separate from the vegetative patch and travel to other organs of the body, causing significant damage (septic emboli). Fungi or more commonly bacteria (particularly alpha-hemolytic streptococcus or *Staphylococcus aureus*) are frequently implicated in infective endocarditis.

Complete antibiotic or antifungal treatment of the causative organism is necessary, and treatment may last 4 to 7 weeks. Prevention of infective endocarditis in the susceptible child with CHD or a valvular disorder is of utmost importance (Greenberg et al., 2005; Yee, 2005).

Nursing Assessment

For a full description of the assessment phase of the nursing process, refer to page 1285. Assessment findings related to endocarditis are discussed below.

Health History

Obtain the health history, noting intermittent, unexplained low-grade fever. Document history of fatigue, anorexia, weight loss, or flu-like symptoms (arthralgia, myalgia, chills, night sweats). Note history of CHD, valve disorder, or heart failure.

Physical Examination

Measure the child's temperature, noting low-grade fever. Observe for edema if heart failure is also present. Note petechiae on the palpebral conjunctiva, the oral mucosa, or the extremities. Inspect for signs of extracardiac emboli:

- Roth's spots: splinter hemorrhages with pale centers on sclerae, palate, buccal mucosa, chest, fingers, or toes

• Janeway lesions: painless flat red or blue hemorrhagic lesions on the palms or the soles
• Osler's nodes: small, tender nodules on the pads of the toes or fingers
• Black lines (splinter hemorrhages) under the nails

Evaluate the electrocardiogram for a prolonged PR interval or dysrhythmias. Auscultate the heart for a new or changing murmur. Auscultate the lungs for adventitious breath sounds. Palpate the abdomen for splenomegaly (Greenberg et al., 2005; Yee, 2005).

Laboratory and Diagnostic Tests

Diagnosis is usually based on the clinical presentation. Laboratory tests may reveal:

• Blood culture: bacteria or fungus
• CBC: anemia, leukocytosis
• Urinalysis: microscopic hematuria
• Echocardiogram: cardiomegaly, abnormal valve function, area of vegetation

Nursing Management

Nursing management focuses on maintaining IV access for at least 4 weeks to appropriately administer the antibiotic or antifungal course of therapy. Monitor the child's temperature and subsequent blood culture results.

Ideally, infective endocarditis in children should be prevented. Children at increased risk for the development of infective endocarditis include those with:

• Valvular dysfunction or prosthetic valves
• Mitral valve prolapse with regurgitation
• Most congenital heart defects (certain simple septal defects are excluded)
• Surgically constructed systemic-to-pulmonary shunts
• Hypertrophic cardiomyopathy

Children at high risk should practice good oral hygiene, including regular tooth brushing and flossing. Instruct parents or the older child to carry emergency medical identification at all times. A wallet card is available from the American Heart Association at http://www.americanheart.org/presenter.jhtml?identifier=3003000. The card may be presented to any health care provider and includes the recommended antibiotic prophylactic regimen. Instruct the parents to notify the primary care provider or cardiologist if the child develops flu-like symptoms or a fever.

High-risk children (as noted above) who are undergoing procedures that increase the risk for the introduction of the types of bacteria responsible for endocarditis should receive prophylaxis as recommended by the American Heart Association. Usual antibiotics for prophylaxis may include ampicillin, amoxicillin, gentamicin, or vancomycin. Box 40.3 lists procedures for which antibiotic prophylaxis in high-risk children is recommended.

BOX 40.3 Procedures for which Infective Endocarditis Prophylaxis is Recommended

Dental Procedures
• Tooth extractions
• Periodontal procedures
• Dental implant placement
• Replacement of avulsed tooth
• Root canal or surgery
• Intraligamentary local anesthetic injections
• Any prophylactic dental procedure during which bleeding is anticipated

Respiratory Tract Procedures
• Tonsillectomy, adenoidectomy
• Rigid bronchoscopy
• Surgery involving the respiratory mucosa

Gastrointestinal Tract Procedures
• Esophageal varices sclerotherapy
• Dilation of esophageal stricture
• Endoscopic retrograde cholangiography for biliary obstruction
• Other biliary tract surgery
• Surgery involving the gastrointestinal mucosa

Genitourinary Tract Procedures
• Cystoscopy
• Urethral dilation
• Surgery involving the prostate

Data from American Heart Association. (2008a). *Bacterial endocarditis.* Retrieved 1/4/08 from http://www.americanheart.org/presenter.jhtml?identifier=4436; Greenberg, J. D., Bonwit, A. M., & Roddy, M. G. (2005). Subacute bacterial endocarditis prophylaxis: A succinct review for pediatric emergency physicians and nurses. *Clinical Pediatric Emergency Medicine, 6*(4), 266–272; and Yee, C. A. (2005). Endocarditis: The infected heart. *Nursing Management, 36*(2), 25–30.

▶ ACUTE RHEUMATIC FEVER

Acute rheumatic fever (ARF) is a delayed sequela of group A streptococcal pharyngeal infection. In the United States this disease occurs more often in school-age children between 5 and 15 years of age in areas where streptococcal pharyngitis is more prevalent, especially during the colder months. It usually develops 2 to 3 weeks after the initial streptococcal infection. Current understanding of the disease process of ARF is that the child develops an antibody response to surface proteins of the bacteria. The antibodies then cross-react with antigens in cardiac muscle and neuronal and synovial tissues, causing carditis, arthritis, and chorea (involuntary random, jerking movements). ARF affects the joints, central nervous system, skin, and subcutaneous tissue and causes chronic, progressive damage to the heart and valves. Most attacks of ARF last 6 to 12 weeks and then are resolved, but rheumatic fever may recur with subsequent streptococcal infections.

Diagnosis of ARF is based on the modified Jones' criteria (Box 40.4). Therapeutic management is directed toward managing inflammation and fever, eradicating the bacteria, preventing permanent heart damage, and preventing recurrences. A full 10-day course of penicillin therapy (or equivalent) as well as corticosteroids and nonsteroidal anti-inflammatory drugs are used. Continuous prophylaxis with monthly intramuscular injections of penicillin G benzathine or daily oral doses of penicillin or erythromycin following the initial illness is recommended to prevent a new streptococcal infection and recurrent ARF. Prophylaxis is continued until adulthood (no valvular disease) or age 40 years (with valvular disease) (Martin & Green, 2006).

Nursing Assessment

Elicit a description of the present illness and chief complaint, noting fever and joint pain. Explore the patient's recent medical history for risk factors such as documented streptococcal infection or sore throat within the past 2 to 3 weeks, or for past history of ARF. Observe the child for Sydenham chorea, a movement disorder of the face and upper extremities. Inspect the skin for evidence of the classic rash, erythema marginatum, a maculopapular red rash with central clearing and elevated edges. Auscultate the heart, noting a murmur. Palpate the surfaces of the wrist, elbows, and knees for firm, painless, subcutaneous nodules. Note prolonged PR interval on the electrocardiogram. Throat culture will provide definitive diagnosis of current streptococcal infection, while streptococcal antibody tests may yield evidence of recent infection. Echocardiogram is required to determine if carditis if present.

Nursing Management

Nursing management of the child with ARF focuses on ensuring compliance with the acute course of antibiotics as well as prophylaxis following initial recovery from ARF. Allow the child to verbalize the frustration he or she may be feeling in relation to chorea symptoms. Offer support for dealing with the abnormal movements. Educate the child and others that the sudden jerky movements of chorea will eventually disappear, though they may last as long as several months. Some children may require a neuroleptic agent such as haloperidol (Haldol) for management of chorea. Administer corticosteroids or nonsteroidal anti-inflammatory agents for control of joint pain and swelling.

▶ CARDIOMYOPATHY

Cardiomyopathy is a condition in which the myocardium cannot contract properly. The incidence of cardiomyopathy among children is increasing; it occurs at a rate of 1.13 per 100,000 (AHA, 2006d). Cardiomyopathy may occur in children with genetic disorders or congenital heart defects, as a result of an inflammatory or infectious process or hypertension, or after cardiac transplantation or surgery, but most commonly it is idiopathic. Cardiomyopathy clusters in infancy and adolescence. Three types of cardiomyopathy exist. Restrictive cardiomyopathy is rare in children and results in atrial relaxation. Dilated cardiomyopathy is the most common type in childhood and may result in heart failure because of ventricular dilatation with decreased contractility. There is some familial tendency toward dilated cardiomyopathy, and it is also associated with Duchenne and Becker muscular dystrophy (Marian et al., 2004). Children with dilated cardiomyopathy may present with heart failure. Hypertrophic cardiomyopathy is more common in adolescence and results in hypertrophy of the heart muscle, particularly the left ventricle, affecting the heart's ability to fill. About two thirds of all cases of hypertrophic cardiomyopathy are familial, with some inherited in an autosomal dominant fashion (Marian et al., 2004; Maron, 2004).

There is no cure for cardiomyopathy, meaning that currently heart muscle function cannot be restored. Therapeutic management is directed toward improving heart function and blood pressure. Mechanical ventilation and

---

BOX 40.4) Modified Jones Criteria (American Heart Association)

Diagnosis of acute rheumatic fever requires the presence of either two major criteria or one major plus two minor criteria.

Major Criteria
• Carditis
• Migratory polyarthritis
• Subcutaneous nodules
• Erythema marginatum
• Sydenham chorea

Minor Criteria
• Arthralgia
• Fever
• Elevated erythrocyte sedimentation rate or C-reactive protein
• Prolonged PR interval

Data from Jaggi, P., & Shulman, S. T. (2006). Group A streptococcal infections. *Pediatrics in Review, 27,* 99–105; and Parrillo, S. J., & Parrillo, C. V. (2006). *Rheumatic fever.* Retrieved 11/13/06 from http://www.emedicine.com/emerg/topic509.htm.

vasoactive medications are needed in many children. ACE inhibitors, beta blockers, or calcium channel blockers may be used. Pacemakers or surgery are helpful in some children. Nearly 40% of children with cardiomyopathy either die or require heart transplantation (Strauss & Lock, 2003).

Nursing Assessment

Explore the health history for risk factors such as:

- Congenital heart defect, cardiac transplantation or surgery
- Duchenne or Becker muscular dystrophy
- History of myocarditis, HIV infection, or Kawasaki disease
- Hypertension
- Drugs, alcohol, or radiation exposure
- Connective tissue, autoimmune, or endocrine disease
- Maternal diabetes
- Familial history of sudden death

Inquire about a history of respiratory distress, fatigue, or poor growth (dilated) or chest pain, dizziness, or syncope (hypertrophic). Observe the child for extremity edema and abdominal distention. Note increased work of breathing. Auscultate the heart, noting tachycardia and irregular rhythm. Evaluate heart rhythm via electrocardiogram, noting dysrhythmias or indications of left ventricular hypertrophy.

Chest x-ray may reveal cardiomegaly or congested lungs. Echocardiogram demonstrates increased heart size, poor contractility, decreased ejection fraction, or asymmetric septal hypertrophy. Cardiac catheterization is usually performed to aid in the diagnosis.

Nursing Management

Many children with cardiomyopathy require intensive care initially. Monitor for complications such as blood clots or arrhythmias, which could lead to cardiac arrest. Refer to the prior section on heart failure for nursing interventions related to heart failure, which may be present with dilated cardiomyopathy. Administer vasoactive and other medications as prescribed, monitoring the child closely for response to these therapies as well as for complications. Support the child in choosing activities that fit within the prescribed restrictions. Provide extensive emotional support to the child and family, who may experience significant stress as they realize the severity of this illness.

▶ HYPERTENSION

Hypertension affects only 1% to 3% of children and adolescents but often leads to long-term health consequences such as cardiovascular disease and left ventricular hypertrophy (Cromwell et al., 2005a). In children, acceptable BP values are based on gender, age, and height. Hypertension is defined as BP persistently greater than the 95th percentile for gender, age, and height. Prehypertension refers to BP that is persistently between the 90th and 95th percentiles. BP is considered normal when the systolic and diastolic values are less than the 90th percentile for gender, age, and height (USDHHS, NHLBI, 2005).

Childhood hypertension may be further defined as primary or secondary. Primary hypertension in children is rare, but its incidence increases with age, so it is more common in adolescence than in early childhood. Hypertension in children most frequently occurs secondary to an underlying medical problem (most often renal disease). Mild to moderate hypertension in childhood is usually asymptomatic and usually is determined only upon BP screening during a well-child visit or during follow-up for known risk factors.

Therapeutic management depends on the extent of the hypertension and the length of time it has existed. Weight reduction, appropriate diet, and increased physical activity are important components of management of prehypertensive and asymptomatic hypertensive children. Some children are candidates for and require antihypertensive medications or diuretics.

Pathophysiology

The balance between cardiac output and vascular resistance determines the BP. An increase in either of these variables, in the absence of a compensatory decrease in the other, increases the mean BP. Factors regulating cardiac output and vascular resistance include changes in electrolyte balance, particularly sodium, calcium, and potassium.

Nursing Assessment

Elicit the health history, determining the presence of risk factors for hypertension such as:

- Family history
- Obesity
- Hyperlipidemia
- Renal disease (including frequent urinary tract infections)
- Systemic lupus erythematosus
- Congenital heart disease
- Neurofibromatosis, Turner syndrome, and other genetic disorders
- Prematurity
- Prolonged neonatal ventilation
- Umbilical artery catheterization
- Diabetes mellitus
- Increased intracranial pressure
- Malignancy
- Solid organ transplant
- Medications known to raise BP

Signs and symptoms reported during the health history might include growth retardation (with certain chronic medical conditions), obesity, and, particularly in older children, headache, subtle behavioral or school performance changes, fatigue, blurred vision, nosebleed, or Bell's palsy.

Determine the child's weight and height/length. Plot these growth parameters on the gender-appropriate chart for the child's age. Note the percentile for height/length, as it will be used to determine the BP percentile (see Appendix F). Measure the BP in all four extremities (to rule out coarctation of the aorta). Ensure that the child is relaxed and sitting or reclined. Refer to Chapter 31 for specific information related to accurate BP measurement in children.

Physical Examination

Inspect the skin for:

- Acne, hirsutism, or striae (associated with anabolic steroid use)
- Café-au-lait spots (associated with neurofibromatosis)
- Malar rash (associated with lupus)
- Pallor, diaphoresis, or flushing (associated with pheochromocytoma)

Observe the extremities for edema (renal disease) or joint swelling (lupus). Inspect the chest for apical heave (ventricular hypertrophy) or wide-spaced nipples (Turner syndrome). Auscultate heart sounds, noting tachycardia (associated with primary hypertension) or murmur (associated with coarctation of the aorta). Palpate the abdomen for a mass or enlarged kidney.

Laboratory and Diagnostic Testing

Though diagnosis of hypertension is based upon BP measurements, additional laboratory or diagnostic tests may be used to evaluate the underlying cause of secondary hypertension, including:

- Urinalysis, blood urea nitrogen, and serum creatinine: may determine presence of renal disease
- Renal ultrasound or angiography: may reveal kidney or genitourinary tract abnormalities
- Echocardiogram: may show left ventricular hypertrophy
- Lipid profile: determines the presence of hyperlipidemia (USDHHS, NHLBI, 2005)

Nursing Management

Salt restriction and potassium or calcium supplements have not been scientifically shown to decrease BP in children (Cook & Daniels, 2005). However, certain children may benefit from salt restriction, as some children seem to be sensitive to salt intake. Assist the child and family to develop a plan for weight reduction if the child is overweight or obese. Encourage the child and family to control portion sizes, decrease the intake of sugary beverages

and snacks, eat more fresh fruits and vegetables, and eat a healthy breakfast (USDHHS, NHLBI, 2005). Consult the nutritionist for additional assistance with meal planning. To increase physical activity, the child should find a sport or type of exercise in which he or she is interested. Aerobic activities involving running, walking, or cycling are particularly helpful. When a child requires antihypertensive therapy, teach the child and family how to administer the medication. Caution the parents about side effects related to antihypertensives. Teach the parent to measure the child's BP as determined by the primary care physician or specialist, as well as to keep appointments for BP follow-up. See Healthy People 2010.

▶ KAWASAKI DISEASE

Kawasaki disease is an acute systemic vasculitis occurring mostly in infants and young children. It is the leading cause of acquired heart disease among children and occurs more frequently in the winter and spring (Newburger et al., 2004). Over 4,000 children are hospitalized annually in the United States with Kawasaki disease, and though it affects all ethnic groups, it occurs more frequently in those of Asian or Pacific descent (Newburger et al., 2004). It is a self-limited syndrome but causes serious cardiovascular sequelae in up to 25% of affected children (Newburger et al., 2004). Coronary artery aneurysm results in myocardial infarction and death in some children (Driscoll, 2006a). Therapeutic management of acute Kawasaki disease focuses on reducing inflammation in the walls of the coronary arteries and preventing coronary thrombosis. Chronic management of children developing aneurysms during the initial phase is directed toward preventing myocardial ischemia (Newburger et al., 2004). In the acute phase, high-dose aspirin in four divided doses daily and a single infusion of intravenous immunoglobulin (IVIG) are used. Children whose fever persists longer than 48 hours after initiation of aspirin therapy may receive a second dose of IVIG. Pulsed-dose corticosteroid therapy may also be used to prevent or halt coronary dilatation and inhibit progression to aneurysm (Dummer & Newburger, 2004).

HEALTHY PEOPLE *2010*	
Objective	Significance
Increase the proportion of persons appropriately counseled about health behaviors	• To prevent development of hypertension, encourage children to maintain a healthy weight and participate in regular exercise.

Pathophysiology

Though the etiology is still unknown, Kawasaki disease may result from an infectious cause. Current thought is that some infectious organism (as yet unidentified) causes disease in genetically susceptible people. Kawasaki disease appears to be an autoimmune response mediated by cytokine-induced endothelial cell surface antigens that leads to vasculitis. Neutrophils, followed by mononuclear cells, T lymphocytes, and immunoglobulin A–producing plasma cells, infiltrate the vessels. Inflammation then occurs in all three layers of the small and medium-sized blood vessels. Edema and smooth muscle necrosis occur in the vessel wall media in severe cases. Generalized systemic vasculitis occurs in the blood vessels throughout the body due to the inflammation and edema. As elastin and collagen fibers fragment, the structural integrity of the vessel wall is impaired. This mechanism leads to coronary dilatation (ectasia) or aneurysm. Some children never develop coronary artery changes, while others develop an aneurysm in either the acute phase or as a long-term sequela. Infants are at the highest risk for coronary aneurysm or ectasia (Newburger et al., 2004).

Nursing Assessment

Nursing assessment consists of determining the health history, physical examination, and laboratory and diagnostic testing.

Health History

Elicit the health history, noting any of the following:

- Fever
- Chills
- Headache
- Malaise
- Extreme irritability
- Vomiting
- Diarrhea
- Abdominal pain
- Joint pain

Of particular note is a history of high fever (39.9°C) of at least 5 days' duration that is unresponsive to antibiotics.

Physical Examination

Observe for significant bilateral conjunctivitis without exudate. Inspect the mouth and throat for dry, fissured lips, strawberry (cracked and reddened) tongue, and pharyngeal and oral mucosa erythema. Note hyperdynamic precordium. Evaluate the skin for:

- Diffuse, erythematous, polymorphous rash
- Edema of the hands and feet
- Erythema and painful induration of the palms and soles
- Desquamation (peeling) of the perineal region, fingers, and toes, extending to the palms and soles
- Possible jaundice

Palpate the neck for cervical lymphadenopathy (usually unilateral) and the joints for tenderness. Palpate the abdomen for liver enlargement. Auscultate the heart, noting tachycardia, gallop, or murmur (Newburger et al., 2004; Rowley, 2004).

Laboratory and Diagnostic Testing

The CBC may reveal mild to moderate anemia, an elevated white blood cell count during the acute phase, and significant thrombocytosis (elevated platelet count [500,000 to 1 million]) in the later phase. The erythrocyte sedimentation rate (ESR) and the C-reactive protein (CRP) level are elevated. Echocardiogram is performed as soon as possible after the diagnosis is confirmed to provide a baseline of a healthy heart or to evaluate for coronary artery involvement. Echocardiograms may be repeated during the illness and as part of long-term follow-up. Occasionally cardiac involvement warrants cardiac catheterization.

Nursing Management

In addition to the administration of aspirin and immunoglobulin, nursing management of the child with Kawasaki disease focuses on monitoring cardiac status, promoting comfort, and providing family education.

Monitoring Cardiac Status

Administer intravenous and oral fluids as ordered, evaluating intake and output carefully. Prepare the child for the echocardiogram. Assess frequently for signs of developing heart failure such as tachycardia, gallop, decreased urine output, or respiratory distress. Evaluate quality and strength of pulses. Provide cardiac monitoring as ordered, reporting arrhythmias.

Promoting Comfort

Provide acetaminophen for fever management and apply cool cloths as tolerated. Keep the environment quiet and cluster nursing care activities to decrease stimulation and hence irritability. Teach parents that irritability is a prominent feature of Kawasaki disease, and support their efforts to console the child. Apply petrolatum jelly or another lubricating ointment to the lips. Encourage the older child to suck on ice chips; the younger child may suck on a cool, moist washcloth. Popsicles are also soothing. Provide comfortable positioning, particularly if the child has joint pain or arthritis.

Providing Patient and Family Education

Teach parents to continue to monitor the child's temperature after discharge until the child has been afebrile for several days. Children with prolonged or recurrent fever may require a second dose of IVIG. Inform parents that irritability may last for up to 2 months after initial diagnosis with Kawasaki disease. Toxic effects of aspirin therapy such as headache, confusion, dizziness, or tinnitus should be reported to the primary care provider. Nonsteroidal anti-inflammatory agents should be avoided while aspirin therapy is ongoing. For children with continued arthritis (which resolves in several weeks), range-of-motion exercises with a morning bath may help to decrease stiffness. Instruct parents to avoid measles and varicella vaccination for 11 months after high-dose IVIG administration (Newburger et al., 2004). It is critical that the family comply with regularly scheduled cardiology follow-up appointments to determine development or progression of coronary artery ectasia or aneurysm. If the child has severe cardiac involvement, teach the parents about infant and/or child cardiopulmonary resuscitation before discharge from the hospital.

◗ HYPERLIPIDEMIA

Hyperlipidemia refers to high levels of lipids (fats/cholesterol) in the blood. High lipid levels are a risk factor for the development of atherosclerosis, which can result in coronary artery disease, a serious cardiovascular disorder occurring in adults. Children with high lipid levels, though remaining asymptomatic, are likely to have high levels as adults, which increases their risk for coronary artery disease. Therefore, detection, screening, and early intervention are important, especially if there is a family tendency toward heart disease (Armstrong, 2007).

Pathophysiology

Cholesterol is a building block for hormones and cell membranes. It occurs naturally in foods derived from animals such as eggs, dairy products, meat, poultry, and seafood. Cholesterol is also manufactured in the body. Together, cholesterol and triglycerides are known as lipids. Very-low-density lipoprotein (VLDL) is a lipoprotein composed mainly of triglycerides with only small amounts of cholesterol, phospholipid, and protein. VLDLs are easily converted to low-density lipoproteins (LDLs). Cholesterol is expressed in terms of LDL cholesterol or high-density lipoprotein (HDL) cholesterol. LDLs contain relatively more cholesterol and triglycerides than they do protein. HDLs contain about 50% protein, with the rest being cholesterol, triglyceride, and phospholipid. High levels of cholesterol and triglycerides place a person at risk for atherosclerosis. Elevated VLDL and LDL levels and decreased HDL levels produce a particular increase in the risk for atherosclerosis.

Therapeutic Management

Screening children for hyperlipidemia is of prime importance for early detection, intervention, and subsequent prevention of adult atherosclerosis. The National Cho-

lesterol Education Program recommends screening for hyperlipidemia in children over 2 years of age if:

- The parent has a total cholesterol level above 240 mg/dL
- There is a family history of cardiovascular disease in a parent or grandparent before age 55 years
- If the family history is unavailable

All children should eat a diet with the appropriate amount of fats (see the section on nursing management below) and should participate in physical activity. When diet and exercise are not enough to lower cholesterol to appropriate levels, medications such as resins, fibric acid derivatives, statins, or niacin may be used.

Nursing Assessment

Elicit the health history, noting risk factors such as family history of hyperlipidemia, early heart disease, hypertension, diabetes or other endocrine abnormality, cerebral vascular accident, or sudden death. Note prior lipid levels if available. Measure the child's height and weight, plotting them on standardized growth charts. Note overweight or obesity, as these are risk factors associated with hyperlipidemia. Typically, there are no other particular physical findings associated with hyperlipidemia. Table 40.3 gives details about the interpretation of cholesterol levels.

Nursing Management

Instruct families that the child must fast for 12 hours before lipid screening (initially and on follow-up samples). Dietary management is the first step in the prevention and management of hyperlipidemia in children over 2 years of age. The diet should consist primarily of fruits, vegetables, low-fat dairy products, whole grains, beans, lean meat and poultry, and fish. As in adults, fat should account for no more than 30% of daily caloric intake. Fat intake may vary over a period of days, as many young children are picky eaters. Limit saturated fats by choosing lean meats, removing skin from poultry before cooking, and avoiding palm, palm kernel, and coconut oils as well as hydrogenated fats. Teach families to read nutrition labels

TABLE 40.3   INTERPRETATION OF CHOLESTEROL LEVELS FOR CHILDREN AGE 2 TO 19 YEARS

Total Cholesterol (mg/dL)	LDL Cholesterol (mg/dL)	Interpretation
<170	<100	Normal
170–200	100–130	Borderline
>200	>130	High

Gidding, S. S., Dennison, B. A., Birch, L. L., et al. (2006). Dietary recommendations for children and adolescents: A guide for practitioners. *Pediatrics, 117,* 544–559.

to determine the content of the food. Limit intake of processed or refined foods as well as high-sugar drinks; these products provide minimal nutrition and significant calories. Children over 2 years of age should have 60 minutes per day of vigorous play or physical activity. Refer parents to "Healthy Habits for Healthy Kids—A Nutrition and Activity Guide for Parents" published by the American Dietetic Association, available at http://www.wellpoint.com/healthy_parenting/index.html.

If medications are required, teach the child and family about the dose, administration, and possible adverse effects. Assist the family to develop a medication dosing plan that is compatible with school and work schedules to increase compliance.

Heart Transplantation

Heart transplantation is indicated in children with end-stage heart disease related to cardiomyopathy or inoperable CHD. Candidates for heart transplantation are infants and children whose medical and surgical options have been exhausted and who have a 12- to 24-month life expectancy (Gabrys, 2005). Between 350 and 390 children have received a heart transplant each year since 1991 (Boucek et al., 2006). The 5-year survival rate is 75% and the 10-year rate is 65% (Gabrys, 2005).

A comprehensive evaluation is performed to determine whether the child is a candidate for heart transplant. The evaluation includes:

- Chest x-ray, electrocardiogram, echocardiogram, exercise stress test, cardiac catheterization, pulmonary function tests
- CBC with differential, prothrombin and partial thromboplastin time, serum chemistries and electrolytes, blood urea nitrogen, and creatinine
- Urinalysis and urine creatinine clearance
- Blood, throat, urine, stool, and sputum cultures for bacteria, viruses, fungi, and parasites
- Epstein-Barr virus, cytomegalovirus, varicella, herpes, hepatitis, and HIV titers
- HLA typing and panel reactive antibody typing and titer
- Computed tomography or MRI scan, electroencephalogram
- Consults with neurology, psychology, genetics, social work, nutritionist, physical and occupational therapy, and financial coordinator or case manager

Children with irreversible lung, liver, kidney, or central nervous system disease, recent malignancy (past 5 years), or chronic viral infection may be excluded as candidates.

Once candidacy is determined, the transplant center registers the child as a potential recipient with the United Network for Organ Sharing (UNOS). Blood type, body size, length of time on the waiting list, and medical urgency are used to evaluate compatibility. Children awaiting transplantation may need continuous or intermittent hospitalization. Coordination of organ procurement and the transplantation procedure is essential (Canter, 2000; Gabrys, 2005).

Surgical Procedure and Postoperative Therapeutic Management

Most transplantation procedures are **orthotopic**, which means that the recipient's heart is removed and the donor heart is implanted in its place in the normal anatomic position. Cardiopulmonary bypass and hypothermia are used to maintain circulation, protect the brain, and oxygenate the recipient during the procedure. Postoperatively, the child may have near-normal heart function and capacity for exercise and may be able to return to school.

Immunosuppressive therapy is necessary for the rest of the child's life to avoid rejection of the transplanted heart. Usually a three-drug regimen is used that includes calcineurin inhibitors (cyclosporine, tacrolimus), cell toxins (mycophenolate mofetil, azathioprine), and corticosteroids. Ongoing follow-up is provided by the cardiologist and transplant surgeon. Complications of heart transplantation include bacterial, fungal, and viral infection and heart rejection. Neoplasm may occur as a result of chronic immunosuppression.

Nursing Management

Preoperative nursing care for the child undergoing a heart transplant is similar for children undergoing other types of heart surgery. In addition, the nurse should assist with the comprehensive pretransplant evaluation. Care for the child in the post-transplant period is intense and complex. Evaluate the family's ability to perform the tasks that will be necessary. Teach families about the evaluation and transplantation process, as well as the waiting period. In the immediate preoperative period, perform a thorough history and physical examination and obtain last-minute blood work. Provide preoperative teaching similar to other cardiac surgeries. Older children, adolescents, and parents may enjoy the book *Future Conditional* by J. Hatton (1996, Yorkshire Art Circus), which was written by one of the first heart transplant survivors.

Postoperatively, provide frequent assessments and routine care for cardiac surgery patients. In addition, monitor the child closely for infection or signs of rejection. Acute rejection may be indicated by low-grade fever, fatigue, tachycardia, nausea, vomiting, abdominal pain, and decreased activity tolerance, though some children will be asymptomatic. Maintain strict handwashing techniques and isolate the child from other children with infections. Though live vaccines are contraindicated in immunosuppressed children, inactivated vaccines should be given as recommended (Centers for Disease Control and Prevention, 2006). Teach children and families that the child may return to school and usual activities about 3 months after the transplant. Provide emotional support to the child related to body image changes such as hair growth, gum hyperplasia, weight gain, moon facies, acne, and rashes that occur due to long-term immunosuppressive therapy.

■■■ Key Concepts

- At birth, when the umbilical cord is cut and the neonate's first breath occurs, the ductus venosus closes with the foramen ovale and the ductus arteriosus closes shortly thereafter. Pulmonary vascular resistance decreases and systemic vascular resistance increases.

- The infant's heart rate averages 120 to 130 beats per minute and decreases throughout childhood, reaching the adult rate in adolescence. Conversely, the infant and child's blood pressure is significantly lower than the adult's, increasing as the child ages.

- Check the infant's apical pulse prior to digoxin administration and hold the dose if the heart rate is less than 90.

- Poor weight gain, failure to thrive, and increased fatigability commonly occur with congestive heart failure.

- Clubbing of the fingernails occurs as a result of chronic hypoxia in the child with severe congenital heart disease.

- Children with cardiac conditions resulting in cyanosis often have baseline oxygen saturations that are relatively low, because of the mixing of oxygenated with deoxygenated blood.

- Document the presence of a murmur by grading its intensity (I–IV), describing where it occurs within the cardiac cycle, and noting the location where the murmur is best heard.

- Congenital heart disease should be suspected in the cyanotic newborn who does not improve with oxygen administration.

- Cardiac catheterization post-procedure care focuses on evaluation of the child's vital signs and condition of the pressure dressing, as well as assessment of the distal pulses bilaterally for presence and quality.

- Congenital heart disorders resulting in decreased pulmonary blood flow (tetralogy of Fallot, tricuspid atresia) result in cyanosis.

- Disorders with increased pulmonary blood flow (patent ductus arteriosus, atrial septal defect, and ventricular septal defect) may result in pulmonary edema if the defect is severe.

- A decrease in the lower extremity pulses or blood pressure as compared with the upper extremities may be indicative of coarctation of the aorta.

- It is important to remain calm when an infant or child demonstrates a hypercyanotic spell. Place the child in a knee-chest position, administer oxygen and/or morphine or propranolol, and supply intravenous fluids.

- Children with certain congenital heart defects and/or heart failure require additional calories in order to display adequate growth.

- Children with hypertrophic cardiomyopathy, certain congenital heart defects, valve dysfunction, or prosthetic valves require prophylaxis for infective endocarditis when undergoing procedures or invasive dental work.

- Hypertension in the child or adolescent often leads to long-term health consequences such as cardiovascular disease and left ventricular hypertrophy.

- Kawasaki disease may result in severe cardiac sequelae, so these children need ongoing cardiac follow-up to screen for development of problems.

- It is important to screen for hyperlipidemia in high-risk children.

- Abrupt cessation of chest tube output, accompanied by an increase in the heart rate and increased filling pressure, may indicate cardiac tamponade.

REFERENCES

Abdallah, H. (2006). *Pediatric cardiac testing.* Retrieved 10/3/06 from http://www.childrenheartinstitute.org/testing/testhome.htm.

Ackley, B. J., & Ladwig, G. B. (2006). *Nursing diagnosis handbook: A guide to planning care* (7th ed.). St. Louis: Mosby.

AGA Medical Corporation. (2007). *Amplatzer® septal occluder for atrial septal defect closure.* Retrieved 1/4/08 from http://www.amplatzer.com/USProducts/ASDDevices/tabid/179/Default.aspx.

American Academy of Pediatrics, National High Blood Pressure Education Program, Working Group on High Blood Pressure in Children and Adolescents. (2004). The fourth report on the diagnosis, evaluation, and treatment of high blood pressure in children and adolescents. *Pediatrics, 114*(2), 555–576.

American Heart Association. (2008a). *Bacterial endocarditis.* Retrieved 1/5/08 from http://www.americanheart.org/presenter.jhtml?identifier=4436.

American Heart Association. (2008b). Bacterial endocarditis wallet card. Retrieved 1/5/08 from http://www.americanheart.org/presenter.jhtml?identifier=3003000.

American Heart Association. (2008c). *Diseases, conditions and treatments.* Retrieved 1/5/08 from http://www.americanheart.org/presenter.jhtml?identifier=3028667.

American Heart Association. (2008d). *Youth and cardiovascular disease–statistics.* Retrieved 1/5/08 from http://www.americanheart.org/presenter.jhtml?identifier=3000943.

Armstrong, C. (2007). Practice guidelines: Cardiovascular risk reduction in children. *American Family Physician, 75*(15), 1873–1874, 1876, 1878.

Balentine, J., & Eisenhart, A. (2005). *Aortic stenosis.* Retrieved 11/19/06 from http://www.emedicine.com/emerg/topic40.htm.

Barbas, K. H., & Kelleher, D. K. (2004). Breastfeeding success among infants with congenital heart disease. *Pediatric Nursing, 30*(4), 285–289.

Beke, D. M., Braudis, N. J., & Lincoln, P. (2005). Management of the pediatric postoperative cardiac surgery patient. *Critical Care Nursing Clinics of North America, 17*(4), 405–416.

Betz, C. L., & Sowden, L. A. (2005). *Mosby pediatric nursing reference* (5th ed.). St. Louis: Mosby.

Bezold, L. I. (2006). Cardiovascular embryology. In J. A. McMillan (Ed.), *Oski's pediatrics: Principles and practice.* Philadelphia: Lippincott Williams & Wilkins.

Boucek, M. M., Waltz, D. A., Edwards, L. B., et al. (2006). Registry of the International Society for Heart and Lung Transplantation: Ninth official pediatric heart transplantation report, 2006. *Journal of Heart and Lung Transplantation, 25*, 893–903.

Bricker, J. T. (2006). Hypertension. In J. A. McMillan (Ed.), *Oski's pediatrics: Principles and practice.* Philadelphia: Lippincott Williams & Wilkins.

Broyles, B. (2006). *Case studies in pediatrics.* Clifton Park, NY: Thomson Delmar Learning.

Cannon, B. C. (2006). Abnormalities in rate and rhythm. In J. A. McMillan (Ed.), *Oski's pediatrics: Principles and practice.* Philadelphia: Lippincott Williams & Wilkins.

Canter, C. E., & American Heart Association Council on Cardiovascular Disease in the Young. (2007). Indication for heart transplantation in pediatric heart disease. *Circulation, 115*(5), 658–676.

Carpenito-Moyet, L. J. (2004). *Nursing care plans & documentation: Nursing diagnoses and collaborative problems.* Philadelphia: Lippincott Williams & Wilkins.

Chamberlain, R. S. (2006). Pediatric cardiovascular disorders. In S. M. Nettina (Ed.), *Lippincott manual of nursing practice.* Philadelphia: Lippincott Williams & Wilkins.

Cheatham, J. P. (2006). Pulmonary stenosis. In J. A. McMillan (Ed.), *Oski's pediatrics: Principles and practice.* Philadelphia: Lippincott Williams & Wilkins.

Chen, C.-W., Li, C.-Y., & Wang, J.-K. (2004). Growth and development of children with congenital heart disease. *Journal of Advanced Nursing, 47*(3), 260–269.

Chen, C.-W., Li, C.-Y., & Wang, J.-K. (2005). Self-concept: Comparison between school-aged children with congenital heart disease and normal school-aged children. *Journal of Clinical Nursing, 14,* 394–402.

Christensen, D. D., Vincente, R. N., & Campbell, R. M. (2005). Presentation of atrial septal defect in the pediatric population. *Pediatric Cardiology, 26*(6), 812–814.

Cilliers, A. M. (2006). Rheumatic fever and its management. *British Medical Journal, 333,* 1153–1156.

Connor, J. A., Arons, R. R., Figueroa, M., & Gebbie, K. M. (2004). Clinical outcomes and secondary diagnoses for infants born with hypoplastic left heart syndrome. *Pediatrics, 114*(2), e160–165. Retrieved 11/18/06 from http://www.pediatrics.org/cgi/ content/full/114/2/e160.

Couch, S. C., & Daniels, S. R. (2005). Diet and blood pressure in children. *Current Opinion in Pediatrics, 17*(5), 642–647.

Cromwell, P. F., Munn, N., & Zolkowski-Wynne, J. (2005a). Evaluation and management of hypertension in children and adolescents (part 1): Diagnosis. *Journal of Pediatric Health Care, 19*(3), 172–175.

Cromwell, P. F., Munn, N., & Zolkowski-Wynne, J. (2005b). Evaluation and management of hypertension in children and adolescents (part 2): Evaluation and management. *Journal of Pediatric Health Care, 19*(5), 309–313.

Cunningham, F. G., Leveno, K. L., Bloom, S. L., et al. (2005). *Williams obstetrics* (22nd ed.). New York: McGraw-Hill Companies.

Driscoll, D. J. (2006a). *Fundamentals of pediatric cardiology.* Philadelphia: Lippincott Williams & Wilkins.

Driscoll, D. J. (2006b). Tricuspid atresia. In J. A. McMillan (Ed.), *Oski's pediatrics: Principles and practice.* Philadelphia: Lippincott Williams & Wilkins.

Dummer, K. B., & Newburger, J. W. (2004). Acute management of Kawasaki disease. *Progress in Pediatric Cardiology, 19*(2), 129–135.

Eidem, B. W. (2006). Hypoplastic left heart syndrome. In J. A. McMillan (Ed.), *Oski's pediatrics: Principles and practice.* Philadelphia: Lippincott Williams & Wilkins.

El-Said, G. M., Baghdady, Y. M. K., & El-Said, H. G. (2006). Rheumatic fever. In J. A. McMillan (Ed.), *Oski's pediatrics: Principles and practice.* Philadelphia: Lippincott Williams & Wilkins.

El-Said, G. M., Baghdady, Y. M. K., & El-Said, H. G. (2006). Rheumatic heart disease. In J. A. McMillan (Ed.), *Oski's pediatrics: Principles and practice.* Philadelphia: Lippincott Williams & Wilkins.

Fernandes, J. R. H. (2005). The experience of a broken heart. *Critical Care Nursing Clinics of North America, 17*(4), 319–327.

Fixler, D. E. (2006). Epidemiology of congenital heart disease. In J. A. McMillan (Ed.), *Oski's pediatrics: Principles and practice.* Philadelphia: Lippincott Williams & Wilkins.

Francis, G. S., Sonnenblick, E. H., Wilson Tang, W. H., & Poole-Wilson, P. (2008). Pathophysiology of heart failure. In Fuster, V., O'Rourke, R. A., Walsh, R., Poole-Wilson, P., King, S. B., Roberts, R., Nash, I., & Prystowsky, E. N., *Hurst's the heart* (12th ed.). New York: McGraw-Hill.

Freeman, A. F. (2006). Kawasaki disease: Summary of the American Heart Association guidelines. *American Family Physician, 74*(7), 1141–1150.

Friedman, R. A., & Starke, J. R. (2006). Infective endocarditis. In J. A. McMillan (Ed.), *Oski's pediatrics: Principles and practice.* Philadelphia: Lippincott Williams & Wilkins.

Freitas-Nichols, J. (2004). Cardiovascular disorders. In C. E. Burns et al., *Pediatric primary care: A handbook for nurse practitioners* (3rd ed.). Philadelphia: W. B. Saunders.

Fulton, D. R., & Freed, M. D. (2004). The pathology, pathophysiology, recognition, and treatment of congenital heart disease. In V. Fuster, R. W. Alexander, & R. A. O'Rourke (Eds.), *Hurst's the heart* (11th ed., pp. 1785–1850). New York: McGraw-Hill Companies.

Fyfe, D. A., & Parks, W. J. (2002). Noninvasive diagnostics in congenital heart disease: Echocardiography and magnetic resonance imaging. *Critical Care Nursing Quarterly, 25*(3), 26–36.

Gabrys, C. A. (2005). Pediatric cardiac transplants: A clinical update. *Journal of Pediatric Nursing, 20*(2), 139–143.

Gidding, S. S., Dennison, B. A., Birch, L. L., et al. (2006). Dietary recommendations for children and adolescents: A guide for practitioners. *Pediatrics, 117,* 544–559.

Green, A. (2004). Outcomes of congenital heart disease: A review. *Pediatric Nursing, 30*(4), 280–284.

Greenberg, J. D., Bonwit, A. M., & Roddy, M. G. (2005). Subacute bacterial endocarditis prophylaxis: A succinct review for pediatric emergency physicians and nurses. *Clinical Pediatric Emergency Medicine, 6*(4), 266–272.

Gumbiner, C. H. (2006). Ventricular septal defect. In J. A. McMillan (Ed.), *Oski's pediatrics: Principles and practice.* Philadelphia: Lippincott Williams & Wilkins.

Hershberger, R. E. (2005). Familial dilated cardiomyopathy. *Progress in Pediatric Cardiology, 20*(2), 161–168.

Huhta, J. C. (2006). Echocardiography and electrocardiography. In J. A. McMillan (Ed.), *Oski's pediatrics: Principles and practice.* Philadelphia: Lippincott Williams & Wilkins.

Jaggi, P., & Shulman, S. T. (2006). Group A streptococcal infections. *Pediatrics in Review, 27,* 99–105.

Karch, A. M. (2008). *Lippincott's nursing drug guide.* Philadelphia: Lippincott Williams & Wilkins.

Kavey, R. E., Allada, V., Daniels, S. R., Hayman, L. L., McCrindle, B. W., Newburger, J. W., Parekh, R. S., & Steinberger, J. (2007). Cardiovascular risk reduction in high-risk pediatric patients. *Journal of Cardiovascular Nursing, 22*(3), 218–253.

Kilian, K. (2006). Left-sided obstructive congenital heart defects. *Newborn and Infant Nursing Reviews, 6*(3), 128–136.

Kopf, G. S., & Mello, D. M. (2006). Cardiovascular surgery in the newborn. In J. A. McMillan (Ed.), *Oski's pediatrics: Principles and practice.* Philadelphia: Lippincott Williams & Wilkins.

Lawoko, S., & Soares, J. J. F. (2006). Psychosocial morbidity among parents of children with congenital heart disease: A prospective longitudinal study. *Heart & Lung, 35*(5), 310–314.

Mahle, W. T., Visconti, K. J., Freier, M. C., et al. (2006). Relationship of surgical approach to neurodevelopmental outcomes in hypoplastic left heart syndrome. *Pediatrics, 117*(1), e90–97.

Marian, A. J., Brugada, R., & Roberts, R. (2004). Cardiovascular disease due to genetic abnormalities. In V. Fuster, R. W. Alexander, & R. A. O'Rourke (Eds.), *Hurst's the heart* (11th ed., pp. 1747–1733). New York: McGraw-Hill Companies.

Marino, B. S., & Fine, K. S. (2007). *Blueprints: Pediatrics* (4th ed.). Philadelphia: Lippincott Williams & Wilkins.

Maron, B. J. (2004). Hypertrophic cardiomyopathy in childhood. *Pediatric Clinics of North America, 51*(5), 1305–1346.

Martin, J. M., & Green, M. (2006). Group A streptococcus. *Seminars in Pediatric Infectious Diseases, 17*(3), 140–148.

McDonagh, J. E. (2005). Growing up and moving on: Transition from pediatric to adult care. *Pediatric Transplantation, 9*(3), 364–372.

Milan, C., & Chandran, L. (2006). What's new in Kawasaki disease? *Contemporary Pediatrics.* [electronic version]. Available at: www.contemporarypediatrics.com.

Molczan, K. (2006). Cardiac anomalies in the neonate: High index of suspicion important. *Journal of Emergency Nursing, 32,* 94–97.

Morriss, M. J. H. (2006). Coarctation of the aorta. In J. A. McMillan (Ed.), *Oski's pediatrics: Principles and practice*. Philadelphia: Lippincott Williams & Wilkins.

Mullins, C. E. (2006a). Patent ductus arteriosus. In J. A. McMillan (Ed.), *Oski's pediatrics: Principles and practice*. Philadelphia: Lippincott Williams & Wilkins.

Mullins, C. E. (2006b). Therapeutic cardiac catheterization. In J. A. McMillan (Ed.), *Oski's pediatrics: Principles and practice*. Philadelphia: Lippincott Williams & Wilkins.

Muscari, M. E. (2004). *Lippincott's review series: Pediatric nursing*. Philadelphia: Lippincott Williams & Wilkins.

Neches, W. H., Park, S. C., & Ettedgui, J. A. (2006a). Tetralogy of Fallot. In J. A. McMillan (Ed.), *Oski's pediatrics: Principles and practice*. Philadelphia: Lippincott Williams & Wilkins.

Neches, W. H., Park, S. C., & Ettedgui, J. A. (2006b). Transposition of the great arteries. In J. A. McMillan (Ed.), *Oski's pediatrics: Principles and practice*. Philadelphia: Lippincott Williams & Wilkins.

Newburger, J. W., Takahashi, M., Gerber, M. A., et al. (2004). Diagnosis, treatment and long-term management of Kawasaki disease: A statement for health professionals from the Committee on Rheumatic Fever, Endocarditis, and Kawasaki Disease, Council on Cardiovascular Disease in the Young, American Heart Association. *Pediatrics, 114*(6), 1708–1733.

Pagana, K. D., & Pagana, T. J. (2006). *Mosby's manual of diagnostic and laboratory tests* (3rd ed.). St. Louis: Mosby.

Park, M. K., Menard S. W., & Schoolfield, J. (2005). Oscillometric blood pressure standards for children. *Pediatric Cardiology, 26*(5), 601–607.

Parrillo, S. J., & Parrillo, C. V. (2006). *Rheumatic fever*. Retrieved 11/13/06 from http://www.emedicine.com/emerg/topic509.htm.

Ressel, G. W. (2004). AAP releases policy statement on the prevention of RSV infections. *American Family Physician, 69*(4), 993–994.

Rhodes, J., Curran, T. J., Camil, L., et al. (2005). Impact of cardiac rehabilitation on the exercise function of children with serious congenital heart disease. *Pediatrics, 116*(6), 1339–1345.

Roos-Hesselink, J. W., Meijboom, F. J., Spitaels, S. E. C., et al. (2004). Outcome of patients after surgical closure of ventricular septal defect at young age: Longitudinal follow-up of 22–34 years. *European Heart Journal, 25*, 1057–1062.

Rosenthal, D., Chrisant, M. R., Edens, E., et al. (2004). International Society for Heart and Lung Transplantation: Practice guidelines for management of heart failure in children. *Journal of Heart and Lung Transplantation, 23*, 1313–1333.

Rowley, A. H. (2004). The etiology of Kawasaki disease: A conventional infectious agent. *Progress in Pediatric Cardiology, 19*(2), 109–113.

Slesnick, T. C., & Kovalchin, J. P. (2006). Truncus arteriosus. In J. A. McMillan (Ed.), *Oski's pediatrics: Principles and practice*. Philadelphia: Lippincott Williams & Wilkins.

Sondheimer, H. M., Yetman, A. T., & Miyamoto, S. D. (2007). Cardiovascular diseases. In W. W. Hay, M. J. Levin, J. M. Sondheimer, & R. R. Deterding (Eds.), *Current pediatric diagnosis and treatment* (18th ed.) New York: McGraw-Hill.

Suddaby, B., & Mowery, B. (2002). Progression of congenital heart disease. *Pediatric Nursing, 28*(1), 69.

Suddaby, E. C. (2001). Contemporary thinking for congenital heart disease. *Pediatric Nursing, 27*(3), 233–238, 270.

Szkutnik, M. (2007). Use of the Amplatzer® muscular ventricular septal defect occlude for closure of perimembranous ventricular septal defects. *Heart, 93*(3), 355–358.

Taketokmo, C. K., Hodding, J. H., & Kraus, D. M. (2007). *Lexi-comp's pediatric dosage handbook* (14th ed.). Hudson, Ohio: Lexi-comp.

Taylor, M. L. (2005). Coarctation of the aorta: A critical catch for newborn well-being. *Nurse Practitioner, 30*(12), 34–44.

Towbin, J. A., & Bowles, N. E. (2006). Cardiomyopathy. In J. A. McMillan (Ed.), *Oski's pediatrics: Principles and practice*. Philadelphia: Lippincott Williams & Wilkins.

Towbin, J. A., Lowe, A. M., Colan, S. D., et al. (2006). Incidence, causes, and outcomes of dilated cardiomyopathy in children. *JAMA, 296*(15), 1867–1876.

U.S. Department of Health and Human Services. (2000). *Healthy people 2010: Understanding and improving health*. Washington, D.C.: Department of Health and Human Services.

U.S. Department of Health and Human Services, National Institutes of Health, National Heart, Lung, and Blood Institute. (2005). *The fourth report on the diagnosis, evaluation, and treatment of high blood pressure in children and adolescents (NIH Publication No. 05-5267)*. Washington, D.C.: Author.

Valente, A. M., Fleishman, C. E., & Talner, N. S. (2006). Cardiovascular disease in the newborn. In J. A. McMillan (Ed.), *Oski's pediatrics: Principles and practice*. Philadelphia: Lippincott Williams & Wilkins.

Vick, G. W., & Bezold, L. I. (2006). Defects of the atrial septum, including the atrioventricular canal. In J. A. McMillan (ed.), *Oski's pediatrics: Principles and practice*. Philadelphia: Lippincott Williams & Wilkins.

Ward, K. E. (2006). Anomalous pulmonary venous connections. In J. A. McMillan (Ed.), *Oski's pediatrics: Principles and practice*. Philadelphia: Lippincott Williams & Wilkins.

Watt, R. H. (2004). Congenital heart disease: An overview of the condition and treatment options. *Lippincott's Case Management, 9*(4), 205–208.

Webb, G. D., Smallhorn, J. F., Therrien, J., & Redington, A. N. (2005). Congenital heart disease. In D. P. Zipes, P. Libby, R. O. Bonow, & E. Braunwald. *Braunwald's heart disease: A textbook of cardiovascular medicine* (7th ed.). St. Louis: Elsevier.

Yee, C. A. (2005). Endocarditis: The infected heart. *Nursing Management, 36*(2), 25–30.

WEBSITES

National Cholesterol Education Program: http://hp2010.nhlbihin.net/ncep.htm

Congenital Heart Information Network: http://tchin.org/

American Heart Association: www.americanheart.org

Children's Heart Foundation (awareness, education, and research for children's heart disease): www.childrensheartfoundation.org

Children's Heart Institute (helps children and parents to understand the defects): www.childrenheartinstitute.org

Children's Cardiomyopathy Foundation (focused on broadening the understanding of pediatric cardiomyopathy): www.childrenscardiomyopathy.org

Pediatric Cardiomyopathy Registry: www.pcmregistry.org

Society of Pediatric Cardiovascular Nurses: www.spcnonline.com

United Network for Organ Sharing: www.unos.org

"Healthy Habits for Healthy Kids—A Nutrition and Activity Guide for Parents": www.wellpoint.com/healthy_parenting/index.html

CHAPTER WORKSHEET

MULTIPLE CHOICE QUESTIONS

1. The nurse is caring for a 5-year-old child with a congenital heart anomaly causing chronic cyanosis. When performing the history and physical examination, what is the nurse least likely to assess?

   a. Obesity from overeating.

   b. Clubbing of the nail beds.

   c. Squatting during play activities.

   d. Exercise intolerance.

2. A 2-day-old infant was just diagnosed with aortic stenosis. What is the most likely nursing assessment finding?

   a. Gallop and rales.

   b. Blood pressure discrepancies in the extremities.

   c. Right ventricular hypertrophy on ECG.

   d. Heart murmur.

3. Sam, age 11, has a diagnosis of rheumatic fever and has missed school for a week. What is the most likely cause of this problem?

   a. Previous streptococcal throat infection.

   b. History of open heart surgery at 5 years of age.

   c. Playing too much soccer and not getting enough rest.

   d. Exposure to a sibling with pneumonia.

4. The nurse is caring for a child after a cardiac catheterization. What is the nursing priority?

   a. Allow early ambulation to encourage activity participation.

   b. Check pulses above the catheter insertion site for strength and quality.

   c. Assess extremity distal to the insertion site for temperature and color.

   d. Change the dressing to evaluate the site for infection.

5. While assessing a 4-month-old infant, the nurse notes that the baby experiences a hypercyanotic spell. What is the priority nursing action?

   a. Provide supplemental oxygen by face mask.

   b. Administer a dose of IV morphine sulfate.

   c. Begin cardiopulmonary resuscitation.

   d. Place the infant in a knee-to-chest position.

CRITICAL THINKING EXERCISES

1. A baby boy was born at 26 weeks' gestation to 15-year-old unmarried parents who abuse drugs. The infant weighed 1.5 kg at birth and was diagnosed with AV canal defect and Down syndrome. Discuss some of the major issues in planning for care. Include a care plan and a list of teaching needs for the family.

2. A 4-year-old boy has parents with little education, and the child has Medicaid coverage. Another child is 7 years old and has well-educated parents with private insurance coverage. Both of these children need a heart transplant, and a heart is available that is a very good match for both children. Discuss some of the issues involved in deciding which child should receive the heart.

3. A 13-year-old boy was diagnosed with hypertension over 2 years ago. He is noncompliant with his anti-hypertensive medication regimen. He is 5 feet tall and weighs 170 pounds. His favorite activity is video games. Develop a teaching plan for this teen, providing creative approaches at the appropriate developmental level.

STUDY ACTIVITIES

1. Teach a class of sixth graders about healthy activities to prevent high cholesterol levels, hypertension, and heart disease. Use visual materials.

2. Spend the day with a nurse practitioner in the pediatric cardiology clinic. Report to the clinical group your observations about the children's quality of life, growth, and development.

3. Observe in the pediatric cardiothoracic intensive care unit or telemetry unit. Note the different cardiac rhythms displayed by children with a variety of cardiovascular disorders.

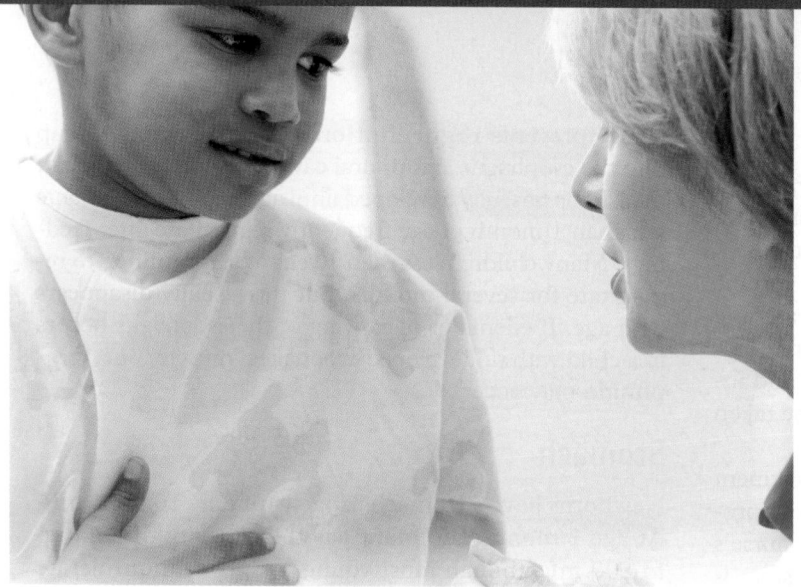

CHAPTER *41*

NURSING CARE OF THE CHILD WITH A GASTROINTESTINAL DISORDER

KEY TERMS

ALTE	dysphagia	lethargy
anal fissure	encopresis	protuberant
anastomosis	enteral	pylorus
atresia	fecal impaction	rebound tenderness
cholestasis	fibrosis	regurgitation
cirrhosis	guarding	steatorrhea
cleft	icteric	

LEARNING OBJECTIVES

Upon completion of the chapter, the learner will be able to:

1. Compare the differences in the anatomy and physiology of the gastrointestinal system between children and adults.
2. Discuss common medical treatments for infants and children with gastrointestinal disorders.
3. Discuss common laboratory and diagnostic tests used to identify disorders of the gastrointestinal tract.
4. Discuss medication therapy used in infants and children with gastrointestinal disorders.
5. Recognize risk factors associated with various gastrointestinal illnesses.
6. Differentiate between acute and chronic gastrointestinal disorders.
7. Distinguish common gastrointestinal illnesses of childhood.
8. Discuss nursing interventions commonly used for gastrointestinal illnesses.
9. Devise an individualized nursing care plan for infants/children with a gastrointestinal disorder.
10. Develop teaching plans for family/patient education for children with gastrointestinal illnesses.
11. Describe the psychosocial impact that chronic gastrointestinal illnesses have on children.

Ethan Richardson, 2 months old, is brought to the clinic by his mother. He has been vomiting for the past 3 days. His mother states she switched formula to see if that would help, but the vomiting worsened. Since last night she has attempted to feed him only Pedialyte. Mrs. Roberts says, "He can't keep anything down and he's very irritable." His weight at birth was 8 lbs 9 ounces, length 21 inches, and head circumference 37 cm. At his 2-month check-up last week he weighed 13 lbs.

Wow

Children instinctively eat to live, and the nurse can help them devour the joys that life brings.

Gastrointestinal (GI) disorders affect children of all ages. The most common result of a GI illness is dehydration, requiring fluid therapy at home or, in more extreme cases, in a hospital setting. GI illnesses range from acute to chronic problems. However, even acute, non-life-threatening illnesses (e.g., diarrhea or vomiting) can become life-threatening without proper nursing assessment and interventions. Therefore, all GI disorders should be taken seriously until symptoms are well controlled.

Patient and family education related to the treatment of GI disorders is key to preventing the illness from progressing to an emergency situation. Therefore, the nurse's knowledge of the disorders that affect the GI system is crucial. Most often, the parents or patient will contact the primary care provider in an outpatient setting to seek help. The nurse is usually the person to triage the phone call to determine the next step in the situation, which may be determining whether the patient should be managed at home, brought to the office for assessment, or sent directly to an emergency room for evaluation. The majority of GI disorders can be handled in an outpatient setting to avoid unnecessary hospitalizations, but some life-threatening problems (e.g., bowel obstruction) require emergency care in the hospital. Again, the knowledge base of the nurse is instrumental in obtaining the proper information by taking a thorough and accurate health history from the caregiver or patient.

Variations in Pediatric Anatomy and Physiology

The GI tract includes all of the structures from the mouth to the anus. The primary functions of the GI system are the digestion and absorption of nutrients and water, elimination of waste products, and secretion of various substances required for digestion. Babies are born with GI tracts that are not fully mature until age 2. Due to this immaturity, there are many differences between the digestive tract of the young child and that of the older child or adult.

Mouth

The mouth is highly vascular, making it a common entry point for infectious invaders. In addition, the infant and young child repeatedly bring objects to their mouths and explore them in that fashion. This behavior increases the infant's and young child's risk for contracting infectious agents via the mouth.

Esophagus

The esophagus provides a passageway from the mouth to the stomach for food. The lower esophageal sphincter (LES) prevents **regurgitation** of stomach contents up into the esophagus and/or oral cavity. The muscle tone of the LES is not fully developed until age 1 month, so infants less than 1 month of age frequently regurgitate after feedings. Many children less than 1 year of age continue to regurgitate for several months, but this usually disappears with age. If edema or narrowing of the esophagus occurs in a child with undeveloped esophageal muscle tone, **dysphagia** may occur.

Stomach

Newborns have a stomach capacity of only 10 to 20 mL. At age 2 months an infant has the capacity to hold up to 200 mL, though most young infants cannot tolerate 200-mL feedings. By age 16, the stomach capacity is 1,500 ml; by adulthood it is 2,000 to 3,000 mL. Hydrochloric acid, which is found in gastric contents to aid in digestion, reaches the adult level by age 6 months.

Intestines

A full-term infant has approximately 250 cm of small intestine; an adult has up to 600 cm. The small intestine is not functionally mature at birth. Fat losses may be up to 20% of intake for a newborn, as opposed to 7% for an adult. Intestinal growth occurs in rapid spurts, usually between the age of 1 and 3 years and again at 15 to 16 years. Infants who have small bowel loss during early infancy have more problems with absorption and diarrhea than adults who have the same amount of small bowel loss.

Biliary System

The liver is relatively large at birth, accounting for 5% of the infant's body weight, compared with 2% in an adult. This allows the smooth edge of the liver to be easily palpated in infancy, as much as 2 cm below the costal margin. The pancreatic enzymes all develop at certain postnatal times, not reaching adult levels until 2 years of age.

Fluid Balance and Losses

Children exhibit differences compared with adults that affect the ways that fluid volume is maintained. These differences are evident in body fluid balance and insensible fluid losses.

Body Fluid Balance

Infants and children have a proportionately greater amount of body water than do adults. Infants and young children require a larger relative fluid intake than adults and excrete a relatively greater amount of fluid. This places them at increased risk for fluid loss with illness compared to adults. Until age 2 years, the extracellular fluid makes up about half of the child's total body water. Since extracellular fluid has a larger proportion of sodium and chloride, when potential fluid-loss states occur, water loss occurs more rapidly and in larger amounts than in adults.

Insensible Fluid Losses

Fever increases fluid loss at a rate of about 7 mL/kg/24-hour period for every sustained 1°C rise in temperature. Since children become febrile with illness more readily and their fevers are higher than those of adults, infants and young children are more apt than adults to experience insensible fluid loss with fever when ill.

Fluid loss via the skin accounts for about two thirds of insensible fluid loss. Infants have a relatively larger body surface area (BSA) than older children and adults. The newborn's BSA is about two or three times greater than the adult's, and the preterm infant's is about five times greater than the adults. This places infants, especially young infants, at increased risk of insensible fluid loss as compared to older children and adults.

The basal metabolic rate in infants and children is higher than that of adults in order to support growth. This higher metabolic rate, even in states of wellness, accounts for increased insensible fluid losses and increased need for water for excretory functions. The young infant's renal immaturity does not allow the kidneys to concentrate urine as well as in older children and adults. This puts infants at particular risk for dehydration or overhydration, depending upon the circumstances.

Common Medical Treatments

There are many different forms of medical treatment for GI disorders. In the hospital setting, most medical treatments will require a physician's order. The most common treatments and medications used for GI disorders are listed in Common Medical Treatments 41.1 and Drug Guide 41.1. Both tables provide essential information about medical treatments and medications used in pediatric GI disorders. These tables should be referred to as needed while completing the remainder of the chapter.

NURSING PROCESS OVERVIEW FOR THE CHILD WITH A GI DISORDER

Nursing care of the child with a GI disorder includes nursing assessment, nursing diagnosis, planning, interventions, and evaluation. Each step of this process must be individualized for each patient. A general understanding of the GI tract and the most common disorders can help the nurse to individualize the nursing care plan.

Remember Ethan, the 2-month-old with vomiting and irritability? What additional health history and physical examination assessment information should you obtain?

Assessment

The assessment of the child with a GI disorder includes a health history, physical examination, and laboratory and diagnostic testing.

Health History

A thorough health history is very important in the assessment of a child with a GI disorder. The health history includes past history (previous illnesses/surgeries), past family history, present illness (when the symptoms began and how this differs from the patient's normal status), and how the patient's symptoms have been managed up to this point (relevant medical records/home treatments). Detailed knowledge of the past medical and surgical history of the patient may reveal bowel resection, previous intestinal infections, and dietary issues and problems. The patient's growth patterns can also be an instrumental part of the health history and may help to generate a timeline for when the current problems appeared. The family history is also extremely important in identifying common genetic/familial GI symptoms or disorders such as irritable bowel syndrome, inflammatory bowel disease, or food allergies. The history of the present illness and symptoms can often distinguish chronic problems from acute disorders. All of these pieces of the health history require descriptive questions and answers from both nurses and patients. The person providing the history must be able to provide accurate details of the health history.

Physical Examination

The physical examination of the child should be done from the least invasive part of the examination to the most invasive. It is important for the child to remain as relaxed as possible during this part of the assessment.

Inspection and Observation

Inspect and observe the child's color, hydration status, abdominal size and shape, and mental status.

Color. First observe the patient's skin, eye, and lip color. Pale skin or lips in a patient with a GI disorder may be a sign of anemia or dehydration. During liver dysfunction, the bilirubin levels can rise, causing the skin to look jaundiced (yellow). The eyes can also become **icteric**, further indicating that the liver is not functioning correctly. Inspect the abdomen for distended veins, which can indicate abdominal or vascular obstruction or distention. As in any part of a physical assessment, watch for areas of ecchymosis, which may be a sign of abuse.

Hydration Status. The child's hydration status often indicates how severe the current GI illness is. Dehydration can occur rapidly in children, especially in infants and young children. The oral mucosa should be pink and moist. Skin turgor should be elastic. Decreased turgor

(text continues on page 1332)

COMMON MEDICAL TREATMENTS 41.1 GASTROINTESTINAL DISORDERS

Treatment	Explanation	Indication	Nursing Implications
Cleansing enema	Insertion of fluid into the rectum to soften the stool and stimulate bowel activity	Fecal impaction, severe constipation	Explain procedure to child prior to enema. With multiple enemas, observe for electrolyte imbalances.
Bowel preparation	Use of highly osmotic fluids to induce severe diarrhea to cleanse the entire bowel	Preparation for colonoscopy or bowel surgery	Some children may need to have a nasogastric tube placed so they can consume the needed amounts of fluids. Observe for signs and symptoms of dehydration/ electrolyte imbalance.
Feeding tubes	Flexible tubes used for enteral feeding when the infant or child is incapable of swallowing safely or for augmenting nutrition. May be orogastric, nasogastric, gastrostomy, or jejunostomy.	Feeding difficulties, failure to thrive, gastro-esophageal reflux disease, chronic illness	Orogastric and nasogastric tubes must be checked for placement prior to each use. If required long term, use a softer, flexible tube intended for long-term use. Stomahesive or Duoderm applied to the cheek may decrease risk of skin breakdown from tape. Gastrostomy tubes vary in type. Keep insertion site clean and dry.
Intravenous therapy	Administration of fluids via a catheter that delivers electrolytes and fluids into the venous system	Dehydration, bowel rest, NPO status	Monitor intravenous site for redness, swelling, and pain. Assess urine output to evaluate hydration status.
Ostomy	A portion of the intestine is brought to the level of the skin to allow passage of stool.	Imperforate anus, gastroschisis, omphalocele, Hirschsprung's disease, necrotizing enterocolitis, Crohn's disease, ulcerative colitis	Ostomy contents may be acidic and irritate the skin. Use Stomahesive or Duoderm under the pouch to avoid tape irritation to the skin. Pouch should fit the stoma correctly. Assess stoma for pinkness and moist appearance.
Oral rehydration therapy	Administration by mouth of fluids that contain certain amounts of electrolytes and glucose to prevent dehydration and/or promote rehydration	Diarrhea, acute gastroenteritis, vomiting	Fluid administration should begin prior to the onset of dehydration. Urine output should be monitored to evaluate hydration status.
Probiotics (lactobacillus, acidophilus)	Food supplement containing dormant bacteria that when activated may alter the intestinal microflora	Treatment/prevention of diarrhea	Particularly helpful in prevention of or decreasing incidence of antibiotic-induced diarrhea.
Total parenteral nutrition (TPN)	Intravenous complete nutrition. Provides glucose, protein, lipids, vitamins, and minerals.	Long-term NPO status, swallowing difficulties, difficulties tolerating enteral feeding (short bowel syndrome, necrotizing enterocolitis)	Higher glucose and protein concentrations and solutions containing calcium require central venous access. Monitor blood glucose levels with initiation, rate changes, and discontinuation. Blood chemistries should be monitored on a regular basis.

DRUG GUIDE 41.1   Common Drugs for GI Disorders

Classification	Action/Indication	Nursing Implications
Histamine-2 blockers (ranitidine, famotidine, cimetidine, nizatidine)	Decreases histamine production, thereby reducing gastric acid secretion. Used for heartburn, esophagitis, GERD, benign duodenal or gastric ulcers.	May cause drowsiness or dizziness
Proton pump inhibitors (omeprazole, lansoprazole, esomeprazole, pantoprazole, rabeprazole)	Blocks the pump that produces gastric acids. Indicated for erosive esophagitis, symptomatic GERD, *H. pylori* eradication.	Adverse effects include headache, nausea, abdominal pain, or diarrhea.
Prokinetics (metoclopramide, cisapride)	Stimulates GI motility to help empty the stomach faster and promote intestinal motility.	Metoclopramide may have central nervous system adverse effects. Cisapride available only in limited-access protocol studies.
Antibacterials/antibiotics (metronidazole, vancomycin)	Treatment of bacterial infections of the GI tract. Used for suspected or proven bacterial infections of the GI tract, such as *C. difficile* or parasitic infections.	May cause GI upset, diarrhea. Very important to finish entire course of treatment.
Immunosuppressants (6-mercaptopurine, azathioprine)	Suppresses the immune system to keep autoimmune disorders in remission such as Crohn's disease, ulcerative colitis, autoimmune hepatitis.	Drug levels should be checked to determine drug metabolite levels and potential for hepatotoxicity or bone marrow suppression.
Stimulants (senna, docusate sodium)	Stimulates peristalsis in the large intestine to produce a bowel movement. Used to relieve constipation.	May cause cramping or diarrhea. Stool patterns should be constantly assessed.
Laxatives (polyethylene glycol, milk of magnesia, lactulose)	Softens the stool to allow for easier passage through the colon. Used to relieve constipation.	Stool patterns should be monitored. Doses may need to be readjusted frequently to find the correct dose for the patient.
Antidiarrheals (loperamide, diphenoxylate/atropine)	Decreases peristalsis, thus prolonging transit time of stool through the intestines. Indicated to treat diarrhea related to short bowel syndrome, chronic nonspecific diarrhea, irritable bowel syndrome.	May cause drowsiness or constipation
Corticosteroids (prednisone)	Acts systemically to reduce inflammation and suppress the normal immune response. Used in inflammatory bowel disease, autoimmune disorders.	Systemic adverse effects include hirsutism, osteoporosis, GI upset, cushingoid appearance, increased intraocular pressure, irritability, and personality changes. Should be taken as directed. Stopping the medication suddenly may cause adrenal insufficiency.
Antiemetics (promethazine, metoclopramide)	Acts on the central nervous system transmitters to prevent nausea and vomiting.	May have central nervous system adverse effects, such as drowsiness or irritability
Anticholinergic/antispasmodics (hyoscyamine, dicyclomine, glycopyrrolate)	Used to control abdominal spasms and cramping associated with irritable bowel syndrome, functional bowel disorders.	May cause excessive thirst or dizziness. Encourage plenty of fluids while taking these medications.
Anti-inflammatory (mesalamine, balsalazide, hydrocortisone enemas/suppositories, olsalazine, sulfasalazine)	Reduces inflammation in the colon associated with ulcerative colitis, proctitis.	Stool output should be monitored to assess for presence of oral medications (indicating poor absorption).

GERD, gastroesophageal reflux disease.

and tenting indicate dehydration. During crying, especially in infants, the absence of tears may indicate dehydration. Assess the amount of urine output the patient has had in the past 24 hours.

Abdominal Size and Shape. Inspect the size and shape of the abdomen while the child is standing and while lying supine. The abdomen should be flat when the child is supine. An especially **protuberant** abdomen suggests the presence of ascites, fluid retention, gaseous distention, or even a tumor, but many children (toddlers in particular) have a prominent "pot-bellied" abdomen as a normal variation of their anatomy. A depressed or concave abdomen could indicate a high abdominal obstruction or dehydration. Inspect the umbilicus for color, odor, discharge, inflammation, and herniation.

Mental Status. Perform a brief mental status examination of all GI patients. Mental status changes can occur in many instances, such as when ammonia levels are elevated with severe liver disease, severe dehydration, anaphylactic reactions to foods/medicines, tumors, and other metabolic disorders. Irritability and restlessness are usually the early signs of mental status changes. **Lethargy** and listlessness can occur much more rapidly in children than in adults and should be identified promptly and emergently treated.

Auscultation

As with all patients, both pediatric and adult, auscultate bowel sounds in all four quadrants. Hyperactive bowel sounds may be noted in children with diarrhea or gastroenteritis. Hypoactive or absent bowel sounds may signify an obstructive process and should be reported to the physician immediately. Absence of bowel sounds can be determined after a 5-minute period of auscultation. This can be extremely difficult to perform with children and infants, who may be uncooperative during the examination.

Percussion

Dullness or flatness is normally found along the right costal margin and 1 to 3 cm below the costal margin of the liver. The area above the symphysis pubis may be dull in young children with full bladders, which is a normal finding. Percussion of the remainder of the abdomen should reveal tympany. Note abnormal findings.

Palpation

Palpation should be reserved for last in the sequence of abdominal examination. First, lightly palpate the abdomen to assess for areas of tenderness, lesions, muscle tone, turgor, and cutaneous hyperesthesia (a finding in acute peritonitis). Then perform deep palpation from the lower quadrants upward to best feel the liver edge, which should be firm and smooth. In infants and children, palpate the liver during inspiration below the right costal margin. The

tip of the spleen may be palpated also during inspiration; it should be 1 to 2 cm below the left costal margin. Palpable kidneys, except in neonates, may indicate tumor or hydronephrosis. The sigmoid colon can be palpated in the left lower quadrant. The cecum may be felt in the right lower quadrant as a soft mass. Areas of firmness or masses may indicate tumor or stool in the abdomen.

Tenderness in the abdomen is not a normal physical finding. Right upper quadrant tenderness could indicate liver enlargement. Right lower quadrant pain, including **rebound tenderness**, can be a warning sign of appendicitis and should be reported to a physician immediately. Palpate the external inguinal canals for presence of inguinal hernias, often elicited by having the child turn the head and cough, or blow up a balloon.

Laboratory and Diagnostic Testing

Common Laboratory and Diagnostic Tests 41.1 gives information about the tests most often ordered by physicians for children with GI illnesses. Some of these tests are ordered in the hospital setting; others are done on an outpatient basis. Typically, the nurse is involved directly in specimen collection while a specifically trained person performs the diagnostic tests. Regardless of who performs the test, nurses must be familiar with preparation guidelines for the patient, how each test is performed, and normal and abnormal findings and their significance so that patient and family education may be provided. Teaching Guidelines 41.1 gives tips on collecting stool specimens.

Nursing Diagnoses, Goals, Interventions, and Evaluation

Upon completion of a thorough assessment, the nurse might identify several nursing diagnoses, including:

- Risk for deficient fluid volume
- Diarrhea
- Constipation
- Risk for impaired skin integrity
- Imbalanced nutrition: less than body requirements
- Pain
- Ineffective breathing pattern
- Risk for caregiver role strain
- Disturbed body image

After completing an assessment on Ethan, you note the following: weight 10 lbs, length 23.5 inches, head circumference 40.75 cm. Head is round with sunken anterior fontanel, eyes appear sunken, mucous membranes are dry, heart rate 158, breath sounds clear with respiratory rate of 42, positive bowel sounds in all four quadrants, difficulty palpating abdomen due to crying. Based on these assessment findings, what would your top three nursing diagnoses be for Ethan?

COMMON LABORATORY AND DIAGNOSTIC TESTS 41.1

Test	Explanation	Indication	Nursing Implications
Abdominal ultrasonography	Visualizes abdominal organs and related vessels	Abdominal pain, vomiting, pregnancy, abnormal liver tests, abdominal mass, enlarged organs on palpation	Barium decreases visualization of organs on ultrasound.
Abdominal x-ray (KUB)	Plain x-ray of the abdomen without contrast media	Constipation, abdominal pain, abdominal distention, ascites, foreign body, palpable mass	Usually ordered as flat and upright to allow for free air and fluid levels in the bowel to be detected.
Amylase (serum)	An enzyme that changes starch to sugar, which enters the blood with inflammation of the pancreas	Acute pancreatitis, pancreatic trauma, acute cholecystitis	Increased levels are seen after 3 to 6 hours of the onset of abdominal pain.
Barium enema	After instillation of barium, fluoroscopically allows visualization of the colon	Constipation, rectal prolapse, bleeding, suspected intussusception	Bowel preparation prior to examination may be ordered. Stool will be light-colored due to barium for a few days.
Electrolytes (serum)	Sodium, potassium, CO_2, chloride, blood urea nitrogen (BUN), creatinine	To determine extent of dehydration	BUN and creatinine may be elevated with dehydration. Sodium, potassium, chloride, and CO_2 levels can be greatly affected with dehydration.
Barium swallow/ upper GI series	Visualizes the form, position, mucosal folds, peristaltic activity, and motility of the esophagus, stomach, and upper GI tract	Foreign body ingestion, abdominal pain, vomiting, dysphagia, malrotation	Females of reproductive age must be screened for pregnancy. Infants may need to be given barium via syringe.
Small bowel series	Done in conjunction with upper GI series to visualize the small intestine contour, position, and motility	Suspected inflammatory bowel disease (bowel wall thickening), intussusception	Very important to encourage large amounts of water/fluids after test to avoid barium-induced constipation.
Endoscopic retrograde cholangio-pancreatography (ERCP)	A fiberoptic endoscope is used to view the hepato-biliary system by instilling contrast to outline the pancreatic and common bile ducts.	Pancreatitis, jaundice, pancreatic tumors, common duct stones, biliary tract disease	Monitor for infection, urinary retention, cholangitis, or pancreatitis after the procedure. Done only occasionally in children.
Esophageal manometry	Tests the esophagus for normal contractile activity and effectiveness of swallowing by measure-ment of intraluminal pres-sures and acid sensors	Abnormal esophageal muscle function, dysphagia, chest pain of unknown cause, esophagitis, vomiting	Often done in conjunction with pH probe. The manometric catheter is placed through the nose into the esophagus. May cause nasal irritation/sore throat.
Esophageal pH probe	A single- or double-channeled probe placed into the esophagus to monitor the pH of the contents that are regurgi-tated into the esophagus from the stomach	Vomiting, gastroesophageal reflux, correlation of symp-toms to gastroesophageal reflux events and high risk for problems, as in asthma, apparent life-threatening event, sinusitis, or choking/gagging episodes	24-hour study is most accurate. Special diet during study is often used. Accurate diary of symptoms and feedings dur-ing the study is essential. May cause nasal irritation/sore throat.

(continued)

COMMON LABORATORY AND DIAGNOSTIC TESTS 41.1 (continued)

Test	Explanation	Indication	Nursing Implications
Gastric emptying scan	Assesses the rate at which the stomach empties food into the small intestine by adding isotopes to food and visualizing with scans	Unexplained nausea, vomiting, diarrhea, abdominal cramping	Medications may alter gastric emptying times. Crying or stress during the examination may cause delay in emptying and should be documented.
Hemoccult	Checks for occult blood in the stool	Crohn's disease, ulcerative colitis, malabsorption syndromes, diarrhea, abdominal pain	Indicates bleeding in the GI tract.
Hepatobiliary scan (HIDA scan)	Visualizes the gallbladder and determines patency of the biliary system by use of a radionuclide. The amount of radionuclide ejected from the gallbladder (ejection fraction) is calculated.	Differentiate between biliary atresia and neonatal hepatitis; assess liver trauma, right upper quadrant pain, and congenital malformations	Intravenous line will be established to give radionuclide. Pain during injection should be assessed and documented.
Lactose tolerance test	After ingesting lactose, this tests the hydrogen levels in the breath, which will increase with lactose build-up in the intestines.	Postprandial diarrhea, gassiness, bloating, abdominal pain	May produce similar symptoms during the test itself. A positive test will require diet modification and education regarding lactose intolerance.
Lipase (serum)	An enzyme that changes fat to fatty acids and glycerol appearing in the blood with pancreatic change	Pancreatitis, pancreatic carcinoma, cholecystitis, peritonitis	Lipase levels stay elevated longer with acute pancreatitis.
Liver biopsy	A test done to evaluate the microscopic hepatic structures	Hyperbilirubinemia, jaundice, chronic liver disease, hepatitis	Monitor after procedure for bleeding complications; must maintain strict bed rest for up to 8 hours.
Liver function tests (LFTs) (AST/ ALT/ GGT)	Enzymes that have high concentrations in the liver	Elevations may indicate the severity of liver disease.	May be affected by drugs or viral illnesses
Lower endoscopy (colonoscopy)	Allows visualization and biopsies of the lower GI tract from the anus to the terminal ileum with a fiberoptic instrument	Rectal bleeding, lower abdominal pain, suspected tumors or strictures, foreign body removal	The child must undergo a bowel cleansing prior to the examination. Encourage fluids to prevent dehydration. Conscious sedation or anesthesia care; monitor for possible complications of perforation, bleeding, increased abdominal pain.
Meckel's scan	A gamma camera is used to identify gastric mucosa seen in the distal portion of the ileum after injection of radiopharmaceuticals.	Rectal bleeding, anemia, used only to identify a Meckel's diverticulum	Gloves are worn by nurse during and after scan when radiopharmaceuticals are given.
Oropharyngeal motility study (OPMS)	A study done with different textures to evaluate the dynamics of swallowing and reveal transient abnormalities	Dysphagia, recurrent aspiration	Usually done in combination with therapists and nutritionist.
Rectal suction biopsy	Biopsy is taken of the rectum at different levels to assess for the presence of ganglion cells.	Absence of ganglion cells indicates Hirschsprung's disease.	Infants/children should be assessed for rectal bleeding after examination.

Test	Explanation	Indication	Nursing Implications
Stool culture	Stool is smeared on culture medium and assessed for growth of bacteria over a period of days.	To determine bacterial cause of diarrhea	Requires minimum of 48 hours for growth, several days to weeks in some cases. Can be done with a small amount of stool.
Stool for ova and parasites (O&P)	Checks for the presence of parasites or their eggs in the stool	To determine cause of diarrhea or abdominal pain	Requires about 2 tablespoons of stool.
Upper endoscopy (EGD)	Allows visualization and biopsies of the upper GI tract (mouth to upper jejunum) with a fiberoptic instrument	Dysphagia, foreign body removal, epigastric/abdominal pain, suspected celiac disease	Conscious sedation or anesthesia care; monitor for complications of perforation/bleeding.
Urea breath test	Used to detect the presence of *Helicobacter pylori* in the exhaled breath	*Helicobacter pylori* infection	Patient must not take proton pump inhibitors for 5 days, all antibiotic therapy and Pepto-Bismol for 14 days.

From Pagana & Pagana, 2006.

Nursing goals, interventions, and evaluation for the child with a GI disorder are based on the nursing diagnoses. Nursing Care Plan 41.1 can be used as a guide in planning nursing care for the child with a GI disorder. The nursing care plan should be individualized based on the patient's symptoms and needs. Refer to Chapter 35 for detailed information about pain management. Additional information will be included later in the chapter as it relates to specific disorders.

B̸ased on your top three nursing diagnoses for Ethan, describe appropriate nursing interventions.

Stool Diversions

Children may undergo stool diversions for a variety of GI disorders. Surgical procedures involve the creation of an ostomy, primarily an *ileostomy* or *colostomy,* by bringing a portion of the small or large intestine to the surface of the abdomen (Fig. 41.1).

Ostomy pouches are worn over the ostomy site to collect stool. The pouch must be of an appropriate size and it should fit around the stoma properly (Fig. 41.2). The pouch may be tucked inside the diaper or underwear or angled to fit outside of the diaper/underwear. Contemporary pouches cannot be seen under most clothing because they are designed to lie flat against the body. Avoid tight or constricting clothing around the stoma site. Teach families to store ostomy supplies in a cool, dry place. Educate parents to inform school staff that the child should be allowed to use the water fountain and the bathroom without restriction, and the school nurse should have extra ostomy supplies available.

Ostomy care for a child can be challenging due to the child's normal growth and development as well as activity. Empty the ostomy pouch and measure for stool output several times per day. The stool may be semisolid to very liquid in consistency depending on the location of the stoma. Liquid stool output can be acidic, causing irritation

(text continues on page 1338)

TEACHING GUIDELINES 41.1

Stool Specimen Collection Variations

- If the child is in diapers, use a tongue blade to scrape a specimen into the collection container.
- If the child has runny stool, a piece of plastic wrap in the diaper may catch the stool specimen. Very liquid stool may require application of a urine bag to the anal area to collect the stool.
- The older ambulatory child may first urinate in the toilet, and then the stool specimen may be retrieved from the new or clean collection container that fits under the seat at the back of the toilet.
- For the bedridden child, collect the stool specimen from a clean bedpan (do not allow urine to contaminate the stool specimen).
- Send the specimen to the laboratory immediately for accuracy of results.

Nursing Care Plan 41.1

OVERVIEW FOR THE CHILD WITH A GI DISORDER

NURSING DIAGNOSIS: Fluid volume, risk for deficit: risk factors may include excessive losses through vomiting or diarrhea, inadequate oral intake, possible NPO status (particularly in the surgical client)

Outcome Identification and Evaluation

Child will maintain adequate fluid volume as evidenced by *elastic skin turgor; moist, pink oral mucosa; presence of tears; urine output 1 mL/kg/hr or more.*

Intervention: Maintaining Fluid Balance

- Maintain IV line and administer IV fluid as ordered *to maintain fluid volume.*
- Offer small amounts of oral rehydration solution frequently *to maintain fluid volume. Small amounts are usually well tolerated by children with diarrhea and vomiting.*
- When symptoms have lessened or resolved, reintroduce regular diet *to reduce number of stools, provide adequate nutrition, and shorten duration of effects of illness.*
- Avoid high-carbohydrate fluids such as Kool-aid and fruit juice, *as they are low in electrolytes, and increased simple carbohydrate consumption can decrease stool transit time.*
- Assess hydration status (skin turgor, oral mucosa, presence of tears) every 4 to 8 hours *to evaluate maintenance of adequate fluid volume.*
- Assess adequacy of urine output *to assess end-organ perfusion.*
- Maintain strict intake and output record and weigh child daily *to evaluate effectiveness of rehydration.*
- Weigh child daily: *accurate weight is one of the best indicators of fluid volume status in children.*
- Discourage milk products and fluids that contain high levels of sugar during the acute phase of illness, *as these products may worsen diarrhea.*

NURSING DIAGNOSIS: Diarrhea; may be related to inflammation of small intestines, presence of infectious agents or toxins, possibly evidenced by loose liquid stools, hyperactive bowel sounds, or abdominal cramping

Outcome Identification and Evaluation

Child will experience decrease in diarrhea: *will have bulkier stool as per normal routine.*

Intervention: Relieving Diarrhea

- Maintain clear liquid diet no longer than 24 hours, *as prolonged clear liquids will result in continued liquid ("starvation") stools.*
- Avoid milk products until diarrhea improves: *temporary poor absorption from villus injury follows viral diarrhea.*
- Encourage complex carbohydrate foods *to bulk up the stools.*
- Add fat to carbohydrates *to increase intestinal transit time to encourage water absorption (bulks up stool).*

NURSING DIAGNOSIS: Constipation, related to GI obstructive lesions, pain on defecation, diagnostic procedures, inadequate toileting, or behavioral stool holding, possibly evidenced by change in character or frequency of stools, feeling of abdominal or rectal fullness or pressure, changes in bowel sounds, and abdominal distention

Outcome Identification and Evaluation

Child will experience improvement in constipation *by passing daily soft bowel movement without pain or straining.*

Intervention: Relieving Constipation

- Palpate for abdominal distention, percuss for dullness, and auscultate for bowel sounds *to assess for signs of constipation.*
- Encourage adequate fluid intake *to soften the stool.*
- Administer medications as ordered *to keep stool moving on daily basis.*
- Encourage activity as tolerated: *immobility contributes to constipation.*
- The child with stool withholding should sit on the toilet twice daily, preferably after breakfast and dinner, *to maximize chances for successful stool passage by taking advantage of the gastrocolic reflex.*
- For behavioral stool holding, use rewards or stickers *to encourage appropriate toileting.*

Nursing Care Plan 41.1 (continued)

NURSING DIAGNOSIS: Skin integrity, risk for impaired: risk factors include frequent loose stools, poor nutritional status, presence of stoma, acidic gastric contents contact with skin if gastrostomy present

Outcome Identification and Evaluation
Infant's skin will remain intact: *buttocks skin will be free from rash, excoriation.*
In the child with an ostomy: skin surrounding stoma will remain intact: *free from redness, rash, excoriation.*

Intervention: Maintaining Skin Integrity
- Change diapers frequently *to limit acidic stool content contact with skin.*
- Use barrier diaper cream *to protect skin.*
- Assess skin integrity at every diaper change *to recognize skin changes early so that corrective measures can begin.*
- Leave diaper area open to air several times a day if redness is present *so that air can circulate and skin healing can be facilitated.*
- Use plain water or only mild soap to cleanse the skin with diaper changes *to avoid pH changes that contribute to diaper area skin breakdown.*
- Avoid diaper wipes that contain fragrance or alcohol if the skin is red or has a rash, *as both alcohol and perfume cause stinging if used on non-intact skin and can worsen skin breakdown.*

For the child with an ostomy:
- Ensure proper fit of the ostomy appliance/pouch *to avoid acidic stool contact with skin.*
- Use a barrier wafer (e.g., Stomahesive or Duoderm) to attach appliance: *avoids repeated pulling of adhesive tape from skin.*
- If redness occurs, use barrier/healing cream or paste on skin around stoma *to promote healing and prevent further skin breakdown.*
- Consult enterostomal therapy nurse as needed *to provide additional support.*

NURSING DIAGNOSIS: Nutrition: imbalanced, less than body requirements; may be related to inability to ingest, digest, or absorb nutrients; intestinal pain after eating; decreased transit time through bowel; or psychosocial factors, possibly evidenced by lack of appropriate weight gain or growth, weight loss, aversion to eating, poor muscle tone, or observed lack of intake

Outcome Identification and Evaluation
Nutritional status will be maximized: *child will maintain or gain weight appropriately.*

Intervention: Maintaining Appropriate Nutrition
- Encourage favorite foods (within prescribed diet restrictions if present) *to maximize oral intake.*
- Administer enteral tube feedings as ordered *to maximize caloric intake.*
- Add butter, gravy, cheese as appropriate to foods (if allowed within diet restrictions) *to increase caloric intake.*
- Encourage high-quality, high-calorie snacks between meals, *so as not to interfere with meal intake.*
- Document response to feeding *to determine feeding tolerance.*
- Limit intake of calorie-free beverages: *beverages should contain nutrients and calories.*
- Consult nutritionist *for appropriate diet supplementation recommendations.*

NURSING DIAGNOSIS: Breathing pattern, ineffective, related to postoperative immobility, abdominal pain interfering with breathing, use of narcotic analgesics as evidenced by increased work of or shallow breathing, tachypnea, decrease lung aeration

Outcome Identification and Evaluation
Child will demonstrate effective breathing pattern: *respiratory rate normal for age, absence of accessory muscle use, adequate aeration with clear breath sounds throughout all lung fields.*

Intervention: Promoting Effective Breathing Patterns
- Turn, cough, deep breathe every 2 hours *to encourage adequate aeration and discourage fluid pooling in lungs.* In the infant or toddler, turn every 2 hours and use percusser or chest physiotherapy *to prevent pooling of secretions.*
- Play games to encourage deep breathing (blow out penlight, blow cotton ball across bedside table with straw, etc.): *children are more likely to cooperate with interventions if play is involved.*
- In the developmentally able child, encourage incentive spirometer use every 2 hours *to improve lung aeration.*
- Demonstrate/encourage use of pillow splinting with coughing *to decrease abdominal pain and stress on incision.*

(continued)

Nursing Care Plan 41.1 (continued)

NURSING DIAGNOSIS: Caregiver role strain, risk for: risk factors may include infant with congenital defect, child with chronic illness, marginal caregiver coping patterns, long-term stress, complexity and quantity of care child requires

Outcome Identification and Evaluation
Caregiver will exhibit emotional health: *verbalizes concerns calmly, participates in child's care, and demonstrates knowledge of resources.*

Intervention: Easing Caregiver Role Strain
- Assess parental behavior *to identify role strain.*
- Provide emotional support and encourage talking about feelings, fears, and concerns: *to promote trust in nurse as a source of emotional support.*
- Arrange for and/or encourage respite care for child: *provides parent with time away from continual care.*
- Consult social services *to identify community resources available for caregiver support (home health, support group, etc.).*
- Encourage parent to meet own needs and find personal time *to increase energy level and self-esteem, ultimately enhancing the quality of care given.*

NURSING DIAGNOSIS: Body image disturbance; may be related to presence of stoma, loss of control of bowel elimination, scars from multiple surgical procedures, or effects of treatment regimen, possibly evidenced by verbalization of negative feelings about body, refusal to look at stoma or participate in care

Outcome Identification and Evaluation
Child or teen will demonstrate acceptance of change in body image *by verbalization of adjustment; looking at, touching, caring for body; returning to previous social involvement.*

Intervention: Promoting Proper Body Image
- Observe child's coping mechanisms *to reinforce their use in times of stress.*
- Acknowledge denial, anger, and other feelings as normal *to support child/teen through difficult transition.*
- Allow child gradual introduction to stoma *to ease transition.*
- Encourage child/teen to participate in care, *as this sense of control will contribute to positive self-esteem.*

---

and severe burn-like areas on the surrounding skin, so special attention to skin care around the ostomy site is essential. Products such as powders and pastes are available to help protect the skin.

The stoma should be moist and pink or red, demonstrating proper circulation to the intestine (Fig. 41.3).

Immediately notify the physician if the stoma is not moist and pink or red. Also notify the provider if the volume of stool output is greatly increased, or if the stoma is prolapsed or retracted.

Perform ostomy care as needed; pouches usually need to be changed every 1 to 4 days. The word "stoma"

Colostomy   Ileostomy

FIGURE 41.1 A colostomy is a stoma from the colon; an ileostomy is a stoma from the ileum.

FIGURE 41.2 Ensure that the ostomy pouch fits closely around the stoma to prevent irritation of the surrounding skin.

can be used as a mnemonic for the steps for changing an ostomy pouch. See Nursing Procedure 41.1.

Structural Anomalies of the GI Tract

Structural anomalies of the GI tract include cleft lip and palate, omphalocele and gastroschisis, hernias (inguinal and umbilical), and anorectal malformations.

▶ CLEFT LIP AND PALATE

Cleft lip and palate (Fig. 41.4) is the most common congenital craniofacial anomaly, occurring once in every 500–550 births (Tolarova & Oh, 2006). It occurs frequently in association with other anomalies and has been identified in more than 300 syndromes. The most com-

FIGURE 41.3 The healthy stoma is pink and moist.

Nursing Procedure 41.1

PERFORMING OSTOMY CARE

1. **S**et up the equipment:
   - Warm, wet washcloths or paper towels
   - Clean pouch and clamp
   - Skin barrier powder, paste, and/or sealant
   - Pencil or pen
   - Scissors
   - Pattern to measure stoma size
2. **T**ake off the pouch (may need to use adhesive remover or wet washcloth to ease pouch removal).
3. **O**bserve the stoma and surrounding skin. Clean the stoma and skin as needed, allowing it to dry thoroughly.
4. **M**easure the stoma, mark the new pouch backing, and cut the new backing to size.
5. **A**pply the new pouch.

Adapted from Children's Healthcare of Atlanta. (2004). *Ostomy care homecare manual.*

---

mon anomalies associated with cleft lip and palate include heart defects, ear malformations, skeletal deformities, and genitourinary abnormality.

Complications of cleft lip and palate include feeding difficulties, altered dentition, delayed or altered speech development, and otitis media. The infant with cleft lip may have difficulty forming an adequate seal around a nipple in order to create the necessary suction for feeding and may also experience excessive air intake. Gagging, choking, and nasal regurgitation of milk may occur in babies with cleft palate. Excessive feeding time, inadequate intake, and fatigue contribute to insufficient growth. Primary or permanent teeth may be missing, malformed, or unusually positioned. Children with cleft palate may have slight delays in speech development, a nasal quality to the speech, and difficulty saying certain consonants correctly. The opening in the cleft palate contributes to build-up of fluid in the middle ear (otitis media with effusion), which can lead to an acute infection (acute otitis media). Long-lasting otitis media with effusion leads to temporary and sometimes permanent hearing loss.

Pathophysiology

Development of the **cleft** occurs early in pregnancy. The tissue that forms the lip ordinarily fuses by 5 to 6 weeks of gestation, and the palate closes between 7 and 9 weeks of gestation. Therefore, if either the lip or palate does not fuse, then the infant is born with a cleft. Cleft lip or cleft palate may occur in isolation from one another, but 30% of infants born with cleft lip also have cleft palate (March of Dimes, 2008). The cleft may be unilateral (the left side is affected more often) or bilateral.

A   **B**

FIGURE 41.4 (**A**) The cleft lip may extend all the way through the vermilion border and up into the nostril, or it may be significantly smaller. (**B**) The cleft palate may be a small opening or may involve the entire palate.

Therapeutic Management

Babies with cleft lip and palate are usually managed by a specialized team that may include a plastic surgeon or craniofacial specialist, oral surgeon, dentist or orthodontist, prosthodontist, psychologist, otolaryngologist, nurse, social worker, audiologist, and speech-language pathologist. Many children's hospitals offer these services in one location, such as a craniofacial specialty center. Historically, cleft lip has been repaired surgically around the age of 2 to 3 months and cleft palate at 9 to 18 months, but in recent years institutions with an experienced craniofacial team have successfully repaired clefts in the neonatal period. Early repair of the cleft lip restores a normal appearance to the child's face and may improve parent–infant bonding. Regardless of the timing of the surgical repair, however, surgical revision of the palate may be required as the child grows.

Nursing Assessment

For a full description of the assessment phase of the nursing process refer to page 1329. Assessment findings pertinent to cleft lip and palate are discussed below.

Health History

For the newborn, explore pregnancy history for risk factors for development of cleft lip and palate, which include:

• Maternal smoking
• Prenatal infection
• Advanced maternal age
• Use of anticonvulsants, steroids, and other medications during early pregnancy

When an infant or child with cleft lip or palate returns for a clinic visit or hospitalization, inquire about feeding difficulties, respiratory difficulties, speech development, and otitis media.

Physical Examination

Observe the infant for the presence of the characteristic physical appearance of cleft lip. The cleft may involve the lip only or extend up into the nostril (Fig. 41.5). Cleft palate may be visualized on examination of the mouth. Palpate with a gloved finger to discover mild clefts.

Laboratory and Diagnostic Tests

Cleft lip may be diagnosed by prenatal ultrasound, but it is diagnosed most commonly at birth by the classic physical appearance.

Nursing Management

Refer to the Nursing Care Plan 41.1 for nursing diagnoses and interventions related to airway maintenance, pain alleviation, fluid balance promotion, and restoration of

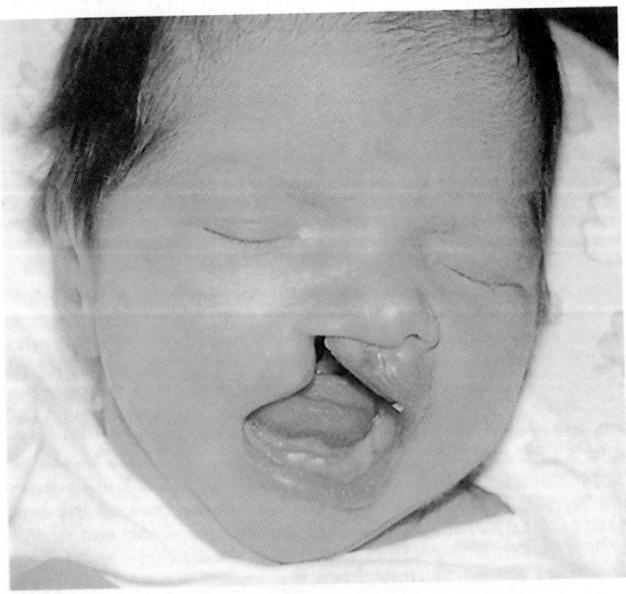

FIGURE 41.5 Cleft lip.

family processes. These should be individualized for the particular situation. In addition to the nursing diagnoses and related interventions discussed in the Nursing Care Plan, interventions common to cleft lip and palate follow.

Preventing Injury to the Suture Line

It is critical to prevent injury to the facial suture line or to the palatal operative sites. Do not allow the infant to rub the facial suture line. To prevent this, position the infant in a supine or side-lying position. It may be necessary to use arm restraints to stop the hands from touching the face or entering the mouth. Clean the suture line as ordered by the surgeon. Possible care options include using petroleum jelly on the facial suture line or a lip-protective device such as a Logan bow (curved thin metal apparatus) or a butter-fly adhesive, both of which protect and maintain the suture line. Protect the palate operative site. Avoid putting items in the mouth that might disrupt the sutures (e.g., suction catheter, spoon, straw, pacifier, or plastic syringe).

Prevent vigorous or sustained crying in the infant, because this may cause tension on either suture line. Ways to prevent crying include administering medications as needed for pain and providing other comfort or distraction measures, such as cuddling, rocking, and anticipation of needs.

Promoting Adequate Nutrition

Preoperatively, the baby with a cleft lip may demonstrate enhanced growth patterns if breastfed. The contour of the breast against the lip may allow for a better seal to be maintained for adequate sucking. Some infants will be fed with a special cleft lip nipple (Fig. 41.6). Parent and surgeon preference will determine the method of feeding. Burp the infant well to expel excess air taken in during difficulty with sucking.

The infant with cleft palate is at risk for aspiration with oral feeding. In some instances a prosthodontic device may be created to form a false palate covering. This device may prevent breast milk or formula from being aspirated. Breastfeeding may be effective in the infant with cleft palate due to the pliability of the breast and the fact that breast tissue may cover the opening in the palate. Post-operatively, some surgeons allow breastfeeding to be resumed almost immediately. In the bottle-fed infant special nipples or feeders may have to be used. When the suture line is healed, ordinary feeding may resume.

Encouraging Infant–Parent Bonding

For some parents, the appearance of a cleft lip is appalling. Encourage parents to hold the medically stable infant immediately after delivery to encourage bonding. Acknowledge normal feelings of guilt, anger, and sadness. Support the parents in providing care for the infant, particularly feeding, which is a viewed as a significant nurturing function. Provide education about the anticipated surgical procedure and eventual normal appearance of the child's lip.

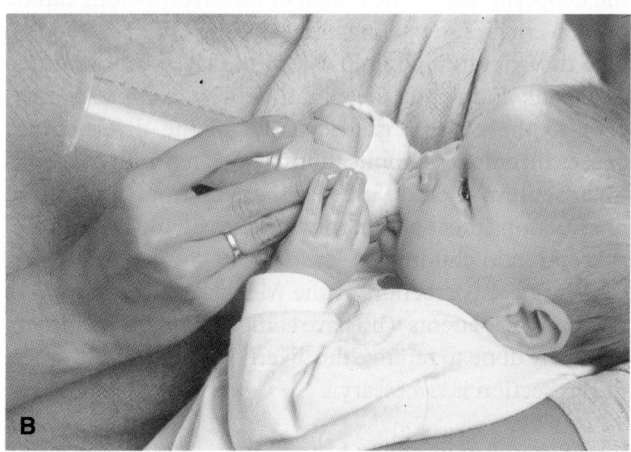

FIGURE 41.6 (**A**) Specialty feeding devices used for infants with cleft lip and cleft palate. (**B**) An infant uses a Haberman Feeder.

Providing Emotional Support

Many families will benefit from support in addition to that received from the craniofacial team. Refer parents to the Cleft Palate Foundation (www.cleftline.org) or a parent-to-parent support network such as www.cleft.org. See Healthy People 2010.

HEALTHY PEOPLE 2010	
Objective	Nursing Significance
Increase the number of states and the District of Columbia that have a system for recording and referring infants and children with cleft lips, cleft palates, and other craniofacial anomalies to craniofacial anomaly rehabilitative teams.	• Ensure that your office, clinic, or hospital participates in such a system. • If it does not, advocate for such participation.

▶ MECKEL'S DIVERTICULUM

Meckel's diverticulum is the result of an incomplete fusion of the omphalomesenteric duct during embryonic development. This causes a fibrous band to connect the small intestine to the umbilicus, known as a Meckel's diverticulum (Fig. 41.7). It is the most common congenital anomaly of the GI tract. The risk of complications from Meckel's diverticulum decreases with advancing age, and most affected patients remain asymptomatic. Thus, infants under the age of 1 year are at the greatest risk for complications (21%). The disorder is more common in males than females (Wyllie, 2004d).

The location of a Meckel's diverticulum is on the anterior mesenteric border of the ileum, 40 to 90 cm from the ileocecal valve. The length of the diverticulum can be up to 5 cm and the diameter up to 2 cm (Wyllie, 2004d). The diverticulum contains all of the layers of the intestinal wall, and peptic ulceration of the ileal mucosa adjacent to the ectopic gastric tissue of the diverticulum causes bleeding. Complications associated with Meckel's diverticulum include bleeding, anemia, and intestinal obstruction (most commonly seen as volvulus and intussusception in children).

Surgical correction of the Meckel's diverticulum is necessary in patients who have complications. The surgery is usually done to remove the diverticulum itself. At times, ileal resection is necessary.

Nursing Assessment

For a full description of the assessment phase of the nursing process refer to page 1329. Assessment findings pertinent to Meckel's diverticulum are discussed below.

FIGURE 41.7 A Meckel's diverticulum is usually found within 100 cm of the ileocecal valve.

Health History

Elicit a description of the present illness and chief complaint. Common signs and symptoms reported during the health history might include:

- Bleeding
- Anemia
- Severe colicky abdominal pain (in children with associated intestinal obstruction)

Physical Examination

Assess the child for an acute abdomen. Observe for abdominal distention, palpate for an abdominal mass, assess for abdominal **guarding** and rebound tenderness, and auscultate for hypoactive bowel sounds.

Laboratory and Diagnostic Tests

Common laboratory and diagnostic tests ordered for assessment of Meckel's diverticulum include:

- Abdominal x-rays to rule out an acute obstructive process
- Meckel's scan (conclusive)
- Stool tests for color, consistency, and occult blood (usually positive in Meckel's diverticulum)
- Complete blood count (CBC) to assess for anemia

Nursing Management

If anemia is significant, administer ordered blood products (packed red blood cells) to stabilize the patient before surgery. Administer intravenous fluids and maintain NPO status for symptomatic patients while further evaluation is being performed. Immediately report an acute abdomen to a physician. Postoperative care will vary depending on the surgery that was performed. Provide patient and family education as necessary to relieve anxiety related to the diagnosis and surgical intervention. Refer to the Nursing Care Plan 41.1 for additional information.

▶ INGUINAL AND UMBILICAL HERNIAS

Inguinal and umbilical hernias are defects that occur during fetal development. They are one of the most common reasons why infants and children are referred to pediatric surgeons.

Inguinal Hernia

Inguinal hernias occur 9 times more frequently in boys than in girls. Premature infants are particularly susceptible, and 5% have inguinal hernias. Boys are 3 to 10 times more likely to have an inguinal hernia than girls (Sondheimer, 2007). In most cases of inguinal hernia, the processus vaginalis fails to completely close, which then allows the abdominal or pelvic viscera to enter the patent processus and travel through the internal inguinal ring into the inguinal canal. The hernia sacs that develop most often contain bowel in males and fallopian tubes or ovaries in females. Surgical correction of the inguinal hernia is usually performed when the infant is several weeks old and has been thriving.

Nursing Assessment

Assess infants and children with an inguinal hernia for the presence of a bulging mass in the lower abdomen or groin area (Fig. 41.8). It may be possible to visualize the mass, but often the mass is seen only during crying or straining, making it difficult to actually identify in the clinic setting.

Nursing Management

If a mass is felt upon palpation, the physician may attempt to reduce the hernia by pushing it back through the external inguinal ring. The nurse may be asked to help assist in a reduction, most likely helping to hold the child in a position that will allow the physician to reduce the hernia. If reduction is not possible even with patient sedation, the hernia could be incarcerated. An incarcerated hernia could eventually lead to bowel strangulation.

FIGURE 41.8 (**A**) Inguinal hernia: note the bulge in the inguinal (groin) area. (**B**) Umbilical hernia: note the protrusion in the umbilical area.

Reduction is only a temporary method of managing inguinal hernias; they must be corrected surgically. The hernia should be manually reduced as needed until the time of the surgery, so teach the family how to reduce the hernia. Instruct the family to contact the surgeon immediately if the hernia becomes irreducible. Routine pre- and postoperative care is expected during inguinal hernia surgical repair. Provide patient and family education to relieve anxiety.

> ▶ **Take** NOTE!
>
> Tell the parents that if the child's inguinal hernia becomes hard, discolored, or painful (inconsolable crying), they should immediately call the physician to determine the next course of action (office visit or emergency room visit).

Umbilical Hernia

Umbilical hernia occurs commonly in preterm infants and much more frequently in African-Americans than Caucasians (Sondheimer, 2007). An umbilical hernia is caused by an incomplete closure of the umbilical ring, allowing intestinal contents to herniate through the opening. Unlike inguinal hernias, most umbilical hernias are not corrected surgically. Most children will have spontaneous closure of the umbilical hernia by age 5. Surgical correction is necessary only for the largest umbilical hernias that have failed to close by age 5 years.

Nursing Assessment

Assess whether the hernia can be reduced. Notify the surgeon if the hernia will not reduce. Incarceration is extremely rare, but when it does occur, the child will report abdominal pain, tenderness, or redness at the umbilicus (see Fig. 41.8).

Nursing Management

Since operative repair is not as likely with umbilical hernias as with inguinal hernias, the aim of nursing management is education. Teach the patient and family how to reduce the hernia. The child may have some self-esteem issues related to the large protrusion of the unrepaired umbilical hernia. Teach the child coping skills to help relieve anxiety.

> ▶ **Take** NOTE!
>
> The use of home remedies to reduce an umbilical hernia should be discouraged because of the risk of bowel strangulation. This includes taping a quarter over a reduced umbilical hernia and the use of "belly bands."

▶ ANORECTAL MALFORMATIONS

Imperforate anus is a congenital malformation of the anorectal opening. The defect is identified in the newborn period. A colostomy must be placed at that time in order to facilitate stool passage (see Chapter 24). Numerous other congenital anomalies may be associated with imperforate anus (Box 41.1). The pediatric nurse may encounter the infant with imperforate anus and an ostomy when the child is admitted to the hospital at several months of age for corrective surgery. Infants often require a staged repair in which the bowel is connected to the anal opening or an anal opening is created (Peña, 2004). When the final repair is achieved, the stoma will be closed and the infant will pass stool through the anal opening.

Nursing Assessment

Perform a thorough physical examination. Note the color, volume, and stool output from the stoma. Ensure that the stoma appears pink and well perfused.

Nursing Management

Preoperatively, provide bowel irrigation as ordered in preparation for the surgery. Maintain NPO status, administer IV fluids as ordered, and monitor fluid volume status.

After the intestinal pull-through procedure is completed, it will be the first time that stool has passed through the anal sphincter. The stool may be quite loose depending on the severity of the imperforate anus. The perianal skin is at significant risk for breakdown, so a barrier cream should be used on that area and it should be cleaned once daily with soap and water. Otherwise, wipe liquid stool off the barrier cream with mineral oil and cotton balls. Most of the barrier cream will remain intact, protecting the infant's perianal area.

> ▶ *Take* NOTE!
>
> *To decrease the drying associated with frequent cleaning, avoid baby wipes and frequent use of soap and water.*

Acute GI Disorders

Acute GI disorders include dehydration, vomiting, diarrhea, oral candidiasis, oral lesions, hypertrophic pyloric stenosis, necrotizing enterocolitis, intussusception, malrotation and volvulus, and appendicitis.

▶ DEHYDRATION

Dehydration occurs more readily in infants and young children than it does in adults. The risk is increased in infants and young children because they have an increased extracellular fluid percentage and a relative increase in body water compared to adults. Increased basal metabolic rate, increased body surface area, immature renal function, and increased insensible fluid loss through temperature elevation also contribute to the increased risk for dehydration in infants and young children as compared to adults. Dehydration left unchecked leads to shock, so early recognition and treatment of dehydration is critical to prevent progression to hypovolemic shock. The goals of therapeutic management of dehydration are to restore appropriate fluid balance and to prevent complications.

Nursing Assessment

For a full description of the assessment phase of the nursing process refer to page 1329. Assessment findings pertinent to dehydration are discussed below.

Health History

Elicit a description of the present illness and chief complaint. Common signs and symptoms reported during the health history are included in Comparison Chart 41.1, which compares the clinical manifestations of mild, moderate, and severe dehydration.

Explore the client's current and past medical history for risk factors for dehydration such as:

- Diarrhea
- Vomiting
- Decreased oral intake
- Sustained high fever
- Diabetic ketoacidosis
- Extensive burns

BOX 41.1 **Anomalies Associated with Anorectal Malformations**

- VACTERL syndrome: vertebral, anorectal, cardiovascular, tracheoesophageal, renal, and limb
- Esophageal atresia
- Intestinal atresia
- Malrotation
- Renal agenesis
- Hypospadias
- Vesicoureteral reflux
- Bladder exstrophy
- Cardiac anomalies
- Skeletal anomalies

COMPARISON CHART 41.1 DEHYDRATION

	Mild	Moderate	Severe
Mental status	Alert	Alert to listless	Alert to comatose
Fontanels	Soft and flat	Sunken	Sunken
Eyes	Normal	Mildly sunken orbits	Deeply sunken orbits
Oral mucosa	Pink and moist	Pale and slightly dry	Dry
Skin turgor	Elastic	Decreased	Tenting
Heart rate	Normal	May be increased	Increased, progressing to bradycardia
Blood pressure	Normal	Normal	Normal, progressing to hypotension
Extremities	Warm, pink, brisk capillary refill	Delayed capillary refill	Cool, mottled or dusky, significantly delayed capillary refill
Urine output	May be slightly decreased	<1 mL/kg/hour	Significantly <1 mL/kg/hour

▶ *Take* NOTE!

Nurses must be able to assess a child's hydration status accurately and intervene quickly. Children are at higher risk than adults for hypovolemic shock. Dehydrated children may deteriorate very quickly and experience shock.

Physical Examination and Laboratory and Diagnostic Tests

Assess the child's hydration status: heart rate, blood pressure, skin turgor, fontanels, oral mucosa, eyes, temperature and color of extremities, mental status, and urine output. Children usually compensate well initially; their heart rate increases in moderate dehydration, but blood pressure remains normal until it decreases in severe dehydration.

Nursing Management

Nursing goals for the infant or child with dehydration are aimed at restoring fluid volume and preventing progression to hypovolemia. Provide oral rehydration to children for mild to moderate states of dehydration (Dale, 2004) (Teaching Guidelines 41.2). Children with severe dehydration should receive intravenous fluids. Initially, administer 20 mL/kg of normal saline or lactated Ringer's, and then reassess the hydration status (refer to Chapter 52 for further specifics regarding hypovolemic shock).

Once initial fluid balance is restored, the physician may order intravenous fluids at the maintenance rate or as much as 1.5 times maintenance. Maintenance fluid requirements refer to the amount needed under conditions of normal hydration. Maintenance fluid requirements may be determined with the use of the formula found in Box 41.2. In the example provided in Box 41.2, a 23-kg child will need maintenance fluid equivalent to 65 mL/hr.

TEACHING GUIDELINES 41.2

Oral Rehydration Therapy

- Oral rehydration solution (ORS) should contain 75 mmol/L sodium chloride and 13.5 g/L glucose (standard ORS solutions include Pedialyte, Infalyte, and Ricelyte).
- Tap water, milk, undiluted fruit juice, soup, and broth are NOT appropriate for oral rehydration.
- Children with mild to moderate dehydration require 50 to 100 mL/kg of ORS over 4 hours.
- After re-evaluation, oral rehydration may need to be continued if the child is still dehydrated.
- When rehydrated, the child can resume a regular diet.

From Koslap-Petraco, 2006.

BOX 41.2 **Formula for Fluid Maintenance**

- 100 mL/kg for first 10 kg
- 50 mL/kg for next 10 kg
- 20 mL/kg for remaining kg
- Add together for total mL needed per 24-hour period.
- Divide by 24 for mL/hr fluid requirement.

Thus, for a 23-kg child:
- $100 \times 10 = 1,000$
- $50 \times 10 = 500$
- $20 \times 3 = 60$
- $1,000 + 500 + 60 = 1,560$

$1,560/24 = 65$ mL/hr

The same anatomic and physiologic differences that make infants and young children susceptible to dehydration also make them susceptible to overhydration. Thus, continuously evaluate hydration status and be aware of the appropriateness of intravenous fluid orders.

▶ VOMITING

Vomiting is the forceful expulsion of gastric contents through the mouth (Ulshen, 2004c). It occurs as a reflex with three different phases:

• Prodromal period: nausea and signs of autonomic nervous system stimulation
• Retching
• Vomiting

Vomiting in infants and children has many different causes and is considered to be a symptom of some other condition. Table 41.1 lists common causes of vomiting.

Therapeutic management of vomiting most often involves slow oral rehydration and at times may require administration of antiemetics.

Nursing Assessment

For a full description of the assessment phase of the nursing process refer to page 1329. Assessment findings pertinent to vomiting are discussed below.

Health History

Elicit a description of the present illness and chief complaint. Note onset and progression of symptoms. The assessment of an infant or child with vomiting should include a history of the vomiting events, including:

• Contents/character of the emesis
• Effort and force of vomiting episodes
• Timing

Contents and character of the vomitus may give clues to the cause of vomiting. Bilious vomiting is never considered normal and suggests an obstruction distal to the ampulla of Vater. Bloody emesis can signify esophageal or GI bleeding. Assess the effort and force of vomiting to identify whether the episodes are effortful and projectile, as with pyloric stenosis, or effortless, as is often seen in gastroesophageal reflux. The timing of the vomiting also is helpful in determining the cause. Vomiting that occurs several hours past meals could signify delayed gastric emptying. When vomiting occurs upon waking or in the middle of the night, particularly if it is associated with headaches, an intracranial lesion or tumor may be suspected. Note any associated events, such as diarrhea or pain.

Diarrhea may occur with viral gastroenteritis or food poisoning. Pain in the epigastric area could signify peptic ulcer disease, pancreatitis, or cholecystitis. Assess the client's past medical history to identify preexisting illnesses, drug abuse, trauma, prescribed medications, and previous abdominal surgery (Ulshen, 2004c). Risk factors for vomiting include exposure to viruses, certain medication use, and overfeeding in an infant.

Physical Examination

Perform a physical examination, noting the child's general appearance. Note hydration status, as well as mental status changes. Note the quality of bowel sounds

TABLE 41.1 CAUSES OF VOMITING BY TEMPORAL PATTERN

Category	Acute	Chronic	Cyclic
Infectious	Gastroenteritis, otitis media, pharyngitis, sinusitis (acute), hepatitis, pyelonephritis, meningitis	*H. pylori, Giardia,* sinusitis (chronic)	Chronic sinusitis
GI	Intussusception, malrotation with volvulus, appendicitis, cholecystitis, pancreatitis	GERD, gastritis, peptic ulcer disease	GERD, malrotation with volvulus
Genitourinary	Ureteropelvic junction obstruction, pyelonephritis	Pregnancy, pyelonephritis	Hydronephrosis
Endocrine/Metabolic	Diabetic ketoacidosis	Adrenal hyperplasia	Diabetic ketoacidosis, Addison's disease, acute intermittent porphyria
Neurologic	Concussion, subdural hematoma, brain tumor	Brain tumor, Arnold-Chiari malformation	Migraines, Arnold-Chiari malformation, brain tumor
Other	Food poisoning, toxic ingestion	Bulimia, rumination	Cyclic vomiting syndrome

GERD, gastroesophageal reflux disease.

upon auscultation. Palpate the abdomen for the presence of abdominal masses, tenderness, or signs of trauma.

Laboratory and Diagnostic Tests

Laboratory studies may be ordered to assess the child's hydration status or to rule out certain causes of vomiting, such as urinary tract infection, pancreatitis, or an acute infectious process. Common laboratory and diagnostic tests ordered for assessment of the cause of vomiting include:

• Abdominal ultrasound
• Upper GI series
• Plain abdominal radiographs

Nursing Management

Nursing management focuses on promoting fluid and electrolyte balance. Oral rehydration is accomplished successfully in most outpatient cases of simple vomiting. Teach the primary caregiver about oral rehydration (refer to Teaching Guidelines 41.2). In the child with mild to moderate dehydration resulting from vomiting, oral feeding should be withheld for 1 to 2 hours after emesis, after which time oral rehydration can begin. Give the infant or child 0.5 to 2 ounces of oral rehydration solution every 15 minutes, depending on the child's age and size. Most infants and children can retain this small amount of fluid if fed the restricted amount every 15 minutes. As the child improves, larger amounts will be tolerated (Dale, 2004).

> ▶ **Take** NOTE!
>
> Homemade oral rehydration solution can be made by combining 1 quart of water (can be water poured from cooking rice if desired), 8 teaspoons sugar, and 1 teaspoon salt.

If oral rehydration is not possible due to continued nausea and vomiting, intravenous fluids will likely be ordered. In some cases, antiemetics may be used to help control the vomiting. Some antiemetics can cause drowsiness or other side effects and should not be used until a definitive diagnosis is made or severe pathologic processes can be excluded. Educate the family regarding the prevention of vomiting and use of antiemetic therapy.

> ▶ **Take** NOTE!
>
> Ginger capsules, ginger tea, and candied ginger are generally useful in reducing nausea, are safe for use in children, and usually produce no side effects. Most commercially produced "ginger ale" no longer contains real ginger and so is of limited usefulness (Gardiner & Kemper, 2005).

▶ DIARRHEA

Diarrhea is either an increase in the frequency or a decrease in the consistency of stool (Ulshen, 2004c). Diarrhea in children can either be acute or chronic. Acute infectious diarrhea (gastroenteritis) remains the leading cause of death for children worldwide. In the United States, over 3.5 million infants experience diarrhea yearly, leading to more than 500,000 office visits and 55,000 hospitalizations (Grupka & Wu, 2006).

Pathophysiology

Acute diarrhea in children is most commonly caused by viruses, but it may also be related to bacterial or parasitic enteropathogens. Viruses injure the absorptive surface of mature villous cells, resulting in decreased fluid absorption and disaccharidase deficiency. Bacteria produce intestinal injury by directly invading the mucosa, damaging the villous surface, or releasing toxins. Acute diarrhea may be bloody or nonbloody. The viral, bacterial, and parasitic causes of acute infectious diarrhea are discussed in Box 41.3. Diarrhea may also occur in relation to antibiotic use. Risk factors for acute diarrhea include recent ingestion of undercooked meats, foreign travel, daycare attendance, and well water use.

Though most cases of diarrhea in children are of acute origin, it may also occur chronically. Chronic diarrhea is diarrhea that lasts for more than 2 weeks. This type of diarrhea is not usually caused by serious illnesses. The causes of chronic diarrhea are listed in Box 41.4 according to age groups.

Since most cases of diarrhea are acute and viral in nature, therapeutic management of diarrhea is usually supportive (maintaining fluid balance and nutrition). Probiotic supplementation may decrease the length and extent of diarrhea (Walker & Isolauri, 2007). Bacterial and parasitic causes of diarrhea may be treated with antibiotics or antiparasitic medications, respectively.

Nursing Assessment

For a full description of the assessment phase of the nursing process refer to page 1329. Assessment findings pertinent to diarrhea are discussed below.

Health History

Elicit a description of the present illness and chief complaint. Important information related to the course of the diarrhea includes:

• Number and frequency of stools
• Duration of symptoms
• Stool volume
• Associated symptoms (abdominal pain, cramping, nausea, vomiting, fever)
• Presence of blood or mucus in the stool

BOX 41.3 Causes of Acute Infectious Diarrhea

Viral	Bacterial	Parasitic
Rotavirus: characterized by acute onset of fever and vomiting, followed by loose, watery stools; most common cause of viral diarrhea	Salmonella: usually from ingestion of poultry, meats, or dairy products. Infants are at highest risk. Bacteria are excreted for up to 1 year. Severe cases are treated with antibiotics.	*Giardia lamblia:* the most common intestinal parasite in the United States; oral–fecal transmission; sudden onset of watery, foul-smelling stool; often causes gassiness and belching; treated with antiparasitic medications
Adenovirus 40 and 41: second most common cause of viral diarrhea illnesses, similar characteristics to rotavirus	*Escherichia coli* 0157:H7: most often associated with gross bloody stools and abdominal cramping; may lead to hemolytic-uremic syndrome	*Entamoeba histolytica:* oral–fecal transmission; more common outside of United States; colitis symptoms common
Norwalk virus: more common in older children and adults; characterized by vomiting, nausea, and cramping abdominal pain	Campylobacter: symptoms vary from mild diarrhea to dysentery; severe cases may be treated with antibiotics	*Cryptosporidium:* spread via farm animals and people; fecal–oral transmission; watery diarrhea, nausea, vomiting, and flu-like symptoms. No definitive treatment.
Caliciviruses: affected age usually 3 months to 6 years, seen in daycare settings	Shigella: high fevers and bloody stools are common; may cause seizures with fever. Treatment with antibiotics is recommended.	
Astrovirus: affected age usually 1 to 3 years, causing vomiting, diarrhea, fever, and abdominal pain	*Clostridium difficile:* usually related to antibiotic use; may cause pseudo-membranous colitis in severe cases. Infants may be carriers of the bacteria and asymptomatic. Treatment with anti-infective medications may be helpful. Probiotic therapy is usually recommended.	
Cytomegalovirus (CMV): causes other medical problems, but may cause diarrhea with colitis	*Yersinia enterocolitica:* usually affects children less than 5 years of age; watery or mucoid diarrhea common, occasionally with gross blood	

BOX 41.4 Causes of Chronic Diarrhea by Age

Infants	Toddlers	School-Age Children
Intractable diarrhea of infancy	Chronic non-specific diarrhea	Inflammatory bowel disease
Milk and soy protein intolerance	Viral enteritis *Giardia*	Appendiceal abscess
Infectious enteritis	Tumors (secretory diarrhea)	Lactase deficiency
Hirschsprung's disease	Ulcerative colitis	Constipation with encopresis
Nutrient malabsorption	Celiac disease	

Explore the client's current and past medical history for risk factors such as:

- Likelihood of exposure to infectious agents (well water, farm animals, daycare attendance)
- Dietary history
- Family history of similar symptoms
- Recent travel
- Patient age (to identify common etiology for that age group)

Physical Examination

Inspection

Assess the child with diarrhea for dehydration. Observe the child's general appearance and color. In mild dehydration, the child may appear normal. In moderate dehydration, the eyes may have decreased tear production or sunken orbits. Mucous membranes may also be dry. Mental sta-

EVIDENCE-BASED PRACTICE 41.1
Effects of Probiotics Use on the Course of Diarrhea

● **Study**

Diarrhea (more than three loose, watery stools in a 24-hour period) occurs frequently in children. Most cases of diarrhea are caused by viruses, and symptomatic treatment is the only available therapy. The authors reviewed 23 randomized controlled studies that included a total of over 1,900 participants. The studies evaluated the use of probiotics as compared with placebo or no treatment in relation to the severity and length of diarrhea.

▲ **Findings**

A variety of probiotics were noted to reduce diarrhea in infants and children as well as adults. Several of the studies demonstrated a shortened course of diarrhea when probiotics were used. The results were statistically significant, leading the authors to determine that probiotic therapy during acute diarrhea may be beneficial.

■ **Nursing Implications**

Probiotics are available as supplements: capsules or powder that may be sprinkled on food. Additionally, live culture yogurt contains probiotics. Recommend these additions to the diet of older infants or children with acute diarrhea.

Allen, S. J., Okoko, B., Martinez, E., Gregorio, G., & Dans, L. F. (2007). Probiotics for treating infectious diarrhoea. *The Cochrane Library 2007, 4.* Indianapolis: John Wiley & Sons.

---

tus may be compromised with moderate to severe dehydration, as evidenced by listlessness or lethargy. Skin may be nonelastic or exhibit tenting, signifying lack of proper hydration. Abdominal distention or concavity may be present. Urine output may also be decreased if the child is dehydrated. Stool output may be available to assess for color and consistency. Inspect the anal area for presence of redness or rash related to increased stool volumes and increased frequency.

Auscultation

Auscultate bowel sounds to assess for presence of hypoactive or hyperactive bowel sounds. Hypoactive bowel sounds may indicate obstruction or peritonitis. Hyperactive bowel sounds may indicate diarrhea/gastroenteritis.

Percussion

Percuss the abdomen. Note any abnormalities; the presence of abnormalities on examination for a diagnosis of acute or chronic diarrhea would indicate a pathologic process.

Palpation

Tenderness in the lower quadrants may be related to gastroenteritis. Rebound tenderness or pain should not be found on palpation; if found, it could indicate appendicitis or peritonitis.

Laboratory and Diagnostic Tests

Common laboratory and diagnostic studies ordered for the assessment of diarrhea include:

- Stool culture: may indicate presence of bacteria
- Stool for ova and parasites (O&P): may indicate the presence of parasites
- Stool viral panel or culture: to determine presence of rotavirus or other viruses
- Stool for occult blood: may be positive if inflammation or ulceration is present in the GI tract
- Stool for leukocytes: may be positive in cases of inflammation or infection
- Stool pH/reducing substances: to see if the diarrhea is caused by carbohydrate intolerance
- Electrolyte panel: may indicate dehydration
- Abdominal x-rays (KUB): presence of stool in colon may indicate constipation or **fecal impaction**; air–fluid levels may indicate intestinal obstruction

Nursing Management

Nursing management of the child with diarrhea focuses on restoring fluid and electrolyte balance and providing family education.

Restoring Fluid and Electrolyte Balance

Continue the child's regular diet if the child is not dehydrated. Initial nursing management of the dehydrated child with diarrhea is focused on fluid and electrolyte balance restoration. Refer to the Nursing Care Plan Overview on page 000. Probiotic supplementation while a child is taking antibiotics for other disorders may reduce the incidence of antibiotic-related diarrhea (Walker & Isolauri, 2007). After rehydration is achieved, it is important to encourage the child to consume a regular diet to maintain energy and growth (Brunell, 2006) (see Common Medical Treatments 41.1).

▶ *Take* NOTE!

Avoid prolonged use of clear liquids in the child with diarrhea because "starvation stools" may result. Also avoid fluids high in glucose, such as fruit juice, gelatin, and soda, which may worsen diarrhea.

FIGURE 41.9 Thick white patches in the infant with oral candidiasis (thrush).

Providing Family Education

Teach the parents the importance of oral rehydration therapy (see Teaching Guidelines 41.2). The physician may order medication therapy. In such instances, teach the importance of finishing all prescribed antibiotic therapy. After the cause of the diarrhea is known, teach the child and family how to prevent further occurrences. As most cases of acute diarrhea are infectious, provide education about proper hand washing techniques and transmission route. Chronic diarrhea is often a result of excessive intake of formula, water, or fruit juice, so teach the parents about appropriate fluid intake.

▶ ORAL CANDIDIASIS (THRUSH)

Oral candidiasis (thrush) is a fungal infection of the oral mucosa. It is most common in newborns and infants. Children at risk for thrush include those with immune disorders and those receiving therapy that suppresses the immune system (e.g., chemotherapy for cancer). Children who use corticosteroid inhalers are also at increased risk for the development of thrush. Antibiotic use may also contribute to thrush. Fungal infection may be transmitted between the infant and breastfeeding mother.

Therapeutic management includes treatment with oral antifungal agents such as Mycostatin (nystatin) or fluconazole.

Nursing Assessment

Assess for risk factors for oral candidiasis such as young age, immune suppression, antibiotic use, use of corticosteroid inhalers, or presence of fungal infection in the mother. Inspect the oral mucosa. Thrush appears as thick white patches on the tongue, mucosa, or palate, resembling curdled milk (Fig. 41.9). Unlike milk retained in the mouth, the patches do not easily wipe off with a swab or washcloth. Also assess for presence of candidal diaper rash (beefy-red rash with satellite lesions). Determine the extent to which the presence of the lesions is interfering with the infant's ability to feed. The lesions may cause significant discomfort.

Diagnosis is usually based on clinical presentation, though a careful scraping of the lesions can be sent out for fungal culture.

Nursing Management

Nursing management of the patient with thrush includes administering medications and providing family education.

Administering Medications

Ensure appropriate administration of oral antifungal agents. Mycostatin suspension should be given four times per day following feeding to allow the medication to remain in contact with the lesions. In the younger infant, Mycostatin can be applied to the lesions with a cotton-tipped applicator. The older infant or child can easily swallow the pleasantly flavored suspension. An advantage of fluconazole is its once-daily dosing, but infants and children receiving it should be monitored for hepatotoxicity. Unlike Mycostatin, fluconazole should be administered with food to decrease the side effects of nausea and vomiting.

Educating the Family

If the mother is also infected, she must receive antifungal treatment as well. Fungal infection of the breast can cause the mother a great deal of pain with nursing, but if appropriately treated breastfeeding can continue without interruption. Appropriate hand washing should be stressed. Bottle nipples and pacifiers need to be kept clean. Infants and young children often mouth their toys, so they should also be cleaned appropriately. Parents of infants with thrush should report diaper rash because fungal infections in the diaper area often occur concomitantly with thrush and also need to be treated.

▶ *Take* NOTE!

Geographic tongue is a benign, non-contagious condition. A reduction in the filiform papillae (bumps on the tongue) occurs in patches that migrate periodically, thus giving a map-like appearance to the tongue, with darker and lighter, higher and lower patches. Do not confuse the lighter patches of geographic tongue with the thick white plaques that form on the tongue with thrush.

▶ ORAL LESIONS

A number of oral lesions may affect infants and children. A few of the most common are aphthous ulcers, gingivostomatitis (from herpes simplex virus), and herpangina. Table 41.2 lists the causes of common oral lesions. Re-gardless of type, oral lesions are often painful and can interfere with the child's ability to eat. Therapeutic management of oral lesions varies depending on the cause.

Nursing Assessment

Explore the health history for the presence of risk factors such as immune deficiency, cancer chemotherapy treatment, exposure to infectious agents, trauma, stress, or celiac or Crohn's disease. Note the onset of the lesion(s) and progression over time. Question the parent or child about presence of sore throat or dysphagia (occurs with herpangina). Inspect the oral cavity, including the tongue, buccal mucosa, palate, and hypoglossal area. Note presence of lesions and their distribution. Refer to Table 41.2 for descriptions and illustrations of various oral lesions. Inspect the pharynx, which may be red with herpangina. Generally the diagnosis is based on the history and clinical presentation, but occasionally oral lesions are cultured for herpes simplex virus (HSV).

TABLE 41.2 ORAL LESIONS

	Aphthous Ulcers	Gingivostomatitis	Herpangina
Cause	Trauma, vitamin deficiency, celiac disease, Crohn's disease	Herpes simplex virus	Enterovirus (Coxsackie)
Appearance	Erythematous border, often yellow appearance to the ulcer, anywhere on oral mucosa or lips	Vesicular lesions on erythematous base, anywhere in oral cavity, including lips	Bright-red ulcers, generally in posterior oral cavity
Fever	Generally absent	May have high fever with initial outbreak	Abrupt onset of high fever (up to 39.4° to 40.6°C), lasting 1 to 4 days
Length of illness	Generally heal within 7 to 14 days; may recur	10 to 12 days initially; may recur with stress, febrile illness, or intense sunlight exposure (as virus lies dormant in system)	Generally resolves within 5 to 7 days
Therapeutic management	Topical corticosteroid in dental paste may help.	Acyclovir	Supportive treatment only

Nursing Management

The primary concerns with oral lesions are pain management and maintenance of hydration. A corticosteroid-containing dental paste used for aphthous ulcers is formulated to "stick" to mucous membranes, so the lesion area should be as dry as possible prior to application of the paste. Children do not care for having the paste applied and will often resist. Older children with herpangina or stomatitis can "swish and spit" various formulations of "magic mouthwash" (typically a combination of liquid diphenhydramine, liquid acetaminophen, and milk of magnesia); they may offer some pain relief. Common over-the-counter medications such as Ambesol, Oragel, and Kanka may be helpful for topical pain relief, though oral analgesics are often necessary.

The child with herpangina is typically a toddler or preschooler. It may be very difficult to coach a young child to drink fluids when his or her mouth is hurting. Playing games and offering favorite fluids and Popsicles may encourage adequate oral intake. Carbonated beverages and citrus juices should be avoided when oral lesions are present as they can cause further stinging and burning.

> ▶ *Take* NOTE!
>
> *Viscous lidocaine should be used with caution as a topical treatment for numbing the lesions or as a swish-and-spit treatment, as younger children may swallow the lidocaine.*

▶ HYPERTROPHIC PYLORIC STENOSIS

Hypertrophic pyloric stenosis is one of the most common conditions requiring surgery in the first 2 months of life. In pyloric stenosis, the circular muscle of the **pylorus** becomes hypertrophied, causing thickness in the luminal side of the pyloric canal (Fig. 41.10). This thickness creates a gastric outlet obstruction, causing nonbilious vomiting. The vomiting becomes more frequent and forceful as time goes on and is often projectile. The incidence is 1 to 8 per 1000 live births and occurs more in males than females (4:1) (Sondheimer, 2007).

The cause of pyloric stenosis is unknown, but a positive family history is present in 13% of patients (Sondheimer, 2007). Infants with pyloric stenosis typically present with symptoms of nonbilious vomiting between weeks 2 and 4 of life.

Pyloric stenosis requires surgical intervention. A pyloromyotomy is performed to cut the muscle of the pylorus and relieve the gastric outlet obstruction (see Fig. 41.10). Postoperative complications are rare.

FIGURE 41.10 (**A**) Hypertrophied pylorus muscle and narrowed stomach outlet. (**B**) In pyloromyotomy, the pylorus is incised, thus increasing the diameter of the pyloric outlet.

Nursing Assessment

For a full description of the assessment phase of the nursing process refer to page 1329. Assessment findings pertinent to hypertrophic pyloric stenosis are discussed below.

Health History

Elicit a description of the present illness and chief complaint. Common signs and symptoms reported during the health history might include:

• Forceful, nonbilious vomiting, unrelated to feeding position
• Hunger soon after vomiting episode
• Weight loss due to vomiting
• Progressive dehydration with subsequent lethargy

Risk factors include a positive family history. The disorder occurs most frequently in first-born males.

Physical Examination and Laboratory and Diagnostic Tests

Palpate for a hard, moveable "olive" in the right upper quadrant (hypertrophied pylorus). If an easily palpable mass is felt, no further testing is necessary and a surgical consult is called. If no mass is identified, a pyloric ultrasound may be ordered to identify a thickened hypoechoic ring in the region of the pylorus. An upper GI series may identify pyloric stenosis as well, but an ultrasound is less invasive and is considered more diagnostic of pyloric stenosis. Assess laboratory values to determine if the infant has metabolic alkalosis resulting from dehydration.

Nursing Management

Preoperative management of infants with pyloric stenosis is aimed at fluid management and correcting abnormal electrolyte values. Family anxiety is high during this time because of the impending surgery for an otherwise healthy infant. Provide emotional support to the family. Teach them about the surgical procedure and what to expect postoperatively. After surgery, infants usually resume oral feedings after 1 to 2 days.

▶ INTUSSUSCEPTION

Intussusception is a process that occurs when a proximal segment of bowel "telescopes" into a more distal segment, causing edema, vascular compromise, and ultimately partial or total bowel obstruction (Fig. 41.11). Intussusception usually occurs in otherwise healthy infants under age 2. It is three times more likely in males than females. Seventy-five percent to 90% of cases of intussusception occur with no specified "lead point" (i.e., pathologic point) that causes the telescoping. When a lead point is identified, it usually occurs in children over age 5. The most common type of lead point is a Meckel's diverticulum, but other lead points may include duplication cysts,

polyps, hemangiomas, tumors, the appendix, or even lymphomas (Wyllie, 2004b). Children with cystic fibrosis, celiac disease, and Crohn's disease may be at higher risk for developing intussusception.

A barium enema is successful at reducing a large percentage of intussusception cases; other cases are reduced surgically. If surgical reduction is unsuccessful or bowel necrosis has occurred, a portion of the bowel must be resected.

Nursing Assessment

For a full description of the assessment phase of the nursing process refer to page 1329. Assessment findings pertinent to intussusception are discussed below.

Health History
Elicit a description of the present illness and chief complaint. Common signs and symptoms reported during the health history might include:

- Sudden onset of intermittent, crampy abdominal pain
- Severe pain (children usually draw up their knees and scream)
- Vomiting
- Diarrhea
- Currant-jelly stools, gross blood, or Hemoccult-positive stools
- Lethargy

Typically, symptoms flare and then regress. Between episodes, children may have no symptoms of intussusception. This return to a normal state is due to the intussusception reducing on its own. The child may be asymptomatic and may appear well when presenting to the pediatrician or emergency room. Again, this may be a sign that the bowel has reduced spontaneously. Assess the severity of pain, length of time the symptoms have been present, presence of vomiting, and stool patterns and color. Immediately report the presence of bilious vomiting, which occurs only in an obstructive situation. Also assess for signs and symptoms of acute peritonitis. Explore the client's current and past medical history for risk factors, such as cystic fibrosis or celiac disease.

Physical Examination
Palpate the abdomen for the presence of a sausage-shaped mass in the upper mid-abdomen: this is a hallmark sign of intussusception. Note any mental status changes.

Laboratory and Diagnostic Tests
Intussusception is usually diagnosed with an air or barium enema. Use of an enema may show the intussusception and also may reduce it, making the enema therapeutic (Wyllie, 2004b). A pediatric surgeon should be available at the time of the enema in case the enema is unsuccessful or perforation (rare) occurs. White blood cell elevation may occur and electrolytes may show signs of dehydration.

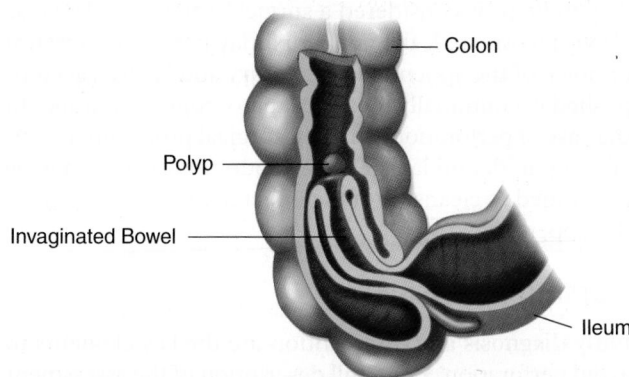

FIGURE 41.11 In intussusception, the intestine telescopes upon itself.

Nursing Management

Administer intravenous fluids and antibiotics before the diagnostic laboratory and radiograph studies are performed. Refer to the Nursing Care Plan 41.1 for nursing management of the postoperative child.

The parents may be very fatigued after dealing with a crying infant. They are often quite anxious about surgery in an otherwise healthy child. Offer emotional support and provide appropriate preoperative and postoperative education to the family.

▶ MALROTATION AND VOLVULUS

Intestinal malrotation occurs during the 10th week of embryonic development. At week 10, the intestine is anchored to the abdominal wall by the base of the mesentery in a specific pattern to avoid kinking or twisting (Wyllie, 2004c). When malrotation occurs, the intestine is abnormally attached and the mesentery narrows, twisting on itself (volvulus). If the volvulus involves the entire small bowel, it is termed a mid-gut volvulus.

The main symptom of malrotation is bilious vomiting. Many children also have abdominal pain, shock symptoms, abdominal distention, tachycardia, and bloody stools. Most cases of malrotation will present in the first few weeks of life, but symptoms may not occur until the patient is well into adulthood.

Therapeutic management of malrotation and volvulus is accomplished surgically. A Ladd procedure is performed, during which the intestine is straightened out and bands contributing to the misalignment are divided. If bowel necrosis has occurred (rare), then an ostomy may be necessary.

Nursing Assessment

For a full description of the assessment phase of the nursing process refer to page 1329. Assessment findings pertinent to malrotation and volvulus are discussed below.

Health History

Elicit a description of the present illness and chief complaint. Common signs and symptoms reported during the health history might include vomiting and abdominal pain. Since obstruction can occur with resulting necrosis of the bowel, immediately inform the physician if obstruction is suspected.

Physical Examination and Diagnostic and Laboratory Tests

Observe for severity of pain, palpate for abdominal guarding and rebound tenderness, and auscultate for hypoactive bowel sounds. Common laboratory and diagnostic studies ordered for the assessment of malrotation and volvulus include:

- KUB to reveal obstruction
- Upper GI series to identify the location of the duodenojejunal junction and corkscrew appearance of the twisted bowel

Nursing Management

When diagnostic testing reveals malrotation/volvulus, administer ordered intravenous fluids and intravenous antibiotics. Often a nasogastric tube is placed to decompress the stomach. Surgery is performed as soon as possible. After surgery, provide postoperative care of the child (see Nursing Care Plan 41.1). Provide continuous emotional support and family education.

▶ APPENDICITIS

Appendicitis, an acute inflammation of the appendix, is the most common cause of emergent abdominal surgery in children. It occurs in all age groups; the median age in the pediatric population is 4 to 15 years (Albanese & Sylvester, 2006).

Pathophysiology

Appendicitis is due to a closed-loop obstruction of the appendix (Fig. 41.12). It is thought that the obstruction is due to fecal material impacted into the relatively narrow appendix, though other causes such as ingested foreign bodies may exist. This causes a subsequent increase in the intraluminal pressure of the appendix, resulting in mucosal edema, bacterial overgrowth, and eventual perforation. Due to the fecal material in the appendix, perforation causes inflammatory fluid and bacterial contents to leak into the abdominal cavity, resulting in peritonitis. Diffuse peritonitis is more likely in younger children. Older children and adolescents have a more developed omentum, which walls off the inflamed or perforated appendix, often causing a focal abscess.

Therapeutic Management

Appendicitis is considered a surgical emergency because if left uncorrected, the appendix may perforate. Surgical removal of the appendix is necessary and is often accomplished via minimally invasive laparoscopic technique. In the case of perforation, an open surgical procedure is usually required, and lavage of the abdominal cavity may be performed to cleanse it of the infected fluid released from the appendix.

Nursing Assessment

Early diagnosis and intervention are the key elements to avoid perforation. For a full description of the assessment phase of the nursing process refer to page 1329. Assessment findings pertinent to appendicitis are discussed below.

A

B

FIGURE 41.12 (**A**) In appendicitis, the lumen of the appendix is obstructed, resulting in edema and compressed blood vessels. (**B**) As appendicitis progresses, pain may become localized at McBurney's point (a point midway between the anterior superior iliac crest and the umbilicus).

Health History

Elicit a description of the present illness and chief complaint. Appendicitis may be gradual, and symptoms usually do not come and go; they remain persistent and intensify. Common signs and symptoms reported during the health history might include:

- Vague abdominal pain in the initial stages, localizing to the right lower quadrant over a few hours
- Nausea and vomiting (which usually develop after the onset of pain)
- Small-volume, frequent, soft stools, often confused with diarrhea
- Fever (usually low grade unless perforation occurs, which results in high fever)

Physical Examination

Children with appendicitis often appear anorexic and ill. They often cannot walk or climb up onto the examination table without assistance. Upon palpation, maximal tenderness occurs over McBurney's point in the right lower quadrant (see Fig. 41.12). Assess the abdomen for

acute peritonitis, as indicated by diffuse abdominal tenderness or distention. Immediately report positive findings to a physician.

> ▶ **Take** NOTE!
>
> *If the child's abdominal pain is suddenly relieved without intervention, suspect perforation and notify the physician immediately.*

Laboratory and Diagnostic Tests

Common laboratory and diagnostic studies ordered for the assessment of appendicitis include:

- Abdominal computed tomography (CT) scan: performed to visualize the appendix for further evaluation
- Laboratory testing: may reveal an elevated white blood cell count
- C-reactive protein: may be elevated

Nursing Management

Provide pre- and postoperative care and patient and family education (see Nursing Care Plan 41.1). Care depends on what was found during surgical exploration. A nonruptured, nongangrenous appendix usually requires no antibiotic therapy, so provide routine surgical care. In addition to routine surgical care, administer 48 to 72 hours of ordered antibiotics to the child with a suppurative or gangrenous (nonperforated) appendix to decrease the risk of postoperative infection. The child with a perforated appendix will require 7 to 14 days of intravenous antibiotic therapy in addition to normal postoperative care. Provide family teaching, because the child is often discharged home while still receiving intravenous antibiotic therapy.

Chronic GI Disorders

Chronic GI disorders include gastroesophageal reflux, peptic ulcer disease, constipation/encopresis, Hirschsprung's disease, short bowel syndrome, inflammatory bowel disease, celiac disease, recurrent abdominal pain, failure to thrive, and chronic feeding problems.

▶ GASTROESOPHAGEAL REFLUX

Gastroesophageal reflux (GER) is passage of gastric contents into the esophagus. It is considered a normal physiologic process that occurs in healthy infants and children. However, when complications develop from the reflux of gastric contents back into the esophagus or oropharynx, it becomes more of a pathologic process known as gastroesophageal reflux disease (GERD). GER occurs frequently during the first year of life; most infants outgrow the reflux by age 6 months. GER is particularly common in premature infants. Other possible diagnoses that can be mistaken for GER include food allergies, formula enteropathies, gastric outlet obstruction, malrotation, cyclic vomiting, or central nervous system lesions.

Pathophysiology

The process of GER occurs during episodes of transient relaxation of the LES, which can occur during swallowing, crying, or other Valsalva maneuvers that increase intra-abdominal pressure. Delayed esophageal clearance and gastric emptying, highly acidic gastric contents, hiatal hernia (protrusion of the stomach upward into the mediastinal cavity through the esophageal hiatus of the diaphragm), or neurologic disease may also be contributing factors associated with reflux.

Symptoms of GERD in infants and children are listed below in the health history section. The signs and symptoms of GERD are often seen as a result of the dam-

aging components of the refluxate (the pH of the gastric contents, bile acids, and pepsin). The longer the pH of the refluxate is below 4, the higher the risk for development of severe GERD.

As a result of GERD, other systems may be at risk for damage. These complications include esophagitis, esophageal stricture, Barrett's esophagus (a precancerous condition), laryngitis, recurrent pneumonia, asthma, or anemia from chronic esophageal erosion.

Therapeutic Management

Conservative medical management begins with appropriate positioning, such as elevating the head of the bed and keeping the infant or child upright for 30 minutes after feeding. Smaller, more frequent feedings may be helpful. If reflux does not improve with these measures, medications are prescribed to decrease acid production and stabilize the pH of the gastric contents. Also, prokinetic agents may be used to help empty the stomach more quickly, minimizing the amount of gastric contents in the stomach that the child can reflux.

If the GERD cannot be medically managed effectively or requires long-term medication therapy, surgical intervention may be necessary. A Nissen fundoplication is the most common surgical procedure performed for antireflux therapy. The gastric fundus is wrapped around the lower 2 to 3 cm of the esophagus (Fig. 41.13). Laparoscopic fundoplications are being performed as a way to minimize the recovery period and reduce potential complications.

Nursing Assessment

For a full description of the assessment phase of the nursing process refer to page 1329. Assessment findings pertinent to gastroesophageal reflux are discussed below.

Health History

Elicit a description of the present illness and chief complaint. Note onset and progression of symptoms. Com-

FIGURE 41.13 In the Nissen fundoplication, the fundus (upper portion of the stomach) is wrapped around the lower segment of the esophagus.

mon signs and symptoms reported during the health history include:

- Recurrent vomiting or regurgitation
- Weight loss or poor weight gain
- Irritability in infants
- Respiratory symptoms (chronic cough, wheezing, stridor, asthma, apnea)
- Hoarseness/sore throat
- Halitosis (mostly in older children)
- Heartburn or chest pains
- Abdominal pain
- Abnormal neck posturing (Sandifer syndrome)
- Hematemesis
- Dysphagia or feeding refusal
- Chronic sinusitis, otitis media
- Poor dentition (caused by acid erosion)

Explore the patient's current and past medical history for risk factors such as:

- Prematurity, noting prolonged ventilator use or chronic lung disease
- Dietary habits (e.g., chocolate, coffee, spicy or fatty foods, caffeine, formula-fed or breastfed, overeating or overfeeding)
- Current medications
- Smoking/alcohol use (older children)
- Food allergies
- Other GI disorders (gastric outlet dysfunction/hiatal hernia) or congenital abnormalities
- Feeding positions and patterns (especially important in infants)
- Sleeping positions/patterns
- Other medical history, such as asthma, recurrent infections/pneumonia

Physical Examination

The physical examination consists of inspection, auscultation, percussion, and palpation.

Inspection

Observe the child's general appearance and color. Infants and children with uncontrolled GER for a period of time may appear underweight or malnourished. Infants may be irritable due to painful regurgitation/reflux events. Note breathing patterns, because reflux-induced asthma may have developed. **Acute life-threatening events** (ALTE) and apnea have been associated with severe GERD. Observe the child for cyanosis, altered mental status, and alterations in tone. Inspect emesis for blood or bile.

Auscultation

Evaluate the lung fields for the presence of complications related to GERD, such as wheezing or pneumonia. No further pathologic findings related to GERD should be auscultated on examination.

Percussion

Perform routine abdominal percussion, noting any abnormalities. No specific findings should be noted.

Palpation

Use caution when palpating the abdomen, especially with infants with GER, because it may induce vomiting. No abnormalities should be palpated.

> ▶ **Take** NOTE!
>
> *Not all infants with GERD actually vomit. Those with "silent" GERD may only demonstrate irritability associated with feeding or posturing (arching back during or after feeding) and grimacing. Episodes of GERD often cause bradycardia, so if the above signs occur, they should be reported to the physician, even if the baby is not vomiting.*

Laboratory and Diagnostic Tests

Common laboratory and diagnostic studies ordered for the assessment of gastroesophageal reflux include:

- Upper GI series: though not sensitive or specific to GER, may show some reflux; used to narrow down the differential diagnosis
- Esophageal pH probe study: quantifies GER episodes as they correlate to symptoms
- Esophagogastroduodenoscopy (EGD): shows esophageal and gastric tissue damage from GERD
- Complete blood count: may demonstrate anemia if chronic esophagitis or hematemesis is present
- Hemoccult: may be positive if chronic esophagitis is present

Nursing Management

As with most GI disorders, initial nursing management is aimed at restoring proper fluid balance and nutrition. Refer to the Nursing Care Plan on page 1336. Additional considerations are reviewed below.

Promoting Safe Feeding Techniques and Positioning

Feeding adjustments are an essential part of reflux management. Give infants smaller, more frequent feedings using a nipple that controls flow well. Frequently burp the infant during feeds to control reflux. Thickening of the formula with products such as rice or oatmeal cereal can significantly help keep the formula and gastric contents down. Positioning after feedings is important. Keep infants upright for 30 to 45 minutes after feeding. For infants, elevate the head of the crib 30 degrees. For older children, elevate the head of the bed as much as possible and restrict meals for several hours before bedtime. While the proper positioning of an infant with GERD for sleep is controversial, infants can be positioned safely on their sides or upright in a car seat to minimize the risk of aspiration while on their backs. However, individual physicians may have specific preferences about sleeping positions for infants with GERD.

Maintaining a Patent Airway

GERD symptoms often involve the airway. Maximize reflux precautions to keep the risk of airway involvement to a minimum. In rare instances, GERD causes apnea or an ALTE. In these cases, use an apnea or bradycardia monitor to monitor for such episodes. The monitor requires a physician's order and can be ordered through a home health company. Teach parents how to deal with these episodes, as their anxiety is very high. Provide CPR instruction to all parents whose children have had an ALTE previously.

Educating the Family and Child

The goals for the infant and child with gastroesophageal reflux are a decrease in symptoms, a decrease in the frequency and duration of reflux episodes, healing of the injured mucosa, and prevention of further complications of GERD. Teach the parents the signs and symptoms of complications. Explain that reflux is usually limited to the first year of life, though in some cases it persists. If medications are prescribed, thoroughly explain their use and their side effects (see Drug Guide 41.1).

Providing Postoperative Care

If the child requires fundoplication, a gastrostomy tube is often placed for use in the immediate postoperative period or for long-term feeding. In the immediate postoperative period, assess for pain, abdominal distention, and return of bowel sounds. If a gastrostomy tube is placed, it is often open to straight drain for a period of time postoperatively to keep the stomach empty and allow for the internal incision to heal. When bowel sounds have returned and the infant or child is stable, introduce feedings slowly (typically via the gastrostomy tube). Assess for tolerance of feedings (absence of abdominal distention or pain, minimal residual, and passage of stool). If the abdomen does become distended or the child has discomfort, open the gastrostomy tube to air to decompress the stomach. Assess the insertion site of the gastrostomy tube for redness, edema, or drainage. Keep the site clean and dry per surgeon or hospital protocol. Teach the parents how to care for the gastrostomy tube and insertion site and how to use the tube for feeding.

Promoting Family and Patient Coping

Parents can feel a great deal of anxiety. Teach the family about all aspects of GERD to help promote coping. School-age children often have reflux episodes exhibited by postprandial vomiting, which can be very embarrassing

for the children. Notify the school about the medical issues related to GER to minimize the situations for the child.

▶ PEPTIC ULCER DISEASE

Peptic ulcer disease (PUD) is a term used to describe a variety of disorders of the upper GI tract that result from the action of gastric secretions (Fig. 41.14). Mucosal inflammation and subsequent ulceration occur as a result of either a primary or a secondary factor. In children, duodenal ulcers are more common than gastric ulcers. Primary peptic ulcers are usually associated with *Helicobacter pylori*, a gram-negative organism that causes mucosal inflammation and in some cases more severe disease. *H. pylori* is found mostly in the duodenum.

Secondary peptic ulcers may occur as a result of an identifiable factor, such as excess acid production, stress, medications, or the presence of other underlying conditions. Secondary ulcers tend to be gastric in location as opposed to duodenal.

Primary PUD is more common in children over age 10. There is a higher incidence of secondary PUD in patients under age 6, though it can be found in children of all ages (Herbst, 2004).

> ▶ **Take** NOTE!
>
> *Severe stress, such as burns or another illness necessitating critical care, can contribute to the development of a peptic ulcer in children.*

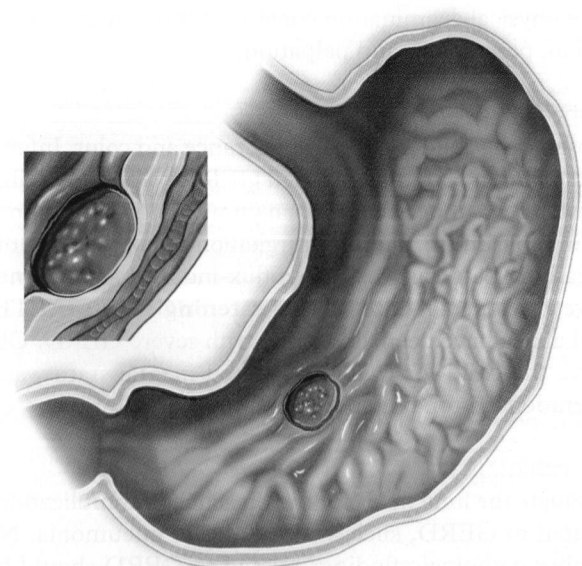

FIGURE 41.14 Peptic ulcer disease.

Therapeutic Management

PUD may be treated with antibiotics (if *H. pylori* is verified), histamine agonists, and/or proton pump inhibitors. If the child presents with a severe esophageal or gastric hemorrhage, a nasogastric tube may be placed to decompress the stomach. The patient may require intravenous infusion of a histamine H2-receptor antagonist or a proton pump inhibitor initially until the bleeding has stopped and the disease is stabilized.

Nursing Assessment

For a full description of the assessment phase of the nursing process refer to page 1329. Assessment findings pertinent to PUD are discussed below.

Health History

Elicit a description of the present illness and chief complaint. Common signs and symptoms reported during the health history might include:

- Abdominal pain
- GI bleeding
- Vomiting

Abdominal pain is the most common complaint of children with PUD. It is important to characterize the abdominal pain, as many other digestive disorders may mimic PUD. The pain tends to be dull and vague, mostly epigastric or periumbilical. Most often, patients with PUD have pain that worsens after meals, and the pain may wake them at night. Vomiting may be noted in preschool and school-age children.

Explore the client's current and past medical history for risk factors such as a family history of PUD or other GI diseases, or chronic salicylate or prednisone use.

▶ **Take** NOTE!

Adolescents at increased risk for the development of PUD include those who use tobacco, alcohol, and caffeine.

Physical Examination and Laboratory and Diagnostic Tests

Palpate the abdomen for the location of the pain, which is usually epigastric or periumbilical. Note the presence of blood in emesis or stools, as GI bleeding may occur (Sondheimer, 2007). Common laboratory and diagnostic studies ordered for the assessment of PUD include the following:

- Laboratory studies: to identify anemia or *H. pylori* antibodies

- Urea breath test: to identify *H. pylori* gastritis
- Upper GI series: to detect presence of ulcerations
- Upper endoscopy: the definitive diagnostic test to look for ulceration and nodularity in the upper GI tract
- Biopsies: to assess for *H. pylori*, granulomas, eosinophils, or corrosive agents to identify the primary cause of the PUD

Nursing Management

Hemodynamic stabilization should be the focus of nursing management if significant GI bleeding occurs. Once patients are stabilized and tolerating oral feeds, they may be discharged to home. Provide discharge instructions on the following topics:

- Medications
- Dietary management (especially when allergic gastroenteropathy is found)
- Safety precautions (in cases of ingested substances)
- Stressors
- Prevention of disease recurrence

▶ CONSTIPATION AND ENCOPRESIS

Constipation is a very common problem seen in a pediatric practice, reportedly representing 3% to 5% of all pediatric outpatient visits. As many as one third of children aged 6 to 12 years experience constipation (Biggs & Dery, 2006).

Constipation is usually defined as failure to achieve complete evacuation of the lower colon. It is usually associated with difficulty in passing hard, dry stools but can sometimes be seen as small stools the size of marbles. Term newborns should pass a meconium stool within the first 24 hours of life. If this does not occur, the newborn is at risk for developing an underlying GI disorder. The bowel habits of both infants and children vary widely, so assess and treat each child on an individual basis. Breastfed infants may produce a stool with each feeding, though some will skip a few days between stools. Most bottle-fed babies will produce a stool one or two times per day, but they may go 2 to 3 days without producing a stool.

Encopresis is a term used to describe soiling of fecal contents into the underwear beyond the age of expected toilet training (4 to 5 years of age). Encopresis is often seen as a result of chronic constipation and withholding of stool. As stool is withheld in the rectum, the rectal muscle can stretch over time, and this stretching of the rectum causes fecal impactions. Patients who have a stretched rectal vault may experience diarrhea, where leakage occurs around a fecal mass. This is often an embarrassing issue that occurs with school-age children, and the child may hide his or her underwear to avoid punishment. Many psychological issues arise from chronic constipation and encopresis.

Pathophysiology

As stool passes through the colon, water is reabsorbed into the colon, resulting in a formed stool by the time it reaches the rectum. At this point, the anal sphincter relaxes to allow the passage of stool from the anus. In constipation, however, this relaxation does not occur.

Most causes of constipation are functional in nature (inorganic). Children with functional constipation usually present with this problem during the toilet-training years. Children have a painful experience during defecation, which in turn creates a fear of defecation, resulting in further withholding of stool. Organic causes of constipation rarely occur in children; however, this may be a sign of a disease such as spina bifida or sacral agenesis. The causes of pediatric constipation are discussed in Box 41.5.

Therapeutic Management

Once any organic process is ruled out as a cause for constipation, it may initially be managed with dietary manipulation such as increasing fiber and fluids. Behavior modification is necessary for most children. Children need to relearn to allow bowel evacuation when stool is present. Children with severe constipation and withholding behaviors may not benefit from dietary management and may require laxative therapy. Sometimes mechanical disimpaction is required initially, followed by the above measures.

Nursing Assessment

For a full description of the assessment phase of the nursing process refer to page 1329. Assessment findings pertinent to constipation/encopresis are discussed below.

Health History

Elicit a description of the present illness and chief complaint. Note the onset of symptoms as described by the parent/child. Common signs and symptoms reported during the health history may include:

- Altered stooling patterns (size, frequency, amount, color)
- Pain with defecation
- Withholding behaviors (postures to try to withhold the stool, such as crossing the legs, squatting or hiding in a corner, or "dancing")
- Complaints of abdominal pain and cramping and poor appetite
- Diarrhea leakage
- Soiling of undergarments

It is important to note the duration of the symptoms to determine an acute onset versus a chronic disorder.

Explore the client's past and current medical history for risk factors such as:

- Family history of GI disorders
- History of rectal bleeding or **anal fissures**
- Report of first meconium stool after 24 hours of age
- History of sexual abuse

An accurate dietary history as well as a history of fluid intake should be taken. Current medication or laxative use should also be explored.

Physical Examination

Physical examination of the child with constipation consists of inspection, auscultation, percussion, and palpation.

BOX 41.5 Causes of Pediatric Constipation by Age

Newborn/Infant	Toddler and Ages 2–4 Years	School Age	Adolescent	Any Age
• Meconium plug • Hirschsprung's disease • Cystic fibrosis • Congenital anorectal malformations • Pseudo-obstruction • Endocrine: hypothyroidism • Metabolic: diabetes insipidus, renal tubular acidosis • Withholding • Dietary changes	• Anal fissures • Withholding • Toilet refusal • Short-segment Hirschsprung's disease • Neurologic disorders • Spinal cord: meningomyelocele, tumors, tethered cord	• Toilet or bathroom access limited or unavailable • Limited ability to recognize physiologic cues, preoccupation with other activities • Tethered cord • Withholding	• Spinal cord injury (accidents, trauma) • Dieting • Anorexia • Pregnancy • Idiopathic slow transit constipation, particularly in females • Laxative abuse • Irritable bowel syndrome, constipation variant	• Medication side effect, dietary, postoperative state • Previous anorectal surgery • Withholding and overflow from chronic rectal distention • Relatively rapid change to sedentary state, dehydration • Hypothyroidism

Inspection

Observe the child's general appearance. Note whether the abdomen appears distended or rounded. Observe the lower back for a deep pilonidal dimple with hair tuft, which is suggestive of spina bifida occulta. Flat buttocks may be suggestive of sacral agenesis. Inspect the anus for signs of fissures or soiling. Inspect the child's underwear for stains or smears, which are indicative of soiling (Ulshen, 2004c).

Auscultation

Auscultate bowel sounds to determine the possibility of an obstruction (hypoactive or absent bowel sounds) in the child with an acute case of constipation.

Percussion

Percuss the abdomen to reveal dullness, which would indicate a fecal mass.

Palpation

Palpate the abdomen for any tenderness or masses. The nurse may assist the physician or practitioner with the performance of a rectal examination to assess for rectal tone and rectal vault size.

Laboratory and Diagnostic Tests

Laboratory and diagnostic tests are not routine with the diagnosis of functional constipation, but if an organic cause is suspected, the following laboratory and diagnostic tests would be ordered:

• Stool for occult blood: the presence of blood could indicate some other disease process
• Abdominal x-ray: large quantities of stool may be seen in the colon
• Sitz marker study: to detect colonic dysmotility
• Barium enema: to rule out a stricture or Hirschsprung's disease
• Rectal manometry: to evaluate rectal musculature dysfunction
• Rectal suction biopsy: to rule out Hirschsprung's disease

Nursing Management

Nursing management for the infant or child with constipation is aimed at educating the patient and family and promoting patient and family coping. Refer to the Nursing Care Plan on page 1336. Additional considerations are reviewed below.

Educating the Family and Patient

Teach parents how to assess for signs of constipation and withholding behaviors. Also provide guidelines on scheduling and supervising bowel habits in reconditioning the child to use the toilet regularly. Teach parents to use positive reinforcement techniques: for example, when the child produces an adequate-volume bowel movement, reward him or her with stickers, extra playtime or television time, and so on (Schmitt, 2004).

Dietary changes may help some children. High-fiber diets help to regulate bowel activity. Increasing fluid intake may also aid in bringing extra water into the bowel, thereby softening the stool. Infants and toddlers with constipation may experience constipation from formula or milk changes. Manipulating the formula or milk may result in better bowel habits.

Educate families about the importance of compliance with medication use, if medication is ordered. Parents often are very anxious about the use of these medications, but stress to them that compliance is essential. Assess for improper laxative use based on the history of stool patterns.

Many children present to their doctor with fecal impaction or partial impaction. Teach parents how to disimpact their children at home; this often requires an enema or stimulation therapy. Nursing Procedure 41.2 gives instructions on enema administration in children. Explain the procedure to the child in developmentally appropriate terms. Enema administration can be uncomfortable, but calming measures, such as distraction and praise, provide a comforting environment. After the impaction is removed, promote regular bowel habits to keep the impaction from recurring.

Promoting Patient and Family Coping

Childhood constipation can be a very stressful process for both the child and family. Behavior modification is

---

Nursing Procedure 41.2

ADMINISTERING AN ENEMA

1. Gather supplies (enema bag, lubricant, enema solution).
2. Wash hands and apply gloves.
3. Position the child:
   • Infant or toddler on abdomen with knees bent
   • Child or adolescent on left side with right leg flexed toward chest
4. Clamp the enema tubing, remove the cap, and apply lubricant to the tip.
5. Insert the tube into the rectum:
   • 2.5 to 4 cm (1 to 1.5 inches) in the infant
   • 5 to 7.5 cm (2 to 3 inches) in the child
6. Unclamp the tubing and administer the prescribed volume of enema solution at a rate of about 100 mL per minute. Recommended volumes:
   • 250 mL or less for the infant
   • 250 to 500 mL for the toddler or preschooler
   • 500 to 1,000 mL for the school-age child
7. Hold the child's buttocks together if needed to encourage retention of the enema for 5 to 10 minutes.

necessary for many children. To facilitate daily bowel evacuation, the child should sit on the toilet twice a day (after breakfast and dinner) for 5 to 15 minutes. Instruct the family to keep a "star" or reward chart to encourage compliance. The star should be awarded for compliance with time sitting on the toilet and should not be reserved for successful bowel movements only. Weeks to months may be required to change the stooling pattern.

Many parents seek counselors to help the entire family deal with the issues. Counseling is geared toward allaying the fears of a child who is afraid to defecate due to pain. Also, children who are older may have behavioral issues that need to be addressed. Psychological evaluation and possible behavioral therapy may need to be implemented if constipation becomes a power struggle.

▶ *Consider* THIS!

Jung Kim, 3 years old, is brought to the clinic by his parents with abdominal pain and a poor appetite. His mother states, "He cries when I put him on the toilet."

What other assessment information would you obtain?

What education and interventions may be necessary for this child and family?

▶ HIRSCHSPRUNG'S DISEASE (CONGENITAL AGANGLIONIC MEGACOLON)

Hirschsprung's disease is the most common cause of neonatal intestinal obstruction (Fig. 41.15). The disease is most commonly characterized by constipation in newborns. This is due to a lack of ganglion cells in the bowel, which causes inadequate motility in part of the intestine. These ganglion cells can be absent from the rectosigmoid colon all the way into the small intestine. Approximately 75% of cases affect only the rectosigmoid colon (short-segment Hirschsprung's), but in 8% of the cases, total colonic involvement is seen (long-segment Hirschsprung's). The incidence is 1 in 5,000, and males are affected three times more than females. Hirschsprung's usually occurs in the absence of other associated anomalies, but there is an association with Down syndrome (Wyllie, 2004a).

Therapeutic Management

Surgical resection of the aganglionic bowel and reanastomosis of the remaining intestine is necessary to promote proper bowel function. There are several types of surgical procedures to correct this, usually performed in stages. The surgical resection requires the child to have an ostomy to divert the stool through a stoma on the abdomen. This allows the area of the resected bowel and anastomosis to heal before it is used. The ostomy is closed at a later date.

Nursing Assessment

For a full description of the assessment phase of the nursing process refer to page 1329. Assessment findings pertinent to Hirschsprung's are discussed below.

Health History

Elicit a description of the present illness and chief complaint. Newborn stool patterns are a key element in recognizing this diagnosis. Assess whether the newborn passed a meconium stool: most children with Hirschsprung's do not pass a meconium stool within the first 24 to 48 hours of life. Also, newborns who required rectal stimulation to pass their first meconium stool or who passed a meconium plug should be evaluated for Hirschsprung's.

Explore the child's current and past medical history for risk factors such as a family history of Hirschsprung's or Down syndrome. Hirschsprung's may also be associated with congenital deafness, malrotation, gastric diverticulum, and intestinal atresia.

Physical Examination

Inspect and palpate the abdomen. The abdomen is typically distended, and often stool masses can be palpated in the abdomen. Perform a rectal examination to assess for rectal tone and the presence of stool in the rectum. Often with Hirschsprung's, no stool is present in the rectum, but at the end of the rectal examination, when the finger is being withdrawn, a child with Hirschsprung's may have a forceful expulsion of fecal material.

Laboratory and Diagnostic Tests

Common laboratory and diagnostic studies ordered for the assessment of Hirschsprung's include:

• Barium enema: to look for a narrowing of the intestine
• Rectal suction biopsy: to demonstrate an absence of ganglion cells (definitive diagnosis)

— Distended sigmoid colon

— Aganglionic Portion
— Rectum

FIGURE 41.15 Enlarged megacolon of Hirschsprung's disease.

Nursing Management

Nursing management includes providing postoperative care, performing ostomy care, and providing patient and family education.

Providing Postoperative and Ostomy Care

Provide routine postoperative care and observe for the complication of enterocolitis (see Nursing Care Plan 41.1). Observe for the following signs and symptoms of enterocolitis:

• Fever
• Abdominal distention
• Chronic diarrhea
• Explosive stools
• Rectal bleeding
• Straining

If any of the above symptoms are noted, immediately notify the physician, maintain bowel rest, and administer intravenous fluids and antibiotics to prevent the development of shock and possibly death.

The patient with Hirschsprung's may have either a colostomy or ileostomy, depending on the extent of disease in the intestine. In either case, perform proper ostomy care to avoid skin breakdown. Accurately measure stool output to assess the child's fluid volume status.

Providing Patient and Family Education

The family may be anxious and fearful about upcoming surgeries and possible complications. Help to relieve their anxiety by providing information about the diagnosis and the stages of surgical procedures the patient will undergo. Provide postoperative teaching to educate parents on proper stoma care as well as medication management (to avoid dehydration, most Hirschsprung's patients will be prescribed medications to slow stool output). Arrange for the family to consult with a wound care nurse to help them deal with the anxieties and care of newly placed stomas. Provide education about possible postsurgical problems, emphasizing the importance of prompt medical treatment for signs of enterocolitis.

▶ SHORT BOWEL SYNDROME

Short bowel syndrome is a clinical syndrome of nutrient malabsorption and excessive intestinal fluid and electrolyte losses that occurs following massive small intestinal loss or surgical resection. The degree of malabsorption is usually related to the extent of resection of small bowel. The most common causes of short bowel syndrome are necrotizing enterocolitis, small intestinal atresia, gastroschisis, malrotation with volvulus, and trauma to the small intestine. A child can lose as much as 75% of the small intestine

without serious long-term problems, as long as the duodenum, terminal ileum, and ileocecal valve are still functioning. However, even a 25% intestinal loss can result in significant problems if the terminal ileum and ileocecal valve are not spared (Jakubik et al., 2000). If the terminal ileum is lost, vitamin B12 deficiency and bile salt malabsorption may occur. If the ileocecal valve is lost, small bowel bacterial overgrowth is likely to occur, as well as poor intestinal motility.

Therapeutic Management

The child with short bowel syndrome is at risk for chronic complications. The goals of therapeutic management are to minimize bacterial overgrowth and to maximize the child's nutritional status. Antibiotics may be used to control bacterial overgrowth. Vitamin and mineral supplementation is necessary because the small intestine is usually where fat-soluble vitamins, calcium, magnesium, and zinc are absorbed. Antidiarrheal agents such as loperamide and gastric acid-suppressive medications may be used to decrease stool output. Many children with short bowel syndrome require TPN for extended periods to achieve adequate growth. Progression to enteral feeding may occur extremely slowly, depending upon the intestine's response. Despite a markedly improved prognosis for these patients, some will not do as well and may ultimately require intestinal and liver transplantation due to irreversible liver damage from long-term use of TPN (Jakubik et al., 2000).

Nursing Assessment

Elicit the health history, noting diarrhea, which is the primary symptom of short bowel syndrome. Note past history of bowel loss or resection as noted above. Assess the child's hydration state. Inspect the stool for consistency, color, odor, and volume. Review laboratory results, particularly chemistries, to evaluate hydration status, and liver function tests, which may reveal evolving **cholestasis** secondary to long-term TPN use.

Nursing Management

Nursing management focuses on encouraging adequate nutrition and promoting effective family coping.

Encouraging Adequate Nutrition

Treatment for short bowel syndrome can be a slow and tedious process. Most patients will require TPN until they can tolerate enteral feeds without significant malabsorption. TPN is usually required for a lengthy time, so most children will require long-term intravenous access. Long-term intravenous access places the child at high risk for infection and resulting sepsis, so closely monitor for signs and symptoms of infection. Immediately report to the physician any fevers or redness or drainage at the intravenous site.

When started, enteral feeding must be administered very slowly to avoid further malabsorption. Usually the feeding is started continuously, 24 hours per day, via a feeding pump. Most patients have long-term feeding tubes, usually gastrostomy tubes. Most of these children will require special formulas to promote absorption. Assess for feeding tube residuals and abdominal distention or discomfort. Strictly monitor intake and output to avoid dehydration. Assess the stool for signs of carbohydrate malabsorption. Administer vitamin and mineral supplementation, antidiarrheals, and antibiotics as ordered. Teach the family about use of enteral feeding tubes, feeding pumps, and medication administration. (Jakubik et al., 2000).

Promoting Effective Family Coping

Children with short bowel syndrome are considered to be medically fragile for a lengthy period. There is much anxiety related to the initial bowel resection that resulted in short bowel. Long-term hospitalization is almost always required, causing parents to miss work and cutting down on the time they have to spend with other children. This can lead to even more anxiety about finances and relationships. Encourage families to become the experts on their child's needs and condition via education and participation in care. Provide teaching so that the family is better able to care for the child in an outpatient setting. Education focuses on information about TPN and central line care, enteral feedings, assessing for hydration status, and managing medications.

> ▶ *Take NOTE!*
>
> *Maintaining long-term central venous access for TPN in infants can present a challenge. One-piece clothing with the central venous line (CVL) tubing exiting and secured on the back of the outfit can help discourage the infant from pulling on (and subsequently dislodging) the line.*

▶ INFLAMMATORY BOWEL DISEASE

Crohn's disease and ulcerative colitis are the two major idiopathic inflammatory bowel diseases of children. The causes are unknown, but they may be due to an abnormal or uncontrolled genetically determined immunologic or inflammatory response to an environmental antigenic trigger, possibly a virus or bacterium. The features of Crohn's disease and ulcerative colitis are listed in Comparison Chart 41.2.

Therapeutic Management

Medication is used to control inflammation and symptoms. Medications commonly used include 5-aminosalicylates, antibiotics, immunomodulators, immunosuppressives, and anti-tumor necrosis antibody therapy. Dietary manipulation is also very important.

Failure to respond to medical therapy may result in surgical intervention. Many patients with ulcerative colitis eventually undergo a total proctocolectomy, with resulting ostomy, as a curative measure. Approximately 70% of Crohn's disease patients will require surgery to relieve obstruction, drain an abscess, or relieve intractable symptoms (Sondheimer, 2007).

Nursing Assessment

For a full description of the assessment phase of the nursing process refer to page 1329. Assessment findings pertinent to Crohn's disease and ulcerative colitis are discussed below.

Health History

Elicit a description of the present illness and chief complaint. Common signs and symptoms reported during the health history include:

• Abdominal cramping
• Nighttime symptoms, including waking due to abdominal pain or urge to defecate
• Fever
• Weight loss
• Poor growth
• Delayed sexual development

Children may be reluctant or unwilling to talk about their bowel movements, so explain the importance of doing so. Assess stool pattern history, including frequency, presence of blood or mucus, and duration of symptoms.

Explore the patient's current and past medical history for risk factors, such as:

• Family history of inflammatory bowel disease
• Family history of colon cancer
• Family history of immunologic disorders

Physical Examination

Assess the child's growth using growth charts to identify any poor growth patterns. Perform a full abdominal examination, noting tenderness, masses, or fullness. Inspect the perianal area to look for skin tags or fissures, which would be highly suspicious for Crohn's disease. Assist the physician in performing a rectal examination to further assess the rectal area for blood or other lesions.

Laboratory and Diagnostic Tests

Laboratory test results may be normal. Results for children with Crohn's disease and ulcerative colitis are found in Comparison Chart 41.2. Common laboratory and diag-

COMPARISON CHART 41.2 FEATURES OF CROHN'S DISEASE AND ULCERATIVE COLITIS

Feature	Crohn's Disease	Ulcerative Colitis
Age at onset	10 to 20 years	10 to 20 years
Incidence	4 to 6 per 100,000	3 to 15 per 100,000
Area of bowel affected	Oropharynx, esophagus, and stomach, rare: small bowel only, 25% to 30%; colon and anus only, 25%; ileocolitis, 40%; diffuse disease, 5%	Total colon, 90%; proctitis, 10%
Distribution	Segmental; disease-free skip areas common	Continuous; distal to proximal
Pathology	Full-thickness, acute, and chronic inflammation; noncaseating granulomas (50%), extraintestinal fistulas, abscesses, stricture, and fibrosis may be present	Superficial, acute inflammation of mucosa with microscopic crypt abscess
X-ray findings	Segmental lesions; thickened, circular folds, cobblestone appearance of bowel wall secondary to longitudinal ulcers and transverse fissures; fixation and separation of loops; narrowed lumen; "sting sign"; fistulas	Superficial colitis; loss of haustra; shortened colon and pseudopolyps (islands of normal tissue surrounded by denuded mucosa) are late findings
Intestinal symptoms	Abdominal pain, diarrhea (usually loose with blood if colon involved), perianal disease, enteroenteric or enterocutaneous fistula, abscess, anorexia	Abdominal pain, bloody diarrhea, urgency, tenesmus
Extraintestinal symptoms:		
Arthritis/arthralgia	15%	9%
Fever	40% to 50%	40% to 50%
Stomatitis	9%	2%
Weight loss	90% (mean 5.7 kg)	68% (mean 4.1 kg)
Delayed growth and sexual development	30%	5% to 10%
Uveitis, conjunctivitis	15% (in Crohn's colitis)	4%
Sclerosing cholangitis	—	4%
Renal stones	6% (oxalate)	6% (urate)
Pyoderma gangrenosum	1% to 3%	5%
Erythema nodosum	8% to 15%	4%
Laboratory findings	High erythrocyte sedimentation rate; microcytic anemia; low serum iron and total iron-binding capacity; increased fecal protein loss; low serum albumin; antineutrophil cytoplasmic antibodies present in 10% to 20%; *Saccharomyces cervisiae* antibodies positive in 60%	High erythrocyte sedimentation rate; microcytic anemia; high white blood cell count with left shift; antineutrophil cytoplasmic antibodies present in 80%

From Sondheimer, 2007.

nostic studies ordered for the assessment of inflammatory bowel disease include:

• Radiologic studies such as upper GI series with small bowel series: may identify evidence of intestinal inflammation, estimate distribution and extent of disease, and help distinguish between Crohn's disease and ulcerative colitis
• CT scan: to rule out suspected abscess
• Colonoscopy: to diagnose inflammatory bowel disease

• Upper endoscopy: to rule out affected mucosal tissue between the mouth and anus in children with upper abdominal complaints

Nursing Management

Nursing management focuses on teaching about disease management, teaching about nutritional management, teaching about medication therapy, and promoting family and child coping.

Teaching About Disease Management

The diagnosis of Crohn's disease or ulcerative colitis can be very difficult for the patient and family to comprehend. Provide teaching about the disease process and medication therapy to help the child and family understand the seriousness of the disease. The physician may discuss surgical options during uncontrolled flare-ups, but the nurse may be the person to whom the family members or patient address their questions regarding surgery. Provide the family with information to help answer some of their questions and allay fears.

Teaching About Nutritional Management

Teach the child and family about nutritional management of the disease. For example, adequate nutrition with a high-protein and high-carbohydrate diet may be recommended; when the disease is active, lactose may be tolerated poorly; and vitamin and iron supplements will most likely be recommended. Explain that in severe cases enteral feeding tubes or TPN may be needed; this is rare but often induces remission.

Teaching About Medication Therapy

Medications are extremely important in controlling inflammatory bowel disease. Provide information about the following common medications used to control the disease:

- 5-aminosalicylates (5-ASA): used to prevent relapse (usually used in ulcerative colitis)
- Antibiotics (usually metronidazole and ciprofloxacin): typically used in patients who have perianal Crohn's disease
- Immunomodulators (usually 6-mercaptopurine [6-MP] or azathioprine): used to help maintain remission. Monitor patients for neutropenia and hepatotoxicity.
- Cyclosporine or tacrolimus: used occasionally in conjunction with 6-MP or azathioprine to maintain remission in fulminant ulcerative colitis
- Methotrexate: sometimes used to manage severe Crohn's disease
- Anti-tumor necrosis antibody therapy: widely used for children with Crohn's disease; occasionally used for children with ulcerative colitis

Promoting Family and Child Coping

Inflammatory bowel disease is a chronic and often debilitating illness. Many children with this diagnosis can lead normal lives, but frequent illnesses can cause school absences, which in turn add stress to the situation. Because schools have become much less tolerant of absences and tardiness, it may be necessary to write letters to the school explaining the frequent absences or in-school needs. Bathroom privileges should be very flexible for children during flare-ups. Children tend to be of small stature due to the illness itself and steroid use, which stunts growth; this may cause psychological issues, especially for older boys.

Children with ostomies as a result of surgical resection may have self-esteem issues related to the presence and care of the ostomy. Arrange for counseling for both the child and family to discuss fears and anxiety related to a chronic disease.

▶ CELIAC DISEASE

Celiac disease, also known as celiac sprue, is an immunologic disorder in which gluten, a product most commonly found in grains, causes damage to the small intestine. The villi of the small intestine are damaged due to the body's immunologic response to the digestion of gluten. The function of the villi is to absorb nutrients into the bloodstream. When the villi are blunted or damaged, malnutrition occurs.

Celiac disease is one of the most common chronic disorders in Europe and the U.S., affecting about 1% of the population. Increased incidence occurs in those with a family history of celiac disease and in persons with autoimmune or genetic disorders (Gelfond & Fasano, 2006).

The only current treatment for celiac disease is a strict gluten-free diet. Eliminating gluten will cause the villi of the intestines to heal and function normally, with subsequent improvement of symptoms. Even very small amounts of gluten introduced back into the diet can cause damage to the villi, so the patient must adhere to the diet throughout life.

Nursing Assessment

For a full description of the assessment phase of the nursing process refer to page 1329. Assessment findings pertinent to celiac disease are discussed below. The child with symptoms of celiac disease often presents for evaluation by age 2.

Health History

Elicit a description of the present illness and chief complaint. The symptoms of celiac disease are very broad and are easily confused with other GI disorders. The classic symptoms of children with celiac disease are:

- Diarrhea
- **Steatorrhea**
- Constipation
- Failure to thrive or weight loss
- Abdominal distention or bloating
- Poor muscle tone
- Irritability and listlessness
- Dental disorders
- Anemia
- Delayed onset of puberty or amenorrhea
- Nutritional deficiencies

Explore the child's current and past medical history for risk factors such as Caucasian European descent and a family history of celiac disease (Allen, 2004).

Physical Examination

Assess for the typical appearance of children with celiac disease: distended abdomen, wasted buttocks, and very thin extremities (Allen, 2004) (Fig. 41.16).

Laboratory and Diagnostic Tests

Common laboratory and diagnostic studies ordered for the assessment of celiac disease include serological antibody screening and intestinal biopsy for confirmation and genetic testing. The serum antibody markers look for antibodies in the bloodstream that are specific to a patient's response to gluten. The intestinal biopsy is taken from the duodenum during an upper endoscopic procedure performed by a gastroenterologist. Pathology from the biopsy

FIGURE 41.16 The child with celiac disease typically displays a distended abdomen and wasted extremities.

reveals partial or subtotal villous atrophy or blunting of the villi of the small intestine. A child undergoing an intestinal biopsy to confirm or rule out celiac disease must not be restricted from consuming gluten for approximately 2 months before the biopsy. However, children may become symptomatic and extremely ill with a gluten challenge; in these cases, biopsies should be obtained sooner. Genetic testing is also available for celiac disease, looking for certain human leukocyte antigen (HLA) types. This may rule out celiac disease with 99% accuracy in people who are genetically predisposed to celiac disease, obviating the need for an intestinal biopsy (Allen, 2004).

Nursing Management

Providing patient and family education is the key nursing role in managing children with celiac disease. The patient must adhere to a strict gluten-free diet for his or her entire life. This is often very challenging, because gluten is found in most wheat products, rye, barley, and possibly oats. Encourage the parents and child to maintain this gluten-free diet. Often, families consult a dietitian to learn about the gluten-free diet (Teaching Guidelines 41.3).

Provide educational materials and resources to the parents. Many resources are available today about celiac disease because it is becoming more commonly diagnosed (Box 41.6).

▶ RECURRENT ABDOMINAL PAIN

Recurrent abdominal pain is a common GI complaint of children and adolescents. It affects children of all ages, and about 2% to 4% of all pediatric outpatient visits are related to recurrent abdominal pain (Saps & Li, 2006). The etiology remains unclear. The Rome Committee is a group of specialists who are focusing on the identification, management, and treatment of both adults and children with these functional GI disorders. The three categories of recurrent abdominal pain in children are functional abdominal pain, nonulcer dyspepsia, and irritable bowel syndrome. Box 41.7 outlines the Rome Committee's criteria for distinguishing different features of irritable bowel syndrome (Saps & Li, 2006).

Pathophysiology

The etiology of recurrent abdominal pain is controversial but most likely multifactorial. It is thought that the autonomic nervous system, which controls the body's response to emotions and stress, and intestinal motility are the two mechanisms. Symptoms may result from an alteration in the transmission of messages between the enteric nervous system and the central nervous system, leading to visceral hypersensitivity. Information from the GI tract is transmitted through bidirectional nerve

TEACHING GUIDELINES 41.3

Dietary Considerations in a Gluten-Free Diet

Foods Allowed

Potato, soy, rice, or bean flour, rice bran, cornmeal, arrowroot, corn or potato starch, sago, tapioca, buckwheat, millet, flax, teff, sorghum, amaranth, quinoa

Plain, fresh, frozen, or canned vegetables made with allowed ingredients

All fruits and fruit juices

All milk and milk products except those made with gluten additives, aged cheese

All meat, poultry, fish, and shellfish, dried peas and beans, nuts, peanut butter, soybean, cold cuts, frankfurters or sausage without fillers

Butter, margarine, salad dressings, sauces, soups, and desserts with allowable ingredients, sugar, honey, jelly, jam, hard candy, plain chocolate, coconut, molasses, marshmallows, meringues, pure instant or ground coffee, tea, carbonated drinks, wine (from the United States)

Foods To Avoid

Wheat flour, rye, triticale, barley, oats, wheat germ or bran, graham, gluten, or durum flour, wheat starch, oat bran, bulgur, farina, spelt, kamut, malt extract, hydrolyzed vegetable protein

Any creamed or breaded vegetables, canned baked beans, some French fries

Some commercial fruit pie fillings and dried fruit

Malted milk, flavored or frozen yogurt

Any meats or poultry prepared with wheat, rye, oats, barley, gluten stabilizers, or fillers for meats, canned meats, self-basting turkey, some egg substitutes

Commercial salad dressings, prepared soups, condiments, sauces, and seasonings made with avoided products, nondairy cream substitutes, flavored instant coffee, alcohol distilled from cereals, licorice

From NDDIC, 2007.

pathways to the brain. Most neurotransmitters are found in both the brain and the gut, suggesting the potential for integrated effects of pain modulation (Saps & Li, 2006). As different possibilities exist for the pathophysiology of recurrent abdominal pain, it is clear that there are no structural or biochemical abnormalities that are identifiable.

Therapeutic management most often focuses on increasing the child's coping skills. Some children may need dietary manipulation or medications to control diarrhea (irritable bowel syndrome).

Nursing Assessment

For a full description of the assessment phase of the nursing process refer to page 1329. Assessment findings pertinent to recurrent abdominal pain are discussed below.

BOX 41.6 **Resources for Parents of Children with Celiac Disease**

• American Celiac Society: 973-325-8837
• Celiac Disease Foundation: www.celiac.org, 818-990-2354
• Celiac Sprue Association: www.csaceliacs.org, 402-558-0600
• Gluten Intolerance Group (GIG): www.gluten.net, 206-246-6652
• R.O.C.K. (Raising Our Celiac Kids) support group: www.celiackids.com, 858-395-5421

These resources can offer information on all aspects of celiac disease, including dietary guidelines and resources for food shopping and eating in restaurants.

BOX 41.7 **Rome Committee Criteria for Irritable Bowel Syndrome**

12 weeks or more of the following symptoms:
• Abdominal pain relieved by defecation
• Onset of pain or discomfort associated with a change in frequency of stool
• Onset of pain or discomfort associated with a change in form of the stool
• No structural or metabolic explanation for this abdominal pain

From Saps & Li, 2006.

Health History

The diagnosis of recurrent abdominal pain is made on a symptom-based approach. Elicit a description of the present illness and chief complaint. The symptom reported mostly commonly during the health history is abdominal pain. The child may have difficulty providing a good description of the pain. It is usually periumbilical and is usually described as attacks of pain. It is uncommon for the child to wake up in the middle of the night with this type of pain. In cases of irritable bowel syndrome, the pain may be relieved by defecation. Because diet may play a large role in the symptoms, obtain a dietary history. Take a detailed medication history, because abdominal pain may be an adverse effect of some medications. Identifying social and school stressors is essential.

Physical Examination

Note the child's body positioning and facial expressions. Interactions with family members during the interview may provide more details regarding social stressors. Palpate the abdomen for tenderness.

Laboratory and Diagnostic Tests

Common laboratory and diagnostic studies ordered for the assessment of recurrent abdominal pain include:

- Complete blood count: to rule out organic causes of abdominal pain
- Erythrocyte sedimentation rate: to rule out organic causes of abdominal pain
- Urinalysis: to rule out organic causes of abdominal pain
- Complete metabolic panel (CMP): to rule out organic causes of abdominal pain
- Stool studies: to assess for routine pathogens

Nursing Management

Once the diagnosis of recurrent abdominal pain with no organic cause is made, the majority of the nursing management is focused on promoting coping skills. Often the physician performs a battery of tests to rule out organic causes, especially when patient and family anxiety is high. After these tests are complete, teach the family about the factors that exacerbate the pain and how to deal with these factors.

Diet changes may need to be implemented. High-fiber diets help with bowel regulation by keeping motility regular.

Often medications are used to relieve abdominal cramps. Antidiarrheals may be used for patients with irritable bowel syndrome that is manifested by diarrhea. Occasionally pain modulators and antidepressants are used to help block the neurotransmitters in the brain–gut connection that cause pain. Encourage compliance with the medication regimen: compliance is needed to achieve beneficial results with many of these medications.

Arrange for counseling, if necessary, for children with social stressors. Children with recurrent abdominal pain may become so debilitated that they cannot function in school, possibly requiring homebound instruction. Provide education to the school, with parental permission, regarding the child's illness and how to best deal with it. Explain that this recurrent abdominal pain is a true pain that children feel and is not "in their minds."

Hepatobiliary Disorders

Hepatobiliary disorders include pancreatitis, gallbladder disease, jaundice, biliary atresia, hepatitis, cirrhosis and portal hypertension, and liver transplantation.

▶ PANCREATITIS

Pancreatitis is increasingly being recognized as a childhood problem. It is classified into two categories: acute and chronic. Acute pancreatitis is an acute inflammatory process that occurs within the pancreas, with variable involvement of localized tissues and remote organ systems. Most common causes of acute pancreatitis include abdominal trauma, drugs and alcohol (though probably rare in children), multisystem disease (such as inflammatory bowel disease or systemic lupus erythematosus), infections (usually viruses such as cytomegalovirus or hepatitis), congenital anomalies (ductal or pancreatic malformations), obstruction (most likely gallstones or tumors in children), or metabolic disorders. Chronic pancreatitis is defined based on the structural and/or functional permanent changes that occur in the pancreas (Werlin, 2004).

When pancreatitis is suspected, the child is placed on immediate bowel rest (NPO). Often, a nasogastric tube placed for suction will be needed to keep the stomach decompressed. Serial monitoring of serum amylase levels will determine when oral feeding may be restarted (Werlin, 2004).

Nursing Assessment

For a full description of the assessment phase of the nursing process refer to page 1329. Assessment findings pertinent to pancreatitis are discussed below.

Health History

Elicit a description of the present illness and chief complaint. Common signs and symptoms reported during the health history include:

- Acute onset of persistent midepigastric and periumbilical abdominal pain, often with radiation to the back or chest
- Vomiting, especially after meals
- Fever

Explore the child's current and past medical history for risk factors such as:

• Cystic fibrosis
• History of gallstones
• Traumatic injury
• Family history of hereditary pancreatitis

Physical Examination

On abdominal assessment, the bowel sounds may be diminished, suggesting peritonitis. The abdomen may be tender, and distention may occur in younger children and infants. In severe cases, jaundice, ascites, or pleural effusions may occur. Bluish discoloration around the umbilicus or flanks is seen in the most severe cases of pancreatitis when hemorrhage is present.

Laboratory and Diagnostic Tests

Common laboratory and diagnostic studies ordered for the assessment and monitoring of pancreatitis include:

• Serum amylase and/or lipase: levels three times the normal values are extremely indicative of pancreatitis (Werlin, 2004)
• Liver profile: often done to check for increased liver functions and/or bilirubin levels
• Blood work: leukocytosis is common with acute pancreatitis. Hyperglycemia and hypocalcemia may also be noted.
• C-reactive protein: levels may be elevated

Diagnostic imaging studies performed to identify malformations or cysts on the pancreas include:

• Plain abdominal x-ray: may show a localized ileus
• Ultrasound: allows direct visualization of the pancreas and the surrounding structures. This is used most frequently with children, as it is less invasive than a CT scan. A CT scan is usually used when there is difficulty in determining the cause of the pancreatitis during ultrasonography.
• Endoscopic retrograde cholangiopancreatography (ERCP): used in some children who may have ductal anomalies, usually with chronic pancreatitis, though complications from this procedure may occur.

Nursing Management

Maintain NPO status and nasogastric tube suction and patency. Administer intravenous fluids to keep the patient hydrated and correct any alterations in fluid and electrolyte balance. Pain management is crucial in children with pancreatitis. If hemorrhagic pancreatitis has occurred, blood products and/or intravenous antibiotics may be needed. Oral feedings are restarted only after the serum amylase level has returned to normal (usually in 2 to 4 days) (Werlin, 2004). Often, pancreatic enzymes are given with oral feedings if pain occurs after oral feeds are restarted.

Surgery is rarely needed in patients with pancreatitis, except in those with severe abdominal trauma or major ductal abnormalities.

Though chronic pancreatitis is rare in children, provide patient and family education regarding the signs and symptoms of recurrence and complications.

▶ GALLBLADDER DISEASE

Cholelithiasis is the presence of stones in the gallbladder. Cholesterol stones are usually associated with hyperlipidemia, obesity, pregnancy, birth control pill use, or cystic fibrosis. They are seen more often in females than males, and increased risk occurs with age and onset of puberty. These stones occur in the gallbladder and may be found in the common bile duct. Pigment stones are found in prepubertal children and occur about equally in males and females. They are usually found in the common bile duct (associated with bacterial or parasitic infections) or the gallbladder itself (associated with hemolytic anemia or liver cirrhosis). Cholecystitis is an inflammation of the gallbladder that is caused by the chemical irritation due to the obstruction of bile flow from the gallbladder into the cystic ducts (Fig. 41.17). This inflammation is typically associated with gallstones in children. The most common complication in children with gallstone disease is pancreatitis (Suchy, 2004).

If cholelithiasis results in symptomatic cholecystitis, then surgical removal of the gallbladder (cholecystectomy) will be necessary. This is often accomplished laparoscopically.

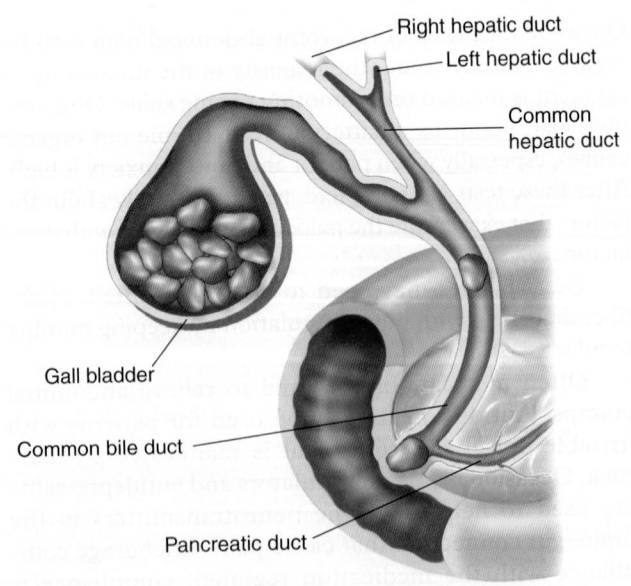

FIGURE 41.17 When gallstones block the flow of bile through the ducts, cholecystitis results.

Nursing Assessment

For a full description of the assessment phase of the nursing process refer to page 1329. Assessment findings pertinent to gallbladder disease are discussed below.

Health History

Elicit a description of the present illness and chief complaint. Common signs and symptoms reported during the health history include:

• Right upper quadrant pain, often radiating substernally or to the right shoulder
• Nausea and vomiting
• Jaundice and fever (with cholecystitis)

Document a detailed diet history as it relates to the presenting symptoms. Pain episodes usually occur after meals (postprandially), especially after the ingestion of fatty or greasy foods. Younger children may present with more nonspecific symptoms, most often due to their lack of ability to communicate their symptoms to others. Explore the patient's current and past medical history for risk factors such as chronic TPN use or sickle cell disease.

Physical Examination

Palpate the abdomen for tenderness. If cholecystitis is present, the gallbladder becomes inflamed, often to the point of causing localized tenderness upon palpation. Assess skin and sclerae color for jaundice. Note presence of fever.

Laboratory and Diagnostic Tests

Common laboratory and diagnostic studies ordered for the assessment of cholecystitis include:

• Liver function tests, bilirubin, and C-reactive protein: values may be elevated if ductal stones are present
• CBC: may reveal leukocytosis
• Amylase and lipase: may be elevated if pancreatitis is also present
• Plain abdominal x-rays: may reveal radiopaque stones
• Ultrasound of the gallbladder and surrounding structures: to assess the intraluminal contents of the gallbladder as well as any anatomic alterations
• ERCP: to rule out ductal stones
• HIDA scan: to evaluate the function of the gallbladder

Nursing Management

The child with symptomatic cholecystitis will usually be hospitalized. Administer intravenous fluids, maintain NPO status and gastric decompression, and administer pain medications. If ordered, administer intravenous antibiotics to treat clinically worsening symptoms of cholecystitis, such as persistent fever. Provide routine postoperative care after cholecystectomy is performed. Provide pre- and postoperative teaching for families of children undergoing gallbladder removal.

▶ BILIARY ATRESIA

Biliary atresia is an absence of some or all of the major biliary ducts, resulting in obstruction of bile flow. The resultant obstruction to bile flow causes cholestasis and progressive fibrosis with end-stage cirrhosis of the liver (Balistreri, 2004). In approximately 80% of the cases, biliary atresia presents around 4 weeks of age in term, healthy infants who have resolved physiologic jaundice. In approximately 20% of cases, biliary atresia presents with persistent jaundice that never disappeared from the physiologic period. This second type of biliary atresia often is associated with other congenital anomalies, such as situs inversus, malrotation, polysplenia, and cardiovascular defects (Balistreri, 2004). The etiology of biliary atresia is unknown, but there are several theories, including infectious, autoimmune, or ischemic causes.

Therapeutic Management

If there is a high suspicion of biliary atresia, the infant will undergo exploratory laparotomy. If biliary atresia is found, a Kasai procedure (hepatoportoenterostomy) is performed to connect the bowel lumen to the bile duct remnants found at the porta hepatis. This procedure is usually successful only for infants up to 8 weeks of age, as bile flow restoration after this age is minimal. Infants who are not identified early enough or those who have failed to respond to the Kasai procedure will need to undergo liver transplantation, usually by age 2.

Nursing Assessment

For a full description of the assessment phase of the nursing process refer to page 1329. Assessment findings pertinent to biliary atresia are discussed below.

Health History

Elicit a description of the present illness and chief complaint. Persistent or recurring jaundice is the most common symptom reported during the health history.

Physical Examination

In the initial assessment of an infant with cholestasis of unknown origin, assess the stool character. In biliary atresia, stools will be acholic (chalky and white due to the lack of bile pigment). Note jaundice of the skin and sclerae (yellow discoloration caused by bile pigment deposition). Palpate the abdomen; the liver will feel enlarged and hardened. Splenomegaly may occur. In the absence of other congenital malformations, the infant will otherwise appear healthy.

Laboratory and Diagnostic Studies

Common laboratory and diagnostic studies ordered for the assessment of biliary atresia include:

- Serum bilirubin, alkaline phosphatase, liver enzymes, GGT: elevated
- Ultrasound: to identify anomalies
- Biliary scan: to distinguish whether the cholestasis is intrahepatic or extrahepatic
- Liver biopsy: to confirm the diagnosis (Balistreri, 2004)

Nursing Management

Nursing management of infants who have biliary atresia will focus on vitamin and caloric support. Administer fat-soluble vitamins A, D, E, and K. Special formulas containing medium-chain triglycerides are used because significant fat malabsorption occurs when cholestasis is present. Administer feedings via nasogastric tube as needed to ensure increased caloric intake. Identify infections as quickly as possible and administer intravenous antibiotics as ordered. Manage ascites with diuretics and dietary restrictions. Preoperative management before a Kasai procedure is focused on preparation for surgery;

infants who have suspected biliary atresia require immediate surgery to optimize outcomes.

Parents and family members of these infants will have extreme anxiety due to the implications of the diagnosis and outcomes. Focus education on the diagnosis and postoperative care. Nursing Care Plan 41.1 gives information about routine postoperative care.

▶ HEPATITIS

Hepatitis is an inflammation of the liver that is caused by a variety of agents, including viral infections, bacterial invasion, metabolic disorders, chemical toxicity, and trauma. The most common viral causes of hepatitis are listed in Table 41.3. Other viruses that may cause hepatitis are cytomegalovirus (CMV), Epstein-Barr virus (EBV), and adenovirus. Fulminant hepatitis is thought to be caused by a non-A, non-B, non-C virus. Children who present with fulminant hepatitis have acute massive hepatic necrosis, resulting in death without liver transplantation. The disease progresses rapidly to severe jaundice, coagu-

TABLE 41.3 **HEPATITIS VIRUSES A–E**

	Hepatitis A (HAV)	Hepatitis B (HBV)	Hepatitis C (HCV)	Hepatitis D (HDV)	Hepatitis E (HEV)
Transmission route	Oral–fecal route, poor sanitation, waterborne	Sexual, intravenous drug use, blood transfusion, perinatally transmitted from mother to infant	Blood product transfusion, intravenous drug use	Same as HBV; HBV markers in serum must be present	Oral–fecal, possible contact
Incubation period	15 to 30 days	50 to 150 days	30 to 160 days	50 to 150 days	15 to 65 days
Signs and symptoms	Flu-like symptoms Preicteric phase: headache, fatigue, fever, anorexia Icteric phase: jaundice, dark urine, tender liver (right upper quadrant pain)	Some cases are asymptomatic; others present with anorexia, abdominal pain, fatigue, rash, slight fever, visible jaundice, enlarged liver.	Chronic cases usually present asymptomatically; others with flu-like symptoms, jaundice, hepatosplenomegaly	Same as HBV	Same as HAV, more severe in pregnant women
Prognosis	Rarely develops into fulminant liver failure; 95% of children recover without sequelae	Chronic disease state likely; increased risk of hepatic cancer	Many will develop chronic hepatitis and cirrhosis.	Same as HBV, but increased likelihood of chronic active hepatitis and cirrhosis	Same as HAV; high mortality in pregnant women

lopathy, elevated ammonia levels, significantly elevated liver enzyme levels (AST and ALT), and progressive coma. Autoimmune hepatitis is a chronic disorder, affecting mostly adolescent females. The clinical presentation of a child with autoimmune hepatitis includes hepatosplenomegaly, jaundice, fever, fatigue, and right upper quadrant pain.

Therapeutic Management

Acute hepatitis is treated with rest, hydration, and nutrition. Control of bleeding may also be necessary. Chronic hepatitis often eventually requires liver transplantation. Corticosteroids and immunosuppressants may be used for autoimmune hepatitis. The child with fulminant hepatitis usually requires intensive care with cardiorespiratory support. See Healthy People 2010.

Nursing Assessment

For a full description of the assessment phase of the nursing process refer to page 1329. Assessment findings pertinent to hepatitis are discussed below. The nursing assessment for any child who presents with suspected hepatitis should be the same.

Health History

Elicit a description of the present illness and the chief complaint. Common signs and symptoms reported during the health history include:

- Jaundice
- Fever
- Fatigue
- Abdominal pain

Explore the patient's current and past medical history for risk factors such as:

- Recent foreign travel
- Sick contacts
- Medication use
- Abdominal trauma

HEALTHY PEOPLE 2010

Objective	Significance
Reduce or eliminate indigenous cases of vaccine-preventable diseases, hepatitis B (persons aged 2 to 18 years). Reduce hepatitis A.	• Educate families about hepatitis B and its transmission. • Encourage routine infant and childhood vaccination against hepatitis A and B as recommended. • For hepatitis A prevention, educate families about appropriate hygiene and hand washing.

- Sexual activity
- Intravenous drug use
- Blood product transfusion

Document onset of symptoms as well as all signs and symptoms the patient has been experiencing.

Physical Examination

Observe the skin for jaundice and the sclerae for icterus. Palpate the abdomen to reveal abnormal liver and spleen size or tenderness.

Laboratory and Diagnostic Studies

Common laboratory and diagnostic studies ordered for the assessment of hepatitis include:

- Liver enzymes, GGT: elevated
- PT/PTT: prolonged
- Ammonia: elevated in the presence of encephalopathy
- Autoimmune studies, such as antinuclear antibodies, anti–smooth muscle antibodies, and liver–kidney microsomal antibodies: may be used to diagnose autoimmune hepatitis
- Viral studies: to identify viral causes of hepatitis, such as hepatitis A–E antigens and antibodies, CMV and EBV
- Ultrasound: to assess liver or spleen abnormalities
- Liver biopsy: to determine the type of hepatitis and to assess for damage that has already been done to the liver

Nursing Management

Acute hepatitis requires rest, hydration, and nutrition. If the child develops vomiting, dehydration, elevated bleeding times (PT/PTT), or mental status changes (encephalopathy), hospitalization may be required. When caring for patients with infectious hepatitis, provide education about transmission and prevention, including proper hygiene, safe sexual activity, careful hand washing techniques, and blood/bodily fluid precautions.

Fulminant hepatitis treatment is aggressive and will require NPO status, nasogastric tube administration of lactulose to decrease ammonia levels that lead to encephalopathic conditions, TPN administration, vitamin K injections to help with coagulopathies, and, ultimately, liver transplantation. Fear and anxiety of the patient and parents will likely be very high. Teach the child and family about the diagnosis and what to expect during treatment. Provide immunoglobulin therapy and vaccinations to close contacts of infectious hepatitis patients.

▶ CIRRHOSIS AND PORTAL HYPERTENSION

Cirrhosis of the liver occurs as a result of the destructive processes that occur during liver damage, leading to the formation of nodules. These nodules can be small (micro-nodular [less than 3 mm]) or large (macronodular [greater than 3 mm]) and distort the vasculature of the liver, leading to further complications. Causes of cirrhosis in children include biliary malformations, alpha-1 antitrypsin deficiency, Wilson's disease, galactosemia, tyrosinemia, chronic active hepatitis, and prolonged TPN use (Sokol & Narkewicz, 2005). Major complications may exist due to cirrhosis of the liver, including portal hypertension. In portal hypertension, the blood flow to, through, or from the liver meets resistance, causing portal blood flow pressures to rise. As these pressures rise, collateral veins form between the portal and systemic venous circulations. The most significant complication of portal hypertension is GI bleeding, from shunting to submucosal veins (varices) in the stomach and esophagus. Esophageal varices may be treated with sclerotherapy during endoscopy to stop acute bleeding. Often blood product administration and vasopressive drugs are needed. In the long term, the only cure for cirrhosis is liver transplantation.

FIGURE 41.18 Esophageal varices.

Nursing Assessment

For a full description of the assessment phase of the nursing process refer to page 1329. Assessment findings pertinent to cirrhosis and portal hypertension are discussed below.

Health History

Elicit a description of the present illness and chief complaint. Common signs and symptoms reported during the health history include:

- Nausea and vomiting
- Jaundice
- Weakness
- Swelling
- Weight loss

Explore the patient's current and past medical history for risk factors such as hepatitis, cystic fibrosis, Wilson's disease, hematochromatosis, and biliary atresia. Assess the past medical history to identify possible causes for liver disease.

Physical Examination

Inspect for jaundice, ascites, spider angiomas, and palmar erythema. Gynecomastia is often seen in males. Palpate the liver; typically it is enlarged and hard, but occasionally it is small and shrunken. Evaluate mental status to determine the presence of hepatic encephalopathy.

Laboratory and Diagnostic Studies

Laboratory and diagnostic testing will be similar to that of a child with hepatitis. Common laboratory and diagnostic studies ordered for the assessment of cirrhosis or portal hypertension include:

- Liver biopsy: reveals regenerating nodules and surrounding **fibrosis**
- Upper endoscopy: reveals varices and bleeding (Fig. 41.18)

Nursing Management

Nursing management is very similar to the care of the patient with hepatitis. In cases of cirrhosis causing portal hypertension and bleeding varices, GI bleeding must be controlled. This is usually done by replacing blood loss and providing vasopressive therapy to constrict the shunted blood flow. As with all liver disorders and GI bleeding, address and manage family and patient anxiety. Be honest about the child's treatment plan and prognosis. Involve the family in the care of the child and educate them as needed.

▶ LIVER TRANSPLANTATION

Hepatobiliary disorders that result in failure of the liver to function result in the need for liver transplantation. Liver transplantation in children has become increasingly successful in the past several years due to advances in immunosuppression, better selection of transplant candidates, and improvements in surgical techniques and postoperative care. Transplant centers now offer both cadaveric and living-related liver transplants for children. Rejection of the transplanted liver is the most significant complication. Most children will require immunosuppressive therapy for a lifetime, putting them at risk for infections.

Nursing Assessment

Many children will be admitted to a transplant center for a preoperative work-up to determine the best possible tissue and blood match for the patient. There is much anxiety among family members when a cadaveric transplant is the only possibility for survival. This puts a child on a waiting list that is prioritized based on several criteria. Because there are a limited number of pediatric liver transplant centers throughout the country, there may be many issues regarding transportation, finances, job loss, and lodging. Assess the need for social work intervention; a social worker is almost always involved with these patients. A liver transplant coordinator will assist with coordinating the care for pre- and post-transplant patients.

Nursing Management

Preoperatively, assist with the transplant work-up and teach the child and family what to expect during and after the liver transplantation. Postoperatively, the child will be in the intensive care unit for several days until he or she is stabilized from the actual surgery (see Nursing Care Plan 41.1). After the child is sent to a regular unit in the hospital, monitor the child for several days to weeks for signs and symptoms of rejection and infection, including fever, increasing liver function test results and GGT, and increasing pain, redness, and swelling at the incision site.

Patient and family education is an important element of nursing management in the post-transplant patient. Assess and reassess medication knowledge throughout the entire hospitalization, as these children usually require medications for a lifetime.

■■■ Key Concepts

- The esophagus of the young child exhibits underdeveloped muscle tone compared with the adult.
- A major difference between children and adults is the reduced stomach capacity in the child and the significantly shorter length of the small intestine (250 cm in the child vs. 600 cm in the adult).
- Infants and children have a proportionately greater amount of body water than adults, resulting in a relatively greater fluid intake requirement than adults and placing infants and children at higher risk for fluid loss as compared with adults.
- The most common result of GI illnesses in infants and children is dehydration.
- The mildly or moderately dehydrated child must be identified and receive rehydration therapy to prevent progression to hypovolemic shock.
- Rehydration is a key medical treatment for dehydration as a result of many different GI disorders. Oral rehydration is most common, but in cases requiring hospitalization intravenous fluid therapy is key.

- Promotion of adequate nutrition is another significant treatment component. The child with a chronic GI disorder may require intravenous TPN or enteral tube feedings to exhibit appropriate growth.
- Surgical intervention is necessary for many acute or congenital GI disorders, such as pyloric stenosis, omphalocele, gastroschisis, cleft lip and palate, appendicitis, Hirschsprung's disease, and intestinal malrotation.
- Abdominal ultrasound is the diagnostic test of choice when evaluating for pyloric stenosis.
- Monitoring the blood count, electrolyte levels, and liver function tests is necessary in many pediatric GI disorders.
- Histamine-2 blockers, proton pump inhibitors, and prokinetic agents are used to treat disorders in which gastric acid is a problem, such as esophagitis, GERD, and ulcers.
- Close monitoring for infection is important in children with inflammatory bowel disease, autoimmune hepatitis, or liver transplant who are being treated with immunosuppressants and/or corticosteroids.
- GI stimulants and laxatives may be necessary for treating constipation and encopresis.
- Diarrhea, vomiting, decreased oral intake, sustained high fever, diabetic ketoacidosis, and extensive burns place the infant or child at risk for the development of dehydration.
- Risk factors for vomiting include exposure to viruses, use of certain medications, and overfeeding in the infant.
- Risk factors for acute diarrhea include recent ingestion of undercooked meats, foreign travel, daycare attendance, and well water ingestion.
- Vomiting is a symptom and should be characterized in terms of volume, color, relation to meals, duration, and associated symptoms.
- Bleeding may occur as a result of a GI disorder, particularly from the intestine with Meckel's diverticulum and from esophageal varices with portal hypertension.
- Acute GI disorders are those that usually have a rapid onset and a short course, which at times may be severe. Examples include dehydration, vomiting, diarrhea, hypertrophic pyloric stenosis, and appendicitis.
- Chronic GI disorders are those that are long lasting or recur over time. Examples include constipation, GER, inflammatory bowel disease, recurrent abdominal pain, and failure to thrive.
- Right lower quadrant pain and rebound tenderness of the abdomen found on physical examination are telltale signs of appendicitis, which is considered a surgical emergency.
- Bilious vomiting is the main symptom of conditions resulting in bowel obstruction, such as malrotation with volvulus.
- The focus of nursing management of the child with diarrhea or vomiting is restoring proper fluid and

electrolyte balance through oral rehydration therapy or intravenous fluids if necessary.

▪ Reduction of inguinal and umbilical hernias should be attempted; if reduction of the hernia is impossible, immediately notify the physician.

▪ Small, frequent, and thickened feedings and proper positioning after feedings are key elements in the treatment of GER.

▪ A crucial nursing intervention related to cleft lip and palate repair is protection of the surgical site while it is healing.

▪ Palpation of the abdomen should be the last part of the physical examination of an infant or child.

▪ A key element of nursing care for the child with a GI disorder is promotion of appropriate bowel elimination.

▪ Maximizing nutritional status is a critical nursing function for the child with a GI disorder.

▪ For the child who has undergone surgical repair or correction of a GI disorder, promoting effective breathing patterns and managing pain are important nursing goals.

▪ Counseling families about how to manage the child with vomiting or diarrhea at home, including oral rehydration therapy, is a key component of patient/family education.

▪ Education of the child and family regarding the importance of medication compliance for management of inflammatory bowel disease is critical.

▪ Behavioral therapy and counseling may be necessary for children who have functional constipation and stool withholding.

▪ The child or adolescent with ineffective bowel control, poor growth, or an ostomy may have poor self-esteem and body image.

REFERENCES

Albanese, C. T., & Sylvester, K. G. (2006). Pediatric surgery. In G. M. Doherty & L. W. Way (Eds.), *Current surgical diagnosis and treatment* (12th ed.). New York: McGraw-Hill.

Allen, P. L. J. (2004). Guidelines for the diagnosis and treatment of celiac disease in children. *Pediatric Nursing, 30*(6), 473–476.

Arguin, A. L., & Swartz, M. K. (2004). Gastroesophageal reflux in infants: A primary care perspective. *Pediatric Nursing, 30*(1), 45–51, 71.

Balistreri, W. F. (2004). Cholestasis. In R. E. Behrman, R. M. Kliegman, & H. B. Jenson (Eds.), *Nelson textbook of pediatrics* (17th ed.). Philadelphia: W. B. Saunders.

Bender, B. J., Skae, C. C., & Ozuah, P. O. (2005). Oral rehydration therapy: The clear solution to fluid loss. *Contemporary Pediatrics, 22*(4), 72–76.

Biggs, W. S., & Dery, W. H. (2006). Evaluation and treatment of constipation in infants and children. *American Family Physician, 73*(3), 469–477.

Bhutani, V. K., Johnson, L. H., & Keren, R. (2005). Treating acute bilirubin encephalopathy before it's too late. *Contemporary Pediatrics, 22*(5), 57–74.

Brunnell, P. A. (2006). Winter vomiting disease, 1929–2006. *Infectious Diseases in Children, 19*(1), 6–7.

Children's Healthcare of Atlanta. (2004). *Ostomy care home care manual.* Atlanta: Children's Healthcare of Atlanta.

Cincinnati Children's Hospital Medical Center. (2005). *Enema administration.* Retrieved 1/6/08, from www.cincinnatichildrens.org/health/info/abdomen/home/enema.htm

ConvaTec. (2008). *Just for kids.* Retrieved 1/6/08 from http://www.convatec.com/convatec/jsp/CVTUSCStaticContent.do?lang=en&country=US&audience=Consumer&channelId=-13838.

Curtin, G. (2004). Cleft lip and cleft palate. In P. L. Jackson & J. A. Vessey (Eds.), *Primary care of the child with a chronic condition* (4th ed.). St. Louis: Mosby.

Dale, J. (2004). Oral rehydration solutions in the management of acute gastroenteritis among children. *Journal of Pediatric Health Care, 18*, 211–212.

Engel, J. (2006). *Pocket guide to pediatric assessment* (5th ed). St. Louis: Mosby.

Ford, D. M. (2007). Fluid, electrolyte, and acid-base disorders & therapy. In W. W. Hay, M. J. Levin, J. M. Sondheimer, & R. R. Deterding, *Current pediatric diagnosis and treatment* (18th ed.). New York: McGraw-Hill.

Gardiner, P., & Kemper, K. J. (2005). For GI complaints, which herbs and supplements spell relief? *Contemporary Pediatrics, 22*(8), 51–55.

Gelfond, D., & Fasano, A. (2006). Celiac disease in the pediatric population. *Pediatric Annals, 35*(4), 275–279.

Gilger, M. A. (2006). Normal gastrointestinal function. In J. A. McMillan (Ed.), *Oski's pediatrics: Principles and practice*. Philadelphia: Lippincott Williams & Wilkins.

Grupka, M. J., & Wu, G. (2006). *Gastroenteritis, viral.* Retrieved 1/4/08 from http://www.emedicine.com/med/topic856.htm

Herbst, J. J. (2004). Primary (peptic) ulcers. In R. E. Behrman, R. M. Kliegman, & H. B. Jenson (Eds.), *Nelson textbook of pediatrics* (17th ed.). Philadelphia: W. B. Saunders.

Holcomb, S. S. (2005). Managing jaundice in full-term infants. *Nurse Practitioner, 30*(1), 6–12.

Hollister Incorporated. (2007). *Caring for your child with an ostomy.* Libertyville, IL: Author.

Howell, L. J. (2004). *Information about specific surgical procedures: ileostomy.* Retrieved 1/4/08, from www.chop.edu/consumer/jsp/division/generic.jsp?id=72368

Jakubik, L. D., Colfer, A., & Grossman, M. B. (2000). Pediatric short bowel syndrome: Pathophysiology, nursing care, and management issues. *Journal of the Society of Pediatric Nurses, 5*(3), 111–121.

Koslap-Petraco, M. B. (2006). Homecare issues in rotavirus gastroenteritis. *Journal of the American Academy of Nurse Practitioners, 18*(9), 422–428.

Kula, K. S., & Josell, S. D. (2006). Oral problems. In J. A. McMillan (Ed.), *Oski's pediatrics: Principles and practice.* Philadelphia: Lippincott Williams & Wilkins.

Long, S. S. (2006). Herpangina. In J. A. McMillan (Ed.), *Oski's pediatrics: Principles and practice.* Philadelphia: Lippincott Williams & Wilkins.

March of Dimes. (2008). *Cleft lip and palate.* Retrieved 1/4/08 from http://www.marchofdimes.com/professionals/14332_1210.asp.

National Digestive Diseases Information Clearinghouse (NDDIC) (2007). *Celiac disease.* http://digestive.niddk.nih.gov/ddiseases/pubs/celiac/index/htm

Nemours Foundation. (2006). *Stool tests.* Retrieved 1/4/08 from http://www.kidshealth.org/parent/general/sick/labtest8.html.

Nuthakki, S., & Schlievert, R. (2007). Child with "burns" on the tongue. *Consultant for Pediatricians, 6*(6), 345–346.

Orenstein, S. R. (2007). Issues in diagnosis and management of pediatric GERD. *Contemporary Pediatrics, 24*(2 Suppl.), 1–6.

Pagana, K. D., & Pagana, T. J. (2006). *Mosby's manual of diagnostic and laboratory tests* (3rd ed.). St. Louis: Mosby.

Peña, A. (2004). Anorectal malformations. In R. E. Behrman, R. M. Kliegman, & H. B. Jenson (Eds.), *Nelson textbook of pediatrics* (17th ed.). Philadelphia: W. B. Saunders.

Pollack, V. P., & Ravenscroft, A. D. (2004). Inflammatory bowel disease. In P. L. Jackson & J. A. Vessey (Eds.), *Primary care of the child with a chronic condition* (4th ed.). St. Louis: Mosby.

Rolstad, B. S., & Erwin-Toth, P. (2004). Peristomal skin complications: Prevention and management. *Ostomy/Wound Management, 50*(9), 68–77.

Saps, M., & Li, B. U. K. (2006). Chronic abdominal pain of functional origin in children. *Pediatric Annals, 35*(4), 246–256.

Schmitt, B. (2002). *Enema: How to give.* Broomfield, CO: McKesson Health Solutions LLC.

Schmitt, B. D. (2004). Toilet training problems: Underachievers, refusers, and stool holders. *Contemporary Pediatrics, 21*(4), 71–80.

Sehgal, S., & Allen, P. L. J. (2004). Hepatitis C in children. *Pediatric Nursing, 30*(5), 409–413.

Shollenberger, D. A., & Small, C. C. (2004). GI care. In E. J. Mills (Ed.), *Nursing procedures*. Philadelphia: Lippincott Williams & Wilkins.

Silbermintz, A., & Markowitz, J. (2006). Inflammatory bowel disease. *Pediatric Annals, 35*(4), 269–274.

Sokol, R., & Narkewicz, M. (2005). Liver & pancreas. In W. W. Hay, M. J. Levin, J. M. Sondheimer, & R. R. Deterding (Eds.), *Current pediatric diagnosis & treatment* (17th ed.). New York: McGraw-Hill.

Sondheimer, J. M. (2007). Gastrointestinal tract. In W. W. Hay, M. J. Levin, J. M. Sondheimer, & R. R. Deterding, *Current pediatric diagnosis and treatment* (18th ed.). New York: McGraw-Hill.

Steiner, M. J., DeWalt, D. A., & Byerley, J. S. (2004). Is this child dehydrated? *Journal of the American Medical Association, 291*(22), 2746–2754.

Stoll, B. J. & Kliegman, P. M. (2004). Neonatal necrotizing enterocolitis (NEC). In R. E. Behrman, R. M. Kliegman, & H. B. Jenson (Eds.), *Nelson textbook of pediatrics* (17th ed.). Philadelphia: W. B. Saunders.

Suchy, F. J. (2004). Diseases of the gallbladder. In R. E. Behrman, R. M. Kliegman, & H. B. Jenson (Eds.), *Nelson textbook of pediatrics* (17th ed.). Philadelphia: W. B. Saunders.

Suwandhi, E., Ton, M. N., & Schwarz, S. M. (2006). Gastroesophageal reflux in infancy and childhood. *Pediatric Annals, 35*(4), 259–266.

Taketokmo, C. K., Hodding, J. H., & Kraus, D. M. (2007). *Lexi-comp's pediatric dosage handbook* (14th ed.). Hudson, Ohio: Lexi-comp.

Tolan, R. W., & Kumar, M. (2007). *Thrush*. Retrieved 1/4/08 from http://www.emedicine.com/ped/topic2245.htm.

Tolarova, M. M., & Oh, H. S. (2006). *Cleft lip and palate*. Retrieved 1/4/08 from http://www.emedicine.com/ped/topic2679.htm.

Ulshen, M. (2004a). Chronic ulcerative colitis. In R. E. Behrman, R. M. Kliegman, & H. B. Jenson (Eds.), *Nelson textbook of pediatrics* (17th ed.). Philadelphia: W. B. Saunders.

Ulshen, M. (2004b). Crohn disease (regional enteritis, regional ileitis, granulomatous colitis). In R. E. Behrman, R. M. Kliegman, & H. B. Jenson (Eds.), *Nelson textbook of pediatrics* (17th ed.). Philadelphia: W. B. Saunders.

Ulshen, M. (2004c). Major symptoms and signs of digestive tract disorders. In R. E. Behrman, R. M. Kliegman, & H. B. Jenson (Eds.), *Nelson textbook of pediatrics* (17th ed.). Philadelphia: W. B. Saunders.

Walker, A., & Isolauri, E. (2007). Understanding the use of probiotics in pediatric populations. *Contemporary Pediatrics, 24*(4 Suppl.), 1–6.

Werlin, S. L. (2004). Pancreatitis. In R. E. Behrman, R. M. Kliegman, & H. B. Jenson (Eds.), *Nelson textbook of pediatrics* (17th ed.). Philadelphia: W. B. Saunders.

Wyllie, R. (2004a). Congenital aganglionic megacolon (Hirschsprung disease). In R. E. Behrman, R. M. Kliegman, & H. B. Jenson (Eds.), *Nelson textbook of pediatrics* (17th ed.). Philadelphia: W. B. Saunders.

Wyllie, R. (2004b). Intussusception. In R. E. Behrman, R. M. Kliegman, & H. B. Jenson (Eds.), *Nelson textbook of pediatrics* (17th ed.). Philadelphia: W. B. Saunders.

Wyllie, R. (2004c). Malrotation. In R. E. Behrman, R. M. Kliegman, & H. B. Jenson (Eds.), *Nelson textbook of pediatrics* (17th ed.). Philadelphia: W. B. Saunders.

Wyllie, R. (2004d). Meckel diverticulum and other remnants of the omphalomesenteric duct. In R. E. Behrman, R. M. Kliegman, & H. B. Jenson (Eds.), *Nelson textbook of pediatrics* (17th ed.). Philadelphia: W. B. Saunders.

WEBSITES

International Foundation for Functional Gastrointestinal Disorders: www.aboutkidsgi.org
American Cleft Palate/Craniofacial Association: www.acpa-cpf.org
Celiac Disease Foundation: www.celiac.org
R.O.C.K. (Raising Our Celiac Kids) support group: www.celiackids.com
Children's Liver Disease Foundation: www.childliverdisease.org
Support for families with cleft lip or palate: www.cleft.org
Cleft Palate Foundation: www.cleftline.org
ConvaTec: www.convatec.com
Celiac Sprue Association: www.csaceliacs.org
Gluten Intolerance Group: www.gluten.net
American Liver Foundation: www.liverfoundation.org
March of Dimes: www.marchofdimes.com
North American Society for Pediatric Gastroenterology, Hepatology and Nutrition: www.naspgn.org
Oley Foundation, a national organization for persons dependent upon intravenous or tube-fed nutrition: www.oley.org
Pull-thru Network: www.pullthrunetwork.org
United Ostomy Associations of America: www.uoaa.org
Wide Smiles, a cleft lip and palate resource: www.widesmiles.org/
Wound, Ostomy and Continence Nurse Society: www.wocn.org

CHAPTER WORKSHEET

MULTIPLE CHOICE QUESTIONS

1. A mother brings her 6-month-old infant to the clinic. The child has been vomiting since early morning and has had diarrhea since the day before. His temperature is 38° C, pulse 140, and respiratory rate 38. He has lost 6 ounces since his well-child visit 4 days ago. He cries before passing a bowel movement. He will not breastfeed today. What is the priority nursing diagnosis?

   a. Thermoregulation alteration

   b. Pain (abdominal) related to diarrhea

   c. Fluid volume deficit related to excessive losses and inadequate intake

   d. Alteration in nutrition, less than body requirements, related to decreased oral intake

2. A child presents with a 2-day history of fever, abdominal pain, occasional vomiting, and decreased oral intake. Which finding would the nurse prioritize for immediate reporting to the physician?

   a. Temperature 101.9° F

   b. Rebound tenderness and abdominal guarding

   c. Parents will be leaving the child alone in the hospital

   d. Child can tolerate only sips of fluid without nausea

3. A 3-day-old infant presenting with physiologic jaundice is hospitalized and placed under phototherapy. Which response indicates to the nurse that the parent needs more teaching?

   a. "My infant is at risk for dehydration."

   b. "My infant needs to stay under the lights, except during feeding time."

   c. "My infant can continue to breastfeed during this time."

   d. "My infant has a serious liver disease."

4. A 3-month-old infant presents with a history of vomiting after feeding. The plan for the infant is to rule out GERD. What information from the history would lead the nurse to believe that this infant may need further intervention?

   a. Poor weight gain

   b. Has small "spits" after feeding

   c. Sleeps through the night

   d. Is difficult to burp

5. The nurse is caring for a child who has had diarrhea and vomiting for the past several days. What is the priority nursing assessment?

   a. Determine the child's weight.

   b. Ask if the family has traveled outside of the country.

   c. Assess circulation and perfusion.

   d. Send a stool specimen to the lab.

CRITICAL THINKING EXERCISES

1. A 6-month-old baby is brought to the pediatrician's office with a history of diarrhea. She has had six watery stools in the past 18 hours. She is vomiting her formula. Her mother states that she has had no fever.

   a. Upon completion of the history and physical examination, what signs and symptoms would you expect to find that would indicate that the baby is experiencing mild dehydration?

   b. What is the priority nursing diagnosis for this infant?

   c. Identify a plan for this nursing diagnosis; include a teaching plan for the mother.

2. A 14-kg child with moderate dehydration has received two boluses of normal saline in the emergency room prior to being admitted to the pediatric nursing unit. The physician orders D5 ½ NS @ 1½ maintenance.

   a. What would the intravenous fluid rate be?

   b. What will the nurse assess for to determine whether the child is becoming overhydrated?

3. An infant requires a temporary colostomy. What discharge instructions would you provide to the parents about how to take care of the colostomy and when to call their health care provider?

STUDY ACTIVITIES

1. In the clinical setting, compare the growth records of a child with celiac disease to those of a similar-aged child without disease.

2. While caring for children in the clinical setting, compare and contrast the medical history, signs and symptoms of illness, and prescribed treatment for a child with Crohn's disease and one with ulcerative colitis.

3. In the clinical setting, observe the behavioral responses of an infant or young child with inorganic failure to thrive.

CHAPTER 42

NURSING CARE OF THE CHILD WITH A GENITOURINARY DISORDER

KEY TERMS

amenorrhea
anasarca
anuria
azotemia
bacteriuria

dysmenorrhea
enuresis
hematuria
hyperlipidemia
menorrhagia

oliguria
proteinuria
sepsis
urgency
urinary frequency

LEARNING OBJECTIVES

Upon completion of the chapter, the learner will be able to:

1. Compare anatomic and physiologic differences of the genitourinary system in infants and children versus adults.
2. Describe nursing care related to common laboratory and diagnostic testing used in the medical diagnosis of pediatric genitourinary conditions.
3. Distinguish genitourinary disorders common in infants, children, and adolescents.
4. Identify appropriate nursing assessments and interventions related to medications and treatments for pediatric genitourinary disorders.
5. Develop an individualized nursing care plan for the child with a genitourinary disorder.
6. Describe the psychosocial impact of chronic genitourinary disorders on children.
7. Devise a nutrition plan for the child with renal insufficiency.
8. Develop patient/family teaching plans for the child with a genitourinary disorder.

Corey Bond, 5 years old, is brought to the clinic by her mother. She presents with fever and lethargy for the past 24 hours. Her mother states, "Corey has had a few accidents in her pants over the past few days, which is unusual for her. She also has been getting up at night more often to use the bathroom."

Wow
A child's essential bodily processes of elimination can be a major event of wonder and creative accomplishment.

Genitourinary (GU) disorders in children and adolescents may occur as a result of abnormalities in fetal development, infectious processes, trauma, neurologic deficit, genetic influences, or other causes. Congenital disorders account for a large proportion of GU disorders in infants, while enuresis and urinary tract infection (UTI) also occur in a significant number of children. Some of the disorders directly involve the kidney from the outset, while others involve other parts of the urinary tract and may have a long-term effect on the kidneys and renal function, particularly if left untreated or treated inadequately. Disorders affecting the reproductive organs often require early diagnosis and management to preserve future reproductive capabilities.

Nurses must be knowledgeable about pediatric GU conditions to provide prompt recognition, nursing care, education, and support to children and their families. Though some disorders are acute and resolve quickly, many have a long-term effect on quality of life and will require more intense, extended support.

Management of acute or common pediatric GU disorders may be provided in the pediatric or family practice outpatient setting, while specialists such as pediatric nephrologists or urologists usually manage chronic involved GU disorders.

Variations in Pediatric Anatomy and Physiology

Though all of the urinary tract and reproductive organs are present at birth, their functioning is immature initially. Many pediatric GU disorders are congenital (present at birth). External GU malformations are easily identified at birth, but internal structural defects may not be identified until later in infancy or childhood when symptoms or complications arise. In children, chronic kidney disease is most often the result of congenital structural defects or infectious, inflammatory, or immune processes that damage the kidney, whereas in adults it usually results from hypertension or diabetes. The infant or child is at increased risk for the development of certain GU disorders because of the anatomical and physiological differences between children and adults.

Urinary Concentration

Blood flow through the kidneys (glomerular filtration rate [GFR]) is slower in the infant and young toddler compared with the adult. The kidney is less able to concentrate urine and reabsorb amino acids, placing the infant and young toddler at increased risk for dehydration during times when fluid loss or decreased fluid intake occurs. The normal range for serum blood urea nitrogen (BUN) and creatinine of the healthy infant or young toddler is usually less than the older child's or adult's. The renal system usually reaches functional maturity at around 2 years of age.

Structural Differences

The kidney is large in relation to the size of the abdomen until the child reaches adolescence. Due to this increased size, the kidneys of the child are less well protected from injury by the ribs and fat padding than they are in the adult. The urethra is naturally shorter in all ages of females than in males, placing them at increased risk for the entrance of bacteria into the bladder via the urethra. In the female infant or young child, this risk is compounded by the physical proximity of the urethral opening to the rectum. The young male's urethra is much shorter than the adult male's, placing the male infant or young child at increased risk of urinary tract infection compared with the adult male.

Urine Output

Bladder capacity is about 30 mL in the newborn; it increases to the usual adult capacity of about 270 mL by 1 year of age. The expected urine output in the infant and child is 0.5 to 2 mL/kg/hour, with the average 1-year-old voiding about 400 to 500 mL per day. The average urine output for a teenager is about 800 to 1,400 mL per day. The infant and toddler may void as often as 9 or 10 times per day. By age 3 the average number of voids per day is the same as the adult's (three to eight).

Reproductive Organ Maturity

The reproductive organs are also immature at birth. The gonads are not mature until adolescence in most children. The hormonal changes that occur with puberty account for some of the reproductive concerns, particularly for female adolescents.

Common Medical Treatments

A variety of medications as well as other medical treatments and surgical procedures are used to treat GU problems in children. Most of these treatments will require a physician's order when the child is in the hospital. The most common treatments and medications are listed in Common Medical Treatments 42.1 and Drug Guide 42.1. The nurse caring for the child with a GU disorder should be familiar with what the procedures are, how the treatments and medications work, and common nursing implications related to use of these modalities.

NURSING PROCESS OVERVIEW FOR THE CHILD WITH A GU DISORDER

Care of the child with a GU disorder includes assessment, nursing diagnosis, planning, interventions, and evaluation. There are a number of general concepts related to the nursing process that may be applied to GU disorders. From a

COMMON MEDICAL TREATMENTS 42.1   GENITOURINARY DISORDERS

Treatment	Explanation	Indications	Nursing Implications
Urinary diversion	Surgical diversion of ureters to the abdominal wall. Continent diversion uses a piece of intestine to create a bladder that can be catheterized. Noncontinent diversion involves a stoma on the abdominal wall that requires use of an ostomy pouch.	Any situation in which the bladder needs to be removed or does not function correctly (bladder exstrophy or prune belly)	Meticulous skin care is necessary to prevent breakdown around stoma. Teach families how to care for ostomy pouch or how to catheterize continent stoma. Expect mucus in urine if intestine is used for urinary reservoir. Monitor for signs of urinary tract infection.
Foley catheter	An indwelling urinary catheter stays in place by means of an inflated balloon.	Usually used only during the postoperative period	Monitor for urethral drainage or irritation. Keep area clean and dry. Monitor color, consistency, clarity, and amount of urine in drainage bag. Monitor for infection, checking results of urinalysis and urine cultures.
Ureteral stent	A thin catheter temporarily placed in the ureter to drain urine. Removed via cystoscopy when it is time for discontinuation.	Urinary tract anomalies	Monitor urine output carefully. Check for bleeding postoperatively.
Nephrostomy tube	Tube placed directly into the kidney to drain urine externally to a bag	Urinary tract anomalies	Monitor urine output carefully.
Suprapubic tube	Catheter placed in the bladder via the abdominal wall above the symphysis pubis	Postoperative urine drainage with reconstructive surgeries	Monitor for blood in urine, adequate urine output. Minimize manipulation of suprapubic tube to avoid triggering bladder spasms.
Vesicostomy	Stoma in the abdominal wall to the bladder	Urinary tract anomalies, neurogenic bladder	Constant urine drainage requires diaper use. Monitor urine output. Assess skin around stoma for breakdown.
Appendicovesicostomy (Mitrofanoff procedure)	Uses appendix to create a stoma on the abdominal wall that allows for catheterization of the bladder	Urinary tract anomalies, neurogenic bladder	Allows for urinary continence, which improves the child's self-esteem. Teach family and child how to catheterize stoma.
Bladder augmentation	Uses a piece of stomach or intestine to enlarge bladder capacity	Decreased bladder capacity	Since a portion of the GI tract is used, urine is often mucus-like.

general understanding of the care involved for a child with urinary, renal, or reproductive dysfunction, the nurse can then individualize the care based on client specifics.

Assessment

Assessment of urinary tract, renal, or reproductive dysfunction includes health history, physical examination, and laboratory and diagnostic testing.

*R*emember Corey, the 5-year-old with fever and lethargy? *What additional health history and physical examination assessment information should you obtain?*

Health History

The health history comprises past medical history, including the mother's pregnancy history, family history,

DRUG GUIDE 42.1 COMMON DRUGS FOR GU DISORDERS

Medication	Action/Indication	Nursing Implications
Anticholinergic agents (oxybutynin, propantheline bromide, belladonna & opium suppository)	Cause smooth muscle relaxation of the bladder, used for urinary tract spasms or contractions related to surgical procedure or use of catheters. Control of nocturnal enuresis.	Increase fluid intake (limit to during the day in the child with nocturnal enuresis). Avoid use in febrile patient.
Antibiotics (oral, parenteral)	Kill bacteria or arrest their growth. Used for urinary tract infection.	Check for antibiotic allergies. Should be given as prescribed for the length of time indicated.
Desmopressin (DDAVP)	Antidiuretic hormone effects by causing renal tubule to absorb more water, decreasing volume of urine in children with nocturnal enuresis.	Nasal spray may cause nasal irritation, nausea, flushing, or headache. Administer at bedtime; alternate nares. Associated with a high relapse rate.
Human chorionic gonadotropin (hCG)	Stimulates production of gonadal steroids to precipitate testicular descent.	Monitor for signs of precocious puberty if used long term.
Corticosteroids	Anti-inflammatory and immunosuppressive action to induce remission and promote diuresis in nephrotic syndrome. High-dose intravenous therapy used when nephrotic syndrome is resistant to conventional doses.	Administer with food to decrease GI upset. May mask signs of infection. Do not stop treatment abruptly, or acute adrenal insufficiency may occur. Monitor for Cushing syndrome. Doses may be tapered over time. Monitor for hypertension during infusion.
Cytotoxic drugs (cyclophos-phamide [Cytoxan] and chlorambucil [Leukeran])	Interfere with normal function of DNA by alkylation. Used to induce prolonged remission in nephrotic syndrome.	Causes bone marrow suppression. Monitor for signs of infection. Cyclophosphamide: administer in the morning; provide adequate hydration; have child void frequently during and after infusion to decrease risk of hemorrhagic cystitis. Chlorambucil: administer with nonspicy, non-acidic foods; rarely seizures occur.
Immunosuppres-sant drugs (cyclosporine A [CyA], azathioprine, tacrolimus, mycopheno-late)	Cause immune suppression to prevent rejection of renal transplants. CyA and tacrolimus may be used for steroid-dependent nephrotic syndrome.	Monitor complete blood count, serum creatinine, potassium, and magnesium. Monitor blood pressure and observe for signs of infection. Blood levels should be drawn prior to morning dose. CyA: do not give with grapefruit juice. Azathioprine and mycophenolate: give on empty stomach; do not open capsule or crush tablet. Tacrolimus: give on empty stomach, assess for development of hyperglycemia. Relapse of nephrotic syndrome may occur after withdrawal of CyA or tacrolimus therapy.
Muromonab-CD3 (Orthoclone OKT3)	Removal of all CD3 molecules from T-lymphocyte surface so it has inability to act . Used for treatment of acute renal transplant rejection.	Monitor for development of pulmonary edema. First-dose effect may cause fever, chills, chest tightness, wheezing, nausea, and vomiting.

Medication	Action/Indication	Nursing Implications
Angiotensin-converting enzyme (ACE) inhibitors (captopril, enalapril)	Potent vasoconstrictor, prevents conversion of angiotensin I to angiotensin II. Used to treat renal causes of hypertension.	Monitor blood pressure frequently. May cause cough, hyperkalemia. Captopril: administer on empty stomach. Enalapril: administer without regard to food.
Imipramine (Tofranil) (tricyclic antidepressant)	Increases the synaptic concentration of serotonin and/or norepinephrine. Treatment of enuresis.	Monitor for urinary retention. May cause decreased appetite.
Diuretics: furosemide (Lasix), hydrochlorothiazide (HCTZ)	Inhibits resorption of sodium and chloride leading to increased excretion of water and electrolytes. Used in nephrotic syndrome, acute glomerulonephritis, hemolytic-uremic syndrome or other instances of fluid overload with renal sufficiency.	Administer with food or milk to decrease GI upset. Monitor blood pressure, renal function, and electrolytes (particularly potassium). May cause photosensitivity.
Vasodilators: hydralazine (Apresoline), minoxidil	Direct vasodilation of arterioles, resulting in decreased systemic resistance. Used to treat renal causes of hypertension.	May cause fluid retention. Hydralazine: administer with food. Monitor heart rate and blood pressure (closely with intravenous use). Minoxidil: may be administered without regard to food. May cause dizziness.
Calcium channel blocker: nifedipine (Procardia)	Prevents calcium from entering voltage-sensitive channels, resulting in coronary vasodilation. Used to treat renal causes of hypertension.	Administer with food; avoid grapefruit juice. Insoluble shell of extended-release tablet may pass in stool. Use caution when administering liquid-filled capsule sublingually or by bite and swallow method, as significant hypotension may occur.
Albumin (intravenous)	Increases intravascular oncotic pressure, resulting in movement of fluid from interstitial to intravascular space. Indicated for fluid volume excess associated with nephrotic syndrome.	May require a filter depending upon brand used. Rapid infusion can result in vascular overload. Monitor vital signs; observe for pulmonary edema and cardiac failure.

and history of present illness (when the symptoms started and how they have progressed), as well as medications and treatments used at home. The past medical history may be significant for maternal polyhydramnios, oligohydramnios, diabetes, hypertension, or alcohol or cocaine ingestion. Neonatal history may include the presence of a single umbilical artery or an abdominal mass, chromosome abnormality, or congenital malformation. Document past medical history of UTI or other problems with the GU tract. Family history may be significant for renal disease or uropathology, chronic UTIs, renal calculi, or a history of parental enuresis. Determine age of successful toilet training, pattern of incontinent episodes (having "accidents"), and toileting hygiene self-care routines. Note myelomeningocele or other spinal disturbance that may affect the child's ability to urinate. Note previous urologic surgeries or ongoing renal interventions (e.g., dialysis). For the adolescent girl, obtain a thorough menstrual history, including sexual behavior and pregnancy history.

When determining the history of the present illness, inquire about the following:

• Burning on urination
• Changes in voiding patterns
• Foul-smelling urine
• Vaginal or urethral discharge
• Genital pain, irritation, or discomfort
• Blood in the urine
• Edema
• Masses in the groin, scrotum, or abdomen
• Flank or abdominal pain

- Cramps
- Nausea and/or vomiting
- Poor growth
- Weight gain
- Fever
- Infectious exposure (particularly streptococcus A or *Escherichia coli*)
- Trauma

Record medications used for acute or chronic conditions, or for contraception.

Physical Examination

Physical examination of the GU system includes inspection and observation, auscultation, percussion, and palpation.

Inspection and Observation

Observe the child's general appearance, noting growth retardation or unusual weight gain. Inspect the skin for presence of pruritus, edema (generalized or periorbital), or bruising. Note pallor of the skin or dysmorphic features (associated with genetic conditions). Document presence of lethargy, fatigue, rapid respirations, confusion, or developmental delay. Observe the external genitalia area for infant diaper rash, constant urine dribble, displaced urethral opening, reddened urethral opening, or discharge. In females note vaginal irritation or labial fusion. In males observe the scrotal sac for enlargement or discoloration. Note the condition of a urinary stoma or diversion if present. With the child lying flat, observe the abdomen for distention, ascites, or slack abdominal musculature.

Auscultation

Listen carefully to heart sounds, as a flow murmur may be present in the anemic child with a renal disorder. Noted elevated heart rate. Auscultate blood pressure with the appropriate-size cuff, noting elevation or depression. In the edematous child, carefully auscultate the lungs, noting presence of adventitious sounds. Note absence of bowel sounds, as this may indicate peritonitis. In the child who receives chronic hemodialysis, auscultate the fistula for presence of a bruit (desired normal finding).

▶ **Take** NOTE!

Use the bell of the stethoscope when auscultating the infant's or child's blood pressure so that you can hear the softer Korotkoff sounds more accurately.

Percussion

Percuss the abdomen. Note unusual dullness or flatness (dullness is usually heard over the spleen at the right costal margin, over the kidneys, and 1 to 3 cm below the left costal margin). A full bladder may yield dullness above the symphysis pubis.

Palpation

Palpate the abdomen. Note presence of palpable kidneys (indicating enlargement or mass, as they are usually difficult to palpate in the older infant or child). Note presence of abdominal masses or a distended bladder. Document tenderness to palpation or along the costovertebral angle. Palpate the scrotum for presence of descended testicles, masses, or other abnormalities. Note whether the foreskin, if present, can be retracted. In the child who receives chronic hemodialysis, palpate the fistula or graft for presence of a thrill (desired normal finding).

Laboratory and Diagnostic Testing

Common Laboratory and Diagnostic Tests 42.1 offers an explanation of the most commonly used laboratory and diagnostic tests used for a child suspected of having a GU disorder. The test results can help the physician to diagnose the disorder or to determine treatment. Laboratory or non-nursing personnel obtain some of the tests, while the nurse might obtain others. In either instance the nurse should be familiar with how the tests are obtained, what they are used for, and normal versus abnormal results. This knowledge will also be necessary when providing patient and family education related to the tests and results.

Urine specimens may be collected using a variety of different methods in infants and children. Suprapubic aspiration is a useful method for obtaining a sterile urine specimen from the neonate or young infant. A sterile needle is inserted into the bladder through the anterior wall of the abdomen and the urine is then aspirated. This method is generally performed by the physician or advanced practitioner. Infants and toddlers who are not toilet trained may require a urine bag for urine collection. A sterile urine bag is required for a urine culture, a clean bag for routine urinalysis. A 24-hour urine-collection bag is also available. Nursing Procedure 42.1 gives details on the use of the urine bag.

Sterile urinary catheterization is performed like that in adults. The size of the catheter varies depending on the size of the child. If a small urinary catheter is not available, a sterile 5 French or 8 French feeding tube works well.

▶ **Take** NOTE!

Use familiar terms such as "pee-pee," "tinkle," or "potty" to explain to the child what is needed and to gain his or her cooperation.

COMMON LABORATORY AND DIAGNOSTIC TESTS 42.1
GENITOURINARY DISORDERS

Test	Explanation	Indication	Nursing Implications
Complete blood count	Evaluate hemoglobin and hematocrit, white blood cell count, and platelet count	Any condition in which anemia, infection, or thrombo-cytopenia is suspected	Normal values vary according to age and gender. White blood cell count differential is helpful in evaluating source of infection.
Blood urea nitrogen (BUN) (serum)	Indirect measurement of renal function and glomerular filtration in the presence of adequate liver function	Nephrotic syndrome, hemolytic-uremic syndrome, renal failure, acute glomerulonephritis or other renal diseases	BUN may be elevated with high-protein diet or dehydration, may be decreased with over-hydration or malnutrition.
Creatinine (serum)	A more direct measurement of renal function, only minimally affected by liver function. Generally, doubling of the creatinine level is suggestive of a 50% reduction in glomerular filtration rate.	Used to diagnose impaired renal function	A diet high in meat may cause a transient though not pronounced increase in creatinine. There are also slight diurnal variations in levels. Draw at same time each day if serial evaluations are ordered.
Creatinine clearance (urine and serum)	A 24-hour urine collection is evaluated for the presence of creatinine, then compared with the serum creatinine level to determine creatinine clearance.	Used to diagnose impaired renal function	Discard the first void and then begin the 24-hour urine collection. Keep the specimen on ice during the collection period. Collect ALL urine passed in the 24-hour period. Ensure that a venous blood sample is drawn during the 24-hour period. The urine specimen should be sent promptly to the laboratory at the end of the 24-hour period.
Potassium (serum)	Measures the concentration of potassium in the blood	Any suspected renal disease; followed routinely in renal failure	Avoid hemolysis and allowing child to open and close the hand with a tourniquet in place, as these can cause elevation in potassium levels. Evaluate the child with increased or decreased potassium levels for cardiac arrhythmias. Immediately notify physician of critically high potassium levels.
Total protein, globulin, albumin (serum)	Protein electrophoresis separates the various components into zones according to their electrical charge.	Used to diagnose, evaluate, and monitor chronic renal disease	Significantly low levels of albumin contribute to extent of edema, as albumin is necessary in the blood to maintain colloidal osmotic pressure.
Calcium (serum)	Measurement of calcium level in the blood; half of all calcium is protein-bound, so the level will decrease with hypoalbuminemia.	Renal diseases associated with hypoalbuminemia and edema	Avoid prolonged tourniquet use during blood draw, as this may falsely increase the calcium level.

(continued)

COMMON LABORATORY AND DIAGNOSTIC TESTS 42.1
GENITOURINARY DISORDERS (continued)

Test	Explanation	Indication	Nursing Implications
Phosphorus (serum)	Measurement of phosphate level in the blood. Phosphorus levels are inversely related to calcium levels (they increase when calcium levels decrease).	Renal disease, ongoing monitoring, particularly in the patient with hypocalcemia	Child should be NPO past midnight prior to the morning of the blood draw. Avoid hemolysis, as it can falsely elevate the phosphate level.
Urinalysis (urine)	Evaluates color, pH, specific gravity, and odor of urine. Also assesses for presence of protein, glucose, ketones, blood, leukocyte esterase, red and white blood cells, bacteria, crystals, and casts.	Reveals preliminary information about the urinary tract. Useful in children with fever, dysuria, flank pain, urgency, or hematuria. Proteinuria may be noted in renal disorders.	Be aware of the many drugs affecting urine color and notify laboratory if child is taking one. Notify laboratory if female is menstruating. Refrigerate specimen if not processed promptly. While proteinuria may occur with various renal disorders, it may also occur as either transient or orthostatic proteinuria, both of which are benign events.
Cystoscopy	Endoscopic visualization of the urethra and bladder	Evaluate hematuria, recurrent urinary tract infection; determine ureteral reflux; measure bladder capacity	Encourage fluids. Monitor vital signs. Child may feel burning with voiding after procedure. Pink tinge to urine is common after procedure.
Urine culture and sensitivity	Urine is plated in the laboratory and evaluated every day for the presence of bacteria. A final report is usually issued after 48 to 72 hours. Sensitivity testing is performed to determine the best choice of antibiotic.	Used to diagnose urinary tract infection	Obtain culture specimen prior to starting antibiotics if at all possible. Avoid contamination of the specimen with stool. May be obtained by catheterization, clean-catch specimen, or sterile U-bag. In some institutions, suprapubic tap is performed in neonates and young infants by the physician or nurse practitioner.
Urodynamic studies	Measure the urine flow during micturition via a urine flow meter	Dysfunctional voiding	The child must have a full bladder. The child then urinates into the urine flow meter. There is no discomfort associated with the test.
Voiding cystourethrogram (VCUG)	The bladder is filled with contrast material via catheterization. Fluoroscopy is performed to demonstrate filling of the bladder and collapsing after emptying.	Hematuria, urinary tract infections, vesicoureteral reflux, suspected structural anomalies	Just prior to the test, insert the Foley catheter. Ensure that the adolescent female patient is not pregnant. After the test, encourage the child to drink fluids to prevent bacterial accumulation and aid in dye elimination.
Intravenous pyelogram (IVP)	Radiopaque contrast material is injected intravenously and filtered by the kidneys. X-ray films are obtained at set intervals to show pas-	Urinary outlet obstruction, hematuria, trauma to the renal system, suspected kidney tumor	Contraindicated in children allergic to shellfish or iodine. If the dye infiltrates at the intravenous site, hyaluronidase (Wydase) may be used to

Test	Explanation	Indication	Nursing Implications
	sage of the dye through the kidneys, ureters, and bladder.		speed absorption of the iodine. Ensure adequate hydration before and after the test. Some institutions require enema or laxative evacuation of the bowel prior to the study to ensure adequate visualization of the urinary tract.
Renal biopsy	Usually a percutaneous specimen is obtained by inserting a needle through the skin and into the kidney. The sample of kidney tissue obtained is then microscopically examined.	Diagnosis of renal disease or assessment of renal transplant rejection	After the biopsy, carefully assess for signs or symptoms of bleeding: increased heart rate, pale color, flank pain or backache, shoulder pain, lightheadedness. Inspect urine for gross hematuria. Child will be on bed rest, preferably supine for 24 hours.
Renal ultrasound	Reflected sound waves allow visualization of the kidneys, ureters, and bladder.	Useful in determining kidney size (as with hydronephrosis and polycystic kidney), presence of cysts or tumors, or rejection of kidney transplant	No fasting is required prior to the procedure. Does not require contrast material. The child should feel no discomfort during the ultrasound.

Nursing Diagnoses and Related Interventions

Upon completion of a thorough assessment, the nurse might identify several nursing diagnoses, such as:

- Impaired urinary elimination
- Fluid volume excess
- Imbalanced nutrition, less (or more) than body requirements
- Risk for infection
- Deficient knowledge of the child or family
- Urinary retention
- Activity intolerance
- Interrupted family process
- Disturbed body image

After completing an assessment of Corey, you note the following: foul-smelling urine, abdominal tenderness, redness in her perineal area, and slightly blood-tinged, cloudy urine. Based on these assessment findings, what would your top three nursing diagnoses be for Corey?

Nursing goals, interventions, and evaluation for the child with a GU disorder are based on the nursing diagnoses. Nursing Care Plan 22.1 can be used as a guide in planning nursing care for the child with a GU disorder. The care plan overview includes nursing diagnoses and interventions for urinary tract disorders as well as genital (or reproductive system) disorders. It should be individualized based on the patient's symptoms and needs. Refer to Chapter 35 for detailed information about pain management. Additional information will be included later in the chapter as it relates to specific disorders.

Based on your top three nursing diagnoses for Corey, describe appropriate nursing interventions.

Urinary Tract and Renal Disorders

The urinary tract and renal disorders discussed below include structural disorders, UTI, enuresis, and acquired disorders that result in altered renal function.

▶ STRUCTURAL DISORDERS

Numerous urologic conditions occur as a result of altered fetal development. Many of these defects are apparent at birth, yet some are not recognized until later in infancy or childhood.

Nursing Procedure 42.1

APPLYING THE URINE BAG

1. Cleanse the perineal area well and pat dry (Fig. 1). If a culture is to be obtained, cleanse the genital area with povidone–iodine (Betadine) or per institutional protocol.
2. Apply benzoin around the scrotum or the vulvar area to aid with urine bag adhesion.
3. Allow the benzoin to dry.
4. Apply the urine bag.
   * For boys: Ensure that the penis is fully inside the bag; a portion of the scrotum may or may not be inside the bag, depending upon scrotal size.
   * For girls: Apply the narrow portion of the bag on the perineal space between the anal and vulvar areas first for best adhesion, then spread the remaining adhesive section (Fig. 2).

5. Tuck the bag downward inside the diaper to discourage leaking.
6. Check the bag frequently for urine (Fig. 3).

Bladder Exstrophy

In classic bladder exstrophy, a midline closure defect occurs during the embryonic period of gestation, leaving the bladder open and exposed outside of the abdomen. The bony pelvis may also be malformed, resulting in an opening in the pelvic arch. Bladder exstrophy may be diagnosed by prenatal ultrasound. Complications include UTI from ascending organisms. Treatment of bladder exstrophy involves surgical repair.

Nursing Assessment

On physical examination of the infant or child, note the red appearance to the bladder seen on the abdominal wall (Fig. 42.1). Draining urine will be visible. Note excoriation of abdominal skin around the bladder resulting from contact with urine. A malformed urethra may be present in females, while males may have an unformed or malformed penis or a normal penis with an epispadias.

Nursing Management

Nursing management consists of preventing infection and skin breakdown, providing postoperative care, and catheterizing the stoma.

Preventing Infection and Skin Breakdown

Bladder exstrophy requires surgical repair. In the preoperative period, care is focused on protecting the exstrophied bladder and preventing infection. Keep the infant in a supine position; keep the bladder moist and cover it with a sterile plastic bag. Change soiled diapers immediately to prevent contamination of the bladder with feces. Sponge-bathe the infant rather than immersing him or her in water to prevent pathogens in the bath water from entering the bladder. Prevent breakdown of the surrounding abdominal skin by applying protective barrier creams. In some instances it may be necessary to consult the ostomy nurse for advice on dealing with the abdominal skin excoriation. If

(text continues on page 1392)

Nursing Care Plan 42.1

OVERVIEW FOR THE CHILD WITH A GENITOURINARY DISORDER

NURSING DIAGNOSIS: Activity intolerance related to generalized edema, anemia, or generalized weakness as evidenced by verbalization of weakness or fatigue, elevated heart rate, respiratory rate, or blood pressure with activity, complaint of shortness of breath with play or activity

Outcome Identification and Evaluation
Child will display increased activity tolerance, desire to play without developing symptoms of exertion.

Intervention: Promoting Activity
- Encourage activity or ambulation per physician's orders: *early mobilization results in better outcomes.*
- Observe child for symptoms of activity intolerance such as pallor, nausea, lightheadedness, or dizziness or changes in vital signs *to determine level of tolerance.*
- If child is on bed rest, perform range-of-motion exercises and frequent position changes, *as negative changes to the musculoskeletal system occur quickly with inactivity and immobility.*
- Cluster nursing care activities and plan for periods of rest before and after exertional activities *to decrease oxygen need and consumption.*
- Refer the child to physical therapy *for exercise prescription to increase skeletal muscle strength.*

NURSING DIAGNOSIS: Excess fluid volume related to decreased protein in the bloodstream, decreased urine output, sodium retention, possible inappropriate fluid intake, or altered hormone levels inducing fluid retention as evidenced by edema, bloating, weight gain, oliguria, azotemia, or changes in heart and lung sounds

Outcome Identification and Evaluation
Child will attain appropriate fluid balance, will lose weight (fluid), edema or bloating will decrease, lung sounds will be clear and heart sounds normal.

Intervention: Encouraging Fluid Loss
- Weigh child daily on same scale in similar amount of clothing; *in children, weight is the best indicator of changes in fluid status.*
- Monitor location and extent of edema (measure abdominal girth daily if ascites present): *decrease in edema indicates positive increase in oncotic pressure.*
- Auscultate lungs carefully to determine presence of crackles (*indicating pulmonary edema*).
- Assess work of breathing and respiratory rate (*increased work of breathing is associated with pulmonary edema*).
- Assess heart sounds for presence or absence of gallop (*presence of S3 may indicate fluid overload*).
- Maintain fluid restriction as ordered *to decrease intravascular volume and workload on the heart.*
- Strictly monitor intake and output *to quickly note discrepancies and provide intervention.*
- Provide sodium-restricted diet as ordered (*restricting sodium in the diet allows for better renal excretion of extra fluid*).
- Administer diuretics as ordered and monitor for side effects of those medications. *Diuretics encourage excretion of fluid and elimination of edema, reduce cardiac filling pressures, and increase renal blood flow. Side effects include electrolyte imbalance as well as orthostatic hypotension.*

(continued)

Nursing Care Plan 42.1 (continued)

NURSING DIAGNOSIS: Imbalanced nutrition: less than body requirements related to anorexia and protein loss as evidenced by weight, length/height, and/or BMI below average for age

Outcome Identification and Evaluation
Child will improve nutritional intake, resulting in steady increase in weight and length/height.

Intervention: Promoting Adequate Nutrition
* Determine body weight and length/height norm for age, *to determine goal to work toward.*
* Assess child for food preferences that fall within dietary restrictions, *as the child will be more likely to consume adequate amounts of foods that he or she likes.*
* Weigh daily or weekly (according to physician order or institutional standard) and measure length/height weekly *to monitor for increased growth.*
* Offer highest calorie meals at the time of day when the child's appetite is the greatest (*to increase likelihood of increased caloric intake*).
* Provide increased calorie shakes or puddings within diet restriction (*high calorie foods increase weight gain*).
* Administer vitamin and mineral supplements as prescribed *to attain/maintain vitamin and mineral balance in the body.*

NURSING DIAGNOSIS: Imbalanced nutrition: more than body requirements related to increased appetite secondary to steroid therapy as evidenced by weight greater than 95th percentile for age or recent increase in weight

Outcome Identification and Evaluation
Child will demonstrate balanced nutritional intake, will maintain current weight or steadily lose excess weight.

Intervention: Encouraging Appropriate Nutritional Intake
* Determine ideal body weight and body mass index for age *to determine goal to work toward.*
* Consult dietitian *for guidance in planning nutrient-rich diet in context of restrictions.*
* Evaluate for emotional/psychological reasons for overeating *to address these concerns.*
* Formulate a contract with the child *to involve him/her in the planning process and encourage compliance with the plan.*
* With the child, plan for daily exercise/activity *to expend excess calories.*
* Instruct the child/parent about appropriate nutrient-rich foods to choose within the constraints of diet and fluid restrictions *to provide basis for ongoing diet management at home.*
* Weigh child twice weekly on same scale *to determine progress toward goal.*

NURSING DIAGNOSIS: Impaired urinary elimination related to urinary tract infection or other urologic condition, or other factors such as ignoring urge to void at appropriate time as evidenced by urinary retention or incontinence, dribbling, urgency, or dysuria

Outcome Identification and Evaluation
Child will maintain continence; will void in the toilet.

Intervention: Promoting Adequate Urinary Elimination
* Assess the child's usual voiding pattern and success within that pattern *to determine baseline.*
* Develop a schedule for bladder emptying *to encourage voiding in the toilet.*
* Maintain adequate hydration, *as dehydration irritates the bladder.*
* Avoid constipation, *as constipation is associated with inability to adequately empty bladder.*
* Teach parents to restrict child's fluid intake after dinner *to avoid bedwetting.*
* Ensure child voids prior to going to bed *to avoid bedwetting.*
* Teach bladder-stretching exercises as prescribed per physician *to increase bladder capacity.*

Nursing Care Plan 42.1 (continued)

NURSING DIAGNOSIS: Urinary retention related to anatomic obstruction, sensory motor impairment or dysfunctional voiding as evidenced by dribbling, inadequate bladder emptying

Outcome Identification and Evaluation
Child's bladder will empty adequately, according to pre-established quantities and frequencies individualized for the child (usual urine output is 0.5 to 2 mL/kg/hour).

Intervention: Promoting Successful Bladder Emptying
- Assess child's ability to adequately empty bladder via history focused on character and duration of lower urinary symptoms *to establish baseline.*
- Assess for history of fecal impaction or encopresis, *as alterations in bowel elimination may have a negative impact on urinary elimination.*
- Assess for bladder distention by palpation or urinary retention by post-void residual obtained via catheterization or bladder ultrasound *to determine extent of retention.*
- Maintain adequate hydration *to avoid irritating effects of dehydration on the bladder.*
- Schedule voiding *to decrease bladder overdistension.*
- In the child with significant urinary retention, teach parents/child the technique of clean intermittent catheterization, *which allows for regular complete bladder emptying.*

NURSING DIAGNOSIS: Disturbed body image related to anatomic differences, short stature, or effects of long-term corticosteroid use as evidenced by verbalization of dissatisfaction with the child's or adolescent's looks

Outcome Identification and Evaluation
Child or adolescent will display appropriate body image, will look at self in mirror and participate in social activities.

Intervention: Promoting Body Image
- Acknowledge feelings of anger over body changes and illness: *venting feelings is associated with less body image disturbance.*
- Support the child's or teen's choices of comfortable, fashionable clothing *that may disguise anatomic abnormalities and dialysis tubing.*
- Involve the child and especially the teen in the decision-making process, *as a sense of control of their own body will improve body image.*
- Encourage children or teens to spend time with others their own age who have short stature or other effects of renal disorders: *a peer's opinions are often better accepted than those of persons in authority, such as parents or health care professionals.*

NURSING DIAGNOSIS: Knowledge deficit related to lack of information regarding complex medical condition, prognosis, and medical needs as evidenced by verbalization, questions, or actions demonstrating lack of understanding regarding child's condition or care

Outcome Identification and Evaluation
Child and parents will verbalize accurate information and understanding about condition, prognosis, and medical needs: *Child and parents demonstrate knowledge of condition and medications and will demonstrate therapeutic procedures the child requires.*

Intervention: Educating the Child and Parents
- Assess child's and parents' willingness to learn: *Child and parents must be open to learning for teaching to be effective.*
- Provide parents with time to adjust to diagnosis: *will facilitate adjustment and ability to learn and participate in child's care.*
- Teach in short sessions: *many short sessions are found to be more helpful than one long session.*
- Repeat information: *allows parents and child time to learn and understand.*
- Individualize teaching to the parents' and child's level of understanding (depends on age of child, physical condition, memory) *to ensure understanding.*
- Provide reinforcement and rewards *to facilitate the teaching/learning process.*
- Use multiple modes of learning involving many senses (written, verbal, demonstration, and videos) when possible: *child and parents are more likely to retain information when presented in different ways using many senses.*

FIGURE 42.1 Note the bright-red color of the bladder exstrophy.

FIGURE 42.2 The abdominal stoma allows for urinary continence and requires catheterization.

an orthopedic surgeon is involved due to the malformed pubic arch, follow through with recommended positioning or bracing to prevent further separation of the pubic arch.

Providing Postoperative Care

Nursing management in the postoperative period focuses on preventing infection. Keep the infant supine and quickly change soiled diapers to prevent contamination of the incision with stool. Surgical reconstruction of the bladder within the pelvic cavity and reconstruction of a urethra are done if enough bladder tissue is present. An indwelling urethral catheter or suprapubic tube will allow urinary drainage, allowing the bladder to rest in the initial postoperative period. Ensure that catheters drain freely and do not become kinked. Sometimes tubes or catheters used in the postoperative period require irrigation. Refer to the institution's policy and the surgeon's orders for specifics related to urinary catheter irrigation.

Manage bladder spasms with oxybutynin (Ditropan) or belladonna and opioid (B & O) suppositories as ordered. Note blood-tinged urine upon return from surgery, with clearing of urine within hours to days.

Catheterizing the Stoma

If bladder tissue is insufficient for repair, then the bladder is removed and a continent urinary reservoir created. The ureters are connected to a portion of the small intestine that is separated from the gastrointestinal (GI) tract, thus creating a urinary reservoir. The intestines are reanastomosed to leave the GI tract intact and separate from the GU tract. A stoma is created on the abdominal wall; it provides access to the urinary reservoir (Fig. 42.2). The stoma is catheterized about four times per day to empty the reservoir of urine. Urine from an intestine-based urinary reservoir tends to be mucus-like and is often cloudier than urine from a urinary bladder. Teach parents the procedure for catheterizing the urinary reservoir and instruct them to call the child's urologist or pediatrician if signs or symptoms of UTI occur.

▶ **Take** NOTE!

About one third of all children with urologic malformations are at high risk for the development of latex allergy. Latex allergy can result in anaphylaxis. Primary prevention of latex allergy is warranted in all children with urologic malformations, so use latex-free gloves, tubes, and catheters in these children.

Hypospadias/Epispadias

Hypospadias is a urethral defect in which the opening is on the ventral surface of the penis rather than at the end of the penis (Fig. 42.3). Epispadias is a urethral defect in which the opening is on the dorsal surface of the penis. In either case, the opening may be near the glans of the

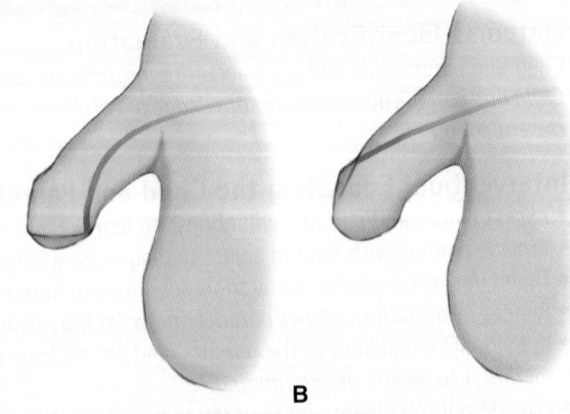

A   **B**

FIGURE 42.3 (**A**) Hypospadias: the urethral opening is located on the ventral side of the penis. (**B**) Epispadias: the urethral opening is located on the dorsal side of the penis.

penis, midway along the penis, or near the base. If left uncorrected, the boy may not be capable of appropriately aiming a urinary stream from a standing position. The abnormal placement of the urethral opening may interfere with the deposition of sperm during intercourse, leaving the man infertile. Also, if left uncorrected, the boy's self-esteem and body image may be damaged by the abnormal appearance of his genitalia. For these reasons, the defect is usually repaired sometime after about 1 year of age. The goal of surgical correction for either condition is to provide for an appropriately placed meatus that allows for normal voiding and ejaculation. The meatus is moved to the glans penis and the urethra is reconstructed as needed. Most repairs are accomplished in one surgery. More extensive reconstructions may require two stages.

Nursing Assessment

Note history of an unusual urine stream. Inspect the penis for placement of the urethral meatus: it may be slightly off center of the glans or may be present somewhere along the shaft of the penis. Inspect for chordee, a fibrous band causing the penis to curve downward. Palpate for presence or absence of testicles in the scrotal sac, because cryptorchidism (undescended testicles) often occurs with hypospadias, as do hydrocele and inguinal hernia.

Nursing Management

The newborn with hypospadias or epispadias should not undergo circumcision until after surgical repair of the urethral meatus. In more extreme cases, the surgeon may need to use some of the excess foreskin while reconstructing the meatus. Nursing management of the infant who has undergone a hypospadias or epispadias repair focuses on providing routine postoperative care and parent education.

Providing Postoperative Care

Postoperatively, assess urinary drainage from the urethral stent or drainage tube, which allows for discharge of urine without stress along the surgical site. Ensure that the urinary drainage tube remains carefully taped with the penis in an upright position to prevent stress on the urethral incision. The penile dressing is usually a compression type, used to decrease edema and bruising. Administer antibiotics if prescribed. Assess for pain, which is usually not extensive, and administer analgesics or antispasmodics (oral oxybutynin or B & O suppository) as needed for bladder spasms.

> ▶ **Take** NOTE!
>
> *Bladder spasms may also be managed effectively through the use of epidural analgesia, which is being used more frequently in the postoperative period in the pediatric population.*

Double diapering is a method used to protect the urethra and stent or catheter after surgery; it also helps keep the area clean and free from infection. The inner diaper contains stool and the outer diaper contains urine, allowing separation between the bowel and bladder output. Nursing Procedure 42.2 details the double-diapering technique. Change the outside (larger) diaper when the child is wet; change both diapers when the child has a bowel movement.

Educating the Family

If the child is to be discharged with the urinary catheter in place (which is common), teach the parents how to care for

---

Nursing Procedure 42.2

DOUBLE DIAPERING

1. Cut a hole or a cross-shaped slit in the front of the smaller diaper.
2. Unfold both diapers and place the smaller diaper (with the hole) inside the larger one.
3. Place both diapers under the child.
4. Carefully bring the penis (if applicable) and catheter/stent through the hole in the smaller diaper and close the diaper.
5. Close the larger diaper, making sure the tip of the catheter/stent is inside the larger diaper.

Cut slit

Larger diaper   Smaller diaper

Pictures and text adapted from Children's Healthcare of Atlanta (2004). *Double diapering.*

the catheter and drainage system. Have parents demonstrate their ability to irrigate the catheter should a mucus plug occur. Tub baths are generally prohibited until it is time to remove the penile dressing. Roughhousing, ride-on toys, or any activity involving straddling is not allowed for 2 to 3 weeks.

Obstructive Uropathy

Obstructive uropathy is an obstruction at any level along the upper or lower urinary tract. This discussion will focus on congenital structural defects, though obstruction can also occur as a result of other disease processes (acquired obstructive uropathy). The most common sites of obstruction are listed in Table 42.1. The defect may be unilateral or bilateral and can cause partial or complete obstruction of urine flow, resulting in dilation of the affected kidney (hydronephrosis). Complications include recurrent UTI, renal insufficiency, and progressive damage to the kidney resulting in renal failure.

Nursing Assessment

For a full description of the assessment phase of the nursing process refer to page 1381. Assessment findings pertinent to obstructive uropathy are discussed below.

Health History

Elicit a description of the present illness and chief complaint. Common signs and symptoms reported during the health history might include:

• Recurrent UTI
• Incontinence
• Fever
• Foul-smelling urine
• Flank pain
• Abdominal pain
• **Urinary frequency**
• Urinary **urgency**
• Dysuria
• **Hematuria**

Explore the child's current and past medical history for risk factors such as:

• "Prune belly" syndrome
• Chromosome abnormalities
• Anorectal malformations
• Ear defects

Physical Examination and Laboratory and Diagnostic Tests

Palpate the abdomen for presence of an abdominal mass (hydronephrotic kidney). Assess the blood pressure; elevation may occur if renal insufficiency is present. Many cases of obstructive uropathy may be diagnosed with prenatal ultrasound if the obstruction has been significant enough to cause hydronephrosis or dilatation elsewhere along the urinary tract.

Nursing Management

Surgical correction is specific to the type of obstruction and generally consists of removal of the obstruction, reimplantation of the ureters as necessary, and occasionally creation of a urinary diversion. Postoperatively, assess urine output via vesicostomy, nephrostomy, suprapubic tube, or urethral catheter for color, clots, clarity, and amount. Encourage fluids once the child can tolerate them orally. Administer analgesics and/or antispasmodics as needed for bladder spasms. Teach parents care of vesicostomy or drainage tubes, with which the child may be discharged.

> ▶ **Take** NOTE!
>
> *Upon return from surgery, most children have intravenous fluids without added potassium infusion. Potassium is withheld from the intravenous fluid until adequate urine output is established post-operatively to avoid the development of hyperkalemia should the kidneys fail to function properly.*

Hydronephrosis

Hydronephrosis is a condition in which the pelvis and calyces of the kidney are dilated (Fig. 42.4). Hydronephrosis may occur as a congenital defect, as a result of obstructive uropathy, or secondary to vesicoureteral reflux. Congenital hydronephrosis may be revealed on prenatal ultrasound. Complications of hydronephrosis include renal insufficiency, hypertension, and eventually renal failure.

Nursing Assessment

For a full description of the assessment phase of the nursing process refer to page 1381. Assessment findings pertinent to hydronephrosis are discussed below.

Health History

Elicit a description of the present illness and chief complaint. The infant may be asymptomatic, but signs and symptoms reported during the health history might include:

• Failure to thrive
• Intermittent hematuria
• Presence of an abdominal mass
• Signs and symptoms associated with a UTI such as fever, vomiting, poor feeding, and irritability

Explore the child's current and past medical history for risk factors such as:

• Maternal oligohydramnios or polyhydramnios (congenital hydronephrosis)
• Elevated levels of serum alpha-fetoprotein (congenital hydronephrosis)

TABLE 42.1 COMMON SITES OF OBSTRUCTIVE UROPATHY

Disorder	Site	Illustration
Ureteropelvic junction (UPJ) obstruction	Junction of the upper ureter with the pelvis of the kidney	Urinary tract with unilateral hydronephrosis and narrowing of the UPJ on that side
Ureterovesical junction (UVJ) obstruction	Junction of the lower ureter and the bladder	Urinary tract with unilateral hydronephrosis and dilated ureters with narrowing of the UVJ on that side
Ureterocele	Ureter swells into the bladder	Bladder with cystic pouch where ureters insert (unilateral)
Posterior urethral valves (males only)	Flaps of tissue in the proximal urethra	Distended proximal urethra, bladder, ureters, and hydronephrosis

FIGURE 42.4 Hydronephrosis.

FIGURE 42.5 Note retrograde flow of urine up the ureter upon bladder contraction.

Physical Examination and Diagnostic and Laboratory Tests

Monitor the blood pressure of infants and children suspected of having hydronephrosis. Palpation of the abdomen may reveal enlarged kidney(s) or a distended bladder. A voiding cystourethrogram (VCUG) will be performed to determine the presence of a structural defect that may be causing the hydronephrosis. Other diagnostic tests, such as a renal ultrasound or an intravenous pyelogram, may also be performed to clarify the diagnosis.

Nursing Management

Teach the parents signs and symptoms of UTI and sepsis, as these complications may occur. The parents should observe the child for adequacy of urine output and hydration status. Teach the parents to perform appropriate perineal hygiene and to avoid using irritants in the genital area. The infant or child with hydronephrosis will need follow-up with a pediatric nephrologist or urologist.

Vesicoureteral Reflux

Vesicoureteral reflux (VUR) is a condition in which urine from the bladder flows back up the ureters. This reflux of urine occurs during bladder contraction with voiding (Fig. 42.5). Reflux may occur in one or both ureters. If reflux occurs when the urine is infected, the kidney is exposed to bacteria and pyelonephritis may result. The increased pressure placed upon the kidney with reflux can cause renal scarring and lead to hypertension later in life and, if severe, renal insufficiency or failure.

Primary VUR results from a congenital abnormality at the vesicoureteral junction that results in incompetence of the valve. Secondary VUR is related to other structural or functional problems such as neurogenic bladder, bladder dysfunction, or bladder outlet obstruction. As many

as 30% to 40% of all children diagnosed with UTI have primary VUR (Thompson et al., 2005).

VUR is graded according to its severity: grade 1 results in minor dilatation of the proximal ureter and grade V is severe dilatation of the ureter and pelvis of the kidney (Wald, 2006). Grade I and II VUR cases usually resolve spontaneously, but grade III to V cases are generally associated with recurrent UTIs, hydronephrosis, and progressive renal damage.

The goal of therapeutic management of VUR is prevention of pyelonephritis and subsequent renal scarring, which may contribute to the development of hypertension later in life (Ellsworth et al., 2000). Management includes antibiotic prophylaxis and hygiene/voiding practices to prevent UTI. Serial urine cultures are used to determine recurrence of UTI. Biannual, annual, or biennial radionuclide VCUGs are performed to determine the status of VUR.

Grade III, IV, and V cases usually warrant surgical intervention. The ureters are resected from the bladder and reimplanted elsewhere in the bladder wall to regain functionality.

> ▶ **Take** NOTE!
>
> *The keys to prevention of long-term sequelae such as hypertension in children with urologic conditions are early diagnosis and intervention, prevention of infection, and close clinical follow-up. Nurses play a key role in monitoring and education.*

Nursing Assessment

For a full description of the assessment phase of the nursing process refer to page 1381. Assessment findings pertinent to VUR are discussed below.

Health History

Elicit a description of the present illness and chief complaint. Common signs and symptoms reported during the health history might include:

- Fever
- Dysuria
- Frequency or urgency
- Nocturia
- Hematuria
- Pain in the back, abdomen, or flank

Explore the child's current and past medical history for risk factors such as:

- Recurrent UTI in the female
- Single episode of UTI in the male
- Congenital defect
- Family history of VUR

For the child who is receiving ongoing follow-up for VUR, determine whether UTIs have occurred since the last visit, as well as the name and dose of prophylactic antibiotic.

Physical Examination

Monitor the blood pressure for elevation. Palpate the abdomen for presence of a mass (if hydronephrosis is present). VCUG may be used to diagnose VUR.

Nursing Management

Nursing management for the child with VUR includes preventing infection and providing postoperative care.

Preventing Infection

When VUR is present, the goal is to avoid urine infection so that infected urine cannot gain access to the kidneys. Initially, most cases of VUR are managed medically. Teach the child to empty the bladder completely. Teach child and parents appropriate perineal hygiene as well as toileting hygiene to prevent recurrence of UTI. Teach parents about the antibiotic therapy prescribed: the child will be maintained on a low daily dose to prevent UTI. The drug is most effective when given at bedtime because of urinary stasis overnight. Inform parents of the schedule for serial urine cultures and follow-up VCUG.

Providing Postoperative Care

If VUR is severe or if UTI is recurrent, surgical correction will be necessary. In the first 24 to 48 hours after surgery, maintain the intravenous fluid rate at 1.5 times maintenance to encourage a high urinary output. Monitor urine output via the Foley catheter; urine should be bloody initially, clearing within 2 to 3 days. If ureteral stents are present, monitor urine output from those as well. Administer analgesics for incisional pain relief and antispasmodics or B & O suppositories as needed for bladder spasms. Encourage ambulation and advancement of diet as ordered to promote return of appropriate bowel function. Teach

parents that prophylactic antibiotics will be given until 1 to 2 months after surgery, when the VCUG demonstrates absence of reflux.

> ▶ *Take* NOTE!
>
> *When caring for the child who has undergone urologic surgery, avoid manipulating the Foley or suprapubic catheter: catheter manipulation contributes to bladder spasms.*

▶ URINARY TRACT INFECTION

UTI occurs most often as a result of bacteria ascending to the bladder via the urethra. UTI is the most common serious bacterial infection in children (Dulczak & Kirk, 2005), with lower tract infection (cystitis) being less serious than upper tract infection (pyelonephritis). As many as 7% of females and 2% of males will experience a UTI by age 6 years (Alper & Curry, 2005). UTI is most common in infants and young children. It occurs more frequently in males than females during infancy, but after 1 year of age is more common in females. One explanation for the more common occurrence in females is that the female's shorter urethra allows bacteria to have easier access to the bladder. The urethra is also located quite close to the vagina and anus in females, allowing spread of bacteria from those areas. The sexually active female adolescent is at risk for the development of cystitis, as bacteria may be forced in to the urethra by pressure from intercourse. The male may be somewhat protected from UTI by the antibacterial properties of prostate secretions.

UTI presents differently in infants than it does in children. Infants may exhibit fever, irritability, vomiting, failure to thrive, or jaundice. Children may also experience fever and vomiting and may have dysuria, frequency, hesitancy, urgency, or pain.

Pathophysiology

E. coli accounts for about 60% to 80% of all UTIs, as it is usually found in the perineal and anal region, close to the urethral opening (Alper & Curry, 2005). Other organisms include *Klebsiella, Staphylococcus aureus, Proteus, Pseudomonas,* and *Haemophilus.* Numerous factors may contribute to bacterial proliferation. Urinary stasis contributes to the development of a UTI once the bacteria have gained entry. Urine that remains in the bladder after voiding allows bacteria to grow rapidly. A decreased fluid intake also contributes to bacterial growth, as the bacteria become more concentrated. If the urine is alkaline, bacteria are better able to flourish. Untreated bladder infection may allow reflux of infected urine up the ureters to the kidneys and result in pyelonephritis, a more serious infection.

Therapeutic Management

UTIs are treated with either oral or intravenous antibiotics, depending on the severity of the infection. Urine culture and sensitivity determines the appropriate antibiotic. A 7- to 14-day course of antibiotics is often prescribed, though 2- to 5-day courses may be as effective (Alper & Curry, 2005). Adequate fluid intake is necessary to flush the bacteria from the bladder. Fever management may also be needed.

Nursing Assessment

For a full description of the assessment phase of the nursing process refer to page 1381. Assessment findings pertinent to UTI are discussed below.

Health History

Elicit a description of the present illness and chief complaint. Common signs and symptoms reported during the health history might include:

- Fever
- Nausea or vomiting
- Chills
- Abdomen, back, or flank pain
- Lethargy
- Jaundice (in the neonate)
- Poor feeding or "just not acting right" (in the infant)
- Urinary urgency or frequency
- Burning or stinging with urination (the infant may cry with urination, the toddler may grab the diaper)
- Foul-smelling urine
- Poor appetite (child)
- Enuresis or incontinence in a previously toilet-trained child
- Blood in the urine

Explore the child's current and past medical history for risk factors such as:

- Previous UTI
- Obstructive uropathy
- Inadequate toileting hygiene (often occurs with preschool girls)
- VUR
- Constipation
- Urine holding or dysfunctional voiding
- Neurogenic bladder
- Uncircumcised male
- Sexual intercourse
- Pregnancy
- Chronic illness

Physical Examination

In the neonate or young infant, observe for jaundice or increased respiratory rate. In infants and children, inspect the perineal area for redness or irritation. Observe the urine for visible blood, cloudiness, dark color, sediment, mucus, or foul odor. Note pallor, edema, or elevated blood pressure. Palpate the abdomen. Note distended bladder, abdominal mass, or tenderness, particularly in the flank area.

Laboratory and Diagnostic Tests

Common laboratory and diagnostic studies ordered for the assessment of UTI include:

- Urinalysis (clean-catch, suprapubic, or catheterized): may be positive for blood, nitrites, leukocyte esterase, white blood cells, or bacteria (bacteriuria)
- Urine culture: will be positive for infecting organism
- Renal ultrasound: may show hydronephrosis if child also has a structural defect
- VCUG: not usually performed until the child has been treated with antibiotics for at least 48 hours, as infected urine tends to reflux up the ureters anyway. VCUG performed once the urine has regained sterility may be positive for VUR.

Renal ultrasound, VCUG, and other nuclear medicine scans such as the DMSA scan may be indicated in certain populations. The physician or nurse practitioner will determine the need for radiologic testing.

Nursing Management

Goals for nursing management include eradicating infection, promoting comfort, preventing complications, and preventing recurrence of infection.

Eradicating Infection

The child who can tolerate oral intake will be prescribed an oral antibiotic. The child who has protracted vomiting related to the UTI or who has suspected pyelonephritis will require hospitalization and intravenous antibiotics. Any infant less than 3 months of age with fever and suspected UTI should also be hospitalized for administration of intravenous antibiotics. Administer oral or intravenous antibiotics as prescribed. Urge the parent to complete the entire course of oral antibiotic at home, even though the child is feeling better. Administer intravenous fluids as ordered or encourage generous oral fluid intake to help flush the bacteria from the bladder.

Promoting Comfort

Administer antipyretics such as acetaminophen or ibuprofen to reduce fever. A heating pad or warm compress may help relieve abdomen or flank pain. If the child is afraid to urinate due to burning or stinging, encourage voiding in a warm sitz or tub bath.

EVIDENCE-BASED PRACTICE 42.1
Antibiotics and Urinary Tract Infections in Children

● Study

Urinary tract infections (UTI) commonly occur in children, causing frequent and painful urination. Traditionally, 7- to 10-day courses have been recommend for treating UTI in children. In the search for options to decrease side effects and improve costs, short courses of antibiotics may provide the solution. The authors included 10 randomized and quasi-randomized trials with a total of 652 participants. Participants included were low-risk, between the ages of 3 months and 18 years with culture-proven UTI. The studies assessed the benefits and harms of short-course (2–4 days) antibiotic treatment compared with that of standard duration (7–14 days).

▲ Findings

The authors found that a 2- to 4-day course of oral antibiotics appears to be as effective as the traditional long course (7–14 days) in eradicating UTI in children. Additionally, there was no statistical significance demonstrated in terms of repeat UTI within 1 to 15 months after the original infection.

■ Nursing Implications

Shorter courses of antibiotic treatment are much easier for families to comply with and complete, yet families may be accustomed to longer courses of antibiotic treatment and need further education. Educate families that the shorter course is indeed effective in treating UTI. Nurses should advocate for short-course antibiotic treatment in low-risk children with UTI.

Michael, M., Hodson, E. M., Craig, J. C., Martin, S., & Voyer, V. A. (2007). Short versus standard duration oral antibiotic therapy for acute urinary tract infection in children. *The Cochrane Library 2007, 4.* Indianapolis: John Wiley & Sons.

Preventing Recurrence of Infection

Encourage the parents to return as ordered for a repeat urine culture after completion of the antibiotic course to ensure eradication of bacteria. Teaching Guidelines 42.1 gives further information on preventing UTI.

TEACHING GUIDELINES 42.1

Preventing Urinary Tract Infection in Females

• Drink enough fluid (to keep urine flushed through bladder).
• Drink cranberry juice to acidify the urine. Avoid colas and caffeine, which irritate the bladder.
• Urinate frequently and do not "hold" urine (to discourage urinary stasis).
• Avoid bubble baths (they contribute to vulvar and perineal irritation).
• Wipe from front to back after voiding (to avoid contaminating the urethra with rectal material).
• Wear cotton underwear (to decrease the incidence of perineal irritation).
• Avoid wearing tight jeans or pants.
• Wash the perineal area daily with soap and water.
• While menstruating, change sanitary pads frequently to discourage bacterial growth.
• Void immediately after sexual intercourse.

► ENURESIS

Enuresis is continued incontinence of urine past the age of toilet training. Box 42.1 gives further definitions related to enuresis. Nocturnal enuresis generally subsides by 6 years of age; if it does not, further investigation and treatment may be warranted. Occasional daytime wetting or dribbling of urine is usually not a cause for concern, but frequent daytime wetting concerns both the child and the parents. Nocturnal enuresis may persist in some children into late childhood and adolescence, causing significant distress for the affected child and family.

In some children, enuresis may occur secondary to a physical disorder such as diabetes mellitus or insipidus, sickle cell anemia, ectopic ureter, or urethral

BOX 42.1 Definitions Related to Enuresis

• **Primary enuresis:** enuresis in the child who has never achieved voluntary bladder control
• **Secondary enuresis:** urinary incontinence in the child who previously demonstrated bladder control over a period of at least 3 to 6 consecutive months
• **Diurnal enuresis:** daytime loss of urinary control
• **Nocturnal enuresis:** nighttime bedwetting

obstruction. Other causes common to both diurnal and nocturnal enuresis include a urine-concentrating defect, UTI, constipation, and emotional distress (sometimes serious). The most frequent cause of daytime enuresis is dysfunctional voiding or holding of urine, though giggle incontinence and stress incontinence also occur. Nocturnal enuresis may be related to a high fluid intake in the evening, obstructive sleep apnea, sexual abuse, a family history of enuresis, or inappropriate family expectations. Physical causes of enuresis must be treated; further management of the disorder focuses on behavioral training, which may be augmented with the use of enuresis alarms or medications.

Nursing Assessment

Elicit a description of the present illness and chief complaint. Determine the age of toilet training and when or if the child achieved successful daytime and nighttime dryness. Inquire about urine-holding behaviors such as squatting, dancing, or staring as well as rushing to the bathroom (diurnal enuresis). Inquire about the amount and types of fluid the child typically consumes before bedtime (nocturnal enuresis). Assess for risk factors such as:

- Family disruption or other stressors
- Chronic constipation (carefully assess bowel movement patterns)
- Excessive family demands related to toileting patterns
- History of being difficult to arouse from sleep
- Family history of enuresis

Assess the child's cognitive status: developmentally delayed children may take significantly longer to achieve urine continence than their typical same-age peers. Assess for short stature or elevated blood pressure, as these may occur when renal abnormalities are present.

Nursing Management

For the child with diurnal enuresis, encourage him or her to increase the amount of fluid consumed during the day in order to increase the frequency of the urge to void. Set a fixed schedule for the child to attempt to void throughout the day. These practices will usually be sufficient to retrain the child's voiding patterns. The child with nocturnal enuresis without a physiologic cause for bedwetting may present a management challenge.

Educating the Child and Family About Nocturnal Enuresis

Teach the family that the child is not lazy, nor does he or she wet the bed intentionally. Encourage the child and family to read books such as *Dry All Night: The Picture Book Technique That Stops Bedwetting* by Alison Mack or *Waking Up Dry: A Guide to Help Children Overcome Bedwetting* by Dr. Howard Bennett. Encourage the parents to

limit intake of bladder irritants such as chocolate and caffeine. Teach parents to limit fluid intake after dinner and ensure that the child voids just before going to bed. Waking the child to void at 11 p.m. may also be helpful. Teach the parents to use bed pads and to make the bed with two sets of sheets and pads to decrease the workload in the middle of the night. When sleeping at home, the child should wear his or her usual underwear or pajamas. If away on a family vacation, pull-ups may decrease the stress on both the child and the parents.

Providing Support and Encouragement

It is important for the child to understand that he or she is not alone. Depending on the child's developmental level, explain that as many as 5 million people have enuresis (this can be done in terms the child can relate to, such as a proportion within a school or 100 times the number of children in one school, etc.). It is not only "little kids" who wet the bed, and all kids who wet the bed need help overcoming this problem. Parents should include the child in plans for nighttime urinary control; this helps to increase the child's motivation to become dry. Parents should set up a reward system for dry nights. Parents should include the child in bed linen changes when he or she does wet the bed, but should do so in a matter-of-fact manner rather than in a punitive way; in fact, punishment for bedwetting should always be avoided.

With patience, consistency, and time, dryness will be achieved. Provide ongoing emotional support and positive reinforcement to the child and family.

Decreasing Nighttime Voiding

Teach the family using an enuresis alarm system how to use the alarm as well as the previously mentioned techniques (Fig. 42.6 and Box 42.2). Most of these devices work by sounding an alarm when the first few drops of urine appear; the child then awakens and stops the urine flow. Over time the child becomes conditioned to either awaken when the bladder is full or stop the urine flow when sleeping.

When behavioral and motivational therapies are unsuccessful, particularly in the older child, medications may be prescribed. Teach the child and parents about the use of medications such as oxybutynin, imipramine, and desmopressin (DDAVP) if these are prescribed (refer to Drug Guide 22.1).

▶ *Take* NOTE!

Enuresis is a source of shame and embarrassment for children and adolescents. It affects the child's life emotionally, behaviorally, and socially. The family's life is also significantly affected. Treatment failures for enuresis have been correlated with adolescent low self-esteem.

FIGURE **42.6** Some children and families find great success with the use of an enuresis alarm. The alarm wakes the child at the first sign of wetness. Over time, the child learns to awaken at night in response to the sensation of a full bladder.

▶ *Consider* THIS!

Antonio Cruise, a 7-year-old boy, is brought to the clinic by his mother for his annual examination. During your assessment the mother brings up concerns that Antonio continues to wet the bed at night. She states, "I was hoping this would end on its own, but now I'm concerned that there is a problem."

What further assessment information would you obtain?

What education and interventions may be necessary for this child and family?

What can you do to provide support and encouragement for Antonio and his family?

▶ ACQUIRED DISORDERS RESULTING IN ALTERED RENAL FUNCTION

A number of acquired disorders are responsible for alterations in renal function. They may occur as an autoimmune response or in relation to a bacterial infection. Renal dysfunction may also occur as a result of obstruc-

BOX 42.2 **Sources for Enuresis Alarms**

- www.bedwettingstore.com (800) 214-9605
- www.dri-sleeper.com (877) 331-2768
- www.nytone.com (801) 973-4090
- www.pottypager.com (800) 497-6573

tive disorders or repeated VUR, as discussed earlier. Left untreated, these disorders may lead to renal failure; even when treated appropriately, sometimes the appropriate response is not achieved and acute or chronic renal failure develops. Renal disorders are the most frequent cause of hypertension in children.

▶ *Take* NOTE!

Severe hypertension (blood pressure higher than the 99th percentile for age and sex) may lead to damage of the eye or vital organs (kidney, brain, or heart), or even death. Pediatric nurses must be adept at accurately measuring blood pressure in children.

Nephrotic Syndrome

Nephrotic syndrome occurs as a result of increased glomerular basement membrane permeability, which allows abnormal loss of protein in the urine. Nephrotic syndrome generally occurs in three forms: congenital, idiopathic, and secondary. Congenital nephrotic syndrome is an inherited disorder; it is rare and occurs primarily in families of Finnish descent. The prognosis is poor, though some success has occurred with early, aggressive treatment and with the advances in kidney transplantation in infants. Nephrotic syndrome may occur secondary to another condition such as systemic lupus erythematosus, Henoch-Schonlein purpura, or diabetes. Idiopathic nephrotic syndrome is the most commonly occurring type in children and is often termed minimal change nephrotic syndrome (MCNS). MCNS occurs more frequently in males than females and is most common in children less than 3 years of age. This discussion will focus primarily on MCNS. Complications of nephrotic syndrome include anemia, infection, poor growth, peritonitis, thrombosis, and renal failure.

Pathophysiology

Increased glomerular permeability results in the passage of larger plasma proteins through the glomerular basement membrane. This results in excess loss of protein (albumin) in the urine (**proteinuria**) and decreased protein and albumin (hypoalbuminemia) in the bloodstream. Protein loss in nephrotic syndrome tends to be almost exclusively albumin. Hypoalbuminemia results in a change in osmotic pressure, and fluid shifts from the bloodstream into the interstitial tissue (causing edema). This decrease in blood volume triggers the kidneys to respond by conserving sodium and water, leading to further edema. The liver senses the protein loss and increases production of lipoproteins. **Hyperlipidemia** then develops as the excess lipids cannot be excreted in the urine. Hyperlipidemia associated with nephrotic syndrome may be quite severe, yet cholesterol levels may decrease when the nephrotic syndrome is in remission, only to rise significantly again with a relapse.

Children with nephrotic syndrome are at increased risk for clotting (thromboembolism) because of the decreased intravascular volume. They are also at increased risk for the development of serious infection, most commonly pneumococcal pneumonia, sepsis, or spontaneous peritonitis. Steroid-resistant nephrotic syndrome may result in acute renal failure.

Therapeutic Management

Medical management of MCNS usually involves the use of corticosteroids. Intravenous albumin may be used in the severely edematous child. Diuretics are also required in the edematous phase. Long-term therapy is usually required to induce remission. The nephrologist will determine the length of therapy based on the child's response. Children who have steroid-responsive MCNS generally have a favorable prognosis. Some children with MCNS exhibit a minimal response to steroid therapy or experience remissions and the MCNS is steroid-resistant. Immunosuppressive therapy such as cyclophosphamide, cyclosporine A, or mycophenolate mofetil may be necessary.

Nursing Assessment

For a full description of the assessment phase of the nursing process refer to page 1381. Assessment findings pertinent to MCNS are discussed below.

Health History

Elicit a description of the present illness and chief complaint. Common signs and symptoms reported during the health history might include:

• Nausea or vomiting (may be related to ascites)
• Recent weight gain
• History of periorbital edema upon waking, progressing to generalized edema throughout the day
• Weakness or fatigue
• Irritability or fussiness

Explore the child's current and past medical history for risk factors such as:

• Intrauterine growth retardation
• Young age (less than 3 years)
• Male sex

Physical Examination

The physical assessment of the child with nephrotic syndrome includes inspection and observation, auscultation, and palpation.

Observe the child for edema (periorbital, generalized [**anasarca**], or abdominal ascites). As the disease progresses, the edema also progresses to become more generalized, eventually becoming severe. Inspect the skin

for a stretched, tight appearance, pallor, or skin breakdown related to significant edema (Fig. 42.7). Document height (or length) and weight. Note increased respiratory rate or increased work of breathing related to ascites and edema.

Note the blood pressure; it may be elevated in the child with nephrotic syndrome, though it is most often either normal or decreased unless the child is progressing to renal failure. Auscultate heart and lung sounds, noting abnormalities related to fluid overload. Palpate the skin, noting tautness. Palpate the abdomen and document presence of ascites.

Laboratory and Diagnostic Tests

Urine dipstick will reveal marked proteinuria. Infrequently, mild hematuria is also present. Serum protein and albumin levels will be low (often markedly so). Serum cholesterol and triglyceride levels are elevated. With continued nephrotic syndrome, creatinine and blood urea nitrogen (BUN) may become elevated.

Nursing Management

Goals for nursing management include promoting diuresis, preventing infection, promoting adequate nutrition, and educating the parents about ongoing care at home. As with other chronic disorders, provide ongoing emotional support to the child and family.

Promoting Diuresis

Administer corticosteroids as ordered. Tapering or weaning doses are required when the time comes to stop corticosteroid therapy. Administer diuretics if ordered, usually furosemide (Lasix). Children may develop hypokalemia because of potassium loss as an adverse effect of furosemide. Those children may require potassium supplementation or a diet higher in potassium-containing foods. Monitor urine output and the amount of protein in the

FIGURE 42.7 Note marked edema associated with nephrotic syndrome.

urine (by dipstick). Weigh the child daily on the same scale either naked or wearing the same amount of clothing. Assess for resolution of edema. Measure pulse rate and blood pressure every 4 hours to detect hypovolemia resulting from excessive fluid shifts. Enforce oral fluid restrictions if ordered.

In cases of severe hypoalbuminemia, intravenous albumin may be administered. Increases in the serum albumin level cause fluid to shift from the subcutaneous spaces back into the bloodstream. A diuretic such as furosemide administered immediately after the albumin infusion allows for optimal diuresis and prevents fluid overload. Refer to Drug Guide 42.1 for the nursing implications related to use of these medications.

Preventing Infection

Monitor the child's temperature. Viral illness may trigger a relapse in children with nephrotic syndrome who have achieved remission. Administer pneumococcal vaccine as prescribed (see Chapter 30 for information on immunizations). Administer prophylactic antibiotics, if prescribed. Live vaccines should be delayed until at least 2 weeks after corticosteroid or other immunosuppressive medication therapy ceases. Teach parents that if the child is unimmunized and is exposed to chickenpox, the pediatrician or nephrologist should be notified immediately so that the child may receive varicella zoster immunoglobulin.

Encouraging Adequate Nutrition and Growth

Encourage a nutrient-rich diet within prescribed restrictions. Fluid restriction is reserved for children with massive edema. Sodium intake may be restricted in the edematous child in an effort to prevent further fluid retention. Consultation with the dietitian is often helpful in meal planning because many of the foods that children like are high in sodium. Encourage protein-rich snacks. Consult with the child and family in planning meals and snacks that the child likes and will be likely to consume. Use of nutritional supplement shakes may be helpful in some children.

Educating the Family

Teach parents how to give medications and monitor for adverse effects. Demonstrate the urine dipstick technique for detecting protein, and encourage the family to keep a chart of dipstick results. The child may return to school but should avoid contact with sick playmates. If the child is exposed to another child with an infectious illness, the parents should monitor temperature and urine dipstick results more frequently to identify a relapse in nephrotic syndrome early so that treatment can begin.

Providing Emotional Support

Nephrotic syndrome is often a chronic condition, and children who are responsive to steroid treatment may enter remission only to experience relapse. This cycle of relapse and remission takes an emotional toll on the child and family. Frequent hospitalizations require the child to miss school and the parents to miss work; this creates further stress for the family. The child may experience social isolation because he or she must avoid exposure to infections or because of self-esteem problems. The child may be dissatisfied with his or her appearance because of edema and weight gain, short stature, and the classic "moon face" associated with chronic steroid use.

Provide emotional support to the child and family. Encourage them in their efforts to maintain the treatment plan. Introduce the child to other youngsters with chronic renal conditions. Refer families to the National Kidney Foundation (www.kidney.org) for information about local support groups and resources.

Acute Glomerulonephritis

Acute glomerulonephritis is a condition is which immune processes injure the glomeruli. Immune mechanisms cause inflammation, which results in altered glomerular structure and function in both kidneys. It often occurs following an infection, usually an upper respiratory or skin infection. The most common form is acute post-streptococcal glomerulonephritis (APSGN), and the following discussion will focus on this type. APSGN is caused by an antibody–antigen reaction secondary to an infection with a nephritogenic strain of group A beta-hemolytic streptococcus. APSGN occurs more frequently in males than females and is most common in children older than 2 years of age. The most serious complication is progression to uremia and renal failure (either acute or chronic).

There is no specific medical treatment for APSGN. Treatment is aimed at maintaining fluid volume and managing hypertension. If there is evidence of a current streptococcal infection, antibiotic therapy will be necessary.

Nursing Assessment

For a full description of the assessment phase of the nursing process refer to page 1381. Assessment findings pertinent to acute glomerulonephritis are discussed below.

Health History

Elicit a description of the present illness and chief complaint. Common signs and symptoms reported during the health history might include:

- Fever
- Lethargy
- Headache
- Decreased urine output
- Abdominal pain
- Vomiting
- Anorexia

Assess the child's current and past medical history for risk factors such as a recent episode of pharyngitis or other streptococcal infection, age over 2 years, or male sex.

Physical Examination and Laboratory
and Diagnostic Tests

Assess the child's blood pressure for elevation, which is common. Note the presence of mild edema. Observe for signs of cardiopulmonary congestion such as increased work of breathing or cough. Auscultate the lungs for crackles and the heart for gallop. The urine dipstick test will reveal proteinuria as well as hematuria. Inspect the urine for gross hematuria, which will cause the urine to appear tea-colored, cola-colored, or even a dirty green color. Serum creatinine and BUN may be normal or elevated, the serum complement level is depressed, and the erythrocyte sedimentation rate is elevated. Laboratory findings specific to streptococcus include an elevated anti-streptolysin (ASO) titer and an elevated DNAase B antigen titer.

Nursing Management

Administer antihypertensives such as labetalol or nifedipine and diuretics as ordered. Monitor blood pressure frequently. Maintain sodium and fluid restrictions as prescribed during the initial edematous phase. Weigh the child daily on the same scale wearing the same amount of clothing. Monitor increasing urine output and note improvement in the urine color. Document resolution of edema. Provide careful neurological evaluation, as hypertension may cause encephalopathy and seizures. Children with APSGN generally are fatigued and choose bed rest during the acute phase. Provide the child with age-appropriate activities and cluster care to allow rest periods.

Some children may be managed at home if edema is mild and they are not hypertensive. Teach the family to monitor urine output and color, take blood pressure measurements, and restrict the diet as prescribed. The child cared for at home should not participate in strenuous activity until proteinuria and hematuria are resolved.

If renal involvement progresses, dialysis may become necessary.

> ▶ **Take** NOTE!
>
> *Avoid use of nonsteroidal anti-inflammatory drugs (NSAIDs) in children with questionable renal function, as the antiprostaglandin action of NSAIDs may cause a further decrease in the glomerular filtration rate.*

Hemolytic–Uremic Syndrome

Hemolytic-uremic syndrome (HUS) is defined by three features: hemolytic anemia, thrombocytopenia, and acute renal failure. In 90% of cases of HUS, an illness featuring diarrhea precedes the onset of the syndrome. Other causes include idiopathic, inherited, drug-related, association with malignancies, transplantation, and malignant hypertension. This discussion will focus on typical HUS, the type preceded by a diarrheal illness. Watery diarrhea progresses to hemorrhagic colitis, then to the triad of HUS. The features of HUS, as well as effects on other organs, are caused primarily by microthrombi and ischemic changes within the organs. The thrombotic events in the small blood vessels of the glomerulus lead to occlusion of the glomerular capillary loops and glomerulosclerosis, resulting in renal failure.

A verotoxin-producing strain of *E. coli*, O157:H7, causes the majority of cases, though *Streptococcus pneumoniae*, *Shigella dysenteriae*, and other bacteria may also be the cause. It is thought that antibiotic treatment for the aforementioned bacteria may contribute to release of the verotoxin. Undercooked ground beef accounts for most cases of *E. coli* O157:H7 infection, but it is also transmitted via the feces of numerous animals as well as unpasteurized dairy and fruit products. Transmission also occurs via human feces, and cases have been linked to public swimming pools. HUS occurs most often in children age 6 months to 4 years. Complications include chronic renal failure, seizures and coma, pancreatitis, intussusception, rectal prolapse, cardiomyopathy, congestive heart failure, and acute respiratory distress syndrome.

Therapeutic management of HUS is directed toward maintaining fluid balance; correcting hypertension, acidosis, and electrolyte abnormalities; replenishing circulating red blood cells; and providing dialysis if needed.

Nursing Assessment

For a full description of the assessment phase of the nursing process refer to page 1381. Assessment findings pertinent to HUS are discussed below.

Health History

Elicit a description of the present illness and chief complaint. Common signs and symptoms reported during the health history might include watery diarrhea accompanied by cramping and sometimes vomiting. After several days, the diarrhea becomes bloody and eventually improves.

Explore the child's current and past medical history for risk factors such as ingestion of ground beef, visits to a water park or to a petting zoo before the onset of the diarrheal illness, or use of antidiarrheal medications or antibiotics.

Physical Examination

Observe the child for pallor, toxic appearance, edema, **oliguria**, or **anuria**. Assess for elevated blood pressure and tenderness in the abdomen. Assess the child for neurologic involvement, which may include irritability, altered level of consciousness, seizures, posturing, or coma.

Laboratory and Diagnostic Tests

Urinalysis may reveal the presence of blood, protein, pus, and/or casts. Serum laboratory abnormalities are numerous and may include:

- Elevated BUN and creatinine
- Moderate to severe anemia (with the presence of Burr cells, schistocytes, spherocytes, or helmet cells), mild to severe thrombocytopenia
- Increased reticulocyte count
- Increased bilirubin and lactic dehydrogenase (LDH) levels
- Negative Coombs' test (except in cases of *S. pneumoniae* infection)
- Leukocytosis with left shift
- Hyponatremia
- Hyperkalemia
- Hyperphosphatemia
- Metabolic acidosis

Nursing Management

Nursing management of the child with HUS focuses on close observation and monitoring of the child's status. Institute and maintain contact precautions to prevent spread of *E. coli* O157:H7 to other children (bacteria are shed for up to 17 days after resolution of the diarrhea). Close attention must be paid to fluid volume status. Prevention of HUS is also an important nursing function.

Maintaining Appropriate Fluid Volume Balance

Maintain strict intake and output monitoring and recording to evaluate the progression toward renal failure. Carefully monitor intravenous infusions and blood chemistries. Administer diuretics as ordered. Assess blood pressure frequently and report elevations to the physician. Administer antihypertensives as ordered and monitor their effectiveness. Encourage adequate nutritional intake within the constraints of prescribed dietary restrictions. Monitor for bleeding as well as for fatigue and pallor. Follow the institutional protocol for transfusion of packed red blood cells and/or platelets (platelets are usually transfused only if active bleeding or severe thrombocytopenia occurs). Report progressive deterioration in laboratory findings to the physician. About 50% of children with HUS will require dialysis for at least several days.

Preventing HUS

Proper hand washing is necessary. Teach children to wash their hands after using the bathroom, before eating, and after petting farm animals. Encourage the use of "swim diapers," which contain feces, for children who are not toilet trained. Teach parents to thoroughly cook all meats to a core temperature of 155° F, or until the meat is gray or brown throughout and the juices from the meat are clear rather than pink. Wash all fruits and vegetables thoroughly. Ensure that drinking water and water used for recreation are appropriately treated. Avoid unpasteurized dairy products and fruit juices (including cider).

▶ RENAL FAILURE

Renal failure is a condition in which the kidneys cannot concentrate urine, conserve electrolytes, or excrete waste products. As in adults, renal failure in children may occur as an acute or chronic condition. Some cases of acute renal failure resolve without further complications, while dialysis is necessary in other children. When acute renal failure continues to progress, it becomes chronic (also known as end-stage renal disease [ESRD]). Dialysis and kidney transplantation are treatment modalities used for ESRD.

Acute Renal Failure

Acute renal failure is defined as a sudden, often reversible, decline in renal function that results in the accumulation of metabolic toxins (particularly nitrogenous wastes) as well as fluid and electrolyte imbalance. Fluid overload may lead to hypertension, pulmonary edema, and congestive heart failure. Additional complications include hyperkalemia, metabolic acidosis, hyperphosphatemia, and uremia. In children, acute renal failure most commonly occurs as a result of decreased renal perfusion, as occurs in hypovolemic or septic shock. It may also occur in children with hemolytic anemia or as a result of nephrotoxicity from medications. Complications include anemia, hyperkalemia, hypertension, pulmonary edema, cardiac failure, and altered level of consciousness or seizures, and acute renal failure may also progress to a chronic state.

Therapeutic management is aimed at treating the underlying cause and managing the fluid and electrolyte disturbances, as well as decreasing blood pressure.

▶ **Take** NOTE!

Medications commonly used in children can reduce renal function. Cephalosporins may cause a transient increase in BUN and creatinine. Truly nephrotoxic drugs often used in children include aminoglycosides, sulfonamides, vancomycin, and nonsteroidal anti-inflammatories (NSAIDs). Make sure that potentially nephrotoxic drugs are administered according to published safe guidelines (dosage, frequency, rate of administration).

Nursing Assessment

For a full description of the assessment phase of the nursing process refer to page 1381. Assessment finding pertinent to acute renal failure are discussed below.

Health History

Elicit a description of the present illness and chief complaint. Common signs and symptoms reported during the health history might include:

- Nausea
- Vomiting
- Diarrhea
- Lethargy
- Fever
- Decreased urine output

Assess the child's current and past medical history for risk factors such as history of shock, trauma, burns, urologic abnormalities, renal disease, use of nephrotoxic medications, or severe blood transfusion reaction.

Physical Examination and Laboratory and Diagnostic Tests

Note decreased skin elasticity, dry mucous membranes, or edema. Auscultate lungs for crackles, which may occur with pulmonary edema. Document tachypnea. Note cardiac rhythm disturbances. Evaluate the child's level of consciousness. Laboratory tests will reveal increased serum creatinine levels and possible electrolyte disturbances, such as hyperkalemia or hypocalcemia. Urinalysis may reveal proteinuria or hematuria.

> ▶ *Take* NOTE!
>
> *Monitor the infant or child with renal failure carefully for signs of congestive heart failure, such as edema accompanied by bounding pulse, presence of an S3 heart sound, adventitious lung sounds, and shortness of breath.*

Nursing Management

Nursing care focuses on managing hypertension, restoring fluid and electrolyte balance, and educating the family.

Managing Hypertension

Carefully monitor the child's blood pressure. Administer antihypertensives as prescribed. When a fast-acting drug such as nifedipine (Procardia) sublingually or labetalol intravenously is used, stay with the child and frequently monitor blood pressure. Immediately notify the physician if high blood pressure is resistant to medication and the blood pressure remains elevated.

Restoring Fluid and Electrolyte Balance

Monitor vital signs frequently and assess urine specific gravity. Maintain strict records of intake and output. Administer diuretics as ordered. When urine output is restored, diuresis may be significant. Monitor for signs of hyperkalemia (weak, irregular pulse; muscle weakness; abdominal cramping) and hypocalcemia (muscle twitching or tetany). Administer polystyrene sulfonate (Kayexalate) as ordered orally, rectally, or through a nasogastric tube to decrease potassium levels. Kayexalate removes potassium primarily by exchanging sodium for it, which is then eliminated in the feces. Administer packed red blood cell transfusions as ordered (may need to be followed by a dose of diuretic). Dialysis may become necessary if oliguria is sustained and leads to significant fluid overload, the electrolyte imbalance reaches dangerous levels, or uremia results in depression of the central nervous system.

Providing Family Education

Educate the family about the plan of care and the need for fluid restriction if ordered. Instruct the family to save all voids for observation and measurement by the nurse. Provide education about the use of dialysis if relevant.

End-Stage Renal Disease

End-stage renal disease (ESRD) is chronic renal failure requiring long-term dialysis or renal transplantation. Chronic renal failure in children most often results from congenital structural defects such as obstructive uropathy. It may also be caused by an inherited condition such as familial nephritis or may result from an acquired problem such as glomerulonephritis; it may follow an infectious process such as pyelonephritis or HUS. This is in contrast to chronic renal failure in adults, which primarily results from diabetes or hypertension. Uremia, hypocalcemia, hyperkalemia, and metabolic acidosis occur. Complications of ESRD are many. Uremic toxins deplete erythrocytes and the failing kidneys cannot produce erythropoietin, so severe anemia results. Hypertension is common and heart failure may occur. Hypocalcemia results in renal rickets (brittle bones). Growth is retarded and sexual maturation may be delayed or absent. Many children with ESRD experience depression, anxiety, impaired social interaction, and poor self-esteem. See Healthy People 2010.

Nursing Assessment

For a full description of the assessment phase of the nursing process refer to page 1381. Assessment finding pertinent to ESRD are discussed below.

HEALTHY PEOPLE 2010	
Objective	**Nursing Significance**
Reduce the rate of new cases of end-stage renal disease (ESRD).	• Encourage compliance with medical regimens related to urinary tract disorders in order to prevent progression to chronic renal failure

Health History

Explore the health history for low birthweight (associated with kidney dysfunction and anatomic alterations), poor growth (weight, length/height, and head circumference), and regimen of dialysis. Note decreased appetite or energy level, dry or itchy skin, or bone or joint pain.

Physical Examination and Laboratory and Diagnostic Tests

Perform a thorough physical assessment, noting any abnormalities (may vary from child to child). If present, assess the peritoneal catheter site for absence of drainage, bleeding, or redness. If the child undergoes hemodialysis, assess the fistula or graft site for the presence of a bruit and a thrill. Laboratory tests may reveal low hemoglobin and hematocrit, increased serum phosphorus and potassium levels, and decreased sodium, calcium, and bicarbonate levels. BUN, uric acid, and creatinine levels will be elevated. A 24-hour urine creatinine clearance test will show increased amounts of creatinine in the urine, reflecting decreasing kidney function.

> ▶ **Take** NOTE!
>
> *Carefully assess children with ESRD for worsening uremia or metabolic acidosis. Uremia may result in central nervous system symptoms such as headache or coma, or gastrointestinal or neuromuscular disturbances. Metabolic acidosis causes lethargy, dull headache, and confusion.*

Nursing Management

Nursing goals for the child with ESRD include promoting growth and development, removing waste products and maintaining fluid balance via dialysis, encouraging psychosocial well-being, and supporting and educating the family.

Promoting Growth and Development

Encourage the child to choose foods he or she likes that are within the imposed dietary restrictions. Daily protein requirements for adequate growth range from 0.9 to 1.5 grams of protein per kilogram of weight. Sodium and/or potassium restrictions may also be necessary. Enforce fluid restrictions if prescribed. Administer medications such as erythropoietin, growth hormone, and vitamin and mineral supplements to augment nutritional status and promote growth. Table 42.2 lists medications and supplements used to support growth.

Encouraging Psychosocial Well-Being

The child with chronic renal failure and particularly ESRD often suffers from depression and anxiety. Refer children and their families to the hospital social worker or counselor as needed for depression or anxiety issues. The chronic need for dialysis (daily with peritoneal dialysis or three or four times per week with hemodialysis) confers long-term stress on the child and family. The child usually demonstrates poor growth and often suffers from body image disturbance. Frequent medical appointments and hospitalizations interfere with the child's scholastic achievements. Introduce the child to other children with ESRD (this often happens anyway at the hemodialysis center).

Ensure that the family is aware of financial and support resources within the community (refer them to the National Kidney Foundation at www.kidney.org). The American Kidney Fund (www.kidneyfund.org) provides financial aid for kidney patients and summer camps for children with renal problems. Camp is an excellent way for children to demonstrate that they have mastered some of the loss-of-control issues related to their disease.

Several websites provide forums for children and teens with kidney failure or transplantation so they can learn about their disease, access resources, and/or communicate with other children. Two of them are:

- www.kidskare.org/: created by children, for children; contains information about organ donation and transplantation
- www.transweb.org: contains information about transplantation and donation

Dialysis and Transplantation

Peritoneal dialysis or hemodialysis is required on a long-term basis for children with chronic renal failure or ESRD. Once the child has progressed to ESRD, kidney transplan-

TABLE 42.2 MEDICATIONS AND SUPPLEMENTS COMMONLY USED TO TREAT ESRD COMPLICATIONS

Medication or Supplement	Purpose
Vitamin D and calcium	Correction of hypocalcemia and hyperphosphatemia
Ferrous sulfate	Treatment of anemia
Bicitra or sodium bicarbonate tablets	Correction of acidosis
Multivitamin	Augment nutritional status
Erythropoietin injections	Stimulate red blood cell growth
Growth hormone injections	Stimulate growth in stature

FIGURE 42.8 The peritoneal dialysis catheter is tunneled under the skin into the peritoneal cavity.

tation is needed for the child to progress with growth and development.

Peritoneal Dialysis

Peritoneal dialysis uses the child's abdominal cavity as a semipermeable membrane to help remove excess fluid and waste products (Figs. 42.8 and 42.9). The parent or caregiver performs peritoneal dialysis at home after completing a training course. The process is either completed overnight with the use of a machine (continuous cyclic peritoneal dialysis) or in increments throughout the day for a total of 4 to 8 hours (continuous ambulatory peritoneal dialysis). Comparison Chart 42.1 compares these two methods of peritoneal dialysis.

The advantages of peritoneal dialysis over hemodialysis include improved growth as a result of more dietary freedom, increased independence in daily activities, and a steadier state of electrolyte balance. However, the risk for infection (peritonitis and sepsis) is a continual concern with peritoneal dialysis. Dialysate exchange proto-

FIGURE 42.9 (**A**) During the "fill" phase of peritoneal dialysis, dialysate fluid is instilled into the peritoneal cavity. (**B**) During the "dwell" phase, the child may be up out of bed with the empty dialysate bag folded up with the tubing under his clothing. (**C**) During the "drain" phase, the old dialysate is drained from the peritoneum by gravity, bringing with it waste products and excess fluid. The dialysate bags are weighed prior to filling and after draining to determine the amount of fluid removed from the child.

COMPARISON CHART 42.1 METHODS OF PERITONEAL DIALYSIS

	Continuous Ambulatory Peritoneal Dialysis (CAPD)	Continuous Cyclic Peritoneal Dialysis (CCPD)
When performed	Throughout the day, with exchanges every 3 to 6 hours. Fluid is usually allowed to dwell overnight to allow child to sleep.	Usually overnight while child is sleeping
Method	Manual instillation and draining and changing of dialysate bags with each exchange	Automated via CCPD machine; bags and tubing are attached when started, then disconnected in the morning
Dwell time	3 to 6 hours	Usually 30 minutes to 1 hour
Mobility	Allows for mobility and permits child to participate in activities between exchanges	Child is confined to bed during the night while CCPD is ongoing but completely mobile while off CCPD during the day.

cols, care of the catheter in the abdomen, and dressing changes must all be performed using sterile technique to avoid introducing microorganisms into the peritoneal cavity. Box 42.3 lists additional risks associated with peritoneal dialysis.

Hemodialysis

Hemodialysis removes toxins and excess fluid from the blood by pumping the child's blood through a hemodialysis machine and then reinfusing the blood into the child. Needles to remove and reinfuse the blood are inserted into an arteriovenous fistula or graft, usually located in the child's arm (Figs. 42.10 and 42.11).

Hemodialysis frees the parent from the need to perform daily dialysis, but the procedure, which takes 3 to 6 hours, must be done two to four times per week (usually three) at a pediatric hemodialysis center. This requires time away from school and other activities for the child and from work and other family responsibilities for the parent. Since hemodialysis is usually performed only every other day, larger amounts of waste products build up in the child's blood (uremia), placing the child at higher risk for seizures. The access site may become infected, and occlusion is also possible. The child must follow a stricter diet between hemodialysis treatments, though dietary restrictions are usually lifted while the child is actually undergoing the treatment.

Nursing Assessment

Refer to the section on nursing assessment of the child with chronic renal failure/ESRD, as it is similar to assessment of the child undergoing dialysis. Assess for alterations in blood pressure and laboratory values following dialysis. Monitor for signs and symptoms of infection.

Assess the child receiving peritoneal dialysis for toleration of the fluid volume instilled within the peritoneum. The abdomen will remain distended while the fluid is indwelling and will be significantly flatter when the fluid is drained. Assess the Tenckhoff catheter site for signs of infection. Monitor the child's temperature. Inspect the dialysate effluent for fibrin or cloudiness, which may indicate infection. Weigh the child daily (in the drain phase if on peritoneal dialysis).

BOX 42.3 **Risks Associated with Peritoneal Dialysis**

- Hypertension and other cardiac complications
- Seizures
- Obstructed catheter
- Dialysate leakage
- Hyperglycemia
- Increased triglyceride levels
- Increased protein loss
- Parental stress and burnout related to repetitive nature of daily intervention

FIGURE 42.10 (**A**) Arteriovenous fistula. (**B**) Arteriovenous graft.

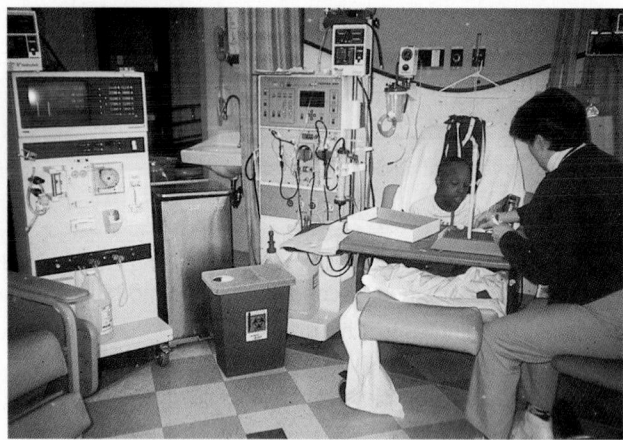

FIGURE 42.11 Pediatric hemodialysis via arteriovenous fistula or graft in left arm.

HEALTHY PEOPLE 2010

Objective	Nursing Significance
Increase the proportion of new hemodialysis patients who use arteriovenous fistulas as the primary mode of vascular access. Increase the proportion of dialysis patients registered on the waiting list for transplantation.	• Educate families about the benefits of an arteriovenous fistula over other methods of hemodialysis access. • Advocate for the patient to obtain an arteriovenous fistula. • Educate families about transplantation, and if no living-related match is available, encourage the family to seek placement on the organ transplant waiting list.

For the child who receives hemodialysis, assess the arteriovenous fistula or graft site with each set of vital signs. Auscultate the site for the presence of a bruit and palpate for the presence of a thrill. Notify the physician immediately if either is absent.

▶ **Take** NOTE!

Avoid taking blood pressure, performing venipuncture, or using a tourniquet in the extremity with the arteriovenous fistula or graft: these procedures may cause occlusion and subsequent malfunction of the fistula or graft. Teach parents and children to inform all health care providers they come in contact with about the presence of the fistula or graft.

Nursing Management

Both peritoneal dialysis and hemodialysis are performed by specially trained and certified nurses. The general pediatric nurse's role is related to the ongoing care of the child. The child undergoing peritoneal dialysis usually is allowed a more liberal diet and intake of fluid than the child undergoing hemodialysis. Peritoneal dialysis removes waste and excess fluids on a daily basis, whereas hemodialysis occurs about every other day. Most routine medications are withheld on the morning that hemodialysis is scheduled, since they would be filtered out through the dialysis process anyway. Administer these medications as soon as the child returns from the dialysis unit. See Healthy People 2010.

Renal Transplantation

Renal transplantation is the optimal treatment for ESRD and offers the best opportunity for the child to live a normal life. Vigilant medication administration is necessary after the transplant to prevent organ rejection. The child may achieve 40% to 80% renal function with the transplant and demonstrate improved growth, enhanced cognitive development, and improved psychosocial development and quality of life (Milliner, 2004).

Kidneys are obtained from a cadaver (a patient declared brain-dead who had previously given consent to organ donation) or from a blood relative (living-related). The transplanted kidney must match the child's blood type and the child's human leukocyte antigens (HLA). The cadaver kidney or living-related kidney is implanted surgically in the abdomen and the blood vessels are anastomosed to the aorta and superior vena cava.

Generally, living-related transplants have a decreased rejection rate compared to cadaver transplants. Living-related kidney donation and subsequent transplantation can be planned ahead and scheduled in advance. In contrast, cadaver kidneys become available suddenly, leaving less time for preoperative preparation. For either type, last-minute blood tissue typing is required before the final decision is made to move forward with transplantation. Often the child's native kidneys are removed before or at the time of the renal transplant because of their association with hypertension in the child.

▶ **Take** NOTE!

Cadaver kidneys are allocated to potential recipients based on the age of the renal failure patient, the time that he or she has been awaiting a transplant, blood type, HLA antibody matching, panel reactive antibodies, and region of the country (so that the donated kidney can be received expeditiously).

Nursing Assessment

A thorough physical assessment is warranted for any renal transplant patient, whether in the initial postoperative period, at a clinic visit, or when admitted to the hospital to rule out transplant rejection. Note recent health history, medications and their doses, and any symptoms the child has been having. In the initial postoperative period, assess the incision for redness, edema, or drainage; if any of these signs of infection or rejection occur, notify the transplant surgeon and nephrologist immediately. Monitor blood pressure and other vital signs closely. Document resolution of edema. Record intake and output accurately. Assess for signs and symptoms of transplant rejection such as malaise, fever, unexplained weight gain, or pain over the transplant area.

Nursing Management

Postoperative care focuses on preventing rejection, monitoring renal function, maintaining fluid and electrolyte balance, and educating the child and family.

> ▶ **Take** NOTE!
>
> *Encourage the child with a renal transplant to wear a medical alert necklace or bracelet, and urge the parents to inform community emergency services of the child's transplant status.*

Preventing Rejection and Promoting Renal Function

Administer immunosuppressants accurately and in a timely fashion. Obtain and monitor serum levels of these medications per protocol. Immediately report significant alterations in vital signs or edema at the surgical site, as they may indicate transplant rejection. Maintain strict documentation of intake and output. Once adequate urine output is established, intake is usually liberalized.

Educating the Child and Family

Develop a schedule to cluster care so that the child may receive the rest needed for recovery despite the many and frequent assessments and interventions. With the family, develop a medication schedule that will be compatible with the family's life at home as well as the restrictions related to some medications. Begin teaching with the family as soon as the child's condition is stable. Accurate medication administration and home monitoring are necessary to prevent rejection. The child may return to school when discharged from the hospital, but the family will need to communicate closely with the school nurse about the child's immunosuppressed status. The American Nephrology Nurses Association has developed a renal transplant fact sheet that can be shared with the school nurse (available at www.annanurse.org).

> ▶ **Take** NOTE!
>
> *Tell the parents to inform their primary care provider about the child's long-term corticosteroid use and/or immunosuppressed status, as the child should not receive any live vaccines.*

Reproductive Organ Disorders

A number of disorders may occur within the female or male genitalia and internal reproductive organs in children. These problems may be structural or infectious.

▶ FEMALE DISORDERS

Disorders of the female reproductive organs that occur in children and adolescents include structural disorders, infectious disorders, and menstrual disorders.

Labial Adhesions

Labial adhesion or labial fusion is partial or complete adherence of the labia minora (Fig. 42.12). UTI may result from urinary stasis behind the labia; if the adhesions are left untreated, the vaginal orifice may become inaccessible, presenting difficulty with sexual intercourse in the future.

FIGURE 42.12 Labial adhesions. Note fusion of the upper portion of the labia minora.

Nursing Assessment

Younger girls have a higher risk of adhesions (3 months to 4 years). Assess the history for dysuria or urinary frequency. Inspect the genitalia for fusion or adherence of the labia minora.

Nursing Management

Administer topical estrogen cream as prescribed, usually once or twice daily. Teach the parents to continue cream application until the labia separate. Encourage use of petroleum jelly daily for 1 month following labial separation to prevent recurrence of adhesion.

Vulvovaginitis

Vulvovaginitis is inflammation of the vulva and vagina. Inflammation may occur as a result of bacterial or yeast overgrowth or from chemical factors such as bubble bath, soaps, or perfumes found in personal care products. Poor hygiene may also cause vulvovaginitis. Tight clothing may cause a heat rash in the perineal area. Persistent scratching of the irritated area may result in the complication of superficial skin infection.

Nursing Assessment

Elicit a description of the present illness and chief complaint. Common signs and symptoms reported during the health history may include itching or burning in the perineal area. Explore the client's current and past medical history for risk factors, which may include:

- Young age (toilet-trained preschooler)
- Poor hygiene
- Sexual activity
- Immune disorders
- Diabetes mellitus

Inspect the perineum for redness, edema, irritation, rash, or vaginal discharge (note color, consistency, and odor).

Nursing Management

Teach appropriate hygiene (daily and toileting). Girls (or their parents) should wash the genital area thoroughly on a daily basis with mild soap and water. Rinse the area well. Encourage girls to wipe after urinating and after bowel movements to wipe in a front-to-back motion. The girl should wear cotton underwear and should change it at least once a day. Administer topical or oral medications as ordered. Table 42.3 lists treatments related to specific types of vulvovaginitis.

▶ MALE DISORDERS

Male reproductive disorders include structural disorders and disorders caused by infection or inflammation. Circumcision will also be discussed below.

Phimosis and Paraphimosis

In phimosis, the foreskin of the penis cannot be retracted. Although this is normal in the newborn, it can be pathologic later. Over time, the prepuce (foreskin) naturally becomes retractable. Local irritation, balanitis, or UTI may occur if urine is retained within the foreskin after voiding. Paraphimosis (Fig. 42.13) is a more serious disorder characterized by retraction of the phimotic prepuce, which causes a constricting band behind the glans of the penis and results in incarceration if left untreated.

TABLE 42.3 **VULVOVAGINITIS: TYPES AND TREATMENTS**

Cause	Assessment Findings	Treatment
Unhygienic practices	Irritation of labia and vaginal opening May have foul brownish-green discharge if infected with bacteria from rectum	Good hygiene Sometimes a mild anti-inflammatory cream is prescribed. Assess for signs and symptoms of UTI, which may occur as a complication.
Candida albicans	Red bumpy perineal rash in infants White cottage-cheese–like discharge Intense itching	Antifungal cream or vaginal suppository Prevent by ingesting probiotics (found in yogurt and kefir) daily and supplementing with a probiotic such as Lactinex when taking antibiotics.
Bordetella, Gardnerella	Thin gray vaginal discharge with fishy odor	Flagyl (metronidazole) orally
Trichomonas vaginalis	Foul yellow-gray or green vaginal discharge	Flagyl (metronidazole) orally. Sexually transmitted, so can be prevented with the use of condoms.

FIGURE 42.13 Paraphimosis: note the swollen prepuce.

Hygiene in the Uncircumcised Male

- The foreskin does not normally retract in the newborn boy, so do not force it to do so.
- Change the diaper frequently and wash the penis daily with water and mild soap.
- When the infant is older and the foreskin easily retracts, gently retract the foreskin and clean around the glans with water and mild soap once a week.
- Dry the area prior to replacing the foreskin.
- Always replace the foreskin after retraction.
- Teach the preschool-age boy to retract the foreskin and clean the penis during each bath or shower.

Topical steroid cream applied twice a day for 1 month may be prescribed for phimosis. Paraphimosis requires reduction of the prepuce or a small dorsal incision to release the foreskin. Circumcision may be used to treat either condition.

Nursing Assessment

Elicit a description of the present illness and chief complaint. Common signs and symptoms reported during the health history might include:

- Irritation or bleeding from the opening of the prepuce (phimosis)
- Dysuria (phimosis)
- Pain (paraphimosis)
- Swollen penis (paraphimosis)

Determine the onset of symptoms and inspect the penis for irritation, erythema, edema, or discharge.

> ▶ *Take* NOTE!
>
> *A swollen, reddened penis (paraphimosis) is a medical emergency and can quickly result in necrosis of the tip of the penis if left untreated.*

Nursing Management

Apply topical steroid medication as prescribed for phimosis, following gentle retraction to stretch the foreskin back. Topical vitamin E cream may also help to soften the phimotic ring. When surgical intervention is necessary, provide routine postprocedural care and pain management (refer to the section on circumcision below). Teach the parents and uncircumcised boy proper hygiene, which will help to prevent phimosis and paraphimosis (Teaching Guidelines 42.2).

Circumcision

Circumcision is the removal of the excess foreskin of the penis. Some newborn boys are circumcised shortly after birth before going home from the hospital. Some parents elect not to have their newborn boy circumcised at that time but may desire it later. Neonatal circumcision may be performed in the newborn nursery, hospital unit treatment room, or outpatient office. Circumcision is indicated later for the conditions of phimosis and paraphimosis. Circumcision done after the newborn period usually requires general anesthesia.

The benefits of circumcision include a decreased incidence of UTI, sexually transmitted diseases, acquired immune deficiency syndrome, and penile cancer, and in female partners a decreased occurrence of cervical cancer. Complications of circumcision include alterations in the urinary meatus, unintentional removal of excessive amounts of foreskin, or damage to the glans penis.

Whether to circumcise or not is a personal decision and often based on religious beliefs or social or cultural customs. Nurses should support and educate the parents in either case.

Nursing Assessment

Prior to the procedure, assess for normal placement of the urinary meatus on the glans penis (in boys with hypospadias, circumcision should be delayed until evaluation by the pediatric urologist). After the circumcision, assess for redness, edema, or active bleeding. Note signs of infection, such as purulent drainage. Assess pain level.

Nursing Management

Nursing care of the boy undergoing circumcision focuses on managing pain, providing postprocedural care, and educating the parents.

Managing Pain

Whether circumcision is performed in the obstetric area of the hospital before newborn discharge or in the outpatient setting at a few days of age, pain management during the procedure must not be neglected. Advocate for appropriate pain management for the infant undergoing circumcision. The American Academy of Pediatrics (AAP) recommends using a subcutaneous ring block with lidocaine or a dorsal nerve block to the penis. The AAP also recommends the use of EMLA (eutectic mixture of local anesthetic) cream topically to decrease pain during the circumcision. Playing calming music during the procedure may also help to soothe the infant, providing distraction. A sucrose-dipped pacifier may also be used as adjuvant therapy for pain management. To increase a sense of comfort during the procedure, restrain the infant in a padded circumcision chair with blankets covering the legs and upper body. This allows the infant to be in a semi-upright position during the procedure while still allowing for a sterile procedural field. If a padded restraint chair is not available, provide atraumatic care by padding the circumcision board and covering the infant as previously described.

Providing Postprocedural Care

Usual care after circumcision depends on the type of appliance used (Gomco or Mogan clamp or Plastibell apparatus). Cleanse the penis with clear water for the first few days and avoid using alcohol-containing wipes. To avoid irritation to the penis, fasten diapers loosely. Notify the physician if excessive redness, active bleeding, or purulent discharge occurs. Assess for the first void following the procedure, or if performed in the outpatient setting instruct parents to call the physician if the infant has not voided by 6 to 8 hours after the circumcision. Apply antibiotic ointment or petroleum jelly to the penile head with each diaper change as prescribed, based on the circumcision method used and the preference of the health care provider.

> ▶ **Take** NOTE!
>
> If excess bleeding occurs after the circumcision, apply direct pressure and notify the health care provider immediately.

Educating the Parents

Instruct parents to give sponge baths until the circumcision is healed. Describe the normal granulation tissue that will be present during the healing process. Teach parents to apply ointment or petroleum jelly if indicated. Instruct the parents to call the health care provider if any of the following occur:

- The infant does not urinate within 6 to 8 hours after the procedure.
- Heavy bleeding occurs (more than small spots on the diaper or bleeding that requires direct pressure to stop it).
- There is purulent or serous drainage from the circumcised area.
- There is redness or swelling of the penile shaft.

> ▶ **Take** NOTE!
>
> If the Plastibell is used, teach parents NOT to use petroleum jelly, as it may cause the ring to be dislodged. A yellowish crust may form that should be allowed to fall off on its own after several days.

Cryptorchidism

Cryptorchidism (also known as undescended testicles) occurs when one or both testicles do not descend into the scrotal sac. Ordinarily the testes, which in the fetus develop in the abdomen, make their descent into the scrotal sac during the seventh month of gestation. The cause for this failure to descend may be mechanical, hormonal, chromosomal, or enzymatic. The disorder may occur unilaterally or bilaterally. Up to 4% of term male infants and as many as 30% of all preterm male infants exhibit cryptorchidism (Burns et al., 2004).

Complications associated with cryptorchidism that is allowed to progress into the school-age years include sterility and an increased risk for testicular cancer in adolescence or the young adult years. Therapeutic management is surgical. An orchiopexy is performed to release the spermatic cord, and the testes are then pulled into the scrotum and tacked into place.

Nursing Assessment

Explore the health history for risk factors such as:

- Prematurity
- First-born child
- Cesarean birth
- Low birthweight
- Hypospadias

Palpate for the presence (or absence) of both testes in the scrotal sac.

> ▶ **Take** NOTE!
>
> A retractile testis is one that may be brought into the scrotum, remains for a time, and then retracts back up the inguinal canal. This should not be confused with true cryptorchidism.

Nursing Management

If the testes are not descended by 6 months of age, the infant should be referred for surgical repair. The AAP recommends that orchiopexy be performed by 1 year of age. Postoperatively, observe the incision for signs of bleeding or infection.

Hydrocele and Varicocele

Hydrocele (fluid in the scrotal sac) is usually a benign and self-limiting disorder. It is usually noted early in infancy and often resolves spontaneously by 1 year of age. Varicocele (a venous varicosity along the spermatic cord) is often noted as a swelling of the scrotal sac. Complications of varicocele include low sperm count or reduced sperm motility, which can result in infertility.

Nursing Assessment

Elicit a description of the present illness and chief complaint. The boy with hydrocele will have an enlarged scrotum that may decrease in size when he is lying down. Inspect the scrotum for a fluid-filled appearance.

The boy with varicocele will have a mass on one or both sides of the scrotum and bluish discoloration. Inspect the scrotum for masses; the spermatic vein feels worm-like on palpation. The boy with varicocele may have pain.

Nursing Management

Both hydrocele and painless varicocele require watchful waiting, as these conditions will usually resolve spontaneously. If they do not resolve, or if the difference in testicular volume is marked in the boy with varicocele, refer the child to a urologist, as surgery may be indicated. Reassure parents that hydrocele is not associated with the development of infertility. Varicocele may lead to infertility if left untreated, so instruct parents to seek care if pain occurs or if there is a large difference in testicular size. Either condition may be surgically corrected on an outpatient basis. Provide routine postoperative care following either surgery.

Testicular Torsion

In testicular torsion, a testicle is abnormally attached to the scrotum and twisted. It requires immediate attention because ischemia can result if the torsion is left untreated, leading to infertility. Testicular torsion may occur at any age but most commonly occurs in boys aged 12 to 18 years (Burns et al., 2004).

Nursing Assessment

Elicit a description of the present illness and chief complaint. Signs and symptoms of testicular torsion include sudden, severe scrotal pain. Inspect the affected side for significant swelling, which may appear hemorrhagic or blue-black.

Nursing Management

Surgical correction is necessary immediately. Administer pain medication prior to surgery. Reassure the child and family that surgery will alleviate the problem and is performed to restore adequate blood flow to the testicle. After surgical repair, provide routine postoperative care.

▶ *Take* NOTE!

Testicular torsion is considered a surgical emergency, as necrosis of the testis may occur and gangrene may set in.

Epididymitis

Epididymitis (inflammation of the epididymis) is caused by infection with bacteria. It is the most common cause of pain in the scrotum. It rarely occurs before puberty, but if it does it may occur as a result of a urethral or bladder infection related to a urogenital anomaly (Burns et al., 2004). Therapeutic management is directed toward eradicating the bacteria. If left untreated, a scrotal abscess, testicular infarction, or infertility may occur.

Nursing Assessment

Note history of painful swelling of the scrotum, which may be gradual or acute. If the boy is sexually active, explore history of sexual encounters prior to the onset of symptoms. Document history of dysuria or urethral discharge. Note fever, which may last from days to weeks. On inspection, note edema and erythema of the scrotum. Gently palpate the scrotum for a hardened and tender epididymis. Note urethral discharge if present. Palpate the inguinal lymph nodes for enlargement. Urinalysis may be positive for bacteria and white blood cells. The culture of urethral discharge may be positive for a sexually transmitted infection such as gonorrhea or *Chlamydia*. The complete blood count may reveal an elevated white blood cell count.

Nursing Management

Encourage the boy to rest in bed with the scrotum elevated. Ice packs to the scrotum may help with pain relief. Administer pain medications such as NSAIDs or other analgesics as needed.

Administer antibiotics as prescribed. Educate the boy and his family to complete the entire course of antibiotics as prescribed to eradicate the infection. Advise the child and family to notify the physician if the condition is not improving or if the pain and swelling worsen.

■■■ Key Concepts

■ The urinary tract is immature in infants and young children, with a slower glomerular filtration rate and a decreased ability to concentrate urine and reabsorb amino acids compared with the adult.

- In children, chronic kidney disease is most often the result of congenital structural defects, or infectious, inflammatory, or immune processes that damage the kidney, whereas in adults it usually results from hypertension or diabetes.
- The short length of the urethra in girls and its proximity to the vagina and anus place the young girl at higher risk for the development of urinary tract infections compared with the adult.
- The expected urine output in the infant and child is 0.5 to 2 mL/kg/hour.
- Though present at birth, the reproductive organs do not reach functional maturity until puberty.
- Obtaining a clean or sterile urine specimen is necessary for accurate urine culture results.
- A urinary catheter must be inserted just prior to the voiding cystourethrogram.
- Close monitoring of serum blood counts and electrolytes is a critical component of nursing care related to renal disorders.
- Certain congenital urologic anomalies may require multiple surgeries as well as urinary diversion; urine drains through a stoma on the abdominal wall that is either pouched or catheterized.
- The treatment for nocturnal enuresis may include the use of desmopressin nasal spray and/or an enuresis alarm to train the child to awaken to the sensation of a filling bladder.
- Nephrotic syndrome results in significant proteinuria and edema.
- Acute glomerulonephritis most often follows a group A streptococcal infection and commonly results in hematuria, proteinuria, and hypertension.
- The most common cause of hemolytic-uremic syndrome is infection with *E. coli* O157:H7. It can be prevented by adequately cooking ground meat, washing hands and produce well, and making sure that an appropriate chemical balance is maintained in public recreational water sources such as swimming pools and water parks.
- Corticosteroids can cause gastrointestinal upset. If used on a long-term basis, they should be tapered rather than discontinued abruptly to avoid adrenal crisis.
- Children taking immunosuppressants for nephrotic syndrome or for renal transplant are at increased risk for the development of overwhelming infection.
- Peritoneal dialysis may be accomplished at home by the parent. Close attention to sterile technique is needed.
- Hemodialysis requires an arteriovenous fistula or graft that is accessed with needles three or four times per week at a hemodialysis center. This is disruptive to their academic, social, and family lives.
- Renal transplantation is the best option for the treatment of end-stage renal disease in children, but vigilant medication administration is needed to prevent organ rejection.
- Children with renal failure experience anemia, poor growth, depression, anxiety, and low self-esteem.
- The diet for a child with a renal disorder must be individualized according to prescribed sodium, fluid, and/or protein restrictions.
- Postoperative care for the child undergoing urologic surgery includes pain management, avoidance or treatment of bladder spasms, and monitoring of urine output.

REFERENCES

Ackley, B. J., & Ladwig, G. B. (2006). *Nursing diagnosis handbook: A guide to planning care* (7th ed.). St. Louis: Mosby.

Alper, B. S., & Curry, S. H. (2005). Urinary tract infection in children. *American Family Physician, 72*(12), 2483–2488.

American Academy of Pediatrics. (2005). *Circumcision policy statement.* Retrieved 12/31/07 from http://aappolicy.aappublications.org/cgi/content/full/pediatrics%3b103/3/686.

American Academy of Pediatrics, Committee on Quality Improvement, Subcommittee on Urinary Tract Infection. (1999). Practice parameter: The diagnosis, treatment, and evaluation of the initial urinary tract infection in febrile infants and young children. *Pediatrics, 103*(4), 843–693.

American Nephrology Nurses' Association. (2005). *Pediatric ESRD renal transplant fact sheet.* Pitman, N.J.: Author.

Anderson, H. (2005). Children on the frontline against *E. coli*: Typical hemolytic uremic syndrome. *Clinical Laboratory Science, 18*(2), 90–99.

Anonymous. (2004). Information from your family doctor: Urinary tract infections in children. *American Family Physician, 69*(1), 155–156.

Balinski, W. (2000). Pediatric end-stage renal disease: Incidence, management and prevention. *Journal of Pediatric Health Care, 14*(6), 304–308.

Bennett, H. J. (2005). Clinical tips for helping patients overcome bedwetting. *Contemporary Pediatrics, 22*(9); available at www.contemporarypediatrics.com/contpeds/article/articleDetail.jsp?id=179973&&pageID=4

Berry, A. (2005). A child with daytime wetting: Three case studies. *Urologic Nursing, 25*(3), 202–205.

Brewer, D. E., & Berry, P. L. (2006). Glomerulonephritis and nephrotic syndrome. In J. A. McMillan (Ed.), *Oski's pediatrics: Principles and practice.* Philadelphia: Lippincott Williams & Wilkins.

Buie, M. E. (2005). Circumcision: The good, the bad and American values. *American Journal of Health Education, 36*(2), 102–108.

Burns, C. E., Dunn, A. M., Brady, M. A., Starr, N. B., & Blosser, C. (2004). *Pediatric primary care: A handbook for nurse practitioners* (3rd ed.). Philadelphia: Saunders.

Camille, C. J., Kuo, R. L., & Wiener, J. S. (2002). Caring for the uncircumcised penis: What parents (and you) need to know. *Contemporary Pediatrics, 19* [Electronic version].

Chiang, D., Ben-Meir, D., Pout, K., & Dewan, P. A. (2005). Management of post-operative bladder spasm. *Journal of Paediatrics and Child Health, 41,* 56–58.

Children's Healthcare of Atlanta. (2004). *Double diapering.* Atlanta: Children's Healthcare of Atlanta.

Cromwell, P. F., Munn, N., & Zolkowski-Wynne, J. (2005). Evaluation and management of hypertension in children and adolescents (Part 1: Diagnosis). *Journal of Pediatric Health Care, 19*(3), 172–175.

Dufour, J. L. (2001). Assessing and treating epididymitis. *Nurse Practitioner, 26*(3), 23–24.

Dulczak, S., & Kirk, J. (2005). Overview of the evaluation, diagnosis, and management of urinary tract infections in infants and children. *Urologic Nursing, 25*(3), 185–192.

Dunlop, A. (2005). Meeting the needs of parents and pediatric patients: Results of a survey on primary nocturnal enuresis. *Clinical Pediatrics, 44,* 297–303.

Farnham, S. B., Adams, M. C., Brock, J. W., & Pope, J. C. (2005). Pediatric urological causes of hypertension. *Journal of Urology, 173,* 697–704.

Frazier, J. P., Parks, D. K., & Yetman, F. J. (2001). Congenital hydronephrosis. *Journal of Pediatric Health Care, 15*(5), 260–262.

Fritz, G., Rockney, R., Bernet, W., Arnold, V., Beitchman, J., Benson, R. S., Bukstein, O., Kinlan, J., McClellan, J., Rue, D., Shaw, J. A., & Stock, S. (2004). Practice parameter for the assessment and treatment of children and adolescents with enuresis. *Journal of the American Academy of Child & Adolescent Psychiatry, 43*(12), 1540–1550.

Gaines, K. K. (2004). Desmopressin (DDAVP) for enuresis, diabetes insipidus, and . . . *Urologic Nursing, 24*(6), 520–523.

Garin, E. H., Olavarrie, F., Nieto, V. G., Valenciano, B., Campos, A., & Young, L. (2006). Clinical significance of primary vesicoureteral reflux and urinary antibiotic prophylaxis after acute pyelonephritis: A multicenter, randomized controlled study. *Pediatrics, 117*(3), 626–632.

Gillespie, R. S. (2005). Management of nephrotic syndrome. *Resident and Staff Physician* [electronic version]. Available at: http://www.residentandstaff.com/issues/articles/2005–08–01.asp.

Hawkins, E. P. (2006). Renal malformations. In J. A. McMillan (Ed.), *Oski's pediatrics: Principles and practice (4th ed.).* Philadelphia: Lippincott Williams & Wilkins.

Herrinton, L. J., Zhao, W., & Husson, G. (2003). Management of cryptorchidism and risk of testicular cancer. *American Journal of Epidemiology, 157*(7), 602–605.

Hinds, A. C. (2004). Obstructive uropathy: Considerations for the nephrology nurse. *Nephrology Nursing Journal, 31*(2), 166–180.

Hornor, G. (2007). Genitourinary assessment: An integral part of a complete physical examination. *Journal of Pediatric Health Care, 21*(3), 162–170.

Lau, K. K., & Wyatt, R. J. (2005). Glomerulonephritis. *Adolescent Medicine Clinics, 16*(1), 67–85.

Kelley, K. (2004). How peritoneal dialysis works. *Nephrology Nursing Journal, 31*(5), 481–490.

Klein, N. J. (2001). Management of primary nocturnal enuresis. *Urologic Nursing, 21*(2), 71–76.

Koester, M. C. (2005). Initial evaluation and management of acute scrotal pain. *Journal of Athletic Training, 35*(1), 76–79.

Landgraf, J. M., Abidari, J., Cilento, B. G., Cooper, C. S., Schulman, S. L., & Ortenberg, J. (2004). Coping, commitment, and attitude: Quantifying the everyday burden of enuresis on children and their families. *Pediatrics, 113,* 334–344.

Lum, G. M. (2005). Kidney and urinary tract. In W. W. Hay, M. J. Levin, J. M. Sondheimer, & R. R. Deterding (Eds.), *Current pediatric diagnosis and treatment* (17th ed.) New York: McGraw-Hill.

Miller, D., Macdonald, D., Kolnacki, K., & Simek, T. (2004). Challenges for nephrology nurses in the management of children with chronic kidney disease. *Nephrology Nursing Journal, 31*(3), 287–295.

Milliner, D. S. (2004). Pediatric renal-replacement therapy: Coming of age. *New England Journal of Medicine, 350*(26), 2637. Retrieved May 12, 2005, from ProQuest database.

Mills, M., White, S. C., Kershaw, D., Flynn, J. T., Brophy, P. D., Thomas, S. E., & Smoyer, W. (2005). Developing clinical protocols for nursing practice: Improving nephrology care for children and their families. *Nephrology Nursing Journal, 32*(6), 599–607.

Nettina, S. M. (2005). *Lippincott manual of nursing practice.* Philadelphia: Lippincott Williams & Wilkins.

Neuhaus, T. J. (2004). Immunization in children with chronic renal failure: A practical approach. *Pediatric Nephrology, 19,* 1334–1339.

Nield, L. S., & Kamat, D. (2004). Enuresis: How to evaluate and treat. *Clinical Pediatrics, 43,* 409–415.

Pagana, K. D., & Pagana, T. J. (2006). *Mosby's manual of diagnostic and laboratory tests* (3rd ed.). St. Louis: Mosby.

Pulsifer, A. (2005). Pediatric GU examination: A clinician's reference. *Urologic Nursing, 25*(3), 163–168.

Razmus, I. S., Dalton, M. E., & Wilson, D. (2004). Pain management for newborn circumcision. *Pediatric Nursing, 30*(5), 414–427.

Robson, W. L. M., Leung, A. K. C., & Van Howe, R. (2005). Primary and secondary enuresis: Similarities in presentation. *Pediatrics, 115*(4), 956–959.

Roth, D. R., & Gonzales, E. T. (2006). Disorders of renal development and anomalies of the collecting system, bladder, penis, and scrotum. In J. A. McMillan (Ed.), *Oski's pediatrics: Principles and practice* (4th ed.). Philadelphia: Lippincott Williams & Wilkins.

Rusk, J. (2006). Proper diagnosis and treatment of UTIs in infants and young children outlined. *Infectious Diseases in Children, 19*(3), 79.

Serna, A., & Boedeker, E. (2008). Pathogenesis and treatment of shiga toxin-producing *Escherichia coli* infections. *Current Opinion in Gastroenterology, 24*(1), 38–47.

Silverstein, D. M. (2004). Enuresis in children: Diagnosis and management. *Clinical Pediatrics, 43*(3), 217–221.

Sparta, G., Kemper, M. J., Gerber, A. C., Goetschel, P., & Neuhaus, T. J. (2004). Latex allergy in children with urological malformation and chronic renal failure. *Journal of Urology, 171,* 1647–1659.

Super, E. A., Kemper, K. J., Woods, C., & Nagaraj, S. (2005). Cranberry use among pediatric nephrology patients. *Ambulatory Pediatrics, 5*(4), 249–252.

Taketokmo, C. K., Hodding, J. H., & Kraus, D. M. (2007). *Lexi-comp's pediatric dosage handbook* (14th ed.). Hudson, Ohio: Lexi-comp.

Thompson, M., Simon, S. D., Sharma, V., & Alon, U. S. (2005). Timing of follow-up voiding cystourethrogram in children with primary vesicoureteral reflux: Development and application of a clinical algorithm. *Pediatrics, 115*(2), 426–434.

Wald, E. R. (2006). Vesicoureteral reflux: The role of antibiotic prophylaxis. *Pediatrics, 117*(3), 919–922.

Zorzanello, M. M. (2004). Peritoneal dialysis and hemodialysis: Similarities and differences. *Nephrology Nursing Journal, 31*(5), 588–589.

WEBSITES

American Organ Transplant Association—helps patients obtain and sustain organ transplantation: aotaonline.org

National Kidney and Urologic Diseases Information Clearinghouse: kidney.niddk.nih.gov

American Association of Kidney Patients—information for kidney patients, resources for dialysis and transplant patients: www.aakp.org

American Academy of Nephrology: www.aan.com

American Kidney Fund—provides financial aid for kidney patients, summer camps for children: www.kidneyfund.org

American Nephrology Nurses Association—resources for nurses specializing in nephrology nursing: www.annanurse.org

American Society of Pediatric Nephrology: www.aspneph.com

American Urologic Association: www.auanet.org

Children's Organ Transplant Association—fundraising for children's transplants, promotion of organ and tissue donation: www.cota.org

Healthy People 2010: www.healthypeople.gov/default.htm

International Transplant Nurses Society: itns.org

National Kidney Foundation—resources for kidney patients: www.kidney.org

Nemours Foundation for Kids' Health (for kids and teens): www.kidshealth.org

A website made by children, for children about organ donation and transplantation: www.kidskare.org/

Organization for Transplant Professionals: www.natco1.org

Society of Urologic Nurses and Associates: www.suna.org

United Network for Organ Sharing—registry for donors and patients needing transplants: www.unos.org

Transplantation and donation: www.transweb.org

CHAPTER WORKSHEET

MULTIPLE CHOICE QUESTIONS

1. The nurse is performing patient education for the parents of an infant with bladder exstrophy. Which statement by the parents would indicate an understanding of the child's future care?

   a. "Care will be no different than that of any other infant."

   b. "My infant will only need this one surgery."

   c. "My child will wear diapers all his life."

   d. "We will need to care for the urinary diversion."

2. A 4-year-old girl presents with recurrent urinary tract infection. A prior workup did not reveal any urinary tract abnormalities. What is the priority nursing action?

   a. Obtain a sterile urine sample after completion of antibiotics.

   b. Teach appropriate toileting hygiene.

   c. Prepare the child for surgery to reimplant the ureters.

   d. Administer antibiotics intramuscularly.

3. A 5-year-old who had a renal transplant 9 months ago and has no history of chickenpox presents to the pediatric clinic for his vaccinations. Which is the most appropriate set to give?

   a. DTaP, IPV.

   b. DTaP, IPV, MMR, Varicella.

   c. DTaP, IPV, Varicella.

   d. IPV only.

4. When the nurse is caring for a child with hemolytic-uremic syndrome or acute glomerulonephritis and the child is not yet toilet trained, which action by the nurse would best determine fluid retention?

   a. Test urine for specific gravity.

   b. Weigh child daily.

   c. Weigh the wet diapers.

   d. Measure abdominal girth daily.

CRITICAL THINKING EXERCISES

1. Devise a meal plan for a 5-year-old child with a renal disorder that requires a 2-g sodium restriction per day. Keep in mind the child's developmental level and feeding idiosyncrasies at this age.

2. Develop a discharge teaching plan for a 3-year-old with nephrotic syndrome who will be taking corticosteroids long term.

3. Devise a developmental stimulation plan for an 11-month-old who has had significant urinary tract reconstruction surgery and is facing a prolonged period of confinement to the crib.

STUDY ACTIVITIES

1. In the clinical setting, compare the growth and development of two children the same age, one with chronic renal failure and one who has been healthy.

2. While caring for children in the clinical setting, compare and contrast the medical history, signs and symptoms of illness, and prescribed treatments for a child with nephrotic syndrome and one with acute glomerulonephritis.

3. Observe peritoneal dialysis in the hospital or hemodialysis in a hospital or outpatient center. Record observations about the children's psychosocial and developmental status.

CHAPTER 43

NURSING CARE OF THE CHILD WITH A NEUROMUSCULAR DISORDER

KEY TERMS

atrophy
clonus
contracture

dystrophy
hypertonicity
hypotonia

neurogenic
spasticity

LEARNING OBJECTIVES

Upon completion of the chapter, the learner will be able to:

1. Compare differences between the anatomy and physiology of the neuromuscular system in children versus adults.
2. Identify nursing interventions related to common laboratory and diagnostic tests used in the diagnosis and management of neuromuscular conditions.
3. Identify appropriate nursing assessments and interventions related to medications and treatments used for childhood neuromuscular conditions.
4. Distinguish various neuromuscular illnesses occurring in childhood.
5. Devise an individualized nursing care plan for the child with a neuromuscular disorder.
6. Develop patient/family teaching plans for the child with a neuromuscular disorder.
7. Describe the psychosocial impact of chronic neuromuscular disorders on the growth and development of children.

Frederick Stevens, 4 years old, seems to be falling often and has started to have difficulty climbing the stairs on his own. His mother states, "Recently he hasn't been able to keep up with his 6-year-old sister when we're playing at the park. He usually ends up sitting on the bench with me." She is concerned about the changes she has seen in her son.

Wow

Enhancing a child's abilities may enhance his or her strength to overcome anything.

A variety of neuromuscular disorders may affect children, but the result of each is muscular dysfunction. Some of the disorders result from a neurologic insult such as trauma or hypoxia to the brain or spinal cord. Others occur as a result of genetic dysfunction or structural abnormality. Still others may be autoimmune in nature, often following a simple viral infection. Many of the neuromuscular disorders are chronic, lasting the child's entire life and resulting in handicaps.

The nurse caring for a child with neuromuscular dysfunction plays an important role in the management of these disorders. Not only must the nurse provide direct intervention in response to health alterations that result, but the nurse is often part of the larger multidisciplinary team and may serve as the coordinator of many specialists or interventions. Understanding the most common responses to these disorders gives the nurse the foundation required to plan care for any child with any neuromuscular disorder.

Variations in Pediatric Anatomy and Physiology

Neuromuscular disorders in children may occur as a congenital malformation or a genetic disorder that is present from birth but may not be identified until later in childhood or adolescence. They may also result from trauma or hypoxia or develop following a viral illness. The neurologic and musculoskeletal systems in infants and children are immature compared with adults, placing them at increased risk for the development of a neuromuscular disorder.

Brain and Spinal Cord Development

Early in gestation, around 3 to 4 weeks, the neural tube of the embryo begins to differentiate into the brain and spinal cord. If the fetus suffers infection, trauma, malnutrition, or teratogen exposure during this critical period of growth and differentiation, brain or spinal cord development may be altered. Compared with the adult, the child's spine is very mobile, especially the cervical spine region, resulting in a higher risk for cervical spine injury. The premature infant's central nervous system is less mature than the term newborn's. Such immaturity in the preterm infant places him or her at a higher risk of central nervous insult within the neonatal period, which may result in delayed motor skill attainment or cerebral palsy.

Myelinization

Though development of the structures of the nervous system is complete at birth, myelinization is incomplete. Myelinization continues to progress and is complete by about 2 years of age. Myelinization proceeds in a cephalo-caudal and proximodistal fashion, allowing the infant to gain head and neck control before becoming able to control the trunk and the extremities. As myelinization proceeds, the speed and accuracy of nerve impulses increase.

Muscular Development

The muscular system, including tendons, ligaments, and cartilage, arises from the mesoderm in early embryonic development. At birth (term or preterm), the muscles, tendons, ligaments, and cartilage are all present and functional. The newborn infant is capable of spontaneous movement but lacks purposeful control. Full range of motion is present at birth. Healthy infants and children demonstrate normal muscle tone; hypertonia or **hypotonia** is an abnormal finding. Deep tendon reflexes are present at birth and are initially brisk in the newborn and progress to average over the first few months. Sluggish deep tendon reflexes indicate an abnormality. As the infant matures and becomes mobile, the muscles develop further and become stronger. The adolescent boy, in response to testosterone release, experiences a growth spurt, particularly in the trunk and legs, and develops bulkier muscles at that time.

Common Medical Treatments

A variety of medications as well as other medical treatments are used to treat neuromuscular disorders in children. Most of these treatments will require a physician's order when the child is in the hospital. The most common treatments and medications are listed in Common Medical Treatments 43.1 and Drug Guide 43.1. The nurse caring for the child with a neuromuscular disorder should become familiar with what these procedures are and how they work as well as common nursing implications related to use of these modalities.

NURSING PROCESS OVERVIEW FOR THE CHILD WITH A NEUROMUSCULAR DISORDER

Care of the child with a neuromuscular disorder includes assessment, nursing diagnosis, planning, interventions, and evaluation. There are a number of general concepts related to the nursing process that may be applied to neuromuscular dysfunction in children. From a general understanding of the care involved for a child with a neuromuscular disorder, the nurse can then individualize the care based on patient specifics.

Assessment

Assessment of neuromuscular dysfunction in children includes health history, physical examination, and laboratory and diagnostic testing.

COMMON MEDICAL TREATMENTS 43.1

Treatment	Explanation	Indication	Nursing Implications
Skeletal or cervical traction	Traction is used to immobilize the cervical spine. Halo traction will be applied in stable injuries and allows the patient greater mobility. Cervical traction is applied by a jacket-like apparatus, and the patient can get out of bed, use a wheelchair, and even ambulate.	To minimize or prevent trauma to the spinal cord	Monitor neurologic status closely. Assess for signs and symptoms of infection or impaired skin integrity. Provide appropriate pin site care.
Physical therapy, occupational therapy, or speech therapy	Physical therapy focuses on attainment or improvement of gross motor skills. Occupational therapy focuses on refinement of fine motor skills, feeding, and activities of daily living. Speech therapy is warranted for the child with a speech impairment or feeding difficulty related to oral muscular issues.	Cerebral palsy, spina bifida, spinal cord injury, muscular dystrophy, spinal muscular atrophy	Provide follow-through with prescribed exercises or supportive equipment. Success of therapy is dependent upon continued compliance with the prescribed regimen. Ensure that adequate communication exists within the interdisciplinary team.
Orthotics, braces	Adaptive positioning devices specially fitted for each child by the physical or occupational therapist or orthotist. Used to maintain proper body or extremity alignment, improve mobility, and prevent contractures.	Cerebral palsy, spinal cord injury, spina bifida, muscular dystrophy, spinal muscular atrophy	Provide frequent assessments of skin covered by the device to avoid skin breakdown. Follow the therapist's schedule of recommended "on" and "off" times. Encourage families to comply with use.

*R*emember Frederick, the 4-year-old who has been falling, having difficulty climbing stairs, and seems to tire easily when playing with his sister? What additional health history and physical examination assessment information should the nurse obtain?

Health History

The health history comprises past medical history, including the mother's pregnancy history, family history, and history of present illness (when the symptoms started and how they have progressed) as well as treatments used at home. The past medical history might be significant for prematurity, difficult birth, infection during pregnancy, changes in gait, falls, delayed development, or poor growth. Family history might be significant for neuromuscular disorders that are genetic. When eliciting the history of the present illness, inquire about the following:

• Changes in gait
• Recent trauma
• Poor feeding
• Lethargy

• Fever
• Weakness
• Alteration in muscle tone

Determine the child's history of attainment of developmental milestones. Note the age that milestones such as sitting, crawling, and walking were attained, and determine whether the pace of attainment of milestones has decreased. Some children may progress normally at first and then demonstrate decreased velocity of development of achievements or even loss of abilities. Obtain a clear description of weakness; is it fatigue, or is the child truly not as strong as he or she was in the past?

Physical Examination

Physical examination of the nervous and musculoskeletal systems consists of inspection, observation and palpation and should also include auscultation of the heart and lungs, as the function of these organs may be affected by certain neuromuscular conditions.

Inspection and Observation

Observe the infant or child playing with toys, crawling, or walking to obtain significant information about cranial

DRUG GUIDE 43.1 COMMON DRUGS FOR NEUROMUSCULAR DISORDERS

Medication	Action/Indications	Nursing Implications
Benzodiazepines (diazepam, lorazepam)	Anticonvulsant; enhance the inhibition of GABA Used adjunctively for relief of skeletal muscle spasm associated with cerebral palsy and paralysis resulting from spinal cord injury	Monitor sedation level. Assess for improvements in spasticity.
Baclofen (oral or intrathecal)	Central-acting skeletal muscle relaxant; precise mechanism unknown Used to treat painful spasms and decrease spasticity in children with motor neuron lesions, such as cerebral palsy and spinal cord injury	Assess motor function. Monitor for a decrease in spasticity. Observe for mental confusion, depression, or hallucinations. Dosage must be tapered before discontinuing because withdrawal symptoms may occur.
Corticosteroids	Anti-inflammatory and immunosuppressive action Duchenne muscular dystrophy, myasthenia gravis, dermatomyositis	Administer with food to decrease GI upset. May mask signs of infection. Do not stop treatment abruptly or acute adrenal insufficiency may occur. Monitor for Cushing syndrome. Dosage may be tapered over time.
Botulin toxin	Neurotoxin produced by *Clostridium botulinum* that blocks neuromuscular conduction Relief of spasticity in cerebral palsy, occasionally for torticollis	Injected into the muscle by an advanced provider. May cause dry mouth.

nerve, cerebellar, and motor function. Observe the child's general appearance, noting any asymmetry in muscle development. Lack of use of extremities leads to muscular **atrophy**, so a shortened limb may indicate chronic hemiparesis. Note symmetry of spontaneous movement of extremities as well as facial muscles. Determine cranial nerve function. Inspect the spine for cutaneous abnormalities such as dimples or hair tufts, which may be associated with spinal cord abnormalities. Observe the child's level of consciousness (LOC), noting decrease or significant changes. Note presence of lethargy. Refer to Chapter 38 for a complete description of evaluation of LOC.

Motor Function. Observe spontaneous activity, posture, and balance, and assess for asymmetrical movements. In the infant, observe resting posture, which will normally be a slightly flexed posture. The infant should be able to extend extremities to a normal stretch. Note position of comfort of the infant's or child's neck.

Reflexes. Note sluggish or brisk deep tendon reflexes. Note persistence of primitive reflexes in the older infant or child, such as Moro or tonic neck. Assess for development of protective reflexes, which is often delayed in infants with motor disorders.

Sensory Function. Alterations in sensory function accompany many neuromuscular disorders. Assess sensory function in a similar fashion to that used in the adult. The sensory functions of light touch, pain, vibration, heat, and cold are distinguishable by a child. In the infant, assess for response to light touch or pain. The usual response to pain will be withdrawal from the stimulus. Always prepare the child for the sensory examination in order to gain cooperation. The pinprick test may be particularly frightening, but most children will cooperate if educated appropriately.

Palpation

Assess muscle strength and tone in the infant or child. Compare strength and tone bilaterally. Evaluate neck tone by pulling the infant from a supine position to a sitting position (Fig. 43.1). By 4 to 5 months the infant should be able to maintain the head in a neutral position. Perform passive range of motion of the neck. Alterations in range of motion may indicate a neuromuscular disorder or torticollis. Note trunk tone in the infant by holding the infant under the axillae and palpating for trunk tone. The hypotonic infant will feel as though he or she is slipping through the examiner's hands. The hypertonic infant will feel rigid, extending the trunk and legs. Assess leg tone in the infant by placing the infant in the vertical position with the feet on a flat surface; the 4-month-old infant should be able to momentarily support his or her weight. Assess the strength of the infant or child by noting ability to move the muscles

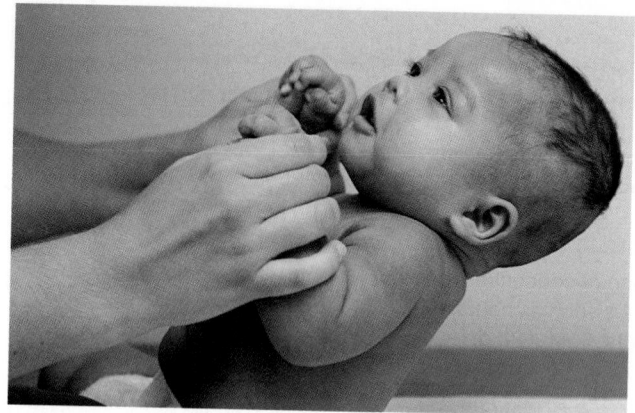

FIGURE 43.1 Assessing neck tone in an infant.

FIGURE 43.2 Assessing leg strength of the child.

against gravity (Fig. 43.2). Note any hypertonia or **spasticity**, which may be an early indication of cerebral palsy or other neuromuscular disorder.

▶ *Take NOTE!*

In cases of trauma or suspected trauma, do not perform any assessment that involves movement of the head and neck until cervical injury is ruled out. Maintain complete immobilization of the cervical spine until that time.

Auscultation

Auscultate the child's lungs; adventitious sounds are often present when respiratory muscle function is impaired.

Laboratory and Diagnostic Testing

Common Laboratory and Diagnostic Tests 43.1 offers an explanation of the laboratory and diagnostic tests most commonly used in neuromuscular disorders. The tests can assist the physician in diagnosing the disorder and/or be used as guidelines in determining ongoing treatment. Laboratory or non-nursing personnel perform some of

COMMON LABORATORY AND DIAGNOSTIC TESTS 43.1

Test	Explanation	Indication	Nursing Implications
Cervical spine x-rays	Radiographic image of the cervical spine	Detection of spinal fractures	In the trauma victim, the cervical spine should remain immobilized until cleared after cervical spine x-rays.
Fluoroscopy	Radiographic examination that uses continuous x-rays to show live, real-time images	Assessment of cervical spine instability during movement	Children may be afraid of the x-ray machine but will need to cooperate with flexion and extension of the neck. Allow a parent or family member to accompany the child.
Myelography	X-ray study of the spinal cord allowing visualization of the cord, nerve roots, and surrounding meninges	Detection of space-occupying lesions of the spinal cord; visualization of neural tube defects; evaluation of traumatic injury	Involves injection of contrast medium into the CSF via lumbar puncture. After procedure, keep head of bed elevated for several hours. Encourage hydration. Observe for signs of meningeal irritation.

(continued)

COMMON LABORATORY AND DIAGNOSTIC TESTS 43.1 (continued)

Test	Explanation	Indications	Nursing Implications
Ultrasound	Use of sound waves to locate the depth and structure within soft tissues and fluid	Assessment of spinal abnormalities	Better tolerated by nonsedated children than CT or MRI. Can be performed with a portable unit at bedside.
Computed tomography (CT)	Noninvasive x-ray study that looks at tissue density and structures. Images a "slice" of tissue.	Evaluation of congenital abnormalities such as neural tube defects, fractures, demyelinization, or inflammation	Machine is large and can be frightening to children. Procedure can be lengthy and child must remain still. If unable to do so, sedation may be necessary. If performed with contrast medium, assess for allergy. Encourage fluids after procedure if not contraindicated.
Magnetic resonance imaging (MRI)	Based on how hydrogen atoms behave in a magnetic field when disturbed by radiofrequency signals. Does not require ionizing radiation. Provides a 3D view of the body part being scanned.	Assessment of inflammation, congenital abnormalities such as neural tube defects	Remove all metal objects from the child. Child must remain motionless for entire scan; parent can stay in room with child. Younger children will require sedation in order to be still. A loud thumping sound occurs inside the machine during the procedure, which can be frightening to children.
Creatine kinase	Reflects muscle damage: it leaks from muscle into plasma as muscles deteriorate	Diagnosis of muscular dystrophy, spinal muscular atrophy	Draw sample before electromyogram or muscle biopsy, as those tests may lead to release of creatine kinase.
Electromyography	A recording electrode is placed in the skeletal muscle and electrical activity is recorded.	Differentiates muscular disorders from those that are neurologic in origin	Requires insertion of short needles into the muscles.
Nerve conduction velocity	Measures the speed of nerve conduction	Differentiation of muscular disorders	Feels like mild electric shocks
Muscle biopsy	Removal of a piece of muscular tissue either by needle or by open biopsy	Determination of type of muscular dystrophy or spinal muscular atrophy	Post-biopsy care is similar to that for other types of biopsy. Involves a small incision with one or two sutures.
Dystrophin	A normal intracellular plasma membrane protein in the muscle	Determination of specific type of muscular dystrophy	Absent in Duchenne muscular dystrophy, decreased in Becker muscular dystrophy
Genetic testing	Tests for presence of the gene for the disease or for carrier status	Determination of disease or carrier status of inherited muscular disorder	Entire family should be tested, even those unaffected, because carrier status should be determined and genetic counseling related to reproduction provided.

the tests, while the nurse might perform others. In either instance the nurse should be familiar with how the tests are performed, what they are used for, and normal versus abnormal results. This knowledge will also be necessary when providing patient and family education related to the testing.

Nursing Diagnoses, Goals, Interventions, and Evaluations

Upon completion of a thorough assessment, the nurse might identify several nursing diagnoses, including:

- Impaired physical mobility
- Imbalanced nutrition, less than body requirements
- Urinary retention
- Constipation
- Self-care deficit
- Risk for impaired skin integrity

- Chronic sorrow
- Risk for injury
- Deficient knowledge
- Family processes, interrupted

After completing an assessment of Fredrick, the nurse noted the following: he started walking at 2 years of age, he has difficulty jumping, his gait has a waddling appearance, and he does not rise from the floor in the usual fashion. Based on these assessment findings, what would your top three nursing diagnoses be for Fredrick?

Nursing goals, interventions, and evaluation for the child with neuromuscular dysfunction are based on the nursing diagnoses (see Nursing Care Plan Overview 43.1). The nursing care plan may be used as a guide in planning

(text continues on page 1428)

Nursing Care Plan 43.1

OVERVIEW FOR THE CHILD WITH A NEUROMUSCULAR DISORDER

NURSING DIAGNOSIS: Impaired physical mobility related to muscle weakness, hypertonicity, impaired coordination, loss of muscle function or control as evidenced by an inability to move extremities, to ambulate without assistance, to move without limitations

Outcome Identification and Evaluation
Child will be able to engage in activities within age parameters and limits of disease: *child is able to move extremities, move about environment, and participate in exercise programs within limits of age and disease.*

Intervention: Maximizing Physical Mobility
- Encourage gross and fine motor activities *to facilitate motor development.*
- Collaborate with physical therapy, occupational therapy, and speech therapy to strengthen muscles and promote optimal mobility *to facilitate motor development.*
- Use passive and active range-of-motion exercises and teach child and family how to perform them *to prevent contractures, facilitate joint mobility and muscle development (active ROM), and help increase mobility.*
- Praise accomplishments and emphasize child's abilities *to improve self-esteem and encourage feeling of confidence and competence.*

NURSING DIAGNOSIS: Nutrition, imbalanced, less than body requirements, related to difficulty feeding secondary to deficient sucking, swallowing, or chewing; difficulty assuming normal feeding position; inability to feed self as evidenced by decreased oral intake, impaired swallowing, weight loss or plateau.

Outcome Identification and Evaluation
Child will exhibit signs of adequate nutrition *as evidenced by appropriate weight gain, intake & output within normal limits, and adequate ingestion of calories.*

Intervention: Promoting Adequate Nutrition
- Monitor height and weight: *insufficient intake will lead to impaired growth and weight gain.*
- Monitor hydration status (moist mucous membranes, elastic skin turgor, adequate urine output): *insufficient intake can lead to dehydration.*

(continued)

Nursing Care Plan 43.1 (continued)

- Use techniques to promote caloric and nutritional intake and teach family about these techniques (e.g., positioning, modified utensils, soft or blended foods, allowing extra time) *to facilitate intake.*
- Assess respiratory system frequently *to assess for aspiration.*
- Assist family to help child assume as normal a feeding position as possible *to help increase oral intake.*

NURSING DIAGNOSIS: Urinary retention related to sensory motor impairment as evidenced by dribbling, inadequate bladder emptying

Outcome Identification and Evaluation
Child's bladder will empty adequately, *according to pre-established quantities and frequencies individualized for the child (usual urine output is 0.5 to 2 mL/kg/hour).*

Intervention: Promoting Successful Bladder Emptying
- Assess child's ability to empty bladder via history focused on character and duration of lower urinary symptoms *to establish baseline.*
- Assess for history of fecal impaction or constipation, *as alterations in bowel elimination may hinder urinary elimination.*
- Assess for bladder distention by palpation or urinary retention by post-void residual obtained via catheterization or bladder ultrasound *to determine extent of retention.*
- Maintain adequate hydration *to avoid irritating effects that dehydration has on the bladder.*
- Schedule voiding to *decrease bladder overdistention.*
- Teach the family (and the child if old enough) with significant urinary retention the technique of clean intermittent catheterization *to allow regular, complete bladder emptying.*

NURSING DIAGNOSIS: Risk for constipation related to immobility, loss of sensation

Outcome Identification and Evaluation
Child will demonstrate adequate stool passage, *will pass soft, formed stool every 1 to 3 days without straining or other adverse effects.*

Intervention: Promoting Appropriate Bowel Elimination
- Assess usual pattern of stooling *to determine baseline and identify potential problems with elimination.*
- Palpate for abdominal fullness and auscultate for bowel sounds *to assess for bowel function and presence of constipation.*
- Encourage fiber intake *to increase frequency of stools.*
- Ensure adequate fluid intake *to prevent formation of hard, dry stools.*
- Encourage activity within child's limits or restrictions: *even minimal activity increases peristalsis.*
- Administer medications or enemas as ordered *to promote bowel training/evacuation (especially in child with myelomeningocele or spinal cord injury).*

NURSING DIAGNOSIS: Self-care deficit related to neuromuscular impairments, cognitive deficits as evidenced by an inability to perform hygiene care and transfer self independently

Outcome Identification and Evaluation
Child will demonstrate ability to care for self within age parameters and limits of disease: *Child is able to feed, dress, manage elimination within limits of disease and age.*

Intervention: Maximizing Self-Care
- Introduce child and family to self-help methods as soon as possible *to promote independence from the beginning.*
- Encourage family and staff to allow child to do as much as possible *to allow child to gain confidence and independence.*
- Teach specific measures for bowel and urinary elimination as needed *to promote independence and increase self-care abilities and self-esteem.*
- Collaborate with physical therapy, occupational therapy, and speech therapy to provide child and family with appropriate tools to modify environment and methods to promote transferring and self-care *to allow for maximum functioning.*
- Praise accomplishments and emphasize child's abilities *to improve self-esteem and encourage feelings of confidence and competence.*
- Balance activity with periods of rest *to reduce fatigue and increase energy for self-care.*

Nursing Care Plan 43.1 (continued)

NURSING DIAGNOSIS: Risk for impaired skin integrity related to immobility, use of braces or adaptive devices

Outcome Identification and Evaluation
Child's skin will remain intact, *without evidence of redness or breakdown.*

Intervention: Promoting Skin Integrity
- Monitor condition of entire skin surface at least daily *to provide baseline and allow for early identification of areas at risk.*
- Avoid excessive friction or harsh cleaning products *that may increase risk of breakdown in child with susceptible skin.*
- Keep child's skin free from stool and urine *to decrease risk of breakdown.*
- Change child's position frequently *to decrease pressure to susceptible areas.*
- Monitor skin condition affected by braces or adaptive equipment frequently *to prevent skin breakdown related to poor fit.*

NURSING DIAGNOSIS: Chronic sorrow related to presence of chronic disability as evidenced by child's or family's expression of sadness, anger, disappointment, or feeling overwhelmed

Outcome Identification and Evaluation
Child and/or family will accept situation; *child/family will appropriately identify feelings, function at a normal developmental level, and plan for the future.*

Intervention: Easing Sorrow
- Assess degree of sorrow *to provide baseline for intervention.*
- Identify problems with eating or sleeping, *often affected when grief or sorrow is present.*
- Spend time with the child and family; *an empathetic presence is valued by suffering families.*
- Encourage the use of positive coping techniques; *taking action, expressing feelings, intentional attempts at coping are helpful techniques.*
- Refer for spiritual counseling as desired; *many families experience grief resolution in a more timely fashion if spiritual needs are addressed.*

NURSING DIAGNOSIS: Risk for injury related to muscle weakness

Outcome Identification and Evaluation
Child will remain free from injury; *child will not fall or experience other injury.*

Intervention: Preventing Injury
- Ensure that side rails of bed are elevated when caregiver is not directly at bedside *to prevent fall from bed.*
- Use appropriate safety restraints with adaptive equipment and wheelchairs *to prevent fall or slipping from equipment.*
- Do not leave child unattended in tub *as weakness may cause the child to slip under the water.*
- Avoid restraint use if at all possible; *close observation is more appropriate.*

NURSING DIAGNOSIS: Deficient knowledge related to lack of information regarding complex medical condition, prognosis, and medical needs as evidenced by verbalization, questions, or actions demonstrating lack of understanding regarding child's condition or care

Outcome Identification and Evaluation
Child and family will verbalize accurate information and understanding about condition, prognosis, and medical needs: *Child and family demonstrate knowledge of condition and prognosis and medical needs, including possible causes, contributing factors, and treatment measures.*

Intervention: Providing Patient and Family Teaching
- Assess child's and family's willingness to learn: *Child and family must be willing to learn for teaching to be effective.*
- Provide family with time to adjust to diagnosis *to facilitate adjustment and ability to learn and participate in child's care.*
- Repeat information *to allow family and child time to learn and understand.*
- Teach in short sessions: *many short sessions are more helpful than one long session.*

(continued)

Nursing Care Plan 43.1 (continued)

- Gear teaching to the level of understanding of the child and family (depends on age of child, physical condition, memory) *to ensure understanding.*
- Provide reinforcement and rewards *to facilitate the teaching/learning process.*
- Use multiple modes of learning involving many senses (provide written, verbal, demonstration and videos) when possible: *child and family are more likely to retain information when it is presented in different ways using many senses.*

NURSING DIAGNOSIS: Family processes, interrupted, related to child's illness, hospitalization, diagnosis of chronic illness in child, and potential long-term effects of illness as evidenced by family's presence in hospital, missed work, demonstration of inadequate coping

Outcome Identification and Evaluation
Family will maintain functional system of support, demonstrate adequate coping, adaptation of roles: *Parents are involved in child's care, ask appropriate questions, express fears and concerns, and are able to discuss child's care and condition calmly.*

Intervention: Promoting Appropriate Family Functioning
- Encourage parents and family to verbalize concerns related to child's illness, diagnosis, and prognosis: *allows the nurse to identify concerns and areas where further education may be needed; demonstrates family-centered care.*
- Explain therapies, procedures, child's behaviors, and plan of care to parents: *understanding of the child's current status and plan of care helps decrease anxiety.*
- Encourage parental involvement in care *to allow parents to feel needed and valued and to have a sense of control over their child's health.*
- Identify support system for family and child: *support system is often needed by stressed families to assist with coping.*
- Educate family and child on additional resources available *to help them develop a wide base of support.*

---

nursing care for the child with a neuromuscular disorder. The care plan includes many nursing diagnoses that are applicable to the child or adolescent. Children's responses to neuromuscular dysfunction and its treatment will vary, and nursing care should be individualized based on the child's and family's responses to illness; see Healthy People 2010. Additional information about nursing management will be included later in the chapter as it relates to specific disorders.

Internet resources for families of children with disabilities include:

- www.acf.hhs.gov/programs/add: Administration on Developmental Disabilities, Department of Health and Human Services
- www.childrensdisabilities.info: Children's Disabilities Information
- www.childrensdefense.org: Children's Defense Fund
- www.familiesusa.org: Families USA
- www.irsc.org: Internet Resources for Special Children
- www.nichcy.org: National Information Center for Children and Youth with Disabilities

Based on your top three nursing diagnoses for Fredrick, describe appropriate nursing interventions.

HEALTHY PEOPLE 2010

Objective	Significance
Increase the proportion of children with special health needs who have access to a medical home.	• Educate the family that specialist care (though often consisting of frequent and multiple visits) does not replace primary care through the medical home. • Encourage families to find a primary care pediatrician with whom they feel comfortable for well-child check-ups and routine childhood illnesses.

Congenital Neuromuscular Disorders

Several disorders with neuromuscular effects are congenital in nature. These include the neural tube defects and genetic neuromuscular disorders. The structural disorders are spina bifida occulta, meningocele, and myelomeningocele (neural tube defects). The genetic neuromuscular disorders include the various types of muscular dystrophy and spinal muscular atrophy. These disorders are not always recognized at birth, as signs and symptoms are not evident until months or even years after birth, but they are still considered to be congenital as they have a genetic basis.

NEURAL TUBE DEFECTS

Neural tube defects account for the majority of congenital anomalies of the central nervous system. The neural tube closes between the third and fourth week of gestation. The cause of neural tube defects is not known, but many factors, such as drugs, malnutrition, chemicals, and genetics, can hinder normal central nervous system development. Strong evidence exists that supplementation of folic acid by the mother before conception decreases the incidence of neural tube defects in pregnancies at risk by 50% (Kliegman et al., 2007). In 1992 the U.S. Public Health Service recommended that all women of childbearing age who are capable of becoming pregnant take 0.4 mg of folic acid daily (CDC, 2007). According to the Centers for Disease Control and Prevention (CDC), the number of pregnancies affected by neural tube defects decreased from 4,000 in 1995–1996 to 3,000 in 1999–2000 (Merereau et al., 2004). Prenatal screening of maternal serum for alpha-fetoprotein (AFP) and ultrasound at 16 to 18 weeks of gestation can help identify fetuses at risk. Neural tube defects primarily affecting spinal cord development include spina bifida occulta, meningocele, and myelomeningocele (Fig. 23.3). Neural tube defects primarily affecting brain development are discussed in Chapter 38.

Spina Bifida Occulta

Spina bifida is a term that is often used to refer to all neural tube disorders that affect the spinal cord. This can be confusing and a cause of concern for parents. There are well-defined degrees of spinal cord involvement, and use of the correct terminology is important for health care professionals.

Spina bifida occulta is a defect of the vertebral bodies without protrusion of the spinal cord or meninges. This defect is not visible externally and in most cases has no adverse affects (see Fig. 43.3). Spina bifida occulta is a common anomaly: it is estimated that it affects one fifth of the population (Spina Bifida Association, 2006). Children with spina bifida occulta need no immediate medical intervention. Complications may include tethered cord, syringomyelia, or diastematomyelia.

Nursing Assessment

In most cases, spina bifida occulta is benign and asymptomatic and produces no neurologic signs; it may be considered a normal variant. The defect, which is usually present in the lumbosacral area, often goes undetected. However, there may be noticeable dimpling, abnormal patches of hair, or discoloration of skin at the defect site. If so, further investigation, including magnetic resonance imaging (MRI), may be warranted.

Nursing Management

Nursing care will focus on educating the family. Inform parents of its presence and what the diagnosis means. Many times parents will confuse this diagnosis with spina bifida cystica, a much more serious defect. Occasionally, children with spina bifida occulta eventually need surgical intervention due to degenerative changes or involvement of the spine and nerve roots resulting in complications such as tethered cord, syringomyelia, or diastematomyelia. When these associated problems occur, the condition is often termed "occult spinal dysraphism" to avoid confusion.

Meningocele

Meningocele, the less serious form of spina bifida cystica, occurs when the meninges herniate through a defect in

FIGURE 43.3 (**A**) Normal spine. (**B**) Spina bifida occulta. (**C**) Meningocele. (**D**) Myelomeningocele

A

B

C

D

the vertebrae. The spinal cord is usually normal and there are typically no associated neurologic deficits. Treatment for meningocele involves surgical correction of the lesion (see Fig. 43.3).

Nursing Assessment

Initial assessment after delivery will reveal a visible external sac protruding from the spinal area. It is most often seen in the lumbar region but can be anywhere along the spinal canal. Most are covered with skin and pose no threat to the patient. However, assessment to ensure that the sac covering is intact remains important. Assess neurologic status carefully: most children will be asymptomatic, with no neurologic deficits. Before surgical correction the infant will be thoroughly examined to determine whether there is any neural involvement or associated anomalies. Diagnostic procedures such as computed tomography (CT), MRI, and ultrasound may be performed.

Nursing Management

If the skin covering the sac is intact, surgical correction may be delayed. However, as in a child with myelomeningocele, immediately report any evidence of leaking cerebrospinal fluid (CSF) to ensure prompt intervention to prevent infection. Nursing management will be supportive. Provide preoperative and postoperative care similar to the child with myelomeningocele to prevent rupture of the sac, to prevent infection, and to provide adequate nutrition and hydration. Monitor for symptoms of constipation or bladder dysfunction that may result due to increasing size of the lesion. Resulting hydrocephalus has been associated with some cases of meningocele; therefore, monitor head circumference and watch for signs and symptoms of increased intracranial pressure (ICP).

Myelomeningocele

Myelomeningocele, the most severe form of neural tube defect, occurs in approximately 1 in 4,000 live births (Kliegman et al., 2007). Myelomeningocele is a type of spina bifida cystica, and clinically the term "spina bifida" is often used to refer to myelomeningocele. It may be diagnosed *in utero* via ultrasound; otherwise it is visually obvious at birth. The newborn with myelomeningocele is at increased risk for meningitis, hypoxia, and hemorrhage.

In myelomeningocele, the spinal cord often ends at the point of the defect, resulting in absent motor and sensory function beyond that point (see Fig. 43.3). Therefore, the long-term complications of paralysis, orthopedic deformities, and bladder and bowel incontinence are often seen in children with myelomeningocele. The presence of **neurogenic** bladder and frequent catheterization puts the child at an increased risk for urinary tract infections, pyelonephritis, and hydronephrosis, which may result in long-term renal damage if managed inappropriately. Accompanying hydrocephalus associated with type II Chiari

defect is seen in 80% of patients with myelomeningocele (Kliegman et al., 2007). Due to the improper development and the downward displacement of the brain into the cervical spine, CSF flow is blocked, resulting in hydrocephalus. The lower the deformity is on the spine, the lower the risk of developing hydrocephalus.

These children usually require multiple surgical procedures and due to frequent catheterizations are at an increased risk of developing a latex allergy. Learning problems and seizures are more common in these children than in the general population, but 70% of those with myelomeningocele have normal intelligence (Kliegman et al., 2007). Ambulation is possible for some children, depending on the level of the lesion. Due to advances in medical treatment the life expectancy of children with this disorder has increased. For children born with a myelomeningocele who receive aggressive treatment, the mortality rate is 10% to 15%; most deaths occur before the age of 4 years old (Kliegman et al., 2007).

Pathophysiology

The cause of myelomeningocele is unknown, but risk factors are consistent with other neural tube defects, such as maternal drug use, malnutrition, and a genetic predisposition. In myelomeningocele, the neural tube fails to close at the end of the fourth week of gestation. As a result, an external sac-like protrusion that encases the meninges, spinal fluid, and in some cases nerves is present on the spine (see Fig. 43.3). A myelomeningocele can be located anywhere along the spinal cord, but 75% are located in the lumbosacral region (Kliegman et al., 2007). The degree of neurologic deficit will depend on the location. An increase in neurologic deficit is seen as the myelomeningocele extends into the thoracic region.

Therapeutic Management

Surgical closure will be performed as soon as possible after birth, especially if a CSF leak is present or if there is a danger of the sac rupturing. The goal of early surgical intervention is to prevent infection and to minimize further loss of function, which can result from the stretching of nerve roots as the meningeal sac expands after birth. A new option is becoming available but remains experimental. *In utero* fetal surgery to repair the myelomeningocele has been performed in the United States. The benefits and risks remain uncertain at this time. Ongoing management of this disorder remains complex; a multidisciplinary approach is needed, involving specialists in neurology, neurosurgery, urology, orthopedics, therapy, and rehabilitation along with intense nursing care. The chronic nature of this disorder necessitates lifelong follow-up.

Nursing Assessment

For a full description of the assessment phase of the nursing process, refer to page 1420. Assessment findings pertinent to myelomeningocele are discussed below.

Health History

High-risk deliveries should be identified. Explore the pregnancy history and past medical history for risk factors such as:

- Lack of prenatal care
- Lack of preconception and/or prenatal folic acid supplementation
- Previous child born with neural tube defect or family history of neural tube defects
- Maternal consumption of certain drugs that antagonize folic acid, such as anticonvulsants (carbamazepine and phenobarbital)

The older infant or child with a history of myelomeningocele requires numerous surgical procedures and lifelong follow-up. In an infant or child returning for a clinic visit or hospitalization, the health history should include questions related to:

- Current mobility status and any changes in motor abilities
- Genitourinary function and regimen
- Bowel function and regimen
- Signs or symptoms of urinary infections
- History of hydrocephalus with presence of shunt
- Signs or symptoms of shunt infection or malfunction (refer to section on hydrocephalus)
- Latex sensitivity
- Nutritional status, including changes in weight
- Any other changes in physical or cognitive state
- Resources available and used by the family

Physical Examination

Initial assessment after delivery will reveal a visible external sac protruding from the spinal area (Fig. 43.4). Observe the baby's general appearance and assess whether the sac covering is intact. Assess neurologic status and look for associated anomalies. Assess for movement of extremities and anal reflex, which will help determine the level of neurologic involvement. Flaccid paralysis, absence of deep tendon reflexes, lack of response to touch and pain stimuli, skeletal abnormalities such as club feet, constant dribbling of urine, and a relaxed anal sphincter may be found.

In the older infant or child, perform a thorough physical examination and focus on the functional assessment. Note level of paralysis or paresthesia. Inspect skin for breakdown. Determine the child's motor capabilities.

Laboratory and Diagnostic Tests

A myelomeningocele may be detected prenatally around 16 to 18 of weeks' gestation by ultrasound, by a blood test that detects AFP increases, or by analysis of amniotic fluid for AFP increases. Common laboratory and diagnostic studies ordered for the assessment of myelomeningocele include:

- MRI
- CT
- Ultrasound
- Myelography

These diagnostic tests are used to evaluate brain and spinal cord involvement (refer to Common Laboratory and Diagnostic Tests 43.1).

Nursing Management

Initial nursing management of the child with myelomeningocele involves preventing trauma to the meningeal sac and preventing infection before surgical repair of the defect. Refer to the Nursing Care Plan Overview in this chapter. Additional considerations are reviewed below.

Preventing Infection

Risk for infection related to the presence of the meningeal sac and potential for rupture is a central nursing concern in the newborn with myelomeningocele. Until surgical intervention occurs, the goal is to prevent rupture or leakage of CSF from the sac. Keeping the sac from drying out is important, as well as preventing trauma or pressure on the sac. Use sterile saline-soaked non-adhesive gauze or antibiotic-soaked gauze to keep the sac moist. Immediately report any seepage of clear fluid from the lesion, as this could indicate an opening in the sac and provide a portal of entry for microorganisms. Position the infant in the prone position or supported on the side to avoid pressure on the sac. To keep the infant warm, place the infant in a warmer or Isolette to avoid the use of blankets, which could exert too much pressure on the sac. Pay special attention while the infant is in a warmer or Isolette because the radiant heat can cause drying and cracking of the sac.

Keep the lesion free of feces and urine to help avoid infection. Position the infant so that urine and feces flow away from the sac (e.g., prone position, or place a folded towel under the abdomen) to help prevent infection. Placing a piece of plastic wrap below the meningocele is another way of preventing feces from coming into contact with the

FIGURE 43.4 Usually a sac covers the deformity of myelomeningocele and is visible at birth.

lesion. After surgery, position the infant in the prone or side-lying position to allow the incision to heal. Continue with precautions to prevent urine or feces from coming into contact with the incision.

Promoting Urinary Elimination

Children with myelomeningocele often have bladder incontinence, though some children may achieve normal urinary continence. The level of the lesion will influence the amount of dysfunction. Myelomeningocele remains one of the most common causes of neurogenic bladder in children. Therefore, evaluation of renal function by a pediatric urologist should be performed on each child with myelomeningocele.

Neurogenic bladder refers to the failure of the bladder to either store urine or empty itself of urine. Children with neurogenic bladder have loss of control over voiding. The spastic type of neurogenic bladder is hyperreflexive and yields frequent release of urine, but with incomplete emptying. The hypotonic neurogenic bladder is flaccid and weak and becomes stretched out; it can hold very large amounts of urine, resulting in continuous dribbling of urine from the urethra. Urinary stasis and retention occur in both types, placing the child at risk for urinary tract infection as well as reflux of bladder contents back up into the ureters and kidneys, resulting in renal scarring and insufficiency.

The goals of neurogenic bladder management are to promote optimal urinary continence and prevent renal complications. Interventions for neurogenic bladder include clean intermittent catheterization to promote bladder emptying; medications such as oxybutynin chloride (Ditropan) to improve bladder capacity; prompt recognition and treatment of infections; and in some children

surgical interventions such as a continent urinary reservoir or vesicostomy to facilitate urinary elimination. Clean intermittent catheterization is addressed below. In the child with a spastic or rigid bladder, teach parents how to administer antispasmodic medications such as oxybutynin. Teach the parents that the medication is used to increase the bladder capacity and reduce the potential for reflux. Refer to Chapter 42 for additional information on nursing care related to the surgical procedures.

Assessing Urinary Function

Determine the child's pattern and success of toilet training, both for bladder and bowel. Assess the child's cognitive/developmental level. Observe the genital area for dribbling of urine from the urethra, noting odor of urine if present. Note redness of the urethra or excoriation in the diaper area. Inspect the abdomen for scars from prior surgeries and the presence of urinary diversion or continent stoma. Palpate the abdomen for presence of distended bladder, fecal mass, or enlarged kidneys. Determine the child's level of paralysis or paresthesia.

Clean Intermittent Catheterization

Depending on the level of paralysis at birth in the child with myelomeningocele, clean intermittent catheterization may be started at that time. In other children with spina bifida and in children who suffer spinal cord injury, catheterization may be started at a later age. Teach parents the technique of clean intermittent catheterization via the urethra, unless a urinary diversion or continent stoma has been created (Teaching Guidelines 43.1).

Teaching the parents the techniques of clean intermittent catheterization is an important step in preserving renal functioning, preventing infection and helping the family gain some control over the child's physical condition. Until

EVIDENCE-BASED PRACTICE 43.1
Self-Intermittent Catheterization Among Female Children With Myelomeningocele and the Potential for Increased Complications

● **Study**
The authors reviewed the medical records of 31 females with myelomeningocele followed from the start of clean intermittent catheterization (CIC). Between all subjects, CIC was used for 459 patient-years. In all cases, the girls used noncoated polyvinyl chloride catheters.

▲ **Findings**
Over the total 459 patient-years, 13 patients experienced a total of 20 episodes of complications among them. These included hematuria, urethral polyps, and difficulties in

catheterization. Complications were increased if assisted CIC was used or if a smaller bore catheter was utilized.

■ **Nursing Implications**
There are few complications occurring in females with myelomeningocele who self-catheterize using clean technique. Encourage the use of large-size noncoated polyvinyl catheters. Teach females when developmentally capable to perform self CIC. This function is safe and yields greater independence in this special population.

Source: Lindehall, B., Abrahamsson, K., Jodal, U., Olsson, I., & Sillen, U. (2007). Complications of clean intermittent catheterization in young females with myelomeningocele: 10 to 19 years of followup. *Journal of Urology, 178*(3), 1053–1055.

TEACHING GUIDELINES 43.1

Clean Intermittent Catheterization

- Wash hands with soap and water.
- Apply water-based lubricant to catheter.
- Perform catheterization. Insert catheter only as far as needed to obtain urine flow.
- Wash reusable catheter after use with soapy water; rinse and allow to dry.
- When dry, store in zip-top plastic bag or other clean storage container.
- Weekly, soak the catheter in a 1:1 vinegar and water solution, rinsing well before next use.
- When developmentally ready, teach the child to self-catheterize.

▶ *Take* NOTE!

Use only latex-free catheters and gloves for catheterization of children with myelomeningocele and/or neurogenic bladder, as these children exhibit a high incidence of latex allergy.

Promoting Adequate Nutrition

The risk for altered nutrition, less than body requirements, related to the restrictions on positioning of the infant before and after surgery is another nursing concern. Assist the family in assuming as normal a feeding position as possible. Preoperatively, the risk of rupture may be too high to warrant holding. Therefore, the infant's head can be turned to the side or the infant can be placed in the side-lying position to facilitate feeding. If the infant is held, special care needs to be taken to avoid pressure on the sac or postoperative incision. Encourage the parents to interact as much as possible with the infant by talking to and touching the infant during feeding to help promote intake. If the mother was planning on breastfeeding the infant, assist her in meeting this goal, if possible. If the infant can be held, encourage her to do this, or assist her in pumping and saving breast milk to be given to the infant via bottle until the infant is able to be held. Feeding an infant in an unusual position can be difficult, and it is the nurse's role to provide support, education, and modeling for the parents and family when needed.

the child is able to self-catheterize, the parents will be responsible for this procedure. Children with normal intelligence and upper extremity motor skills usually learn to self-catheterize at the age of 6 years. Urinary incontinence is associated with poor self-esteem, particularly as the child gets older. Educating the child to self-catheterize the urethra or stoma as appropriate empowers the child, gives him or her a sense of control, and allows for appropriate urinary elimination when the child is away from the parents (e.g., at school).

Offer support and appropriate referrals to the child and family. Refer families to vendors in the local area for catheterization supplies.

▶ *Take* NOTE!

Over time, bacterial colonization of the bladder may occur; however, antibiotic prophylaxis is not recommended for these children because of the increased risk for development of antibiotic resistance.

Promoting Bowel Elimination

Children with myelomeningocele often have bowel incontinence as well; the level of the lesion affects the amount of dysfunction. Many children with myelomeningocele can achieve some degree of bowel continence. Bowel training with the use of timed enemas or suppositories along with diet modifications can allow for defecation at predetermined times once or twice a day. Although bowel incontinence can be difficult for children as they grow older due to social concerns and self-esteem and body image disturbances, it does not pose the same health risks as urinary incontinence.

Preventing Latex Allergic Reaction

Sensitivity to latex or natural rubber is very common among children with myelomeningocele. They are at an increased risk of developing an allergy to latex related to the multiple exposures to latex products during surgical procedures and bladder catheterizations. Research has shown that at least 70% of children who require repeat surgeries due to spina bifida are sensitive to latex (Noble, 2005). A latex-free environment should be created for all procedures performed on children with myelomeningocele to prevent latex allergy. Therefore, children at high risk for or with a known latex allergy must be identified and managed in a latex-free environment. Ensure that these children do not come into direct contact with latex or equipment and supplies that contain latex. Be familiar with those products and equipment at your facility that contain latex and those that are latex-free. The Food and Drug Administration now requires that all medical supplies be labeled if they contain latex, but this is not the case for consumer products. Many resources exist that list products that are latex-free, and each hospital should have such a list readily available to health care professionals. For an updated list of latex-containing products and other helpful information for parents regarding consumer products, contact the Spina Bifida Association of America (www.sbaa.org; 4590 MacArthur Blvd. NW, Suite 250, Washington D.C. 20007; 1-800-621-3141 or 202-944-3295).

Children who are at a high risk for latex sensitivity should wear medical alert identification. Education programs regarding latex sensitivity and ways to prevent it need to be directed at those who care for high-risk children, including teachers, school nurses, relatives, babysitters, and all health care professionals.

Maintaining Skin Integrity

Address the risk for altered skin integrity related to the infant's prone position and impaired mobility. The prone position puts constant pressure on the knees and elbows, and it may be difficult to keep the infant clean of urine and feces. Diapering may be contraindicated preoperatively to avoid pressure on the sac. Therefore, ensure that the infant is kept as clean and dry as possible. This is made more difficult by the constant dribbling of stool and urine that may be present. Placing a pad beneath the diaper area and changing it frequently is important. Perform meticulous skin care. Place the infant on a special care mattress and place synthetic sheepskin under the infant to help reduce friction. Special attention to the infant's legs needs to occur when positioning them, since paralysis may be present. Using a folded diaper between the legs can help reduce pressure and friction from the legs rubbing together.

Educating and Supporting the Child and Family

Myelomeningocele is a serious disorder that affects multiple body systems and produces varying degrees of deficits. It is a disorder that has lifelong effects. Thanks to medical advances and technology most children born with myelomeningocele can expect to live a normal life, but challenges remain for the family and child as they learn to cope and live with this physical condition. Adjusting to the demands this condition places on the child and family is difficult. Parents may need time to accept their infant's condition, but as soon as possible they should be involved in the infant's care.

Teaching should begin immediately in the hospital. Teaching should include positioning, preventing infection, feeding, promoting urinary elimination through clean intermittent catheterization, preventing latex allergy, and the signs and symptoms of complications like increased ICP. Due to the chronic nature of this condition, long-term planning needs to begin in the hospital. These children usually require multiple surgical procedures and hospitalizations, and this can place stress on the family and their finances. The nurse has an important role in providing ongoing education about the illness and its treatments and the plan of care. As the family becomes more comfortable with the condition, they will become the experts in the child's care. Respect and recognize the family's changing needs. Providing intense daily care can take its toll on a family, and continual support and en-

couragement are needed. Referral to the Spina Bifida Association and a local support group for families of children with myelomeningocele is appropriate. See Healthy People 2010.

▶ **Consider THIS!**

A newborn has an obvious defect on his spine. Upon assessment, the nurse notes flaccid extremities and a distended bladder. The parents are devastated.

Identify additional assessments the nurse should make.

Describe nursing care for this neonate.

What teaching will the nurse do with this infant's family?

MUSCULAR DYSTROPHY

Muscular **dystrophy** refers to a group of inherited conditions that result in progressive muscle weakness and wasting. The muscles affected are primarily the skeletal (voluntary) muscles. Nine types of muscular dystrophy exist. All include muscle weakness over the lifetime; it is progressive in all cases but more severe in others. The various muscular dystrophies are most often diagnosed in childhood and affect a variety of muscle groups. The inheritance pattern for muscular dystrophy differs for each type but may be X-linked, autosomal dominant, or recessive. The genetic mutation in muscular dystrophy results in absence or decrease of a specific muscle protein that prevents normal function of the muscle. The skeletal muscle fibers are affected, yet there are no structural abnormalities in the spinal cord or the peripheral nerves. Table 43.1 gives specifics related to the various types of muscular dystrophy.

Duchenne muscular dystrophy, the most common neuromuscular disorder of childhood, is universally fatal (usually by the teens or twenties). The incidence is about 1 in 3,500 live male births (Balaban et al., 2005). For these reasons, this discussion will focus on Duchenne muscular dystrophy.

HEALTHY PEOPLE 2010

Objective	Significance
Increase the proportion of children and youth with disabilities who spend at least 80% of their time in regular education programs.	• Become familiar with local schools' offerings and capabilities so that you can refer families to an educational site appropriate for their child.

TABLE 43.1 **Types of Muscular Dystrophy**

Type	Onset	Inheritance	Muscle Involvement
Duchenne (pseudohypertrophic)	Early childhood	X-linked recessive	Generalized weakness, muscle wasting (limb and trunk first)
Becker	Adolescence or adulthood	X-linked recessive	Similar but less severe than Duchenne
Congenital	At birth	Autosomal dominant or recessive	Generalized muscular weakness, possible joint deformities
Emery-Dreifuss	Childhood to early teens	X-linked recessive	Weakness, wasting of shoulder, upper arm, and shin muscles
Limb-girdle	Childhood to middle age	Autosomal or X-linked recessive	Weakness, wasting of shoulder and pelvic girdles first
Facioscapulohumeral	Childhood to early adulthood	Autosomal dominant	Facial muscles weaken first, then shoulders and upper arms
Myotonic	Childhood to middle age	Autosomal dominant	Generalized weakness, wasting of face, feet, hands, and neck first Delayed relaxation of muscles after contraction
Oculopharyngeal	Early adulthood to middle age	Autosomal dominant	Affects muscles of eyelid and throat first
Distal	40 to 60 years of age	Autosomal dominant	Weakness, wasting of hand, forearm, lower leg muscles

Data from www.mda.org

Pathophysiology

The gene mutation in Duchenne muscular dystrophy results in the absence of dystrophin, a protein that is critical for maintenance of muscle cells. The gene is X-linked recessive, meaning that mainly boys are affected and they receive the gene from their mothers (women are carriers but have no symptoms). Absence of dystrophin leads to generalized weakness of voluntary muscles, and the weakness progresses over time. The hips, thighs, pelvis, and shoulders are affected initially; as the disease progresses, all voluntary muscles as well as cardiac and respiratory muscles are affected. Rarely, males with Duchenne muscular dystrophy may survive beyond the early 30s (Muscular Dystrophy Association, 2006b).

Boys with Duchenne muscular dystrophy are often late in learning to walk. As toddlers, they may display pseudohypertrophy (enlarged appearance) of the calves. During the preschool years they fall often and are quite clumsy. The affected child has difficulty climbing stairs and running and cannot get up from the floor in the usual fashion. The school-age child walks on the toes or balls of the feet with a rolling or waddling gait. Balance is disturbed significantly, and the child's belly may stick out when the shoulders are pulled back to stay upright and keep from falling over. During the school-age years it also becomes difficult for the child to raise his or her arms. Sometime between the ages of 7 and 12 years nearly all boys with Duchenne muscular dystrophy lose the ability to ambulate, and by the teen years any activity of the arms, legs, or trunk requires assistance or support. Most boys with Duchenne muscular dystrophy have normal intelligence, but many may exhibit a specific learning disability (Cotton et al., 2005).

Therapeutic Management

Though there is no cure for Duchenne muscular dystrophy, the use of corticosteroids may slow the progression of the disease. It is thought that prednisone helps by protecting muscle fibers from damage to the sarcolemma (defective in the absence of dystrophin). Numerous studies have shown that boys treated with prednisone demonstrate improved strength and function. The side effects of corticosteroids are many, including weight gain, osteoporosis, and mood changes (Palmieria & Sblendorio, 2007). Calcium supplements are prescribed to prevent osteoporosis, and antidepressants may be helpful when depression occurs related to the chronicity of the disease and/or as an effect of corticosteroid use; see Healthy People 2010. Braces or orthoses and mobility and positioning aids are necessary.

As the muscles deteriorate, joints may become fixated, resulting in **contractures**. Contractures restrict flexibility and mobility and cause discomfort. Sometimes contractures require surgical tendon release. Spinal curvatures result over time. The boy with Duchenne muscular dystrophy who can still walk may develop lordosis. More frequently, scoliosis or kyphosis develops with this disorder. Surgical spinal fixation with rod implantation is often required by the age of 11 to 13 years. Additional complications include pulmonary, urinary, or systemic infections, depression, learning or behavioral disorders, aspiration pneumonia (as oropharyngeal muscles become affected), cardiac dysrhythmias, and eventually respiratory insufficiency and failure (as weakness of the chest muscles and diaphragm progresses).

Nursing Assessment

For a full description of the assessment phase of the nursing process, refer to page 1420. Assessment findings pertinent to Duchenne muscular dystrophy are discussed below.

Health History

Examine the health history for a family history of neuromuscular disorders. Note pregnancy and delivery history, as this information may be useful in ruling out a pregnancy problem or birth trauma as a cause for the motor dysfunction. Determine status of developmental milestone achievement. Boys with Duchenne muscular dystrophy learn to walk but over time become unable to do so. If the child was previously diagnosed with muscular dystrophy, determine progression of disease. Inquire about functional status and need for assistive or adaptive equipment such as braces or wheelchairs. Determine skills related to activities of daily living. Note history of cough or frequent respiratory infections, which occur as the respiratory muscles weaken. While talking with the child and family, determine whether psychosocial issues such as decreased self-esteem, depression, alterations in socialization, or altered family processes might be present.

Physical Examination

Perform a thorough physical examination on the child with suspected muscular dystrophy or the child with known history of the disorder. Particular findings related to inspection, observation, auscultation, and palpation are presented below.

Inspection and Observation

Observe the child's ability to rise from the floor. A hallmark finding of Duchenne muscular dystrophy is the presence of Gowers' sign: the child cannot rise from the floor in standard fashion because of increasing weakness (Fig. 43.5). Observe the child's gait. Determine effectiveness of cough.

Auscultation and Palpation

Auscultate the heart and lungs. Note tachycardia, which develops as the heart muscle weakens. Note adequacy of breath sounds, which may diminish with decreasing respiratory function. Note muscle strength with resistance testing. Palpate muscle tone.

Laboratory and Diagnostic Tests

Electromyography (EMG) demonstrates that the problem lies in the muscles, not in the nerves. Serum creatine kinase levels are elevated early in the disorder, when significant muscle wasting is actively occurring. Muscle biopsy provides definitive diagnosis, demonstrating the absence of dystrophin. DNA testing reveals the presence of the gene.

Nursing Management

Nursing management is aimed at promoting mobility, maintaining cardiopulmonary function, preventing complications, and maximizing quality of life. Interventions directed at maintaining mobility and cardiopulmonary function also help to prevent complications. Refer to Nursing Care Plan Overview 43.1, and individualize nursing care based upon the child's and family's response to the illness. Additional specifics related to care of the child with muscular dystrophy are discussed below.

Promoting Mobility

Administer corticosteroids and calcium supplements as ordered. Encourage at least minimal weight-bearing in a standing position to promote improved circulation, healthier bones, and a straight spine. Boys with Duchenne muscular dystrophy may use a standing walker or standing frame to maintain an upright position. Perform passive stretching or strengthening exercises as recommended by the physical therapist. These exercises preserve mobility and may help to prevent muscle atrophy. Use orthotic supports such as hand braces or ankle–foot orthoses (AFOs) to prevent contractures of joints. Schedule activities during the part of the day when the child has the most energy. Teach parents the use of positioning, exercises, orthoses, and adaptive equipment.

Maintaining Cardiopulmonary Function

Assess respiratory rate, depth of respirations, and work of breathing. Auscultate the lungs to determine whether aeration is sufficient and to assess clarity of breath sounds. Position the child for maximum chest expansion, usually in

FIGURE 43.5 Gower's sign; (**A**) First the child must roll onto his hands and knees.
(**B**) Then he must bear weight by using his hands to support some of his weight, while
raising his posterior. (**C–E**) The boy then uses his hands to "walk" up his legs to
assume an upright position.

the upright position. Teach the child and family deep-breathing exercises to strengthen or maintain respiratory muscles and encourage coughing to clear the airways. Perform chest physical therapy or assist with chest percussion. Monitor the results of pulmonary function testing. Use of intermittent positive-pressure ventilation and mechanically assisted coughing will become necessary in the teen years for some boys, possibly later for others. Teach parents monitoring and use of these modalities in conjunction with the respiratory therapist. Monitor cardiac status closely to identify heart failure early. Assess for edema, weight gain, or crackles. Strictly monitor fluid intake and output.

Maximizing Quality of Life

Long periods of bed rest may contribute to further weakness. Work with the family and child to develop a schedule for diversional activities that provide appropriate developmental stimulation but avoid overexertion or frustration (related to inability to perform the activity). Periods of adequate rest must be balanced with activities. Walking or riding a stationary bike is appropriate for the child who has upper extremity involvement. For the child with lower extremity involvement, a wheelchair may become necessary for mobility, and the child may participate in crafts, drawing, and computer activities. Participating in the Special Olympics may be appropriate for some children (www.specialolympics.org).

Provide emotional support to the child and family. Long-term direct care is stressful for families and becomes more complex as the child gets older. Families often need respite from continual caregiving duties. When a child is hospitalized, the caregiver may feel comfortable allowing nurses and other health care professionals to assume more of the child's daily care; this can be an opportunity for the caregiver to obtain respite from daily care. Respite care may also be offered in the home by various community services, so explore these resources with families.

Assess the child's educational status. Some children attend school; others may opt for home-schooling.

Administer antidepressants as ordered: managing depression may increase the child's desire to participate in activities and self-care.

Refer the child and family to the Muscular Dystrophy Association (www.mda.org), which provides multidisciplinary care via clinics located throughout the United States. The association is also a clearinghouse for resources for individuals with muscular dystrophy.

Ensure that families receive genetic counseling for family planning purposes as well as determining which family members may be carriers for muscular dystrophy.

▶ SPINAL MUSCULAR ATROPHY

Spinal muscular atrophy (SMA) is a genetic motor neuron disease that affects the spinal nerves' ability to communi-cate with the muscles. It is inherited via an autosomal recessive mechanism. The motor neuron protein SMN (survival of motor neurons) is deficient as a result of a faulty gene on chromosome 5. The motor neurons are located mostly in the spinal cord. Without adequate SMN, the signals from the neurons to the muscles instructing them to contract are ineffective, so the muscles lose function and over time atrophy. The proximal muscles, those closer to the body's center, are usually more affected than the distal muscles. Emotional and mental development as well as sensation are unaffected by the disease (Muscular Dystrophy Association, 2006c).

There are several types of SMA: type 1 (Werdnig-Hoffmann disease, infantile SMA), type 2 (intermediate), and type 3 (Kugelberg-Welander disease or juvenile SMA). Table 43.2 compares these three types, their usual progression, and their prognosis.

Respiratory muscle weakness may occur with all types of SMA and is usually the cause of death in type 1 and type 2 SMA. Upper respiratory tract infections and aspiration related to dysphagia or gastroesophageal reflux often develop into pneumonia and eventual respiratory failure, as the affected child cannot effectively cough independently in order to clear the airway. Many children with severe type 1 SMA are ventilator dependent. Pectus excavatum develops in children with type 1 and 2 SMA who exhibit paradoxical breathing (use of the diaphragm without intercostal muscle support). The chest becomes funnel-shaped and the xiphoid process is retracted (pectus excavatum), further restricting respiratory development. Inability to appropriately suck and swallow leads to difficulty feeding in the child with type 1 SMA. Weak back muscles affect the developing spine, resulting in the complication of scoliosis, kyphosis, or both.

Therapeutic management of SMA is supportive, aimed at promoting mobility, maintaining adequate nutrition and pulmonary function, and preventing complications. Spinal fusion may be performed in older children with significant scoliosis. Supplementation with creatine and/or coenzyme Q10 is under investigation (Muscular Dystrophy Association, 2006c).

Nursing Assessment

Note history of attainment of developmental milestones, as well as loss of milestones. In the infant or child with known SMA, assess for recent hospitalizations or respiratory illness. Determine the respiratory support regimen used at home (if any). Note level of motor ability, and identify the orthoses or adaptive equipment used. Elicit history related to feeding patterns at home. Assess for floppy appearance in the infant with SMA (Fig. 43.6). Note decreased ability to initiate spontaneous muscle movement. In the infant or young child with SMA, note narrow chest with decreased excursion, relatively protuberant abdomen, and paradoxical breathing pattern (Fig. 43.7). Observe chest for formation of pectus exca-

TABLE 43.2   FEATURES OF SPINAL MUSCULAR ATROPHY

Features	Type 1 SMA (Werdnig-Hoffman disease, infantile SMA)	Type 2 SMA (Intermediate SMA)	Type 3 SMA (Kugelberg-Welander disease, juvenile SMA)
Onset	Before birth to 6 months of age	6 to 18 months of age	After 18 months of age; child has started walking or has taken at least five independent steps
Symptoms	• Generalized weakness; cannot sit without support • Weak cry • Difficulty sucking, swallowing, and breathing	• Weakness that is most severe in the shoulders, hips, thighs, and upper back • Respiratory muscles may be involved. • Scoliosis may occur.	• Weakness that is most severe in the shoulders, hips, thighs, and upper back • Respiratory muscles may be involved. • Scoliosis may occur.
Progression	Rapidly progresses to early childhood death. Use of ventilators and gastrostomy feeding tubes may prolong life expectancy.	Slower progression. Survival into adulthood common if respiratory status maintained appropriately.	Slow progression. Life span usually unaffected. Walking ability maintained until at least adolescence; may need wheelchair later in life.

Data from Muscular Dystrophy Association, 2006.

vatum. Auscultate lungs for diminished or adventitious breath sounds. Monitor laboratory testing, which may include:

• Creatine kinase (CK): elevated when muscular damage is occurring
• Genetic testing: identifies presence of gene for SMA
• Muscle biopsy: shows the muscle abnormality

• Nerve conduction velocity test and electromyelogram: to determine extent of involvement

Nursing Management

Nursing management of type 2 and type 3 SMA focuses on promoting mobility, maintaining pulmonary function, and preventing complications. Children with type 1 SMA need

FIGURE 43.6 Note the hypotonic (floppy) posture of this infant with type 1 SMA (rotated arms, frog legged lower extremities). (Graphic courtesy of the Muscular Dystrophy Association, www.mda.org.)

FIGURE 43.7 Note the very narrow chest, beginning xiphoid depression, and relatively enlarged appearance of the abdomen in this infant with type 1 SMA.

additional interventions related to prevention of complications from immobility and assistance with nutrition. Refer to Nursing Care Plan Overview 43.1 for interventions related to these areas. Individualize the nursing plan of care based on the individual child's responses to the disorder.

Promote mobility through the use of range-of-motion exercises, lightweight orthotics, standing frames, and wheelchair use as appropriate. Support parents in their efforts to comply with physical and occupational therapy regimens. Older children may exercise with assistance in a warm pool. Position the child in a fashion that maintains appropriate body alignment (Fig. 43.8).

Provide chest percussion to assist with coughing and clearance of secretions. In collaboration with respiratory therapy, teach families the use of noninvasive ventilation support, in which positive pressure is delivered to the lungs through a mask or mouthpiece (Fig. 43.9). Provide routine tracheostomy care if the child has a tracheostomy (refer to tracheostomy section of Chapter 40).

Administer gastrostomy tube feedings if ordered, and teach families gastrostomy tube care. Use bracing as prescribed to prevent spinal curvature (Fig. 43.10). Make frequent inspections for skin breakdown in areas affected by bracing.

Cerebral Palsy

Cerebral palsy is a term used to describe a range of non-specific clinical symptoms characterized by abnormal motor pattern and postures caused by nonprogressive ab-

FIGURE 43.9 Use of noninvasive positive-pressure monitoring via a mask can maximize respiration and may help prevent pulmonary complications.

normal brain function. The majority of causes occur before or during delivery and are often associated with brain anoxia (Box 43.1); see Healthy People 2010. Many times no specific cause can be identified. Cerebral palsy is the most common movement disorder of childhood; it is a lifelong condition and one of the most common causes of physical disability in children. The incidence is about 2.5 in every 1,000 live births (Hirtz et al., 2007). The incidence is higher in premature and twin births.

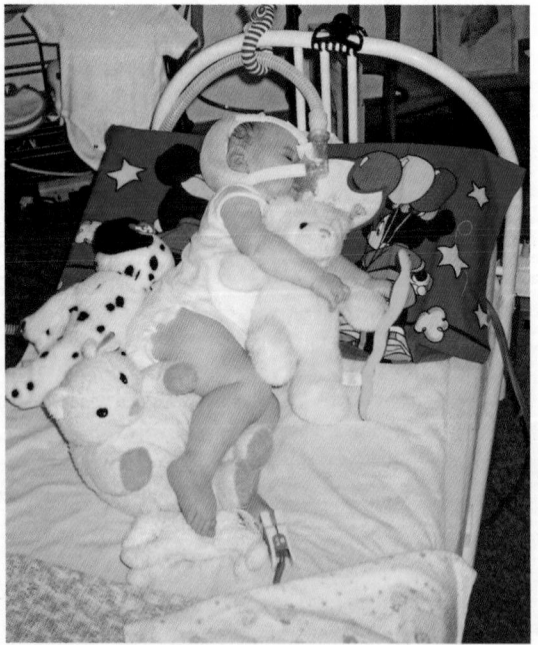

FIGURE 43.8 Position the infant with SMA to maintain appropriate body alignment, propping extremities as needed. (Graphic courtesy of the Muscular Dystrophy Association, www.mda.org.)

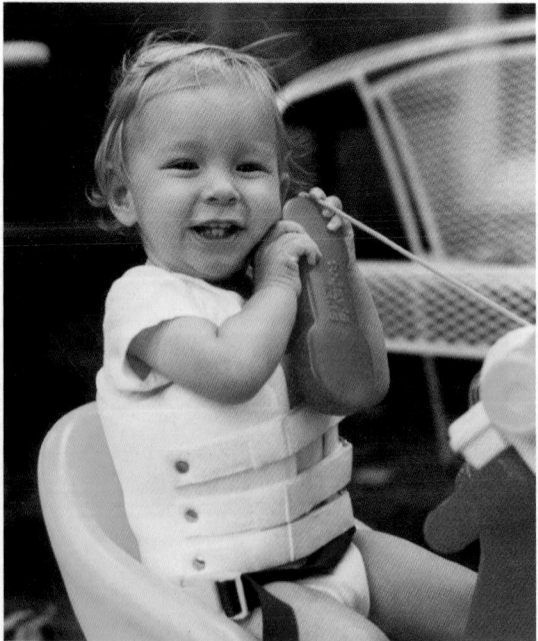

FIGURE 43.10 Bracing may be necessary in the young child with SMA to either prevent scoliosis from developing or prevent its progression. (Graphic courtesy of the Muscular Dystrophy Association, www.mda.org.)

BOX 43.1 Causes of Cerebral Palsy

Prenatal
- Congenital malformation
- Maternal seizures
- Maternal bleeding
- Exposure to radiation
- Environmental toxins
- Genetic abnormalities
- Intrauterine growth restriction
- Intrauterine infection, such as cytomegalovirus and toxoplasmosis
- Nutritional deficits
- Pre-eclampsia
- Multiple births
- Prematurity
- Low birthweight
- Malformation of brain structure
- Abnormalities of blood flow to the brain

Perinatal
- Prematurity (<32 weeks)
- Asphyxia
- Hypoxia
- Breech position
- Sepsis or central nervous system infection
- Placental complications
- Electrolyte disturbance
- Cerebral hemorrhage
- Kernicterus (a type of brain damage that may result from neonatal hyperbilirubinemia)
- Chorioamnionitis (infection of the placental tissues and amniotic fluid)

Postnatal
- Head trauma (e.g., motor vehicle accidents, abuse)
- Seizures
- Toxins
- Viral or bacterial infection of the central nervous system (e.g., meningitis)

HEALTHY PEOPLE 2010

Objective	Significance
Reduce preterm births.	• Encourage appropriate birth control use among adolescents to decrease the incidence of teen pregnancy (teens have an increased incidence of preterm delivery). • If an adolescent does become pregnant, encourage early appropriate prenatal care. • Discourage substance use among pregnant teens. • Teach pregnant teens about an appropriate diet.

Most affected children will develop symptoms in infancy or early childhood. There is a large variation in symptoms and disability. For some children it may be as mild as a slight limp; for others it may result in severe motor and neurologic impairments. Primary signs include motor impairments such as spasticity, muscle weakness, and ataxia. Complications include mental impairments, seizures, growth problems, impaired vision or hearing, abnormal sensation or perception, and hydrocephalus. Most children can survive into adulthood but may suffer substantial impairments in function and quality of life.

Pathophysiology

Cerebral palsy is a disorder caused by abnormal development of, or damage to, the motor areas of the brain. It results in a disruption in the brain's ability to control movement and posture. It is difficult to establish an exact location of the neurologic lesion, and the lesion itself does not change; thus, the disorder is considered nonprogressive since the brain injury does not progress. However, the clinical manifestations of the lesion change as the child grows. Some children may improve, but many either plateau in their attainment of motor skills or demonstrate worsening of motor abilities, as it is difficult to maintain the ability to move over time.

Cerebral palsy is classified in several ways. One common way is by the type of movement disturbance (Table 43.3).

Therapeutic Management

Management involves multiple disciplines, including a primary physician, specialty physicians such as neurologist and orthopedic surgeon, nurses, physical therapists, occupational therapists, speech therapists, dietitian, psychologist, counselors, teachers, and parents. Spasticity management will be a primary concern and will be determined by clinical findings. There is no standard treatment for all children. The overall focus of therapeutic management will be to assist the child to gain optimal development and function within the limits of the disease. Treatment is mainly symptomatic, preventive, and supportive.

Medical management is focused on promoting mobility through the use of therapeutic modalities and medications. Many children will require surgical procedures to correct deformities related to spasticity. Multiple corrective surgeries may be required; they usually are orthopedic or neurosurgical. Surgery may be used to correct contractures that are severe enough to cause movement limitations. Common orthopedic procedures include tendon lengthening procedures, correction of hip and adductor muscle spasticity, and fusion of unstable joints to help improve locomotion, correct bony deformities, decrease painful spasticity, and maintain, restore, or stabilize a spinal deformity.

TABLE 43.3 **CLASSIFICATION OF CEREBRAL PALSY**

Types	Description	Characteristics
Spastic	Hypertonicity and permanent contractures; different types based on which limbs are affected: • Hemiplegia: both extremities on one side • Quadriplegia: all four extremities • Diplegia or paraplegia: lower extremities	• Most common form • Poor control of posture, balance, and movement • Exaggeration of deep tendon reflexes • Hypertonicity of affected extremities • Continuation of primitive reflexes • In some children, failure to progress to protective reflexes
Athetoid or dyskinetic	Abnormal involuntary movements	• Infant is limp and flaccid. • Uncontrolled slow worm-like, writhing, or twisting movements • Affects all four extremities and possible involvement of face, neck, and tongue • Movements increase during periods of stress. • Dysarthria and drooling may be present.
Ataxic	Affects balance and depth perception	• Rare form • Poor coordination • Unsteady gait • Wide-based gait
Mixed	Combination of the above	Most common is spastic and athetoid.

Neurosurgical interventions may include placement of a shunt in children who have developed hydrocephalus, or surgical interventions to decrease spasticity. Selective dorsal root rhizotomy is used to decrease spasticity in the lower extremities by reducing the amount of stimulation that reaches the muscles via nerves. The effectiveness of this surgery is controversial, and research is ongoing.

Physical, Occupational, and Speech Therapy

The use of therapies such as physical therapy, occupational therapy, and speech therapy will be essential in promoting mobility and development in the child with CP. The earlier the treatment begins, the better chance the child has of overcoming developmental disabilities.

Physical therapists work with children to assist in the development of gross motor movements such as walking and positioning, and they help the child develop independent movement. They also assist in preventing contractures, and they instruct children and caregivers in the use of assistive devices such as walkers and wheelchairs. Occupational therapists may be responsible for fashioning orthotics and splints. AFOs are the most common orthotic used by children with cerebral palsy (Fig. 43.11). AFOs help prevent deformity from conditions such as contractures and help reduce the effects of existing deformities. They can help improve a child's mobility by assisting in control of alignment and helping to increase the efficiency of the child's gait. Spinal orthotics such as braces are used in young children with cerebral palsy to combat scoliosis that develops due to spasticity. These braces are used to delay surgical management of the scoliosis until

the child reaches skeletal maturity. Splinting is used to maintain muscle length. Serial casting may also be used to increase muscle and tendon length.

Occupational therapy also assists in the development of fine motor skills and will help the child to perform opti-

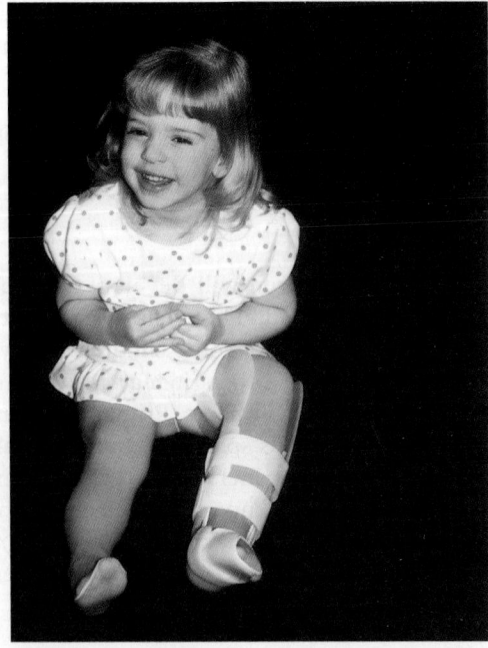

FIGURE 43.11 The child with cerebral palsy may benefit from wearing ankle–foot orthotics (AFOs) to provide support needed for independent or assisted walking.

mal self-care by working on skills such as activities of daily living. Speech therapy assists in the development of receptive and expressive language and addresses the use of appropriate feeding techniques in the child who has swallowing problems. Speech therapists may teach augmented communication strategies to children who are nonverbal or who have articulation problems. Many children may not communicate verbally but can use alternative means such as communication books or boards to make their desires known or to participate in conversation.

Pharmacologic Management

Various pharmacologic options are available to manage spasticity. Medications are also used to treat seizure disorders in children with cerebral palsy (refer to Chapter 38 for information related to seizure management). Oral medications used to treat spasticity include baclofen and diazepam (see Drug Guide 43.1). Patients with athetoid cerebral palsy may be given anticholinergics to help decrease abnormal movements.

Parenterally administered medications such as botulin toxins and baclofen are also used to manage spasticity. Botulinum toxin is injected into the spastic muscle to balance the muscle forces across joints and to decrease spasticity. It is useful in managing focal spasticity in which the spasticity is interfering with function, producing pain, or contributing to a progressive deformity. Botulin toxin injection is performed by the physician or advanced practitioner and can be done in the clinic or outpatient setting.

Intrathecal administration of baclofen has been shown to decrease tone, but it must be infused continuously due to its short half-life. Surgical placement of a baclofen pump will be considered in children with general spasticity that is limiting function, comfort, activities of daily living, and endurance. To test whether it is a suitable option, an intrathecal test dose of baclofen will be administered. If the trial is successful, a baclofen pump will be implanted. Once inserted, delivery of the drug can be individualized to meet the patient's unique needs. The pump needs to be replaced every 5 to 7 years and must be refilled with medication approximately every 3 months, depending on the type of pump. Complications with baclofen pump placement include infection, rupture, dislodgement, or blockage of the catheter.

Nursing Assessment

For a full description of the assessment phase of the nursing process, refer to page 1420. Assessment findings pertinent to cerebral palsy are discussed below.

Health History

Elicit a description of the present illness and chief complaint. Obtain a detailed account of gestation and perinatal events (refer to Box 43.1). Common signs and symptoms reported during the health history of the undiagnosed child might include:

- Intrauterine infections
- Prematurity with intracranial hemorrhage
- Difficult, complicated, or prolonged labor and delivery
- Multiple births
- History of possible anoxia during prenatal life or birth
- History of head trauma
- Delayed attainment of developmental milestones
- Muscle weakness or rigidity
- Poor feeding
- Hips and knees feel rigid and unbending when pulled to a sitting position
- Seizure activity
- Subnormal learning
- Abnormal motor performance, scoots on back instead of crawling on abdomen, walks or stands on toes

Children known to have cerebral palsy are often admitted to the hospital for corrective surgeries or other complications of the disease, such as aspiration pneumonia and urinary tract infections. The health history should include questions related to:

- Respiratory status: Has a cough, sputum production, or increased work of breathing developed?
- Motor function: Has there been a change in muscle tone, increase in spasticity?
- Presence of fever
- Feeding and weight loss
- Any other changes in physical state or medication regimen

Physical Examination

Observe general appearance. Pay close attention to the neurologic assessment and motor assessment. Assess for delayed development, size for age, and sensory alterations like strabismus, vision problems, and speech disorders. Abnormal postures may be present. While lying supine, the infant may demonstrate scissor crossing of the legs with plantar flexion. In the prone position the infant may raise his or her head higher than normal due to arching of the back, or the opisthotonic position may be noted. The infant may also abnormally flex the arms and legs under the trunk. Primitive reflexes may persist beyond the point at which they disappear in a healthy infant. Evolution of protective reflexes may be delayed. Watch the infant or child play, crawl, walk, or climb to determine motor function and capability. Note any movement disorder. Infants with cerebral palsy may demonstrate abnormal use of muscle groups such as scooting on their back instead of crawling or walking.

Assess active and passive range of motion. Pay particular attention to muscle tone. Though an increased or decreased resistance may be noted with passive movements, **hypertonicity** is most often seen. Increased resistance to dorsiflexion and passive hip abduction are the most common early signs. Sustained **clonus** may be present after forced dorsiflexion. Lift the child by placing your hands in the infant's or child's axillary area to assess shoulder girdle function and tone. Infants with cerebral palsy often demonstrate prolonged standing on their toes when supported in an upright standing position in this fashion. Lift the young child off the ground while the child holds your thumbs to test hand strength. Observe for presence of limb deformity, as decreased use of an extremity (as in the case of hemiparesis) may result in shortening of the extremity compared to the other one.

Laboratory and Diagnostic Tests

A complete history, physical examination, and ancillary investigations are the primary modality for establishing a diagnosis of cerebral palsy. Common supplementary laboratory and diagnostic studies ordered for the diagnosis and assessment of cerebral palsy include:

- Electroencephalogram: usually abnormal but the pattern is highly variable
- Cranial x-rays or ultrasound: may show cerebral asymmetry
- MRI or CT: may show area of damage or abnormal development but may be normal
- Screening for metabolic defects and genetic testing may be performed to help determine the cause of cerebral palsy.

These tests will help determine whether cerebral palsy is the likely cause or whether another condition may be the cause of the child's symptoms. These tests also will be important in evaluating the severity of the child's physical disabilities.

Nursing Management

Nursing management focuses on promoting growth and development by promoting mobility and maintaining optimal nutritional intake. Providing support and education to the child and family is also an important nursing function. In addition to the nursing diagnoses and related interventions discussed in the Nursing Care Plan Overview, interventions common to caring for a child with cerebral palsy follow.

Promoting Mobility

Mobility is critical to childhood development. Treatment modalities to promote mobility include physiotherapy, pharmacologic management, and surgery. Surgical procedures are discussed above. Physical or occupational therapy as well as medications may be used to address musculoskeletal abnormalities, to facilitate range of motion, to delay or prevent deformities such as contractures, to provide joint stability, to maximize activity, and to encourage the use of adaptive devices. The nurse's role in relation to the various therapies is to provide ongoing follow-through with prescribed exercises, positioning, or bracing.

▶ **Take** NOTE!

Therapeutic horseback riding has been demonstrated to improve gross motor function in children with cerebral palsy. If available in the local area, refer the child and family to the North American Riding for the Handicapped Association (NARHA) (Sterba, 2004; Sterba, 2007).

When casting, splinting, or orthotics are used, assess skin integrity frequently. Pain management may also be necessary. Nursing management of children receiving botulin toxin focuses on assisting with the procedure and providing education and support to the child and family. Nursing interventions related to baclofen include assisting with the test dose and providing preoperative and postoperative care if a pump is placed, as well as providing support and education to the child and family. Teaching Guidelines 43.2 gives information related to baclofen pump insertion.

Promoting Nutrition

Children with cerebral palsy may have difficulty eating and swallowing due to poor motor control of the throat, mouth, and tongue. This may lead to poor nutrition and problems with growth. The child may require a longer time to eat because of poor motor control. Special diets, such as soft or puréed, may make swallowing easier.

TEACHING GUIDELINES 43.2

Baclofen Pump: Patient/Family Education

- Check the incisions daily for redness, drainage, or swelling.
- Notify the physician if the child has a temperature greater than 101.5° F, or if the child has persistent incision pain.
- Avoid tub baths for 2 weeks.
- Do not allow the child to sleep on the stomach for 4 weeks after pump insertion.
- Discourage twisting at the waist, reaching high overhead, stretching, or bending forward or backward for 4 weeks.
- When the incisions have healed, normal activity may be resumed.
- Wear loose clothing to prevent irritation at the incision site.
- Carry implanted device identification and emergency information cards at all times.

Proper positioning during feeding is essential to facilitate swallowing and reduce the risk of aspiration. Speech or occupational therapists can assist in working on strengthening swallowing muscles as well as assisting in developing accommodations to facilitate nutritional intake. Consult a dietitian to ensure adequate nutrition for children with cerebral palsy. In children with severe swallowing problems or malnutrition, a feeding tube such as a gastrostomy tube may be placed.

Providing Support and Education

Cerebral palsy is a lifelong disorder that can result in severe physical and cognitive disability. In some cases disability may require complete intensive daily care of the child. Adjusting to the demands of this multifaceted illness is difficult. Children are frequently hospitalized and need numerous corrective surgeries, which places strain on the family and its finances. From the time of diagnosis, the family should be involved in the child's care. It is important to include parents in the planning of interventions and care of this child. In most cases they are the primary caregivers and will assist the child in development of functioning and skills as well as providing daily care. They will provide essential information to the health care team and will be advocates for their child throughout his or her life. It is important that nurses provide ongoing education for the child and family.

As the child grows, the needs of the family and child will change. Recognize and respect these needs. Providing daily intense care can be demanding and tiring. When a child with cerebral palsy is admitted to the hospital, this may serve as a time of respite for family and primary caregivers. Encourage respite care and provide support and encouragement. Because cerebral palsy is a lifelong condition, children will need meaningful education programs that emphasize independence in the least restrictive educational environment. Refer caregivers to local resources, including education services and support groups. United Cerebral Palsy, a national organization, can be accessed at www.ucp.org/ (1660 L Street, NW, Suite 700, Washington, D.C. 20036; 800-872-5827/202-776-0406). Easter Seals is an organization that helps children with disabilities and special needs and provides support to families (www.easterseals.com).

Refer children under age 3 years to the local early intervention service. Early intervention provides case management of developmental services for children with special needs. Each state has a coordinator for early intervention. The office of the early intervention coordinator can then direct the health care professional to the local or district early intervention office.

Additional resources for families of young children with special needs are available at www.zerotothree.org. For additional reading, recommend the book *Children with Cerebral Palsy: A Parent's Guide* by E. Geralis (published by Woodbine House).

Acquired Neuromuscular Disorders

A number of neuromuscular disorders may be acquired during childhood or adolescence. These include disorders resulting from trauma as well as those that are autoimmune and infectious in nature. Trauma or unintentional injury is a leading cause of childhood morbidity and mortality in the United States. Injuries are the leading cause of death in children younger than 1 year of age and account for a significant percentage of childhood morbidity. The child is at increased risk for trauma based on the developmental factors of physical and emotional immaturity; additionally, adolescents display belief of invincibility. The developing neuromuscular system, if injured, may be irreparable, so the injury may result in life-threatening or lifelong effects. Neuromuscular trauma includes spinal cord injury and birth trauma (addressed in Chapter 18). Autoimmune neuromuscular disorders include Guillain-Barré syndrome, myasthenia gravis, and dermatomyositis. Botulism, though uncommon in developed countries, is an important neuromuscular disorder resulting from infection.

▶ SPINAL CORD INJURY

Spinal cord injury is damage to the spinal cord that results in loss of function. Frequent causes are trauma, such as car accidents, falls, diving into shallow water, gunshot or stab wounds, sports injuries, child abuse, or birth injuries. Spinal cord injuries are relatively uncommon in children, but when they do occur they have a devastating impact on the child's physical and functional status, social and emotional development, and family functioning. More spinal cord injuries are seen in adolescents due to their increased incidence of accidents, particularly motor vehicle accidents.

Spinal cord injury is a medical emergency and immediate medical attention is required. Cervical traction is often used initially and surgical intervention is sometimes necessary. Ongoing medical treatment will be based on the child's age and overall health and the extent and location of the injury. Therapeutic management focuses on rehabilitation and prevention of complications. Spinal cord injury in children is managed similarly to that in adults.

Nursing Assessment

Symptoms vary based on the location and severity of the injury. Common signs and symptoms associated with spinal cord injury include:

• Inability to move or feel extremities
• Numbness
• Tingling
• Weakness

The higher the injury in the spinal cord, the more extensive the damage and the greater the loss of function. High cervical injury will result in damage to the phrenic nerve, which innervates the diaphragm. Damage to this nerve will leave the child unable to breathe without assistance. Paralysis depends on the location of the injury to the spinal cord.

The diagnosis of spinal cord injury is made by clinical signs and diagnostic tests, which may include x-rays, CT, and MRI.

Nursing Management

Any child who requires hospitalization due to trauma should be considered at risk for a spinal cord injury, and immobilization of the spine is essential until full evaluation of the injury is complete and spinal cord damage is ruled out. Nursing management will be similar to management of the adult with a spinal cord injury and will focus on optimizing mobility, promoting bladder and bowel management, promoting adequate nutritional status, preventing complications associated with extreme immobility such as contractures and muscle atrophy, managing pain, and providing support and education to the child and family. Refer to the myelomeningocele section of this chapter for information related to urinary and bowel elimination.

The nurse plays an important role not only in the acute care of children with spinal cord injury but also during rehabilitation. Recovery from a spinal cord injury requires long-term hospitalization and rehabilitation. An interdisciplinary team of physicians, nurses, therapists, social workers, and case managers will work to manage the child's complex and long-term needs. Promoting communication among the interdisciplinary team is essential and will be a key nursing function. Rehabilitation will need to focus on the ever-changing developmental needs of the child as he or she grows.

Prevention of spinal cord injuries is an important nursing consideration. Educate the public on vehicular safety, including seat belt use and the proper use of age-appropriate safety seats. Additional education topics include bicycle, sports, and recreation safety, prevention of falls, violence prevention including gun safety, and water safety, including the risk of diving. This education can help decrease the incidence of spinal cord injury in children.

▶ GUILLAIN-BARRÉ SYNDROME

Guillain-Barré syndrome (also called acute inflammatory demyelinating polyradiculoneuropathy or polyneuropathy) is an uncommon disorder in which an immune response within the body attacks the peripheral nervous system but does not usually affect the brain or spinal cord. Guillain-Barré syndrome results in inflammation and demyelinization of the peripheral nerves. It is not fully understood why this occurs, but it is believed to be an autoimmune condition that most commonly is triggered by a previous viral or bacterial infection, usually described as an influenza-like upper respiratory tract infection or an acute gastroenteritis with fever. In rare cases it has occurred after the patient has had an immunization. In most cases the causative agent remains unidentified.

Therapeutic Management

Treatment of Guillain-Barré syndrome is symptomatic and focuses on lessening the severity and speeding recovery. Plasma exchange and administration of intravenous immunoglobulins may occur, especially in severe cases. The goal of treatment is to keep the body functioning until the nervous system recovers. Guillain-Barré syndrome is a life-threatening condition, and some children will die during the acute phase due to respiratory failure. Most children will make a full recovery, but a few may have residual damage.

Nursing Assessment

Early diagnosis and prompt treatment are essential since the disorder can quickly lead to respiratory failure and death from muscle paralysis. For a full description of the assessment phase of the nursing process, refer to page 1420. Assessment findings pertinent to Guillain-Barré syndrome are discussed below.

Health History

Elicit a description of the present illness and chief complaint. The clinical presentation is fairly similar in children and adults. It can occur a few days or weeks after the causative infection or event. Guillain-Barré syndrome has a quick onset and begins with muscle weakness and paresthesias such as numbness and tingling. Classically it initially affects the legs and progresses in an ascending manner. Occasionally it affects the arms or face first and proceeds in a descending manner. Progression is usually complete in 2 to 4 weeks, followed by a stable period leading to the recovery phase, which lasts for a few weeks to months in most cases but can take years. Severity of the disorder ranges from mild weakness to total paralysis.

In children, pain, especially of the lower extremities, as the initial presentation preceding motor involvement has been reported. Other symptoms seen during the course of the illness include:

- Fairly symmetrical flaccid weakness or paralysis
- Ataxia
- Sensory disturbances

Physical Examination and Laboratory and Diagnostic Tests

Physical examination findings may include decreased or absent tendon reflexes. Facial weakness or difficulty swallowing may also be present. Diagnosis is usually based on clinical findings of paralysis. CSF analysis may reveal an increased level of protein, but this may not be evident until after the first week of the illness.

> ▶ **Take** NOTE!
>
> *Tickling may be a successful technique for assessing the level of paralysis in the child with Guillain-Barré syndrome, either initially or in the recovery phase.*

Nursing Management

Nursing management is supportive. In severe cases the child may require intensive nursing care along with mechanical ventilation. Observe the child closely for the extent of paralysis and monitor for respiratory involvement. Nursing care focuses on the same concerns as in any patient with extreme immobility or paralysis.

Prevention of complications associated with immobility is a central concern and involves maintaining skin integrity, preventing respiratory complications and contractures, maintaining adequate nutrition, and managing pain. Interventions include turning and repositioning every 2 hours, assessing the skin for redness or breakdown, performing range-of-motion exercises, keeping the skin clean and dry, encouraging intake of fluids to maintain hydration status, and encouraging coughing and deep breathing every 2 hours and as needed. Enteral feeding or parenteral nutrition may be indicated if swallowing becomes impaired. Physical therapy may be helpful in preventing complications and promoting motor skill recovery. Provide support and education to the parent and child. The rapid onset and long recovery can be difficult and can cause strain on the family and its finances. If residual disability occurs, the family will need help adjusting and caring for their child.

> ▶ **Take** NOTE!
>
> *Serial measurement of tidal volumes may reveal respiratory deterioration in the child with Guillain-Barré syndrome.*

▶ MYASTHENIA GRAVIS

Myasthenia gravis is an autoimmune disease that may be triggered by a viral or bacterial infection or by the thymus gland. The acetylcholine receptor at the neuromuscular junction is affected, inhibiting normal neuromuscular transmission. The result is progressive weakness and fatigue of the skeletal muscles. Though no gene has been discovered as responsible for myasthenia gravis, autoimmune diseases do demonstrate a genetic predisposition. Myasthenia gravis occurs in three forms: neonatal, congenital, and acquired.

Therapeutic management generally involves the use of anticholinesterase medications such as pyridostigmine, which blocks the breakdown of acetylcholine at the neuromuscular junction. Additional medications may include corticosteroids and other immunosuppressants, plasmapheresis, intravenous immunoglobulin, and, in children who have reached puberty, thymectomy (Parr & Jayawant, 2007). Myasthenia gravis usually reaches maximum severity within 1 to 3 years of onset, and with proper treatment children can remain physically active (Muscular Dystrophy Association, 2006d). It may be aggravated by stress, exposure to extreme temperatures, and infections, resulting in a myasthenic crisis.

Nursing Assessment

Note history of fatigue and weakness; difficulty chewing, swallowing, or holding up the head; or pain with muscle fatigue. In the verbal child, note complaints of double vision. Observe the child for ptosis (droopy eyelids) or altered eye movements from partial paralysis. The neonate may display inadequate suck, weak cry, floppy extremities, and, possibly, respiratory insufficiency. Note increased work of breathing. Laboratory testing may involve the edrophonium (Tensilon) test, in which a short-acting cholinesterase inhibitor is used. Acetylcholine receptor (AchR) antibodies may be present in elevated quantities in the serum.

Nursing Management

Administer anticholinergic or other medications as ordered, teaching children and families about the use of these drugs. Anticholinergic drugs should be given 30 to 45 minutes before meals, on time and exactly as ordered. Encourage families to seek prompt medical treatment for suspected infections. Encourage appropriate stress management and avoidance of extreme temperatures. Teach families that physical activities should be performed during times of peak energy; rest periods are needed for energy conservation. Teach families to call their neurologist immediately if signs and symptoms of myasthenic crisis or cholinergic crisis appear. Encourage children to wear a medical alert bracelet.

> ▶ **Take** NOTE!
>
> *Signs and symptoms of myasthenic crisis include severe muscle weakness, respiratory difficulty, tachycardia, and dysphagia. Signs and symptoms of cholinergic crisis include severe muscle weakness, sweating, increased salivation, bradycardia, and hypotension.*

▶ DERMATOMYOSITIS

Dermatomyositis is an autoimmune disease that results in inflammation of the muscles or associated tissues. It occurs more often in girls and is generally diagnosed between the ages of 5 and 14 years. The autoimmune response may be triggered by exposure to a virus or to certain medications. As with other autoimmune diseases, a genetic predisposition is present. The inflammatory cells of the immune system cause a vasculitis that affects the skin, muscles, kidneys, retinas, and gastrointestinal tract.

Therapeutic management involving the use of corticosteroids or other immunosuppressants is necessary to prevent the complications of painful calcium deposits under the skin, as well as joint contractures. With appropriate treatment, children may recover completely, though some children experience relapses (Muscular Dystrophy Association, 2006a).

Nursing Assessment

Elicit a health history, which commonly involves history of fever, fatigue, and rash, usually followed by muscle pain and weakness. Determine onset and progression of muscle weakness. Inspect the skin for presence of rash involving the upper eyelids and extensor surfaces of the knuckles, elbows, and knees. The rash is initially a reddish-purplish color, and then progresses to scaling with resulting roughness of the skin. Test muscle strength, noting particularly weakness in the pelvic and shoulder girdles. Laboratory and diagnostic testing may include muscle enzyme levels, a positive ANA test, and an electromyelogram to distinguish muscular weakness from other causes.

Nursing Management

Administer medications as ordered and teach families about their use; instruct them to monitor for side effects. Educate the family about the importance of maintaining the medication regimen in order to prevent calcinosis (calcium deposits) and joint deformity in the future. Encourage compliance with physical therapy regimens. Ensure that children are excused from physical education classes while the disease is active.

▶ BOTULISM

Botulism is a disease that is caused by a toxin produced in the immature intestines of young children resulting from infection with the bacterium *Clostridium botulinum*. It is rare but can cause serious paralytic illness. Botulism is mainly a food-borne infection but can also be contracted through wound infections or intestinal infections in infants. *C. botulinum* is common in soil and can also be found in a variety of foods, such as improperly preserved home-canned foods. It generally occurs in infants less than 6 months of age. It has been associated with feeding honey and corn syrup to infants; thus, these should be avoided in children less than 1 year of age. The disease is not infectious; to become infected, the child must ingest the bacterial spores. These spores then multiply in the intestinal tract and produce the toxin, which is absorbed in the immature intestines of the infant. It is generally not a problem for older children because the bacteria do not grow well in mature intestines due to the presence of the normal intestinal flora. Prognosis is good, but if treatment is not initiated, paralysis of the arms, legs, trunk, and respiratory system can develop. Therapeutic management is usually supportive but may involve administration of botulinum toxin.

Nursing Assessment

For a full description of the assessment phase of the nursing process, refer to page 1420. Assessment findings pertinent to botulism are discussed below.

Health History

Elicit a description of the present illness and chief complaint. Signs and symptoms usually occur soon after ingestion of the bacteria. Common signs and symptoms in infants reported during the health history might include:

• Constipation
• Poor feeding
• Listlessness
• Generalized weakness
• Weak cry

Common signs and symptoms in older children reported during the health history might include:

• Double vision
• Blurred vision
• Drooping eyelids
• Difficulty swallowing
• Slurred speech
• Muscle weakness

Physical Examination and Laboratory and Diagnostic Tests

Assess for a diminished gag reflex, which is indicative of botulism. Diagnostic tests include cultures of stool and serum. Botulism is a rare disease and is difficult to diagnose since its symptoms are similar to those of other neuromuscular diseases. Therefore, assessment may include diagnostic tests to help rule out other diseases, such as Guillain-Barré syndrome, stroke, and myasthenia gravis.

Nursing Management

Treatment is mainly supportive and focuses on maintaining respiratory status and nutritional status. If ordered, administer botulinum toxin early in the disease to reduce its severity and progression.

∎∎∎ Key Concepts

∎ Muscles, tendons, ligaments, and cartilage are all present and functional at birth, though intentional, purposeful movement develops only as the infant matures.

∎ The spine is very mobile in the newborn and infant, especially the cervical spine region, resulting in a high risk for cervical spine injury.

∎ The nurse's role in laboratory and diagnostic testing for neuromuscular disorders is mainly that of educating the child and family about and preparing the child for the test or procedure.

∎ Assessment of range of motion and muscle tone is critical in the child with a neuromuscular disorder. Hypertonia or hypotonia is an abnormal finding in the infant or child.

∎ Determining attainment of developmental milestones and subsequent progression or loss of those milestones is useful in distinguishing various neuromuscular disorders.

∎ The nurse reinforces and carries out the exercise plans and adaptive equipment use as prescribed by the physical or occupational therapist in order to maintain neuromuscular function and to prevent complications.

∎ Nursing management of a child with myelomeningocele focuses on preventing infection, promoting bowel and urinary elimination, promoting adequate nutrition, preventing latex allergy reaction, maintaining skin integrity, providing education and support to the family, and recognizing complications, such as hydrocephalus or increased ICP, associated with the disorder.

∎ Cerebral palsy may result in significant motor impairment. Children with cerebral palsy require ongoing physical therapy as well as nutritional intervention.

∎ Boys with Duchenne muscular dystrophy initially learn to walk but later lose this ability.

∎ Respiratory compromise occurs in muscular dystrophy and spinal muscular atrophy and eventually leads to death.

∎ Children with spinal cord injury require intense nursing management and lengthy rehabilitation to maintain or regain function.

∎ Children with neuromuscular disorders often suffer depression related to the chronic nature of the disorder.

∎ School attendance and participation in activities such as the Special Olympics are important for children with neuromuscular dysfunction.

REFERENCES

Atkinson, S. B. (2006). The challenges of managing and treating Guillain-Barré syndrome during the acute phase. *Dimensions of Critical Care Nursing, 25*(6), 256–263.

Balaban, B., Matthews, D. J., Clayton, G. H., & Carry, T. (2005). Corticosteroid treatment and functional improvement in Duchenne muscular dystrophy: Long-term effect. *American Journal of Physical Medicine and Rehabilitation, 84,* 843–850.

Birse, J. (2006). Pilot testing of the Starship Infant Neurological Assessment tool. *Journal of Neuroscience Nursing, 38*(4), 206–211.

Blann, L. E. (2005). Early intervention for children and their families with special needs. *Maternal Child Nursing, 30*(4), 263–267.

Centers for Disease Control and Prevention. (2007). *Why folic acid is so important.* Retrieved October 20, 2007 from http://www.cdc.gov/ncbddd/folicacid/overview.htm.

Cooley, W. C. (2004). Providing a primary care medical home for children and youth with cerebral palsy. *Pediatrics, 114*(4), 1106–1113.

Cotton, S. M., Voudouris, N. J., & Greenwood, K. M. (2005). Association between intellectual functioning and age in children and young adults with Duchenne muscular dystrophy: Further results from a meta-analysis. *Developmental Medicine and Child Neurology, 47*(4), 257–265.

Darras, B. T. (2006). Muscular dystrophies. *Continuum: Lifelong Learning in Neurology, 12*(3), 33–75.

Emory University School of Medicine, Department of Pediatrics. (2007). *Baclofen pump implants (intrathecal): Home care.* Retrieved October 20, 2007 from http://www.pediatrics.emory.edu/divisions/neurology/baclofen.html.

Hayes, J. S., & Arriola, T. (2005). Pediatric spinal injuries. *Pediatric Nursing, 31*(6), 464–469.

Hirtz, D., Thurman, D. J., Gwinn-Hardy, K., Mohamed, M., Chaudhuri, A. R., & Zalutsky, R. (2007). How common are the "common" neurologic disorders? *Neurology, 68*(5), 326–337.

Hollister, J. R. (2007). Rheumatic diseases. In W. W. Hay, M. J. Levin, J. M. Sondheimer, & R. R. Deterding (Eds.), *Current pediatric diagnosis & treatment* (18th ed.). New York: McGraw-Hill.

Kliegman, R., Behrman, R., Jenson, H., & Stanton, B. (2007). *Nelson textbook of pediatrics* (18th ed.). Philadelphia: Saunders.

Koman, L. A., Smith, B. P., & Shilt, J. S. (2004). Cerebral palsy [electronic version]. *Lancet, 363*(9421), 1619–1632. Retrieved 6/23/04 from Proquest database.

Komelasky, A. (2005). Pediatric neurologic disorders. In S. M. Nettina (Ed.), *Lippincott manual of nursing practice.* Philadelphia: Lippincott Williams & Wilkins.

Lee, L., Chuang, Y., Yang, B., Hsus, M., & Liu, Y. (2004). Botulinum toxin for lower limb spasticity in children with cerebral palsy. *American Journal of Physical Medicine & Rehabilitation, 83*(10), 766–773.

Merereau, P., Kilker, K., Carter, H., Fassett, E., et al. (2004). Spina bifida and anencephaly before and after folic acid mandate— United States, 1995–1996 and 1999–2000 [electronic version]. *Morbidity and Mortality Weekly Report, 53*(17), 362–365. Retrieved 6/19/04 from Proquest database.

Moe, P. G., & Benke, T. A. (2005) Neurologic and muscular disorders. In W. W. Hay, M. J. Levin, J. M. Sondheimer, & R. R. Deterding (Eds.), *Current pediatric diagnosis & treatment* (17th ed.). New York: McGraw-Hill.

Morantz, C., & Torrey, B. (2004). Immunotherapy in patients with Guillain-Barré syndrome [electronic version]. *American Family Physician, 69*(4), 997–999.

Muscular Dystrophy Association. (2006a). *Dermatomyositis.* Retrieved April 8, 2007 from http://www.mda.org/disease/pmdm-d.html.

Muscular Dystrophy Association. (2006b). *Duchenne muscular dystrophy (DMD).* Retrieved April 8, 2007 from http://www.mda.org/disease/dmd.html.

Muscular Dystrophy Association. (2006c). *Facts about spinal muscular atrophy (SMA).* Retrieved April 8, 2007 from http://www.mda.org/publications/fa-sma-qa.html.

Muscular Dystrophy Association. (2006d). *Myasthenia gravis.* Retrieved April 8, 2007 from http://www.mda.org/disease/mg.html.

National Institute of Neurological Disorders and Stroke. (2007). *Guillain-Barré syndrome fact sheet.* Retrieved October 20, 2007 from http://www.ninds.nih.gov/disorders/gbs/detail_gbs.htm.

Noble, K. A. (2005). The patient with latex allergy. *Journal of Perianesthesia Nursing, 20*(4), 285–288.

Palmieria, B., & Sblendorio, V. (2007). Duchenne muscular dystrophy: An update, part II. *Journal of Clinical Neuromuscular Disease, 8*(3), 122–151.

Parr, J. R., & Jayawant, S. (2007). Childhood myasthenia: Clinical subtypes and practical management. *Developmental Medicine & Child Neurology, 49*(8), 629–635.

Petrone, A., Pavone, M., Testa, M. B., Petreschi, F., Bertini, E., & Cutrera, R. (2007). Noninvasive ventilation in children with spinal muscular atrophy types 1 and 2. *American Journal of Physical Medicine & Rehabilitation, 86*(3), 216–221.

Ropper, A. H., & Brown, R. H. (2005). *Adams and Victor's principles of neurology.* New York: McGraw-Hill.

Simonds, A. K. (2007). Respiratory support for the severely handicapped child with neuromuscular disease: Ethics and practicality. *Seminars in Respiratory & Critical Care Medicine, 28*(3), 342–354.

Spina Bifida Association. (2006). *An overview of spina bifida occulta.* Retrieved October 20, 2007 from http://www.sbaa.org/site/c.gpILKXOEJqG/b.2021299/k.5080/An_Overview_of_Spina_Bifida_Occulta.htm.

Sterba, J. A. (2004). Effect of horseback riding therapy on Gross Motor Function Measure for each level of disability for children with cerebral palsy. *Developmental Medicine and Child Neurology, 46,* 47.

Sterba, J. A. (2007). Does horseback riding therapy or therapist-directed hippotherapy rehabilitate children with cerebral palsy? *Developmental Medicine & Child Neurology, 49*(1), 68–73.

Taillac, P. P., & Kim, J. (2006). *Botulism.* Retrieved October 20, 2007 from http://www.emedicine.com/emerg/topic64.htm.

Zickler, C. F., & Richardson, V. (2004). Achieving continence in children with neurogenic bowel and bladder. *Journal of Pediatric Health Care, 18*(6), 276–283.

WEBSITES

American Academy for Cerebral Palsy and Developmental Medicine—multidisciplinary scientific society devoted to the study of cerebral palsy, focusing on improving quality of life: www.aacpdm.org/index

American Association of Spinal Cord Injury Nurses: www.aascin.org/

Administration on Developmental Disabilities, Department of Health and Human Services: www.acf.dhhs.gov/programs/add

Cerebral Palsy Connection—network for parents of children with cerebral palsy: www.cpconnection.com

Children's Defense Fund: www.childrensdefense.org

Children's Medical Services program—provides family-centered, multidisciplinary, case-managed care to children with special health care needs through age 21, coordinated through offices throughout the United States: www.cms-kids.com

Families USA: www.familiesusa.org

Foundation for Spinal Cord Injury Prevention, Care & Cure: www.fscip.org

March of Dimes—research to prevent birth defects.: www.marchofdimes.com

Muscular Dystrophy Association—research, support, resources, education, regional multidisciplinary clinics throughout the United States: www.mda.org/

Muscular Dystrophy Canada: www.muscle.ca

Muscular Dystrophy Family Foundation—resources and assistance for families: www.mdff.org/

National Information Center for Children and Youth with Disabilities: www.nichcy.org

National Spinal Cord Injury Association: www.spinalcord.org/

Parent Project Muscular Dystrophy—an organization for parents of boys with Duchenne and Becker muscular dystrophy, providing education, resources, research, and advocacy: www.parentprojectmd.org/

Spina Bifida Association—dedicated to improving the lives of children with spina bifida: www.sbaa.org/

Spina Bifida and Hydrocephalus Association of Canada—resources and education: www.sbhac.ca/beta/index.php

Spinal Cord Injury Information Network: www.spinalcord.uab.edu/

Spinal Cord Injury Network International: www.spinalcordinjury.org

Spinal Cord Injury Resource Center: www.spinalinjury.net/

United Cerebral Palsy—research, resources, education: www.ucp.org

Zero to Three: www.zerotothree.org

CHAPTER WORKSHEET

MULTIPLE CHOICE QUESTIONS

1. A boy with Duchenne muscular dystrophy is admitted to the pediatric unit. He has an ineffective cough. Lung auscultation reveals diminished breath sounds. What is the priority nursing intervention?

   a. Apply supplemental oxygen.

   b. Notify the respiratory therapist.

   c. Monitor pulse oximetry.

   d. Position for adequate airway clearance.

2. A 7-year-old child with cerebral palsy has been admitted to the hospital. Which information is most important for the nurse to obtain in the history?

   a. Age that the child learned to walk

   b. Parents' expectations of the child's development

   c. Functional status related to eating and mobility

   d. Birth history to identify cause of cerebral palsy

3. The nurse is caring for a 2-year-old with myelomeningocele. When teaching about care related to neurogenic bladder, what response by the parent would indicate that additional teaching is required?

   a. "Routine catheterization will decrease the risk of infection from urine staying in the bladder."

   b. "I know it will be important for me to catheterize my child for the rest of her life."

   c. "I will make sure that I always use latex-free catheters."

   d. "I will wash the catheter with warm soapy water after each use."

4. The nurse is caring for a child with cerebral palsy who requires a wheelchair to attain mobility. Which intervention would help the child achieve a sense of normality?

   a. Encourage follow-through with physical therapy exercises.

   b. Restrict the child to a special needs classroom.

   c. Encourage after-school activities within the limits of the child's abilities.

   d. Ensure the school is aware of the child's capabilities.

5. What is the priority nursing intervention for the child recently admitted with Guillain-Barré syndrome?

   a. Perform range-of-motion exercises.

   b. Take temperature every 4 hours.

   c. Monitor respiratory status closely.

   d. Assess skin frequently.

CRITICAL THINKING EXERCISES

1. A 5-year-old girl, diagnosed with myelomeningocele, is admitted to the hospital for a corrective surgical procedure. Choose four questions from below that the nurse should ask when obtaining the health history that would assist in planning the child's care.

   a. What is the child's current mobility status?

   b. Is there a family history of myelomeningocele?

   c. What is the child's genitourinary and bowel function and regimen?

   d. Does this child have a history of hydrocephalus with presence of shunt?

   e. Does she have known latex sensitivity?

   f. Were there any complications during the pregnancy or birth of this child?

   g. Did the mother take prenatal folic acid supplementation?

2. Based on the case in the above question, develop a nursing care plan for the child with myelomeningocele.

3. A 5-year-old child is admitted to the pediatric unit with a history of cerebral palsy sustained at birth. The child is admitted for a scheduled tendon lengthening procedure. Based on your knowledge about the effects of cerebral palsy, list three priorities to focus on when planning her care. Compare this to a child admitted for surgical correction of a broken femur with no significant past medical history.

STUDY ACTIVITIES

1. In the clinical setting, compare the growth of a child with muscular dystrophy, spinal muscular atrophy, or cerebral palsy to the growth of a similar-age child who has been healthy. What differences or similarities

do you find? What are the explanations for your findings?

2. Identify the role of the registered nurse in the multidisciplinary care of the child with a debilitating neuromuscular disorder.

3. In the clinical setting, interview the parent of a child with Duchenne muscular dystrophy, myelomeningo-cele, spinal muscular atrophy, or severe cerebral palsy. Determine the parent's feelings about the ongoing care that he or she is responsible for. Reflect upon this interview in your clinical journal.

4. In the clinical setting, compare the cognitive abilities of two children with a severe neuromuscular disorder. What are the reasons for the similarities or differences that you find?

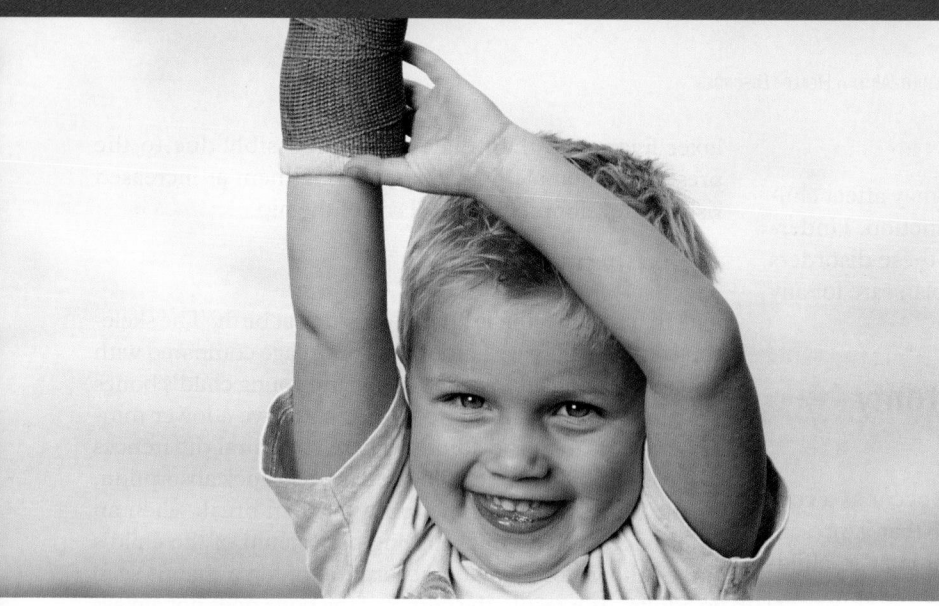

NURSING CARE OF THE CHILD WITH A MUSCULOSKELETAL DISORDER

KEY TERMS

compartment
  syndrome
distraction
epiphysis

external fixation
immobilize
kyphosis
lordosis

ossification
splint
traction
Trendelenburg gait

LEARNING OBJECTIVES

Upon completion of the chapter, the learner will be able to:

1. Compare the anatomy and physiology of the musculoskeletal system in children versus adults.
2. Identify nursing interventions related to common laboratory and diagnostic tests used in the diagnosis and management of musculoskeletal disorders.
3. Identify appropriate nursing assessments and interventions related to medications and treatments for common childhood musculoskeletal disorders.
4. Distinguish various musculoskeletal disorders occurring in childhood.
5. Devise an individualized nursing care plan for the child with a musculoskeletal disorder.
6. Develop patient/family teaching plans for the child with a musculoskeletal disorder.
7. Describe the impact of chronic musculoskeletal disorders on the growth and development of children.

Dakota Dawes, 2 years old, is brought to the clinic by his mother. She states, "Last night Dakota said his arm hurt, but he didn't have any complaints during the day. Today when he was playing I noticed he wasn't using his right arm."

WOW

Nursing care that heals children to take wobbly steps, run, jump, fall, and get up again provides life itself in a child's world.

A variety of musculoskeletal disorders may affect children, but the result of each is motor dysfunction. Understanding the most common responses to these disorders gives the nurse the foundation required to plan care for any child with any musculoskeletal disorder.

Variations in Pediatric Anatomy and Physiology

Musculoskeletal disorders in children may occur as a congenital malformation or a genetic disorder that is present from birth but may not be identified until later in childhood or adolescence. Some disorders are developmental; others result from trauma. The infant and young child have resilient soft tissue, so sprains and strains are less common in this age group. Older school-age children and adolescents often participate in sports, resulting in an increased risk of injuries such as sprains, fractures, and torn ligaments. The musculoskeletal system in infants and children is immature compared with adults; thus, when a musculoskeletal problem occurs in childhood, the child's growth may be hindered. The immobility associated with most musculoskeletal disorders may affect the child's development and acquisition of motor skills.

Myelinization

Myelinization of the central nervous system continues to progress after birth and is complete by about 2 years of age. Myelinization proceeds in a cephalocaudal and proximal–distal fashion, allowing voluntary muscle control to progress as myelinization occurs. As myelinization proceeds, the speed and accuracy of nerve impulses increase. Primitive reflexes are replaced with voluntary movement.

Muscle Development

The muscular system, including tendons, ligaments, and cartilage, arises from the mesoderm in early embryonic development. At birth (term or preterm), the muscles, tendons, ligaments, and cartilage are all present and functional. The newborn infant is capable of spontaneous movement but lacks purposeful control. Full range of motion is present at birth. Healthy infants and children demonstrate normal muscle tone. As the infant matures and becomes mobile, the muscles develop further and become stronger and their mass increases. The infant's muscles account for approximately 25% of total body weight, as compared with the adult's muscle mass, which accounts for about 40% of total body weight. Muscles grow rapidly in adolescence; this contributes to clumsiness, which places the teen at increased risk for injury. In response to testosterone release, the adolescent boy experiences a growth spurt, particularly in the trunk and legs, and develops bulkier muscles. Female infants tend to have

laxer ligaments than male infants, possibly due to the presence of female hormones, placing them at increased risk for developmental dysplasia of the hip.

Skeletal Development

The infant's skeleton is not fully ossified at birth. The skeleton contains increased amounts of cartilage compared with adolescents and adults. The infant and young child's bones are more flexible and more porous and have a lower mineral content than the adult's. These structural differences of a young child's bones allow for greater shock absorption, so the bones will often bend rather than break when an injury occurs. The thick, strong periosteum of the child's bones allows for a greater absorption of force than is seen in adults. As a result, the cortex of the bone does not always break, sometimes buckling or bending only. **Ossification** and conversion of cartilage to bone continue throughout childhood and are complete at adolescence.

During fetal development the spine displays **kyphosis**. Cervical **lordosis** develops as the infant starts to hold the head up. When the infant or toddler assumes an upright position, the primary and secondary curves of the spine begin to develop. The balance of the curves allows the head to be centered over the pelvis. During the toddler years, the period of early walking, lumbar lordosis may be significant (also termed toddler lordosis), and the toddler appears quite swaybacked and potbellied. As the child develops, the spine takes on more adult-like curves. During adolescence thoracic kyphosis may become evident. This is most often a postural effect, and as the teen matures, the posture appears similar to that of an adult.

Growth Plate

The ends of the bones in young children are composed of the **epiphysis** and the physis, in combination termed the growth plate. In infants, the epiphyses are cartilaginous and ossify over time. In children, the epiphysis is the secondary ossification center at the end of the bone. The physis is a cartilaginous area between the epiphysis and the metaphysis. Growth of the bones occurs primarily in the epiphyseal region. This area is vulnerable and structurally weak. Traumatic force applied to the epiphysis during injury may result in fracture in that area of the bone. Epiphyseal injury may result in early, incomplete, or partial closure of the growth plate, leading to deformity or shortening of the bone. Epiphyseal growth continues until skeletal maturity is reached during adolescence. Production of androgens in adolescence gradually causes the growth plates to fuse, and thus long bone growth is complete (Fig. 44.1).

Bone Healing

The child's bones have a thick, strong periosteum with an abundant blood supply. Bone healing occurs in the same fashion as in the adult, but because of the rich nutrient supply to the periosteum, it occurs more quickly in children. Children's bones produce callus more rapidly and in

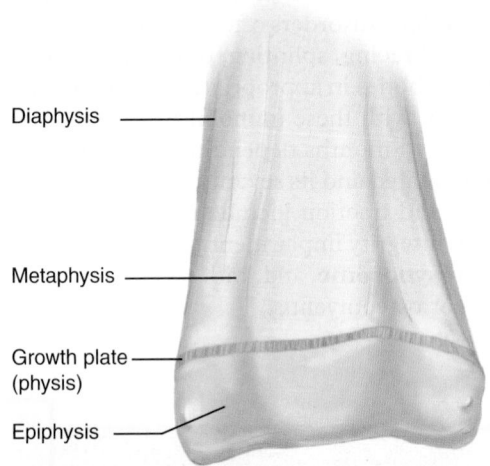

FIGURE 44.1 Anatomic areas of growing bone.

Diaphysis

Metaphysis

Growth plate (physis)

Epiphysis

larger quantities than do adults'. As new bone cells quickly form, a bulge of new bone growth occurs at the site of the fracture. The younger the child, the more quickly the bone heals. Also, the closer the fracture is to the growth plate (epiphysis), the more quickly the fracture heals. The capacity for remodeling (the process of breaking down and forming new bone) is increased in children as compared with adults. This means that straightening of the bone over time occurs more easily in children.

Positional Alterations

The lower extremities of the infant tend to have a bowed appearance, attributed to *in utero* positioning. *In utero*, the fetus' hips are usually flexed, abducted, and externally rotated, with the knees also flexed and the lower limbs inwardly rotated (Fig. 44.2). This normal developmental variation is termed internal tibial torsion. The legs

FIGURE 44.2 Internal tibial torsion with metatarsus adductus—normal findings in the infant.

FIGURE 44.3 Genu valgum (knock-knees): note knees touching at midline and outward angle of the lower half of the legs.

straighten with passive motion, and internal tibial torsion should not be confused with "bowlegs." Internal tibial torsion usually resolves independently some time in the second or third year of life as the toddler bears weight and the lower extremity muscles and bones mature. The bow-legged appearance is sometimes also referred to as genu varum. As internal tibial torsion or genu varum resolves, physiologic genu valgum occurs. Children usually demonstrate symmetric genu valgum (knock-knees) by the age of 2 to 3 years. In genu valgum, when the knees are touching the ankles are significantly separated, with the lower portion of the legs angled outward (Fig. 44.3). By age 7 or 8 years, genu valgum gradually resolves in most children.

The newborn's feet also display in-toeing (metatarsus adductus) as a result of *in utero* positioning (see Fig. 44.2). The feet remain flexible and may be passively moved to midline and in a straight position. This also resolves as the infant's musculoskeletal system matures. Pes planus (flat feet) is noted in infants when they begin to walk. The long arch of the foot is not yet developed and makes contact with the floor, resulting in a medial bulge. As the child grows and the muscles become less lax, the arch generally develops. Some children may continue with flexible flat feet, and this is considered a normal variation.

▶ *Take* NOTE!

Fractures are rare in children less than 1 year of age. The infant who presents with a fracture should be carefully evaluated for child abuse or an underlying musculoskeletal disorder.

Common Medical Treatments

A variety of medications as well as other medical treatments are used to treat musculoskeletal disorders in children. Most of these treatments will require a physician's order when the child is in the hospital. The most common treatments and medications are listed in Common Medical Treatments 44.1 and Drug Guide 44.1. The nurse caring for the child with a musculoskeletal disorder should become familiar with what the procedures are, how they work, as well as common nursing implications

related to use of these modalities. The treatment of musculoskeletal disorders often involves immobilization via casting, bracing, splinting, or traction to allow healing with the bones in appropriate alignment. The length of treatment with these immobilization methods varies from weeks to months depending on the type of disorder being treated and its severity. Complications related to casting and traction include neurovascular compromise, skin integrity impairment, soft tissue injury, **compartment syndrome**, and, with skeletal traction, pin site infection or osteomyelitis.

COMMON MEDICAL TREATMENTS 44.1

Treatment	Explanation	Indication	Nursing Implications
Traction	Application of a pulling force on an extremity or body part	Fracture reduction, dislocations, correction of deformities	To maintain even, constant traction: • Ensure weights hang free at all times and ropes remain in the pulley grooves. • Keep weights out of child's reach. • Maintain prescribed weight. • Elevate head or foot of bed only with physician order. Monitor for complications: • Perform neurovascular checks at least every 4 hours. • Assess for skin impairment.
Casting	Application of plaster or fiberglass material to form a rigid apparatus to immobilize a body part	Fracture reduction, dislocations, correction of deformities	Assess frequently for neurovascular compromise, skin impairment at cast edges. Protect cast from moisture. Teach family how to care for cast at home.
Splinting	Temporary stiff support of injured area	Temporary fracture reduction, immobilization and support of sprains	Similar to cast care. Some splints are removable and are replaced when the child is up out of bed. Teach family appropriate use of splints.
Fixation	Surgical reduction of a fracture or skeletal deformity with an internal or external pin or fixation device	Fractures, skeletal deformities	No additional care for internal fixation. External fixation: perform pin care as prescribed by the surgeon. Assess for excess drainage or pin slippage, notifying physician if this occurs. Velcro or snaps on sleeves and pant legs help with dressing.
Cold therapy	Application of ice bags, commercial cold packs, or cold compresses	Most often used in acute injuries to cause vasoconstriction, thereby decreasing pain and swelling	Apply for 20 to 30 minutes, then remove for 1 hour, then reapply for 20 to 30 minutes. Discontinue when numbness occurs. Place a towel between the cold pack and the skin to prevent thermal injury.
Crutches	Ambulatory devices that transfer body weight from lower to upper extremities	Used whenever weight bearing is contraindicated	Top of crutch should reach 2 to 3 fingerbreadths below the axillae to prevent nerve palsy. Teach child appropriate ambulation with crutches or reinforce teaching if performed by physical therapist.

Treatment	Explanation	Indication	Nursing Implications
Physical therapy, occupational therapy	Physical therapy focuses on attainment or improvement of gross motor skills. Occupational therapy focuses on refinement of fine motor skills, feeding, and activities of daily living.	Restore function after injury or surgery; promote developmental activities when limb use is compromised, as in limb deficiency	Provide follow-through with prescribed exercises or supportive equipment. Success of therapy is dependent upon continued compliance with the prescribed regimen. Ensure adequate communication exists within the interdisciplinary team.
Orthotics, braces	Adaptive positioning devices specially fitted for each child by the physical or occupational therapist or orthotist. Used to maintain proper body or extremity alignment, improve mobility, and prevent contractures.	Used to immobilize a body part or prevent deformity through positioning. Used to treat developmental dysplasia of the hip and scoliosis; also may be used for a period of time after cast removal.	Provide frequent assessments of skin covered by the device to avoid skin breakdown. Cotton undergarment worn under the brace helps to maintain skin integrity. Follow the therapist's schedule of recommended "on" and "off" times. Encourage families to comply with use.

DRUG GUIDE 44.1 COMMON DRUGS FOR MUSCULOSKELETAL DISORDERS

Medication	Action	Indication	Nursing Implications
Benzodiazepines (diazepam, lorazepam)	Antianxiety drugs that also have the effect of skeletal muscle relaxation	Treatment of muscle spasms associated with traction or casting	Monitor sedation level. May cause dizziness. Paradoxical excitement may occur. Assess for improvements in spasms.
Acetaminophen	Blocks pain impulses in response to inhibition of prostaglandin synthesis	Relief of mild pain if used alone, moderate or severe pain if used with a narcotic analgesic	Often combined with a narcotic such as codeine or oxycodone for increased analgesic effect. Monitor pain levels and response to medication.
Narcotic analgesics	Act on receptors in the brain to alter perception of pain	Relief of moderate to severe pain associated with injuries, orthopedic procedures	Assess pain location, quality, intensity, and duration. Assess respiratory rate prior to and periodically after administration. Monitor sedation level. May cause nausea, vomiting, constipation, pupil constriction.
Nonsteroidal anti-inflammatory drugs (NSAIDs: ibuprofen, ketorolac)	Inhibit prostaglandin synthesis, having a direct inhibitory effect on pain perception	Relief of mild to moderate pain, treatment of Legg-Calvé-Perthes disease	Monitor for nausea, vomiting, diarrhea, constipation. Administer with water or food to decrease GI upset.
Bisphosphonate: IV—pamidronate, zoledronic acid; oral—alendronate, risedronate	Increase bone mineral density	Decrease incidence of fractures in moderate to severe osteogenesis imperfecta	IV: given at 4-month intervals, causes a decrease in serum calcium level, influenza-like reaction with first IV dose. Oral: side effects include heartburn, regurgitation, upper abdominal discomfort.

Casts

Casts are used to **immobilize** a bone that has been injured or a diseased joint. When a fracture has occurred, a cast serves to hold the bone in reduction, thus preventing deformity as the fracture heals. Casts are constructed of a hard material, traditionally plaster but now more commonly fiberglass. The hard nature of the cast keeps the bone aligned so that healing may occur more quickly. In a fracture that would heal on its own without specific immobilization, a cast may be used to reduce pain and to allow the child increased mobility. The choice of cast material and type of cast will be determined by the pediatrician or orthopedic surgeon. Table 44.1 shows selected casts used in children.

Traction

Traction, another common method of immobilization, may be used to reduce and/or immobilize a fracture, to align an injured extremity, and to allow the extremity to be restored to its normal length. Traction may also reduce pain by decreasing the incidence of muscle spasm. In running traction, the weight pulls directly on the extremity in only one plane. This may be achieved with either skin or skeletal traction. In balanced suspension traction, additional weights are used to provide a counterbalance to the force of traction. This allows for constant pull on the extremity even if the child changes position somewhat. Comparison Chart 44.1 discusses skin versus skeletal traction.

External Fixation

External fixation may be used for complicated fractures, especially open fractures with soft tissue damage. A series of pins or wires are inserted into bone and then attached to an external frame. The fixator apparatus may be adjusted as needed by the health care provider. Once the desired level of correction is achieved, no further adjustment occurs and the bone is allowed to heal. Advantages of external fixation include increased patient

TABLE 44.1   SELECTED CASTS USED IN CHILDREN

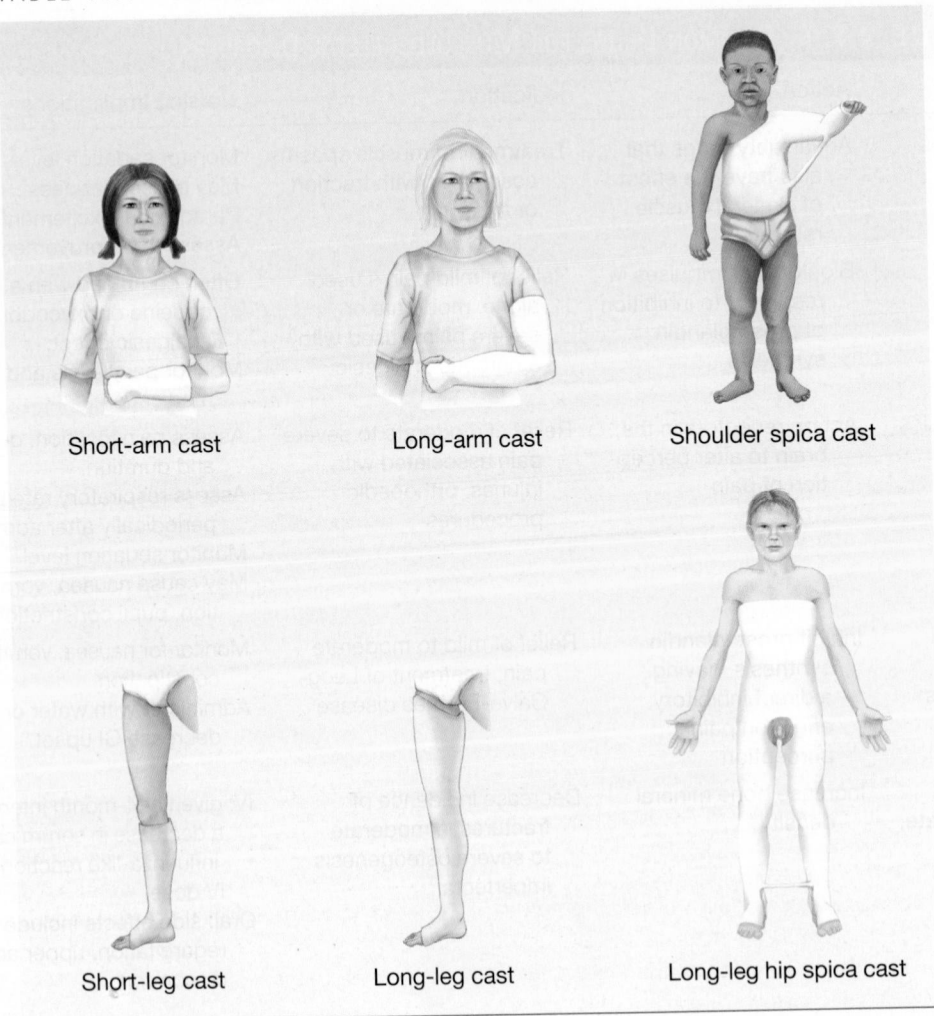

Short-arm cast

Long-arm cast

Shoulder spica cast

Short-leg cast

Long-leg cast

Long-leg hip spica cast

COMPARISON CHART 44.1 SKIN VERSUS SKELETAL TRACTION

	Skin Traction	Skeletal Traction
Application of force	To the skin via strips or tapes secured with Ace bandages or traction boots	To the body part directly by fixation into or through the bone
Length of treatment	Usually limited	Allows for longer periods of traction
Amount of force	Less	More

comfort and improved function of muscles and joints when complicated fracture occurs.

NURSING PROCESS OVERVIEW FOR THE CHILD WITH A MUSCULOSKELETAL DISORDER

Care of the child with a musculoskeletal disorder includes assessment, nursing diagnosis, planning, interventions, and evaluation. There are a number of general concepts related to the nursing process that may be applied to musculoskeletal dysfunction in children. The nursing care of immobilized children is similar to that of adults, yet developmental and age-appropriate effects must be taken into account. Prevention of complications is a key nursing function. Nursing Care Plan Overview 44.1 gives interventions related to prevention of complications. Particular care related to casts, traction, and fixators is discussed below.

Assessment

Assessment of musculoskeletal dysfunction in children includes health history, physical examination, and laboratory and diagnostic testing.

Remember Dakota, the 2-year-old with right arm pain and refusal to use his arm? What additional health history and physical examination assessment information should the nurse obtain?

Health History

The health history comprises past medical history, family history, and history of present illness (when the symptoms started and how they have progressed) as well as treatments used at home. The past medical history might be significant for musculoskeletal congenital anomaly or orthopedic injury during the birthing process. Breech delivery may be associated with developmental dysplasia of the hip. Determine history related to attainment of developmental milestones, such as walking and whether or not the child participates in sports. Inquire about the child's usual level of physical activity, participation in sports, and use of

protective equipment. Family history may be positive for orthopedic problems. When eliciting the history of the present illness, inquire about the following:

• Limp or other changes in gait
• Recent trauma (determine the mechanism of injury)
• Recent strenuous exercise
• Fever
• Weakness
• Alteration in muscle tone
• Areas of redness or swelling

Physical Examination

Physical examination of the musculoskeletal system consists of inspection, observation, and palpation.

Inspection and Observation

Observe the child's posture and alignment of the trunk. Inspect extremities for symmetry and positioning and for absence, duplication, or webbing of any digits. Note any obvious extremity deformity or limb-length discrepancy. Inspect skin for redness, warmth, bruises, and puncture sites. Observe gait in the child who has achieved the developmental skill of walking. Note refusal to walk, limp, in-toeing, out-toeing, or foot slap. Inspect injured joints for ecchymosis or swelling. In the injured extremity, note color of fingertips or toes. Observe spontaneous range of motion. Perform scoliosis screening to determine spinal alignment. Note symmetry of thigh folds.

Palpation

Palpate the clavicles in the newborn or young infant for tenderness or a bump that indicates callus formation with clavicle fracture. Perform active range of motion to determine if a joint position is fixed (e.g., clubfoot). Palpate the affected joint or extremity to detect warmth or tenderness. In the injured child or the child with a cast or splint, thoroughly assess the neurovascular status of the affected extremities. Palpate the fingers or toes for warmth. Determine the capillary refill time. Note presence of sensation or motion. Evaluate muscle strength. Palpate pulses distal to the injury, noting their strength and quality. Perform the Ortolani and Barlow maneuvers to assess for developmental dysplasia of the hip.

(text continues on page 1462)

Nursing Care Plan 44.1

OVERVIEW FOR THE CHILD WITH A MUSCULOSKELETAL DISORDER

NURSING DIAGNOSIS: Impaired physical mobility related to injury, pain, or weakness as evidenced by inability to move an extremity, to ambulate, or to move without limitations

Outcome Identification and Evaluation
Child will engage in physical activities within limits of injury or disease: *child will assist with transfers and positioning in bed and/or participate in prescribed bed exercises.*

Intervention: Maximizing Physical Mobility
- Assess child's ability to move based upon injury or disease and within limits of prescribed treatment *to determine baseline.*
- Prior to prescribed exercise or major position changes, ensure that pain medication is given: *relief of pain increases child's ability to tolerate and participate in activity.*
- Use passive and active range-of-motion exercises and teach child and family how to perform them *to facilitate joint mobility and muscle development (active ROM) and to help increase mobility (within limits of restrictions related to injury or prescribed treatment).*
- Praise accomplishments and emphasize child's abilities *to improve self-esteem and encourage feelings of confidence and competence.*
- Teach child and family necessary care related to mobility issues *so the family can continue with these measures at home.*

NURSING DIAGNOSIS: Risk for constipation related to immobility and/or use of narcotic analgesics

Outcome Identification and Evaluation
Child will demonstrate adequate stool passage, *will pass soft, formed stool every 1 to 3 days without straining or other adverse effects.*

Intervention: Promoting Appropriate Bowel Elimination
- Assess usual pattern of stooling *to determine baseline and identify potential problems with elimination.*
- Palpate for abdominal fullness and auscultate for bowel sounds *to assess for bowel function and presence of constipation.*
- Encourage fiber intake *to increase frequency of stools.*
- Ensure adequate fluid intake *to prevent formation of hard, dry stools.*
- Encourage activity within child's limits or restrictions *as even minimal activity increases peristalsis.*

NURSING DIAGNOSIS: Self-care deficit related to immobility as evidenced by inability to perform hygiene care and transfer self independently

Outcome Identification and Evaluation
Child will demonstrate ability to care for self within age parameters and limits of disease: *child is able to feed, dress, and manage elimination within limits of injury or disease and age.*

Intervention: Maximizing Self-care
- Introduce child and family to self-help methods as soon as possible *to promote independence from the beginning.*
- Encourage family and staff to allow child to do as much as possible *to allow child to gain confidence and independence.*
- Collaborate with physical therapy and occupational therapy as needed to provide child and family with appropriate tools to modify environment and methods to promote transferring and self-care *to allow for maximum functioning.*
- Praise accomplishments and emphasize child's abilities *to improve self-esteem and encourage feelings of confidence and competence.*
- Balance activity with periods to rest *to reduce fatigue and increase energy available for self-care.*

Nursing Care Plan 44.1 (continued)

NURSING DIAGNOSIS: Risk for impaired skin integrity related to immobility, casting, traction, use of braces or adaptive devices

Outcome Identification and Evaluation
Child's skin will remain intact, *without evidence of redness or breakdown.*

Intervention: Promoting Skin Integrity
- Monitor condition of entire skin surface at least daily *to provide baseline and allow for early identification of areas at risk.*
- Avoid excessive friction or harsh cleaning products *that may increase risk of breakdown in child with susceptible skin.*
- Keep child's skin free from stool and urine *to decrease risk of breakdown.*
- Keep linen free from food crumbs and wrinkles *to prevent pressure areas from forming.*
- Change child's position frequently *to decrease pressure on susceptible areas.*
- Monitor condition of skin affected by braces or adaptive equipment frequently *to prevent skin breakdown related to poor fit.*

For the child in traction:
- Pad bony prominences with cotton padding before applying traction *to protect skin from injury.*
- Gently massage child's back and sacrum with lotion *to stimulate circulation.*

For the child in a spica cast:
- Apply plastic wrap to the perineal edges of the cast *to prevent soiling of cast edges, which can contribute to cast breakdown.*
- Use a fracture bedpan *to facilitate toileting without soiling cast.*
- For the child still in diapers, tuck a smaller diaper under the perineal edges of cast and cover with a larger diaper *to prevent cast soiling.*

NURSING DIAGNOSIS: Deficient knowledge related to cast care, activity restrictions, or other prescribed treatment as evidenced by verbalization, questions, or actions demonstrating lack of understanding regarding child's condition or care

Outcome Identification and Evaluation
Child and family will demonstrate accurate understanding about condition and course of treatment *through verbalization and return demonstration.*

Intervention: Providing Patient and Family Teaching
- Assess child's and family's willingness to learn: *child and family must be willing to learn for teaching to be effective.*
- Provide teaching at an appropriate level for the child and family (depends on age of child, physical condition, memory) *to ensure understanding.*
- Teach in short sessions: *many short sessions are more helpful than one long session.*
- Repeat information *to give family and child time to learn and understand.*
- Provide reinforcement and rewards *to facilitate the teaching/learning process.*
- Use multiple modes of learning involving many senses (provide written, verbal, demonstration, and videos) when possible: *child and family are more likely to retain information when presented in different ways using many senses.*

NURSING DIAGNOSIS: Risk for delayed development related to immobility, alterations in extremities

Outcome Identification and Evaluation
Development will be enhanced; *child will make continued progress toward developmental milestones and will not show regression in abilities.*

Intervention: Promoting Development
- Screen for developmental capabilities *to determine child's current level of functioning.*
- Offer age-appropriate toys, play, and activities (including gross motor) *to encourage further development.*
- Perform exercises or interventions as prescribed by physical or occupational therapist: *repeat participation in those activities helps to promote function and acquisition of developmental skills.*
- Provide support to families: *immobility and extremity deficits may lead to slow progress in achieving developmental milestones, so ongoing motivation is needed.*

▶ *Take* NOTE!

Assess the injured site last, and do so gently.

Laboratory and Diagnostic Testing
Common Laboratory and Diagnostic Tests 44.1 explains the laboratory and diagnostic tests most commonly used when considering musculoskeletal disorders. The tests can assist the physician in diagnosing a disorder and/or be used as guidelines in determining ongoing treatment. Some of the tests are obtained by laboratory or non-nursing personnel, while others might be obtained by the nurse. In either instance the nurse should be familiar with how the tests are obtained, what they are used for, and normal versus abnormal results. This knowledge will also be necessary when providing patient and family education related to the tests.

Nursing Diagnoses, Goals, Interventions, and Evaluation
Upon completion of a thorough assessment, the nurse might identify several nursing diagnoses, including:

• Pain (see Chapter 35)
• Impaired physical mobility
• Risk for constipation
• Self-care deficit
• Risk for impaired skin integrity
• Deficient knowledge
• Risk for developmental delay

After completing an assessment of Dakota, the nurse noted the following: the history revealed he had been sledding with his older brother the day before. Upon examination, bruising and swelling of the right arm are noted, with point tenderness at the wrist. Based on the assessment findings, what would your top three nursing diagnoses be for Dakota?

Nursing goals, interventions, and evaluation for the child with musculoskeletal dysfunction are based on the nursing diagnoses (see Nursing Care Plan Overview 44.1). The nursing care plan may be used as a guide in planning nursing care for the child with a musculoskeletal disorder. The care plan includes many nursing diagnoses that are applicable to the child or adolescent. Children's responses to musculoskeletal dysfunction and its treatment will vary, and nursing care should be individualized based on the child's and family's responses to illness.

The nursing care of immobilized children is similar to that of adults but developmental and age-appropriate effects must be taken into account. Prevention of complications is a key nursing function. Refer to Nursing Care

Plan 44.1 for interventions related to prevention of complications. Additional information about nursing care related to certain disorders will be included later in the chapter as it relates to specific disorders. Refer to Chapter 35 for nursing interventions related to pain management. Particular care related to casts, traction, and external fixation is discussed below.

Based on your top three nursing diagnoses for Dakota, describe appropriate nursing interventions.

Assisting with Cast Application
Before cast or splint application, perform baseline neurovascular assessment for comparison after immobilization. Include:

• Color (note cyanosis or other discoloration)
• Movement (note inability to move fingers or toes)
• Sensation (note whether loss of sensation is present)
• Edema
• Quality of pulses

Enlist the cooperation of the child and reduce his or her fear by showing the child the cast materials and using an age-appropriate approach to describe cast application. Premedicate as ordered to reduce pain when manual traction is applied to align the bone. Use **distraction** throughout cast application and assist with application of the cast or splint (Fig. 44.4).

▶ *Take* NOTE!

Modern fiberglass cast materials are available in a variety of colors, as well as a few patterns. Allowing the child to choose the color will increase the child's cooperation with the procedure.

After the cast or splint is applied, drying time will vary based on the type of material used. Splints and fiberglass casts usually take only a few minutes to dry and will cause a very warm feeling inside the cast, so warn the child that it will begin to feel very warm. Plaster requires 24 to 48 hours to dry. Take care not to cause depressions in the plaster cast while drying, as those may cause skin pressure and breakdown. Instruct the child and family to keep the cast still, positioning it with pillows as needed.

Caring for the Child With a Cast
Perform frequent neurovascular checks of the casted extremity to identify signs of compromise early. These signs include:

• Increased pain
• Increased edema
• Pale or blue color

COMMON LABORATORY AND DIAGNOSTIC TESTS 44.1

Test	Explanation	Indication	Nursing Implications
X-rays	Radiographic image; usually two views are obtained of the affected extremity (lateral and anteroposterior)	To detect fractures and other anomalies	Child must cooperate and hold still. Enlist the family's help in calming the child.
Ultrasound	Use of sound waves to locate the depth and structure within soft tissues and fluid	To diagnose toxic synovitis, Legg-Calvé-Perthes disease, slipped capital femoral epiphysis, osteomyelitis, fractures, ligament or soft tissue injuries. Monitoring and follow-up of fractures and remodeling.	Better tolerated by nonsedated children than CT or MRI. Can be performed with a portable unit at bedside.
Computed tomography (CT)	Noninvasive x-ray study that looks at tissue density and structures. Images a "slice" of tissue.	To evaluate the extent of osteomyelitis, Legg-Calvé-Perthes disease, or slipped capital femoral epiphysis or to rule out other problems	Machine is large and can be frightening to children. Procedure can be lengthy and child must remain still. If unable to do so, sedation may be necessary. If performed with contrast medium, assess for allergy. Encourage fluids after the procedure if not contraindicated.
Magnetic resonance imaging (MRI)	Based on how hydrogen atoms behave in a magnetic field when disturbed by radio-frequency signals. Does not require ionizing radiation. Provides a 3D view of the body part being scanned.	To assess hard and soft tissue, as well as bone marrow, to evaluate extent of osteomyelitis, Legg-Calvé-Perthes disease, or slipped capital femoral epiphysis, or to rule out other problems	Remove all metal objects from the child. Child must remain motionless for entire scan; parent can stay in room with child. Younger children will require sedation in order to be still. A loud thumping sound occurs inside the machine during the scan procedure, and this can be frightening to children.
Arthrography	X-ray of a joint after direct injection with a radiopaque substance	To assess ligaments, muscles, tendons, and cartilage, particularly after injury	Should not be performed if joint infection is present. Apply cold therapy afterward and assess for swelling and pain. Crepitus may be present in the joint for 1 to 2 days after procedure.
Complete blood count	Evaluates hemoglobin and hematocrit, white blood cell count, platelet count	To evaluate hemoglobin and hematocrit with fracture with potential bleeding. To determine infection in osteomyelitis, septic arthritis, and toxic synovitis.	Normal values vary according to age and gender. White blood cell count differential is helpful in evaluating for infection. May be affected by myelosuppressive drugs.
Erythrocyte sedimentation rate	Nonspecific test used to determine presence of infection or inflammation	To evaluate for osteomyelitis or septic arthritis	Send sample to laboratory immediately; if allowed to stand for longer than 3 hours, may produce falsely low result.

(continued)

COMMON LABORATORY AND DIAGNOSTIC TESTS 44.1 (continued)

Test	Explanation	Indications	Nursing Implications
C-reactive protein	Measures acute-phase reactant protein indicative of inflammatory process	To evaluate for osteomyelitis or septic arthritis	Anti-inflammatory drugs may cause decreased levels. More sensitive and rapidly responsive than erythrocyte sedimentation rate.
Blood culture	To determine presence of bacteria in blood	May be positive with septic arthritis or osteomyelitis	Transport specimen to laboratory within 30 minutes. Avoid skin contamination of specimen while obtaining it. Cultures should usually be drawn before starting antibiotics, as partial antibiotic treatment may result in negative culture.
Joint fluid aspiration	Aspirated joint fluid is examined for presence of pus and white blood cells; culture is performed.	To evaluate for septic arthritis	Use cold therapy to decrease swelling after aspiration. Apply pressure dressing to prevent hematoma formation or fluid re-collection. Assess for fever and joint pain or edema, which may indicate infection. Positive fluid culture indicates a bacterial infection in the joint. May also be used to relieve pressure in the joint space.

• Skin coolness
• Numbness or tingling
• Prolonged capillary refill
• Decreased pulse strength (or absence of pulse)

Notify the physician of changes in neurovascular status or odor or drainage from the cast.

Fiberglass casts usually have a soft fabric edge, so they usually do not cause skin rubbing at the edges of the cast. On the other hand, plaster casts require special treatment of the cast edge to prevent skin rubbing. This may be accomplished through a technique called petaling: cut rounded-edge strips of moleskin or another soft material with an adhesive backing and apply them to the edge of cast, as shown in Figure 44.5.

► **Take** NOTE!

Persistent complaints of pain may indicate compromised skin integrity under the cast.

FIGURE 44.4 Assist with cast application by distracting or comforting the child.

To petal a cast:

1. Cut several strips of adhesive tape or moleskin three to four inches in length. Use one inch tape for smaller areas (e.g., infant's foot) and two inch tape for larger areas (e.g., adolescent's waist).

2. Round one end of each strip to keep the corners from rolling.

3. Apply the first strip by tucking the straight end inside the cast and by bringing the rounded end over the cast edge to the outside.

4. Repeat the procedure, overlapping each additional strip, until all rough edges are completely covered.

FIGURE 44.5 Petaling the cast.

Position the child with the casted extremity elevated on pillows. Ice may be applied during the first 24 to 48 hours after casting if needed. Teaching the child to use crutches is an important nursing intervention for any child with lower extremity immobilization so that the child can maintain mobility (Fig. 44.6). Provide home care instructions to the family about cast care (Teaching Guidelines 44.1).

Assisting With Cast Removal

Children may be frightened by cast removal. Prepare the child using age-appropriate terminology:

- The cast cutter will make a loud noise (Fig. 44.7).
- The skin or extremity will not be injured (demonstrate by touching the cast cutter lightly to your palm).
- The child will feel warmth or vibration during cast removal.

Teaching Guidelines 44.2 gives instructions related to skin care after cast removal.

Caring for the Child in Traction

Nursing care of the child in any type of traction focuses not only on appropriate application and maintenance of traction but also on promoting normal growth and development and preventing complications (see Table 44.2). Apply skin traction over intact skin only so that the pull of the traction is effective. Prepare the skin with an appropriate adhesive before applying the traction tapes to ensure that the tapes adhere well, preventing skin friction. After application of the traction tapes, apply the elastic bandage

FIGURE 44.6 Reinforce appropriate crutch walking for children with lower extremity immobilization.

TEACHING GUIDELINES 44.1

Home Cast Care

- For the first 48 hours, elevate the extremity above the level of the heart and apply cold therapy for 20 to 30 minutes, then off 1 hour, and repeat.
- Assess for swelling, and have the child wiggle the fingers or toes hourly.
- For itching inside the cast:
  - Never insert anything into the cast for the purposes of scratching.
  - Blow cool air in from a hair dryer set on the lowest setting.
  - Do not use lotions or powders.
- Check the skin at the cast edges daily for irritation.
- Protect the cast from wetness.
- Apply a plastic bag around cast and tape securely for bathing or showering.
- Call the physician if:
  - The casted extremity is cool to the touch.
  - The child cannot move the fingers or toes.
  - Severe pain occurs when the child attempts to move the fingers or toes.
  - Persistent numbness or tingling occurs.
  - Drainage or a foul smell comes from under the cast.
  - Severe itching occurs inside the cast.
  - The child runs a fever greater than 101.5° F for longer than 24 hours.
  - Skin edges are red and swollen or exhibit breakdown.
  - The cast gets wet or is cracked, split, or softened.

Modified from DiFazio, R., & Atkinson, R. (2005). Extremity fractures in children: When is it an emergency? *Journal of Pediatric Nursing, 20*(4), 298–304.

or use the foam boot. Attach the traction spreader block and then apply the prescribed amount of weight via a rope attached to the spreader block. Ensure that the rope moves without obstruction and that the weights hang freely without touching the floor.

In skeletal traction, apply weight via ropes attached to the skeletal pins. The pin sites should be treated as surgical wounds (see section on pin site care). Protect the exposed ends of the pins to avoid injury. Whether skin or skeletal traction is used, be sure that constant and even traction is maintained.

▶ **Take** NOTE!

Avoid sudden bumping or movement of the bed: this can disturb traction alignment and cause additional pain to the child as the weights are jostled.

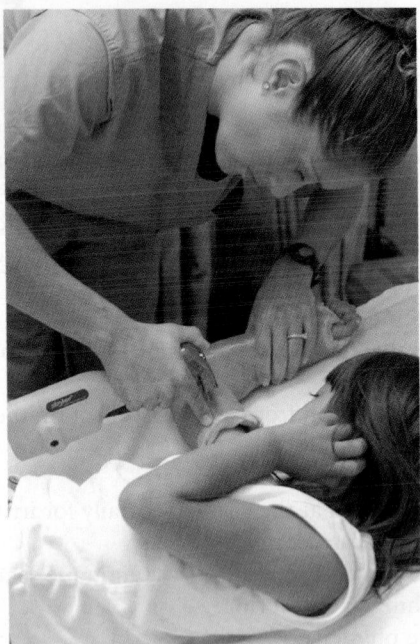

FIGURE 44.7 The loud noise of the cast saw may frighten the child.

Preventing Complications

Refer to Nursing Care Plan 44.1 for interventions related to pain management and prevention of complications of immobility such as skin integrity impairment. To prevent contractures and atrophy that may result from disuse of muscles, ensure that unaffected extremities are exercised. Assist the child to exercise the unaffected joints and to use the unaffected extremity if this does not disrupt traction alignment. Promote use of a trapeze if not contraindicated to involve the child in repositioning and assist with movement. Encourage deep-breathing exercises to prevent the pulmonary complications of long-term immobilization.

TEACHING GUIDELINES 44.2

Skin Care After Cast Removal

- Brown, flaky skin is normal and occurs as dead skin and secretions accumulate under the cast.
- Soak with warm water daily.
- Wash with warm soapy water, avoiding excessive rubbing, which may traumatize the skin.
- Discourage the child from scratching the dry skin.
- Apply moisturizing lotion to relieve dry skin.
- Encourage activity to regain strength and motion of extremity.

Promote normal growth and development by:

- Placing age-appropriate toys within the child's reach
- Encouraging visits from friends
- Providing diversional activities such as drawing, coloring, or video games (Fig. 44.8)

> ▶ **Take** NOTE!
>
> *Ongoing, careful neurovascular assessments are critical in the child with a cast or in skeletal traction. Notify the physician immediately if these signs of compartment syndrome occur: extreme pain (out of proportion to the situation), pain with passive range of motion of digits, distal extremity pallor, inability to move digits, loss of pulses.*

Caring for the Child With an External Fixator

In addition to routine neurovascular assessment, elevate the extremity to prevent swelling. The fixator may be moved by grasping the frame, as the fixator can tolerate ordinary movement. Encourage weight bearing as prescribed. Provide appropriate education to the child and family. Encourage the child to look at the apparatus.

Providing Pin Care

Whether pins are inserted for skeletal traction or as part of an external fixator (see section on fractures), keeping the pin sites clean is important to prevent infection. Perform pin site care according to institutional policy or the physician's orders. Cleaning of the pin sites prevents infection by promoting comfort and preventing healing skin from adhering to the metal pin. Notify the orthopedic surgeon if signs of pin site infection are present or if pin slippage occurs.

Thus far, attempts to obtain evidence supporting the various types of pin site care have been unsuccessful. Certain physicians prefer the site to be cleaned with normal saline; others choose a solution with antibacterial properties. Some institutions recommend removal of all crusts formed on the skin around the pin; others do not. The rationale for crust removal is to promote free drainage and prevent the surrounding skin from adhering to the pin. A keyhole dressing may be necessary around the pin if drainage is present. No matter which procedure is ordered or preferred, perform pin care as necessary to prevent infection at the pin site. The Ilizarov fixator uses wires that are thinner than ordinary pins, so simply cleansing by showering is usually sufficient to keep the pin site clean. If drainage is present, the skin around the wires can be cleansed with a dry gauze pad.

TABLE 44.2 TYPES OF TRACTION AND NURSING IMPLICATIONS

Type of Traction	Description	Nursing Implications
Bryant's traction Knees slightly flexed Buttocks slightly elevated and clear of bed	Both legs are extended vertically, with child's weight serving as countertraction. Skin traction is applied to both legs. Used for infants with femur fracture or developmental dysplasia of the hip.	Maintain appropriate position. Ensure heels and ankles are free from pressure. Rewrap elastic bandages as ordered.
Russell's traction Buck's traction 	Skin traction for femur fracture, hip and knee contractures. Uses a knee sling. In split Russell's traction, a portion of the traction weight may be redistributed via a pulley from the sling to the head of the bed (used for femur fracture, Legg-Calvé-Perthes disease, slipped capital femoral epiphysis). Skin traction for hip and knee contractures, Legg-Calvé-Perthes disease, slipped capital femoral epiphysis. Traction force delivered in straight line.	Wrap bandages from ankle to thigh on children less than age 2 years, from ankle to knee on children older than 2 years. Use a foot support to prevent foot drop. Ensure heel is free from bed. Assess popliteal region for skin breakdown from the sling. Mark leg to ensure proper replacement of sling. Remove traction boot every 8 hours to assess skin. Leg may be slightly abducted.
Cervical skin traction 	Skin traction applied with a skin strap (head halter). Used for neck sprains/strains, torticollis, or nerve trauma.	Ensure that head halter or skin strap does not place pressure on ears or throat. Limit of 5 to 7 pounds weight.
Side-arm 90-90 	Skin traction for humerus fractures and injuries to the shoulder girdle. Used to treat fractures of the humerus and injuries in or around the shoulder girdle.	Maintain elbow flexed at 90 degrees. Fingers and hand may feel cool because of elevation. Child may turn to affected side only.

(continued)

TABLE 44.2 TYPES OF TRACTION AND NURSING IMPLICATIONS (continued)

Type of Traction	Description	Nursing Implications
Dunlop side-arm 00-90	Skeletal traction through an olecranon screw or pin in distal humerus. Lower arm is held in balanced suspension.	See side-arm 90-90. In addition, provide appropriate pin site care.
90-90 traction	For femur fracture reduction when skin traction is inadequate. Skeletal traction with force applied through pin in distal femur.	A foam boot may be used for suspension of the lower leg. Force of traction applied to femur via the pin. The amount of weight used is just enough to hold lower limb suspended.
Cervical skeletal tongs	Tongs attached to skull via pins. Used with fractures or dislocations of the cervical or high thoracic vertebrae.	Assess frequently for increased pain, respiratory distress, and cranial nerve or brachial plexus injury. Place on Stryker frame or specially equipped bed to ease positioning without disruption of alignment.
Halo traction	Metal halo attached to skull via pins. Used for cervical or high thoracic vertebrae fracture or dislocation and for postoperative immobilization following cervical fusion.	Refer to nursing implications for cervical tongs. Tape small wrench to front of brace so that front panel can be quickly removed in an emergency. May become ambulatory in this type of traction; will be top-heavy so may need assistance with balance.
Balanced suspension traction	Used for femur, hip, or tibial fracture. Thomas splint suspends the thigh while the Pearson attachment allows knee flexion and supports the leg below the knee.	Avoid pressure to popliteal area.

FIGURE 44.8 Provide age-appropriate diversional activities and schoolwork for children confined to bed in traction.

Congenital and Developmental Disorders

Congenital anomalies of the musculoskeletal system are usually readily identified at birth. Congenital structural anomalies involving the skeleton include pectus excavatum, pectus carinatum, limb deficiencies, polydactyly or syndactyly, metatarsus adductus, congenital clubfoot, and osteogenesis imperfecta. A developmental anomaly that may be diagnosed at birth or later in life is developmental dysplasia of the hip. A muscular condition, torticollis, most often presents as a congenital condition but may also de-velop after birth. Tibia vara is a developmental disorder affecting young children. Rarely, a developmental positional alteration such as genu varum, genu valgum, or pes planus will persist past the usual age of resolution or cause the child pain. If those situations occur, bracing, orthotics, or surgical correction may become necessary.

▶ PECTUS EXCAVATUM

Pectus excavatum and pectus carinatum are anterior chest wall deformities. Pectus excavatum, a funnel-shaped chest, accounts for 87% of anterior chest wall deformities (Goretsky et al., 2004). A depression that sinks inward is apparent at the xiphoid process (Fig. 44.9). Pectus carinatum, a protuberance of the chest wall, accounts for only 5% of anterior chest wall deformities. The remainder are mixed deformities.

Pectus excavatum does not resolve as the child grows; rather, it progresses with growth. The chest depression may be minimal or marked. When the pectus is more pronounced, cardiac and pulmonary compression occurs. Symptoms of this compression most often present during puberty, when the pectus quickly worsens. Children may complain of shortness of breath, withdraw from physical activities, and have a poor body image.

Therapeutic Management

Therapeutic management of pectus excavatum involves surgical correction, preferably before puberty, when the

---

EVIDENCE-BASED PRACTICE 44.1
Pin Site Cleaning Methods and Infection Prevention

● **Study**
External fixation (metal pins) is used to immobilize bones while fractures heal. By the nature of pin insertion into the bone, pin sites place the child at risk for development of an infection. Numerous studies have been conducted to evaluate the effectiveness of pin site care. To date, pin site care is usually determined by physician or institution preference. The authors reviewed randomized controlled studies that evaluated the management of pin sites. The interventions reviewed included any type of cleaning method versus no cleaning, sterile versus non-sterile technique, use of massage, and whether or not a dressing was used.

▲ **Findings**
The results were inconclusive. No particular method of pin site care was determined to be statistically significant in reducing infection from orthopedic pins.

■ **Nursing Implications**
Despite the lack of clear insight from this study, it remains important for nurses to continue vigilance regarding pin site care. Ongoing assessment of pin sites for signs of infection and monitoring of the child's temperature are particularly important. Provide pin site care according to the physician's preference or institution's protocol. With the lack of conclusive evidence related to pin site care, nurses caring for pediatric orthopedic patients are in a prime position to develop and execute a well-designed research study related to pin site care.

Temple, J. & Santy, J. (2007). Pin site care for preventing infections associated with external bone fixators and pins. *The Cochrane Library 2007, 4.* Indianapolis: John Wiley & Sons.

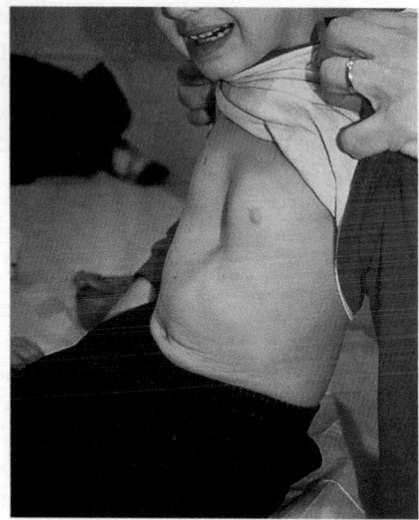

FIGURE 44.9 Pectus excavatum: note the depression in the chest wall at the xiphoid process.

skeleton is more pliable. Various surgical techniques may be used and generally involve either the placement of a surgical steel bar or using a piece of bone in the rib cage to lift the depression. This discussion will focus on care of the child who undergoes surgical steel bar placement for pectus correction.

Nursing Assessment

Elicit the health history, noting progression of the defect and effects on the child's cardiopulmonary function. Note shortness of breath, exercise intolerance, or chest pain. Observe the child's chest for anterior wall deformity, noting depth and severity. Auscultate the lungs to determine the adequacy of aeration. X-rays, computed tomography (CT), or magnetic resonance imaging (MRI) may be used to determine the extent of the anomaly and compression of inner structures.

Nursing Management

Prepare the child preoperatively by allowing a tour of the surgical area and the pediatric intensive care unit. Introduce the child to the pain scale that will be used in the postoperative period.

Postoperatively, nursing management focuses on assessment, protection of the surgical site, and pain management. Auscultate lung sounds frequently to determine the adequacy of aeration and to monitor for development of the complication of pneumothorax. Assess for signs of wound infection that would necessitate removal of the curved bar. Do not allow the child to lie on either side and do not log-roll the child (these positions may disrupt the bar's position). Administer analgesics as needed either intravenously or via the epidural catheter. Teach families that the child will not be allowed to lie on his or her side at home for 4 weeks after the surgery to ensure that the band does not shift. Encourage aerobic activity at home after cleared by the surgeon (this will increase the child's vital capacity, previously hindered by the pectus). The bar will be removed 2 to 4 years after the initial placement.

▶ LIMB DEFICIENCIES

Limb deficiencies, either complete absence of a limb or a portion of it or deformity, occur as the fetus is developing. These defects are attributed to an amniotic band constricting the limb, resulting in either incomplete development or amputation of the limb. Many children born with limb deformities also have developmental craniofacial abnormalities (Morrissy et al., 2006).

Therapeutic management is aimed at improving the child's functional ability. Physical therapy and occupational therapy may be helpful. Adaptive equipment such as a prosthesis may also be prescribed.

Nursing Assessment

Note the extent of limb deformity, providing an accurate description of the presence or absence of a portion of the arm or leg, or missing fingers or toes. Assess the child's ability to use the extremity as a helper (arms) or in ambulation (legs). Determine status of acquisition of developmental skills.

Nursing Management

Reinforce prescribed activities that are meant to improve the child's function. Provide activities in which the child is capable of participating. If the limb deficiency is significant, refer the infant to the local early intervention office as soon as possible after birth. Early intervention, available in all 50 states, is designed to promote development from birth to age 3 years. Absence of a limb or a significant portion of a limb will have a considerable impact on the child's ability to meet developmental milestones as expected.

▶ POLYDACTYLY/SYNDACTYLY

Polydactyly is the presence of extra digits on the hand or foot (Fig. 44.10). It occurs equally in both genders and affects African-Americans more frequently than Caucasians. One third of the time, polydactyly occurs in

FIGURE 44.10 Note additional digits (toes) of polydactyly.

FIGURE 44.11 Metatarsus adductus: note medial deviation of the forefoot.

both the hand and foot (Gore & Spencer, 2004). It usually involves digits at the border of the hand or foot, near the fifth finger or toe. Syndactyly is webbing of the fingers and toes.

Treatment includes tying off the additional digit until it falls off or surgical removal of the digit. No treatment is usually required for syndactyly, though surgical repair is sometimes performed for cosmetic reasons.

Nursing Assessment

Inspect the hands and feet for the presence of extra digits. Note whether the additional digits are soft (without bone) or are full or partial digits with bone present. Note location of webbing.

Nursing Management

If the digit is tied off, observe for expected necrosis of tissue and eventually loss of the extra digit. When surgical removal is necessary, provide routine pre- and postoperative care as appropriate.

▶ METATARSUS ADDUCTUS

Metatarsus adductus, a medial deviation of the forefoot, is one of the most common foot deformities of childhood (Fig. 44.11). It occurs as a result of *in utero* positioning. It occurs as often as once in every 100 live births (Hart et al., 2005). Type I and Type II are usually benign deformities, resolving spontaneously by the age of 3 years. Children with type III deformity usually require manipulation and serial casting, preferably before the age of 8 months. Surgical intervention is rarely needed.

Nursing Assessment

The deformity is usually noted at birth. Note inward deviation of the forefoot. The great and second toes might be separated. Determine forefoot flexibility. Range of motion of the ankle, hindfoot, and midfoot is normal in all

three types. Box 44.1 describes the three types based on flexibility of the forefoot.

Nursing Management

Nursing care for children with type I and II metatarsus adductus is aimed at education and reassurance of the parents. The nursing care for the child with type III is similar to that of the child with clubfoot (see below).

▶ CONGENITAL CLUBFOOT

Congenital clubfoot (also termed congenital talipes equinovarus) is a congenital anomaly that occurs in one to two of 1,000 live births (Hart et al., 2005). Clubfoot consists of:

- Talipes varus (inversion of the heel)
- Talipes equinus (plantarflexion of the foot; the heel is raised and would not strike the ground in a standing position)
- Cavus (plantarflexion of the forefoot on the hindfoot)
- Forefoot adduction with supination (the forefoot is inverted and turned slightly upward)

BOX 44.1   Types of Metatarsus Adductus

- Type I: Forefoot is flexible past neutral actively and passively.
- Type II: Forefoot is flexible passively past neutral, but only to midline actively.
- Type III: Forefoot is rigid and does not correct to midline even with passive stretching.

FIGURE 44.12 Note inverted heel, ankle equinus, and forefoot adduction in this infant with bilateral clubfoot.

The foot resembles the head of a golf club (Fig. 44.12). Half of all cases occur bilaterally. Males are affected two and a half times more frequently than females. The exact etiology of clubfoot is unknown.

Clubfoot may be classified into four categories: postural, neurogenic, syndromic, and idiopathic. Postural clubfoot often resolves with a short series of manipulative casting. Neurogenic clubfoot occurs in infants with myelomeningocele. Clubfoot in association with other syndromes (syndromic) is often resistant to treatment. Idiopathic clubfoot occurs in otherwise normal healthy infants. The approach to treatment is similar regardless of the classification.

Therapeutic Management

The goal of therapeutic management of clubfoot is achievement of a functional foot; treatment starts as soon after birth as possible. Weekly manipulation with serial cast changes is performed; later, cast changes occur every 2 weeks. This approach is successful in about half of all cases. The other infants require corrective shoes or bracing; in some infants, surgical release of soft tissue may be necessary. Following surgery, the foot is immobilized with a cast for up to 12 weeks, and then ankle–foot orthoses or corrective shoes are used for several years.

Complications of clubfoot and its treatment include residual deformity, rocker-bottom foot, awkward gait, weight bearing on the lateral portion of the foot if uncorrected, and disturbance to the epiphysis.

Nursing Assessment

Note family history of foot deformities and obstetric history of breech position. Inspect the foot for position at rest. Perform active range of motion, noting inability to move foot into normal positioning at midline. X-rays are obtained to determine bony abnormality and note progress during treatment.

Nursing Management

Perform neurovascular assessment and cast care as for any disorder requiring casting. Provide emotional support, as treatment often begins in the newborn period and families may have a difficult time adjusting to the diagnosis and treatment required for their new baby. Teach families cast care and later the use of orthotics or braces as prescribed.

▶ OSTEOGENESIS IMPERFECTA

Osteogenesis imperfecta is a genetic bone disorder that results in low bone mass, increased fragility of the bones, and other connective tissue problems such as joint hypermobility, resulting in instability of the joints that may further contribute to fracture occurrence. Dentinogenesis imperfecta may also occur: the tooth enamel wears easily and the teeth become discolored.

The disorder usually occurs as a result of a defect in the collagen type 1 gene, usually through an autosomal recessive or dominant inheritance pattern. The types of osteogenesis imperfecta range from mild to severe connective tissue and bone involvement (Table 44.3). In children with

TABLE 44.3 CLASSIFICATION OF OSTEOGENESIS IMPERFECTA

Classification	Characteristics
I	Common and mild Autosomal dominant Blue sclera Fragile bones, early fractures (by preschool age) Type A without dentinogenesis imperfecta, type B with dentinogenesis
II	Lethal in perinatal period Autosomal recessive Dark-blue sclera
III	Severe Autosomal recessive Normal sclera Fractures at birth with progressive deformity
IV	Moderately severe Autosomal dominant Normal sclera Fragile bones Type A without dentinogenesis imperfecta, type B with dentinogenesis

Zaleske, D. J. (2006). Metabolic and endocrine abnormalities. In R. T. Morrissy & S. L. Weinstein (Eds.), *Lovell & Winter's pediatric orthopaedics* (6th ed.). Philadelphia: Lippincott Williams & Wilkins.

moderate to severe disease, fractures are more likely to occur, and short stature is common. In addition to multiple fractures, additional complications include early hearing loss, acute and chronic pain, scoliosis, and respiratory problems.

> ▶ **Take** NOTE!
>
> *Blue sclera is not diagnostic of osteogenesis imperfecta, but it is a common finding. The sclerae of newborns tend to be bluish, progressing to white over the first few weeks of life. There are some individuals with blue sclerae who do not have osteogenesis imperfecta.*

Therapeutic Management

The goal of medical and surgical management is to decrease the incidence of fractures and maintain mobility. Bisphosphonate administration is used for moderate to severe disease. Fracture care is often required. Physical therapy and occupational therapy prevent contractures and maximize mobility. Standing with bracing is encouraged. Lightweight splints or braces may allow the child to bear weight earlier. Severe cases may require surgical insertion of rods into the long bones.

Nursing Assessment

Elicit a health history, which may reveal a family history of osteogenesis imperfecta, a pattern of frequent fractures, or screaming associated with routine care and handling of the newborn. Inspect the eyes for sclerae that have a blue, purple, or gray tint. Note abnormalities of the primary teeth. Inspect skin for bruising and note joint hypermobility with active range of motion. Laboratory tests may include a skin biopsy (which reveals abnormalities in type 1 collagen) or DNA testing (locating the genetic mutation).

Nursing Management

Handle the child carefully and teach the family to avoid trauma (Teaching Guidelines 44.3). Refer families to the Osteogenesis Imperfecta Foundation (www.oif.org), which provides access to multiple resources as well as clinical trials. An excellent book for families of children with osteogenesis imperfecta is *Children with OI: Strategies to Enhance Performance* by H. L. Cintas and L. H. Gerber.

Encourage safe mobility. Reinforce physical and occupational therapists' recommendations for promotion of fine motor skills and independence in activities of daily living, as well as use of adaptive equipment and appropriate promotion of mobility. Adapted physical education is important to promote mobility and maintain bone and

TEACHING GUIDELINES 44.3

Preventing Injury in Children With Osteogenesis Imperfecta

- Never push or pull on an arm or leg.
- Do not bend an arm or leg into an awkward position.
- Lift a baby by placing one hand under the legs and buttocks and one hand under the shoulders, head, and neck.
- Do not lift a baby's legs by the ankles to change the diaper.
- Do not lift a baby or small child from under the armpits.
- Provide supported positioning.
- If fracture is suspected, handle the limb minimally.

muscle mass. If the child is ambulatory, even with adaptive equipment use, walking is a good form of exercise. Swimming and water therapy are appropriate, allowing independent movement with little fracture risk.

> ▶ **Take** NOTE!
>
> *Use caution when inserting an intravenous line or taking a blood pressure measurement, as pressure on the arm or leg can lead to bruising and fractures.*

▶ DEVELOPMENTAL DYSPLASIA OF THE HIP

Developmental dysplasia of the hip (DDH) refers to abnormalities of the developing hip that include dislocation, subluxation, and dysplasia of the hip joint. In DDH, the femoral head has an abnormal relationship to the acetabulum. Frank dislocation of the hip may occur, in which there is no contact between the femoral head and acetabulum. Subluxation is a partial dislocation, meaning that the acetabulum is not fully seated within the hip joint. Dysplasia refers to an acetabulum that is shallow or sloping instead of cup-shaped. DDH may affect just one or both hips. The dysplastic hip may be provoked to subluxation or dislocated and then reduced again. DDH affects females eight times more often than males (Fig. 44.13).

Pathophysiology

While dislocation may occur during a growth period *in utero*, the laxity of the newborn's hip allows dislocation and relocation of the hip to occur. The hip can develop normally

FIGURE 44.13 Developmental dysplasia of the hip.

only if the femoral head is appropriately and deeply seated within the acetabulum. If subluxation and periodic or continued dislocation occur, then structural changes in the hip's anatomy occur. Continued dysplasia of the hip leads to limited abduction of the hip and contracture of muscles. DDH is more common in females, probably because female hormones contribute to laxity of the ligaments. Mechanical factors such as breech positioning or the presence of oligohydramnios also contribute to the development of DDH. Genetic factors also play a role: there is an increased incidence of DDH among persons of Native American and Lapp descent, with very low rates among people of African or southern Chinese heritage. Complications of DDH include avascular necrosis of the femoral head, loss of range of motion, recurrently unstable hip, femoral nerve palsy, leg-length discrepancy, and early osteoarthritis.

Therapeutic Management

The goal of therapeutic management is to maintain the hip joint in reduction so that the femoral head and acetabulum can develop properly.

Treatment varies based upon the child's age and the severity of DDH. Infants younger than 6 months of age may be treated with a Pavlik harness, which reduces and stabilizes the hip by preventing hip extension and adduction. The Pavlik harness is successful in the treatment of DDH in the majority of infants less than 6 months of age if it is used on a full-time basis and applied properly (Weinstein, 2006). Children from 6 months to 2 years of age often require closed reduction. Skin or skeletal traction may be used first to gradually stretch the associated soft tissue structures. Closed reduction occurs under general anesthesia, with the hip being gently maneuvered back into the acetabulum. A spica cast worn for 12 weeks maintains reduction of the hip. After the cast is removed, the child must wear an abduction brace full-time (except for baths) for 2 months. Then the brace is worn at night and during naps until development of the acetabulum is normal. Children over 2 years of age or those who have failed to respond to prior treatment require an open surgical reduction followed by a period of casting (Weinstein, 2006).

Nursing Assessment

Nursing assessment of children with DDH includes obtaining a health history and inspecting, observing, and palpating for findings common to DDH.

Health History

Assess the health history for risk factors such as:

• Family history of DDH
• Female gender
• Oligohydramnios or breech birth
• Native American or Laplander descent
• Associated lower limb deformity or other congenital musculoskeletal deformity

Previously undiagnosed older children may complain of hip pain.

Physical Assessment

The physical examination for DDH includes inspection, observation, and palpation. Since DDH is a developmental process, ongoing screening assessments are required throughout at least the first several months of the infant's life.

Inspection and Observation

Ensure that the infant is on a flat surface and is relaxed. Note asymmetry of thigh or gluteal folds with the infant in a prone position. Document shortening of affected femur observed as limb-length discrepancy. Older children may exhibit **Trendelenburg gait**. Figure 44.14 illustrates these assessments.

Palpation

Note limited hip abduction when passive range of motion is performed. Abduction should ordinarily occur to 75 degrees and adduction to within 30 degrees with the infant's pelvis stabilized. Perform Barlow and Ortolani tests, noting a "clunk" as the femoral head dislocates or reduces back into the acetabulum. Force is not necessary when performing the Barlow and Ortolani maneuvers (see Fig. 44.14).

▶ ***Take*** NOTE!

A higher-pitched "click" may occur with flexion or extension of the hip. When assessing for DDH, do not confuse this benign, adventitial sound with a true "clunk."

Diagnostic Testing

Ultrasound of the hip allows for visualization of the femoral head and the outer edge of the acetabulum. Plain hip x-rays may be used in the infant or child over 6 months of age.

A. Assess for asymmetry of thigh and gluteal folds.

B. Assess for unequal knee height related to femur shortening.

C. Note limitation in hip abduction.

D. Positive Trendelenburg sign: note pelvis/hip drops when leg is raised.

E. Assess for "clunk" with the Ortolani maneuver.

FIGURE 44.14 Assessment techniques for developmental dysplasia of the hip.

Nursing Management

Earlier recognition of hip dysplasia with earlier harness use results in better correction of the anomaly. Excellent assessment skills and reporting of any abnormal findings are critical. Initially, the infant will need to wear the Pavlik harness continuously (Fig. 44.15). The physician makes all appropriate adjustments to the harness when applied so that the hips are held in the optimal position for appropriate development. Teach parents use of the harness and assessment of the baby's skin. If started early, harness use usually continues for about 3 months (Teaching Guidelines 44.4). Breastfeeding can continue throughout the harness treatment period, but creative positioning of the infant may be needed.

For infants or children diagnosed later than 6 months of age or those who do not improve with harness use, surgical reduction may be performed after a period of traction. Postoperative casting followed by bracing or orthotic use is common. Caring for the child in the postoperative period is similar to care of any child in a cast. Pain management and monitoring for bleeding are priority activities. Teach families care of the cast at home.

▶ TIBIA VARA (BLOUNT'S DISEASE)

Tibia vara (Blount's disease) is a developmental disorder affecting young children. The normal physiologic bowing or genu varum becomes more pronounced in the child with tibia vara. The cause of tibia vara is unknown, but it is considered to be a developmental disorder as it occurs most frequently in children who are early walkers. Most cases occur in African-Americans. In addition to early walking, obesity is also a risk factor. If left untreated, the growth plate of the upper tibia ceases bone production. Asymmetric growth at the knee then occurs and the bowing progresses. Severe degenerative arthritis of the knee is an additional long-term complication.

Therapeutic management is aimed at stopping the progression of the disease through bracing or surgical

FIGURE 44.15 Pavlik harness for treatment of developmental dysplasia of the hip.

TEACHING GUIDELINES 44.4

Caring for a Child in a Pavlik Harness

• Do not adjust the straps without checking with the physician first.
• Until your physician instructs you to take the harness off for a period of time each day, it must be used continuously (for the first week or sometimes longer).
• Change your baby's diaper while in the harness.
• Place your baby to sleep on his or her back.
• Do not place clothes under the harness during the period of continuous use.
• Once the baby is permitted to be out of the harness for a short period, you may bathe your baby while the harness is off.
• Long knee socks and an undershirt are recommended to prevent rubbing of the skin against the brace.
• Note location of the markings on the straps for appropriate placement of the harness.
• Wash the harness with mild detergent by hand and air dry. If using the dryer, use *only* the air fluffing setting (no heat).

treatment. Medical or surgical treatment should begin early, before 4 years of age.

Nursing Assessment

Elicit a health history and determine the age at which the child started walking. Assess growth parameters to determine whether the risk factor of obesity is present. Note significant bowing of the legs in standing and while ambulating (Fig. 44.16).

Nursing Management

Bracing may include a modified knee–ankle–foot orthosis that relieves the compression forces on the growth plate, allowing bone growth resumption and correction of bowlegs. To be successful, bracing must be continued for months to years and the brace must be worn 23 hours per day. Compliance is the most significant barrier to successful treatment. Parents have a difficult time forcing their toddler to stay in a brace that inhibits mobility for the bulk of the day (particularly a bilateral brace). Support

parents by encouraging and praising their compliance with bracing. Teach parents to assess for potential skin impairment from brace rubbing.

When surgical treatment is required, the leg(s) will be immobilized in a long-leg bent knee or spica cast after the osteotomy is performed. Perform routine cast care. Refer to Nursing Care Plan 44.1 for additional interventions related to care of the immobilized child.

▶ TORTICOLLIS

Torticollis is a painless muscular condition presenting in infants or in children with certain syndromes. Congenital muscular torticollis may result from *in utero* positioning or difficult birth. Preferential turning of the head to one side while in the supine position after birth may also lead to torticollis. Torticollis results from tightness of the sternocleidomastoid muscle, resulting in the infant's head being tilted to one side.

Medical treatment involves passive stretching exercises, which are effective in 90% of affected infants (Luther, 2002). Botulinum toxin injection has been used recently with success in cases of torticollis that have not improved with stretching exercises. Plagiocephaly may result from the continued pressure on the side of the skull to which the neck is turned.

FIGURE 44.16 Note extreme bowing of the legs in tibia vara.

FIGURE 44.17 Note wry-neck or head tilt in the infant with torticollis.

Nursing Assessment

Note history of head tilt and infant's lack of desire to turn the head in the opposite direction. Observe the infant for wry-neck (tilting of the head to one side; Fig. 44.17). Note limited movement of the neck when passive range of motion is performed. Palpate the neck, noting a mass in the sternocleidomastoid muscle on the affected side. Examine the head for evidence of plagiocephaly.

Nursing Management

Teach parents gentle neck-stretching exercises to be performed several times a day. While immobilizing the shoulder on the affected side, gently sustain a side-to-side stretch toward the unaffected side, holding the stretch for 10 to 30 seconds. Repeat 10 to 15 times per session. Perform an ear-to-shoulder stretch in a similar fashion. To prevent the development of torticollis in the unaffected infant, positional plagiocephaly must be prevented. Prevent flatness of one side of the head by varying the baby's head position, and do not always turn the head to one side while in the infant seat or swing or lying supine. Refer families to

the National Infant Torticollis Foundation (www.infant-torticollis.org), a parent support network.

Acquired Disorders

Several acquired musculoskeletal disorders may affect children. Nutritional deficits or malabsorption of fats may lead to rickets. Slipped capital femoral epiphysis and Legg-Calvé-Perthes disease affect mainly school-age and adolescent boys. Osteomyelitis, septic arthritis, and toxic synovitis are common infectious musculoskeletal disorders. Spinal curvature may occur as a result of a neuromuscular disorder or idiopathically.

▶ RICKETS

Rickets is a condition in which there is softening or weakening of the bones. Childhood rickets may occur as a result of nutritional deficiencies such as inadequate consumption of calcium or limited exposure to sunlight (required for adequate production of vitamin D). Rickets may also occur if the body cannot regulate calcium and phosphorus in the appropriate balance, such as in chronic renal disease. Gastrointestinal disorders in which fat absorption is altered (e.g., Crohn's disease and cystic fibrosis) may lead to rickets, as vitamin D is a fat-soluble vitamin. Vitamin D regulates calcium absorption from the small intestine and levels of calcium and phosphate in the bones. Calcium is primarily laid down in the bones of the fetus during the third trimester. Premature infants miss this period of calcium accumulation and also suffer from inadequate calcium intake in the neonatal period and often demonstrate rickets of prematurity. When calcium and phosphate levels in the blood are imbalanced, then calcium is released from the bones into the blood, resulting in loss of the supportive bony matrix. Rickets is most likely to occur during periods of rapid growth.

Therapeutic Management

Treatment of rickets is aimed at correcting the calcium imbalance so that the skeleton may develop properly and without deformity. Calcium and phosphorus supplements are given, and some children also require vitamin D supplements. If rickets is not corrected while the child is still growing, permanent skeletal deformities and short stature may result.

> ▶ **Take** *NOTE!*
>
> *Children who do not receive adequate daily exposure to sunlight require supplementation with 5 micrograms of vitamin D per day.*

Nursing Assessment

Obtain a health history, determining risk factors such as:

- Limited exposure to sunlight
- Strict vegetarian diet or lactose intolerance (either one without milk product ingestion)
- Exclusive breastfeeding by a mother who has a vitamin D deficiency
- Dark-pigmented skin
- Prematurity
- Malabsorptive gastrointestinal disorder
- Chronic renal disease

Note history of fractures or bone pain. Observe for dental deformities and bowlegs. Decreased muscle tone may also be present. Note low serum calcium and phosphate levels and high alkaline phosphatase levels. X-rays may show changes in the shape and structure of the bone.

Nursing Management

Administer calcium and phosphorus supplements at alternate times to promote proper absorption of both of these supplements. Encourage exposure to moderate amounts of sunlight and administer vitamin D supplements as prescribed. Teach families that good dietary sources of vitamin D are fish, liver, and processed milk.

▶ SLIPPED CAPITAL FEMORAL EPIPHYSIS

Slipped capital femoral epiphysis (SCFE) is a condition in which the femoral head dislocates from the neck and shaft of the femur at the level of the epiphyseal plate.

The epiphysis slips downward and backward. SCFE occurs most frequently in obese males, 9 to 16 years of age; it is more common in African-American boys than in Caucasians (Leung & Lemay, 2004). The exact cause is unknown, but it is thought that during the teenage growth spurt the femoral growth plate weakens and becomes less resistant to stressors. Hormonal alterations during this period may also play a role.

SCFE is classified based upon its severity and whether the slip is acute or chronic. Chronic SCFE may lead to shortening of the affected leg and thigh atrophy.

Therapeutic Management

Promptly refer the child with SCFE to an orthopedic surgeon, as early surgical intervention will decrease the risk of long-term deformity. The goals of therapeutic management are to prevent further slippage, minimize deformity, and avoid the complications of cartilage necrosis (chondrolysis) and avascular necrosis of the femoral head. Surgical intervention may include in situ pinning, in which a pin or screw is inserted percutaneously into the femoral head to hold it in place. Osteotomy may be used for more severe cases. Osteoarthritis may be a long-term complication of SCFE.

Nursing Assessment

Elicit a health history, determining the onset and extent of pain. In acute SCFE, the pain is usually sudden in onset and results in inability to bear weight. Chronic SCFE may present with an insidious onset of pain and limp. Note risk factors of age 9 to 16 years, African-American race, and obesity. Observe ambulation, noting Trendelenburg gait. Assess for pain that is in the hip or that is referred to the groin, medial thigh, or knee. Note decreased range of motion in the affected hip with external rotation. X-rays will be obtained to confirm the diagnosis (anteroposterior and lateral frog-leg views of hips). Bone scan can rule out avascular necrosis, and CT scan helps define the extent of slippage.

> ▶ **Take** *NOTE!*
>
> *Do not attempt to perform passive range of motion to determine the extent of limitation in the child with SCFE; this may cause worsening of the condition.*

Nursing Management

Enforce bed rest and activity restriction. If traction is used for a period before surgery, perform routine traction care and neurovascular assessments. Assess pain and administer analgesics as needed. After in situ pinning, assist the child with crutch walking. Teach the family that weight bearing is usually resumed about a week after the surgery and that the pin will be removed later. Prolonged immobility may isolate the adolescent from usual peer interactions, so encourage phone calls and visits with friends. Provide books, games, electronic devices, and magazines for distraction during the period of immobility. Provide family support.

▶ LEGG-CALVÉ-PERTHES DISEASE

Legg-Calvé-Perthes disease is a self-limiting condition that involves avascular necrosis of the femoral head. It most often affects children aged 4 to 8 years, but can occur as early as 18 months, until skeletal maturity (Hoffmeister, 2008). The disease affects girls much less frequently. The etiology is unknown, but the interruption of the blood supply to the femoral head results in bone death, and the spherical shape of the femoral head may be lost. Swelling of the soft tissues around the hip may occur. As new blood vessels develop, the area is supplied with circulation, allowing bone resorption and deposition to take place. During this period of revascularization, which takes 18 to 24 months, the bone is soft and more likely to fracture. Over time, the femoral head reforms.

Therapeutic Management

The goal of therapeutic management is to maintain normal femoral head shape and to restore appropriate motion. Treatment of Legg-Calvé-Perthes disease includes anti-inflammatory medication to decrease muscle spasms around the hip joint and to relieve pain. Activity limitation may be prescribed, and sometimes bracing is recommended to contain the femoral head. Serial x-ray follow-up determines progress of the disease. If surgery becomes warranted, then osteotomy may be performed. Complications include joint deformity, early degenerative joint disease, persistent pain, loss of hip motion or function, and gait disturbance.

Nursing Assessment

Explore the health history for short stature, delayed bone maturation, or a family history of Legg-Calvé-Perthes disease. Note painless limp, which may be intermittent over a period of months. Mild hip pain may result and may be referred to the knee or the thigh. Pain may be aggravated by exercise. Observe the child walking and note Trendelenburg gait. Perform range of motion, noting internal rotation of the hip and limited abduction. Muscle spasm may result with hip extension and rotation. Hip x-rays are obtained to evaluate the extent of epiphyseal involvement. MRI or bone scan may also be used to differentiate Legg-Calvé-Perthes disease from other disorders.

Nursing Management

Nursing care of Legg-Calvé-Perthes disease is highly variable and depends on the stage of the disease and its severity. Administer anti-inflammatory medications, noting their effect on pain. If activities are restricted, exercise the unaffected body parts. Assist families with use of the brace if prescribed. The brace may be wiped with a damp cloth if it becomes dirty. Some children will be prescribed no treatment other than avoidance of contact or high-impact sports. Swimming and bicycle riding help to maintain range of motion with little risk. If mobility equipment is needed, educate the child and family on its use. If osteotomy is performed, provide routine postoperative care, with education and support of the child and family.

▶ OSTEOMYELITIS

Osteomyelitis is a bacterial infection of the bone and soft tissue surrounding the bone. The long bone metaphysis is the most common location, with *Staphylococcus aureus* being the most common infecting organism (Eilert, 2007). Additional causes in infants include group B streptococcus and *Escherichia coli*; in children, *Streptococcus pyogenes* and *Haemophilus influenzae* are also implicated. Children usually present for evaluation within a few days to a week of onset of symptoms, though some may present later.

Osteomyelitis is acquired hematogenously. Bacteria from the bloodstream mainly invade the most rapidly growing portion of the bone. The invading bacteria trigger an inflammatory response, formation of pus and edema, and vascular congestion. Small blood vessels thrombose and the infection extends into the metaphyseal marrow cavity. As the infection progresses, the inflammation extends throughout the bone and blood supply is disrupted, resulting in death of the bone tissues (Fig. 44.18).

Therapeutic Management

Treatment includes a 4- to 6-week course of antibiotics. Some children may receive 1 to 2 weeks of intravenous antibiotics and then be switched to oral antibiotics for the remainder of the course. Surgical débridement is rarely necessary. Early treatment may prevent the complications of bone destruction, fracture, and growth arrest. Additional complications include recurrent infection, septic arthritis, and systemic infection.

Nursing Assessment

For a full description of the assessment phase of the nursing process, refer to page 1459. Assessment findings pertinent to osteomyelitis are discussed here. Explore the health

FIGURE 44.18 In osteomyelitis, bacterial invasion leads to infection within the bone.

history for risk factors and symptoms. Risk factors include impetigo, infected varicella lesions, furunculosis, infected burns, and prolonged intravenous line use. Note history of irritability, lethargy, possible fever, and onset of pain or change in activity level. The child usually refuses to walk and demonstrates decreased range of motion in the affected extremity. Inspect the affected extremity for swelling. Palpate for local warmth and tenderness. Note point tenderness over affected bone.

Laboratory and diagnostic testing may reveal:

- Elevated white blood cell count, erythrocyte sedimentation rate, and C-reactive protein level
- Positive blood cultures
- Deep soft tissue swelling on x-ray
- Changes on ultrasound or CT scan

Nursing Management

Nursing management of the child with osteomyelitis focuses on assessment, pain management, and maintenance of intravenous access for administration of antibiotics. Individualize care based on the child's and family's response to the illness; see Nursing Care Plan Overview 44.1. Maintain bed rest initially to prevent injury and promote comfort. Administer antipyretics as ordered if the child is febrile in the initial stage of the illness. Encourage use of unaffected extremities by providing developmentally appropriate toys and games. Instruct child and family on safe and proper use of crutches or walker if prescribed. Some children will be discharged home on intravenous antibiotics, while others will finish an oral antibiotic course. Teach par-

ents proper administration of medications and maintenance of a peripherally inserted central catheter or central line at home if the child is finishing the antibiotic course intravenously.

▶ SEPTIC ARTHRITIS

Acute septic arthritis is a condition in which bacteria invade the joint space, most often the hip. It usually occurs in children less than 10 years old, with 3- to 7-year-olds being most frequently affected. Bacteria gain access to the joint in one of three ways:

- Directly from a puncture of the joint or via venipuncture or wound infection
- Seeding from a distal infection site (e.g., otitis media or respiratory infection)
- Compression of the joint capsule from adjacent osteomyelitis

S. aureus, H. influenzae type B, and various streptococci are the most commonly responsible organisms. Sepsis of the hip joint may cause avascular necrosis of the femoral head due to pressure on blood vessels and cartilage within the joint space. Septic arthritis is considered a medical emergency, as this destruction may occur within just a few days. Additional complications of septic arthritis include permanent deformity, leg-length discrepancy, and long-term decreased range of motion and disability.

The goals of treatment of septic arthritis are to prevent destruction of the joint cartilage and maintain function, motion, and strength. Septic arthritis is treated rapidly with joint aspiration or arthrotomy, followed by intravenous antibiotic therapy while in the hospital and oral antibiotics at home.

Nursing Assessment

Note history of predisposing factors such as respiratory infection or otitis media, skin or soft tissue infections, or, in the neonate, traumatic puncture wounds and femoral venipunctures. The history is usually significant for sudden onset of fever and moderate to severe pain.

Upon physical examination, the infant or child appears ill. Note extent of fever, refusal to bear weight or straighten the hip, and limited range of motion (the child usually maintains the joint in flexion and will not allow the leg to be straightened). Palpate the affected joint for warmth and swelling.

Laboratory findings may include:

- White blood cell count normal or elevated with elevated neutrophil counts
- Elevated erythrocyte sedimentation rate and C-reactive protein levels

- Fluid from joint aspiration demonstrates elevated white blood cell count; culture determines responsible organism.
- Joint x-ray may show subtle soft tissue changes or increase in the joint space.
- Positive blood culture for the causative organism (15% of cases)

Nursing Management

Refer to Nursing Care Plan Overview 44.1 for interventions related to musculoskeletal disorders. Assess aspiration wound for signs of infection. Monitor vital signs for resolution of fever. Pain management with ibuprofen or acetaminophen will be sufficient for some children; others may initially require codeine or morphine. Assess the affected joint for decrease in swelling, increasing range of motion, and decreasing or absent pain. The child may be discharged after 72 hours of intravenous antibiotics following joint aspiration if he or she is improving and can tolerate oral antibiotics. At discharge, if the child cannot ambulate, physical therapy may be consulted for short-term use of crutches or a wheelchair. Teach families how to assess for signs and symptoms of wound infection, how to administer oral antibiotics and pain medication, and how to assist their child with crutch walking.

▶ TRANSIENT SYNOVITIS OF THE HIP

Transient synovitis of the hip (also termed toxic synovitis) is the most common cause of hip pain in children (Eilert, 2007). It occurs in children as young as 9 months of age through adolescence, most commonly affecting children 3 to 8 years old. Boys are affected twice as often as girls and African-Americans exhibit the lowest incidence. The exact cause is unclear, but it is thought to be associated with recent or active infection or with trauma. A self-limiting disease, most cases resolve within a week, but it may last as long as 4 weeks. Therapeutic management involves nonsteroidal anti-inflammatory medications and bed rest to relieve weight bearing on the affected hip joint.

Nursing Assessment

Explore the health history for risk factors such as antecedent trauma, concurrent or recent upper respiratory tract infection, pharyngitis, or otitis media. Note sudden acute onset of moderate to severe pain of one hip. Sometimes pain is referred to the anterior thigh or knee. Pain is usually the worst upon arising in the morning, and the child refuses to walk, with pain decreasing throughout the day. Temperature will be normal or low-grade (<38°C). Observe for a limp or for refusal to bear weight. Observe position of the affected hip: it will be held in a flexed and externally rotated position. Note restricted range of motion for abduction and internal rotation.

Nursing Management

Nursing care focuses on educating the family. Parents are very concerned when their child refuses to walk, and they will need significant support and reassurance.

Scoliosis

Scoliosis is a lateral curvature of the spine that exceeds 10 degrees. It may be congenital, associated with other disorders, or idiopathic. Table 44.4 explains the types of scoliosis. Idiopathic scoliosis accounts for 65% of all cases of scoliosis, with the majority of those occurring during adolescence (Zak, 2005). Hence, this discussion will focus on adolescent idiopathic scoliosis. The etiology of idiopathic scoliosis is not known, but genetic factors, growth abnormalities, and bone, muscle, disk, or central nervous system disorders may contribute to its development. Early screening and detection of scoliosis result in improved outcomes.

Pathophysiology

In the rapidly growing adolescent, the involved vertebrae rotate around a vertical axis, resulting in lateral curvature. The vertebrae rotate to the convex side of curve, with the spinous processes rotating toward the concave side. Wedge-shaped vertebral bodies and disks develop because growth is suppressed on the concave side of the curve (Newton & Wenger, 2006). As the curve progresses, the shape of the thoracic cage changes and respiratory and cardiovascular compromise may occur (the main complications of severe scoliosis).

TABLE 44.4   **TYPES OF SCOLIOSIS**

Type	Associated Factors
Idiopathic	Unknown cause Infantile: occurs in the first 3 years of life Juvenile: diagnosed between age 4 and 10 years, or prior to adolescence Adolescent: age 11 to 17 years
Neuromuscular	Associated with neurologic or muscular disease such as cerebral palsy, myelomeningocele, spinal cord tumors, spinal muscular atrophy
Myopathic	Associated with certain types of muscular dystrophy
Congenital	Results from anomalous vertebral development

> **BOX 44.2** **Types of Braces Used to Treat Scoliosis**
>
> • Underarm (Boston, Wilmington): less conspicuous, no visible neckpiece
> • Milwaukee: traditional standard, has a visible neckpiece
> • Nighttime bending (Charleston): creates a curve so severe that walking is not possible, so can be worn only at night

Therapeutic Management

Treatment of scoliosis is aimed at preventing progression of the curve and decreasing the impact on pulmonary and cardiac function. Treatment is based on the age of the child, expected future growth, and severity of the curve. Observation with serial examinations and spine x-rays is used to monitor curve progression. For curves of 20 to 50 degrees, bracing may be sufficient to decrease progression of the curve. Box 44.2 describes types of scoliosis braces and Figure 44.19 shows examples. The choice of brace will depend on the location and severity of the curve. Some curves will progress despite appropriate bracing and compliance.

Surgical correction is often required for curves greater than 45 degrees; it is achieved with rod placement and bone grafting. Partial spinal fusion accompanies many of the corrective surgeries. Multiple surgical approaches and techniques exist for fusion and rod placement. The surgical approach may be anterior, posterior, or both. Traditional rod placement (Harrington rod) involved a single rod fused to the vertebrae, resulting in curve correction but also a flat-backed appearance. Newer rod instrumentations allow for scoliosis curve correction with maintenance of normal back curvature. The rods are shorter, and several are wired or grafted to the appropriate vertebrae to achieve correction. Figure 44.20 shows one example of surgical rod instrumentation.

Nursing Assessment

For a full description of the assessment phase of the nursing process, refer to page 1459. Assessment findings pertinent to scoliosis are discussed below.

Health History
Determine why the child is presenting for evaluation of scoliosis. Commonly the child or adolescent will not report back pain, as only mild discomfort is associated with idiopathic scoliosis until the curve becomes severe. Often the family recognizes asymmetry in the hips or shoulders or the child is screened for scoliosis at school and determined to be at risk. Explore the client's current and past medical history for risk factors such as:

• Family history of scoliosis
• Recent growth spurt
• Physical changes related to puberty

Determine the age of development of secondary sex characteristics and the age of menarche, as these signs of pubertal development indicate the expected velocity and length of remaining growth.

Physical Examination
The physical assessment of a child with possible or actual scoliosis involves mainly inspection and observation.

A   B   C

FIGURE 44.19 (**A**) Boston brace. (**B**) Milwaukee brace. (**C**) Nighttime bending brace.

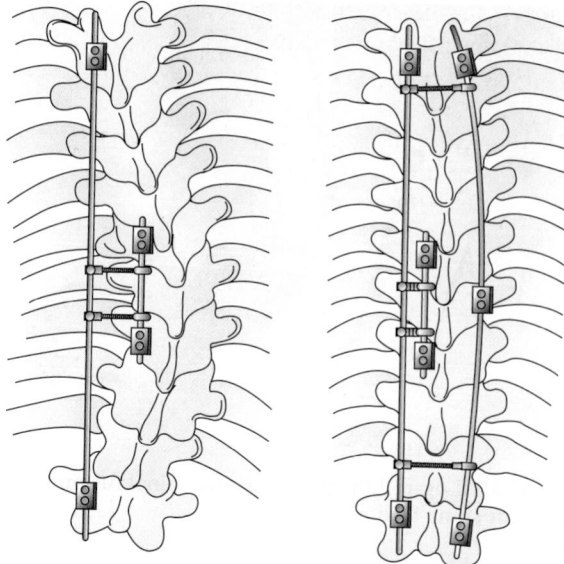

FIGURE 44.20 Rods are fused to the vertebrae and connected to a distracting rod to rotate the vertebral column (Cotrel-Dubousset method is shown).

Auscultate the heart and lungs to determine compromise related to severe curvature.

Observe the child at rest, sitting, and standing for evidence of poor posture. Inspect the child's back in a standing position. Note asymmetries such as shoulder elevation, prominence of one scapula, uneven curve at the waistline, or a rib hump on one side. Measure shoulder levels from the floor to the acromioclavicular joints. Note the difference between the height of the high and low shoulder in centimeters. Measure heights of anterior and posterior iliac spines and note the difference in centimeters. View the patient from the side, noting abnormalities in the spinal curve. With the child bending forward, arms hanging freely, note asymmetry of the back (pronounced hump on one side). Figure 44.21 shows scoliosis noted upon visual inspection. Note leg-length discrepancy if present. During the neurologic examination, balance, motor strength, sensation, and reflexes should all be normal.

Laboratory and Diagnostic Tests

Full-spine x-rays are necessary to determine the degree of curvature. The radiologist will determine the extent of the curve based on specific formulas and techniques of measurement.

Nursing Management

Nursing Care Plan 44.1 lists general interventions; nursing care should be tailored based on the adolescent's response to the disease and its treatment. Additional nursing interventions specific to scoliosis are discussed here.

Encouraging Compliance With Bracing

Bracing is intended to prevent progression of the curve but does not correct the current curve. Although modern braces display an improved appearance, with no visible neckpiece, and can be worn under clothes, many adolescents are not compliant with brace wear. The brace must be worn 23 hours per day to prevent curve progression. Many factors may contribute to noncompliance, including the discomfort associated with brace

FIGURE 44.21 (**A**) Note right shoulder, scapula, and hip elevation as well as discrepancy in waist curvature. (**B**) Note right upper back hump.

wear such as pain, heat, and poor fit. The family environment may not be conducive to compliance with brace wear, and teenagers are very concerned about body image.

Inspect the skin for evidence of rubbing by the brace that may impair skin integrity. Teach families appropriate skin care and recommend they check the brace daily for fit and breakage. Encourage the teen to shower during the 1 hour per day that the brace is off and to ensure that the skin is clean and dry before putting the brace back on. Wearing a cotton T-shirt under the brace may decrease some of the discomfort associated with brace wear. Exercises to strengthen back muscles may prevent muscle atrophy from prolonged bracing and maintain spine flexibility.

Promoting Positive Body Image

Encourage the teen to express his or her feelings or concerns about wearing the brace. Give the teen ways to explain scoliosis and its treatment to his or her peers. Wearing stylish baggy clothes may help the teen to conceal the brace if desired. Refer teens and their families to the National Scoliosis Foundation (www.scoliosis.org) for additional support.

Providing Preoperative Care

If the curve progresses despite bracing or causes pulmonary or cardiac compromise, surgical intervention will be warranted. In the preoperative period, teach the teen the importance of turning, coughing, and deep breathing in the postoperative period. Explain the tubes and lines that will be present immediately after the surgery. Review positioning guidelines: back flexion or extension will not be allowed. Introduce the child to the patient-controlled analgesia pump and explain pain scales. There is a high risk for significant blood loss with spinal fusion and instrumentation, so if possible arrange for preoperative autologous blood donation.

Providing Postoperative Care

The goal of nursing management in the postoperative period after spinal fusion with or without instrumentation is to avoid complications. Perform neurovascular checks with each set of vital signs. When turning the child, use the log-roll technique to avoid flexion of the back (Fig. 44.22). Administer prophylactic intravenous antibiotics if ordered. Assess for drainage from the operative site and for excess blood loss via the Hemovac or other drainage tube. Maintain Foley patency, as the child will be confined to bed for the first couple of days. Maintain strict recording of fluid intake and output. Administer transfusions of packed red blood cells if ordered. Ambulation, once ordered, should be done slowly to avoid orthostatic hypotension. Assist the family with arrangements to continue the teen's school work while hospitalized and/or arrange for home tutoring during the several-week recovery period.

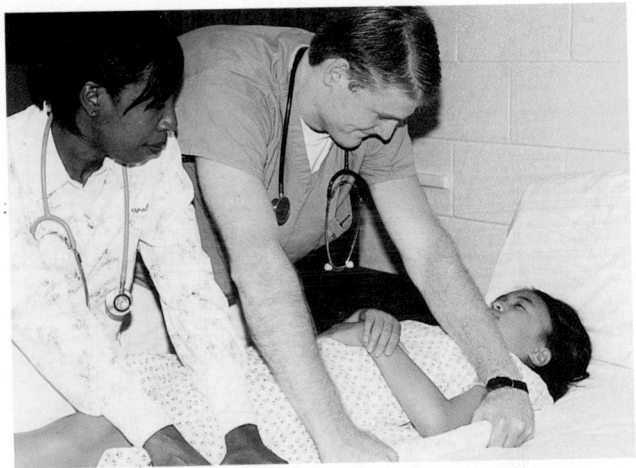

FIGURE 44.22 Log-roll the postoperative spinal fusion patient to prevent spine flexion.

▶ **Consider** THIS!

Angela Hernandez, a 15-year-old girl, is being seen in the clinic after she was found to be at high risk for scoliosis during a school screening. Upon assessment the nurse notes asymmetry of the hips, with shoulder elevation and prominence of one scapula. She is visibly upset and wants to know what caused this and what can be done. How would you address her concerns?

Angela's plan of care will include wearing of a brace. What education will be necessary and how can you promote compliance?

Describe nursing care for Angela if surgical correction is necessary.

Injuries

Injuries throughout childhood are inevitable. Trauma often occurs as a result of motor vehicle injury. The bulk of trauma resulting from physical activity or sports in children is due to running, skateboarding, and climbing trees. Only about one third of sports injuries in children occur during organized sports; the rest occur in physical education class or non-organized sports (Busch, 2006). Younger children tend to suffer contusions, sprains, and simple upper extremity fractures; adolescents more frequently experience lower-extremity trauma. As the number of children participating in youth sports increases and the intensity of training and the level of competition also increase, the incidence of injury is also likely to increase.

Many types of musculoskeletal injuries exist. This discussion will focus on fractures, sprains, overuse syndromes, and dislocated radial head.

▶ *Take* NOTE!

Fracture in the newborn or infant should raise a high index of suspicion for abuse, as fractures are very unusual in children who cannot yet walk.

▶ *Take* NOTE!

Spiral femur fractures and humerus fractures, particularly in the child less than 2 years of age, should always be thoroughly investigated to rule out the possibility of child abuse.

▶ FRACTURE

Fractures occur frequently in children and adolescents; 40% of boys and 25% of girls will suffer a fracture by age 16 years. About 50% of fractures occur in the distal forearm and hand. Greenstick and buckle fractures account for about half of pediatric fractures, and only about 20% of childhood fractures require reduction (Price et al., 2006).

▶ *Take* NOTE!

Do not attempt to straighten or manipulate an injured limb.

Pathophysiology

Fractures result most frequently from accidental trauma (DiFazio & Atkinson, 2005). Nonaccidental trauma (child abuse) and other disease processes are the other causes of fractures. The growth plate is the most vulnerable portion of the child's bone and is frequently the site of injury. The Salter-Harris classification system is used to describe fractures involving the growth plate (Table 44.5). The thicker, more elastic periosteum in children yields to the force encountered with trauma, resulting more frequently in nondisplaced fractures in children. The increased vascularity and decreased mineral content make the child's bones more flexible. Plastic or bowing deformities and buckle and greenstick fractures are the result. Complete fractures do occur in children, but they tend to be more stable than in the adult, resulting in improved healing and function. Spiral, pelvic, and hip fractures are rare in children. Table 44.6 explains common types of fractures in children.

Plastic deformity and Salter-Harris type IV fractures may result in an angular deformity. Though healing of fractures is usually quick and without incident in children, delayed union, nonunion, or malunion can occur. Additional complications include infection, avascular necrosis, bone shortening from epiphyseal arrest, vascular or nerve injuries, fat embolism, reflex sympathetic dystrophy, and compartment syndrome, which is an orthopedic emergency. Later in life, osteoarthritis may occur as a long-term complication from childhood fracture.

Therapeutic Management

The vast majority of childhood fractures would heal well with splinting only, but casting of these fractures is performed to provide further comfort to the child and to allow for increased activity while the fracture is healing. Displaced fractures require manual traction to align the bones, followed by casting. More severe fractures may require traction for a period of time, usually followed by casting. Severe or complicated fractures may alternatively require open reduction and internal fixation for healing to occur. Complex fractures are often treated with external fixation (Fig. 44.23).

▶ *Take* NOTE!

Significant swelling may occur initially after immobilization with a splint. Splinting and then delaying casting for a few days provides time for some of the swelling to subside, allowing for successful casting a few days after the injury.

Nursing Assessment

For a full description of the assessment phase of the nursing process, refer to page 1459. Assessment findings pertinent to fractures are discussed below.

Health History

Elicit a description of the present illness and chief complaint. Common signs and symptoms reported during the health history might include recent trauma or fall, complaint of pain, difficulty bearing weight, limp, or refusal to use an extremity. Young children often demonstrate sudden onset of irritability and refusal to bear weight. Ask about the mechanism of injury and obtain a description of the traumatic event. Be alert to inconsistencies between the history and the clinical picture or mechanism of injury, as such inconsistency may be an indicator of child abuse. Explore the patient's current and past medical history for risk factors such as:

• Rickets
• Renal osteodystrophy
• Osteogenesis imperfecta
• Participation in sports, particularly contact sports

TABLE 44.5 THE SALTER–HARRIS CLASSIFICATION SYSTEM

Type	Description	Illustration
I	Fracture is through the physis, widening it.	
II	Fracture is partially through the physis, extending into the metaphysis.	
III	Fracture is partially through the epiphysis, extending into the epiphysis.	
IV	Fracture is through the metaphysis, physis, epiphysis.	
V	Crushing injury to the physis	

TABLE 44.6   TYPES OF FRACTURES IN CHILDREN

Fracture Type	Description	Illustration
Plastic or bowing deformity	Significant bending without breaking of the bone	
Buckle fracture	Compression injury; the bone buckles rather than breaks	
Greenstick fracture	Incomplete fracture of the bone	
Complete fracture	Bone breaks into two pieces	

- Failure to use protective equipment as recommended for various physical activities and sports (e.g., wrist guards while rollerblading)

Physical Examination

Perform the physical examination of the child with a potential fracture carefully, so as not to cause further pain or trauma. The physical examination particular to fractures includes inspection, observation, and palpation.

Inspection and Observation

Inspect the skin for bruising, erythema, or swelling. Observe the extremities for deformity. Note neglect of an extremity or inability to bear weight. If ambulating, note any limp.

Palpation

Carefully palpate the joint or injured part. Distract the young child with a toy or activity while palpating. Note point tenderness, which is a reliable indicator of fracture in children. Assess neurovascular status, noting distal extremity temperature, spontaneous movement, sensation, numbness, capillary refill time, and quality of pulses. The neurovascular assessment is critical to providing a baseline so that any changes associated with compartment syndrome can be quickly identified.

Laboratory and Diagnostic Tests

Usually plain x-ray films are all that is required to identify a simple fracture. Complicated fractures that require surgical intervention may require further evaluation with CT or MRI.

Nursing Management

Immediately after the injury, immobilize the limb above and below the site of injury in the most comfortable position with a splint. Use cold therapy to reduce swelling in the first 48 hours after injury. Elevate the injured extremity above the level of the heart. Perform frequent neurovascular checks. Assess pain level and administer

FIGURE 44.23 (A) External fixation is required for complicated fractures. (B) The Ilizarov fixator is a circular apparatus usually used for complicated lower extremity fractures. The pins are smaller in diameter, more like wires, than those used in other fixators.

pain medications as needed. Administer tetanus vaccine in the child with an open fracture if he or she has not received a tetanus booster within the past 5 years.

> ▶ **Take** NOTE!
>
> *Assess the injured, splinted, or casted extremity frequently for the "5 P's," which may indicate compartment syndrome: pain (increased out of proportion), pulselessness, pallor, paresthesia, paralysis. Report these findings immediately.*

Providing Family Education

Unless bed rest is prescribed, children with upper extremity casts and "walking" leg casts can resume increased levels of activity as the pain subsides. Children who require crutches while in a cast may return to school, but those in spica casts will be at home for several weeks. Providing distraction and finding ways to keep up with school work are important. Families must also learn to care for the cast (see Teaching Guidelines 44.1).

Preventing Fractures

Discourage risky behavior such as climbing trees and performing tricks on bicycles. Provide appropriate supervision, particularly with outdoor activity. Encourage appropriate use of protective equipment, such as wrist guards with rollerblading and shin guards with soccer. Ensure that playground equipment is in good working order and intact; there should not be protruding screws or unbalanced portions of equipment, which may increase the risk for falling.

▶ SPRAINS

Sprains result from a twisting or turning motion of the affected body part. The tendons and ligaments stretch excessively and may tear slightly. They may occur at any joint, but the most common are ankle and knee sprains. Therapeutic management of sprains includes rest, ice, compression, and elevation (RICE). On initial evaluation, sprains need to be differentiated from torn ligaments and meniscal tears, as those conditions are more serious and may require surgical intervention.

Nursing Assessment

Elicit a health history, determining the mechanism of injury (whether it occurred during sports or simply a misstep or fall). Determine what treatment the family has used so far. Inspect the affected body part for edema, which is frequently present, and bruising, which some-

times occurs. Note limp or inability to bear weight. Do not attempt to perform passive range of motion on the affected body part. Assess neurovascular status distal to the injury (usually normal).

Nursing Management

Instruct the child and family in appropriate treatment of sprains, which includes:

• Rest: limit activity.
• Ice: apply cold packs for 20 to 30 minutes, remove for 1 hour, and repeat (for the first 24 to 48 hours).
• Compression: apply an Ace wrap or other elastic bandage or brace; check skin for alterations when rewrapping.
• Elevation: elevate the injured extremity above the level of the heart to decrease swelling (Fig. 44.24).

The child may require instruction in crutch walking as well. Teach families that to prevent sprains during sports, it is important for the child to perform appropriate stretching and warm-up activities.

> ▶ **Take** NOTE!
>
> *If the child's fingers or toes become increasingly swollen or discolored, remove the Ace wrap immediately.*

▶ OVERUSE SYNDROMES

The term "overuse syndrome" refers to a group of disorders that result from repeated force applied to normal tissue. The connective tissues fail in response to repetitive stress, leading to a small amount of tissue breakdown. They develop over the course of weeks to months. There is usually no identifiable injury associated with overuse syndromes. Pain is usually associated with the activity and worsens with continued participation in the activity. Table 44.7 gives details on several common overuse syndromes. Therapeutic management is aimed at reassurance, pain management, and limiting rather than eliminating activity.

Nursing Assessment

Elicit a health history to determine the extent of involvement in sports. Note onset of pain, duration, intensity, aggravating factors, and treatments used at home. Examine the painful part, noting findings similar to those noted for each syndrome in Table 44.7.

RICE

Rest

Ice

Compression

Elevation

FIGURE 44.24 RICE (rest, ice, compression, elevation) is the appropriate treatment for sprains.

TABLE 44.7 OVERUSE DISORDERS

Disorder	Anatomic Area Affected	Most Commonly Occurs in	Symptoms
Osgood-Schlatter disease	Partial avulsion of the ossification center of the tibial tubercle	Active adolescents, most often boys. Most frequently during periods of rapid growth.	• Mild to moderate pain, activity-related. • Tibial tubercle is tender when palpated. • Painful swelling or prominence of the anterior portion of the tibial tubercle.
Epiphysiolysis of proximal humerus	Proximal humerus (widening of growth plate)	Occurs with rigorous upper extremity activity, such as baseball pitching	• Tenderness in the shoulder or proximal humerus. • Pain with active internal rotation. • Full shoulder range of motion continues.
Epiphysiolysis of distal radius	Distal radius (widening of growth plate)	Occurs with overuse of the distal radius, such as in gymnasts	• Wrist pain that worsens with activity.
Sever's disease (calcaneal apophysitis)	Calcaneus (heel)	Usually in 9- to 14-year-olds	• Pain over the posterior aspect of the calcaneus. • Limited active and passive dorsiflexion of foot.
Shin splints	Refers to a variety of overuse syndromes associated with the shin (stress fracture, tibial stress, muscular issues)	Occurs with activities that place repeated exertion on the lower leg, as in runners, ballerinas, elite soccer players	• Exercise-induced pain of the anterior aspect of the middle part of the lower leg. • May be sharp pain • Worsens with exercise • With stress fracture, may have a limp that worsens with activity.

Nursing Management

Initially, apply ice when pain is severe. Anti-inflammatory medications such as ibuprofen may be helpful. The child should limit exercise and participate in a different activity. After a few weeks, most overuse syndromes resolve; at that point, the athlete may resume the prior activity. Osgood-Schlatter disease is the exception and may require 12 to 18 months to resolve. Using pads or braces that are appropriate to the painful body part is also helpful. Supporting the arm with a sling may relieve stress on the proximal humerus when epiphysiolysis occurs. Heel cups used in athletic shoes help relieve stress on the heels associated with Sever's disease. To prevent overuse syndromes, encourage athletes to perform appropriate stretching exercises during a 20- to 30-minute warm-up period before each practice or game. Also encourage several weeks of conditioning training before the season begins.

> ▶ *Take* NOTE!
>
> *"Energy healing" such as therapeutic touch and Reiki may provide a non-pharmacologic adjunct to pain management for musculoskeletal injuries.*

▶ DISLOCATED RADIAL HEAD

Dislocation of the radial head ("nursemaid's elbow") occurs when a pulling motion on the arm causes the ligament surrounding the radial head to become entrapped within the joint. It usually occurs in children less than 7 years of age and is a common injury in children aged 1 to 4. To reduce the injury, the elbow is flexed to 90 degrees and then the forearm is fully and firmly supinated, causing the ligament to snap back into place. With appropriate reduction of the radial head, no complications result.

Nursing Assessment

The child will hold the arm slightly flexed at the side and refuse to move it. When the arm is still, the child apparently has no discomfort. Assess neurovascular status (intact).

Nursing Management

After treatment, usually hyperpronation to reduce the dislocation, assess the child's ability to use the arm without pain. Teach parents to avoid pulling up on the child's arm, particularly in an abrupt jerking fashion, to prevent recurrence.

■■■ Key Concepts

- The bones of the infant and young child are more flexible and have a thicker periosteum and more abundant blood supply than the adult's; as a result, bending occurs more frequently than breaking of the bone, and the fractured bone heals more quickly.
- The epiphysis of long bones is the growth center of the bones in children. Injury to this area may result in long-term extremity deformity.
- Rapid muscle growth in the adolescent years places the teenager at increased risk for injury compared with other age groups.
- Plain radiographs are usually sufficient for diagnosing injuries in children. If CT or MRI scans are required, the nurse may need to help the child stay calm and still during the procedure.
- Apply a pressure dressing following joint aspiration to prevent hematoma formation or fluid recollection.
- Perform frequent assessments of pain status and the effect of pain medication in the child with a musculoskeletal disorder.
- Diazepam (Valium) may be helpful in relieving muscle spasm associated with traction.
- Fractures may occur as a result of unintentional or intentional injury, or because the bones are fragile, as in rickets or osteogenesis imperfecta.
- Congenital or developmental disorders such as DDH or clubfoot require bracing or casting for correction and to prevent deformity later in life.
- Sprains, fractures, and overuse syndromes occur frequently in young athletes. Appropriate warm-up and stretching may help prevent some of these injuries.
- Assessment of neurovascular status is an essential component of care for a child with a neuromuscular disorder.
- To prevent complications after a spinal fusion for scoliosis correction, use the log-roll method for turning the child so that back flexion is avoided.
- Rest, ice, compression, and elevation is the appropriate treatment for sprains.
- Maintain traction and the appropriate amount of weight as ordered.
- The bulk of cast care occurs in the home. Teach the family of a child with a cast to perform neurovascular assessments, prevent the cast from getting wet, and care for the skin appropriately.
- Torticollis may be treated by teaching the family to perform daily neck muscle stretching exercises.
- Children with chronic disorders such as osteogenesis imperfecta may demonstrate slower or lesser growth than other children and may also be unable to participate in certain activities because of bone fragility.

REFERENCES

Ackley, B. J., & Ladwig, G. B. (2006). *Nursing diagnosis handbook: A guide to planning care* (7th ed.). St. Louis: Mosby.

Allard, P., Chavet, P., Barbier, F., Gatto, L., Labelle, H., & Sadeghi, H. (2004). Effect of body morphology on standing balance in adolescent idiopathic scoliosis. *American Journal of Physical Medicine and Rehabilitation, 83,* 689–697.

American Academy of Pediatrics, Committee on Quality Improvement, Subcommittee on Developmental Dysplasia of the Hip. (2000). Clinical practice guideline: Early detection of developmental dysplasia of the hip. *Pediatrics, 105*(4), 896–905.

Bahr, R. (2007). Prevention of ankle sprains in adolescent athletes. *Clinical Journal of Sport Medicine, 17*(4), 334–335.

Bonner, S. M. (2007). Fixate on pin site care. *Nursing Made Incredibly Easy!, 5*(4), 22–25.

Bradin, S. A., & Leung, A. K. C. (2007). What's your diagnosis? *Consultant for Pediatricians, 6*(7), 413–416.

Brown, D., & Fisher, E. (2004). Femur fractures in infants and young children. *American Journal of Public Health, 94*(4), 558–560.

Busch, M. T. (2006). Sports medicine in children and adolescents. In R. T. Morrissy & S. L. Weinstein (Eds.), *Lovell & Winter's pediatric orthopaedics* (6th ed.). Philadelphia: Lippincott Williams & Wilkins.

Cady, R. B. (2006). Developmental dysplasia of the hip: Definition, recognition, and prevention of late sequelae. *Pediatric Annals, 35*(2), 90–100.

DiFazio, R., & Atkinson, R. (2005). Extremity fractures in children: When is it an emergency? *Journal of Pediatric Nursing, 20*(4), 298–304.

DiNucci, E. M. (2005). Energy healing: A complementary treatment for orthopaedic and other conditions. *Orthopaedic Nursing, 24*(4), 259–269.

Eilert, R. E. (2007). Orthopedics. In W. W. Hay, M. J. Levin, J. M. Sondheimer, & R. R. Deterding (Eds.), *Current pediatric diagnosis and treatment* (18th ed.). New York: McGraw-Hill.

Gore, A. I., & Spencer, J. P. (2004). The newborn foot. *American Family Physician, 69*(4), 865–872.

Goretsky, M. J., Kelly, R. E., Croitoru, D., & Nuss, D. (2004). Chest wall anomalies: Pectus excavatum and pectus carinatum. *Adolescent Medicine Clinics, 15*(3), 455–471 [electronic version]. Accessed 10/1/05.

Gris, M., Van Nieuwenhove, O., Gehanne, C., Quintin, J., & Burny, F. (2004). Treatment of supracondylar humeral fractures in children using external fixation. *Orthopedics, 27*(11), 1146–1150.

Hart, E. S., Grottkau, B. E., Rebello, G. N., & Albright, M. B. (2005). The newborn foot: Diagnosis and management of common conditions. *Orthopaedic Nursing, 24*(5), 313–323.

Hoffmeister, E. (2008). Research sheds greater light on Legg-Calve-Perthes disease. *Lippincott's Bone & Joint Newsletter, 14*(1), 1, 4–5.

Howard, A. W., MacArthur, C., Willan, A., Rothman, L., Moses-McKeag, A., & MacPherson, K. (2005). The effect of safer play equipment on playground injury rates among school children. *Canadian Medical Association Journal, 172*(11), 1443–1446.

Katz, D. A. (2006). Slipped capital femoral epiphysis: The importance of early diagnosis. *Pediatric Annals, 35*(2), 102–111.

Kocher, M. W., Lee, B., Dolan, M., Weinberg, J., & Shulman, S. T. (2006). *Pediatric Annals, 35*(2), 112–122.

Koester, M., & Mangus, B. C. (2004). Heads up for soccer injuries! What you need to know. *Contemporary Pediatrics, 22*(5), 75–88.

Lazzarini, L., Mader, J. T., & Calhoun, J. H. (2004). Current concepts review: Osteomyelitis in long bones. *Journal of Bone and Joint Surgery, 86*(10), 2305–2318.

Leung, A. K. C., & Lemay, J. F. (2004). The limping child. *Journal of Pediatric Health Care, 18,* 219–223.

Listernick, R. (2007). A 13-year-old girl with a history of weight loss and fatigue. *Pediatric Annals, 36*(8), 451–458

Luther, B. L. (2002). Congenital muscular torticollis. *Orthopedic Nursing, 21*(3), 21–28.

Mayrl, J. M., Grechenig, W., & Hollwarth, M. E. (2004). Musculoskeletal ultrasound in pediatric trauma. *European Journal of Trauma, 3,* 150–160 [electronic version]. Accessed 10/1/05 via Proquest database.

Metzl, J. D., & Metzl, J. A. (2004). Shin pain in an adolescent soccer player: A case-based look at "shin splints." *Contemporary Pediatrics, 21*(9), 36–48.

Moreland, M. S. (2001). Special concerns of the pediatric athlete. In F. H. Fu & D. A. Stone (Eds.), *Sports injuries: Mechanisms, prevention, treatment* (2nd ed.). Philadelphia: Lippincott Williams & Wilkins.

Morrissy, R. T., Giavedoni, B. J., & Coulter-O'Berry, C. (2006). The limb-deficient child. In R. T. Morrissy & S. L. Weinstein (Eds.),

Lovell & Winter's pediatric orthopaedics (6th ed.). Philadelphia: Lippincott Williams & Wilkins.

Newton, P. O., & Wenger, D. R. (2006). Idiopathic and congenital scoliosis. In R. T. Morrissy & S. L. Weinstein (Eds.), *Lovell & Winter's pediatric orthopaedics* (6th ed.). Philadelphia: Lippincott Williams & Wilkins.

Pagana, K. D., & Pagana, T. J. (2006). *Mosby's manual of diagnostic and laboratory tests* (3rd ed.). St. Louis: Mosby.

Parikh, S. N., Crawford, A. H., & Choudhury, S. (2004). Magnetic resonance imaging in the evaluation of infantile torticollis. *Orthopedics, 27*(5), 509–515.

Paton, E. (2007). Evaluating the child with a limp. *Advanced Emergency Nursing Journal, 29*(1), 68–72.

Price, C. T., Phillips, J. H., & Devito, D. P. (2006). Management of fractures. In R. T. Morrissy & S. L. Weinstein (Eds.), *Lovell & Winter's pediatric orthopaedics* (6th ed.). Philadelphia: Lippincott Williams & Wilkins.

Rauch, F., & Glorieux, F. H. (2004). Osteogenesis imperfecta. *Lancet, 363,* 1377–1385.

Ryan, L. M., DePiero, A. D., Sadow, K. B., Warmink, C. A., Chamberlin, J. M., Teach, S. J., & Johns, C. M. S. (2004). Recognition and management of pediatric fractures by pediatric residents. *Pediatrics, 114*(6), 1530–1533.

Sakkers, R., Kok, D., Engelbert, R., van Dongen, A., Jansen, M., Pruijs, H. Verbout, A., Schweitzer, D., & Uiterwaal, C. (2004). Skeletal effects and functional outcome with olpadronate in children with osteogenesis imperfecta: A 2-year randomized placebo-controlled study. *Lancet, 363,* 1427–1431.

Samaddar, K. (2007). Vitamin D deficiency rickets. *Consultant for Pediatricians, 6*(7), 408–412.

Stellwagen, L. M., Hubbard, E., & Vaux, K. (2004). Look for the 'stuck baby' to identify congenital torticollis. *Contemporary Pediatrics, 21*(5), 55 [electronic version]. Available at www.contemporarypediatrics.com.

Swoveland, B., Medvick, C., Kirsh, M., Thompson, K., & Nuss, D. (2001). The Nuss procedure for pectus excavatum correction. *AORN Journal, 74*(6), 827–850.

Taketokmo, C. K., Hodding, J. H., & Kraus, D. M. (2004). *Lexi-comp's pediatric dosage handbook* (11th ed.). Hudson, Ohio: Lexi-comp.

Tice, A., Rehm, S. J., Dalovisio, J. R., Bradley, J. S., Martinelli, L. P., Graham, D. R., Gainer, R. B., Kunkel, M. J., Yancey, R. W., & Williams, D. N. (2004). Practice guidelines for outpatient parenteral antimicrobial therapy. *Journal of Infusion Nursing, 27*(5), 339–359.

Weinstein, S. L. (2006). Developmental hip dysplasia and dislocation. In R. T. Morrissy & S. L. Weinstein (Eds.), *Lovell & Winter's pediatric orthopaedics* (6th ed.). Philadelphia: Lippincott Williams & Wilkins.

Zak, M. (2005). Pediatric orthopedic problems. In S. M. Nettina (Ed.), *Lippincott manual of nursing practice.* Philadelphia: Lippincott Williams & Wilkins.

Zaleske, D. J. (2006). Metabolic and endocrine abnormalities. In R. T. Morrissy & S. L. Weinstein (Eds.), *Lovell & Winter's pediatric orthopaedics* (6th ed.). Philadelphia: Lippincott Williams & Wilkins.

WEBSITES

National Infant Torticollis Association: www.infant-torticollis.org/

March of Dimes (birth defects foundation): www.marchofdimes.com

Youth sports information for parents: www.momsteam.com

National Institute of Arthritis and Musculoskeletal and Skin Diseases—sports injuries information: www.niams.nih.gov/Health_Info/Sports_Injuries/child_sports_injuries.asp

Osteogenesis Imperfecta Foundation: www.oif.org

Pediatric orthopedics and pediatric sports medicine for parents: www.orthoseek.com/

United Kingdom pectus excavatum and pectus carinatum information site: www.pectus.org/

Pediatric orthopedic surgery resource site: www.peds-ortho.com/

Pediatric orthopedic information from the Southern California Orthopedic Institute: www.scoi.com/peds.htm

Information on nonsurgical correction of scoliosis: www.scoliosis.com

National Scoliosis Foundation: www.scoliosis.org/

National Center for Sports Safety: www.sportssafety.org/

USA Safe Kids: www.usa.safekids.org/

CHAPTER WORKSHEET

MULTIPLE CHOICE QUESTIONS

1. The nurse is evaluating a parent's understanding of treatment for torticollis. Which response best indicates that the parent understands the appropriate treatment?

   a. Encourages the infant to turn the head to the unaffected side.

   b. States that prone positioning for sleep will be needed.

   c. Places the infant on the affected side.

   d. Stretches the infant's neck to the opposite side and holds it for 5 seconds.

2. The nurse is providing patient education related to use of a brace that the orthopedic surgeon has ordered as treatment for idiopathic scoliosis in an adolescent girl. Which statement by the teen best indicates an understanding of appropriate use of the brace?

   a. "I can take my brace off only for special occasions."

   b. "I will take my brace off for only 1 hour per day, for showering."

   c. "I do not need to wear my brace at night while I am sleeping."

   d. "It is most important for me to wear my brace during the day, while I am upright."

3. The nurse is caring for orthopedic patients who are in the postoperative period following spinal fusion. What is the most appropriate activity to delegate to unlicensed assistive personnel?

   a. Ambulate the children twice daily to promote mobility.

   b. Encourage commode use to promote bowel function.

   c. Provide diversionary activities, as the children must stay flat on their backs.

   d. Assist with log-rolling the children every 2 hours.

4. The nurse is caring for a child with a fractured left femur who has been in skeletal traction for several days. Upon assessment, she notes that the left foot is pale, with a nonpalpable pedal pulse. What is the priority nursing intervention?

   a. Release the traction, as there may be too much weight on it.

   b. Nothing; alterations in circulation are expected with skeletal traction.

   c. Immediately notify the physician of this abnormal finding.

   d. Massage the foot immediately to increase circulation.

CRITICAL THINKING EXERCISES

1. Develop a teaching plan for the family of an infant with developmental dysplasia of the hip or clubfoot.

2. Develop a discharge teaching plan for a 2-year-old who will be in a hip spica cast for 10 more weeks at home.

3. Devise a developmental/education plan for a child who will be confined to traction for 6 weeks. Choose a child in the clinical area whom you have cared for or choose a particular age group and develop the plan.

STUDY ACTIVITIES

1. In the clinical setting, compare the growth and development of a child with osteogenesis imperfecta or rickets with that of typical healthy child. What differences or similarities do you find? What are the explanations for your findings?

2. Attend a pediatric orthopedic clinic or the local clinic of Children's Medical Services. Identify the role of the registered nurse in this setting.

NURSING CARE OF THE CHILD WITH AN INTEGUMENTARY DISORDER

KEY TERMS

annular
dermatitis
erythema

macule
papule
pruritus

scaling
vesicle

LEARNING OBJECTIVES

Upon completion of the chapter, the learner will be able to:

1. Compare anatomic and physiologic differences of the integumentary system in infants and children versus adults.
2. Describe nursing care related to common laboratory and diagnostic tests used in the medical diagnosis of integumentary disorders in infants, children, and adolescents.
3. Distinguish integumentary disorders common in infants, children, and adolescents.
4. Identify appropriate nursing assessments and interventions related to pediatric integumentary disorders.
5. Develop an individualized nursing care plan for the child with an integumentary disorder.
6. Describe the psychosocial impact of a chronic integumentary disorder on children or adolescents.
7. Develop patient/family teaching plans for the child with an integumentary disorder.

Eva Lopez, 1 year old, is brought to the clinic by her mother, who states, "Eva has dry patches of skin, her wrists bleed from her scratching, and she's having trouble sleeping at night."

Wow

To a nurse the child's skin is life's gift wrapping, but to the child the skin is the space suit for life.

Integumentary disorders occur often in children, and if they are severe or chronic they can have a significant impact on the child. Infants and children are exposed to a multitude of infectious microorganisms and allergens, and their skin is sometimes affected by these exposures. Some integumentary disorders are as mild and self-limited as a minor abrasion, while others, such as atopic dermatitis, are chronic. Any skin disorder that is severe or could become so can have a major impact on the child's physiologic or psychological status. Nurses who care for children need to be familiar with common skin disorders of infancy, childhood, and adolescence so they can effectively intervene with children and their families.

Variations in Pediatric Anatomy and Physiology

Skin is the largest organ of the body and serves to protect the underlying tissues from trauma and invasion by microorganisms. The skin's health reflects the internal well-being of the body. The skin is also important for the perception of pain, heat, and cold and for the regulation of body temperature.

Differences in the Skin Between Children and Adults

The infant's epidermis is thinner than the adult's, and the blood vessels lie closer to the surface because there is a decreased amount of subcutaneous fat. Thus, the infant loses heat more readily through the skin's surface than the older child or adult does. The thinness of the infant's skin also allows substances to be absorbed through the skin more readily than they would be in an adult. Bacteria can gain access via the infant's and younger child's skin more readily than they can through the adult's skin. The infant's skin contains more water than in adults, and the epidermis is loosely bound to the dermis. This means that friction may easily cause separation of the layers, resulting in blistering or skin breakdown. The infant's skin is also less pigmented than that of the adult (in all races), placing the infant at increased risk of skin damage from ultraviolet radiation. Over time, the infant's skin toughens and becomes less hydrated and thus is less susceptible to microorganism invasion. The skin thickness and characteristics reach adult levels in the late teenage years (Starr, 2004).

Differences in Dark-Skinned Children

Children with dark skin tend to have more pronounced cutaneous reactions compared to children with lighter skin (Starr, 2004). Hypopigmentation or hyperpigmentation in the affected area following healing of a dermatologic con-

FIGURE 45.1 Keloid formation is more common in dark-skinned than light-skinned children.

dition is common in dark-skinned children. This change in pigmentation may be temporary (a few months following a superficial skin disorder) or permanent (following a more involved skin condition). Dark-skinned children tend to have more prominent papules, follicular responses, lichenification, and vesicular or bullous reactions than lighter-skinned children with the same disorder. Hypertrophic scarring and keloid formation (Fig. 45.1) occur more often in dark-skinned children.

Sebaceous and Sweat Glands

Sebaceous glands function immaturely at birth. The sebum secreted serves to lubricate the skin and hair. Sebum production increases in the preadolescent and adolescent years, which is why acne develops at that time. The infant's eccrine sweat glands are somewhat functional and will produce sweat as a response to emotional stimuli and heat. They become fully functional in the middle childhood years. Until that time, temperature regulation is less effective compared to older children and adults. The apocrine sweat glands are small and nonfunctional in the infant. They mature during puberty, at which time body odor develops in response to the fluid secreted by these glands.

Common Medical Treatments

A variety of medications as well as other medical treatments are used to treat integumentary disorders in children. Most of these treatments will require a physician's order when the child is in the hospital. The most common treatments and medications are listed in Common Medical Treatments 45.1 and Drug Guide 45.1. The nurse caring for the child with an integumentary disorder should be familiar with the procedures and medications, how they work, as well as common nursing implications related to their use.

COMMON MEDICAL TREATMENTS 45.1

Treatment	Explanation	Indications	Nursing Implications
Wet dressing	Dressing moistened with lukewarm water (sterile water may be required in certain cases)	In the presence of itching, crusting, or oozing—helps to remove crusts	May use Burow's, Domeboro, or saline solutions in certain cases. Provide atraumatic care by giving premedication before dressing change.
Sunscreen	Lotion, gel, or cream with a sun-protective factor (SPF)	All children over 6 months of age	Use a fragrance-free, para-aminobenzoic acid (PABA)–free preparation with an SPF of 15 or higher. Apply at least 30 minutes prior to sun exposure. Reapply at least every 2 hours while exposed (every 60 to 80 minutes while in the water). Sweat- and water-resistant preparations are available yet still require reapplication as noted above. Use daily in summer and in warm climates, even on overcast and cloudy days.
Bathing	Use of lukewarm water (with or without soap) to bathe	Itchy and irritating skin conditions	Recommend fragrance-free, dye-free soaps such as Dove, Aveeno, Basis, Lubriderm. Colloid (oatmeal baths) are especially helpful. Pat the child dry; do not rub the skin. Leave the child moist before applying medication, dressing, or moisturizer.

NURSING PROCESS OVERVIEW FOR THE CHILD WITH A INTEGUMENTARY DISORDER

Nursing management of the child with an integumentary disorder requires astute assessment skills, development of accurate nursing diagnoses and expected outcomes, implementation of appropriate interventions, and evaluation of the entire process. Many skin rashes may be associated with other, often serious, illnesses, so the nurse must use comprehensive and excellent assessment skills when evaluating rashes in children. Certain integumentary conditions are chronic and require ongoing care related to health maintenance, education, and psychosocial needs.

Assessment

Nursing assessment of the child with an integumentary disorder includes obtaining the health history and performing a physical examination. Assisting with or obtaining laboratory tests may also be necessary.

Remember Eva, the 1-year-old with the dry patches, itching, and trouble sleeping? What additional health history and physical examination assessment information should the nurse obtain?

Health History

Determine the child's or parent's chief complaint, which is most often related to pruritus, **scaling**, or a cosmetic disruption. Document the history of the present illness, noting onset, location, duration, characteristics, other symptoms and relieving factors, particularly as related to a rash or lesion. Also ask about the quantity and quality of any discharge from the rash or lesions. Document accompanying symptoms. Note the child's general state of health, history of chronic medical conditions, recent surgeries, hospitalizations, medications, or immunizations. Has there been a recent change in the child's food intake or environment? Is there a family history of chronic or acute skin conditions? Does anyone in the home have a similar concern at this time? Does the family have pets that go outdoors? Does the child play in the woods or garden? Note usual skin care routines, as well as types of soaps, cosmetics, or other skin care products used. Determine the amount of daily sun exposure and whether the child consistently uses sunscreen.

Physical Examination

Perform a complete physical examination, noting any abnormalities. Perform a focused and thorough examination of the skin. The best lighting for examination of the skin is natural daylight. Look at the skin in general, noting distribution of any obvious lesions. Inspect the mucous

DRUG GUIDE 45.1 COMMON DRUGS FOR INTEGUMENTARY DISORDERS

Medication	Action/Indication	Nursing Implications
Antibiotics (topical)	Decrease skin colonization with bacteria. Indicated for mild acne vulgaris, impetigo, folliculitis.	Apply as prescribed to clean skin or a cleansed wound. Be alert for neomycin allergy.
Antibiotics (systemic)	Bactericidal or bacteriostatic against a variety of organisms, depending on the preparation. Used for moderate to severe acne vulgaris, extensive impetigo, cellulitis, scalded skin syndrome.	Check for medication allergies prior to administration. Teach families to finish entire course of antibiotics.
Corticosteroids (topical)	Anti-inflammatory effect in atopic dermatitis and certain kinds of contact dermatitis.	Do not use moderate- or high-potency corticosteroid preparations on the face or genitals. Do not cover with an occlusive dressing. Absorption is increased in the young infant.
Antifungals (topical)	Fungicidal used to treat tinea, candidal diaper rash.	Apply a thin layer as prescribed. Comply with length of treatment as prescribed to prevent reemergence of the rash.
Antifungals (systemic): griseofulvin, ketoconazole	Kills fungus; binds to human keratin, making it resistant to fungus. Indicated for tinea capitis and severe or widespread fungal skin infections.	Griseofulvin: give with fatty food to increase absorption. Requires minimum 4-week course. Monitor liver function tests and CBC. May cause photosensitivity. Ketoconazole: administer with food to decrease GI upset.
Benzoyl peroxide	Decreases colonization of *P. acnes* in mild acne vulgaris.	Available in combination with topical antibiotics. Apply sparingly. Shake before application. Avoid contact with eyes and mucous membranes.
Retinoids (topical): tretinoin, adapalene, tazarotene	Anticomedogenic activity in moderate to severe acne vulgaris.	Adverse effects: dryness, burning, photosensitivity. Instruct child to use SPF 15 or higher sunscreen.
Topical immune modulators (tacrolimus, pimecrolimus)	Inhibits T-lymphocyte action at the skin level. Used for moderate to severe atopic dermatitis, or in conditions resistant to topical steroids.	Use only in children over 2 years old. Avoid sunlight exposure. May cause burning, pruritus, flu-like symptoms, or headache.
Antihistamines (diphenhydramine, chlorpheniramine, hydroxyzine)	Antihistaminic effect, results in sedation. Indicated for hypersensitivity reactions, atopic dermatitis or contact dermatitis that is severely pruritic.	May give three or four times a day unless sedation effect interferes with activities of daily living or school.
Systemic corticosteroids (prednisone, dexamethasone, methylprednisolone)	Anti-inflammatory and immunosuppressive action. Used in severe contact dermatitis.	Administer with food to decrease GI upset. May mask signs of infection. Monitor blood pressure, urine for glucose. Do not stop treatment abruptly or acute adrenal insufficiency may occur. Monitor for Cushing syndrome. Doses may be tapered over time.
Isotretinoin (Accutane)	Reduces sebaceous gland size, decreases sebum production, and regulates cell proliferation and differentiation. Indicated for cystic acne or severe acne that is resistant to 3 months of treatment with oral antibiotics.	Ensure that the adolescent girl is not pregnant and does not become pregnant. Monitor CBC, lipid profiles, liver function tests, and beta-human chorionic gonadotropin monthly. Monitor for suicide risk.

Medication	Action and Indications	Nursing Implications
Coal tar preparations	Antipruritic and anti-inflammatory effect. Useful in psoriasis, atopic dermatitis.	May stain fabrics; strong and unpleasant odor. Apply at bedtime and rinse off in the morning to improve compliance.
Silver sulfadiazine 1%(Silvadene)	Bactericidal against gram-positive and gram-negative bacteria and yeasts. Indicated for burns.	Cover with occlusive dressing. Apply BID. Do not use in patients with sulfa allergy. Forms a gel on the burn that is painful to remove. May cause transient neutropenia. Do not use on the child's face or on an infant less than 2 months of age.

membranes, noting and describing lesions if present. Examine all surfaces of the skin and scalp carefully. Note temperature, moisture, texture, and fragility of the skin. If a rash or lesions are present, note their location and provide a detailed description of them. Describe whether a rash is macular, papular, pustular, or vesicular. Provide a description of vascular lesions if present (refer to Chapter 31 for additional information on vascular lesions). Describe lesions according to the following criteria:

• Linear: in a line
• Shape: Are the lesions round, oval, **annular** (ring around central clearing)?
• Morbilliform: a rosy, maculopapular rash
• Target lesions: like a bull's-eye

If lesions are present on the scalp, has hair loss in that region occurred? If drainage is present, describe it as clear, purulent, honey-colored, or otherwise. Note scaling or lichenification of the skin. Palpate for regional lymphadenopathy.

Laboratory and Diagnostic Testing
Common Laboratory and Diagnostic Tests 45.1 details the laboratory and diagnostic tests most commonly used when considering integumentary disorders. The tests can assist the physician or nurse practitioner in diagnosing the disorder or can be used as guidelines in determining ongoing treatment. Some of the tests are obtained by laboratory or non-nursing personnel, while others might be obtained by the nurse. In either instance the nurse should be familiar with how the tests are obtained, what they are used for, and normal versus abnormal results. This knowledge will also be necessary when providing patient and family education related to the testing.

Nursing Diagnoses and Related Interventions
Upon completion of a thorough assessment, the nurse might identify several nursing diagnoses, such as:

• Impaired skin integrity
• Pain

• Risk for infection
• Disturbed body image
• Risk for fluid volume deficit
• Altered nutrition

After completing an assessment of Eva, the nurse noted the following: hypopigmentation of the skin behind her knees, dry patches on her wrists and face, and slight wheezing heard bilaterally on auscultation. Based on these assessment findings, what would your top three nursing diagnoses be for Eva?

Desired outcomes and interventions are based on the nursing diagnoses. Nursing Care Plan 45.1 can be used as a guide in planning nursing care for the child with an integumentary disorder. Individualize the plan of care based on the child's and family's responses to the health alteration; see Chapter 35 for information about pain management. Additional information will be included later in the chapter as it relates to specific disorders.

Based on your top three nursing diagnoses for Eva, describe appropriate nursing interventions.

Infectious Disorders

Infectious disorders of the skin include those caused by viral, bacterial, or fungal infection. The viral exanthems are discussed in Chapter 36. Bacterial and fungal infections of the skin are discussed below.

▶ BACTERIAL INFECTIONS

Bacterial infections of the skin include bullous and non-bullous impetigo, folliculitis, cellulitis, and staphylococcal scalded skin syndrome. These bacterial skin infections

COMMON LABORATORY AND DIAGNOSTIC TESTS 45.1

Test	Explanation	Indications	Nursing Implications
Complete blood count (CBC) with differential	Evaluate hemoglobin and hematocrit, WBC count (particularly the percentage of individual WBCs), and platelet count	Infection or inflammatory process	Normal values vary according to age and gender. WBC differential is helpful in evaluating source of infection. May be affected by myelosuppressive drugs. Eosinophils may be elevated in the child with atopic dermatitis.
Erythrocyte sedimentation rate (ESR)	Nonspecific test used to detect presence of infection or inflammation	Infection or inflammatory process	Send sample to laboratory immediately; if allowed to stand for longer than 3 hours, may result in falsely low result.
Potassium hydroxide (KOH) prep	Reveals branching hyphae (fungus) when viewed under microscope	To identify fungal infection	Place skin scrapings on a microscope slide and add KOH 20% drop.
Culture of wound or skin drainage	Allows for microbial growth and organism identification	Identification of specific organism	Note sensitivities.
Immunoglobulin E (IgE)	Measurement of serum IgE	Atopic dermatitis	Often elevated in allergic or atopic disease, though this is a nonspecific finding. May be increased if the child takes systemic corticosteroids.
Patch or skin testing	Needle prick testing with allergens	Atopic or contact dermatitis	Have emergency equipment available in the event of anaphylaxis (rare).

are often caused by *Staphylococcus aureus* and group A beta-hemolytic streptococcus, which are ordinarily normal flora on the skin. Impetigo, folliculitis, and cellulitis are usually self-limited disorders that rarely become severe.

Impetigo is a readily recognizable skin rash (Fig. 45.2). Nonbullous impetigo generally follows some type of skin trauma or may arise as a secondary bacterial infection of another skin disorder, such as atopic dermatitis. Bullous impetigo demonstrates a sporadic occurrence pattern and develops on intact skin, resulting from toxin production by *S. aureus*.

Folliculitis, infection of the hair follicle, most often results from occlusion of the hair follicle. It may occur as a result of poor hygiene, prolonged contact with contaminated water, maceration, or a moist environment or from use of occlusive emollient products.

Cellulitis is a localized infection and inflammation of the skin and subcutaneous tissues and is usually preceded by skin trauma of some sort (Fig. 45.3).

Staphylococcal scalded skin syndrome results from infection with *S. aureus* that produces a toxin, which then causes exfoliation. It has an abrupt onset and results in diffuse erythema and skin tenderness. Scalded skin syndrome is most common in infancy and rare beyond 5 years of age (Marino & Fine, 2007).

Of particular concern are bacterial skin infections caused by methicillin-resistant *S. aureus* (MRSA). In chil-

dren these infections most commonly occur after an insect or spider bite or other cause of cellulitis (Siberry, 2005). Additional risk factors for community-acquired MRSA are turf burns, towel-sharing, shaving, improper disinfection of sports protective equipment and locker rooms, and poor hygiene (Romero et al., 2006). Community outbreaks of MRSA became widespread throughout the United States by 2004 (Siberry, 2005). If the child presents with a moderate to severe skin infection or with an infection that is not responding as expected to therapy, it is important to culture the infected area for MRSA.

Therapeutic management of bacterial skin infections includes topical or systemic antibiotics and appropriate hygiene (Table 45.1).

Nursing Assessment

Obtain the history as noted in the nursing process overview section. Note history of skin disruption such as a cut, scrape, or insect or spider bite (nonbullous impetigo and cellulitis). Note body piercing in the adolescent, which can lead to impetigo or cellulitis. Measure the child's temperature: fever may occur with bullous impetigo or cellulitis and is common with scalded skin syndrome. Inspect the skin, noting abnormalities, documenting their location and distribution, and describing drainage if present. Table 45.1 gives specific clinical manifestations of

Nursing Care Plan 45.1

OVERVIEW FOR THE CHILD WITH AN INTEGUMENTARY DISORDER

NURSING DIAGNOSIS: Impaired skin integrity related to infectious process, hypersensitivity reaction, injury, or mechanical factors as evidenced by rash, inflammation, abrasion, laceration, or disrupted epidermis

Outcome Identification and Evaluation

Integrity of skin surface will be restored; *rash, abrasion, laceration, or other skin disruption will heal.*

Interventions: Restoring Skin Integrity

- Assess site of skin impairment *to determine extent of involvement and plan care.*
- Monitor skin impairment every shift for changes in color, warmth, redness, or other signs of infection *to identify problems early.*
- Determine the child's and family's skin care practices to *establish need for education related to skin care.*
- Individualize the child's skin care regimen depending on the child's particular skin condition *to most appropriately care for skin in light of the child's disorder.*
- In the immobile child, use a risk assessment tool (such as a modified Norton or Braden scale) *to identify risk for skin breakdown.*
- Position the child on the opposite side of the skin impairment *to avoid further skin breakdown.*
- Encourage appropriate nutritional intake *as adequate nutrients are necessary for appropriate immune function and skin healing.*
- Consult the wound and ostomy care nurse specialist *to determine best approach for individualized wound care.*
- Provide dressing change and wound care as prescribed *to promote wound or burn healing.*

NURSING DIAGNOSIS: Risk for infection related to disruption in protective skin barrier

Outcome Identification and Evaluation

Child will remain free of local or systemic infection, will remain afebrile, *without additional redness or warmth at skin disruption site.*

Interventions: Preventing Infection

- Use appropriate hand hygiene *to decrease transmission of infectious organisms.*
- Assess the skin impairment site for increased warmth, redness, discharge, or new purulence *to identify infection early.*
- Assess temperature every 4 hours or more frequently if needed, *as children develop fever quickly in response to infection.*
- Note WBC and culture results, reporting unexpected values to the primary care provider *so that appropriate treatment may be started.*
- Follow prescribed therapies for skin alteration *to maintain skin moisture and prevent further breakdown, which may lead to infection.*
- Encourage appropriate nutritional intake *as adequate nutrients are necessary for appropriate immune function and skin healing.*

NURSING DIAGNOSIS: Disturbed body image related to chronic skin changes caused by disease process, burns, or other skin alteration as evidenced by child's verbalization, reluctance to participate in activities, or social withdrawal

Outcome Identification and Evaluation

Child will verbalize or demonstrate acceptance of alteration in body, *will return to previous level of social involvement.*

Interventions: Promoting Appropriate Body Image

- Assess child or teen for feelings about alteration in skin *to determine baseline.*
- Acknowledge feelings of anger or depression related to skin changes *to provide an outlet for feelings.*
- Encourage the child or teen to participate in skin care *to give some sense of control over what is occurring.*
- Help the child or teen to accept self *as the perception of self is tied to knowing oneself and identifying what the self values.*

(continued)

Nursing Care Plan 45.1 (continued)

NURSING DIAGNOSIS: Risk for deficient fluid volume related to burns

Outcome Identification and Evaluation

Fluid volume status will be balanced, *child will maintain urine output of 1 to 2 mL/kg/hour, oral mucosa will be moist and pink, heart rate will remain within age- and situation-specific parameters.*

Interventions: Promoting Fluid Balance

• Assess fluid volume status at least every shift, more frequently if disrupted, *to obtain baseline for comparison.*
• Strictly monitor intake and output *to detect imbalance or need for additional fluid intake.*
• Weigh the child daily on the same scale, at the same time, in the same amount of clothing *as changes in weight are an accurate indicator of fluid volume status in children.*
• Provide intravenous fluid resuscitation in initial period, followed by encouragement of oral fluid intake in the burned patient, *to compensate for fluid loss through burned areas.*

NURSING DIAGNOSIS: Imbalanced nutrition, less than body requirements, related to increased metabolic state (burns) as evidenced by poor wound healing, difficulty gaining or maintaining body weight

Outcome Identification and Evaluation

Child will demonstrate balanced nutritional state, *will maintain or gain weight as appropriate for situation, will demonstrate improvement in wound healing.*

Interventions: Promoting Nutrition

• Assess the child's food preferences and ability to eat *to provide a baseline for planning nursing care.*
• Consult the nutritionist *because nutritional needs are increased related to altered metabolic state as a result of burns.*
• Collaborate with the nutritionist, child, and parents to plan meals that appeal to the child *to increase the child's intake.*
• Administer vitamin and mineral preparations as prescribed *to supplement nutrients.*
• Provide smaller, more frequent meals and snacks *to promote increased intake.*
• Weigh the child daily *to determine progress.*

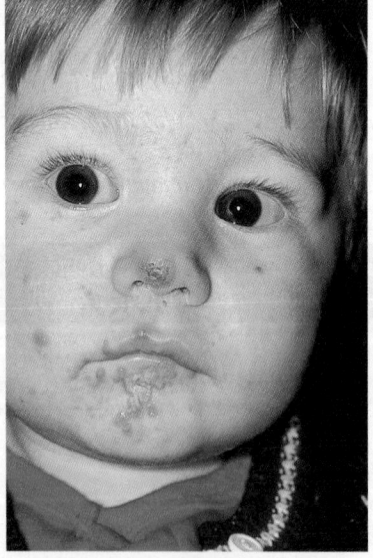

FIGURE 45.2 Note honey-colored crusting with impetigo.

FIGURE 45.3 Note erythema and edema associated with cellulitis.

TABLE 45.1 BACTERIAL SKIN INFECTIONS

Disorder	Skin Findings	Usual Treatment
Nonbullous impetigo	• **Papules** progressing to vesicles, then painless pustules with a narrow erythematous border • Honey-colored exudate when the vesicles or pustules rupture, which forms a crust on the ulcer-like base (see Fig. 45.2)	• Limited amount: treat topically with mupirocin ointment. • If numerous lesions, oral first-generation cephalosporin is indicated (Marino & Fine, 2007). • Clindamycin may be needed for MRSA. • Remove honey-colored crust with cool compresses BID.
Bullous impetigo	• Red macules and bullous eruptions on an erythematous base • Size may be from a few millimeters to several centimeters.	• Oral first-generation cephalosporin • Good hygiene
Folliculitis	• Red, raised hair follicles	• Treat with aggressive hygiene: warm compresses after washing with soap and water several times a day. • Topical mupirocin is indicated; occasionally oral antibiotics are required.
Cellulitis	• Localized reaction: **erythema**, pain, edema, warmth at site of skin disruption (see Fig. 45.3)	• Mild cases are usually treated with cephalexin or amoxicillin/clavulanic acid. • More severe cases and periorbital or orbital cellulitis require IV cephalosporins.
Staphylococcal scalded skin syndrome	• Flattish bullae that rupture within hours • Red, weeping surface is left, most commonly on face, groin, neck, and axillary region	• Mild to moderate cases are treated with oral cephalexin, dicloxacillin, or amoxicillin/clavulanic acid. • Severe cases are managed similar to burns with aggressive fluid management and IV oxacillin or clindamycin.

the various bacterial skin infections. Palpate for regional lymphadenopathy, which may be present with impetigo or cellulitis. Blood cultures are indicated in the child with cellulitis with lymphangitic streaking and in all cases of periorbital or orbital cellulitis.

Nursing Management

Administer antibiotics topically or systemically as prescribed. Teach the family about antibiotic administration and care of the lesions or rash. Soak impetiginous lesions with cool compresses or Burow's solution to remove crusts before applying topical antibiotics. Though impetigo is considered a contagious disorder among vulnerable populations, removal from school or day care is not necessary unless the condition is widespread or actively weeping (Watkins, 2005). Prevent transmission of nosocomial MRSA by appropriately isolating children according to the institution's policy when the child is hospitalized. In children with scalded skin syndrome, the risk of scarring may be reduced by minimal handling, avoidance of corticosteroids, and application of soothing ointments as the skin heals (Starr, 2004).

Educate the family about prevention of bacterial skin infections. Stress the importance of cleanliness and hygiene. Teach the family to keep the child's fingernails cut short and to clean the nails with a nail brush at bath time. When a skin disruption such as a cut, scrape, or insect bite occurs, teach the family to clean the area well to prevent the development of cellulitis. Folliculitis may be prevented with diligent hygiene and avoidance of occlusive emollients. Table 45.1 gives additional information about specific treatments for bacterial skin infections.

▶ FUNGAL INFECTIONS

Fungi also cause infections on children's skin. *Tinea* is a fungal disease of the skin occurring on any part of the body. The part of the body affected determines the second word in the name; for instance, tinea pedis refers to a fungal infection on the feet. The three organisms most often responsible for tinea are *Epidermophyton, Microsporum,* and *Trichophyton,* though *Malassezia furfur* causes tinea versicolor. *Candida albicans* may cause an infection of the skin, particularly in a warm, moist area such as the diaper area; in fact, 80% of diaper rashes lasting longer than 4 days are colonized with *C. albicans* (Marino & Fine, 2007). All fungal skin infections may occur year-round, but tinea versicolor is more common in warm weather.

Therapeutic management of fungal infections involves appropriate hygiene and administration of an antifungal agent. Table 45.2 gives further information about treatment.

Nursing Assessment

Elicit the health history, noting exposure to another person with a fungal infection or exposure to a pet (fungi are often carried by pets). Note onset of the rash and whether it is itchy. Determine if the child has recently visited the barber (tinea capitis). Note contact with damp areas such as locker rooms and swimming pools, use of nylon socks or nonbreathable shoes, or minor trauma to the feet (tinea pedis). Document a history of wearing tight clothing or participating in a contact sport such as wrestling (tinea cruris). Inspect the skin and scalp, noting the location, description, and distribution of the rash or lesions (Figs. 45.4, 45.5, and 45.6). Table 45.2 describes the clinical findings associated with various types of tinea.

Scraping and KOH preparation show branching hyphae. For tinea capitis, Wood's lamp will fluoresce yellow-green if it is caused by *Microsporum,* but not with *Trichophyton.* A fungal culture of a plucked hair is more reliable for diagnosis of tinea capitis.

FIGURE 45.4 Tinea corporis: note raised scaly border with clearing in center.

Nursing Management

Maintain appropriate hygiene and administer antifungal agents as prescribed (see Table 45.2). Additional specifics related to the individual fungal disorders are as follows:

• Tinea corporis is contagious, but the child may return to daycare or school once treatment has begun. Identify and treat family members or other contacts.

TABLE 45.2 MANIFESTATIONS AND MANAGEMENT OF FUNGAL INFECTIONS

Disorder	Skin Findings	Usual Treatment
Tinea corporis (ringworm)	• Annular lesion with raised peripheral scaling and central clearing (looks like a ring) (see Fig. 45.4)	• Topical antifungal cream is required for at least 4 weeks.
Tinea capitis	• Patches of scaling in the scalp with central hair loss • Risk of kerion development (inflamed, boggy mass that is filled with pustules) (see Fig. 45.5)	• Oral griseofulvin for 4 to 6 weeks. • Selenium sulfide shampoo may be used to decrease contagiousness (adjunct only). • No school or daycare for 1 week after treatment initiated.
Tinea versicolor	• Superficial tan or hypopigmented oval scaly lesions, especially on upper back and chest and proximal arms • More noticeable in the summer with tanning of unaffected areas	• Apply selenium sulfide shampoo all over body (from face to knees) and allow to stay on skin overnight, rinsing in the morning, once a week for 4 weeks (this may cause skin irritation). • Topical antifungals in the imidazole family may be used instead.
Tinea pedis (athlete's foot)	• Red, scaling rash on soles and between the toes	• Topical antifungal cream, powder, or spray. • Appropriate foot hygiene.
Tinea cruris	• Erythema, scaling, maceration in the inguinal creases and inner thighs (penis/scrotum spared)	• Topical antifungal preparation for 4 to 6 weeks.
Diaper candidiasis (also called monilial diaper rash)	• Fiery red lesions, scaling in the skin folds, and satellite lesions (located further out from the main rash) (see Fig. 45.6)	• Topical nystatin with diaper changes for several days. • See section on diaper dermatitis for additional information.

FIGURE 45.5 Note hair breakage and loss with tinea capitis.

FIGURE 45.6 A bright red rash with satellite lesions occurs with diaper candidiasis.

- Counsel the child with tinea capitis and parents that hair will usually regrow in 3 to 12 months. Wash sheets and clothes in hot water to decrease the risk of the infection spreading to other family members.
- Instruct the child with tinea pedis to keep the feet clean and dry. Feet should be rinsed with water or a water/vinegar mixture and dried well, especially between the toes. The child should wear cotton socks and shoes that allow the feet to breathe. Going barefoot at home is allowed, but flip-flops should be worn around swimming pools and in locker rooms.
- Inform the child with tinea versicolor that return to normal skin pigmentation may take several months.
- Counsel the boy with tinea cruris to wear cotton underwear and loose clothing. It is important to maintain good hygiene, particularly after sports practice or a sporting event.

- For management of diaper candidiasis, follow the suggestions listed below in the section on diaper dermatitis.

Hypersensitivity Reactions

Skin disorders caused by hypersensitivity reactions include diaper dermatitis, atopic dermatitis, contact dermatitis, erythema multiforme, and urticaria. Drug reactions may result in skin rashes, or as erythema multiforme or urticaria.

▶ DIAPER DERMATITIS

Diaper dermatitis is an inflammatory reaction of the skin in the area covered by a diaper (Nield & Kamat, 2006).

EVIDENCE-BASED PRACTICE 45.1
Effectiveness of Various Systemic Antifungal Drugs in Treating Tinea Capitis in Children

● **Study**
Tinea capitis (fungal infection of the scalp) affects a large number of children. Traditionally, a 6- to 8-week course of oral griseofulvin was required to eradicate the infection. The authors evaluated 21 randomized controlled studies that included a total of 1,812 participants. The studies determined the effectiveness of terbinafine, itraconazole, fluconazole, and griseofulvin at eradicating dermatophytes in tinea capitis.

▲ **Findings**
The authors found that shorter courses (2 to 4 weeks) with terbinafine, itraconazole, or fluconazole were as effective

at treating tinea capitis as the traditional longer course with griseofulvin.

■ **Nursing Implications**
Shorter courses of treatment will improve compliance, although the drugs may be more expensive. Educate families that the shorter course will be simpler to complete and result in fewer side effects and decreased need for laboratory evaluation of their child. Assist families with any paperwork needed to encourage insurance coverage for these drugs if needed.

González, U., Seaton, T., Bergus, G., Jacobson, J., & Martínez-Monzón, C. (2007). Systemic antifungal therapy for tinea capitis in children. *The Cochrane Library 2007, 4.* Indianapolis: John Wiley & Sons.

It is a nonimmunologic response to a skin irritant that results in skin cell hydration disturbance (Allen, 2004). Prolonged exposure to urine and feces may lead to skin breakdown (Fig. 45.7). Diaper wearing increases the skin's pH, activating fecal enzymes that further contribute to skin maceration.

Nursing Assessment

Determine from the history whether the infant or child wears diapers. Ask about the onset and progression of the rash, as well as any treatments and response. Inspect the skin in the diaper area for erythema and maceration (see Fig. 45.7). Ordinary diaper dermatitis does not usually result in a bumpy rash, but starts as a flat red rash in the convex skin creases. It may appear red and shiny and may or may not also have papules. Untreated, it may become more widespread or severe. Some cases of diaper dermatitis are caused by overgrowth of *C. albicans* (see Fig. 45.6 and the section on fungal infections).

Nursing Management

Prevention is the best management. Topical products such as ointments or creams containing vitamins A, D, and E, zinc oxide, or petrolatum are helpful to provide a barrier to the skin. Teaching Guidelines 45.1 gives further information on diaper dermatitis. See above for treatment of diaper rash caused by *C. albicans* infection.

> ▶ *Take* NOTE!
>
> *Discourage parents from using any type of baby powder to avoid the risk of aspiration, which may result in pneumonitis.*

FIGURE 45.7 Diaper dermatitis.

TEACHING GUIDELINES 45.1

Diaper Dermatitis

- Change diapers frequently. Stool-soiled diapers should be changed as soon as possible.
- Gently wash the diaper area with a soft cloth, avoiding harsh soaps.
- Baby wipes may be used in most children, but avoid wipes that contain fragrance or preservatives.
- Once the rash has occurred, allow the infant or child to go diaperless for a period of time each day to allow the rash to heal.
- Blow-dry the diaper area with the dryer set on the warm (not hot) setting for 3 to 5 minutes.
- Avoid rubber pants.

▶ ATOPIC DERMATITIS

Atopic dermatitis (eczema) is one of the disorders in the atopy family (along with asthma and allergic rhinitis). Atopic dermatitis affects 10% of the population as a whole (Marino & Fine, 2007). About half of the children who have atopic dermatitis also have asthma (Marino & Fine, 2007). Seventy-five percent of persons with atopic dermatitis have a family history of the disorder, and as many as 60% to 65% of children with the disorder show signs of it in the first year of life (Garfunkel et al., 2007). Ninety percent of children with atopic dermatitis develop symptoms before 5 years of age (Peterson & Chan, 2007).

The chronic itching associated with atopic dermatitis causes a great deal of psychological distress. The child's self-image may be affected, particularly if the rash is extensive. Difficulty sleeping may occur because of the itching. The child is irritable and has difficulty concentrating, and family life is disrupted. Parents' stress related to the child's condition may increase the child's anxiety and lead to an increase in itching and scratching. The child may outgrow atopic dermatitis, its severity may decrease as the child approaches adulthood, or the child may continue to have difficulties into the adult years. Bacterial superinfection may occur as a complication.

Therapeutic management includes good skin hydration, application of topical corticosteroids or immune modulators, oral antihistamines for sedative effects, and antibiotics if secondary infection occurs.

Pathophysiology

Atopic dermatitis is a chronic disorder characterized by extreme itching and inflamed, reddened, and swollen skin. It has a relapsing and remitting nature. The skin reaction occurs in response to specific allergens, usually food (especially eggs, wheat, milk, and peanuts) or environmental triggers (e.g., molds, dust mites, and cat dander). Other factors, such as high or low ambient temperatures, perspiring, scratching, skin irritants, or stress, may contribute to flare-ups. When the child encounters a triggering antigen, antigen-presenting cells stimulate interleukins to begin the inflammatory process. The skin begins to feel pruritic and the child starts to scratch. The sensation of itchiness comes first, and then the rash becomes apparent. The scratching causes the rash to appear. Sweating causes atopic dermatitis to worsen, as does excessively humid or dry environments.

Nursing Assessment

For a full description of the assessment phase of the nursing process, refer to page 1495. Assessment findings pertinent to atopic dermatitis are discussed below.

Health History

Elicit a description of the present illness and chief complaint. Common signs and symptoms reported during the health history might include:

• Wiggling or scratching
• Dry skin
• Scratch marks noticed by the parents
• Disrupted sleep
• Irritability

Explore the child's current and past medical history for risk factors such as:

• Family history of atopic dermatitis, allergic rhinitis, or asthma
• Child's history of asthma or allergic rhinitis
• Food or environmental allergies

Determine the onset of the rash, its location, progression, severity, and response to treatments used so far. Note medications used to treat the rash, as well as other medications the child may be taking.

Physical Examination

Physical examination consists of inspection and observation and auscultation.

Inspection and Observation

Observe whether the infant is wiggling or the child is actively scratching. Carefully inspect the skin. Document dry, scaly, or flaky skin, as well as hypertrophy and lichenification (Fig. 45.8). If lesions are present they may be dry lesions or weepy papules or vesicles. In children under 2 years old, the rash is most likely to occur on the face, scalp, wrists, and extensor surfaces of the arms or legs. In older children it may occur anywhere on the skin, but is found more commonly on the flexor areas. Note erythema or warmth, which may indicate associated sec-

FIGURE 45.8 Atopic dermatitis rash is red, dry, and scaly.

ondary bacterial infection. Document areas of hyperpigmentation or hypopigmentation, which may have resulted from a prior exacerbation of atopic dermatitis or its treatment. Inspect the eyes, nose, and throat for symptoms of allergic rhinitis.

Auscultation

Auscultate the lungs for wheezing (commonly found in the associated condition of asthma).

Laboratory and Diagnostic Tests

Serum IgE levels may be elevated in the child with atopic dermatitis. Skin prick allergy testing may determine the food or environmental allergen to which the child is sensitive.

Nursing Management

Nursing management of the child with atopic dermatitis focuses on promoting skin hydration, maintaining skin integrity, and preventing infection.

Promoting Skin Hydration

First and foremost, avoid hot water and any skin or hair product containing perfumes, dyes, or fragrance. Bathe the child twice daily in warm (not hot) water. Use a mild soap to clean only the dirty areas. Recommended mild soaps or cleansing agents include:

• Unscented Dove or Dove for sensitive skin
• Tone
• Caress
• Oil of Olay
• Cetaphil
• Aquanil

Slightly pat the child dry after the bath, but do not rub with the towel. Leave the child moist. Apply topical ointments or creams as prescribed to the affected area. Apply fragrance-free moisturizer over the prescribed topical medication and all over the child's body. Recommended moisturizers include:

- Eucerin, Moisturel, Curel (cream or lotion)
- Aquaphor
- Vaseline
- Crisco

Apply moisture multiple times throughout the day. Avoid clothing made of synthetic fabrics or wool. Avoid triggers known to exacerbate atopic dermatitis.

Evening primrose oil and other essential fatty acid supplements over a period of at least 6 weeks may produce an improvement in the atopic dermatitis. Headache and nausea are rare adverse effects of these supplements and if they occur are usually mild (Magin et al., 2006). Chamomile preparations for topical use may also be effective and are generally considered safe.

▶ *Take NOTE!*

Vaseline or generic petrolatum is an inexpensive, readily available moisturizer.

Maintaining Skin Integrity and Preventing Infection

Cut the child's fingernails short and keep them clean. Avoid tight clothing and heat. Use 100% cotton bed sheets and pajamas. In addition to keeping the child's skin well moisturized, it is extremely important to prevent the child from scratching. Scratching causes the rash to appear and further scratching may lead to secondary infection. Antihistamines given at bedtime may sedate the child enough to allow him or her to sleep without awakening because of itching.

During the waking hours, behavior modification may help to keep the child from scratching. Have the parent keep a diary for 1 week to determine the pattern of scratching. Help the parent to determine specific strategies that may raise the child's awareness of scratching. A hand-held clicker or counter may help to identify the scratching episode for the child, thus raising awareness. The use of diversion, imagination, and play may help to distract the child from scratching. The parent and child may create a game together that results in the child participating in a behavior rather than scratching. Pressing the skin or clenching the fist may replace scratching. It is important for the child to stay active to distract his or her mind from the itching. The parent should positively reinforce and reward the desired behaviors (Buchanan, 2001).

▶ CONTACT DERMATITIS

Contact dermatitis is a cell-mediated response to an antigenic substance exposure. The first exposure is the sensitization phase. The antigen attaches to cells that migrate to regional lymph nodes and have contact with T lymphocytes, where recognition of antigen is developed. During the second phase, elicitation, contact with the antigen results in T-lymphocyte proliferation and release of inflammatory mediators. An allergic response occurs within 24 to 48 hours after contact with the substance (Allen, 2004).

One of the more common causes of contact dermatitis in children results from exposure to highly allergenic plants and thus will be the focus of this discussion. *Toxicodendron radican* (poison ivy), *Toxicodendron quercifolium* (Eastern poison oak), *Toxicodendron diversilobum* (Western poison oak), and *Toxicodendron vernix* (poison sumac) are the typical offenders. Contact with the plant's oil (urushiol), which is found in the leaves, stems, and roots, results in an allergic reaction in 50% to 70% of people (Allen, 2004). Even contact with dormant plants or plants perceived to be dead may cause an allergic response. The rash is extremely pruritic and may last for 2 to 4 weeks, and lesions continue to appear during the illness.

Contact dermatitis is not contagious and does not spread either to other parts of the affected child's skin or to other people. Scratching does not spread the rash, but it may cause skin damage or secondary infection. Complications of contact dermatitis include secondary bacterial skin infections and lichenification or hyperpigmentation, particularly in dark-skinned people.

Therapeutic management is directed toward management of itching and the use of topical corticosteroids. Moderate-potency topical glucocorticoid cream or ointment is used for mild to moderate contact dermatitis, and high-potency preparations are used for more severe cases. Some severe cases of contact dermatitis may require the use of systemic steroids.

Nursing Assessment

Elicit the health history, noting time spent in the woods or noncultivated areas within 1 to 2 days before the onset of the rash. Note contact with a family pet that spends time outdoors. Note onset, description, location, and progression of the rash, which will be intensely pruritic in most children (Fig. 45.9). Document treatment used thus far, and the child's response to it. Examine the skin, noting an erythematous papulovesicular rash at the site of contact. Some lesions may be weeping; others erupt and form a crust. The lesions are often distributed in an asymmetric linear pattern on exposed body parts. If the child's shirt came in contact with the plant and then the shirt was removed by pulling it over the head, there may be widespread lesions over both sides of the face. Lesions near the eyes often cause significant eyelid edema.

FIGURE 45.9 Note vesicular rash in linear formation characteristic of poison ivy.

▶ **Take** NOTE!

Nickel dermatitis may occur from contact with jewelry, eyeglasses, belts, or clothing snaps. Infants may display a small red circle with scaling at the site of contact with sleeper snaps.

Nursing Management

Contact dermatitis may be prevented by avoiding contact with the allergen. When the condition does occur, nursing management focuses on relieving the discomfort associated with the rash. Administer topical or systemic corticosteroids as prescribed and teach the family about use of the medications. Teaching Guidelines 45.2 gives more information about the treatment and prevention of contact dermatitis.

▶ ERYTHEMA MULTIFORME

Erythema multiforme, though uncommon in children, is an acute, self-limiting hypersensitivity reaction. It may occur in response to viral infections, such as adenovirus or Epstein-Barr virus, *Mycoplasma pneumoniae* infection, or a drug (especially sulfa drugs, penicillins, or immunizations) or food reaction. Stevens-Johnson syndrome is the most severe form of erythema multiforme and most often occurs in response to certain medications or to *Mycoplasma* infection (Box 45.1). Therapeutic management of erythema multiforme is generally supportive, as it resolves on its own.

TEACHING GUIDELINES 45.2

Prevention and Treatment of Contact Dermatitis

Prevention

- Wear long sleeves and long pants on outings in the woods.
- Identify and remove offending plants in the yard by using a commercial weed or underbrush killer.
- Vinyl gloves (not rubber or latex) are an effective barrier.
- The plant's oil residue may be on clothes, pets, garden and sports equipment, and toys; wash those well with soap and water.
- If contact occurs, wash vigorously with soap and water within 10 minutes of contact.
- Zanfel and Tecnu Oak-N-Ivy Outdoor Skin Cleanser (both soap mixtures) may prevent rash if used to wash the skin soon after exposure.
- Ivy Block (an organoclay) is the only FDA-approved preventive treatment for contact dermatitis related to poison ivy, oak, or sumac (www.enviroderm.com). It is applied to the skin before possible exposure.

Treatment

- Wash lesions daily with mild soap and water.
- Mildly débride crusted lesions.
- Tepid baths (colloidal oatmeal such as Aveeno) are helpful to decrease itching.
- Avoid hot baths or showers, as they aggravate itching.
- Apply corticosteroid preparations topically as directed (if using high-potency preparations, do not cover with an occlusive dressing).
- Weeping lesions may be wrapped lightly; avoid occlusion.
- Burow's or Domeboro solutions with a dressing applied twice daily for 20 minutes may help to dry weepy lesions.
- Over-the-counter preparations such as calamine lotion or Ivy Rest may reduce itching and help the lesions to dry.
- Do not use topical antihistamines, benzocaine, or neomycin because of the potential for sensitization.

Data from Allen, P. L. J. (2004). Leaves of three, let them be: If it were only that easy! *Pediatric Nursing, 30*(2), 129–135; and Guin, J. D., & Bruckner, A. L. (2005). Compendium on poison ivy dermatitis: The insidious plants, the resulting lesions, the treatment options. *Contemporary Pediatrics, 22*(1 suppl.), 4–15.

BOX 45.1 **Stevens-Johnson Syndrome**

• 1- to 14-day history of fever, malaise, headache, generalized aching, emesis, and diarrhea
• Sudden onset of high fever with rash appearing
• Rash is characteristic of erythema multiforme with the addition of inflammatory bullae on at least two types of mucosa (lips, oral mucosa, bulbar conjunctivae, or anogenital region)
• Mortality rate of 10% (Marino & Fine, 2007), particularly when the genitourinary, gastrointestinal, and respiratory tracts are involved
• Treatment: hospitalization, isolation, fluid and electrolyte support, treatment of secondary infection of the lesions
• Ophthalmologic consult to determine if corneal ulceration, keratitis, uveitis, or panophthalmitis is present

Nursing Assessment

Note history of fever, malaise, and achiness (myalgia). Determine onset and progression of rash, and presence of **pruritus** and burning. Document the child's temperature upon assessment. Inspect the skin for lesions, which most commonly occur over the hands and feet and extensor surfaces of the extremities, with spread to the trunk. Lesions progress from erythematous macules to papules, plaques, vesicles, and target lesions over a period of days (hence the name *multiforme*) (Fig. 45.10).

Nursing Management

Discontinue the medication or food if it is identified as the cause. Ensure that treatment for *Mycoplasma* is instituted if present. Encourage oral hydration. Administer analgesics and antihistamines as needed to promote comfort. If oral lesions are present, encourage soothing mouthwashes or

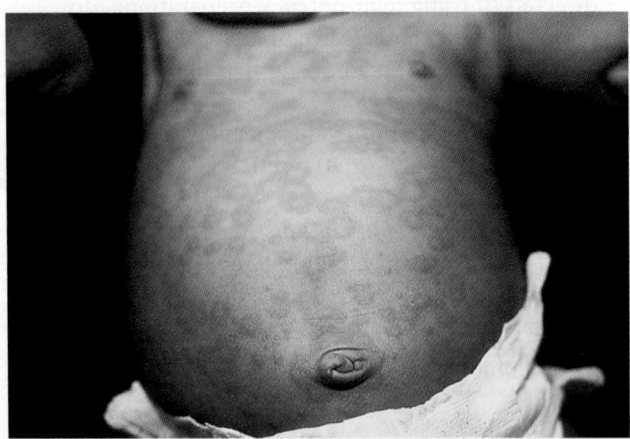

FIGURE 45.10 Erythema multiforme.

use of topic oral anesthetics in the older child or teen. Oral lesions may be débrided with hydrogen peroxide.

▶ URTICARIA

Urticaria, commonly called hives, is a type I hypersensitivity reaction caused by an immunologically mediated antigen–antibody response of histamine release from mast cells. Vasodilation and increased vascular permeability result, and erythema and wheals then occur. Urticaria usually begins rapidly and may disappear in a few days or may take up to 6 or 8 weeks to resolve. The most common causes of this reaction are foods, drugs, animal stings, infections, environmental stimuli (e.g., heat, cold, sun, tight clothes), and stress. Therapeutic management focuses on identifying and removing the cause as well as providing antihistamines or steroids.

Nursing Assessment

Obtain a detailed history of new foods, medications, symptoms of a recent infection, changes in environment, or unusual stress. Inspect the skin, noting raised, edematous hives anywhere on the body or mucous membranes. The hives are pruritic, blanch when pressed, and may migrate. Angioedema may also be present and is identifiable as subcutaneous edema and warmth, occurring most frequently on the extremities, face, or genitalia. Carefully assess airway and breathing, as hypersensitivity reactions may affect respiratory status.

Nursing Management

Identify and remove the offending trigger. Discontinue antibiotics. Administer antihistamines, corticosteroids, and topical antipruritics as prescribed. Inform the child and family that the episode should resolve within a few days. If it lasts up to 6 weeks, the child should be re-evaluated. Advise the family to obtain a medical alert bracelet for the child if the reaction is severe.

▶ *Take* NOTE!

In an emergency situation when airway and breathing are compromised, subcutaneous epinephrine followed by IV diphenhydramine and steroids is necessary.

Seborrhea

Seborrhea is a chronic inflammatory dermatitis that may occur on the skin or scalp. In infants it occurs most often on the scalp and is commonly referred to as cradle cap. Infants may also manifest seborrhea on the nose or eyebrows, behind the ears, or in the diaper area. It usually resolves completely by 8 to 12 months of age (Krowchuk & Tunnessen, 2006). Adolescents manifest seborrhea on the scalp (dandruff) and on the eyebrows and eyelashes, behind the ears, and between the shoulder blades. Skin lesions are treated with corticosteroid creams or lotions. Anti-dandruff shampoos containing selenium sulfide, ketoconazole, or tar are used to treat the scalp. It is thought that seborrhea is an inflammatory reaction to the fungus *Pityrosporum ovale* and is worsened by sebaceous involvement related to maternal hormones in the infant and androgens in the adolescent (Krowchuk & Tunnessen, 2006).

Nursing Assessment

Elicit the health history, determining onset and progression of skin and scalp changes. Note response to treatment used so far. In the infant, inspect the scalp and forehead, behind the ears, and the neck, trunk, and diaper area for thick or flaky greasy yellow scales (Fig. 45.11). In the adolescent, note mild flakes in the hair with yellow greasy scales on the scalp, forehead, and eyebrows, behind the ears, or between the scapulae.

Nursing Management

Wash or shampoo the affected areas with a mild soap. Apply anti-inflammatory cream to skin lesions if prescribed. In the infant, apply mineral oil to the scalp, massage it in well with a washcloth, and then shampoo 10 to 15 minutes later, using a brush to gently lift the crusts; do not forcibly remove the crusts. If needed, selenium sulfide shampoo may safely be used on the infant, following the aforementioned procedure. The adolescent may require daily shampooing with an anti-dandruff shampoo.

FIGURE 45.11 Severe cradle cap (yellow, greasy-appearing plaques).

Psoriasis

Psoriasis is a chronic skin disease with periods of remission and exacerbation (Marino & Fine, 2007). Control is possible with conscientious therapy. Psoriasis does occur in children, but the peak onset is between 15 and 25 years of age (Wong & Rogers, 2006). Psoriasis demonstrates a multifactorial inheritance pattern (Marino & Fine, 2007), with up to 50% of patients having a family history of psoriasis (Wong & Rogers, 2006).

Hyperproliferation of the epidermis occurs, with a rash developing at sites of mechanical, thermal, or physical trauma. Therapeutic management includes skin hydration, use of tar preparations, ultraviolet light, or tazarotene (a topical retinoid). Narrow-band ultraviolet light has been used with some success in children with severe psoriasis (Wong & Rogers, 2006).

Nursing Assessment

Note family history of psoriasis. Determine onset and progression of rash, as well as treatments used and the response to treatment. Question the child about pruritus, which is usually absent with psoriasis. Inspect the skin for erythematous papules that coalesce to form plaques, most frequently found on the scalp, elbows, genital area, and knees. Facial plaques may also occur and are more common in children than adults (Wong & Rogers, 2006). The plaques have a silvery or yellow-white scale and sharply demarcated borders. Layers of scale may be present, which, when removed, result in pinpoint bleeding (referred to as the Auspitz sign). Plaques on the scalp may result in alopecia. Examine the palms and soles, noting fissures and scaling. Skin biopsy, though rarely needed for diagnosis, will show hyperplastic epidermis, with thinning of the papillary dermis (Marino & Fine, 2007).

Nursing Management

Exposure to sunlight may promote healing, but take care not to allow the child to become sunburned. Apply skin moisturizers or emollients daily to prevent dry skin and flare-ups. Apply topical anti-inflammatory creams as prescribed during flare-ups. Apply tar shampoos or skin preparations. Use mineral oil and warm towels to soak and remove thick plaques.

Acne

Acne, the most common skin condition occurring in childhood, is a disorder that affects the pilosebaceous unit. It affects males and females, as well as all ethnic groups. Overall, males tend to have more severe disease than females, probably because of the androgen influence. Acne that persists past the usual course of time for infantile or adolescent acne may be caused by endocrine abnormalities. It may also occur in response to the use of certain types of drugs such as corticosteroids, androgens, phenytoin, and others. The usual presentation and nursing management of acne neonatorum and acne vulgaris is presented below.

▶ ACNE NEONATORUM

Acne neonatorum occurs as a response to the presence of maternal androgens and affects about 20% of newborns (Holmes & Krusinski, 2006). It generally appears between 2 and 4 weeks of age and lasts up to 4 to 6 months, sometimes lasting until 2 to 3 years of age. Neonatal acne affects boys more often than girls and tends to be more severe in boys. Usually no treatment is necessary, but in severe cases there is a risk of scarring, so a topical preparation may be prescribed.

Nursing Assessment

Note oily face or scalp. Examine the face (especially the cheeks), upper chest, and back for inflammatory papules and pustules. Document absence of fever.

Nursing Management

Instruct parents to avoid picking or squeezing the pimples; to do so places the infant at risk for secondary bacterial infection and cellulitis. Teach parents to wash the affected areas daily with clear water. Avoid using fragranced soaps or lotions on the area with acne. Inform the parents that as the newborn's hormones stabilize over time, the acne usually resolves without additional intervention.

▶ ACNE VULGARIS

Acne vulgaris affects about 85% of adolescents between the ages of 12 and 16 years, and endogenous androgens play a role (Morelli & Burch, 2007). It may start as early as between 7 and 10 years of age, with peak onset between 15 and 18 years of age (Silverberg et al., 2005). Acne vulgaris may also continue into the 20s and 30s. It occurs most frequently on the face, chest, and back. Risk factors for the development of acne vulgaris include preadolescent or adolescent age, male gender (due to the presence of androgens), an oily complexion, Cushing syndrome, or another disease process resulting in increased androgen production (Marino & Fine, 2007).

Pathophysiology

The sebaceous gland produces sebum and is connected by a duct to the follicular canal that opens on the skin's surface. Androgenous hormones stimulate sebaceous gland proliferation and production of sebum. These hormones exhibit increased activity during the pubertal years. Abnormal shedding of the outermost layer of the skin (the stratum corneum) occurs at the level of the follicular opening, resulting in a keratin plug that fills the follicle. The sebaceous glands increase sebum production. Bacterial overgrowth of *Proprionibacterium acnes* occurs because the presence of sebum and keratin in the follicular canal creates an excellent environment for growth. Inflammation occurs as the follicular wall perforates, allowing the contents to leak into nearby tissue.

Therapeutic Management

Therapeutic management focuses on reducing *P. acnes*, decreasing sebum production, normalizing skin shedding, and eliminating inflammation. The skin should be cleansed gently twice a day. Medication therapy may include a combination of benzoyl peroxide, salicylic acid, retinoids, and topical or oral antibiotics. Isotretinoin (Accutane) may be used in severe cases. Drug Guide 45.1 gives further information on these medications. In girls, oral contraceptives may help lessen acne by decreasing the effects of androgens on the sebaceous glands (Keri, 2006). Diode laser or blue ultraviolet light therapy may also be used. CO_2 lasers and dermabrasion may be used to treat pitted scarring (Silverberg et al., 2005).

Nursing Assessment

Note history of onset of acne lesions, as well as family history of acne. Determine medication use; certain medications may hasten the onset of acne or worsen it when already present. In particular, note use of corticosteroids, androgens, lithium, phenytoin, and isoniazid. Document history of an endocrine disorder, particularly one that results in hyperandrogenism. In girls, note worsening of acne 2 to 7 days before the start of the menstrual period. Inspect the skin for lesions (particularly on the face and upper chest and back, which are the areas of highest sebaceous activity). Note presence, distribution, and extent of noninflammatory lesions, such as open and closed comedones, as well as inflammatory lesions such as papules, pustules, nodules, or cysts (open comedones are commonly referred to as blackheads and closed comedones as whiteheads; see Fig. 45.12). Examine the skin for hypertrophic scarring resulting from inflammatory lesions. Table 45.3 explains the acne classification. Note oily skin and oily hair, which result from increased sebum production. Determine remedies that have been used and the extent of success of those treatments. Assess the child's or teen's feelings about the disorder.

Nursing Management

Avoid oil-based cosmetics and hair products, as their use may block pores, contributing to noninflammatory lesions. Look for cosmetic products labeled as noncomedogenic. Headbands, helmets, and hats may exacerbate the lesions

FIGURE 45.12 Acne vulgaris.

by causing friction. Dryness and peeling may occur with acne treatment, so encourage the child to use a humectant moisturizer. Mild cleansing with soap and water twice daily is appropriate. Avoid excessive scrubbing and harsh chemical or alcohol-based cleansers (Berson, 2005). Avoid picking or squeezing the lesions. Using a noncomedogenic sunscreen with an SPF of 30 or higher may reduce the risk of postinflammatory discoloration from acne lesions (Silverberg et al., 2005). Teach adolescents that the prescribed topical medications must be used daily and that it may take 4 to 6 weeks to see results. Avoid the use of over-the-counter preparations because they are irritating and aggravate the drying effect of prescription acne treatments. Boys should shave gently and avoid using dull razors, so as not to further irritate the condition. Adolescent girls taking isotretinoin (Accutane) who are sexually active must be on a pregnancy prevention program because the drug causes defects in fetal development (Box 45.2).

Patients interested in complementary medicine approaches may try topical use of a tea tree oil preparation. Fewer adverse effects may occur with tea tree oil preparations than with benzoyl peroxide preparations, but local reactions may still occur.

TABLE 45.3 CLASSIFICATION OF ACNE

Classification	Manifestations
Mild acne	Primarily noninflammatory lesions (comedones)
Moderate acne	Comedones plus inflammatory lesions such as papules or pustules (localized to face or back)
Severe acne	Lesions similar to moderate acne, but more widespread, and/or presence of cysts or nodules. Associated more frequently with scarring.

BOX 45.2 Decreasing Risk of Fetal Exposure to IsoTretinoin: iPLEDGE

- As of 2006, physicians, pharmacists, and patients are required to register in the iPLEDGE program before they prescribe, dispense, or receive isotretinoin (Accutane).
- The iPLEDGE program is a central registry requiring monthly input as noted below in order to continue isotretinoin treatment.
- Monthly input includes the following:
  - Females of childbearing age are using two forms of contraception.
  - Pregnancy test results are negative.
  - Isotretinoin users do not donate blood during or for 1 month after completion of treatment.
- Additional information is available at http://www.fda. gov/cder/drug/infopage/accutane/default.htm

Data from Cuzzell, J. Z. (2005). FDA approves mandatory risk management program for isotretinoin. *Dermatology Nursing, 17*(5), 383; and U.S. Food and Drug Administration, Center for Drug Evaluation and Research. (2007).

If the acne is severe, depression may occur as a result of body image disturbances. Provide emotional support to adolescents undergoing acne therapy. Refer teens for counseling if necessary.

▶ **Take** NOTE!

Chocolate, skim milk, and French fries have not been proven to contribute to the incidence or severity of acne. However, advise teens to wash their hands after eating greasy finger foods to avoid spreading additional oil to the surface of the face.

▶ **Consider** THIS!

Paxton Herman, age 16, comes to the clinic with complaints of acne on his face and back. What assessment information should the nurse obtain? What education will be important for Paxton?

Injuries

Children, by their inquisitive natures, developmental immaturity, and skin's properties, are prone to experience a variety of skin injuries. Pressure ulcers are most likely to occur in hospitalized or otherwise immobile children.

Typical healthy, active children are likely to suffer cuts, abrasions, and foreign body penetration, burns and other thermal injuries, bites, and stings.

▶ PRESSURE ULCERS

Skin breakdown involves changes in intact skin, which may range from blanchable erythema to deep pressure ulcers. The term "pressure ulcer" refers to damage to the skin resulting in skin loss and development of a crater that may be mild or deep (Suddaby et al., 2006). The incidence of pressure ulcers in children remains unknown. Pressure ulcers develop from a combination of factors, including immobility or decreased activity, decreased sensory perception, increased moisture, impaired nutritional status, inadequate tissue perfusion, and the forces of friction and shear. Common sites of pressure ulcers in hospitalized children include the occiput and toes, while children who require wheelchairs for mobility have pressure ulcers in the sacral or hip area more frequently.

Nursing Assessment

Note history of immobility (chronic, related to a condition such as paralysis) or lengthy hospitalization, particularly in intensive care. Inspect the skin for areas of erythema or warmth. Note ulceration of the skin. Use the facility's wound assessment scale to document the extent of the ulcer. Take a photo of the ulcer if possible.

Nursing Management

Position the child to alleviate pressure on the area of the ulcer. Use specialized beds or mattresses to prevent further pressure areas from developing. Perform prescribed wound care meticulously, noting the formation of granulation tissue as the ulcer begins to heal. Prevent pressure ulcers in the child who is hospitalized for long periods of time by turning the child frequently, assessing the entire surface of the child's skin at least every shift, using pressure-alleviating beds and mattresses, and maintaining the child's nutritional status.

▶ MINOR INJURIES

Children suffer minor injuries very frequently. These include minor cuts and abrasions, as well as skin penetration of foreign bodies such as splinters or glass fragments. Because of their developmental immaturity and inquisitive nature, children often attempt tasks they are not yet capable of or take risks that an adult would not, often resulting in a fall or other accident. The break in the skin allows an entry point for bacteria, and the complication of cellulitis

may occur. Treatment is directed at cleaning the wound and preventing infection.

Nursing Assessment

Obtain the history from the child or caregiver to determine whether dirt or a foreign object may be present in the wound. Inspect the wound, noting depth of injury, a foreign body, and bleeding.

Nursing Management

Cleanse the wound with mild soap and water or with an antibacterial cleanser. Wet gauze helps to scrub away fine and large sand particles. Remove pieces of loose skin with sterile scissors, foreign particles with sterile forceps, and road tar with petrolatum. Small abrasions and minor, well-approximated cuts may be left open to the air. Apply a small amount of antibacterial ointment and cover large abrasions with a loose dressing. Change the dressing 12 hours later and redress after cleaning the wound. Leave it open to air after 24 hours have passed from the time of injury.

Calendula preparations are presumed to be safe for topical use and may speed wound healing. Chamomile may help to dry a weeping wound, and allergic reactions to the herb are rare (Gardiner et al., 2001).

Assess the wound daily for signs of infection, which include purulence, warmth, edema, increasing pain, and erythema that extends past the margin of the cut or abrasion.

▶ BURNS

Over 1 million people experience a burn injury each year in the United States, and 35% of those burn injuries are to children (Shriners Hospital for Children, 2005). Burns are the second-leading cause of death from unintentional injury in children between 1 and 4 years of age and the third-leading cause in all persons under 19 years old. Children less than 6 years of age are at highest risk for burns (Schweich, 2006), and the mortality rate from burns in young children is twice that of older children (National Safe Kids Campaign, 2004).

Most pediatric burn-related injuries do not result in death, but injuries from burns often cause extreme pain and extensive burns can result in serious disfigurement. While most pediatric burns are tragic unintentional injuries, about 75% of them could have been prevented, and child abuse is the cause of about 15% to 30% of serious pediatric burns (American Medical Student Association, 2006). See Healthy People 2010.

Carbon monoxide poisoning often occurs in conjunction with burns as a result of smoke inhalation, and infants and children are at greater risk for carbon monoxide poisoning than adults.

Great advances have been made in the care of children with serious burns. As a result of improved burn care, children who in the past would have died as a result of burns over large body surface areas have a much greater chance of survival.

Conventional wisdom is that children with severe burns should be transferred to a specialized burn unit. The Committee on Trauma of the American College of Surgeons (1999) has developed the following criteria for referral of burned persons to a burn unit:

• Partial thickness burns greater than 10% of total body surface area
• Burns that involve the face
• Burns that involve the hands and feet, genitalia, perineum, or major joints
• Electrical burns, including lightning injury
• Chemical burns
• Inhalation injury
• Burn injury in patients who have pre-existing conditions that might affect their care
• Persons with burns and traumatic injuries
• Persons who will require special social, emotional, or long-term rehabilitative care
• Burned children in a hospital without qualified personnel or equipment for the care of children

Burns are classified according to the extent of injury. Superficial burns involve only epidermal injury and usually heal without scarring or other sequelae within 4 to 5 days. In partial-thickness burns, injury occurs not only to the epidermis but also to portions of the dermis. These burns usually heal within about 2 weeks and carry a minimal risk of scar formation. Deep partial-thickness burns take longer to heal, may scar, and result in changes in nail and hair appearance as well as sebaceous gland function in the affected area. They may require surgical intervention. Full-thickness burns result in significant tissue damage as they extend through the epidermis, dermis, and hypodermis. Extensive scarring results, as hair follicles and sweat glands are destroyed. Full-thickness burns require a significant time to heal. If underlying tendons and/or bone are involved, the burn may be termed fourth degree. Contractures and limited function may occur as a complication of full-thickness burns. Skin grafting is usually necessary. Full or partially circumferential burns may re-sult in ischemia from loss of blood flow related to progressive swelling of the area.

Pathophysiology

Burned tissue begins to coagulate after the injury, and direct coagulation and microvascular reactions in the adjacent dermis may extend the burn. The blood vessels demonstrate increased capillary permeability, resulting in vasodilatation. This leads to increased hydrostatic pressure in the capillaries, causing water, electrolytes, and protein to leak out of the vasculature and result in significant edema. Edema forms very rapidly in the first 18 hours after the burn, peaking at around 48 hours. Capillary permeability then returns to normal between 48 and 72 hours after the burn and the lymphatics can reabsorb the edema fluid. Diuresis occurs, ridding the body of the excess fluid. Fluid loss from burned skin occurs at an amount that is 5 to 10 times greater than that from undamaged skin, and this fluid loss continues until the damaged surface is healed or grafted (Merz et al., 2003).

Initially, the severely burned child experiences a decrease in cardiac output, with a subsequent hypermetabolic response during which cardiac output increases dramatically. During this heightened metabolic state, the child is at risk for insulin resistance and increased protein catabolism. Children who are burned during an indoor or chemical fire are at an increased risk of respiratory injury. Children who have aspirated hot liquids are particularly at risk for airway-altering edema.

Therapeutic Management

Therapeutic management of burns focuses on fluid resuscitation, wound care, prevention of infection, and restoration of function. Burn infections are treated with antibiotics specific to the causative organism. If invasive burn damage occurs, surgery may be necessary.

Nursing Assessment

For a full description of the assessment phase of the nursing process, refer to page 1495. Upon arrival, the pediatric burn client should be evaluated to determine if he or she will require intensive management. Remove any smoldering clothing. Obtain a brief history of the burn circumstances while you are assessing the child and providing care.

Health History

If the burn is severe or there is a potential for respiratory compromise, obtain a brief history while simultaneously evaluating the child and providing emergency care. If the burn does not appear to pose an immediate life-threatening risk, obtain an in-depth history. Elicit a description of how the burn occurred, noting date, time, and cause. Determine if smoke inhalation or an associated fall may have occurred. Document treatment that the parent or caregiver has provided to the child's burn so far. Note the child's recent health status, current medications, recent or chronic illness, and immunization status, in particular noting the date of the most recent tetanus vaccination. Determine whether the history being given sounds consistent with the type of burn injury that has occurred. Inquire about what caused the burn and if the event was witnessed by anyone. Spatter-type burns resulting from the child pulling a source of hot fluid onto himself or herself usually yield a nonuniform, asymmetric distribution of injury. In contrast, intentional scald injuries usually yield a uniform "sock" or "glove" distribution when the child's extremity is held under very hot water as punishment. It is important for the nurse to pick up on clues in the health history that may indicate that the burn is a result of child abuse, rather than an accident (Box 45.3). Children are also burned by curling irons, gasoline, fireworks, room heaters, ovens, and ranges. Obtain a detailed history about the circumstances surrounding these types of burns. Ask the parent what the home hot water heater temperature is.

Physical Examination

Emergency examination of the burned child consists of a primary survey followed by a secondary survey. The primary survey includes evaluation of the child's airway, breathing, and circulation; the secondary survey focuses on evaluation of the burns and other injuries. Box 45.4 gives information about emergency assessment of the burned child. Inspect the child's skin, noting erythema, blistering, weeping, or eschar (charred skin).

BOX 45.4   Emergency Assessment of the Burned Child

Primary Survey
- Assess the child's airway, noting whether it is patent, maintainable, or unmaintainable.
  - Suspect airway injury from burn or smoke inhalation if any of the following are present: burns around the mouth, nose, or eyes; carbonaceous (black-colored) sputum; hoarseness or stridor.
- Evaluate the child's skin color, respiratory effort, symmetry of breathing, and breath sounds.
- Determine the pulse strength, perfusion status, and heart rate. Note extent and location of edema.

Secondary Survey
- Determine burn depth.
- Estimate burn extent by determining the percentage of body surface area affected. Use a chart for estimation (see Fig. 45.16) or rapidly estimate by using the child's palm size, which is equivalent to about 1% of the child's body surface area.
- Inspect the child for other traumatic injuries (children who have jumped or fallen from a house fire may suffer cervical spine or internal injuries).

The old terms used to describe the depth of burns as first, second, and third degree have been replaced by the contemporary terminology. Classify the burn according to its severity. Superficial burns are painful, red, dry and possibly edematous (Fig. 45.13). Partial-thickness and

---

BOX 45.3   Signs of Child Abuse–Induced Burns

- Inconsistent history given when caregivers are interviewed separately
- Delay in seeking treatment by caregiver
- Uniform appearance of the burn, with clear delineation of burned and nonburned area (as with a hot object applied to the skin)
- In the case of a scald-induced burn, lack of spattering of water but evidence of so-called "porcelain-contact sparing," where the portion of the child's skin that was in contact with the tub or sink is not burned (commonly seen with a forced immersion in extremely hot water used as punishment)
- Flexor-sparing burns or burns that involve the dorsum of the hand
- A stocking/glove pattern on the hands or feet (circumferential ring appearing around the extremity, resulting from a caregiver forcefully holding the child under extremely hot water)

FIGURE 45.13 Superficial burn—painful but without blisters.

FIGURE 45.14 Partial-thickness burn—very painful, with blistering.

deep partial-thickness burns are very painful and edematous and have a wet appearance or blisters (Fig. 45.14). Full-thickness burns may be very painful or numb or pain-free in some areas. They appear red, edematous, leathery, dry, or waxy and may display peeling or charred skin (Fig. 45.15). Note whether the burn is circumferential (encircling a body part) or partially circumferential.

> ▶ *Take* NOTE!
>
> *Due to overlying blistering, it is difficult to accurately distinguish between partial- and full-thickness burns. In addition, in the case of third-degree burns, it is difficult to estimate burn depth during the initial evaluation.*

Laboratory and Diagnostic Tests

In the child with more extensive burns, electrolytes and complete blood count are used to measure fluid and elec-

FIGURE 45.15 Full-thickness burn—color ranges from red to charred, or white, minimal pain, marked edema.

trolyte balance and to determine the possibility of infection, respectively. If wound infection is suspected, culture of the drainage will determine the particular bacteria. Nutritional indices such as albumin, transferrin, carotene, retinol, copper, cholesterol, calcium, thiamine, riboflavin, pyridoxine, and iron may be evaluated when the child has severe or extensive burns. Pulmonary status may be evaluated via pulse oximetry and end-tidal CO_2 monitoring, arterial blood gases, carboxyhemoglobin levels, and chest x-ray. Fiberoptic bronchoscopy and xenon ventilation–perfusion scanning may be used to evaluate inhalation injury. Electrocardiographic monitoring is important for the child who has suffered an electrical burn to identify cardiac arrhythmias, which can be noted for up to 72 hours after a burn injury.

Nursing Management

Nursing management of the child who has been burned focuses first on stabilizing the child. Place the child on a cardiac/apnea monitor, measure the child with the Broselow tape, monitor pulse oximetry, and apply an end-tidal CO_2 monitor if the child is ventilated. Further management focuses on cleansing the burn, pain management, and prevention and treatment of infection. Fluid status and nutrition are important components of burn care, particularly in the early stages. Rehabilitation of the child with severe burns is also an important nursing function. Providing patient and family education about the prevention of burns as well as care of burns at home is critical. Nursing Care Plan 45.1 gives additional interventions related to fluid and nutritional management.

Promoting Oxygenation and Ventilation

Institute emergency airway management as needed. If the child requires intubation, make sure that the tracheal tube is taped in a very secure manner, as reintubations in these patients will become increasingly difficult as the edema spreads. The burned child's respiratory status warrants vigilant evaluation and re-evaluation, as airway edema that is secondary to a burn may not become evident until 2 days after the injury. All children with severe burns should receive 100% oxygen via nonbreather mask or bag-valve-mask ventilation. Continue to reassess the child's pulmonary status, adjusting the interventions as necessary (refer to Chapter 52 for further information about respiratory emergency care).

> ▶ *Take* NOTE!
>
> *High levels of carboxyhemoglobin as a result of smoke inhalation may contribute to falsely high pulse oximetry readings.*

Restoring and Maintaining Fluid Volume

Several formulas are available for the calculation of resuscitative fluids in children. Most experts recommend that pediatric burn therapy include:

- Fluid calculation based on the body surface area burned (Fig. 45.16)
- Use of a crystalloid (Ringer's lactate) during the first 24 hours; in smaller children, a small amount of dextrose may be added
- Administration of most of the volume during the first 8 hours (amounts and timing of fluid volume resuscitation will vary from child to child)
- Reassessment of the child and adjustment of the fluid rate accordingly; fluid requirements greatly de-

crease after 24 hours and should be adjusted to reflect this
- Administration of a colloid fluid later in therapy once capillary permeability is less of a concern
- Monitoring of the child's urine output as part of ongoing assessment of response to therapy, expecting at least 1 mL/kg per hour
- Daily weights obtained at the same time each day (the best indicator of fluid volume status)
- Monitoring of electrolyte levels (particularly sodium and potassium) for their return to normal levels

Preventing Hypothermia

Due to the loss of the protective dermis, children who are burned are at high risk for hypothermia and secondary

EXAMPLE

Calculating TBSA By Age
(Total Body Surface Area)

Color Code
Red - 3º
Blue - 2º

Area	Birth 1 yr	1-4 yrs	5-9 yrs	10-14 yrs	15 yrs	Adult	2	3	Total
Head	19	17	13	11	9	7	-	8	8.0
Neck	2	2	2	2	2	2	-	1	1.0
Ant. Trunk	13	13	13	13	13	13	1	12	13.0
Post. Trunk	13	13	13	13	13	13	-	-	-
R. Buttock	2 1/2	2 1/2	2 1/2	2 1/2	2 1/2	2 1/2	-	-	-
L. Buttock	2 1/2	2 1/2	2 1/2	2 1/2	2 1/2	2 1/2	-	-	-
Genitalia	1	1	1	1	1	1	-	-	-
R.U. Arm	4	4	4	4	4	4	-	3.5	3.5
L.U. Arm	4	4	4	4	4	4	1	2.5	3.5
R.L. Arm	3	3	3	3	3	3	-	3	3
L.L. Arm	3	3	3	3	3	3	-	3	3
R. Hand	2 1/2	2 1/2	2 1/2	2 1/2	2 1/2	2 1/2	-	2.5	2.5
L. Hand	2 1/2	2 1/2	2 1/2	2 1/2	2 1/2	2 1/2	-	2.5	2.5
R. Thigh	5 1/2	6 1/2	8	8 1/2	9	9 1/2	1	2	3
L. Thigh	5 1/2	6 1/2	8	8 1/2	9	9 1/2	-	2	2
R. Leg	5	5	5 1/2	6	6 1/2	7	-	-	-
L. Leg	5	5	5 1/2	6	6 1/2	7	-	-	-
R. Foot	3 1/2	3 1/2	3 1/2	3 1/2	3 1/2	3 1/2	-	-	-
L. Foot	3 1/2	3 1/2	3 1/2	3 1/2	3 1/2	3 1/2	-	-	-
Total							3%	42%	45%

FIGURE 45.16 Calculate total body surface area (TBSA) affected by using the child's age and the area affected, as well as whether the burned area is second degree (partial thickness) or third degree (full thickness).

infection. Therefore, care should be taken to keep the child warm. Warm intravenous fluids prior to their administration. Maintain a neutral thermal environment and monitor the child's temperature frequently.

Cleansing the Burn

Initially, burning must be stopped, so remove charred clothing. Wash and rinse the burn thoroughly with mild soap and water from the tap. Cool water may be used, but ice should never be applied. Children who are burned with tar require special care. Tar can be removed with cool water and mineral oil. Blisters that are intact should not routinely be removed as they provide a protective barrier; however, débridement is recommended in certain cases where large blisters impede wound care. Wounds that are open require débridement. Débridement involves the removal of loose skin and eschar (dead, charred skin). This procedure is usually performed with sterile scissors and a pair of forceps or with a gauze sponge. The burned area should be gently cleansed; there is no advantage to aggressive scrubbing, and this technique only makes the pain more intense for the child. The nurse should wear a gown, mask, head covering, and gloves during dressing changes. Débridement is a necessary but often excruciatingly painful procedure, so the pain management needs of the child are of utmost importance (refer to the pain management section below).

When children return for evaluation of a wound that was previously seen in your facility, the dressing must be removed. Soak the dressing in lukewarm tap water to ease the removal of gauze, which may be stuck to the wound. The nurse plays an important role in ensuring that the dressing change goes smoothly. Be sure to:

• Have all dressing supplies ready.
• Provide pain medication as ordered.
• Promote good infection control technique among your colleagues.
• Assist with restraining young children, using the positions of comfort previously discussed in relation to atraumatic care.
• Encourage participation by the child's parents.
• Talk soothingly to the child, explain what you are going to do, and provide distraction during the procedure.

Preventing Infection

Prevention of infection is critical to successful outcomes for burned children. If the child's immunization status is unknown or if it has been 5 years or longer since the last tetanus vaccine, administer the tetanus vaccine. If the child has never received tetanus vaccination, also give 250 units tetanus human immunoglobulin intravenously. Apply antibiotic ointment in conjunction with burn dressing changes. Refer to Drug Guide 45.1 for information about topical antibiotics. Membrane dressings such as porcine xenograft and hydrocolloid dressings are alternatives to

topical antibiotics and sterile dressings. Evaluate the child's wound during dressing changes, looking for wound redness, swelling, odor, or drainage. Strictly adhere to infection control procedures and hand hygiene to decrease the risk of burn infection. Maximize the child's nutritional status to decrease his or her susceptibility to a burn infection. Monitor the child's temperature for the development of fever. Upon discharge, instruct the parents about the signs of a wound infection.

Managing Pain

Pain management is of the utmost importance, and several options are available for the treatment of burn-related pain. Local anesthesia, sedatives, and systemic analgesics are commonly used. Children who have less severe burns that are managed at home can be given oral medications such as acetaminophen with codeine 30 to 45 minutes before dressing changes. In burns that result in more severe pain, the child should be hospitalized and given intravenous pain control with medications such as morphine sulfate. Midazolam (a sedative) may be used in conjunction with pain medication for pain reduction during dressing changes.

Pain may also occur at any time of the day or night, not just in relation to dressing changes. Assess the child's pain status frequently using an age-appropriate pain assessment scale. Administer pain medications as prescribed and/or use nonpharmacologic techniques to alleviate or decrease the child's perception of pain. Nontraditional therapies such as virtual-reality therapy have been shown to alleviate pain during dressing changes. Virtual-reality therapy programs allow the child to immerse himself or herself in a three-dimensional computer-generated world, an extremely effective method of distraction from the pain (Hoffman, 2004).

Treating Infected Burns

The potential for burn infection increases if the child has a large, open burn wound and if there are other sources of infection, such as multiple intravenous lines. In addition, children who are immunocompromised have an increased risk of burn infection. *S. aureus* is the usual bacterium implicated in burn cellulitis and burn impetigo, though *Pseudomonas aeruginosa* may also cause cellulitis. In burn wound cellulitis, the area around the burn becomes increasingly red, swollen, and painful early in the course of burn management. With invasive burn cellulitis, the burn develops a dark brown, black, or purplish color, with a discharge and foul odor. Burn impetigo is characterized by multifocal small superficial abscesses. Burn impetigo causes marked destruction of skin-grafted areas.

When an infection is suspected, antibiotics are usually started, pending wound culture results. Administer antibiotics as prescribed (or antifungals if an extensive burn injury becomes infected with a fungus).

Providing Burn Rehabilitation

Children who have suffered a significant burn injury face a myriad of physical and psychological challenges that extend well beyond the acute injury phase. These children may display regression behaviors because of injury, pain, fear, or anxiety. Skin grafting or special burn dressings are required for some children (Box 45.5). Children who have suffered extensive burns often require multiple skin-grafting surgeries. Figures 45.17 and 45.18 show healed skin grafts. Extensive burns may also result in the need for pressure garments to decrease the risk of extensive scarring. Pressure garments are not comfortable and they must be worn continuously for at least 1 year, sometimes 2, but they have been shown to be very effective in reducing hypertrophic scarring resulting from significant burn injury.

Physical therapy will usually be initiated in the critical care setting and will continue long after hospital discharge, sometimes throughout life. Positioning, exercise, and range of motion are necessary to maintain joint flexibility.

Nurses play a key role in smoothing the transition from the acute care phase of life-saving interventions and frequent dressing changes to normal activities such as school and play. Body image considerations may have a significant impact on the child when he or she returns to school and should be addressed. Children with altered body image as a result of a burn might benefit from regular counseling and group therapy. Parents often need assistance with the behavioral challenges of caring for a child who is recovering from a burn injury. Various websites are available for support of persons who are burned:

- www.burnsupportgroupsdatabase.com: Burn Support Group Database
- burnsurvivor.com: Burn Resource Center
- www.survivingburns.org: mentor services for burn survivors

FIGURE 45.17 Healed mesh graft.

Navigating through life after suffering a serious burn injury can be difficult for the child and family, and a skilled nurse can provide valuable assistance to families during the equally important but less acute phase of the journey.

Preventing Burns and Carbon Monoxide Poisoning

Instruct parents about prevention of burns. All homes should have working smoke detectors, and batteries should be changed yearly. All homes should be equipped with fire extinguishers, and adults and older teenagers should be taught how to operate them. Children should sleep in fire-retardant sleepwear. Parents should not smoke in the house or the car, and they should keep lighters and matches out of children's reach. Young children are

---

BOX 45.5 Skin Grafting and Special Burn Care

- Biologic skin coverings are used for extensive burns or in cases of no donor.
- Autograft allows for permanent coverage of a deep partial-thickness or full-thickness burn.
- Consists of patient's own skin
- Split-thickness consists of epidermis and superficial layers of dermis. The donor site heals completely.
- Full-thickness consists of full dermal thickness. Cover the donor site with fine-mesh gauze or synthetic wound coverings to allow the site to heal.
- Kaltostat (calcium alginate dressing) is a brown seaweed extract that is spun into a fiber that is highly absorbent. It reacts with exudate on the wound to form a protective gel.

FIGURE 45.18 Extensive grafting to the face.

particularly susceptible to burns that occur in the kitchen, such as scalds from hot liquids and foods and burns from contact with hot burners or oven doors. Caution parents about the extreme danger that fireworks present to children. Teaching Guidelines 45.3 gives additional information for parents related to burn prevention. The booklet "Burn Prevention Tips," which includes a coloring book, is available from the Shriners Hospitals for Children (www.shrinershq.org).

Children are at significant risk for burns related to hot water. Scald burns can occur when hot water comes into contact with the child's skin, even for a relatively short time. Since hot water presents such a serious risk to children, the temperature on all hot water heaters should be 120° F or lower. Figure 45.19 is a graph that shows how long a child can be exposed to water of various temperatures before a burn occurs. For example:

- If the water is 150°, a child can receive a third-degree burn within 2 seconds.
- If the water is 140°, it takes 6 seconds of exposure to cause a significant burn.
- If the water is 130°, a child can be burned significantly in only 30 seconds.
- At 120°, the recommended maximal home hot water heater temperature, it takes as long as 5 minutes of exposure to burn a person (plenty of time to get out of the tub!).

Instruct parents about prevention of carbon monoxide poisoning. All homes should have working carbon monoxide detectors, and batteries should be changed yearly. Teach parents the signs of carbon monoxide poi-

Hot Water Burn & Scalding Graph

FIGURE 45.19 Length of hot water exposure that results in significant burns based on water temperature.

soning: headaches, dizziness, disorientation, and nausea. If the carbon monoxide detector sounds, turn off any potential sources of combustion, if possible, and evacuate all occupants immediately. Do not attempt to re-enter the home until a qualified professional repairs the source of the carbon monoxide leak.

Providing Burn Care at Home

Teach parents about proper burn care in the home. Seek medical attention for burns when:

- The child has a second- or third-degree burn.
- Burns result from a fire, an electrical wire or socket, or chemicals.
- The child has a burn on the face, scalp, hands, feet, or genitals or over the joints.
- The burn appears to be infected.
- The burn is causing prolonged and significant pain.
- Concern exists that the burn was a result of abuse.

If the burn is very extensive, even if it appears to be a first-degree burn, seek medical attention immediately. Teaching Guidelines 45.4 gives specific information about burn care at home.

▶ SUNBURN

Sunburn occurs as a result of overexposure to the ultraviolet (UV) rays of the sun. The erythema and eventual blisters occur as a result of the skin's blood flow changes as well as alterations in cell kinetics and pigment products in response to UV exposures. Erythema may occur

---

TEACHING GUIDELINES 45.3

Burn Prevention

- Keep hot water heater temperature lower than 120° F.
- Test bath water temperature before bathing children.
- Keep children away from open flames, stoves, and candles.
- Cook with pots on the inside of the stove with the handles turned in.
- Keep children away from the stove while cooking.
- Place hot liquids out of reach of children.
- Avoid drinking hot beverages while holding a child.
- Keep curling irons out of reach of children.
- Teach older children how to safely get out of the house in case of fire.
- Practice fire drills.
- Teach children to "stop, drop, and roll" if their clothes catch on fire.

TEACHING GUIDELINES 45.4

Providing Burn Care

For First-Degree (Superficial) Burns

- Run cool water over the burned area until the pain lessens.
- Do not apply ice to the skin.
- Do not apply butter, ointment, or cream.
- Cover the burn lightly with a clean, non-adhesive bandage.
- Administer acetaminophen or ibuprofen for pain.
- Have the child seen by the primary care provider within 24 hours.
- Ongoing care: clean in tub or shower with fragrance-free mild soap; pat or air dry.
  - Apply a thin layer of antibiotic ointment.
  - Cover with a nonadherent dressing such as Adaptic, and then cover with dry gauze.

For More Extensive Burns

- Remove clothing only if it comes off easily or if it is still smoldering.
- Check the child's ABCs and perform CPR if necessary.
- Do not apply butter, ointment, or any other type of cream.
- Cover the burn with a clean, lint-free bandage or sheet.
- Avoid applying large, wet sheets, as this can cause the child to become too cold.
- Do not attempt to break any blisters.
- If the child appears to be in shock, elevate the legs while protecting the burn and call 911.

Data from Frank, K. (2005). *Preventing and treating burns.* Retrieved 1/4/08 from www.kidsgrowth.com/resources/articledetail.cfm?id=2029; and Nemours Foundation. (2005). Burns. Retrieved 1/4/08 from http://www.kidshealth.org/teen/safety/first_aid/burns_sheet.html.

within 4 hours and blisters within 6 hours (Krowchuk & Tunnessen, 2006). Excessive sun exposure has been linked to the development of skin cancer later in life. See Healthy People 2010.

Sunburn is usually treated with cool compresses, cooling lotions, and oral nonsteroidal anti-inflammatory agents.

Nursing Assessment

Obtain the health history, noting recent sun exposure. Determine length of exposure and whether any type of sunscreen or sun block product was used. Note redness of the skin on the exposed areas. More severe areas will

HEALTHY PEOPLE 2010

Objective	Nursing Significance
(Developmental) Increase the proportion of adolescents in grades 9 through 12 who follow protective measures that may reduce the risk of skin cancer.	• Encourage use of sunscreen in all children over 6 months of age, to form a lifelong habit. • Discourage sun exposure between 10 a.m. and 2 p.m. • Inform teens of the hazards of ultraviolet light (even artificial) and discourage the use of tanning beds.

have a darker red, slightly purple hue. Blisters may be noted with more severe sunburn.

Nursing Management

Cool compresses may help to cool the burn. Aloe vera gel applied topically may provide significant soothing. Rarely are adverse effects reported with the use of aloe vera gel. Administer a nonsteroidal anti-inflammatory such as ibuprofen. Discourage hot showers or baths. Instruct the child to wear loose clothing and to ensure that burned areas are covered when going outside (until they are healed). If skin flaking occurs, discourage the child from "peeling" the flaked skin in order to prevent further injury. Refer to Chapter 30 for further information about safe sun exposure.

▶ COLD INJURY

The term "frostbite" implies freezing of the tissues. It is described on a continuum from first to fourth degree. When a child is exposed to an extremely cold environment, changes in cutaneous circulation help to maintain the core body temperature. As circulation is shunted to the core, the most peripheral body parts are those at highest risk for frostbite. Local damage occurs when the tissue temperature drops to 32° F (0° C). Initially skin sensation is lost, the vasculature constricts, and plasma leakage occurs. Ice crystals develop in the extracellular fluid, and eventually vascular stasis leads to endothelial cell damage, necrosis, and sloughing of dead tissue (Nield & Nanda, 2005).

Nursing Assessment

Note history of cold exposure. Inquire about pain or numbness. Examine the skin for indications of frostbite. First-degree frostbite results in superficial white plaques with surrounding erythema. Second-degree frostbite demonstrates blistering with erythema and edema. In third-degree frostbite, hemorrhagic blisters occur, progressing to tissue necrosis and sloughing in fourth-degree frostbite (Nield & Nanda, 2005).

Nursing Management

Remove wet or tight clothing. Avoid vigorous massage to decrease the chance of damaging the skin further. Immerse the affected part in 104° F water for 15 to 30 minutes. Thawing may cause significant pain, so administer analgesics. Keep the thawed part loosely covered, warm, and dry. Splinting may be used to help decrease associated edema. Consult the wound care specialist or plastic surgeon for further management.

Preventing frostbite may be achieved by:

• Dressing warmly in layers, and keeping warm and dry
• Avoiding exertion
• Not playing outside when wind chill advisories are in effect, and locking doors with high locks to prevent toddlers from going outside (Nield & Nanda, 2005)

► HUMAN AND ANIMAL BITES

About 1% of emergency department visits yearly are due to bites from mammals (Starr, 2006). Children may be bitten by other children, or animals that are pets or strays such as dogs, cats, or ferrets. The hand and face are common locations for animal bites. A dog is most often provoked to bite a child when the child is playing with the dog or when the child hits, kicks, hugs, grabs, or chases the dog (Melnick, 2005).

Therapeutic management involves cleansing and irrigation of the wound, wound suturing or stapling if necessary, and topical and/or systemic antibiotic therapy. Rabies prophylaxis is indicated if the rabies status of the dog is unknown. Secondary bacterial infection of the bite wound with streptococci, staphylococci, or *Pasteurella multocida* may occur. Cat and human bites are the most likely to become infected.

Nursing Assessment

Determine the history of the attack and whether it was provoked. Determine the child's tetanus vaccination status. Inspect the bite to determine the extent of laceration, avulsion, or crushing injury.

Nursing Management

Provide rabies immunoprophylaxis and a tetanus booster vaccination if indicated. Thoroughly cleanse the wound with soap and water or a povidone–iodine solution. Irrigate the wound well with normal saline after cleansing (Villani, 2006). If the animal may be rabid, cleanse the wound for at least 10 minutes with a virucidal agent such as povidone–iodine solution (Behrman, 2004). Administer antibiotics as prescribed.

Prevention of animal bites is important. Teach children the following:

• Never provoke a dog with teasing or roughhousing.
• Get adult permission before interacting with a dog, cat, or other animal that is not your pet.
• Do not bother an eating, sleeping, or nursing dog.
• Avoid high-pitched talking or screaming around dogs.
• Display a closed fist first for the dog to sniff.
• Keep ferrets away from the face.
• If a cat hisses or lashes out with the paw, leave it alone (American Veterinary Medical Association, 2006; Melnick, 2005).

Never leave a child under 5 years of age alone with a dog. Contact the local humane society for a dog bite prevention program that is appropriate for school-age children.

Children may suffer significant emotional distress after being bitten. Nightmares and increased anxiety are common (Villani, 2006). Help children through this period by talking about the incident or reading books about this type of event.

► INSECT STINGS AND SPIDER BITES

Members of the Hymenoptera class of insects sting. This class includes bees, wasps, ants, yellow jackets, and hornets. Spiders inject their venom when they bite. Stings and bites usually result in a local reaction. A systemic or anaphylactic reaction to a Hymenoptera sting may also occur, possibly resulting in airway compromise (refer to Chapter 47 for additional information on anaphylaxis). Serious reactions may occur with brown recluse or black widow spider bites. This discussion will focus on local reactions.

Local reactions to insect stings and spider bites include pruritus, pain, and edema. A hypersensitivity reaction thought to be mediated by immunoglobulin E occurs in response to the venom. This may be a physiological response to the antigens present in the insect's or spider's saliva and other fluids that are transmitted during stinging or biting. Bacterial superinfection may occur as a complication and as a result of scratching (Bircher, 2005).

Therapeutic management includes antihistamines to decrease itching and in some cases corticosteroids to decrease inflammation and swelling.

Nursing Assessment

Obtain the history of the bite or sting. Children are usually acutely aware when they have been stung by an insect, but spiders are generally not observed before the bite. Inspect the bite or sting, noting an urticarial wheal or papular reaction. A large local reaction may be mistaken for cellulitis. Note whether a stinger remains present. Assess the child's work of breathing to determine if a systemic reaction or anaphylaxis is occurring (refer to Chapter 47).

Nursing Management

Remove jewelry or constrictive clothing if the sting is on an extremity. Cleanse the wound with mild soap and water. If the stinger is present, scrape it away with your fingernail or a credit card. Apply ice intermittently to decrease pain and edema. Administer diphenhydramine as soon as possible after the sting in an attempt to minimize the reaction.

Prevent insect stings and spider bites by wearing protective clothing and shoes when outdoors. Use insect repellants (with a maximum concentration of 30% DEET in infants and children older than 2 months). Teach children never to disturb a bee or wasp nest or an ant hill.

▪▪▪ Key Concepts

- The infant's epidermis is thinner, loses heat more readily, absorbs substances more easily, and is more accessible to bacterial invasion than the skin of the adult. The increased water content of the infant's skin compared with the adult places the infant at increased risk of blister development and other skin alterations.
- The child's skin thickness and characteristics reach adult levels in the late teenage years.
- Children with dark skin tend to have more pronounced cutaneous reactions than children with lighter skin.
- Sebum production increases in the preadolescent and adolescent years, contributing to the development of acne at that time.
- Skin scrapings placed on a slide and prepared with potassium chloride may be evaluated microscopically to determine the presence of fungus.
- Most bacterial skin infections are caused by *Staphylococcus aureus* and group A beta-hemolytic streptococcus.
- Fungal skin infections, referred to collectively as tinea, may require up to several weeks of treatment.
- Contact dermatitis and atopic dermatitis both present as pruritic rashes, whereas psoriasis is generally nonpruritic.
- Hypersensitivity responses may result in erythema multiforme or urticaria.
- Scaling may occur with atopic dermatitis and psoriasis, whereas honey-colored crusting is common with impetigo. Erythema is a common finding with many skin disorders in children.
- Burns may result in significant weeping and fluid loss.
- Keeping the skin well moisturized is a key intervention in the management of atopic dermatitis and psoriasis.
- Appropriate hygiene is of particular importance in integumentary disorders.
- Pain management, prevention of infection, and rehabilitation are the focus of nursing management for the burned child.

- The constant itch–rash–itch cycle of atopic dermatitis may have a considerable impact on the child's sleep, school functioning, and self-esteem.
- Acne vulgaris, particularly if moderate or severe, may have a significant negative effect on the teen's self-esteem.
- Teach children with chronic disorders such as atopic dermatitis, psoriasis, and acne (and their parents) to cleanse and moisturize the skin properly, avoid particular skin irritants, and use medications appropriately.
- Many skin disorders are preventable. Teach families how to prevent contact dermatitis, burns, sunburn, frostbite, and bites and stings.
- Educate children and families about the importance of good soap-and-water cleansing of all minor skin injuries.

REFERENCES

Accurate Building Inspectors. (2007). *Water temperature thermometry*. Retrieved January 4, 2008 from www.accuratebuilding.com/services/legal/charts/hot_water_burn_scalding_graph.pdf.

Allen, P. L. J. (2004). Leaves of three, let them be: If it were only that easy! *Pediatric Nursing, 30*(2), 129–135.

American Medical Student Association. (2007). *Child abuse and neglect*. Retrieved May 19, 2007 from http://www.amsa.org/programs/gpit/child.cfm.

American Veterinary Medical Association. (2006). *Don't worry, they won't bite*. Retrieved July 23, 2006 from http://www.avma.org/pubhlth/dogbite/dogbitebroc.asp.

Behram, R. E., Kliegman, R. M. & Jenson, H. B. (2004). *Nelson's textbook of pediatrics* (17th ed.). Philadelphia: Saunders.

Berson, D. S. (2005). Cosmetic management of patients with acne vulgaris and acne rosacea. *Pediatric News (supplement), 7–8*, 12.

Bircher, A. (2005). Systemic immediate allergic reactions to arthropod stings and bites. *Dermatology, 210*, 119–127.

Borkowski, S. (2004). Diaper rash care and management. *Pediatric Nursing, 30*(6), 467–470.

Brown, K. M. (2007). Dermatoses of summer. *Contemporary Pediatrics, 24*(6 Suppl.), 13–18.

Buchanan, P. I. (2001). Behavior modification: A nursing approach for young children with atopic eczema. *Dermatology Nursing, 13*(1), 15–16, 18, 21–25.

Casale, T. B., & Stokes, J. R. (2006). Urticaria and angioedema. In J. A. McMillan (Ed.), *Oski's pediatrics: Principles and practice* (pp. 2410–2416). Philadelphia: Lippincott Williams & Wilkins.

Chen, N., & Cunningham, B. B. (2001). Psoriasis: Finding the right approach for your patients. *Contemporary Pediatrics, 18*(8), 86–93.

Cohen, B. (2004). A baby, a cutaneous lesion—and an efficient approach to recognition and management. *Contemporary Pediatrics, 21*(7), 28–48.

Committee on Trauma, American College of Surgeons. (1999). Guidelines for the operation of burn units. In *Resources for optimal care of the injured patient* (pp. 55–62). Chicago: Author.

Cuzzell, J. Z. (2005). FDA approves mandatory risk management program for isotretinoin. *Dermatology Nursing, 17*(5), 383.

Drago, D. A. (2005). Kitchen scalds and thermal burns in children five years and younger. *Pediatrics, 115*(1), 10–16.

Esselman, P. C., Thombs, B. D., Magyar-Russell, G., & Fauerbach, J. (2006). Burn rehabilitation: State of the science. *American Journal of Physical Medicine & Rehabilitation, 85*(4), 383–413.

Findlay, J. (2007). Treating atopic dermatitis. *Contemporary Pediatrics, 24*(6 suppl.), 4–12.

Frank, K. (2005). *Preventing and treating burns*. Retrieved 7/16/06 from www.kidsgrowth.com/resources/articledetail.cfm?id=2029.

Garfunkel, L. C., Kaczorowski J., & Christy, C. (Eds). (2007). *Mosby's pediatric clinical advisor: instant diagnosis and treatment*. (2nd ed.) St. Louis: Mosby.

Guin, J. D., & Bruckner, A. L. (2005). Compendium on poison ivy dermatitis: The insidious plants, the resulting lesions, the treatment options. *Contemporary Pediatrics, 22*(1 suppl.), 4–15.

Hoffman, H. G. (2004). Virtual reality therapy. *Scientific American, 291*(2), 58–65.

Holmes, T. E., & Krusinski, P. A. (2006). Dermatologic diseases. In J. A. McMillan (Ed.), *Oski's pediatrics: Principles and practice* (p. 462). Philadelphia: Lippincott Williams & Wilkins.

Kaplan, D. L. (2004). A photo quiz to hone dermatologic skills. *Consultant for Pediatricians, 3*(4), 169–176.

Keri, J. E. (2006). Acne: Improving skin and self-esteem. *Pediatric Annals, 35*(3), 174–179.

Klein, G. L., & Herndon, D. N. (2004). Burns. *Pediatrics in Review, 25*(12), 411–416.

Krowchuk, D. P., & Tunnessen, W. W. (2006). Pediatric dermatology. In J. A. McMillan (Ed.), *Oski's pediatrics: Principles and practice* (pp. 827–878). Philadelphia: Lippincott Williams & Wilkins.

Lee, P. J. (2004). Preschooler with slowly progressing rash on one arm. *Consultant for Pediatricians, 3*(3), 114–116.

Leung, A. K. C., & Kao, C. P. (2004). What's your diagnosis? *Consultant for Pediatricians, 3*(4), 188–191.

Lyder, C. H. (2006). Effective management of pressure ulcers: A review of proven strategies. *Advances for Nurse Practitioners, 14*(7), 32–38.

Magin, P. J., Adams, J., Heading, G. S., Pond, D. C., & Smith, W. (2006). Complementary and alternative medicine therapies in acne, psoriasis, and atopic eczema. *Journal of Alternative and Complementary Medicine, 12*(5), 451–457.

Mannenbach, M., & Bechtel, K. (2005). Patterns of injury that should raise suspicion for child abuse. *Pediatric Emergency Medicine Reports.* Retrieved 4/10/06 from Health and Wellness Resource Center.

Marino, B. S., & Fine, K. S. (2007). *Blueprints: Pediatrics.* Philadelphia: Lippincott Williams & Wilkins.

McGuinness, T. M. (2006). Teens and body art. *Journal of Psychosocial Nursing & Mental Health Services, 44*(4), 13–16.

Melnick, A. (2005). "Dog bites man" is news: How pediatricians can spread the word to parents and patients. *Contemporary Pediatrics* [electronic version] Available www.contemporarypediatrics.com.

Mondozzi, M. (2006). *Burns.* Retrieved 1/4/08 from http://www.kidshealth.org/parent/firstaid_safe/emergencies/burns.html.

Morelli, J. G., & Burch, J. M. (2007). Skin. In W. W. Hay, M. J. Levin, J. M. Sondheimer, & R. R. Deterding (Eds.), *Current pediatric diagnosis and treatment* (18th ed.) New York: McGraw-Hill.

National Institute of Arthritis and Musculoskeletal and Skin Diseases. (2006). *Questions and answers about acne.* Retrieved 7/8/06 from http://www.niams.nih.gov/hi/topics/acne/acne.htm.

National SAFE KIDS Campaign (2004). *Burn injury fact sheet.* Washington, DC: Author.

Nemours Foundation. (2005). Burns. Retrieved 1/4/08 from http://www.kidshealth.org/teen/safety/first_aid/burns_sheet.html.

Nield, L. S., & Kamat, D. M. (2006). Diaper dermatitis: From 'A' to 'Pee.' *Consultant for Pediatricians, 5*(6), 373–380.

Nield, L. S., & Nanda, S. (2005). Cold injuries: A guide to preventing and treating hypothermia and frostbite. *Consultant for Pediatricians, 4*(9), 427–434.

Peterson, J. D., & Chan, L. S. (2006). A comprehensive management guide for atopic dermatitis. *Dermatology Nursing, 18*(6), 531–543.

Reed, J. L., & Pomerantz, W. J. (2005). Emergency management of pediatric burns. *Pediatric Emergency Care, 21*(2), 118–129.

Romero, D. V., Treston, J., & O'Sullivan, A. L. (2006). Hand-to-hand combat: Preventing MRSA. *Nurse Practitioner, 31*(3), 16–23.

Safe Kids. (2008). *Preventing childhood burns.* Retrieved 1/4/08 from http://www.usa.safekids.org/content_documents/Burn_tips.pdf.

Schweich, P. J. (2006). Selected topics in emergency medicine. In J. A. McMillan (Ed.), *Oski's pediatrics: Principles and practice.* Philadelphia: Lippincott Williams & Wilkins.

Siberry, G. K. (2005). Fighting a rising tide of MRSA infection in the young. *Contemporary Pediatrics, 22*(7), 44–53.

Silverberg, N. B., Silverberg, J. I., & Silverberg, A. I. (2005). Eradicating acne vulgaris of puberty: What makes for optimal therapy? *Contemporary Pediatrics, 22*(10, suppl.), 12–22.

Sockrider, M. M. (2006). Respiratory complications of burns and smoke inhalation (respiratory burns). In J. A. McMillan (Ed.), *Oski's pediatrics: Principles and practice.* Philadelphia: Lippincott Williams & Wilkins.

Starr, N. B. (2004). Dermatologic diseases. In C. E. Burns, A. M. Dunn, M. A. Brady, et al. (Eds.), *Pediatric primary care: a handbook for nurse practitioners* (3rd ed.). Philadelphia: Saunders.

Suddaby, E. C., Barnett, S., & Facteau, L. (2006). Skin breakdown in acute care pediatrics. *Dermatology Nursing, 18*(2), 155–161.

Tanghetti, E. A. (2005). The importance of vehicle in acne therapy. *Pediatric News (supplement)*, 1–3.

U.S. Fire Administration. (2006). Exposing an invisible killer: The dangers of carbon monoxide. Retrieved 1/4/08 from http://www.usfa.dhs.gov/safety/co/fswy17.shtm.

U.S. Food and Drug Administration, Center for Drug Evaluation and Research. (2007). *iPledge.* Retrieved 1/4/08 from http://www.fda.gov/cder/drug/infopage/accutane/iPLEDGE200710.htm.

Villani, N. M. (2006). Treating dog and cat bites. *Advance for Nurse Practitioners, 14*(7), 44–45.

Watkins, P. (2005). Impetigo: Aetiology, complications and treatment options. *Nursing Standard, 19*(36), 50–54.

Weed, R. O., & Berens, D. E. (2005). Basics of burn injury: Implications for case management and life care planning. *Lippincott's Case Management, 10*(1), 22–29.

Willock, J., & Maylor, M. (2004). Pressure ulcers in infants and children. *Nursing Standard, 24*(18), 56–62.

Wong, L., & Rogers, M. (2006). Psoriasis: Varied presentations, individualized treatment. *Contemporary Pediatrics, 23*(1), 33–39.

WEBSITES

Acne Net (comprehensive online acne information resource): www.skincarephysicians.com/acnenet/FAQ.html

American Academy of Dermatology: www.aad.org

American Botanical Council and Herb Research Foundation (a peer-reviewed journal of herbal medical research): www.herbalgram.org

Burn Resource Center: www.burnsurvivor.com

Burn Support Group Database: www.burnsupportgroupsdatabase.com

HerbMed, an interactive electronic database of information on herbs: www.herbmed.org

Mentor services for burn survivors: www.survivingburns.org

National Eczema Association: www.nationaleczema.org

National Eczema Society: www.eczema.org

National Psoriasis Foundation: www.psoriasis.org

SafeKids: www.safekids.org

CHAPTER WORKSHEET

MULTIPLE CHOICE QUESTIONS

1. The nurse is teaching about skin care for atopic dermatitis. Which statement by the parent indicates that further teaching may be necessary?

   a. "I will use Vaseline or Crisco to moisturize my child's skin."

   b. "A hot bath will soothe my child's itching when it is severe."

   c. "I will buy cotton rather than wool or synthetic clothing for my child."

   d. "I will apply a small amount of the prescribed cream after the bath."

2. The nurse is caring for a child who has received significant partial-thickness burns to the lower body. What is the priority assessment in the first 24 hours after injury?

   a. Fluid balance.

   b. Wound infection.

   c. Respiratory arrest.

   d. Separation anxiety.

3. The nurse is caring for a child in the emergency department who was bitten by the family dog, who is fully immunized. What is the priority nursing action?

   a. Administer rabies immunoglobulin.

   b. Refer the child to a counselor.

   c. Assess the depth and extent of the wound.

   d. Administer a tetanus booster.

4. The nurse is caring for an infant on the pediatric unit who has a very red rash in the diaper area, with red lesions scattered on the abdomen and thighs. What is the priority nursing intervention?

   a. Administer griseofulvin with a fatty meal.

   b. Institute contact isolation precautions.

   c. Apply topical antibiotic cream.

   d. Apply topical antifungal cream.

5. A varsity high-school wrestler presents with a "rug burn" type of rash on his shoulder that is not healing as expected, despite use of triple antibiotic cream. Two other wrestlers on his team have a similar abrasion. What infection should the nurse be most concerned about, based on the history?

   a. Tinea cruris.

   b. MRSA.

   c. Impetigo.

   d. Tinea versicolor.

CRITICAL THINKING EXERCISES

1. A 4-year-old presents with his mother for evaluation of a yellowish, runny sore on his head. What questions would be most appropriate to ask the mother when taking the history? Should this child be placed in isolation? If so, why?

2. An 11-month-old comes to the primary care office with his mother for evaluation of a significant flaking red rash on both cheeks. The child is diagnosed with atopic dermatitis. What additional information should be obtained in the health history? What information should be included in the teaching plan for this family?

STUDY ACTIVITIES

1. Plan an educational activity:

   a. For parents of babies about the treatment and prevention of diaper dermatitis

   b. For parents of school-age children about prevention of contact dermatitis (related to poison ivy)

2. During your clinical rotation, spend a day with the wound and ostomy care nurse in a children's hospital. Report to the clinical group about what you learned that day.

3. Talk to teenagers with severe acne, atopic dermatitis, or psoriasis about their feelings about their skin's appearance. Reflect on this information in your clinical journal.

NURSING CARE OF THE CHILD WITH A HEMATOLOGIC DISORDER

KEY TERMS

anemia
chelation therapy
erythropoietin
hematocrit
hemoglobin
hemosiderosis

hypochromic
macrocytic
microcytic
platelet
platelet count
poikilocytosis

polycythemia
purpura
red blood cell
splenomegaly
thrombocytopenia
white blood cell (WBC)

LEARNING OBJECTIVES

Upon completion of the chapter, the learner will be able to:

1. Identify major hematologic disorders that affect children.
2. Determine priority assessment information for children with hematologic disorders.
3. Identify priority interventions for children with hematologic disorders.
4. Analyze laboratory data in relation to normal findings and report abnormal findings.
5. Provide nursing diagnoses appropriate for the child and family with hematologic disorders.
6. Develop a teaching plan for the family of children with hematologic disorders.
7. Identify resources for children and families with hematologic disorders or nutrition deficits.

*S*haun O'Malley, 10 months old, is being admitted to the pediatric unit after being brought to the clinic by his father for a small laceration that he thought needed stitches. His father states, "I didn't think the cut was very deep. I was surprised by how long it bled."

WOW

Blood is just red to the child, but to the nurse, blood is life.

The hematologic system consists of the blood and blood-forming tissues of the body. These typically function together in a balance that affects the metabolism of the body. The three categories of cells are erythrocytes, or **red blood cells** (RBCs); thrombocytes, or **platelets**; and leukocytes, or **white blood cells** (WBCs). RBCs are responsible for transporting nutrients and oxygen to the body tissues and waste products from the tissues. The platelets are responsible for clotting. WBCs are responsible for fighting infection. WBCs are further divided into granulocytes (neutrophils, eosinophils, and basophils) and agranulocytes (lymphocytes and monocytes) (Kimball, 2007).

All blood cells originate from a single type of cell called a multipotent stem cell, which goes on to differentiate into the various types of blood cells. Thrombopoietin (TPO) and interleukin-7 (IL-7) act on the cell and differentiate the cell into either myeloid or lymphoid progenitor cells. The lymphoid cells either, under the influence of IL-6, become B lymphocytes, or change directly into T lymphocytes. The myeloid cells are differentiated in one of two ways, either by the action of **erythropoietin** (EPO) or granulocyte–monocyte colony-stimulating factor (GM-CSF). When the cell is acted upon by EPO, which is produced by the kidneys, the cell becomes the megakaryocyte, also known as the erythroid progenitor cell. The megakaryocyte is acted on by either EPO, to become the red blood cell, or TPO and IL-11, to become a megakaryocyte that goes on to form platelets. GM-CSF influences the cell to become the granulocyte, also known as the macrophage progenitor cell. These cells further differentiate under various influences to become the WBCs (Kimball, 2007) (Fig. 46.1).

Certain conditions may cause problems to develop within this system. These problems are related to either the production of the blood cells (too much or too little) or loss and destruction of these cells.

Nursing care for the child with a hematologic disorder is often multifaceted. A child who has iron deficiency anemia requires adequate oxygenation and may require packed red blood cells; a child with hemophilia requires factor replacement and monitoring for safety. Each condition may be life-threatening but requires different interventions.

Variations in Pediatric Anatomy and Physiology

Many factors are involved in the development of hematologic disorders, ranging from genetic causes to disorders resulting from injury, infection, or nutritional deficit. In the absence of a congenital defect, the hematologic system is intact and functional at birth. RBC and hemoglobin production as well as iron stores undergo changes

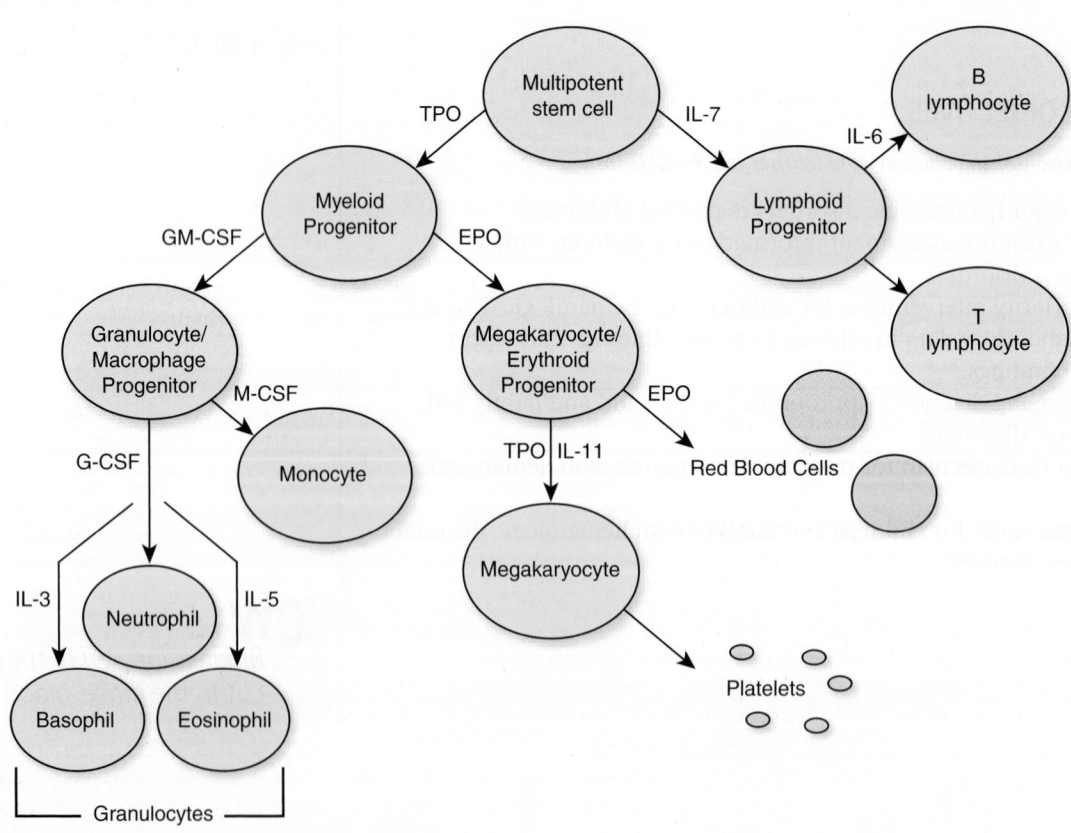

FIGURE 46.1 Process of blood cell formation.

in the first few months of life; after this time, hematologic function is stable.

RBC Production

The production of blood cells in the embryo begins by 8 weeks' gestation. In the embryo, blood cells primarily form in the liver; this continues until a few weeks before delivery. Some cell production, lymphoid cells in particular, takes place in the spleen of the embryo, and the thymus is a site for some transient lymphocyte production. EPO, the hormone that regulates RBC production, is derived primarily from the liver in the fetus, and after birth the kidneys take over this production.

Hemoglobin

Three types of normal **hemoglobin** (Hgb) are present at any given time in the blood: Hgb A, Hgb F or fetal, and Hgb A_2. After 6 months of age, Hgb A is the predominant type. In the neonatal period, the largest difference is with the RBCs. Fetal hemoglobin, which has a much shorter cell life, is present in higher quantities, putting the infant at risk for anemia and leading to problems with the oxygen-carrying capacity of the blood. As the production of the cells transfers from the liver to the bone marrow of the long and flat bones, the balance between oxygenation and production is affected.

Iron

The fetus receives iron through the placenta from the mother. The preterm infant misses out on the final weeks or months of transplacental iron transfer, putting him or her at increased risk for anemia. In the term infant, a period of physiologic anemia occurs between the age of 2 and 6 months. The infant demonstrates rapid growth and an increase in blood volume over the first several months of life, and maternally derived iron stores are depleted by age 4 to 6 months. Sufficient iron intake is critical for the appropriate development of hemoglobin and RBCs, so the infant must ingest adequate quantities of iron either from breast milk or from iron-fortified formula in early infancy and other food sources in later infancy. Adolescence is also a time of rapid growth, and intake of iron must increase.

Common Medical Treatments

Various medications as well as other medical treatments are used to treat hematologic disorders in children. Most of these treatments will require a physician's order when the child is in the hospital. The most common treatments and medications are listed in Common Medical Treatments 46.1 and Drug Guide 46.1. The nurse caring for the child with a hematologic disorder should be familiar with the procedures are used, how the medications work, and common nursing implications related to their use.

NURSING PROCESS OVERVIEW FOR THE CHILD WITH A HEMATOLOGIC DISORDER

Care of the child with a hematologic disorder includes assessment, nursing diagnosis, planning, interventions, and evaluation. There are a number of general concepts related to the nursing process that may be applied to hematologic dysfunction in children.

Development of a plan of care will depend upon which component of the blood is altered. A decrease in hemoglobin will necessitate evaluation of oxygen-carrying capacity and effects of hypoxia on the tissues. A reduction in platelet production will lead the nurse to evaluate for prolonged bleeding, hemorrhage, and shock. An elevation in WBCs would require an evaluation for infection.

Remember Shaun, the 10-month-old with the laceration and prolonged bleeding? What additional health history and physical examination assessment information should you obtain?

Assessment

Signs of changes in the hematologic system are often insidious and overlooked. Skin color changes such as pallor, bruising, and flushing are often the first signs that a problem is developing. Changes in mental status such as lethargy can indicate a decrease in Hgb and a decreased amount of oxygen being delivered to the brain. Nursing assessment must include a thorough systems approach.

Health History

Elicit the birth and maternal history, noting low birthweight or gestational diabetes and ascertaining whether vitamin K was given after birth. The past medical history might be significant for recent illnesses that may contribute to a change in blood cell distribution. Determine the child's sleep/wake patterns and bowel elimination patterns, which may be affected by alterations in circulating blood volume or changes in oxygenation. Explore the family history for inherited disorders such as hemophilia, sickle cell disease, and thalassemia. Evaluate the child's typical diet for nutritional deficits. Determine risk for lead exposure based on the use of a standard questionnaire. When eliciting the history of the present illness, inquire about:

- Fatigue or malaise
- Pallor of the skin
- Unusual bruising
- Excessive bleeding or difficulty stopping bleeding
- Pain: location, onset, duration, quality, relieving factors

COMMON MEDICAL TREATMENTS 46.1

Treatment	Explanation	Indication	Nursing Implications
Blood product transfusion	Intravenous administration of whole blood, packed red blood cells (PRBCs), platelets, or plasma	PRBCs: severe anemia, thalassemia, sickle cell disease Whole blood: acute hemorrhage or trauma Fresh-frozen plasma: hemophilia	Follow institution's transfusion protocol. Double-check blood type and product label with a second nurse. Use only leukodepleted, CMV-negative blood products in the child with a hemoglobinopathy. Monitor vital signs and assess child frequently to detect adverse reaction to blood transfusion. If adverse reaction is suspected, immediately discontinue transfusion, run normal saline IV, reassess the child, and notify the physician. Some children require premedication with diphenhydramine and/or acetaminophen before receiving blood products.
Supplemental oxygen	Administration of oxygen via mask, cannula, or blow-by	Hypoxia associated with sickle cell crisis or severe anemia	Frequently monitor work of breathing, oxygen saturation via pulse oximetry, cardiopulmonary status, and level of consciousness.
Splenectomy	Surgical removal of the spleen	Life-threatening or recurrent splenic sequestration of sickle cell disease; thalassemia	Provide immunization against the following organisms, because they place the child at risk for overwhelming infection: *Streptococcus pneumoniae, Neisseria meningitidis,* and *Haemophilus influenzae* type B. Monitor carefully for signs of infection. Administer prophylactic antibiotics. Instruct child or teen to wear medical alert bracelet. Teach families to seek medical treatment at first sign of infection or fever.
Hematopoietic stem cell transplantation	Bone marrow transplant: transfer of healthy bone marrow into a child with disease; the transplanted cells can then develop into functional cells. Stem cell transplant: Peripheral stem cells are removed from the donor via apheresis, or stem cells are retrieved from the umbilical cord and placenta. The stem cells are then transplanted into the recipient.	Sickle cell disease, aplastic anemias, thalassemia	Maintain medical asepsis and protective isolation to prevent infection. Monitor closely for graft-versus-host disease. Provide meticulous oral care. Avoid taking rectal temperatures and inserting suppositories. Encourage appropriate nutrition. Administer immunosuppressive medications as ordered.

DRUG GUIDE 46.1 COMMON DRUGS FOR HEMATOLOGIC DISORDERS

Medication	Action and Indications	Nursing Implications
Iron supplements (ferrous sulfate, ferrous fumarate)	Supplemental iron in deficient child Iron deficiency anemia	Dosage is based on mg of elemental iron. Do not administer with milk or milk products. May color stools and urine black Liquid can stain the teeth; mix with a small amount of juice; drinking with straw decreases tooth staining. May cause constipation; increase fiber and fluid intake
Deferoxamine (Desferal)	Binds with iron, which is removed via the kidneys Iron toxicity	Rotate subcutaneous injection sites to decrease local reactions. Apply corticosteroid cream to irritation.
Factor (VIII or IX) replacement	Replaces deficient clotting factors Hemophilia	Use filter needle to draw up medication. Administer IV when bleeding occurs.
Penicillin VK	Kills susceptible bacteria Prophylaxis of infection in asplenia	Determine whether penicillin allergy is present. Monitor renal and hematologic function during prolonged use.
Folic acid	Replaces the vitamin Folic acid deficiency; questionable use with sickle cell anemia	Administer without regard to meals. Monitor hematologic function.
Intravenous immune globulin (IVIG) (multiple manufacturers)	Provides exogenous IgG antibodies Idiopathic thrombocytopenic purpura	Do not mix with IV medications or with other IV fluids. Do not give IM or SQ. Monitor vital signs and watch for adverse reactions frequently during infusion. Child may require antipyretic or antihistamine to prevent chills and fever during infusion. Have epinephrine available during infusion.
Chelating agents: dimercaprol (BAL), edentate calcium disodium (CaEDTA), succimer (Chemet)	Remove lead from soft tissues and bone, allowing for its excretion via the renal system Used for blood lead levels >45 mcg/dL	Monitor intake and output closely to ensure adequacy of renal system. Encourage adequate oral hydration or provide IV hydration if required. Follow lead levels as prescribed. Ensure that lead is being removed from the child's home.

Physical Examination

A child's general appearance gives great insight into his or her health and can indicate problems such as malnutrition or lead poisoning. Physical examination of the child with a hematologic disorder includes inspection and observation, palpation, and auscultation.

Inspection and Observation

Note the child's general appearance, including thin or emaciated appearance or obesity, as well as color. Measure weight and height (or length) and plot on standardized growth charts. Observe the nail beds, palms, and soles for pallor. Evaluate the fingertips for clubbing, which occurs with chronic decreases in oxygen. Document the location and extent of bruises, petechiae, or

purpura. Count the respiratory rate and observe for work of breathing. Obtain a pulse oximeter reading to determine oxygen saturation of tissues. Note conjunctival color as well as color and moisture of oral mucosa. Determine urinary output, which may be altered with decreases in circulatory blood volume or inadequate oxygenation. Note the child's responsiveness to stimuli, movement of extremities, and quality of gait.

Auscultation

Auscultate breath sounds, noting adequacy of air movement and depth of respiration. Note adventitious sounds or absence of breath sounds (which would occur in an area of the lung filled with blood). Auscultate heart sounds, listening closely for murmurs (which can develop with changes in blood viscosity and volume). Note the rate and rhythm of the heart tones. Auscultate bowel sounds, noting presence and normalcy.

Palpation

Measure blood pressure, which may change with alterations in blood volume. Palpate the peripheral pulses for strength and equality. Determine capillary refill time, which may be prolonged when the circulating blood volume is decreased. Carefully palpate the abdomen for tenderness, hepatomegaly, or **splenomegaly** (increased spleen size). Note temperature of the skin. Determine elasticity of skin, noting decreased turgor. Palpate the joints for tenderness. Assess range of motion.

Laboratory and Diagnostic Testing

The nurse must understand the main elements of the complete blood count (CBC; hemogram) to recognize critical values and intervene as appropriate. The components of the CBC are:

- RBC count: the actual number of counted RBCs in a certain volume of blood
- Hgb: measure of the protein made up of heme (iron surrounded by protoporphyrin) and globin, alpha and beta-polypeptide chains, primarily responsible for the transport of nutrients and oxygen to the tissues
- **Hematocrit** (Hct): an indirect measure of red blood cells (number and volume)
- RBC indices
  - MCV: average size of the RBC
  - Mean corpuscular hemoglobin (MCH): a calculated value of the oxygen-carrying capacity of the Hgb in the RBCs
  - MCHC: a calculated value that reflects the concentration of Hgb inside the RBC
  - Red cell distribution width (RDW): a calculated value that is a measure of the width of RBCs
- WBC count: actual count of the number of WBCs in a volume of blood
- **Platelet count**: number of platelets per blood volume
  - Mean platelet volume (MPV): a measurement of the size of the platelets

Tables 46.1 and 46.2 provide age-related values for the CBC and leukocyte count (Carey et al., 2005). When evaluating the CBC, the nurse must take into account the presenting clinical picture of the child. For instance, the RBC count may be truly elevated (erythrocytosis or **polycythemia**) in certain diseases or in the case of dehydration from diarrhea or burns. When anemia is present, the RBC count is low. When the mean corpuscular volume (MCV) is elevated, the RBCs are larger than normal (**macrocytic**). When the MCV is decreased, the RBCs are smaller than normal (**microcytic**). A decrease in the mean corpuscular hemoglobin concentration (MCHC) means that the Hgb is diluted in the cell and less of the red color is present (**hypochromic**). When the Hgb concentration

is increased in the RBC, then the pigmentation (red color) is increased (hyperchromic).

WBCs are the body's defense against infection or injury. The specific types of WBCs are discussed in Chapter 36. Platelets are necessary for clot formation, and if changes occur, problems may develop: elevations can indicate an increase in clotting, while decreases can put the child at risk for increased bleeding. Decreases can result if the platelets are being used up when bleeding is present, if an inherited disorder is present, or if the spleen holds them, as in hypersplenism. Platelets are larger when they are new; thus, an elevation in the mean platelet volume indicates that an increased number of platelets are being produced in the bone marrow (Carey et al., 2005).

Common Laboratory and Diagnostic Tests 46.1 explains the most commonly used laboratory and diagnostic tests used in children with hematologic disorders. The tests can assist the physician in diagnosing the disorder and/or be used as guidelines in determining ongoing treatment. Laboratory or non-nursing personnel obtain some of the tests, while the nurse might obtain others. In either instance the nurse should be familiar with how the tests are obtained, what they are used for, and normal versus abnormal results. This knowledge will also be necessary when providing patient and family education related to the testing.

Nursing Diagnoses, Goals, Interventions, and Evaluation

Upon completion of a thorough assessment, the nurse might identify several nursing diagnoses, including:

- Fatigue
- Pain
- Impaired physical mobility
- Ineffective health maintenance
- Anxiety
- Ineffective family coping

You have finished assessing Shaun and your findings include the following. The history revealed he bled with all four of the teeth he has cut. Upon examination numerous bruises are noted. Based on the assessment findings, what would your top three nursing diagnoses be for Shaun?

Nursing goals, interventions, and evaluation for the child with hematologic dysfunction are based on the nursing diagnoses. Nursing Care Plan Overview 46.1 may be used as a guide in planning nursing care for the child with a hematologic disorder. Children's responses to hematologic disorders and their treatments will vary, and nursing care should be individualized based on the child's and family's responses to illness. Other conditions may contribute to these nursing diagnoses and must also

TABLE 46.1 NORMAL HEMOGRAM VALUES

Age	WBC (×10³/mm³)	RBC (×10⁶/mm³)	Hgb (g/dL)	Hct (%)	MCV (fL)	MCH (pg/cell)	MCHC (g/dL)	Platelets (×10³/mm³)	RDW (%)	MPV (fL)
Birth–2 weeks	9.0–30.0	4.1–6.1	14.5–24.5	44–54	98–112	34–40	33–37	150–450	—	—
2–8 weeks	5.0–21.0	4.0–6.0	12.5–20.5	39–59	98–112	30–36	32–36	—	—	—
2–6 months	5.0–19.0	3.8–5.6	10.7–17.3	35–49	83–97	27–33	31–35	—	—	—
6 months–1 year	5.0–19.0	3.8–5.2	9.9–14.5	29–43	73–87	24–30	32–36	—	—	—
1–6 years	5.0–19.0	3.9–5.3	9.5–14.1	30–40	70–84	23–29	31–35	—	—	—
6–16 years	4.8–10.8	4.0–5.2	10.3–14.9	32–42	73–87	24–30	32–36	—	—	—
16–18 years	4.8–10.8	4.2–5.4	11.1–15.7	34–44	75–89	25–31	32–36	—	—	—
>18 years (males)	5.0–10.0	4.5–5.5	14.0–17.4	42–52	84–96	28–34	32–36	140–400	11.5–14.5	7.4–10.4
>18 years (females)	5.0–10.0	4.0–5.0	12.0–16.0	36–48	84–96	28–34	32–36	140–400	11.5–14.5	7.4–10.4

Data from Fischbach, F. T. (2004). *A manual of laboratory and diagnostic tests* (7th ed., p. 47). Philadelphia: Lippincott Williams & Wilkins.

TABLE 46.2 NORMAL DIFFERENTIAL FOR LEUKOCYTES (WHITE BLOOD CELL DIFFERENTIAL)

Age	Bands/Stab (%)	Segs/Polys (%)	Eos (%)	Basos (%)	Lymphs (%)	Monos (%)
Birth– 1 week	10–18	32–62	0–2	0–1	26–36	0–6
1–2 weeks	8–16	19–49	0–4	0	38–46	0–9
2–4 weeks	7–15	14–34	0–3	0	43–53	0–9
4–8 weeks	7–13	15–35	0–3	0–1	41–71	0–7
2–6 months	5–11	15–35	0–3	0–1	42–72	0–6
6 months– 1 year	6–12	13–33	0–3	0	46–76	0–5
1–6 years	5–11	13–33	0–3	0	46–76	0–5
6–16 years	5–11	32–54	0–3	0–1	27–57	0–5
16–18 years	5–11	34–64	0–3	0–1	25–45	0–5
>18 years	3–6	50–62	0–3	0–1	25–40	3–7

Data from Fischbach, F. T. (2004). *A manual of laboratory and diagnostic tests* (7th ed., p. 51). Philadelphia: Lippincott Williams & Wilkins.

be considered when prioritizing care. Additional information about nursing management will be included later in the chapter as it relates to specific disorders.

Based on your top three nursing diagnoses for Shaun, describe appropriate nursing interventions.

Anemia

Anemia is a condition in which levels of RBCs and Hgb are lower than normal. Hgb levels vary throughout childhood and should be monitored to ensure that adequate growth and development will be achieved. Anemia may develop as a result of decreased production of RBCs or loss and destruction of RBCs. The loss of production can be related to lack of dietary intake of the nutrients needed to produce the cells, alterations in the cell structure, or malfunctioning tissues, such as the bone marrow. Anemia related to nutritional deficiency includes iron deficiency, folic acid deficiency, and pernicious anemia. Anemia may also result from toxin exposure (lead poisoning) or as an adverse reaction to a medication (aplastic anemia). Blood loss may result from surgery or trauma, and destruction of cells occurs in certain genetic and cellular development disorders.

Anemia caused by the alteration or destruction of the RBC is termed hemolytic anemia. There are several types of hemolytic anemia, such as sickle cell disease and thalassemia; these two disorders are discussed under "Hemoglobinopathies."

Anemia related to insufficient intake of specific nutrients is the most common type of anemia in children. Nutrient intake may be reduced in children due to food dislikes or conditions that produce malabsorption.

▶ IRON DEFICIENCY ANEMIA

Iron deficiency anemia occurs when the body does not have enough iron to produce Hgb. In the United States, 3% to 8% of children and adolescents have iron deficiency anemia. One of the factors that contributes to iron deficiency anemia in older infants is the consumption of cow's milk: infants between the ages of 9 and 12 months who drank more than 500 g of cow's milk per day had reduced Hgb levels (Zetterstrom, 2004).

▶ **Take** NOTE!

Dietary intake of more than 500 g/day of cow's milk in children has been shown to produce decreased Hgb levels (Gunnarsson et al., 2004). This study also found that children with lower iron levels had increased weight gain from birth to 2 years of age.

The heme portion of Hgb consists of iron surrounded by protoporphyrin. When not enough iron is available to the bone marrow, Hgb production is reduced. Adequate dietary intake of iron is required for the body to make enough Hgb. As Hgb levels decrease,

COMMON LABORATORY AND DIAGNOSTIC TESTS 46.1

Test	Explanation	Indication	Nursing Implications
Blood type and cross-match	Determines ABO blood type as well as presence of antigens. Cross-match is performed on RBC-containing products to avoid transfusion reaction.	Trauma victim or any person in whom blood loss is suspected, in preparation for transfusion	Avoid hemolysis of specimen. Appropriately sign and date specimen. Apply "type and cross" or "blood band" to child at the time of blood draw if indicated by the institution. Most type and cross-match specimens expire after 48 to 72 hours.
Clotting studies	Prothrombin time (PT), partial thromboplastin time (PTT), activated partial thromboplastin time (aPTT), International Normalized Ratio (INR)	Evaluation of common pathway in clotting mechanism PT, INR: evaluation of extrinsic system PTT, aPTT: evaluation of intrinsic system	Apply pressure to venipuncture site. Assess for bleeding (gums, bruising, blood in urine or stool).
Coagulating factor concentration	Measures concentration of specific coagulating factors in the blood	Hemophilia, DIC	Apply pressure to venipuncture site. Assess for bleeding (gums, bruising, blood in urine or stool). Deliver specimen to laboratory as soon as possible (unstable at room temperature).
Complete blood count (CBC) with differential	Evaluates hemoglobin and hematocrit, WBC count (particularly the percentage of individual WBCs), and platelet count	Anemia, infection, bleeding disorder, clotting disorder	Normal values vary according to age and gender. WBC differential is helpful in evaluating source of infection. May be affected by certain medications
Hemoglobin electrophoresis	Measures percentage of normal and abnormal hemoglobin in the blood	Sickle cell anemia, thalassemia	Blood transfusions within the previous 12 weeks may alter test results.
Iron	Evaluates iron metabolism	Iron deficiency anemia, hemosiderosis with chronic transfusion or hemoglobinopathies	Recent blood transfusions increase level. Child should fast for 12 hours before the test. Avoid hemolysis (will falsely elevate result).
Lead	Measures level of lead in blood	Lead poisoning	Normal amount in blood is zero.
Reticulocyte count	Measures the amount of reticulocytes (immature RBCs) in the blood	Indicates bone marrow's ability to respond to anemia with production of RBCs	Rises quickly in response to iron supplementation in the iron-deficient child
Serum ferritin	Measures the level of ferritin (the major iron storage protein) in the blood	Most sensitive test for determining iron deficiency anemia	Elevated in hemolytic disease and if transfused recently Iron supplementation increases ferritin levels.

the oxygen-carrying capacity of the blood is decreased, resulting in weakness and fatigue. In addition to delayed growth, iron deficiency anemia has been associated with cognitive delays and behavioral changes (Brotanek et al., 2007).

Therapeutic Management

Iron supplements are usually provided in the form of ferrous sulfate or ferrous fumarate and are available

(text continues on page 1536)

Nursing Care Plan 46.1

OVERVIEW FOR THE CHILD WITH A HEMATOLOGIC DISORDER

NURSING DIAGNOSIS: Fatigue related to decreased oxygen supply in the body as evidenced by lack of energy, increased sleep requirements, or decreased interest in play

Outcome Identification and Evaluation
Child will display increased endurance, desire to play without developing symptoms of exertion.

Intervention: Decreasing Fatigue
- Cluster nursing care activities and plan for periods of rest before and after exertion *to decrease oxygen need and consumption.*
- Encourage activity or ambulation per physician's orders; *early mobilization results in better outcomes.*
- Observe child for signs of activity intolerance such as pallor, nausea, lightheadedness, or dizziness or changes in vital signs *to determine level of tolerance.*
- If child is on bed rest, perform range-of-motion exercises and frequent position changes: *negative changes to the musculoskeletal system occur quickly with inactivity and immobility.*
- Refer the child to physical therapy *for exercise prescription to increase skeletal muscle strength.*

NURSING DIAGNOSIS: Impaired physical mobility related to pain from sickle cell crisis or acute bleeds or imposed activity restrictions, as evidenced by guarding of painful extremity, resistance to activity

Outcome Identification and Evaluation
Child will be able to engage in activities within age parameters and limits of disease: *child is able to move extremities, move about environment, and participate in exercise programs within limits of age and disease.*

Intervention: Promoting Physical Mobility
- Encourage gross and fine motor activities as able within constraints of pain/bleed *to facilitate motor development.*
- Collaborate with physical therapy to strengthen muscles and promote mobility *to facilitate motor development.*
- Use passive and active range-of-motion exercises and teach child and family how to perform them *to prevent contractures and facilitate joint mobility and muscle development (active ROM) to help increase mobility.*
- Praise accomplishments and emphasize child's abilities *to improve self-esteem and encourage feelings of confidence and competence.*

NURSING DIAGNOSIS: Ineffective health maintenance related to knowledge and skill acquisition regarding nutritional and medical treatment of anemia, prevention of infection, home administration of intravenous clotting factors, or protection from injury as evidenced by new diagnosis and inability to verbalize appropriate treatment regimen or demonstrate medication administration skills

Outcome Identification and Evaluation
Child's health will be maintained; *child will receive supplements, medications as prescribed and will eat an appropriate diet.*

Intervention: Educating Parents About Effective Health Maintenance
- Educate the family about iron-rich foods to be promoted in the child with iron deficiency anemia and limited in the child with thalassemia.
- Limit cow's milk intake in the child with iron deficiency anemia *to decrease risk of microscopic GI bleeding and increase appetite for other foods.*
- Provide ongoing evaluation of nutritional intake *to ensure that appropriate dietary restrictions are followed.*
- Ensure that parents can verbalize understanding of home medication regimen: iron or folic acid supplementation for anemia, prophylactic antibiotics for sickle cell anemia, chelation for thalassemia and factor replacement for hemophilia.
- Have parents provide return demonstration of subcutaneous infusion of deferoxamine or intravenous factor as appropriate *to ensure accuracy and independence in the home environment.*
- Educate families about when to call or visit medical provider *to ensure timely intervention when signs and symptoms develop.*

Nursing Care Plan 46.1 (continued)

NURSING DIAGNOSIS: Anxiety related to diagnostic testing as evidenced by parent verbalization, child resistance or crying with procedures

Outcome Identification and Evaluation

Child's anxiety will be minimized; *child will verbalize less fear, experience less pain with procedures.*

Intervention: Relieving Anxiety

- Use topical anesthetic creams or agents for non-emergency lab draws *to decrease stress related to needlesticks or venipunctures.*
- Maintain a quiet and calm environment *to reduce the child's stress.*
- Educate the child, as appropriate, and the family regarding the need for laboratory specimens *to alleviate anxiety related to the unknown.*
- Identify the need for the specific test and explain the procedure before obtaining the specimen *to decrease the anxiety and time required for the procedure.*
- Provide developmentally appropriate activities for the child; *activities can reduce stress and also provide stimulus for children; serves as a model for the family.*

NURSING DIAGNOSIS: Ineffective family coping related to hospitalization of child or chronic, possibly life-threatening genetic disorder as evidenced by excessive tearfulness or denial statements, withdrawal, or verbalization of inadequate coping skills

Outcome Identification and Evaluation

Child and/or family will demonstrate adequate coping skills, *will verbalize feeling supported and demonstrate healthy family interactions.*

Intervention: Promoting Effective Family Coping

- Provide emotional support to the child and family *to improve coping abilities.*
- Actively listen to the child's and family's concerns *to validate their feelings and establish trust.*
- Encourage parents to talk about their child and the illness *to bring feelings out in the open.*
- Validate feelings of guilt, shock, frustration, resentment, or depression *to promote trust and begin appropriate coping.*
- Provide open communication with the child and siblings: *children appreciate honesty about their illness, and coping is improved.*
- Refer families to community resources such as parent support groups, grief counseling *to improve coping abilities.*
- Encourage role-playing and play activities *to identify the child's fears and work through feelings.*

NURSING DIAGNOSIS: Risk for injury related to alteration in peripheral sensory perception, decreased platelet count, deficient coagulation factor, or excessive iron load

Outcome Identification and Evaluation

Child will not experience hemorrhage; *will experience decreased bruising or episodes of prolonged bleeding.*

Intervention: Preventing Injury

- Assess for petechiae, purpura, bruising, or bleeding *to provide baseline data for comparison; if present, may warrant intervention.*
- Encourage quiet activities or play *to avoid trauma with active play.*
- Avoid rectal temperatures and examinations. Post sign at head of bed "no rectal temperatures or medications" *to avoid rectal mucosa damage resulting in bleeding.*
- Avoid intramuscular injections and lumbar puncture if possible *to decrease risk of bleeding from a puncture site.*
- If bone marrow aspiration must be performed, apply pressure dressing to site *to prevent bleeding.*
- Teach families about preferred physical activities for the child with ITP or hemophilia *to provide safe physical activities and decrease risk for injury.*

HEALTHY PEOPLE 2010	
Objective	**Significance**
Reduce iron deficiency among young children and females of child-bearing age.	• Encourage use of iron-fortified formulas and infant cereal. • Encourage iron supplementation in the second half of infancy for the breast-fed infant. • Educate parents about iron-containing foods. • Encourage adolescent females to consume a diet high in iron-rich foods.

over the counter. Dosage is based on the amount of elemental iron. The recommended amounts of elemental iron are:

• For prophylaxis: 1 to 2 mg/kg/day, up to a maximum of 15 mg elemental iron per day
• Mild to moderate iron deficiency: 3 mg/kg/day of elemental iron in one or two divided doses
• Severe iron deficiency anemia: 4 to 6 mg/kg/day of elemental iron in three divided doses

In more severe cases, blood transfusions may be indicated. Transfusion of packed red blood cells (PRBCs) is reserved for the most severe cases. When PRBC administration is warranted, follow specific blood bank guidelines for administration. Monitor subsequent laboratory results for improvement.

Nursing Assessment

For a full description of the assessment phase of the nursing process, refer to page 1527. Assessment findings pertinent to iron deficiency anemia are discussed below.

Health History
Elicit a description of the current illness and chief complaint. Common signs and symptoms reported during the health history may include irritability, headache, dizziness, weakness, shortness of breath, pallor, and fatigue. Other symptoms may be subtle and difficult for the clinician to identify; these include difficulty feeding, pica, muscle weakness, or unsteady gait.

Explore the health history for risk factors such as:

• Maternal anemia during pregnancy
• Poorly controlled diabetes during pregnancy
• Prematurity, low birthweight, or multiple birth
• Cow's milk consumption before 12 months of age
• Excessive cow's milk consumption (greater than 24 ounces a day)
• Infant consumption of low-iron formula
• Lack of iron supplementation after age 6 months in breastfed infants

• Excessive weight gain
• Chronic infection or inflammation
• Chronic or acute blood loss
• Restricted diets
• Use of medication interfering with iron absorption, such as antacids
• Low socioeconomic status
• Recent immigration from a developing country

Evaluate the child's diet for adequate intake of iron-rich foods. Recommended dietary daily intake for iron in children is:

• 0 to 6 months: 6 mg
• 6 to 12 months: 10 mg
• 1 to 10 years: 10 mg
• Boys 11 to 18 years: 12 mg
• Girls 11 to 18 years: 15 mg (Abrams et al., 2006)

Physical Examination
Observe the child for fatigue and lethargy. Inspect the skin, conjunctivae, oral mucosa, palms, and soles for pallor. Note spooning of the nails (concave shape) (Fig. 46.2). Obtain a pulse oximeter reading. Evaluate the heart rate for tachycardia. Auscultate the heart for a flow murmur. Palpate the abdomen for splenomegaly.

Laboratory and Diagnostic Tests
Laboratory evaluation will reveal decreased Hgb and Hct, decreased reticulocyte count, microcytosis, hypochromia, decreased serum iron and ferritin levels, and an increased free erythrocyte protoporphyrin (FEP) level.

Nursing Management

Nursing management of the child with iron deficiency focuses on promoting safety, ensuring adequate iron intake, and educating the family.

Promoting Safety
The child with anemia is at risk for changes in neurologic functioning related to the decreased oxygen supply to the

FIGURE 46.2 Note the concave shape of nails ("spooning") that occurs with iron deficiency anemia.

brain. This can lead to fatigue and inability to eat enough. Neurologic effects may be manifested when the child's ability to sit, stand, or walk is impaired. Provide close observation of the anemic child. Assist the older child with ambulation. Educate the parents on how to protect the child from injury due to an unsteady gait or dizziness.

Providing Dietary Interventions

Ensure that iron-deficient infants are fed only formulas fortified with iron. Interventions for breastfed infants include beginning iron supplementation around the age of 4 or 5 months. Iron supplementation may range from adding iron-fortified cereals to the child's diet to giving iron-containing drops. Encourage breastfeeding mothers to increase their dietary intake of iron or take iron supplements when breastfeeding so that the iron may be passed on to the infant. For children over 1 year of age, limit cow's milk intake to 24 ounces per day. Limit fast-food consumption and encourage intake of iron-rich foods such as red meats, tuna, salmon, eggs, tofu, enriched grains, dried beans and peas, dried fruits, leafy green vegetables, and iron-fortified breakfast cereals (iron from red meat is the easiest for the body to absorb).

Teach the parents about dietary intake, and encourage them to provide a variety of foods for iron support and vitamins and other minerals necessary for growth. A big problem for toddlers is their "picky" eating. This often becomes a means of control for the child, and parents should guard against getting involved in a power struggle with their child. Referring parents to a developmental specialist who can assist them in their approach to diet may prove beneficial. Refer families who meet the financial limits and who have children age 5 and under to the Women, Infants and Children (WIC) program, which provides for supplementation of infant's and children's diets.

▶ *Take* NOTE!

Parents are often concerned that a diagnosis of iron deficiency anemia or referral to the WIC program may lead to interventions from children's services. Assure the family that as long as appropriate measures are taken to address the anemia, referrals of this nature are not generally made.

Teaching About Iron Supplement Administration

The use of iron supplements in infants begins with the use of formula fortified with iron in the formula-fed infant. Oral supplements may be necessary as well if the baby's iron levels are extremely low. Oral supplements or multivitamin formulas that contain iron are often dark in color, as the iron is pigmented. Teaching the parents to measure

precisely the amount of iron to be administered is an important nursing role. Parents should place the liquid behind the teeth, as iron in liquid form can stain the teeth. Iron supplementation can also cause constipation. In some cases reducing the amount of iron can resolve this problem, but stool softeners may be necessary to control painful or difficult-to-pass stools. Encourage parents to increase their child's fluid intake and include adequate dietary fiber to avoid constipation.

▶ OTHER NUTRITIONAL CAUSES OF ANEMIA

Other forms of anemia related to nutritional deficit include folic acid deficiency and pernicious anemia. Comparison Chart 46.1 discusses the causes, assessment, and management of these disorders.

▶ LEAD POISONING

Lead poisoning is not as common as it once was, yet in 2002 there were 310,000 children in the United States with elevated blood lead levels (EPA, 2007). Lead exerts toxic effects on the bone marrow, erythroid cells, nervous system, and kidneys. The presence of lead in the bloodstream interferes with the enzymatic processes of the biosynthesis of heme. The process results in hypochromic, microcytic anemia, and children may exhibit classic signs of anemia. Risk factors for lead poisoning are related to lead exposure in the home, school, or local environment. Sources of lead include:

• Paint in homes built before 1978, at which time lead was banned as an additive to paint used in houses
• Dust from windowsills, walls, and plaster in older homes
• Soil where cars that used leaded gas have been in the past (lead was removed from all gasoline in the United States as of 1996)
• Glazed pottery
• Stained glass products
• Lead pipes supplying water to the home
• On the clothing of parents who work in certain manufacturing jobs (battery makers, cable makers)
• Certain folk remedies, such as *greta* or *arzacon*
• Old painted toys or furniture (EPA, 2007)

Complications of lead poisoning include behavioral problems and learning difficulties and, with higher lead levels, encephalopathy, seizures, and brain damage.

Treatment for high blood levels of lead involves **chelation therapy**, either orally or intramuscularly. Drug Guide 46.1 gives further information on chelating agents.

COMPARISON CHART 46.1 FOLIC ACID DEFICIENCY VERSUS PERNICIOUS ANEMIA

	Folic Acid Deficiency	Pernicious Anemia
Cause	Low dietary intake of green leafy vegetables, liver, and citrus Malabsorption from medication such as phenytoin (Dilantin) or parasitic infection	Deficiency in vitamin B12
Assessment	Determine risk factors such as prematurity, low socioeconomic status, and history of malabsorption disease. Determine dietary history, noting dislike of fresh vegetables or fruit, ingestion of overcooked foods, or lack of family purchase of fruits and vegetables. Note history of fatigue, headache, poor growth, anorexia, or diarrhea. Inspect the skin for pallor or jaundice, and note presence of a sore on the mouth or tongue.	Note history of anorexia, irritability, or chronic diarrhea. Observe the skin or conjunctivae for pallor and the tongue for smooth texture and bright-red color.
Laboratory analysis	RBC, Hgb, Hct	RBC, Hgb, Hct, low vitamin B12 level
Management	Encourage parents to include green leafy vegetables, liver, and citrus in diet. Ensure that parents comply with dietary changes.	Administer monthly injections of vitamin B12. Inform parents injections will be required throughout the child's life. Provide emotional support related to the chronic nature of this disorder.

Nursing Assessment

Explore the health history for subtle signs such as anorexia, fatigue, or abdominal pain. Determine whether behavioral problems, irritability, hyperactivity, or lack of ability to meet developmental milestones have occurred in recent months. Screen children for risk of exposure to lead in the home. Refer to Chapter 30 for a simple screening questionnaire that can be used to determine the need for lead screening in young children. Blood levels of lead greater than 10 mcg/dL require conscientious follow-up. Note pallor of the skin.

Nursing Management

Prevention of elevated lead levels is critical. Screen children for lead exposure risk. The American Academy of Pediatrics recommends screening in high-risk children at ages 12 and 24 months. Table 46.3 gives recommendations for appropriate follow-up depending on lead levels.

Removing old paint is the best way to eliminate the most significant source of lead exposure for a large number of children. If the family rents or lives in public housing, the landlord or owner is responsible for following the guidelines set forth by local and state governmental agencies to correct the problem. The Enterprise Foundation has made recommendations for healthy and affordable housing (www.enterprisefoundation.org) (Proscio, 2005).

Educate families about how to prevent exposure to lead, particularly in young children. Additional resources for families include:

- Coalition to End Childhood Lead Poisoning: www.leadsafe.org/
- National Lead Awareness Program: www.epa.gov/lead/index.html
- National Lead Information Program: 1-800-424-5323 (LEAD)
- Alliance for Healthy Homes: www.afhh.org
- Childhood Lead Poisoning Prevention Program: www.cdc.gov/nceh/lead/lead.htm
- Community Environmental Health Resource Center: www.cehrc.org
- U.S. Department of Housing and Urban Development, 1-800-HUDS-FHA, www.hud.gov

If the child is undergoing chelation therapy, ensure adequate fluid intake and monitor intake and output closely. Refer children with elevated lead levels and developmental or cognitive deficits to developmental centers. These children may need an early intervention program for further evaluation and treatment of developmental delays.

HEALTHY PEOPLE 2010

Objective	Significance
Eliminate elevated blood lead levels in children.	• Appropriately screen infants and young children for lead exposure at each health care visit.

TABLE 46.3 INTERVENTIONS BASED ON BLOOD LEAD LEVEL

Blood Lead Level (in mcg/dL)	Recommended Action
<10	None required
10–14	Confirm with repeat test in 1 month and educate parents to decrease lead exposure. Repeat test within 3 months.
15–19	Confirm with repeat test in 1 month and educate parents to decrease lead exposure. Repeat test within 2 months.
20–44	Confirm with repeat test within 1 week and educate parents to decrease lead exposure. Refer to local health department for investigation of home for lead reduction, with referrals for support services.
45–69	Confirm with repeat test within 2 days and educate parents to decrease lead levels. Begin chelation therapy and refer to health department as above.
>70	Hospitalize child and begin chelation therapy. Ensure lead is removed from the home.

Adapted from American Academy of Pediatrics, Committee on Environmental Health. (1998). Screening for elevated blood lead levels. *Pediatrics, 101*(6), 1172–1178.

▶ APLASTIC ANEMIA

Aplastic anemia (failure of the bone marrow to produce cells) is characterized by bone marrow aplasia and pancytopenia (decreased numbers of all blood cells). Most cases are acquired, but there are a few rare types of inherited aplastic anemias. The inherited types present as congenital bone marrow failure; the best known is Fanconi's anemia, an autosomal recessive disorder. Acquired aplastic anemia is thought to be an immune-mediated response. Most cases are idiopathic, meaning the trigger remains unidentified. Other causes include exposure to environmental toxins, viruses, myelosuppressive drugs, or radiation.

Aplastic anemia may be classified as severe or nonsevere. In the severe form, the granulocyte count is less than 500, the platelet count is less than 20,000, and the reticulocyte count is less than 1%. In nonsevere aplastic anemia, the granulocyte count is about 500, the platelet count is over 20,000, and the reticulocyte count is over 1%. Complications of aplastic anemia include severe overwhelming infection, hemorrhage, and death. Therapeutic management of aplastic anemia in children involves hematopoietic stem cell transplantation from an HLA-matched sibling donor; if one is not available, immunosuppressive therapy or high-dose cyclophosphamide can be given.

Nursing Assessment

Determine history of exposure to myelosuppressive medications or radiation therapy. Obtain a detailed family, environmental, and infectious disease history. Note history of epistaxis, gingival oozing, or increased bleeding with menstruation. Anemia may lead to headache and fatigue. On physical examination, note ecchymoses, petechiae or purpura, oral ulcerations, tachycardia, or tachypnea. In addition to suppression of all blood cells, laboratory and diagnostic testing may reveal:

- Guaiac-positive stool
- Blood in the urine
- Severe decrease in or absence of hematopoietic cells on bone marrow aspiration

Nursing Management

Safety is of the utmost concern in children with aplastic anemia. Injury must be prevented to avoid hemorrhage. Stool softeners may be used to prevent anal fissures associated with constipation. Administer only irradiated and leukocyte-depleted packed red blood cells or platelet transfusions as necessary. This limits exposure to HLA antigens should the child require bone marrow transplantation in the future. If the child does require hematopoietic stem cell transplantation, refer to Chapter 49 for additional nursing management information.

Refer families whose child has only mild or moderate disease to the Aplastic Anemia and Myelodysplastic Syndrome International Foundation (www.aamds.org).

Hemoglobinopathies

Hemoglobinopathy is a condition in which abnormal hemoglobin is present. A large percentage of the newborn's hemoglobin is fetal hemoglobin (Hgb F). Hgb F can exchange oxygen molecules at lower oxygen tensions compared to adult hemoglobin. Over the first several months of life, Hgb F levels fall as it is replaced with Hgb A (adult hemoglobin). The healthy older infant then displays Hgb AA. In hemoglobinopathies, this normal hemoglobin configuration is disturbed. Causes of hemoglobinopathies are genetic and include sickle cell anemia, hemoglobin SC disease, alpha-thalassemia, and beta-thalassemia. This discussion will focus on sickle cell disease and beta-thalassemia (Cooley's anemia).

► SICKLE CELL DISEASE

Sickle cell disease is a group of inherited hemoglobinopathies in which the RBCs do not carry the normal adult hemoglobin, but rather a less effective type. In the United States, the most common types of sickle cell disease are hemoglobin SS disease (sickle cell anemia), hemoglobin SC disease, and hemoglobin sickle–beta thalassemia. Among the sickle cell diseases, sickle cell anemia is the most common and will be the focus of this discussion.

Sickle cell anemia is a severe chronic blood disorder that affects 2,000 infants born in the United States each year. It is most common in individuals of African, Mediterranean, Middle Eastern, and Indian decent (AAP, 2006). One in 500 African-Americans has sickle cell anemia (Human Genome Management Information System, 2005). Instead of Hgb AA, individuals with sickle cell anemia have Hgb SS. In hemoglobin S, glutamic acid is replaced with valine in the hemoglobin molecule. This results in an elongated RBC with a shortened life span. The elongated cell is more rigid than a normal cell and becomes sickled in shape (Fig. 46.3). Persons with heterozygous representation (Hgb AS) are said to have sickle cell trait and are carriers for the disorder. One in 12 African-Americans has sickle cell trait (Human Genome Management Information System, 2005). Generally, persons with sickle cell trait have only minimal health problems.

The recessive genes for sickle cell are passed on from both parents who have the gene or trait. Each parent has the gene Hgb AS. Hgb A refers to normal adult hemoglobin and Hgb S refers to sickle hemoglobin. These recessive genes for sickle cell may be passed on to the child. The risk for developing Hgb SS is one in four, or 25%, in each child from this union. With each pregnancy the risk is 25% that the child will have disease, 25% that the child will have normal hemoglobin, and 50% that the child will have the trait (Hgb AS) and will be a carrier. Figure 46.4 illustrates the inheritance probability. Infants with sickle cell anemia are usually asymptomatic until 3 to 4 months of age because Hgb F protects against sickling.

Complications of sickle cell anemia include recurrent vaso-occlusive pain crises, stroke, sepsis, acute chest syndrome, splenic sequestration, reduced visual acuity related to decreased retinal blood flow, chronic leg ulcers, cholestasis and gallstones, delayed growth and development, delayed puberty, and priapism (the sickled cells prevent blood from flowing out of an erect penis) (National Heart, Lung and Blood Institute, 2007). Children with sickle cell anemia have an increased incidence of enuresis because the kidneys cannot concentrate urine effectively. As children reach adulthood, multiple organ dysfunction is common.

Pathophysiology

Significant anemia may occur when the RBCs sickle. Sickling may be triggered by any stress or traumatic event, such as infection, fever, acidosis, dehydration, physical exertion, excessive cold exposure, or hypoxia. As the cells sickle, the blood becomes more viscous because the sickled cells clump together and prevent normal blood flow to the tissues of that area. The sickle-shaped RBCs cannot pass through the smaller capillaries and venules of the circulatory system (Fig. 46.5). This vaso-occlusive process leads to local tissue hypoxia followed by ischemia and may result in infarction. Pain crisis results as circulation is

FIGURE 46.3 This peripheral blood smear demonstrates the elongated sickle-shaped red blood cell seen in sickle cell disease.

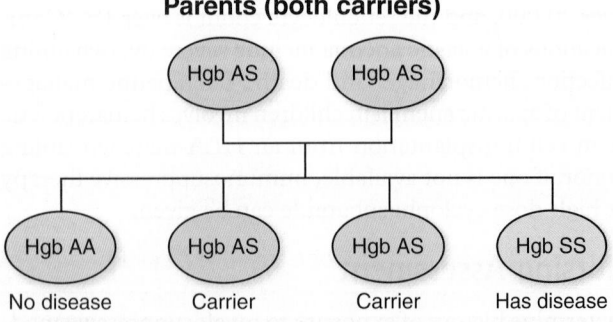

Parents (both carriers)

FIGURE 46.4 Simplified genetic scheme for sickle cell disease. A denotes adult hemoglobin; S denotes sickle hemoglobin. Hemoglobin AA = normal hemoglobin, hemoglobin AS = sickle cell trait, hemoglobin SS = sickle cell disease.

FIGURE 46.5 Clumping of sickle-shaped cells.

decreased to the area. Pain can occur in any part of the body but is most common in the joints. Pain causes increased metabolic need by resulting in tachycardia and sometimes tachypnea, which leads to further sickling. Clumping of cells in the lungs (acute chest syndrome) results in decreased gas exchange, producing hypoxia, which leads to further sickling. Sequestration of blood in the spleen leads to splenomegaly and abdominal pain. Hemolysis follows sickling and leads to further anemia. The increased activity of the spleen related to RBC hemolysis leads to splenomegaly, then fibrosis and atrophy. Functional asplenia may develop as early as 3 months of age (AAP, 2006).

Therapeutic Management

The therapeutic management of children with sickle cell anemia focuses on preventing sickling crisis and infection as well as other complications. Prevention of infection is critical because the child with sickle cell anemia is at increased risk for serious infection related to alterations in splenic function. Functional asplenia (decrease in the ability of the spleen to function appropriately) places the child at significant risk for serious infection with *Streptococcus pneumoniae* or other encapsulated organisms. Prophylactic antibiotics in the young child and appropriate immunization in all children with sickle cell anemia can reduce the risk of serious infection.

Treatment of sickle cell crisis focuses on pain control. Oxygen administration is necessary during episodes of crisis to prevent additional cell sickling. Adequate hydration with intravenous fluids is critical. Close monitoring of Hgb, Hct, and reticulocytes determines the point at which transfusion of packed red blood cells becomes necessary. Electrolyte analysis is also necessary to ensure that appropriate amounts of electrolytes are present in the serum. When RBCs are administered, there is the potential for hemolysis of the cells, thus increasing the potassium level in the serum. Antibiotic therapy is necessary when infection

is present. Box 46.1 describes additional medical treatments that are needed in some children.

Nursing Assessment

Children with sickle cell anemia experience a significant number of acute and chronic manifestations of the condition (Comparison Chart 46.2). For a full description of the assessment phase of the nursing process, refer to page 1527. Assessment findings pertinent to sickle cell anemia are discussed below.

Health History

Elicit the health history, noting growth and development, frequency and extent of vaso-occlusive crises, past hospitalizations, and treatment for pain crises. Note history of immunizations, including pneumococcal, flu, and meningococcal vaccinations. Determine history of blood transfusions. Document the current medication regimen. Note history of recurrent infections. Determine history of the present illness that results in a precipitating event, such as hypoxia, infection, or dehydration. Note onset, character, and quality of pain, as well as relieving factors.

Physical Examination

Perform a thorough physical examination, because sickling, hypoxia, and tissue ischemia affect most areas of the body (Fig. 46.6). Note the physical findings discussed below that may be detected using inspection, observation, auscultation, and palpation.

Inspection and Observation

Inspect the conjunctivae, palms, and soles for pallor and the skin for pallor, lesions, or ulcers. Note jaundice of the skin or scleral icterus. Document color and moisture of oral mucosa. Measure temperature to evaluate for infection (which can precipitate a sickling crisis). Note blood pressure, which may be decreased with severe anemia or increased with sickle cell nephropathy. Determine baseline mental status. Perform a neurologic assessment frequently, as about 8% to 17% of children with sickle cell anemia experience a stroke.

Auscultation

Auscultate heart sounds for a murmur. The heart rate is often elevated with pain, hyperthermia, or dehydration. Listen to breath sounds, noting the rate and depth of respiration as well as the adequacy of aeration. Adventitious breath sounds may be present if a respiratory infection has triggered the sickle cell crisis or in the case of acute chest syndrome.

Palpation

Palpate the joints for warmth, tenderness, and range of motion. Palpate the abdomen for areas of tenderness. Note hepatomegaly or splenomegaly.

EVIDENCE-BASED PRACTICE 46.1
Prophylactic Antibiotics and Pneumococcal Infection in Children With Sickle Cell Disease

● **Background**

Children with sickle cell disease are prone to infection, particularly respiratory infections and sepsis. *Streptococcus pneumoniae* is one of the most common causes of respiratory infection and sepsis in all young children. Though pneumococcal vaccines are available, they do not prevent infection by all strains of pneumococci. Prophylactic antibiotics are routinely prescribed for infants and young children (less than 5 years of age) with sickle cell disease in an attempt to prevent overwhelming pneumococcal infection.

▲ **Study**

To determine the effect that prophylactic antibiotic treatment has upon the prevention of pneumococcal infection in children with sickle cell disease, the authors of this review searched for randomized or quasi-randomized controlled trials comparing prophylactic antibiotics to no treatment or placebo. Three trials were analyzed, comprising just under 900 young children. Both authors independently reviewed the studies and documented the results.

■ **Findings**

In all three trials, the incidence of pneumococcal infection was reduced in young children with sickle cell disease who received prophylactic penicillin. Overall pneumococcal infection rates were reduced by 50% to 100% in treated children. Adverse drug reactions

were rare and minor. No deaths occurred in any of the trials as a result of pneumococcal infection. The authors concluded that antibiotic prophylaxis for pneumococcal infection in children less than 5 years of age with sickle cell disease is an appropriate approach to treatment and recommend its continuation as standard of practice.

● **Nursing Implications**

Nurses are in an optimal position to educate parents about the importance of daily administration of antibiotic prophylaxis of pneumococcal infection in young children with sickle cell anemia. The occurrence of antibiotic resistance was minimal in the trials but did exist, so providers must weigh the risks and benefits of antibiotic prophylaxis. Review the medication regimen at each clinic visit and with each hospitalization. Ensure that prescriptions are being filled; if insurance or payment is an issue, refer the family for financial assistance. Educate families about the need to continue antibiotic prophylaxis even if the child has been immunized against *S. pneumoniae*. Encourage families to comply with the recommendations for 7-valent conjugate vaccine in children under 2 years of age and 23-valent polysaccharide vaccine after 2 years of age. Educate families and provide reassurance about the decreased risk for overwhelming pneumococcal infection after age 5 years, as they may be fearful of discontinuing the antibiotics at that time.

Hirst, C., & Owusu-Ofori, S. (2007). Prophylactic antibiotics for preventing pneumococcal infection in children with sickle cell disease. *Cochrane Database of Systematic Reviews.* Retrieved November 2, 2007, from Ovid–EBM Review Database.

▶ *Take* NOTE!

Immediately report symmetric swelling of the hands and feet in the infant or toddler. Termed dactylitis, *aseptic infarction occurs in the metacarpals and metatarsals. This is often the first vaso-occlusive event seen (Fig. 46.7).*

Laboratory and Diagnostic Testing

Newborn screening for sickle cell anemia is required by law or rule in all of the 50 United States. Screening by Sickledex or sickle cell prep does not distinguish between sickle cell disease and sickle cell trait. If the screening test result indicates the possibility of sickle cell anemia or sickle cell trait, Hgb electrophoresis is performed promptly to confirm the diagnosis. Hgb electrophoresis is the only accurate test for sickle cell disease. Hgb electrophoresis will

demonstrate the presence of Hgb S and Hgb F only in the young infant; in the older infant or child, the result will be Hgb SS.

Common laboratory and diagnostic studies ordered for the assessment of sickle cell anemia include:

• Hemoglobin: baseline is usually 7 to 10 mg/dL; will be significantly lower with splenic sequestration, acute chest syndrome, or aplastic crisis
• Reticulocyte count: greatly elevated
• Peripheral blood smear: presence of sickle-shaped cells and target cells
• Platelet count: increased
• Erythrocyte sedimentation rate: elevated
• Abnormal liver function tests with elevated bilirubin

X-ray studies or other scans may be performed to determine the extent of organ or tissue damage resulting from vaso-occlusion.

<table>
<tr><td colspan="2">

BOX 46.1 Additional Medical Treatments for Some Children With Sickle Cell Anemia

</td></tr>
</table>

- Cholecystectomy may become necessary if gallstones develop.
- Splenectomy may be performed to prevent recurrence of splenic sequestration if it is life-threatening.
- Considered investigational, administration of hydroxyurea may increase the percentage of fetal hemoglobin; a large clinical trial in children is ongoing.
- Blood transfusions, though not routinely given to children with sickle cell disease, are indicated in children with prolonged or widespread pain, aplastic crisis, or splenic sequestration.
- Partial exchange transfusion may be used to rapidly lower the circulating amount of Hgb SS in the event of stroke or acute chest syndrome.
- Hematopoietic stem cell transplantation is usually reserved for children with an identical HLA-matched sibling (risk of death and incidence of graft-versus-host disease is high).

Nursing Management

Nursing care of the child with sickle cell anemia focuses on preventing vaso-occlusive crises, providing education to the family and child, managing pain episodes, and providing psychosocial support to the child and family. All children with sickle cell anemia need ongoing evaluation of growth and development to maximize their potential in those areas.

COMPARISON CHART 46.2 ACUTE VERSUS CHRONIC MANIFESTATIONS OF SICKLE CELL ANEMIA

Acute	Chronic
*Acute chest syndrome	Anemia
*Aplastic crisis	Avascular necrosis of the hip
*Bacterial sepsis or meningitis	Cardiomegaly, functional murmur
	Cholelithiasis
Bone infarction	Delayed growth and development
Dactylitis	Delayed puberty
Hematuria	Functional asplenia
Recurrent pain episodes	Hyposthenuria (low urine specific
Pain crisis	gravity) and enuresis
*Splenic sequestration	Jaundice
*Stroke	Leg ulcers
Priapism	Proteinuria
	*Pulmonary hypertension
	*Restrictive lung disease
	Retinopathy

*Often life-threatening.

Monitor school performance to detect neurodevelopmental problems and seek intervention early. The nursing diagnoses and interventions provided in Nursing Care Plan Overview 46.1 should be individualized based on the child's and family's response to the disorder. Specifics related to sickle cell disease are discussed below.

Educating the Family and Child

Education should begin immediately after the diagnosis of sickle cell anemia is confirmed. Initially, teach the family about the genetics of the disease and encourage family members to be tested for carrier status. Educate families about the disease process. Emphasize the importance of regularly scheduled health maintenance visits and immunizations. Teach families how to administer prophylactic penicillin. Encourage families to seek medical evaluation urgently for any febrile illness. Educate families about how to prevent and recognize vaso-occlusive events (Teaching Guidelines 46.1). Discuss complications such as delayed growth and development, delayed puberty, stroke, cholelithiasis, retinopathy, avascular necrosis, priapism, and leg ulcers.

Managing Pain Crisis

Initiate pain assessment with a standardized pain scale upon admission. Provide frequent evaluations of pain. Always believe the child's report of pain: only the person suffering the pain knows what it feels like. Moderate to severe pain usually requires opioid medication. To bring the pain under control, initially administer analgesics routinely rather than on an "as needed" (PRN) basis. Once the pain is better managed, medications may be moved to PRN status. Monitor patient-controlled analgesia (PCA) in the child or adolescent. Addiction to narcotics is rarely a concern in the child with sickle cell anemia if the narcotic is used to alleviate severe pain. Nonsteroidal anti-inflammatory medications and acetaminophen are often used for less severe pain. Adequate pain management helps to decrease the child's stress level; elevated stress may contribute to further sickling and additional pain. Use nonpharmacologic pain management techniques such as relaxation or hypnosis, music, massage, play, guided imagery, therapeutic touch, or behavior modification to augment the pain medication regimen. Box 46.2 provides a summary of sickle cell pain management.

> ▶ **Take** NOTE!
>
> *Avoid repeated use of meperidine (Demerol) for pain management during sickle cell crisis because it has been associated with an increased risk of seizures when used in children with sickle cell anemia (Sickle Cell Disease Care Consortium, 2002).*

Infarction
Pneumonia
Chest syndrome
Pulmonary hypertension

Atelectasis

Congestive
heart failure

Hemolysis

↓

Anemia

CVA (stroke)
Paralysis
Death

Retinopathy
Blindness
Hemorrhage

Hepatomegaly
Gallstones
Splenomegaly
Splenic sequestration
Autosplenectomy

Hematuria
Hyposthenuria
(dilute urine)

Abdominal pain

Dactylistis
(Hand foot syndrome)

Priapism
Pain
Osteomyelitis

Chronic ulcers

FIGURE 46.6 Effects of sickle cell anemia on various parts of the body.

FIGURE 46.7 Swelling of the hands and feet (dactylitis) in a toddler.

Managing Sickle Cell Crisis

Treat any underlying conditions such as infection or injury. Deficient fluid volume occurs as a result of decreased intake, increased fluid requirements during sickle cell crisis, and the kidney's inability to concentrate urine. Increasing fluid intake will dilute the blood and decrease

HEALTHY PEOPLE 2010

Objective	Significance
(Developmental) Ensure appropriate newborn blood-spot screening, follow-up testing, and referral to services.	• Follow up with state agencies at first contact with infant to ascertain results of newborn screening. • If screening not done at birth, ensure Hgb electrophoresis obtained.

TEACHING GUIDELINES 46.1

Prevention or Early Recognition of Vaso-occlusive Events

- Seek immediate attention for ANY febrile illness.
- Obtain vaccinations and penicillin prophylaxis.
- Encourage adequate fluid intake daily.
- Avoid temperatures that are too hot or too cold.
- Avoid overexertion or stress.
- Have 24-hour access to medical provider or facility familiar with sickle cell care.
- Contact medical provider promptly if you suspect a pain crisis is developing.
- Seek medical attention immediately if any of the following develop:
  - Child is pale and listless
  - Abdominal pain
  - Limp or swollen joints
  - Cough, shortness of breath, chest pain
  - Increasing fatigue
  - Unusual headache, loss of feeling, or sudden weakness
  - Sudden vision change
  - Painful erection that won't go down (priapism)

its viscosity. To promote hemodilution, provide 150 mL/kg of fluids per day or as much as double maintenance, either orally or intravenously. Maintain appropriate electrolyte and pH balance.

Risk for ineffective tissue perfusion related to the effects of RBC sickling and infarction of tissues is another concern. Frequently evaluate respiratory and circulatory status. Administer supplemental oxygen if the pulse oxime-

BOX 46.2   ABCs of Managing Sickle Cell Pain

A: Assess the pain (use a pain assessment tool).
B: Believe the child's report of pain.
C: Complications or cause of pain (look for complications)
D: Drugs and distraction: pain medication (opiates and NSAIDs, if no contraindications); use fixed dosing; give on a timed schedule; no PRN dosing for pain medications; distraction with music, TV, relaxation techniques
E: Environment (rest in quiet area with privacy)
F: Fluids (hypotonic—D5W or D5 with 0.25 normal saline solution)

Adapted from Platt, A., Eckman, J. R., Beasley, J., & Miller, G. (2002). Treating sickle cell pain: An update from the Georgia Comprehensive Sickle Cell Center. *Journal of Emergency Nursing, 28*(4), 297–303, with permission.

try reading is 90% or less to promote adequate oxygenation. Supplementation with oxygen in the absence of hypoxia is unnecessary and may inhibit erythropoiesis. Monitor level of consciousness and immediately report changes.

▶ **Take** NOTE!

The child's temperature should be maintained as close to normal as possible without the use of cooling mattresses; a cooling mattress can cause localized circulation reduction or shivering, which may lead to increased metabolic needs and sickling of the red blood cells.

Preventing Infection

To prevent severe infection in the child with sickle cell anemia, a variety of interventions are necessary. By 2 months of age, begin administration of oral penicillin V potassium as prophylaxis against pneumococcal infection. In the penicillin-allergic child, erythromycin may be used. Continue prophylaxis until at least age 5 years (AAP, 2006). Administer childhood immunizations according to the currently recommended schedule. To prevent overwhelming sepsis or meningitis as a result of infection with *S. pneumoniae,* the child should receive not only the 7-valent pneumococcal vaccine series in infancy but also the 23-valent pneumococcal conjugate vaccine annually after age 2 years. Meningococcal vaccination is also warranted (refer to Chapter 30 for additional information on these vaccines). Provide influenza immunization annually before the onset of flu season (after 6 months of age).

Supporting the Family and Child

As with any chronic illness, families of children with sickle cell anemia need significant support. They often feel guilty or responsible for the disease. Reassure the family and provide education. Refer families to a regional sickle cell disease center for multidisciplinary care. Additional resources for families include:

- Sickle Cell Information Center, P.O. Box 109, Grady Memorial Hospital, 80 Jesse Hill Jr. Drive, SE, Atlanta, GA 30303 (www.scinfo.org)

HEALTHY PEOPLE 2010

Objective	Significance
Reduce stroke deaths.	• Educate families appropriately to decrease incidence of vaso-occlusive episodes in children with sickle cell anemia.

- Sickle Cell Disease Association of America, 16 S. Calvert Street, Suite 600, Baltimore, MD 21202; 410-528-1555 or 1-800-421-8453 (www.sicklecell disease.org)
- SickleCellKids.org, 740 Drewry Street, Atlanta, GA, 30306 (www.sicklecellkids.org/)
- American Sickle Cell Anemia Association, 10300 Carnegie Avenue, Cleveland Clinic, Cleveland, OH 44106; 1-216-229-8600 (www.ascaa.org)

▶ *Consider* THIS!

A 3-year-old boy with sickle cell disease is being admitted to the pediatric unit. He has had a runny nose, slight fever, and vomiting over the past 2 to 3 days. He has not been eating well and is complaining of pain in the right leg and refusing to walk. On assessment you find his vital signs to be temperature 101.7°F, pulse 132, respirations 32, blood pressure 88/52. He is coughing, he has slightly dusky mucous membranes, and his capillary refill is 4 seconds.

1. *List nursing assessment findings in order of priority.*
2. *Identify at least three nursing interventions, prioritize them, and list the rationale for the prioritization and the intervention itself.*
3. *List teaching you will perform with this family.*

▶ THALASSEMIA

Thalassemia is a genetic disorder that most often affects those of African descent, but it also affects individuals of Caribbean, Middle Eastern, South Asian, and Mediterranean descent (Marengo-Rowe, 2007). The genetics of thalassemia are similar to those of sickle cell disease in that it is inherited via an autosomal recessive process. Children with thalassemia have reduced production of normal hemoglobin.

There are two basic types of thalassemia, alpha and beta. In alpha-thalassemia, synthesis of the alpha chain of the hemoglobin protein is affected. Problems with the beta chain occur more often, and the condition beta-thalassemia can be divided into three subcategories based on severity:

- Thalassemia minor (also called beta-thalassemia trait): leads to mild microcytic anemia; often no treatment is required
- Thalassemia intermedia: child requires blood transfusions to maintain adequate quality of life
- Thalassemia major: to survive the child requires ongoing medical attention, blood transfusions, and iron removal (chelation therapy) (Marengo-Rowe, 2007)

The focus of this discussion will be on beta-thalassemia major (Cooley's anemia).

In beta-thalassemia major, the beta-globulin chain in hemoglobin synthesis is reduced or entirely absent. A large number of unstable globulin chains accumulate, causing the RBCs to be rigid and hemolyzed easily. The result is severe hemolytic anemia and chronic hypoxia. In response to the increased rate of RBC destruction, erythroid activity is increased. The increased activity causes massive bone marrow expansion and thinning of the bony cortex. Growth retardation, pathologic fractures, and skeletal deformities (frontal and maxillary bossing) result.

Hemosiderosis (excessive supply of iron) is an additional complication of significant concern. It occurs as a result of rapid hemolysis of RBCs, the decrease in hemoglobin production, and the increased absorption of dietary iron in response to the severely anemic state. The excess iron is deposited in the body's tissues, causing bronze pigmentation of the skin, bony changes, and altered organ function, particularly in the cardiac system. Additional complications include splenomegaly, endocrine abnormalities, osteoporosis, liver and gallbladder disease, and leg ulcers.

Left untreated, beta-thalassemia major is fatal, but the use of chelation therapy has increased the life expectancy of these children to beyond their teen years (Marengo-Rowe, 2007).

Therapeutic Management

The therapeutic management for children with beta-thalassemia includes monitoring hemoglobin and hematocrit and transfusing packed red blood cells at regular intervals. Blood iron levels are monitored and iron chelation therapy is provided.

Nursing Assessment

Infants are usually diagnosed by 1 year of age and have a history of pallor, jaundice, failure to thrive, and hepatosplenomegaly. Determine the history of the present illness or whether the child is presenting for a routine blood transfusion. Note medications taken at home and any concerns that have arisen since the last visit. Inspect the skin, oral mucosa, conjunctivae, soles, and/or palms for pallor. Note icteral sclerae or jaundice of the skin. Measure weight and height (or length) and plot on an appropriate growth chart. Observe the child for bony deformities and frontal bossing (prominent forehead) (Fig. 46.8). Measure oxygen saturation via pulse oximetry. Evaluate neurologic status, determining level of consciousness and developmental abilities.

Laboratory testing may reveal the following:

- Hemoglobin and hematocrit are significantly decreased.
- Peripheral blood smear shows prominence of target cells, hypochromia, microcytosis and extensive anisocytosis and **poikilocytosis** (variation in the size and shape of the RBCs, respectively).

FIGURE 46.8 Iron overload related to thalassemia leads to bony changes such as frontal bossing and maxillary prominence.

- Bilirubin levels are elevated.
- Hgb electrophoresis shows presence of Hgb F and Hgb A_2 only.
- Iron level is elevated.

Nursing Management

The nursing care of the child with thalassemia is primarily aimed at supporting the family and minimizing the effects of the illness. This includes administering blood transfusions and educating the family.

Administering Packed Red Blood Cell Transfusions

Administer packed red blood cell transfusions as prescribed to maintain an adequate level of hemoglobin for oxygen delivery to the tissues and to suppress erythrocytosis in the bone marrow. Monitor for reactions to the transfusions.

Excess iron (hemosiderosis) is removed by chelation therapy. Administer the chelating agent Desferal (deferoxamine) with the transfusion. Deferoxamine binds to the iron and allows it to be removed through the stool or urine. Oral deferasirox (Exjade) may also be prescribed and is generally well tolerated, with minimal gastrointestinal side effects.

Educating the Family

Educate the child and family about the recommended regimen. Ensure that families understand that adhering to the prescribed blood transfusion and chelation therapy

schedule is essential to the child's survival. Chelation therapy must be maintained at home to continuously decrease the iron levels in the body. Teach family members to administer deferoxamine subcutaneously with a small battery-powered infusion pump over a several-hour period each night (usually while the child is sleeping). If oral deferasirox is prescribed, instruct the family to dissolve the tablet in juice or water and administer it once daily.

Refer the family for genetic counseling and family support as needed. Resources for families of children with thalassemia include:

- Cooley's Anemia Foundation: 1-800-522-7222 (www. thalassemia.org)
- Thalassemia Action Group, 129-09 26th Avenue, #203, Flushing, NY 11354; 1-800-522-7222

Glucose-6-Phosphate Dehydrogenase (G6PD) Deficiency

G6PD is an enzyme that is responsible for maintaining the integrity of RBCs by protecting them from oxidative substances. G6PD deficiency is an X-linked recessive disorder that occurs when the RBCs have insufficient G6PD, or the enzyme is abnormal and does not function properly. The RBCs are then affected by oxidative stress more easily. Triggers that may result in oxidative stress and hemolysis include bacterial or viral illness or exposure to certain substances such as medications (e.g., sulfonamides, sulfones, malaria-fighting drugs [such as quinine], or methylene blue [for treating urinary tract infections]), naphthalene (an agent in mothballs), or fava beans (Frank, 2005).

G6PD deficiency is most common in males of African decent. Other groups with G6PD deficiency are from the Mediterranean basin, including Italians, Greeks, Arabs, and Sephardic Jews. The condition tends to be less severe in those of African decent and more severe in those of Mediterranean decent. Complications include prolonged neonatal jaundice and life-threatening acute episodes of hemolysis. Therapeutic management is primarily aimed at avoiding triggers that cause oxidative stress.

Nursing Assessment

Note health history, including fatigue. Determine the parents' understanding of the disorder and the medications and foods to avoid. Inspect the skin for pallor or jaundice. Evaluate neurologic status, which may also be affected. Measure heart rate and respiratory rate, noting elevations. Determine oxygen saturation via pulse oximeter or blood gas analysis. Note tea-colored urine. Palpate the abdomen for splenomegaly. Laboratory studies will reveal anemia (Frank, 2005).

Nursing Management

Administer oxygen and treat the symptoms. Once the triggering agent is removed or the child recovers from an illness, the child will improve. Provide further education to the child and family about triggers and advise them that the child should avoid contact with these agents.

Clotting Disorders

Clotting is a process that occurs after injury. The blood clotting system requires certain factors in the blood and platelets to perform adequately. Individuals with deficiencies of these factors or platelets tend to bleed; they do not bleed more easily than people without these conditions, but it is just more difficult for the clot to form, and bleeding cannot be stopped easily. Factors that are most often involved in problems with clotting include factor VIII, factor IX, and factor XI. Each plays a role in clot formation. Platelets also play a role in the clotting cascade and are necessary for clot formation. Some processes can lead to destruction of the platelets and may lead to a reduction in clotting. Bleeding times are prolonged when a clotting disorder is present. Table 46.4 provides usual values for clotting studies.

Conditions affecting clotting include idiopathic thrombocytopenia purpura, Henoch-Schonlein purpura, disseminated intravascular coagulation, and factor deficiencies such as hemophilia A (factor VIII deficiency), von Willebrand disease, hemophilia B (Christmas disease, factor IX deficiency), and hemophilia C (factor XI deficiency). Table 46.5 reviews the proteins involved in coagulation.

▶ IDIOPATHIC THROMBOCYTOPENIA PURPURA

Idiopathic thrombocytopenia purpura (ITP) is thought to be an immune response following a viral infection that produces antiplatelet antibodies. These antibodies destroy platelets, which then leads to the development of petechiae, purpura, and excessive bruising. Petechiae are pinpoint hemorrhages that occur anywhere on the body and do not blanch to pressure (Fig. 46.9). **Purpura** are larger areas of hemorrhage in which blood collects under the tissues; they are purplish (see Fig. 46.9). ITP usually develops about 1 to 4 weeks after a viral infection. Remission is seen in 80% to 90% of the children in 6 to 9 months (Panepinto, 2005). Complications include severe hemorrhage and bleeding into vital organs and intracranial hemorrhage, although these rarely occur.

For children with platelet counts below 20,000/mm^3, corticosteroids or intravenous immunoglobulin (IVIG) may be used. Prednisone or prednisolone is administered for 2 to 3 weeks, or until platelet counts increase above 30,000/mm^3. IVIG will be infused for 1 to 3 days. Platelet transfusions are not indicated unless a life-threatening condition such as intracranial hemorrhage is present. Refer the child for follow-up care with a pediatric hematologist. ITP is usually self-limiting, but if it persists for a year or longer, splenectomy may be indicated (Panepinto, 2005).

Nursing Assessment

Elicit the child's health history (usually a previously healthy child who recently has developed increased bruising, epistaxis, or bleeding of the gums). Note history of blood in the stool. Note risk factors such as recent viral illness, recent MMR immunization, or ingestion of medications that can cause thrombocytopenia. Inspect for petechiae, purpura, and bruising, which may progress rapidly within the first 24 to 48 hours of the illness. Document the size and location of each lesion. Inspect the lips and buccal mucosa for petechiae. The remainder of the physical examination is usually within normal limits.

Usual laboratory findings include an extremely low platelet count (less than 50,000), normal WBC count and differential, and normal hemoglobin and hematocrit unless hemorrhage has occurred (this is rare). Bone marrow aspiration may be performed to rule out leukemia.

Nursing Management

Many children require no medical treatment except observation and re-evaluation of laboratory values. Educate the family about avoiding aspirin, nonsteroidal anti-inflammatory drugs (NSAIDs), and antihistamines because these medications may precipitate the development of anemia in these children. The use of acetaminophen for pain control is more appropriate when necessary. Teach the family to prevent trauma by avoiding activities that may cause injury, such as contact sports; activities such as swimming provide physical activity with less risk of trauma. Parents also need to know the signs and symptoms of serious bleeding and whom to call if it is suspected.

TABLE 46.4 CLOTTING STUDIES

Test	Measure
Prothrombin time (PT)	11.0–13.0 seconds (may vary by laboratory)
Partial thromboplastin time (PTT), activated partial thromboplastin time (aPTT)	21–35 seconds
International Normalized Ratio (INR) (used to evaluate coagulation)	2.0–3.0 usual target in thromboembolic conditions

Data from Fischbach, F. T. (2004). *A manual of laboratory and diagnostic tests* (7th ed.). Philadelphia: Lippincott Williams & Wilkins.

TABLE 46.5 SELECT PROTEINS INVOLVED IN COAGULATION (FACTORS)

Protein	Synonym	Concentration in Plasma (mg/dL)	Function
Fibrinogen	Factor I	200–400	Converts fibrin along with platelets to form clot
Factor II	Prothrombin	10–15	Is converted to thrombin (IIa), splits fibrinogen into fibrin
Factor V	Proaccelerin; labile factor	0.5–1.0	Supports Xa activation of II to IIa
Factor VII	Stable factor; proconvertin	0.2	Activates X
Factor VIII:C	Antihemophilic factor (AHF); platelet cofactor I	1.0–2.0	Supports IXa activation of X
Factor IX	Christmas factor; plasma thromboplastin component (PTC)	0.3–0.4	Activates X
Factor X	Stewart-Prower factor (AVTD prothrombin III)	0.6–0.8	Activates II
Factor XI	Plasma thromboplastin antecedent (antihemophilic factor C)	0.4	Activates XII and prekallikrein
Factor XII	Hageman factor	2.9	Activates XI and prekallikrein
Factor XIII	Fibrin-stabilizing factor; Laki-Lorand factor	2.5	Cross-links fibrin and other proteins
von Willebrand factor	Factor VIII–related antigen (VIII:VWD)	1.0	Stabilizes VIII, mediates platelet adhesion

Data from Fischbach, F. T. (2004). *A manual of laboratory and diagnostic tests* (7th ed.). Philadelphia: Lippincott Williams & Wilkins.

▶ HENOCH-SCHONLEIN PURPURA

Henoch-Schonlein purpura is a condition that in children develops in association with a viral or bacterial infection; in adults, drugs or toxins usually cause it. The classic presentation is vasculitis with IgA-dominant immune deposits affecting small vessels. These small vessels are generally in the skin, gut, and kidney (Roberts et al., 2007). In most children the course of the disease is benign and the prognosis is good. In a few, however, ongoing nephrotic syndrome may occur as a result of renal injury, and those children may have hypertension. Pulmonary, cardiac, and neurologic complications can also occur.

No specific treatment exists for Henoch-Schonlein purpura, since most of the cases resolve without treatment. Treatment with corticosteroids, such as prednisone, is reserved for children with persistent symptoms. If renal injury occurs, children may require renal function testing, and evaluation for hypertension and treatment when present.

Nursing Assessment

Note history of viral or bacterial infection. Determine the onset of the complaint and how it has progressed or changed. Note history of joint or abdominal pain. Measure blood pressure. Inspect the skin for a purpuric palpable rash, and document the size and location of lesions. Palpate the rash to determine its extent (Fig. 46.10). Gently palpate the joints for tenderness. Palpate the abdomen for tenderness. Note visible or occult blood in the stool. Note cherry- or tea-colored urine, indicating the presence of blood in the urine; urinalysis can verify the amount of blood present in the urine. Serum IgA levels may be elevated (Roberts et al., 2007).

FIGURE 46.9 Pinpoint hemorrhages (petechiae) and large purplish areas of discoloration (purpura) in an infant with ITP.

FIGURE 46.10 Palpable purpura on an adolescent's arm.

Nursing Management

Treatment of the symptoms is the focus. In patients with severe joint or abdominal pain, administer analgesics as prescribed and note the response to pain medications. If the child has normal renal function, maintaining hydration is the most important intervention. Monitor intake and output. Note the color of urine. Administer corticosteroids and anticoagulants, alone or together, if ordered to reduce renal impairment (Roberts et al., 2007). Teach the child and family about the therapy, such as management of hypertension with medications, and sodium restriction. Teach them about signs of renal injury, such as blood in the urine and changes in weight, as well as frequency and volume of urine output.

▶ DISSEMINATED INTRAVASCULAR COAGULATION

Disseminated intravascular coagulation (DIC) is a complex condition that leads to activation of coagulation; it usually occurs in critically ill children. Common triggers of DIC include septic shock, presence of endotoxins and viruses, tissue necrosis or injury, and cancer treatment. In DIC, thrombin is generated, fibrin is deposited in the circulation, and platelets are consumed. Deficiencies of coagulation and anticoagulation pathways occur. Hemorrhage and organ tissue damage result and can be irreversible if not recognized and treated immediately (Franchini & Manzato, 2004).

Therapeutic management of children with DIC requires careful consideration of the etiology. Initial treatment focuses on treating the underlying cause. For exam-

ple, if DIC occurs secondary to an infection, appropriate antibiotics would be used to treat the infection. Heparin is also used at lower doses to counteract the deficiency in the coagulation/anticoagulation pathway. Heparin reduces consumption of the platelets, resulting in improved platelet counts. Since heparin is an anticoagulant, there is an increased risk of bleeding.

Nursing Assessment

Because DIC occurs as a secondary condition, it may occur in a child hospitalized for any reason. DIC may affect any body system, so a thorough physical examination is warranted. Inspect for signs of bleeding such as petechiae or purpura, blood in the urine or stool, or persistent oozing from venipuncture or from the umbilical cord in the newborn. Evaluate respiratory status and determine the level of tissue oxygenation via pulse oximetry. Perform a complete circulatory assessment and note signs of circulatory collapse such as poor perfusion, tachycardia, prolonged capillary refill, and weak distal pulses. Note altered level of consciousness and decreased urine output. Careful abdominal palpation may reveal hepatomegaly or splenomegaly.

Laboratory testing may reveal prolonged prothrombin time (PT), partial thromboplastin time (PTT) or activated partial thromboplastin time (aPTT), bleeding time, and thrombin time and decreased levels of fibrinogen, platelets, clotting factors II, V, VIII, and X, and antithrombin III. Increases will be noted in levels of fibrinolysin, fibrinopeptide A, positive fibrin split products, and D-dimers (Fischbach, 2004).

Nursing Management

Continue to provide nursing care related to the triggering event. Assess the child's status frequently. If bleeding is observed, apply pressure to the area along with cold compresses. Elevate the affected body part if this does not affect the child's overall stability. If neurologic deficits are assessed, report the findings immediately so that treatment to prevent permanent damage can be started. Administer anticoagulation therapy (even though hemorrhage is a concern) to interrupt the coagulation process that is present in this condition. Provide ventilatory support as needed and provide continuous cardiac monitoring. Administer clotting factors, platelets, and cryoprecipitate as prescribed to prevent severe hemorrhage (Franchini & Manzato, 2004). Report changes in laboratory values to the physician. Changes can occur rapidly, and vigilance is necessary to prevent further tissue damage to the affected system.

▶ HEMOPHILIA

Hemophilia is a group of X-linked recessive disorders that result in deficiency in one of the coagulation factors in the blood. X-linked recessive disorders are transmitted by carrier mothers to their sons, so usually only males are affected by hemophilia. The coagulation factors in the blood are essential for clot formation either spontaneously or from an injury, and when factors are absent bleeding will be difficult to stop. There are several types of hemophilia, including factor VIII deficiency (hemophilia A), factor IX deficiency or Christmas disease (hemophilia B), and factor XI deficiency (hemophilia C) (Curry, 2004; Miller, 2004). The most common, hemophilia A, will be the focus of this discussion. Hemophilia A occurs when there is a deficiency of factor VIII in an individual. Factor VIII is essential in the activation of factor X, which is required for the conversion of prothrombin into thrombin, resulting in an inability of the platelets to be used in clot formation.

Hemophilia is classified according to the severity of the disease, ranging from mild to severe. The more severe the disease, the more likely it is that there will be bleeding episodes. When bleeding occurs the vessels constrict and a platelet plug forms, but because of the deficient factor the fibrin will not solidify, and thus bleeding continues (Miller, 2004).

Therapeutic Management

The primary goal is to prevent bleeding. This is best accomplished by having the child avoid activities with a high potential for injury (e.g., football, riding motorcycles, skateboarding) and instead participating in those with the least amount of contact (e.g., swimming, running, tennis). Limiting activities does not mean the child should do nothing; activities that promote health without increased exposure to injury are best.

If bleeding or injury occurs, factor administration is prescribed; this practice has been common in outpatient facilities or the patient's home for many years. Once the deficient factor is replaced, clotting factors return to fairly normal levels for a period of time. Factor replacement should be given prior to any surgeries or other traumas that can lead to bleeding, such as intramuscular injections and dental care.

Nursing Assessment

For a full description of the assessment phase of the nursing process, refer to page 1527. Assessment findings pertinent to hemophilia in children are discussed below.

Health History

Elicit the health history, determining the nature of the bleeding episode or bruise. Include in the history any hemorrhagic episodes in other systems, such as the gastrointestinal tract (e.g., black tarry stools, hematemesis) or as a result from injury resulting in joint hemorrhage, or hematuria (Fig. 46.11). Inquire about length of bleeding and amount of blood loss. Because hemophilia A results

FIGURE 46.11 Significant swelling and discoloration associated with a bleeding episode in a hemophiliac's knee.

in difficulty with clotting, the child may bleed for a longer period when injury occurs.

Physical Examination

Focus the physical examination on identification of any bleeding. This is of particular concern after injury, but a nosebleed or other spontaneous bleed can occur if factor levels are extremely low. Assess circulation by evaluating pulses and heart sounds if severe or prolonged bleeding is identified; without intervention, hypovolemia could follow, leading to shock. Note chest pain or abdominal pain, which may indicate internal bleeding. Report these findings immediately so that the underlying condition can be diagnosed and treated rapidly.

Laboratory and Diagnostic Testing

Laboratory findings may include decreased hemoglobin and hematocrit if bleeding is prolonged or severe. Factor levels may be quantified with blood testing.

Nursing Management

Nursing management includes preventing bleeding episodes, managing bleeding episodes, and providing education and support.

Preventing Bleeding Episodes

All patients with hemophilia should attempt to prevent bleeding episodes. Major bleeds into the joints may limit range of motion and function, eventually decreasing physical abilities and crippling some boys. Teach children and families that regular physical activity or exercise helps to keep the muscles and joints stronger, and children with stronger joints and muscles have fewer bleeding episodes (see Teaching Guidelines 46.2). Refer the child with moderate to severe hemophilia to a pediatric hematologist and/or a comprehensive hemophilia treatment center (Miller, 2004).

Managing a Bleeding Episode

Administer factor VIII replacement as prescribed. Factor replacement is pooled from multiple blood donors, so families may be concerned about transmission of viruses via the product (specifically hepatitis and HIV). Dry heat is now used to treat the factor, and there have been no cases of hepatitis or HIV transmission since this practice began (Meeks & Josephson, 2006). Factor replacement has also been produced using recombinant DNA technology.

Administer factor replacement by slow IV push. Document the product name, number of units, lot number, and expiration date. Doses are based on the severity of the bleeding and the weight of the child. Specific dosing guidelines can be obtained from the product insert (Curry, 2004). In mild cases of hemophilia A, desmopressin may be effective in stopping bleeding (see below in the nursing management section of von Willebrand disease for additional information).

If external bleeding develops, apply pressure to the area until bleeding stops. If it is inside a joint, apply ice or cold compresses to the area and elevate any injured extremities, except when contraindicated by further injury. Make sure that all cases of bleeding are followed up to identify whether factor replacement is necessary.

TEACHING GUIDELINES 46.2

Preventing Bleeding in the Child With Hemophilia

- Protect toddlers with soft helmets, padding on the knees, carpets in the home, and softened or covered corners.
- Children should stay active: swimming, baseball, basketball, and bicycling (wearing a helmet) are good physical activities.
- Avoid intense contact sports such as football, wrestling, soccer, and high diving.
- Avoid trampoline use and riding all-terrain vehicles (ATVs).
- Arrange premedication with Amicar if oral surgery is indicated.

Providing Education

Inform the family that the child should wear a health alert bracelet. Families should notify the school nurse and teachers of the child's diagnosis and share precautions with them; they should be instructed to call the parent immediately if the child sustains a head, abdominal, or orbit injury at school. Teach parents and caregivers how to administer the intravenous infusion of factor VIII. Administration in the home is the preferred method for factor infusion, as the child will be able to receive treatment in the most timely and efficient manner when a bleeding episode occurs. Alternatives to the parent giving the infusion is to arrange for a home care nursing visit or for the family to keep their own supply of factor VIII that they take to the local emergency room for infusion if bleeding occurs.

Involve children as developmentally appropriate in the infusion process. Young children may hold and apply the Band-Aid; older children may assist with dilution and mixing of the factor; and teens should be taught to administer their own factor infusions.

Children with severe hemophilia may need factor infusions so often that implantation of a central venous access port is warranted. Teach the family access, care, and flushing of the implanted port.

Providing Support

Children with hemophilia may be able to lead a fairly normal life, with the exception of avoiding a few activities. However, accepting the diagnosis of a bleeding disorder in their child is very difficult for parents. They fear the worst (bleeding that won't stop) as well as complications such as infection with blood-borne viruses. Reassure parents that since 1986, when factor replacement began to be treated with heat, there have been no reports of virus transmission from factor infusion. Educate and support the parents. Factor replacement is expensive and bleeding episodes often cause parents to miss work, both of which create financial strains. Refer families to the National Hemophilia Foundation (116 West 32nd Street, 11th Floor, New York, NY 10001; 1-800-42-HANDI or 1-212-328-3700; www.hemophilia.org/). Children may benefit from the services provided by NHF Youthworld (www.nhfyouthworld.org/), which offers support, education, youth leadership, scholarships, and a directory of camps for children with hemophilia and other bleeding disorders.

▶ VON WILLEBRAND DISEASE

Von Willebrand disease (vWD) is a genetically transmitted bleeding disorder that may affect both genders and all races. The disorder is a deficiency in von Willebrand factor (vWF). Under ordinary circumstances vWF serves two functions: to bind with factor VIII, protecting it from breakdown, and to serve as the "glue" that attaches platelets to the site of injury. Deficiency in this factor results in a mild bleeding disorder. Children with vWD bruise easily, have frequent nosebleeds (epistaxis), and tend to bleed after oral surgery. Pubescent girls often have menorrhagia.

Therapeutic management of vWD is similar to that of hemophilia. Prevention of injury is important. When bleeding or injury does occur, vWF is administered. Desmopressin may also be used to release the factors necessary for clotting. Desmopressin (DDAVP) raises the plasma level from stores in the endothelium of blood vessels (Curry, 2004); this releases factor VIII and vWF from these stores into the bloodstream. These may also be administered prior to dental work or surgery.

Nursing Assessment

Nursing assessment of the child with vWD is similar to the assessment of the child with hemophilia, though severe bleeding occurs much less frequently.

Nursing Management

Nursing management is also similar to the management of the child with hemophilia. The major difference is the administration of desmopressin. Administer desmopressin nasal spray as prescribed when a bleeding episode occurs. Desmopressin may also be given via an intravenous infusion or subcutaneously (less common). Stimate is the only brand of desmopressin nasal spray that is used for controlling bleeding; the other brands are used for homeostasis and enuresis (Curry, 2004). Desmopressin is an antidiuretic hormone, so closely monitor fluid balance. It should be used for 3 days in a row only, as lessening of the response (tachyphylaxis) occurs with frequent use. vWD may also be treated with intravenous infusion of vWF, similar to factor VIII infusion for hemophilia A. Teach children and their families how to avoid or minimize bleeding episodes (see Teaching Guidelines 46.2).

■■■ Key Concepts

- The major forms of anemia affecting children are iron deficiency anemia, lead poisoning, folic acid deficiency, pernicious anemia, sickle cell anemia, thalassemia, and G6PD deficiency.
- The major bleeding disorders affecting children are idiopathic thrombocytopenic purpura, Henoch-Schonlein purpura, disseminated intravascular coagulation, and hemophilia and von Willebrand disease.
- Assess for hypoxia, fatigue, and pallor in the child with anemia.
- Nursing assessment for the child with a bleeding disorder focuses on determining its extent and severity.
- Supplementation with iron is the key intervention for the child with iron deficiency anemia.
- All young children should be screened for lead exposure.

- Prevention of infection and vaso-occlusive episodes takes priority in children with sickle cell anemia.
- Multimodal pain management and astute physical assessment for serious complications are critical in the nursing care of the child having a sickle cell crisis.
- The priority intervention for management of thalassemia is chronic transfusion of packed red blood cells and chelation of iron.
- Idiopathic thrombocytopenic purpura and Henoch-Schonlein purpura are usually self-limiting diseases.
- Administration of factor VII or desmopressin is the key nursing intervention when a bleeding episode occurs in the child with hemophilia or von Willebrand disease.
- Significant anemia may result in hypoxia to the tissues.
- Prolonged bleeding times place the child at risk for hemorrhage.
- Prevention of injury is key for all children with hematologic disorders.
- Patient and family teaching for anemias resulting from nutritional deficiencies focuses on promotion of a diet high in the deficient nutrients.
- Patient and family teaching for bleeding disorders focuses on the prevention of injury.
- Numerous nationwide and local resources are available to children with hematologic disorders or nutritional deficits. These organizations offer a wide range of services, including education, support, multidisciplinary care (as appropriate), and financial assistance in caring for the disease.

REFERENCES

Abrams, A. C., Pennington, S. S., & Lammon, C. B. (2006). *Clinical drug therapy: Rationales for nursing practice* (8th ed.). Philadelphia: Lippincott Williams & Wilkins.

Ackley, B. J., & Ladwig, G. B. (2008). *Nursing diagnosis handbook: An evidence-based guide to planning care* (8th ed.). St. Louis: Mosby.

Ambruso, D. R., Hays, T., Lane, P. A., & Nuss, R. (2007). Hematologic disorders. In W. W. Hay, M. J. Levin, J. M. Sondheimer, & R. R. Deterding (Eds.), *Current pediatric diagnosis and treatment* (18th ed.). New York: McGraw-Hill.

American Academy of Pediatrics, Committee on Environmental Health. (1998). Screening for elevated blood lead levels. *Pediatrics, 101*(6), 1172–1178.

American Academy of Pediatrics. (1999). Iron fortification of infant formulas. *Pediatrics, 104*(1), 119–123.

American Academy of Pediatrics. (2005). Breastfeeding and the use of human milk. *Pediatrics, 115*, 496–506.

American Academy of Pediatrics. (2005). Lead exposure in children: prevention, detection, and management. *Pediatrics, 116*(4), 1036–1046.

American Academy of Pediatrics. (2005). *Recommendations for preventive pediatric health care*. Available online at www.aap.org.

American Academy of Pediatrics. (2006). *Health supervision for children with sickle cell disease*. Retrieved November 2, 2007, from http://aappolicy.aappublication.org/cgi/content/abstract/pediatrics; 109/3/546.

Anderson, N. (2006). Hydroxyurea therapy: Improving the lives of patients with sickle cell disease. *Pediatric Nursing, 32*(6), 541–543.

Balik, S. J., Forman, J. A., Johnson, C. L., & Roberts, J. R. (2007). Safeguarding kids from environmental hazards. *Contemporary Pediatrics, 24*(3), 64–78.

Brotanek, J. M., Gosz, J., Weitzman, M., & Flores, G. (2007). Iron deficiency in early childhood in the United States: Risk factors and racial/ethnic disparities. *Pediatrics, 120*(3), 568–575.

Carey, R. G., Dufour, R., Farkas, D. H., et al. (2005). Complete blood count. Retrieved November 2, 2007, from http://labtests online.org/understanding/analytes/cbc/glance.html.

Cunningham, F. G., Leveno, K. L., Bloom, S. L., Hauth, J. C., Gilstrap, L. C., & Wenstrom, K. D. (2005). Fetal growth and development. In F. G. Cunningham, K. L. Leveno, S. L. Bloom, J. C. Hauth, L. C. Gilstrap, & K. D. Wenstrom (Eds.), *Williams obstetrics* (22nd ed.). New York: McGraw-Hill.

Curry, H. (2004). Bleeding disorder basics. *Pediatric Nursing, 30*(5), 402–429.

Environmental Protection Agency. (2007). *Lead in paint, dust, and soil.* Retrieved November 2, 2007, from http://www.epa.gov/lead/index.html.

Fischbach, F. T. (2004). *A manual of laboratory and diagnostic tests* (7th ed.). Philadelphia: Lippincott Williams & Wilkins.

Franchini, M., & Manzato, F. (2004). Update on the treatment of disseminated intravascular coagulation. *Hematology, 9*(2), 81–85.

Frank, J. E. (2005). Diagnosis and management of G6PD deficiency. *American Family Physician, 72*(7), 1277–1282.

Gunnarsson, B. S., Thorsdottir, I., & Palsson, G. (2004). Iron status in 2-year-old Icelandic children and associations with dietary intake and growth. *European Journal of Clinical Nutrition, 58,* 901–906.

Holcomb, S. S. (2005). Recognizing and managing anemia. *Nurse Practitioner, 30*(12), 16–18.

Human Genome Management Information System. (2005). *Genetic disease profile: Sickle cell anemia.* Retrieved November 2, 2007, from http://www.ornl.gov/sci/techresources/Human_Genome/posters/chromosome/sca.shtml.

Jones, R. J., & Brodsky, R. A. (2005). Aplastic anemia. *Lancet, 365,* 1647–1656.

Kimball, J. W. (2007). Blood. Retrieved November 2, 2007, from http://users.rcn.com/jkimball.ma.ultranet/BiologyPages/B/Blood.html.

Kleinmann, R. E., and the American Academy of Pediatrics, Committee on Nutrition. (2003). *Pediatric nutrition handbook* (5th ed.). Elk Grove Village, IL: American Academy of Pediatrics.

Marengo-Rowe, A. J. (2007). The thalassemias and related disorders. *Baylor University Medical Center Proceedings, 20*(1), 27–31.

Martin, P. L., & Pearson, H. A. (2006). Hemoglobinopathies and thalassemias. In J. A. McMillan et al. (Eds.), *Oski's pediatrics: Principles and practice* (4th ed.). Philadelphia: Lippincott Williams & Wilkins.

Meeks, S. L., & Josephson, C. D. (2006). Should hemophilia treaters switch to albumin-free recombinant factor VIII concentrates? *Current Opinion in Hematology, 13*(6), 457–461.

Miller, K. L. (2004). Factor products in the treatment of hemophilia. *Journal of Pediatric Health Care, 18,* 156–157.

National Heart, Lung and Blood Institute (NHLBI) of the National Institutes of Health, Diseases and Conditions Index. (2007). *What is sickle cell anemia?* Retrieved November 2, 2007, from http://www.nhlbi.nih.gov/health/dci/Diseases/Sca/SCA_WhatIs.html.

National Newborn Screening and Genetics Resource Center. (2007). *National newborn screening and status report.* Retrieved November 2, 2007, from http://genes-r-us.uthscsa.edu/nbsdisorders.pdf.

Pagana, K. D., & Pagana, T. J. (2006). *Mosby's manual of diagnostic and laboratory tests* (3rd ed.). St. Louis: Mosby, Inc.

Panepinto, J. A. (2005). Acute idiopathic thrombocytopenic purpura of childhood—diagnosis and therapy. *Pediatric Emergency Care, 21*(10), 691–698.

Platt, A., & Beasley, J. (2005). Puzzled about sickle-cell disease? *Nursing Made Incredibly Easy!, 3*(6), 60–64.

Platt, A., & Beasley, J. (2007). How much do you know about sickle-cell disease? *LPN, 3*(4), 32–37.

Platt, A., Eckman, J. R., Beasley, J., & Miller, G. (2002). Treating sickle cell pain: An update from the Georgia Comprehensive Sickle Cell Center. *Journal of Emergency Nursing, 28*(4), 297–303.

Proscio, T. (2005). *Healthy housing, healthy families: Toward a national agenda for affordable healthy homes.* Retrieved Nov. 2, 2007, from http://www.practitionerresources.org/showdoc.html?id=56273.

Roberts, P. F., Waller, T. A., Brinker, T. M., Riffe, I. Z., Sayre, J. W., & Bratton, R. L. (2007). Henoch-Schonlein purpura: A review article. *Southern Medical Journal, 100*(8), 821–824.

Ruble, K. (2005). Pediatric hematologic disorders. In S. M. Nettina (Ed.), *Lippincott manual of nursing practice.* Philadelphia: Lippincott Williams & Wilkins.

Segal, G. B., & Palis, J. (2006). Hematology of the newborn. In M. A. Lichtman et al. (Eds.), *Williams' hematology* (7th ed.). New York: McGraw-Hill.

Sickle Cell Disease Care Consortium. (2002). *Outpatient evaluation and management of pain in child with sickle cell disease.* Retrieved November 2, 2007, from http://www.scinfo.org/protpainOP.htm.

Taketokmo, C. K., Hodding, J. H., & Kraus, D. M. (2007). *Lexi-comp's pediatric dosage handbook* (14th ed.). Hudson, OH: Lexi-comp.

Tomlinson, D., & Kline, N. E. (Eds.) (2005). *Pediatric oncology nursing.* New York: Springer.

Trigg, M. E. (2004). Hematopoietic stem cells. *Pediatrics, 113*(4), 1051–1057.

Zetterstrom, R. (2004). Iron deficiency and iron deficiency anaemia during infancy and childhood. *Acta Paediatrica, 93,* 436–439.

WEBSITES

Alliance for Healthy Homes (resources for the prevention of lead poisoning): www.affh.org

American Sickle Cell Anemia Association (resources, education, and support): www.ascaa.org

American Society of Hematology (information related to blood, blood-forming tissues, and blood diseases): www.hematology.org

Aplastic Anemia and Myelodysplasia International Foundation (resources for patient assistance and emotional support): www.aplastic.org

Centers for Disease Control and Prevention (CDC): www.cdc.gov

Coalition to End Childhood Lead Poisoning: www.leadsafe.org/

Community Environmental Health Resource Center (resources for prevention of lead poisoning): www.cehrc.org

Cooley's Anemia Foundation (education, resources, and support): www.thalassemia.org

Enterprise Foundation (resources for lead removal from homes): www.enterprisefoundation.org

Healthy People 2010: www.healthypeople.gov

Iron Disorders Institute (mission is to reduce pain, suffering, and death related to disorders involving iron): www.irondisorders.org

National Heart, Lung, and Blood Institute (education and research related to heart, blood vessel, lung, and blood diseases): www.nhlbi.nih.gov

National Hemophilia Foundation (resources, education, research, and support): www.hemophilia.org/

National Hemophilia Foundation Youthworld (website for children with bleeding disorders): www.nhfyouthworld.org/

National Lead Awareness Program: www.epa.gov/lead/index.html

Sickle Cell Disease Association of America (resources, support, and education): www.sicklecelldisease.org

Sickle Cell Information Center (patient and professional education, news, research updates, and sickle cell resources): www.scinfo.org

Sickle Cell Kids: www.sicklecellkids.org

U.S. Department of Housing and Urban Development (resources for lead removal from homes): www.hud.gov

Women, Infants and Children program of the Food and Nutrition Service of the U.S. Department of Agriculture (provides supplemental foods to low-income children up to 5 years of age): www.fns.usda.gov/wic/

CHAPTER WORKSHEET

MULTIPLE CHOICE QUESTIONS

1. A child on the pediatric unit has morning laboratory results of Hgb 10.0, Hct 30.2, WBC 24,000, platelets 20,000. What is the priority nursing assessment?

   a. Assess for pallor, fatigue, and tachycardia.

   b. Monitor for fever.

   c. Assess for bruising or bleeding.

   d. Determine intake and output.

2. A child with hemophilia fell while riding his bicycle. He was wearing a helmet and did not lose consciousness. He has a mild abrasion on his knee that is not oozing. He is complaining of abdominal pain. What is the priority nursing assessment?

   a. Perform neurologic checks.

   b. Assess ability to void frequently.

   c. Carefully assess abdomen.

   d. Examine his knee frequently.

3. A 14-year-old with thalassemia asks for your assistance in choosing her afternoon snack. Which choice is the most appropriate?

   a. Peanut butter with rice cake

   b. Small spinach salad

   c. Apple slices with cheddar cheese

   d. Small burger on wheat bun

4. The nurse is caring for a child who has just been admitted to the pediatric unit with sickle cell crisis. He is complaining that his right arm and leg hurt. What is the priority nursing intervention?

   a. Administer pain medication every 3 hours intravenously until pain is controlled.

   b. Perform passive range of motion of the arm and leg to maintain function.

   c. Try acetaminophen for pain first, moving up to opioids only if needed.

   d. Use narcotic analgesics and warm compresses as needed to control the pain.

CRITICAL THINKING EXERCISES

1. Develop a discharge teaching plan for the parent of a toddler who has just been diagnosed with hemophilia and received factor infusion treatment for a bleeding episode.

2. An 8-year-old girl has been diagnosed with iron deficiency anemia. Formulate a nutrition plan for this child.

3. A 5-year-old with beta-thalassemia is resistant to nightly chelation therapy at home. Devise a developmentally appropriate teaching plan for this child.

4. Develop a nursing care plan for a child with sickle cell disease who experiences frequent vaso-occlusive crises.

STUDY ACTIVITIES

1. Visit your local WIC office. Meet with the staff and learn about the services offered for prevention of and nutritional support for anemia. Provide a written report of your learning experience or provide a presentation to your classmates.

2. In the clinical setting, compare the growth and development of a child with sickle cell disease to that of a similarly aged child who has been healthy.

3. Talk to a teenager with hemophilia about his life experiences and feelings about his disease and his health. Reflect upon this conversation in your clinical journal.

4. Visit a public health clinic that provides primary care to children. Spend time with the registered nurse, the advanced practice nurse, and the unlicensed assistive personnel. Write a summary of the roles of the registered nurse in screening for and managing hematologic disorders in children, noting roles that are reserved for the advanced practice nurse and activities that the RN would delegate to unlicensed assistive personnel.

NURSING CARE OF THE CHILD WITH AN IMMUNOLOGIC DISORDER

KEY TERMS

antibodies
antigen
autoantibodies
B cells
cellular immunity
chemotaxis
complement

graft-versus host disease
humoral immunity
immunity
immunodeficiency
immunoglobulins
immunosuppressive
lymphocyte

neutrophil
opsonization
phagocytosis
stem cells
T cells

LEARNING OBJECTIVES

Upon completion of the chapter, the learner will be able to:

1. Explain anatomic and physiologic differences of the immune system in infants and children versus adults.
2. Describe nursing care related to common laboratory and diagnostic testing used in the medical diagnosis of pediatric immune and autoimmune disorders.
3. Distinguish immune and autoimmune disorders common in infants, children, and adolescents.
4. Identify appropriate nursing assessments and interventions related to medications and treatments for pediatric immune, autoimmune, and allergic disorders.
5. Develop an individualized nursing care plan for the child with an immune or autoimmune disorder.
6. Describe the psychosocial impact of chronic immune disorders on children.
7. Devise a nutrition plan for the child with immunodeficiency.
8. Develop patient/family teaching plans for the child with an immune or autoimmune disorder.

Lakeisha Harris, 15 years old, is brought to the clinic by her mother. She presents with complaints of pain and swelling in her joints, weight gain, and fatigue. Lakeisha states, "I'm just very tired all the time, and my knees and ankles ache."

Wow
Resistance to disease can be a child's battle for life.

Immunodeficiency, autoimmune, and allergic disorders have a significant impact on the lives of affected children. Infants and children are exposed to many infectious microorganisms and allergens and thus need a functional immune system to protect themselves. Temporary immune deficiencies may follow a common viral infection, surgery, or a blood transfusion. They may also be caused by malnutrition or smoking. Temporary immune depression resolves over a period of time. Primary or secondary immune deficiencies are the focus of this discussion, along with allergy and anaphylaxis. These immune disorders are chronic, and affected children have more infections than healthy children do. Recurrent viral or bacterial infections may cause the child to miss significant amounts of school or playtime with other children. Many immunodeficiencies require chronic and frequent clinic visits as well as daily medications. This can be a stress on the family as well. Autoimmune disorders are also chronic, causing significant disruption to the child's and family's life. Allergic disorders in some children may cause significant stress for the child and family. Nurses who care for children need to be familiar with common immunodeficiencies, autoimmune disorders, and allergies to intervene effectively with children and their families.

Variations in Pediatric Anatomy and Physiology

Normal immune function is a complex process involving **phagocytosis**, **humoral immunity**, **cellular immunity**, and activation of the **complement** system. The lymphatic system and the white blood cells (WBCs) are the primary "players" in the immune response. Though these structures and cells are present at birth, the healthy full-term infant's immune system is still immature. The newborn exhibits a decreased inflammatory response to invading organisms, and this increases his or her susceptibility to infection. Cellular immunity is generally functional at birth, and as the infant is exposed to various substances over time, humoral immunity develops. Comparison Chart 47.1 provides more information on humoral and cellular immunity.

Lymph System

Lymph nodes in the newborn are relatively small, soft, and difficult to palpate. As the infant is exposed to various germs or illnesses, the lymph system passively filters plasma for bacteria or other foreign material before returning it to the bloodstream and back to the heart. As WBCs infiltrate the lymph nodes to attack the foreign substance, the nodes enlarge. Young children have frequent episodes of localized enlarged lymph nodes because of their repeated exposure to viral illnesses. The spleen is functional at birth and also filters the blood for foreign cells. The thymus, responsible for the production of **lymphocyte T cells** as well as for the development and maturation of peripheral lymphoid tissue, is quite enlarged at birth and remains so until about 10 years of age. It then involutes slowly throughout adulthood. The tonsils are also often enlarged throughout early childhood. The bone marrow is functional at birth, producing **stem cells** capable of differentiating into various blood cells.

Phagocytosis

Under conditions of stress, the newborn and infant exhibit decreased phagocytic activity. The complement system, which is responsible for **opsonization** and **chemotaxis**, is immature in the newborn but reaches adult levels of activity by 3 to 6 months of age. The infant's phagocytic cells (**neutrophils** and monocytes) demonstrate decreased chemotaxis, reaching adult levels when the child is several years old. With complement levels being only 50% to 75% of adult levels in the full-term infant, decreased opsonization may be responsible for decreased phagocytic activity compared with adults.

Cellular Immunity

Maternal T cells do not cross the placenta, so the fetal thymus begins production of T cells early in gestation, and the newborn demonstrates a relative lymphocytosis compared with the adult, probably due to increased amounts of T-cell lymphocytes. Though cellular immunity does not cross the placenta, the fetal T cells may become

COMPARISON CHART 47.1 **HUMORAL VERSUS CELLULAR IMMUNITY**

Humoral Immunity (antibody protection)	Cellular Immunity (cell-mediated immune response)
• Lymphocytes: B cells	• Lymphocytes: T cells
• Secrete antibodies to viruses and bacteria	
• Recognize antigens	• Do not recognize antigens
• Antibodies mark the antigen cell for destruction	• Direct and regulate immune response (helper T cells)
• Do not destroy the foreign cell	• Attack infected or foreign cells (killer T cells and natural killer cells)
• Crosses the placenta in the form of IgG	• Does not cross the placenta

sensitized to antigens that do cross the placenta. Viral infection, hyperbilirubinemia, and drugs taken by the mother late in pregnancy may contribute to depressed T-cell function in the newborn. Since delayed hypersensitivity reactions are mediated by T cells rather than antibodies, skin test responses (such as PPD for tuberculosis detection) are diminished until about 1 year of age, probably due to the infant's decreased ability to mount an inflammatory response.

Humoral Immunity

The newborn's **B cells** do not respond as well to infection as do adults'. B cells are responsible for the formation of **antibodies** (specific immunity). The antibodies bind to the **antigen**, thus disabling the specific toxin. The fetus is normally in an antigen-free environment and so produces only trace amounts of IgM. Most of the newborn's IgG is acquired transplacentally from the mother. Hence, the newborn exhibits passive **immunity** to antigens to which the mother had developed antibodies. These antibodies wane over the first months of life as the transplacental IgG is catabolized, having a half-life of only about 25 days. The newborn begins to make IgG but ordinarily experiences a physiologic hypogammaglobulinemia between 2 and 6 months of age until self-production of IgG reaches higher levels. The breastfed infant will acquire passive

transfer of maternal immunity via the breast milk and will be better protected during the physiologic hypogammaglobulinemia phase. By 1 year of age IgG is 70% of the adult level, and by 8 years of age it should reach the adult level.

IgA, IgD, IgE, and IgM do not cross the placenta; they require an antigenic challenge for production. IgD and IgE constitute a very small percentage of the **immunoglobulins** in all ages. IgA increases slowly to about 30% of the adult level at 1 year of age, reaching the adult level by age 11 years. IgM is close to the adult level by 1 year of age.

Common Medical Treatments

A variety of medications and other medical treatments are used to treat immune deficiencies and autoimmune problems in children. Most of these treatments will require a physician's order when the child is in the hospital. The most common treatments and medications are listed in Common Medical Treatments 47.1 and Drug Guide 47.1. The nurse caring for the child with an immune deficiency or autoimmune disorder should be familiar with what the procedures and medications are, how they work, and common nursing implications related to use of these modalities.

COMMON MEDICAL TREATMENTS 47.1

Treatment	Explanation	Indications	Nursing Implications
Immunizations	Killed or modified microorganisms, or components of them, cause the immune system to develop antibodies to the microorganism without developing disease.	Prevention of certain viral and bacterial infections	Do not administer live vaccines to immunosuppressed persons. Refer to the individual vaccine for method of administration and contraindications. Report adverse reactions via the Vaccine Adverse Reaction (VAR) reporting system.
Bone marrow or stem cell transplantation	Bone marrow transplant: Transfer of healthy bone marrow into the bones of a person with immune malfunction; the transplanted cells can then develop into functional B and T cells. Stem cell transplant: Peripheral stem cells are removed from the donor via apheresis or stem cells are retrieved from the umbilical cord and placenta. The stem cells are then transplanted into the recipient.	Wiskott-Aldrich syndrome, SCID	Administer immunosuppressive medications as ordered. Maintain medical asepsis and protective isolation to prevent infection. Monitor closely for graft-versus-host disease. Provide meticulous oral care. Avoid rectal temperatures and suppositories. Encourage appropriate nutrition.

DRUG GUIDE 47.1 COMMON DRUGS FOR IMMUNOLOGIC DISORDERS

Medication	Action/Indication	Nursing Implications
Intravenous immune globulin (IVIG); multiple manufacturers	Provides exogenous IgG antibodies. Indicated for primary immune deficiencies, HIV infection	Do not mix with IV medications or with other IV fluids. Do not give IM or SQ. Monitor vital signs and watch for adverse reactions frequently during infusion. May require antipyretic or antihistamine to prevent chills and fever during infusion. Have epinephrine available during infusion.
Nucleoside analogue reverse transcriptase inhibitors (NRTIs): abacavir, lamivudine, zidovudine	Inhibits reverse transcription of the viral DNA chain. For treatment of HIV-1 infection as part of a 3-drug regimen. Zidovudine is also used to prevent perinatal transmission of HIV.	Notify physician of muscle weakness, shortness of breath, headache, insomnia, rash, or unusual bleeding. Give IV zidovudine over 1 hour. Fatal hypersensitivity reaction may occur with abacavir.
Non-nucleoside analogue reverse transcriptase inhibitors (NNRTIs): efavirenz, nevirapine	Binds to HIV-1 reverse transcriptase, blocking DNA polymerase activity and disrupting the virus life cycle. Used for treatment of HIV-1 infection as part of a 3-drug regimen.	*Nevirapine:* Avoid St. John's wort. Shake suspension gently before administration. Observe for symptoms of Stevens-Johnson syndrome. *Efavirenz:* May cause drowsiness
Protease inhibitors: amprenavir, atazanavir, indinavir, lopinavir, nelfinavir, ritonavir, saqinavir	Inhibits protease activity in the HIV-1 cell, resulting in immature, noninfectious viral particles. Used for treatment of HIV-1 infection as part of a 3-drug regimen.	Multiple drug interactions. Review specific medication for adverse effects and administration implications.
Nonsteroidal anti-inflammatory drugs (NSAIDs): aspirin, trisalicylate, ibuprofen, naproxen, others	Inhibits prostaglandin synthesis, anti-inflammatory action. Indicated for juvenile idiopathic arthritis	Administer with food to decrease GI upset. May cause gastric bleeding, increased liver enzymes, decreased renal function. Monitor liver enzymes. Do not crush or chew extended-release or timed-release preparations. *Aspirin and trisalicylate:* Follow serum salicylate levels. Observe for signs of toxicity, including hyperventilation with heavy breathing, drowsiness, nausea, vomiting, bruising, tinnitus, hearing loss.
Corticosteroids	Anti-inflammatory and immunosuppressive action. Used for juvenile idiopathic arthritis, SLE, and immunosuppression in bone marrow or stem cell transplant patients.	Administer with food to decrease GI upset. May mask signs of infection. Monitor blood pressure, urine for glucose. Do not stop treatment abruptly or acute adrenal insufficiency may occur. Monitor for Cushing syndrome. Doses may be tapered over time. *Intravenous pulse:* Monitor for hypertension during infusion.
Cytotoxic drugs (cyclophosphamide [Cytoxan])	Interferes with normal function of DNA by alkylation. For treatment of severe SLE.	Causes bone marrow suppression. Monitor for signs of infection. *Cyclophosphamide:* Administer in the morning. Provide adequate hydration and have child void frequently during and after infusion to decrease risk of hemorrhagic cystitis.

(continued)

DRUG GUIDE 47.1 COMMON DRUGS FOR IMMUNOLOGIC DISORDERS (continued)

Medication	Action/Indication	Nursing Implications
Immunosuppressant drugs (cyclo-sporine A [CyA], azathioprine)	Inhibition of production and release of interleukin II (CyA). Antagonizes purine metabolism (azathio-prine). Used for severe steroid-resistant autoimmune disease.	Monitor CBC, serum creatinine, potassium, and magnesium. Monitor blood pressure and watch for signs of infection. Draw blood levels before morning dose. *CyA:* Do not give with grapefruit juice.
Antimalarial drugs: hydroxychloroquine sulfate (Plaquenil)	Impairs complement-dependent antigen–antibody reactions to prevent flares in SLE and juvenile arthritis.	Funduscopic eye exam and visual field testing every year
Disease-modifying antirheumatic drugs (DMARDs): methotrexate, etanercept	Methotrexate: antimetabolite that depletes DNA precursors, inhibits DNA and urine synthesis. Etanercept: binds to tumor necrosis factor (TNF), rendering it ineffective. Used for severe polyarticular juvenile arthritis.	*Methotrexate:* Do not give oral form with dairy products. Approximate time to benefit in treatment of arthritis is 3 to 6 weeks. Salicylates may delay clearance. Protect IV preparation from light. Monitor CBC, renal and liver function, and symptoms of infection. *Etanercept:* Monitor closely for infection. Do not give live vaccines. Give SQ, twice weekly; effect in 1 week to 3 months.

Refer to Chap. 15 for a thorough explanation of assessment and management of pain.

NURSING PROCESS OVERVIEW FOR THE CHILD WITH AN IMMUNOLOGIC DISORDER

Care of the child with an immunologic or allergic disorder includes assessment, nursing diagnosis, planning, interventions, and evaluation. There are a number of general concepts related to the nursing process that may be applied to immunodeficiencies and autoimmune disorders. From a general understanding of the care involved for a child with immune dysfunction, the nurse can then individualize the care based on patient specifics.

Assessment

Assessment of children with immunodeficiency, autoimmune disorders, or allergy includes health history, physical examination, and laboratory and diagnostic testing.

Remember Lakeisha, the 15-year-old with joint pain and swelling, fatigue, and weight gain? What additional health history and physical examination assessment information should you obtain?

Health History

The health history comprises past medical history, including the mother's pregnancy history, family history, and history of present illness (when the symptoms started and how they have progressed), as well as medications and treatments used at home. The past medical history may be significant for maternal HIV infection; frequent, recurrent infections such as otitis media, sinusitis, or pneumonia; chronic cough; recurrent low-grade fever; two or more serious infections in early childhood; recurrent deep skin or organ abscesses; persistent thrush in the mouth; extensive eczema; or growth failure. Family history may be positive for primary immune deficiency or autoimmune disorder. Document history of known allergy. Note the response that occurs when the child encounters the allergen.

Physical Examination

Physical examination of the child with immunodeficiency or autoimmune disorder includes inspection and observation, auscultation, percussion, and palpation.

Inspection and Observation

Plot weight and length or height on appropriate growth charts. Inspect the oropharynx for tonsillar size. Note eczematous or other skin lesions, which may occur with allergic diseases or Wiskott-Aldrich syndrome. Document presence of thrush, which occurs frequently in children with immunodeficiency. Observe gait for unexplained ataxia (neurologic alterations occur with HIV infection).

Auscultation, Percussion, and Palpation

Auscultate the lungs for adventitious sounds, which may be present with a concurrent respiratory infection or as wheezing with an allergic reaction. Percuss the abdomen and determine liver span. Palpate for unusually enlarged lymph nodes, particularly in nonadjacent locations. Palpate the abdomen for enlarged spleen or liver.

Laboratory and Diagnostic Testing

Common Laboratory Diagnostic Tests 47.1 explains the laboratory and diagnostic tests most commonly used when considering immune disorders. Results of these tests may assist the physician in diagnosing the disorder and/or be used as guidelines in determining ongoing treatment. Laboratory or non-nursing personnel obtain some of the tests, while the nurse might obtain others. In either instance the nurse should be familiar with how the tests are obtained, what they are used for, and normal versus abnormal results. This knowledge will also be necessary when providing patient and family education related to the testing.

Nursing Diagnoses and Related Interventions

Upon completion of a thorough assessment, the nurse might identify several nursing diagnoses. These may include:

• Ineffective protection
• Imbalanced nutrition, less than body requirements
• Pain
• Impaired skin integrity
• Activity intolerance
• Delayed growth and development

After completing an assessment of Lakeisha, you note the following: alopecia, abdominal tenderness, and oral ulcers. Based on these assessment findings, what would your top three nursing diagnoses be for Lakeisha?

Nursing goals, interventions, and evaluation for the child with an immunologic disorder are based on the nursing diagnoses. Nursing Care Plan Overview 47.1 can be used as a guide in planning nursing care for the child with an immunologic disorder, autoimmune disorder, or allergic response. It should be individualized based on the patient's symptoms and needs. Additional information will be included later in the chapter as it relates to specific disorders.

Based on your top three nursing diagnoses for Lakeisha, describe appropriate nursing interventions.

Primary Immunodeficiencies

More than 100 primary immunodeficiencies have been identified. They are mostly hereditary or congenital. About half of primary immunodeficiencies are humoral deficiencies. The remainder are combined (B- and T-cell deficiencies), phagocytic system defects, and T-cell defects (cellular immunity deficiencies), with only 2% related to complement deficiencies (Petry et al., 2004). This discussion will focus on a few of the more common and/or severe primary immunodeficiencies in children. Box 47.1 lists 10 warning signs that a child may need further evaluation for the possibility of primary **immunodeficiency**.

▶ HYPOGAMMAGLOBULINEMIA

Hypogammaglobulinemia refers to a variety of conditions in which the child does not form antibodies appropriately. It results in low or absent levels of one or more of the immunoglobulin classes or subclasses. Table 47.1 provides an overview of several types of hypogammaglobulinemia. Therapeutic management of most types of hypogammaglobulinemia is periodic administration of intravenous immunoglobulin (IVIG).

Nursing Assessment

Note history of recurrent respiratory, gastrointestinal, or genitourinary infections. Palpate for enlarged lymph nodes and spleen in the child with X-linked hyper-IgM syndrome. In children presenting for routine administration of IVIG, determine whether any infections have occurred since the previous infusion.

Nursing Management

Nursing management of hypogammaglobulinemia involves IVIG administration and the provision of education and support to the child and family.

Administering IVIG

Determine the amount of IVIG to be given and reconstitute the product according to the manufacturer's directions (available on the package insert). Some IVIG preparations are provided as a solution, requiring no reconstitution (Fig. 47.1). Others are packaged as two vials, one of IVIG powder and one of sterile diluent. After the diluent is added to the powder, gently roll the vial between your hands to mix. Reconstituted IVIG may be refrigerated overnight but should be brought to room temperature prior to infusion. Assess baseline serum blood urea nitrogen (BUN) and creatinine, as acute renal insufficiency

Test	Explanation	Indication	Nursing Implications
Complete blood count (CBC) with differential	Evaluate hemoglobin and hematocrit, WBC count (particularly the percentage of individual WBCs), and platelet count.	Infection, inflammatory process, immunosuppression	Normal values vary according to age and gender. WBC count differential is helpful in evaluating source of infection. May be affected by myelosuppressive drugs.
Immunoglobulin electrophoresis	Determines level of individual immunoglobulins (IgA, IgD, IgE, IgG, IgM) in the blood	Immune deficiency, autoimmune disorders	Normal levels vary with age. IVIG administration and steroids alter levels.
IgG subclasses	Measures the levels of the 4 subclasses of IgG (1, 2, 3, and 4)	Determine immune deficiency	Normal levels vary with age. IVIG administration and steroids alter levels.
Lymphocyte immunophenotyping T-cell quantification	Measures level of T cells (T-helper [CD4], T-suppressor [CD8]), B cells, and natural killer cells in the blood	Ongoing monitoring of progressive depletion of CD4 T lymphocytes in HIV disease	Do not refrigerate specimen. Steroids may elevate and immunosuppressive drugs may depress lymphocyte levels.
Delayed hypersensitivity skin test	Measures the presence of activated T cells that recognize certain substances	Immune disorders	Administered intradermally. Read and document size of reaction at 48 to 72 hours (tuberculosis, mumps, candida, tetanus).
Human immunodeficiency virus (HIV) antibodies	Used to detect antibodies to HIV	Determining HIV infection when suspected	ELISA method detects only antibodies, so may remain negative for several weeks up to 6 months (false-negative). False-positive may result with autoimmune disease. Requires serial testing. HIV test results are confidential.
Polymerase chain reaction (PCR)	Used to detect HIV DNA and RNA	Diagnosis of HIV infection in children over 1 month old	Sensitive and specific for presence of HIV in blood. Poor accuracy on samples obtained at birth. Sequential testing needed to determine perinatal transmission.
Complement assay (C3 and C4)	Measures the level of total complement in the blood, as well as levels of C3 and C4	Monitor SLE. Determine complement deficiency.	Send to laboratory immediately (unstable at room temperature). Usually sent out to a reference laboratory.
Erythrocyte sedimentation rate (ESR)	Nonspecific test used to determine presence of infection or inflammation	Immune disorder initial workup, ongoing monitoring of autoimmune disease	Send to laboratory immediately; if allowed to stand >3 hours, falsely low result may occur.
Rheumatoid factor (RF)	Determines the presence of RF in the blood	Juvenile idiopathic arthritis, SLE	Positive RF is also sometimes seen in chronic infectious disorders.
Antinuclear antibody (ANA)	Tests for presence of autoantibodies that react against cellular nuclear material	SLE	Check for signs of infection at venipuncture site. Steroid use can cause false-negative result. May be weakly positive in about 20% of healthy individuals.

Nursing Care Plan 47.1

OVERVIEW FOR THE CHILD WITH AN IMMUNOLOGIC DISORDER

NURSING DIAGNOSIS: Ineffective protection related to inadequate body defenses, inability to fight infection as evidenced by deficient immunity

Outcome Identification and Evaluation
Child will not experience overwhelming infection, *will be infection-free or able to recover if he or she becomes infected.*

Intervention: Preventing Infection
- Maintain meticulous hand washing procedures (include family, visitors, staff) *to minimize spread of infectious organisms.*
- Maintain isolation as prescribed *to minimize exposure to infectious organisms.*
- Clean frequently touched surfaces with an appropriate cleanser *to minimize spread of infectious organisms.*
- Educate family and visitors that child should be restricted from contact with known infectious exposures (in hospital and at home) *to encourage cooperation with infection control.*
- Strictly observe medical asepsis *to avoid unintentional introduction of microorganisms.*
- Promote nutrition and appropriate rest *to maximize body's potential to heal.*
- Educate family to contact health care provider if child has known exposure to chickenpox or measles *so that preventive measures (e.g., VZIG) can be taken.*
- Administer vaccines (not live) as prescribed *to prevent common childhood communicable diseases.*
- Administer prophylactic antibiotics as prescribed *to prevent infection with opportunistic organisms.*

NURSING DIAGNOSIS: Imbalanced nutrition, less than body requirements, related to poor appetite, chronic illness, debilitated state, concurrent illness as evidenced by poor growth, weight gain and stature increases less than expected, poor head growth

Outcome Identification and Evaluation
Child will consume adequate intake, *will demonstrate appropriate weight gain and growth of length/height and/or head circumference.*

Intervention: Promoting Adequate Nutritional Intake
- Monitor growth (weight and height/length weekly) *to determine progress toward goal.*
- Determine realistic goal for weight gain for age (consulting dietitian if necessary) *to have a specific outcome to work toward.*
- Observe child's physical ability to eat *(if pain from candidiasis or motor impairment is present, will need additional interventions).*
- Provide nutrient-rich meals and snacks *to maximize caloric intake.*
- Supplement milkshakes with protein powder or other additives *to maximize caloric intake.*
- Provide child's favorite foods *to encourage increased intake.*
- Provide smaller, more frequent meals *to reduce sensation of fullness and increase overall intake.*
- If vomiting is an issue, administer antiemetics as ordered prior to meals *to provide optimal state for success at mealtime.*

NURSING DIAGNOSIS: Impaired skin integrity related to disease process or photosensitivity as evidenced by skin rash or alopecia

Outcome Identification and Evaluation
Skin integrity will be maintained; *secondary infection will not occur, rash will not increase.*

Intervention: Preventing Skin Impairment
- Assess and monitor extent and location of rash *to provide baseline information and evaluate success of interventions.*
- Keep skin clean and dry *to prevent secondary infection.*
- For the child with eczema, apply topical medications as ordered *to decrease inflammatory response.*
- For the child with limited mobility, turn frequently and use specialty mattress or bed *to prevent pressure ulcers.*
- Implement a written plan of care directed toward topical treatment of skin integrity impairment *to provide consistency of care and documentation.*
- Educate child and family to limit direct sun exposure and use sunscreen *to prevent sun damage.*

(continued)

Nursing Care Plan 47.1 (continued)

NURSING DIAGNOSIS: Activity intolerance related to joint pain, fatigue or weakness, concurrent illness as evidenced by dyspnea, lack of desire to participate in play, inability to maintain usual routine

Outcome Identification and Evaluation

Child will participate in activities; *will demonstrate easy work of breathing and participate in daily routine and play.*

Intervention: Promoting Activity

- Cluster care *to decrease disturbances and allow for longer uninterrupted rest periods.*
- Pace activities and encourage regular rest periods *to conserve energy.*
- Administer early morning warm bath *to ease AM stiffness (juvenile arthritis).*
- Use assistive devices such as splints and orthotics *to improve physical function.*
- Plan developmentally appropriate activities that the child can participate in while in bed *to encourage play and continued development.*
- Schedule activities for time of day child usually has the most energy *to encourage successful participation.*

NURSING DIAGNOSIS: Delayed growth and development related to physical effects of chronic illness, or physical disability (juvenile arthritis) as evidenced by delay in meeting expected milestones

Outcome Identification and Evaluation

Development will be enhanced: *child will make continued progress toward expected developmental milestones.*

Intervention: Enhancing Growth and Development

- Screen for developmental capabilities *to determine child's current level of functioning.*
- Offer age-appropriate toys, play, and activities (including gross motor) *to encourage further development.*
- Encourage peer contact through telephone, e-mail, or letters *to promote/continue socialization.*
- Perform interventions as prescribed by physical or occupational therapist: *repeat participation in those activities helps child improve function and acquire developmental skills.*
- Provide support to families of children with developmental delay *(progress in achieving developmental milestones can be slow, and ongoing motivation is needed).*
- Encourage child to continue schoolwork *so that child will not fall behind.*
- Reinforce positive attributes in the child *to maintain motivation.*

BOX 47.1 **Ten Warning Signs of Primary Immunodeficiency**

- 8 or more episodes of acute otitis media in 1 year
- 2 or more episodes of severe sinusitis in 1 year
- Treatment with antibiotics for 2 months or longer with little effect
- 2 or more episodes of pneumonia in 1 year
- Failure to thrive
- Recurrent deep skin or organ abscesses
- Persistent oral thrush or skin candidiasis after 1 year of age
- History of infections that do not clear with IV antibiotics
- 2 or more serious infections
- Family history of primary immunodeficiency

From the Jeffrey Modell Foundation, 2007.

may occur as a serious adverse reaction. Though less common in children than adults, assess for risk factors associated with a thromboembolic event, such as history of stroke, hypertension, diabetes, hypercholesterolemia, impaired cardiac output, monoclonal gammopathy, clotting disorder, obesity, or immobility.

 ▶ *Take* NOTE!

Do not shake the IVIG, as this may lead to foaming and may cause the immunoglobulin protein to degrade.

Ensure that the child is well hydrated prior to the infusion to decrease the risk for rate-related reactions and aseptic meningitis after the infusion. Premedication with diphenhydramine or acetaminophen may be indicated in children who have never received IVIG, have not had an infusion in more than 8 weeks, have had a recent bacterial infection, have a history of serious infusion-related adverse

TABLE 47.1   TYPES OF HYPOGAMMAGLOBULINEMIA

Type	Definition	Characteristics	Treatment
Selective IgA deficiency	Serum IgA <7 mg/dL, normal IgG and IgM	May be asymptomatic. Child is more prone to allergies due to lack of the mucosal protection that IgA offers. Recurrent infections of respiratory, gastrointestinal, and genitourinary tracts, development of auto-immune disorders.	No specific gammaglobulin treatment available. Treat infections or autoimmune disorders. Severe anaphylactic reaction can occur if child receives transfusion of blood containing IgA and IgA antibodies.
X-linked agammaglobulinemia	Markedly reduced or absent IgG, IgM, and IgA. Absence of B cells.	Males only. Recurrent respiratory and gastrointestinal infections.	Routine IVIG. Treat infections.
X-linked hyper-IgM syndrome	Defect in protein found on T-cell surface, resulting in decreased IgG and IgA levels with significant increase in IgM levels	Males only. Recurrent respiratory infections, diarrhea, malabsorption. Neutropenia, autoimmune disorders.	Routine administration of IVIG. Subcutaneous granulocyte colony-stimulating factor (G-CSF) when neutropenic. Bone marrow transplantation. Treatment of autoimmune disorders.
IgG subclass deficiency	Low levels of one or more of the subclasses of IgG	Recurrent respiratory infections. Some children outgrow this condition.	Treatment of respiratory infections. Administration of IVIG is helpful in some children.

reactions, or are diagnosed with agammaglobulinemia or hypogammaglobulinemia.

The rate for infusion of IVIG is generally prescribed as milligrams of IVIG per kilogram of body weight per minute. Carefully calculate the infusion rate. Obtain a baseline physical assessment and set of vital signs. Begin the infusion slowly, increasing to the prescribed rate as tolerated (see Fig. 47.1). Assess vital signs and check for adverse reactions every 15 minutes for the first hour, then every 30 minutes throughout the remainder of the infusion (the frequency of assessments may vary according to institutional protocol). IVIG is a plasma product, so observe closely for signs of anaphylaxis such as headache, facial flushing, urticaria, dyspnea, shortness of breath, wheezing, chest pain, fever, chills, nausea, vomiting, increased anxiety, or hypotension. If these symptoms occur, discontinue the infusion and notify the physician or nurse practitioner. The infusion may be restarted after the symptoms have subsided. Have oxygen and emergency medications such as epinephrine, diphenhydramine, and intravenous corticosteroids available in case of anaphylactic reaction. If the child complains of discomfort at the intravenous site, a cold compress may be helpful (Murphy et al., 2005).

FIGURE 47.1 Intravenous IVIG.

▶ *Take* NOTE!

Many children who have had previous reactions to IVIG can tolerate the infusion without reaction if they are premedicated and if the infusion is given at a slower rate.

Providing Education and Support

Provide education and support to the child and family. An excellent book for children with an immune deficiency is *Our Immune System* (1993) by Sara le Bien (available from the Immune Deficiency Foundation at www.primary immune.org).

FIGURE 47.2 Boys with Wiskott-Aldrich syndrome often have worsening of eczema over time.

▶ WISKOTT-ALDRICH SYNDROME

Wiskott-Aldrich syndrome is an X-linked genetic disorder that results in immunodeficiency, eczema, and thrombocytopenia. It affects males only. The defective gene responsible for this disorder has been identified recently and is called the Wiskott-Aldrich syndrome protein (WASp). Complications include autoimmune hemolytic anemia, neutropenia, skin or cerebral vasculitis, arthritis, inflammatory bowel disease, and renal disease.

Autoimmune disease may require high-dose steroids, azathioprine, or cyclophosphamide. Splenectomy may be performed to correct thrombocytopenia. The only cure is bone marrow or cord blood stem cell transplantation.

Nursing Assessment

Note history of petechiae, bloody diarrhea, or bleeding episode in the first 6 months of life. Note any history of hematemesis or intracranial or conjunctival hemorrhages. Observe the skin for eczema, which usually worsens with time and tends to become secondarily infected (Fig. 47.2). Laboratory findings include low IgM concentration, elevated IgA and IgE concentrations, and normal IgG concentrations.

> ▶ **Take** NOTE!
>
> *An episode of prolonged bleeding such as after circumcision may be the first sign of Wiskott-Aldrich syndrome in the male infant.*

Nursing Management

Administer IVIG as ordered to help decrease the frequency of bacterial infections. Perform good skin care and frequently assess eczematous areas to detect secondary infection (refer to Chapter 45 for care of eczema). If the patient undergoes splenectomy, in addition to providing routine postoperative care, be aware of the additional risk for development of infection in the asplenic patient. Explain to the patient that severe cutaneous papillomavirus infection may occur after stem cell transplantation (even years later).

▶ SEVERE COMBINED IMMUNE DEFICIENCY

Severe combined immune deficiency (SCID) is a rare X-linked or autosomal recessive disorder; it can occur in girls or boys. SCID is characterized by absent T-cell and B-cell function. There are at least five types of SCID, classified according to the exact genetic defect. Infants with SCID normally present in the first 2 to 7 months of life, when maternally acquired immunity wanes. SCID is a potentially fatal disorder requiring emergency intervention at the time of diagnosis. Gene therapy provides some promise for the future treatment of SCID, but until then bone marrow or stem cell transplantation is necessary. IVIG infusions may help decrease the number of infections until bone marrow or stem cell transplantation can be done. Certain children with SCID (adenosine deaminase enzyme deficiency) may benefit from ongoing subcutaneous adenosine deaminase enzyme replacement. These injections will be required throughout life. Long-term antibiotic therapy helps to contain chronic infections.

Nursing Assessment

Note history of chronic diarrhea and failure to thrive. Note history of severe infections beginning early in infancy. Inspect the mouth for persistent thrush. Auscultate the lungs, noting adventitious sounds related to pneumonia. Laboratory findings include very low levels of all of the immunoglobulins.

Nursing Management

Prevention of infection is critical. Teach the family to practice good hand washing. The child must not be exposed to persons outside the family, particularly young children. Instruct families to administer prophylactic antibiotics if prescribed. Encourage adequate nutrition; supplemental enteral feedings may be necessary in the child with poor appetite. Administer IVIG infusions as prescribed and monitor for adverse reactions (refer to the nursing management section for hypogammaglobulinemia for further information related to IVIG administration). If the child receives a bone marrow transplant (HLA-matched sibling is preferred), provide post-transplant care as outlined in Chapter 49. Refer the family for genetic counseling. Provide ongoing support; this is a difficult situation for families to cope with and the therapy required is lifelong.

> ▶ **Take** NOTE!
>
> *Monitor the bone marrow or stem cell transplant patient closely for a maculopapular rash that usually starts on the palms and soles; this is an indication that **graft-versus-host disease** (GVHD) is developing. Use only cytomegalovirus (CMV)-negative, irradiated blood or platelets if transfusion is necessary in the infant with SCID. CMV-positive blood could cause an infection in the infant, and T lymphocytes in blood products may cause fatal GVHD to occur.*

Secondary Immunodeficiencies

Secondary immunodeficiency may occur as a result of chronic illness, malignancy, use of **immunosuppressive** medication, malnutrition or protein-losing state, prematurity, or HIV infection. This discussion will focus on HIV infection.

▶ HIV INFECTION

Worldwide, 3.2 million children less than 15 years old are living with HIV infection and an additional 1,800 to 2,000 become infected with HIV each day (UNICEF, 2006). More than 10,000 children in the United States have HIV infection or AIDS, and at least 100 of those children die each year (Moylett & Shearer, 2006). Infants primarily become infected through their mothers, whereas adolescents primarily contract HIV infection through sexual activity.

Pathophysiology

HIV affects immune function via alterations mainly in T-cell function, but it also affects B-cells, natural killer cells, and monocyte/macrophage function. HIV infects the CD4 (T-helper) cells. The virus replicates itself via the CD4 cell and renders the cell dysfunctional. Immune deficiency results as the number of normal, functioning CD4 cells drops. Initially, as CD4 counts decrease, the T-suppressor (CD8) counts increase, but as the disease progresses, CD8 counts also fall. The helper T-cell function declines even in asymptomatic infants and children who have not experienced significant decreases in the CD4 cell count. The T cells lose response to recall antigens, and this loss is associated with an increased risk of serious bacterial infection.

B-cell defects also occur in HIV-infected children, contributing to high rates of serious bacterial infections. The B-cells demonstrate impaired response to mitogens and antigens. They also exhibit defective antibody production in response to antigen exposure or vaccination. Also, infants lack a pool of memory B cells for recall antigens (simply from lack of exposure). Natural killer cells also are affected by HIV infection, as they are dependent upon cytokines secreted by the CD4 cells for development of functionality. Functional killer cells play a role in fighting viruses and are critical to immunity in the newborn while the T-cell line develops. Decreased function of the natural killer cells then contributes to increased severity of viral infection in the HIV-infected child or infant. Though the virus does not destroy monocytes and macrophages, their function is affected. Macrophages in the HIV-infected child exhibit decreased chemotaxis and the antigen-presenting capability of the monocytes is defective.

Without appropriate T-cell, B-cell, natural killer cell, monocyte, and macrophage function, the infant's or child's immune system cannot fight infections it ordinarily could. Recurrent infection with ordinary organisms occurs more frequently in children with HIV infection, and the infections are more severe than in noninfected children. Opportunistic infections also occur in HIV-infected children, similar to those in adults with HIV.

HIV rapidly invades the central nervous system in infants and children and is responsible for progressive HIV encephalopathy. As a result of encephalopathy, acquired microcephaly, motor deficits, or loss of previously achieved developmental milestones may occur. In children with progressive HIV encephalopathy, neurologic symptoms may present before immune suppression. Currently, there is no cure for HIV infection.

Children acquire HIV either vertically or horizontally. Vertical transmission refers to perinatal (*in utero* or during birth) transmission or via breast milk. Vertical transmission accounts for 93% of all cases of pediatric HIV infection (Plowfield, 2007). Horizontal transmission refers to transmission via nonsterile needles (as in intravenous drug use or tattooing) or via intimate sexual contact. With nationwide screening of blood products, HIV transmission via transfused blood products has become rare.

The Centers for Disease Control and Prevention (CDC) has developed a classification system for HIV infection in children entitled "The 1994 Revised Classification System for Human Immunodeficiency Virus Infection in Children Less Than 13 years of Age." The classification ranges from the HIV-exposed newborn to the infant or child with AIDS and is based on the severity of the child's clinical symptoms as well as extent of immunologic suppression. The system is useful for determining the severity of illness and for choosing the medication regimen. The classification system may be viewed online at www.cdc.gov/mmwr/preview/mmwrhtml/00032890.htm.

Therapeutic Management

Current recommendations for treatment of HIV infection in children include the use of a combination of antiretroviral drugs. Medication therapy ranges from single-drug therapy in the asymptomatic HIV-exposed newborn to highly active antiretroviral therapy (HAART), consisting of a combination of antiretroviral drugs. Medications are prescribed based on the severity of the child's illness using the CDC classification system (see below). One of the goals of HAART is to prevent or arrest progressive HIV encephalopathy.

Nursing Assessment

For a full description of the assessment phase of the nursing process, refer to page 1560. Assessment findings pertinent to HIV infection and AIDS in children are discussed below.

Health History
Elicit a description of the present illness and chief complaint. Common signs and symptoms reported during the health history might include:

- Failure to thrive
- Recurrent bacterial infections
- Opportunistic infections
- Chronic or recurrent diarrhea
- Recurrent or persistent fever
- Developmental delay
- Prolonged candidiasis

These signs and symptoms may be present in either the child who is undergoing initial diagnosis or the child with known HIV infection. Explore the child's current and past medical history for risk factors such as maternal HIV infection or AIDS, receipt of blood transfusions before current nationwide screening policies, adolescent or childhood sexual abuse, substance use or abuse (including intravenous drug use), or participation in vaginal or anal sex without the use of a condom. Document who the

primary caregiver is, as many children with HIV have lost their parents to the disease. In addition, for the child with known HIV infection, determine the child's medications and dosages as well as the outcome of any recent health care visits or hospitalizations.

Physical Examination
A thorough and complete physical examination should be performed on the child with AIDS or suspected HIV infection.

Inspection and Observation
Note presence of fever. Measure weight, height or length, and head circumference (in children less than 3 years old) and plot this information on standard growth charts, noting whether the measurements fall within the average or below the lower percentiles. Perform a developmental screening test to detect developmental delay. Inspect the oral cavity for candidiasis. Observe work of breathing (may be increased if pneumonitis or pneumonia is present). Determine level of consciousness (may be depressed if HIV encephalopathy is present).

Auscultation and Palpation
Auscultate the lungs, noting adventitious breath sounds associated with pneumonia or pneumonitis. Palpate for the presence of enlarged lymph nodes (lymphadenopathy) or swollen parotid glands. Palpate the abdomen, noting hepatosplenomegaly.

Laboratory and Diagnostic Tests
Common laboratory and diagnostic studies ordered for the assessment of HIV infection include:

- Polymerase chain reaction test (PCR): positive in infected infants over 1 month of age. PCR is the preferred test to determine HIV infection in infants and to exclude HIV infection as early as possible. Box 47.2 gives recommendations for testing.
- Enzyme-linked immunosorbent assay (ELISA) test: positive in infants of HIV-infected mothers because of transplacentally received antibodies. These antibodies may persist and remain detectable up to 24 months of age, making the ELISA test less accurate at detecting HIV infection in infants and toddlers than the PCR.

BOX 47.2 Virologic Testing for HIV-Exposed Infants (with PCR)

- At birth
- 4 to 7 weeks of age
- 8 to 16 weeks of age
- Serologic testing at 12 months of age or older to document disappearance of the HIV-1 antibody

- Platelet count: above 500,000 (in severe HIV infection)
- CD4 counts (low in HIV infection)

Nursing Management

Nursing care of the child with HIV infection or AIDS is directed at avoiding infection, promoting compliance with the medication regimen, promoting nutrition, providing pain management and comfort measures, educating the child and caregivers, and providing ongoing psychosocial support. Children with HIV infection may access health services through funding provided by the Ryan White Comprehensive AIDS Resources Emergency Act. This federal funding provides for primary health care and other services to persons with HIV infection. The Nursing Care Plan Overview lists appropriate nursing diagnoses and interventions. In addition, nursing management specific to HIV infection is covered below.

Preventing HIV Infection in Children

All pregnant women should be offered routine HIV counseling and voluntary testing. Depending upon the stage of pregnancy, the mother should be treated with an antiretroviral drug if she is HIV positive. Children born to HIV-positive mothers should receive a 6-week course of zidovudine (ZDV) therapy. Discourage breastfeeding in the HIV-infected mother and instruct her about safe alternatives to breastfeeding. Early recognition of infection is crucial so that treatment can begin and progression to AIDS can be prevented. Educate sexually active adolescents about HIV transmission and urge them to use condoms. Counsel teens about the increased risk of HIV transmission with all forms of sexual activity, with vaginal and anal sex being even riskier than oral sex. Urge teens to limit the number of sexual partners. Discourage substance use, as the effects of drugs and alcohol often impair the teen's ability to make wise choices about sexual conduct (Morrison-Beedy et al., 2005). Warn teens of the risk of contracting HIV infection via shared needles (as with intravenous drug use). See Healthy People 2010.

Promoting Compliance With Antiretroviral Therapy

Before HAART was available as a treatment option, progressive HIV encephalopathy was inevitably fatal, usually within 2 years of diagnosis. To prevent progression of HIV disease and prevent encephalopathy, compliance with the HAART regimen is required. Educate the family about the importance of complying with the medication regimen. Help the caregivers develop a schedule for medication administration that is compatible with the family's home routine. See Healthy People 2010.

Reducing Risk for Infection

In the newborn whose mother is infected with tuberculosis, syphilis, toxoplasmosis, cytomegalovirus, hepatitis B

HEALTHY PEOPLE 2010	
Objective	**Nursing Significance**
(Developmental) Reduce new cases of perinatally acquired HIV infection. (Developmental) Increase the proportion of pregnant females screened for sexually transmitted diseases (including HIV infection and bacterial vaginosis) during prenatal health care visits, according to recognized standards.	• Encourage sexually active adolescents to seek appropriate reproductive health care and screening. • For the pregnant adolescent, encourage HIV testing to determine status. • Encourage the HIV-positive pregnant adolescent to comply with HIV treatment as prescribed.

or C, or herpes simplex virus, testing and treatment should be provided. To prevent infection with *Pneumocystis jiroveci*, administer prophylactic antibiotics as prescribed in any HIV-exposed infant in whom HIV infection has not yet been excluded. Provide tuberculosis screening and childhood immunization in accordance with national guidelines.

> ▶ **Take** NOTE!
>
> *Do not administer live vaccines to the immunocompromised child without the express consent of the infectious disease or immunology specialist. Immunosuppression is a contraindication to vaccination with live vaccines.*

Promoting Nutrition

For the infant, provide increased-calorie formula as tolerated. For the child, provide high-calorie, high-protein meals and snacks. Supplements may be added to milk-

HEALTHY PEOPLE 2010	
Objective	**Nursing Significance**
(Developmental) Reduce the number of cases of HIV infection among adolescents and adults. (Developmental) Reduce HIV infections in adolescent and young adult females aged 13 to 24 years that are associated with heterosexual contact.	• Encourage abstinence in adolescents. • If adolescents are sexually active, educate about the risks of HIV transmission; encourage condom use with all sexual activity.

EVIDENCE-BASED PRACTICE 47.1
Does Patient Education and Support Promote Adherence to Highly Active Antiretroviral Therapy (HAART) for HIV/AIDS?

● Study

The key determinant of degree and length of viral suppression in HIV infection is high adherence to HAART. Conversely, poor adherence leads to treatment failure. Children potentially have a significant number of years of life for which they will need to remain compliant with HAART. Each period of noncompliance further contributes to cross-resistance, limiting future treatment options. The authors evaluated a large number of randomized controlled trials that examined the effectiveness of patient education and support in improving HAART adherence.

■ Nursing Implications

HAART adherence is critical to the potential life of an HIV-infected child. Despite numerous medication side effects and the stigma associated with HIV infection, nurses can make a difference in these children's lives. Educate parents at every opportunity about the importance of HAART adherence. Provide families with ideas for managing unpleasant side effects of antiretroviral drugs. Involve children in medication administration. Provide developmentally appropriate education to children and adolescents. Praise families' and children's efforts at HAART adherence.

▲ Findings

Education and support interventions are effective in improving HAART adherence. The most effective interventions are those delivered over a 12-week period or longer, targeting individuals rather than groups, and that provide practical medication-management skills.

Reuda, S., Park-Wyllie, L. Y., Bayoumi, A. M., Tynan, A. M., Antoniou, T. A., Rourke, S. B., & Glazier, R. H. (2007). Patient support and education for promoting adherence to highly active antiretroviral therapy for HIV/AIDS. *The Cochrane Library 2007, 4.* Indianapolis: John Wiley & Sons.

shakes to increase the protein intake. Ensure that the child is able to choose foods that he or she prefers from the hospital menu. Document growth through weekly measurements of weight and height/length.

Promoting Comfort

Children with HIV infection experience pain from infections, encephalopathy, adverse effects of medications, and the numerous procedures and treatments that are required, such as venipuncture, biopsy, or lumbar puncture. Refer to Chapter 35 for detailed information about pain assessment and management.

HEALTHY PEOPLE 2010

Objective	Nursing Significance
Reduce deaths from HIV infection. (Developmental) Extend the interval of time between an initial diagnosis of HIV infection and AIDS diagnosis in order to increase years of life of an individual infected with HIV.	• Educate families about the importance of complying with medication therapy (HAART) and receiving regularly scheduled medical evaluations.

Providing Family Education and Support

Educate caregivers about the medication regimen, the ongoing follow-up that is needed, and when to call the infectious disease provider. Families of HIV-infected children experience a significant amount of stress from many sources: the diagnosis of an incurable disease, financial difficulties, multiple family members with HIV, HIV-associated stigmas, desire to keep HIV infection confidential, and multiple medical appointments and hospitalizations. Parents of HIV-infected children often die of AIDS themselves, leaving care of the child to another relative or foster parent. The daycare center or school that the child attends will need education about HIV, which can be provided only if the parent or caretaker consents to divulging the child's diagnosis to that agency. Provide education to the school or daycare center about how the infection is transmitted (i.e., not through casual contact).

Disclosure of the diagnosis of HIV to the child is another source of stress for the family. The timing of this disclosure will vary considerably depending on the child's and family's situation. Generally, children over 6 years of age will eventually need to have their diagnosis disclosed to them in an age-appropriate manner. They begin to ask questions and often seem to sense that something is going on other than what they've been told so far. When made aware of the diagnosis and educated about the disease, the child may exhibit a variety of reactions. Anger, depression,

BOX 47.3 Resources for HIV-Infected Children and their Families

- www.hivpositive.com—information on HIV infection
- www.pedaids.org: Elizabeth Glaser Pediatric AIDS Foundation—resources for HIV-infected children and their families
- www.vachss.com/help_text/hiv_aids_ped.html—Pediatric HIV infection and AIDS resources
- www.womenchildrenhiv.org/: Women, Children and HIV—resources for prevention and treatment

or school problems may occur. The child may experience a spiritual dilemma. The nurse should continue to provide emotional support to the child and family. If the disclosure results in significant emotional turmoil, refer the child and caregivers to a counselor, social worker, or psychologist.

Anticipatory grieving also may occur. Parents or caregivers may express guilt or anger over the diagnosis of HIV infection. At the other end of the spectrum, families may use denial as their method for coping. Use therapeutic communication with open-ended questions to discover the family's thoughts and fears. Provide emotional support and allow for crying and verbalization. If needed, refer the caregivers to the appropriate professional for additional psychological and emotional intervention.

Many children with HIV have psychosocial, emotional, and cognitive problems. These contribute to a lower quality of life. They are affected by the stigma of their diagnosis and often by the social isolation associated with it. They may suffer multiple losses within the family related to deaths caused by HIV infection. Children with HIV infection need significant psychosocial support and intervention. Resources for families of HIV-infected children are listed in Box 47.3.

▶ **Consider** THIS!

Jake Reddington, a 2-year-old diagnosed with HIV infection, is brought to the clinic by his aunt for his regular check-up. His aunt has recently taken over the care of Jake since his mother is too ill with HIV infection to care for him.

What education will be important for Jake's aunt and her family?

Discuss some of the psychosocial issues and concerns that face a child with HIV and his or her family.

▶ **Take** NOTE!

Family-centered care of the HIV-exposed child and HIV-infected mother may involve a multidisciplinary approach and can result in improved outcomes for both the mother and the child.

Autoimmune Disorders

Autoimmune disorders result from the immune system's malfunction. The body manufactures T cells and antibodies against its own cells and organs (**autoantibodies**). The development of an autoimmune disorder is thought to be multifactorial. Potential influencing factors include heredity, hormones, self-marker molecules, and environmental influences such as viruses and certain drugs.

▶ SYSTEMIC LUPUS ERYTHEMATOSUS

Systemic lupus erythematosus (SLE) is a multisystem autoimmune disorder that affects both humoral and cellular immunity. SLE can affect any organ system, so the onset and course of the disease are quite variable. SLE is usually diagnosed after age 5 years (usually between 15 and 45 years of age), but onset can occur at any age. The female-to-male ratio for persons affected by SLE is 8:1 (Cassidy, 2006). SLE is more common in non-Caucasians, and typically black and Hispanic patients experience more severe effects from SLE than other racial or ethnic groups.

Pathophysiology

In SLE, autoantibodies react with the child's self-antigens to form immune complexes. The immune complexes accumulate in the tissues and organs, causing an inflammatory response resulting in vasculitis. Injury to the tissues and pain occur. Since SLE may affect any organ system, the potential for alterations or damage to tissues anywhere in the body is significant. In some cases, the autoimmune response may be preceded by a drug reaction, an infection, or excessive sun exposure. In children, the most common initial symptoms are hematologic, cutaneous, and musculoskeletal in origin. The disease is chronic, with periods of remission and exacerbation (flares). Common complications of SLE include ocular or visual changes, cerebrovascular accident (CVA), transverse myelitis, immune complex–mediated glomerulonephritis, pericarditis, valvular heart disease, coronary artery disease, seizures, and psychosis.

Therapeutic Management

Therapeutic management focuses on treating the inflammatory response. NSAIDs, corticosteroids, and antimalarial agents are often prescribed for the child with mild to moderate SLE. The child with severe SLE or frequent flare-ups of symptoms may require high-dose (pulse) corticosteroid therapy or immunosuppressive drugs. When end-stage renal failure develops as a result of glomerulonephritis, dialysis becomes necessary.

Nursing Assessment

For a full description of the assessment phase of the nursing process, refer to page 1560. Assessment findings pertinent to SLE in children are discussed below.

Health History

Elicit a description of the present illness and chief complaint. Common signs and symptoms reported during the health history are history of fatigue, fever, weight changes, pain or swelling in the joints, numbness, tingling or coolness of extremities, or prolonged bleeding. Assess for risk factors, which include female sex; family history (only 10% of cases); African, Native American, or Asian descent; recent infection; drug reaction; or excessive sun exposure.

Physical Examination

Measure temperature and document the presence of fever. Observe the skin for malar rash (a butterfly-shaped rash over the cheeks); discoid lesions on the face, scalp, or neck; changes in skin pigmentation; or scarring (Fig. 47.3). Document alopecia. Inspect the oral cavity for painless ulcerations and the joints for edema. Measure blood pressure, as hypertension may occur with renal involvement. Auscultate the lungs; adventitious breath sounds may be present if the pulmonary system is involved. Palpate the joints, noting tenderness. Palpate the abdomen and note areas of tenderness (abdominal involvement is more common in

FIGURE 47.3 The malar or butterfly rash (erythema over the cheeks in the shape of a butterfly) is typical in SLE.

children with SLE than in adults). Box 47.4 lists common clinical findings in SLE.

Laboratory and Diagnostic Findings

Laboratory findings may include decreased hemoglobin and hematocrit, decreased platelet count, and low WBC count. Complement levels, C3 and C4, will also be decreased. Though not specific to SLE, the ANA is usually positive in patients with SLE.

Nursing Management

Nursing management of the child or adolescent with SLE is long term and supportive. Management focuses on preventing and monitoring for complications. Educate the child and family about the importance of a healthy diet, regular exercise, and adequate sleep and rest. Administer NSAIDs, corticosteroids, and antimalarial agents as ordered for the child with mild to moderate SLE and pulse corticosteroid therapy or immunomodulators to the child with severe SLE or frequent flare-ups. Refer families to support services such as the Lupus Alliance of America (www.lupusalliance.org) and the Lupus Foundation of America (www.lupus.org).

Preventing and Monitoring for Complications

Teach families to apply sunscreen (minimum SPF 15) to their child's skin daily to prevent rashes resulting from photosensitivity. Instruct the child and family to protect against cold weather by layering warm socks and wearing gloves when outdoors in the winter. If the child is outside for extended periods during the winter months, the fingers and toes should be inspected for discoloration. Watch for the development of nephritis by evaluating blood pressure, serum BUN and creatinine levels, and urine output and monitoring for hematuria or proteinuria.

BOX 47.4 **Most Common Clinical Manifestations of SLE**

- Alopecia
- Anemia
- Arthralgia
- Arthritis
- Fatigue
- Lupus nephritis
- Photosensitivity
- Pleurisy
- Raynaud's phenomenon
- Seizures
- Skin rashes, including malar rash
- Stomatitis
- Thrombocytopenia

Ensure that yearly vision screening and ophthalmic examinations are performed to preserve visual function should changes occur.

> ▶ *Take* NOTE!
>
> *Avascular necrosis (lack of blood supply to a joint, resulting in tissue damage) may occur as an adverse effect of long-term or high-dose corticosteroid use. Teach families to report new onset of joint pain, particularly with weight bearing, or limited range of motion to their physician or nurse practitioner.*

▶ JUVENILE IDIOPATHIC ARTHRITIS

Juvenile idiopathic arthritis is an autoimmune disorder in which the autoantibodies mainly target the joints. Inflammatory changes in the joints cause pain, redness, warmth, stiffness, and swelling. Stiffness usually occurs after inactivity (as in the morning, after sleep). Some forms also affect the eyes or other organs. Table 47.2 explains the three most common types. Juvenile idiopathic arthritis is a chronic disease: the child may experience healthy periods alternating with flare-ups. In some children the disease resolves as they approach adolescence or adulthood, while others will have more severe disease that continues throughout the adult years. Juvenile idiopathic arthritis was formerly termed "juvenile rheumatoid arthritis," but unlike adult rheumatoid arthritis, few types of juvenile arthritis actually demonstrate a positive rheumatoid factor.

Therapeutic management focuses on inflammation control, pain relief, promotion of remission, and maintenance of mobility. NSAIDs, corticosteroids, and antirheumatic drugs such as methotrexate and etanercept are prescribed, depending on the type and severity of the disease. NSAIDs are helpful with pain relief, but disease-modifying (antirheumatic) drugs are necessary to prevent disease progression.

Nursing Assessment

Note history of irritability or fussiness, which may be the first sign of this disease in the infant or very young child. Note complaints of pain, though children do not always communicate this. Document history of withdrawal from play or difficulty getting the child out of bed in the morning (joint stiffness after inactivity). Inquire about history of fever (above 39.5°C for 2 weeks or more in systemic disease).

Measure temperature (fever is present with systemic disease). Inspect skin for evanescent, pale red, nonpruritic macular rash, which may be present at diagnosis of systemic disease. Observe the gait, noting limping or guarding of a joint or extremity. Document growth, which may be delayed. Inspect and palpate each joint for edema, redness, warmth, and tenderness (Fig. 47.4). Note positioning of joints (usually flexed in position of comfort). Mild to moderate anemia and an elevated erythrocyte sedimentation rate are common. Young children with the pauciarticular form may demonstrate a positive antinuclear antibody, and adolescents with polyarticular disease may have a positive rheumatoid factor.

Nursing Management

Nursing management focuses on managing pain, maintaining mobility, and promoting a normal life. Refer the child to a pediatric rheumatologist to ensure that he or she receives the most up-to-date treatment. Disease-modifying medications approved for use in children may produce better long-term outcomes than were possible in the past. Clinical research trial information is available through the Childhood Arthritis & Rheumatology Research Alliance. Encourage regular eye examinations and

TABLE 47.2 TYPES OF JUVENILE IDIOPATHIC ARTHRITIS

Type	Definition	Non-Joint Manifestations	Complications
Pauciarticular	Involvement of four or fewer joints; quite often the knee is involved. Most common type.	Eye inflammation, malaise, poor appetite, poor weight gain	Iritis, uveitis, uneven leg bone growth
Polyarticular	Involvement of five or more joints; frequently involves small joints and often affects the body symmetrically.	Malaise, lymphadenopathy, organomegaly, poor growth	Often a severe form of arthritis; rapidly progressing joint damage, rheumatoid nodules
Systemic	In addition to joint involvement, fever and rash may be present at diagnosis.	Enlarged spleen, liver, and lymph nodes; myalgia; severe anemia	Pericarditis, pericardial effusion, pleuritis, pulmonary fibrosis

FIGURE 47.4 Note the swollen, reddened joints of this child with juvenile arthritis.

vision screening to allow for early treatment of visual changes and to prevent blindness.

Managing Pain and Maintaining Mobility

Administer medications as prescribed to control inflammation and prevent disease progression. Refer to Drug Guide 47.1 for information related to NSAIDs, corticosteroids, and disease-modifying antirheumatic drugs. Maintain joint range of motion and muscle strength via exercise (physical or occupational therapy). Swimming is a particularly useful exercise to maintain joint mobility without placing pressure on the joints. Teach families appropriate use of splints prescribed to prevent joint contractures. Monitor for pressure areas or skin breakdown with splint or orthotic use.

Promoting Normal Life

Chronic pain and decreased mobility may impact the child's psychological and emotional status significantly, both during childhood and adulthood. Providing adequate pain relief and promoting compliance with the disease-modifying medication regimen may allow the child to have a more normal life in the present as well as in the future. In addition to measures described in the previous section, encourage adequate sleep to allow the child to cope better with symptoms and to function better in school. Sleep may be promoted by a warm bath at bedtime and warm compresses to affected joints or massage. To prevent social isolation, encourage the child to attend school and ensure that teachers, the school nurse, and classmates are educated about the child's disease and any limitations on activity. Having two sets of books (one at school and one at home) allows the child to do homework without having to carry heavy books home. Modifications such as allowing the child to leave the classroom early in order to get to the next class on time may seem small but can have a significant impact on the child's life.

Encourage children and families to become involved with local support groups so they can see that they are not alone. Assist children to set and achieve goals to increase their sense of hopefulness. Special summer camps for children with juvenile arthritis allow the child to socialize and belong to a group and have been shown to promote self-esteem in the child with chronic illness. Encourage appropriate family functioning and refer the family to support groups such as those sponsored by the American Juvenile Arthritis Organization. See Healthy People 2010.

Allergy and Anaphylaxis

Allergy is an immune-mediated response resulting in an adverse physiologic event or reaction (Sampson & Eggleston, 2006). Allergy affects about 20% to 25% of the U.S. population; the extent of the allergic response is determined by the duration, rate, and amount of exposure to the allergen as well as environmental and host factors (American College of Allergy, Asthma and Immunology, 2006). IgE-mediated allergy will be the focus of this discussion. This type of allergic response is mediated by antigen-specific IgE antibodies. When the antibody is exposed to the antigen (allergen), rapid cell activation occurs and potent mediators and cytokines are released, resulting in changes in the blood vessels, bronchi, and mucus-secreting glands. In addition to the atopic diseases (asthma, allergic rhinitis, atopic dermatitis), urticaria, digestive allergy, and systemic anaphylaxis are also IgE-mediated (Sampson & Eggleston, 2006). Though any allergen has the potential to trigger an anaphylactic response, food and insect sting allergies are most common.

▶ FOOD ALLERGIES

A true food hypersensitivity or allergy is defined as an immunologic reaction resulting from the ingestion of a food or food additive (Ozol & Mete, 2008). This type of reaction is an IgE-mediated response to a particular food. Food allergy affects approximately 2% to 8% of children and can lead to significant medical complications (Bollinger et al.,

HEALTHY PEOPLE 2010	
Objective	Nursing Significance
(Developmental) Increase the proportion of persons with arthritis who have had effective, evidence-based arthritis education as an integral part of the management of their condition.	• Educate children and families about juvenile arthritis, its treatments, and interventions for improving mobility. Begin at diagnosis and provide continual reinforcement.

2006). During the first few years of life, the most common food allergens are milk, eggs, peanuts, tree nuts, fish and shellfish, wheat, and soy. Typically, allergies to these foods are acquired in childhood, and for most children only allergies to peanuts, tree nuts, and fish and shellfish persist into adulthood. Most reactions occur within minutes of exposure, but they may occur up to 2 hours after ingestion. Signs and symptoms of a food allergy reaction include hives, flushing, facial swelling, mouth and throat itching, and runny nose. Many children also have a gastrointestinal reaction, including vomiting, abdominal pain, and diarrhea. In extreme cases, swelling of the tongue, uvula, pharynx, or upper airway may occur. Wheezing can be an ominous sign that the airway is edematous. Rarely, cardiovascular collapse occurs. Though the risk for anaphylaxis is small, parents, caregivers, and health care providers should be vigilant when caring for children with food allergies.

Therapeutic Management

Therapeutic management involves verifying the food allergy, avoiding the allergen, and treating the reaction with epinephrine or antihistamines. Preventing the development of food allergies is also a key intervention.

It is important to discern a true food allergy from intolerance to certain foods. "Food intolerance" is a general term that describes an abnormal physiologic response to an ingested food or food additive that has not been proven to be immunologic. Often a milk allergy is confused with lactose intolerance. Therefore, a detailed dietary history is important when distinguishing a true allergy versus intolerance.

To prevent the development of food allergies, infants should be breastfed for at least the first 6 months of life and the following common food allergens should be avoided in children under 1 year of age (Chamberlain, 2006; Muraro et al., 2004):

- Cow's milk
- Eggs
- Peanuts
- Tree nuts
- Sesame seeds
- Kiwi fruit
- Fish and shellfish

Nursing Assessment

Patients with food allergy reactions must be assessed accurately. In the initial nursing assessment, the child should be immediately assessed for airway, breathing, or circulation problems (see Chapter 52). If the child's condition is stable, the nurse should finish the assessment. The history should include a detailed food history and documentation of the reaction, including the food suspected of causing the reaction, the quantity of food ingested, the length of time between ingestion and development of symptoms,

the symptoms, what treatment has been administered, and the subsequent response. Note gastrointestinal symptoms such as:

- Burning in the mouth or throat
- Bloating
- Nausea
- Diarrhea

Assess for risk factors such as previous exposure to the food, history of poorly controlled asthma, or an increase in atopic dermatitis flare-ups in relation to food intake.

Inspect the skin for color, rash, hives, or edema. Auscultate the heart and lungs to determine heart rate and to assess for wheezing.

The American College of Allergy, Asthma & Immunology's new practice parameter recommends food-specific IgE testing if the child has a history of food allergy. Food avoidance is recommended for those who have a highly predictive reaction to testing or a history of anaphylactic response. If the child has episodic symptoms, an oral challenge may be appropriate. If symptoms are chronic, a trial elimination diet may be indicated. If symptoms resolve without the food, true allergy may be present (American College of Allergy, Asthma & Immunology, 2006). On an elimination diet, the child should stop eating all suspicious foods for 1 to 2 weeks and then retry the foods one at a time, over a period of several days, to see whether a similar reaction occurs. Often this is done in the pediatrician's office or hospital setting if severe reactions have occurred in the past. If a similar reaction occurs, it is very suggestive of a food allergy. Allergy skin prick tests and RAST blood tests are widely used by pediatricians to look for reactions. However, these tests may have false-positive results, and children may need to avoid many foods unnecessarily.

Nursing Management

Initial nursing management is aimed at stabilizing the child's condition if an acute reaction to a food allergen is present (see Chapter 52). Medications used in the treatment of a food allergy reaction include histamine blockers and, in anaphylactic reactions, epinephrine. Teach the child (if appropriate) and the parents how and when to use these medications during an allergic reaction. Since these reactions can be so sudden (unknown ingestion of allergen) and severe, it is helpful for the family to have an emergency written plan in case of a reaction.

Managing the Child's Diet

Dietary teaching is aimed at educating the family on how to avoid the offending foods. Families should be extremely careful when reading food labels. A dietitian may be helpful in this teaching process. Teaching Guidelines 47.1 gives information about hidden allergens in

TEACHING GUIDELINES 47.1

Allergens Hidden in Food

If Child is Allergic to:	Teach Families to Avoid:	Unexpected Locations of Common Ingredients
Milk	Artificial butter flavor, casein, lactalbumin, nougat, pudding, whey, yogurt, ghee	Some deli meats and hot dogs, nondairy products, coffee whiteners
Wheat	Cereal extract, couscous, durum, semolina, spelt	
Eggs	Albumin, globulin, ovalbumin	
Peanuts	Fast food cooked in peanut oil, many Asian foods, baked goods with nuts or processed on equipment that also processes peanuts	Brown gravy, barbeque sauce, meat sauce, egg rolls, enchilada sauce, hot chocolate

Data from Munoz-Furlong, A. (2003). Daily coping strategies for patients and their families. *Pediatrics,* *111*(6), 1654–1661; and Vadas, P. (2003). Food allergens and anaphylaxis. *Canadian Journal of Dietetic Practice and Research, 64*(2), insert.

food. Teach the parents what "safe" foods can be substituted for offensive ones (Box 47.5). Children with peanut allergy should also avoid tree nuts.

Having a child with a food allergy can be very anxiety-producing for parents: they often live in fear that the child may accidentally ingest an allergen. Educating the child and family about allergic reactions may help to decrease their anxiety. Teach the child and family how to recognize the signs and symptoms of an allergic reaction. The nurse may need to provide information to daycare providers as well as schoolteachers, staff, and camp counselors (Munoz-Furlong, 2003). Refer families to the Food Allergy & Anaphylaxis Network (www.foodallergy.org).

◆ ANAPHYLAXIS

Anaphylaxis is an acute IgE-mediated response to an allergen that involves many organ systems and may be

BOX 47.5 Food Substitutions

- Replace milk with water, fruit juice, rice milk, or soy milk.
- Replace each egg with 1.5 tablespoons each of water and oil and 1 teaspoon baking powder; OR 1 packet plain gelatin with 2 tablespoons warm water added at time of use; OR 1 teaspoon yeast and a quarter-cup warm water.
- Replace peanuts or tree nuts with raisins, dates, or crispy cereal.

Munoz-Furlong, A. (2003). Daily coping strategies for patients and their families. *Pediatrics, 111*(6), 1654–1661.

life-threatening (Sampson, 2006). As many as 1% to 2% of the population is at risk for anaphylaxis due to food allergies or insect stings (McIntyre et al., 2005). In addition to nuts, shellfish, eggs, and bee or wasp stings, drugs such as penicillin and NSAIDs, radiopaque dyes, and latex are the leading causes of anaphylaxis (Lane & Bolte, 2007). The reaction is severe and usually starts within 5 to 10 minutes of exposure, though delayed reactions are possible. Histamines and secondary mediators are released from the mast cells and eosinophils in response to contact with an allergen. Cutaneous, cardiopulmonary, gastrointestinal, and neurologic symptoms occur. Vasodilation results in a rapid decrease in plasma volume, leading to the risk of circulatory collapse (Dreskin, 2005). Prolonged resuscitation may be needed, and death may occur.

Therapeutic management focuses on assessment and support of the airway, breathing, and circulation. Epinephrine is usually required, and intramuscular or intravenous diphenhydramine is used secondarily. Late-onset reactions can be prevented with corticosteroids.

Nursing Assessment

Assess patency of the airway and adequacy of breathing. Determine if circulation is sufficient. Note level of consciousness. Obtain a brief history, inquiring specifically about allergen exposure. Determine whether the child has received any medication (e.g., epinephrine or diphenhydramine) since the onset of the reaction and what effect the medication had on the symptoms. Table 47.3 gives additional signs and symptoms of anaphylaxis.

Nursing Management

Nursing management initially focuses on supporting airway, breathing, and circulation. Provide supplemental oxygen by mask or bag-valve-mask ventilation. Ensure that bronchodilator inhalation treatment (albuterol) is

TABLE 47.3 CLINICAL MANIFESTATIONS OF ANAPHYLAXIS

Body Area or System	Manifestation
Oral	• Lip, tongue, or palate pruritus • Lip or tongue edema
Cutaneous	• Urticaria (hives), flushing, pruritus, angioedema
Respiratory	• Nasal pruritus, congestion, sneezing, rhinorrhea • Stridor, tightness in the throat, dysphagia, dysphonia, hoarseness • Shortness of breath, dyspnea, tight chest, wheeze
Cardiovascular	• Tachycardia, chest pain, arrhythmia, hypotension
Neurologic	• Syncope, feeling faint, aura of doom, lethargy, disorientation
Gastrointestinal	• Bloating, abdominal pain, diarrhea, vomiting

Data from Clark, A. T., & Ewan, P. W. (2003). Food allergy in childhood. *Archives of Disease in Childhood, 88*(1), 79–81; Sampson, H. A. (2003). Anaphylaxis and emergency treatment. *Pediatrics, 111*(6), 1601–1908; Dreskin, S.C. (2005). Anaphylaxis. Available at http:www.emedicine.com/med/topic/28.htm.

given if bronchospasm is present. Administer intravenous fluids to provide volume expansion. Administer epinephrine, diphenhydramine, and/or corticosteroids as ordered to reverse the allergic process (Lane & Bolte, 2007).

Preventing and Managing Future Episodes

Education of the family about preventing and managing future episodes is critical. Teach the family how to use injectable epinephrine in case of subsequent allergen exposure. Intramuscular epinephrine may be given via the Epipen or Epipen Jr. Dosage is based on the child's weight. The gray safety release on the Epipen should never be removed until just before use. The thumb, fingers, or hand should not be placed over the black tip. Nursing Procedure 47.1 gives further instructions related to Epipen use. Instruct the child and family to call 911 and seek immediate medical attention after using the Epipen. Warn the child that the epinephrine may make him or her feel as if the heart is racing.

Daycare providers, school nurses, teachers, and staff who interact with the child must know how to recognize an anaphylactic event. In 2004, Public Law No. 108-377, Asthmatic Schoolchildren's Treatment and Health Management Act, was passed by the U.S. Congress. This law is intended to ensure that students with severe allergies can carry prescribed medications (i.e., Epipen) with them. All children with allergies should have an action plan in place at the school or daycare center (Frost & Chalin, 2005). Advise the child to wear a medical alert bracelet or necklace at all times (Lane & Bolte, 2007).

Teach children and families to avoid known food allergens. Avoid stings from bees and wasps (Hymenoptera) by being alert when eating outdoors, wearing long sleeves and pants when in fields, and removing hives or

nests. Desensitization is available for children with severe penicillin allergy. Avoid use of cephalosporins in children with severe penicillin allergy (Lane & Bolte, 2007).

▶ LATEX ALLERGY

Latex allergy is an IgE-mediated response to exposure to latex, a natural rubber product used in many common items (especially gloves in the health care setting). The pathophysiology of latex allergy is similar to that of food allergy. Avoidance of latex products is recommended for those who are allergic to it. An immediate allergic reaction may occur if a latex-allergic child comes in to contact with latex. Latex allergy can also result in anaphylaxis (refer to section above on anaphylaxis).

Nursing Assessment

Screen all children who visit a health care facility of any kind for latex allergy. Ask if the child is allergic to rubber gloves or has ever developed hives after exposure to them. Ask the parent if the child has symptoms such as coughing, wheezing, or shortness of breath after glove exposure. Has the child ever had swelling in the mouth or complained that the mouth itched after a dental examination? Determine whether the child has ever had allergic symptoms after eating foods with a known cross-reactivity to latex, such as pear, peach, passion fruit, plum, pineapple, kiwi, fig, grape, cherry, melon, nectarine, papaya, apple, apricot, banana, chestnut, carrot, celery, avocado, tomato, or potato. For the child who has come into contact with latex, assess for symptoms

Nursing Procedure 47.1

USE OF THE EPIPEN OR EPIPEN JR.

1. Grasp the Epipen or Epipen Jr. with the black tip pointing downward, forming a fist.
2. With the other hand, pull off the gray safety release.

3. Swing and jab the epipen firmly into the outer thigh at a 90-degree angle and hold firmly there for 10 seconds

4. Remove the Epipen and massage the thigh for 10 seconds.

Adapted from the Epipen website (www.epipen.com/howtouse/aspx).

of a reaction such as hives; wheeze; cough; shortness of breath; nasal congestion and rhinorrhea; sneezing; nose, palate, or eye pruritus; or hypotension.

Nursing Management

Nursing management of latex allergy focuses on preventing exposure to latex products. Instruct children and their families to avoid foods with a known cross-reactivity to latex such as those listed above. If the child is exposed to latex, remove the irritating substance and cleanse the area with soap and water. Assess for the need for resuscitation and perform it if needed. Become familiar with your institution's latex allergy policy. Know which products contain latex and which do not. Document latex allergy on the chart, patient identification band, the medication administration record, and the physician's order sheet. Refer families to resources for persons with latex allergy, such as:

• www.latexallergyresources.org: American Latex Allergy Association

• latexallergylinks.tripod.com/: comprehensive listing of latex allergy websites and documents

■■■ Key Concepts

■ Waning of maternal antibodies in early infancy while humoral immunity is developing leads to physiologic hypogammaglobulinemia, placing the young infant at risk for overwhelming infection.

■ Infants and young children have large lymph nodes, tonsils, and thymus compared with adults.

■ Infants have decreased phagocytic activity, placing them at higher risk for serious infection.

■ Children with immune disorders often show a decreased or absent response to delayed hypersensitivity skin testing (e.g., the tuberculosis test).

■ The enzyme-linked immunosorbent assay (ELISA) test for HIV detects only antibodies to HIV (which in the infant may be maternal in origin), whereas the polymerase chain reaction test (PCR) for HIV tests for HIV genetic material, making it the more accurate test for HIV infection in infants and young children.

■ Primary immune deficiencies such as SCID and Wiskott-Aldrich syndrome are congenital and serious; they can be cured only by bone marrow or stem cell transplantation.

■ Systemic lupus erythematosus is a chronic autoimmune disorder that can affect any organ system, primarily causing vasculitis.

■ Juvenile idiopathic arthritis results in chronic pain and affects growth and development as well as school performance.

■ Various forms of hypogammaglobulinemia may be treated with exogenous immunoglobulin administered intravenously every several weeks, allowing children to lead a healthier life with fewer infections.

■ Nasal, palatal, or throat pruritus and difficulty breathing may indicate an anaphylactic reaction.

■ Children with severe allergy or previous anaphylactic episodes must avoid contact with allergens.

■ Nursing management of lupus focuses on preventing flare-ups and complications.

■ Managing pain, maintaining mobility, and administering disease-modifying medications are key nursing interventions in the management of juvenile idiopathic arthritis.

■ HIV infection may be prevented in infants by prenatal screening and maternal treatment, as well as postnatal treatment with zidovudine.

■ HIV infection in children often results in encephalopathy and developmental delay.

■ Spread of HIV infection can be prevented in adolescence by avoiding high-risk behaviors.

■ For children with immune deficiency or autoimmune disease, prevention of infection is a primary nursing concern.

■ A chronic illness such as immune deficiency, SLE, or juvenile arthritis has a significant impact on the family as well as the child.

■ When planning care for the child with an immune deficiency or autoimmune disorder, the nurse should include the child and the family.

■ To promote proper growth, encourage the child with an immune or autoimmune disorder to eat a balanced diet.

■ Teach families of children with immune deficiencies about infection prevention.

■ Teach the family of the child with juvenile arthritis about ways to decrease pain while increasing or maintaining the child's mobility.

■ Teach families of children with allergy how to avoid allergens and how to use the Epipen. Staff at the child's school or daycare center should be aware of the allergy. The child should wear medical alert identification.

REFERENCES

Ackley, B. J., & Ladwig, G. B. (2006). *Nursing diagnosis handbook: A guide to planning care* (7th ed.). St. Louis: Mosby.

American Academy of Pediatrics. (2007). Increasing antiretroviral drug access for children with HIV infection. *Pediatrics, 119,* 838–845.

American College of Allergy, Asthma, & Immunology (ACAAI). (2006). Food allergy: A practice parameter. *Annals of Allergy, Asthma, & Immunology, 96*(3 Suppl. 2), S1–S68.

Anderson, V. L. (2006). Uncovering a pediatric immunodeficiency, part 1. *Journal for Nurse Practitioners, 2*(3), 186–193.

AORN. (2004). AORN latex guideline. *AORN, 79*(3), 653–672.

Bader-Meunier, B., Armengaud, J. B., Haddad, E., Salomon, R., Desche'nes, G., Kone-Paut, I., et al. (2005). Initial presentation of childhood-onset systemic lupus erythematosus: A French multicenter study. *Journal of Pediatrics, 146,* 648–653.

Baxter Healthcare Corporation. (2006). *Primary immunodeficiency (e-textbook).* Accessed 4/29/06 at www.immunedisease.com/US/hcp/etextbook/index.html.

Berrien, V. M., Salazar, J. C., Reynolds, E., & McKay, K. (2004). Adherence to antiretroviral therapy in HIV-infected pediatric patients improves with home-based intensive nursing intervention. *AIDS Patient Care and STDs, 18*(6), 355–363.

Buckley, R. H. (2006). Combined immunodeficiency diseases. In J. A. McMillan (Ed.), *Oski's pediatrics: Principles and practice* (4th ed.). Philadelphia: Lippincott Williams & Wilkins.

Camm, J. (2005). Allergic reaction. *Community Practitioner, 78*(7), 234–235.

Casale, T. B., & Stokes, J. R. (2006). Urticaria and angioedema. In J. A. McMillan (Ed.), *Oski's pediatrics: Principles and practice* (4th ed.). Philadelphia: Lippincott Williams & Wilkins.

Cassidy, J. T. (2006). Rheumatic diseases of childhood. In J. A. McMillan (Ed.), *Oski's pediatrics: Principles and practice* (4th ed.). Philadelphia: Lippincott Williams & Wilkins.

Centers for Disease Control & Prevention (1994). *1994 Revised classification system for human immunodeficiency virus infection in children less than 13 years of age* [electronic version]. Available at www.cdc.gov/mmwr/preview/mmwrhtml/00032890.htm.

Chamberlain, J. (2006). Preventing food allergies in children: Some effective measures, but many unknown. *Infectious Diseases in Children, 19*(2), 72.

Chiappini, E., Galli, L., Gabiano, C., Tovo, P., & de Martino, M. (2006). Early triple therapy vs. mono or dual therapy for children with perinatal HIV infection. *Journal of the American Medical Association, 295*(6), 626–628.

Chiriboga, C. A., Fleishman, J. S., Champion, S., Gaye-Robinson, L., & Abrams, E. J. (2005). Incidence and prevalence of HIV encephalopathy in children with HIV infection receiving highly active anti-retroviral therapy (HAART). *Journal of Pediatrics*, 402–407.

Connelly, T. W. (2005). Family functioning and hope in children with juvenile rheumatoid arthritis. *Maternal Child Nursing*, 30(4), 245–250.

Domek, G. J. (2006). Social consequences of antiretroviral therapy: Preparing for the unexpected futures of HIV-positive children. *Lancet*, 367, 1367–1369.

Dominguez, K. L. (2006). Prophylaxis for exposure to human immunodeficiency virus. In J. A. McMillan (Ed.), *Oski's pediatrics: Principles and practice* (4th ed.). Philadelphia: Lippincott Williams & Wilkins.

Elder, J. S. (2006). Latex gloves: Time for a change. *The Journal of Urology*, 175(4), 1193–1194.

Ellaurie, M. (2004). Thrombocytosis in pediatric HIV infection. *Clinical Pediatrics*, 43(7), 627–629.

Farland, E. J. (2005). Human immunodeficiency virus infection. In W. W. Hay, M. J. Levin, J. M. Sondheimer, & R. R. Deterding (Eds.), *Current pediatric diagnosis & treatment* (17th ed.). New York: McGraw-Hill.

Frost, D. W., & Chalin, C. G. (2005). The effect of income on anaphylaxis preparation and management plans in Toronto primary schools. *Canadian Journal of Public Health*, 96(4), 250–253.

Gelfand, E. W. (2005). Critical decisions in selecting an intravenous immunoglobulin product. *Journal of Infusion Nursing*, 28(6), 366–374.

Gillespie, C. A., Woodgate, R. L., Chalmers, K. I., & Watson, W. T. A. (2007). "Living with risk": Mothering a child with food-induced anaphylaxis. *Journal of Pediatric Nursing*, 22(1), 30–42.

Golden, D. B. K. (2007). What is anaphylaxis? *Current Opinion in Allergy & Clinical Immunology*, 7(4), 331–336.

Grimshaw, K. E. (2006). Dietary management of food allergy in children. *Proceedings of the Nutrition Society*, 65(4), 412–417.

Hashkes, P. J., & Laxer, R. M. (2005). Medical treatment of juvenile idiopathic arthritis. *Journal of the American Medical Association*, 294, 1671–1684.

Hayward, A. R. (2005). Immunodeficiency. In W. W. Hay, M. J. Levin, J. M. Sondheimer, & R. R. Deterding (Eds.), *Current pediatric diagnosis & treatment* (17th ed.). New York: McGraw-Hill.

Health Resources and Services Administration, The HIV/AIDS Bureau. (2006). *Ryan White CARE Act*. Washington, DC: United States Department of Health and Human Services.

Hollister, J. R. (2005). Rheumatic diseases. In W. W. Hay, M. J. Levin, J. M. Sondheimer, & R. R. Deterding (Eds.), *Current pediatric diagnosis & treatment* (17th ed.) New York: McGraw-Hill.

Houck, J. (2005). HIV disease and AIDS. In S. M. Nettina (Ed.), *Lippincott manual of nursing practice*. Philadelphia: Lippincott Williams & Wilkins.

Hughes, W. T., Dankner, W. M., Yogev, R., Huange, S., Paul, M. E., Flores, M. S., et al. (2005). Comparison of atovaquone and azithromycin with trimethoprim-sulfamethoxazole for the prevention of serious bacterial infections in children with HIV infection. *Clinical Infectious Diseases*, 40, 136–145.

Immune Deficiency Foundation. (2005). *IDF patient and family handbook for the primary immune deficiency diseases* (3rd ed.). Retrieved 3/12/06 from http://www.primaryimmune.org/pubs/book_pats/book_pats.htm.

Jones, K., & Walsek, C. (2005). Pediatric immunologic disorders. In S. M. Nettina (Ed.), *Lippincott manual of nursing practice*. Philadelphia: Lippincott Williams & Wilkins.

King, S. M. (2004). Evaluation and treatment of the human immunodeficiency virus-1-exposed infant. *Pediatrics*, 114(2), 497–505.

Laffort, C., Le Deist, F., Favre, M., Caillat-Zucman, S., Radfore-Weiss, I., Debre, M., et al. (2004). Severe cutaneous papillomavirus disease after haemopoietic stem-cell transplantation. *Lancet*, 363, 2051–2054.

Lane, R. D., & Bolte, R. G. (2007). Pediatric anaphylaxis. *Pediatric Emergency Care*, 23(1) 49–60.

Lederman, H. M. (2006). Primary immunodeficiency diseases. In J. A. McMillan (Ed.), *Oski's pediatrics: Principles and practice* (4th ed.). Philadelphia: Lippincott Williams & Wilkins.

Lederman, H. M. (2006). Disorders of humoral immunity. In J. A. McMillan (Ed.), *Oski's pediatrics: Principles and practice* (4th ed.). Philadelphia: Lippincott Williams & Wilkins.

Lederman, H. M. (2006). The immune system. In J. A. McMillan (Ed.), *Oski's pediatrics: Principles and practice* (4th ed.). Philadelphia: Lippincott Williams & Wilkins.

Lee, G. M., Gortmaker, S. L., McIntosh, K., Hughes, M. D., Oleske, J. M., & Pediatric AIDS Clinical Trials Group Protocol 219C Team. (2006). Quality of life for children and adolescents: Impact of HIV infection and antiretroviral treatment. *Pediatrics, 117*(2), 273–283.

McIntyre, C. L., Sheetz, A. H., Carroll, C. R., & Young, M. C. (2005). Administration of epinephrine for life-threatening allergic reactions in school settings. *Pediatrics, 116*(5), 1134–1140.

McKinney, R. E. (2006). Antiretroviral therapy in pediatric acquired immunodeficiency syndrome. In J. A. McMillan (Ed.), *Oski's pediatrics: Principles and practice* (4th ed.). Philadelphia: Lippincott Williams & Wilkins.

Miller-Hoover, S. (2005). Juvenile idiopathic arthritis: Why do I have to hurt so much? *Journal of Infusion Nursing, 28*(6), 385–391.

Morantz, C., & Torrey, B. (2004). Treatment of infants with HIV-1 infection. *American Family Physician, 70*(6), 1171–1172.

Morrison-Beedy, D., Nelson, L. E., & Volpe, E. (2005). HIV risk behaviors and testing rates in adolescent girls: Evidence to guide clinical practice. *Pediatric Nursing, 31*(6), 508–512.

Moylett, E. H., & Shearer, W. T. (2006). Pediatric human immunodeficiency virus infection. In J. A. McMillan (Ed.), *Oski's pediatrics: Principles and practice* (4th ed.). Philadelphia: Lippincott Williams & Wilkins.

Munoz-Furlong, A. (2003). Daily coping strategies for patients and their families. *Pediatrics, 111*(6), 1654–1661.

Muraro, A., Dreborg, S., Halken, S., Host, A., Niggemann, B., Aalberse, R., et al. (2004). Dietary prevention of allergic diseases in infants and small children, part III: Critical review of published peer-reviewed observational and interventional studies and final recommendations. *Pediatric Allergy and Immunology, 15,* 291–307.

Murphy, E., Martin, S., & Patterson, J. V. (2005). Developing practice guidelines for the administration of intravenous immunoglobulin. *Journal of Infusion Nursing, 28*(4), 265–272.

Niggeman, B., & Beyer, K. (2007). Diagnosis of food allergy in children: Toward a standardization of food challenge. *Journal of Pediatric Gastroenterology & Nutrition, 45*(4), 399–404.

Noble, K. A. (2005). The patient with latex allergy. *Journal of PeriAnesthesia Nursing, 20*(4), 285–288.

Ozol, D. & Mete, E. (2008). Asthma and food allergy. *Current Opinion in Pulmonary Medicine, 14*(1), 9–12.

Pagana, K. D., & Pagana, T. J. (2006). *Mosby's manual of diagnostic and laboratory tests* (3rd ed.). St. Louis: Mosby.

Patrick, C. C. (2006). Opportunistic infections in the compromised host. In J. A. McMillan (Ed.), *Oski's pediatrics: Principles and practice* (4th ed.). Philadelphia: Lippincott Williams & Wilkins.

Petry, L., Mathur, A., & Kamat, D. M. (2004). Immunodeficiency disorders: What should primary care providers know? *Consultant for Pediatricians, 3*(5), 228–232.

Plowfield, L. A. (2007). HIV disease in children 25 years later. *Pediatric Nursing, 33*(3), 273–278.

Read, J. S. (2007). Diagnosis of HIV-1 infection in children younger than 18 months in the United States. *Pediatrics, 120*, e1547–e1562.

Sampson, H. A. (2006). Food allergies. In J. A. McMillan (Ed.), *Oski's pediatrics: Principles and practice* (4th ed.). Philadelphia: Lippincott Williams & Wilkins.

Sampson, H. A., & Eggleston, P. A. (2006). General considerations of allergies in childhood. In J. A. McMillan (Ed.), *Oski's pediatrics: Principles and practice* (4th ed.). Philadelphia: Lippincott Williams & Wilkins.

Shah, I. (2005). Age-related clinical manifestations of HIV infection in Indian children. *Journal of Tropical Pediatrics, 51*(5), 300–303.

Symmons, D. (2005). Juvenile idiopathic arthritis: Issues of definition and causation. *International Journal of Epidemiology, 34,* 671–672.

Taketokmo, C. K., Hodding, J. H., & Kraus, D. M. (2007). *Lexi-comp's pediatric dosage handbook* (14th ed.). Hudson, OH: Lexi-comp.

Tretheway, P. (2004). Systemic lupus erythematosus. *Dimensions in Critical Care Nursing, 23*(3), 111–115.

UNICEF. (2006). *The state of the world's children 2007: Executive summary*. New York: Author.

United States House of Representatives. (2004). *Public Law No. 108-377 Asthmatic Schoolchildren's Treatment and Health Management Act of 2004*. Washington, DC: Library of Congress.

Watson, D. C., & Counts, D. R. (2004). Growth hormone deficiency in HIV-infected children following successful treatment with highly active antiretroviral therapy. *Journal of Pediatrics*, 549–551.

Weglarz, M., & Boland, M. (2005). Family-centered nursing care of the perinatally infected mother and child living with HIV infection. *Journal for Specialists in Pediatric Nursing*, *10*(4), 161–170.

Working Group on Antitetroviral Therapy and Medical Management of HIV-Infected Children. (2005). *Guidelines for the use of antiretroviral agents in pediatric HIV infection* [electronic version]. Available at http://aidsinfo.nih.gov/.

Wysocki, L. (2007). Anaphylaxis doesn't have to be a shock. *Nursing Made Incredibly Easy!*, *5*(6), 9–13.

WEBSITES

U.S. Department of Health and Human Services offers information on HIV/AIDS treatment, prevention, and research: http://aidsinfo.nih.gov/

American Academy of Allergy, Asthma, & Immunology: www.aaaai.org

Asthma & Allergy Foundation of America: www.aafa.org

Allergy & Asthma Network Mothers of Asthmatics: www.aanma.org

Anaphylaxis Canada: www.anaphylaxis.org

Arthritis Foundation—education, research, resources for patients, local chapters, and a juvenile arthritis division: American Juvenile Arthritis Organization: www.arthritis.org

Childhood Arthritis & Rheumatology Research Alliance: www.carragroup.info/

Centers for Disease Control's National Prevention and Information Network: www.cdcnpin.org/

Coordinating center for the Pediatric Rheumatology Collaborative Research Group (PRCRG)—research and clinical trials: www.cincinnatichildrens.org/Research/Divisions/Rheumatology/default.htm

Canadian Society of Allergy and Clinical Immunology: www.csaci.medical.org

American Dietetic Association: www.eatright.org

Food Allergy & Anaphylaxis Network—focuses on education, advocacy, research, and awareness: www.foodallergy.org

HIV infection information: www.hivpositive.com/

National Primary Immunodeficiency Research Center—increasing public awareness: www.info4pi.org

Jeffery Modell Foundation—dedicated to research, physician and patient education, patient support, and public awareness: www.jmfworld.org

Lupus Alliance of America—support, education, and resources for lupus patients: www.lupusalliance.org

Lupus Foundation of America—support, education, resources for lupus patients, local support chapters: www.lupus.org

MedicAlert Foundation: www.medicalert.org

National Institute of Arthritis and Musculoskeletal and Skin Diseases through the National Institutes of Health—health information, research, and training: www.niams.nih.gov/

Elizabeth Glaser Pediatric AIDS Foundation—resources for HIV-infected children and their families: www.pedaids.org

Immune Deficiency Foundation—a national organization dedicated to research, education, and advocacy for the primary immune deficiency diseases; has patient and family resources: www.primaryimmune.org

American College of Rheumatology—educational materials, guidelines, and referrals: www.rheumatology.org

Education, support, resources on severe combined immunodeficiency: www.scid.net

Complete HIV/AIDS resource: www.thebody.com/

Pediatric HIV infection and AIDS resources: www.vachss.com/help_text/hiv_aids_ped.html

Resources for prevention and treatment of HIV infection: www.womenchildrenhiv.org/

CHAPTER WORKSHEET

MULTIPLE CHOICE QUESTIONS

1. The nurse is caring for a 6-year-old with juvenile idiopathic arthritis. The mother states that she has trouble getting her daughter out of bed in the morning and believes the girl's behavior is due to a desire to avoid going to school. What is the best advice by the nurse?

   a. Refer the girl to a psychologist for evaluation of school phobia related to chronic illness.

   b. Administer a warm bath every morning before school.

   c. Give the child her prescribed NSAIDs 30 minutes before getting out of bed.

   d. Allow her to stay in bed some mornings if she wants.

2. A 14-year-old with systemic lupus erythematosus wants to know how to care for her skin. What should the nurse teach this adolescent?

   a. Careful sun tanning will give your skin an attractive color.

   b. No special skin care is needed.

   c. Use sunscreen daily to avoid rashes.

   d. Use makeup to camouflage the butterfly rash on her face.

3. The mother of a child with hypogammaglobulinemia reports that her child had a fever and slight chills with an intravenous gammaglobulin infusion last month. She wants to know what other course of treatment might be available. What is the best response by the nurse?

   a. Administration of acetaminophen or diphenhydramine prior to the next infusion may decrease the incidence of fever or chills.

   b. Giving the gammaglobulin intramuscularly is recommended to prevent a reaction.

   c. Talk to her physician about alternative medications that may be used to boost the gamma-globulin level in the blood.

   d. If the child is no longer experiencing frequent infections, then the IV infusions may not be necessary.

4. A 4-month-old infant born to an HIV-infected mother is going into foster care because the mother is too ill to care for the child. The foster mother wants to know if the infant is also infected. What is the best response by the nurse?

   a. "It's too early to know; we have to wait until the infant has symptoms."

   b. "Since the mother is so ill, it's likely the child is also infected with HIV."

   c. "The ELISA test is positive, so the child is definitely infected."

   d. "The PCR test is positive; this indicates HIV infection, which may or may not progress to AIDS."

5. A mother has received instructions about avoiding wheat and soy allergens. Which response by the mother would indicate that further education is needed?

   a. "I will not feed my child any breads made with wheat flour."

   b. "I will allow my child to eat semolina pasta, the kind he loves."

   c. "I will not feed my child shakes made with soy protein."

   d. "I will read labels to be sure I am avoiding wheat and soy."

CRITICAL THINKING EXERCISES

1. Develop a discharge teaching plan for a 14-year-old with systemic lupus erythematosus who will be taking corticosteroids long term.

2. Devise a developmental stimulation plan for a 22-month-old with HIV infection and encephalopathy with developmental delay (to the level of a 9-month-old).

3. Determine an appropriate nursing plan of care for an infant who has undergone bone marrow transplantation for severe combined immune deficiency.

4. Develop a prioritized list of nursing diagnoses for a child with HIV infection, candidiasis, poor growth, and pneumonia requiring oxygen.

5. A child with recurrent infections is being evaluated. Other than information about onset of symptoms and events leading up to this present episode, what other types of information would the nurse ask while obtaining the history?

STUDY ACTIVITIES

1. In the clinical setting, compare the growth and development of two children the same age, one with HIV infection and one who has been healthy.

2. Attend an outpatient clinic that provides care to children with HIV infection. Observe the physician or nurse practitioner during office visits and attend a multidisciplinary planning meeting. Identify the role of the registered nurse in providing family education, coordination of care, and referrals.

3. Conduct an Internet search to determine the educational material available to children and their families related to immune deficiencies, autoimmune disorders, or allergies.

4. Research your clinical institution's policies related to latex allergy, alternative products available at the institution, and how to obtain them for a latex-allergic patient. Provide a presentation to your clinical group about your findings.

NURSING CARE OF THE CHILD WITH AN ENDOCRINE DISORDER

KEY TERMS

adrenarche
beta cells
constitutional delay
diabetic ketoacidosis
  (DKA)
exophthalmos
gland
glucose
glycosylated hemoglobin

goiter
gonad
hirsutism
hormone
hyperfunction/
  hypersecretion
hypofunction/
  hyposecretion
ketoacidosis

ketone
Kussmaul respiration
menarche
polydipsia
polyphagia
polyuria
tetany

Carlos Rodriguez, 12 years old, is seen in the clinic today with complaints of weakness, fatigue, blurred vision, and headaches. His mother states, "Carlos' teacher has noticed mood changes and is concerned about his behavior at school. He's always been a good boy. I'm not sure what's going on."

LEARNING OBJECTIVES

Upon completion of the chapter, the learner will be able to:

1. Describe the major components and functions of a child's endocrine system.
2. Differentiate between the anatomic and physiologic differences of the endocrine system in children versus adults.
3. Identify the essential assessment elements, common diagnostic procedures, and laboratory tests associated with the diagnosis of endocrine disorders in children.
4. Identify the common medications and treatment modalities used for palliation of endocrine disorders in children.
5. Distinguish specific disorders of the endocrine system affecting children.
6. Link the clinical manifestations of specific disorders in the endocrine system of a child with the appropriate nursing diagnoses.
7. Establish the nursing outcomes, evaluative criteria, and interventions for a child with specific disorders in the endocrine system.
8. Develop child/family teaching plans for the child with an endocrine disorder.

WOW

Endocrine disorders in children often elude the medical radar screen.

The endocrine system consists of various **glands**, tissues, or clusters of cells that produce and release hormones. **Hormones** are chemical messengers that stimulate and/or regulate the actions of other tissues, organs, or other endocrine glands that have specific receptors to a hormone. Along with the nervous system, the endocrine milieu influences all physiologic effects such as growth and development, metabolic processes related to fluid and electrolyte balance and energy production, sexual maturation and reproduction, and the body's response to stress. The release patterns of the hormones vary, but the level in the body is maintained within specified limits to preserve health.

Problems develop in the endocrine system when there is a deficiency (**hypofunction**) or excess (**hyperfunction**) of a specific hormone. In children, endocrine conditions often develop insidiously and result from an insufficient production of hormones. If the problem is not diagnosed and treated early, delayed growth and development, cognitive impairments, or death may result. Generally, the treatment plan involves correction of the underlying reason for the dysfunction, such as surgical removal of a tumor, and supplementation of missing hormones or adjustment of specific hormone levels. This allows most children to live normal lives.

Variations in Anatomy and Physiology

The organs or tissues of the endocrine system include the hypothalamus, pituitary gland, thyroid gland, parathyroid glands, adrenal glands, gonads, and the islets of Langerhans located in the pancreas. Figure 48.1 shows the location of the organs or tissues involved in the endocrine system. Typically, most endocrine glands begin to develop during the first trimester of gestation, but their development is incomplete at birth. Thus, complete hormonal control is lacking during the early years of life, and the infant cannot appropriately balance fluid concentration, electrolytes, amino acids, **glucose**, and trace substances.

Hormone Production and Secretion

The hypothalamic-pituitary axis produces a number of releasing and inhibiting hormones that regulate the function of many of the other endocrine glands, including the thyroid gland, the adrenal glands, and the male and female gonads. Some glands regulate their function in connection with the nervous system, such as the islets of Langerhans in the pancreas and the parathyroid glands. Many other cells in the body secrete hormones such as the pineal gland, the scattered epithelial cells in the gastrointestinal tract, and the thymus. Disorders related to these other cells as well as gonad dysfunction are discussed in other chapters in this textbook.

Figure 48.1 shows the major glands, the hormones produced by the glands, and the effect each hormone has on the target cell, tissue, or organ. The process of hormone production and secretion involves the principle of feedback control. One gland produces a hormone that affects another endocrine gland. Once the physiologic effect is achieved, this gland, known as the target organ, inhibits the further release of the original hormone. The reverse occurs when the first gland detects low levels of the target gland hormone. If the original gland does not release enough of the hormone, the inhibition process stops so that the gland increases the production of the hormone. The endocrine system and the nervous system work closely together to maintain an optimal internal environment for the body, known as homeostasis.

Common Medical Treatments

Primarily, the treatment of endocrine disorders involves decreasing hormone production (in cases of hypersecretion) or replacing the hormones (in cases of hypofunction). The first step in treating many of these disorders is to screen for potential problems, especially when familial patterns are present. Since the proper functioning of the endocrine system is critical to growth and development, the child's growth is affected by endocrine dysfunction and lack of treatment may lead to mental retardation. Early treatment is often associated with better prognosis and prevention of long-term problems. The next step in treatment involves identifying underlying causes for the dysfunction (e.g., a tumor or growth that requires surgical removal or irradiation). The use of supplemental hormone in cases of hypofunction is generally successful in children, as is the use of inhibiting substances in cases of hyperfunction.

Common Medical Treatments 48.1 describes the common treatments used in children with endocrine disorders. The table explains and gives indications for each treatment as well as relevant nursing implications. Advances in technology and our understanding of molecular biology continue to increase our knowledge of these disorders and the modalities needed to prevent them or improve quality of life for affected children. These advances are vital, since the whole body is influenced by the endocrine milieu.

Drug Guide 48.1 lists the medications most commonly used to treat endocrine disorders. The table gives the actions and indications of each drugs, as well as pertinent nursing implications. Many of the medications are synthetic preparations of the actual hormones. It is important to maintain specific blood levels of the drugs to mimic the actual hormone in the body. Nurses must monitor for side effects of too little or too much of the hormone in the child's system. Most endocrine disorders in children require treatment and follow-up with a pediatric endocrinologist as well as a multidisciplinary team that includes a registered nurse who specializes in this area.

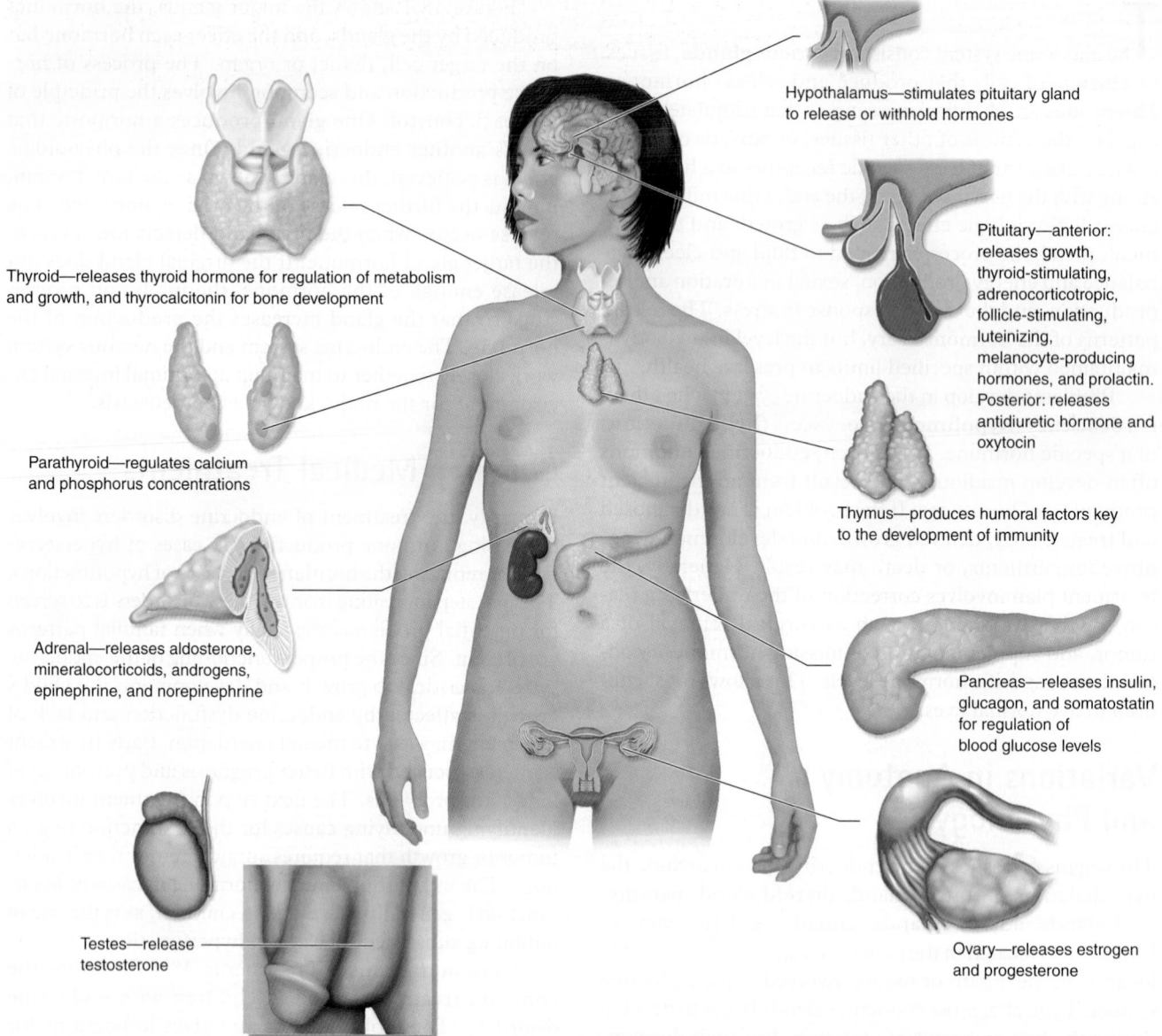

Hypothalamus—stimulates pituitary gland to release or withhold hormones

Pituitary—anterior: releases growth, thyroid-stimulating, adrenocorticotropic, follicle-stimulating, luteinizing, melanocyte-producing hormones, and prolactin. Posterior: releases antidiuretic hormone and oxytocin

Thyroid—releases thyroid hormone for regulation of metabolism and growth, and thyrocalcitonin for bone development

Parathyroid—regulates calcium and phosphorus concentrations

Thymus—produces humoral factors key to the development of immunity

Adrenal—releases aldosterone, mineralocorticoids, androgens, epinephrine, and norepinephrine

Pancreas—releases insulin, glucagon, and somatostatin for regulation of blood glucose levels

Testes—release testosterone

Ovary—releases estrogen and progesterone

FIGURE 48.1 Location of the endocrine glands in the body, with the major effects of the glands listed.

NURSING PROCESS OVERVIEW FOR THE CHILD WITH AN ENDOCRINE DISORDER

The nursing care of the child with an endocrine disorder requires astute assessment skills, accurate nursing diagnoses and expected outcomes, skilled interventions, and evaluation of the entire process. Children, especially very young ones, easily develop imbalances such as fluid and electrolyte disturbances that can cause further problems. Most of the endocrine disorders are chronic conditions that require ongoing care related to health maintenance, education, developmental issues, and psychosocial needs.

These conditions are sometimes complex and range from mild to profound. Early diagnosis and treatment can improve the long-term outcomes for these children.

Remember Carlos, the 12-year-old with weakness, fatigue, blurred vision, headaches, and mood changes? What additional health history and physical examination assessment information should the nurse obtain?

Assessment

Nursing assessment of a child with endocrine dysfunction includes obtaining a thorough health history, performing a physical assessment, and assisting with or obtaining

COMMON MEDICAL TREATMENTS 48.1

Treatment	Explanation	Indications	Nursing Implications
Newborn metabolic screening programs	Newborn blood testing to identify certain disorders	Identification of newborns so that treatment can begin early to prevent impact of disorder, such as severe cognitive impairment or death	• Refer to each state's protocol for fetal/newborn screening for endocrine disorders. • Explain to family the rationale and procedure. • Infant should be feeding for 24 hours prior to collection. • Collect blood sample accurately. • IV antibiotic use in newborn may affect results. • Ensure screening is done for early discharges.
Surgery	Surgical removal of tumors or cysts	Any endocrine malfunction caused by the presence of a mass	• Provide routine preoperative and postoperative care, depending on location and extent of surgery. • Keep family informed of choices.
Irradiation/ radioactive iodine	Radiation is used to influence the hormone secretion of a gland; it is less invasive than surgery.	Hyperfunction of an endocrine gland; may be used when surgery is not possible	• Prepare child for specific procedures following protocols. • Explain the procedure. • Check to ensure child has no sensitivity to iodine preparations.
Glucose monitoring	Fingerstick blood sample several times per day	Monitoring of glucose control	• Teach family appropriate procedure. • Refer family to sources for equipment and supplies. • Assist family to develop a system of record-keeping that works for them.
Dietary interventions	Restriction or manipulation of dietary intake	Diabetes mellitus	• Refer family to a dietitian specializing in pediatric diabetes mellitus. • Reinforce teaching related to special diets.

laboratory and diagnostic tests. The clinical manifestations of endocrine disorders occur as a result of the altered control of the bodily processes normally regulated by the gland or hormone. These manifestations present in many areas of the body because of the diverse functions associated with the endocrine system.

Health History

Focus the health history on the possibility of a family history of an endocrine disorder, prenatal history, history of chronic childhood disease, and growth and development patterns. Use a genogram or family tree to detail the information about the family history in a clear and concise manner.

Endocrine disorders often cause problems in normal growth and development as well as behavioral changes.

Question the parent or caregiver about prior growth patterns, achievement of developmental milestones, and the child's behavior. Have the child and family describe the child's activities on a typical day, including school performance, to identify subtle variations in the child's behavior or moods. For example, a child who is typically quiet might ordinarily be less active than average children of that age, and the child with decreased endocrine function also often displays inactivity and fatigue. By having the family and child describe a typical day, the nurse can distinguish between what is appropriate for that child and what may be a change related to endocrine dysfunction.

In addition, obtain a history of dietary and elimination habits. Note extreme thirst, excessive appetite, vomiting, or frequent voiding. Children with endocrine disorders

DRUG GUIDE 48.1   Common Drugs for Endocrine Disorders

Medication	Action/Indication	Nursing Implications
Insulin	Used diabetes mellitus to replace body's natural insulin, which is necessary for proper glucose use	• Monitor vital signs and blood glucose levels. • Educate child and family on proper techniques, actions, and adverse effects. • Rotate site of injections to prevent adipose hypertrophy.
Oral hypoglycemic drugs (glipizide, glyburide, metformin)	Assists body's production of insulin by stimulating beta cells to secrete more insulin. Indicated for diabetes mellitus type 2.	• Monitor vital signs and glucose levels. • Administer with food to minimize gastric upset. • Instruct child and family on use of drug and adverse effects. • Warn family that some over-the-counter or other drugs may increase hypoglycemic effect.
Growth hormone (GH)/somatropin (Humatrope)	Stimulates linear bone, skeletal muscle, and organ growth. Used for GH deficiency, growth failure related to inadequate pituitary hormone.	• Monitor blood sugar and electrolyte levels. • Administer before epiphyses are fused. • Monitor growth with accurate measurements. • Instruct child and family on appropriate route and method of administration. • Periodic thyroid function tests will be needed. • May interact with glucocorticoid therapy • Monitor for limping or complaints in knee or hip related to slipped epiphysis.
Octreotide acetate (Sandostatin)	Suppresses GH release Acromegaly	• Monitor for biliary tract abnormalities, glucose tolerance, and hypothyroidism. • Give subcutaneous injections between meals to decrease gastric effects. • Refer family to www.pap.novartis.com for assistance with covering cost of drug.
Corticosteroids (dexamethasone or hydrocortisone)	Cortisol replacement in congenital adrenal hyperplasia, absence of adrenal glands. Also used to close epiphyseal plates in hyperpituitarism.	• Give with milk or food. • May need to increase dose if child is ill or runs fever • Monitor for edema, weight gain, glycosuria, signs of infection, and symptoms of peptic ulcer development. • Do not decrease dose or abruptly stop drug to avoid adrenal crisis.
Desmopressin acetate (DDAVP)	Synthetic antidiuretic hormone that promotes reabsorption of water by action on renal tubules. Used to control diabetes insipidus.	• Contraindicated in nephrogenic diabetes insipidus. • Monitor for water intoxication and adverse effects such as nasal irritation, headache, nausea, increased blood pressure. • Record input and output and weigh child daily. • Titrate dose until appropriate output is obtained. • Instruct child and family in proper intranasal administration. • Avoid over-the-counter cough/hay fever preparations, as they may decrease the drug response. • Store in refrigerator.

Medication	Action/Indication	Nursing Implications
Levothyroxine (Synthroid)	Thyroid hormone replacement for hypothyroidism.	• Check blood pressure and pulse before each dose. • Monitor input and output and daily weights. • Watch for thyroid storm. • Report irritability or anxiety. • Instruct child and family to avoid over-the-counter preparations with iodine or foods such as soybeans, iodized salt, tofu, turnips. • Administer at same time each day.
Methimazole, propylthiouracil	Antithyroid drug; blocks synthesis of T3 and T4. Indicated for hyperthyroidism.	• Check pulse and blood pressure before each dose. • Monitor input and output, daily weights, serum T3 and T4 levels; watch for edema, leukopenia, thrombocytopenia, or agranulocytosis. • Administer with meals to decrease gastric upset. • Give at the same time each day. • Store in light-resistant container. • Instruct child and family to report sore throat, mouth lesions, unusual bleeding or bruising. • Signs of overdose: periorbital edema, cold intolerance, mental depression • Signs of inadequate dose: tachycardia, diarrhea, fever, or irritability
Mineralocorticoid (Florinef)	Promotes reabsorption of Na and K, water from distal renal tubules. Used in adrenal insufficiency.	• Monitor daily weights, blood pressure, intake and output. • Observe for potassium depletion. • Titrate dose to lowest effective dose. • Adverse effects include flushing, sweating, headache, increased blood pressure.

may have some of these symptoms. Table 48.1 lists the types of questions to ask or areas to review when obtaining a health history on a child with possible endocrine dysfunction.

Physical Examination

Table 48.2 lists key physical examination findings that may be present in the child with endocrine dysfunction.

Inspection and Observation

Note a fatigued appearance, cool or dry skin, poor muscle tone, sweatiness, faintness, nervousness, or confusion. Inspect the head and face, noting coarse or brittle hair, excessive hair growth, a rounded face, a protuberant tongue, drooping eyelids, or **exophthalmos** (protrusion of the eyeballs). On inspection of the mouth, note delayed dentition or a fruity breath odor. Note early, excessive, or delayed growth of the genitals. Plot the child's height and weight on growth charts to determine abnormal growth velocity, which occurs in many of these disorders.

Auscultation

Auscultate the heart and lungs. Note tachycardia or irregular heart rhythm. During auscultation of the lungs, note labored respiratory effort, such as Kussmaul breathing, which occurs in diabetic ketoacidosis. Document the blood pressure.

Percussion and Palpation

Percuss and then palpate the abdomen. Dull (nontympanic) sounds or the presence of masses may indicate constipation or a tumor of the ovaries.

Laboratory and Diagnostic Testing

Common Laboratory and Diagnostic Tests 48.1 describes the diagnostic tests and procedures frequently used in identifying and monitoring endocrine disorders in children. Serum and urine hormone and other levels are used to determine whether amounts are adequate, deficient, or excessive. Radiographic studies are used to evaluate bone

TABLE 48.1 HEALTH HISTORY QUESTIONS RELATED TO ENDOCRINE DISORDERS

General Demographics	Gender, Age
Present illness	Gradual or sudden onset of symptoms Changes in child's lifestyle, physical appearance, sleep patterns, appetite, thirst, vision, bowel and urinary habits, or nausea and vomiting Recent increases or decreases in weight and height, muscle weakness, cramps, twitching, or headaches
Past medical history	Birth: any neonatal screening done and results, trauma during birth, birth size, feeding difficulties Prenatal history: maternal factors that may affect growth and development such as substance abuse, use of tobacco or alcohol, Graves' disease Past health: treated for any endocrine problem in the past, recent gastroenteritis or viral syndrome Current immunization status
Allergies	History of allergies to medications, foods, milk or formula
Current medications	Prescribed, over-the-counter, or home remedies
Family history	Any endocrine disorders or growth and development difficulties
Environmental exposure	Exposure to exogenous steroids or gonadotropins
Social history	Normal daily activities; activity level; family resources such as insurance and support systems to maintain long-term treatment regimen
Growth and development milestones	History of growth patterns Presence of learning disabilities, cognitive delays, early or late development of secondary sexual characteristics

TABLE 48.2 KEY PHYSICAL EXAMINATION FINDINGS RELATED TO ENDOCRINE PROBLEMS

Height and weight	Below third percentile or above 90th percentile (pituitary, thyroid, adrenal, or diabetes mellitus)
Hair	Coarse, brittle, excessive (hypothyroidism) Abnormal distribution (adrenal disorders)
Face	Round with hair growth (Cushing's syndrome) Deformities or abnormal features (hypoparathyroidism)
Eyes	Blurred or changes in vision (diabetes mellitus, pituitary tumors, precocious puberty)
Mouth	Delayed dentition (hypocalcemia, hypopituitarism) Fruity breath (ketoacidosis)
Neck	Goiter (hyperthyroidism)
Skin	Cool to touch, dry (hypothyroidism) Changes in color or texture (pituitary disorders) Easy bruising, striae (Cushing's syndrome)
Chest	Tachycardia (hyperthyroidism) Palpitations, sweating (thyroid disorders) Deep, labored breathing (ketoacidosis) Hypertension (Cushing's syndrome)
Abdomen	Extreme weight loss (diabetes mellitus) Extreme fat (Cushing's syndrome) Changes in bowel habits (SIADH, diabetes insipidus, diabetes mellitus)
Fingers	Trembling (hyperthyroidism, parathyroid disorders)
Genitals	Excessive growth (adrenogenital syndrome) Early growth (precocious puberty) Delayed growth (hypopituitarism)

COMMON LABORATORY AND DIAGNOSTIC TESTS 48.1

Diagnostic Test or Procedure	Explanation	Indication	Nursing Implications
Random serum hormone levels	Serum levels of various hormones; immunoassay measures levels with very small amounts of blood	High or low levels are used to evaluate the function of the specific gland.	• May need to draw specimens at specific times. • Keep child NPO after midnight before test if ordered. • Diurnal variations and episodic secretion of many hormones may require special directions or further testing.
Genetic testing	Identify DNA sequencing	Determines genetic involvement of any disorder	• Explain procedure and the expense involved. • Refer for genetic counseling if needed.
Serum chemistry levels	Serum blood urea nitrogen (BUN), creatinine, sodium, potassium, glucose, calcium, phosphorus, alkaline phosphatase, etc.	To rule out chronic renal failure or other chronic illnesses; to monitor effects of treatment	• BUN levels may be elevated with high-protein diet or dehydration, may be decreased with overhydration or malnutrition. • A diet high in meat may cause a transient but not pronounced increase in creatinine. There are also slight diurnal variations in levels. • Avoid hemolysis of specimen, as this may cause elevation in potassium levels. • Calcium and phosphorus: avoid prolonged tourniquet use during blood draw, as this may falsely increase levels. Child should be NPO past midnight prior to the morning of the blood draw.
Growth hormone stimulation	Stimulate release of GH in response to administration of insulin, arginine, or clonidine	Evaluate and diagnose GH deficiency	• Keep child NPO for specified time. • Obtain serial blood samples at specific times. • Monitor blood glucose levels during study. • Observe for signs of hypoglycemia, diaphoresis, somnolence. • Provide cookies and punch at end of test.
Water deprivation study	Child is deprived of fluids for several hours, and serum sodium and urine osmolality are monitored.	Diabetes insipidus	• Stop test if child exhibits extreme weight loss or changes in vital signs or neurologic status. • Weigh child before, during, and after test. • Rehydrate child after test. • Monitor for orthostatic hypotension.

(continued)

COMMON LABORATORY AND DIAGNOSTIC TESTS 48.1 (continued)

Diagnostic Test or Procedure	Explanation	Indication	Nursing Implications
Bone age radiograph	Radiographic study of wrist or hand to determine bone maturation compared to national standards	Determine if bone age is consistent with chronologic age to rule out GH deficiency or excess or hypothyroidism	• Explain procedure to child because child must hold still for the x-ray. • Allow family to accompany child. Enlist the family's help if needed to calm child during x-ray.
Other nuclear medicine studies	Contrast media uptake is assessed with serial radiographs.	To visualize an ectopic, enlarged, absent, or nodular gland	• Assess child for allergy to iodine or shellfish. • Explain procedure to child.
Computed tomography or magnetic resonance imaging of brain	Noninvasive imaging methods to identify abnormalities of brain or other areas as necessary	Evaluate presence of tumors, cysts, or structural abnormalities that may affect specific gland or structure	• Machine is large and can be frightening to children. • Scan may be lengthy and the child must remain still, so sedation may be necessary. • If contrast medium is to be used, assess for allergy. • Encourage fluids after procedure if not contraindicated.
Ultrasonography	Noninvasive sound waves are used to visualize structures such as thyroid or pelvic region.	Evaluate presence of tumors or cysts in specific gland, such as the adrenal glands or ovaries, to rule out disorders	• Requires full bladder if in pelvic region.

maturation and growth potential as well as density or tissue calcification. Genetic studies may be used to determine enzyme deficiencies or chromosome defects. Stimulation studies provide a more accurate or definitive test for identifying the disorder after preliminary serum levels are abnormal. Serial blood sampling identifies peak or trough levels of hormones. Computed tomography (CT) scans, magnetic resonance imaging (MRI), nuclear medicine studies, and ultrasonography are used to look for tumors, cysts, or structural defects.

Nursing Diagnoses, Goals, Interventions, and Evaluation

After completing the assessment, the nurse identifies nursing diagnoses with related goals/outcomes, interventions, and evaluations. The nursing diagnoses for a child with endocrine dysfunction may include:

• Delayed growth and development
• Disturbed body image
• Deficient knowledge
• Interrupted family processes
• Imbalanced nutrition: less than or more than body requirements
• Deficient or excess fluid volume
• Noncompliance

After completing an assessment of Carlos, the nurse noted the following: history reveals Carlos has had episodes of bedwetting over the past month and has had polydipsia and polyphagia. His weight continues to be greater than the 95th percentile on the growth chart. Based on these assessment findings, what would your top three nursing diagnoses be for Carlos?

Because of the gradual, insidious onset of many of these disorders, the child may first be seen in an acute situation. It may be easier for the child and family to work with short-term goals until they accept the chronic situation. A major goal will be to achieve compliance with medical management. The goals for the child with a disorder of the endocrine system generally include re-establishing homeostasis, promoting adequate growth and development, establishing appropriate body image, promoting health-seeking behaviors, and providing education so the family can manage the condition.

Nursing Care Plan 48.1 can be used as a guide in planning care for the child with a disorder of the endocrine system. Of course, this plan will need to be individualized based on the child's symptoms, needs, and disorder as well as the family's requirements. A key element to include in

(text continues on page 1596)

Nursing Care Plan 48.1

OVERVIEW FOR THE CHILD WITH AN ENDOCRINE DISORDER

NURSING DIAGNOSIS: Delayed growth and development related to hypo- or hyperfunction of gland/hormone as evidenced by weight and/or height less than expected for age, failure to meet expected age-appropriate developmental milestones

Outcome Identification and Evaluation
Nutritional status will be maximized and development will be enhanced: *child will maintain or gain weight appropriately and will make continued progress toward expected developmental milestones.*

Interventions: Enhancing Growth and Development
- Monitor growth parameters using standard growth charts.
- Encourage favorite foods (within prescribed diet restrictions if present) *to maximize oral intake.*
- Consult dietitian *for appropriate diet supplementation recommendations.*
- Encourage compliance with hormone supplementation *to enhance ability to achieve appropriate growth.*
- Provide care related to any complications of dysfunction *such as correcting fluid and electrolyte imbalances or diarrhea.*
- Screen for developmental capabilities *to determine child's current level of functioning.*
- Offer age-appropriate toys, play, and activities (including gross motor) *to encourage further development.*
- Provide support to families of children with developmental delay *(progress in achieving developmental milestones can be slow and ongoing motivation is needed).*
- Reinforce positive attributes in the child *to maintain motivation.*

For the child with diabetes mellitus:
- Provide a calorie-appropriate, nonrestricted, well-balanced diet *to maintain appropriate growth.*
- Encourage three meals with two or three snacks with consistent carbohydrates *to maintain appropriate blood glucose levels and promote growth.*

NURSING DIAGNOSIS: Disturbed body image related to abnormal growth and development/changes in physical appearance due to hormone dysfunction as evidenced by verbalization of dissatisfaction with the child's or adolescent's looks

Outcome Identification and Evaluation
Child demonstrates appropriate self-esteem in relation to body image; *expresses positive feelings about self and participates in social activities.*

Interventions: Promoting Healthy Body Image
- Provide opportunities for child to explore feelings related to appearance: *venting feelings is associated with less body image disturbance.*
- Relate to child on age level, not appearance level: *"babying" a child who looks younger due to his or her small size reduces self-image.*
- Involve the child and especially the teen in the decision-making process: *a sense of control will improve body image.*
- Encourage the child to spend time with peers who have similar endocrine disorders: *peers' opinions are often better accepted than those of persons in authority, such as parents or health care professionals.*
- Refer to counseling or support groups *to further support the child.*

(continued)

Nursing Care Plan 48.1 (continued)

NURSING DIAGNOSIS: Deficient knowledge related to therapeutic regimen as evidenced by questions about endocrine disorder and self-management

Outcome Identification and Evaluation
Child and family will demonstrate sufficient understanding and skills for self-management; *verbalize information about disorder, complications/adverse effects, home care regimen, and long-term needs, and provide return demonstrations of medication administration or other procedures.*

Interventions: Promoting Knowledge Required for Self-management
- Assess child's developmental level and family's ability to absorb instruction *to determine how to approach teaching sessions.*
- Establish teaching plan with child and family *to gain cooperation and involvement.*
- Teach and give printed instructions on disorder, complications, home care, and follow-up requirements *so family has a source to refer to at home.*
- Evaluate teaching with return demonstrations *to determine whether child/family is skilled enough for home management of the disorder.*

For the child with diabetes mellitus:
- First teach "survival skills" (e.g., glucose and urine testing, administering insulin, record-keeping, food guidelines, when to call physician) *to provide initial base of knowledge for self-management.*
- Implement second-phase home management program with more extensive instruction; *providing additional teaching over time is necessary for management of a significant chronic illness.*
- Monitor outcomes of teaching with every contact *to ensure progress with patient/family education.*

NURSING DIAGNOSIS: Interrupted family processes or adjustment issues related to lifestyle changes required to manage chronic illness and possible lifestyle changes as evidenced by family's presence in the hospital, missed work, demonstration of inadequate coping

Outcome Identification and Evaluation
Family will maintain functional system of support; demonstrate adequate coping, adaptation of roles and functions, and decreased anxiety: *Parents are involved in child's care, ask appropriate questions, express fears and concerns, identify needs, seek appropriate resources and support, can discuss child's care and condition calmly.*

Interventions: Encouraging Healthy Family Processes
- Encourage parents and family members to verbalize concerns related to child's illness, diagnosis, and prognosis: *allows the nurse to identify concerns and areas where further education may be needed.*
- Explain treatments, medications, procedures, child's behaviors, and plan of care to parents: *Understanding of the child's current status and plan of care helps decrease anxiety.*
- Identify support system for family and child: *helps nurse identify needs and resources available for coping.*
- Provide family with information about support groups, financial resources, and special clinics in the area for the particular type of disorder *to provide family with a wide base of support.*
- Encourage parents to become involved in care: *allows parents to feel needed and valued and gives them a sense of control over their child's health.*
- Evaluate coping processes on follow-up visits *to determine restoration of family processes.*

Nursing Care Plan 48.1 (continued)

NURSING DIAGNOSIS: Imbalanced nutrition: less than or more than body requirements related to pathophysiology of dysfunction as evidenced by growth parameters significantly less or more than expected for age

Outcome Identification and Evaluation
Child's nutritional status is balanced; *child adheres to nutritional guidelines, demonstrates adequate growth (weight and height) pattern within normal range for age and gender or, in the child who has difficulty growing, a progressive increase over time.*

Interventions: Maintaining Adequate Nutrition
- Determine body weight and length/height norm for age or what the child's pretreatment measurements were *to determine goal to work toward.*
- Weigh daily or weekly (according to physician order or institutional standard) and measure length/height weekly *to monitor for appropriate growth.*
- Determine child's food preferences and provide favorite foods as able *to increase the likelihood that the child will consume appropriate amounts of foods.*
- Instruct child and family about nutritional requirements *so that they are involved and are prepared for home care.*
- Refer to dietitian *for more detailed information and assistance.*

For the child who needs to gain weight:
- Offer highest-calorie meals at the time of day when the child's appetite is the greatest *to increase likelihood of increased caloric intake.*
- Provide increased-calorie shakes or puddings within dietary restrictions *(high-calorie foods increase weight gain).*
- Administer vitamin and mineral supplements as prescribed *to attain/maintain vitamin and mineral balance in the body.*

NURSING DIAGNOSIS: Deficient or excess fluid volume related to pathophysiology of endocrine dysfunction as evidenced by signs and symptoms of dehydration (deficient fluid volume) or edema and excessive urine output (excess fluid volume)

Outcome Identification and Evaluation
Child will maintain adequate fluid volume *as evidenced by elastic skin turgor; absence of edema; moist, pink oral mucosa; presence of tears; urine output 1 mL/kg/hr or more; vital signs within normal range for age; and normal electrolyte/hormone serum levels.*

Interventions: Maintaining Adequate Fluid Volume
- Assess hydration status (skin turgor, oral mucosa, presence of tears) every 4 to 8 hours *to evaluate maintenance of adequate fluid volume.*
- Assess adequacy of urine output *to evaluate end-organ perfusion.*
- Maintain strict intake and output record *to evaluate effectiveness of rehydration.*
- Weigh child daily: *accurate weight is one of the best indicators of fluid volume status in children.*
- Administer specific hormone, fluid, and electrolyte requirements as ordered *to aid in fluid balance.*

Fluid volume deficit:
- Maintain IV line and administer IV fluid as ordered *to maintain fluid volume.*

Fluid volume excess:
- Maintain fluid restriction as ordered *to restore homeostasis.*

(continued)

Nursing Care Plan 48.1 (continued)

NURSING DIAGNOSIS: Noncompliance related to long-term/complex management of some disorders as evidenced by failure to keep appointments, development of complications or exacerbation of symptoms, or child/family verbalization of inability to maintain treatment plan

Outcome Identification and Evaluation
Child and family will comply with treatment regimen; *child and family will list treatment expectations and agree to follow through.*

Interventions: Encouraging Compliance
- Listen nonjudgementally while child/family describe reasons for noncompliance; *assessment of problem should begin with nonthreatening discussion.*
- Help child/family develop a schedule for medication administration and other home regimens that works best for them; *involving child and family in planning care will increase compliance by making them feel respected and valued.*
- Work with the child and family to develop a written treatment plan or schedule that best suits their needs *to provide support for maintenance of treatment plan.*
- Establish follow-up visits to fit family's situation *to promote compliance.*
- Encourage monitoring with pediatric endocrinologist and specialists: *multidisciplinary involvement has been shown to increase compliance.*
- Recognize that behavioral change comes slowly; *allows time for child and family to adjust to chronic nature of illness.*

---

any care plan for the child with an endocrine disorder involves preparing the child, based on his or her developmental needs, for invasive procedures and tests. Provide an opportunity for the family and child to express their concerns and fears during diagnosis and treatment. Reinforce realistic expectations for treatment and prospects for improvement with the family and child. The care plan also needs to address developmental, acute, chronic, and home care issues as well as patient and family education. Families will need assistance with managing the condition from a multidisciplinary team.

Based on your top three nursing diagnoses for Carlos, describe appropriate nursing interventions.

Pituitary Disorders

Because of the close anatomic and functional relationships between the hypothalamus and pituitary gland, we will discuss them together. The hypothalamus affects the pituitary by releasing and inhibiting hormones and may be the cause of pituitary disorders. In general, disorders of the pituitary fall into two major groups: the anterior pituitary hormones and the posterior pituitary hormones. Anterior pituitary primary disorders in children include growth hormone deficiency, hyperpituitarism, and precocious puberty. Posterior pituitary disorders include diabetes insipidus and syndrome of inappropriate antidiuretic hormone secretion.

▶ GROWTH HORMONE DEFICIENCY

Growth hormone deficiency, also known as hypopituitarism or dwarfism, is characterized by poor growth and short stature. It is generally a result of the failure of the anterior pituitary to produce sufficient growth hormone (GH). GH is vital for postnatal growth. It is released throughout the day, with most secreted during sleep. GH stimulates linear growth, bone mineral density, and growth in all body tissues.

GH deficiency occurs in approximately 1 in 3,500 children (Hardin et al., 2007). Although it occurs with the same frequency in both genders, society often expects boys to be a certain height, and as a result families may more often request an evaluation in boys. Often this condition is first identified when the health care provider assesses growth patterns. Children may start with a normal birthweight and length, but within a few years the child is less than the third percentile on the growth chart.

Possible complications related to GH deficiency and its treatment include slipped capital femoral epiphysis, pseudotumor cerebri, increased glucose levels, infection at the injection site, edema, and sodium retention. Recent reports have found no evidence linking GH therapy to higher rates of neoplastic diseases.

Pathophysiology

Primary causes of GH deficiency include an injury or destruction of the anterior pituitary gland because of a tumor such as craniopharyngioma, infection, infarction, or irradiation. Secondary causes of GH deficiency include primary hypothalamic dysfunction related to a deficiency of the hypothalamic releasing or inhibitory factors or insulin-like growth factor (IGF-1) deficiency. A genetic factor such as a dominant or recessive inheritance or genetic mutation may also play a role. For example, mutations in growth hormone–releasing hormone (GHRN) occur in larger numbers in individuals from Pakistan, India, and Brazil (Parks, 2007).

> ▶ *Take* NOTE!
>
> *Psychosocial dwarfism results from emotional deprivation that causes suppression of production of the pituitary hormones, resulting in decreased growth hormone. The child is withdrawn, has bizarre eating and drinking habits such as drinking from toilets, and has primitive speech. The treatment involves removing the child from the dysfunctional environment and providing normal dietary intake. With normalized eating and behavioral habits, pituitary secretion is restored and the child dramatically catches up in growth parameters.*

Therapeutic Management

Treatment of primary GH deficiency involves the use of supplemental GH. Secondary GH deficiency requires removal of any tumors that might be the underlying problem, followed by GH therapy. Biosynthetic GH, derived from recombinant DNA, is given by subcutaneous injection. The weekly dosage is 0.18 to 0.3 mg/kg, divided into equal doses given daily for best growth. The first year of treatment results in 8 to 10 cm of growth, followed by normal growth (Kemp, 2006).

Nursing Assessment

The focus of the evaluation for GH deficiency is to rule out chronic illnesses such as renal failure, liver disorders, and thyroid dysfunction. For a full description of the assessment phase of the nursing process, refer to page 1586. Assessment findings pertinent to GH deficiency are discussed below.

Health History

The health history may reveal a familial pattern of short stature or a prenatal history of maternal disorders such as malnutrition. The past history may be significant for birth history of intrauterine growth retardation or past history of severe head trauma or a brain tumor such as craniopharyngioma. Evaluate previous and current growth patterns. Note history of chronic illness such as cardiac, kidney, or intestinal disorders that may contribute to a decreased growth pattern. Assess the child's feelings about being short.

Physical Examination

In addition to the linear height being at or below the third percentile on standard growth charts, the physical assessment findings may show that the child has a higher weight-to-height ratio (Fig. 48.2). Other physical findings may include prominent subcutaneous deposits of abdominal fat, a childlike face with a large, prominent forehead, a high-pitched voice, delayed sexual maturation (e.g., micropenis and undescended testes in boys), delayed dentition, and decreased muscle mass.

> ▶ *Take* NOTE!
>
> *Infants with congenital defects of the pituitary gland or hypothalamus may present as a neonatal emergency. The symptoms include apnea, cyanosis, severe hypoglycemia with possible seizures, and prolonged jaundice.*

Laboratory and Diagnostic Testing

The child will undergo laboratory tests to rule out chronic illnesses such as renal failure or liver and thyroid dysfunc-

FIGURE 48.2 The child with growth hormone deficiency displays short stature.

tion. Laboratory and diagnostic tests used in children with suspected GH deficiency include:

• Bone age (as shown by radiographs) will be two or more deviations below normal.
• CT or MRI rules out tumors or structural abnormalities.
• Pituitary function testing confirms the diagnosis. This test consists of providing a GH stimulant such as glucagon, clonidine, insulin, arginine, or L-dopa to stimulate the pituitary to release a burst of GH. Peak GH levels below 7 to 10 ng/mL in at least two tests confirm the diagnosis.

Nursing Management

Nursing management for the child with GH deficiency focuses on promoting growth, enhancing the child's self-esteem related to short stature, and providing appropriate education about the disorder.

Promoting Growth

The goal of growth promotion is for the child to demonstrate an improved growth rate, as evidenced by at least 3 to 5 inches in linear growth in the first year of treatment without complications. With early diagnosis and treatment, the child has a better prognosis for reaching a normal adult height. Growth is usually excellent in the first year of therapy compared to later years. Treatment stops when the epiphyseal growth plates fuse.

At the beginning of treatment, monitor for height increase and possible side effects related to the medications. Measure the child's height at least every 6 months and plot growth over time on standardized growth charts. Provide information to the child and family about normal development and growth rates, bone age, and growth potential. Explore with the family and child the expectations and their understanding of what is normal so they will have realistic expectations of treatment. Consult a dietitian if the child and family need assistance in providing adequate nutrition for growth and development.

> ► **Take** NOTE!
>
> *Many children are measured inaccurately in primary care centers. Improved accuracy, especially in performing linear measurements, could yield earlier detection and diagnosis of growth disorders (Lipman et al., 2004).*

Enhancing the Child's Self-Esteem

The child with GH deficiency often has younger-looking features and is shorter than his or her peers. Encourage the child to express positive feelings about his or her self-

image, as shown by comments during health care visits as well as involvement with peers. Encourage the child to voice concerns. Emphasize the child's strengths and assets. Provide information about community support groups or websites related to GH deficiency. Evaluate for long-term learning problems that may develop if the child had a tumor and surgery or irradiation to remove it. Unidentified learning problems can have a negative impact on the child's self-esteem. Treat and communicate with the child in an age-appropriate manner even though he or she may appear younger.

Educating the Family

GH is a powder that is mixed with packaged diluents. Explain how to prepare it and give the correct dosage. Have the family provide a return demonstration to make sure they understand correct dilution and administration of GH. Instruct the family to report headaches, rapid weight gain, or painful hip joints as possible adverse reactions. The child should visit the pediatric endocrinologist every 3 to 6 months to monitor for potential adverse effects and for compliance with therapy; the family should know that these frequent visits will be needed. Stress the importance of complying with the GH replacement therapy and frequent supervision by a pediatric endocrinologist. Educate the family about the financial costs of therapy, which may be around $15,000 to treat a child weighing 20 kg (Behrman et al., 2004); the family may need help in obtaining assistance and require referral to social services.

Guide the family and child in setting realistic goals and expectations based on age, personal abilities and strengths, and the effectiveness of the GH replacement therapy. For example, the family may want to encourage the child to choose sports that are not dependent on height. Encourage the family to dress the child according to age, not size. Refer the child and family to counseling if indicated. Inform families about support groups such as the Short Stature Foundation (1-800-243-9273) or the Human Growth Foundation (www.hgfound.org/, 1-800-451-6434).

► HYPERPITUITARISM (PITUITARY GIGANTISM)

Hyperpituitarism, an extremely rare disorder in children, results from an excessive secretion of GH that leads to an increased growth rate greater than the 97th percentile (Lifshitz, 2007). The cause of this overproduction of GH is most often a tumor of the anterior pituitary, a pituitary adenoma, or, if combined with precocious puberty, a tumor of the hypothalamus. If this overproduction occurs before the epiphyseal plates close, the child may grow to 7 to 8 feet in height. If the overproduction occurs after they close, acromegaly occurs. Acromegaly is an enlargement of the bones of the head and soft parts of the feet and hands. Being tall is valued in today's society, so assessment for accelerated growth is often delayed, especially in boys.

Therapeutic management includes removing the tumor, restoring the GH patterns to normal, and preventing recurrence. Treatment depends on the cause and may involve surgery, radiation therapy, radioactive implants, or pituitary hormone replacement after surgery. Alternatively, treatment may involve administration of somatostatin analogs to suppress GH production.

Complications of hyperpituitarism include hypogonadism, visual loss, and heart failure.

Nursing Assessment

In addition to excessive height, physical findings include coarse facial features and enlarged hands and feet. Some patients display behavioral and visual problems. Typically, the condition presents at puberty, but it has been found as early as the newborn period. Increased levels of IGF-1 establish the diagnosis of hyperpituitarism. The gold standard for making the diagnosis of GH excess is failure to suppress serum GH levels after an oral glucose challenge test. A bone scan determines whether the epiphyseal plates are closed. Radiologic studies, including MRI, are used to detect any tumors.

Nursing Management

Nursing management depends on which treatment the child undergoes. If surgical removal of a tumor is required, provide routine pre- and postoperative care. Administer somatostatin analog (e.g., octreotide acetate) if ordered. It is usually given as a subcutaneous injection every 12 hours; refer to Drug Guide 48.1 for further information. Treat the child according to chronologic age rather than according to height. Assess the child's self-image, teach the child and family about the disorder and the treatment plan, and provide emotional support. Monitor for and report signs of potential complications such as hypogonadism, visual loss, or heart failure.

▶ PRECOCIOUS PUBERTY

In precocious puberty, the child develops sexual characteristics before the usual age of pubertal onset. Puberty, also known as sexual maturation, occurs when the gonads produce increased amounts of sex hormones. Typically, this occurs around 10 to 12 years of age for girls and 11 to 14 years of age for boys. In precocious puberty, breasts develop before age 7 years in white girls or before age 6 years in African-American girls, or secondary sex characteristics develop in boys younger than 9 years. The incidence appears to be 0.1 to 0.5 per 1,000 children; the disorder is five times more common in girls, and 95% of

the cases have idiopathic etiologies (Burg et al., 2006). Other causes include benign hypothalamic tumor, brain injury or radiation, a history of infectious encephalitis, meningitis, congenital adrenal hyperplasia, and tumors of the ovary, adrenal gland, or testes.

Pathophysiology

True precocious puberty develops as a result of premature activation of the hypothalamic-pituitary-gonadal axis that results in the production of gonadotropin-releasing hormone (GnRH), which stimulates the pituitary to produce luteinizing hormone (LH) and follicle-stimulating hormone (FSH). These hormones in turn stimulate the gonads to secrete the sex hormones (estrogen or testosterone). The child develops sexual characteristics, shows increased growth and skeletal maturation, and has reproductive capability. Pseudoprecocious puberty presents with no early secretion of gonadotropin or maturation of gonads but rather early overproduction of sex hormones. The condition results in increased end-organ sensitivity to low levels of circulating sex hormones and leads to premature pubic hair and breast development. If left untreated, the child may become fertile. In addition, the hormones stimulate the closure of the epiphyseal plates, which results in overall short stature.

Therapeutic Management

The clinical treatment for precocious puberty first involves determining the cause. For example, if the etiology is a tumor of the central nervous system, the child undergoes surgery, radiation, or chemotherapy. The treatment for central precocious puberty involves administering a GnRH analog. This is available as a depot injection given every 3 to 4 weeks, a subcutaneous injection given daily, or an intranasal compound given two or three times each day. This analog stimulates gonadotropin release initially but when given on a long-term basis will suppress gonadotropin release. With this treatment, the growth rate slows and secondary sexual development stabilizes or regresses. When treatment is discontinued, puberty resumes according to appropriate developmental stages. Medroxyprogesterone (Depo-Provera) reduces secretion of gonadotropins and prevents menstruation. The overall aim of treatment is to halt or even reverse sexual development and rapid growth as well as promote psychosocial well-being.

Nursing Assessment

For a full description of the assessment phase of the nursing process, refer to page 1586. Pertinent assessment findings related to precocious puberty are discussed below.

Health History

The health history may reveal complaints of headaches, nausea, vomiting, and visual difficulties due to the circulating hormones. The psychosocial development is typical for the child's age, but the child may show emotional lability, aggressive behavior, and mood swings. Information from the child and family may also reveal risk factors such as exposure to exogenous hormones, history of central nervous system trauma or infection, or a family history of early puberty.

Physical Examination

Physical examination may reveal acne and an adult-like body odor. The child will present with an accelerated rate of growth. The Tanner staging of breasts, pubic hair, and genitalia reveals advanced maturation for the child's age, but the child does not typically display sexual behavior.

Laboratory and Diagnostic Testing

Radiologic examinations and pelvic ultrasound identify advanced bone age, increased uterus size, and development of ovaries consistent with the diagnosis of precocious puberty. Laboratory studies include screening radioimmunoassays for LH, FSH, estradiol, or testosterone. The child's response to GnRH stimulation confirms the diagnosis of central precocious puberty versus gonadotropin-independent puberty. This test involves administering synthetic GnRH intravenously and drawing serial blood levels, about every 2 hours, of LH, FSH, and estrogen or testosterone. A positive result is defined as pubertal or adult levels of these hormones in response to the GnRH administration. CT, MRI, or skull radiography reveals any lesions in the central nervous system.

Nursing Management

In general, nursing management of the child with precocious puberty focuses on administering medications, helping the child to deal with self-esteem issues related to the accelerated growth and development of secondary sexual characteristics, and educating the child and family. Goals of nursing management include appropriate physical development and pubertal progression appropriate for age. Refer to Nursing Care Plan 48.1, and individualize care based on the child's and family's response to this disorder.

Nursing care involves assessing and documenting the physical changes the child is experiencing and administering medications. Demonstrate correct administration of medication and observe for potential adverse effects (teach this information to the family as well). Encourage the family to comply with follow-up appointments, which typically occur every 6 months and include scheduled stimulation tests. Inform families that pharmacologic intervention stops when the child reaches the age appropriate for pubertal development. Provide appropriate sex education, but reassure parents that precocious puberty does not usually involve precocious sexual behavior.

Dealing With Self-Esteem Issues

Often these children develop self-esteem issues and anxiety related to body image disturbances and impaired social interactions. The goal is for the child to exhibit normal psychosocial development and understand the physical and emotional changes that occur with early onset of puberty. Communicate with the child on an age-appropriate level, even when physical characteristics make the child appear older. Maintain a calm, supportive atmosphere and provide for privacy during examinations. Refer the child and family for counseling if behavioral or psychological disturbances develop. Since the child may have issues with self-image and may be self-conscious, encourage him or her to express his or her feelings about the changes, and use role-playing to show the child how to handle teasing from other children. Let the child know that everyone develops sexual characteristics in time.

▶ DELAYED PUBERTY

Delayed puberty is a condition of delayed secondary sexual development. In girls, it exists if the breasts have not developed by age 13, pubic hair has not appeared by age 14, or **menarche** has not occurred by age 16. In boys, it exists when no testicular enlargement or scrotal changes have occurred by age 14 or pubic hair has not appeared by age 15 followed by testicular enlargement. The most common cause for delayed puberty is a hereditary condition known as **constitutional delay** (Burg et al., 2006). Hypogonadism also may result when there is decreased stimulation of the gonads due to dysfunction in the hypothalamus or pituitary gland as well as from tumors, irradiation, or genetic syndromes such as Turner or Klinefelter syndrome. Another common cause is a chronic condition such as anorexia or cystic fibrosis.

Management involves administering testosterone or estradiol in low dosages if there is no underlying situation to address. This is usually necessary for only a short time to get puberty started.

Nursing Assessment

Assessment involves obtaining a health history to identify the indications for this condition. Assessment of the growth pattern using correct techniques and standards for comparison is essential. On physical assessment, note absence of secondary sex characteristics as noted above. Laboratory and diagnostic testing rules out other causes for delayed puberty. Blood levels of reproductive hormones may also be evaluated.

Nursing Management

In addition to the general interventions presented in Nursing Care Plan 48.1, instruct the child and family about the medication therapy. Educate the child and family about the different stages of puberty. Help the family develop a home management schedule for the administration of medication. Answer the family's questions about the condition or potential complications (e.g., infertility), depending on the cause of the condition.

▶ DIABETES INSIPIDUS

Diabetes insipidus is a disorder of the posterior pituitary gland resulting from a deficiency in the secretion of antidiuretic hormone (ADH). This hormone, also known as vasopressin, is produced in the hypothalamus and stored in the pituitary gland. ADH is involved in concentrating the urine from the kidneys by stimulating reabsorption of water in the renal collecting tubules through increased membrane permeability. This conserves water and maintains normal osmolality. With a deficiency in ADH, the kidney loses massive amounts of water and retains sodium in the serum.

Typically, this disorder occurs in children as a result of complications from head trauma or cranial surgery to remove hypothalamic-pituitary tumors such as craniopharyngioma. Other causes include granulomatous disease, infections such as meningitis or encephalitis, vascular anomalies, congenital malformations, infiltrative disease such as leukemia, or drug administration; 10% of the cases in children are idiopathic (Breault & Majzoub, 2004a). A rare variant, nephrogenic diabetes insipidus, tends to be transmitted genetically (e.g., sex-linked, autosomal dominant, or autosomal recessive forms); it is not associated with the pituitary gland and displays vasopressin insensitivity at the level of the kidneys (Breault & Majzoub, 2004a).

Diabetes insipidus is usually permanent and requires treatment throughout life.

Therapeutic Management

Unless a tumor is present (in which case it is removed by surgery), the usual treatment involves daily replacement of ADH in older children. In neonates and young infants, the treatment is fluid therapy at 3 L/m^2 per 24 hours (Behrman et al., 2004). The drug of choice for home treatment is desmopressin acetate (DDAVP), 25 to 300 mcg, a long-acting vasopressin analog. It is given intranasally, subcutaneously, or orally every 8 to 12 hours. The dose depends on the child's age, urine output, and urine specific gravity. The use of DDAVP in infants is controversial. In the hospital, the child receives aqueous vasopressin, 8-arginine vasopressin (Pitressin), intravenously. This is a short-acting drug, so the dosage can be quickly adjusted. Both types of the medication decrease urinary output and thirst but need to be titrated.

For nephrogenic diabetes insipidus, the treatment involves diuretics, high fluid intake, and restricted sodium intake as well as a high-protein diet.

Nursing Assessment

For a full description of the assessment phase of the nursing process, refer to page 1586. Assessment findings pertinent to diabetes insipidus are discussed below.

Health History
Nursing assessment involves obtaining a history of any conditions that led to the development of the disorder. This review includes information about the neonatal period as well as a current history of infections such as meningitis, diseases such as leukemia, or familial patterns. Most symptoms of endocrine disorders develop slowly, but the onset of this disorder is abrupt. The health history usually elicits the cardinal symptoms as well as complaints representing the early signs of dehydration.

The most common initial symptoms reported are polyuria and polydipsia. Except for unconscious patients, the child typically maintains adequate perfusion by drinking water. The parent or child may report frequent trips to the bathroom, nocturia, or enuresis. When the child cannot compensate for the excessive loss of water by increasing fluid intake, other symptoms will be reported, such as weight loss or signs of dehydration. For example, irritability may be due to the early signs of dehydration or the frustration the child feels at being unable to quench his or her thirst. Other signs may be intermittent fever, vomiting, and constipation.

Physical Examination
Observation and inspection may reveal weight loss or failure to thrive in the young infant. Inspection may also reveal signs of dehydration, such as dry mucous membranes or decreased tears. The child may excrete greater than 3 L/m^2 of urine per day. On auscultation, tachycardia or increased respiratory rate may be signs of compensation for the decrease in fluid volume. Palpation reveals slightly depressed fontanels or decreased skin turgor.

▶ **Take** *NOTE!*

*The cardinal signs of diabetes insipidus are **polyuria** (excessive urination) and **polydipsia** (excessive thirst).*

Laboratory and Diagnostic Testing
Diagnostic tests used to evaluate diabetes insipidus include:

- Radiographic studies such as CT scan or ultrasound of the skull and kidneys to determine whether a lesion or tumor is present
- Urinalysis: urine is dilute, osmolarity is less than 3000 mOsm/L, specific gravity is less than 1.005

- Serum osmolality is greater than 300 mOsm/L.
- Serum sodium is elevated.
- Fluid deprivation test measures vasopressin release from the pituitary in response to water deprivation. Normal results will show decreased urine output, increased urine specific gravity, and no change in serum sodium.

▶ *Take* NOTE!

During a fluid deprivation test, the child may be irritable and frustrated because fluid is being withheld. Don't drink in front of the child.

Nursing Management

Refer to Nursing Care Plan 48.1, and individualize the plan of care based on the child's and family's response to the illness. Specific interventions related to nursing care of the child with diabetes insipidus are discussed below.

Promoting Hydration

The goal of treatment is to achieve hourly urine output of 1 to 2 mL/kg and urine specific gravity of at least 1.010. Maintain fluid intake regimens as ordered. Monitor fluid status by measuring vital signs, fluid intake and output, and daily weights (using the same scale at the same time of day). If fluids are stopped too soon, the child may become hypernatremic, which can lead to seizures. Feed infants more frequently, since they excrete more dilute urine, consume larger volumes of free water, and secrete lower amounts of vasopressin than older children. Monitor for signs and symptoms of dehydration during the fluid deprivation test as well as when starting the treatment regimen. If the child is unconscious or has brain injury, maintain hydration and nutrition with nasogastric or gastrostomy feedings.

▶ *Take* NOTE!

Monitor blood pressure closely when initiating vasopressin.

▶ *Take* NOTE!

Notify the physician if the urine output is greater than 1,000 mL per hour for two consecutive voids.

Promoting Activity

Establish appropriate activity for the child, and allow time for him or her to regain strength and the desire to increase level of activity. Assess the child's abilities daily, schedule frequent bathroom breaks, keep fluids the child likes available at all times, and fit the treatment plan to the child's activity.

Educating the Family

Involve the family in development of the fluid intake regimens. A journal or daily log is essential in maintaining the regimen and identifying problems. Children with intact thirst centers can self-regulate their need for fluids, but if this is not the situation, help the family develop a plan for 24-hour fluid replacement. This may require instruction on nasogastric or gastrostomy feedings. Infants will need fluid intake at night. Educate the family about the symptoms of water intoxication and dehydration. Help the family develop a plan to inform the school and other individuals in the child's life about the need for liberal bathroom privileges and extra fluids to prevent accidents or dehydration. Teaching Guidelines 48.1 gives tips on educating the family about the medication regimen. Recommend that the family obtain a medical alert bracelet or necklace for the child. Encourage compliance with follow-up appointments, which will probably be every 6 months.

▶ SYNDROME OF INAPPROPRIATE ANTIDIURETIC HORMONE (SIADH)

SIADH occurs when ADH (vasopressin) is secreted in the presence of low serum osmolality because the feedback mechanism that regulates ADH does not function

TEACHING GUIDELINES 48.1

DDAVP Administration

- Keep DDAVP in the refrigerator at all times.
- Clear the nostrils (the medication may be poorly absorbed if the child has nasal congestion).
- Insert the measuring tube into the bottle.
- Fill to proper dosage and hold the top of the tube closed while inserting the medication-filled end into the nostril.
- Blow the liquid out of the tubing into the nostril.
- If the child sneezes, repeat the dosage.
- Measure urine specific gravity to monitor effectiveness of the drug.

properly. ADH continues to be released, and this leads to water retention, decreased serum sodium due to hemodilution, and extracellular fluid volume expansion. SIADH is often caused by central nervous system infections such as meningitis, head trauma, brain tumors, intracranial surgery, and certain medication such as analgesics, barbiturates, or chemotherapy. SIADH may also result from excessive administration of vasopressin during the treatment of diabetes insipidus (Breault & Majzoub, 2004b).

Management of SIADH includes correcting the underlying disorder in addition to fluid restriction and intravenous sodium chloride administration to correct hyponatremia and increase serum osmolality.

Nursing Assessment

Obtain a health history, noting history of a central nervous system infection or tumor, intracranial surgery, head trauma, or use of the above-mentioned medications. Note symptoms such as decreased urine output and weight gain, or gastrointestinal symptoms such as anorexia, nausea, and vomiting. Assess neurologic status, noting lethargy, behavioral changes, headache, altered level of consciousness, seizure, or coma. Neurologic signs develop as the sodium level decreases. Diagnostic tests reveal low serum sodium and osmolality, as well as decreased urea, creatinine, uric acid, and albumin levels. Urine samples demonstrate elevated osmolality, high sodium concentrations, and specific gravity greater than 1.030. Adrenal, thyroid, and renal function studies may be used to rule out other causes of hyponatremia.

Nursing Management

Nursing goals focus on restoring fluid balance and preventing injury. Institute safety precautions if altered level of consciousness, confusion, or seizures are present. Notify the physician if headache or irritability is present. Monitor intake and output and weigh the child daily. An indwelling urinary catheter may be needed to allow for hourly monitoring of urine volume and specific gravity. Help the child cope with fluid restriction by offering sugarless candy, a

wet washcloth, or maybe ice chips. Administer electrolyte replacement as necessary to correct imbalances.

Comparison Chart 48.1 compares diabetes insipidus with SIADH.

Disorders of Thyroid Function

Disorders of the thyroid gland are relatively common in infancy and childhood. These disorders can be serious because thyroid hormones are important for growth and development: they regulate metabolism of nutrients and energy production.

▶ CONGENITAL HYPOTHYROIDISM

Congenital hypothyroidism, also known as cretinism, usually results from failure of the thyroid gland to migrate during fetal development. This results in malformation or malfunction of the thyroid gland, which leads to insufficient production of the thyroid hormones that are required to meet the body's metabolic and growth and development needs. Congenital hypothyroidism leads to low concentrations of circulating thyroid hormones (T3 and T4).

Congenital hypothyroidism occurs in 1 in 4,000 live births (Eugster et al., 2004). It occurs over a wide range of ethnic groups, though less among African-Americans (Lifshitz, 2007).

Pathophysiology

Congenital hypothyroidism is due to a defect in the development of the thyroid gland in the fetus due to a spontaneous gene mutation, an inborn error of thyroid hormone synthesis resulting from an autosomal recessive trait, pituitary dysfunction, or failure of the central nervous system–thyroid feedback mechanism to develop. Transient primary hypothyroidism may also occur; it results from transplacental transfer of maternal antithyroid drugs,

COMPARISON CHART 48.1 DIABETES INSIPIDUS VERSUS SIADH

Diabetes Insipidus	Syndrome of Inappropriate Antidiuretic Hormone
• "High and dry"	• "Low and wet"
• Increased urination	• Decreased urination
• Hypernatremia	• Hyponatremia
• Serum osmolality > 300 mOsm/kg	• Serum osmolality < 280 mOsm/kg
• Urine specific gravity < 1.005	• Urine specific gravity > 1.030
• Decreased urine osmolality	• Increased urine osmolality
• Dehydration, thirst	• Fluid retention, weight gain, and hypertension

topical iodine exposure, or maternal thyroid-blocking anti-bodies (Eugster et al., 2004).

Therapeutic Management

To prevent mental retardation and restore normal growth and motor development, thyroid hormone replacement with sodium L-thyroxine (Synthroid, synthetic thyroxine or Levothroid) begins. The recommended starting dosage is 10 to 15 mcg/kg per day; infants and younger children typ-ically require a higher dosage per unit of body weight (Burg et al., 2006). There are no adverse effects with physiologic doses, but thyroid function tests are performed initially every 2 weeks to closely monitor for effects and to ensure proper dosing. Since thyroid hormone is vital to the infant's developing central nervous system, the goal is to normalize thyroid function as quickly as possible. This treatment will be needed lifelong to maintain normal metabolism and normal physical and mental growth and development.

Nursing Assessment

Nursing assessment of the child with congenital hypo-thyroidism includes health history, physical examination, and laboratory testing.

Health History

Determine whether the neonatal metabolic screening test was performed early or whether it was not performed shortly after birth. Inquire about maternal history that may indicate a connection to hypothyroidism, such as maternal exposure to iodine. Additional history findings may in-clude sensitivity to cold, constipation, feeding problems, or lethargy. Since parents like babies to sleep well, the parents may not complain that the baby is sleeping too much; rather, they may remark that it is difficult to keep the baby awake.

Physical Examination

Most infants are asymptomatic until the first month, when they begin to develop clinical signs. Inspection and observation reveal a lethargic baby or a child with hypo-tonia, hypoactivity, and a dull expression. A combina-tion of lethargy and irritability may exist, with an overall delayed mental responsiveness. Measurements of weight and height may reveal delayed growth. Other findings may include a persistent open posterior fontanel, coarse facies with short neck and limbs, periorbital puffiness, enlarged tongue, and poor sucking response (Fig. 48.3). The skin may appear pale with mottling or yellow from prolonged jaundice, or it may be cool, dry, and scaly to the touch, with sparse hair development on the older child. Auscul-tation of the chest might reveal bradycardia. Signs of res-piratory distress and decreased pulse pressure may also be present. On palpation of the abdomen, there may be evi-dence of an umbilical hernia or a mass due to constipation.

FIGURE 48.3 Newborn with congenital hypothyroidism.

Laboratory and Diagnostic Testing

States mandate newborn screening for thyroid hormone levels before discharge from the hospital or 2 to 6 days after birth. When the test is performed within the first 24 to 48 hours along with other metabolic screenings, the result may be inaccurate because of the immediate increase in thyroid-stimulating hormone (TSH) shortly after birth. Radioimmunoassay is used to measure levels of thyroxine (T4), which accurately reflects the child's thyroid status. If the T4 level is less than 6.5 µU/mL (normal is 6.5 to 13 µU/mL), then a second confirming laboratory test is performed, as well as determining whether the TSH is greater than 5 µU/mL through a non-isotopic, time-released fluoroimmunoassay (TR-FIA). A thyroid scan may also be used to check for the absence or ectopic place-ment of the gland. In addition to serum measurement of T4, other diagnostic tests include serum T3, radioiodine uptake, thyroid-bound globulin, and ultrasonography.

Nursing Management

The overall goal of nursing management of the infant or child with congenital hypothyroidism is to establish a normal growth pattern without complications such as men-tal retardation or failure to thrive. Individualize the nursing care plan based on the infant's responses to the illness.

Promoting Appropriate Growth

Measure and record growth at regular intervals. Thyroid levels are measured every 2 to 4 weeks until the target range is reached on a stabilized dose of medication. Tests are then obtained every 3 to 4 months for the first several years of life, changing to every 6 to 12 months during adolescence. Monitor for signs of hypo- or hyperfunc-tion, including changes in vital signs, thermoregulation, and activity level. Provide adequate rest periods and meet thermoregulation needs. If the infant's tongue is unusu-ally large, observe feeding ability, prevent airway obstruc-tion, and position the infant on the side. Fluid restrictions or a low-salt diet may be ordered.

> ▶ *Take* NOTE!
>
> *Observe for signs of thyroid hormone overdose (irritability, rapid pulse, dyspnea, sweating, fever) or ineffective treatment (fatigue, constipation, decreased appetite).*

Educating the Family

Since many infants are asymptomatic, the diagnosis may be unexpected, so reassure and convey realistic expectations to the family. Developmental screening may be required if the child showed any symptoms initially or as the child gets older to ensure that drug therapy is appropriate. Educate the family about the disorder, the medication and method of administration, and adverse effects such as increased pulse rate (which may indicate an overdose of thyroid hormone). Instruct the family to check the pulse before giving the medication.

L-Thyroxine is an oral medication that is available as a pill. It must be crushed for infants and young children. It can be mixed with a small amount of formula and placed in the nipple, but it should not be placed in a full bottle of formula because the infant will not ingest all the medication if he or she does not finish the bottle. The medication can also be mixed with a small amount of liquid and given with a dropper. Medication absorption is affected by soy-based formulas and iron preparations, so carefully evaluate before starting the infant on formulas such as Alsoy, Isomil, Nursoy, ProSobee, and Soyalac. If the child vomits within 1 hour of administration, instruct the family to repeat the dose, since many missed doses may lead to developmental delays and poor growth.

Inform the family that this medication will be needed throughout the child's life. Tell them that frequent blood tests will be needed to evaluate thyroid function and the child's growth rate; genetic counseling may be needed. Current recommendations include monitoring by a pediatric endocrinologist every 1 to 2 months for the first year of life, every 2 to 3 months between 1 and 3 years of age, and every 2 to 12 months until growth is completed (Lafranchi, 2004). The nurse may need to help the family to find a laboratory nearby or to handle financial issues related to the therapy. Educate the family about infant stimulation programs if the child shows cognitive problems, retarded physical growth, or slow intellectual development. Some information may need to be reinforced during school-age or adolescent stages of development. Finally, encourage the family to obtain a medical identification bracelet or necklace for the child.

> ▶ *Consider* THIS!
>
> *Asha Virani, 1 week old, is brought to the clinic. Her newborn screening test was positive for hypothyroidism. Her parents are shocked and upset by the news. Her mother states, "My daughter's been doing so well since she came home from the hospital. She seems to be doing everything she should be. She's a great sleeper. I just can't believe anything's wrong with her."*
>
> 1. *How would you address the parents' concerns?*
> 2. *What teaching will be appropriate for this family?*

▶ ACQUIRED HYPOTHYROIDISM

Hypothyroidism also occurs as an acquired condition. This disorder most commonly results from an autoimmune chronic lymphocytic thyroiditis thyroiditis (Lafranchi, 2004). As a genetic condition, antibodies develop against the thyroid gland, causing the gland to become inflamed, infiltrated, and progressively destroyed. It occurs more often in girls during childhood and adolescence (Lafranchi, 2004). Less common etiologies include hypothyroidism associated with pituitary or hypothalamic dysfunction or exposure to drugs or substances such as lithium that interfere with thyroid hormone synthesis.

Management involves oral sodium L-thyroxine, which is given at 2 to 5 mcg/kg per day to maintain T4 in the upper half of the normal range and to suppress TSH.

Nursing Assessment

Interview the family and child to determine activity tolerance and behavior changes. The symptoms may develop over a period of time and may be subtle. Note vague complaints of fatigue, weakness, weight gain, cold intolerance, constipation, and dry skin. The severity of symptoms depends on the length of time that the hormone deficiency has existed and its extent. Reviewing the growth pattern may reveal a slowed or arrested growth rate (height) and increased weight.

Physical examination may reveal a **goiter** (enlargement of the thyroid gland). Deep tendon reflexes may be sluggish and the face, eyes, and hands may be edematous. Note thinning or coarse hair, muscle hypertrophy with muscle weakness, and signs of delayed or precocious puberty. The diagnostic evaluation involves serum thyroid function studies (TSH, T3, and T4) as well as serum thyroid antibodies to confirm autoimmune thyroiditis. MRI and a thyroid uptake test and scan may also be necessary.

Nursing Management

Work with the family to establish a daily schedule for administering L-thyroxine, which should be taken 30 to 60 minutes before a meal for optimal absorption. Explain to the family that growth is related to the child's response to the treatment, and there are no specific strategies to aid in this growth. The family should understand the diagnosis, should be able to recognize signs and symptoms of hypo- and hyperfunction, and should know when to notify the physician. The family and child may need assistance in accepting the therapy as well as the experience of catch-up growth that may occur at the beginning of therapy. The child with chronic or severe hypothyroidism may be at risk for adverse effects such as restlessness, insomnia, or irritability. The child's thyroid levels should be evaluated every 3 to 6 months by a pediatric endocrinologist.

▶ HYPERTHYROIDISM

Hyperthyroidism is the result of hyperfunction of the thyroid gland. This leads to excessive levels of circulating thyroid hormones. This condition is uncommon in children; the peak incidence in children occurs in adolescence as a result of Graves' disease (Lifshitz, 2007). Graves' disease is an autoimmune disorder that causes excessive amounts of thyroid hormone to be released in response to human thyroid stimulator immunoglobulin (TSI). It occurs five times more often in girls than in boys. A goiter usually develops in this condition. There is a genetic marker in the individuals, with 60% of affected persons having a family history of autoimmune thyroid problems (Lifshitz, 2007). A congenital form, neonatal thyrotoxicosis, occurs in infants of mothers with Graves' disease. This neonatal condition, which can be life-threatening, is a self-limiting disorder lasting 2 to 4 months. Less common causes are thyroiditis, thyroid hormone–producing tumors, and pituitary adenomas.

Management is aimed at decreasing thyroid hormone levels. Current treatment involves antithyroid medication, radioactive iodine therapy, and subtotal thyroidectomy. First-line treatment involves propylthiouracil (PTU) or methimazole (MTZ, Tapazole), which blocks the production of T3 and T4. Adjunct therapy with beta-adrenergic blockers (Inderal) may also be used if the child has marked symptoms. Radioactive iodine therapy is becoming acceptable for children as a long-term therapy (Lifshitz, 2007). This therapy is administered orally and results in tissue damage and destruction of the thyroid gland within 6 to 18 weeks, but it can result in hypothyroidism. Subtotal thyroidectomy is used when drug therapy is not possible or other treatments have failed. Risks include hypothyroidism, hypoparathyroidism, or laryngeal nerve damage.

▶ *Take NOTE!*

The sudden release of high levels of thyroid hormones results in thyroid storm, which progresses to heart failure and shock. Immediately report the signs of thyroid storm: sudden onset of severe restlessness and irritability, fever, diaphoresis, and tachycardia (Burg et al., 2006).

Nursing Assessment

Most of these children are seen in the outpatient setting with a history of a problem with sleep, school performance, and distractibility. They become easily frustrated and overheated and fatigued during physical education class. The child may complain of diarrhea, excessive perspiration, and muscle weakness. The history may also reveal hyperactivity, heat intolerance, emotional lability, and insomnia. Initially, the symptoms are mild and often overlooked. Physical examination of the older child may reveal an increased rate of growth; weight loss despite an excellent appetite; hyperactivity; warm, moist skin; tachycardia; fine tremors; an enlarged thyroid gland or goiter; and ophthalmic changes (exophthalmos, which is less pronounced in children; proptosis; lid lag and retraction; staring expression; periorbital edema; and diplopia) (Fig. 48.4). Elevated pulse and blood pressure may also be noted. Serum T4 and T3 levels are markedly elevated. TSH levels are suppressed.

FIGURE 48.4 Adolescent with Graves' disease.

> ▶ *Take* NOTE!
>
> *Infants with neonatal thyrotoxicosis present with low birthweight, failure to gain weight, hyperphagia, microcephaly, irritability, tachycardia, tachypnea, ophthalmopathy, enlarged thyroid, vomiting, diarrhea, jaundice, hepatosplenomegaly, and thrombocytopenia. Cardiac failure and dangerous central nervous system sequelae result if treatment is delayed.*

Nursing Management

Once the treatment plan is initiated, educate the family and child about the medication and potential adverse effects, the goals of treatment, and possible complications. Monitor for adverse effects such as rash, mild leukopenia, loss of taste, sore throat, gastrointestinal disturbances, and arthralgia. If surgical intervention is chosen, provide appropriate preoperative teaching and postoperative care. Provide supportive measures such as fluid maintenance, nutritional support, and electrolyte correction. Monitor red blood cell count and liver function tests. Provide family education related to the medication. If the medication is given two or three times a day, teach the family to use a pill dispenser and alarm clock. Inform the family of the need for routine blood tests and follow-up visits with the pediatric endocrinologist every 2 to 4 months until normal levels are reached; then visits may be decreased to once or twice a year. Instruct the parents to contact the health care provider if the child has tachycardia or extreme fatigue.

Help the child and family to cope with symptoms such as heat intolerance, emotional lability, or eye problems. Ensure that this information is passed on to school or daycare personnel. The child should take more frequent rest breaks, in a cool environment, and should avoid physical education classes until normal hormone levels are attained. Encourage the family to have the child consume a healthy diet with an appropriate level of calories; the child may need to eat five or six meals a day. Provide community referrals such as to the National Graves' Disease Foundation (www.ngdf.org/ or 1-877-NGDF123). Encourage the family to obtain a medical identification bracelet or necklace.

Comparison Chart 48.2 compares hypothyroidism and hyperthyroidism.

Disorders Related to Parathyroid Gland Function

The parathyroid glands secrete parathyroid hormone (PTH), which, along with vitamin D and calcitonin, regulates calcium/phosphate homeostasis by increasing

COMPARISON CHART 48.2 HYPOTHYROIDISM VERSUS HYPERTHYROIDISM

Hyperthyroidism	Hypothyroidism
• Nervousness/anxiety	• Tiredness/fatigue
• Diarrhea	• Constipation
• Heat intolerance	• Cold intolerance
• Weight loss	• Weight gain
• Smooth, velvety skin	• Dry, thick skin; edema of face, eyes, and hands
	• Decreased growth

osteoclastic activity, absorption of calcium and excretion of phosphate by the kidneys, and absorption of calcium in the gastrointestinal tract. The two disorders associated with this gland are hypoparathyroidism and hyperparathyroidism.

▶ HYPOPARATHYROIDISM

Hypoparathyroidism is the result of a deficiency in PTH secretion, which usually functions to maintain serum calcium. The impaired secretion affects calcium and phosphorus metabolism, leading to hypocalcemia and hyperphosphatemia. It is a very uncommon disorder in children and can be congenital (the result of aplasia or hypoplasia of the parathyroid gland) or acquired (due to inadvertent removal of the glands during thyroidectomy). It may occur in the newborn as a result of maternal hyperparathyroidism, maternal diabetes mellitus, or a diet of formula with a high phosphate-to-calcium ratio (Behrman et al., 2004).

Emergency treatment involves giving intravenous calcium gluconate 10% solution at a dose of 1 to 3 mL slowly, followed by a continuous intravenous infusion of 20 to 50 mg of elemental calcium per kilogram over 24 hours (Burg et al., 2006). The goal is to maintain normal serum calcium and phosphate levels without complications. The treatment for less acute situations involves oral calcium gluconate and vitamin D with supplemental magnesium to help normalize PTH secretion (Burg et al., 2006).

Nursing Assessment

Determine health history, noting poor eating, lethargy, muscle cramps progressing to numbness, and tingling in the hands and feet or around the mouth. The child may be irritable, have a history of unexplained convulsions, or complain of constipation, nausea, vomiting, or diarrhea. Physical examination may reveal **tetany**, stridor, Chvostek's sign (facial muscle spasm elicited by tapping the facial nerve), Trousseau's sign (carpopedal spasm that results from oxygen deficiency), papilledema, and dental enamel hypoplasia. The skeleton is affected over time, which may lead to permanent bone deformities and limited growth.

On palpation the child may complain of vague bone pain or abdominal discomfort. Skin may be dry, scaly, and coarse with eruptions. Laboratory testing reveals decreased serum calcium and PTH levels and increased serum phosphorus levels, which confirms the diagnosis. Bone age radiographs are usually normal, but if the condition has existed long term there may be evidence of increased bone density and suppressed growth.

▶ *Take* NOTE!

The neonate with hypoparathyroidism presents with jittery movements, convulsions, and apnea.

Nursing Management

Administer intravenous calcium gluconate for acute or severe tetany. Monitor the child for the development of cardiac arrhythmias. Ensure that the intravenous site is patent; if extravasation occurs, tissue damage or cardiac arrhythmias may result. Monitor fluid and electrolyte status, weigh the child daily, and measure urinary calcium excretion to prevent nephrocalcinosis. Institute seizure precautions and reduce environmental stimuli (e.g., loud or sudden noises, bright lights, or stimulating activities). Observe for signs and symptoms of laryngospasm (e.g., stridor, hoarseness, or a feeling of tightness in the throat). Teach the child and family about the need for continuous daily administration of calcium salts and vitamin D. Have the family observe for vitamin D toxicity by observing for signs such as weakness, fatigue, lassitude, headache, nausea and vomiting, and diarrhea.

▶ HYPERPARATHYROIDISM

Hyperparathyroidism is an extremely rare disorder in children; the most common cause is an adenomatous disorder of the parathyroid gland (Behrman et al., 2004). Chronic renal disease or congenital anomalies of the urinary tract are the causes of secondary hyperparathyroidism.

Management depends on the cause of the disorder. Surgery may be done to remove a tumor, and an attempt is made to place half of the parathyroid gland in the forearm to maintain normal calcium homeostasis. Intravenous fluids are given as well as furosemide at a dosage of 1 mg/kg

every 6 hours may be given in an attempt to decrease calcium (Lifshitz, 2007).

Nursing Assessment

The health history includes determining whether the child has a history of renal failure or congenital anomalies of the urinary tract. Note history of failure to thrive, headaches, poor school performance, and irritability. Inspection and observation may identify somnolence, stupor, or difficulty concentrating. Auscultation may reveal irregular heart rate, possibly related to cardiac dysrhythmias. Palpation of the abdomen may elicit pain, a mass due to constipation, or flank pain related to renal stones. Testing range of motion and strength may reveal muscle weakness. Blood studies are used to identify elevated calcium and decreased phosphorus levels. Serum measurements of PTH and radiographic studies are used to identify specific causes.

Nursing Management

Increase the child's fluid intake to minimize renal calculi formation. Provide fruit juices to maintain low urinary pH, acidity of body fluids, and calcium absorption. Strain the urine for renal casts. Monitor for safety by placing the child on seizure precautions, checking for fractures, and assessing the child's level of muscular weakness. If the child develops renal rickets (osteodystrophy), long-term braces may be required, so provide family education and encourage compliance. Keep the diet low in phosphorus and watch for hypocalcemia after surgery.

Disorders Related to Adrenal Gland Function

Disorders of the adrenal gland include acute and chronic adrenal insufficiency and disorders of hyperfunction such as Cushing syndrome. The adrenal cortex is the site of production of glucocorticoids, mineralocorticoids, and androgenic and estrogenic steroid compounds. The adrenal medulla is the site of production of the catecholamines and is under neuroendocrine control. When production of these compounds is altered, disease results.

▶ CONGENITAL ADRENAL HYPERPLASIA

Congenital adrenal hyperplasia (CAH) is a group of autosomal recessive inherited disorders in which there is an insufficient supply of the enzymes required for the synthesis of cortisol and aldosterone. The incidence is about 1 in 15,000 to 20,000 live births (Behrman et al., 2007). Many children with CAH do not synthesize aldosterone; this results in adrenal crisis with hyponatremia and shock fairly soon after birth (Sperling, 2002). Other complications of CAH include hypertension, hypoglycemia, short adult stature, and adult testicular tumor in males.

Pathophysiology

More than 90% of the cases of CAH are caused by a deficiency of 21-hydroxylase (21-OH) enzyme (Behrman et al., 2007). This defect results in the reduction of cortisol, which leads to increased ACTH production by the anterior pituitary. Prolonged oversecretion of ACTH causes enlargement or hyperplasia of the adrenal glands and excess production of androgens.

In males, the enzyme deficiency of 21-OH with excessive androgen secretion leads to a slightly enlarged penis, which may become adult-sized by school age, and a hyperpigmented scrotum. The female fetus develops male secondary sexual characteristics; thus, CAH causes pseudohermaphroditism, or ambiguous genitalia, in girls. The clitoris is enlarged and may resemble the penis, the labia have a rugated appearance, and the labial folds are fused, but the ovaries, fallopian tubes, and uterus are normal. The atypical form of 21-OH deficiency becomes evident later, in the toddler or preschool years, with premature **adrenarche**, pubic hair development, accelerated growth velocity, advanced bone age, early closure of the epiphyseal plates, acne, and hirsutism.

Therapeutic Management

The goal of treatment is to stop excessive adrenal secretion of androgens while maintaining normal growth and development. Most children with 21-OH deficiency will take a glucocorticoid such as hydrocortisone and the mineralocorticoid fludrocortisone (Florinef) for life. Infants may also require sodium supplementation. When the medications are taken at physiologic doses there are no adverse effects, but if the levels become elevated, hypertension, growth impairment, and acne become a problem. Regular follow-up care and appropriate titration maintain the dose at appropriate levels to allow normal growth and development.

In the past when girls were born with ambiguous genitalia, standard medical treatment was to correct the external genitalia and establish adequate sexual functioning. Typically, a reduction of the clitoris and opening of the labial folds were done within the first few months of life, with further surgeries at puberty. There is a trend today, however, to wait until the child can make the decision, since the surgery often results in a loss of nerve endings in the clitoris, which impairs sexuality and sexual experiences (Levine & White, 2004). The decision to intervene immediately or to delay treatment is a complex one that raises many concerns for the family.

Nursing Assessment

Nursing assessment of the child with CAH includes health history, physical examination, and laboratory and

FIGURE 48.5 Newborn with ambiguous genitalia.

diagnostic testing. Specific findings related to CAH are presented below.

Health History and Physical Examination

Obtain the health history, noting history of abnormal genitalia at birth in the infant.

In the toddler or preschooler, note history of accelerated growth velocity and signs of premature adrenarche. Upon inspection of the infant's genitalia, note a large penis in the boy and ambiguous genitalia in the girl (Fig. 48.5). When observing the toddler or preschooler, note pubic hair development, acne, and hirsutism.

Laboratory and Diagnostic Testing

The most common type of CAH, 21-OH enzyme deficiency, is detected by newborn metabolic screening. If this test has not been done or the results are unavailable, random hormone levels or levels associated with ACTH stimulation may be obtained. Bone age is advanced and premature closure of epiphyseal plates is noted on radiographs of the long bones. See Healthy People 2010.

Nursing Management

In addition to the common interventions associated with endocrine disorders in childhood (see Nursing Care Plan 48.1), nursing management of the infant or child with CAH focuses on helping the family to under-

HEALTHY PEOPLE 2010

Objective	Significance
(Developmental) Ensure appropriate newborn bloodspot screening, follow-up testing, and referral to services.	• Follow up with state agencies at first contact with infant to ascertain results of newborn screening.

stand the child's response to disease and the importance of maintaining hormone supplementation. Supporting the family is also a key nursing focus. Provide ongoing assessment of the ill or hospitalized child with a history of CAH to recognize the development of life-threatening acute adrenal crisis. If signs and symptoms of adrenal crisis develop, the child will receive fluid resuscitation with an intravenous bolus of 0.9% normal saline (20 mL/kg). Further rehydration will occur with D5NS at twice the recommended maintenance rate. Intravenous hydrocortisone will also be given.

> ▶ *Take* NOTE!
>
> *Signs and symptoms of acute adrenal crisis include persistent vomiting, dehydration, hyponatremia, hyperkalemia, hypotension, tachycardia, and shock. Monitor children with CAH and notify the physician if adrenal crisis is suspected.*

Educating the Family

Medication will be required throughout the child's life, as cortisone is necessary to sustain life. Teach the family the appropriate oral dosages of hydrocortisone and fludrocortisone. It is critical to maintain tight control over the levels of these medications in the bloodstream, as either underdosing or overdosing may lead to short adult stature. Low levels of the hormones may also result in adrenal crisis. These drugs are usually given orally but in some instances will need to be given via intramuscular injections. Teach families how to give hydrocortisone intramuscularly if the child is vomiting and cannot keep down oral medication. If the child becomes ill, is under stress, or needs surgery, additional doses of medications may be required. Encourage the family to obtain an identification bracelet or necklace for the child.

> ▶ *Take* NOTE!
>
> *Families must keep extra Solu-Cortef (injectable form) at home to give during an emergency (Burg et al., 2006).*

Providing Family Support

Make sure the family of a newborn with ambiguous genitalia feels comfortable asking questions and exploring their feelings. There are many issues to consider, such as whether the family will reassign the child's sex or raise the child with the original assignment at birth. The birth certificate may pose a problem if the state requires iden-

tification of sex. Cultural attitudes, the parents' expectations, and the extent of family support influence the family's response to the child and the decision-making process related to sex assignment and surgical correction. If corrective surgery is immediately decided upon, then typical surgical concerns for newborns will need to be addressed.

In general, laypeople do not understand adrenal function and what this diagnosis may mean to the family. Provide families with privacy to discuss these issues, and offer emotional support. When referring to the infant, use terms such as "your baby" instead of the pronouns "he," "she," or "it" and describe the genitals as "sex organs" instead of "penis" or "clitoris." Refer families to the CARES (Congenital Adrenal Hyperplasia Research, Education, and Support) Foundation (www.caresfoundation.org, 1-866-227-3737) and the Magic Foundation (www.magicfoundation.org, 1-800-362-4423) for additional support and resources. Local parent-to-parent support groups are also helpful.

▶ ADDISON'S DISEASE

Addison's disease (primary adrenal insufficiency) is rare in children. It results from damage or destruction of the adrenal glands caused by infections such as tuberculosis, fungal infections, or HIV-related infections; hemorrhage or surgical removal of both glands; or dysfunction of the hypothalamus or pituitary gland. Generally, the etiology in children is an autoimmune process that is familial or sporadic (Levine & White, 2004). Destruction of the adrenal glands by the circulating antibodies leads to deficiency in the adrenal steroids, glucocorticoids (cortisol), and mineralocorticoids (aldosterone).

Management involves replacing deficient or absent hormones. In the acute situation this is accomplished with intravenous hydrocortisone, as well as restoring and maintaining fluid, electrolyte, and glucose balance (Levine & White, 2004). Treatment for the chronic form of Addison's disease is oral hydrocortisone at a dosage of 10 to 15 mg/m^2 in three divided doses and Florinef at 0.05 to 0.30 mg as necessary to maintain renin levels (Levine & White, 2004). This is a lifelong condition, and illness, stress, or surgery will require adjustment in the medication dosage to meet the body's physiologic needs. Potential complications include diabetes, thyrotoxicosis, reproductive malfunction, hypoparathyroidism, and pernicious anemia.

Nursing Assessment

Note history of gradual onset of weight loss, fatigue, anorexia, syncope, nausea, vomiting, and diarrhea. Observe the skin for hyperpigmentation and note decreased blood pressure. Addisonian crisis is an acute onset that presents during a febrile illness, infection, extreme stress, or any condition that results in increase adrenal steroid release. It is potentially life-threatening; the symptoms include sudden penetrating pain in the lower back, abdomen, or legs with severe weakness, vomiting and diarrhea, dehydration, hypotension, electrolyte imbalances, decreased cardiac output, fever, mental status changes, and hypoglycemia.

Laboratory testing reveals low serum sodium, elevated serum potassium, and low fasting glucose levels. Blood urea nitrogen and creatinine levels are increased. The blood test that confirms the diagnosis is a low fasting morning cortisol level 30 to 60 minutes after stimulation with intravenous synthetic ACTH (Levine & White, 2004). In addition, the adrenal antibodies are positive in Addison's disease but negative with other causes for the condition.

Nursing Management

Nursing management of Addison's disease is similar to that of congenital adrenal insufficiency. A critical aspect of the education plan for this disorder, however, is to teach the parents to increase the dosage of cortisol during periods of illness and to use the injectable form of hydrocortisone during periods of extreme nausea or vomiting. Information about the child's condition should always be available to emergency personnel.

► CUSHING'S SYNDROME

Cushing's syndrome is characterized by a cluster of signs and symptoms resulting from excess levels of glucocorticoids (excessive circulating free cortisol). Usually this condition is due to a small ACTH-producing pituitary adenoma. There are two to five new cases of Cushing's syndrome for every 1 million people each year, with about 10% of these new cases occurring in children or teenagers (National Institute of Child Health and Human Development, 2007). The most common cause in older children is prolonged or excessive use of corticosteroid therapy (Levine & White, 2004). Excessive cortisol suppresses the release of GH, so linear growth is decreased in these patients.

Management varies depending on the cause. The goal is to restore hormone balance and reverse Cushing's syndrome. If the cause is an adrenal or pituitary tumor, then surgical removal of the tumor alone or the entire adrenal gland is performed. If the cause is long-term steroid therapy, then the corticosteroid dose is reduced to the lowest dose that is effective in treating the underlying disorder. Ketoconazole may also be given to suppress adrenocortical function.

Nursing Assessment

Note history of rapid weight gain, decreased velocity of linear growth, fatigue, irritability, and sleep disturbance. The child may also have a history of long-term corticosteroid use, water retention, poor wound healing, frequent infections, and in teenage girls, missed menstrual periods. Upon observation of the child's general status, note weight gain around the abdomen, round face (moon face), and a cervical fat pad (buffalo hump) developing over time (Fig. 48.6). The skin may be thin and fragile, with a tendency to bruise. Acne and hirsutism may be present. Note reddish-purple striae on the abdomen. Test muscle strength, noting weakness. Measure the blood pressure, noting hypertension.

Laboratory testing reveals reduced serum levels of potassium and phosphorus, elevated serum calcium and sodium levels, increased 24-hour urinary levels of free cortisol and 17-hydroxycorticosteroid (17-OHCs), loss of diurnal rhythm in serum cortisol levels, chronic hyperglycemia, and elevated glycosylated hemoglobin levels. The adrenal suppression test using low-dose dexamethasone is used initially to screen for adrenocortical hyperfunction. CT and MRI are used to detect tumors in the adrenal and pituitary glands that may cause Cushing's syndrome.

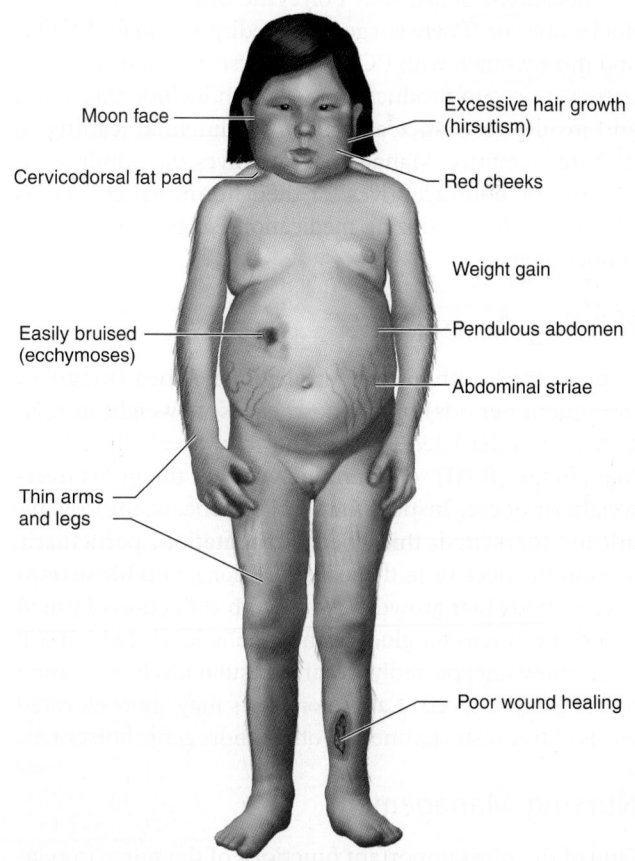

Moon face

Cervicodorsal fat pad

Easily bruised (ecchymoses)

Thin arms and legs

Excessive hair growth (hirsutism)

Red cheeks

Weight gain

Pendulous abdomen

Abdominal striae

Poor wound healing

FIGURE **48.6** Cushing's syndrome.

Nursing Management

Provide routine yet individualized nursing interventions as outlined in Nursing Care Plan 48.1. In addition, counsel the family that the cushingoid appearance is reversible with appropriate treatment. Be alert for signs of adrenal insufficiency if the child has surgery or if corticosteroid withdrawal occurs quickly.

> ▶ *Take* NOTE!
>
> *Watch for signs of shock if the adrenal gland is removed, since without epinephrine from the adrenal gland, the body's ability to maintain blood pressure is severely compromised.*

Polycystic Ovary Syndrome

Polycystic ovary syndrome (PCOS), also referred to as functional ovarian hyperandrogenism or ovarian androgen excess, is an endocrine order that produces a variety of symptoms in adolescent girls and women. Testosterone production by the ovaries and adrenal cells is excessive, causing hirsutism, balding, acne, increased muscle mass, and decreased breast size. Polycystic ovaries may or may not be present. There is a genetic predisposition for PCOS, and most women with PCOS are obese. Complications of excess androgen production in women include infertility, and insulin resistance and hyperinsulinemia, leading to diabetes mellitus. Management involves the administration of oral contraceptives for their hormonal effects, as well as insulin-sensitizing medications such as metformin (Glucophage).

Nursing Assessment

Explore the health history for oligomenorrhea (irregular, infrequent periods) or amenorrhea. Note weight in relation to standardized growth charts and calculate body mass index (BMI) to determine whether the girl is overweight or obese. Inspect the skin for acne, acanthosis nigricans (darkened, thickened pigmentation, particularly around the neck or in the axillary region), and **hirsutism** (excess body hair growth). Assist with collection of timed blood specimens for glucose and insulin levels (which will often show unexpectedly elevated insulin levels in relation to the glucose level). Laboratory tests may show elevated levels of free testosterone and other androgenic hormones.

Nursing Management

One of the most important functions of the nurse in relation to PCOS is to assist with early recognition and treat-ment. Educate the adolescent girl about the use of oral contraceptives to normalize hormone levels, which will decrease androgenic effects. Support the teen in her efforts to diet and exercise to lose weight. Oral insulin-sensitizing drugs such as metformin (Glucophage) may be prescribed, and the teen should be encouraged to comply with the medication regimen. Routinely measure weight to determine progress with weight loss. Measure blood pressure to screen for hypertension, which may develop as a complication of PCOS. Online support groups and education are available at:

- www.kidshealth.org/teen/sexual_health/girls/pcos.html (Nemours Foundation)
- www.youngwomenshealth.org/pcos_resources.html (Children's Hospital Boston)
- www.pcosupport.org (Polycystic Ovarian Syndrome Foundation)

Diabetes Mellitus

In the most common disorder of the pancreas, the islets of Langerhans, specifically the **beta cells**, fail to produce adequate insulin. This results in diabetes mellitus (DM). DM is a chronic disorder in which carbohydrate, protein, and lipid metabolism is impaired. It is one of the leading health problems in the United States and now the most common childhood endocrine disorder (Behrman et al., 2004; Burg et al., 2002). "Primarily, DM represents a spectrum of insulin dysfunction, ranging from an autoimmune destruction of insulin-secreting beta cells (Type 1) at one end to a lack of tissue responsiveness to circulating insulin (Type 2) at the other" (Perkin et al., 2003, p. 529). If the condition goes unrecognized, **diabetic ketoacidosis (DKA)** or fat catabolism develops, resulting in anorexia, nausea and vomiting, presence of **ketones** in urine, sweet-smelling breath, Kussmaul respirations, air hunger, and, if left untreated, coma and death. Approximately 30% to 40% of children with type 1 DM present with DKA on initial evaluation (Burg et al., 2002). Eventually, the lack of insulin and resulting problems produce structural abnormalities in various tissues and organs. Long-term complications of DM include failure to grow, poor wound healing, recurrent infections, retinopathy, neuropathy, vascular complications, nephropathy, microaneurysms, and cardiovascular disease.

> ▶ *Take* NOTE!
>
> *Signs and symptoms of DKA include lethargy, stupor, decreased skin turgor, abdominal pain, Kussmaul respirations and air hunger, and tachycardia.*

▶ DIABETES MELLITUS TYPE 1

DM type 1 is an autoimmune disorder that occurs in genetically susceptible individuals who may also be exposed to one of several environmental factors, such as chemicals, viruses, or other toxic agents implicated in the development process. The long arm of chromosome 14 at the 14q24 locus is the type 1 diabetes-11 marker. Approximately 5% of children have a first- or second-degree relative with DM type 1 (ADA, 2008). The incidence is 0.14 to 0.17 per 1,000 children under 20 years old in North America, with a higher incidence in African-American and Hispanic children (Alemzadeh & Wyatt, 2004). There is equal distribution between the genders, with the peak incidence occurring in school-age children.

As the genetically susceptible individual is exposed to environmental factors, the immune system begins a T-lymphocyte–mediated process that damages and destroys the beta cells of the pancreas, resulting in inadequate insulin secretion. Insulin cannot alter peripheral cells to transport glucose across the cell membrane. The end result is hyperglycemia, glucose accumulation in the blood, and the body's inability to use its main source of fuel efficiently. By the time symptoms are present and the diagnosis is made, 90% of the beta cells have been destroyed. Immunologic markers, islet cells antibodies (ICA), insulin autoantibodies (IAA), and other antibodies may be present for years before the child develops signs and symptoms (Alemzadeh & Wyatt, 2004).

▶ DIABETES MELLITUS TYPE 2

In DM type 2 the pancreas usually produces insulin but the body is resistant to the insulin or there is an inadequate compensatory insulin secretion response. Eventually, insulin production decreases, with a result similar to DM type 1. Historically, DM type 2 occurred mostly in adults, with only 2% to 3% of cases occurring in children. Since the early 1990s, however, the incidence has increased: today, 8% to 45% of children with newly diagnosed diabetes have type 2 (Alemzadeh & Wyatt, 2004). Many of these children have a relative with DM type 2 or they are overweight or from an African-American, Hispanic-American, Asian-American, or Native American background (Alemzadeh & Wyatt, 2004). See Healthy People 2010.

▶ SECONDARY DIABETES MELLITUS

Secondary DM, or exacerbation of insulin deficiency and resistance forms, develops as a result of conditions such as diseases of the exocrine gland (e.g., cystic fibrosis), endocrine pathologies (e.g., Cushing's syndrome), drug-induced problems (e.g., corticosteroid overuse), genetic defects of insulin action (e.g., congenital lipodystrophy), infection (e.g., congenital rubella), and gestational diabetes (Alemzadeh & Wyatt, 2004).

HEALTHY PEOPLE 2010

Objective	Significance
Prevent diabetes. Reduce the overall rate of diabetes that is clinically diagnosed.	• Screen all children periodically for the development of overweight and obesity using body mass index on the CDC growth charts. • Educate families about appropriate diet and exercise beginning in toddlerhood in order to prevent the development of obesity.

Therapeutic Management

Treatment involves a multidisciplinary health care team, with the family and child as a central part of that team. In the past the children would be admitted to the hospital for 3 to 5 days for stabilization and education, but today the trend is toward treating children on an outpatient basis. The general goals for therapeutic management include:

- Achieving normal growth and development
- Promoting optimal serum glucose regulation, including fluid and electrolyte levels and near-normal **glycosylated hemoglobin** levels
- Preventing complications
- Promoting positive adjustment to the disease, with ability to self-manage in the home

The key to success is to educate the child and family so they can self-manage this chronic condition. Treatment involves blood glucose monitoring; daily injections of insulin for DM type 1 or oral hypoglycemic medications for DM type 2; a realistic diet; an exercise program; and self-management and decision-making skills.

Glucose Monitoring

With the advent of home blood glucose monitoring in the late 1970s, daily glucose monitoring replaced urine testing for glucose levels. Urine testing does not supply enough quantitative data to make adequate decisions about insulin doses. Glucose monitoring allows for tighter glucose control because supplemental insulin can be used to correct or prevent hyperglycemia; it also enables patients and health care providers to provide better management. The frequency of blood glucose monitoring is based on the patient's goals. Children who are in the hospital for management of their DM require blood glucose monitoring before meals, at bedtime, and at 2 a.m., if not more frequently. Additional glucose checks, such as mid-morning or mid-afternoon, should be made if glycemic control has not occurred (Alemzadeh & Wyatt, 2004).

FIGURE 48.7 The subcutaneous injector uses pressure jets to deliver insulin safely and accurately.

Insulin Replacement Therapy

Insulin replacement therapy is the cornerstone of management of DM type 1. Insulin is administered daily by subcutaneous injections into adipose tissue over large muscle masses using a traditional insulin syringe or a subcutaneous injector (Fig. 48.7). U-100 insulin may also be administered using a portable insulin pump. The frequency, dose, and type of insulin are based on how much the child needs to achieve a normal, average blood glucose concentration and to prevent hypoglycemia. Typically, two or four daily injections are commonly used, with newly diagnosed children receiving 1 unit of insulin per kilogram of body weight per day, but the dosage depends on the needs of the child (Alemzadeh & Wyatt, 2004). The dose may need to be increased during the pubertal growth spurt.

> ▶ **Take** NOTE!
>
> *An insulin pump is a device that administers a continuous infusion of rapid-acting insulin. It comprises a computer, a reservoir of rapid-acting insulin, thin tubing through which the insulin is delivered, and a small needle inserted into the abdomen. A continuous basal rate of insulin is maintained, and a bolus of insulin can be delivered if glucose testing results show it is needed.*

Types of insulin include rapid-acting, short-acting, intermediate-acting, long-acting, and fixed combinations (Table 48.3). They can be kept at room temperature but should be discarded 1 month after opening even if refrigerated. The child may receive only one type or a mixture of short-acting and intermediate-acting. Again, this depends on the child's needs. Insulin is either animal (pork) or synthetic human, produced through recombinant DNA technology, which is better for children.

> ▶ **Take** NOTE!
>
> *Lantus is usually given in a single dose at bedtime. Lantus may not be mixed with other insulins.*

Oral Hypoglycemic Medications

In DM type 2, oral hypoglycemic medications such as sulfonylureas and meglitinides are used to increase insulin response to glucose. Another group, the biguanides, reduces glucose production from the liver, but because this group causes hypoglycemia it is not used as often in children. Insulin sensitizers improve the body's ability to use insulin in the liver and skeletal tissues. Common adverse effects of these oral agents include headache, dizziness, edema, and liver enzyme elevation. If the oral hypoglycemics fail to maintain a normal glucose level, then insulin injections will be required. These children may also be prescribed antilipidemic medication since hyperglycemia results in transient hyperlipidemia (Alemzadeh & Wyatt, 2004).

Other Therapies

Other therapies involve diet and exercise protocols and management of complications. The American Dietetic Association in conjunction with the American Diabetes Association recommends goals that do not exclude any foods and reflect the growth needs of the child. The recommendations suggest that approximately 50% to 60% of calories come from carbohydrates, such as grains, breads, fruit, milk, and vegetables; 12% to 20% from

TABLE 48.3 INSULIN TYPE, ACTION, AND DURATION

Type	Onset	Peak	Duration
Lispro: ultra-short-acting	15–30 minutes	60–90 minutes	3–4 hours
Regular: short-acting	30 minutes	2–3 hours	3–6 hours
NPH or Lente: intermediate-acting	Lente: 1–2.5 hours NPH: 1–1.5 hours	7–15 hours 6–10 hours	12–24 hours 10–18 hours
Ultralente: long-acting	4–8 hours	Variable; 10–16 hours	24–36 hours
Lantus	1–2 hours	Does not truly peak; offers continual steady coverage	20–24 hours

EVIDENCE-BASED PRACTICE 48.1
The Daily Experience of Parents Who Manage Their Children's Diabetes With an Insulin Pump

● Study

Children with Type I diabetes mellitus require multiple daily insulin injections to manage their glucose levels. This presents difficulties for many families in a number of ways. The authors performed a qualitative descriptive study to determine what life is like for parents whose children's diabetes is managed with a continuous subcutaneous insulin pump as opposed to multiple daily injections. Twenty-one parents of 16 children were included in the study. The parents participated in lengthy interviews with questions structured to determine how life was experienced before and after the pump. The verbatim transcripts were then rigorously analyzed.

▲ Findings

Parents varied in the amount of time it took for them to become comfortable with using the pump and eventually confident with its use (up to several months). They identified the transition period as a little scary at times. Parents reported improved day-to-day diabetes management, flexibility, and quality of life when the insulin pump is used compared with the previous regimen of multiple daily injections.

■ Nursing Implications

Educate families on the use of the continuous subcutaneous insulin pump and the improved glucose control that it may allow them to have. Involve children over 6 years of age in management of their diabetes. Provide ongoing emotional support to families as they make the transition to using the insulin pump.

Sullivan-Bolyai, S., Knafl, K., Tamborlane, W., et al. (2004). Parents' reflections on managing their children's diabetes with insulin pumps. *Journal of Nursing Scholarship, 36,* 316–323.

protein, such as meat, beans, eggs, cheese, and legumes; and 30% from fats, such as butter, oil, or mayonnaise (Alemzadeh & Wyatt, 2004).

Exercise has an important influence on the hypoglycemic effects of insulin, so the child should maintain or increase his or her activity levels. If the child is taking insulin, the family should know how to change the dosage or add food to maintain blood glucose control. Children with DM type 2 are often overweight, so the exercise plan is very important in helping the child to lose weight as well as assisting with the hypoglycemic effects of the medications.

Nursing Assessment

Assessment involves understanding the ever-changing needs of children as they grow and develop. The first phase of assessment involves identifying the child who may have DM. The second phase involves identifying problems that might develop in the child with DM. The nurse should always be aware of this when observing for complications or management problems and should always be alert for opportunities to provide education that will expand the understanding and skills of the child and family.

Health History and Physical Examination

During the initial diagnosis of DM, obtain a detailed history of family patterns and problems in school related to some of the mental and behavior changes that may occur in a hyperglycemic state (e.g., weakness, fatigue, mood changes). The child may also complain of blurred vision, headaches, or bedwetting. The child with DM type 1 may have a history of poor growth. Comparison Chart 48.3 gives information about common history and physical examination findings in children with type 1 versus type 2 DM.

In the child who is known to have DM, the health history includes any problems with hyperglycemia or hypoglycemia, diet, activity and exercise patterns, and ability to administer insulin and monitor blood glucose levels. Perform a thorough physical examination, noting any abnormal findings.

Laboratory and Diagnostic Testing

A random glucose level above 200 mg/dL, a fasting glucose level above 126 mg/dL, and a 2-hour postprandial blood glucose level above 200 mg/dL are laboratory criteria for the diagnosis of DM. Other laboratory and diagnostic tests include glycosylated hemoglobin; hemoglobin A_{1c}, which reflects the percentage of hemoglobin to which glucose is attached; and serum measurements of islet cell antibodies. Serum levels of urea nitrogen, creatinine, calcium, magnesium, phosphate, and electrolytes such as potassium and sodium may be drawn. Additional tests include a complete blood count, urinalysis, and immunoassay to measure levels of C-peptides

COMPARISON CHART 48.3 TYPE 1 VERSUS TYPE 2 DIABETES MELLITUS

History and Physical Findings Usually Present at Diagnosis	Type 1	Type 2
Polydipsia, polyuria, **polyphagia**	Yes	Yes
Weight	Possibly weight loss	Obese
Age of onset	Usually younger children	Usually pubertal children
Incidental finding on screening urinalysis	Rare	Common
Antecedent flu-like illness	Common	Possible
Autoimmune antibodies	Yes	No
Diabetic ketoacidosis	Common	Possible
Hypertension	No	Common
Acanthosis nigricans	No	Common
Vaginal infection	No	Common
Dyslipidemia	No	Common

Pinhas-Hamiel, O., & Zeitler, P. (2001). Type 2 diabetes: Not just for grownups anymore. *Contemporary Pediatrics, 1,* 102 [electronic version]. Available at www.contemporarypediatrics.com.

after a glucose challenge to verify endogenous insulin secretion.

Nursing Management

Nursing management is focused on regulating glucose control, monitoring for complications, and educating and supporting the child and family. Individualize the general nursing care discussed in Nursing Care Plan 48.1 based on the child's and family's response to illness. Additional nursing care topics related to DM are discussed below.

Regulating Glucose Control

If the child presents with DKA, monitor the glucose level hourly to prevent it from falling more than 100 mg/dL per hour. A too-rapid decline in blood glucose predisposes the child to cerebral edema. Administration of regular insulin, given intravenously, is preferred during DKA; a bolus dose of 0.1 unit/kg is given, followed by a continuous infusion of 0.1 unit/kg per hour. Usually the child with DKA is treated in the pediatric intensive care unit.

The subcutaneous route of insulin administration is used once the serum glucose level reaches 250 mg/dL, serum pH is 7.35, dehydration is corrected, and the child is no longer NPO. Many times the regimen consists of three injections of intermediate-acting insulin, with the addition of rapid-acting insulin before breakfast and dinner. Insulin doses are typically ordered on a sliding scale related to the serum glucose level and how the insulin works. Two thirds of the dose is usually given before breakfast and one third before dinner (Perkin et al., 2003).

Teach the child and family to use proper subcutaneous injection techniques to avoid injecting into muscle

or vascular spaces. Figure 48.8 shows appropriate sites for subcutaneous injection of insulin. Sites should be rotated to avoid adipose hypertrophy (fatty lumps that absorb insulin poorly).

> ▶ *Take* NOTE!
>
> *When giving a combination of short- and long-acting insulin, draw up the clear (short-acting) insulin first to prevent contamination with the long-acting insulin. Rotate the vial instead of shaking it to prevent air bubbles.*

Monitoring for Complications

While the child is in the hospital, monitor for signs of complications such as acidosis, coma, hyperkalemia or hypokalemia, hypocalcemia, cerebral edema, or hyponatremia and assess for the development of hypoglycemia or hyperglycemia every 2 hours (Comparison Chart 48.4). Monitor the child's status closely during peak times of insulin action. Perform blood glucose testing as ordered or as needed if the child develops symptoms.

When the child is having a hypoglycemic reaction, administer glucagon (a hormone produced by the pancreas and stored in the liver) either subcutaneously or intramuscularly. Children under 7 years of age receive 0.5 mg; children over 7 years of age receive 1 mg. Dextrose (50%) may be given intravenously if needed. If the child is coherent, glucose paste or tablets may be used. Offer 10 to 15 g of a

FIGURE **48.8** Insulin injection sites.

simple carbohydrate such as orange juice if the child feels some symptoms and glucose monitoring indicates a drop. Follow this with a more complex carbohydrate such as peanut butter and crackers to maintain the glucose level.

The hyperglycemic child requires insulin; the dosage is usually based on a sliding scale or determined after consultation with the physician.

> ▶ *Take* NOTE!
>
> *Double-check all insulin doses against the order sheet and with another nurse to ensure accuracy.*

Educating the Family

Education is the priority intervention because it will enable the child and family to self-manage this chronic condition. The child and family first need time to adjust to the diagnosis of a chronic illness that will require self-management. DM is a lifelong condition that requires regular follow-up visits (three or four times a year) to a diabetes specialty clinic. Because approximately 150,000 school-age children and adolescents have diabetes, this becomes a health issue for the community, especially the schools (National Institutes of Health, National Diabetes Education Program, 2006). With appropriate management, involvement of the community, and confidence and compliance by the family, the child can maintain a happy, productive life. See Healthy People 2010.

COMPARISON CHART 48.4 HYPOGLYCEMIA VERSUS HYPERGLYCEMIA

Hypoglycemia	Hyperglycemia
Behavioral changes, confusion, slurred speech, belligerence	Mental status changes, fatigue, weakness
Diaphoresis	Dry, flushed skin
Tremors	Blurred vision
Palpitations, tachycardia	Abdominal cramping, nausea, vomiting, fruity breath odor

HEALTHY PEOPLE 2010

Objective	Significance
Increase the proportion of persons with diabetes who receive formal diabetes education.	• Begin diabetes education with child and family upon knowledge of diagnosis. • Use developmentally appropriate education with children. • Increase the self-management skills taught as the child progresses in age and cognitive development.

Challenges related to educating children with diabetes include:

- Children lack the maturity to understand the long-term consequences of this serious chronic illness.
- Children do not want to be different from their peers, and having to make lifestyle changes may result in anger or depression.
- Poor families may not be able to afford appropriate food, medication, transportation, and telephone service.
- Families may demonstrate unhealthy behaviors, making it difficult for the child to initiate change because of the lack of supervision or role modeling.
- Family dynamics are affected because management of diabetes must occur all day, every day.

▶ *Take* NOTE!

Children with diabetes mellitus have significantly higher rates of depression than the general population and may have other comorbid conditions, such as eating disorders, adjustment disorders, or anxiety disorder (Alemzadeh & Wyatt, 2004).

The initial goal of education is for the family to develop basic management and decision-making skills. Assess the family's ability to learn the basic concepts, and offer psychological support. Teach about specific topics in sessions lasting 15 to 20 minutes for the children and 45 to 60 minutes for the caregivers. Teaching must be geared toward the child's level of development and understanding (Table 48.4).

Among the topics to include when teaching children and their families about diabetes management are:

- Fingerstick method and blood glucose measurement (Fig. 48.9)
- Urine ketone testing
- Medication use (Fig. 48.10)
  Oral hypoglycemic agents
  Subcutaneous insulin injection or insulin pump use
  Subcutaneous site selection and rotation
  When to alter insulin dosages
  Use of glucagon
- Signs and symptoms of hypoglycemia and hyperglycemia
- Complications
- Sick-day instructions
- Laboratory testing and follow-up care

Teaching Guidelines 48.2 presents information to cover when teaching the family about blood glucose monitoring. Teach families how to give insulin, how to use the

TABLE 48.4 DEVELOPMENTAL ISSUES RELATED TO DIABETES MELLITUS

Age Group	Child and Family Implications	Nursing Implications
Infants and toddlers	Management falls on parents/caretakers; signs and symptoms are sometimes difficult to assess in infants and young toddlers.	Attempt to achieve consistent dietary intake. Let toddler choose foods. Get toddler to find a word or phrase to use to describe feelings when hypoglycemic. Establish rituals/routines with home management.
Preschoolers	Increased motor maturity; widening social circle, so the child will notice that he or she is "different." Magical thinking presents some issues. Some children can began to perform blood glucose testing with the newer devices.	Use simple explanations and play therapy when instructing or preparing for a procedure.
School-age children	Can perform finger/blood glucose testing, choose injection sites and give injections, perform ketone testing, recognize need to eat and treat for hypoglycemia. Must incorporate management into school day, and plan for field trips.	Use concise and concrete terms when instructing. Allow child to proceed at his or her own rate. Assist family to incorporate the testing and injections into school day and plan for field trips. Involve the school nurse in helping with the school plan.
Adolescents	Conflicts develop with self-management, body image, and peer group acceptance; must assume more of the care with supervision. Teens do not always foresee the consequences of their activity.	Slowly care is turned over to the adolescent with minor supervision from the family. Watch for depression.

FIGURE 48.9 The school-age child has developed the psycho-motor skills needed for blood glucose monitoring and insulin injection.

insulin pump, and how to rotate injection sites (see above). Sick-day instructions may include the following:

• Contact the physician.
• Perform blood glucose monitoring more often.
• Use a sliding scale to calculate the insulin dosage.

A dietitian can help the family with detailed meal planning and dietary guidelines. Review basic nutritional information with the child and family and provide sample meals. Incorporate the family's cultural preferences when planning meals. Encourage the child and family to keep a food diary. For the child who needs to lose weight, suggest low-carbohydrate snacks and encourage appropriate daily physical activity (Teaching Guidelines 48.3).

Supporting the Child and Family

Children with diabetes and their families may have difficulty coping if they lack confidence in their self-management skills. Assess the ability of the child and family to handle situations. Role-play specific situations

FIGURE 48.10 The school-age child may first practice insulin injections on a doll.

TEACHING GUIDELINES 48.2

Blood Glucose Monitoring

• Obtain glucose levels before meals and bedtime snacks.
• Perform monitoring more often during prolonged exercise, if you are ill, if you have eaten more food than usual, or if you suspect nighttime hypoglycemia.
• Use the manufacturer's recommendations and perform quality control measures as directed.
• Look for patterns. For example, 3 to 4 days of a consistent pattern of glucose values above 200 mg/dL before dinner indicates a need to adjust the insulin dose.
• Blood glucose measurements are the best way to determine daily insulin dosages.
• Normal levels are as follows: nondiabetics, 70 to 110 mg/dL; children with type 1 DM, 80 to 150 mg/dL; infants and toddlers, 100 to 200 mg/dL.

TEACHING GUIDELINES 48.3

Diet and Exercise for Children With Diabetes Mellitus

• Provide sufficient calories and good nutrition for normal growth and development. The diet should be low in saturated fats and concentrated carbohydrates (1,000 kcal/day + 100 kcal for each year, up to 2,500 kcal).
• Learn to identify carbohydrate, protein, and fat foods.
• Make adjustments during periods of rapid growth and issues such as travel, school parties, and holidays.
• Consult a dietitian with expertise in diabetes education as needed.
• Provide three meals per day and mid-afternoon and bedtime snacks. Consistency of intake can help prevent complications and maintain near-normal blood glucose levels.
• Encourage the child to exercise routinely to help the body use insulin efficiently, thus reducing the insulin requirement.
• Encourage the child to participate in age-appropriate sports.
• When exercising, monitor insulin dose and nutritional and fluid intake, and observe for hypoglycemic reactions. Add an extra snack containing 15 to 30 g carbohydrate for each 45 to 60 minutes of exercise. Avoid exercising excessively when insulin is peaking.

related to symptoms or complications to help them see different ways to solve problems. Work with the child and family to enhance their conflict resolution skills. Provide opportunities for them to express their feelings. Observe for signs of depression, especially in adolescents.

To enhance the child's confidence and promote feelings of mastery and inclusion, refer him or her to a special camp for children with diabetes (see www.diabetescamps.org/ or www.childrenwithdiabetes.com/camps/). Also refer families to local support groups, parent-to-parent networks, or one of many national support resources and foundations, such as:

• www.diabetes.org: American Diabetes Association
• www.childrenwithdiabetes.com/index_cwd.htm: Children with Diabetes (online community)
• www.mychildhasdiabetes.com/ (parenting and diabetes resources)
• www.jdf.org/: Juvenile Diabetes Research Foundation International

■■■ Key Concepts

■ The endocrine system consists of cells, tissues, and glands that produce and/or secrete hormones (chemical messengers) in response to a negative feedback system involving the hypothalamus and nervous system.

■ Hormones (chemical messengers), along with the nervous system, play an intricate role in reproduction, growth and development, energy production and use, as well as maintenance of the internal homeostasis.

■ The pituitary, along with the hypothalamus connection, is considered the "control center," producing hormones that stimulate many glands to produce other hormones or to inhibit the process.

■ Hormonal control is immature at birth; this is partly why the infant has trouble maintaining an appropriate balance of fluid concentration, electrolytes, amino acids, glucose, and trace substances.

■ Linear growth and cognitive development may be impaired by untreated endocrine dysfunction in the infant or child.

■ A thorough health history of the child with a known or potential endocrine disorder often reveals poor growth, school or learning problems, and inactivity or fatigue.

■ Serial measurement of growth parameters is a key part of the physical assessment for children with endocrine dysfunction.

■ Close monitoring of the child's status is critical during a hormone stimulation test or water deprivation study.

■ Hormone supplementation is required lifelong for many of the endocrine disorders.

■ The key nursing functions related to hormone supplementation are educating the child and family about medication use and monitoring for therapeutic results and adverse effects.

■ Children with adrenocortical dysfunction will require additional hormone supplementation during times of stress such as fever, infection, or surgery.

■ Growth hormone deficiency is characterized by poor growth and short stature as a result of failure of the anterior pituitary to produce sufficient growth hormone. Early treatment enables the child to reach normal growth.

■ Precocious puberty involves early development of secondary sex characteristics as a result of premature activation of the hypothalamic-pituitary-gonad axis.

■ Diabetes insipidus is characterized by water intoxication as a result of a deficiency in the antidiuretic hormone that leads to the cardinal signs of polyuria and polydipsia, resulting in hypernatremic dehydration.

■ Key findings in congenital hypothyroidism are a thickened protuberant tongue, an enlarged posterior fontanel, feeding difficulties, hypotonia, and lethargy.

■ Early diagnosis and treatment of hypothyroidism can prevent impaired growth and severe cognitive impairment.

■ Congenital adrenal hyperplasia results from a genetic defect that causes a breakdown in steroid synthesis and an overproduction of androgens that can lead to ambiguous genitalia in females.

■ Diabetes mellitus is the most common endocrine disorder now seen in children. The incidence of DM type 2 has risen dramatically.

■ DM type 1 is an autoimmune disorder resulting from damage and destruction of the beta cells in the islets of Langerhans in the pancreas; the end result is insulin insufficiency. Peak onset occurs in childhood.

■ DM type 2 results in an insensitivity or resistance to insulin. It is occurring at an alarming rate in children, especially in those who are obese and from certain ethnic groups.

■ Diabetic ketoacidosis is a medical emergency. The child will usually be admitted to a pediatric intensive care unit.

■ Critical areas in the nursing management of children with endocrine dysfunction include maintaining appropriate nutrition and fluid balance and promoting growth and development.

■ The nurse provides ongoing assessment and education of the child and family, imparting to them the knowledge and skills required for self-management.

■ Encouraging the child to have a healthy body image and working with the family in establishing healthy family processes are also key nursing functions.

■ The focus of diabetes management is regulation of glucose control, which is accomplished by medications, diet, and exercise.

■ Diabetes education involves instruction in glucose monitoring, administration of insulin or oral hypoglycemics, meal planning, and promotion of a healthy lifestyle.

References

Alemzadeh, R., & Wyatt, D.T. (2004). Diabetes mellitus in children. In R.E. Behrman, R.M. Kliegman, & H.B. Jensen (Eds.), *Nelson textbook of pediatrics* (17th ed.). Philadelphia: Saunders.

Amer, K. S. (2005). Advances in assessment, diagnosis, and treatment of hyperthyroidism in children. *Journal of Pediatric Nursing, 20*(2), 119–126.

American Diabetes Association. (2008). All about diabetes. Retrieved 1/6/08 from www.diabetes.org/about-diabetes.jsp.

American Diabetes Association. (2008). Standards of medical care in diabetes—2008. *Diabetes Care, 32,* S12–S54.

Breault, D.T. , & Majzoub, J.A. (2004a). Diabetes insipidus. In R.E. Behrman, R.M. Kliegman, & H.B. Jensen (Eds.), *Nelson textbook of pediatrics* (17th ed.). Philadelphia: Saunders.

Breault, D.T., & Majzoub, J.A. (2004b). Other abnormalities of arginine vasopressin metabolism and action. In R.E. Behrman, R.M. Kliegman, & H.B. Jensen (Eds.), *Nelson textbook of pediatrics* (17th ed.). Philadelphia: Saunders.

Burg, F.D., Ingelfinger, J.R., Polin, R.A., & Gershon, A.A. (2006). *Current pediatric therapy* (18th ed.). Philadelphia: Saunders.

Cohen, P. (2004). Hyperpituitarism, tall stature, and overgrowth syndromes. In R.E. Behrman, R.M. Kliegman, & H.B. Jensen (Eds.), *Nelson textbook of pediatrics,* 17th ed. Philadelphia: Saunders.

Doyle, D.A., & DiGeorge, A.M. (2004). Disorders of the parathyroid. In R.E. Behrman, R.M. Kliegman, & H.B. Jensen (Eds.), *Nelson textbook of pediatrics* (17th ed.). Philadelphia: Saunders.

Edwards, E. (2004). Addison's disease, case study. Retrieved 5/21/04 from www.pens.org/articles/edwards-3.htm.

Eugster, E. A., LeMay, D., Zern, M., & Pescovitz, O. H. (2004). Definitive diagnosis in children with congenital hypothyroidism. *Journal of Pediatrics, 144*(5), 643–646.

Everly, D., Kaplan, B. S., & Meyers, K. (2006) *Treating NDI: Emphasizing the first year of life.* Retrieved 1/6/08 from www.diabetesinsipidus.org/4di_treating_ndi_firstyear.htm.

Farthing, N., & Sadler, J. (2004). Working together with diabetes. *Pediatric Nursing, 16*(4), 20. Retrieved 5/17/04 from ProQuest database.

Gaines, K. K. (2004). Desmopressin (DDAVP®) for enuresis diabetes insipidus. *Urologic Nursing, 24*(6), 520–523.

Garibaldi, L. (2004). Disorders of pubertal development. In R.E. Behrman, R.M. Kliegman, & H.B. Jensen (Eds.), *Nelson textbook of pediatrics* (17th ed.). Philadelphia: Saunders.

Hanberg, A. (2005). Common disorders of the pituitary gland: Hyposecretion versus hypersecretion. *Journal of Infusion Nursing, 28*(1), 36–44.

Hardin, D.S., Kemp, S.F., & Allen, D. (2007). Twenty years of recombinant human growth hormone in children: Relevance to pediatric care providers. *Clinical Pediatrics, 46*(4), 279–286.

Kemp, S. (2006). *Growth hormone deficiency.* Retrieved 1/6/08 from http://www.emedicine.com/ped/topic1810.htm.

Klingensmith, G., Kaufman, F., Schatz, D., & Clarke, W. (2004). Diabetes care in the school and day care setting. *Diabetes Care, 27,* S122. Retrieved 5/17/2004 from ProQuest database.

Lafranchi, S. (2004). Disorders of the thyroid gland. In R.E. Behrman, R.M. Kliegman, & H.B. Jensen (Eds.), *Nelson textbook of pediatrics* (17th ed.). Philadelphia: Saunders.

Leonard, B. J., Garwick, A., & Adwan, J. Z. (2005). Adolescents' perceptions of parental role involvement in diabetes management. *Journal of Pediatric Nursing, 20*(6), 405–414.

Levine, L.S., & White, P.C. (2004). Disorders of the adrenal glands. In R.E. Behrman, R.M. Kliegman, & H.B. Jensen (Eds.), *Nelson textbook of pediatrics* (17th ed.). Philadelphia: Saunders.

Lifshitz, F. (2007). *Pediatric endocrinology.* New York: Informa Healthcare.

Lipman, T. H., Hench, K. D., Benyi, T., et al. (2004). A multicentre randomized controlled trial of an intervention to improve the accuracy of linear growth measurement. *Archives of Diseases of Childhood, 89*(4), 342–346.

National Institute of Child Health & Human Development. (2007). *Cushing's syndrome.* Retrieved 1/6/08 from http://www.nichd.nih.gov/health/topics/cushingssyndrome.cfm.

National Institutes of Health, National Diabetes Education Program (2006). Retrieved 1/6/08 from http://ndep.nih.gov/diabetes/youth/youth_FS.htm.

O'Neal, K. J., Jonnalagadda, S. S., Hopkins, B. L., & Kicklighter, J. R. (2005). Quality of life and diabetes knowledge of young persons with type 1 diabetes: Influence of treatment modalities and demographics. *Journal of the American Dietetic Association, 105*(1), 85–91.

Pagana, K. D., & Pagana, T. J. (2006). *Mosby's manual of diagnostic and laboratory tests* (3rd ed.). St. Louis: Mosby.

Parks, J.S. (2004). Hypotpituitarism. In R.E. Behrman, R.M. Kliegman, & H.B. Jensen (Eds.), *Nelson textbook of pediatrics* (17th ed.). Philadelphia: Saunders.

Pediatric Endocrinology Nursing Society. (2007). *Children with diabetes at school.* [electronic version]. Available https://www.pens.org/.

Preston, A., Storch, E. A., Lewin, A., Geffken, G. R., Baumeister, A. L., Strawser, M. S., et al. (2005). Parental stress and maladjustment in children with short stature. *Clinical Pediatrics, 44,* 327–331.

Ramchandani, N. (2004). Type 2 diabetes in children. *American Journal of Nursing, 104*(3), 65–68.

Sechrist, B. (2005). Who's helping the children? Successful practices in pediatric practices in pediatric diabetes. *Lippincott's Case Management, 10*(1), 53–56.

Sullivan-Bolyai, S., Knafl, K., Tamborlane, W., et al. (2004). Parents' reflections on managing their children's diabetes with insulin pumps. *Journal of Nursing Scholarship, 36,* 316–323.

Taketokmo, C. K., Hodding, J. H., & Kraus, D. M. (2007). *Lexi-comp's pediatric dosage handbook* (14th ed.). Hudson, OH: Lexi-comp.

Wise-Faberowski, L., Soriano, S. G., Ferrari, L., et al. (2004) Perioperative management of diabetes insipidus in children. *Journal of Neurosurgical Anesthesiology, 16*(2), 14–19.

WEBSITES

CARES (Congenital Adrenal Hyperplasia Research, Education, and Support) Foundation, Inc.: www.caresfoundation.org

Children with Diabetes (online community for kids, families, and adults with diabetes; multiple resources): www.childrenwithdiabetes.com/index_cwd.htm

American Diabetes Association (resources for diabetes information): www.diabetes.org

Maintains current catalog of commercially available and research-based tests for genetic disorders: www.genetests.org

Healthy People 2010: www.healthypeople.gov

Human Growth Foundation (research, education, support, and advocacy for children with disorders of growth): www.hgfound.org/

Hormone Foundation (the education affiliate of the Endocrine Society): www.hormone.org

Juvenile Diabetes Research Foundation International: www.jdf.org

Resources for families with long-term conditions: www.magicfoundation.org

Parenting and diabetes resources: www.mychildhasdiabetes.com/

National Diabetes Education Program (information and resources on diabetes in children): www.ndep.nih.gov/

Maria I. New Children's Hormone Foundation: www.newchf.org/

National Graves' Disease Foundation: www.ngdf.org/

Pediatric Endocrinology Nursing Society: www.pens.org

Resource for octreotide acetate: www.us.sandostatin.com

CHAPTER WORKSHEET

MULTIPLE CHOICE QUESTIONS

1. A young mother brings her new baby, diagnosed with congenital hypothyroidism, to the clinic so she can learn how to administer levothyroxine. The nurse should include which of the following instructions?

   a. Crush the medication and place it in a full bottle of formula to disguise the taste.

   b. Administer the medication every other day.

   c. Use an oral dispenser syringe or nipple to give the crushed medication mixed with a small amount of formula.

   d. Tell the mother that the medication will not be needed after the age of 7.

2. The nurse is instructing a 14-year-old boy about the different types of insulin. Since he takes NPH insulin every morning at 7:30 a.m., at what time could he possibly have an insulin reaction?

   a. When he goes to school at 9 a.m.

   b. When he takes a test at 11 a.m.

   c. When he eats lunch at noon

   d. When he works out after school at 3 p.m.

3. A child diagnosed with Graves' disease begins to take propylthiouracil (PTU). What symptoms should the parents and child observe for to determine if the dose is too high?

   a. Weight loss.

   b. Lethargy.

   c. Difficulty in school.

   d. Tachycardia.

4. Which endocrine disorder is considered the most common one observed in early childhood?

   a. Hypothyroidism.

   b. Hyperthyroidism.

   c. Diabetes mellitus.

   d. Cushing's disease.

5. When should growth hormone be given in a child who has growth hormone deficiency?

   a. Before meals.

   b. After meals.

   c. At bedtime.

   d. First thing in the morning.

CRITICAL THINKING EXERCISES

1. A 12-year-old boy with DM type 1 has the flu. His mother calls the diabetes clinic to report that he stayed home from school and does not have an appetite, so he is not eating. The mother asks the nurse how much insulin the boy should take. He is currently taking three injections daily with Regular and NPH in the morning before breakfast, Regular and NPH in the evening after dinner, and Regular before bedtime. What questions should the nurse ask before answering the mother's question? Based on the answers to these questions, how would you instruct the mother?

2. The mother of Robin, a 5-year-old girl, reports that Robin has a body odor. She is developing breasts and some pubic hair and was teased when she had a sleepover with friends. The review of her growth charts reveals that Robin went from the 50th percentile to the 93rd percentile in the past 6 months. Based on this information, what are the three major nursing diagnoses to begin establishing a plan of care for the child and family? What are the expected outcomes and major interventions associated with the nursing diagnosis of knowledge deficit?

3. A mother brings her baby to the clinic after receiving a phone message from the clinic saying there was a problem with the baby's thyroid test. She says the trip on the bus took a long time, but the infant slept the entire way. She says that the baby is sleeping much of the time and does not want to eat very much. The baby was discharged from the hospital 2 weeks ago. The birth was without difficulty and there were no problems during labor. Why is this visit urgent? What would the test show if the disorder was due to a pituitary gland problem and not the thyroid gland?

STUDY ACTIVITIES

1. During your clinical experiences, ask to be on an inpatient unit that provides care for children with alterations in endocrine function. Compare and contrast the health histories, assessments, laboratory tests, diagnostic procedures, and plans of care for these children with those for the care of children on other units. Participate in the teaching plan for these children and their families.

2. Attend an outpatient clinic that provides care to children with endocrine disorders. Identify the role of the registered nurse in providing coordination of care, health teaching, and referrals for these children and their families.

3. Shadow a diabetes nurse educator to observe the teaching methods and strategies he or she uses to provide an education plan for a child with diabetes mellitus. Observe how the nurse educator includes the family in the plan. Are there any differences between the teaching plans for type 1 and type 2 DM?

4. Conduct a literature review for one of the common endocrine disorders to research current management practices. Are there evidence-based practice guidelines for nursing interventions?

5. Conduct an Internet search to research the information that is available to children and their families related to diabetes mellitus.

NURSING CARE OF THE CHILD WITH A NEOPLASTIC DISORDER

KEY TERMS

biopsy
biotherapy
chemotherapy

clinical trial
extravasation
malignant

metastasis
neoplastic
staging

LEARNING OBJECTIVES

Upon completion of the chapter, the learner will be able to:

1. Compare childhood and adult cancers.
2. Describe nursing care related to common laboratory and diagnostic testing used in the medical diagnosis of pediatric cancer.
3. Identify types of cancer common in infants, children, and adolescents.
4. Identify appropriate nursing assessments and interventions related to medications and treatments for pediatric cancer.
5. Develop an individualized nursing care plan for the child with cancer.
6. Describe the psychosocial impact of cancer on children and their families.
7. Devise a nutrition plan for the child with cancer.
8. Develop patient/family teaching plans for the child with cancer.

John Shaw, 4 years old, is brought to the clinic by his parents with a fever. His father states, "John seems to get fevers and colds more often than our other children. He's also very tired these days. He hardly ever wants to go out and play with his friends. He complains of headaches frequently and just doesn't really seem like himself."

Wow

Be inspired by the courage of a child with cancer and reflect it in the care you provide.

Cancer accounts for the most deaths from disease in children over age 1 year. Cure has been achieved in some children with childhood leukemia and other cancers, but there is no universal long-term cure available for any of the childhood cancers. The 5-year survival rate for all cancers in children approaching 75% (Eiser, 2007).

Cancer is a life-threatening illness that involves emotional distress, fear of the unknown, and changes in life priorities for the child and family. Children with cancer are at a significant risk for depression because they have a life-threatening illness and must undergo frequent and stressful tests and treatments (Eiser, 2007). Initial and ongoing diagnostic testing and the adverse effects of chemotherapy, radiation, or other treatments are often painful as well.

Treatment for cancer has a significant psychosocial impact on the child or adolescent. The child often feels isolated from his or her peers, and the adolescent may have difficulty achieving independence, which is the core developmental task of the teenage years. Children and teens with cancer often demonstrate poorer school performance than healthy peers (Hokkanen et al., 2004). Nurses caring for children with cancer need to be knowledgeable about the medical treatment of the disease and must also be particularly aware of the psychosocial and emotional impact of cancer on the child and family.

Childhood Cancer Versus Adult Cancer

Cancers in children differ greatly from cancers in adults. Pediatric cancers most often arise from primitive embryonal (mesodermal) and neuroectodermal tissues, resulting in leukemias, lymphomas, sarcomas, or central nervous system (CNS) tumors. This is in direct contrast to adult cancers, which mostly arise from epithelial cells, resulting in carcinomas. The most common childhood cancers, in order of frequency, are leukemia, CNS tumors, lymphoma, neuroblastoma, rhabdomyosarcoma, Wilms' tumor, bone tumors, and retinoblastoma. Comparison Chart 49.1 explains how cancer is different in children versus adults.

In children, warning signs of cancer are most often related to changes in blood cell production or as a result of compression, infiltration, or obstruction caused by the tumor. Changes in blood cell production may result in fatigue, pallor, frequent or severe infection, or easy bruising. Infiltration, obstruction, or compression by a tumor may result in bone or abdominal pain, pain elsewhere, swelling, or unusual discharge.

> ▶ **Take** *NOTE!*
>
> *Research is underway to determine whether a statistically significant link exists between the use of supplemental oxygen in the neonatal period and the development of childhood cancer. Studies thus far have proven to be equivocal.*

Common Medical Treatments

Deciding on a course of medical treatment for cancer in a developing child is complicated. Some of the treatments can impair the child's growth and development. Many pediatric oncologists and cancer treatment centers are active members of the Children's Oncology Group (COG), a National Cancer Institute–supported group that approves and administers clinical trials devoted exclusively to childhood and adolescent cancer research. A **clinical trial** is a carefully designed research study that assesses

COMPARISON CHART 49.1   CHILDHOOD CANCER VERSUS ADULT CANCER

	Childhood Cancer	Adult Cancer
Cancer usually affects	Tissues	Organs
Histologic type	Embryonal, leukemia, lymphoma	Epithelial in origin
Most common sites	Blood, lymph, brain, bone, kidney, muscle	Breast, lung, prostate, bowel, bladder
Environmental and lifestyle factors	Only a small amount of environmental influence proven	Strong influence on cancer development
Cancer prevention	Little known	80% preventable
Detection	Usually incidental or accidental	Very early detection possible if screening recommendations followed
Latent period	Relatively short	Can be very long (20 years or greater)
Extent of disease	Metastasis often present at diagnosis	Metastasis less often present at diagnosis
Response to treatment	Very responsive	Less responsive

HEALTHY PEOPLE 2010

Objective	Significance
Increase the proportion of persons who use at least one of the following protective measures that may reduce the risk of skin cancer: avoid the sun between 10 a.m. and 4 p.m., wear sun-protective clothing when exposed to sunlight, use sunscreen with a sun-protective factor (SPF) of 15 or higher, and avoid artificial sources of ultraviolet light.	• Educate families to start skin protection from the sun in childhood to reduce the risk of skin cancer as an adult. • Teach parents to use PABA-free sunscreen (formulated specifically for children) after age 6 months with an SPF of 15 or greater and to reapply sunscreen frequently while the child is out of doors. • Advocate for schools to encourage a sun-safe environment.

BOX 49.1 **American Academy of Pediatrics, Committee on Bioethics, Recommendations Regarding Pediatric Assent**

• Give consideration to each child's developmental capacity, rationality, and autonomy.
• Help each child to achieve a developmentally appropriate understanding of the illness.
• Tell the child what s/he can expect regarding testing procedures and treatments.
• Assess the child's understanding of the situation and how s/he is responding.
• Note if there is inappropriate pressure to assent to testing or treatment.
• Seriously solicit the child's expression of willingness to accept the proposed plan of care.

the effectiveness of a treatment as well as its acute and long-term effects on the patient. Current cancer care in children is a result of the knowledge gained through clinical trials. A clinical trial may include existing medications or treatments in combination with new drugs or may involve a different approach to sequencing or dosing of medications and treatment.

To provide optimal outcomes, the child with cancer should be treated at an institution with multidisciplinary cancer care specialists that can provide the most advanced care available. Each case of pediatric cancer should be considered individually, with the oncology health care team and the family reaching treatment decisions together, whether the treatment plan is standard or involves enrollment in a clinical trial.

In the child with cancer, particularly advanced disease, the decision to provide treatment ("let's do everything we can") or to withhold treatment in the event of an extremely poor prognosis is extraordinarily challenging in an ethical sense. A mature older child or adolescent may have a strong desire to continue or discontinue treatment, and sometimes this desire conflicts with the parents' desires or choices. The American Academy of Pediatrics, Committee on Bioethics (1995), recommends that decision making for older children and adolescents should include the assent of the patient (Box 49.1).

Hospice or palliative care may be needed for the child with cancer. Children facing the end of life experience the same effects that adults do, such as pain, fatigue, nausea, and dyspnea. Standards for end-of-life care are still in development, but all dying children have the right to die comfortably and with palliation of symptoms, as has been well established in adult hospice programs. Children's Hospice International (CHI) has demonstration models in several U.S. states that focus on enhancing the quality of life of children with life-threatening conditions. Formerly, only children with a life expectancy of less than 6 months

had access to hospice care, and they were required to forego curative care to enroll in hospice. CHI's goal is to provide a comprehensive, interdisciplinary continuum of care to the child and family from the time of diagnosis with a life-threatening condition through the time of death, if cure is not achieved. For further information related to nursing care of the dying child, refer to Chapter 33.

A variety of medications and treatments are used to treat **neoplastic** disorders in children. Most of these treatments will require a physician's order when the child is in the hospital. The most common treatments and medications are listed in Common Medical Treatments 49.1 and Drug Guide 49.1. Commonly, chemotherapy and radiation therapy are used to treat childhood cancers. In some instances, hematopoietic stem cell transplantation is used. The nurse caring for the child with cancer should be familiar with the procedures, how the treatments and medications work, and common nursing implications related to use of these modalities.

Chemotherapy

To understand how **chemotherapy** works to destroy cancer cells, it is necessary to review the normal cell cycle. All

(text continues on page 1631)

HEALTHY PEOPLE 2010

Objective	Significance
Reduce the overall cancer death rate. Increase the proportion of cancer survivors who are living 5 years or longer after diagnosis.	• Teach adolescent boys testicular self-examination. • Reinforce the importance of this self-screening measure at subsequent visits.

COMMON MEDICAL TREATMENTS 49.1

Treatment	Explanation	Indication	Nursing Implications
Biopsy	A small piece of the tumor is removed with a needle or via an open incision.	Solid tumors	Monitor for bleeding at the needle biopsy site. Provide routine incision care for open biopsy site.
Surgical removal of tumor	The tumor is completely or partially resected surgically.	Solid tumors	Provide routine postoperative nursing care based on the location of the tumor excision.
Leukapheresis	Whole blood is removed from the body, the WBCs are extracted, and then the blood is retransfused into the child.	Hyperviscosity with leukemia (WBC > 100,000)	Performed by specially trained personnel. Monitor blood pressure and other vital signs.
Blood product transfusion	Administration of whole blood, packed red blood cells, platelets, or plasma intravenously.	Anemia, thrombocytopenia, bleeding	Follow institution's transfusion protocol. Double-check blood type and product label with a second nurse. Use only irradiated, leukodepleted, CMV-negative blood products in the pediatric cancer patient. Monitor vital signs and assess child frequently to detect adverse reaction to blood transfusion. If adverse reaction is suspected, immediately discontinue transfusion, run normal saline IV, reassess child, and notify physician. Some children require premedication with diphenhydramine and/or acetaminophen before receiving blood products.
Radiation therapy	Ionizing radiation (high-energy x-ray) is delivered to the cancerous area. The radiation damages all cells in the locally treated area (normal and cancerous), but the normal cells are able to repair themselves. Usually administered several times a week for several weeks (a short rest between treatments allows the normal cells time to regenerate). The lowest possible dose of radiation is used and it is directed to a specific area.	Solid tumors, before or after surgical resection, leukemia, lymphoma	Do not wash off radiation marking. Keep skin clean and dry. Fatigue is a common side effect. Skin at the site of radiation may become red, dry, or pruritic or may peel; eventually may become moist and red. Mucositis, dry mouth, and loss of taste may occur if head or neck radiated. Radiation may also have adverse affects on the organ irradiated, such as the brain; monitor for changes.
Hematopoietic stem cell transplantation	*Bone marrow transplant:* transfer of healthy bone marrow into a child with cancer. The transplanted cells can then develop into functional cells. *Stem cell transplant:* peripheral stem cells are removed from the donor via apheresis, or stem cells are retrieved from the umbilical cord and placenta. The stem cells are then transplanted into the recipient.	Leukemia, lymphoma, other cancers	Maintain medical asepsis and protective isolation to prevent infection. Monitor closely for GVHD. Provide meticulous oral care. Avoid rectal temperatures and suppositories. Encourage appropriate nutrition. Administer immunosuppressive medications as ordered.

COMMON MEDICAL TREATMENTS 49.1 (continued)

Treatment	Explanation	Indication	Nursing Implications
Central venous catheter (Fig. 49.1)	IV catheters inserted into the central circulation for the purpose of administering medications, total parenteral medication, or blood products.	Any child with cancer who will require long-term IV medications or parenteral nutrition	Complaints of shortness of breath or chest pain may indicate air entry into the central venous catheter. Have child lie on left side, and notify physician immediately. Keep dressing clean and dry. Perform sterile dressing change per institution policy or physician order. Monitor for fever. Monitor insertion site for erythema or drainage. Maintain sterile technique when accessing line, performing dressing change, or administering any fluid through catheter.
Implanted port (Fig. 49.2)	A needle-accessible port is implanted under the skin, usually on the chest. The port has a thin catheter exiting it that is tunneled under the skin into the superior vena cava or subclavian vein.	Any child with cancer who will require long-term IV medications or parenteral nutrition	Flush non-accessed port with prescribed heparin dose per institution policy. Use sterile technique to access port with Huber needle. Monitor port site for erythema or warmth.

DRUG GUIDE 49.1 COMMON DRUGS FOR NEOPLASTIC DISORDERS

Medication	Action/Indications	Nursing Implications
Chemotherapy		
Alkylating agents: busulfan, carboplatin, cisplatin, ifosfamide, temozolomide, thiotepa. Nitrosoureas: carmustine, lomustine. Nitrogen mustard: chlorambucil, cyclophosphamide, mechlorethamine, melphalan.	Interferes with DNA replication and RNA transcription by alkylation (replacing the hydrogen ion with an alkyl group), cross-links DNA. Cell cycle–nonspecific. The nitrosoureas are highly lipid-soluble and easily cross the blood–brain barrier. Used in a variety of cancer protocols.	Causes myelosuppression, nausea, vomiting, alopecia, mucositis. Monitor for signs of infection. Provide adequate hydration. Cyclophosphamide, ifosfamide: administer in the morning, provide adequate hydration, and have child void frequently during and after infusion to decrease risk of hemorrhagic cystitis. Cisplatin, mechlorethamine, melphalan: avoid extravasation. Temozolomide: avoid opening capsules. Thiotepa: if contact with skin occurs, wash thoroughly with soap and water.
Antitumor antibiotics: bleomycin, dactinomycin, daunorubicin, doxorubicin, idarubicin, mitomycin, mitoxantrone	Interfere with cellular metabolism, causing disruptions in DNA and/or RNA synthesis. Cell cycle–nonspecific. Indicated in a variety of cancer protocols.	May cause alopecia, nausea, vomiting, myelosuppression. Bleomycin: fever and chills may occur 20 hours after infusion. Dactinomycin, mitomycin: avoid extravasation. Daunorubicin, doxorubicin, idarubicin: may turn urine red-orange, monitor for arrhythmias, congestive heart failure; avoid extravasation. Mitoxantrone: may color urine, sweat, tears, skin, sclera blue-green; monitor for arrhythmias, congestive heart failure.

Medication	Action/Indications	Nursing Implications
Antimetabolites: cladribine, cytarabine, fludarabine, fluorouracil, mercaptopurine, methotrexate, thioguanine	Substitute for a natural metabolite in the molecule, altering the cell's function and ability to replicate. Cell cycle–specific (S phase), cladribine is cell cycle–nonspecific. Used in a variety of cancer protocols.	May cause alopecia, nausea, vomiting, mucositis, and myelosuppression. Cladribine: monitor for fever. Cytarabine: use corticosteroid eye drops to prevent conjunctivitis with high doses. Fludarabine: monitor for visual changes and neurotoxicity; maintain adequate hydration. Fluorouracil: maintain adequate hydration; may cause photosensitivity. Mercaptopurine: do not give oral doses with meals; may cause drug fever; avoid extravasation. Methotrexate: intensive hydration with high doses; may cause photosensitivity. Thioguanine: maintain hydration; administer on empty stomach.
Antimicrotubulars: paclitaxel	Inhibits mitotic cellular function in late G2 and M phases of cell cycle Indicated for refractory leukemia, recurrent Wilms' tumor.	May cause alopecia, nausea, vomiting, mucositis, myelosuppression. May cause drowsiness. Avoid extravasation.
Miscellaneous: asparaginase, pegaspargase	Inhibits protein synthesis by depriving tumor cells of the essential amino acid asparagine. Used in acute lymphocytic leukemia, lymphomas.	May cause alopecia, nausea, vomiting, and myelosuppression. Monitor for vital signs during infusion and for signs of anaphylaxis. Have emergency equipment, oxygen, epinephrine, antihistamines, and steroids available at bedside.
Miscellaneous: dacarbazine, procarbazine	Inhibits DNA and RNA synthesis via cross-linking or suppression of mitosis Indicated in a variety of cancer protocols.	May cause alopecia, nausea, vomiting, myelosuppression. Monitor for flu-like symptoms. Dacarbazine: photosensitivity may occur; avoid extravasation.
Mitotic inhibitors: etoposide, vinblastine, vincristine	Inhibits mitotic activity by inhibiting DNA topoisomerase (etoposide). Causes metaphase arrest by binding to the mitotic spindle (vinblastine, vincristine). Used in a variety of cancer protocols.	May cause alopecia, nausea, vomiting, myelosuppression (only minimal with vincristine). Etoposide: monitor for anaphylaxis; have emergency equipment, oxygen, epinephrine, antihistamines, and steroids available at bedside. Vinblastine, vincristine: maintain hydration; administer allopurinol; avoid extravasation.
Topoisomerase inhibitors: irinotecan, topotecan	Binds to DNA complex, preventing religation of single-strand DNA breaks Indicated for refractory solid tumors.	May cause alopecia, nausea, vomiting, myelosuppression, severe diarrhea (irinotecan), hypotension (topotecan). Maintain hydration. Avoid extravasation. Monitor blood pressure during topotecan infusion.
Corticosteroids: prednisone, dexamethasone	Suppresses immune system by decreasing lymphatic activity and volume. Also decreases edema caused by tumor or tumor necrosis. Indicated for leukemia and some other cancers.	Administer with food to decrease GI upset. May mask signs of infection. Monitor blood pressure; monitor urine for glucose. Do not stop treatment abruptly or acute adrenal insufficiency may occur. Monitor for Cushing syndrome. Doses may be tapered over time.

(continued)

DRUG GUIDE 49.1 COMMON DRUGS FOR NEOPLASTIC DISORDERS (continued)

Medication	Action/Indications	Nursing Implications
Biotherapy		
Colony-stimulating factors: darbepoetin alfa, epoetin alfa, filgrastim, sargramostim	Stimulates production of red blood cells (epoetin) or granulocytes (filgrastim, sargramostim) Used to counteract myelosuppressive effects of chemotherapy.	Administer SC or IV. Filgrastrim, sargramostim: may cause bone pain. Sargramostim may cause hypotension and a first-dose reaction.
Interleukins: aldesleukin	Recombinant DNA interleukin-2 product that recruits T, B, and natural killer cells Indicated for non-Hodgkin's lymphoma.	Adverse effects are dose-dependent. May cause capillary leak syndrome within 2 to 12 hours of start of treatment: hypotension and decreased organ perfusion result.
Tumor necrosis factor (protein cytokine)	Increases effectiveness of immune cells, stops cancer cells from dividing, damages tumor blood vessels. Used in a variety of cancer protocols.	May cause fever, chills, rigors, nausea, vomiting.
Monoclonal antibodies: rituximab, gemtuzumab	Binds to CD20 antigen on B lymphocytes Indicated in CD20-positive non-Hodgkin's lymphoma, post-transplant lymphoproliferative disorder.	Monitor blood pressure for hypotension. Monitor for anaphylaxis and infusion-related reaction. Have epinephrine, antihistamines, and steroids available at bedside for treatment of reaction.
Interferons: alpha, gamma	Alter cancer cell proliferation (alpha), stimulate macrophage production to fight bacteria and fungus (gamma) Indicated in a variety of cancer protocols.	May cause flu-like symptoms. Maintain adequate hydration.
Allopurinol	Decreases production of uric acid. Use to treat secondary hyperuricemia occurring during leukemia or tumor treatment.	Give PO after meals with plenty of food. Cardiovascular adverse effects may occur with IV administration. Maintain adequate hydration.
Antibiotics (oral, parenteral)	Treatment of documented bacterial infections. Also used as prophylaxis of *Pneumocystis jiroveci* and in the neutropenic patient.	Check for antibiotic allergies. Should be given as prescribed for the length of time prescribed. Start IV antibiotics as soon as possible in the neutropenic child admitted with fever.
Antiemetics: promethazine, metoclopramide, ondansetron	Acts on the CNS transmitters to prevent vomiting.	May cause CNS side effects, such as drowsiness or irritability. Ondansetron: may cause dry mouth.
Antifungal agents: nystatin, amphotericin B (conventional and lipid complex)	Invades fungal cell wall, enabling its destruction. Indicated for mucositis, or systemic fungal infection.	Nystatin: administer after meals. Amphotericin B: may cause fever, chills, rigors, cardiovascular adverse effects; monitor patient closely throughout infusion; note dose differences between conventional and lipid complex.
Immunosuppressant drugs: cyclosporine A (CyA), mycophenolate, tacrolimus	Inhibition of production and release of interleukin II (CyA). Inhibition of T- and B-cell proliferation (mycophenolate). Inhibition of T-cell activation (tacrolimus). Used for treatment of GVHD after HSCT.	Monitor CBC, serum creatinine, potassium, and magnesium. Monitor blood pressure and for signs of infection. Draw blood levels prior to morning dose. CyA: do not give with grapefruit juice. Mycophenolate: give on empty stomach; do not open capsule or crush tablet. Tacrolimus: give on empty stomach; monitor for anaphylaxis with first IV dose.

(continued)

Medication	Action/Indications	Nursing Implications
Mesna	Binds with and detoxifies cyclophos- phamide and ifosfamide metabolites in the urinary bladder to prevent hemor- rhagic cystitis	Maintain adequate hydration. Administer concurrently and after cyclophos- phamide or ifosfamide. May cause hypotension.
Methotrexate anti- dote: leucovorin	Reduces toxic effects of methotrexate.	May cause skin disturbances, wheezing, throm- bocytosis. Dose depends on methotrexate level. Dose increased with increased creatinine levels.

cells progress through this cycle (Fig. 49.3). The cell cycle comprises five phases:

- G0 phase: the resting phase; lasts from a few hours to a few years; cells have not started to divide
- G1 phase: cell makes more protein in preparation for dividing; lasts 18 to 30 hours
- S phase: chromosomes are copied so that newly formed cells have the appropriate DNA; lasts 18 to 20 hours
- G2 phase: just before the cell splits into two cells; lasts 2 to 10 hours
- M phase: mitosis, the actual splitting of the cell into two new cells; lasts 30 minutes to 1 hour

Chemotherapy drugs work in two different ways in relation to the cell cycle. Cell cycle–specific agents exert their actions during a specific phase of the cell cycle. Cell cycle–nonspecific drugs exert their effect on the cells regardless of which phase the cell is in. Chemotherapy protocols often call for a combination of drugs that act on different phases of the cell cycle, thus maximizing the de-struction of cancer cells.

Chemotherapeutic medications disrupt the cell cycle of not only cancer cells but also normal rapidly di-viding cells, resulting in a significant number of adverse effects. The cells most likely to be affected by chemo-therapy are those in the bone marrow, the digestive tract (especially the mouth), the reproductive system, and hair follicles.

Chemotherapy drugs are divided into classes that exert slightly different actions and have an effect on dif-ferent portions of the cell cycle. Drug Guide 49.1 gives further explanation about the different classes of chemo-therapy drugs.

A

Huber needle
port reservoir
catheter

B

FIGURE 49.2 **(A)** The implanted port consists of a reservoir under the skin for ready access. The catheter exiting the port is threaded into the subclavian vein or right atrium. **(B)** A 90-degree Huber needle is used to access the port.

FIGURE 49.1 The central venous access catheter is tunneled under the skin and secured with a cuff.

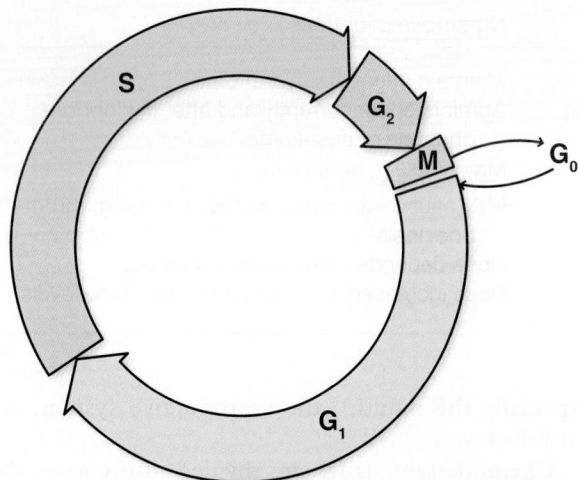

FIGURE 49.3 Phases of the cell cycle.

Adverse effects common to chemotherapeutic drugs include immunosuppression, infection, myelosuppression, nausea, vomiting, constipation, oral mucositis, alopecia, and pain (Woolery et al., 2006). Long-term complications include microdontia and missing teeth as a result of damage to developing permanent teeth; hearing and vision changes; hematopoietic, immunologic, or gonadal dysfunction; endocrine dysfunction, including altered growth and precocious or delayed puberty; various alterations of the cardiorespiratory, gastrointestinal, and genitourinary systems; as well as a second cancer as an adolescent or adult.

▶ *Take* NOTE!

Acupuncture as an adjuvant therapy has been demonstrated to significantly decrease nausea, vomiting and aversion to chemotherapy (Rheingans, 2007).

Radiation Therapy

Radiation therapy uses high-energy radiation to damage or kill cancer cells. Radiant energy in either a gamma or particle form is emitted during the treatment (Tomlinson & Kline, 2005). Radiation affects not only cancer cells but also any rapidly growing cells that they are in contact with. It may be used as a curative, adjuvant, or palliative treatment, either alone or in combination with chemotherapy. Radiation therapy is also used to shrink a tumor prior to surgical resection. The area to be treated is marked carefully to minimize damage to normal cells.

Adverse effects of radiation therapy include fatigue, nausea, vomiting, oral mucositis, myelosuppression, and alterations in skin integrity at the site of irradiation. Long-term complications are related to the area of the body that was irradiated and include alterations in growth; hormone dysfunction; hearing and vision alterations; learning problems; cardiac dysfunction; pulmonary fibrosis; hepatic, sexual, or renal dysfunction; osteoporosis; and development of secondary cancer (particularly at the site of irradiation).

EVIDENCE-BASED PRACTICE 49.1
Nonpharmacologic Therapies for Symptom Management in Childhood Cancer

● **Study**
Even with significant advances in childhood cancer surgery and treatment, troublesome symptoms remain a large problem. Children report that the most upsetting aspect of cancer treatment is the numerous side effects they suffer. The author performed a systematic review of research studies that evaluated the use of complementary and alternative therapies for cancer treatment side effect management. Forty-one studies were reviewed that addressed such topics as procedural pain, distress, fear and anxiety, nausea/vomiting, anxiety, distress, and depression. Nonpharmacologic adjunctive therapies evaluated in the studies included hypnosis, distraction, cognitive behavioral therapies, relaxation, imagery, breathing, music therapy, play, self-hypnosis, acupuncture, art therapy, coping skills training, handholding, humor, and nonessential touch.

▲ **Findings**
Many of the nonpharmacologic adjuvant therapies studies were found to be effective for symptom relief. Cognitive behavioral therapy, distraction, and hypnosis were particularly helpful. Although safety concerns for various therapies were not reported, the author proposed that further rigorous research on these modalities is necessary.

■ **Nursing Implications**
Many families will be seeking nonpharmacologic or complementary/alternative therapies for relieving the distressing symptoms associated with cancer treatment. Nurses must keep an open mind about these therapies. When families have questions about using these treatments, they should be directed to authorities in the area. Nurses are in a perfect position to initiate additional rigorous research to determine the effectiveness and long-term safety of these therapies.

Rheingans, J.I. (2007). A systematic review of nonpharmacologic adjunctive therapies for symptom management in children with cancer. *Journal of Pediatric Oncology Nursing, 24*(2), 81-94.

Hematopoietic Stem Cell Transplantation

Hematopoietic stem cell transplantation (HSCT), also called bone marrow transplantation, is a procedure in which hematopoietic stem cells are infused intravenously into the patient. This follows a period of purging of abnormal cells in the patient that is accomplished through high-dose chemotherapy or irradiation. The use of high-dose chemotherapy and total body irradiation kills the tumor cells but also destroys the child's bone marrow. The transplanted cells migrate to the empty spaces in the child's bone marrow and re-establish normal hematopoiesis in the child.

HSCT is used for a variety of childhood cancers, including leukemia, lymphoma, brain tumors, neuroblastoma, and other solid tumors. For most pediatric cancers, it is not the first line of treatment but is used for refractory or advanced disease.

Autologous HSCT is achieved through harvest and treatment of the child's own bone marrow, followed by infusion of the treated stem cells. Risk for relapse of the original disease is highest in autologous HSCT. Allogenic HSCT refers to transplantation using stem cells from another individual that are harvested from the bone marrow, peripheral blood, or umbilical cord blood. Allogenic HSCT requires human leukocyte antibody (HLA) matching for antigen-specific sites on the leukocytes. Closely matched HLA donors may be difficult to find from a donor listing, and sibling donors are often the closest match. The degree of match is inversely related to the risk for graft rejection and the development of graft-versus-host disease (GVHD). In other words, the lesser the degree of HLA matching in the donor, the higher the risk for graft rejection and GVHD. GVHD occurs to at least some extent in up to 70% of all allogenic HSCT recipients (Graham et al., 2005).

In addition to graft rejection and GVHD, additional initial complications of HSCT are infection, electrolyte imbalance, bleeding, and organ, skin, and mucous membrane toxicities. Long-term complications include impaired growth and fertility related to endocrine dysfunction, developmental delay, cataracts, pulmonary and cardiac disease, avascular necrosis of the bone, and the development of secondary malignancies.

NURSING PROCESS OVERVIEW FOR THE CHILD WITH A NEOPLASTIC DISORDER

Care of the child with a neoplastic disorder includes assessment, nursing diagnosis, planning, interventions, and evaluation. There are a number of general concepts related to the nursing process that may be applied to cancers in children. From a general understanding of the care involved for a child with cancer, the nurse can then individualize the care based on patient specifics. Children with cancer often suffer many physical effects as a result of the disease and its treatment. The nurse must be diligent when assessing for these effects and should involve the parents as a reliable source for reporting the child's physical symptoms.

Assessment

Assessment of children with neoplastic disorders includes health history, physical examination, and laboratory and diagnostic testing.

Remember John, the 4-year-old with fever, fatigue, and headaches? What additional health history and physical examination assessment information should you obtain?

Health History

Determine current medical history. Note history of recurrent fever or frequent infections. Inquire about bleeding tendencies, such as unusual bruising or petechiae. Note early-morning headache with nausea or vomiting, gait or behavior changes, or visual disturbances. Inquire about changes in bowel or bladder habits or decrease in appetite. Note history of bone fractures unrelated to trauma. Explore the health history for the presence of risk factors such as previous malignancy and treatment; synthetic chemical exposures; parental exposure to radiation, chemicals, or chemotherapeutic agents; and a family history of malignancy (especially childhood), immune disorder, or genetic disorders such as neurofibromatosis or Down syndrome.

Physical Examination

A complete physical examination should be performed on any child with or suspected of having cancer. Note particular findings as discussed below.

Inspection and Observation

Observe the child's overall appearance and energy level. Note thin, frail appearance, fatigue, or altered level of consciousness. Document visible masses or asymmetry of the face, thorax, abdomen, or extremities. Note difficulty breathing. Inspect the skin for pallor, bruising, or petechiae. Examine the oral cavity for bleeding gums or pale mucous membranes. Observe the child's gait, noting ataxia or limp. Note rectal bleeding or vaginal discharge.

Auscultation, Percussion, and Palpation

Auscultate the heart, lungs, and abdomen, noting any abnormalities. Percuss the abdomen, noting dullness over a mass if present. Palpate for lymphadenopathy; in particular, note nontender or firm lymph nodes. Palpate any unusual area of swelling anywhere on the body, noting size and absence of tenderness. Palpate the abdomen, noting organomegaly or presence of a mass. Note limited range of motion or pain upon palpation of extremities.

Psychosocial Assessment

Assess the child's and family's psychosocial status, using open-ended questions. It is particularly important to determine the child's self-esteem, level of anxiety or stress, and coping mechanisms. Determine the spiritual status of the child and family. Ongoing medical procedures and the fear of dying take a toll on the child and family. Ask the child how things are going at home; how does he or she get along with brothers, sisters, and parents? If the child is school age, ask how school is going. Does the child have friends that he or she gets to spend time with? Ask the child what he or she does in his spare time; are there any hobbies? These types of queries will provide the nurse with information about how well the child is coping.

Assess the parents' status as well. Ask about the marital relationship and how the other children are doing. Determine whether certain stressors may need to be addressed.

Laboratory and Diagnostic Testing

Common Laboratory and Diagnostic Tests 49.1 explains the laboratory and diagnostic tests most commonly used

COMMON LABORATORY AND DIAGNOSTIC TESTS 49.1

Test	Explanation	Indication	Nursing Implications
Complete blood count (CBC) with differential	Evaluate hemoglobin and hematocrit, WBC count (particularly the percentage of individual WBCs), and platelet count	Infection, immuno-suppression, to determine neutropenia in myelo-suppression	Normal values vary according to age and gender. WBC count differential is helpful in evaluating source of infection. May be affected by myelo-suppressive drugs.
Alpha-fetoprotein (AFP)	Produced by the fetal liver and yolk sac; normally decreases to very low levels by 1 year of age	May be elevated in Hodgkin's disease and other cancers. Used to determine tumor burden	No food or fluid restriction required.
Urine catechol-amines (VMA, HVA)	Catabolism of catechol-amines causes elevated levels in urine	Diagnosis of neuroblastoma (produces catecholamines)	24-hour urine collection. Levels may be altered with certain foods and drugs or vigorous exercise.
Chest x-ray	Radiograph of the chest	Identify tumor or metastasis in the thorax	Chest must be held stationary for a brief time.
Computed tomography (CT scan)	Multiple films taken in successive layers to provide a 3D view of the body part being scanned	Identify tumor location or metastasis	Some CT scans are done with oral or IV contrast (notify physician if child has iodine or shellfish allergy). May require a several-hour period of NPO if contrast is used (contrast may cause nausea). Encourage fluid intake after scan to facilitate excretion of contrast dye.
Magnetic resonance imaging (MRI)	Based on how hydrogen atoms behave in a magnetic field when disturbed by radiofrequency signals. Does not require ionizing radiation. Provides a 3D view of the body part being scanned	Identify extent of tumor or metastatic spread	Remove all metal objects from the child. Child must remain motionless for entire scan; parent can stay in room with child. Younger children will require sedation to keep still. A loud thumping sound occurs inside the machine during the scan procedure; this can be frightening to children.

Test	Explanation	Indication	Nursing Implications
Bone scan	Administration of IV radio-nuclide material, which is taken up by the bone and is visible on the scans	Identifies metastasis to bone	Requires patent IV for injection. Encourage fluid intake after injection to increase uptake of injected radionuclide. Scan will be performed 1 to 3 hours after injection.
Ultrasound	High-frequency sound waves are directed at internal organs and structures, and an image is made of the waves as they are reflected back through the tissues	Identify tumor presence, especially in abdomen or on kidney	Fasting for a few hours may be required when certain organs are to be visualized.
Bone marrow aspiration and biopsy	A needle is inserted through the cortex of the bone into the bone marrow (most often the iliac spine), bone marrow is aspirated, and the cells are evaluated	Evaluation for leukemia or metastasis of other cancers to bone marrow	Use EMLA or lidocaine to decrease pain with procedure. Often performed under conscious sedation. Apply a pressure dressing to arrest bleeding. Assess for tenderness or erythema. May require mild analgesia for post-procedure pain.
Lumbar puncture (LP)	A needle is placed in the sub-arachnoid space of the spinal column, below the base of the cord, and cerebrospinal fluid is withdrawn for analysis	Evaluation of tumor or metastasis to brain or spinal cord. Also used to administer intrathecal medications	Use EMLA before the procedure to decrease pain. May be performed under conscious sedation. Position child appropriately. Use distraction techniques in the older child or teen. Encourage child to recline for up to 12 hours after LP.

for neoplastic disorders. The tests can assist the physician in diagnosing the disorder or can be used as guidelines in determining treatment. Laboratory or non-nursing personnel obtain some of the tests, while the nurse might obtain others. In either instance the nurse should be familiar with how the tests are obtained, what they are used for, and normal versus abnormal results. This knowledge will also be necessary when providing patient and family education about the testing.

Nursing Diagnosis, Goals, Interventions, and Evaluation
Upon completion of a thorough assessment, the nurse might identify several nursing diagnoses, including:

• Risk for infection
• Pain
• Impaired oral mucous membranes
• Nausea
• Imbalanced nutrition

• Constipation
• Diarrhea
• Risk for impaired skin integrity
• Activity intolerance
• Disturbed body image
• Situational low self-esteem
• Compromised family coping
• Anticipatory grieving

After completing an assessment of John, you note the following: history of recurrent infections, unusual bruising, and enlarged lymph nodes. Based on the assessment findings, what would your top three prioritized nursing diagnoses be for John?

Nursing goals, interventions, and evaluation for the child with cancer are based on the nursing diagnoses. Nursing Care Plan 49.1 may be used as a guide in planning

(text continues on page 1640)

Nursing Care Plan 49.1

OVERVIEW FOR THE CHILD WITH A NEOPLASTIC DISORDER

NURSING DIAGNOSIS: Risk for infection related to neutropenia and immunosuppression

Outcome Identification and Evaluation
Child will not experience overwhelming infection; *will be free from infection or able to recover if becomes infected.*

Interventions: Preventing Infection
- Assess for fever, pain, cough, tachypnea, adventitious breath sounds, skin ulceration, stomatitis, and perirectal fissures *to identify potential infection.*
- Administer antibiotics for temperature >38.4° C *to decrease likelihood of overwhelming sepsis.*
- Maintain meticulous handwashing procedures (include family, visitors, staff) *to minimize spread of infectious organisms.*
- Maintain isolation as prescribed *to minimize exposure to infectious organisms.*
- Avoid rectal temperatures and examinations, intramuscular injections, and urinary catheterization when child is neutropenic *to decrease possibility of introducing microorganisms.*
- Educate family and visitors that child should be restricted from contact with known infectious exposures (in hospital and at home) *to encourage cooperation with infection control.*
- Strictly observe medical asepsis *to avoid unintentional introduction of microorganisms.*
- Promote nutrition and appropriate rest *to maximize body's potential to heal.*
- Inform family to contact provider if child has known exposure to chickenpox or measles *so that preventive measures (e.g., VZIG) can be taken.*
- Administer vaccines (not live) as prescribed (after clearance with oncologist) *to prevent common childhood communicable diseases.*
- Teach family to monitor for fever at home and report temperature elevations to oncologist immediately *so that antibiotic therapy may be instituted as soon as possible.*

NURSING DIAGNOSIS: Pain related to invasive diagnostic testing, surgical procedure, neuropathy, disease progression, or adverse effects of treatment as evidenced by verbalization of pain, elevated pain scale ratings, guarding, withdrawal from play or refusal to participate in activities of daily living, or physiologic indicators such as elevated heart rate, diaphoresis, muscle tension or rigidity

Outcome Identification and Evaluation
Child will demonstrate pain relief, i*n amount sufficient to allow participation in play, activities of daily living, or therapeutic interventions. Use the age-appropriate pain scale to set the goal and set a time frame for achievement of the goal.*

Interventions: Promoting Comfort
- Determine level of pain using child interview, pain scale, and assessment of physiologic variables *to determine baseline.*
- Document location, intensity, description of pain *to determine baseline.*
- Discuss with the child and parent techniques that have helped alleviate pain in the past *to incorporate successful interventions into the plan of care.*
- Administer acetaminophen for mild pain *(avoid salicylate and nonsteroidal anti-inflammatory drugs due to increased risk for bleeding).*
- Administer medications as ordered using the least invasive method possible *to avoid pain (intramuscular, subcutaneous, and rectal route should be avoided in the child with thrombocytopenia).*
- Monitor frequently for adverse effects (particularly respiratory effects) of opioid analgesics, *as opioids reduce responsiveness of carbon dioxide receptors in the brain's respiratory center.*
- Use nonpharmacologic measures such as play therapy, games, TV, guided breathing, imagery, hypnosis, or meditation as appropriate *(distracts child's attention from the pain).*
- Use massage, positioning, or heat *to relieve pain in a particular area.*
- Use EMLA before needlesticks and conscious sedation with lumbar puncture and bone marrow aspiration *to reduce recurrent acute painful episodes associated with frequent blood draws and diagnostic/treatment procedures.*
- Have the child lie flat for 30 minutes after a lumbar puncture and increase fluid intake for 24 hours after the procedure *to decrease incidence of headache.*

Nursing Care Plan 49.1 (continued)

NURSING DIAGNOSIS: Impaired oral mucous membranes related to chemotherapy, radiation therapy, immunocompromise, decreased platelet count, malnutrition, or dehydration as evidenced by oral lesions, ulcers, plaques, hyperemia or bleeding, difficulty eating or swallowing, or complaint of oral discomfort

Outcome Identification and Evaluation
Child will maintain intact, moist mucosa, *free from redness, ulceration, or debris.*

Interventions: Restoring Healthy Oral Mucosa
- Frequently assess oral cavity for redness, lesions, ulcers, plaques, or bleeding *to provide baseline for comparison and identify alterations early.*
- Offer ice chips frequently while NPO *to maintain hydration of mucosa.*
- Use only a soft toothbrush or toothette for dental care, avoiding excessive pressure with brushing, *to decrease incidence of bleeding with mouth care.*
- Keep lips lubricated with petroleum jelly or fragrance-free lip balm *to maintain moist, hydrated lips.*
- Rinse with salt solution or mouthwash every 1 to 2 hours *to keep oral cavity clean and moist.*
- Administer glutamine and/or beta-carotene supplements, *which have been shown to decrease the incidence and severity of mucositis.*
- Have child swish and spit 1:1 Benadryl/Maalox solution *to decrease pain.*
- Administer antifungal solution *to prevent or treat oral candidiasis.*
- Avoid spicy, acidic, or very hot or very cold foods *to decrease pain.*
- Administer pain medication (usually acetaminophen or codeine) as ordered *to decrease pain.*

NURSING DIAGNOSIS: Nausea related to adverse effects of chemotherapy or radiation therapy as evidenced by verbalization of nausea, increased salivation, swallowing movements, or vomiting

Outcome Identification and Evaluation
Child will experience decreased nausea, *will verbalize symptom relief and will be free from vomiting.*

Interventions: Alleviating Nausea and Vomiting
- Administer antiemetics prior to chemotherapy and as needed thereafter *to decrease frequency of nausea.*
- Assess frequency of vomiting and level of hydration *to provide baseline data and recognize alterations early.*
- Offer frequent, smaller meals or snacks; *smaller amounts are less likely to be vomited.*
- Avoid spicy foods *to avoid stomach upset.*
- Allow bubbles to dissipate from carbonated beverages before they are ingested *(carbonation may contribute to nausea).*
- Remove cover from meal tray before entering child's room *(this will allow the food odor to dissipate outside of the room; food odors may trigger nausea and vomiting).*

NURSING DIAGNOSIS: Imbalanced nutrition: less than body requirements related to anorexia, nausea, vomiting, or mucosal irritation associated with chemotherapy or radiation as evidenced by decreased oral intake and weight, length/height, and/or BMI below average for age or individual child's usual measures

Outcome Identification and Evaluation
Child will improve nutritional intake, resulting in *steady increase in weight and length/height.*

Interventions: Promoting adequate nutrition
- Determine body weight and length/height norm for age or find out what the child's pretreatment measurements were *to determine goal to work toward.*
- Determine child's food preferences and provide favorite foods as able *to increase the likelihood that the child will consume adequate amounts of foods.*
- Administer antiemetics as ordered *to increase the likelihood that the child will retain the food he or she ingests.*
- Weigh child daily or weekly (according to physician order or institutional standard) and measure length/height weekly *to monitor for growth.*
- Offer highest-calorie meals at the time of day when the child's appetite is the greatest *(to increase likelihood of increased caloric intake).*
- Provide increased-calorie shakes or puddings within diet restriction *(high-calorie foods increase weight gain).*
- Administer vitamin and mineral supplements as prescribed *to attain/maintain vitamin and mineral balance in the body.*
- Administer total parenteral nutrition and intravenous lipids as ordered *to provide adequate nutrition for healing.*

(continued)

Nursing Care Plan 49.1 (continued)

NURSING DIAGNOSIS: Constipation related to effects of vinca alkaloids, opioid use, decreased activity, and dietary changes as evidenced by hard stool or stool that is difficult to pass

Outcome Identification and Evaluation
Child's bowel function will return to usual pattern, *child will pass a formed, soft stool every day (or modify this criterion according to child's usual pattern).*

Interventions: Preventing or Managing Constipation
- Ensure that child increases fluid intake *to provide enough water in the intestines for soft stool formation.*
- Increase fiber in the diet *to provide bulk for stool formation.*
- Administer stool softeners such as mineral oil, docusate sodium; *these help soften the stool, aiding in passage.*
- Provide motivator laxatives such as magnesium hydroxide, lactulose, or sorbitol *to stimulate stool passage.*
- Use stimulant laxatives such as senna or bisacodyl only intermittently rather than on a daily basis *to avoid dependency and diarrhea.*

NURSING DIAGNOSIS: Diarrhea related to effects of radiation therapy as evidenced by loose or watery stools, possibly frequent

Outcome Identification and Evaluation
Child's bowel function will return to usual pattern, *child will pass a formed, soft stool daily (or modify this criterion according to child's usual pattern).*

Interventions: Managing Diarrhea
- Assess frequency of diarrhea and level of hydration *to provide data about severity.*
- Obtain weight daily on same scale *to determine extent of fluid loss.*
- Maintain accurate intake and output records *to determine extent of fluid loss.*
- Administer oral rehydration solutions or intravenous fluids as ordered *to maintain or restore adequate hydration.*
- Restrict roughage and residue in diet *to decrease likelihood of diarrhea.*
- Avoid milk products during acute diarrheal phase *(lactose often worsens diarrhea).*
- Provide an elemental diet to relieve symptoms *(absorbed in the upper small bowel).*
- Provide meticulous perineal care *to avoid skin breakdown related to frequent or loose stools.*
- Administer antidiarrheal medications if ordered *to decrease frequency of stools.*
- If severe and related to radiation therapy, may require a 3- to 4-day rest period from radiation *to begin recovery of normal absorptive capabilities of bowel.*

NURSING DIAGNOSIS: Risk for impaired skin integrity related to radiation therapy

Outcome Identification and Evaluation
Child's skin will remain intact, *areas of redness in radiation field will not progress to desquamation.*

Interventions: Promoting Skin Integrity
- Assess skin frequently for erythema, erosions, ulcers, or blisters *to provide baseline data and intervene early if skin is impaired.*
- Use a mild soap for cleansing and pat dry rather than rubbing *to avoid skin irritation.*
- Use aloe vera lotion *to moisturize the skin.*
- Avoid perfumed lotions, soaps, heat, cold, or sun, *as these will further irritate the skin in the irradiated area.*
- Do not scrub ink from marked radiation field, and avoid adhesive tape in that area, *to avoid further skin irritation.*
- Administer diphenhydramine or apply hydrocortisone 1% cream *to reduce itching and urge to scratch.*
- For areas of desquamation related to radiation, apply Silvadene cream once or twice a day *to hasten skin repair.*

Nursing Care Plan 49.1 (continued)

NURSING DIAGNOSIS: Activity intolerance related to treatment adverse effects, anemia, or generalized weakness as evidenced by verbalization of weakness or fatigue, elevation of heart rate, respiratory rate, or blood pressure with activity, complaint of shortness of breath with play or activity

Outcome Identification and Evaluation
Child will display increased activity tolerance, *desire to play without developing symptoms of exertion.*

Interventions: Promoting Activity
- Encourage activity or ambulation per physician's orders; *early mobilization results in better outcomes.*
- Observe child for symptoms of activity intolerance such as pallor, nausea, lightheadedness or dizziness, or changes in vital signs *to determine level of tolerance.*
- If child is on bed rest, perform range-of-motion exercises and frequent position changes: *negative changes to the musculoskeletal system occur quickly with inactivity and immobility.*
- Cluster nursing care activities and plan for periods of rest before and after exertion *to decrease oxygen need and consumption.*
- Refer the child to physical therapy *for exercise prescription to increase skeletal muscle strength.*

NURSING DIAGNOSIS: Disturbed body image related to hair loss as evidenced by verbalization of dissatisfaction with appearance

Outcome Identification and Evaluation
Child or adolescent will display appropriate body image, *will look at self in mirror and participate in social activities.*

Interventions: Promoting Body Image
- Acknowledge child's feelings of anger over body changes and illness; *venting feelings is associated with less body image disturbance.*
- Encourage the child or teen to choose a wig or hats and scarves *to involve the child in making decisions about appearance.*
- Support the child's or teen's choices of comfortable, fashionable clothing *to disguise weight loss or scarring while promoting self-esteem.*
- Involve the child in the decision-making process, *as a sense of control will improve body image.*
- Encourage the child to spend time with peers who have experienced hair, limb, or weight loss, *as peers' opinions are often better accepted than those of persons in authority, such as parents or health care professionals.*

NURSING DIAGNOSIS: Risk for situational low self-esteem related to loss of control and inability to progress with quest for independence (adolescents)

Outcome Identification and Evaluation
Adolescent will maintain or increase self-esteem, *will display increased coping responses and verbalize control as appropriate as well as discuss plans for future.*

Interventions: Promoting Self-Esteem
- Identify the adolescent's positive abilities *to promote self-esteem.*
- Give genuine and honest positive feedback, *as the child or adolescent desires honesty.*
- Explore strengths and weaknesses with the adolescent: *helps the teen to see similarities and differences with healthy peers of the same age.*
- Encourage the teen to perform self-care as possible *to promote independence.*
- Offer emotional support *(reduces psychological distress and increases coping abilities).*
- Encourage participation in a support group *to allow teens to discuss body changes and the reactions they perceive in others.*
- When the adolescent is physically able, encourage attendance at camp or an adventure/wilderness event *(these programs have been shown to improve mental health and coping skills).*

(continued)

Nursing Care Plan 49.1 (continued)

NURSING DIAGNOSIS: Compromised family coping related to potentially life-threatening illness and stressors involved with cancer treatment

Outcome Identification and Evaluation
Child and/or family will demonstrate adequate coping skills, *will verbalize feeling supported and demonstrate healthy family interactions.*

Interventions: Promoting Child and Family Coping
- Provide emotional support to child and family *(improves coping abilities).*
- Actively listen to the child's and family's concerns *(validates their feelings, establishes trust).*
- Provide open communication with the child and siblings; *children appreciate honesty about their illness, and coping is improved.*
- Refer families to community resources such as parent support groups and grief counseling *(such support improves coping abilities).*
- Give terminally ill children the permission to discuss their feelings about their illness, *allowing them to conquer fears and express love for their family and friends.*
- Encourage families to be honest with siblings about the treatment and prognosis of the child with cancer *(children often sense what is going on and cope better when they are prepared and are given an honest explanation of events).*
- Prepare siblings for the death of the child with cancer, using the child life specialist and chaplain as necessary: *the bereavement period is eased when siblings are prepared.*

NURSING DIAGNOSIS: Anticipatory grieving (family) related to diagnosis of cancer in a child and impending loss of child as evidenced by crying, disbelief of diagnosis, and expressions of grief

Outcome Identification and Evaluation
Family will express feelings of grief; *seek help in dealing with feelings, plan for future one day at the time.*

Intervention: Supporting the Grieving Family
- Use therapeutic communication with open-ended questions *to encourage an open and trusting relationship for better communication.*
- Actively listen to family's expression of grief; *just being present and listening conveys support.*
- Encourage the family to cry and express feelings away from the child *to work through feelings while not upsetting the child.*
- Assess for spiritual distress *and refer the family to the hospital chaplain or clergy of choice for support.*
- Educate the family about the child's condition honestly: *knowing what is going on, what is to be expected, and what the treatment plan is gives the family a sense of control.*
- Support the family through discussions with the child about anticipated death *when the illness is deemed terminal.*

---

nursing care for the child with a neoplastic disorder. The care plan includes many nursing diagnoses that are applicable to the child or adolescent, but not all children will have the same effects from cancer and its treatment. Nursing care should be individualized based on the child's and family's responses to illness. Additional information about nursing management related to specific types of cancer will be included later in the chapter as it relates to specific disorders.

Provide education to families of all children with cancer as outlined in Teaching Guidelines 49.1.

*B*ased on your top three nursing diagnoses for John, describe appropriate nursing interventions.

Administering Chemotherapy
All chemotherapy medications have the potential to cause toxicities in the child as well as the persons handling or preparing the medication. General guidelines related to the preparation and administration of chemotherapy include:

- Chemotherapy should be prepared and administered only by specially trained personnel.
- Personal protective equipment (PPE) in the form of double gloves and nonpermeable gowns should be worn when preparing or administering chemotherapy. If splashing is possible or a spill occurs, then a face shield and/or mask may also be necessary.
- Dispose of all equipment used in chemotherapy preparation and administration in a puncture-resistant container.

TEACHING GUIDELINES 49.1

Education for Families of Children With Cancer

- Obtain a printed or written copy of the child's treatment plan.
- Keep a calendar of all appointment times, blood count lab draw days, and phone numbers of all physicians, home care companies, laboratory, and hospital.
- Seek medical care IMMEDIATELY if the child's temperature is 38.3° C (101° F) or higher.
- Call the oncologist or seek medical care if any of the following occur:
  - Cough or rapid breathing
  - Increased bruising, bleeding or petechiae, pallor or increased levels of fatigue
  - Earache, sore throat, nuchal rigidity
  - Blisters, rashes, ulcers
  - Red, irritated skin on the child's buttocks
  - Abdominal pain, difficulty or pain with eating, drinking or swallowing
  - Constipation or diarrhea
  - For children with central venous catheters:
    - Pus, redness, or swelling at the site
    - Breakage of the catheter
- Do not give the child aspirin.

Kline, 2004.

FIGURE 49.4 A child who weighs 13.2 kg and is 140 cm tall has a BSA of 0.80 m².

It is critical to calculate the chemotherapy dose correctly. Chemotherapy medication doses in children are based on body surface area (BSA). A nomogram is a commonly used device for determining BSA. To use the nomogram, draw a straight line between the child's height on the left and the child's weight on the right. The point at which the straight line crosses the center is the child's BSA expressed in meters squared (Fig. 49.4).

An alternative to using the nomogram is to use the following formula: BSA (m²) = the square root of (height [in centimeters] × weight [in kilograms] divided by 3,600). For example, for a child 140 cm tall and weighing 30 kg: 140 × 30 = 4,200; 4,200/3,600 = 1.167; and the square root of 1.167 is 1.08. The BSA would be 1.08.

Managing Adverse Effects of Chemotherapy

Chemotherapy can result in multiple adverse effects. Myelosuppression leads to low blood counts in all cell lines, placing the child at risk for infection, hemorrhage, and anemia. Nausea, vomiting, and anorexia may hinder the child's growth. Alopecia and facial changes may affect the child's self-esteem (Fig. 49.5). Nursing interventions related to the effects of myelosuppression, nausea, vomiting, and anorexia are discussed below. Refer to Nursing Care Plan 49.1 for nursing interventions related to altered body image.

▶ *Take* NOTE!

Cooling the scalp during chemotherapy administration with the use of a cooling cap may decrease hair loss. (Tomlinson & Kline, 2005).

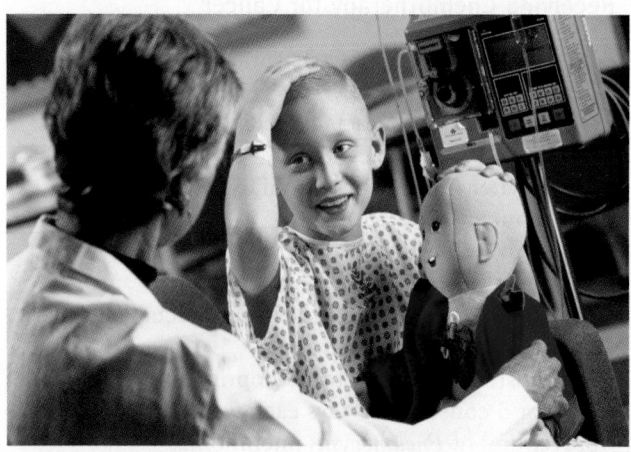

FIGURE 49.5 Chemotherapy often causes alopecia.

Preventing Infection

Many chemotherapeutic drugs cause significant bone marrow suppression and decreased amounts of circulating mature neutrophils ("segs," or segmented neutrophils). Administer granulocyte colony-stimulating factor (GCSF) as ordered to promote neutrophil growth and maturation. Administer varicella zoster immunoglobulin (VZIG) within 72 hours of exposure to active chickenpox. If the child is actively infected with chickenpox, administer intravenous acyclovir as ordered. Children receiving treatment for acute lymphoblastic leukemia are at risk for opportunistic infection with *Pneumocystis jiroveci*, as most children are colonized with this fungus. Administer prophylactic antibiotics as ordered and teach the parents to administer them at home. Teaching Guidelines 49.2 gives further information about infection prevention at home.

As neutrophils are the primary means of fighting bacterial infection, when the neutrophil count is low, the chance for developing an overwhelming bacterial infection is high. Each drug that causes bone marrow suppression has a point of nadir. *Nadir* is the time after administration of the drug when bone marrow suppression is expected to be at its greatest and the neutrophil count is expected to be at its lowest (neutropenia). Nadir is individual for each drug and ranges from 7 to 28 days after dosing. An absolute neutrophil count (ANC) below 500 places the child at greatest risk, although an ANC below 1,500 usually warrants evaluation (Box 49.2).

Depending on institutional policy, precautions for neutropenia will be followed if the ANC is depressed. Precautions related to neutropenia generally include:

• Perform hand hygiene before and after each patient contact.
• Place the child in a private room.

TEACHING GUIDELINES 49.2

Prevention of Infection in Children Receiving Chemotherapy for Cancer

• Practice meticulous hygiene (oral, personal, perianal).
• Avoid known ill contacts, especially persons with chickenpox.
• Immediately notify physician if exposed to chickenpox.
• Avoid crowded areas.
• Do not let the child receive live vaccines.
• Do not take the child's temperature rectally or give medications by the rectal route.
• Administer twice-daily trimethoprim-sulfamethoxazole for 3 consecutive days each week as ordered for prevention of *Pneumocystis* pneumonia.

BOX 49.2 Calculating the Absolute Neutrophil Count (ANC)

1. Add together the percentage of banded and segmented neutrophils reported on the complete blood count with differential (CBC with diff).
2. Multiply the total number of white blood cells reported on the CBC by the sum above. This yields the ANC (total number of neutrophils present).

Example: Bands 5%, Segs 15%, WBCs 2,500
5% + 15% = 20% (0.20)
2,500 × 0.20 = 500
ANC = 500

• Monitor vital signs every 4 hours.
• Assess for signs and symptoms of infection at least every 8 hours.
• Avoid rectal suppositories, enemas, or examinations; urinary catheterization; and invasive procedures.
• Restrict visitors with fever, cough, or other signs/symptoms of infection.
• Do not permit raw fruits or vegetables or fresh flowers or live plants in the room.
• Place a mask on the patient when he or she is being transported outside of the room.
• Perform dental care with a soft toothbrush if the platelet count is adequate.

Children with neutropenia and fever must be started on intravenous broad-spectrum antibiotics without delay to avoid overwhelming sepsis.

Preventing Hemorrhage

Assess for petechiae, purpura, bruising, or bleeding. Determine changes from baseline that warrant intervention. Encourage quiet activities or play to avoid trauma. Avoid rectal temperatures and examinations to avoid rectal mucosal damage that results in bleeding. Post a sign at the head of the bed stating "no rectal temperatures or medications." Avoid intramuscular injections and lumbar puncture if possible to decrease the risk of bleeding from a puncture site. If bone marrow aspiration must be performed, apply a pressure dressing to the site to prevent bleeding.

For active or uncontrolled bleeding, transfuse platelets as ordered to control bleeding.

Preventing Anemia

To maintain blood volume, limit blood draws to the minimum volume required. Encourage the child to eat an appropriate diet that includes adequate iron. Administer erythropoietin injections as ordered. Teach families to give the injections at home if prescribed.

Managing Nausea, Vomiting, and Anorexia

Many chemotherapeutic drugs produce the adverse effect of nausea and vomiting. The cycle of nausea, vomiting, and anorexia is difficult to break once it begins. Prevent nausea by administering antiemetics prior to the administration of chemotherapy and on a routine schedule around the clock for the first 1 to 2 days rather than on an as-needed (PRN) basis. Bright lights and noise may worsen nausea, so the child's environment should be dimly lit and calm. Relaxation therapy and guided imagery may also be helpful in preventing or treating nausea and vomiting. Refer to Nursing Care Plan 49.1 for additional interventions.

> ▶ *Take NOTE!*
>
> *Ginger capsules, ginger tea, and candied ginger have been used as a nausea remedy for centuries. (Ginger ale is usually artificially flavored, so it would not have the same effect.) Though ginger is considered safe, instruct families to check with the oncologist before using this remedy.*

Taste alterations are common in children who have received chemotherapy. During or after chemotherapy, children may develop an aversion to a food that was previously their favorite (Tomlinson & Kline, 2005).

> ▶ *Take NOTE!*
>
> *Foot massage has been demonstrated to decrease the nausea and pain associated with chemotherapy.*

Monitoring the Child Receiving Radiation Therapy

Radiation causes damage to the cells in a localized area, which may include normal cells in addition to the cancerous ones. Assess the child's skin daily, particularly at the treatment site. Provide good hygiene, but gently. Encourage moisture retention in the skin by applying aqueous creams or moisturizers. Do not apply deodorants or perfumed lotions on the radiation treatment site. Avoid the use of heat or ice packs at the site. Instruct the child and family that clothing should fit loosely so as not to irritate the site. During and for 8 weeks after the radiation treatment, the skin will be more photosensitive. Protect the skin with a high-SPF sunscreen.

Providing Care to the Child Undergoing Stem Cell Transplantation

Stem cell transplantation is performed at limited specialty centers in the United States, and special training is re-quired for all personnel caring for the transplanted child. The intent of this discussion is to provide only a brief introduction to and overview of nursing management related to HSCT.

Care may be divided into three phases: the pretransplant phase, the post-transplant phase, and the lengthy supportive care phase. Nursing management of each phase is briefly discussed below.

Pretransplant Phase

In the pretransplant phase, the child is being prepared to receive the transplant. The child's own bone marrow cells are eradicated through high-dose chemotherapy and total body irradiation. This phase usually occurs over 7 to 10 days. The child will be hospitalized because he or she is at extreme risk for serious infection. Maintain protective isolation in a positive-pressure room and limit visitors. Administer gammaglobulin, acyclovir, or antibiotics as ordered to prevent or treat infection. Lymphohematopoietic rescue occurs with infusion of the donor or autologous cells.

Post-transplant Phase

The post-transplant phase is also a time of high risk for the child. Monitor closely for symptoms of GVHD such as severe diarrhea and maculopapular rash progressing to redness or desquamation of the skin (especially palms or soles) (Fig. 49.6). If GVHD occurs, administer immunosuppressive drugs such as cyclosporine, tacrolimus, or mycophenolate (which place the child at further risk for infection).

Supportive Care

During the supportive care phase, which lasts several months after the transplant, continue to monitor for and prevent infection. Administer packed red blood cells or platelets and granulocyte colony-stimulating factor as needed.

FIGURE 49.6 The first sign of GVHD may be a maculopapular rash.

Families and children who undergo HSCT need prolonged and extensive emotional and psychosocial support. A medical social worker and psychologist or counselor are usually members of the transplant team and are excellent resources for these families' needs.

Promoting a Normal Life

Children and teens want to be normal and to experience the things that other children their age do. The child should attend school when he or she is well enough and the white blood cell counts are not dangerously low. Children, their families, and their teachers should be aware that cancer and its treatment can affect scholastic abilities. Learning disabilities, difficulty with memory, attention disorders, and cognitive deficits can occur (Spencer, 2006).

Maintain other activities if the child is able and if platelet counts are within normal limits. Special camps are available for children with cancer. These camps offer an opportunity for children and adolescents to experience a variety of activities safely and to network with youngsters who are experiencing similar physical and emotional challenges. The Children's Oncology Camping Association (http://www.coca-intl.org/membercamps/1_usa.html) and the Candlelighter's Childhood Cancer Foundation (http://www.candlelighters.org/supportcamps.stm) provide lists of camps throughout the United States and Canada and internationally for children and teens with cancer.

Promoting Growth

Promote growth in children with cancer by encouraging an appropriate diet and preventing nausea and vomiting and also by addressing concerns such as diarrhea and constipation. Chronic diarrhea related to radiation therapy may prevent the child from gaining weight and growing properly (see Nursing Care Plan 49.1). The use of vinca alkaloids and opioids, as well as the decreased activity level of the child with cancer, may contribute to constipation. Constipation increases the pain experience, contributes to the child's malaise, and decreases quality of life. It directly affects the child's ability to grow by increasing anorexia, nausea, and vomiting (Tomlinson & Kline, 2005). Nursing Care Plan 49.1 details interventions related to preventing and managing constipation.

Preventing and Treating Oncologic Emergencies

Oncologic emergencies may occur as an effect of the disease process itself or from cancer treatment. As progress is made in chemotherapy and radiation treatment, children with cancer have an increased survival rate, but they still face the risk of developing an oncologic emergency. Nurses caring for children with cancer need to be familiar with signs and symptoms of oncologic emergencies as well as with their treatment. All of these problems warrant careful, frequent monitoring of respiratory, cardiovascular, neurologic, and renal status. Table 49.1 provides information about oncologic emergencies.

TABLE 49.1 ONCOLOGIC EMERGENCIES

Emergency	Associated with	Signs and Symptoms	Laboratory or Diagnostic Test Findings	Management
Sepsis	Neutropenia resulting from bone marrow suppression due to chemotherapy	• Fever or low temperature • Respiratory distress • Poor perfusion • Altered level of consciousness	• ANC < 500 • Positive blood culture • Increased BUN, creatinine, potassium, clotting times • Decreased platelet count • Metabolic acidosis	• Airway and ventilation maintenance • Fluid volume resuscitation • Inotropic support • Broad-spectrum antibiotics and antifungals • Dialysis if needed
Tumor lysis syndrome	ALL, lymphoma, neuroblastoma	• Nausea, vomiting, diarrhea, anorexia • Lethargy • Increased heart rate and blood pressure • Decreased or absent urine output • Altered level of consciousness	• Hyperuricemia • Hyperkalemia • Hyperphosphatemia • Hypocalcemia • Hypoxia	• Prevent by giving allopurinol for several days prior to chemotherapy (also treat with allopurinol) • Double IV fluid maintenance • Sodium bicarbonate

Emergency	Associated with	Signs and Symptoms	Laboratory or Diagnostic Test Findings	Management
Hyperleuko-cytosis	Leukemia with high WBC count	• Respiratory distress • Murmur, increased heart rate	• WBC count > 100,000 • Hyperkalemia, hyperphospha-temia • Hyperuricemia • Decreased pH and bicarbonate	• Leukapheresis • Respiratory support • Double IV fluid maintenance with sodium bicarbonate added • Diuretics
Typhlitis (neutropenic enterocolitis)	Inflammatory process of GI tract occurring with induction phase of leukemia chemotherapy	• Acute abdominal pain • Nausea, vomiting • Bloody diarrhea and emesis • Fever • Anorexia	• KUB: scarcity of bowel gas, possibly ileus • CT (abdominal): inflammation, bowel wall thickening, peritoneal fluid	• Bowel rest (NPO status) • IV nutrition • Assess for bowel perforation/shock. • Broad-spectrum antibiotics and antifungals • Comfort measures
Superior vena cava syndrome	Compression on the SVC by NHL or other mediastinal mass, such as neuroblastoma	• Dyspnea and cyanosis • Large cervical lymph nodes • Wheezing, diminished breath sounds	• Chest x-ray or CT shows mediastinal mass. • Pleural effusion	• Intubation and ventilation • Comfort measures • Treat cause (usually surgical removal of mass)
Spinal cord compression	Tumor or metastasis compresses spinal cord	• Back, neck, or leg pain • Sensory or autonomic dysfunction • Extremity weakness or paralysis	• MRI reveals location of tumor or metastasis to epidural space.	• Dexamethasone • Careful assessment • Radiation therapy • Comfort measures
Increased intracranial pressure	Brain tumor or metastasis to brain causing compression of brain; may result in herniation	• Headache, visual disturbances • Morning vomiting • Infants: increased head circumference • Altered level of consciousness • Cushing's triad • Seizure activity	• Head CT or MRI reveals extent of mass.	• Frequent, careful neurologic assessment • Limit fluids • Dexamethasone • Anticonvulsants • Tumor resection, radiation or chemotherapy • Comfort measures
Massive hepatomegaly	Obstruction caused by neuroblastoma filling a large portion of the abdominal cavity	• Distended, enlarged abdomen • Respiratory distress, hypoxia • Poor perfusion • Tachycardia, hypotension	• Abdominal CT reveals extent of tumor • Coagulopathy	• Tumor resection or debulking • Mechanical ventilation, inotropic support • Nasogastric decompression • Position to minimize abdominal pressure • Blood transfusions • Comfort measures

Caring for the Dying Child

Of the 12,000 children diagnosed with cancer annually in the United States, about 2,200 will die from the disease each year (Houlahan et al., 2006). A "do not resuscitate" (DNR) order for the child with progressive cancer is obtained in many situations. This order helps to optimize care in the terminal phase of cancer (Postovksy et al., 2004). Nurses serve as patient and family advocates, clarifying terminology and providing support as needed during the discussion of DNR orders and throughout the rest of the terminal phase.

Children with terminal cancer often experience a great deal of pain, particularly when death is imminent. Pain is often accompanied by agitation and dyspnea, which further contribute to the child's discomfort. Whether the child has a DNR order or the status remains that of "full code," pain management is central to the nursing care of the child who is dying from cancer. The Association of Pediatric Oncology Nurses' position paper entitled "Pain Management for the Child with Cancer in End-of-Life Care" outlines the following recommendations for managing children's pain at the end of life:

• Prevention and alleviation of pain is a primary goal of care in the child dying of cancer.
• Children and parents are equal partners with members of the health care team in managing the patient's pain.
• Children dying of cancer may require aggressive dosing of analgesics. Medications that do not have a dose maximum should be escalated, sometimes rapidly, to achieve adequate pain control or to maintain pain control when tolerance has occurred.
• The nurse's role in caring for children who are in pain at the end of life includes assessment, identifying expected outcomes, and planning, performing, and evaluating interventions (Hooke et al., 2002).

Interventions related to pain management may be found in Nursing Care Plan 49.1. Further discussion related to care of the dying child is found in Chapter 13.

Leukemia

Leukemia is a primary disorder of the bone marrow in which the normal elements are replaced with abnormal white blood cells. Normally, lymphoid cells grow and develop into lymphocytes, and myeloid cells grow and develop into red blood cells, granulocytes, monocytes, and platelets. Leukemia may develop at any time during the usual stages of normal lymphoid or myeloid development. Leukemia may be classified as acute or chronic, lymphocytic or myelogenous. Acute leukemias are rapidly progressive diseases affecting the undifferentiated or immature cells; the result is cells without normal function. Chronic leukemias progress more slowly, permitting maturation and differentiation of cells so that they retain

some of their normal function. Acute leukemias, including acute lymphoblastic leukemia (ALL) and acute myelogenous leukemia (AML), account for about 95% of all cases of leukemia in children and adolescents (Mahoney, 2006; Airewele & Steuber, 2006), so they will be the focus of the discussion below.

Complications of leukemia include metastasis to the blood, bone, CNS, spleen, liver, or other organs and alterations in growth. Late effects include problems with neurocognitive function and ocular, cardiovascular, or thyroid dysfunction. With advances in treatment over the past 50 years, most cases of childhood leukemia are curable, though children who experience relapse or present with advanced disease have a poorer prognosis (Mahoney, 2006).

▶ ACUTE LYMPHOBLASTIC LEUKEMIA

ALL is the most common form of cancer in children. It most often occurs in children between 2 and 10 years of age (Albano et al., 2005). It is more common in white children than in other races. ALL is classified according to the type of cells involved: T cell, B cell, early pre-B cell, or pre-B cell. Most children will achieve initial remission if appropriate treatment is given. The overall cure rate of ALL is 65% to 75%. Relapse is rare after 7 years from diagnosis.

Prognosis is based upon the white blood cell (WBC) count at diagnosis, the type of cytogenetic factors and immunophenotype, the age at diagnosis, and the extent of extramedullary involvement. Generally, the higher the WBC at diagnosis, the worse the prognosis. Children ages 2 to 10 years at diagnosis usually have the best prognosis. Infants less than 12 months of age at diagnosis generally have a poorer prognosis. When a child experiences a relapse, the prognosis becomes poorer. Complications include infection, hemorrhage, poor growth, and CNS, bone, or testicular involvement.

▶ **Take** NOTE!

Growth hormone replacement therapy using recombinant human growth hormone may improve the long-term growth of children with leukemia.

Pathophysiology

The exact cause of ALL remains unknown. Genetic factors and chromosome abnormalities may play a role in its development. In ALL, abnormal lymphoblasts abound in the blood-forming tissues. The lymphoblasts are fragile and immature, lacking the infection-fighting capabilities of the normal WBC. In ALL, the growth of lymphoblasts is excessive and the abnormal cells replace the normal cells in the bone marrow. The proliferating leukemic cells demonstrate massive metabolic needs, depriving normal body cells of needed nutrients and resulting in fatigue, weight loss or growth arrest, and muscle wasting. The bone marrow becomes unable to maintain normal levels of red blood cells, WBCs, and platelets, so anemia, neutropenia, and thrombocytopenia result. As the bone marrow expands or the leukemic cells infiltrate the bone, joint and bone pain may occur. The leukemic cells may permeate the lymph nodes, causing diffuse lymphadenopathy, or the liver and spleen, resulting in hepatosplenomegaly. With spread to the CNS, vomiting, headache, seizures, coma, vision alterations, or cranial nerve palsies may occur.

> ▶ *Take* NOTE!
>
> *Changes in behavior or personality, headache, irritability, dizziness, persistent nausea or vomiting, seizures, gait changes, lethargy, or altered level of consciousness may indicate CNS infiltration with leukemic cells. Immediately report these findings to the pediatric oncologist.*

Therapeutic Management

Therapeutic management of the child with ALL focuses on giving chemotherapy to eradicate the leukemic cells and restore normal bone marrow function. Treatment is divided into three stages. CNS prophylaxis is provided at each stage; without CNS prophylaxis, leukemia would spread to the CNS in up to 50% of children with ALL. The length of treatment and choice of medications are based on the child's age, risk category, and subtype determined by bone marrow analysis. Table 49.2 discusses the stages of leukemia treatment. For relapsed or less responsive leukemia, HSCT may be necessary.

Nursing Assessment

For a full description of the assessment phase of the nursing process, refer to page 1633. Assessment findings pertinent to ALL are discussed below.

Health History

Elicit a description of the present illness and chief complaint. Common signs and symptoms reported during the health history might include:

- Fever (may be persistent or recurrent, with unknown cause)
- Recurrent infection
- Fatigue, malaise, or listlessness
- Pallor
- Unusual bleeding or bruising
- Abdominal pain
- Nausea or vomiting
- Bone pain
- Headache

Explore the child's current and past medical history for risk factors such as:

- Male gender
- Age 2 to 5 years
- Caucasian race
- Down syndrome, Shwachman syndrome, or ataxia-telangiectasia
- X-ray exposure *in utero*
- Previous radiation-treated cancer

Determine the child's history of varicella zoster immunization or disease. Chickenpox infection in the

TABLE 49.2 **STAGES OF LEUKEMIA TREATMENT**

Stage	Purpose	Length	Usual Medications
Induction	Rapid induction of complete remission	3 to 4 weeks	Oral steroids, IV vincristine, IM L-asparaginase, daunomycin (high-risk)
Consolidation (intensification)	Strengthen remission, reduce leukemic cell burden	Varies	High-dose methotrexate, 6-mercaptopurine; possibly cyclophosphamide, cytarabine, asparaginase, thioguanine, epipodophyllotoxins
Maintenance	Eliminate all residual leukemic cells	2 to 3 years	Low-dose: daily 6-mercaptopurine, weekly methotrexate, intermittent IV vincristine and oral steroids
CNS prophylaxis	Reduce risk of development of CNS disease	Given periodically in all stages	Intrathecal chemotherapy; cranial radiation is used infrequently

leukemic child may lead to disseminated, overwhelming infection.

Physical Examination

Take the child's temperature (fever may be present), and look for petechiae, purpura, or unusual bruising (due to decreased platelet levels). Inspect the skin for signs of infection. Auscultate the lungs, noting adventitious breath sounds, which may indicate pneumonia (present at diagnosis or due to immunosuppression during treatment). Note location and size of enlarged lymph nodes. Palpate the liver and spleen for enlargement. Document tenderness on abdominal palpation.

Laboratory and Diagnostic Tests

Common laboratory and diagnostic studies ordered for the assessment of ALL include:

- Abnormal complete blood counts: low hemoglobin and hematocrit, decreased red blood cell count, decreased platelet count, and elevated, normal, or decreased WBC count
- Peripheral blood smear may reveal blasts.
- Stained smear from bone marrow aspiration will show greater than 25% lymphoblasts. Bone marrow aspirate is also examined for immunophenotyping (lymphoid vs. myeloid, and level of cancer cell maturity) and cytogenetic analysis (determines abnormalities in chromosome number and structure). Immunophenotyping and cytogenetic analysis are used in the classification of the leukemia, which helps guide treatment.
- Lumbar puncture will reveal whether leukemic cells have infiltrated the CNS.
- Liver function tests and blood urea nitrogen (BUN) and creatinine levels determine liver and renal function, which if abnormal may preclude treatment with certain chemotherapeutic agents.
- Chest x-ray may reveal pneumonia or a mediastinal mass.

Nursing Management

Nursing care of children with ALL focuses on managing disease complications such as infection, pain, anemia, bleeding, and hyperuricemia and the many adverse effects related to treatment. Many children require blood product transfusion for the treatment of severe anemia or low platelet levels with active bleeding.

Individualize nursing care based on the diagnoses, interventions, and outcomes presented in Nursing Care Plan 49.1, depending on the child's response to the disease and chemotherapy. Refer to the nursing process overview section for further information related to managing the adverse effects of chemotherapy.

> ▶ **Take** NOTE!
>
> Blood products administered to children with any type of leukemia should be irradiated, cytomegalovirus (CMV) negative, and leukodepleted. This treatment of blood products before transfusion will decrease the amount of antibodies in the blood, an important factor in preventing GVHD should HSCT become necessary at a later date.

Reducing Pain

Children and teens with leukemia suffer pain related to the disease as well as the treatment. Chemotherapy drugs commonly used in leukemia may cause peripheral neuropathy and headache. Lumbar puncture and bone marrow aspiration, which are periodically performed throughout the course of treatment, also cause pain. The most common areas of pain are the head and neck, legs, and abdomen (probably from protracted vomiting with chemotherapy). Distraction techniques such as listening to music, watching TV, or playing games may take the child's mind off the pain. Administer mild analgesics such as acetaminophen for acute episodes of pain. The use of EMLA cream prior to venipuncture, port access, lumbar puncture, and bone marrow aspiration may decrease procedure-related pain events. Application of heat or cold to the painful area is usually acceptable. Narcotic analgesics may be used for episodes of acute severe pain or for palliation of chronic pain.

▶ ACUTE MYELOGENOUS LEUKEMIA

AML is the second most common type of leukemia in children. Its incidence peaks during the adolescent years. AML affects the myeloid cell progenitors or precursors in the bone marrow, resulting in malignant cells. The French-American-British (FAB) classification system identifies eight subtypes of AML (MO to M7), depending on myeloid lineage involved and the degree of cell differentiation. These subtypes are useful for determining treatment. The overall cure rate for childhood AML is about 50%. Complications include treatment resistance, infection, hemorrhage, and metastasis.

The induction phase of AML requires intense bone marrow suppression and prolonged hospitalization because AML is less responsive to treatment than ALL. Toxicity from treatment is more common in AML and is likely to be more serious than with ALL. Empiric broad-spectrum antibiotics and prophylactic platelet transfusions may be prescribed. After remission is achieved, children require intensive chemotherapy to prolong the duration of remission. HSCT is often required in children with AML, depending on the subtype.

> ▶ *Take* NOTE!
>
> *At the time of diagnosis, about 25% of children with AML present with a WBC count above 100,000 (hyperleukocytosis); this results in venous stasis and backup of blast cells in small vessels, causing hypoxia, hemorrhage, and lung or brain infarction. Hyperleukocytosis is a medical emergency. These children require leukapheresis to decrease hyperviscosity by quickly decreasing the number of circulating blasts.*

Nursing Assessment

Explore the health history for common signs and symptoms, including recurrent infections, fever, or fatigue. Explore the medical history for risk factors, such as Hispanic race, previous chemotherapy, and genetic abnormalities such as Down syndrome, Fanconi anemia, neurofibromatosis type I, Shwachman syndrome, Bloom syndrome, and familial monosomy 7.

Perform a thorough physical examination. Note skin pallor and salmon-colored or blue-gray papular lesions. Palpate the skin for subcutaneous rubbery nodules. Palpate for lymphadenopathy. Note headache, visual disturbance, or signs of increased intracranial pressure, such as vomiting, that may indicate CNS involvement. Upon diagnosis of AML, the child's WBC count is typically extremely elevated. Bone marrow aspiration will reveal greater than 30% blast cells.

Nursing Management

Nursing management of the child with AML is similar to that of the child with ALL. Nursing interventions focus on managing the adverse effects of treatment and preventing infection. Refer to the nursing process overview section and to Nursing Care Plan 49.1 for appropriate interventions.

Lymphomas

Lymphomas, or tumors of the lymph tissue (lymph nodes, thymus, spleen), account for about 10% to 15% of cases of childhood cancer (Maloney et al., 2007). Lymphomas may be divided in to two categories: Hodgkin's disease (or Hodgkin's lymphoma) and non-Hodgkin's lymphoma (NHL), which includes more than a dozen types. Hodgkin's disease tends to affect lymph nodes located closer to the body's surface, such as those in the cervical, axillary, and inguinal areas, whereas NHL tends to affect lymph nodes located more deeply inside the body.

▶ HODGKIN'S DISEASE

In Hodgkin's disease, malignant B lymphocytes grow in the lymph tissue, usually starting in one general area of lymph nodes. The presence of Reed-Sternberg cells (giant transformed B lymphocytes with one or two nuclei) differentiates Hodgkin's disease from other lymphomas. As the cells multiply, the lymph nodes enlarge, compressing nearby structures, destroying normal cells, and invading other tissues. The cause of Hodgkin's disease is still being researched, but there appears to be a link with Epstein-Barr virus infection. Hodgkin's disease is rare in children under 5 years of age and is most common in adolescents and young adults; it is more common in boys than girls.

In addition to the traditional **staging** (I through IV, depending on the amount of spread; Table 49.3), Hodgkin's is also classified as A (asymptomatic) or B (presence of symptoms of fever, night sweats, or weight loss of 10% or more). Prognosis depends on the stage of the disease, tumor bulk, and A or B classification (disease classified as A generally carries a better prognosis). Overall, children with Hodgkin's disease have a 75% 20-year survival rate (Maloney et al., 2007). Complications of Hodgkin's disease include liver failure and secondary cancer such as acute non-lymphocytic leukemia and NHL.

Chemotherapy, usually with a combination of drugs, is the treatment of choice for children with Hodgkin's disease. Radiation therapy may also be necessary. In the child with disease that does not go into remission or in the child who experiences relapse, HSCT may be an option.

Nursing Assessment

Explore the health history for common signs and symptoms, which may include recent weight loss, fever, drenching night sweats, anorexia, malaise, fatigue, or pruritus. Elicit the health history, determining risk factors such as prior Epstein-Barr virus infection, family history of Hodgkin's disease, genetic immune disorder, or HIV infection.

TABLE 49.3 **STAGING OF HODGKIN'S DISEASE**

Stage	Clinical Findings
I	One group of lymph nodes is affected.
II	Two or more groups on the same side of the diaphragm are affected.
III	Groups of lymph nodes above and below the diaphragm are affected.
IV	Metastasis to organs such as the liver, bone, or lungs

Evaluate respiratory status, as the presence of a mediastinal mass may compromise respiration. Palpate for enlarged lymph nodes; they may feel rubbery and tend to occur in clusters (most common sites are cervical and supraclavicular). Palpate the abdomen for hepatomegaly or splenomegaly, which may be present with advanced disease. The chest x-ray may reveal a mediastinal mass. The complete blood count may be normal or reflect anemia. Tissue sampling will reveal Reed-Sternberg cells.

> ▶ **Take** NOTE!
>
> *Significant pain in the affected lymph nodes has sometimes been noted after alcohol ingestion.*

Nursing Management

Nursing management of the child with Hodgkin's lymphoma focuses on addressing the adverse effects of chemotherapy or radiation. Refer to the nursing process overview section and Nursing Care Plan 49.1 to develop an individualized nursing care plan based on the child's response to treatment.

▶ NON-HODGKIN'S LYMPHOMA

NHL results from mutations in the B and T lymphocytes that lead to uncontrolled growth. NHL tends to affect lymph nodes located more deeply within the body. NHL spreads by the bloodstream and in children is a rapidly proliferating, aggressive malignancy that is very responsive to treatment. Prognosis depends on the cell type involved and the extent of the disease at diagnosis. Seventy percent to 90% of children with treated NHL have disease-free long-term survival (Maloney et al., 2007). Complications include metastasis and the development of a secondary malignancy later in life.

Remission is induced with chemotherapy and followed with a maintenance phase of chemotherapy lasting about 2 years. NHL tends to spread easily to the CNS, so CNS prophylaxis similar to that used in leukemia is warranted. Autologous bone marrow transplantation may be used in some children.

Nursing Assessment

Children with NHL are usually symptomatic for only a few days or a few weeks before diagnosis because the disease progresses so quickly. Note onset and location of pain or lymph node swelling. Document history of abdominal pain, diarrhea, or constipation. Explore the health history for risk factors such as congenital or acquired immune deficiency.

Observe for increased work of breathing, facial edema, or venous engorgement (mediastinal mass). Palpate for the presence of lymphadenopathy and palpate the abdomen for the presence of a mass. Lymph node biopsy and bone marrow aspiration determine the diagnosis. CT scan, chest x-ray, and bone marrow results may be used to determine the extent of metastasis.

> ▶ **Take** NOTE!
>
> *Cough, dyspnea, orthopnea, facial edema, or venous engorgement may indicate mediastinal disease in the child with NHL. This is an emergency requiring rapid treatment.*

Nursing Management

As with Hodgkin's lymphoma, nursing management of NHL is directed toward managing the adverse effects of chemotherapy. Refer to the Nursing Process Overview section and Nursing Care Plan 49.1 to plan nursing care for the child and family based on the responses they exhibit.

Brain Tumors

Brain tumors are the most common form of solid tumor and the second most common type of cancer in children (Maloney et al., 2007). Slightly more than half of brain tumors arise in the posterior fossa (infratentorial); the rest are supratentorial in origin. The cause of brain tumors in children is unknown. Some tumors are localized, while others are of higher grade and more invasive. The prognosis depends on the location and extent of tumor. Low-grade tumors and those that are fully resectable have a better prognosis than tumors that are located deeper within the brain, making them difficult to resect. For example, low-grade astrocytomas have a 5- to 10-year survival rate of 60% to 90% (Albano et al., 2005), but the rate for the highly malignant medulloblastoma is not as positive. There are many different types of childhood brain tumors; Table 49.4 explains the most common ones.

Complications of brain tumors include hydrocephalus, increased intracranial pressure, brain stem herniation, and negative effects of radiation such as neuropsychological, intellectual, and endocrinologic sequelae.

Pathophysiology

Though the cause of brain tumors is generally not known, the effects of brain tumors are predictable. As the tumor grows within the cranium, it exerts pressure on the brain tissues surrounding it. The tumor mass may compress vital

TABLE 49.4   **CHILDHOOD BRAIN TUMORS**

Tumor	Location	Characteristics
Medulloblastoma (most common)	Cerebellum	Invasive, highly malignant, grows rapidly. Less favorable outcome with disseminated disease. Progresses quickly to increased intracranial pressure, seeds on CNS pathways. Half occur in children <6 years old.
Brain stem glioma	Brain stem	Aggressive, difficult to resect, resistant to chemotherapy. Spreads widely within the brain stem but rarely extends outside of brain stem area. Affects cranial nerve function.
Ependymoma	Frequently arises from floor of fourth ventricle	Varying speed of growth. Often causes hydrocephalus. Usually diagnosed before it spreads to other parts of the brain or spinal cord.
Astrocytoma	Cerebellum, cerebral hemispheres, thalamus, hypothalamus	Slow course with insidious onset. Responsive to chemotherapy, often resectable. Causes slowly increasing intracranial pressure. Low-grade tumor may be removed completely. High-grade tumors have poor prognosis.

structures in the brain, block cerebrospinal fluid flow, or cause edema in the brain. The result is an increase in intracranial pressure. Presenting symptoms vary according to location and type of tumor.

Therapeutic Management

The type of tumor may be identified at the time of surgery. The location of the tumor within the brain will determine the extent to which it can safely be resected. Children with hydrocephalus may require a ventriculoperitoneal shunt (see Chapter 37 for further information on hydrocephalus). Radiation is reserved for children over age 2 years because it can have long-term neurocognitive effects. Chemotherapy is being used increasingly in the treatment of pediatric brain tumors in an attempt to avoid the use of radiation therapy.

Nursing Assessment

For a full description of the assessment phase of the nursing process, refer to page 1633. Assessment findings pertinent to CNS tumors are discussed below.

Health History

Elicit a description of the present illness and chief complaint. Common signs and symptoms reported during the health history might include:

- Nausea or vomiting
- Headache
- Unsteady gait
- Blurred or double vision
- Seizures
- Motor abnormality or hemiparesis
- Weakness, atrophy
- Swallowing difficulties

- Behavior or personality changes
- Irritability, failure to thrive or developmental delay (in very young children)

Explore the patient's current and past medical history for risk factors such as history of neurofibromatosis, tuberous sclerosis, or prior treatment for CNS leukemia.

Physical Examination

Inspection and Observation

Observe for strabismus or nystagmus, "sunsetting" eyes, head tilt, alterations in coordination, gait disturbance, or alterations in sensation. Note alteration in gag reflex, cranial nerve palsy, lethargy, or irritability. Note the child's posture. Check pupillary reaction, noting size, equality, reaction to light, and accommodation.

Palpation

Measure blood pressure, which may decrease with increasing intracranial pressure. In the infant, palpate the anterior fontanel for bulging. Assess deep tendon reflexes, noting hyperreflexia.

 ▶ ***Take*** NOTE!

A fixed and dilated pupil is a neurosurgical emergency.

Laboratory and Diagnostic Tests

Common laboratory and diagnostic studies ordered for the assessment of CNS tumors include:

- CT, MRI, or positron-emission tomography (PET) will demonstrate evidence of the tumor and its location within the intracranial cavity.

- Lumbar puncture with cerebrospinal fluid cell evaluation may show tumor markers or the presence of alpha-fetoprotein or human chorionic gonadotropin, which may assist in the diagnosis.

Nursing Management

Nursing management of the child with a brain tumor includes preoperative and postoperative care, as well as interventions to manage adverse effects related to chemotherapy and radiation. Refer to the nursing process overview section for a discussion of nursing interventions related to chemotherapy adverse effects. Nursing Care Plan 49.1 provides additional interventions that may be individualized depending on the child's response to the brain tumor and its treatment.

Providing Preoperative Care

Preoperatively, care focuses on monitoring for additional increases in intracranial pressure and avoiding activities that cause transient increases in intracranial pressure. Administer dexamethasone as prescribed to decrease intracranial inflammation. Prevent straining with bowel movements by use of a stool softener. Assess the child's pain level as well of level of consciousness, vital signs, and pupillary reaction to determine subtle changes as soon as possible. Provide a tour of the intensive care unit, which is where the child will wake up after the surgery. Instruct the child and family about the possibility of intubation and ventilation in the postoperative period. If a ventriculoperitoneal shunt will be placed for the treatment of hydrocephalus caused by the tumor, provide education about shunts to the child and family (see Chapter 37).

Shave the portion of the head as determined by the neurosurgeon. Some children may choose to have the entire head shaved. Sometimes children with long hair may feel better about losing it if they donate it to Locks of Love (www.locksoflove.org), an organization that provides hairpieces for financially disadvantaged children.

Providing Postoperative Care

Regulate fluid administration, as excess fluid intake may cause or worsen cerebral edema. Administer mannitol or hypertonic dextrose to decrease cerebral edema. Assess vital signs frequently, along with checking pupillary reactions and determining level of consciousness. Extreme lethargy or coma may be present for several days postoperatively. Increases in temperature may indicate infection or may be caused by cerebral edema or disturbance of the hypothalamus. Treat hyperthermia with antipyretics such as acetaminophen and with sponge baths, as increases in temperature increase metabolic need. Reduce the temperature slowly.

Monitor for signs of increased intracranial pressure. Headache is common in the postoperative period. Assess pain level and provide analgesics as prescribed. Minimize environmental stimuli, providing a calm and quiet atmo-

sphere. Check the head dressing for cerebrospinal fluid drainage or bleeding. Assess for and document the extent of head, face, or neck edema. Administer eye lubricant if edema prevents complete closure of the eyelids. Apply cool compresses to the eyes to decrease swelling.

As the child begins to regain consciousness, he or she may be confused or combative. Restrain the child if needed to keep him or her in bed and prevent dislodging of tubes and lines.

Positioning the Child in the Postoperative Period

Position the child on the unaffected side with the head of the bed flat or at the level prescribed by the neurosurgeon. Side positioning is usually preferred, as the child may have difficulty handling oral secretions if the level of consciousness is decreased. Do not elevate the foot of the bed, as this may increase intracranial pressure and contribute to bleeding. When changing the child's position, maintain the head in alignment with the remainder of the body. Children with paralyzed or spastic extremities will need additional positioning support.

▶ **Take** NOTE!

Observe preoperatively and postoperatively for signs of brain stem herniation such as opisthotonos (see Fig. 37.13), nuchal rigidity, head tilt, sluggish pupils, increased blood pressure with widening pulse pressure, change in respirations, bradycardia, irregular pulse, and changes in body temperature.

▶ **Consider** THIS!

Alice Tice, 6 years old, is scheduled to receive chemotherapy for a brain tumor. As the nurse caring for her, how can you prepare Alice for this? What nursing interventions are important when caring for a child receiving chemotherapy (discuss reducing pain, reducing risk of infection, promoting adequate nutrition, and managing nausea and vomiting)?

Neuroblastoma

Neuroblastoma, a tumor that arises from embryonic neural crest cells, is the most common extracranial solid tumor in children. It most frequently occurs in the abdomen, mainly in the adrenal gland, but it may occur anywhere along the paravertebral sympathetic chain in the chest or retroperitoneum. By the time of diagnosis, the neuroblastoma has usually already metastasized. Neuroblastoma is the second most frequently occurring solid tumor in children; and 90% of cases are diagnosed before the age of 5 years (Maloney et al., 2007).

Staging of the tumor at diagnosis determines the course of treatment and prognosis. Table 49.5 discusses the staging of neuroblastomas. Survival rates range from 40% to 90%. Prognosis depends on the tumor stage, age at diagnosis, location of tumor, and location of **metastasis**. Infants less than 12 months of age and children with stage I disease have the best survival rates. Children with tumors above the diaphragm tend to have a better prognosis than those with abdominal tumors. Metastasis to the bone is a worse prognostic factor than metastasis to the skin, liver, or bone marrow. Children who relapse after initial treatment also tend to have a dismal prognosis. In addition to metastasis, complications may include nerve compression, resulting in neurologic deficits.

The neuroblastoma must be surgically removed. Radiation and chemotherapy are administered to all children with neuroblastoma except those with stage I disease, in whom the tumor is completely resected.

Nursing Assessment

For a full description of the assessment phase of the nursing process, refer to page 1633. Assessment findings pertinent to neuroblastoma are discussed below.

Health History
Presenting signs and symptoms of neuroblastoma depend on the location of the primary tumor and the extent of metastasis. Often parents are the first to notice a swollen or asymmetric abdomen. Elicit the health history, documenting bowel or bladder dysfunction, especially watery diarrhea, neurologic symptoms (brain metastasis), bone pain (bone metastasis), anorexia, vomiting, or weight loss.

TABLE 49.5   STAGING OF NEUROBLASTOMA

Stage	Clinical Findings
I	Tumor confined to organ or structure of origin
II	Tumor extends beyond organ or structure, not beyond midline, and regional nodes on the same side may be involved
III	Tumor invasively extends beyond the midline with bilateral lymph node involvement
IV	Metastasis to bone, bone marrow, other organs, distant lymph nodes
IV-S	Tumor would have been considered a stage I or II, but remote metastasis to one or more sites (liver, skin, or bone marrow) has occurred, but does not involve skeleton

Physical Examination
Note neck or facial swelling, bruising above the eyes, or edema around the eyes (metastasis to skull bones). Inspect the skin for pallor or bruising (bone marrow metastasis) and document cough or difficulty breathing. Auscultate the lungs for wheezing. Palpate for lymphadenopathy, especially cervical. Palpate the abdomen, noting a firm, nontender mass. Palpate for and note hepatomegaly or splenomegaly if present.

Laboratory and Diagnostic Testing
Laboratory and diagnostic testing may reveal the following:

- CT scan or MRI to determine site of tumor and evidence of metastasis
- Chest x-ray, bone scan, and skeletal survey to identify metastasis
- Bone marrow aspiration and biopsy to determine metastasis to the bone marrow
- 24-hour urine collection for homovanillic acid (HVA) and vanillylmandelic acid (VMA); levels will be elevated.

Nursing Management

Postoperative nursing care depends on the site of tumor removal, which is most often the abdomen. Routine care after abdominal surgery will be needed. Refer to the nursing process overview section and Nursing Care Plan 49.1 related to the effects of chemotherapy and radiation. As the disease has often metastasized significantly by the time of diagnosis, these children and families will need emotional support and possibly referrals to help them cope with the poor prognosis.

Bone and Soft Tissue Tumors

Bone and soft tissue tumors account for about 10% to 15% of malignant tumors in children (National Cancer Institute, 2008). Bone tumors are most often diagnosed in adolescence, whereas soft tissue tumors tend to occur in younger children. This discussion will focus on the most common bone and soft tissue tumors occurring in childhood. The most common bone tumors in children are osteosarcoma and Ewing sarcoma. These bone tumors often initially go undiagnosed, as adolescents frequently seek care for traumatic events and the pain suffered with a bone tumor may initially be attributed to trauma (DeGroot, 2008). Rhabdomyosarcoma is the most common soft tissue tumor in childhood.

▶ OSTEOSARCOMA

Osteosarcoma is the most common **malignant** bone cancer in children, occurring most frequently in adolescents at the peak of the growth spurt (Maloney et al.,

2007). Osteosarcoma occurs slightly more often in females and is rare among African-Americans. It presumably arises from the embryonic mesenchymal tissue that forms the bones. The most common sites are in the long bones, particularly the proximal humerus, proximal tibia, and distal femur. Survivors of retinoblastoma who suffer a secondary malignancy are most frequently diagnosed with osteosarcoma. Complications include metastasis, particularly to the lungs and other bones, and recurrence of disease within 3 years, primarily affecting the lungs.

Surgical removal of the tumor is necessary. Chemotherapy is often administered before surgery to decrease the size of the tumor; it is usually administered after surgery to treat or prevent metastasis. The type of surgery performed depends on the tumor size, extent of disease outside of the bone, distant metastasis, and skeletal maturity. Radical amputation may be performed, but often teens undergo a limb salvage procedure. Radical amputation may include the entire extremity or the entire affected bone. Limb-sparing surgery entails removing only the affected portion of the bone, replacing it with either an endoprosthesis or cadaver bone.

Nursing Assessment

Obtain the health history, ascertaining when pain, limp, or limitation of motion was first noticed. Dull bone pain may be present for several months, eventually progressing to limp or gait changes.

Inspect the affected limb for erythema and swelling. Palpate the affected area for warmth and tenderness and to determine the size of the soft tissue mass, if present. As with other pediatric cancers, a thorough physical examination is warranted to detect other abnormalities that may indicate metastasis.

Laboratory and diagnostic testing may include:

- CT scan or MRI to determine the extent of the lesion and to identify metastasis
- Bone scan to determine the extent of malignancy
- Elevated alkaline phosphatase levels: these may or may not be helpful, as the quickly growing adolescent often normally has elevated levels as a response to rapid bone growth

Nursing Management

The adolescent will generally be quite anxious about the possibility of amputation and even about the limb salvage procedure. Present preoperative teaching at the adolescent's developmental level and ensure that he or she is included in planning treatment. Regardless of the type of surgery performed, provide routine orthopedic postoperative care. Educate the adolescent and parents on the care of the stump, if amputation is necessary, and ensure that the teen becomes competent in crutch

walking. A prosthesis may be ordered. The adolescent will need time to adjust to these significant body image changes and may benefit from talking with another teen who has undergone a similar procedure. Support the teen in choosing clothing that may camouflage the prosthesis while still allowing the teen to appear fashionable. Provide emotional support, as the teen's maturity level allows him or her to understand the severity of the disease. Peer support groups are often helpful, as teens value their peers' opinions and enjoy being part of a group. Examples of comprehensive online support groups are www.teenslivingwithcancer.org/ and www.grouploop.org/default_flash.php.

▶ EWING SARCOMA

Ewing sarcoma is a highly malignant bone tumor. It is rarer than osteosarcoma, accounting for only about 10% of childhood bone tumors (Maloney et al., 2007). It occurs most frequently in the pelvis, chest wall, vertebrae, and long bone diaphyses (midshaft). About 25% of children demonstrate metastasis; the lung, bone, and bone marrow are the most common sites (Maloney et al., 2007). The prognosis depends on the extent of metastasis. Only about 30% of children with metastasis survive, despite traditional chemotherapy and surgery or augmentation with total body irradiation and HSCT (Miser et al., 2004).

Radiation, chemotherapy, and surgical excision are usually used in combination. Treatment varies depending on the site of the primary tumor and the extent of metastasis at diagnosis. Myeloablative chemotherapy (which destroys the child's marrow) may be used for metastatic disease, followed by a stem cell rescue transplant.

Nursing Assessment

Explore the history for intermittent pain that progressively worsens. Note a possible history of fever. Eventually the pain becomes constant and severe, sometimes interrupting sleep.

Note the presence of swelling or erythema at the tumor site. CT scan or MRI of the affected area will reveal the extent of the tumor. Serum LDH levels are usually elevated. CT scan of the chest, bone scan, and bilateral bone marrow aspiration with biopsy determine the extent of metastasis.

Nursing Management

Before treatment begins, discourage active play or weight bearing on the affected extremity to avoid pathologic fracture at the tumor site. Nursing management focuses on addressing the adverse effects of treatment (refer to the nursing process overview section). Teens with Ewing sarcoma need honest and direct answers to questions about their disease. These children will undergo intensive therapy and spend a great deal of time in the hospital. Depending on the age of the child, fantasy play, art or pet therapy, drama, writing, humor, and/or music may help the child to work through the psychological impact of this disease. Refer to Nursing Care Plan 49.1 for additional interventions, which should be individualized depending on the child's and family's response to the disease process and treatment.

▶ RHABDOMYOSARCOMA

Rhabdomyosarcoma is a soft tissue tumor that usually arises from the embryonic mesenchymal cells that would ordinarily form striated muscle. The most common locations for the tumor are the head and neck, genitourinary tract, and extremities (Fig. 49.7). The tumor is highly ma-

lignant and spreads via local extension or through the venous or lymphatic system, with the lung being the most common site for metastasis. Diagnosis is usually made between 2 and 5 years of age, with 70% of all rhabdomyosarcomas diagnosed by age 10 years (Maloney et al., 2007). The prognosis is based on the stage of the disease at diagnosis. Box 49.3 explains the staging of rhabdomyosarcoma. Prognosis is generally favorable for stage I disease (Stevens et al., 2005). Children with metastatic disease have about a 40% survival rate (Breneman et al., 2003). Complications of rhabdomyosarcoma include metastasis to lung, bone, or bone marrow and direct extension into the CNS, resulting in brain stem compromise or cranial nerve palsy.

Surgical removal of the primary tumor is generally performed. At the time of the surgery, the lesion is biopsied and the stage of disease determined. Radiation and chemotherapy may be used to shrink the tumor to avoid disability, depending on the site and size of the tumor (especially head, neck, and pelvis).

Nursing Assessment

The child or parent will often discover an asymptomatic mass and seek medical attention at that time. Obtain a health history, noting recent illness, when the mass was discovered, and whether it has changed since first noted. Examine the history for risk factors such as parental smoking, exposure to environmental chemicals, family history of cancer, or neurofibromatosis. Note respiratory effort and cough, and auscultate the lungs for adventitious sounds. Palpate for lymphadenopathy. Palpate the abdomen for a mass or hepatosplenomegaly. Abnormalities found on physical examination depend on the location of the rhabdomyosarcoma (Table 49.6).

Laboratory and diagnostic testing may include:

- CT scan or MRI of primary lesion and the chest for metastasis
- Open biopsy of the primary tumor for definitive diagnosis
- Bone marrow aspiration and biopsy, bone scan, and skeletal survey to determine metastasis

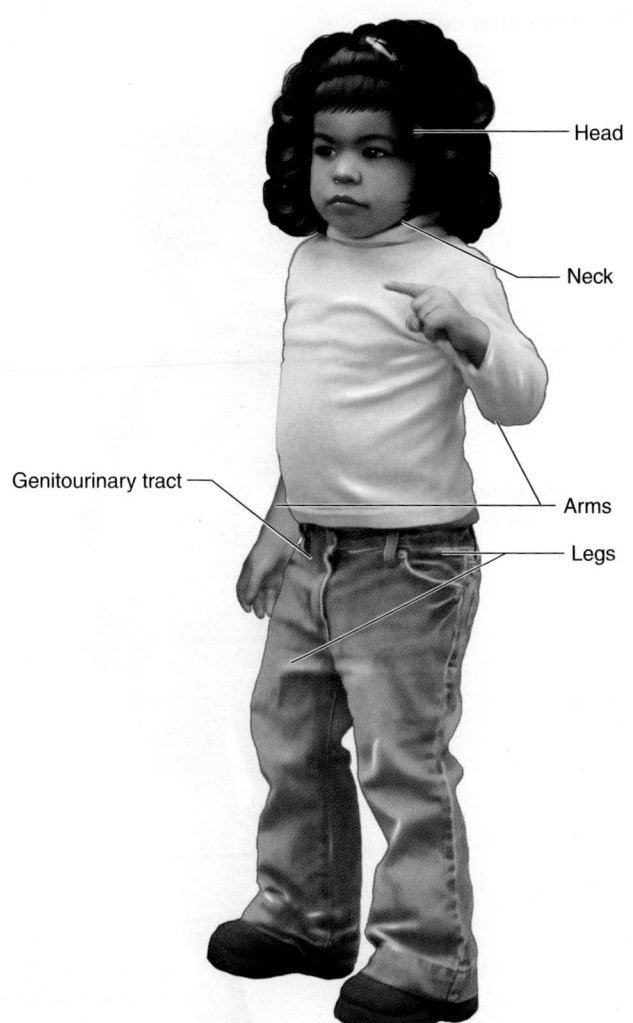

Head

Neck

Genitourinary tract

Arms

Legs

FIGURE 49.7 The most common sites of rhabdomyosarcoma.

BOX 49.3 **Staging of Rhabmomyosarcoma**

- Stage I: completely resectable localized tumor
- Stage II: after local tumor resection, microscopic residual disease remains
- Stage III: after local tumor resection, gross residual disease remains
- Stage IV: metastasis present at diagnosis

TABLE 49.6   PRESENTING SIGNS AND SYMPTOMS RELATED TO LOCATION OF RHABDOMYOSARCOMA

Location of Tumor	Presenting Signs and Symptoms
Orbit	Proptosis
Middle ear	Drainage, pain, facial nerve palsy
Sinuses	Discharge, pain, sinusitis, facial swelling
Nasopharynx	Pain, epistaxis, dysphagia, nasal quality to speech, airway obstruction
Neck	Dysphagia, hoarseness
Thorax, testicle, extremities	Enlarging mass, painless
Retroperitoneum	Gastrointestinal and urinary tract obstruction, pain, weakness, paresthesia
Bladder, prostate	Hematuria, urinary obstruction
Vagina	Mass, vaginal bleeding or chronic discharge

▶ *Take* NOTE!

Primary tumors arising in the neck region may compress the child's airway. Assess work of breathing and lung sounds.

Nursing Management

Provide routine postoperative care, depending on the site of surgery. Assess for adverse effects of high-dose radiation, which is generally used to treat the primary tumor as well as metastatic sites. Administer chemotherapy as ordered and assess for adverse effects. Refer to the nursing process overview section and Nursing Care Plan 49.1 to determine an individualized plan of care based on the child's response to the treatment.

Wilms' Tumor

Wilms' tumor is the most common renal tumor in children, accounting for 5% to 7% of all childhood cancers. Peak incidence occurs between the ages of 4 and 5 years (Amin, 2007). It usually affects only one kidney (Fig. 49.8). The etiology is unknown, but some cases occur via genetic inheritance. Associated anomalies may occur with Wilms' tumor. Wilms' tumor demonstrates rapid growth and is usually large at diagnosis. Metastasis occurs via direct extension or through the bloodstream. Wilms' tumor most commonly metastasizes to the perirenal tissues, liver, diaphragm, lungs, abdominal muscles, and lymph nodes. The prognosis depends on staging at diagnosis and the extent of metastasis (Box 49.4). The overall survival rate is about 90%. Complications include metastasis or complications from radiation therapy such as liver or renal damage, female sterility, bowel obstruction, pneumonia, or scoliosis.

Therapeutic Management

Surgical removal of the tumor and affected kidney (nephrectomy) is the treatment of choice and also allows for accurate staging and assessment of tumor spread. Radiation or chemotherapy may be administered either before or after surgery.

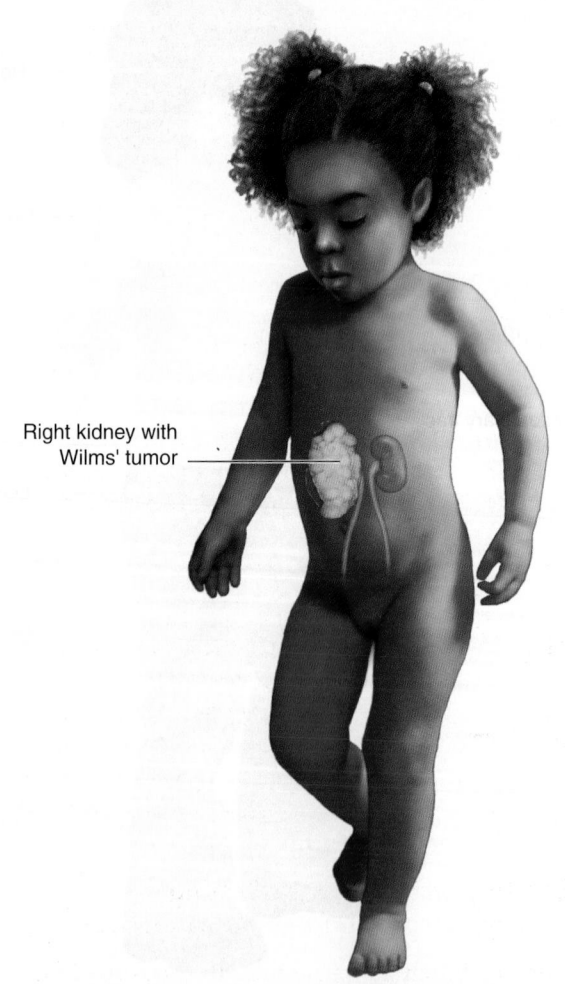

Right kidney with Wilms' tumor

FIGURE 49.8 Wilms' tumor is usually unilateral.

> ### BOX 49.4   Staging of Wilms' Tumor
>
> - Stage I: unilateral, limited to kidney, completely resectable
> - Stage II: unilateral, tumor extends beyond kidney but is completely resectable
> - Stage III: unilateral, tumor has spread outside of kidney, located in abdominal cavity only, not fully removed
> - Stage IV: unilateral with metastasis in liver, lung, bone, or brain
> - Stage V: bilateral kidney involvement

Nursing Assessment

For a full description of the assessment phase of the nursing process, refer to page 1633. Assessment findings pertinent to Wilms' tumor are discussed below.

Health History

Parents typically initially observe the abdominal mass associated with Wilm's tumor and then seek medical attention. Elicit the health history, noting when the mass was discovered. Note abdominal pain, which may be related to rapid tumor growth. Document history of constipation, vomiting, anorexia, weight loss, or difficulty breathing. Determine risk factors such as hemihypertrophy of the spine, Beckwith-Wiedemann syndrome, genitourinary anomalies, absence of the iris, or family history of cancer.

Physical Examination

Measure blood pressure: hypertension occurs in 25% of children with Wilms' tumor (Maloney et al., 2007). Inspect the abdomen for asymmetry or a visible mass. Observe for associated anomalies as noted above. Auscultate the lungs for adventitious breath sounds associated with tumor metastasis. Palpate for lymphadenopathy.

> ▶ **Take** NOTE!
>
> *Avoid palpating the abdomen after the initial assessment preoperatively. Wilms' tumor is highly vascular and soft, so excessive handling of the tumor may result in tumor seeding and metastasis.*

Laboratory and Diagnostic Testing

Laboratory and diagnostic testing may include:

- Renal or abdominal ultrasound to assess the tumor and the contralateral kidney
- CT scan or MRI of the abdomen and chest to determine local spread to lymph nodes or adjacent organs, as well as any distant metastasis
- Complete blood count, BUN, and creatinine: usually within normal limits
- Urinalysis: may reveal hematuria or leukocytes
- 24-hour urine collection for HVA and VMA to distinguish the tumor from neuroblastoma (levels will not be elevated with Wilms' tumor)

Nursing Management

Postoperative care of the child with Wilms' tumor resection is similar to that of children undergoing other abdominal surgery. Assessment of remaining kidney function is critical. The child may have adverse effects related to chemotherapy or radiation. Refer to the nursing process overview section and Nursing Care Plan 49.1 to individualize care for the child based on the child's response to therapy.

> ▶ **Take** NOTE!
>
> *To avoid injuring the remaining kidney, children with a single kidney should not play contact sports.*

Retinoblastoma

Retinoblastoma is a congenital, highly malignant tumor that arises from embryonic retinal cells. It accounts for 5% of cases of blindness in children (Maloney et al., 2007). Most children are diagnosed by age 3, and the overall survival rate is 90%. Retinoblastoma may be hereditary or nonhereditary. Nonhereditary retinoblastoma may be associated with advanced paternal age and always presents with unilateral involvement. Hereditary retinoblastoma is inherited via the autosomal dominant mode. These cases may be unilateral or bilateral. The tumor may grow forward into the vitreous cavity of the eye or extend into the subretinal space, causing retinal detachment. The tumor may extend into the choroid, the sclera, and the optic nerve.

Complications include spread to the brain and the opposite eye, as well as metastasis to lymph nodes, bone, bone marrow, and liver. Second tumors, most often sarcomas, may also occur in children who have been treated for retinoblastoma. Table 49.7 explains the staging of retinoblastoma.

The goals of treatment are to eradicate the tumor, preserve vision, and provide a good cosmetic outcome. Retinoblastoma may be treated with radiation, chemotherapy, laser surgery, cryotherapy, or a combination. Moderate vision may be preserved for most children without advanced

TABLE 49.7 STAGING OF RETINOBLASTOMA

A	Small tumors (<3 mm; about 0.1 inch) confined to the retina
B	Larger tumors confined to the retina
C	Localized seeding of the vitreous or under the retina <6 mm (0.2 inches) from the original tumor
D	Widespread vitreous or subretinal seeding, may have total retinal detachment
E	No visual potential, eye cannot recover

From American Cancer Society. (2006). How is retinoblastoma staged? Available online at http://www.cancer.org/docroot/CRI/content/CRI_2_4_3X_How_is_retinoblastoma_staged_37.asp?sitearea=.

disease. In advanced disease or in the case of a massive tumor with retinal detachment, enucleation (removal of the eye) is necessary.

Nursing Assessment

Parents are often the first to notice the "cat's eye reflex" or "whitewash glow" to the child's affected pupil. Obtain the health history, determining when other associated symptoms such as strabismus, orbital inflammation, vomiting, or headache began. Inquire about risk factors such as a family history of retinoblastoma or other cancer or the presence of chromosomal anomalies. Assess pupils for size and reactivity to light. Note presence of leukocoria ("cat's eye reflex," a whitish appearance of the pupil) in the affected eye (Fig. 49.9). Assess the eyes for associated signs, which may include erythema, orbital inflammation, or hyphema.

Diagnostic evaluation includes an ophthalmologic examination under anesthesia. CT, MRI, or ultrasound of the head and eyes will help to visualize the tumor. The infant or toddler may also undergo lumbar puncture and bone marrow aspiration to determine the presence and extent of metastasis.

FIGURE 49.9 Note the whitish appearance of this child's pupil (leukocoria). (Photo courtesy of The Childhood Eye Cancer Trust of the United Kingdom.)

Nursing Management

Provide routine postoperative care to the infant or toddler. If the eye is enucleated, observe the large pressure dressing on the eye socket for bleeding. Dressing changes to the socket may include sterile saline rinses and/or antibiotic ointment application. If disease occurs outside of the eye or if metastasis is present, inform the parents that chemotherapy will be necessary. Monitor for side effects of chemotherapy (see the nursing process overview section). Follow-up will include eye examinations every 3 to 6 months until age 6 and then annually to check for further tumor development. If the eye is enucleated, several weeks after removal, a prosthetic eye will be fitted. Teach families use of the prosthetic eye; it does not require daily removal.

Provide parents with support and encouragement. Refer the family for genetic counseling. Subsequent children will need ophthalmologic examination under anesthesia at 2 months of age and frequent examinations until age 3 years. Children treated for retinoblastoma will also need genetic counseling as they reach puberty, as about half of the offspring of children with retinoblastoma have bilateral disease.

> ▶ **Take** NOTE!
>
> *Educate parents about protecting vision in the remaining eye: routine eye checkups, protection from accidental injury, use of safety goggles during sports, and prompt treatment of eye infections. Generally, children with one eye should not participate in contact sports.*

Screening for Reproductive Cancers in Adolescents

Increasingly, reproductive cancers are being diagnosed in adolescents. Cervical cancer and testicular cancer may be discovered early with appropriate screening, and earlier discovery leads to better outcomes. Starting screening in the teenage years may also instill a lifelong healthy habit in the adolescent.

▶ CERVICAL CANCER

Risk factors for cervical cancer include young age at first intercourse, infection with a sexually transmitted disease, and a history of multiple sex partners, and more and more teenagers are presenting with these risk factors. Counsel all sexually active adolescents to seek reproductive care, which is available without parental consent in most states. The screening Papanicolaou (Pap) smear is efficient and

Objective	Significance
Increase the proportion of women who receive a Pap test.	• When an adolescent girl makes the decision to become sexually active, counsel her about the importance of getting annual Pap smears.

reliable at determining abnormal cervical cells and is a key part of screening for cervical cancer (if cancer is present, the parent will have to be notified). Cervical cancer has a very high response to therapy and rate of cure if treated in its early stages, so nurses should encourage teenage girls to be responsible for their sexual health by seeking appropriate examination and screening.

▶ TESTICULAR CANCER

Although uncommon in teens, testicular cancer is the most frequently diagnosed cancer in males age 15 to 35. It is one of the most curable cancers if diagnosed early. To get into the habit of screening for testicular lumps, adolescent boys should begin performing testicular self-examinations monthly (Teaching Guidelines 49.3).

TEACHING GUIDELINES 49.3

Testicular Self-Examination

- Perform the examination once a month, after a shower.
- Be familiar with the size and weight of your testicles.
- Roll the testicle between your fingers. The small ropelike structure is the epididymis; this is normal.
- Report any lump, swelling, or heaviness of one testicle to your health care provider.

■■■ Key Concepts

- Childhood cancer tends to develop from embryonal tissue; in general it is more responsive to therapy than adult cancers, which tend to be derived from epithelial tissue.
- In adults, cancer is influenced to a large extent by environmental factors. Cancer in children is not, so there are no routine screening measures or prevention strategies for childhood cancer.
- The pain associated with lumbar puncture or bone marrow aspiration may be minimized with the use of topical anesthetics or conscious sedation.
- CT scans and MRI are used extensively in the diagnosis and follow-up of childhood cancer. The young child may have difficulty holding still for these scans and may need short-term sedation.
- Leukemia often presents in children with a history of fever, infection, and fatigue. Bone pain or CNS symptoms may be present if metastasis to the bone or brain has occurred.
- Lymphomas in children present similarly to those in adults, often with an enlarged, nontender lymph node.
- Symptoms of brain tumors depend on the location of the tumor; commonly they present with signs and symptoms of increased intracranial pressure, such as headache, nausea, and vomiting.
- Neuroblastoma has often significantly metastasized at diagnosis. It most commonly presents as a mass in the abdomen.
- Shortness of breath or chest pain in the child with cancer is a medical emergency; it may indicate superior vena cava syndrome or a tumor in the mediastinal region.
- Retinoblastoma may be identified by the presence of leukocoria in one or both eyes. Retinoblastoma occurs in early infancy up until early childhood.
- Bone cancer does not necessarily require amputation; it may be treated with a combination of limb salvage procedure, radiation, and chemotherapy.
- The symptoms of rhabdomyosarcoma depend on the location of the tumor.
- Avoid abdominal palpation preoperatively in the child with Wilms' tumor; palpation may cause seeding of the tumor and metastasis.
- Radiation therapy may result in fatigue, nausea and vomiting, and long-term cognitive sequelae (if directed to the cranium).
- Nursing care of the child receiving treatment for cancer focuses on preventing or treating adverse effects such as fatigue, nausea, vomiting, alopecia, mucositis, and infection.
- The neutropenic child with fever should receive medical attention as soon as possible so that intravenous antibiotics may be started immediately.
- Cancer is a significant stressor for children and families. Families need support and education throughout

the diagnostic process, treatment and cure, or palliative care.

■ The child with cancer should lead as near normal a life as possible. When physically able and cleared by the oncologist, the child should resure usual activities such as school. Camps for children with cancer provide an excellent opportunity for children to enjoy everyday activities and meet children experiencing similar alterations in their lives.

■ Nutrition may be optimized for children with cancer by managing nausea and vomiting with antiemetics, providing favorie foods, and possibly using total parenteral nutrition.

■ Teach adolescents appropriate screening techniques for reproductive cancers.

■ Educate the child and family about the adverse effects of cancer treatments.

■ Teach parents how to avoid infection in the child receiving chemotherapy, the signs and symptoms of infection, and when to seek medical treatment.

REFERENCES

Ackley, B. J., & Ladwig, G. B. (2006). *Nursing diagnosis handbook: A guide to planning care* (7th ed.). St. Louis: Mosby.

Airewele, G. E., & Steuber, C. P. (2006). Acute myeloid leukemia. In J. A. McMillan (Ed.), *Oski's pediatrics: Principles and practice* (pp. 918–923). Philadelphia: Lippincott Williams & Wilkins.

American Academy of Pediatrics, Committee on Bioethics. (1995). Informed consent, parental permission, and assent in pediatric practice. *Pediatrics, 95*(2), 314–317.

American Cancer Society. (2006). *How is retinoblastoma staged?* Retrieved 1/1/08 from http://www.cancer.org/docroot/CRI/content/CRI_2_4_3X_How_is_retinoblastoma_staged_37.asp?sitearea=.

Amin, N. (2008). Young child with hematuria and dysuria. *Consultant for Pediatricians, 6*(7), 419–422.

Ballard, K. (2004). Meeting the needs of siblings of children with cancer. *Pediatric Nursing, 30*(5), 394–401.

Clerici, C. A., Ferrari, A., Massimino, M., Terenziani, M., Casanova, M., Luksch, R., et al. (2004). Five questions for assessing psychological problems in pediatric patients cured of neoplastic disease. *Pediatric Hematology and Oncology, 21*, 481–487.

Colby-Graham, M. F., & Chordas, C. (2003). The childhood leukemias. *Journal of Pediatric Nursing, 18*(2), 87–95.

College of Medicine, Baylor University. (2008). *Cancer pain management in children.* Retrieved 1/1/08 from http://www.childcancerpain.org/.

Cordier, S., Monfort, C., Filippini, G., Preston-Martin, S., Lubin, F., Mueller, B. A., et al. (2004). Parental exposure to polycyclic aromatic hydrocarbons and the risk of childhood brain tumors. *American Journal of Epidemiology, 159*(12), 1109–1116.

DeGroot, H. (2008). *Metastatic tumors in bone.* Retrieved January 3, 2008 from http://www.bonetumor.org/tumors/pages/page60.html.

Eiser, C. (2007). Beyond survival: Quality of life and follow-up after childhood cancer. *Journal of Pediatric Psychology, 32*(9), 1140–1150.

Feudtner, C. (2004). Perspective on quality at the end of life. *Archives of Pediatric and Adolescent Medicine, 158*, 415–418.

Florin, T. A., & Hinkle, A. S. (2005). A guide to caring for cancer survivors. *Contemporary Pediatrics, 22*(8), 31–48.

Haut, C. (2005). Oncological emergencies in the pediatric intensive care unit. *AACN Clinical Issues, 16*(2), 232–245.

Heiferty, C. M. (2004). Spiritual development and the dying child: The pediatric nurse practitioner's role. *Journal of Pediatric Health Care, 18*, 271–275.

Hendershot, E. (2005). Treatment approaches for metastatic Ewing's sarcoma: A review of the literature. *Journal of Pediatric Oncology Nursing, 22*(6), 339–352.

Hokkanen, H., Eriksson, E., Ahonen, O., & Salantera, S. (2004). Adolescents with cancer: Experience of life and how it could be made easier. *Cancer Nursing, 27*(4), 325–335.

Hooke, C., Hellsten, M. B., Stutzer, C., & Forte, K. (2002). Pain management for the child with cancer in end-of-life: APN position paper. *Journal of Pediatric Oncology Nursing, 19*, 43–47.

Houlahan, K. E., Branowicki, P. A., Mack, J. W., Dinning, C., & McCabe, M. (2006). Can end-of-life care for the pediatric patient suffering with escalating and intractable symptoms be improved? *Journal of Pediatric Oncology Nursing, 23*, 45–51.

Hugger, L. (2005). The psychological treatment of children recovering from leukemia. *Journal of Infant, Child, and Adolescent Psychotherapy, 4*(4), 408–423.

Hurwitz, C. A., Duncan, J., & Wolfe, J. (2004). Caring for the child with cancer at the close of life: "There are people who make it, and I'm hoping I'm one of them." *Journal of the American Medical Association, 292*(17), 2141–2149.

Iwamoto, Y. (2007). Diagnosis and treatment of Ewing's sarcoma. *Japanese Journal of Clinical Oncology, 37*(2), 79–89.

Keating, A. K., Giller, R. H., &quinines, R. R. (2007). Hematopoietic stem cell transplantation. In W. W. Hay, M. J. Levin, J. M. Sondheimer, & R. R. Deterding (Eds.), *Current pediatric diagnosis and treatment* (18th ed.). New York: McGraw-Hill.

Kingston, J. (2005). Thyroid cancer after neck irradiation during childhood. *Lancet, 365*, 1987–1988.

Kline, N. E. (2004). *Essentials of pediatric oncology nursing: A core curriculum* (2nd ed.). Glenview, IL: Association of Pediatric Hematology/Oncology Nurses.

Koontz, B. F. (2006). Palliative radiation therapy for metastatic Ewing sarcoma. *Cancer, 106*(8), 1790–1793.

Kreitler, S., & Arush, M. W. B. (eds.). (2004). *Psychosocial aspects of pediatric oncology.* West Sussex, England: John Wiley and Sons.

Kushner, B. H., & Cheung, N. V. (2005). Neuroblastoma: From genetic profiles to clinical challenge. *New England Journal of Medicine, 353*(21), 2215–2217.

Kutluk, M. T., Yalcin, B., Akyuz, C., Varan, A., Ruacan, S., & Buyukpamukcu, M. (2004). Treatment results and prognostic factors in Ewing sarcoma. *Pediatric Hematology and Oncology, 21*, 597–610.

Larouceh, S. S., & Chin-Peuckert, L. (2006). Changes in body image experienced by adolescents with cancer. *Journal of Pediatric Oncology Nursing, 23*, 200–209.

Lievkovsky, Y. E., Donaldson, S. S., Torres, M. A., Wong, R. M., Amylon, M. D., Link, M. P., & Agarwal, R. (2004). High-dose therapy and autologous hematopoietic stem-cell transplantation for recurrent or refractory pediatric Hodgkin's disease: Results and prognostic indices. *Journal of Clinical Oncology, 22*(22), 4532–4540.

Lund, A. E. (2005). Cancer therapies in childhood can damage developing teeth. *Journal of the American Dental Association, 10*, 1370.

Mabbott, D. J., Speigler, B. J., Greenberg, M. L., Rutka, J. T., Hyder, D. J., & Bouffet, E. (2005). Serial evaluation of academic and behavioral outcome after treatment with cranial radiation in childhood. *Journal of Clinical Oncology, 23*(10), 2256–2263.

Mahoney, D. H. (2006). Acute lymphoblastic leukemia. In J. A. McMillan (Ed.), *Oski's pediatrics: Principles and practice* (pp. 918–923). Philadelphia: Lippincott Williams & Wilkins.

Maloney, K., Greffe, B. S., Foreman, N. K., et al. (2007). Neoplastic disease. In W. W. Hay, M. J. Levin, J. M. Sondheimer, & R. R. Deterding (Eds.), *Current pediatric diagnosis and treatment* (18th ed.). New York: McGraw-Hill.

Marcoux, K. K. (2005). Management of increased intracranial pressure in the critically ill child with acute neurological injury. *AACN Clinical Issues, 16*(2), 212–231.

Marinsek, Z. P. (2006). Ewing sarcoma/PNET: 27 years of experience in Slovenia. *Pediatric Hematology and Oncology, 23*(4), 355–367.

McCaffrey, C. N. (2006). Major stressors and their effect on the well-being of children with cancer. *Journal of Pediatric Nursing, 21*(1), 59–66.

Melamud, A., Palekar, R., & Singh, A. (2006). Retinoblastoma. *American Family Physician, 73*(6), 1039–1044.

Metzler, L. J., & Rourke, M. T. (2005). Oncology summer camp: Benefits of social comparison. *Children's Health Care, 34*(4), 305–314.

Miller, V. A. & Nelson, R. M. (2006). A developmental approach to child assent for nontherapeutic research. *Journal of Pediatrics, 149,* S25–S30.

Miser, J. S., Krailo, M. D., Tarbell, N. J., Link, M. P., Fryer, J. H., Pritchard, D. J., et al. (2004). Treatment of metastatic Ewing's sarcoma or primitive neuroectodermal tumor of bone: Evaluation of combination ifosfamide and etoposide: A Children's Cancer Group and Pediatric Oncology study. *Journal of Clinical Oncology, 22*(14), 2873–2876.

Mosher, R. B. (2006). This is the best life yet: Life at Camp Friendship. *Pediatric Nursing, 32*(1), 84–87.

National Cancer Institute. (2008). *Types of cancer.* Retrieved January 3, 2008 from http://www.cancer.gov/cancertopics.

Nelson, M. B., & Meeske, K. (2005). Recognizing health risks in childhood cancer survivors. *Journal of the American Academy of Nurse Practitioners, 17*(3), 96–103.

Pagana, K. D., & Pagana, T. J. (2006). *Mosby's manual of diagnostic and laboratory tests* (3rd ed.). St. Louis: Mosby.

Paulino, A. C., & Fowler, B. Z. (2005). Secondary neoplasms after radiation for a childhood solid tumor. *Pediatric Hematology and Oncology, 22,* 89–101.

Postovsky, S., Levenzon, A., Ofir, R., & Arush, M. W. B. (2004). "Do not resuscitate" orders among children with solid tumors at the end of life. *Pediatric Hematology and Oncology, 21,* 661–668.

Quimby, E. L. (2007). The use of herbal therapies in pediatric oncology patients: Treating symptoms of cancer and side effects of standard therapies. *Journal of Pediatric Oncology Nursing, 24,* 35–40.

Rheingans, J. I. (2007). A systematic review of nonpharmacologic adjunctive therapies for symptom management in children with cancer. *Journal of Pediatric Oncology Nursing, 24*(2), 81–94.

Ruble, K. (2005). Pediatric oncology. In S. M. Nettina (Ed.), *Lippincott manual of nursing practice.* Philadelphia: Lippincott Williams & Wilkins.

Spector, L. G., Klebanoff, M. A., & Feusner, J. H. (2005). Childhood cancer following neonatal oxygen supplementation. *Journal of Pediatrics, 147,* 27–31.

Speigler, B. J., Bouffet, E., Greenberg, M. L., Rutka, J. T., & Mabbott, D. J. (2004). Change in neurocognitive functioning after treatment with cranial radiation in childhood. *Journal of Clinical Oncology, 22*(4), 706–713.

Spencer, J. (2006). The role of cognitive remediation in childhood cancer survivors experiencing neurocognitive late effects. *Journal of Pediatric Oncology Nursing, 23,* 321–325.

Stevens, M. C. G., Rey, A., Bouvet, N., Ellershaw, C., Flamant, F., Habrand, J. L., et al. (2005). Treatment of nonmetastatic rhabdomyosarcoma in childhood and adolescence: Third study of the International Society of Pediatric Oncology. *Journal of Clinical Oncology, 23*(12), 2618–2628.

Susman, E. (2005). Cancer pain management guidelines issues for children; adult guidelines updated. *Journal of the National Cancer Institute, 97*(10), 711–719.

Taketokmo, C. K., Hodding, J. H., & Kraus, D. M. (2007). *Lexi-comp's pediatric dosage handbook* (14th ed.). Hudson, Ohio: Lexi-comp.

Tomlinson, D., & Kline, N. E. (Eds.) (2005). *Pediatric oncology nursing.* New York: Springer.

Trigg, M. E. (2004). Hematopoietic stem cells. *Pediatrics, 113*(4), 1051–1057.

Turkoski, B. B. (2005). When a child's treatment decisions conflict with the parents. *Home Healthcare Nurse, 23*(2), 123–126.

Ulster, A. A., & Antle, B. J. (2005). In the darkness there can be light: A family's adaptation to a child's blindness. *Journal of Visual Impairment & Blindness, 99*(4), 209–218.

Van Cleve, L., Bossert, W., Beecroft, P., Adlard, K., Alvarez, O., & Savedra, M. C. (2004). The pain experience of children with leukemia during the first year after diagnosis. *Nursing Research, 53*(1), 1–10.

Van Larebeke, N. A., Birnbaum, L. S., Boogaerts, M. A., Bracke, M., Davis, D. L., Demarini, D. M., et al. (2005). Unrecognized or potential risk factors for childhood cancer. *International Journal of Occupational and Environmental Health, 11*(2), 199–201.

Wohlschlaeger, A. (2004). Prevention and treatment of mucositis: A guide for nurses. *Journal of Pediatric Oncology Nursing, 21*(5), 281–287.

Woodgate, R. L. (2005). Adolescents' experiences with cancer. *Cancer Nursing, 28*(1), 8–15.

Woolery, M., Carroll, E., Fenn, E., Weiland, H., Jarosinski, P., Corey, B., & Wallen, E. R. (2006). A constipation assessment scale for use in pediatric oncology. *Journal of Pediatric Oncology Nursing, 23*(2), 65–73.

WEBSITES

Information for teen boys on testicular self-examination: kidshealth.org/teen/sexual_health/guys/tse.html

Pediatric Oncology Branch of the National Cancer Institute; clinical protocol childhood cancer treatment on the NIH campus in Bethesda, MD: home.ccr.cancer.gov/oncology/pediatric

Pediatric Oncology Resource Center: www.acor.org/ped-onc

Alliance for Childhood Cancer, a forum of national patient advocacy groups interested in advancing research, public education, survivorship of children and teens with cancer: www.allianceforchildhoodcancer.org

Association of Pediatric Oncology Nursing: www.apon.org

American Society of Pediatric Hematology and Oncology: www.aspho.org

Bear Necessities Pediatric Cancer Foundation (patient and family services, research and support): www.bearnecessities.org

Camp Mak-a-Dream, a cost-free camp in Montana for children with cancer: www.campdream.org

National Cancer Institute of the U.S. National Institutes of Health: www.cancer.gov

American Cancer Society (research, education, referrals, help finding a pediatric cancer center): www.cancer.org

Candlelighters Childhood Cancer Foundation (support and education for children with cancer and their families): www.candlelighters.org

Children's Brain Tumor Foundation (education, research, and parent-to-parent network for family support): cbtf.org/cms

Childhood Eye Cancer Trust (United Kingdom), charity for those with retinoblastoma: www.chect.org.uk/index.php

Childhood Brain Tumor Foundation (public awareness, research, improvement of quality of life): www.childhoodbraintumor.org

Children's Cause for Cancer Advocacy (resources for research and treatment, addresses needs and concerns of survivors): www.childrenscause.org/

Children's Hospice and Palliative Care Coalition: www.childrenshospice.org/coalition

Children's Oncology Group (cancer treatment clinical trials): www.childrensoncologygroup.org

Children's Hospice International (hospice and palliative care support for children through pediatric care facilities, hospice and home care programs): www.chionline.org

Ewing sarcoma and pediatric cancer support group resources page from the "Cure Our Children" Foundation (extensive resources and links): www.cureourchildren.org

Combined effort of the National Childhood Cancer Foundation and the Children's Oncology Group for prevention and treatment of childhood cancers: www.curesearch.org

Florida's Enhanced Awareness of Retinoblastoma: www.florida FEAR.org

The Wellness Community (national cancer support, education and hope for teens): www.grouploop.org/default_flash.php

Healthy People 2010: www.healthypeople.gov

Education, support, and advocacy for children with cancer and their families: www.hopestreetkids.org

Leukemia and Lymphoma Society (research, education and patient services): www.leukemia.org

Leukemia Research Foundation: www.leukemia-research.org

Locks of Love (provides hairpieces to financially disadvantaged children): www.locksoflove.org

National Marrow Donor Program (information and resources for donors, patients, and physicians about bone marrow and stem cell transplantation): www.marrow.org

Partnership for Parents–Spanish site for the Children's Hospice and Palliative Care Coalition: www.padrescompadres.org/

Penguin cold cap therapy: www.msc-worldwide.com

Memorial Sloan Kettering Cancer Center (information on diseases, treatment, and resources): www.mskcc.org/mskcc/html/2715.cfm

National Children's Cancer Society (financial and in-kind assistance, advocacy, support services and education): www.nationalchildrenscancersociety.com

Cancer resource sponsored by Abramson Cancer Center of the University of Pennsylvania: www.oncolink.org

Pediatric Brain Tumor Consortium (multidisciplinary cooperative research organization focusing on central nervous system tumors of childhood): www.pbtc.org

Canadian resources for retinoblastoma: www.retinoblastoma.ca

Retinoblastoma International (education, research, resources, focusing on early diagnosis and treatment): www.retinoblastoma.net

Starlight, Starbright Children's Foundation (dedicated to brightening the lives of seriously ill children and their families): www.starbright.org

Saint Jude Children's Research Hospital: www.stjude.org

Brain Tumor Society (education, research, support, family networking): www.tbts.org

Melissa's Living Legacy Foundation/Helping Teens Live with Cancer: www.teenslivingwithcancer.org

Make-A-Wish Foundation (granting wishes of children with life-threatening illnesses): www.wish.org

CHAPTER WORKSHEET

MULTIPLE CHOICE QUESTIONS

1. A 5-year-old has been diagnosed with Wilms' tumor. What is the priority nursing intervention for this child?

   a. Educate the parents about dialysis, as the kidney will be removed.

   b. Measure abdominal girth every shift.

   c. Avoid palpating the child's abdomen.

   d. Monitor BUN and creatinine every 4 hours.

2. A child with leukemia has the following a.m. laboratory results: Hgb 8.0, Hct 24.2, WBC 8,000, platelets 150,000. What is the priority nursing assessment?

   a. Monitor for fever.

   b. Assess for bruising or bleeding.

   c. Determine intake and output.

   d. Assess for pallor, fatigue, tachycardia.

3. A child with leukemia received chemotherapy about 10 days ago. She presents today with a temperature of 100.4° F, an absolute neutrophil count of 500, and mild bleeding of the gums. What is the priority nursing intervention?

   a. Administer IV antibiotics as ordered.

   b. Provide vigorous oral care frequently with a firm toothbrush.

   c. Monitor pulse and blood pressure for changes.

   d. Administer packed red blood cell transfusion.

4. A child with cancer is receiving chemotherapy, and his mother is concerned that the nausea and vomiting associated with chemotherapy are reducing his ability to eat and gain weight appropriately. What is the most appropriate nursing action?

   a. Administer an antiemetic at the first hint of nausea.

   b. Offer the child's favorite foods to encourage him to eat.

   c. Start antiemetic drugs prior to the chemotherapy infusion.

   d. Maintain IV fluid infusion to avoid dehydration.

CRITICAL THINKING EXERCISES

1. Develop a discharge teaching plan for a child who has just completed the induction phase of chemotherapy for acute lymphocytic leukemia.

2. A 17-year-old girl has recently been diagnosed with osteosarcoma. She is worried about how treatment will affect her plans for college, marriage, and children. How will you respond to her concerns?

3. A 3-year-old is going to be starting chemotherapy for rhabdomyosarcoma. Develop an age-appropriate teaching plan for this child.

4. Develop a nursing care plan for an adolescent with cancer who is undergoing radiation and chemotherapy and experiencing a significant number of adverse effects from his treatment.

STUDY ACTIVITIES

1. While in the clinical area, care for a young child who has undergone therapy for a brain tumor. Compare this child's growth and development to those of a healthy similar-age child who you know or have cared for.

2. During your clinical rotation, care for a child who has received several chemotherapy treatments. After establishing a therapeutic relationship, talk with the child about his or her understanding of the disease and the experience the child has had with diagnosis and treatment thus far. If time allows, ask the child to draw a picture describing this experience. Record your observations in your clinical journal and reflect on the emotions you feel about this experience.

3. Attend the pediatric oncology clinic. Determine the role of the advanced practice nurse (nurse practitioner or clinical nurse specialist), compared to the role of the registered nurse in the outpatient care of children with cancer. Determine which activities the nurse appropriately delegates to unlicensed assistive personnel in that setting.

4. Talk to the hospital chaplain about his or her experiences with dying children. Reflect on this conversation in your clinical journal.

NURSING CARE OF THE CHILD WITH A GENETIC DISORDER

KEY TERMS

chromosomal abnormality
gene testing
genetics

inborn errors of
metabolism
newborn screen

neurocutaneous disorders
trisomy 21

LEARNING OBJECTIVES

Upon completion of the chapter, the learner will be able to:

1. Discuss the nurse's role and responsibilities when caring for a child diagnosed with a genetic disorder and his her family.
2. Identify nursing interventions related to common laboratory and diagnostic tests used in the diagnosis and management of genetic conditions.
3. Distinguish various genetic disorders occurring in childhood.
4. Devise an individualized nursing care plan for the child with a genetic disorder.
5. Develop patient/family teaching plans for the child with a genetic disorder.

*J*ulie Woods, a 5-year-old, is brought to the clinic for her annual examination. Her mother states, "She's so much smaller than all of the other kindergartners."

Wow

When a woman discovers that she is pregnant she must remember to protect and nourish the fetus by making wise choices.

1664

Genetics is the study of heredity and its variation (Venes, 2005). Many disorders of childhood have a genetic or inherited cause. Common disorders suspected to be caused or influenced by genetic factors include birth defects, chromosomal abnormalities, neurocutaneous disorders, mental retardation, many types of short stature, connective tissue disorders, and inborn errors of metabolism. According to the Centers for Disease Control and Prevention, birth defects and genetic disorders are a significant cause of morbidity and mortality in infancy and childhood: "Twenty-five to thirty-nine percent of admissions to children's hospitals involve children with genetically determined or partially genetically determined disorders; 11% of all deaths in childhood are related to an underlying genetic condition" (Behrman et al., 2004, p. 367).

Our ability to diagnose genetic conditions is far superior to our ability to cure or treat them. However, accurate diagnosis leads to improved treatment and outcomes. Nurses should have a basic knowledge of genetics, common genetic disorders in children, genetic testing, and genetic counseling so that they can provide support and information to families and can promote an improved quality of life. Refer to Chapter 10 for further information regarding patterns of inheritance and genetic evaluation and counseling.

Nurse's Role and Responsibilities

Pediatric nurses will encounter children with genetic disorders in every clinical specialty area. This includes clinics, hospitals, schools, and community-based centers. Talking with families who have recently been diagnosed with a genetic disorder or who have had a child born with congenital anomalies is very difficult. Many times the nurse is the one who has first contact with these parents and will be the one to provide follow-up care.

Genetic disorders are significant, life-changing, and possibly life-threatening situations. The information is highly technical and the field is still evolving, so in most cases the family should be referred to a health care provider who specializes in genetics. The nurse should understand who will benefit from genetic counseling and should be able to discuss the role of the genetic counselor with families. Families at risk should be informed that genetic counseling is available before they attempt to have another baby. Nurses play an essential role in providing emotional support to the family throughout this challenging time. Nurses should also refer the family to appropriate agencies, support groups, and resources.

Common Medical Treatments

A variety of medications and other medical treatments are used to treat the symptoms of genetic disorders in children. Genetic disorders do not have specific treatments

and there is no cure, so treatment focuses on the specific symptoms of each disorder. Genetic disorders often involve multiple organ systems and the patients have complex medical needs, so a multidisciplinary approach and good communication are imperative. See below for a discussion on common genetic disorders and their management.

NURSING PROCESS OVERVIEW FOR THE CHILD WITH A GENETIC DISORDER

Care of the child with a genetic disorder includes assessment, nursing diagnosis, planning, interventions, and evaluation. There are a number of general concepts related to the nursing process that may be applied to the care of children with genetic disorders. From a general understanding of the care involved for a child with a genetic disorder, the nurse can then individualize the care based on patient specifics.

Assessment

Assessment of the child with a genetic disorder includes health history, physical examination, and laboratory and diagnostic testing.

Remember Julie, the 5-year-old brought in for her annual examination? What additional health history and physical examination information should you obtain?

Health History

The health history comprises past medical history, including the mother's pregnancy history, family history, neonatal history, history of present illness (when the symptoms started and how they have progressed), as well as treatments used at home. Explore the patient's current and past medical history for risk factors such as:

- Family history of genetic disorders
- Any complications during the prenatal, perinatal, or postnatal periods
- Changes in developmental status or delays in developmental milestones

The pregnancy history can be extremely relevant when identifying a genetic disorder. The pregnancy history may be significant for maternal age over 35 years, repeated premature births, breech delivery, congenital hip dysplasia, abnormalities found on ultrasound, abnormalities in prenatal blood screening tests (e.g., triple/quadruple screen, alpha fetoprotein), amniotic fluid abnormalities (polyhydramnios, oligohydramnios), multiple births, exposure to medications and known teratogens, and decreased fetal movement.

A focused neonatal history can also help identify a genetic problem. The neonatal history may be significant for symmetric intrauterine growth restriction, large for gestational age without a reason, hearing impaired, persistent hyperbilirubinemia, poor adaptation to the extrauterine environment (demonstrated by temperature and heart rate instability and poor feeding), hypotonia or hypertonia, seizures, and abnormal newborn screening results.

The family history plays a critical role in identifying genetic disorders. Data should be gathered for three generations. If there is a positive family history, the likelihood of a genetic disorder in the patient is increased. It is helpful to create a family pedigree (refer to Chapter 10 for genetic evaluation and counseling). The family history may be significant for major congenital anomalies, mental retardation, genetic diseases, metabolic disorders, multiple miscarriages or stillbirths, developmental delays, significant learning disabilities, psychiatric problems, consanguinity, and chronic serious illness (e.g., diabetes, hypertension, renal disease, hearing impairment, blindness, asthma, seizures, and unexplained death).

When eliciting the history of the present illness, inquire about:

- Developmental delay
- Seizures
- Hypotonia or hypertonia
- Feeding problems
- Lethargy
- Failure to thrive
- Septic appearance
- Vomiting

Children known to have a genetic disorder are often admitted to the hospital for other health-related issues or complications and management of the genetic disorder. The health history should include questions related to:

- Age when the disorder was diagnosed
- Developmental delay
- Complications of the disorder (e.g., thyroid problems, cardiac problems, respiratory problems, leukemia, seizures, cognitive impairment)
- Medications the child takes for complications associated with the disorder
- Dietary restrictions
- Compliance with management regimen

Once complications have been identified, further investigation into their severity, frequency, and management is essential to the care of this child while in the hospital.

Physical Examination

Physical examination of the child with a genetic disorder includes inspection and observation, palpation, and auscultation.

BOX 50.1 Major Congenital Anomalies

- Cleft lip
- Cleft palate
- Congenital heart disease, structural and conduction disorders
- Neural tube defects
- Brain anomalies
- Omphalocele
- Hepatosplenomegaly
- Asymmetry of face, skeleton, or limb
- Generalized dysmorphism
- Specific skin lesions, such as café-au-lait macules, hypopigmented macules, or cutaneous hemangiomas

Adapted from Siegel, B., & Milunsky, J. (2004). When should the possibility of a genetic disorder cross your radar screen? *Contemporary Pediatrics, 21*(5), 37.

Inspection and Observation

Inspect and observe for congenital anomalies, either major or minor. A major anomaly is an anomaly or malformation that creates significant medical problems and requires surgical or medical management (Box 50.1). Minor anomalies are features that vary from those seen in the general population but do not cause an increase in morbidity in and of themselves (Box 50.2).

BOX 50.2 Minor Congenital Anomalies

- Flat occiput
- Prominent occiput
- Widow's peak
- Triple hair whorl
- Flat-bridged nose
- Nostrils anteverted
- Ear lobe crease
- Ear lobe notched
- Forward displacement or protruding ears
- Cleft uvula
- Webbed neck
- Extra nipples
- Single umbilical artery
- Umbilical hernia
- Tapered fingers
- Overlapping digits
- Broad thumb or great toe
- Increased space between toes
- Syndactyly
- Polydactyly

Adapted from Siegel, B., & Milunsky, J. (2004). When should the possibility of a genetic disorder cross your radar screen? *Contemporary Pediatrics, 21*(5), 37.

▶ *Take* NOTE!

Low-set ears are associated with numerous genetic dysmorphisms. If noted, assess thoroughly for other abnormalities.

When three or more minor anomalies are present, the risk for a major anomaly or mental retardation is approximately 20% (Siegel & Milunsky, 2004). When one major anomaly is present, the possibility of a genetic cause must be investigated. In children with three or more minor anomalies, selected major anomalies, a recognized pattern of anomalies, or a combination of major and minor anomalies, a genetic diagnostic workup is recommended (Siegel & Milunsky, 2004).

▶ *Take* NOTE!

Cleft lip and cleft palate are associated with many syndromes. If noted, assess for other anomalies.

Inspect and observe for an abnormal or foul odor of the child's excretions, as certain metabolic disorders or inborn errors of metabolism are associated with specific odors (Table 50.1).

Auscultation

Physical examination includes auscultation of the heart. Murmurs or dysrhythmias may have a genetic cause. In a patient with a congenital heart problem (e.g., ventricular septal defect) and a strong family history of cardiac structural problems, a genetic cause needs to be considered. Approximately 3% of all cases of congenital heart disease are caused by a single mutant gene, and 5% of congenital heart defects are caused by chromosomal abnormalities (Siegel & Milunsky, 2004).

TABLE 50.1 INBORN ERRORS OF METABOLISM AND ASSOCIATED ODOR

Inborn Error of Metabolism	Associated Odor
Phenylketonuria	Mousy or musty
Maple syrup urine disease	Maple syrup
Tyrosinemia	Cabbage-like, rancid butter
Trimethylaminuria	Rotting fish

Palpation

Palpation can be used to detect hepatosplenomegaly (an enlarged spleen and liver), but because this requires skill and experience, this assessment may be performed by advanced practitioners or physicians. Hepatosplenomegaly may indicate a metabolic disorder.

Laboratory and Diagnostic Testing

Common Laboratory and Diagnostic Tests 50.1 explains the laboratory and diagnostic tests used most commonly to detect genetic disorders. Refer to Chapter 10 for further information regarding common laboratory and diagnostic tests to detect genetic disorders in utero. The tests can assist the physician in diagnosing the disorder or can be used as guidelines in determining treatment. Laboratory or non-nursing personnel obtain some of the tests, while the nurse might obtain others. In either instance the nurse should be familiar with how the tests are obtained, what they are used for, and normal versus abnormal results. This knowledge will also be necessary when providing patient and family education related to the testing. Due to the nature of the information, a referral to genetic counseling before testing may be appropriate. Advances in genetic technology, including information obtained from the Human Genome Project, have led to dramatic increases in the number of diagnostic and screening tests.

Nursing Diagnoses, Goals, Interventions, and Evaluation

Upon completion of an assessment, the nurse might identify several nursing diagnoses, including:

• Deficient knowledge
• Decisional conflict
• Risk for delayed growth and development
• Fear
• Interrupted family processes

*A*fter completing an assessment of Julie, the nurse noted the following: short stature for age and a low posterior hairline. Based on these assessment findings, what would your top three nursing diagnoses be for Julie?

Nursing goals, interventions, and evaluation for the child with a genetic disorder are based on the nursing diagnoses. Nursing Care Plan 50.1 provides a general guide for planning care for a child with a genetic disorder. Additional information about nursing management will be included later in the chapter as it relates to specific disorders.

No matter what the genetic abnormality is, the news may be shattering to the family. It is difficult for nurses to even begin to understand what the family is going through. When providing support and education to families of

(text continues on page 1671)

COMMON LABORATORY AND DIAGNOSTIC TESTS 50.1

Test	Explanation	Indications	Nursing Implications
Gene testing	Gene testing is currently available for over 950 inherited diseases. It involves analysis of DNA, RNA, chromosomes, proteins, metabolites, and biochemical agents. Specimens for gene testing can be obtained from numerous sources; leukocytes from blood are the most common and easily obtained site, during pregnancy, amniocentesis and chorionic villus sampling, and fetal tissue or products of conception after a miscarriage Most common use is DNA or chromosomes isolated from blood Direct detection of abnormalities in genes and chromosomes is performed using DNA-based tests or cytogenetic tests (which look at chromosome) and other methods. Cytogenetic tests also include a relatively new technology, fluorescent in situ hybridization (FISH), to assist in detecting chromosomal abnormalities such as duplication, deletion, rearrangements and translocations.	To detect abnormalities that may indicate actual disease or predict future disease. Indicated in the evaluation of congenital anomalies, mental retardation, growth retardation, recurrent miscarriage to determine reason for the loss of a fetus, prenatal diagnosis of genetic disease.	Provide support, information, and resources to family. Refer to genetic counseling before and after test.
Newborn screening	Blood screening performed shortly after birth, used to identify many life threatening genetic illnesses that have no immediate visible effects but can lead to physical problems, mental retardation and even death.	Every U.S. state routinely screens all newborns, but each state dictates which disorders to screen for, so components of the screening vary from state to state.	Ideally performed after 24 hours of age; obtain specimen as close to time of discharge from newborn or labor and delivery unit as possible and no later than 7 days of age. The test is less accurate if done before 24 hours of age and should be repeated by 2 weeks of age if the newborn is less than 24 hours old. Ensure appropriate follow-up with newborn screening results; results are available in 2 to 3 weeks.

Nursing Care Plan 50.1

OVERVIEW FOR THE CHILD WITH A GENETIC DISORDER

NURSING DIAGNOSIS: Deficient knowledge related to lack of information regarding complex, technical medical condition, prognosis, and medical needs as evidenced by verbalization, questions, or actions demonstrating lack of understanding about child's condition or care

Outcome Identification and Evaluation

Child and family will verbalize accurate information and understanding about condition, prognosis, and medical needs: *Child and family demonstrate knowledge of condition, prognosis, and medical needs, including possible causes, contributing factors, and treatment measures.*

Intervention: Providing Patient and Family Teaching

- Assess child's and family's willingness to learn: *child and family must be willing to learn for teaching to be effective.*
- Provide family with time to adjust to diagnosis: *will facilitate adjustment and ability to learn and participate in child's care.*
- Repeat information: *allows family and child time to learn and understand.*
- Teach in short sessions: *many short sessions are more helpful than one long session.*
- Gear teaching to the child and family's level of understanding (depends on age of child, physical condition, memory) *to ensure understanding.*
- Provide reinforcement and rewards: *facilitates the teaching/learning process.*
- Use multiple modes of learning involving many senses (written, verbal, demonstration, and videos) when possible: *child and family are more likely to retain information when presented in different ways using many senses.*
- Refer child and family to a genetics specialist: *genetic information is highly technical; the field is advancing at a rapid pace, and information needs to be the most current and accurate. A genetic specialist can provide this along with expertise, support, and resources.*

NURSING DIAGNOSIS: Decisional conflict related to treatment options, conflicting values, and ethical, legal, and social issues surrounding genetic testing as evidenced by verbalization of uncertainty about choices, verbalization of undesired consequences of alternative actions being considered, delayed decision making, physical signs of stress

Outcome Identification and Evaluation

Family will state they are able to make an informed decision: *Family will state advantages and disadvantages of choices and share fears and concerns regarding choices.*

Intervention: Providing Decision-Making Support

- Give family time and encourage them to express their feelings associated with decision making: *the decision-making process becomes more difficult if feelings are not expressed.*
- Encourage family to list advantages and disadvantages of each alternative: *aids in problem solving and helps family recognize all alternatives.*
- Initiate health teaching and referral to genetic specialist when needed: *genetic testing information is often technical and complex. Families need accurate and up-to-date information to aid in decision making.*
- Maintain a nondirective manner: *this is a difficult decision that the family must make for themselves; the nurse should provide all the necessary information while maintaining an unobtrusive role.*
- Validate the family's feelings regarding the decisional conflict: *Validation is a therapeutic communication technique that promotes the nurse–patient relationship.*

(continued)

Nursing Care Plan 50.1 (continued)

NURSING DIAGNOSIS: Risk for delayed growth and development related to physical disability, cognitive deficits, activity restrictions secondary to genetic disorder

Outcome Identification and Evaluation

Child's growth and development will be enhanced; child will demonstrate adequate growth patterns within parameters of disease, child will make continued progress toward attainment of developmental milestones and will not suffer regression in abilities.

Child will demonstrate developmental milestones within age parameters and limits of disease.

Child will make steady gains in growth patterns (e.g., height and weight) within disease parameters. Child expresses interest in the environment and people around him or her, interacts with environment appropriately for developmental level.

Intervention: Promoting Growth and Development

- Screen for developmental capabilities *to determine child's current level of functioning.*
- Offer age-appropriate toys, play, and activities (including gross motor) *to encourage further development.*
- Perform exercises or interventions as prescribed by physical or occupational therapist: *these activities promote function and developmental skills.*
- Provide support to families: *due to immobility and extremity deficits, the child's progress toward developmental milestones may be slow.*
- Use therapeutic play and adaptive toys *to facilitate developmental functioning.*
- Provide stimulating environment when possible *to maximize potential for growth and development.*
- Praise accomplishments and emphasize child's abilities *to improve self-esteem and encourage feelings of confidence and competence.*
- Monitor height and weight and plot on growth chart *to identify growth patterns and deviations in these patterns.*

NURSING DIAGNOSIS: Fear related to outcome of genetic testing as evidenced by reports of apprehension and increased tension

Outcome Identification and Evaluation

Family will state they can cope with the results of the genetic testing or demonstrate reduced fear. *Family accurately discusses chances of offspring having genetic disease, demonstrates positive coping, asks questions about genetic testing and meaning of results.*

Intervention: Managing Fear

- Empathize with the family and avoid false reassurances; be truthful: *allows family to recognize that fear is a reasonable response. Giving false information or reassurance will actually increase fear.*
- Explore coping skills used previously by the family to cope with fear. Reinforce these skills and explore other outlets, such as relaxation, breathing, and physical activity: *encourages use of coping mechanisms that help control fear.*
- Encourage verbalization of feelings and concerns about genetic testing. Allow time for questions: *provides a safe outlet to express feelings and encourages open communication between the family members.*
- Explain all procedures and review results as available: *Knowledge deficit contributes to fear.*
- Refer to appropriate support groups and genetic counseling: *talking with families who have gone through similar situations can help decrease fear and provide methods of coping. Genetic counseling provides information along with support and additional resources.*

Nursing Care Plan 50.1 (continued)

NURSING DIAGNOSIS: Family processes, interrupted, related to child's illness, hospitalization, diagnosis of genetic illness in child, and potential long-term effects of illness as evidenced by family's presence in hospital and clinic, missed work, demonstration of inadequate coping

Outcome Identification and Evaluation

Family will maintain functional system of support, demonstrate adequate coping, adaptation of roles and functions, and decreased anxiety. *Parents are involved in child's care, ask appropriate questions, express fears and concerns, and can discuss child's care and condition calmly.*

Intervention: Promoting Family Coping

- Encourage family to verbalize concerns about child's illness, diagnosis, and prognosis: *allows the nurse to identify concerns and areas where further education may be needed and demonstrates family-centered care.*
- Explain therapies, procedures, child's behaviors, and plan of care to parents: *Understanding the child's current status and plan of care helps decrease anxiety.*
- Encourage parental involvement in care: *allows parents to feel needed and valued and gives them a sense of control over their child's health.*
- Identify support system for family and child: *helps nurse identify needs and resources available for coping.*
- Educate family about resources available *to help them develop a wide base of support.*

---

children with serious genetic abnormalities, use these guiding principles:

- Build a trusting relationship.
- Stress the authenticity of the parents' feelings.
- Reject your own personal biases.
- Recognize that individuals cope in various ways; the family's behavior may not be what you would expect.
- Help the family to identify their own strengths and supports, building on those as able.
- Know that the family's emotions may exhaust and disorganize them.
- Assist the family members to maintain open communication among themselves.
- Provide referrals to local parent groups or other families with a child with a similar disorder.
- Allow the family to verbalize their emotions and ask questions.
- Always ask the parents how *they* are doing (Lashley, 2005).

B̶ased on your top three nursing diagnoses for Julie, describe appropriate nursing interventions.

Common Chromosomal Abnormalities

Chromosomal abnormalities, which result from a mutation that changes the number of chromosomes or the structure of the chromosomes, are seen in 1 in 150 babies (March of Dimes, 2007). Many children with chromosomal abnormalities have associated mental retardation, learning disabilities, behavioral problems, and distinct features, including physical birth defects. The risk for autosomal trisomies increases with advanced maternal age. The most common chromosomal abnormalities will be discussed below. New techniques in chromosome analysis have made it possible to identify tiny abnormalities that could not be seen before. Therefore, more chromosomal abnormalities are being identified in children (Table 50.2).

▶ TRISOMY 21 (DOWN SYNDROME)

Trisomy 21 (Down syndrome) is a genetic disorder caused by the presence of all or part of an extra 21st chromosome. It is the most common chromosomal abnormality associated with mental retardation. One in 800 live births result in trisomy 21 (Chen, 2007). Approximately 75% of trisomy 21 conceptions result in spontaneous abortion (Chen, 2007). Trisomy 21 is seen in all ages, races, and socioeconomic levels, but a higher incidence is found with a maternal age above 35 years: the likelihood of having a baby with Down syndrome is 1 in 400 at age 35, 1 in 60 at age 42, and 1 in 12 by age 49 (National Institutes of Health, 2006).

Trisomy 21 is associated with some degree of mental retardation, characteristic facial features (e.g., slanted eyes and depressed nasal bridge), and other health problems (e.g., cardiac defects, visual and hearing impairment,

TABLE 50.2 LESS COMMON CHROMOSOMAL ABNORMALITIES

Chromosomal Abnormality	Features
Prader-Willi syndrome	Severe hypotonia, obesity, short stature, small hands and feet, hypogonadism, hyperphagia, and mental retardation (varies from mild to severe)
Angelman syndrome	Hypotonia, microbrachycephaly, fair hair, midface hypoplasia, deep-set eyes, large mouth with tongue protrusion, seizures, jerky ataxic movements (resembling a puppet gait), uncontrolled bouts of laughter/smiling, happy demeanor, easily excitable personality, developmental delay and speech impairment, and severe mental retardation www.angelman.org: Angelman Syndrome Foundation, Inc.
Cri-du-chat syndrome	Hypotonia, short stature, slow growth, low birthweight, characteristic weak, cat-like cry, microcephaly with protruding metopic suture, moon-like round face, bilateral epicanthal folds (folds of skin over the eyelids), high-arched palate, wide and flat nasal bridge, micrognathia (small receding chin), simian crease, and mental retardation www.fivepminus.org: 5p- Society
Velocardiofacial/DiGeorge syndrome	Hypoplasia or agenesis of the thymus and parathyroid glands, hypoplasia of auricle and external auditory canal, cardiac anomalies, cleft palate, short stature, distinctive facial appearance (elongated face, almond-shaped eyes, wide nose, small ears), and learning, speech, feeding, and behavioral problems www.vcfsef.org/: Velo-Cardio-Facial Syndrome Educational Foundation, Inc.

intestinal malformations, and an increased susceptibility to infections). The severity of these problems varies.

The prognosis has been improving over the past few decades. Fundamental changes in the care of these children have resulted in longer life expectancy (around 55 years of age) and an improved quality of life.

Pathophysiology

Trisomy 21 is a disorder caused by nondisjunction (an error in cell division) prior to or at conception. Each egg and sperm cell normally contains 23 chromosomes. When they join, this results in 23 pairs or 46 chromosomes. Sometimes, due to nondisjunction, a cell contributes an extra critical portion of chromosome number 21, resulting in an embryo with three chromosome 21s in all cells (Fig. 50.1). This results in the characteristic features and birth defects of Down syndrome. This error in cell division and the presence of three chromosome 21s in all cells is responsible for 95% of cases of Down syndrome (Behrman et al., 2004).

In approximately 1% of cases of Down syndrome, the nondisjunction occurs after fertilization and a mixture of two cell types is seen (Behrman et al., 2004). In these cases some cells have 47 chromosomes (due to three chromosome 21s), while others have the normal 46 chromosomes (with the normal two chromosome 21s present). This is referred to as the mosaic form of Down syndrome. Children with mosaic Down syndrome may have a milder form of the disorder, but this is not a general finding.

About 4% of Down syndrome cases involve a translocation, in which part of the number 21 chromosome

breaks off during cell division prior to or at conception and attaches to another chromosome. The cells will remain with 46 chromosomes, but this extra portion of the number 21 chromosome results in the clinical findings of Down syndrome. Cases of translocation are not associated with older maternal age, as is the situation with nondisjunction errors, and 25% of cases are the result of a hereditary translocation (Chen, 2007).

Therapeutic Management

Management of Down syndrome will involve multiple disciplines, including a primary physician, specialty physicians such as a cardiologist, ophthalmologist, and gastroenterologist, nurses, physical therapists, occupational therapists, speech therapists, dietitian, psychologist, coun-

FIGURE 50.1 Down syndrome karyotype. Note the third chromosome located at chromosome 21.

selors, teachers, and of course the parents. There is no standard treatment for all children, and there is no cure or prevention. The overall focus of therapeutic management will be to promote the child's optimal growth and development and function within the limits of the disease. Treatment is mainly symptomatic and supportive.

Managing Complications

Children with Down syndrome need the usual immunizations, well-child care, and screening recommended by the American Academy of Pediatrics. In addition, medical management will focus on complications associated with Down syndrome.

Congenital heart disease occurs in 40% to 50% of children with Down syndrome (Chen, 2007). Cardiac problems vary from minor defects that respond to medication therapy to major defects that require surgical intervention. The risk of acute leukemia is 56 times that of children without Down syndrome, with one in 150 children with Down syndrome developing leukemia (Chen, 2007).

Children with Down syndrome also have an increased incidence of gastrointestinal disorders. These disorders vary from those that can be managed by dietary manipulation, such as celiac disease and constipation, to intestinal malformations such as Hirschsprung disease and imperforate anus, which require surgical intervention.

Hearing and vision impairments also are common. More than 60% of children with Down syndrome have a hearing loss (Chen, 2007), so regular evaluation of vision and hearing is essential.

Obstructive sleep apnea is present in 50% to 75% of children with Down syndrome (American Academy of Pediatrics, 2007). Often parents are unaware their child is having sleep disturbances, so baseline testing in young children may be warranted (Shott et al., 2006).

Children with Down syndrome have a higher incidence of thyroid disease, which can affect growth and cognitive function. Most of these children have hypothyroidism (an underactive thyroid), but sometimes hyperthyroidism (an overactive thyroid) occurs. Periodic thyroid testing may be warranted.

Atlanto-axial instability (increased mobility of the cervical spine at the first and second vertebrae) is seen in about 14% of children with Down syndrome (Chen, 2007). In most cases these children are asymptomatic, but symptoms may appear if spinal cord compression occurs. Screening for atlanto-axial instability may be appropriate, especially if the child is involved in sports.

▶ **Take** NOTE!

If neck pain, unusual posturing of the head and neck (torticollis), change in gait, loss of upper body strength, abnormal reflexes, or change in bowel or bladder functioning is noted in the child with Down syndrome, immediate attention is required.

Children with Down syndrome also have a higher susceptibility to infection and a higher mortality rate from infectious diseases, so precautions to prevent and monitor for infection are needed.

Due to their increased risk for certain congenital anomalies and diseases, children with Down syndrome will need to be monitored closely, and regular medical care is essential.

Early Intervention Therapy

Early intervention refers to a variety of specialized programs and resources available to young children with developmental delay or other impairment. These programs may involve an array of health care professionals such as physical, occupational, and speech therapists, special educators, and social workers. The programs focus on providing stimulation and encouragement to children with Down syndrome. They help encourage and accelerate development and may help to prevent some developmental delays. The earlier the intervention can begin, the more beneficial it will be. The programs are individualized to meet the specific needs of each child.

Children with Down syndrome progress through the same developmental stages as typical children, but they do so on their own timetable. For example, children with Down syndrome will learn to walk, but the average child with Down syndrome walks at 24 months (versus 12 months for a child without Down syndrome). Conditions such as hypotonia, ligament laxity, decreased strength, enlarged tongue, and short arms and legs are common in children with Down syndrome, and early intervention can help in the development of gross and fine motor skills, language, and social and self-care skills.

Parents also benefit from early intervention programs in terms of support, encouragement, and information. Early intervention programs teach parents how to interact with their child while meeting the child's specific needs and encouraging development.

Nursing Assessment

For a full description of the assessment phase of the nursing process, refer to page 000. Assessment findings pertinent to Down syndrome are discussed below.

Health History

Down syndrome is often diagnosed prenatally using perinatal screening and diagnostic tests. If not diagnosed prenatally, most cases are diagnosed in the first few days of life based on the physical characteristics associated with Down syndrome. High-risk deliveries should be identified. Explore the pregnancy history and past medical history for risk factors such as:

• Lack of prenatal care
• Abnormal prenatal screening or diagnostic tests for Down syndrome (e.g., triple/quadruple screen, ultrasound, amniocentesis)
• Maternal age over 35 years

EVIDENCE-BASED PRACTICE 50.1
Testing Children With Down Syndrome for Obstructive Sleep Apnea

Children with Down syndrome are at greater risk for development of obstructive sleep apnea syndrome (OSAS). Previous research evaluating children with Down syndrome has found the incidence of OSAS to be 100%. OSAS leads to sleep pattern abnormalities such as sleep fragmentation and sleep arousals. The significance of these are just beginning to be understood. With this high incidence of OSAS, should all children with Down syndrome be objectively evaluated for OSAS? If so, what is an appropriate age for this evaluation?

● Study

A prospective cohort study was performed over a 5-year period to determine the incidence of OSAS in children aged 2 to 4 years with Down syndrome. In addition, the parents' ability to predict sleep abnormalities in this patient population was examined. The study began with 65 children with Down syndrome, in which otolaryngologic problems seen in Down syndrome were evaluated. The study was conducted at a children's hospital, and 56 of the 65 children enrolled were able to complete a full sleep study or polysomnogram. Prior to the sleep study, 35 participants' parents completed a survey regarding their child's sleep behaviors.

▲ Findings

Fifty-seven percent (n=32) of the children had abnormal sleep study results as defined by an abnormal obstructive index, hypoventilation with hypercarbia, and/or hypoxemia; if an abnormal or elevated arousal index is included, the incidence increases to 80% (n=45). The significance of an elevated arousal state in an otherwise normal sleep study has not yet been fully established. Polysomnography in children is a developing field. The evaluation of sleep abnormalities in children has been based on standard adult definitions. Due to the anatomic differences in children and adults alone, these definitions may not be accurate. For example, children tend to have significant oxygen desaturation after shorter periods of apnea compared with adults due to their smaller functional residual capacity and increased respiratory rate. There is a need to develop appropriate criteria to evaluate sleep abnormalities in children.

Sixty-nine percent of parents reported no sleep problems in their children, yet 54% of these children had an abnormal sleep study. Overall, it was found that parents of children with Down syndrome underestimated the severity of their child's sleep disturbances.

■ Nursing Implications

Obstructive sleep apnea syndrome has been associated with various morbidities such as pulmonary hypertension and cor pulmonae. It has also been linked to neurocognitive abnormalities. Hypoxemia associated with OSAS has correlated with lower IQ testing and behavior problems. Sleep fragmentation, related to increased arousal and decreased REM, is just beginning to be understood but has been linked to symptoms associated with sleep deprivation, such as daytime sleepiness, lack of energy, and lack of initiative. The American Academy of Pediatrics currently recommends questioning parents of children with Down syndrome about possible sleep disorders when the children are 5 years or older, but no recommendations for specific testing are made at this time. Nurses need to be aware of recent research recommending baseline sleep studies in children aged 3 to 4 with Down syndrome even if the parents report no sleep problems in their child. Nurses need to assess for signs and symptoms of OSAS in children with Down syndrome at any age.

Shott, S.R., Amin, B. Chini, C. Heubi, Hotze, S. & Akers, R. (2006). Obstructive sleep apnea: Should all children with Down syndrome be tested? *Archive of Otolaryngology Head & Neck Surgery, 132*(4), 432–436.

The older infant or child known to have Down syndrome is often admitted to the hospital for corrective surgeries or other complications of the disease, such as infections. Elicit a description of the present illness and chief complaint. In an infant or child returning for a clinic visit or hospitalization, the health history should include questions related to:

- Cardiac defects or disease (treatment regimen, surgical repair)
- Hearing or vision impairment (last hearing and vision evaluation, any corrective measures)
- Developmental delays (speech, gross and fine motor skills)
- Sucking or feeding problems
- Cognitive abilities (degree of mental retardation)
- Gastrointestinal disorders such as vomiting or absence of stools (special dietary management, surgical interventions)
- Thyroid disease
- Leukemia
- Atlanto-axial instability
- Seizures
- Infections such as recurrent or chronic respiratory infections, otitis media
- Growth (height and weight changes, feeding problems, unexplained weight gain)
- Signs and symptoms of sleep apnea, such as snoring, restlessness during sleep, daytime sleepiness
- Any other changes in physical state or medication regimen

Physical Examination

The initial assessment after birth may reveal certain physical features characteristic of Down syndrome (Box 50.3 and Fig. 50.2).

Observe the child's general appearance. Note lack of muscle tone and loose joints; this is usually more pronounced in infancy, and the infant has a floppy appearance. Observe growth and development. Plot growth on appropriate growth charts. Because children with Down syndrome grow at a slower rate, special growth charts have been developed (see http://thepoint.lww.com for an example).

When assessing achievement of developmental milestones in children with Down syndrome, it may be more useful to look at the sequence of milestones rather than the age at which they were achieved. Each milestone represents a skill that is needed for the next stage of development.

Perform a subjective assessment of hearing and refer the child for further evaluation if indicated. Assess vision, especially for cataracts. Assess respiratory status and cardiac status. Auscultate for murmurs and pulmonary changes, which can indicate congenital heart disease. Chronic or recurrent respiratory infections, such as pneumonia and otitis media, may be found.

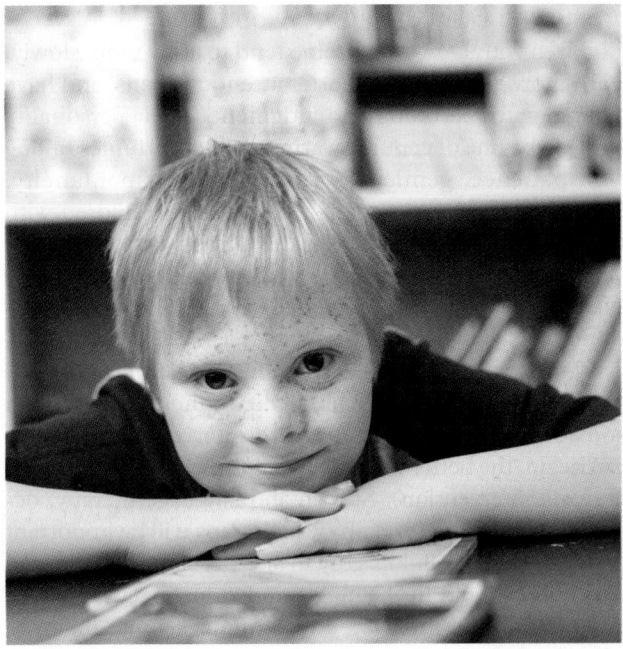

FIGURE 50.2 Child with Down syndrome.

Laboratory and Diagnostic Tests

Down syndrome can be detected prenatally around 16 to 18 weeks of gestation using ultrasound, a blood test to detect increases in alpha fetoprotein, or analysis of amniotic fluid or tissue from chorionic villi to detect chromosomal abnormalities. Down syndrome can be confirmed after birth using chromosome analysis (see Common Laboratory and Diagnostic Tests 50.1).

Common laboratory and diagnostic studies ordered for the diagnosis and assessment of complications associated with Down syndrome include:

• Echocardiogram: to detect cardiac defects
• Vision and hearing screening: to detect vision and hearing impairments
• Thyroid hormone level: to detect thyroid disease
• Cervical x-rays: to assess for atlanto-axial instability
• Ultrasound: to assess gastrointestinal malformations

These tests will be important in evaluating the severity of the child's physical disabilities.

Nursing Management

Due to the high incidence of Down syndrome and the complex medical needs of these children, most pediatric nurses are likely to care for these children in their practice. Nursing management focuses on providing supportive measures such as promoting growth and development, preventing complications, promoting nutrition, and providing support and education to the child and family. In addition to the nursing diagnoses and related interventions discussed in Nursing Care Plan 50.1, additional considerations are reviewed below.

> BOX 50.3 **Common Clinical Manifestations of Down Syndrome**

• Flattened occiput
• Small (brachycephalic) head
• Flat facial profile
• Depressed nasal bridge and small nose
• Oblique palpebral fissures (an upward slant to the eyes)
• Brushfield spots (white spots on the iris of the eye)
• Low-set ears
• Abnormally shaped ears
• Small mouth
• Protrusion of tongue; tongue is large compared to mouth size
• Arched palate
• Hands with broad, short fingers
• A single deep transverse crease on the palm of the hand (simian crease)
• Congenital heart defect
• Short neck, with excessive skin at the nape
• Hyperflexibility and looseness of joints (excessive ability to extend the joints)
• Dysplastic middle phalanx of fifth finger (one flexion furrow instead of two)
• Epicanthal folds (small skin folds on the inner corner of the eyes)
• Excessive space between large and second toe
• Hypotonia

Promoting Growth and Development

Children with Down syndrome tend to grow more slowly, learn more slowly, have shorter attention spans, and have trouble with reasoning and judgment. Their personality tends to be one of genuine warmth and cheerfulness along with patience, gentleness, and a natural spontaneity. Growth and developmental milestones for children with Down syndrome have been developed as a guide for health care providers. Table 50.3 gives examples of the average age at which these children reach selected milestones versus typical children.

Nurses play a key role in connecting families with appropriate resources that can facilitate the child's growth and development. The sooner early intervention programs can begin, the better for the child (see the above discussion on early intervention). Speech and language therapy, occupational therapy, and physical therapy will be important in promoting the child's growth and development. Special education should fit the child's individual needs, and the child should be integrated into mainstream education whenever possible.

Preventing Complications

Children with Down syndrome are at risk for certain health problems (see above). Even though most nurses will encounter a child with Down syndrome in their practice, only a few nurses will become experts in their care. The needs of these children are complex, and guidelines have been established that can help the nurse care for these children and their families (these guidelines can be reviewed at http://www.ndscenter.org/resources/healthcare.

pdf). Nurses also play a key role in educating parents and caregivers about how to prevent the complications of Down syndrome (Teaching Guidelines 50.1 and Fig. 50.3).

Promoting Nutrition

Children with Down syndrome may have difficulty sucking and feeding due to lack of muscle tone. They tend to have small mouths; a smooth, flat, large tongue; and due to the underdeveloped nasal bone, chronically stuffy noses. This may lead to poor nutritional intake and problems with growth. These problems usually improve as the child gains tongue control. Use of a bulb syringe, humidification, and changing the infant's position can lessen the problem. Breastfeeding a baby with Down syndrome is usually possible, and the antibodies in breast milk can help the child fight infections. The caregiver's hand can be used to provide additional support of the chin and throat. Speech or occupational therapists can work on strengthening muscles and assisting in feeding accommodations. Other feeding problems and failure to thrive can be related to cardiac defects and usually improve after medical management is initiated or corrective surgery performed.

Children with Down syndrome do not need a special diet unless underlying gastrointestinal disease is present, such as celiac disease. A balanced, high-fiber diet and regular exercise are important. Research has suggested that children with Down syndrome have lower basal metabolic rates, which can lead to problems with obesity, so it is important in the early years to develop appropriate eating habits and a regular exercise routine. High fiber intake is important for children with Down syndrome because their

TABLE 50.3 AVERAGE AGE OF SKILL ACQUISITION IN CHILDREN WITH DOWN SYNDROME

Developmental Milestone	Average Age of Acquisition, Children with Down Syndrome	Average Age of Acquisition, Typical Children
Smile	2 months	1 month
Roll over	6 months	4 months
Sit alone	9 months	7 months
Crawl	11 months	9 months
Walk	21 months	13 months
Speak words	14 months	10 months
Speak in sentences	24 months	21 months
Feed self with fingers	12 months	8 months
Use spoon	20 months	13 months
Bladder training	48 months	32 months
Bowel training	42 months	29 months
Undress	40 months	32 months
Put on clothes	58 months	47 months

Adapted from Pueschel, S. M. (2001). *A parent's guide to Down syndrome: Toward a brighter future.* Baltimore: Paul H. Brookes Publishing Company, Inc.

TEACHING GUIDELINES 50.1

Health Guidelines for Children With Down Syndrome

- Have your child evaluated by a pediatric cardiologist before 3 months of age, including an echocardiogram.
- Take your child for routine vision and hearing tests.
- Make sure your child gets regular medical care, including a yearly thyroid test.
- Have your child follow a regular diet and exercise routine.
- Make sure all family members perform proper hand hygiene to prevent infection.
- Monitor for signs and symptoms of respiratory infections, such as pneumonia and otitis media.
- Discuss with your pediatrician the use of pneumococcal, respiratory syncytial virus, and influenza vaccines.
- Begin early interventions, therapy, and education as soon as possible.
- Make sure your child brushes his or her teeth regularly. He or she should visit the dentist every 6 months.
- Make sure the child gets a cervical x-ray between 3 to 5 years of age to screen for atlanto-axial instability.

lack of muscle tone may decrease gastric motility, leading to constipation.

Providing Support and Education for the Child and Family

Down syndrome is a lifelong disorder that can result in health problems and cognitive disability. The diagnosis is usually made prenatally or shortly after birth. Parents and caregivers will need support and education during this difficult time. The range of mental impairment varies from mild to moderate; severe deficits occur occasionally. Some families may see having a child with Down syndrome as a lifelong tragedy; others may view it as a positive growing experience. Evaluate how the family defines and manages this experience. Base the plan of care on each individual family's values, beliefs, strengths, and resources.

Family members may have trouble meeting the demands of caring for a child with Down syndrome. These children have complex medical needs, which place strain on the family and its finances. From the time of diagnosis, the family should be involved in the child's care. Include parents in planning interventions and care for the child. In most cases they are the primary caregivers and will provide daily care as well as assisting the child in the development of functioning and skills. They can provide essential infor-

mation to the health care team and will be advocates for their child throughout his or her life.

As the child grows, the needs of the family and child will change. Recognize and respect these needs and provide ongoing education and support for the child and family. Children with Down syndrome will need meaningful education programs. Many children with Down syndrome begin formal education in infancy and continue through high school. Full integration is recommended when possible.

The outlook is brighter than it once was for children with Down syndrome. Many go on in adulthood to obtain jobs, to receive secondary education, and to live on their own or in semi-independent housing. Be familiar with local and national resources for families of children with Down syndrome so that you can help them fulfill their potential (Box 50.4).

▶ *Consider* THIS!

Charles Faust, a 10-month-old with Down syndrome, is seen in the clinic for a well-child examination. The parents have questions about his growth and development. They are concerned because Charles can't pick up finger foods such as Cheerios and put them in his mouth.

How would you address their concerns?

Discuss ways the family can encourage Charles's growth and development.

In addition to usual well-child care, what other medical management will you want to discuss with the family to prevent complications associated with Down syndrome?

▶ TRISOMY 18 AND TRISOMY 13

Trisomy 18 (also known as Edwards syndrome) and trisomy 13 (also known as Patau syndrome) are two other common trisomies. The incidence of trisomy 18 (the presence of three number 18 chromosomes) is 1 in 6,000 births; the incidence of trisomy 13 (the presence of three number 13 chromosomes) is 1 in 10,000 births (Behrman et al., 2004). As in Down syndrome, they usually result from nondisjunction (failure of a chromosome pair to separate) during cell division. Trisomy 18 and trisomy 13 can be present in all cells or may occur in mosaic forms. Both are associated with a characteristic set of anomalies and mental retardation.

The prognosis for trisomy 18 and trisomy 13 is usually poor; these children usually do not survive beyond the first year of life. There is no cure for trisomy 18 or trisomy 13. Therapeutic management will focus on

Sheet #1: Birth to Age 12 Years

Name: _____   **Birthday:** _____

	Age, in years																
Medical Issues	At Birth or at Diagnosis	6-mo	1	1-1/2	2	2-1/2	3	4	5	6	7	8	9	10	11	12	
Karotype & Genetic Counseling	___																
Usual Preventative Care	___	___															
Cardiology	Echo																
Audiologic Evaluation	ABR or OAE	___															
Ophthalmologic Evaluation	Red reflex																
Thyroid (TSH & T$_4$)	State screening																
Nutrition	___	___															
Dental Exam[1]																	
Celiac Screening[2]																	
Parent Support	___	___															
Developmental & Educational Services	Early Intervention																
Neck X-rays & Neurological Exam[3]							X-ray										
Pneumococcal Conjugate Vaccine Series																	

Instructions: Perform indicated exam/screening and record date in blank spaces. The grey or shaded boxes mean no action is to be taken for those ages.

[1]Begin Dental Exams at 2 years of age, and continue every 6 months thereafter.

[2]IgA antiendomysium antibodies and total IgA.

[3]Cervical spine x-rays: flexion, neutral and extension, between 3-5 years of age. Repeat as needed for Special Olympics participation. Neurological examination at each visit.

Figure 50.3 Down Syndrome health care guidelines (1999 revision) record sheet. (Reprinted from *Down Syndrome Quarterly,* Volume 4, Number 3, September 1999.)

Resources for Families of Children with Down Syndrome

- March of Dimes, 1275 Mamaroneck Avenue, White Plains, NY 10605
  1-888-MODIMES (1-888-663-4637)
  http://www.marchofdimes.com/
- National Association for Down Syndrome, P.O. Box 206, Wilmette, IL 60091
  1-630-325-9112
  http://www.nads.org/
- National Down Syndrome Congress, 1370 Center Drive, Suite 102, Atlanta, GA 30338
  1-800-232-6372
  http://www.ndsccenter.org
- National Down Syndrome Society, 666 Broadway, New York, NY 10012
  1-800-221-4602
  http://www.ndss.org/
- Canadian Down Syndrome Society, 811- 14 Street NW, Calgary, Alberta T2N 2A4
  1-800-883-5608
  http://www.cdss.ca

FIGURE 50.4 Trisomy 18.

managing the various congenital anomalies and health issues associated with the disorders.

Nursing Assessment

Nursing assessment will include a general observation for characteristic anomalies (Table 50.4 and Figs. 50.4 and 50.5).

Prenatal screening and diagnostic tests for trisomy 18 and 13 exist. If not diagnosed during the prenatal period, most cases are diagnosed in the first few days of life based on the physical characteristics associated with the disorders.

Nursing Management

Nursing management will be mainly supportive. This will be a difficult time for the family, so providing support and resources for the family will be an important nursing function. SOFT is a support organization for families who have had a child with a chromosome abnormality; they can be reached at http://www.trisomy.org/; 2982 South Union Street, Rochester, NY 14624; (800) 716-SOFT (7638).

▶ TURNER SYNDROME

Turner syndrome is a common abnormality of the sex chromosome. The phenotype is female. It occurs in about 1 in 4,000 live female births (Behrman et al., 2004). Affected fetuses are often aborted spontaneously. The abnormality is due to a loss of all or part of one of the sex chromosomes. About half of the affected individuals have only one X chromosome; the other half have a variety of abnormalities of one of their sex chromosomes and may present with the mosaic form. In about 5% to 10% of cases of Turner syndrome the individual presents with some Y chromosome material in some or all of her cells (Behrman et al., 2004). These females may present

TABLE 50.4   CLINICAL MANIFESTATIONS OF TRISOMY 18 AND TRISOMY 13

Chromosomal Abnormality	Clinical Manifestations
Trisomy 18	Prominent occiput, low-set ears, short eyelid fissures, severe mental retardation, severe hypotonia, webbing, clenched fist with index finger over third digit and fifth digit overlapping the fourth, hypoplasia of fingernails, narrow hips with limited abduction, short sternum, congenital cardiac defects
Trisomy 13	Microcephalic head, wide sagittal suture and fontanels, malformed ears, small eyes, extra digits, severe hypotonia, severe mental retardation, congenital heart defects, cleft lip, cleft palate

FIGURE 50.5 Trisomy 13.

FIGURE 50.6 Note the webbed neck of the child with Turner syndrome.

with some masculinization. The risk of recurrence in future pregnancies is not increased, as Turner syndrome appears to be a sporadic event.

There is no cure for Turner syndrome. Therapeutic management will focus on managing the health issues associated with the syndrome. Children with Turner syndrome are more prone to cardiovascular problems, kidney and thyroid problems, skeletal disorders such as scoliosis and osteoporosis, hearing and eye disturbances, and obesity. They have normal intelligence, although 70% have some learning disability (Sybert & McCauley, 2004). Infertility is usually present, but some women with mosaic Turner syndrome may be fertile. Growth hormone administration is a standard of care and usually begins when the child's height falls below the fifth percentile for healthy girls. Hormone replacement therapy may also be given to initiate puberty and complete growth.

Nursing Assessment

On assessment, note patterns of growth; short stature and slow growth will be a characteristic finding and often the first indication. Other physical characteristics include a webbed neck, low posterior hairline, wide-spaced nipples, edema of the hands and feet, amenorrhea, no development of secondary sex characteristics, sterility, and perceptual and social skill difficulties (Fig. 50.6).

Turner syndrome can be suspected prenatally by ultrasound findings such as fetal edema or redundant nuchal skin or by abnormal results of the triple screen. It can be diagnosed by chromosomal analysis, either prenatally or after birth. Most children are diagnosed at birth or in early child-

hood when slow growth or growth failure is noted. Some cases will not be diagnosed until the pubertal growth spurt does not occur.

Nursing Management

Nursing management is mainly supportive. Provide education and support to the family; they need to understand that short stature and infertility are likely. Explain that mental retardation is unlikely, but some learning disabilities may be present. Emphasize that with medical supervision and support, girls with Turner syndrome may lead healthy, satisfying lives. Counseling about infertility is important. Parents may be upset that their daughter will not be able to reproduce, so explain that many alternatives for reproduction, such as in vitro fertilization and adoption, are available.

Providing support and resources for the family is an important nursing function. The Turner Syndrome Society of the United States provides assistance, support, and education to individuals with Turner syndrome and their families and can be accessed at http://www.turner-syndrome.org/about/ or 10960 Millridge North Drive 214 A, Houston, TX 77070, (800) 365-9944.

▶ KLINEFELTER SYNDROME

Klinefelter syndrome is the most common chromosomal abnormality. It is an abnormality of the sex chromosome: the karyotype and phenotype are male, but one or more extra X chromosomes is present. The abnormality is usually caused by nondisjunction during meiosis, but mosaic forms do present. The incidence of Klinefelter syndrome is 1 in 1,000 males (Wattendorf & Muenke, 2005). Males present with some female-like physical features that are caused by testosterone deficiency. The risk of recurrence in future pregnancies is not increased.

There is no cure for Klinefelter syndrome. Therapeutic management will focus on interventions to enhance masculine characteristics, such as testosterone replacement. Early recognition and hormonal treatment are important to improve quality of life and prevent serious consequences. Cosmetic surgery may be performed to minimize female characteristics such as gynecomastia (increased breast size).

Nursing Assessment

Due to nonspecific findings during childhood, the diagnosis is not usually made until adolescence or adulthood. Prenatal diagnosis is rare unless amniocentesis was performed for genetic testing. Many males with Klinefelter syndrome go through life without being diagnosed. The diagnosis is confirmed by chromosomal analysis.

On assessment, lack of development of secondary sex characteristics may be found. The individual may have decreased facial hair, gynecomastia, decreased pubic hair, and hypogonadism or underdeveloped testes, which leads to infertility. The individual may be taller than average by

FIGURE 50.7 Klinefelter syndrome.

5 years of age, with long legs and a short torso (Fig. 50.7). Mental retardation is not present, but cognitive impairments of varying degree, such as motor delay, speech or language difficulties, attention deficits, and learning disabilities, may be found.

Nursing Management

Nursing management will be mainly supportive. Provide education and support to the family. The American Association for Klinefelter Syndrome Information & Support can be accessed at http://www.aaksis.org or at 1-888-466-KSIS, the Klinefelter Syndrome Support Group at http://klinefeltersyndrome.org/, or Klinefelter Syndrome and Associates at http://genetic.org.

Counseling about infertility is important. Educate patients and families that marriage and sexual relations are possible. Parents may be upset that their son will not be able to reproduce, so explain that many alternatives for reproduction are available and technology is advancing in the field of infertility.

▶ FRAGILE X SYNDROME

Fragile X syndrome is the most common inherited cause of mental retardation (National Institute of Child Health & Human Development, 2006). It is the outcome of a mutation of a gene (FMR1 [fragile X mental retardation]) on the X chromosome. This mutation essentially "turns off" the gene, triggering fragile X syndrome. The exact number of children affected by the mutation or premutation is not known. Males and females are both affected, but females usually have milder symptoms. The inheritance of fragile X is complex and is less straightforward than single-gene or Mendelian inheritance. Some carrier females are affected, and not all males with the gene abnormality show symptoms. Males and females are both fertile and can transmit the disorder to their offspring, so genetic counseling is appropriate. The prognosis for individuals with fragile X is good, and they tend to live a normal life span.

There is no cure for fragile X syndrome. Therapeutic management will be multidisciplinary and aimed at interventions to improve cognitive, emotional, and behavioral impairments.

Nursing Assessment

During childhood, clinical manifestations are subtle, with minor dysmorphic features and developmental delay. Problems with sensation, emotion, and behavior often are the first signs. A delay in attaining developmental milestones will most likely be the first clue found on assessment. Intellectual impairment can range from subtle learning disabilities to severe mental retardation and autistic-like behaviors. In adolescence, boys tend to present with characteristic features such as an elongated face, prominent jaw, large, protruding ears, large size, macro-orchidism (large testes), and a range of behavioral abnormalities and cognitive deficits (Fig. 50.8). There is a characteristic pattern to the cognitive deficits, with problems in abstract reasoning, sequential processing, and mathematics. Typical behavior problems include attention deficits, hand flapping and biting, hyperactivity, shyness, social isolation, low self-esteem, and gaze aversion. In females the clinical manifestations are similar but are more varied and often present in a milder form.

The average age at diagnosis is 8 years. Diagnosis is confirmed by molecular genetic testing. Fragile X can be diagnosed prenatally if inheritance is suspected.

Nursing Management

Nursing management will be mainly supportive. Early diagnosis and intervention with developmental therapies and an individualized education plan are ideal. Care of these children will be the same as care of other children with mental retardation (see Chapter 51 for further information on mental retardation).

Provide education and support to the family. The National Fragile X Foundation provides education and emotional support and works to increase awareness and advance research for fragile X (http://www.fragilex.org/).

FIGURE 50.8 Fragile X syndrome.

Neurocutaneous Disorders

Neurocutaneous disorders, also referred to as hamartoses, are a group of disorders characterized by abnormalities of both the skin and the central nervous system. Many neurologic conditions are associated with cutaneous manifestations, since the skin and the nervous system share a common embryologic origin. They are complex conditions and most also affect other organ systems such as eyes, bones, heart, and kidneys. Most are hereditary and follow an autosomal dominant inheritance pattern or sporadic occurrence. Neurofibromatosis is a common neurocutaneous syndrome and will be discussed in detail below. Table 50.5 provides information on other neurocutaneous syndromes.

▶ NEUROFIBROMATOSIS

Neurofibromatoses are neurocutaneous genetic disorders of the nervous system that primarily affect the development and growth of neural cell tissues. There are two distinct types: neurofibromatosis 1 and neurofibromatosis 2. Neurofibromatosis 1 (von Recklinghausen disease) is the more common type. This disorder causes tumors to grow on nerves and produce other abnormalities such as skin changes and bone deformities. Complications associated with neurofibromatosis include scoliosis, cardiac defects, hypertension, seizures, vision and hearing loss, learning disabilities, attention deficit disorder, abnormalities of speech, and a higher risk for neoplasms. In lay circles this is often referred to as "Elephant Man" disease, but health care providers should avoid this term. Many assume that the disease will result in horrible disfigurement, but in reality most patients present with fairly mild disease.

Although many affected persons inherit the disorder, nearly half of the cases are due to a new mutation. The inheritance pattern is autosomal dominant; therefore, offspring of affected individuals have a 50% chance of inheriting the altered gene and presenting with symptoms. Neurofibromatoses are due to a mutation of the neurofibromin gene on chromosome 17. The estimated prevalence is 1 in 3,000 live births (Behrman et al., 2004; Jones, 2006).

There is no cure for neurofibromatosis. Therapeutic management is aimed at controlling symptoms. Surgical intervention can help reduce some of the bone malformations and remove painful or disfiguring tumors. The American Academy of Pediatrics recommends that these children have a yearly physical, including blood pressure, scoliosis screening, and an ophthalmology examination, developmental screening, and a neurologic examination (Behrman et al., 2004).

TABLE 50.5   OTHER NEUROCUTANEOUS SYNDROMES

Disorder	Incidence	Clinical Manifestations	Nursing Considerations
Tuberous sclerosis	1 in 6,000 (Behrman et al., 2004)	Benign tumors present in the brain and skin. Presents most often as a generalized seizure disorder. Tumors can also involve heart, kidney, eyes, lung, and bones. Developmental delay and behavioral problems may be noted. Usually evident in early childhood. Wide clinical spectrum from severe mental retardation with incapacitating seizures to normal intelligence and no seizures.	Treatment will be mainly symptomatic. Seizure control will be a primary concern. Provide support and education to the family. Referral for genetic counseling (it follows an autosomal dominant inheritance pattern and half the cases are due to a new mutation) and appropriate resources. www.tsalliance.org: Tuberous Sclerosis Alliance
Sturge-Weber syndrome	1 in 50,000 (Behrman et al., 2004)	Facial nevus (port wine stain) most often seen on the forehead and on one side of the face, seizures, hemiparesis, intracranial calcifications. In many cases mental retardation, behavioral and emotional problems, and learning disabilities are present. Seizures usually begin in infancy and may worsen with age. Convulsions are usually noted on the side of the body opposite the facial nevus. Muscle weakness may be present on the same side. Most affected individuals have glaucoma at birth or will develop it later in life.	Treatment will be mainly symptomatic. Seizure control will be a primary concern (use of anticonvulsants or surgery). Seizures due to Sturge-Weber are often difficult to control. Laser treatment may be used to lighten or remove the facial nevus. Surgery may be performed on more serious cases of glaucoma. Physical therapy should be considered for infants and children with muscle weakness. Educational therapy is often prescribed for those with mental retardation or developmental delays. Provide support and education to the family. Refer to appropriate resources. Genetic counseling may be appropriate (inheritance is unclear and sporadic). www.sturge-weber.org: Sturge-Weber Foundation

The disease is progressive and symptoms usually worsen over time, but it is difficult to predict the course. Most affected individuals develop mild to moderate symptoms, with non-life-threatening complications, and live a normal, productive life.

Nursing Assessment

On assessment the nurse may find café-au-lait spots (light-brown macules), which are the hallmark of neurofibromatosis (Fig. 50.9). These are usually present at birth but can appear during the first year of life and usually increase in size, number, and pigmentation. They are present all over the body, particularly the trunk and extremities, while usually sparing the face. Pigmented nevi, axillary freckling, slow-growing cutaneous, subcutaneous, or dermal neuro-

FIGURE 50.9   Café-au-lait spots associated with neurofibromatosis.

fibromas, which are benign tumors, are other signs of neurofibromatosis. Many children with neurofibromatosis have larger-than-normal head circumference and are shorter than average. Enough features are usually present by 6 years of age to make a diagnosis. The severity of symptoms varies greatly, but the diagnosis is made if two or more of the clinical signs in Box 50.5 are present.

▶ **Take** NOTE!

If more than six café-au-lait spots are present, neurofibromatosis should be suspected.

Nursing Management

Nursing management will be mainly supportive. Early detection of treatable conditions and complications is a priority. Provide support and education to the child and family. Discuss genetic counseling with the family. Referral to appropriate resources is essential. The Children's Tumor Foundation can be accessed at http:// www.ctf. org/ or 95 Pine Street, 16th Floor, New York, NY 10005, (800) 323-7938. Neurofibromatosis, Inc. can be accessed at http://www.nfinc.org/ or P.O. Box 18246, Minneapolis, MN 55418, (800) 942-6825.

Other Genetic Disorders

Thousands of genetic disorders are known, and new ones are being discovered, but most of them are rare. Table 50.6 lists other genetic disorders that the pediatric nurse may encounter. Nursing management of these disorders will be mainly supportive and will focus on providing support

---

BOX 50.5 Clinical Signs of Neurofibromatosis

Diagnosis is made if two or more of the following are present:
• Six or more café-au-lait macules (light brown spots) >5 mm in diameter in children and >15 mm in diameter in adolescents and adults
• Two or more neurofibromas (benign tumors) or one plexiform neurofibroma (tumor that involves many nerves)
• Freckling in the armpit or groin
• Presence of an optic glioma (a tumor on the optic nerve)
• Two or more growths on the iris of the eye (Lisch nodules or iris hamartomas)
• Abnormal development of the spine (scoliosis), the temple bone of the skull, or the tibia
• A first-degree relative (parent, sibling, or child) with neurofibromatosis 1

---

and education to the family and child, with an emphasis on developmental and educational needs. Referral to genetic counseling and appropriate resources is an important nursing function.

▶ **Take** NOTE!

Children with VATER syndrome who have only one kidney should not play contact sports.

Inborn Errors of Metabolism

Inborn errors of metabolism are a group of hereditary disorders. They are collectively common but individually rare. Most follow an autosomal recessive inheritance pattern. They are caused by gene mutations that result in abnormalities in the synthesis or catabolism of proteins, carbohydrates, or fats. The body cannot convert food into energy as it normally would. Most inborn errors are due to a defect in an enzyme or transport protein that results in a block in the metabolic pathway. The blocked metabolic pathway allows for accumulation of the damaging byproduct of the impaired metabolic process or may be responsible for a deficiency or absence of a necessary product. Presentation can occur at any time, even in adulthood, but many affected individuals exhibit signs in the newborn period or shortly after. Most inborn errors of metabolism presenting in the neonatal period are lethal if specific treatment is not initiated immediately.

Newborn screening is used to detect these disorders before symptoms develop. Recent developments in screening techniques (tandem mass spectrometry) allow dozens of metabolic disorders to be detected from a single drop of blood. A child who tests positive will require additional testing to confirm the diagnosis (see Chapter 30 for more information on newborn screening).

Therapeutic management of these disorders varies depending on the cause of the error of metabolism, but dietary management is often a key component.

Nursing Assessment

Clinical signs and symptoms vary with each disorder. Table 50.7 gives information on some common inborn errors of metabolism seen in children.

▶ **Take** NOTE!

If the blood sample for the newborn screening was obtained within the first 24 hours after birth, the American Academy of Pediatrics recommends that a repeat sample be obtained within 2 weeks (Goodin, 2006).

(text continues on page 1687)

TABLE 50.6   OTHER GENETIC DISORDERS, SYNDROMES, AND ASSOCIATIONS

Disorder	Inheritance/Cause	Signs and Symptoms	Management
CHARGE syndrome (a recognizable pattern of congenital anomalies seen) **C:** **C**oloboma **H:** **H**eart disease **A:** **A**tresia (choanal) **R:** **R**etarded growth and development and/or CNS anomalies **G:** **G**enital anomalies, hypogonadism **E:** **E**ar anomalies and deafness Incidence is 1 in 10,000 to 12,000 (Griffin et al., 2004).	Autosomal dominant inheritance; most cases are due to new mutation of the gene. Mutations in the gene CDH7 have been indicated in some cases.	Coloboma is a lesion or defect of the eye, usually a fissure or cleft in the iris, ciliary, or choroid; can also see microphthalmos (small eyes) and cryptophthalmos (absent eye). Can lead to vision impairments. Heart anomaly can include any type but most common are aortic arch anomalies and tetralogy of Fallot. Atresia (choanal) is blocked or narrowed passages from the nose to the throat, which can lead to aspiration. Retarded growth or cognitive development can range from mild to severe. Genital anomaly may include micropenis, undescended testes, and hypoplastic labia. Ear anomalies include short, wide ears with little or no lobe, prominent inner fold, floppy appearance, asymmetry; can have hearing impairment. Each feature occurs in a spectrum from absent to severe; no single feature is present in all individuals.	Focus is on identifying and treating all defects; early diagnosis is important. www.chargesyndrome.org: CHARGE Syndrome Foundation
Marfan syndrome: disorder of connective tissue Incidence is 1 in 5,000 to 10,000 (Behrman et al., 2004).	Autosomal dominant inheritance; caused by a mutation in the gene fibrillin-1, which results in changes in connective tissue	Tall stature with long slim limbs, minimal subcutaneous fat, muscle hypotonia, loose joints, long and narrow face, abnormalities of skeletal system (e.g., pectus excavatum [funnel chest] or pectus carinatum [pigeon breast]), ocular system (e.g., enlarged cornea or lens subluxation), and cardiovascular system (e.g., dilation of the aorta or mitral valve prolapse). Delayed achievement of gross and fine motor milestones may occur.	Focus is on preventing complications. www.marfan.org: National Marfan Foundation www.marfan.ca: Canadian Marfan Association

(continued)

TABLE 50.6   Other Genetic Disorders, Syndromes, and Associations (continued)

Disorder	Inheritance/Cause	Signs and Symptoms	Management
VATER association (not a diagnosis, but refers to a non-random association of defects found to occur together) **V: V**ertebral defects **A: A**nal atresia **TE: T**racheo**E**sophageal fistula with esophageal atresia **R**adial and **R**enal dysplasia May also occur as VACTERL association, with **C: C**ardiac anomalies **L: L**imb abnormalities added	Sporadic inheritance. Cause is unknown. Can occur with other chromosomal abnormalities such as trisomy 18. Frequently seen in the offspring of diabetic mothers.	3 or more anomalies are present. Anomalies seen include hypoplastic (small) vertebrae or hemivertebra (only half the bones are formed). These anomalies lead to an increased risk of scoliosis. With imperforate anus or anal atresia, the anus does not open to the outside of the body. Incomplete formation of one or more kidneys, obstruction of urine flow out of kidneys, or severe reflux back into kidneys can all lead to kidney failure later in life. Cardiac anomalies: most common are ventricular septal defects, atrial septal defects, and tetralogy of Fallot. Absent or displaced thumb, polydactyly (extra digits), syndactyly (fusion of digits). A single umbilical artery at birth is often present. Failure to thrive and slow development in early infancy due to anomalies. Usually normal intelligence.	Focus is on identifying and treating all defects. www.tefvater.org: TEF VATER National Support Network
Apert syndrome (named for the French physician who described the syndrome) Incidence is 1 in 65,000 live births (Jones, 2006).	Autosomal dominant inheritance. Cases are sporadic and have been associated with older paternal age.	Craniosynostosis, bilateral symmetrical syndactyly, and craniofacial anomalies such as prominent forehead, midface hypoplasia resulting in sunken appearance, short anteroposterior diameter, down-slanting eyelids. Small nasopharynx can lead to upper airway obstruction and sleep apnea. Learning disabilities and mental deficiency.	Early surgery for craniosynostosis when increased intracranial pressure is noted. Vigorous early management should occur with a multidisciplinary approach to address multiple anomalies. www.aboutfaceusa.org: About Face USA www.ccakids.com: Children's Craniofacial Association www.faceit.org: Let's Face It, Inc. www.faces-cranio.org: National Craniofacial Association www.nffr.org: National Foundation for Facial Reconstruction

Disorder	Inheritance/Cause	Signs and Symptoms	Management
Achondroplasia (most common chondro-dysplasia [diseases resulting in dis-ordered growth]) Incidence is 1 in 15,000 (Jones, 2006).	Autosomal dominant inheritance pattern. Caused by mutations in fibroblast growth factor receptor 3 (FGFR3). 90% new gene mutation. Older paternal age may be a contributing factor.	Characterized by abnormal body proportion. Small stature (average adult height is 4 feet for both men and women), short limbs with normal-size torso, low nasal bridge with prominent fore-head. Midface hypoplasia, caudal narrowing of spinal canal, megalocephaly, small foramen magnum; hands are short and stubby with separa-tion between middle and ring finger ("trident hand"). Delayed motor skills, problems with persistent middle ear dys-function and infections, and bowing of lower legs. Less common complications in-clude hydrocephalus, cranio-cervical junction compression, upper airway obstruction, and thoracolumbar kyphosis. Usually present with normal intel-ligence and lead independent, productive lives.	Medical management of symptoms. Monitor height, weight, and head circum-ference. Manage and prevent complications (careful and thorough neuro-logic exam, assess-ment for sleep apnea). Growth hormone therapy is controversial and still experimental. Limb-lengthening surger-ies may be performed. www.lpaonline.org: Little People of America, Inc. www.shortsupport.org: Short Persons Support

Because of newborn screening and early identifica-tion and management, it is rare to see an untreated newborn with clinical signs and symptoms of the dis-ease. If seen, in many cases a newborn who was healthy at birth will present with lethargy, poor feeding, apnea or tachypnea, recurrent vomiting, altered conscious-ness, failure to thrive, seizures, septic appearance, or developmental delay. Physical changes that may be seen include dysmorphology, cardiomegaly, rashes, cataracts, retinitis, optic atrophy, corneal opacity, deafness, skele-tal dysplasia, macrocephaly, hepatomegaly, jaundice, or cirrhosis.

▶ **Take** NOTE!

When a previously healthy newborn presents with a history of deterioration, an inborn error of metabolism should be suspected.

The diagnostic workup usually requires a variety of specific laboratory studies and may include:

• Glucose: may be elevated
• Ammonia: may be elevated

• Blood gases: may have low bicarbonate and low pH, metabolic acidosis (respiratory alkalosis may also be seen, especially when high ammonia levels are present)

Early diagnosis is the key to saving and improving the lives of these children.

When a child who has previously been diagnosed with an inborn error of metabolism is hospitalized, the nurse must determine the prescribed diet and medications so these may be continued while in the hospital setting.

▶ **Take** NOTE!

If an inborn error of metabolism is suspected, feedings will usually be stopped until the test results are received.

Nursing Management

Ensure that the diet prescribed for the infant or child is followed. For amino acid disorders (e.g., phenylketonuria [PKU]), urea cycle defects (e.g., tyrosinemia type I), and organic acidemia (e.g., maple syrup urine disease),

(text continues on page 1690)

TABLE 50.7   INBORN ERRORS OF METABOLISM

Disorder/Explanation	Incidence*	Clinical Manifestations	Management
Phenylketonuria (PKU): deficiency in a liver enzyme leading to inability to process the essential amino acid phenylalanine properly. Phenyl-alanine accumula-tion can lead to brain damage un-less PKU is de-tected soon after birth and treated.	>1 in 25,000	No symptoms at birth. Most cases are identified before symptoms are present due to newborn screening (PKU is screened for in all states). If undiagnosed, newborn may present with vomiting, irri-tability, eczema-like rash, and mousy odor to urine.	Low-phenylalanine diet. Phenylalanine is found mostly in protein-containing foods such as meat and milk (including breast milk and formula). www.pkunetwork.org: Children's PKU Network www.pku-allieddisorders. org: National Coalition for PKU & Allied Disorders www.pkunews.org: National PKU News
Galactosemia: defi-ciency in the liver enzyme needed to convert galactose, the breakdown product of lactose, which is commonly found in dairy products, into glucose. Galactose accumulation leads to damage to vital organs.	>1 in 50,000	No symptoms at birth. If un-diagnosed, newborn will have jaundice, diarrhea, and vomiting and will not gain weight. If untreated, can lead to liver disease, blindness, severe mental retardation, and death.	Ingestion of galactose can produce sepsis in an affected child; therefore, septic workup and anti-biotics may be necessary in a child if galactose ingestion has occurred. Elimination of galactose and lactose from the diet is the only treatment. Therefore, milk and dairy products will be elimi-nated for life. www.galactosemia.org: Parents of Galactosemic Children
Maple sugar urine disease: affects the metabolism of amino acids. A deficiency in the enzyme that metabolizes leucine, isoleucine, and va-line, which are com-ponents of protein often referred to as the branch chain amino acids. These amino acids then accumulate in the blood and cause damage to the brain.	<1 in 100,000	No symptoms at birth, but if untreated newborns soon begin to show neurologic signs, vomiting, poor feed-ing, increased reflex action, and seizures. If untreated, can lead to life-threatening neurologic damage.	Special low-protein diet, will vary based on severity of symptoms. Thiamine supplements may be given. Diet must be continued throughout life. www.msud-support.org: Maple Syrup Urine Disease Family Support Group

Disorder/Explanation	Incidence*	Clinical Manifestations	Management
Biotinidase deficiency: lack of the enzyme biotinidase results in biotin deficiency	>1 in 75,000	No symptoms at birth; in first weeks or months of life, symptoms such as hypotonia, uncoordinated movement, seizures, developmental delay, alopecia, seborrheic dermatitis, hearing loss, optic nerve atrophy, and mental retardation develop. Metabolic acidosis can lead to death.	Daily oral free biotin www.kumc.edu/gec/support/metaboli.html: Association for Neuro-Metabolic Diseases
Medium-chain acyl-CoA dehydrogenase deficiency (MCAD): lack of an enzyme required to metabolize fatty acids	>1 in 25,000	Recurrent episodes of metabolic acidosis and hypoglycemia, lethargy, seizures, liver failure, brain damage, coma, and cardiac arrest. Can lead to serious and fatal illness in children not eating well.	Avoid fasting; have frequent meals. Special considerations during illness. If unable to tolerate food, IV dextrose is required. www.fodsupport.org: Fatty Oxidation Disorders (FOD) Family Support Group
Homocystinuria: deficiency in the enzyme needed to digest a component of food called methionine (an amino acid)	<1 in 100,000	If undetected and untreated can lead to mental retardation, psychiatric disturbances, developmental delays, displacement of the lens of the eye, abnormal thinning and weakness of bones, and formation of thrombi in veins and arteries that can lead to life-threatening complications such as stroke.	Methionine-restricted diet and cystine supplements; vitamin B6 and B12 supplements and possibly other supplements, such as betaine and folic acid. www.rarediseases.org: National Organization for Rare Disorders
Tyrosinemia: deficiency in an enzyme essential in the metabolism of tyrosine; accumulation of the byproducts results in liver and kidney damage	<1 in 100,000	Symptoms usually appear in the first months of life: poor weight gain, enlarged liver and spleen, increased bleeding tendency, distended abdomen, jaundice, cirrhosis, and liver failure.	Diet low in phenylalanine, methionine, and tyrosine. www.liverfoundation.org: American Liver Foundation

(continued)

TABLE 50.7 INBORN ERRORS OF METABOLISM (continued)

Disorder/Explanation	Incidence*	Clinical Manifestations	Management
Tay-Sachs: caused by insufficient activity of an enzyme called hexosaminidase A, which is necessary for the breakdown of certain fatty substances in brain and nerve cells	Occurs more frequently among persons of Central and Eastern European and Ashkenazi Jewish descent. ~1 in every 27 Jews is a carrier, whereas in the general population 1 in 250 people is a carrier (National Human Genome Research Institute, 2007). Non-Jewish French Canadians from the East St. Lawrence River Valley of Quebec and members of the Cajun population in Louisiana are also at an increased risk. These groups have about a 100 times higher incidence than other ethnic groups (March of Dimes, 2006b).	Infants appear normal and healthy for the first few months of life. Then, as harmful quantities of the fatty substances (called gangliosides) build up in tissues and nerve cells and cause damage, mental and physical deterioration occurs. The child becomes blind, deaf, and unable to swallow; muscles begin to atrophy; and paralysis sets in. Dementia, seizures, and an increased startle reflex may be seen. There is a late-onset type of Tay-Sachs seen in persons in their 20s and early 30s, but this is much rarer.	No treatment or cure. Medical management will focus on managing symptoms and maintaining comfort. Anticonvulsants may be given to control seizures. Death usually occurs in early childhood, by age 4 or 5. Carriers can be identified by a blood test and prenatal testing is available. www.ntsad.org: National Tay-Sachs & Allied Diseases Association

*Incidence data from March of Dimes (2006c). *Recommended newborn screening tests: 29 disorders.* Retrieved on March 1, 2006, from http://www.marchofdimes.com/professionals/14332_15455.asp.
Saving Babies through Screening Foundation, Inc. (2005). *Disease description.* Retrieved on March 1, 2006, at http://www.savebabies.org/diseasedescriptions.php

nutritional therapy is the major intervention. Dietary intake of specific amino acids is restricted according to the disorder. Ensure that overall protein and calorie needs are still met, as children need sufficient calories for proper growth. In children with urea cycle defects and organic acidemia, anorexia is common and severe, and the child may need gastrostomy tube feeding supplementation. In fatty acid oxidation disorders (e.g., medium-chain acyl-CoA dehydrogenase deficiency), the goal is to avoid prolonged periods of fasting and to provide frequent feeds when the child is sick. Supplementation with specific vitamins may also be important in the treatment of these disorders. Strict adherence to the diet is necessary and will require close supervision by registered dietitians, physicians, and nurses and the cooperation of both the parent and child.

Nursing management will focus on education and support for the family, who will need thorough knowledge about the child's disease and management. Referral to a dietitian and appropriate resources, including support groups, will be important. The nurse should also monitor the child's developmental progress and begin therapies as soon as a concern arises.

■■ Key Concepts

■ The purpose of a genetic consultation is to confirm or rule out genetic conditions, identify medical management issues, calculate and communicate genetic risks to a family, discuss ethical and legal issues, and provide psychosocial support.

■ Nurses play an important role in the counseling process. Many times the nurse is the one who has first contact with these parents and is the one to provide follow-up care.

■ The nurse must be able to identify those who could benefit from genetic counseling and must be able to discuss the role of the genetic counselor with families. Families at risk must be aware that genetic counseling is available before they attempt to have another baby.

- Nurses play an essential role in providing emotional support and referrals to appropriate agencies, support groups, and resources when caring for families with suspected or diagnosed genetic disorders.
- Referral for genetic counseling prior to genetic testing may be appropriate.
- Many children with chromosomal abnormalities have mental retardation, learning disabilities, behavioral problems, and distinct features, including birth defects.
- Trisomy 21 (Down syndrome) is associated with some degree of mental retardation, characteristic facial features (e.g., slanted eyes and depressed nasal bridge), and other health problems, such as cardiac defects, visual and hearing impairments, intestinal malformations, and an increased susceptibility to infections.
- In Turner syndrome, short stature and slow growth are characteristic findings.
- Klinefelter syndrome is usually diagnosed in adolescence or adulthood due to a lack of development of secondary sex characteristics.
- Fragile X syndrome's clinical manifestations are subtle during childhood, with minor dysmorphic features and developmental delay. Problems with sensation, emotion, and behavior often are the first signs.
- Café-au-lait spots (light-brown macules) are the hallmark of neurofibromatosis.
- Inborn errors of metabolism are caused by gene mutations that result in abnormalities in the synthesis or catabolism of proteins, carbohyhrdates, or fats. Most inborn errors of metabolism presenting in the neonatal period are lethal if specific treatment is not initiated immediately.
- Nurses should have a basic knowledge of genetics, common genetic disorders in children, genetic testing, and genetic counseling so they can provide support and information to families and can help improve their quality of life.
- Genetic disorders usually result in a lifelong complex medical condition. Nurses must provide ongoing education and support for the child and family about the disorder, treatment, and management as well as available resources.

REFERENCES

Ackley, B. J., & Ladwig, G. B. (2006). *Nursing diagnosis handbook: A guide to planning care*. (7th ed.). St. Louis: Mosby.

American Academy of Pediatrics, Committee on Genetics. (2006). Newborn screening fact sheets. *Pediatrics, 118*(3), e934–e963.

American Academy of Pediatrics, Committee on Genetics. (2007). Health supervision for children with Down syndrome. *Pediatrics, 107*(2), 442–449.

Behrman, R. E., Kliegman, R. M., & Jenson, H. B. (2004). *Nelson's textbook of pediatrics* (17th ed.). Philadelphia: Saunders.

CHARGE Syndrome Foundation. (2008). *About CHARGE*. Retrieved May 16, 2008, from http://www.chargesyndrome.org/about-charge.asp.

Chen, H. (2007) *Down syndrome*. Retrieved May 16, 2008 from http://www.emedicine.com/ped/TOPIC615.HTM.

Cohen, W. (1999). *Health care supervision guidelines for individuals with Down syndrome: 1999 revision*. Retrieved May 16, 2008 from http://www.ndsccenter.org/resources/healthcare.pdf.

Dolan, S. M. & Moore, C. (2007). Linking family history in obstetric and pediatric care: Assessing risk for genetic disease and birth defects. *Pediatrics, 120*, 66–70.

Doswell, B. H., Visootsak, J A., Brady, N. and Graham Jr. J. M. (2006) Turner syndrome: An update and review for the primary pediatrician. *Clinical Pediatrics, 45*(4), 301–313.

Goodin, B. (2006). An overview of expanded newborn screening for inborn errors of metabolism. *Practical Gastroenterology*. Retrieved on November 27, 2007 at http://www.healthsystem.virginia.edu/internet/digestive-health/nutritionarticles/Aug2006.pdf.

Griffin, H. C., Davis, M. L., & Williams, S. C. (2004). CHARGE Syndrome: Educational and technological interventions. *RE:view: Rehabilitation and Education for Blindness and Visual Impairment, 35*(4), 149–158.

Jones, K. L. (2006). *Smith's recognizable patterns of human malformation* (6th ed.). Philadelphia: Elsevier Saunders.

Kam, J. R., & Helm, T. N. (2005). Neurofibromatosis. *eMedicine*. Retrieved May 16, 2008, from http://www.emedicine.com/DERM/topic287.htm.

Lashley, F. R. (2005). *Clinical genetics in nursing practice*. New York: Springer Publishing.

Leung, A. K. C. & Robson, W. L. M. (2006). A young girl with café au lait spots. *Consultant for Pediatricians, 5*(4), 229–232.

March of Dimes. (2008a). *Chromosomal abnormalities*. Retrieved May 16, 2008 from http://www.marchofdimes.com/professionals/14332_1209.asp.

March of Dimes. (2008b). *Recommended newborn screening tests: 29 disorders*. Retrieved May 16, 2008 from http://www.marchofdimes.com/professionals/14332_15455.asp.

March of Dimes. (2008c). *Tay-Sachs disease*. Retrieved May 16, 2008 from http://www.marchofdimes.com/professionals/14332_1227.asp.

National Human Genome Research Institute. (2007). *Learning about Tay-Sachs disease*. Retrieved April 22, 2007 from http://www.genome.gov/10001220.

National Institute of Child Health and Human Development. (2006) *Fragile X syndrome*. Retrieved November 13, 2007 at http://www.nichd.nih.gov/health/topics/fragile_x_syndrome.cfm.

National Institutes of Health, National Institute of Child Health and Human Development. (2006). *Facts about Down syndrome*. Retrieved July 22, 2006, from http://www.nichd.nih.gov/publications/pubs/downsyndrome/down.htm#TheOccurrence.

National Institute of Neurological Disorders and Stroke (2007). *Neurofibromatosis fact sheet*. Retrieved May 16, 2008, from www.ninds.nih.gov/disorders/neurofibromatosis/detail_neurofibromatosis.htm.

National Institute of Neurological Disorders and Stroke (2007). *NINDS Tay-Sachs disease information page*. Retrieved May 16, 2008, from www.ninds.nih.gov/disorders/taysachs/taysachs.htm.

Pagana, K. D., & Pagana, T. J. (2006). *Mosby's manual of diagnostic and laboratory tests* (3rd ed.). St. Louis: Mosby.

Pueschel, S. M. (2001). *A parent's guide to Down syndrome: Toward a brighter future*. Baltimore: Paul H. Brookes Publishing Company, Inc.

Saving Babies through Screening Foundation, Inc. (2007). *Disease descriptions*. Retrieved May 16, 2008, from http://www.savebabies.org/diseasedescriptions.php.

Seibert, D. (2007). Newborn screening: As testing choices expands, so must your knowledge. *Advance for Nurse Practitioners, 15*(4), 55.

Shott, S. R., Amin, B. Chini, C. Heubi, Hotze, S. & Akers, R. (2006). Obstructive sleep apnea: Should all children with Down syndrome be tested? *Archives of Otolaryngology Head & Neck Surgery, 132*(4), 432–436.

Siegel, B., & Milunsky, J. (2004). When should the possibility of a genetic disorder cross your radar screen? *Contemporary Pediatrics, 21*(5), 30–45.

Skinner, D., & Schaffer, R. (2005). Families and genetic diagnoses in the genomic and internet age. *Infants and Young Children, 19*(1), 16–24.

Sybert, V. P., & McCauley, E. (2004). Turner's syndrome. *New England Journal of Medicine, 351*(12), 1227–1241.

Trotter, T. L., Hall, J. G., & American Academy of Pediatrics Committee on Genetics. (2005). Health supervision for children with achondroplasia. *Pediatrics, 116*(3), 771–784.

Van Cleve, S. N. & Cohen, W. I. (2006). Part I: Clinical practice guidelines for children with Down syndrome: Birth to 12 years. *Journal of Pediatric Health Care, 20*(1), 47–54.

Van Cleve, S. N., Cannon, S. & Cohen, W. I. (2006). Part II: Clinical practice guidelines for adolescents and young adults with Down syndrome: 12 to 21 years. *Journal of Pediatric Health Care, 20*(3), 198–205.

Venes, D. (2005). *Taber's cyclopedic medical dictionary* (20th ed.). Philadelphia: F. A. Davis.

Wattendorf, D. J., & Muenke, M. (2005). Klinefelter syndrome. *American Family Physician, 72*(11), 2259–2263.

Wattendorf, D. J., & Muenke, M. (2005). Diagnosis and management of fragile X syndrome. *American Family Physician, 72*(1), 111–114.

Weiner, D. L. (2005). Pediatrics, inborn errors of metabolism. *eMedicine.* Retrieved July 22, 2006, from http://www.emedicine.com/emerg/topic768.htm.

WEBSITES

About Face USA: www.aboutfaceusa.org

Angelman Syndrome Foundation, Inc.: www.angelman.org

Children's Craniofacial Association: www.ccakids.com

Canadian Down Syndrome Society: www.cdss.ca

CHARGE Syndrome Foundation: www.chargesyndrome.org

Children's Tumor Foundation (dedicated to neurofibromatosis research): www.ctf.org/

Let's Face It, Inc.: www.faceit.org

National Craniofacial Association: www.faces-cranio.org

5p- Society (cri-du-chat syndrome): www.fivepminus.org

Fatty Oxidation Disorders (FOD) Family Support Group: www.fodsupport.org

National Fragile X Foundation: www.fragilex.org/

Parents of Galactosemic Children: www.galactosemia.org

Association for Neuro-Metabolic Diseases: www.kumc.edu/gec/support/metaboli.html

American Liver Foundation: www.liverfoundation.org

Little People of America, Inc.: www.lpaonline.org

March of Dimes (information on birth defects, genetic disorders and inborn errors of metabolism): www.marchofdimes.com/

Canadian Marfan Association: www.marfan.ca

National Marfan Foundation: www.marfan.org

Maple Syrup Urine Disease Family Support Group: www.msud-support.org

National Association for Down Syndrome: www.nads.org/

National Down Syndrome Congress: www.ndsccenter.org/

National Down Syndrome Society: www.ndss.org/

National Foundation for Facial Reconstruction: www.nffr.org

Neurofibromatosis, Inc. (dedicated to education, advocacy, and research): www.nfinc.org/

National Tay-Sachs & Allied Diseases Association: www.ntsad.org

Children's PKU Network: www.pkunetwork.org

National PKU News: www.pkunews.org

National Organization for Rare Disorders: www.rarediseases.org

Short Persons Support: www.shortsupport.org

Sturge-Weber Foundation: www.sturge-weber.com

TEF VATER National Support Network: www.tefvater.org

Support Organization for Trisomy 18, 13, and Related Disorders: www.trisomy.org/

Tuberous Sclerosis Alliance: www.tsalliance.org

Turner Syndrome Society of the United States: www.turner-syndrome-us.org/about/

Velo-Cardio-Facial Syndrome Educational: www.vcfsef.org/

CHAPTER WORKSHEET

MULTIPLE CHOICE QUESTIONS

1. The nurse is caring for a child with Down syndrome. What should the nurse's focus be?

   a. Teaching hygiene skills to the child in order to increase self-esteem

   b. Screening for anomalies and teaching about prevention of respiratory infection

   c. Finding opportunities to increase socialization for the child and family

   d. Expecting walking at age 1 year and toilet training completion at age 2 years

2. The nurse is caring for a child with Turner syndrome admitted to the unit for treatment of a kidney infection. What characteristics associated with this syndrome may the nurse expect to find upon assessment?

   a. Microcephaly, polydactyly

   b. Low-set ears, cleft lip

   c. Short stature, webbed neck

   d. Gynecomastia, taller than average

3. A child born with a single transverse palmar crease, a short neck with excessive skin at the nape, a depressed nasal bridge, and cardiac defects is most likely to have which autosomal abnormality?

   a. Trisomy 21

   b. Trisomy 18

   c. Trisomy 14

   d. Trisomy 13

4. A mother brings her 4-day-old infant to the clinic with vomiting and poor feeding. The newborn was healthy at birth. The nurse should suspect:

   a. Sturge-Weber syndrome

   b. An inborn error of metabolism

   c. Trisomy 18

   d. Turner syndrome

CRITICAL THINKING EXERCISES

1. An 8-month-old is seen in the clinic. On assessment the nurse finds eight café-au-lait spots on the child's trunk and extremities. What other assessment findings may be pertinent?

2. A child's newborn screen came back positive for phenylketonuria. After further testing, the diagnosis is confirmed. What instructions would you give the parents regarding care of their child?

3. A 6-year-old boy with Down syndrome is admitted to the hospital with pneumonia. Choose three pieces of information that the nurse should seek when obtaining the health history:

   a. Presence of cardiac defects or disease

   b. Last hearing and vision evaluation

   c. Mother's pregnancy history

   d. Presence of thyroid disease

   e. Mother's immunization history

STUDY ACTIVITIES

1. Develop a nursing care plan for a child with Down syndrome.

2. Shadow a genetic counselor. Identify ways he or she helps families understand and cope with genetic disorders.

3. Attend a meeting of an ethics committee at a local hospital. Identify some of the ethical, legal, and social issues in health care that they discuss, particularly related to genetic testing and genetic disorders.

NURSING CARE OF THE CHILD WITH A COGNITIVE OR MENTAL HEALTH DISORDER

KEY TERMS

abuse
affect
anxiety

bingeing
comorbidity
neglect

purging
suicide
violence

LEARNING OBJECTIVES

Upon completion of the chapter, the learner will be able to:

1. Discuss the impact of alterations in mental health upon the growth and development of infants, children, and adolescents.
2. Describe techniques used to evaluate the status of mental health in children.
3. Identify appropriate nursing assessments and interventions related to therapy and medications for the treatment of childhood and adolescent mental health disorders.
4. Distinguish mental health disorders common in infants, children, and adolescents.
5. Develop an individualized nursing care plan for the child with a mental health disorder.
6. Develop patient/family teaching plans for the child with a mental health disorder.

*J*ohn Howard, age 6 years, is brought to the clinic for his annual examination. His father states, *"John has frequent emotional outbursts and his mood seems to switch from happy to sad rather quickly. His teachers have said his performance at school has been poor."*

Wow

A child's sense often exceeds all human intellect.

Mental health issues make up the bulk of the "new morbidity" of children. Such issues include academic difficulties, psychiatric disorders, **violence**, school hostility, substance abuse, and adverse effects of the media (Reasor & Farrell, 2004). As many as 13 million children may be suffering from mental health-related problems (American Academy of Pediatrics [AAP], 2000). Up to 80% of children with social, emotional, or behavioral problems fail to receive the services they need, leading to further academic and social difficulties. Mental illness manifested in the early years increases the risk of adolescent emotional issues, use of firearms, reckless driving, substance abuse, and promiscuous sexual activity. Some cognitive or neurobehavioral disorders may have a genetic or physiologic cause, whereas others result from family or environmental stressors.

Usually children with cognitive or mental health disorders are treated in the community or on an outpatient basis, but sometimes the disorder has such a significant impact on the child and family that hospitalization is required. Many hospitalized children also suffer from cognitive or mental health disorders. When a child is diagnosed with a neurobehavioral disorder, the family may become overwhelmed by the multifaceted services that he or she requires.

The scope of mental health issues among children, adolescents, and their families has become so extensive that the U.S. Surgeon General has published a "National Agenda for Action." The Surgeon General's Conference on Children's Mental Health has set the following goals:

1. Promote public awareness of children's mental health issues and reduce the stigma associated with mental illness.
2. Continue to develop, disseminate, and implement scientifically proven prevention and treatment services in the field of children's mental health.
3. Improve the assessment of and recognition of mental health needs in children.
4. Eliminate racial/ethnic and socioeconomic disparities in access to mental health care services.
5. Improve the infrastructure for children's mental health services, including support for scientifically proven interventions across professions.
6. Increase access to and coordination of quality mental health care services.
7. Train front-line providers to recognize and manage mental health issues, and educate mental health care providers about scientifically proven prevention and treatment services.
8. Monitor the access to and coordination of quality mental health care services (U.S. Public Health Service, 2004).

Mental health problems in children are real and painful and can be severe. For affected children to have a chance at a healthy future, nurses must participate in the early identification and referral of children with potential cognitive deficits or other mental health issues.

Effects of Mental Health Issues on Health and Development

Children's behavior is influenced by biologic or genetic characteristics, nutrition, physical health, developmental ability, environmental and family interactions, the child's individual temperament, and the parents' or caregiver's responses to the child's behavior (Goldson & Reynolds, 2007). The changes that occur with normal growth and development are often a source of stress for children, and in some children they may lead to dysfunction. Children progress at very different rates, so it is often difficult to identify subtle abnormalities. When stress, fatigue, or pain occurs in children, they may quickly regress to earlier patterns of behavior. These regressive behaviors may continue if a mental health concern is present. It is possible that stress placed on developing neurons leads to decreased coping abilities later in life. Children learn through their experiences; therefore, they may develop maladaptive behaviors through life interactions.

Common Medical Treatments

A variety of medications and other medical treatments are used to treat mental health disorders in children. Most of these treatments will require a physician's order when the child is in the hospital. The most common medications are listed in Drug Guide 51.1. The nurse caring for the child with a mental health disorder should become familiar with how the treatments and medications work, as well as medication adverse effects to monitor for. Many mental health disorders are treated with some type of therapy. Table 51.1 reviews the types of therapies commonly used. These therapies are generally carried out only by specially trained personnel.

Behavior management techniques are also used to help children alter negative behavior patterns. The methods may be used outside of therapy sessions, in the hospital, clinic, or classroom. Behavior management techniques include the following:

- Set limits with the child, holding him or her responsible for his or her behavior.
- Do not argue, bargain, or negotiate about the limits once established.
- Provide consistent caregivers (unlicensed assistive personnel and nurses for the hospitalized child) and establish the child's daily routine.
- Use a low-pitched voice and remain calm.
- Redirect the child's attention when needed.
- Ignore inappropriate behaviors.
- Praise the child's self-control efforts and other accomplishments.
- Use restraints only when necessary

DRUG GUIDE 51.1 DRUGS USED FOR PEDIATRIC MENTAL HEALTH DISORDERS

Medication	Action/Indication	Nursing Implications
Psychostimulants: methylphenidate (Ritalin), dextro-amphetamine (Adderall), lisdexamfetamine (Vyronase), pemoline (Cylert), long-acting methylphenidate (Concerta, Focalin XR, Metadate CD, Ritalin LA), long-acting dextroamphet-amine (Dexedrine Spansules, Adderall XR)	Increases synaptic levels of dopamine and norepinephrine ADHD	• Methylphenidate has a short half-life; give TID (a.m., mid-day at school, at home after school). • Long-acting preparations are given once daily in the a.m. • Adverse effects: decreased appetite, headache, abdominal pain, difficulty sleeping, irritability, social withdrawal, motor tics. If dose is too high, child may have flat affect. • Vyronase—if chest pain and fainting occurs notify physician at once. • Pemoline is only rarely used because of hepatotoxicity.
Antianxiety agent: buspirone (BuSpar)	Highly blocks reuptake of dopamine Anxiety, rage, mania, psychosis, depression, Tourette syndrome	• Administer in consistent relation to food (either with or without). • May cause drowsiness • Monitor for disinhibition, agitation, confusion, depression.
Antimanic agent: lithium (Eskalith, Lithobid)	Influences reuptake of serotonin and/or norepinephrine Bipolar disorder, depression, hyperaggression	• Monitor closely. • May cause polyuria, polydipsia, tremor, nausea, weight gain, diarrhea
Selective serotonin reuptake inhibitors: fluoxetine (Prozac), paroxetine (Paxil), sertraline (Zoloft)	Potentiates serotonin activity in the brain Depression, obsessive-compulsive disorder, anxiety	• Observe for irritability, insomnia, GI distress, nausea, headache. • Monitor BP for increase.
Atypical antidepressants: trazodone (Desyrel)	Inhibits reuptake of serotonin Depression	• Monitor BP for postural hypotension. • Observe for sedation and drowsiness; avoid alcohol use. • Administer after meals or with a snack.
Nonstimulant norepinephrine reuptake inhibitors: atomoxetine (Straterra)	Enhances norepinephrine activity ADHD	• Administer without regard to food once or twice daily. • Monitor weight, height, BP, heart rate. • May cause dizziness, dry mouth.
Alpha-agonist antihypertensive agents: clonidine (Catapres), guan-facine (Tenex)	Activates inhibitory neurons in the brain stem ADHD, Tourette syndrome, self-abuse, aggression	• Clonidine is strongly sedating. • Monitor BP and pulse. • Observe for dry mouth, confusion, depression, urinary retention, constipation.

Medication	Action/Indication	Nursing Implications
Antipsychotic agents: thioridazine (Mellaril), chlorpromazine (Thorazine), haloperidol (Haldol)	Reversibly block type 2 dopamine receptors in the central nervous system Psychosis, mania, self-harm, violent or destructive behavior	• May cause drowsiness. • Monitor for anticholinergic effects, drowsiness and dystonia (extrapyramidal effects), dizziness. • Evaluate for the development of orthostatic hypotension, tachycardia. • Observe closely for the development of tardive dyskinesia, particularly early in treatment.
Atypical antipsychotics: risperidone (Risperdal), clozapine (Clozaril), olanzapine (Zyprexa)	Reversibly block type 2 dopamine receptors in the central nervous system Psychosis, bipolar disorder, autism spectrum disorder, Tourette syndrome	• Monitor for seizures, agitation, headache, nausea, sedation. • Olanzapine may cause weight gain. • Note WBC.
Tricyclic anti-depressants: amitriptyline (Elavil), desipramine (Norpramin), imipramine (Tofranil), nortriptyline (Pamelor)	Enhances synaptic concentration of serotonin and/or norepinephrine Depression, ADHD, tics, anxiety	• Monitor for anticholinergic effects, weight loss. • Check blood levels. • Monitor ECG for arrhythmias.

TABLE 51.1 TYPES OF THERAPY

Treatment	Explanation
Behavioral therapy	Uses stimulus and response conditioning to manage or alter behavior. Reinforces desired behaviors, replacing the inappropriate ones. Consistency is of utmost importance.
Play therapy	Designed to change emotional status. Encourages the child to act out feelings of sadness, fear, hostility, or anger.
Cognitive therapy	Teaches children to change reactions so that automatic negative thought patterns are replaced with alternative ones.
Family therapy	Exploration of the child's emotional issue and its effect on family members.
Group therapy	May be conducted in a school, hospital, treatment facility, neighborhood center. Feelings are expressed and participants gain hope, feel a part of something, and benefit from role modeling. Takes advantage of peer relationships as developmental focus in preteen and teen groups.
Milieu therapy	A specially structured setting designed to promote the child's adaptive and social skills. A safe and supportive environment for those at risk of self-harm or those who are very ill or very aggressive.
Individual therapy	The child and therapist work together to resolve the conflicts, emotions, or behavior problems. Trust is central. Structured based on the child's developmental level (e.g., may use play therapy for a younger child).
Hypnosis	Deep relaxation with suggestibility remarks.

EVIDENCE-BASED PRACTICE 51.1
Behavioral and Cognitive Behavioral Therapy for Children and Adolescents With Obsessive Compulsive Disorder

● **Study**

Behavioral or cognitive-behavioral therapy (BT/CBT) is often recommended for children and adolescents with obsessive-compulsive disorder (OCD). The authors reviewed studies comparing BT/CBT with no treatment or in combination with pharmacotherapeutics for OCD. Four studies with 222 total participants were included in the review.

▲ **Findings**

Participants who underwent BT/CBT demonstrated better post-treatment functioning and reduced risk of continuing with OCD as compared with those receiving no BT/CBT.

Evidence surfaced that BT/CBT combined with medication was superior to treatment with medication alone. The dropout rate during therapy was low, indicating acceptance by participants and their families.

■ **Nursing Implications**

Encourage families to explore the possibility of adding BT/CBT to the treatment plan. Assist families with finding an appropriate provider of BT/CBT in their local area. Praise children and families for ongoing dedication to BT/CBT. Continue to offer emotional support to all members of the family throughout the treatment process.

O'Kearne, R. T., Ansley, K. J., & von Sanden, C. (2006). Behavioural and cognitive behavioural therapy for obsessive compulsive disorder in children and adolescents. *The Cochrane Library 2006, 4.* Indianapolis: John Wiley & Sons.

NURSING PROCESS OVERVIEW FOR THE CHILD WITH A MENTAL HEALTH DISORDER

Care of the child with a mental health disorder includes assessment, nursing diagnosis, planning, interventions, and evaluation. There are a number of general concepts related to the nursing process that may be applied to mental health concerns in children. From a general understanding of the care involved for a child with a mental health disorder, the nurse can then individualize the care based on patient specifics.

Assessment

A careful and thorough health history forms the basis of the nursing assessment of a child with a mental health or cognitive disorder. The physical examination may yield clues to the type of disorder but is often completely normal.

> ▶ *Take* NOTE!
>
> *Observe a child's play or drawings; if you suspect cognitive or psychological issues from the play or artwork, refer the child for further mental health evaluation.*

Health History

Elicit the health history, noting the child's prenatal and birth history, past medical history, including previously diagnosed cognitive or mental health disorders, history of neurologic injury or disease, and family history of mental health disorder. Perform a developmental history, noting age of attainment (or loss) of milestones. Question the child and/or parent about behavior changes such as:

• Altered sleep
• Difference in eating patterns, weight loss or gain, change in appetite
• Problems at school
• Participation in risk-taking behaviors
• Alterations in friendships
• Changes in extracurricular activity participation

Note results of any developmental testing performed. Ask the family about progression of the child's skills. Note any unusual deficits or capabilities. Question the family about recent stress, trauma, or change in family structure; are any family members chronically ill? Note medications the child takes routinely, and any allergies to food, drugs, medications, or environmental agents.

Interview the child at an age-appropriate level to determine his or her self-perception, future plans, and stressors and how he or she copes with them. Determine the child's perception of his relationship with his parents, siblings, friends, peers, pets, inanimate objects, and transitional or security objects. What is the child's predominant mood? Determine whether the child likes himself or herself, asking such questions as "What do you like most about yourself?" and "What would you like to change about yourself?" Determine the child's gender identity status. Does the child have a sense of pride in his or her accomplishments? Has the child developed an appropriate conscience (with understanding of right and wrong)?

Note history of complaints that may be associated with certain mental health disorders, such as sore throat, difficulty swallowing, or genital burning or itching. Document if the child displays any of the following during the health interview:

- Hallucinations
- Aggression
- Impulsivity
- Distractibility
- Intolerance to frustration
- Lack of sense of humor or fun
- Inhibition
- Poor attention span
- Potential cognitive or learning disabilities
- Unusual motor activities

*R*emember John, the 6-year-old brought in for his annual examination? What additional health history and physical examination assessment information should the nurse obtain?

Physical Examination

Observe the child's clothing, noting whether it is appropriate for age, developmental level, and setting. Note the child's facial expression and response to the parent or caretaker and the nurse. Does the child make appropriate eye contact? Determine the child's level of consciousness and extent of interest in and interaction with surroundings. Note the child's posture, **affect**, and mood. How appropriate to the situation are the child's emotional reactions? Does the child communicate well?

Measure the child's weight and height/length, as well as head circumference if he or she is less than 3 years old. Perform a thorough physical examination, noting any physical abnormalities or signs of other physical health disorders. Note abnormal findings that may be associated with particular mental health disorders, such as bruising, burns, contusions, cuts, abrasions, unusual skin marks, soft/sparse body hair, split fingernails, inflamed oropharynx, eroded tooth enamel, reddened gums, or genitourinary discharge or bleeding.

Laboratory and Diagnostic Testing

Mental health disorders are generally diagnosed based upon clinical features. Brain imaging such as computed tomography or magnetic resonance imaging may be used to evaluate for a congenital abnormality or alterations in the brain tissue that may lead to developmental delay. A blood or urine toxicology panel is useful in the diagnosis of drug abuse or overdose, or instances of bizarre behavior.

Nursing Diagnoses and Related Interventions

The overall goal of nursing management of cognitive and mental health disorders in children is to help the child and family to reach an optimal level of functioning. This may be achieved through interventions designed to decrease the impact of stressors upon the child's life. Upon completion of a thorough assessment of the child and family, the nurse might identify several nursing diagnoses, including:

- Impaired social interaction
- Delayed growth and development
- Ineffective individual coping
- Hopelessness
- Imbalanced nutrition, less than body requirements
- Disturbed thought processes
- Caregiver role strain

*A*fter completing an assessment of John, the nurse noted the following: difficulty sitting still for the examination, easily distracted, and frustrated, labile mood. Based on the assessment findings, what would your top three nursing diagnoses be for John?

Nursing goals, interventions, and evaluation for the child with a mental health disorder are based on the nursing diagnoses. Nursing Care Plan Overview 51.1 provides a general guide for planning care for a child with a mental health disorder. Children's responses to a mental health issue and its treatment will vary, and nursing care should be individualized based on the child's and family's responses to illness. Additional information about nursing management will be included later in the chapter as it relates to specific disorders. See Healthy People 2010.

*B*ased on your top three nursing diagnoses for John, describe appropriate nursing interventions.

Developmental and Behavioral Disorders

Developmental and behavioral disorders make up a large proportion of mental health disorders in children. They include learning disabilities, mental retardation, autism spectrum disorder, and attention-deficit/hyperactivity disorder.

▶ LEARNING DISABILITIES

About 15 million children and adolescents have learning disabilities (Prasher & Kadapia, 2006). About half of the children with a learning disability have at least one other co-morbid condition (usually a mental health or behavioral disorder). The National Center for Learning Disabilities

Nursing Care Plan 51.1

OVERVIEW FOR THE CHILD WITH A MENTAL HEALTH DISORDER

NURSING DIAGNOSIS: Impaired social interaction related to altered social skills as evidenced by impulsivity, intrusive behavior, inability to follow through, anxiety, depressed mood, feelings of unattractiveness or unworthiness

Outcome Identification and Evaluation
The child will demonstrate socially acceptable skills, *interacting successfully with peers and in the educational setting, completing tasks as required.*

Interventions: Promoting Appropriate Social Interaction
- Identify factors that may aggravate the child's performance *to minimize stimuli that exacerbate the child's undesired behaviors.*
- Modify the environment to decrease distracting stimuli *as child's ability to deal with external stimuli may be impaired.*
- Ensure that the child hears his name and makes eye contact prior to conversing or instructions *so that child is engaged and has increased ability to follow through.*
- State expectations for tasks or behaviors clearly *as understanding is necessary to ensure completion.*
- Provide positive feedback for appropriate behaviors or task completion, *encouraging the child to adopt expectations into his behaviors and routine.*

NURSING DIAGNOSIS: Ineffective individual coping related to inability to deal with life stressors as evidenced by few or no meaningful friendships, inability to empathize or give/receive affection, low self-esteem, or maladaptive coping behaviors such as substance abuse

Outcome Edentification and Evaluation
The child will demonstrate improved coping, *verbalize feelings, socially engage, demonstrate problem-solving skills.*

Interventions: Promoting Coping Skills
- Encourage discussion of thoughts and feelings, *as this is an initial step toward learning to deal with them appropriately.*
- Provide positive feedback for appropriate discussion, *as this increases the likelihood of continuing performance.*
- Demonstrate unconditional acceptance of the child as a person *to increase self-esteem in the child who has been feeling rejection.*
- Set clear limits on behavior as needed *so the child has a structure to adhere to.*
- Teach the child problem-solving skills *as an alternative to acting-out behaviors.*
- Role-model appropriate social and conversation skills *so the child can see what is expected in a nonthreatening manner.*

NURSING DIAGNOSIS: Imbalanced nutrition, less than body requirements, related to intake insufficient to meet metabolic needs as evidenced by weight loss, failure to gain weight, less-than-expected increases in stature and weight, loss of appetite, or refusal to eat

Outcome Identification and Evaluation
The child or adolescent will demonstrate appropriate growth, *making gains in weight and stature as appropriate.*

Interventions: Improving Nutritional Intake
- Provide favorite foods *to encourage the child with poor appetite to eat more.*
- Assist families to choose nutrient-rich foods *so that the food the child does eat is most beneficial.*
For the child with an eating disorder:
- Mutually establish a contract related to treatment *to promote the child's sense of control.*
- Provide mealtime structure, *as clear limits let the child know what the expectations are.*
- Encourage the child to choose foods and timing of meals *to develop independence in eating habits.*
- Ensure the eating environment is pleasant and relaxed, with minimal distractions, *to minimize the child's anxiety and guilt about not eating.*
- Withdraw attention if child refuses to eat *(secondary gain is minimized if refusal to eat is ignored).*
- Provide continuous supervision during the meal and for 30 minutes following it *so that the child cannot conceal or dispose of food or induce vomiting.*

Nursing Care Plan 51.1 (continued)

NURSING DIAGNOSIS: Delayed growth and development related to disability, behavioral disorder, or altered nutrition as evidenced by lack of attainment of age-appropriate skills, regression in skills, or altered intellectual functioning

Outcome Identification and Evaluation
Child will demonstrate progress toward developmental milestones: *Child expresses interest in the environment and people around him, interacts with environment in an age-appropriate way.*

Interventions: Promoting Development
- Use therapeutic play and adaptive toys *to facilitate developmental functioning.*
- Provide stimulating environment when possible *to maximize potential for growth and development*
- Praise accomplishments and emphasize child's abilities *to improve self-esteem and encourage feeling of confidence and competence.*
- Follow through with physical, occupational, and speech therapists' recommendations *to maximize exposure to exercises designed to increase the child's skills.*
- Determine parents' expectations of child's future achievement *to help them work toward these goals.*

NURSING DIAGNOSIS: Disturbed thought processes related to behavioral disorder, depression, anxiety, abusive situation, or substance abuse as evidenced by distractibility, non–reality-based thinking, hypervigilance, or inaccurate interpretation of interactions of others

Outcome Identification and Evaluation
Child's thought processes will improve; *child will demonstrate appropriate orientation, remain free from physical harm, and perform activities of daily living as able.*

Interventions: Improving Thought Processes
- Observe for causes of altered thought processes *to provide a baseline for assessment and intervention.*
- Perform an age-appropriate mental status examination *to determine extent of altered thinking.*
- Adjust communication style based on child's cues *to improve communication.*
- Listen carefully and seek clarification *to determine basis for child's agitation or other behaviors.*
- Provide validation of the child's thoughts and feelings *to improve trust in the relationship.*
- Establish a daily routine *to provide the child with a sense of security.*

NURSING DIAGNOSIS: Hopelessness related to child's perception of his life situation, negative life view, or alteration in mental well-being as evidenced by passivity, verbalization, alterations in sleep, or lack of initiative

Outcome Identification and Evaluation
Child will display a sense of hope, *will verbalize feelings, participate in care, make positive statements.*

Interventions: Promoting Hope
- Monitor and document potential for suicide, *as hopelessness often leads to suicidal ideation.*
- Assist the child to identify reasons for hope and for living, *so the nurse is aware of the child's values.*
- Help the child to set goals that are important to him *to allow the child to see possibilities.*
- Encourage simple decision making on a daily basis, *as hopelessness often occurs as a response to loss of control.*
- Assist the child to identify positive qualities in himself and his life *to facilitate the development of hope.*
- Involve parents or others the child loves in the child's care *as social support is critical to the development of hope.*

(continued)

Nursing Care Plan 51.1 (continued)

NURSING DIAGNOSIS: Caregiver role strain related to long-term care of the child with a chronic mental health disorder as evidenced by fatigue, inattention to own needs, conflict, or ambivalence

Outcome Identification and Evaluation

The child's caregiver will participate in the child's care, *verbalizing the child's needs and treatment plan and demonstrating skills necessary for care.*

Interventions: Decreasing Role Strain

- Teach the parent or caregiver about the child's illness, treatments, and medications *to clarify expectations for the child and parent.*
- Role-model appropriate interaction behaviors with the child *so the parent can learn these techniques by watching.*
- Encourage structure in daily routines *to allow the parent to meet own needs and allow for adequate rest.*
- Gradually increase the parent's responsibility related to care of the child *to help the parent feel less overwhelmed.*
- Allow the parent to move at his or her own pace in assuming care *to enhance the chances for success.*
- Help the parent to identify a back-up caregiver *so the parent has times of respite from constant involvement with the child.*

(2007) defines a learning disability as "a neurological disorder that affects the brain's ability to receive, process, store, and respond to information." Learning disabilities become evident when a child of average intelligence has difficulty mastering basic academic skills. Learning disabilities can affect the child's ability to listen, speak, read, write, and perform mathematics:

- Children with dyslexia have difficulty with reading, writing, and spelling.
- Dyscalculia leads to problems with mathematics and computation.
- Problems with manual dexterity and coordination result when a child has dyspraxia.
- Children with dysgraphia have difficulty producing the written word (composition, spelling, and writing).

Sensory integration dysfunction may be mistaken for a learning disability, but it is not and should be treated differently. Box 51.1 provides additional information.

Nursing Assessment

Elicit the health history, noting risk factors such as a family history of learning disability, problems during pregnancy or birth, prenatal alcohol or drug use, low birthweight, premature or prolonged labor, head injury, poor nutritional status or failure to thrive, or lead poisoning. Obtain detailed information about the educational difficulties the child is experiencing (e.g., he seems to do fine in math but always reverses letters when reading). A thorough physical examination may reveal clues to comorbid conditions. Ensure that the child has undergone a comprehensive education evaluation with assessment testing to diagnose the specific learning disability. Testing may be performed by a school, educational, developmental, or clinical psychologist, occupational therapist, speech and language therapist, or other

HEALTHY PEOPLE 2010

Objective	Significance
(Developmental) Increase the proportion of children with mental health problems who receive treatment.	• Screen all children and adolescents for mental health problems. • Encourage children and adolescents to participate in treatment planning as is developmentally appropriate, allowing them to make choices about intervention as possible.

BOX 51.1 Sensory Integration Dysfunction (Also Called Sensory Processing Disorder)

- A neurologic disorder in which the child cannot organize sensory input used in daily living
- Hyposensitivity or hypersensitivity to sensory input
- Results in overreaction to different textures, decreasing the child's ability to participate in the world
- Preterm and low-birthweight infants are at increased risk compared with typical infants.
- Occupational and other therapies may increase the child's ability to function.

developmental specialist, depending on the areas of learning with which the child is experiencing difficulty.

> ▶ **Take** NOTE!
>
> *If a child cannot speak in sentences by 30 months of age, does not have understandable speech 50% of the time by age 3 years, cannot sit still for a short story by 3 to 5 years of age, or cannot tie shoes, cut, button, or hop by 5 to 6 years of age, refer the child to be evaluated for a learning disability.*

Nursing Management

Ensure that families are aware of their child's rights under the Individuals with Disabilities Act (IDEA), which was reapproved in 2004. IDEA offers protection from discrimination and the right to assistance in the school or workplace. Each child will need an individualized education plan (IEP) that reflects his or her particular needs, which then must be provided for through the school system. Offer encouragement and support to families as they advocate for their child. Follow up at subsequent health care visits to determine that the child is receiving the services he or she needs to optimize his or her potential for success. Refer families for additional resources through the National Center for Learning Disabilities (www.ncld.org), Learning Disabilities Online (www.ldonline.org), or the Center for Learning Differences (www.centerforlearning differences.org).

▶ MENTAL RETARDATION

Mental retardation refers to a functional state in which significant limitations in intellectual status and adaptive behavior (functioning in daily life) develop before the age of 18 years. Up to 3% of the population may be designated as mentally retarded (Accardo et al., 2006; Wickham, 2004).

As defined by the American Association on Intellectual and Developmental Disabilities (AAIDD, 2007), mental retardation includes:

• Deviations in IQ of two or more standard deviations (IQ of less than 70 to 75)
• Coexisting deficits in at least two adaptive skills: communication, community use, functional academics, health and safety, home living, leisure, self-care, self-direction, social skills, and work
• Occurring before the age of 18 years

Long ago mentally retarded persons were confined to institutions and were thought to be harmful to soci-

ety. In the early 21st century, most children with mental retardation are receiving their education in public schools with their peers and living at home with their families or elsewhere in the community. Only the most severely affected individuals require separate classrooms or schools.

Pathophysiology

In many instances of mental retardation the exact cause remains unknown. Prenatal errors in central nervous system development may be responsible, or an insult or damage to the brain may occur in the prenatal, perinatal, or postnatal period from a variety of causes. Motor problems such as hypotonia, tremor, ataxia, or clumsiness, visual motor problems, or other issues may occur concomitantly with mental retardation. When a learning disability or sensory processing impairment is also present, functioning at a higher intellectual level may be prevented. Mental retardation is generally categorized according to severity:

• Mild: IQ 50 to 70
• Moderate: IQ 35 to 50
• Severe: IQ 20 to 35
• Profound: IQ less than 20

Therapeutic Management

The primary goal of therapeutic management of children with mental retardation is to provide appropriate educational experiences that allow the child to achieve a level of functioning and self-sufficiency needed for existence in the home, community, work, and leisure settings. The child's conceptual, social, practical, and intellectual abilities will drive school placement and the focus of the educational experience. The student's success is also dependent upon community and family influences. The majority of mentally retarded individuals require only minimal support, and these individuals are able to achieve some level of self-sufficiency. Only a few children and adults with mental retardation require extensive support.

Nursing Assessment

Perform developmental screening at each health care visit to identify developmental delays early. Elicit the health history, determining the mental and adaptive capacities of the child's parents and other family members. Obtain a detailed pregnancy and birth history. Document sequence and age of attainment of developmental milestones. Note history of motor, visual, or language difficulties. Assess the child's health history for risk factors such as preterm or postterm birth, low birthweight, birth injury, prenatal or neonatal infection, prenatal alcohol or drug exposure, genetic syndrome, chromosomal alteration, metabolic disease, exposure to toxins (e.g., lead), head injury or other trauma, nutritional deficiency, cerebral malformation, and other brain disease or mental health disorder. Note history of or concomitant seizure disorder, orthopedic problems, speech problems, or vision or hearing deficit.

For the child with known mental retardation, assess language, sensory, and psychomotor functioning. Determine the child's ability to toilet, dress, and feed himself or herself. Ask the parents about involvement with school and community services and support.

On physical examination note dysmorphic features (possibly very mild) consistent with certain syndromes (e.g., fetal alcohol syndrome; Box 51.2). Evaluate the newborn or metabolic screening results. Computed tomography or magnetic resonance imaging of the head may be performed to evaluate the brain structure. Thyroid function tests may be ordered to rule out thyroid problems leading to developmental delay.

> ▶ *Take* NOTE!
>
> *Due to the extent of cognition required to understand and produce speech, the most sensitive early indicator of intellectual disability is delayed language development.*

Nursing Management

When children with mental retardation are admitted to the hospital (usually for some other physical or medical condition), it is important for the nurse to continue the child's usual home routine. Follow through with feeding and motor supports that the child uses. Ensure that the child is closely supervised and remains free from harm. Allow parents time to verbalize frustrations or fears. For some families the caretaking burden is extensive and lifelong; arrange for respite care as available. Support the child's strengths, and assist the child and family to follow through with therapy or treatment designed to enhance the child's functioning. Assist with the development of the child's IEP as appropriate.

BOX 51.2 **Fetal Alcohol Syndrome**

- Results from in utero alcohol exposure
- Typical facial features include low nasal bridge with short upturned nose, flattened midface, long philtrum with narrow upper lip
- Poor coordination, skeletal abnormalities
- Microcephaly
- Failure to thrive
- Hearing loss

▶ AUTISM SPECTRUM DISORDER

Autism spectrum disorder (ASD), also termed pervasive developmental disorder, has its onset in infancy or early childhood. One child in 500 is diagnosed with autism (Choueiri & Bridgemohan, 2005), though some sources estimate the incidence to be as frequent as 1 in 250 children (Dumont-Mathieu et al., 2005). The spectrum of autism disorder ranges from mild (e.g., Asperger syndrome) to severe. Autistic behaviors may be first noticed in infancy as developmental delays or between the age of 12 and 36 months when the child regresses or loses previously acquired skills. Parental concerns about development may be sensitive indicators of the development of autism (Beauchesne & Kelly, 2004).

Pathophysiology

The exact etiology of autism continues to elude scientists, but it may be due to genetic makeup, brain abnormalities, altered chemistry, a virus, or toxic chemicals. Children with ASD display impaired social interactions and communication as well as perseverative or stereotypic behaviors. They may fail to develop interpersonal relationships and experience social isolation. Most children with autism are mentally retarded, requiring lifelong supervision (Choueiri & Bridgemohan, 2005), though some are gifted.

Therapeutic Management

There are no medications or treatments available to cure autism. Each child's treatment is individualized; behavioral and communication therapies are very important. Children with ASD respond very well to highly structured educational environments. Stimulants may be used to control hyperactivity, and antipsychotic medications are sometimes helpful in children with repetitive and aggressive behaviors.

Many families are drawn to the use of complementary and alternative medical therapies in attempts to treat their autistic child. They may use vitamins and nutritional supplements, herbs or restrictive diets, music therapy, art therapy, and sensory integration techniques. To date, these therapies have not been scientifically proven to improve autism.

The goal of therapeutic management is for the child to reach optimal functioning within the limitations of the disorder.

Nursing Assessment

Elicit the health history, noting delay or regression in developmental skills, particularly speech and language abilities. The child may be mute, utter only sounds (not words), or repeat words or phrases over and over. The parent may report that the infant or toddler spends hours in repetitive activity and demonstrates bizarre motor and stereotypic behaviors. The infant may resist cuddling, lack eye contact, be indifferent to touch or affection, and have little change in facial expression. Toddlers may display hyperactivity, aggression, temper tantrums, or self-injury behaviors, such as head-banging or hand-biting. The history may also reveal hypersensitivity to touch or hyposensitivity to pain. Assess the child's functional status, including behavior, nutrition, sleep, speech and language, education needs, and developmental or neurologic limitations (Giarelli et al., 2005). Assist with screening, using an approved autism screening tool such as:

• Checklist for Autism in Toddlers (CHAT)
• Modified Checklist for Autism in Toddlers (M-CHAT)
• Social Communication Questionnaire (SCQ)
• Pervasive Developmental Disorders Screening Test-II (PDDST-II)

Perform a thorough physical examination. Observe the infant or toddler for lack of eye contact, failure to look at objects pointed to by the examiner, failure to point to himself, failure to let his needs be known, perseverative play activities, and unusual behavior such as hand-flapping or spinning. Measure growth parameters, in particular noting head circumference (macrocephaly or microcephaly may be associated with ASD). Note the presence of large, prominent, or posteriorly rotated ears. Examine the skin for hypo- or hyperpigmented lesions. Note asymmetry of nerve function or palsy, hypertonia, hypotonia, alterations in deep tendon reflexes, toe-walking, loose gait, or poor coordination. Obtain hearing screening results and ascertain that lead screening has been performed.

> ▶ *Take* NOTE!
>
> *Screen all infants and toddlers for warning signs of autism:*
> • *Not babbling by 12 months*
> • *Not pointing or using gestures by 12 months*
> • *No single words by 16 months*
> • *No two-word utterances by 24 months*
> • *Losing language or social skills at any age*

Nursing Management

When children are initially diagnosed with autism, parents need an extensive amount of emotional support, professional guidance, and education about the disorder while they are attempting to adjust to the diagnosis (Giarelli et al., 2005). Assess the "fit" between the child's developmental needs and the treatment plan. Help parents overcome barriers to obtain appropriate education, developmental, and behavioral treatment programs. Ensure that the child younger than 36 months of age receives services via the local early intervention program and children 3 years and over have an IEP in place if enrolled in the public school

system. Stress the importance of rigid, unchanging routines, as children with ASD often act out when their routine changes (which is likely to occur if the child must be hospitalized for another condition). Many special schools exist for children with significant developmental disorders, though some are extremely expensive. Assess the parents' need for respite care and make referrals accordingly. Provide positive feedback to parents for their perseverance in working with their child.

▶ ATTENTION-DEFICIT/ HYPERACTIVITY DISORDER

Attention-deficit/hyperactivity disorder (ADHD) is one of the most common mental health disorders diagnosed in childhood: it affects 3% to 7% of all children, and up to 70% of children with ADHD will manifest symptoms throughout adulthood (DeNisco et al., 2005). ADHD is characterized by inattention, impulsivity, distractibility, and hyperactivity. Three subtypes of ADHD exist: hyperactive–impulsive, inattentive, and combined. The child with ADHD has a disruption in learning ability, socialization, and compliance, placing significant demands on the child, parents, teachers, and community. About two thirds of children with ADHD also have a **comorbidity** such as oppositional defiant disorder, conduct disorder, an anxiety disorder, depression, a less severe developmental disorder, an auditory processing disorder, or learning or reading disabilities (DeNisco et al., 2005; Vlam, 2006). Comparison Chart 51.1 gives information about oppositional defiant disorder and conduct disorder to distinguish them from ADHD.

Pathophysiology

Though the exact cause of ADHD remains unidentified, current thought includes as its etiology an alteration in the dopamine and norepinephrine neurotransmitter system. The symptoms of impulsivity, hyperactivity, and inattention begin before 7 years of age and persist longer than 6 months. Symptoms exist in the school and home settings, impairing family and social interactions. Children and teens with ADHD experience frustration, labile moods, emotional outbursts, peer rejection, poor school performance, and low self-esteem. They may also have poor metacognitive abilities such as organization, time management, and the ability to break a project down into a series of smaller tasks. They are not lazy or unmotivated, but simply have poor skills in these areas. Box 51.3 provides criteria for the diagnosis of ADHD.

Therapeutic Management

Medication management of ADHD includes the use of psychostimulants, nonstimulant norepinephrine reuptake inhibitors, and/or alpha-agonist antihypertensive

COMPARISON CHART 51.1

Oppositional Defiant Disorder	Conduct Disorder
• Excessive arguing with adults • Frequent temper tantrums • Active defiance • Revenge-seeking behaviors • Frequent resentment or anger • Touchiness; easily annoyed • Noncompliance with adult requests or limits • Blaming of others for misbehavior or mistakes	• Bullying and threatening of others • Initiation of physical fights • Weapon use to cause others harm • Physical cruelty to animals or people • Destruction of property or arson • Lying and stealing • Serious violation of rules: staying out past curfew, truancy, running away • Use of force in sexual activity

agents. These medications are not a cure for ADHD, but help to increase the child's ability to pay attention and decrease the level of impulsive behavior. The child's activity level is not usually affected. Since ADHD manifests into young adulthood, treatment should continue throughout adolescence (Barbaresi et al., 2006). Concomitant disorders, such as anxiety, should also be treated. Behavior therapy and classroom restructuring may be useful.

BOX 51.3 Diagnosis of ADHD

Presence of six or more of the following:
• Failure to pay close attention
• Careless mistakes on schoolwork
• Difficulty paying attention to tasks or play
• Doesn't listen
• Doesn't follow through
• Doesn't complete tasks
• Doesn't understand instructions
• Poorly organized
• Avoids, dislikes, or fails to engage in activities requiring mental effort
• Loses things needed for task completion
• Easily distracted
• Forgetful
Presence of six or more of the symptoms of hyperactivity or impulsivity:
• Fidgety or squirmy
• Often out of seat
• Activity inappropriate to the situation
• Cannot engage in quiet play
• Always on the go
• Talks excessively
• Blurts out answers
• Has difficulty waiting his turn
• Often interrupts or intrudes on others (Stevens, 2005)

Nursing Assessment

For a full description of the assessment phase of the nursing process, refer to page 1698. Assessment findings pertinent to ADHD are discussed below.

Health History

Elicit a description of the behavioral issue or school performance problem. Explore the child's history for risk factors such as head trauma, lead exposure, cigarette smoke exposure, prematurity, or low birthweight. The past history may also reveal a larger-than-usual number of accidents. Determine if there is a family history of ADHD. Question the parent about school behavior. The school-age child may be unable to stay on task, talks out of turn, leaves his desk frequently, and either neglects to complete in-class and homework assignments or forgets to turn them in. The adolescent may be inattentive in school, poorly organized, and forgetful.

Several behavioral checklists are available that may assist in the diagnosis of ADHD. They may be completed by the child's teacher and/or parent and focus on behavior patterns related to conduct or learning problems, social competence, anxiety, activity level, and attention. Obtain the completed behavioral checklists (usually one from the parent and one from the teacher) as well as any school records or testing performed.

Physical Examination

Perform vision and hearing screening to rule out vision or hearing impairment as the cause of poor school performance. Observe the preschool child's behavior, noting quickness, agility, fearlessness, and the desire to touch or explore everything in the room.

Laboratory and Diagnostic Tests

No definitive laboratory or diagnostic test is available for the identification of ADHD. A complete blood count may be performed to rule out anemia, and thyroid hormone levels may be drawn to determine whether they are normal.

Nursing Management

Having a child with ADHD can be frustrating as the child's inattention, high activity level, impulsivity, and distractibility are often very difficult to deal with. Parents may doubt their ability to be effective parents or may view their child as somehow defective. Children with ADHD may also feel they are bad, faulty, stupid, or retarded. Provide emotional support, allowing enough time for the family to air their concerns. Work with the child and family to develop goals such as completion of homework, improved communication, or increasing independence in self-care.

Assist the family to advocate for their child's needs through the public school system. The child is entitled to a developmentally appropriate education via an IEP as necessary (refer to Chapter 13 for additional information about special education). The IEP should be updated as needed. Ensure coordination of health and school services. Flag the child's chart and set up a schedule for systematic communication with the family and school. Teach families and school personnel to use behavioral techniques such as time-out, positive reinforcement, reward or privilege withdrawal, or a token system. The token system rewards appropriate behavior with a token and results in a token being taken away if inappropriate behavior occurs. At the end of a specified period of time, the tokens may be exchanged for a prize or privilege. Refer families to local support groups and the national ADHD support group www.chadd.org.

Stimulant medications should be taken in the morning to decrease the adverse effect of insomnia. Some children may experience decreased appetite, so giving the medication with or after the meal may be beneficial. The child may feel "different" from his peers if he has to visit the school nurse for a lunchtime dose of ADHD medication; this may lead to noncompliance and a subsequent increase in ADHD symptoms, with deterioration in schoolwork. In this situation, encourage the family to explore with their physician the option of one of the newer extended-release or once-daily ADHD medications.

Tourette Syndrome

Tourette syndrome is estimated to affect about 1% of children (Zinner, 2004a). Its onset is before 18 years of age. The syndrome consists of multiple motor tics and one or more vocal tics occurring either simultaneously or at different times. Children are not tic-free for longer than 3 months. Tics are defined as sudden rapid recurrent stereotypical movements and/or sounds over which the child appears to have no control. Comorbid conditions such as ADHD and obsessive-compulsive disorder occur in 90% of children with Tourette syndrome (Zinner, 2004a). The exact pathophysiologic mechanism of Tourette syndrome has yet to be identified, though genetics does seem to play a part. Therapeutic management is highly individualized and involves psychopharmacology and behavioral therapies. Habit reversal training may help in some children.

Nursing Assessment

Evaluate the health history for the occurrence of tics. The child may be embarrassed or ashamed about the tics and the parents may feel fearful, angry, or guilty. Determine the presence of comorbid symptoms. Elicit the child's past health history, noting a family history of tics. Assess the child's psychosocial history to determine the extent to which the tics interfere with friendship, school performance, and self-esteem. Observe the child for simple or complex motor tics. Vocal tics such as sniffling, grunting, clicking, or word utterance may occur. Perform a thorough physical examination, which is usually normal.

Nursing Management

Inform families that the tics become more noticeable or severe during times of stress and less pronounced when the child is focused on an activity such as watching TV, reading, or playing a video game. Help the family to build on the child's functional behaviors and adaptive skills to improve the child's self-esteem. Encourage the family to pursue classroom accommodations such as allowing for "tic breaks," taking untimed tests or tests in another room, or using note-takers or tape recording. Support the family's decisions related to medication use and provide appropriate education about the particular drugs. "Teaching the Tiger" by M. P. Dornbush and S. K. Pruitt (Hope Press) is useful for teachers of the child with Tourette syndrome. For additional support refer families to www.tsa-usa.org (Tourette Syndrome Association), www.tourette.ca (Tourette Syndrome Foundation of Canada), or www.tourette syndrome.net (Tourette Syndrome Plus).

Eating Disorders

Eating disorders affect a significant number of children, especially adolescents. Pica, which occurs most frequently in 2- to 3-year-olds, is an eating disorder in which the child ingests (over at least a 1-month period) a nonnutritive material such as paint, clay, or sand. Rumination is an eating disorder occurring in infants in which the baby regurgitates partially digested food or formula and expels or swallows it. The numbers of children affected by pica and rumination is not known.

Anorexia nervosa and bulimia are common eating disorders affecting primarily adolescents, though younger children may also be affected. In American society, being thin is highly valued, compounding the problem. Anorexia nervosa occurs in about 1 of 200 adolescent females; bulimia affects about 1% to 3% (Marino & Fine, 2007). Anorexia nervosa is characterized by dramatic weight loss as a result of decreased food intake and sharply increased physical exercise. Bulimia refers to a cycle of normal food intake, followed by binge-eating and then purging; the adolescent remains at a near-normal weight. Complications include fluid and electrolyte imbalance, decreased blood volume, cardiac arrhythmias, esophagitis, rupture of the esophagus or stomach, tooth loss, and menstrual problems. The mortality rate for anorexia is about 4% (Marino & Fine, 2007).

Nursing Assessment

Determine the health history, noting risk factors such as family history, female gender, Caucasian race, preoccupation with appearance, obsessive traits, or low self-esteem. Adolescents with anorexia may have a history of constipation, syncope, secondary amenorrhea, abdominal pain, and periodic episodes of cold hands and feet. Parents usually note the chief complaint as weight loss. Note history of depression in the child with bulimia. Evaluate the child's self-concept, noting multiple fears, high need for acceptance, disordered body image, and perfectionism. Perform a thorough physical examination. The anorexic is usually severely underweight, with a body mass index (BMI) less than 17. Note cachetic appearance, dry sallow skin, thinning scalp hair, soft sparse body hair, and nail pitting. Measure vital signs, noting low temperature, bradycardia, or hypotension. Auscultate the heart, noting murmur as a result of mitral valve prolapse (occurs in about one third of patients). The adolescent with bulimia will be of normal weight or slightly overweight. Inspect the hands for calluses on the backs of the knuckles and split fingernails. Inspect the mouth and oropharynx for eroded dental enamel, red gums, and inflamed throat from self-induced vomiting. Careful evaluation of serum electrolytes and electrocardiogram is needed in anorexics, as severe electrolyte disturbances and cardiac arrhythmias often occur.

Nursing Management

Most children with eating disorders can be treated successfully on an outpatient basis. Those with anorexia who display severe weight loss, unstable vital signs, food refusal, or arrested pubertal development or who require enteral nutrition will need to be hospitalized. Refeeding syndrome (cardiovascular, hematologic, and neurologic complications) may occur in the severely malnourished patient if rapid nutritional replacement is given, so slow refeeding is essential to avoid complications. Give phosphorus supplements as ordered. Assess vital signs frequently for orthostatic hypotension, irregular and decreased pulse, or hypothermia.

Consult the nutritionist for assistance with calculating caloric needs and determining an appropriate diet. Aim for a weight gain goal of 0.5 to 2 pounds per week. Instruct the child and family to keep a daily journal of intake, bingeing and purging behaviors, mood, and exercise. The journal may be used as an assessment tool as well as to document progress toward recovery. Assist the child and family to plan a suitably structured routine for the child that includes meals, snacks, and appropriate physical activity.

Use the physical findings associated with anorexia to educate the child about the consequences of malnutrition and how they can be remedied with adequate nutrient intake. Behavior or group therapy may also be needed. Assess the child's need for intervention for concomitant depression or **anxiety** (some anorexics also require psychotropic medications). Provide emotional support and positive reinforcement to the child and family. Refer the family to local support groups or online resources such as the Academy for Eating Disorders (www.aedweb.org) or the National Eating Disorders Association (www. national eatingdisorders.org). See Healthy People 2010.

> ▶ *Consider* THIS!

> *Nicole Ashton, 16 years old, is seen in your clinic due to weight loss. Her mother states that she has lost noticeable weight over the past few months and has stopped menstruating. What additional assessment information would be necessary?*
>
> *After further examination it is determined that Nicole has anorexia nervosa. Her treatment is to take place on an outpatient basis beginning immediately. Discuss ways the family can encourage and assist in Nicole's recovery.*

Mood Disorders

Mood disorders in children include depressive disorders and bipolar disorder. About 5% of children may suffer from depression at any one time. Children may experience major depressive disorder or dysthymic disorder. Girls are twice as likely to be affected as boys; particularly during the teenage years. Bipolar disorder refers to a condition of alternating manic and depressive episodes. During the manic episode, mood is significantly elevated and the patient displays excess energy.

Depression may cause significant alterations in school performance and social relationships. Anxiety disorders and disruptive behavior may occur together with depres-

HEALTHY PEOPLE 2010

Objective	Significance
(Developmental) Reduce the relapse rate for persons with eating disorders, including anorexia nervosa and bulimia nervosa.	• Provide appropriate follow-up for all children recovering from anorexia or bulimia. • Ensure that psychotherapy is available to children with eating disorders.

sion. Substance abuse also occurs about 25% of the time with depression. Divorce and serious family issues may contribute to the development of depression because of the ongoing stress they place on the child and their strong psychological impact (Pompili et al., 2005).

Depressed children are at risk for suicide, which is the third leading cause of death among teens age 15 to 19 years (CDC, 2007). The 2005 Centers for Disease Control and Prevention Youth Risk Behavior Surveillance Report revealed that nearly 17% of teens had seriously considered suicide and 8.4% had attempted it (CDC, 2006).

Pathophysiology

Both norepinephrine and dopamine play a role in mood. Norepinephrine is considered to be important in the areas of energy and alertness, dopamine in the areas of pleasure and motivation. When alterations in the neurotransmission of norepinephrine and dopamine occur, the symptoms of depression (apathy, loss of interest and pleasure) result. Decreased levels of serotonin have also been implicated in depressive symptoms. In addition, circadian rhythm disturbances may play a role in the development of depression.

Therapeutic Management

Children with mood disorders usually benefit from psychotherapy. This helps the child to deal with the psychosocial consequences of his or her behavior on his or her interpersonal relationships with others. Crisis management, parental counseling, and individual, group, or family therapy may be useful. Major depressive disorder warrants the use of pharmacologic antidepressants. Bipolar disorder may be treated with neuroleptic agents or mood stabilizers.

Nursing Assessment

Children with untreated depression are at high risk for suicide as well as the development of comorbid disorders such as anxiety, substance abuse, and disruptive behavioral disorders. The nurse must screen all children for the development of depression.

Health History

Obtain a health history from the child and separately from the parent. Evaluate the child for history of recent changes in behavior, changes in peer relationships, alterations in school performance, withdrawal from previously enjoyed activities, sleep disturbances, changes in eating behaviors, increase in accidents, or sexual promiscuity. If possible, use a standardized depression screening questionnaire; there are many available.

Ask about potential stressors such as school concerns, conflicts with parents, dating issues, and **abuse** (physical or sexual). When bipolar disorder is suspected, the history may reveal rapid, pressured speech, increased energy, decreased sleep, flamboyant behavior, or irritability during the manic episodes.

Note history of weight loss, failure to thrive, or increased incidence of infections in the infant. For the toddler, note delay or regression in developmental skills, increase in nightmares, or parental reports of clinginess. The preschooler may have a history of loss of interest in newly acquired skills; manifest encopresis, enuresis, anorexia, or binge-eating; or make frequent negative self-statements. The parents of a school-age child may report that he or she has a depressed, irritable, or aggressive mood.

Assess for risk factors for suicide, which include:

- Previous suicide attempt (Pompili et al., 2005)
- Change in school performance, sleep, or appetite
- Loss of interest in formerly favorite school or other activities
- Feelings of hopelessness or depression
- Statements about thoughts of suicide (Pompili et al., 2005)

Physical Examination

Observe the infant for weepiness, withdrawn behaviors, or a frozen facial expression. Note a sad or expressionless face in the toddler or preschooler. In any age child, observe for apathy. Inspect the entire body surface for self-inflicted injuries, which may or may not be present. The remainder of the physical examination is generally normal unless the depressed child also has a chronic medical condition.

Nursing Management

Nursing management of children and adolescents with mood disorders focuses on education, support, and prevention.

Educating and Supporting the Child and Family

Teach families that mood disorders are biologic conditions, not personality flaws. Teach families how to administer antidepressant medication and to monitor for adverse effects. Encourage and praise their efforts at following through with cognitive and behavioral therapies. Support the family throughout the process, as sometimes treatment may be lengthy. Refer parents to local support resources or to the Depression and Bipolar Support Alliance (http://www.ndmda.org) or the Child and Adolescent Bipolar Foundation (www.bpkids.org).

Preventing Depression and Suicide

Establish a trusting relationship with the children and adolescents with whom you interact, particularly in the primary care setting, school, or chronic illness clinic. This trusting relationship may encourage children or adolescents to confide feelings or problems earlier than they may do with their parents. Screen all healthy and chronically ill preteens and teens for the development of depression. Use standardized screening tools such as those listed in Box 51.4. When a potential problem is identified, immediately refer the child for mental health assessment and intervention. It is important to identify depression early so that treatment can start. When a grief-inducing event is impending (such as the death of a family member), begin preventive intervention to help the child to deal with it. Provide appropriate observation for any child exhibiting suicidal ideation. See Healthy People 2010.

▶ *Take* NOTE!

Closely observe children taking antidepressants for the development of presuicidal behavior.

Anxiety Disorders

Anxiety disorders are the most commonly diagnosed psychiatric conditions among children and adolescents (Bothe & Olness, 2007). As many as 6% to 20% of children experience at least one anxiety disorder (American Academy of Child and Adolescent Psychiatry, 2007a). Anxiety often occurs together with other mental health disorders, especially depression. Normal children experience fear, worry, and shyness. Infants fear loud noises,

being startled, and strangers. Toddlers are afraid of the dark and of separation. Preschoolers fear imaginary creatures and body mutilation. School-age children worry about injury and natural events, whereas adolescents are anxious about school and social performance. These normal fears produce a certain level of anxiety that is tolerated by most children, but it is important to distinguish normal developmentally appropriate anxiety from problematic anxiety.

Anxiety is considered to be a reaction to a perceived or actual threat. The threat may or may not be distorted by the child, and emotional distress leads to behavioral responses. The "fight-or-flight" response results in tachycardia, increased blood pressure, sweating, enhanced arousal and reactivity, tremors, and increased blood flow to the muscles.

Types of Anxiety Disorders

Generalized anxiety disorder (GAD) is characterized by unrealistic concerns over past behavior, future events, and personal competence. Social phobia may result, in which the child or teen demonstrates a persistent fear of speaking or eating in front of others, using public restrooms, or speaking to authorities. Selective mutism may also occur. Separation anxiety is more common in children than adolescents; the child may need to remain close to the parents, and the child's worries focus on separation themes. Obsessive-compulsive disorder (OCD) is characterized by compulsions (repetitive behaviors such as cleaning, washing, checking something), which the child performs to reduce anxiety about obsessions (unwanted and intrusive thoughts). Post-traumatic stress disorder (PTSD) is an anxiety disorder that occurs after a child experiences a traumatic event, later experiencing physiologic arousal when a stimulus triggers memories of the event.

Pathophysiology

Anxiety disorders are thought to occur as a result of disrupted modulation within the central nervous system. Underactivation of the serotonergic system and overactivation of the noradrenergic system are thought to be responsible for dysregulation of physiologic arousal and the resulting emotional experience. Disruption of the gamma-butyric acid (GABA) system may also play a role. Recently, the role of corticosteroids in behaviors related to stress and the way the brain processes fear-inducing stimuli have been explored.

Therapeutic Management

Therapeutic management of anxiety disorders generally involves the use of pharmacologic agents and psychological therapies. Anxiolytics or antidepressants are the most common pharmacologic approaches. Cognitive-behavioral therapy, individual, family, or group psychotherapy, and

HEALTHY PEOPLE 2010	
Objective	Significance
(Developmental) Reduce the rate of suicide attempts by adolescents.	• Screen all children and adolescents for the development of depression. • When depression or excess stress is present, refer the child to the appropriate support.

other behavioral interventions such as relaxation techniques may also be useful.

Nursing Assessment

Children and adolescents do not usually express anxiety directly, so it is very important for the nurse to evaluate somatic complaints and perform a careful history.

Health History

Explore the patient's current and past medical history for risk factors such as depression, anxious temperament, family history of anxiety disorders, certain environmental or life experiences (such as parental dysfunction or significant stressful event or trauma), or unstable parental attachment. Elicit the health history, noting history of social inhibition, panic, or "heart racing." Young children may display overactivity, acting out, sleep difficulties, or separation issues. Older children may describe feelings of nervousness, anger, fear, or tension and may display disruptive behavior. Ask the child to choose a number on a scale from 0 to 10 to describe how much he or she worries about things. Have the parent rank the child's worry in the same fashion, and ask the parent what the child worries about most. Determine frequency of headaches and stomachaches. Use a standardized screening tool such as:

- Multidimensional Anxiety Scale for Children (MASC), available at http://harcourtassessment.com
- Spence Children's Anxiety Scale (SACS), available at http://www2.psy.uq.edu.au/%7Esues/scas/
- Preschool Anxiety Scale, available at http://www2.psy.uq.edu.au/%7Esues/scas/preschool.html
- Beck Anxiety Inventory for Youth, available at http://harcourtassessment.com

Physical Examination

Perform a complete physical examination to rule out physiologic causes of the child's symptoms. Note patches of hair loss that occur with repetitive hair twisting or pulling associated with anxiety. Evaluate for evidence of nail biting, sucking blisters, or skin erosion from finger-rubbing. Inspect the entire body for signs of self-injury, which may or may not be present.

Nursing Management

Screen children at well-child or other health care visits, as well as upon admission to the hospital, for anxiety symptoms. If an anxiety disorder is suspected, refer the child to the appropriate mental health provider for further evaluation. When the child is diagnosed with an anxiety disorder and medication is prescribed, teach families about medication administration and adverse effects. Encourage and praise them for follow-through related to cognitive and behavioral therapy or psychotherapy. Provide emotional support to the child and family. Assess the family for the presence of parental anxiety or insecure attach-

ment. Note parenting style and parent–child interactions. Not only the child but also the family will benefit from interventions that improve parent–child relationships, decrease parental anxiety, and foster parenting skills that promote autonomy in the child. Thus, ensure that concurrent family therapy occurs if needed.

Abuse and Violence

Abuse and violence contribute significantly to mental illness in children. Children may suffer from physical or sexual abuse, Münchausen syndrome, or substance abuse.

▶ PHYSICAL AND SEXUAL ABUSE

Physical abuse refers to injuries that are intentionally inflicted and that result in morbidity or mortality. Sexual abuse refers to involvement of the child in any activity meant to provide sexual gratification to an adult. **Neglect** is defined as failure to provide a child with appropriate food, clothing, shelter, medical care, and schooling. A history of childhood abuse is associated with the development of depressive disorders, suicidal ideation and attempts, and alcohol and drug use (Child Welfare Information Gateway, 2006). The Youth Risk Behavior Surveillance Survey reveals some startling statistics about the extent of abuse and violence in the United States:

- 6% of youths have not gone to school on at least one occasion because they thought they would be unsafe.
- Almost 14% have been involved in a physical fight at school.
- 8% have been threatened with a weapon one or more times on school property.
- 9% of youths have been slapped, hit, or intentionally physically hurt by their boyfriend or girlfriend.
- 7.5% have been physically forced to have sexual intercourse when they did not want to (CDC, 2006).

Statistics related to family violence as well as child physical and sexual abuse are difficult to determine, as the perpetrator usually forces the victim into silence. Children usually do not want to admit that their parent or relative has hurt them, partly from feelings of guilt and partly because they do not want to lose that parent. Abuse and violence occur across all socioeconomic levels but are more prevalent among the poor. Despite the lack of adequate statistics, it is well known that the problem of abuse and violence is widespread. Infants represent almost half of all children brought for medical treatment related to abuse (Marino & Fine, 2007). Parents, boyfriends of the child's mother, and stepparents are the most frequent perpetrators. Abuse places children at risk for low self-esteem, depressive disorders, and poor academic achievement. Long-term sequelae of abuse and violence include mood and anxiety disorders, post-traumatic stress disorder, reactive attachment disorder, later substance abuse, perpetuation of the violence cycle, and unknown neurobiologic effects.

Therapeutic management of victims of abuse and violence involves physical treatment of the injury, palliative care in some cases, and intervention to preserve or restore the child's mental well-being as well as family functioning. To protect children, all states require by law that health care professionals report suspected cases of abuse or neglect.

Nursing Assessment

Elicit the health history, noting the chief complaint and timing of onset. Pay particular attention to statements made by the child's parent or caretaker. Is the history given consistent with the injury? Identify abuse and violence by screening all children and families using these questions:

- Questions for children:
  Are you afraid of anyone at home?
  Who could you tell if someone hurt you or touched you in a way that made you uncomfortable?
  Has anyone hurt you or touched you in that way?
- Ask parents:
  Are you afraid of anyone at home?
  Do you ever feel like you may hit or hurt your child when frustrated? (Melnyk et al., 2003)

Note inappropriate sexual behavior for developmental age, such as seductiveness, as this may indicate sexual abuse. Determine if the child has a history of hurting self or others, running away, attempting suicide, or being involved in high-risk behaviors. Assess for risk factors such as poverty, prematurity, cerebral palsy, chronic illness, or mental retardation. Risk factors in parents or caretakers include a history of being abused themselves, alcohol or substance abuse, or extreme stress. Note history of chronic sore throat or difficulty swallowing, which may occur with forced oral sex or sexually transmitted infections. Document history of genital burning or itching (associated with sexual abuse).

> ▶ *Take NOTE!*
>
> *A delay in seeking medical treatment, a history that changes over time, or a history of trauma that is inconsistent with the observed injury all suggest child abuse.*

Physical Examination

Perform a gentle but thorough physical examination, using a soft touch and calm voice. Observe the parent–child interaction, noting fear or an excessive desire to please. Note the infant's level of consciousness. Vigorous shaking in the infant leads to intracranial hemorrhage and shaken baby syndrome. Inspect the skin for bruises, burns, cuts, abrasions, contusions, scars, and any other unusual or suspicious marks. Current or healed scratches or cuts may be found on parts of the body ordinarily covered by clothing in the child who self-mutilates. Burns that occur in a stocking or glove pattern, or only to the soles or palms, are highly suspicious for inflicted burns. Injuries in various stages of healing are also indicative of abuse. Bruises on the chest, head, neck, or abdomen are suspicious for abuse. Nonambulatory children infrequently experience bruises or fractures. Figure 51.1 shows injury sites usually indicative of abuse; Figure 51.2 is a photograph of a child who was beaten with an electric cord. Observe for inflammation of the oropharynx (may occur with forced oral sex). Inspect the anus and penis or vaginal area for bleeding or discharge (sexual abuse).

Laboratory and Diagnostic Tests

Common laboratory and diagnostic studies ordered for the assessment of abuse include:

- Radiographic skeletal survey or bone scan: current or past fractures
- Computed tomography scan of the head: intracranial hemorrhage
- Rectal, oral, vaginal, urethral specimens: sexually transmitted infections such as gonorrhea or Chlamydia

Common nonaccidental injury sites

FIGURE 51.1 Injury sites that are suspicious for abuse.

FIGURE 51.2 Note the mark left from a looped electric cord.

Nursing Management

Refer suspected cases of neglect or abuse to the local child protection agency. In the hospital, contact the social worker. In addition to physical or palliative care needed for the injuries, abused children need to re-develop a sense of trust in adults. Provide consistent care to the abused child by assigning a core group of nurses. Role-model appropriate caretaking activities to the parent or caregiver. Call attention to normal growth and development activities noted in the infant or child, as sometimes parents have expectations of child behavior that may be unrealistic based on the child's age, leading to the abuse. Praise parents and caretakers for taking appropriate steps toward getting help and for providing appropriate care to the child. Refer parents to Parents Anonymous, an organization dedicated to the prevention of child abuse through strengthening of the family (www.parentsanonymous.org). If the child is removed from the family temporarily or permanently, provide the foster or adoptive family with education necessary to assume the child's care.

▶ MÜNCHAUSEN SYNDROME BY PROXY

Münchausen syndrome by proxy (MSBP) is a type of child abuse in which the parent creates physical and/or psychological symptoms of illness or impairment. The adult meets her own psychological needs by having an ill child. MSBP is difficult to detect and may remain hidden for years. In most cases, the biological mother is the perpetrator (Mason, 2007).

Nursing Assessment

Determine the health history, using quotations to document the parent's responses. Observe the mother's behavior with the child, spouse or partner, and staff. Use of covert video surveillance may reveal maternal actions causing illness in the child. Warning signs of MSBP include:

• Child with one or more illnesses that do not respond to treatment or that follow a puzzling course; a similar history in siblings
• Symptoms that do not make sense or that disappear when the perpetrator is removed or not present; the symptoms are witnessed only by the caregiver (e.g., cyanosis, apnea, seizure)
• Physical and laboratory findings that do not fit with the reported history
• Repeated hospitalizations failing to produce a medical diagnosis, transfers to other hospitals, discharges against medical advice
• Parent who refuses to accept that the diagnosis is not medical

Nursing Management

Management of MSBP is complex. Detailed documentation of the history and physical examination is the basis for determining that MSBP is present. Observe the caregiver–child interactions closely, using covert video surveillance if available. When an actual abusive activity is identified, notify the social services and risk management departments of the hospital. Ensure that the local child protection team and the caregiver's family or support system is present when the caregiver is confronted. Inform the caregiver of the plan of care for the child and of the availability of psychiatric assistance for the caregiver.

▶ SUBSTANCE ABUSE

According to the Youth Risk Behavior Survey, over 40% of students drink alcohol, and 25% of them take their first alcoholic drink before age 13. Among youths, 20% use marijuana, almost 8% use some form of cocaine, and about 2% use injectable illegal drugs. In addition, youths report having used heroin, hallucinogenic drugs, methamphetamines, inhalants, and Ecstasy (CDC, 2006). Twenty-five percent of children under 18 years of age are exposed to alcohol abuse in their families (Melnyk et al., 2003).

Nursing Assessment

Note risk factors for substance abuse, such as family history, current parental substance use, dysfunctional family relationships, concurrent mental health disorder, negative life events, or peers who use substances. Determine the child's history, noting altered school performance or attendance, changes in peer group participation, frequent mood swings, changes in physical appearance, or an altered relationship with or perception of parents. Document history of insomnia, appetite loss, excessive itching, sleepiness or extreme fatigue, dry mouth, or shakiness. Note violent behavior, drunkenness, stupor, blank expression, drowsiness, lack of coordination, confusion, incoherent speech, extremes in emotions, aggressive behavior, silly behavior, or rapid speech. Observe for an odor of alcohol or marijuana smoke. Assess the eyes, noting wateriness or dilated pupils. Inspect the nares, noting rhinorrhea or absence of nasal hair. Inspect the fingers for glue smears or discoloration and the skin for needle marks or tracks. Palpate the hands and feet for coolness. Toxicology studies such as urine screening can determine the presence of stimulants, sedative-hypnotics, barbiturates, Quaaludes, opiates, cocaine, and marijuana.

Nursing Management

Help the adolescent to acknowledge that he or she has a problem. Explain the negative consequences of substance use and raise the teen's awareness of risks. Remain empathetic, yet leave responsibility with the adolescent.

Promoting Participation in Treatment Programs

Refer the adolescent to a substance abuse program. Outpatient or day treatment programs are useful in most situations. Family-based programs produce the highest level of recovery. Self-help or 12-step groups are an important element in the recovery process. Serious addiction, the presence of one or more comorbid psychiatric conditions, or suicidal ideation requires residential treatment or hospitalization. See Healthy People 2010.

Preventing Substance Abuse

Teach all children, beginning at the elementary school level, that all chemicals have the potential to be harmful to the body, including tobacco, alcohol, and illicit drugs. Help children to learn problem-solving skills that they can call upon in the future rather than relying on drugs or other substances. Teach children to "just say no." Reinforce that they are the ones who have control over their body and

what they expose it to. Educate children and adolescents that no matter which administration route is used, the drug still enters the body and affects it. Encourage children to participate in the local DARE program (Drug Abuse Resistance Education) and praise them for completing it.

■■■ Key Concepts

- Mental health and behavioral disorders account for the bulk of the "new morbidity" among children and adolescents.
- The child with behavioral problems or mental health issues often has difficulty in the areas of school, peer relationships, and the family, all of which may worsen the child's self-concept, further hindering his or her emotional health.
- Developmental screening is a key component in the evaluation of a child's mental health.
- Various screening tools are available for depression, ADHD, and anxiety.
- Children with autism spectrum disorder often have impaired social interactions as well as altered communication.
- Learning disabilities and ADHD have a significant negative impact on the child's potential for appropriate education.
- Individualized education plans help children with learning disabilities, mental retardation, and ADHD receive the educational support they require to optimize their educational capacity.
- Provide support and education to children with mood or anxiety disordes and their families.
- Educating parents about medication administration and its adverse effects is a critical aspect of nursing management of the child with a mental health disorder.
- Provide nutritional replacement at the appropriate pace in the child with anorexia nervosa. Monitor the child closely for the development of refeeding syndrome.
- A key nursing function is screening all children and their families for abuse and violence.
- Report suspected cases of child abuse to the appropriate authorities.
- Educate children about the dangers associated with substance abuse. Reward and praise children and adolescents who do not experiment with or use alcohol or illicit drugs.

HEALTHY PEOPLE 2010

Objective	Significance
(Developmental) Increase the proportion of persons with co-occurring substance abuse and mental disorders who receive treatment for both disorders.	• Screen all children and adolescents with mental health disorders for the coexistence of substance abuse (and vice versa). • Refer clients to appropriate treatment programs and therapy.

REFERENCES

Accardo, P. J., Accardo, J. A., & Capute, A. J. (2006). Mental retardation. In J. A. McMillan (Ed.), *Oski's pediatrics: Principles and practice.* Philadelphia: Lippincott Williams & Wilkins.

American Academy of Child and Adolescent Psychiatry. (2007a). Practice parameter for the assessment and treatment of children and adolescents' anxiety disorders. *Journal of the American Academy of Child and Adolescent Psychiatry, 46*(2), 267–283.

American Academy of Child and Adolescent Psychiatry. (2007b). Practice parameter for the assessment and treatment of children and adolescents with oppositional defiant disorder. *Journal of the American Academy of Child and Adolescent Psychiatry, 46*(1), 126–141.

American Academy of Pediatrics. (2000). Insurance coverage of mental health and substance abuse service of children and adolescents: a consensus statement. *Pediatrics, 106,* 860–862.

American Association on Intellectual and Developmental Disability. (2007). The AAMR definition of mental retardation. Retrieved January 22, 2007, from http://www.aamr.org/Policies/faq_mental_retardation.shtml.

Barbaresi, W. J., Katusic, S. K., Colligan, R. C., et al. (2006). Long-term stimulant medication treatment of attention-deficit/ hyperactivity disorder: Results from a population-based study. *Journal of Developmental and Behavioral Pediatrics, 27*(1), 1–10.

Beauchesne, M. A., & Kelly, B. R. (2004). Evidence to support parental concerns as an early indicator of autism in children. *Pediatric Nursing, 30*(1), 57–67.

Bothe, D. & Olness, K. (2007). Worried sick: Anxiety among youth, part 1. *Contemporary Pediatrics, 24*(7), 58–63.

Bothe, D. & Olness, K. (2007). Worried sick: Anxiety among youth, part 2. *Contemporary Pediatrics, 24*(8), 82–89.

Centers for Disease Control and Prevention. (2007). *Youth suicide.* Retrieved October 20, 2007 from http://www.cdc.gov/ncipc/dvp/Suicide/youthsuicide.htm.

Centers for Disease Control and Prevention. (2006). Youth risk behavior surveillance—United States, 2005. *Morbidity and Mortality Weekly Report, 55*(SS-5), 1–112.

Child Welfare Information Gateway. (2006). *Long-term consequences of child abuse and neglect.* Retrieved October 20, 2007 from http://www.childwelfare.gov/pubs/factsheets/long_term_consequences.cfm.

Choueiri, R., & Bridgemohan, C. (2005). To make the biggest difference, screen early for autism spectrum disorders. *Contemporary Pediatrics, 22*(10), 54–64.

Compton, S.N., Kratochvil, C.J., & March, J.S. (2007). Pharmacotherapy for anxiety disorders in children and adolescents: An evidence-based medicine review. *Pediatric Annals, 36*(9), 586–598.

Davis, D. W., Burns, B., Snyder, E., et al. (2004). Parent–child interaction and attention regulation in children born prematurely. *Journal for Specialists in Pediatric Nursing, 9*(3), 85–94.

DeNisco, S., Tiago, C., & Kravitz, C. (2005). Evaluation and treatment of pediatric ADHD. *Nurse Practitioner, 30*(8), 14–23.

Dumont-Mathieu, T., Fein, D., & Kleinman, J. (2005). *Screening for autism in young children: The modified checklist for autism in toddlers (M-CHAT).* Retrieved December 27, 2006, from www.dbpeds.org/articles/detail.cfm?TextID=377.

Ellis, C. R., & Schnoes, C. J. (2006). *Eating disorder: Pica.* Retrieved February 18, 2007, from www.emedicine.com/ped/topic1798.htm.

Ellis, C. R., & Schnoes, C. J. (2006). *Eating disorder: Rumination.* Retrieved February 18, 2007, from http://www.emedicine.com/ped/topic2652.htm.

Erickson, C.A., Posey, D.J., Stigler, K.A., & McDougle, C.J. (2007). Pharmacologic treatment of anxiety and related disorders. *Pediatric Annals, 36*(9), 575–585.

Ferren, P. M. (2006). Demystifying the black box warning on antidepressants: A protocol for safe prescribing in your office. *Contemporary Pediatrics, 23*(2), 28–35.

Ford-Martin, P. (2006). Stanford-Binet intelligence scales. *Gale encyclopedia of medicine, vol. 4* (3rd ed., pp. 3517–3518). Detroit: Gale.

Giarelli, E., Souders, M., Pinto-Martin, J., et al. (2005). Intervention pilot for parents of children with autistic spectrum disorder. *Pediatric Nursing, 31*(5), 389–398.

Goldson, E., & Reynolds, A. (2007). Child development and behavior. In W. W. Hay, M. J. Levin, J. M. Sondheimer, & R. R. Deterding, *Current pediatric diagnosis and treatment* (8th ed.). New York: McGraw-Hill.

Harris, J. C. (2006). Depression in childhood and adolescence. In J. A. McMillan (Ed.), *Oski's pediatrics: Principles and practice.* Philadelphia: Lippincott Williams & Wilkins.

Harris, J. C. (2006). Disruptive behavior disorders. In J. A. McMillan (Ed.), *Oski's pediatrics: Principles and practice.* Philadelphia: Lippincott Williams & Wilkins.

Harris, J. C. (2006). Emotional disorders with childhood onset. In J. A. McMillan (Ed.), *Oski's pediatrics: Principles and practice.* Philadelphia: Lippincott Williams & Wilkins.

Harris, J. C. (2006). Mental disorders and psychological stress. In J. A. McMillan (Ed.), *Oski's pediatrics: Principles and practice.* Philadelphia: Lippincott Williams & Wilkins.

Harris, J. C. (2006). Pervasive developmental disorder and autistic disorder. In J. A. McMillan (Ed.), *Oski's pediatrics: Principles and practice.* Philadelphia: Lippincott Williams & Wilkins.

Harris, J. C. (2006). Psychosocial interview. In J. A. McMillan (Ed.), *Oski's pediatrics: Principles and practice.* Philadelphia: Lippincott Williams & Wilkins.

Harris, J. C. (2006). Suicide. In J. A. McMillan (Ed.), *Oski's pediatrics: Principles and practice.* Philadelphia: Lippincott Williams & Wilkins.

Kellogg, N.D., American Academy of Pediatrics, Committee on Child Abuse and Neglect. (2007). Evaluation of suspected child abuse. *Pediatrics, 119*(6), 1232–1241.

Kreipe, R. E. (2006). Eating disorders. In J. A. McMillan (Ed.), *Oski's pediatrics: Principles and practice.* Philadelphia: Lippincott Williams & Wilkins.

Lansford, A. H. (2005). The importance of recognizing a child with bipolar disorder. *Contemporary Pediatrics, 22*(2), 69–78.

Lemmon, K.M., & Stafford, W.M. (20007). Recognizing and responding to child and adolescent stress: The role of the pediatrician, *Pediatric Annals, 36*(4), 225–234.

Malatack, J. J, Consolini, D., Mann, K., & Rabb, C. (2006). Taking on the parent to save a child: Munchausen syndrome by proxy. *Contemporary Pediatrics, 23*(6), 50–63.

Marino, B. S., & Fine, K. S. (2007). *Blueprints: Pediatrics.* Philadelphia: Lippincott Williams & Wilkins.

Mason, J.D. (2007). Munchausen syndrome by proxy. Retrieved October 20, 2007 from http://www.emedicine.com/emerg/topic830.htm.

McClain, N. (2003). Adolescent suicide attempt: Undisclosed secrets. *Pediatric Nursing, 29*(1), 52–53.

Melnyk, B. M., Brown, H. E., Jones, D. C., et al. (2003). Improving the mental/psychosocial health of U.S. children and adolescents: Outcomes and implementation strategies from the national KySS summit. *Journal of Pediatric Health Care, 17*(6), S1–S24.

National Center for Learning Disabilities. (2007). *Mission and history.* Retrieved October 20, 2007 from http://www.ncld.org/content/view/402/458/.

Newcorm, J.H., & Ivanov, I. (2007). Psychopharmacologic treatment of attention-deficit/hyperactivity disorder and disruptive behavior disorders. *Pediatric Annals, 36*(9), 564–574.

Newton, A.W. (2007). Update on child maltreatment. *Current Opinion in Pediatrics, 19*(2), 223–229.

Pinto-Martin, J. A., Souders, M. C., Giarelli, E., & Levy, S. E. (2005). The role of nurses in screening for autistic spectrum disorder in pediatric primary care. *Journal of Pediatric Nursing, 20*(3), 163–169.

Pompili, M., Mancinelli, I., Girardi, P., et al. (2005). Childhood suicide: A major issue in pediatric health care. *Issues in Comprehensive Pediatric Nursing, 28,* 63–68.

Prasher, V.P. & Kapadia, H.M. (2006). Epidemiology of learning disability and comorbid conditions. *Psychiatry, 5*(9), 302–305.

Reasor, J. E., & Farrell, S. P. (2004). Early childhood mental health: Services that can save a life. *Journal of Pediatric Nursing, 19*(2), 140–144.

Scarpa, A., & Raine, A. (2004). The psychophysiology of child misconduct. *Pediatric Annals, 33*(5), 297–304.

Schultz, J. M., & Videbeck, S. L. (2005). *Lippincott's manual of psychiatric nursing care plans.* Philadelphia: Lippincott Williams & Wilkins.

Smith, F. (2007). Safeguarding children: Every nurse's responsibility. *Nursing in Practice: The Journal for Today's Primary Care Nurse, 33,* 40–42.

Smoot, L.C. & Boothby, L.A., & Gillett, R.C. (2007). Clinical assessment and treatment of ADHD in children. *International Journal of Clinical Practice, 61*(10), 1730–1738.

Stevens, S. (2005). Attention deficit/hyperactivity disorder: Working the system for better diagnosis and treatment. *Journal of Pediatric Nursing, 20*(1), 47–51.

U.S. Public Health Service. (2004). Report of the Surgeon Generals' Conference on Children's Mental Health: A national action agenda. Washington, D.C.: Department of Health and Human

Services. Retrieved January 2, 2007, from www.surgeongeneral. gov/topics/cmh/childreport.htm.

Vlam, S. L. (2006). Attention-deficit/hyperactivity disorder: Diagnostic assessment methods used by advanced practice registered nurses. *Pediatric Nursing, 31*(1), 18–24.

Wickham, P. (2004). Retardation. In P. S. Fass (Ed.), *Encyclopedia of children and childhood in history and society, vol. 2* (pp. 712–714). New York: Macmillan.

Zinner, S. H. (2004a). Tourette syndrome—much more than tics: Management tailored to the entire patient. *Contemporary Pediatrics, 21*(8), 38–49.

Zinner, S. H. (2004b). Tourette syndrome—much more than tics: Moving beyond misconceptions to a diagnosis. *Contemporary Pediatrics, 21*(8), 22–36.

Zinner, S. H. (2006c). Tourette syndrome in infancy and early childhood. *Infants and Young Children, 19*(4), 353–370.

WEBSITES

American Academy of Child and Adolescent Psychiatry: www. aacap.org

American Association of Intellectual and Developmental Disability: www.aamr.org

Academy for Eating Disorders: www.aedweb.org

American Foundation for Suicide Prevention: www.afsp.org

American Autism Society: www.autism-society.org

Autism Online: www.autismonline.org

Child and Adolescent Bipolar Foundation: www.bpkids.org

Center for Learning Differences: www.centerforlearningdifferences.org

Children and Adults with Attention-Deficit/Hyperactivity Disorder: www.chadd.org

Child Abuse Prevention Network: http://child-abuse.com

Child Welfare Information Gateway: www.childwelfare.gov

Developmental and Behavioral Pediatrics Online: www.dbpeds.org

National Center on Education, Disability, and Juvenile Justice: www.edjj.org

Office of Safe and Drug-Free Schools: www.ed.gov/about/offices/list/osdfs/index.html

Family Violence Prevention Fund: http://endabuse.org

To order the Pervasive Developmental Disorders Screening Test-II (PDDST-II): www.harcourtassessment.com

Help Autism Now Society: www.helpautismnow.com

Learning disabilities and ADHD: www.ldonline.org

Association of Child and Adolescent Psychiatric Nurses: www.ispn-psych.org/html/acapn.html

Substance Abuse and Mental Health Services Administration's (SAMHSA) National Mental Health Information Center: http://mentalhealth.samhsa.gov/child/childhealth.asp

Alcohol and drug information from Prevention Online: http://ncadi.samhsa.gov

Depression and bipolar support alliance: http://www.ndmda.org/

National Eating Disorders Association: www.nationaleating disorders.org

National Center for Learning Disabilities: www.ncld.org

National Center for Mental Health and Juvenile Justice: www.ncmhjj.com

National Child Traumatic Stress Network: www.nctsnet.org/nccts/nav.do?pid5hom_main

National Institute on Alcohol Abuse and Alcoholism: www.niaaa.nih.gov

National Institute of Mental Health: www.nimh.nih.gov

Parents Anonymous (child abuse prevention): www.parents anonymous.org

Prevent Child Abuse U.S.A.: www.preventchildabuse.org

Shaken Baby Alliance: www.shakenbaby.com

Stop Family Violence: www.stopfamilyviolence.org

CHAPTER WORKSHEET

MULTIPLE CHOICE QUESTIONS

1. The nurse is caring for a child with ADHD. Which behavior would the nurse *not* expect the child to display?

   a. Moody, morose behavior with pouting.

   b. Interruption and inability to take turns.

   c. Forgetfulness and easy distractibility.

   d. Excessive motor activities and fidgeting.

2. An adolescent girl who has been receiving treatment for anorexia nervosa has failed to gain weight over the past week despite eating all of her meals and snacks. What is the priority nursing intervention?

   a. Increase the teen's daily caloric intake by at least 500 calories.

   b. Ensure that the teen's entire fluid intake includes calories.

   c. Supervise the teen for 2 hours after all meals and snacks.

   d. Assess the teen's anxiety level to determine need for medication.

3. A 15-year-old patient has been making demands all day, exaggerating her every need. She is now crying, saying she has nothing to live for and threatening to kill herself. What is the priority nursing action?

   a. Ignore her continued exaggerated and melodramatic behavior.

   b. Consult with the physician to increase her antidepressant dose.

   c. Leave the girl alone for a little while until she composes herself.

   d. Take the girl's suicidal threat seriously and provide close supervision.

4. When trying to manage aggressive or impulsive behaviors in children or adolescents, what is the best nursing intervention?

   a. Train the child to be assertive.

   b. Provide consistency and limit-setting.

   c. Allow the child to negotiate the rules.

   d. Encourage the child to express feelings.

5. The nurse is caring for an adolescent who says, 'I'm sick of this, I wish I weren't alive anymore." What is the best response by the nurse?

   a. "I often feel sad and sick of things."

   b. "Have you thought about hurting yourself?"

   c. "Are you trying to escape your problems?"

   d. "Do your parents know about this feeling?"

CRITICAL THINKING EXERCISES

1. A mother tells you that her son's behavior is unmanageable, and she is having difficulty coping with it. The boy is argumentative and is bullying others. He is struggling with his schoolwork because he has difficulty staying on task, gets out of his chair often, and frequently distracts others. What additional assessments should you obtain? What interventions would be helpful in managing the boy's behavior?

2. A 14-year-old moderately retarded boy is able to feed himself but is incontinent. Discuss the issues his family must deal with.

STUDY ACTIVITIES

1. Explore several of the websites related to child abuse prevention listed at the end of this chapter. Develop a list of resources for families in your local area.

2. Attend a group therapy session during your pediatric clinical rotation. Observe the children's verbal and nonverbal communication, noting inconsistencies or other interesting observations.

3. Visit a school for autistic children. Spend time with the various specialists who work with children with ASD, determining their roles and the effect the treatment they are providing has on the children. Report your findings to your classmates.

4. Attend a local CHADD meeting. Talk to parents about having a child with ADHD.

NURSING CARE DURING A PEDIATRIC EMERGENCY

KEY TERMS

asystole
barotrauma
bradycardia
cardioversion
cricoid pressure
defibrillation

hypercapnia
hyperventilation
hypocapnia
hypoventilation
intubation
periodic breathing

tachycardia
tachypnea
tracheal (endotracheal)
tube

LEARNING OBJECTIVES

Upon completion of the chapter, the learner will be able to:

1. Identify various factors contributing to emergency situations among infants and children.
2. Discuss common treatments and medications used during pediatric emergencies.
3. Conduct a health history of a child in an emergency situation, specific to the emergency.
4. Perform a rapid cardiopulmonary assessment.
5. Discuss common laboratory and other diagnostic tests used during pediatric emergencies.
6. Integrate the principles of the American Heart Association (AHA) and Pediatric Advanced Life Support (PALS) in the comprehensive management of a pediatric emergency.

Alma Anderson, age 8 years, has been admitted to the pediatric unit. Her mother calls the nurse into the room, stating, "Alma's having trouble breathing!"

WoW
A nurse must possess the knowledge and skills to aid an acutely ill child.

Children are uniquely vulnerable to a range of emergency situations. These situations are often life-threatening if not treated in an efficient manner. Because of their developmental level, children are at a greater risk for traumatic injury, near-drowning, and poisoning than adults. Most pediatric cardiopulmonary arrests result from respiratory failure or shock. Data suggest that children who have a cardiopulmonary arrest requiring resuscitative measures rarely fare well. For these reasons, the American Heart Association (AHA) has delineated two distinct "chains of survival," one for adults and one for children, that should be followed during a life-threatening situation.

The adult chain of survival is:

1. Early emergency medical system (EMS) activation
2. Early cardiopulmonary resuscitation (CPR)
3. Early defibrillation
4. Early access to advanced care

In contrast, the pediatric chain of survival is:

1. Prevention of cardiac arrest and injuries
2. Early CPR
3. Early access to emergency response system
4. Early advanced care

Considering the special risks that threaten children, the AHA has also developed specific guidelines for Pediatric Advanced Life Support (PALS). Courses in PALS are offered for health care professionals so that they can provide expert care for children in emergencies. This chapter emphasizes the principles of PALS in its discussion of the nurse's role in the management of pediatric emergencies.

▶ *Take* NOTE!

New PALS guidelines published in 2005 define "pediatric patient" as any child up to about 16 to 18 years of age. Children in this age group should be managed using the PALS guidelines rather than those for adults (AHA, 2005f).

HEALTHY PEOPLE 2010

Objective	Significance
Increase the number of states and the District of Columbia that have implemented guidelines for pre-hospital and hospital pediatric care.	• Become politically active in your local area and at the national level. • Advocate for optimal care for infants, children, and adolescents.

Common Medical Treatments

A variety of medications and other medical treatments are used in pediatric emergencies. Most of these treatments will require a physician's order when the child is in the hospital, though some emergency departments and pediatric units may have standing orders for pediatric emergencies. The most common medical treatments and medications used in pediatric emergencies are listed in Common Medical Treatments 52.1 and Drug Guide 52.1. The nurse should be familiar with these procedures and medications, how they work, and nursing implications.

▶ *Take* NOTE!

*Certain emergency drugs for children may be given via a **tracheal tube** (a tube inserted into the trachea that serves to maintain the airway and facilitate artificial respiration). Use the mnemonic LEAN (lidocaine, epinephrine, atropine, and naloxone) to remember which drugs may be given via the tracheal route (AHA, 2007). In certain cases, when an emergency drug is given via a tracheal tube, the dosage must be increased. In addition, drugs given via this route should usually be diluted with 2 to 5 mL of sterile saline and followed by multiple positive-pressure ventilations to ensure that the drugs are delivered.*

NURSING PROCESS OVERVIEW FOR THE CHILD IN AN EMERGENCY SITUATION

The nurse may encounter a pediatric emergency in a variety of settings. As a member of a trauma team at a pediatric hospital, the nurse may participate in the stabilization of a child who has suffered a near-drowning or trauma. The emergency department nurse may encounter a child who has just been injured, such as from a fall, accident, or sports. On the hospital unit, a child with asthma may suffer respiratory distress or stop breathing. Regardless of the setting or how the emergency developed, the principles for managing pediatric emergencies are the same.

Care of the child in an emergency includes all components of the nursing process: assessment, nursing diagnosis, planning, interventions, and evaluation. In an emergency, the nurse must act quickly, intervening immediately when an abnormality is determined upon assessment. When evaluating a child who presents emergently, always follow the AHA's guidelines for basic life support: evaluate airway, then breathing, then circulation. No matter what the cause of the emergency, the general approach

COMMON MEDICAL TREATMENTS 52.1 PEDIATRIC EMERGENCIES

Treatment	Explanation	Indication	Nursing Implications
Suctioning (oropharyngeal, nasopharyngeal, tracheal, or tracheostomy)	Removal of secretions via bulb syringe or suction catheter	Excessive airway secretions affecting airway patency	Use caution and suction only as far as recommended for age, tracheal tube size, or tracheostomy tube size or until coughing or gagging occurs.
Oxygen	Supplementation via mask, nasal cannula, hood, or tent or via tracheal/nasotracheal tube	Hypoxemia, respiratory distress, shock, trauma	Monitor response via color, work of breathing, respiratory rate, oxygen saturation levels via pulse oximetry, and level of consciousness.
Bag-valve-mask ventilation	Provision of ventilation via a bag-valve-mask device, manual ventilation	Apnea, ineffective ventilation and oxygenation with spontaneous breaths, extremely slow respiratory rate	Ensure adequate chest rise with ventilation. Do not overventilate or bag aggressively to avoid barotrauma. Maintain a seal on the child's face with the appropriate-sized mask. Ensure the oxygen supply tubing is connected to 100% oxygen.
Intubation	Insertion of a tube into the trachea to provide artificial ventilation	Apnea, airway that is not maintainable, need for prolonged assisted ventilation	Determine adequacy of breath sounds with bagging immediately upon insertion of the tracheal tube. Assess for symmetrical chest rise. Tape tube securely in place and note number marking on the tube. Connect to ventilator when available.
Needle thoracotomy	Insertion of a needle between the ribs into the pleural space to remove air	Tension pneumothorax	There should be a rush of air as the needle reaches the air space. Monitor breath sounds, work of breathing, pulse oximetry. Ensure patency of IV catheter.
IV fluid therapy	Administration of crystalloid or colloid solutions to provide hydration or improve perfusion	Altered perfusion states such as respiratory distress, shock, trauma, cardiac disturbances	Use intraosseous route if a peripheral IV cannot be obtained quickly in the young child in shock. Reassess respiratory and circulatory status frequently after each IV fluid bolus and during continuous infusion.
Blood product transfusion	Administration of whole blood, packed red blood cells, platelets, or plasma intravenously	Trauma, hemorrhage	Follow institution's transfusion protocol. Double-check blood type and product label with a second nurse.

Treatment	Explanation	Indication	Nursing Implications
			Monitor vital signs and assess child frequently to identify adverse reaction to blood transfusion. If adverse reaction is suspected, immediately discontinue transfusion, infuse normal saline solution IV, reassess the child, and notify the physician.
Cervical stabilization	Maintenance of the cervical spine in an immobile position	Trauma, near-drowning	Use the jaw-thrust maneuver without head tilt to open the airway. Maintain cervical stabilization until the cervical spine x-rays are cleared by the physician or radiologist.
Defibrillation and synchronized cardioversion	Provision of electrical current to alter the heart's electrical rhythm	Defibrillation: ventricular fibrillation and pulseless ventricular tachycardia Synchronized cardioversion: supraventricular tachycardia and ventricular tachycardia with a pulse	In the pulseless client, always ensure CPR is ongoing while the defibrillator is being readied. Ensure adequate oxygenation. Provide lidocaine or epinephrine if indicated before defibrillation. Sedate the child if time allows.

to managing the child is universal, with minimal specific variations. Once the child's cardiopulmonary status is stabilized or the child is resuscitated, assessment and management will vary depending on the cause of the emergency.

Assessment

Nursing assessment of the child who presents emergently includes health history, physical examination, and laboratory and diagnostic testing. However, the initial history may be focused and very brief if the child is critically ill; the nurse may need to proceed immediately to rapid cardiopulmonary assessment. Once a child is stabilized, a more comprehensive history is obtained. Laboratory tests, while often important, should never take priority over cardiopulmonary and hemodynamic stabilization.

Remember Alma, the 8-year-old with breathing trouble? What additional health history and physical examination assessment information should the nurse obtain?

Health History

Obtain the health history rapidly while simultaneously evaluating the child and providing life-saving interventions. A brief history is needed initially, followed by a more thor-

ough history after the child is stabilized. The parents or caregiver will provide information about the child's chief complaint. Record the information using the caregiver's own words. For example, the caregiver might say, "He's been having trouble breathing" if the child is presenting in respiratory distress. If the child was injured in a bicycle accident, the caregiver might say, "She was riding her bike down the hill and lost control." This brief statement provides guidance for obtaining more in-depth information about the emergency.

Ask about any significant past history that may affect the care of the child. For example, children who are medically fragile, who were born prematurely, or who have a significant genetically linked disease (e.g., sickle cell anemia) may require special consideration when planning and implementing care.

Physical Examination

In an emergency, the nurse must perform a rapid cardiopulmonary assessment and intervene immediately if alterations are noted. The remainder of the physical examination then follows.

Rapid Cardiopulmonary Assessment

As the brief history is being obtained, begin to evaluate the ABCs of the rapid cardiopulmonary assessment: A, airway; B, breathing; and C, circulation. Since pediatric

DRUG GUIDE 52.1 COMMON MEDICATIONS USED IN PEDIATRIC EMERGENCIES

Medication	Action/Indication	Nursing Implications
Adenosine (antiarrhythmic)	Slows conduction through AV node, restoring normal sinus rhythm Supraventricular tachycardia (SVT)	• Administer IV at a dose ranging from 0.05 to 0.1 mg/kg. • Administer very rapidly (1 to 2 seconds) followed by a rapid, generous saline flush. • Repeat every 1 to 2 minutes, increasing by 0.05 to 0.1 mg/kg with each dose (maximum dose 0.3 mg/kg). • Monitor for shortness of breath, dyspnea, worsening of asthma.
Atropine (anticholinergic)	Increases cardiac output, dries secretions, inhibits serotonin and histamine Sinus bradycardia, asystole, pulseless electrical activity	• Administer via IV, IO, or ET route at a dose of 0.02 mg/kg (maximum dose 0.5 mg child, 1 mg adolescent). • Repeat every 5 minutes PRN. • Give undiluted over 30 seconds for IV or IO route. • Dilute with 3 to 5 mL normal saline for ET route; follow with five positive-pressure ventilations. • Do not mix with sodium bicarbonate (incompatible).
Dobutamine (synthetic catecholamine)	Beta-adrenergic agent primarily affecting beta-1 receptors; increases myocardial contractility and heart rate Ongoing short-term management of shock (hypovolemic and cardiogenic)	• Administer via IV or IO route at 2 to 20 mcg/kg/minute via a continuous infusion. Monitor for development of ventricular arrhythmias. • Expect to titrate infusion rate based on cardiac output and BP. • Administer via central line if possible due to risk of extravasation. • Monitor child closely, preferably in an ICU setting.
Dopamine (inotropic)	Increases cardiac output, BP, and renal perfusion (beta-adrenergic agonist) Bradycardia, hypotension, and poor cardiac output	• Administer via IV or IO route at a dose of 2 to 20 mcg/kg/minute via continuous infusion. • Ensure that child has received adequate fluid resuscitation prior to administration. • Due to risk of extravasation, give via central line if possible. • Monitor child closely, preferably in an ICU setting. • Assess for ventricular arrhythmias.
Epinephrine (adrenergic)	Stimulates alpha- and beta-adrenergic receptors, increasing heart rate and systemic vascular resistance Bradycardia, anaphylaxis	• Administer via IV or IO route at a dose of 0.01 mg/kg (0.1 mL/kg of 1:10,000 solution) or via ET route at 0.1 mg/kg (0.1 mL/kg of 1:1,000 solution). • During CPR, repeat every 3 to 5 minutes. • Monitor for ventricular arrhythmias. • High doses may cause tachycardia in newborns. • Due to risk of extravasation and subsequent tissue necrosis, give through a central line if possible. • May also be used as a bronchodilator IV or via inhalation (racemic epinephrine)

Medication	Action/Indication	Nursing Implications
Glucose	Increases blood glucose level Hypoglycemia	• Administer via IV or IO route at a dose of 1 to 2 mL/kg (D50%); maximum dose 2 to 4 mL/kg. • When administering via a peripheral IV line, dilute 1:1 with sterile water to make D25%. Monitor IV site for infiltration and tissue extravasation. • Monitor blood glucose levels closely.
Lidocaine (anti-dysrhythmic)	Decreases automaticity of conduction tissues of the heart Ventricular arrhythmias	• Administer via IV or IO route at a dose of 1 mg/kg; administer via ET route at dose 2 times IV dose diluted with 3 to 5 mL normal saline, followed by positive-pressure ventilation. Maximum dose 5 mg/kg or 100 mg/dose. • Monitor ECG continuously. • Contraindicated in complete heart block • With larger-than-normal doses, monitor for hypotension or seizures.
Naloxone (Narcan)	Antagonizes action of narcotic agents Reversal of respiratory depression related to narcotic effects	• Administer via IV, IO, SC, or ET route at a dose of 0.01 to 0.1 mg/kg in children <5 years old or <20 kg or at a dose of 2 mg in children >5 years old or >20 kg. Onset of action is within 2 to 5 minutes. • May repeat dose as necessary; narcotic effects outlast therapeutic effects of naloxone.

arrests are usually related primarily to airway and breathing, and usually only secondarily to the heart, focus the assessment and interventions using the ABCs of resuscitation. Always perform the assessment and interventions in that order. In most circumstances, if a child's airway is properly managed and breathing is assisted, the child may not experience a full arrest requiring chest compressions.

▶ **Take** NOTE!

Assessment and management of the airway of a pre-arresting or arresting child is ALWAYS the first intervention in a pediatric emergency. Intervene if there is an airway problem before moving on to assessment of breathing. If an intervention for breathing is required, start it before proceeding to assessment of circulation.

A: Airway Evaluation and Management

First evaluate the airway. Assess its patency. If cervical spine injury is not suspected, position the airway in a manner that promotes good air flow. If secretions are obstructing the airway, suction the airway to remove them. If the child is unconscious or has just been injured, open

the airway using the head tilt–chin lift maneuver. Place the fingertips on the bony prominence of the child's chin and lift the chin to open the airway. Simultaneously, place one hand on the forehead and tilt the child's head back (Fig. 52.1). If the airway is not maintainable, reposition the airway for appropriate airflow. Place the child immediately on oxygen at 100% and apply a pulse oximeter to monitor oxygen saturation levels.

▶ **Take** NOTE!

If cervical spine injury is a possibility, do not use the head tilt–chin lift maneuver; use only the jaw-thrust technique for opening the airway (see trauma section for explanation and illustration).

B: Breathing Evaluation and Management

After establishing an open airway, look for signs of respiration. Turn your head and place your ear over the child's mouth to "look, listen, and feel" for spontaneous respirations. Look to see if the child's chest is rising, listen for air escaping, and note if you feel any air coming out of the child's nose or mouth. If the child is breathing, evaluate the quality of the respirations: Is ventilation effective, or is the child simply gasping ineffectively for air? Count the

FIGURE 52.1 Head tilt–chin lift maneuver in a child.

respiratory rate. Observe the child's color. Note depth of respiration, chest rise, adequacy of air flow in all lung fields, and presence of adventitious sounds. Evaluate for increased work of breathing and the use of accessory muscles.

When signs of respiratory distress are noted, immediately place the child on oxygen at 100% and apply a pulse oximeter to monitor oxygen saturation levels. If the child is breathing shallowly and has poor respiratory effort, attempt to reposition the airway to promote better airflow. For the child receiving 100% oxygen who does not improve with repositioning, begin assisted ventilation with a bag-valve-mask (BVM) device. A need for ongoing BVM ventilation may require airway **intubation** (process by which a breathing tube, such as a tracheal tube, is inserted into a child's airway to assist with breathing).

▶ *Take* NOTE!

Attempts to insert a tracheal tube should last no longer that 20 to 30 seconds each. After each attempt, the child should receive multiple ventilations by the BVM method using 100% oxygen.

C: Circulation Evaluation and Management

The next step is to evaluate C, circulation. During this phase, evaluate the heart rate, pulses, perfusion, skin color and temperature, blood pressure, cardiac rhythm, and level of consciousness. Determine the heart rate via direct auscultation or palpation of central pulses. Radial and brachial pulses are more difficult to palpate, espe-

cially in infants and young children. If perfusion is poor, such as with shock or cardiac arrest, the child may have a weak pulse or no pulse. In the young infant, check the brachial artery for a pulse. In the child and adolescent, evaluate the carotid pulse. If there is a pulse, note its quality: Is it barely palpable or weak? Is it strong or bounding? Compare the strength and quality of central and peripheral pulses. Assess capillary refill time.

▶ *Take* NOTE!

ALWAYS evaluate the presence of a heart rate by auscultation of the heart or by palpation of central pulses. NEVER use the cardiac monitor to determine if the child has a heart rate. The presence of a cardiac rhythm is not a reliable way to evaluate the ability to perfuse the body. In certain circumstances a rhythm continues but there is no pulse (pulseless electrical activity). If the child has no heart rate (pulse) despite adequate respiratory interventions, begin cardiac compressions.

Evaluate the child's perfusion by noting skin temperature and color. Is the skin pink? Is it warm to the touch? The child's skin may be cool to the touch and may appear pale, mottled, or cyanotic. As the child's condition worsens with developing shock and cardiovascular compromise, note a line of demarcation of skin temperature. In this situation, the distal extremities will feel cooler than the proximal regions of the body. Measure the blood pressure (BP) and place the child on a cardiac monitor to evaluate the cardiac rhythm. Note the child's sensorium or level of consciousness; if circulation is poor, the child will demonstrate an altered level of consciousness as perfusion to the brain becomes diminished.

▶ *Take* NOTE!

According to PALS, calculate minimum acceptable systolic BP by using this formula: 70 + (2 times the age in years). For example, a 4-year-old should have a minimal systolic BP of 78: 70 + (2 × 4) = 78.

If the circulation or perfusion is compromised, then fluid resuscitation is necessary. Establish large-bore intravenous (IV) access immediately and administer isotonic fluid rapidly. Provide 20 mL/kg of normal saline (NS) or lactated Ringer's (LR) as an IV bolus (if the infant is less than 1 month old, administer 10 mL/kg). If peripheral IV access cannot be obtained in the child with altered perfusion within three attempts or 90 seconds, assist with insertion of an intraosseous needle for fluid administration (refer to shock section for further information about intraosseous access). Central venous lines or cutdown access may also be used, but these measures take longer to accomplish.

Additional Physical Examination Components

In addition to assessing and stabilizing the child's airway, breathing, and circulation, perform a thorough physical examination and assess pain.

Neurologic Evaluation

Quickly evaluate the sensorium in an older child. Ask the child to state his or her name. Ask what happened to the child. Does the child know what day it is? Is the child aware of where he or she is?

If the child is an infant, evaluate his or her interest in the environment and response to parents. An infant who is not interested in the environment or seems unable to recognize his or her parents is a cause for concern. In contrast, an infant who enjoys sucking on a finger and making eye contact with the nurse during the assessment is reassuring.

Evaluate the child's head. In the infant or young toddler, palpate the anterior fontanel to determine if it is normal (soft and flat), depressed, or full. A sunken fontanel is associated with volume depletion from dehydration or blood loss. If the fontanel is full, note if it is bulging or tense, which may indicate increased intracranial pressure. Next assess the eyes. Are they open or closed? If closed, do they open spontaneously, to voice, to pain? Does the child focus on and follow your movements? Evaluate the pupils for equality and reactivity. Sluggish pupillary reaction may occur with increased intracranial pressure.

> ▶ **Take** NOTE!
> A nonreactive pupil is an ominous sign indicating a need for immediate relief of increased intracranial pressure.

Evaluate the child's face. Does the child smile or cry? Does the child react to playfulness with a laugh? Does the young infant cry vigorously? Are facial movements equal? In a child, a normal or near-normal neurologic examination can be a reassuring sign. Conversely, obtunded or muted responses to environmental stimuli are a cause for concern.

Next evaluate for spontaneous movement of the extremities. Young infants cannot walk, so assess their ability to move their arms and legs and grossly evaluate the tone of their extremities. Does the infant vigorously and equally move the arms and legs? Is the muscle tone nor-

mal, or does the infant appear floppy or flaccid? When evaluating the older child, note whether he or she is ambulatory alone, ambulatory with assistance, or unable to walk. Note whether the child has use of the upper extremities. In the case of trauma, the child may arrive immobilized on a backboard. In this scenario, evaluate the child's motor responsiveness and sensation in each extremity, comparing findings bilaterally while the child is in the supine position. Ask the child if he or she feels you touching each extremity. Ask the child to squeeze your fingers and to wiggle the toes. This will provide information about cerebral integrity and perfusion, cerebellar health, and spinal cord integrity.

The Pediatric Glasgow Coma Scale may also be used to evaluate the neurologic status in children. Chapter 37 provides a more in-depth discussion of this scale.

Skin and Extremity Evaluation

Remove the child's clothing and thoroughly examine the skin for bruising, lesions, or rashes. If the child has a rash, note the size, shape, color, configuration, and location. Apply pressure to the rash with the fingertips to see whether it blanches. Inspect the trunk, abdomen, and extremities for abrasions or deformities.

> ▶ **Take** NOTE!
> Rashes that do not blanch may be classified as petechiae or purpura. This type of rash may be associated with certain serious conditions, such as meningococcemia. Report this finding to the physician or nurse practitioner immediately.

Pain Assessment

In emergencies, children may experience pain as a direct result of the injury or disease, and life-saving interventions such as resuscitation, insertion of IV lines, and administration of medications may cause further pain. The child's pain may also be exaggerated by light, noise, movement of the stretcher or bed, and the sensations of cold or heat. Nurses play a key role in minimizing the child's pain, and this may decrease the child's future distress (Johnston et al., 2005; Probst et al., 2005). If the child is awake and verbal, use an age-appropriate pain assessment scale to determine the child's pain level. If the child is sedated or unconscious, assess pain with a standardized scale that relies on physiologic measurements as well as behavioral parameters. Refer to Chapter 35 for additional information on pain assessment in children.

Laboratory and Diagnostic Testing

A number of laboratory and diagnostic tests may be ordered in a pediatric emergency. Laboratory tests can help to distinguish the cause of the emergency or additional problems that need to be treated. Standard laboratory tests obtained in most emergency departments include:

- Arterial blood gases (ABG), obtained initially and then serially to assess for changes
- Electrolytes and glucose levels
- Complete blood count (CBC)
- Blood cultures
- Urinalysis

If an ingestion is suspected, then a toxicology panel will be obtained. In suspected sepsis, erythrocyte sedimentation rate (ESR), C-reactive protein (CRP), and urine and spinal fluid cultures may also be obtained. The pediatric trauma victim may have additional laboratory tests performed, including amylase, liver enzymes, and blood type and cross-match.

Diagnostic tests may include radiologic tests, computed tomography (CT) scanning, and magnetic resonance imaging (MRI). One advantage of radiologic diagnostic testing is that the tests are relatively noninvasive. A disadvantage of CT and MRI scans is that before they can be performed, the patient must be stabilized. Common Laboratory and Diagnostic Tests 52.1 discusses the tests most commonly used in pediatric emergencies.

After completing an assessment of Alma, the nurse noted the following: a patent airway, anxious but able to speak in short sentences, and skin temperature cool on the extremities. Based on these assessment findings, what would your top three nursing diagnoses be for Alma? Describe appropriate nursing interventions.

Nursing Diagnoses and Related Interventions

After completing a thorough assessment and initial stabilization of the child, the nurse might identify several nursing diagnoses, including:

- Airway clearance, ineffective
- Breathing pattern, ineffective
- Gas exchange, impaired
- Fluid volume, deficient
- Cardiac output, decreased
- Tissue perfusion (cardiopulmonary, peripheral cerebral, or renal), ineffective
- Knowledge, deficient
- Fear
- Family processes, interrupted

Specific nursing goals, interventions, and evaluation for the child in an emergency are based on the nursing diagnoses. Additional information about nursing management will be included later in the chapter as it relates to specific disorders.

Providing Cardiopulmonary Resuscitation

Always evaluate and manage the airway first, unless this is an out-of-hospital, witnessed, sudden collapse of a child. Call for help and assign someone to obtain the automatic external defibrillator (AED). Open the airway and assess for adequate breathing. If the child is not breathing, begin rescue breathing. Check for a pulse. In the child, the carotid or femoral pulses are easiest to assess. In the past, it was recommended that the brachial pulse be checked in the infant, but this is often difficult, so an alternative is to check the femoral pulse. Carefully assess for signs of a pulse, but do not spend more than 10 seconds checking the pulse. If there is not a pulse or if the heart rate is less than 60 beats per minute, begin chest compressions.

> ▶ *Take* NOTE!
>
> *When an arrest occurs out of the hospital and is a witnessed, sudden collapse, initial management is slightly different than that for other arrests. In these sudden, witnessed events, phone first, get the AED, and return to start CPR.*

Table 52.1 presents the AHA's most recent recommendations for ratios of breaths and compressions. These recommendations stress the importance of properly performed chest compressions. Therefore, several changes have been made to the guidelines:

- Rescuers must provide compressions of adequate rate and depth.
- Chest recoil should be allowed.
- Minimal interruption of chest compressions should be the goal.
- For infant CPR, two-person infant CPR can be performed by encircling the chest with two thumbs and simultaneously using the hands to provide a thoracic squeeze.
- For two-person CPR, no pauses should occur for ventilation, with the compressing health care provider giving continuous compressions.

Providing Defibrillation or Synchronized Cardioversion

In some cases, the child has an abnormal life-threatening cardiac rhythm or an arrhythmia that does not respond to pharmacologic therapy or leads to hemodynamic instability. In these cases, electrical therapy, in the form of defibrillation or synchronized cardioversion, may be needed.

Defibrillation is the use of electrical energy to depolarize the cells of the myocardium to terminate an abnormal life-threatening cardiac rhythm, such as ventricular fibrillation. Defibrillation is used in conjunction with oxygen, CPR, and medications. The effects of defibrillation are

COMMON LABORATORY AND DIAGNOSTIC TESTS 52.1 PEDIATRIC EMERGENCIES

Test	Explanation	Indications	Nursing Implications
Chest x-ray	Radiograph used to evaluate heart and lung structures	To identify: • Infections (e.g., pneumonia) • Foreign body • Injury • Endotracheal tube placement • Central line placement • Pneumothorax Re-evaluation of lungs after chest tube placement	• X-rays can be obtained quickly during resuscitation; usually available in emergency department. • Assist the child to lie still if necessary.
Computed tomography (CT)	Use of high radiation (equivalent to about 100 to 150 chest x-rays) with computer processing targeting specific body areas	Rapid evaluation of tissues and skeletal areas Superior test for the evaluation of internal bleeding	• Expect the child to be transported out of the area for the study. • Accompany the child to provide continued observation and management, especially if child's condition is unstable.
Magnetic resonance imaging (MRI)	Incorporation of responses of hydrogen protons to a dynamic magnetic field	Superior test for the evaluation of the spinal cord and the cerebrospinal fluid spaces; less useful in emergency situations	• Administer sedation as ordered. • Assist child in remaining still; MRI requires child to remain still for a longer period than for a CT. • Assist the conscious child to deal with fear related to loud banging noise of the machine.
Arterial blood gases (ABG)	Evaluation of blood pH and arterial blood levels of oxygen and carbon dioxide	Evaluation of quality of respiration and evaluation of acid–base balance	• Anticipate serial ABGs to assess for status changes. • Never delay resuscitation efforts pending blood gas results.
Serum electrolytes	Evaluation of electrolyte levels, such as sodium, potassium, and chloride, in the blood	Useful for determining baseline and if dehydration is hypertonic or isotonic	• Hemolysis of specimen may lead to falsely elevated potassium levels.
Glucose	Evaluation of glucose level in the blood	Valuable for determining need for supplementation, as in the case of hypoglycemia	• Use Accucheck or other rapid glucose test at the bedside or obtain serum blood specimen. • Elevated glucose levels can be associated with stress or with use of corticosteroids.
Toxicology panel (blood and/ or urine)	Determination of most commonly abused mood-altering medications, as well as commonly ingested drugs	Drug abuse, overdose, or poisoning	• Standard toxicology panel varies with the agency. • Follow agency protocol; may require special handling or labeling of specimen. • Use a blood specimen that is best for determining overdose or poisoning.

(continued)

COMMON LABORATORY AND DIAGNOSTIC TESTS 52.1 PEDIATRIC EMERGENCIES (continued)

Test	Explanation	Indications	Nursing Implications
Complete blood count (CBC)	Evaluation of hemoglobin and hematocrit, white blood cell count, and platelet count	Any condition in which anemia, infection, or thrombocytopenia is suspected Trauma if blood loss is suspected	• Be aware of normal values and how they vary with age and gender. • Hemoglobin and hematocrit may be elevated secondary to hemoconcentration in the case of hypovolemia.
Blood type and cross-match	Determination of ABO blood typing as well as presence of antigens Cross-match is performed on RBC-containing products to avoid transfusion reaction.	Trauma victim or any person with suspected blood loss as preparation for transfusion	• Handle specimen gently to avoid hemolysis. • Ensure that specimen request and label are appropriately signed and dated. • Apply "type and cross" or "blood band" to child at time of specimen collection if required by agency. • Most type and cross-match specimens expire after 48 to 72 hours.
Urinalysis	Evaluation of color, pH, specific gravity, and odor of urine Assessment for protein, glucose, ketones, blood, leukocyte esterase, RBCs, WBCs, bacteria, crystals, and casts	Clients with fever, dysuria, flank pain, urgency, or hematuria or those who have experienced trauma to provide information about the urinary tract	• Many drugs can affect urine color; notify the laboratory if the child is taking one. • Notify the laboratory and document on the laboratory form if the client is menstruating. • Refrigerate the specimen if it is not processed promptly. • Specimen may be obtained by catheterization, clean-catch voiding sample, or a U-bag.

enhanced in an oxygen-rich environment coupled with good artificial circulation (CPR). **Cardioversion**, another means of applying electrical current to the heart, is used when the child has supraventricular tachycardia (SVT) or ventricular tachycardia with a pulse. Cardioversion may also be enhanced with medications. Cardioversion is deliv-

ered synchronized—that is, the electrical current is applied on the R wave of the electrocardiogram (ECG).

The basic defibrillator is equipped with adult- and pediatric-sized paddles. A switch turns the machine on and controls are used to select the amount of energy (joules). Typically, the initial energy amount is 2 joules/kg; it can be

TABLE 52.1 RATIOS OF BREATHS TO COMPRESSIONS

Age	One-Person CPR	Two-Person CPR
Infant	• 30 compressions to 2 breaths • Hand placement: two fingers, placed one fingerbreadth below the nipple line	• 15 compressions to 2 breaths • Hand placement: two thumbs encircling the chest at the nipple line
Child	• 30 compressions to 2 breaths • Hand placement: heel of hand or two hands (adult position in larger child), pressing on the sternum at the nipple line	• 15 compressions to 2 breaths • Hand placement: heel of one hand or two hands (adult position in larger child), pressing on the sternum at the nipple line

American Heart Association. (2005e). Part 11: Pediatric basic life support. *Circulation, 112,* 156–166.

increased up to 4 joules/kg for defibrillation. Energy for cardioversion is delivered at 0.5 to 1 joule/kg.

When the defibrillator is being used in an acute care setting, the leader of the code team will take charge of defibrillator use. He or she is responsible for ensuring that only the patient receives the energy from the defibrillator. The code team leader will count to 4 before delivering a shock to the patient to ensure that all personnel and other equipment are clear of the bed to avoid accidental shock.

Using Automated External Defibrillation

In cases of sudden, witnessed, out-of-hospital collapse, an arrhythmia is often the cause. Therefore, the AHA has revised its recommendations about the use of an AED. An AED is an alternative to manually defibrillating a patient. The AED device consists of electrodes that are applied to the chest. These electrodes are used to monitor the heart rhythm and deliver the electrical current. AED devices are readily available in a variety of locations, such as airports, sports facilities, and businesses. Traditionally, the AED was designed for use in adults, but newer AEDs with smaller pads and the ability to alter energy delivery are now more readily available. Therefore, the AHA has recommended that an AED be used for children who are older than age 1 year who have no pulse and have suffered a sudden, witnessed collapse.

The AED is designed to be used by persons in the prehospital setting. Once the AED is turned on, the machine uses auditory commands to guide laypersons and health care professionals alike through the correct placement of the electrodes and the administration of energy. The AED periodically evaluates the victim's cardiac rhythm and instructs the user about checking the pulse, continuing CPR, and delivering shocks. Nurses who care for children should be able to operate an AED and be prepared to use it in nontraditional settings.

Determining Medication Doses and Equipment Sizes

Many pediatric acute care facilities prepare code reference sheets when a child is admitted. This sheet uses the child's actual weight to determine medication doses and equipment sizes. The reference sheet is kept on a clipboard at the child's bedside or taped on the wall at the head of the bed. An additional copy is placed in the child's chart.

Ambulatory care providers often use the Broselow tape to estimate the child's weight based on the child's length (Fig. 52.2). The tape is color-coded and emergency equipment for a child of that size is stored in corresponding color-coded packages or in color-coded drawers on the pediatric emergency cart (DeBoer et al., 2005). Medication doses and equipment sizes are also located on the tape. The most accurate calculation for code medications

---

EVIDENCE-BASED PRACTICE 52.1
The Role of Automated External Defibrillators (AEDs) in Cardiac Resuscitation of Children

● Background
Primary cardiac arrest resulting from arrhythmia or commotio cordis is rare in children and adolescents but often has a very poor outcome. Also, sudden death during sporting events has occurred in children and adolescents. Traditionally, manual defibrillation has been the only form of defibrillation used in children. With the newer technology available in AEDs, the question arose as to whether they could be used effectively to treat arrhythmia in children.

▲ Study
Cecchin et al. (2001) performed a study of over 600 children to determine the specificity and sensitivity of automated external defibrillation in children.

■ Findings
The researchers found that AEDs can be sensitive and specific for detecting and treating arrhythmia by defibrilla-

tion in children over 1 year of age. Salib et al. (2005) report a positive and healthy outcome after an AED was used at the scene on a 13-year-old who suffered a baseball blow to the chest resulting in commotio cordis. As a result of these and many other studies, in 2005 the American Heart Association recommended changes in the pediatric basic life support guidelines to include the use of AEDs in sudden witnessed collapse in children.

● Nursing Implications
For nurses working in hospitals, ensure that witnessed collapse in children includes assessing for the need for defibrillation. Outside the hospital, nurses should advocate for AEDs to be placed in all high school gymnasiums and at all parks and ball fields.

Cecchin, F., Jorgenson, D. B., Berul, C. I., et al. (2001). Is arrhythmia detection by automatic external defibrillator accurate for children? Sensitivity and specificity of an automatic external defibrillator algorithm in 696 pediatric arrhythmias. *Circulation, 103,* 2438–2483; Salib, E. A., Cyran, S. E., Cilley, R. E., Maron, B. J., & Thomas, N. J. (2005). Efficacy of bystander cardiopulmonary resuscitation and out-of-hospital automated external defibrillation as life-saving therapy in commotio cordis. *Journal of Pediatrics, 147,* 863–869.

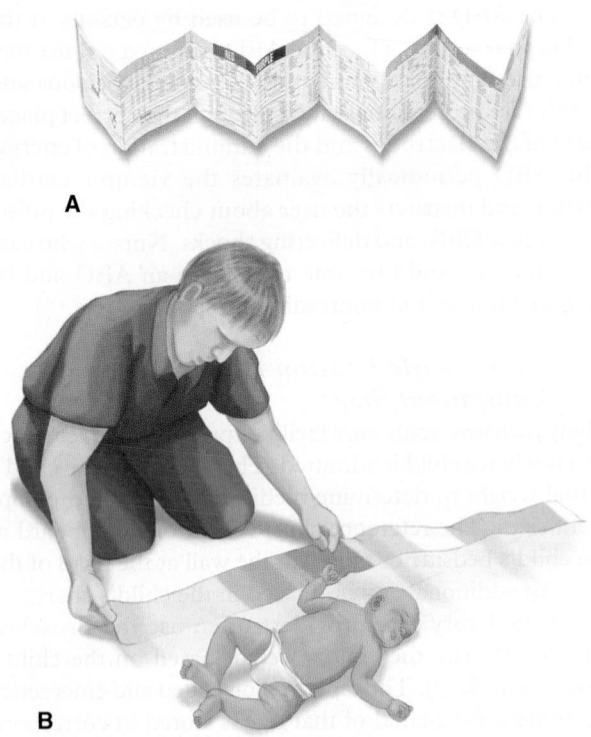

FIGURE 52.2 (**A**) Broselow tape. (**B**) Measure the child's length with the Broselow tape to determine medication doses and tracheal tube size.

is based on the child's weight, but in numerous research studies, use of the Broselow tape for estimating the weight has been shown to be successful except in the case of very obese children (Hashikawa et al., 2007).

Managing Pain

Depending on the child's status and pain level, individualize pain management interventions. For the alert child, nonpharmacologic measures may be used in addition to medications. Provide atraumatic care for procedures and use aggressive pharmacologic treatments to manage pain as the child's condition allows. Refer to Chapter 35 for additional information on pain management strategies.

Ensuring Stabilization

After a child has been resuscitated, the nurse plays a key role in stabilization and transport. Thoroughly document the interventions that were performed as well as the ongoing assessment of the child's response to the interventions. Provide continued monitoring of the child while awaiting transport. Copy and assemble any pertinent documentation, such as the resuscitation record, nurse's notes, and laboratory test results, that will be given to the receiving institution. Ensure that all lines are taped securely and that vascular access sites are dressed and labeled with the date and time of insertion. As soon as possible, bring the child's family in to visit with the child. Provide explanations about the IV lines, monitoring equipment, and other med-

ical equipment and devices. Encourage the family to talk to and touch the child.

Providing Support and Education to the Child and Family

The experience of respiratory distress, oxygen deprivation, and an emergency situation is a frightening one for persons of all ages. The life-saving interventions that take place during an emergency can be especially intimidating and upsetting to children. Infants and young children cannot understand explanations about these interventions, and older children and adolescents may feel frightened and angry about the loss of control. The caregivers may feel fear, anger, guilt, and sadness. They may be concerned about the very real possibility that their child might die.

Resuscitation of a child is often a perplexing and frightening event for laypersons to observe. Therefore, traditionally family members have been excluded during the resuscitation of children. Recently, however, there has been a trend to allow family members to be present during pediatric resuscitation. Current evidence-based practice guidelines recommend individual evaluation of each family to determine whether allowing their presence during the resuscitation will be beneficial (Nibert & Ondrejka, 2005).

Considering the highly technical nature of resuscitation, the rapidity with which interventions occur, and the fear associated with a life-threatening event, nurses can play a crucial role in providing understandable explanations to families, coupled with empathic support. During the acute phase, the nurse should give brief explanations as life-saving interventions are being provided. Examples of these types of explanations include:

- When applying the pulse oximeter sensor: "I need to put this little light on Johnny to check his oxygen level; it won't hurt."
- When connecting the child to the cardiac monitor: "We're going to put these sticky patches on Johnny and connect them so we can monitor his heart rate on this screen."
- When preparing for intubation and ventilation: "Johnny can't breathe on his own right now, so we're going to give him some extra help with this tube. This tube will go through his breathing passage and this machine will help him to breathe."

The nurse plays a key role in providing empathy and support. Do not provide false reassurance and say, for example, "He's going to be alright." The outcome is never certain. Rather, communicate empathically. For example, say, "This must be very difficult for you. We're doing everything we can to help Johnny." Provide honest answers in a reassuring manner. Respect each family's diversity and observe their strengths and weaknesses. Be nonjudgmental in all interactions with families, even when the child's emergency situation may have resulted from family neglect.

Parents often feel helpless when their child is in a high-tech environment. Suddenly overwhelmed with the equipment and monitoring devices, they no longer are the persons who are the most skilled in caring for their child. Integrate the child's parents into the health care team. Suggest ways the parents can make the hospital experience more normal for their child. For example, simply allowing a father to read a story to his daughter or encouraging a mother to hold her child's hand is therapeutic both for the child and the parents. Be aware of this dramatic change and how it affects the parents. Always ensure that they feel like they are a welcome part of their child's care.

Providing the child with familiar comfort objects helps to decrease stress. Once the intubated child is alert and stabilized, assist him or her with communication. Some children can lift one finger for yes and two fingers for no. If the child is old enough to write, provide paper and pencil. Play is essential to the work of the child, and even if he or she is immobile, play is still possible. Puppets at the bedside and books help give the child a more normal experience in a scary situation that is far from the norm. Teenagers may enjoy listening to music through headphones. Even children who are comatose should be talked to and allowed to listen to familiar music.

Even if the outcomes are serious, the nurse can provide critical support to children and families. Whether hugging a crying mother or playing "peek-a-boo" with an intubated child, the nurse will be the one who can make a difference during a frightening experience.

Nursing Management of Children in Emergencies

Nurses must be adept at identifying the beginning stages of an emergency so they can quickly and appropriately intervene to prevent deterioration to cardiopulmonary arrest. Assessment and management of the most common types of emergencies in children are discussed below. The topics covered include respiratory arrest, shock, cardiac arrhythmias and arrest, near-drowning, traumatic injury, and poisoning.

▶ RESPIRATORY ARREST

Respiratory emergencies may lead to respiratory failure and eventual cardiopulmonary arrest in children. Infants and young children are at greater risk for respiratory emergencies than adolescents and adults because they have smaller airways and underdeveloped immune systems, resulting in a diminished ability to combat serious respiratory illnesses. Young children often lack coordination, making them susceptible to choking on foods and small objects, which may also lead to cardiopulmonary arrest. In addition, sudden infant death syndrome (SIDS) is a leading cause of cardiopulmonary arrest in young infants

and thus is one of the leading causes of post-neonatal mortality in the United States. For these reasons, nurses must be skilled at recognizing the signs of pediatric respiratory distress so they can prevent progression to cardiopulmonary arrest. Table 52.2 lists some of the more common causes of pediatric respiratory arrest.

TABLE 52.2 CAUSES OF RESPIRATORY ARREST IN CHILDREN

Condition	Cause
Upper airway	Burns Croup Epiglottitis Foreign body aspiration Reflux Strangulation or near-strangulation Tracheomalacia Vascular ring
Lower airway	Asthma Bronchiolitis Burns Foreign body aspiration Pertussis infection Pneumonia Pneumothorax Reflux
Nonrespiratory origins	Septic shock HIV
Neurologic	CNS infection Guillain-Barré syndrome Poliomyelitis Seizures Sleep apnea Spinal cord trauma Sudden infant death
Chronic illness	Complications of severe prematurity Cystic fibrosis Bone marrow transplant Neutropenia
Metabolic/ endocrine disorders	Diabetic ketoacidosis Mitochondrial disorders
Cardiac conditions	Arrhythmia Congenital cardiac problems Acquired cardiac problems
Traumatic/ unintentional/ intentional injury	Asphyxia Child abuse/"shaken baby syndrome" Drowning Electrocution Gunshot wound Toxic ingestion Vehicular-related trauma

Adapted from Balwin, G. (2001). *Handbook of pediatric emergencies.* Philadelphia: Lippincott Williams & Wilkins; Behrman, R. E., Kliegman, R. M., & Jenson, H. B. (2004). *Nelson's textbook of pediatrics* (17th ed.). Philadelphia: Saunders.

Nursing Assessment

If the child has severe respiratory compromise, obtain a brief history while simultaneously providing respiratory interventions. To obtain the history, use the following questions as a guide:

• When did the symptoms begin and when do they occur?
• Did the symptoms have a sudden onset (as with a foreign body aspiration)?
• How have the symptoms progressed?
• Is the cough continual, intermittent, or worse at night or with exercise?
• Has there been any stridor? (Stridor is heard upon inhalation and may be associated with swelling of the trachea [as with croup] or with a foreign body in the upper airway.)
• Is there wheezing? If so, is the wheezing on inspiration or on expiration, or both?
• What makes the symptoms better and what makes them worse?
• Does drinking from a bottle induce the symptoms (as with gastroesophageal reflux–induced aspiration)?
• Is the child taking any medication for the symptoms? Does the child or do any members of the immediate family have a history of chronic respiratory disease, such as asthma?
• Are the child's immunizations up to date?
• Was the child born prematurely? If so, did the child require mechanical ventilation? For how long?
• Were there any respiratory problems during the first few days of life?
• When did the child last eat? (This question is important because a recent meal will increase the child's risk of aspiration in the event of a respiratory arrest. In addition, the presence of food in the stomach will increase the risk of aspiration during tracheal intubation.)

If the child can communicate, ask how he or she is feeling. Is he or she short of breath? Does his or her chest hurt? Observe the child while speaking. Children who are in respiratory distress may speak in short sentences with gasping between words.

Physical Examination

In an emergency, physical examination is often limited to inspection, observation, and auscultation. First, quickly survey the respiratory status. Determine if the child is breathing.

Inspection and Observation

Establish if the airway is patent, maintainable, or unable to be maintained. The child with a patent airway is breathing without signs of obstruction. The maintainable airway remains patent independently by the child or with interventions such as a towel roll under an infant's neck

or the insertion of a nasal trumpet. The airway that cannot be maintained does not remain patent unless a more aggressive intervention, such as the insertion of a tracheal tube, is performed.

Look at the child's posture. Is the child sitting up, leaning forward, and drooling, as with epiglottitis? Observe the child's face: does he or she appear anxious or relaxed? Children in respiratory distress often appear anxious. Look at the nose and mouth. Are the nares patent? Is there noticeable nasal congestion or mucus coming from the nose? Note nasal flaring or mouth breathing. Observe for head bobbing. Listen for audible expiratory grunting or inspiratory stridor. Note the child's color. Does the child appear pale, mottled, dusky, or cyanotic? Children may appear mottled in response to poor oxygenation, hypothermia, or stress. Children with severe respiratory compromise may appear dusky. Look for cyanosis around the mouth or on the trunk. Cyanosis is a late and often ominous sign of respiratory distress. Central cyanosis is more likely to be associated with respiratory or cardiac compromise. In contrast, peripheral cyanosis is more likely to be associated with circulatory alteration.

> ▶ *Take NOTE!*
>
> *Closely inspect the color of the area around the mouth. Circumoral pallor is a sign of poor oxygenation.*

Evaluate the pattern and quality of respiration, noting the respiratory rate. **Tachypnea** (increased respiratory rate) is often noted in children in respiratory distress. However, seriously ill children grunt and may have normal or subnormal respiratory rates. **Hypoventilation**, a decrease in the depth and rate of respirations, is noted in very ill children or children who have central respiratory depression secondary to narcotics. If the child is a young infant (less than 2 months) or premature, periodic breathing may occur. **Periodic breathing** is regular breathing with occasional short pauses (brief periods of apnea). After the apneic pause, the infant will breathe rapidly (up to 60 breaths per minute) for a short period and then will resume a normal respiratory rate. In general, the infant who has periodic breathing looks pink and has a normal heart rate. Observe for the use of accessory muscles in the neck or retractions in the chest, determining the extent and severity of the retractions.

Auscultation

Auscultate the lungs with the diaphragm of the stethoscope. Breath sounds over the tracheal region are higher-pitched and are described as "vesicular," while breath sounds over the peripheral lung fields tend to be lower-pitched, known as "bronchial." Instruct the child to take deep breaths with the mouth open. To encourage the young child to exhale strongly, instruct him or her to "blow out" the penlight (as with a candle) or to blow on a tissue. Encourage the child not to breathe more rapidly than normal (to prevent **hyperventilation** [increased depth and rate of respirations]) and to avoid making any noises with the mouth.

> ▶ *Take* NOTE!
>
> *Significant upper respiratory congestion often interferes with assessment of the lower airways because the sound is easily transmitted throughout the chest. Differentiate between the upper and lower airway noises by listening with the stethoscope over the nose. You may be able to determine whether the noise is nasal or bronchial by using this technique.*

Auscultate the child's chest systematically. Listen in all anterior, axillary, and posterior regions, comparing the left to the right sides. Note any decreased or absent breath sounds, which may be the result of bronchial obstruction (as with mucous infection) or air trapping (as in children with asthma). Unilateral absent breath sounds are associated with foreign body aspiration and pneumothorax.

> ▶ *Take* NOTE!
>
> *Sometimes a child's respiratory status is so severely compromised that little or no air movement is noted. This commonly occurs during a severe asthma exacerbation. Minimal or no air movement requires immediate intervention.*

Note the presence and location of adventitious breath sounds such as crackles, wheezes, or rhonchi. Document the presence of a pleural friction rub (a low-pitched, grating sound), a sound resulting from inflammation of the pleura (RNCeus, 2006).

Palpation

Palpate the chest for any abnormalities. In the older, less severely ill, and cooperative child, assess for tactile fremitus. Using the palm of the hand, palpate over the lung regions in the same manner as for auscultation and percussion while the child says, "ninety-nine." Increased vibrations elicited during this maneuver are associated with consolidating conditions, such as pneumonia.

Percussion

Percuss the interspaces of the chest between the ribs in the same systematic fashion as with auscultation. Nor-

mally, percussion over an air-filled lung reveals resonant sounds. Note the presence of hyperresonance, which may indicate an acute problem such as a pneumothorax or a chronic disease such as asthma. In contrast, percussion sounds will be dull over a lobe of the lung that is consolidated with fluid, infectious organisms, and blood cells, as in the case of pneumonia.

Laboratory and Diagnostic Testing

Use continuous pulse oximetry if respiratory status is a concern. Note and report oxygen saturation levels below 95%. (See Chapter 39 for additional information about use of the pulse oximeter.)

Additional tests may reveal:

- Arterial or capillary blood gases: hypoxemia, hypercarbia, altered pH
- Chest x-ray: alterations in normal anatomy or lung expansion, or evidence of pneumonia, tumor, or foreign body
- Metal detector: evidence of metallic foreign body. Novel as it may sound, metal detectors have been found to be highly accurate (99%) in detecting the presence of ingested coins in children (Lee et al., 2005).

> ▶ *Take* NOTE!
>
> *Children with cardiac conditions resulting in cyanosis often have baseline oxygen saturations that are relatively low because of the mixing of oxygenated with deoxygenated blood.*

Nursing Management

The basic principle of pediatric emergency care and PALS is prevention of cardiopulmonary arrest. Therefore, the nurse must rapidly assess and appropriately manage children who have signs of respiratory distress. Nursing management of the child in respiratory distress involves maintaining a patent airway, providing supplemental oxygen, monitoring for changes in status, and in some cases assisting ventilation. In addition to providing these lifesaving measures and monitoring the child's progress, offer support and education to the child and family.

Maintaining a Patent Airway

When a child exhibits signs of respiratory distress, make a quick decision about whether it will be safe to allow the child to stay with the parent or whether the child must be placed on the examination table or bed. For example, in the case of croup, the child will often breathe more comfortably and experience less stridor while in the comfort of the parent's lap. Many children in respiratory distress often are most comfortable sitting upright, as this position helps to decrease the work of breathing by allowing appropriate diaphragmatic movement. In contrast, a child with a decreasing level of consciousness may need to be placed in the supine position to facilitate positioning of the airway.

The infant will benefit from a small sheet or towel folded under the shoulders. This will facilitate positioning the infant's airway in the "sniff" position, as is recommended by AHA's Basic Cardiac Life Support (BCLS) guidelines (Fig. 52.3). Avoid neck flexion or hyperextension, which may completely occlude the infant's airway. In children over age 1 year, the optimal method for opening the airway is to hyperextend the neck, as recommended by AHA BCLS. If a cervical spine injury is not suspected, use the head tilt–chin lift technique to open the airway. If the child has suffered head or neck trauma and cervical spine instability is a concern, use the jaw-thrust maneuver by placing three fingers under the child's lower jaw and lifting the jaw upward and outward (Fig. 52.4). In either case, never place the hand under the neck to open the airway.

Often the nurse encounters an acutely ill child who cannot maintain an airway independently but may be able to do so with some assistance. For example, sometimes simply opening the airway and moving the tongue away from the tracheal opening is all that is required to regain airway patency. In certain conditions, a nasopha-

Figure 52.4 Jaw-thrust technique for opening the airway.

ryngeal or oropharyngeal airway may be necessary for airway maintenance. Comparison Chart 52.1 provides additional information about these types of airways.

Assisting Ventilation

The child in respiratory distress may ventilate poorly, hypoventilate, or tire and become apneic. In this case, the child may require assistance with ventilation through BVM ventilation, tracheal intubation, or a laryngeal mask airway. Table 52.3 explains these methods.

Providing Bag-Valve-Mask Ventilation

BVM ventilation is used in the management of children who cannot ventilate or oxygenate effectively on their own. This technique is a more efficient way of ensuring ventilation than using only supplemental oxygen. In addition, resuscitating a child in this manner is superior to mouth-to-mouth resuscitation as it provides higher oxygen concentrations and protects the nurse from exposure to oral secretions. However, this technique requires proper training and practice. The proper procedure involves appropriate opening of the airway followed by providing breaths with the BVM.

Ventilation with the BVM may be performed with either one or two rescuers. First, choose an appropriate-sized bag and a corresponding face mask that fits the infant or child. Self-inflating bags are usually available in neonatal, infant, child, and adult sizes. Corresponding masks are available. Choose a face mask that properly fits the child's face and that provides a seal over the nose and mouth and excludes the eyes, thus preventing any pressure on the eyes (Fig. 52.5).

Figure 52.3 (A) The infant and young child's prominent occiput encourages flexion of the neck and may result in airway occlusion. (B) Putting a towel roll under the shoulders helps to open the infant's or young child's airway by placing it in the neutral or "sniff" position.

► **Take** *NOTE!*

Face masks should be clear so that the nurse can see the child's lip color and identify any emesis during resuscitation. Older face masks, which were black, should no longer be used.

COMPARISON CHART 52.1 OROPHARYNGEAL VERSUS NASOPHARYNGEAL AIRWAYS

Oropharyngeal airway (used only in unconscious children)	• Consists of a simple plastic curved body that has a central air channel to allow for aeration • Is used when an unconscious child has difficulty maintaining airway patency due to upper airway obstruction, such as from the tongue • Allows for oral suction • Determine the correct size of the airway by placing it next to the child's cheek with the tip pointing down. An airway that is too large will extend past the angle of the child's mandible and can obstruct the glottic opening when inserted. • Choose the airway that best fits the child to decrease the risk of injury to the structures of the mouth.
Nasopharyngeal airway (may be used in conscious children and children who have an intact gag reflex)	• Consists of a flexible curved tube that is inserted nasally • Is used when the child has difficulty maintaining airway patency due to tongue obstruction or palate problems, when neurologic impairment causes poor pharyngeal tone, or in the child with impaired consciousness • Allows for nasopharyngeal suction • When selecting this airway, keep in mind that the diameter of the airway should not be so large that it puts too much pressure on the internal nasal tissue. There are two common methods for measuring this airway: 1) Measure the distance from the end of the child's nose to the tragus of the ear; 2) Look at the child's fifth digit, which is usually the approximate diameter of the nasopharyngeal airway. • Monitor for mucosal irritation, nasal septum swelling, and laceration of the adenoids. • Do not use this type of airway in children with a history of bleeding disorders and basilar skull fractures. • This airway's small diameter can easily become obstructed with secretions and blood.

Connect the BVM via the tubing to the oxygen source and turn on the oxygen. When resuscitating infants and children, set the flow rate at approximately 10 L/minute. For an adolescent who is adult-sized, set the flow rate at 15 L/minute or higher to compensate for the larger-volume bag. Check to make sure that the oxygen is flowing through the tubing to the bag. Self-inflating bags do not provide "free-flow" oxygen out of the face mask; manual pumping of the bag is necessary. However, the bags have a corrugated plastic tail that allows oxygen to freely flow. Therefore, check over the tail for oxygen flow through the bag.

After opening the airway appropriately (see above), place the mask over the child's face. When one rescuer is providing ventilation (commonly referred to as "bagging"), the person must provide a seal with the mask over the child's face with one hand and use the other hand to manipulate the resuscitator bag. The hand used to provide the mask seal will simultaneously maintain the airway in an open position. Generally, use the left thumb and index finger to hold the mask on the child's face. While maintaining a good seal with the mask, use upward pressure on the jaw angle while pressing downward on the mask below the child's mouth to keep the mouth open (Fig. 52.6). Take care not to put pressure on the neck with the fourth and fifth fingers.

If adequate personnel are available, a more desirable situation involves one person standing behind the child's head to maintain an open airway and to provide a seal of the mask over the face with a hand on each side (usually the thumbs and second fingers). A second rescuer stands on one side of the child and compresses the bag to ven-tilate the child using both hands. If the child is more difficult to ventilate, the two-rescuer method allows the ventilating nurse to provide better ventilation than with the one-rescuer method. In addition, the two-rescuer method ensures the best possible mask seal, as the rescuer holding the mask can use both hands to maintain the seal.

Regardless of the number of persons present, proper placement of the face mask is critical, and a good seal must be maintained throughout the resuscitation. In addition, during ventilation, use only the force and tidal volume necessary to cause a chest rise, no more. If a good chest rise is not observed, attempt to open the airway again. It may be necessary to adjust the position of the airway a few times to achieve a patency conducive to ventilation.

Compress the bag to deliver breaths at the amount recommended in infants and children. Initially, provide two rescue breaths and observe for a chest rise. Rescue breaths should not overinflate the lungs. Breaths should be delivered over 1 second. After the first two rescue ventilations, perform rescue breathing at a rate of one breath every 3 to 5 seconds, or about 12 to 20 breaths per minute. Delivering each breath should be a steady, one-inhalation-to-one-exhalation ratio. This means that the amount of time delivering the inspiratory ventilation is equal to the amount of time that expiration is allowed. While ventilating the infant or child, work with, not against, any spontaneous respiratory effort; in other words, if the child is breathing out, do not attempt to force air in at the same time.

If the child is unconscious and a third rescuer is available, that person can apply cricoid pressure. **Cricoid pressure** (also known as the Sellick maneuver) is the use

TABLE 52.3 AIRWAY AND VENTILATION METHODS

Method	Description	Comments
Anesthesia bag or flow-inflating ventilation systems	A small, collapsible bag that consists of a reservoir bag, an overflow port, and a fresh gas inflow port	• Adjustment of the oxygen flow and of the outlet control valve is necessary. • Useful in providing positive end-expiratory pressure (PEEP) or continuous positive airway pressure (CPAP) • Adequate training and significant skill are needed to properly operate this device. • Hypercapnia and barotrauma may result with improper use. • Used more commonly in the post-anesthesia care unit (PACU) and in the neonatal intensive care unit
Bag-valve-mask device or manual resuscitator	A self-inflating oxygen delivery bag that does not require an oxygen source for resuscitation and ventilation. The bag can be connected to oxygen to provide higher oxygen levels than room air. When the child exhales, the non-rebreathing valve closes, allowing exhaled, deoxygenated air to escape.	• Effective in providing oxygen to a child who is in severe respiratory distress or who has suffered a respiratory arrest • A more efficient method of respiratory resuscitation than mouth-to-mouth resuscitation; decreased rescuer exposure to communicable disease • Most medical personnel can be trained to perform resuscitation with this method. • Possibly tiring for the rescuer when used to ventilate a child for long periods of time (see discussion on bag-mask ventilation)
Laryngeal mask airway	An inflatable silicone mask and rubber connecting tube that is inserted blindly into the airway, forming a seal	• The airway is introduced into the pharynx and advanced until it meets resistance; balloon cuff is then inflated. • Easier insertion than a tracheal tube • Usually used in the unconscious child who benefits from bag-valve-mask ventilation but does not require intubation • Improvement in client comfort
Tracheal intubation	A plastic tube inserted in the trachea to establish and maintain an airway when the airway cannot be maintained effectively using other measures (e.g., nasal trumpet or bag-valve-mask ventilation)	• Skilled medical professional (physician, nurse practitioner, respiratory specialist, EMT, or physician's assistant) necessary for insertion • The nurse acts as a valuable assistant during the intubation procedure.

of gentle pressure to occlude the esophagus, preventing air from entering the stomach (Fig. 52.7). Cricoid pressure may help to prevent vomiting secondary to gastric distention. Vomiting during resuscitative efforts can complicate the situation because the child is at risk of aspirating abdominal contents.

Monitoring Effectiveness of Ventilation
During the resuscitation, continually reassess the child's response to the resuscitative efforts, noting:

• Adequacy of chest rise
• Absence or minimal presence of abdominal distention
• Improved heart rate and pulse oximetry readings
• Improved color

• Capillary refill less than 3 seconds with strengthening pulses

If the child's status deteriorates and he or she becomes pulseless, then CPR must be started. In addition, periodically and briefly stop ventilating to evaluate for spontaneous respirations.

Preventing Complications Related to Bag-Valve-Mask Ventilation
During resuscitation, health care personnel usually exhibit high energy levels, a normal physiologic response that facilitates resuscitative efforts as the rescuers act quickly. However, this heightened state can lead to overzealousness while ventilating an infant or child. Health care providers

FIGURE 52.5 The mask should form a seal over the nose and mouth, across the chin and nose bridge.

may inadvertently ventilate the child too rapidly using too much tidal volume, leading to excessive ventilation volume and increased airway pressure. This poor technique can be detrimental to the child, causing:

• Reduced cardiac output (due to increased intrathoracic pressure and increased cardiac afterload)

FIGURE 52.6 Proper hand placement for maintaining airway and adequate mask seal using one-rescuer technique.

FIGURE 52.7 Applying cricoid pressure.

• Air trapping
• **Barotrauma** (trauma caused by changes in pressure)
• Air leak (thus reducing the oxygen delivered to the child)

In addition, children with head injury who receive excessive ventilation volumes and high rates may develop:

• Decreased cerebral blood flow
• Cerebral edema
• Neurologic damage (adapted from AHA, Pediatric Advanced Life Support, 2001b)

Thus, nurses must be mindful of their technique during bagging, not exceeding the recommended respiratory rate or providing too much tidal volume to the child. Ventilate the child in a controlled and uniform manner, providing just enough volume to result in a chest rise.

Assisting With Tracheal Intubation

Tracheal intubation is needed if the infant or child does not have a maintainable airway or will require artificial ventilation for a prolonged time. Intubation of infants and children is a procedure that requires great skill and therefore should be performed by only the most qualified and experienced personnel. Children are most commonly intubated orally, rather than nasally, in acute situations.

Nurses are an essential part of the intubation team, usually assisting a physician, nurse practitioner, respiratory therapist, or physician's assistant during the intubation procedure (Nursing Procedure 52.1). The nurse may set up the equipment, prepare and administer intubation medications, or assist with suctioning the oral secretions and preparing the tape to secure the tracheal tube. In a child in full arrest, the nurse might be responsible for performing ongoing chest compressions while other team members manage the child's airway.

Setting Up Equipment

Appropriate setup and preparation of equipment is essential (Table 52.4). The tracheal tube size used depends on the child's size. To calculate tracheal tube size, divide the child's age by 4 and add 4. The resulting number will in-

Nursing Procedure 52.1

ASSISTING WITH TRACHEAL INTUBATION

1. Prepare equipment and supplies.
2. Draw up medications (for rapid sequence intubation).
3. Turn up the volume on the cardiac monitor so that members of the team can easily hear the audible QRS indication of the child's heart rate and note any bradycardia with the procedure.
4. Turn on the suction. Make sure that suction is working by placing your hand over the tubing before you attach the suction catheter.
5. Continue to ventilate the child with the BVM and 100% oxygen as the team prepares to intubate the child.
6. When there is no suspected cervical spine injury, in the child over age 2 years, place a small pillow under the child's head to facilitate opening of the airway; this step is unnecessary in children younger than age 2 due to the prominence of their occiput.
7. When assisting with the intubation, stand beside the patient's head and prepare to assist with suctioning of oral secretions, applying cricoid pressure during the insertion of the tube, providing BVM as needed, and assisting with securing the tube with tape.
8. Before the initial intubation attempt and after each subsequent attempt to intubate, provide several inhalations of 100% oxygen via the BVM ventilation method (optimally for a few minutes).
9. Administer premedication and medications for sedation.
10. Administer paralyzing medication.
11. Observe as the health care professional who is intubating the child follows the recommended procedure for intubation using the laryngoscope to visualize the vocal cords.
12. As the tracheal tube is inserted, apply gentle cricoid pressure (too much pressure can block the trachea) if appropriate.

dicate the size of the tracheal tube in millimeters. For example, if the child is 2 years old, the proper-sized tube would be 4.5 ([2/4] + 4 = 4.5). Always have one size smaller ready also, so have a 4.0 and a 4.5 tracheal tube for this child.

Administering Medications

Several medications are often given to facilitate intubation of children. Premedicating a child before passing a tracheal tube aids in the following:

• Reducing pain and anxiety (consistent with the concept of atraumatic care)

• Minimizing the effects of passing the tracheal tube down the airway (vagal stimulation leading to **bradycardia** [decrease in heart rate])
• Preventing hypoxia
• Reducing intracranial pressure
• Preventing airway trauma and aspiration of stomach contents

The use of medications during the intubation process is known as rapid sequence intubation (Table 52.5). Typically, these medications are used in controlled settings such as the emergency department or the intensive care unit. Rapid sequence intubation is done only in children who are not experiencing cardiac arrest. If the intubation is expected to be particularly difficult, paralyzing medication should not be used.

The nurse must be aware of the differences in the various medication classes, their advantages, disadvantages, and adverse effects. The nurse must also be able to distinguish between medications that produce sedation and ones that produce analgesia. Children who are paralyzed and sedated may be suffering severe pain. The pain control needs of children who are acutely ill are of paramount importance and cannot be overstated. Do not mistake a child who is immobilized as a result of sedative and paralytic medications for a child who is pain-free.

Ensuring and Maintaining Correct Tube Placement

To assess for correct placement once the tracheal tube is inserted, observe for symmetrical chest rise and auscultate over the lung fields for equal breath sounds. Inspect the tracheal tube for the presence of water vapor on the inside, indicating that the tube is in the trachea. To rule out accidental esophageal intubation, auscultate over the abdomen while the child is being ventilated: there should not be breath sounds in the abdomen. Note improvement in the oxygen saturation level via pulse oximetry.

Once tracheal tube placement is verified, mark the tube with an indelible pen at the level of the child's lip and secure it with tape. Document the number on the tracheal tube at the level of the child's mouth. Anticipate a chest x-ray to confirm correct placement of the tracheal tube.

After placement is confirmed, the tracheal tube is connected to the ventilator by respiratory personnel. The ventilator will provide continuous artificial ventilation and oxygenation. Exhaled CO_2 monitoring is recommended as it provides an indication of appropriate ventilation (Box 52.1). If an exhaled CO_2 monitor is being used, the exhaled CO_2 should be yellow.

The nurse plays a key role in ensuring that the tracheal tube remains taped securely in place by doing the following:

• Using soft wrist restraints if necessary to prevent the child from removing the tracheal tube
• Providing sedative and/or paralyzing medications
• Using caution when moving the child for x-rays, changing linens, and performing other procedures

TABLE 52.4 EQUIPMENT AND SUPPLIES FOR TRACHEAL INTUBATION

Laryngoscope blades	Straight blades (Miller) are usually used for infants and young children. A curved-blade laryngoscope (Macintosh) may be used for older children and adolescents. The blade has a little light bulb attached to it for visualization of the trachea. The light bulb should be bright and attached securely.
Tracheal tubes	Three sizes should be readily available: the estimated size, a size smaller, and a size larger. A stylet may be used to guide the tube through the child's vocal cords (it is then removed after the intubation procedure).
Oxygen	100% oxygen is provided using a bag-valve-mask before intubation and after unsuccessful intubation attempts.
Suction	Properly working wall or portable suction with appropriate-sized suction catheters (that fit the tracheal tube) should be prepared; the package is opened, leaving the sterile-tipped end inside the package and connecting the other end to the suction tubing. A Yankauer suction catheter (large catheter) should also be available if copious secretions are present in the mouth that interfere with the ability to visualize the airway.
Monitors	Pulse oximeter and cardiac monitor with an audible tone indicating the QRS complex should be in place. Exhaled CO_2 device is needed to detect increased CO_2 levels after the intubation.
Nasogastric tube	Placing a nasogastric (NG) tube will help to mitigate abdominal distention. Clients who are manually ventilated typically have some abdominal distention as some air passes into the stomach.
Personal protective equipment	Usually just gloves, goggles, and a mask are necessary to protect health care workers. In the case of copious bleeding, health care workers should wear gowns also.
Tape, etc.	Tape should be prepared for securing the tube. Benzoin, a sticky substance, is usually applied under the tape for enhanced security of the tape. For children who have had multiple intubations, a protective barrier (as used to protect the skin around an ostomy) may be applied under the tape to protect the skin. Gauze pads should be available to clean up excess secretions that may interfere with taping the tracheal tube.

Monitoring the Child Who Is Intubated

Provide ongoing and frequent monitoring of the intubated child to determine adequacy of oxygenation and ventilation as noted earlier. Once the child is intubated, the ventilatory support being provided should result in improvement in oxygen saturation and vital signs. If the child begins to exhibit signs of poor oxygenation, perform a quick assessment. Auscultate the lungs for equal air entry and determine the heart rate. Are the breath sounds equal? Is the heart rate normal for age? Perform a quick survey of the equipment and look for any disconnected tubes or kinks in the tubing. Determine oxygen saturation levels via pulse oximeter and evaluate the end-tidal CO_2 color (see Box 52.1). Use the PALS mnemonic "DOPE" for troubleshooting when the status of a child who is intubated deteriorates:

D = Displacement. The tracheal tube is displaced from the trachea.

O = Obstruction. The tracheal tube is obstructed (e.g., with a mucus plug).

P = Pneumothorax. Usually a pneumothorax results in a sudden change in the child's assessment. The signs of a pneumothorax include decreased breath sounds and decreased chest expansion on the side of the pneumothorax. Subcutaneous emphysema may be noted over the chest. In the case of tension pneumothorax, there may be a sudden drop in heart rate and blood pressure.

E = Equipment Failure. Relatively simple problems as previously discussed, such as a disconnected oxygen supply, can cause the child to deteriorate. Culprits such as a leak in the ventilator circuit or a loss of power are other types of equipment failure that may be responsible.

Make sure all equipment is appropriately connected and functional. When obstruction with secretions is suspected, suction the tracheal tube. If the tracheal tube is displaced from the trachea, remove the tube if it remains in the child's mouth and begin BVM ventilation. In the case of pneumothorax, prepare to assist with needle thoracotomy.

Preparing the Intubated Child for Transport

Once the child is stabilized with a secure tracheal tube in place, prepare to transport the child. The child will be moved by stretcher to an intensive care unit in the acute care facility or by air or land ambulance to another facility that specializes in the care of acutely ill children.

TABLE 52.5 Medications for Rapid Sequence Intubation

Medications	Desired Effects	Undesirable Effects
Anticholinergic: atropine	Decreases respiratory secretions and mitigates the vagal affects of intubation, thus decreasing the risk of bradycardia	Doses that are too low (<0.1 mg) can cause a paradoxical bradycardia. Young infants are more prone to the bradycardic effects of atropine, so its use is generally contraindicated in this population.
Sedatives: barbiturates— thiopental (short-acting barbiturate)	Has very rapid onset and short duration of action; reduces intracranial pressure and oxygen demand	Hypotensive effects of this drug are more severe in the dehydrated client. When given in combination with narcotics, respiratory depression is potentiated.
Sedatives: benzodiazepines— midazolam (Versed)	Has a slightly slower onset than thiopental but is associated with fewer adverse effects Also causes amnesia Can be titrated up or down (at lower doses it causes conscious sedation; at higher doses it can induce anesthesia)	When given in combination with narcotics, respiratory depression is potentiated.
Anesthetic agent: ketamine	Has a rapid onset with sedative, amnesic, and analgesic affects. Can be dissociative (child is awake but unaware). May improve BP and cause bronchodilation (helpful for children with status asthmaticus).	Ketamine can cause increased intracranial pressure and increased ocular pressure. Therefore, children who have suffered head trauma or globe injury should not receive this medication. Because of ketamine's sympathetic effects, hypertension can result from its use. Ketamine tends to cause increased secretions, often necessitating the concomitant use of atropine to counteract this adverse affect. May cause hallucinations and is therefore contraindicated in children with psychiatric problems.
Anesthetic agent: lidocaine	Can decrease intracranial pressure at higher doses Has an advantage when used in the management of hypovolemia because it is less likely to cause hypotension	Lidocaine can cause adverse cardiac effects (bradycardia, hypotension, dysrhythmias) in high doses. May be associated with CNS depression and seizures
Narcotic analgesic: fentanyl citrate (Sublimaze)	A highly concentrated opioid that causes fewer adverse effects (e.g., pruritus) than other opioids Also exerts a less hypotensive effect	Constipation and urinary retention (as is common with opioids) may occur. Increases risk for respiratory depression, increased intracranial pressure, and hypotension Chest wall rigidity is common with this drug and may cause difficulty with ventilation.

Medications	Desired Effects	Undesirable Effects
Paralyzing or neuromuscular blocking agents: rocuronium (Zemuron), succinylcholine (Anectine), vercuron (Norcuron)	Used for short-term paralysis during the intubation process. May be used for extended paralysis in ICU for clients in whom movement would be detrimental. For example, a child with epiglottitis has a very precarious airway and must remain intubated until the epiglottis decreases in size. In certain respiratory conditions, spontaneous respiratory effort would interfere with the ventilation of a client and therefore prolonged paralysis is desirable.	Succinylcholine (a depolarizing agent) has always been the gold standard for paralysis because it has a relatively rapid onset and is short-acting. However, it has a greater risk of adverse effects (bradycardia, hyperkalemia, hypertension, increased intracranial and ocular pressure) and is contraindicated in a variety of clinical conditions. The contemporary approach to paralysis involves the use of longer-acting agents, such as rocuronium and vercuron, because clients have fewer adverse effects with these medications. In addition, rocuronium and vercuron may be used for extended paralysis (not an option with succinylcholine).

Make sure that all tubes are securely taped. During transport, use portable oxygen and manually ventilate with the BVM. As the "sending" nurse, ensure that all laboratory results are obtained and provided to your "receiving" colleagues. If the child is going to another facility, complete a detailed summary of the resuscitation or provide a copy of the nurse's and/or progress notes. Complete the appropriate transfer forms as determined by the institution.

If the child is being transported by ambulance, the parents may not be able to accompany their child. In this case, find out as much as possible about the transport and assist the parents by giving directions to the receiving institution.

BOX 52.1 Exhaled CO$_2$ Monitoring or End-Tidal CO$_2$ Monitoring

- Device that connects to the child's ventilator circuit to detect CO$_2$ in the tubing. CO$_2$ should be noted in the tubing after six ventilations.
- Devices are usually color-coded. In the case of tracheal intubation, observe the color on the device change from purple to tan to yellow.
- The AHA's Pediatric Advanced Life Support (2007) suggests the following method to remember how the colors on the end-tidal CO$_2$ device correspond with tracheal tube placement:
  - Purple = Problem (little or no CO$_2$ detected)
  - Tan = Think about a problem.
  - Yellow = Yes, CO$_2$ is definitely detected and the tube is in the trachea.

▶ SHOCK

Shock is defined as a "clinical state characterized by inadequate tissue perfusion resulting in delivery of oxygen and metabolic substrates that is insufficient to meet tissue metabolic demands," according to the AHA (2007). If shock is left untreated, cardiopulmonary arrest will result. Shock, which may be classified as compensated or decompensated, is due to a variety of clinical problems. Compensated shock occurs when poor perfusion exists without a decrease in BP. In decompensated shock, inadequate perfusion is accompanied by a drop in BP. Unchecked decompensated shock leads to cardiac arrest and death. The principles of PALS stress the early evaluation and management of children in compensated shock with the goal of preventing decompensated shock. Once the child in shock is hypotensive, organ perfusion is dramatically impaired and a dire clinical scenario ensues.

Pathophysiology

Shock is the result of dramatic respiratory or hemodynamic compromise. Shock is caused by impaired cardiac output or impaired systemic vascular resistance (SVR) or a combination of both. Cardiac output (CO) is equal to heart rate (HR) times ventricular stroke volume (SV) (CO = HR × SV). Stroke volume is how much blood is ejected from the heart with each beat. Stroke volume is related to left ventricular filling pressure, the impedance to ventricular filling, and myocardial contractility. Left ventricular filling pressure is also known as preload, and the impedance to ventricular filling is commonly called afterload. Young children and infants have relatively small stroke volumes compared to older children and adults. Therefore, infants and young children differ from their adult counterparts in that their cardiac output depends on their heart rate, not their stroke volume. Clinically, in cases of circulatory compromise and compensated shock in infants and children, the heart rate is increased. The exception to this is a paradoxical phenomenon in neonates, who may have bradycardia rather than tachycardia.

Systemic vascular resistance or afterload is the impediment to the heart's ventricular ejection. Increased SVR will result in a decrease in blood flow unless the ventricular pressure increases. Increased vascular resistance is a common problem in shock. In children who have shock-related increased SVR, cardiac output will fall unless the ventricle can compensate by increasing pressure. In cardiac insufficiency, the child's heart will have impaired ability to compensate for the increased afterload.

Types of Shock

The most common types of shock are hypovolemic, septic, cardiogenic, and distributive. Hypovolemic shock, the most common type of shock in children, occurs when systemic perfusion decreases as a result of "inadequate intravascular volume in relation to vascular space" (AHA, 2007). Children commonly have hypovolemic shock that occurs in association with fluid losses. For example, hypovolemic shock may occur with gastroenteritis that results in vomiting and diarrhea, medications such as diuretics, and heat stroke. Other causes of hypovolemia in children include blood loss, such as from a major injury, and third spacing of fluid, such as with burns.

Septic shock is related to a systemic inflammatory response in which there may be increased cardiac output with a low SVR, known as "warm shock." More commonly in children, septic shock results in a decrease in cardiac output with an increase in SVR, known as "cold shock."

Cardiogenic shock results from an ineffective pump, the heart, with a resultant decrease in stroke volume. Children who have congenital or acquired cardiac abnormalities with a poorly functioning heart are at risk for cardiogenic shock.

Distributive shock is the result of a loss in the SVR. A relative hypovolemia occurs, most often with neurogenic injury-related shock and anaphylaxis. In relative hypovolemia, the vascular compartment expands due to systemic vasodilation. This results in a relatively larger vasculature requiring more fluid to maintain cardiac output despite no actual loss of fluid.

Lastly, toxic drug ingestions may also lead to shock.

Altered microcirculatory status is common in all types of shock. Compensatory mechanisms are activated in response to decreased blood flow. Sympathetic nervous system response results in marked contraction of larger vessel sphincters and arterioles. This compression results in dramatically impaired capillary blood flow. Blood is redirected away from less important body systems, such as the skin and the kidneys, to the vital organs (the heart and brain). During compensated shock, the body can main-

tain some level of blood flow to the vital organs. Peripheral vasoconstriction, the body's compensatory response to diminished blood flow, often results in the child's ability to maintain a normal or near-normal BP. As shock continues, capillary beds become obstructed by cellular debris, and platelets and white blood cells aggregate. Endothelial damage occurs as a result of capillary congestion. Poor blood flow to the capillaries results in anaerobic metabolism. Lactic acid accumulates, and this can lead to acidosis. In addition, children with septic shock sustain marked endothelial damage as a result of exposure to bacterial toxins.

The cumulative effect of capillary obstruction and dramatically impaired blood flow is tissue ischemia. As tissue ischemia progresses, the child will show signs of altered perfusion to vital organs. For example, as blood flow to the brain is diminished, the child will demonstrate an altered level of consciousness. Altered blood flow to the kidneys will result in decreased urine output or absence of urine output (oliguria). Commonly, the heart rate will increase in the early stages of shock, but as the heart becomes compromised as a result of poor perfusion, the child will become bradycardic. The child will demonstrate an increased respiratory rate in the initial phase of shock. Tachypnea is seen in septic shock as well. In fact, the child may demonstrate marked hyperventilation in an effort to "blow off" carbon dioxide in response to the acidosis that is associated with septic shock.

Nursing Assessment

Nursing assessment of the child in shock includes the health history and physical examination as well as laboratory and diagnostic testing. The nursing assessment must be performed quickly and accurately so that resuscitation can be expedited.

Health History

In shock, the health history is based on the child's presentation. Children with shock are critically ill and require emergent intervention. Therefore, the history is obtained as life-saving interventions are provided. Determine when the child first became ill and treatments that have been given thus far. Inquire about sources of volume loss, such as:

- Vomiting
- Diarrhea
- Decreased oral intake
- Blood loss

Ask when the child last urinated. Investigate for other related symptoms such as behavioral changes or lethargy. Has the child had a fever or rash, complained of headache, or been exposed to anyone with similar symptoms? Inquire about daycare attendance and whether the family has recently traveled outside of the country. Determine if the child has a history of a congenital heart defect or other heart condition or if the child has severe allergies. Ask the parent about accidental ingestion of medications or other substances and, for the older child or adolescent, about the possibility of illicit substance use.

Physical Examination

The key to successful shock management is early recognition of the signs and symptoms. Obtain vital signs, noting any alterations. Measure BP, although this is not a reliable method of evaluating for shock in children. Children tend to maintain a normal or slightly less-than-normal BP in compensated shock while sacrificing tissue perfusion until the child suffers a cardiopulmonary arrest. Therefore, other components of the circulatory evaluation will be more valuable when assessing a child.

> ▶ *Take* NOTE!
>
> *Bradycardia is a serious sign in neonates and may occur with respiratory compromise, circulatory compromise, and/or overwhelming sepsis.*

As with any emergency, evaluate the airway first. Is it patent? Then determine if the child is breathing. The child in shock will often demonstrate signs of respiratory distress, such as grunting, gasping, nasal flaring, tachypnea, and increased work of breathing. Auscultate breath sounds to determine the adequacy of air entry and airflow. If the child shows signs of respiratory distress, manage the airway and breathing problem first, as discussed earlier in the chapter.

Assess the skin color. Palpate the skin temperature and determine quality of pulses. Except in special cases, such as distributive shock, the child in shock will generally have darker and cooler extremities with delayed capillary refill. Note the line of demarcation if present. This refers to the point on the distal extremity where cool temperature begins (the proximal portion of the extremity may continue to be warm). In distributive shock, the initial assessment will reveal full and bounding pulses and warm, erythemic skin. Evaluate the pulse quality. Distal pulses will likely be weaker than central pulses.

Evaluate the child's hydration state and check skin turgor. Decreased elasticity is associated with hypovolemic states, though this is usually a late sign. Observe the child's face; in compensated shock the child may be awake but obtunded and demonstrate signs of distress. The child in decompensated shock may have his or her eyes closed and may be responsive only to voice or other stimulation. Evaluate pupillary responses. Determine urinary output, which will be decreased in the child with shock.

After having evaluated and provided initial life-saving management for airway, breathing, and circulation, evaluate the child's entire body for other disabilities. Injuries warrant vigilant evaluation for ongoing blood loss, although they may also produce internal blood loss (e.g., a femur fracture). Look for signs of malforma-tion, swelling, redness, or pain of the extremities, which may suggest internal blood loss. Also inspect for any open wounds and active sites of bleeding. Children with abdominal injuries also may lose copious amounts of blood internally. Inspect the abdomen for redness, skin discoloration, or distention. Auscultate for bowel sounds in all four quadrants.

Laboratory and Diagnostic Testing

As the child is being resuscitated, laboratory tests and radiographs will be ordered and obtained. However, no diagnostic test should replace the priority of respiratory support, vascular access, and fluid administration. Laboratory results will guide ongoing management. Common laboratory and diagnostic tests used for children with shock include:

- Blood glucose levels: usually performed at the bedside using a glucose meter (e.g., Chem-strip or Accucheck) to obtain a rapid result
- Electrolytes: to evaluate for electrolyte abnormalities
- CBC with differential: to assess for viral or bacterial infection (septic shock) and to evaluate for anemia and platelet abnormalities
- Blood culture: to evaluate for sepsis; preliminary results will not be available for 1 to 2 days
- C-reactive protein: to evaluate for infection
- Arterial blood gases: to assess oxygen and carbon dioxide levels and to provide information about acid–base balance
- Toxicology panel (if ingestion is suspected)
- Lumbar puncture: to evaluate the cerebrospinal fluid for meningitis
- Urinalysis: to evaluate for glucose, ketones, and protein; concentration (specific gravity) is increased in dehydration states
- Urine culture: to evaluate for urinary tract or kidney infection
- Radiographs: to evaluate heart size, to evaluate the lungs for pneumonia or pulmonary edema (present with cardiogenic shock)

Nursing Management

Signs of shock in children warrant an emergent response. Always evaluate and manage the airway and breathing and check for pulses. Initiate CPR if the child is pulseless. All children who have signs and symptoms of shock should receive 100% oxygen via mask. If the child has poor respiratory effort or is apneic, administer 100% oxygen via BVM or tracheal tube (refer to the section on respiratory emergencies for more specific information about management of airway and breathing). As part of ongoing monitoring, institute cardiac and apnea monitoring and assess oxygen saturation levels via pulse oximetry.

Obtaining Vascular Access

Once the airway and breathing are addressed, nursing management of shock focuses on obtaining vascular access and restoring fluid volume. Children with signs of shock should receive generous amounts of isotonic IV fluids rapidly. However, obtaining vascular access in critically ill children can be challenging. Vascular access must be obtained using the quickest route possible in children whose condition is markedly deteriorated, such as those in decompensated shock.

Various forms of vascular access available for the management of the critically ill child include:

- Peripheral IV route: A large-bore catheter is used to give large amounts of fluid. This route may not be feasible in children with significant vascular compromise.
- Central IV route: Central lines can be inserted into the jugular vein and threaded into the superior vena cava. The femoral route is best for obtaining central venous access while CPR is in progress because the insertion procedure will not interfere with life-saving interventions involving the airway and cardiac compressions. The subclavian vein, located under the clavicle, is an alternative route for central access.
- Saphenous vein: The saphenous vein (found in the ankle) is an alternative route for venous access that is obtained using a surgical incision.
- Intraosseous access: Intraosseous access, obtained by cannulating the bone marrow, is recommended in cases of decompensated shock or cardiac arrest if IV access cannot be attained rapidly. The preferred site is the anterior tibia. Special intraosseous needles are used (generally a 15-gauge needle for older children, 18-gauge for younger children). The needle is inserted using a firm twisting motion slightly away from the growth plate. Any medications or fluids that can be administered using an IV site can be given using this route. Alternative sites include the femur, the iliac crest, the sternum, and the distal tibia.

Restoring Fluid Volume

Administer IV isotonic fluids, such as Ringer's lactate or normal saline (the isotonic fluids of choice) rapidly. Administer 20 mL/kg of the prescribed fluid as a bolus, infusing the fluid as rapidly as possible. In general a large-bore syringe, such as a 35- to 60-cc syringe attached to a three-way stopcock, is the preferred method for rapid fluid delivery in children. Infusing the fluid via gravity is too slow. The fluid bolus may be repeated up to two times (for a total of three times) if required.

▶ **Take** NOTE!

Dextrose solutions are contraindicated in shock because of the risk of complications such as osmotic diuresis, hypokalemia, hyperglycemia, and worsening of ischemic brain injury.

Children in septic shock will often require larger volumes of fluid as a result of the increased capillary permeability. Children in shock due to trauma will usually receive a colloid, such as blood, when there is an inadequate response to crystalloid isotonic fluid. After each fluid bolus, reassess the child for signs of positive response to the fluid administration.

Insert an indwelling urinary catheter to allow for accurate and frequent measurement of urine output.

Indicators of improvement include:

- Improved cardiovascular status: The central and peripheral pulses are stronger. The line of demarcation of extremity coolness is diminishing and capillary refill is improved (time is decreased). BP is improved.
- Improved mental status: The child is more alert. For example, the child's eyes are open and watching personnel. If the child is younger, he or she may be pulling at the IV line.
- Improved urine output: This may not be noted initially but should be noted over the next few hours; the goal is 1 to 2 mL/kg/hour.

The process of fluid resuscitation involves giving the fluid, assessing and reassessing the child, and documenting findings. Children in shock may require as much as 100 to 200 mL/kg of resuscitative fluid during the initial hours of shock management. Most children in shock need and can tolerate this large volume of fluid. Continued reassessment will determine if the child is beginning to experience fluid overload in the form of pulmonary edema (this is rare but may occur in children with pre-existing cardiac conditions or severe chronic pulmonary disease) (AHA, 2007; Prentiss et al., 2007).

▶ **Take** NOTE!

Do not focus solely on the child's circulatory status; you may overlook signs and symptoms of respiratory deterioration.

Administering Medications

In some circumstances, such as septic shock or distributive shock, fluid alone does not adequately improve the child's status and adjunctive medications may be ordered. Vasoactive medications are used either alone or in combination to improve cardiac output, to increase SVR or to decrease SVR. The selection of medications is dictated by the child's cardiac and vascular status. For example, dobutamine is a medication with significant beta-adrenergic effects and thus can improve cardiac contractility. Epinephrine, which affects the heart muscle, is also a powerful vasoconstrictor. Dopamine affects the heart at lower doses but increasingly affects the vasculature with increased doses. These medications may be given as a loading dose, followed by a continuous infusion. When vasoactive drugs are administered, monitor for improvement in heart rate, BP, perfusion, and urine output.

◆ CARDIAC ARRHYTHMIAS AND ARREST

Unlike adults, in whom cardiopulmonary arrest is most often caused by a primary cardiac event, children typically have healthy hearts and thus rarely experience primary cardiac arrest. More commonly they experience cardiopulmonary arrest from gradual deterioration of respiration and/or circulation (AHA, 2005f). In particular, children experiencing a respiratory emergency or shock may deteriorate and eventually demonstrate cardiopulmonary arrest. Thus, the standard of care for managing a child in this situation is vastly different from that for an adult.

Nurses should be skilled in evaluating and managing respiratory alterations and shock in children, as discussed in previous sections. Overwhelming evidence suggests that if primary respiratory compromise or shock is identified and treated in the critically ill child, a secondary cardiac arrest can be prevented. Rare exceptions do exist, however. For example, electrolyte abnormalities and toxic drug ingestions are primary insults to the cardiovascular system that may lead to a sudden cardiac arrest rather than a gradual progression. Other exceptions in which the child is at risk for a primary and sudden cardiac arrest include:

- History of a serious primary congenital or acquired cardiac defect
- Potentially lethal arrhythmias, such as prolonged QT syndrome
- Hyper- or hypotrophic cardiomyopathy
- Traumatic cardiac injury or a sharp blow to the chest, known as "commotio cordis" (e.g., when a high-velocity ball hits the chest)

The overwhelming majority of children rarely experience cardiac arrhythmias, so it is beyond the scope of this chapter to discuss the myriad of possible complex rhythm disturbances. Therefore, this discussion will be limited to the management of emergent cardiac conditions that are more typically found in children.

Pathophysiology

The AHA has simplified the nomenclature used to describe pediatric cardiac compromise and has established three major categories of cardiac rhythm disturbances:

"Slow": bradyarrhythmias
"Fast": tachyarrhythmias
"Absent": pulseless, cardiovascular collapse

The pathophysiology, causes, and therapeutic management of each of the categories of rhythm disturbances are discussed below.

Bradyarrhythmias

Bradycardia is a heart rate significantly slower than the normal heart rate for age. Bradycardia in children is most commonly "sinus bradycardia"—in other words, there is not a cardiac nodal abnormality associated with the slowed heart rate. In sinus bradycardia, the P waves and QRS complex remain normal on the ECG. Brief dips in heart rates can be normal, such as when the child sleeps. Children are also susceptible to brief drops in heart rate that are associated with vagal stimulation. For example, passing an orogastric tube down the esophagus of a young infant may induce a temporary bradycardic response. These normal decreases in the child's heart rate should recover with or without stimulation and are not normally associated with signs of altered perfusion.

Less commonly, children manifest bradycardia as a result of cardiac abnormalities and heart block. Infants with bradycardia related to heart block may exhibit poor feeding and tachypnea, whereas older children may demonstrate fatigue, dizziness, and syncope. Comparison Chart 52.2 compares the causes of sinus bradycardia and heart block in children.

In contrast, the child with a serious and possibly life-threatening bradyarrhythmia will have a heart rate below 60 beats per minute, with signs of altered perfusion. The most common causes of profound bradycardia in children are respiratory compromise, hypoxia, and shock. Sustained bradycardia is commonly associated with arrest. It is an ominous sign and should be taken seriously.

Tachyarrhythmias

Children normally have faster heart rates than adults, and fever, fear, and pain are common explanations for significant increases in the heart rate of a child (**tachycardia**). This normal elevation in heart rate is known as sinus tachycardia. However, once the fever is reduced, the child is comforted, or the pain is managed, the heart rate should return close to the child's baseline. Hypoxia and hypovolemia are pathological reasons for tachycardia in the child. The signs, symptoms, and management of these concerns were discussed in previous sections. If the child

COMPARISON CHART 52.2 CAUSES OF SINUS BRADYCARDIA VERSUS HEART BLOCK

	Sinus Bradycardia	Heart Block
Causes	• Pathologic: medications such as digoxin, hypoxia, hypothermia, head injury • Nonpathologic: well-conditioned athlete	• Congenital: associated with cardiac anomalies • Acquired: endocarditis, rheumatic fever, Kawasaki disease

has sinus tachycardia that results from any of these causes, the focus is on the underlying cause. It is inappropriate and dangerous to treat sinus tachycardia with medications aimed at decreasing the heart rate or with a defibrillation device.

Tachyarrhythmias in children that are associated with cardiac compromise have unique characteristics that present differently from sinus tachycardia. Examples of these include supraventricular tachycardia (SVT) and ventricular tachycardia. SVT is a cardiac conduction problem in which the heart rate is extremely rapid and the rhythm is very regular, often described as "no beat-to-beat variability." Comparison Chart 52.3 explains the differences between SVT and sinus tachycardia. The most common cause of SVT is a re-entry problem in the cardiac conduction system. Commonly, SVT is the result of a genetic cardiac conduction problem such as Wolff-Parkinson-White syndrome. SVT may also be associated with medications such as caffeine and theophylline. Children often can tolerate the characteristically higher heart rate that is associated with SVT for short periods of time. However, the increased demand that is placed on the cardiovascular system usually overtaxes the child and results in signs of congestive heart failure if the SVT continues unchecked for a prolonged time.

Ventricular tachycardia is a rhythm involving an elevation of the heart rate and a wide QRS (greater than 0.08 seconds) that is the result of an abnormal, rapid firing of one or both of the ventricles. Ventricular tachycardia is a rare arrhythmia in children and usually is associated with a congenital or acquired cardiac abnormality. In addition, prolonged QT syndrome is a conduction abnormality that can result in ventricular tachycardia and sudden death in children. Less commonly, ingestion of medications and toxins, acidosis, hypocalcemia, abnormalities of potassium, and hypoxemia have been associated with the development of ventricular tachycardia in children.

Collapsed Rhythms (Pulseless Rhythms)

A collapsed rhythm, as defined by PALS, is one that produces cardiac arrest with no palpable pulse and no signs of perfusion (cardiac arrest). Typically, the most common pulseless arrest rhythms in children are asystole or pulseless electrical activity (PEA). **Asystole** occurs when there is no cardiac electrical activity, commonly referred to as "a straight line" on the ECG. The child with PEA has some appreciable rhythm on the ECG but no palpable pulses. PEA may be caused by hypoxemia, hypovolemia, hypothermia, electrolyte imbalance, tamponade, toxic ingestion, tension pneumothorax, or thromboembolism. Ventricular tachycardia may also present as pulseless. Ventricular fibrillation, once thought to be rare in children, occurs in serious cardiac conditions in which the ventricle is not pumping effectively. It may develop from ventricular tachycardia. Ventricular fibrillation is characterized by variable, high-amplitude waveforms (coarse VF) or a finer, lower-amplitude waveform with no discernible cardiac rhythm (fine VF). In either case, cardiac output is insufficient.

Nursing Assessment

Nursing assessment of the child with a cardiac emergency includes the health history and physical examination as well as laboratory and diagnostic testing. The nursing assessment must be performed quickly and accurately so that resuscitation can be instituted if needed.

Health History

Obtain a brief health history of the child with a cardiac emergency while simultaneously assessing the child and providing life-saving interventions. Key areas to inquire about include:

- History of cardiac problems, asthma, chromosomal anomaly, delayed growth
- Symptoms such as syncope, dizziness, palpitations or racing heart, chest pain, coughing, wheezing, increased work of breathing
- Activity tolerance with play or feeding: Does the child get out of breath, turn blue, or squat during play? Can the child keep up with playmates? Does the infant tire with feedings?
- Precipitating illness, fever, unexplained joint pains, ingested medications
- Participation in a sport before the cardiac event occurred or injury to the chest
- Family history of cardiac problems, sudden death from a cardiac condition, heart attacks at a young age, chromosomal abnormalities

Determine treatment measures performed at the scene. Was CPR initiated? Was an AED used?

Physical Examination

Quickly establish the child's status. A child who is obviously in distress or is arresting must receive emergent life-saving

COMPARISON CHART 52.3	DISTINGUISHING SVT FROM SINUS TACHYCARDIA	
	SVT	Sinus Tachycardia
Rate (bpm)	Infants >220, children >180	Infants <220, children <180
Rhythm	Abrupt onset and termination	Beat-to-beat variability
P waves	Flattened	Present and normal
QRS	Narrow (<0.08 seconds)	Normal
History	Usually no significant history	Fever, fluid loss, hypoxia, pain, fear

interventions. Briefly perform the assessment while simultaneously providing life-saving interventions.

Inspection and Observation

Assess the child's airway patency and efficiency of breathing. Observe the child's color, noting circumoral pallor or duskiness or central pallor, mottling, duskiness, or cyanosis. Note any increased work of breathing, grunting, head bobbing, or apnea. Inspect the chest for barrel shape, which may be associated with chronic pulmonary or cardiac disease. Observe the pericardium for the presence of lifts or heaves. Note diaphoresis, anxious appearance, or dysmorphic features (50% of children with Down syndrome also have a congenital cardiac defect). Determine if neck vein distention is present. Inspect the fingertips for clubbing, which is indicative of chronic tissue hypoxemia.

Auscultation

Auscultate the breath sounds, noting any crackles or wheezes. Auscultate the heart rate. If the child does not have an adequate pulse, initiate CPR. If the child has a strong, perfusing pulse, complete the cardiac assessment. Auscultate with the diaphragm of the stethoscope first and then listen with the bell. Evaluate all of the auscultatory areas, listening first over the second right interspace (aortic valve) and then over the second left interspace (pulmonic valve); next move to the left lower sternal border (tricuspid area); and finally auscultate over the fifth interspace, midclavicular line (mitral area). Evaluate the rate and rhythm of the heart. Listen for any extra sounds or murmurs. Note and describe the quality, intensity, and location of any cardiac murmurs.

> ► **Take** NOTE!
>
> *Murmurs are most often systolic and can be benign or associated with pathology. Murmurs that radiate to the back and are grade III or louder are more likely to be due to a cardiac defect. True diastolic murmurs are rare and almost always have a pathologic origin.*

Percussion and Palpation

Percuss between the costal interspaces and note the heart's size. Palpate the heart to find the point of maximal impulse (PMI) and to evaluate for an associated thrill. A thrill feels like a fluttering under the fingers and is associated with cardiac pathology. Palpate and note the quality of the pulses. Evaluate each of the pulses bilaterally and note whether they are absent, faint, normal, or bounding. Compare the quality of pulses on each side of the body and also those of the upper and lower body. Note the skin temperature and evaluate the capillary refill.

Laboratory and Diagnostic Testing

The major diagnostic test used is the ECG. Identify the arrhythmia according to the ECG reading (Fig. 52.8).

Nursing Management

Provide oxygen at 100%. Institute cardiac monitoring and assess oxygen saturation levels via pulse oximetry. Obtain the child's preprinted code drug sheet or use the Broselow tape to obtain the child's height to estimate the tracheal tube sizes and medication dosages that are appropriate for the child. Always remember to intervene in this order: first airway, then breathing, then circulation. The remainder of this discussion will assume that the nurse has initiated interventions for airway and breathing as discussed earlier in the chapter.

> ► **Take** NOTE!
>
> *Pay attention to the rhythm on the monitor, but continually monitor the child's pulse. If the child does not have a pulse or has a pulse of less than 60 bpm, perform cardiac compressions despite the monitor reading.*

Managing Bradyarrhythmias

The management of sinus bradycardia is focused on remedying the underlying cause of the slow heart rate. Since hypoxia is the most common cause of sustained bradycardia, oxygenation and ventilation are necessary. The newborn is particularly susceptible to bradycardia in relation to hypoxemia. Continue to reassess the child to determine if the bradycardia improves with adequate oxygenation and ventilation. If bradycardia persists, administer epinephrine and/or atropine as ordered. Epinephrine is the drug of choice for the treatment of persistent bradycardia.

Other causes of bradycardia such as hypothermia, head injury, and toxic ingestion are managed by addressing the underlying condition. Warming the hypothermic child may restore a normal sinus rhythm. Patients with head injury may have bradycardia without any cardiac involvement, and with successful management of the head injury, the bradycardia will resolve. Antidotes to toxins may be necessary in children whose bradycardia is the result of a toxic ingestion.

Managing Tachyarrhythmias

The tachyarrhythmias include SVT (stable or unstable) and ventricular tachycardia with a pulse. Examine the ECG to determine if the child is experiencing ventricular tachycardia or SVT. Clinically, determine whether the child in SVT is showing signs that require emergent intervention or if the child is stable. In compensated SVT, the child will appear to be alert, breathing comfortably, and well perfused. The child who is demonstrating signs of

A

B

C

D

FIGURE 52.8 Arrhythmias. (**A**) Sinus tachycardia: normal QRS and P waves, mild beat-to-beat variability. (**B**) Supraventricular tachycardia: note rate above 220, abnormal P waves, no beat-to-beat variability. (**C**) Ventricular tachycardia: rapid and regular rhythm, wide QRS without P waves. (**D**) Coarse ventricular fibrillation: chaotic electrical activity.

TABLE 52.6 MANAGING TACHYARRHYTHMIAS

Tachyarrhythmia	Signs and Symptoms	Management
Compensated SVT	• Tachycardia, heart rate >220 • Abnormal P waves • Alert, well-perfused client • Possible complaints of headache and dizziness in older children	• Vagal maneuvers such as ice to face or blowing through a straw that is obstructed • Adenosine if vagal maneuvers fail
Uncompensated SVT	• Tachycardia, heart rate >220 • Abnormal P waves • Signs of shock: altered level of consciousness, poor perfusion, weak pulses	• Adenosine or synchronized cardioversion
Ventricular tachycardia	• Rate may range from normal to 200 bpm. • Wide QRS • No P waves • Pulse present, poor perfusion	• Synchronized cardioversion • IV amiodarone • Treatment of underlying causes

compromise, such as a change in consciousness, respiratory status, and perfusion, is considered to be in uncompensated SVT. Uncompensated SVT requires emergent intervention. The child who has ventricular tachycardia with a pulse will have poor perfusion and also requires immediate intervention. The evaluation and approaches to the tachyarrhythmias are discussed in Table 52.6.

▶ **Take** NOTE!

Adenosine has a rapid onset of action and an extremely short half-life. Administer it extremely rapidly with a generous amount of IV flush; otherwise, it will be ineffective.

Managing Collapsed Rhythms

As in any pediatric emergency, support the ABCs by managing the airway, providing oxygen, and giving fluids. In addition, if the child is pulseless or has a heart rate less than 60 bpm, initiate cardiac compressions. The pulseless rhythms include ventricular tachycardia, ventricular fibrillation, asystole, and PEA. ECG characteristics and management of these rhythms are summarized in Table 52.7. Also treat the underlying causes of the arrhythmia, if known.

The AHA emphasizes the importance of cardiac compressions in pulseless clients with arrhythmias. Give compressions before and immediately after defibrillation. In the past it was recommended that clients who required defibrillation be given three shocks in a row, but recent research findings have shown that the client should be de-

TABLE 52.7 ECG CHARACTERISTICS AND MANAGEMENT OF PULSELESS RHYTHMS

Pulseless Arrhythmia	ECG Characteristics	Management
Ventricular tachycardia	Wide QRS, no P waves	• CPR • Defibrillation • Epinephrine; also possibly amiodarone, lidocaine, or magnesium • Treat underlying causes.
Ventricular fibrillation	• Chaotic ventricular activity • No P waves, no QRS, no T waves	• CPR • Defibrillation • Epinephrine; also possibly amiodarone, lidocaine, or magnesium • Treat underlying causes.
Asystole	Flat line	• Check lead placement. • CPR if no pulse • Epinephrine
Pulseless electrical activity	Electrical activity that is not consistent with ventricular tachycardia or ventricular fibrillation	• Check lead placement. • CPR if no pulse • Treat underlying cause. • Epinephrine

fibrillated only once, followed by five cycles of CPR. For defibrillation to be most effective, cardiac compressions must be performed effectively with minimal interruptions (AHA, 2006).

> ▶ *Take* NOTE!

Previously, multiple doses of epinephrine were given in pediatric emergency situations. Recently, however, the AHA has recommended against this practice, as multiple doses of epinephrine have not been shown to be helpful and may actually cause harm to the child.

▶ NEAR-DROWNING

Water can be a great source of fun and exercise for children and adolescents, but drowning is the second-leading cause of preventable death in children and adolescents in the United States and worldwide (World Health Organization, 2008). In warm-weather states where swimming pools are more common, drowning is the primary cause of death in young people. Most drowning deaths are preventable, and the World Health Organization (2008) notes that "lapse in adult supervision is the single most important contributory cause for drowning."

Near-drowning is defined as a submersion injury in which the child survives. Traditionally, children experiencing cold-water submersion were expected to fare better than those drowning in warmer water. Survival and neurologic outcome depend on early and appropriate resuscitation. In recent years, with appropriate resuscitation efforts and treatment, children have demonstrated better neurologic outcomes. Currently, there are no factors to predict whether the child's long-term neurologic status will be affected after surviving a near-drowning incident (Minto & Woodward, 2005).

Typically, a child who is drowning will struggle to breathe and eventually will aspirate water. Aspiration of relatively small amounts of water leads to poor oxygenation, with retention of carbon dioxide. Alveolar surfactant is depleted during the drowning event and pulmonary edema commonly occurs. Hypoxemia results in increased capillary permeability and resultant hypovolemia. Even small amounts of aspirated water may lead to pulmonary edema within a 24- to 48-hour period after the near-drowning episode. A near-drowning survivor is also at risk for renal complications due to altered renal perfusion during the hypoxemic state.

Nursing Assessment

Nursing assessment of the near-drowning survivor is crucial and must take place quickly and accurately.

Health History

Obtain the history rapidly while providing life-saving interventions. Ask about the circumstances of the event:

• Where did the incident occur? Was the child in a lake, river, ocean, or swimming pool? Was the child submerged in a toilet, bucket, or bathtub?
• Did someone witness the child's entry into the water?
• Was the water fresh or salty? Cold or warm?
• Is it likely the water was contaminated?
• Were there any extenuating circumstances, such as a diving or automobile accident, associated with the near-drowning?
• What was the approximate length of time of the submersion? Was the child conscious or unconscious when rescued?
• What was done at the scene? Was CPR initiated? If so, when?
• If a cervical spine injury was suspected, was the cervical spine immobilized?
• Was an AED used?
• When did the child last eat (to prepare for possible intubation)?

Physical Examination

Evaluate airway patency and breathing. Auscultate all lung fields for signs of pulmonary edema, such as coarseness or crackles. Evaluate the heart rate, pulses, and perfusion. Note the cardiac rhythm on the monitor and report evidence of arrhythmias. Evaluate the child's neurologic status. Use a pen light to determine pupillary reaction. Use the pediatric coma score to further assess the neurologic status. Does the child open the eyes spontaneously, to stimuli, or not at all? Is there any spontaneous movement? Is the younger child crying? Can the older child speak? Measure the child's temperature, as hypothermia often occurs with near-drowning.

Laboratory and Diagnostic Testing

While awaiting laboratory and diagnostic testing results, continue resuscitative efforts as addressed below. Laboratory and diagnostic tests typically include the following:

• Arterial blood gases: hypoxemia, acidosis
• ECG: cardiac arrhythmias
• Chest x-ray: pulmonary edema, infiltrates
• Serum electrolytes: imbalance related to development of shock

Nursing Management

Because of the potentially devastating effects that drowning-related hypoxia has on the child's brain, airway interventions must be initiated immediately after retrieving a child from the water. Every second counts. Initial interventions in a near-drowning event are always focused on airway, breathing, and circulation; commonly, resuscitative efforts have begun before the child arrives at the acute care facility.

If a cervical spine injury is suspected (as in the case of a diving accident), provide stabilization either manually or with a cervical collar. As with any suspected neck injury, do not remove the cervical collar until injury to the cervical spine has been ruled out through an x-ray and clinical evaluation. Suction the airway to ensure airway patency. The child may have aspirated particles from a contaminated water source or emesis, a relatively common complication associated with near-drowning. A large-bore suction catheter (e.g., Yankauer) is an effective tool for clearing the upper airway. Administer supplemental oxygen at 100%. Children who have poor or absent respiratory effort most likely will require intubation. Insert a nasogastric tube to decompress the stomach and prevent aspiration of stomach contents. Initiate chest compressions if a pulse is not present.

Usually, the child exhibits some degree of hypothermia and will require warming. Generally, the core body temperature should be raised slowly, as warming a drowning victim too quickly may have deleterious effects. Remove any wet clothing, dry the child, and cover him or her with warmed blankets. Warm IV fluids and use other warming methods as prescribed.

▶ **Consider** THIS!

> Teva Dawson, a 2-year-old girl, is rushed to the emergency room by ambulance after experiencing a near-drowning in the family swimming pool. Eva was resuscitated at the scene and is now breathing spontaneously. She is lethargic and coughs occasionally.
>
> What health history information would you obtain from the parents or caregivers? What immediate management is necessary?
>
> What education may be necessary for this family?

▶ POISONING

Emergency care of the pediatric poisoning victim consists of rapid nursing assessment and prompt management.

▶ **Take** NOTE!

> If a normally healthy child (particularly a young child) suddenly deteriorates without a known cause, suspect a toxic ingestion.

Nursing Assessment

Nursing assessment of the poisoning victim focuses on a thorough health history, followed by physical examination and laboratory and diagnostic testing.

Health History

Obtain the health history from the parents or caregiver or, in the case of an older child or teenager, from the child. Inquire about the approximate time of poisoning and the nature of the toxin. Was the toxin ingested, inhaled, or applied to the skin? In the case of pill ingestion, does the caregiver have the medication bottle? Did the child experience nausea, vomiting, anorexia, abdominal pain, or neurologic changes such as disorientation, slurred speech, or altered gait? Determine the progression of the symptoms. Did the parent or caregiver call the poison control center? Has any treatment been given? In the case of older children and teens, inquire about any history of depression or threatened suicide.

Physical Examination

Ingestion of medications or chemicals may result in a wide variety of clinical manifestations. Perform a thorough physical examination, noting alterations that may occur with particular ingestions, such as:

- Hyper- or hypotension
- Hyper- or hypothermia
- Respiratory depression or hyperventilation
- Miosis (pupillary contraction) or mydriasis (pupillary dilatation)

Pay particular attention to the child's mental status, skin moisture and color, and bowel sounds (Barry, 2005).

Laboratory and Diagnostic Testing

The suspected poison may direct the laboratory and diagnostic testing. A variety of blood tests may be performed:

- Chemistry panel: to detect hypoglycemia or metabolic acidosis and assess renal function
- ECG: to identify arrhythmias or conduction delay
- Liver function tests: to assess for liver injury
- Urine and blood toxicology screens (available for a limited number of medications; may vary per institution)
- Specific drug levels if the substance ingested is known or highly suspected

Nursing Management

Management should focus on prevention of poisoning, but when poisoning does occur, give priority to airway, breathing, and circulation, treating alterations as discussed earlier in this chapter. Monitor vital signs frequently and provide supportive care. Few specific antidotes are available for medications or other toxins. Ipecac is rarely used in the health care setting to induce vomiting and is no longer recommended for use in the home setting. Gastric lavage, administration of activated charcoal (binds with the chemical substance in the bowel), or whole bowel irrigation with polyethylene glycol electrolyte solutions may be used. Occasionally, dialysis is required to lower the level of toxin in the bloodstream. The intervention is based on the source of the ingestion. For example, activated charcoal is an effective method for preventing the absorption of many medications but is not effective in the case of an iron overdose.

If opiate or other narcotic ingestion is suspected, administer naloxone to reverse the respiratory depression or altered level of consciousness. Treatment of seizures and alterations in thermoregulation may also be needed.

Specific treatment of the poisoning will be determined when the toxin is identified and poison control is queried. Maintain ongoing assessment of the poisoned child because many toxins exhibit very late effects.

> ▶ *Take* NOTE!
>
> *The National Poison Control number is 1-800-222-1222.*

▶ TRAUMA

The leading cause of death in persons between 3 and 33 years of age is unintentional injuries (Centers for Disease Control and Prevention [CDC], 2007d). Childhood trauma results from such events as automobile accidents, pedestrian accidents, falls, sporting injuries, and firearm use. Falls are the most common cause of pediatric injury. Children of varying ages are susceptible to various forms of injury due to their developmental level as well as their environmental exposure. Young children rely on their caregivers to promote their safety. Young children also are not developmentally equipped to be able to recognize dangerous situations.

Automobile accidents continue to cause the deaths of about five children daily, with significant numbers experiencing injury (National Highway Traffic Safety Administration, 2006). Pedestrian injuries cause 25% of traffic-related deaths in children (CDC, 2005), and annually about 280,000 children are evaluated in emergency rooms following bicycle accidents (SafeKids, 2006). Because pediatric injury is so common, nurses must become adept at assessment and intervention in the pediatric trauma victim.

Nursing Assessment

The trauma survey includes a brief health history as the child is being assessed and life-saving measures are being instituted.

Health History

Begin the health history by asking when the injury happened. If the child sustained a motor vehicle–related injury, ask how fast the vehicle was going. Determine if the child was appropriately restrained in the automobile. If the child was riding a bicycle, skateboarding, or using in-

line skates, was he or she wearing a helmet, knee pads, and wrist guards? Determine what interventions were performed at the scene. Was the child immobilized on a backboard to protect the cervical spine? If the child is bleeding, ask the person who transported the child to estimate the amount of blood lost.

If the child experienced a fall, ask if the fall was witnessed and the height from which the child fell. Did the child fall onto a hard surface such as concrete? How did the child land: on the head or back, or did the child catch himself or herself with the hands? Younger children and boys are at higher risk for injuring their head. Did the child lose consciousness at the scene? What kind of behavior did the child exhibit after the fall? Since the fall, has the child complained of a headache or been vomiting?

While obtaining a detailed history about the fall, think about the child's developmental stage. For example, does it seem plausible that a toddler might fall down the stairs? In contrast, what is the likelihood that a 2-month-old would suffer a fractured femur from a fall? Keep in mind the possibility of child abuse. Critically evaluate the reported circumstances and try to determine if the history, developmental stage of the child, and the type of injury sustained match. In addition, evaluate the type of injury that the child sustained and the history given by the caregiver. For example, children who fall from significant heights often suffer skeletal fractures, but abdominal and chest injuries rarely result from falling from significant heights.

Physical Examination

Physical examination of the child with a traumatic injury should be approached with an evaluation of the ABCs (primary survey) first. Assess the patency of the airway and establish the effectiveness of breathing (as discussed earlier in the chapter). Examine the child's respiratory effort, breath sounds, and color. Next, evaluate the circulation. Note the pulse rate and quality. Observe the color, skin temperature, and perfusion. If bleeding has occurred, the child's circulation may become compromised.

After assessing and intervening for airway, breathing, and circulation, proceed to the secondary survey. Assess for disability. Rapidly assess critical neurologic function. Determine the level of consciousness, pupillary reaction, and verbal and motor responses to auditory and painful stimuli. If the patient is a young infant, palpate the anterior fontanel: a full and bulging fontanel signals increased intracranial pressure. The traumatized child's neurologic status may range from completely normal to comatose.

> ▶ *Take* NOTE!
>
> *Unequal pupils or a fixed and dilated pupil is considered a neurosurgical emergency. Immediately report this finding.*

Following the ABCs and D (disability) is E (exposure). Expose the child to observe the entire body for signs of injury, whether blunt or penetrating. Perform a systematic, thorough inspection of the child's body. Note active bleeding and extremity deformity, as well as any lacerations and abrasions. Observe for movement and any complaints of immobility or pain with movement. Inspect the abdomen for redness, skin discoloration, or distention. Auscultate for bowel sounds in all four quadrants. If the child is verbal, ask if he or she has any pain in the stomach. If the child is younger, ask, "Do you have a tummy ache?" If the child reports abdominal pain, ask the child to point to where it hurts. Note any guarding of the abdomen, which is an indication of abdominal pain. If bowel injury is a possibility, only light palpation is acceptable. Always assess the least tender areas first and palpate the more sensitive areas last.

Laboratory and Diagnostic Testing

As in other pediatric emergencies, never delay life-saving measures to wait for laboratory or diagnostic test results. In addition to routine laboratory tests, common laboratory and diagnostic tests for the pediatric trauma victim include:

• Type and cross-match: to assess the child's blood type before blood products are given
• Prothrombin time and partial thromboplastin time: to evaluate for clotting dysfunction
• Amylase and lipase: to identify pancreatic injury
• Liver function tests: to assess for liver injury
• Pregnancy test (in any female who has reached puberty)
• CT scan, ultrasound, or MRI of the head, abdomen, or extremities: to evaluate the extent of the injury

Nursing Management

Nursing management of the pediatric trauma victim focuses initially on the ABCs.

Providing Immediate Care

If head or spinal injury is suspected, open the airway using the jaw-thrust maneuver with cervical spine stabilization (see Fig. 52.4). The revised AHA guidelines for basic life support recommend that if the airway cannot be opened using the jaw-thrust maneuver, it may be opened using the head tilt–chin lift maneuver. The rationale for this change in guidelines is that the jaw thrust is often a difficult maneuver to perform. Since opening the airway is the priority, AHA has made this allowance even if the cervical spine is at risk (AHA, 2005e). In addition, new AHA recommendations advise that the head and neck of a trauma victim should be stabilized manually rather than with an immobilization device.

▶ *Take* NOTE!

Infants and young children require unique cervical spine management because they have prominent occiputs that result in flexion of the neck in the supine position. To maintain the optimal neutral spinal position in the young child, use a special pediatric backboard with a head indentation, or use a folded towel to elevate the child's torso.

Clear the airway of obstruction using a large-bore suction device such as a Yankauer. If the child is breathing on his or her own, give oxygen at the highest flow possible (such as with a non-rebreathing mask). If the child is not breathing on his or her own, intervene using the AHA guidelines discussed earlier in this chapter.

If a BVM device is available, connect it to the oxygen source and use the bag to ventilate the child. Observe the chest rise and be careful not to overventilate, as this results in abdominal distention. Deliver breaths at the rate recommended by the AHA, one breath every 3 seconds. Do not hyperventilate. In the not-too-distant past, head injury in children was managed using hyperventilation. This resulted in **hypocapnia** (decreased amounts of carbon dioxide in the blood). The physiologic effect of hypocapnia is the induction of vasoconstriction, which in turn results in tissue ischemia. Therefore, current management of head injury in children does not use hyperventilation. The only exception to this rule is in an acute situation, if the child is showing signs of a possible brain stem herniation, hyperventilation may be used initially and briefly.

Assess the child for a strong central pulse. If the child has no pulse, initiate CPR immediately. When perfusion is compromised, administer IV fluid resuscitation. Trauma victims are more likely to require colloids or blood products due to blood loss from the injury.

▶ *Take* NOTE!

Clients with head injury who have signs of shock such as poor perfusion and bradycardia should receive fluid volume resuscitation.

■■■ Key Concepts

■ Young children's smaller airways and immature respiratory and immune systems place them at higher risk for respiratory distress than older children and adults. Children generally have healthy hearts and cardiovascular systems and thus rarely present with primary cardiac arrest. Younger children and adolescents are at higher risk for injury due to normal development at those ages.

■ Children present with a variety of emergencies and injuries and must be evaluated and treated in an appropriate and timely fashion to achieve a positive outcome. The health history is obtained rapidly while life-saving measures are performed simultaneously.

■ Assess the airway, then breathing, then circulation, providing interventions for alterations before moving on to the next assessment. Provide continuous reassessment, as children respond quickly to interventions and deteriorate quickly as well.

■ Pulse oximetry and capnometry can be useful tools for evaluating respiratory status. Never delay intervention pending laboratory results if the child's clinical status warrants immediate action.

■ Provide support and education to the child and family involved in an emergency. Teach families why certain procedures are being done, explaining technical medical interventions in simple terms and, for the child, at his or her developmental level.

■ Small amounts of edema or secretions can contribute to significant respiratory effort in infants and young children.

■ Children dehydrate more quickly than adults and experience alterations in perfusion related to hypovolemia.

■ Children in respiratory distress and shock require supplemental oxygen. Intubation is necessary for the apneic child or the child whose airway is not maintainable.

■ Accurate assessment of perfusion status and appropriate fluid resuscitation are critical in the prevention and treatment of shock in children.

■ Life-threatening arrhythmias in children, though uncommon, often must be quickly treated with defibrillation or synchronized cardioversion in addition to CPR.

■ In the case of near-drowning, maintain ongoing assessment and intervention of pulmonary status.

■ Maintain airway, breathing, and circulation in the child has experienced an accidental ingestion and prepare for gastric lavage or administration of activated charcoal.

■ In addition to intervening for airway, breathing, and circulation problems in the pediatric trauma victim, assess for altered neurologic status and extent of bleeding or injury.

REFERENCES

Agarwal, S., Swanson, S., Murphy, A., et al. (2005). Comparing the utility of a standard pediatric resuscitation cart with a pediatric resuscitation cart based on the Broselow tape: A randomized, controlled, crossover trial involving simulated resuscitation scenarios. *Pediatrics, 116*(3), 741.

Alterman, D. M., Daley, B. J., Kennedy, A. P., et al. (2006). *Considerations in pediatric trauma.* Retrieved 10/16/06 from http://www.emedicine.com/med/topic3223.htm.

American Academy of Pediatrics. (2007a). *The injury prevention program: A guide to safety counseling in office practice.* Retrieved 12/30/07 from http://www.aap.org/family/tippmain.htm.

American Academy of Pediatrics. (2007b). *Summer safety tips: Part I.* Retrieved 12/30/07 from http://www.aap.org/advocacy/releases/summertips.htm.

American Academy of Pediatrics. (2007c). *Summer safety tips: Part II.* Retrieved 12/30/07 from http://www.aap.org/advocacy/releases/summertips-p2.htm.

American Academy of Pediatrics, Committee on Injury, Violence, and Poison Prevention. (2007). *Policy statement: Poison treatment in the home.* Available at http://aappolicy.aappublications.org/cgi/content/full/pediatrics;112/5/1182.

American Association of Critical Care Nurses. (2006). *Core curriculum for pediatric critical care nursing* (2nd ed.). St. Louis: Mosby.

American Heart Association. (2005a). *Basic cardiac life support for healthcare providers.* Dallas: American Heart Association.

American Heart Association. (2005b). Highlights of the 2005 American Heart Association guidelines for cardiopulmonary resuscitation and emergency cardiovascular care. *Currents in Emergency Cardiovascular Care, 16,* 4.

American Heart Association. (2005c). Part 6: Pediatric basic and advanced life support, *Circulation, 112,* III-73-III-90. Retrieved 1/24/06 from http://circ.ahajournal.org/cgi/content/full/112/22_ suppl/III-73.

American Heart Association. (2005d). Part 10.3: Drowning. *Circulation, 112,* 133–135.

American Heart Association. (2005e). Part 11: Pediatric basic life support. *Circulation, 112,* 156–166.

American Heart Association. (2005f). Part 12: Pediatric advanced life support. *Circulation, 112,* 167–187.

American Heart Association. (2006). 2005 AHA guidelines for cardiopulmonary resuscitation (CPR) and emergency cardiovascular care (ECC) of pediatric and neonatal clients: Pediatric advanced life support. *Pediatrics, 117*(5), e1005–e1028.

American Heart Association. (2007). *Pediatric advanced life support provider manual.* Dallas: American Heart Association.

American Medical Student Association. (2007). *Child abuse and neglect.* Retrieved 12/30/07 from http://www.amsa.org/programs/gpit/child.cfm.

Atkins, D. L., & Kenney, M. A. (2004). Automated external defibrillators: Safety and efficacy in children and young adolescents. *Pediatric Clinics of North America, 51*(5), 1443–1462.

Barry, J. D. (2005). Diagnosis and management of the poisoned child. *Pediatric Annals, 34*(12), 936–946.

Behrman, R. E., Kliegman, R. M., & Jenson, H. B. (2004). *Nelson textbook of pediatrics* (17th ed.). Philadelphia: W. B. Saunders.

Belville, R. G., & Seupaul, R. A. (2005). MD pain measurement in pediatric emergency care: A review of the Faces Pain Scale-Revised. *Pediatric Emergency Care, 21*(2), 90–93.

Berger, S., Utech, L., & Hazinski, M. F. (2004). Lay rescuer automated external defibrillation programs for children and adolescents. *Pediatric Clinics of North America, 51*(5), 1463–1478.

Brophy, M., Sinclair, S. A., Hostetler, G., & Xiang, H. (2006). Pediatric eye injury-related hospitalizations in the United States. *Pediatrics, 117*(6), 2267.

Centers for Disease Control and Prevention, National Center for Health Statistics. (2005). *Emergency department visit data from the National Hospital Ambulatory Medical Care Survey.* Retrieved 6/24/06 from http://www.cdc.gov/nchs/about/otheract/injury/injury_emergency.htm.

Centers for Disease Control and Prevention, National Center for Injury Prevention and Control. (2006). *Tips to prevent poisoning.* Retrieved 12/30/07 from http://www.cdc.gov/ncipc/factsheets/poisonprevention.htm.

Centers for Disease Prevention and Control, National Center for Injury Prevention and Control. (2007a). *Injuries among children and adolescents.* Retrieved 12/30/07 from http://www.cdc.gov/ncipc/factsheets/children.htm.

Centers for Disease Control and Prevention, National Center for Injury Prevention and Control. (2007b). *National Child Passenger Safety Week, September 16–22, 2007.* Retrieved 12/30/07 from www.cdc.gov/ncipc/duip/spotlite/chldseat.htm#airbag.

Centers for Disease Control and Prevention, National Center for Injury Prevention and Control. (2007c). *Water-related injuries: Fact sheet.* Retrieved 12/30/07 from http://www.cdc.gov/ncipc/factsheets/drown.htm.

Centers for Disease Control and Prevention, National Center for Injury Prevention and Control. (2007d). *WISQARS injury mortality reports, 1999–2004.* Retrieved 12/30/07 from http://webappa.cdc.gov/sasweb/ncipc/mortrate10_sy.html.

Common Sense about Kids and Guns. (2007). *Fact file.* Retrieved 12/20/07 from http://www.kidsandguns.org/study/fact_file.asp.

Crain, E. F., & Gershal, J. C. (2004). *Clinical manual of emergency pediatrics* (4th ed.). New York: McGraw-Hill.

Davis, D. P. (2005). Quantitative capnometry as a critical resuscitation tool. *Journal of Trauma Nursing, 12*(2), 40–42.

DeBoer, S., Seaver, M., & Broselow, J. (2005). Color coding to reduce errors—the Broselow-Luten system streamlines pediatric emergency treatment. *American Journal of Nursing, 105*(8), 68–71.

Decina, L. E., Lococo, K. H., & Block, A. W. (2005). *Misuse of restraints: Results of a workshop to review field data results.* Retrieved 9/29/05 from http://www.nhtsa.dot.gov/people/injury/research/TSF_MisuseChildRetraints/809851.html.

Doniger, S. J., & Sharieff, G. Q. (2006). Pediatric dysrhythmias. *Pediatric Clinics of North America, 53*(1), 85–106.

Donoghue, A., Baren, J., & Winograd, S. M. (2004). Rapid sequence intubation in pediatrics. *Pediatric Emergency Medicine Reports, 105*(12). Retrieved 4/10/06 from Health Reference Center Academic via Thomson Gale.

Fallot, A. (2005). Respiratory distress: Evaluating and treating common pulmonary emergencies in the office. *Pediatric Annals, 34*(11), 885–891.

Farah, M. (2006). *Pediatrics, tachycardia.* Retrieved 1/24/06 from http://www.emedicine.com/emerg/topic408.htm.

Fish, F. A. (2004). Ventricular fibrillation: Basic concepts. *Pediatric Clinics of North America, 51*(5), 1211–1222.

Fortenberry, J. D., & Mariscalco, M. (2006). General principles of poisoning management. In J. A. McMillan (Ed.), *Oski's pediatrics: Principles and practice.* Philadelphia: Lippincott Williams & Wilkins.

Frost, P. (2005). Pediatric resuscitation: Recognizing and managing children at risk. *Nursing Spectrum/Nurseweek CE: Course NW0560.*

Frost, P., & Wise, B. (2006). *Kids in crisis: Pediatric emergencies.* Retrieved 6/24/06 from http://www2.nursingspectrum.com/CE/Self-Study_modules/syllabus.html?CCID=1089.

Garzon, D. L. (2005). Contributing factors to preschool unintentional injury. *Journal of Pediatric Nursing, 20*(6), 441–447.

Glassbrenner, D. (2005). *Child restraint use in 2004, overall results.* Retrieved 10/29/06 from http://www-nrd.nhtsa.dot.gov/pdf/nrd-30/NCSA/RNotes/2005/809845.pdf.

Hashikawa, A., Juhn, Y., Homme, J., & Gardner, B. (2007). Dose length-based resuscitation tape accurately place pediatric patients into appropriate color-coded zones? *Pediatric Emergency Care, 23*(12), 856–861.

Hazinski, M. F. (2005). Major changes in the 2005 AHA guidelines for CPR and ECC: Reaching the tipping point for change. *Circulation, 112,* 206–211.

Himle, M. B., & Miltenberger, R. G. (2004). Preventing unintentional firearm injury in children: The need for behavioral skills training. *Education & Treatment of Children, 27*(2), 161–177.

Johnston, C. C., Bournaki, M. C., Gagnon, A. J., et al. (2005). Self-reported pain intensity and associated distress in children aged 4–18 years on admission, discharge, and one-week follow up to emergency department. *Pediatric Emergency Care, 21*(5), 342–346.

Langlois, J. A., Rutland-Brown, W., & Thomas, K. E. (2005). The incidence of traumatic brain injury among children in the United States: Differences by race. *Journal of Head Trauma Rehabilitation, 20*(3), 229–238.

Lee, J., Ahmad, S., & Gale, C. (2005). Detection of coins ingested by children using a handheld metal detector: A systematic review. *Emergency Medicine Journal, 22*(12), 839–844.

Mace, S. E. (2005). The fifth vital sign: Pulse oximetry in noninvasive respiratory monitoring. *Pediatric Emergency Medicine Reports, 10*(3), 25–35.

Madden, M. A. (2005). Pediatric poisonings: Recognition, assessment, and management. *Critical Care Nursing Clinics of North America, 17*(4), 395–404.

Mannenbach, M., & Bechtel, K. (2005). Patterns of injury that should raise suspicion for child abuse. *Pediatric Emergency Medicine Reports.* Retrieved 4/10/06 from Health and Wellness Resource Center.

Marino, B. S., & Fine, K. S. (2007). *Blueprints pediatrics* (4th ed.). Philadelphia: Lippincott Williams & Wilkins.

Mariscalco, M. M. (2006). Shock. In J. A. McMillan (Ed.), *Oski's pediatrics: Principles and practice.* Philadelphia: Lippincott Williams & Wilkins.

Matteucci, M. J. (2005). One pill can kill: Assessing the potential for fatal poisonings in children. *Pediatric Annals, 34*(12), 965–968.

McGahey-Oakland, P. R., Lieder, H. S., Young, A., & Jefferson, L. S. (2007). Family experiences during resuscitation at a children's hospital emergency department. *Journal of Pediatric Health Care, 21*(4), 217–225.

McKiernan, C. A., & Lieberman, S. A. (2005). Circulatory shock in children: An overview. *Pediatrics in Review, 26*(12), 451–460.

Minto, G., & Woodward, W. (2005). Drowning and immersion injury. *Anaesthesia and Intensive Care Medicine, 6*(9), 321–323.

Monachino, A. M. (2005). Pediatric code readiness: Practice is the key. *Journal for Nurses in Staff Development, 21*(3), 126–131.

Moses, S. (2005). *Fluid resuscitation in trauma.* Retrieved 1/9/06 from http://www.fpnotebook.com/ER46.htm.

Nadkarni, V., Larkin, G., Peberdy, M., et al. (2006). First documented rhythm and clinical outcome from in-hospital cardiac arrest among children and adults. *Journal of the American Medical Association, 29*(1), 50–57.

National Highway Traffic Safety Administration. (2006). *2004 motor vehicle occupant protection facts.* Retrieved May 16, 2008 from http://www.nhtsa.dot.gov/people/injury/airbags/MVOP2004/images/2004MVOPFactsLo.pdf.

National SAFE KIDS Campaign. (NSKC) (2004a). *Drowning fact sheet.* Washington, DC: Author.

National SAFE KIDS Campaign. (NSKC) (2004b). *Falls fact sheet.* Washington, DC: Author.

National SAFE KIDS Campaign. (NSKC) (2004c). *Poisoning fact sheet.* Washington, DC: Author.

Nibert, L., & Ondrejka, D. (2005). Family presence during pediatric resuscitation: An integrative review for evidence-based practice. *Journal of Pediatric Nursing, 20*(2), 145–146.

Osterhoudt, K. C., Durbin, D., Alpern, E. R., & Henretig, F. M. (2004). Risk factors for emesis after therapeutic use of activated charcoal in acutely poisoned children. *Pediatrics, 113*(4), 806–810.

Perondi, M. B. M., Reis, A. G., Paiva, E. F., et al. (2004). A comparison of high-dose and standard-dose epinephrine in children with cardiac arrest. *New England Journal of Medicine, 350,* 1722–1730.

Prentiss, K. A., Mick, N. W., Cummings, B. M., et al. (2007). *Emergency management of the pediatric client.* Philadelphia: Lippincott Williams & Wilkins.

Probst, B. D., Lyons, E., Leonard, D., et al. (2005). Factors affecting emergency department assessment and management of pain in children. *Pediatric Emergency Care, 21*(5), 298–305.

Rezendes, J. L. (2006). Bicycle helmets: Overcoming barriers to use and increasing effectiveness. *Journal of Pediatric Nursing, 21*(1), 35–44.

RNCeus. (2006). *Abnormal breath sounds.* Retrieved 10/25/06 from www.rnceus.com/resp/respabn.html.

Robertson, J., & Shilkofski, N. (2005). *The Harriet Lane handbook* (17th ed.). Philadelphia: Mosby.

Rosman, N. P. (2006). Acute head trauma. In J. A. McMillan (Ed.), *Oski's pediatrics: Principles and practice.* Philadelphia: Lippincott Williams & Wilkins.

Ross, J. (2006). *Summer injuries: Near drowning.* Retrieved 4/25/06 from http://rnweb.com/rnweb/article/articleDetail.jsp?id=168160.

SafeKids. (2006). *Poisoning safety.* Retrieved 6/20/06 from http://www.safekids.org/tips/tips_poison.html.

Samson, R. A., Berg, R. A., Bingham, R., et al. (2003). Use of automated external defibrillators in children: An update: An advisory statement from the Pediatric Advanced Life Support Task Force, International Liaison Committee on Resuscitation. *Circulation, 107,* 3250–3255.

Schweich, P. J. (2006). Selected topics in emergency medicine. In J. A. McMillan (Ed.), *Oski's pediatrics: Principles and practice.* Philadelphia: Lippincott Williams & Wilkins.

Stephenson, M. (2005). Danger in the toy box. *Journal of Pediatric Health Care, 19,* 187–189.

Strange, G., Ahrens, W., McQuillen, K., et al. (2004). *Pediatric emergency medicine: Just the facts.* New York: McGraw-Hill.

Taketokmo, C. K., Hodding, J. H., & Kraus, D. M. (2007). *Lexi-comp's pediatric dosage handbook* (14th ed.). Hudson, Ohio: Lexi-comp.

Wilson, M. H., & Levin-Goodman, R. (2006). Injury control and prevention. In J. A. McMillan (Ed.), *Oski's pediatrics: Principles and practice*. Philadelphia: Lippincott Williams & Wilkins.

World Health Organization. (2008). *Drowning*. Retrieved May 16, 2008 from http://www.who.int/violence_injury_prevention/other_injury/drowning/en/.

WEBSITES

American Academy of Pediatrics safety information: www.aap.org/healthtopics/safety.cfm

American Association of Poison Control Centers: www.aapcc.org

Centers for Disease Control and Prevention, National Center for Injury Prevention and Control, Child Passenger Safety Fact Sheet: www.cdc.gov/ncipc/factsheets/childpas.htm

Centers for Disease Control and Prevention, National Center for Injury Prevention and Control, Teen Drivers Fact Sheet: www.cdc.gov/ncipc/factsheets/teenmvh.htm

Kidspace @ the Internet Public Library: www.ipl.org/div/kidspace/poisonsafe/kjump.html

National Highway Traffic Safety Administration: http://www.nhtsa.dot.gov/

Nemours Foundation: www.kidshealth.org

Nursing CEUs and information: www.rnceus.com/index.html#_parent#_parent

Poison Prevention Week Council: www.poisonprevention.org/materials.htm

Safe Kids Worldwide: www.safekids.org

U.S. Consumers Product Safety Commission, Poison Prevention Publications: www.cpsc.gov/cpscpub/pubs/pois_prv.html

CHAPTER WORKSHEET

MULTIPLE CHOICE QUESTIONS

1. An unresponsive toddler is brought to the emergency department. Assessment reveals mottled skin color, respiratory rate of 10 breaths per minute, and a brachial pulse of 52 bpm. What is the priority nursing action?

   a. Prepare the defibrillator and draw up code medications.

   b. Provide 100% oxygen with a bag-valve-mask and start chest compressions.

   c. Start chest compressions and provide 100% oxygen via non-rebreather mask.

   d. Begin an IV fluid infusion and administer epinephrine IV.

2. A 10-year-old child in respiratory distress requires intubation. Which sizes of tracheal tubes will the nurse prepare?

   a. 9.5 mm and 10.0 mm

   b. 8.5 mm and 9.0 mm

   c. 6.0 mm and 6.5 mm

   d. 6.5 mm and 7.0 mm

3. A preschooler presents to the emergency department with a history of vomiting, diarrhea, and fever over the past few days. She is receiving 100% oxygen via non-rebreather mask. Vital signs are temperature 104.5°F, pulse 144 bpm, respiratory rate 22 breaths per minute, and BP 70/50 mm Hg. She is listless and difficult to arouse and has weak peripheral pulses and prolonged capillary refill. What nursing intervention takes priority?

   a. Administering acetaminophen rectally for the high fever

   b. Administering IV antibiotics for the infection

   c. Preparing the child for tracheal intubation

   d. Giving an IV bolus of normal saline 20 mL/kg

4. Assessment of a 12-year-old who crashed his bicycle without a helmet reveals the following: temperature 99.2°F, pulse 100 bpm, respiratory rate 24 breaths per minute with easy work of breathing, and BP 102/70 mm Hg. What is the priority action by the nurse?

   a. Assess neurologic status while observing for obvious injuries.

   b. Administer IV fluid bolus of normal saline at 20 mL/kg.

   c. Remove the cervical collar if he complains that it bothers him.

   d. Listen for bowel sounds while assessing for pain.

5. An 18-month-old child is brought to the emergency department via ambulance after an accidental ingestion. What is the priority nursing action?

   a. Take the child's vital signs.

   b. Give oral syrup of ipecac.

   c. Insert a nasogastric tube.

   d. Start an IV line.

CRITICAL THINKING EXERCISES

1. A school-age child presents to the emergency department for evaluation. He had been feeling faint off and on and today fainted at school. On the cardiac monitor an abnormal cardiac rhythm is noted. At present the child is stable. What questions would be most appropriate for the nurse to ask when obtaining the child's health history? What objective assessments should the nurse make?

2. Charlie is a 2-year-old who is admitted to the hospital after accidentally ingesting a medication. His mother, who brought Charlie to the hospital, is upset and crying. How does Charlie's age and stage of development affect his risk for accidental ingestion? How should the nurse respond to the mother's distress? Develop a discharge teaching plan for Charlie and his family related to poison prevention.

3. A 7-month-old is brought to the acute care facility with a chief complaint of difficulty breathing. The infant's mother says that his cold has gotten worse and he won't eat. What additional questions should the nurse ask about the infant's health history? How would the nurse appropriately manage this infant's airway?

STUDY ACTIVITIES

1. Spend a day in the pediatric emergency department or urgent care center and document the role of the triage nurse.

2. Observe the pediatric emergency medical team at work or observe a pediatric code in the hospital. Compare and contrast the measures performed for the child with those that would be performed for an adult in a similar emergency situation.

3. Develop a teaching project related to injury prevention and present it at a local elementary, middle, or high school. Ensure that the education is geared toward the children's developmental level.

4. Interview the parents of a child who has experienced an emergency situation about how they felt during and after the emergency. Present the information to your classmates.

5. When providing care to a child in an emergency, the nurse performs the following assessments. Place them in the proper sequence.

   a. Pupillary reaction

   b. Presence of cough or sputum

   c. Heart rate and capillary refill

   d. Presence of bruises and abrasions

   e. Work of breathing

APPENDIX

STANDARD LABORATORY VALUES

Pregnant and Nonpregnant Women

Values	Nonpregnant	Pregnant
Hematologic		
Complete Blood Count (CBC)		
Hemoglobin, g/dL	12–16*	11.5–14*
Hematocrit, PCV, %	37–47	32–42
Red cell volume, mL	1600	1900
Plasma volume, mL	2400	3700
Red blood cell count, million/mm³	4–5.5	3.75–5.0
White blood cells, total per mm³	4500–10,000	5000–15,000
Polymorphonuclear cells, %	54–62	60–85
Lymphocytes, %	38–46	15–40
Erythrocyte sedimentation rate, mm/h	≤	30–90
MCHC, g/dL packed RBCs (mean corpuscular hemoglobin concentration)	30–36	No change
MCH (mean corpuscular hemoglobin per picogram)	29–32	No change
MCV/μm³ (mean corpuscular volume per cubic micrometer)	82–96	No change
Blood Coagulation and Fibrinolytic Activity†		
Factors VII, VIII, IX, X		Increase in pregnancy, return to normal in early puerperium; factor VIII increases during and immediately after delivery
Factors XI, XIII		Decrease in pregnancy
Prothrombin time (protime)	60–70 sec	Slight decrease in pregnancy
Partial thromboplastin time (PTT)	12–14 sec	Slight decrease in pregnancy and again during second and third stage of labor (indicates clotting at placental site)

(continued)

Values	Nonpregnant	Pregnant
Bleeding time	1–3 min (Duke) 2–4 min (Ivy)	No appreciable change
Coagulation time	6–10 min (Lee/White)	No appreciable change
Platelets	150,000 to 350,000/mm³	No significant change until 3–5 days after delivery, then marked increase (may predispose woman to thrombosis) and gradual return to normal
Fibrinolytic activity		Decreases in pregnancy, then abrupt return to normal (protection against thromboembolism)
Fibrinogen	250 mg/dL	400 mg/dL
Mineral and Vitamin Concentrations		
Serum iron, μg	75–150	65–120
Total iron-binding capacity, μg	250–450	300–500
Iron saturation, %	30–40	15–30
Vitamin B₁₂, folic acid, ascorbic acid	Normal	Moderate decrease
Serum protein		
Total, g/dL	6.7–8.3	5.5–7.5
Albumin, g/dL	3.5–5.5	3.0–5.0
Globulin, total, g/dL	2.3–3.5	3.0–4.0
Blood sugar		
Fasting, mg/dL	70–80	65
2-hour postprandial, mg/dL	60–110	Under 140 after a 100-g carbohydrate meal is considered normal
Cardiovascular		
Blood pressure, mm Hg	120/80‡	114/65
Peripheral resistance, dyne/s · cm⁻⁵	120	100
Venous pressure, cm H₂O		
Femoral	9	24
Antecubital	8	8
Pulse, rate/min	70	80
Stroke volume, mL	65	75
Cardiac output, L/min	4.5	6
Circulation time (arm-tongue), sec	15–16	12–14
Blood volume, mL		
Whole blood	4000	5600
Plasma	2400	3700
Red blood cells	1600	1900
Plasma renin, units/L	3–10	10–80
Chest x-ray studies		
Transverse diameter of heart	—	1–2 cm increase
Left border of heart	—	Straightened
Cardiac volume	—	70-mL increase
Electrocardiogram	—	15° left axis deviation
V₁ and V₂	—	Inverted T-wave
kV₄	—	Low T
III	—	Q + inverted T
aVr	—	Small Q

Values	Nonpregnant	Pregnant
Hepatic		
Bilirubin total	Not more than 1 mg/dL	Unchanged
Cephalin flocculation	Up to 2+ in 48 h	Positive in 10%
Serum cholesterol	110–300 mg/dL	↑ 60% from 16–32 weeks of pregnancy; remains at this level until after delivery
Thymol turbidity	0–4 units	Positive in 15%
Serum alkaline phosphatase	2–4.5 units (Bodansky)	↑ from week 12 of pregnancy to 6 weeks after delivery
Serum lactate dehydrogenase		Unchanged
Serum glutamic-oxaloacetic transaminase		Unchanged
Serum globulin albumin	1.5–3.0 g/dL 4.5–5.3 g/dL	↑ slight ↓ 3.0 g by late pregnancy
A/G ratio		Decreased
α_2-globulin		Increased
β-globulin		Increased
Serum cholinesterase		Decreased
Leucine aminopeptidase		Increased
Sulfobromophthalein (5 mg/kg)	5% dye or less in 45 min	Somewhat decreased
Renal		
Bladder capacity	1300 mL	1500 mL
Renal plasma flow (RPF), mL/min	490–700	Increase by 25%, to 612–875
Glomerular filtration rate (GFR), mL/min	105–132	Increase by 50%, to 160–198
Nonprotein nitrogen (NPN), mg/dL	25–40	Decreases
Blood urea nitrogen (BUN), mg/dL	20–25	Decreases
Serum creatinine, mg/kg/24 hr	20–22	Decreases
Serum uric acid, mg/kg/24 hr	257–750	Decreases
Urine glucose	Negative	Present in 20% of gravidas
Intravenous pyelogram (IVP)	Normal	Slight to moderate hydroureter and hydronephrosis; right kidney larger than left kidney
Miscellaneous		
Total thyroxine concentration	5–12 μg/dL thyroxine	↑ 9–16 μg/dL thyroxine (however, unbound thyroxine not greatly increased)
Ionized calcium		Relatively unchanged
Aldosterone		↑ 1 mg/24 hr by third trimester
Dehydroisoandrosterone	Plasma clearance 6–8 L/24 hr	↑ plasma clearance tenfold to twentyfold

* At sea level. Permanent residents of higher levels (e.g., Denver) require higher levels of hemoglobin.

From Scott, J. R., et al. (2000). *Obstetrics and gynecology*. Philadelphia: Lippincott Williams & Wilkins.

† Pregnancy represents a hypercoagulable state.

‡ For the woman about 20 years of age.

10 years of age: 103/70.

30 years of age: 123/82.

40 years of age: 126/84.

APPENDIX

CLINICAL PATHS

LABOR AND DELIVERY CLINICAL PATH—LABOR: EXPECTED OUTCOMES

	Active Phase	Expulsion/Pushing	Recovery 1st Hour Post Partum
PATIENT EDUCATION	Patient coping with labor support Patient utilizing appropriate labor options Patient verbalizes satisfaction with plan Management interventions	Patient demonstrates effective pushing technique. Patient coping effectively with pushing. Support person coping effectively with labor.	Bonding appropriately with baby

PATIENTS STATUS	Cervix dilated 5 cm—complete
	Contraction regularly with progressive cervical change.
	Maternal/fetal well-being maintained
	Hydration maintained
	If indicated: FSE and/or IUPC placed
	    IV Pitocin started
	    Epidural placed/WE encouraged
	    Medicate with prn pain meds
		Vaginal birth	Placenta delivered
			Fundus firm
			Lochia small–moderate
			Without clots
			Perineum intact/repaired
			Hemodynamically stable
			EBL <500 cc

CONTINUUM OF CARE	Prenatal record available after 32 weeks Prenatal labs WNL Pre-registered to hospital Pediatrician identified Support after hospitalization identified Discharge plan discussed with patient/family Communicates understanding of hospital and community resources		

	Interventions		
ASSESSMENT/ TREATMENT	Assess: Continuous EFM or auscultation Q 15 of 30 minutes as indicated. Vital signs hourly/Temp Q4 hr if intact membranes/Q 2 hr if membranes ruptured Uterine by monitor or palpation Bladder for distention Hydration status Cervical dilation, effacement, station	Assess: Q 15 minutes monitoring of fetal well being (Low-Risk) and Q 5 minutes (High-Risk) Vital signs hourly Temp. Q 2–4 hr depending on membrane status Bladder for distention Hydration status Pushing effectiveness Descent of presenting part Caput	Assess: Uterus—fundus Vital signs Lochia Bladder Perineum Placenta
PATIENT EDUCATION	Reinforce comfort measures Encourage use of labor options Inform patient/support person of plan of care	Teaching of upright pushing positions Discourage prolonged maternal breath holding Encourage to assume position of choice Inform patient of progress	Baby status Breast feeding
TESTS/ PROCEDURES	Hgb or Hct (if not done recently) T & S (if ordered) VE as indicated IV therapy AROM by M.D. or CNM: assess for color, amount and odor, as appropriate FSE/IUPC placement if indicated	AROM: assess for color, amount and odor, as appropriate	Cord blood or Rhogam workup if appropriate Cord blood if O+ Mom
THERAPIES	Comfort measures/birthing ball/ambulate/telemetry/ shower IV therapy Amnio infusion for variable decelerations If appropriate, Pain Mgmt. reviewed	Perineal massage Warm soaks to perineal area Allow to rest until feels urge to push Frequent position changes Cool cloth/ice chips	Ice pack to perineum Warm blankets
MEDS	Antibiotics as indicated for + GBS Pitocin if indicated PRN pain medication (encourage WE if requesting this)	Pitocin if indicated	Pitocin IV
ACTIVITY/ SAFETY	Labor option usage Position changes	Provide wedge if supine Promote effective position for pushing: i.e., squatting, side lying, upright Breathing technique patient/ support person most comfortable with	Assist with ambulate to bathroom Infant care Assist with positioning for breast feeding Infant ID bands present

(continued)

LABOR AND DELIVERY CLINICAL PATH—LABOR: EXPECTED OUTCOMES (continued)

Interventions		
NUTRITION Clear liquids Ice chips OTHER	Clear liquids Ice chips	Return to previous diet

(Left vertical label: **UNIQUE PATIENT NEEDS**)

INTEGRATED PLAN OF CARE FOR CESAREAN DELIVERY

	Expected Patient Outcomes			
	Phase 1 Preadmission (Cesarean Delivery)	Phase 2 Surgery/ Immediate Postop/ Day of Surgery	Phase 3 Postop Day 1	
Usual time in Phase	**N/A Date Started:**	Up to 23 hours	1 day	1–2 days
Assessment / Potential Complications	VS WNL for patient Hgb or Hct/values within normal SLH antepartum range	VS WNL for patient Systems assessment: Skin warm, dry Clear → Alert & oriented → Neg. Homans' sign → Breast soft/nipples intact → Lungs clear → Bowel sounds present → Fundus firm u/u or u 1–2 (–/+) Lochia sm—mod Dsg dry and intact No signs infiltration IV site Verbalizes comfort using pain rating scale 0–10	VS WNL for patient Afebrile Voiding without foley → Passing flatus Incision without redness or drainage Lochia small amount Fundus firm u/1–2 Verbalizes comfort using pain scale 0–10 on oral pain meds	Incision well approximated, without drainage or redness Passing flatus Lochia sm/mod amt Fundus firm u/1–2 Verbalizes comfort using pain medication as described

Expected Patient Outcomes				
	Phase 1 Preadmission (Cesarean Delivery)	Phase 2 Surgery/ Immediate Postop/ Day of Surgery	Phase 3 Postop Day 1	
Patient / Family Knowledge	**Date All Above Met** Verbalizes understanding of condition and need for surgery Verbalizes understanding of all pre-op teaching	**Date All Above Met** Verbalizes correct use of PCA/Fentanyl pump and when to request pain medication Turn, cough & deep breath appropriately	**Date All Above Met** Can state criteria for when to call doctor for problems post discharge → ↑ bleeding ↑ Temperature → incision redness, odor or drainage →	**Date All Above Met** Verbalizes follow-up appointment date and time Verbalizes proper dosing of pain medication
ADL's / Activity	**Date All Above Met** Verbalizes understanding of NPO status	**Date All Above Met** Able to ambulate with minimal assistance Tolerating clear/full liquid diet Bonding observed with newborn— Taking-in phase →	**Date All Above Met** Ambulating without assistance Tolerating soft to regular diet	**Date All Above Met** Ambulating in hall
Unique Patient Needs	**Date All Above Met**	**Date All Above Met**	**Date All Above Met**	**Date All Above Met**
	Date All Above Met Entire Phase Outcomes Met; Progress patient to next phase	**Date All Above Met Entire Phase Outcomes Met; Progress patient to next phase**	**Date All Above Met Entire Phase Outcomes Met; Progress patient to next phase**	**Date All Above Met Entire Phase Outcomes Met; Progress patient to next phase**

Plan of Care				
	#1 Preadmission	#2 Surgery/ Immediate Postop/ Day of Surgery	#3 Postop Day 1	#4 Postop Day 2- Discharge
Assessments	Vital Signs Fetal status immediately prior to surgery	VS per PACU then q 4 hr Systems assessment: *Skin, LOC, FROM, Homans' sign *Breasts, Lungs, Fundus, Incision *Lochia, bladder, bowel sounds, IV and site	VS q 6 hr Assess pain control 0–10 scale Incision Foley-volding Fundus/lochia Homans' sign IV site Breasts ID band on mother Activity	Assess pain control 0–10 scale Incision Volding Fundus lochia Homans' sign IV site as needed ID band on mother Activity

(continued)

INTEGRATED PLAN OF CARE FOR CESAREAN DELIVERY (continued)

		Plan of Care		
	#1 Preadmission	#2 Surgery/ Immediate Postop/ Day of Surgery	#3 Postop Day 1	#4 Postop Day 2- Discharge
		*I & O q shift *Assess pain control 0–10 scale *Assess Rhogam status *Assess Rubella titer status *ID band on mother		
Consults	Anesthesia	Social Work as needed, Anesthesia, Lactation, Dietitian as needed	Social Work, Lactation, Dietitian as needed	Social Work, Lactation, Dietitian as needed
Patient / Family Education Discharge Planning	— Need for surgery — Review Cesarean Delivery — Review procedure, postop expectations — Demonstrate/ Discuss equipment—PCA, Fentanyl pump — Tour of OR area & Nsy	Review postop expectations Review equipment us prn Instruct pt on: Hospital/Infant security systems Unity orientation Newborn orientation/care/feeding (if breastfeeding problems see decision trees)	Review dietary needs post surgery Review Bleeding/ Lochia Precautions post cesarean delivery Review follow-up care and doctor Appointments Review incision care, peri care Infant care Infant feeding	Verify follow-up appointment date and time Activity restrictions Follow-up for staple removal as needed Offer home follow-up care Discuss birth control
Tests and Procedures	PAT; Hgb or Hct (if not done recently—within one month) T & S (if ordered)			
Pharmacologic Needs		IV fluids as ordered Pain control: PCA, Fentanyl pump, IM to PO	IV lock PO pain meds Give Rhogam if indicated Give Rubella if indicated	DC IV lock as ordered

	Plan of Care			
	#1 Preadmission	#2 Surgery/ Immediate Postop/ Day of Surgery	#3 Postop Day 1	#4 Postop Day 2- Discharge
Activity / Rehabilitation	Patient's usual	Change position q 2 hr while in bed, OOB stand at bedside post-op night/dangle and transfer to chair Progress to pt. endurance Observe bonding with infant Observe family support system (if inadequate consult SW)	Progress endurance/ begin Ambulation in hall OOB in AM May shower	Ambulate in halls without assistance
Nutrition / Elimination		NPO then clear liquids to DAT Foley empty q shift	DAT to regular or pre-vious diet at home Foley DC'd	
Miscellaneous Interventions		TCDB q 2 hr while awake	Dressing removed by MD or RN with MD request	
Unique Patient Needs				

CERVICAL DILATION CHART

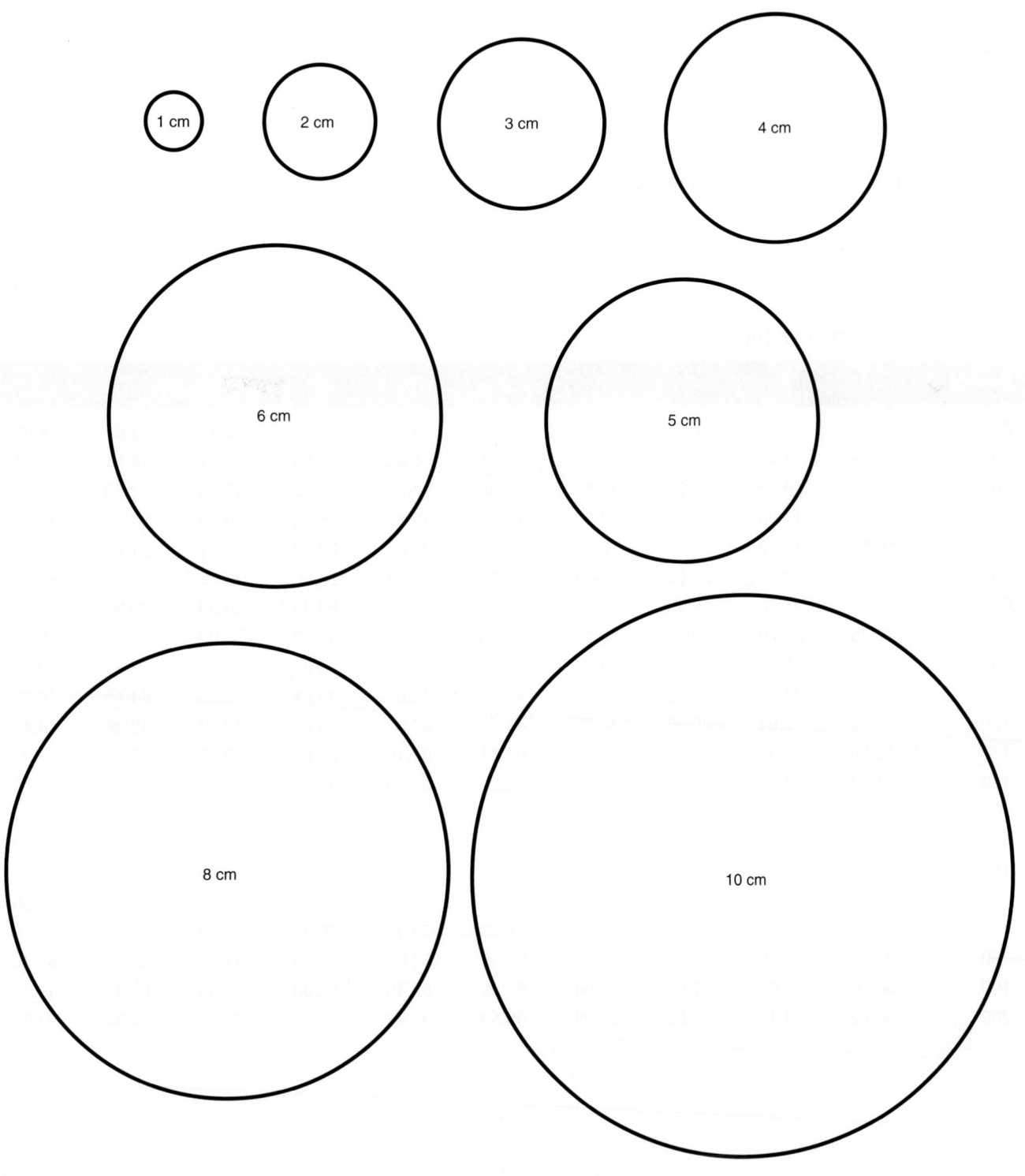

WEIGHT CONVERSION CHARTS

CONVERSION OF POUNDS TO KILOGRAMS

Pounds	0	1	2	3	4	5	6	7	8	9
0	—	0.45	0.90	1.36	1.81	2.26	2.72	3.17	3.62	4.08
10	4.53	4.98	5.44	5.89	6.35	6.80	7.25	7.71	8.16	8.61
20	9.07	9.52	9.97	10.43	10.88	11.34	11.79	12.24	12.70	13.15
30	13.60	14.06	14.51	14.96	15.42	15.87	16.32	16.78	17.23	17.69
40	18.14	18.59	19.05	19.50	19.95	20.41	20.86	21.31	21.77	22.22
50	22.68	23.13	23.58	24.04	24.49	24.94	25.40	25.85	26.30	26.76
60	27.21	27.66	28.12	28.57	29.03	29.48	29.93	30.39	30.84	31.29
70	31.75	32.20	32.65	33.11	33.56	34.02	34.47	34.92	35.38	35.83
80	36.28	36.74	37.19	37.64	38.10	38.55	39.00	39.46	39.91	40.37
90	40.82	41.27	41.73	42.18	42.63	43.09	43.54	43.99	44.45	44.90
100	45.36	45.81	46.26	46.72	47.17	47.62	48.08	48.53	48.98	49.44
110	49.89	50.34	50.80	51.25	51.71	52.16	52.61	53.07	53.52	53.97
120	54.43	54.88	55.33	55.79	56.24	56.70	57.15	57.60	58.06	58.51
130	58.96	59.42	59.87	60.32	60.78	61.23	61.68	62.14	62.59	63.05
140	63.50	63.95	64.41	64.86	65.31	65.77	66.22	66.67	67.13	67.58
150	68.04	68.49	68.94	69.40	69.85	70.30	70.76	71.21	71.66	72.12
160	72.57	73.02	73.48	73.93	74.39	74.84	75.29	75.75	76.20	76.65
170	77.11	77.56	78.01	78.47	78.92	79.38	79.83	80.28	80.74	81.19
180	81.64	82.10	82.55	83.00	83.46	83.91	84.36	84.82	85.27	85.73
190	86.18	86.68	87.09	87.54	87.99	88.45	88.90	89.35	89.81	90.26
200	90.72	91.17	91.62	92.08	92.53	92.98	93.44	93.89	94.34	94.80

CONVERSION OF POUNDS AND OUNCES TO GRAMS FOR NEWBORN WEIGHTS

Pounds	Ounces															
	0	1	2	3	4	5	6	7	8	9	10	11	12	13	14	15
0	—	28	57	85	113	142	170	198	227	255	283	312	340	369	397	425
1	454	482	510	539	567	595	624	652	680	709	737	765	794	822	850	879
2	907	936	964	992	1021	1049	1077	1106	1134	1162	1191	1219	1247	1276	1304	1332
3	1361	1389	1417	1446	1474	1503	1531	1559	1588	1616	1644	1673	1701	1729	1758	1786
4	1814	1843	1871	1899	1928	1956	1984	2013	2041	2070	2098	2126	2155	2183	2211	2240
5	2268	2296	2325	2353	2381	2410	2438	2466	2495	2523	2551	2580	2608	2637	2665	2693
6	2722	2750	2778	2807	2835	2863	2892	2920	2948	2977	3005	3033	3062	3090	3118	3147
7	3175	3203	3232	3260	3289	3317	3345	3374	3402	3430	3459	3487	3515	3544	3572	3600
8	3629	3657	3685	3714	3742	3770	3799	3827	3856	3884	3912	3941	3969	3997	4026	4054
9	4082	4111	4139	4167	4196	4224	4252	4281	4309	4337	4366	4394	4423	4451	4479	4508
10	4536	4564	4593	4621	4649	4678	4706	4734	4763	4791	4819	4848	4876	4904	4933	4961
11	4990	5018	5046	5075	5103	5131	5160	5188	5216	5245	5273	5301	5330	5358	5386	5415
12	5443	5471	5500	5528	5557	5585	5613	5642	5670	5698	5727	5755	5783	5812	5840	5868
13	5897	5925	5953	5982	6010	6038	6067	6095	6123	6152	6180	6209	6237	6265	6294	6322
14	6350	6379	6407	6435	6464	6492	6520	6549	6577	6605	6634	6662	6690	6719	6747	6776
15	6804	6832	6860	6889	6917	6945	6973	7002	7030	7059	7087	7115	7144	7172	7201	7228

Breast-Feeding and Medication Use

General Considerations

- Most medications are safe to use while breast-feeding; however, the woman should always check with the pediatrician, physician, or lactation specialist before taking any medications, including over-the-counter and herbal products.
- Inform the woman that she has the right to seek a second opinion if the physician does not perform a thoughtful risk-versus-benefit assessment before prescribing medications or advising against breast-feeding.
- Most medications pass from the woman's bloodstream into the breast milk. However, the amount is usually very small and unlikely to harm the baby.
- A preterm or other special needs neonate is more susceptible to the adverse effects of medications in breast milk. A woman who is taking medications and whose baby is in the neonatal intensive care unit or special care nursery should consult with the pediatrician or neonatologist before feeding her breast milk to the baby.
- If the woman is taking a prescribed medication, she should take the medication just after breast-feeding. This practice helps ensure that the lowest possible dose of medication reaches the baby through the breast milk.
- Some medications can cause changes in the amount of milk the woman produces. Teach the woman to report any changes in milk production.

Lactation Risk Categories (LRC)

Location Category	Risk	Rationale
L1	Safest	Clinical research or long-term observation
L2	Safer	of use in many breast-feeding women has not demonstrated risk to the infant. Limited clinical esearch has not demonstrated an increase in adverse effects in the infant.
L3	Moderately safe	There is possible risk to the infant; however, the risks are minimal or nonthreatening in nature. These medications should be given only when the potential benefit outweighs the risk to the infant.
L4	Possibly hazardous	There is positive evidence of risk to the infant; however, in life-threatening situations or for serious diseases, the benefit might outweigh the risk.

(continued)

Location Category	Risk	Rationale
L5	Contraindicated	The risk of using the medication clearly outweighs any possible benefit from breast-feeding.

Potential Effects of Selected Medication Categories on the Breast-Fed Infant

Narcotic Analgesics

- Codeine and hydrocodone appear to be safe in moderate doses. Rarely the neonate may experience sedation and/or apnea. (LRC: L3)
- Meperidine (Demerol) can lead to sedation of the neonate. (LRC: L3)
- Low to moderate doses of morphine appear to be safe. (LRC: L2)
- Trace-to-negligible amounts of fentanyl are found in human milk. (LRC: L2)

Non-narcotic Analgesics and NSAIDs

- Acetaminophen and ibuprofen are approved for use. (LRC: L1)
- Naproxen may cause neonatal hemorrhage and anemia if used for prolonged periods. (LRC: L3 for short-term use and L4 for long-term use)
- The newer COX2 inhibitors, such as celecoxib (Celebrex), appear to be safe for use. (LRC: L2)

Antibiotics

- Levels in breast milk are usually very low.
- The penicillins and cephalosporins are generally considered safe to use. (LRC: L1 and L2)
- Tetracyclines can be safely used for short periods but are not suitable for long-term therapy (e.g., for treatment of acne). (LRC: L2)
- Sulfonamides should not be used during the neonatal stage (the first month of life). (LRC: L3)

Antihypertensives

- A high degree of caution is advised when antihypertensives are used during breast-feeding.
- Some beta blockers can be used.
- Hydralazine and methyldopa are considered to be safe. (LRC: L2)

- ACE inhibitors are not recommended in the early postpartum period.

Sedatives and Hypnotics

- Neonatal withdrawal can occur when antianxiety medications, such as lorazepam, are taken. Fortunately withdrawal is generally mild.
- Phenothiazines, such as Phenergan and Thorazine, may lead to sleep apnea and increase the risk for sudden infant death syndrome.

Antidepressants

- The risk to the baby often is higher if the woman is depressed and remains untreated, rather than taking the medication.
- The older tricyclics are considered to be safe; however they cause many bothersome side effects, such as weight gain and dry mouth, which may lead to noncompliance on the part of the woman.
- The selective serotonin uptake inhibitors (SSRIs) also are considered to be safe and have a lower side effect profile, which makes them more palatable to the woman. (LRC: L2 and L3)

Mood Stabilizers (Antimanic Medication)

- Lithium is found in breast milk and is best not used in the breast-feeding woman. (LRC: L4)
- Valproic acid (Depakote) seems to be a more appropriate choice for the woman with bipolar disorder. The infant will need periodic lab studies to check platelets and liver function.

Corticosteroids

- Corticosteroids do not pass into the milk in large quantities.
- Inhaled steroids are safe to use because they don't accumulate in the bloodstream.

Thyroid Medication

- Thyroid medications, such as levothyroxine (Synthroid), can be taken while breast-feeding.
- Most are in LRC category L1.

Medications That Usually Are Contraindicated for the Breast-Feeding Woman

- Amiodarone
- Antineoplastic agents
- Chloramphenicol

- Doxepin
- Ergotamine and other ergot derivatives
- Iodides
- Methotrexate and immunosuppressants
- Lithium

- Radiopharmaceuticals
- Ribavirin
- Tetracycline (prolonged use—more than 3 weeks)
- Pseudoephedrine (found in many over-the-counter medications)

Material in this Appendix was adapted from information found on the American Academy of Pediatrics website (www.aap.org) and from Riordan, J. (2005). *Breastfeeding and human lactation* (3rd ed.). Boston: Jones and Bartlett Publishers; Hale, T. W. (2004). *Medications and mother's milk* (11th ed.). Amarillo, TX: Pharmasoft Publishing.

APPENDIX ℱ

GROWTH CHARTS

Birth to 36 months: Boys
Length-for-age and Weight-for-age percentiles

NAME _____

RECORD # _____

AGE (MONTHS)

95
90
75
50
25
10
5

95
90
75
50
25
10
5

AGE (MONTHS)

	12	15	18	21	24	27	30	33	36	kg	lb

Mother's Stature _____ Gestational
Father's Stature _____ Age: _____ Weeks   Comment

Date	Age	Weight	Length	Head Circ.
	Birth			

Birth   3   6   9

Published May 30, 2000 (modified 4/20/01).
SOURCE: Developed by the National Center for Health Statistics in collaboration with
the National Center for Chronic Disease Prevention and Health Promotion (2000).
http://www.cdc.gov/growthcharts

SAFER · HEALTHIER · PEOPLE™

Birth to 36 months: Boys
Head circumference-for-age and
Weight-for-length percentiles

NAME _____

RECORD # _____

HEAD CIRCUMFERENCE

AGE (MONTHS)

Birth 3 6 9 12 15 18 21 24 27 30 33 36

in cm — 52 50 48 46 44 42 40 38 36 34 32 30

95 90 75 50 25 10 5

WEIGHT

LENGTH

LENGTH																			
64	66	68	70	72	74	76	78	80	82	84	86	88	90	92	94	96	98	100	cm
26		27	28	29	30	31	32	33	34	35	36	37	38	39	40	41			in

Date	Age	Weight	Length	Head Circ.	Comment

cm	46 48 50 52 54 56 58 60 62
in	18 19 20 21 22 23 24

Published May 30, 2000 (modified 10/16/00).
SOURCE: Developed by the National Center for Health Statistics in collaboration with
the National Center for Chronic Disease Prevention and Health Promotion (2000).
http://www.cdc.gov/growthcharts

SAFER·HEALTHIER·PEOPLE™

Birth to 36 months: Girls
Length-for-age and Weight-for-age percentiles

NAME _____

RECORD # _____

AGE (MONTHS)

Birth 3 6 9 12 15 18 21 24 27 30 33 36

LENGTH

WEIGHT

AGE (MONTHS)

12 15 18 21 24 27 30 33 36 kg lb

Birth 3 6 9

Mother's Stature _____		Gestational		Comment
Father's Stature _____		Age: _____ Weeks		
Date	Age	Weight	Length	Head Circ.
	Birth			

Published May 30, 2000 (modified 4/20/01).
SOURCE: Developed by the National Center for Health Statistics in collaboration with
the National Center for Chronic Disease Prevention and Health Promotion (2000).
http://www.cdc.gov/growthcharts

SAFER · HEALTHIER · PEOPLE™

Birth to 36 months: Girls
Head circumference-for-age and
Weight-for-length percentiles

NAME _____

RECORD # _____

AGE (MONTHS)

Birth 3 6 9 **12** 15 18 21 **24** 27 30 33 **36**

HEAD CIRCUMFERENCE

in cm

—20 —52

—19 —50

—48

—18 —46

—17 —44

—16 —42

—15 —40

—14 —38

—36

—13 —34

—12 —32

—30

95
90
75
50
25
10
5

cm in

—52

—50 —20

—48 —19

—46 —18

—44

—42 —17

HEAD CIRCUMFERENCE

WEIGHT

—50
—22 —48
—21 —46
—20 —44
—19 —42
—18 —40
—17 —38
—16 —36
—15 —34
—14 —32
—13 —30
—12 —28
—11 —26
—11 —24
—10 —22
—9 —20
—8 —18
—7 —16
—6 —14
—5 —12
kg —lb

95
90
75
50
25
10
5

WEIGHT

in cm
—24 —11
—22 —10
—20 —9
—18 —8
—16 —7
—14 —6
—12 —5
—10 —4
—8 —3
—6 —2
—4
—2 —1
lb —kg

LENGTH

cm 64 66 68 70 72 74 76 78 80 82 84 86 88 90 92 94 96 98 100
in 26 27 28 29 30 31 32 33 34 35 36 37 38 39 40 41

cm 46 48 50 52 54 56 58 60 62
in 18 19 20 21 22 23 24

Date	Age	Weight	Length	Head Circ.	Comment

Published May 30, 2000 (modified 10/16/00).
SOURCE: Developed by the National Center for Health Statistics in collaboration with
the National Center for Chronic Disease Prevention and Health Promotion (2000).
http://www.cdc.gov/growthcharts

SAFER·HEALTHIER·PEOPLE™

2 to 20 years: Boys
Stature-for-age and Weight-for-age percentiles

NAME _____

RECORD # _____

Mother's Stature _____ Father's Stature _____

Date	Age	Weight	Stature	BMI*

*To Calculate BMI: Weight (kg) ÷ Stature (cm) ÷ Stature (cm) x 10,000
or Weight (lb) ÷ Stature (in) ÷ Stature (in) x 703

AGE (YEARS)

STATURE

WEIGHT

AGE (YEARS)

Published May 30, 2000 (modified 11/21/00).
SOURCE: Developed by the National Center for Health Statistics in collaboration with
the National Center for Chronic Disease Prevention and Health Promotion (2000).
http://www.cdc.gov/growthcharts

SAFER · HEALTHIER · PEOPLE™

2 to 20 years: Boys
Body mass index-for-age percentiles

NAME _____

RECORD # _____

Date	Age	Weight	Stature	BMI*	Comments

*To Calculate BMI: Weight (kg) ÷ Stature (cm) ÷ Stature (cm) x 10,000
or Weight (lb) ÷ Stature (in) ÷ Stature (in) x 703

BMI

95
90
85
75
50
25
10
5

BMI

27
26
25
24
23
22
21
20
19
18
17
16
15
14
13
12

kg/m²

AGE (YEARS)

kg/m²

BMI
35
34
33
32
31
30
29
28
27
26
25
24
23
22
21
20
19
18
17
16
15
14
13
12

2 3 4 5 6 7 8 9 10 11 12 13 14 15 16 17 18 19 20

Published May 30, 2000 (modified 10/16/00).

SOURCE: Developed by the National Center for Health Statistics in collaboration with
the National Center for Chronic Disease Prevention and Health Promotion (2000).
http://www.cdc.gov/growthcharts

SAFER · HEALTHIER · PEOPLE™

2 to 20 years: Girls
Stature-for-age and Weight-for-age percentiles

NAME _____

RECORD # _____

Mother's Stature _____		Father's Stature _____		
Date	Age	Weight	Stature	BMI*

*To Calculate BMI: Weight (kg) ÷ Stature (cm) ÷ Stature (cm) x 10,000
or Weight (lb) ÷ Stature (in) ÷ Stature (in) x 703

AGE (YEARS)

12 13 14 15 16 17 18 19 20

STATURE

WEIGHT

AGE (YEARS)

2 3 4 5 6 7 8 9 10 11 12 13 14 15 16 17 18 19 20

Published May 30, 2000 (modified 11/21/00).
SOURCE: Developed by the National Center for Health Statistics in collaboration with
the National Center for Chronic Disease Prevention and Health Promotion (2000).
http://www.cdc.gov/growthcharts

SAFER · HEALTHIER · PEOPLE™

2 to 20 years: Girls
Body mass index-for-age percentiles

NAME _____

RECORD # · _____

Date	Age	Weight	Stature	BMI*	Comments

*To Calculate BMI: Weight (kg) ÷ Stature (cm) ÷ Stature (cm) x 10,000
or Weight (lb) ÷ Stature (in) ÷ Stature (in) x 703

BMI

AGE (YEARS)

kg/m² · · · · · · · kg/m²

Published May 30, 2000 (modified 10/16/00).
SOURCE: Developed by the National Center for Health Statistics in collaboration with
the National Center for Chronic Disease Prevention and Health Promotion (2000).
http://www.cdc.gov/growthcharts

SAFER · HEALTHIER · PEOPLE™

DENVER II DEVELOPMENT ASSESSMENT

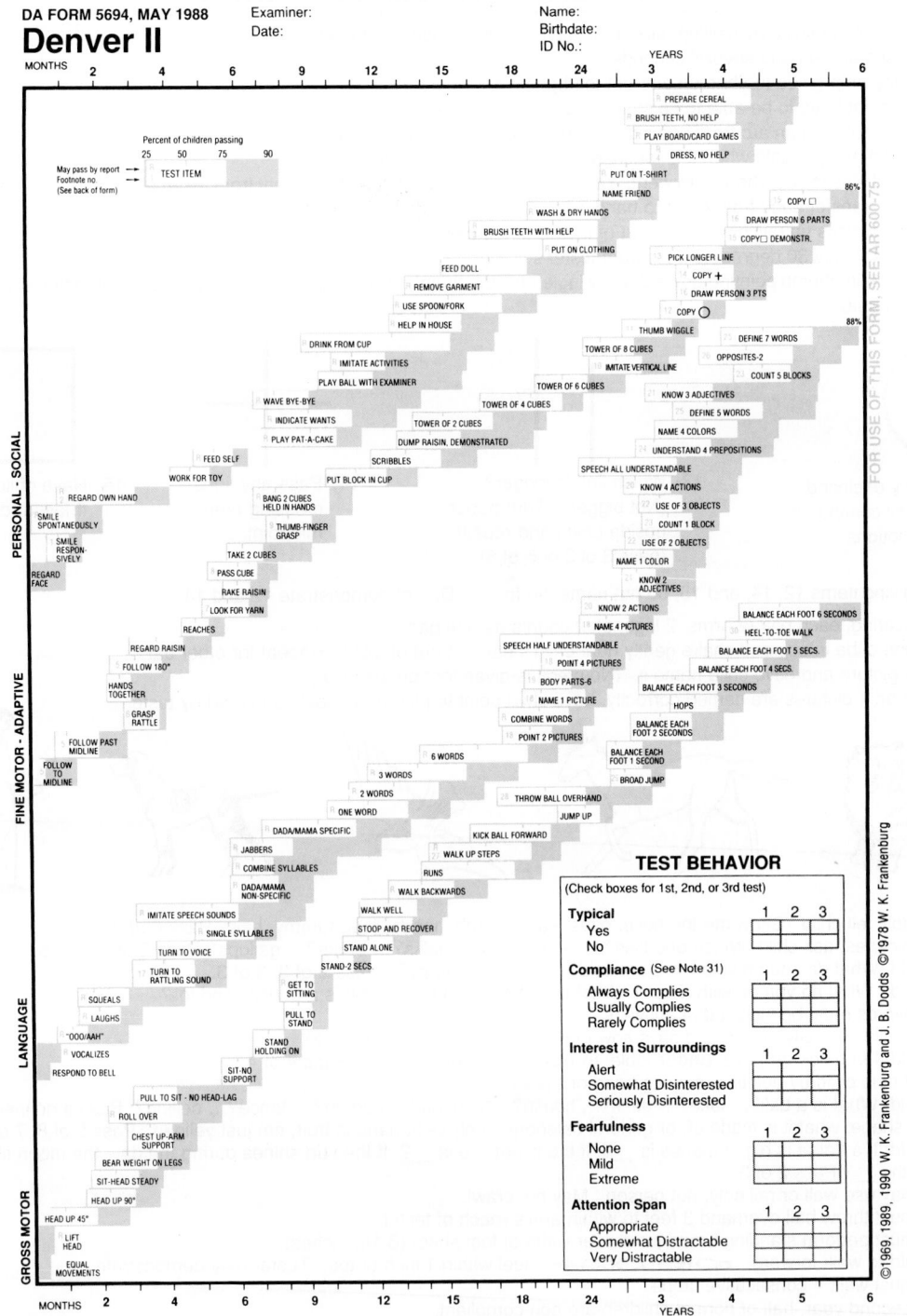

DA FORM 5694, MAY 1988

Denver II

Examiner:
Date:

Name:
Birthdate:
ID No.:

DIRECTIONS FOR ADMINISTRATION

1. Try to get child to smile by smiling, talking or waving. Do not touch him/her.
2. Child must stare at hand several seconds.
3. Parent may help guide toothbrush and put toothpaste on brush.
4. Child does not have to be able to tie shoes or button/zip in the back.
5. Move yarn slowly in an arc from one side to the other, about 8" above child's face.
6. Pass if child grasps rattle when it is touched to the backs or tips of fingers.
7. Pass if child tries to see where yarn went. Yarn should be dropped quickly from sight from tester's hand without arm movement.
8. Child must transfer cube from hand to hand without help of body, mouth, or table.
9. Pass if child picks up raisin with any part of thumb and finger.
10. Line can vary only 30 degrees or less from tester's line.
11. Make a fist with thumb pointing upward and wiggle only the thumb. Pass if child imitates and does not move any fingers other than the thumb.

12. Pass any enclosed form. Fail continuous round motions.

13. Which line is longer? (Not bigger.) Turn paper upside down and repeat. (pass 3 of 3 or 5 of 6)

14. Pass any lines crossing near midpoint.

15. Have child copy first. If failed, demonstrate.

When giving items 12, 14, and 15, do not name the forms. Do not demonstrate 12 and 14.

16. When scoring, each pair (2 arms, 2 legs, etc.) counts as one part.
17. Place one cube in cup and shake gently near child's ear, but out of sight. Repeat for other ear.
18. Point to picture and have child name it. (No credit is given for sounds only.)
    If less than 4 pictures are named correctly, have child point to picture as each is named by tester.

19. Using doll, tell child: Show me the nose, eyes, ears, mouth, hands, feet, tummy, hair. Pass 6 of 8.
20. Using pictures, ask child: Which one flies?… says meow?… talks?… barks?… gallops? Pass 2 of 5, 4 of 5.
21. Ask child: What do you do when you are cold?… tired?… hungry?   Pass 2 of 3, 3 of 3.
22. Ask child: What do you do with a cup? What is a chair used for? What is a pencil used for?
    Action words must be included in answers.
23. Pass if child correctly places <u>and</u> says how many blocks are on paper. (1, 5).
24. Tell child: Put block **on** table; **under** table; **in front of** me, **behind** me. Pass 4 of 4.
    (Do not help child by pointing, moving head or eyes.)
25. Ask child: What is a ball?… lake?… desk?… house?… banana?… curtain?… fence?… ceiling? Pass if defined in terms of use, shape, what it is made of, or general category (such as banana is fruit, not just yellow). Pass 5 of 8, 7 of 8.
26. Ask child: If a horse is big, a mouse is __? If fire is hot, ice is __? If the sun shines during the day, the moon shines during the __? Pass 2 of 3.
27. Child may use wall or rail only, not person. May not crawl.
28. Child must throw ball overhand 3 feet to within arm's reach of tester.
29. Child must perform standing broad jump over width of test sheet (8 1/2 inches).
30. Tell child to walk forward, ⚏⚏⚏⟶ heel within 1 inch of toe. Tester may demonstrate.
    Child must walk 4 consecutive steps.
31. In the second year, half of normal children are non-compliant.

OBSERVATIONS:

THE FOOD GUIDE PYRAMID

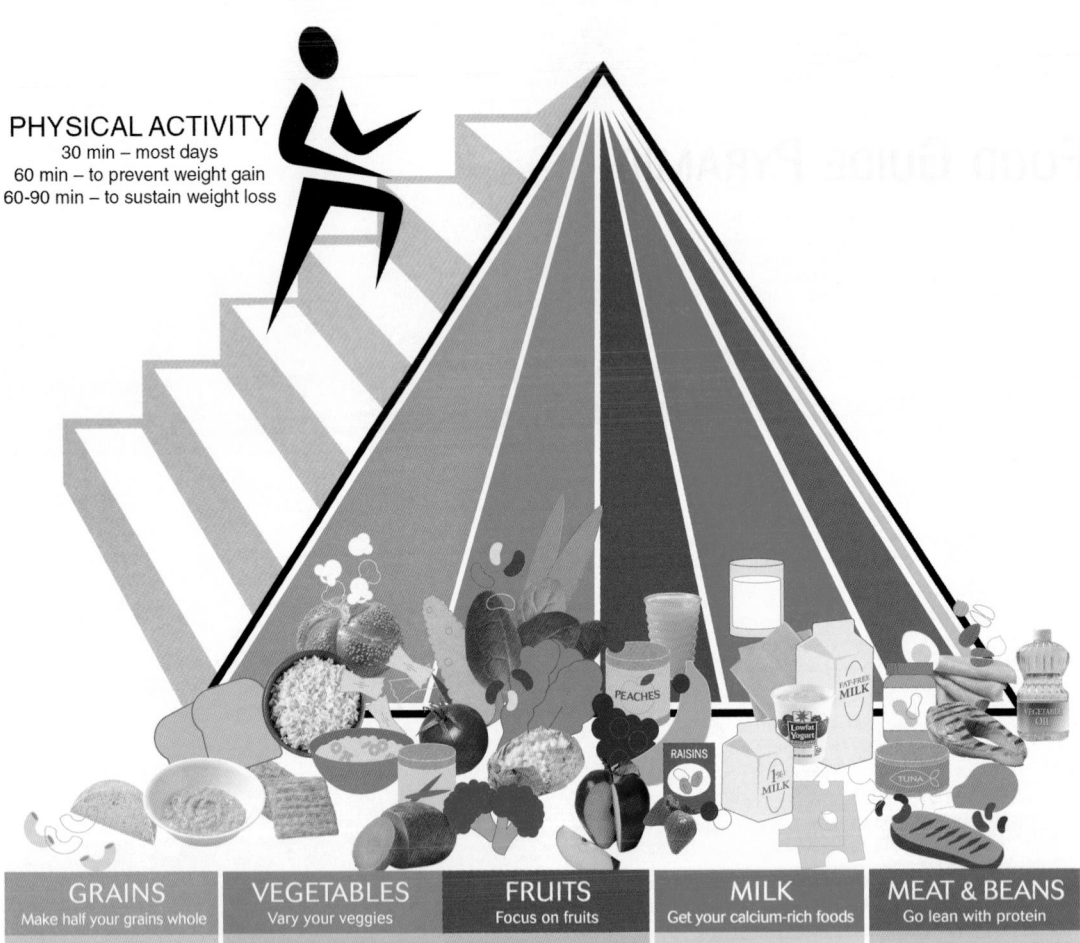

PHYSICAL ACTIVITY
30 min – most days
60 min – to prevent weight gain
60-90 min – to sustain weight loss

GRAINS	VEGETABLES	FRUITS	MILK	MEAT & BEANS
Make half your grains whole	Vary your veggies	Focus on fruits	Get your calcium-rich foods	Go lean with protein
Eat at least 3 oz. of whole-grain cereals, breads, crackers, rice, or pasta every day	Eat more dark-green veggies like broccoli, spinach, and other dark leafy greens	Eat a variety of fruit	Go low-fat or fat-free when you choose milk, yogurt, and other milk products	Choose low-fat or lean meats and poultry
1 oz. is about 1 slice of bread, about 1 cup of breakfast cereal, or ½ cup of cooked rice, cereal, or pasta	Eat more orange vegetables like carrots and sweetpotatoes	Choose fresh, frozen, canned, or dried fruit	If you don't or can't consume milk, choose lactose-free products or other calcium sources such as fortified foods and beverages	Bake it, broil it, or grill it
	Eat more dry beans and peas like pinto beans, kidney beans, and lentils	Go easy on fruit juices		Vary your protein routine — choose more fish, beans, peas, nuts, and seeds

For a 2,000-calorie diet, you need the amounts below from each food group. To find the amounts that are right for you, go to MyPyramid.gov.

Eat 6 oz. every day	Eat 2½ cups every day	Eat 2 cups every day	Get 3 cups every day; for kids aged 2 to 8, it's 2	Eat 5½ oz. every day

Find your balance between food and physical activity
- Be sure to stay within your daily calorie needs.
- Be physically active for at least 30 minutes most days of the week.
- About 60 minutes a day of physical activity may be needed to prevent weight gain.
- For sustaining weight loss, at least 60 to 90 minutes a day of physical activity may be required.
- Children and teenagers should be physically active for 60 minutes every day, or most days.

Know the limits on fats, sugars, and salt (sodium)
- Make most of your fat sources from fish, nuts, and vegetable oils.
- Limit solid fats like butter, margarine, shortening, and lard, as well as foods that contain these.
- Check the Nutrition Facts label to keep saturated fats, *trans* fats, and sodium low.
- Choose food and beverages low in added sugars. Added sugars contribute calories with few, if any, nutrients.

Blood Pressure Charts for Children and Adolescents

TABLE I.1 BLOOD PRESSURE LEVELS FOR BOYS BY AGE AND HEIGHT PERCENTILE

Age (Year)	BP Percentile ↓	Systolic BP (mmHg) ← Percentile of Height →							Diastolic BP (mmHg) ← Percentile of Height →						
		5th	10th	25th	50th	75th	90th	95th	5th	10th	25th	50th	75th	90th	95th
1	50th	80	81	83	85	87	88	89	34	35	36	37	38	39	39
	90th	94	95	97	99	100	102	103	49	50	51	52	53	53	54
	95th	98	99	101	103	104	106	106	54	54	55	56	57	58	58
	99th	105	106	108	110	112	113	114	61	62	63	64	65	66	66
2	50th	84	85	87	88	90	92	92	39	40	41	42	43	44	44
	90th	97	99	100	102	104	105	106	54	55	56	57	58	58	59
	95th	101	102	104	106	108	109	110	59	59	60	61	62	63	63
	99th	109	110	111	113	115	117	117	66	67	68	69	70	71	71
3	50th	86	87	89	91	93	94	95	44	44	45	46	47	48	48
	90th	100	101	103	105	107	108	109	59	59	60	61	62	63	63
	95th	104	105	107	109	110	112	113	63	63	64	65	66	67	67
	99th	111	112	114	116	118	119	120	71	71	72	73	74	75	75
4	50th	88	89	91	93	95	96	97	47	48	49	50	51	51	52
	90th	102	103	105	107	109	110	111	62	63	64	65	66	66	67
	95th	106	107	109	111	112	114	115	66	67	68	69	70	71	71
	99th	113	114	116	118	120	121	122	74	75	76	77	78	78	79
5	50th	90	91	93	95	96	98	98	50	51	52	53	54	55	55
	90th	104	105	106	108	110	111	112	65	66	67	68	69	69	70
	95th	108	109	110	112	114	115	116	69	70	71	72	73	74	74
	99th	115	116	118	120	121	123	123	77	78	79	80	81	81	82
6	50th	91	92	94	96	98	99	100	53	53	54	55	56	57	57
	90th	105	106	108	110	111	113	113	68	68	69	70	71	72	72
	95th	109	110	112	114	115	117	117	72	72	73	74	75	76	76
	99th	116	117	119	121	123	124	125	80	80	81	82	83	84	84
7	50th	92	94	95	97	99	100	101	55	55	56	57	58	59	59
	90th	106	107	109	111	113	114	115	70	70	71	72	73	74	74
	95th	110	111	113	115	117	118	119	74	74	75	76	77	78	78
	99th	117	118	120	122	124	125	126	82	82	83	84	85	86	86
8	50th	94	95	97	99	100	102	102	56	57	58	59	60	60	61
	90th	107	109	110	112	114	115	116	71	72	72	73	74	75	76
	95th	111	112	114	116	118	119	120	75	76	77	78	79	79	80
	99th	119	120	122	123	125	127	127	83	84	85	86	87	87	88
9	50th	95	96	98	100	102	103	104	57	58	59	60	61	61	62
	90th	109	110	112	114	115	117	118	72	73	74	75	76	76	77
	95th	113	114	116	118	119	121	121	76	77	78	79	80	81	81
	99th	120	121	123	125	127	128	129	84	85	86	87	88	88	89
10	50th	97	98	100	102	103	105	106	58	59	60	61	61	62	63
	90th	111	112	114	115	117	119	119	73	73	74	75	76	77	78
	95th	115	116	117	119	121	122	123	77	78	79	80	81	81	82
	99th	122	123	125	127	128	130	130	85	86	86	88	88	89	90
11	50th	99	100	102	104	105	107	107	59	59	60	61	62	63	63
	90th	113	114	115	117	119	120	121	74	74	75	76	77	78	78
	95th	117	118	119	121	123	124	125	78	78	79	80	81	82	82
	99th	124	125	127	129	130	132	132	86	86	87	88	89	90	90
12	50th	101	102	104	106	108	109	110	59	60	61	62	63	63	64
	90th	115	116	118	120	121	123	123	74	75	75	76	77	78	79
	95th	119	120	122	123	125	127	127	78	79	80	81	82	82	83
	99th	126	127	129	131	133	134	135	86	87	88	89	90	90	91

TABLE I.1   (continued)

Age (Year)	BP Percentile ↓	Systolic BP (mmHg)							Diastolic BP (mmHg)						
		← Percentile of Height →							← Percentile of Height →						
		5th	10th	25th	50th	75th	90th	95th	5th	10th	25th	50th	75th	90th	95th
13	50th	104	105	106	108	110	111	112	60	60	61	62	63	64	64
	90th	117	118	120	122	124	125	126	75	75	76	77	78	79	79
	95th	121	122	124	126	128	129	130	79	79	80	81	82	83	83
	99th	128	130	131	133	135	136	137	87	87	88	89	90	91	91
14	50th	106	107	109	111	113	114	115	60	61	62	63	64	65	65
	90th	120	121	123	125	126	128	128	75	76	77	78	79	79	80
	95th	124	125	127	128	130	132	132	80	80	81	82	83	84	84
	99th	131	132	134	136	138	139	140	87	88	89	90	91	92	92
15	50th	109	110	112	113	115	117	117	61	62	63	64	65	66	66
	90th	122	124	125	127	129	130	131	76	77	78	79	80	80	81
	95th	126	127	129	131	133	134	135	81	81	82	83	84	85	85
	99th	134	135	136	138	140	142	142	88	89	90	91	92	93	93
16	50th	111	112	114	116	118	119	120	63	63	64	65	66	67	67
	90th	125	126	128	130	131	133	134	78	78	79	80	81	82	82
	95th	129	130	132	134	135	137	137	82	83	83	84	85	86	87
	99th	136	137	139	141	143	144	145	90	90	91	92	93	94	94
17	50th	114	115	116	118	120	121	122	65	66	66	67	68	69	70
	90th	127	128	130	132	134	135	136	80	80	81	82	83	84	84
	95th	131	132	134	136	138	139	140	84	85	86	87	87	88	89
	99th	139	140	141	143	145	146	147	92	93	93	94	95	96	97

BP, blood pressure

* The 90th percentile is 1.28 SD, 95th percentile is 1.645 SD, and the 99th percentile is 2.326 SD over the mean.

U.S. Department of Health and Human Services, National Institutes of Health, National Heart, Lung, and Blood Institute (NHLBI).

TABLE I.2   BLOOD PRESSURE LEVELS FOR GIRLS BY AGE AND HEIGHT PERCENTILE

Age (Year)	BP Percentile ↓	Systolic BP (mmHg) ← Percentile of Height →							Diastolic BP (mmHg) ← Percentile of Height →						
		5th	10th	25th	50th	75th	90th	95th	5th	10th	25th	50th	75th	90th	95th
1	50th	83	84	85	86	88	89	90	38	39	39	40	41	41	42
	90th	97	97	98	100	101	102	103	52	53	53	54	55	55	56
	95th	100	101	102	104	105	106	107	56	57	57	58	59	59	60
	99th	108	108	109	111	112	113	114	64	64	65	65	66	67	67
2	50th	85	85	87	88	89	91	91	43	44	44	45	46	46	47
	90th	98	99	100	101	103	104	105	57	58	58	59	60	61	61
	95th	102	103	104	105	107	108	109	61	62	62	63	64	65	65
	99th	109	110	111	112	114	115	116	69	69	70	70	71	72	72
3	50th	86	87	88	89	91	92	93	47	48	48	49	50	50	51
	90th	100	100	102	103	104	106	106	61	62	62	63	64	64	65
	95th	104	104	105	107	108	109	110	65	66	66	67	68	68	69
	99th	111	111	113	114	115	116	117	73	73	74	74	75	76	76
4	50th	88	88	90	91	92	94	94	50	50	51	52	52	53	54
	90th	101	102	103	104	106	107	108	64	64	65	66	67	67	68
	95th	105	106	107	108	110	111	112	68	68	69	70	71	71	72
	99th	112	113	114	115	117	118	119	76	76	76	77	78	79	79
5	50th	89	90	91	93	94	95	96	52	53	53	54	55	55	56
	90th	103	103	105	106	107	109	109	66	67	67	68	69	69	70
	95th	107	107	108	110	111	112	113	70	71	71	72	73	73	74
	99th	114	114	116	117	118	120	120	78	78	79	79	80	81	81
6	50th	91	92	93	94	96	97	98	54	54	55	56	56	57	58
	90th	104	105	106	108	109	110	111	68	68	69	70	70	71	72
	95th	108	109	110	111	113	114	115	72	72	73	74	74	75	76
	99th	115	116	117	119	120	121	122	80	80	80	81	82	83	83
7	50th	93	93	95	96	97	99	99	55	56	56	57	58	58	59
	90th	106	107	108	109	111	112	113	69	70	70	71	72	72	73
	95th	110	111	112	113	115	116	116	73	74	74	75	76	76	77
	99th	117	118	119	120	122	123	124	81	81	82	82	83	84	84
8	50th	95	95	96	98	99	100	101	57	57	57	58	59	60	60
	90th	108	109	110	111	113	114	114	71	71	71	72	73	74	74
	95th	112	112	114	115	116	118	118	75	75	75	76	77	78	78
	99th	119	120	121	122	123	125	125	82	82	83	83	84	85	86
9	50th	96	97	98	100	101	102	103	58	58	58	59	60	61	61
	90th	110	110	112	113	114	116	116	72	72	72	73	74	75	75
	95th	114	114	115	117	118	119	120	76	76	76	77	78	79	79
	99th	121	121	123	124	125	127	127	83	83	84	84	85	86	87
10	50th	98	99	100	102	103	104	105	59	59	59	60	61	62	62
	90th	112	112	114	115	116	118	118	73	73	73	74	75	76	76
	95th	116	116	117	119	120	121	122	77	77	77	78	79	80	80
	99th	123	123	125	126	127	129	129	84	84	85	86	86	87	88
11	50th	100	101	102	103	105	106	107	60	60	60	61	62	63	63
	90th	114	114	116	118	118	119	120	74	74	74	75	76	77	77
	95th	118	118	119	121	122	123	124	78	78	78	79	80	81	81
	99th	125	125	126	128	129	130	131	85	85	86	87	87	88	89
12	50th	102	103	104	105	107	108	109	61	61	61	62	63	64	64
	90th	116	116	117	119	120	121	122	75	75	75	76	77	78	78
	95th	119	120	121	123	124	125	126	79	79	79	80	81	82	82
	99th	127	127	128	130	131	132	133	86	86	87	88	88	89	90

TABLE I.2   (continued)

Age (Year)	BP Percentile ↓	Systolic BP (mmHg) ← Percentile of Height →							Diastolic BP (mmHg) ← Percentile of Height →						
		5th	10th	25th	50th	75th	90th	95th	5th	10th	25th	50th	75th	90th	95th
13	50th	104	105	106	107	109	110	110	62	62	62	63	64	65	65
	90th	117	118	119	121	122	123	124	76	76	76	77	78	79	79
	95th	121	122	123	124	126	127	128	80	80	80	81	82	83	83
	99th	128	129	130	132	133	134	135	87	87	88	89	89	90	91
14	50th	106	106	107	109	110	111	112	63	63	63	64	65	66	66
	90th	119	120	121	122	124	125	125	77	77	77	78	79	80	80
	95th	123	123	125	126	127	129	129	81	81	81	82	83	84	84
	99th	130	131	132	133	135	136	136	88	88	89	90	90	91	92
15	50th	107	108	109	110	111	113	113	64	64	64	65	66	67	67
	90th	120	121	122	123	125	126	127	78	78	78	79	80	81	81
	95th	124	125	126	127	129	130	131	82	82	82	83	84	85	85
	99th	131	132	133	134	136	137	138	89	89	90	91	91	92	93
16	50th	108	108	110	111	112	114	114	64	64	65	66	66	67	68
	90th	121	122	123	124	126	127	128	78	78	79	80	81	81	82
	95th	125	126	127	128	130	131	132	82	82	83	84	85	85	86
	99th	132	133	134	135	137	138	139	90	90	90	91	92	93	93
17	50th	108	109	110	111	113	114	115	64	65	65	66	67	67	68
	90th	122	122	123	125	126	127	128	78	79	79	80	81	81	82
	95th	125	126	127	129	130	131	132	82	83	83	84	85	85	86
	99th	133	133	134	136	137	138	139	90	90	91	91	92	93	93

BP, blood pressure
* The 90th percentile is 1.28 SD, 95th percentile is 1.645 SD, and the 99th percentile is 2.326 SD over the mean.
U.S. Department of Health and Human Services, National Institutes of Health, National Heart, Lung, and Blood Institute (NHLBI).

Down Syndrome Health Care Guidelines

TABLE J.1   DOWN SYNDROME HEALTH CARE GUIDELINES (1999 REVISION) RECORD SHEET
SHEET #1: BIRTH TO AGE 12 YEARS

Name:_____   Birthday:_____

Medical Issues	At Birth or at Diagnosis	Age, in years														
		6-mo	1	1½	2	2½	3	4	5	6	7	8	9	10	11	12
Karyotype & Genetic Counseling																
Usual Preventative Care																
Cardiology	Echo															
Audiologic Evaluation	ABR or OAE															
Ophthalmologic Evaluation	Red reflex															
Thyroid (TSH & T_4)	State screening															
Nutrition																
Dental Exam[1]																
Celiac Screening[2]																
Parent Support																
Developmental & Educational Services	Early Intervention															
Neck X-rays & Neurological Exam[3]							X-ray									
Pneumococcal Conjugate Vaccine Series																

Instructions: Perform indicated exam/screening and record date in blank spaces. The grey or shaded boxes mean no action is to be taken for those ages.

[1]Begin Dental Exams at 2 years of age, and continue every 6 months thereafter.

[2]IgA antiendomysium antibodies and total IgA.

[3]Cervical spine x-rays: flexion, neutral and extension, between 3–5 years of age. Repeat as needed for Special Olympic participation. Neurological examination at each visit.

TABLE J.2 DOWN SYNDROME HEALTH CARE GUIDELINES (1999 REVISION) RECORD SHEET
SHEET #2: 13 YEARS TO ADULTHOOD

Name:_____ Birthday:_____

Medical Issues	Age, in years							
	13	14	15	16	17	18	19	20–29
Usual Preventative Care								
Audiologic Evaluation								
Ophthalmologic Evaluation								
Thyroid (TSH & T_4)								
Nutrition								
Dental Exam[1]								
Parent Support								
Developmental & Educational Services								
Neck X-rays & Neurological Exam[2]								
Pelvic exam[3]								
Assess Contraceptive Need[3]								

Instructions: Perform indicated exam/screening and record date in blank spaces. The shaded boxes mean no action is to be taken for those ages.

[1]Begin Dental Exams at 2 years of age, and continue every 6 month thereafter.

[2]Cervical spine x-rays: flexion, neutral and extension, between 3–5 years of age. Repeat as needed for Special Olympics participation. Neurological examination at each visit.

[3]If sexually active.

INDEX

Note: A *b* following a page number indicates a boxed features; *d* indicates a display; *f* indicates a figure; *t* indicates a table.